DIAGNOSTIC IMAGING
BRAIN
SECOND EDITION

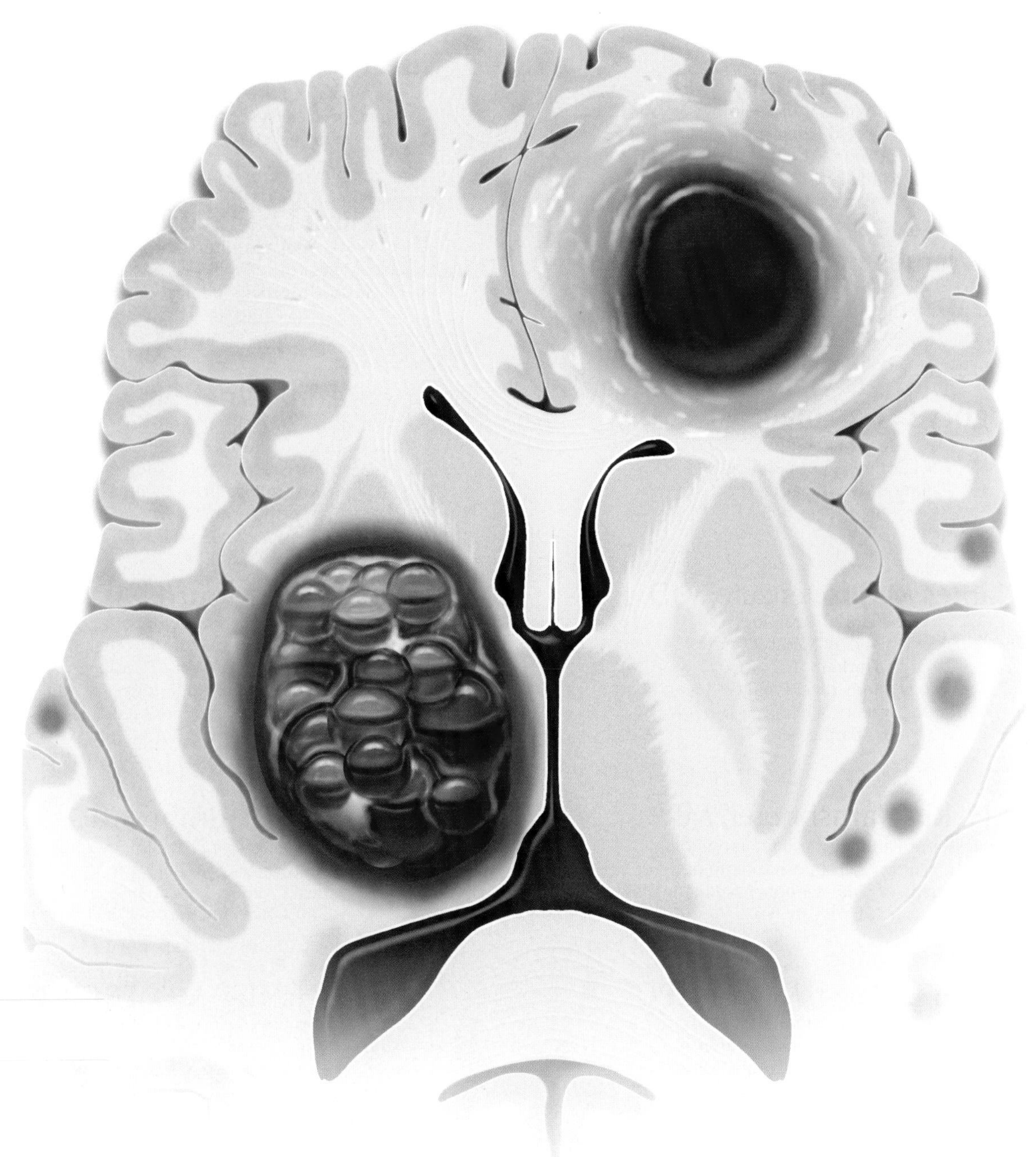

DIAGNOSTIC IMAGING
BRAIN
SECOND EDITION

Anne G. Osborn, MD, FACR
University Distinguished Professor
Professor of Radiology
William H. and Patricia W. Child
Presidential Endowed Chair in Radiology
University of Utah School of Medicine
Salt Lake City, UT

Karen L. Salzman, MD
Associate Professor of Radiology
Leslie W. Davis Endowed Chair in Neuroradiology
University of Utah School of Medicine
Salt Lake City, UT

A. James Barkovich, MD
Professor of Radiology, Neurology, Pediatrics and Neurosurgery
University of California at San Francisco
San Francisco, CA

Gregory L. Katzman, MD, MBA
Neuroradiologist
Section of Neuroradiology
SimonMed Imaging, Inc.
Scottsdale, AZ

James M. Provenzale, MD
Professor of Radiology
Duke University Medical Center
Durham, NC
Professor of Radiology, Biomedical Engineering and Oncology
Emory University School of Medicine
Atlanta, GA

H. Ric Harnsberger, MD
Professor of Radiology and Otolaryngology
R.C. Willey Chair in Neuroradiology
University of Utah School of Medicine
Salt Lake City, UT

Susan I. Blaser, MD, FRCPC
Staff Neuroradiologist
The Hospital for Sick Children
Associate Professor of Neuroradiology
University of Toronto
Ontario, Canada

Chang Y. Ho, MD
Assistant Professor of Radiology
Director of Pediatric Neuroradiology
Riley Hospital for Children
Indiana University School of Medicine
Indianapolis, IN

Bronwyn E. Hamilton, MD
Associate Professor of Radiology
Oregon Health & Science University
Portland, OR

Miral D. Jhaveri, MD
Assistant Professor
Department of Diagnostic Radiology & Nuclear Medicine
Rush University Medical Center
Chicago, IL

Anna Illner, MD
Pediatric Neuroradiologist
Texas Children's Hospital
Assistant Professor of Radiology
Baylor College of Medicine
Houston, TX

Kevin R. Moore, MD
Pediatric Neuroradiologist
Primary Children's Medical Center
Adjunct Associate Professor of Radiology
Section of Neuroradiology
University of Utah School of Medicine
Salt Lake City, UT

Majda M. Thurnher, MD
Associate Professor of Radiology
Department of Radiology
Medical University of Vienna
Vienna, Austria

Sheri L. Harder, MD, FRCPC
Assistant Professor of Radiology
Loma Linda University Medical Center
Loma Linda, CA

Blaise V. Jones, MD
Division Chief, Neuroradiology
Cincinnati Children's Hospital Medical Center
Associate Professor of Radiology and Pediatrics
University of Cincinnati College of Medicine
Cincinnati, OH

Laurie A. Loevner, MD
Professor of Radiology & Otolaryngology: Head & Neck Surgery
Neuroradiology Division
University of Pennsylvania School of Medicine
Philadelphia, PA

Gary M. Nesbit, MD
Professor of Radiology, Neurology, Neurological Surgery
and the Dotter Interventional Institute
Oregon Health & Science University
Portland, OR

Gilbert Vézina, MD
Director, Program in Neuroradiology
Children's National Medical Center
Professor of Radiology and Pediatrics
The George Washington University School of Medicine and
Health Sciences
Washington, DC

Gary L. Hedlund, DO
Adjunct Professor of Radiology
University of Utah School of Medicine
Pediatric Neuroradiologist
Department of Medical Imaging
Primary Children's Medical Center
Salt Lake City, UT

Charles Raybaud, MD, FRCPC
Head of the Division of Neuroradiology
The Hospital for Sick Children
Professor of Radiology
University of Toronto
Toronto, Ontario

P. Ellen Grant, MD
Associate Professor in Radiology, Harvard Medical School
Founding Director, Center for Fetal-Neonatal Neuroimaging &
Developmental Science
Director of Fetal and Neonatal Neuroimaging Research
Children's Hospital Boston Chair in Neonatology
Children's Hospital Boston
Member of the Affiliated Faculty of the Harvard-MIT Division of
Health Sciences and Technology
Children's Hospital Boston
Boston, MA

Perry P. Ng, MBBS (Hons), FRANZCR
Assistant Professor, Department of Radiology
Interventional Neuroradiologist
University of Utah School of Medicine
Salt Lake City, UT

Yoshimi Anzai, MD, MPH
Professor, Department of Radiology
University of Washington Medical Center
Seattle, WA

John H. Rees, MD
Neuroradiologist,
Progressive Radiology
Assistant Professor of Radiology,
Georgetown University
Visiting Scientist,
Armed Forces Institute of Pathology
Washington, DC

Edward P. Quigley, III, MD, PhD
Assistant Professor of Radiology
Division of Neuroradiology
University of Utah School of Medicine
Salt Lake City, UT

Jeffrey S. Anderson, MD, PhD
Assistant Professor of Neuroradiology and Bioengineering
University of Utah School of Medicine
Salt Lake City, UT

Lubdha M. Shah, MD
Assistant Professor of Radiology
Division of Neuroradiology
University of Utah School of Medicine
Salt Lake City, UT

Ulrich A. Rassner, MD
Assistant Professor of Radiology
Division of Neuroradiology
University of Utah School of Medicine
Salt Lake City, UT

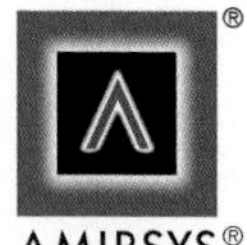

AMIRSYS®
Names you know. Content you trust.®

Second Edition

Printed in Canada by Friesens, Altona, Manitoba, Canada

ISBN: 978-1-931884-72-3

Notice and Disclaimer

The information in this product ("Product") is provided as a reference for use by licensed medical professionals and no others. It does not and should not be construed as any form of medical diagnosis or professional medical advice on any matter. Receipt or use of this Product, in whole or in part, does not constitute or create a doctor-patient, therapist-patient, or other healthcare professional relationship between the copyright holders and any recipient. This Product may not reflect the most current medical developments, and the copyright holders (individually and jointly), make no claims, promises, or guarantees about accuracy, completeness, or adequacy of the information contained in or linked to the Product. The Product is not a substitute for or replacement of professional medical judgment. The copyright holders, and their affiliates, authors, contributors, partners, and sponsors, individually and jointly, disclaim all liability or responsibility for any injury and/or damage to persons or property in respect to actions taken or not taken based on any and all Product information.

In the cases where drugs or other chemicals are prescribed, readers are advised to check the Product information currently provided by the manufacturer of each drug to be administered to verify the recommended dose, the method and duration of administration, and contraindications. It is the responsibility of the treating physician relying on experience and knowledge of the patient to determine dosages and the best treatment for the patient.

To the maximum extent permitted by applicable law, the copyright holders provide the Product AS IS AND WITH ALL FAULTS, AND HEREBY DISCLAIMS ALL WARRANTIES AND CONDITIONS, WHETHER EXPRESS, IMPLIED OR STATUTORY, INCLUDING BUT NOT LIMITED TO, ANY (IF ANY) IMPLIED WARRANTIES OR CONDITIONS OF MERCHANTABILITY, OF FITNESS FOR A PARTICULAR PURPOSE, OF LACK OF VIRUSES, OR ACCURACY OR COMPLETENESS OF RESPONSES, OR RESULTS, AND OF LACK OF NEGLIGENCE OR LACK OF WORKMANLIKE EFFORT. ALSO, THERE IS NO WARRANTY OR CONDITION OF TITLE, QUIET ENJOYMENT, QUIET POSSESSION, CORRESPONDENCE TO DESCRIPTION OR NON-INFRINGEMENT, WITH REGARD TO THE PRODUCT. THE ENTIRE RISK AS TO THE QUALITY OF OR ARISING OUT OF USE OR PERFORMANCE OF THE PRODUCT REMAINS WITH THE READER.

The respective copyright holders, individually and jointly, disclaim all warranties of any kind if the Product was customized, repackaged or altered in any way by any third party.

Library of Congress Cataloging-in-Publication Data

Diagnostic imaging. Brain / [edited by] Anne G. Osborn, Karen L. Salzman, A. James Barkovich. -- 2nd ed.
p. ; cm.
Includes bibliographical references and index.
ISBN 978-1-931884-72-3
1. Brain--Imaging--Handbooks, manuals, etc. I. Osborn, Anne G., 1943- II. Salzman, Karen L. III. Barkovich, A. James, 1952- IV. Title: Brain.
[DNLM: 1. Brain--radiography. 2. Central Nervous System Diseases--diagnosis. 3. Diagnosis, Differential. 4. Neuroradiography--methods. WL 141 D5347 2009]

RC386.6.D52D53 2009
616.8'04754--dc22

2009038951

To the intrepid Amirsys "Brain Team"

You put your collective bodies into the harness and pulled unbelievably hard to get this one across the finish line in record time. Wouldn't have happened without you! We did it!

AGO

PREFACE

Welcome to one of the first volumes in the series of brand-new *Diagnostic Imaging*, second edition books. The response to the first editions was overwhelmingly positive. The gorgeous graphics, Key Facts boxes, high-resolution images, and "don't waste any words" philosophy behind the synoptic text bullets met with great success. We on the "Brain Team" loved writing the first edition. You clearly loved the new templated style and have asked for more. So we've rounded up our stellar team once again and produced what we think is an even better, more robust second edition.

What's new? In a nutshell, lots! We've improved but kept the basic layout so that the same information is in the same place—every time, in every volume. We've added over one hundred *new diagnoses*, thousands of *new images*, and a bunch more of our *signature color graphics*. The references have all been updated to within a few weeks of publication. What else makes the second edition significantly different? We've added prose (yes, prose!) introductions to each section. These almost literally "take you by the hand," leading you through an overview and orientation to the specific diagnoses that really can't be conveyed any other way.

The introduction to the section on neoplasms covers the newest World Health Organization (WHO) classification and grading schema. Other introductions provide an approach to understanding brain malformations, toxic/metabolic disorders, trauma, infections, etc. New tables, charts, diagrams, and pathology images have been added for your delectation and reading delight.

We've loved hearing from you. We appreciate—and pay close attention to—your ideas and input on what new diagnoses or information you'd like to see included. Thanks also for the beautiful cases that some of you have shared with us. We've chosen to include images from some of them in this second edition with our grateful acknowledgement.

You, the reader, are the reason we "do what we do." We want *Diagnostic Imaging: Brain*, second edition, to be your favorite neuroradiology text—used, worn, dog-eared, and loved. Any ideas/thoughts/comments/suggestions? Email them to feedback@amirsys.com, and I'll answer personally.

Thanks again for making the books in our *Diagnostic Imaging* series the bestsellers they so quickly became. We hope you enjoy the sequels!

Anne G. Osborn, MD, FACR
University Distinguished Professor
Professor of Radiology
William H. and Patricia W. Child
Presidential Endowed Chair in Radiology
University of Utah School of Medicine
Salt Lake City, UT

ACKNOWLEDGEMENTS

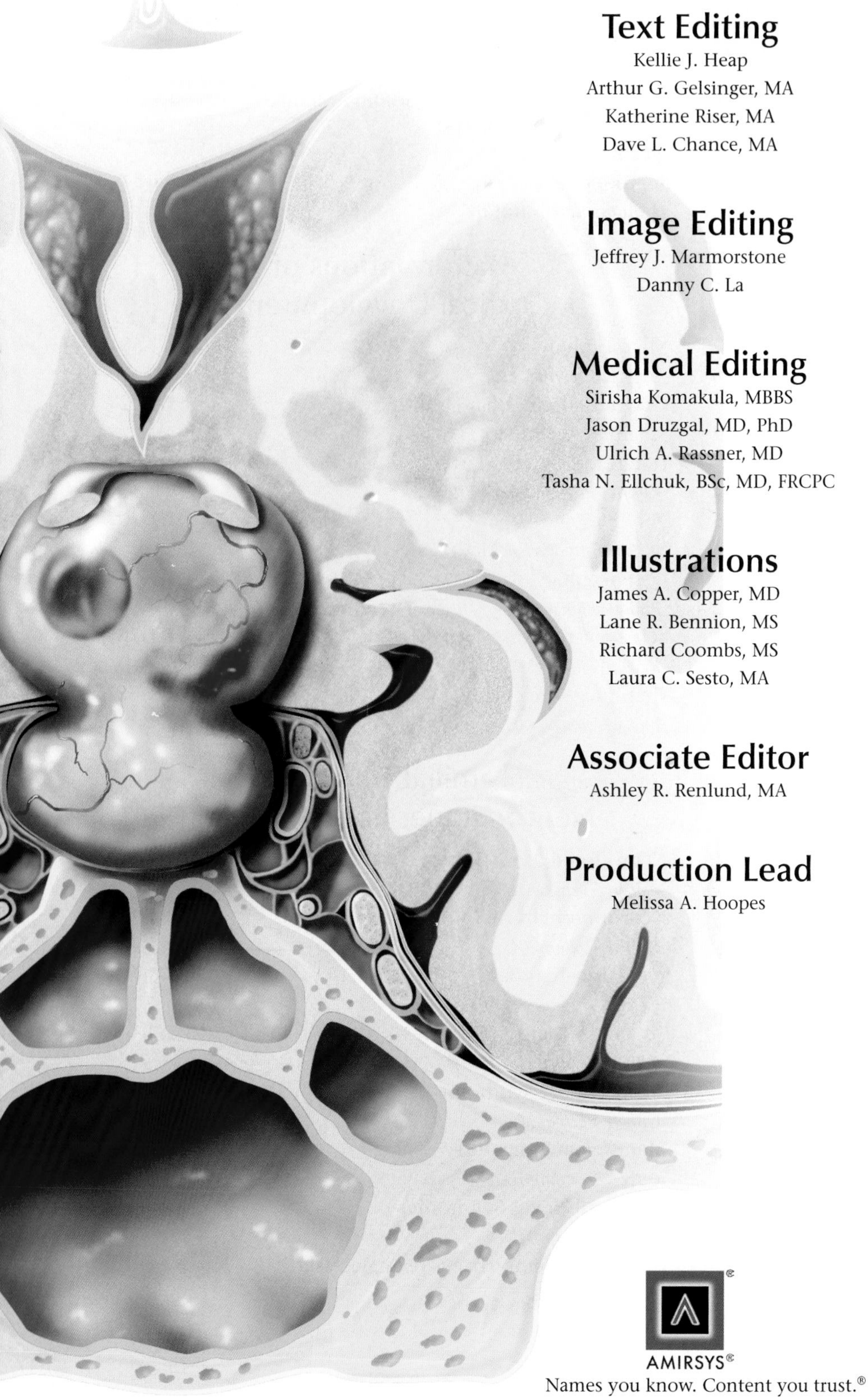

Text Editing
Kellie J. Heap
Arthur G. Gelsinger, MA
Katherine Riser, MA
Dave L. Chance, MA

Image Editing
Jeffrey J. Marmorstone
Danny C. La

Medical Editing
Sirisha Komakula, MBBS
Jason Druzgal, MD, PhD
Ulrich A. Rassner, MD
Tasha N. Ellchuk, BSc, MD, FRCPC

Illustrations
James A. Copper, MD
Lane R. Bennion, MS
Richard Coombs, MS
Laura C. Sesto, MA

Associate Editor
Ashley R. Renlund, MA

Production Lead
Melissa A. Hoopes

AMIRSYS®
Names you know. Content you trust.®

TABLE OF CONTENTS

PART I
Pathology-based Diagnoses

SECTION 1
Congenital Malformations

Introduction and Overview

Hindbrain Herniations, Miscellaneous Malformations

Hindbrain Malformations

Disorders of Diverticulation/Cleavage

Malformations of Cortical Development

Familial Tumor/ Neurocutaneous Syndromes

SECTION 2 Trauma

Introduction and Overview

Primary Effects of CNS Trauma

Secondary Effects of CNS Trauma

SECTION 3 Subarachnoid Hemorrhage and Aneurysms

Introduction and Overview

Subarachnoid Hemorrhage

Aneurysms

SECTION 4 Stroke

Introduction and Overview

Nontraumatic Intracranial Hemorrhage

Atherosclerosis and Carotid Stenosis

Nonatheromatous Vasculopathy

Cerebral Ischemia and Infarction

SECTION 5
Vascular Malformations

Introduction and Overview

CVMs with AV Shunting

CVMs without AV Shunting

SECTION 6
Neoplasms

Introduction and Overview

Astrocytic Tumors, Infiltrating

Astrocytic Tumors, Localized

Oligodendroglial and Miscellaneous Tumors

Ependymal Tumors

Choroid Plexus Tumors

Neuronal and Mixed Neuronal-Glial Tumors

Pineal Parenchymal Tumors

Embryonal and Neuroblastic Tumors

Tumors of Cranial/Peripheral Nerves

Blood Vessel and Hemopoietic Tumors

Germ Cell Tumors

Metastatic Tumors and Remote Effects of Cancer

SECTION 7
Primary Nonneoplastic Cysts

Introduction and Overview

Primary Nonneoplastic Cysts

SECTION 8
Infectious and Demyelinating Disease

Introduction and Overview

Peroxisomal Disorders

Organic and Aminoacidopathies

Miscellaneous

SECTION 10
Acquired Toxic/Metabolic/ Degenerative Disorders

Introduction and Overview

Toxic, Metabolic, Nutritional, Systemic Diseases with CNS Manifestations

Dementias and Degenerative Disorders

PART II
Anatomy-based Diagnoses

SECTION 1
Ventricles and Cisterns

Introduction and Overview

Normal Variants

Hydrocephalus

SECTION 2
Sella and Pituitary

Introduction and Overview

Congenital

Neoplasms

Miscellaneous

SECTION 3
CPA-IAC

Introduction and Overview

Congenital

Inflammatory

Vascular

Neoplasms

SECTION 4
Skull, Scalp, and Meninges

Introduction and Overview

Congenital

Trauma

Nonneoplastic and Tumor-like Disorders

Neoplasms

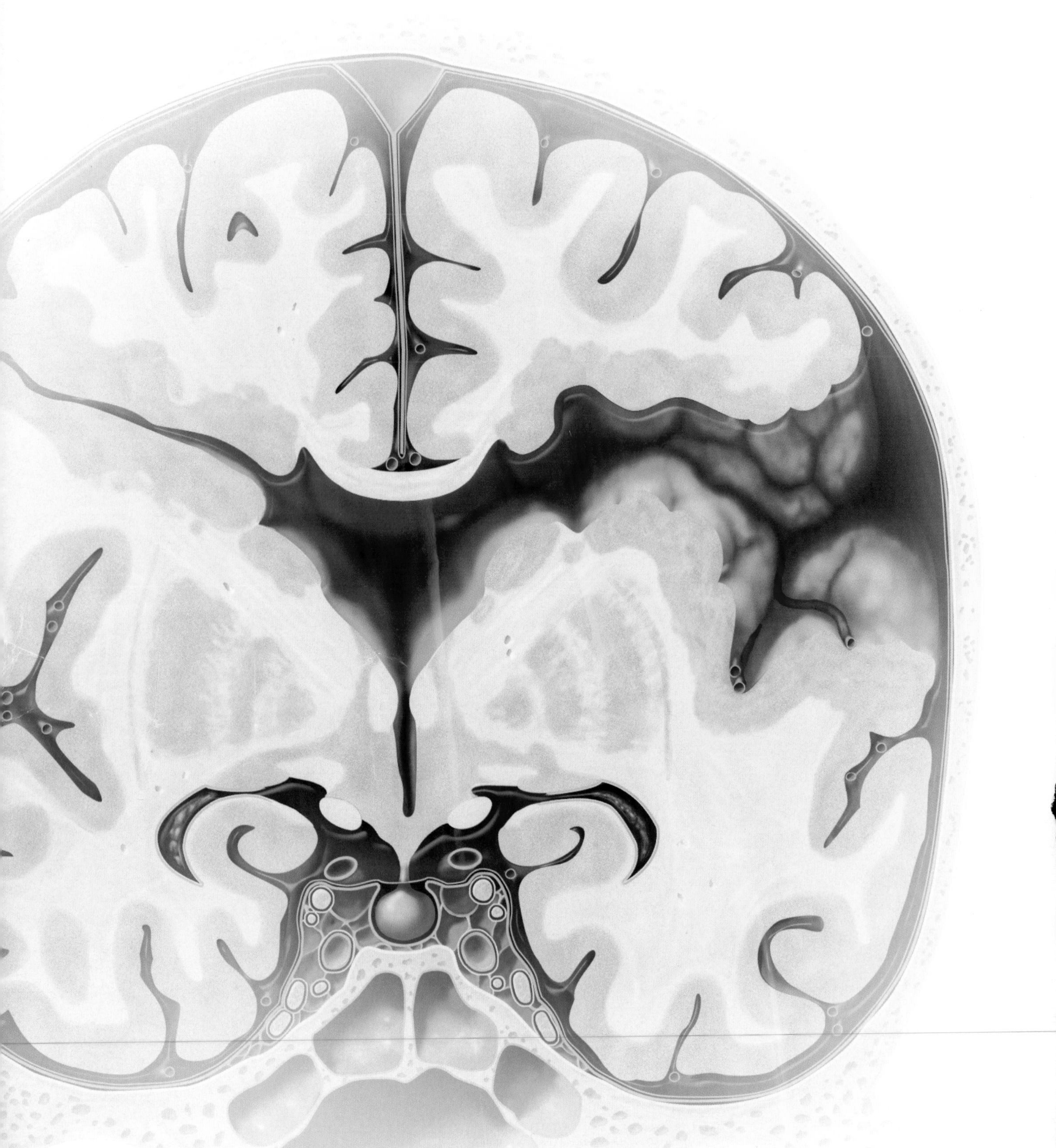

SECTION 1
Congenital Malformations

Introduction and Overview

Hindbrain Herniations, Miscellaneous Malformations

Hindbrain Malformations

Disorders of Diverticulation/Cleavage

Malformations of Cortical Development

Familial Tumor/Neurocutaneous Syndromes

A General Imaging Approach to Brain Malformations

Whenever an infant or child is referred for imaging because of either seizures or delayed development, a brain malformation is a possible cause. If the child appears dysmorphic in any way (low set ears, abnormal facies, hypotelorism), the likelihood of an underlying brain malformation is even higher. In all such cases, imaging should be geared toward showing a structural abnormality. The imaging sequences should maximize contrast between gray matter and white matter, have high spatial resolution, and should be acquired as volumetric data whenever possible so that images can be reformatted in any plane or as a surface rendering. The high resolution and ability to reformat will aid in the diagnosis of subtle abnormalities. High-resolution T1-weighted volumetric images are essential for this purpose. If possible, volumetric T2-weighted images can be acquired, but the images must have excellent spatial resolution and sharp contrast between gray matter and white matter, which is not currently easy to achieve with volumetric T2-weighted sequences. If contrast between gray and white matter is poor with volumetric acquisition, acquire 2 dimensional sequences (2D) in at least 2 planes and with relatively thin (3-4 mm) section size. FLAIR images are not particularly useful in looking for malformations, as the contrast between gray matter and white matter is often poor. Diffusion-weighted images are not currently of diagnostic utility, although the use of diffusion tensor imaging (DTI) to acquire color fractional anisotropy (FA) maps and perform tractography is useful to better understand the connectivity of the malformed brain and may become clinically useful in the near future.

After acquisition of appropriate images, image analysis must take place in an orderly manner. The midline structures (including cerebral commissures, septum pellucidum, nose and rhinencephalon, pituitary gland, and hypothalamus), the cerebral cortex (cortical thickness, gyral pattern, and cortical-white matter junction), cerebral white matter (myelination, presence of nodules or clefts), the basal ganglia, the ventricular system (are all ventricles completely present and normally shaped), the interhemispheric fissure, and the midbrain hindbrain structures (brain stem and cerebellum) should all be scrutinized in every patient.

Evaluate the midline structures first, as many disease processes of children take place in the midline, including anomalies of the cerebral commissures (corpus callosum, anterior commissure, and hippocampal commissure), midline tumors (suprasellar, pineal, brain stem, and 4th ventricle), anomalies of the cerebellar vermis, and anomalies of the craniocervical junction. Anomalies of the cerebral commissures are the most common of brain malformations; more than 130 syndromes involving hem have been described. Many of these are associated ith anomalies of the hypothalamus, so remember always look at the hypothalamus and pituitary nd to ensure that the posterior pituitary gland is he sella turcica and not in the median eminence e hypothalamus. The midline leptomeninges are tant in commisural development, so make sure for other anomalies associated with abnormal leptomeninges, such as interhemispheric lipomas rhemispheric cysts when the commissures are absent or dysmorphic. Remember that large cerebrospinal fluid (CSF) spaces in the posterior fossa (mega cisterna magna) are often associated with anomalies of the cerebellum. The reason for this has only recently been discovered. Several cerebellar growth factors derive from the overlying leptomeninges. Therefore, abnormalities of the cerebellar leptomeninges may result in anomalies of the cerebellum itself, as well as abnormalities of the surrounding CSF spaces. This is the basis of development of the Dandy-Walker malformation: It requires abnormal development of the cerebellum itself and of the overlying leptomeninges. Looking at the midline image also gives an idea of the relative head size by assessing the craniofacial ratio. In the normal neonate, the ratio of the cranial vault to the face on midline images is 5:1 or 6:1. By the age of 2 years, it should be 2.5:1, and by age 10 years, it should be about 1.5:1.

After looking at the midline, evaluate the brain from outside to inside. Start with the cerebral cortex. Is the thickness normal (2-3 mm)? If it is too thick, think of pachygyria or polymicrogyria. Is the cortical-white matter junction smooth or irregular? If it is irregular, think of polymicrogyria or the cobblestone cortex seen associated with congenital muscular dystrophies such as muscle-eye-brain disease. The location of these abnormalities is important as well. Pachygyria more severe in the parietal and occipital lobes suggests a mutation of *LIS1* or *TUBA1A*, whereas pachygyria worst in the frontal lobes suggests a mutation of *DCX*. Similarly, there are many different polymicrogyria syndromes that depend upon the location of the polymicrogyria: Bilateral frontal polymicrogyria is a different entity than bilateral perisylvian polymicrogyria or bilateral parasagittal parieto-occipital polymicrogyria; it is important to be specific in reporting the location of the abnormality. If the cortex is abnormally thin, one should think of a prenatal injury (infectious or ischemic), particularly if the thinning is focal or multifocal.

After the cortex, look at the cerebral white matter. Make sure myelination is appropriate for age (there are many sources of normal myelination charts, including journal articles and textbooks). Then, look for areas of abnormal myelination within the deep white matter. Diffuse layers of hypomyelination or amyelination associated with overlying polymicrogyria should raise suspicion for congenital cytomegalovirus infection. More localized foci of delayed or absent myelination are often seen in deep white matter of patients with congenital muscular dystrophy and in the subcortical white matter of those with focal cortical dysplasias (FCDs). With FCDs, the absent myelination may be localized to a gyrus or may extend centrally as a curvilinear cone-shaped abnormality coursing from the cortex to the superolateral margin of a lateral ventricle (this is known as the "transmantle" sign). Also, look for nodules of heterotopic gray matter in the periventricular or deep white matter. Subcortical heterotopia typically extend from the cortex all the way to the lateral ventricular wall, while periventricular nodular heterotopia are more localized to the immediate subependymal/periventricular region. Heterotopia might be difficult to differentiate from unmyelinated or injured white matter on T1-weighted images, so be sure to look at T2-weighted images or FLAIR images to ensure that the lesion is isointense to gray matter on all sequences.

The basal ganglia are sometimes abnormal in disorders of neuronal migration, as they are formed from neurons

Brain Anomaly Imaging Checklist

Anomaly	*Findings*
Anomalies of the Cerebral Cortex	
Agyria/pachygyria	Thick cortex, smooth inner margin, few shallow sulci
Polymicrogyria	Thin undulating cortex, irregular inner margin
Cobblestone cortex	Thick cortex, irregular inner margin, abnormal myelin
Focal cortical dysplasia	Blurred gray-white junction, ± abnormal myelination
White Matter Abnormalities with Cortical Malformation	
Polymicrogyria	Enlarged perivascular spaces
Cobblestone cortex	Delayed myelination, patchy hypomyelination
Congenital cytomegalovirus	Deep layers of hypomyelination/gliosis
Focal cortical dysplasia	Focal subcortical hypomyelination
Malformations Associated with Absent Septum Pellucidum	
Septooptic dysplasia	
Holoprosencephaly	
Bilateral schizencephaly	
Bilateral polymicrogyria	
Rhombencephalosynapsis	
Malformations with prolonged severe hydrocephalus	

generated in the medial and lateral ganglionic eminences, the same germinal zones that produce GABAergic neurons that migrate to the cerebral cortex. In particular, the basal ganglia tend to be dysmorphic in appearance in patients with subcortical heterotopia. In addition, the hippocampi are often abnormal in malformations of cortical development. In patients with lissencephaly, in particular, the hippocampi are incompletely folded. Sometimes, the only structural abnormalities in children with developmental delay are hippocampal; always look to make sure that they are fully folded and not too round.

Always look at the entire interhemispheric fissure (IHF); if the cerebral hemispheres are continuous across the midline, holoprosencephaly should be diagnosed. In severe holoprosencephalies, the interhemispheric fissure is completely absent, whereas in milder forms of holoprosencephaly certain areas of the interhemispheric fissure will be absent (anterior IHF in semilobar holoprosencephaly, central IHF in syntelencephaly). Look at the septum pellucidum; absence of the septum is seen in corpus callosum dysgenesis/agenesis, septo-optic dysplasia, and in some cases of schizencephaly or bilateral polymicrogyria. While checking the septum, look at the lateral ventricles to ensure that they are normal in size and shape. Abnormally enlarged trigones and temporal horns are often associated with callosal anomalies and pachygyria. Enlarged frontal horns are often seen in bilateral frontal polymicrogyria.

Don't forget to look carefully at the posterior fossa; anomalies of the brain stem and cerebellum are commonly overlooked. Make sure that the 4th ventricle and cerebellar vermis are normally sized. In newborns, the vermis should extend from the inferior colliculi to the obex, while infants and older children should have a vermis that extends from the intercollicular sulcus to the obex. Also, make sure you see normal vermian fissures. If the fissuration of the vermis looks abnormal, look at an axial or coronal image to make sure the vermis is present; if the cerebellar hemispheres are continuous without a vermis between them, make a diagnosis of rhombencephalosynapsis. If the 4th ventricle has an abnormal rectangular shape (with a horizontal superior margin) with a narrow isthmus and small vermis, think about a molar tooth malformation. To confirm this diagnosis, look for the "molar tooth" sign of the lower midbrain, consisting of large, horizontal superior cerebellar peduncles extending posteriorly toward the cerebellum, and a longitudinal cleft in the superior vermis. Make sure that the components of the brain stem are of normal size; in a child, the height of the pons should be double that of the midbrain on the midline sagittal image. An important clue can be provided by looking at the size of the pons compared to that of the cerebellar vermis. Since much of the anterior pons is composed of the decussation of the middle cerebellar peduncles, development hypoplasia of the cerebellum is nearly always associated with hypoplasia of the ventral pons. If the pons is normal in the setting of a small cerebellum, it is most likely that the cerebellum lost volume near the end of gestation or after birth. Remember that a small posterior fossa, intracranial **hypo**tension, **or** intracranial **hyper**tension can result in descent of the cerebellum below the foramen magnum. Look for causes of a small posterior fossa (clival anomaly, anomaly of the craniovertebral junction), intracranial hypertension (space-occupying mass, hydrocephalus), or evidence of intracranial hypotension (large dural venous sinuses, large pituitary gland, "slumping" brain stem) before making a diagnosis of Chiari 1 malformation. Finally, remember to look at the size of the CSF spaces in the posterior fossa, enlargement of which may be a sign of abnormal leptomeningeal development.

(Left) *Midline analysis using sagittal T1WI MR shows significant commissural anomaly with only a small corpus callosum remnant ➔ and another small remnant, probably of hippocampal commissure ➔. A large anterior commissure ➔ is present, possibly partly compensating for the small corpus.* ***(Right)*** *Sagittal T1WI MR shows corpus callosum hypogenesis in addition to a 2nd midline anomaly, an interhemispheric lipoma ➔. Lipomas form secondary to midline mesenchymal dysgenesis.*

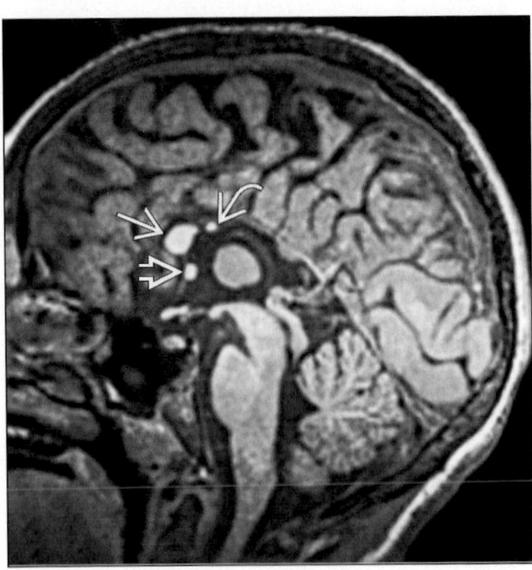

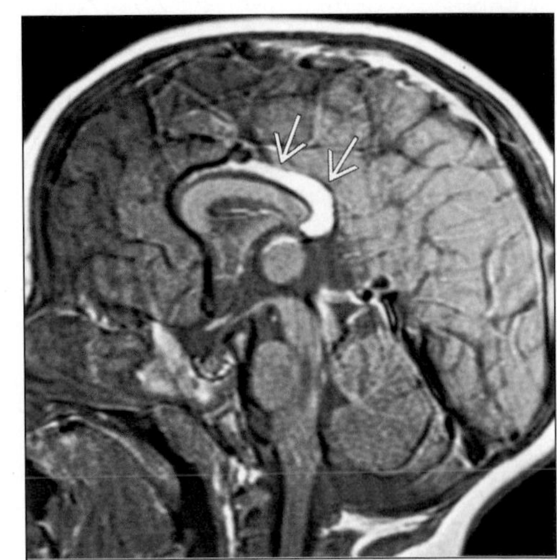

(Left) *Axial T2WI MR shows a very thickened cerebral cortex with a small cell-sparse zone ➔ and markedly diminished sulcation. This patient has anterior pachygyria and posterior agyria, suggesting lissencephaly secondary to a LIS1 mutation. Note the enlarged lateral ventricles.* ***(Right)*** *This axial T2WI MR also shows thickened cortex, but this has a much different appearance than agyria-pachygyria. The affected cortex is undulating ➔, establishing a diagnosis of right frontal polymicrogyria.*

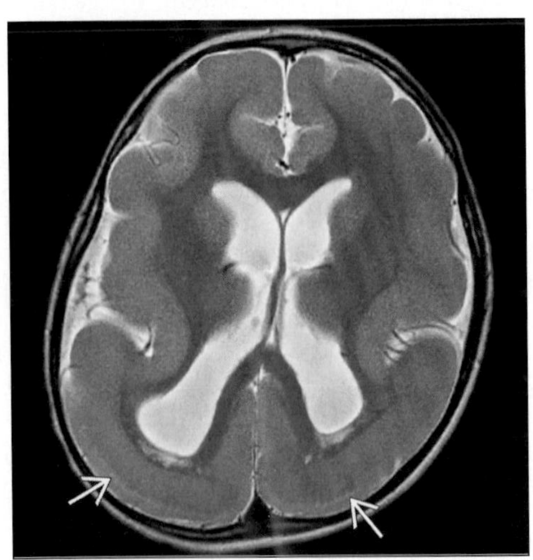

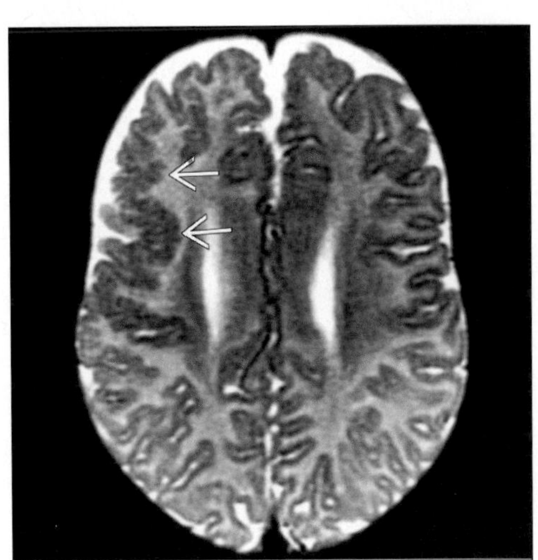

(Left) *Axial T1WI MR in this patient with epilepsy shows gray matter intensity curvinodular regions ➔ in the right temporal deep and periventricular white matter. The thinned overlying cortex establishes that this is subcortical heterotopia.* ***(Right)*** *Axial FLAIR MR in a teenager with partial epilepsy shows a focus of hyperintense white matter ➔ in the subcortical white matter of the left parietal obe. The overlying cortex is lso hyperintense in this case focal cortical dysplasia.*

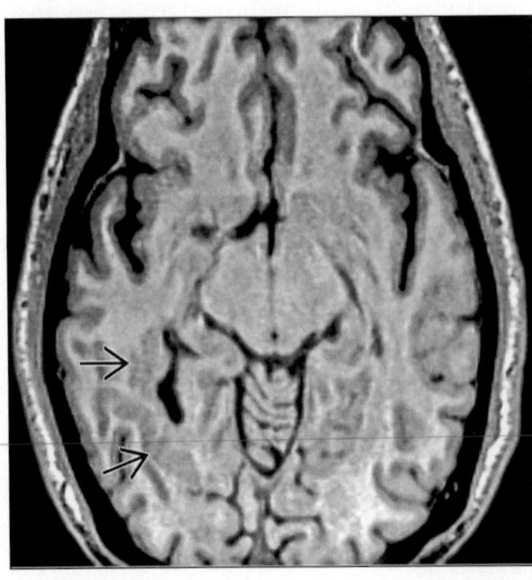

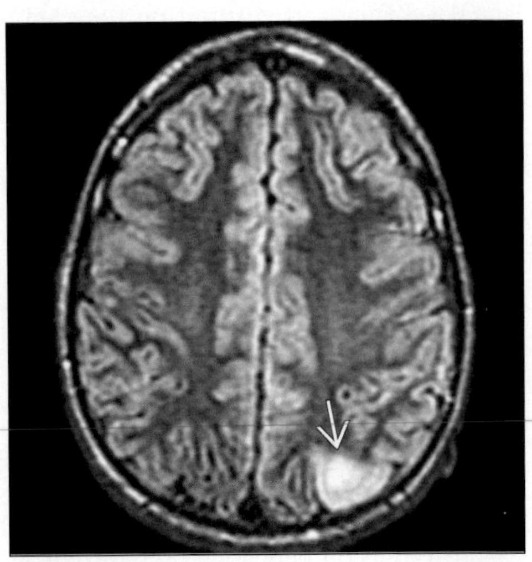

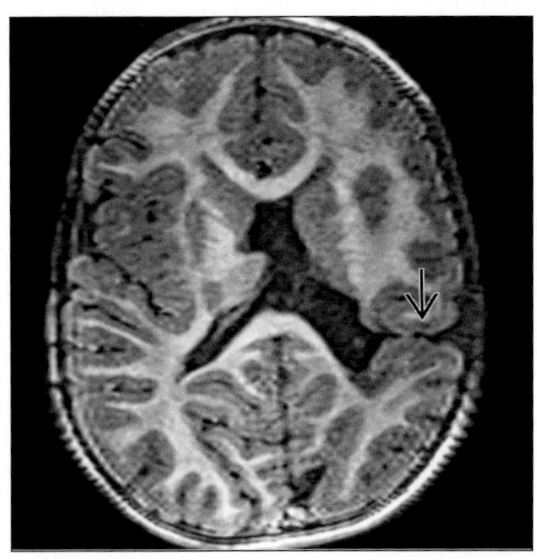

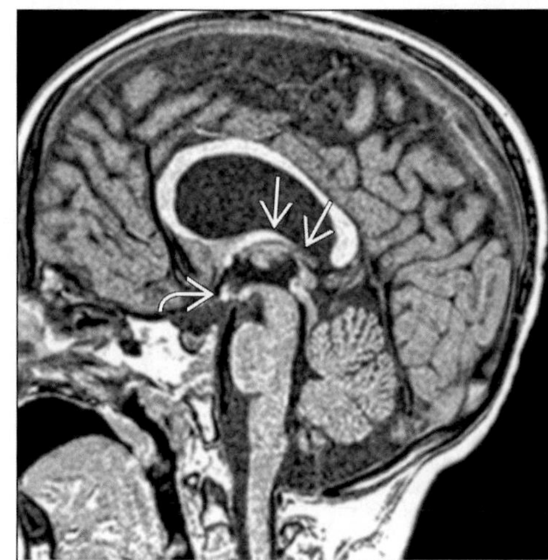

(Left) *On this axial T1WI MR, a gray matter lined cleft → is seen extending from the cortex into the enlarged trigone of the left lateral ventricle, giving a diagnosis of schizencephaly. Note the absence of the midline septum pellucidum, a common finding in bilateral schizencephaly.* ***(Right)*** *Sagittal T1WI MR shows low fornices ➡, suggesting absent septum pellucidum. Looking at the (commonly affected) hypothalamus allows diagnosis of ectopic posterior pituitary gland ➡.*

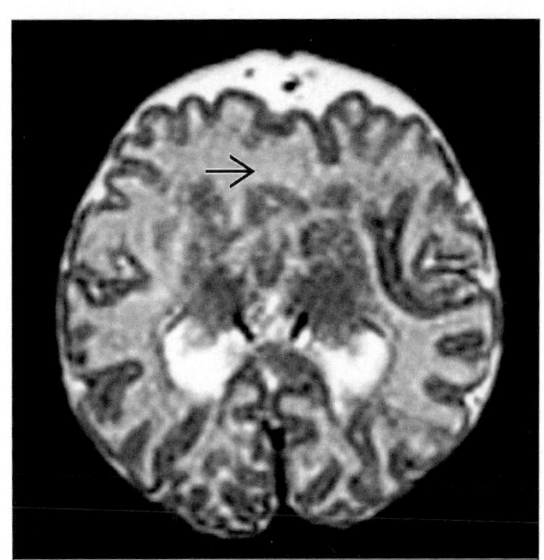

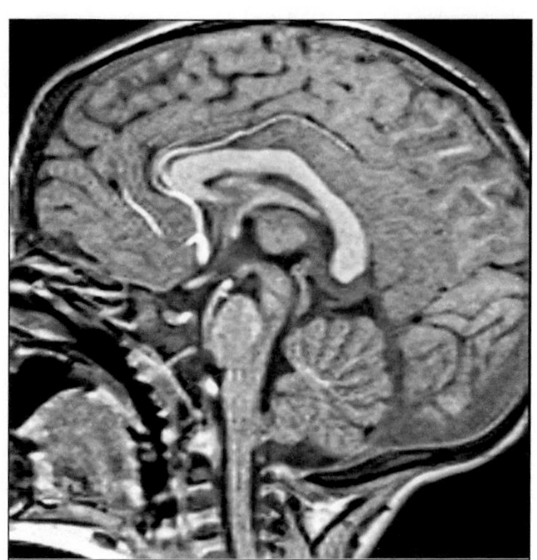

(Left) *Axial T2WI MR allows analysis of midline and shows absent interhemispheric fissure in frontal lobes (white matter continuous across midline →). This finding, plus the absence of frontal horns, gives the diagnosis of holoprosencephaly.* ***(Right)*** *Analysis of midline posterior fossa on sagittal T1WI MR shows abnormal fissures in the vermis of this 18-month-old child with ataxia. The diagnosis of vermian dysgenesis could not be established without careful observation of the vermian fissures.*

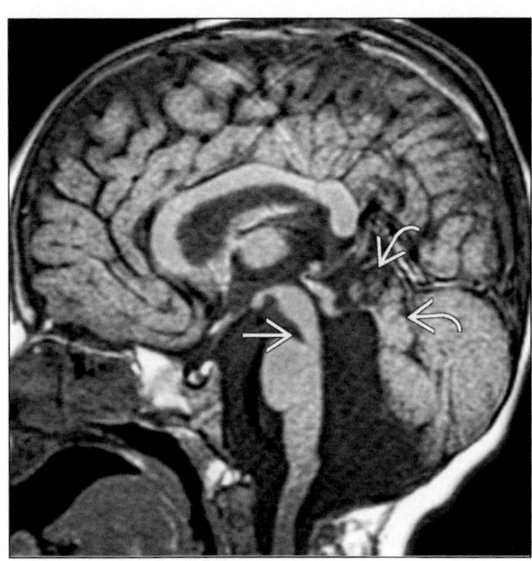

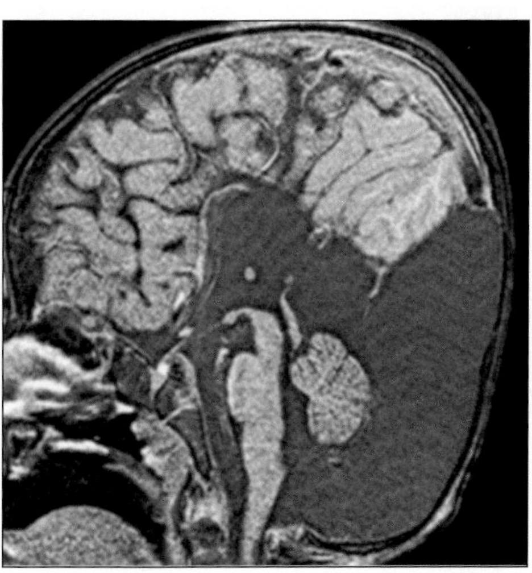

(Left) *Sagittal T1WI MR shows too much CSF in the posterior fossa. Careful analysis shows a very small vermis ➡ with a large, almost rectangular 4th ventricle. These findings, plus a very small isthmus ➡, help to establish the diagnosis of molar tooth malformation.* ***(Right)*** *Sagittal T1WI MR shows multiple midline anomalies. Corpus callosum and anterior commissure are absent, cerebellar vermis and pons are small, and the posterior fossa CSF spaces ("cisterna magna") are markedly enlarged.*

CHIARI 1

Key Facts

Terminology

- Chiari type 1 malformation (Ch 1)
- Caudal protrusion of elongated peg-shaped cerebellar tonsils below foramen magnum (FM)

Imaging

- Cerebellar tonsils ≥ 5 mm below FM, ± syringohydromyelia
- Morphology more important than extent of descent (pointed, triangular, peg-like)
- Tonsillar impaction in FM without caudal herniation may be symptomatic
- Craniovertebral segmentation/fusion anomalies are common
- Protocol: Thin sagittal T2WI MR of craniovertebral junction; ± CSF flow studies
- Image spine to detect syrinx, low/tethered cord, ± fatty filum

Pathology

- "Mismatch" between posterior fossa size (small), cerebellum (normal) → tonsillar "ectopia"

Clinical Issues

- Pediatric symptoms
  - Headache
  - Neck pain
  - Syrinx and scoliosis
- Adult symptoms
  - Neck pain and drop attacks
- Symptoms in infant/very young child may include impaired oropharyngeal function or apnea
- Treatment aim: Restore normal CSF flow at FM
- Controversial: International consensus states "no intervention for asymptomatic Chiari 1 unless syrinx"

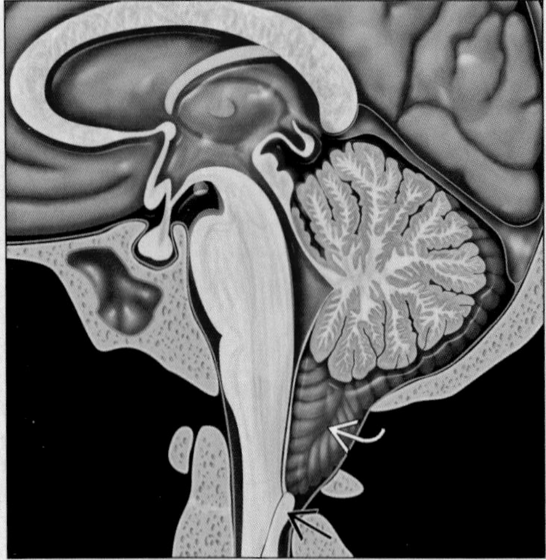

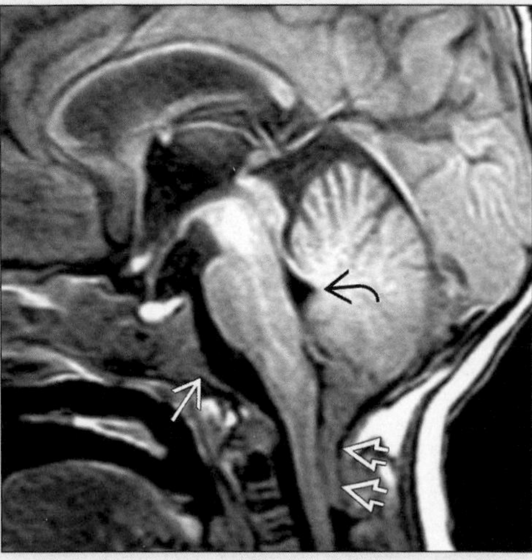

(Left) *Sagittal graphic shows low nucleus gracilis ➔ marking the obex. The compressed, pointed cerebellar tonsils ➔ protrude through foramen magnum and completely fill the cisterna magna.* ***(Right)*** *Sagittal T1WI MR in an infant reveals a compressed, slender, peg-like herniated cerebellar tonsil ➔, closely applied to the dorsal surface of the cervical spinal cord. The 4th ventricle ➔ is small but normally located. The clivus ➔ is short and scalloped.*

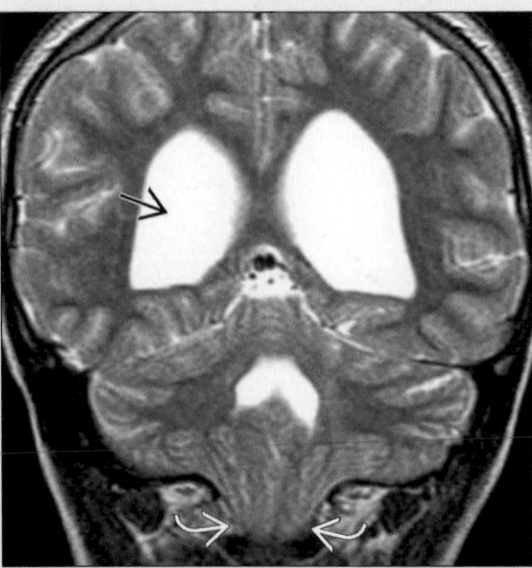

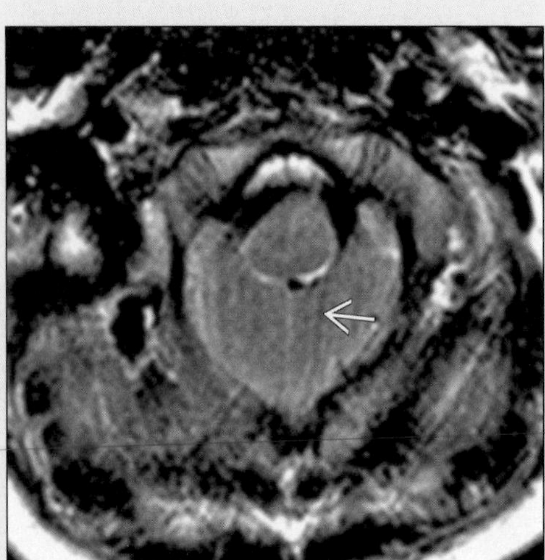

(Left) *Coronal T2WI MR in another child with symptomatic Chiari 1 malformation demonstrates ventriculomegaly ➔. The cerebellar tonsils ➔ protrude well below the obstructed foramen magnum. Consideration should be given here to a diagnosis of hydrocephalus with tonsillar herniation.* ***(Right)*** *Axial T2WI MR confirms cerebellar tonsils filling the foramen magnum and effacing the cisterna magna and basal cisterns. Note the vertical (rather than horizontal) array of cerebellar folia ➔.*

TERMINOLOGY

Abbreviations
- Chiari type 1 malformation (Ch 1)

Synonyms
- Tonsillar ectopia

Definitions
- Caudal protrusion of elongated peg-shaped cerebellar tonsils below foramen magnum (FM)

IMAGING

General Features
- Best diagnostic clue
  - Pointed cerebellar tonsils ≥ 5 mm below FM, ± syringohydromyelia
  - Oblique or vertical (not horizontal) sulci
  - Compressed/absent cisterna magna
- Location
  - Craniovertebral junction (CVJ)
- Size
  - Classically ≥ 5 mm below FM, but morphology more important than extent of descent
- Morphology
  - Pointed, triangular-shaped (peg-like) tonsils
  - Tonsillar impaction in FM without caudal herniation may be symptomatic
    - Absent cisterna magna, posteriorly angled odontoid with compressed brainstem, short posterior arch C1, short clivus, syrinx

Radiographic Findings
- Radiography
  - 4th occipital sclerotome syndromes (> 50%)
    - Craniovertebral segmentation/fusion anomalies, pro-atlas remnants, atlas assimilation, odontoid retroflexion
    - Small occipital enchondral skull: Basiocciput/clivus, exocciput, supraocciput
    - Posteriorly tilted odontoid process (more common in females) → ↑ symptoms
  - Suspect syrinx if enlarged cervical spinal canal on lateral film

CT Findings
- NECT
  - Small posterior fossa (PF) → low torcular, effaced PF cisterns
  - "Crowded" FM
  - Lateral/3rd ventricles usually normal (89%)

MR Findings
- T1WI
  - Sagittal: Pointed, triangular-shaped (peg-like) tonsils ≥ 5 mm below FM
  - "Tight" FM, effaced cisterns
  - Short clivus → "apparent" descent 4th ventricle
  - ± Elongated 4th ventricle, low nucleus gracilis
- T2WI
  - Look for upper cervical cord edema, syrinx (15-75%)
  - Vertical or oblique tonsillar folia (like "sergeant's chevron")
  - Syringohydromyelia (14-75%)
- Phase-contrast cine MR or bSSFP shows pulsatile systolic tonsillar descent, obstructed CSF flow through FM

Ultrasonographic Findings
- Color Doppler
  - Loss of bidirectional CSF flow, peak velocity of 3-5 cm/s, and waveform that exhibits vascular and respiratory variations

Imaging Recommendations
- Best imaging tool
  - Thin sagittal MR views of CVJ
- Protocol advice
  - MR ± CSF flow studies
  - Spine MR to detect syrinx, low/tethered cord, ± fatty filum

DIFFERENTIAL DIAGNOSIS

Normal Age-Related Tonsil Descent Below "Opisthion-Basion Line"
- 1st decade (6 mm); most pronounced at ~ 4 years, then tonsils "retreat"
- 2nd-3rd decades (5 mm)
- 4th-8th decades (4 mm)
- 9th decade (3 mm)

Acquired Tonsillar Ectopia/Herniation
- "Pull from below"
  - Lumbar puncture or (LP) shunt ⇒ intracranial hypotension
    - "Sagging" brainstem, acquired tonsillar herniation
  - Spontaneous intracranial hypotension
- "Push from above"
  - Chronic ventriculo-peritoneal shunt (thick skull, premature sutural fusion, lumbar arachnoidal adhesions)
  - Tonsillar herniation 2° ↑ intracranial pressure, mass effect, or tumor

PATHOLOGY

General Features
- Etiology
  - "Mismatch" between posterior fossa size (small), cerebellum (normal) → tonsillar "ectopia"
  - Hydrodynamic theory of symptomatic Chiari 1
    - Systolic piston-like descent of impacted tonsils/medulla → abnormal intraspinal CSF pressure-wave
    - Hydrosyringomyelia develops as secondary phenomenon
- Genetics
  - Syndromic/familial
    - Craniosynostoses, midline anomalies
    - Mutated *LHX4* gene (Chr 1q25)
      - Posterior pituitary ectopia, Chiari 1
    - Macrencephaly syndromes
      - Neurofibromatosis type 1, Sotos, Proteus, hemimegalencephaly

- Associated abnormalities
  - CVJ bony anomalies frequent
    - 4th occipital sclerotome anomalies, underdeveloped basichondrocranium, Klippel-Feil, Sprengel deformity, platybasia
  - Embryology
    - Underdeveloped occipital enchondrium → small PF vault → crowded PF → downward herniated hindbrain → obstructed FM → lack of communication between cranial/spinal CSF compartments

Staging, Grading, & Classification

- 1 = asymptomatic (14-50%), treatment controversial
- 2 = brainstem compression
- 3 = hydrosyringomyelia

Gross Pathologic & Surgical Features

- Herniated, sclerotic tonsillar pegs
- Tonsils grooved by impaction against opisthion
- Arachnoid adhesions between cerebellar tonsils, medulla
- Thickened leptomeninges &/or thickened dura mater at CVJ

Microscopic Features

- Purkinje/granular cell loss

CLINICAL ISSUES

Presentation

- Most common signs/symptoms
  - Up to 50% asymptomatic
  - Prevalence of symptoms ↑ if spinal canal diameter < 19 mm
  - "Chiari 1 spells": Cough or sneezing → acute ↑ intrathecal pressure due to obstructed CSF flow → headache or syncope
  - Symptomatic brainstem compression
    - Hypersomnolence/central apnea/sudden death (infant)
    - Bulbar signs (e.g., lower CN palsies)
    - Neck or back pain, torticollis, ataxia
  - Symptomatic syringohydromyelia
    - Paroxysmal dystonia, unsteady gait, incontinence
    - Atypical scoliosis (progressive, painful, atypical curve)
    - Dissociated sensory loss/neuropathy (hand muscle wasting)
  - Other: Hiccoughs, trigeminal facial pain; may mimic multiple sclerosis
- Clinical profile
  - Infant/very young child: Impaired oropharyngeal function common
  - Child: Headache, neck pain, syrinx, and scoliosis
  - Adult: Neck pain and drop attacks

Demographics

- Age
  - Very young child: Mean 3.3 years
  - Pediatric: Mean 11 years (range in 1 series: 2 months to 20 years)
  - Adult: Mean 34 years
- Gender
  - M:F = 1:1.3
- Epidemiology
  - 0.01% of population

Natural History & Prognosis

- Increasing ectopia + ↑ time → ↑ likelihood of symptoms
- Children respond better than adults; treat early
- Postoperative complications
  - Cerebellar ptosis
  - Regrowth/ossification of resected bone

Treatment

- Controversial: International consensus states "no intervention for asymptomatic Chiari 1 unless syrinx"
  - Most will also intervene if scoliosis, even in absence of syringohydromyelia **or** central apnea
  - Syrinx shunted only if syrinx persists or progresses post suboccipital decompression
- Treatment aim = restore normal CSF flow at FM
  - Suboccipital decompression/resection posterior arch C1; ± duraplasty, cerebellar tonsil resection **or** endoscopic suboccipital decompression
    - > 90% → ↓ brainstem signs
    - > 80% → ↓ syringohydromyelia
    - Scoliosis arrests (improves in younger patients)
    - Progression of spinal deformity post suboccipital decompression ↑ with older age, severity of initial symptoms, double scoliosis curve, thoracic kyphosis, rotation, large curve

DIAGNOSTIC CHECKLIST

Consider

- If spine imaged 1st, remember to image brain: Hydrocephalus & brain tumors "push" tonsils down

Image Interpretation Pearls

- Low tonsils with normal rounded shape are usually asymptomatic
- Tonsils with peg/triangular shape + obliteration of surrounding CSF are abnormal at any level below opisthion-basion line

SELECTED REFERENCES

1. Aitken LA et al: Chiari type I malformation in a pediatric population. Pediatr Neurol. 40(6):449-54, 2009
2. Milhorat TH et al: Association of Chiari malformation type I and tethered cord syndrome: preliminary results of sectioning filum terminale. Surg Neurol. 72(1):20-35, 2009
3. Tisell M et al: Long-term outcome after surgery for Chiari I malformation. Acta Neurol Scand. Epub ahead of print, 2009
4. Novegno F et al: The natural history of the Chiari Type I anomaly. J Neurosurg Pediatr. 2(3):179-87, 2008
5. Tubbs RS et al: Surgical experience in 130 pediatric patients with Chiari I malformations. J Neurosurg. 99(2):291-6, 2003
6. Ventureyra EC et al: The role of cine flow MRI in children with Chiari I malformation. Childs Nerv Syst. 19(2):109-13, 2003

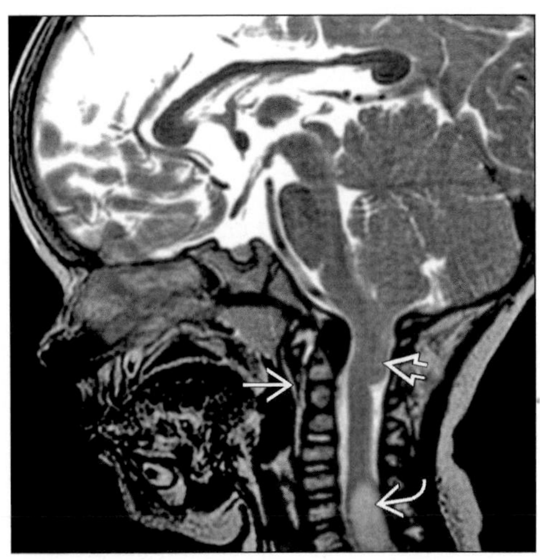

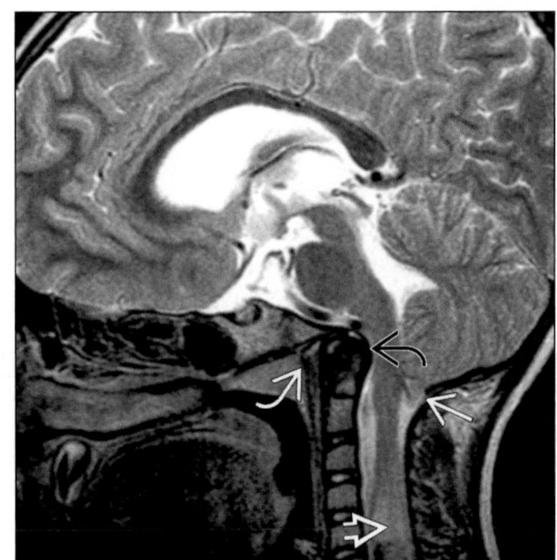

(Left) *Sagittal T2WI MR in a child with Crouzon disease shows spinal segmentation anomalies, syringohydromyelia, Chiari 1 with caudal protrusion of cerebellar tonsils, and obliteration of the cisterna magna. Mild odontoid retroversion contributes to compression of the cervicomedullary cord.* ***(Right)*** *Sagittal T2WI MR in a child reveals platybasia with an abnormal clival-axial angle, retroverted dens, syringohydromyelia, and Chiari 1 malformation.*

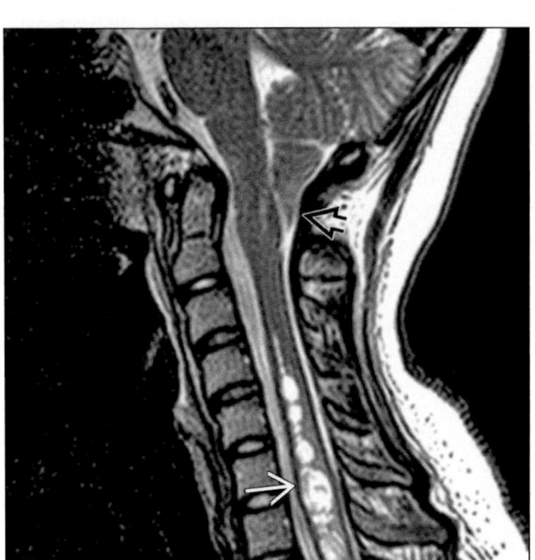

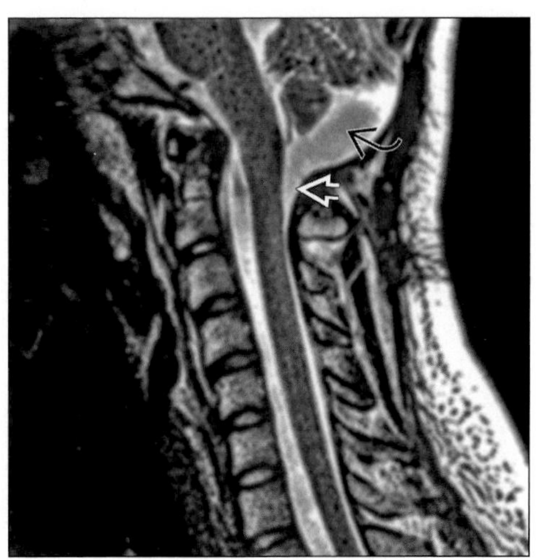

(Left) *Sagittal T2WI MR in a teenage girl with headaches reveals pointed cerebellar tonsils extending well below the foramen magnum. Extensive syringohydromyelia is also seen.* ***(Right)*** *Sagittal T2WI MR in the same teenager, following foramen magnum decompression with duraplasty and removal of posterior arch of C1, demonstrates resolution of syringohydromyelia, a widely patent foramen magnum, and an open cisterna magna.*

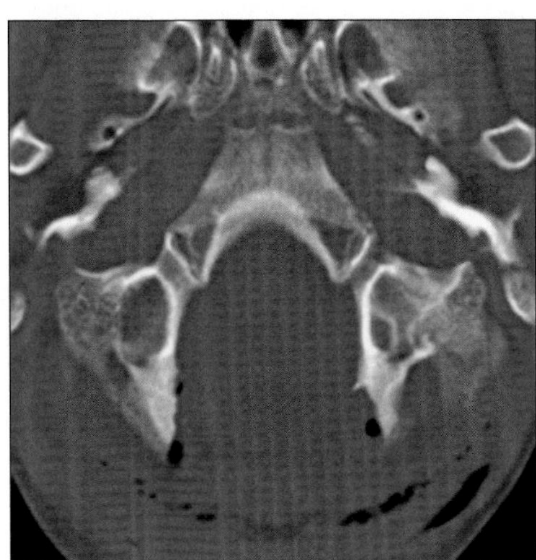

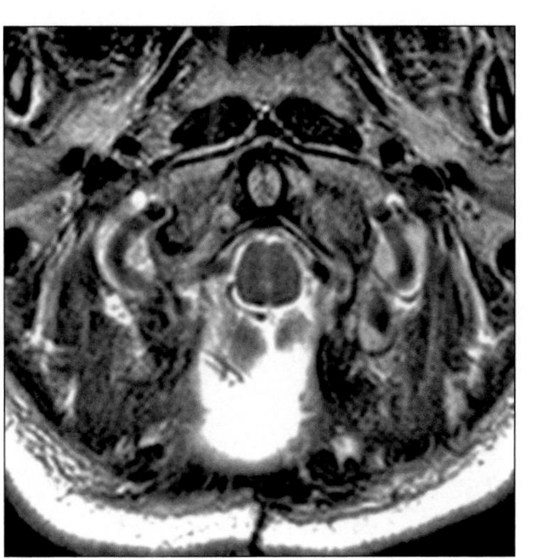

(Left) *Axial bone CT of the foramen magnum in a 6-year-old patient immediately after a foramen magnum decompression shows postoperative appearance, consisting of a wide resection of the opisthion and adjacent bony margin of the foramen magnum.* ***(Right)*** *Axial T2WI MR in a teenager, following suboccipital craniectomy/foramen magnum decompression for symptomatic Chiari 1 malformation, demonstrates expected wide bony defect filled with CSF at the level of the foramen magnum.*

CHIARI 2

Key Facts

Terminology

- Arnold-Chiari malformation (AC2), Chiari 2 (Ch 2)
- Complex malformation of hindbrain, virtually 100% associated with neural tube closure defect (NTD), usually lumbar myelomeningocele (MMC)

Imaging

- "Cascade" or "waterfall" of tissue behind medulla
- Fenestrated/hypoplastic falx ⇒ interdigitated gyri
- "Beaked" (sagittal) or heart-shaped (axial) tectum
- Chiari-shaped lateral ventricles: Pointed anterior horns, colpocephaly
- Periventricular nodular heterotopia (usually in trigone) in 10-15%
- Concave clivus and temporal bones
- "Lacunar" skull (Lückenschädel)

Pathology

- Basic abnormality = small PF with herniated hindbrain, hydrocephalus
- Neurogenic, renal, and orthopedic complications are the norm
- Pathogenesis
  - Abnormal neurulation →
  - CSF escapes through NTD →
  - Failure to maintain 4th ventricular distention →
  - Hypoplastic PF chondrocranium →
  - Displaced/distorted PF contents

Diagnostic Checklist

- Imaging features due to long-term effects of mechanical distortion
- Brainstem compression may cause sedation and anesthesia risks

(Left) Sagittal graphic shows hydrocephalus with enlarged anterior recesses of the 3rd ventricle →, small posterior fossa, large massa intermedia →, "beaked" tectum →, callosal hypogenesis, elongated 4th ventricle with inferiorly herniating cerebellum and choroid plexus →, and medullary spur →. (Right) Axial T2WI MR in an infant with myelomeningocele and Chiari 2 malformation reveals prominent massa intermedia →, colpocephaly, and a heterotopic gray matter nodule in the dilated posterior horn →.

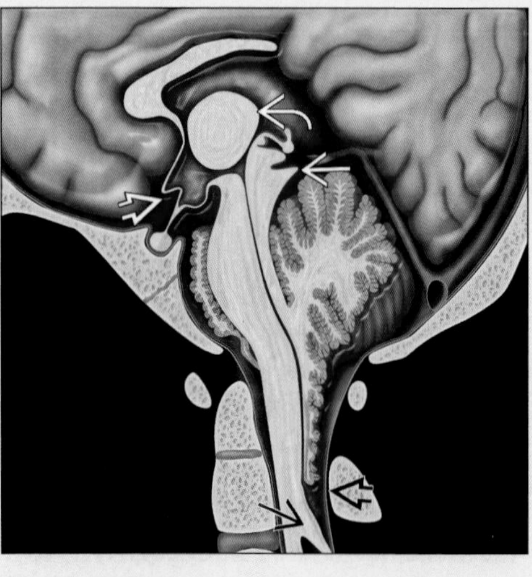

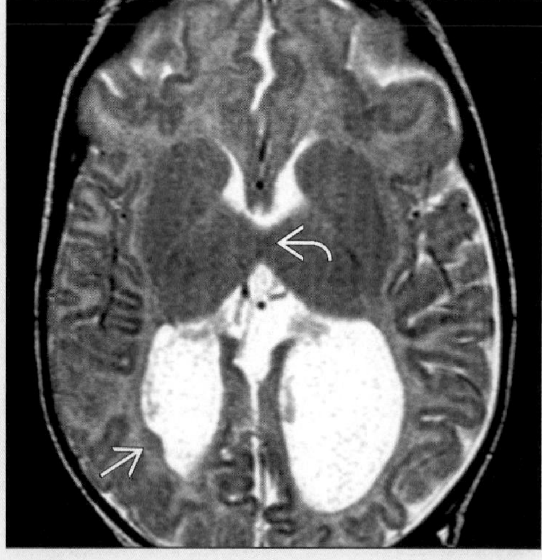

(Left) Sagittal T2WI MR in a teenager shows a truncated, malformed corpus callosum →, "beaked" tectum →, caudally displaced pons → and cerebellar tissue →, prominent massa intermedia →, and volume loss of the medial parietal cortex. (Right) Coronal T2WI MR in another child reveals volume loss of the medial parietooccipital cortex with gyral interdigitation →. Note the towering cerebellum → projecting through the widened tentorial incisura.

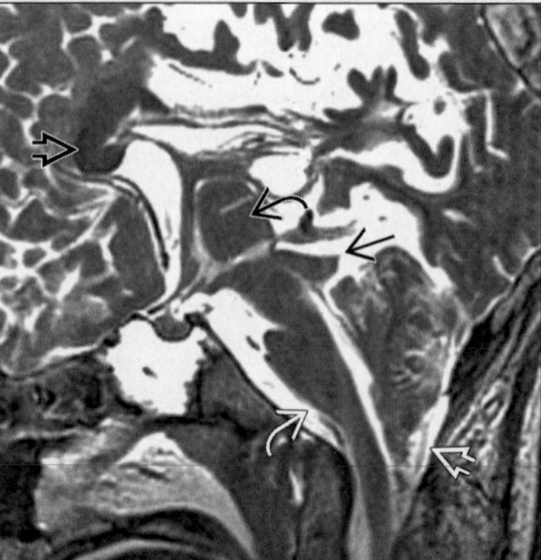

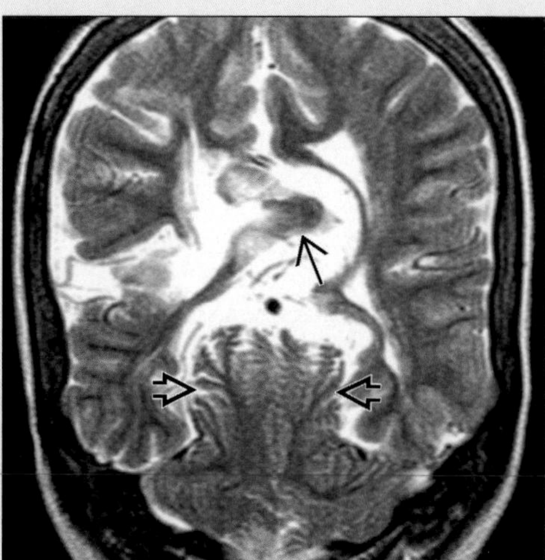

TERMINOLOGY

Synonyms
- Arnold-Chiari malformation (AC2), Chiari 2 (Ch 2)

Definitions
- Complex malformation of hindbrain, virtually 100% associated with neural tube closure defect (NTD), usually lumbar myelomeningocele (MMC)

IMAGING

General Features
- Best diagnostic clue
  - Presence of MMC and hindbrain herniation
- Location
  - Hindbrain
- Size
  - Small posterior fossa
- Morphology
  - "Cascade" of tissue herniates through foramen magnum behind upper cervical cord
    - Vermis (nodulus)
    - Choroid plexus of 4th ventricle
    - Medullary "spur"

Radiographic Findings
- Radiography
  - "Lacunar" skull (Lückenschädel)
    - Universal at birth; largely resolves by 6 months
    - Craniolacunia involves inner, outer tables (squamous bones)
    - Caused by mesenchymal defect (not ↑ ICP)
  - Incorporation of accessory frontal bone → transient "bifrontal foramina"
  - Widened upper cervical canal (Chiari malformation ± syrinx)

CT Findings
- NECT
  - Small posterior fossa (PF)
    - Low-lying tentorium/torcular inserts near foramen magnum
    - Large, funnel-shaped foramen magnum
    - "Scalloped" petrous pyramid, "notched" clivus
  - Dural abnormalities
    - Fenestrated/hypoplastic falx → interdigitated gyri
    - Heart-shaped incisura
    - Absent falx cerebelli

MR Findings
- T1WI
  - Small PF → contents shift down into cervical canal, herniate upward through incisura
    - Cerebellar (CBLL) hemispheres/tonsils "wrap" anteriorly around medulla
    - Compressed, elongated, low-lying 4th ventricle often lacks fastigial recess, may pouch into cervical canal
    - "Towering" cerebellum protrudes up through incisura, compresses tectum
  - Associated abnormalities: Dysgenetic corpus callosum (CC) (90%)
  - "Beaked" (sagittal) or heart-shaped (axial) tectum
- T2WI
  - Ventricles
    - Lateral: Pointed anterior horns, colpocephaly, periventricular nodular heterotopia in 10-15%
    - 3rd: Large massa intermedia
    - 4th: Elongated, straw-like without fastigial recess
  - Small PF
    - Concave clivus, temporal bones
    - Obliterated basal cisterns
  - "Cascade" or "waterfall" of tissue behind medulla
    - Vermian nodulus (± abnormal ↑ signal)
    - Choroid plexus
    - Medulla
      - "Heaps up" over cord tethered by dentate ligaments → kink-spur, Z-shaped cervico-medullary junction in 70%
- MRV
  - Torcular, transverse sinuses extremely low
- MR spine
  - Open dysraphism, MMC almost 100% (lumbar >> cervical)
  - Hydrosyringomyelia (20-90%)
  - Posterior arch C1 anomalies (66%)
  - Diastematomyelia (5%)

Ultrasonographic Findings
- Grayscale ultrasound
  - Fetal ultrasound
    - MMC defined as early as 10 weeks on US
    - AC2 ("lemon" or "banana" signs) recognized as early as 12 weeks gestation
    - Lacunar skull identified by irregular echogenicity of calvarium

Angiographic Findings
- Descent posterior inferior cerebellar arteries (PICA), depressed basilar tip

Nonvascular Interventions
- Myelography
  - Tethered cord
  - Nerve roots pass horizontal or even upward

Imaging Recommendations
- Best imaging tool
  - Magnetic resonance imaging
- Protocol advice
  - Image entire brain and spine
  - Follow-up for
    - Symptoms of brainstem compression
    - Increasing ventricular size
    - Increasing spinal symptoms

DIFFERENTIAL DIAGNOSIS

Severe, Chronic Shunted Congenital Hydrocephalus
- May cause collapsed brain and upward herniated cerebellum, but no spina bifida

Other Chiari Malformations
- Chiari 1: Herniated CBLL tonsils
- Chiari 3: Chiari 2 with encephalocele

- Chiari 4: Controversial, not just hypoplastic cerebellum
  - Some reserve term for severe hypoplasia of cerebellum in association with Chiari 2

PATHOLOGY

General Features

- Etiology
  - Embryology
    - Origins during 4th fetal week
    - Abnormal neurulation → CSF escapes through NTD → failure to maintain 4th ventricular distention → hypoplastic PF chondrocranium → displaced/distorted PF contents
  - New studies demonstrate that vimentin is focally upregulated in ependyma in dysgenetic regions
- Genetics
  - 4-8% recurrence risk if 1 child affected
  - Methylene-tetra-hydrofolate-reductase (*MTHFR*) mutations (especially C677T) associated with abnormal folate metabolism
  - *MTHFR* mutations + folate deficiency ⇒ ↑ risk NTD
  - Decreases in serum folate are seen with anti-epileptic drugs, oral contraceptives, and smoking
- Associated abnormalities
  - 4th ventricular glial or arachnoidal cysts, choroidal nodules, and subependymoma
    - Situated in roof of 4th ventricle, closely associated with choroid plexus
    - Rarely identified on imaging
  - Neurogenic, renal, and orthopedic complications are often present

Staging, Grading, & Classification

- Hydrocephalus, brain malformation relate to
  - Size of PF
  - Degree of hindbrain descent

Gross Pathologic & Surgical Features

- Basic abnormality = small PF with herniated hindbrain, hydrocephalus
- Associated abnormalities
  - "Polygyria" (too many small crowded gyri) with normal 6-layer lamination
  - ± absent septum pellucidum/fused forniceal columns
  - Heterotopias
  - Aqueduct stenosis

Microscopic Features

- Purkinje cell loss
- Variable sclerosis of herniated tissues

CLINICAL ISSUES

Presentation

- Most common signs/symptoms
  - Neonate: MMC
- Clinical profile
  - MMC
  - Enlarging head
  - Lower extremity paralysis, sphincter dysfunction
  - Bulbar signs

Demographics

- Age
  - Identified in utero or at birth
    - Fetal screening: ↑ α-fetoprotein
- Gender
  - Slight female predominance
- Ethnicity
  - ↑ incidence in Mexico
    - Probably associated with high prevalence of *MTHFR* mutation
- Epidemiology
  - 0.44 in 1,000 births, decreasing with folate replacement and elective termination of affected fetus

Natural History & Prognosis

- AC2 most common cause of death in MMC
  - Brainstem compression/hydrocephalus
  - Intrinsic brainstem "wiring" defects

Treatment

- Folate supplements given to mothers
  - From pre-conception to 6 weeks post-conception ↓↓ (but does not eradicate) risk of MMC
- CSF diversion/shunting
- Chiari decompression
- Fetal repair of MMC in selected patients may ameliorate severity of AC2

DIAGNOSTIC CHECKLIST

Consider

- Brainstem compression may cause sedation and anesthesia risks

Image Interpretation Pearls

- Imaging features due to long-term effects of mechanical distortion
  - "Too small" PF
  - Cerebellar contents herniate upward and downward

SELECTED REFERENCES

1. Hirose S et al: Fetal surgery for myelomeningocele. Clin Perinatol. 36(2):431-8, xi, 2009
2. Sarnat HB: Regional ependymal upregulation of vimentin in Chiari II malformation, aqueductal stenosis, and hydromyelia. Pediatr Dev Pathol. 7(1):48-60, 2004
3. McLone DG et al: The Chiari II malformation: cause and impact. Childs Nerv Syst. 19(7-8):540-50, 2003
4. Tulipan N: Intrauterine myelomeningocele repair. Clin Perinatol. 30(3):521-30, 2003
5. Coley BD: Ultrasound diagnosis of luckenschadel (lacunar skull). Pediatr Radiol. 30(2):82-4, 2000
6. Northrup H et al: Spina bifida and other neural tube defects. Curr Probl Pediatr. 30(10):313-32, 2000
7. Mutchinick OM et al: High prevalence of the thermolabile methylenetetrahydrofolate reductase variant in Mexico: a country with a very high prevalence of neural tube defects. Mol Genet Metab. 68(4):461-7, 1999

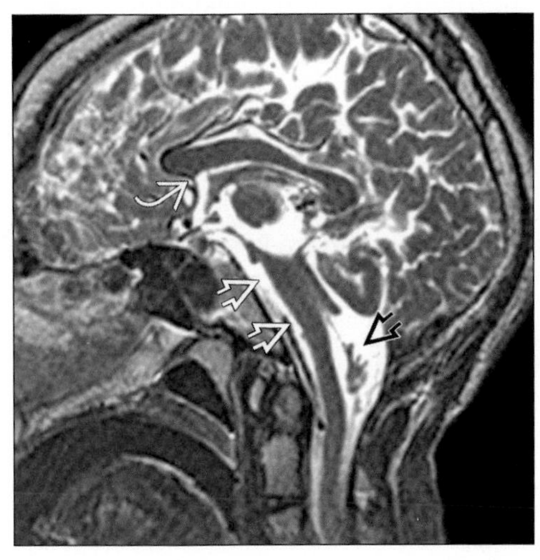

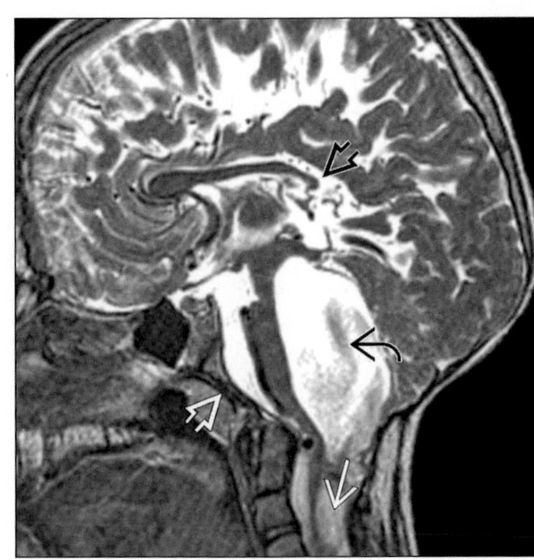

(Left) *Sagittal T1WI FS MR demonstrates truncation of the rostral corpus callosum ➔, marked thinning of the brainstem ➔, a thinned tectal plate, and a "disappearing" cerebellum ➔.* ***(Right)*** *Sagittal T2WI MR in another child demonstrates truncation of the rostrum and absence of the splenium ➔ of the corpus callosum. The 4th ventricle ➔ is isolated, syringohydromyelia ➔ is present, the brainstem is thinned, and the clivus ➔ appears scalloped.*

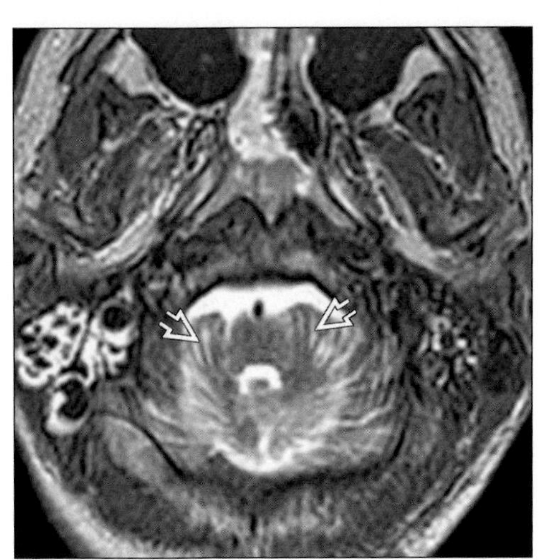

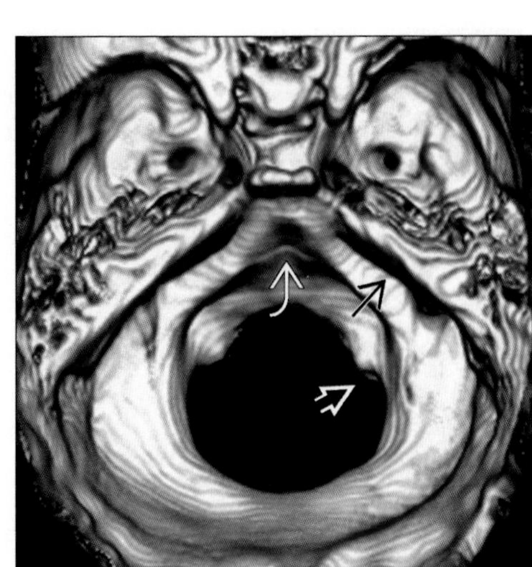

(Left) *Axial T2WI MR reveals enlargement of the foramen magnum and typical "wrapping" of the medulla by the cerebellar tonsils ➔. Sinus and mastoid mucosal swelling is incidental.* ***(Right)*** *Axial 3D reconstruction of the skull base demonstrates a large, funnel-shaped foramen magnum ➔, petrous scalloping ➔, and a clival notch or clival scalloping ➔. These are believed to result from pressure effects of normal-sized posterior fossa structures in a small posterior fossa.*

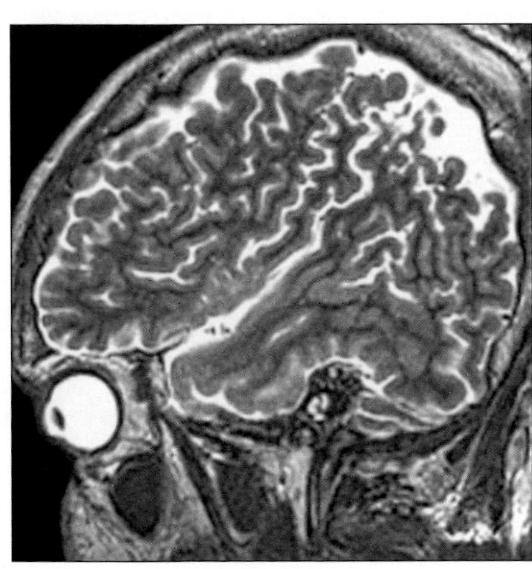

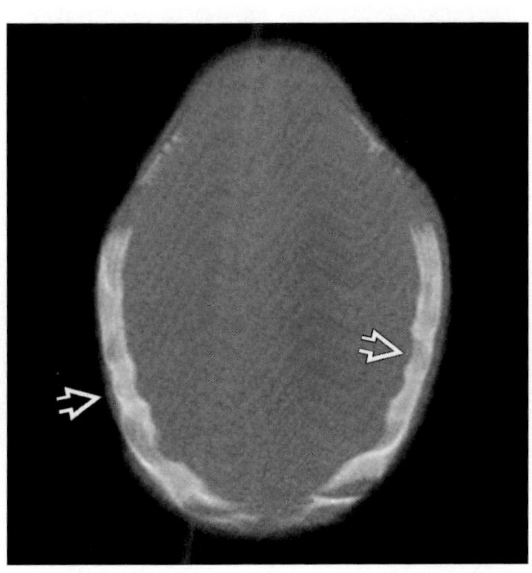

(Left) *Sagittal T2WI MR reveals the appearance of "too many gyri," also called stenogyria or polygyria. This condition is believed to result from pressure effects upon the cortical sulci from congenital hydrocephalus, compounded by CSF diversion.* ***(Right)*** *Axial bone CT in a newborn reveals a lemon-shaped calvarium with extensive Lückenschädel ➔ or "lacunar" skull. The lacunar skull is also believed to result from intracranial hypotension in utero. It resolves by age 6 months.*

CHIARI 3

Key Facts

Terminology

- Chiari type 3 malformation (Ch 3)
- Synonym: Rhombencephalocele
- Chiari described herniation of cerebellum and brain stem through spina bifida at C1-C2
- Many currently classify as meningoencephalocele involving posterior foramen magnum + intracranial Chiari 2 malformation

Imaging

- Sac contents: Meninges, ± cerebellum, ± brainstem
- Occipital poles and upper cervical cord may be "pulled into defect"
- Contents may also include cisterns, 4th ventricle, dural sinuses
- Enlarged foramen magnum at site of opisthion
- Defect in ventral chondral portion of supraoccipital bone

Pathology

- Contents: Disorganized (neuronal migration anomalies, cortical dysplasias) and gliotic tissue

Clinical Issues

- Symptoms and prognosis proportional to amount and type of herniated tissue
- Mechanical traction brainstem, respiratory deterioration, lower cranial nerve dysfunction
- Developmental delay, spasticity, hypotonia, seizures
- Occipital/upper cervical cephalocele, microcephaly

Diagnostic Checklist

- Beware of venous structures and brainstem!
- If it does not involve the opisthion, it's not classical Chiari 3

*(**Left**) Sagittal T1WI MR in a neonate with prenatally diagnosed cephalocele shows a large meningoencephalocele composed of meninges, CSF, cerebellum, brain stem, and upper cervical spinal cord, herniated through a defect in the lower occipital bone and upper cervical spine. (**Right**) Bone CT surface rendering of the posterior calvarium/upper cervical spine in the same patient shows a large defect ➔ of the ventral chondral and squamous supraoccipital bones, with upper cervical spina bifida.*

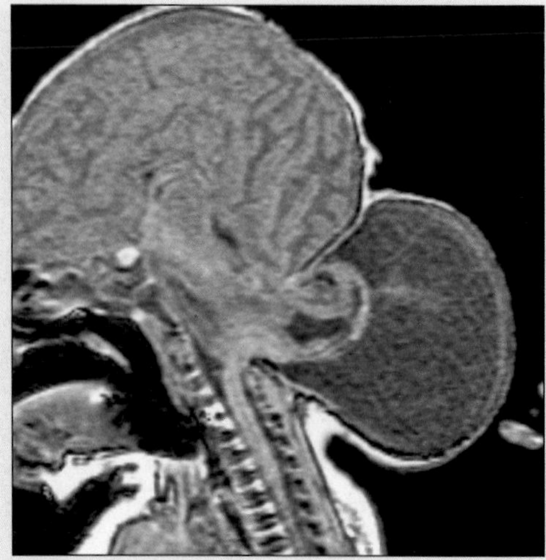

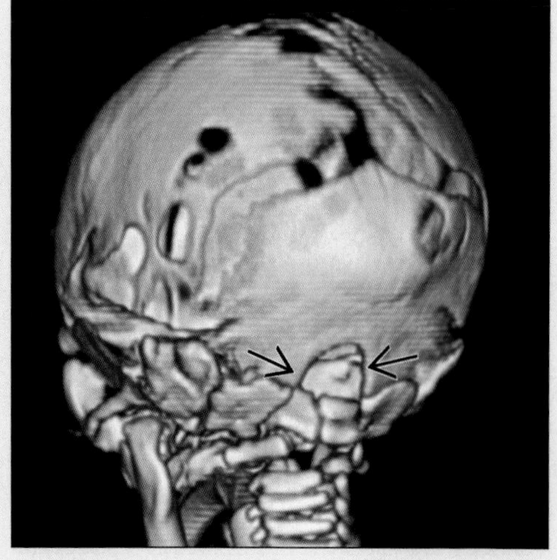

*(**Left**) Sagittal T1WI MR demonstrates very large occipital meningocele containing little residual cerebellar tissue. Calvarial defect extends downward from the region of the inion to the opisthion. A small amount of residual cerebellar vermis ➔ remains. The upper cervical vertebrae are nonsegmented ➔. (**Right**) Sagittal MRV demonstrates typical venous abnormalities of Chiari 3. The straight sinus ➔ is severely hypoplastic. Occipital sinuses ➔ are present, rather than transverse sinuses.*

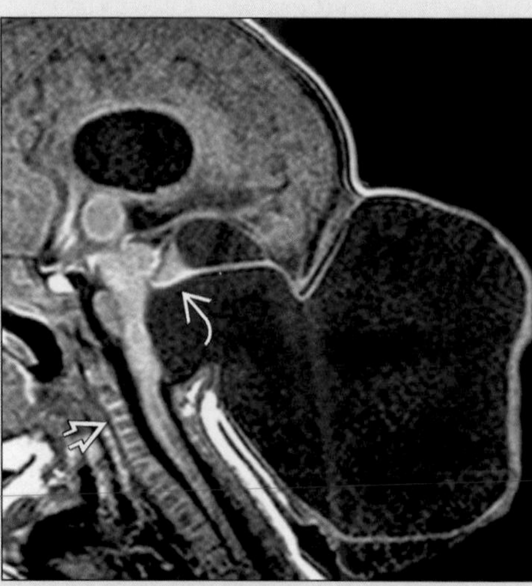

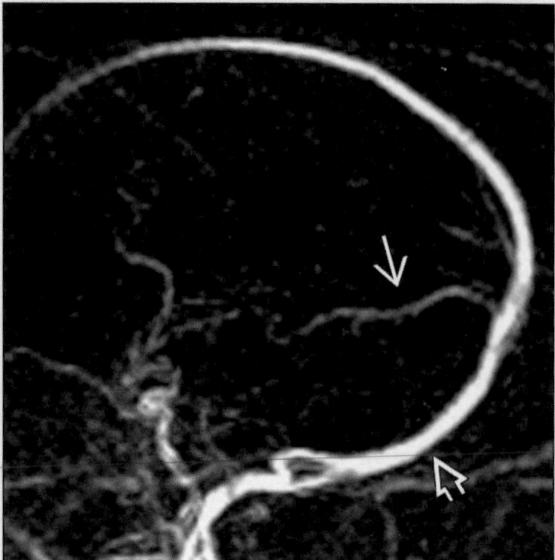

TERMINOLOGY

Abbreviations
- Chiari type 3 malformation (Ch 3)

Synonyms
- Rhombencephalocele

Definitions
- Professor Chiari described herniation of cerebellum and brain stem through spina bifida at C1-C2
- Many currently classify as meningoencephalocele involving posterior foramen magnum + intracranial Chiari 2 malformation

IMAGING

General Features
- Best diagnostic clue
  - Low occipital, high cervical meningoencephalocele
  - Cranium bifidum below inion
  - Upper cervical spina bifida
- Location
  - Ventral chondral portion of supraoccipital bone, opisthion of foramen magnum
  - May extend to involve squamous portion of supraoccipital bone
  - May extend to involve posterior arch of upper cervical vertebrae
- Size
  - Variable
- Morphology
  - Large skin-covered, sac-like mass protruding from craniovertebral junction (CVJ)

Radiographic Findings
- Radiography
  - Enlarged foramen magnum
  - Defect in ventral chondral portion of supraoccipital bone
  - Low cranium bifidum

CT Findings
- NECT
  - Opisthion and ventral chondral supraoccipital bone defect
    - Absent Kerckring ossicle
    - Absent cerebellar falx and inferior internal occipital crest
  - Bony features of Chiari 2
    - Small posterior cranial fossa, scalloped clivus, lacunar skull
- CECT
  - CTV: Veins/dural sinuses within sac
    - Anomalous &/or ptotic veins/dural sinuses
- CTA
  - Basilar artery "pulled" into defect with brainstem herniation into sac

MR Findings
- T1WI
  - Sac contents
    - Meninges, ± cerebellum, ± brainstem, ± upper cervical cord
    - Occipital poles may be "pulled" into defect
    - Cisterns, 4th ventricle, dural sinuses (50%)
  - Hydrocephalus
  - ± occasionally "absent ventricles" if massive brain herniation into defect
- T2WI
  - Tissues in sac may be bright (gliosis) or strand-like (necrotic)
- T1WI C+
  - Contrast may clarify location of veins, choroid plexus
- MRV
  - ± durovenous structures in cephalocele
  - ± anomalous course of transverse sinuses

Imaging Recommendations
- Best imaging tool
  - MR
- Protocol advice
  - Sagittal T1WI, sagittal T2WI, sagittal FIESTA, and MR venogram

DIFFERENTIAL DIAGNOSIS

Isolated Occipital Encephalocele
- Lack intracranial findings of Chiari 2

Other Occipital Encephaloceles
- High occipital encephalocele, sparing foramen magnum
- Iniencephaly
  - Occipital defect, ectatic foramen magnum ± encephalocele, dorsal medullary cleft, cervical dysraphism/Klippel-Feil, severe cervicothoracic lordosis, fixed retroflexion of head
- Syndromic occipital encephalocele
  - Meckel-Gruber: Occipital encephalocele, multicystic kidney, polydactyly
  - Dandy-Walker malformation
  - Goldenhar-Gorlin
  - MURCS (Müllerian, renal, cervical-spine)
  - Walker-Warburg
  - Amniotic band

PATHOLOGY

General Features
- Etiology
  - Etiologies of neural tube defects (NTD)
    - Maternal dietary folate deficiency; folate antagonists (antiepileptics)
    - Toxins: *Tripterygium wilfordii* (Chinese herbs), arsenic
    - Maternal hyperthermia
- Genetics
  - Nearly half of NTD cases have 677C ⇒ T mutation on methylene-tetra-hydrofolate reductase (*MTHFR*) gene
    - Especially occipital encephalocele or extensive spina bifida
    - Leads to ↑ amniotic homocysteine levels
- Associated abnormalities

- High cervical-occipital meningoencephalocele with herniated cerebellar tissue and posterior/caudal displacement of brainstem
- Embryology-anatomy theories
  - Failure of enchondral bone induction by incomplete closure of neural tube
  - Failure of fusion of ossification centers
  - Squamous supraoccipital or parietal extension: Faulty induction or pressure erosion by sac

Staging, Grading, & Classification

- Classify severity by contents
  - Meninges, cerebellum, brainstem ± cervical cord, ± occipital poles, ± vasculature
- Encephalocele not involving opisthion of foramen magnum is not Chiari 3

Gross Pathologic & Surgical Features

- Sac contents: Meninges, cerebellum, brainstem ± cervical cord, ± occipital poles, ± vasculature

Microscopic Features

- Tissues in sac
  - Disorganized (neuronal migration anomalies, cortical dysplasias)
  - Gliotic tissue
- Lining of sac may show gray matter heterotopias

CLINICAL ISSUES

Presentation

- Most common signs/symptoms
  - Occipital/upper cervical cephalocele, microcephaly
  - Discovered by fetal ultrasound/MR or at birth
- Other signs/symptoms
  - Mechanical traction brainstem, respiratory deterioration, lower cranial nerve dysfunction
- Clinical profile
  - Developmental delay, spasticity, hypotonia, seizures

Demographics

- Age
  - Newborns
- Gender
  - Girls overrepresented (as in all NTDs) in most series
- Epidemiology
  - Rare form of Chiari malformations
  - 1-4.5% of all Chiari cases

Natural History & Prognosis

- Proportional to amount and type of herniated tissue

Treatment

- Cerebrospinal fluid diversion
  - Diversion pre-resection sac may allow decreased tension on brainstem
- Resect or repair sac (most structures in sac are nonfunctioning)
  - Beware of venous structures and brainstem!
- If amount CNS tissue in sac > intracranial ⇒ not surgical candidate

DIAGNOSTIC CHECKLIST

Consider

- Chiari 3 in newborn with low occipital encephalocele

Image Interpretation Pearls

- If it does not involve the opisthion, it's not classically Chiari 3

Reporting Tips

- Comment on location of venous structures and brainstem

SELECTED REFERENCES

1. Furtado SV et al: Repair of Chiari III malformation using cranioplasty and an occipital rotation flap: technical note and review of literature. Surg Neurol. 72(4):414-7, 2009
2. Işik N et al: Chiari malformation type III and results of surgery: a clinical study: report of eight surgically treated cases and review of the literature. Pediatr Neurosurg. 45(1):19-28, 2009
3. Chaudhari AM et al: Unique defect representing features of Chiari type III and IV malformations. Pediatr Neurosurg. 44(6):513-4, 2008
4. Menezes AH: Craniocervical developmental anatomy and its implications. Childs Nerv Syst. 24(10):1109-22, 2008
5. Jaggi RS et al: Chiari malformation type III treated with primary closure. Pediatr Neurosurg. 43(5):424-7, 2007
6. Muzumdar D et al: Type III Chiari malformation presenting as intermittent respiratory stridor: a neurological image. Pediatr Neurosurg. 43(5):446-8, 2007
7. Caldarelli M et al: Chiari type III malformation. Childs Nerv Syst. 18(5):207-10, 2002
8. Castillo M et al: Chiari III malformation: imaging features. AJNR Am J Neuroradiol. 13(1):107-13, 1992
9. Cohen MM Jr et al: Syndromes with cephaloceles. Teratology. 25(2):161-72, 1982

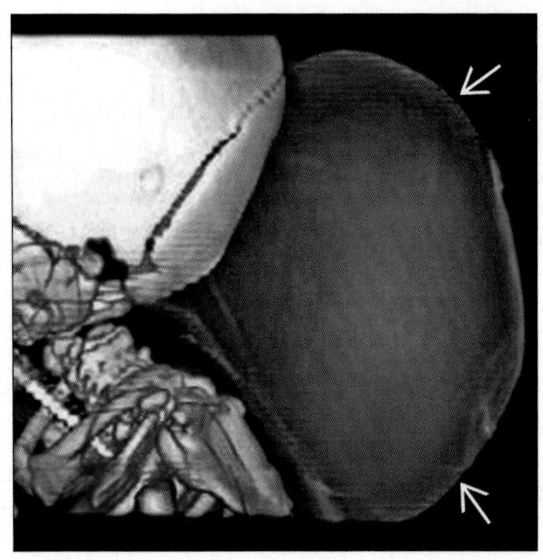

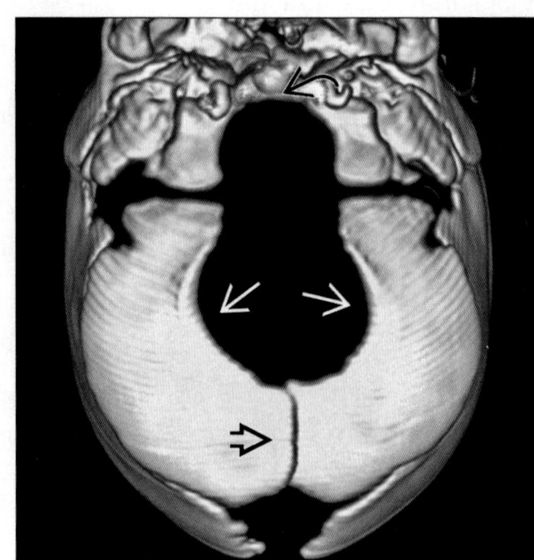

*(**Left**) Sagittal 3D reconstruction of Chiari 3 reveals a very large meningocele sac ➡. This 3D reconstruction has rendered the skin-covered sac transparent in order to demonstrate its relationship to subjacent bony structures. (**Right**) Axial 3D reconstruction in the same infant demonstrates an enlarged foramen magnum with a defect of opisthion ↪ and ventral chondral supraoccipital bone ➡. The squamous portion is split by a persistent median occipital suture ⇨.*

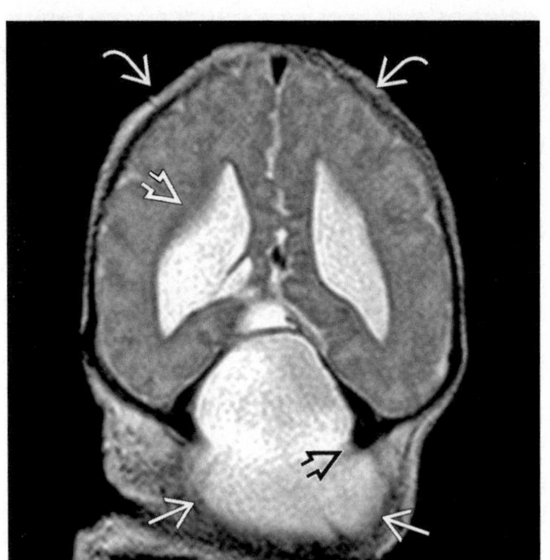

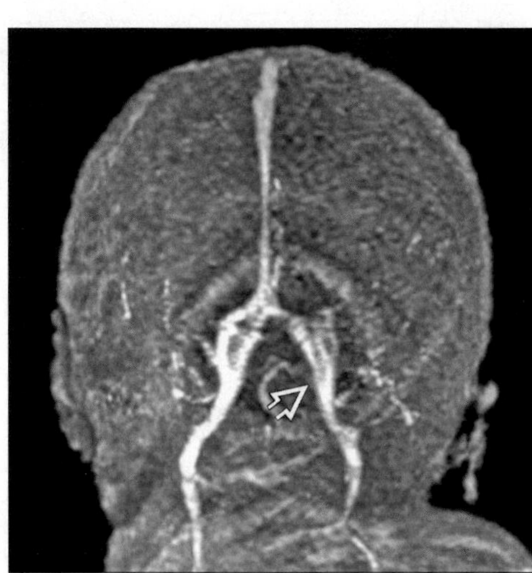

*(**Left**) Coronal T2WI MR demonstrates typical Chiari-shaped ventricles ⇨ and head ↪. Note the splaying of the walls of the foramen magnum/occipital defect ⇨ by a large fluid-filled encephalocele ➡. (**Right**) Coronal MRV in the same patient demonstrates a lack of transverse sinuses. The occipital sinuses ⇨ are usually more closely approximated when present; however, they are displaced laterally in this infant by the protruding encephalocele.*

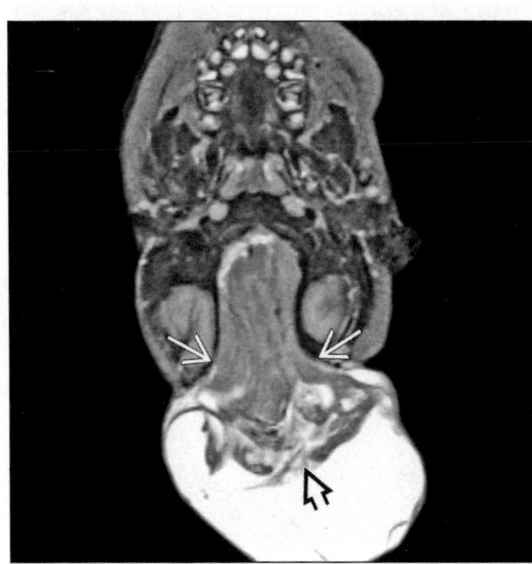

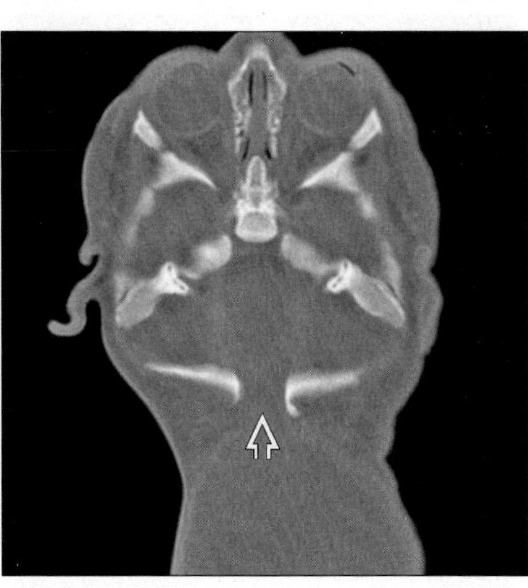

*(**Left**) Axial T2WI MR in this infant reveals hindbrain tissue ➡ protruding through a large defect of the posterior margin of the foramen magnum. The cerebellar tissue within the encephalocele sac is heterogeneous ⇨ due to gliosis and atrophy. (**Right**) Axial NECT in another infant with Chiari 3 demonstrates the defect ⇨ of the posterior aspect of the foramen magnum. Note the typical size discrepancy between the small bony defect and the very large encephalocele sac.*

CALLOSAL DYSGENESIS

Key Facts

Terminology
- Partial or complete absence of corpus callosum and hippocampal commissure

Imaging
- Absent corpus callosum on sagittal, coronal
- Atrium/occipital horns dilated ("colpocephaly")
- On CT, colpocephaly key to diagnosis
- DTI: Callosal fiber tracts form Probst bundles instead of crossing, where CC is absent
- Vertical/posterior course of ACA (no genu to sweep around)

Pathology
- Most common feature seen in CNS malformations
  - > 130 syndromes
- May be complete or variably partial
- May have interhemispheric dysplasia: Meningeal cysts, lipomas
- May be part of syndrome

Clinical Issues
- Any age, classically identified in early childhood, most common malformation found in fetuses
- Seizures, developmental delay, cranial deformity/ hypertelorism
- Sporadic/isolated ACC: Normal/near normal at 3 years (75%), but subtle cognitive defects apparent with increasing complexity of school tasks
- ACC with associated/syndromic anomalies = worst

Diagnostic Checklist
- Look for absent/incomplete CC rather than indirect signs
- Fully assess for associated lesions

*(**Left**) Coronal graphic shows lack of of transverse corpus callosum and separate lateral ventricles. The interhemispheric fissure extends to the 3rd ventricle. The bundles of Probst ➔ contain the parasagittally re-routed callosal fibers. (**Right**) Midline sagittal T2WI MR shows complete absence of both corpus callosum and hippocampal commissure. The anterior commissure ➔ is normal. Note the vertical-posterior course of the ACA ➔ and the radiating cingulate sulci ➔.*

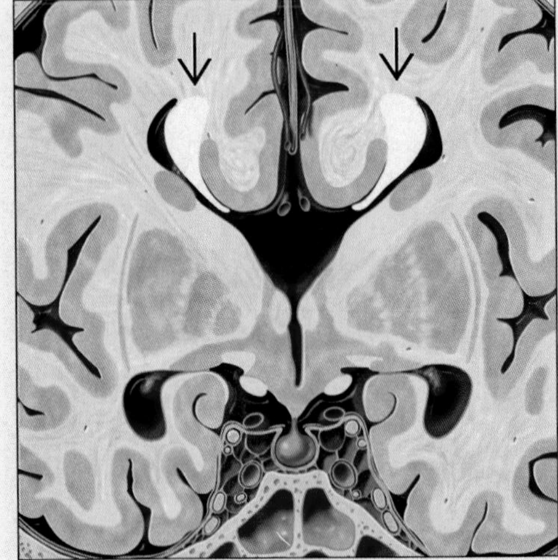

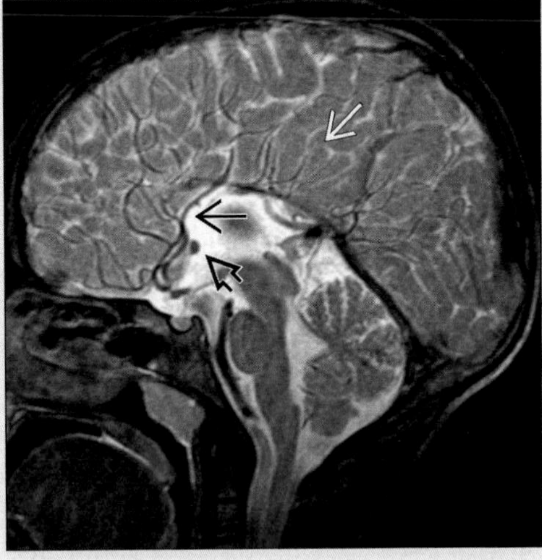

*(**Left**) Coronal T2WI MR shows separated ventricular bodies, away from the midline. The ventricular lumen is compressed medially by the leaf of the septum pellucidum ➔ that contains re-routed callosal fibers (Probst bundle) above and forniceal column below. Falx cerebri and interhemispheric fissure extend to the 3rd ventricular roof. Rounded hippocampi are surrounded by large temporal horns ➔. (**Right**) Axial T2WI MR shows dilated trigones/occipital horns ➔ (colpocephaly).*

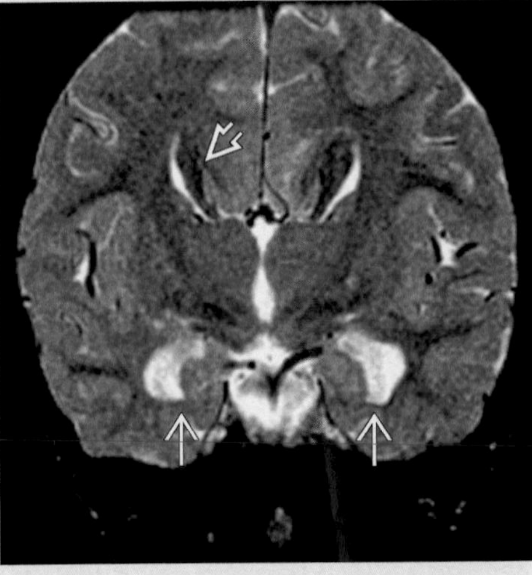

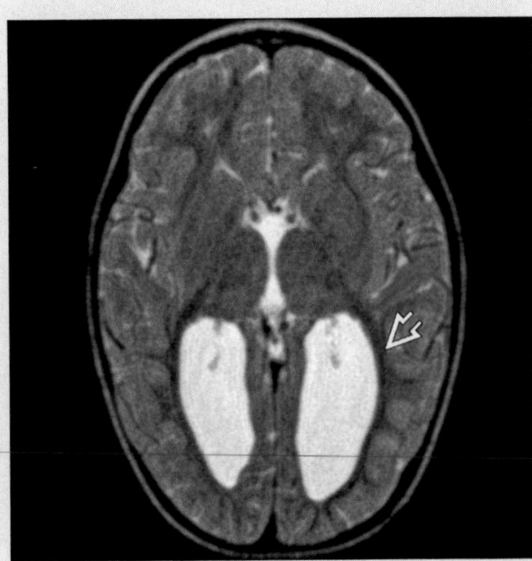

CALLOSAL DYSGENESIS

TERMINOLOGY

Abbreviations

- Agenesis/dysgenesis corpus callosum (ACC)

Synonyms

- Callosal agenesis/dysgenesis, commissural agenesis/dysgenesis

Definitions

- Partial or complete absence of corpus callosum and hippocampal commissure

IMAGING

General Features

- Best diagnostic clue
  - Partially or completely absent corpus callosum on midline sagittal and coronal planes
  - Lateral ventricles separate and parallel (axial), "bull's-head," "trident," "Viking helmet," "moose head" appearances (coronal)
- Size
  - When present CC remnants vary in size, extent, shape
    - Prior to myelin maturation, may be difficult to define (T2WI is better)
- Morphology
  - Commissural plate, clockwise
    - Anterior commissure
    - Lamina rostralis and rostrum
    - Genu, body and isthmus, splenium
    - Hippocampal commissure below splenium and behind septum pellucidum

CT Findings

- NECT
  - On axial CT, lateral ventricles key to diagnosis
    - Parallel and separate
    - Atrium/occipital horns dilated ("colpocephaly")
- CTA
  - Anterior cerebral arteries (ACAs) course directly upward in interhemispheric fissure

MR Findings

- T1WI
  - Sagittal
    - Absent or incomplete commissural plate, expanded 3rd ventricular roof
    - Abnormal cingulate gyrus: Radiating sulcal pattern
    - Anterior commissure may be absent, small, or normal
  - Coronal
    - Interhemispheric fissure extends down to 3rd ventricular roof
    - Probst bundles: Medial parasagittal white matter tracts, brighter than other myelin on T1WI, indent lateral ventricles ("bull's head," etc.)
    - Bifid temporal horns and rounded hippocampi
  - Axial
    - Parallel separate lateral ventricles, colpocephaly
- T2WI
  - Same morphology as on T1WI
    - Probst bundles darker than rest of white matter
  - Variants and associated malformations
    - High-riding 3rd ventricle
    - Partial agenesis usually affects posterior CC and hippocampal commissure
    - Multiple interhemispheric cysts (meningeal dysplasia)
    - Lipomas: Nodular, curvilinear
    - MCD: Polymicrogyria-like cortical malformation (often along midline cysts), subcortical or periventricular nodular heterotopia
    - Malformation of eyes, hindbrain (Dandy-Walker), hypothalamus-pituitary, cord, heart
- DWI
  - DTI: Callosal fiber tracts form Probst bundles instead of crossing, where CC is absent
- MRA
  - Vertical/posterior course of ACA (no genu to sweep around), ± azygous ACA
- MRV
  - Occasional midline venous anomalies, persistent falcine sinus

Ultrasonographic Findings

- Grayscale ultrasound
  - Coronal
    - Absent CC, "bull's-head" lateral ventricles, separated lateral ventricles, colpocephaly
  - Sagittal
    - Radially arranged gyri "point to" 3rd ventricle
- Color Doppler
  - Abnormal posterior ACA course

Imaging Recommendations

- Best imaging tool
  - MR
- Protocol advice
  - Multiplanar MR (look for associated malformations)
  - If MR unavailable, multiplanar CT will diagnose ACC
  - In fetuses, use ultrafast single-shot T2WI in 3 planes

DIFFERENTIAL DIAGNOSIS

Destruction of Corpus Callosum

- Surgery (callosotomy), trauma
- Hypoxic ischemic encephalopathy, infarcts, hemorrhages
- Metabolic (Marchiafava-Bignami) with necrosis, longitudinal splitting of CC

Stretched Corpus Callosum

- Thinned CC (e.g., hydrocephalus) but all parts present

Hypoplastic Corpus Callosum

- CC thin but all parts present

Immature Corpus Callosum

- Premyelinated CC may be difficult to confirm; look for cingulate gyrus

CALLOSAL DYSGENESIS

PATHOLOGY

General Features

- Etiology
  - Axons fail to form
    - Rare: CRASH syndrome/*L1CAM* gene defect, cobblestone lissencephaly
  - Axons not guided to midline (mutations in adhesion molecules)
  - Axons reach midline but fail to cross (absence or malfunction of midsagittal guiding "substrate")
    - Turn and form large, aberrant, parasagittal Probst bundles
  - Miscellaneous
    - Toxic: Fetal alcohol exposure may affect L1CAM
    - Infection: In utero cytomegalovirus (CMV)
    - Inborn errors of metabolism: Nonketotic hyperglycinemia, pyruvate dehydrogenase deficiency, maternal phenylketonuria (PKU), Zellweger
- Genetics
  - Genetics of associated/syndromic CC anomalies
    - Most common abnormality seen as part of CNS malformations: > 130 syndromes
    - Chiari 2, frontonasal dysplasia, syndromic craniosynostoses, MCD, etc.
    - Aicardi syndrome: X-linked ACC, PMG and heterotopia, infantile spasms, retinal lacunae, developmental delay
- Associated abnormalities
  - MCD: Heterotopias, lissencephaly, schizencephaly, etc.
  - Ocular/hypothalamic-pituitary/cord/facial anomalies
  - Heart, limbs
  - ACC may be malformation in itself or feature of many malformative syndromes

Staging, Grading, & Classification

- May be isolated or part of syndrome; complete or partial
- May have interhemispheric dysplasia: Meningeal cysts, lipomas
- May be part of syndrome (> 130)

Gross Pathologic & Surgical Features

- Leaves of septum pellucidum laterally displaced, contain Probst bundles
- Probst bundles contain parasagittal callosal bundle
  - Only form if callosal neurons present
  - Variable-sized bundles smaller than normal CC
- Associated dysgenetic brain lesions

CLINICAL ISSUES

Presentation

- Most common signs/symptoms
  - Seizures, developmental delay, cranial deformity-hypertelorism
  - Hypopituitarism-hypothalamic malfunction
- Clinical profile
  - None specific

Demographics

- Age
  - Any age, classically identified in early childhood, most common malformation found in fetuses
- Gender
  - M > F, if isolated finding
- Epidemiology
  - 0.5-70 per 10,000 live births
  - 4% of CNS malformations
  - Can be isolated (often males) or part of other CNS malformations

Natural History & Prognosis

- Sporadic/isolated ACC: Normal/near normal at 3 years (75%), but subtle cognitive defects apparent with increasing complexity of school tasks
- ACC with associated/syndromic anomalies = worst

DIAGNOSTIC CHECKLIST

Consider

- Syndromic associations common

Image Interpretation Pearls

- Look for absent/incomplete CC rather than indirect signs
- Fully assess for associated lesions

SELECTED REFERENCES

1. Hopkins B et al: Neuroimaging aspects of Aicardi syndrome. Am J Med Genet A. 146A(22):2871-8, 2008
2. Miller E et al: The old and the new: supratentorial MR findings in Chiari II malformation. Childs Nerv Syst. 24(5):563-75, 2008
3. Lee SK et al: Diffusion tensor MR imaging visualizes the altered hemispheric fiber connection in callosal dysgenesis. AJNR Am J Neuroradiol. 25(1):25-8, 2004
4. Küker W et al: Malformations of the midline commissures: MRI findings in different forms of callosal dysgenesis. Eur Radiol. 13(3):598-604, 2003
5. Moutard ML et al: Agenesis of corpus callosum: prenatal diagnosis and prognosis. Childs Nerv Syst. 19(7-8):471-6, 2003
6. Sato N et al: MR evaluation of the hippocampus in patients with congenital malformations of the brain. AJNR Am J Neuroradiol. 22(2):389-93, 2001
7. Giedd JN et al: Development of the human corpus callosum during childhood and adolescence: a longitudinal MRI study. Prog Neuropsychopharmacol Biol Psychiatry. 23(4):571-88, 1999
8. Pirola B et al: Agenesis of the corpus callosum with Probst bundles owing to haploinsufficiency for a gene in an 8 cM region of 6q25. J Med Genet. 35(12):1031-3, 1998
9. Kier EL et al: The lamina rostralis: modification of concepts concerning the anatomy, embryology, and MR appearance of the rostrum of the corpus callosum. AJNR Am J Neuroradiol. 18(4):715-22, 1997
10. Dobyns WB: Absence makes the search grow longer. Am J Hum Genet. 58(1):7-16, 1996
11. Kier EL et al: The normal and abnormal genu of the corpus callosum: an evolutionary, embryologic, anatomic, and MR analysis. AJNR Am J Neuroradiol. 17(9):1631-41, 1996
12. Pujol J et al: When does human brain development end? Evidence of corpus callosum growth up to adulthood. Ann Neurol. 34(1):71-5, 1993

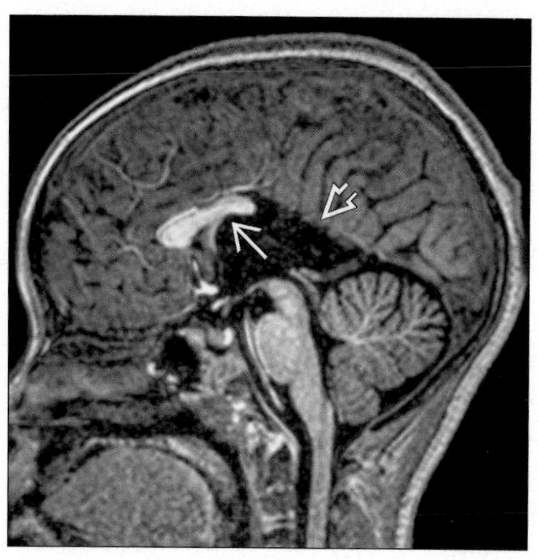

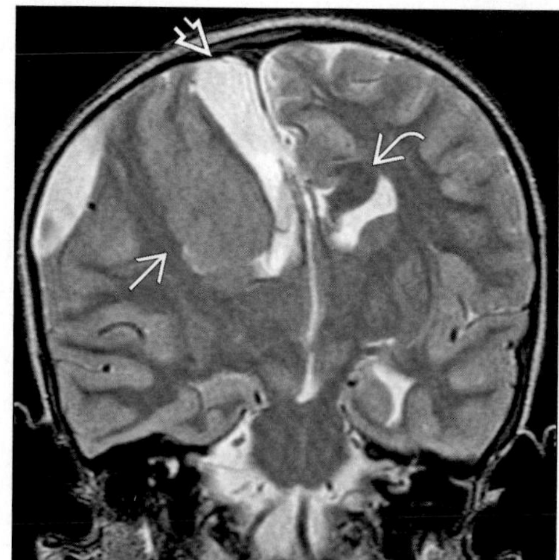

(Left) Sagittal T1WI MR shows pure partial ACC. The posterior portion of the corpus callosum is missing ➡, but the junction with the fornix ➡ seems preserved. Posterior coronals would show Probst bundles, whereas anterior images would appear normal. (Right) Coronal T2WI MR shows ACC with (shunted) interhemispheric meningeal cysts ➡. Note the massive nodular heterotopia on the right ➡. A Probst bundle has formed on the left ➡ but not on the right.

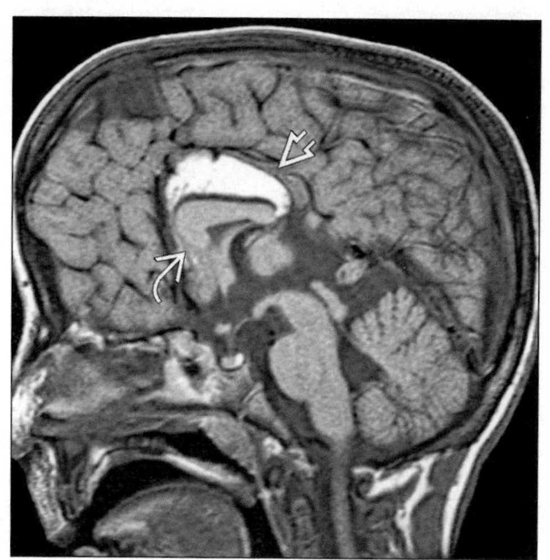

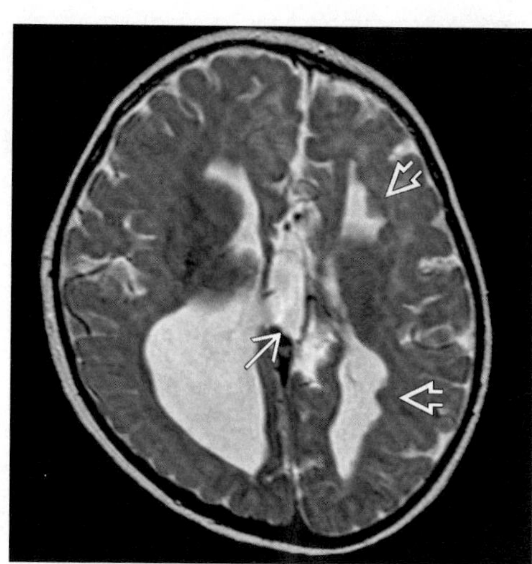

(Left) Sagittal T1WI MR shows interhemispheric lipoma ➡ with partial posterior ACC ➡. Lipoma is mostly above the CC; it may wrap around the corpus or be located behind and in the choroid plexuses. ACA branches are commonly dysplastic. (Right) Axial T2WI MR of a girl with infantile spasms and Aicardi syndrome. Note ACC, interhemispheric cysts ➡, periventricular nodular heterotopia ➡, and hemispheric asymmetry. Eye colobomas and choroid plexus tumors are common.

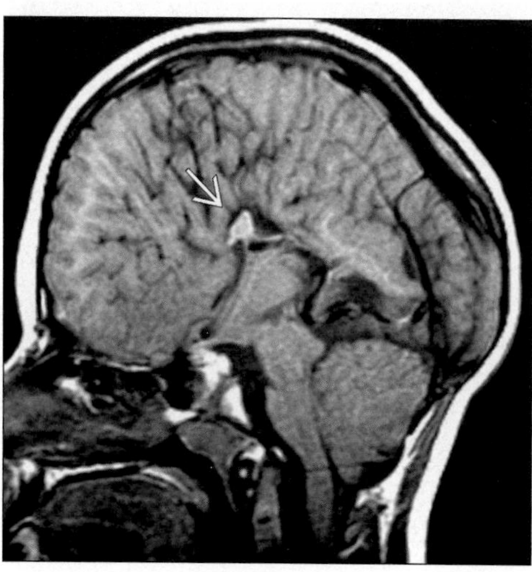

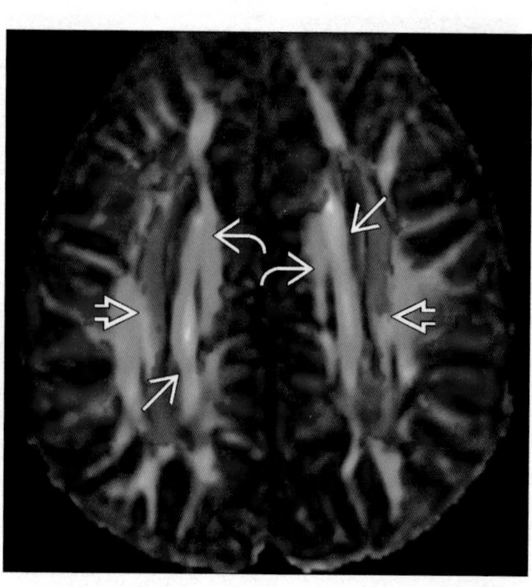

(Left) Sagittal T1WI MR in a child with Chiari 2. ACC in Chiari 2 is always partial ➡; Probst bundles are never seen. Note the multiple supra- and infratentorial Chiari 2 features. (Right) Axial DTI of a child with complete callosal agenesis. Transverse is red, dorso-ventral green, and craniocaudal blue. Probst bundles (uncrossed callosal fibers ➡) form a thick dorso-ventral bundle on each side of the midline, medial to the corona radiata ➡ and lateral to the cingulum ➡.

LIPOMA

Key Facts

Terminology
- Intracranial lipoma (ICL)
- Mass of mature nonneoplastic adipose tissue
- CNS lipomas are congenital malformations, not true neoplasms

Imaging
- Well-delineated lobulated extraaxial mass with fat attenuation/intensity
- 80% supratentorial
  - 40-50% interhemispheric fissure (over corpus callosum; may extend into lateral ventricles, choroid plexus)
  - 15-20% suprasellar (attached to infundibulum, hypothalamus)
  - 10-15% tectal region (usually inferior colliculus/ superior vermis)
- 20% infratentorial
- Cerebellopontine angle (may extend into internal auditory canal, vestibule)
- Lobulated pial-based fatty mass that may encase vessels and cranial nerves
- CT: -50 to -100 HU (fat density)
- Ca++ varies from none to extensive
- Standard SE MR: Hyperintense on T1WI
- Becomes hypointense with fat suppression

Top Differential Diagnoses
- Teratoma
  - Locations similar to lipoma
  - Tissue from all 3 embryonic germ layers

Diagnostic Checklist
- When in doubt, use fat-saturation sequence
- Could high signal on T1WI be due to other substances with short T1 (e.g., subacute hemorrhage)?

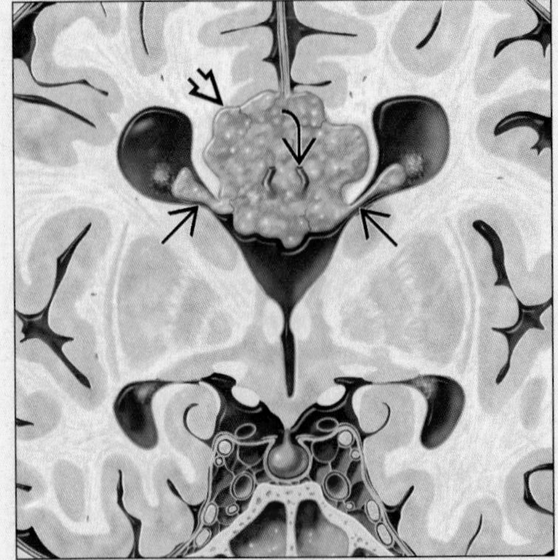

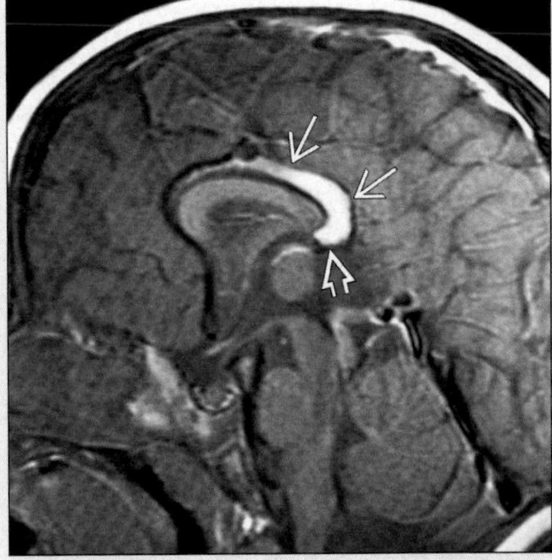

***(Left)** Coronal graphic shows callosal agenesis with a bulky tubulonodular interhemispheric lipoma ➯ that encases the arteries ➚ and extends into the lateral ventricles ➔. **(Right)** Sagittal T1WI MR shows a rather thin curvilinear interhemispheric lipoma in a 9 month old. Note that the hyperintense lipoma ➔ is thicker posteriorly than anteriorly. It wraps around the back of the corpus callosum, and it extends beneath the corpus ➯ into the velum interpositum.*

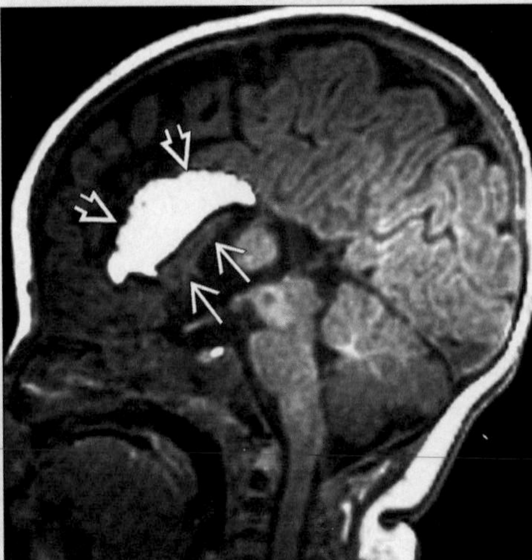

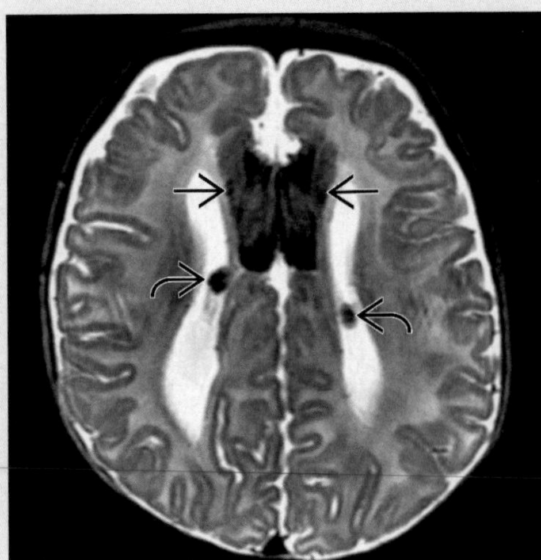

***(Left)** Sagittal T1WI MR in a neonate shows a large, tubulonodular, interhemispheric lipoma ➯ dorsal to a wedge-shaped callosal remnant ➔. The brain is otherwise normal. **(Right)** Axial T2WI MR in the same patient shows the lipoma ➔ as hypointense, lying between the 2 cerebral hemispheres. The lipoma extends through the choroidal fissures into the lateral ventricles ➚ where it is in the stroma of the choroid plexuses.*

TERMINOLOGY

Abbreviations

- Intracranial lipoma (ICL)

Synonyms

- Lipomatous hamartoma

Definitions

- Mass of mature nonneoplastic adipose tissue
  - CNS lipomas are congenital malformations, not true neoplasms
  - Lipoma variants in CNS include angiolipoma, hibernoma, osteolipoma

IMAGING

General Features

- Best diagnostic clue
  - Well-delineated lobulated extraaxial mass with fat attenuation/intensity
- Location
  - Midline location common
  - 80% supratentorial
    - 40-50% interhemispheric fissure (over corpus callosum [CC]; may extend into lateral ventricles, choroid plexus)
    - 15-20% suprasellar (attached to infundibulum, hypothalamus)
    - 10-15% tectal region (usually inferior colliculus/ superior vermis)
    - Uncommon: Meckel cave, lateral cerebral fissures, middle cranial fossa
  - 20% infratentorial
    - Cerebellopontine angle (may extend into internal auditory canal, vestibule)
    - Uncommon: Jugular foramen, foramen magnum
- Size
  - Varies from tiny to very large
- Morphology
  - Lobulated pial-based fatty mass that may encase vessels and cranial nerves
  - 2 kinds of interhemispheric lipoma
    - Curvilinear type (thin ICL curves around callosal body, splenium)
    - Tubulonodular type (bulky mass; frequent Ca++, usually associated with callosal agenesis)

Radiographic Findings

- Radiography
  - Usually normal
  - Very large interhemispheric lipomas may show low density
  - Tubulonodular lipomas may show rim Ca++

CT Findings

- NECT
  - -50 to -100 Hounsfield units (HU); fat density
  - Ca++ varies from none to extensive
    - Present in 65% of bulky tubulonodular CC lipomas
    - Rare in posterior fossa, parasellar lesions
- CECT
  - Does not enhance
- CTA
  - May demonstrate aberrant pericallosal artery course in interhemispheric lipoma associated with callosal dysgenesis

MR Findings

- T1WI
  - Hyperintense mass
  - Becomes hypointense with fat suppression
  - Chemical shift artifact in frequency-encoding direction
- T2WI
  - Hypointense with striking chemical shift artifact
    - Round/linear "filling defects" present where vessels, cranial nerves pass through lipoma
    - May show low signal intensity foci (Ca++)
  - FSE: Iso- to hyperintense (J-coupling)
- PD/intermediate
  - Iso- to hyperintense (depending on repetition and echo times)
    - Striking chemical shift artifact
- STIR
  - Hypointense
- FLAIR
  - Hyperintense
- DWI
  - Diffusion tensor imaging visualizes altered fiber connections if associated callosal dysgenesis present
- T1WI C+
  - Does not enhance

Ultrasonographic Findings

- Grayscale ultrasound
  - Generally hyperechoic
  - May show other fetal anomalies (CC agenesis, etc.)

Imaging Recommendations

- Best imaging tool
  - MR
- Protocol advice
  - Add fat-suppression sequence for confirmation

DIFFERENTIAL DIAGNOSIS

Dural Dysplasia

- Fat often in falx, cavernous sinuses
- Metaplastic ossified dura may contain fat

Dermoid

- Density usually 20 to 40 HU
- Signal intensity usually more heterogeneous
- Rupture with cisternal fat droplets common
- Usually no associated malformations (common with lipoma)
- Dermoids often calcify; lipomas in locations other than interhemispheric do not

Teratoma

- Locations similar to lipoma
- Tissue from all 3 embryonic germ layers
- Imaging appearance usually more heterogeneous
  - May show foci of contrast enhancement

LIPOMA

Lipomatous Differentiation of Neoplasm

- May occur occasionally in PNETs, ependymoma, gliomas
- Cerebellar liponeurocytoma
  - Primarily hypointense on T1WI, mixed with hyperintense foci
  - Patchy, irregular enhancement
- Meningiomas, schwannomas, metastases rarely have lipomatous transformation

Subacute Hemorrhage

- T1 shortening can be confused with lipoma
- Use T2* (hemorrhage blooms), fat saturation (hemorrhage does not suppress)

PATHOLOGY

General Features

- Etiology
  - Persistent maldevelopment of embryonic meninx primitiva
    - Normally differentiates into leptomeninges, cisterns
    - Maldifferentiates into fat instead
  - Developing pia-arachnoid invaginates through embryonic choroid fissure
    - Explains frequent intraventricular extension of interhemispheric lipomas
- Genetics
  - No known defects in sporadic ICL
- Associated abnormalities
  - Most common: Interhemispheric lipoma + corpus callosum anomalies
  - Other congenital malformations: Cephaloceles, closed spinal dysraphism
  - Encephalocraniocutaneous lipomatosis → Fishman syndrome
  - Pai syndrome → facial clefts, skin lipomas; occasional ICLs, usually interhemispheric

Gross Pathologic & Surgical Features

- Yellow lobulated fatty mass attached to leptomeninges, sometimes adherent to brain
- Cranial nerves, arteries/veins pass through lipoma

Microscopic Features

- Identical to adipose tissue elsewhere
- Cells vary in shape/size, measure up to 200 μm
- Occasional nuclear hyperchromasia; mitoses rare/absent
- Liposarcoma = extremely rare malignant intracranial adipose tumor

CLINICAL ISSUES

Presentation

- Most common signs/symptoms
  - Usually found incidentally at imaging, autopsy
  - Rare: Cranial neuropathy (vestibulocochlear dysfunction, facial pain), seizures (associated with other congenital anomalies)
  - Seizures associated with lipomas over (dysmorphic) cortex

Demographics

- Age
  - Any age
- Gender
  - M = F
- Ethnicity
  - None known
- Epidemiology
  - < 0.5% of all intracranial masses (not true neoplasm)

Natural History & Prognosis

- Benign, usually stable
- May expand with corticosteroids
  - High-dose, long-term administration may result in neural compressive symptoms

Treatment

- Generally not a surgical lesion
  - Surgery has high morbidity/mortality
- Reduce/eliminate steroids

DIAGNOSTIC CHECKLIST

Consider

- Could high signal on T1WI be due to other substances with short T1 (e.g., subacute hemorrhage)?

Image Interpretation Pearls

- When in doubt, use fat-saturation sequence

SELECTED REFERENCES

1. Kemmling A et al: A diagnostic pitfall for intracranial aneurysms in time-of-flight MR angiography: small intracranial lipomas. AJR Am J Roentgenol. 190(1):W62-7, 2008
2. Loddenkemper T et al: Intracranial lipomas and epilepsy. J Neurol. 253(5):590-3, 2006
3. Yildiz H et al: Intracranial lipomas: importance of localization. Neuroradiology. 48(1):1-7, 2006
4. Gaskin CM et al: Lipomas, lipoma variants, and well-differentiated liposarcomas (atypical lipomas): results of MRI evaluations of 126 consecutive fatty masses. AJR Am J Roentgenol. 182(3):733-9, 2004
5. Kurt G et al: Hypothalamic lipoma adjacent to mamillary bodies. Childs Nerv Syst. 18(12):732-4, 2002
6. Tankéré F et al: Cerebellopontine angle lipomas: report of four cases and review of the literature. Neurosurgery. 50(3):626-31; discussion 631-2, 2002
7. Feldman RP et al: Intracranial lipoma of the sylvian fissure. Case report and review of the literature. J Neurosurg. 94(3):515-9, 2001
8. Ickowitz V et al: Prenatal diagnosis and postnatal follow-up of pericallosal lipoma: report of seven new cases. AJNR Am J Neuroradiol. 22(4):767-72, 2001
9. Amor DJ et al: Encephalocraniocutaneous lipomatosis (Fishman syndrome): a rare neurocutaneous syndrome. J Paediatr Child Health. 36(6):603-5, 2000
10. Kieslich M et al: Midline developmental anomalies with lipomas in the corpus callosum region. J Child Neurol. 15(2):85-9, 2000

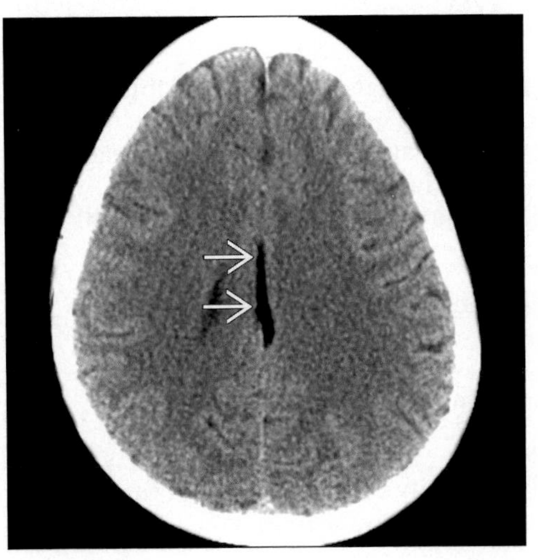

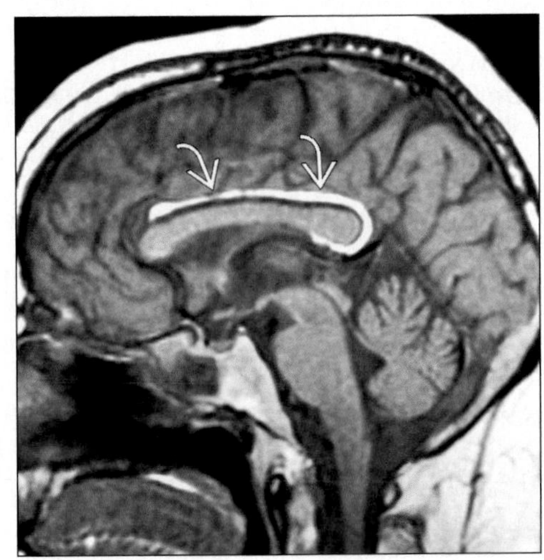

(Left) *Axial NECT in a young woman studied for an unrelated headache shows a hypodense linear structure ➡ in the midline.* ***(Right)*** *Sagittal T1WI MR in the same patient shows that the linear structure ➡ is a curvilinear interhemispheric lipoma that wraps around the posterior aspect of a hypogenetic corpus callosum and courses into the posterior part of the velum interpositum. The callosal genu and splenium are incompletely formed.*

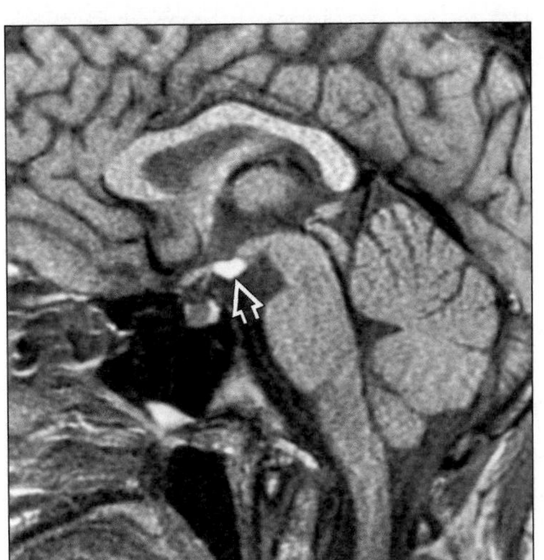

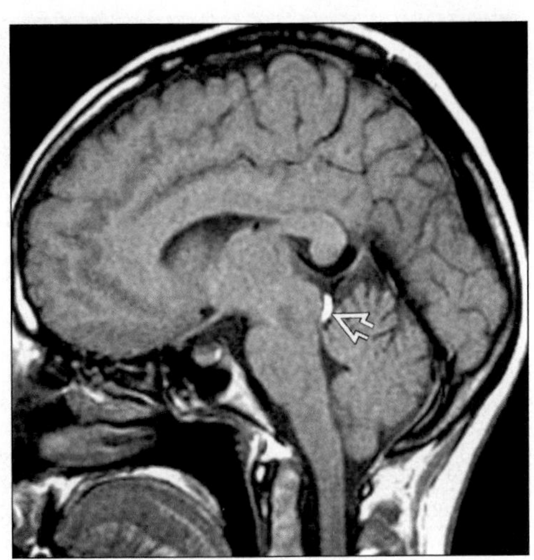

(Left) *Sagittal T1WI MR in a 25-year-old man with unrelated symptoms shows a hypothalamic lipoma ➡, which is located in the tuber cinereum of the hypothalamus (between the infundibulum and the mamillary bodies).* ***(Right)*** *Sagittal T1WI MR shows a tectal lipoma ➡, situated immediately posterior to the inferior tectum and between the inferior colliculus and the superior surface of the cerebellar vermis. This is a very common location for lipomas.*

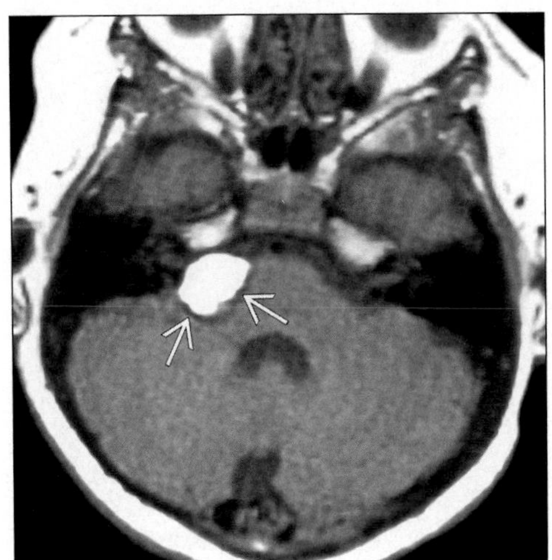

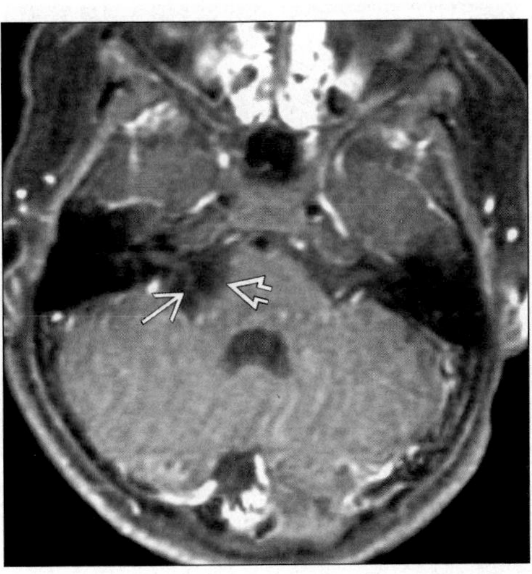

(Left) *Axial T1WI MR shows a round lipoma ➡ in the right cerebellopontine angle cistern, adjacent to the IAC. Lipomas do not cause hearing loss and should not be resected.* ***(Right)*** *Axial T1WI FS MR + C shows that the mass ➡ becomes very hypointense after the fat-suppression pulse is applied. With fat signal suppressed, the 8th cranial nerve ➡ can be seen, coursing through the lipoma in the cerebellopontine angle cistern to the internal auditory canal.*

DANDY-WALKER CONTINUUM

Key Facts

Terminology

- DWS represents broad spectrum of cystic posterior fossa (PF) malformations
  - Dandy-Walker spectrum (DWS)/complex (DWC)
  - "Classic" DW malformation (DWM)
  - Hypoplastic vermis with rotation (HVR)
  - Persistent Blake pouch cyst (BPC)
  - Mega cisterna magna (MCM)

Imaging

- "Classic" DWM
  - Cystic dilatation of 4th ventricle → enlarged PF
  - Vermis hypoplastic, rotated superiorly
- HVR
  - Variable vermian hypoplasia
  - PF/brainstem normal-sized
  - No or small cyst, "keyhole" vallecula
- BPC
  - "Open" 4th ventricle communicates with cyst
  - Fastigial recess, primary fissure, PF/brainstem normal
- MCM
  - Enlarged pericerebellar cisterns communicate with basal subarachnoid spaces
- Occipital bone may appear scalloped/remodeled with **all** DWS types (including MCM)
- Routine MR imaging (thin sagittal views crucial)

Pathology

- Most severe to mildest: DWM with 4th ventriculocele → classic DWM → HVR → BPC → MCM
- Numerous syndromes associated with DWS

Clinical Issues

- Marked heterogeneity in genetic, clinical findings
- DWM: 80% diagnosed by 1 year

(Left) *Sagittal graphic of classic Dandy-Walker malformation shows an enlarged posterior fossa, elevated torcular herophili →, superior rotation of hypoplastic cerebellar vermis →, an overexpanded 4th ventricle with a thin wall →, and a dilated ventricle (hydrocephalus).* ***(Right)*** *Sagittal T2WI MR shows Dandy-Walker with a hypoplastic, rotated vermis →, lack of fastigial crease, and incomplete vermian lobulation of the posterior lobules beyond the primary fissure →. The cyst wall is faintly seen →.*

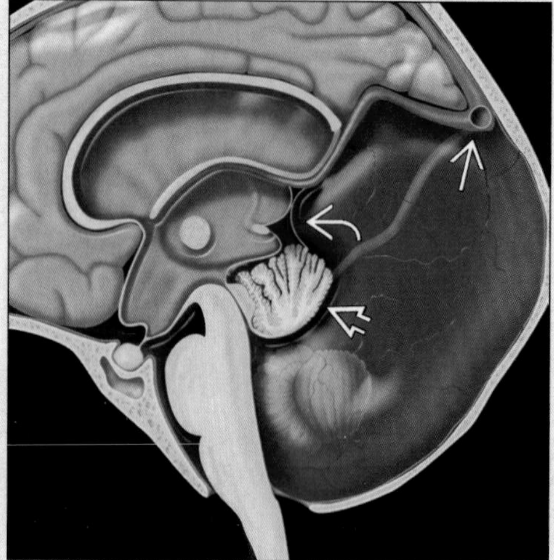

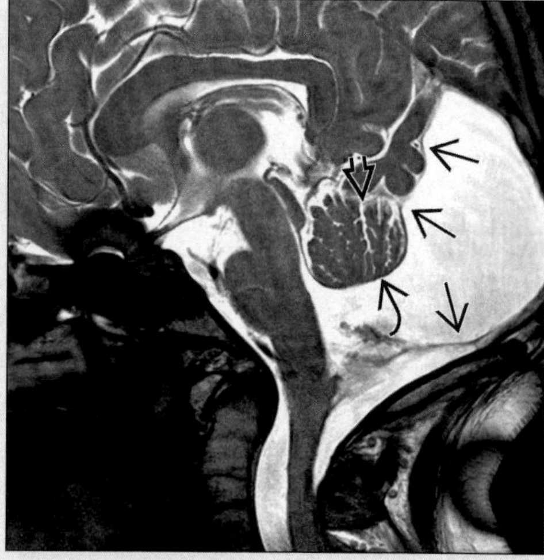

(Left) *Sagittal MRV demonstrates torcular-lamboid inversion. The transverse sinuses → angle upward toward the torcular → as the cyst has prevented normal fetal torcular descent. Note the persistent fetal occipital sinus →.* ***(Right)*** *Coronal T2WI MR demonstrates a huge, fluid-filled posterior fossa. Again, notice that the transverse sinuses → are angled upward toward the torcular herophili →.*

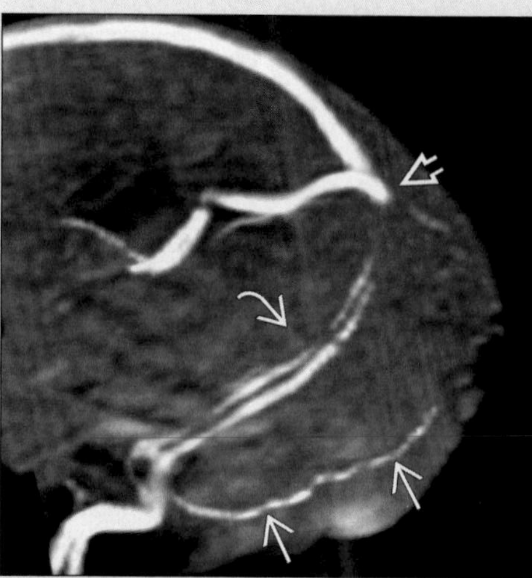

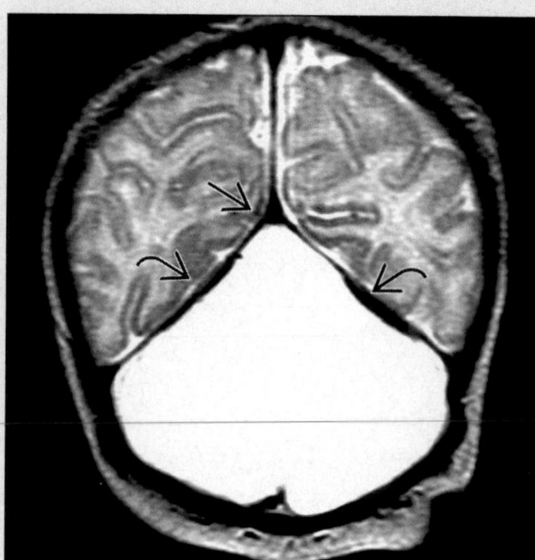

DANDY-WALKER CONTINUUM

TERMINOLOGY

Abbreviations

- Dandy Walker (DW) spectrum (DWS), DW complex (DWC), "classic" DW malformation (DWM)
- Hypoplastic vermis with rotation (HVR), formerly DW variant (DWV)
- Persistent Blake pouch cyst (BPC), mega cisterna magna (MCM)

Definitions

- DWS represents broad spectrum of cystic posterior fossa (PF) malformations

IMAGING

General Features

- Best diagnostic clue
  - DWM: Large PF + cerebrospinal fluid (CSF) cyst, normal 4th ventricle (V) absent
  - HVR, BPC: Failure of "closure" of 4th ventricle
- Location
  - Posterior fossa
- Size
  - Variable
- Morphology
  - DWS (from most to least severe)
    - 4th ventriculocele (10-15% of cases)
      - DWM + large 4th ventricle erodes occipital bone → "encephalocele"
    - "Classic" DWM
      - Cystic dilatation of 4th V → enlarged PF, superiorly rotated hypoplastic vermis
      - Torcular-lambdoid inversion: Cyst mechanically hinders normal fetal caudal migration of torcular
    - HVR (formerly DW variant)
      - Variable vermian hypoplasia, no or small cyst, normal-sized PF/brainstem, "keyhole" vallecula
    - BPC
      - "Open" 4th ventricle communicates with cyst, normal fastigial recess, and primary fissure
    - MCM
      - Enlarged pericerebellar cisterns communicate with basal subarachnoid spaces
      - Cistern crossed by falx cerebelli, tiny veins
      - Normal vermis/4th ventricle

Radiographic Findings

- Radiography
  - Enlarged calvarium, particularly posterior fossa
  - DWM: Lambdoid-torcular inversion (transverse sinus grooves elevated above lambda)
    - Sinuses are originally above lambda in fetus; cyst mechanically hinders descent

CT Findings

- NECT
  - DWM: Large posterior fossa
    - Variable-sized cyst communicates with 4th V
    - Torcular-lambdoid inversion (torcular above lambdoid suture)
  - Occipital bone may appear scalloped, remodeled with all DWS types, including MCM

MR Findings

- T1WI
  - Sagittal DWM
    - Floor 4th ventricle present
    - 4th V opens dorsally to variable-sized CSF cyst
    - Cyst wall difficult to discern
    - Vermian remnant (± fastigium, fissures) rotated up, over cyst
    - ± remnant fused to tentorium
    - Elevated torcular with high/steeply sloping tentorium (classic)
  - Sagittal HVR
    - Smaller PF ± cyst
    - 4th V "open" with partial rotation vermis, presence of fastigium, and fissures variable
  - Sagittal BPC
    - Rotated but normal-appearing vermis
    - Free communication of 4th V with prominent inferior CSF space
    - Basal cisterns compressed posteriorly or effaced
  - Sagittal MCM
    - Normal vermis (not rotated/hypoplastic)
    - 4th ventricle is "closed"
- T2WI
  - Associated anomalies
    - Cortical dysplasia, heterotopias, myelination delays (syndromic DWS)
- FLAIR
  - ± very slight signal difference between cyst, CSF
  - ± compressed basal cisterns
- DWI
  - Very slight restriction may be seen if reduced fluid motion
- MRV
  - Elevated torcular herophili (DWM)

Nonvascular Interventions

- Cisternography delineates cyst wall

Imaging Recommendations

- Best imaging tool
  - MR best characterizes severity, associated anomalies
- Protocol advice
  - Routine MR imaging (thin sagittal views crucial)

DIFFERENTIAL DIAGNOSIS

Dandy-Walker Spectrum

- "In-between" cases common

Posterior Fossa Arachnoid Cyst (AC)

- Location: Retrocerebellar, supravermian, or in cerebellopontine angle
- Included in DW spectrum by some authors
- Normal 4th V compressed or displaced
- AC not traversed by falx cerebelli, tiny veins
- ACs lined by arachnoid cells/collagen

Molar Tooth Deformity

- Prototype = Joubert anomaly

DANDY-WALKER CONTINUUM

- Episodic hyperpnea, oculomotor apraxia, retinal dystrophy, ± renal cysts, hepatic fibrosis
- Split vermis, "bat-wing" 4th V, mesencephalon is shaped like molar tooth

Isolated 4th Ventricle

- Inferior 4th ventricle "closed" vs. "open" in DWM/DWV on sagittal view

PATHOLOGY

General Features

- Etiology
  - Rhombencephalic roof divides into cephalic (anterior membranous area [AMA]) and caudal (posterior membranous area [PMA])
    - AMA invaded by neural cells → becomes cerebellum
    - PMA expands then disappears to form outlet foramina of 4th V
  - Hindbrain development arrested
    - Defective AMA and PMA → DWM and HVR
    - Defective PMA only → BPC and MCM
- Genetics
  - Majority sporadic, X-linked DWM reported
    - Some have interstitial deletions of 3q2 which encompass *ZIC1* and *ZIC4* genes
  - Many, many syndromes with DWS
    - Chromosomal or midline anomalies; PHACES (facial hemangiomas, coarctation, DWS in 81%)
- Associated abnormalities
  - 2/3 have associated CNS/extracranial anomalies
    - Craniofacial, cardiac/urinary tract anomalies, polydactyly, orthopedic ± respiratory problems
- Embryology
  - Common association DWM/HVR with facial, cardiovascular anomalies suggests onset between formation, migration of neural crest cells (3rd-4th postovulatory week)

Staging, Grading, & Classification

- Spectrum: DWM with 4th ventriculocele (most severe) → classic DWM → HVR → BPC → MCM (mildest)

Gross Pathologic & Surgical Features

- DWM: Large PF with big CSF-containing cyst
  - Inferior margin vermian remnant continuous with cyst wall
  - 4th V choroid plexus absent or displaced into lateral recesses

Microscopic Features

- DWM: Outer cyst wall layer continuous with leptomeninges
  - Intermediate stretched neuroglial layer is continuous with vermis
  - Inner layer of glial tissue lined with ependyma/ependymal nests
  - Anomalies of inferior olivary nuclei/corticospinal tract crossings

CLINICAL ISSUES

Presentation

- Most common signs/symptoms
  - DWM: Macrocephaly, bulging fontanel, etc.
  - MCM: Incidental finding
- Clinical profile
  - Marked heterogeneity in genetic, clinical findings

Demographics

- Age
  - DWM: 80% diagnosed by 1 year
- Gender
  - M ≤ F
- Epidemiology
  - 1:25,000-100,000 births
  - Accounts for 1-4% of all hydrocephalus cases

Natural History & Prognosis

- Classic DWM: Early death common (up to 44%)
- Cognitive outcome dependent upon associated syndromes or supratentorial anomalies/hydrocephalus and completeness of residual vermis
  - Intelligence normal in 35 to 50% of patients with classic DWM
    - Small remnant without fissures or fastigium
      - Seizures
      - Cognitive delay
      - Poor motor skills/balance
    - Large remnant, normal lobulation and fastigium, normal supratentorial brain
      - Better cognition
      - Better skills/balance

Treatment

- CSF diversion **if** hydrocephalus: VP shunt ± cyst shunt/marsupialization

DIAGNOSTIC CHECKLIST

Consider

- Many associated syndromes, mimics

Image Interpretation Pearls

- Presence of fastigium/vermian lobulation predicts cognitive outcome
- Thin sagittal views crucial for delineation, diagnosis

Reporting Tips

- Is fastigium/vermian lobulation normal?

SELECTED REFERENCES

1. Aldinger KA et al: FOXC1 is required for normal cerebellar development and is a major contributor to chromosome 6p25.3 Dandy-Walker malformation. Nat Genet. 41(9):1037-42, 2009
2. Walbert T et al: Symptomatic neurocutaneous melanosis and Dandy-Walker malformation in an adult. J Clin Oncol. 27(17):2886-7, 2009
3. Elsen GE et al: Zic1 and Zic4 regulate zebrafish roof plate specification and hindbrain ventricle morphogenesis. Dev Biol. 314(2):376-92, 2008
4. Millen KJ et al: Cerebellar development and disease. Curr Opin Neurobiol. 18(1):12-9, 2008

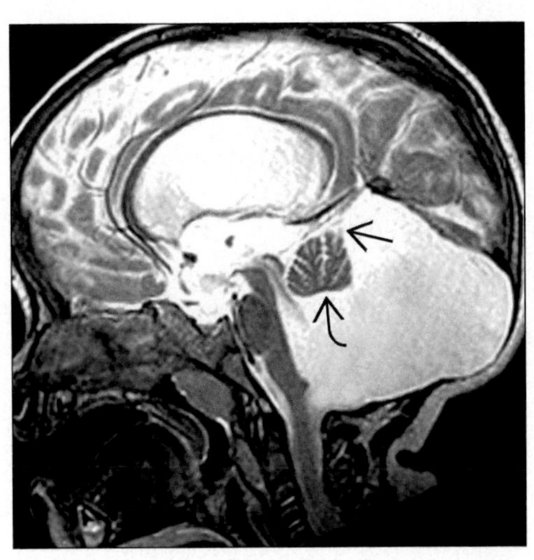

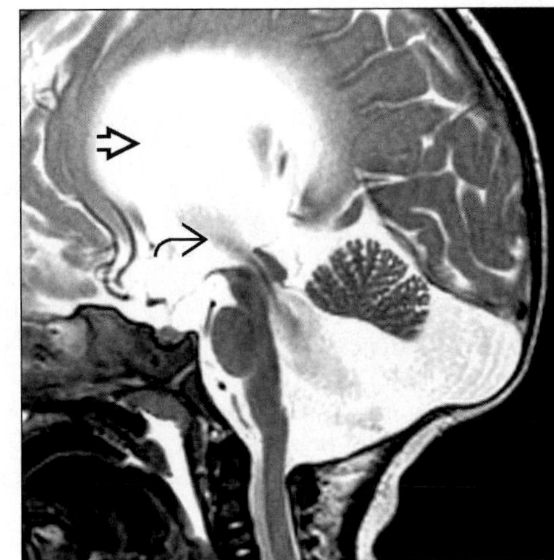

(Left) *Sagittal T2WI MR in a patient with DWM demonstrates hydrocephalus, a large posterior fossa, cephalad rotation of a small, incompletely lobulated vermis with a very shallow fastigial crease ⮳, and a very thin cyst wall →.* ***(Right)*** *Sagittal T2WI MR in HVR shows ventriculomegaly ⇨, patent aqueduct with prominent flow void ⮳, and a large posterior fossa. There is no torcular-lambdoid inversion. There is better lobulation of the vermis and less PF enlargement than in the previous patient.*

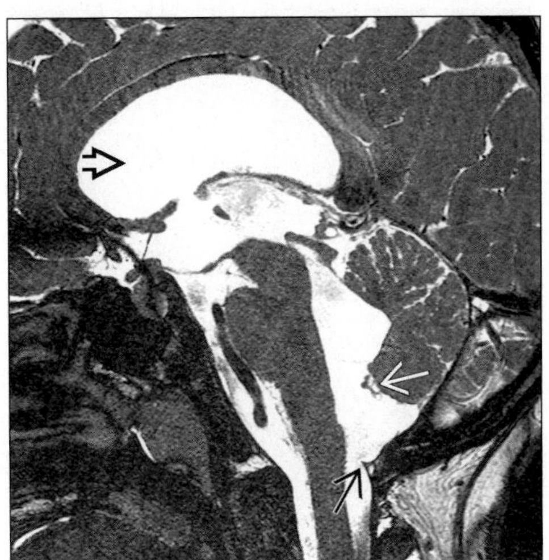

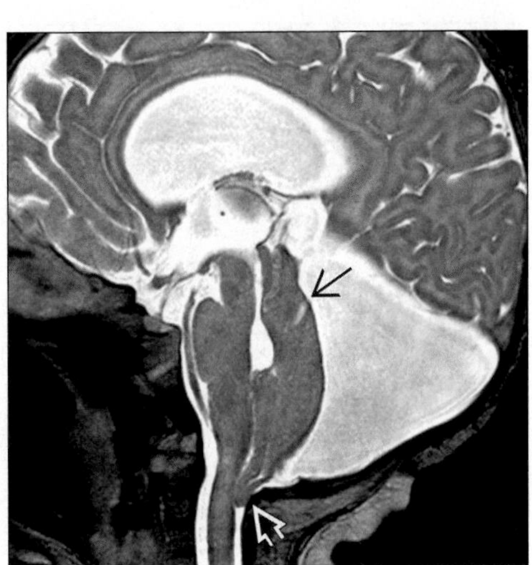

(Left) *Sagittal bSSFP demonstrates ventriculomegaly ⇨ and a patent and open inferior 4th ventricle. There is cyst wall visualization inferiorly →. The posteriorly displaced choroid plexus ➡ suggests Blake pouch cyst. Fastigial recess, primary fissure, and vermian lobulation are intact.* ***(Right)*** *Sagittal bSSFP shows a closed inferior 4th ventricle with acquired Chiari 1 ➡. The primary fissure → and the vermis are compressed by the wall of the retrocerebellar cyst.*

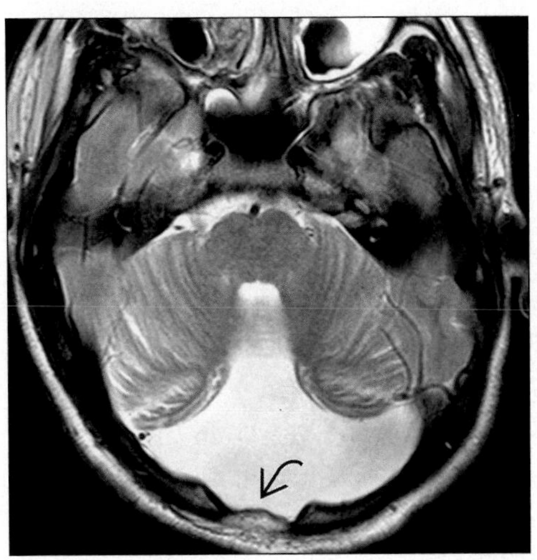

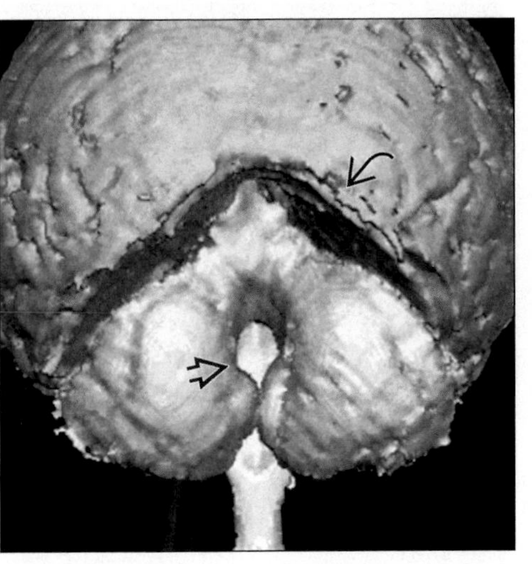

(Left) *Axial T2WI MR in a patient with DWM reveals relative hypoplasia of the cerebellar hemispheres and nonvisualization of the vermis at its usual location. There is a focal calvarial ⮳ defect at the site of a prior occipital encephalocele.* ***(Right)*** *Coronal 3D surface reconstruction of the brain (viewed from the inferoposterior aspect) from T1 gradient echo sequence shows the typical elevation of the tentorium ⮳ and separation of the cerebellar hemispheres ⇨ without intervening vermis.*

RHOMBENCEPHALOSYNAPSIS

Key Facts

Terminology
- Congenital continuity (lack of division) of cerebellar hemispheres
  - Usually with fusion of dentate nuclei and superior cerebellar peduncles
  - May be partial, affecting inferior portions of hemispheres only

Imaging
- Small, single hemisphere cerebellum with continuous white matter (WM) tracts crossing midline
  - Diamond or keyhole-shaped 4th ventricle
  - Absent primary fissure
  - ± aqueductal stenosis ⇒ hydrocephalus
  - ± corpus callosum dysgenesis (especially posterior)

Top Differential Diagnoses
- Molar tooth malformations
- Lhermitte-Duclos syndrome
- Vermian hypoplasia
- Diffuse cerebellar cortical dysplasia

Pathology
- Failure of vermian differentiation
  - Differentiation of vermis required to separate cerebellar hemispheres

Diagnostic Checklist
- Remember to define associated supratentorial anomalies
- Can be mimicked by mechanically induced cerebellar deformation in chronically shunted patients

*(**Left**) Coronal graphic of rhombencephalosynapsis shows that no vermis is present in the midline of the cerebellum. Instead, the folia, interfoliate sulci, and cerebellar white matter ➔ are continuous across the cerebellar midline. (**Right**) Coronal FLAIR MR clearly shows the continuity of the cerebellar white matter tracts and folia across the midline ➔ secondary to absence of the vermis and subsequent failure of cerebellar hemisphere separation.*

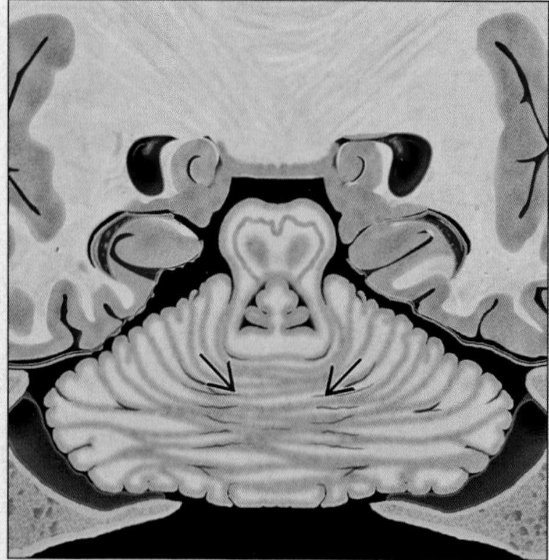

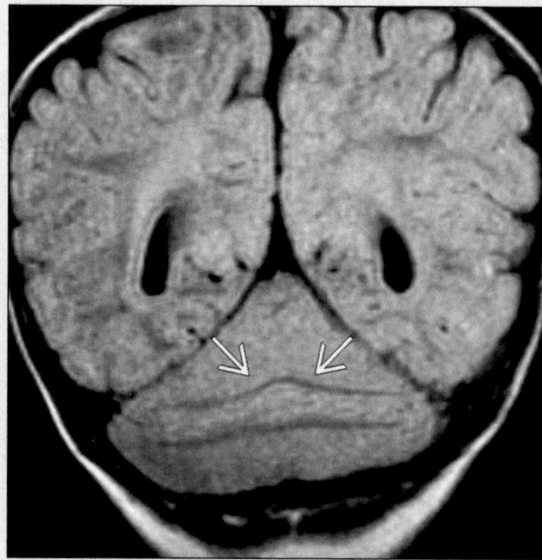

*(**Left**) Axial T2WI MR shows the single continuous cerebellar hemisphere at the level of the otic capsules. The small size of the posterior fossa has allowed inferior displacement of the occipital lobes ➔, which lie lateral to the cerebellum at the level of the medulla. (**Right**) Axial T2WI MR in another child with rhombencephalosynapsis shows the characteristic diamond-shaped 4th ventricle ➔ that results from lack of separation of the cerebellar dentate nuclei.*

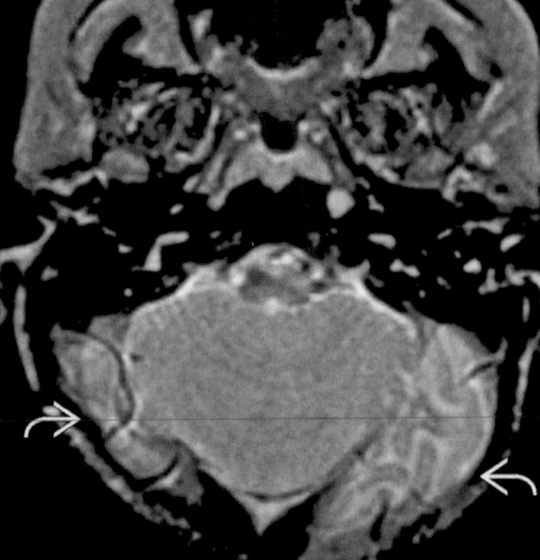

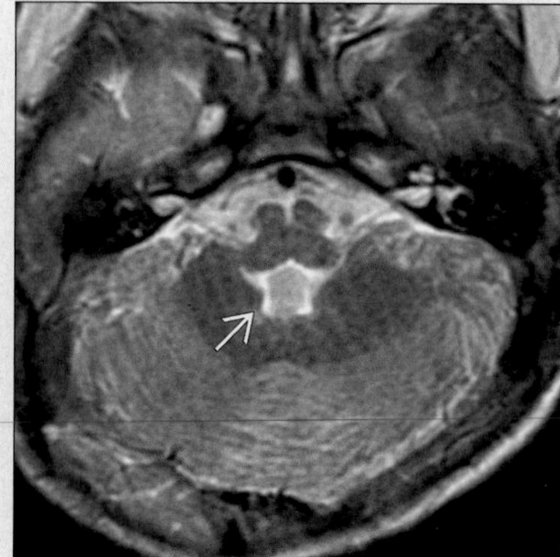

TERMINOLOGY

Abbreviations

- Rhombencephalosynapsis (RES)

Definitions

- Congenital continuity (lack of division) of cerebellar hemispheres
  - Usually with fusion of dentate nuclei and superior cerebellar peduncles
  - Complete or subtotal vermian agenesis
  - May be partial, affecting inferior portions of hemispheres only
  - Classified by Patel and Barkovich as "focal cerebellar dysplasia"

IMAGING

General Features

- Best diagnostic clue
  - Small, single hemisphere cerebellum with continuous white matter (WM) tracts crossing midline
- Location
  - Midline posterior fossa
- Size
  - Posterior fossa typically smaller than usual
- Morphology
  - Round or oval solitary cerebellar hemisphere

Radiographic Findings

- Radiography
  - Bilateral lambdoid synostosis ⇒ "flattened" occiput

CT Findings

- NECT
  - Cerebellar hemispheric fusion
  - Diamond- or keyhole-shaped 4th ventricle
  - Narrowed transverse diameter of cerebellum

MR Findings

- T1WI
  - Sagittal
    - Absent primary fissure
    - ± upwardly rounded fastigial recess of 4th ventricle
      - Nodulus preserved if fastigial recess present
    - ± aqueductal stenosis ⇒ hydrocephalus
    - ± corpus callosum dysgenesis (especially posterior)
  - Axial
    - ± collicular fusion
    - ± supratentorial cortical dysplasias
- T2WI
  - Coronal
    - Fused cerebellar hemispheres ⇒ total or partial
      - Continuous WM tracts across midline
      - Midline superior "tenting" of WM
    - Absent or severely hypoplastic vermis
    - Transverse folia
    - ± absent septum pellucidum
    - ± fused thalami and fornices
  - Fetal
    - Can be identified on fetal MR
      - Typically performed to investigate hydrocephalus seen on US
    - Abnormal shape of 4th ventricle and absence of vermis most reliable signs

Ultrasonographic Findings

- Grayscale ultrasound
  - Occasionally identified on fetal sonography

Imaging Recommendations

- Best imaging tool
  - MR
- Protocol advice
  - High resolution FSE T2WI in multiple imaging planes
    - T2WI more clearly defines posterior fossa structures in neonate and infant

DIFFERENTIAL DIAGNOSIS

Molar Tooth Malformations

- Joubert syndrome
  - Vermian dysplasia with prominent superior cerebellar peduncles
  - 4th ventricle has "bat wing" shape

Lhermitte-Duclos Disease

- Dysplastic cerebellar gangliocytoma
- Striated cerebellar hemisphere
- Associated with Cowden syndrome

Vermian Hypoplasia

- Small vermis without hemispheric fusion
- Vermis develops enough to separate hemispheres, then arrests

Single Hemisphere Cerebellar Hypoplasia

- Often secondary to in utero insult

Diffuse Cerebellar Cortical Dysplasia

- May be associated with congenital muscular dystrophies
- Type 2 lissencephaly

PATHOLOGY

General Features

- Etiology
  - Unknown: 2 major theories
    - Failure of vermian differentiation
      - Based on evidence that hemispheres develop as unpaired structure from cerebellar primordium
      - Differentiation of vermis required to separate cerebellar hemispheres
      - Better explains cases of partial rhombencephalosynapsis
    - Vermian agenesis allowing hemisphere continuity
      - Based on theory that hemispheres form separately from rhombic lips
      - Absence of vermian development allows hemispheres to become apposed and then fuse in midline
- Genetics

- *FGF8* and *Lmx1a* genes may influence expression of isthmic organizer
    - Isthmic organizer
        - Controls/influences patterning of midbrain and anterior hindbrain
        - Located within neuroepithelium of isthmic constriction at midbrain-hindbrain boundary
- Associated abnormalities
    - Absent septum pellucidum
    - Callosal and anterior commissure dysgenesis
    - Forniceal &/or thalamic fusion
    - Collicular fusion
    - Hydrocephalus associated with aqueductal stenosis
    - Prosencephalic and midline facial anomalies
    - Gomez-Lopez-Hernandez syndrome
        - Cerebello-trigeminal-dermal dysplasia
        - RES, parietooccipital alopecia, trigeminal anesthesia
        - Craniofacial dysmorphisms, short stature
    - Occasional associated extracranial anomalies
        - Segmentation and fusion anomalies in spine
        - Cardiovascular (conotruncal) anomalies reported
        - Variable respiratory, GU anomalies reported
        - Musculoskeletal anomalies common: Phalangeal and radial-ray

Staging, Grading, & Classification

- Partial fusion
    - Fused inferiorly, separated superiorly
- Presence or absence of supratentorial anomalies

Gross Pathologic & Surgical Features

- Typical
    - Fused cerebellar hemispheres
    - Fused cerebellar white matter ⇒ large corpus medullare
    - Absent posterior cerebellar incisura, vallecula
    - Horseshoe-shaped dentate nuclei
    - Agenesis or hypogenesis anterior vermis, velum medullare anterior, and nuclei fastigii
    - Hypoplastic posterior vermis
        - Nodulus may form
- Rare
    - Aventriculy (also called "synencephaly" or "telencephalosynapsis")
    - Encysted 4th ventricle

CLINICAL ISSUES

Presentation

- Most common signs/symptoms
    - Variable neurological signs
        - Ataxia, gait abnormalities, seizures
        - Developmental delay
        - RES discovered in near-normal patients at autopsy

Demographics

- Age
    - Usually found during early infancy or childhood
    - Rarely an incidental finding
- Epidemiology
    - Rare but increasingly recognized on MR

Natural History & Prognosis

- Developmental delay
- Psychiatric disorders (self-injurious, bipolar, hyperactive)
- Additional midline supratentorial anomalies and hydrocephalus ⇒ worse prognosis

Treatment

- Treat related hydrocephalus, monitor hypothalamic-pituitary axis

DIAGNOSTIC CHECKLIST

Consider

- Isolated rhombencephalosynapsis is less common than rhombencephalosynapsis with supratentorial anomalies

Image Interpretation Pearls

- Can be mimicked by mechanically induced cerebellar deformation in chronically shunted patients

Reporting Tips

- Remember to define associated supratentorial anomalies

SELECTED REFERENCES

1. Alkan O et al: Malformations of the midbrain and hindbrain: a retrospective study and review of the literature. Cerebellum. 8(3):355-65, 2009
2. Dill P et al: Fetal magnetic resonance imaging in midline malformations of the central nervous system and review of the literature. J Neuroradiol. 36(3):138-46, 2009
3. Jellinger KA: Rhombencephalosynapsis with and without associated malformations. Acta Neuropathol. 117(2):219, 2009
4. Michael GA et al: Reactivity to visual signals and the cerebellar vermis: Evidence from a rare case with rhombencephalosynapsis. Behav Neurosci. 123(1):86-96, 2009
5. Pasquier L et al: Rhombencephalosynapsis and related anomalies: a neuropathological study of 40 fetal cases. Acta Neuropathol. 117(2):185-200, 2009
6. Poretti A et al: Cognitive outcome in children with rhombencephalosynapsis. Eur J Paediatr Neurol. 13(1):28-33, 2009
7. Elliott R et al: Rhombencephalosynapsis associated with autosomal dominant polycystic kidney disease Type 1. J Neurosurg Pediatr. 2(6):435-7, 2008
8. Demaerel P et al: Partial rhombencephalosynapsis. AJNR Am J Neuroradiol. 25(1):29-31, 2004
9. Patel S et al: Analysis and classification of cerebellar malformations. AJNR Am J Neuroradiol. 23(7):1074-87, 2002
10. Toelle SP et al: Rhombencephalosynapsis: clinical findings and neuroimaging in 9 children. Neuropediatrics. 33(4):209-14, 2002
11. Brocks D et al: Gomez-Lopez-Hernandez syndrome: expansion of the phenotype. Am J Med Genet. 94(5):405-8, 2000

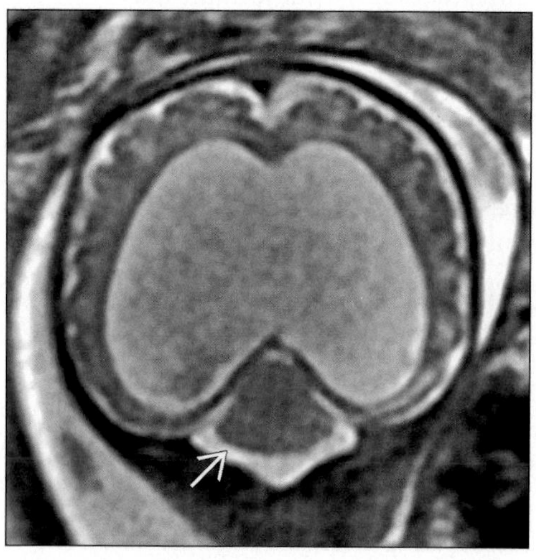

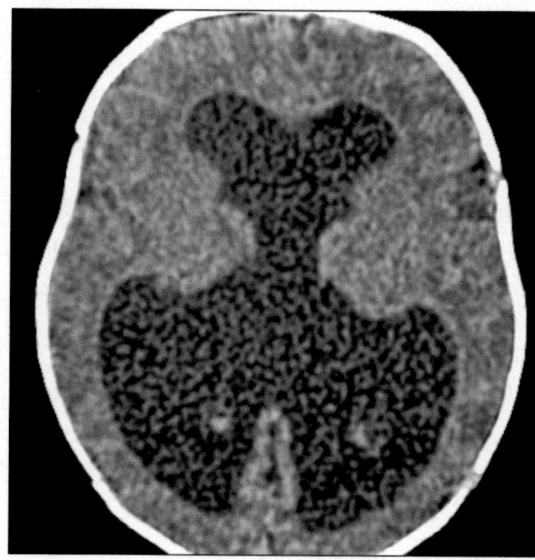

(Left) *Coronal T2WI fetal MR acquired at 22 weeks gestation shows midline continuity of the cerebellar hemispheres ➡. Septum pellucidum is absent. Marked supratentorial hydrocephalus is secondary to aqueductal stenosis.* **(Right)** *Postnatal axial NECT in same child shows hydrocephalus and absence of septum pellucidum. The supratentorial abnormalities associated with rhombencephalosynapsis may be more clinically significant than the cerebellar malformation.*

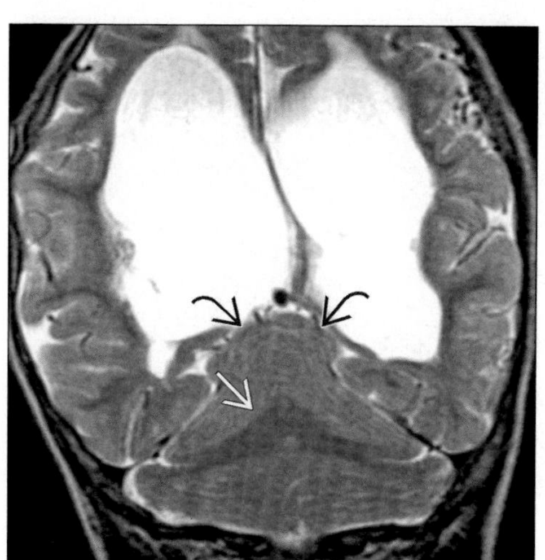

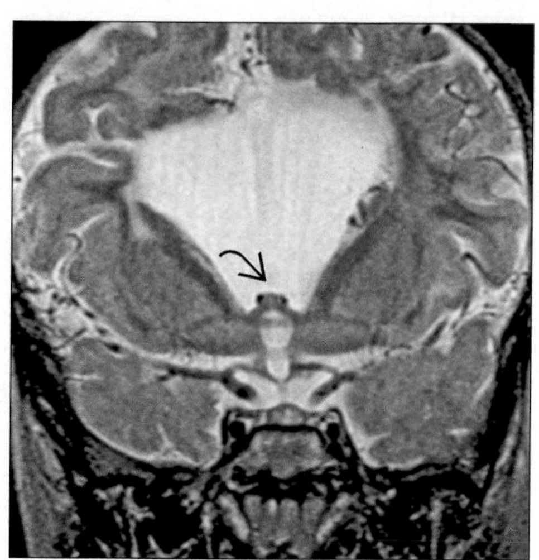

(Left) *Coronal T2WI MR in a child with rhombencephalosynapsis and shunted hydrocephalus shows upward herniation of the cerebellum ➡ through low-lying tentorial incisura. Note the superior tenting of cerebellar white matter tracts ➡ that are continuous across the midline.* **(Right)** *Coronal T2WI MR in the same child at the level of the anterior commissure shows midline forniceal fusion ➡ and absence of the septum pellucidum and corpus callosum.*

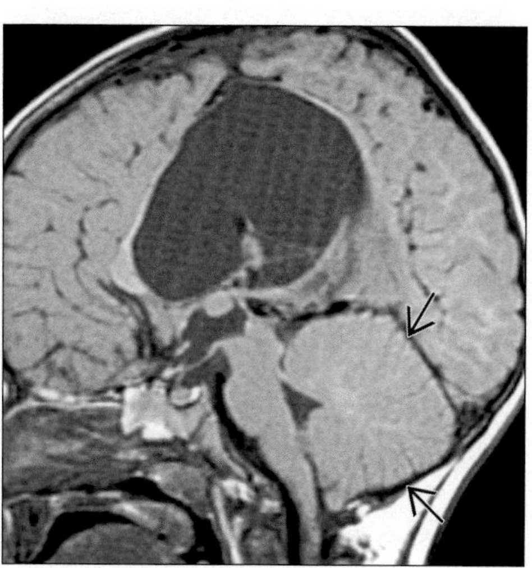

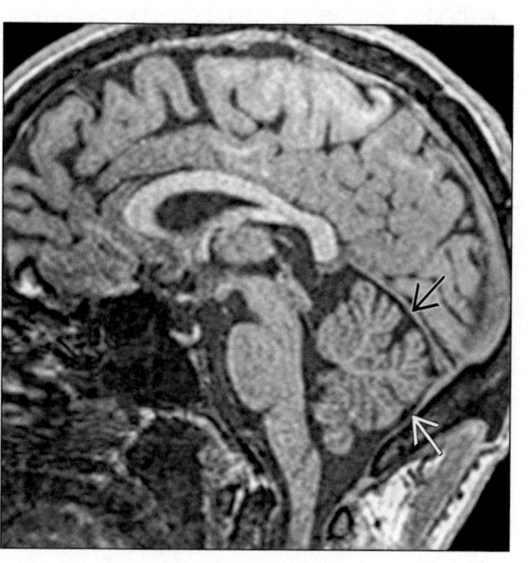

(Left) *Sagittal T1WI MR in the same child with rhombencephalosynapsis and shunted hydrocephalus is notable for ventricular enlargement, dysmorphic corpus callosum, and absence of the primary and prepyramidal fissures of the cerebellar vermis, which should be located at the arrows ➡. Abnormal midline cerebellar morphology is a clue to the diagnosis.* **(Right)** *Sagittal T1WI MR in a teenager clearly shows the normal primary ➡ and prepyramidal ➡ fissures.*

UNCLASSIFIED CEREBELLAR DYSPLASIAS

Key Facts

Terminology

- Focal or diffuse dysplasias of cerebellar hemispheres or vermis not associated with other known malformations or syndromes

Imaging

- Asymmetry or focal disruption of cerebellar folial and sulcal morphology
- Bumpy gray-white matter interface in cerebellum
- Lack of normal arborization of white matter
- Abnormal hyperintense signal in subcortical white matter ⇒ cyst-like foci
- Cerebellar gray matter heterotopia
- Enlarged and vertically oriented fissures
- Disordered foliation

Pathology

- Cerebellar cortex does not assume adult-like histology prior to age 1
- In 1 study of 147 normal infants, minor cerebellar dysplasias were identified in close to 85%
  - Some minor dysplasias involute after 9 months of age

Clinical Issues

- Hypotonia, microcephaly, speech delay

Diagnostic Checklist

- Assess for "cobblestone" lissencephaly and congenital muscular dystrophy when considering diagnosis of isolated cerebellar dysplasia
- Look for and document associated posterior fossa and supratentorial lesions

*(**Left**) Coronal FLAIR MR in a 5 year old with developmental delay and right hemiparesis shows agenesis of the corpus callosum with focal dysplasia of the left cerebellar hemisphere. Note the abnormal foliation in the small affected hemisphere ➡ compared to the normal right side. (**Right**) Axial T2WI MR in the same patient shows the distorted and disorganized pattern of white matter in the dysplastic left hemisphere in comparison with the normal right cerebellum (folia should be parallel to calvarium in axial plane).*

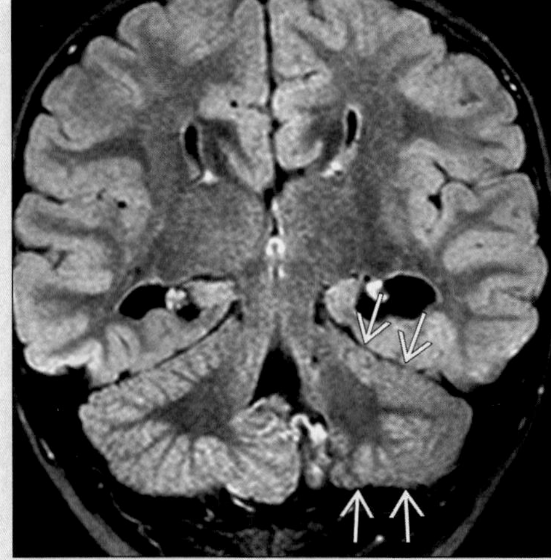

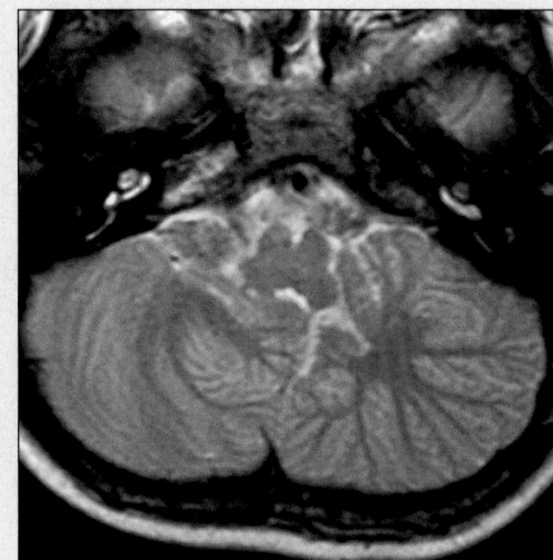

*(**Left**) Coronal T2WI MR in a child with vermian hypoplasia shows disordered foliation ➡ in the right hemisphere and a prominent vertical fissure on the left ➡. These disorders are thought to most likely be disruptions due to prenatal injury. (**Right**) Coronal T2WI MR in a 4-year-old boy with global developmental delay shows a very abnormal cerebellum with vertically oriented folia ➡ and fissures along with nodular areas of gray matter ➡, likely cerebellar heterotopia.*

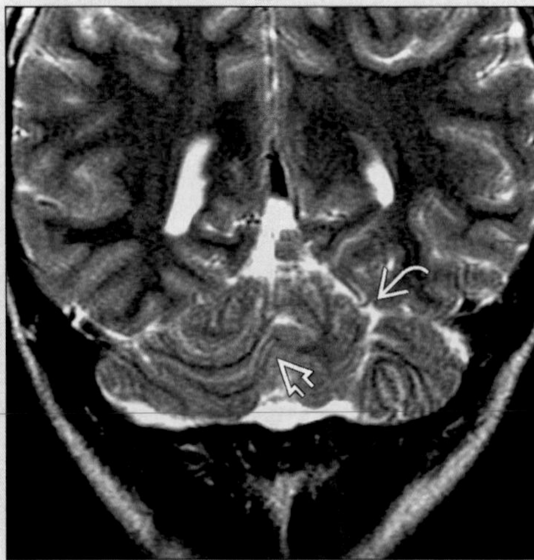

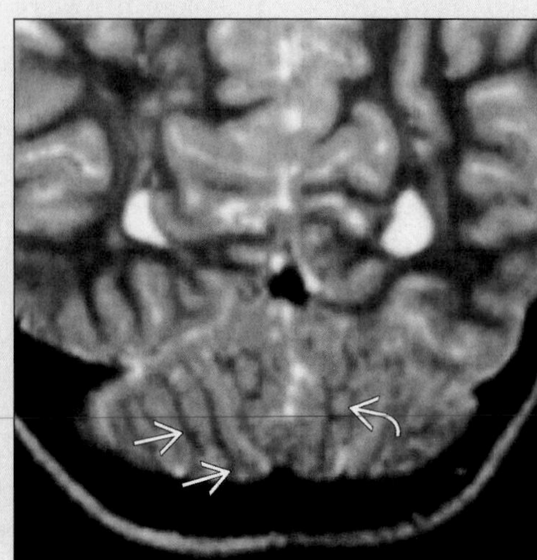

UNCLASSIFIED CEREBELLAR DYSPLASIAS

TERMINOLOGY

Synonyms

- Diffuse cerebellar dysplasia
- Cerebellar cortical dysplasia

Definitions

- Focal or diffuse dysplasias of cerebellar hemispheres or vermis not associated with other known malformations or syndromes
  - Excludes Dandy-Walker spectrum, Lhermitte-Duclos disease, rhombencephalosynapsis, molar tooth malformations, and congenital muscular dystrophies

IMAGING

General Features

- Best diagnostic clue
  - Asymmetry or focal disruption of cerebellar folia and sulcal morphology
- Location
  - Variable
- Size
  - Variable
- Morphology
  - Variable

CT Findings

- Irregular morphology of 4th ventricle or cisterna magna

MR Findings

- T1WI
  - Bumpy gray-white matter interface in cerebellum
  - Lack of normal arborization of white matter
- T2WI
  - Cyst-like foci in subcortical white matter
  - Gray matter heterotopias, disordered foliation
  - Enlarged and vertically oriented fissures

Imaging Recommendations

- Best imaging tool
  - MR
- Protocol advice
  - Use thin slice profile T2WI in axial and coronal planes to define cerebellar morphology

DIFFERENTIAL DIAGNOSIS

Rhombencephalosynapsis

- Fused cerebellar hemispheres with vermian hypo-/aplasia

Molar Tooth Malformations (Joubert)

- "Bat-wing" 4th ventricle

Cerebellar Dysplasia Associated with Lissencephalies

- Congenital muscular dystrophies

PATHOLOGY

General Features

- Cerebellar cortex does not assume adult-like histology prior to age 1
- In 1 study of 147 normal infants, minor cerebellar dysplasias were identified in close to 85%
  - Some minor dysplasias involute after 9 months of age

Gross Pathologic & Surgical Features

- Dysmorphic foliation, hemispheres often small
- Primitive foliation
- Mega cisternal magna

Microscopic Features

- Fusing of apposed molecular layers
- Small cavities with meningeal vessels
- Nodules of Purkinje cells
- Deficient/absent granular layer

Associated Findings

- Cerebral cortical dysplasia
- Agenesis/dysgenesis of corpus callosum
- Macro-/microscopic heterotopia

CLINICAL ISSUES

Presentation

- Most common signs/symptoms
  - Hypotonia, microcephaly, speech delay
- Other signs/symptoms
  - Ataxia, facial malformations, abnormal eye movements, motor delay

DIAGNOSTIC CHECKLIST

Consider

- Assess for "cobblestone" lissencephaly and congenital muscular dystrophy when considering diagnosis of isolated cerebellar dysplasia

Reporting Tips

- Look for and document associated posterior fossa and supratentorial lesions

SELECTED REFERENCES

1. Bolduc ME et al: Neurodevelopmental outcomes in children with cerebellar malformations: a systematic review. Dev Med Child Neurol. 51(4):256-67, 2009
2. Poretti A et al: Cerebellar cleft: a form of prenatal cerebellar disruption. Neuropediatrics. 39(2):106-12, 2008
3. Demaerel P: Abnormalities of cerebellar foliation and fissuration: classification, neurogenetics and clinicoradiological correlations. Neuroradiology. 44(8):639-46, 2002
4. Soto-Ares G et al: Cerebellar cortical dysplasia: MR findings in a complex entity. AJNR Am J Neuroradiol. 21(8):1511-9, 2000

MOLAR TOOTH MALFORMATIONS (JOUBERT)

Key Facts

Terminology

- Hindbrain anomaly characterized by dysmorphic vermis, lack of decussation of superior cerebellar peduncle, central pontine tracts, corticospinal tracts

Imaging

- "Molar tooth" appearance of midbrain on axial images
- Midline vermian clefting
- Thick, horizontal (perpendicular to brainstem), superior cerebellar peduncles
- Midline depression of 4th ventricular floor at isthmus (thin isthmus on midline)
- High-definition T2 (CISS/FIESTA) provides exquisite structural analysis
- HASTE allows clear identification of "molar tooth" sign in fetuses
- DTI is useful complementary technique

Top Differential Diagnoses

- Dandy-walker continuum
- Vermian and pontocerebellar hypoplasia
- Rhombencephalosynapsis
- Cerebellar vermian atrophy

Pathology

- *AHI1* gene at 6q23 (part of *JBST3* locus), *NPHP1* gene at 2q13
- Loci at 9q34.3 (*JBTS1*), 11p11.2-q12.3 (*JBTS2*), and 6q23 (*JBST3*) identified
- Absence of decussation of superior cerebellar peduncles
- Near total absence of pyramidal decussation

Clinical Issues

- Ataxia, developmental delay, oculomotor and respiratory abnormalities

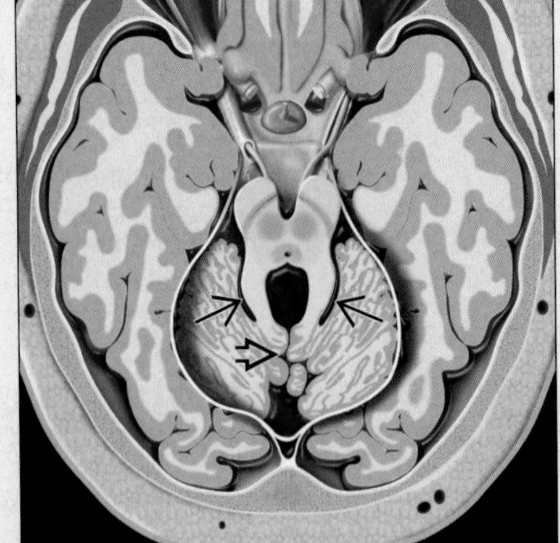

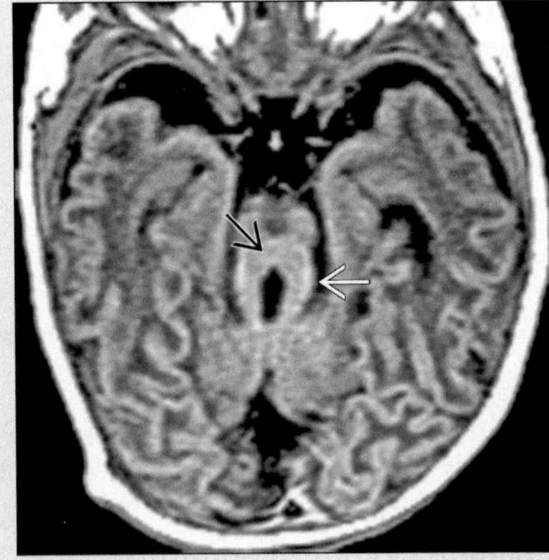

(Left) *Axial graphic depicts Joubert malformation. Thickened superior cerebellar peduncles ⇨ around the elongated 4th ventricle form the classic "molar tooth" seen in this anomaly. Note the cleft cerebellar vermis ⇨* ***(Right)*** *Axial T1WI MR at the midbrain/pons junction (isthmus) shows the 4th ventricle pointed anteriorly ⇨, explaining the sagittal thinning of the isthmus. It is flanked on both sides by thick, elongated, in-plane superior cerebellar peduncles ➡, forming the "molar tooth."*

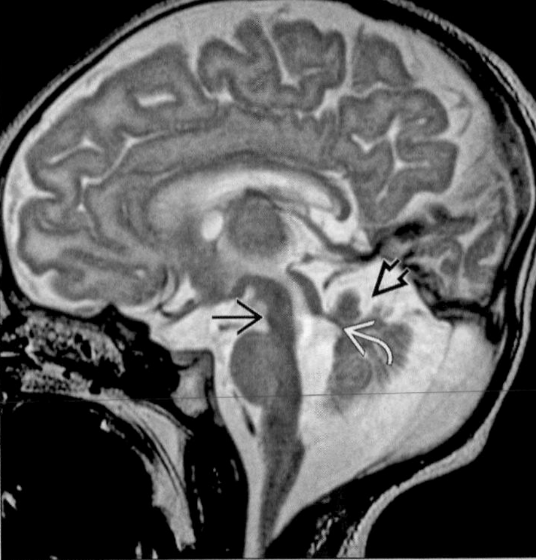

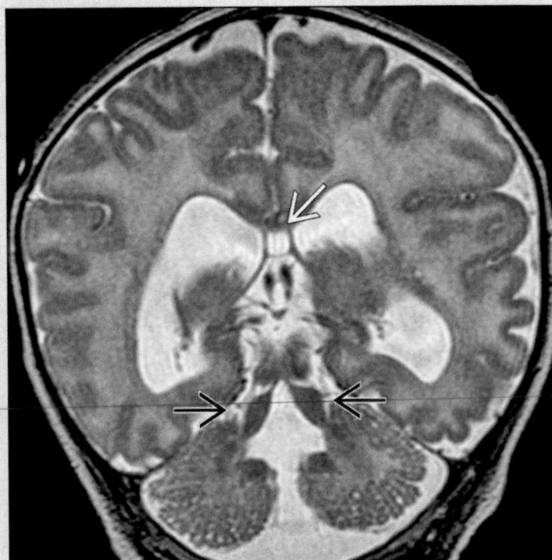

(Left) *Sagittal T2WI MR of a neonate with ocular and breathing disorder shows a very small, dysmorphic vermis ⇨. The 4th ventricle is large and upwardly convex ➡; the midbrain ⇨ appears thin and elongated. CSF spaces are enlarged over the convexity.* ***(Right)*** *Coronal T2WI MR in the same patient demonstrates the thick, horizontal superior cerebellar peduncles ⇨. Note also the ventriculomegaly, with persisting cavum vergae ➡ between the corpus callosum and the hippocampal commissure.*

MOLAR TOOTH MALFORMATIONS (JOUBERT)

TERMINOLOGY

Abbreviations

- Molar tooth malformation (MTM)
- Joubert syndrome related disorders (JSRD)
  - Include Joubert, Dekaban-Arima, COACH, Senior-Loken, Varadi-Papp, Joubert-polymicrogyria syndromes

Definitions

- Hindbrain anomaly characterized by dysmorphic vermis, lack of decussation of superior cerebellar peduncle, central pontine tracts, corticospinal tracts
  - Sagittal clefting of cerebellar vermis
  - Abnormal brainstem nuclei

IMAGING

General Features

- Best diagnostic clue
  - "Molar tooth" appearance of midbrain on axial images
  - Midline vermian clefting
- Location
  - Brainstem isthmus (pontomesencephalic)
  - Vermis and superior (efferent) cerebellar peduncle
- Morphology
  - Hard to identify vermis with midline sagittal cleft
    - Dorsal 4th ventricle has dysmorphic, irregular fastigium
  - Thick, horizontal (perpendicular to brainstem), superior cerebellar peduncles
  - Midline depression of 4th ventricular floor at isthmus (thin isthmus on midline)

CT Findings

- NECT
  - Vermis clefting
  - 4th ventricle has "bat wing" configuration

MR Findings

- T1WI
  - Sagittal
    - Normal midline appearance of vermis lost
    - Dysmorphic roof of 4th ventricle with fastigial point lost
    - Large CSF spaces, but tentorium in normal location
  - Coronal
    - Vermian clefting above "apposed hemispheres" (cleft lined with cortex)
  - Axial: Vermian clefting, "molar tooth" appearance
    - Anteriorly pointed ventricular floor at pons-midbrain junction (thin isthmus)
    - Prominent, in-plane, parallel superior cerebellar peduncles (molar roots)
- T2WI
  - Same findings as T1WI
    - Better contrast than T1WI
    - Prominent CSF spaces common
    - Abnormal myelination sometimes
  - High-definition T2 (CISS/FIESTA) provides exquisite structural analysis
  - HASTE allows clear identification of "molar tooth" sign in fetuses

Ultrasonographic Findings

- Prenatal ultrasound shows small vermis, large cisterna magna
  - May show supernumerary digits, heart disease, kidney disease, etc.

Imaging Recommendations

- Best imaging tool
  - MR
- Protocol advice
  - Use high definition; posterior fossa structures are small
  - DTI is useful complementary technique

DIFFERENTIAL DIAGNOSIS

Dandy-Walker Continuum

- Agenetic vermis (not clefting)
- 4th ventricular cyst lined with ependyma, not cortex
- Elevated tentorium

Vermian and Pontocerebellar Hypoplasia

- Vermis is small, no clefting
- Variable abnormalities of pons, medulla, midbrain

Rhombencephalosynapsis

- Cerebellar hemispheres/dentates are fused without differentiated midline vermis

Cerebellar Vermian Atrophy

- Midbrain, cerebellar peduncles normal; normal vermian foliation with enlarged fissures
- Causal context (prematurity, metabolic, etc.)

PATHOLOGY

General Features

- Etiology
  - Thought to result from mutations of ciliary/centrosomal proteins that can affect cell migration, axonal pathway, other still unknown mechanisms
    - Referred to as "ciliopathy"
    - Related to Meckel-Gruber syndrome
- Genetics
  - *AHI1* gene at 6q23 (part of *JBST3* locus), *NPHP1* gene at 2q13
    - *NPHP1* mutations have more subtle neuroimaging findings, severe renal disease
    - *AHI1* mutations have severe cerebellar and midbrain-hindbrain malformation, ± polymicrogyria
  - 7 other loci identified (9q34.3, 11p12-q13.3, 12q21.3, 8q21.13-q22.1, 16q12.2, 3q11.2, 4p15.3)
  - Malformation complex probably result of several different processes
    - Frequent anomalies of kidneys, eyes, extremities, liver/bile ducts
- Associated abnormalities
  - Polymicrogyria; renal, retinal, hepatic abnormalities
    - Prominent CSF spaces and ventriculomegaly

- Rarely: Meningoencephaloceles, microcephaly, lissencephaly, agenesis of corpus callosum
- Hypothalamic hamartomas
- Juvenile nephronophthisis or multicystic dysplastic kidney
- Ocular anomalies (retinal dysplasias and colobomata)
- Hepatic fibrosis and cysts, heart disease, polydactyly

Gross Pathologic & Surgical Features

- Midbrain-hindbrain malformation characterized by
  - Dysmorphic vermis with midline cleft
  - Thick horizontal superior cerebellar peduncles
  - Absent cerebellar decussation in midbrain
  - Multiple decussation defects

Microscopic Features

- Absence of decussation of superior cerebellar peduncles
- Near total absence of pyramidal decussation
- Dysplasias and heterotopia of cerebellar nuclei
- Structural anomalies in multiple locations
  - Inferior olivary nuclei, descending trigeminal tract, solitary fascicle, dorsal column nuclei

CLINICAL ISSUES

Presentation

- Most common signs/symptoms
  - Ataxia, developmental delay, oculomotor and respiratory abnormalities
- Other signs/symptoms
  - Neonate: Nystagmus, alternating apnea, hyperpnea (Joubert syndrome), seizures
  - Characteristic facial features
    - Large head
    - Prominent forehead
    - High, rounded eyebrows
    - Epicanthal folds
    - Upturned nose with evident nostrils
    - Tongue protrusion and rhythmic tongue motions
  - Retinal anomalies
    - Congenital retinal dystrophy
    - Pigmentary retinopathy
    - Chorioretinal colobomata
    - Fundus flavus

Demographics

- Age
  - Infancy and childhood; isolated oculomotor apraxia may present later
- Gender
  - M = F

Natural History & Prognosis

- Early death in affected infants
- Older children → problems with temperament, hyperactivity, aggressiveness, and dependency
  - Most affected children are severely impaired

Treatment

- Genetic counseling, physical therapy, occupational therapy

DIAGNOSTIC CHECKLIST

Consider

- Consider MTM whenever scanning infants/children with severe hypotonia and ocular anomalies

Image Interpretation Pearls

- If vermis not recognized on sagittal and dysmorphic 4th ventricle
  - Look for vermian cleft and "molar tooth" on axials

SELECTED REFERENCES

1. Gunay-Aygun M et al: MKS3-related ciliopathy with features of autosomal recessive polycystic kidney disease, nephronophthisis, and Joubert Syndrome. J Pediatr. 155(3):386-92, 2009
2. Kuchukhidze G et al: Hypoplasia of deep cerebellar nuclei in joubert syndrome. Pediatr Neurol. 40(6):474-6, 2009
3. Zaki MS et al: The molar tooth sign: a new Joubert syndrome and related cerebellar disorders classification system tested in Egyptian families. Neurology. 70(7):556-65, 2008
4. Fluss J et al: Molar tooth sign in fetal brain magnetic resonance imaging leading to the prenatal diagnosis of Joubert syndrome and related disorders. J Child Neurol. 21(4):320-4, 2006
5. Parisi MA et al: AHI1 mutations cause both retinal dystrophy and renal cystic disease in Joubert syndrome. J Med Genet. 43(4):334-9, 2006
6. Valente EM et al: AHI1 gene mutations cause specific forms of Joubert syndrome-related disorders. Ann Neurol. 59(3):527-34, 2006
7. Widjaja E et al: Diffusion tensor imaging of midline posterior fossa malformations. Pediatr Radiol. 36(6):510-7, 2006
8. Chodirker BN et al: Another case of Varadi-Papp Syndrome with a molar tooth sign. Am J Med Genet A. 136(4):416-7, 2005
9. Kroes HY et al: Cerebral, cerebellar, and colobomatous anomalies in three related males: Sex-linked inheritance in a newly recognized syndrome with features overlapping with Joubert syndrome. Am J Med Genet A. 135(3):297-301, 2005
10. Valente EM et al: Distinguishing the four genetic causes of Jouberts syndrome-related disorders. Ann Neurol. 57(4):513-9, 2005
11. Gleeson JG et al: Molar tooth sign of the midbrain-hindbrain junction: occurrence in multiple distinct syndromes. Am J Med Genet A. 125(2):125-34; discussion 117, 2004
12. Kumandas S et al: Joubert syndrome: review and report of seven new cases. Eur J Neurol. 11(8):505-10, 2004
13. Marsh SE et al: Neuroepithelial cysts in a patient with Joubert syndrome plus renal cysts. J Child Neurol. 19(3):227-31, 2004
14. Valente EM et al: Description, nomenclature, and mapping of a novel cerebello-renal syndrome with the molar tooth malformation. Am J Hum Genet. 73(3):663-70, 2003
15. Maria BL et al: Molar tooth sign in Joubert syndrome: clinical, radiologic, and pathologic significance. J Child Neurol. 14(6):368-76, 1999
16. Quisling RG et al: Magnetic resonance imaging features and classification of central nervous system malformations in Joubert syndrome. J Child Neurol. 14(10):628-35; discussion 669-72, 1999
17. Satran D et al: Cerebello-oculo-renal syndromes including Arima, Senior-Loken and COACH syndromes: more than just variants of Joubert syndrome. Am J Med Genet. 86(5):459-69, 1999

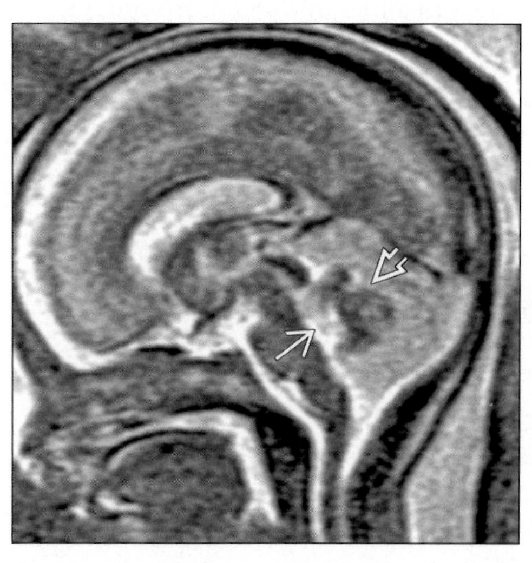

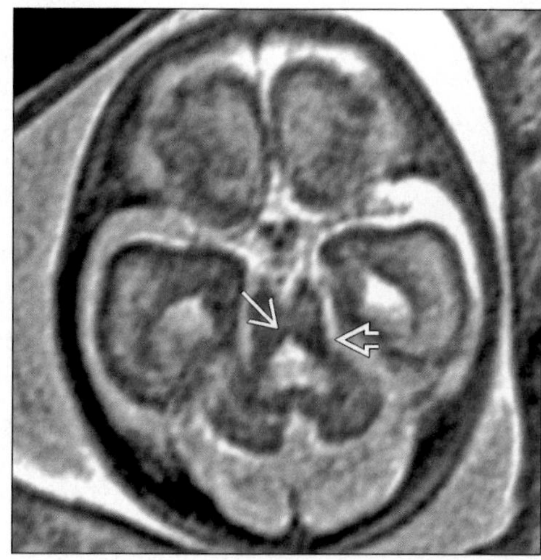

(Left) *Sagittal T2WI MR (HASTE) of a 27-week fetus shows a dysmorphic 4th ventricle ➔ with a hardly recognizable vermis ➔ (abnormal shape, no normal fissures identified). The posterior fossa cisterns are markedly enlarged. Supratentorial structures are normal.* ***(Right)*** *Axial T2WI MR (HASTE) in the same 27-week fetus demonstrate an anteriorly pointed 4th ventricle ➔ and thick superior cerebellar peduncles ➔, giving an appearance like a molar tooth.*

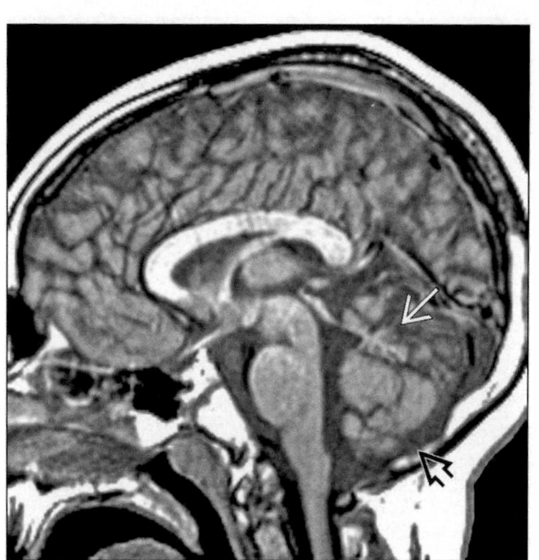

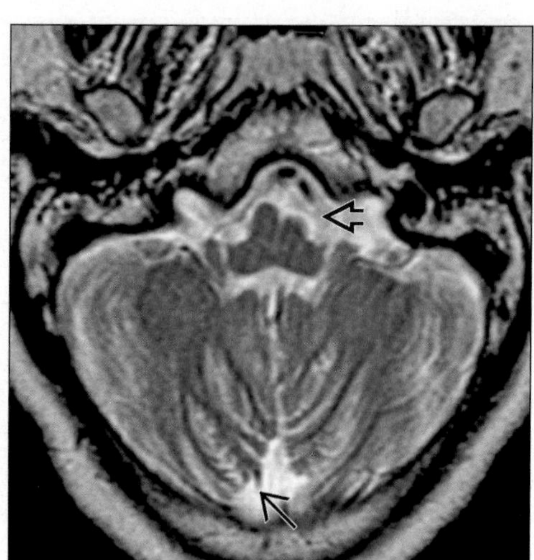

(Left) *Sagittal T1WI MR shows the characteristic appearance of the Joubert ("molar tooth") malformation with a tiny, dysplastic vermis ➔ located too far superiorly and the medial aspect of the cerebellar hemispheres ➔ in the midline below.* ***(Right)*** *Axial T2WI MR of the same patient demonstrates an asymmetric medulla with hypoplasia of the pyramidal tract on the left ➔, medial hemispheres apposing in the midline, and an unusual orientation of the cerebellar hemispheric folia ➔.*

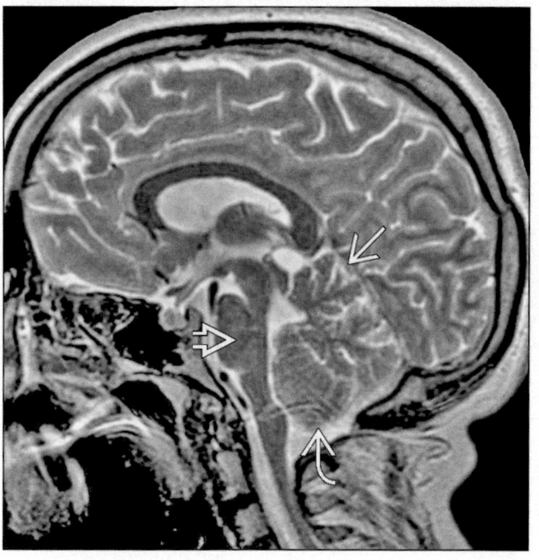

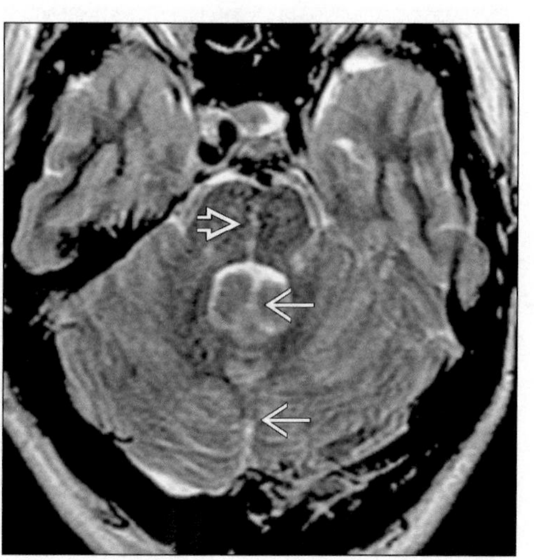

(Left) *Sagittal T2WI MR demonstrates a small, ill-formed superior vermis ➔ and medial cerebellar hemisphere in the midline below ➔. Note the small size of the posterior fossa, large foramen magnum, and thinning of the brainstem ➔.* ***(Right)*** *Axial T2WI MR shows clefting of the nodulus and posterior vermis ➔, as well as flattening of the brainstem with a midline sagittal line of bright signal ➔. Although of uncertain significance, this could suggest poor decussation.*

HOLOPROSENCEPHALY

Key Facts

Terminology
- Formerly called arrhinencephaly

Imaging
- Single ventricle
- Absent or partial hemispheric and basal cleavage with absent interhemispheric fissure/falx
- Azygous ACA
- ± associated facial defects

Top Differential Diagnoses
- Syntelencephaly or middle interhemispheric variant (MIH) of HPE
- Septo-optic dysplasia (fornices fused but present)
- Schizencephaly (hemispheric clefts, fornices present)
- Torn septum pellucidum: Severe, usually congenital hydrocephalus

Pathology
- Cytogenetic abnormalities in 25-50%: Trisomy 13, 18q-, 18p-, 3p, 7-, trisomy 9, 1q15q, 11q12-q13 (*DHCR7* gene mutation = Smith-Lemli-Opitz)
- Sonic hedgehog *SHH* (7q36), SIX3 (2p21), *TGIF1* (18p11.3) all ⇒ ventrodorsal gradient ⇒ non-cleavage anterobasal midline, disorganized neocortex (anterior)
- *SHH* also controls neural crest (midface) and oligodendrocytic (myelination) development

Clinical Issues
- Mentally retarded microcephalic infant with hypotelorism

Diagnostic Checklist
- Not all cases of missing septum pellucidum are single ventricle

*(**Left**) Oblique 3D reconstruction in a child with semilobar HPE. The major finding is absence of anterior interhemispheric fissure. The gyral pattern is almost normal, but the sylvian fissure ⇨ is shallow and vertical (due to frontal lobe hypoplasia). (**Right**) Axial T1WI MR shows lack of hemispheric division. Sylvian fissures ➡ are anteromedial due to frontal hypoplasia. The anterobasal striatum ⇨ and medial thalamus ➡ are not divided, and the ventricular atria open posteriorly into the dorsal cyst.*

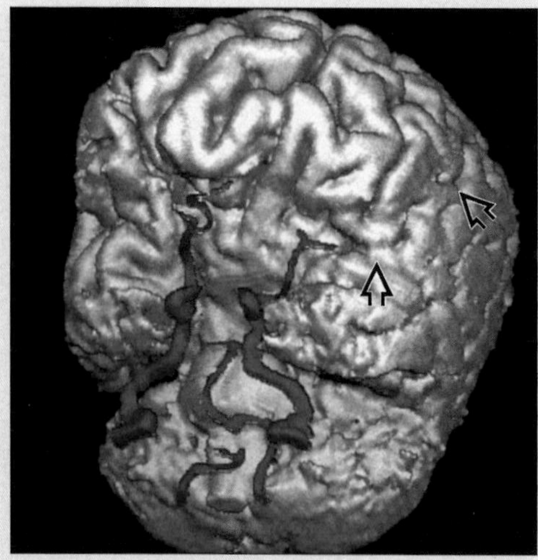

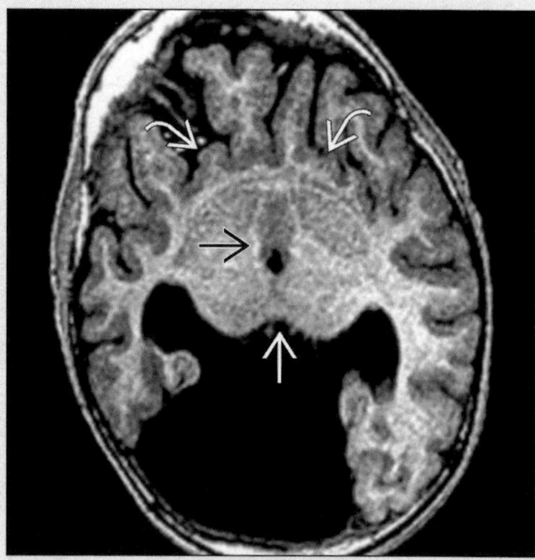

*(**Left**) Sagittal T2WI MR shows small, single frontal lobe ⇨ with single undivided anterobasal striatum ➡ and the widely expanded tela choroidea forming the prosencephalic dorsal cyst ⇨. (**Right**) Oblique posterior view of surface rendering 3D T1 gradient echo sequence shows the large dorsal cyst ➡. Note that the temporal ⇨ cortex shows no normal recognizable gyral pattern. The cerebellum appears normal.*

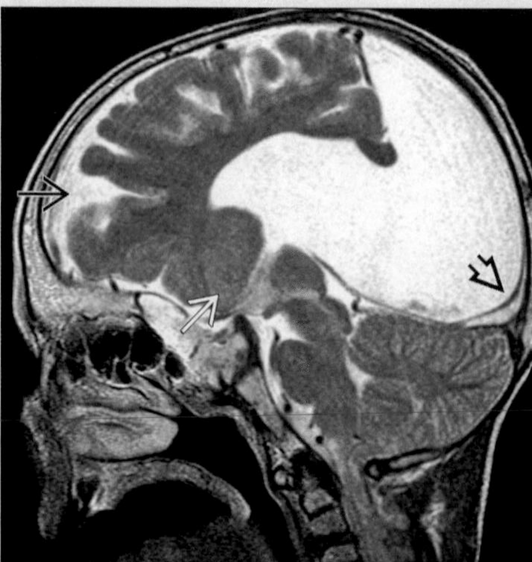

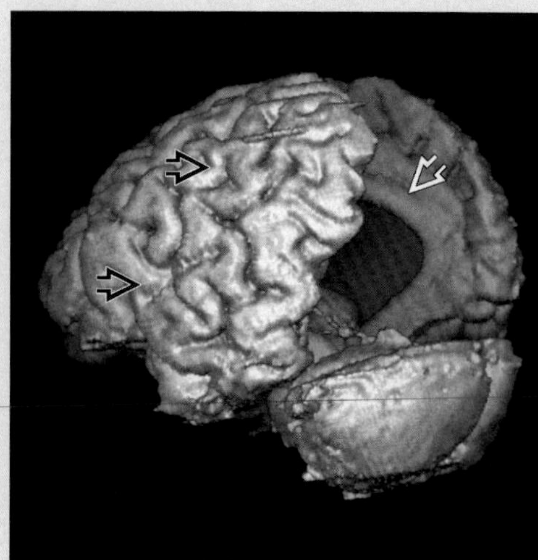

HOLOPROSENCEPHALY

TERMINOLOGY

Abbreviations
- Holoprosencephaly (HPE)

Synonyms
- Formerly called arrhinencephaly

Definitions
- Failure to delineate normal prosencephalic midline with absent/incomplete hemispheric and basal cleavage

IMAGING

General Features
- Best diagnostic clue
  - Single ventricle
  - Absent or partial hemispheric and basal cleavage with absent/incomplete interhemispheric fissure/ falx
  - Azygous anterior cerebral artery (ACA)
  - ± associated facial defects
- Location
  - Forebrain ± midface
- Morphology
  - Single forebrain vesicle (ventricle): HPE
  - Anomaly and severity defined by degree of forebrain cleavage

Radiographic Findings
- Radiography
  - Hypotelorism, ± single orbit, missing midface, single frontal "plate" of bone, microcephaly

CT Findings
- NECT
  - Single ventricle without septum pellucidum
  - Uncleaved basal nuclei
  - Variable extent of posterior interhemispheric fissure
  - Variable degree of aplasia of midface, nasal cavity, and paranasal sinuses (all derived from neural crest)

MR Findings
- T1WI
  - 3-planar, high definition
  - Evaluates severity: Alobar, semilobar, or lobar HPE
    - Degree of differentiation of single ventricular cavity, presence of dorsal cyst
      - 3rd ventricle identified when thalami are separated
    - Hemispheric cleavage (extent of interhemispheric fissure [IHF], falx) defines anatomic severity
      - Alobar: No fissure
      - Semilobar: Divided temporal lobes around midbrain
      - Lobar: Fissure extends anteriorly to frontal lobes, posterior callosum present
      - All intermediate degrees can be encountered
    - Gyration variably developed, from agyria to well convoluted
    - Variable extent of basal cleavage: Thalami, striatum, hypothalamus
  - Sylvian angle (SA) reflects frontal development, hence severity of HPE as well
    - Superiorly tilted sylvian fissures (↑ SA) = less developed frontal lobes, more severe HPE
- T2WI
  - Same as T1WI
  - In addition, evaluates myelin maturation, optic nerves/globes, olfactory nerves, pituitary
- DWI
  - DTI helps in identifying white matter (WM) tracts
- MRA
  - Azygous anterior cerebral artery (ACA)
    - May present with early fan-like array of branching arteries over surface of single frontal lobe
- MRV
  - Absent venous sinuses correlate falx/tentorium malformations

Ultrasonographic Findings
- Grayscale ultrasound
  - HPE diagnosable on fetal ultrasound and MR
- Color Doppler
  - Abnormal arterial and venous pattern

Angiographic Findings
- Azygous ACA

Imaging Recommendations
- Best imaging tool
  - MR
- Protocol advice
  - Multiplanar MR imaging with special attention to midline

DIFFERENTIAL DIAGNOSIS

Syntelencephaly or Middle Interhemispheric Variant (MIH) of HPE
- Single ventricular cavity: No septum pellucidum, no fornix, no 3rd ventricular roof
- Azygous ACA
- Noncleavage of anterior-inferior basal ganglia (BG)
- Interhemispheric cortical continuity usually in posterior frontal-parietal area
- Anterior &/or posterior corpus callosum found

Absent Septum Pellucidum
- False single ventricular cavity and paired ACA
- Septo-optic dysplasia (fornices fused but present)
- Schizencephaly (hemispheric clefts, fornices present)

Torn Septum Pellucidum
- Severe, usually congenital hydrocephalus
- Typically macrocephalic (HPE usually microcephalic), fornices present

PATHOLOGY

General Features
- Etiology

- Cytogenetic abnormalities in 25-50%: Trisomy 13, 18q-, 18p-, 3p, 7-, trisomy 9, 1q15q, 11q12-q13 (*DHCR7* gene mutation = Smith-Lemli-Opitz)

- Genetics
  - 12 genomic regions spread over 11 chromosomes may contain HPE candidate genes (HPE 1-12)
    - Classic HPE
      - Sonic hedgehog *SHH* (7q36), *SIX3* (2p21), *TGIF1* (18p11.3) all ⇒ ventrodorsal gradient ⇒ non-cleavage anterobasal midline, disorganized neocortex (anterior)
      - *SHH* also controls neural crest (midface) and oligodendrocytic (myelination) development
    - Middle interhemispheric (MIH) variant: *ZIC2* (13q32) ⇒ dorsoventral gradient, dorsal midline
  - In addition: Environmental/maternal factors: Diabetes (1% HPE in diabetic mothers), alcohol, retinoid acid, plant alkaloids (*Veratrum californicum*)
- Associated abnormalities
  - HPE mostly sporadic, sometimes familial, 25% syndromic
  - 80% of facial anomalies; correlate with severity of HPE
    - Cyclopia, proboscis; single nare; single nasal bone/absent internasal suture
    - Midline cleft lip or palate; premaxillary agenesis
    - Single maxillary central incisor; absent superior lingual frenulum

Staging, Grading, & Classification

- Class 1 HPE spectrum: All ranges of decreasing severity may be found in same pedigree
  - Alobar
    - No lateral separation of hemispheres, single prosencephalic vesicle/ventricle, midface essentially absent, cyclopia, no olfactory nerves
  - Semilobar
    - Temporal lobe separated
  - Lobar
    - Single frontal lobe, callosal splenium present, small or normal olfactory nerves
  - Midfacial abnormalities without overt brain malformation
    - Flat face, maxillary hypoplasia, midline cleft lip/palate, hypotelorism
  - Isolated single maxillary central incisor (SMCI)
    - Often associated with, but not always an indicator of, HPE
- Class 2 syntelencephaly, or MIH variant of HPE
  - Posterior frontal-parietal cortical continuity across midline; both callosal genu and splenium often present

Gross Pathologic & Surgical Features

- Variable hypoplasia of cortex, variable gyral development
- Variable degree of separation of diencephalon and BG with incorporation into upper brainstem
- Dorsal cyst represents posteriorly located tela choroidea of single ventricle

CLINICAL ISSUES

Presentation

- Most common signs/symptoms
  - Facial malformation (hypotelorism +++)
  - Seizures (50%) and developmental delays
  - Hypothalamic/pituitary malfunction (75%, mostly diabetes insipidus), poor body temperature regulation
  - Dystonia and hypotonia: Severity correlates with degree of BG nonseparation
- Clinical profile
  - Mentally retarded microcephalic infant with hypotelorism

Demographics

- Age
  - Presentation in infancy or early childhood
    - Can be diagnosed with fetal US or MR
- Gender
  - M:F = 1.4:1
- Epidemiology
  - 1.3/10,000 live births, but 1 in 250 conceptuses

Natural History & Prognosis

- Over represented in fetal demise, stillbirths
- Clinical severity and life expectancy relate to degree of hemispheric and deep gray nuclei nonseparation (alobar HPE = worst)

Treatment

- Treat seizures and endocrine dysfunction

DIAGNOSTIC CHECKLIST

Consider

- Whenever HPE in doubt, look at basal forebrain for cleavage failure

Image Interpretation Pearls

- Not all cases of missing septum pellucidum are single ventricles

SELECTED REFERENCES

1. Fernandes M et al: The ups and downs of holoprosencephaly: dorsal versus ventral patterning forces. Clin Genet. 73(5):413-23, 2008
2. Richieri-Costa A et al: Single maxillary central incisor, holoprosencephaly, and holoprosencephaly-like phenotype. Am J Med Genet A. 140(23):2594-7, 2006
3. Hayashi M et al: Neuropathological evaluation of the diencephalon, basal ganglia and upper brainstem in alobar holoprosencephaly. Acta Neuropathol. 107(3):190-6, 2004
4. Barkovich AJ et al: Analysis of the cerebral cortex in holoprosencephaly with attention to the sylvian fissures. AJNR Am J Neuroradiol. 23(1):143-50, 2002
5. Blaas HG et al: Brains and faces in holoprosencephaly: pre- and postnatal description of 30 cases. Ultrasound Obstet Gynecol. 19(1):24-38, 2002
6. Plawner LL et al: Neuroanatomy of holoprosencephaly as predictor of function: beyond the face predicting the brain. Neurology. 59(7):1058-66, 2002
7. Simon EM et al: The middle interhemispheric variant of holoprosencephaly. AJNR Am J Neuroradiol. 23(1):151-6, 2002

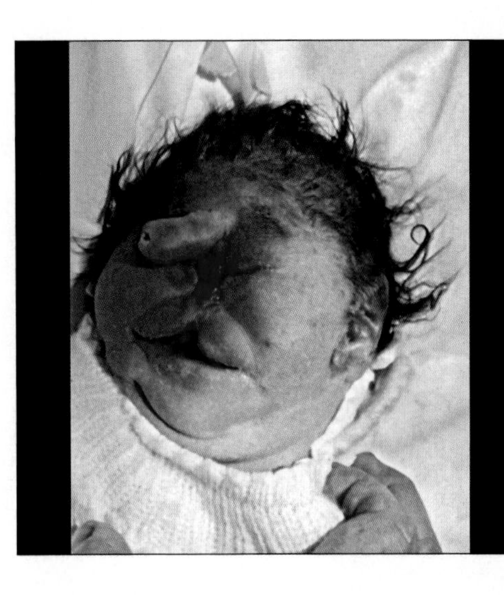

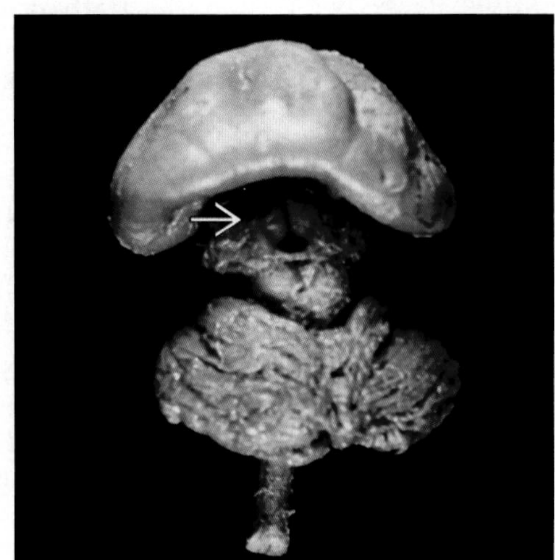

(Left) *Clinical photograph of a neonate with midfacial aplasia, midline orbital fusion, proboscis with single primordium of nare and midline cleft lip. Note also microcephaly and malformed outer ear.* ***(Right)*** *Gross pathology demonstrates the pancake-like single forebrain vesicle of alobar HPE. The dorsal cyst was removed to obtain a direct view of the basal diencephalic region with thalamic fusion →. The cerebral cortex is lissencephalic with hardly any appearance of sulcation.*

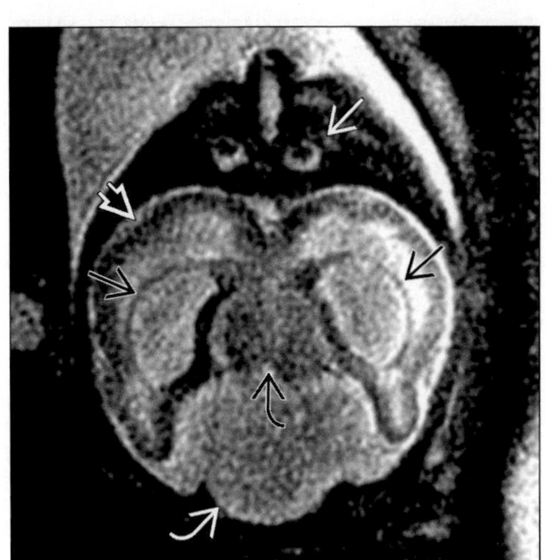

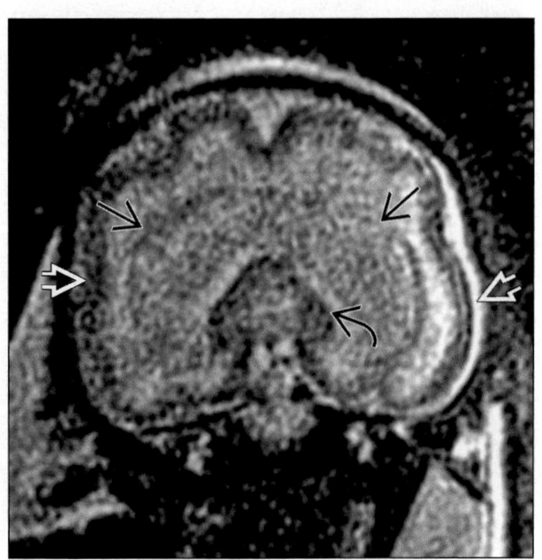

(Left) *Axial T2WI MR in a 35-week fetus shows the striking hypotelorism with microphthalmic globes →. The surface of the brain has a smooth appearance → for fetal age of 35 weeks. Note also the dorsal cyst →, nonseparated thalami →, and large ventricular cavity →.* ***(Right)*** *Coronal T2WI MR of the same fetus shows the single ventricular cavity → surrounding a small round ball → of deep gray nuclei. Note also the nearly agyric cortex → and the absence of IHF.*

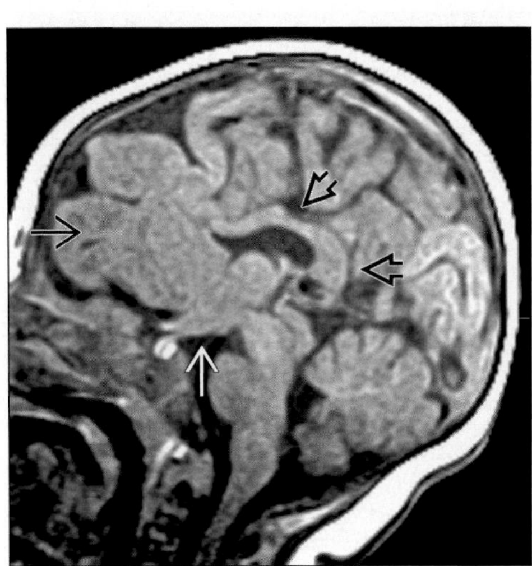

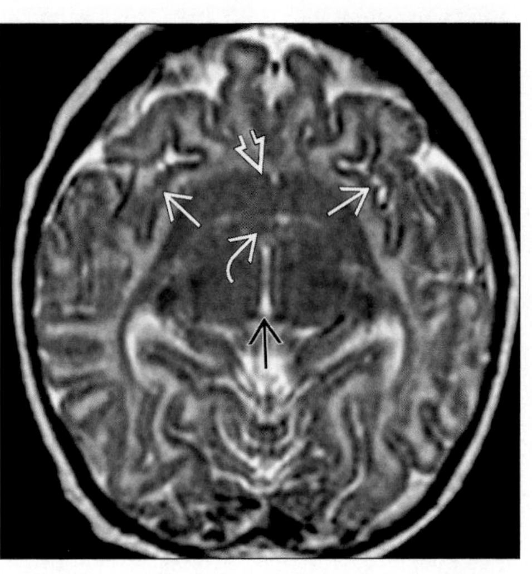

(Left) *Sagittal T1WI MR in 7 week old shows small, dysmorphic anterobasal frontal lobes → with no true callosal genu. Sulcation and callosal structures → are more normal posteriorly between the posterior frontal, parietal, and occipital lobes →. Note the anterior 3rd ventricle obliterated by the undivided hypothalamus →.* ***(Right)*** *Axial T2WI MR shows striatal → and hypothalamic → fusion, but separate thalami →. Frontal lobes are small, sylvian fissures → located anteromedially.*

HOLOPROSENCEPHALY VARIANTS

Key Facts

Terminology
- Solitary median maxillary central incisor (SMMCI)
- Middle interhemispheric variant of holoprosencephaly (MIH) (syntelencephaly)
- SMMCI: 1 of several microforms of autosomal dominant holoprosencephaly (HPE)

Imaging
- MIH: Interhemispheric fusion of posterior frontal/parietal lobes + normal separation of frontal/occipital poles
- SMMCI: Findings range from isolated dental abnormality to alobar HPE
  - Up to 90% have congenital nasal atresia/stenosis

Top Differential Diagnoses
- Hypodontia: Congenital absence of teeth
- Mesiodens: Supernumerary tooth
- Classic holoprosencephaly

Pathology
- MIH: Linked to *ZIC2* mutation at 13q32
- *SHH* and *TGIF* mutations identified in SMMCI

Clinical Issues
- SMMCI: 1:50,000; MIH: Rare
- SMMCI prognosis: Determined by CNS involvement; isolated SMMCI or other microforms, good to excellent
- Clinical profile MIH most similar to lobar HPE

Diagnostic Checklist
- SMMCI: Inspect nose for nasal stenosis
- SMMCI can be microform HPE, and further MR evaluation of brain should be performed

(Left) Axial NECT 3D reconstruction shows hypotelorism and an unerupted solitary median maxillary central incisor (SMMCI) ➔. (Right) Axial NECT in the same patient shows the precise midline location of the SMMCI ➔. In addition to the prominent mid-palatal ridge ➔, the hard palate appears transversely narrow and V-shaped. Although some cases of SMMCI are isolated, many are microforms of holoprosencephaly, and further evaluation with brain MR should be performed.

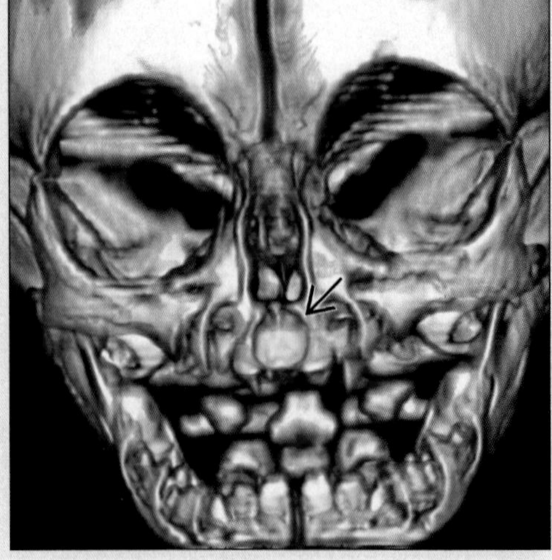

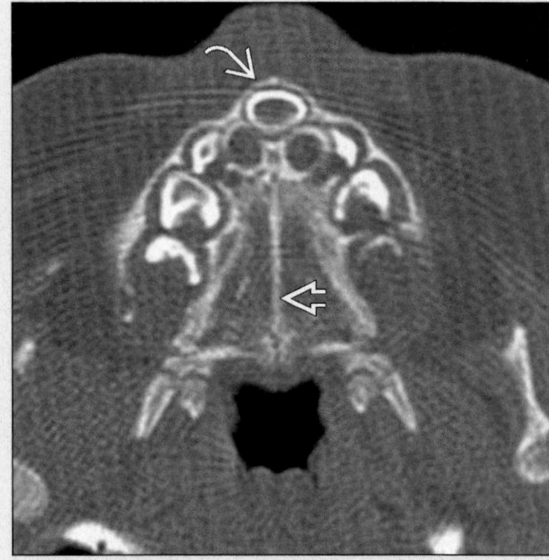

(Left) Coronal NECT performed in a newborn for nasal obstruction shows the solitary median maxillary central incisor (SMMCI) ➔. The brain was normal. (Right) Axial NECT in the same patient shows pyriform aperture stenosis ➔ causing nasal obstruction. Up to 90% of patients with SMMCI have nasal obstruction 2° to choanal atresia, mid-nasal stenosis, or pyriform aperture stenosis and are thus identified in the newborn period. Approximately 60% of patients with pyriform aperture stenosis have SMMCI.

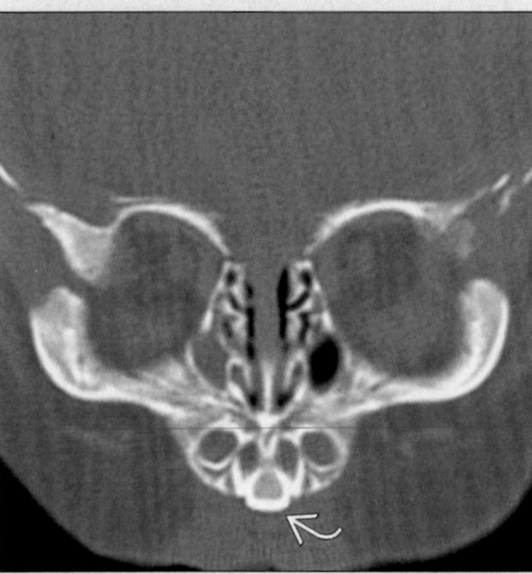

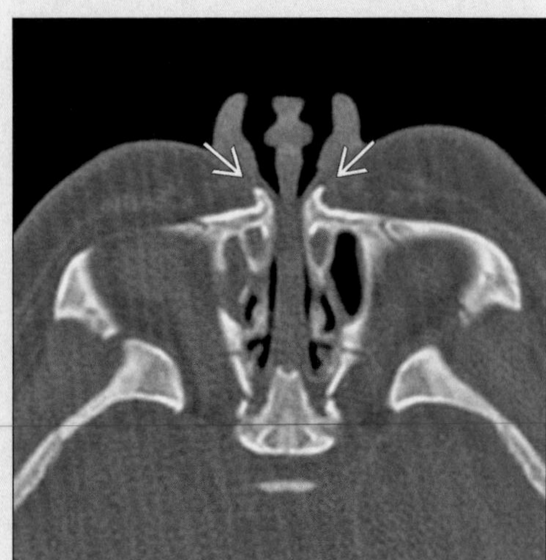

HOLOPROSENCEPHALY VARIANTS

TERMINOLOGY

Abbreviations

- Solitary median maxillary central incisor (SMMCI)
- Middle interhemispheric variant of holoprosencephaly (MIH)

Synonyms

- Syntelencephaly

Definitions

- SMMCI: 1 of several microforms of autosomal dominant holoprosencephaly (HPE)
- MIH: HPE variant characterized by dorsal telencephalic fusion

IMAGING

General Features

- Best diagnostic clue
  - SMMCI: Single, midline central maxillary incisor
  - MIH: Midline continuity of posterior frontal/parietal lobes + normal separation of frontal/occipital poles
- Location
  - SMMCI: Midline, superior alveolar ridge
  - MIH: Posterior frontal and parietal lobes
- Size
  - SMMCI: Equivalent to normal central incisor
- Morphology
  - SMMCI: Symmetric crown
- MIH
  - Features distinguishing MIH from classic HPE
    - Continuity of posterior frontal and parietal lobes across midline
    - Normal separation of frontal poles with present anterior interhemispheric fissure (IHF)/falx
    - Callosal (CC) dysgenesis characterized by presence of genu and splenium with absent body
    - Normal separation of hypothalamus, basal ganglia
  - Frequent features of MIH
    - Continuity of sylvian fissures across midline
    - Incomplete thalamic separation (33%)
    - Cortical dysplasia/heterotopia
  - Occasional features of MIH
    - Cerebellar abnormalities (20%): Cerebellar hypoplasia, Chiari 1 and 2, cephalocele
  - Features in common with classic HPE
    - Absent septum pellucidum
    - Azygous anterior cerebral artery

CT Findings

- NECT
  - SMMCI
    - Single, midline central maxillary incisor
    - Midpalatal vomerine ridge
    - V-shaped palate
    - Up to 90% have choanal atresia, midnasal stenosis, or pyriform aperture stenosis
  - MIH
    - Interhemispheric isodense band of brain ± sylvian fissure (SF)
- CTA
  - MIH
    - Azygous anterior cerebral artery
    - Middle cerebral artery branches identified in abnormal SF

MR Findings

- T1WI
  - SMMCI
    - Findings range from isolated dental abnormality to alobar HPE
    - Frequent microcephaly, hypotelorism
    - Occasional pituitary/stalk hypoplasia
  - MIH
    - Fused posterior frontal, parietal lobes isointense to brain on all pulse sequences; ± SF fusion
    - Frequent heterotopia/cortical dysplasia along fusion
    - Normal myelin maturation (in contrast to classic HPE)
    - Dysgenetic CC (genu > splenium present, absent body)
- T2WI
  - MIH: 25% hyperintense dorsal cyst
    - Occurs with thalamic noncleavage ⇒ obstructs 3rd ventricle
- MRA
  - MIH
    - Azygous anterior cerebral artery
    - Middle cerebral artery branches identified in abnormal SF

Prenatal US/MR

- MIH can be identified in 2nd trimester
- SMMCI can be identified on prenatal MR

Imaging Recommendations

- Best imaging tool
  - SMMCI: Maxillofacial CT
  - MIH: MR with multiplanar 3D T1 gradient echo sequence
- Protocol advice: Follow-up brain MR for SMMCI

DIFFERENTIAL DIAGNOSIS

Hypodontia

- Congenital absence of teeth
- 2nd premolars, 3rd molars, and maxillary lateral incisors most commonly affected

Mesiodens

- Supernumerary permanent tooth between central maxillary incisors
- Conical, slightly off midline

Classic Holoprosencephaly

- Failure of basal forebrain structures to cleave
- Severity of malformation related to degree of anterior brain development
  - Alobar (least differentiated): Absent IHF, falx, and CC with pancake-like mass of brain
  - Semilobar: IHF/falx formed posteriorly; splenium CC present; fused caudate heads
  - Lobar (most differentiated): IHF/falx extend anteriorly; genu CC aplastic/hypoplastic; minimal frontal lobe fusion

HOLOPROSENCEPHALY VARIANTS

PATHOLOGY

General Features

- Etiology
  - Theory for SMMCI: Lack of midline cell division and lateral growth of dental lamina by day 35-38 gestation → fusion of left and right dental lamina into single midline incisor
  - MIH: Impaired expression of roof plate properties by week 3-4 gestation alters mitosis/apoptosis → faulty IHF formation and fusion of cerebral hemispheres
- Genetics
  - SMMCI: Microform of autosomal dominant HPE (ADHPE); fewer reported sporadic cases
    - Most common genetic mutations ADHPE: SHH 7q36, ZIC2 13g32, SIX3 2p21, TGIF 18p11.3
    - *SHH* and *TGIF* mutations identified in SMMCI
    - Variable expression of ADHPE accounts for wide range of phenotypes (alobar HPE → microforms)
    - 70% penetrance of ADHPE ⇒ risk of SMMCI or other microform in offspring obligate carrier = 13-14%
    - Risk of severe (semilobar/alobar) HPE in offspring obligate carrier ADHPE = 16-21%
  - Mutations of SMMCI not associated with HPE: 22q11 deletion, ring chr 18, 47XXX
  - MIH: Linked to *ZIC2* mutation at 13q32
    - In mice, ZIC2 plays role in differentiation of embryonic roof plate; mutations cause neural tube defects, HPE
    - In contrast to other genes linked to classic HPE, *ZIC2* is not involved in ventral patterning of neuraxis ⇒ accounts for lack of severe midline facial dysmorphisms in MIH
- Associated abnormalities
  - SMMCI: VACTERL, CHARGE, velocardiofacial syndrome, ectodermal dysplasia, Duane syndrome, cardiac anomalies (25%), vertebral anomalies
  - MIH: Report of 5 patients with *ZIC2* mutations with limb, renal, and genital anomalies

Gross Pathologic & Surgical Features

- MIH: IHF present in frontal, occipital poles; hemispheric fusion of posterior frontal and parietal lobes; fused SF
- MIH: Foci of undifferentiated cortex, subependymal gray matter heterotopia

Microscopic Features

- MIH: Callosal fibers identified anteriorly, posteriorly

CLINICAL ISSUES

Presentation

- Most common signs/symptoms
  - SMMCI
    - Neonatal nasal obstruction (choanal atresia, midnasal stenosis, or pyriform aperture stenosis)
    - Eruption deciduous SMMCI at 7-8 months; absent upper labial frenulum
  - MIH
    - Spasticity, hypotonia, seizures, developmental delay
- Other signs/symptoms
  - SMMCI
    - Short stature (50%), hypotelorism, microcephaly
      - 33% short stature 2° to ↓ growth hormone
    - Other microforms of ADHPE: Cleft lip, mid-face hypoplasia, microcephaly, coloboma, choanal atresia, midnasal stenosis, pyriform aperture stenosis, developmental delay, learning difficulties
    - SMMCI with severe HPE (alobar) uncommon
  - MIH
    - Mild facial dysmorphisms frequent: Hypertelorism, cleft lip/palate, SMMCI
    - Severe facial dysmorphisms (as with classic HPE) do not occur
    - Endocrine disorders uncommon
- Clinical profile
  - SMMCI
    - Infant with SMMCI, short stature, hypotelorism
    - Isolated SMMCI in mother and offspring with classic HPE
  - MIH
    - Infant/young child with spasticity

Demographics

- Age
  - SMMCI: Eruption of deciduous incisor at 7-8 months
- Gender
  - Isolated SMMCI more common in females
- Epidemiology
  - SMMCI: 1:50,000
  - MIH: Rare

Natural History & Prognosis

- Prognosis
  - SMMCI: Determined by CNS involvement; isolated SMMCI or other microforms, good to excellent
  - MIH: Mild/moderate psychomotor delay, seizures
    - Clinical profile of MIH most similar to lobar HPE

Treatment

- SMMCI: No treatment for isolated dental abnormality
  - Hormone replacement, corrective surgery for other microforms of ADHPE
- MIH: Antiepileptics

DIAGNOSTIC CHECKLIST

Image Interpretation Pearls

- SMMCI: Inspect nose for nasal stenosis

Reporting Tips

- SMMCI can be microform HPE and further MR evaluation of brain should be performed

SELECTED REFERENCES

1. Atalar MH et al: holoprosencephaly associated with bilateral perisylvian polymicrogyria. Pediatr Int. 50(2):241-4, 2008

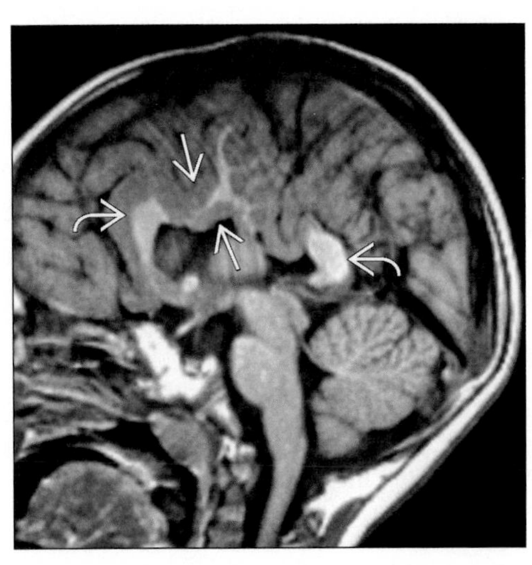

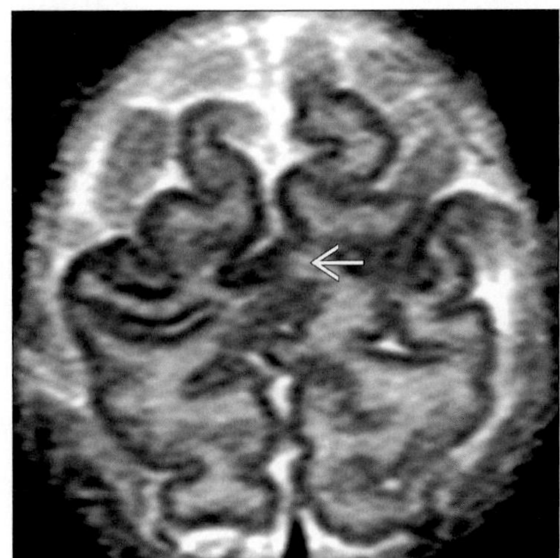

(Left) *Sagittal T1WI MR shows middle interhemispheric variant (MIH) of holoprosencephaly (HPE). GM & WM are continuous across midline at the posterior frontal/parietal lobe levels. Heterotopia/ cortical dysplasia cross the midline ➔. In contrast to classic HPE, the callosal body is absent with present genu & splenium ➔. The pituitary/ hypothalamus are usually normal in MIH.* ***(Right)*** *Axial T2WI MR in a patient with MIH shows posterior frontal/ parietal continuity across the midline ➔.*

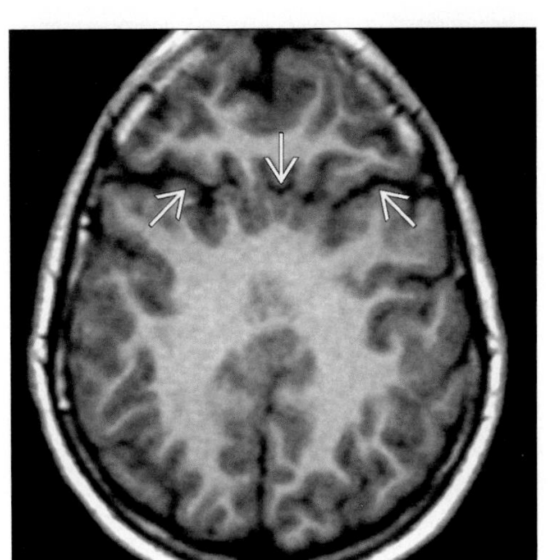

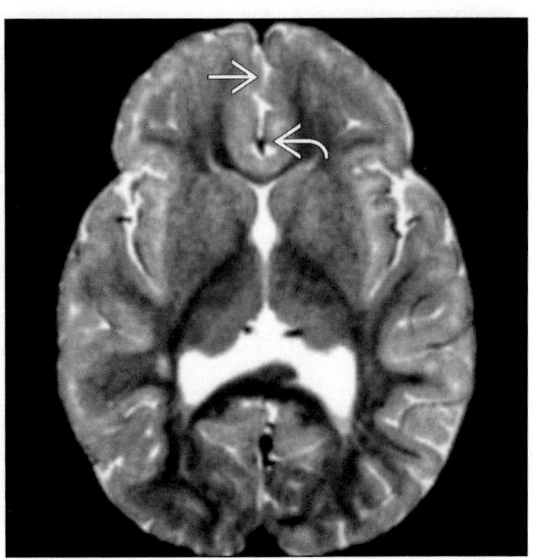

(Left) *Axial T1WI MR shows continuity of frontal white matter & sylvian fissures ➔ across the midline. Sylvian fissure continuity is an inconstant finding but fairly specific for MIH when present.* ***(Right)*** *Axial T2WI FS MR shows absent septum pellucidum and an azygous anterior cerebral artery ➔ as seen in classic HPE. In contrast to classic HPE, the anterior interhemispheric fissure ➔ & falx are formed and the basal ganglia are separated. Incomplete thalamic separation occurs in 33% of patients.*

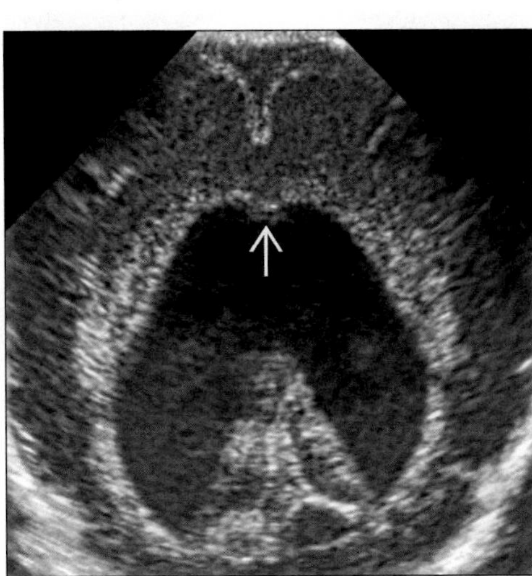

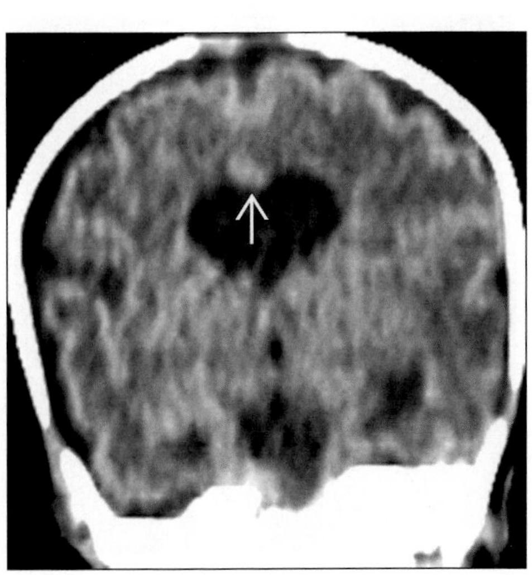

(Left) *Cranial ultrasound in a premature newborn with MIH nicely demonstrates abnormal continuity of the cerebral hemispheres across midline at the mid cranial level. Note the gray matter nodule ➔ in the midline.* ***(Right)*** *Coronal reconstruction from axial NECT in the same patient confirms MIH. In the location of the posterior frontal and parietal lobes, there is continuity of gray and white matter across the midline. Characteristic of MIH is the gray matter nodule in the midline ➔.*

SYNTELENCEPHALY (MIDDLE INTERHEMISPHERIC VARIANT)

Key Facts

Terminology

- Syntelencephaly; middle interhemispheric variant of holoprosencephaly (MIHV)

Imaging

- Single ventricular cavity (100%)
- Fused dorsal mid-hemispheric cortex (100%) (by definition)
- Azygous anterior cerebral artery (ACA) (100%)
- Abnormal sylvian fissure (SF) spans both hemispheres (86%)
- Heterotopia, cortical malformations (86%)
- Dysgenetic corpus callosum (CC)
- Bilateral perisylvian polymicrogyria (PMG)

Top Differential Diagnoses

- Classic holoprosencephaly
- Septooptic dysplasia
- Bilateral schizencephaly

Pathology

- High occurrence of syntelencephaly (as well as other forms of HPE) has been observed in babies born from diabetic mothers
- *ZIC2* mutation at 13q32 is observed in 5-6% of patients

Clinical Issues

- Spasticity (86%), hypotonia (57%), dystonia (50%), seizures (40%), developmental delay (common)
- Mild facial dysmorphisms frequent: Hypertelorism, cleft lip/palate

Diagnostic Checklist

- Look at ventricle
- Look at bridging cortex lining upper surface of pseudo-corpus callosum

*(**Left**) Axial graphic depicts classic findings of syntelencephaly, with an anomalous coronal fissure ⇨ and both gray matter (GM) and white matter (WM) bridges → crossing the interhemispheric fissure in several locations. The gray matter in the cortical bridges appears thickened and dysplastic. (**Right**) Axial T1WI MR shows white and gray matter crossing the interhemispheric fissure in the midline →, creating several interhemispheric cortical bridges.*

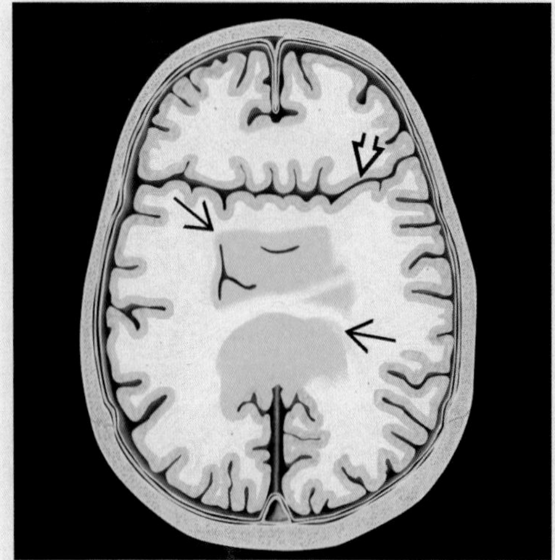

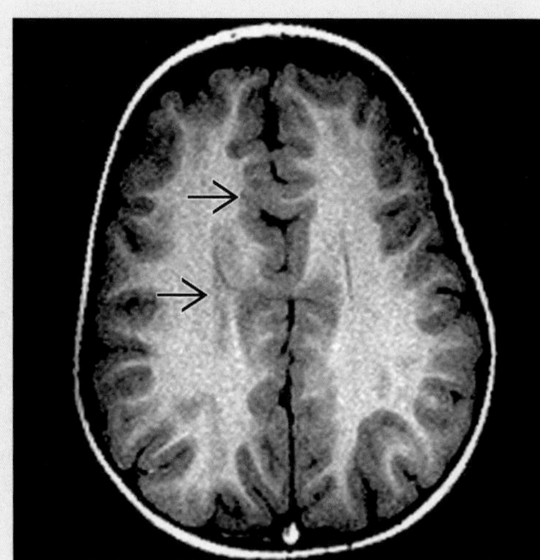

*(**Left**) Sagittal T1WI MR shows posterior frontal interhemispheric fusion. Note well-developed callosal splenium →/posterior body, azygous ACA ➔, heterotopic GM bulging into the ventricle under the interhemispheric fusion ➔. (**Right**) Coronal T1WI MR in the same case shows thick layer of cortex ⇨ crossing the interhemispheric fissure; some GM ➔ protrudes into the ventricular lumen. Note the parasagittal bright T1 signal bundle of WM ⇨ on each side, which may represent misdirected callosal fibers.*

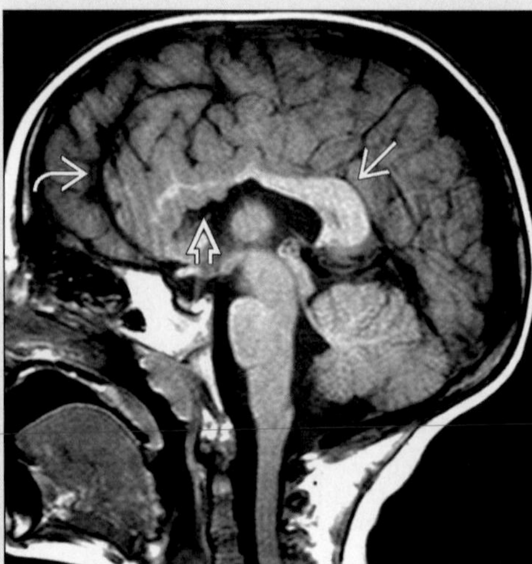

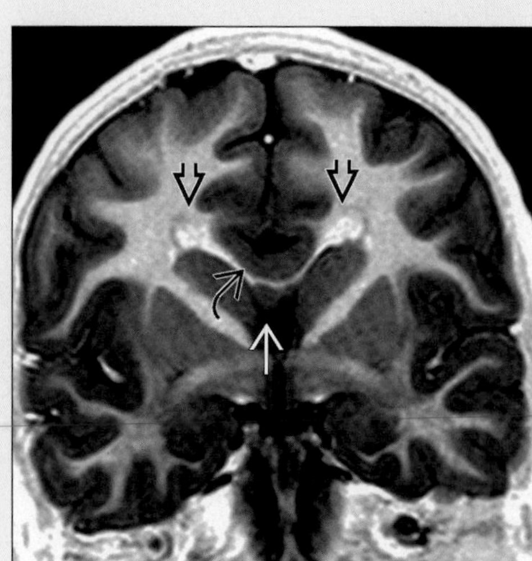

SYNTELENCEPHALY (MIDDLE INTERHEMISPHERIC VARIANT)

TERMINOLOGY

Synonyms

- Syntelencephaly
- Middle interhemispheric variant (MIHV) of holoprosencephaly

Definitions

- Variant of holoprosencephaly (HPE) characterized by lack of separation of midportion of hemispheres

IMAGING

General Features

- Best diagnostic clue
  - Midline continuity of posterior frontal/parietal cortex with normal separation of frontal/occipital poles
  - Single ventricular cavity
- Location
  - Midline
- Size
  - Typically normocephalic
- Morphology
  - Noncleavage of dorsal aspect of cerebral hemispheres, usually posterior frontal lobes
  - Single ventricular cavity
  - Single (azygous) anterior cerebral artery (ACA)
  - Mostly normal ventral hemispheres, basal ganglia, and hypothalamus

CT Findings

- Axial view: Absent septum pellucidum
- Sagittal reformats: Segmented corpus callosum (typically, only genu and splenium present)
- Coronal reformats: Cortical bridge between midportion of hemispheres
- Bone algorithms of facial bones: Cleft lip, cleft palate, hypertelorism
  - Never hypotelorism (unlike true HPE)

MR Findings

- T1WI
  - Hemispheres
    - Fused dorsal mid-hemispheric cortex (100%) (by definition)
    - Single ventricular cavity (100%)
    - Single abnormal sylvian fissure (SF) spans both hemispheres dorsally (86%)
    - Heterotopia, cortical malformations (86%)
      - Thick cortex lining anterior interhemispheric fissure
      - Heterotopic gray matter nodules often situated on top of lateral ventricle bodies
    - Dysgenetic corpus callosum (CC)
      - Genu and splenium only (61%)
      - Genu or splenium (22%)
      - Genu, splenium, and some of body (20%)
    - Olfactory sulci normal (57%), olfactory bulbs (64%)
    - Hippocampi poorly developed
  - Deep gray matter
    - Lentiform nuclei normal, anterobasal caudate fused (11%)
    - Hypothalamus usually normal
    - Thalami fused (33%)
  - Midbrain
    - Incomplete segmentation diencephalon-mesencephalon (18%)
  - Posterior fossa
    - Chiari malformation, cerebellar hypoplasia possible
  - Meninges
    - Dorsal cyst (25%), may require CSF diversion
    - Rarely, cephaloceles overlying unseparated portion of hemispheres
  - Others
    - No endocrinopathy (unlike HPE)
    - Normal thermoregulation (unlike HPE)
- T2WI
  - Brain morphology
    - Similar to T1WI
  - Brain maturation
    - Myelination is normal, in keeping with patient age (unlike in classic HPE)
- MRA
  - Azygous anterior cerebral artery (ACA) (100%)

Imaging Recommendations

- Best imaging tool
  - MR
- Protocol advice
  - Multisequence triplanar
  - T1-weighted IR, MPRAGE/SPGR provide exquisite gray/white contrast
  - DTI may help in understanding white matter organization

Ultrasonographic Findings

- Grayscale ultrasound
  - Absent septum pellucidum
  - Absence of middle portion of interhemispheric fissure
- Color Doppler
  - Azygous anterior cerebral artery

DIFFERENTIAL DIAGNOSIS

Classic Holoprosencephaly

- Single hemisphere and ventricle
- Failure of cleavage
  - Hypothalamus
  - Basal ganglia
  - Prefrontal cerebrum

Septooptic Dysplasia

- Absent/incomplete septum pellucidum
- Well-separated cerebral hemispheres
- Well-separated basal ganglia and thalami
- Normal corpus callosum
- Bilateral ACA

Bilateral Schizencephaly

- Clefts communicate with ventricles
- Well-separated cerebral hemispheres

SYNTELENCEPHALY (MIDDLE INTERHEMISPHERIC VARIANT)

- Bilateral ACA

Bilateral Perisylvian Polymicrogyria (PMG)
- Well-divided hemispheres and ventricles
- Bilateral ACA

PATHOLOGY

General Features
- Etiology
  - Mitosis/apoptosis of embryonic roof plate form interhemispheric fissure (IHF) after neural tube closure (fetal weeks 3-4)
    - Impaired expression of roof plate properties alters mitosis and apoptosis → faulty dorsal IHF formation, poor cleavage of cerebral hemispheres
  - High occurrence of syntelencephaly (as well as other forms of HPE) has been observed in babies born from diabetic mothers
- Genetics
  - Presumably linked to dorsal induction genes
    - Genes linked to classic HPE (e.g., sonic hedgehog [*SHH*]) affect ventral induction mostly
      - May explain importance of facial defects in classic HPE
    - By contrast, dorsal induction disorder is predominant in syntelencephaly
      - May explain lack of severe midline facial dysmorphisms
      - Presumably induction of neural crest that forms midfacial skeleton proceeds normally
    - *ZIC2* mutation at 13q32 is observed in 5-6% of patients
      - Involved in differentiation of embryonic roof plate
- Associated abnormalities
  - Hypertelorism
  - Cleft lips, palate

Staging, Grading, & Classification
- Classic spectrum of HPEs from alobar to lobar
- Syntelencephaly considered milder end of spectrum
  - Clinically severe, however, although less than complete HPE

Gross Pathologic & Surgical Features
- IHF present at frontal, occipital poles
  - Hemispheric fusion posterior frontal and parietal lobes
- Lentiform nuclei normal, caudate fused
- Thalami fused in 1/3
- Hypothalamus not fused

CLINICAL ISSUES

Presentation
- Most common signs/symptoms
  - Developmental disorders
    - Spasticity (86%)
    - Hypotonia (57%)
    - Dystonia (50%)
    - Seizures (40%)
    - Developmental delay (speech, etc.) (100%)
- Other signs/symptoms
  - Mild facial dysmorphisms frequent
    - Hypertelorism
    - Cleft lip/palate
- Clinical profile
  - Developmental delay
  - Spasticity
  - Seizures

Demographics
- Age
  - Presents in infancy

Natural History & Prognosis
- Static course

Treatment
- Rehabilitation

DIAGNOSTIC CHECKLIST

Image Interpretation Pearls
- Look at ventricle
- Look at bridging cortex lining upper surface of pseudo-corpus callosum

SELECTED REFERENCES

1. Dheen ST et al: Recent studies on neural tube defects in embryos of diabetic pregnancy: an overview. Curr Med Chem. 16(18):2345-54, 2009
2. Dubourg C et al: Holoprosencephaly. Orphanet J Rare Dis. 2:8, 2007
3. Cheng X et al: Central roles of the roof plate in telencephalic development and holoprosencephaly. J Neurosci. 26(29):7640-9, 2006
4. Picone O et al: Prenatal diagnosis of a possible new middle interhemispheric variant of holoprosencephaly using sonographic and magnetic resonance imaging. Ultrasound Obstet Gynecol. 28(2):229-31, 2006
5. Hahn JS et al: Endocrine disorders associated with holoprosencephaly. J Pediatr Endocrinol Metab. 18(10):935-41, 2005
6. Biancheri R et al: Middle interhemispheric variant of holoprosencephaly: a very mild clinical case. Neurology. 63(11):2194-6, 2004
7. Lewis AJ et al: Middle interhemispheric variant of holoprosencephaly: a distinct cliniconeuroradiologic subtype. Neurology. 59(12): 1860-5, 2002
8. Marcorelles P et al: Unusual variant of holoprosencephaly in monosomy 13q. Pediatr Dev Pathol. 5(2):170-8, 2002
9. Simon EM et al: The middle interhemispheric variant of holoprosencephaly. AJNR Am J Neuroradiol. 23(1): 151-6, 2002
10. Robin NH et al: Syntelencephaly in an infant of a diabetic mother. Am J Med Genet. 66(4):433-7, 1996
11. Barkovich AJ et al: Middle interhemispheric fusion: an unusual variant of holoprosencephaly. AJNR Am J Neuroradiol. 14(2):431-40, 1993

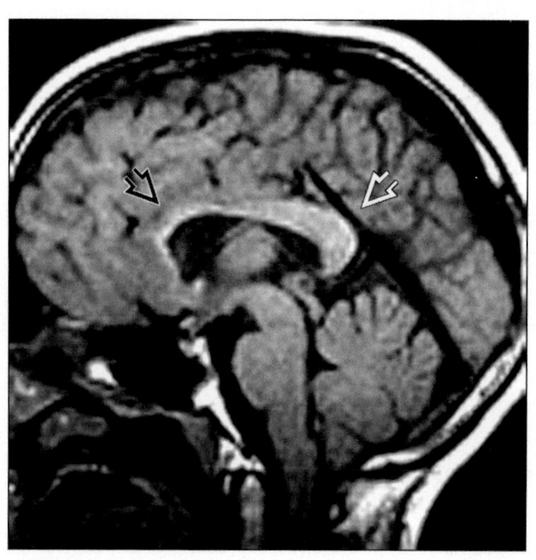

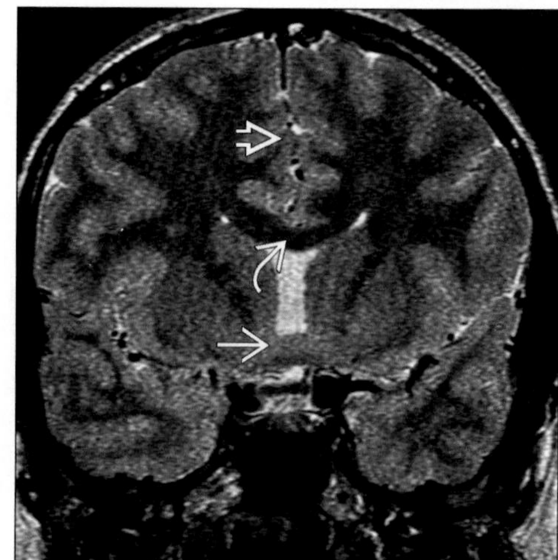

(Left) *Sagittal T1WI MR in a patient with frontal interhemispheric fusion. The posterior CC is well developed ➡, but the anterior portion is attenuated ➡.* ***(Right)*** *Coronal thin section T2WI MR shows a continuous bridge of cortex ➡ anteriorly between the frontal lobes, with an interhemispheric fissure ➡ present dorsally. A single ventricular cavity is present, without a septum pellucidum or forniceal columns. Note fusion of the anterobasal caudate (nucleus accumbens) ➡.*

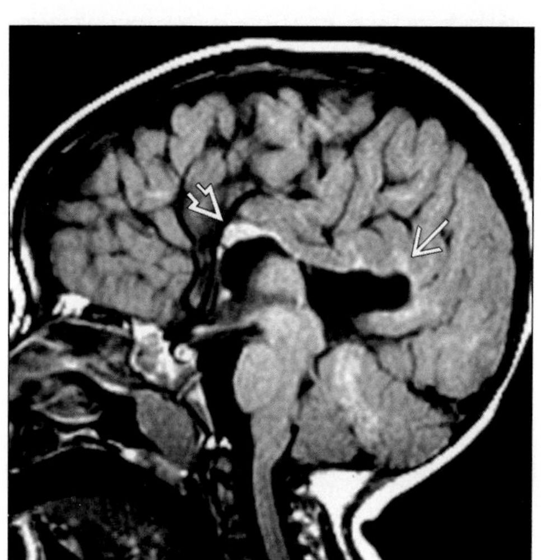

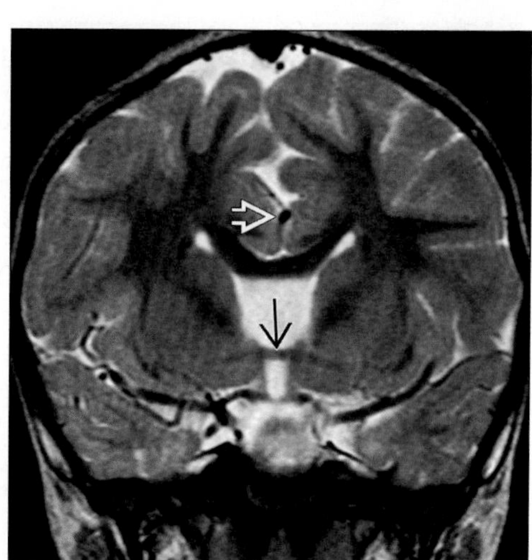

(Left) *Sagittal T1WI MR shows a patient with a more posterior hemispheric fusion. No frank callosal splenium can be seen, although some white matter fibers ➡ appear to be crossing the midline just above the lateral ventricles. The genu is present ➡, although hypoplastic.* ***(Right)*** *Coronal T2WI MR shows clearly separate frontal lobes with azygous ACA ➡. No septum pellucidum can be identified. The anterior commissure ➡ appears normal. The hypothalamus is well divided above the chiasm.*

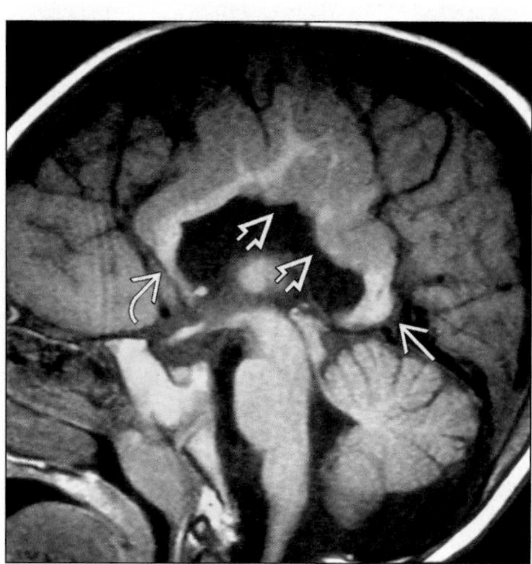

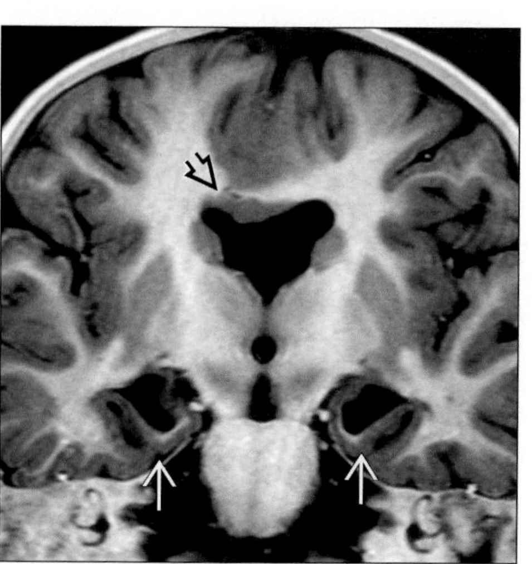

(Left) *Sagittal T1WI MR shows middle hemispheric fusion. The splenium ➡ and rostrum ➡ are well delineated. In the area of interhemispheric continuity, gray matter encroaches on the ventricular lumen ➡. Interhemispheric fissure was normal in the anterior frontal and the parietooccipital areas.* ***(Right)*** *Coronal T1WI MR shows a single ventricular cavity and interhemispheric cortical continuity. Note the heterotopic gray matter on the ventricular roof ➡ & the poorly developed hippocampi ➡.*

CENTRAL INCISOR SYNDROME/SOLITARY MEDIAN MAXILLARY CENTRAL INCISOR

Key Facts

Terminology
- Solitary median maxillary central incisor (SMMCI) syndrome

Imaging
- Triangular-shaped palate with solitary maxillary incisor tooth
- Look for stenosis of pyriform aperture or choanal atresia
- Consider MR imaging to evaluate brain for midline anomalies

Top Differential Diagnoses
- Congenital nasal pyriform aperture stenosis (CNPAS)
  - Solitary central incisor in 60%
- Choanal atresia
  - Most common congenital abnormality of nasal cavity

Pathology
- ~ 1:50,000 live births
- Presence of solitary incisor can be considered predictor or risk factor for HPE or gene carrier status
- Associated with mutations in human sonic hedgehog gene
- Also seen with 18p mutations

Clinical Issues
- Difficulty feeding
  - Nasal passage stenosis hampers breathing when infant feeds

Diagnostic Checklist
- Look for SMMCI, CNPAS, or choanal atresia when imaging neonates with feeding/breathing difficulties
- Be sure to check for findings of HPE

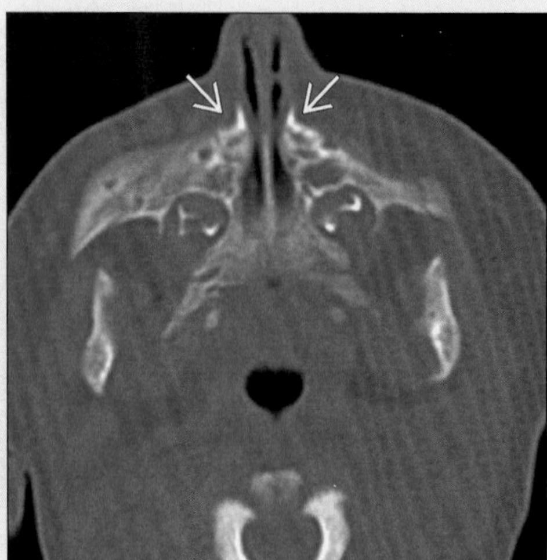

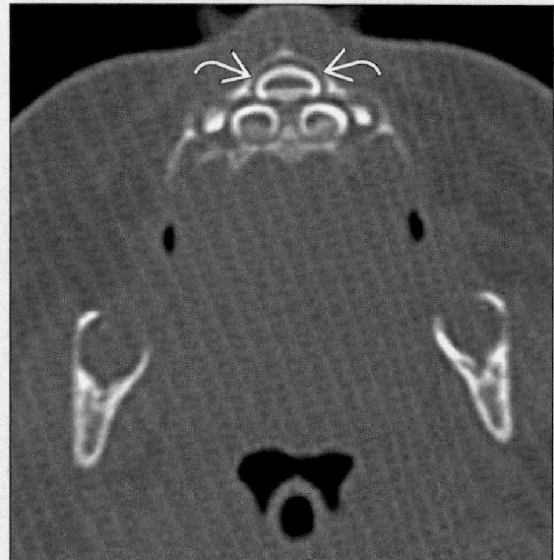

(Left) *Axial NECT shows bilateral and symmetric stenosis of the pyriform aperture of the nose ➡. More than 60% of children with pyriform aperture stenosis have an associated solitary central maxillary incisor.* ***(Right)*** *Axial NECT through the anterior-inferior maxilla of the same patient shows the solitary unerupted central incisor ➡. In the infant with unerupted milk teeth, the clinical findings of SMMCI can be quite subtle.*

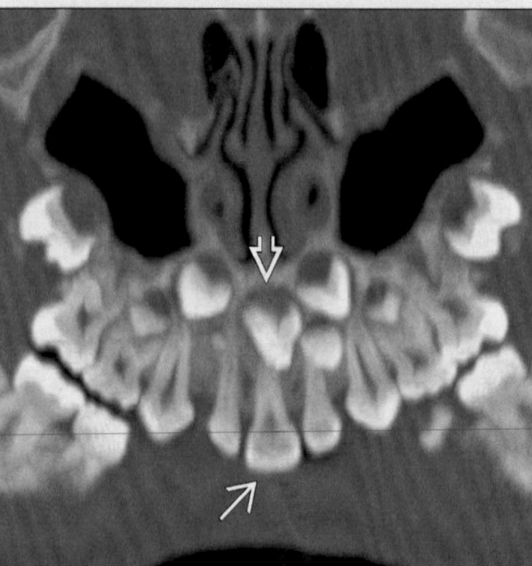

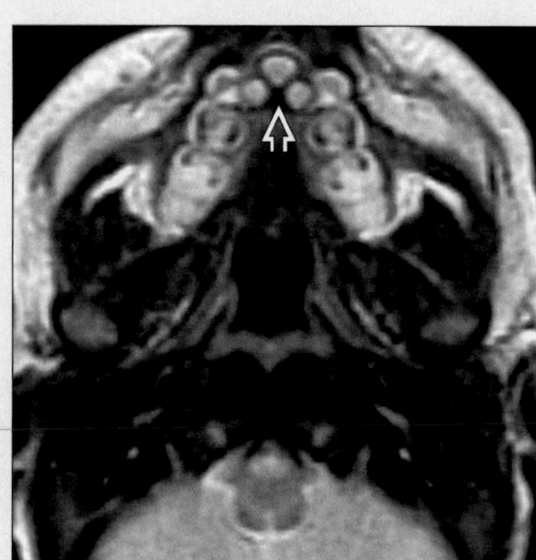

(Left) *Bone CT with curved reformatting along the maxillary alveolar ridge in the same patient shows the solitary central incisor ➡ and the unerupted permanent solitary central incisor superior to it ➡.* ***(Right)*** *Axial T2WI MR through the hard palate in a neonate with pyriform aperture stenosis shows the solitary central incisor ➡. When pyriform aperture stenosis is found or the palate has an abnormal triangular shape, look for a single central incisor.*

CENTRAL INCISOR SYNDROME/SOLITARY MEDIAN MAXILLARY CENTRAL INCISOR

TERMINOLOGY

Abbreviations

- Solitary median maxillary central incisor (SMMCI) syndrome

Synonyms

- Solitary median maxillary central incisor, short stature, choanal atresia/midnasal stenosis syndrome
- Monosuperoincisivodontic dwarfism

IMAGING

General Features

- Best diagnostic clue
  - Triangular-shaped palate with solitary maxillary incisor tooth
- Location
  - Maxilla

CT Findings

- Narrow anterior palate
  - Triangular-shaped
- Single maxillary incisor
  - May be unerupted

MR Findings

- Findings often more confusing on MR
  - Tooth buds appear more crowded
- Prenatal MR diagnosis has been reported

Imaging Recommendations

- Best imaging tool
  - NECT with bone algorithm
- Protocol advice
  - Look for stenosis of pyriform aperture or choanal atresia
  - Consider MR imaging to evaluate brain for midline anomalies

DIFFERENTIAL DIAGNOSIS

Congenital Nasal Pyriform Aperture Stenosis

- Solitary central incisor in 60%

Choanal Atresia

- Most common congenital abnormality of nasal cavity
  - 1:5,000-8,000 births

Mesiodens

- Midline supernumerary tooth

PATHOLOGY

General Features

- Genetics
  - Associated with mutations in human Sonic hedgehog gene and in chromosome 18p
    - Sonic hedgehog mutations are most frequent etiology of holoprosencephaly (HPE)
    - Presence of solitary incisor can be considered predictor or risk factor for HPE or gene carrier status
- Associated abnormalities
  - CHARGE (ocular **c**oloboma, **h**eart defects, choanal **a**tresia, developmental **r**etardation, **g**enital/urinary anomalies, **e**ar abnormalities)
  - VACTERL (**v**ertebral defects, **a**nal atresia, **c**ardiovascular defects, **t**racheo**e**sophageal fistula, **r**adial ray or renal anomalies, **l**imb defects)
  - Velocardiofacial, Duane, Goldenhar, DiGeorge syndromes
  - Clavicle hypoplasia, holoprosencephaly, pituitary insufficiency, microcephaly, oromandibular-limb hypogenesis syndrome type 1, ectodermal dysplasia

Gross Pathologic & Surgical Features

- Absent labial frenulum and incisive papilla
- Absent intermaxillary suture, prominent midpalatal ridge

CLINICAL ISSUES

Presentation

- Most common signs/symptoms
  - Difficulty feeding
    - When associated with pyriform aperture or midnasal stenosis or choanal atresia/stenosis
    - Nasal passage stenosis hampers breathing when infant feeds
    - Clinical mimic of nasolacrimal duct mucocele
- Other signs/symptoms
  - Hypotelorism, microcephaly, hypopituitarism

Demographics

- ~ 1:50,000 live births

Treatment

- Directed toward relief of associated nasal stenosis
  - Surgical enlargement and stenting

DIAGNOSTIC CHECKLIST

Image Interpretation Pearls

- Look for SMMCI, congenital nasal pyriform aperture stenosis, or choanal atresia when imaging neonates with feeding/breathing difficulties
- Be sure to check for findings of HPE

SELECTED REFERENCES

1. Bolan M et al: Solitary median maxillary central incisor. J Dent Child (Chic). 76(1):82-6, 2009
2. El-Jaick KB et al: Single median maxillary central incisor: new data and mutation review. Birth Defects Res A Clin Mol Teratol. 79(8):573-80, 2007
3. Hall RK: Solitary median maxillary central incisor (SMMCI) syndrome. Orphanet J Rare Dis. 1:12, 2006
4. Garavelli L et al: Solitary median maxillary central incisor syndrome: clinical case with a novel mutation of sonic hedgehog. Am J Med Genet A. 127A(1):93-5, 2004

SEPTOOPTIC DYSPLASIA

Key Facts

Terminology

- Septooptic dysplasia (SOD)
- De Morsier syndrome

Imaging

- Absent septum pellucidum, small optic chiasm
- Optic nerves, pituitary gland, septum pellucidum
- Coronal imaging shows
  - Flat-roofed ventricles
  - Downward pointing anterior horns
- 3 orthogonal planes crucial to identify all findings
  - Absent septum pellucidum, flat roof of frontal horns, small optic chiasm

Clinical Issues

- Newborns: Hypoglycemic seizures, apnea, cyanosis, hypotonia, prolonged conjugated jaundice, and (in boys) microphallus
- Abnormal endocrine function (60%): Look for multiple pituitary deficiencies
- Normal endocrine function (40%): Often have schizencephaly, seizures
- Child with short stature, endocrine dysfunction
- Normal or color blindness, visual loss, nystagmus, strabismus
- ± mental retardation, spasticity, microcephaly, anosmia
- 75-90% have brain abnormalities; 45% have pituitary insufficiency
- Bilateral optic nerve hypoplasia (70%)

Diagnostic Checklist

- SOD in small stature pediatric patient with absent septum pellucidum
- Small optic nerves, + ectopic posterior pituitary lobe, + absent septum pellucidum

(Left) Coronal graphic depicts flat-roofed anterior horns and the absence of a midline septum pellucidum. The anterior horns are draped inferiorly around the fornices ➪, and the optic chiasm ➡ is small. (Right) Sagittal T1WI MR shows absent septum pellucidum (note low-lying fornices ➡) and the ectopic posterior lobe of the pituitary gland ➡ at the median eminence. Note that the pituitary gland is small for an adolescent, and the infundibulum is not seen.

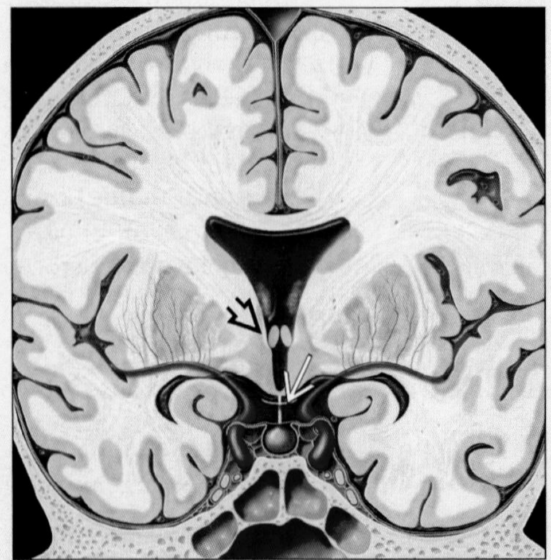

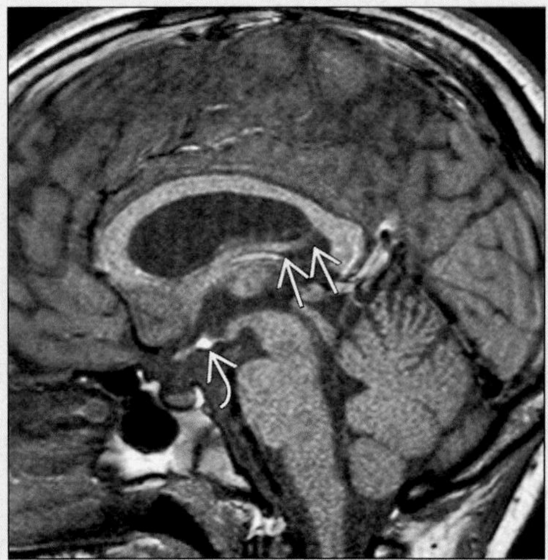

(Left) Coronal T2WI FSE MR shows the absence of septum pellucidum and pointing ➡ of the inferior margins of the frontal horns, draped over fornices. Note that the optic chiasm ➪ is normal in size, as is often the case in septooptic dysplasia. (Right) Coronal T2WI FSE MR in the same patient at the level of the intraorbital optic nerves shows unilateral optic nerve hypoplasia. The right optic nerve ➡ is tiny, running through a small optic nerve sheath. The left optic nerve ➡ is normal.

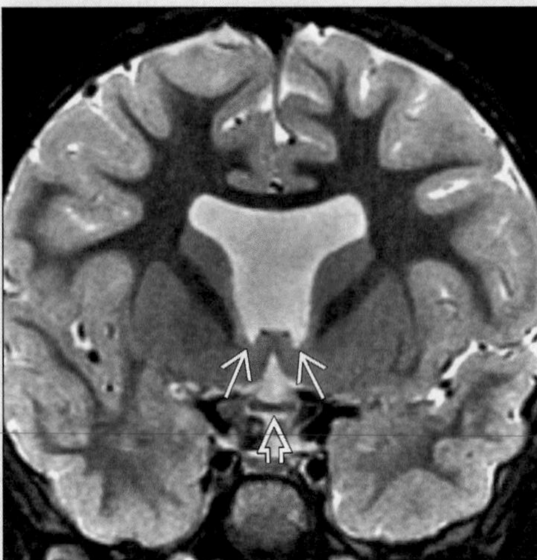

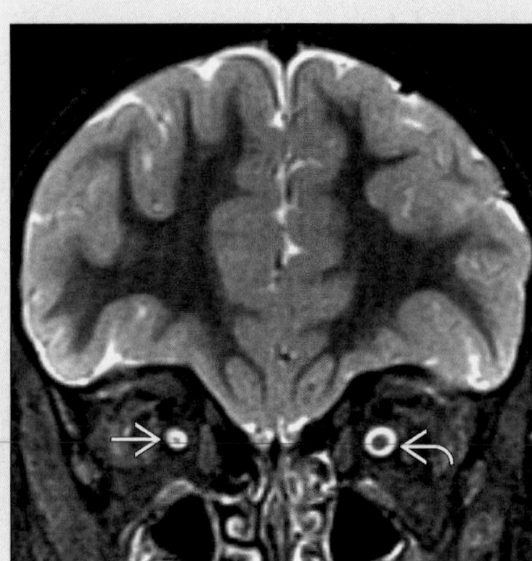

SEPTOOPTIC DYSPLASIA

TERMINOLOGY

Abbreviations

- Septooptic dysplasia (SOD)

Synonyms

- De Morsier syndrome
- Kaplan-Grumbach-Hoyt syndrome
- Suprasellar dysgenesis
- Septooptic-pituitary dysgenesis

Definitions

- Heterogeneous disorder characterized by optic nerve hypoplasia (ONH), absent septum pellucidum, hypothalamic-pituitary dysfunction
  - De Morsier (1956): Described 7 patients with SOD
  - Hoyt (1978): Described association of SOD with hypopituitarism
- Some authors consider SOD and lobar holoprosencephaly to be the same disorder
- SOD plus: Abnormal optic nerves/chiasm, septum pellucidum, pituitary gland, + cortical dysplasias

IMAGING

General Features

- Best diagnostic clue
  - Absent septum pellucidum, small optic chiasm
- Location
  - Optic nerves, pituitary gland, septum pellucidum
- Size
  - Small optic nerves
  - Small pituitary gland with ectopic posterior lobe
  - Absent septum pellucidum
- Morphology
  - Coronal imaging shows
    - Flat-roofed ventricles
    - Downward-pointing anterior horns

CT Findings

- NECT
  - Absent septum pellucidum
  - Large lateral ventricles
  - Small bony optic foramina on axial and coronal imaging

MR Findings

- T1WI
  - 3 orthogonal planes crucial to identify all findings
    - Absent septum pellucidum (remnants may be present)
    - Flat roof of frontal horns, pointed inferior aspect of frontal horns
    - Small optic chiasm/nerves (fat saturation aides visualization of optic nerves)
    - ± thin pituitary stalk
    - Posterior pituitary ectopia
    - Callosal-forniceal continuation or fused midline fornices
    - Thin corpus callosum
    - Vertical hippocampi
    - ± hypoplastic/absent olfactory nerves
    - ± schizencephaly
    - ± heterotopia, polymicrogyria
- T2WI
  - Deficient falx (especially anteriorly) ± hypomyelination
- T1WI C+
  - Enhancement of infundibulum, ectopic posterior pituitary lobe
  - Delayed enhancement of anterior pituitary lobe on dynamic MR

Angiographic Findings

- Conventional

Imaging Recommendations

- Best imaging tool
  - MR
- Protocol advice
  - Coronal, sagittal thin sections through sella/orbits
  - Use fat saturation or CISS/FIESTA to better see optic nerves

DIFFERENTIAL DIAGNOSIS

Syndromes Overlapping with Septooptic Dysplasia

- Optic-infundibular dysplasia, normal septum
- Schizencephaly with absent septum

Kallmann Syndrome

- Absent olfactory nerves
- ± visual, septal, pituitary abnormalities

Holoprosencephaly

- Similar to SOD
  - Many consider it same disorder as SOD

Isolated Ectopic Posterior Pituitary Lobe

- Normal chiasm/nerves, septum pellucidum

PATHOLOGY

General Features

- Etiology
  - Theories
    - Midline heritable defect (mild holoprosencephaly variant)
    - Or secondary degeneration of optic nerve fibers due to cerebral lesion
    - Or vascular disruption (field defect) during brain development
    - Damage to cerebral and optic nerve around 6th week gestation
    - Teratogens: Cytomegalovirus, antiepileptic drugs, alcohol, maternal diabetes
- Genetics
  - Most are sporadic
  - Some are autosomal dominant or recessive
  - Some cases have mutations in *HESX1* gene
    - Homozygous mutations = full syndrome
    - Heterozygous mutations = milder pituitary phenotypes

SEPTOOPTIC DYSPLASIA

- Inactivation of *HESX1* (3p21.2-3p21.2) by Arg53Cys substitution leads to deficient anterior pituitary lobe (does not occur in sporadic SOD)
- Associated abnormalities
  - Frequently associated with other cerebral anomalies
    - Most common = schizencephaly
    - Perisylvian polymicrogyria
    - Midline malformations (callosal dysgenesis, etc.)
    - Ocular anomalies (coloboma, anophthalmia, microphthalmia)
    - Olfactory tract/bulb hypoplasia
    - Incomplete hippocampal rotation
  - Overlapping syndromes with optic, septal, frontal lobe, midline, olfactory deficiencies

Staging, Grading, & Classification

- Isolated optic nerve hypoplasia (ONH): Visual defect only; intelligence and growth normal
- ONH and septal deficiency: Same as isolated
- ONH and septal and pituitary deficiency: May have developmental delay
- Complete septal agenesis: Worse developmental prognosis
- Intrauterine or perinatal insult (especially meningitis) as cause of optic nerve, chiasmatic, and hypothalamic deficiency

Gross Pathologic & Surgical Features

- Small optic chiasm/nerves
- Small or absent geniculate nucleus
- Deficient/absent septum pellucidum
- Forniceal columns (± fused) ⇒ run along roof of 3rd ventricle
- Common: Hypoplasia pituitary, olfactory lobes

Microscopic Features

- Optic nerves, chiasm have sparse or absent myelinated fibers
- Geniculate nucleus (if found): Disorganized layering of small neurons

CLINICAL ISSUES

Presentation

- Most common signs/symptoms
  - Newborns: Hypoglycemic seizures, apnea, cyanosis, hypotonia, prolonged conjugated jaundice, and (in boys) microphallus
  - Abnormal endocrine function (60%): Look for multiple pituitary deficiencies
  - Normal endocrine function (40%): Often have schizencephaly, seizures
- Clinical profile
  - Child with short stature, endocrine dysfunction
  - Normal or color blindness, visual loss, nystagmus, strabismus
  - ± mental retardation, spasticity, microcephaly, anosmia

Demographics

- Age
  - Generally detected in infants
  - More common among younger mothers & 1st born child
- Gender
  - M = F
- Epidemiology
  - 1 in 50,000 worldwide
  - Optic nerve hypoplasia
    - 60% have brain abnormalities (not just schizencephaly); 62-88% have pituitary insufficiency
      - 30% have both
    - 25-50% have absent septum pellucidum
  - Septooptic dysplasia
    - 75-90% have brain abnormalities; 45% have pituitary insufficiency
    - Bilateral optic nerve hypoplasia (70%)

Natural History & Prognosis

- Hypothalamic and pituitary crises; sudden death (hypocortisolism)
- Depends upon severity of associated brain and pituitary malformations

Treatment

- Hormonal replacement therapy

DIAGNOSTIC CHECKLIST

Consider

- SOD in small stature pediatric patient with absent septum pellucidum

Image Interpretation Pearls

- Small optic nerves, + ectopic posterior pituitary lobe, + absent septum pellucidum

SELECTED REFERENCES

1. Volpe P et al: Disorders of prosencephalic development. Prenat Diagn. 29(4):340-354, 2009
2. Borchert M et al: The syndrome of optic nerve hypoplasia. Curr Neurol Neurosci Rep. 8(5):395-403, 2008
3. Hung JH et al: Prenatal diagnosis of schizencephaly with septo-optic dysplasia by ultrasound and magnetic resonance imaging. J Obstet Gynaecol Res. 34(4 Pt 2):674-9, 2008
4. Riedl S et al: Refining clinical phenotypes in septo-optic dysplasia based on MRI findings. Eur J Pediatr. 167(11):1269-76, 2008
5. Camino R et al: Septo-optic dysplasia plus. Lancet Neurol. 2(7):436, 2003
6. Wakeling EL et al: Septo-optic dysplasia, subglottic stenosis and skeletal abnormalities: a case report. Clin Dysmorphol. 12(2):105-7, 2003
7. Antonini SR et al: Cerebral midline developmental anomalies: endocrine, neuroradiographic and ophthalmological features. J Pediatr Endocrinol Metab. 15(9):1525-30, 2002
8. Dattani ML et al: Molecular genetics of septo-optic dysplasia. Horm Res. 53 Suppl 1:26-33, 2000
9. Miller SP et al: Septo-optic dysplasia plus: a spectrum of malformations of cortical development. Neurology. 54(8):1701-3, 2000
10. Barkovich AJ et al: Septo-optic dysplasia: MR imaging. Radiology. 171(1):189-92, 1989

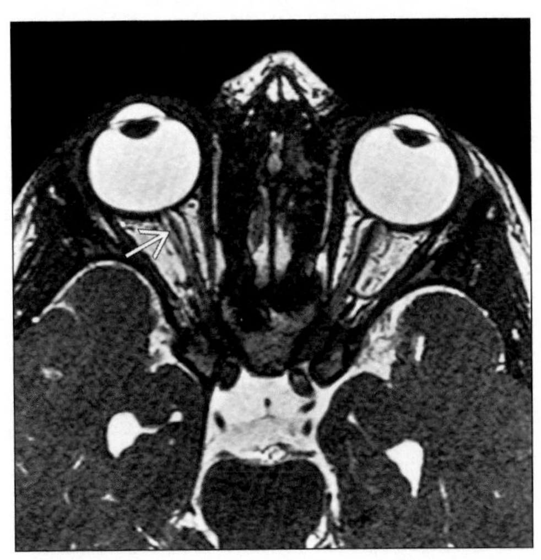

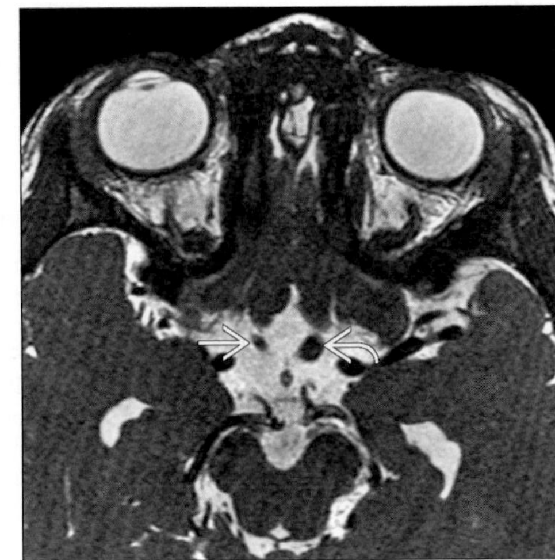

(Left) *Axial steady state acquisition (FIESTA) MR with 1 mm sections shows that the right intraorbital section of the optic nerve ➡ is extremely thin. Steady state magnetization sequences are excellent for assessing the optic nerve, both in the intraorbital and intracranial segments.* ***(Right)*** *Axial steady state acquisition (FIESTA) MR with 1 mm sections in the same patient shows the small intracranial right optic nerve ➡. Compare this with the normal left optic nerve ➡.*

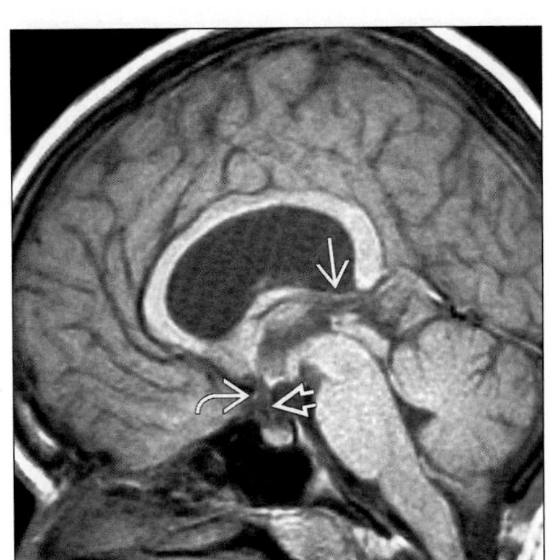

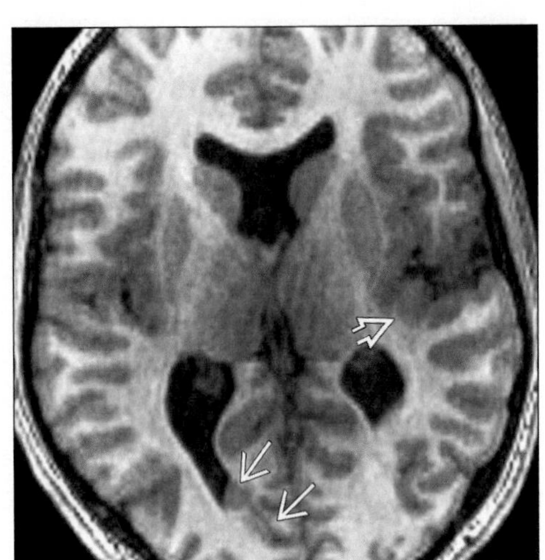

(Left) *Sagittal T1WI MR in a young boy shows stretched corpus callosum and low-lying fornix ➡ to suggest absent septum. The optic chiasm ➡ is tiny, and the pituitary infundibulum ➡ is very attenuated.* ***(Right)*** *Axial T1WI MR in the same patient confirms absent septum pellucidum and brain anomalies, such as left posterior sylvian polymicrogyria ➡ and transmantle column of heterotopic gray matter ➡ extending from the tip of right occipital horn to medial occipital cortex.*

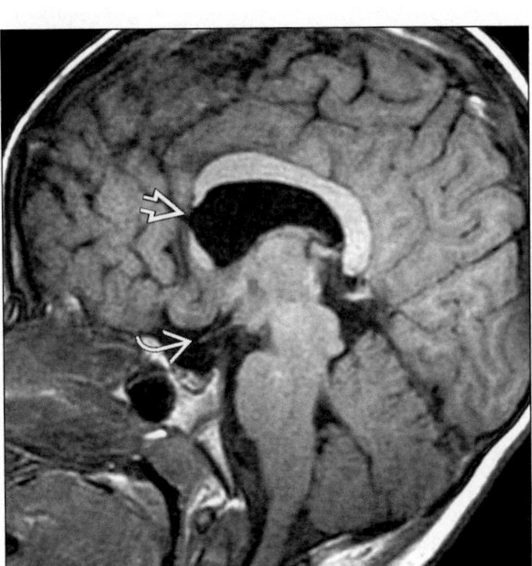

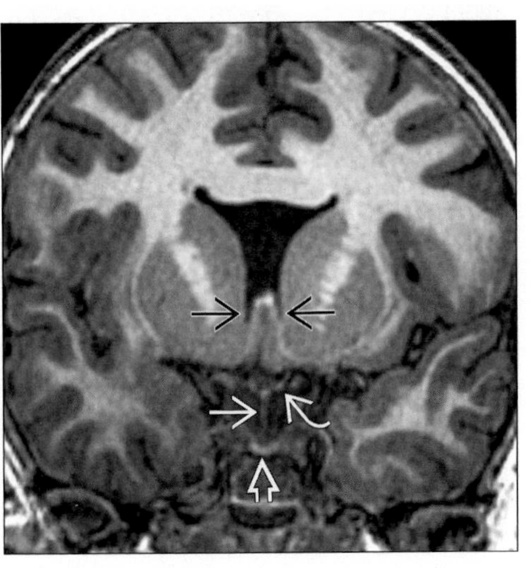

(Left) *Sagittal T1WI MR shows anomalous corpus callosum with discontinuous genu ➡ and an abnormally thick, flat, callosal body. The optic chiasm ➡ is unusually thin, the pituitary infundibulum is not seen, and the anterior lobe of the pituitary gland is too small.* ***(Right)*** *Coronal T1WI MR in the same patient shows tiny optic tracts ➡, infundibulum ➡, and anterior lobe of the pituitary gland ➡. The inferior aspects of frontal horns ➡ are pointed, curving around the fornices.*

MICROCEPHALY

Key Facts

Terminology

- Microcephaly with simplified gyral pattern (MSG)
- Primary (genetic) microcephaly, secondary (nongenetic) microcephaly

Imaging

- Imaging findings dictated by cause of microcephaly
- Consider supplemental use of NECT to detect Ca++
- MR brain: SWI or GRE T2* (blood and Ca++), 3D T1 gradient echo (brain topography), FLAIR for detecting subdurals
- Ca++ in TORCH and pseudo-TORCH syndromes

Top Differential Diagnoses

- Antenatal: Preeclampsia, maternal infection (TORCH), maternal diabetes, fetal alcohol syndrome
- Perinatal: Hypoxic-ischemic encephalopathy (HIE), infection
- Postnatal: Prolonged status epilepticus, HIE, hypoglycemia, meningeo-encephalitis, neurodegenerative, abusive head injury

Pathology

- With every cause, there is reduced growth of brain, ↓ proliferation of glia and neurons
- Simple gyral pattern (oligogyria)

Clinical Issues

- Criteria for diagnosis of microcephaly: Head circumference > 3 SDs below mean for age and sex

Diagnostic Checklist

- If midline anomalies accompany microcephaly, consider fetal alcohol syndrome

(Left) Sagittal T1WI MR demonstrates slanting of the frontal bone ➔ and marked decrease in cranial-to-facial proportions. Note the large occipital cephalocele ➔, which are more common in white populations of Europe and North America and rarely syndrome related. (Right) Axial T2WI MR of a 14-month-old microcephalic child demonstrates bifrontal shallow sulci and simplified gyri ➔. Note the delay in hemispheric myelination ➔, findings characteristic of MSG group 2.

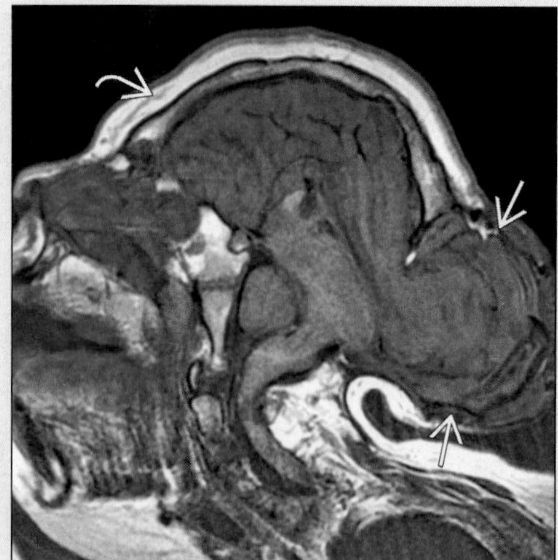

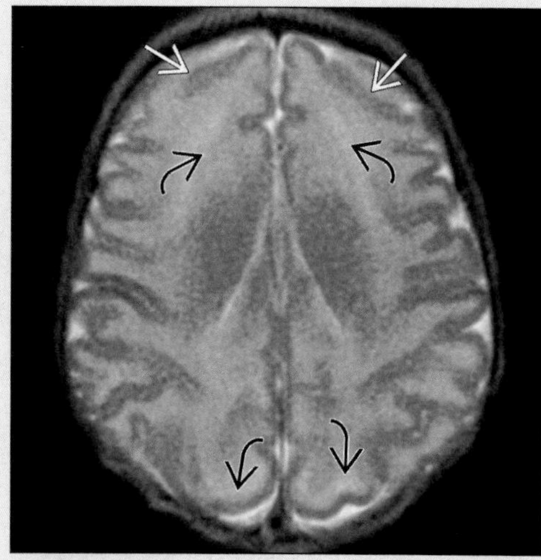

(Left) Coronal T2WI MR of a neonate with MSG group 5 and a head circumference > 3 standard deviations below the mean shows the brain surface is smooth, with reduced white matter volume, and an indistinct appearance of the cortical-white matter junction ➔. (Right) Axial T2WI MR of a microcephalic infant with classical lissencephaly (type 1, LIS1) shows a thick inner band of cortex ➔, cell sparse zone ➔, thin outer cortex, shallow sylvian fissures ➔, and an "hourglass" configuration of the brain.

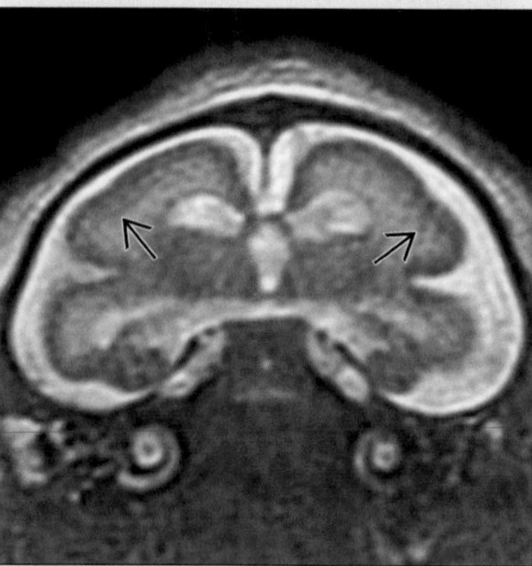

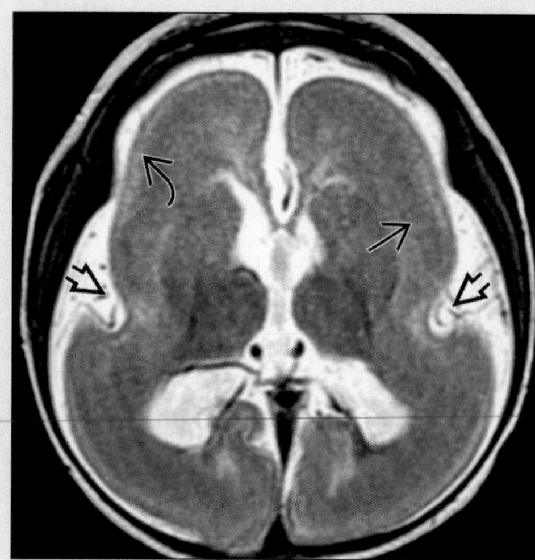

MICROCEPHALY

TERMINOLOGY

Abbreviations

- Microcephaly (MCPH)
  - Primary (genetic) MCPH
  - Secondary (nongenetic) MCPH

Synonyms

- Microcephaly with simplified gyral pattern (MSG)

Definitions

- Primary (genetic): Mendelian inheritance **or** associated with genetic syndrome
  - MSG: Head circumference > 3 standard deviations (SDs) below mean, simplified gyri, shallow sulci
  - Microlissencephaly: Head circumference > 3 SDs below mean, pachy- or agyria
- Secondary (nongenetic): Noxious agent affecting fetal, neonatal, or infant brain growth

IMAGING

General Features

- Best diagnostic clue
  - ↓ craniofacial proportions, suture overlap, simplified gyri, shallow sulci
  - Imaging findings dictated by the cause of microcephaly
  - Microcephaly with simplified gyral pattern (MSG)
    - Group 1: Small, grossly normal brain, simplified gyri, shallow sulci, normal myelination
    - Group 2: Same as group 1 except delayed myelination
    - Group 3: Fewer gyri and sulci than groups 1 and 2, ± heterotopias and arachnoid cysts
    - Group 4: Significant perinatal problems, polyhydramnios, imaging similar to group 1
    - Group 5: Microlissencephaly, profound micrencephaly, smooth brain
- Imaging: Dictated by cause of microcephaly
  - Primary (genetic) microcephaly, MSG (groups 1-5)
    - Small, but grossly normal brain ⇔ gyral simplification, ± myelination delay OR
    - More profound sulcal gyral simplification → lissencephaly
  - Secondary (nongenetic) microcephaly
    - Hypoxic-ischemic encephalopathy (HIE): ± cortical, white matter, or basal ganglia volume loss
    - TORCH infection: Ca++, abnormal white matter, neuronal migration anomalies, germinolytic cysts
    - Abusive head injury: Encephalomalacia, chronic subdurals, ± parenchymal lacerations
- Lateral radiograph, CT scout, or sagittal MR: ↓ craniofacial proportions
  - Normal craniofacial ratios: Preterm (5:1), term (4:1), 2 years (3:1), 3 years (2.5:1), 12 years (2:1), adult (1.5:1)

Radiographic Findings

- Radiography
  - ↓ craniofacial ratio, slanted forehead, closely apposed or overlapping calvarial sutures

CT Findings

- NECT
  - Small cranial vault: Sutures closely apposed, overlapping ± secondary craniosynostosis
  - Ca++ in TORCH and pseudo-TORCH syndromes
  - Cortical surface: Normal ⇔ simplified ⇔ migrational abnormalities ⇔ microlissencephaly

MR Findings

- T1WI
  - Primary (genetic) microcephaly, MSG, or microlissencephaly
    - Small yet normal brain ⇔ simplified gyral pattern (oligogyria) ⇔ microlissencephaly
    - Normal myelination ⇔ hypomyelination ⇔ demyelination
  - Secondary (nongenetic) microcephaly
    - Destructive changes: Encephalomalacia, ± Ca++ TORCH infections, ± subdural collections
- T2WI
  - Primary (genetic) microcephaly, MSG, or microlissencephaly
    - Sulci (1/4-1/2 normal depth), simplified cortex ⇔ pachygyria ⇔ heterotopia ⇔ microlissencephaly
    - White matter maturation: Normal ⇔ hypomyelinated ⇔ demyelinated
    - Possible midline anomalies: Absent corpus callosum, holoprosencephaly
  - Secondary (nongenetic) microcephaly
    - White matter: Gliosis, cavitation, demyelination, diminished volume, ± hypointensity (Ca++)
    - Cortex: Normal ⇔ simplified ⇔ polymicrogyria (TORCH)
    - May see thick calvarium, subdurals from shrinking brain
- PD/intermediate
  - Gliosis (↑ signal) and Ca++ (↓ signal) more common in secondary microcephaly (infection)
- FLAIR
  - Periventricular: Cavitation (↓ signal), gliosis (↑ signal), ± hyperintense chronic subdural collections
- T2* GRE
  - Sequelae to nonaccidental trauma: Hypointensities from hemorrhagic parenchymal shear injury
- DWI
  - T2 shine-through associated with gliosis or demyelination
- MRS
  - ↓ NAA; myoinositol and choline may be ↑ in states of ongoing demyelination and neurodegeneration

Ultrasonographic Findings

- Grayscale ultrasound
  - ± basal ganglia or thalamic Ca++ (TORCH or HIE), ± germinolytic cysts (TORCH)

Imaging Recommendations

- Best imaging tool
  - NECT detects: Ca++ (TORCH, pseudo-TORCH, HIE), encephalomalacia, and subdural collections in abusive head injury
  - MR depicts: Gyral pattern, cortical organization/ migration, myelination, midline anomalies, gliosis, hemorrhage

MICROCEPHALY

- Protocol advice
  - Consider supplemental use of NECT to detect Ca++
  - MR brain: SWI or GRE T2* (blood and Ca++), 3D T1 gradient echo (brain topography), FLAIR for detecting subdurals

DIFFERENTIAL DIAGNOSIS

Secondary (Nongenetic) Microcephaly

- Antenatal
  - Preeclampsia, maternal infection (TORCH), maternal diabetes, fetal alcohol syndrome
- Perinatal
  - Hypoxic-ischemic encephalopathy, infection

PATHOLOGY

General Features

- Etiology
  - From any cause, there is reduced growth of brain, ↓ proliferation of glia and neurons
- Genetics
  - Primary (genetic) microcephaly is typically autosomal recessive (example: Familial form → 1/40,000 births)
  - Syndrome associations
    - MCPH genetic heterogeneity: Mutations *MCPH5* (1q31) most prevalent
    - Down (21-trisomy), Edward (18-trisomy), Cri-du-chat (5p-), Cornelia de Lange, Rubinstein-Taybi

Staging, Grading, & Classification

- MSG groups 1-5
  - MSG 1: Spasticity, normal myelination
  - MSG 2: Seizures, recurrent vomiting, delayed myelination, gastrointestinal disease
  - MSG 3: Seizures, spasticity, heterotopia, cysts
  - MSG 4: Profound neonatal encephalopathy, prenatal brain injury
  - MSG 5: Microlissencephaly

Gross Pathologic & Surgical Features

- Extreme microcephaly (as low as 300 grams, head circumference = 5-10 SDs below mean)
- Simple gyral pattern (oligogyria), short central sulcus, enlarged sulcus parietooccipitalis (simian fissure)
- Island of Reil remains uncovered (incomplete operculization)

Microscopic Features

- *MCPH5*: No evidence of abnormal neuronal migration or architecture
- Other forms may occur with 4 layer cortex (lissencephalic)

CLINICAL ISSUES

Presentation

- Most common signs/symptoms
  - Severe mental retardation, ± seizures, developmental delay
- Criteria for diagnosis of microcephaly: Head circumference > 3 SDs below mean for age and sex

Demographics

- Age
  - Primary (genetic) microcephaly often detected in utero or shortly after birth
  - Secondary (nongenetic) microcephaly usually results from insults within 1st 2 years of life
- Gender
  - Variable based upon type: Primary (autosomal recessive inheritance) vs. secondary (nongenetic)
- Ethnicity
  - Common genetic forms ≈ pan-ethnic; certain syndromic causes of microcephaly may show ethnic preference
- Epidemiology
  - Incidence of microcephaly in general population: 0.06-0.16%
  - Incidence of genetically determined microcephaly: Familial 1/40,000, Down syndrome 1/800

Natural History & Prognosis

- Dictated by cause of microcephaly, variable seizures, mental retardation, and motor handicap

Treatment

- Supportive; genetic testing available for some microcephalic disorders

DIAGNOSTIC CHECKLIST

Consider

- Presence of cerebellar hypoplasia more common in primary microcephaly
- If midline anomalies accompany microcephaly, consider fetal alcohol syndrome

Image Interpretation Pearls

- MR provides most sensitive tool for investigating simplified cortex in microcephaly

SELECTED REFERENCES

1. Berger I: Prenatal microcephaly: can we be more accurate? J Child Neurol. 24(1):97-100, 2009
2. Abdel-Salam GM et al: Microcephaly, malformation of brain development and intracranial calcification in sibs: pseudo-TORCH or a new syndrome. Am J Med Genet A. 146A(22):2929-36, 2008
3. Bond J et al: ASPM is a major determinant of cerebral cortical size. Nat Genet. 32(2):316-20, 2002
4. Jackson AP et al: Identification of microcephalin, a protein implicated in determining the size of the human brain. Am J Hum Genet. 71(1):136-42, 2002
5. Custer DA et al: Neurodevelopmental and neuroimaging correlates in nonsyndromal microcephalic children. J Dev Behav Pediatr. 21(1):12-8, 2000
6. Barkovich AJ et al: Microlissencephaly: a heterogeneous malformation of cortical development. Neuropediatrics. 29(3):113-9, 1998

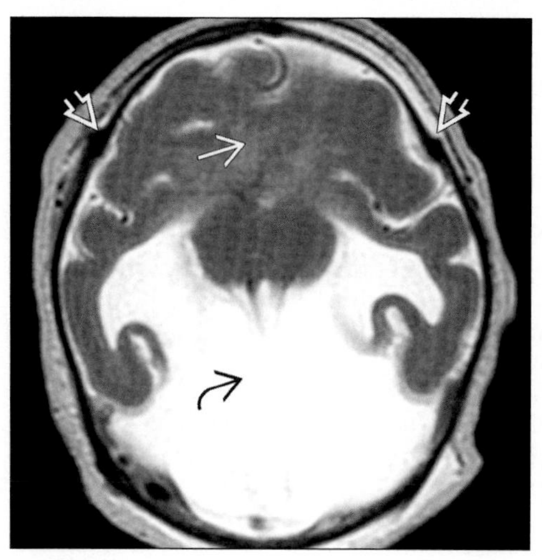

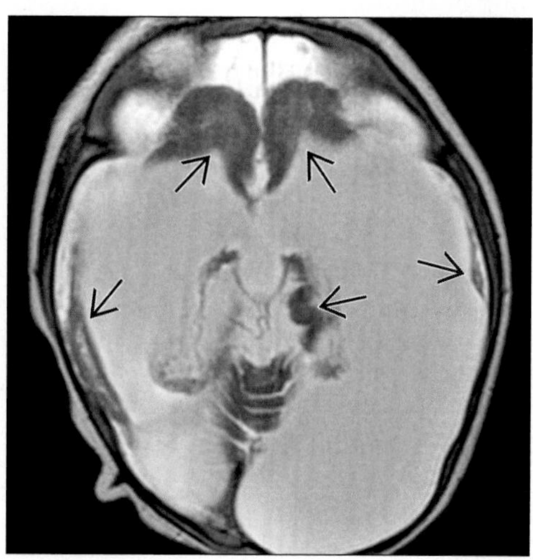

(Left) *Axial T2WI MR of a microcephalic neonate with alobar holoprosencephaly shows fused anterior cerebral tissue* ➔. *The monoventricle is uncovered posteriorly (dorsal cyst)* ➔. *The coronal suture overlap* ➔ *reflects micrencephaly.* ***(Right)*** *Axial T2WI MR in a profoundly microcephalic newborn with hydranencephaly shows that the obliteration of tissue is in the carotid arterial distributions. Note the small residual islands of cerebral tissue* ➔ *from the frontal and temporal lobes.*

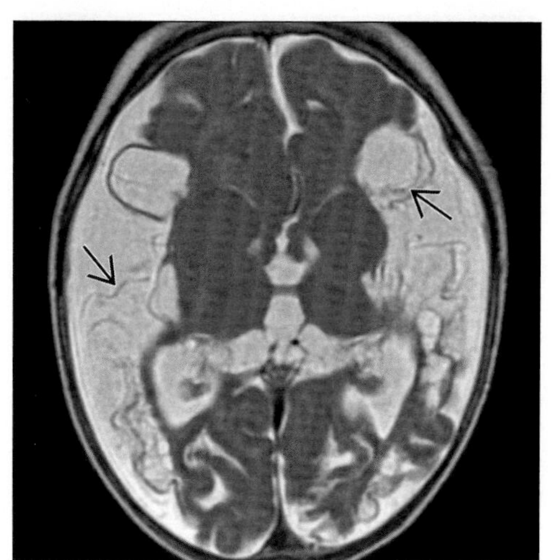

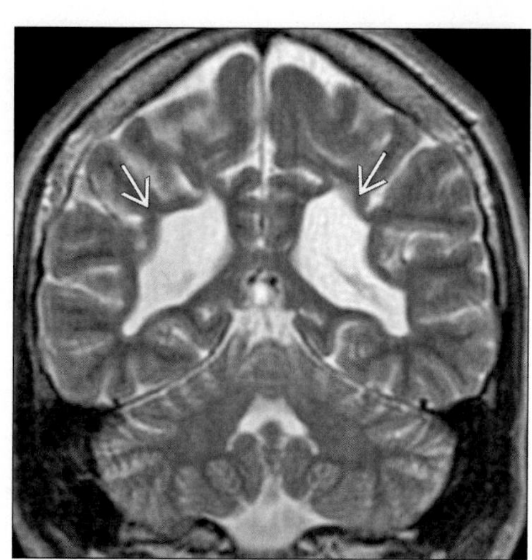

(Left) *Axial T2WI MR in an infant with microcephaly resulting from in utero middle cerebral artery territory infarctions shows extensive hemispheric cystic encephalomalacia* ➔. ***(Right)*** *Coronal T2WI MR in a premature microcephalic infant with a maternal history of chorioamnionitis demonstrates marked reduction of periventricular and deep white matter* ➔. *Axial FLAIR (not shown) revealed findings of periventricular gliosis. These findings reflect a remote perinatal brain injury.*

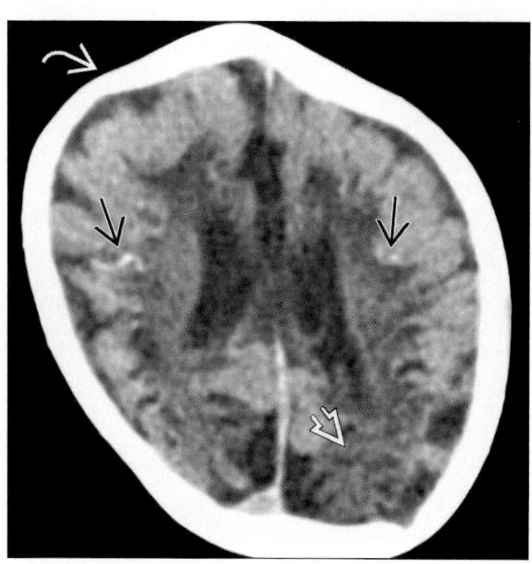

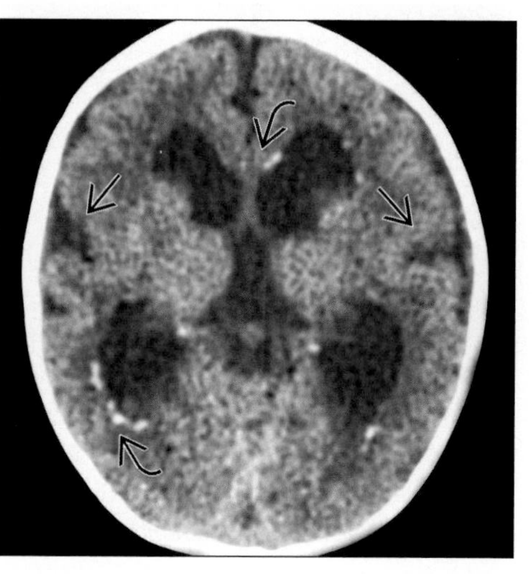

(Left) *Axial NECT in a microcephalic infant, who was the product of a precipitous birth following placental abruption, shows scattered focal subcortical calcifications* ➔, *cerebral cortical atrophy* ➔, *and overlapping of the right coronal suture* ➔, *reflecting micrencephaly.* ***(Right)*** *Axial NECT in a microcephalic infant with a congenital CMV infection shows scattered periventricular calcifications* ➔. *Note the shallow sylvian fissures* ➔ *and associated simplified gyri (polymicrogyria seen on MR).*

CONGENITAL MUSCULAR DYSTROPHY

Key Facts

Terminology

- CMDs = heterogeneous group of autosomal recessive myopathies presenting at birth with hypotonia

Imaging

- Cobblestone brain with myelination defects and Z-shaped brainstem in hypotonic infant
  - Look for enlarged tectum
- Polymicrogyria, abnormal myelin, cysts cerebellum

Pathology

- Mutations in molecules (merosin: Laminin-α2) with roles in cell migration and connection
- Skeletal muscle extracellular matrix protein that binds dystrophin-associated glycoprotein complex utilized in migration of oligodendrocyte precursors
- Autosomal recessive
- CMDs with brain anomalies have hypoglycosylation of α-dystroglycan ⇒ neurons overmigrate through gaps in external lamina; "pebbled" brain surface
- Marked phenotypic overlap amongst Fukuyama CMD, Walker-Warburg, and MEB
- Muscle biopsy: Mild to moderate dystrophic changes, ± inflammatory infiltrate, ± absent staining laminin-α2

Clinical Issues

- Hypotonia, developmental delay, poor vision, seizures
- "Floppy" newborn

Diagnostic Checklist

- Not all Z-shaped brainstems are CMD
- Not all CMD have Z-shaped brainstems (e.g., merosin[-] CMD)

(Left) Reformatted MR surface rendering of microcephalic 10-day-old boy with Walker-Warburg syndrome demonstrates total absence of sulci beyond a shallow sylvian fissure and a bumpy appearance of the surface ("cobblestone" brain). (Right) Sagittal T1WI MR in a macrocephalic neonate shows hydrocephalus (note very enlarged anterior recesses of 3rd ventricle ➔), abnormal kinked brain stem with a very large tectum ➔, small pons, and a very small cerebellum.

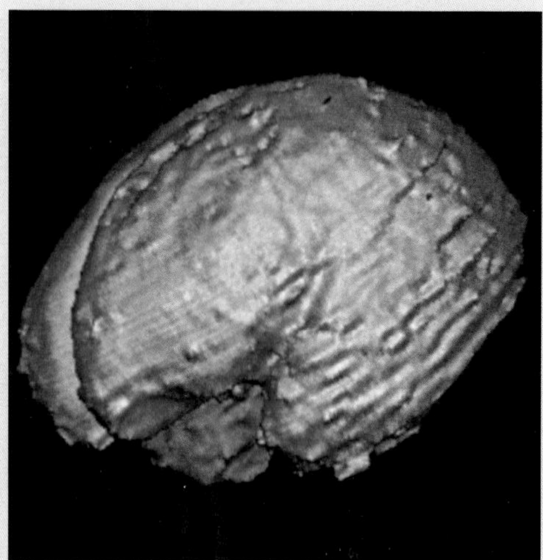

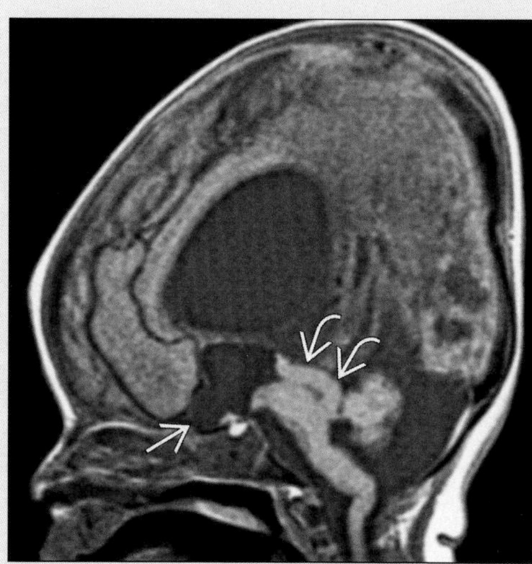

(Left) Axial T2WI MR in the same macrocephalic neonate shows markedly enlarged lateral ventricles with very abnormal sulcation. The cortex is abnormally thick and shows radially oriented collections of neurons extending into the underlying white matter ➔ and separated by strands of white matter. (Right) Coronal T2WI MR in the same patient shows hydrocephalus and thinned white matter, in addition to the "cobblestone" cortex. Note the very small, dysmorphic cerebellar hemispheres.

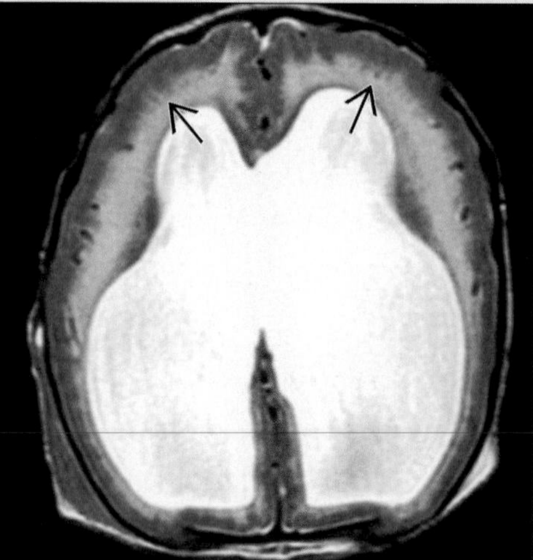

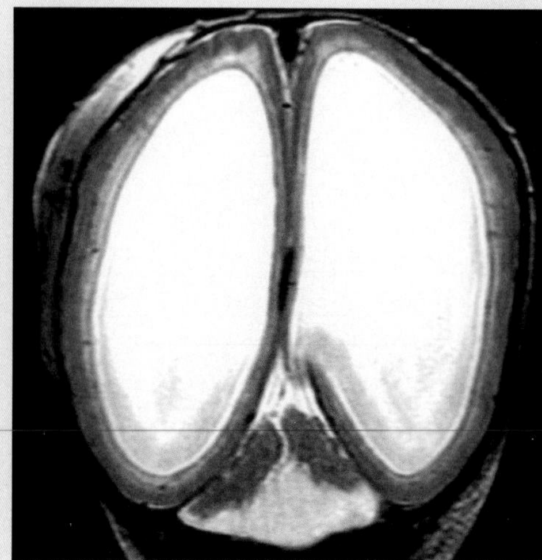

CONGENITAL MUSCULAR DYSTROPHY

TERMINOLOGY

Abbreviations

- Congenital muscular dystrophy (CMD)

Synonyms

- Dystroglycanopathies
- CMD 1: Merosin(+) or merosin(-) CMD
- CMD 2-4: "Cobblestone" lissencephaly (LIS2); CMD with severe CNS malformations

Definitions

- CMDs = heterogeneous group of autosomal recessive myopathies presenting at birth with hypotonia
- CMDs without major brain malformations are either merosin(+) or merosin(-)
  - CMD 1 merosin(+) normal laminin-α2 expression: Normal/very mild imaging findings (cerebellar hypoplasia, nonspecific white matter [WM] changes, focal PMG)
  - CMD 1 merosin(-) deficient laminin-α2 expression: Significant dys-/hypomyelination of WM
- CMD 2-4 with major brain abnormalities (50%) variably associated ("cobblestone" brain, abnormal WM signal, ocular and cerebellar anomalies)
  - CMD 2: Fukuyama CMD (FCMD) least severe
  - CMD 3: Santavuori muscle-eye-brain (MEB) (Finnish type)
  - CMD 4: Walker-Warburg syndrome (WWS) most severe
- Mixed patterns may occur: Merosin(-) CMD with brain malformations

IMAGING

General Features

- Best diagnostic clue
  - "Cobblestone" brain and Z-shaped brainstem in hypotonic infant
- Morphology
  - CMDs with major brain malformations (WWS most severe)
    - "Cobblestone" brain ± ventriculomegaly ± posterior cephalocele
    - Agenesis/hypogenesis of corpus callosum
    - Flat or Z-shaped brainstem or notched pons, hypoplastic vermis

CT Findings

- NECT
  - All imaging findings most severe in WWS
    - Huge ventriculomegaly, shallow or absent sulci
    - ↓ attenuation WM
    - Vermian hypoplasia (Dandy-Walker-like) ± posterior cephalocele

MR Findings

- T1WI
  - Thin, dysplastic, polymicrogyric (PMG) or "pebbled" hemispheric cortex, ± ventriculomegaly
  - ± callosal, septal, or vermian hypogenesis
  - Flat, deeply clefted, notched, Z-shaped brainstem with large tectum
- T2WI
  - PMG, abnormal myelin, cysts cerebellum
    - CMD merosin(-): Dysmyelination centrum semiovale ≤ subcortical WM
    - FCMD, MEB: WM abnormalities in 50%
    - WWS: Severe WM hypomyelination

Imaging Recommendations

- Best imaging tool
  - MR
- Protocol advice
  - Multiplanar, multisequence for white matter, brainstem, and cerebellar changes

DIFFERENTIAL DIAGNOSIS

Multiple Disorders with Brainstem Clefting

- Joubert (mesencephalon and vermian hypoplasia); midline clefting syndromes

Horizontal Gaze Palsy Associated with Progressive Scoliosis (HGPS): Chr 11q23

- Also: Brainstem hypoplasia/clefting, mild cerebellar atrophy

CEDNIK Syndrome

- Mutation of *SNAP29* on 22q11.2

PATHOLOGY

General Features

- Etiology
  - Mutations in molecules (merosin: Laminin-α2)) with roles in cell migration and connection
    - Skeletal muscle extracellular matrix protein that binds dystrophin-associated glycoprotein complex utilized in migration of oligodendrocyte precursors
- Genetics
  - Autosomal recessive
  - CMD 1 merosin(+): Genetic defect(s) unknown
  - CMD 1 merosin(-): Mutation in gene for laminin-α2 on Chr 6
  - CMDs with brain anomalies have hypoglycosylation of α-dystroglycan ⇒ neurons overmigrate through gaps in external lamina; "pebbled" brain surface
    - FCMD: Mutation in gene encoding fukutin (*FCMD* at 9q31)
    - MEB: O-Mannoside N-acetyl-glucosaminyl-transversae (POMGnT1 at 1p32-p34)
    - WWS: O-Mannosyltransferase gene (*POMT1*)
  - Mutations in *FKRP* (fukutin-related protein gene) may cause congenital or late-onset phenotypes
  - Other CMD variants with known defects
    - CMD with mutation integrin-α7 gene on Chr 12
    - CMD with familial junctional epidermolysis bullosa (plectin gene on Chr 8)
    - CMD with spine rigidity (linked to Chr 1 in some)
  - Mixed patterns and intermediate forms occur
    - CMD merosin(-) with brain anomalies, cerebellar cysts, vermis hypoplasia, mental retardation
- Associated abnormalities
  - Some associated features in CMD variants with "not yet found" mutations: Occipito-temporal PMG,

occipital agyria, calf-hypertrophy, arthrogryposis, ptosis, adducted thumbs

Staging, Grading, & Classification

- CMD 1: Abnormal WM varies from mild (CMD 1 merosin[+]) to more severe (CMD 1 merosin[-])
- CMD 2: FCMD: Moderate dysplasia of cerebral neocortex and cerebellum, abnormal WM
  - Frontal PMG, occipital cobblestone cortex, "peripheral 1st" myelination pattern
- CMD 3: Finnish-type MEB, less severe than CMD 4
  - Ventriculomegaly, vermian hypogenesis, dysplastic cortex, patchy abnormal WM, ± callosal dysgenesis
- CMD 4: Walker-Warburg, most severe
  - "Cobblestone" brain, massive ventriculomegaly with absent/abnormal callosum, no myelin, kinked pons-midbrain, vermian hypoplasia ± cephalocele

Gross Pathologic & Surgical Features

- CMDs with brain malformations
  - Supratentorial: Coarse gyri, agyric regions, ± ventriculomegaly and focal interhemispheric fusion
  - Brainstem: Variable degrees of pontine hypoplasia and fused colliculi; flat, cleft, or Z-shaped brainstem
  - Cerebellum: Cerebellar hypoplasia, PMG, and cysts ± encephalocele
  - Ocular: Retinal/optic nerve dysplasias, microphthalmia, buphthalmos, glaucoma, anterior chamber dysplasias, cataracts
- Marked phenotypic overlap amongst FCMD, Walker-Warburg, and MEB

Microscopic Features

- Cortical disorganization, cerebral and cerebellar PMG
- Fibroglial proliferation of leptomeninges (→ "pebbled" surface and trapped CSF "cysts")
- Hypoplasia of white matter
- Muscle biopsy: Mild to moderate dystrophic changes, ± inflammatory infiltrate, ± absent staining laminin-$\alpha 2$

CLINICAL ISSUES

Presentation

- Most common signs/symptoms
  - Hypotonia, developmental delay, poor vision, seizures
- Clinical profile
  - "Floppy" newborn

Demographics

- Age
  - CMD with brain malformations can be diagnosed in utero via US and MR, otherwise in early infancy
  - FCMD: High percentage spontaneous abortions
- Gender
  - M = F usually (some M > F or M < F variants)
- Ethnicity
  - FCMD most common in Japan (carrier state 1:88)
  - MEB more prevalent in Finland
  - WWS has worldwide distribution
- Epidemiology
  - 7-12 per 100,000 children in Japan; incidence elsewhere uncertain

Natural History & Prognosis

- CMD 1 (merosin[+]): Mild or nonprogressive; most can sit, some can walk; intellect usually normal
- CMD 1 (merosin[-]): More severe; intellect usually normal; some have seizures
- FCMD: Early contractures, rarely learn to walk, death < 20 years
- MEB: May survive to 20 years but spasticity and contractures
- WWS: Lethal in infancy

Treatment

- No treatment other than supportive

DIAGNOSTIC CHECKLIST

Consider

- Typical brainstem and cerebellar findings should prompt diagnosis even if eyes and supratentorial cortex radiographically normal

Image Interpretation Pearls

- Not all Z-shaped brainstems are CMD
- Not all CMD have Z-shaped brainstems (e.g., merosin[-] CMD)
- Look for large tectum

SELECTED REFERENCES

1. Muntoni F et al: Muscular dystrophies due to glycosylation defects. Neurotherapeutics. 5(4):627-32, 2008
2. Sprecher E et al: A mutation in SNAP29, coding for a SNARE protein involved in intracellular trafficking, causes a novel neurocutaneous syndrome characterized by cerebral dysgenesis, neuropathy, ichthyosis, and palmoplantar keratoderma. Am J Hum Genet. 77(2):242-51, 2005
3. Triki C et al: Merosin-deficient congenital muscular dystrophy with mental retardation and cerebellar cysts, unlinked to the LAMA2, FCMD, MEB and CMD1B loci, in three Tunisian patients. Neuromuscul Disord. 13(1):4-12, 2003
4. Zolkipli Z et al: Occipito-temporal polymicrogyria and subclinical muscular dystrophy. Neuropediatrics. 34(2):92-5, 2003
5. Mercuri E et al: Early white matter changes on brain magnetic resonance imaging in a newborn affected by merosin-deficient congenital muscular dystrophy. Neuromuscul Disord. 11(3):297-9, 2001
6. Philpot J et al: Brain magnetic resonance imaging abnormalities in merosin-positive congenital muscular dystrophy. Eur J Paediatr Neurol. 4(3):109-14, 2000
7. Barkovich AJ: Neuroimaging manifestations and classification of congenital muscular dystrophies. AJNR Am J Neuroradiol. 19(8):1389-96, 1998
8. Santavuori P et al: Muscle-eye-brain disease: clinical features, visual evoked potentials and brain imaging in 20 patients. Eur J Paediatr Neurol. 2(1):41-7, 1998

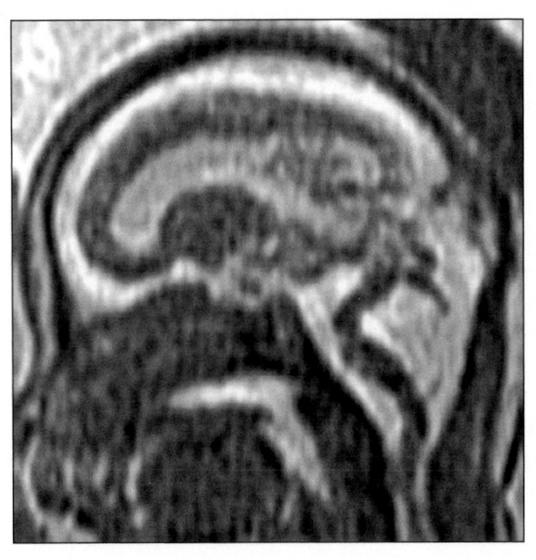

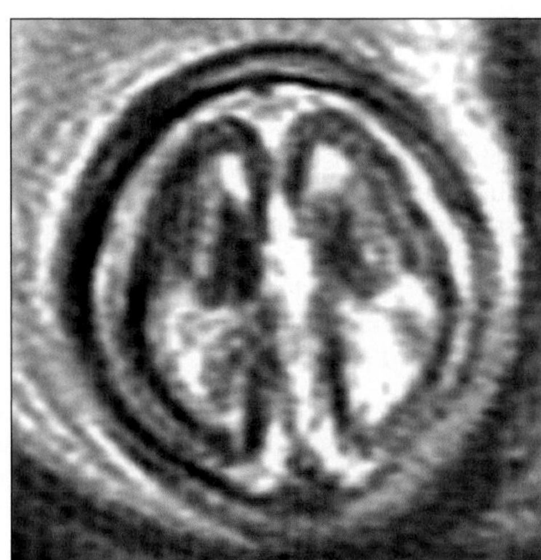

(Left) *Sagittal T2WI MR (ultrafast single shot) in a 20-week-old fetus shows kinked brainstem, dilated 4th ventricle, and hypoplastic vermis. At GA 20 weeks, the abnormal hindbrain is the most significant diagnostic feature of WWS (confirmed postnatally).* **(Right)** *Axial T2WI (ultrafast single shot) MR shows an agyric brain; sylvian fissure at this GA should be apparent. No corpus callosum as well as ventriculomegaly without hydrocephalus are consistent with poor development of WM.*

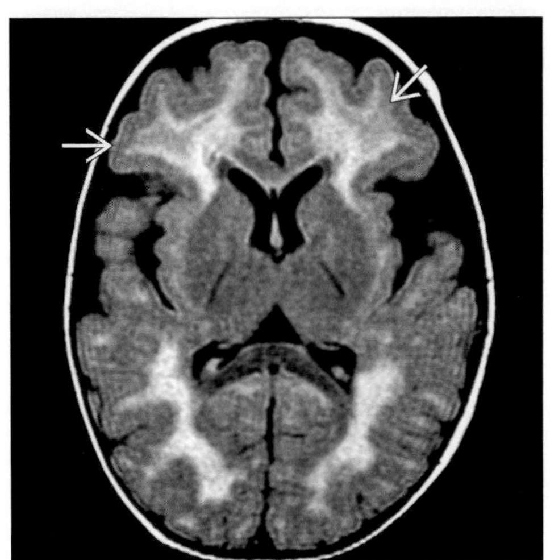

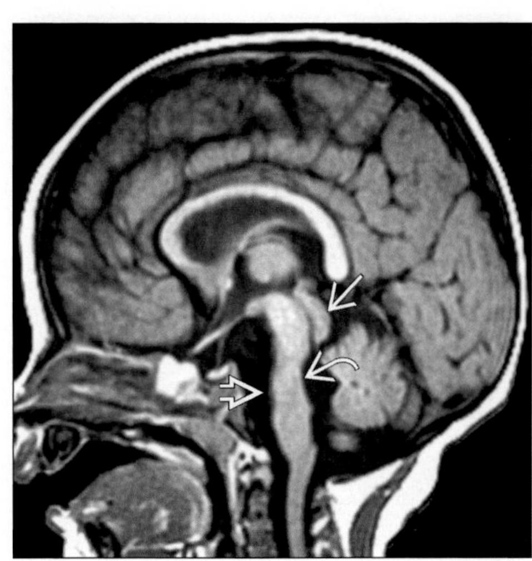

(Left) *Axial FLAIR MR in 9-month-old girl, whose brother has MEB, shows prominent CSF spaces and irregular sulcation. Myelination is extensively abnormal ➔ in subcortical, deep, and periventricular WM, with more normal posterior limb of the internal capsule and callosum.* **(Right)** *Sagittal T1WI MR in MEB shows grossly normal forebrain and commissural morphology. Cerebellar vermis is small with microcysts. Note the large tectum ➔ and small pons (flat ventrally ➔ and excavated dorsally ➔).*

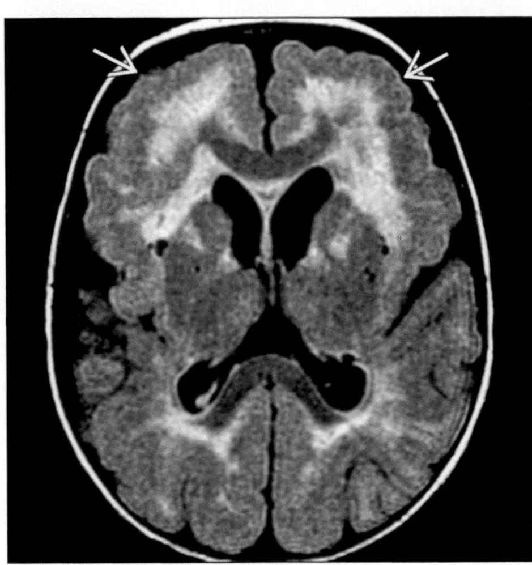

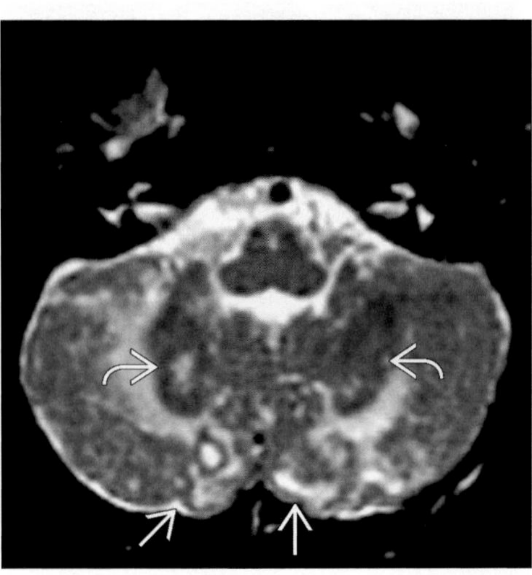

(Left) *Axial FLAIR MR in 1-year-old girl with FCMD. Note the large pericerebral spaces, mild ventriculomegaly, and abnormal myelination sparing the corpus callosum. Bilateral frontal polymicrogyria ➔ is a relatively specific finding.* **(Right)** *Axial T2WI MR in FCMD shows a cerebellar cortex that appears blurred due to polymicrogyria. Note the poor myelination of arbor vitae with prominence of dentate nuclei ➔. Multiple high T2-signal cortical microcysts ➔ are typical of FCMD.*

HETEROTOPIC GRAY MATTER

Key Facts

Terminology

- Heterotopia (HTP)
- Arrested/disrupted migration of groups of neurons from periventricular germinal zone (GZ) to cortex

Imaging

- Ectopic nodule or ribbon, isointense with gray matter (GM) on every MR sequence
- Periventricular, subcortical/transcerebral, molecular layer
- Subependymal HTP located next to periventricular white matter (GZ of cerebral mantle) but not in corpus callosum (fiber tract) or next to basal ganglia (GZ of ganglionic eminence)
- Variable: From tiny to huge, isolated to diffuse
- Thin slice, high-definition 3D acquisition, heavily weighted T1 provides optimal contrast and definition
- Large nodular HTP: Often thinned, polymicrogyric-looking overlying cortex

Top Differential Diagnoses

- Tuberous sclerosis
- "Closed-lip" schizencephaly
- Tumors

Pathology

- Nodular periventricular HTP often genetic
    - *FLNA* gene commonly involved (required for cell migration to cortex) on Xq28
- Band HTP: Mild form of type 1 (classic) lissencephaly (agyria/pachygyria/double cortex)
    - Predominantly posterior lissencephaly/band HTP: Deletion *LIS1* located on 17p13.3
    - Predominantly anterior lissencephaly/band HTP: Deletion *DCX* = double cortin on Xq22.3-q23

*(**Left**) Axial T2WI MR in a 6-year-old girl with refractory epilepsy shows massive right posterior subcortical HTP containing cortex-like GM, WM, CSF spaces ➔, and blood vessels ➔. The mass may suggest a tumor, but the hemisphere is small. Note the thin overlying cortex. (**Right**) Axial DTI color FA map in the same patient depicts the complete disorganization of the WM in and around the nodular subcortical HTP ➔. Red indicates R-L, green A-P, blue S-I fiber orientation. Other hues imply intermediate directions.*

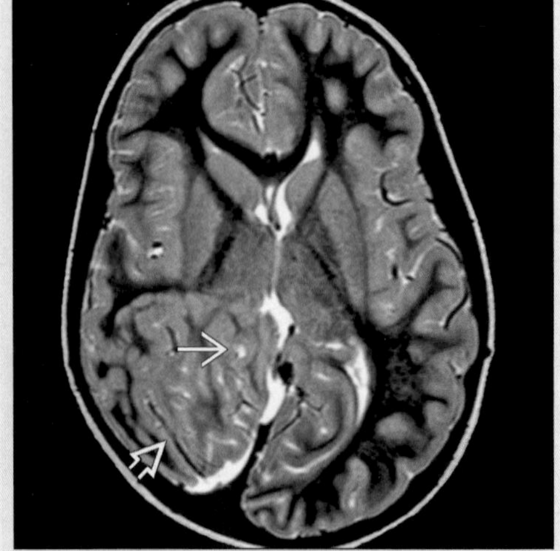

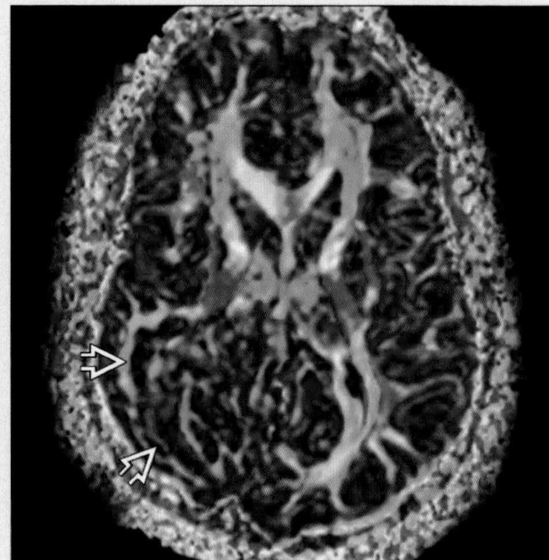

*(**Left**) Axial 3D T2WI MR shows subcortical band heterotopia in a 12-year-old boy. The symmetric HTP lies below an intermediate layer of WM. It is thicker posteriorly, in keeping with LIS1 mutation (autosomal recessive). Overlying cortex looks essentially normal. (**Right**) Axial T1WI MR in the same patient coregistered with magnetoencephalography (MEG) shows that the MEG spikes (triangles) originate from HTP, yet both the HTP and overlying cortex participate in the epileptogenic loop.*

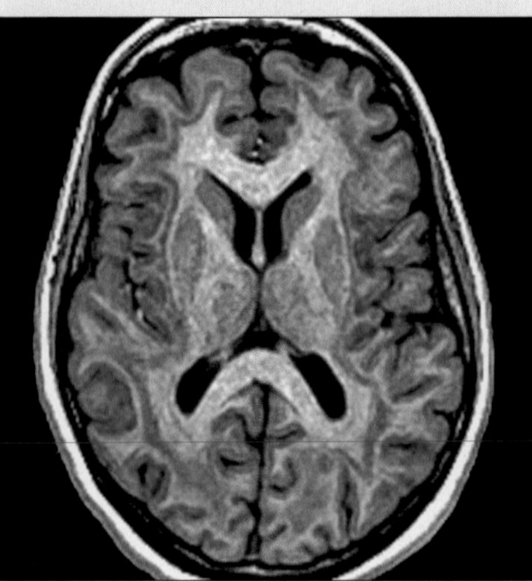

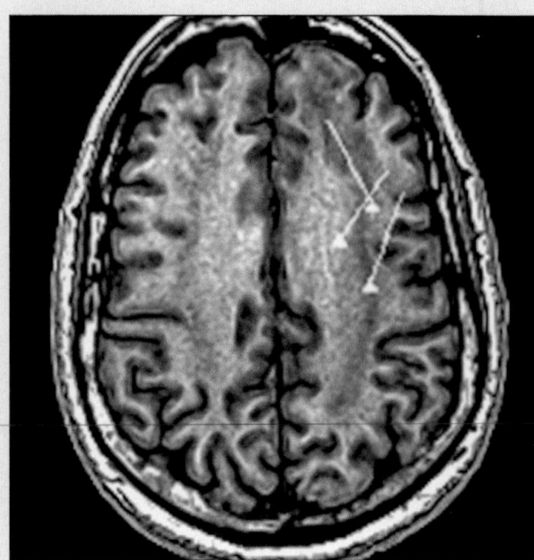

HETEROTOPIC GRAY MATTER

TERMINOLOGY

Abbreviations

- Heterotopia (HTP)

Synonyms

- Gray matter heterotopia; double cortex = band HTP

Definitions

- Arrested/disrupted migration of groups of neurons from periventricular germinal zone (GZ) to cortex

IMAGING

General Features

- Best diagnostic clue
  - Nodule or ribbon isointense with gray matter (GM) on every MR sequence, but in wrong place
- Location
  - Anywhere from ependymal to pial lining
    - Periventricular, subcortical/transcerebral, molecular layer
      - Subependymal HTP always found in periventricular white matter (GZ of cerebral mantle) but not in corpus callosum (fiber tract) or next to basal ganglia (GZ of ganglionic eminence)
- Size
  - Variable: From tiny to huge, isolated to diffuse
- Morphology
  - Periventricular nodular heterotopia (most common)
    - Focal/multifocal asymmetric GM indentation of ventricle
  - Band heterotopia = laminar HTP, double cortex
    - Thick symmetric subcortical GM band + thin cortex
  - Nodular subcortical heterotopia
    - Focal HTP nodules, often single
      - Large nodular HTP: Often thinned, polymicrogyria-like overlying cortex
    - Swirling GM mass continuous both with cortex and ventricular surface; contain GM, white matter (WM), sometimes pia, vessels, and CSF
  - Associated subcortical and periventricular HTP

CT Findings

- NECT
  - Isodense with GM (extremely rare dysplastic Ca++)
- CECT
  - No enhancement

MR Findings

- T1WI
  - Imaging characteristics match GM
  - Well demarcated
- T2WI
  - Imaging characteristics match GM
  - If subcortical, look for continuity with cortex and ventricular surface
    - Small ipsilateral hemisphere, large ipsilateral ventricle common (poor WM development)
- FLAIR
  - GM signal
- DWI
  - DTI shows connectivity patterns

Ultrasonographic Findings

- Grayscale ultrasound
  - Fetal US and MR have documented periventricular heterotopia

Nuclear Medicine Findings

- PET
  - Band HTP: Glucose uptake similar to or greater than normal cortex
- SPECT (HMPAO-SPECT)
  - Perfusion similar to normal cortex; HTP included in brain circuitry

Imaging Recommendations

- Best imaging tool
  - MR imaging
- Protocol advice
  - Thin slice and high-definition 3D acquisition, heavily weighted T1 provides optimal contrast and definition

DIFFERENTIAL DIAGNOSIS

Tuberous Sclerosis

- Subependymal nodules of tuberous sclerosis bulge into ventricular lumen, along thalamo-caudate groove, or over caudate
  - Often calcify; may enhance; associated with tubers, subependymal giant cell astrocytoma

"Closed-Lip" Schizencephaly

- Gray matter extending from cortex to ventricle lines cleft (look for "kissing" ventricle)
  - Transcerebral HTP may be associated with, even contralateral to, schizencephalic cleft

Tumors

- Ependymal seeding

Cytomegalovirus

- Periventricular calcifications

PATHOLOGY

General Features

- Etiology
  - Genetic: Mutations alter molecular interactions at multiple migration points → migration arrest → HTP
    - Complete/partial deletion/mutation of genes that govern specific stages of neuronal migration
  - Acquired (rare): Toxins/infections → reactive gliosis/ macrophage infiltration → disturbed neuronal migration/cortical positioning
- Genetics
  - Nodular periventricular HTP often genetic
    - *FLNA* gene commonly involved (required for cell migration to cortex) on Xq28
    - Other periventricular HTP localizing to 5p15.1, 5p15.33, 7q11.23
    - Microcephaly and nodular periventricular HTP: *ARFGEF2*

HETEROTOPIC GRAY MATTER

- Band HTP is mild form of classic lissencephaly (agyria/pachygyria/double cortex)
  - Predominantly posterior lissencephaly/band HTP: Deletion *LIS1* located on 17p13.3
  - Predominantly anterior lissencephaly/band HTP: Deletion *DCX* = double cortin on Xq22.3-q23
- Associated abnormalities
  - Gray matter HTP common in certain malformations
    - Agenesis of corpus callosum, classic: Nodular periventricular HTP common
    - Agenesis of corpus callosum with interhemispheric cysts (e.g., Aicardi syndrome): Nodular subcortical HTP nearly always present
    - Chiari 2 malformation: Nodular periventricular HTP in almost half of cases
    - Periventricular HTP with large cisterna magna
- Embryology
  - Cellular migration: Cell-cycle control, cell-cell adhesion, growth factor, neurotransmitter release, interaction with matrix proteins
    - Pyramidal cell progenitors produced in periventricular GZ (mantle) migrate toward surface, guided by radial glia
    - Stop-signal from Cajal-Retzius cells in molecular layer (future cortical layer 1)
    - Inside-out process: Young neurons more superficial
    - Migration essentially finished by week 20
  - Abnormal migration
    - ⇒ GZ (periventricular HTP), ⇒ mantle but below cortex (subcortical HTP), ⇒ molecular layer, beyond pia ⇒ meninges (leptomeningeal HTP = "cobblestone" brain)

Staging, Grading, & Classification

- Classification by location, type, and size; phenotype may predict genotype
  - Nodular periventricular HTP
    - Isolated, multiple, diffuse, uni-/bilateral
  - Band HTP (laminar HTP, double cortex) part of lissencephaly type 1
    - Lesser form of agyria, agyria/pachygyria spectrum
  - Leptomeningeal HTP
    - Seen in "cobblestone" brain (with congenital muscular dystrophies)

Gross Pathologic & Surgical Features

- Variable gray matter masses

Microscopic Features

- Multiple cell types, immature/dysplastic cells
  - Excitatory exceeds inhibitory

CLINICAL ISSUES

Presentation

- Most common signs/symptoms
  - Cognitive function, seizure onset/severity depend on location/degree of abnormalities
- Clinical profile
  - Young child with developmental delay, seizures

Demographics

- Age
  - Severe cases present in infancy with seizure and severe motor and cognitive dysfunction
  - In milder cases, epilepsy may appear in 2nd decade and tends to become severe
- Gender
  - Males with X-linked disorders have significantly worse brain malformation and outcome
- Epidemiology
  - 17% of neonatal CNS anomalies at autopsy
  - Found in up to 40% of patients with intractable epilepsy

Natural History & Prognosis

- Variable life span dependent on extent of malformation and severity of epilepsy
- Can be incidental on imaging/autopsy

Treatment

- Palliative surgery reserved for intractable seizures

DIAGNOSTIC CHECKLIST

Consider

- Gray matter HTP is common and commonly associated with other anomalies

Image Interpretation Pearls

- Gray matter HTP does not enhance or calcify
  - Extremely rare dystrophic Ca++

SELECTED REFERENCES

1. Guerrini R et al: Abnormal development of the human cerebral cortex: genetics, functional consequences and treatment options. Trends Neurosci. 31(3):154-62, 2008
2. Widjaja E et al: Evaluation of subcortical white matter and deep white matter tracts in malformations of cortical development. Epilepsia. 48(8):1460-9, 2007
3. Barkovich AJ et al: A developmental and genetic classification for malformations of cortical development. Neurology. 65(12):1873-87, 2005
4. Eriksson SH et al: Exploring white matter tracts in band heterotopia using diffusion tractography. Ann Neurol. 52(3):327-34, 2002
5. Barkovich AJ et al: Gray matter heterotopia. Neurology. 55(11):1603-8, 2000
6. Barkovich AJ: Morphologic characteristics of subcortical heterotopia: MR imaging study. AJNR Am J Neuroradiol. 21(2):290-5, 2000
7. Gressens P: Mechanisms and disturbances of neuronal migration. Pediatr Res. 48(6):725-30, 2000
8. Hannan AJ et al: Characterization of nodular neuronal heterotopia in children. Brain. 122 (Pt 2):219-38, 1999
9. Morioka T et al: Functional imaging in periventricular nodular heterotopia with the use of FDG-PET and HMPAO-SPECT. Neurosurg Rev. 22(1):41-4, 1999
10. Marsh L et al: Proton magnetic resonance spectroscopy of a gray matter heterotopia. Neurology. 47(6):1571-4, 1996
11. Shimodozono M et al: Functioning heterotopic grey matter? Increased blood flow with voluntary movement and sensory stimulation. Neuroradiology. 37(6):440-2, 1995
12. De Volder AG et al: Brain glucose utilization in band heterotopia: synaptic activity of "double cortex". Pediatr Neurol. 11(4):290-4, 1994

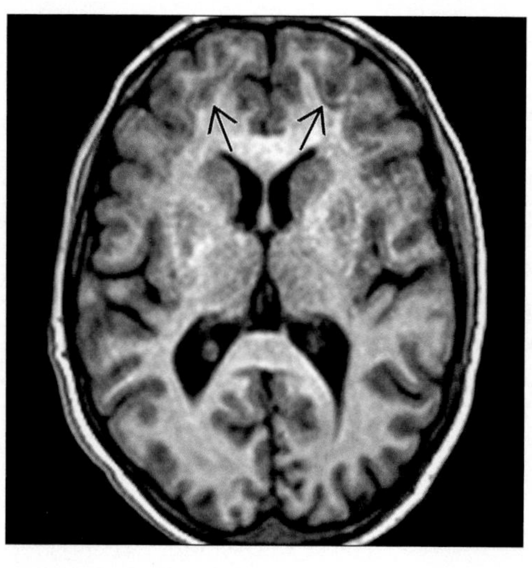

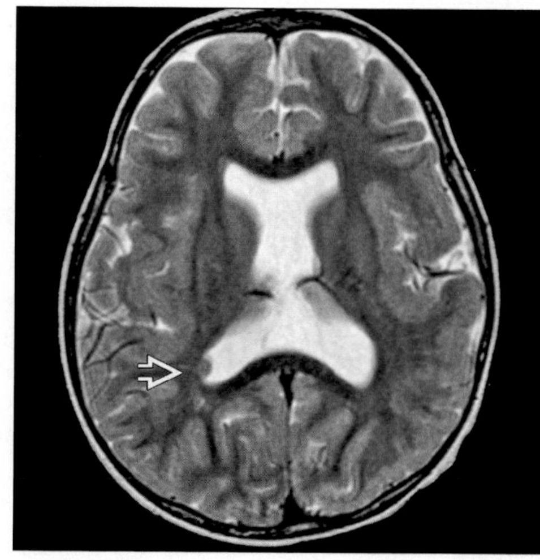

(Left) *Axial T1WI MR in a 15-year-old girl with severe epilepsy. Small, bilateral, frontal band HTP* ➔ *can be seen under a normal-looking cortex. The anterior location of the HTP suggests a DCX gene defect.* ***(Right)*** *Axial T2WI MR in a 2-year-old girl with optic atrophy disclose bilateral perisylvian polymicrogyria, absent septum pellucidum, and a single nodular periventricular HTP* ➔*, iso-intense to cortex. Heterotopia are rarely seen beneath polymicrogyria.*

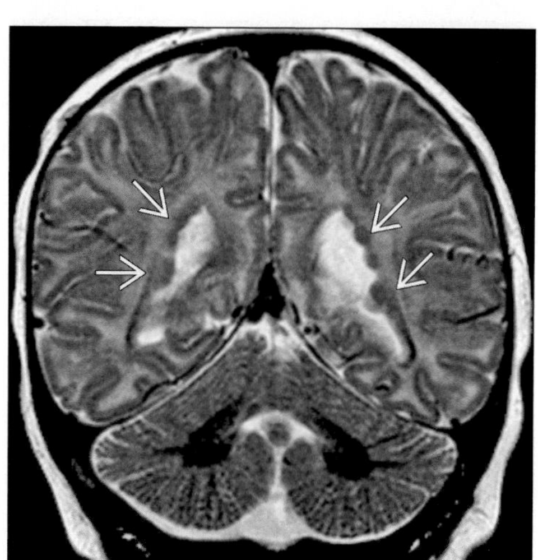

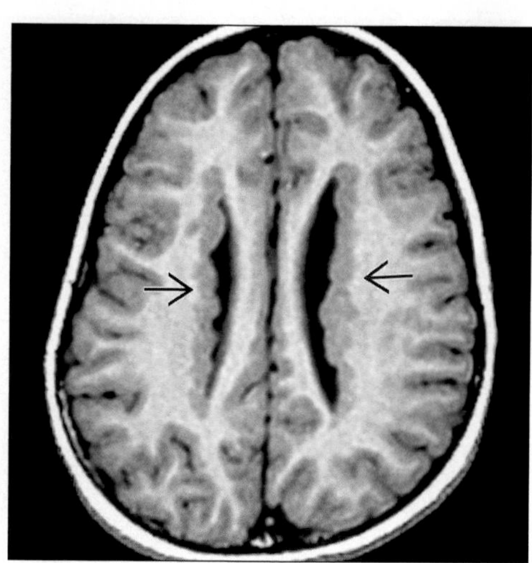

(Left) *Coronal T2WI MR in a 5-month-old boy shows mild ventriculomegaly with multiple nodular periventricular HTP* ➔ *lining the ventricular atria. A mega cisterna magna was also present.* ***(Right)*** *Axial T1WI MR of a 9-year-old girl with headaches (no seizures) reveals extensive bilateral periventricular nodules, isointense to gray matter* ➔ *that continuously line the lateral ventricles. Bilateral diffuse nodular periventricular HTP is often related to a FLNA mutation (Xq28).*

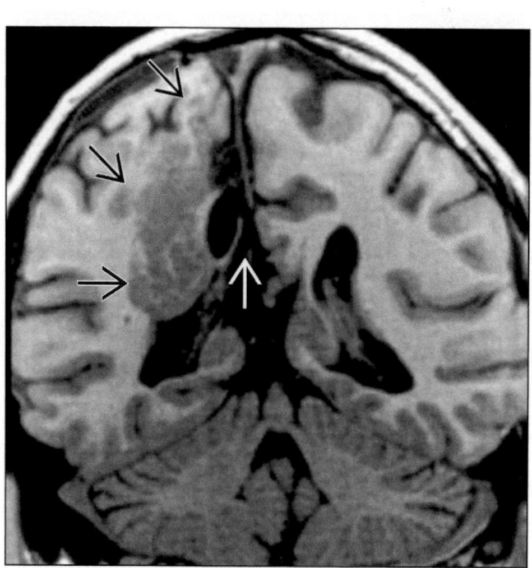

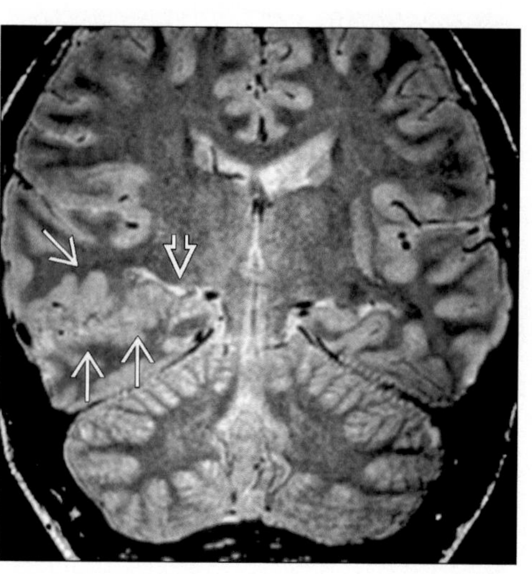

(Left) *Coronal T1WI MR in a 15-year-old boy with epilepsy shows ACC with interhemispheric meningeal cysts and a massive nodular subcortical HTP* ➔*, located on the medial aspect of the hemisphere, adjacent to previously drained cysts* ➔*.* ***(Right)*** *Coronal T2WI MR with surface coil in a 14-year-old boy with intractable mesial temporal epilepsy. A large nodular subcortical HTP* ➔ *extends to where the hippocampus should have been* ➔*. A normal right hippocampus cannot be identified.*

POLYMICROGYRIA

Key Facts

Terminology

- Malformation due to abnormality in late neuronal migration and cortical organization
- Result is cortex containing multiple small sulci that often appear fused on gross pathology and imaging
- Neurons reach cortex but distribute abnormally forming multiple small undulating gyri

Imaging

- Excessively small and prominent convolutions
- Predilection for perisylvian regions; when bilateral, often syndromic
- Small irregular gyri, but cortex appears normal or thick on MR
- May appear as deep infolding of thick cortex
- MR comprehensively assesses malformation; NECT for suspected Ca++ (TORCH)
- Best Sequence: Volume 3D SPGR (T1-weighted) in mature brain; thin section T2WI if unmyelinated

Top Differential Diagnoses

- Microcephaly with simplified gyral pattern (MSG)
- Hemimegalencephaly (HME)
- Congenital cytomegalovirus
- Pachygyria
- Dystroglycanopathies ("cobblestone" malformations)

Clinical Issues

- Polymicrogyria most commonly → developmental delay, seizure
- Onset and severity of seizures, neurological deficits relate to extent of malformation, presence of associated anomalies

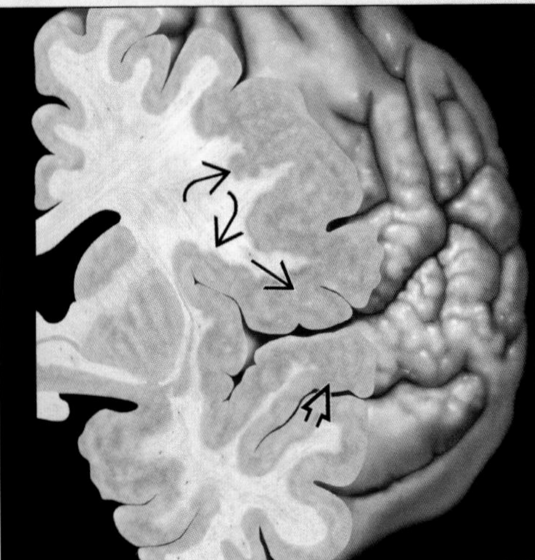

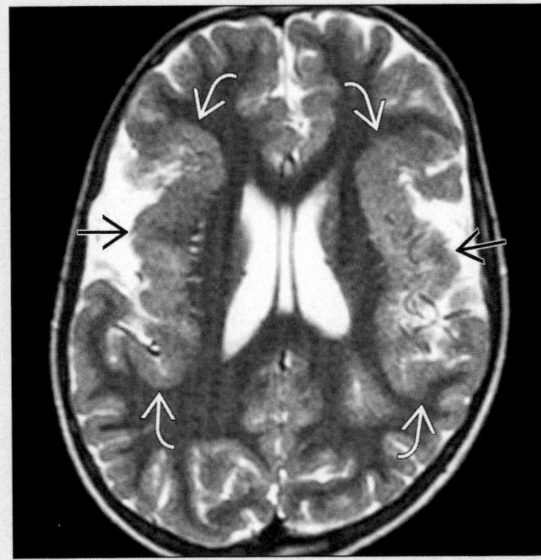

*(**Left**) Coronal oblique graphic shows the thickened "pebbly" gyri of polymicrogyria involving the frontal ➔ and temporal ➔ opercula. Note the abnormal sulcation and the irregular cortical-white matter interface ➔ in the affected regions. (**Right**) Axial T2WI MR of a patient with bilateral perisylvian polymicrogyria shows a thickened, irregular cortex in the insulae ➔, as well as frontal and parietal opercula ➔. Incidental cavum septi pellucidi is also seen.*

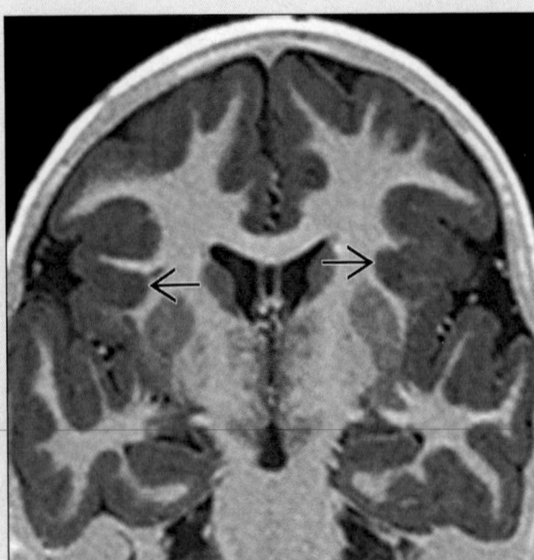

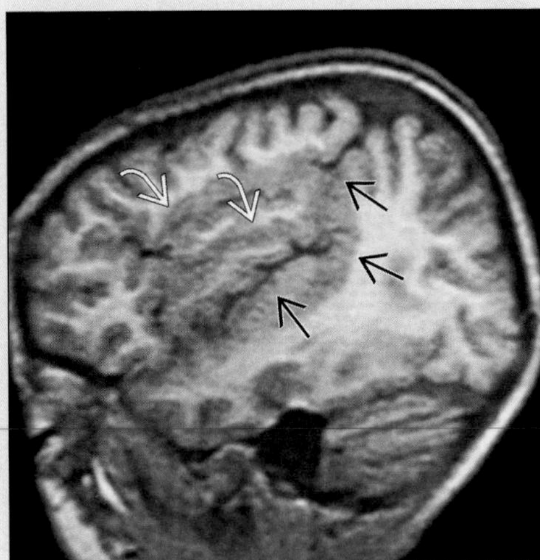

*(**Left**) Coronal T1WI MR of the same patient shows thickened, deeply undulating insulae ➔ and opercula around the abnormal sylvian fissures. PMG is often more poorly characterized in the coronal plane. The microgyri are not as well seen. (**Right**) Sagittal T1WI MR shows the characteristic continuation of the perisylvian PMG posteriorly into the superior parietal lobule ➔, which establishes the diagnosis. Other abnormal horizontal sulci with thick, irregular cortex ➔ are present.*

POLYMICROGYRIA

TERMINOLOGY

Abbreviations

- Polymicrogyria (PMG), sometimes referred to as cortical dysplasia

Definitions

- Malformation due to abnormality in late neuronal migration and cortical organization
  - Neurons reach cortex but distribute abnormally, forming multiple small undulating gyri
  - Result is cortex containing multiple small sulci that often appear fused on gross pathology and imaging
    - May give false impression of several large, thick gyri

IMAGING

General Features

- Best diagnostic clue
  - Excessively small gyri and prominent convolutions
- Location
  - Predilection for perisylvian regions; when bilateral, often syndromic
- Morphology
  - Small irregular gyri, but cortex looks normal or thick
  - May appear as deep infolding of thick cortex

Radiographic Findings

- Radiography
  - Polymicrogyric newborns, infants often microcephalic

CT Findings

- NECT
  - Look for altered sulcation pattern; suggests PMG
  - Excessive small convolutions difficult to detect on CT due to poor contrast resolution
  - Will detect periventricular Ca++ if secondary to cytomegalovirus (CMV)

MR Findings

- T1WI
  - Irregular cortical surface, often seen best on parasagittal images
  - May appear as arc of thick (5-7 mm) cortex with irregular cortex-white matter junction, without normal sulci
  - May appear as deep infolding of irregular, thick cortex
- T2WI
  - Polymicrogyria (2 imaging patterns)
    - < 12 months: Small, fine undulating cortex with normal thickness (3-4 mm)
    - > 18 months: Thick, bumpy cortex (6-8 mm), ± large perivascular spaces, ± cortical infolding
- STIR
  - Less useful due to poor spatial resolution
- FLAIR
  - May be difficult to see microgyri because of poor contrast between cortex and white matter
  - Allows differentiation between dilated perivascular spaces (common in PMG) and abnormal myelination (suggests dystroglycanopathy/"cobblestone" malformation or prenatal infection such as CMV)
- T2* GRE
  - Hypointense foci of periventricular Ca++ → CMV
- T1WI C+
  - Amplifies dysplastic leptomeningeal veins (when present) overlying regions of polymicrogyria
- MRV
  - Demonstrates large leptomeningeal veins overlying abnormal cortex
- MRS
  - ↓ NAA at seizure-precipitating, atrophic, &/or hypomyelinated sites

Angiographic Findings

- May see large veins in clefts of PMG

Nuclear Medicine Findings

- PET
  - Increased metabolism during ictus
  - Hypometabolic interictally

Other Modality Findings

- Fetal MR and US: Agyric cortex normal up to 26 weeks
- Prenatal MR can detect PMG and other anomalies of cortical development as early as 22 weeks

Imaging Recommendations

- Best imaging tool
  - MR comprehensively assesses malformation; NECT for suspected Ca++ (TORCH)
- Protocol advice
  - Volume 3D SPGR (T1-weighted) in mature brain; thin-section T2WI if unmyelinated

DIFFERENTIAL DIAGNOSIS

Malformations Secondary to Inborn Errors of Metabolism

- Mitochondrial and pyruvate metabolism disorders
- Zellweger syndrome: Deficiency of peroxisomes, severe hypomyelination, cortical malformations

Microcephaly with Simplified Gyral Pattern (MSG)

- Disorder of stem cell proliferation, head circumference < 3 SDs below mean
- MSG has normal cortical thickness, smooth inner cortical margin, normal primary and secondary sulci

Hemimegalencephaly (HME)

- Disorder of neuronal proliferation, migration, and differentiation
- In HME, affected hemisphere is large; in unilateral PMG, affected hemisphere is small

Congenital Cytomegalovirus

- Association with polymicrogyria; NECT for detection of periventricular Ca++

Pachygyria

- Thicker cortex (8-10 mm), smooth cortex-white matter junction

POLYMICROGYRIA

Dystroglycanopathies ("Cobblestone" Malformations)

- Associated with hypomyelination, cerebellar dysgenesis, pontine hypoplasia

PATHOLOGY

General Features

- Etiology
  - Causes → intrauterine infection, ischemia, toxins, or gene mutations
    - Timing: 2nd half of 2nd trimester
- Genetics
  - Mutations of Xq28, Xq21.33-q23 (SRPX2),16q12.2-21, 1p36, and 22q11.2, and genetic loci on chromosomes 1p36.3, 2p16.1-p23, 4q21.21-q22.1, 6q26-q27, and 21q21.3-22.1 have been identified
- Associated abnormalities
  - Congenital bilateral perisylvian syndrome (Foix-Chavany-Marie)
  - Aicardi, Zellweger, Delleman, Warburg micro syndromes

Staging, Grading, & Classification

- Polymicrogyria → unlayered or 4-layered cytoarchitecture

Gross Pathologic & Surgical Features

- Multiple small gyri that lie in haphazard orientation
- Fusion of molecular layer (cortical layer 1)
- Multiple appearances and locations
  - Unilateral: Focal, perisylvian, or hemispheric
  - Bilateral symmetrical: Perisylvian, frontal, frontoparietal, lateral parietal, medial parasagittal parietooccipital
  - Bilateral asymmetrical

Microscopic Features

- Range of histology reflecting derangement of 6-layered lamination of cortex
  - Cortical layers 4 and 5 most involved
  - Leptomeningeal embryonic vasculature overlies malformation
  - Myelination within subcortical or intracortical fibers changes cortical appearance on T2-weighted images

CLINICAL ISSUES

Presentation

- Most common signs/symptoms
  - Polymicrogyria most commonly ⇒ developmental delay, seizure
    - Bilateral perisylvian PMG may cause faciopharyngoglossomasticatory diplegia
    - Unilateral PMG ⇒ often hemiparesis
- Clinical profile
  - Onset and severity of seizures, neurological deficits relates to extent of malformation

Demographics

- Age
  - Signs and symptoms vary with severity of gene mutation and resultant phenotypic expression
- Gender
  - No gender preference
- Ethnicity
  - Found in all populations
- Epidemiology
  - Malformations of cortical development found in ~ 40% of children with intractable epilepsy

Natural History & Prognosis

- Variable based on severity of genetic mutation, resultant malformation, associated anomalies

Treatment

- Options, risks, complications
  - Focal PMG may be resected in refractory epilepsy
  - Corpus callosotomy if bilateral or diffuse unresectable lesions

DIAGNOSTIC CHECKLIST

Consider

- Polymicrogyria always seen with schizencephaly
- Look for PMG in congenital hemiplegia with epilepsy

Image Interpretation Pearls

- Sylvian region most common location for PMG
- Open sylvian fissures with thick cortex → polymicrogyria

SELECTED REFERENCES

1. Mosca AL et al: Polymicrogyria in a child with inv dup del(9p) and 22q11.2 microduplication. Am J Med Genet A. 149A(3):475-81, 2009
2. Brandão-Almeida IL et al: Congenital bilateral perisylvian syndrome: familial occurrence, clinical and psycholinguistic aspects correlated with MRI. Neuropediatrics. 39(3):139-45, 2008
3. Barkovich AJ et al: A developmental and genetic classification for malformations of cortical development. Neurology. 65(12):1873-87, 2005
4. Piao X et al: Genotype-phenotype analysis of human frontoparietal polymicrogyria syndromes. Ann Neurol. 58(5):680-7, 2005
5. Wieck G et al: Periventricular nodular heterotopia with overlying polymicrogyria. Brain. 128(Pt 12):2811-21, 2005
6. Mirzaa G et al: Megalencephaly and perisylvian polymicrogyria with postaxial polydactyly and hydrocephalus: a rare brain malformation syndrome associated with mental retardation and seizures. Neuropediatrics. 35(6):353-9, 2004
7. Righini A et al: Early prenatal MR imaging diagnosis of polymicrogyria. AJNR Am J Neuroradiol. 25(2):343-6, 2004
8. Takanashi J et al: The changing MR imaging appearance of polymicrogyria: a consequence of myelination. AJNR Am J Neuroradiol. 24(5):788-93, 2003

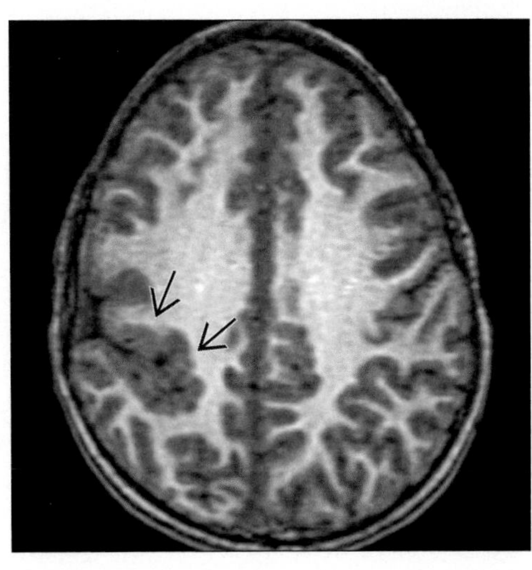

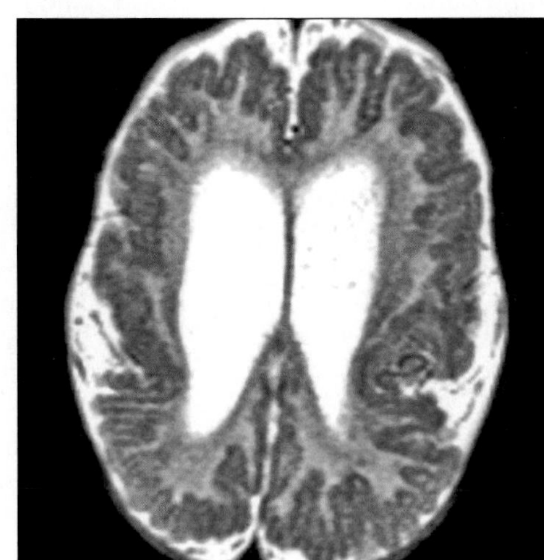

(Left) *Axial T1WI MR shows a large infolding of thickened cortex ⇨ with irregularity of the cortical-white matter junction in the posterior right frontal lobe. This is a characteristic appearance of focal polymicrogyria.* ***(Right)*** *Axial T2WI FSE MR shows diffuse polymicrogyria. Distinct microgyri can be seen in the individual gyri, but this particular case is also characterized by abnormally thin gyri separated by abnormally deep sulci.*

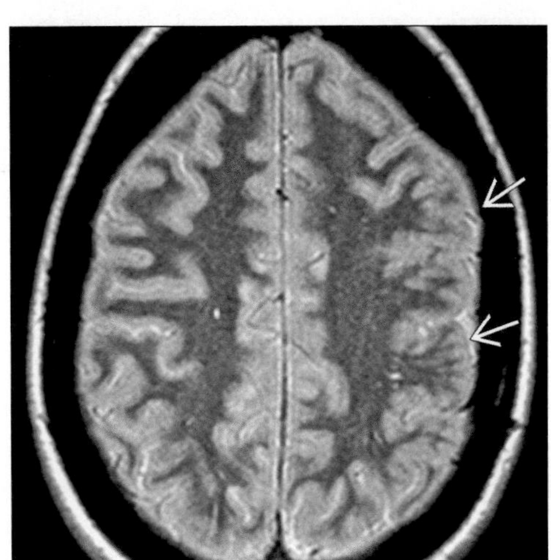

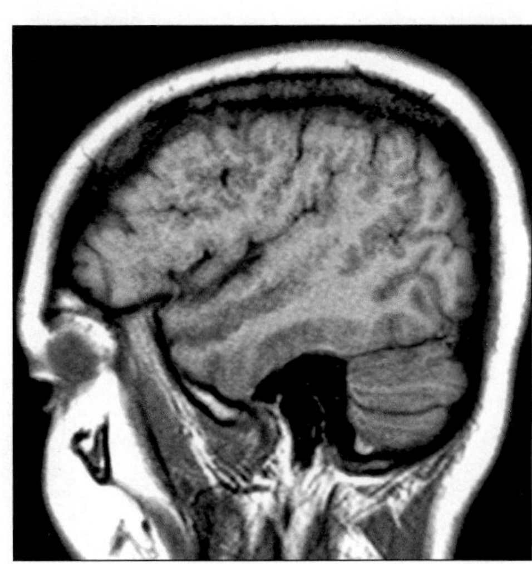

(Left) *Axial proton density MR in an asymptomatic adult shows multiple, small delicate gyri ➡ in the posterior left frontal and parietal lobes. Compare with the coarse appearance of the prior image. PMG can have a spectrum of appearances on MR.* ***(Right)*** *Sagittal T1WI MR in the same patient shows the extent of the PMG, involving most of the frontal & parietal lobes, as well as the superior temporal lobe. Most hemispheric PMG is centered in the sylvian fissure region.*

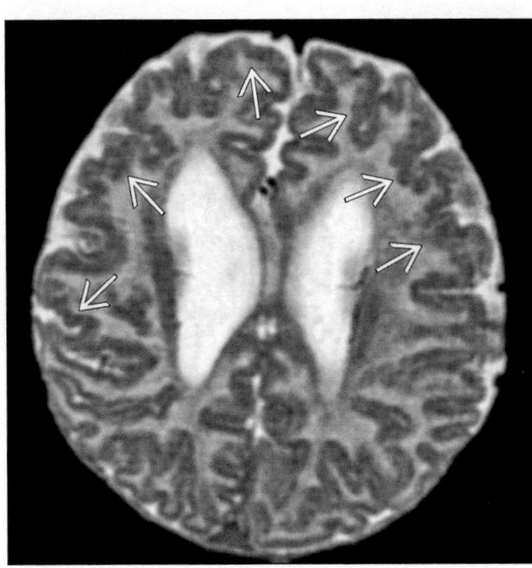

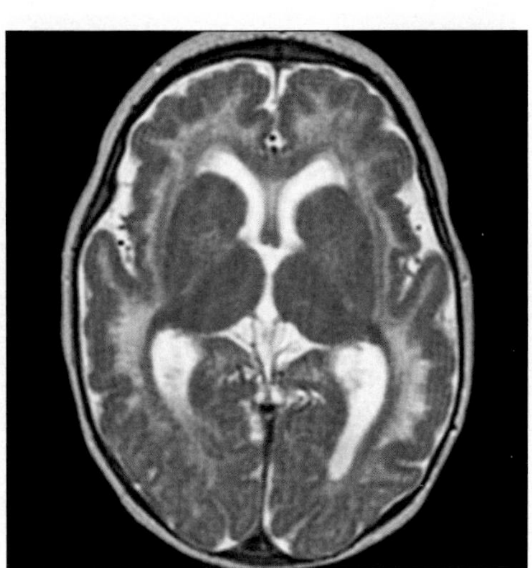

(Left) *Axial T2WI MR of a patient with bilateral frontal polymicrogyria shows multiple tiny irregularities ➡ at the junction of the cortex and white matter throughout the frontal lobes. Volume of frontal white matter is diminished, and the frontal horns are large.* ***(Right)*** *Axial T2WI MR shows a patient with congenital CMV infection. PMG is present throughout much of the lateral frontal and temporal lobes with abnormally hyperintense underlying white matter.*

LISSENCEPHALY

Key Facts

Terminology

- Disorders of cortical formation caused by arrested neuronal migration, resulting in thick 4-layer cortex and smooth brain surface
- Significant overlap with band heterotopia (BH)

Imaging

- "Hourglass" or "figure eight" shape of cerebral hemispheres
- Truncated arborization of white matter
- 3 layers may be distinguished on T2WI in neonate
  - Outer cellular layer → may be relatively thin, smooth
  - Intervening cell-sparse layer
  - Deeper thick layer of arrested neurons mimicking band heterotopia
- Posterior > anterior brain involvement in *LIS1*

Top Differential Diagnoses

- Band heterotopia
- Microcephaly with simplified gyral pattern
- Immature brain
- "Cobblestone" lissencephalies (type 2 lissencephaly)
  - Congenital muscular dystrophies

Pathology

- Caused by variety of gene alterations, resulting in spectrum of phenotypes
- *LIS1* gene → 17p13.3
  - Miller-Dieker syndrome
- *DCX* gene → Xq22.3-q23
- *RELN* gene → 7q22
  - Norman-Roberts syndrome
- *ARX* gene → Xp21.1
- *TUBA1A* gene → 12q12-q14.3

*(**Left**) Axial NECT in a child with type 1 lissencephaly shows the classic "hourglass" configuration of the cerebral hemispheres due to a smooth cortical surface and wide shallow sylvian fissures ➡. (**Right**) Coronal T2WI MR shows complete absence of cerebral sulcation, but the cerebellum is unaffected. A hyperintense cell sparse zone ➡ separates the thin cortical ribbon from the thicker band of disorganized neurons, which is in turn separated from the ventricles by white matter.*

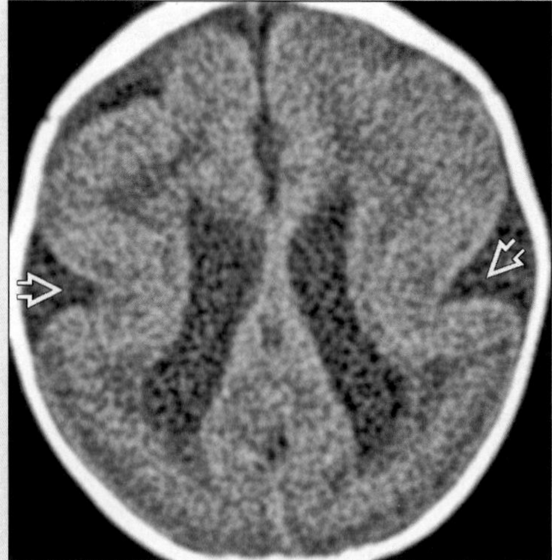

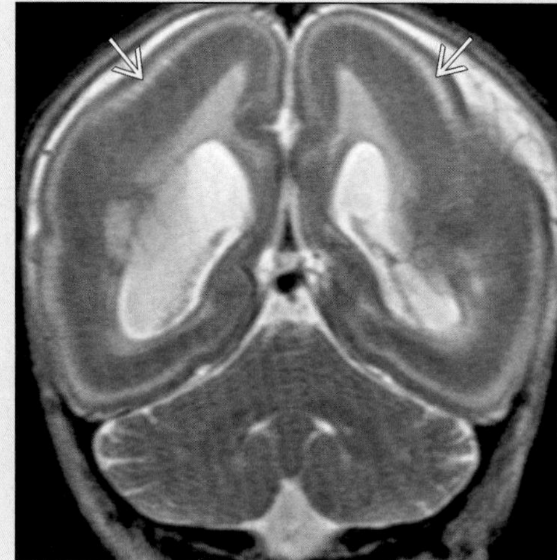

*(**Left**) Midline sagittal T1WI MR clearly shows relatively normal sulcation at frontal and occipital poles, with fewer sulci in between. Note the characteristic 90° angle ➡ between the callosal body and splenium. (**Right**) Anterosuperior perspective of a volume rendered surface-shaded reconstruction in the same infant shows the relative preservation of sulcation anteriorly ➡ with many fewer cortical sulci over the vertex further posteriorly ➡.*

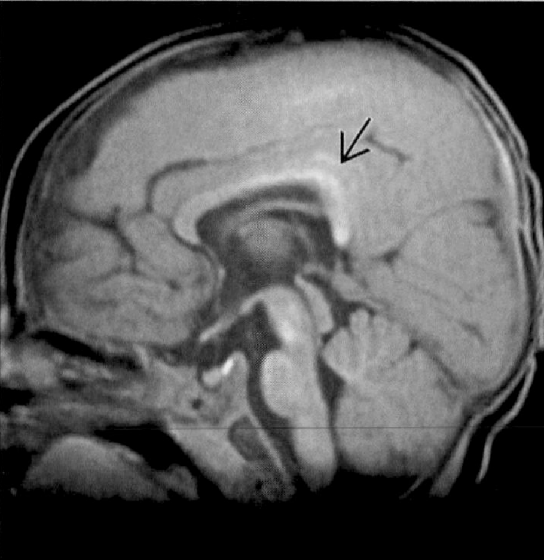

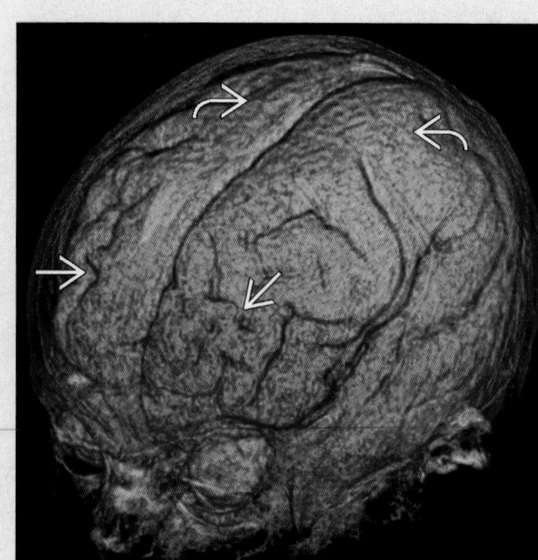

LISSENCEPHALY

TERMINOLOGY

Synonyms

- Classical lissencephaly, type 1 lissencephaly (LIS1), pachygyria-agyria complex, X-linked lissencephaly

Definitions

- Disorders of cortical formation caused by arrested neuronal migration, resulting in thick 4-layer cortex and smooth brain surface
- Significant overlap with band heterotopia (BH)
  - BH → overwhelmingly female, associated with *DCX* gene mutations
  - Outer cortical layer in BH has relatively normal sulcation and thickness

IMAGING

General Features

- Best diagnostic clue
  - Absence or diminished number of cortical sulci throughout cerebral hemispheres with thick cortex
  - "Hourglass" or "figure eight" shape of cerebral hemispheres
- Location
  - Cerebral hemispheres
- Size
  - Normocephalic to microcephalic

CT Findings

- NECT
  - Thick band of disorganized neurons often appears better defined than gray matter in normal infants
  - May see small midline calcifications in Miller-Dieker syndrome
  - May see periventricular calcifications in CMV-associated lissencephaly
- CECT
  - Large vessels in sylvian fissures

MR Findings

- T1WI
  - Small number of shallow sulci with broad intervening gyri
    - Smooth cortical surface
  - Mildly to moderately enlarged ventricles
  - Truncated arborization of white matter
  - Thick deep band of gray matter may resemble myelinated white matter
- T2WI
  - Best sequence for distinction of cortical layers in neonate
    - 3 layers may be distinguished
      - Outer cellular layer → may be relatively thin, smooth
      - Intervening cell-sparse layer
      - Deeper thick layer of arrested neurons mimicking band heterotopia
  - Prominent vessels in shallow sylvian fissures
- T2* GRE
  - Midline calcification in Miller-Dieker
  - Periventricular and subcortical white matter calcifications in CMV-related lissencephaly
- MRS
  - ↓ N-acetylaspartate (NAA) in affected cortex

Ultrasonographic Findings

- Grayscale ultrasound
  - Late intrauterine documentation possible

Nuclear Medicine Findings

- PET
  - Inner cellular layer has higher glucose utilization than outer layer (fetal pattern)

Imaging Recommendations

- Best imaging tool
  - MR
- Protocol advice
  - Utilize T2WI for best distinction of cortical layers in neonate
  - Multiplanar reconstructed volume T1WI ideal in child with completed myelination
  - Surface-shaded volume rendering may provide unique perspective on undersulcation for clinicians

DIFFERENTIAL DIAGNOSIS

Band Heterotopia

- Double cortex
  - Band of smooth gray matter separated from cortex by layer of normal-appearing white matter (WM)
    - Overlying cortex has shallow sulci
- Complete or partial
- Overwhelmingly female

Microcephaly with Simplified Gyral Pattern

- Head circumference ≤ 3 standard deviations below normal
- Too few gyri and abnormally shallow sulci
- No tertiary sulci

"Cobblestone" Lissencephalies (Type 2 Lissencephaly, LIS2)

- Congenital muscular dystrophies
  - Fukuyama CMD, Walker-Warburg syndrome, muscle-eye-brain disease
- "Pebbly" surface of brain, cerebellar and ocular abnormalities, congenital muscular dystrophy

Immature Brain

- Sulci do not fully develop until ~ 40 weeks gestation

PATHOLOGY

General Features

- Etiology
  - Genetic or acquired
    - Mutations of genes encoding for proteins required for normal neuronal migration
    - CMV-infected cells can fail to migrate or arrest
    - Toxin exposure (alcohol/irradiation) in utero can lead to abnormal migration
- Genetics
  - Caused by variety of gene alterations, resulting in spectrum of phenotypes

LISSENCEPHALY

- *LIS1* gene ⇒ 17p13.3
  - Regulates microtubule motor protein cytoplasmic dynein
  - Defects lead to parietooccipital agyria, classical lissencephaly
  - Miller-Dieker syndrome → large *LIS1* deletions
- *DCX* gene → Xq22.3-q23
  - Encodes for doublecortin (microtubule-binding) and stabilizing protein
  - Mutation in males leads to frontal agyria
  - Mutation in females leads to band heterotopia
- *RELN* gene → 7q22
  - Encodes for reelin, extracellular matrix protein that regulates neuronal migration and synaptic plasticity
  - Mutations lead to Norman-Roberts syndrome → small cerebellum, hypoplastic brainstem, mild decrease of cortical sulci gyri
- *ARX* gene → Xp21.1
  - Homeobox-containing gene
  - Mutations lead to frontal pachygyria, parietooccipital agyria, agenesis of corpus callosum, and ambiguous genitalia
- *TUBA1A* gene → 12q12-q14.3
  - Encodes for microtubule constituent proteins
  - Mutations lead to perisylvian pachygyria, posterior pachygyria, dysgenetic internal capsule, cerebellar hypoplasia

- Associated abnormalities
  - Miller-Dieker syndrome
    - Cardiac, GI, and renal anomalies
    - Characteristic facial features → prominent forehead, upturned nares, thickened upper lip, hypertelorism, low ears, small jaw
  - Norman-Roberts syndrome
    - Low sloping forehead, prominent nasal bridge

Microscopic Features

- 4-layer cortex (*LIS1* and *DCX*)
  - Superficial molecular or marginal layer
  - Thin outer cortical layer of neurons (large, abnormal position)
  - "Cell-sparse" WM zone
  - Thick deep cortical layer of neurons (lack orderly arrangement)
- Hypoplastic corticospinal tracts

CLINICAL ISSUES

Presentation

- Most common signs/symptoms
  - Developmental delay and seizures
- Clinical profile
  - Global developmental delay and seizures
    - Severe and diffuse involvement → diagnosis in infancy
    - Limited involvement → diagnosed in later childhood
  - Females with BH may be minimally symptomatic, mild seizures only

Demographics

- Age
  - Usually diagnosed early in life
  - Mild/partial cases may have delayed presentation
  - BH may be asymptomatic
- Gender
  - *DCX* gene mutations
    - Mothers → band heterotopia
      - BH > 90% female
    - Sons → lissencephaly
- Epidemiology
  - 1-4:100,000 live births

Natural History & Prognosis

- Significant mental retardation, motor deficits, seizures, early demise
- Exception → focal subcortical BH often lead normal life

Treatment

- Treat seizures (corpus callosotomy = option for intractable epilepsy)
- Supportive

DIAGNOSTIC CHECKLIST

Consider

- Patterns of gyral abnormalities may provide insight into genetic defect

Image Interpretation Pearls

- When suspecting lissencephaly in neonate, verify gestation age
  - Especially important in assessing fetal MR or US
    - Agyric (smooth) cortex is normal up to 26 weeks
  - Look for specific signs on fetal studies
    - Presence or absence of parietooccipital fissure; poor development of sylvian fissure

Reporting Tips

- Be very hesitant to use term "band heterotopia" in males
- Describe regions of involvement to help in clinical management, classification
- "Pachygyria" is useful as descriptive term, not as diagnostic label

SELECTED REFERENCES

1. Morris-Rosendahl DJ et al: Refining the phenotype of alpha-1a Tubulin (TUBA1A) mutation in patients with classical lissencephaly. Clin Genet. 74(5):425-33, 2008
2. Reiner O et al: Lissencephaly 1 linking to multiple diseases: mental retardation, neurodegeneration, schizophrenia, male sterility, and more. Neuromolecular Med. 8(4):547-65, 2006
3. Sicca F et al: Mosaic mutations of the LIS1 gene cause subcortical band heterotopia. Neurology. 61(8):1042-6, 2003

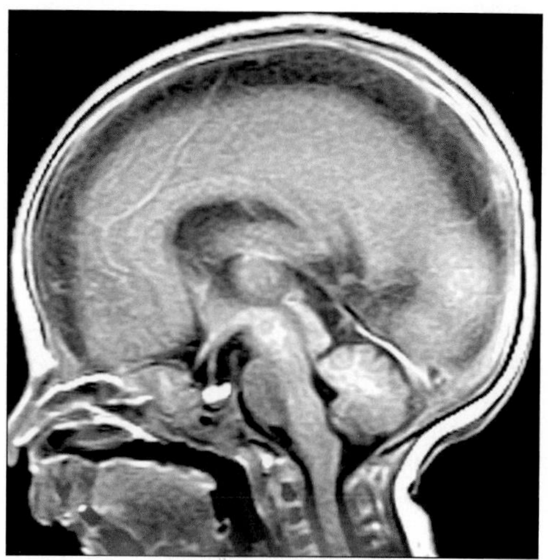

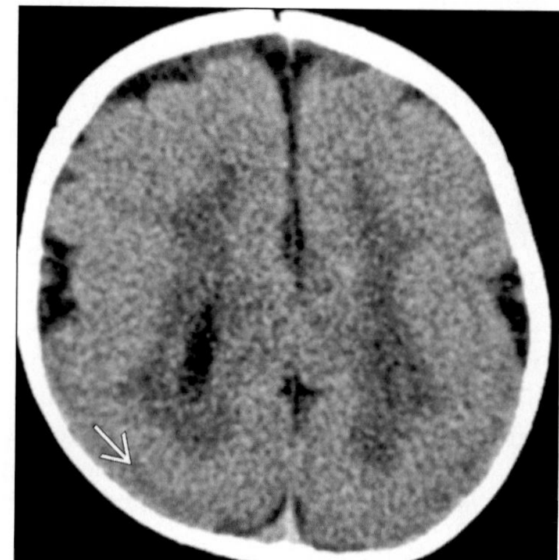

(Left) *Sagittal T1WI MR shows a smooth and featureless cortex in the supratentorial brain with a normal cerebellum and brainstem in this infant with the Miller-Dieker syndrome, caused by larger deletions of the LIS1 gene.* ***(Right)*** *Axial NECT in another child with classic lissencephaly shows the lack of arborization of the otherwise clearly delineated white matter. Note the subtle low attenuation of the "cell-sparse" zone ➔ in the right occipital pole.*

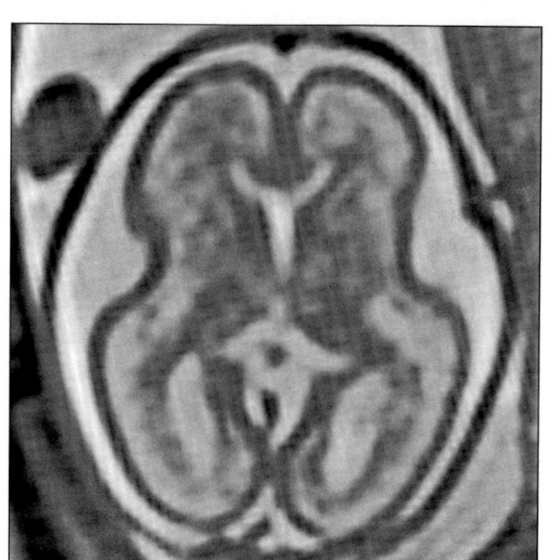

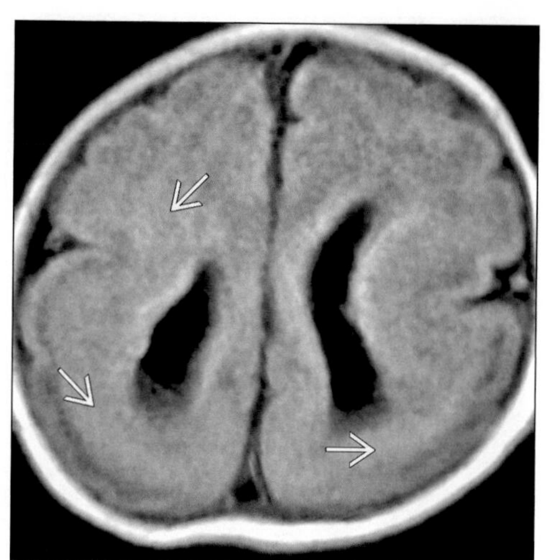

(Left) *Axial T2WI from a fetal MR exam at 22 weeks gestation shows an "hourglass" configuration of the cerebrum reminiscent of type 1 lissencephaly. However, this is normal at 22 weeks gestational age.* ***(Right)*** *Axial T1WI MR in another neonate with lissencephaly shows narrower but equally shallow sylvian fissures compared to the fetal MR. The slightly hyperintense signal deep to the cortex ➔ represents the deep zone of disorganized neurons.*

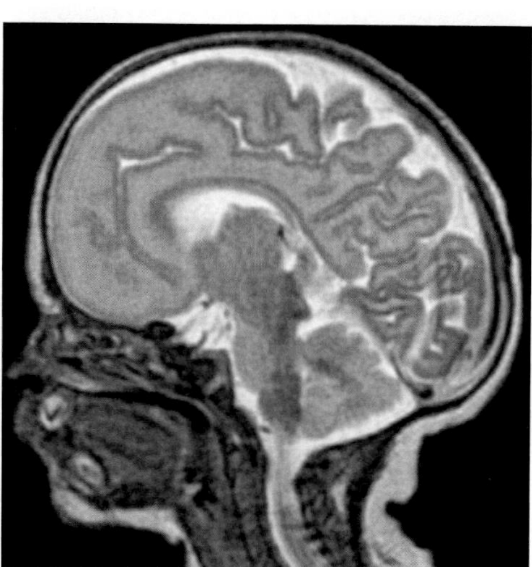

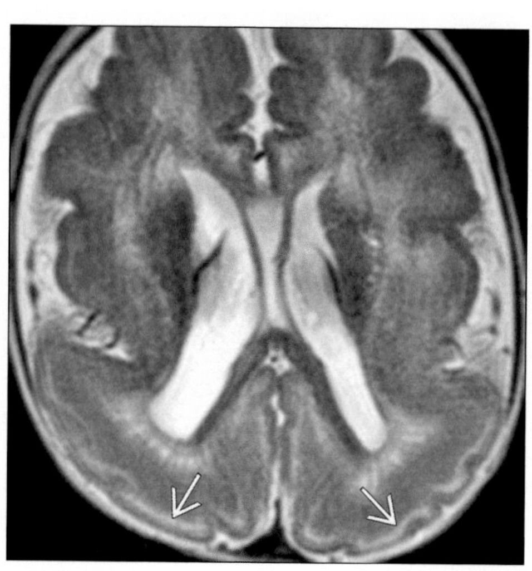

(Left) *Sagittal T2WI MR clearly shows the frontal predominance of pachygyria in this child with lissencephaly. The frontal pattern is characteristically seen in cases caused by mutations of the DCX gene.* ***(Right)*** *Axial T2WI MR in another child shows parieto-occipital predominance of pachygyria, a pattern seen with TUBA1A & LIS1 gene mutations. Bright signal can be seen in the cell-sparse zone ➔ between the thick subcortical band of disorganized neurons & thin superficial cortex.*

SCHIZENCEPHALY

Key Facts

Imaging

- Transmantle gray matter lining clefts
  - Look for dimple in wall of ventricle if cleft is narrow/closed
- Up to 1/2 of schizencephalies are bilateral
  - When bilateral, 60% are "open-lipped" on both sides
- Gray matter lining clefts may appear hyperdense
- Ca++ when associated with CMV
- Prior to myelination T2WI more clearly defines lesion

Top Differential Diagnoses

- Encephaloclastic porencephaly
  - Lined by gliotic WM, not dysplastic GM
- Hydranencephaly
  - Residual tissue is supplied by posterior circulation
- Semilobar holoprosencephaly
  - Can mimic bilateral "open-lip" schizencephaly

Pathology

- Can be result of acquired in utero insult affecting neuronal migration
- 1/3 of children with schizencephaly have non-CNS abnormalities
- Infection (CMV), vascular insult, maternal trauma, toxin

Clinical Issues

- Unilateral: Seizures or mild motor deficit
- Bilateral: Developmental delay, paresis, microcephaly, spasticity
- Seizure more common with unilateral clefts
- Size of clefts and presence of associated malformative lesions govern severity of impairment

(Left) Axial T2WI MR in a neonate with seizures shows "open-lipped" schizencephaly ➔ at the left temporal-parietal junction, with dysplastic GM extending anteriorly in the left temporal lobe. Note GM heterotopion in the anterior right temporal lobe ➔. (Right) Coronal FLAIR MR in the same infant shows a right parietal "open-lipped" cleft ➔ and the anterior part of the left-sided cleft ➔. Close to 50% of schizencephalies are bilateral; the majority of these are "open-lipped."

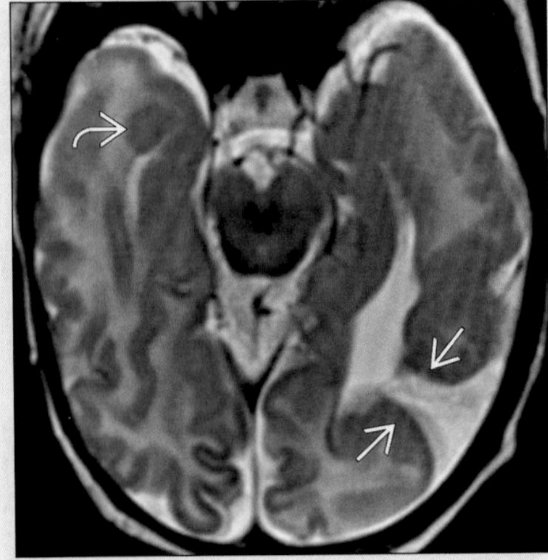

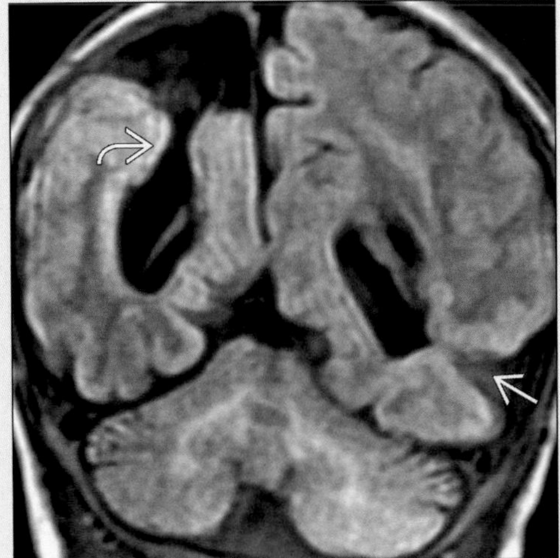

(Left) Sagittal T1WI MR shows a "closed-lip" schizencephaly at the right frontal-parietal junction. The dysplastic gray matter lining the cleft has an irregular interface with the underlying white matter ➔ compared to the smooth interface of the normal gray matter in the occipital lobe ➔. (Right) Coronal T1WI MR in the same patient shows the enlargement and distortion of the occipital horn where the schizencephalic cleft enters and the thickened gray matter ➔ lines it.

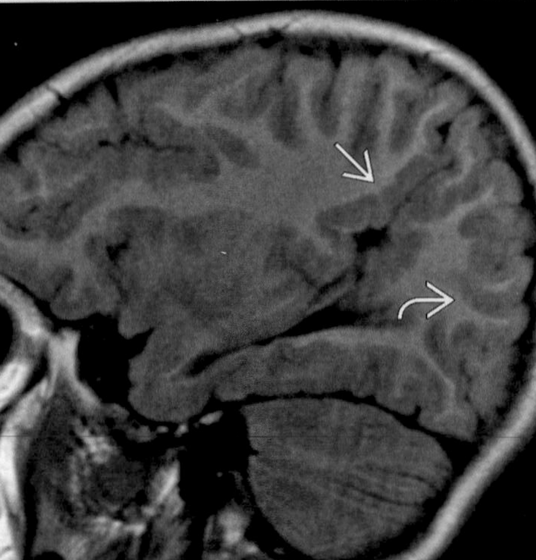

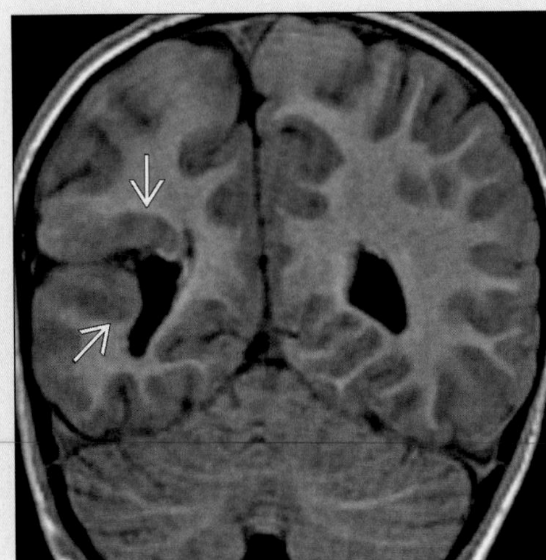

SCHIZENCEPHALY

TERMINOLOGY

Synonyms

- Agenetic porencephaly

Definitions

- Clefts in brain parenchyma that extend from cortical surface to ventricle (pia to ependyma), lined by dysplastic gray matter (GM)

IMAGING

General Features

- Best diagnostic clue
  - Transmantle gray matter lining clefts
    - Look for dimple in wall of ventricle if cleft is narrow/closed
- Location
  - Frontal and parietal lobes near central sulcus
- Size
  - "Closed-lip" (small defect) or "open-lip" (large defect)
- Morphology
  - Up to 1/2 of schizencephalies are bilateral
    - When bilateral, 60% are "open-lipped" on both sides

CT Findings

- NECT
  - Cleft of CSF density (in "open-lip" schizencephaly)
  - GM lining clefts may appear hyperdense
  - Dimple on lateral wall of lateral ventricle indicating ependymal margin of cleft
  - Ca++ when associated with cytomegalovirus (CMV)
  - Thinning and expansion of calvarium can be seen with large "open-lipped" clefts
- CECT
  - Large, primitive-appearing veins near cleft

MR Findings

- T1WI
  - Distinction of GM lining cleft can be difficult prior to myelination
  - "Closed-lip" → irregular tract of GM extending from cortical surface to ventricle
    - Lining GM can appear dysplastic → lumpy/bumpy on margin of cleft or at gray-white interface
  - "Open lip" → can be wide and wedge-shaped or with nearly parallel walls
    - GM lining cleft may be harder to discern than in "closed-lip"
- T2WI
  - Infolding of gray matter along transmantle clefts
    - Prior to myelination T2WI more clearly defines lesion
- FLAIR
  - Gliotic foci present in later insults
- T2* GRE
  - May show Ca++ when associated with CMV
- MRV
  - Developmental venous anomalies (DVAs) overlying cleft
- 3D surface rendered MR
  - Clearly shows relationship of adjacent gyri/sulci to cleft in cerebral mantle
- fMR: Functional reorganization of undamaged hemisphere reported

Ultrasonographic Findings

- Grayscale ultrasound
  - Diagnosable by fetal ultrasound and fetal MR; progressive changes have been reported

Nuclear Medicine Findings

- PET
  - Normal or ↑ glucose metabolism and perfusion of wall of cleft (normal gray matter activity)

Imaging Recommendations

- Best imaging tool
  - MR
- Protocol advice
  - Younger than 9 months → rely on T2WI
  - Older than 9 months → rely on T1WI
  - Volumetric acquisitions that allow multiplanar reformatting and surface rendering

DIFFERENTIAL DIAGNOSIS

Encephaloclastic Porencephaly

- Cleft in brain due to insult after migration complete
- Lined by gliotic white matter (WM), not dysplastic GM

Hydranencephaly

- Destruction of tissue in middle and anterior cerebral artery territory
  - Residual tissue is supplied by posterior circulation → posterior fossa, occipital poles, medial temporal lobes
- Severe schizencephaly with hydrocephalus can strongly mimic; may be a continuum

Semilobar Holoprosencephaly

- Can mimic bilateral "open-lip" schizencephaly

PATHOLOGY

General Features

- Etiology
  - Can be result of acquired in utero insult affecting germinal zone prior to neuronal migration
    - Infection (CMV), vascular insult, maternal trauma, toxin
    - Reported with alloimmune thrombocytopenia
    - Experimental schizencephaly induced by mumps virus
- Genetics
  - *EMX2* (gene locus 10q26.1) has been reported in some familial cases
    - Regulatory gene with role in structural patterning of developing forebrain
    - Expressed in germinal matrix of developing neocortex
  - Multiple other studies have shown no association with *EMX2* mutations
- Associated abnormalities

- Septooptic dysplasia (SOD), de Morsier syndrome
  - Heterogeneous disorder characterized by hypoplasia of optic nerves and absent septum pellucidum
    - 45% have pituitary insufficiency
  - Schizencephaly seen in up to 35%, usually bilateral
  - Septum pellucidum is absent in large percentage of schizencephaly cases, especially bilateral schizencephaly
- Frontal lobe dysplasia
- Hippocampal and callosal anomalies

Staging, Grading, & Classification

- Type 1 ("closed-lip")
  - 15-20%
- Type 2 ("open-lip")
  - 80-85%

Gross Pathologic & Surgical Features

- Transmantle clefts with separated or apposed gray matter lining
- Thalami, corticospinal tracts may be atrophied or not formed

Microscopic Features

- Little if any glial scarring
- Loss of normal laminar architecture
- Pachygyria, polymicrogyria, or heterotopic gray matter

CLINICAL ISSUES

Presentation

- Most common signs/symptoms
  - Unilateral: Seizures or mild motor deficit ("congenital" hemiparesis)
  - Bilateral: Developmental delay, paresis, microcephaly, spasticity
    - Seizure more common with unilateral clefts
- Other signs/symptoms
  - Psychiatric disorders
  - Perisylvian syndrome
    - Pseudobulbar palsy

Demographics

- Epidemiology
  - 1.54/100,000
  - 1/3 of children with schizencephaly have non-CNS abnormalities
    - > 50% likely due to vascular disruption
      - Gastroschisis, bowel atresias, and amniotic band disruption sequence

Natural History & Prognosis

- Malformation is stable; development of epilepsy common
- Size of clefts and presence of associated malformative lesions govern severity of impairment

Treatment

- Treat seizures and hydrocephalus
  - Lesionectomy, hemispherectomy

DIAGNOSTIC CHECKLIST

Consider

- Image to confirm etiology of "congenital hemiparesis"
  - Perinatal stroke vs. unilateral schizencephaly

Image Interpretation Pearls

- Multiplanar imaging to avoid "in-plane" oversight of "closed-lip" clefts
  - If plane of imaging is same as plane of cleft, abnormality may be overlooked
- Contours of lateral walls of lateral ventricles should be smooth
  - Dimples may indicate subtle "closed-lip" schizencephaly
- Absence of septum pellucidum should prompt thorough investigation for schizencephaly &/or polymicrogyria
- Consider large bilateral "open-lip" schizencephaly when diagnosis semilobar holoprosencephaly or hydranencephaly

SELECTED REFERENCES

1. da Rocha FF et al: Borderline personality features possibly related to cingulate and orbitofrontal cortices dysfunction due to schizencephaly. Clin Neurol Neurosurg. 110(4):396-9, 2008
2. Heuer GG et al: Anatomic hemispherectomy for intractable epilepsy in a patient with unilateral schizencephaly. J Neurosurg Pediatr. 2(2):146-9, 2008
3. Merello E et al: No major role for the EMX2 gene in schizencephaly. Am J Med Genet A. 146A(9):1142-50, 2008
4. Vinayan KP et al: A case of congenital bilateral perisylvian syndrome due to bilateral schizencephaly. Epileptic Disord. 9(2):190-3, 2007
5. Witters I et al: Prenatal diagnosis of schizencephaly after inhalation of organic solvents. Ultrasound Obstet Gynecol. 29(3):356-7, 2007
6. Huang WM et al: Schizencephaly in a dysgenetic fetal brain: prenatal sonographic, magnetic resonance imaging, and postmortem correlation. J Ultrasound Med. 25(4):551-4, 2006
7. Curry CJ et al: Schizencephaly: heterogeneous etiologies in a population of 4 million California births. Am J Med Genet A. 137(2):181-9, 2005
8. Cecchi C: Emx2: a gene responsible for cortical development, regionalization and area specification. Gene. 291(1-2):1-9, 2002
9. Dale ST et al: Neonatal alloimmune thrombocytopenia: antenatal and postnatal imaging findings in the pediatric brain. AJNR Am J Neuroradiol. 23(9):1457-65, 2002
10. Vandermeeren Y et al: Functional relevance of abnormal fMRI activation pattern after unilateral schizencephaly. Neuroreport. 13(14):1821-4, 2002
11. Takano T et al: Experimental schizencephaly induced by Kilham strain of mumps virus: pathogenesis of cleft formation. Neuroreport. 10(15):3149-54, 1999

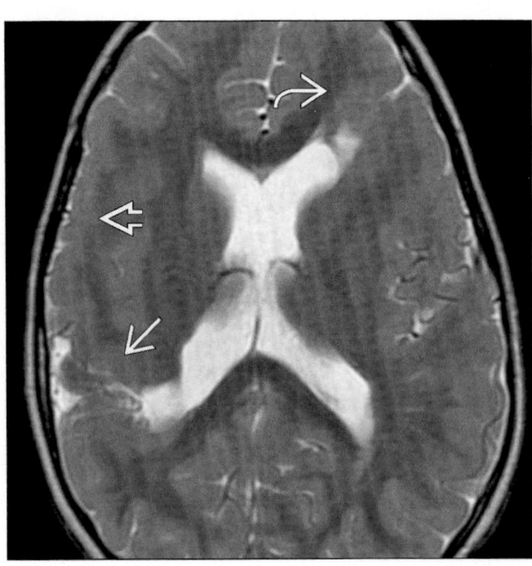

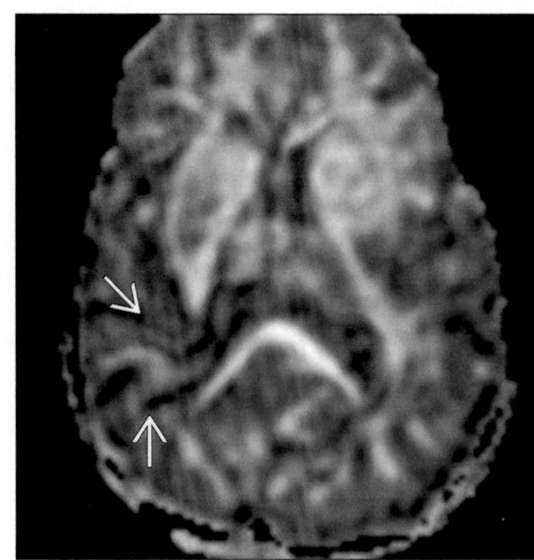

(Left) *Axial T2WI MR in a 2 year old with seizures and developmental delay shows 2 "closed-lip" schizencephalic clefts, 1 in the right parietal lobe and 1 in the left frontal lobe. Note additional cortical dysplasia extending anteriorly along the frontal lobe from the right-sided cleft.* ***(Right)*** *Axial fractional anisotropy map from DTI in the same child shows disruption of WM tracts at the site of the right parietal cleft. This image is inferior to the WM distortion on the left.*

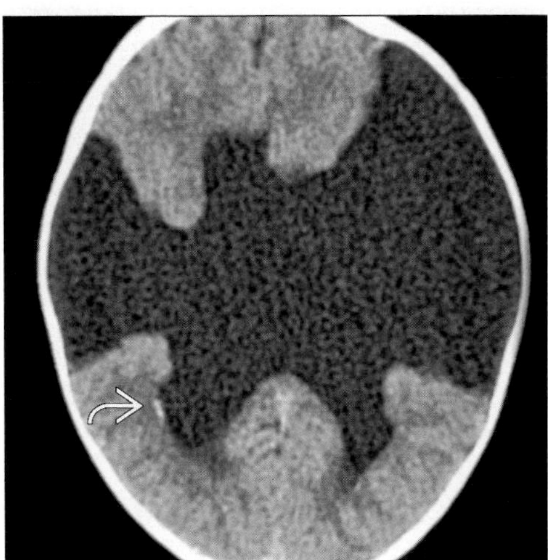

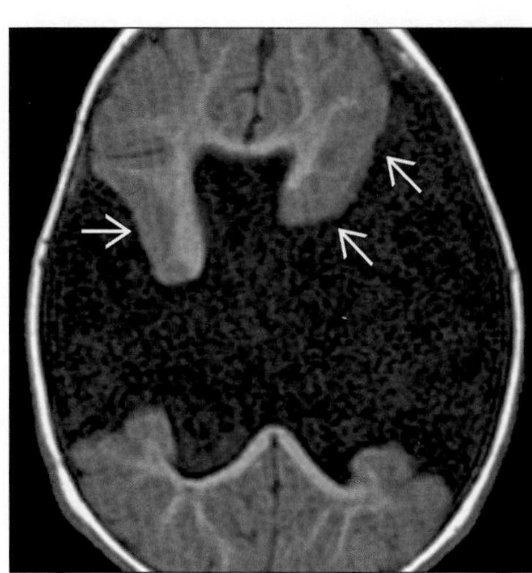

(Left) *Axial NECT shows a "bat wing" configuration of the lateral ventricles due to bilateral large "open-lipped" schizencephaly. Note the dystrophic calcification bordering the right lateral ventricle wall, suggesting a history of intrauterine CMV infection as the source of this child's migrational abnormality.* ***(Right)*** *Axial T1WI MR in the same child shows the abnormally thick and featureless cortex lining the schizencephalic clefts, as well as absence of the septum pellucidum.*

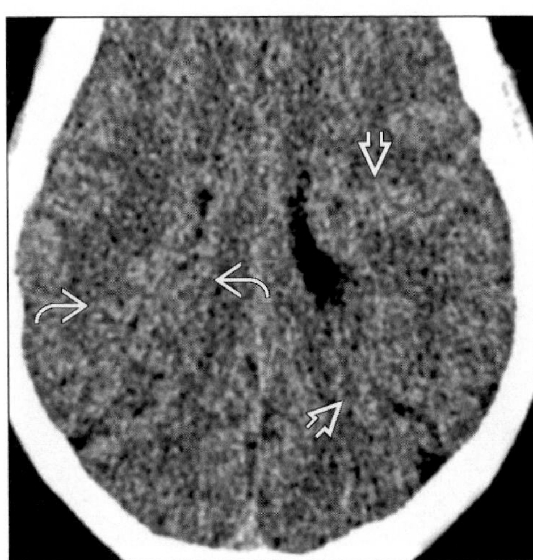

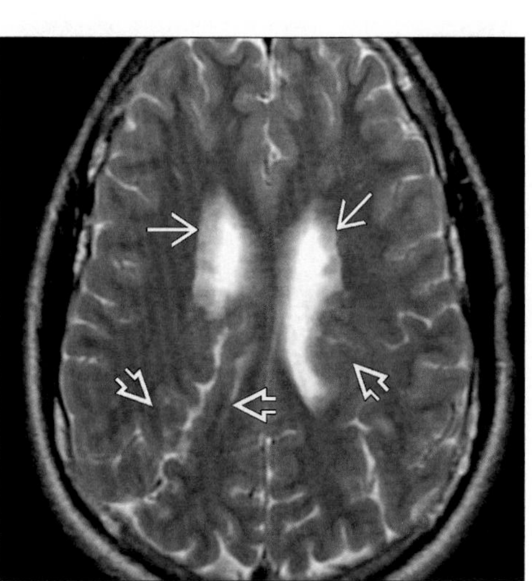

(Left) *Axial NECT in a 9 year old with seizures shows abnormal gray matter extending from the hemispheric surface to the lateral ventricle at the right frontal-parietal junction. Additional regions of abnormal gray matter can be seen on the left.* ***(Right)*** *Axial T2WI MR in the same child shows more clearly that the thickened, irregular gray matter lines schizencephalic clefts in each hemisphere. Additional foci of heterotopic gray matter can be seen in each lateral ventricle.*

HEMIMEGALENCEPHALY

Key Facts

Terminology
- Hamartomatous overgrowth of part/all of hemisphere
- Defect of cellular organization, neuronal migration

Imaging
- Large cerebral hemisphere, hemicranium
  - Posterior falx and occipital pole "swing" to contralateral side
  - Lateral ventricle is large with abnormally shaped frontal horn
- Frequently increased WM signal
  - "Accelerated myelination" → mineralization; disorganized heterotopic neurons cause T1/T2 shortening
- Lateral ventricle is usually large and frontal horn is pointed
- Size and signal intensity of affected hemisphere change over time
  - May atrophy and become hypointense with constant seizure activity
- Serial imaging may be required to document full extent of abnormality
- Status of contralateral hemisphere key for clinical decision-making

Pathology
- Giant neurons, balloon cells, hypertrophic/atypical cells
- White matter hypertrophy and gliosis

Clinical Issues
- Anticonvulsants usually ineffective
- Anatomic or functional hemispherectomy
  - Anatomic hemispherectomy may require shunting of surgical cavity

*(**Left**) Axial T2WI MR shows a thickened and hypointense insular cortex, abnormal hyperintense signal in the basal ganglia and external capsule, and nodular foci of dysplastic gray matter lining the left lateral ventricle ➔ in this child with left-sided hemimegalencephaly. Heterogeneity of pathology is characteristic of this entity, making the etiology uncertain. (**Right**) Axial F-18 FDG PET in the same patient shows decreased glucose metabolism throughout the affected left hemisphere.*

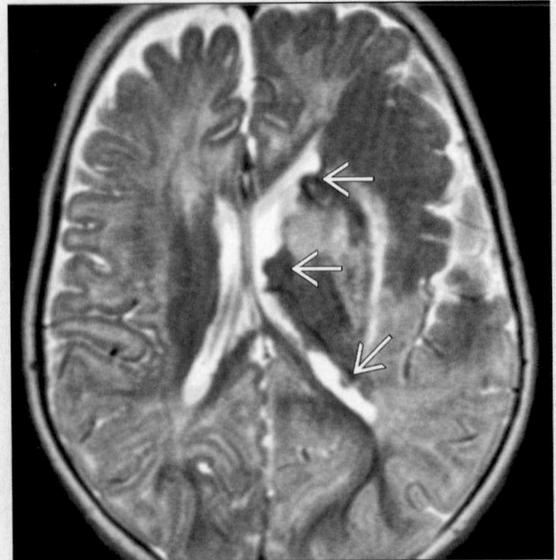

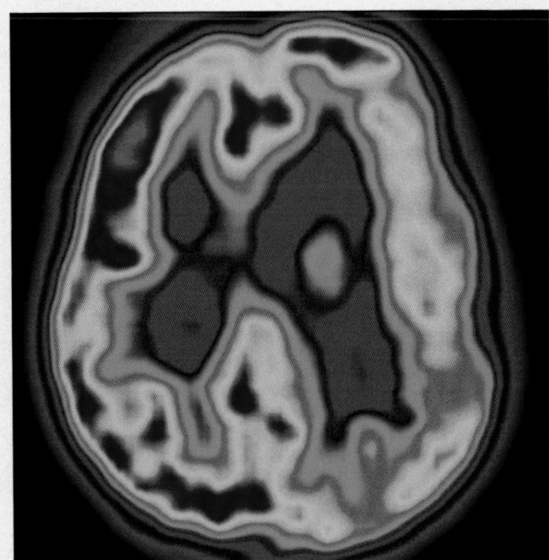

*(**Left**) Axial T2WI MR of a 33-week fetus shows enlargement of the entire left cerebral hemisphere with an associated enlarged occipital horn. Note the primitive venous structure ➔ overlying the sylvian fissure. (**Right**) Axial FLAIR MR shows extensive bright signal in the white matter of the abnormal left hemisphere, reflecting gliosis and disorganized neuronal and glial elements. Hemimegalencephaly is the only disorder that enlarges both the cerebral hemisphere and the ipsilateral ventricle.*

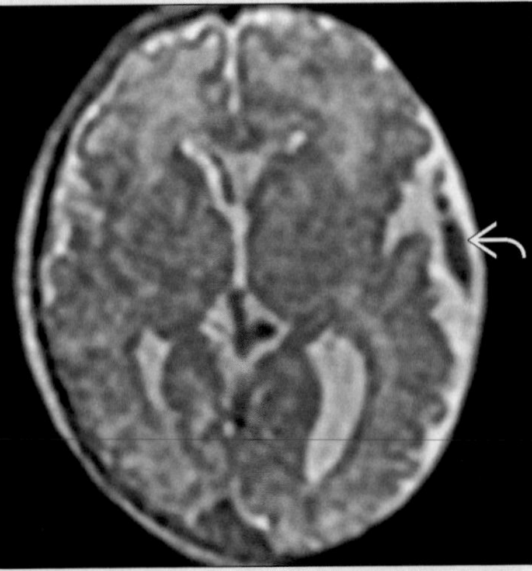

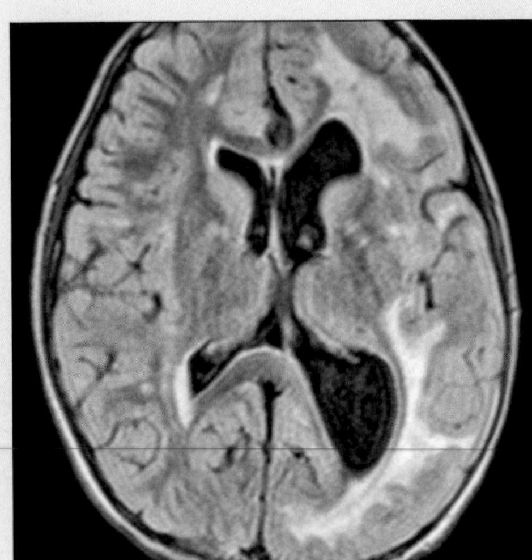

HEMIMEGALENCEPHALY

TERMINOLOGY

Abbreviations

- Hemimegalencephaly (HME)

Synonyms

- Unilateral megalencephaly
- Focal megalencephaly

Definitions

- Hamartomatous overgrowth of part/all of hemisphere
- Defect of cellular organization, neuronal migration

IMAGING

General Features

- Best diagnostic clue
  - Mild, moderate, or markedly enlarged dysplastic hemisphere
  - Dysplastic cortex, abnormal gyri
  - Displaced posterior falx
  - Large lateral ventricle with abnormally shaped frontal horn
- Location
  - Occipital common (any lobe may be involved)
    - Infrequently involves ipsilateral cerebellum
- Size
  - Usually grossly enlarged, can be subtle
- Morphology
  - Variable, usually broad gyri, shallow sulci

CT Findings

- NECT
  - Large cerebral hemisphere, hemicranium
  - Posterior falx and occipital pole "swing" to contralateral side
  - Lateral ventricle is large with abnormally shaped frontal horn
  - Dystrophic Ca++ of white matter (WM) or of thickened cortex
- CECT
  - Large vessels common

MR Findings

- T1WI
  - Thickened cortex
  - Frequently increased WM signal
    - "Accelerated myelination" → mineralization; disorganized heterotopic neurons cause T1 shortening
  - Neuronal heterotopias, subependymal, ± scattered throughout hemisphere
  - Lateral ventricle is usually large and frontal horn is pointed
  - ± Chiari 1 (bulky supratentorial brain tissue displaces tonsils)
- T2WI
  - Pachygyria, polymicrogyria
  - Size and signal intensity of affected hemisphere change over time
    - May atrophy and become hypointense with constant seizure activity
  - Margins between gray-white matter often blurred
    - Dysplastic neurons scattered throughout white matter
  - ± cerebellar hemiovergrowth, heterotopias
- FLAIR
  - Gliosis-like bright signal in white matter
- T2* GRE
  - Dystrophic calcifications
- DWI
  - DTI can show abnormal fiber tracts connecting hemispheres
    - Helpful for assessing residual connections after functional hemispherectomy
- T1WI C+
  - May have bizarre enhancement
  - Enhancement of primitive cortical veins, developmental venous anomalies
- MRS
  - With seizures, progressive ↓ NAA and ↑ creatine, choline, and myoinositol
- Magnetoencephalography (MEG)
  - Somatosensory maps predict severity of cortical lamination defects

Ultrasonographic Findings

- Grayscale ultrasound
  - Diagnosis can be made in fetus and neonate

Nuclear Medicine Findings

- PET
  - Glucose hypometabolism in 50%
- SPECT
  - Increased or decreased tracer uptake in affected side

Imaging Recommendations

- Best imaging tool
  - Multiplanar MR
- Protocol advice
  - Serial imaging may be required to document full extent of abnormality
    - Abnormal regions become more apparent with myelination of normal areas
  - Abnormal signal in WM may be best indicator of extent of abnormality
  - Status of contralateral hemisphere key for clinical decision-making

DIFFERENTIAL DIAGNOSIS

Type 1 Lissencephaly

- Bilateral agyria & pachygyria without true overgrowth
- Overlap with band heterotopia

Rasmussen Encephalitis

- Unilateral encephalitis with progressive atrophy
- Almost always unilateral

Tuberous Sclerosis (TS)

- HME of lobe or hemisphere = occasional manifestation
- Heavy burden of tubers can mimic HME
  - Bilaterally distributed

Gliomatosis Cerebri

- Diffusely infiltrating glioma

- Rare in children
  - Multicentric glioma more common

PATHOLOGY

General Features

- Etiology
  - Abnormal proliferation, migration, and differentiation of neurons
  - Embryology
    - Insult to developing brain causes development of too many synapses, persistence of supernumerary axons, and potential for white matter overgrowth
    - Localized epidermal growth factor (EGF) in cortical neurons and glial cells may lead to excessive proliferation
      - Variable patterns of overgrowth, gliosis reflect variability in timing of precipitating insult
- Genetics
  - Significant overlap with tuberous sclerosis
  - Syndromic hemimegalencephaly with somatic hemihypertrophy (30%)
    - Klippel-Trenaunay-Weber
    - Proteus syndrome
    - Hypomelanosis of Ito
- Associated abnormalities
  - Optic nerve (ipsilateral) enlargement
  - Ipsilateral brainstem enlargement
  - Cerebellar enlargement and dysplasia

Gross Pathologic & Surgical Features

- Large hemisphere, shallow sulci, fused and disorganized gyri
- Regional polymicrogyria, pachygyria, and heterotopias

Microscopic Features

- Giant neurons, loss of horizontal layering of neurons
- Balloon cells, hypertrophic/atypical cells
  - Few lysosomes, microfilaments, microtubules
  - Variable reactivity for neuronal and glial proteins
  - Abundant lipofuscin granules
- White matter hypertrophy and gliosis
- Dystrophic calcifications
- Contralateral hemisphere may harbor occult heterotopias and cortical dysplasia
- Platelet-activating factor (role in neuronal migration) reported absent in hemimegalencephaly specimens

CLINICAL ISSUES

Presentation

- Most common signs/symptoms
  - Seizures, developmental delay
  - Macrocrania
- Other signs/symptoms
  - Hemiparesis, hemihypertrophy
- Clinical profile
  - Early seizures
  - Severe developmental delay and contralateral hemiparesis common

Demographics

- Age
  - Usually diagnosed during 1st year of life
- Epidemiology
  - ~ 3% of cortical dysplasias that are diagnosed by imaging

Natural History & Prognosis

- Intractable seizures with progressive hemiparesis
- Poor outcome → intractable seizures and developmental delay

Treatment

- Anticonvulsants usually ineffective
- Anatomic or functional hemispherectomy
  - Confirm normal contralateral hemisphere first!
  - Anatomic hemispherectomy may require shunting of surgical cavity
    - Significant risk of shunt malfunctions

DIAGNOSTIC CHECKLIST

Consider

- Involved hemisphere may atrophy (effect of chronic seizures)

Image Interpretation Pearls

- Serial imaging shows remarkable signal transformation with myelin maturation
- Hemimegalencephaly is only condition in which increase in parenchymal volume is associated with increase in ipsilateral ventricle volume

Reporting Tips

- Goals of imaging → identify/quantify lesion, identify contralateral abnormalities

SELECTED REFERENCES

1. Guerra MP et al: Intractable epilepsy in hemimegalencephaly and tuberous sclerosis complex. J Child Neurol. 22(1):80-4, 2007
2. Di Rocco C et al: Hemimegalencephaly: clinical implications and surgical treatment. Childs Nerv Syst. 22(8):852-66, 2006
3. Soufflet C et al: The nonmalformed hemisphere is secondarily impaired in young children with hemimegalencephaly: a pre- and postsurgery study with SPECT and EEG. Epilepsia. 45(11):1375-82, 2004
4. Flores-Sarnat L et al: Hemimegalencephaly: part 2. Neuropathology suggests a disorder of cellular lineage. J Child Neurol. 18(11):776-85, 2003
5. Flores-Sarnat L: Hemimegalencephaly: part 1. Genetic, clinical, and imaging aspects. J Child Neurol. 17(5):373-84; discussion 384, 2002
6. Ishibashi H et al: Somatosensory evoked magnetic fields in hemimegalencephaly. Neurol Res. 24(5):459-62, 2002
7. Di Rocco F et al: Hemimegalencephaly involving the cerebellum. Pediatr Neurosurg. 35(5):274-6, 2001
8. Hoffmann KT et al: MRI and 18F-fluorodeoxyglucose positron emission tomography in hemimegalencephaly. Neuroradiology. 42(10):749-52, 2000

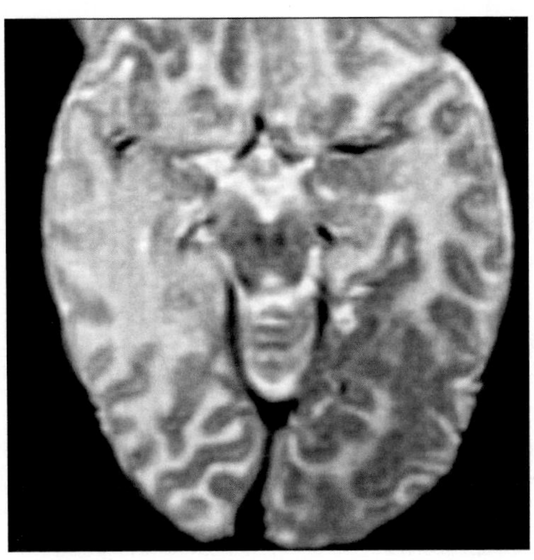

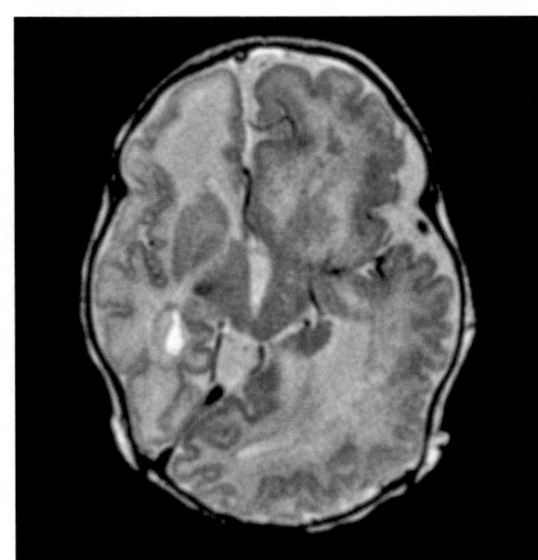

(Left) *Axial T2WI MR in a neonate with seizures shows overgrowth of the left occipital pole with abnormal sulcation and abnormal hypointense signal, reflecting focal megalencephaly.* ***(Right)*** *Axial T2WI MR in another neonate with hemimegalencephaly shows a dramatic rightward "swing" of the posterior falx due to overgrowth of the left temporal and occipital lobes. The "dirty" appearance of the unmyelinated white matter in the left hemisphere reflects the presence of heterotopic and dysplastic neurons.*

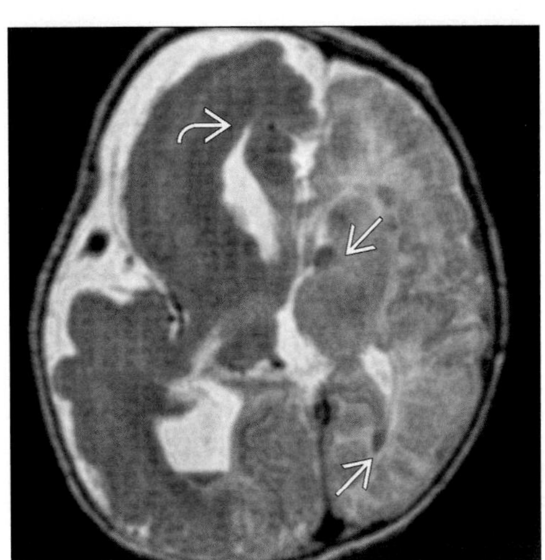

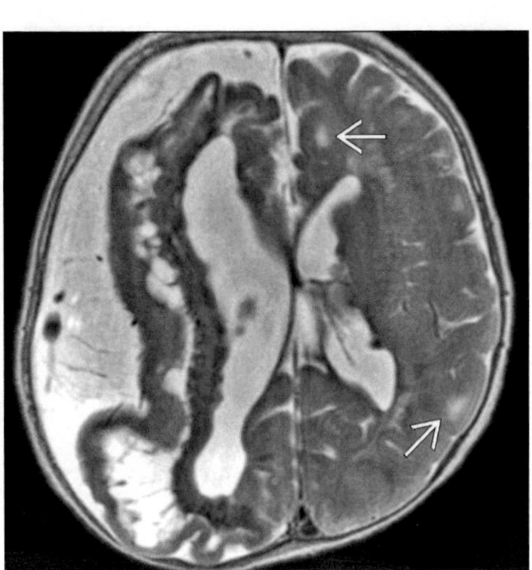

(Left) *Axial T2WI MR in a neonate with tuberous sclerosis shows HME of right cerebrum, with a thickened cortex and characteristic pointing of the frontal horn ↪. Note the subependymal nodules in the left lateral ventricle →. TS is 1 of several overgrowth syndromes associated with HME.* ***(Right)*** *Axial T2WI MR in the same patient 1 year later shows dramatic atrophy of the right cerebral hemisphere secondary to unremitting seizure activity. Subcortical tubers in the left hemisphere → are now more evident.*

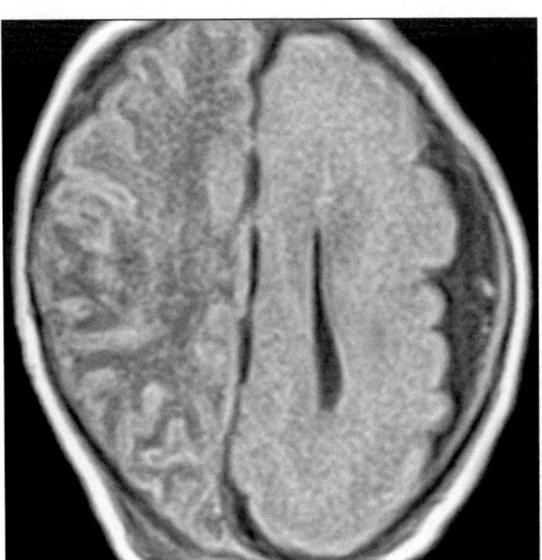

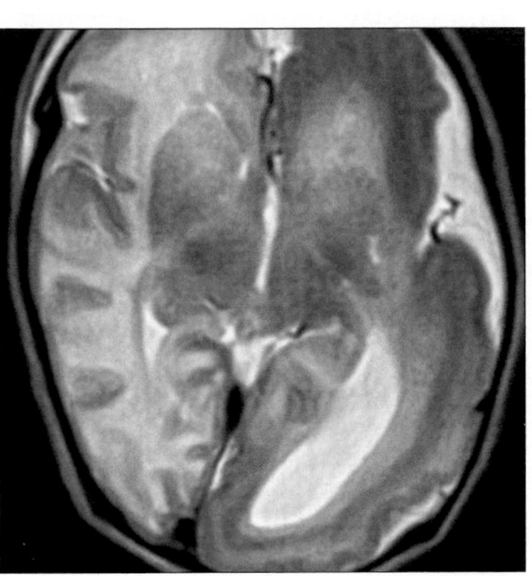

(Left) *Axial T1WI MR in a neonate with hemimegalencephaly shows a lack of gray-white differentiation in the affected left hemisphere, despite the "accelerated myelination" in the white matter. The increased signal may not represent myelin deposition.* ***(Right)*** *Axial T2WI MR in a child with left hemisphere hemimegalencephaly shows alternating bands of hypo- and hyperintense signal reminiscent of band heterotopia in the occipital lobe. The morphology of HME varies considerably.*

NEUROFIBROMATOSIS TYPE 1

Key Facts

Terminology

- NF1, von Recklinghausen disease, peripheral neurofibromatosis

Imaging

- FASI on T2WI in 70-90% of preteen children
- Plexiform neurofibromas
- Optic pathway gliomas
- Parenchymal gliomas
- Sphenoid wing and occipital bone dysplasia found in association with plexiform tumors
- WM lesions may also involve cerebellar white matter, globus pallidus, thalamus, brainstem
- WM lesions are hyperintense and typically poorly defined; no mass effect
- Vascular dysplasias → stenosis, moyamoya, aneurysm

Pathology

- Autosomal dominant; gene locus is chromosome 17q12
- *NF* gene product is neurofibromin (negative regulator of RAS protooncogene)
  - Neurofibromin also regulates neuroglial progenitor function
  - Required for normal glial and neuronal development
- Foci of myelin vacuolization, proliferation of protoplasmic astroglia, microcalcifications

Clinical Issues

- ~ 50% have macrocephaly; in part 2° ↑ WM volume
- OPG can cause progressive vision loss
- Café au lait spots are earliest finding
- Most common neurocutaneous and inherited tumor syndrome

*(Left) Axial graphic shows enlarged right middle cranial fossa, dysplastic sphenoid wing, and a large orbital/periorbital plexiform neurofibroma. Note the exophthalmos and buphthalmos of the involved globe ➲. **(Right)** Axial T2WI FS MR shows an extensive plexiform neurofibroma ➔ of the right orbit and temporal region. The right sphenoid wing is eroded, with resulting exophthalmos of the right globe ➲. The affected right globe is enlarged (bupthlalmos).*

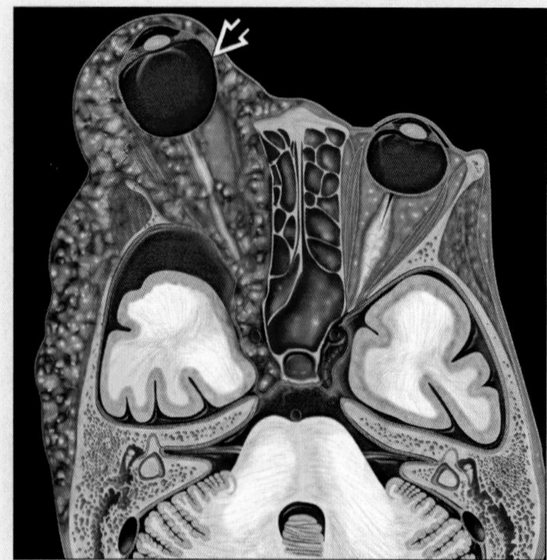

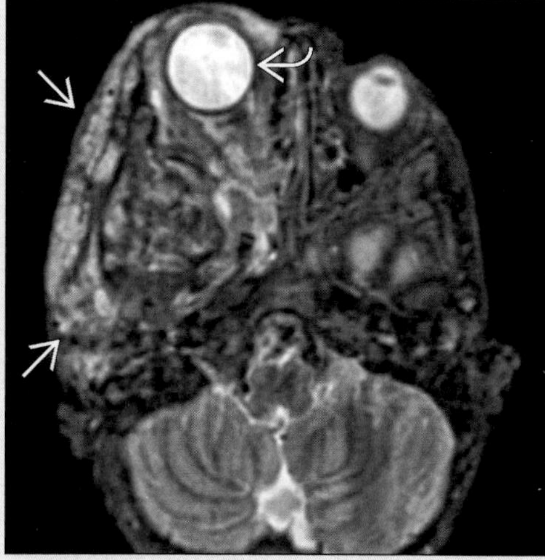

*(Left) Axial T2WI MR shows an optic pathway glioma infiltrating the chiasm ➔, the optic tracts ➔ within the suprasellar cistern, and the medial temporal lobes ➲. The tumor was identified at the time of a screening MR exam of the brain of this 21-month-old infant with newly diagnosed NF1. **(Right)** Axial T1WI MR of the same patient reveals near complete enhancement of the chiasmatic and optic tract ➔ components. Enhancement of the temporal lobe components is incomplete.*

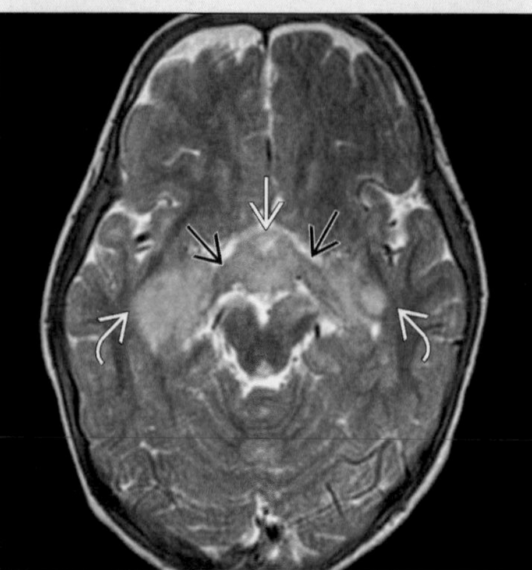

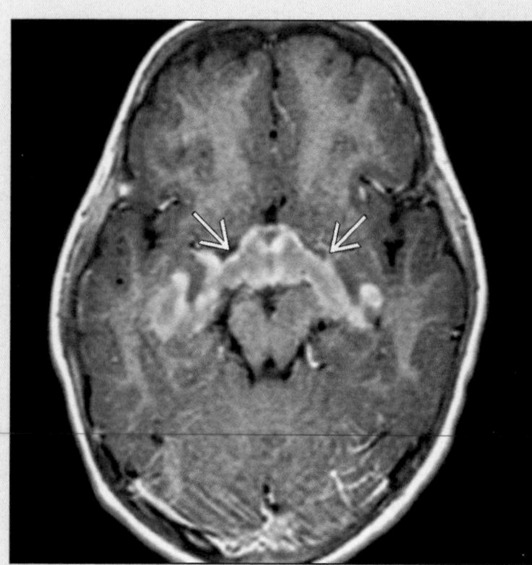

NEUROFIBROMATOSIS TYPE 1

TERMINOLOGY

Abbreviations

- Neurofibromatosis type 1 (NF1)

Synonyms

- von Recklinghausen disease, peripheral neurofibromatosis

Definitions

- Neurocutaneous disorder (phakomatosis) characterized by
  - Waxing/waning dysplastic white matter (WM) lesions
    - Sometimes called focal areas of signal intensity (FASI), nonspecific bright foci, unidentified bright objects (UBOs)
  - Optic nerve glioma (ONG)
  - Optic pathway glioma (OPG): Chiasm/tract ± nerve
  - Other gliomas: Brainstem, cerebral hemisphere, basal ganglia
  - Neurofibromas/plexiform neurofibromas (PNF)
  - Vascular dysplasias
  - Hyperpigmented macules (café au lait spots)
  - Dysplastic skeletal lesions

IMAGING

General Features

- Best diagnostic clue
  - FASI on T2WI in 70-90% of preteen children
  - Plexiform neurofibromas
  - Optic pathway gliomas
- Location
  - WM lesions may also involve cerebellar white matter, globus pallidus, thalamus, brainstem
  - Plexiform lesions often apparent on brain imaging
    - Scalp lesions over occiput
    - Skull base lesions extending into retropharynx
    - Orbital lesions extending from cavernous sinus through orbit into periorbital soft tissues
  - OPG in 15% → intraorbital optic nerves (ON), chiasm/hypothalamus, optic tracts; rarely into radiations
- Size
  - WM lesions: 2-20 mm
  - Chiasmatic glioma: 3-50 mm
  - Brainstem can show moderate to marked enlargement ("hamartoma")
    - Probably result of vacuolation
    - Less T1 hypointense and T2 hyperintense than brain stem glioma
    - Resolves in teen years/young adulthood
  - Plexiform lesions can be massive
- Morphology
  - WM lesions: Spherical/ovoid, often amorphous
  - ONG: Conform to and enlarge ON and chiasm; can be spherical in chiasm and hypothalamus

Radiographic Findings

- Radiography
  - Sphenoid wing and occipital bone dysplasia found in association with plexiform tumors

CT Findings

- NECT: Sphenoid dysplasia with associated enlargement of middle cranial fossa, ipsilateral proptosis
  - Enlarged optic nerve/chiasm
- CTA: Vascular dysplasias → stenosis, moyamoya, aneurysm

MR Findings

- T1WI
  - WM lesions usually isointense to surrounding tissue
    - Irregular hyperintensity may reflect myelin clumping or microcalcification
- T2WI
  - WM lesions are hyperintense and typically poorly defined; no mass effect
    - T2WI may be more sensitive than FLAIR for WM lesions in cerebellum
  - ONG iso-/hyperintense to normal parenchyma
  - ↑ T2 signal and mild-moderate enlargement of hippocampi (uni- or bilateral)
- STIR
  - Excellent definition of plexiform/paraspinal neurofibromas
- DWI
  - ↑ ADC values in FASI compared to normal-appearing white matter (NAWM)
  - ↑ ADC values in NF NAWM compared to controls
    - Reflects accumulation of fluid or vacuolation within myelin sheath
  - ↓ FA in adult NF1 brains compared to healthy brains
- T1WI C+
  - WM lesions/FASI do not enhance
    - Enhancement raises concern for neoplasm
  - Plexiform lesions have variable enhancement
    - Less well defined than on STIR images
  - Visual pathway gliomas have variable enhancement
    - Significance of ↓ enhancement in response to treatment uncertain
- T1WI C+ FS
  - Best sequence for evaluation of ONG
- MRA
  - Useful in evaluation of vascular lesions
- MRS
  - Benefit in evaluation of WM lesions to distinguish from visual pathway glioma
    - WM lesions have relative preservation of NAA
    - Glioma have ↓ NAA with elevated choline

Angiographic Findings

- Most vascular lesions non-CNS, caused by vascular intimal proliferation
  - Aneurysms/AVMs, renal artery stenosis, aortic stenosis/coarctation; moyamoya

Imaging Recommendations

- Best imaging tool
  - MR
    - Benefit of routine surveillance imaging controversial
    - Coronal STIR sequences essential when imaging spine or head and neck
- Protocol advice
  - Include fat-saturated post-contrast imaging of orbits

- Consider MRA if moyamoya suspected

DIFFERENTIAL DIAGNOSIS

Demyelinating Disease

- Lesions of acute disseminated encephalomyelitis or multiple sclerosis mimic WM lesions of NF1

Viral Encephalitis

- Ebstein-Barr (EBV), cytomegalovirus (CMV)

Gliomatosis Cerebri

- If FASI are extensive

Mitochondrial Encephalopathies

- Pantothenate kinase-associated neurodegeneration (PKAN, Hallervorden-Spatz), Leigh syndrome, glutaric acidurias, Kearns-Sayre syndrome
- Often have lesions in basal ganglia or thalami that resemble WM lesions of NF1

Krabbe Disease (Globoid Cell Leukodystrophy)

- Can cause optic nerve enlargement mimicking ONG

PATHOLOGY

General Features

- Etiology
  - *NF* gene product is neurofibromin (negative regulator of RAS protooncogene)
    - Inactivated in NF1 → tissue proliferation, tumor development
  - Neurofibromin also regulates neuroglial progenitor function
    - Required for normal glial and neuronal development
  - Oligodendrocyte myelin glycoprotein also embedded in *NF1* gene
- Genetics
  - AD; gene locus on chromosome 17q12
    - Penetrance = 100%
  - ~ 50% new mutations

Staging, Grading, & Classification

- 2 or more of following fulfills diagnostic criteria for NF1
  - 6+ café au lait spots measuring ≥ 15 mm in adults or 5 mm in children
  - 2+ neurofibromas or 1 plexiform neurofibroma
  - Axillary/inguinal freckling
  - Visual pathway glioma
  - 2+ Lisch nodules
  - Distinctive bony lesion (sphenoid wing dysplasia, thinning of long bone ± pseudoarthrosis)
  - 1st-degree relative with NF1

Gross Pathologic & Surgical Features

- Gliomas usually pilocytic astrocytomas
  - Frankly malignant in < 20%
- Slight ↑ incidence of medulloblastoma/ependymoma
- Rare subependymal glial nodules
  - Can result in CSF obstruction

Microscopic Features

- WM lesions (FASI)
  - Foci of myelin vacuolization, proliferation of protoplasmic astroglia, microcalcifications
  - No demyelination or inflammation

CLINICAL ISSUES

Presentation

- Most common signs/symptoms
  - Café au lait spots are earliest finding
  - ~ 50% have macrocephaly; in part 2° ↑ WM volume
  - OPG can cause progressive vision loss

Demographics

- Epidemiology
  - Incidence is 1:3,000-5,000
  - Most common neurocutaneous syndrome
  - Most common inherited tumor syndrome

Natural History & Prognosis

- Morbidity related to specific manifestations
  - OPG → vision loss/blindness, hypothalamic dysfunction
  - Plexiform NF → risk of sarcomatous degeneration
  - Paraspinal NF → kyphoscoliosis
  - Vascular stenoses → hypertension (renal artery), stroke
- FASI increase in number/size in 1st decade of life, regress afterwards; rarely seen in adults
- NF1-related learning disability in 40-60%
- Visual pathway gliomas in NF1 often have more indolent clinical course than sporadic optic glioma

Treatment

- Clinical observation
- Chemotherapy and radiation for OPG

DIAGNOSTIC CHECKLIST

Consider

- Absence of visible stigmata does not exclude NF1
- Be aware of potential for vascular lesions

SELECTED REFERENCES

1. Cairns AG et al: Cerebrovascular dysplasia in neurofibromatosis type 1. J Neurol Neurosurg Psychiatry. 79(10):1165-70, 2008
2. van Engelen SJ et al: Quantitative differentiation between healthy and disordered brain matter in patients with neurofibromatosis type I using diffusion tensor imaging. AJNR Am J Neuroradiol. 29(4):816-22, 2008
3. Hegedus B et al: Neurofibromatosis-1 regulates neuronal and glial cell differentiation from neuroglial progenitors in vivo by both cAMP- and Ras-dependent mechanisms. Cell Stem Cell. 1(4):443-57, 2007
4. Hyman SL et al: The nature and frequency of cognitive deficits in children with neurofibromatosis type 1. Neurology. 65(7):1037-44, 2005

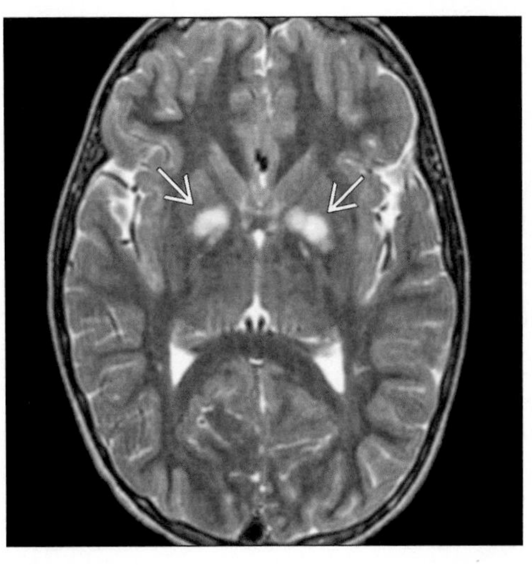

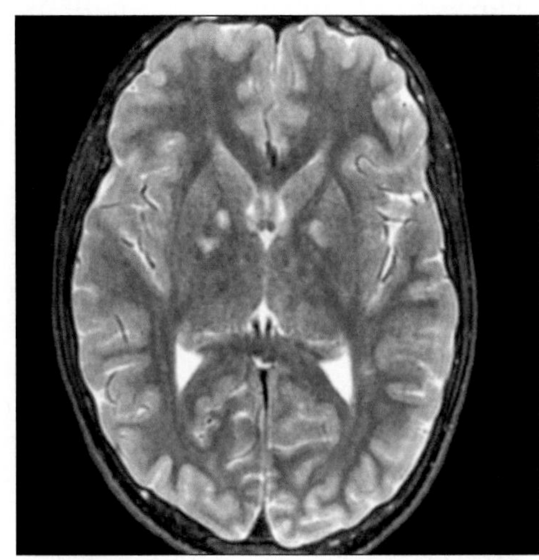

(Left) *Axial T2WI MR shows characteristic T2 bright foci encountered in pediatric patients with NF1. Note the hyperintensity ➔ in the bilateral globi pallidi of this 7-year-old child. Little or no mass effect is appreciable. No abnormal enhancement was seen on the T1 C+ images.* ***(Right)*** *Axial T2WI FS MR in the same patient 4 years later shows the characteristic T2 bright foci within the globi pallidi are smaller, suggesting that a reparative/"healing" process is on-going.*

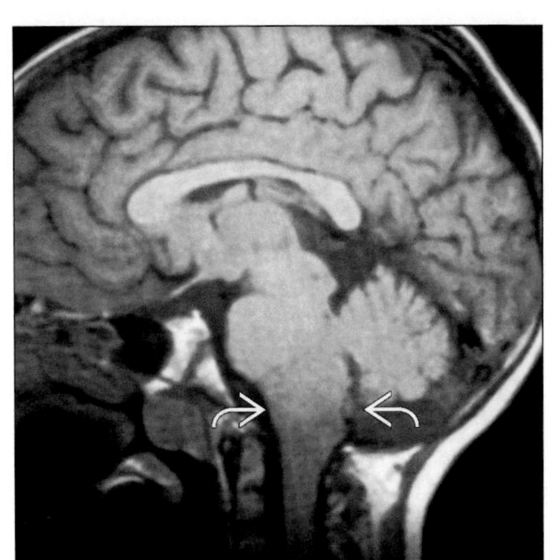

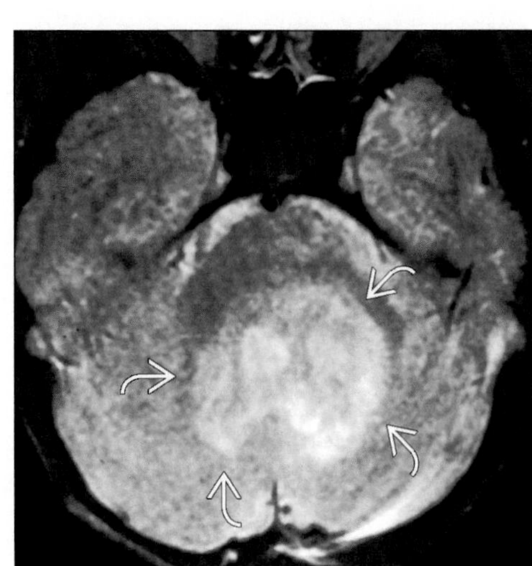

(Left) *Sagittal T1WI MR of a 10-year-old boy with NF1 reveals massive enlargement of the brainstem (mostly pons and medulla ➔). The T1 signal is near identical to other white matter structures.* ***(Right)*** *Axial T2WI MR of the same patient shows abnormal thickening and T2 hyperintensity ➔ around the 4th ventricle, especially in the left middle cerebellar peduncle. A 20-year MR follow-up (not shown) has demonstrated slow normalization of the T2 hyperintensity of this presumed "hamartoma."*

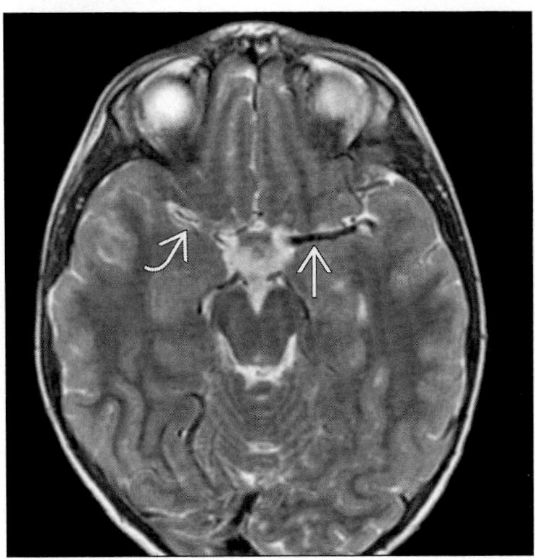

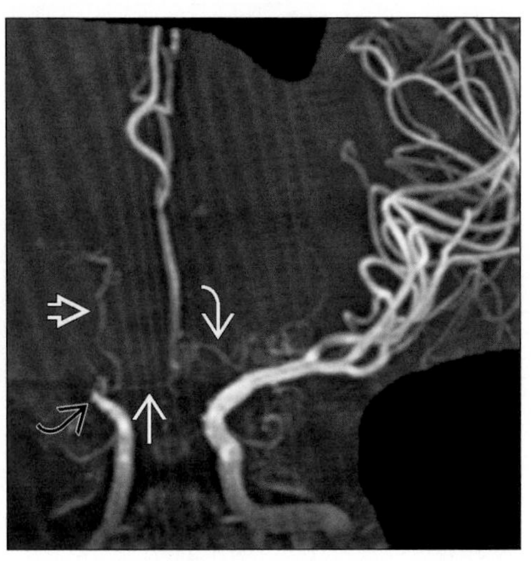

(Left) *Axial T2WI MR shows a well-defined left MCA flow void ➔. The flow voids of the A1 segments of the anterior cerebral arteries and of the right MCA ➔ are very small.* ***(Right)*** *Coronal MRA (reformatted from a 3D TOF study) confirms the diagnosis moyamoya vasculopathy. The distal left ICA and left MCA are normal. The right ICA terminus ➔ tapers. The right MCA is not identified; the right ➔ and left ➔ A1 segments are tiny. A collateral vessel is seen on the right ➔.*

NEUROFIBROMATOSIS TYPE 2

Key Facts

Terminology
- Multiple intracranial schwannomas, meningiomas, and ependymomas

Imaging
- Bilateral vestibular schwannomas
- Schwannomas of cranial nerves (CN) and spinal nerve roots
- Meningiomas on dural surfaces (up to 50%)
- Ependymomas in spinal cord and brainstem (6%)
- Use high resolution T1 C+ through basal cisterns with fat saturation to evaluate cranial nerves

Top Differential Diagnoses
- Schwannomatosis
- Multiple meningiomas
- Metastases

Pathology
- All NF2 families have chromosome 22q12 abnormalities
- *NF2* gene encodes for Merlin protein

Clinical Issues
- Usually presents between 2nd and 4th decade with hearing loss, ± vertigo
- Incidence: 1:25,000-30,000
- Life span substantially shortened by presence of meningiomas and by complications related to lower cranial neuropathies (i.e., aspiration)

Diagnostic Checklist
- Carefully evaluate other cranial nerves in any new diagnosis of vestibular schwannoma

*(**Left**) Axial graphic shows bilateral CPA schwannomas pathognomonic of NF2. The tumor ⇨ on the right is large and several small schwannomas → are seen on the left vestibulocochlear nerves. (**Right**) Axial T1WI C+ FS MR shows bilateral, intensely enhancing masses in the cerebellopontine angles, extending into enlarged internal auditory canals ➔; this is pathognomonic of NF2. The masses compress and deform the adjacent middle cerebellar peduncles, more so on the left.*

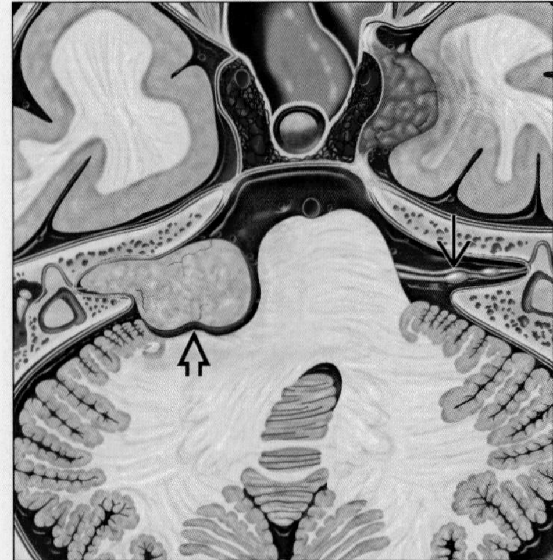

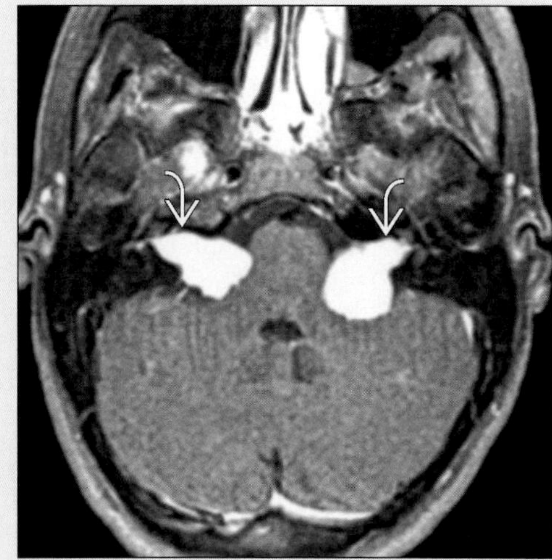

*(**Left**) Coronal T1WI C+ MR of a 17-year-old patient shows bilateral vestibular schwannomas extending into the internal auditory canals ➡. A mass in the right jugular foramen ➔ is indicative of a schwannoma of a lower cranial nerve (9, 10, &/or 11.) The cranial nerve of origin cannot be differentiated by imaging. (**Right**) Axial T1WI C+ FS MR in the same patient reveals additional schwannomas ↷ of the bilateral 5th cranial nerves, as well as some subcutaneous ones ➔.*

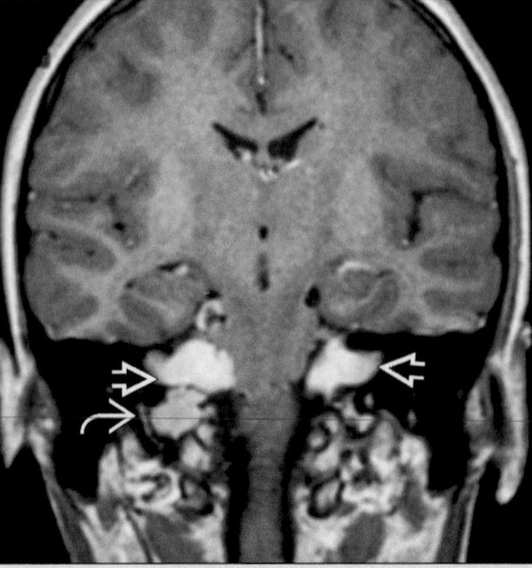

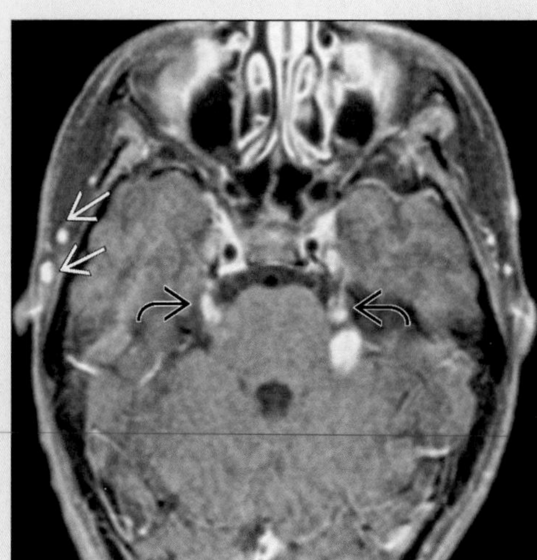

NEUROFIBROMATOSIS TYPE 2

TERMINOLOGY

Abbreviations
- Neurofibromatosis type 2 (NF2)

Synonyms
- Acoustic neurofibromatosis, central neurofibromatosis
- Multiple intracranial schwannomas, meningiomas, and ependymomas (MISME)

Definitions
- Hereditary syndrome causing multiple cranial nerve schwannomas, meningiomas, and spinal tumors

IMAGING

General Features
- Best diagnostic clue
  - Bilateral vestibular schwannomas
- Location
  - Multiple extraaxial tumors
    - Schwannomas of cranial nerves (CN) and spinal nerve roots
    - Meningiomas on dural surfaces (up to 50%)
  - Intraaxial tumors
    - Ependymomas in spinal cord and brainstem (6%)
- Size
  - Cranial nerve tumors typically symptomatic while still small but can achieve great size
- Morphology
  - Tumors grow spherically but accommodate to bony canals, e.g., internal auditory canal (IAC)
- Multiplicity of lesions
  - Schwannomas of other cranial nerves in 50%
    - CN5 most common; also CN3, CN12 common
  - Schwannoma of spinal nerves (up to 90%)
  - Meningiomas (often multiple)
  - Intramedullary ependymomas (spinal cord)
  - Cerebral calcifications
  - Posterior lens opacities (juveniles, in 60-80%)
  - Meningioangiomatosis
  - Glial microhamartomas

CT Findings
- NECT
  - Vestibular schwannoma
    - Cerebellopontine angle (CPA) mass ± widened IAC
    - Isodense to hyperdense
    - Rarely cystic/necrotic
  - Meningioma
    - High-density dural-based mass(es)
  - Nonneoplastic cerebral Ca++ (uncommon)
    - Extensive choroid plexus Ca++
    - Cortical surface
    - Ventricular lining
- CECT
  - Cranial nerve tumor enhancement
  - Meningioma enhancement

MR Findings
- T1WI
  - Schwannomas
    - Hypointense to isointense
    - Rare cystic change
  - Meningiomas
    - Isointense to hypointense
    - Occasional hyperintense foci from Ca++
- T2WI
  - Schwannomas
    - Small intracanalicular lesions can be shown on high-resolution T2WI
  - Meningiomas
    - May incite significant adjacent edema
- T2* GRE
  - Shows nonneoplastic Ca++ to best advantage
- DWI
  - Some meningiomas have restricted diffusion
    - Characteristic of atypical or malignant meningioma
- T1WI C+
  - Schwannomas
    - Diffuse enhancement
    - Usually homogeneous
    - T1 C+ with fat saturation and thin slice profile essential for identification of small CN tumors
    - Vestibular schwannomas typically "bulge" into CPA cistern from IAC
  - Meningiomas
    - Diffuse enhancement of tumor, may be plaque-like
- MRS
  - Meningioma
    - Absent NAA peak, ↑ alanine, ± lactate
  - Schwannoma
    - Absent NAA peak, ↑ myoinositol, usually no lactate

Nonvascular Interventions
- Myelography
  - Will demonstrate multiple spinal tumorlets
    - Replaced by contrast-enhanced MR

Imaging Recommendations
- Best imaging tool
  - Contrast-enhanced MR
- Protocol advice
  - Use high resolution T1 C+ through basal cisterns with fat saturation to evaluate cranial nerves
  - Evaluation for spinal disease is critical

DIFFERENTIAL DIAGNOSIS

Schwannomatosis
- Multiple schwannomas without vestibular tumors
- No cutaneous stigmata or meningiomas

Cerebellopontine Angle (CPA) Masses
- Arachnoid cyst
  - Follows CSF on all sequences
- Epidermoid
  - DWI easily distinguish from arachnoid cyst
- Aneurysm
  - PICA/AICA/VA aneurysms may project into CPA
  - Pulsation artifact in phase-encoding direction
- Ependymoma

NEUROFIBROMATOSIS TYPE 2

- Extends into CPA from 4th ventricle

Multiple Meningiomas
- Recurrent or metastatic
- Secondary to radiation therapy

Metastases
- CNS primary
  - Glioblastoma, PNET-MB, germinoma, ependymoma
- Non-CNS primary

Inflammatory Disease
- Granulomatous disease: Sarcoidosis, tuberculosis
- Neuritis: Bell palsy, Lyme disease

PATHOLOGY

General Features
- Etiology
  - 50% known family history of NF2; 50% new mutations
  - Mutations cause truncated, inactivated Merlin protein
  - Tumor cells are usually hemizygous or homozygous for *NF2* mutations
- Genetics
  - Autosomal dominant
  - All NF2 families have chromosome 22q12 abnormalities
  - Germline, somatic *NF2* gene mutations
    - *NF2* gene encodes for Merlin protein (**m**eosin-**er**zin-**r**axidin-**l**ike prote**in**)
    - *NF2* gene functions: Links cytoskeleton and cell membranes; also a tumor suppressor gene
- Multiple schwannomas, meningiomas, ependymomas

Staging, Grading, & Classification
- NF2-associated schwannomas are WHO grade I
- Diagnostic criteria
  - Bilateral vestibular schwannomas or
  - 1st-degree relative with NF2 and 1 vestibular schwannoma or
  - 1st-degree relative with NF2 and 2 of following
    - Neurofibroma
    - Meningioma
    - Glioma
    - Schwannoma
    - Posterior subcapsular lenticular opacity

Gross Pathologic & Surgical Features
- Schwannomas are round-ovoid encapsulated masses
- Meningiomas are unencapsulated but sharply circumscribed

Microscopic Features
- NF2-related schwannomas have higher proliferative activity than sporadic tumors but not necessarily more aggressive course

CLINICAL ISSUES

Presentation
- Most common signs/symptoms
  - Usually presents between 2nd and 4th decade with hearing loss, ± vertigo
  - 1/3 of children with NF2 present with hearing loss, 1/3 present with other cranial nerve symptoms
- Other signs/symptoms
  - Scoliosis, paraplegia, or neck pain from spinal lesions
- Clinical profile
  - Wishart type: Early onset, rapid progression before adulthood, more severe presentation
  - Gardner type: Later onset, less severe manifestations

Demographics
- Epidemiology
  - 1:25,000-30,000

Natural History & Prognosis
- Life span substantially shortened by presence of meningiomas and by complications related to lower cranial neuropathies (i.e., aspiration)

Treatment
- Complete resection of CN8 schwannoma if feasible
  - Can be difficult as NF2 tumors tend to splay/ envelop CNs instead of displacing them
- Subtotal microsurgical resection with functional cochlear nerve preservation in last hearing ear

DIAGNOSTIC CHECKLIST

Consider
- Carefully evaluate other cranial nerves in any new diagnosis of vestibular schwannoma
  - Be highly suspicious if < 30 years
- Study entire neuraxis in suspected cases (multiple small, asymptomatic schwannomas on cauda equina common)

Image Interpretation Pearls
- Coronal thin slice T1WI C+ with fat saturation to assess cranial nerves

SELECTED REFERENCES

1. Hanemann CO: Magic but treatable? Tumours due to loss of merlin. Brain. 131(Pt 3):606-15, 2008
2. Fisher LM et al: Distribution of nonvestibular cranial nerve schwannomas in neurofibromatosis 2. Otol Neurotol. 28(8):1083-90, 2007
3. Bosch MM et al: Optic nerve sheath meningiomas in patients with neurofibromatosis type 2. Arch Ophthalmol. 124(3):379-85, 2006
4. Omeis I et al: Meningioangiomatosis associated with neurofibromatosis: report of 2 cases in a single family and review of the literature. Surg Neurol. 65(6):595-603, 2006
5. Neff BA et al: Current concepts in the evaluation and treatment of neurofibromatosis type II. Otolaryngol Clin North Am. 38(4):671-84, ix, 2005
6. Ruggieri M et al: Earliest clinical manifestations and natural history of neurofibromatosis type 2 (NF2) in childhood: a study of 24 patients. Neuropediatrics. 36(1):21-34, 2005
7. Otsuka G et al: Age at symptom onset and long-term survival in patients with neurofibromatosis Type 2. J Neurosurg. 99(3):480-3, 2003

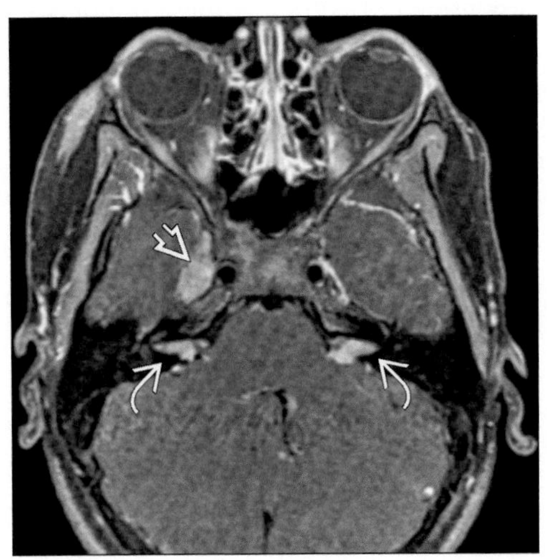

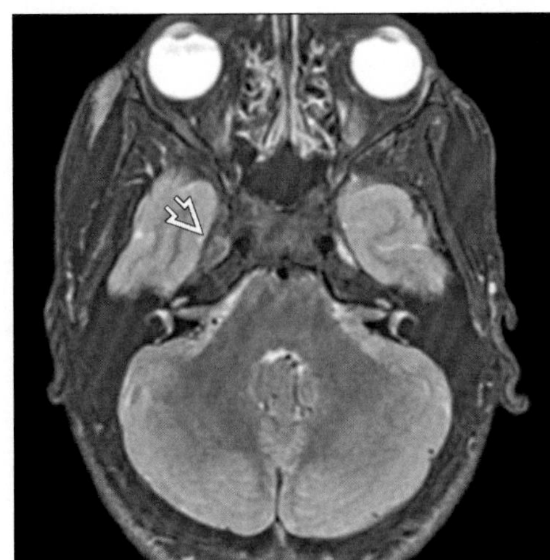

(Left) *Axial T1 C+ FS MR of a 9 year old reveals small enhancing vestibular schwannomas* ↷ *in the IAC-CPA bilaterally. An enhancing mass is also demonstrated in the right trigeminal cistern* ⇨ *and found to be a trigeminal schwannoma.* ***(Right)*** *Axial T2WI FS MR in the same patient shows expansion and T2 hypointense signal* ⇨ *in the right trigeminal cistern. The IAC/CPA masses are not well appreciated. This child was asymptomatic for these lesions.*

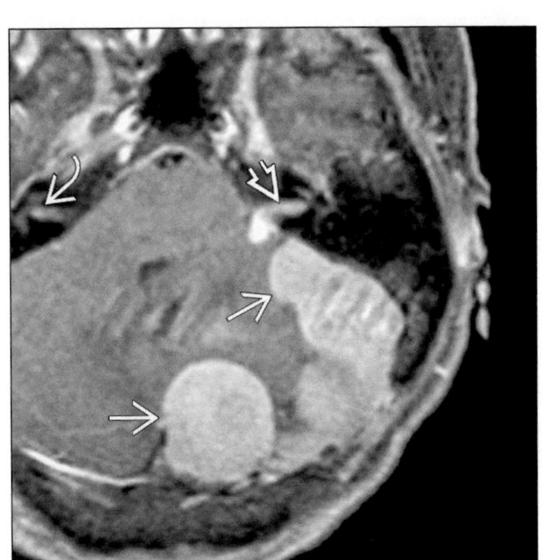

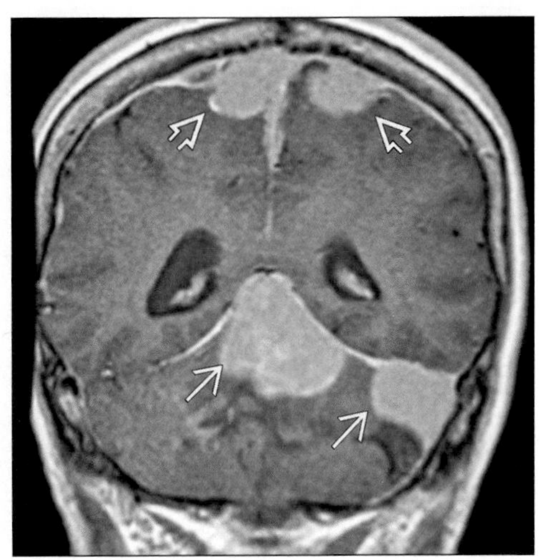

(Left) *Axial T1WI C+ MR of a 70-year-old woman with NF2 shows extensive meningiomatosis with dural-based masses* ➔ *in the posterior fossa. There is a small enhancing mass in the left IAC-CPA* ⇨ *and a tiny, almost imperceptible one* ↷ *at the fundus of the right internal auditory canal.* ***(Right)*** *Coronal T1WI C+ MR shows the dural-based meningiomas in the posterior fossa* ➔ *and along the falx and convexities* ⇨*. In this patient, the meningiomatosis predominates over the schwannomas.*

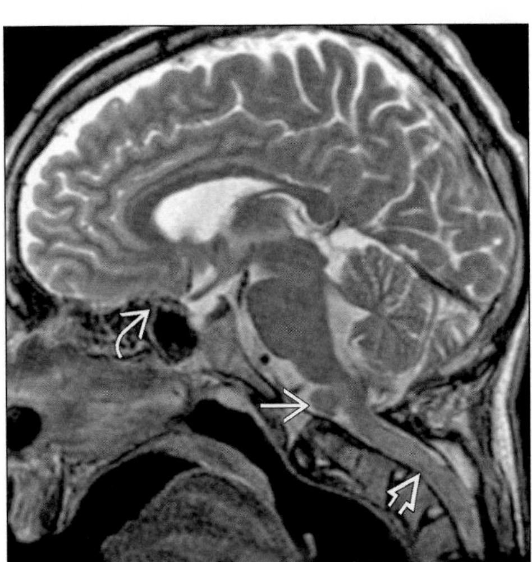

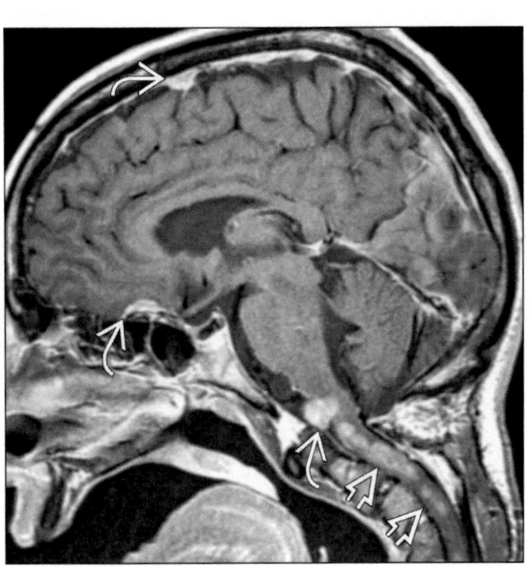

(Left) *Sagittal T2WI FS MR of the brain and upper cervical spine shows "blistering" of the planum sphenoidale* ↷*, an extraaxial mass in front of the medulla at the foramen magnum* ➔*, and an enlarged, hyperintense cervical spinal cord* ⇨*.* ***(Right)*** *Sagittal T1 C+ MR in the same patient shows multiple enhancing meningiomas* ↷ *and enhancing ependymoma of the upper cervical cord* ⇨*. A "swan neck" deformity is noted in the upper neck, from prior multilevel laminectomies.*

VON HIPPEL-LINDAU

Key Facts

Terminology

- Autosomal dominant familial syndrome with hemangioblastomas (HGBLs), clear cell renal carcinoma, cystadenomas, pheochromocytomas

Imaging

- 2 or more CNS HGBLs or 1 HGBL + visceral lesion or retinal hemorrhage
- HGBLs vary from tiny mass to very large with even larger associated cysts

Top Differential Diagnoses

- Vascular metastasis
- Solitary hemangioblastoma
- Pilocytic astrocytoma
- Hemispheric medulloblastoma in teenager or young adult
- Multiple AVMs in vascular neurocutaneous syndrome

Pathology

- Posterior distribution of HGBLs = result of tumor development during embryogenesis

Clinical Issues

- Phenotypes based on absence or presence of pheochromocytoma
- Earliest symptom in VHL often visual
- Nearly 75% of symptom-producing tumors have associated cyst, peritumoral edema
- HGBLs → multiple periods of tumor growth (usually associated with increasing cyst size) separated by periods of arrested growth

Diagnostic Checklist

- Follow NIH screening rules
- Look for ELS tumors in VHL patients with dysequilibrium, hearing loss, or aural fullness

*(**Left**) Sagittal graphic shows 2 HGBLs in VHL. In this case, the spinal cord tumor has an associated cyst ⇨ and would cause myelopathy. The small cerebellar HGBL would be asymptomatic. (**Right**) Sagittal T1 C+ MR of the craniocervical junction reveals 3 HGBLs. Two arise from the dorsal medulla ➡ and have small associated cysts, while the 3rd consists of a tiny enhancing nodule ↷ at C4 with a large associated cyst that severely compresses and expands the cervical spinal cord.*

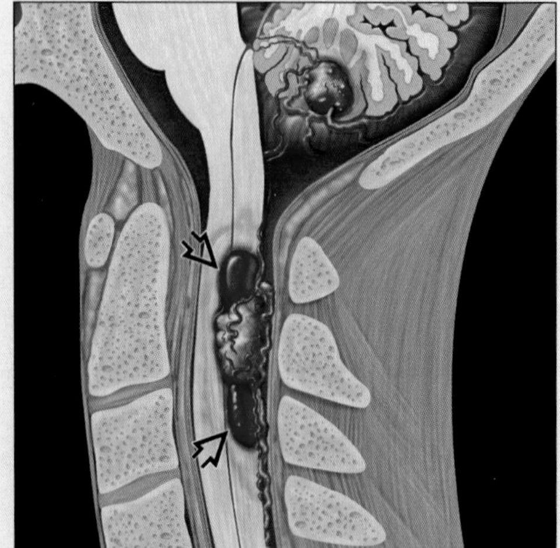

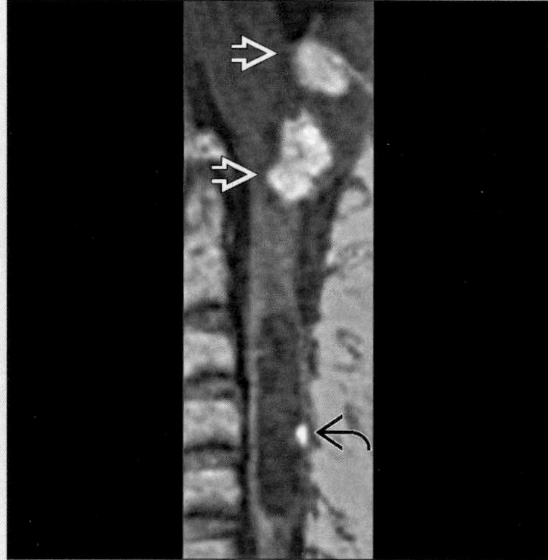

*(**Left**) High-resolution axial NECT of a 14-year-old patient with VHL shows a destructive mass (endolymphatic sac tumor ➦) in the medial aspect of the right petrous bone. The mass is centered in the expected location of the endolymphatic sac and vestibular aqueduct. (**Right**) Axial T1 C+ MR in the same patient reveals multiple tiny, enhancing cerebellar lesions ➡, which represent HGBLs. The endolymphatic sac tumor ➦ in the right petrous bone shows bright T1 signal.*

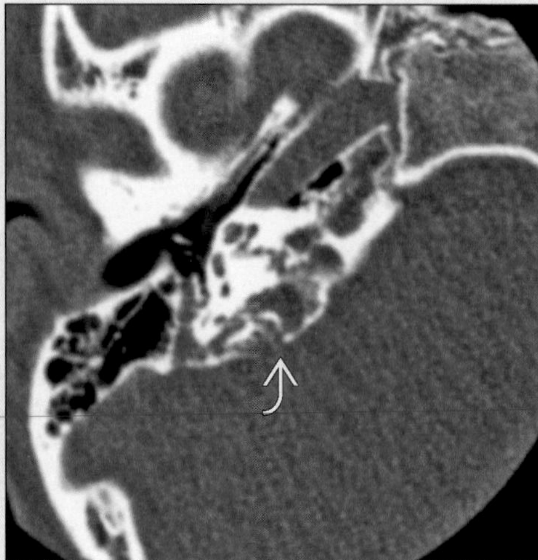

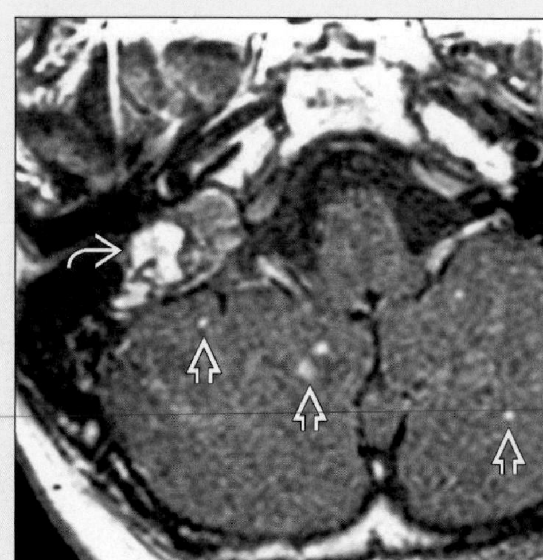

VON HIPPEL-LINDAU

TERMINOLOGY

Abbreviations

- von Hippel-Lindau (VHL) syndrome

Definitions

- Autosomal dominant familial syndrome with hemangioblastomas (HGBLs), clear cell renal carcinoma, cystadenomas, pheochromocytomas
  - Affects 6 different organ systems, including eye, ear, and central nervous system (CNS)
  - Involved tissues often have multiple lesions
  - Lesions → benign cysts, vascular tumors, carcinomas

IMAGING

General Features

- Best diagnostic clue
  - 2 or more CNS HGBLs; or 1 HGBL + visceral lesion or retinal hemorrhage
- Location
  - HGBLs in VHL in 60-80% of patients
    - Typically multiple
    - 40-50% in spinal cord (posterior half)
    - 44-72% cerebellum (posterior > anterior half)
    - 10-25% brainstem (posterior medulla)
    - 1% supratentorial (along optic pathways, in cerebral hemispheres)
  - Ocular angiomas
    - Found in 25-60% of *VHL* gene carriers
    - Cause retinal detachment, hemorrhage
  - Cystadenoma of endolymphatic sac (ELS)
    - Large; located posterior to internal auditory canal
- Size
  - HGBLs vary from tiny mass to very large with even larger associated cysts

CT Findings

- NECT
  - HGBL: 2/3 → well-delineated cerebellar cyst + nodule
    - Nodule typically abuts pial surface
    - 1/3 solid, without cyst
  - Cystadenoma of ELS → destructive changes in petrous bone
- CECT
  - Intense enhancement of tumor nodule

MR Findings

- T1WI
  - HGBL: Mixed iso- to hypointense nodule, ± "flow voids"
  - Associated cyst slightly hyperintense to cerebrospinal fluid (CSF)
  - Cystadenoma of ELS: Heterogeneous hyper-/hypointense
- T2WI
  - HGBL: Hyperintense nodule, cyst
  - Cystadenoma of ELS: Hyperintense mass
- FLAIR
  - HGBL: Hyperintense cyst with variable edema
  - Cystadenoma of ELS: Hyperintense mass
- T2* GRE
  - HGBL: "Blooms" if hemorrhage present
- T1WI C+
  - HGBL: Tumor nodule enhances strongly; cyst wall does not enhance
  - May detect tiny asymptomatic enhancing nodules
  - Cystadenoma of ELS: Heterogeneous enhancement

Angiographic Findings

- Conventional
  - HGBL: DSA shows intensely vascular mass, prolonged stain
  - A-V shunting (early draining vein) common

Imaging Recommendations

- Best imaging tool
  - Brain: MR ± contrast
- Protocol advice
  - Scan entire brain and spine
- NIH recommendations
  - Contrast-enhanced MR of brain/spinal cord from age 11 years, every 2 years
  - US of abdomen from 11 years, yearly
  - Abdominal CT from 20 years, yearly/every other
  - MR of temporal bone if hearing loss/tinnitus/vertigo

DIFFERENTIAL DIAGNOSIS

Vascular Metastasis

- Usually solid, not cyst + nodule
- Some tumors (e.g., renal clear cell carcinoma) can resemble HGBL histopathologically

Solitary Hemangioblastoma

- 25-40% of HGBLs occur in VHL
- No *VHL* mutations, family history, other tumors or cysts

Pilocytic Astrocytoma

- Usually younger than VHL patients
- Tumor nodule lacks vascular flow voids (more characteristic of HGBL)
- Tumor nodule often does not abut pial or ependymal surface

Hemispheric Medulloblastoma in Teenager or Young Adult

- Rare; occur in peripheral cerebellar hemisphere
- May appear extraparenchymal
- Solid, gray matter intensity on T2WI

Multiple AVMs in Vascular Neurocutaneous Syndrome

- Osler-Weber-Rendu, Wyburn-Mason, etc.
- Small AVMs may resemble HGBL at angiography

PATHOLOGY

General Features

- Genetics
  - Autosomal dominant inheritance with high penetrance, variable expression
    - 20% of cases due to new mutation
  - Germline mutations of *VHL* tumor suppressor gene

VON HIPPEL-LINDAU

- Chromosome 3p25-26
- Gene product: pVHL; inactivation of pVHL results in overexpression of hypoxia inducible mRNA's, including VGEF (vascular endothelial growth factor)
- Involved in cell cycle regulation, angiogenesis
- Disease features vary depending on specific *VHL* mutations
- Posterior distribution of HGBLs = result of tumor development during embryogenesis
  - Tumors are derived from embryonic multipotent cells
- VHL characterized by development of
  - Capillary hemangioblastomas of CNS and retina
  - ELS tumors
  - Cysts, renal clear cell carcinoma
  - Pancreatic cysts, islet cell tumors
  - Pheochromocytoma
  - Epididymal cysts, cystadenomas

Staging, Grading, & Classification

- Capillary hemangioblastoma: WHO grade I

Gross Pathologic & Surgical Features

- HGBL seen as well-circumscribed, very vascular, reddish nodule
  - 75% at least partially cystic; fluid is amber-colored

Microscopic Features

- 2 components in HGBL
  - Rich capillary network
  - Large vacuolated stromal cells with clear cytoplasm

CLINICAL ISSUES

Presentation

- Most common signs/symptoms
  - VHL is clinically very heterogeneous; phenotypic penetrance: 97% at 65 years
  - Retinal angiomas
    - Earliest symptom in VHL often visual
    - Retinal detachment, vitreous hemorrhages
  - Cerebellar HGBLs
    - Headache (obstructive hydrocephalus)
    - Nearly 75% of symptom-producing tumors have associated cyst, peritumoral edema
  - Spinal cord HGBLs
    - Progressive myelopathy
    - 95% associated syrinx
- Clinical profile
  - Phenotypes based on absence or presence of pheochromocytoma
    - Type 1: Without pheochromocytoma
    - Type 2A: With both pheochromocytoma, renal cell carcinoma
    - Type 2B: With pheochromocytoma, without renal cell carcinoma
  - Diagnosis of VHL: Capillary hemangioblastoma in CNS/retina and 1 of typical VHL-associated tumors or previous family history

Demographics

- Age
  - VHL presents in young adults: Mean age of presentation
    - Retinal angioma: 25 years
    - Cerebellar angioma, pheochromocytoma: 30 years
    - Endolymphatic sac tumor: 31 years
    - Renal carcinoma: 33 years
- Epidemiology
  - 1:35,000-50,000

Natural History & Prognosis

- Renal carcinoma proximal cause of death in 15-50%
- HGBLs → multiple periods of tumor growth (usually associated with increasing cyst size) separated by periods of arrested growth
- On average, new lesion develops every 2 years in VHL

Treatment

- Ophthalmoscopy yearly from infancy
- Physical/neurological examination yearly
- Surgical resection of symptomatic cerebellar/spinal hemangioblastoma
- Stereotactic radiosurgery may control smaller, noncystic lesions
- Laser treatment of retinal angiomata

DIAGNOSTIC CHECKLIST

Consider

- Follow NIH screening rules
- Look for ELS tumors in VHL patients with dysequilibrium, hearing loss, or aural fullness

Image Interpretation Pearls

- Solitary HGBL in young patient may indicate VHL

SELECTED REFERENCES

1. Lonser RR et al: Pituitary stalk hemangioblastomas in von Hippel-Lindau disease. J Neurosurg. 110(2):350-3, 2009
2. Jagannathan J et al: Surgical management of cerebellar hemangioblastomas in patients with von Hippel-Lindau disease. J Neurosurg. 108(2):210-22, 2008
3. Ammerman JM et al: Long-term natural history of hemangioblastomas in patients with von Hippel-Lindau disease: implications for treatment. J Neurosurg. 105(2):248-55, 2006
4. Fisher C et al: Central nervous system hemangioblastoma and von Hippel-Lindau syndrome: a familial presentation. Clin Pediatr (Phila). 45(5):456-62, 2006
5. Choo D et al: Endolymphatic sac tumors in von Hippel-Lindau disease. J Neurosurg. 100(3):480-7, 2004
6. Wanebo JE et al: The natural history of hemangioblastomas of the central nervous system in patients with von Hippel-Lindau disease. J Neurosurg. 98(1):82-94, 2003
7. Conway JE et al: Hemangioblastomas of the central nervous system in von Hippel-Lindau syndrome and sporadic disease. Neurosurgery. 48(1):55-62; discussion 62-3, 2001
8. Friedrich CA: Genotype-phenotype correlation in von Hippel-Lindau syndrome. Hum Mol Genet. 10(7):763-7, 2001

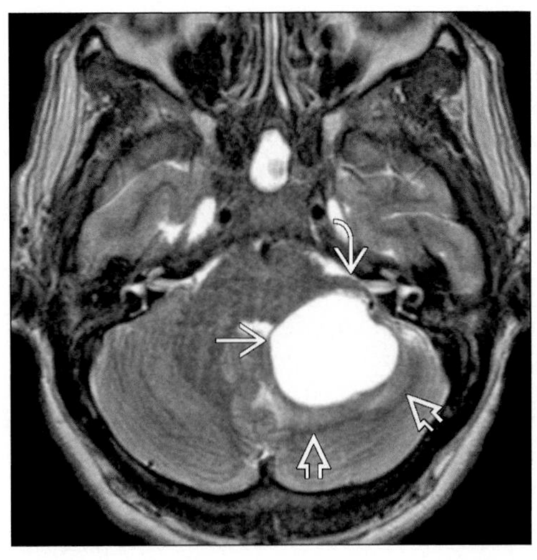

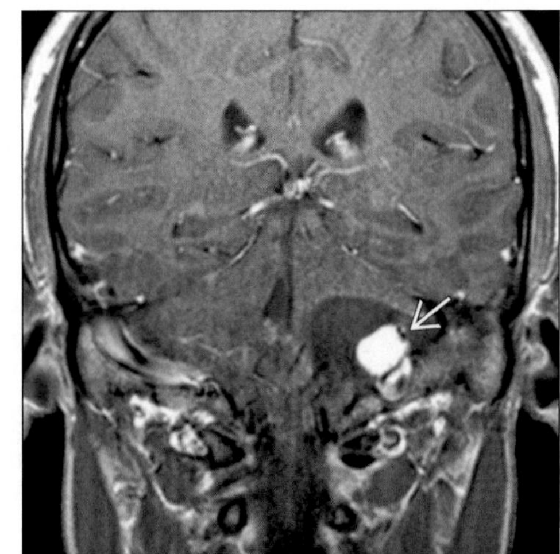

(Left) *Axial T2WI MR shows a typical cerebellar hemisphere hemangioblastoma in a 42-year-old patient. A T2 hyperintense cyst in the deep left cerebellar hemisphere causes mass effect on the adjacent middle cerebellar peduncle, which narrows the adjacent cerebellopontine angle. The tumor elicits mild surrounding edema.* ***(Right)*** *Coronal T1 C+ FS MR in the same patient reveals the solid, avidly enhancing nodule along the inferior lateral aspect of the cyst.*

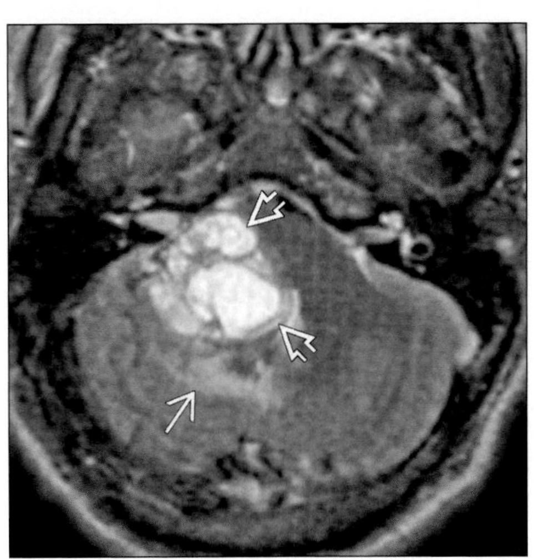

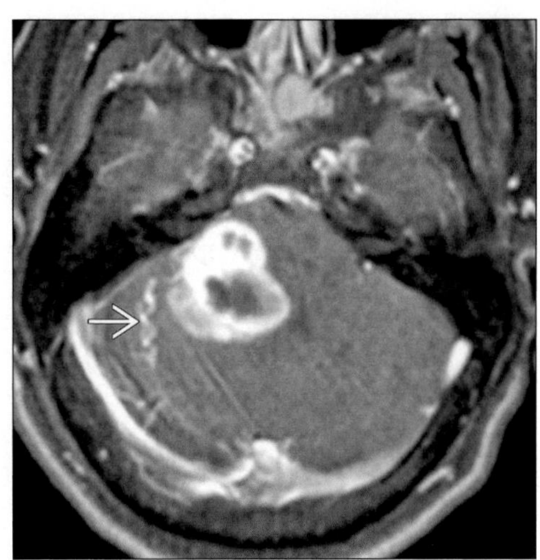

(Left) *Axial T2WI MR shows a mixed solid-cystic HGBL centered in the right middle cerebellar peduncle. The cystic components are evident as well-marginated T2 hyperintense foci. Mild interstitial edema surrounds the mass.* ***(Right)*** *Axial T1 C+ FS MR in the same patient shows intense enhancement of the solid portions of the tumor. Multiple associated enlarged feeding arteries/draining veins are evident and indicate the highly vascular nature of this tumor.*

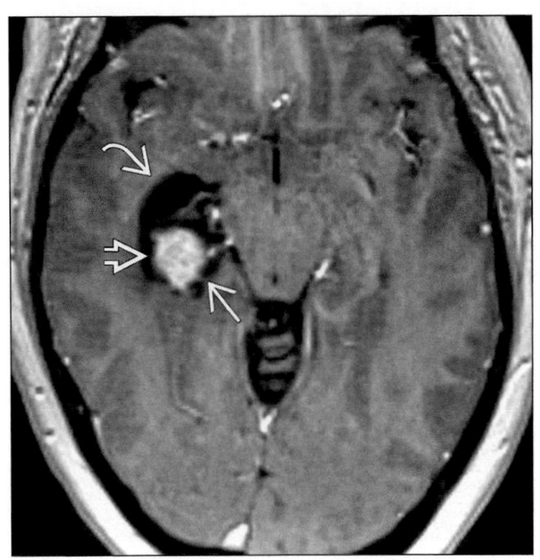

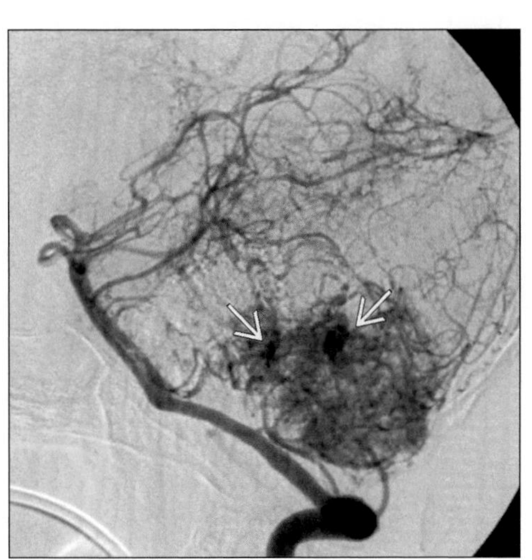

(Left) *Axial T1 C+ MR shows an HGBL in the right medial temporal lobe. The mass enhances strongly and contains cystic as well as solid components. The temporal horn is trapped by the tumor.* ***(Right)*** *Lateral angiography projection of a different patient (mid-arterial phase of a VA injection) shows a hypervascular mass (HGBL) in the lower posterior fossa. The mass is fed by enlarged feeders from the AICA and PICA. Two ill-defined nodules are evident superiorly.*

TUBEROUS SCLEROSIS COMPLEX

Key Facts

Terminology
- Tuberous sclerosis complex (TSC)
- Synonym: Bourneville-Pringle syndrome
- Inherited tumor disorder with multiorgan hamartomas

Imaging
- Calcified subependymal nodules (SEN) (hamartomas)
- Subependymal giant cell astrocytoma (SEGA) (15%); most located at foramen of Monro
- Cortical/subcortical tubers (95%)
- White matter radial migration lines
- Cyst-like white matter lesions (cystoid brain degeneration)
- Cortical/subcortical tubers: Early T1 ↑ but variable after myelin maturation
- SEN enhancement more visible on MR than on CT
- AMT-PET distinguishes epileptogenic from nonepileptogenic tubers

Top Differential Diagnoses
- X-linked subependymal heterotopia
- Cytomegalovirus (CMV): Periventricular Ca++, typical WM lesions, polymicrogyria
- Taylor type cortical dysplasia (FCD type 2)

Pathology
- Abnormal differentiation/proliferation of germinal matrix cells
- Mutations in TSC tumor suppressor genes cause abnormal cellular differentiation, proliferation

Diagnostic Checklist
- FLAIR and T1 MT most sensitive sequences for diagnosis
- SEN (< 1.3 cm) vs. SEGA (> 1.3 cm)

*(**Left**) Axial graphic of typical brain involvement in tuberous sclerosis complex shows a giant cell astrocytoma ➡ in the left foramen of Monro, subependymal nodules ⇨, radial migration lines ⮫, and cortical/subcortical tubers →. (**Right**) Axial T1WI C+ MR shows a mass at the level of the left foramen of Monro extending into the frontal horn of the left lateral ventricle. The mass, a SEGA, enhances intensely and uniformly and mimics a choroid plexus papilloma.*

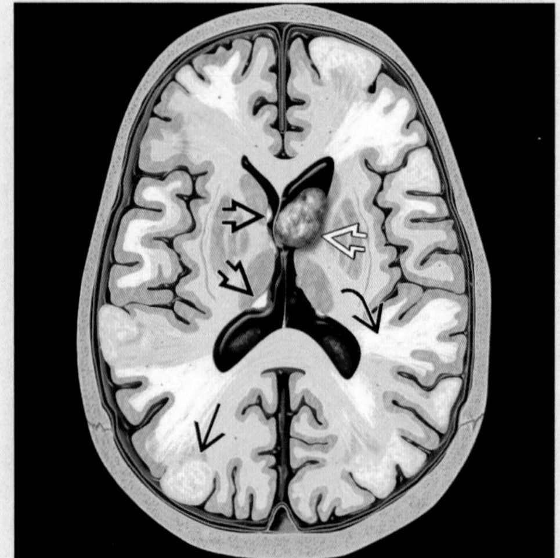

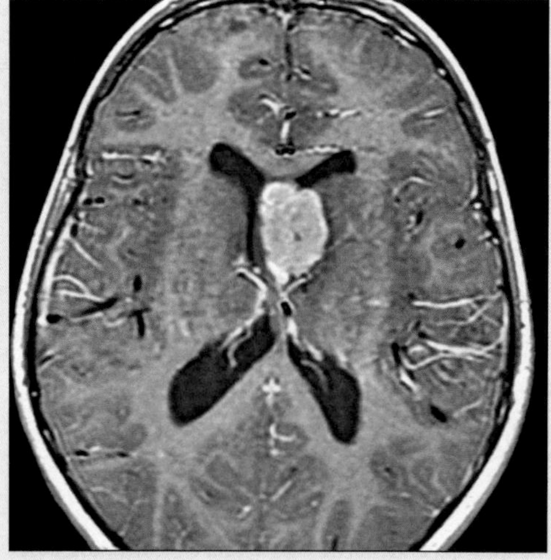

*(**Left**) Axial T1WI MR with magnetization transfer (MT) in a 13 month old shows classic findings of TS: Multiple cortical/subcortical tubers ➡ and white matter radial migration lines ➡. These lesions are well demonstrated as the signal from normal white matter is suppressed by the MT pulse. (**Right**) Corresponding axial T2WI MR demonstrates tubers as T2 hyperintense lesions beneath expanded ("clubbed") gyri. The white matter radial migration lines are not well appreciated.*

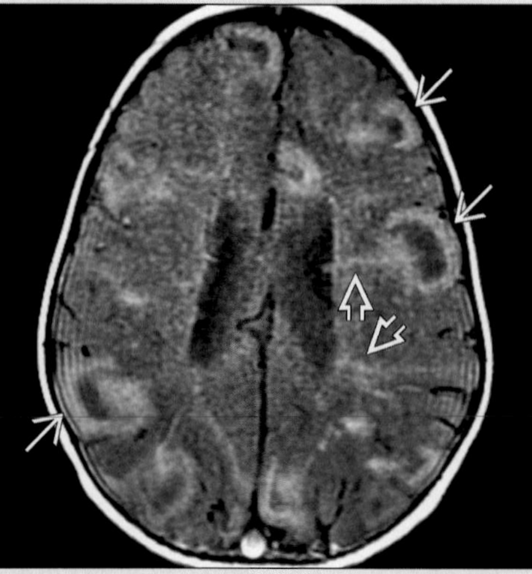

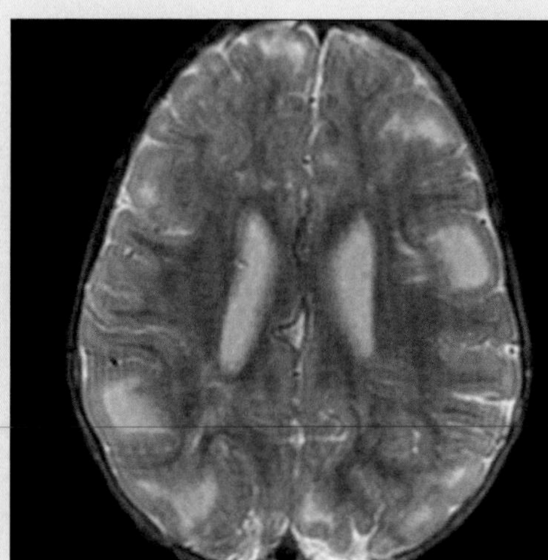

TUBEROUS SCLEROSIS COMPLEX

TERMINOLOGY

Abbreviations
- Tuberous sclerosis complex (TSC)

Synonyms
- Bourneville-Pringle syndrome

Definitions
- Inherited tumor disorder with multiorgan hamartomas
  - Spectrum of central nervous system (CNS) hamartomas, all contain giant (balloon) cells

IMAGING

General Features
- Best diagnostic clue
  - Calcified subependymal nodules (hamartomas)
    - 98% have subependymal nodules (SENs)
- Location
  - Subependymal giant cell astrocytoma (SEGA) arise in 15%; most located at foramen of Monro
  - Cortical/subcortical tubers (95%)
    - Frontal > parietal > occipital > temporal > cerebellum
    - ↑ number tubers → ↑ neurologic symptoms
  - White matter radial migration lines (WMRMLs)
    - Represent heterotopic glia + neurons along path of cortical migration from ventricle to cortex
  - Cyst-like white matter lesions (cystoid brain degeneration)
- Size
  - Thickened cortex, enlarged gyri associated with cortical/subcortical tubers
  - SEN that grows over time and measures > 1.3 cm = SEGA
- Morphology
  - Pyramidal-shaped gyral expansion
  - 20% have "eye-of-potato" central depression

Radiographic Findings
- Radiography
  - Bone islands (skull)
  - Undulating periosteal new bone

CT Findings
- NECT
  - SENs
    - Along caudothalamic groove > atrial > > temporal
    - 50% Ca++ (progressive after 1 year)
  - Tubers
    - Early: Low-density/Ca++ cortical/subcortical mass
    - Later: Isodense/Ca++ (50% by 10 years)
  - Ventriculomegaly common even without SEGA
- CECT
  - Enhancing/enlarging SEN suspicious for SEGA

MR Findings
- T1WI
  - Cortical/subcortical tubers: Early T1 ↑ but variable after myelin maturation
  - Focal lacune-like cysts (vascular etiology)
  - WMRMLs, tubers: Bright signal with magnetization transfer (MT) imaging
- T2WI
  - Variable signal (relative to myelin maturation)
- FLAIR
  - WMRMLs: Streaky linear or wedge-shaped ↑ signal
  - FLAIR becomes more positive with age
- T2* GRE
  - Ca++ SEN more readily discerned
- DWI
  - ↑ ADC values in epileptogenic tubers
  - ↑ ADC, ↓ FA in normal-appearing white matter (WM) on DTI
- T1WI C+
  - SEN enhancement more visible on MR than on CT
    - 30-80% enhance (enlarging SEN at foramen of Monro: SEGA)
    - Other enhancing lesions followed (unless growing or obstructing CSF)
  - 3-4% tubers enhance
- MRA
  - Rare aneurysms and dysplasias/moyamoya
- MRS
  - ↓ NAA/Cr, ↑ mI/Cr in subcortical tubers, SENs

Ultrasonographic Findings
- Grayscale ultrasound
  - Fetal documentation of rhabdomyoma: TSC confirmed in 96%
    - Identified as early as 20 weeks gestation

Nuclear Medicine Findings
- PET
  - ↓ glucose metabolism in lateral temporal gyri in TSC with autism
  - α-11C-methyl-L-tryptophan (AMT PET) distinguishes epileptogenic from nonepileptogenic tubers
- Brain SPECT: ↓ uptake quiescent tubers; ictal SPECT ↑ uptake tubers with active seizure focus
  - Helps localize for surgery

Imaging Recommendations
- Best imaging tool
  - MR with contrast
- Protocol advice
  - MR with contrast, ± NECT (document Ca++ SENs)
  - Yearly surveillance imaging if incompletely calcified SEGA or enhancing SEGA
    - Look for rapid growth, ± ventricular obstruction

DIFFERENTIAL DIAGNOSIS

X-linked Subependymal Heterotopia
- Isointense to gray matter (GM) T1/T2+

(S)TORCH
- Cytomegalovirus (CMV): Periventricular Ca++, typical WM lesions, polymicrogyria

Taylor Type Cortical Dysplasia (FCD Type 2)
- Considered *forme fruste* TSC

TUBEROUS SCLEROSIS COMPLEX

PATHOLOGY

General Features

- Etiology
  - Abnormal differentiation/proliferation of germinal matrix cells
  - Migrational arrest of dysgenetic neurons
- Genetics
  - ~ 50% of TSC cases inherited
    - Autosomal dominant, high but variable penetrance
    - De novo: Spontaneous mutation/germ-line mosaicism (60-85%)
  - Mutations in TSC tumor suppressor genes cause activation of mTOR protein → ↑ protein synthesis + cell proliferation
    - 2 distinct loci: *TSC1* (9q34) encodes "hamartin"; *TSC2* (16p13.3) encodes "tuberin"
- Associated abnormalities
  - Renal: Angiomyolipoma and cysts (40-80%)
  - Cardiac: Rhabdomyomas (50-65%); majority involute over time
  - Lung: Cystic lymphangiomyomatosis/fibrosis
  - Solid organs: Adenomas, leiomyomas
  - Skin: Ash-leaf spots (majority), including scalp/hair; facial angiofibromas; shagreen patches
  - Extremities: Subungual fibromas (15-20%), cystic bone lesions, undulating periosteal new bone formation
  - Ocular: "Giant drusen" (50%), retinal astrocytomas (which may regress)
  - Dental pitting of permanent teeth in most adults

Staging, Grading, & Classification

- SEGA: WHO grade I

Gross Pathologic & Surgical Features

- Firm cortical masses ("tubers") with dimpling ("potato-eye")

Microscopic Features

- Cortical dysplasia with balloon cells, ectopic neurons
- Myelin loss, vacuolation, and gliosis

CLINICAL ISSUES

Presentation

- Most common signs/symptoms
  - Classic clinical triad
    - Facial angiofibromas (90%), mental retardation (50-80%), seizures (Sz) (80-90%)
      - All 3 ("epiloia"): 30%
- Clinical profile
  - Sz (infantile type spasms in very young), facial angiofibroma, hypopigmented skin lesions, mental retardation
  - Infant/toddler: Infantile spasms (20-30%), autism → bad prognosis
    - Infantile spasms occur before development of facial lesions, shagreen patches
  - Diagnostic criteria: 2 major or 1 major + 1 minor
    - Major: Facial angiofibroma/forehead plaque, sub-/periungual fibroma, ≥ 3 hypomelanotic macules, shagreen patch, multiple retinal nodular hamartomas, cortical tuber, SEN, SEGA, cardiac rhabdomyoma, lymphangioleiomyomatosis, renal angiomyolipoma
    - Minor: Dental enamel pits, hamartomatous rectal polyps, bone cysts, cerebral WM radial migration lines (> 3 = major sign), gingival fibromas, nonrenal hamartoma, retinal achromic patch, confetti skin lesions, multiple renal cysts

Demographics

- Age
  - Diagnosed at any age
    - 1st year of life if infantile spasms or surveillance for positive family history
    - Child: Autistic-like behavior, mental retardation, seizures, or skin lesions
    - Adult diagnoses reported with demonstration of symptomatic SEGA on brain imaging
- Epidemiology
  - 1:6,000 live births

Treatment

- Surveillance MR every 1-3 years during childhood/adolescence
- Treat seizures: Infantile spasms respond to vigabatrin
- Resect isolated tubers if seizure focus or if able to identify seizure focus among many tubers
- SEGAs resected if obstructing foramen of Monro
- Oral rapamycin (inhibitor of mTOR protein signaling pathway) reported to cause regression of SEGA

DIAGNOSTIC CHECKLIST

Image Interpretation Pearls

- FLAIR and T1 MT most sensitive sequences for diagnosis
- T1WI readily documents early white matter abnormalities (pre-myelin maturation)
- SEN differs from SEGA based on size
  - SEN < 1.3 cm
  - SEGA > 1.3 cm

SELECTED REFERENCES

1. Baskin HJ Jr: The pathogenesis and imaging of the tuberous sclerosis complex. Pediatr Radiol. 38(9):936-52, 2008
2. Luat AF et al: Neuroimaging in tuberous sclerosis complex. Curr Opin Neurol. 20(2):142-50, 2007
3. Makki MI et al: Characteristics of abnormal diffusivity in normal-appearing white matter investigated with diffusion tensor MR imaging in tuberous sclerosis complex. AJNR Am J Neuroradiol. 28(9):1662-7, 2007
4. Jansen FE et al: Diffusion-weighted magnetic resonance imaging and identification of the epileptogenic tuber in patients with tuberous sclerosis. Arch Neurol. 60(11):1580-4, 2003
5. Christophe C et al: MRI spectrum of cortical malformations in tuberous sclerosis complex. Brain Dev. 22(8):487-93, 2000
6. Baron Y et al: MR imaging of tuberous sclerosis in neonates and young infants. AJNR Am J Neuroradiol. 20(5):907-16, 1999
7. Griffiths PD et al: White matter abnormalities in tuberous sclerosis complex. Acta Radiol. 39(5):482-6, 1998

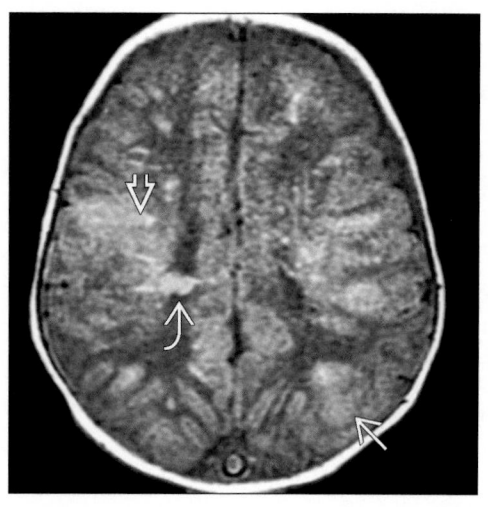

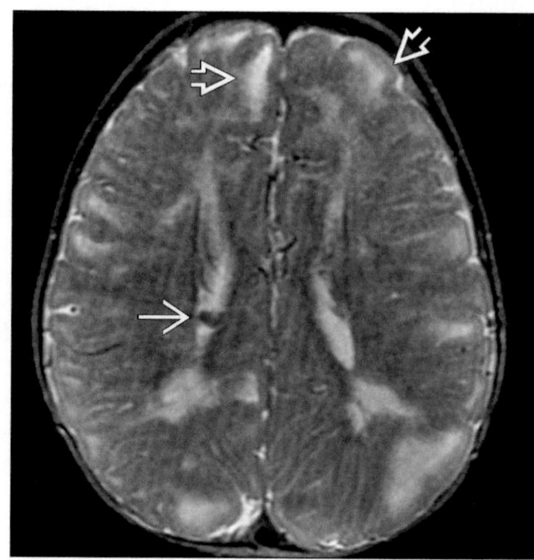

(Left) *Axial T1WI MR in a 13 day old nicely demonstrates multiple T1 bright subcortical tubers, white matter radial migration lines, and a hyperintense subependymal nodule (SEN). The unaffected, unmyelinated white matter is hypointense.* ***(Right)*** *Axial T2WI MR in the same patient at 1 year of age shows T2 hypointense SEN and multiple T2 bright tubers. Some abnormalities evident on the prior scan are not appreciated; some tubers not previously evident are now seen.*

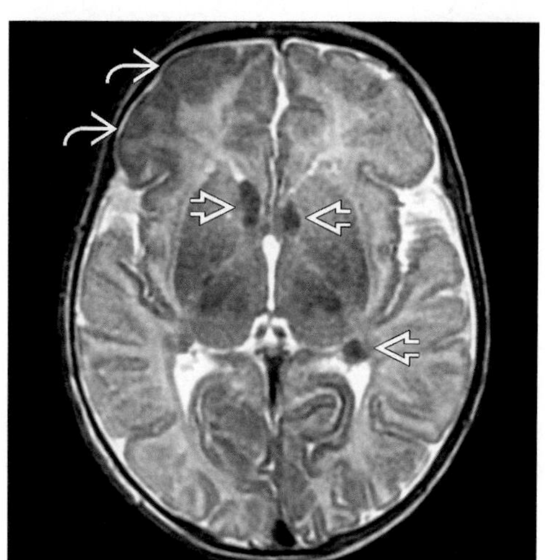

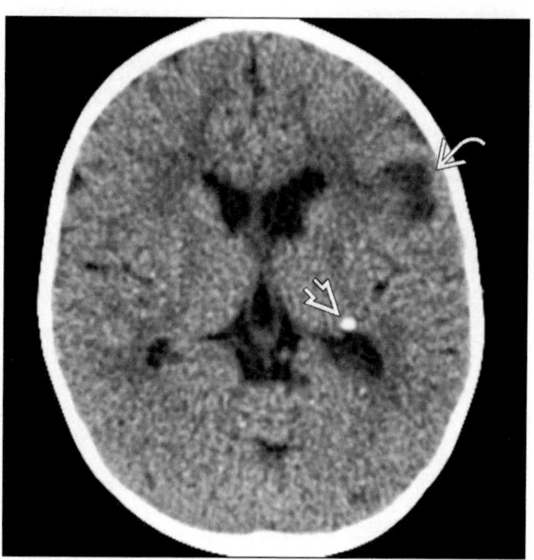

(Left) *Axial T2WI MR in a 1 month old shows multiple T2 hypointense SENs originating from the walls of the lateral ventricles. The cortex of the right frontal lobe is thickened and probably diffusely dysplastic.* ***(Right)*** *Axial NECT of a different patient demonstrates a calcified SEN along the anterior margin of the atrium of the left lateral ventricle. A hypodense, probably cystic tuber is appreciated in the inferior left frontal lobe.*

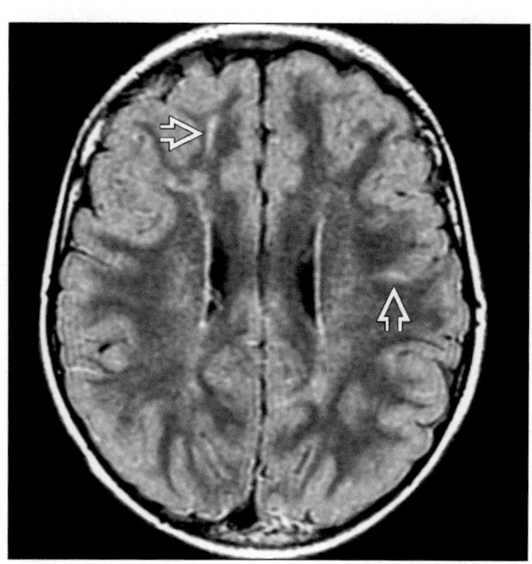

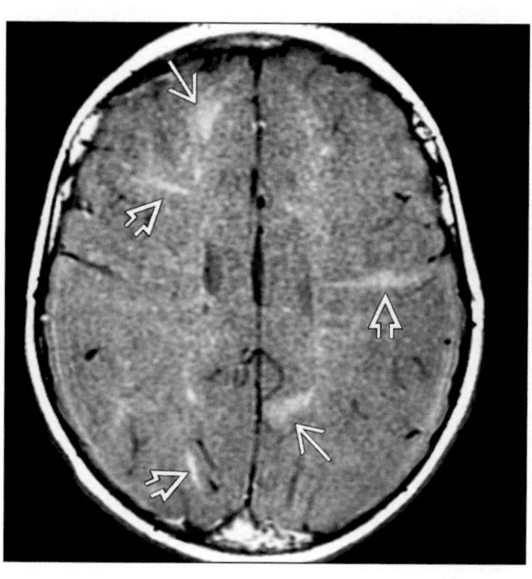

(Left) *Axial FLAIR MR shows multiple ill-defined, hyperintense bands extending radially from the cortex to the lateral ventricle in this 6-year-old child.* ***(Right)*** *Axial T1WI MR with magnetization transfer (MT) in the same patient demonstrates multiple T1 bright lesions pathognomonic for subcortical tubers and radial migration lines. The diagnosis of TS is much more easily and confidently made with the T1 + MT images than with the FLAIR images.*

STURGE-WEBER SYNDROME

Key Facts

Terminology

- Synonyms: Sturge-Weber-Dimitri, encephalotrigeminal angiomatosis
- Usually sporadic congenital (but not inherited) malformation in which fetal cortical veins fail to develop normally
- Imaging features are sequelae of progressive venous occlusion and chronic venous ischemia

Imaging

- Cortical Ca++, atrophy, and enlarged ipsilateral choroid plexus
- Pial angiomatosis unilateral (80%), bilateral (20%)
- "Tram-track" calcification
- Early: Transient hyperperfusion → "accelerated" myelin maturation
- Late: Increased signal in region of gliosis and decreased cortical signal in regions of calcification
- Early: Serpentine leptomeningeal enhancement, pial angiomatosis of subarachnoid space
- Amount of CE increases if MR performed during ictal period; mimics disease progression

Clinical Issues

- "Port wine stain," seizures, hemiparesis
- Rare: 1:20,000-50,000
- ↑ extent of lobar involvement and atrophy leading to increased likelihood of seizures
- Seizures cause further brain injury

Diagnostic Checklist

- FLAIR C+ most sensitive sequence to detect leptomeningeal angioma, especially in infancy
- T2 hypointensity of white matter underlying angioma is clue to early diagnosis

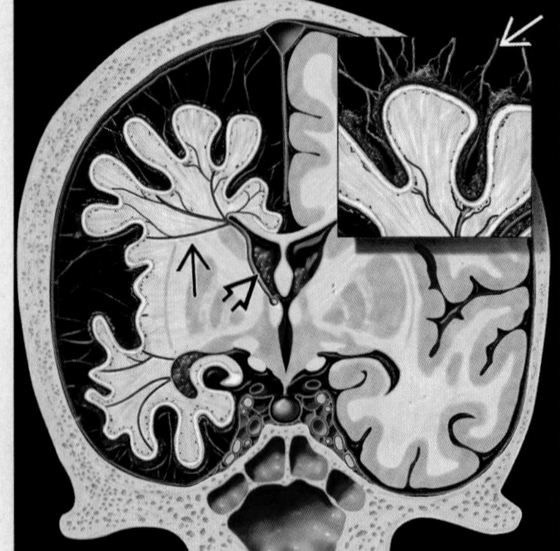

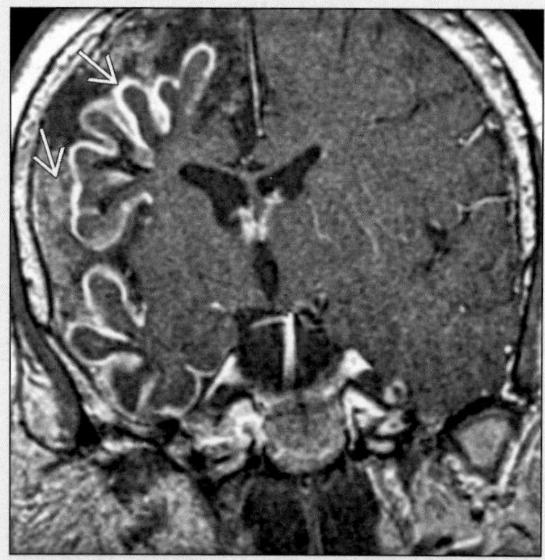

(Left) *Coronal graphic shows extensive pial angiomatosis ➔ surrounding affected gyri, prominent deep medullary collaterals ➔ shunt venous blood to deep system, enlarged ipsilateral choroid plexus ➔, and atrophy of the right cerebral hemisphere.* ***(Right)*** *Coronal T1WI C+ MR shows extensive serpentine enhancement of thickened pia ➔ (pial angiomatosis) and enlarged subarachnoid space over the right cerebral hemisphere. Severe right-sided hemiatrophy is evident.*

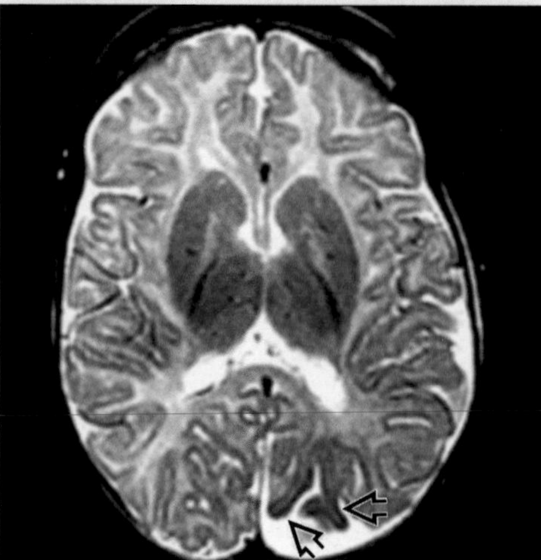

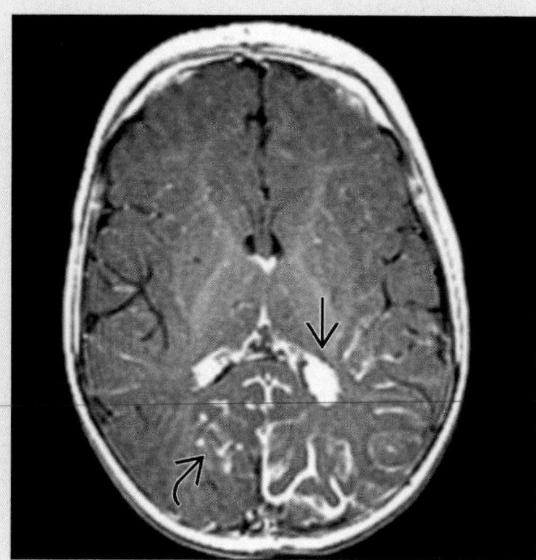

(Left) *Axial T2WI MR in a 4-month-old infant with SW demonstrates volume loss in the posterior left hemisphere and hypointense white matter, "pseudo-acceleration" of myelin maturation. Decreased cortical signal ➔ is also evident.* ***(Right)*** *Axial T1WI C+ MR in the same patient reveals leptomeningeal enhancement on the left side and less severe involvement of the right medial occipital lobe ➔. Bilateral enlargement of the choroid plexus is observed, worse on the left ➔ than on the right.*

STURGE-WEBER SYNDROME

TERMINOLOGY

Abbreviations

- Sturge-Weber syndrome (SWS)

Synonyms

- Sturge-Weber-Dimitri, encephalotrigeminal angiomatosis

Definitions

- Usually sporadic congenital (but not inherited) malformation in which fetal cortical veins fail to develop normally
  - Imaging features are sequelae of progressive venous occlusion and chronic venous ischemia

IMAGING

General Features

- Best diagnostic clue
  - Cortical Ca++, atrophy, and enlarged ipsilateral choroid plexus
- Location
  - Pial angiomatosis unilateral (80%), bilateral (20%)
  - Occipital > parietal > frontal/temporal lobes > diencephalon/midbrain > cerebellum

Radiographic Findings

- Radiography
  - "Tram-track" calcification

CT Findings

- NECT
  - Gyral/subcortical white matter (WM) Ca++
    - Ca++ not in leptomeningeal angioma
    - Progressive, generally posterior to anterior
  - Late
    - Cerebral atrophy
    - Hyperpneumatization of paranasal sinuses
    - Thick diploe
- CECT
  - Serpentine leptomeningeal enhancement
  - Ipsilateral choroid plexus enlargement usual
    - Choroidal fissure if frontal involvement
    - Trigonal glomus if posterior involvement

MR Findings

- T1WI
  - Early: ↑ WM volume subjacent to pial angiomatosis
  - Late: Atrophy of WM and gray matter
- T2WI
  - Early: Transient hyperperfusion → "accelerated" myelin maturation
  - Late: Increased signal in region of gliosis and decreased cortical signal in regions of calcification
- FLAIR
  - Late: Gliosis in involved lobes
- T2* GRE
  - "Tram-track" gyral calcifications
- DWI
  - Restricted diffusion in acute ischemia
- T1WI C+
  - Early: Serpentine leptomeningeal enhancement, pial angiomatosis of subarachnoid space
    - Amount of CE increases if MR performed during ictal period; mimics disease progression
  - Late: "Burnt out" → decreased pial enhancement, increased cortical/subcortical Ca++; atrophy
  - Engorged, enhancing choroid plexus
  - Susceptibility weighted imaging (SWI) superior to T1 C+ for identification of enlarged transmantle and periventricular veins
- MRA
  - Rare high-flow arteriovenous malformations
- MRV
  - Progressive sinovenous occlusion
    - Lack of superficial cortical veins
    - ↑ ↑ prominence deep collateral (medullary/subependymal) veins
- MRS
  - ↑ choline, ↓ NAA in affected areas
- Fat saturation: Orbital enhancement > 50%, best seen with T1 C+ fat saturation
  - Choroidal angioma, periorbital soft tissues, bony orbit, and frontal bone

Ultrasonographic Findings

- Pulsed Doppler
  - ↓ middle cerebral artery velocity

Angiographic Findings

- Conventional
  - Pial blush, rare arteriovenous malformation
  - Findings mostly venous: Paucity of normal cortical veins, extensive medullary and deep collaterals

Nuclear Medicine Findings

- PET
  - Progressive hypoperfusion, progressive glucose hypometabolism
- SPECT: Transient hyperperfusion (early), hypoperfusion (late)
  - Pattern inconsistent; may be smaller or larger than abnormality detected on CT/MR

Imaging Recommendations

- Best imaging tool
  - Enhanced MR
- Protocol advice
  - NECT to evaluate for calcification (may be more extensive than recognized on MR)
  - MR with contrast (assess extent, uni-/bilaterality, orbital involvement)
    - FLAIR + contrast improves conspicuity of leptomeningeal angiomatosis
    - Perfusion may predict progression

DIFFERENTIAL DIAGNOSIS

Other Vascular Phakomatoses (Neurocutaneous Syndromes)

- Blue rubber bleb nevus syndrome
  - Multiple small, cutaneous venous malformations plus intracranial developmental venous anomalies
- Wyburn-Mason syndrome

STURGE-WEBER SYNDROME

- Facial vascular nevus; visual pathway &/or brain arteriovenous malformation (AVM)
- Klippel-Trenaunay-Weber syndrome
  - Osseous/soft tissue hypertrophy, extremity vascular malformations
  - May be combined with some features of SWS
- PHACES
  - **P**osterior fossa malformations, **h**emangiomas, **a**rterial anomalies, **c**oarctation of aorta, cardiac, **e**ye, and **s**ternal anomalies
- Meningioangiomatosis
  - Ca++ common; variable leptomeningeal enhancement; atrophy usually absent
  - May invade brain through Virchow-Robin perivascular spaces

Leptomeningeal Enhancement

- Meningitis, leptomeningeal metastases, and leukemia; encephalocraniocutaneous lipomatosis

PATHOLOGY

General Features

- Etiology
  - Persistent fetal vasculature → deep venous occlusion/stasis → anoxic cortex
- Genetics
  - Usually sporadic: Probable somatic mutation or cutaneous mosaicism
    - Fibronectin (found in SWS "port wine"-derived fibroblasts and SWS surgical brain samples) regulates angiogenesis and vasculogenesis
  - Very rarely familial but occasionally with other vascular phakomatosis
- Associated abnormalities
  - 50% have extracranial "port wine stains" (torso or extremities), so evaluate for other vascular phakomatoses
- Cutaneous nevus flammeus CNV1 and CNV2, ± visceral angiomatosis
- Embryology
  - 4-8 weeks: Embryonic cortical veins fail to coalesce and develop → persistent primordial vessels
  - Visual cortex adjacent to optic vesicle and upper fetal face

Staging, Grading, & Classification

- Roach scale
  - Type 1: Facial, choroid + leptomeningeal
  - Type 2: Facial only, ± glaucoma
  - Type 3: Leptomeningeal angioma only (5% of all)

Microscopic Features

- Pial angioma = multiple, thin-walled vessels in enlarged sulci
- Cortical atrophy, Ca++
- Occasional underlying cortical dysplasia

CLINICAL ISSUES

Presentation

- Most common signs/symptoms
  - CNV1 facial nevus flammeus ("port wine stain") (98%), ± V2, V3
  - Eye findings especially with upper and lower lid nevus flammeus
    - Choroidal angioma (70%) → increased intraocular pressure/congenital glaucoma → buphthalmos
    - Retinal telangiectatic vessels, scleral angioma, iris heterochromia
  - Seizures (75-90%), hemiparesis (30-66%)
  - Stroke-like episodes, neurological deficit, migraines
- Clinical profile
  - "Port wine stain," seizures, hemiparesis

Demographics

- Age
  - Facial lesion visible at birth
    - Pial angiomatosis may be occult if no facial lesion and no seizures to prompt imaging
  - Seizures develop in 1st year of life
    - Infantile spasms → tonic/clonic, myoclonic
- Epidemiology
  - Rare: 1:20,000-50,000

Natural History & Prognosis

- ↑ extent of lobar involvement and atrophy leading to increased likelihood of seizures
- Seizures cause further brain injury
- Progressive hemiparesis (30%), homonymous hemianopsia (2%)

Treatment

- Aggressive seizure management, ± resect affected lobes (hemisphere)
- Low-dose aspirin may decrease frequency of stroke-like episodes

DIAGNOSTIC CHECKLIST

Consider

- Child with facial nevus flammeus who reaches 2 years of age with normal neurological and MR exams probably does not have brain involvement

Image Interpretation Pearls

- FLAIR C+ most sensitive sequence to detect leptomeningeal angioma, especially in infancy

SELECTED REFERENCES

1. Hu J et al: MR susceptibility weighted imaging (SWI) complements conventional contrast enhanced T1 weighted MRI in characterizing brain abnormalities of Sturge-Weber Syndrome. J Magn Reson Imaging. 28(2):300-7, 2008
2. Comi AM: Sturge-Weber syndrome and epilepsy: an argument for aggressive seizure management in these patients. Expert Rev Neurother. 7(8):951-6, 2007
3. Di Rocco C et al: Sturge-Weber syndrome. Childs Nerv Syst. 22(8):909-21, 2006
4. Evans AL et al: Cerebral perfusion abnormalities in children with Sturge-Weber syndrome shown by dynamic contrast bolus magnetic resonance perfusion imaging. Pediatrics. 117(6):2119-25, 2006
5. Comi AM et al: Increased fibronectin expression in sturge-weber syndrome fibroblasts and brain tissue. Pediatr Res. 53(5):762-9, 2003

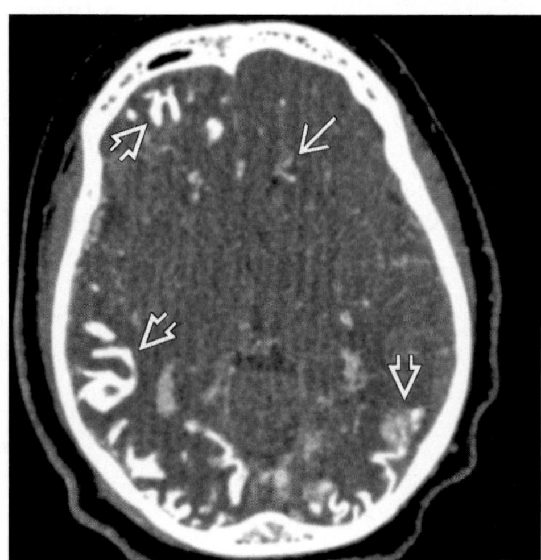

(Left) *Axial T1 C+ MR of a 5 year old reveals extensive bilateral leptomeningeal angiomatosis. The choroid plexuses are enlarged bilaterally, and prominent subependymal/ intraventricular veins are seen as foci of signal void → near the ventricles.* ***(Right)*** *Axial CECT of the same patient 7 years later reveals extensive bilateral cortical calcification →, but relatively little atrophy given the extent of the angiomatosis. Prominent enhancing → subependymal veins are faintly seen.*

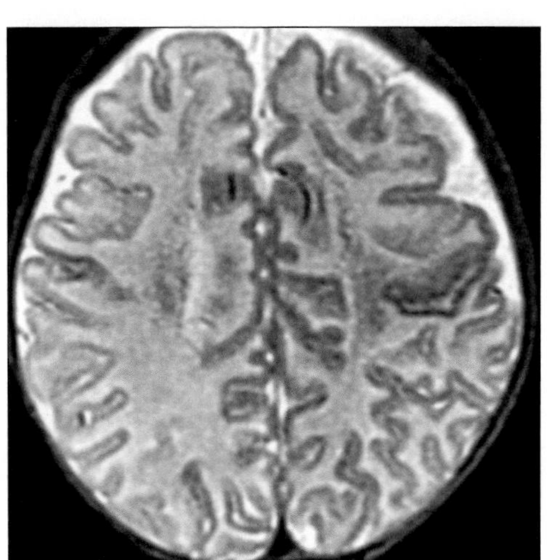

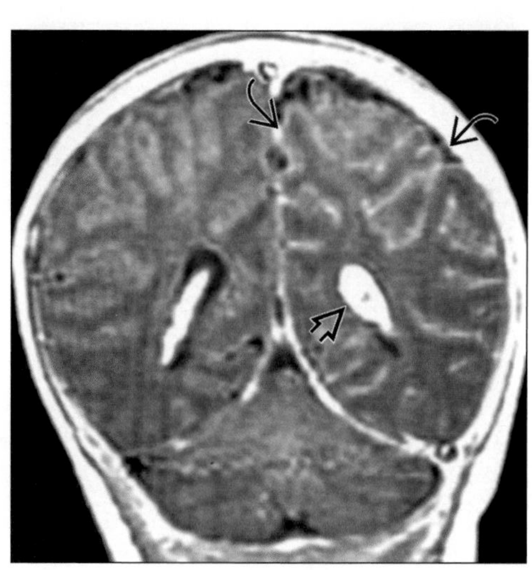

(Left) *Axial T2WI MR of a 5-week-old infant with a left facial "port wine stain" reveals no abnormality.* ***(Right)*** *Coronal T1WI MR of the same patient shows subtle contrast enhancement of the left parietooccipital leptomeninges → and increased volume of the left choroid plexus →. This case nicely demonstrates the importance of contrast-enhanced images to properly evaluate for SWS in infants, at a time when cerebral atrophy may not be present.*

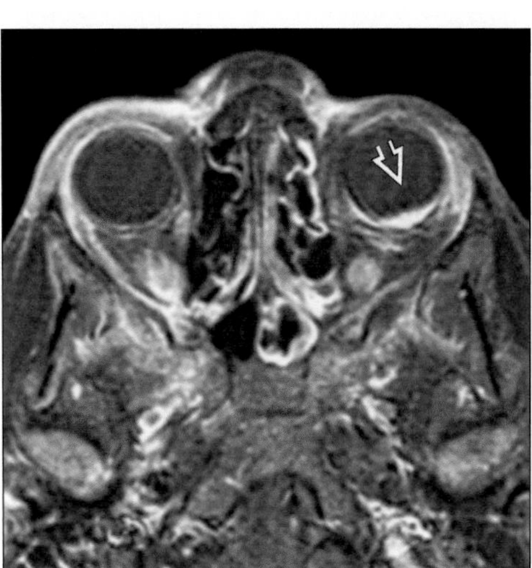

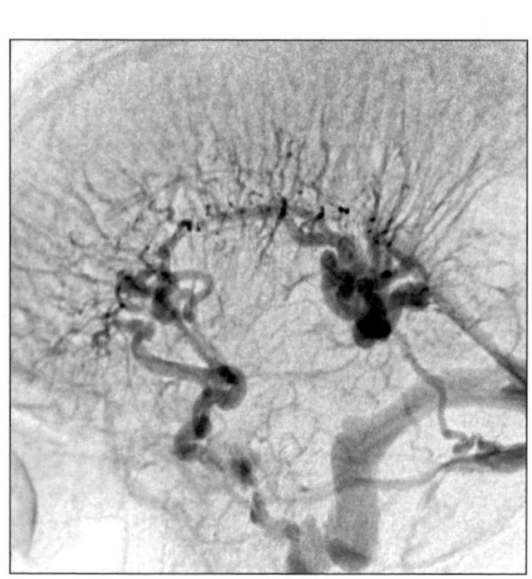

(Left) *Axial T1 C+ FS MR of a 10 year old demonstrates orbital involvement by choroidal angioma, revealed as crescentic enhancement → of the posterior left choroid. One should look for orbital enhancement, as it denotes patients at risk for increased intraocular pressure and glaucoma.* ***(Right)*** *Lateral view, catheter angiogram during the venous phase of carotid injection shows extensive medullary venous collateral drainage and lack of normal superficial drainage in a child with Sturge-Weber syndrome.*

MENINGIOANGIOMATOSIS

Key Facts

Terminology

- Rare, hamartomatous cortical/leptomeningeal malformation

Imaging

- Cortical mass with calcification
- Cortex (frontal and temporal lobes)
- Slight enhancement

Top Differential Diagnoses

- Lesions with calcification and cysts
- Meningioma
- Oligodendroglioma
- Granulomatous meningitis
- Parasitic diseases (cysticercosis)
- Ganglioglioma
- Sturge-Weber disease
- Dysembryoplastic neuroepithelial tumor

Pathology

- Uncertain
  - Hamartoma? meningioma invading brain? vascular malformation?
- Neurofibromatosis found in 1/2 of patients (particularly NF2)
- Features of meningioma and angioma
- Slow-growing tumor
- Confined to cortex, ± involvement of leptomeninges
- Cortical meningovascular proliferation, ± leptomeningeal calcification
- No malignant degeneration

Clinical Issues

- Gross total resection for treatment of seizure disorder; excellent prognosis with excision

*(**Left**) Axial T2WI MR shows a serpiginous peripheral right frontal lobe mass ➔ with cortical hypointensity and subcortical hyperintensity. The hypointense region corresponds to a site of calcification detected on NECT (not shown). (**Right**) Axial T1WI C+ MR shows incomplete, moderate cortical enhancement ➔. The overlying gyrus is deformed ("clubbed"), mimicking a balloon cell dysplasia; however, there is significant enhancement and no extension of abnormality into deeper white matter.*

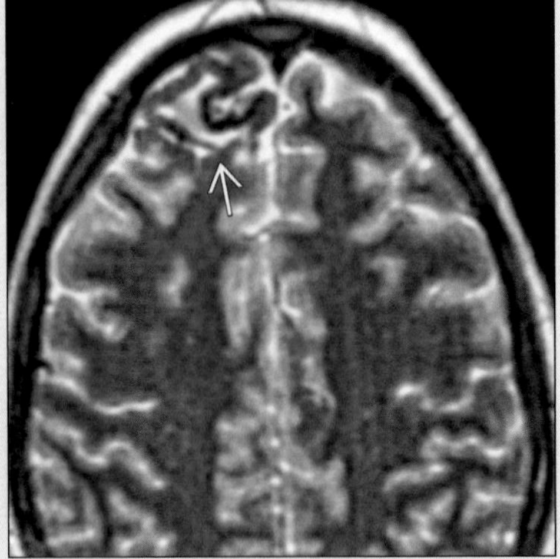

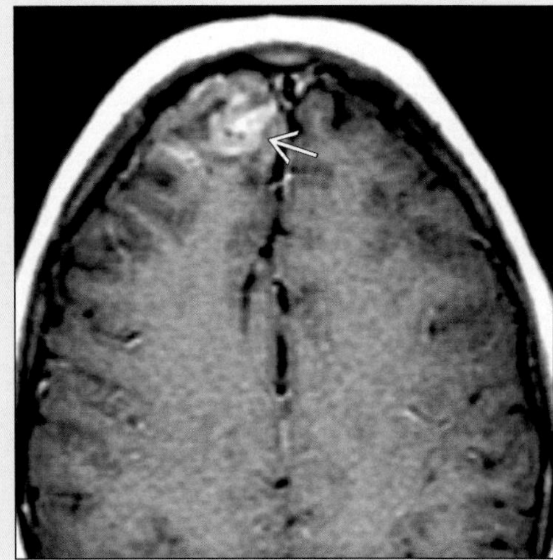

*(**Left**) Axial NECT in a 16-year-old patient with a longstanding seizure disorder shows fine, gyriform increased attenuation in the suprainsular region on the right ➔, representing calcification. (**Right**) Axial FLAIR MR in the same patient shows increased signal in the subarachnoid space ➔. Decreased signal in the subcortical white matter ➔ may be caused by excessive myelination or by iron accumulation within subcortical axons due to interrupted iron transport to the neuronal bodies.*

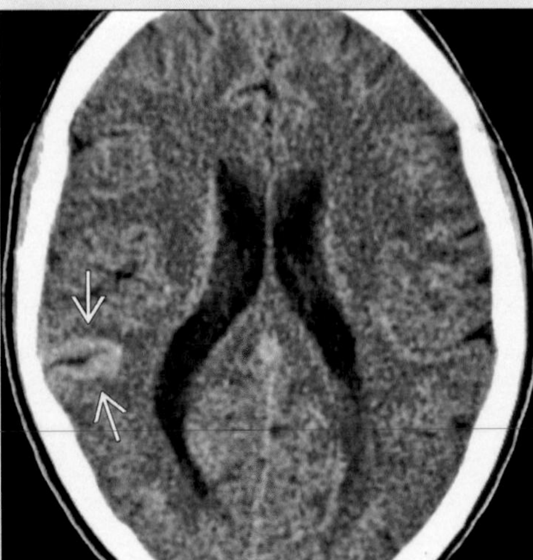

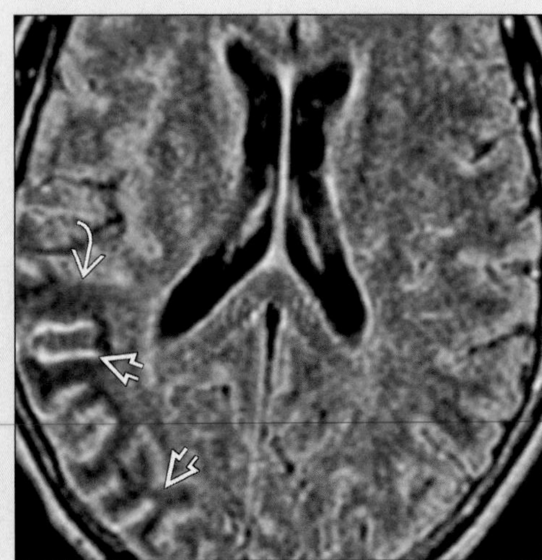

MENINGIOANGIOMATOSIS

TERMINOLOGY

Definitions

- Rare, hamartomatous cortical/leptomeningeal malformation

IMAGING

General Features

- Best diagnostic clue
  - Cortical mass with calcification
- Location
  - Cortex (frontal and temporal lobes)
  - Rarely in 3rd ventricle, thalami, brainstem, cerebellum
- Size
  - Generally small lesions (1-3 cm)

CT Findings

- NECT
  - Solitary or multiple cortical mass(es) and Ca++
    - Calcification: Nodular, linear, or gyriform
  - Occasional: Hemorrhage and cysts
  - No or little mass effect
- CECT
  - Little or no enhancement

MR Findings

- T1WI
  - Isointense with areas of signal void (Ca++)
  - Hypointense cysts
- T2WI
  - Hyperintense with areas of signal void (Ca++)
  - Target-like lesions, central hyperintensity
  - Hyperintense cysts
- PD/intermediate
  - Slightly hyperintense, areas of signal void (Ca++)
- T2* GRE
  - Accentuates calcification
- T1WI C+
  - Slight enhancement

Imaging Recommendations

- Best imaging tool
  - MR and CT
- Protocol advice
  - Noncontrast CT to look for calcium; contrast-enhanced MR to look at cysts, edema, and parenchymal enhancement

DIFFERENTIAL DIAGNOSIS

Lesions with Calcification and Cysts

- Meningioma
- Oligodendroglioma
- Granulomatous meningitis
  - Sarcoid, tuberculosis
- Parasitic diseases (cysticercosis)
- Ganglioglioma
- Sturge-Weber disease
- Dysembryoplastic neuroepithelial tumor

PATHOLOGY

General Features

- Etiology
  - Uncertain
    - Hamartoma? meningioma invading brain? vascular malformation?
- Associated abnormalities
  - Neurofibromatosis found in 1/2 of patients (particularly NF2)
  - Meningioma
  - Oligodendroglioma
  - Arteriovenous malformation
  - Encephalocele
  - Meningeal hemangiopericytoma

Gross Pathologic & Surgical Features

- Features of meningioma and angioma
- Generally solitary but may be multiple
- Slow-growing tumor
- Psammomatous Ca++ or dense osteoid
- Serpentine blood vessels overlying lesion

Microscopic Features

- Confined to cortex, ± involvement of leptomeninges
- Cortical meningovascular proliferation, ± leptomeningeal calcification
- Ca++, fibrocartilage, &/or bone formation
- Gliotic cortex
- No malignant degeneration

CLINICAL ISSUES

Presentation

- Most common signs/symptoms
  - Intractable seizures, headaches
  - Can be found incidentally (particularly NF2)
- Clinical profile
  - Children, young adults with seizure disorder

Treatment

- Gross total resection for treatment of seizure disorder; excellent prognosis with excision

DIAGNOSTIC CHECKLIST

Image Interpretation Pearls

- Calcified cortical mass ± cysts

SELECTED REFERENCES

1. Kim NR et al: Allelic loss on chromosomes 1p32, 9p21, 13q14, 16q22, 17p, and 22q12 in meningiomas associated with meningioangiomatosis and pure meningioangiomatosis. J Neurooncol. 94(3):425-30, 2009
2. Jallo GI et al: Meningioangiomatosis without neurofibromatosis: a clinical analysis. J Neurosurg. 103(4 Suppl):319-24, 2005
3. Kim NR et al: Childhood meningiomas associated with meningioangiomatosis: report of five cases and literature review. Neuropathol Appl Neurobiol. 28(1):48-56, 2002

BASAL CELL NEVUS SYNDROME

Key Facts

Terminology

- Basal cell nevus syndrome (BCNS), nevoid basal cell carcinoma syndrome (NBCCS), Gorlin syndrome, Gorlin-Goltz syndrome
- BCNS: Hereditary tumor syndrome characterized by multiple basal cell epitheliomas (BCE)/basal cell carcinomas (BCC), odontogenic keratocysts, palmoplantar pits, dural Ca++, ± medulloblastoma

Imaging

- Multiple jaw cysts, prominent dural Ca++, macrocephaly
- Odontogenic keratocysts (OKC) in 80-90%
- Large, uni-/multilocular sharply marginated cysts containing unerupted teeth
- Early Ca++ of falx cerebri, tentorium, peri-clinoid ligaments (dural bridging), dura, pia, choroid plexus, and basal ganglia

Top Differential Diagnoses

- Prominent dural calcifications (physiologic, metabolic)
- Maxillary/mandibular cyst(s)
  - Ameloblastoma
  - Dentigerous or aneurysmal bone cyst
  - Cherubism
  - Giant reparative granuloma
  - Odontogenic myxoma
  - Maxillary sinus mucocele

Pathology

- Desmoplastic medulloblastoma seen in 4-20% (1-2% of patients with medulloblastomas have BCNS)

Clinical Issues

- Most patients with BCNS have OKC; 5% of patients with OKC have BCNS

(Left) *Coronal T2WI MR of a classic BCNS show a large, unilocular T2 hyperintense cyst arising from the left maxillary alveolar ridge. The cyst bulges into the maxillary sinus, displacing the floor of the sinus and secretions superiorly ➔. Distinguishing a sinus mucous retention cyst from an alveolar ridge/dental cyst is best done on coronal images.* ***(Right)*** *Coronal T1WI MR shows a T1 hypointense cystic mass. The floor of the sinus is less well characterized than on the coronal T2 image.*

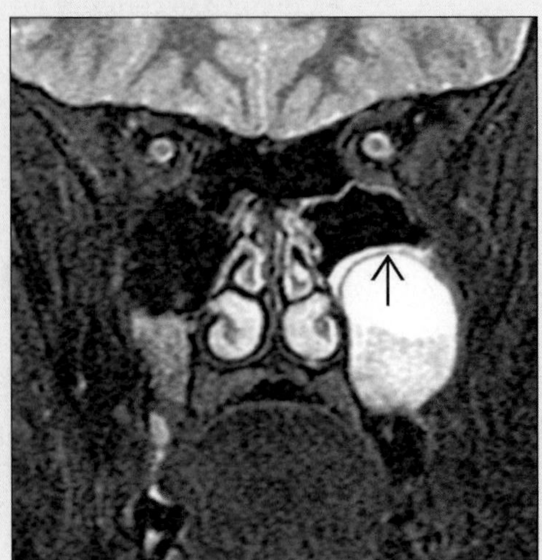

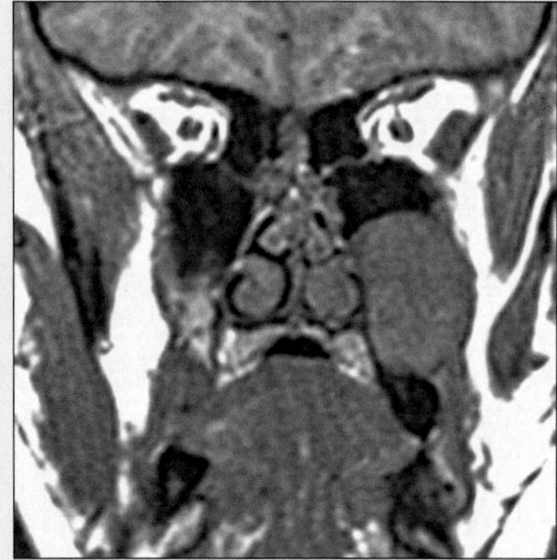

(Left) *Axial NECT of a 16 year old with BCNS reveals extensive lamellar calcifications of the falx cerebri ➔ and the tentorium cerebelli ↷. A defect is evident in the right temporal lobe secondary to the resection of a convexity meningioma.* ***(Right)*** *Axial bone CT demonstrates a well-defined, expansile lesion in the angle of the mandible on the left ↶. At surgery, pathologic exam showed the lesion to be an odontogenic keratocyst.*

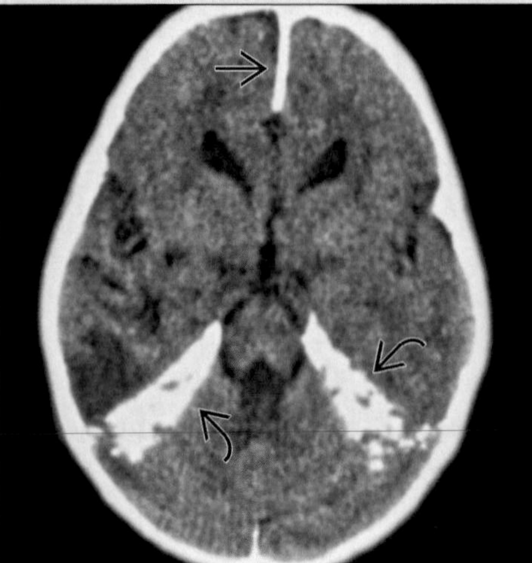

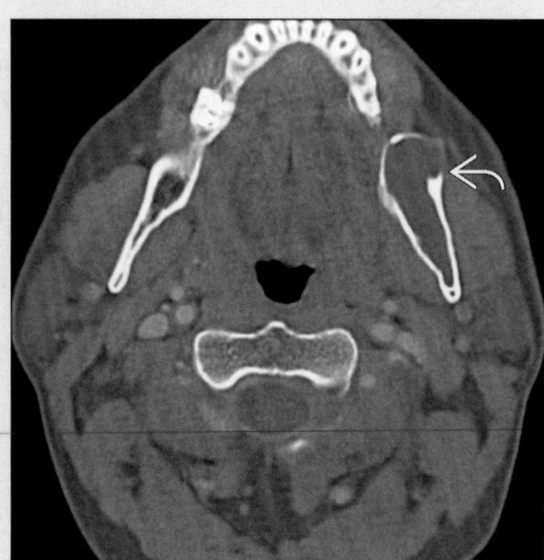

BASAL CELL NEVUS SYNDROME

TERMINOLOGY

Abbreviations

- Basal cell nevus syndrome (BCNS)

Synonyms

- Nevoid basal cell carcinoma syndrome (NBCCS), Gorlin syndrome, Gorlin-Goltz syndrome

Definitions

- Hereditary tumor syndrome characterized by multiple basal cell epitheliomas (BCE)/basal cell carcinomas (BCC), odontogenic keratocysts, palmoplantar pits, dural Ca++, ± medulloblastoma

IMAGING

General Features

- Best diagnostic clue
  - Multiple jaw cysts, prominent dural Ca++, macrocephaly
  - Other skeletal features: Hyperaerated paranasal sinuses, splayed/fused/bifid ribs, kyphoscoliosis, platybasia, Sprengel deformity of scapulae
- Location
  - Cysts: Mandible, maxilla
  - Ca++: Intracranial dura
- Size
  - Variable enlargement of mandible, maxilla

Radiographic Findings

- Radiography
  - Diffuse, tiny, lytic (kerato) cysts of bones (35%), especially jaws
  - Other
    - Thick calvarium with platybasia
    - Rib anomalies (bifid ribs; splayed, fused, or misshapen)
    - Short 4th metacarpals
    - Spina bifida occulta, vertebral segmentation anomalies

CT Findings

- NECT
  - Odontogenic keratocysts (OKC) in 80-90%
    - Large, uni-/multilocular, sharply marginated cysts containing unerupted teeth
    - Mandible > maxilla
  - Early Ca++ of falx cerebri, tentorium, peri-clinoid ligaments (dural bridging), dura, pia, choroid plexus, and basal ganglia
  - ± ventriculomegaly
  - ± callosal dysgenesis
  - Cysts of all kinds common
- CECT
  - Look for
    - Desmoplastic medulloblastoma
    - Meningioma
    - Colloid cyst

MR Findings

- T1WI
  - OKC are hypointense to isointense, contain hypointensity representing unerupted tooth
  - Dural Ca++ difficult to observe on MR
- T2WI
  - OKC are hyperintense, contain hypointensity representing unerupted tooth
- T1WI C+
  - Cysts may show thin peripheral enhancing rim
  - Look for perineural spread of head and neck BCC using fat-saturated images

Nuclear Medicine Findings

- Bone scan
  - May show ↑ uptake

Imaging Recommendations

- Best imaging tool
  - MR to screen for medulloblastoma (until 7th year of life), cystic jaw lesions
  - CT of face for oral surgery planning
- Protocol advice
  - Low mA 2-3 mm axial CT of face, including mandible, coronal reformats
  - Fat-saturated T2 and T1 C+ to diagnose jaw cysts, perineural BCC spread

DIFFERENTIAL DIAGNOSIS

Prominent Dural Calcifications

- Physiologic (usually less striking than BCNS)
- Metabolic (hyperparathyroidism, long-term hemodialysis)

Odontogenic Keratocyst (Maxillary/ Mandibular Cysts)

- Ameloblastoma
  - Bubbly appearing, solitary lesion may contain unerupted tooth
  - When large, associated enhancing soft tissue mass nearly always present
  - May have enhancing solid mural nodule
- Dentigerous cyst
  - Unilocular cyst surrounding tooth crown
  - No enhancing soft tissue
- Cherubism
  - Symmetrical cystic fibrous dysplasia of mandible
- Aneurysmal bone cyst
  - Multilocular, multiseptated mass in mandible
  - Enhancing soft tissues inside and outside of bony rim
- Giant reparative granuloma
  - Solitary mass, generally solid, does not contain unerupted tooth
- Odontogenic myxoma
  - Radiolucent areas with bony trabeculations
  - Well or poorly defined margins, aggressive growth; benign histology
- Miscellaneous maxillary masses
  - Maxillary sinus mucocele: Contains no cysts or septae; smooth expansion of sinus walls
  - Incisor canal cyst: Small; found in midline anterior maxilla, posterior to incisors; water density/ intensity
  - Globulomaxillary cyst: Small; located between lateral incisor and canine

BASAL CELL NEVUS SYNDROME

PATHOLOGY

General Features

- Etiology
  - PATCHED (*PTCH*) gene encodes Sonic hedgehog (SHH) receptor and tumor suppressor protein defective in BCNS
- Genetics
  - Autosomal dominant: Complete penetrance, variable expression
  - de novo mutations (40%)
    - New mutations ↑ with advanced paternal age
  - Mutation inactivated tumor suppressor genes *PTCH1* and *PTCH2* (9q22.3-q31)
- Associated abnormalities
  - Associated neoplasms (mutation inactivated tumor suppressor genes)
    - Rare ameloblastoma and squamous cell cancer
    - Desmoplastic medulloblastoma: Seen in 4-20% (1-2% of patients with medulloblastomas have BCNS)
    - Cardiac, abdominal, and pelvic mesenchymal tumors
- 3x more common in mandible than in maxilla
  - Mainly in premolar and retromolar triangle area
- Usually multiple, small or large, unilocular or multilocular
- May cross midline

Staging, Grading, & Classification

- Need either 2 major or 1 major/2 minor criteria for diagnosis
- Major criteria: > 2 (or 1 < 30 years) basal cell carcinomas; > 10 basal cell nevi; odontogenic keratocyst or polyostotic bone cyst; ≥ 3 palmar/ plantar pits; lamellar or (< 20 years) falx Ca++; family history
- Minor criteria: Rib or vertebral anomalies, macrocrania/frontal bossing; cardiac or ovarian fibromas; mesenteric cysts; facial clefting (5-13%), hand (long fingers, short 4th metacarpal, polydactyly) or ocular anomalies; bridging of sella turcica, medulloblastoma

Gross Pathologic & Surgical Features

- OKC: Expansile mandible &/or maxillary cysts with unerupted tooth
  - Satellite cyst formation is common; may involve coronoid process
  - Maxillary canine/premolar area > retromolar

Microscopic Features

- OKC: Parakeratinized lining and ↑ epithelial growth factor receptor

CLINICAL ISSUES

Presentation

- Most common signs/symptoms
  - Jaw and maxilla deformity with pain
- Desmoplastic medulloblastoma in boys 2 years and younger (before syndrome apparent)
  - Beware: Irradiation induced ↑ ↑ number BCC
- BCE (75%) onset at puberty, resemble nevi or skin tags; BCC by 40 years
- Skin (other): Epidermal (kerato) cysts (55%), milia, fibromas, lipomas
- Palmar and plantar pits (> 85%): Usually noticed after childhood
- Multiple OKC that may fracture or become infected
- Dysmorphic facies, large head/brow, everted mandibular angle, hypertelorism, lip clefts common, macrosomia, tall stature
- Cognition normal if no malformations/tumors and no prior irradiation (mental retardation in 5%)

Demographics

- Age
  - Usually diagnosed during 1st decade of life
    - OKC usually forms before 7 years of age
- Gender
  - No predilection
- Ethnicity
  - No predilection
- Epidemiology
  - 1 in 57,000 (1 in 200 with BCC have syndrome, 1 in 5 if < 19 years old)
  - Most patients with BCNS have OKC; 5% of patients with OKC have BCNS

Natural History & Prognosis

- Develop enormous numbers of BCCs
  - Especially fair skin, sun exposure, irradiation
  - Darkly pigmented skin protective, has smaller numbers of BCC

Treatment

- Surgery for OKC; surgery/chemotherapy, avoid radiotherapy for medulloblastoma

DIAGNOSTIC CHECKLIST

Consider

- When precocious dural Ca++ and OKC are detected

Image Interpretation Pearls

- Multiple mandibular cysts containing teeth or parts of teeth

SELECTED REFERENCES

1. Garrè ML et al: Medulloblastoma variants: age-dependent occurrence and relation to Gorlin syndrome--a new clinical perspective. Clin Cancer Res. 15(7):2463-71, 2009
2. Lo Muzio L: Nevoid basal cell carcinoma syndrome (Gorlin syndrome). Orphanet J Rare Dis. 3:32, 2008
3. Kimonis VE et al: Radiological features in 82 patients with nevoid basal cell carcinoma (NBCC or Gorlin) syndrome. Genet Med. 6(6):495-502, 2004
4. Palacios E et al: Odontogenic keratocysts in nevoid basal cell carcinoma (Gorlin's) syndrome: CT and MRI evaluation. Ear Nose Throat J. 83(1):40-2, 2004
5. Stavrou T et al: Intracranial calcifications in childhood medulloblastoma: relation to nevoid basal cell carcinoma syndrome. AJNR Am J Neuroradiol. 21(4):790-4, 2000
6. Wicking C et al: De novo mutations of the Patched gene in nevoid basal cell carcinoma syndrome help to define the clinical phenotype. Am J Med Genet. 73(3):304-7, 1997

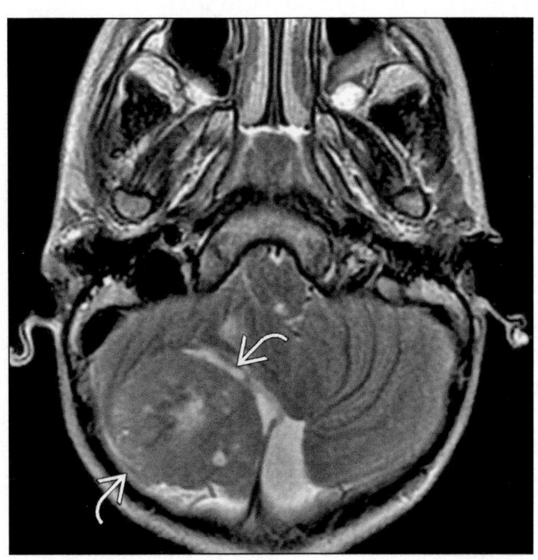

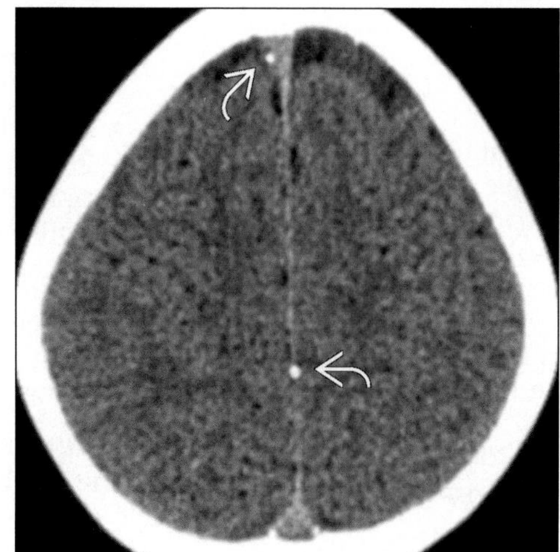

(Left) *Axial T2WI MR in a 3-year-old boy shows a well-defined T2 hypointense mass in the posterior right cerebellar hemisphere. Only slight edema surrounds the mass, which was proven to be a medulloblastoma at pathology.* **(Right)** *Axial NECT in the same patient, obtained preoperatively, reveals 2 small dural-based calcifications. Such calcifications are not normal in a child of this age and should prompt a work-up for BCNS. BCNS was confirmed with a molecular genetic test.*

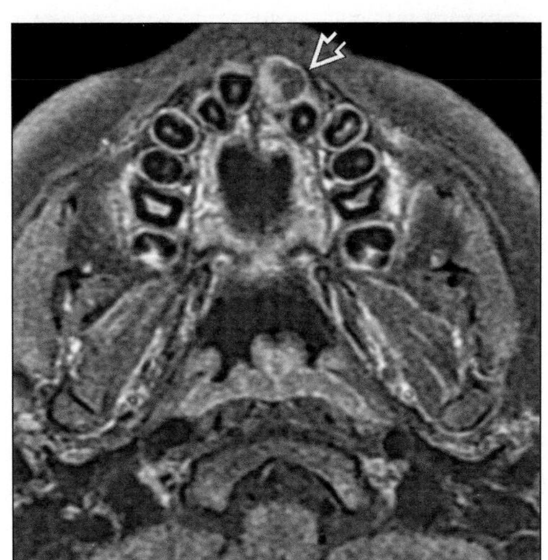

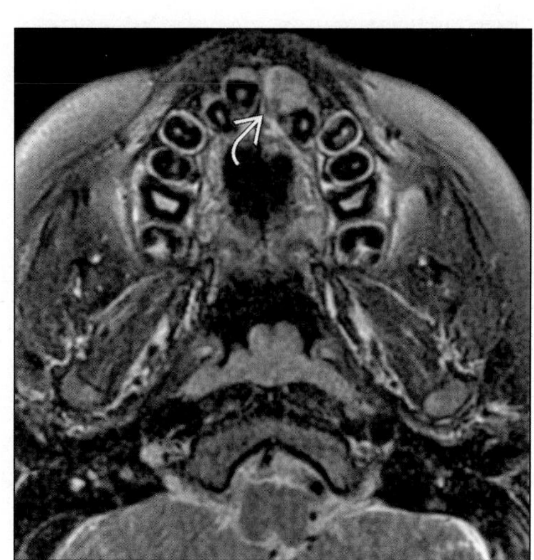

(Left) *Axial T1WI C+ FS MR in a 6-year-old child with known BCNS shows a small cystic mass in the anterior left maxillary ridge, consistent with an odontogenic keratocyst. The cyst has a thin, faintly enhancing rim and an unerupted tooth medially. The MR was performed as a screening test for medulloblastoma.* **(Right)** *Axial T2WI FS MR in the same patient shows moderate hyperintensity of the lesion contents and a hypointense unerupted tooth medial to the lesion.*

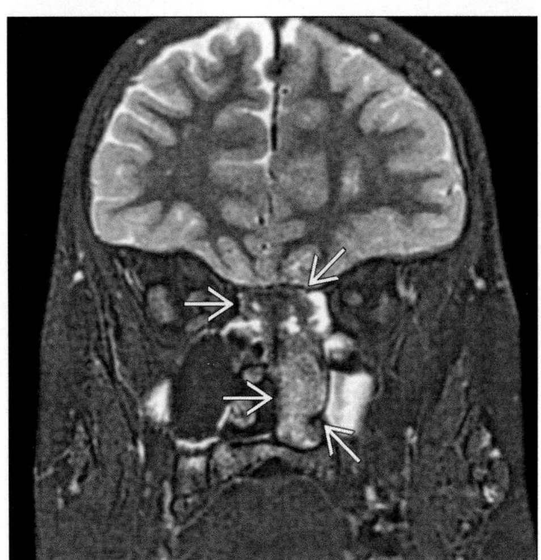

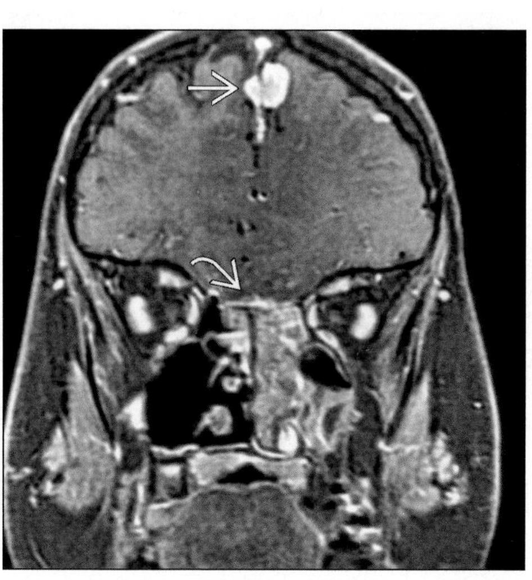

(Left) *Coronal T2WI FS MR reveals a T2 hypointense mass filling the left nasal cavity and extending into ethmoid air cells. This 19 year old with BCNS was radiated for medulloblastoma and developed a radiation-induced rhabdomyosarcoma.* **(Right)** *Coronal T1 C+ FS MR shows moderate enhancement of the nasal mass, which infiltrates the dura above the roof of the ethmoid air cells. A falx meningioma is also evident, poorly seen on the corresponding coronal T2 image.*

HEREDITARY HEMORRHAGIC TELANGIECTASIA

Key Facts

Terminology

- Hereditary hemorrhagic telangiectasia (HHT)
- Synonyms: Rendu-Osler, Rendu-Osler-Weber, Osler-Weber-Rendu syndrome

Imaging

- Intracranial vascular malformations (AVM/AVF, DVA, telangiectasia) may be multiple and occur anywhere; less common in children
- Capillary telangiectasias: Scalp, nasopharynx, orbit
- Brain: MR contrast, T2* useful to show tiny abnormalities
- Baseline screening of brain in all patients with HHT or family highly recommended (cAVMs may be devastating)
- Brain: MR with contrast, T2* GRE, MRA
- Useful: Multislice CT/CTA of lungs and liver

Pathology

- Abnormal TGF-β signal transduction affects vasculogenesis, angiogenesis, endothelial cell properties
- Type 1 HHT: Endoglin gene (9q33-q34) mutation
- Type 2 HHT: *ALK1* gene (12q11-q14) mutation
- Smallest telangiectasias = focal dilatations of post-capillary venules that enlarge and extend through capillaries toward arterioles → AVF/AVM

Clinical Issues

- Telangiectasias: Lips, mouth, tongue, around nails
- Recurrent epistaxis from nasal mucosal telangiectasias

Diagnostic Checklist

- Brain abscess, ischemia uncommon but serious complication in HHT patients with pAVMs

(Left) Sagittal T2WI MR of a 3-month-old boy with hydrocephalus demonstrates a huge, vascular-looking mass within the posterior fossa ➡, causing major brainstem compression ➡ and obstructive hydrocephalus. Note the dilated vein of Galen ➡. This child had a family history of HHT. *(Right)* Coronal T2WI MR in the same child shows the posterior fossa mass ➡ displacing the brain stem ➡, causing massive hydrocephalus. There is a right choroid-thalamic cluster of vessels ➡ suggesting a choroidal AVM.

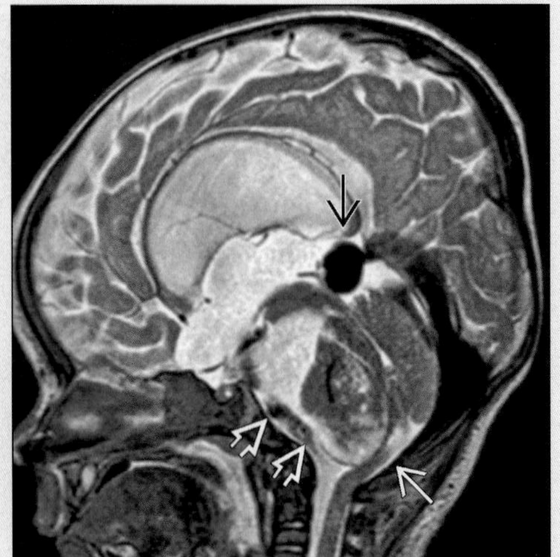

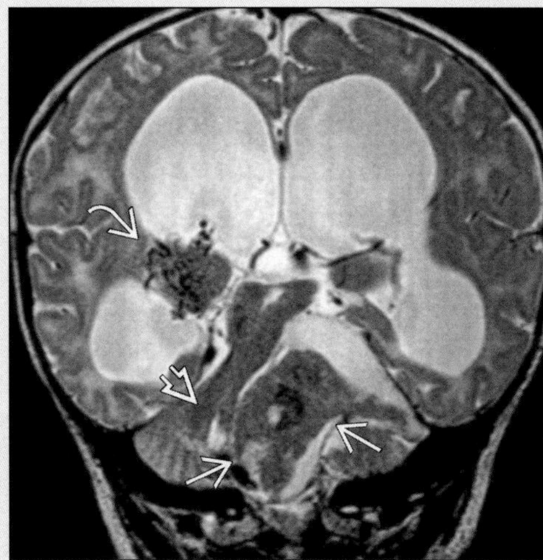

(Left) Lateral right vertebral DSA in the same child confirms that the mass seen on MR is a venous varix fed by a single high-flow fistula ➡ from the right vertebral artery, lateral to the medulla. It drained through 2 stenotic channels toward the straight and the left transverse sinuses. *(Right)* Anteroposterior right carotid DSA confirms nidus ➡ of the choroidal AVM fed by the right choroidal arteries and draining toward the dilated vein of Galen ➡.

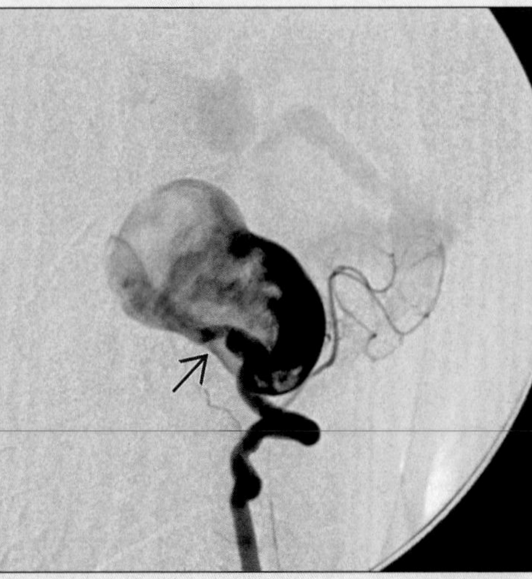

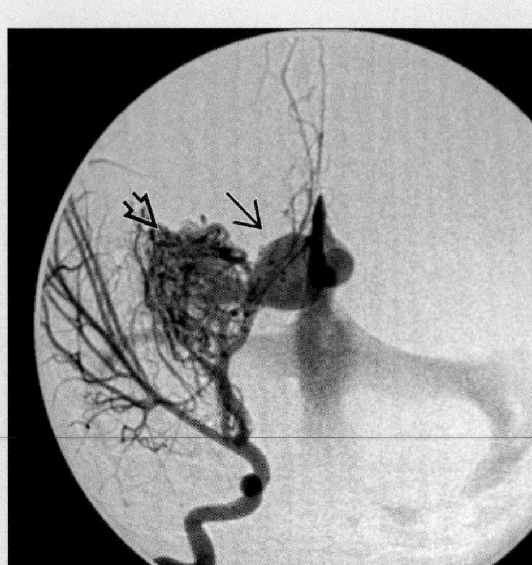

TERMINOLOGY

Abbreviations

- Hereditary hemorrhagic telangiectasia (HHT)

Synonyms

- Rendu-Osler, Rendu-Osler-Weber, Osler-Weber-Rendu syndrome

Definitions

- Autosomal dominant disorder with widely distributed, multisystem angiodysplastic lesions
  - Mucocutaneous, visceral telangiectasias
  - Arteriovenous malformations (AVMs)/arteriovenous fistulas (AVFs), telangiectasias of lungs, brain, GI tract, liver

IMAGING

General Features

- Best diagnostic clue
  - Multiple pulmonary (pAVM) or cerebral (cAVM) arteriovenous malformations in patient with recurrent epistaxis
- Location
  - Capillary telangiectasias: Scalp, nasopharynx, orbit
  - Intracranial vascular malformations (AVM/AVF, DVA, telangiectasia) may be multiple and occur anywhere; less common in children
- Size
  - cAVMs in HHT usually small and often incidental
- Morphology
  - Dilated tangle of vessels, "blooming" artifacts

CT Findings

- NECT
  - Brain
    - AVM = isodense serpentine vessels
    - Abscess = low-density mass, iso-/hyperdense rim
- CECT
  - Brain
    - Strong, uniform, vascular nidus enhancement
    - Ring enhancement of abscesses (late cerebritis, early capsule stage)
    - DVA not rare (8%)
- CTA
  - Demonstrates feeders and draining veins of AVMs, AVFs
  - Visceral evaluation also needed

MR Findings

- T1WI
  - cAVM: Flow voids common, ± hemorrhage
  - Telangiectasia, DVA not visualized
- T2WI
  - cAVM: Flow voids ± hemorrhage, edema, mass effect, gliosis
- FLAIR
  - Nest of flow voids, gliosis
- T2* GRE
  - "Blooming" artifacts of capillary telangiectasias; useful in detecting microhemorrhages
- T1WI C+
  - Slow-flow vascular malformations (e.g., DVAs) enhance
  - Good demonstration of AVM nidus, feeding arteries, and draining veins
- MRA
  - Demonstrates intermediate to large cAVMs
  - "Micro" AVM/telangiectasia/DVA usually not visualized
- MRV
  - May demonstrate DVA

Angiographic Findings

- Vascular malformations shown in brain and nasal mucosa
  - Only 10-20% > 10 mm

Imaging Recommendations

- Best imaging tool
  - Brain: MR contrast, T2* useful to show tiny abnormalities
    - Baseline screening of brain in all patients with HHT or family highly recommended (cAVMs may be devastating)
- Protocol advice
  - Brain: MR with contrast, T2* GRE, MRA
    - Lungs, liver: Multislice CT/CTA useful

DIFFERENTIAL DIAGNOSIS

Nasal Mucosal "Blush"

- Prominent but normal nasal mucosal "blush" can mimic capillary telangiectasia

Multiple Intracranial AVMs without HHT

- 50% associated with other vascular neurocutaneous syndrome (Wyburn-Mason, etc.)

Multiple Intracranial DVAs

- Less common than in blue rubber bleb nevus syndrome (BRBN)

Multiple Capillary Telangiectasias

- Can be found incidentally without HHT
- Capillary telangiectasias in HHT more common outside brain than in it!

Multiple Cavernous Malformations

- Multiple cavernoma syndrome

PATHOLOGY

General Features

- Etiology
  - Abnormal TGF-β signal transduction affects
    - Vasculogenesis
    - Angiogenesis
    - Endothelial cell properties
- Genetics
  - Autosomal dominant: Inheritance; 2 main mutations
    - Type 1 HHT: Endoglin gene (9q33-q34) mutation
      - Telangiectasias, early onset of epistaxis, pAVMs
    - Type 2 HHT: *ALK1* gene (12q11-q14) mutation
      - Lower penetrance, milder disease, GI bleeds

HEREDITARY HEMORRHAGIC TELANGIECTASIA

Staging, Grading, & Classification

- Most cAVMs in HHT are low grade (Spetzler-Martin 1 or 2)

Gross Pathologic & Surgical Features

- Multiple telangiectasias of mucosa, dermis, viscera
- AVMs, AVFs only in certain forms of HHT
  - Most pAVMs are actually AVFs (direct connection between artery and vein through thin-walled aneurysm)
  - Hepatic AV shunts less common, often numerous

Microscopic Features

- Smallest telangiectasias = focal dilatations of post-capillary venules that enlarge and extend through capillaries toward arterioles → AVF/AVM

CLINICAL ISSUES

Presentation

- Most common signs/symptoms
  - Recurrent epistaxis from nasal mucosal telangiectasias
- Other signs/symptoms
  - Telangiectasia locations
    - Lips
    - Mouth
    - Tongue
    - Around nails
- Clinical profile
  - HHT diagnosis based on combination of findings (Shovlin criteria)
    - Mucocutaneous telangiectasias, spontaneous/recurrent episodes of epistaxis, visceral involvement, family history
  - 70% of patients with pAVMs have HHT
    - 5-15% of HHT patients have pAVMs
  - > 50% of patients with multiple cAVMs have HHT
    - 5-13% of HHT patients have cAVMs (usually late in life)
  - 2-17% of HHT patients have hepatic AVMs (depends on kindred)
- Neurologic symptoms common
  - Intracranial bleed from AVM/AVF
  - TIA, stroke, abscess secondary to pAVMs

Demographics

- Age
  - Epistaxis typically begins by age 10
  - Most HHT patients are symptomatic by 21 years old
  - Skin lesions appear later (most by 40 years old)
- Epidemiology
  - Rare: 1-2:10,000

Natural History & Prognosis

- Epistaxis
  - Increases in frequency and severity
- HHT cAVMs have lower bleeding risk than sporadic AVMs
  - Rare cases may regress spontaneously
  - Significant lifetime risk of brain abscess or stroke if pAVM present
- GI bleeding limits lifespan when < 50 years old
  - Many require multiple transfusions and endoscopies
  - Heart failure with hepatic AVM: Poor prognosis

Treatment

- pAVMs: Excellent results with embolization
- cAVMs: Embolization vs. radiosurgery depending on size and location
- Mucosal telangiectasias (nose, GI tract): Laser coagulation
- Prophylactic antibiotics prior to all dental work if pAVM present
- IV iron useful if oral iron fails to maintain satisfactory level

DIAGNOSTIC CHECKLIST

Consider

- Screening brain MR in family members of HHT patients

Image Interpretation Pearls

- Most common intracranial vascular malformation in HHT patients is AVM, not telangiectasia
- Brain abscess and ischemia uncommon but serious complication in HHT patients with pAVMs

SELECTED REFERENCES

1. Govani FS et al: Hereditary haemorrhagic telangiectasia: a clinical and scientific review. Eur J Hum Genet. 17(7):860-71, 2009
2. Giordano P et al: HHT in childhood: screening for special patients. Curr Pharm Des. 12(10):1221-5, 2006
3. Krings T et al: Hereditary hemorrhagic telangiectasia in children: endovascular treatment of neurovascular malformations: results in 31 patients. Neuroradiology. 47(12):946-54, 2005
4. Jaskolka J et al: Imaging of hereditary hemorrhagic telangiectasia. AJR Am J Roentgenol. 183(2):307-14, 2004
5. Berg J et al: Hereditary haemorrhagic telangiectasia: a questionnaire based study to delineate the different phenotypes caused by endoglin and ALK1 mutations. J Med Genet. 40(8):585-90, 2003
6. Kuwayama K et al: Central nervous system lesions associated with hereditary hemorrhagic telangiectasia--three case reports. Neurol Med Chir (Tokyo). 43(9):447-51, 2003
7. Marchuk DA et al: Vascular morphogenesis: tales of two syndromes. Hum Mol Genet. 12 Spec No 1:R97-112, 2003
8. Sabba C et al: Hereditary hemorrhagic teleangiectasia (Rendu-Osler-Weber disease). Minerva Cardioangiol. 50(3):221-38, 2002
9. Shah RK et al: Hereditary hemorrhagic telangiectasia: a review of 76 cases. Laryngoscope. 112(5):767-73, 2002
10. Byard RW et al: Osler-Weber-Rendu syndrome--pathological manifestations and autopsy considerations. J Forensic Sci. 46(3):698-701, 2001
11. Dong SL et al: Brain abscess in patients with hereditary hemorrhagic telangiectasia: case report and literature review. J Emerg Med. 20(3):247-51, 2001
12. Willemse RB et al: Bleeding risk of cerebrovascular malformations in hereditary hemorrhagic telangiectasia. J Neurosurg. 92(5):779-84, 2000

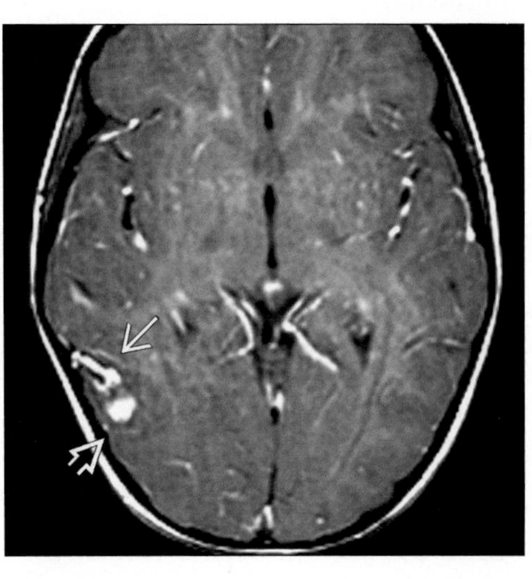

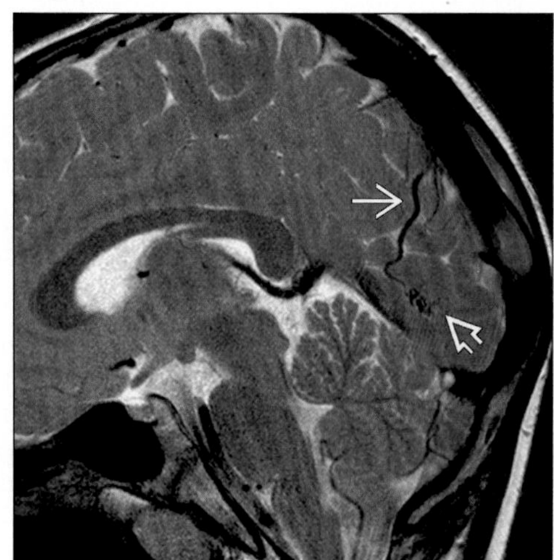

(Left) *Axial T1WI C+ MR demonstrates a venous pouch ➡ in the right posterior temporal lobe with an adjacent dilated artery ➡ in a child with documented HHT. The suspected diagnosis of pial AV fistula was confirmed on MRA (not shown).* **(Right)** *Sagittal T2WI MR in a child screened for brain lesions in the context of familial HHT demonstrates a small, silent medial occipital AVF/AVM ➡ with its dilated draining vein ➡ coursing toward the superior sagittal sinus.*

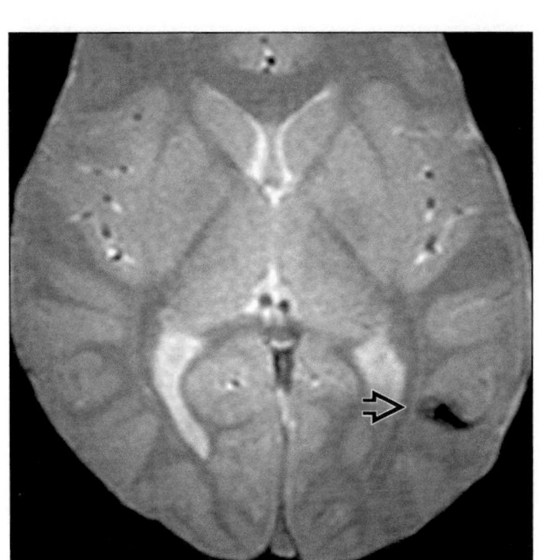

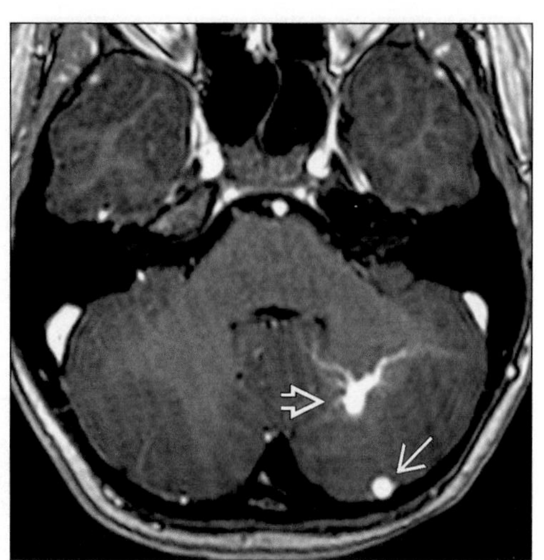

(Left) *Axial T2* GRE MR of a child with diagnosed HHT. Hypointensity is seen in the left parietooccipital region ➡ due to susceptibility effects of a pial telangiectasia. Similar lesions were seen in the right cerebellum and left middle temporal sulci (not shown).* **(Right)** *Axial T1WI C+ SPGR MR in a child with diagnosed HHT shows a left cerebellar DVA ➡ draining into a posterior pial vein ➡. Although not specific, DVAs are more common in HHT than in the general population.*

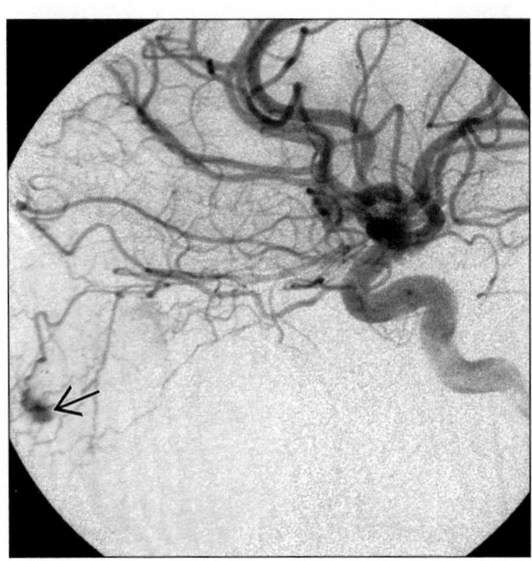

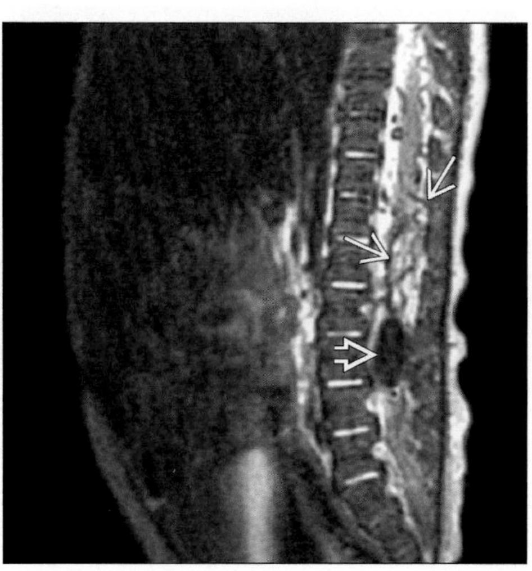

(Left) *Lateral DSA of a left internal carotid artery injection in a patient with multiple nasal mucosal telangiectasias and recurrent epistaxis shows that the ophthalmic artery supplies an inferior orbital conjunctival telangiectasia ➡.* **(Right)** *Sagittal T2WI of the spine and cord in a 1-year-old boy with HHT demonstrates a rare example of juvenile-type AVM of the cord, with multiple tortuous feeding arteries ➡ and a large draining venous pouch ➡.*

ENCEPHALOCRANIOCUTANEOUS LIPOMATOSIS

Key Facts

Terminology
- Rare congenital neurocutaneous syndrome characterized by ipsilateral scalp, eye, and brain abnormalities

Imaging
- Unilateral cerebral hemispheric atrophy ipsilateral to scalp lipoma
- Intracranial (IC) lipomas in ~ 2 out of 3 patients
- Spinal lipomas/lipomatosis frequent; cervicothoracic > lumbar
- Polymicrogyria of temporal, parietal, &/or occipital lobes
- ± diffuse, ipsilateral leptomeningeal enhancement
- Scalp/intracranial lipomas

Top Differential Diagnoses
- Sturge-Weber syndrome
- Oculocerebrocutaneous syndrome
- Epidermal nevus syndrome
  - Ipsilateral epidermal nevus, hemimeganencephaly, facial lipoma, and hemihypertrophy
- Proteus syndrome
  - Progressive asymmetric, bilateral trunk/limb hypertrophy

Pathology
- Defect in development of mesenchymal tissues

Clinical Issues
- Nevus psiloliparus: Sharply demarcated focus of scalp alopecia overlying scalp lipoma
- Hallmark of ECCL
- Newborn with nevus psiloliparus, scleral mass, and periocular papules
- Rare; ~ 54 reported cases (likely underreported)

*(**Left**) Color photograph of a scalp shows the typical appearance of "nevus psiloliparus," a well-circumscribed area of scalp alopecia. The nevus overlies a lipoma and is the hallmark of encephalocraniocutaneous lipomatosis. (**Right**) Sagittal T1WI MR at the level of the posterior fossa shows craniocervical ➦ and cerebellopontine angle ➡ lipomas. The severe ventriculomegaly is likely secondary to CSF obstruction at foramen magnum and cerebral atrophy.*

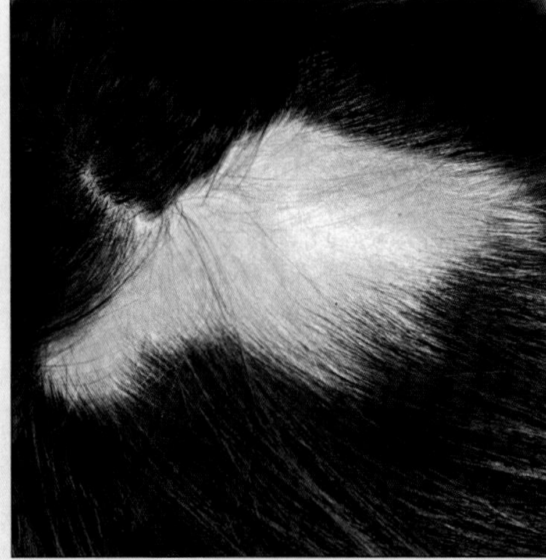

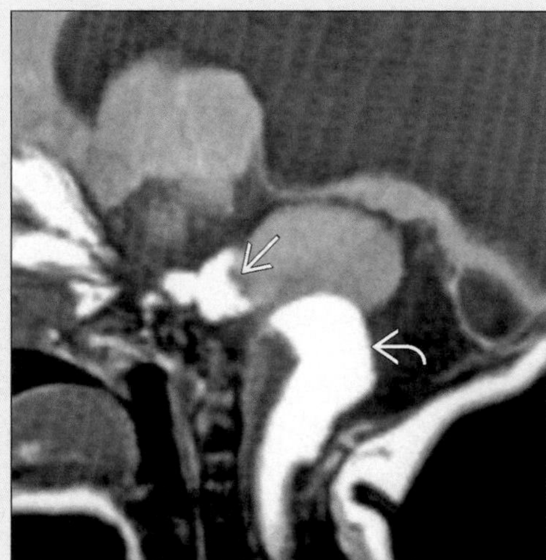

*(**Left**) Coronal T1WI MR shows mild thickening of the right-sided subcutaneous fat ➦ in this 3 month old with an orbital dermoid (not shown) and prominence of right frontal scalp tissues. The ipsilateral cerebral hemisphere is atrophic, with enlargement of the ipsilateral lateral ventricle and subarachnoid spaces. (**Right**) Axial T1 C+ FS MR demonstrates abnormal thickening and enhancement of the meninges over the right lateral convexity ➡. The right occipital horn ➡ is enlarged.*

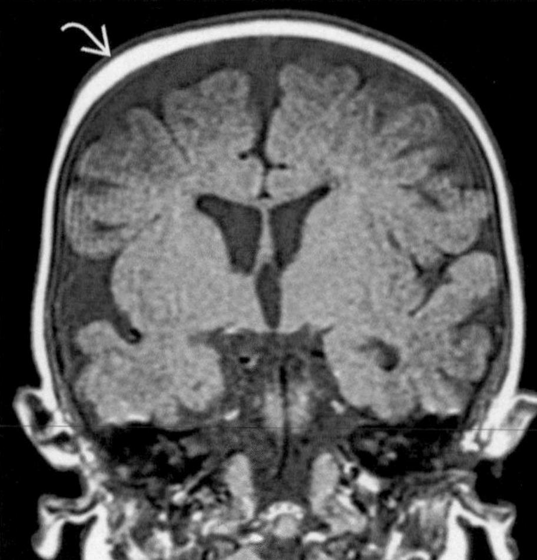

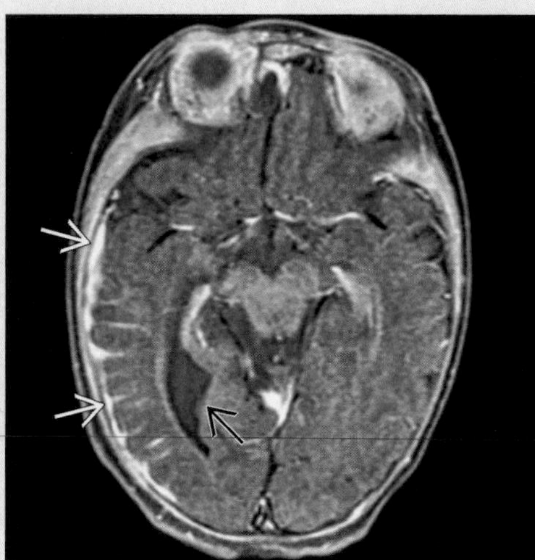

ENCEPHALOCRANIOCUTANEOUS LIPOMATOSIS

TERMINOLOGY

Abbreviations

- Encephalocraniocutaneous lipomatosis (ECCL)

Synonyms

- Haberland syndrome, Fishman syndrome

Definitions

- Rare congenital neurocutaneous syndrome characterized by ipsilateral scalp, eye, and brain abnormalities
- 1st described in 1970 by Catherine Haberland

IMAGING

General Features

- Best diagnostic clue
  - Unilateral cerebral hemispheric atrophy ipsilateral to scalp lipoma
  - Other frequent ipsilateral CNS abnormalities
    - Middle cranial fossa arachnoid cyst
    - Cortical dysplasia
    - Cortical Ca++
  - Intracranial (IC) lipomas in ~ 2 out of 3 patients
  - Spinal lipomas/lipomatosis frequent; cervicothoracic > lumbar
  - Rarely, CNS abnormalities limited to IC lipoma
- Location
  - Intracranial lipomas
    - CP angle, Meckel cave, foramen magnum
    - Usually ipsilateral to scalp lipoma; occasionally contra- or bilateral
  - All other CNS anomalies ipsilateral to scalp lipoma
- Morphology
  - Focal occipital lobe atrophy and occipital horn enlargement characteristic

CT Findings

- NECT
  - Hemispheric atrophy, ventriculomegaly
    - Ventriculomegaly primarily due to volume loss although hydrocephalus occasionally present
  - Low-density scalp lipoma (may be difficult to identify, particularly if at vertex)
  - ± cortical Ca++
    - Identified as early as 1st month of life, progressive
  - ± focal calvarial enlargement
    - Usually underlies scalp lipoma
- CECT
  - ± diffuse, ipsilateral leptomeningeal (LM) enhancement
- CTA
  - Arterial ectasias, pouches, and aneurysms described in older patients

MR Findings

- T1WI
  - Scalp/intracranial lipomas
  - Polymicrogyria of temporal, parietal, &/or occipital lobes
  - Scleral choristoma occasionally visible; heterogeneous with focal areas of hyperintensity
- T2WI
  - Cortical Ca++ hypointense
  - Lipomas hyperintense on FSE T2
  - Arachnoid cysts isointense to CSF
- FLAIR
  - Nulling of signal from arachnoid cyst
- T2* GRE
  - "Blooming" of cortical Ca++
- DWI
  - Arachnoid cyst isointense to CSF
- T1WI C+
  - ± diffuse, ipsilateral leptomeningeal enhancement
- MRA
  - Arterial ectasias, pouches, and aneurysms described in older patients

Ultrasonographic Findings

- Ventriculomegaly reported on 3rd trimester US

Angiographic Findings

- Conventional
  - Arterial ectasias, pouches, and aneurysms described in older patients

Imaging Recommendations

- Best imaging tool
  - Contrast-enhanced MR
- Protocol advice
  - Multiplanar MR with fat saturation to identify scalp lipoma (may be missed on CT)
  - MRA may disclose vascular abnormalities

DIFFERENTIAL DIAGNOSIS

Sturge-Weber Syndrome (SWS)

- Unilateral hemispheric cerebral atrophy and cortical Ca++, LM enhancement ipsilateral to forehead port-wine nevus
  - CNS findings frequently posterior

Oculocerebrocutaneous Syndrome (OCCS)

- Characterized by unique cutaneous striated muscle hamartoma, cystic microphthalmia, and giant tectum absent vermis malformation
- Cortical dysplasia, agnesis of corpus callosum, and Dandy-Walker malformation frequently present
- Cutaneous, eye, and CNS anomalies usually ipsilateral but less consistently than ECCL

Epidermal Nevus Syndrome (ENS)

- Ipsilateral epidermal nevus, hemimeganencephaly, facial lipoma, and hemihypertrophy
- Occasional scleral choristoma

Proteus Syndrome

- Progressive asymmetric, bilateral trunk/limb hypertrophy
- Osteomas, lipomas, and pigmented nevi common
- CNS anomalies uncommon; hemimeganencephaly most common

ENCEPHALOCRANIOCUTANEOUS LIPOMATOSIS

PATHOLOGY

General Features

- Etiology
  - Defect in development of mesenchymal tissues
    - Affects mostly neural crest cells surrounding brain and forming vessels
- Genetics
  - Sporadic
  - May survive autosomal lethal gene by somatic mosaicism
- ECCL considered distinct entity; however, some clinical/imaging overlap with SWS, OCCS, ENS, and proteus syndrome
- Embryology-anatomy
  - 3rd week gestation: Embryonic disc consists of ectoderm, mesoderm, entoderm
  - Neural tube develops from ectoderm during 3rd week gestation
  - 4th and 5th week gestation: Mesoderm forms mesenchymal sheath over brain and spinal cord → precursor blood vessels, bone, cartilage, and fat

Gross Pathologic & Surgical Features

- Brain: Cortical atrophy, white matter hypoplasia, ventriculomegaly, polymicrogyria, wallerian degeneration brainstem
  - Arterial ectasias, pouches, aneurysms described in older patients
- Leptomeninges: Thick, gray, gelatinous with excess underlying arteries, veins, and varicose capillaries
- Skull: Macrocranium with focal hyperostosis
- Scalp: Focal lipomatous thickening with overlying circumscribed alopecia
- Face: Multiple, tiny, white/purple/yellow periocular > perinasal papules

Microscopic Features

- Brain: Abnormal 4-layered cytoarchitecture, mineral concretions outer cortical lamina, scattered glial nodules
- Leptomeninges: Lipoangiomatosis
- Skull: Diploic replacement with mature fat cells
- Scalp: Benign lipoma > fibrolipoma expanding into dermis; absent hair follicles with preserved erector pili muscles
- Skin: Subcutaneous angiofibroma, fibrolipoma, or lipoma
- Eye: Corneal limbus/scleral choristoma
  - Other ocular abnormalities: Persistent hyaloid vasculature, coloboma, cloudy cornea, lens dislocation, ectopic pupils

CLINICAL ISSUES

Presentation

- Most common signs/symptoms
  - Nevus psiloliparus: Sharply demarcated focus of scalp alopecia overlying scalp lipoma
    - Hallmark of ECCL
- Other signs/symptoms
  - Ipsilateral ocular choristomas and periocular > perinasal papules; epibulbar dermoid
  - Macrocranium (unrelated to hydrocephalus)
  - Seizures, psychomotor delay, spastic hemiparesis
  - Infrequent scoliosis, foot deformities, sensorimotor deficits (2° to spinal lipoma)
- Clinical profile
  - Newborn/infant with nevus psiloliparus, scleral mass, and periocular papules; seizures in infants

Demographics

- Age
  - Newborn > infant presentation
  - Rare presentation teen/adult with cutaneous, ocular lesions
- Gender
  - M = F
- Ethnicity
  - No racial or geographic predilection
- Epidemiology
  - Rare; ~ 54 reported cases (likely underreported)

Natural History & Prognosis

- Natural history
  - Reported growth lipomas and ocular choristomas; remaining congenital abnormalities static
  - Abnormal vasculature, aneurysms later in life
- Prognosis
  - Majority with variable degrees of psychomotor impairment and dependency
  - Few reports neurologically normal patients with nevus psiloliparus; nonsyndromic nevus psiloliparus vs. ECCL with minimal CNS involvement

Treatment

- Antiepileptics
- Shunt placement for hydrocephalus

DIAGNOSTIC CHECKLIST

Image Interpretation Pearls

- Considerable imaging overlap with SWS → search for scalp lipoma
- Low-density IC lipoma may be difficult to distinguish from CSF on CT

SELECTED REFERENCES

1. Prontera P et al: Encephalocraniocutaneous lipomatosis (ECCL) in a patient with history of familial multiple lipomatosis (FML). Am J Med Genet A. 149A(3):543-5, 2009
2. Gokhale NR et al: Encephalocraniocutaneous lipomatosis: a rare neurocutaneous syndrome. Indian J Dermatol Venereol Leprol. 73(1):40-2, 2007
3. Moog U et al: Brain anomalies in encephalocraniocutaneous lipomatosis. Am J Med Genet A. 143A(24):2963-72, 2007
4. Hunter AG: Oculocerebrocutaneous and encephalocraniocutaneous lipomatosis syndromes: blind men and an elephant or separate syndromes? Am J Med Genet A. 140(7):709-26, 2006
5. Lasierra R et al: Encephalocraniocutaneous lipomatosis: neurologic manifestations. J Child Neurol. 18(10):725-9, 2003
6. Parazzini C et al: Encephalocraniocutaneous lipomatosis: complete neuroradiologic evaluation and follow-up of two cases. AJNR Am J Neuroradiol. 20(1):173-6, 1999

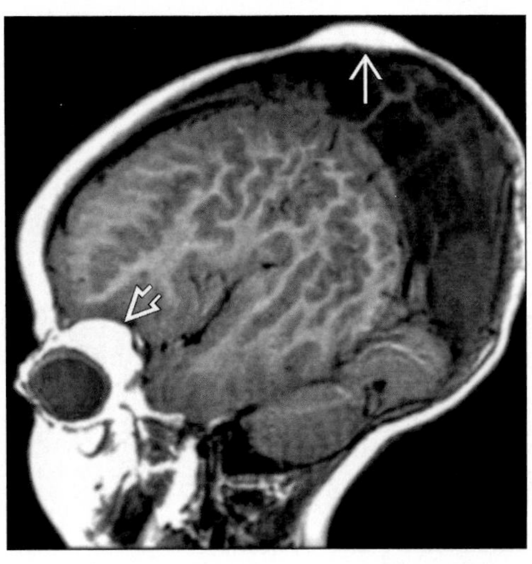

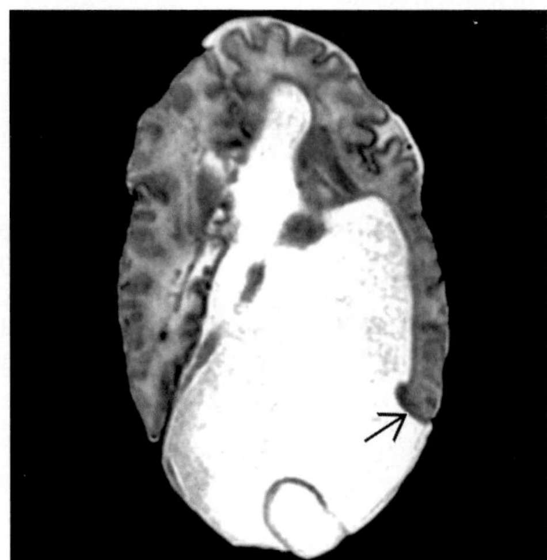

(Left) Sagittal T1WI MR shows an ipsilateral scalp ➡ and orbital ➡ lipoma. The globe is buphthalmic with a scleral lipodermoid. *(Right)* Axial T2WI MR shows marked left ventriculomegaly with herniation of the ventricle through the choroidal fissure and hemispheric volume loss. The herniated ventricle is displacing the posterior aspect of the cerebral hemisphere ➡ anteriorly, thereby compressing and distorting the hemispheric parenchyma.

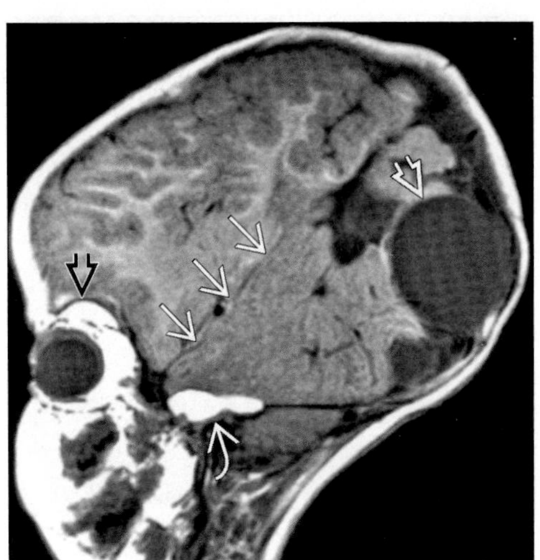

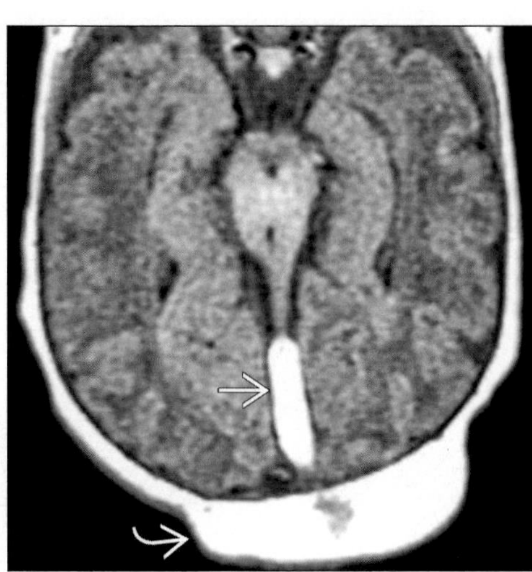

(Left) Sagittal T1WI MR shows ipsilateral orbital ➡ and middle cranial fossa ➡ lipomas. The cerebral cortex ➡ is distorted by the enlarged lateral ventricle. Note the intracranial cyst ➡. *(Right)* Axial T1WI MR shows an intracranial lipoma in the interhemispheric fissure ➡ and an extracranial lipoma ➡ in subcutaneous fat. There is no hemispheric atrophy or ventriculomegaly. The patient is clinically normal. The findings may represent a forme fruste of ECCL.

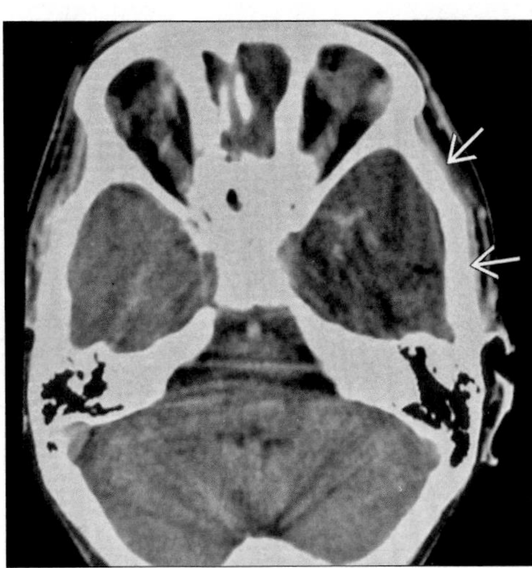

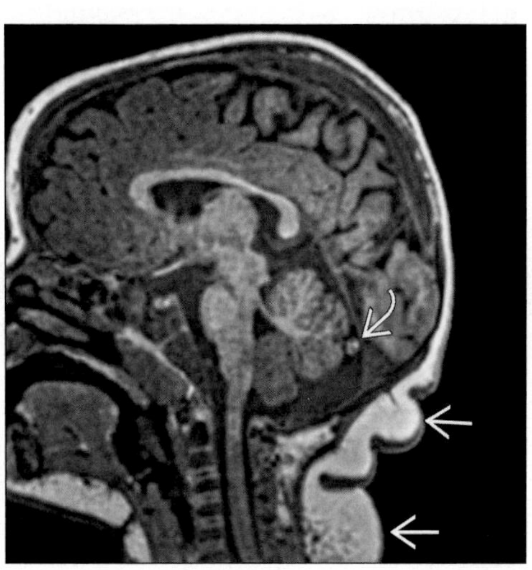

(Left) Axial NECT shows a middle cranial fossa arachnoid cyst in a patient with ECCL. Note the expansion of the left middle cranial fossa ➡ by the cyst. The cyst is ipsilateral to hemispheric atrophy and a scalp lipoma. Scalp lipoma is sometimes poorly seen by imaging. *(Right)* Sagittal T1WI MR shows large subcutaneous lipomas ➡ in the upper neck and the occipital area of the scalp. Note the small lipoma ➡ immediately behind the cerebellar vermis.

LHERMITTE-DUCLOS DISEASE

Key Facts

Terminology

- Benign cerebellar lesion; unclear if neoplastic, malformative, or hamartomatous
- Multiple hamartoma syndrome (MHAM) → autosomal dominant, mutation in *PTEN* gene, associated with increased incidence of malignancy
- LDD now considered neurological manifestation of MHAM and part of new neurocutaneous syndrome
- MHAM = Cowden syndrome; COLD (Cowden plus Lhermitte-Duclos) = MHAM + LDD

Imaging

- Relatively well-defined cerebellar mass with striated/ corduroy/tigroid/gyriform pattern
- LDD always in cerebellum and may be large → mass effect, tonsillar herniation, hydrocephalus

Top Differential Diagnoses

- Subacute cerebellar infarction
- Cerebellitis
- Unclassified cerebellar dysplasias
- Ganglioglioma
- Medulloblastoma
- Meningeal metastases
- Meningeal granulomatous disease

Clinical Issues

- Most common presentation: Headache, nausea and vomiting, ataxia, blurred vision
  - Can present in coma
- Surgical resection is treatment of choice
- If LDD, screen for MHAM; if MHAM, screen for LDD
- Long-term cancer screening needed, especially thyroid and breast (↑ malignancy in MHAM)

*(**Left**) Axial graphic shows thickened and irregular cerebellar folia in the right cerebellar hemisphere. This results in the enlargement of the hemisphere and mass effect upon the brain stem that are typical of LDD. (**Right**) Coronal T2WI MR shows a striated thickening of isointense cortex with hyperintense intervening white matter composing the right cerebellar mass ➡ that extends into the vermis and herniates ➡ across the cerebellar midline.*

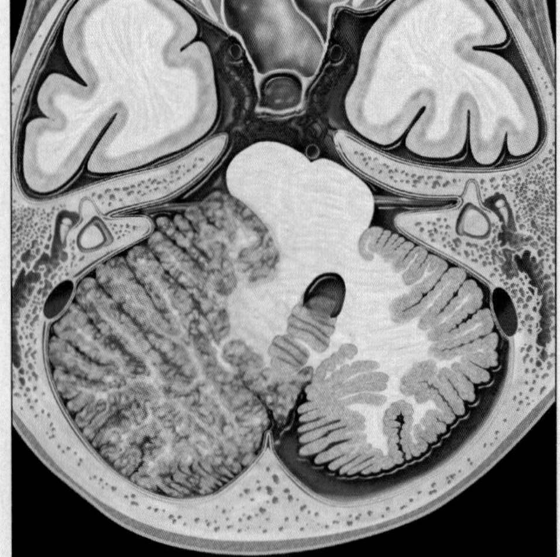

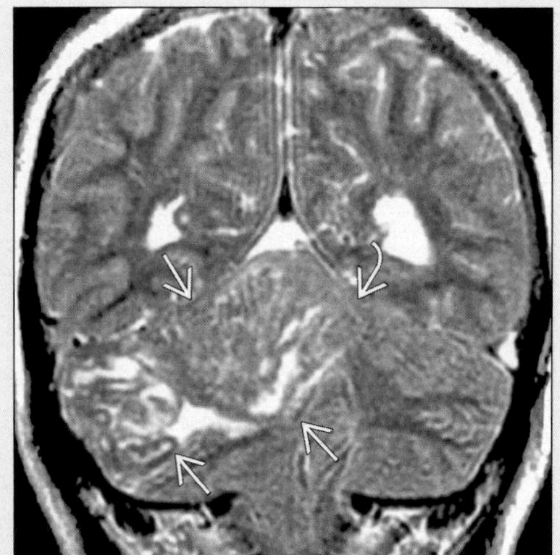

*(**Left**) Axial T2WI MR shows a large left cerebellar mass ➡ that compresses and distorts the brainstem ➡ and crosses the cerebellar midline ➡. (**Right**) Axial T1 C+ MR in the same patient shows subtle enhancement ➡, possibly due to enlarged leptomeningeal veins, within the striated iso- and hypointense left cerebellar mass. This should be differentiated from a cerebellar tumor, in which the parenchyma typically enhances.*

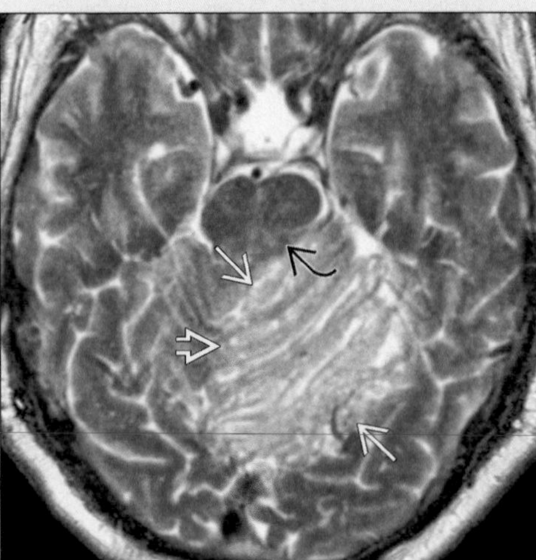

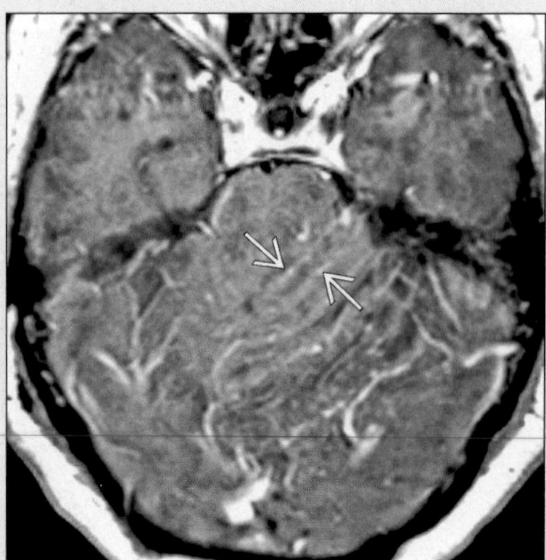

LHERMITTE-DUCLOS DISEASE

TERMINOLOGY

Synonyms

- Lhermitte-Duclos disease (LDD)
  - Dysplastic cerebellar gangliocytoma, gangliocytoma dysplasticum, hamartoma of cerebellum
  - Hamartoblastoma, cerebelloparenchymal disorder 6, granule cell hypertrophy, granular cell hypertrophy, granulomolecular hypertrophy
  - Diffuse ganglioneuroma of cerebellar cortex, diffuse cerebellar hypertrophy, neurocytic blastoma, myelinated neurocytoma, purkingeoma
- Multiple hamartoma syndrome (MHAM)
  - Multiple hamartoma-neoplasia syndrome, Cowden disease, Cowden syndrome (CS), Cowden-Lhermitte-Duclos syndrome (COLD)

Definitions

- Lhermitte-Duclos disease → neurological manifestation of MHAM
  - Benign cerebellar lesion but unclear if neoplastic, malformative, or hamartomatous
  - Association between LDD and MHAM probably represents new neurocutaneous syndrome
- Multiple hamartoma syndrome
  - Autosomal dominant, variable expression, typically mutation in *PTEN* gene
  - Hamartomatous neoplasms of skin (90-100%), mucosa, GI tract, bones, CNS, eyes, and GU tract
  - Associated with increased incidence of malignancy

IMAGING

General Features

- Best diagnostic clue
  - Widened cerebellar folia, "gyriform" pattern
- Location
  - Always in cerebellum, usually unilateral
  - Often involves vermis, rarely brainstem
- Size
  - Size variable, may be large → mass effect, tonsillar herniation, hydrocephalus
- Morphology
  - Infiltrative but well demarcated

Radiographic Findings

- ± thinning of skull

CT Findings

- NECT
  - Normal to high attenuation with striations
  - Occasionally cystic areas &/or calcifications
- CECT
  - ± enhancement

MR Findings

- T1WI
  - Iso- to hypointense with striations
  - Rarely calcifications may cause ↑ signal
- T2WI
  - ↑ signal with characteristic iso- to hypointense striations
  - May have bizarre gyriform appearance
  - Newborns may not have obvious striations since cerebellar WM not fully myelinated
- FLAIR
  - ↑ signal with striations
  - May have hypointense cysts
- T2* GRE
  - Veins between folia
- DWI
  - ↑ signal on DWI usually due to ↑ T2 signal
  - Low to ↑ ADC; ↑ ADC in white matter, cysts
  - May have ↑ fractional anisotropy (FA) in white matter
- PWI
  - May show areas of ↑ rCBV and rCBF
- T1WI C+
  - ± enhancement (increased vascularity in molecular layer and leptomeninges, predominantly venous)
- MRS
  - ↓ NAA, ↓ choline, ↓ myoinositol
  - Variable lactate, may be increased

Nuclear Medicine Findings

- PET
  - ↑ uptake FDG PET and 11C-methionine PET
  - Report of ↑ CBF, ↓ OEF, and similar $CMRO_2$ compared to normal cerebral hemisphere

Imaging Recommendations

- Best imaging tool
  - MR with DWI, MRS, and contrast
- Protocol advice
  - Coronal T2 may be helpful
  - If LDD, initiate workup for MHAM and screen for malignancies
  - If it enhances, consider differential diagnosis carefully

DIFFERENTIAL DIAGNOSIS

Subacute Cerebellar Infarction

- Mass effect, ↑ signal on DWI but vascular territory

Cerebellitis/Vasculitis

- Acute onset of symptoms

Unclassified Cerebellar Dysplasias

- Do not progress, hydrocephalus rare

Ganglioglioma

- May have bizarre appearance simulating LDD

Tuberous Sclerosis Complex

- Rarely mass-like cerebellar dysplastic lesions but other features of tuberous sclerosis complex

Medulloblastoma

- Lateral "desmoplastic" type may have somewhat striated appearance
- ↑ signal on DWI but most have marked ↑ Cho/NAA

Meningeal Metastases

- Nodular leptomeningeal enhancement

Meningeal Granulomatous Disease

- Nodular leptomeningeal enhancement

LHERMITTE-DUCLOS DISEASE

PATHOLOGY

General Features

- Etiology
  - Unclear, but evidence of nonproliferation/absence of malignant transformation favors hamartomatous nature
- Genetics
  - Many have mutations of *PTEN/MMAC 1* gene at 10q23.31 (tumor suppressor gene)
  - Activation of PTEN/AKT/mTOR pathway suggests role for mTOR in pathogenesis
- Associated abnormalities
  - Most patients with LDD likely have MHAM

Staging, Grading, & Classification

- WHO grade I

Gross Pathologic & Surgical Features

- Markedly enlarged cerebellar hemisphere/vermis with thick folia
- Mass appears pale

Microscopic Features

- Widening of molecular cell layer → occupied by abnormal ganglion cells
- Absence of Purkinje cell layer
- Hypertrophy of granule cell layer
- ↓ volume of white matter
- Histologically may be confused with ganglion cell tumor

CLINICAL ISSUES

Presentation

- Most common signs/symptoms
  - Headache, nausea and vomiting, papilledema, unsteady gait, upper limb ataxia and dysmetria, blurred vision, lower cranial nerve palsies
- Other signs/symptoms
  - Sensory motor deficits, vertigo, neuropsychological deficits
- Clinical profile
  - If LDD, screen for MHAM; if MHAM, screen for LDD

Demographics

- Age
  - Any; most common between 20-40 years
- Gender
  - M ≈ F
- Ethnicity
  - No known predilection
- Epidemiology
  - ↑ degree of penetrance in family members

Natural History & Prognosis

- Many do not grow or grow only slowly
- If mass effect is not relieved prognosis is poor
- Post-surgery recurrences are rare but do occur

Treatment

- Options, risks, complications
  - Borders of lesion blend into normal surrounding cerebellum → total resection difficult
  - Surgical resection in symptomatic patients

DIAGNOSTIC CHECKLIST

Consider

- Search for other features of MHAM when LDD is diagnosed and vice versa
- Long-term cancer screening needed (especially breast in women, thyroid in men and women)

Image Interpretation Pearls

- Relatively well-defined cerebellar mass with striated "tigroid" or gyriform pattern

SELECTED REFERENCES

1. Shinagare AB et al: Case 144: Dysplastic cerebellar gangliocytoma (Lhermitte-Duclos disease). Radiology. 251(1):298-303, 2009
2. Cianfoni A et al: Morphological and functional MR imaging of Lhermitte-Duclos disease with pathology correlate. J Neuroradiol. 35(5):297-300, 2008
3. Thomas B et al: Advanced MR imaging in Lhermitte-Duclos disease: moving closer to pathology and pathophysiology. Neuroradiology. 49(9):733-8, 2007
4. Van Calenbergh F et al: Lhermitte-Duclos disease: 11C-methionine positron emission tomography data in 4 patients. Surg Neurol. 65(3):293-6; discussion 296-7, 2006
5. Padma MV et al: Functional imaging in Lhermitte-Duclose disease. Mol Imaging Biol. 6(5):319-23, 2004
6. Buhl R et al: Dysplastic gangliocytoma of the cerebellum: rare differential diagnosis in space occupying lesions of the posterior fossa. Acta Neurochir (Wien). 145(6):509-12; discussion 512, 2003
7. Capone Mori A et al: Lhermitte-Duclos disease in 3 children: a clinical long-term observation. Neuropediatrics. 34(1):30-5, 2003
8. Klisch J et al: Lhermitte-Duclos disease: assessment with MR imaging, positron emission tomography, single-photon emission CT, and MR spectroscopy. AJNR Am J Neuroradiol. 22(5):824-30, 2001
9. Ogasawara K et al: Blood flow and oxygen metabolism in a case of Lhermitte-Duclos disease: results of positron emission tomography. J Neurooncol. 55(1):59-61, 2001
10. Robinson S et al: Cowden disease and Lhermitte-Duclos disease: characterization of a new phakomatosis. Neurosurgery. 46(2):371-83, 2000
11. Murata J et al: Dysplastic gangliocytoma (Lhermitte-Duclos disease) associated with Cowden disease: report of a case and review of the literature for the genetic relationship between the two diseases. J Neurooncol. 41(2):129-36, 1999
12. Awwad EE et al: Atypical MR appearance of Lhermitte-Duclos disease with contrast enhancement. AJNR Am J Neuroradiol. 16(8):1719-20, 1995

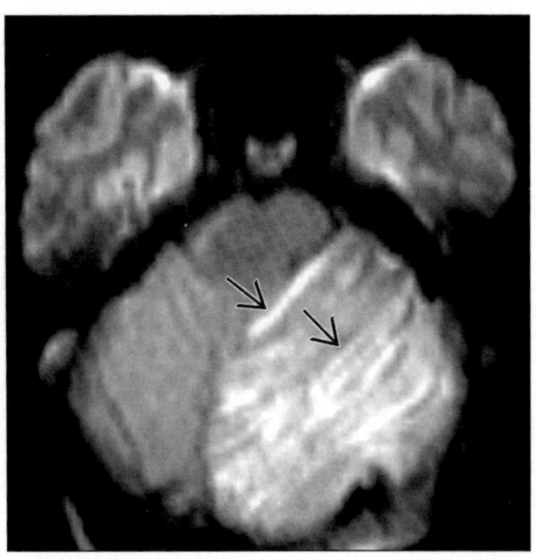

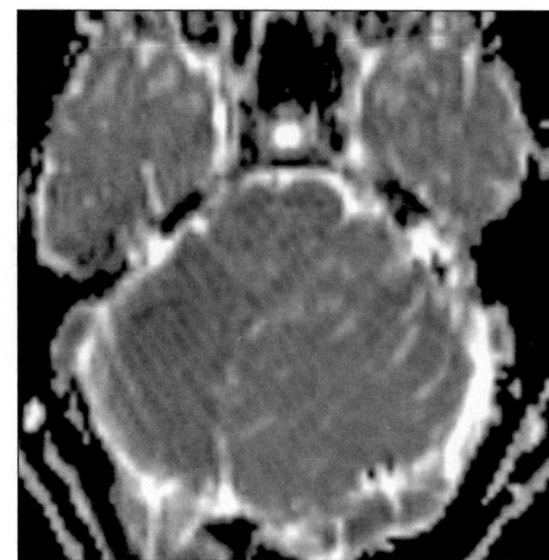

(Left) *Axial DTI, DWI image shows streaks of increased signal* ➔ *interspersed with streaks of isointense signal in the involved left cerebellar hemisphere.* ***(Right)*** *Corresponding axial DTI ADC map shows absence of hypointensity (reduced diffusivity), indicating that the hyperintense DWI signal is due to increased T2 signal. Note that, on the ADC map, there is overall increased signal within the involved left cerebellar hemisphere.*

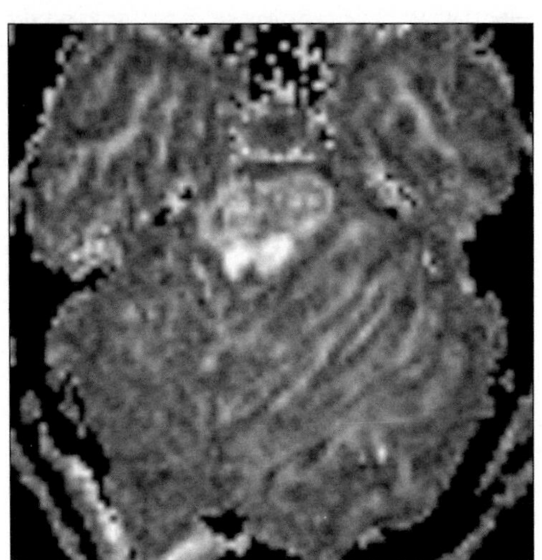

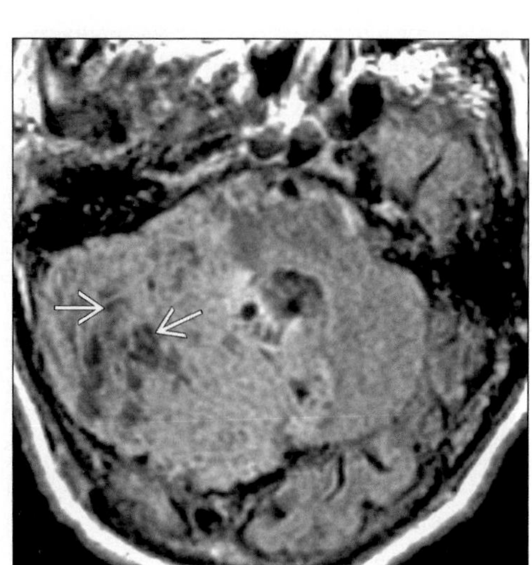

(Left) *Corresponding axial DTI, fractional anisotropy (FA) map in the same case shows hyperintensity (increased FA) within the involved left cerebellar hemisphere. The reason for the increased FA is unknown.* ***(Right)*** *Axial FLAIR MR in a patient with LDD shows multiple low signal cyst-like lesions* ➔ *in the affected right cerebellar hemisphere. Such cysts are occasionally identified within the involved cerebellum in LDD.*

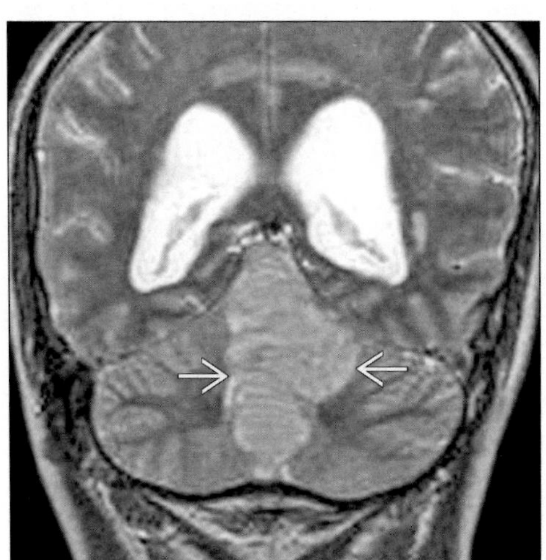

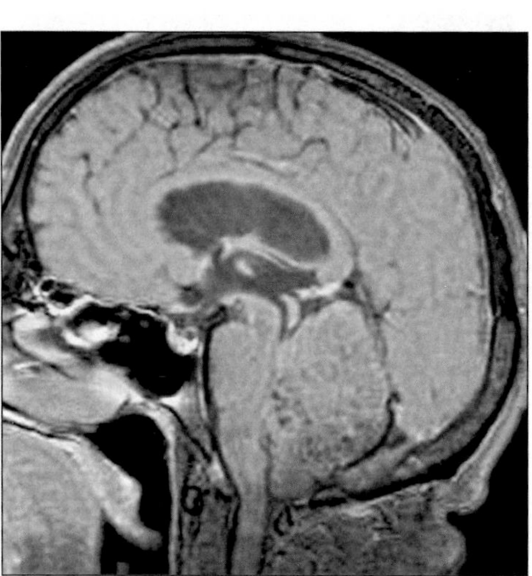

(Left) *Coronal T2WI MR shows involvement largely limited to the cerebellar vermis* ➔*. As is typical in LDD, the involved region of the cerebellum is sharply marginated, striated in appearance, and demonstrates moderate mass effect.* ***(Right)*** *Sagittal T1WI MR in the same patient shows effacement of the 4th ventricle and mass effect on the brain stem with effacement of the prepontine cistern. The cerebellar tonsils are herniated through the foramen magnum.*

NEUROCUTANEOUS MELANOSIS

Key Facts

Terminology
- Congenital phakomatosis characterized by giant or multiple cutaneous melanocytic nevi (GCMN) and benign and malignant melanotic lesions of CNS
- Leptomeningeal melanosis (LMs): Excess of benign melanotic cells in leptomeninges
- Leptomeningeal melanoma (LMm): Malignant melanoma of leptomeninges

Imaging
- GCMN + foci of T1 hyperintensity (parenchymal melanosis) in amygdala or cerebellum
- GCMN + diffuse leptomeningeal (LM) enhancement

Pathology
- Focal or diffuse proliferation of melanin-producing cells in both skin and leptomeninges
- Results from error in morphogenesis of embryonic neuroectoderm
- Hydrocephalus (seen in 2/3 of symptomatic NCM): Obstruction of CSF flow at basal cisterns and arachnoid granulations
- Strong association: Dandy-Walker spectrum (10%)
- Melanocytes normally present in pia mater over convexities, base of brain, ventral brainstem, upper cervical cord, and lumbosacral spinal cord

Clinical Issues
- Sx NCM manifests by 2-3 years of age
- Asx NCM: Parenchymal melanosis often stable
- GCMN (isolated or NCM): 5-15% lifetime risk of malignant degeneration (melanoma)

Diagnostic Checklist
- Normal MR does not exclude diagnosis NCM
- LMs cannot be distinguished from LMm by imaging
- Clinically irrelevant since sx LMs and LMm have equally poor prognosis

(Left) Graphic shows localized dark (melanotic) pigmentation of the leptomeninges. Inset demonstrates extension of melanosis into the brain substance along the Virchow-Robin spaces ➔. (Right) Axial T1WI MR of a 6 year old with benign parenchymal and leptomeningeal melanosis. Multiple foci of T1 shortening (hyperintense signal) are evident in the amygdala ➔ (indicates parenchymal involvement), and in the right ambient cistern ➔ (indicates leptomeningeal disease).

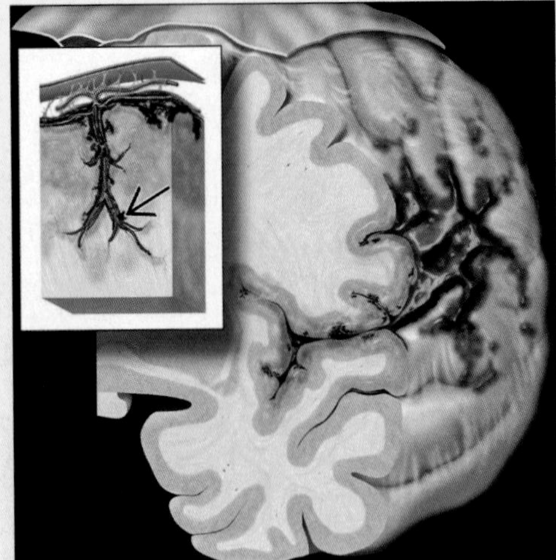

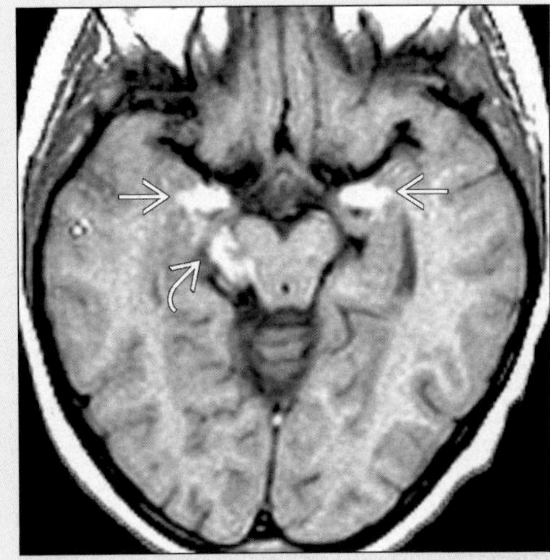

(Left) Axial T2WI MR in the same patient reveals T2 shortening (hypointense signal) of the mass lesions in the amygdala ➔ and the ambient cistern ➔. Note that the abnormal signal is more difficult to see on T2-weighted images. (Right) Axial T1 C+ MR in the same patient demonstrates enhancement of the leptomeningeal lesion ➔. The parenchymal lesions ➔ do not enhance, and are actually slightly less conspicuous, as is often the case following contrast injection.

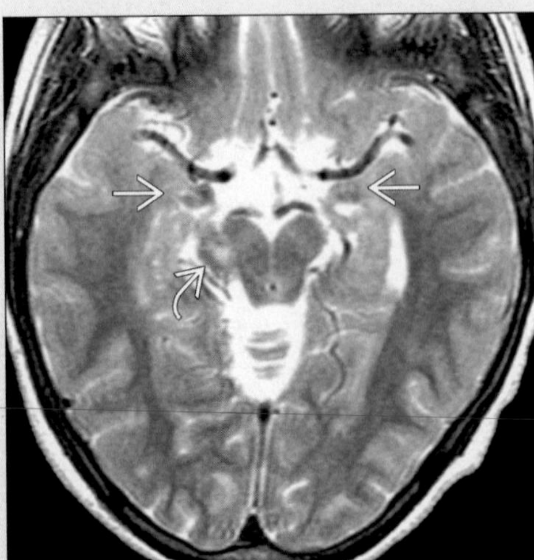

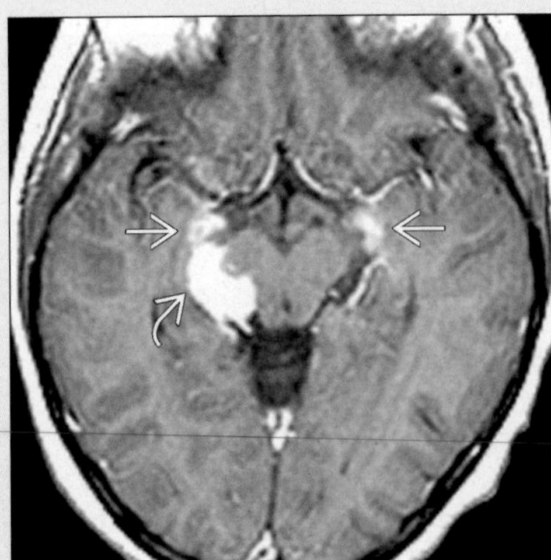

NEUROCUTANEOUS MELANOSIS

TERMINOLOGY

Abbreviations

- Neurocutaneous melanosis (NCM)

Definitions

- Congenital phakomatosis characterized by giant or multiple cutaneous melanocytic nevi (GCMN) and benign and malignant melanotic lesions of CNS
  - CNS disease: Parenchymal
    - Melanosis: Focal collection of benign melanotic cells
    - Malignant melanoma (MM)
  - CNS disease: Leptomeningeal
    - Leptomeningeal melanosis (LMs): Excess of benign melanotic cells in leptomeninges
    - Leptomeningeal melanoma (LMm): Malignant melanoma of leptomeninges

IMAGING

General Features

- Best diagnostic clue
  - GCMN + foci of T1 hyperintensity (parenchymal melanosis) in amygdala or cerebellum
  - GCMN + diffuse leptomeningeal (LM) enhancement
- Location
  - Parenchymal melanosis: Amygdala, cerebellum, basis pontis, thalami, base of frontal lobes
  - LMs or LMm: Diffuse LM involvement; rarely focal
  - MM: Temporal lobe most common
- Size
  - Parenchymal melanosis: < 1 cm
  - MM: Typically several cms
- Morphology
  - Parenchymal melanosis: Round or oval lesions
  - LMs/LMm: Linear or nodular (bulky)
  - MM: Large, round mass
- 64% symptomatic (sx), patients with NCM (MM, LMm, ± LMs) have hydrocephalus
  - Communicating > noncommunicating
- Arachnoid cysts occasionally identified
- Spinal involvement (LM enhancement, syrinx, arachnoiditis) in 20%
- Stable free radicals in melanin responsible for MR appearance

CT Findings

- NECT
  - Parenchymal melanosis: Normal or hyperdense
  - MM: Hyperdense mass with edema, mass effect; frequent necrosis/hemorrhage
- CECT
  - Parenchymal melanosis: No enhancement
  - LMs: Normal or diffuse LM enhancement
  - LMm: Diffuse LM enhancement
  - MM: Avid enhancement, often heterogeneous

MR Findings

- T1WI
  - Parenchymal melanosis: Hyperintense
  - LMs/LMm: Sulci/cisterns normal, iso- or hyperintense
  - MM: Mixed signal intensity; frequently hyperintense
- T2WI
  - Parenchymal melanosis: Mixed signal intensity, frequently hypointense; no edema, mass effect
  - LMs/LMm: Sulci/cisterns normal, iso- or hypointense
  - MM: Mixed signal intensity with edema, mass effect; frequent necrosis, hemorrhage
- FLAIR
  - LMm/LMs: Variable leptomeningeal hyperintensity
- T2* GRE
  - "Blooming" of hemorrhage and melanin
- T1WI C+
  - Parenchymal melanosis: No enhancement
  - LMs: Normal or diffuse LM enhancement
  - LMm: Diffuse LM enhancement
  - MM: Avid enhancement, often heterogeneous

Imaging Recommendations

- Best imaging tool
  - MR C+ brain and spine
- Protocol advice
  - MR screen for asymptomatic (asx) infants with GCMN

DIFFERENTIAL DIAGNOSIS

T1 Hyperintense Mass

- Lipoma: Chemical shift artifact, extraaxial (subarachnoid) location
- Dermoid: Chemical shift artifact, extraaxial location, sharply demarcated, exerts mass effect
- Acute/subacute hemorrhage: Marked T2 hypointensity, mass effect/edema, neurological deficit
- Hemorrhagic, nonmelanotic neoplasms: Areas of marked T2 hypointensity, mass effect/edema

Diffuse Leptomeningeal Enhancement

- Carcinomatous meningitis/CSF seeding: History 1° malignancy, linear/nodular LM enhancement
- Infectious meningitis (routine bacterial, TB, coccidioidomycosis): Basal cisterns, linear enhancement, signs/symptoms of meningitis; (+) CSF cultures
- Noninfectious inflammation (sarcoidosis, Wegener granulomatosis): Linear/nodular enhancement

PATHOLOGY

General Features

- Etiology
  - Focal or diffuse proliferation of melanin-producing cells in both skin and leptomeninges
  - Pathological presence of melanotic cells in VR spaces
  - Results from error in morphogenesis of embryonic neuroectoderm
  - LMm/MM: Degeneration (anaplasia) melanotic cells
  - Hydrocephalus (seen in 2/3 of symptomatic NCM): Obstruction of CSF flow at basal cisterns and arachnoid granulations
- Genetics

- Sporadic: May survive autosomal lethal gene by somatic mosaicism
- Deregulation hepatocyte growth factor/scatter factor and receptor (Met) may play role

• Associated abnormalities
  - Strong association with Dandy-Walker spectrum (10%)
    - Abnormal meningeal cells causally related to hindbrain malformation

• Embryology
  - Neural crest derived primordial cells migrate, differentiate into melanocytes in pia mater and basal layer of epidermis
  - Melanocytes in epidermis at 8-10 weeks gestation
  - Melanocytes in pia mater at 23 weeks gestation

• Anatomy
  - Melanocytes normally present in pia mater over convexities, base of brain, ventral brainstem, upper cervical cord, and lumbosacral spinal cord
  - Melanocytes normally surround blood vessels but do not extend into Virchow-Robin (VR) spaces

Staging, Grading, & Classification

• Criteria for diagnosis
  - Giant or multiple (≥ 3) cutaneous melanocytic nevi
    - Child: 6 cm body, 9 cm head maximal diameter
    - Adult: 20 cm maximal diameter
  - Cutaneous melanoma only in patients with benign meningeal lesions
  - Leptomeningeal melanoma only in patients with benign cutaneous lesions

Gross Pathologic & Surgical Features

• Parenchymal melanosis: Focal, abnormal pigmentation within brain

• LMs/LMm: Darkly pigmented, thickened pia mater

• MM: Pigmented mass, ± necrosis, hemorrhage

• GCMN: Giant or multiple pigmented, hairy nevi
  - Giant nevi comprise 66% (in NCM)
    - Lumbosacral > occipital, upper back
    - Involvement of head and neck occurs in 94%
    - Patients with nevi ≥ 50 cm at highest risk NCM
  - Multiple nevi comprise 34%

Microscopic Features

• Parenchymal melanosis: Melanotic cells and melanin-laden macrophages in VR spaces, parenchyma

• Benign LMs difficult to differentiate from LMm histologically
  - Indicators of malignancy: Necrosis, hemorrhage, basal lamina invasion, cellular atypia, frequent mitoses, presence of annulate lamellae

• GCMN: Melanocytic nevi > compound nevi

CLINICAL ISSUES

Presentation

• Most common signs/symptoms
  - ↑ intracranial pressure (seizures, vomiting, headache, macrocranium, CN6 palsy, lethargy)
  - Other signs/symptoms
    - Focal neurological deficit, psychiatric disturbance in rare older child/young adult presentation

• Clinical profile
  - Asymptomatic infant with GCMN (parenchymal melanosis)
    - Parenchymal melanosis may causes seizures
  - Infant/child with GCMN + signs/symptoms ↑ intracranial pressure (LMm, ± LMs, MM)
    - Histologically benign disease (LMs) may be symptomatic

• CSF (sx NCM): ↑ protein, ↓ glucose, ± benign/malignant melanotic cells

Demographics

• Age
  - Sx NCM manifests by 2-3 years of age

• Epidemiology
  - NCM: Rare; 100+ reported cases
    - 64% patients with proven NCM have LMm
  - GCMN: 1:20,000 live births
    - Sx NCM: < 3% patients with GCMN
    - ~ 30% patients with GCMN have parenchymal melanosis (asx NCM)

Natural History & Prognosis

• Natural History
  - Asx NCM: Parenchymal melanosis often stable
    - Few reports of regression, and degeneration into MM
  - GCMN (isolated or NCM): 5-15% lifetime risk of malignant degeneration (melanoma)

• Prognosis
  - Asx NCM: Unknown; at risk developing sx NCM
  - Sx NCM: Dismal; median survival 6.5 months after symptom onset
    - Prognosis equally poor for histologically benign (LMs) or malignant (LMm, MM) sx NCM

Treatment

• Asx NCM: Screening with MR beginning 6 months of age

• Sx NCM: Shunt hydrocephalus (filter prevents peritoneal seeding)
  - Surgery, XRT, systemic/intrathecal chemotherapy
    - Palliative; no significant alteration course of NCM

DIAGNOSTIC CHECKLIST

Image Interpretation Pearls

• Normal MR does not exclude diagnosis of NCM

• LMs cannot be distinguished from LMm by imaging
  - Clinically irrelevant since sx LMs and LMm have equally poor prognosis

SELECTED REFERENCES

1. Schreml S et al: Neurocutaneous melanosis in association with Dandy-Walker malformation: case report and literature review. Clin Exp Dermatol. 33(5):611-4, 2008
2. Acosta FL Jr et al: Neurocutaneous melanosis presenting with hydrocephalus. Case report and review of the literature. J Neurosurg. 102(1 Suppl):96-100, 2005
3. Di Rocco F et al: Neurocutaneous melanosis. Childs Nerv Syst. 20(1):23-8, 2004
4. Hayashi M et al: Diffuse leptomeningeal hyperintensity on fluid-attenuated inversion recovery MR images in neurocutaneous melanosis. AJNR Am J Neuroradiol. 25(1):138-41, 2004

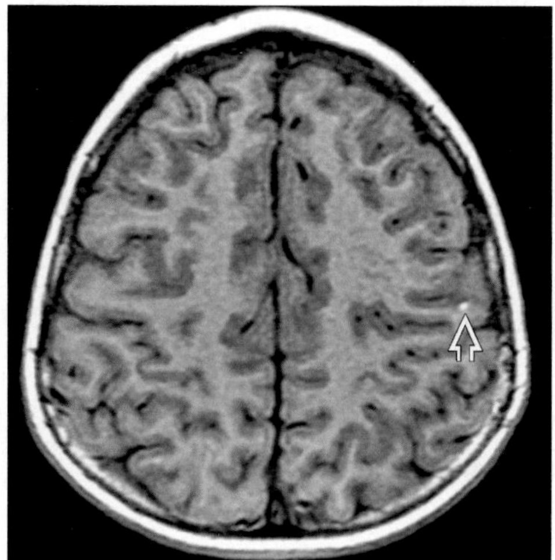

(Left) *Axial T1WI MR of a 4-year-old child with NCM reveals 2 small deposits of T1 hyperintense melanin on the surface of the right cerebellar hemisphere.* **(Right)** *Axial T1WI MR of the same patient reveals another small T1 hyperintense nodule in the posterior left frontal cortex. These lesions were poorly seen on magnetization transfer T1 images and on contrast-enhanced T1 images (not shown), illustrating the importance of unenhanced T1 images in this patient population.*

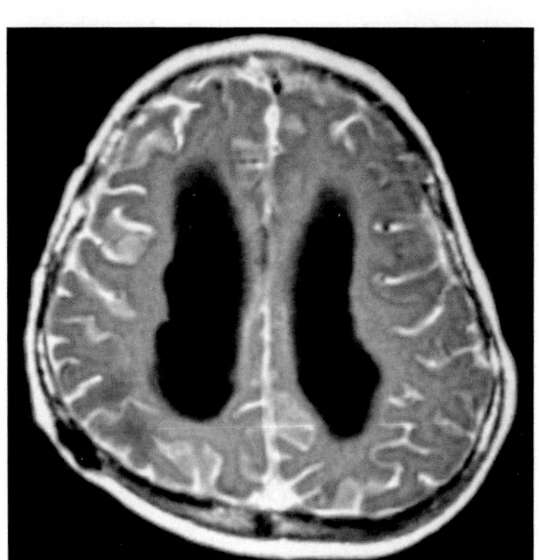

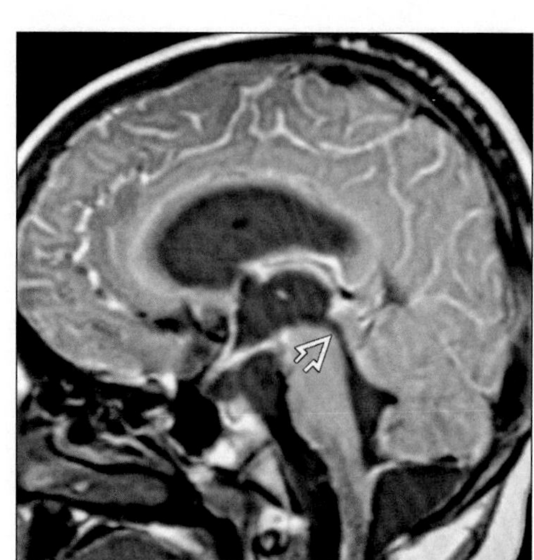

(Left) *Axial T1 C+ MR shows diffuse neurocutaneous melanosis in a 6-year-old child. The pial melanosis involves virtually the entire surface of the brain and enhances strongly and uniformly. Moderate to severe lateral ventriculomegaly is evident.* **(Right)** *Sagittal T1WI MR in the same patient reveals patent aqueduct of Sylvius and enlarged basilar cisterns. Thus, the hydrocephalus is of the extraventricular obstructive type. Diffusely abnormal leptomeningeal enhancement is evident.*

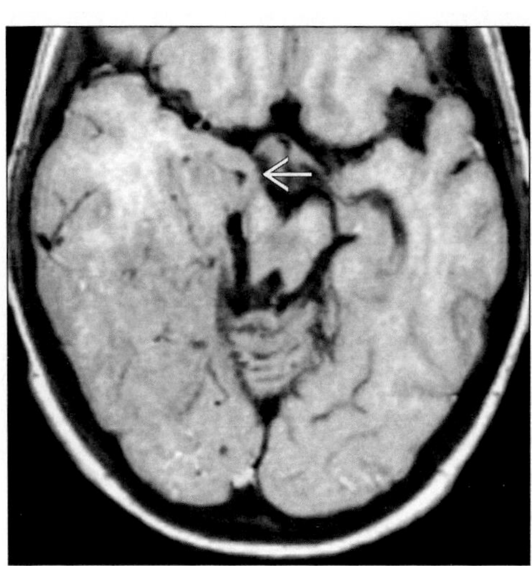

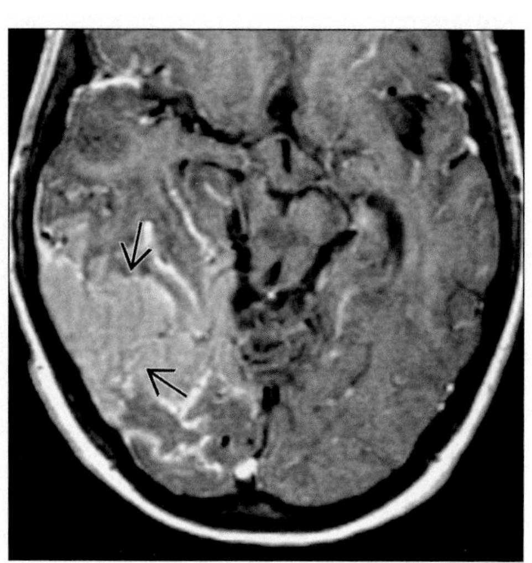

(Left) *Axial T1WI MR shows significant mass effect in the right posterior temporal and occipital lobes with effacement of the surface sulci. The uncus is herniated. Only minimal hyperintensity is evident. Surgery disclosed extensive melanosis that had invaded the brain via the perivascular spaces.* **(Right)** *Axial T1WI C+ MR in the same patient shows a strongly enhancing superficial mass that fills the adjacent sulci and extends deeply into the underlying brain parenchyma.*

AICARDI SYNDROME

Key Facts

Terminology
- Classic triad of callosal dysgenesis, infantile spasms, and chorioretinal lacunae, but more complex with other major features

Imaging
- Callosal agenesis: Complete (70%), partial (30%)
- Polymicrogyria: Frontal or perisylvian (~ 100%)
- Heterotopia: Periventricular (100%), subcortical (30%)
- Intracranial cysts: Midline > intraventricular; other extraaxial sites; choroid plexus; intraparenchymal
- Ocular coloboma
- Choroid plexus papillomas
- Hemispheric asymmetry
- Hypoplastic/dysplastic cerebellar hemispheres or vermis

Top Differential Diagnoses
- Congenital toxoplasmosis
- Congenital CMV

Pathology
- Likely X-linked dominant with lethality in hemizygous male (not yet confirmed)

Clinical Issues
- Infantile spasms or other early-onset epilepsy, typically poorly controlled
- Chorioretinal lacunae: Only true pathognomonic feature (may be unilateral)
- 91% function at < 1 year level, 21% able to walk, 4% able to communicate
- Many need surgery for scoliosis

*(**Left**) Coronal T2WI MR in a young girl shows absence of the corpus callosum ⇒ with bundles of Probst ➡, right insular and temporal polymicrogyria ➡, and both periventricular nodular ➡ and subcortical heterotopia ➡. Scattered foci of increased T2 white matter and a small extraaxial cyst at the foramen of Luschka were also present. (**Right**) Axial T2WI MR in a newborn girl shows extensive right hemispheric polymicrogyria ➡ and a left interhemispheric extraaxial cyst ➡.*

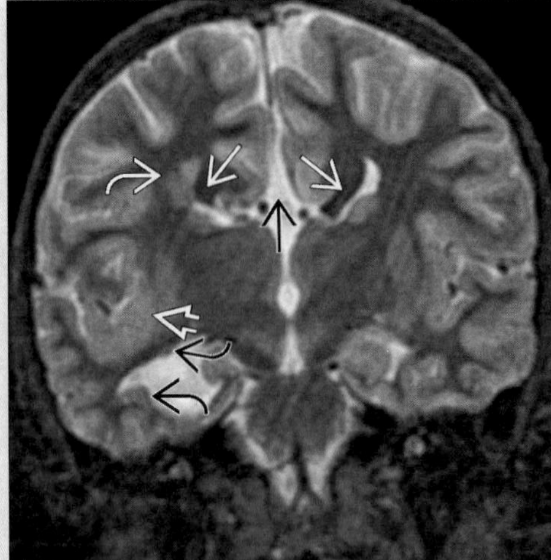

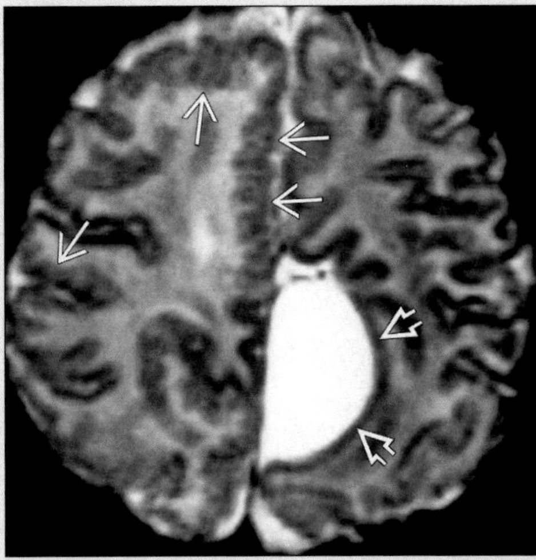

*(**Left**) Axial T2WI MR in an infant with infantile spasms shows multiple findings that are characteristic of Aicardi syndrome: Callosal agenesis, interhemispheric cyst ➡, periventricular nodular heterotopia ➡, and polymicrogyria ⇒. (**Right**) Axial T2WI MR shows a hypoplastic left cerebellar hemisphere ⇒ and vermis (not seen well here), as well as an extraaxial cyst ➡ that was associated with the choroid plexus, suggesting this is a choroid plexus papilloma.*

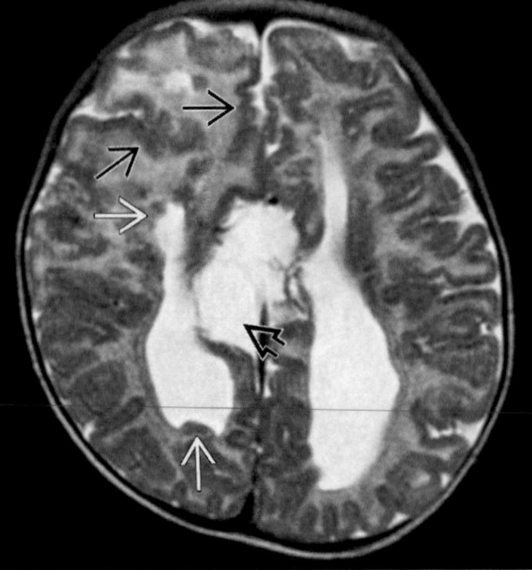

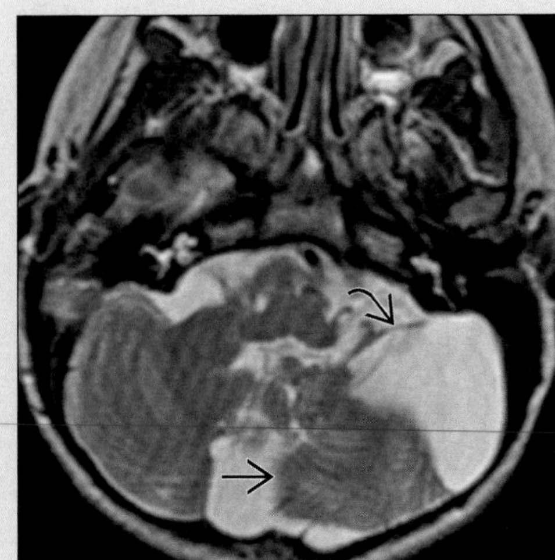

AICARDI SYNDROME

TERMINOLOGY

Abbreviations

- Aicardi (AIC) syndrome

Definitions

- Classic triad of callosal dysgenesis, infantile spasms, and chorioretinal lacunae; but more complex, other major features

IMAGING

General Features

- Best diagnostic clue
  - Major features
    - Callosal agenesis: Complete (70%), partial (30%)
    - Polymicrogyria: Frontal or perisylvian (~ 100%)
    - Heterotopia: Periventricular (100%), subcortical (30%)
    - Intracranial cysts: Midline > intraventricular; other extraaxial sites; choroid plexus; intraparenchymal
    - Ocular coloboma
    - Choroid plexus papillomas
  - Supporting features
    - Vertebral or rib abnormalities
    - Microphthalmia
    - Hemispheric asymmetry
  - Other reported CNS imaging findings
    - Hypoplastic/dysplastic cerebellar hemispheres or vermis
    - Enlarged cisterna magna
    - Increased tectal size
    - Optic nerve hypoplasia
    - Delayed myelination

Imaging Recommendations

- Best imaging tool
  - MR
- Protocol advice
  - Volumetric T1 in myelinated brains
  - High resolution T2 in infants
  - Contrast to diagnose choroid plexus papillomas

CT Findings

- NECT
  - No calcifications

DIFFERENTIAL DIAGNOSIS

Congenital Toxoplasmosis

- Calcifications, no polymicrogyria or heterotopia

Congenital Cytomegalovirus

- Calcifications, no heterotopia

Other Genetic Syndromes

- Microphthalmia with linear skin defects (MLS) shares some features, but eye lesions are not lacunae

PATHOLOGY

General Features

- Etiology
  - Unknown
- Genetics
  - Likely X-linked dominant with lethality in hemizygous male (not yet confirmed)
    - Xp22.3 in some
  - Almost all reported cases are sporadic, making linkage analysis impossible
- Associated abnormalities
  - Scoliosis secondary to costovertebral anomalies, often requiring surgery
  - ± distinct facial phenotype, ~ 25% microphthalmia
  - ± cleft lip and palate
  - Probable increased incidence of benign and malignant extra-CNS tumors
  - Probable increased incidence of vascular malformations/tumors

CLINICAL ISSUES

Presentation

- Most common signs/symptoms
  - Infantile spasms or other early onset epilepsy, typically poorly controlled
  - Chorioretinal lacunae: Only true pathognomonic feature (may be unilateral)
  - Majority have severe psychomotor retardation

Demographics

- Age
  - Most present in infancy; range is 3 days to 12 years
- Gender
  - Female almost exclusively, rare male 47 XXY
- Epidemiology
  - Early lethality in males → spontaneous abortion
  - Almost exclusively female after 2nd trimester

Natural History & Prognosis

- Median age of survival 18.5 ± 4 years

Treatment

- Symptomatic only

SELECTED REFERENCES

1. Steffensen TS et al: Cerebellar migration defects in aicardi syndrome: an extension of the neuropathological spectrum. Fetal Pediatr Pathol. 28(1):24-38, 2009
2. Hopkins B et al: Neuroimaging aspects of Aicardi syndrome. Am J Med Genet A. 146A(22):2871-8, 2008
3. Glasmacher MA et al: Phenotype and management of Aicardi syndrome: new findings from a survey of 69 children. J Child Neurol. 22(2):176-84, 2007
4. Grosso S et al: Aicardi syndrome with favorable outcome: case report and review. Brain Dev. 29(7):443-6, 2007
5. Palmér L et al: Aicardi syndrome: presentation at onset in Swedish children born in 1975-2002. Neuropediatrics. 37(3):154-8, 2006
6. Aicardi J: Aicardi syndrome. Brain Dev. 27(3):164-71, 2005

LI-FRAUMENI SYNDROME

Key Facts

Terminology

- Li-Fraumeni syndrome (LFS)
- Li-Fraumeni-like (LFL) syndromes
- Hereditary cancer syndrome conferring high susceptibility to breast cancer, sarcomas, and childhood malignancies, including brain tumors

Imaging

- Astrocytoma: Cerebrum > cerebellum > spine
- Choroid plexus carcinoma: Lateral ventricle > > > 4th ventricle

Top Differential Diagnoses

- Hereditary syndromes causing familial cancers, including brain tumors
- Tuberous sclerosis
- von Hippel-Lindau
- Medulloblastoma
- Basal cell nevus syndrome
- Turcot
- Neurofibromatosis type 1
- Carney complex
- Melanoma-astrocytoma syndrome

Pathology

- Mutation in *TP53* suppressor gene (17p13); AD
- p53: Transcription factor important in apoptosis, cell cycle control; frequently mutated in tumors
- Breast cancer (24-30%), soft tissue sarcoma (12-18%), brain tumors (12-14%), bone sarcoma (12-13%), adrenocortical carcinoma (6%)

Clinical Issues

- Propensity to develop additional primary neoplasms
- BTs: High prevalence below 10 years of age

*(**Left**) Axial T2WI MR demonstrates a massive tumor centered in the body of the left lateral ventricle in an 18-month-old infant. Satellite tumors are evident in the right frontal ➔ and occipital horns ➔. The tumor is iso- to hypointense, consistent with dense cellularity. Histology revealed choroid plexus carcinoma. (**Right**) Axial T1WI C+ MR of the same patient shows the large enhancing tumor centered in the body of the left lateral ventricle with satellite tumors in the frontal horns ➔.*

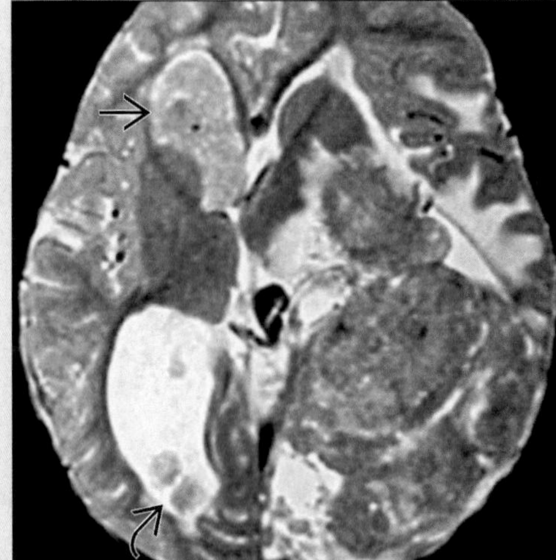

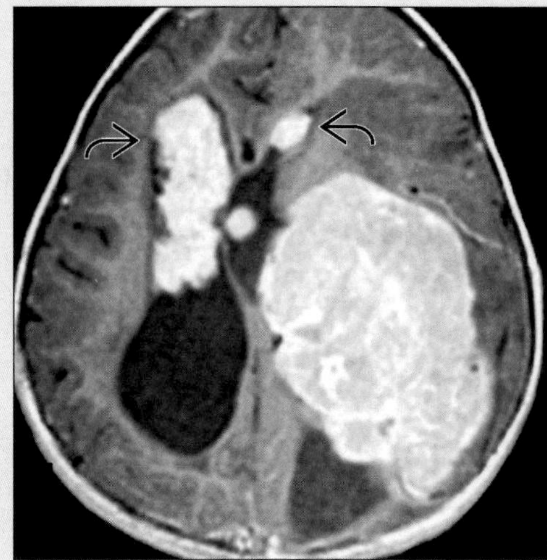

*(**Left**) Sagittal T1WI MR shows an intramedullary enhancing tumor (a PNET at pathology) in a 2-year-old child presenting with acute leg weakness. Heterogeneous enhancement is evident in the expanded lower spinal cord ➔. Edema/swelling is evident above and below. The patient's mother had recently passed away from breast cancer. (**Right**) Axial T2WI MR through the enhancing portion of the PNET shows expansion of the lower thoracic cord ➔ and heterogeneously increased T2 signal.*

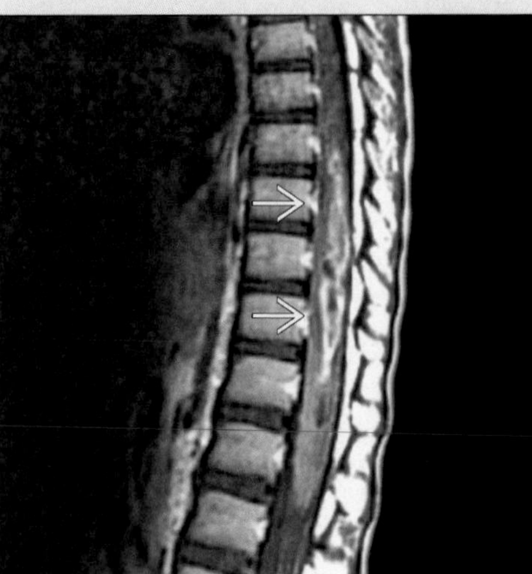

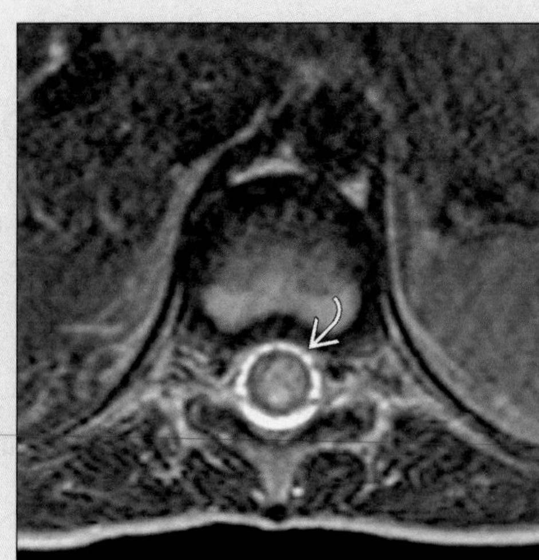

LI-FRAUMENI SYNDROME

TERMINOLOGY

Abbreviations

- Li-Fraumeni syndrome (LFS)
- Li-Fraumeni-like (LFL) syndromes

Synonyms

- Sarcoma, breast, leukemia, and adrenal syndrome

Definitions

- Hereditary cancer syndrome conferring high susceptibility to breast cancer, sarcomas, and childhood malignancies, including brain tumors (BTs)

IMAGING

General Features

- Best diagnostic clue
  - CNS tumor in child with two 1st and 2nd degree relatives with cancer
- Location
  - Astrocytoma: Cerebrum > cerebellum > spine
  - Choroid plexus carcinoma (CPC): Lateral ventricle > > > 4th ventricle

Imaging Recommendations

- Best imaging tool
  - MR with contrast

DIFFERENTIAL DIAGNOSIS

Hereditary Syndromes Causing Familial Cancers, Including Brain Tumors

- Neurofibromatosis type 1
  - Neurofibroma, optic glioma, astrocytoma
  - Rhabdomyosarcoma, parathyroid adenoma, pheochromocytoma, others
- Tuberous sclerosis
  - Ependymoma, giant cell astrocytoma
  - Renal angiomyolipoma/carcinoma
- von Hippel-Lindau
  - Hemangioblastoma (cerebellum, spinal cord)
  - Hemangioblastoma (pancreas, kidney); renal cell carcinoma, pheochromocytoma, papillary cystadenoma (epididymis)
- Basal cell nevus syndrome
  - Medulloblastoma
  - Basal cell nevi/carcinoma, ovarian carcinoma
- Carney complex
  - Melanotic schwannoma
  - Myxoma (eyelid, atrium), Sertoli cell tumor, pheochromocytoma, pituitary adenoma
- Melanoma-astrocytoma syndrome
  - Cerebral astrocytoma, other CNS tumors
  - Cutaneous malignant melanoma
- Turcot
  - Medulloblastoma, glioblastoma multiforme, astrocytoma, ependymoma
  - Colon cancer, basal cell carcinoma, gastric cancer

PATHOLOGY

General Features

- Etiology
  - Mutation in *TP53* suppressor gene (17p13); AD
- Genetics
  - *TP53* gene encodes p53 protein, 55-kDa, 393 amino-acid phosphoprotein
    - Transcription factor important in apoptosis, cell cycle control; frequently mutated in tumors
  - Germ line mutations: LFS (55-75%), LFL (20-35%)

Staging, Grading, & Classification

- LFS: Proband with sarcoma diagnosed < 45 years **and** two 1st degree relatives with any cancer < 45 years
- LFL: 3 different schemes; most predictive is Chompet
  - Proband with sarcoma, brain tumor, breast cancer, or adrenocortical carcinoma (ACC) < 36 years
  - **And** one 1st/2nd degree relative with cancer < 46 years
  - **Or** proband with multiple primary tumors, 2 of which are sarcoma, brain tumor, breast cancer, or ACC

Gross Pathologic & Surgical Features

- Breast cancer (24-30%), soft tissue sarcoma (12-18%), BT (12-14%), bone sarcoma (12-13%), ACC (6%)
- Less frequent tumors: Lung, hematopoietic system, stomach, colorectum, skin, ovary

Microscopic Features

- Astrocytoma (50%), CPC (15%)
- Medulloblastoma, PNET less common

CLINICAL ISSUES

Demographics

- Age
  - BTs: High prevalence below 10 years of age
- Epidemiology
  - Frequency of p53 germline mutations could be as high as 1:20,000

Natural History & Prognosis

- Propensity to develop additional primary neoplasms

Treatment

- Total resection of tumors ± chemotherapy
- Avoid radiation: Risk of radiation-induced tumors

DIAGNOSTIC CHECKLIST

Consider

- Nearly all CPC have p53 germline mutations

SELECTED REFERENCES

1. Gonzalez KD et al: Beyond Li Fraumeni Syndrome: clinical characteristics of families with p53 germline mutations. J Clin Oncol. 27(8):1250-6, 2009
2. Melean G et al: Genetic insights into familial tumors of the nervous system. Am J Med Genet C Semin Med Genet. 129C(1):74-84, 2004

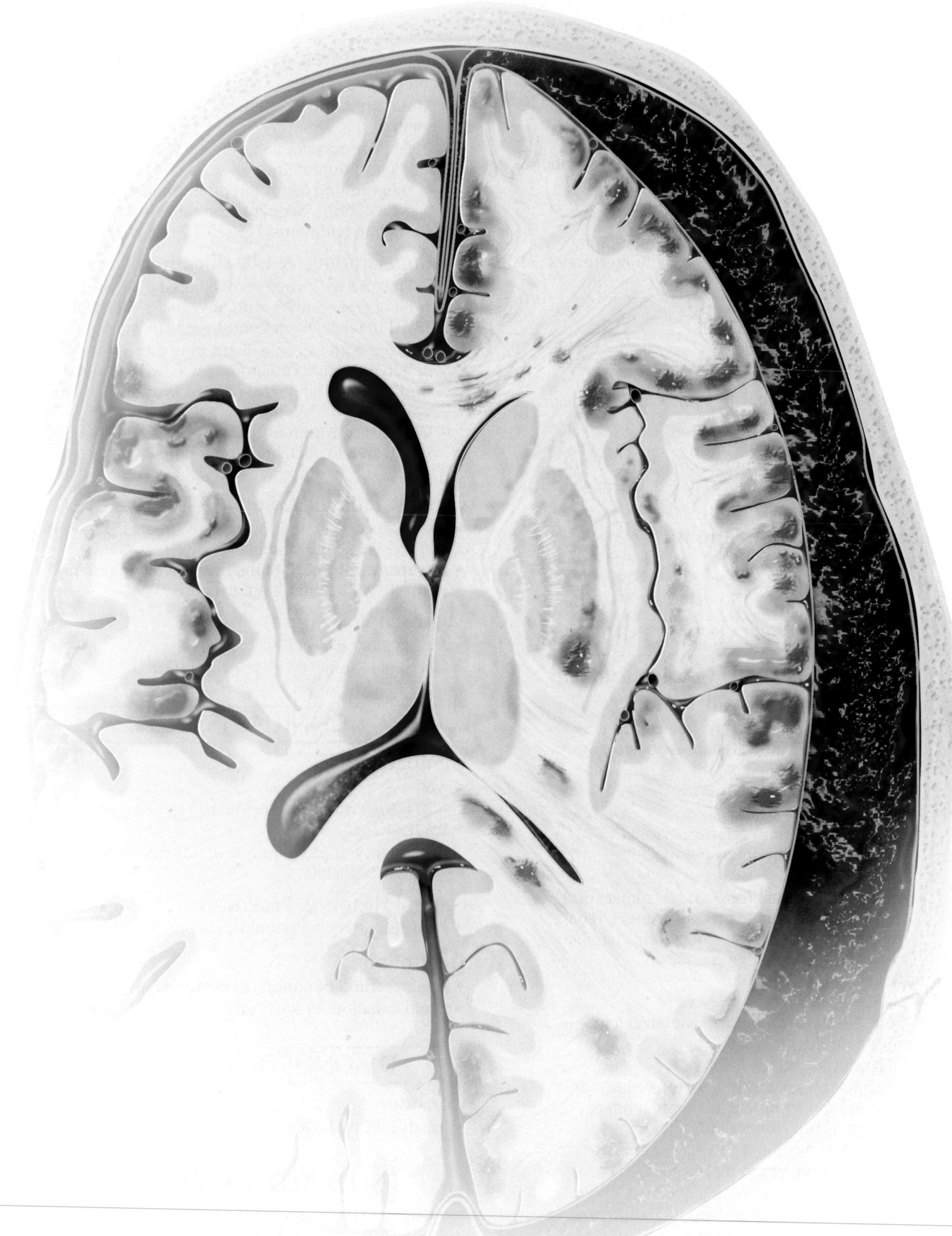

SECTION 2
Trauma

Introduction and Overview

Primary Effects of CNS Trauma

Secondary Effects of CNS Trauma

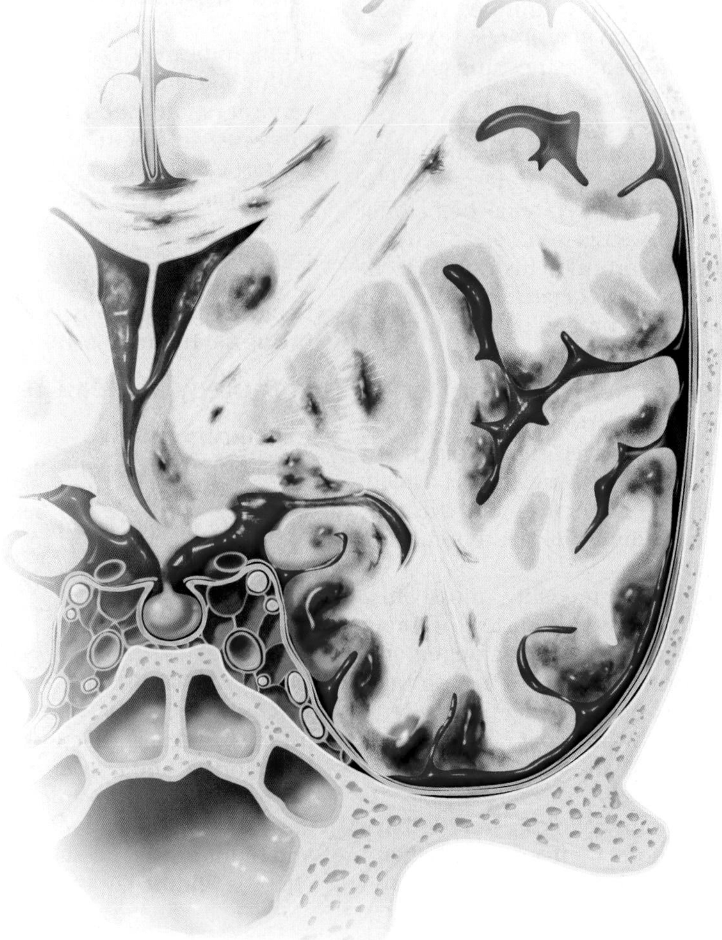

Approach to Head Trauma

General Considerations

Epidemiology. Trauma is the most common worldwide cause of death and disability in children and young adults. In these patients, neurotrauma is responsible for the vast majority of cases. In the USA and Canada, emergency departments (ED) treat more than 8,000,000 patients with head injuries, representing 6-7% of all ED visits.

The vast majority of patients with head trauma are classified as having minimal or minor injury. Minimal head injury is defined as no neurologic alteration or loss of consciousness (LOC). Minor head injury or concussion is epitomized by a walking, talking patient with a Glasgow Coma Score (GCS) of 13-15 who has experienced LOC, amnesia, or disorientation.

Of all head-injured patients, approximately 10% sustain fatal brain injury while another 5-10% of neurotrauma survivors have permanent serious neurologic deficits. A number have more subtle deficits ("minimal brain trauma"), while 20-40% of patients have moderate disability.

Mechanisms of Injury

Missile vs. non-missile injury. Trauma can be a missile or non-missile injury. Missile injury results from penetration of the skull, meninges, &/or brain by an external object, such as a bullet.

While direct impact and penetrating injuries often fracture the skull as well as cause significant brain damage, non-missile closed head injury (CHI) is a more common cause of neurotrauma. High-speed accidents exert significant acceleration/deceleration forces, causing the brain to move within the skull and forcibly impact the calvarium or dura, resulting in gyral contusion. Rotation and changes in angular momentum may also cause serious nonimpact injuries by deforming and stretching axons.

Vascular injuries. Large arteries, such as the internal carotid, vertebral, and middle meningeal arteries, can be injured either directly or indirectly. Cortical arteries can also be lacerated. Arterial injury results in a spectrum of findings, ranging from epidural hematoma to intimal flaps, dissection/transection, and cerebral ischemia/infarction. Bridging cortical veins can be torn, resulting in subdural hematoma. Moderate to severe brain injuries are almost uniformly accompanied by traumatic subarachnoid hemorrhage.

Imaging Acute Head Trauma

Modality. Since its introduction over 35 years ago, CT has gradually but completely replaced skull radiographs as the "workhorse" of trauma imaging. CT is widely (although not universally) accessible, fast, and effective. It is now the worldwide screening tool for the imaging evaluation of head trauma.

MR is generally a secondary modality, most often used in the late acute or subacute stages of brain injury. It is helpful in detecting focal/regional/global perfusion alterations, assessing the extent of hemorrhagic and nonhemorrhagic injuries, and assisting in long-term prognosis. MR should also be considered if nonaccidental trauma is suspected either clinically or on the basis of initial CT scan findings.

Appropriateness criteria. Many clinical studies have attempted to determine "whom to image and when." The American College of Radiology has delineated and published updated appropriateness criteria for imaging head trauma. While NECT in mild/minor CHI (GCS ≥ 13) without risk factors or neurologic deficit is "known to be low yield," it is rated as 7 out of 9 in appropriateness. Early post-injury NECT in mild/minor CHI, with a focal neurologic deficit &/or other risk factors, is deemed as very appropriate, as is imaging-traumatized children under 2 years of age.

The New Orleans Criteria (NOC) and Canadian CT Head Rule (CCHR) also attempt to cost effectively triage patients with minimal/mild head injuries. Although a GCS of 15 without any of the New Orleans Criteria is a highly sensitive negative predictor of clinically important brain injury or the need for neurosurgical intervention, many emergency department physicians still routinely order CT scans of all patients with head trauma regardless of clinical findings.

Between 6-7% of patients with minor head injury have positive findings on head CT scans; most all also have headache, vomiting, drug or alcohol intoxication, seizure, short-term memory deficits, or physical evidence of trauma above the clavicles. CT should be used liberally in these cases as well as in patients over 60 years of age and in children under the age of 2 with trauma indicated.

Technique. Nonenhanced CT scans (5 mm thick) from the foramen magnum to the vertex with both soft tissue and bone algorithm should be performed. "Subdural" windowing (e.g., window width of 150-200 H) of the soft tissue images on PACS (or film, if PACS is not available) is highly recommended.

"Scout" views should be included and examined for foreign objects, cervical spine abnormalities, and jaw/facial trauma. Because many patients with moderate to severe head trauma also have cervical spine injuries, MDR CT with both brain and cervical imaging is often indicated. Soft tissue and bone algorithm with multiplanar reformatted images (coronal, sagittal) of the cervical spine should be obtained. If the transverse processes are fractured or the facet joints subluxed, CTA for suspected vascular injury may also be indicated.

Repeat CT of patients with head injury should be obtained if there is sudden clinical deterioration, regardless of initial imaging findings. Delayed development or enlargement of both extra- and intraaxial hemorrhages typically occurs within 36 hours following the initial traumatic event.

Pathology of Head Trauma

Classification

Brain trauma can be divided into primary and secondary injury. Primary head injuries occur at the time of initial trauma, whereas secondary injuries typically present later. Secondary responses to primary injury include edema with or without brain herniation, metabolic and perfusion alterations, and a variety of other induced effects.

Primary Head Injury

Overview. Primary traumatic lesions include scalp injuries, skull fractures, extraaxial hemorrhages/hematomas, and a spectrum of intraaxial injuries.

Scalp injuries. Bruising, laceration, and scalp hematoma are common in patients with both penetrating missile and blunt impact head injury. Some scalp soft tissue mass effect is almost always seen with a skull fracture and is a good indication of its presence. A linear lucent line in the calvarium that is not associated with overlying scalp swelling is probably a suture, not a fracture.

Skull fractures. Skull fractures are classified into 3 types: (1) linear, (2) depressed, and (3) diastatic fractures. Skull fractures can be asymptomatic or cause serious injury to vessels (arteries, veins, and dural venous sinuses) and cranial nerves, as well as the underlying brain. Fractures can tear the dura and arachnoid, cause pneumocephalus, and result in CSF leaks. Approximately 1/3 of patients with moderate to severe brain injury have **no** imaging evidence of a skull fracture; about 25% of autopsies on people with fatal head injuries show no skull fracture.

Extraaxial hemorrhages and hematomas. Extraaxial hemorrhage can occur in any compartment. Epidural hematomas (EDH) arise between the calvarium and the outer (periosteal) dural layer. Subdural hematomas (SDH) occur between the inner (meningeal) layer of the dura and the arachnoid. Traumatic subarachnoid hemorrhage (tSAH) is found within the sulci and subarachnoid cisterns.

An **EDH** is uncommon but potentially fatal. The classic textbook "lucid interval" is seen in less than 1/2 of all cases. Mortality and morbidity can be low if an EDH is promptly recognized and appropriately treated. Most EDHs are unilateral, supratentorial, and biconvex in shape. Most are caused by arterial laceration (usually damage to the middle meningeal artery) but 10-15% are associated with tearing of a dural venous sinus. The "vertex" EDH is caused by tearing of the superior sagittal sinus, may develop late, and can be difficult to see on axial NECT scans.

SDHs are much more common than EDHs. Most are associated with other significant injuries, such as cortical contusions, brain lacerations, and tSAH. Approximately 1/2 are caused by bridging vein rupture and the other 1/2 are associated with torn cortical arteries. Most SDHs spread diffusely over the brain and, at surgery or autopsy, appear as a purplish "currant jelly" clot under the bulging dura. Bilateral SDHs and "contrecoup" injuries are common.

tSAH is the most common extraaxial hemorrhage associated with head injury. While tSAH may result in focal/regional alterations in cerebral blood flow, diffusion/perfusion changes are more often incidental to, and caused by, injuries such as contusions and edema. In contrast to aneurysmal SAH, tSAH tends to spare the suprasellar cisterns and is more often seen along the superficial sulci and within sylvian fissures adjacent to cortical contusions. Subtle tSAH in head-injured patients can sometimes be seen as blood layering in the dependent portion of the interpeduncular notch.

Intraaxial injuries. These include cortical contusions and lacerations, diffuse axonal injury (DAI), intracerebral hematomas in the subcortical gray matter and basal ganglia, brainstem injuries, and intraventricular hemorrhages.

Cortical contusions and lacerations are the most common types of parenchymal injury. Contusions are gyral "crest" injuries (basically superficial "brain bruises"). Gyri impact bone or a hard, knife-like edge of dura (i.e., the falx cerebri or tentorium cerebelli). More than 90% are multiple and bilateral. The cerebral hemispheres are more commonly involved than the cerebellum. The anterior-inferior temporal and frontal lobes are most commonly affected. The dorsolateral corpus callosum may be suddenly forced against the inferior free margin of the falx and contused by the "shake, rattle, and roll" that occurs in severe CHI. Cortical contusions typically evolve with time; the initial head CT does not reveal the full extent of injury in up to 1/2 of all cases, so follow-up imaging is recommended.

Diffuse axonal injury is the 2nd most common parenchymal lesion seen in traumatic brain injury. DAIs are nonimpact injuries, resulting from the inertial forces of rotation and differential brain acceleration/deceleration. Most DAIs are not caused by immediate axonal "shearing." A "secondary axotomy" that causes impaired axoplasmic transport, swelling, and disconnection is more common. The injured axons undergo traumatic depolarization and ion fluxes, and they cause spreading depression in the adjacent parenchyma. Axonal swellings or "retraction balls" form, leaving microscopic gaps in the white matter. Microglial reaction ensues within a few weeks.

Most DAIs are microscopic and nonhemorrhagic. MR with T2* (GRE or SWI imaging) is the most useful technique for imaging hemorrhagic DAI.

Secondary Head Injury

Overview. Secondary head injuries are common following initial brain trauma. Brain swelling, increased intracranial pressure, and herniations are common. Traumatic cerebral ischemia with focal, regional, or global perfusion alterations may follow. When intracranial pressure exceeds intraarterial pressure, brain death may ensue.

Herniation syndromes and the Monro-Kellie doctrine. Once the sutures fuse and the fontanelles close, brain, CSF, and blood coexist in a rigid, unyielding "bone box." Cerebral blood volume, perfusion, and CSF exist in a delicate balance. Any increase in intracranial contents (blood, edema, tumor, etc.) requires compensatory decrease in other contents. CSF in the sulci is initially squeezed out. The lateral ventricles may decrease in size. If the expanding volume in 1 brain compartment overwhelms the compensatory mechanisms, brain and accompanying blood vessels are displaced (herniated) in a variety of predictable ways.

Subfalcine herniation is the most common type of cerebral herniation. The cingulate gyrus and pericallosal branches of the anterior cerebral artery herniate from 1 side to the other under the inferior free margin of the falx cerebri. The ipsilateral ventricle is compressed; the choroid plexus in the contralateral ventricle continues to produce CSF, so the ventricle enlarges.

Descending transtentorial herniation (DTH) is the 2nd most common type of brain displacement. Initially the uncus is displaced medially into the suprasellar cistern. The hippocampus soon follows. The posterior cerebral artery is displaced inferiorly through the U-shaped tentorial incisura and may occlude if the herniation becomes severe. Periaqueductal necrosis, midbrain (Duret) hemorrhage, and "Kernohan notch" with displacement of the contralateral cerebral peduncle against the tentorium may ensue. A posterior fossa mass may cause **tonsillar herniation**, the 3rd most common type.

Uncommon cerebral herniations include **ascending transtentorial herniation**, caused by a posterior fossa mass forcing the cerebellum superiorly through the incisura, and is much less common than DTH.

TRAUMA OVERVIEW

New Orleans Criteria in Minor Head Injury

CT indicated if GCS = 15 plus any of following

- Headache
- Vomiting
- Patient > 60 years
- Intoxication (drugs, alcohol)
- Short-term memory deficits (anterograde amnesia)
- Visible trauma above clavicles
- Seizure

Canadian Head CT Rule in Minor Head Injury

Clinical assessment and head CT indications

- CT if GCS 13-15 and witnessed LOC, amnesia, or confusion
  - High risk for neurosurgical intervention
    - GCS < 15 at 2 hours
    - Suspected open/depressed skull fracture
    - Clinical signs of skull base fracture
    - 2 or more vomiting episodes
    - Age ≥ 65 years
  - Medium risk for brain injury detected by head CT
    - Antegrade amnesia ≥ 30 minutes
    - "Dangerous mechanism" (i.e., auto-pedestrian, ejected, etc.)

Modified, adapted from Stiell IG et al., Comparison of the Canadian CT head rule and the New Orleans criteria in patients with minor head injury. JAMA 294(12): 1511-1518, 2005

Transalar herniation, can be superior (caused by upward displacement of the temporal lobe over the greater sphenoid wing) or inferior (displacement of the frontal lobe posteriorly). **Transdural/transcranial herniations** (sometimes called "brain fungus" by the neurosurgeons) occur when increased intracranial pressure is severe. Brain extrudes through torn dura into the epidural space. If a skull fracture or burr hole is present, extruded brain may extend under the galea and scalp.

Cerebral edema, ischemia. Traumatic cerebral edema occurs in 10-20% of moderate to severe brain injuries. Diffuse brain swelling develops, typically between 24 and 48 hours after trauma. Children and young adults are most commonly affected. Swollen hemispheres with low-density brain showing decreased gray-white differentiation is typical. Sulci and subarachnoid spaces are compressed and may become completely effaced.

Perfusion and metabolic alterations. Metabolic derangements are common in TBI. A complex cascade of events causes vascular dysautoregulation with oxidative tissue damage, elevated reactive nitrogen species, and inflammation. Perfusion alterations are also common and may reflect the disordered autoregulation. They can be local, regional, or generalized and vary in severity from focal cortical ischemia to frank infarction and laminar cortical necrosis. The most severe perfusion reduction results from markedly elevated intracranial pressure and may result in brain death.

Brain death. When intracranial pressure exceeds intraarterial pressure, complete and irreversible cessation of brain function may ensue. Legal criteria for brain death vary with jurisdiction. In general, imaging may confirm but does not substitute for clinical criteria.

Vascular injuries. Vascular manifestations of trauma include both primary effects (such as vessel laceration, dissection, thrombosis, pseudoaneurysm, or AV shunting) and secondary injuries. Brain herniation may cause vascular occlusion and infarction. The posterior cerebral artery territory is most commonly affected and is caused by unilateral DTH. With severe brain swelling and complete bilateral DTH, perforating arteries from the circle of Willis may occlude, causing multifocal infarcts in the basal brain.

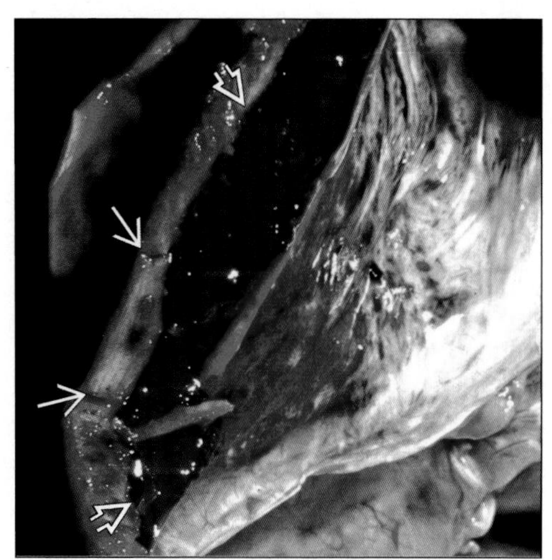

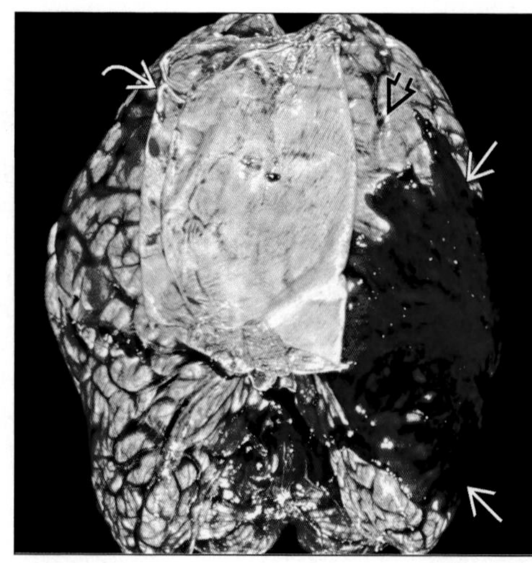

(Left) *Axial gross pathology of fatal epidural hematoma. The brain has been removed to show the comminuted depressed fracture of the squamous temporal bone →. The acute epidural hematoma is seen as a biconvex, dark purple, "currant jelly" clot →.* ***(Right)*** *Autopsied brain shows acute subdural hematoma → spreading diffusely over the brain between the dura → and the thin, veil-like arachnoid →. (Courtesy E.T. Hedley-Whyte, MD.)*

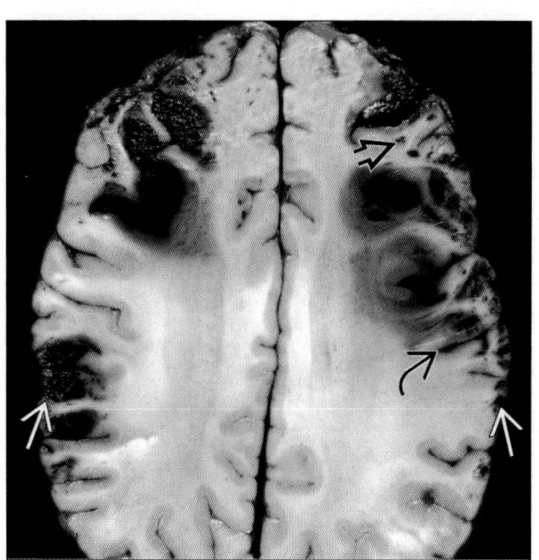

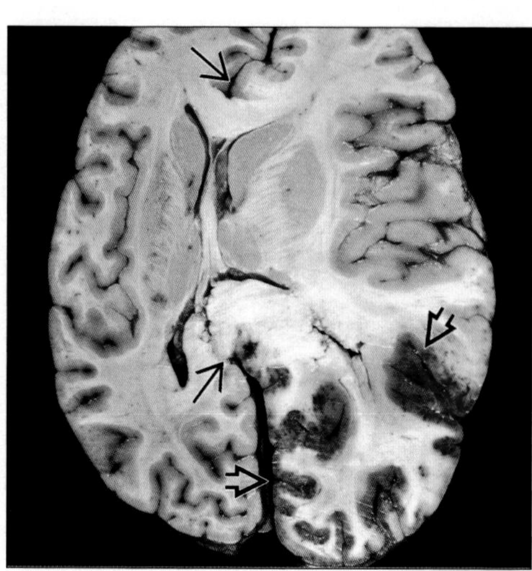

(Left) *Autopsied brain shows multifocal cortical contusions → with traumatic subarachnoid hemorrhage in the overlying sulci →. Several foci of hemorrhagic axonal injury can be seen in the subcortical white matter →. (Courtesy R. Hewlett, PhD.)* ***(Right)*** *Subfalcine herniation of the cingulate gyri and lateral ventricles → was caused by a large SDH (not shown). Descending transtentorial herniation caused secondary PCA occlusion and hemorrhagic infarction →. (Courtesy R. Hewlett, PhD.)*

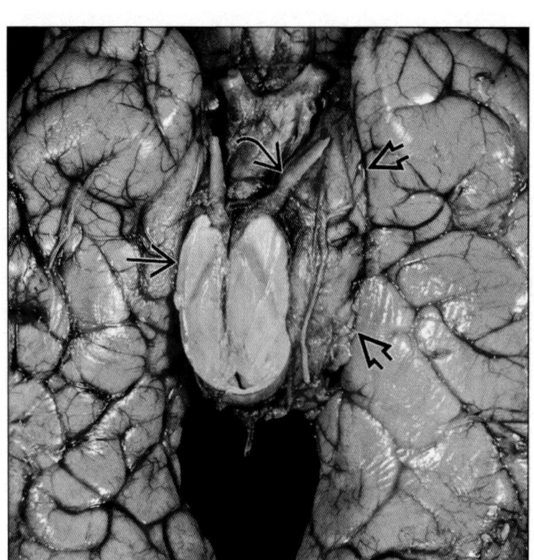

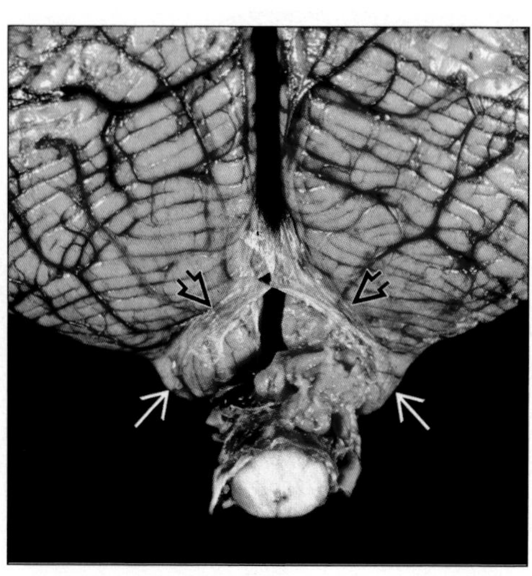

(Left) *Gross pathology shows descending transtentorial herniation. "Grooving" of the temporal lobe is caused by compression against the tentorial incisura →. The 3rd nerve is compressed →; the contralateral cerebral peduncle is smashed against the tentorium →, causing a "Kernohan notch." (Courtesy R. Hewlett, PhD.)* ***(Right)*** *Gross pathology shows tonsillar herniation →. "Grooving" → of the cerebellar hemispheres is caused by compression against the foramen magnum. (Courtesy R. Hewlett, PhD.)*

MISSILE AND PENETRATING INJURY

Key Facts

Terminology
- Impalement injury

Imaging
- Single or multiple intracranial foreign bodies, missile tract, pneumocephalus, entry ± exit wound
- Extent of injury extremely variable depending on
  - Size, shape, and number of projectiles
  - Projectile velocities
  - Entry/exit site(s) and course through brain
- Entry site → embedded bullet and bone fragments
- Epidural, subdural, subarachnoid hemorrhage
- Hemorrhagic tract through brain
- Intracerebral, intraventricular hemorrhage
- Ischemia and infarction
- Brain herniation
- Nuclear medicine brain death scanning with cerebral perfusion agents can be confirmatory test
- Best imaging tool → NECT ± CTA
- Vascular injury

Clinical Issues
- Prognosis ranges from brain death to full recovery
- High morbidity and mortality

Diagnostic Checklist
- Injury is most severe when
  - Missile is large and traveling at high velocities
  - If it fragments through tissue early in its path
- Reporting tips
  - Determine entry site
  - Assess missile path
  - Evaluate for exit site and secondary ricochet paths
  - Consider vascular injury

(Left) Axial NECT shows a small-caliber, low-velocity injury. A bullet fragment is present in the left temporal lobe → with minimal adjacent hemorrhage. A narrow hemorrhagic tract extends through the midbrain → with a 2nd fragment imbedded in the right temporal lobe →. Regional subarachnoid and intraventricular blood are also seen. *(Right)* Axial bone CT demonstrates the tiny entry site in the squamous temporal bone →, with a focus of underlying intracranial air →.

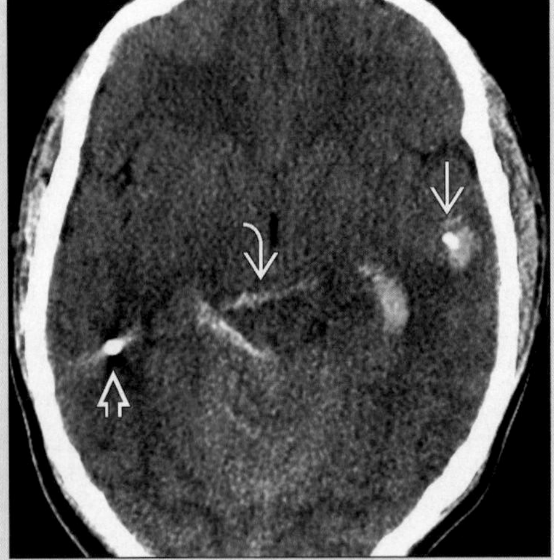

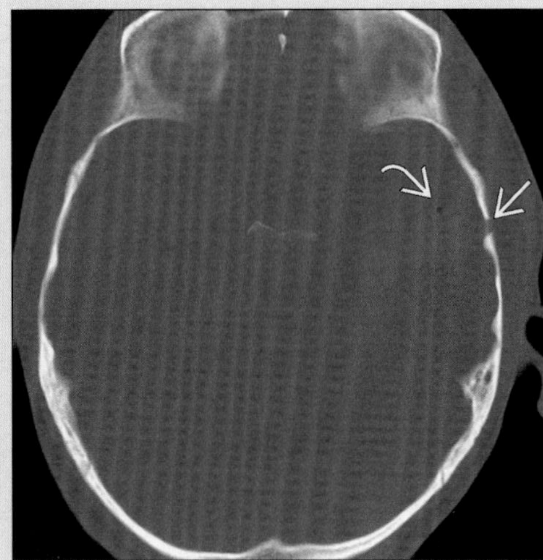

(Left) Axial NECT shows a large-caliber, high-velocity injury with a frontal entry site → and a wide oblique hemorrhagic tract → that extends to the left temporoparietal region. There is sulcal effacement and midline shift to the right. *(Right)* Axial bone CT shows the frontal entry site → and left parietal fracture →. Multiple bone and bullet fragments and foci of air are noted along the tract. Ricocheted metallic fragments → are seen posteriorly, away from the primary trajectory.

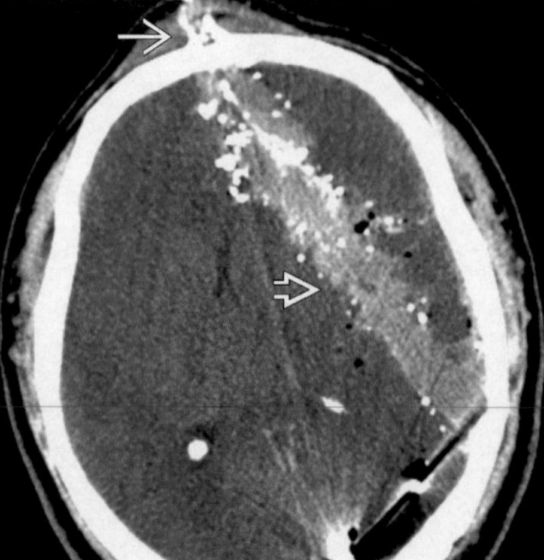

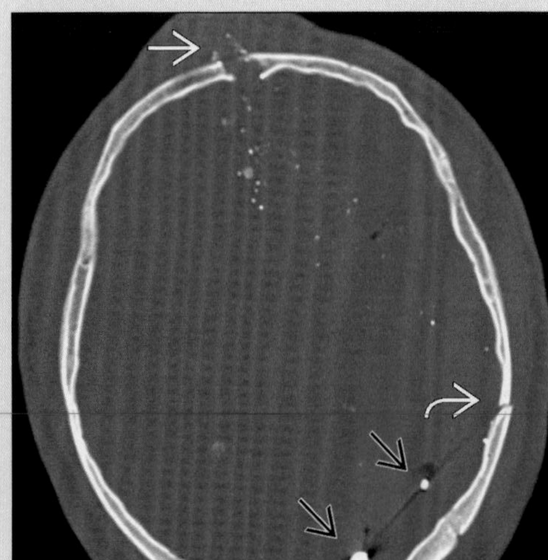

MISSILE AND PENETRATING INJURY

TERMINOLOGY

Synonyms

- Impalement injury
- Stabbing injury

Definitions

- Cranial trauma from high-velocity projectile (typically gunshot wound [GSW]) or impalement with sharp object

IMAGING

General Features

- Best diagnostic clue
  - Single or multiple intracranial foreign bodies, missile tract, pneumocephalus, entry ± exit wound
- Location
  - Supra- or infratentorial, affecting cerebral/cerebellar hemispheres or brainstem
- Size
  - Small linear tract if small caliber and low velocity
  - Large linear tract if large caliber and high velocity
- Morphology
  - Extremely variable depending on
    - Size, shape, number of projectiles
    - Projectile velocities
    - Entry/exit site(s), course through brain
  - Skull fracture(s)
    - Entry site → embedded bullet and bone fragments
    - Exit site → if high enough velocity
    - Pneumocephalus
  - Intracranial hemorrhage
    - Epidural, subdural, subarachnoid hemorrhage
    - Hemorrhagic tract through brain
    - Intracerebral, intraventricular hemorrhage
  - Vascular injury
    - Pseudoaneurysm, dissection, arteriovenous fistula (AVF), spasm
  - CSF leak
  - Secondary effects
    - Ischemia and infarction
    - Brain herniation

CT Findings

- NECT
  - Best assessment of extent of soft tissue injury
  - Identify entrance and exit wounds
- Bone CT
  - Osseous entry and exit sites and pneumocephalus shown to better advantage
  - Metallic fragments easier to evaluate
- CTA
  - Evaluate for pseudoaneurysm, dissection, or traumatic AVF

MR Findings

- T1WI
  - Variable signal (hemorrhage, foreign bodies, air)
- T2WI
  - Edema from pressure wave
  - Variable signal (hemorrhage, foreign bodies, air)
- T2* GRE
  - "Blooming" from hemorrhage, as well as susceptibility artifact from foreign bodies, air
- DWI
  - Secondary infarction
- MRA
  - Evaluate for pseudoaneurysm, dissection, or traumatic AVF
- MRV
  - Venous injury or thrombosis if missile tract crosses or tears interdural veins or lacerates sinus
  - Dural sinus thrombosis → reported incidence < 5% with penetrating trauma

Angiographic Findings

- Conventional
  - Traumatic intracranial aneurysms in atypical locations
    - Proximal to or beyond circle of Willis and major arterial bifurcations
  - Extracranial pseudoaneurysms vary in size, configuration
    - Small saccular lesions
    - Fusiform dilatations
    - Large paravascular collections with huge cavitating hematomas
  - Other possible injuries
    - Traumatic direct carotid cavernous fistulas, dural AVFs involving meningeal vessels
    - Extracranial AVFs
    - Arterial dissection
  - Vascular spasm from projectile velocity or subarachnoid hemorrhage

Nuclear Medicine Findings

- Nuclear medicine brain death scanning with cerebral perfusion agents can be confirmatory test

Imaging Recommendations

- Best imaging tool
  - NECT
- Protocol advice
  - NECT ± CTA
  - Consider MR/MRA/MRV
  - Conventional cerebral angiography depending on type of trauma and degree of injury

DIFFERENTIAL DIAGNOSIS

Nonprojectile Intracranial Injury

- Contusion
- Axonal injury

PATHOLOGY

General Features

- Etiology
  - Pressure wave in front of missile crushes/stretches/disintegrates tissue, creates temporary cavitation
- General pathology comments
  - Appearance and degree of injury highly variable
  - Traumatic aneurysms account for < 1% of all intracranial aneurysms

MISSILE AND PENETRATING INJURY

Gross Pathologic & Surgical Features

- Highly variable depending on severity of trauma

Microscopic Features

- Highly variable
  - Ranges from axonal transection to axonal edema
  - Vascular transection to luminal injury

CLINICAL ISSUES

Presentation

- Most common signs/symptoms
  - Highly variable depending on type and degree of traumatic injury
    - Motor deficits
    - Cranial nerve palsies
    - Visual field defects
- Other signs/symptoms
  - Post-traumatic seizures

Demographics

- Age
  - Any age can be affected, but younger patients involved more often
- Gender
  - M > F
- Ethnicity
  - Some studies document higher frequency of intentional assault injury among certain minority groups
- Epidemiology
  - Highly variable → incidence higher in inner cities and combat situations
    - May be influenced by regional legislation and social attitudes toward gun control
  - Accidental
  - Intentional
    - Self-inflicted/suicidal
      - Percent increase with age
    - Assault/homicidal intent

Natural History & Prognosis

- Prognosis ranges from brain death to full recovery
  - High morbidity and mortality
    - Most fatalities occur within 1st day
- Poor outcomes associated with
  - Transventricular or bihemispheric central type of trajectory → predictive of high morbidity/mortality
  - Low Glasgow Coma Scale (GCS) value at presentation
  - High head Abbreviated Injury Score (AIS)
  - Pupil irregularity
  - Low blood pressure
  - Older patient
- Good outcomes associated with tangential gunshot wounds
  - Bullet fragments do not penetrate inner table of skull
    - Skull fracture and intracranial hemorrhage can still be present

Treatment

- Options, risks, complications
  - Dependent upon type and degree of injury
- Debridement
  - Penetrating objects may be left in place
- Decompressive craniectomy
- CSF diversion to control hydrocephalus
  - Especially in setting of infratentorial injury
- Intracranial pressure control

DIAGNOSTIC CHECKLIST

Consider

- Could there be associated vascular injury and aneurysm formation?
- Post-traumatic pseudoaneurysm may be overlooked on CT → often obscured by hemorrhagic contusion

Image Interpretation Pearls

- Injury is most severe when missile is large and traveling at high velocity and if it fragments through tissue early in its path

Reporting Tips

- Determine entry site
- Assess missile path
  - Determine extent of wound, including bone fragmentation and ricochet paths
- Evaluate for exit site and secondary ricochet paths
- Consider vascular injury

SELECTED REFERENCES

1. Finley CJ et al: The demographics of significant firearm injury in Canadian trauma centres and the associated predictors of inhospital mortality. Can J Surg. 51(3):197-203, 2008
2. Kim H et al: Intentional traumatic brain injury in Ontario, Canada. J Trauma. 65(6):1287-92, 2008
3. McNett M: A review of the predictive ability of Glasgow Coma Scale scores in head-injured patients. J Neurosci Nurs. 39(2):68-75, 2007
4. Aryan HE et al: Gunshot wounds to the head: gang- and non-gang-related injuries and outcomes. Brain Inj. 19(7):505-10, 2005
5. Coşar A et al: Craniocerebral gunshot wounds: results of less aggressive surgery and complications. Minim Invasive Neurosurg. 48(2):113-8, 2005
6. Kim KA et al: Vector analysis correlating bullet trajectory to outcome after civilian through-and-through gunshot wound to the head: using imaging cues to predict fatal outcome. Neurosurgery. 57(4):737-47; discussion 737-47, 2005
7. Murano T et al: Civilian craniocerebral gunshot wounds: an update in predicting outcomes. Am Surg. 71(12):1009-14, 2005
8. Hackam DJ et al: Mechanisms of pediatric trauma deaths in Canada and the United States: the role of firearms. J Trauma. 56(6):1286-90, 2004
9. Thiex R et al: Delayed oedema in the pyramidal tracts remote from intracerebral missile path following gunshot injury. Neuroradiology. 46(2):140-3, 2004

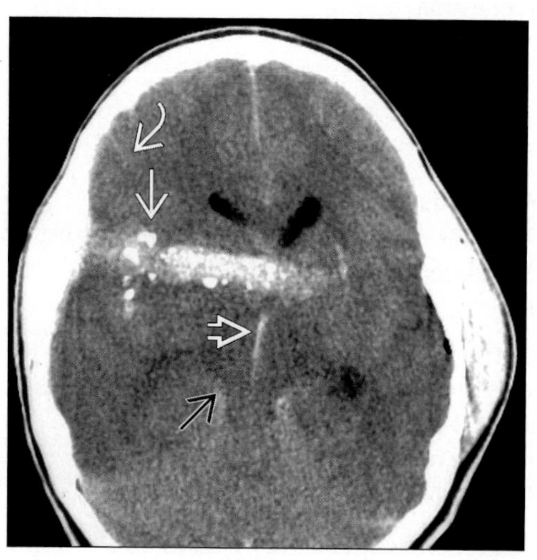

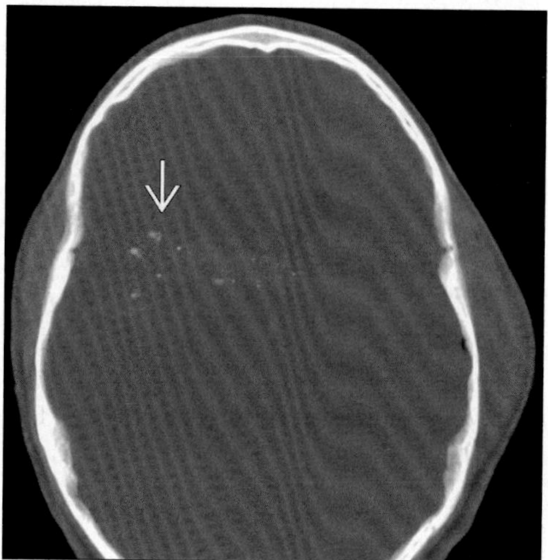

(Left) *Axial NECT shows extensive hemorrhage along the small-caliber missile trajectory from right to left ➡, crossing both basal ganglia. Scattered subarachnoid blood ➡ and minimal intraventricular blood ➡ are seen, along with diffuse sulcal effacement and early transtentorial herniation →.* ***(Right)*** *Axial bone CT in the same patient confirms the presence of intracranial bullet and bone fragments on the right ➡ near the entry site.*

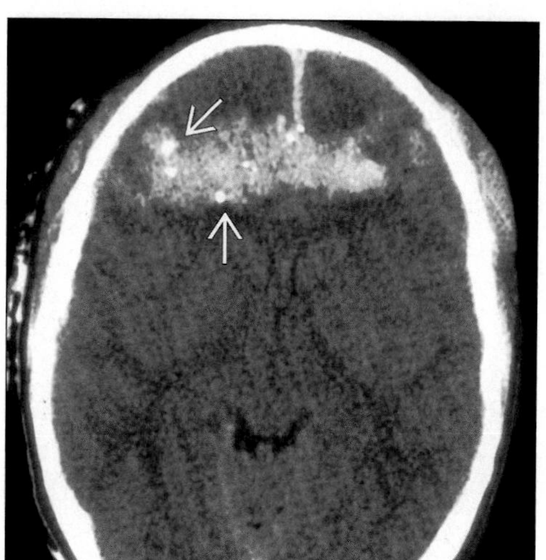

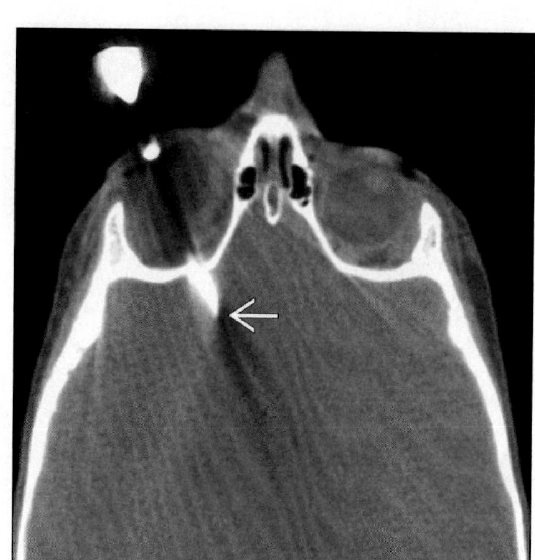

(Left) *Axial NECT shows the trajectory of the injury across the frontal lobes, with extensive hemorrhage and small hyperdense foci that represent bullet &/or bone fragments ➡.* ***(Right)*** *Axial bone CT shows the tip of a screwdriver embedded in the right frontal lobe ➡.*

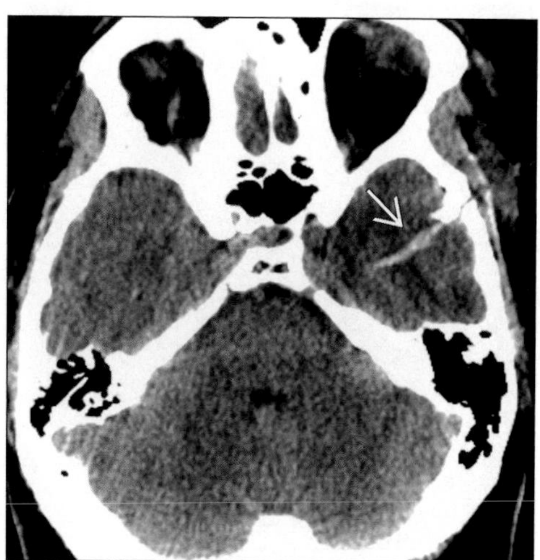

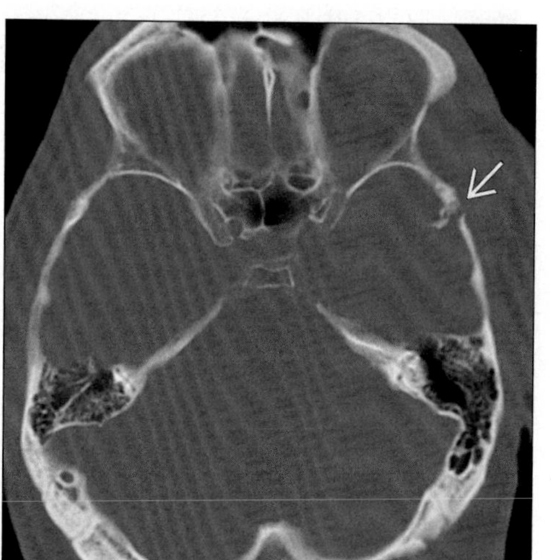

(Left) *Axial NECT demonstrates findings related to a stabbing injury. The knife has been removed, but there is a linear hemorrhagic tract in the left temporal lobe ➡ showing the knife's course through the brain. (Courtesy N. Wycliffe, MD.)* ***(Right)*** *Axial bone CT in the same patient shows a defect ➡ in the left squamous temporal bone. (Courtesy N. Wycliffe, MD.)*

EPIDURAL HEMATOMA

Key Facts

Terminology
- Blood collection in space between skull, dura

Imaging
- Use NECT for traumatic cases
  - Hyperdense biconvex extraaxial collection
  - Does not cross sutures unless sutural diastasis/ fracture present
  - Compresses/displaces underlying brain, subarachnoid space
  - Low-density "swirl" sign: Active/rapid bleeding with unretracted clot
- 1/3 to 1/2 have other significant lesions
  - Skull fracture (> 95%)
  - > 95% unilateral; bilateral rare (2.58%)
- Supratentorial (90-95%), posterior fossa (5-10%)

Top Differential Diagnoses
- Subdural hematoma
- Neoplasm
- Infection/inflammation
- Extramedullary hematopoiesis

Pathology
- Arterial 90%, venous 10%
- Arterial EDH most often near MMA groove fracture
- Venous EDH related to fractures near dural sinus attachments

Clinical Issues
- Classic "lucid interval": Approximately 50% of cases
- Good outcome if promptly recognized and treated
- EDH < 1 cm may be managed nonoperatively; consider endovascular adjunct treatment

(Left) Coronal graphic illustrates swirling acute hemorrhage from a laceration of the middle meningeal artery by an overlying skull fracture. The epidural hematoma displaces the dura inward as it expands. (Right) Axial NECT reveals a classic biconvex epidural hematoma ➔. Note heterogeneity within the hematoma, the "swirl" sign ➢ that suggests active bleeding. There is also a thin posterior falcine subdural hematoma ↪.

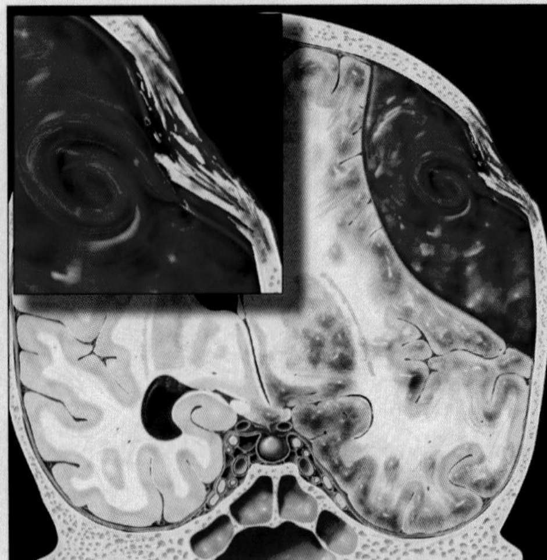

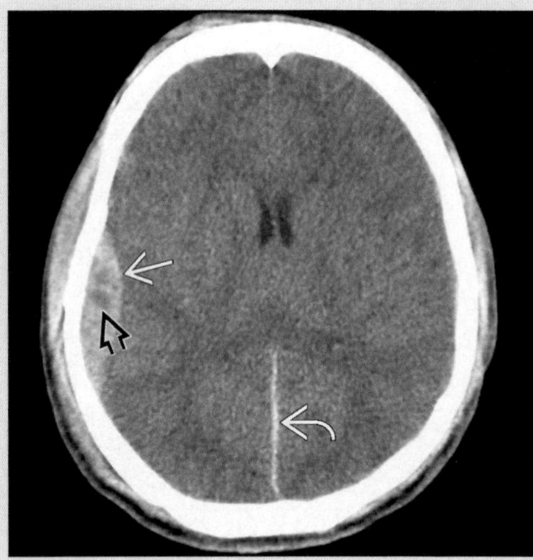

(Left) Axial bone CT shows a severely comminuted calvarial fracture with depressed components ↪. Even with bone algorithm, an associated epidural hematoma is evident ➔, although it is better seen in the next image. (Right) Axial NECT reveals a right, frontoparietal, biconvex, hyperdense lesion ➔ with mass effect. Note the relatively hypodense foci ➢ within the rapidly expanding epidural hematoma. Some traumatic subarachnoid hemorrhage is also present ➢.

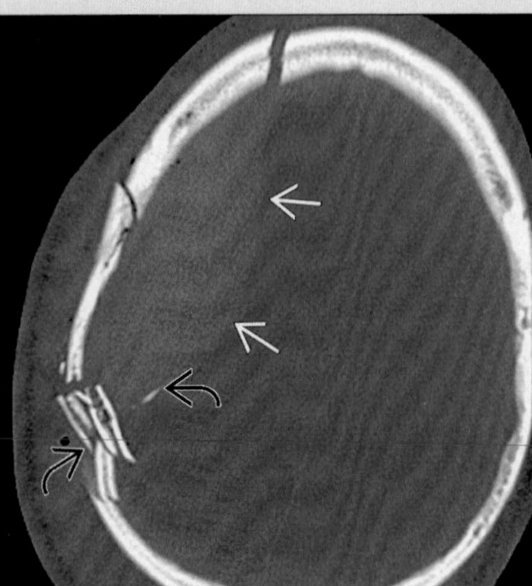

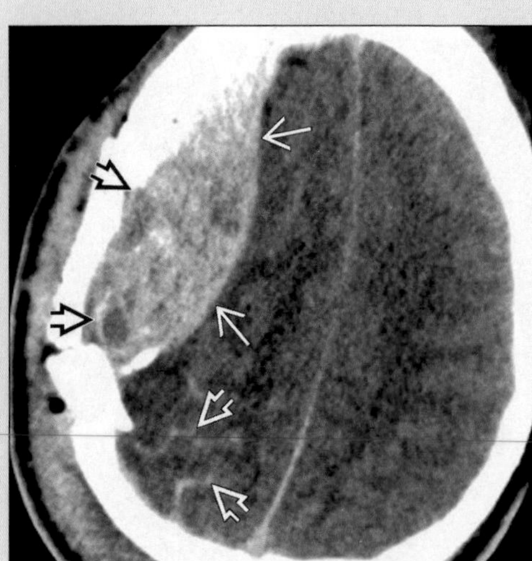

EPIDURAL HEMATOMA

TERMINOLOGY

Abbreviations

- Epidural hematoma (EDH)

Definitions

- Blood collection in space between inner table of skull and outer layer of dura

IMAGING

General Features

- Best diagnostic clue
  - Hyperdense biconvex extraaxial collection on NECT
- Location
  - Epidural space between skull, dura
  - Nearly all EDH occur at impact (coup) site
  - > 95% unilateral; bilateral rare (2.58%)
  - Supratentorial (90-95%)
    - Temporoparietal (65%), frontal or parietooccipital (30%)
    - Rarely at vertex
  - 5-10% in posterior fossa
  - Venous EDH adjacent to venous sinus
- Size
  - Variable; rapid expansion typical
    - Attains maximum size within 36 hours
  - Slower accumulation of blood in venous EDH
- Morphology
  - Biconvex or lentiform extraaxial collection
  - Does not cross sutures unless sutural diastasis/ fracture present
  - Compresses/displaces underlying brain, subarachnoid space
  - Venous EDH
    - Straddles multiple cranial compartments
    - Sinus transgressed by fracture line
    - Dural sinus displaced, usually not occluded
    - Can cross falx, tentorium
  - 1/3 to 1/2 have other significant lesions
    - Skull fracture (> 95%)
    - Mass effect, secondary herniations common
    - Contrecoup subdural hematoma
    - Cerebral contusions

Radiographic Findings

- Radiography
  - Skull fracture in 95%

CT Findings

- NECT
  - Acute: 2/3 hyperdense, 1/3 mixed density
    - Low-density "swirl" sign: Active/rapid bleeding with unretracted clot
    - Acute extravasation: 30-50 Hounsfield units (HU); coagulated: 50-80 HU
    - Medial hyperdense margin: Displaced dura
  - Air in EDH (20%) suggests sinus or mastoid fracture
  - Vertex EDH easily overlooked
  - Bilateral (rare) → "hourglass" brain
  - Chronic EDH → hypo-/mixed density
  - CT "comma" sign
    - EDH plus subdural hematoma
    - Often temporoparietal or temporoparietooccipital
    - Important to identify → treated as 2 different surgical entities
- CECT
  - Acute: Rarely contrast extravasation
  - Chronic: Peripheral dural enhancement from neovascularization, granulation

MR Findings

- T1WI
  - Acute: Isointense
  - Subacute/early chronic: Hyperintense
  - Black line between EDH & brain: Displaced dura
- T2WI
  - Acute: Variable hyper- to hypointense
  - Early subacute: Hypointense
  - Late subacute/early chronic: Hyperintense
  - Black line between EDH & brain: Displaced dura
- T1WI C+
  - Venous EDH: Displaced dural sinus by hematoma
  - Spontaneous (nontraumatic) EDH: Enhancement of hemorrhagic epidural mass
- MRV
  - Assess for patency of venous sinus
  - Displaced venous sinus flow by hematoma

Angiographic Findings

- Diagnostic
  - Avascular mass effect; displaced cortical arteries
  - ± lacerated middle meningeal artery (MMA)
    - If forms AV fistula → "tram-track" sign
    - Simultaneous opacification of artery, vein
  - Venous EDH: Displaced dural sinus
- Interventional: Consider endovascular treatment as adjunct in patients who may not require surgery

Imaging Recommendations

- Best imaging tool
  - NECT for traumatic cases, MR if nontraumatic
- Protocol advice
  - Traumatic: Consider MR if EDH straddles dural compartments or sinuses on NECT
  - Nontraumatic: Enhanced MR

DIFFERENTIAL DIAGNOSIS

Subdural Hematoma

- Usually crescentic, may also be biconvex
- Crosses sutures, does not cross falx
- No displaced dura

Neoplasm

- Meningioma
- Soft tissue component (subperiosteal) of osseous mass
  - Metastasis, lymphoma, primary sarcoma
- Dural-based mass
  - Metastases, lymphoma, mesenchymal tumor

Infection/Inflammation

- Subperiosteal extension of osseous inflammatory lesion
- Epidural empyema secondary to osteomyelitis
- Soft tissue from granulomatous osseous lesion

- Tuberculosis

Extramedullary Hematopoiesis

- History of blood dyscrasia

PATHOLOGY

General Features

- Etiology
  - Trauma most common
    - Arterial (90%), venous (10%)
    - Arterial EDH most often near MMA groove fx
    - Venous EDH usually related to fractures near dural sinus attachments
  - Nontraumatic
    - Coagulopathy, thrombolysis, vascular malformation, neoplasm, epidural anesthesia, Paget disease of skull
    - "Spontaneous" EDH are rare; may arise from skull metastases
- Associated abnormalities
  - Skull fracture in 95%, may cross MMA groove
  - Subdural/subarachnoid hemorrhage, contusion

Staging, Grading, & Classification

- Type 1: Acute EDH, arterial bleeding (58%)
- Type 2: Subacute EDH (31%)
- Type 3: Chronic EDH, venous bleeding (11%)

Gross Pathologic & Surgical Features

- Subperiosteal hematoma (outer layer of dura is periosteum of inner table of skull)
- May cross midline, dural attachments
- Hematoma collects between calvarium, outer dura
  - Rarely crosses sutures
    - Exception: Large hematoma with diastatic fx
- "Vertex" EDH (rare)
  - Usually venous: Linear or diastatic fracture crosses superior sagittal sinus
- 20% have blood in both epidural and subdural spaces at surgery or autopsy

Microscopic Features

- Tear/laceration of adjacent vessel

CLINICAL ISSUES

Presentation

- Most common signs/symptoms
  - Classic "lucid interval": Approximately 50% of cases
    - Initial brief loss of consciousness (LOC)
    - Subsequent asymptomatic time between LOC and symptom/coma onset
  - Headache, nausea, vomiting, seizures, focal neurological deficits (field cuts, aphasia, weakness)
  - Mass effect/herniation common
    - Pupil-involving CN3 palsy, somnolence, ↓ consciousness, coma
- Clinical profile
  - Alcohol, other intoxications associated with ↑ incidence of EDH

Demographics

- Age
  - More common < 20 years; extremely rare in elderly
  - Uncommon in infants
- Gender
  - M:F = 4:1
- Epidemiology
  - 1-4% of imaged head trauma patients
  - 5-15% of patients with fatal head injuries

Natural History & Prognosis

- Factors affecting rate of growth
  - Arterial vs. venous flow rate, arterial spasm
  - Decompression through fracture into scalp
  - Tamponade
- Delayed development or enlargement common
  - 10-25% of cases within 1st 36 hours
- Epidural abscess may develop if bacteria colonize EDH via fracture site
- Good outcome if promptly recognized and treated
  - Overall mortality approximately 5%
  - Bilateral EDH have higher mortality and morbidity
    - 15-20% mortality rate
- Increased mortality in posterior fossa EDH (26%)
  - Can have delayed symptom onset 2° slower expansion from lower venous pressure

Treatment

- Complications: Mass effect causing herniations
- Prompt recognition, appropriate treatment essential
  - Poor outcome often related to delayed referral, diagnosis, or operation
- Nearly always requires surgical evacuation
  - Additional EDH may be unmasked post-procedure
- EDH < 1 cm thick may be managed nonoperatively
  - Unless there is concomitant cerebral edema
  - Consider endovascular adjunct treatment
  - Repeat CT in 1st 36 hours to monitor for change
    - 23% enlarge within 36 hours
    - Mean enlargement: 7 mm
  - Failure of nonoperative management has no adverse effect on outcome

DIAGNOSTIC CHECKLIST

Image Interpretation Pearls

- NECT highly sensitive
- If MR unavailable, coronal CT reconstructions to evaluate vertex EDH

SELECTED REFERENCES

1. Kanai R et al: Spontaneous epidural hematoma due to skull metastasis of hepatocellular carcinoma. J Clin Neurosci. 16(1):137-40, 2009
2. Ross IB: Embolization of the middle meningeal artery for the treatment of epidural hematoma. J Neurosurg. 110(6):1247-9, 2009
3. De Souza M et al: Nonoperative management of epidural hematomas and subdural hematomas: is it safe in lesions measuring one centimeter or less? J Trauma. 63(2):370-2, 2007

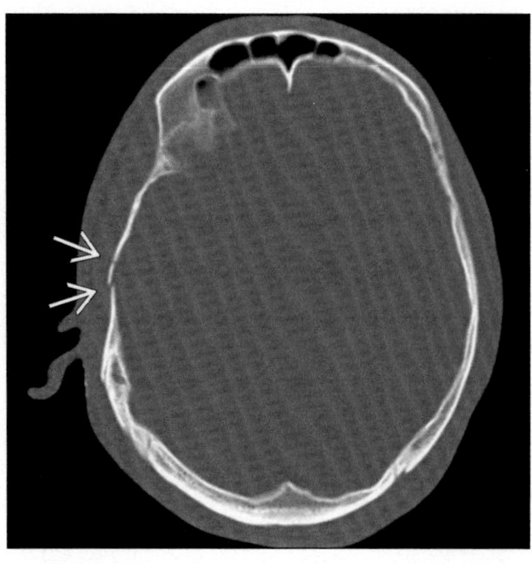

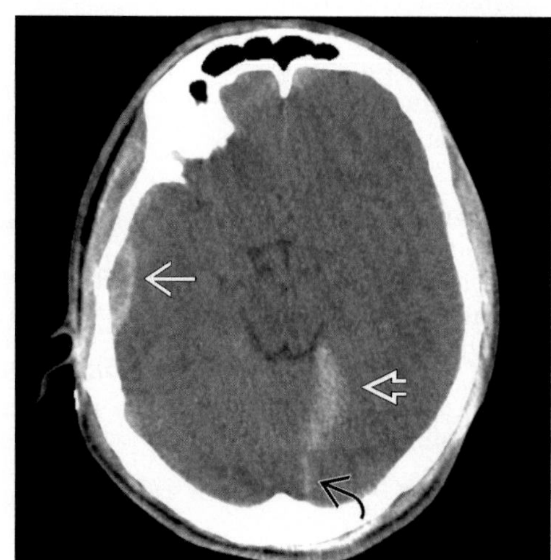

(Left) *Axial bone CT demonstrates a portion of a comminuted fracture about the pterion ➡.* ***(Right)*** *Axial NECT reveals a small yet classic biconvex epidural hematoma ➡ underlying the skull fracture seen on the previous image. There is also a posterior falcine subdural hematoma ↷ extending to involve the leftward tentorium ⇨.*

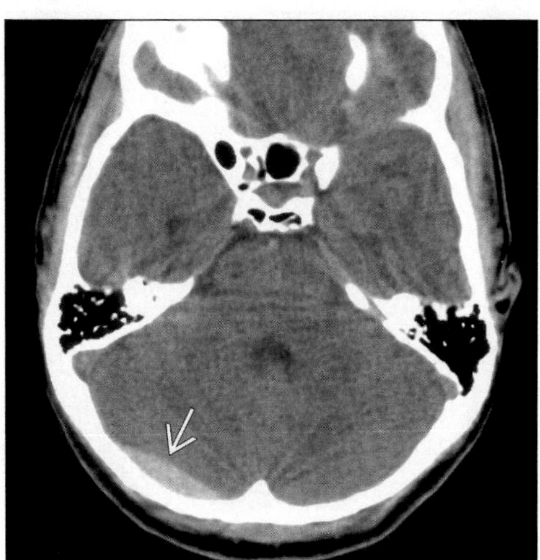

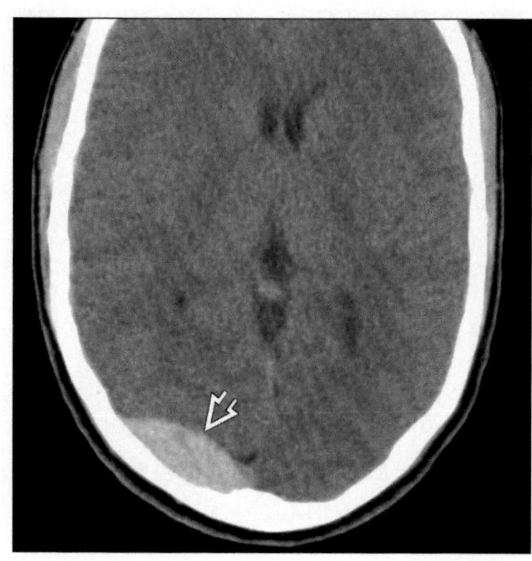

(Left) *Axial NECT demonstrates a biconvex venous epidural hematoma that extends both below ➡ the tentorium as well as above it, as demonstrated in the next image.* ***(Right)*** *Axial NECT demonstrates a biconvex venous epidural hematoma that extends both above ⇨ the tentorium as well as below it.*

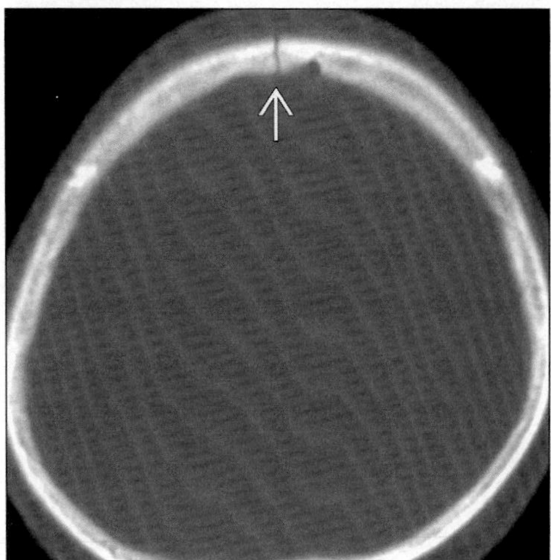

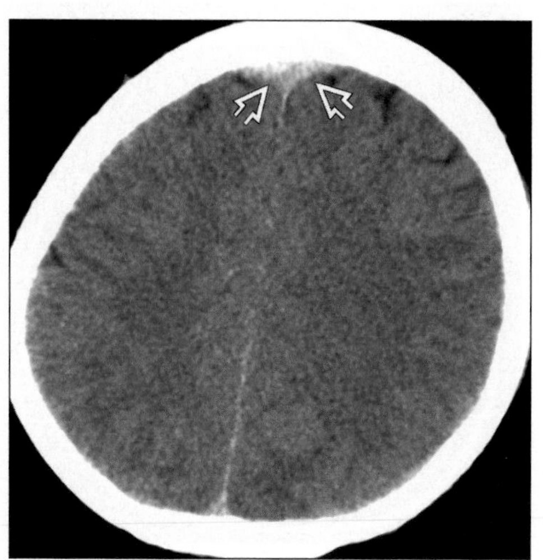

(Left) *Axial bone CT reveals a nondisplaced midline linear frontal bone fracture ➡.* ***(Right)*** *Axial NECT demonstrates a subtle and somewhat ill-defined, biconvex, hyperdense, venous epidural hematoma ⇨ in the expected location of the anterior superior sagittal sinus and underlying the nondisplaced fracture seen in the previous image.*

ACUTE SUBDURAL HEMATOMA

Key Facts

Imaging
- CT: Crescentic hyperdense extraaxial collection spread diffusely over convexity
- Between arachnoid and inner layer of dura
- Supratentorial convexity most common
- May cross sutures, not dural attachments
- NECT as initial screen
- Inward displacement of cortical veins
- Presence of tears in pia-arachnoid membrane can lead to CSF leakage into SDH collections; may also alter signal intensity by CSF dilution

Top Differential Diagnoses
- Hygroma
  - Clear CSF, no encapsulating membranes
- Effusion
  - Xanthochromic fluid secondary to extravasation of plasma from membrane; 1-3 days post-trauma; near CSF density/intensity
- Empyema
  - Peripheral enhancement, hyperintensity on FLAIR and DWI; restricted diffusion
- Acute epidural hematoma
  - Biconvex extraaxial collection, may cross dural attachments, limited by sutures

Pathology
- Trauma most common cause

Diagnostic Checklist
- Important to inform responsible clinician if unsuspected finding
- Wide window settings for CT increases conspicuity of subtle SDH
- FLAIR, T2* usually most sensitive sequences for SDH

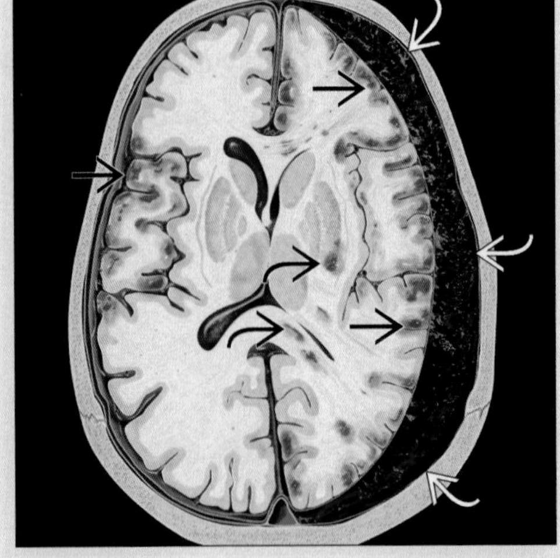
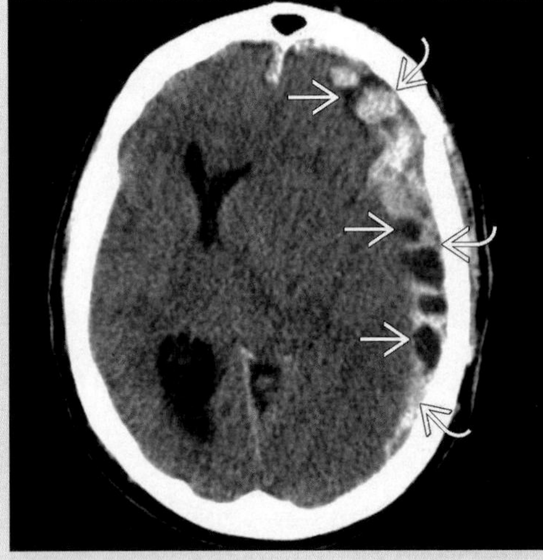

(Left) *Axial graphic shows an acute subdural hematoma (SDH) ➔ compressing the left hemisphere and lateral ventricle, resulting in midline shift. Note also the hemorrhagic contusions ➔ and diffuse axonal injuries ➔. Additional traumatic lesions are common in patients with subdural hematomas.* ***(Right)*** *Axial NECT shows multiple low-attenuation foci ➔ within this hyperacute SDH ➔, findings consistent with active extravasation. Note the significant associated midline shift.*

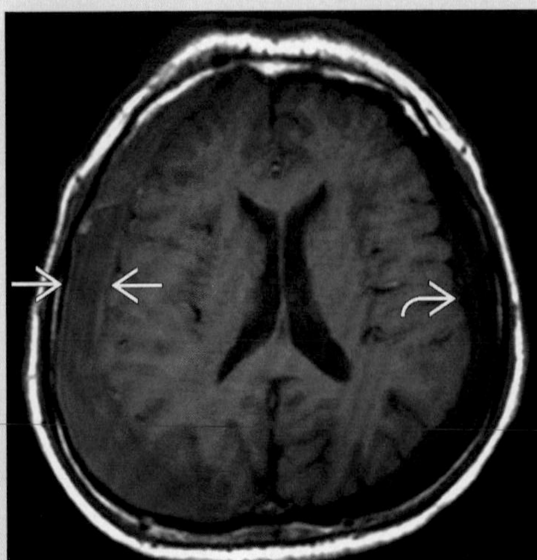
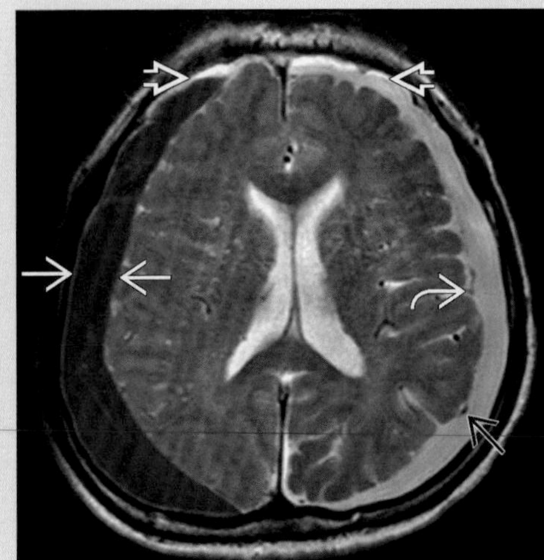

(Left) *Axial T1WI MR shows an acute right subdural hematoma with early mild T1 hyperintensity ➔. The left-sided subdural hematoma ➔ is hyperacute and more closely follows CSF signal intensity.* ***(Right)*** *Axial T2WI MR of an aSDH in the same patient shows marked hypointensity ➔, typical for deoxyhemoglobin. The left-sided subdural hematoma ➔ is hyperacute, close to CSF signal. Pial vessels are displaced inward ➔ by the collection. Note layering fluid levels ➔ anteriorly in both.*

ACUTE SUBDURAL HEMATOMA

TERMINOLOGY

Abbreviations

- Acute subdural hematoma (aSDH)

Definitions

- Acute hemorrhagic collection in subdural space

IMAGING

General Features

- Best diagnostic clue
  - CT: Crescentic hyperdense extraaxial collection spread diffusely over affected hemisphere
- Location
  - Between arachnoid and inner layer of dura
  - Supratentorial convexity most common
- Morphology
  - Crescent-shaped extraaxial fluid collection
  - May cross sutures, not dural attachments
  - May extend along falx, tentorium, and anterior and middle fossa floors

CT Findings

- NECT
  - Hyperacute SDH (≤ 6 hours) may have heterogeneous density or hypodensity
  - aSDH (6 hours to 3 days)
    - aSDH: 60% homogeneously hyperdense
    - 40% mixed hyper-, hypodense with active bleeding ("swirl" sign), torn arachnoid with CSF accumulation, clot retraction
    - Rarely isodense → coagulopathy, anemia (Hgb < 8-10 g/dL)
    - If no new hemorrhage, density decreases ± 1.5 HU/day
- CECT
  - Inward displacement of cortical veins
  - Dura and membranes enhance when subacute; useful to visualize loculations

MR Findings

- T1WI
  - Hyperacute (< 12 hours): Iso- to mildly hyperintense
  - Acute (12 hours to 2 days): Mildly hypointense
- T2WI
  - Hyperacute: Mildly hyperintense
  - Acute: Hypointense
- FLAIR
  - Typically hyperintense to CSF
  - Signal intensity varies depending on relative T1 and T2 effects
    - Acute hematomas can be isointense to CSF due to T2 shortening effects of intracellular methemoglobin
  - Often most conspicuous sequence
- T2* GRE
  - Hypointense unless hyperacute
- DWI
  - Heterogeneous signal (nonspecific)
  - May differentiate extraaxial empyema (marked central hyperintensity) from hemorrhage
- T1WI C+
  - Enhancement of displaced bridging veins
  - Enhancement within SDH predictive of subsequent growth
- MR signal of SDH quite variable
  - Often evolves in similar fashion to intraparenchymal hemorrhage
  - Recurrent hemorrhage common; results in acute and chronic blood products even at initial exam
  - SDH signal is variable due to recurrent hemorrhage; difficult to age accurately
  - Pia-arachnoid membrane tears can lead to CSF leakage into SDH collections and may alter signal intensity by CSF dilution

Angiographic Findings

- Conventional
  - Displacement, mass effect from extraaxial collection; veins displaced from inner table of skull
  - Perform if underlying vascular lesion suspected

Imaging Recommendations

- Best imaging tool
  - NECT as initial screen
  - MR more sensitive to detect and determine extent of SDH and additional findings of traumatic brain injury

DIFFERENTIAL DIAGNOSIS

Other Subdural Collections

- Subdural hygroma
  - Clear CSF, no encapsulating membranes
- Subdural effusion
  - Xanthochromic fluid secondary to extravasation of plasma from membrane; 1-3 days post-trauma; near CSF density/intensity
- Empyema: Peripheral enhancement, hyperintensity on FLAIR; restricted diffusion on DWI

Epidural Hematoma

- Biconvex extraaxial collection
- Often associated with fracture
- May cross dural attachments, limited by sutures

Pachymeningopathies (Thickened Dura)

- Chronic meningitis (may be indistinguishable)
- Neurosarcoid: Nodular, "lumpy-bumpy"
- Postsurgical (e.g., shunt)
- Intracranial hypotension
  - "Slumping" midbrain, tonsillar herniation

Tumor

- Meningioma, lymphoma, leukemia, metastases
- Dural-based, enhancing masses
- ± skull and extracranial soft tissue involved

Peripheral Infarct

- Cortex involved, not displaced
- Hyperintense DWI

Chemical Shift Artifact

- Marrow or subcutaneous fat may "shift," can appear intracranial, mimic T1 hyperintense SDH
  - Seen with ↑ field of view or ↓ bandwidth

- Worse with higher field strength MR

PATHOLOGY

General Features

- Etiology
  - Trauma most common cause
    - Tearing of bridging cortical veins as they cross subdural space to drain into dural sinus
    - Nonimpact (falls) as well as direct injury
    - Trauma may be minor, particularly in elderly; often recurrent with initial episodes subclinical
  - Less common etiologies
    - Dissection of intraparenchymal hematoma into subarachnoid, then subdural space
    - Aneurysm rupture
    - Vascular malformations: Dural arteriovenous fistula, arteriovenous malformation (AVM), cavernoma
      - Typically other hemorrhages present (parenchymal &/or subarachnoid)
    - Moyamoya (greater propensity for hemorrhage in adults, ischemia in children)
    - Dural invasion by tumor with secondary hemorrhage (prostate cancer)
    - Spontaneous hemorrhage with severe coagulopathy
  - Predisposing factors
    - Atrophy
    - Shunting (→ increased traction on superior cortical veins)
    - Coagulopathy (e.g., alcohol abuse) and anticoagulation
- Associated abnormalities
  - > 70% have other significant associated traumatic lesions

Gross Pathologic & Surgical Features

- Hematoma
- Delayed development of membranes/granulation tissue

Microscopic Features

- Outer membrane of proliferating fibroblasts and capillaries
- Fragile capillaries hypothesized as source of recurrent hemorrhage (chronic SDH)
- Inner membrane (made up of dural fibroblasts or border cells) forms fibrocollagenous sheet

CLINICAL ISSUES

Presentation

- Most common signs/symptoms
  - Most commonly following trauma
  - Varies from asymptomatic to loss of consciousness
    - "Lucid" interval in aSDH: Initially awake, alert patient loses consciousness a few hours after trauma
    - Patients with early symptomatic presentation (< 4 hours) and advanced age have poor prognosis
  - Other symptoms (focal deficit, seizure) from mass effect, diffuse brain injury, secondary ischemia
  - Coagulopathy or anticoagulation increase risk and extent of hemorrhage

Demographics

- Any age, more common in elderly
- No gender predilection
- Epidemiology
  - Found in 30% of autopsy cases following craniocerebral trauma

Natural History & Prognosis

- Can grow slowly with increased mass effect if untreated
- Compresses and displaces underlying brain
- Recurrent hemorrhage common; in children, raises suspicion of nonaccidental trauma

Treatment

- Poor prognosis (35-90% mortality)
  - Emergency preoperative high-dose mannitol may improve outcome
- Hematoma thickness, midline shift > 20 mm correlate with poor outcome
- Lethal if hematoma volume > 8-10% of intracranial volume

DIAGNOSTIC CHECKLIST

Consider

- NECT initial screen
- MR if degree of mass effect &/or symptoms greater than expected for size of SDH
  - Helps identify extent of traumatic brain injury
  - MR to evaluate nontraumatic causes
- In child with recurrent or mixed-age hemorrhage, suspect nonaccidental trauma!

Image Interpretation Pearls

- Wide window settings for CT increases conspicuity of subtle SDH
- FLAIR, T2* usually most sensitive sequences for SDH
- CT density and MR intensity vary with age and degree of recurrent hemorrhage and contribution of CSF (arachnoid tears)

SELECTED REFERENCES

1. Kim KH: Predictors for functional recovery and mortality of surgically treated traumatic acute subdural hematomas in 256 patients. J Korean Neurosurg Soc. 45(3):143-50, 2009
2. Fernando S et al: Neuroimaging of nonaccidental head trauma: pitfalls and controversies. Pediatr Radiol. 38(8):827-38, 2008
3. Morais DF et al: Clinical application of magnetic resonance in acute traumatic brain injury. Arq Neuropsiquiatr. 66(1):53-8, 2008
4. Sawauchi S et al: The effect of haematoma, brain injury, and secondary insult on brain swelling in traumatic acute subdural haemorrhage. Acta Neurochir (Wien). 150(6):531-6; discussion 536, 2008

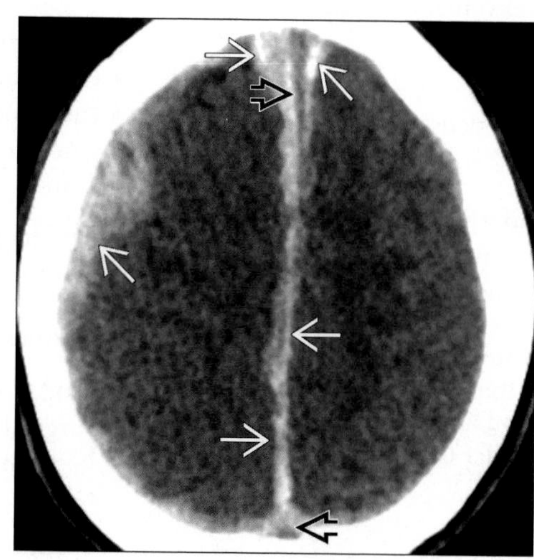

(Left) Axial NECT shows a large, heterogeneous, acute left hemispheric subdural hematoma that is predominantly hyperdense but also contains irregular hypodense areas ➔, indicative of active bleeding ("swirl" sign). Significant mass effect and midline shift are also seen. **(Right)** Axial NECT shows an acute subdural hematoma along the right hemisphere and falx bilaterally ➔. Note the normal appearance of the less dense venous blood within the superior sagittal sinus ⇨.

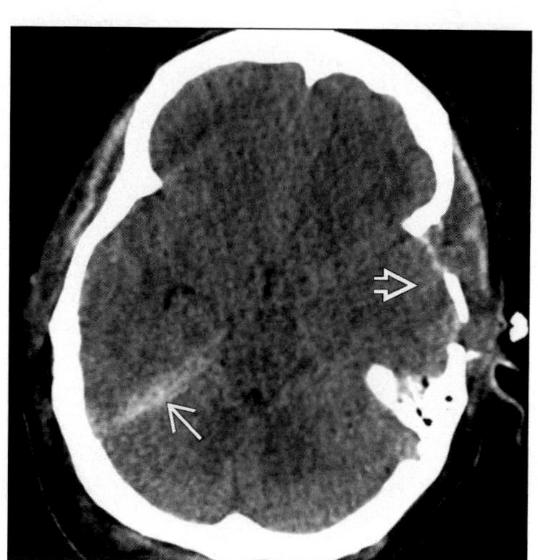

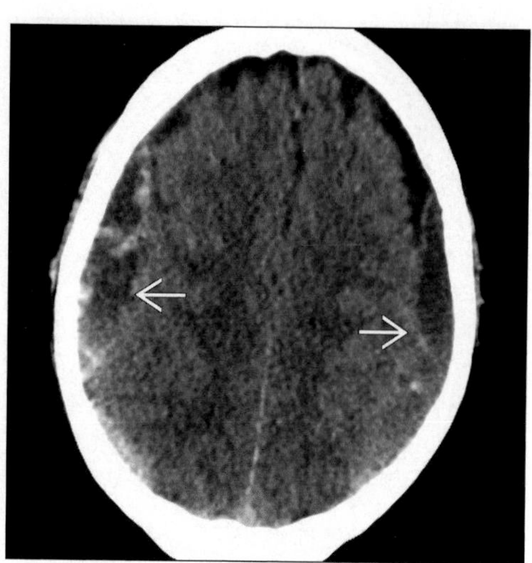

(Left) Axial NECT shows a right tentorial aSDH ➔, reflecting contrecoup injury. The patient had an injury to the left head, where a craniectomy defect ⇨ was present, which predisposed the patient to intracranial injury despite only minor trauma. There was a large intraparenchymal hematoma in the left frontal lobe (not shown). **(Right)** Axial NECT demonstrates a bilateral aSDH ➔ with internal mixed attenuation. Linear areas of high attenuation may reflect acute blood products &/or septations.

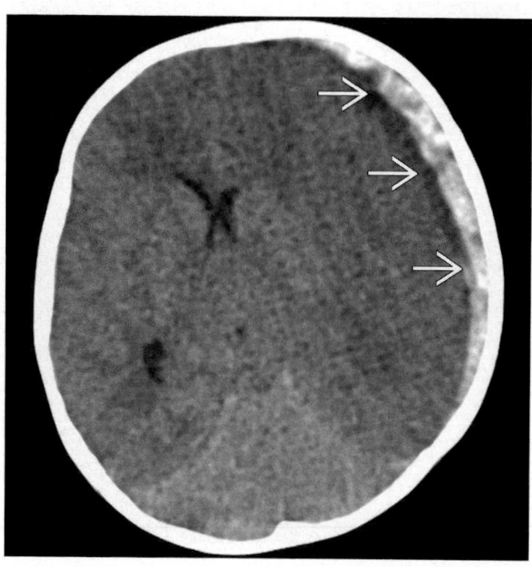

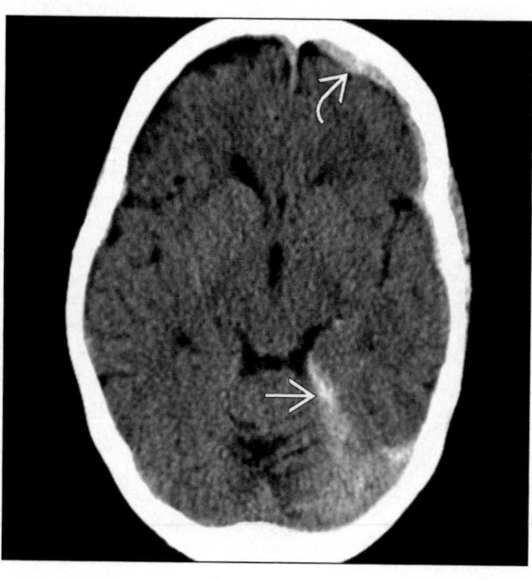

(Left) Axial NECT shows an aSDH ➔ in an infant victim of nonaccidental trauma. Always consider nonaccidental trauma in a child with a recurrent or mixed subdural hematoma. **(Right)** Axial NECT shows an acute frontal ↗ and a tentorial ➔ SDH in a patient with no history of trauma. Concurrent intraparenchymal hematoma (not shown) raised the question of AVM, which was confirmed on subsequent angiography. An underlying vascular lesion should be considered in nontraumatic patients with an aSDH.

SUBACUTE SUBDURAL HEMATOMA

Key Facts

Terminology

- Subacute (~ 3 days to 3 weeks) hemorrhagic collection in subdural space

Imaging

- Crescent-shaped, iso- to hypodense on CT, extraaxial collection that spreads diffusely over affected hemisphere
- May be same density as underlying cortex
- May cross sutures, not dural attachments
- Typically T1 hyperintense (methemoglobin) in both early and late subacute
- Most sSDH are DWI hypointense; presence of hyperintensity may alter surgical approach
- General imaging recommendations
  - NECT initial screen; consider CECT for membranes/loculations
  - MR more sensitive for SDH and additional findings of traumatic brain injury

Top Differential Diagnoses

- Other subdural collections
- Pachymeningopathies (thickened dura)
- Chronic dural sinus thrombosis
- Tumor

Pathology

- Traumatic stretching and tearing of bridging cortical veins as they cross subdural space
- Trauma may be minor, particularly in elderly

Clinical Issues

- Surgical drainage indicated if growing/symptomatic
- "Separated" morphology have highest rehemorrhage rates

(Left) Axial graphic shows a typical subacute SDH ➔. Inset shows the traversing "bridging" vein ➔ and developing membranes ➔. These are often related to relatively minor trauma in the elderly. (Right) Axial NECT show almost perfectly isodense bilateral subdural hematomas ➔. They are barely perceptible, as they are almost exactly the same attenuation as the underlying gray matter. However, the displaced gray-white matter interface toward the midline helps make the accurate diagnosis.

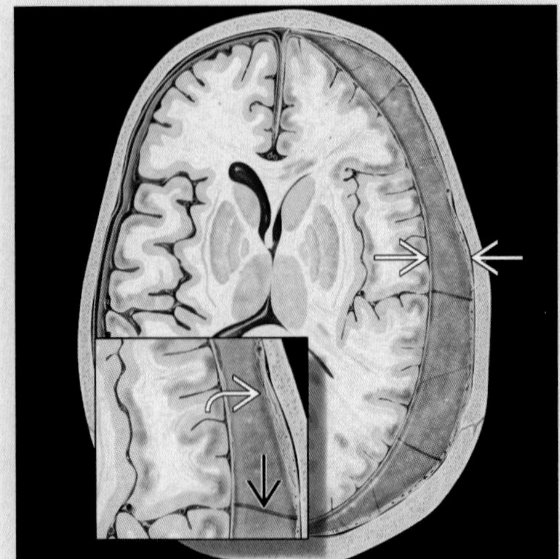

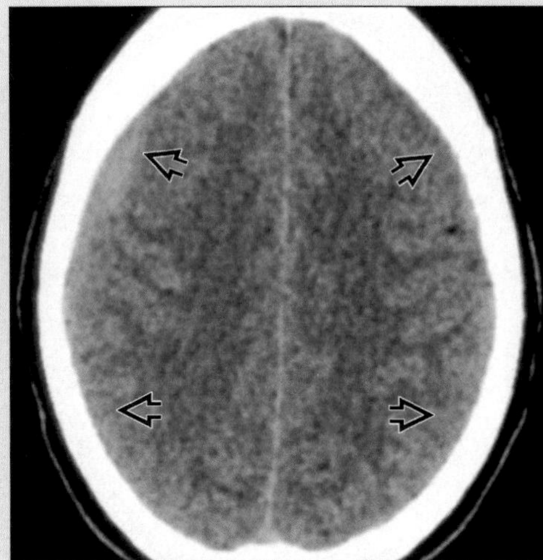

(Left) Axial T1WI MR shows a slightly hyperintense SDH ➔ related to an early subacute hemorrhage. Note the displaced sulci, brain, and vessels away from the calvarium ➔. Note the smaller right SDH ➔. (Right) Axial T2WI MR in the same patient shows the SDH has a large hypointense ➔ portion (intracellular methemoglobin). A smaller right SDH ➔ is predominantly bright (late subacute). SDH MR signal is variable but generally evolves in a pattern similar to parenchymal blood.

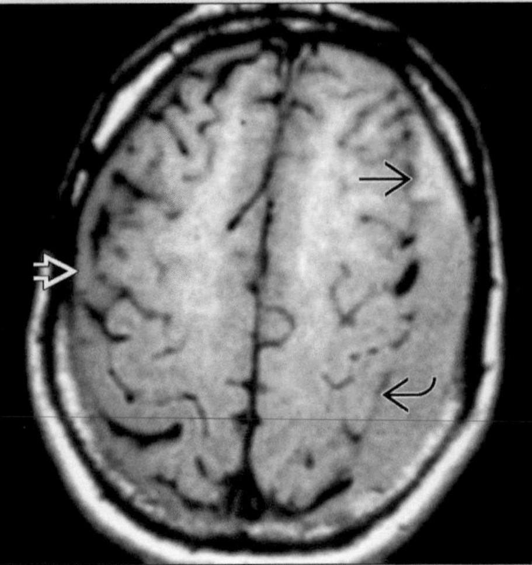

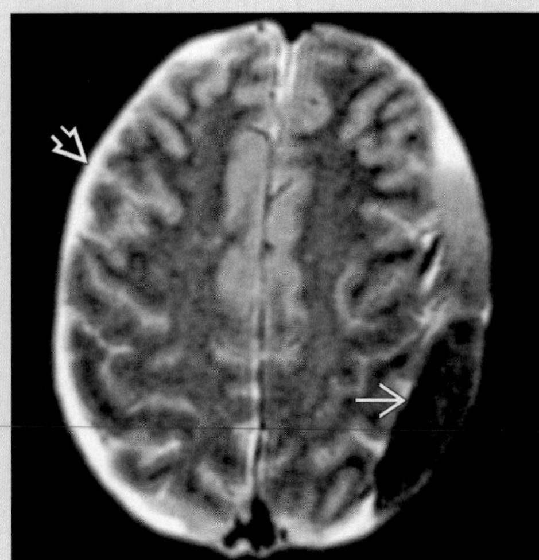

SUBACUTE SUBDURAL HEMATOMA

TERMINOLOGY

Abbreviations

- Subacute subdural hematoma (sSDH)

Definitions

- Subacute (~ 3 days to 3 weeks) hemorrhagic collection in subdural space

IMAGING

General Features

- Best diagnostic clue
  - Crescent-shaped, iso- to hypodense on CT, extraaxial collection that spreads diffusely over affected hemisphere
- Location
  - Between arachnoid and inner layer of dura
- Morphology
  - Crescent-shaped extraaxial fluid collection
  - May cross sutures, not dural attachments
  - May extend along falx and tentorium
  - Compresses & displaces underlying brain surface, cortical vessels, and subarachnoid space fluid
    - Sulci are often effaced
  - Recurrent, mixed-age hemorrhage common; in children, raises suspicion of nonaccidental trauma!
  - CT density and MR signal intensity vary with age and organization of hemorrhage

CT Findings

- NECT
  - Iso- to hypodense; may be same density as underlying cortex
  - Gray-white junction displaced medially
  - Surface sulci do not reach inner calvarial table
  - May see line of displaced/compressed sulci as "dots" of CSF
  - Density varies, depending on stage of evolution
    - Progression from hyperdense acute SDH to iso- (subacute) to hypodense chronic SDH over ~ 3 weeks
    - Recurrent hemorrhage can result in mixed density hematomas
- CECT
  - Dura and membranes enhance
  - Inward displacement of enhancing cortical vessels

MR Findings

- T1WI
  - Typically hyperintense (methemoglobin) in both early and late subacute
- T2WI
  - Hypointense for early subacute (intracellular methemoglobin) typical
    - May see T2 and FLAIR hyperintensity in early subacute
  - Hyperintense for late subacute (extracellular methemoglobin)
  - May see linear hypointensity due to membranes that predispose to repeated hemorrhage
- PD/intermediate
  - Signal variable: Iso- to hyperintense, depending on protein content or re-bleed into collection and relative T1 and T2 contributions
- FLAIR
  - Hyperintense often (usually most conspicuous sequence) in more commonly seen late subacute SDH (extracellular methemoglobin)
    - FLAIR signal varies depending on relative contribution of T1 and T2 effects
    - Prominent T1 shortening often results in bright FLAIR signal
    - May be hypointense (early subacute) due to T2 shortening effects
    - Early subacute hematomas, if small, can therefore be "invisible" on FLAIR
      - Look carefully for mass effect, sulcal effacement, &/or vessel displacement
- T2* GRE
  - May show susceptibility: "Blooming"
- DWI
  - Most sSDH are hypointense; presence of hyperintensity may alter surgical approach
    - Hyperintense foci suggest solid clots
    - Subdural hyperintense band indicates relatively fresh bleeding from outer membrane
- T1WI C+
  - Enhancing and thickened dura common
  - May see enhancing membranes
    - Suggest unstable SDH, prone to re-hemorrhage
    - Delayed scans may show contrast diffusion into SDH
- Signal on MR often parallels that of intracerebral hematoma
  - Exceptions reported for early subacute hematomas
  - T2/FLAIR may be hyperintense in early subacute
- Early MR favored as most concurrent injuries are more conspicuous in early subacute phase

Imaging Recommendations

- Best imaging tool
  - NECT as initial screen; consider CECT for membranes/loculations
  - MR more sensitive for SDH and additional findings of traumatic brain injury
  - Recommendations for nonaccidental trauma evaluation in children
    - NECT initial screen
    - Early MR, including DWI, if NECT abnormal or if clinical concerns persist
- Protocol advice
  - Add FLAIR, DWI, and GRE to MR protocol for hemorrhage/trauma indications

DIFFERENTIAL DIAGNOSIS

Other Subdural Collections

- Effusion
  - MR: Typically follows CSF signal
  - Often related to meningitis, post-op, intracranial hypotension
- Empyema
  - MR: Peripheral enhancement; DWI+

SUBACUTE SUBDURAL HEMATOMA

- Often related to sinus infection or penetrating injury
- Hygroma
  - MR: Follows CSF signal, no membranes
  - Result from tear in arachnoid; without hemorrhage

Pachymeningopathies (Thickened Dura)
- Chronic meningitis (may be indistinguishable)
- Postsurgical (shunt, etc.)
- Intracranial hypotension
  - "Slumping" midbrain, tonsillar herniation
- Sarcoid (nodular, "lumpy-bumpy")

Chronic Dural Sinus Thrombosis
- Diffuse dural thickening and enhancement

Tumor
- Meningioma, lymphoma, leukemia, metastases
- Dural-based, enhancing mass ± skull involvement

Chemical Shift Artifact
- Marrow or subcutaneous fat may "shift" → can appear intracranial, mimic T1 hyperintense SDH

PATHOLOGY

General Features
- Etiology
  - Traumatic stretching and tearing of bridging cortical veins as they cross subdural space
  - Trauma may be minor, particularly in elderly
  - Mechanisms of enlargement
    - Re-hemorrhage
    - Serum protein exudation

Gross Pathologic & Surgical Features
- Membranes: Granulation tissue, with resorbing blood products
- Outer membrane related to hematoma enlargement with repetitive hemorrhages
- Inner membrane related to liquefaction of subdural hematoma

CLINICAL ISSUES

Presentation
- Most common signs/symptoms
  - Varies; range from asymptomatic to loss of consciousness
- Other signs/symptoms
  - Headaches, seizures, focal neurological deficit

Demographics
- Age
  - Young and elderly
- Gender
  - M > F
- Epidemiology
  - SDH found in 10-20% of patients imaged and 30% of autopsy cases following craniocerebral trauma

Natural History & Prognosis
- Can spontaneously resolve or enlarge
- Older age and brain atrophy are contributory factors in conversion of traumatic SDH into subacute and chronic SDH
- Recurrence rate higher for skull base location SDH compared to convexity SDH

Treatment
- Surgical drainage indicated if growing/symptomatic
- Resection of membranes, if present
- "Separated" morphology have highest re-hemorrhage rates

DIAGNOSTIC CHECKLIST

Consider
- Contrast enhancement if suspected isodense subdural to look for membrane formation/loculations
- MR with DWI to assess for presence of membranes

Image Interpretation Pearls
- Remember: MR signal of SDH quite variable
  - Generally evolve in pattern similar to intracerebral hemorrhage (but not always!)
- Enhancement helpful to differentiate subacute and chronic SDH from pachymeningopathies

SELECTED REFERENCES

1. Kemp AM et al: What neuroimaging should be performed in children in whom inflicted brain injury (iBI) is suspected? A systematic review. Clin Radiol. 64(5):473-83, 2009
2. Duhem R et al: [Main temporal aspects of the MRI signal of subdural hematomas and practical contribution to dating head injury.] Neurochirurgie. 52(2-3 Pt 1):93-104, 2006
3. Kuwahara S et al: Diffusion-weighted imaging of traumatic subdural hematoma in the subacute stage. Neurol Med Chir (Tokyo). 45(9):464-9, 2005
4. Kuwahara S et al: Subdural hyperintense band on diffusion-weighted imaging of chronic subdural hematoma indicates bleeding from the outer membrane. Neurol Med Chir (Tokyo). 45(3):125-31, 2005
5. Tomlin JM et al: Transdural metastasis from adenocarcinoma of the prostate mimicking subdural hematoma: case report. Surg Neurol. 58(5):329-31; discussion 331, 2002
6. Mori K et al: Delayed magnetic resonance imaging with GdD-DTPA differentiates subdural hygroma and subdural effusion. Surg Neurol. 53(4):303-10; discussion 310-1, 2000
7. Yamashima T: The inner membrane of chronic subdural hematomas: pathology and pathophysiology. Neurosurg Clin N Am. 11(3):413-24, 2000
8. Kaminogo M et al: Characteristics of symptomatic chronic subdural haematomas on high-field MRI. Neuroradiology. 41(2):109-16, 1999
9. Okuno S et al: Falx meningioma presenting as acute subdural hematoma: case report. Surg Neurol. 52(2):180-4, 1999
10. Fujisawa H et al: Serum protein exudation in chronic subdural haematomas: a mechanism for haematoma enlargement? Acta Neurochir (Wien). 140(2):161-5; discussion 165-6, 1998
11. Wilms G et al: CT and MR in infants with pericerebral collections and macrocephaly: benign enlargement of the subarachnoid spaces versus subdural collections. AJNR Am J Neuroradiol. 14(4):855-60, 1993

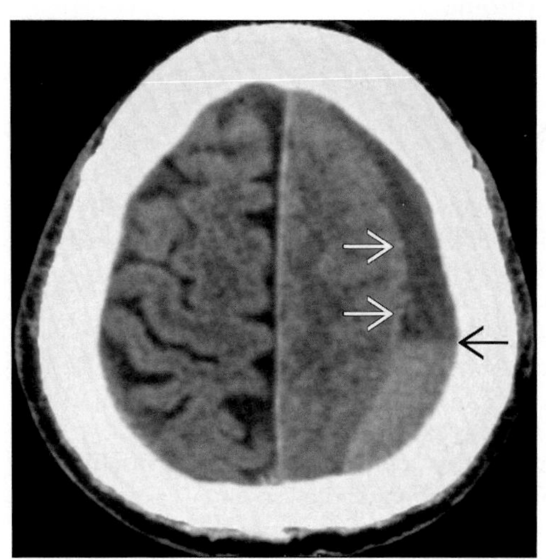

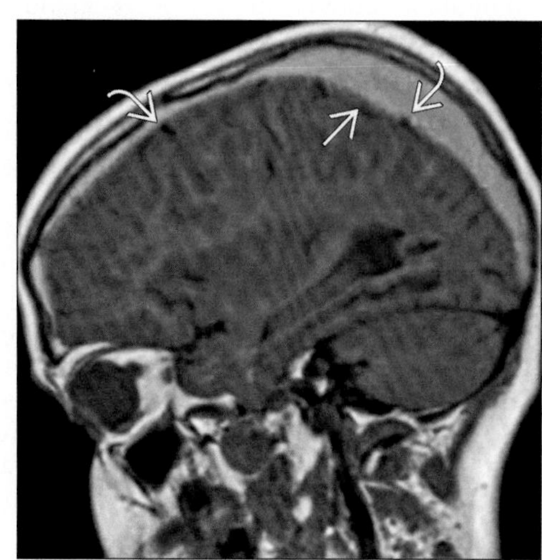

(Left) *Axial NECT shows a mixed density subacute SDH with a blood/hematocrit level. Note the displaced cortical vessels or "dot" sign.* **(Right)** *Sagittal T1WI MR shows a hyperintense SDH over the cerebral convexities related to subacute blood products (methemoglobin). Note the displacement of the cerebral gyri and surface vessels away from the inner calvarium. MR is more sensitive for SDH and for the often additional findings of traumatic brain injury.*

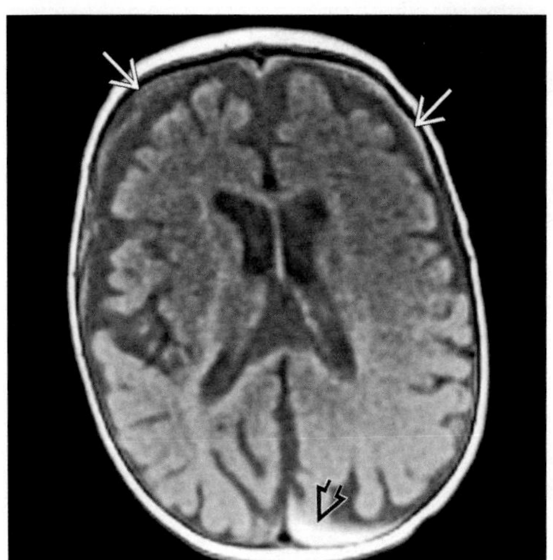

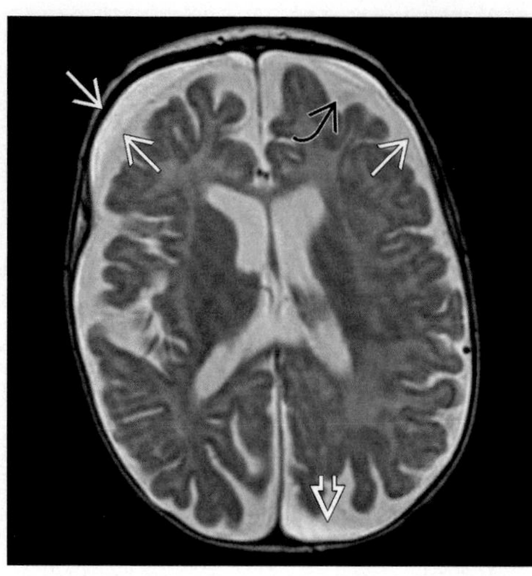

(Left) *Axial T1WI MR in an infant with suspected nonaccidental trauma shows a bilateral SDH, with largely hyperintense blood products. Signal intensity in the posterior left collection is brighter, suggesting a slightly more recent age.* **(Right)** *Axial T2WI MR in the same patient shows a bilateral T2 hyperintense (late subacute) SDH. CSF is relatively hypointense by comparison. The CSF spaces are large in this patient due to atrophy. The posterior left SDH was seen only on MR.*

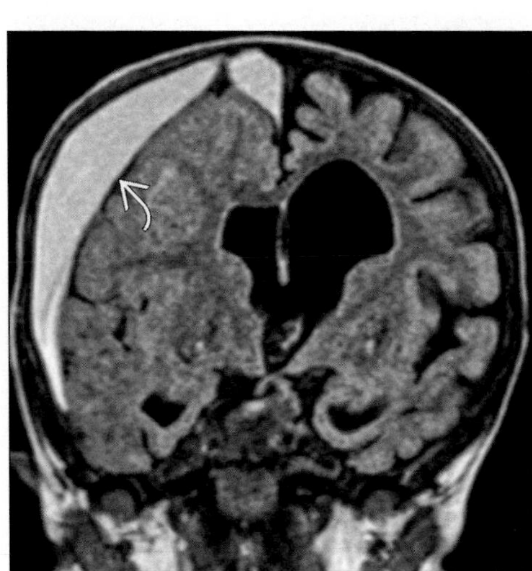

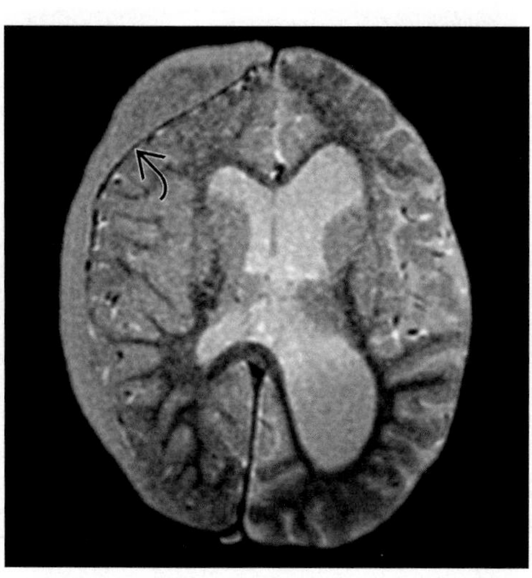

(Left) *Coronal FLAIR MR in an infant shows a diffusely hyperintense subdural collection related to prominent T1 effects of this subacute SDH. FLAIR is often the most sensitive sequence for identifying subacute subdural hematomas. Note the prominent atrophy.* **(Right)** *Axial T2* GRE MR in the same patient shows no significant susceptibility within the subacute subdural hematoma. Although GRE will often show "blooming," lack of blooming does not exclude the diagnosis.*

CHRONIC SUBDURAL HEMATOMA

Key Facts

Terminology
- Chronic (> 3 wks) collection of blood products in subdural space

Imaging
- Crescent-shaped, multiseptated, extraaxial collection with enhancing surrounding membranes, spreads diffusely over affected hemisphere
- cSDH often septated, with internal membranes
- May cross sutures, not dural attachments
- Imaging recommendations
  - NECT good initial screen
  - Use wide window settings (150-200 HU)
  - MR better demonstrates cSDH: Often hyperintense (due to methemoglobin) on T1, T2, PD, FLAIR
- Recurrent, mixed-age hemorrhage common; in children, raises suspicion of nonaccidental trauma!

Top Differential Diagnoses
- Subdural hygroma
- Subdural effusion
- Subdural empyema

Clinical Issues
- Treatment
  - Surgical drainage with resection of membranes
- Older age and brain atrophy are contributory factors in conversion of traumatic SDH into cSDH
- Recurrence risk of cSDH varies with type
  - "Separated" is highest; thickened or calcified membrane almost never re-hemorrhages
- Recurrence rate higher for skull base location SDH compared to convexity SDH
- If no trauma history, consider underlying vascular lesion or dural metastases

*(**Left**) Axial graphic shows a chronic subdural hematoma with the formation of internal membranes ➡. Note the intact "bridging" veins, normally traversing the subdural space ⇨. There is mild mass effect and effacement of the left lateral ventricle. (**Right**) Axial CECT scan shows hypodense extra-axial fluid collection in the left posterior frontoparietal area. Note thickened, enhancing membranes and septations ➡ that loculate the fluid collection. The underlying sulci are compressed.*

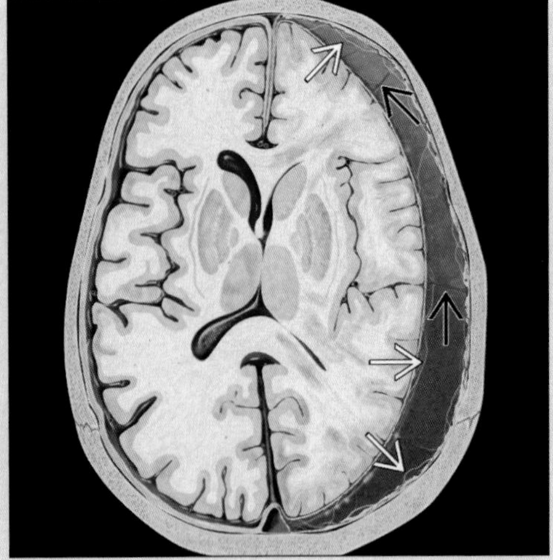

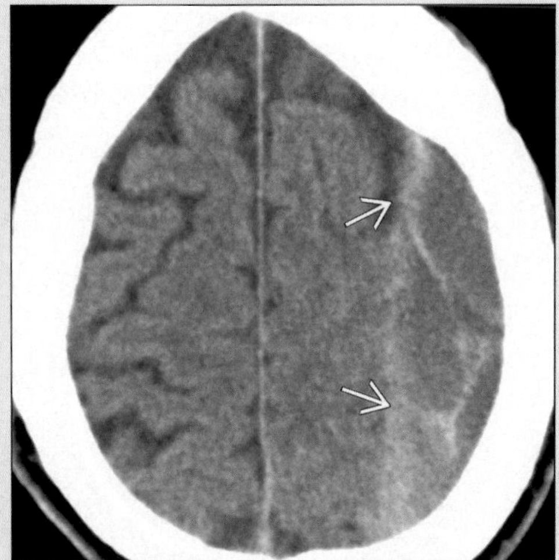

*(**Left**) Axial T1WI MR shows a chronic, 2-month-old SDH ➡ with signal intensity similar to CSF. MR signal intensity is variable but typically evolves similar to a parenchymal hemorrhage. (**Right**) Coronal FLAIR C+ MR shows a chronic SDH ➡ with dark signal intensity following that of CSF. It is important to correlate with conventional T2 images, as early subacute blood with intrinsic T2 shortening may also be dark on FLAIR. Note also the typical dural thickening and enhancement ↪.*

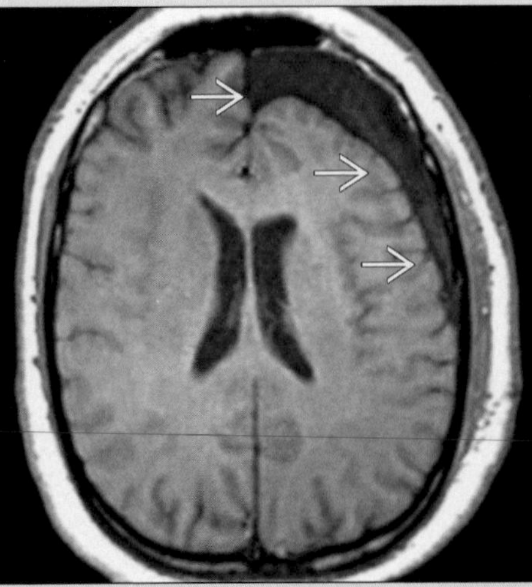

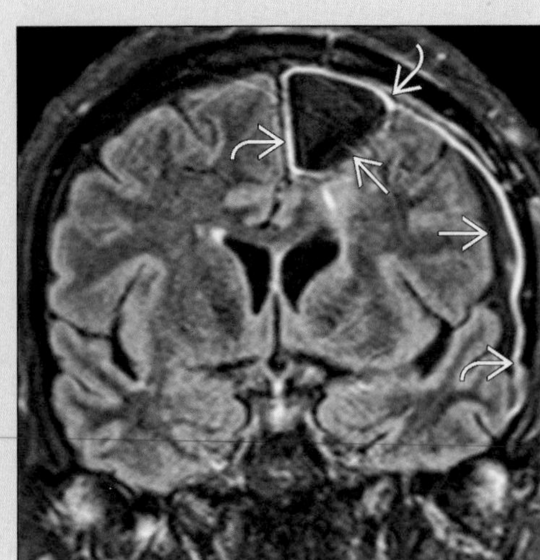

CHRONIC SUBDURAL HEMATOMA

TERMINOLOGY

Abbreviations

- Chronic subdural hematoma (cSDH)

Definitions

- Chronic (> 3 weeks) collection of blood products in subdural space

IMAGING

General Features

- Best diagnostic clue
  - Crescent-shaped, multiseptated, extraaxial collection with enhancing surrounding membranes that spreads diffusely over affected hemisphere
- Location
  - Potential space between inner layer of dura mater and arachnoid
  - Supratentorial convexity most common
- Morphology
  - Crescent-shaped extraaxial fluid collection
  - May cross sutures, not dural attachments
  - May extend along falx and tentorium
  - Compresses and displaces underlying brain surface, cortical vessels, and subarachnoid space fluid
  - Often septated, with internal membranes
  - Calcification in 1-2%
  - Enhancement of encapsulating membranes
  - Recurrent, mixed-age hemorrhage common; in children, raises suspicion of nonaccidental trauma!
  - CT density and MR signal intensity vary with age and organization of hemorrhage

CT Findings

- NECT
  - Density varies, depending on stage of evolution
    - Typically follows cerebrospinal fluid density
    - Progression from hyperdense acute SDH to iso- (subacute) to hypodense cSDH over ~ 3 weeks
    - Progressive increase in density &/or size of cSDH from 3 weeks to 3 months; likely from re-bleed of fragile neocapillaries in outer membrane
    - Eventual resorption in most cSDH > 3 months (outer membrane "stabilizes" and thus not prone to re-bleed)
  - Calcification can be seen along periphery of chronic collections, typically those present for many years
- CECT
  - Inward displacement of enhancing cortical vessels
  - Enhancement of dura and membranes

MR Findings

- T1WI
  - Variable depending on stage of evolution
    - Isointense to CSF if stable/chronic
    - Hyperintense with re-bleed or ↑ protein
- T2WI
  - Variable depending on stage of evolution
    - Isointense to CSF if stable/chronic
    - Hypointense with re-bleed
  - T2 hypointense signal seen in majority of cSDHs (73%); related to repeat hemorrhage
  - Membranes usually hypointense
- PD/intermediate
  - Iso- to hyperintense, depending on protein content or re-bleed into collection
- FLAIR
  - Hyperintense to CSF in most cases
    - Depends on inherent T1 and T2 signal characteristics &/or presence of protein
  - Usually most sensitive sequence for detection of SDH
- T2* GRE
  - Hypointense signal from subacute-chronic blood products
  - May be hyperintense from T2 effects
- DWI
  - Variable signal
  - Hyperintense outer membranes suggest predisposition to repeated hemorrhage
- T1WI C+
  - Peripheral &/or dural enhancement
  - Delayed scans show contrast diffusion into SDH
- Signal of SDH quite variable on MR
  - Generally evolves in pattern similar to intracerebral hemorrhage

Imaging Recommendations

- Best imaging tool
  - NECT good initial screen
  - MR better demonstrates cSDH
    - cSDH frequently hyperintense (due to methemoglobin) on T1, T2, PD, FLAIR
  - MR uniquely suited to evaluate nonaccidental trauma cases, since differing ages of blood products are better characterized
    - Membranes and clot better demonstrated on MR
      - Thickened or extensive neomembranes or clot with mass effect are indications for cSDH evacuation and membranectomy
- Protocol advice
  - Use wide window settings (150-200 HU) to identify small SDH

DIFFERENTIAL DIAGNOSIS

Subdural Hygroma

- Clear CSF (surgery, trauma tears arachnoid)
- No blood
- No encapsulating membranes
- No enhancement

Subdural Effusion

- Usually occurs as complication of meningitis
- Plasma exudate, not CSF

Subdural Empyema

- Pus accumulates in subdural space
- Peripheral enhancement
- Restricted diffusion (hyperintense) centrally

Pachymeningopathies (Thickened Dura)

- Chronic meningitis (may be indistinguishable)
- Postsurgical (shunt, etc.)

CHRONIC SUBDURAL HEMATOMA

- Intracranial hypotension ("slumping" midbrain, tonsillar herniation)
- Sarcoid (nodular, "lumpy-bumpy")

Tumors

- Meningioma, lymphoma, leukemia, metastases
- Metastatic lesions may also result in SDH, particularly breast and prostate cancer and melanoma metastases
- Dural based, enhancing mass
- ± skull involvement

Chemical Shift Artifacts

- Marrow or subcutaneous fat may "shift"; can appear intracranial, mimic T1 hyperintense SDH
- Seen with ↑ field of view or ↓ bandwidth

PATHOLOGY

General Features

- Etiology
  - SDH most commonly results from traumatic stretching & tearing of bridging cortical veins as they cross subdural space to drain into dural sinus
  - Chronic SDH
    - Develops over 2-3 weeks
    - May continue to enlarge
    - May resolve spontaneously if membrane stabilizes
    - DWI may show hyperintense band that suggests fresh hemorrhage and propensity for enlargement
  - Mechanisms for SDH enlargement
    - Re-hemorrhage
    - Serum protein exudation
- Associated abnormalities
  - Trauma is most common cause

Staging, Grading, & Classification

- Blood in subdural space incites tissue reaction resulting in organization & resorption of hematoma
- Chronic SDH may be classified by internal architecture
  - Homogeneous/laminar
    - Homogeneous content; may be laminar with thin layer of fresh blood along inner membrane
  - Separated
    - Hematocrit level
    - Sometimes content gradually changes ("gradated")
  - Trabecular
    - Heterogeneous with internal septae
    - Thickened or calcified capsule

Gross Pathologic & Surgical Features

- Serosanguineous fluid
- Encapsulated by granulation tissue: "Neomembranes" with fragile capillaries
- 5% multiloculated with fluid-blood density levels
- Cycle of recurrent bleeding → coagulation → fibrinolysis

Microscopic Features

- Outer membrane formed by proliferating fibroblasts and capillaries; fragile capillaries hypothesized as source of recurrent hemorrhage in cSDH
- Inner membrane formed by dural fibroblasts or border cells, forms fibrocollagenous sheet

CLINICAL ISSUES

Presentation

- Most common signs/symptoms
  - Varies from asymptomatic to loss of consciousness
    - "Lucid" interval in acute SDH: Initially awake, alert patient who loses consciousness a few hours after trauma
  - Other symptoms from mass effect, diffuse brain injury, secondary ischemia

Demographics

- Age
  - Any age, more common in elderly
- Epidemiology
  - SDH found in 10-20% of patients who are imaged and 30% of autopsy cases following head trauma

Natural History & Prognosis

- Older age and brain atrophy are contributory factors in conversion of traumatic SDH into cSDH
- Recurrence rate higher for skull base location SDH compared to convexity SDH
- Recurrence high for separated SDH, low for trabeculated SDH
- Extent of primary brain injury most important factor that affects outcome

Treatment

- Surgical drainage with resection of membranes
- Recurrence risk of cSDH varies with type
  - "Separated" has highest risk; thickened or calcified membrane almost never re-hemorrhages

DIAGNOSTIC CHECKLIST

Image Interpretation Pearls

- Enhancement may help differentiate chronic SDH from pachymeningopathies
- If no trauma history, consider underlying vascular lesion or dural metastases

SELECTED REFERENCES

1. Fernando S et al: Neuroimaging of nonaccidental head trauma: pitfalls and controversies. Pediatr Radiol. 38(8):827-38, 2008
2. Torihashi K et al: Independent predictors for recurrence of chronic subdural hematoma: a review of 343 consecutive surgical cases. Neurosurgery. 63(6):1125-9; discussion 1129, 2008
3. Amirjamshidi A et al: Glasgow Coma Scale on admission is correlated with postoperative Glasgow Outcome Scale in chronic subdural hematoma. J Clin Neurosci. 14(12):1240-1, 2007
4. Rocchi G et al: Membranectomy in organized chronic subdural hematomas: indications and technical notes. Surg Neurol. 67(4):374-80; discussion 380, 2007
5. Kuwahara S et al: Subdural hyperintense band on diffusion-weighted imaging of chronic subdural hematoma indicates bleeding from the outer membrane. Neurol Med Chir (Tokyo). 45(3):125-31, 2005
6. Burger P et al: Surgical Pathology of the Nervous System and Its Coverings. 4th Ed. New York: Churchill Livingstone, 2002

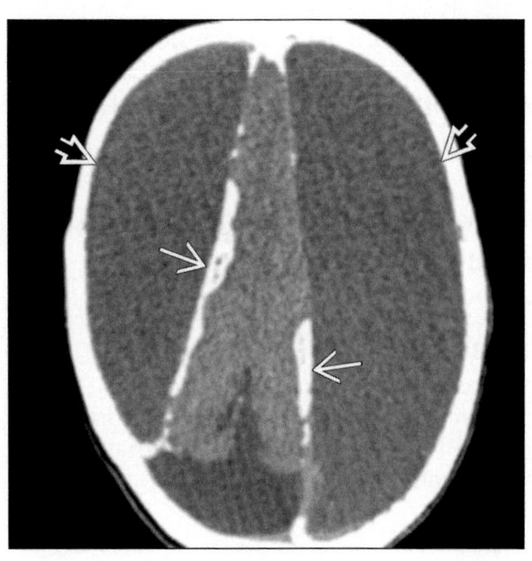

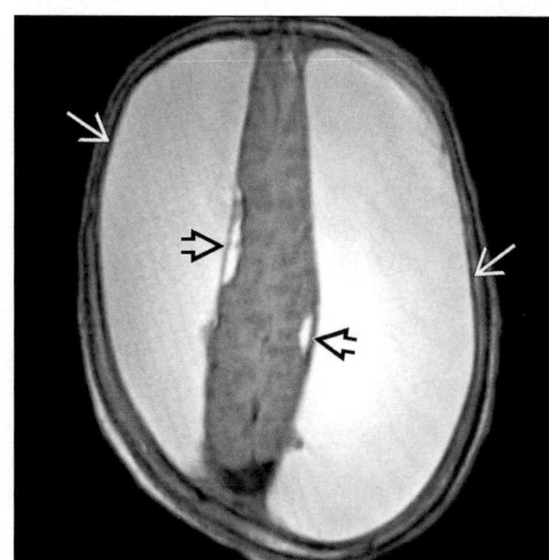

(Left) *Axial NECT shows a bilateral chronic SDH ➲ with calcified margins ➔. The brain is squeezed toward the midline by the SDH.* ***(Right)*** *Axial T1WI MR in the same patient shows a large hyperintense bilateral SDH ➔ bordered medially by dense calcifications, reflecting osseous metaplasia. Note the intrinsic high T1 signal due to marrow fat ➲. Although chronic SDHs usually follow CSF signal, T1 hyperintensity related to methemoglobin, re-bleeds, or increased protein content may be seen.*

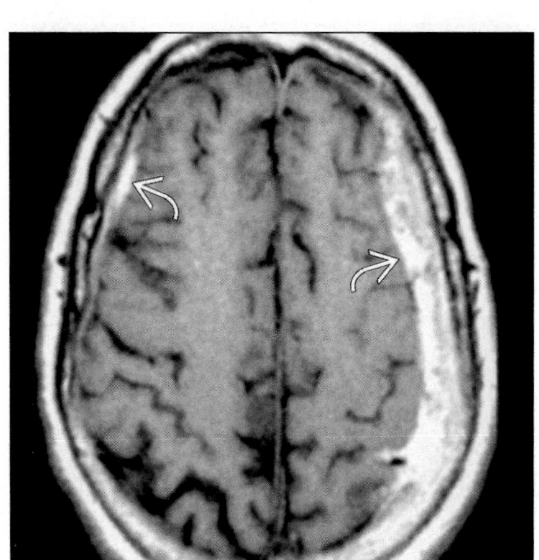

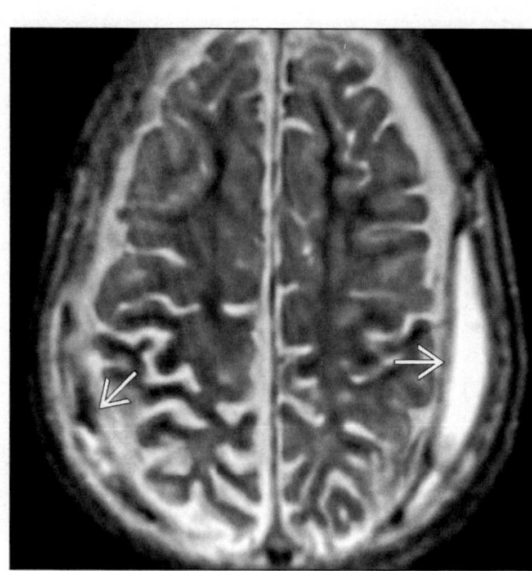

(Left) *Axial T1WI MR shows bilateral chronic subdural hematomas ➔. The hyperintensity in this patient is related to repeat hemorrhage. Chronic SDHs are more common in the elderly and may be related to a relatively minor traumatic event.* ***(Right)*** *Axial T2WI MR shows bilateral SDHs ➔ with differing signal characteristics. Though variable signal characteristics are present, these had been present and unchanged for many years on successive scans. MR signal of chronic SDH often follows CSF signal.*

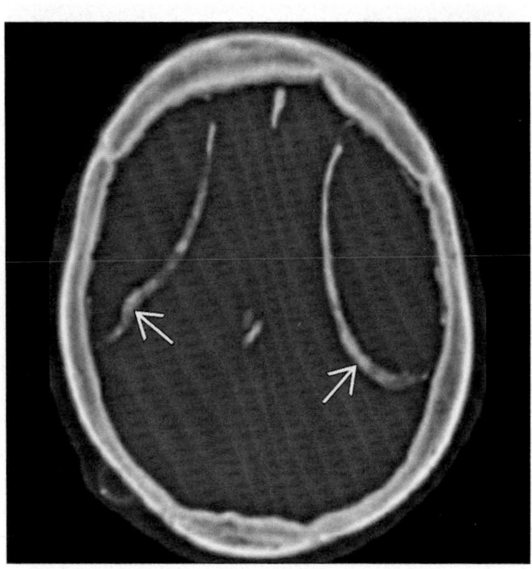

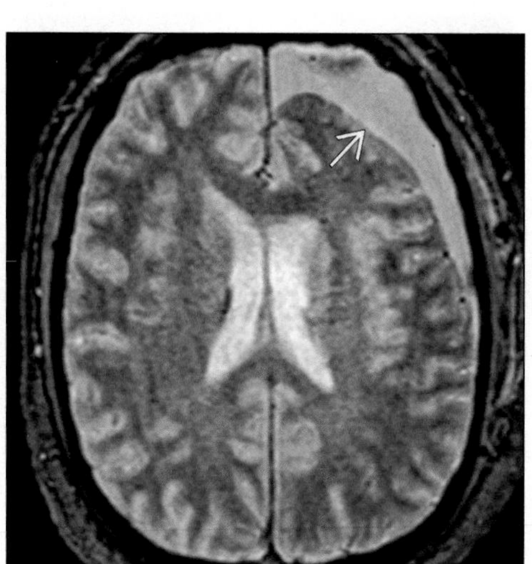

(Left) *Axial bone CT shows bilateral chronic subdural collections with dense calcifications along the inner membranes ➔. These calcified SDHs are often seen in patients with chronically shunted hydrocephalus, as in this case.* ***(Right)*** *Axial T2* GRE MR shows a frontal chronic SDH ➔ with local mass effect. GRE MR may show hypointense signal related to chronic hemosiderin. However, bright signal is often seen on GRE sequence related to the T2 effects of the fluid collection.*

MIXED SUBDURAL HEMATOMA

Key Facts

Terminology

- Hemorrhage of differing ages/evolution in subdural space, often bilateral

Imaging

- Imaging recommendations
  - NECT initial screen
  - MR more sensitive: Bleed age, extent of injuries
- General features
  - Crescentic, mixed density/signal intensity, extraaxial convexity collection
  - Often septated, with enhancing internal membranes (biconvex)
  - May cross sutures but not dural attachments
  - Inward displacement of cortical veins
  - Variable heterogeneous density
  - Loculated: Hypo- and hyperdense components

Pathology

- Re-hemorrhage into preexistent SDH
- > 70% of SDH: Significant associated lesions
- Mixed SDH may be acute: Low-density foci ("swirl sign") reflect unclotted blood, serum, or CSF leak

Clinical Issues

- Recurrent, mixed-age hemorrhages common
- Suspect nonaccidental trauma in children!
- Surgical evacuation if symptomatic or growing
- Can spontaneously resolve or enlarge

Diagnostic Checklist

- Consider contrast to demonstrate internal membranes, sign predictive of future re-hemorrhage
- Mixed density SDH are prone to re-hemorrhage and are usually best drained surgically

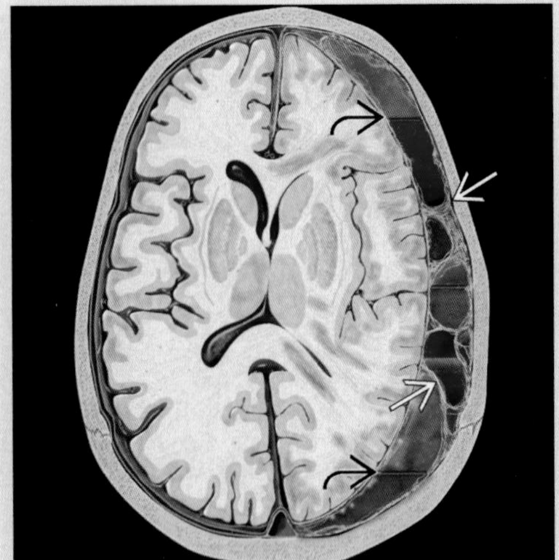

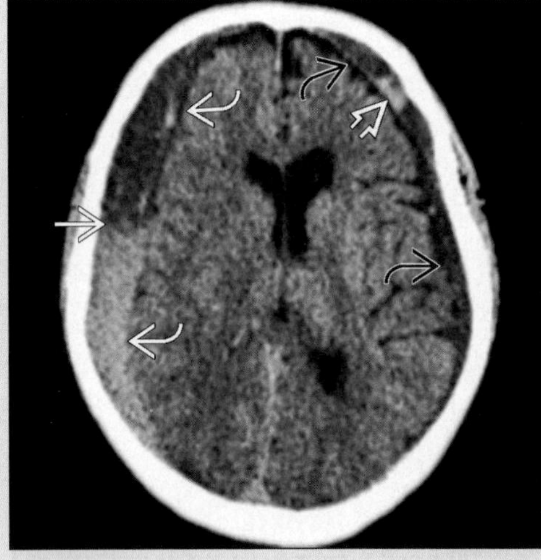

(Left) *Axial graphic shows hemorrhage of multiple ages in this mixed SDH with numerous loculations from multiple membranes ➡. Repeat hemorrhage within mixed hematomas is common, as seen here, with acute blood levels ⇨. These mixed hematomas are usually related to acute re-hemorrhage.* ***(Right)*** *Axial NECT shows a dependent hyperdense fluid collection ➡ due to acute hemorrhage in a chronic right SDH ➡ and a mixed density in a left chronic SDH ⇨ with a small acute hemorrhage ➡.*

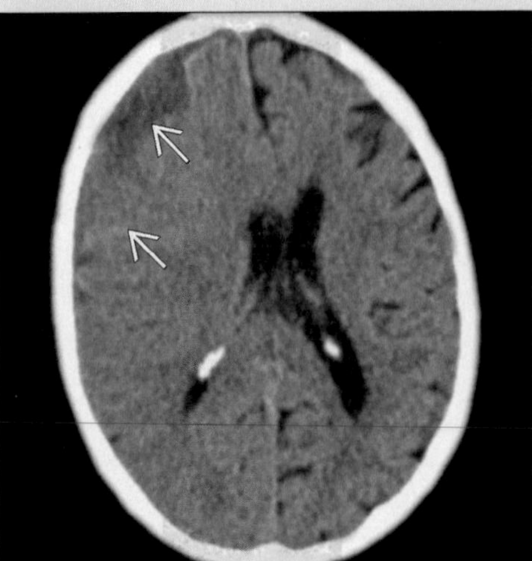

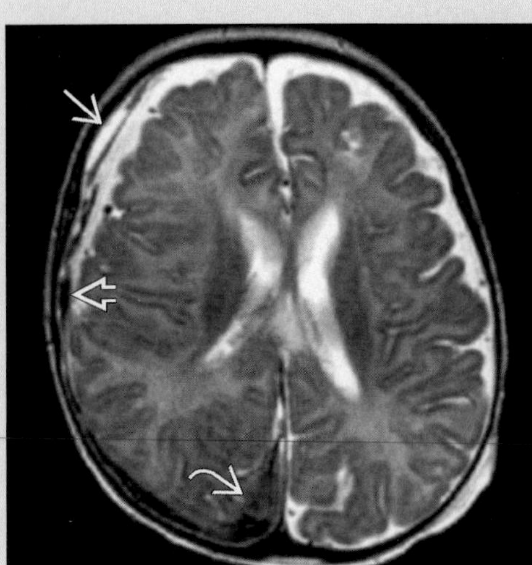

(Left) *Axial NECT shows mixed density within this SDH ➡ that was rapidly expanding on successive CT scans.* ***(Right)*** *Axial T2WI MR show a mostly hyperintense SDH ➡, but the posterior aspect ➡ is hypointense, indicating a more recent hemorrhage. Additional recent hemorrhage ➡ is also seen. At least 2 separate episodes of hemorrhage are present. MR can be very helpful in detecting mixed-age subdural hematomas, particularly in nonaccidental trauma.*

MIXED SUBDURAL HEMATOMA

TERMINOLOGY

Abbreviations

- Subdural hematoma (SDH)

Definitions

- Hemorrhage of differing ages &/or evolution in subdural space

IMAGING

General Features

- Best diagnostic clue
  - Crescentic, mixed density/signal intensity (SI), extraaxial convexity collection
- Location
  - Potential space between inner dura layer and arachnoid
  - Supratentorial convexity most common
- Morphology
  - Crescentic, extraaxial fluid collection
  - May cross sutures but not dural attachments
  - Often septated, with internal membranes (biconvex)

CT Findings

- NECT
  - Variable heterogeneous density
    - Dependent layering: Hyperdense posteriorly
    - Loculated: Hypo- and hyperdense components
  - Bilateral isodense SDH: Medial displacement of corticomedullary junctions
    - Sulci & lateral ventricles small; ventricles parallel
    - Central herniation: Nonvisualization of suprasellar cistern; 3rd ventricle posterior to sella
- CECT
  - Inward displacement of cortical veins
  - Enhancement of dura and membranes

MR Findings

- T1WI
  - Mixed signal: Hyperintense (hemorrhage > 3 days)
- T2WI
  - Mixed signal: Hypointense (hemorrhage < 5 days)
- FLAIR: Mixed signal; hyperintense to CSF
- Mixed signal due to blood of differing ages (often re-bleed)
- Loculations: Regions of different SI related to blood products of different ages

Imaging Recommendations

- Best imaging tool
  - NECT initial screen
  - MR more sensitive to help age bleed and evaluate extent of injuries
- Protocol advice
  - Wide window settings (150-200 HU)

DIFFERENTIAL DIAGNOSIS

Other Subdural Collections

- Acute traumatic effusion, empyema, hygroma

Acute Epidural Hematoma

- CT hyperdense biconvex extraaxial mass

Pachymeningopathies (Thickened Dura)

- Chronic meningitis: Granulomatous
- Postsurgical (e.g., shunt)
- Intracranial hypotension

Tumor

- Meningioma, lymphoma, leukemia, metastases

PATHOLOGY

General Features

- Etiology
  - Re-hemorrhage into preexistent SDH typical
  - Mixed SDH may be acute: Low-density foci ("swirl sign") reflect unclotted blood, serum, or CSF leak
- Associated abnormalities
  - > 70% of SDH: Significant associated lesions

CLINICAL ISSUES

Presentation

- Most common signs/symptoms
  - Headache, loss of consciousness
  - Patient may be asymptomatic

Demographics

- Age
  - Usually > 70 years of age
  - In young children, related to nonaccidental trauma
- Epidemiology
  - 10-20% of patients with SDH, 30% of autopsy cases following head trauma

Natural History & Prognosis

- Can spontaneously resolve or enlarge
- Onset 2 days to 2 weeks after trauma
  - Recurrent, mixed-age hemorrhages common
  - Suspect nonaccidental trauma in children!

Treatment

- Surgical evacuation if symptomatic or growing

DIAGNOSTIC CHECKLIST

Consider

- Contrast to demonstrate internal membranes, a sign predictive of future re-hemorrhage

Image Interpretation Pearls

- Mixed density SDH are prone to re-hemorrhage and are usually best drained surgically

SELECTED REFERENCES

1. Tung GA et al: Comparison of accidental and nonaccidental traumatic head injury in children on noncontrast computed tomography. Pediatrics. 118(2):626-33, 2006

TRAUMATIC SUBARACHNOID HEMORRHAGE

Key Facts

Terminology

- Blood within subarachnoid spaces
  - Contained between pia, arachnoid membranes

Imaging

- High density on CT, hyperintensity on FLAIR

Top Differential Diagnoses

- Nontraumatic SAH
- Meningitis: Cellular and proteinaceous debris
- Carcinomatosis meningitis
- Pseudosubarachnoid hemorrhage
- Gadolinium administration
- High-inspired oxygen

Pathology

- Associated with contusions, subdural or epidural hematoma, diffuse axonal injury

Clinical Issues

- Headache, emesis, decreased consciousness
- Trauma most common cause of SAH
- Presence of tSAH is marker of more severe brain injury
- Outcome related in logistic regression analysis to
  - Admission Glasgow Coma Scale score
  - Amount of subarachnoid blood
- Poor prognosis if associated with other intracranial injuries
- Vasospasm develops earlier than w/aneurysmal SAH
- Associated with ↓ neuropsychologic profiles, worse vocational outcomes in 1 year follow-up

Diagnostic Checklist

- Isolated supratentorial sulcal blood common
- Hyperdense blood in interpeduncular cistern may be only manifestation of subtle SAH

*(**Left**) Coronal graphic depicts findings in a severe traumatic brain injury. Closed head trauma has resulted in multiple gyral contusions and subarachnoid hemorrhage. Most tSAH ⇒ occurs adjacent to parenchymal brain injuries and is found centered around the sylvian fissures, inferior frontotemporal and convexity sulci. (**Right**) Axial NECT in a patient with head trauma and tSAH demonstrates focal hyperdense collections in a few left posterior frontal sulci bordering the interhemispheric fissure ⇒.*

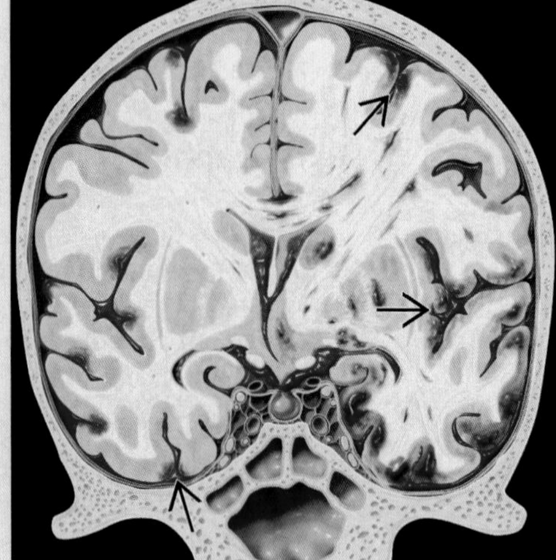

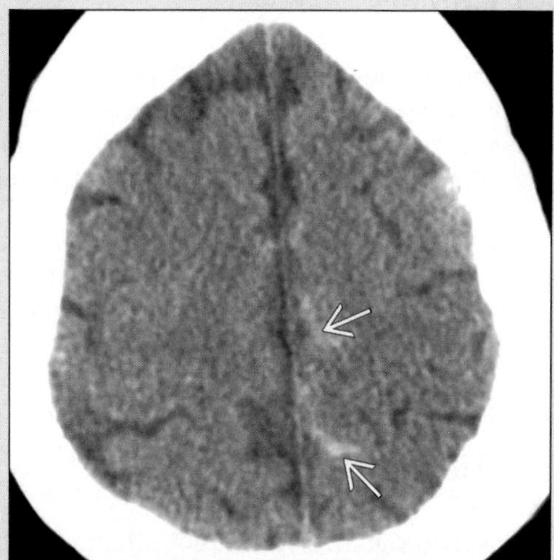

*(**Left**) Axial FLAIR MR shows abnormal hyperintensity within bilateral sulci, right more than left ⇒. There is also T2 hyperintensity suggesting cerebral contusion ⇒, as well as calvarial and soft tissue injuries ⇒. (**Right**) Axial NECT reveals a tSAH within the convexity sulci ⇒ in association with a large epidural hematoma ⇒, skull fractures ⇒, and soft tissue injury ⇒.*

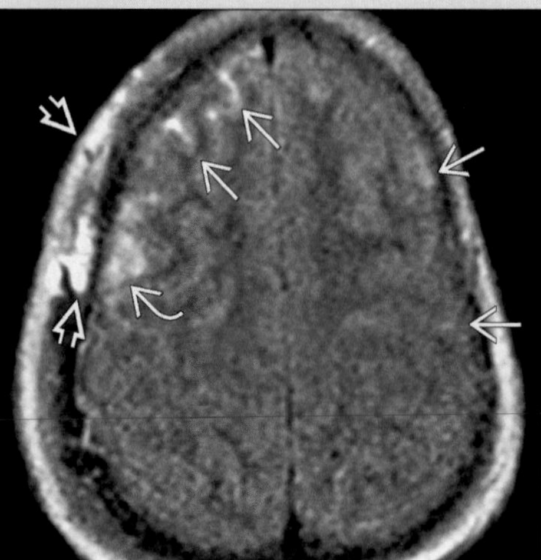

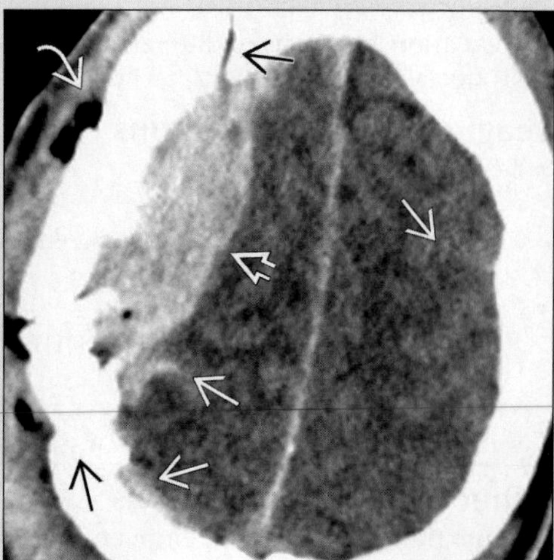

TERMINOLOGY

Abbreviations

- Traumatic subarachnoid hemorrhage (tSAH)

Definitions

- Blood within subarachnoid spaces
  - Contained between pia, arachnoid membranes

IMAGING

General Features

- Best diagnostic clue
  - High density on NECT
  - Sulcal-cisternal FLAIR hyperintensity (in trauma patient)
- Location
  - Can be focal or diffuse
    - Focal SAH adjacent to contusion, subdural/ epidural hematoma, fracture, laceration
      - Sylvian fissure, inferior frontal subarachnoid spaces most common
      - Isolated convexity sulci (adjacent to contusion)
    - Diffusely in subarachnoid space &/or basal cisterns
    - Layering on tentorium

CT Findings

- NECT
  - High density in subarachnoid space(s)/cisterns
  - Hyperdense blood in interpeduncular cistern may be only manifestation of subtle SAH
  - Identical to aneurysmal SAH except location
    - Adjacent to contusions, subdural hematoma
    - Convexity sulci > basal cisterns

MR Findings

- T1WI
  - Hyperintense to ventricular CSF ("dirty" CSF)
- T2WI
  - Isointense to CSF (not detected)
- FLAIR
  - Hyperintense sulci/cisterns; more sensitive, less specific than CT
- T2* GRE
  - Occasionally hypointense
- DWI
  - Evaluation of tSAH-induced spasm
    - Restricted diffusion in areas of ischemia

Angiographic Findings

- Conventional DSA
  - Exclusion of aneurysm, evaluation of tSAH-induced spasm: CTA replaces DSA
  - "Beaded" appearance of spasm-involved vessels
    - From 2-3 days → 2 weeks after trauma

Imaging Recommendations

- Best imaging tool
  - NECT; FLAIR for subtle SAH

DIFFERENTIAL DIAGNOSIS

Nontraumatic SAH (ntSAH)

- Ruptured aneurysm
  - Causes 80-90% of all ntSAH
  - Aneurysm identified on DSA, CTA, MRA in > 90%
- Ruptured dissecting aneurysm
- Arteriovenous malformation (AVM)
  - Account for 15% of ntSAH
  - Identified on DSA, CTA, MRA
- Perimesencephalic venous hemorrhage
  - Limited to basal cisterns: Clot around basilar artery
  - Normal DSA, CTA, MRA
- Cerebral infarction with reperfusion hemorrhage
  - Presence of known infarct
- Anticoagulation therapy
  - Long-term warfarin (Coumadin) therapy; usually unrecognized mild head trauma
  - Alcohol abuse as cause of abnormal coagulation
- Blood dyscrasia
  - Usually known preexisting entity
- Eclampsia (pregnancy-induced hypertension)
  - Reported complication, eclampsia symptomatology
- Spinal vascular malformation
  - Spontaneous
  - Negative initial and repeat cerebral DSA
  - MR: Spinal SAH, cord edema
  - MRA and DSA to establish diagnosis

Meningitis: Cellular & Proteinaceous Debris

- Dirty CSF on CT
- Hyperintensity on FLAIR due to T1 shortening and failure of signal nulling

Carcinomatosis Meningitis

- Cellular CSF prevents FLAIR CSF nulling

Pseudosubarachnoid Hemorrhage

- Severe cerebral edema → diffusely hypodense brain
- Dura, circulating blood in arteries/venous sinuses look relatively hyperdense compared to adjacent brain

Gadolinium Administration

- IV contrast for routine-enhanced MR may cause FLAIR hyperintensity
  - Stroke, high-grade gliomas, or meningiomas (neoplasm surfaces contact subarachnoid spaces/ ventricles)
  - CSF changes more evident close to pathology &/or hemisphere involved

High-Inspired Oxygen

- 100% O_2 during general anesthesia
  - May cause incomplete nulling of subarachnoid CSF
  - Hyperintense sulcal CSF on FLAIR
  - Ventricular CSF not affected

PATHOLOGY

General Features

- Etiology
  - Tearing of vessels in subarachnoid space

TRAUMATIC SUBARACHNOID HEMORRHAGE

- Traumatic dissecting aneurysm → basal cisternal SAH
  - Most often from vertebral artery dissection
  - Suspect with basilar skull fracture
  - Mimics aneurysmal SAH
- Genetics
  - *APOE* ε4 allele predisposes to poor outcome after traumatic brain injury (TBI), SAH, and hemorrhagic stroke
- Associated abnormalities
  - Contusions, subdural or epidural hematoma, diffuse axonal injury

Staging, Grading, & Classification

- Grade 1: Thin tSAH ≤ 5 mm
- Grade 2: Thick tSAH > 5 mm
- Grade 3: Thin tSAH with mass lesion(s)
- Grade 4: Thick tSAH with mass lesion(s)

Gross Pathologic & Surgical Features

- Acute blood in sulci/cisterns
- Autopsy studies show
  - Bleeding from cortical arteries/veins
  - Leakage from surface contusions

Microscopic Features

- Evolutionary hemoglobin changes different than described for intracerebral hematoma
  - Much slower progression, delayed degradation
  - Most likely secondary to high ambient oxygen tension of subarachnoid CSF

CLINICAL ISSUES

Presentation

- Most common signs/symptoms
  - Headache, emesis, decreased consciousness
- Other signs/symptoms
  - May ↑ risk of corrected QT prolongation on ECG, ventricular tachycardia, sudden death
- Clinical profile
  - Trauma, not ruptured aneurysm, most common cause of SAH!

Demographics

- Age
  - Median = 43 years (standard deviation = 21.1 years)
- Gender
  - M:F = 2:1, for sustaining traumatic brain injury
- Epidemiology
  - 33% with moderate TBI, 60% with severe TBI
  - Nearly 100% at autopsy (typically mild)
  - tSAH-associated vasospasm in 2-10% of cases
- Risk factors for TBI
  - Young age, low income, chronic alcohol/substance abuse
  - Prior episodes of TBI

Natural History & Prognosis

- Natural history: Breakdown and resorption from CSF
- Presence of tSAH is early marker of severe brain injury
- Outcome related in logistic regression analysis to
  - Admission Glasgow Coma Scale score
  - Amount of subarachnoid blood
- Poor prognosis if associated with other intracranial injuries
  - Amount of tSAH on initial CT correlates with delayed ischemia, poor outcome
  - 46-78% of moderate-to-severe TBI associated with tSAH result in
    - Increased morbidity, leading to severe disability and persistent vegetative state
    - Increased mortality as high as 2x
- Acute hydrocephalus
  - Rare; usually obstruction of aqueduct or 4th ventricular outlet by clotted SAH
  - Obstructive, noncommunicating hydrocephalus
    - Asymmetric ventricular dilatation
- Delayed hydrocephalus
  - Arachnoid granulation defect in CSF resorption
  - Obstructive communicating hydrocephalus
    - Symmetric ventricular dilatation
  - Observed in 11.96% of TBI patients after 3-month follow-up interval
  - No correlation between location of tSAH and development of hydrocephalus
- Vasospasm
  - Develops earlier with tSAH than with aneurysmal SAH
  - Peaks 7-10 days after injury
  - Threat remains up to 2 weeks
  - Uncommon cause of post-traumatic infarct
- Associated with ↓ neuropsychologic profiles, worse vocational outcomes in 1 year follow-up

Treatment

- Supportive therapy is primary treatment
  - Intubation, supplemental oxygen, IV fluids, therapy of altered vital signs
  - Sedatives; medications for pain, nausea, and vomiting
  - Anticonvulsants for seizures
- Nimodipine (calcium channel blocker) may prevent vasospasm and its complications

DIAGNOSTIC CHECKLIST

Image Interpretation Pearls

- tSAH often accompanied by additional injuries
- Isolated supratentorial sulcal blood common
- Hyperdense blood in interpeduncular cistern may be only manifestation of subtle SAH

SELECTED REFERENCES

1. Compagnone C et al: Patients with moderate head injury: a prospective multicenter study of 315 patients. Neurosurgery. 64(4):690-6; discussion 696-7, 2009
2. Steyerberg EW et al: Predicting outcome after traumatic brain injury: development and international validation of prognostic scores based on admission characteristics. PLoS Med. 5(8):e165; discussion e165, 2008
3. Tian HL et al: Risk factors related to hydrocephalus after traumatic subarachnoid hemorrhage. Surg Neurol. 69(3):241-6; discussion 246, 2008

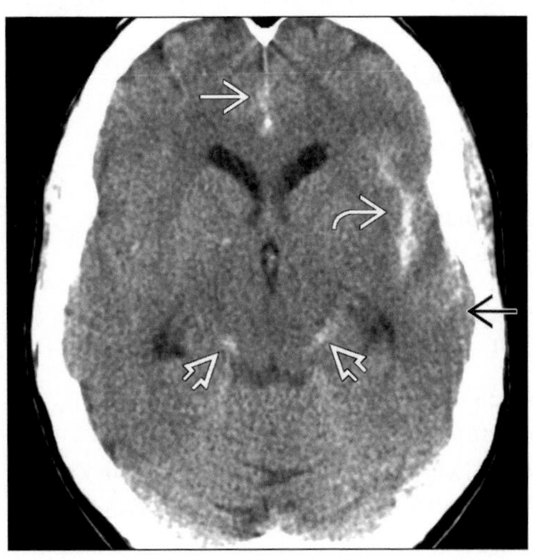

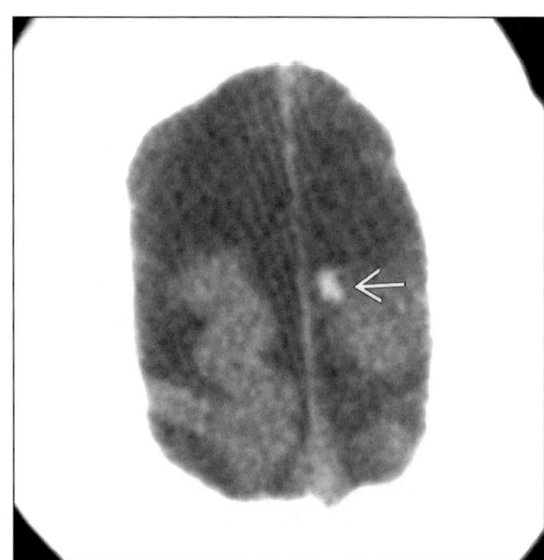

(Left) *Axial NECT shows hyperdense traumatic subarachnoid hemorrhage within the sulci ➙, left sylvian fissure ➙, ambient cisterns ➙, and interhemispheric fissure ➙.* ***(Right)*** *Axial NECT reveals a small collection of hyperdensity ➙ along a left frontal medial sulcus, representing traumatic subarachnoid hemorrhage.*

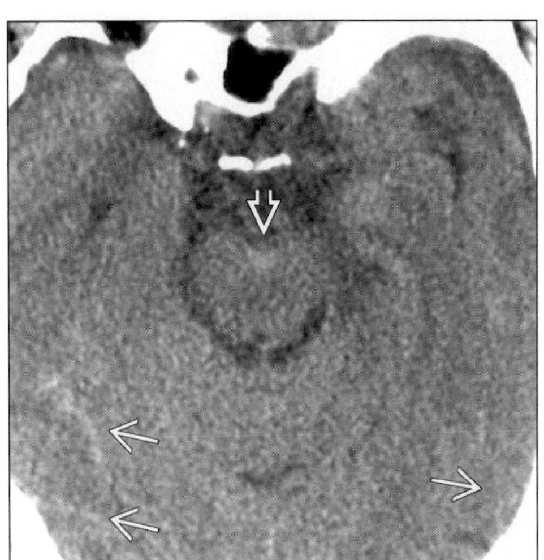

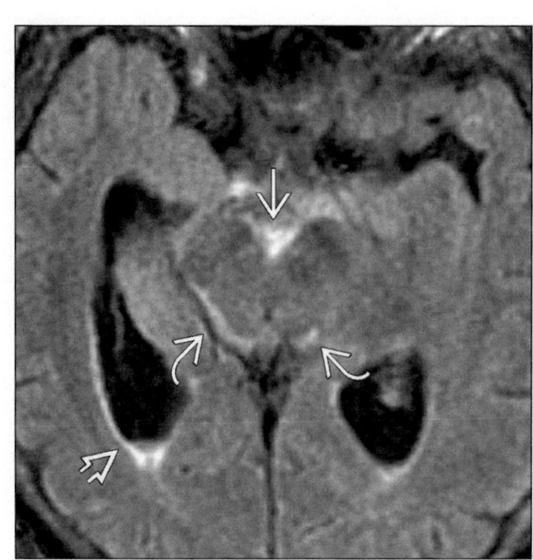

(Left) *Axial NECT demonstrates collections of hyperdensity within a few sulci ➙ and the interpeduncular cistern ➙ from traumatic subarachnoid hemorrhage.* ***(Right)*** *Axial FLAIR MR shows abnormal CSF hyperintensity within the interpeduncular cistern ➙ and ambient/quadrigeminal cisterns ➙. It also reveals a small amount of layering-dependent hemorrhage within the right occipital horn ➙.*

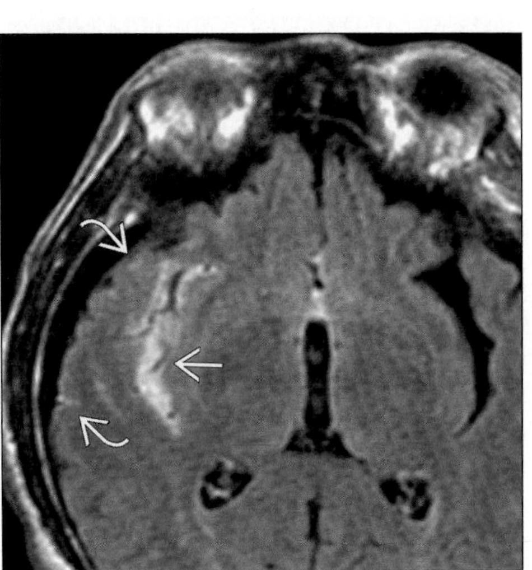

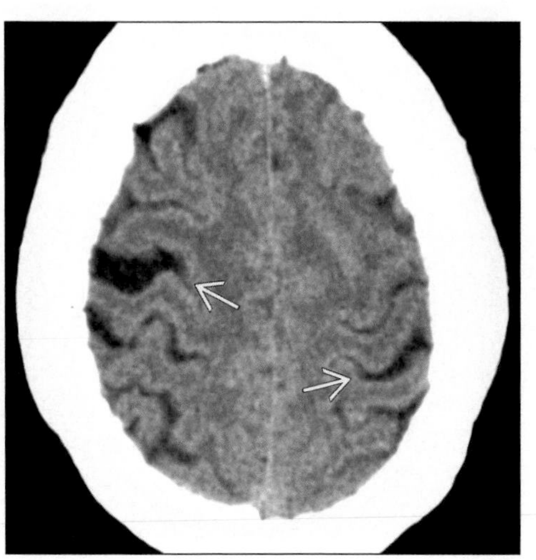

(Left) *Axial FLAIR MR demonstrates traumatic subarachnoid hemorrhage as an abnormal CSF hyperintensity within the right sylvian fissure ➙, as well as within a few right sulci ➙.* ***(Right)*** *Axial NECT shows widening of bilateral sulci, right more than left, by a CSF-isodense process ➙ due to subacute-to-chronic subarachnoid hemorrhage.*

CEREBRAL CONTUSION

Key Facts

Terminology
- Brain surface injuries involving gray matter and contiguous subcortical white matter

Imaging
- Best diagnostic clue: Patchy hemorrhages within edematous background
- Characteristic locations: Adjacent to irregular bony protuberance or dural fold
- Anterior inferior frontal lobes and anterior inferior temporal lobes most common
- FLAIR: Best for hyperintense cortical edema and subarachnoid hemorrhage
- GRE: Hypointense hemorrhagic foci "bloom"
- Best imaging tool
  - CT to detect acute hemorrhagic contusions, other intracranial lesions, and herniations
  - MR to detect presence & delineate extent of lesions
- Coup: Direct injury to brain beneath impact site
- Contrecoup: Injury opposite impact site; usually more severe than coup

Top Differential Diagnoses
- Infarct
- Venous sinus thrombosis
- Cerebritis
- Low-grade neoplasm
- Transient postictal changes

Pathology
- Inflammation → worsening/enlarging lesions

Clinical Issues
- Initial symptom: Confusion → obtundation
- Central goal: Prevent and treat secondary injury
- Mass effect and herniation may require evacuation

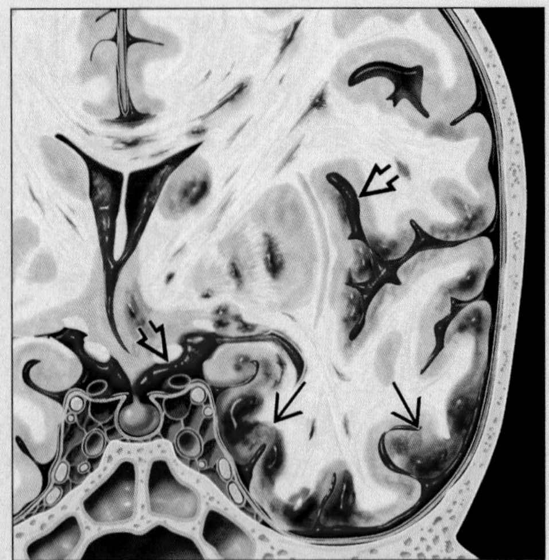

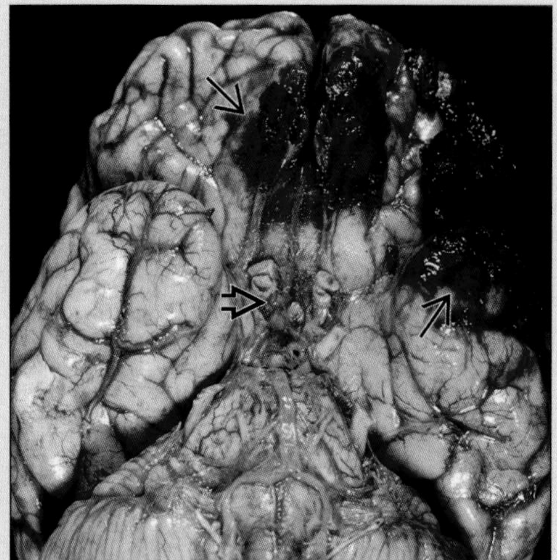

(Left) Coronal graphic illustrates the pathology of closed head injury. Note hemorrhagic foci involving gray matter of several contused gyri ➔, axonal and deep gray injuries, and traumatic subarachnoid hemorrhage ⇨ in basal cisterns and sylvian fissure. (Right) Gross pathology of the brain from a patient who died with closed head injury shows bifrontal, temporal hemorrhagic contusions ➔, as well as traumatic subarachnoid hemorrhage in the suprasellar cistern ⇨. (Courtesy R. Hewlett, PhD.)

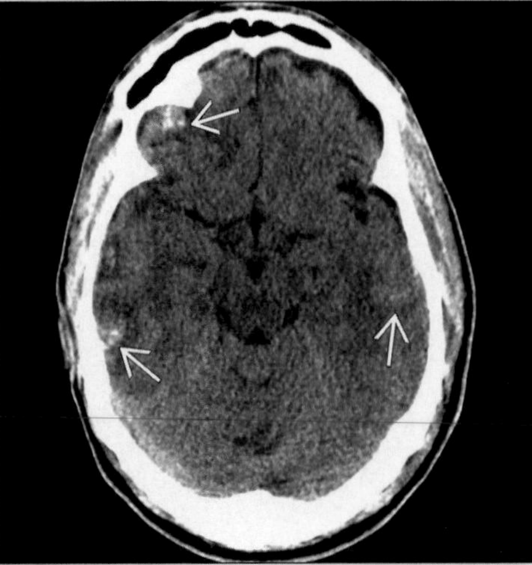

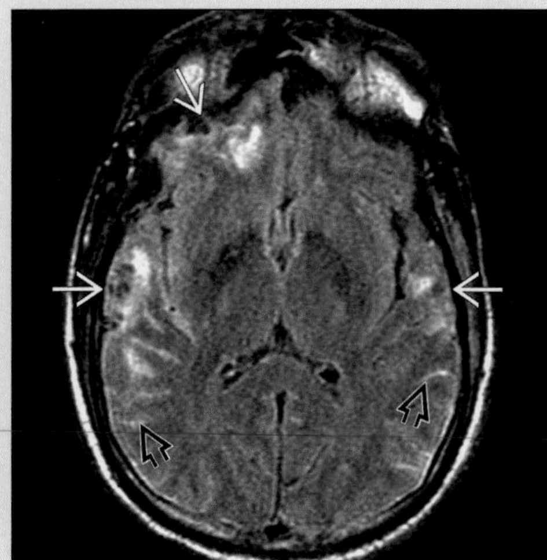

(Left) Axial NECT demonstrates the classic findings of hemorrhagic contusions (hyperdense blood within hypodense contusions) involving the bitemporal and inferior right frontal lobes ➔. (Right) Axial FLAIR in the same patient better demonstrates the hemorrhagic contusions as containing hypointense hemorrhage within hyperintense contusions ➔. These contusions "bloomed" on T2 GRE (not shown). Also note the presence of hyperintense subarachnoid hemorrhage within several sulci ⇨.*

CEREBRAL CONTUSION

TERMINOLOGY

Definitions

- Brain surface injuries involving gray matter and contiguous subcortical white matter

IMAGING

General Features

- Best diagnostic clue
  - Patchy hemorrhages within edematous background
- Location
  - Characteristic locations: Adjacent to irregular bony protuberance or dural fold
    - Anterior inferior frontal lobes and anterior inferior temporal lobes most common
    - 25% parasagittal ("gliding" contusions)
  - Less common locations
    - Parietal/occipital lobes, posterior fossa
  - Coup: Direct injury to brain beneath impact site
  - Contrecoup: Injury opposite impact site; usually more severe than coup
- Morphology
  - Early: Patchy, ill-defined, superficial foci of punctate or linear hemorrhage along gyral crests
  - 24-48 hours: Existing lesions enlarge and become more hemorrhagic; new lesions may appear
  - Chronic: Encephalomalacia with volume loss
  - Multiple, bilateral lesions in 90% of cases

CT Findings

- NECT
  - Early: Patchy, ill-defined, low-density edema with small foci of hyperdense hemorrhage
  - 24-48 hours
    - Edema, hemorrhage, & mass effect often increase
    - New foci of edema and hemorrhage may appear
    - Petechial hemorrhage may coalesce
  - Chronic
    - Become isodense, then hypodense
    - Encephalomalacia with volume loss
  - Secondary lesions
    - Herniations/mass effect with secondary infarction
    - Hydrocephalus due to hemorrhage
- Perfusion CT
  - More sensitive than NECT in detection of cerebral contusions (87.5% vs. 39.6%, respectively)

MR Findings

- T1WI
  - Acute: Inhomogeneous isointensity and mass effect
  - Chronic: Focal or diffuse atrophy
- FLAIR
  - Acute: Best for hyperintense cortical edema and subarachnoid hemorrhage (SAH)
  - Chronic
    - Hyperintense demyelination and microglial scarring
    - Hypointense hemosiderin staining
    - Hypointense cavitation (cystic encephalomalacia)
- T2* GRE
  - Acute: Hypointense hemorrhagic foci "bloom"
  - Chronic: Hypointense hemosiderin deposits
- DWI
  - Hyperintense in areas of cell death: Apparent diffusion coefficient (ADC) decreased
  - Isointense in vasogenic edema: ADC increased
  - DTI can show white matter damage in minor head trauma when CT and routine MR are normal
- MRS
  - ↓ NAA, ↑ choline

Nuclear Medicine Findings

- SPECT Tc-99m HMPAO imaging
  - Depicts focal changes in 53% with mild injury
  - Negative in 1st month predicts good outcome
    - Positive can predict poor clinical outcome

Imaging Recommendations

- Best imaging tool
  - CT to detect acute hemorrhagic contusions, other intracranial lesions, & herniations
  - MR to detect presence and delineate extent of lesions
- Protocol advice
  - FLAIR for edema and SAH; GRE for hemorrhagic foci

DIFFERENTIAL DIAGNOSIS

Infarct

- No trauma history
- Characteristic acute onset focal neurologic deficit
- Vascular distribution: Spares frontal & temporal poles

Venous Sinus Thrombosis

- Edema and hemorrhage adjacent to occluded sinus

Cerebritis

- No trauma history
- Herpes typically involves medial temporal lobe

Low-Grade Neoplasm

- No trauma history
- Solitary nonhemorrhagic lesion
- No predilection for anterior frontal or temporal lobes

Transient Postictal Changes

- No trauma history
- Preceding or ongoing seizure activity
- May be hyperintense on DWI; can enhance acutely

PATHOLOGY

General Features

- Etiology
  - Stationary head struck by object
    - Direct injury beneath impact site
    - Contusion is rare without fracture
  - Moving head: Motor vehicle crash, falls
    - Differential accel-/deceleration & rotational forces on portions of brain with different densities
    - Gliding injury: Cortex anchored to dura by arachnoid granulations; subcortical tissue glides more than cortex
  - Traffic injuries main cause in young adults (20-40)
  - Falls are main cause in infants (0-4) & elderly (≥ 70)

CEREBRAL CONTUSION

- Associated abnormalities
  - Soft tissue injuries in 70% of patients
  - Subdural hematoma (SDH), traumatic SAH, intraventricular hemorrhage
  - Skull fracture at coup site

Gross Pathologic & Surgical Features

- Contusions
  - Edema along gyral crests
  - Petechial hemorrhages (most evident in 24-48 hours)
  - Small hemorrhages may coalesce into hematoma
  - Delayed hematomas may develop 24-48 hours later
- Lacerations
  - Intracerebral hematoma with "burst" lobe
  - SDH communicates with hematoma via lacerated brain, torn pia-arachnoid
- Liquefaction & encephalomalacia in chronic phase

Microscopic Features

- Capillary disruption → blood extravasation: RBCs cause visible hemorrhage, plasma leads to edema
- Perivascular hemorrhage, ↑ pinocytic activity of endothelial cells, & cytotoxic edema of astroglial cells
- Higher levels of serum protein S100B & IL-6 correlate with ultrastructural changes of endothelial cells

Cellular Features

- Chemokine, nitric oxide activation occurs early
  - Inflammatory response → neutrophil oxidative burst → proteolytic and neurotoxic enzyme release
  - Neuroinflammation mediated by cyto-/chemokines, complement
    - Contributes to secondary ischemic damage, contusion enlargement
  - CNS cells synthesize distinct chemokines
    - Chemokine CCL2 is highly expressed early in pericontusional area
    - Chemokine CXCL8 (a.k.a. IL-8) is highly expressed as late inflammatory mediator
  - Inflammatory processes contribute to pericontusional cytotoxic injury via astrocytic activation with capillary vessel compression and leukocyte accumulation → microvascular occlusion
- Blood-brain barrier failure aided by proinflammatory factor activation and matrix metalloproteinases
- Injured cortex upregulates peroxisome proliferator-activated receptor α (PPAR-α) binding activity and protein expression
  - Peaks 24-72 hours post-injury; PPAR-α agonists protect against excessive oxidative stress and inflammation in traumatic brain injury (TBI) and stroke

CLINICAL ISSUES

Presentation

- Most common signs/symptoms
  - Initial symptom: Confusion → obtundation
  - ± Cerebral dysfunction, seizures

Demographics

- Age
  - Children:adults = 2:1; highest risk 15-24 years
- Gender
  - M:F = 3:1
- Epidemiology
  - Annual cerebral contusion incidence is 200 per 100,000 brain trauma-related hospitalizations
  - Contusion is 2nd most common primary traumatic neuronal injury (44%); DAI is most common
  - 1.4 million suffer TBI each year in USA; 50,000 die and 80,000 experience long-term disability
  - TBI causes 6.5% of deaths in USA (32 per 100,000)

Natural History & Prognosis

- Varies with extent of primary injury
- Outcome is critically dependent on extent of brain damage that evolves after initial insult
  - Secondary lesions: Hypoxia, hypotension, ischemia, brain edema, & ↑ intracranial pressure
- Highest mortality rate: Elderly population
  - Linear increase of 40-50% in odds of poor outcome for every 10 years of age
- 90% of patients survive injury
  - ~ 25% have significant residual complaints
- Temporal and especially brain stem contusions are independent risk factors for poor outcome
- In severe TBI, 63% have good clinical outcome, 32% have excellent clinical outcome

Treatment

- Central goal: Prevent or rapidly treat secondary injury
- Mass effect and herniation may require evacuation
  - Focal hematoma more amenable to surgery than hemorrhagic contusion
  - Removing damaged tissue shown to prevent increase of molecular cascades triggered by secondary injury
- Mitigate secondary effects of ↑ intracranial pressure, perfusion disturbances
- Ventricular catheter to monitor and control intracranial pressure
- Long-term (5 days) mild hypothermia significantly improves outcome of severe TBI patients with cerebral contusion and intracranial hypertension

DIAGNOSTIC CHECKLIST

Consider

- Repeat exam recommended if initial exam negative but symptoms persist for 24-48 hours

Image Interpretation Pearls

- Inferior anterior frontal lobes most often injured
- Mixed-density contusions can be mistaken for common artifacts caused by orbital roof

SELECTED REFERENCES

1. Feng D et al: Cortical expression of peroxisome proliferator-activated receptor-alpha after human brain contusion. J Int Med Res. 36(4):783-91, 2008
2. Stefini R et al: Chemokine detection in the cerebral tissue of patients with posttraumatic brain contusions. J Neurosurg. 108(5):958-62, 2008

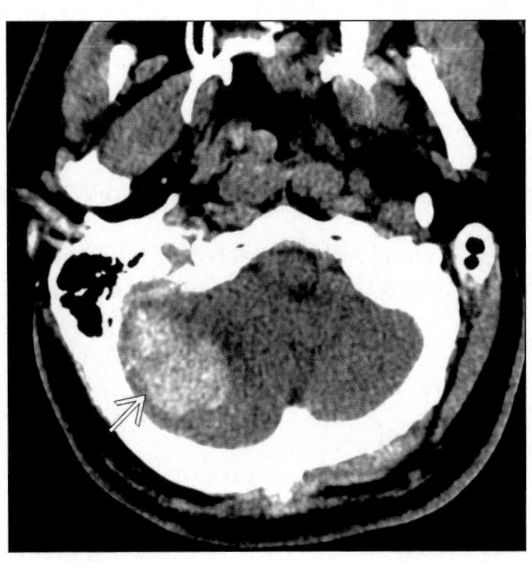

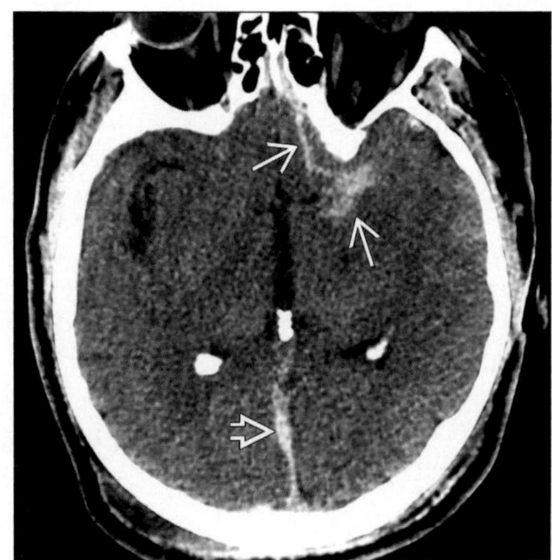

(Left) *Axial NECT reveals a coup hemorrhagic contusion of the right cerebellar hemisphere. The contusion has coalesced into a hematoma ➔.* ***(Right)*** *Axial NECT in the same patient reveals a larger contrecoup hemorrhagic contusion involving the left inferior and periorbital frontal brain ➔. Note that morphology may be linear along gyral crests or focal; both are seen in this example. There is also an associated subdural hematoma of the posterior falx ➔.*

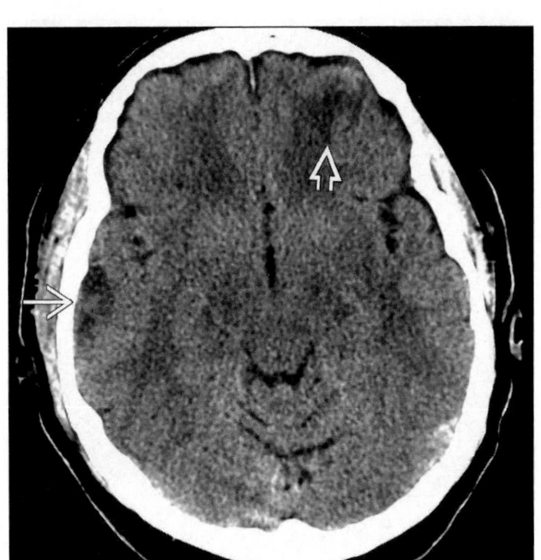

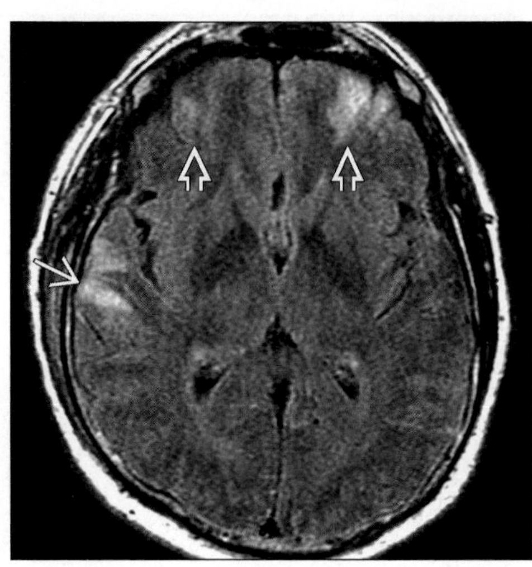

(Left) *Axial NECT shows both a larger contrecoup left frontal lobe contusion ➔ and a smaller temporal lobe coup contusion ➔. Contrecoup lesions are usually more severe than coup.* ***(Right)*** *Axial FLAIR in the same patient redemonstrates the right temporal lobe coup contusion ➔ but reveals the contrecoup lesion as both larger and bifrontal ➔. FLAIR is the most sensitive technique for visualizing the presence and extent of cerebral contusion-related edema.*

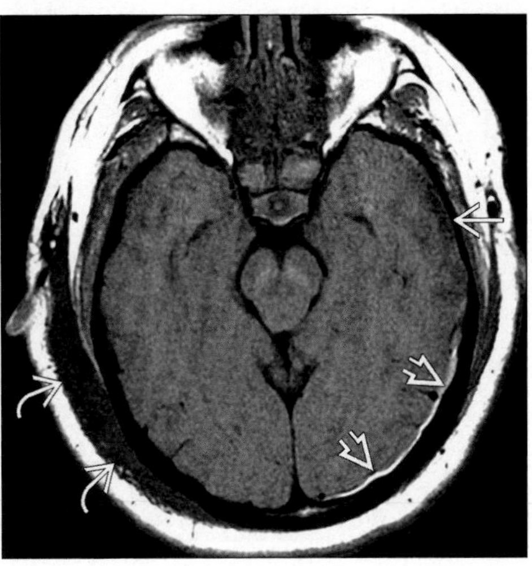

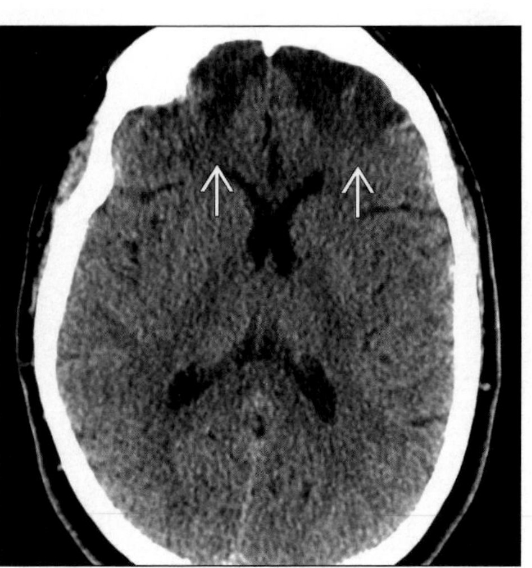

(Left) *Axial T1WI MR demonstrates the loss of gray-white interface from a contrecoup nonhemorrhagic hypointense contusion involving the left temporal lobe ➔. There is also a thin hyperintense subdural hematoma ➔ that was not visible on CT. Soft tissue swelling and injury is apparent at the primary impact, or coup, site ➔.* ***(Right)*** *Axial NECT shows the evolutionary findings of significantly hypodense, bifrontal contusions as they progress to encephalomalacia ➔.*

DIFFUSE AXONAL INJURY (DAI)

Key Facts

Terminology
- Traumatic axonal stretch injury

Imaging
- Gray-white matter junction (67%)
  - Corpus callosum (20%) (splenium)
  - Deep WM, brainstem
  - ↑ severity correlates with deeper brain involvement
- General features
  - Hemorrhagic or nonhemorrhagic
  - NECT often normal (50-80%)
- MR
  - FLAIR: Nonhemorrhagic DAI → hyperintense foci
  - GRE: Hypointense foci secondary to hemorrhage
  - SWI: Depicts significantly more DAI foci than GRE
  - May show restricted diffusion and ↓ ADC

Top Differential Diagnoses
- Multifocal nonhemorrhagic lesions
- Multifocal hemorrhagic lesions

Pathology
- Closed head injury → sudden deceleration, change in angular momentum
- Cortex rotates at different speed in relation to WM, deep brain structures
  - Axons stretched (rarely disconnected or "sheared")
  - Especially at interface between tissues of differing density
- 80% of lesions are microscopic, nonhemorrhagic
  - Visible lesions are "tip of iceberg"

Diagnostic Checklist
- Consider DAI if symptoms are disproportionate to imaging findings

__(Left)__ Sagittal graphic illustrates multiple diffuse axonal injury hemorrhagic foci within the corpus callosum and brainstem. __(Right)__ Sagittal T2WI MR demonstrates hyperintense diffuse axonal injury lesions involving the corpus callosum ➔ as well as the central midbrain ⇨.

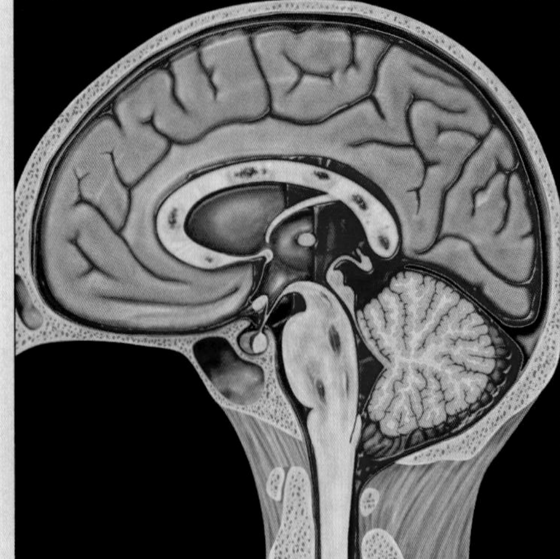

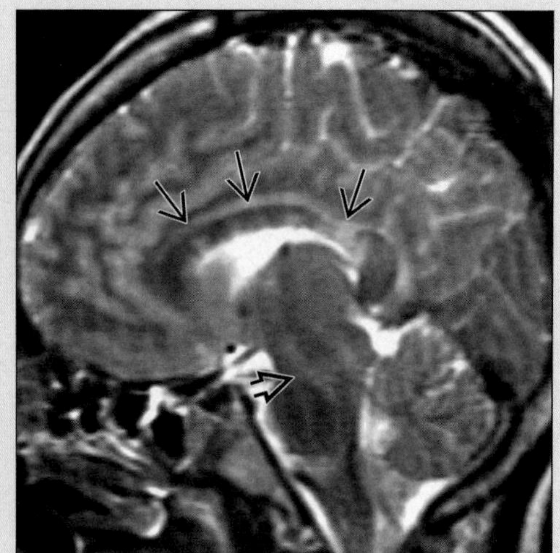

__(Left)__ Axial gross pathology section shows DAI with multiple punctate and linear hemorrhages in the subcortical and deep cerebral white matter ➔. Traumatic subarachnoid hemorrhage ⇨ and diffuse cerebral edema are also seen. (Courtesy R. Hewlett, PhD.) __(Right)__ Axial SWI in a patient with severe DAI shows multifocal cortical/ subcortical microhemorrhages ➔. The sensitivity of SWI for detecting microhemorrhage from DAI is impressive when compared to NECT or GRE. (Courtesy K. Tong, MD.)

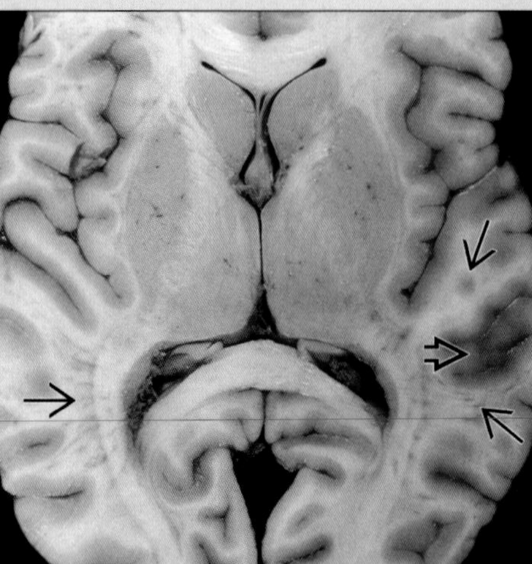

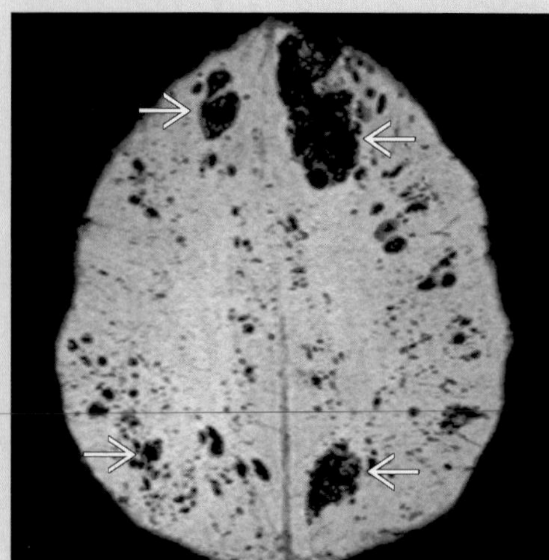

DIFFUSE AXONAL INJURY (DAI)

TERMINOLOGY

Abbreviations

- Diffuse axonal injury (DAI)
- Closed head injury (CHI)

Definitions

- Traumatic axonal stretch injury

IMAGING

General Features

- Best diagnostic clue
  - Punctate lesions at corticomedullary junction, corpus callosum, deep gray matter, brainstem
- Location
  - Gray-white matter (GM-WM) interface (67%), especially frontotemporal lobes
  - Corpus callosum (20%); 3/4 involve splenium/ undersurface of posterior body
  - Brainstem, especially dorsolateral midbrain and upper pons (poor prognosis)
  - Less common
    - Deep GM, internal/external capsule, tegmentum, fornix, corona radiata, cerebellar peduncles
- Size
  - Punctate to 15 mm
- Morphology
  - Punctate, round, ovoid foci; often hemorrhagic
  - Nearly always multiple bilateral lesions

CT Findings

- NECT
  - Often normal (50-80%)
    - > 30% with negative CT have positive MR
  - Nonhemorrhagic: Small hypodense foci
  - Hemorrhagic: Small hyperdense foci (20-50%)
  - 10-20% evolve to focal mass lesion with hemorrhagic/edema admixture
  - Repeat scans may reveal "new" lesions

MR Findings

- T1WI
  - Usually normal
  - If > 1 cm & hemorrhagic, hyperintense for 3-14 days
- T2WI
  - Nonhemorrhagic: Hyperintense foci
  - Hemorrhagic: Hypointense foci
- FLAIR
  - Nonhemorrhagic DAI: Hyperintense foci
  - Hemorrhagic DAI: Hypointense foci
- T2* GRE
  - Hypointense foci secondary to susceptibility from blood products
  - Multifocal hypointense foci may remain for years
  - Most sensitive "routine" sequence; microbleeds may be visible only on GRE
  - Number of GRE lesions correlates with intracranial hypertension and outcome
- DWI
  - May show hyperintense foci of restricted diffusion: ↓ apparent diffusion coefficient (ADC)
  - Diffusion tensor imaging (DTI)
    - Fractional anisotropy (FA) maps document integrity & direction of white matter tracts
    - Damage to white matter reduces anisotropy
      - Visible on FA maps
    - DTI "tractograms" allow delineation of white matter tract disruption pattern
      - Detect abnormalities when routine imaging, including GRE, is normal
- MRS
  - Normal-appearing brain
    - ↓ N-acetyl aspartate in WM 2° to neuronal injury
    - ↑ choline in GM suggestive of inflammation
  - Abnormal NAA/Cr and Cho/Cr accurately predicts outcomes in
    - Normal-appearing brain (85%)
    - Visibly injured brain (67%)
- SWI
  - Depicts significantly more DAI foci than GRE
  - Still not "routine" sequence, but becoming more common

Nuclear Medicine Findings

- PET
  - Hypometabolism in cingulate gyrus, lingual gyrus, and cuneus
    - Dysfunction of above regions plays key role in neuropsychologic deficits
- SPECT
  - May show focal perfusion abnormalities

Imaging Recommendations

- Best imaging tool
  - MR for detection
- Protocol advice
  - Nonhemorrhagic: FLAIR and DWI
  - Hemorrhagic: SWI best, but GRE best "routine" sequence

DIFFERENTIAL DIAGNOSIS

Multifocal Nonhemorrhagic Lesions

- Aging: No trauma history; leukoaraiosis & lacunes
- Demyelinating disease: Ovoid, may enhance
- Marchiafava-Bignami syndrome: Splenium lesion in patients with chronic alcoholism & poor nutrition
- Radiation therapy: May cause focal lesions of splenium

Multifocal Hemorrhagic Lesions

- Cerebral amyloid angiopathy: Elderly, normotensive
- Chronic hypertension: Older, hypertensive
- Cavernous malformations: Mixed-age hemorrhages
- Hemorrhagic tumors: Enhancing masses

PATHOLOGY

General Features

- Etiology
  - Overlying cortex moves at different speed in relation to underlying deep brain structures
    - Results in axonal stretching, particularly where brain tissues of different density intersect
  - Trauma-induced forces of inertia

DIFFUSE AXONAL INJURY (DAI)

  - Differential acceleration/deceleration and rotational/angular forces
  - Head impact not required
- Axons stretched, rarely disconnected or "sheared" (only in most severe injury)
- Effect on nondisruptively injured axons
  - Traumatic depolarization, ion fluxes, spreading depression, and excitatory amino acid release
  - Metabolic alterations with accelerated glycolysis and lactate accumulation
  - Cellular swelling, cytotoxic edema, and apoptosis
- Corpus callosum injury
  - Believed due to rotational shear/strain forces
  - Posterior falx prevents tissue displacement, allowing greater tensile stresses locally

- Genetics
  - Significant genomic responses to brain trauma
    - Induction of "immediate early genes"
    - Activation of signal transduction pathways
    - Apolipoprotein E (apoE) genotype, amyloid deposition may influence clinical outcome

Staging, Grading, & Classification

- Adams and Gennarelli staging
  - Stage 1: Frontal and temporal lobe GM/WM interface lesions (mild traumatic brain injury [TBI])
  - Stage 2: Lesions in lobar WM and corpus callosum (moderate TBI)
  - Stage 3: Lesions of dorsolateral midbrain and upper pons (severe TBI)
- Increasing severity of traumatic force correlates with deeper brain involvement

Gross Pathologic & Surgical Features

- Multiple, small, round, ovoid, linear lesions

Microscopic Features

- 80% of lesions are microscopic, nonhemorrhagic
  - Visible lesions are "tip of iceberg"
- Impaired axoplasmic transport, axonal swelling
- Axonal swelling 2° "axotomy" & "retraction" balls
- Microglial clusters
- Macro-, microbleeds (torn penetrating vessels)
- Wallerian degeneration

CLINICAL ISSUES

Presentation

- Most common signs/symptoms
  - Transient LOC, retrograde amnesia in mild TBI
  - LOC at moment of impact: Moderate to severe TBI
  - Immediate coma typical
    - Persistent vegetative state in severe cases
    - Slow recovery in many cases
  - Greater impairment than with cerebral contusions, intracerebral hematoma, extraaxial hematomas
- Clinical profile
  - Suggestive in patient with clinical symptoms disproportionate to imaging findings
  - Most common primary traumatic neuronal injury (48%)
    - Usually in setting of high velocity MVA
    - Admission GCS may not correlate with outcome

Demographics

- Age
  - Any, but most common in 15-24 year olds
  - May occur in utero if pregnant woman subjected to sufficient force
- Gender
  - Men 2x as likely to sustain traumatic brain injury; peaks at 20-24 years
- Epidemiology
  - 2,000,000 traumatic brain injuries annually in USA
  - Leading cause of death/disability in children and young adults
  - Approximately 50% of all primary intraaxial traumatic brain lesions in moderate and severe TBI
  - 80-100% autopsy prevalence in fatal injuries
  - Survivors incur annual cost of more than $40,000,000,000 ~ 0.5% of GNP

Natural History & Prognosis

- Spectrum of severity: Mild to severe
  - Mild TBI most common: Clinical abnormalities may persist for months or longer
    - Headache, memory & mild cognitive impairment, personality change (post-concussion syndrome)
- Severe DAI rarely causes death
  - > 90% remain in persistent vegetative state (brainstem spared)
  - Prognosis worsens as number of lesions increases
- 10% of patients who return to normal function do so within 1 year
  - May experience prolonged symptoms
- Brainstem damage (pontomedullary rent) associated with immediate or early death
- Neurocognitive deficits thought to persist in
  - 100% severe, 67% moderate, and 10% mild TBI
    - Figures may significantly underestimate sequelae of mild and moderate TBI

Treatment

- No real treatment; supportive therapy
- Treatment of comorbidities: Herniation, hemorrhage(s), hydrocephalus, seizures

DIAGNOSTIC CHECKLIST

Consider

- Consider DAI if symptoms are disproportionate to imaging findings

Image Interpretation Pearls

- Best detected by FLAIR (nonhemorrhagic) or SWI (hemorrhagic)

SELECTED REFERENCES

1. Yanagawa Y et al: Relationship between maximum intracranial pressure and traumatic lesions detected by T2*-weighted imaging in diffuse axonal injury. J Trauma. 66(1):162-5, 2009

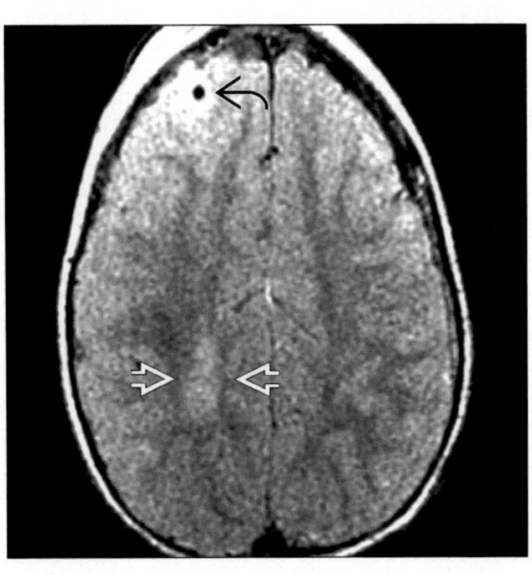

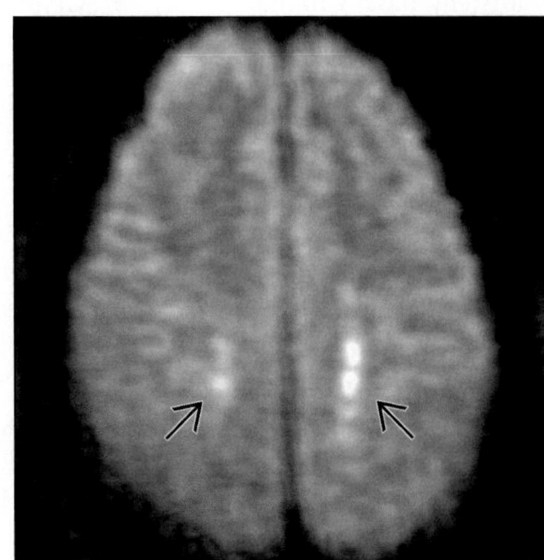

(Left) *Axial FLAIR MR shows a large, nonhemorrhagic, hyperintense diffuse axonal injury lesion with a more ovoid morphology ➡. An artifact from a ventriculostomy tube is also present ↪.* ***(Right)*** *Axial DWI MR reveals restriction within several bilateral diffuse axonal injury lesions, evidence of altered anisotropy ➡.*

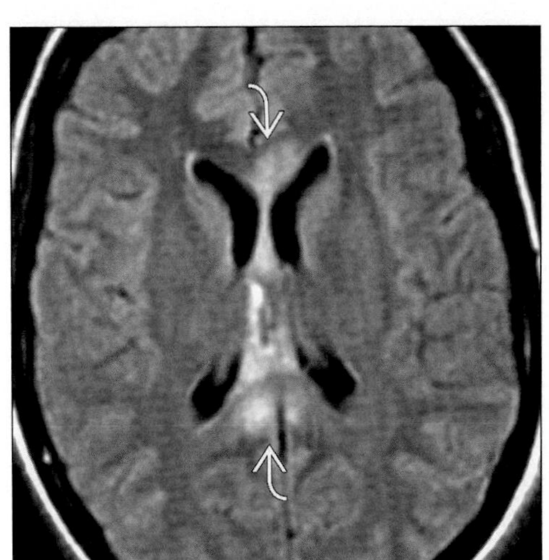

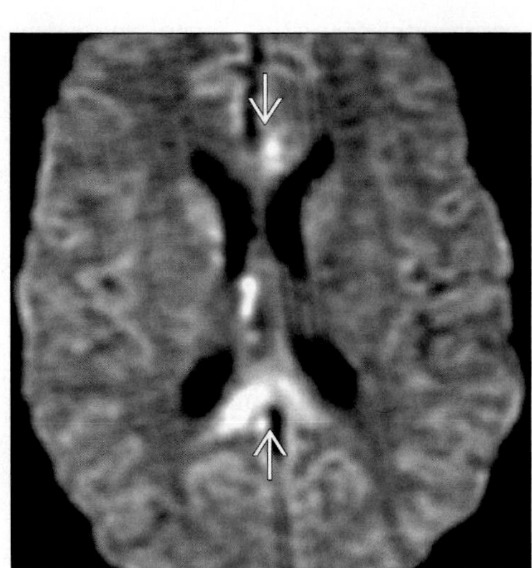

(Left) *Axial FLAIR MR reveals extensive traumatic injury involving nearly the entire corpus callosum ↪. There was also deeper midbrain injury (not shown).* ***(Right)*** *Axial DWI MR in the same patient demonstrates restriction within the corpus callosal lesions, evidence of altered anisotropy ➡.*

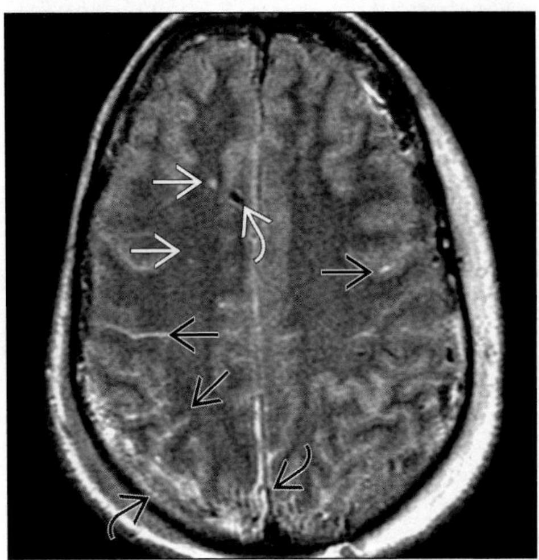

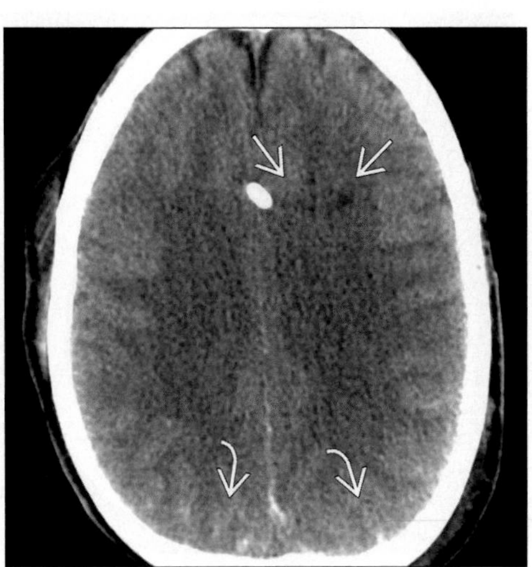

(Left) *Axial FLAIR MR shows nonhemorrhagic hyperintense foci of DAI ➡. These foci were not evident on GRE, although GRE revealed hemorrhagic DAI in the left frontal lobe that is not apparent on FLAIR. Note the subarachnoid hemorrhage ➡, subdural hematoma ↪, and ventriculostomy ↪.* ***(Right)*** *Axial NECT may show nonhemorrhagic DAI as focal hypodense abnormalities ➡ corresponding to T2 hyperintense edematous foci. Note the hyperdense subarachnoid hemorrhage ↪.*

SUBCORTICAL INJURY

Key Facts

Terminology
- SCI: Deep DAI lesions of brainstem, basal ganglia, thalamus, and regions around 3rd ventricle
- IVH: Hemorrhage within ventricular system
- CH: Hemorrhage localized to choroidal tissues

Imaging
- SCI: FLAIR most sensitive → hyperintense foci
- IVH: Hyperdense intraventricular blood; fluid-heme level common
- CH: Localized hyperdense choroidal hemorrhage

Top Differential Diagnoses
- SCI: Cavernous malformation, lacunar infarcts, small vessel ischemia
- IVH: None
- CH: Normal calcification may mask small hemorrhages

Pathology
- SCI: Most commonly induced by shear-strain forces that disrupt penetrating &/or choroidal vessels
- IVH: Disruption of subependymal veins
- CH: Traumatic shear forces damage to choroid tissue

Clinical Issues
- SCI: Profound neurologic deficits
- IVH: Obtundation, seizures
- CH: Can lead to IVH
- Treatment = supportive therapies; considerations of indirect/associated abnormalities (herniation, hematoma, hydrocephalus, seizures, etc.)

Diagnostic Checklist
- SCI: MR is superior to CT
- IVH/CH: CT is superior to MR

*(**Left**) Axial NECT shows a hyperdense hemorrhagic subcortical diffuse axonal injury lesion of the right middle cerebellar peduncle/cerebellar hemisphere ➔. (**Right**) Axial FLAIR MR reveals hyperintense subcortical injury of the tectum (on this slice, inferior colliculi) ➔ and adjacent vermis ➔. There is also a right temporal lobe hemorrhagic contusion ➔, as well as subarachnoid hemorrhage within many of the sulci ➔ and the interpeduncular fossa ➔.*

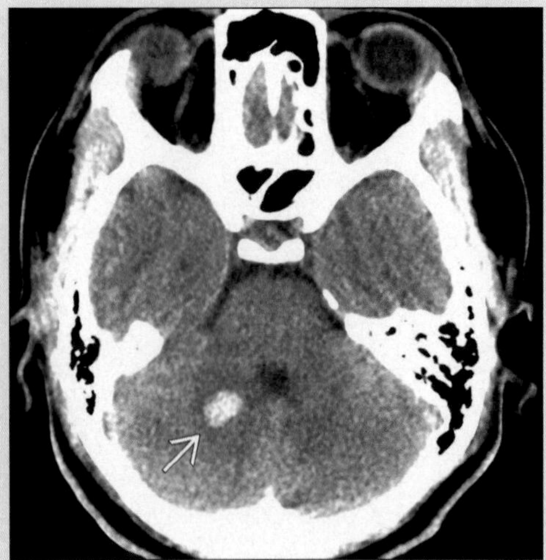

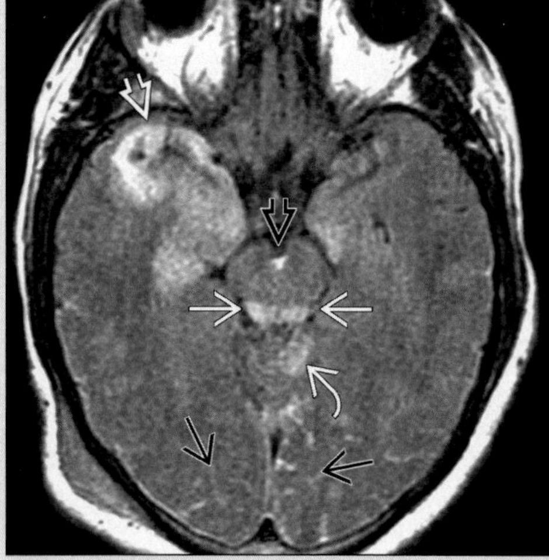

*(**Left**) Axial NECT shows a hyperdense choroidal hemorrhage within choroid plexus substance of both ventricles ➔. Note the subarachnoid hemorrhage ➔, corpus callosum DAI ➔, left caudate hemorrhagic DAI ➔, and a ventriculostomy tube tip ➔. (**Right**) Axial T2WI MR in the same patient shows hypointense hemorrhage distending the choroidal substance ➔. Note that the larger right choroidal hemorrhage bows the septum to the left ➔. A left caudate hemorrhagic DAI ➔ is again seen.*

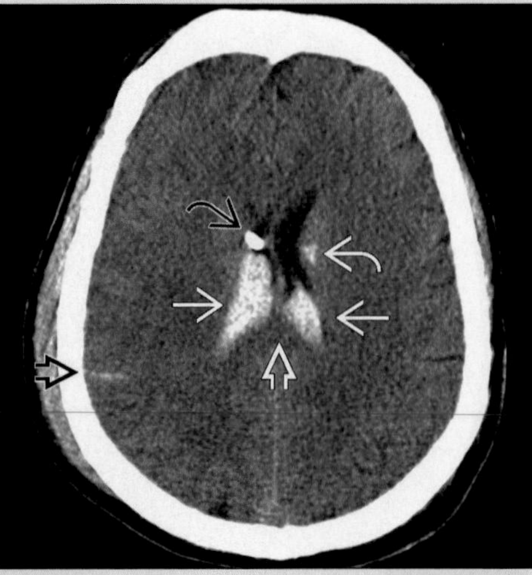

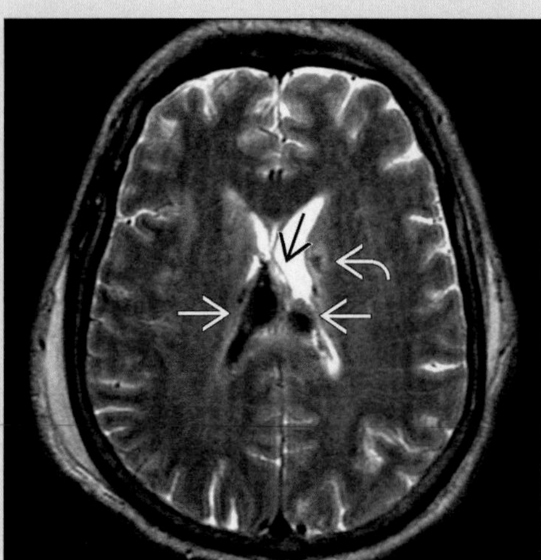

SUBCORTICAL INJURY

TERMINOLOGY

Abbreviations

- Subcortical injury (SCI)

Definitions

- Traumatic lesions of brainstem (BS), basal ganglia (BG), thalamus, and ventricles, composed of
  - Deep diffuse axonal injury type SCI lesions
  - Intraventricular hemorrhage (IVH)
  - Choroid hemorrhage (CH)

IMAGING

General Features

- Best diagnostic clue
  - SCI: Punctate hemorrhages
  - IVH: Hyperdense intraventricular CSF on NECT, fluid-heme level common
  - CH: Hyperdense, enlarged choroid on NECT
- Location
  - SCI = BS, BG, thalamus, and regions around 3rd ventricle
    - Most within thalamus and putamen
  - IVH: Intraventricular spaces
  - CH: Localized within choroid tissue
- Size
  - SCI: Limited to size of structure involved
  - IVH: Can fill/expand ventricles
  - CH: Limited to size of choroid involved
- Morphology
  - SCI: Petechial, linear, globular
  - IVH: Can cast ventricle
  - CH: Shape of choroid involved

CT Findings

- NECT
  - SCI: Often normal; petechial hyperdense foci
    - Deep nuclei, dorsolateral BS, periaqueductal
    - Rarely overt hemorrhage
  - IVH
    - Hyperdense intraventricular blood
    - May fill, even expand, ventricle
    - Fluid-heme level common
  - CH: Localized hyperdense choroidal hemorrhage

MR Findings

- T1WI
  - SCI: Acutely isointense
  - IVH: Fluid-heme level common
- T2WI
  - SCI: Acutely hyperintense
  - IVH: Fluid-heme
- FLAIR
  - SCI: Most sensitive sequence → hyperintense foci
  - IVH: Detection comparable to CT in acute stage
- T2* GRE
  - SCI: Susceptibility of petechial hemorrhage
- DWI
  - SCI: Foci of restricted diffusion
    - ↓ apparent diffusion coefficient (ADC)
    - Damage to white matter reduces anisotropy: Visible on FA maps
    - DTI "tractograms" allow delineation of pattern of white matter tract disruption
    - Detects abnormalities when routine imaging, including GRE, are normal
- SWI
  - Depicts significantly more DAI foci than GRE
  - Still not a "routine," may not alter care/prognosis

Imaging Recommendations

- Best imaging tool
  - SCI: MR > > > CT
    - Protocol analogous to DAI
  - ICH/CH: NECT > MR
    - Protocol analogous to subarachnoid hemorrhage
- Protocol advice
  - SCI: FLAIR and GRE
  - ICH/CH
    - CT = NECT
    - MR = FLAIR and GRE

DIFFERENTIAL DIAGNOSIS

Subcortical Injury

- Cavernous malformation: Symptoms without trauma
- Lacunar infarcts: Located in central tegmentum of pons/BS
- Small vessel ischemia

Intraventricular Hemorrhage

- ± choroid plexus hemorrhage

Choroid Hemorrhage

- Normal calcification may mask small hemorrhages

PATHOLOGY

General Features

- Etiology
  - SCI: Most commonly induced by shear-strain forces that disrupt penetrating &/or choroidal vessels
    - Usually very small, typically nonhemorrhagic
  - SCI: Less commonly
    - Dorsolateral BS impacts tentorial incisura with violent brain motion
    - Anterorostral BS damaged with sudden craniocaudal brain displacement
  - IVH
    - Disruption of subependymal veins (most common)
    - Bleeding from choroid plexus
    - Shearing injuries
    - Basal ganglia/intracerebral hemorrhage with rupture into ventricles
    - Isolated IVH in absence of parenchymal hematoma is unusual
  - CH: Traumatic shear forces damage to choroid tissue
- Associated abnormalities
  - SCI: All stages of DAI present (without exception), cerebral contusion, intracranial hemorrhages
  - IVH: DAI, deep GM/BS/intracerebral hemorrhage, SAH, cerebral contusion, hydrocephalus
  - CH: DAI, SAH, cerebral contusion

SUBCORTICAL INJURY

Staging, Grading, & Classification

- SCI: BS injury (BSI)
  - Primary injury: Direct result of trauma
    - DAI; most common primary BSI
    - Direct laceration/contusion; rare
    - Multiple primary petechial hemorrhages; not associated with more superficial DAI
    - Pontomedullary rent or separation; may occur without widespread brain injury
  - Secondary injury: Indirect result of trauma, most common cause of BSI; usually herniation
- SCI: When BSI → BS hemorrhage
  - Group 1: Midline rostral anterior BS, posterior to interpeduncular cistern (69%)
    - Associated with anterior impact; 71% survival
  - Group 2: Misc foci of acute BS hemorrhage (18%)
    - Associated with transtentorial herniation and BS compression; 88% survival
  - Group 3: Any BS hemorrhage
    - Associated with transtentorial herniation and BS compression; 100% mortality

Gross Pathologic & Surgical Features

- SCI
  - Usually nonhemorrhagic, yet more often hemorrhagic than other 1° intraaxial injuries
  - 2° to rich network of perforating vessels in basal ganglia and thalamus
- IVH
  - Gross blood collected within ventricular system
  - Blood-CSF level common
    - Layering, rather than clot formation, likely relates to intrinsic antithrombotic CSF properties due to high concentrations of fibrinolytic activators
  - May cast/expand involved ventricle
- CH: Hemorrhagic choroid tissue

Microscopic Features

- SCI: Petechial hemorrhages
- IVH: Expected evolutionary hemoglobin changes different than described for intracerebral hematoma
  - High ambient CSF, O_2 tension delays progression
- CH: Blood extravasated into choroid tissue

CLINICAL ISSUES

Presentation

- Most common signs/symptoms
  - SCI: Profound neurologic deficits
    - Low initial Glasgow coma scale scores; coma
  - IVH: Obtundation, seizures

Demographics

- Age
  - Any, but most common in 15-24 year olds
- Gender
  - Men 2x as likely to sustain traumatic brain injury (TBI); peaks at 20-24 years
- Epidemiology
  - SCI: In 5-10% TBI, 3rd most common 1° traumatic neuronal injury
  - IVH: Present in 60% of patients with corpus callosal DAI, 12% in patients without

Natural History & Prognosis

- SCI: Severely injured patients
  - Poor prognosis, often die soon after trauma
  - Regain consciousness very slowly and retain permanent neurological impairment/disability
- SCI: May proceed to BS hemorrhage
  - Associated with high mortality
- IVH
  - Gradually clears as resorbed, although patients > 20 cc of blood do poorly
  - Hydrocephalus rare manifestation
    - Early: CSF outlet obstruction
      - Obstructive, noncommunicating
      - Asymmetric ventricular dilatation
    - Late: Arachnoid dysfunction of CSF resorption
      - Obstructive, communicating hydrocephalus
      - Symmetric ventricular dilatation
  - Hemorrhagic dilation of 4th ventricle: Ominous predictor with 100% reported mortality
  - At baseline, predicts 2x increase in mortality
    - Does not predict functional outcome
- CH: Can lead to IVH

Treatment

- SCI
  - Supportive therapy
  - Treatment considerations of indirect/associated abnormalities: Herniation, hematoma, hydrocephalus, seizures, etc.
- IVH
  - Ventriculostomy
  - Excellent results following r-TPA thrombolytic therapy
    - Effective and safe, despite preexisting multiple hemorrhagic intracranial injuries
  - Repeat NECT to evaluate for hydrocephalus, treatment complications

DIAGNOSTIC CHECKLIST

Consider

- Patients with SCI have experienced severe trauma and are often highly complex cases with a multitude of abnormal findings
  - When you think you have finished reviewing the case, look at everything 1 more time!

Image Interpretation Pearls

- SCI: MR is superior to CT
- IVH/CH: CT is superior to MR

SELECTED REFERENCES

1. Mamere AE et al: Evaluation of delayed neuronal and axonal damage secondary to moderate and severe traumatic brain injury using quantitative MR imaging techniques. AJNR Am J Neuroradiol. 30(5):947-52, 2009
2. Tian HL et al: Risk factors related to hydrocephalus after traumatic subarachnoid hemorrhage. Surg Neurol. 69(3):241-6; discussion 246, 2008

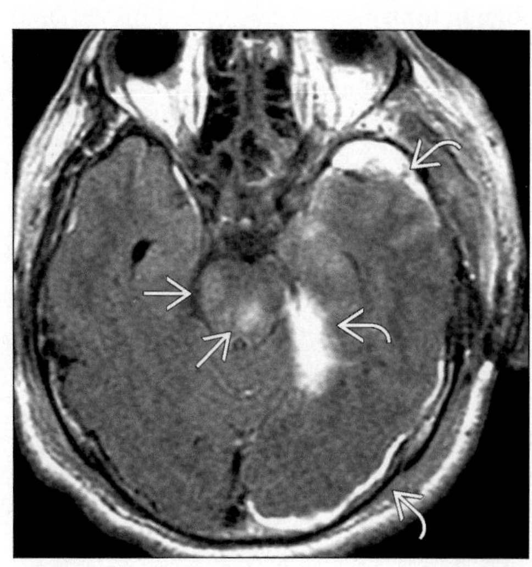

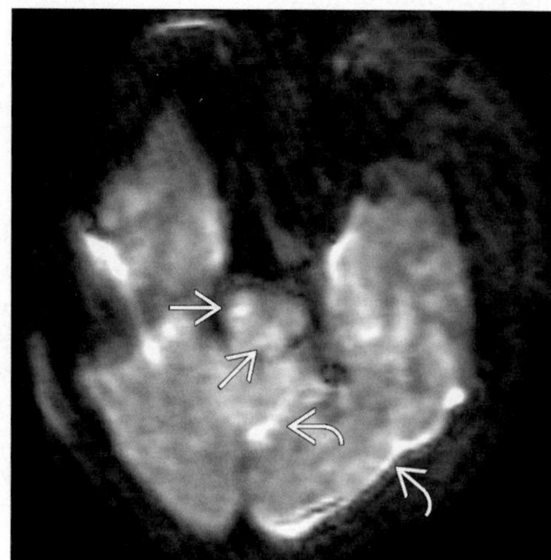

(Left) *Axial FLAIR MR demonstrates subcortical injury DAI lesions in the midbrain →. There are also subdural hematomas ↶. Not shown are DAI of bilateral cerebral peduncles, as well as the left caudate, internal capsule, and anterior lentiform nuclei. Also not seen are bifrontal and bitemporal hemorrhagic cortical contusions.* ***(Right)*** *Axial DWI MR in the same patient shows diffusion abnormality of the midbrain SCI DAI lesions →. Note the subdural hematomas ↶.*

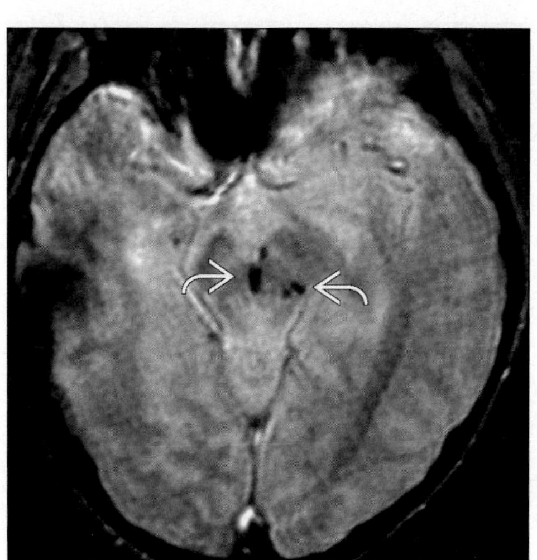

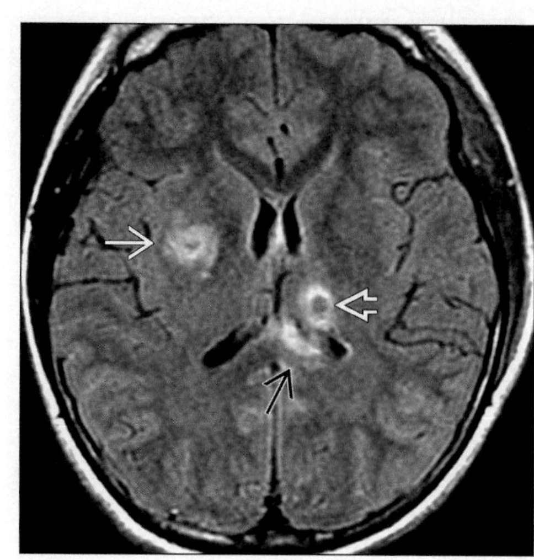

(Left) *Axial T2* GRE MR shows susceptibility of SCI DAI hemorrhage involving the midbrain and left cerebral peduncle ↶. The patient had corresponding hemiplegia.* ***(Right)*** *Axial FLAIR MR in the same patient reveals more SCI DAI lesions involving the right lentiform nuclei →, left thalamus ⇨, and corpus callosum →.*

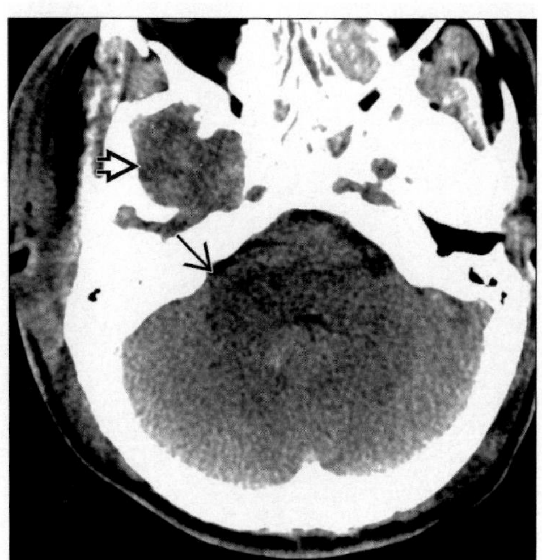

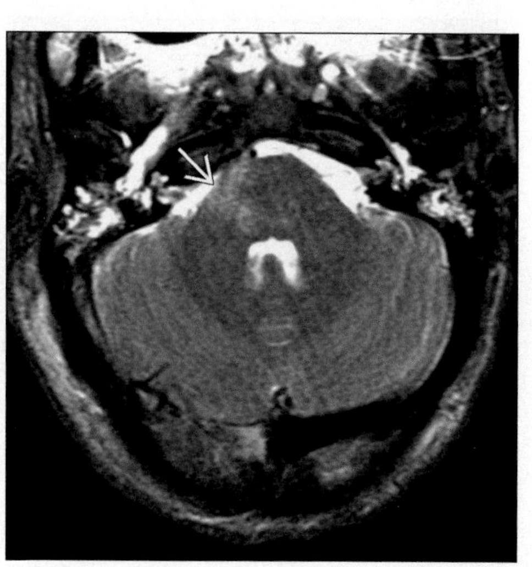

(Left) *Axial NECT reveals SCI DAI as subtle CT hypodense abnormality involving the right middle cerebellar peduncle and pons →. There is also abnormal hypodensity from a right temporal contusion ⇨. Not shown are additional lesions of the midbrain, right thalamus, and corpus callosum, as well as bifrontal and left occipital lobe contusions.* ***(Right)*** *Axial T2WI MR in the same patient better shows the right middle cerebellar peduncle/pontine lesion →.*

BIRTH TRAUMA

Key Facts

Terminology

- Birth trauma = injury sustained by infant during labor and delivery due to mechanical forces

Imaging

- Caput succedaneum
- Subgaleal hematoma
- Cephalohematoma
- Fracture
- Sutural diastasis
- Epidural hematoma
- Subdural hematoma
- Subarachnoid hemorrhage
- Contusion
- MR T2* SWI for blood products; DWI for cellular injury; MRV to rule out venous thrombosis

Top Differential Diagnoses

- Hypoxic ischemic injury
- Arterial ischemic stroke
- Venous thrombosis/edema/infarct
- Vascular anomaly
- Coagulopathy

Clinical Issues

- M > F
- Birth trauma incidence = 2.6 per 1,000 live births reported in USA in 2004 (based on hospital records)
- Subgaleal hematoma may be associated with significant blood loss; check for coagulopathy
- Subdural hematomas reported in 46% of asymptomatic neonates (parafalcine > occipital > tentorial and posterior fossa) based on MR

*(**Left**) Oblique NECT in this 1 day old delivered by spontaneous vaginal delivery shows a hyperintense cephalohematoma ➔ that is lens-shaped and does not cross suture lines. A serosanguinous subgaleal hematoma ➔ is also present. Note that the subgaleal collection crosses suture in the midline. (**Right**) Axial bone CT in a 4 day old shows a linear fracture ➔ in the right parietal bone. A cephalohematoma ➔ overlies the fracture. Note that the cephalohematoma does not cross the sutures.*

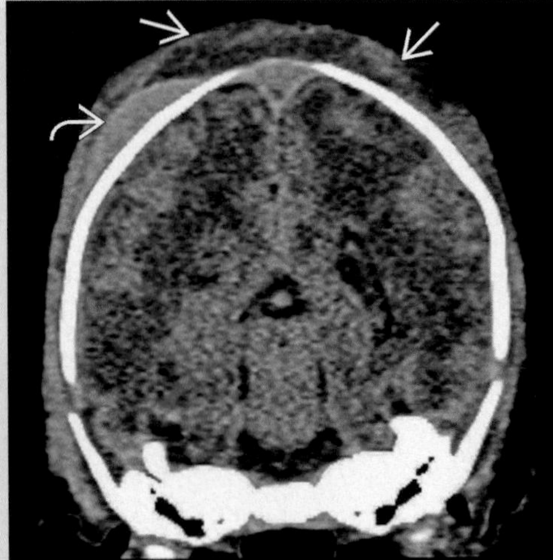

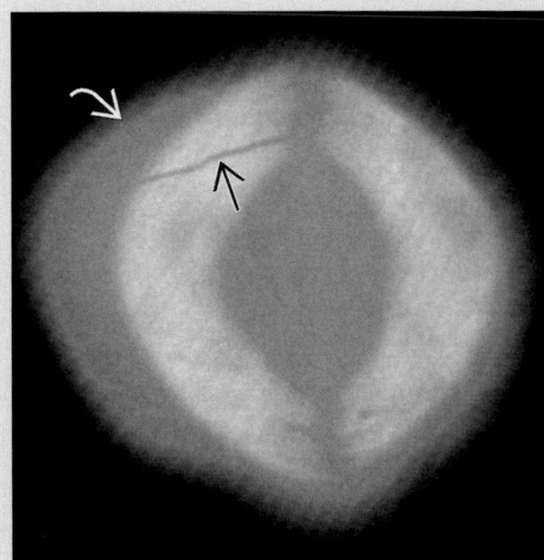

*(**Left**) Axial T2* SWI MR in 3 day old after vacuum extraction shows multifocal subarachnoid hemorrhage ➔ and parenchymal hemorrhage ➔. A subgaleal ➔ and small subdural ➔ hematoma are present. (**Right**) Axial DWI MR in the same 3 day old shows multifocal hyperintensity ➔ that corresponded to decreased diffusivity on ADC map (not shown). Low signal is seen in the subarachnoid space ➔ due to the subarachnoid hemorrhage with the T2 effects of blood dominating the signal.*

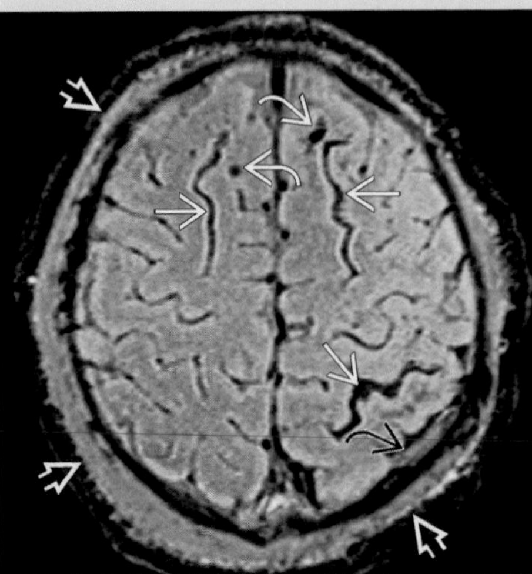

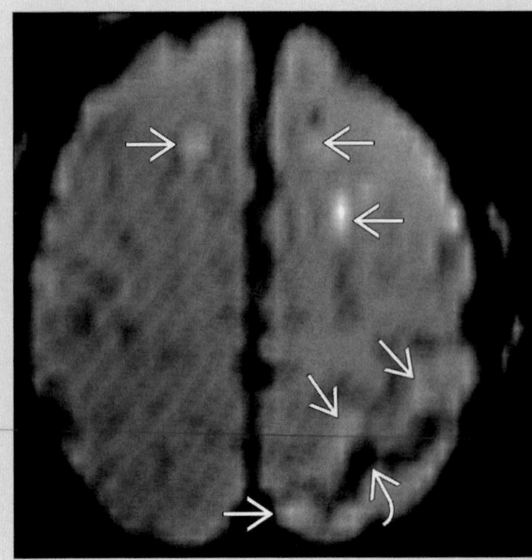

TERMINOLOGY

Definitions

- Injury sustained by infant during labor and delivery due to mechanical forces

IMAGING

General Features

- Best diagnostic clue
  - Imaging shows evidence of injuries caused by mechanical forces
- Location
  - Soft tissues
    - Caput succedaneum
    - Subgaleal hematoma
  - Skull
    - Cephalohematoma
    - Fracture
    - Sutural diastasis
  - Extracerebral/intracranial hemorrhage
    - Epidural hematoma
    - Subdural hematoma (SDH)
    - Subarachnoid hemorrhage
    - Subpial hemorrhage
  - Brain parenchymal injury
    - Hemorrhage/contusion
- Morphology
  - Caput succedaneum
    - Superficial serosanguineous collection that crosses suture lines
  - Subgaleal hematoma
    - Hemorrhage beneath aponeurosis of scalp that crosses suture lines
  - Cephalohematoma
    - Hemorrhage beneath periosteum that does not cross sutures
    - Check for skull fracture
  - Fracture
    - Linear (usually parietal) or depressed ("ping-pong" lesion with inward buckling)
    - Check for associated intracranial hemorrhage and brain injury
  - Sutural diastasis
    - Separation of calvarial bones ("molding")
  - Epidural hematoma
    - Lens-shaped extraaxial collection of blood
    - Often associated with cephalohematoma or skull fracture
  - Subdural hematoma
    - Crescent-shaped
  - Subarachnoid hemorrhage
    - Follows sulci
  - Subpial hemorrhage
    - Immediately adjacent to cortex without expected spread of subarachnoid hemorrhage
  - Parenchymal hemorrhage/contusion
    - Blood products, edema, or ischemia in peripheral cerebral or cerebellar parenchyma

Imaging Recommendations

- Best imaging tool
  - CT for fractures
  - MR for soft tissue and intracranial injuries
  - US underestimates or misses lesions
- Protocol advice
  - Reformats with minimum intensity projections for CT to differentiate fracture from suture variants
  - MR T2* SWI for blood products
  - DWI for cellular injury
  - MRV if hemorrhage to rule out venous thrombosis

DIFFERENTIAL DIAGNOSIS

Hypoxic Ischemic Injury

- Bilateral, typically symmetric, bright DWI and low ADC
- Rarely hemorrhage
- Etiology is global transient lack of arterial blood flow and oxygen
  - Not directly caused by, but may be associated with, birth trauma

Arterial Ischemic Stroke

- If small, difficult to differentiate from contusion/venous ischemic necrosis caused by birth trauma
- Rarely associated with hemorrhage

Venous Edema/Hemorrhage/Infarct

- Etiology unclear as venous thrombosis not always detected; mechanical compression is possible cause

Vascular Anomaly

- If parenchymal hemorrhage but no signs of trauma, consider arteriovenous malformation or cavernous malformation

Coagulopathy

- Can be primary or secondary to large hemorrhage
- If hemorrhage, consider coagulopathy screen

Metabolic Disorders

- Rarely hemorrhagic
- Consider if severity of parenchymal injury out of proportion to clinical history

CLINICAL ISSUES

Presentation

- Most common signs/symptoms
  - Majority asymptomatic
  - Signs/symptoms may be predominantly from associated injuries
    - Hypoxic ischemic injury
    - Arterial ischemic stroke
  - Severe birth trauma may cause
    - Seizures
    - Apnea
    - ↑ ICP (bulging fontanelles)
  - Subgaleal hematoma
    - May cause significant blood loss
    - Check for coagulopathy
  - Subdural hematoma
    - Occipital osteodiastasis → severe, life-threatening hemorrhage (rare)

BIRTH TRAUMA

Demographics

- Gender
  - M > F
- Epidemiology
  - Birth trauma incidence = 2.6 per 1,000 live births reported in USA in 2004 (based on hospital records)
  - Birth trauma causes ~ 2% of all neonatal deaths
  - Can be seen in normal spontaneous births but higher incidence in
    - Neonates > 4500 g
    - Instrumental deliveries (midcavity forceps, vacuum extraction)
    - Vaginal breech delivery
    - Excessive traction during delivery
    - Prolonged or rapid delivery
  - Subgaleal hematoma incidence 0.6 per 1,000 deliveries, 4.6 per 1,000 vacuum-assisted deliveries
  - Cephalohematoma occurs in 1-2% of spontaneous vaginal deliveries
  - Sutural diastasis has unknown incidence and significance
  - Intracranial hemorrhage (ICH) reported as low as 5-6 live births per 10,000; more recent MR-based studies indicate incidence up to 46% following spontaneous vaginal delivery
  - Subdural hematomas reported in 46% of asymptomatic neonates (parafalcine > occipital > tentorial and posterior fossa) based on MR

Natural History & Prognosis

- Caput succedaneum
  - Resolves in days, typically no sequelae
- Subgaleal hematoma
  - Resolves in 2-3 weeks, typically no sequelae
  - Most patients do well but potential for significant blood loss and secondary coagulopathy
- Cephalohematoma
  - Resolves in weeks to months, typically no sequelae
  - Resolves by calcification, skull remodeling
    - Do not mistake for fibrous dysplasia
- Sutural diastasis
  - Incidence and significance unclear
  - Occipital osteodiastasis associated with severe SDH
- Epidural hematoma
  - Associated with difficult delivery, breech delivery, and instrumental delivery in nulliparous women
  - If small, resolve without sequelae
- Subdural hematoma
  - Probably caused by tentorial laceration (tentorial SDH), occipital osteodiastasis (posterior fossa SDH), falx laceration (falx SDH), superficial cerebral vein laceration (convexity SDH)
  - Can occur in cesarian section without labor
  - Asymptomatic SDH very common in spontaneous vaginal delivery
  - Vast majority of asymptomatic SDH < 3 mm do not rebleed and resolve by 4 weeks with no sequelae
  - If large, monitor closely due to risk of posterior fossa compression
  - Associated with cephalohematomas
  - Associated with prolonged 2nd stage of labor
  - 60-80% of symptomatic SDH have normal outcome
- Subarachnoid hemorrhage
  - Due to rupture of bridging veins or involuting anastomoses between leptomeningeal arteries and therefore self limited
  - Not due to large vessel arterial rupture, as is more common in adults
  - Associated with skull fractures
  - In isolation, excellent prognosis
- Subpial hemorrhage
  - Unique to neonates due to more fragile pial-brain adhesion
  - Probably occur secondary to extension of parenchymal hemorrhage
    - Prognosis depends on severity of associated parenchymal hemorrhage
- Parenchymal hemorrhage/contusion
  - Primary hemorrhage/hemorrhagic venous infarction or compressive cellular injury
  - Associated with subarachnoid hemorrhage, subpial hemorrhage, cephalohematoma
  - Often no associated skull fracture but may be associated with sutural diastasis
  - Typically volume loss/encephalomalacia on follow-up

Treatment

- Vast majority require no treatment
- Depressed skull fractures may require surgical intervention
- Large hemorrhages may require surgical intervention for decompression

DIAGNOSTIC CHECKLIST

Image Interpretation Pearls

- Small SDH, frequently identified in spontaneous vaginal delivery, of no consequence

Reporting Tips

- Reserve term "birth trauma" for injuries due to mechanical forces

SELECTED REFERENCES

1. Doumouchtsis SK et al: Head trauma after instrumental births. Clin Perinatol. 35(1):69-83, viii, 2008
2. Rooks VJ et al: Prevalence and evolution of intracranial hemorrhage in asymptomatic term infants. AJNR Am J Neuroradiol. 29(6):1082-9, 2008
3. Volpe JJ: Injuries of extracranial, cranial, intracranial, spinal cord and peripheral nervous system structures. In: Neurology of the Newborn. 5th ed. Philadelphia: W.B. Saunders. 959-985, 2008
4. Eichler F et al: Magnetic resonance imaging evaluation of possible neonatal sinovenous thrombosis. Pediatr Neurol. 37(5):317-23, 2007
5. Looney CB et al: Intracranial hemorrhage in asymptomatic neonates: prevalence on MR images and relationship to obstetric and neonatal risk factors. Radiology. 242(2):535-41, 2007
6. Noetzel MJ: Perinatal trauma and cerebral palsy. Clin Perinatol. 33(2):355-66, 2006
7. Huang AH et al: Spontaneous superficial parenchymal and leptomeningeal hemorrhage in term neonates. AJNR Am J Neuroradiol. 2004 Mar;25(3):469-75. Erratum in: AJNR Am J Neuroradiol. 35(4):666, 2004

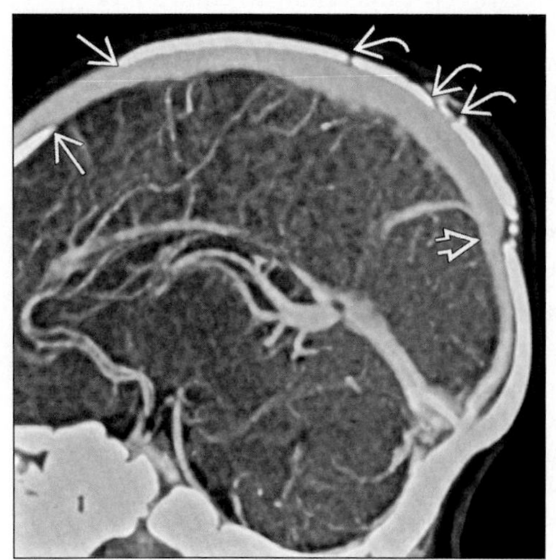

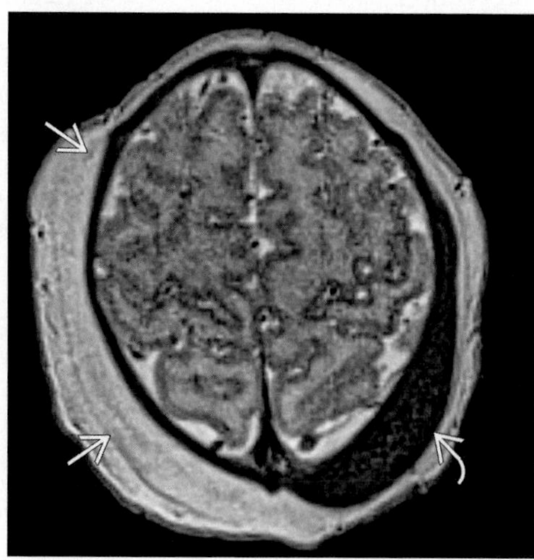

(Left) *Sagittal CTV in this 2-day-old neonate after induced vaginal delivery shows coronal sutural diastasis → and parietal skull fractures ⤻. Note the normal narrowing of the superior sagittal sinus at the lambda ⇨; this narrowing is always seen when neonates lie supine for imaging.* ***(Right)*** *Axial T2WI MR in this 1 day old after forceps delivery shows a left cephalohematoma ⤻ that does not cross suture lines and a large right serosanguineous subgaleal hematoma →.*

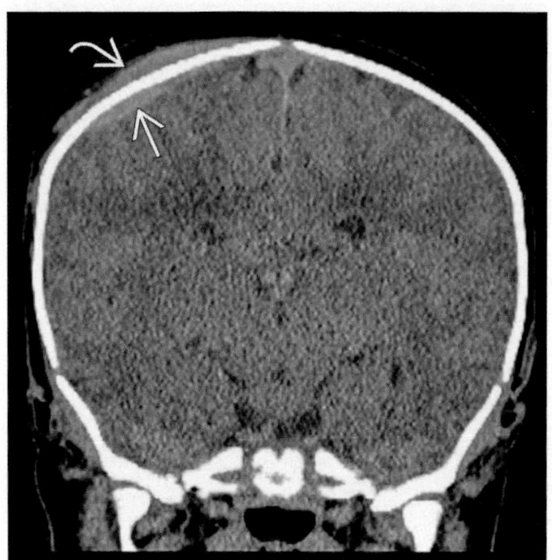

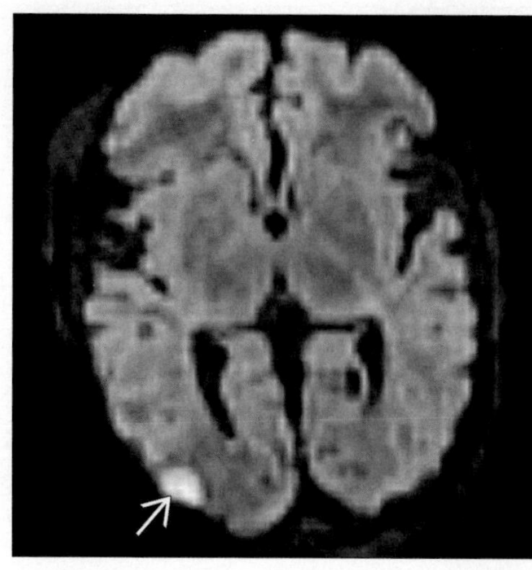

(Left) *Coronal reformat of NECT in a 4 day old shows a cephalohematoma ⤻ and adjacent epidural hematoma →. The associated linear skull fracture was evident on the bone windows (not shown).* ***(Right)*** *Axial DWI MR in this 1 day old after forceps delivery shows a focus of increased signal → that corresponded to decreased diffusion on the corresponding ADC map (not shown). This lesion was immediately below the diastased lambdoid suture and is likely a contusion.*

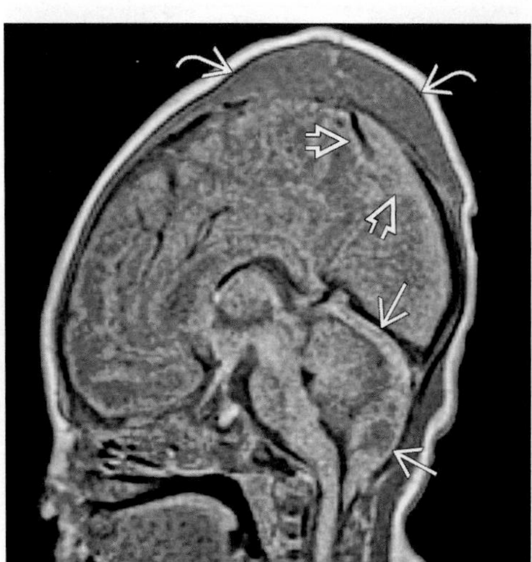

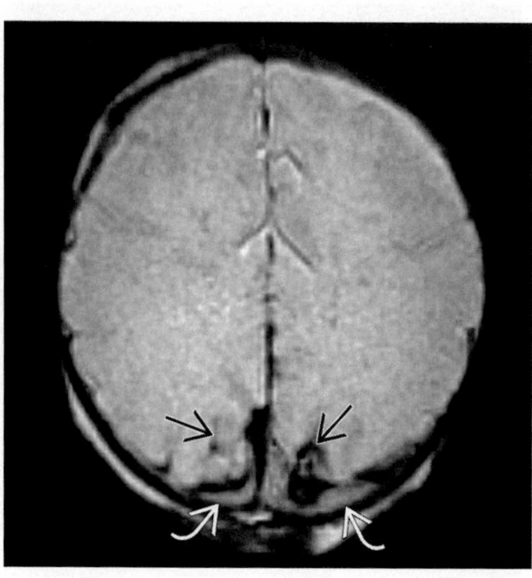

(Left) *Sagittal T1WI MR in a 2 day old with a history of oligohydramnios and precipitous delivery shows a large isointense posterior fossa subdural hematoma (SDH) → and a large subgaleal hematoma that crosses suture lines ⤻. The interhemispheric SDH is difficult to see on this sequence ⇨.* ***(Right)*** *Axial T2* GRE MR in a 2 day old with a history of oligohydramnios and precipitous delivery shows bilateral parietal SDHs ⤻ and adjacent subarachnoid and subpial blood →.*

CHILD ABUSE

Key Facts

Imaging
- Multiple brain injuries disproportionally severe relative to proffered history
- NECT is primary imaging tool in initial evaluation of child abuse
  - Highly sensitive in detection and characterization of intracranial hemorrhage
  - Sensitive in detection and characterization of fractures
- Delayed (24-72 hours) MR may be most sensitive for detection of parenchymal injuries
  - Sagittal T1WI helpful for detecting small SDH along tentorium
  - PD/intermediate sequence is very sensitive in detection of small SDH
  - DWI is key sequence for identification of parenchymal insult

Pathology
- Direct impact injury: Direct blow to cranium or impact of skull on object
  - Skull fractures and injury to immediately underlying brain
- Shaking injury: Violent "to and fro" shaking of head
  - Diffusely distributed subdural hematomas
- Ischemic injury
  - Varies from global hypoxic brain injury to individual vascular territory infarction

Clinical Issues
- 17-25:100,000 annual incidence
  - Most common cause of traumatic death in infancy: 1,200 deaths per year in USA
- 1/3 of perpetrators under influence of alcohol or drugs
- Mortality = 15-38% (60% if coma at presentation)

__(Left)__ Axial NECT in this 12 week old with rib, skull, and humerus fractures and a duodenal hematoma shows a moderate subdural hematoma over the right cerebral hemisphere ➔, with a small amount of subdural blood on the left, causing a pseudo "empty delta" sign of the sagittal sinus ⇨. __(Right)__ Axial bone CT in a 4 month old shows multiple fractures ➔ in the right parietal bone. Fractures that cross suture lines or are comminuted are more suspicious for NAT than linear nondisplaced fractures.

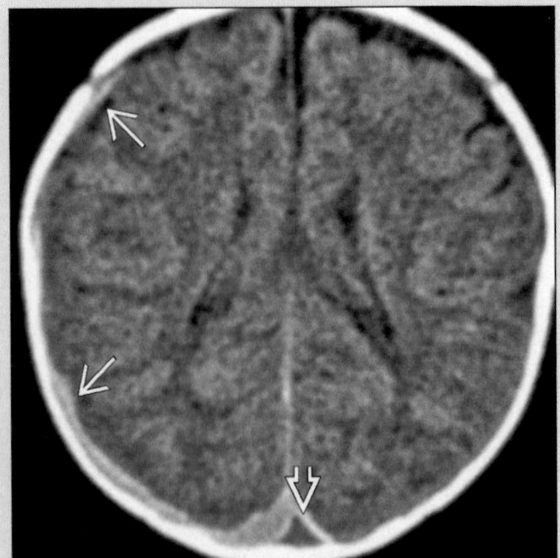

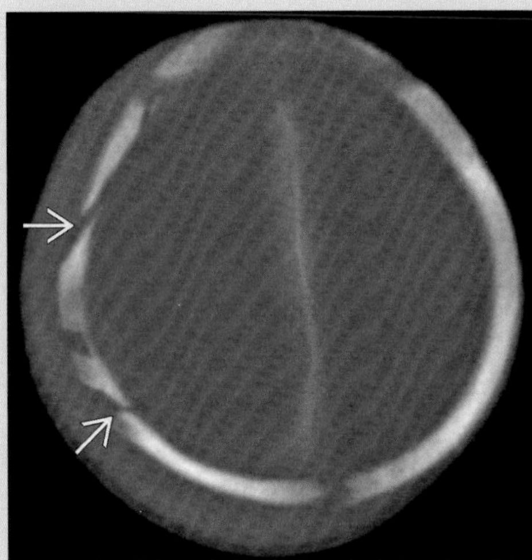

__(Left)__ Axial PD/intermediate MR in this 4 month old shows symmetric subdural collections over each frontal lobe that are hyperintense compared to CSF. A darker rim of normal CSF ➔ separates the hematomas from the underlying brain parenchyma. __(Right)__ Axial T1WI MR in a 3 month old approximately 5 days after presentation with bifrontal subdural hematomas shows blood layering in the subdural space over the occipital poles ➔ and hemorrhagic staining of infarcted cortex on the left ⇨.

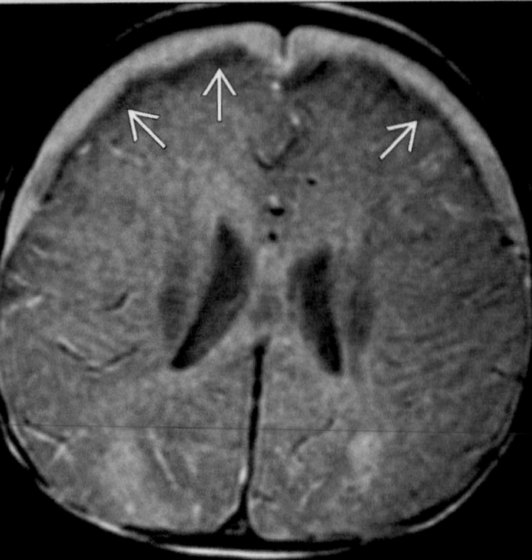

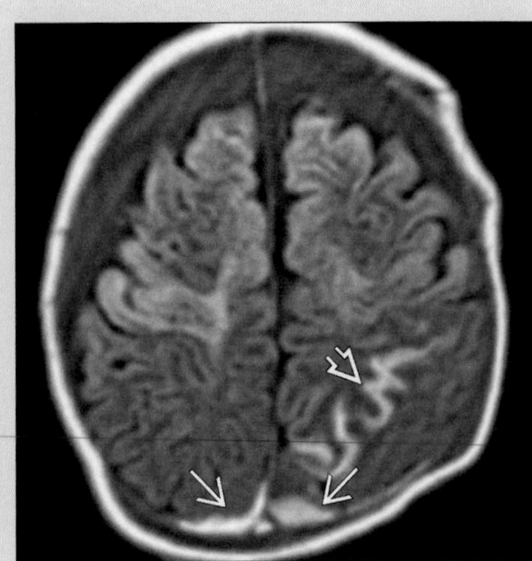

CHILD ABUSE

TERMINOLOGY

Abbreviations

- Nonaccidental trauma (NAT), nonaccidental injury (NAI), shaken-baby syndrome (SBS), nonaccidental head injury (NAHI), rule out parental abuse (ROPA)

Synonyms

- Caffey-Kempe syndrome, whiplash shaken-infant syndrome, trauma-x
  - Multiple synonyms and acronyms reflect sensitivity to social and criminal ramifications of diagnosis

Definitions

- Intentionally inflicted brain injury

IMAGING

General Features

- Best diagnostic clue
  - Multiple brain injuries disproportionally severe relative to proffered history
    - Spectrum of findings, including scalp injuries, skull fractures, intracranial hemorrhages, cerebral contusions, shear injuries, ischemic brain injury

Radiographic Findings

- Radiography
  - Sensitive for detection of skull fractures
    - Generally obtained as part of skeletal survey

CT Findings

- NECT
  - Primary imaging tool in initial evaluation of child abuse
  - Sensitive in detection and characterization of fractures
    - Helical technique with multiplanar reformatting essential in order to detect fractures in axial plane
  - Highly sensitive in detection and characterization of intracranial hemorrhage
    - Subdural hemorrhage (SDH): > 50% of cases
      - Dominant feature of shaking injury
      - Over cerebral convexities, in interhemispheric fissure, overlying tentorium
    - Subarachnoid hemorrhage (SAH): ≤ 50% of cases
      - More common in sulci over convexities; differs from SAH associated with aneurysms, which is more common in basal cisterns
    - Intraventricular hemorrhage (IVH)
    - Epidural hemorrhage (EDH) uncommon in child abuse
    - Shear injuries
      - Typical locations include corticomedullary junction, brainstem, corpus callosum
      - May not be hemorrhagic
    - Cortical contusions
      - Surface of frontal and temporal lobes
      - Hyperattenuating; develop "halo" of edema over 1st few days
      - Focal atrophy chronically
  - Ischemic injury
    - Varies from global hypoxic brain injury to individual vascular territory infarction
    - Actual etiology uncertain
    - Reversal sign: White matter appears more dense than gray matter
      - Indicates severe (irreversible) injury
  - Subdural hygromas can develop 12-36 hours after injury
    - CSF-density subdural collections of CSF that leak from subarachnoid space
    - Resolve without direct treatment
- CTA
  - Helpful in detection of arterial injuries complicating abuse
    - Vascular injuries may manifest in delayed fashion

MR Findings

- T1WI
  - Variable signal of blood products
    - SDH most often bright
    - Sagittal T1WI helpful for detecting small SDH along tentorium
  - May see hyperintensity of cortical ribbon → petechial hemorrhage vs. laminar necrosis
- T2WI
  - Ischemic insult in neonates and infants manifest as loss of cortical ribbon
- PD/intermediate
  - Very sensitive in detection of small SDH
  - Often identifies periventricular injury better than FLAIR or T2WI in neonates and infants
- T2* GRE
  - Highly sensitive for presence of chronic blood products
    - May help detect sites of prior injury
- DWI
  - Key sequence for identification of parenchymal insult
- MRA
  - May identify/characterize arterial injury
- MRS
  - ↓ NAA, ↑ Cho/Cr ratio, ↓ Cr, ↑ lactate/lipid peaks poor prognostic indicators
    - May be normal in 1st 24 hours
- May be difficult to obtain MR in acute setting
  - More difficult to monitor unstable patient
  - Requires sedation/anesthesia
- Delayed (24-72 hours) MR may be most sensitive for detection of parenchymal injuries

Nuclear Medicine Findings

- Bone scan
  - Occasionally used to document associated skeletal injury
    - Can miss skull fractures, metaphyseal injuries

Imaging Recommendations

- Best imaging tool
  - NECT for acute assessment
- Protocol advice
  - Use multiplanar reformats to assess for fractures
  - MR at 24-72 hours
    - Use DWI to assess parenchymal injury
    - Use PD/intermediate sequence to look for white matter (WM) injury and small SDH in infants
    - MRA/MRV to assess vascular injury

CHILD ABUSE

DIFFERENTIAL DIAGNOSIS

Accidental Trauma
- Appropriate history for degree of injury

Mitochondrial Encephalopathies
- Glutaric acidurias (types 1 & 2), Menkes syndrome

Overshunting
- "Passive" subdurals secondary to collapse of ventricular system

Meningitis
- Subdural empyemas or sympathetic effusions

Coagulopathies
- Intracranial hemorrhage from normal activities

Neuroblastoma
- May present with "raccoon eyes," mimicking skull base fracture
- Epidural metastatic disease can mimic SDH

PATHOLOGY

General Features
- Etiology
  - Injuries can be divided into 2 major groupings
    - Direct impact injury: Direct blow to cranium or impact of skull on object
      - Skull fractures and injury to immediately underlying brain
    - Shaking injury: Violent "to and fro" shaking of head
      - Diffusely distributed subdural hematomas

CLINICAL ISSUES

Presentation
- Most common signs/symptoms
  - Discordance between stated history and degree of injury
    - "Killer couch": Injuries commonly attributed to infant rolling off couch onto floor
  - Retinal hemorrhage in up to 96%
- Other signs/symptoms
  - Presentation with "apnea" (33-45%), unexplained seizures, "unable to rouse"

Demographics
- Age
  - Median age 2.2-4.6 months old
- Epidemiology
  - 17-25:100,000 annual incidence
  - Most common cause of traumatic death in infancy: 1,200 deaths per year in USA
  - Risk factors
    - < 1 year, prematurity, twin, male, physical handicap, stepchild
    - Young parents, ↓ socioeconomic status
      - 1/3 of perpetrators under influence of alcohol or drugs

Natural History & Prognosis
- Mortality = 15-38% (60% if coma at presentation)
- Neurologic deficits include acquired microcephaly (93%), early post-traumatic seizures (79%), late post-traumatic epilepsy (> 20%), poor visual outcome (20-65%)

Treatment
- Notification to local Child Protection Agency mandated in USA/Canada/Australia/some European countries
  - Multidisciplinary child abuse team intervention

DIAGNOSTIC CHECKLIST

Consider
- Inborn error of metabolism or bleeding dyscrasia may simulate nonaccidental injury
  - Appropriately investigating these possibilities both improves patient care and clarifies criminal investigation

Image Interpretation Pearls
- Look for combination of hemispheric brain edema and bilateral or interhemispheric SDH

Reporting Tips
- Avoid use of vague or imprecise language in reports
  - Hampers medical care and legal investigation
  - More susceptible to challenges in court

SELECTED REFERENCES

1. Altinok D et al: MR imaging findings of retinal hemorrhage in a case of nonaccidental trauma. Pediatr Radiol. 39(3):290-2, 2009
2. Foerster BR et al: Neuroimaging evaluation of non-accidental head trauma with correlation to clinical outcomes: a review of 57 cases. J Pediatr. 154(4):573-7, 2009
3. Kemp AM et al: What neuroimaging should be performed in children in whom inflicted brain injury (iBI) is suspected? A systematic review. Clin Radiol. 64(5):473-83, 2009
4. Dan B et al: Repeated diffusion-weighted magnetic resonance imaging in infantile non-haemorrhagic, non-accidental brain injury. Dev Med Child Neurol. 50(1):78-80, 2008
5. McKinney AM et al: Unilateral hypoxic-ischemic injury in young children from abusive head trauma, lacking craniocervical vascular dissection or cord injury. Pediatr Radiol. 38(2):164-74, 2008
6. Barnes PD et al: Imaging of the central nervous system in suspected or alleged nonaccidental injury, including the mimics. Top Magn Reson Imaging. 18(1):53-74, 2007
7. Eltermann T et al: Magnetic resonance imaging in child abuse. J Child Neurol. 22(2):170-5, 2007
8. Suh DY et al: Nonaccidental pediatric head injury: diffusion-weighted imaging findings. Neurosurgery. 49(2):309-18; discussion 318-20, 2001
9. Ewing-Cobbs L et al: Acute neuroradiologic findings in young children with inflicted or noninflicted traumatic brain injury. Childs Nerv Syst. 16(1):25-33; discussion 34, 2000

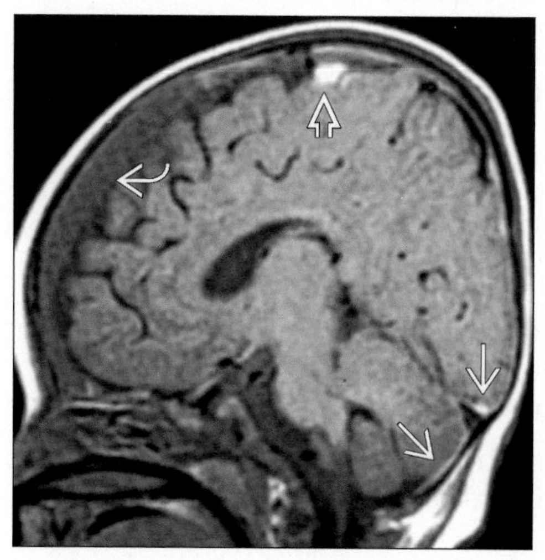

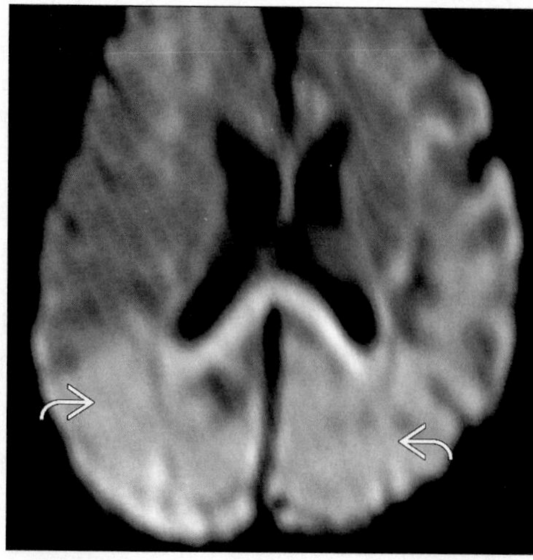

(Left) *Sagittal T1WI MR shows subdural blood ➢ over the frontal lobe that is hypointense to the brain, smaller subdurals ➔ over the cerebellum that are hyperintense to the brain, and a focal hyperintense clot of blood ➯ at the vertex.* ***(Right)*** *Axial DWI MR in the same child shows extensive reduced diffusion in the parietooccipital regions ➢ and splenium of the corpus callosum. Brain swelling secondary to a hypoxic injury is the cause of death in 80% of fatal cases of child abuse.*

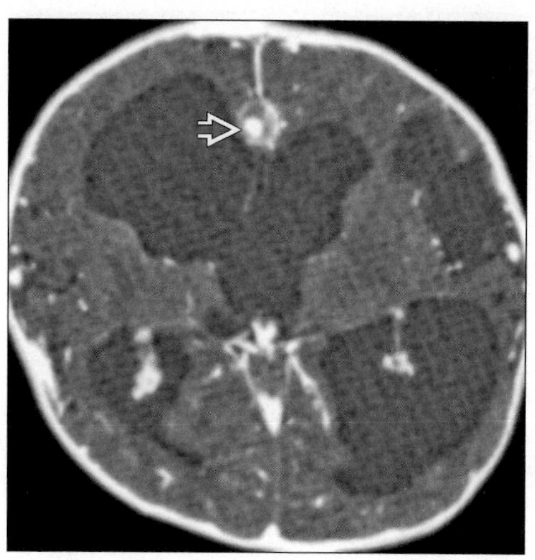

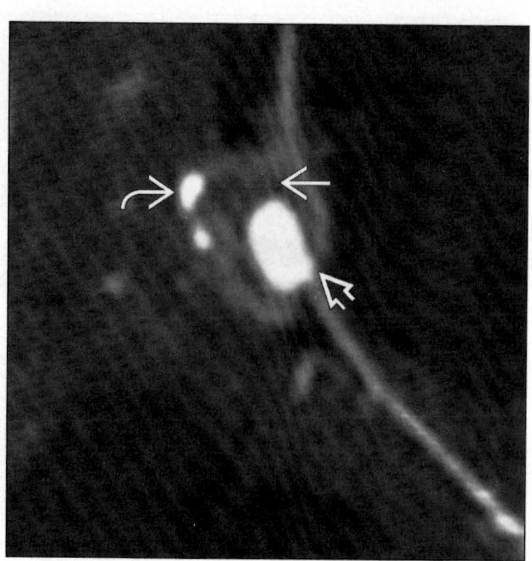

(Left) *Axial CTA shows a focal collection of contrast ➯ at the pericallosal artery in this child with hydrocephalus and multifocal encephalomalacia secondary to shaking injury.* ***(Right)*** *Sagittal reconstructed MIP from the same CTA study in the same child shows a post-traumatic pseudoaneurysm ➯ arising from the pericallosal artery, with a shell of nonenhancing thrombus ➔ and focal calcification on the outer wall ➢.*

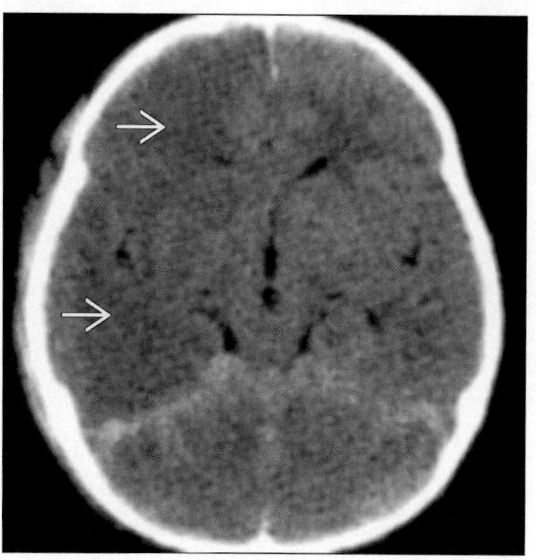

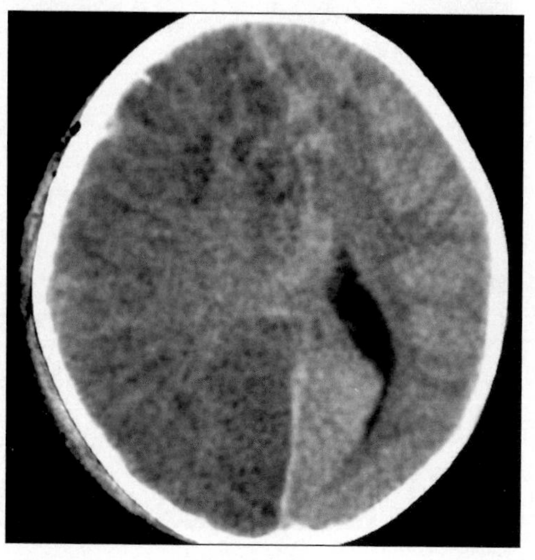

(Left) *Axial NECT shows global injury to the right cerebral hemisphere ➔ and SDH along the tentorium in this 18 month old who presented to the hospital with a history of falling out of bed. Abdominal CT showed liver laceration, rib fractures, and a pneumothorax.* ***(Right)*** *Axial NECT in the same child 24 hours later shows the "reversal" sign on the right, with the white matter more dense than the overlying gray matter. A normal gray-white contrast relationship is maintained on the left.*

INTRACRANIAL HERNIATION SYNDROMES

Key Facts

Terminology

- Brain displaced from 1 compartment into another

Imaging

- Subfalcine herniation
  - Cingulate gyrus displaced under falx
  - Ipsilateral ventricle compressed and displaced across midline
  - Contralateral ventricle dilated
- Unilateral descending transtentorial herniation (DTH)
  - Temporal lobe displaced medially into incisura
  - Encroaches on, then effaces suprasellar cistern
- Bilateral DTH ("central herniation")
  - Both temporal lobes herniated into tentorial hiatus
  - Diencephalon crushed against skull base
  - Suprasellar cistern, CSF spaces obliterated
  - Midbrain/pons displaced inferiorly
- Ascending transtentorial herniation
  - Cerebellum displaced up through incisura
  - Quadrigeminal cistern, tectum flattened
- Tonsillar herniation
  - Tonsils impacted into foramen magnum
  - Cisterna magna obliterated
- Transalar herniation
  - Ascending (middle fossa mass) or descending (frontal mass)
  - Brain, MCA herniated across sphenoid wing
- Transdural/transcranial herniation
  - Brain extruded through dural/skull defect

Top Differential Diagnoses

- Intracranial hypotension

Diagnostic Checklist

- DWI, T2* for ischemic, hemorrhagic complications

*(**Left**) Axial gross pathology section through the ventricles, in a patient who died of multiple traumatic injuries, shows findings of severe subfalcine herniation. Ventricles are displaced across the midline, and the cingulate gyrus ⇒ is herniated under the falx. Left PCA infarct occurred secondary to descending transtentorial herniation. (Courtesy R. Hewlett, PhD.) (**Right**) Axial NECT in severe trauma shows subfalcine herniation with severely compressed left and slightly dilated right lateral ventricle.*

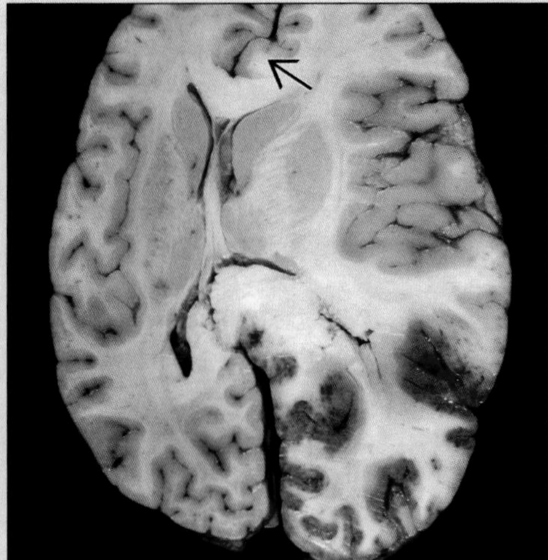

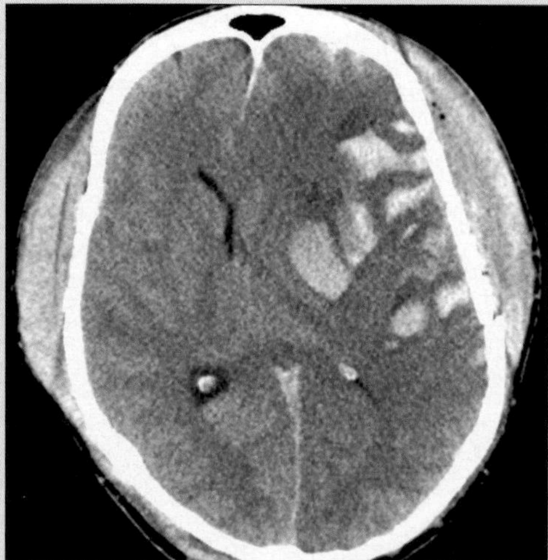

*(**Left**) Submentovertex gross pathology shows findings of unilateral descending transtentorial herniation. Undersurface of herniated temporal lobe shows "grooving" ⇒ from impaction against the tentorium. Note the 3rd nerve compression ⇒ & midbrain displacement. (Courtesy R. Hewlett, PhD.) (**Right**) Axial NECT in a patient with CHI shows changes of left descending transtentorial herniation, with uncus ➡ & hippocampus ➡ herniated into the suprasellar cistern. The right side of the cistern is preserved.*

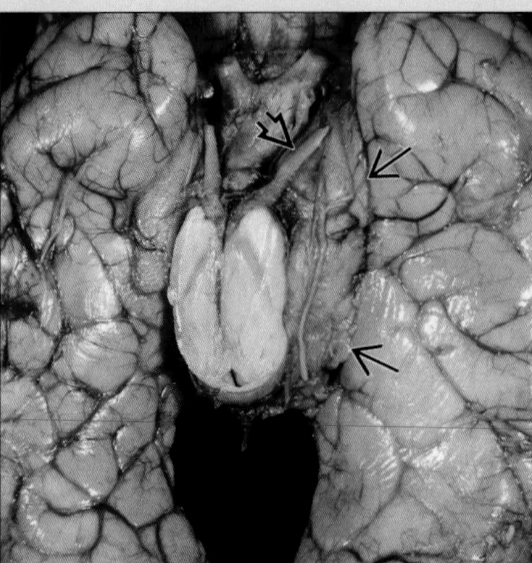

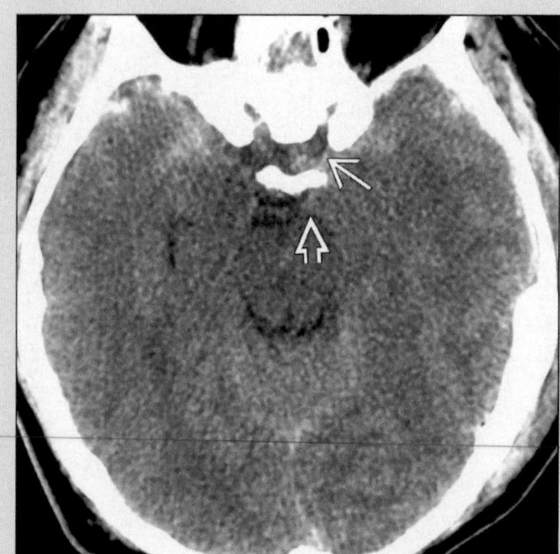

INTRACRANIAL HERNIATION SYNDROMES

TERMINOLOGY

Abbreviations

- Subfalcine herniation (SFH)
- Descending transtentorial herniation (DTH)

Definitions

- Herniation of brain from 1 compartment (normally separated by calvarial &/or dural boundaries) to another

IMAGING

General Features

- Best diagnostic clue
  - Several herniation types (findings vary)
    - SFH: Lateral, 3rd ventricles displaced across midline
    - DTH: Temporal lobe displaced over and into tentorial incisura
- Subfalcine herniation
  - Most common herniation
  - Cingulate gyrus displaced under falx
  - Ipsilateral ventricle compressed and displaced across midline
  - Complications
    - Early: Contralateral ventricle enlarged 2° to obstruction at foramen of Monro
    - Late: Anterior cerebral arteries (ACAs) displaced → compressed against free edge of falx → occlusion → 2° infarct
- Unilateral DTH
  - 2nd most common herniation
  - Medial temporal lobe displaced medially into incisura
    - Early/mild DTH: Uncus effaces ipsilateral suprasellar cistern
    - Moderate DTH: Hippocampus effaces ipsilateral quadrigeminal cistern
      - Displaces, mildly compresses midbrain
    - Severe DTH: Medial temporal lobe, temporal horn displaced inferiorly into upper CPA cistern
      - Suprasellar cistern obliterated
  - Complications
    - Contralateral midbrain compressed against tentorium, may cause "Kernohan notch"
      - Ipsilateral hemiplegia ("false localizing" sign)
      - Supratentorial mass causes compression of **contralateral** peduncle against tentorial edge
    - Midbrain (Duret) hemorrhages
    - Posterior cerebral artery (PCA) displaced inferiorly over free edge of tentorium
      - PCA kinking/occlusion leads to 2° occipital infarct
- Bilateral DTH ("central herniation")
  - Less common; seen with severe supratentorial mass effect(s)
  - Both temporal lobes herniated into tentorial hiatus
  - Optic chiasm/diencephalon crushed against skull base
  - Midbrain displaced inferiorly
    - Anterior inferior 3rd ventricle displaced posteriorly behind dorsum sella
    - Angle between midbrain and pons becomes more acute
  - Complications
    - Penetrating basal arteries occlusion → basal infarcts
- Ascending transtentorial herniation
  - Less common than descending herniation
  - Cerebellum displaced up through incisura
  - Quadrigeminal cistern compressed, tectum flattened
  - Complications
    - Aqueduct obstruction → hydrocephalus
- Tonsillar herniation
  - Most common herniation seen with posterior fossa mass
  - Tonsils pushed inferiorly, impacted into foramen magnum
    - Displacement > 5 mm
    - Tonsil folia become vertically oriented
  - Cisterna magna obliterated
  - Complications
    - 4th ventricle obstruction → hydrocephalus
- Transalar herniation
  - Rare
  - Brain, MCA herniated across sphenoid wing
  - Ascending or descending
    - Ascending: Middle cranial fossa/temporal lobe mass displaces sylvian fissure, MCA, up/over sphenoid wing
    - Descending: Anterior fossa/frontal lobe mass forces gyrus rectus posteroinferiorly over sphenoid wing, displaces sylvian fissure/MCA backwards
  - Complication
    - MCA compressed against sphenoid → infarct
- Transdural/transcranial herniation
  - Rare
    - Sometimes called "brain fungus"
    - Can be life threatening
  - Brain, vessels herniated through dural &/or skull defect
  - Trauma (skull fracture lacerates dura), craniotomy
  - ↑ ICP forces brain through dura ± subgaleal extension

CT Findings

- NECT
  - Ventricles displaced; sulci/cisterns obliterated

MR Findings

- T1WI
  - Best anatomic definition
- T2WI
  - Best for complications (edema, infarcts, hydrocephalus)
- T2* GRE
  - Best for hemorrhagic foci (e.g., Duret hemorrhages)
- DWI
  - Secondary ischemia/infarcts
- DTI
  - ± corticospinal tract disruption
  - Kernohan notch → loss of FA

Imaging Recommendations

- Best imaging tool
  - NECT best rapid screen

- Multiplanar MR for complications
- Protocol advice
  - Add DWI, T2* (GRE), SWI for ischemic, hemorrhagic complications

DIFFERENTIAL DIAGNOSIS

Intracranial Hypotension

- Brain "pulled," not "pushed" down
- Pituitary gland often engorged
- Dural thickening, enhancement often present

Chiari 1

- Congenital anomaly with low-lying tonsils
- Brain otherwise normal

PATHOLOGY

General Features

- Etiology
  - Trauma most common clinical setting
  - Mass lesions, large infarcts, and inflammatory lesions
  - Hemorrhage, extracellular fluid, or added tissue accumulate within closed space
  - CSF spaces (cisterns, ventricles) initially compressed
  - Intracranial volume cannot be accommodated
    - Gross mechanical displacement of brain, vessels → herniation
  - Secondary effects exacerbate severity of primary injuries
  - Herniations, ↑ ICP, altered cerebral hemodynamics → ischemia and infarction
    - PCA occlusion → occipital infarct most common
    - ACA occlusion → distal (cingulate gyrus) infarcts
    - Perforating vessels → basal ganglia, capsule infarcts
    - Midbrain Duret hemorrhage can occur from stretching/tearing of pontine perforators
- Associated abnormalities
  - Secondary obstructive hydrocephalus
  - Ischemia, hemorrhage, necrosis

Gross Pathologic & Surgical Features

- Grossly swollen, edematous brain
- Gyri compressed and flattened against calvarium
- Sulci effaced

CLINICAL ISSUES

Presentation

- Most common signs/symptoms
  - Focal neurologic deficit
    - Contralateral hemiparesis
    - Ipsilateral pupil-involving CN3 palsy
    - Ipsilateral hemiplegia
      - Kernohan notch → compression of opposite cerebral peduncle against tentorium
      - "False localizing" signs
  - Decreased mental status or obtundation

Natural History & Prognosis

- Brain death if ICP continues to rise, mass effect progresses unabated

Treatment

- Mitigate secondary effects
- Removal of mass or decompressive craniectomy
- Prolonged post-traumatic brain hypersensitivity
  - May offer potential "therapeutic window"
  - Possible use of neuroprotective agents

DIAGNOSTIC CHECKLIST

Consider

- Intracranial hypotension (IH) syndrome
  - Can mimic some features of herniations caused by supratentorial mass
    - Common features
      - "Slumping" midbrain
      - "Closed" midbrain-pontine angle
      - Tonsillar herniation
      - ± subdural hematomas
    - Distinguishing features in IH
      - Brain appears "sucked" down, not "pushed" down
      - Dural thickening, enhancement
      - Pituitary engorgement

Image Interpretation Pearls

- Use DWI, T2* sequences in brain trauma, suspected herniation

SELECTED REFERENCES

1. Kalita J et al: Brain herniations in patients with intracerebral hemorrhage. Acta Neurol Scand. 119(4):254-60, 2009
2. Hussain SI et al: Brainstem ischemia in acute herniation syndrome. J Neurol Sci. 268(1-2):190-2, 2008
3. Marupaka SK et al: Atypical Duret haemorrhages seen on computed tomography. Emerg Med Australas. 20(2):180-2, 2008
4. Timms C et al: Brainstem distortion from postoperative cerebellar herniation through a dural and bony defect. J Clin Neurosci. 15(9):1050-1, 2008
5. Yoo WK et al: Kernohan's notch phenomenon demonstrated by diffusion tensor imaging and transcranial magnetic stimulation. J Neurol Neurosurg Psychiatry. 79(11):1295-7, 2008
6. Parizel PM et al: Brainstem hemorrhage in descending transtentorial herniation (Duret hemorrhage). Intensive Care Med. 28(1):85-8, 2002
7. Server A et al: Post-traumatic cerebral infarction. Neuroimaging findings, etiology and outcome. Acta Radiol. 42(3):254-60, 2001
8. Mastronardi L et al: Magnetic resonance imaging findings of Kernohan-Woltman notch in acute subdural hematoma. Clin Neurol Neurosurg. 101(2):122-4, 1999

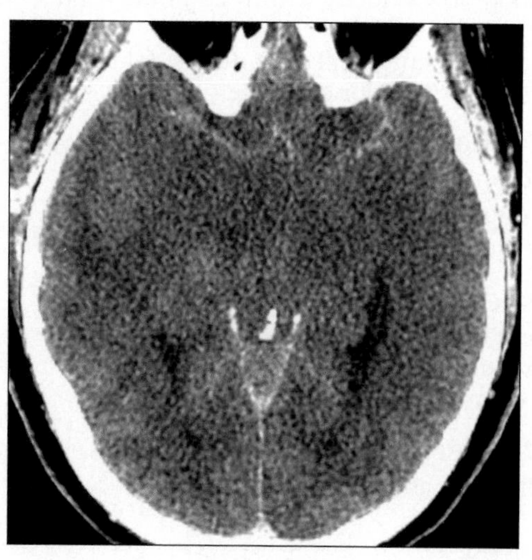

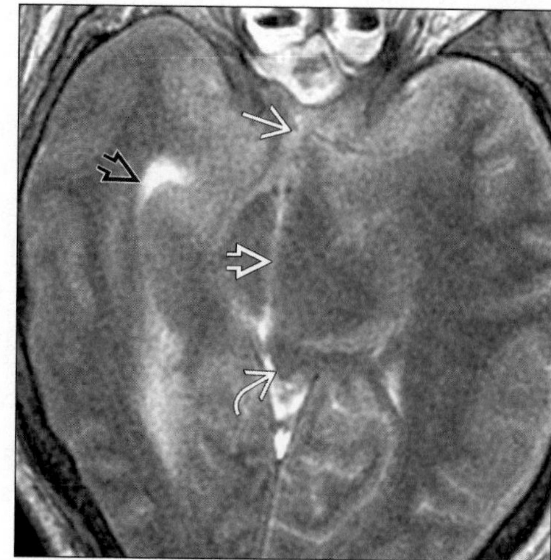

(Left) *Axial NECT in a trauma patient with severe diffuse brain swelling and complete bilateral (central) descending herniation shows total obliteration of all basal CSF spaces by the edematous brain.* ***(Right)*** *Axial T2WI MR shows severe DTH with herniation of the left uncus ➔ and hippocampus ➔ into the suprasellar and quadrigeminal cisterns, respectively. Note the downward displacement of the 3rd ventricle ➔ and dilatation of the contralateral temporal horn ➔.*

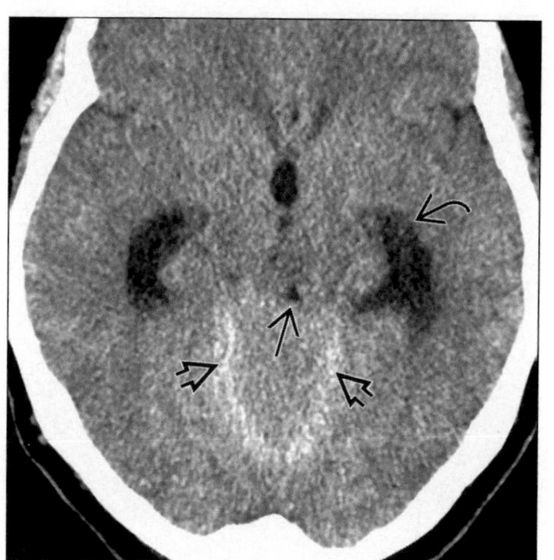

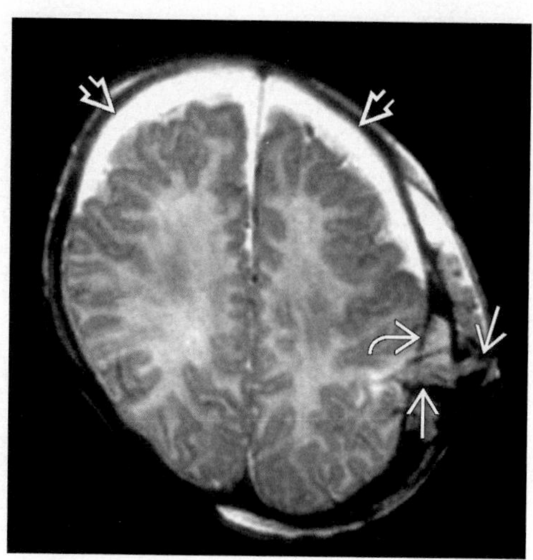

(Left) *Axial NECT shows findings of ascending transtentorial herniation. The vermis is displaced superiorly through the tentorial incisura ➔, flattening and compressing the tectal plate ➔. The aqueduct is obstructed, causing acute hydrocephalus with transependymal CSF flow ➔.* ***(Right)*** *Axial T2WI MR in an infant with a left parietal skull fracture shows transcalvarial herniation of the brain and accompanying vessels ➔ through torn dura ➔. Bilateral chronic SDHs are present ➔.*

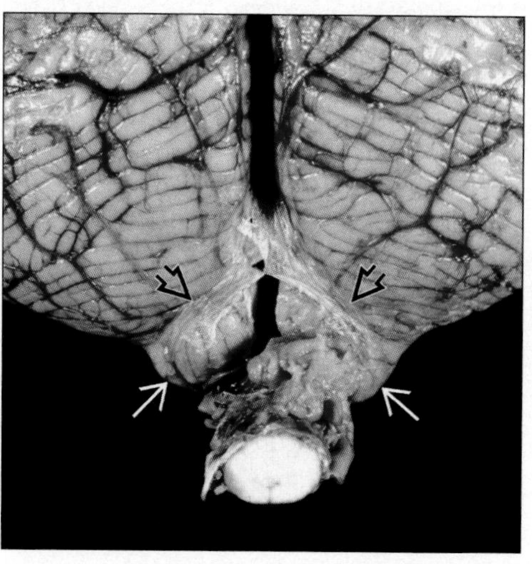

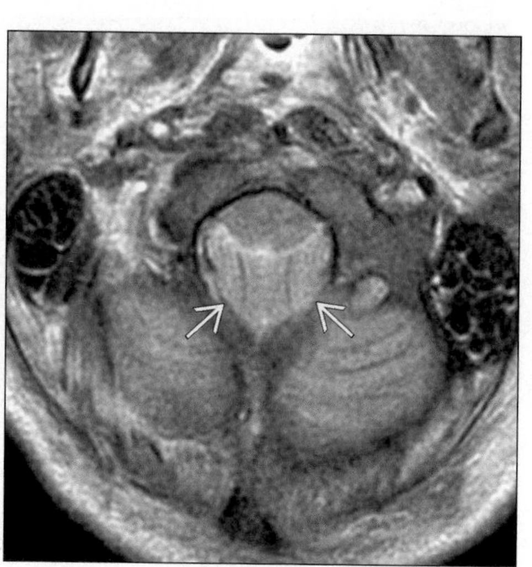

(Left) *Gross pathology of an autopsied brain seen posteriorly shows bilateral tonsillar herniation. Note the grooving of tonsils ➔ from impaction against the foramen magnum as the tonsils ➔ are forced inferiorly into the upper cervical spine. (Courtesy R. Hewlett, PhD.)* ***(Right)*** *Axial T2WI MR shows severe tonsillar herniation, with both tonsils ➔ displaced inferiorly, filling the cisterna magna and displacing the upper cervical spinal cord anteriorly.*

TRAUMATIC CEREBRAL EDEMA

Key Facts

Terminology
- Vasogenic edema (VE), cytotoxic edema (CTE), cerebral edema (CE), diffuse brain swelling (DBS)
- 2 basic forms of brain edema in trauma: VE and CTE ⇒ often coexist
  - VE: Extracellular edema, follows blood-brain barrier (BBB) breakdown
  - CTE: Intracellular (closed barrier) edema

Imaging
- Compressed ventricles, effaced sulci
- Vasogenic more prominent in WM, cytotoxic more prominent in GM
- Secondary effects of CE
  - Brain herniation(s)
  - Vascular compression ⇒ infarction
- DWI together with ADC differentiates VE from CTE
- Brain edema accompanied by ↑ ICP, ↑ pulsatility index, ↓ blood flow velocity within 24 hours ⇒ poor prognosis
- Disturbed cerebral autoregulation during 1st 48 hours correlates with poor outcome

Top Differential Diagnoses
- Anoxic encephalopathy
- Metabolic encephalopathy
- Pressure-related edema

Clinical Issues
- Goal = maintain cerebral perfusion pressure (CPP) without inducing hydrostatic vasogenic edema
- DBS more common in children than adults

Diagnostic Checklist
- Consider hypoxia as contributing factor

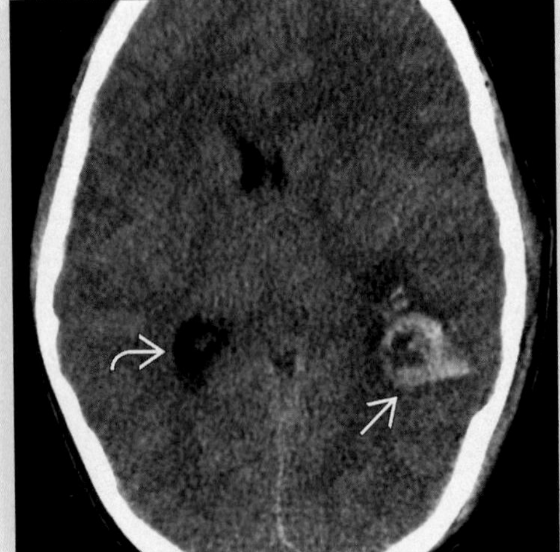

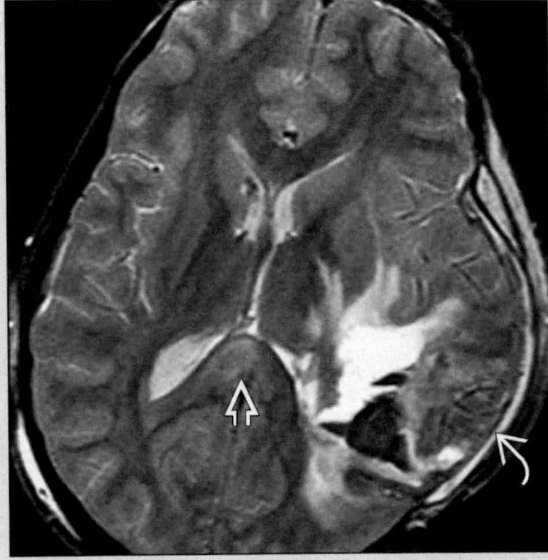

*(**Left**) Axial NECT demonstrates acute left periatrial hemorrhage ➡ with minimal surrounding vasogenic edema. Note diffuse sulcal effacement, midline shift to the right, and early trapping of the right lateral ventricle ↪. (**Right**) Axial T2WI MR in the same patient demonstrates left periatrial hemorrhage with increased surrounding edema. Interval left craniectomy is noted with extracalvarial herniation of brain parenchyma ↪. Edema related to the splenium of the corpus callosum ⇨ is also noted.*

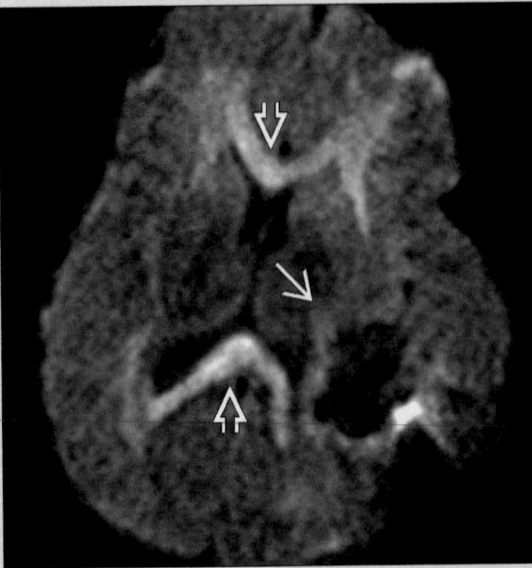

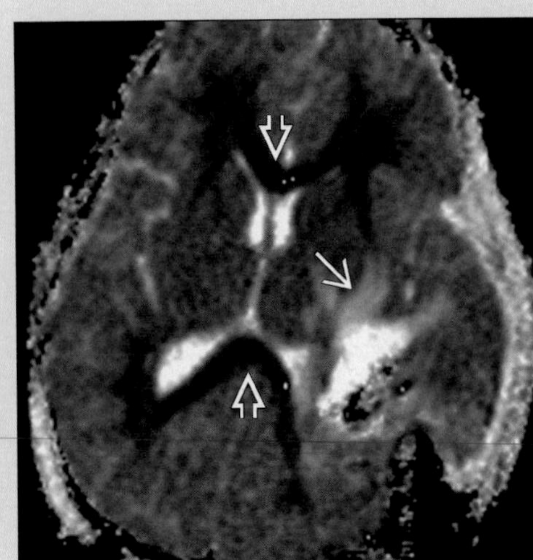

*(**Left**) Axial DWI MR demonstrates increased signal in the corpus callosum and cerebral white matter ⇨, consistent with edema. Edema is also noted around the left periatrial hematoma ➡. (**Right**) Axial ADC in the same patient demonstrates corresponding hypointensity in the corpus callosum and cerebral white matter ⇨, confirming cytotoxic edema. Hyperintensity surrounding the left periatrial hemorrhage reflects vasogenic edema ➡.*

TERMINOLOGY

Synonyms

- Vasogenic edema (VE), cytotoxic edema (CTE), cerebral edema (CE), diffuse brain swelling (DBS)

Definitions

- Brain, CSF, and blood coexist in closed intracranial compartment
  - To maintain normal ICP, ↑ in 1 compartment must be balanced by ↓ in others (Monro-Kellie)
- CE (secondary effect of trauma, ischemia) is dynamic process involving glutamate-mediated excitotoxicity, cell damage
- 2 basic forms of brain edema in trauma: VE and CTE often coexist
  - VE: Extracellular edema, follows blood-brain barrier (BBB) breakdown
  - CTE: Intracellular (closed barrier) edema

IMAGING

General Features

- Best diagnostic clue
  - Compressed ventricles, effaced sulci due to focal or diffuse increase in brain water
- Location
  - Vasogenic more prominent in white matter (WM); cytotoxic more prominent in gray matter (GM)
  - Often coexist
- Morphology
  - Compressed ventricles, effaced sulci
  - Secondary effects of CE
    - Brain herniation(s)
    - Vascular compression ⇒ infarction

Radiographic Findings

- Radiography
  - ± fractures, split sutures

CT Findings

- NECT
  - Compressed ventricles, effaced sulci
  - Low-attenuation brain parenchyma: WM > GM
    - Subcortical WM less resistant to fluid accumulation than GM
    - Loss of GM-WM interfaces
  - Vasogenic edema more prominent in WM
  - Cytotoxic edema more prominent in GM
  - ↓ supratentorial perfusion with preservation of infratentorial perfusion ⇒ "white cerebellum" sign
  - Multifocal hemorrhages often present
- CECT
  - Usually no enhancement unless BBB disrupted
- Xenon CT
  - Edema major contributor to brain swelling
  - Cerebral blood volume actually decreases in proportion to cerebral blood flow

MR Findings

- T1WI
  - Hypointense edema
- T2WI
  - Hyperintense edema
- FLAIR
  - Hyperintense edema
  - Less useful in newborn due to normally ↑ water content of neonatal brain
- T2* GRE
  - ± blood products
- DWI
  - DWI together with ADC differentiates VE from CTE
    - VE: Increased extracellular brain water (↑ ADC)
    - CTE: Cellular swelling (↓ ADC)
  - Diffusion tensor imaging (DTI): ↓ diffusion anisotropy early, when MR/DWI still normal
  - DTI identifies traumatic penumbra, potentially salvageable brain
- T1WI C+
  - Patchy enhancement if BBB breakdown
- MRA
  - ± decreased flow ("thinned" arteries)
  - Vascular obstruction (compression or dissection during herniation) ⇒ post-traumatic infarction
- MRV
  - Sinus compression with severe edema
- MRS
  - ↓ NAA, elevated Cho (membrane breakdown), presence of lactate predict poor prognosis
- Perfusion: ↓ brain perfusion with progressive ↑ ICP

Ultrasonographic Findings

- Pulsed Doppler
  - Brain edema accompanied by ↑ ICP, ↑ pulsatility index, ↓ blood flow velocity within 24 hours ⇒ poor prognosis
  - Moving correlation index between mean arterial BP and ICP = PRx (measures cerebral vasomotor reactivity)
    - PRx < 0.3 = intact reactivity; PRx > 0.3 = impaired reactivity
    - Disturbed cerebral autoregulation during 1st 48 hours correlates with poor outcome

Angiographic Findings

- Conventional
  - Slow arteriovenous transit if ↑ ICP

Nuclear Medicine Findings

- PET
  - PET/SPECT: ↓ rCBV, hypometabolism (dependent upon timing)

Imaging Recommendations

- NECT performed due to accessibility in critically ill trauma patients
- DWI with ADC maps (or DTI) important to differentiate VE, CTE
- Multiplanar MR allows characterization of acquired cerebral herniations
  - Subfalcine (cingulate), tonsillar, uncal, transtentorial (central ascending, central descending, lateral), transalar, external

TRAUMATIC CEREBRAL EDEMA

DIFFERENTIAL DIAGNOSIS

Anoxic Encephalopathy

- Hypoxic-ischemic encephalopathy, drowning, cardiopulmonary arrest

Metabolic Encephalopathy

- Uremia, mitochondrial disorders

Pressure-related Edema

- Posterior reversible encephalopathy syndrome
  - Hypertensive encephalopathy, cyclosporine/FK506 encephalopathy, L-asparaginase, eclampsia
  - Predominantly VE in subcortical WM parieto-occipital regions
- Venous obstruction with ↑ venous pressure

Meningitis/Encephalitis

- Diffuse sulcal effacement, leptomeningeal ± parenchymal enhancement

PATHOLOGY

General Features

- Etiology
  - Vasogenic edema
    - ↑ BBB permeability
    - Endothelial tight junctions disrupted ⇒ leakage of proteins/Na++/water ⇒ fluid shift into extracellular spaces
    - Primarily WM, myelin (major association bundles, relative sparing of commissural/projection fibers)
  - Cytotoxic edema
    - Intracellular (closed barrier) edema
    - Energy failure ⇒ loss of Na++/K homeostasis
    - Intracellular water uptake causes cell swelling, compression of extracellular space
  - Other brain water disturbances
    - Hydrocephalic (interstitial)
    - Hydrostatic (congestive)
    - Hypo-osmotic
- Genetics
  - Differential expression of genes controlling destructive and neuroprotective cascades determine cellular response to injury

Gross Pathologic & Surgical Features

- ↑ brain water, obliteration of cisterns/ventricles/sulci

Microscopic Features

- Extracellular fluid of cortex neuropil ⇒ swelling and shrinkage of pre-/postsynaptic structures, synaptic disassembly
- Effects of hypoxia and cell death

CLINICAL ISSUES

Presentation

- Most common signs/symptoms
  - Altered consciousness
  - Coma
- Clinical profile
  - < 2 years old: Inflicted injury in 80%
  - Teens and adults: Motor vehicle crash, assaults
  - > 65 years old: Accidental falls

Demographics

- Age
  - DBS more common in children than adults
- Gender
  - M:F 1.6-2:1
- Ethnicity
  - African-American, Native Americans overrepresented
- Epidemiology
  - 1.5 million traumatic brain injury per year (USA)
    - Highest incidence in children < 5 years old

Natural History & Prognosis

- Slowly expanding lesions can be accommodated without elevated ICP
- Rapid expansion (trauma, rapid tumor growth, abscess) ⇒ rapid rise of ICP
  - Followed by "cascade" of sequelae (e.g., excitotoxin release) ⇒ cell death
- Post-traumatic edema generally resolves within 2 weeks, atrophy (due to cellular death) ensues

Treatment

- Goal = maintain cerebral perfusion pressure (CPP) without inducing hydrostatic vasogenic edema
  - ↑ CPP in selected patients with intact cerebral vasomotor reactivity
- Decompressive surgery
- Osmotherapy, neuroprotective agents, steroids, all controversial

DIAGNOSTIC CHECKLIST

Consider

- Hypoxia as contributing factor

Image Interpretation Pearls

- Image timing crucial: VE (1st hours) replaced by CTE

SELECTED REFERENCES

1. Greve MW et al: Pathophysiology of traumatic brain injury. Mt Sinai J Med. 76(2):97-104, 2009
2. Tollard E et al: Experience of diffusion tensor imaging and 1H spectroscopy for outcome prediction in severe traumatic brain injury: Preliminary results. Crit Care Med. 37(4):1448-55, 2009
3. Galloway NR et al: Diffusion-weighted imaging improves outcome prediction in pediatric traumatic brain injury. J Neurotrauma. 25(10):1153-62, 2008
4. Morgalla MH et al: Do long-term results justify decompressive craniectomy after severe traumatic brain injury? J Neurosurg. 109(4):685-90, 2008
5. Park E et al: Traumatic brain injury: can the consequences be stopped? CMAJ. 178(9):1163-70, 2008
6. Rutgers DR et al: Diffusion tensor imaging characteristics of the corpus callosum in mild, moderate, and severe traumatic brain injury. AJNR Am J Neuroradiol. 29(9):1730-5, 2008
7. Splavski B et al: Transcranial doppler ultrasonography as an early outcome forecaster following severe brain injury. Br J Neurosurg. 20(6):386-90, 2006

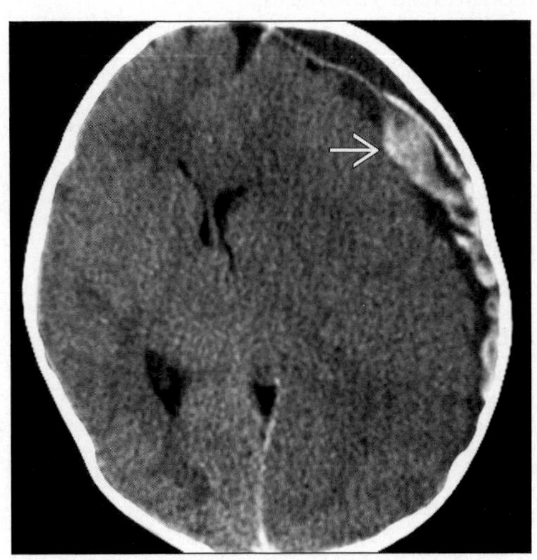

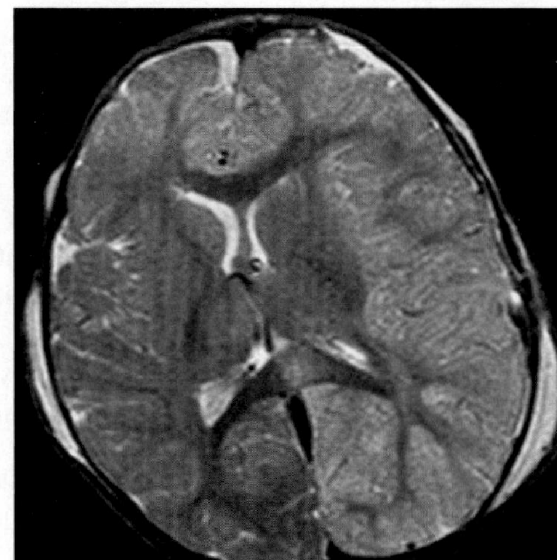

*(**Left**) Axial NECT shows a mixed density, left subdural hematoma ➔ with underlying left cerebral edema. There is effacement of the left lateral ventricle and sulci, midline shift to the right, and early entrapment of the right lateral ventricle. (**Right**) Axial T2WI MR in the same patient shows edema related to the left cerebral hemisphere and the right ACA territory.*

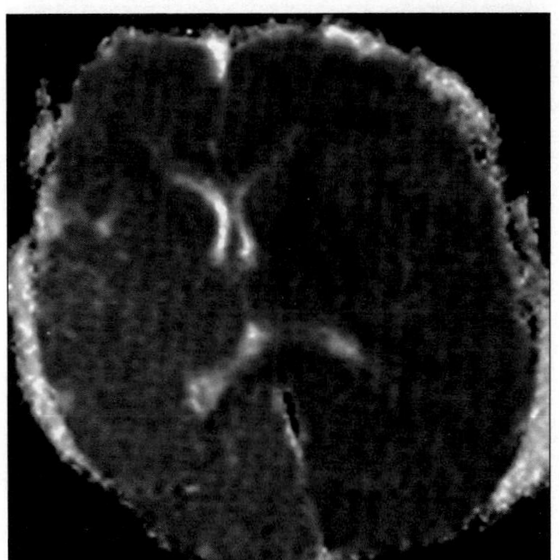

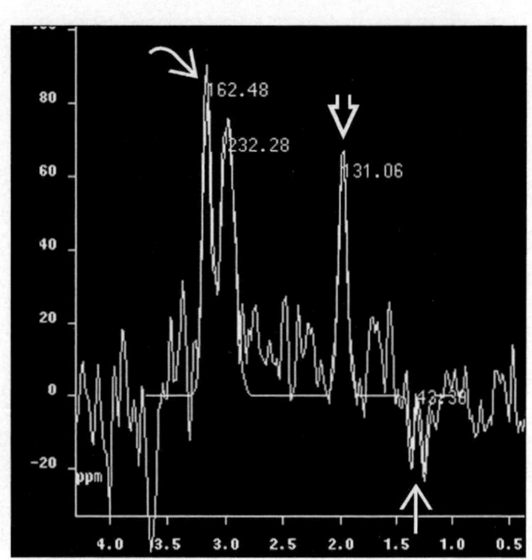

*(**Left**) Axial ADC map shows findings of cytotoxic edema with corresponding hypointensity in the left cerebral hemisphere and right ACA territory. (**Right**) MRS obtained from the left cerebral hemisphere in this same patient demonstrates diminished NAA ➔ in keeping with neuronal loss or dysfunction. Presence of lactate ➔ is a poor prognostic indicator and is consistent with ischemia. Elevated choline ➔ is also noted, reflecting membrane breakdown.*

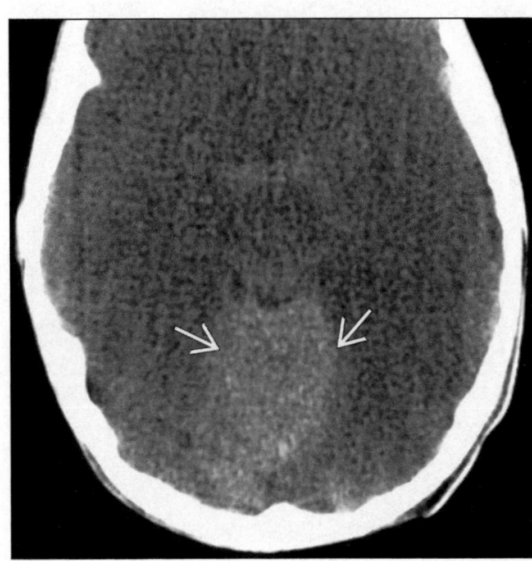

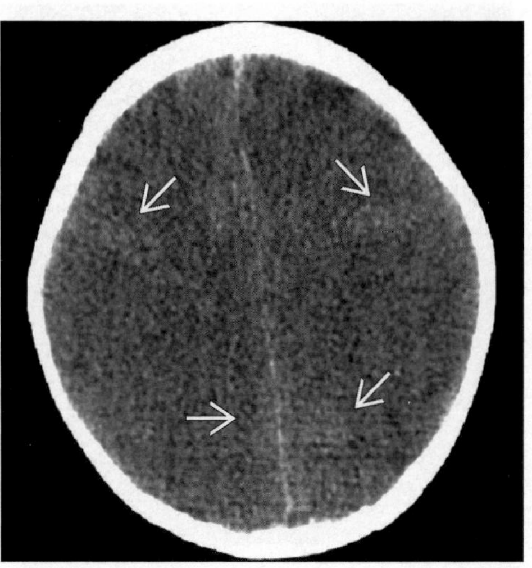

*(**Left**) Axial NECT shows diffuse cerebral edema. A so-called "cerebellar reversal" sign is present. Here the cerebellum ➔ appears unusually dense. This is a relative finding in which the diffusely low-density cerebral hemispheres make the unaffected cerebellum appear more dense. (**Right**) Axial NECT shows diffuse loss of gray-white matter differentiation and sulcal effacement. However, this is not yet complete, as there are small patchy areas of cortex that remain slightly brighter ➔.*

TRAUMATIC CEREBRAL ISCHEMIA

Key Facts

Terminology
- Hemodynamic alterations induced by traumatic brain injury (TBI)
  - Can be local, regional, generalized perfusion alteration(s)

Imaging
- Best diagnostic clue: Restricted diffusion
- Most commonly occurs in PCA vascular distribution
  - MCA, ACA, vertebrobasilar relatively common
  - Less common: Perforating, cerebellar arteries
- Best imaging tool: MR + DWI/ADC
  - Diffusion most sensitive sequence
  - Midsagittal imaging to evaluate for herniation

Top Differential Diagnoses
- Nontraumatic ischemia/infarction
- Vascular (multi-infarct) dementia
- Atherosclerotic occlusion
- Subarachnoid-induced vasospasm

Pathology
- Primary TBI = direct damage at time of trauma
- Secondary brain injury occurs after initial trauma
  - Due to systemic responses to initial injuries
  - PTCI may be most common cause of secondary brain injury in setting of severe TBI
  - 2° injuries often more devastating than 1° TBI
  - 2° injury can occur after negative initial imaging

Clinical Issues
- Most common sign: GCS ≤ 8
- Symptoms often delayed 12-24 hours to several weeks
- PTCI occurs in 1.9-10.4% of craniocerebral trauma
- Ischemic damage present in 90% of fatal TBI deaths

*(**Left**) Axial NECT following an assault shows bilateral uncal herniation ➔ and normal-appearing occipital lobes. (**Right**) Axial NECT in the same patient performed 10 days later for clinical deterioration shows hypodensity within the bilateral occipital lobes from PCA ischemia ➔. Note the basilar cisterns ➔ are completely effaced. Severe cerebral edema and mass effect from large bifrontal hemorrhagic contusions were also seen (not shown).*

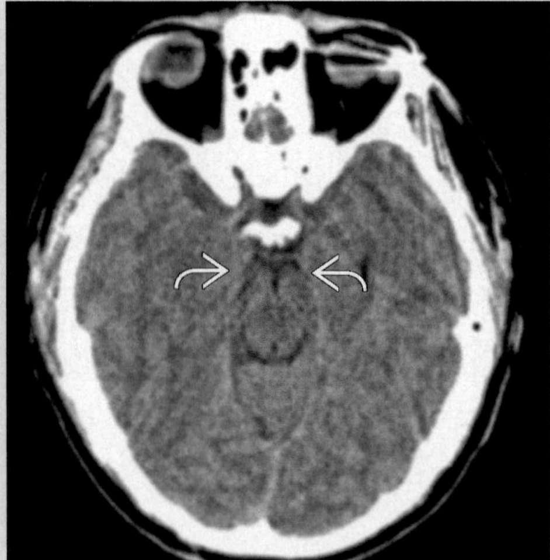

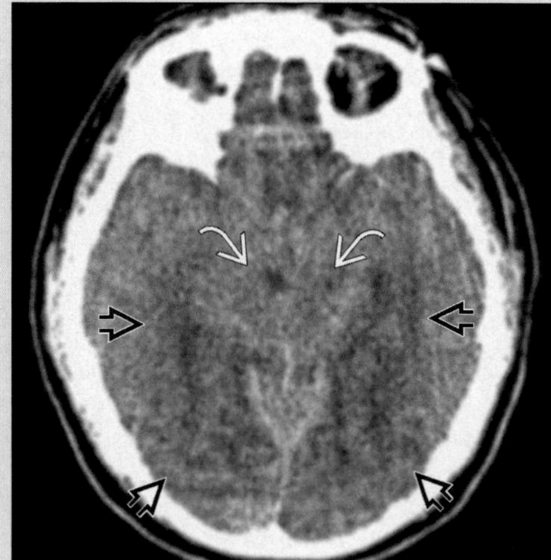

*(**Left**) Axial DWI MR performed 6 days after admission for clinical deterioration shows bilateral ACA distribution acute ischemia ➔. Cerebral edema and mass effect from prior large bifrontal hemorrhagic contusions were also seen (not shown). (**Right**) Axial FLAIR MR in an 11 year old with TBI, performed 4 days after admission following an anoxic event, shows gyral swelling with hyperintensity ➔ secondary to hypoxia. Note the residual subarachnoid hemorrhage ➔.*

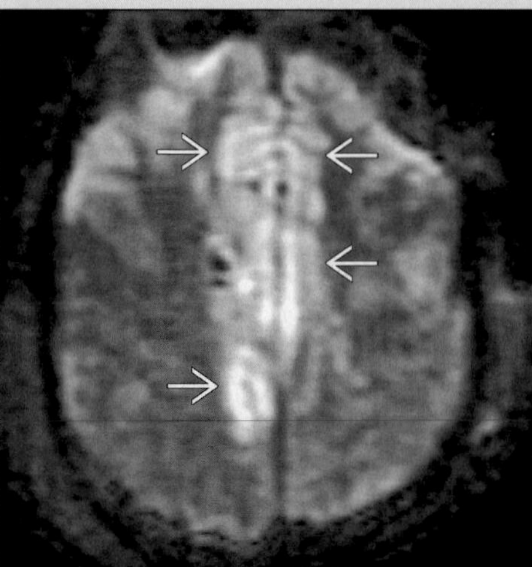

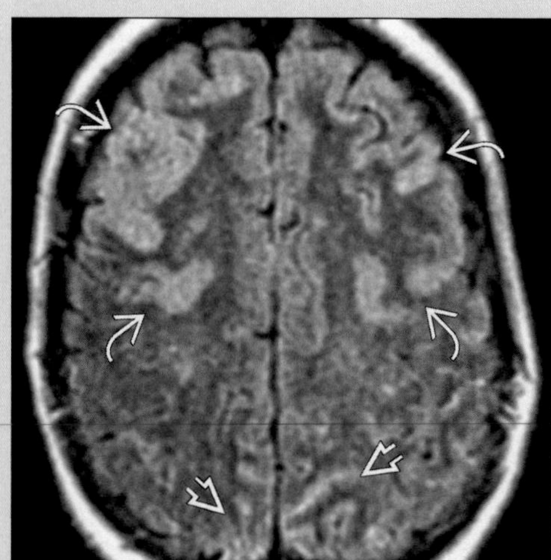

TERMINOLOGY

Abbreviations

- Post-traumatic cerebral ischemia (PTCI)

Definitions

- Hemodynamic alterations induced by traumatic brain injury (TBI)
  - Can be local, regional, generalized perfusion alteration(s)

IMAGING

General Features

- Best diagnostic clue
  - Restricted diffusion
- Location
  - Most commonly occurs in PCA vascular distribution
    - MCA, ACA, vertebrobasilar relatively common
    - Less common: Perforating arteries, cortical/ subcortical, cerebellar

CT Findings

- NECT
  - Initial primary lesions of TBI
    - Hyperdense traumatic subarachnoid hemorrhage, subdural hematoma, &/or epidural hematoma
    - Hypodense contusion, ± dense hemorrhagic foci
    - Diffuse axonal injury
    - Calvarial fractures
  - Subsequent secondary hypodense ischemia
    - Downward tentorial herniation → PCA occlusion
    - Subfalcine → ACA occlusion
    - Central → basal perforating vessel occlusions
- CT perfusion
  - May reveal changes in CBF, CBV, time to peak, &/or mean transit time

MR Findings

- T1WI
  - Acute ischemia: Hypointense
  - Sagittal best to evaluate for herniation(s)
- T2WI
  - Acute ischemia: Hyperintense
- FLAIR
  - Acute ischemia: Hyperintense
- T2* GRE
  - Best for imaging any hemorrhagic foci
- DWI
  - Restricted diffusion with matching ↓ ADC
  - Often multiple; may separate DWI negative moderate TBI from DWI positive severe TBI
- T1WI C+
  - Subacute ischemia will enhance
- MRA
  - Vessel occlusion, regional hypoperfusion
- MRV
  - Occlusion, displacement (e.g., from epidural)
- MRS
  - TBI: ↓ NAA/Cr & ↑ lactate; persistent abnormalities prognostic
- MR perfusion
  - T2* sensitive echo-planar MR with 1st-pass gadolinium bolus
    - May reveal hypoperfusion changes in relative CBF, CBV, time to peak, &/or mean transit time

Ultrasonographic Findings

- Transcranial Doppler
  - Trauma-induced vasospasm: ↑ peak MCA velocity

Angiographic Findings

- Conventional
  - DSA may show vasospasm from traumatic SAH

Nuclear Medicine Findings

- SPECT: Tc-99m-HMPAO-SPECT
  - Very sensitive for cortical ischemia
  - Demonstrates high sensitivity and specificity within initial 48 hours for infarction
- Oxygen-15 PET
  - Coexistence of ischemia and hyperemia shown in some TBI patients
  - Mismatch of perfusion to oxygen use in PTCI
  - ↑ ischemic brain volume acutely correlates with poor Glasgow outcome score 6 months after injury

Imaging Recommendations

- Best imaging tool
  - MR + DWI/ADC
- Protocol advice
  - Diffusion most sensitive sequence
  - Midsagittal imaging to evaluate for herniation

DIFFERENTIAL DIAGNOSIS

Nontraumatic Ischemia/Infarction

- Appears identical; no trauma history

Vascular (Multi-Infarct) Dementia

- Elderly; no trauma history

Atherosclerotic Occlusion

- Elderly; typical location in proximal ICA

SAH-Induced Vasospasm

- Usually in setting of ruptured aneurysm

PATHOLOGY

General Features

- Etiology
  - Motor vehicle accidents: Most common cause of closed head injuries and PTCI
  - Variety of mechanisms account for PTCI
    - Direct vascular compression by mass effects
    - Systemic hypoperfusion
    - Vascular injury, embolization
    - Cerebral vasospasm from traumatic SAH
    - Venous congestion at craniectomy site
  - 2 most common mechanisms
    - Mechanical shift of brain with herniation across falx &/or tentorium → 80-90% of PTCI
    - Result of intracranial space-occupying lesion
  - PTCI relationship with inciting brain injury
    - Primary TBI = direct damage at time of trauma

TRAUMATIC CEREBRAL ISCHEMIA

- Secondary brain injury occurs after initial trauma
  - Due to systemic responses to initial injuries
  - Most 2° injuries result from ↑ ICP, cerebral herniations
  - 2° injuries often more devastating than those sustained from primary injuries
  - PTCI may be most common cause of secondary brain injury in setting of severe TBI
- Genetics
  - Auto-protective mechanisms are induced; production of heat shock proteins, anti-inflammatory cytokines, endogenous antioxidants
  - High expression of chemokine CXCL8 induces neutrophil-dependent microvascular damage
- Associated abnormalities
  - Intracranial hemorrhages, calvarial fractures, contusions, diffuse axonal injury

Gross Pathologic & Surgical Features

- Profound global or regional cerebral hypoperfusion occur in most patients with Glasgow Coma Scores (GCS) ≤ 8
- Specific infarctions (in order of prevalence)
  - PCA: Compression of PCA against rigid tentorial edge from medial temporal lobe herniation
  - ACA: Subfalcine herniation of cingulate gyrus compresses 1 or both ACAs &/or their branches
  - MCA: Gross herniation or severe cerebral edema
  - Lenticulostriate, thalamoperforating: Gross mass effects cause stretching and attenuation of these small perforating vessels
  - Cortical/subcortical: Direct compression from overlying masses; 2 mechanisms
    - Direct pressure effects limit arterial flow
    - Local venous drainage compression occurs
    - Both often result in hemorrhagic infarcts
  - Superior cerebellar artery: Ascending or descending transtentorial herniation compresses artery against tentorium
  - PICA: Compression of artery from tonsillar herniation
- In children, TBI may have intracranial and systemic effects combined → global cerebral ischemia

Microscopic Features

- Blood-brain barrier disruption with vasogenic edema
- Excitatory amino acids induce cellular swelling → cytotoxic edema
- Overproduction of free radicals and apoptosis
- Neurotransmitter release, metabolic perturbation, and membrane depolarization → ion dysfunction
  - PTCI impedes return of ion homeostasis, contributing to development of ↑ ICP
- Inflammatory processes → massive astrocytic activation with leukocyte accumulation & capillary vessel compression → microvascular occlusion

CLINICAL ISSUES

Presentation

- Most common signs/symptoms
  - Most common sign: GCS ≤ 8
  - No reliable clinical findings indicate presence of traumatic cerebral ischemia
  - Neurological signs from brain injury obscure focal findings that may be from secondary ischemia
- Clinical profile
  - Symptoms often delayed 12-24 hours to several weeks
  - Varies greatly with type of injury

Demographics

- Age
  - Children:adults = 2:1 (aged 15-24 at highest risk)
- Gender
  - M:F = 2:1
- Epidemiology
  - TBI: Leading cause of death and disability in children and adults
  - 2,000,000 traumatic brain injuries annually in USA
  - Survivors incur annual cost of > $40 billion ~ 0.5% of GNP
  - TBI causes ~ 50,000 deaths and 235,000 hospitalizations annually in USA
  - PTCI occurs in 1.9-10.4% of craniocerebral trauma
  - Ischemic damage present in 90% of fatal TBI deaths

Natural History & Prognosis

- Poor prognosis: Presence of subdural hematoma, brain swelling/edema, traumatic SAH
- Good prognosis: Patients with none or only 1 poor prognostic factor
- Presence of blunt cerebral vascular injury and treatment with factor VIIa are risk factors for developing PTCI
- Outcome: 50% die or are left in persistent vegetative state

Treatment

- Treatment of comorbidities: Herniation, hemorrhage(s), hydrocephalus, seizures
- Cerebral perfusion **must** be monitored to detect secondary cerebral ischemia following TBI
- Herniation &/or diffuse swelling may require craniectomy

DIAGNOSTIC CHECKLIST

Consider

- Cause of ischemia
- May occur hours to days or even weeks after admission

Image Interpretation Pearls

- Secondary brain injury can occur after negative primary radiologic evaluation

SELECTED REFERENCES

1. Botteri M et al: Cerebral blood flow thresholds for cerebral ischemia in traumatic brain injury. A systematic review. Crit Care Med. 36(11):3089-92, 2008
2. Stefini R et al: Chemokine detection in the cerebral tissue of patients with posttraumatic brain contusions. J Neurosurg. 108(5):958-62, 2008
3. Tawil I et al: Posttraumatic cerebral infarction: incidence, outcome, and risk factors. J Trauma. 64(4):849-53, 2008

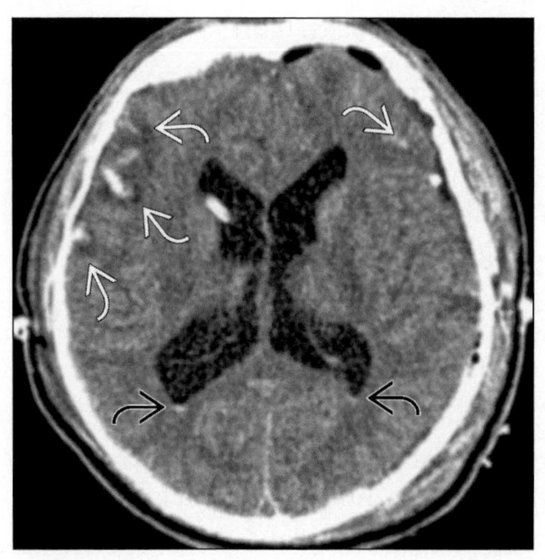

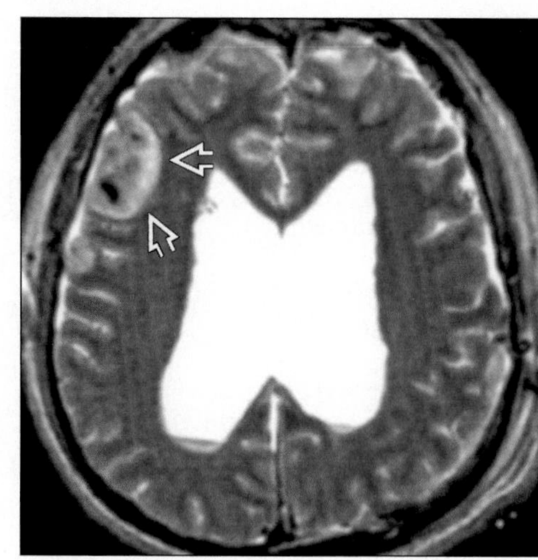

(Left) *Axial NECT following left-sided subdural evacuation shows 2 right and 1 left frontal hemorrhagic contusions ➡. Note the intraventricular hemorrhage ➡ and hydrocephalus.* ***(Right)*** *Axial T2WI MR in the same patient better illustrates the mass effect caused by the anterior right contusion effacing the local sulci and compressing the adjacent parenchyma ➡.*

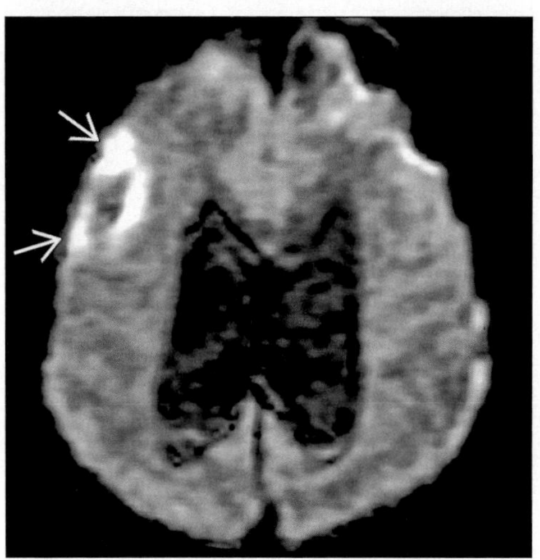

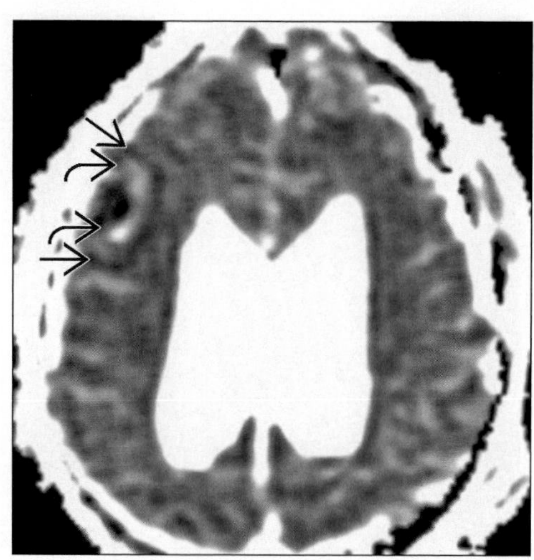

(Left) *Axial DWI MR in the same patient reveals hyperintensity at the periphery of the anterior right contusion ➡, which could be vasogenic edema or ischemia depending on the ADC.* ***(Right)*** *In the same patient, careful evaluation reveals vasogenic edema closest to the hemorrhagic core (bright on both DWI and ADC ➡) but with restricted diffusion of local ischemia at the periphery (bright on DWI but dark on ADC ➡).*

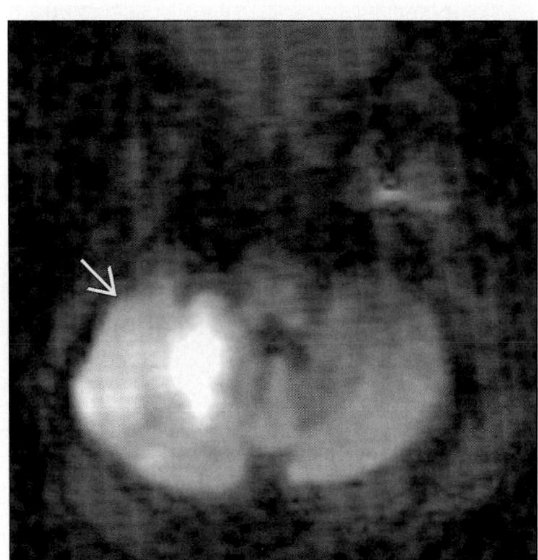

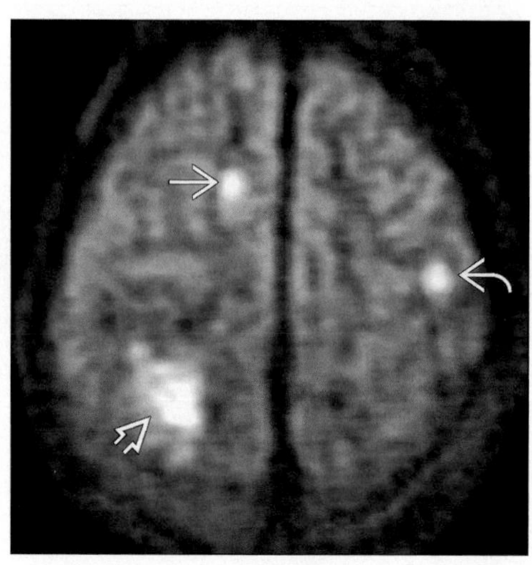

(Left) *Axial DWI MR obtained following an anoxic event on the 7th day of hospitalization shows restriction in the right superior cerebellar artery distribution ➡, which also involved the vermis (not shown), both confirmed with ADC.* ***(Right)*** *Axial DWI MR in the same patient reveals additional ischemic foci in the right frontal white matter ➡, posterior right frontal cortices ➡, and along the left frontal cortex ➡, all confirmed by ADC.*

BRAIN DEATH

Key Facts

Terminology
- Brain death (BD)
- Complete, irreversible cessation of brain function

Imaging
- No flow in intracranial arteries or venous sinuses on radionuclide scan or lack of intravascular enhancement on CT or MR
- Diffuse cerebral edema, effacement of gray-white matter borders
- EEG plus bedside scintigraphy (Neurolite)
- Evoked potentials enables neurofunctional evaluation of comatose patient
- Gyri swollen, ventricles/cisterns compressed

Top Differential Diagnoses
- Reversible diffuse cerebral edema
  - Drug overdose
  - Status epilepticus: Clinically can mimic BD
- Technical difficulty
  - Missed bolus (nuclear study, CTA)
  - Dissection (catheter angiography)
  - Vasospasm (catheter angiography)
- Massive cerebral infarction/edema

Pathology
- Severe cell swelling, ↑ intracranial pressure (ICP)

Clinical Issues
- Imaging may confirm but does not substitute for clinical criteria!
- Reversible causes of coma must be excluded!
- Remember: BD is primarily clinical diagnosis, legal criteria vary
- Clinical diagnosis of BD highly reliable with experienced examiners using established criteria

*(**Left**) Axial NECT shows complete loss of gray-white matter differentiation and diffuse sulcal and gyral effacement in this patient with diffuse cerebral edema and clinical brain death. The lateral ventricles are also effaced posteriorly ➡. (**Right**) Anteroposterior Tc-99m HMPAO scan shows the classic "light bulb" ➢ and "hot nose" signs ➡ related to lack of intracerebral blood flow in brain death. No radionuclide is seen in the intracranial arteries or veins. (Courtesy B. Vomocil, MD.)*

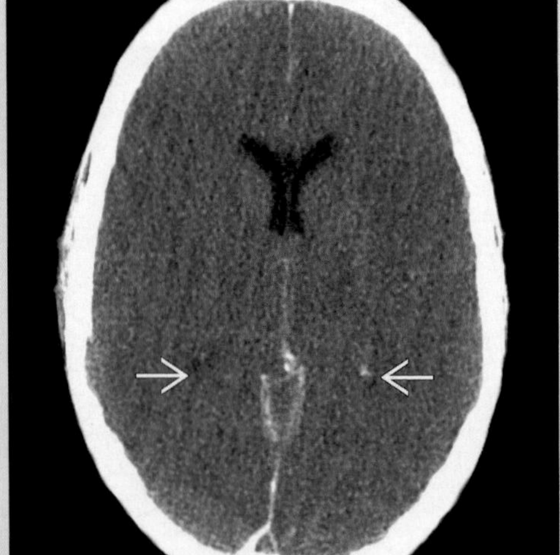

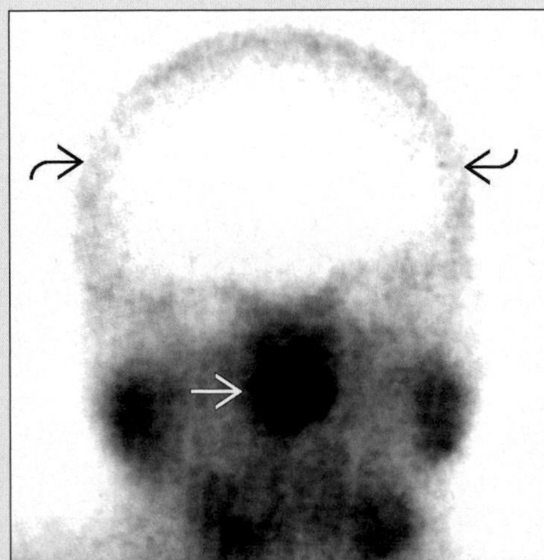

*(**Left**) Lateral DSA shows a common carotid injection with opacification of only the ECA branches ➢ and no contrast filling the intracranial ICA. No intracranial flow supports the clinical diagnosis of brain death. CTA is another modality now also being used to help diagnose brain death. (**Right**) Axial T1WI C+ FS MR shows lack of expected vascular ➢ and sinus mucosal ➡ enhancement. There is reflux of contrast in the cavernous sinus ➡. DWI MR has been found to improve sensitivity for predicting poor outcome.*

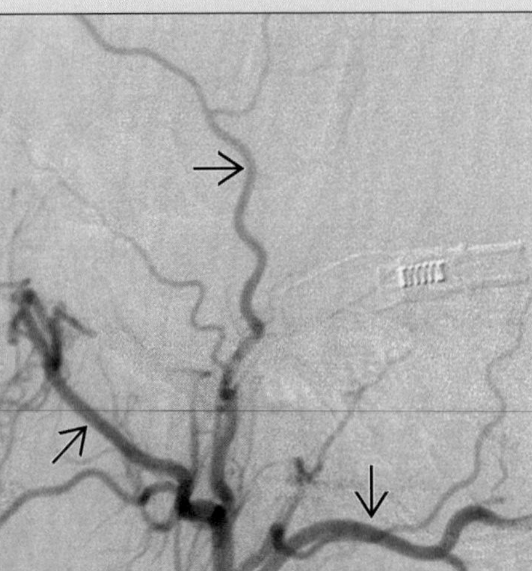

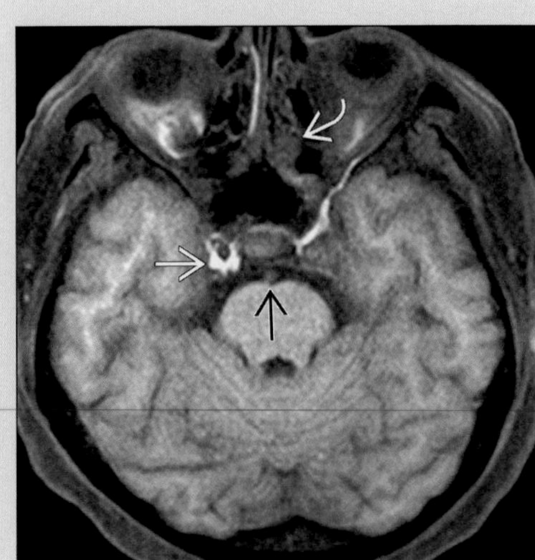

TERMINOLOGY

Abbreviations

- Brain death (BD)

Definitions

- Complete, irreversible cessation of brain function

IMAGING

General Features

- Best diagnostic clue
  - No flow in intracranial arteries or venous sinuses on Tc-99m ECD (Neurolite)
- Imaging may confirm but does not substitute for clinical criteria!

CT Findings

- NECT
  - Diffuse cerebral edema (GM-WM borders effaced)
    - "Reversal" sign (density of cerebellum > > hemispheres)
    - "Pseudosubarachnoid" appearance due to venous congestion in effaced sulci
  - Swollen gyri; compressed ventricles/cisterns
- CTA
  - No intravascular enhancement
    - Lack of opacification of MCA cortical branches and internal cerebral veins (ICVs) highly specific to confirm brain death

MR Findings

- T1WI
  - Hypointense, gray-white matter differentiation lost
  - Complete central brain herniation
- T2WI
  - Cortex hyperintense, gyri swollen
- DWI
  - Hemispheric high signal, severe ADC drop
    - DWI improves sensitivity for predicting poor outcome by 38%; in combination with 72-hour neuro exam, it is 100% specific
  - Diffusion anisotropy diminishes 1-12 hours after BD

Ultrasonographic Findings

- Orbital Doppler
  - Absence/reversal of end-diastolic flow in ophthalmic, central retinal arteries
  - Markedly increased arterial resistive indices
- Transcranial Doppler
  - Oscillating "to and fro" signal
  - Caution: 20% have ICA flow demonstrated despite cerebral circulatory arrest

Angiographic Findings

- Conventional
  - No intracranial flow
  - Contrast stasis (ECA fills, supraclinoid ICA does not)

Nuclear Medicine Findings

- Tc-99m-labeled exametazime scintigraphy
  - Absent intracranial uptake ("light bulb" sign)
  - Increased extracranial activity ("hot nose" sign)

Other Modality Findings

- EEG isoelectric

Imaging Recommendations

- Best imaging tool
  - EEG plus bedside scintigraphy (Neurolite)
  - Evoked potentials enables neurofunctional evaluation of comatose patient

DIFFERENTIAL DIAGNOSIS

Reversible Diffuse Cerebral Edema

- Drug overdose
- Status epilepticus: Clinically can mimic BD

Technical Difficulty

- Missed bolus (Nuclear study, CTA)
- Dissection (catheter angiography)
- Vasospasm (catheter angiography)

Massive Cerebral Infarction/Edema

- "Malignant" MCA infarct can mimic BD

PATHOLOGY

General Features

- Etiology
  - Severe cell swelling, ↑ intracranial pressure (ICP)
  - Markedly elevated ICP, ↓ cerebral blood flow
    - If ICP > end-diastolic pressure in cerebral arteries, diastolic reversal occurs
    - If ICP > systolic pressure, blood flow ceases

Gross Pathologic & Surgical Features

- Markedly swollen brain with severely compressed sulci
- Bilateral descending transtentorial herniation
  - Downward displacement of diencephalon
  - "Grooving" of temporal lobes by tentorial incisura

CLINICAL ISSUES

Presentation

- Most common signs/symptoms
  - Profound coma (GCS = 3) is "known cause"
  - Reversible causes of coma must be excluded!
- Clinical profile
  - Clinical diagnosis of BD highly reliable with experienced examiners using established criteria
  - Brain death is primarily a clinical diagnosis; legal criteria vary
  - Ancillary studies help confirm clinical diagnosis

SELECTED REFERENCES

1. Frampas E et al: CT Angiography for Brain Death Diagnosis. AJNR Am J Neuroradiol. Epub ahead of print, 2009
2. Wijman CA et al: Prognostic value of brain diffusion-weighted imaging after cardiac arrest. Ann Neurol. 65(4):394-402, 2009

TRAUMATIC INTRACRANIAL DISSECTION

Key Facts

Terminology
- Dissection
  - Intramural hematoma extends along vessel wall
- Dissecting aneurysm
  - Dissection + aneurysmal dilation contained by adventitia
- Pseudoaneurysm
  - Lumen contained by thrombus outside vessel wall

Imaging
- General findings
  - At contact between artery, falx/tentorium/skull
  - At region of significant motion
  - Vertebral arteries most common (72%)
  - Other: Peripheral vessels (A2/M2/P2; A3/A4, etc.)
- NECT: Basal subarachnoid hemorrhage
  - Looks like aneurysmal SAH
  - In unusual locations, more extensive than traumatic SAH
- MR: Hyperintense mural hematoma + central flow void on T1/T2WI
  - "Target" or "crescent" sign
  - SAH → sulcal/cisternal hyperintensity on FLAIR
- CTA/MRA/DSA
  - Enlarged vessel due to dissecting aneurysm or mural thrombus
  - Long segment narrowing or tapered occlusion
  - Intraluminal flap (± on DTA/MRA; best seen on DSA)
  - ± Dissecting aneurysm (irregular, wide-neck; at side wall, usually not at vessel bifurcations)

Clinical Issues
- May cause acute emboli
- Rupture (dissecting aneurysm/pseudoaneurysm)

*(**Left**) Axial T2WI MR shows enlarged bilateral intracranial vertebral arteries with heterogeneous signal on the right with an intramural hematoma and fluid level ➔, indicative of dissection with near or total occlusion. (**Right**) Anteroposterior angiography of the left vertebral artery shows reflux into the dissected right vertebral artery that has only a small residual patent lumen ➔. A distal embolus from the dissected vertebral artery is seen in the right posterior cerebral artery ➔.*

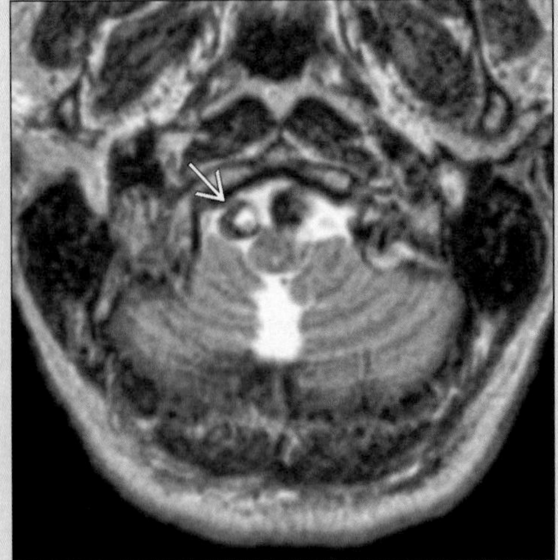

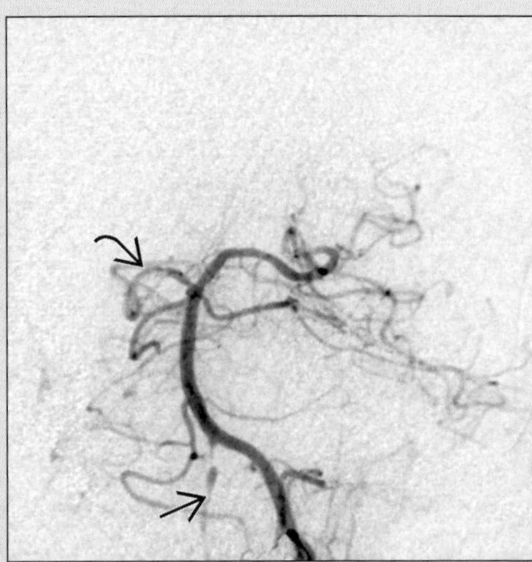

*(**Left**) Lateral angiography of the right internal carotid artery shows a pseudoaneurysm of a pericallosal artery branch at the genu of the corpus callosum ➔, with widening of the vessel and no discernible neck ➔. Locations near the falx, tentorium, and attachment points of the vessels are the most common locations from traumatic dissection and dissecting aneurysms. (**Right**) Axial NECT in the same patient shows hemorrhage ➔ within the corpus callosum due to the pseudoaneurysm.*

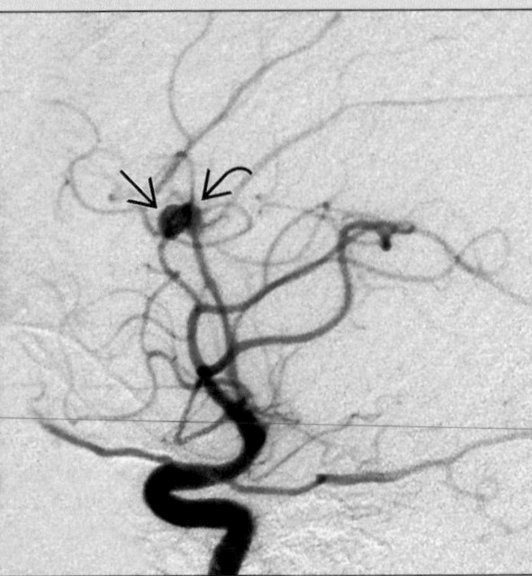

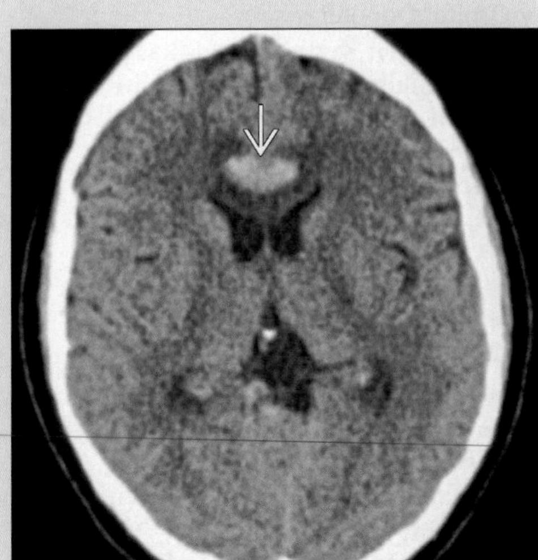

TERMINOLOGY

Synonyms
- Traumatic dissection and pseudoaneurysm

Definitions
- Dissection: Intramural hematoma extends along vessel
- Intimal extension
  - Intimal flap
  - True and false lumen
- Arterial transection
  - Extension through adventitia
- Dissecting aneurysm: Aneurysmal dilation of vessel due to dissection, contained only by adventitia
  - Hematoma between media/adventitia common
- Pseudoaneurysm: Lumen contained only by thrombus outside vessel wall

IMAGING

General Features
- Best diagnostic clue
  - NECT: Basal extensive subarachnoid hemorrhage (SAH) mimics aneurysmal SAH but often more extensive than traumatic SAH or in unusual locations
  - MR: Hyperintense crescent in vessel wall with central or eccentric flow void on axial T1WI and T2WI ("target" or "crescent" sign)
    - Subarachnoid hyperintensity on FLAIR due to hemorrhage
    - Enlarged vessel due to dissecting aneurysm or mural thrombus
  - MRA, CTA, DSA
    - Long segment narrowing or tapered occlusion
    - Intraluminal flap on MRA/CTA source images
    - ± irregular, eccentric side-wall dissecting aneurysm
      - Usually not at bifurcation
- Location
  - Vertebral arteries most common (72%)
  - Otherwise, usually more peripheral (A2, M2, P2, and beyond)
  - Often occurs at contact points with falx, skull, tentorium, or at region of significant motion
  - Basilar artery
  - Posterior inferior cerebellar artery (PICA)
  - Superior cerebral artery (SCA)
  - Posterior cerebral artery (PCA)
  - Anterior cerebral artery (ACA) (A2)
  - Middle cerebral artery (MCA)
- Morphology
  - Tapered stenosis with occlusion
  - Irregular vessel narrowing
  - Fusiform irregular dilatation or focal dissecting aneurysm
  - Intimal flap and double (true and false) lumen
  - Intramural hematoma

CT Findings
- NECT
  - Basal SAH mimics aneurysmal SAH but is more extensive than typical traumatic SAH
    - Atypical SAH located in upper interhemispheric fissure, along tentorium
  - Acute embolic infarct
    - Hypodensity in vascular distribution
    - Hemorrhagic conversion, gyral hyperdensity
  - Basal skull fracture in some cases
- CTA
  - Tapered narrowing &/or occlusion
  - False lumen and flap visible in minority of cases
  - CTA source images show intraluminal flap and vessel wall thickening
  - Irregular dissecting aneurysm: Fusiform or wide-neck

MR Findings
- T1WI
  - Acute thrombus within vessel may be hypointense on T1WI
  - Subacute = hyperintense crescentic intramural hematoma
  - Absent or decreased flow void
- T2WI
  - "Target" or "crescent" sign: Central or eccentric hypointense flow void surrounded by hyperintensity in vessel wall
  - Acute infarct hyperintense
    - ± hemorrhagic conversion (hypointense on T2WI, T2*)
- FLAIR
  - Hyperintense CSF: SAH
  - Hyperintense acute infarct
- DWI
  - Hyperintensity in acute infarct
- MRA
  - Amorphous mild hyperintensity in wall of vessel (intramural hematoma) partially surrounds more marked flow-related hyperintensity but may obscure detail
    - PC MRA may better characterize lumen
  - Decreased flow may be manifested by decreased caliber and intensity of lumen of vessels distal to dissection, especially on 3D TOF

Angiographic Findings
- Conventional
  - Tapered narrowing or occlusion
  - Irregular lumen or intimal flap
  - Focal aneurysmal dilatation is usually wide-neck, irregular, triangular in shape, occurring in unusual locations
  - Embolic occlusion of distal branches

Imaging Recommendations
- Best imaging tool: MR and MRA
- Protocol advice
  - Initial NECT important to assess for SAH
  - MR/MRA → CTA if MRA equivocal
  - Conventional angiography indicated when clinical suspicion is high, but MR/MRA is negative, &/or for therapeutic intervention

TRAUMATIC INTRACRANIAL DISSECTION

DIFFERENTIAL DIAGNOSIS

Atherosclerosis

- Luminal irregularity and stenosis most marked in cavernous carotid artery, vertebral and basilar arteries
  - No aneurysmal dilatation
- Focal and eccentric when involves pial branches
- Mural calcification on NECT, CTA, or MRA source images

Vasospasm

- Smooth narrowing usually centered at vessel bifurcation
- Most severe where SAH is greatest
- No aneurysmal dilatations

Vasculitis

- Short or long segment smooth narrowing not centered on vessel bifurcations
- Regions of narrowing alternate with normal vessel lumen or mild aneurysmal dilatation
- Isolated aneurysmal dilatation less common

Fibromuscular Dysplasia (FMD)

- Rarely intracranial, virtually always in association with extracranial involvement
  - Internal carotid artery opposite C2 in 2/3 of cases
- Alternating zones of focal narrowing and aneurysmal dilatation
  - Corrugated pipe appearance
- Long segment stenosis or aneurysmal dilatation
- May be cause of spontaneous dissection
  - Visualization of vessel wall on MR needed to differentiate between FMD and dissection ± FMD
  - FMD produces focal vessel wall thickening without hemorrhage or calcification

Spontaneous (Nontraumatic) Basal SAH

- Ruptured aneurysm
- Benign perimesencephalic SAH

PATHOLOGY

General Features

- Etiology
  - Skull base fracture, subdural hematoma: Clinically severe head injury
  - Minor injury often overlooked in history
  - Direct injury to intracranial vessel from contact with falx, tentorium, skull
  - Shearing type injury at motion segments: Supraclinoid ICA, MCAs
- Associated abnormalities
  - Fibromuscular dysplasia, arterial fenestrations
  - Collagen disorders, rheumatoid arthritis
  - Metabolic/genetic disorders: Angiolipomatosis, Marfan, α-1-antitrypsin deficiency

CLINICAL ISSUES

Presentation

- Most common signs/symptoms
  - Headache, obtundation, CN3 palsy

Demographics

- Epidemiology
  - 1.5-10% of SAH

Natural History & Prognosis

- If vessel patent, may resolve spontaneously
- Acute emboli is common complication in acute phase
- Rupture is very common with dissecting aneurysm or pseudoaneurysm

Treatment

- Anticoagulation to prevent progressive thrombosis and embolization with distal infarction
- Angioplasty and stent treatment for severely stenotic lesion
- Endovascular occlusion usually of parent vessel or stent/coils or stent graft without adequate collaterals
- Surgical occlusion, wrapping, or bypass

DIAGNOSTIC CHECKLIST

Consider

- Dissection when young patient presents with acute "spontaneous" infarction
  - Inquire about mild trauma or falls in 24 hours prior to onset of symptoms
- Dissecting aneurysm at unusual locations: Pericallosal, distal MCA, distal PCA, not at branch points

Image Interpretation Pearls

- Look for "target" sign in internal carotid or vertebral artery on images at or just below skull base

SELECTED REFERENCES

1. Ansari SA et al: Endovascular treatment of distal cervical and intracranial dissections with the neuroform stent. Neurosurgery. 62(3):636-46, 2008
2. Santos-Franco JA et al: Dissecting aneurysms of the vertebrobasilar system. A comprehensive review on natural history and treatment options. Neurosurg Rev. 31(2):131-40; discussion 140, 2008
3. Ahn JY et al: Endovascular treatment of intracranial vertebral artery dissections with stent placement or stent-assisted coiling. AJNR Am J Neuroradiol. 27(7):1514-20, 2006
4. Benninger DH et al: Mechanism of ischemic infarct in spontaneous carotid dissection. Stroke. 35(2):482-5, 2004
5. Chen CJ et al: Multisection CT angiography compared with catheter angiography in diagnosing vertebral artery dissection. AJNR Am J Neuroradiol. 25(5):769-74, 2004
6. Luo CB et al: Endovascular management of the traumatic cerebral aneurysms associated with traumatic carotid cavernous fistulas. AJNR Am J Neuroradiol. 25(3):501-5, 2004
7. Mizutani T et al: Healing process for cerebral dissecting aneurysms presenting with subarachnoid hemorrhage. Neurosurgery. 54(2):342-7; discussion 347-8, 2004
8. Anxionnat R et al: Treatment of hemorrhagic intracranial dissections. Neurosurgery. 53(2):289-300; discussion 300-1, 2003

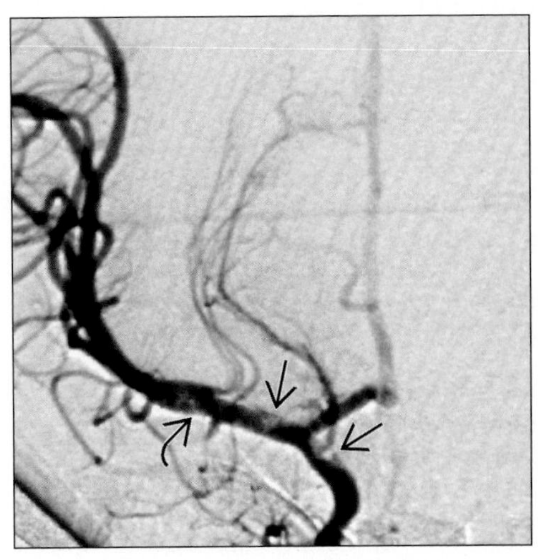

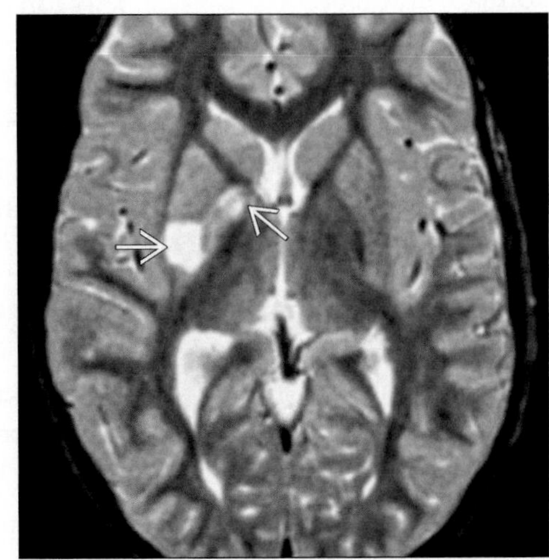

(Left) *Anteroposterior angiography shows irregular narrowing of the supraclinoid ICA and proximal MCA due to intraluminal thrombus → with an intimal flap of the distal M1 segment ↗. This dissection occurred where the ICA passes from its relatively fixed position within the skull to a more mobile location inside the dura and extended distally.* ***(Right)*** *Axial T2WI MR in the same patient shows infarcts in the globus pallidus and posterior putamen → from lenticulostriate occlusion of the proximal M1.*

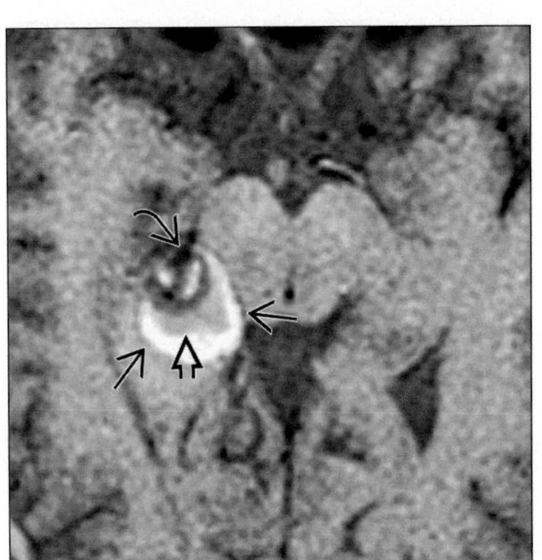

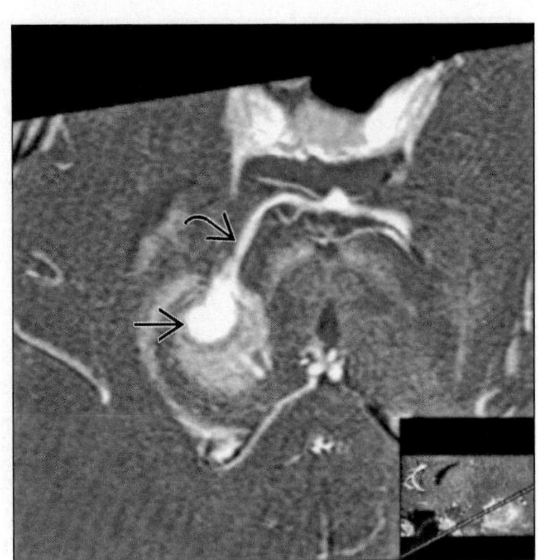

(Left) *Axial T1WI MR shows a mixed signal intensity mass with peripheral hyperintensity of a subacute hematoma →, central isointensity ⇨ due to slow flow or more recent thrombus, and a small "flow void" ↗ representing the residual lumen.* ***(Right)*** *Axial MRA with contrast in the same patient shows a strongly enhancing area of a traumatic pseudoaneurysm → of the P2 segment ↗. The damage in this location is due to the direct injury from its proximity with the midbrain and tentorium.*

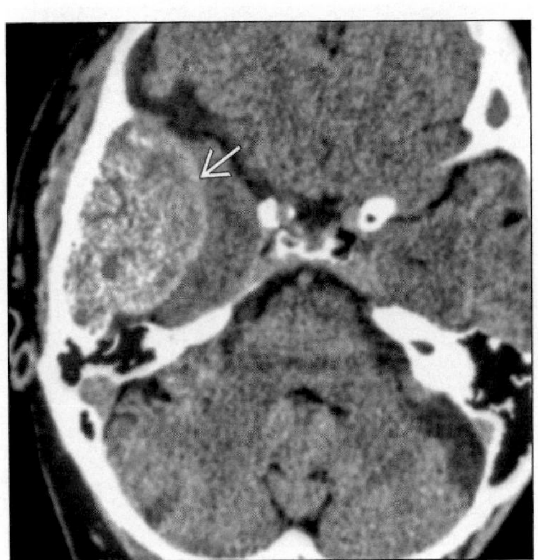

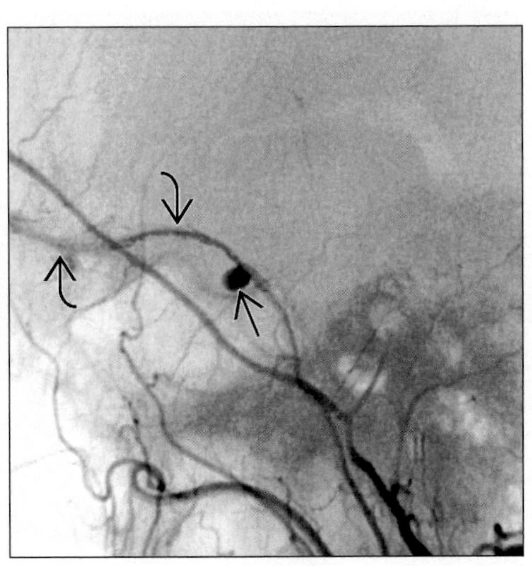

(Left) *Axial NECT shows a biconvex hyperdense epidural hematoma →. A linear skull fracture crossed the middle meningeal artery groove on bone windows.* ***(Right)*** *Lateral DSA in the same patient shows a traumatic pseudoaneurysm of the right middle meningeal artery (MMA) →. The lacerated MMA has also fistulized to the middle meningeal veins, causing a "tram-track" appearance with opacified artery surrounded by the 2 middle meningeal veins that accompany the MMA ↗. (Courtesy C. Looney, MD).*

TRAUMATIC EXTRACRANIAL DISSECTION

Key Facts

Terminology
- Traumatic intramural hemorrhage of ICA or VA

Imaging
- Location: At sites unusual for atherosclerosis
  - ICA: From upper internal carotid bulb to skull base or petrous segment
  - VA dissection most common at C1-2 level
  - Clot between adventitia-media or media-intima
  - 15% involve multiple vessels
- MR
  - "Target" or "crescent" sign
  - Crescentic hyperintense intramural hematoma
  - Surrounds flow void of patent lumen
- CTA/DSA/MRA
  - Tubular narrowing or focal dilatation
  - Linear intraluminal intimal flap
  - Segmental tapered narrowing ("string" sign)
  - ± segmental dilatation (pseudoaneurysm)

Top Differential Diagnoses
- Fibromuscular dysplasia
- Marfan, type 4 Ehlers-Danlos
- Vasospasm, thrombosis, ASVD

Clinical Issues
- Headache, neck pain
  - 60-90% of patients with cervical ICA dissection
  - Onset often delayed, from hours to 3-4 weeks
- Focal cerebral ischemic symptoms (TIA, infarct)
  - Often delayed hours to weeks post injury

Diagnostic Checklist
- Early screening via CTA or MR/MRA of severely injured patients for detection of occult dissection
- MR/MRA in any young or middle-aged patient with unrelenting headache or cervical pain

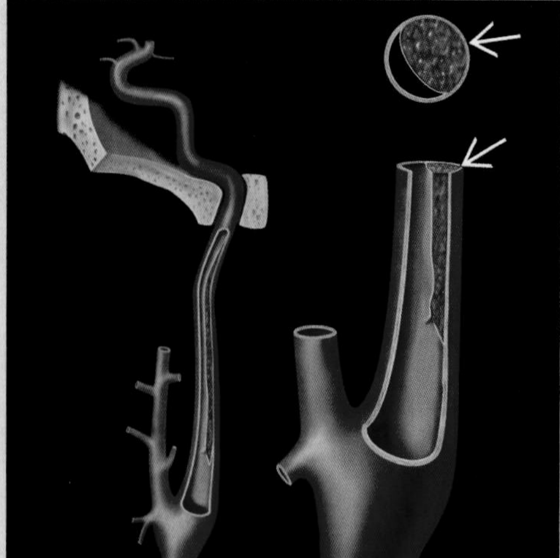

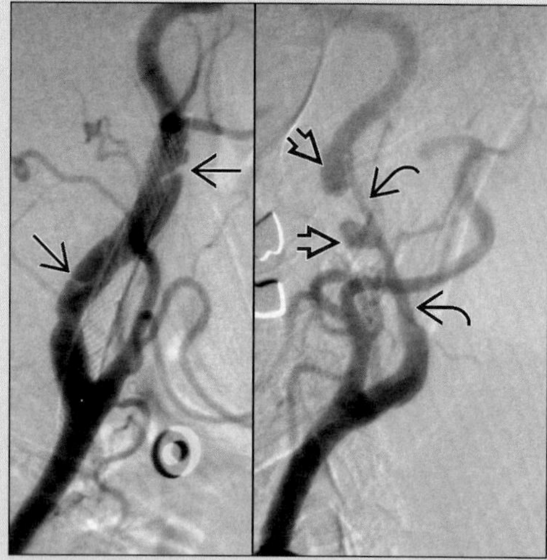

(Left) *Graphic depicts dissection of the cervical internal carotid artery (ICA) with subintimal thrombus ➔. Note the sparing of the carotid bulb. Dissection ends at the skull base.* ***(Right)*** *Oblique DSA of the right and left carotid arteries shows linear intimal flaps and vascular enlargement of the right ➔ ICA and tapered stenosis ➔ with focal pseudoaneurysms ➔ of the left ICA. This patient with traumatic dissections suffered small bilateral strokes on anticoagulation and was treated with bilateral carotid stenting.*

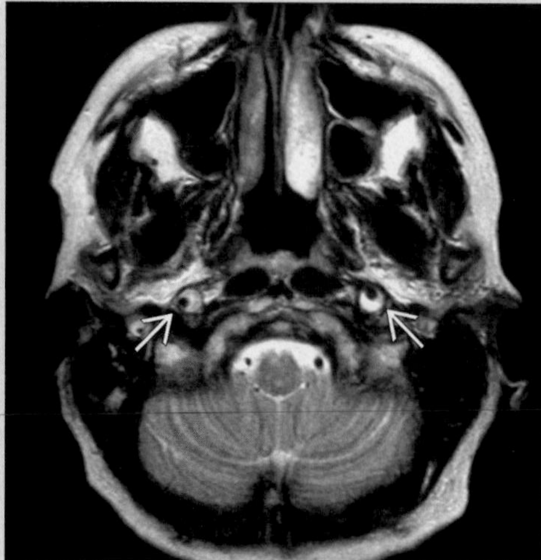

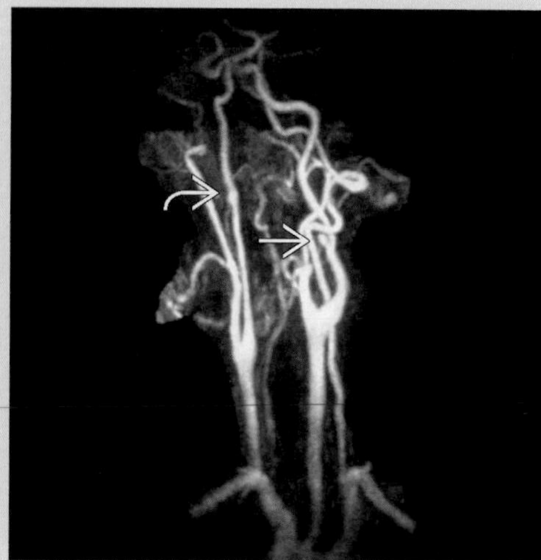

(Left) *Axial T2WI MR shows hyperintense bilateral intramural thrombus in both upper cervical ICAs ➔ with eccentric narrowed flow voids ("crescent" sign) in this patient with acute bilateral dissection.* ***(Right)*** *Oblique MRA in the same patient 1 year later, treated with anticoagulation, shows near complete healing of the dissection with only small residual pseudoaneurysms of the proximal left ➔ and upper mid right ➔ cervical ICA without significant narrowing.*

TRAUMATIC EXTRACRANIAL DISSECTION

TERMINOLOGY

Synonyms

- Cervicocephalic arterial dissection

Definitions

- Traumatic intramural hemorrhage of internal carotid artery (ICA) or vertebral artery (VA)

IMAGING

General Features

- Best diagnostic clue
  - Tubular narrowing or focal dilatation in sites unusual for atherosclerosis
  - Linear intraluminal intimal flap
  - Crescentic, hyperintense, intramural hematoma surrounding flow void on T1WI or T2WI
    - "Target" or "crescent" sign
- Location
  - Between adventitia-media or media-intima
  - Traumatic dissection: ICA > VA
    - ICA dissection: From upper internal carotid bulb to skull base or petrous segment
    - VA dissection most common at C1-2 level
  - 15% involve multiple vessels
- Size
  - Intramural hematoma propagates distally for variable distance
- Morphology
  - Pseudoaneurysm or long stenosis
  - Secondary embolic infarct common

Radiographic Findings

- Radiography
  - Fracture of skull base or cervical spine, often involving arterial foramen

CT Findings

- NECT
  - Usually normal
  - Enlarged hyperdense ICA, carotid space mass (pseudoaneurysm)
  - Brain may show arterial territorial low density secondary to infarction
  - Fracture of skull base or cervical spine, often involving arterial foramen
- CECT
  - Linear luminal filling defect: Intimal flap or false lumen
  - Thin rim of contrast enhancement surrounding mural hematoma secondary to vasa vasorum

MR Findings

- Intramural hematoma ("target" or "crescent" sign)
  - Curvilinear, crescentic, band-like or small focus adjacent to lumen
  - Usually circumferential and eccentric
  - Widens external diameter of artery
  - Surrounds normal/narrow flow void
  - Signal characteristics
    - Acute: Isointense/slightly hyperintense on T1WI, hypointense on T2WI
    - Subacute: Hyperintense on T1WI and T2WI
- Intimal flap
  - Thin curvilinear hypointense partition separating true and false lumen
- Flow void in residual lumen
  - Eccentrically narrowed
  - Absent flow void 2° to slow flow or occlusion

Ultrasonographic Findings

- Color Doppler
  - Echogenic intimal flap (most specific sign)
  - Echogenic thrombus
  - Abrupt smooth tapering of arterial lumen
  - False lumen occasionally seen with color Doppler

Angiographic Findings

- DSA/CTA/MRA
  - Segmental tapered narrowing ("string" sign)
  - Segmental dilatation of vessel (pseudoaneurysm)
    - Oval, parallel to artery, variable size
    - Extraluminal pouch at midportion of stenotic segment
    - "Pearl and string" sign at distal margin of stenotic region
  - Intimal flap at proximal margin of dissection
    - Source MRA/CTA images, less common on DSA
  - Double lumen: True and false lumen (intramural dissection)
    - Uncommon, particularly in VA
  - True lumen may be completely occluded
  - Slow flow in parent artery
  - Distal branch occlusions due to embolization
  - CTA and dynamic gadolinium MRA: Independent of flow phenomena
    - Shows small residual lumen & pseudoaneurysms
    - MRA: Amorphous mild hyperintensity (intramural hematoma) partially engulfs hyperintense lumen (flow)

Imaging Recommendations

- Best imaging tool
  - MR and MRA of head and neck with overlapping imaging volumes
- Protocol advice
  - MR with fat-suppressed T1WI, MRA
  - CTA in acute dissection or if MR/MRA equivocal
  - DSA for equivocal cases and endovascular intervention

DIFFERENTIAL DIAGNOSIS

"Spontaneous" Dissection

- Underlying vasculopathy common
  - Fibromuscular dysplasia
    - "String of beads" appearance > long tubular stenosis
  - Marfan syndrome, type 4 Ehlers-Danlos syndrome
- Familial ICA dissection
- Hypertension in 1/3 of patients
- Delayed presentation of undiagnosed blunt artery injury (occult dissection)

TRAUMATIC EXTRACRANIAL DISSECTION

Arterial Thrombosis

- Often difficult to establish whether underlying dissection is present

Atherosclerosis

- Typically occurs at carotid bifurcation or VA origin
- Irregular > smooth tapered narrowing
- Ca++ often present

Proximal ICA Stenosis

- Severe extracranial arterial stenosis → slow flow in intracranial segment, simulating intracranial dissection ("pseudodissection")
  - Can produce periarterial rim of abnormal signal that is not due to hematoma
  - T1WI isointense, T2WI hyperintense; no marked T1WI or T2WI hyperintensity in wall

Vasospasm

- Catheter-placement induced
- Transient; resolves within minutes

PATHOLOGY

General Features

- Etiology
  - Penetrating injury (gunshot wound or stabbing) may injure common carotid, ICA, or VA
  - Blunt trauma may affect extracranial ICA
    - Motor vehicle crashes (high acceleration/ hyperextension or direct trauma from shoulder belt)
    - Direct blow to neck; may be mild & overlooked
    - Falls, strangulation digital carotid compression, iatrogenic (VA dissection in 5% of facet joint surgeries)
    - Rapid neck rotation or flexion; diving injuries
    - Chiropractic manipulation (stretching/torsion) affects VA > ICA
  - Potential mechanisms of injury
    - Sudden, severe stretch of artery over upper cervical spine in hyperextension & lateral flexion
    - Stretching of ICA over transverse processes of upper cervical vertebrae
    - Compression of ICA between angle of mandible and upper cervical vertebral bodies
    - Stretching of VA over C1-2 vertebral bodies, primarily during head rotation
    - Combination of head, facial, & cervical injuries
- Associated abnormalities
  - Asymptomatic dissection of 2nd artery (15%)
    - Usually accompanies symptomatic VA dissection
  - Severe trauma to cervical spine
  - Patients evaluated for blunt aortic trauma 10x more likely to have blunt carotid injury

Gross Pathologic & Surgical Features

- Intimal disruption or vasa vasorum hemorrhage
- Hemorrhage between intima-media → luminal stenosis
- Hemorrhage between adventitia-media → pseudoaneurysm formation

CLINICAL ISSUES

Presentation

- Most common signs/symptoms
  - Headache, neck pain
    - 60-90% of patients with cervical ICA dissection
    - Onset often delayed, from hours to 3-4 weeks
  - Focal cerebral ischemic symptoms (TIA, infarct)
    - Often delayed hours to weeks post injury
  - Horner syndrome
    - Stretching or injury of sympathetic nerves adjacent to ICA
    - May be incomplete (only miosis, ptosis)
- Other signs/symptoms
  - Uncommon
    - Cranial nerve palsy (CN12 > 9, 10, 11)
    - Carotid bruits, pulsatile tinnitus
- Clinical profile
  - Unrelenting headache or cervical pain in young or middle-aged adults

Demographics

- Age
  - Uncommon in children, adolescents (7% of cases)
- Gender
  - ICA dissection (all causes): M:F = 1.5:1
  - VA dissection (all causes): M:F = 1:3
- Epidemiology
  - Incidence of ICA dissection in blunt trauma patients: 0.08-0.4%
  - Dissection accounts for 0.4-2.5% of all infarcts
    - Common cause of infarcts in patients < age 40
      - 20% of infarcts in young patients

Natural History & Prognosis

- Delayed diagnosis of blunt carotid injury common
- Traumatic vs. spontaneous dissection
  - Traumatic dissection less likely to spontaneously improve
    - More likely to lead to residual neurologic deficits
- More than 2/3 of patients have complete recovery

Treatment

- Anticoagulation with heparin followed by warfarin (Coumadin)
- Endovascular intervention: Occlusion, angioplasty, stenting
- Delayed onset after relatively minor trauma or chiropractic treatment may obscure diagnosis

DIAGNOSTIC CHECKLIST

Consider

- Early screening via CTA or MR/MRA of severely injured patients for detection of occult dissection
- MR/MRA in any young or middle-aged patient with unrelenting headache or cervical pain

SELECTED REFERENCES

1. Chamoun RB et al: Extracranial traumatic carotid artery dissections in children: a review of current diagnosis and treatment options. J Neurosurg Pediatr. 2(2):101-8, 2008

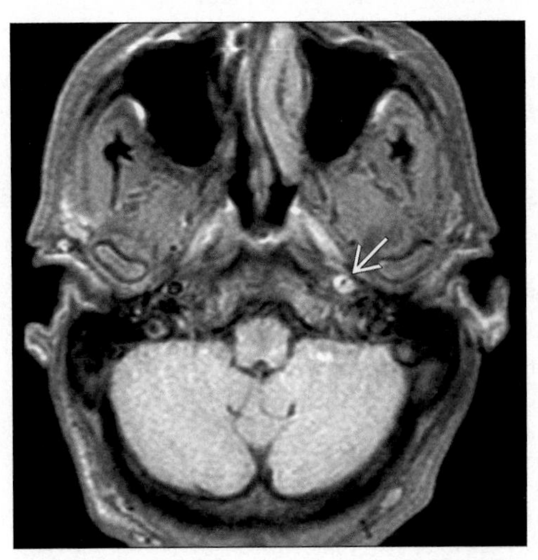

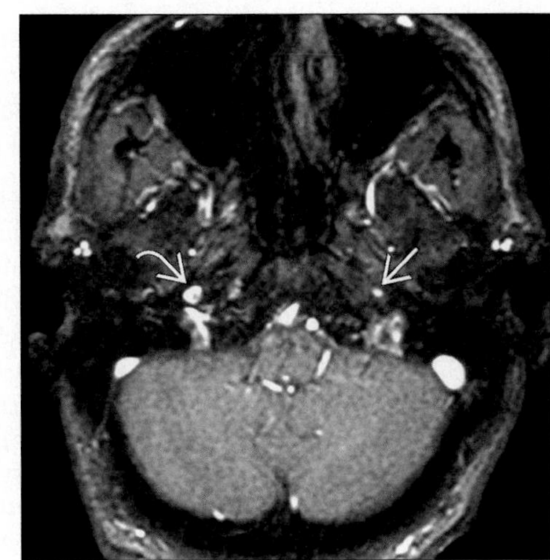

(Left) *Axial T1WI FS MR shows T1 hyperintense thrombus surrounding the central flow void ("target" sign) ➡ in this patient with a traumatic upper cervical carotid dissection.* ***(Right)*** *Axial MRA source image through the same region demonstrates flow signal in the stenotic true lumen ➡. Flow artifact ➡ in the normal right carotid artery can sometimes be misinterpreted as dissection. These artifacts are most commonly seen at course changes, especially in the petrous and cavernous ICA segments.*

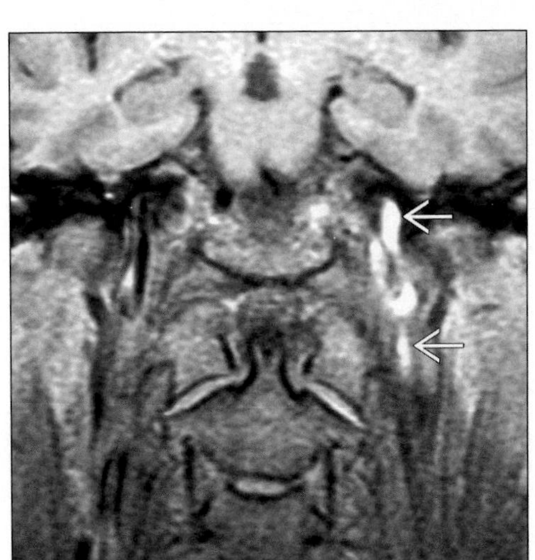

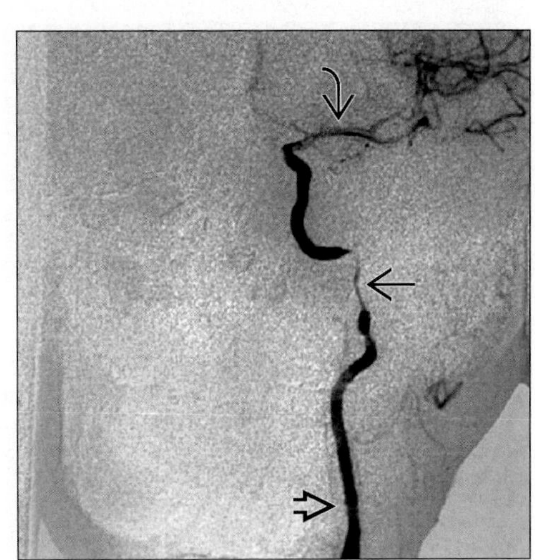

(Left) *Coronal T1WI FS MR demonstrates T1 hyperintense thrombus in the upper cervical and lateral petrous segments of the left ICA ➡ due to traumatic dissection.* ***(Right)*** *Frontal DSA of the left ICA in the same patient shows irregular high-grade stenosis of the same segments due to traumatic dissection ➡. Inflow from the posterior communicating artery creates a pseudo-dissection of the distal ICA and M1 segment ➡, and the proximal ICA has a sawtooth margin due to a traumatic vasospasm ➡.*

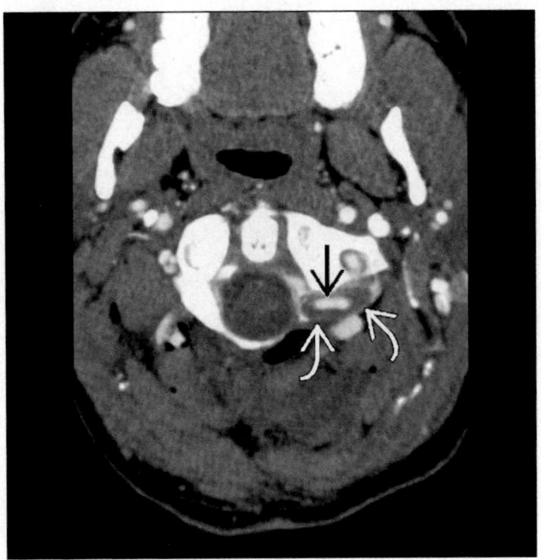

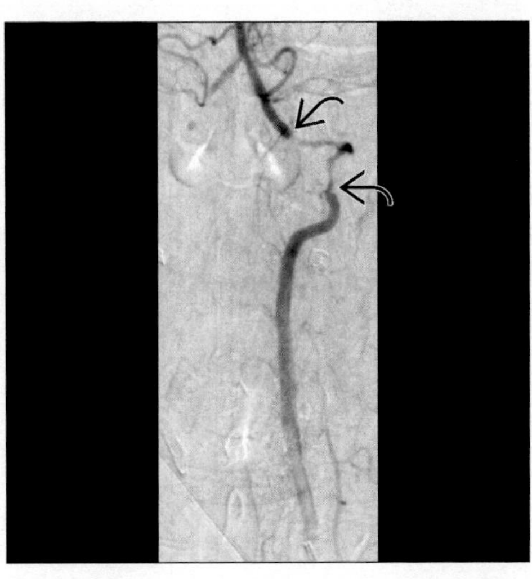

(Left) *Axial CTA shows a narrowed enhancing lumen ➡ surrounded by low-density intramural thrombus and enhancing vasa vasorum ➡ due to traumatic vertebral artery dissection.* ***(Right)*** *Anteroposterior DSA shows an irregular dissection of the left vertebral artery from the C1-2 junction to the dural insertion ➡. Traumatic vertebral dissections often occur where the vertebral artery penetrates the dura, in the highly mobile C1-2 segment, or near fractures involving the transverse foramina.*

TRAUMATIC CAROTID CAVERNOUS FISTULA

Key Facts

Terminology

- Direct CCF, high-flow CCF
- Single-hole tear/transection of cavernous ICA with arteriovenous shunt into cavernous sinus

Imaging

- General features
  - Proptosis, dilated superior ophthalmic vein (SOV) and CS, extraocular muscle (EOM) enlargement
  - Skull base fracture involving sphenoid bone/ carotid canal? ↑ likelihood of ICA injury!
- MRA: ↑ flow-related signal in CS and SOV
- CT/CTA may be suggestive; should proceed to DSA to confirm and treat
- DSA is definitive
  - Early filling of CS + outflow pathways including retrograde filling of SOV, angular + facial veins
  - Reduced or absent antegrade flow in ICA beyond fistula depending on size of ICA tear

Top Differential Diagnoses

- Indirect CCF
  - "Low-flow CCF," CS dural arteriovenous fistula (dAVF)

Clinical Issues

- Bruit, pulsating exophthalmos, orbital edema/ erythema, ↓ vision, glaucoma, headache
- Hemispheric ischemia if ↓ flow in ICA beyond CCF
- Focal deficits → cranial nerves 3-6
- Endovascular treatment options include
  - Transarterial-transfistula detachable balloon embolization
  - Transvenous embolization
  - Covered stent placement
  - ICA sacrifice

*(**Left**) Axial T1WI of proptosis developed after a basisphenoid fracture shows dilatation of both superior ophthalmic veins ➔ as well as the angular veins ➔. The latter may be catheterized via the anterior facial vein to achieve access to the cavernous sinus embolization if access via the inferior petrosal sinus is not possible. (**Right**) Anteroposterior DSA of the left ICA shows early filling of the cavernous sinuses bilaterally ➔. Note filling of the circular sinus ➔ and filling defect within the right cavernous sinus ➔, representing the ICA.*

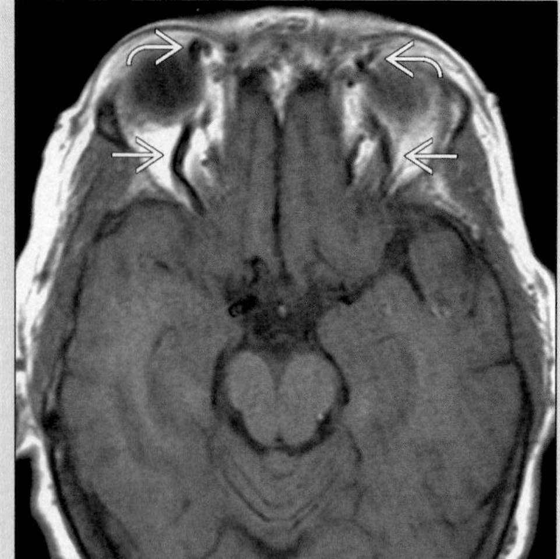

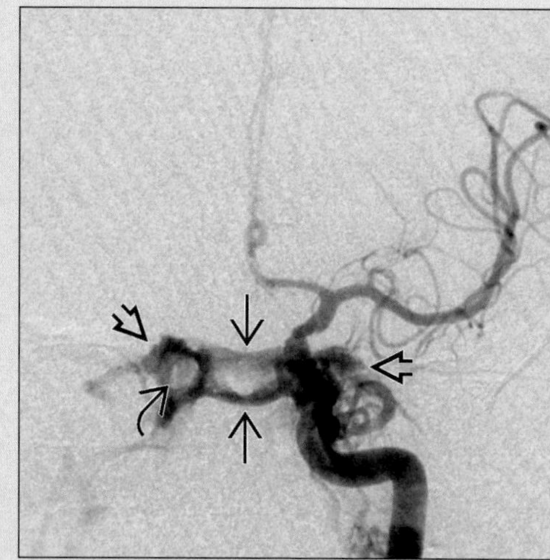

*(**Left**) Lateral DSA shows opacification of the cavernous sinus in the arterial phase. Also outlined are many of the venous outflow pathways of the cavernous sinus, including the superior ophthalmic veins ➔, superior and inferior petrosal sinuses ➔, and pterygoid and pharyngeal venous plexi ➔. (**Right**) Lateral DSA of the left internal carotid artery after coiling ➔ of the fistula shows complete obliteration. Note the preservation of cavernous ICA and all its distal branches.*

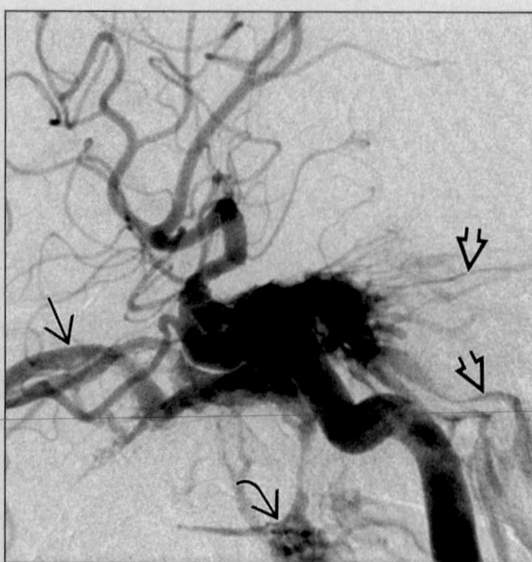

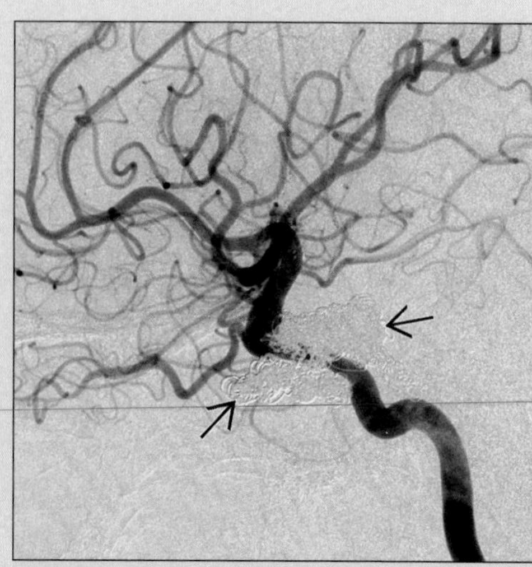

TRAUMATIC CAROTID CAVERNOUS FISTULA

TERMINOLOGY

Abbreviations
- Carotid cavernous fistula (CCF)

Synonyms
- Direct CCF, high-flow CCF

Definitions
- Single-hole tear/transection of cavernous internal carotid artery (ICA) with arteriovenous shunt into cavernous sinus (CS)

IMAGING

General Features
- Best diagnostic clue
  - Proptosis, dilated superior ophthalmic vein (SOV) and CS, extraocular muscle (EOM) enlargement

CT Findings
- NECT
  - Skull base fracture involving sphenoid bone/carotid canal ↑ likelihood of ICA injury
  - Proptosis, enlarged SOV, CS, and EOMs
    - "Dirty" orbital fat secondary to edema
  - Subarachnoid hemorrhage (SAH) from associated trauma or arterialized flow into cortical veins
- CECT
  - Dilated SOV and CS
  - ↑ enhancement of EOMs, patchy enhancement of intraorbital fat

MR Findings
- T1WI C+
  - Same as CECT
- MRA
  - ↑ flow-related signal in CS and SOV
  - Signal loss in ICA secondary to turbulent flow

Ultrasonographic Findings
- Doppler: Reversal of flow in dilated SOV (intra- to extracranial)

Angiographic Findings
- Conventional
  - Early filling of CS + outflow pathways including
    - Retrograde filling of SOV, angular + facial veins
    - Contralateral CS
    - Petrosal sinuses → internal jugular vein(s)
  - Reduced or absent antegrade flow in ICA beyond fistula depending on size of ICA tear

Imaging Recommendations
- Best imaging tool
  - DSA is definitive
  - CT/CTA may be suggestive: Should proceed to DSA to confirm and treat
- Protocol advice
  - DSA: Magnification, high frame rate to visualize exact site of shunt
  - CTA: Thin section scans with reformations

DIFFERENTIAL DIAGNOSIS

Indirect CCF
- a.k.a. "low-flow CCF," CS dural arteriovenous fistula (dAVF)

EOM Enlargement
- Grave disease, inflammatory pseudotumor, neoplasm

PATHOLOGY

General Features
- Etiology
  - Skull base fracture with bony fragment injuring ICA
  - Stretch injury of vessel wall between fixed points at foramen lacerum and anterior clinoid process
- Associated abnormalities
  - Arterialized flow in CS with retrograde venous reflux
    - Superior/inferior ophthalmic veins → proptosis, chemosis, ↑ intraocular pressure → ↓ retinal perfusion pressure → blindness
    - Cortical veins → increased SAH risk
  - Reduced antegrade flow in ICA beyond fistula → hemispheric ischemia

CLINICAL ISSUES

Presentation
- Most common signs/symptoms
  - May present days to weeks post-trauma
  - Bruit, pulsating exophthalmos, orbital edema/ erythema, ↓ vision, glaucoma, headache
  - Hemispheric ischemia if ↓ flow in ICA beyond CCF
  - Severe/rapid vision loss, SAH → emergency
  - Focal deficits → cranial nerves 3-6

Natural History & Prognosis
- Endovascular options include
  - Transarterial-transfistula detachable balloon embolization
  - Transvenous embolization
  - Covered stent placement across tear in ICA
  - ICA sacrifice with coils or detachable balloons (if patient tolerates lack of antegrade flow beyond fistula or passes balloon test occlusion)

DIAGNOSTIC CHECKLIST

Image Interpretation Pearls
- Enlarged SOV & CS, proptosis, intraorbital edema

Reporting Tips
- CT/MR may be suggestive, but DSA is required for definitive diagnosis and treatment

SELECTED REFERENCES

1. Gemmete JJ et al: Endovascular techniques for treatment of carotid-cavernous fistula. J Neuroophthalmol. 29(1):62-71, 2009

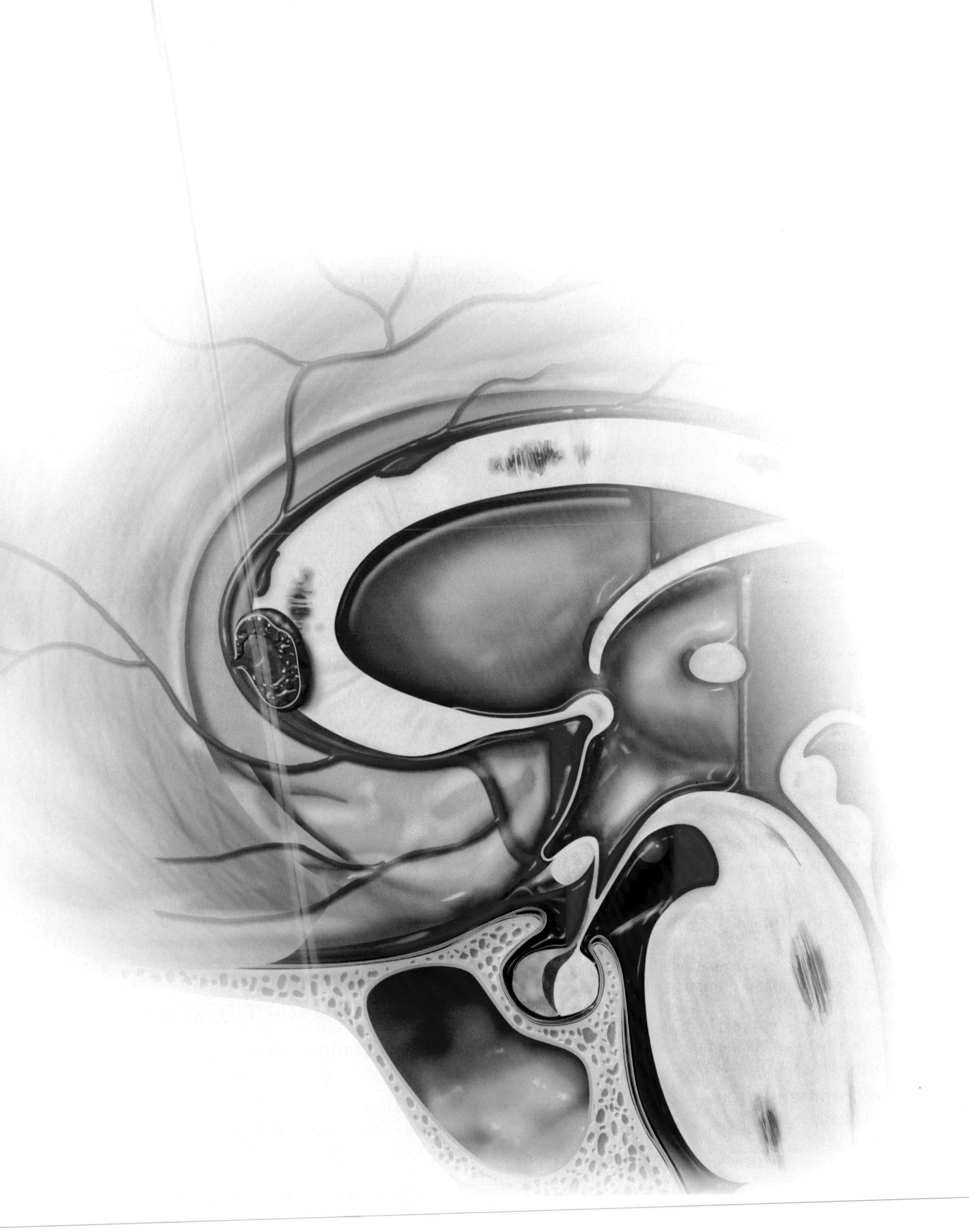

SECTION 3
Subarachnoid Hemorrhage and Aneurysms

Introduction and Overview

Subarachnoid Hemorrhage

Aneurysms

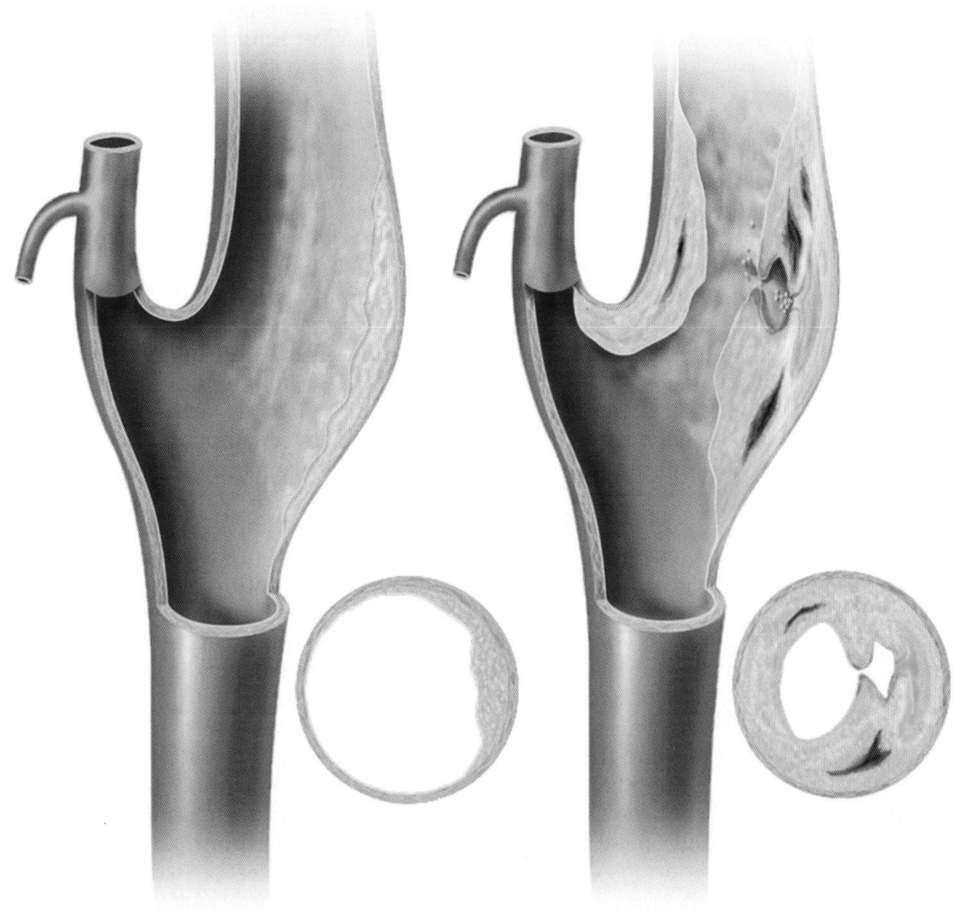

Subarachnoid Hemorrhage

Overview. The subarachnoid spaces (SASs) are CSF-filled spaces between the arachnoid (on the outside) and the pia (on the inside). Focal expansions of the SASs at the base of the brain and around the brainstem, tentorial incisura, and foramen magnum form the brain cisterns.

The SASs are anatomically unique as they surround the entire brain, spinal cord, and spinal nerve roots and contain all the major brain arteries and cortical veins.

Acute extravasation of blood into the CSF spaces between the arachnoid membrane and pia can be caused by arterial leaks or torn veins. Blood can also extend into the SASs from parenchymal hemorrhage that ruptures through the cortex and pia, spilling into the adjacent SAS.

Trauma, "burst" aneurysm, vascular malformations, and amyloid angiopathy are potential causes of subarachnoid hemorrhage (SAH). The most common cause of SAH is trauma. Traumatic subarachnoid hemorrhage (tSAH) occurs when hemorrhage from contused brain or lacerated cortical vessels extends into sulci adjacent to the injury. tSAH is discussed in the trauma section of this book.

Aneurysmal subarachnoid hemorrhage (aSAH). Nontramautic "spontaneous" SAH represents about 5% of all acute "strokes." The most common cause of nontraumatic SAH is a ruptured intracranial saccular ("berry") aneurysm (aSAH). Because most saccular aneurysms are located either on the circle of Willis or at the middle cerebral artery bifurcation, the most common locations for aSAH are the suprasellar cistern and sylvian fissures.

Aneurysmal SAH can be focal or diffuse. Attempts to determine the precise anatomic location of a suspected intracranial aneurysm based on the distribution of SAH are necessarily imprecise. Anterior interhemispheric aSAH is typically associated with rupture of a superiorly directed ACoA aneurysm. aSAH seen primarily in the posterior fossa cisterns &/or 4th ventricle suggests a PICA aneurysm. MCA bi- or trifurcation aneurysm may cause focal hemorrhage in the adjacent sylvian fissure.

Subarachnoid blood in the suprasellar cistern can be found with many aneurysms, especially those arising at the internal carotid-posterior communicating artery junction or the tip of the basilar artery. Focal hematomas are also common adjacent to a ruptured saccular aneurysm and, when present, are generally a much more accurate predictor of aneurysm location than aSAH pattern.

Perimesencephalic nonaneurysmal subarachnoid hemorrhage (pnSAH). An uncommon but important cause of SAH, pnSAH is a clinically benign variant that is probably venous in origin. pnSAH is confined to the cisterns around the midbrain and anterior to the pons.

Superficial siderosis (SS). Chronic, recurrent SAH results in hemosiderin deposition on the pia and cranial nerves. The brain, brainstem, cerebellum, and spinal cord can all be affected, although the posterior fossa is most commonly involved.

The classic clinical presentation of SS is in an adult with a history of trauma or surgery, who presents with ataxia and bilateral sensorineural hearing loss. A history of aSAH is uncommon. SS is best identified on T2* (GRE or SWI).

Aneurysms and Arterial Ectasias

Terminology and overview. The word "aneurysm" comes from the combination of 2 Greek words meaning "across" and "broad." Hence, brain arterial aneurysms are widenings or dilatations of intracranial arteries.

Intracranial aneurysms are generally classified by their phenotypic appearance. Saccular or "berry" aneurysms are the most common type. Fusiform aneurysms are focal dilatations that involve the entire circumference of a vessel and extend for relatively short distances. Ectasias refer to generalized arterial enlargement without focal dilatation and are not true aneurysms; they are nonetheless discussed in this section.

Saccular aneurysm. As the name implies, saccular aneurysms (SAs) are focal sac- or berry-like arterial dilatations. The vast majority are acquired lesions, the result of an underlying genetically based susceptibility plus superimposed mechanical stresses on vessel walls. SAs lack the 2 strongest layers of blood vessel walls, the internal elastic lamina and the muscular layer. The aneurysm sac itself consists of only intima and adventitia.

Most SAs arise at major blood vessel bifurcations, where hemodynamic stresses are highest. The vast majority of intracranial aneurysms are located on the circle of Willis plus the middle cerebral artery bi- or trifurcation. 90% are "anterior circulation" aneurysms, i.e., on the internal carotid artery and its branches. The posterior communicating artery is considered part of the anterior circulation; the vertebrobasilar artery and branches constitute the "posterior circulation."

Pseudoaneurysm. Pseudoaneurysms (PAs) are focal arterial dilatations not contained by layers of the normal arterial wall. They are often irregularly shaped and generally arise on vessels distal to the circle of Willis.

A pseudoaneurysm develops when a completely disrupted blood vessel hemorrhages. A paravascular hematoma forms and then cavitates, establishing a communication with the parent vessel wall. The wall of a PA thus consists only of organized clot. Pseudoaneurysms are much less common than either SAs or fusiform aneurysms. PAs are acquired lesions caused by trauma, infection or inflammation ("mycotic" aneurysm), drug abuse, and neoplasm ("oncotic" aneurysm).

Blood blister-like aneurysm. Blood blister-like aneurysms (BBAs) are eccentric hemispherical outpouchings that can develop at any location. Most commonly found on the greater curvature of the supraclinoid internal carotid artery, they are lined only by a thin layer of adventitia. They are difficult to detect, difficult to treat, and prone to rupture at smaller size and younger age than typical saccular aneurysms.

Fusiform aneurysms. Fusiform aneurysms can be atherosclerotic (common) or nonatherosclerotic (rare). They involve long, nonbranching vessel segments and are seen as more focal circumferential outpouchings from an ectatic vessel. Fusiform aneurysms are more common in the vertebrobasilar (posterior) circulation.

Vertebrobasilar dolichoectasia. Fusiform enlargement or ectasia, also called arteriectasis, is commonly seen in patients with advanced atherosclerotic disease. Less commonly, fusiform ectasias occur with collagen-vascular disorders and non-ASVD arteriopathies.

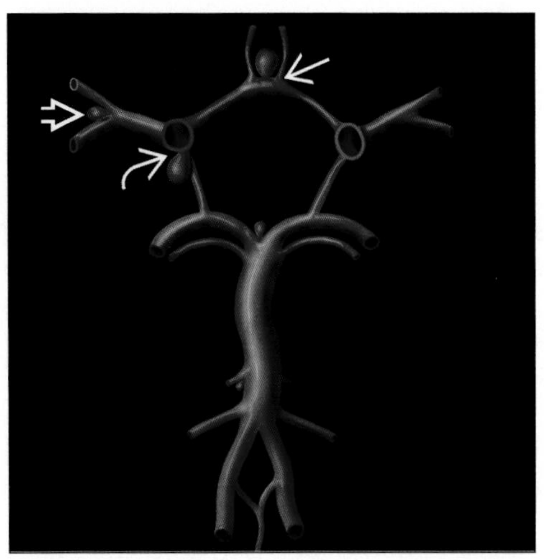

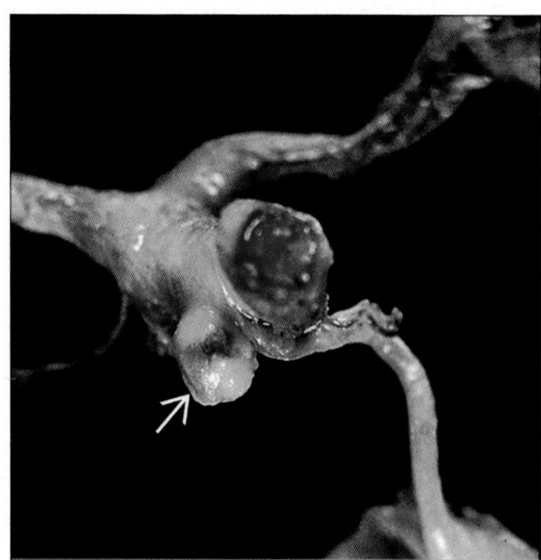

*(**Left**) Diagram depicts the circle of Willis with relative prevalence of intracranial saccular aneurysms. Most are "anterior circulation" with 1/3 occurring on the ACoA → and 1/3 at the internal carotid/PCoA junction →. 15-20% are found at the MCA bi- or trifurcation →. Only 10% occur on the "posterior circulation." (**Right**) Circle of Willis dissected from an autopsied brain shows a classic unruptured IC-PCoA saccular aneurysm →. (Courtesy B. Horten, MD.)*

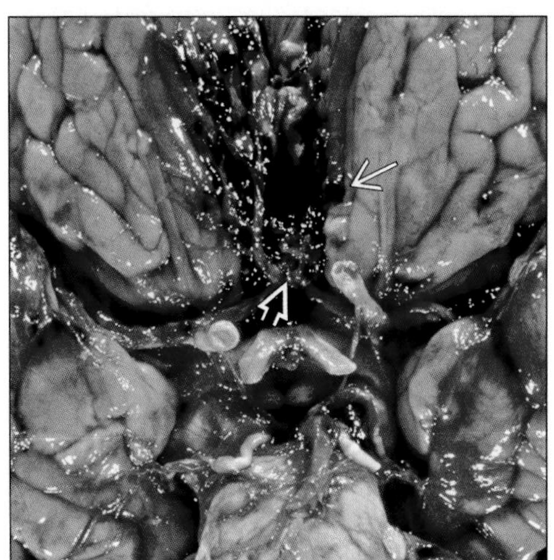

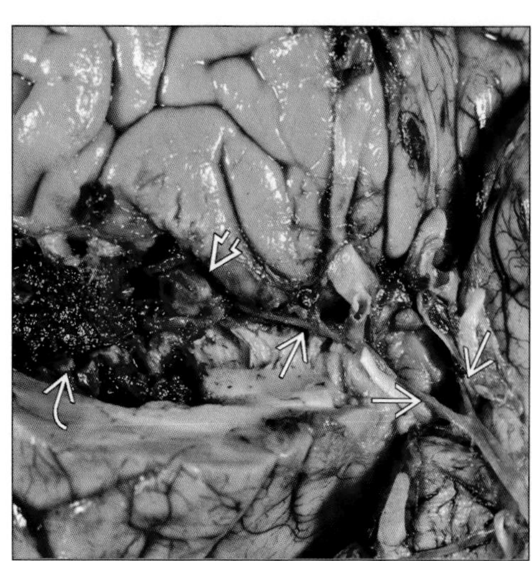

*(**Left**) Autopsied brain shows a small ruptured ACoA aneurysm → with extensive focal clot in the interhemispheric fissure →. Diffuse SAH is also present. (Courtesy B. Horten, MD.) (**Right**) This patient died of cerebral ischemia several days after rupture of a saccular MCA aneurysm →, which is surrounded by clot in the sylvian fissure →. Note the extreme narrowing of the M1 MCA segment and both posterior cerebral arteries, indicative of severe vasospasm →. (Courtesy R. Hewlett, PhD.)*

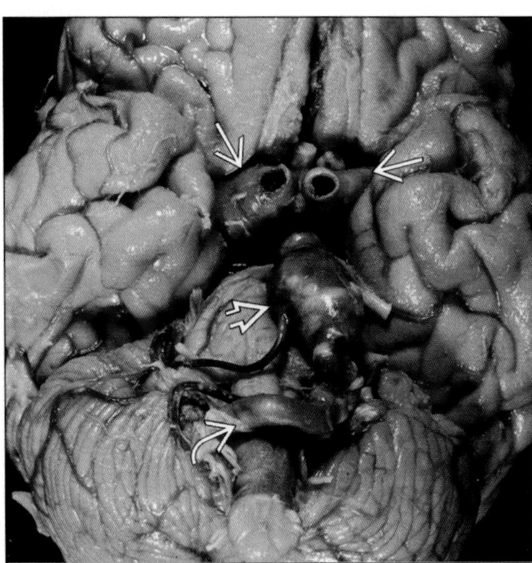

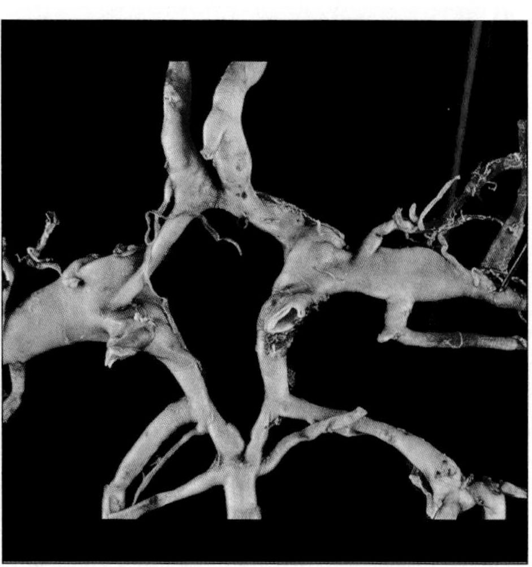

*(**Left**) Gross pathology shows atherosclerotic fusiform ectasias of the vertebrobasilar system →, as well as both internal carotid arteries and M1 MCA segments →. Focal enlargement of the basilar artery represents a fusiform aneurysm → caused by ASVD. (Courtesy R. Hewlett, PhD.) (**Right**) Nonatherosclerotic fusiform ectasias of the M1, A1, A2, and PCoAs are seen in a patient with HIV-associated vasculopathy. (Courtesy L. Rourke, MD.)*

ANEURYSMAL SUBARACHNOID HEMORRHAGE

Key Facts

Terminology

- SAH caused by ruptured aneurysm (aSAH)
  - Saccular (SA) > > dissecting aneurysm (DA)

Imaging

- CT/CTA
  - Hyperdense sulci on NECT
  - Distribution depends on aneurysm location
  - "Culprit" aneurysm sometimes seen as filling defect within hyperdense aSAH
  - SA: Intradural ICA bifurcations, circle of Willis, MCA bifurcation most common sites
  - DA: Intradural vertebral artery most common
  - CTA 90-95% positive if aneurysm ≥ 2 mm
- MR/MRA
  - FLAIR hyperintense (nonspecific)
  - TOF MRA 85-95% sensitive for aneurysms ≥ 3 mm
- DSA
  - "4-vessel angiogram" = gold standard; use if CTA negative for aneurysm in patient with aSAH

Top Differential Diagnoses

- Nonaneurysmal SAH
- "Pseudo-SAH"
- Reversible cerebral vasoconstriction syndrome (RCVS)

Clinical Issues

- Sudden onset severe headache
  - "Thunderclap/worst headache of life"
- 50% mortality, 20% rebleed within 1st 2 weeks
  - Vasospasm 1-3 weeks post aSAH
- Treatment
  - Clipping vs. coil embolization ("coiling")
  - Coiling death/dependence at 1 year = 23.7% vs. 30.7% with clipping

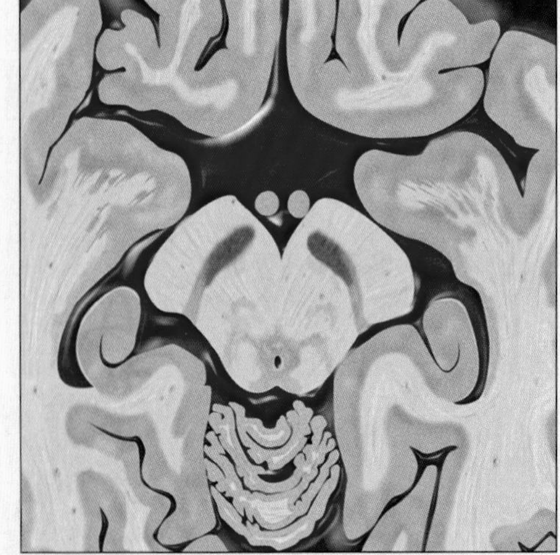

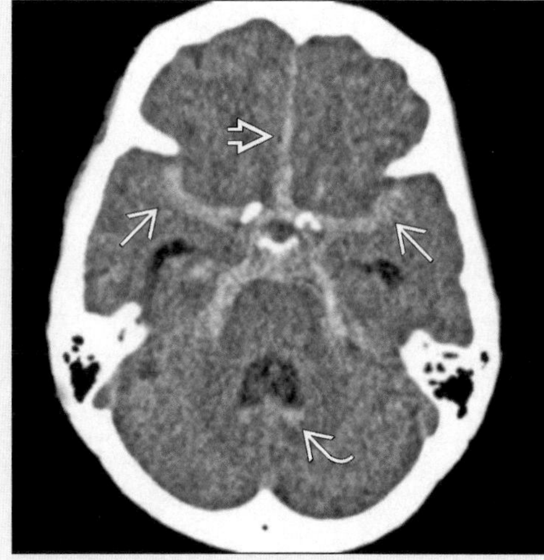

(Left) Axial graphic through the midbrain depicts SAH in red throughout the basal cisterns. Given the diffuse distribution of SAH without focal hematoma, statistically the most likely location of the ruptured aneurysm is the ACoA. (Right) Axial CECT shows diffuse SAH in the basal cisterns, anterior interhemispheric fissure ➡, and sylvian fissures ➡ in a patient with a ruptured ACoA aneurysm. Note hydrocephalus of the lateral and 4th ventricles, as well as intraventricular hemorrhage within the 4th ventricle ➡.

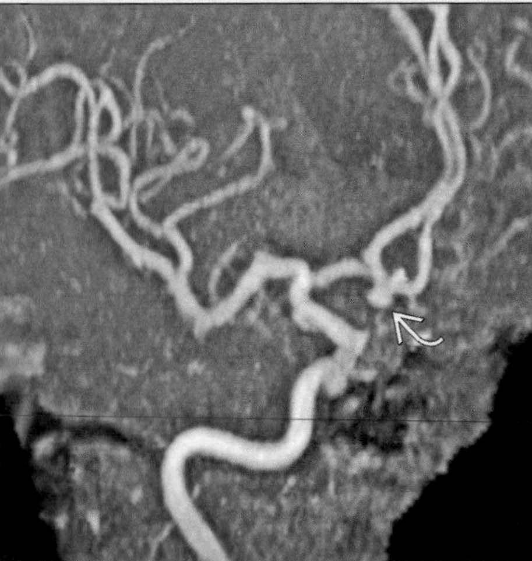

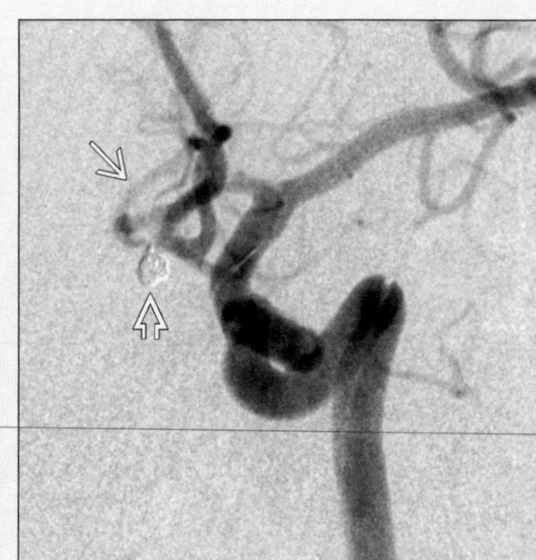

(Left) TOF MRA in the same patient shows a small ACoA aneurysm directed inferiorly ➡. (Right) Oblique left ICA DSA during coil embolization shows complete aneurysm occlusion after placement of the 2nd coil ➡. Note the preservation of the parent ACoA with flash filling of the right ACA ➡. The patient subsequently developed vasospasm and was treated with balloon angioplasty and intraarterial (IA) verapamil infusion but had no permanent neurological sequela.

ANEURYSMAL SUBARACHNOID HEMORRHAGE

TERMINOLOGY

Abbreviations
- Aneurysmal subarachnoid hemorrhage (aSAH)

Definitions
- Subarachnoid hemorrhage caused by ruptured aneurysm

IMAGING

General Features
- Best diagnostic clue
  - Hyperdense sulci on NECT
- Location
  - Suprasellar, basal, sylvian, interhemispheric cisterns
    - ± intraventricular hemorrhage (IVH)
  - aSAH distribution depends on location of saccular aneurysm (SA)
    - aSAH highest near site of rupture
      - Anterior communicating artery (ACoA) aneurysm → anterior interhemispheric fissure
      - Middle cerebral artery (MCA) aneurysm → sylvian fissure
      - Basilar tip, superior cerebellar artery (SCA), posterior inferior cerebellar artery (PICA) SA, or vertebral artery (VA) dissecting aneurysm (DA) → prepontine cistern, foramen magnum, 4th ventricle
    - "Culprit" aneurysm sometimes seen as filling defect within hyperdense aSAH
  - SAs typically located at bifurcation points along intradural ICA, circle of Willis (COW), MCA
    - 90% anterior circulation: ACoA, posterior communicating artery (PCoA), MCA, carotid terminus, carotid-ophthalmic, superior hypophyseal
    - 10% posterior circulation: Basilar tip, PICA, anterior inferior cerebellar artery (AICA), SCA
  - DAs: Intradural V4 VA segment most common
  - Blood-blister aneurysm (BBA)
    - Dorsal supraclinoid ICA
    - Rarely MCA, basilar artery

CT Findings
- NECT
  - 95% positive in 1st 24 hours, < 50% by 1 week
  - "Effaced" sylvian fissure if subacute, filled with isodense SAH
  - Hydrocephalus common, may occur early
  - ± intraparenchymal hemorrhage at site of ruptured aneurysm
- CTA
  - 90-95% positive if aneurysm ≥ 2 mm

MR Findings
- T1WI
  - Acute aSAH is isointense to CSF
  - CSF may appear mildly hyperintense ("dirty")
- T2WI
  - Difficult to see on T2WI (hyperintense), GRE
- FLAIR
  - Hyperintense
    - More sensitive than CT but less specific
- DWI
  - May see foci of restricted diffusion if vasospasm
- MRA
  - TOF MRA 85-95% sensitive for aneurysms ≥ 3 mm

Angiographic Findings
- Conventional "4-vessel angiogram" = gold standard
  - Must image
    - Both ICA circulations
    - Both VAs or dominant VA + reflux to contralateral PICA
  - SA
    - Saccular outpouching at arterial branch point
    - Look for Murphy teat = site of rupture
    - Look for additional aneurysms (20% multiple)
      - If > 1 aneurysm, then biggest, most irregular ± adjacent vasospasm is likely source of bleed
  - DA
    - Irregular ± dilated or stenotic V4 segment of VA
  - BBA
    - Smooth/irregular bleb/dome-shaped outpouching
    - Not associated with major vessel branch point
    - Most common along supraclinoid ICA
  - DSA negative in 15% of aSAH; repeat positive < 5%
    - Evaluate ECAs (to exclude dural AV fistula [dAVF])
    - SA may not be seen on initial DSA if optimal projection not obtained, spontaneous partial or complete aneurysm thrombosis, &/or presence of vasospasm
    - Consider repeating DSA in 5-7 days

Imaging Recommendations
- Best imaging tool
  - NECT + multiplanar CTA
- Protocol advice
  - Proceed to DSA if NECT consistent with aSAH but CTA negative
  - Consider MR if DSA + CTA negative

DIFFERENTIAL DIAGNOSIS

Nonaneurysmal SAH
- Perimesencephalic SAH
  - Small SAH, localized to interpeduncular cistern
  - Presumed venous etiology with low recurrence rate
- Traumatic subarachnoid hemorrhage
  - Adjacent to contusions, subdural hematomas
  - Rarely from intracranial dissection or rupture of traumatic pseudoaneurysm
- Subarachnoid hemorrhage, NOS
  - Vascular malformation: Arteriovenous malformation (AVM), cavernous hemangioma

Reversible Cerebral Vasoconstriction Syndrome (RCVS)
- Clinical: "Thunderclap" headache
- SAH typically in cortical sulci vs. basal cisterns with aSAH

"Pseudo-SAH"
- Hypodense brain: Severe cerebral edema
- Hyperdense CSF: Intrathecal contrast; meningitis

ANEURYSMAL SUBARACHNOID HEMORRHAGE

PATHOLOGY

General Features

- Etiology
  - Saccular aneurysms
    - Berry aneurysms: Congenital deficiency of internal elastic lamina and tunica media at arterial branch points → focal vessel wall weakness
      - ↑ risk: Familial intracranial aneurysms (5% of cases), adult polycystic kidney disease, aortic coarctation
    - May be related to high-flow arteriopathy along feeding vessel of AVM or less commonly dAVF
    - ↑ aneurysm rupture risk if female, smoker, HTN
  - Fusiform aneurysms
    - Dissection from trauma, hypertension, ASVD
    - Underlying arteriopathy including fibromuscular dysplasia (FMD), Marfan, Ehlers-Danlos, infection
    - Mycotic
  - Blood-blister aneurysm: All layers absent (contained in fibrous cap)
- Associated abnormalities
  - Vasospasm
    - Caused by blood breakdown products, apolipoprotein E genotype, endothelin-1 release from CSF leukocytes
    - 70% develop angiographic evidence of vasospasm
    - 30% have clinically apparent vasospasm
    - Starts ~ day 3-4 post SAH; peaks ~ 7-9 days, lasts ~ 12-16 days
  - Cerebral salt-wasting syndrome
    - Excessive renal Na+ excretion → hyponatremia, hypovolemia
  - Terson syndrome
    - Intraocular (retinal, vitreous) hemorrhage associated with SAH secondary to rapid ↑ intracranial pressure

Staging, Grading, & Classification

- Clinical grading: Hunt and Hess (H&H) grade 0-5
  - 0 = no SAH (unruptured aneurysm)
  - 1 = no symptoms, minimal headache, slight nuchal rigidity
  - 2 = moderate to severe headache, nuchal rigidity
    - No neurologic deficit except CN palsy
  - 3 = drowsy, minimal neurologic deficit
  - 4 = stuporous, moderate/severe hemiparesis
  - 5 = coma, decerebrate rigidity, moribund appearance
- WFNS clinical grading system: Based on GCS and presence/absence of major focal neurological deficit
- Fisher CT grading
  - 1 = no SAH visible
  - 2 = diffuse, thin layer (< 1 mm)
  - 3 = localized clot or thick layer (> 1 mm)
  - 4 = intraventricular blood

Gross Pathologic & Surgical Features

- Blood in basal cisterns, sulci, and ventricles

CLINICAL ISSUES

Presentation

- Most common signs/symptoms
  - Sudden "thunderclap/worst headache of life"
  - 10% preceded by "sentinel hemorrhage" = self-limiting SAH + headache in preceding days/weeks

Demographics

- Age
  - Peak = 40-60 years
- Gender
  - M:F = 1:2
- Epidemiology
  - Aneurysms cause 85% of spontaneous SAHs
  - Incidence ~ 9.9/100,000 population

Natural History & Prognosis

- 50% mortality; 20% rebleed within 1st 2 weeks
- Clinical outcome inversely proportional to initial H&H or WFNS grade
- Vasospasm + ischemia → delayed morbidity, mortality
  - Severity correlates with amount of SAH (Fisher CT grade); inverse correlation with patient age
- 90% hydrocephalus at presentation
  - ~ 10% require permanent CSF diversion

Treatment

- Ruptured aneurysm
  - Microneurosurgical clipping
    - Proven effective over decades but invasive, higher morbidity/mortality compared with coiling
    - 1 study: Death or dependence at 1 year = 23.7% with coiling vs. 30.7% with clipping
  - Coil embolization ("coiling"), if anatomy favorable
    - Platinum coils ± bioactive coating to reduce recurrence rate
    - Aneurysm recurrence > surgical clipping but low risk of recurrent SAH
- Vasospasm
  - Ca++ antagonists, "triple-H" therapy (hypervolemia, hemodilution, hypertension)
  - Endovascular: Intraarterial Ca++ antagonist ("chemical angioplasty"), balloon angioplasty
- Hydrocephalus
  - Temporary or permanent CSF diversion
- Cerebral salt-wasting syndrome
  - Na+ tablets or IV hypertonic saline

DIAGNOSTIC CHECKLIST

Consider

- Nonaneurysmal SAH if characteristic blood distribution (e.g., perimesencephalic SAH, RCVS)
- Look for multiple aneurysms and decide which most likely bled

Image Interpretation Pearls

- Isodense SAH: Anterior 3rd ventricle and temporal horns are only CSF density structures at base of brain, absence of sylvian fissure(s)

SELECTED REFERENCES

1. Nael K et al: 3-T contrast-enhanced MR angiography in evaluation of suspected intracranial aneurysm: comparison with MDCT angiography. AJR Am J Roentgenol. 190(2):389-95, 2008

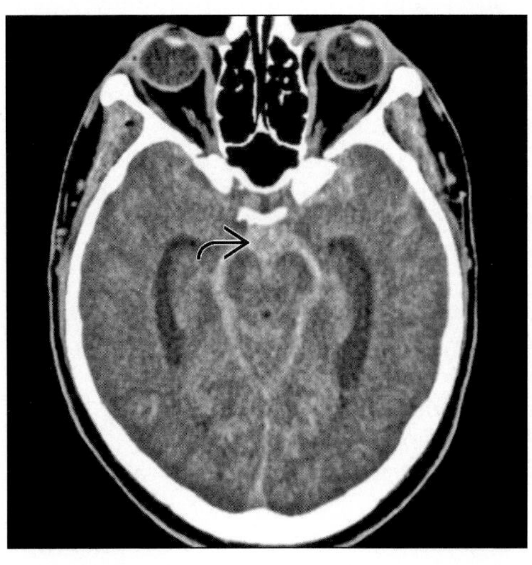

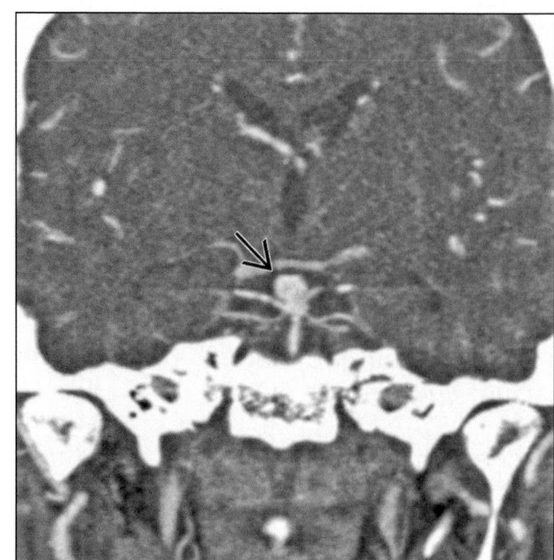

(Left) *Axial NECT in a patient with a ruptured basilar tip aneurysm shows diffuse SAH concentrated in the interpeduncular and ambient cisterns, as well as hydrocephalus. Note the filling defect anterior to the midbrain representing the aneurysm outlined by high-density SAH.* ***(Right)*** *Coronal CTA clearly depicts the basilar apex aneurysm and adjacent vessels. The aneurysm appears to have a relatively narrow neck that would be amenable to coil embolization.*

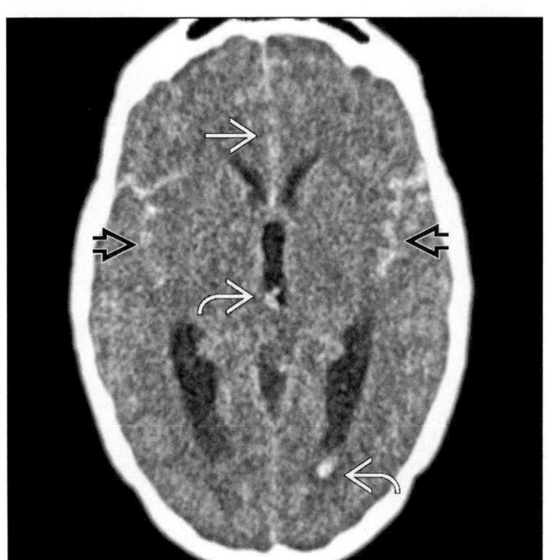

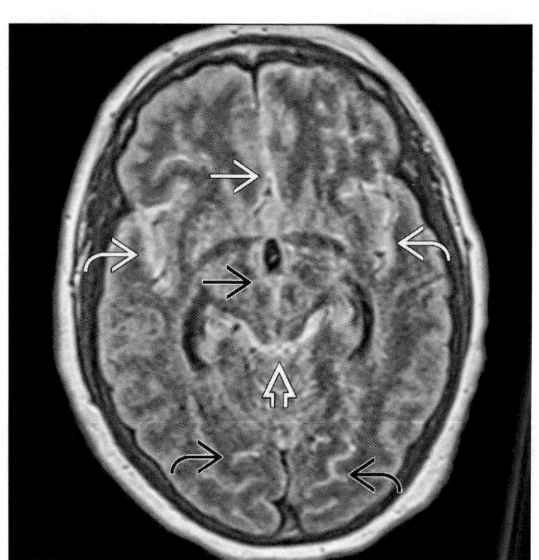

(Left) *Axial NECT shows diffuse SAH in the sylvian fissures and anterior interhemispheric fissure, as well as IVH in the 3rd and lateral ventricles. Note mild hydrocephalus.* ***(Right)*** *Axial FLAIR MR at a more caudal section shows SAH as high signal within the sylvian fissures, anterior interhemispheric fissure, and quadrigeminal plate cistern. SAH is also present in the occipital lobe sulci. A fluid-fluid level is seen in the 3rd ventricle due to IVH.*

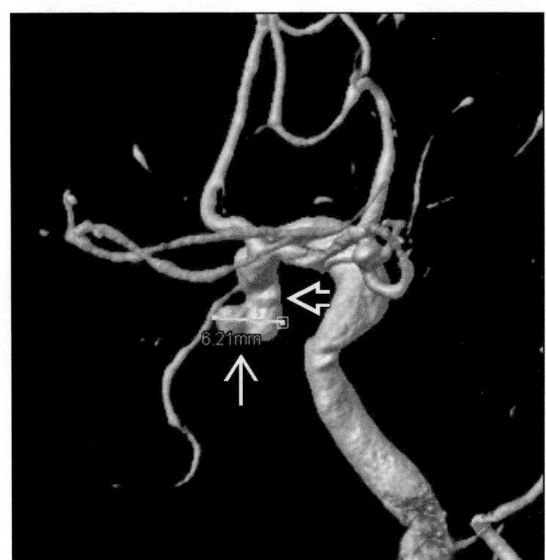

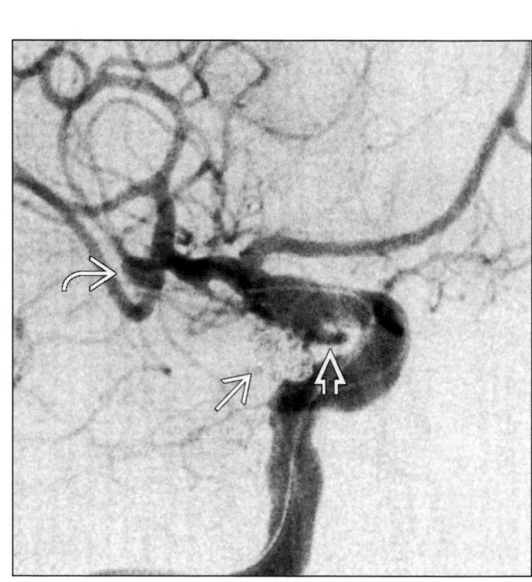

(Left) *3D rotational DSA in the same patient shows a 6.2 mm boot-shaped PCoA aneurysm. The aneurysm has a wide neck at its junction with the ICA.* ***(Right)*** *Oblique DSA during coil embolization shows a dense coil packing within the PCoA aneurysm. Note the preservation of the PCoA arising from the aneurysm neck. A 3 mm MCA aneurysm is also seen. Multiple aneurysms are found in 20% of patients.*

PERIMESENCEPHALIC NONANEURYSMAL SAH

Key Facts

Terminology

- Clinically benign SAH confined to perimesencephalic, prepontine cisterns
- No source demonstrated at angiography

Imaging

- CT: Hyperdense prepontine, perimesencephalic CSF
- T1: Iso-/hyperintense, T2 variable (hypo-/iso-/hyper-) intensity CSF
- FLAIR: Hyperintense prepontine, perimesencephalic CSF
  - May be mimicked by CSF pulsation artifact or in ventilated patients with > 50% O_2 concentration
- Normal DSA required to exclude aneurysm or other cause and confirm diagnosis
- MR/MRA may confirm alternative diagnosis and negate need for repeat DSA

Pathology

- Most likely cause: Ruptured perimesencephalic/ prepontine vein
- Other nonaneurysmal causes: Intracranial dissection, vasculitis, trauma, dural AV fistula, spinal vascular malformation; have less benign course
- Posterior circulation aneurysms may have perimesencephalic nonaneurysmal SAH (pnSAH) pattern

Clinical Issues

- Benign course: Rebleed rare (< 1%); no vasospasm
- Headache (usually Hunt/Hess grade 1 or 2), often intra-/post coitus
- May develop hydrocephalus, intraventricular extension, in more extensive bleeds

(Left) Axial graphic shows a classic pnSAH. Hemorrhage is confined to the interpeduncular fossa and ambient (perimesencephalic) cisterns ➔. The source is usually venous in pnSAHs, unlike in aneurysmal SAHs. (Right) Axial NECT shows subarachnoid hemorrhage in the suprasellar, interpeduncular, and perimesencephalic cisterns ➔ with mild hydrocephalus. Angiography, performed because of a small amount of intraventricular blood, revealed vertebral artery dissection, an uncommon cause for pnSAH.

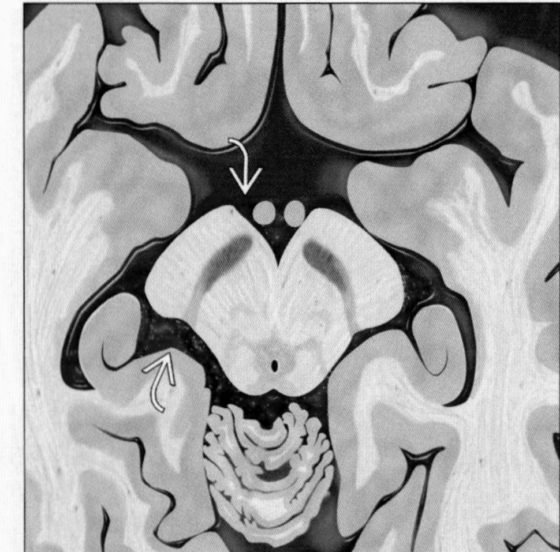

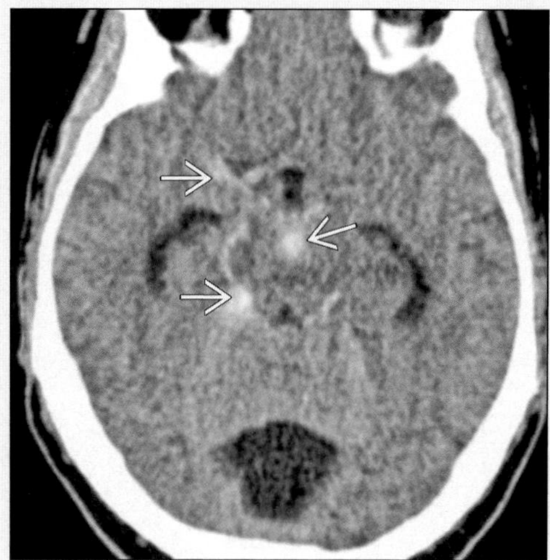

(Left) Axial FLAIR shows striking increased intensity in the suprasellar, perimesencephalic, quadrigeminal plate, and left MCA cisterns ➔ with intraventricular blood ➔. Angiography was negative in this patient, although about 5% of cases with this pattern of subarachnoid hemorrhage have a basilar tip aneurysm. (Right) Sagittal T1WI MR shows iso-/hyperintensity anterior and posterior ➔ to the midbrain with extension along the prepontine cistern ➔ in this patient with negative angiography.

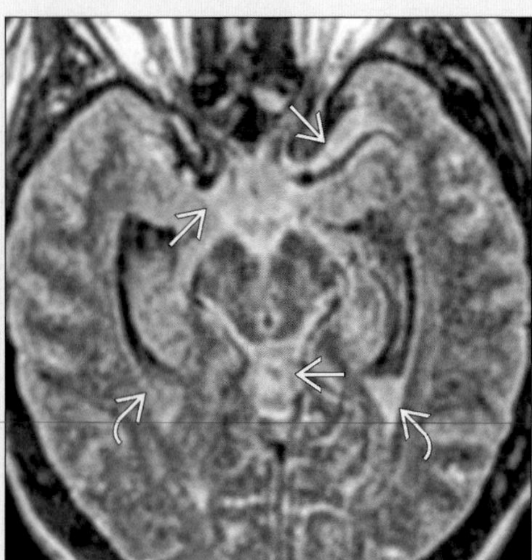

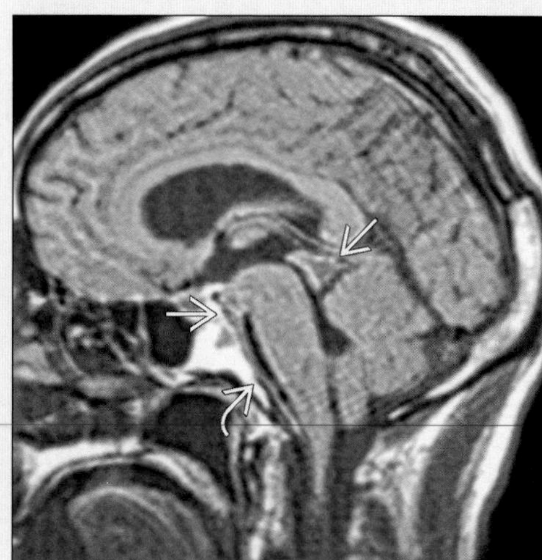

PERIMESENCEPHALIC NONANEURYSMAL SAH

TERMINOLOGY

Abbreviations
- Perimesencephalic nonaneurysmal SAH (pnSAH)

Synonyms
- Benign perimesencephalic SAH

Definitions
- Clinically benign SAH confined to perimesencephalic, prepontine cisterns
- No source demonstrated at angiography

IMAGING

General Features
- Best diagnostic clue
  - Hyperdense prepontine, perimesencephalic CSF
- Location
  - Subarachnoid cisterns around midbrain and anterior to pons

CT Findings
- NECT
  - High attenuation anterior to pons and around midbrain
  - No supratentorial extension

MR Findings
- T1WI
  - Iso- to hyperintense CSF around midbrain
  - Focal clot around basilar artery
- T2WI
  - Iso- to hypointense thrombus in CSF
- FLAIR
  - Hyperintense CSF is more extensive than on T1/T2
    - Mimicked by CSF pulsation artifact
- T2* GRE
  - Hypointense thrombus in CSF

Angiographic Findings
- CTA/MRA/DSA
  - No source of hemorrhage identified
  - Normal DSA required to confirm diagnosis

Imaging Recommendations
- Best imaging tool
  - NECT best screening for pnSAH
  - DSA to exclude aneurysm
  - MR/MRA may confirm SAH or cause; may negate need for repeat DSA
- Protocol advice
  - NECT with CTA
  - MR/MRA may help confirm diagnosis
  - Consider cervical MR to exclude rare spinal vascular source

DIFFERENTIAL DIAGNOSIS

Aneurysmal SAH
- More extensive hemorrhage
- Posterior circulation aneurysms may have pnSAH pattern

Traumatic SAH
- Perisylvian, convexity more common than perimesencephalic pattern

Artifact: FLAIR
- Incomplete CSF suppression
- > 50% O_2 concentration

PATHOLOGY

General Features
- Etiology
  - Most likely cause: Ruptured perimesencephalic/ prepontine vein
  - Other nonaneurysmal causes have less benign course
    - Intracranial dissection, vasculitis, trauma, dural AV fistula, spinal cord vascular malformation
  - Posterior fossa aneurysms may have pnSAH pattern

Gross Pathologic & Surgical Features
- Clotted blood in perimesencephalic cisterns
- Similar to aneurysmal SAH

CLINICAL ISSUES

Presentation
- Most common signs/symptoms
  - Headache (usually Hunt/Hess grade 1 or 2)
    - Often post coitus

Demographics
- Age: 40-60 years
- Gender: M = F
- Epidemiology
  - Majority of angiogram-negative SAH

Natural History & Prognosis
- Benign course: Rebleed rare (< 1%); no vasospasm
- May develop hydrocephalus or intraventricular extension in more extensive bleeds

Treatment
- Monitoring and treatment of rare secondary hydrocephalus, vasospasm

DIAGNOSTIC CHECKLIST

Consider
- Occult trauma, vertebral dissection, vasculitis, dural AV fistula, or spinal vascular malformation

Image Interpretation Pearls
- DSA needed to exclude aneurysm, other vascular cause
- Perimesencephalic thrombus and focal clot around basilar artery on MR

SELECTED REFERENCES

1. Kang DH et al: Does non-perimesencephalic type non-aneurysmal subarachnoid hemorrhage have a benign prognosis? J Clin Neurosci. 16(7):904-8, 2009

SUPERFICIAL SIDEROSIS

Key Facts

Terminology

- Superficial siderosis: Recurrent subarachnoid hemorrhage (SAH) causes hemosiderin deposition on surface of brain, brainstem, and cranial nerve leptomeninges

Imaging

- Nonenhanced CT findings
  - Slightly hyperdense rim over brain surface
  - Brainstem high-density line most evident
  - **Caveat**: Do not mistake high-density rim on brain surfaces as subarachnoid hemorrhage!
- MR findings
  - In diffuse disease, ventricle surfaces, brain, brainstem, cerebellum, and cervical spine all have hypointense hemosiderin rim
  - Contours of brain and cranial nerves outlined by hypointense rim on T2 or T2* GRE MR images
  - CN8 appears darker and thicker than normal
  - GRE: Most sensitive to hemosiderin deposition on CNS surfaces ("blooming" dark signal)
- Once diagnosis of SS is made, search for cause of recurrent SAH must commence
  - Whole brain MR with contrast and MRA 1st
  - Total spine MR if brain negative for underlying lesion

Pathology

- Repeated SAH deposits hemosiderin on meningeal lining of CNS
- Affects brain, brainstem, cerebellum, cranial nerves, and spinal cord
- Causes of recurrent SAH pathologies
  - Traumatic nerve root avulsion
  - Bleeding CNS neoplasm
  - Vascular malformations and aneurysms
  - Surgical sites (brain or spine)

*(**Left**) Axial graphic shows darker brown hemosiderin staining on all surfaces of the brain, meninges, and cranial nerves. Notice that cranial nerves 7 and 8 in the cerebellopontine angle-internal auditory canal ➔ are particularly affected. (**Right**) Axial T2WI MR reveals superficial siderosis in the posterior fossa. Both vestibulocochlear nerves (CN8) are seen as very low signal lines in the cerebellopontine angle cisterns ➔. Also observe low signal along the surface of the cerebellar folia ➔.*

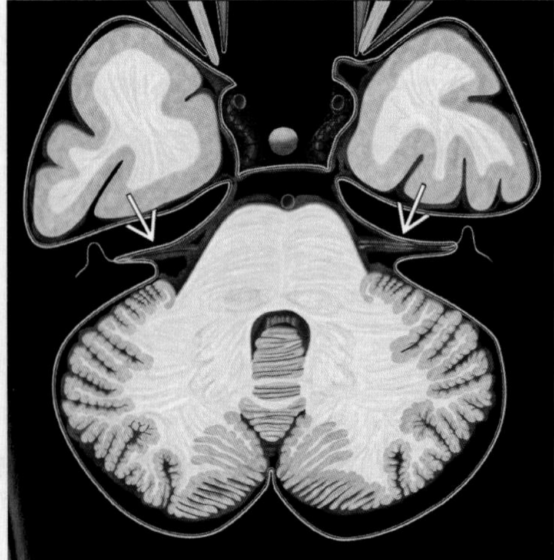

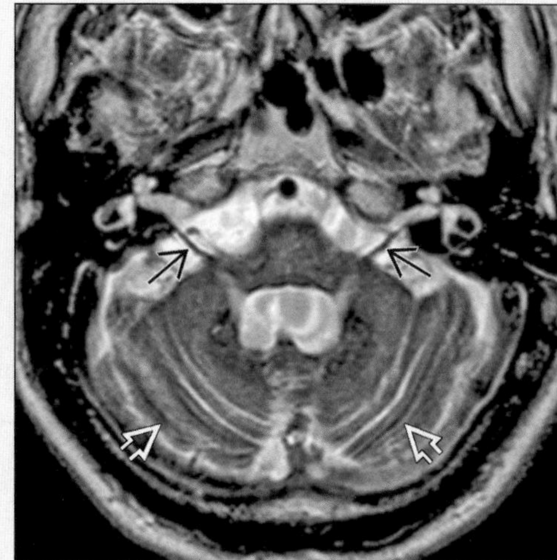

*(**Left**) Axial NECT demonstrates findings of superficial siderosis as a high-density right vestibulocochlear nerve ➔. CT is often normal in this disease as the fine siderosis coating on the cranial nerves, brain, and brainstem may not be dense enough to see. (**Right**) Axial NECT in this patient with superficial siderosis shows linear high density along the surface of the midbrain ➔. This is not an artifact or subarachnoid hemorrhage but hemosiderin deposition on the surface of the midbrain.*

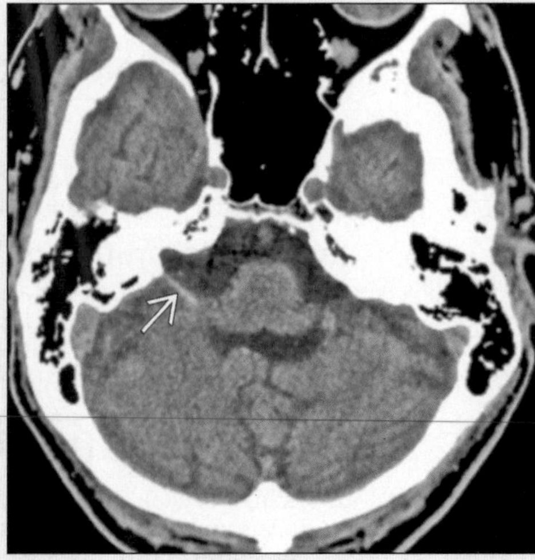

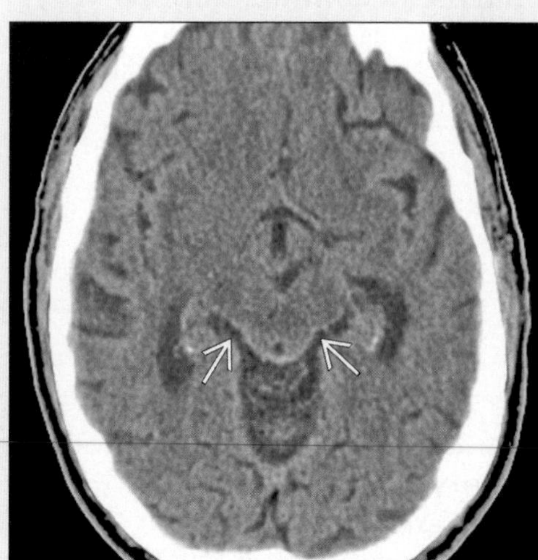

SUPERFICIAL SIDEROSIS

TERMINOLOGY

Abbreviations

- Superficial siderosis (SS)

Synonyms

- Siderosis, central nervous system siderosis

Definitions

- Recurrent subarachnoid hemorrhage (SAH) causes hemosiderin deposition on surface of brain, brainstem, and cranial nerve (CN) leptomeninges

IMAGING

General Features

- Best diagnostic clue
  - Contours of brain and cranial nerves outlined by hypointense rim on T2 or T2* GRE MR images
- Location
  - Cerebral hemispheres, cerebellum, brainstem, cranial nerves, and spinal cord may all be affected
- Size
  - Linear low signal along CNS surfaces varies in thickness but usually ≤ 2 mm
- Morphology
  - Curvilinear dark lines on CNS surfaces

CT Findings

- NECT
  - Cerebral and cerebellar atrophy
    - Especially marked in posterior fossa
      - Cerebellar sulci often disproportionately large
  - CN8 may be hyperdense
  - Slightly hyperdense rim over brain surface
    - Brainstem changes most evident
    - CT relatively insensitive to SS compared to MR
    - **Caveat**: Do not mistake high-density rim on brain surfaces as subarachnoid hemorrhage!
- CECT
  - No enhancement typical

MR Findings

- T1WI
  - Hyperintense signal may be seen on CNS surfaces
- T2WI
  - High-resolution, thin-section T2 MR of CPA-IAC
    - CN8 appears darker and thicker than normal
    - Adjacent cerebellar structures and brainstem show low signal surfaces
    - Less easily seen than on T2* GRE images
  - In diffuse disease, ventricle, brain, brainstem, cerebellum, and cervical spine surfaces all have hypointense hemosiderin rim
  - Vermian and cerebellar atrophy most prominent
- FLAIR
  - Dark border on local surface of brain, brainstem, cerebellum, and cranial nerves
- T2* GRE
  - Most sensitive to hemosiderin deposition on CNS surfaces than T2 sequence
  - "Blooming" dark signal
    - Makes SS appear more conspicuous, thicker
- T1WI C+
  - Surface of CNS does not enhance
- MR findings do not correlate with severity of disease

Imaging Recommendations

- Best imaging tool
  - Brain MR
    - Once diagnosis of SS is made, search for cause of recurrent SAH must commence
    - Whole brain MR with contrast and MRA 1st
    - Then total spine MR if brain negative for underlying lesion
- Protocol advice
  - Brain MR
    - Unenhanced MR with FLAIR initially
    - If SS suspected, add T2* GRE sequences to confirm

DIFFERENTIAL DIAGNOSIS

"Bounce Point" Artifact

- Mismatch between repetition time (TR) and inversion time (TI) on inversion recovery T1 and FLAIR sequences
- Imaging clue: Not present on all sequences

Brain Surface Vessels

- Normal or abnormal surface veins
- Linear, focal area of low signal on brain surface

Neurocutaneous Melanosis

- Congenital syndrome
- Large or multiple congenital melanocytic nevi
- Benign or malignant pigment cell tumors of leptomeninges may be low signal on surface of brain
- T1 high signal diffusely in pia-arachnoid
- T2 low signal diffusely in pia-arachnoid

Meningioangiomatosis

- Hamartomatous proliferation of meningeal cells via intraparenchymal blood vessels into cerebral cortex
- Leptomeninges are thick and infiltrated with fibrous tissue
- May be calcified

PATHOLOGY

General Features

- Etiology
  - Repeated SAH deposits hemosiderin on meningeal lining of CNS
    - Affects brain, brainstem, cerebellum, cranial nerves, and spinal cord
  - Hemosiderin is cytotoxic to neurons
    - "Free" iron with excess production of hydroxyl radicals is best current hypothesis explaining cytotoxicity
  - CN8 is extensively lined with CNS myelin, which is supported by hemosiderin-sensitive microglia
    - Increased exposure in CPA cistern
- Associated abnormalities
  - Causes of recurrent SAH pathologies
    - Traumatic nerve root avulsion
    - Bleeding CNS neoplasm

- Arteriovenous or cavernous malformation
- Aneurysm
- Intradural surgical sites (brain or spine)
- Hemosiderin staining of meninges

Gross Pathologic & Surgical Features

- Dark brown discoloration of leptomeninges, ependyma, and subpial tissue
- Causes of recurrent SAH found in ~ 70%
  - Dural pathology (70%)
    - Traumatic cervical nerve root avulsion
    - CSF cavity lesion (surgical cavity) with "fragile" neovascularity most common
  - Bleeding neoplasms (20%)
    - Ependymoma, oligodendroglioma, astrocytoma, etc.
  - Vascular abnormalities (10%)
    - Arteriovenous malformation (AVM) or aneurysm
    - Multiple cavernous malformations near brain surface

Microscopic Features

- Hemosiderin staining of meninges and subpial tissues to 3 mm depth
- Thickened leptomeninges
- Cerebellar folia: Loss of Purkinje cells and Bergmann gliosis

CLINICAL ISSUES

Presentation

- Most common signs/symptoms
  - Bilateral sensorineural hearing loss (SNHL) in 95%
- Clinical profile
  - Past history of trauma or intradural surgery common
    - Past history of SAH rare
  - Classic presentation is adult patient with bilateral SNHL and ataxia
  - Seen less commonly as late complication of treated childhood cerebellar tumor
- Laboratory
  - CSF from lumbar puncture
    - High protein (100%)
    - Xanthochromic (75%)
- Other symptoms
  - Ataxia (88%)
  - Bilateral hemiparesis
  - Hyperreflexia, bladder disturbance, anosmia, dementia, and headache
  - Presymptomatic phase averages 15 years

Demographics

- Age
  - Broad range: 14-77 years
- Gender
  - M:F = 3:1
- Epidemiology
  - Rare chronic progressive disorder
  - 0.15% of patients undergoing MR

Natural History & Prognosis

- Bilateral worsening SNHL and ataxia within 15 years of onset
- Deafness almost certain if unrecognized
- 25% bedridden in years after 1st symptom
  - Result of cerebellar ataxia, myelopathic syndrome, or both

Treatment

- Treat source of bleeding
  - Surgically remove source of bleeding (surgical cavity, tumor)
  - Endovascular therapy for AVM and aneurysm
- Cochlear implantation for SNHL

DIAGNOSTIC CHECKLIST

Consider

- Remember that SS is effect, not a cause
- Look for source of recurrent SAH in spine or brain
- MR findings do not correlate with severity of patient's symptoms
  - MR diagnosis may be made in absence of symptoms

Image Interpretation Pearls

- CNS surfaces including cranial nerves appear "outlined in black" on T2 MR

Reporting Tips

- Describe individual findings of SS
- Describe any possible sites of chronic SAH
- If no site of SAH visible, recommend full spine MR in search of SAH site
  - Treatment of SAH site may arrest progression of associated symptoms

SELECTED REFERENCES

1. Koeppen AH et al: The pathology of superficial siderosis of the central nervous system. Acta Neuropathol. 116(4):371-82, 2008
2. Kumar N: Superficial siderosis: associations and therapeutic implications. Arch Neurol. 64(4):491-6, 2007
3. Kumar N et al: Superficial siderosis. Neurology. 66(8):1144-52, 2006
4. Dhooge IJ et al: Cochlear implantation in a patient with superficial siderosis of the central nervous system. Otol Neurotol. 23(4):468-72, 2002
5. Hsu WC et al: Superficial siderosis of the CNS associated with multiple cavernous malformations. AJNR Am J Neuroradiol. 20(7):1245-8, 1999
6. Lemmerling M et al: Secondary superficial siderosis of the central nervous system in a patient presenting with sensorineural hearing loss. Neuroradiology. 40(5):312-4, 1998
7. Castelli ML et al: Superficial siderosis of the central nervous system: an underestimated cause of hearing loss. J Laryngol Otol. 111(1):60-2, 1997
8. Offenbacher H et al: Superficial siderosis of the central nervous system: MRI findings and clinical significance. Neuroradiology. 38 Suppl 1:S51-6, 1996
9. Bracchi M et al: Superficial siderosis of the CNS: MR diagnosis and clinical findings. AJNR Am J Neuroradiol. 14(1):227-36, 1993

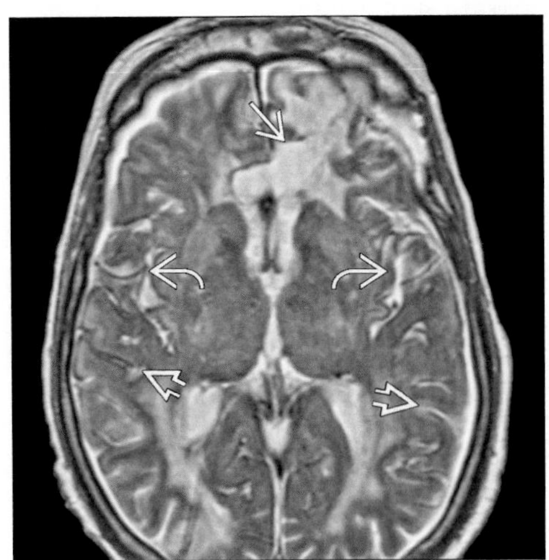

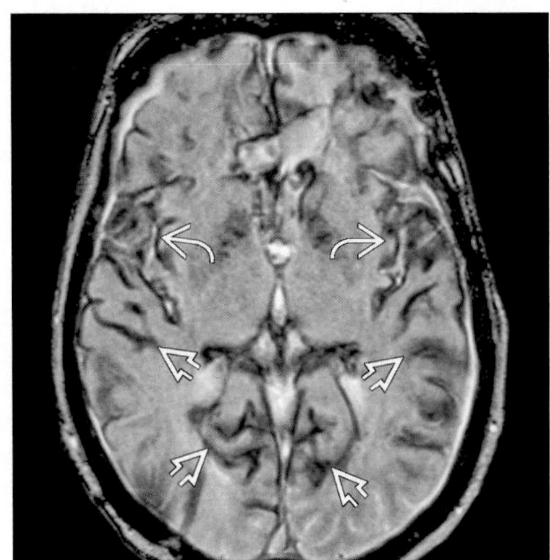

(Left) *Months after the surgical removal of a frontal lobe melanoma metastasis in this patient, axial T2WI MR shows the surgical cavity ➡ and subtle low signal lining the sulci ➡ and sylvian fissures ➡, secondary to superficial siderosis.* ***(Right)*** *Axial T2* GRE MR in the same patient demonstrates much more obvious siderosis involving the sylvian fissures ➡ and sulci ➡. GRE T2* sequences cause hemosiderin deposits to "bloom," increasing the conspicuity of this disease.*

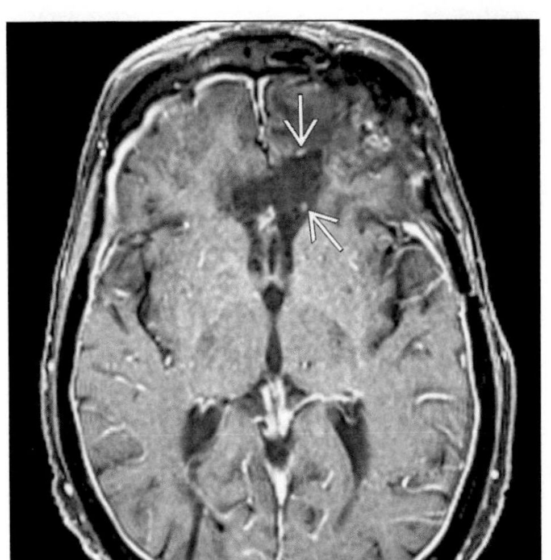

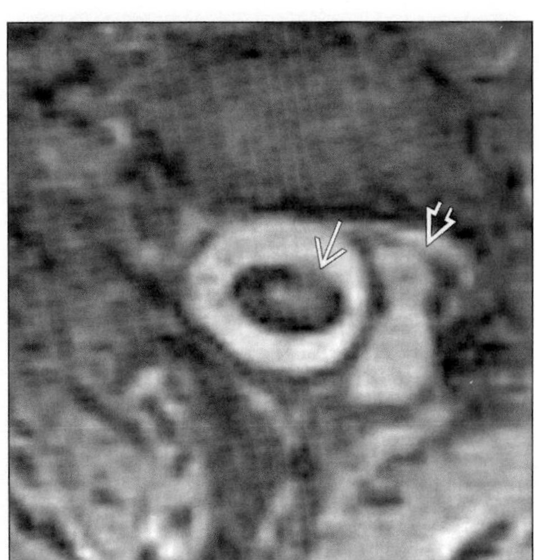

(Left) *Axial T1WI C+ FS MR in same patient reveals focal areas of enhancement in the surgical cavity ➡. These are granulation tissue foci along the margin of the surgical site that likely continue to chronically ooze blood, causing superficial siderosis.* ***(Right)*** *Axial T2WI MR in a patient with cervical trauma shows interruption of hemosiderin hypointense rim ➡ due to the absence of spinal cord pia mater at the root avulsion site. Note the pseudomeningocele ➡. (Courtesy N. Kumar, MD.)*

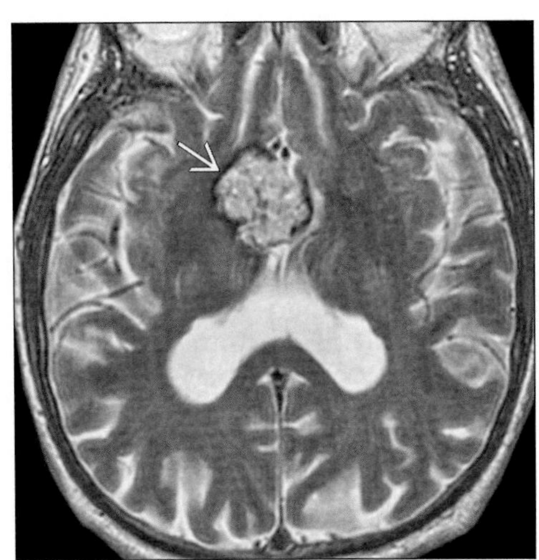

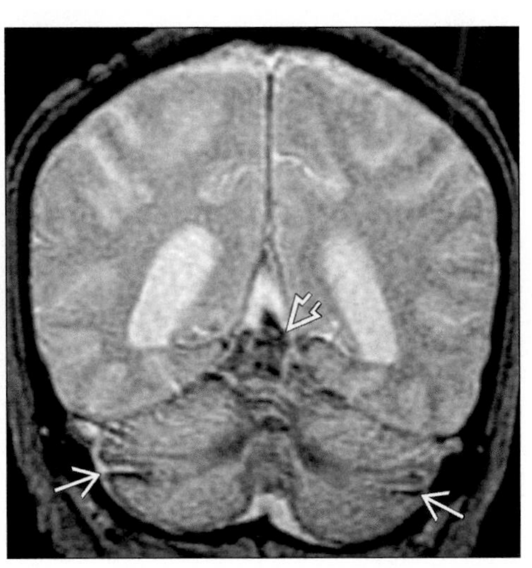

(Left) *Axial T2WI MR reveals the "popcorn ball" appearance of a classic Zabramski type 2 cavernous malformation ➡. A complete hemosiderin rim surrounds the lesion as a hypointense line.* ***(Right)*** *Coronal T2* GRE in the same patient demonstrates extensive superficial siderosis in the posterior fossa. "Blooming" of the hemosiderin on the surfaces is seen as a hypointense outline. The superior vermis ➡ as well as the cerebellar folia ➡ are involved.*

SACCULAR ANEURYSM

Key Facts

Terminology

- Intracranial saccular aneurysm (SA)
- Outpouching affecting only part of arterial circumference
  - Lacks internal elastic lamina ± tunica media

Imaging

- Round/lobulated arterial outpouching
  - Usually arises from bifurcations of circle of Willis (COW), supraclinoid ICA, MCA, cerebellar arteries
  - 90% occur in anterior circulation
  - 10% posterior circulation: Basilar tip, cerebellar arteries (PICA most common)
  - Rare (< 1%): Trigeminal artery, vertebrobasilar junction fenestration
- Ruptured SAs result in SAH
- May have mural Ca++
- Sensitivity of multislice CTA > 95% for SA > 2 mm
- 3D TOF: > 90% sensitive for aneurysms ≥ 3 mm

Top Differential Diagnoses

- Vessel loop
- Vessel infundibulum
- Fusiform aneurysm
- Flow void MR mimic (e.g., aerated anterior clinoid)

Clinical Issues

- Vast majority of unruptured SAs are asymptomatic
  - 2-6% incidental finding at autopsy, imaging
- 80-90% of nontraumatic SAH caused by ruptured SA
- Treatment
  - Endovascular coiling vs. surgical clipping
  - 22.6% relative, 6.9% absolute risk ↓ for coiling vs. surgery for ruptured aneurysms
  - ↓ morbidity, mortality, and hospital costs; quicker recovery for unruptured aneurysms

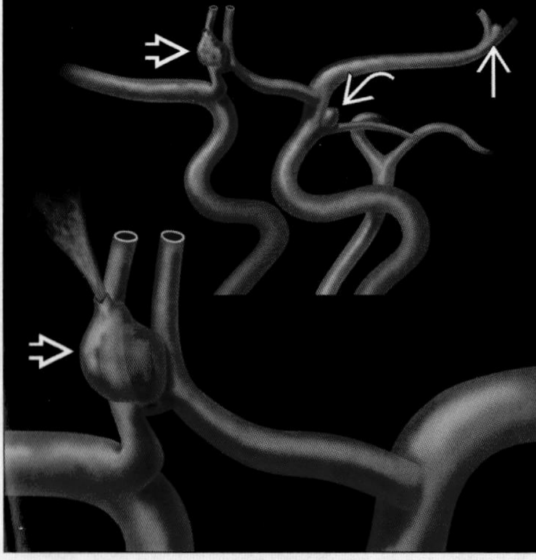

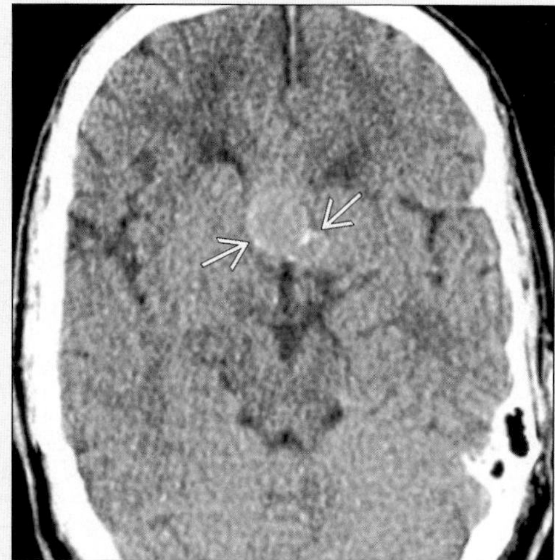

(Left) *LAO graphic of the major arteries at the level of the skull base shows an SA of the anterior communicating artery ⇨ with active extravasation from a superiorly directed bleb (Murphy teat). Note the additional posterior communicating artery SA ↪ and tiny bleb at the left MCA bifurcation →. Patients with SAs have a 20% chance of having > 1 aneurysm.* ***(Right)*** *Axial NECT in a patient with bitemporal hemianopsia shows a slightly hyperdense, lobulated, suprasellar mass just anterior to the 3rd ventricle. Note the mural Ca++ →.*

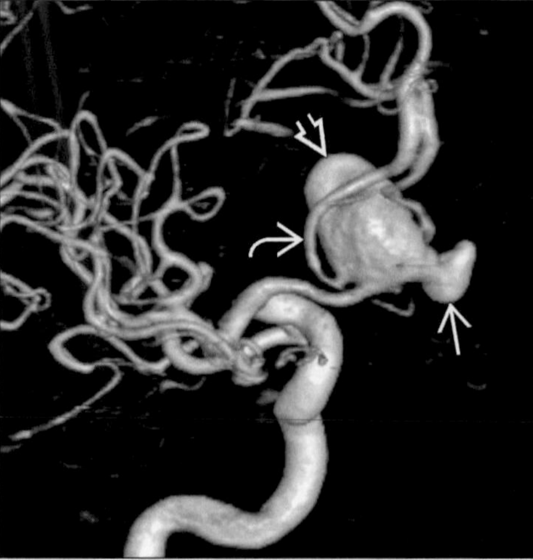

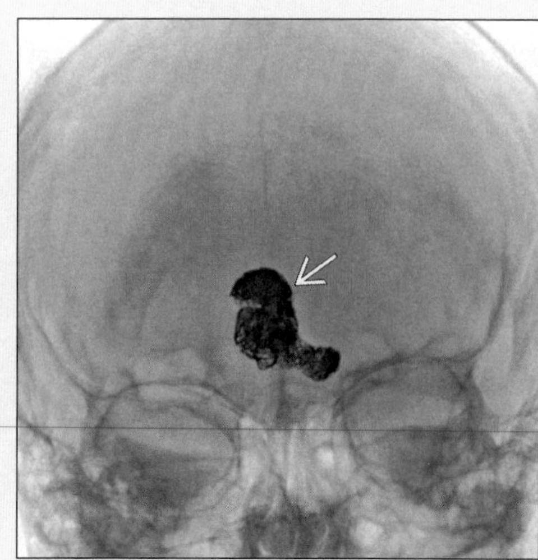

(Left) *3D SSD rotational DSA in the same patient shows a giant anterior communicating artery SA ⇨ with a daughter lobule → worrisome as a potential site for future rupture. The right A2 segment ↪ arises from the aneurysm base, precluding complete aneurysm occlusion with coils. Likelihood of morbidity with clipping is high given the SA's large size and proximity to lenticulostriate perforators.* ***(Right)*** *After placement of 40 embolization coils →, dense packing of both lobes of the anterior coordinating artery SA is seen.*

SACCULAR ANEURYSM

TERMINOLOGY

Abbreviations

- Intracranial saccular aneurysm (SA)

Synonyms

- Berry aneurysm, true aneurysm

Definitions

- Arterial outpouching affecting only part of arterial circumference
  - Lacks internal elastic lamina ± tunica media

IMAGING

General Features

- Best diagnostic clue
  - Round/lobulated arterial outpouching
    - Usually arises from bifurcations of circle of Willis (COW), supraclinoid ICA, MCA, cerebellar arteries
- Location
  - 90% occur in anterior circulation
    - ACoA, PCoA, MCA bifurcation, carotid terminus most common sites
    - Other: Paraclinoid ICA, superior hypophyseal, anterior choroidal artery (AChA)
  - 10% posterior circulation: Basilar tip, cerebellar arteries (PICA most common)
  - Rare (< 1%): Trigeminal artery, vertebrobasilar junction fenestration
  - Vessel bifurcation > side wall aneurysm (e.g., blood blister-like aneurysm)
- Size
  - Small (< 3 mm) to giant (> 2.5 cm)
- Morphology
  - Round, ovoid daughter lobe(s)
  - Narrow or wide necked
  - Branch vessel may be incorporated into aneurysm neck (can preclude coil embolization)

CT Findings

- NECT
  - Ruptured SAs result in subarachnoid hemorrhage (SAH)
    - Pattern of SAH may help localize SA location
  - If SA contains thrombus → hyperdense to brain
  - May have mural Ca++
- CECT
  - Lumen of patent SA enhances uniformly
  - Completely thrombosed SA may have rim enhancement
- CTA
  - Sensitivity of multislice CTA > 95% for SA > 2 mm
  - Look for more than 1 aneurysm, as SA is multiple in 20% of patients
  - Look for associated SAH vasospasm if ruptured SA

MR Findings

- T1WI
  - Patent aneurysm (signal varies)
    - 50% have flow void
    - 50% iso-/heterogeneous signal (slow/turbulent flow, saturation effects, phase dispersion)
  - Partially/completely thrombosed aneurysm
    - Signal depends on age of thrombus
    - Common: Mixed signal, laminated thrombus
    - Hypointense + "blooming" on susceptibility sequences (GRE, SWI)
- T2WI
  - Typically hypointense (flow void)
  - May be laminated with very hypointense rim
- FLAIR
  - Acute SAH: High signal in sulci, cisterns
- DWI
  - May see restricted diffusion secondary to ischemia from SAH vasospasm
  - Thromboembolic events from intraaneurysmal thrombus (rare)
- T1WI C+
  - Slow flow in patent lumen may enhance
  - Increased phase artifact in patent SAs
- MRA
  - 3D TOF: > 90% sensitive for aneurysms ≥ 3 mm
  - Short T1 substances, such as subacute hemorrhage, may simulate flow on TOF MRA

Angiographic Findings

- Conventional DSA
  - Technique
    - Bilateral carotid + dominant vertebral artery injections with reflux to contralateral PICA or "4 vessel" cerebral DSA required
    - Cross-compression of contralateral carotid may be needed for evaluation of ACoA
    - Rotational DSA with 3D surface shaded display (SSD) reconstructions may be helpful but prone to artifact depending on window settings
  - Rare: Contrast extravasation with active SAH
  - Look for Murphy teat (bleb at site of recent rupture) vs. daughter lobe (smaller outpouching from aneurysm fundus, likely indicating focal wall weakness, ↑ future rupture risk)

Imaging Recommendations

- Best imaging tool
  - NECT + CTA for work-up of SAH
  - CTA or MRA for screening of high-risk groups
- Protocol advice
  - Dual energy direct bone removal CT angiography for evaluation of skull base/paraclinoid SA
  - 3D SSD reconstructions helpful to visualize ACoA and MCA bifurcation

DIFFERENTIAL DIAGNOSIS

Vessel Loop

- Use multiple projections

Vessel Infundibulum

- < 3 mm, conical, vessel arises directly from apex
- Commonly at posterior communicating artery (PCoA) and anterior choroidal artery (AChA) origins

Fusiform Aneurysm

- Sausage-shaped morphology with separate inflow, outflow pathways
- Long segment, usually located distal to COW

SACCULAR ANEURYSM

- Can be secondary to ASVD
- Often pseudoaneurysm etiology
  - Trauma, mycotic, vasculitic, connective tissue disease

Flow Void (MR Mimic)

- Aerated anterior clinoid or supraorbital cell

PATHOLOGY

General Features

- Etiology
  - SA development and rupture risk reflect complex combination of inherited susceptibility + acquired mechanically mediated vessel wall stresses
  - Abnormal vascular hemodynamics → ↑ wall stress
    - Flow-related "bioengineering fatigue" in vessel wall more likely with asymmetric COW → ↑ development of SA at site of anomaly
      - e.g., aplastic A1 segment, persistent trigeminal artery, vertebrobasilar fenestration
- Genetics
  - Familial intracranial aneurysms (FIAs)
    - No known heritable connective tissue disorder
    - Occur in "clusters" (1st-order relatives)
    - Younger patients, no female predominance compared to sporadic SAs
    - Consider screening with CTA or MRA
- Associated abnormalities
  - ↑ SA incidence in patients with
    - Fibromuscular dysplasia (FMD): Autosomal dominant, sporadic
  - Bicuspid aortic valve
  - Autosomal dominant polycystic kidney disease (10% have SA)
  - Intracranial AVM: Feeding pedicle ("flow-related") aneurysms in 30%
    - May regress after treatment of AVM

Gross Pathologic & Surgical Features

- Round/lobulated sac, thin or thick wall, ± SAH

Microscopic Features

- Disrupted/absent internal elastic lamina
- Muscle layer absent
- May have "teat" of fragile adventitia

CLINICAL ISSUES

Presentation

- Most common signs/symptoms
  - Vast majority of unruptured SA are asymptomatic
    - Cranial neuropathy uncommon (e.g., pupil-involving CN3 palsy from PCoA aneurysm)
    - TIA/stroke from thromboembolic events secondary to intraaneurysmal thrombus (rare)
  - 80-90% of nontraumatic SAH caused by ruptured SA
    - Headache (typical = "thunderclap")
- Clinical profile
  - 2 common scenarios
    - Middle-aged patient with "worst headache of my life" from ruptured SA → SAH
    - Incidental finding on imaging performed for unrelated symptoms in patient of any age

Demographics

- Age
  - ↑ incidence of SA with age; rare in children
- Gender
  - M < F (especially with multiple aneurysms)
- Epidemiology
  - 2-6% incidental finding of unruptured SA at autopsy
  - Annual risk of de novo aneurysm formation = 0.8% in patients with previous SA

Natural History & Prognosis

- Rupture risk
  - Size: Low risk of SA rupture if < 7 mm
  - Estimated risk of rupture: 1-2% per year cumulative for unruptured aneurysms
  - ~ 20% of ruptured unsecured SA rebleed within 2 weeks, 50% in 6 months
  - Shape: Daughter lobe likely ↑ risk of future SAH; Murphy teat = site of recent rupture and possible rebleed if untreated
  - ↑ in females with history of HTN, smoking

Treatment

- Endovascular coiling
  - Ruptured SA: 22.6% relative, 6.9% absolute risk ↓ for coiling vs. surgery (1 study)
  - Unruptured SA: Coiling vs. clipping
    - ↓ morbidity, mortality, and hospital costs; shorter hospital stay; quicker recovery
- Surgical clipping
  - Lower SA recurrence risk compared with coiling, although rebleeding risk is low with either Rx
  - May have advantage in MCA and other SA where branch vessel arising from SA must be preserved

DIAGNOSTIC CHECKLIST

Consider

- Blood blister-like aneurysm if negative CTA in patient with SAH → perform DSA
- Perimesencephalic bleed in patient with blood localized to interpeduncular cistern

Image Interpretation Pearls

- Diffuse SAH without focal hematoma → ACoA is most likely site of ruptured SA
- Absence of sylvian fissures may be clue to subacute (isodense) SAH

SELECTED REFERENCES

1. Brunken M et al: Coiling vs. Clipping: Hospital Stay and Procedure Time in Intracranial Aneurysm Treatment. Rofo. Epub ahead of print, 2009
2. Héman LM et al: Incidental intracranial aneurysms in patients with internal carotid artery stenosis: a CT angiography study and a metaanalysis. Stroke. 40(4):1341-6, 2009
3. Wiebers DO et al: Unruptured intracranial aneurysms: natural history, clinical outcome, and risks of surgical and endovascular treatment. Lancet. 362(9378):103-10, 2003

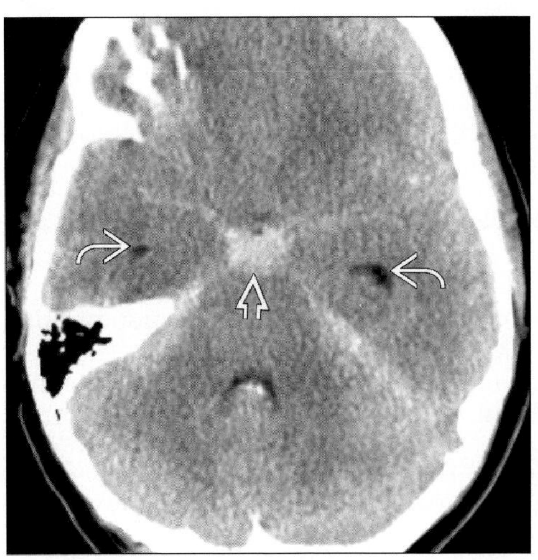

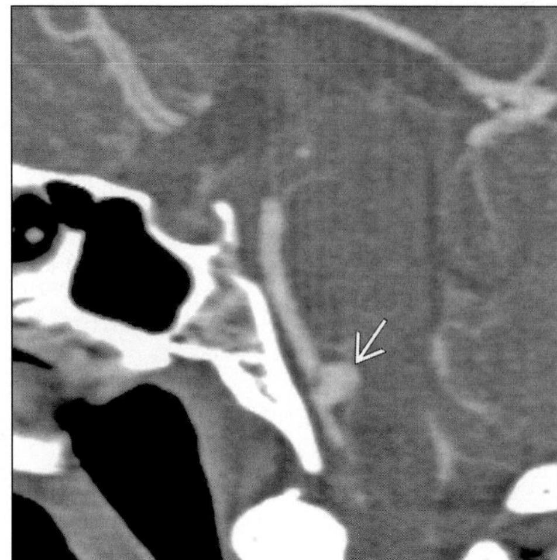

***(Left)** Axial NECT shows diffuse subarachnoid hemorrhage (SAH) in the prepontine cistern ➡ and mild hydrocephalus with dilatation of the temporal horns of the lateral ventricle ➡. The location of the SAH is highly suggestive of a posterior circulation SA rupture. **(Right)** Sagittal CTA in the same patient confirms a posterior circulation SA at the level of the pontomedullary junction ➡. This SA would be difficult to clip surgically due to its intricate relationship to the brainstem perforating vessels.*

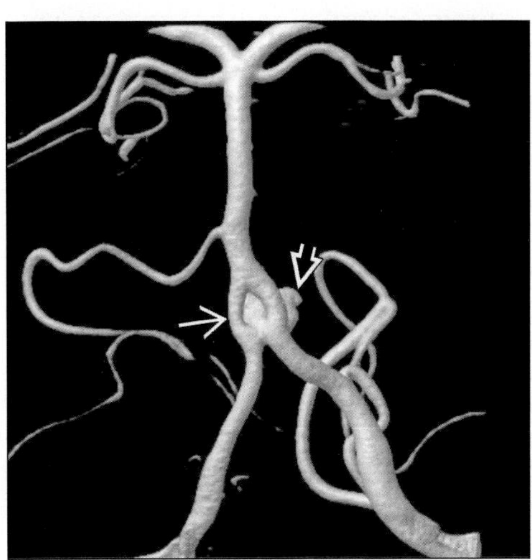

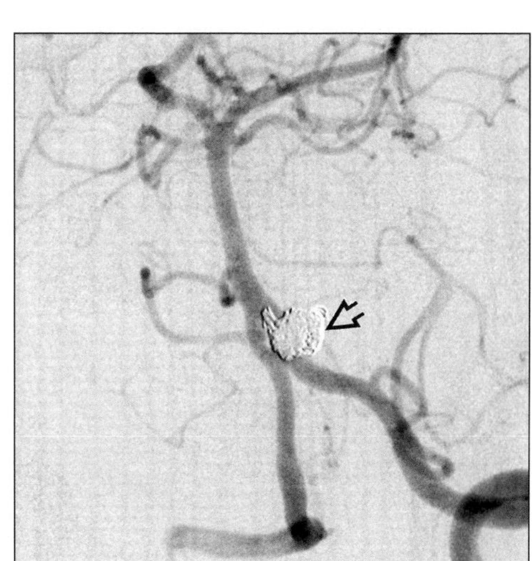

***(Left)** Anteroposterior 3D DSA SSD in the same patient confirms an SA associated with a vertebrobasilar junction fenestration ➡. Note the irregular Murphy teat directed superiorly ➡, which likely represents the site of rupture. **(Right)** Oblique DSA following coil embolization shows a dense coil packing within the SA, including the Murphy teat ➡ with no residual aneurysm filling. The patient was discharged from the hospital neurologically intact a week later.*

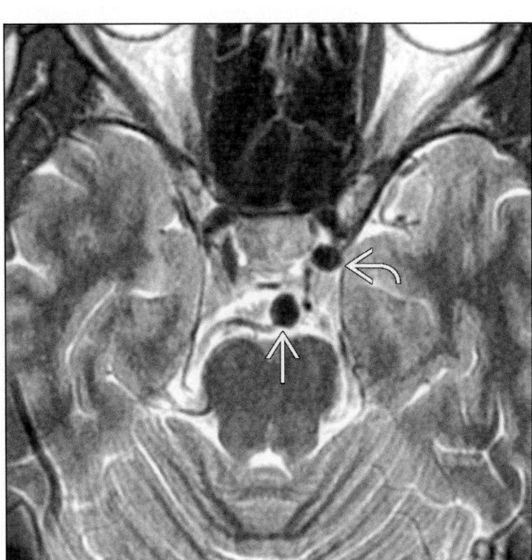

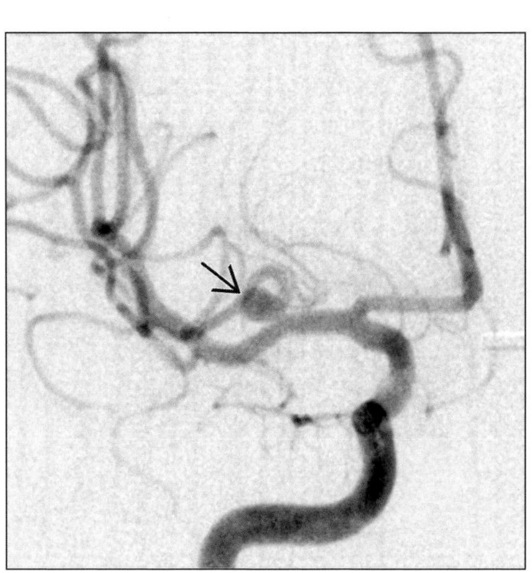

***(Left)** Axial T2WI MR in a middle-aged woman shows 2 rounded flow voids that represent basilar apex ➡ and left posterior communicating artery ➡ SAs, later confirmed with catheter DSA. **(Right)** AP DSA in the same patient shows an additional SA at the right MCA bifurcation ➡. This was treated by endovascular coiling and balloon-remodeling technique without incident. The patient actually also had a left MCA aneurysm. Multiple SAs occur in 20% of patients. Females are much more commonly affected than males.*

PSEUDOANEURYSM

Key Facts

Terminology

- Focal arterial dilatation not contained by layer(s) of normal arterial wall

Imaging

- Irregular, often fusiform arterial outpouching
  - At site, atypical for true (saccular) aneurysm
- NECT: Focal hematoma adjacent to vessel
- CTA: Focal dilatation of vessel diameter vs. adjacent segment of normal vessel
- T1WI: Hematoma signal varies with clot age
- GRE: Hypointense

Top Differential Diagnoses

- Saccular aneurysm
- Dissecting aneurysm

Pathology

- Etiology
  - Trauma (penetrating or blunt)
  - Infection, inflammation ("mycotic" aneurysm)
  - Drug abuse, neoplasm ("oncotic" aneurysm)
  - Spontaneous dissection, underlying vasculopathy
  - XRT, surgery for H&N cancer ("carotid blow-out")

Clinical Issues

- Presentation: Delayed ischemia/infarction, SAH/ parenchymal bleed if ruptures
- Incidence: 3% of patients with infective endocarditis, 1-2% with CHI
- Treatment: Endovascular or surgical vessel occlusion vs. bypass/stent

Diagnostic Checklist

- Enhancing focus within hematoma may represent pseudoaneurysm

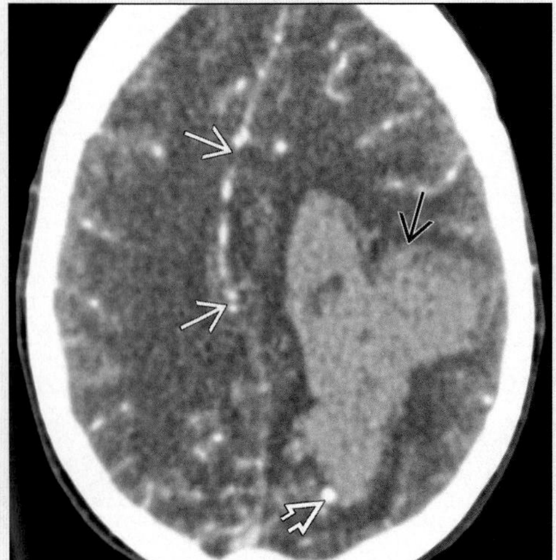

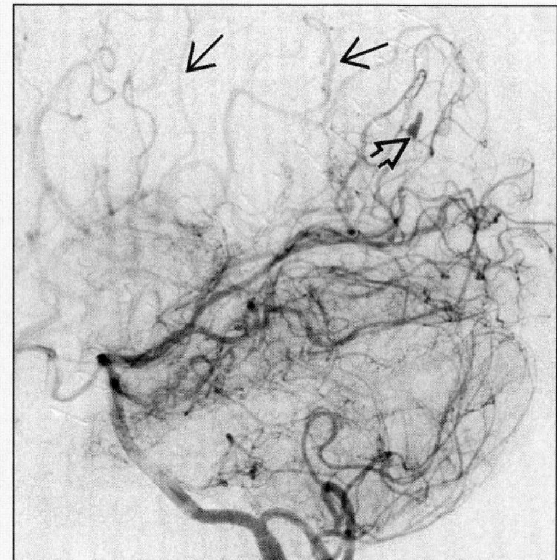

(Left) *Axial CTA shows a large left frontoparietal lobe hematoma → with mass effect and ACA displacement →. A small enhancing focus ⇨ is seen to be contiguous with the posterior aspect of the hematoma.* ***(Right)*** *Vertebral DSA in the same patient shows a bilobed pseudoaneurysm ⇨ of the parietooccipital artery. Note the mass effect on the MCA branches (filling via the PCoA) from the hematoma →. The patient had bacterial endocarditis of the mitral valve and multiple mycotic pseudoaneurysms.*

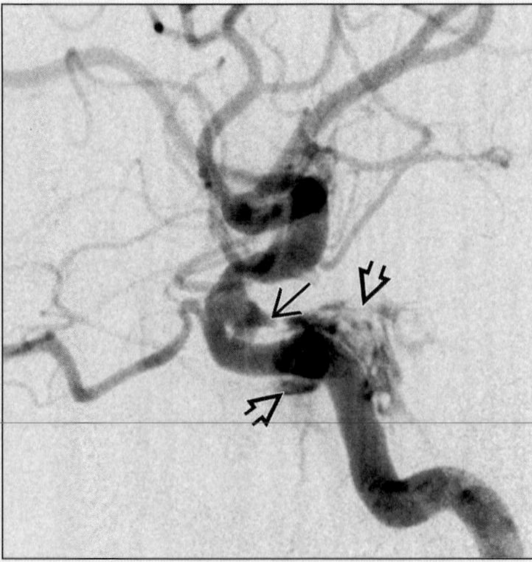

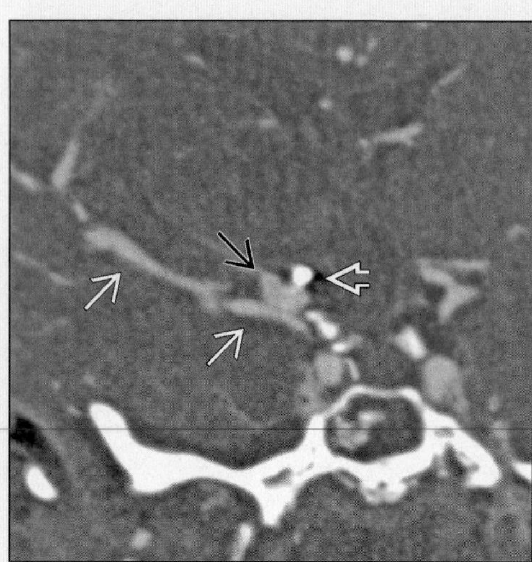

(Left) *Lateral DSA of the ICA in a patient with a closed head injury shows a multilobulated pseudoaneurysm → of the paraclinoid ICA segment and adjacent stenosis, likely due to associated traumatic dissection. Note the direct carotid-cavernous fistula ⇨.* ***(Right)*** *Coronal CTA shows a gunshot wound as a mildly lobulated pseudoaneurysm at the right carotid terminus →. Note the adjacent metallic fragment ⇨ and severe MCA vasospasm → from associated subarachnoid hemorrhage. The pseudoaneurysm enlarged over 2 weeks.*

PSEUDOANEURYSM

TERMINOLOGY

Definitions

- Focal arterial dilatation not contained by layer(s) of normal arterial wall

IMAGING

General Features

- Best diagnostic clue
  - Irregular, often fusiform arterial outpouching at atypical site for true aneurysm formation
- Location
  - Intracranial
    - Distal MCA, ACA, PCA, distal to circle of Willis
    - Petrous/cavernous ICA , vertebral artery (VA)
  - Extracranial
    - Cervical ICA, vertebral artery, ECA branches
- Morphology
  - Often irregular ± fusiform shape

CT Findings

- NECT
  - Focal hematoma adjacent to vessel
  - Base of skull fx ± other CT signs of trauma (e.g., contusion, DAI, extraaxial hemorrhage)
  - Pseudoaneurysm rupture: Subarachnoid hemorrhage, parenchymal hematoma, corpus callosum fistula
- CTA
  - Focal dilatation of vessel diameter vs. adjacent segment of normal vessel
  - Extravascular enhancement confined by adjacent hematoma

MR Findings

- T1WI
  - Hematoma signal varies with clot age
  - ± associated flow void within hematoma
- T2WI
  - Varies with age of hematoma
- T2* GRE
  - Hypointense
- T1WI C+
  - Pseudoaneurysm enhances strongly
- MRA
  - T1 shortening from subacute hematoma may obscure pseudoaneurysm with TOF MRA
  - Contrast-enhanced MRA recommended

Angiographic Findings

- Conventional
  - Lobulated or fusiform arterial outpouching
  - Pseudoaneurysm, distal parent vessel may fill/empty slowly → decreased perfusion
  - ± avascular mass effect (hematoma)

Imaging Recommendations

- Best imaging tool
  - Fine cut CTA with multiplanar recons ± shaded surface display (SSD) for initial investigation
  - DSA for definitive diagnosis ± endovascular Rx

DIFFERENTIAL DIAGNOSIS

Saccular Aneurysm

- Circle of Willis > VA or distal ICA branches

Dissecting Aneurysm

- VA > ICA
- Contained by vessel wall (media, adventitia)

Active Extravasation (Other Causes)

- CTA shows focal enhancement within hematoma but often not contiguous with adjacent vessels

PATHOLOGY

General Features

- Etiology
  - Trauma (penetrating or blunt)
  - Infection, inflammation ("mycotic" aneurysm)
  - Drug abuse, neoplasm ("oncotic" aneurysm)
  - Spontaneous dissection, underlying vasculopathy
  - XRT, surgery for H&N cancer ("carotid blow-out")

CLINICAL ISSUES

Presentation

- Most common signs/symptoms
  - Delayed ischemia/infarction
  - Pseudoaneurysm rupture → SAH, parenchymal bleed
- Clinical profile
  - Patient with delayed stroke/SAH/parenchymal bleed following closed head injury (CHI)

Demographics

- Epidemiology
  - 1-2% of CHI cases
  - 3% of patients with infective endocarditis

Treatment

- Endovascular
  - Pseudoaneurysm ± parent artery occlusion with coils, liquid embolics; covered stent
- Surgical
  - Parent artery sacrifice ± vascular bypass vs. wrapping/patch + preserve parent artery

DIAGNOSTIC CHECKLIST

Consider

- Pseudoaneurysm in patient who develops delayed hematoma following CHI

Image Interpretation Pearls

- Enhancing focus within hematoma may represent pseudoaneurysm

SELECTED REFERENCES

1. DuBose J et al: Endovascular stenting for the treatment of traumatic internal carotid injuries: expanding experience. J Trauma. 65(6):1561-6, 2008

VERTEBROBASILAR DOLICHOECTASIA

Key Facts

Imaging

- General findings
  - Irregular, tortuous VBA ± long segment nonfocal fusiform arterial enlargement
  - Usually 6-12 mm, can be giant (> 2.5 cm)
  - Focal arterial dilatation = fusiform aneurysm
- CT
  - Hyperdense tortuous enlarged vessel, Ca++ common
  - Enlarged lumen enhances, intramural thrombus does not
- MR
  - Signal varies with flow, presence/age of thrombus
  - Dynamic CE MRA best
  - 3D TOF inadequate (slow flow saturation effects)

Top Differential Diagnoses

- Fusiform aneurysm, ASVD
- Giant serpentine aneurysm
- Nonatherosclerotic fusiform vasculopathy
- Dissecting aneurysm

Clinical Issues

- Peak age = 7th, 8th decade
- Often asymptomatic
  - Vertebrobasilar TIAs
  - Cranial neuropathy (e.g., trigeminal neuralgia) less common

Diagnostic Checklist

- Slow complex flow →heterogeneous signal, TOF artifact
- Dynamic contrast-enhanced CTA/MRA or DSA necessary to delineate true lumen

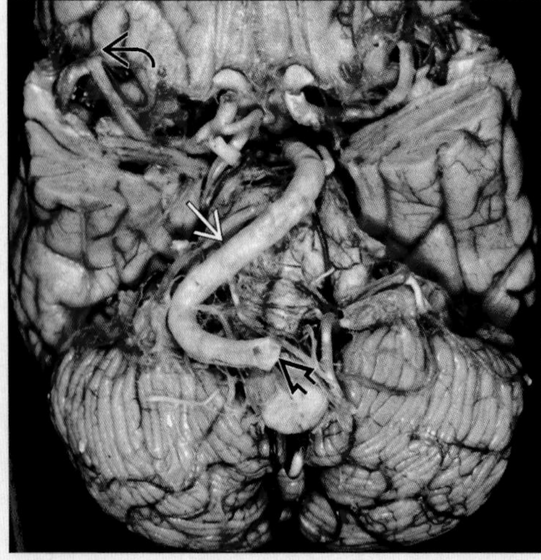

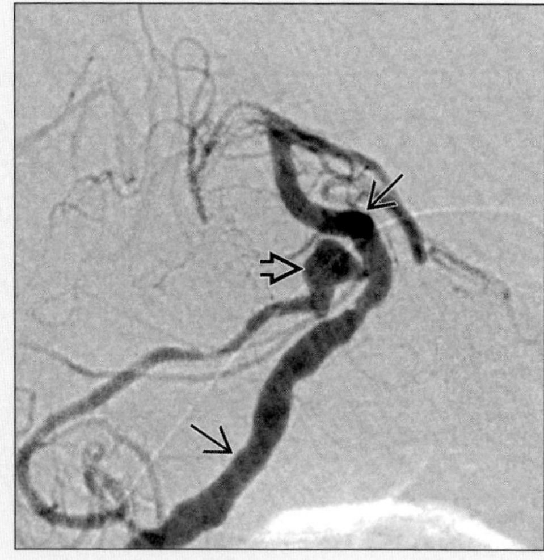

(Left) *Submentovertex view of autopsied brain from an elderly patient shows striking vertebrobasilar dolichoectasia ➔. The basilar artery is uniformly enlarged without aneurysmal outpouching. Note the yellow discoloration from atherosclerotic plaques ⇨. Some ectasia of the middle cerebral artery is also present ↶. (Courtesy R. Hewlett, PhD.)* ***(Right)*** *DSA in a 78-year-old man shows an elongated, ectatic, irregular vertebrobasilar artery with severe atherosclerosis →. Note the fusiform PICA aneurysm ⇨.*

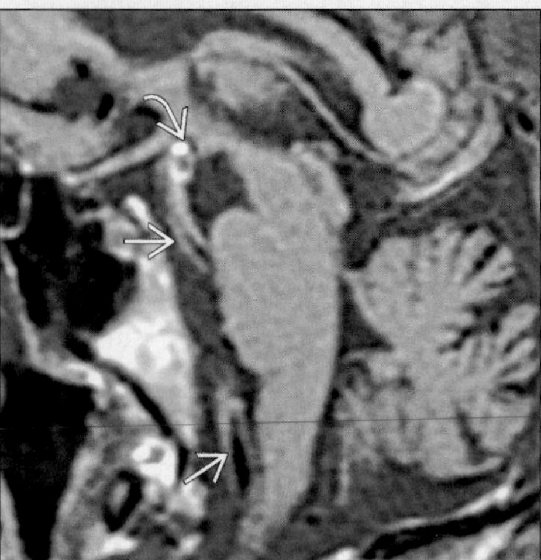

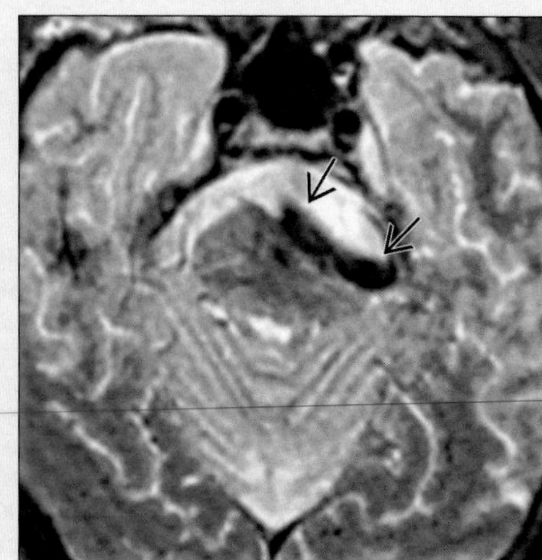

(Left) *Sagittal T1WI MR shows an elongated basilar artery with a thickened wall ➔. Note the mass effect on the hypothalamus and anterior 3rd ventricle caused by the ectatic artery ➔, common with vertebrobasilar dolichoectasia.* ***(Right)*** *Axial T2WI MR in the same patient shows that the flow void of the ectatic artery → compresses the pons with no abnormal pontine signal. Vertebrobasilar dolichoectasia is 1 of the most common manifestations of intracranial atherosclerosis.*

VERTEBROBASILAR DOLICHOECTASIA

TERMINOLOGY

Abbreviations

- Vertebrobasilar dolichoectasia (VBD)

Synonyms

- Fusiform vertebrobasilar ectasia

Definitions

- Extensive ectatic, elongated vertebrobasilar artery (VBA)

IMAGING

General Features

- Best diagnostic clue
  - Irregular, tortuous VBA ± long segment nonfocal fusiform arterial enlargement
    - Focal arterial dilatation = fusiform aneurysm
- Location
  - Basilar > dominant vertebral or both vertebral arteries
    - Other arteries (e.g., PICA, often involved)
- Size
  - Usually moderate (6-12 mm)
    - May be giant (> 2.5 cm diameter)
- Morphology
  - Diffuse or multifocal ectatic vessel
    - ± focal dilatation = fusiform aneurysm

CT Findings

- NECT
  - Hyperdense tortuous enlarged vessel
    - Thickened walls, Ca++ common
    - Thrombus common
- CECT
  - Enlarged lumen enhances
    - Intramural thrombus/plaque does not
- CTA
  - Enlarged tubular ± focal fusiform vertebrobasilar arteries with tortuosity

MR Findings

- T1WI
  - Signal varies with flow, presence/age of thrombus
- T2WI
  - Lumen, thrombus hypointense
- T1WI C+
  - Lumen enhances intensely
    - Pulsation artifact common
- MRA
  - Dynamic CE MRA best
  - 3D TOF inadequate (slow-flow saturation effects)

Imaging Recommendations

- Best imaging tool
  - Dynamic contrast-enhanced CTA/MRA
- Protocol advice
  - CTA/MRA (2D TOF &/or contrast-enhanced) for vessel delineation
  - T2/FLAIR for brainstem delineation

DIFFERENTIAL DIAGNOSIS

Fusiform Aneurysm

- Focal elongated aneurysmal outpouching
- Often superimposed on VBD

Giant Serpentine Aneurysm

- Round/oval mass
- Tortuous lumen, variable thrombus
- Delineation of outer wall morphology on T1, T2, or CT is crucial

Nonatherosclerotic Fusiform Vasculopathy

- Younger patient with inherited vasculopathy, inflammatory disease
- Anterior > posterior circulation

Dissecting Aneurysm

- Vertebral > basilar artery
- Lacks changes of ASVD, Ca++
- Usually more focal or with narrowing

PATHOLOGY

Gross Pathologic & Surgical Features

- Generalized ASVD with diffuse arterial ectasia, tortuosity

CLINICAL ISSUES

Presentation

- Most common signs/symptoms
  - Often asymptomatic
  - Vertebrobasilar TIAs
  - Cranial neuropathy (e.g., trigeminal neuralgia) less common

Demographics

- Peak age = 7th, 8th decade

Natural History & Prognosis

- Slow progressive increasing ectasia
  - May become symptomatic or develop symptoms of other ASVD
- Subarachnoid hemorrhage uncommon
  - Usually with associated focal fusiform aneurysm
  - Parenchymal hemorrhage related to HTN

DIAGNOSTIC CHECKLIST

Image Interpretation Pearls

- Slow complex flow may have heterogeneous signal, saturation artifacts
- Dynamic contrast-enhanced CTA/MRA or DSA necessary to delineate true lumen

SELECTED REFERENCES

1. Takeuchi S et al: Dolichoectasia involving the vertebrobasilar and carotid artery systems. J Clin Neurosci. 16(10):1344-6, 2009

ASVD FUSIFORM ANEURYSM

Key Facts

Terminology

- Atherosclerotic fusiform aneurysm (ASVD FA)
  - Aneurysmal dolichoectasia

Imaging

- Exaggerated arterial ectasia(s) + focal fusiform/ saccular enlargement
  - Long segment irregular fusiform or ovoid arterial dilatation
  - Usually large (> 2.5 cm), may be giant
  - Vertebrobasilar > carotid circulation
- CT: Hyperdense, Ca++ common
  - May present as CPA mass
- MR: Signal varies with degree of flow, presence/age of hematoma
  - Lumen, intramural clot often hypointense on T2WI, but heterogeneous
  - Residual lumen enhances, intramural clot does not
  - Prominent phase artifact common
- Noncontrast 3D TOF inadequate due to flow saturation, phase dispersion
- Dynamic contrast-enhanced MRA for aneurysm delineation, T2 for brainstem delineation

Clinical Issues

- Slow but progressively increasing ectasia, enlargement, thrombosis, symptoms
- Vertebrobasilar TIAs > cranial neuropathy

Diagnostic Checklist

- DSA or contrast-enhanced CTA/MRA necessary to delineate patent lumen
- Slow/complex flow in residual lumen → heterogeneous signal
- Consider dissecting aneurysm, non-ASVD etiology if younger patient

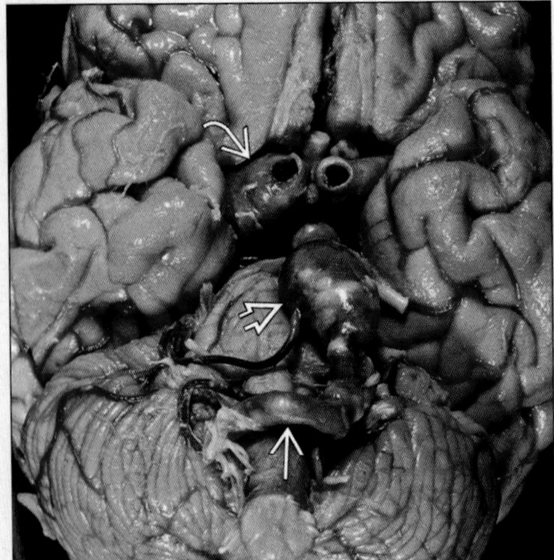

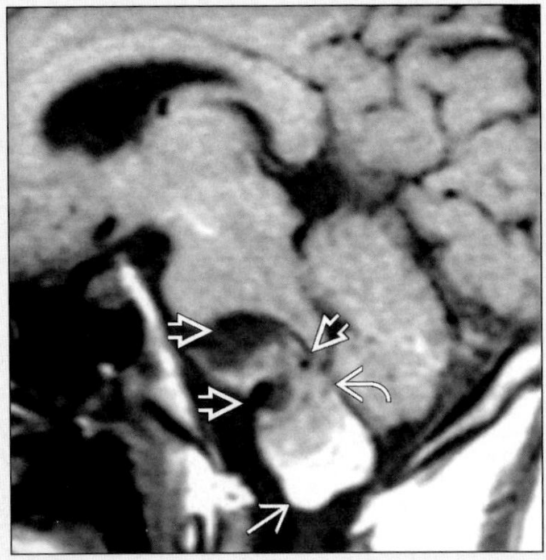

(Left) *Severe ectasia of the internal carotid ➡ and vertebrobasilar ➡ artery shows a giant, partially thrombosed atherosclerotic fusiform aneurysm ➡. (Courtesy R. Hewlett, PhD.)* ***(Right)*** *Sagittal T1WI MR shows a large heterogeneous fusiform atherosclerotic aneurysm of the basilar artery with hyperintense thrombus inferiorly ➡ and isointense material, which may represent slow flow or more acute thrombus superiorly ➡. Only small residual flow voids are seen ➡.*

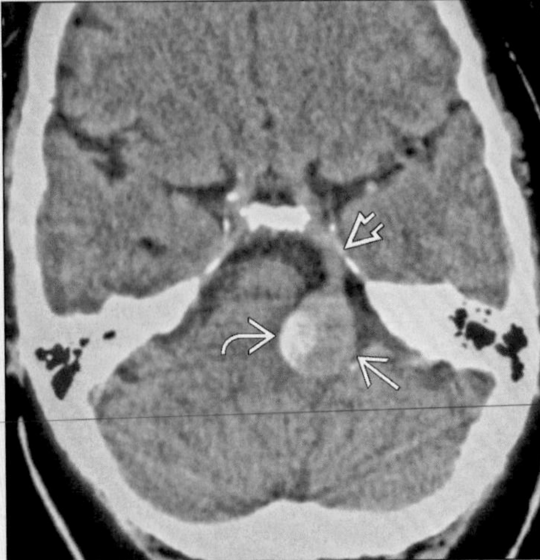

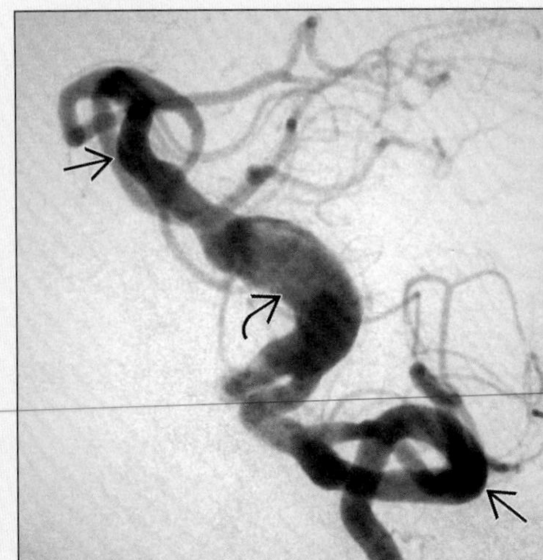

(Left) *Axial NECT shows a hyperintense thrombus ➡ and modestly hyperintense residual lumen ➡ of a fusiform aneurysm with mild dolichoectasia of the adjacent basilar artery ➡.* ***(Right)*** *Oblique DSA in the same patient 2 years later shows dolichoectasia of the proximal vertebral, distal basilar arteries ➡. A fusiform ASVD aneurysm lies between the arterial ectasias. The residual lumen is indicated ➡. The aneurysm had enlarged but also partially thrombosed, leading to mild TIAs.*

ASVD FUSIFORM ANEURYSM

TERMINOLOGY

Abbreviations

- Atherosclerotic fusiform aneurysm (ASVD FA)
  - Aneurysmal dolichoectasia

Definitions

- ASVD → ectasia + elongated aneurysmal outpouching

IMAGING

General Features

- Best diagnostic clue
  - Long segment fusiform/ovoid arterial dilatation
- Location
  - Vertebrobasilar > carotid circulation
- Size
  - Usually large (> 2.5 cm), may be giant
- Morphology
  - Solitary/multifocal generalized dolichoectasia
  - Focal fusiform aneurysmal dilatation

CT Findings

- NECT
  - Hyperdense thrombus, isodense residual lumen
    - Ca++ common
    - May present as CPA mass
- CECT
  - Residual lumen enhances; intramural clot does not
- CTA
  - Exaggerated arterial ectasia(s) + focal fusiform enlargement

MR Findings

- T1WI
  - Signal varies with degree of flow, presence/age of hematoma
- T2WI
  - Lumen, intramural clot often hypointense but heterogeneous
- T1WI C+
  - Residual lumen enhances intensely
    - Prominent phase artifact common
- MRA
  - Noncontrast 3D TOF inadequate due to slow flow, saturation, phase dispersion effects

Imaging Recommendations

- Best imaging tool
  - Dynamic contrast-enhanced MRA or CTA
- Protocol advice
  - Dynamic contrast-enhanced MRA
  - T2, DWI (brainstem compression/edema, infarcts)

DIFFERENTIAL DIAGNOSIS

Atherosclerotic Dolichoectasia

- No focal fusiform/saccular dilatation
- Posterior circulation most commonly affected

Giant Serpentine Aneurysm (GSA)

- Large, partially thrombosed mass with layered clot, no definable neck
- More common in MCA or PCA vs. BA

Nonatherosclerotic Fusiform Vasculopathy

- Younger patient with inherited vasculopathy, immune disorder

Dissecting Aneurysm

- Vertebral > basilar artery
- Lacks changes of ASVD in other vessels

PATHOLOGY

General Features

- Etiology
  - ASVD usual cause of basilar FA in older adults

Gross Pathologic & Surgical Features

- Generalized ASVD with focally dilated fusiform arterial ectasia(s)

Microscopic Features

- Plaques of foam cells with thickened intima, organized thrombus

CLINICAL ISSUES

Presentation

- Most common signs/symptoms
  - Vertebrobasilar TIAs > cranial neuropathy
- Other signs/symptoms
  - Headache, rare subarachnoid hemorrhage

Demographics

- Peak age: 7th to 8th decades

Natural History & Prognosis

- Slow but progressively increasing ectasia
- Progressive enlargement, thrombosis → ↑ TIAs, stroke

Treatment

- Combined surgical, endovascular treatment is option
- Antiplatelet therapy for TIA

DIAGNOSTIC CHECKLIST

Consider

- Dissecting aneurysm, non-ASVD etiology if younger patient

Image Interpretation Pearls

- Slow/complex flow in residual lumen may give heterogeneous signal
- DSA or contrast-enhanced CTA/MRA necessary to delineate patent lumen

SELECTED REFERENCES

1. Chihara Y et al: Fusiform aneurysm of the basilar artery presenting as a cerebellopontine angle mass. Eur Arch Otorhinolaryngol. 266(1):151-2, 2009

NON-ASVD FUSIFORM ANEURYSM

Key Facts

Terminology

- Fusiform enlargement of intracranial vessel(s) caused by inherited/acquired vasculopathy

Imaging

- Long, nonbranching vessel segments; vertebrobasilar > carotid circulation
- Hyperdense; Ca++ common
- Mixed signal intensity (varies with flow, presence/ age of hematoma)
- May require dynamic contrast-enhanced MRA for accurate delineation
- Long segment of tubular, fusiform, or ovoid arterial dilatation in absence of ASVD
- Can be solitary or multifocal
- Elongated, ectatic vessel ± more focal aneurysmal outpouching
- May have significant thrombotic component
- T2WI delineates outer wall of aneurysm and intraluminal or mural thrombus
- DWI may show restriction from distal embolic complications

Pathology

- Collagen vascular disorders (i.e., SLE)
- Viral, other infectious agents (e.g., varicella, HIV)
- Inherited (e.g., Marfan, Ehlers-Danlos, neurofibromatosis type 1, arterial anomalies)

Clinical Issues

- Pain, SAH > TIA, cranial neuropathy in dissection etiology
- Commonly asymptomatic or presents with TIA/ stroke in viral and neurocutaneous etiology
- Treatment depends upon underlying cause, expected natural history, location, and anatomy

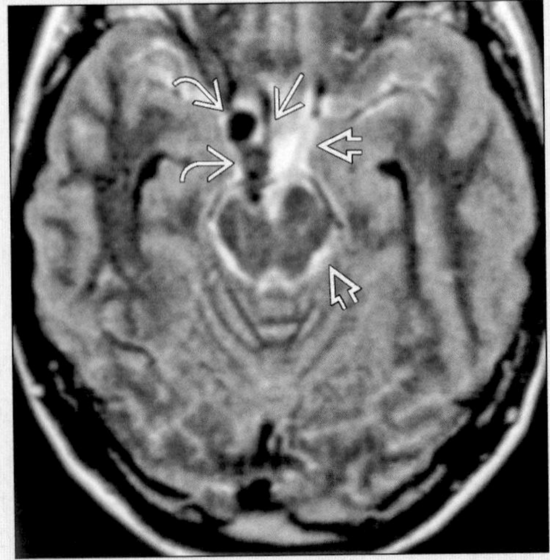

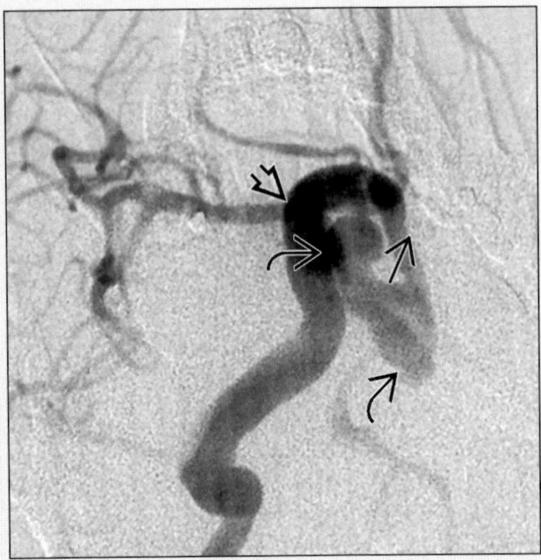

***(Left)** Axial FLAIR MR shows an oddly shaped, elongated flow void → and aneurysm → surrounded by hyperintense SAH that fills the suprasellar and perimesencephalic cisterns →. **(Right)** Submentovertex angiography in the same patient shows an anomalous elongated supraclinoid ICA → and a multilobulated fusiform aneurysm → prior to the MCA-ACA bifurcation → overlapping the ICA. Complex arterial anomalies such as this are commonly associated with saccular or fusiform aneurysms.*

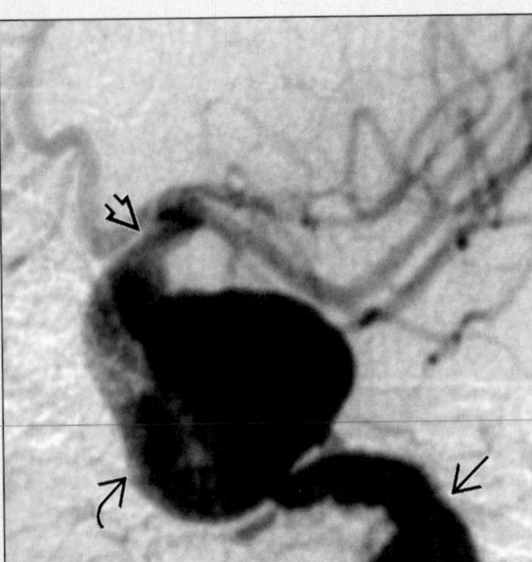

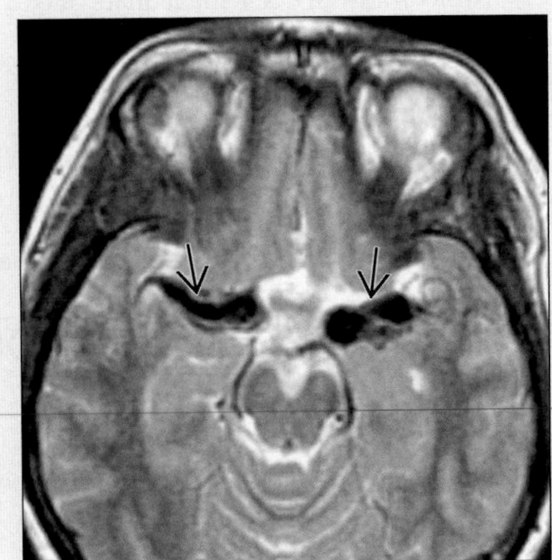

***(Left)** Anteroposterior angiography shows an extensive fusiform aneurysm that involves the entire petrous →, cavernous →, and supraclinoid → internal carotid artery in this patient with Ehlers-Danlos type 4. **(Right)** Axial T2WI MR shows unusually enlarged, bizarre-appearing middle cerebral arteries → in this patient with HIV fusiform arteriopathy. Whether it is the HIV or an associated opportunistic infection that causes the arteriopathy is unknown. Most HIV fusiform aneurysm cases are seen in children.*

NON-ASVD FUSIFORM ANEURYSM

TERMINOLOGY

Abbreviations

- Non-ASVD fusiform aneurysm/vasculopathy (FA)

Definitions

- Fusiform enlargement of intracranial vessel(s) caused by inherited/acquired vasculopathy

IMAGING

General Features

- Best diagnostic clue
  - Long segment of tubular, fusiform, or ovoid arterial dilatation in absence of atherosclerotic vascular disease (ASVD)
- Location
  - Long, nonbranching vessel segments; vertebrobasilar > carotid circulation, depending upon type
- Size
  - Varies from a few mm to several cms

CT Findings

- NECT
  - Hyperdense; Ca++ common
- CECT
  - Lumen enhances strongly, clot does not

MR Findings

- T1WI
  - Elongated, tortuous flow void
  - Mixed signal intensity common, varies with
    - Flow velocity, direction, turbulence
    - ± clot (laminated layers of organized thrombus)
- T2WI
  - Mixed signal intensity (varies with flow, presence/age of hematoma)
- FLAIR
  - Clot usually hyperintense
- DWI
  - May show restriction from distal embolic complications
- T1WI C+
  - Residual lumen enhances strongly
- MRA
  - May require dynamic contrast-enhanced MRA for accurate lumen delineation

Angiographic Findings

- Conventional
  - Solitary/multifocal ectasias, ± focal aneurysmal outpouchings

Imaging Recommendations

- Best imaging tool
  - MR + contrast-enhanced MRA

DIFFERENTIAL DIAGNOSIS

Vertebrobasilar Dolichoectasia

- Older patient with ASVD in other cranial vessels

Giant Serpentine Aneurysm

- Large, partially thrombosed mass

Atypical Saccular Aneurysm

- Looks identical to fusiform aneurysm

Pseudoaneurysm

- May look identical to fusiform aneurysm

PATHOLOGY

General Features

- Etiology
  - Collagen vascular disorders (i.e., SLE)
  - Viral, other infectious agents (e.g., varicella, HIV)
  - Inherited (e.g., Marfan, Ehlers-Danlos, neurofibromatosis type 1)

Staging, Grading, & Classification

- Type 1: Typical dissecting aneurysm
- Type 2: Segmental ectasias due to viral, neurocutaneous syndrome, radiation
- Type 3: Dolichoectatic dissecting aneurysms
- Type 4: Atypically located saccular aneurysm (i.e., lateral wall, unrelated to branching zones)

Gross Pathologic & Surgical Features

- Focally dilated fusiform arterial ectasia(s)

CLINICAL ISSUES

Presentation

- Most common signs/symptoms
  - Pain, SAH > TIA, cranial neuropathy in dissection from collagen disorder etiology
  - Commonly asymptomatic or TIA/stroke in viral and neurocutaneous etiology

Natural History & Prognosis

- Type 1: Rebleed common
- Type 2: Benign clinical course
- Type 3: Slow but progressive enlargement
- Type 4: Rerupture risk high

Treatment

- Dependent upon underlying cause, expected natural history, location, and anatomy
- Often combined surgical, endovascular measures

DIAGNOSTIC CHECKLIST

Consider

- Non-ASVD fusiform aneurysm in young patient with dilated intracranial vessels

SELECTED REFERENCES

1. Bonkowsky J et al: Cerebral vasculopathy with aneurysm formation in HIV-infected young adults. Neurology. 68(8):623; author reply 623, 2007

BLOOD BLISTER-LIKE ANEURYSM

Key Facts

Terminology
- Blood blister-like aneurysm (BBA)
  - Broad-based bulge at nonbranch point

Imaging
- Half-dome or blood blister-like shape
- Supraclinoid ICA most common site
  - Rarely MCA, ACA, ACoA, basilar artery
  - Usually small (< 6 mm; mean = 3 mm)
- NECT: SAH
- CTA: Often difficult to see → CTA negative
- Best imaging tool: High-resolution DSA
  - Obtain multiple obliques ± 3D DSA

Top Differential Diagnoses
- Saccular aneurysm (SA)
- Vasospasm
- Atherosclerotic vascular disease (ASVD)
- Vessel infundibulum

Pathology
- Focal arterial wall defect covered with fibrous tissue
  - ± thin layer of adventitia (pseudoaneurysm)

Clinical Issues
- Middle-aged patient, angio negative SAH ± h/o HTN
  - Higher rebleed rate compared with SA
- Difficult to treat
  - Tend to rupture earlier, at smaller size than SA
  - Small size, wide neck makes coiling difficult
  - High risk of BBA rupture, ICA laceration during surgery

Diagnostic Checklist
- Angiogram negative SAH may be caused by BBA
- Look for subtle dome or bulging of supraclinoid ICA when SA not seen in patient with SAH

*(**Left**) Oblique projection of a left ICA DSA shows a broad-based BBA arising from the dorsal supraclinoid ICA ➡. A large but normal PCoA ⇨ arises from the opposite (ventral) wall of the ICA. (**Right**) Coronal CTA of the same patient shows no definite aneurysm. There is a suggestion of a broad-based bleb ➡ along the left supraclinoid ICA corresponding to the DSA image. BBAs can be extremely difficult to identify on CTA despite multiplanar reformats.*

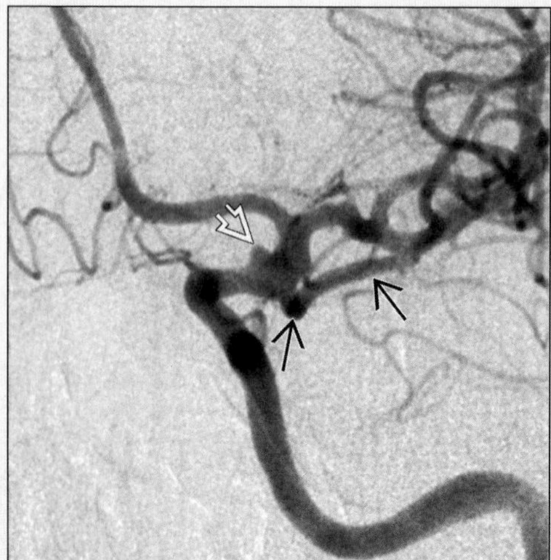

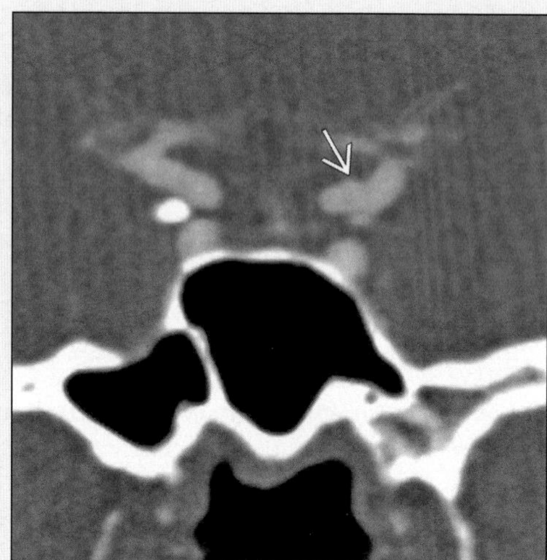

*(**Left**) Lateral right ICA DSA shows a small hemispherical bulge ➡ along the ventral paraclinoid ICA in a patient with SAH. Adjacent irregularity of the ICA lumen more distally likely reflects associated dissection or ASVD ➡. There is vasospasm involving the ACA ⇨ and a PCoA infundibulum ⇗. (**Right**) 3D DSA in the same patient shows a corresponding bleb ➡ along the ventral paraclinoid segment. Note bleb-like appearance of the PCoA infundibulum ➡, which should not be confused with a BBA.*

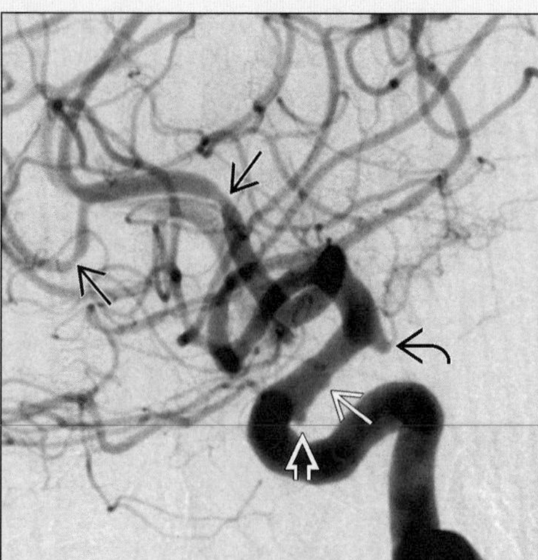

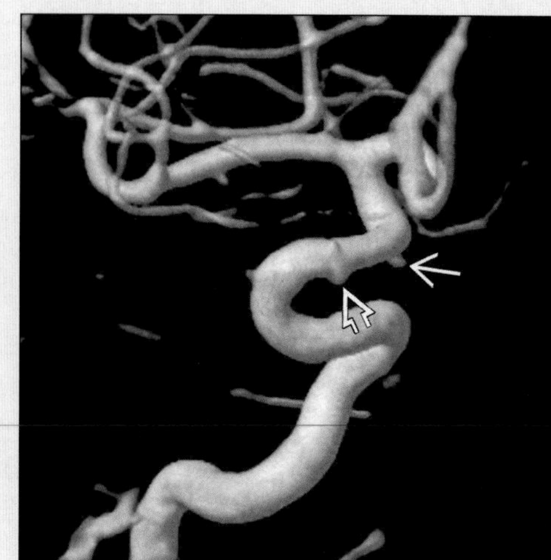

BLOOD BLISTER-LIKE ANEURYSM

TERMINOLOGY

Abbreviations

- Blood blister-like aneurysm (BBA)

Definitions

- Broad-based bulge at non-branch point
  - Supraclinoid ICA > > MCA, ACA, basilar artery

IMAGING

General Features

- Best diagnostic clue
  - Small, broad-based, hemispherical bulge on anterosuperior (dorsal) wall of supraclinoid ICA
  - Rapid change in size/morphology on follow-up angiograms
- Location
  - Supraclinoid ICA is most common site (dorsal wall > ventral)
  - MCA (M1), ACA (A1), anterior communicating artery, basilar artery (rare)
- Size
  - Usually small (< 6 mm; mean = 3 mm)
- Morphology
  - Half-dome or blood blister-like shape

CT Findings

- NECT
  - Aneurysmal subarachnoid hemorrhage (aSAH)
- CTA
  - ± asymmetric bulging of supraclinoid ICA
  - Often difficult to see → CTA negative

MR Findings

- FLAIR
  - Hyperintense CSF if SAH present
- MRA
  - ± visualized on high-resolution MRA

Angiographic Findings

- Conventional DSA
  - BBAs often small, subtle
  - Slight irregularity/small focal hemispherical bulge of arterial wall at characteristic location
  - Multiple projections ± 3D DSA helpful

Imaging Recommendations

- Best imaging tool
  - High-resolution DSA
    - Obtain multiple obliques ± 3D DSA

DIFFERENTIAL DIAGNOSIS

Saccular Aneurysm (SA)

- True aneurysm, typically at arterial bifurcation

Vasospasm

- Usually symmetrical, concentric narrowing of vessel

Atherosclerotic Vascular Disease (ASVD)

- Common in patients with BBA, difficult to distinguish

Vessel Infundibulum

- Funnel-shaped vessel origin; < 3 mm
- Common at posterior communicating artery (PCoA), anterior choroidal artery (AChA) origins

PATHOLOGY

General Features

- Etiology
  - ASVD with ulceration, hematoma formation
  - ICA dissection, arteriosclerosis, HTN

Gross Pathologic & Surgical Features

- Focal arterial wall defect covered with fibrous tissue
  - ± thin layer of adventitia (pseudoaneurysm)

CLINICAL ISSUES

Presentation

- Most common signs/symptoms
  - "Thunderclap" headache 2° to SAH
- Clinical profile
  - Middle-aged patient, angio negative SAH ± h/o HTN

Demographics

- Gender
  - M:F = 1:2
- Epidemiology
  - 1-6% of all intracranial aneurysms resulting in SAH

Natural History & Prognosis

- Tend to rupture earlier, at smaller size than SA
- Higher rebleed rate compared with SA

Treatment

- Endovascular
  - Small size, wide neck makes coiling difficult
  - ↑ risk of intraprocedural rupture, aneurysm regrowth + rebleeding
- Surgical clipping/wrapping
  - High risk of BBA rupture during dissection (45%)
    - BBA avulsion, ICA laceration
- ICA sacrifice → high risk of postoperative ischemic stroke

DIAGNOSTIC CHECKLIST

Consider

- Angiogram negative SAH may be caused by BBA
- Early repeat DSA if 1st angio negative as BBAs often rapidly change in size, shape → ↑ rebleed risk

Image Interpretation Pearls

- Look for subtle dome or bulging of supraclinoid ICA when SA not seen in patient with SAH

SELECTED REFERENCES

1. Meling TR et al: Blood blister-like aneurysms of the internal carotid artery trunk causing subarachnoid hemorrhage: treatment and outcome. J Neurosurg. 108(4):662-71, 2008

SECTION 4
Stroke

Introduction and Overview

Nontraumatic Intracranial Hemorrhage

Atherosclerosis and Carotid Stenosis

Nonatheromatous Vasculopathy

Cerebral Ischemia and Infarction

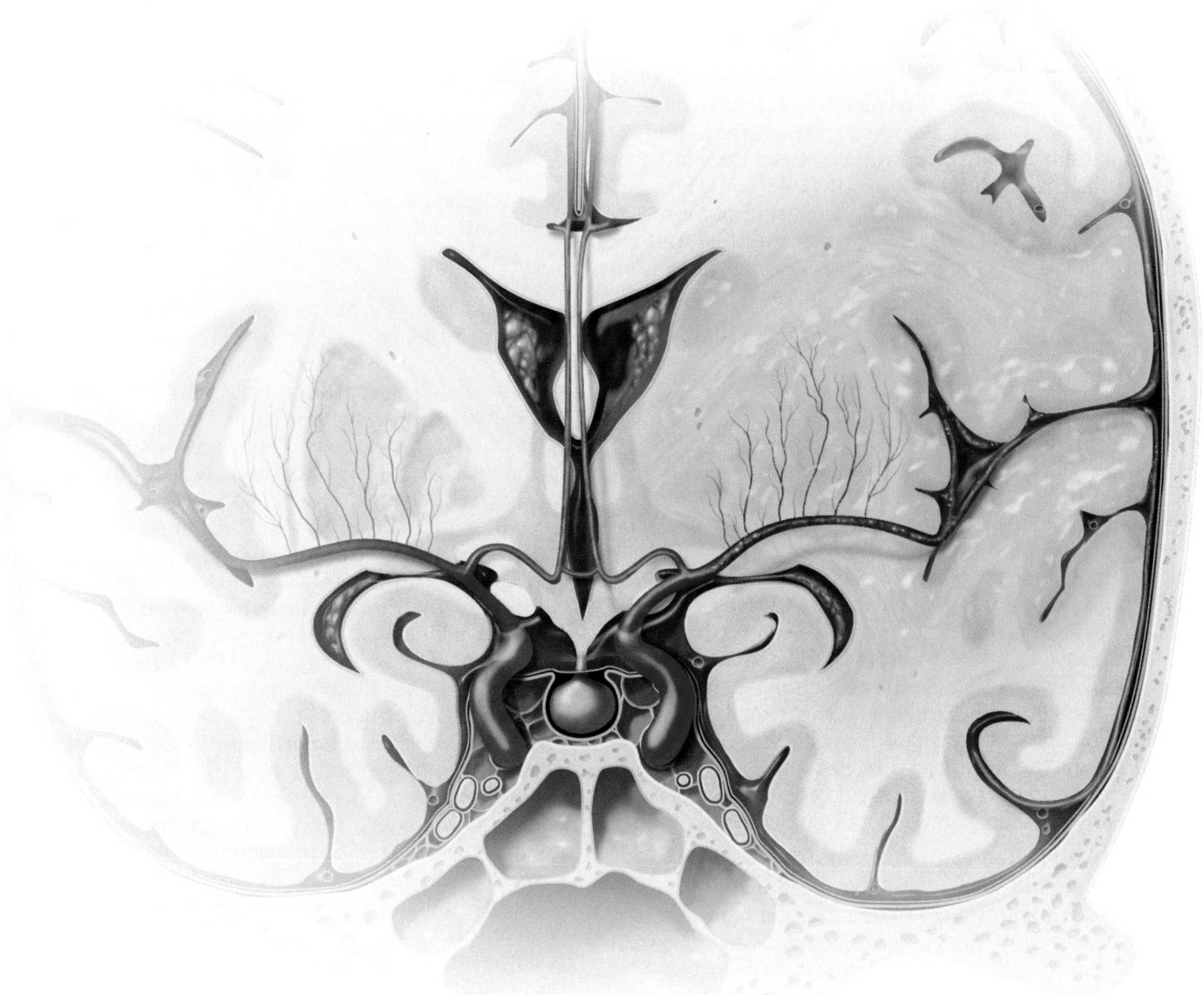

STROKE OVERVIEW

Introduction

Stroke is a lay term that describes the clinical event of a sudden onset of neurologic deficit secondary to cerebrovascular disease. Stroke has 4 main etiologies, including cerebral infarction (80%), intraparenchymal hemorrhage (15%), nontraumatic subarachnoid hemorrhage (5%), and venous infarction (approximately 1%). Clinically, ischemic infarction is the most common etiology and will be the main topic of this introduction. The principal cause of cerebral infarction is atherosclerosis and its sequelae.

Ischemic Infarction

There are 3 major clinical ischemic stroke subtypes based upon the classification from a multicenter clinical trial (trial of drug Org. 10172 in acute stoke treatment). These 3 subtypes include large artery/atherosclerotic infarctions, cardioembolic infarctions, and small vessel occlusion (lacunar) infarctions.

Large artery/atherosclerotic strokes represent ~ 40% of strokes and can arise from thrombosis at the site of a plaque or from emboli produced at the plaque that lodge downstream. The most common site of atherosclerotic plaque is at the carotid bifurcation with involvement of the distal common carotid artery and the 1st 2 cm of the internal carotid artery. Other common locations for atherosclerotic plaque include the carotid siphon and proximal anterior and middle cerebral arteries. The vertebral and basilar arteries are also commonly involved by atherosclerosis.

Cardioembolic disease accounts for 15-25% of ischemic strokes. Risk factors include myocardial infarction, ventricular aneurysm, atrial fibrillation or flutter, cardiomyopathy, and valvular heart disease.

Lacunar infarcts are small in size (< 15 mm), typically in the basal ganglia and thalamus, and account for 15-30% of all strokes. They are often multiple and are due to embolic, atheromatous, or thrombotic lesions in the single penetrating end arterioles that supply the deep gray nuclei, including the lenticulostriate and thalamoperforating arteries. Other common locations for lacunar infarcts include the internal capsule, pons, and corona radiata.

Intraparenchymal Hemorrhage

Intraparenchymal hemorrhage represents about 15% of all strokes and includes multiple etiologies. Hypertensive hemorrhage is the most common etiology, representing about 40-60% of all primarily intracranial hemorrhages. Other etiologies include amyloid angiopathy in elderly patients, as well as vascular malformations, vasculitis, drugs, and bleeding diathesis.

Risk factors for hemorrhagic stroke include increasing age, hypertension, smoking, excessive alcohol consumption, prior ischemic stroke, abnormal cholesterol, and anticoagulant medications.

Although the MR physics related to hemorrhage are complex, the stages are generally accepted as hyperacute, acute, early subacute, late subacute, and chronic.

Nontraumatic Subarachnoid Hemorrhage

Nontraumatic subarachnoid hemorrhage is typically related to an aneurysm (75%) or a vascular malformation such as an AVM or cavernous angioma. Nonaneurysmal "perimesencephalic" subarachnoid hemorrhage is uncommon.

Venous Infarction

Dural sinus or cerebral vein occlusion is rare, representing less than 1% of strokes. Venous thrombosis risk factors include pregnancy, trauma, dehydration, infection, oral contraceptives, coagulopathies, malignancies, collagen vascular diseases, and protein C and S deficiencies. Venous infarcts occur in only about 50% of venous thrombosis cases, and can be differentiated from arterial infarcts by the location of the ischemia. Superior sagittal sinus thrombosis typically results in T2/FLAIR hyperintense parasagittal lesions, while thrombosis of the transverse sinus often results in T2/FLAIR hyperintensities in the posterior temporal lobe. Additionally, venous infarcts more commonly present with associated hemorrhage. Contrast-enhanced CT is useful to identify the "empty-delta" sign representing thrombus within a major dural sinus, typically the superior sagittal or transverse sinus.

Approach to Stroke Imaging

Cerebral ischemia results from significantly decreased blood flow to selected areas or the entire brain. Stroke progresses in stages from ischemia to actual infarction. In the most common situation, middle cerebral artery (MCA) occlusion, there is a densely ischemic central core and a less densely ischemic "penumbra." The central core is usually irreversibly damaged unless reperfusion is quickly established, whereas the cells within the penumbra may remain viable but at risk for several hours. Current stroke therapies attempt to rescue the "at-risk" cells.

Currently, acute stroke protocols vary among different institutions. The exact protocol is often based on the availability of CT versus MR, technology/software, time of stroke, physician expertise, and the possibility of neurointervention. Typically, stroke neurologists work with neuroradiologists to devise a plan that best serves the patient's needs.

Most stroke protocols begin with a noncontrast head CT to evaluate for hemorrhage or mass, which directly affects treatment decisions. Additionally, > 1/3 MCA territory hypodensity at presentation is considered by most to be a contraindication to thrombolysis, as it is associated with a greater risk of fatal hemorrhage. CTA is useful to evaluate for large vessel occlusion. When available, CT perfusion is an excellent way to evaluate for large vessel ischemia.

MR with diffusion-weighted imaging (DWI) is particularly useful for acute ischemia when CT perfusion is negative and the clinical suspicion for stroke remains. MR is also the primary imaging tool when the clinical question includes a posterior fossa or brainstem lesion. MR with perfusion imaging (PWI) has been found extremely helpful in guiding therapy when available.

Most stroke protocols use 3 hour and 6 hour windows for treatment of nonhemorrhagic, ischemic stroke. If the patient presents within 6 hours after the initial onset of symptoms, an unenhanced CT is the initial study of choice to exclude a mass or hemorrhage. If there is a hemorrhage or mass, no thrombolytic therapy is initiated. If there is no hemorrhage or mass, and the patient is within 3 hours after onset of symptoms, the patient is eligible for intravenous (IV) thrombolysis. If the patient is between 3 and 6 hours of onset, either a CTA with CT perfusion or an MR with DWI and PWI is performed

Five Stages of Intraparenchymal Hemorrhage

Stage	*Time (Range)*	*Blood Products*	*T1*	*T2*
Hyperacute	< 24 hours	Oxyhemoglobin	Isointense	Bright
Acute	1-3 days (hours to days)	Deoxyhemoglobin	Isointense	Dark
Early subacute	> 3 days (days to 1 week)	Intracellular methemoglobin	Bright	Dark
Late subacute	> 7 days (1 week to months)	Extracellular methemoglobin	Bright	Bright
Chronic	> 14 days (≥ months)	Hemosiderin	Dark	Dark

to determine if they are eligible for treatment. If the patient has an intracranial thrombus with a penumbra, intraarterial (IA) therapy is recommended. If there is no penumbra, IA therapy may not benefit the patient, so each case is evaluated individually.

The effective therapeutic window for the posterior circulation is thought to be longer than the 3-6 hour window, but the exact time is variable and depends on collateral circulation. Therefore, patients with vertebrobasilar thrombosis are evaluated individually for risk vs. benefit of IA thrombolysis.

Ischemic Penumbra

Ischemic stroke results in a core of tissue which has undergone irreversible injury. The ischemic penumbra is the area of brain which may be salvageable with appropriate therapy. The penumbra typically surrounds the ischemic core & is supported by collateral circulation.

The ischemic penumbra can be identified by a combination of MR diffusion (DWI) and perfusion imaging (PWI). DWI is the most reliable estimate of the ischemic core and generally correlates with irreversible injury. However, with early reperfusion following thrombolysis, some reversal of DWI can be observed. PWI evaluates the presence of a penumbra. With MR, the mismatch between the DWI and PWI defines the penumbra. This model provides a practical means to estimate the ischemic penumbra. In general, if there is no diffusion/perfusion mismatch, therapy may be ineffective.

With the urgency of acute stroke, MR may be impractical. With the newer CT perfusion techniques, an ischemic penumbra may also be measured with CT.

CT Perfusion (pCT)

Cerebral perfusion refers to the tissue level blood flow in the brain. This flow is evaluated by 3 main parameters at pCT: Cerebral blood flow (CBF), cerebral blood volume (CBV), and mean transit time (MTT).

CBF is defined as the volume of blood moving through a given unit volume of brain per unit time. CBF uses units of milliliters of blood per 100 g of brain tissue per minute. Studies suggest that CBF is a reasonable marker for the ischemic penumbra.

CBV is defined as the total volume of blood in a given unit volume of brain. This includes blood in the tissues as well as blood in the large-capacitance vessels, such as arteries, arterioles, capillaries, venules, and veins. CBV uses units of milliliters of blood per 100 g of brain tissue. Some studies suggest that CT perfusion-acquired CBV is a reasonably reliable marker of the ischemic core.

MTT is defined as the average of the transit time of blood through a given brain region. The transit time of blood through the brain parenchyma varies depending on the distance traveled between arterial inflow and venous outflow. MTT = CBV/CBF.

CBF/CBV mismatch correlates with stroke enlargement in untreated or unsuccessfully treated patients. Those patients with a CBF/CBV match or those with early complete recanalization do not exhibit progression of the ischemic stroke.

General treatment guidelines for CTP: If there is a CBF/CBV mismatch, with a larger CBF suggesting an ischemic penumbra, the patient is likely a good candidate for therapy. Many treatment guidelines suggest that a 20% or greater CBF/CBV mismatch should be present to consider thrombolysis. Some authors propose that if there is no mismatch between CBV and CBF, treatment is unlikely to benefit the patient.

CT Perfusion Interpretation Pearls

The MTT is the most sensitive parameter for perfusion deficits. Although it is generally elevated due to a thromboembolic process, it may be elevated in a patient with significant arterial atherosclerotic narrowing. In early ischemia, MTT is elevated and CBF is decreased. However, the CBV can be preserved or even elevated due to capillary bed dilatation in very early ischemia. Once a CBF threshold is reached, CBV starts to decline. This results in the ischemic core, which has a matched decrease in CBF and CBV, whereas a mismatch between CBF and CBV suggests a penumbra.

Differential Diagnosis

When considering stroke in a child or young adult, several possible etiologies should be addressed, including arterial dissection, vascular malformation with hemorrhage, drug abuse, or clotting disorder. In young children other possibilities include congenital heart disease with emboli and idiopathic progressive arteriopathy of childhood (moyamoya disease).

In a middle-aged or older adult, the typical stroke etiologies include arterial thromboembolism, hypertensive hemorrhage, and cerebral amyloid angiopathy.

When evaluating a hemorrhagic stroke, etiologies include vascular lesions, neoplasm, vasculitis, cerebral amyloid angiopathy, drug abuse, dural sinus/cerebral venous occlusion, and coagulopathy.

References

1. Kim JT et al: Early outcome of combined thrombolysis based on the mismatch on perfusion CT. Cerebrovasc Dis. 28(3):259-65, 2009
2. Konstas AA et al: Theoretic basis and technical implementations of CT perfusion in acute ischemic stroke, part 1: Theoretic basis. AJNR Am J Neuroradiol. 30(4):662-8, 2009

STROKE OVERVIEW

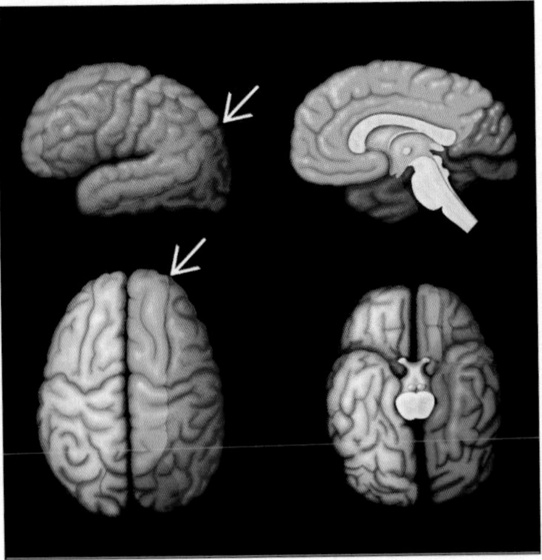

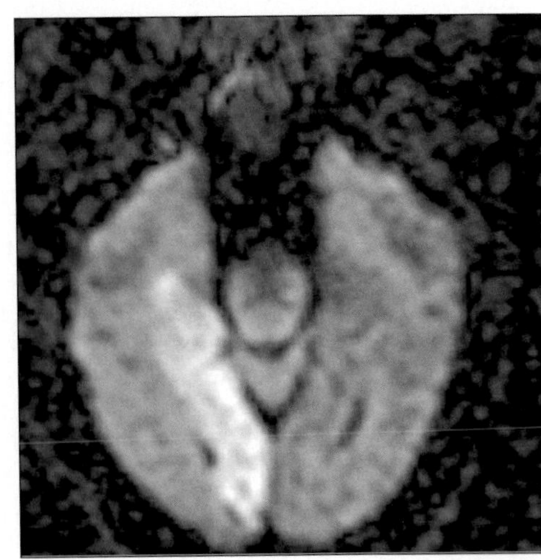

(Left) *Whole brain graphics show the major arterial supply to the hemispheres. The MCA (red) supplies the lateral aspects of the frontal and temporal lobes. The ACA (green) supplies the medial hemispheres. The PCA (purple) supplies the occipital lobes and inferior temporal lobes. The "watershed zone" ➔ is the border between the major vascular territories.* ***(Right)*** *Axial DWI MR shows restriction in the medial occipital and temporal lobes related to PCA ischemia. DWI is the most sensitive MR sequence for acute ischemia.*

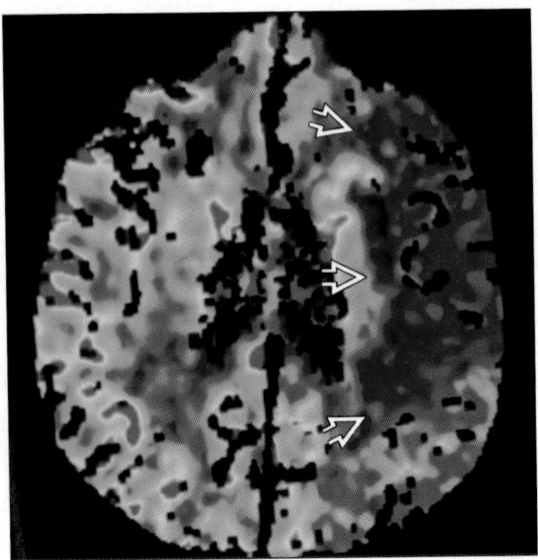

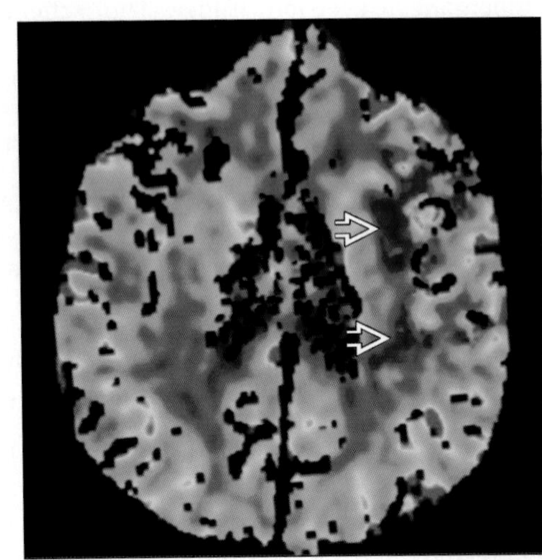

(Left) *Axial CT perfusion CBF color map shows a large area of decreased blood flow ➔ in the left hemisphere related to hyperacute MCA ischemia.* ***(Right)*** *Axial CT perfusion CBV color map in the same patient shows a much smaller area of decreased blood volume ➔. The CBV is a marker for the ischemic core. This CBF/CBV mismatch correlates with the presence of a large ischemic penumbra, which suggests the patient would benefit from thrombolytic therapy.*

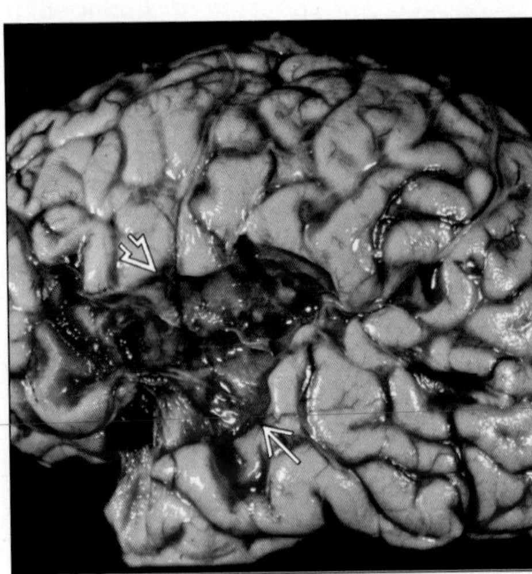

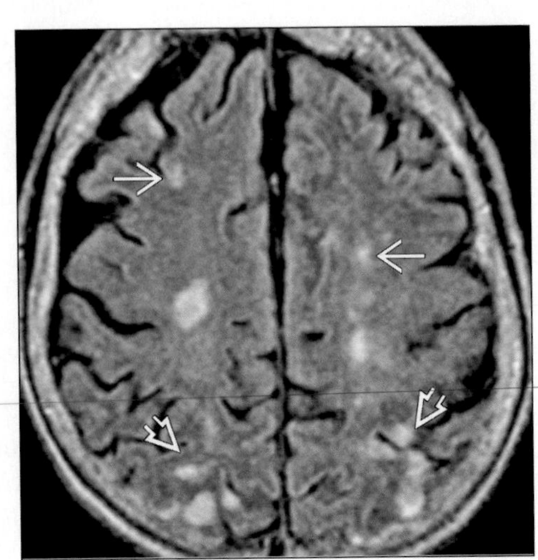

(Left) *Lateral gross pathology shows a chronic MCA infarct with hemorrhage and encephalomalacia in the frontal operculum ➔ and temporal lobe ➔.* ***(Right)*** *Axial FLAIR MR shows multiple hyperintense foci ➔ in the watershed zones between the major cerebral artery territories (MCA, PCA, and ACA) related to acute ischemia from hypoperfusion. The posterior confluence where all 3 vascular distributions meet together at the vertex ➔ is especially vulnerable to cerebral hypoperfusion.*

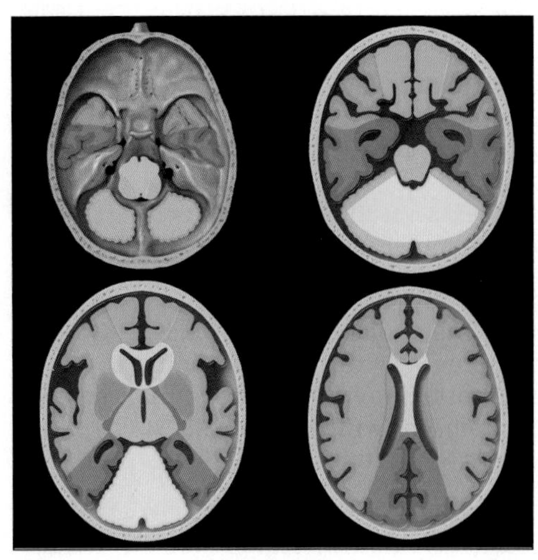

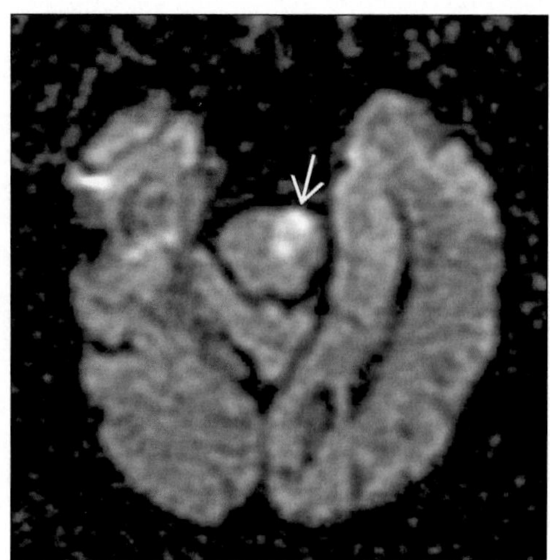

(Left) Axial graphic shows the major penetrating artery distributions. The pontine & thalamic perforating arteries (light purple) as well as the medullary perforators (aqua) arise from the vertebrobasilar system. The medial (light green) and lateral (blue) lenticulostriate arteries arise from the anterior circulation & supply the basal ganglia. The choroidal arteries are shown in magenta. ***(Right)*** Axial DWI MR shows restriction related to acute ischemia ➡ in a pontine-perforating artery distribution.

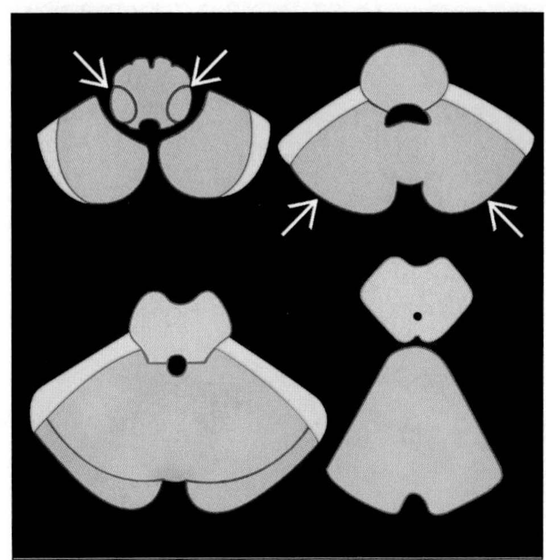

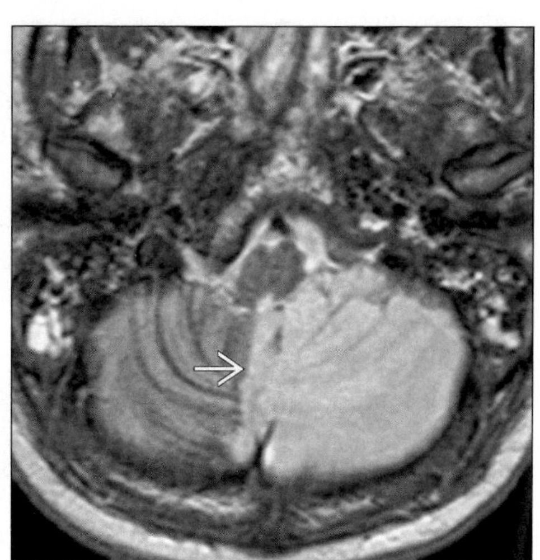

(Left) Axial graphic shows the cerebellar artery distributions. The superior cerebellar artery (SCA) (green) supplies the superior cerebellum. The posterior inferior cerebellar artery (PICA) (peach) ➡ supplies the majority of the inferior cerebellum and lateral medulla. The anterior inferior cerebellar artery (AICA) (yellow) supplies the petrosal surface of the cerebellum. ***(Right)*** Axial T2WI MR shows hyperintensity in the left inferior cerebellum ➡ related to an acute PICA infarct.

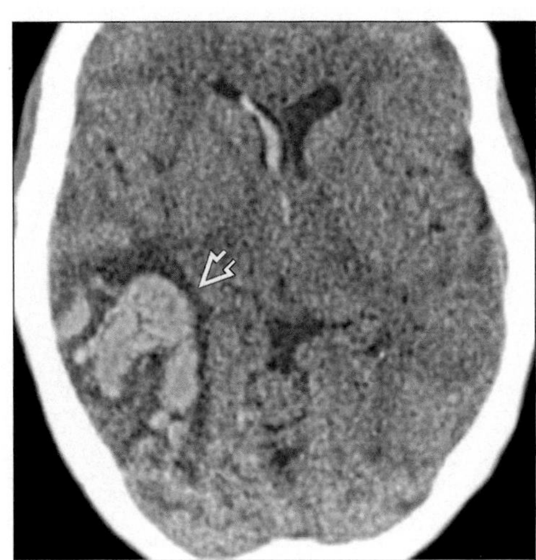

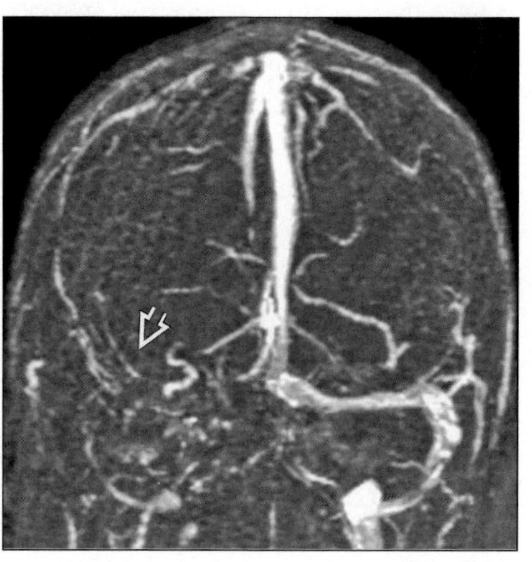

(Left) Axial NECT shows a posterior temporal hemorrhage ➡ in this young adult with headaches and venous infarct related to a transverse sinus occlusion. Differential considerations include trauma, drug abuse, & an underlying vascular or neoplastic mass. Note the associated intraventricular hemorrhage in the right frontal horn. ***(Right)*** Coronal MRV reformatted image shows lack of flow in the right transverse sinus ➡ related to occlusion. Only 50% of patients with sinus thrombosis progress to infarct.

EVOLUTION OF INTRACRANIAL HEMORRHAGE

Key Facts

Imaging

- Hyperdense (50-70 HU) mass on CT; peripheral edema develops over 1st days
- Hematoma matures more slowly in center (core) than in periphery (body)
- MR: Intracranial hemorrhage (ICH) staging based on T1 and T2 signal characteristics
  - MR as sensitive as CT in hyperacute phase and more sensitive in subacute and chronic phase

Pathology

- Very common: HTN, cerebral amyloid angiopathy, trauma, hemorrhagic vascular malformations

Clinical Issues

- Incidence: ~ 30-40 per 100,000
- HTN, ↑ age most important risk factors
- Prognosis depends on size, initial level of consciousness, and location
  - 35-52% dead at 1 month (50% of whom died in 1st 2 days); 59% dead at 1 year
- ICH with warfarin use correlates with higher mortality (2x as high at 3 months)
- Rate of anticoagulant-related ICH has increased over last decades (up to 20%)
- Large hematoma (> 30 mL) and swirl sign on NECT → higher mortality
- Active contrast extravasation and post-contrast enhancement → higher mortality

Diagnostic Checklist

- Marked heterogeneity of acute hematoma on CT predicts hematoma growth and ↑ mortality
- Swirl sign, contrast extravasation, and enhancement indicate hematoma growth and ↑ mortality
- Fluid-fluid levels → question of underlying coagulopathy

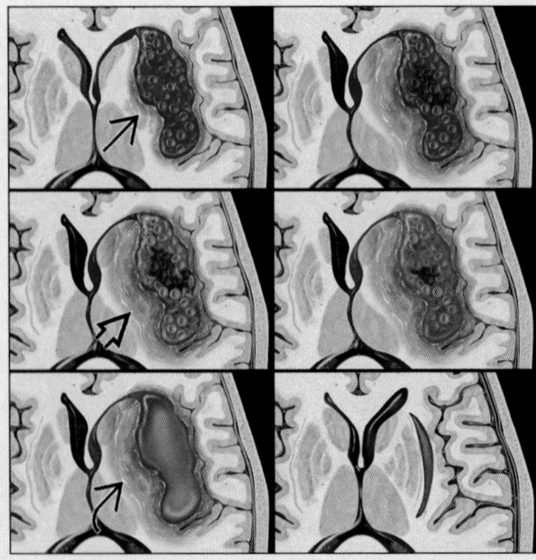

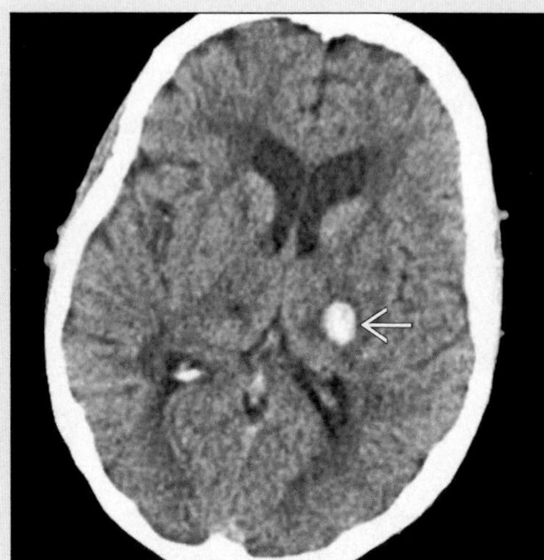

(Left) *Axial graphic shows the evolution of parenchymal hemorrhage from hyperacute ➔ (intracellular oxy-Hgb) to acute (intracellular deoxy-Hgb with surrounding edema). Early ➔ and late subacute (intra- and extracellular met-Hgb respectively) are followed by a chronic cystic cavity ➔ with a hemosiderin stain.* ***(Right)*** *Axial NECT shows an acute left thalamic hemorrhage ➔ with minimal surrounding edema in a patient with multiple cavernous malformations.*

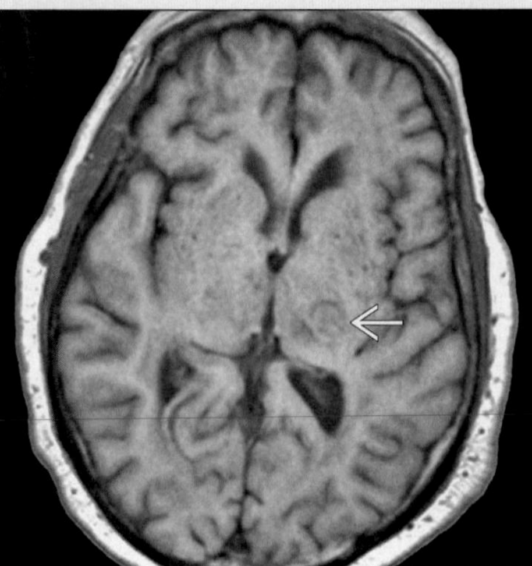

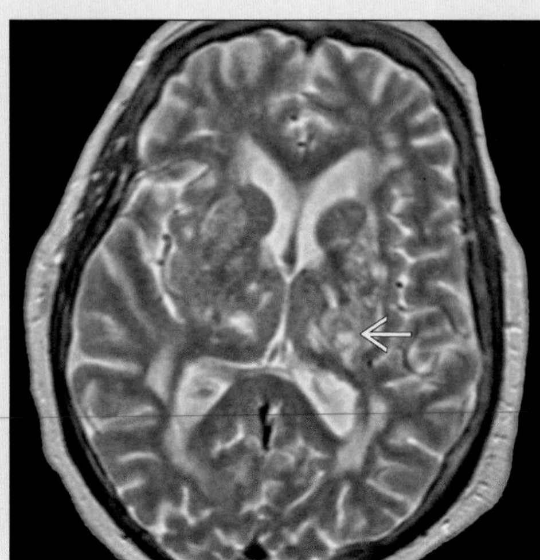

(Left) *Axial T1WI MR in the same patient shows that the thalamic hemorrhage ➔ is isointense to the adjacent brain, indicating hyperacute/acute hemorrhage.* ***(Right)*** *Axial T2WI MR in the same patient shows intermediate to high signal ➔ consistent with hyperacute/acute hemorrhage. No intraventricular extension or abnormal flow voids are seen to suggest an underlying vascular mass. Intracerebral hemorrhage evolves from peripheral to central, with the central core maturing more slowly.*

EVOLUTION OF INTRACRANIAL HEMORRHAGE

TERMINOLOGY

Abbreviations

- Intracerebral hematoma (ICH)

Synonyms

- Intraparenchymal hemorrhage

IMAGING

General Features

- Best diagnostic clue
  - Hyperdense (50-70 HU) mass on CT; peripheral edema develops over 1st few days
  - Hematoma matures more slowly in center (core) than in periphery (body)
  - MR: ICH staging based on T1 and T2 signal
  - MR as sensitive as CT in hyperacute phase and more sensitive in subacute and chronic phases
- Location
  - Supratentorial > infratentorial brain
- Size
  - Near microscopic to very large; solitary > multiple
- Morphology
  - Ovoid; larger hematomas have more irregular shape and heterogeneous attenuation

CT Findings

- NECT
  - Hyperacute and acute: Hyperdense mass (0-3 days)
    - Immediate: Heterogeneous with 40-60 HU
    - CT density increases to 60-80 HU over 1st few hours secondary to clot formation and retraction
    - Clot maturation can increase density to 80-100 HU in hematoma core
    - Isodense if Hgb < 8-10 (hemophilia, renal failure)
    - Fluid-fluid levels seen in larger hematomas, mostly with coagulopathies or anticoagulation
    - Edema and mass effect initially mild (< 3 hours)
    - Swirl sign: Extraaxial collection with hyperdense clot and smaller hypodense area in swirled configuration (active bleeding)
  - Subacute: 3-10 days
    - Progressive attenuation loss (↓ 1.5 HU/day)
      - Decrease in attenuation usually does not correspond to decrease in mass effect
    - Edema peaks at ~ 5 days
    - Isodense in 1-4 weeks, dependent on original size
  - Chronic: > 10 days
    - Residua: ↓ attenuation foci (37%), no visible residua (27%), slit-like lesions (25%), Ca++ (10%)
- CECT
  - Active bleeding: Contrast pooling; CTA "spot" sign
  - Subacute-chronic: Rim enhancement (3 days to 1 month)
  - Chronic: Enhancement disappears (2-6 months)

MR Findings

- T1WI
  - Hyperacute: Isointense to mildly hypointense
  - Acute: Isointense to mildly hypointense
  - Early subacute: ↑ signal periphery, isointense center
  - Late subacute/early chronic: Diffuse ↑ signal
  - Late chronic: Iso- to hypointense
- T2WI
  - Hyperacute: Hyperintense, may have subtle hypointense rim, hyperintense peripheral edema
  - Acute: Markedly hypointense, increased edema
  - Early subacute: ↓ hypointensity, ↑ edema
  - Late subacute/early chronic: Progressive central signal increase, peripheral hypointensity
  - Late chronic: Hypointense rim or cleft, no edema
- FLAIR
  - Same as on T2WI
- T2* GRE
  - Hyperacute: Typically hypointense margin; differentiates hemorrhage from other masses
    - Most sensitive technique for assessing acute ICH
  - Acute: Marked diffuse hypointensity
  - Early subacute: Hypointensity (> T2WI & FLAIR)
  - Late subacute/early chronic: Increasing low signal rim
  - Late chronic: Persistent marked hypointense nodule or cleft due to glial hemosiderin staining
- DWI
  - Signal on DWI strongly affected by underlying T2 signal (T2 "shine through" and T2 "black out")
  - ADC shows diffusion restriction in core during hyperacute, acute, and early subacute phase
  - Increased ADC in perihematoma edema
- T1WI C+
  - Peripheral enhancement can develop within a few days and persist for months
- MRA
  - May show underlying vascular malformation
- MRV
  - May show underlying venous sinus thrombosis
- SWI (susceptibility weighted imaging)
  - ↑ sensitivity for microscopic hemorrhage than GRE

Imaging Recommendations

- Best imaging tool
  - Initial diagnosis: NECT or MR
  - Staging/work-up: MR, MRA/MRV, or CTA/CTV
  - Angiography if no clear cause, or in young, normotensive, stable surgical candidates

DIFFERENTIAL DIAGNOSIS

Fat-Containing Lesions

- Dermoid, lipoma
- Mimics subacute ICH (↑ T1WI, ↑ T2WI)
- Chemical shift artifact, lack of edema, loss of intensity on fat-saturated images confirm diagnosis

Calcified Lesions

- Hypointense on T2WI and GRE, variable on T1WI

Proteinaceous Fluid Collections

- Mildly hyperintense on T1WI, hypointense on T2WI

PATHOLOGY

General Features

- Etiology

EVOLUTION OF INTRACRANIAL HEMORRHAGE

- Very common: HTN, cerebral amyloid angiopathy, trauma, hemorrhagic vascular malformations
- Common: Infarct with reperfusion, coagulopathy, blood dyscrasia, drug abuse, tumor (high-grade glioma, metastases)
- Less common: Dural sinus thrombosis, eclampsia, endocarditis with septic emboli, fungal infection (aspergillosis, mucormycosis), encephalitis

- Genetics
  - ICH can occur sporadically or with familial syndromes (familial cerebral amyloid angiopathy, familial cavernous malformations)
- Associated abnormalities
  - Vasogenic edema forms rapidly, peaks at ~ 5 days
  - May decompress into ventricles/subarachnoid space

Staging, Grading, & Classification

- No consistent definition of hematoma stages for MR
  - Hyperacute: < 6 to < 24 hours; acute: 6-24 hours to 2-3 days; early subacute: 2-7 days; late subacute: 4-7 to 7-14 days

Gross Pathologic & Surgical Features

- Acute to early subacute: Blood-filled cavity surrounded by vasogenic edema, inflammation
- Early subacute to early chronic: Organizing clot, vascularized wall
- Late chronic: Hemosiderin scar with gliosis

Microscopic Features

- Immediate
  - Water-rich liquid hematoma; 95-98% oxy-Hgb
- Hyperacute
  - RBCs contain diamagnetic oxy-Hgb
  - High water content (↑ T2 and ↓ T1)
  - Beginning peripheral vasogenic edema
- Acute
  - Deoxy-Hgb in intact RBCs
    - Paramagnetic deoxy-Hgb with 4 unpaired electrons in intact RBC causes field gradient across cell membrane → ↓ T2WI and GRE
    - Paramagnetic center of Hgb inaccessible to water molecules → no T1 shortening
  - Severe edema
- Early subacute
  - Deoxy-Hgb in intact RBCs oxidized to paramagnetic met-Hgb with 5 unpaired electrons
    - Susceptibility induced gradient across cell membrane → T2WI and GRE hypointensity
  - Met-Hgb formation begins at hematoma periphery → T1 hyperintensity initially seen at margin
- Late subacute-early chronic
  - RBC lysis → release met-Hgb into extracellular space → loss of gradient across RBC membrane
    - Loss of magnetic heterogeneity and increased water content → ↑ T2WI and FLAIR intensity
  - Persistent dipole diploe interaction → T1 shortening
  - Edema and mass effect decrease
- Chronic
  - Lysed RBCs and clot taken up by macrophages
  - Met-Hgb converted into ferritin and hemosiderin
  - Residual cysts and clefts with hemosiderin scar, which persists indefinitely in areas with intact blood-brain barrier
  - Edema, inflammation resolve

CLINICAL ISSUES

Presentation

- Most common signs/symptoms
  - HTN (90%), vomiting, (50%), ↓ consciousness (50%), headache (40%), seizures (10%)
- Clinical profile
  - HTN, ↑ age most important risk factors
  - Increasing incidence of anticoagulation-related ICH

Demographics

- Incidence
  - About 30/100,000 (USA); 37/100,000 (Europe)
- Age
  - Risk increases with age (mean 63 [USA], 70 [Europe])
- Gender
  - Men < 65 years have 3.4x higher risk; > 65 years: No significant gender difference
- Ethnicity
  - Higher risk of ICH for blacks (3.8x higher risk) and Hispanics (2.6x higher risk) compared with whites

Natural History & Prognosis

- 1 or more rebleeds occur in 1/4 of cases
  - Rebleed: Increased mortality
    - 70% died with 2nd or 3rd ICH
- Prognosis depends on size, initial level of consciousness, and location
  - 35-52% dead at 1 month (1/2 of whom died in 1st 2 days); 59% dead at 1 year
  - Higher mortality with posterior fossa and lobar hemorrhage than with deep hemorrhage
  - Ventricular extension: Higher mortality for lobar hemorrhage, but lower mortality for thalamic bleeds
  - ICH with warfarin use correlates with higher mortality (2x as high at 3 months)
- 20% independent at 6 months

Treatment

- Surgical evacuation as needed

DIAGNOSTIC CHECKLIST

Image Interpretation Pearls

- MR more sensitive, more accurate staging of ICH
- Large area of surrounding vasogenic edema more commonly seen with underlying neoplasm
- Marked heterogeneity of acute hematoma on CT predicts hematoma growth and mortality
- Fluid-fluid levels: Question of underlying coagulopathy

SELECTED REFERENCES

1. Silvera S et al: Spontaneous intracerebral hematoma on diffusion-weighted images: influence of T2-shine-through and T2-blackout effects. AJNR Am J Neuroradiol. 26(2):236-41, 2005
2. Parizel PM et al: Intracranial hemorrhage: principles of CT and MRI interpretation. Eur Radiol. 11(9):1770-83, 2001
3. Bradley WG Jr: MR appearance of hemorrhage in the brain. Radiology. 189(1):15-26, 1993

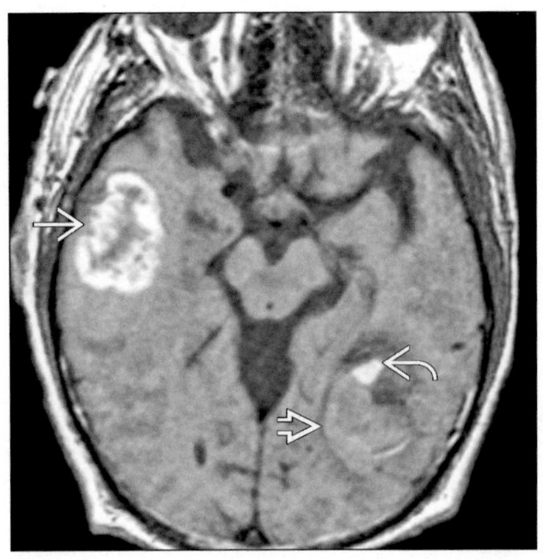

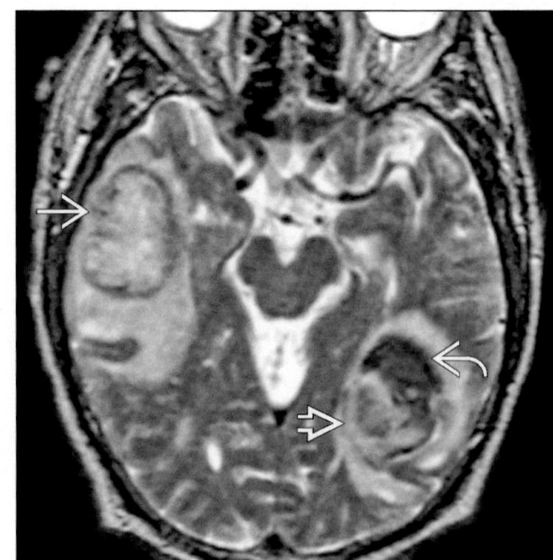

(Left) *Axial T1WI MR shows hemorrhages in an amyloid angiopathy patient. There is a hyperacute* ➯ *(isointense) and an acute/early subacute* ➦ *(hyperintense) left posterior hemorrhage, as well as a late subacute (hyperintense) right temporal hemorrhage* ➔. ***(Right)*** *Axial T2WI MR shows heterogeneous bright signal in the hyperacute* ➯ *portion and low signal in the acute/early subacute* ➦ *portion of the posterior hemorrhage. The late subacute* ➔ *hemorrhage has bright T1 and T2 signal intensity.*

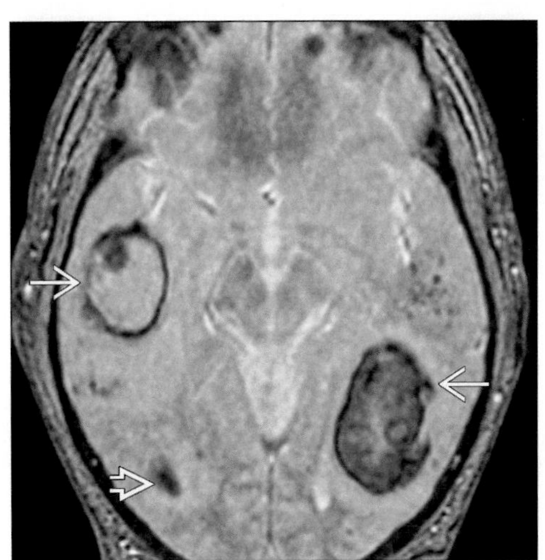

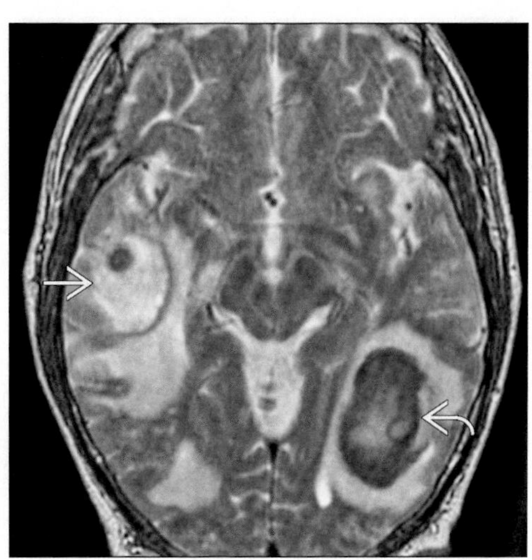

(Left) *Axial T2* GRE MR at 21 hours after the prior 2 images shows central signal of hemorrhages determined by T2 characteristics with peripheral blooming* ➔. *Due to a different slice plane, a 3rd lesion in the right occipital lobe is seen* ➯. ***(Right)*** *Axial T2WI MR 21 hours after initial imaging shows evolution of hemorrhage from hyperacute to the acute stage, with associated loss of T2 signal* ➦. *The right temporal late subacute hemorrhage* ➔ *shows no significant change and remains hyperintense.*

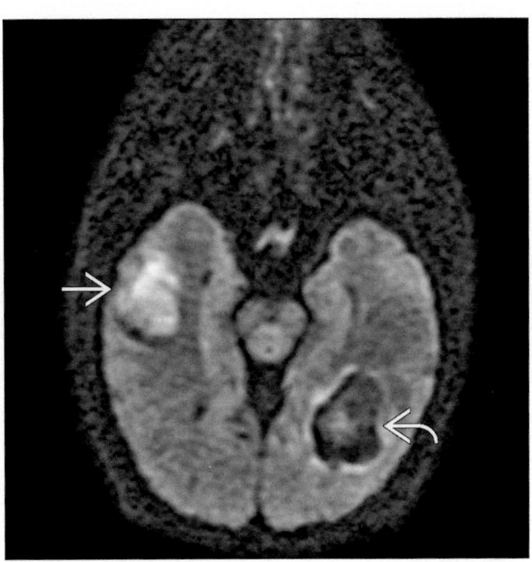

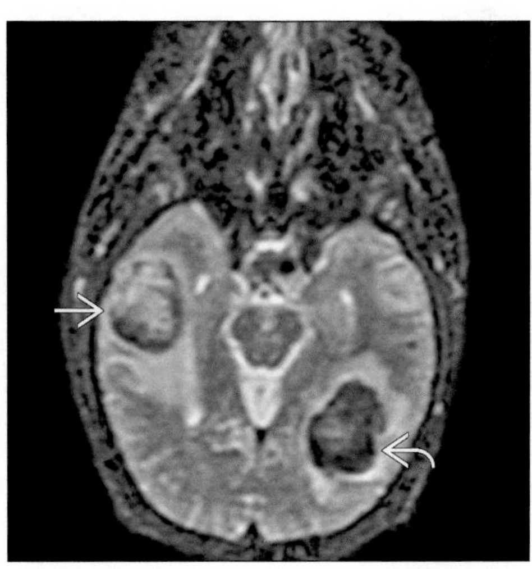

(Left) *Axial DWI MR 21 hours after initial imaging shows that the signal on DWI is mostly determined by underlying T2 effects with T2 "shine through"* ➔ *in the right subacute hemorrhage and T2 blackout* ➦ *in the acute/early subacute hemorrhage.* ***(Right)*** *Axial ADC shows that signal on DWI is mostly determined by underlying T2 effects. Only the acute/early subacute hemorrhage shows low signal on ADC* ➦, *while increased diffusivity is seen in the late subacute right temporal hemorrhage* ➔.

SPONTANEOUS NONTRAUMATIC INTRACRANIAL HEMORRHAGE

Key Facts

Terminology

- Primary intraparenchymal hemorrhage
- Acute nontraumatic intracranial hemorrhage (ICH)

Imaging

- Acute round or oval intracerebral hematoma
- Sub-centimeter "microbleeds" to massive
- Peripheral edema
- Hematoma location for common causes of pICH
  - HTN: Basal ganglia, thalamus, pons, cerebellum
  - Amyloid angiopathy: Lobar
  - Arteriovenous malformation: Any location
  - Cavernous malformation: Any location
  - Venous sinus thrombosis: Subcortical white matter
  - Neoplasm: Any location
- May have fluid-fluid level: Coagulopathy, brisk bleeding, underlying cystic mass
- Recommended imaging protocol
  - If HTN with striatocapsular hematoma → stop
  - Atypical hematoma or unclear history: MR (T2*, DWI, T1 C+)
  - If MR shows atypical hematoma → CTA or MRA
  - If standard study suggests vascular etiology → MRA
  - If venous infarction in DDx → MRV
  - Follow-up: Repeat MR if etiology unclear ± DSA if initial MRA/CTA negative

Pathology

- Patients < 45 years old: AVM, drug abuse, venous infarct, vasculitis
- Patients > 45 years old: HTN, amyloid, venous infarct, neoplasm, coagulopathy

Clinical Issues

- Causes 15-20% of acute strokes
- Control of ICP, hydrocephalus
- Surgical evacuation when clinically indicated

(Left) Axial gross pathology, sectioned through the middle of the cerebellum, shows an acute spontaneous intraparenchymal hemorrhage ⇒. Note the atherosclerosis in the basilar artery ⇒. No underlying lesion was identified in this patient with chronic hypertension. (Courtesy R. Hewlett, PhD.) (Right) Axial NECT shows a large hyperdense hemorrhage in the left external capsule and putamen ⇒ in this classic hypertensive bleed. Intraventricular extension of hemorrhage is present ⇒.

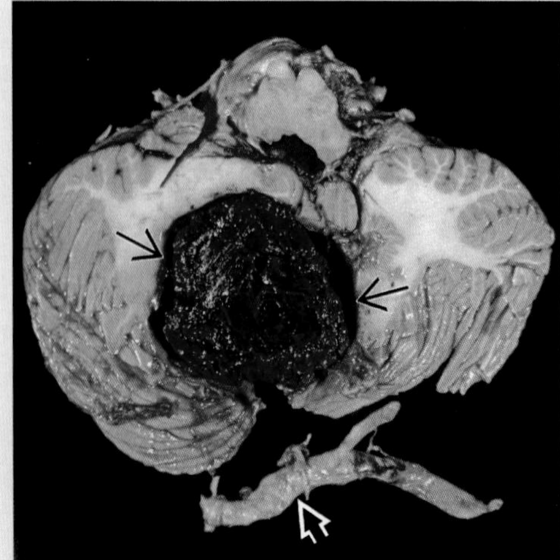

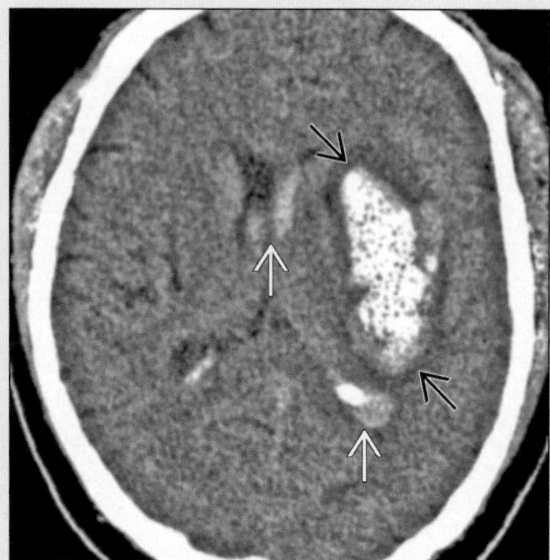

(Left) Axial NECT shows a hyperdense hemorrhage in the left midbrain ⇒. Extensive hypodensity and loss of gray-white differentiation in the posteromedial right temporal lobe and right occipital lobe are consistent with acute stroke. These findings were due to basilar tip thrombosis. (Right) Anteroposterior DSA from a left vertebral artery injection shows clot in the basilar tip ⇒. The clot extended into the right PCA and SCA, which are not opacified. Note the left PCA ⇒ and left SCA ⇒.

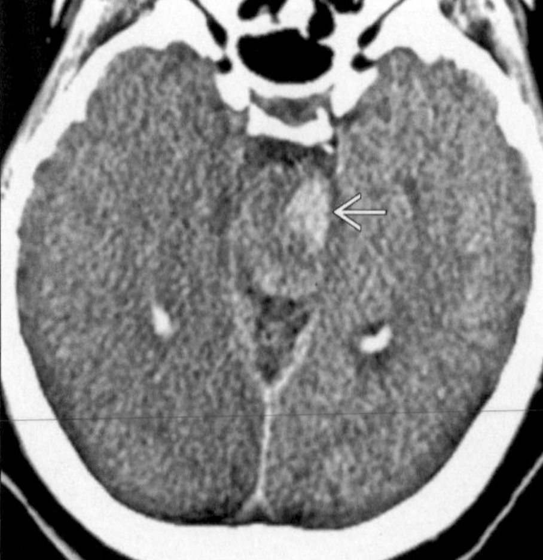

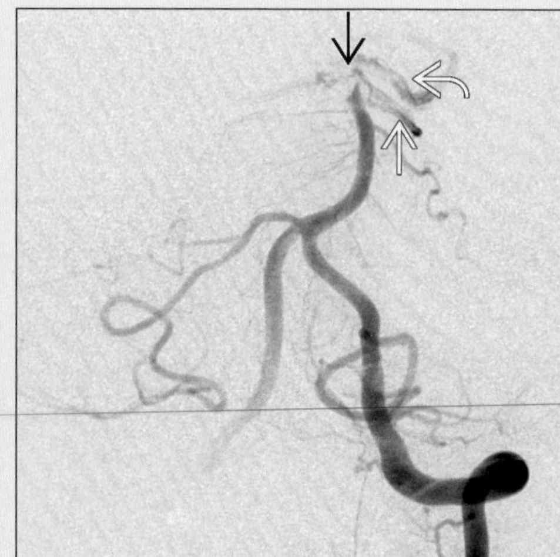

SPONTANEOUS NONTRAUMATIC INTRACRANIAL HEMORRHAGE

TERMINOLOGY

Synonyms

- Primary intraparenchymal hemorrhage (pICH), stroke

Definitions

- Acute nontraumatic intracranial hemorrhage (ICH)
  - Etiology often initially unknown

IMAGING

General Features

- Best diagnostic clue
  - Acute nontraumatic intracerebral hematoma
- Location
  - Varies with etiology
    - Hypertension (HTN): Deep gray matter (basal ganglia, thalamus), pons, cerebellar hemisphere
    - Amyloid angiopathy: Lobar
    - Arteriovenous malformation (AVM): Any location
    - Cavernous malformation: Any location, common in brainstem
    - Venous sinus thrombosis: Subcortical white matter adjacent to occluded sinus
    - Neoplasm: Any location
- Size
  - Sub-centimeter "microbleeds" to massive hemorrhage
- Morphology
  - Typically round or oval; often irregular when large
  - Patterns with HTN and amyloid angiopathy
    - Acute parenchymal hematoma
    - Multiple subacute/chronic "microbleeds" in deep gray matter (HTN > amyloid) &/or subcortical white matter (amyloid > HTN)
    - Microbleeds often seen only on GRE MR

CT Findings

- NECT
  - Acute hyperdense round/elliptical mass
  - May be mixed iso-/hyperdense
  - May have fluid-fluid level
    - Coagulopathy
    - Brisk bleeding
    - Bleed into cystic mass
  - Peripheral low density (edema)
  - Deep (ganglionic) ICH may rupture into lateral ventricle
- CTA
  - Often nonrevealing
  - ± underlying vascular malformation
  - Look for dural sinus venous thrombosis

MR Findings

- T1WI
  - Hyperacute (< 6 hours)
    - Isointense center (oxygenated Hgb)
    - Isointense periphery (deoxygenated Hgb, clot-tissue interface)
    - Hypointense rim (vasogenic edema)
- T2WI
  - Hyperacute (< 6 hours)
    - Iso-/hyperintense, heterogeneous center
    - Hypointense periphery
    - Hyperintense rim of edema
- T2* GRE
  - Hypointense
  - Multifocal hypointense lesions ("black dots")
    - Basal ganglionic suggests HTN
    - Subcortical WM suggests amyloid angiopathy
- DWI
  - T2 "shine through" common
- T1WI C+
  - May enhance if underlying neoplasm, vascular malformation
- MRA
  - Often normal
- MRV
  - Look for dural sinus thrombosis

Angiographic Findings

- DSA, often negative
  - Look for dural sinus occlusion, "stagnating vessels" (thrombosed AVM)

Imaging Recommendations

- Best imaging tool
  - Screening: NECT
    - If patient with HTN and striatocapsular hematoma → stop
  - Standard MR (include T2*, DWI)
    - If no clear cause of hemorrhage, or atypical appearance on CT
    - If T2* shows multifocal "black dots" → stop
    - T1WI C+ to assess for underlying tumor
    - If standard study suggests vascular etiology → MRA
  - Follow-up: Repeat MR if etiology unclear ± DSA if initial MRA/CTA negative
- Protocol advice
  - Atypical hematoma or unclear history: MR (with T2*, DWI, T1WI C+)
  - Add MRV if venous infarction in DDx

DIFFERENTIAL DIAGNOSIS

Hypertensive Intracranial Hemorrhage

- Patients usually older
- Basal ganglionic hematoma most common

Cerebral Amyloid Angiopathy

- Older patients (70 years old, normotensive)
- Usually lobar
- Microbleeds ("black dots") on T2*

Underlying Neoplasm

- Causes 2-15% of nontraumatic ICHs
- Primary (glioblastoma multiforme) or metastasis
- May show enhancement

Vascular Malformation

- AVM, cavernous malformation most common
- ICH rate in AVMs of basal ganglia or thalamus (9.8% per year) much higher than AVMs in other locations

Cortical Venous Thrombosis

- Adjacent dural sinus often thrombosed

SPONTANEOUS NONTRAUMATIC INTRACRANIAL HEMORRHAGE

Anticoagulation
- "Growing" hematoma, fluid-fluid levels common
- Check history

Drug Abuse
- May have hypertensive striatocapsular hemorrhage
- Uncommon = pseudoaneurysm rupture into cerebrum

Vasculitis
- Less common cause of spontaneous ICH
- Patients usually younger

Dural AVF (with Cortical Venous Drainage)
- Dilated venous "flow voids"

Ruptured Pseudoaneurysm
- Mycotic (endocarditis)
- Traumatic
- Vasculopathy

PATHOLOGY

General Features
- Etiology
  - Patients < 45 years old: Vascular malformation, drug abuse, venous thrombosis, vasculitis
  - Patients > 45 years old: HTN, amyloid, venous infarct, neoplasm (primary or metastatic), coagulopathy
- Genetics
  - MMP-9, cytokine gene expression ↑ after acute spontaneous ICH

Staging, Grading, & Classification
- Clinical "ICH score" correlates with 30-day mortality
  - Admission GCS
  - > 80 years old, ICH volume
  - Infratentorial
  - Presence of intraventricular hemorrhage

Gross Pathologic & Surgical Features
- Findings range from petechial "microbleeds" to gross parenchymal hematoma

Microscopic Features
- Coexisting microangiopathy common in amyloid, HTN

CLINICAL ISSUES

Presentation
- Most common signs/symptoms
  - 90% of patients with recurrent pICH are hypertensive
  - Large ICHs present with sensorimotor deficits, impaired consciousness

Demographics
- Age
  - Perinatal through elderly
- Epidemiology
  - Causes 15-20% of acute strokes

Natural History & Prognosis
- Prognosis related to location, size of ICH
- Hematoma enlargement common in 1st 24-48 hours
  - Risk factors: EtOH, low fibrinogen, coagulopathy, irregularly shaped hematoma
- Edema associated with poor outcome
- Mortality: 30-55% in 1st month
- 30% rebleed within 1 year
- Most survivors have significant deficits

Treatment
- Control of ICP, hydrocephalus
- Surgical evacuation when clinically indicated

DIAGNOSTIC CHECKLIST

Consider
- Consider underlying etiology for hemorrhage (AVM, amyloid, neoplasm, drug use, etc.)

Image Interpretation Pearls
- Unexplained ICH → search for microbleeds on T2* MR
- Fluid-fluid level, iso-/mildly hyperdense clot may indicate coagulopathy

SELECTED REFERENCES

1. Hanley DF: Intraventricular hemorrhage: severity factor and treatment target in spontaneous intracerebral hemorrhage. Stroke. 40(4):1533-8, 2009
2. Jeffree RL et al: Warfarin related intracranial haemorrhage: a case-controlled study of anticoagulation monitoring prior to spontaneous subdural or intracerebral haemorrhage. J Clin Neurosci. 16(7):882-5, 2009
3. Kumar R et al: Spontaneous intracranial hemorrhage in children. Pediatr Neurosurg. 45(1):37-45, 2009
4. Tejero MA et al: [Multiple spontaneous cerebral haemorrhages. Description of a series and review of the literature.] Rev Neurol. 48(7):346-8, 2009
5. Walsh M et al: Developmental venous anomaly with symptomatic thrombosis of the draining vein. J Neurosurg. 109(6):1119-22, 2008
6. Harden SP et al: Cranial CT of the unconscious adult patient. Clin Radiol. 62(5):404-15, 2007
7. Chao CP et al: Cerebral amyloid angiopathy: CT and MR imaging findings. Radiographics. 26(5):1517-31, 2006
8. Finelli PF: A diagnostic approach to multiple simultaneous intracerebral hemorrhages. Neurocrit Care. 4(3):267-71, 2006
9. Leach JL et al: Imaging of cerebral venous thrombosis: current techniques, spectrum of findings, and diagnostic pitfalls. Radiographics. 26 Suppl 1:S19-41; discussion S42-3, 2006
10. Thanvi B et al: Sporadic cerebral amyloid angiopathy--an important cause of cerebral haemorrhage in older people. Age Ageing. 35(6):565-71, 2006
11. Chalela JA et al: Multiple cerebral microbleeds: MRI marker of a diffuse hemorrhage-prone state. J Neuroimaging. 14(1):54-7, 2004
12. Skidmore CT et al: Spontaneous intracerebral hemorrhage: epidemiology, pathophysiology, and medical management. Neurosurg Clin N Am. 13(3):281-8, v, 2002
13. Qureshi AI et al: Spontaneous intracerebral hemorrhage. N Engl J Med. 344(19):1450-60, 2001

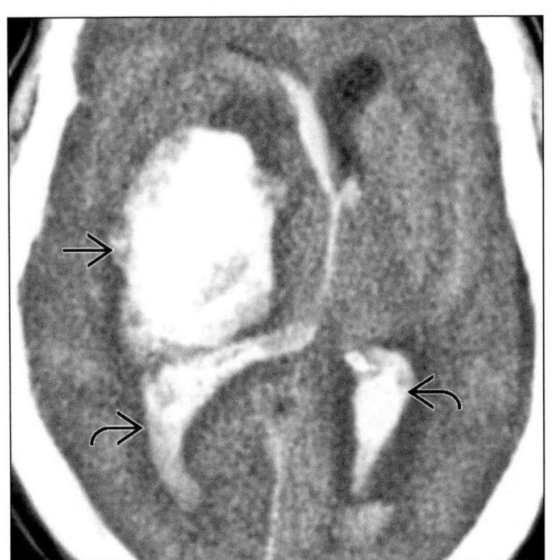

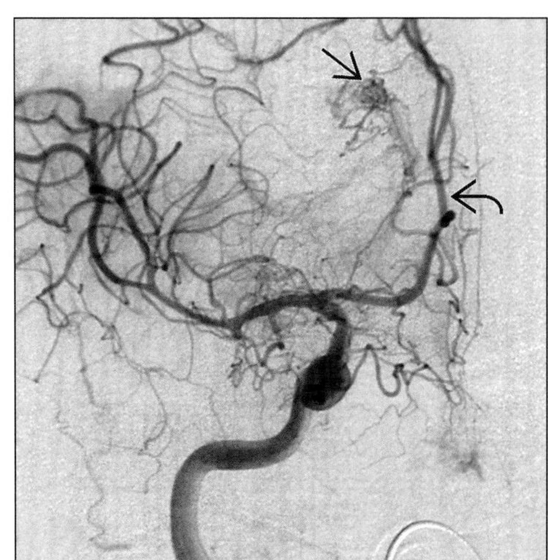

*(**Left**) Axial NECT of what appears to be a classic hypertensive striatocapsular hemorrhage → with intraventricular extension ↪. However, in this young patient underlying etiologies must be considered. (**Right**) Anteroposterior DSA from a right internal carotid artery injection shows an avascular mass in the basal ganglia (hematoma) with midline shift of the anterior cerebral artery ↪. There is a cluster of abnormal arteries (AVM) → fed by a large, medially displaced anterior choroidal artery.*

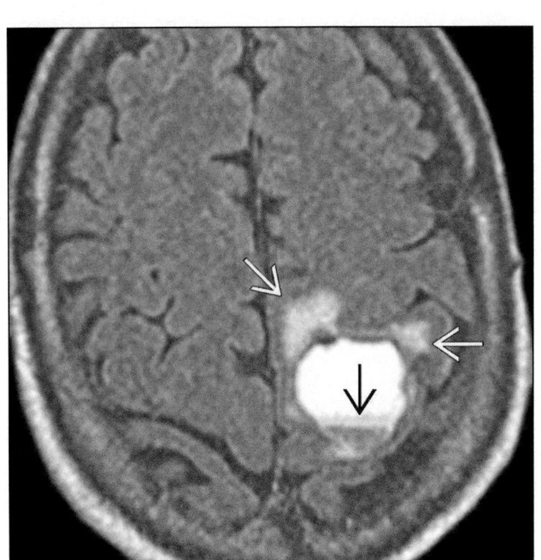

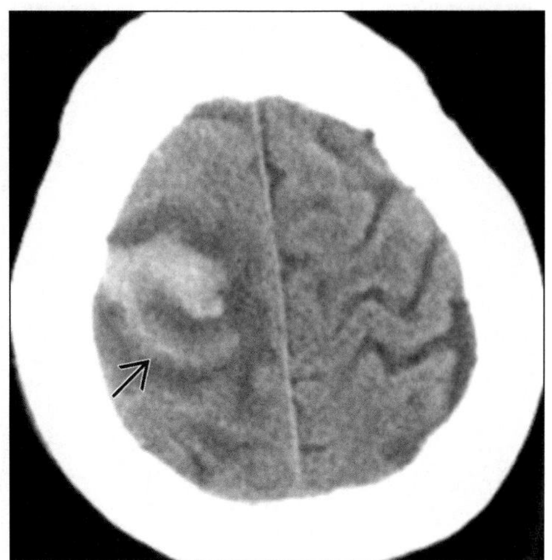

*(**Left**) Axial FLAIR MR shows an oval, demarcated mass in the left parietal lobe. Note the fluid-hemorrhage level → and surrounding white matter vasogenic edema ➔. This was metastatic melanoma. (**Right**) Axial NECT shows a right frontal lobar hematoma in this 74-year-old patient with amyloid angiopathy. There is associated subarachnoid hemorrhage → and mass effect with sulcal effacement. MR GRE (not shown) revealed numerous "black dots," consistent with old micro-hemorrhages.*

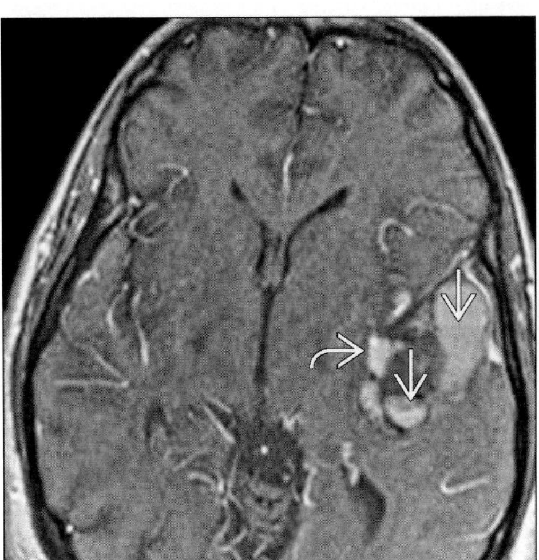

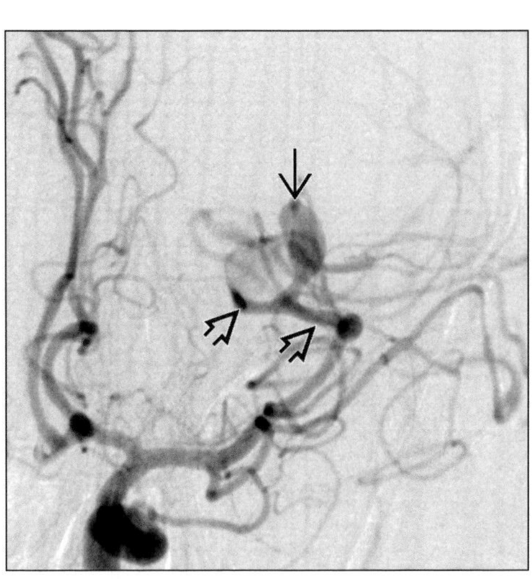

*(**Left**) Axial T1WI C+ MR shows lobular cerebral hematoma in the left temporal lobe. Note fluid-fluid levels ➔ in the hematoma from brisk bleeding. The more avidly enhancing region in sulcus represented pseudoaneurysm ↪. (**Right**) Anteroposterior DSA of selective left internal carotid injection shows fusiform mycotic aneurysm → arising from a distal left middle cerebral artery branch. Note the mass effect on middle cerebral artery branches from the associated cerebral hematoma ⇨.*

HYPERTENSIVE INTRACRANIAL HEMORRHAGE

Key Facts

Terminology
- Hypertensive intracranial hemorrhage (hICH)
- Acute nontraumatic ICH 2° to systemic hypertension
- 2nd most common cause of stroke

Imaging
- Initial screen = NECT in patients with HTN
- CT: Acute round or oval hyperdense mass
  - Striatocapsular: Putamen/external capsule (60-65%)
  - Thalamus (15-25%)
  - Pons, cerebellum (10%)
- Multifocal "microbleeds" (1-5%)
- Heterogeneous density if coagulopathy or active bleeding
- Other findings
  - Intraventricular extension
  - Mass effect: Hydrocephalus, herniation
- MR signal intensity (varies with age of clot)
  - Hyperacute (< 6 hrs): T1WI iso-hypo/T2WI hyper
  - Acute (7 hrs-3 days): T1WI iso-hyper/T2WI hypo
  - Subacute (days): T1WI hyper/T2WI hypo-hyper
  - Chronic (weeks-months): T1WI hyper/T2WI hypo

Top Differential Diagnoses
- Vascular malformation
- Drug abuse (especially in young patient)
- Deep cerebral venous thrombosis
- Hemorrhagic neoplasm
- Amyloid angiopathy (multiple microbleeds)

Clinical Issues
- 10-20% of stroke patients have hICH
- 50% of nontraumatic ICHs caused by hICH
- HTN most common cause of spontaneous ICH in patients 45-70 years old

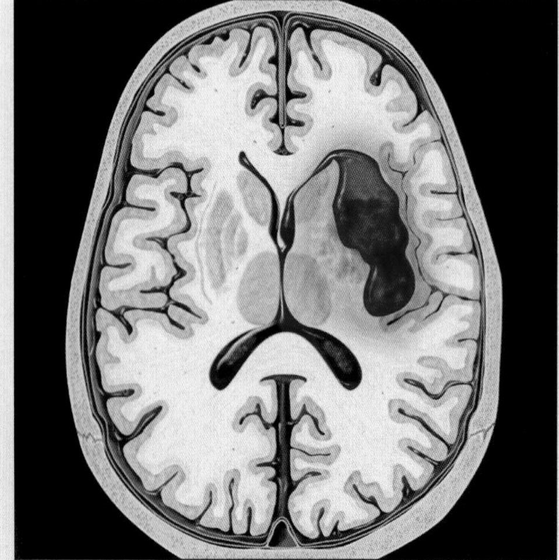

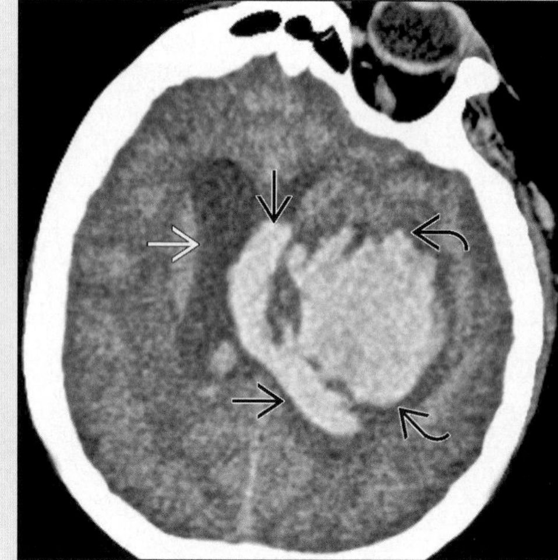

(Left) *Axial graphic shows acute hypertensive basal ganglionic/external capsule hemorrhage with dissection into the lateral ventricle. Hemorrhage extends through the foramen of Monro to the 3rd ventricle.* ***(Right)*** *Axial NECT shows a massive hypertensive hemorrhage in the left basal ganglia ↶. Secondary findings include intraventricular extension →, mass effect including compression of the left lateral ventricle, left-to-right midline shift, and dilatation of the right lateral ventricle →.*

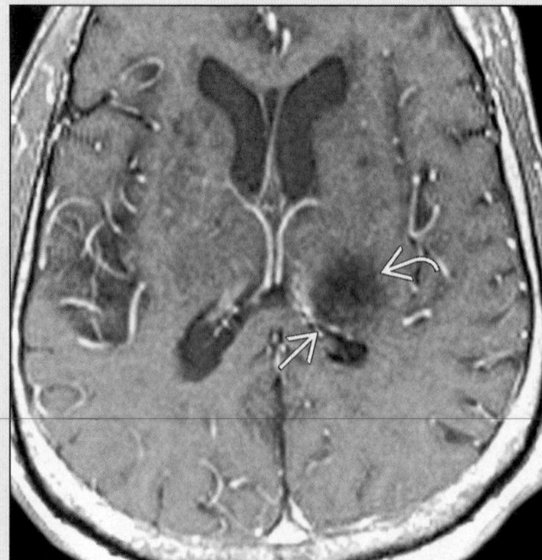

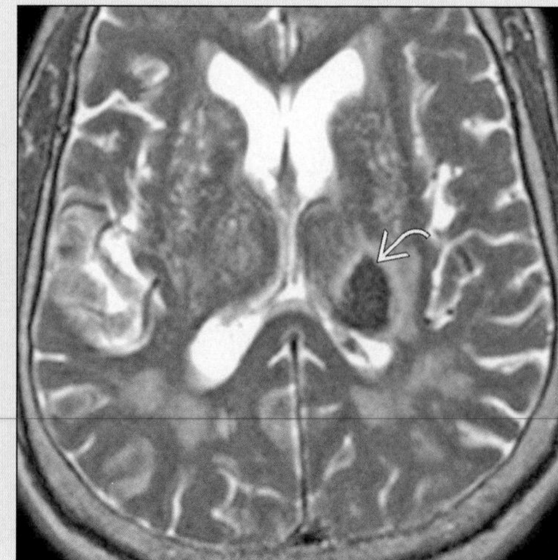

(Left) *Axial T1WI C+ MR in a patient with acute hypertensive hemorrhage shows a slightly hypointense mass in the left thalamus ↶. There is no enhancement and mild mass effect upon the left lateral ventricle →.* ***(Right)*** *Axial T2WI MR shows hypointensity in the left thalamic acute hematoma ↶. Note the numerous foci of T2 hyperintensity in the bilateral basal ganglia, thalami, and deep white matter consistent with sequela of microvasculopathy in this patient with longstanding systemic hypertension.*

HYPERTENSIVE INTRACRANIAL HEMORRHAGE

TERMINOLOGY

Abbreviations

- Hypertensive intracranial hemorrhage (hICH)

Synonyms

- Stroke

Definitions

- Acute nontraumatic ICH secondary to systemic hypertension (HTN)

IMAGING

General Features

- Best diagnostic clue
  - Round or oval hyperdense mass in putamen/external capsule or thalamus in patients with hypertension
- Location
  - Striatocapsular: Putamen/external capsule (60-65%)
  - Thalamus (15-25%)
  - Pons, cerebellum (10%)
  - Lobar (5-10%)
- Size
  - Sub-centimeter ("microbleeds") to several centimeters
- Morphology
  - Typically rounded or oval-shaped
  - 2 distinct patterns seen with hICH
    - Acute focal hematoma
    - Multiple subacute/chronic "microbleeds" (1-5%)

CT Findings

- NECT
  - Round or oval hyperdense parenchymal mass
  - Heterogeneous density if coagulopathy or active bleeding
  - Other: Intraventricular extension
    - Mass effect: Hydrocephalus, herniation
- CECT
  - No enhancement in acute hICH
- CTA
  - Avascular mass effect in acute hICH

MR Findings

- T1WI
  - Varies with age of clot
    - Hyperacute hematoma (< 6 hours)
      - Oxyhemoglobin (Hgb) (iso-/hypointense)
    - Acute hematoma (7 hours to 3 days)
      - DeoxyHgb (iso-/hyperintense)
    - Subacute hematoma (several days)
      - Intracellular metHgb (hyperintense)
    - Chronic hematoma (week to months)
      - Extracellular metHgb (hyperintense)
- T2WI
  - Appearance of hematoma varies with stage
    - Hyperacute hematoma (< 6 hours)
      - OxyHgb (hyperintense)
    - Acute hematoma (7 hours to 3 days)
      - DeoxyHgb (hypointense)
    - Subacute hematoma (3-7 days)
      - Intracellular metHgb (hypointense)
    - Late subacute hematoma (7 days to 3 weeks)
      - Extracellular metHgb (hyperintense)
    - Chronic hematoma (> 3 weeks to months)
      - Hemosiderin (hypointense)
    - Remote hematoma (months to years)
      - Hypointense hemosiderin scar ± central hyperintense cavity
  - "White matter hyperintensities" are hICH risk markers
- T2* GRE
  - Multifocal hypointense lesions ("black dots") on T2*
  - Common with longstanding HTN
  - Also commonly seen with amyloid angiopathy
- DWI
  - Hypo- or mixed hypo-/hyperintense (early hematoma)
- T1WI C+
  - Typically no enhancement with acute hematoma
  - Contrast extravasation = active hemorrhage
- MRA
  - Negative

Angiographic Findings

- Conventional
  - DSA usually normal if history of HTN + deep ganglionic hemorrhage
    - May show avascular mass effect
    - Rare: "Bleeding globe" microaneurysm on lenticulostriate artery (LSA)
  - Coexisting vascular abnormalities
    - Increased prevalence of unruptured intracranial aneurysms
    - More common in females

Imaging Recommendations

- Best imaging tool
  - If older patient with HTN and suspected hICH, NECT
  - If hyperacute ischemic "stroke" suspected, MR + T2* and DWI
  - If MR shows classic hematoma + coexisting multifocal "black dots," stop
  - If MR shows atypical hematoma, MRA or CTA
  - If MRA or CTA inconclusive, consider DSA

DIFFERENTIAL DIAGNOSIS

Cerebral Amyloid Angiopathy

- Lobar > > basal ganglionic
- Usually elderly, often normotensive
- Only 5-10% of hICHs are lobar, but HTN is so common that it is always consideration

Vascular Malformation

- Patients usually normotensive, younger
- Most common = cavernous malformation
  - Look for "black dots" (multiple lesions) on T2* (GRE, SWI) scans
- Less common = thrombosed hemorrhagic AVM or dAVF

Drug Abuse

- Cocaine may cause sudden ↑ ↑ HTN

HYPERTENSIVE INTRACRANIAL HEMORRHAGE

- Be suspicious if unexplained basal ganglionic bleed in young patient

Coagulopathy
- Elderly patients on anticoagulant therapy

Venous Thrombosis
- May have history of dehydration, "flu," pregnancy/ birth control pills
- Cause lobar hematomas
- Look for hyperdense dural sinus (not always present)

Deep Cerebral Venous Thrombosis
- Less common than dural sinus or cortical vein thrombosis
- Look for hypodense bilateral thalami
- Look for hyperdense internal cerebral veins, intraventricular hemorrhage

Hemorrhagic Neoplasm
- Secondary (metastasis) and primary (GBM)

PATHOLOGY

General Features
- Etiology
  - Chronic HTN with atherosclerosis, fibrinoid necrosis, abrupt wall rupture ± pseudoaneurysm formation
  - "Bleeding globe" (penetrating LSA aneurysm)
  - Diffuse "microbleeds" common
  - Striatocapsular hematoma most common autopsy finding

Gross Pathologic & Surgical Features
- Large ganglionic hematoma ± IVH
- Subfalcine herniation, hydrocephalus (common)
- Coexisting small chronic hemorrhages, ischemic lesions (common)

Microscopic Features
- Fibrous balls (fibrosed miliary aneurysm)
- Severe arteriosclerosis with hyalinization, pseudoaneurysm (lacks media/IEL)

CLINICAL ISSUES

Presentation
- Most common signs/symptoms
  - 10-20% of stroke patients have hICH
  - Large ICHs present with sensorimotor deficits, impaired consciousness
- Clinical profile
  - Major risk factor = HTN (increases risk of ICH 4x)

Demographics
- Age
  - Elderly
- Gender
  - Males
- Ethnicity
  - Higher incidence in African-Americans
- Epidemiology
  - 50% of primary nontraumatic ICHs caused by hypertensive hemorrhage
  - HTN most common cause of spontaneous ICH in patients 45-70 years
  - 10-15% of all stroke cases; associated with highest mortality rate
  - 10-15% of hypertensive patients with spontaneous ICH have underlying aneurysm or AVM

Natural History & Prognosis
- Bleeding can persist for up to 6 hours following ictus
- Neurologic deterioration common within 48 hours
  - Increasing hematoma, edema
  - Hydrocephalus
  - Herniation syndromes
- Recurrent hICH in 5-10% of cases, usually different location
- Prognosis related to location, size of hICH
- 80% mortality in massive hICH with IVH
- 1/3 of survivors are severely disabled

Treatment
- Control of ICP and hydrocephalus

DIAGNOSTIC CHECKLIST

Consider
- Does patient have history of poorly controlled systemic HTN?
- Could there be underlying coagulopathy, hemorrhagic neoplasm, or vascular malformation?
- Consider substance abuse in young patients with unexplained hICH

Image Interpretation Pearls
- Underlying cause of lobar intracerebral hemorrhage (ICH) is often difficult to determine
- Subarachnoid extension of hematoma on CT is usually indicative of nonhypertensive etiology; consider lobar ICH caused by vascular abnormality

SELECTED REFERENCES

1. Bogucki J et al: A new CT-based classification of spontaneous supratentorial intracerebral haematomas. Neurol Neurochir Pol. 43(3):236-44, 2009
2. Waran V et al: A new expandable cannula system for endoscopic evacuation of intraparenchymal hemorrhages. J Neurosurg. Epub ahead of print, 2009
3. Narotam PK et al: Management of hypertensive emergencies in acute brain disease: evaluation of the treatment effects of intravenous nicardipine on cerebral oxygenation. J Neurosurg. 109(6):1065-74, 2008
4. Lee GY et al: Hypertensive intracerebral hematoma after aneurysmal subarachnoid hemorrhage. J Clin Neurosci. 14(12):1233-5, 2007
5. Shah QA et al: Acute hypertension in intracerebral hemorrhage: pathophysiology and treatment. J Neurol Sci. 261(1-2):74-9, 2007
6. Hiroki M et al: Link between linear hyperintensity objects in cerebral white matter and hypertensive intracerebral hemorrhage. Cerebrovasc Dis. 18(2):166-73, 2004

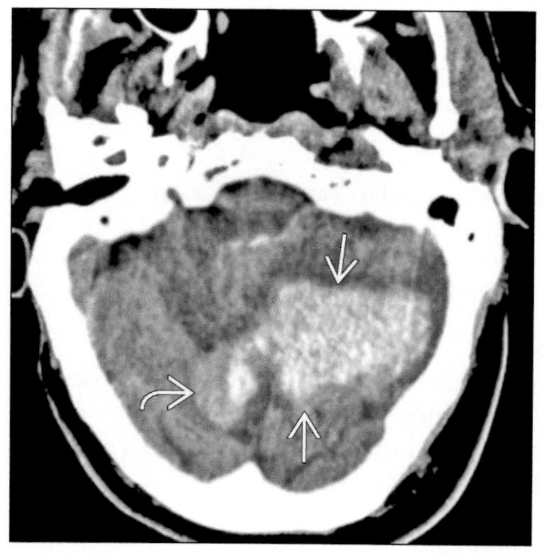

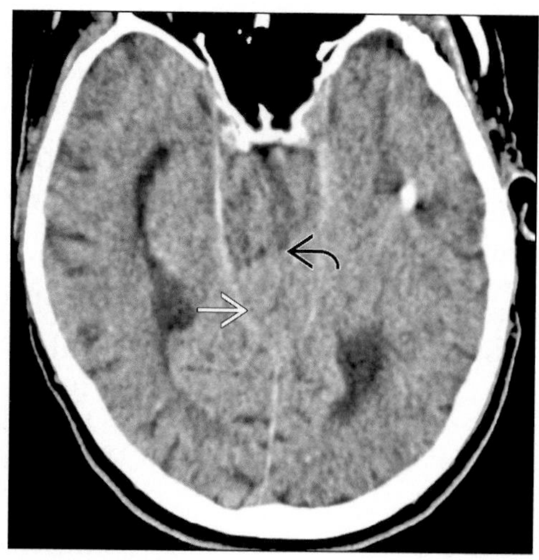

(Left) *Axial NECT shows a large hyperdense acute bleed in the left cerebellum ➡. Adjacent areas of slightly lesser increased attenuation ➡ reflect active bleeding. Note the compression of the 4th ventricle.* ***(Right)*** *Axial NECT in the same patient shows ascending herniation of the cerebellum ➡ through the tentorial incisura with brainstem compression ➡. Note the ventricular dilatation. Though less common, hypertensive bleeds in the posterior fossa are frequently devastating.*

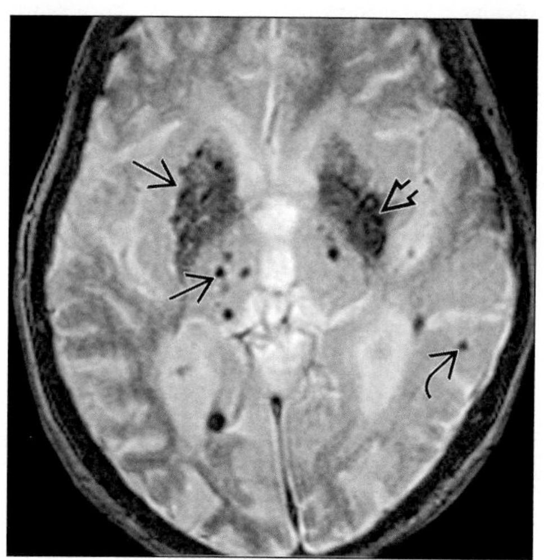

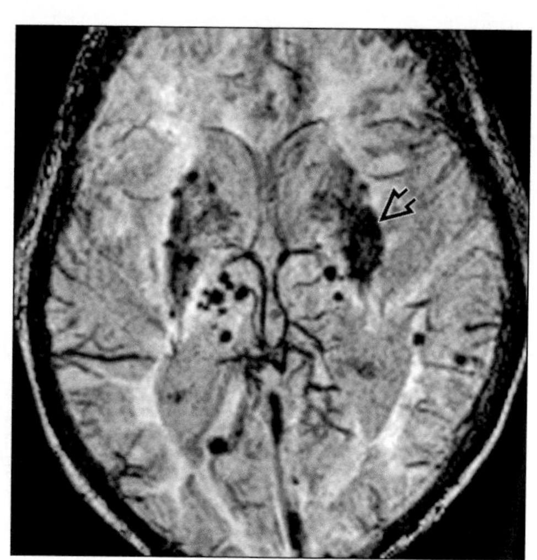

(Left) *Axial T2* GRE MR in a patient with a remote history of hypertensive hemorrhage in the left putamen & external capsule ➡ shows multifocal "black dots" in the basal ganglia & thalami ➡ with only a few lesions in the cortex ➡.* ***(Right)*** *MIP SWI in the same case shows the old hypertensive hemorrhage ➡. The multiple "black dots" (microbleeds) are even more apparent on this sequence than on the standard T2* GRE. Very few of the microhemorrhages were identified on T2WI (not shown).*

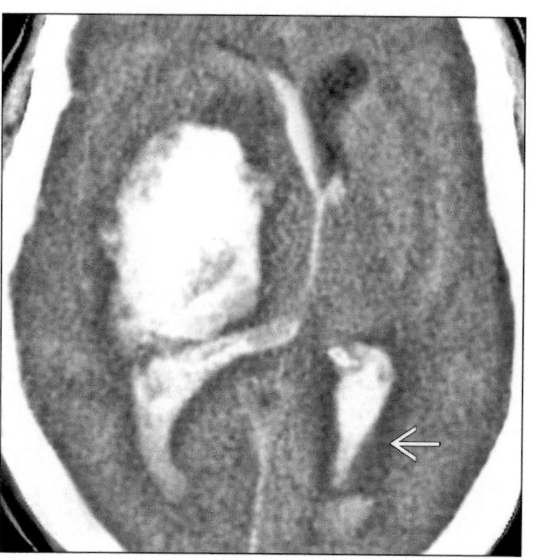

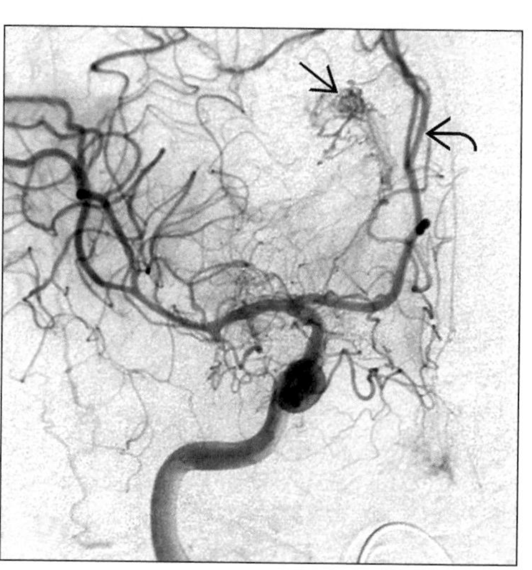

(Left) *Axial NECT shows a spontaneous basal ganglia hemorrhage with intraventricular extension, midline shift, dilatation of the left lateral ventricle, and transependymal flow of CSF ➡. In a young or middle-aged patient, etiologies other than HTN must be considered.* ***(Right)*** *Anteroposterior angiography (DSA) shows an avascular mass in the basal ganglia with a "round" midline shift of the anterior cerebral artery ➡. There is an AVM ➡ fed by an enlarged anterior choroidal artery.*

Key Facts

Terminology
- Remote cerebellar hemorrhage (RCH)
  - Following supratentorial craniotomy
  - Less often after spinal surgery
  - Remote to primary surgical site
  - No underlying pathologic lesion

Imaging
- General features
  - "Zebra" sign (blood layered over cerebellar folia)
  - Location varies (in/over hemisphere, vermis)
  - Subarachnoid vs. superficial parenchymal bleed
  - Contralateral to side of surgery (29%)
  - Ipsilateral (22%)
  - Bilateral (33%)
  - Isolated vermian (9%)
- Imaging recommendations
  - NECT initial screen
  - MR without/with contrast, MRA
  - Include T2* (GRE ± SWI)

Top Differential Diagnoses
- Hypertensive hemorrhage
- Coagulopathy-related spontaneous hemorrhage

Pathology
- CSF drainage → cerebellar "sagging" → vein stretching, bleeding
- RCH usually seen in immediate postoperative period
- Most occur within hours to 1 day postoperatively

Clinical Issues
- True incidence unknown (estimated at 0.3-4% of supratentorial craniotomies)
- Occasionally asymptomatic, occult (not imaged)
- Death/disability in ~ 50% of cases

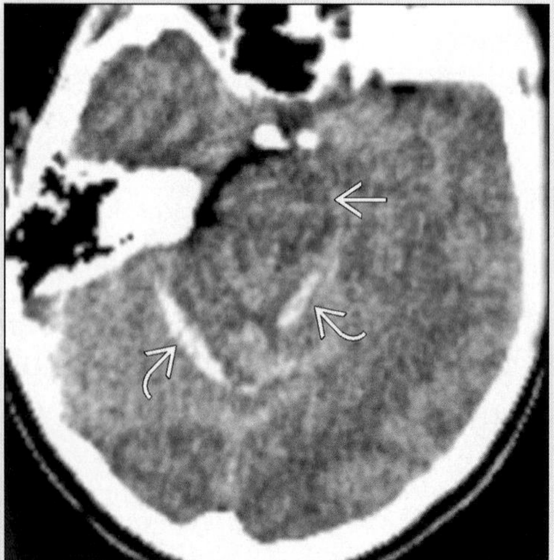
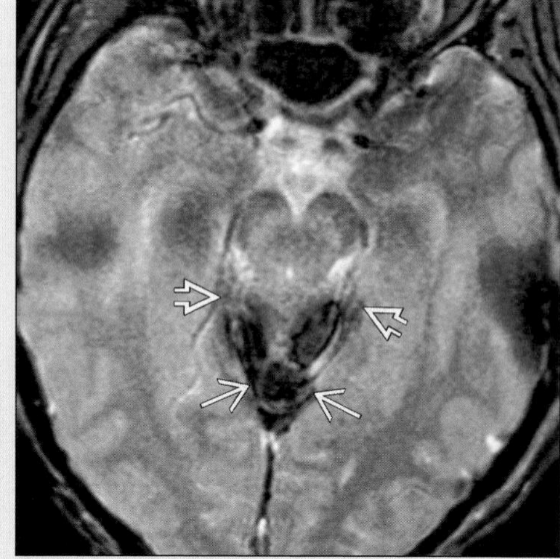

(Left) *Axial NECT in a patient doing poorly immediately after surgery to resect a meningioma shows linear hemorrhages ("zebra" sign) bilaterally along the vermis ➡. This is a common pattern seen in remote cerebellar hemorrhage (RCH). Cisternal effacement is also present ➡.* ***(Right)*** *Axial T2* GRE MR in the same patient demonstrates bilateral "blooming" areas layering along the vermis ➡ and in folia of the superior cerebellar hemispheres ➡ corresponding to the hemorrhage seen on prior CT.*

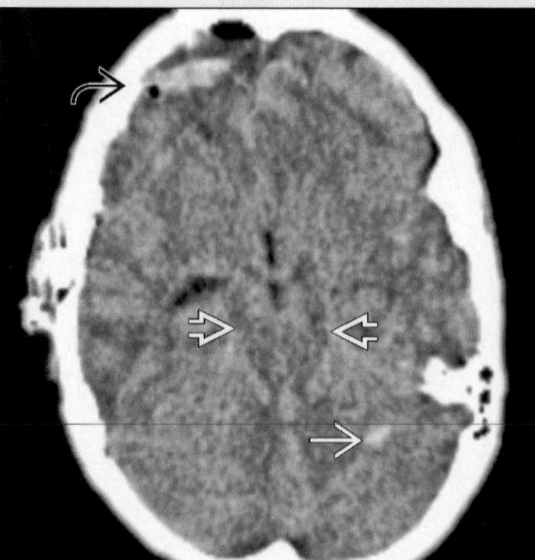
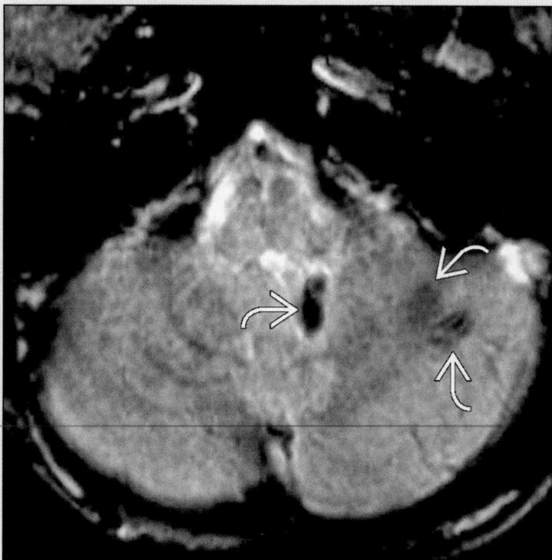

(Left) *Axial NECT reveals a small focus of hemorrhage in the left cerebellum ➡, contralateral and infratentorial to the site of recent craniotomy ➡. Note the associated cisternal effacement ➡ suggesting possible cerebrospinal fluid hypovolemia, a common associated finding in RCH and a likely predisposing factor.* ***(Right)*** *Axial T2* GRE MR in the same patient shows "blooming" of 3 separate hemorrhagic foci ➡. MR with T2* sequences (GRE or SWI) depicts cerebellar hemorrhages better than CT.*

REMOTE CEREBELLAR HEMORRHAGE

TERMINOLOGY

Abbreviations

- Remote cerebellar hemorrhage (RCH)

Definitions

- Cerebellar hemorrhage following cerebral surgery
  - Remote to primary surgical site
  - No underlying pathologic lesion
  - CSF drainage → cerebellar "sagging" → vein stretching, bleeding

IMAGING

General Features

- Best diagnostic clue
  - "Zebra" sign (blood layered over cerebellar folia)
    - Following supratentorial craniotomy or spinal surgery
- Location
  - Sublocation in cerebellum varies
  - Subarachnoid &/or superficial parenchymal bleed
- Morphology
  - Superior cerebellar folia most common pattern

CT Findings

- NECT
  - Hyperdense

MR Findings

- T1WI
  - Varies with age/stage of hematoma
- T2WI
  - Usually mixed hypo-/hyperintense
- T2* GRE
  - Useful to confirm hemorrhage ("blooms")
    - T2* most sensitive for parenchymal blood
    - SWI more sensitive than GRE
- DWI
  - Varied signal intensity depending on age
- T1WI C+
  - No enhancement
- MRA
  - Negative

Angiographic Findings

- DSA negative for underlying vascular etiology
- No cortical venous/dural sinus occlusion

Imaging Recommendations

- Best imaging tool
  - NECT initial screen
  - MR with and without contrast, MRA
    - Include GRE and SWI
- Protocol advice
  - MRI with T2*, gadolinium, plus vascular imaging (MRA &/or DSA)

DIFFERENTIAL DIAGNOSIS

Hypertensive Hemorrhage

- Cerebellar location common
- Lobar > superficial/foliar pattern

Neoplasm with Hemorrhage

- Metastases > primary neoplasm
- Vasogenic edema, nodular enhancement, additional lesions are clues

Vascular Malformation

- Cavernous malformation
- AVM, dAVF

Cerebral Amyloid Angiopathy

- Rarely involves cerebellum

Coagulopathy-related Spontaneous Hemorrhage

- Iatrogenic: Warfarin, heparin, aspirin
- Disseminated intravascular coagulation

PATHOLOGY

General Features

- Etiology
  - CSF (cerebrospinal fluid) hypovolemia?
    - May lead to "brain sagging," occlusion/tearing of bridging veins
    - Result = hemorrhagic venous infarct

Gross Pathologic & Surgical Features

- Hemorrhagic necrosis without underlying vascular malformation or tumor

CLINICAL ISSUES

Presentation

- Most common signs/symptoms
  - ↓ consciousness, seizures
  - Cerebellar signs
    - From primary bleed or herniation (less common)
  - Can be asymptomatic
    - Discovered incidentally on postoperative imaging

Treatment

- Intervention for RCH rarely indicated

DIAGNOSTIC CHECKLIST

Consider

- MR initial evaluation after screening NECT

Image Interpretation Pearls

- Cerebellar bleed in patient with history of craniotomy or spinal surgery probably represents RCH

SELECTED REFERENCES

1. Figueiredo EG et al: Remote cerebellar hemorrhage (zebra sign) in vascular neurosurgery: pathophysiological insights. Neurol Med Chir (Tokyo). 49(6):229-33; discussion 233-4, 2009
2. Huang CY et al: Remote cerebellar hemorrhage after supratentorial unruptured aneurysm surgery: report of three cases. Neurol Res. Epub ahead of print, 2009

GERMINAL MATRIX HEMORRHAGE

Key Facts

Imaging

- Cerebral: Blood products in subependymal region, usually involving caudothalamic notch
- Cerebellar: Blood products on cerebellar surface
- Ultrasound (US) is standard of care: Sensitive but not specific and user dependent
- MR most sensitive and specific; important though to weigh risks of transport

Top Differential Diagnoses

- Deep venous thrombosis with hemorrhage
- Arterial ischemic infarction
- Isolated choroid plexus hemorrhage
- Isolated intraventricular hemorrhage

Pathology

- GMH: Rupture of gray matter capillaries
- PHI: Venous hemorrhagic infarction likely due to GMH ± IVH compressing terminal vein
- Hydrocephalus
- Periventricular leukomalacia (high association with GMH + IVH)
- Selective neuronal necrosis (pontine > thalamus, basal ganglia, hippocampus)
- Grade 1: GMH (typically caudothalamic notch)
- Grade 2: GMH + IVH
- Grade 3: GMH + IVH + ventriculomegaly
- Grade 4 (PHI): GMH + IVH + ventriculomegaly + parenchymal extension

Clinical Issues

- Most common < 32 weeks gestation age, < 1,500 g
- Rare > 34 weeks GA
- ~ 90% GM bleeds occur ≤ 3 days
- Maximal extent reached ≤ 5 days

*(**Left**) Coronal gross pathology section shows a left GMH ➔ with intraventricular extension ➔ and associated PHI ➔ in both the left frontal and temporal lobes. Note the clotted blood extending outward from the left lateral ventricle into the medullary veins ➔. (**Right**) Sagittal transfontanelle ultrasound in a premature infant shows a focus of increased echogenicity ➔ in the caudothalamic notch without intraventricular extension, consistent with a grade 1 GMH.*

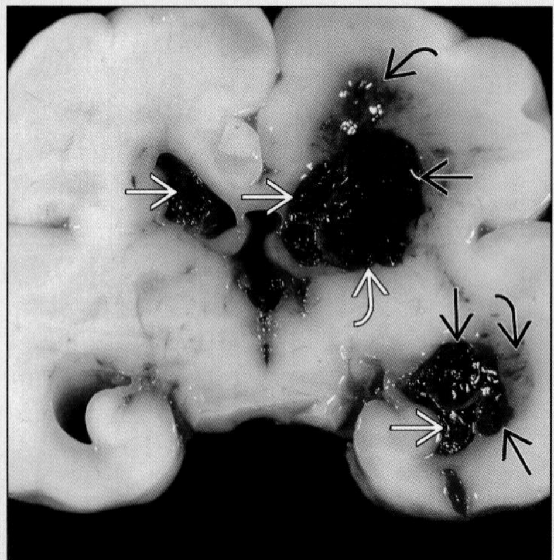

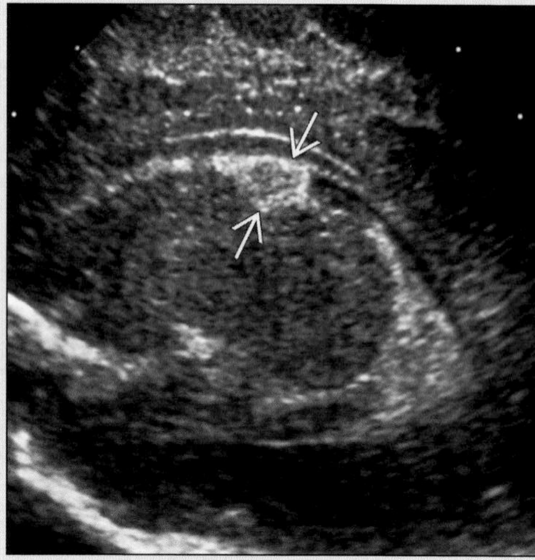

*(**Left**) Axial T2WI MR in a premature infant shows a small focus of hypointense signal ➔ in the wall of the right lateral ventricle due to a small hemorrhage in the GM. (**Right**) Sagittal T1WI MR in the same premature infant shows the small GMH as a focus of increased T1 signal ➔. Note the intraventricular extension ➔ into the occipital horn, consistent with a grade 2 GMH. The US performed on the same day (not shown) was normal.*

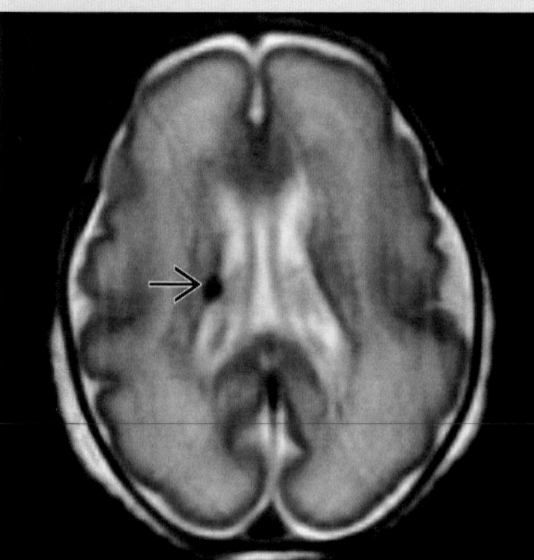

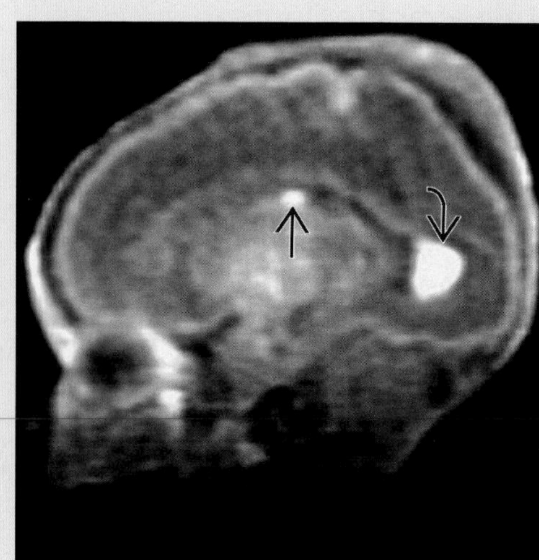

GERMINAL MATRIX HEMORRHAGE

TERMINOLOGY

Abbreviations

- Germinal matrix hemorrhage (GMH)
- Intraventricular hemorrhage (IVH)
- Periventricular hemorrhagic infarction (PHI)

Synonyms

- Grade 4 GMH = periventricular hemorrhagic infarction
- Cerebellar GMH = external granular layer hemorrhage
- Germinal matrix = ventricular + subventricular zone (SVZ)

Definitions

- Germinal matrix
  - Highly vascular, neural-tube derived structure
    - Dynamic; varies both temporally, spatially
  - Contains multiple cell types
    - Neural stem cells
    - Restricted neural progenitor cells
    - Ependymal cells
    - Premigratory/migrating neurons, glia

IMAGING

General Features

- Best diagnostic clue
  - Cerebral: Blood products in subependymal region, usually involving caudothalamic notch
    - ± intraventricular hemorrhage
    - ± choroid plexus bleed (often associated with GMH + IVH)
    - ± ventriculomegaly
    - ± periventricular hemorrhagic infarction
  - Cerebellar: Blood products on cerebellar surface
- Location
  - Cerebral GMH: Hemorrhage into GM along lateral ventricular wall, most commonly caudothalamic notch
  - Cerebellar GMH: Hemorrhage into cerebellar GM over cerebellar hemisphere + vermian surface
  - PHI: Hemorrhage in periventricular white matter adjacent to GM in caudothalamic notch in venous distribution
- Size
  - Variable

CT Findings

- NECT
  - High attenuation due to blood products

MR Findings

- T1WI
  - Blood products initially isointense but become hyperintense after ~ 3 days
- T2WI
  - Blood products hypointense (hyperacute blood that is hyperintense on T2 not currently reported due to typical delay in MR > 12 hours)
  - Become centrally hyperintense with hypointense rim as they evolve
- T2* GRE
  - Blood products "bloom"
- DWI
  - DWI signal variable (low T2 drives signal down, low ADC drives signal up)
  - ADC low due to clotted blood

Ultrasonographic Findings

- Grayscale ultrasound
  - Subependymal mass with ↑ echogenicity
    - Typically caudothalamic notch
    - ± intraventricular echogenicity, ventriculomegaly
- Color Doppler
  - Helps differentiate echogenic choroid plexus from avascular echogenic hemorrhage

Imaging Recommendations

- Best imaging tool
  - Ultrasound (US) is standard of care: Sensitive but not specific and user dependent
  - MR most sensitive and specific; important, though, to weigh risks of transport
- Protocol advice
  - US: High frequency probe, multiple focal points

DIFFERENTIAL DIAGNOSIS

Deep Venous Thrombosis with Hemorrhage

- Typically > 34 weeks gestation age (GA)
- Hemorrhage can occur in caudothalamic notch at site where terminal vein joins choroid vein to form internal cerebral vein

Arterial Ischemic Infarction

- No blood products on MR, arterial vascular distribution

Isolated Choroid Plexus Hemorrhage

- No blood products in ventricular wall

Isolated Intraventricular Hemorrhage

- Typically > 34 weeks GA; no blood products in ventricular wall

White Matter Injury of Prematurity

- Involves periventricular and deep white matter; no "blooming" on gradient echo imaging

Ventriculitis

- No blood products on MR

PATHOLOGY

General Features

- Etiology
  - GMH: Rupture of GM capillaries may occur in relation to many factors
    - Altered CBF caused by
      - Rapid volume expansion
      - Hypercarbia
      - ↑ hemoglobin or blood glucose
      - Hypoxic ischemic events
    - Increase in cerebral venous pressure (delivery, heart failure, positive pressure ventilation, etc.)
    - Coagulopathy

GERMINAL MATRIX HEMORRHAGE

  - Capillary fragility
  - Deficient vascular support
  - Increased fibrinolytic activity
  - Hypoxic ischemic injury
 - PHI: Venous hemorrhagic infarction likely due to GMH ± IVH compressing terminal vein
- Associated abnormalities
 - Hydrocephalus
 - Periventricular leukomalacia (high association with GMH + IVH)
 - Selective neuronal necrosis (pontine > thalamus, basal ganglia, hippocampus)

Staging, Grading, & Classification

- Papile (based on head ultrasound)
 - Grade 1: GMH (typically caudothalamic notch)
 - Grade 2: GMH + IVH
 - Grade 3: GMH + IVH + ventriculomegaly
 - Grade 4: GMH + IVH + ventriculomegaly + parenchymal extension (PHI)
- Volpe (based on head ultrasound)
 - Grade 1: GMH + IVH < 10% ventricular area on parasagittal view
 - Grade 2: GMH + IVH 10-50% ventricular area on parasagittal view
 - Grade 3: GMH + IVH > 50% ventricular area on parasagittal view
 - Periventricular echodensity (probable PHI)

Gross Pathologic & Surgical Features

- GMH originates in subependymal GM
- PHI = venous hemorrhagic infarction

Microscopic Features

- Normally 2.54 ± 0.56 mm thick at 23-24 weeks GA, decreasing to 1.73 ± 0.71 mm at 29-30 weeks GA , and only 0.50 ± 0.26 mm at 35-36 weeks GA
- Subependymal hemorrhage in GM, typically caudothalamic notch if > 28 weeks GA
- Hemorrhage occurs in prominent endothelial-lined vessels similar to capillary-venule or small venule
- ± obliterative arachnoiditis secondary to IVH and spread into subarachnoid space

CLINICAL ISSUES

Presentation

- Most common signs/symptoms
 - Silent > stuttering decline > catastrophic decline
  - Stuttering over hours to days: Altered consciousness, hypotonia, abnormal eye movements, abnormal respirations
  - Catastrophic over minutes to hours: Coma, flaccid &/or fixed pupils, apnea, seizures, decerebrate posturing
 - Most common presentation of GMH + IVH is premature infant with respiratory distress syndrome with mechanical ventilation
- Other signs/symptoms
 - Drop in hematocrit

Demographics

- Age
 - Most common < 32 weeks GA, < 1,500 g
 - Rare > 34 weeks GA
 - Can occur in utero

Natural History & Prognosis

- > 20 weeks GM gives rise to oligodendrocytes and astrocytes
- Blood products have adverse effect on maturing SVZ cells on oligodendrocyte precursors
- ~ 90% of GM bleeds occur ≤ 3 days
- Maximal extent reached ≤ 5 days
- Short term prognosis
 - Grades 1 and 2: Mortality and incidence of posthemorrhagic ventriculomegaly < 15% if > 750g
 - Grade 3: Mortality < 35% and incidence of posthemorrhagic ventriculomegaly > 75%
 - PHI: Mortality up to 45% and incidence of posthemorrhagic ventriculomegaly > 80%
- Incidence of long-term neurological sequelae
 - Grade 1: 15%
 - Grade 2: 25%
 - Grade 3: 50%
 - PHI: 75%

Treatment

- Supportive, rarely shunting of secondary hydrocephalus
- Current emphasis on prevention

SELECTED REFERENCES

1. O'Leary H et al: Elevated cerebral pressure passivity is associated with prematurity-related intracranial hemorrhage. Pediatrics. 124(1):302-9, 2009
2. Roze E et al: Risk factors for adverse outcome in preterm infants with periventricular hemorrhagic infarction. Pediatrics. 122(1):e46-52, 2008
3. Volpe JJ. Neurology of the Newborn. 5th ed. Philadelphia, PA: Saunders, 2008
4. Bassan H et al: Neurodevelopmental outcome in survivors of periventricular hemorrhagic infarction. Pediatrics. 120(4):785-92, 2007
5. Kadri H et al: The incidence, timing, and predisposing factors of germinal matrix and intraventricular hemorrhage (GMH/IVH) in preterm neonates. Childs Nerv Syst. 22(9):1086-90, 2006
6. Morioka T et al: Fetal germinal matrix and intraventricular hemorrhage. Pediatr Neurosurg. 42(6):354-61, 2006
7. Folkerth RD: Neuropathologic substrate of cerebral palsy. J Child Neurol. 20(12):940-9, 2005
8. Kinoshita Y et al: Volumetric analysis of the germinal matrix and lateral ventricles performed using MR images of postmortem fetuses. AJNR Am J Neuroradiol. 22(2):382-8, 2001
9. Blankenberg FG et al: Sonography, CT, and MR imaging: a prospective comparison of neonates with suspected intracranial ischemia and hemorrhage. AJNR Am J Neuroradiol. 21(1):213-8, 2000
10. Felderhoff-Mueser U et al: Relationship between MR imaging and histopathologic findings of the brain in extremely sick preterm infants. AJNR Am J Neuroradiol. 20(7):1349-57, 1999
11. Blankenberg FG et al: Neonatal intracranial ischemia and hemorrhage: diagnosis with US, CT, and MR imaging. Radiology. 199(1):253-9, 1996
12. Szymonowicz W et al: Ultrasound and necropsy study of periventricular haemorrhage in preterm infants. Arch Dis Child. 59(7):637-42, 1984

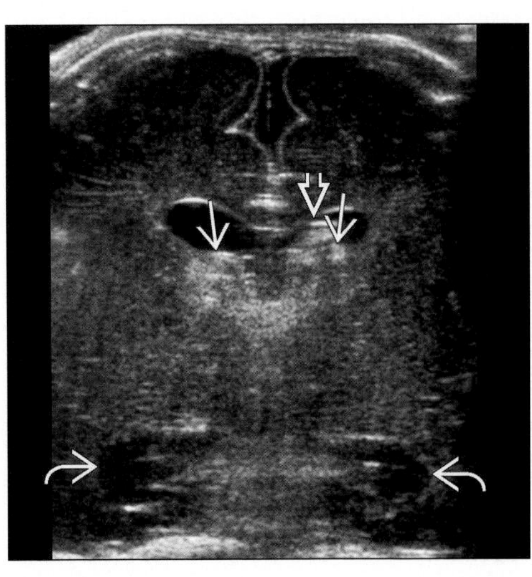

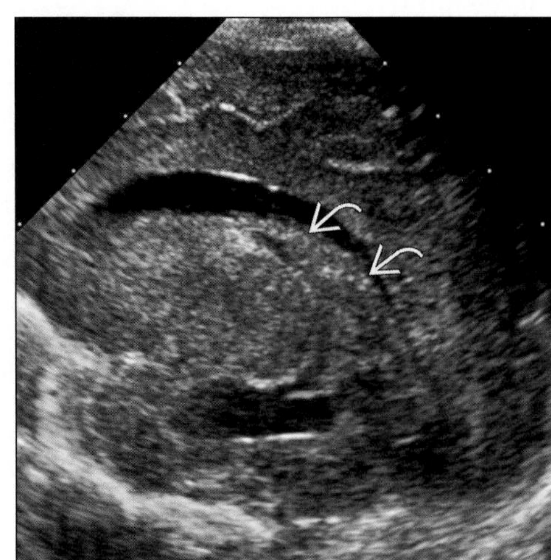

*(**Left**) Coronal ultrasound in a premature infant shows increased echogenicity in the bilateral caudothalamic notch due to GMH, intraventricular extension of blood, and enlargement of the lateral ventricles, including the temporal horns, diagnostic of a grade 3 GMH. (**Right**) Longitudinal ultrasound in the same infant shows an echogenic clot in the enlarged lateral ventricle. These findings allow the diagnosis of a grade 3 GMH to be made.*

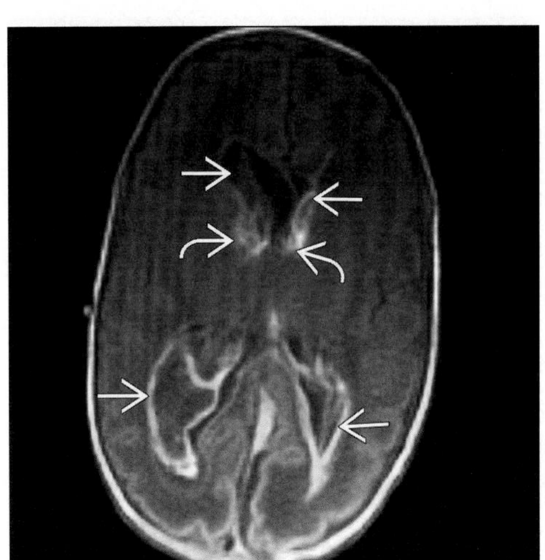

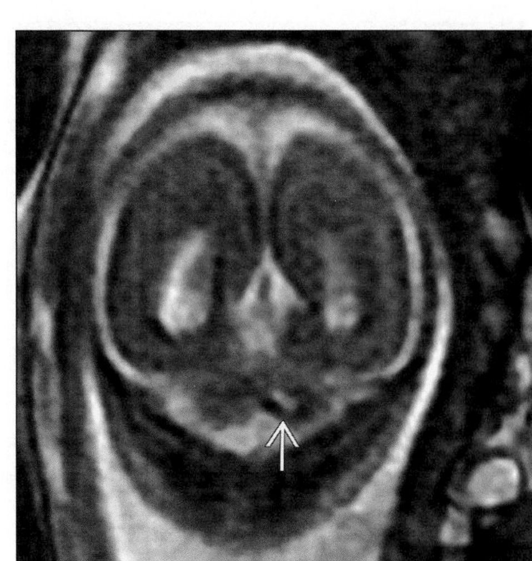

*(**Left**) Axial T1WI MR in the same premature infant with grade 3 hemorrhage 1 week later shows large bilateral germinal matrix hemorrhages and an extensive mixed intensity intraventricular clot with persistent right lateral ventricle enlargement. (**Right**) Coronal T2WI MR (HASTE) in a fetus of 23 weeks gestation age shows decreased signal along the inferomedial surface of the left cerebellar hemisphere, consistent with a cerebellar GMH.*

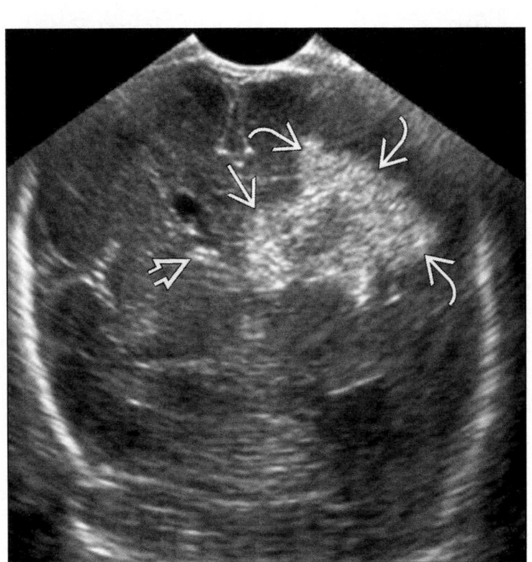

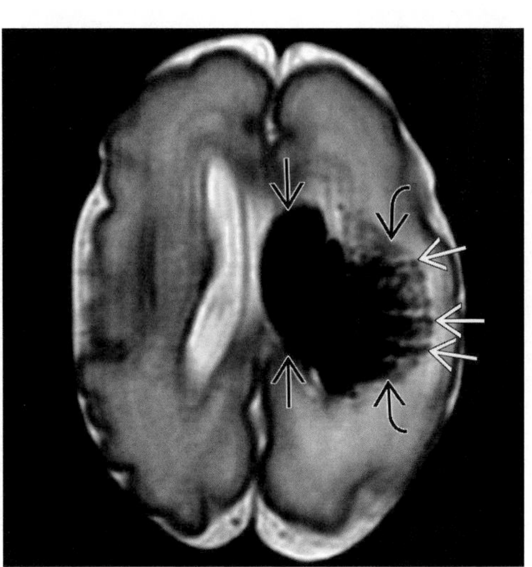

*(**Left**) Coronal transfontanelle ultrasound in a premature infant shows a small increased echogenicity due to GMH in the right caudothalamic notch. The GMH on the left is obscured by the intraventricular extension and very echogenic associated PHI. (**Right**) Axial T2WI MR in the same infant shows hypointense hemorrhage in the ventricle and the associated PHI. Note the radiating pattern of the medullary venous thrombosis in the PHI.*

INTRACRANIAL ATHEROSCLEROSIS

Key Facts

Terminology
- Common: Stenosis secondary to ASVD
  - Eccentric, irregular ± ulceration, Ca++
- Less common: Dolichoectasia
  - Enlargement/tortuosity without stenosis

Imaging
- Stenotic intracranial artery on CTA/MRA/DSA
  - Distal basilar (BA) or internal carotid artery (ICA)
- MDR CTA has high sensitivity/specificity
  - For > 50% stenosis or occlusion of large arteries

Top Differential Diagnoses
- Vasculitis/arteritis
- Vasospasm
- Moyamoya
- Dissection
- Nonocclusive thrombus or embolus

Pathology
- NASCET criteria (used in cervical disease) > 70% stenosis considered flow limiting

Clinical Issues
- Transient ischemic attack, due to emboli, severe stenosis, progressive occlusion
- Plaque rupture usually leads to stroke

Diagnostic Checklist
- Imaging recommendations
  - CTA &/or MRA as excellent screening tool
  - DSA gold standard, allows potential intervention
- Determining status of collaterals important
  - Patients with developed collaterals tolerate stenosis/occlusion better

*(**Left**) Coronal graphic shows atherosclerotic plaques involving the major intracranial arteries and their branches. Inset shows penetrating (lenticulostriate) arteries and lacunar infarcts. (**Right**) Anteroposterior MRA shows lack of flow in the distal left M1 segment, representing either high-grade stenosis or occlusion. There is stenosis of the post-communicating right MCA branches. Dolichoectasia, a less common manifestation of atherosclerosis, of the cavernous left ICA is also seen.*

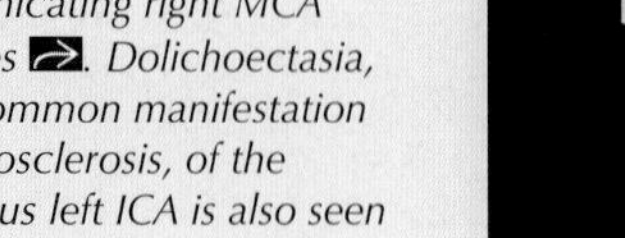

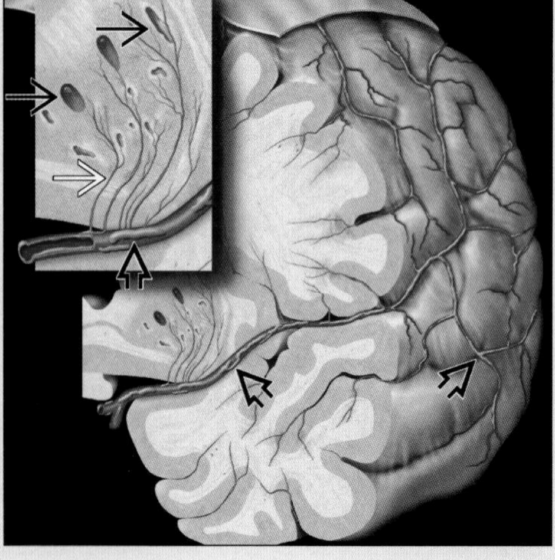

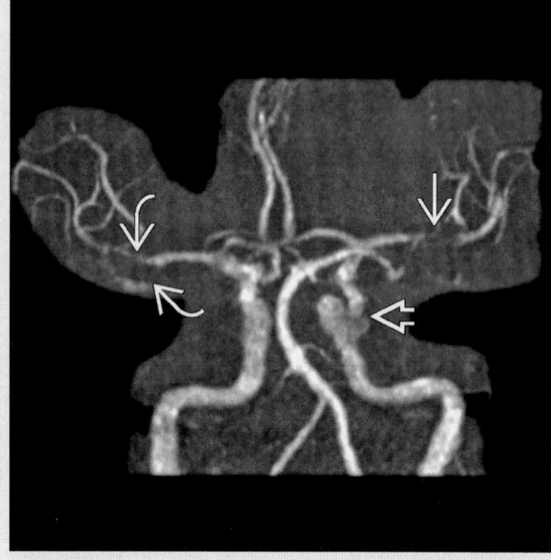

*(**Left**) Axial T2WI in a middle-aged woman with TIAs shows an absent flow void in the right ICA. (**Right**) Axial T2WI in the same patient shows multifocal white matter hyperintensities in a nearly straight line (rosary-like pattern), caused by low pressure in the deep white matter watershed between the junction of the deep penetrating cortical pial vessels and long, unpaired penetrating branches from the circle of Willis. MRA (not shown) revealed occluded right ICA and high-grade stenosis of left cervical ICA.*

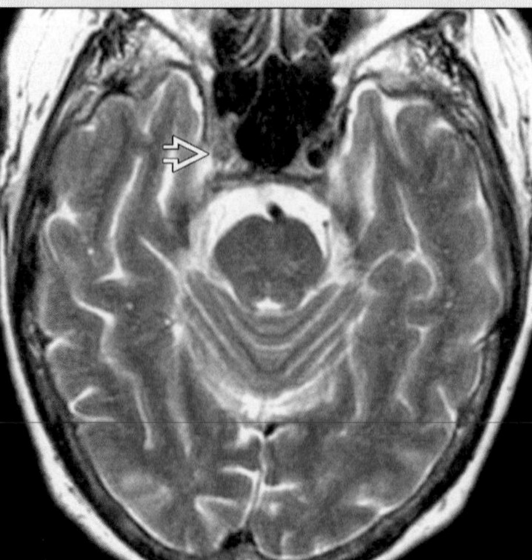

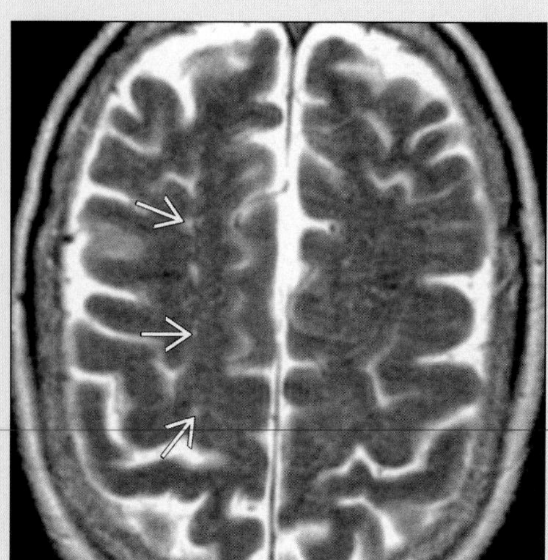

INTRACRANIAL ATHEROSCLEROSIS

TERMINOLOGY

Abbreviations

- Intracranial atherosclerotic vascular disease (ASVD), stenosis

Definitions

- Narrowing or ectasia of intracranial arteries secondary to ASVD

IMAGING

General Features

- Best diagnostic clue
  - Stenotic intracranial artery on CTA/MRA/DSA
  - Less common: Dolichoectasia
    - Enlargement/tortuosity without stenosis
- Location
  - Distal basilar artery (BA), cavernous/supraclinoid ICA most common
  - Less common sites
    - Circle of Willis (COW)
    - MCA rare (2% of cases) **but** high stroke risk
- Morphology
  - Usually eccentric, irregular ± ulceration

CT Findings

- NECT
  - Mural Ca++
- CTA
  - MDR CTA has high sensitivity/specificity
    - In patients with > 50% stenosis or occlusion of large arteries
    - Caveat: Mural Ca++ may ↓ specificity

MR Findings

- T1WI
  - Decreased/absent flow void
  - Also seen in slow flow
    - Proximal (extracranial) stenosis, dissection
- T2WI
  - Decreased/absent flow void
- FLAIR
  - Slow flow or occlusion may appear hyperintense
    - "Dot" sign
- MRA
  - 3D TOF (time of flight) contrast-enhanced MRA
  - Focal stenosis, ectasia, or irregularity
    - 3D TOF may overestimate stenosis
      - Secondary to spin saturation
      - Poor evaluation for slow, in-plane flow
    - Enhanced MRA less affected by spin saturation (also faster)
    - Combined with CTA, sensitivity/specificity ~ DSA
  - CTA > MRA for evaluation of in-stent restenosis
  - Dolichoectasia may also cause reduced flow

Ultrasonographic Findings

- Transcranial Doppler (TCD): Increased velocities

Angiographic Findings

- DSA may show
  - Focal stenosis, luminal irregularities
  - Thrombosis, occlusion
  - Ectasia/elongation
  - "Giant" serpentine/fusiform aneurysms (less common)
- DSA most sensitive/specific test; goals include
  - Grade extracranial stenosis, criteria standardized by NASCET (North American Symptomatic Carotid Endarterectomy Trial)
  - Identify "tandem" lesions
  - Assess collateral status
  - Potential assessment of plaque ulceration
  - Potential intervention (angioplasty ± stenting)
  - Best for post-stenting evaluation

Imaging Recommendations

- Best imaging tool
  - Gold standard is DSA
- Protocol advice
  - CTA or MRA followed by DSA if equivocal
  - CTA or MRA for proximal intracranial stenoses

DIFFERENTIAL DIAGNOSIS

Vasculitis/Arteritis

- Usually involves smaller (tertiary) branches
- More likely associated with hemorrhage
- Can be primary or secondary
- Often associated with systemic disease
- Elevated ESR, autoimmune parameters

Vasospasm

- Subarachnoid hemorrhage related, maximal 7 days post-bleed
- Drug-related (sympathomimetics)

Moyamoya

- Usually involves distal ICA and proximal COW with relative sparing of basilar artery
- Frequently bilateral

Dissection

- Smooth tapering
- T1 hyperintense crescent = thrombus, best seen with fat-sat sequences
- Younger patients
- Can have minimal or no history of trauma

Nonocclusive Thrombus or Embolus

- Appearance of rounded, central nonopacification with peripheral enhancing rim on contrast study

PATHOLOGY

General Features

- Etiology
  - Probably multiple etiologies
    - Lipid hypothesis
      - High plasma LDL leads to LDL-cholesterol deposition in intima
    - Response to injury hypothesis
      - Focal endothelial change or intimal injury leads to platelet aggregation and plaque formation
    - Unifying hypothesis

- Endothelial injury leads to increased permeability of LDL; plaques grow by thrombus formation on plaque surface and transendothelial leakage of plasma lipids
  - Smoking associated with intracranial atherosclerosis
  - Atherosclerosis is systemic, multifactorial disease
  - Intracranial atherosclerosis associated with atherosclerosis of carotids, coronaries, aorta, renal arteries, iliofemoral system
- Associated abnormalities
  - Anatomy
    - Most often involves arterial bifurcations, e.g., ICA and BA
    - May involve distal arterioles leading to vasculitis pattern of alternating stenosis and dilatation

Staging, Grading, & Classification

- NASCET criteria (used in cervical disease) > 70% stenosis considered flow limiting

Gross Pathologic & Surgical Features

- Earliest macroscopic finding: Intimal fatty streaks
- Fibrous atheromatous plaques contain
  - Smooth muscle cells, monocytes, other leukocytes
  - Connective tissue: Collagen, elastic fibers, proteoglycans
  - Intra- and extracellular lipid deposits
  - Angiogenesis produces new capillaries at plaque periphery
    - Leads to intraplaque hemorrhage and ulceration
    - Hemorrhage leads to dystrophic ferrocalcinosis (seen as calcification on CT, as iron on MR)
- Arterial narrowing due to plaque
  - Flow limiting beyond 70% stenosis (based on diameter ratios)
  - Ischemic symptoms depend on collaterals
    - Slow occlusion leads to more collaterals, fewer symptoms
    - Rapid occlusion (from thrombosis or emboli) does not permit time for collaterals to develop, infarct likely
- Arterial irregularity from disrupted endothelium may form thrombogenic surface leading to thrombosis or emboli

Microscopic Features

- Earliest findings
  - Lipid deposition, cellular reaction in intima
- Later findings and determinants of stability in atherosclerotic plaques (MR holds promise for characterization of intraplaque composition)
  - Lipid core
  - Fibrous cap (thicker cap is more stable and less likely to rupture)
  - Inflammatory changes

CLINICAL ISSUES

Presentation

- Most common signs/symptoms
  - Transient ischemic attack, due to emboli, severe stenosis, progressive occlusion
  - Plaque rupture usually leads to stroke
  - Vascular stenosis leads to stuttering ischemia from intermittent thrombosis

Demographics

- Age
  - Older age
- Gender
  - M = F
- Epidemiology
  - 3rd most common cause of thromboembolic stroke, after carotid and cardiac sources
  - Basis for cerebral thromboembolism in over 90%
  - Most common cause of intracranial vascular stenosis in adults
- More common in Western countries
- Higher risk of concurrent intra- and extracranial involvement in Asians

Natural History & Prognosis

- Progressive disease unless treated aggressively
- Poor prognosis without treatment, better prognosis with treatment

Treatment

- Low saturated fat and cholesterol diet and exercise
- Cholesterol lowering drugs ("statins") if lifestyle interventions are insufficient
- Plaque stabilization ("statins") may decrease stroke
- Angioplasty &/or stenting in some cases

DIAGNOSTIC CHECKLIST

Consider

- CTA &/or MRA as excellent screening tool
- DSA gold standard, allows potential intervention

Image Interpretation Pearls

- Status of collaterals important; patients with developed collaterals tolerate stenosis/occlusion better

SELECTED REFERENCES

1. Kassab MY et al: Extent of intra-arterial calcification on head CT is predictive of the degree of intracranial atherosclerosis on digital subtraction angiography. Cerebrovasc Dis. 28(1):45-8, 2009
2. Man BL et al: Lesion patterns and stroke mechanisms in concurrent atherosclerosis of intracranial and extracranial vessels. Stroke. 40(10):3211-5, 2009
3. Nguyen-Huynh MN et al: How accurate is CT angiography in evaluating intracranial atherosclerotic disease? Stroke. 39(4):1184-8, 2008
4. Suwanwela NC et al: Risk factors for atherosclerosis of cervicocerebral arteries: intracranial versus extracranial. Neuroepidemiology. 22(1):37-40, 2003
5. Hirai T et al: Prospective evaluation of suspected stenoocclusive disease of the intracranial artery: combined MR angiography and CT angiography compared with digital subtraction angiography. AJNR Am J Neuroradiol. 23(1):93-101, 2002
6. Beneficial effect of carotid endarterectomy in symptomatic patients with high-grade carotid stenosis: North American Symptomatic Carotid Endarterectomy Trial Collaborators. N Engl J Med. 325(7):445-53, 1991

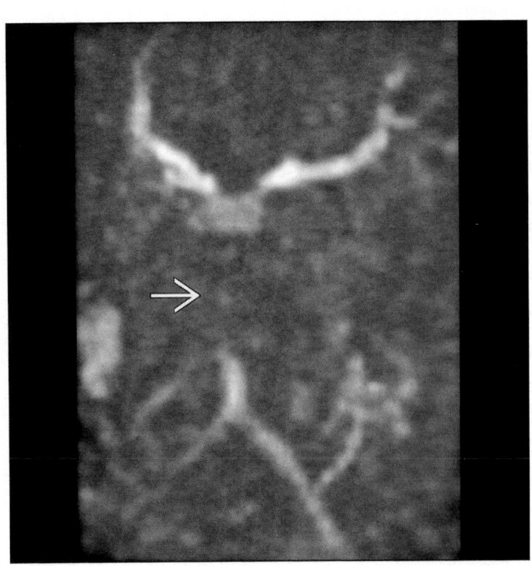

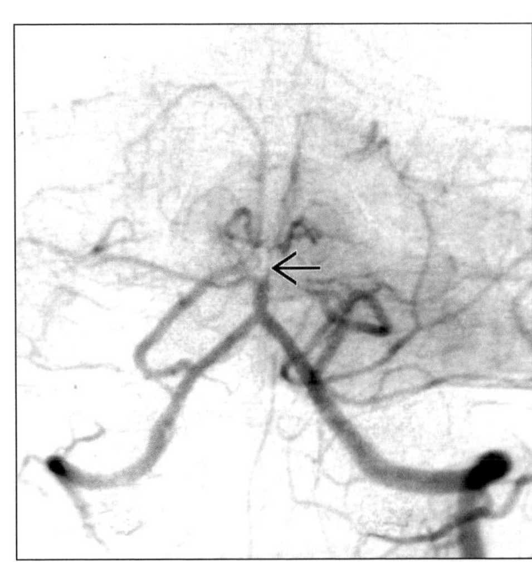

(Left) *Anteroposterior MRA 2D TOF demonstrates lack of flow-related enhancement in the mid and distal basilar artery ➡, related to either very slow flow in a high-grade stenosis or basilar occlusion.* ***(Right)*** *Anteroposterior angiography during arterial phase in the same patient confirms occlusion of the distal basilar artery →.*

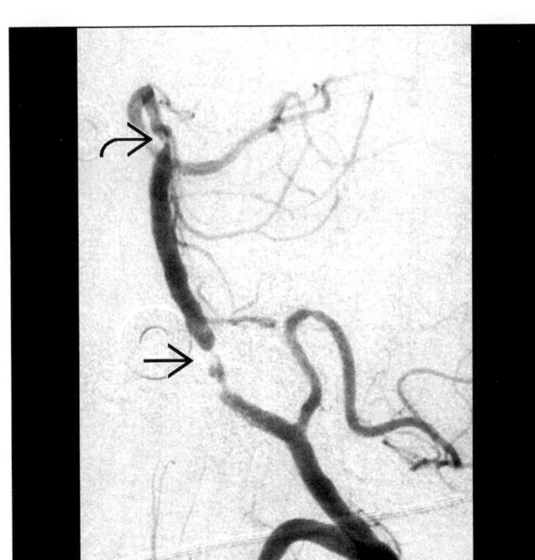

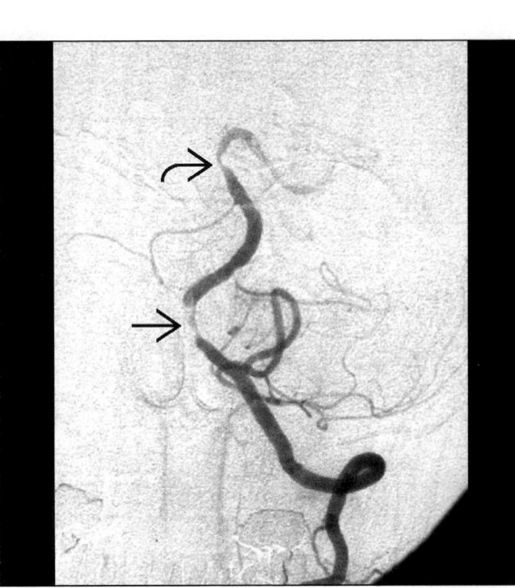

(Left) *Lateral angiography during arterial phase shows severe focal stenosis in the proximal basilar artery →. Note the tandem stenosis ↗ in the distal basilar artery.* ***(Right)*** *Lateral angiography during arterial phase in the same patient shows nonocclusive severe atheromatous narrowing of the basilar artery proximally → and distally ↗. It is important to confirm stenoses using at least 2 projections.*

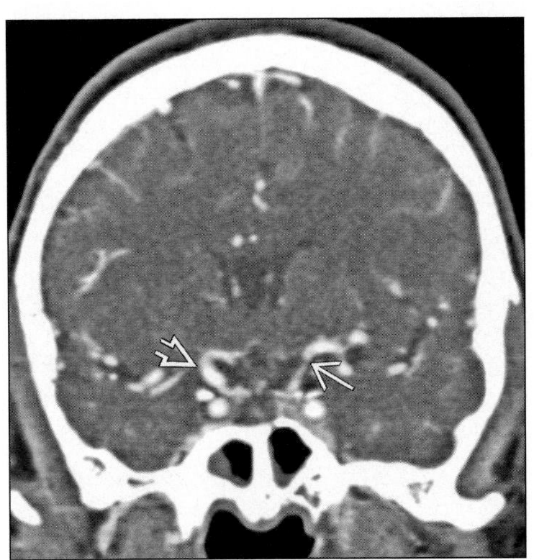

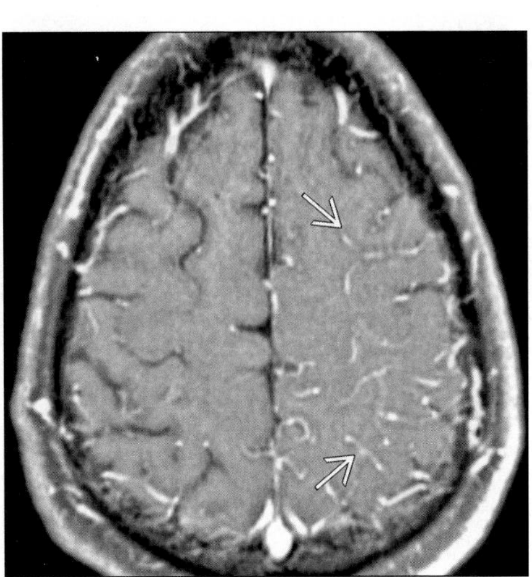

(Left) *Coronal CTA in a patient with TIAs and negative NECT scan in the emergency department shows high-grade stenosis of the distal left ICA ➡ compared to the normal right supraclinoid ICA ➡.* ***(Right)*** *T1WI C+ MR in the same patient shows enhancing sulci ➡. FLAIR scan (not shown) revealed hyperintensity in the left hemispheric sulci. Slow antegrade or retrograde flow through pial cortical branches may cause the appearance of hyperintense sulci on FLAIR and enhancement on T1 C+ scans.*

EXTRACRANIAL ATHEROSCLEROSIS

Key Facts

Terminology

- Degenerative process resulting from plasma lipid deposition in arterial walls

Imaging

- Smooth/irregular narrowing of proximal ICA
- Ca++ in arterial walls
- ICA, vertebrobasilar arteries most common sites
- Protocol advice
  - Color Doppler US as initial screen
  - CTA/MRA or contrast MRA
  - Consider DSA prior to carotid endarectomy, in equivocal cases or if CTA/MRA shows "occlusion"

Pathology

- NASCET method: % stenosis = (normal lumen - minimal residual lumen)/normal lumen, x 100
- Mild (< 50%), moderate (50-70%), severe (70-99%)

Clinical Issues

- CEA if symptomatic carotid stenosis ≥ 70% (NASCET)
- Symptomatic moderate stenosis (50-69%) also benefits from CEA (NASCET)
- Asymptomatic patients benefit even with stenosis of 60% (ACAS)
- Carotid stenting depends on preop risk factors
- Signs/symptoms (can be asymptomatic)
  - Carotid bruit, TIA, stroke (may be silent)

Diagnostic Checklist

- DSA remains "gold standard" but acceptable noninvasive preoperative imaging includes any 2 of
  - US, CTA, TOF, or contrast-enhanced MRA
- Late-phase DSA important to rule out "pseudo-occlusion"
  - High-grade stenosis with "string" sign

*(**Left**) Graphic shows the mild form (A) of ASVD with "fatty streaks" & slight intimal thickening. The severe form (B) is characterized by intraplaque hemorrhage, ulceration, & platelet thrombi. NASCET calculation for % of stenosis = (b-a)/b x 100 where b = normal ICA lumen & a = minimal residual ICA lumen. (**Right**) Coronal CTA oblique reconstruction shows a stenotic, irregular carotid bulb ➩ & calcified plaque at both the bulb & proximal internal carotid artery ➔ with excellent filling of the distal cervical ICA ➦.*

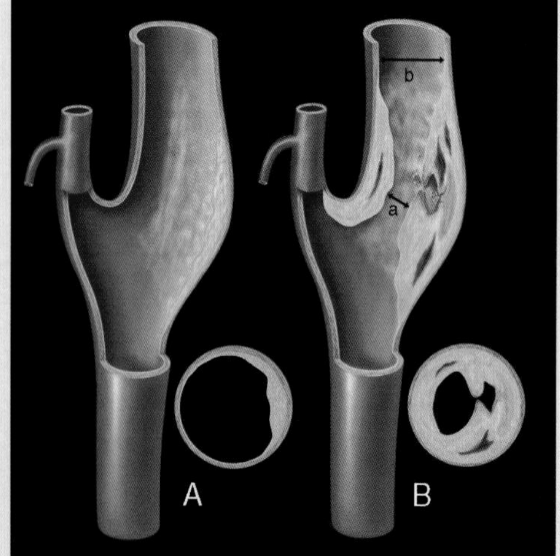

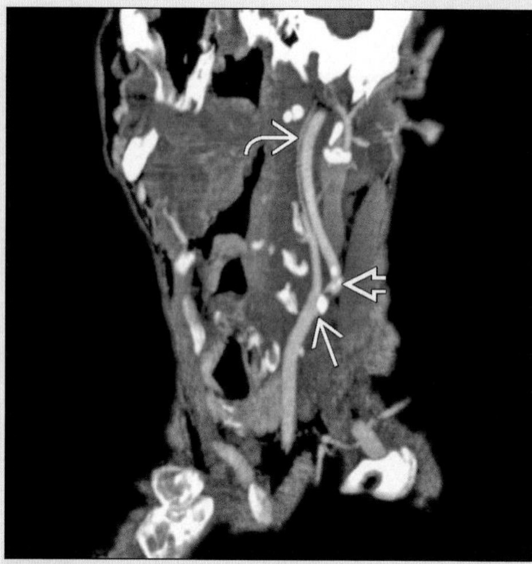

*(**Left**) Coronal oblique MRA shows a "flow gap" in the left internal carotid artery ➩ indicating severely restricted flow. The patient underwent an emergency left carotid endarterectomy. (**Right**) Axial T1WI C+ FS MR shows thickening of the internal carotid artery wall ➔ with only a small residual lumen ➩. Atherosclerotic plaques often have neovascularity, which may cause intraplaque hemorrhage.*

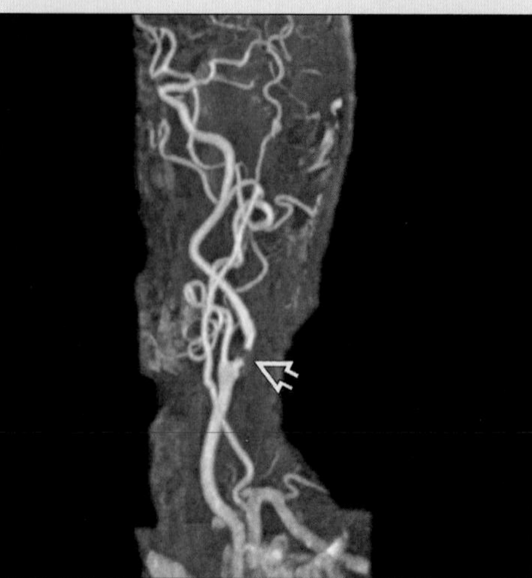

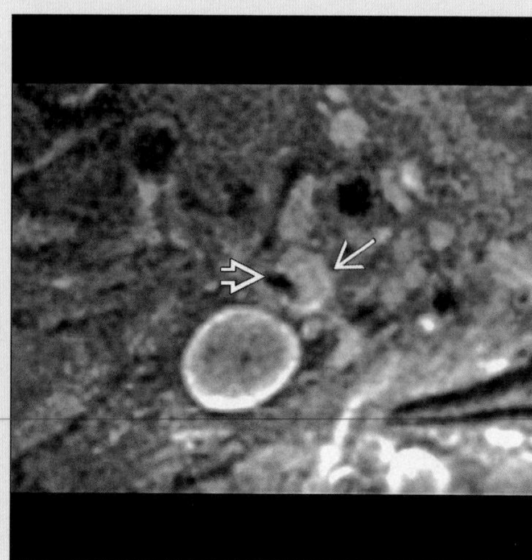

EXTRACRANIAL ATHEROSCLEROSIS

TERMINOLOGY

Abbreviations

- Atherosclerotic vascular disease (ASVD)

Definitions

- Degenerative process resulting from plasma lipid deposition in arterial walls

IMAGING

General Features

- Best diagnostic clue
  - Smooth or irregular narrowing of proximal ICA
  - Ca++ deposition in arterial walls
- Location
  - ICA, vertebrobasilar arteries most common sites
  - Affects large/medium/small arteries, arterioles
- Size
  - Ranges from microscopic lipid deposition to fatty streaks to gross plaque
    - Generally 0.3-1.5 cm in diameter
    - Fatty streaks may coalesce to form larger masses
- Morphology
  - Begins initially as smooth, slight eccentric thickening of vessel intima
  - Progresses to more focal and prominent eccentric thickening (subintimal macrocyte and smooth muscle cell deposition)
  - Subintimal hemorrhage from "new vessels" further narrows lumen
  - Ulceration with rupture of fibrous cap and intima occurs, resulting in "ulcerated plaque"

CT Findings

- NECT
  - Ca++ in vessel walls
  - Large plaques may show low-density foci (soft plaque)
  - Ectasia, tortuosity, fusiform vessel dilatation
- CECT
  - Opacifies vessel lumen
    - Can ↓ ability to visualize calcified plaque
- CTA
  - Visualizes degree of stenosis vs. occlusion
  - CTA can characterize plaque composition
    - Shows hemorrhage, ulceration, fibrous cap
    - Optimal coverage = 20 mm coverage each side
    - Use MIP and MPR reconstructions
      - MPR: Better interobserver agreement
    - Detection of ulceration: Up to 94% sensitivity, 99% specificity
      - Best using axials and volume rendering

MR Findings

- T1WI
  - Wall thickening, luminal narrowing
  - Absence of "flow void"
    - May occur if vessel occluded or severely stenotic
- FLAIR
  - Look for secondary signs of extracranial ASVD in brain (i.e., lacunes, infarcts)
- T1WI C+ FS
  - High-resolution ICA imaging with dedicated surface coils can characterizes plaque composition
  - Hemorrhage/plaques with a higher percentage of lipid-rich/necrotic core
    - Independently associated with a thin or ruptured fibrous cap ("at risk" plaque)
- MRA
  - 2D TOF or contrast enhanced
  - Degree of stenosis visualized
  - Signal loss may occur if high-grade (> 95%) stenosis
  - Severe narrowing causes "flow gap"

Ultrasonographic Findings

- Grayscale imaging allows visualization of noncalcified (hypoechoic) or calcified (hyperechoic) plaque in vessel wall
- Hypoechoic plaques are independent risk factors for stroke; strong correlation with ↑ lipoprotein(s)
- Doppler measures flow velocity; peak systolic velocity is best single velocity parameter for quantifying stenosis
- Spectral analysis allows evaluation of waveform; morphologic changes in waveform occur with increasing stenosis
- Color Doppler may detect high-grade occlusions more reliably than conventional Doppler

Angiographic Findings

- Conventional
  - Identifies degree of stenosis, morphology of plaque, tandem stenoses, potential collateral pathways as coexisting pathology (i.e., aneurysm)
  - Plaque surface irregularity associated with increased risk of stroke at all degrees of stenosis
  - Tandem lesions (distal stenoses) present in ~ 2% of patients with significant cervical ICA lesions
  - Hemodynamic effect of tandem stenoses additive: If both lesions are severe enough to ↓ flow separately
    - If only 1 tandem lesion is critical, flow is governed by more severe lesion
  - Late phase DSA important in high-grade stenosis or suspected occlusion to rule out "pseudo-occlusion"

Imaging Recommendations

- Best imaging tool
  - DSA for evaluating ICA stenosis; ≥ 4 projections recommended (AP, lateral, both obliques)
  - DSA remains gold standard → acceptable noninvasive preoperative imaging includes any 2 of following: US, CTA, TOF, or contrast MRA
    - Exception: Late-phase DSA remains important in suspected high-grade stenosis or occlusion to rule out pseudo-occlusion
- Protocol advice
  - Color Doppler US as initial screen
  - CTA/MRA or contrast MRA
  - Consider DSA prior to carotid endarterectomy in equivocal cases or if CTA/MRA shows "occlusion"

DIFFERENTIAL DIAGNOSIS

Dissection

- Typically spares carotid bulb; no calcification
- Seen in young or middle-aged groups

EXTRACRANIAL ATHEROSCLEROSIS

- Smoother, longer narrowing without intracranial involvement

Fibromuscular Dysplasia

- "String of beads" > > long-segment stenosis

Vasospasm

- Usually iatrogenic (catheter-induced), transient

PATHOLOGY

General Features

- Etiology
  - 3 main hypotheses
    - Lipid hypothesis: Relates ASVD to high plasma LDL levels causing LDL-cholesterol deposits in arterial intima
    - Response to injury hypothesis: ASVD is initiated by focal endothelial damage that initiates platelet aggregation and plaque formation
    - Unifying theory: Suggests that endothelial injury is accompanied by increased permeability to macromolecules, such as LDL
  - Other factors include diet, genes, mechanical stress (e.g., wall shear, anatomic variations), inflammation, hyperhomocysteinemia
  - Complex, multifactorial process; pathogenesis remains controversial
  - Probably no single cause, no single initiating event, and no exclusive pathogenetic mechanism
  - Irregular plaques correlate with higher stroke risk
  - Good collaterals correlates with lower stroke risk
  - Significant ICA narrowing seen in 20-30% of ICA territory strokes vs. 5-10% of general population
- Genetics
  - Probably multigenic

Staging, Grading, & Classification

- Methods for calculating degree of stenosis vary: NASCET, ACAS, ECST, and VACSG
- NASCET method: % stenosis = (normal lumen - minimal residual lumen)/normal lumen, x 100
  - Mild (< 50%), moderate (50-70%), severe (70-99%)

Gross Pathologic & Surgical Features

- 2 well-accepted lesions described: Atheromatous plaque and fatty streak
  - Atheromatous plaque: Most important, principal cause of arterial narrowing in adults
  - Fatty streak: Precursor of atheromatous plaque; present universally in children, even in 1st year
- Intimal fatty streaks are earliest macroscopically visible lesions
- Plaques are whitish-yellow, protrude intraluminally, vary in size

Microscopic Features

- Fibroatheromatous plaques, develop after lipid deposition
- Plaques contain cells (monocytes/macrophages, leukocytes, smooth muscle), connective tissue, intra-/ extracellular lipid deposits
- Necrotic core of lipid, cholesterol, cellular debris, lipid-laden foam cells, and fibrin form within plaque
- Neovascularization may lead to vessel rupture, intraplaque hemorrhage, and ulceration
- Atheromatous plaque may rupture (fibrous cap weakens and fractures); may lead to distal embolization

CLINICAL ISSUES

Presentation

- Most common signs/symptoms
  - Variable: Asymptomatic, carotid bruit, TIA, stroke (may be silent)
- Clinical profile
  - Stroke risk factors: Smoking, hypertension, diabetes, obesity, hypercholesterolemia, advanced age

Demographics

- Age
  - Usually middle-aged to elderly
- Gender
  - M > F
- Ethnicity
  - African-Americans at highest risk for ASVD
- Epidemiology
  - Leading cause of morbidity, mortality in USA
  - Ischemic stroke → up to 40% of deaths in elderly
  - Stroke occurs in > 70% of patients with ICA occlusion
  - 90% of large, recent infarcts are caused by thromboemboli
  - Epidemiological, experimental evidence that increased dietary lipid (cholesterol, saturated fat) and smoking correlate with atherosclerosis

Treatment

- Carotid endarterectomy (CEA) if symptomatic carotid stenosis ≥ 70% (NASCET)
- Symptomatic moderate stenosis (50-69%) also benefits from CEA (NASCET)
- Asymptomatic patients benefit even with stenosis of 60% (ACAS)
- ICA stenting depends on preoperative risk factors

DIAGNOSTIC CHECKLIST

Consider

- To calculate degree of stenosis on DSA, ≥ 2 projections are required to profile plaque adequately
- For patients undergoing CEA, adequacy of collateral circulation is critical; consider MRA or DSA
- Pseudo-occlusion (very high-grade stenosis) may be seen only on late-phase DSA; CEA still option if ICA patent

SELECTED REFERENCES

1. Babiarz LS et al: Contrast-enhanced MR angiography is not more accurate than unenhanced 2D time-of-flight MR angiography for determining > or = 70% internal carotid artery stenosis. AJNR Am J Neuroradiol. 30(4):761-8, 2009
2. Chen CJ et al: Multi-Slice CT angiography in diagnosing total versus near occlusions of the internal carotid artery: comparison with catheter angiography. Stroke. 35(1):83-5, 2004

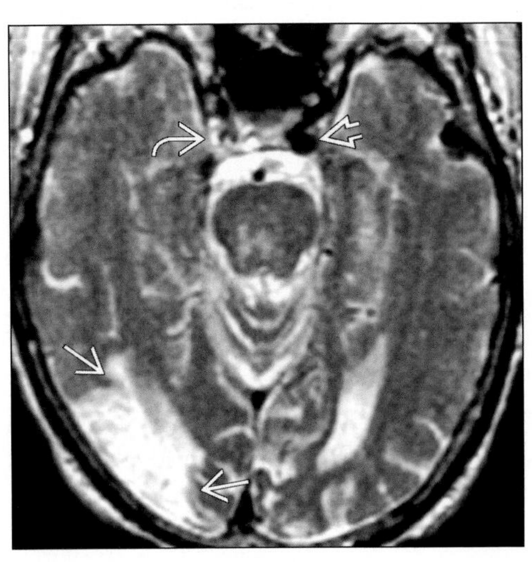

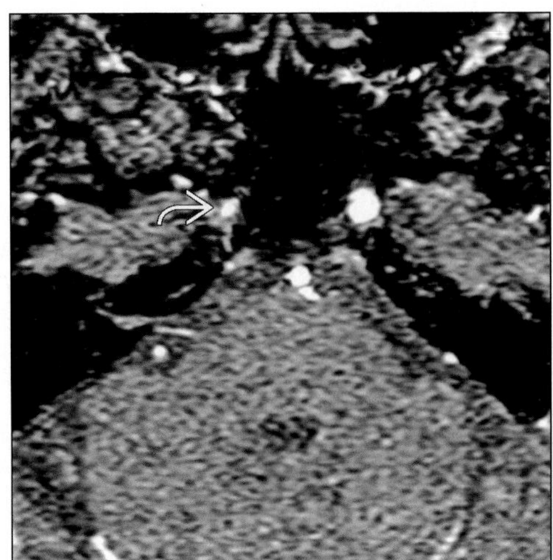

(Left) *Axial T2WI MR shows posterior encephalomalacia ➡, likely remote watershed ischemia. Note loss of the right cavernous ICA flow void ➡ compared to the left ➡.* **(Right)** *Axial MRA source image in the same patient shows a tiny but patent right ICA ➡, illustrating the difficulty of differentiating a completely occluded ICA from a high-grade stenosis using conventional MR. Absent flow voids may reflect slow flow or occlusion and should be confirmed angiographically.*

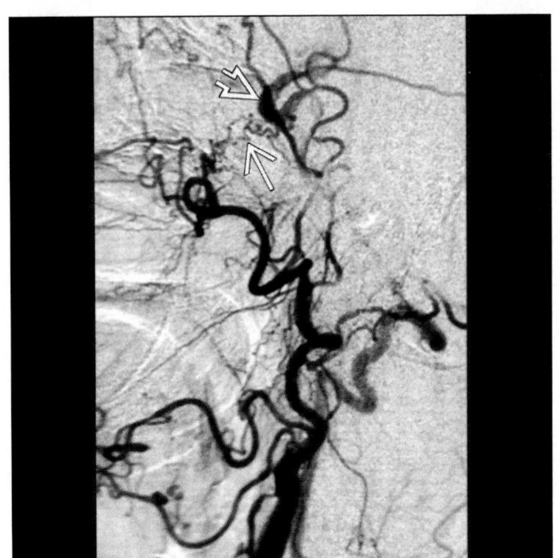

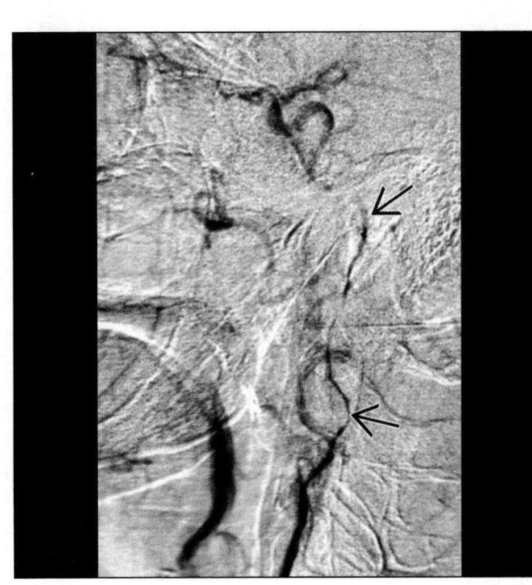

(Left) *Lateral DSA mid-arterial phase in the same patient shows filling of the right ECA and branches. The cervical ICA is not seen but reconstitutes distally in the cavernous sinus ➡ by collaterals from the internal maxillary artery to the lateral mainstem trunk ➡.* **(Right)** *Lateral angiography, late arterial phase in the same patient shows a "string" sign: A trickle of contrast fills a small, irregular cervical ICA ➡ with antegrade flow. This patient may be a candidate for carotid endarterectomy.*

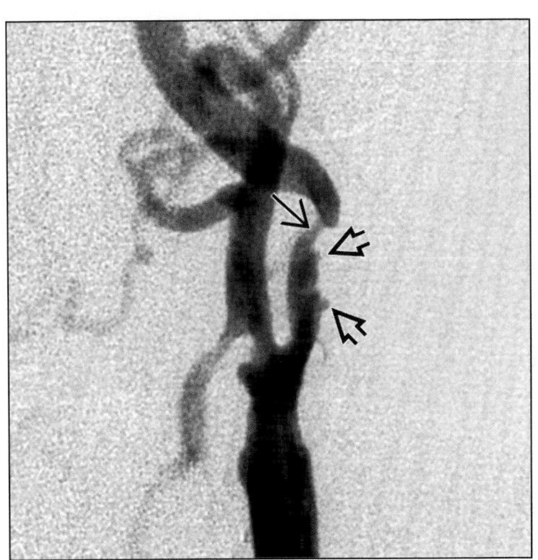

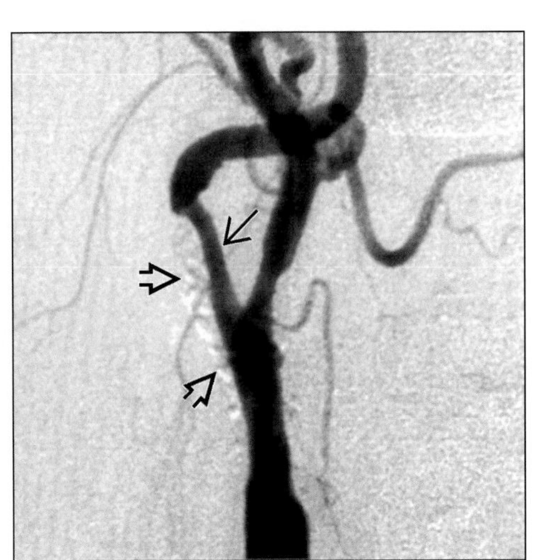

(Left) *Lateral angiography in a patient with left hemisphere TIAs shows a high-grade stenosis ➡ distal to the left ICA bulb. Multiple irregularities in the atherosclerotic plaque are seen here as outpouchings of contrast ➡. Irregularity is an independent risk factor for thromboembolic stroke, making this an "at risk" plaque.* **(Right)** *Lateral angiography in the same patient shows long-segment stenosis of the right ICA origin ➡. Note the subtraction artifact from dense wall calcification ➡.*

ARTERIOLOSCLEROSIS

Key Facts

Terminology
- Sclerosis of small-sized arteries (arterioles)
  - Common with chronic HTN &/or diabetes
  - May lead to vascular dementia

Imaging
- Multifocal white matter (WM) rarefaction on CT
- Patchy/confluent ↑ T2/FLAIR hyperintensities
  - Broad or confluent base with ventricles
  - Periventricular > deep > juxtacortical involvement
- Findings nonspecific
  - Large number of causes other than arteriopathy
  - Demyelination, infection, inflammatory, drug related, metabolic
- Caused by several types of arteriopathy
  - Arteriolosclerosis
  - Chronic hypertension (more basal ganglia, periventricular white matter involvement)
  - Diabetes mellitus (more peripheral involvement)
  - Cerebral autosomal dominant arteriopathy with subcortical infarcts and leukoencephalopathy (CADASIL)
  - Cerebral amyloid angiopathy (peripheral WM, cortex, meninges)

Clinical Issues
- Clinical and radiographic picture overlaps
  - Multi-infarct (vascular) dementia (VaD)
  - Subcortical arteriosclerotic encephalopathy (SAE; Binswanger disease)
- VaD caused by arteriolosclerosis or multiple cortical/ subcortical infarcts

Diagnostic Checklist
- Use FLAIR, T2* (GRE, SWI) sequences in all elderly patients
  - Look for microbleeds (HTN, CAA)

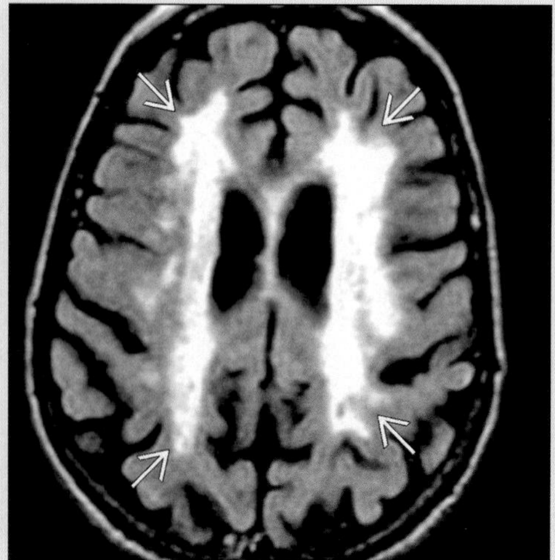
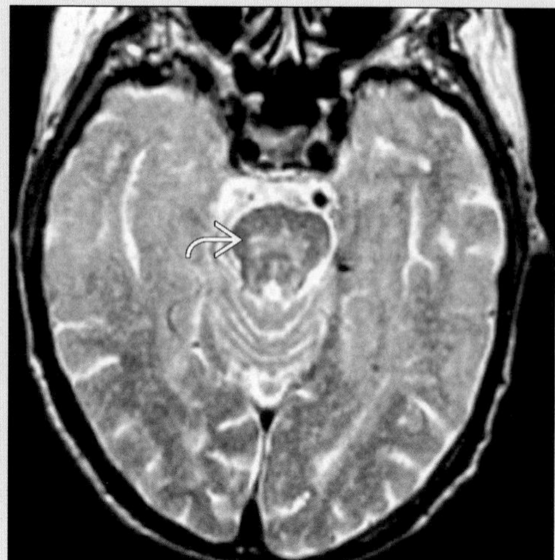

(Left) *Axial FLAIR MR shows moderate atrophy and confluent hyperintensity in the periventricular and deep white matter* ➔ *with mild juxtacortical involvement, rather typical for severe arteriolosclerosis in this elderly, demented, hypertensive patient.* ***(Right)*** *Axial T2WI MR in the same patient shows typical patchy central hyperintensity in the pons* ➔ *due to arteriolosclerosis. Note sparing of white matter around the corpus callosum, a common location for demyelinating lesions.*

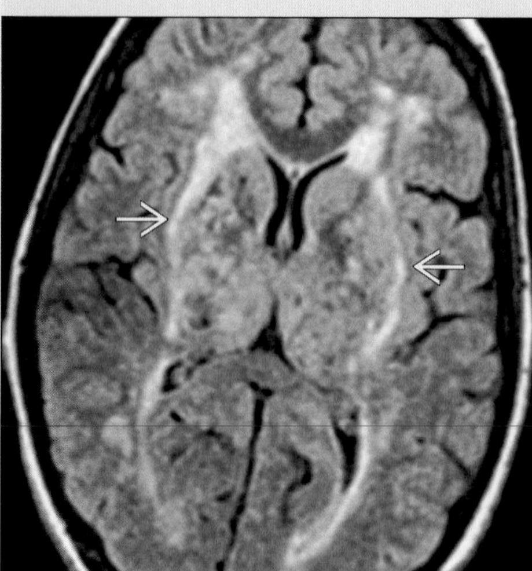
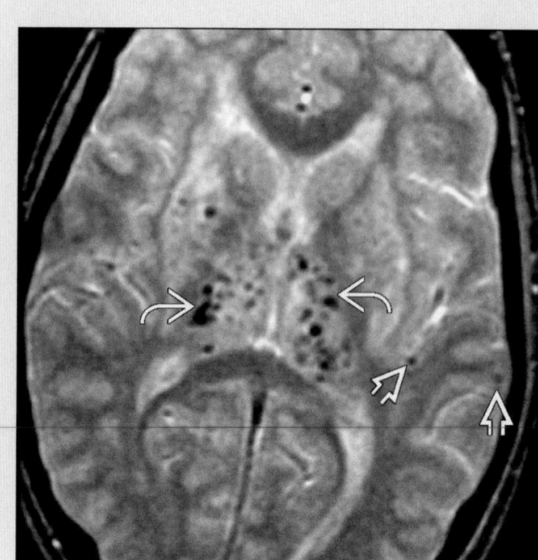

(Left) *Axial FLAIR MR shows multiple areas of increased signal in the basal ganglia, subinsular white matter* ➔*, and the deep and periventricular white matter, typical for modest changes of arteriolosclerosis.* ***(Right)*** *Axial T2* GRE MR in the same patient shows multiple areas of "blooming" in the basal ganglia* ➔ *and few peripheral hypointensities* ➔ *typical of the microbleeds of chronic hypertension. GRE is very helpful in determining the underlying cause as a microbleed site is diagnostic.*

TERMINOLOGY

Synonyms

- Small vessel disease, microangiopathy
- Imaging correlate = leukoaraiosis or periventricular leukoencephalopathy

Definitions

- Sclerosis of small-sized arteries (arterioles)
  - Commonly from chronic HTN &/or diabetes mellitus (DM)
  - May lead to vascular dementia

IMAGING

General Features

- Best diagnostic clue
  - White matter (WM) rarefaction on CT
  - Patchy/confluent hyperintensity on T2WI/FLAIR
- Location
  - Periventricular white matter (PVWM), deep WM
    - Broad or confluent base with ventricle
    - Periventricular > deep > juxtacortical involvement
  - Basal ganglia
    - More basal ganglia involvement with chronic HTN
    - More peripheral WM involvement
      - Diabetes mellitus, cerebral amyloid angiopathy (CAA)
- Size
  - Varies, progresses with age
- Morphology
  - Bilateral patchy or confluent

CT Findings

- NECT
  - Multifocal/confluent ill-defined hypodense areas ≥ 5 mm
  - Broad or confluent base with ventricles
    - Periventricular > deep > juxtacortical involvement
- CECT
  - No enhancement

MR Findings

- T1WI
  - Patchy or confluent PVWM hypointense foci
- T2WI
  - Ill-defined hyperintensities ≥ 5 mm
- PD/intermediate
  - Patchy or confluent PVWM hyperintense foci
- FLAIR
  - Most conspicuous sequence for PVWM hyperintensities
  - Significance of PVWM hyperintensities is controversial
    - Findings nonspecific
    - Likely due to several types of arteriopathy, many of which are combined
      - Arteriolosclerosis
      - Chronic hypertension &/or diabetes mellitus
      - Cerebral amyloid angiopathy
      - Cerebral autosomal dominant arteriopathy with subcortical infarcts and leukoencephalopathy (CADASIL)
- T2* GRE
  - Multifocal "black dots" on T2* are seen, more commonly with chronic hypertension, amyloid angiopathy
- DWI
  - No associated restriction, unless acute lesion
- T1WI C+
  - Nonenhancing
- MRS
  - Reduced N-acetyl aspartate (NAA), NAA/Cr
- ± generalized atrophy (large ventricles, sulci)
- Extensive/confluent lesions found in 2-6% of normal elderly

Angiographic Findings

- Conventional
  - Small and larger vessel arterial stenoses common

Nuclear Medicine Findings

- PET/SPECT: In absence of atrophy, rCBF/rMRGlu usually normal

Imaging Recommendations

- Best imaging tool
  - MR
- Protocol advice
  - NECT screening, MR with FLAIR + GRE

DIFFERENTIAL DIAGNOSIS

Age-Related White Matter Changes

- Significant overlap with normal vs. demented elderly
- Normal rCBF
- Other risk factors (hypertension, DM) common

Perivascular (Virchow-Robin) Spaces (PVSs)

- Variable size, well delineated
- Most common around anterior commissure, deep white matter
- Signal, attenuation like CSF
- Peripheral high signal on FLAIR can be seen with both lacunar infarcts and perivascular spaces

Demyelinating Disease

- MS > ADEM
- Usually ovoid, periventricular
- Callososeptal interface involved (rare with ASVD)

Vascular Dementia (VaD) Overlaps with Arteriolosclerotic Disease

- Cognitive impairment
  - Multi-infarct dementia (MID)
  - Subcortical arteriosclerotic encephalopathy (Binswanger-type vascular dementia)
    - Clinical (not imaging) diagnosis
      - Longstanding hypertension, progressive decline in mental function, gait disturbances, ± minor strokes
- Large, small infarcts
- Decreased rCBF

CADASIL

- Younger patient (≤ 40) with PVWM hyperintensities
- Stronger predilection for anterior temporal lobe involvement than other PVWM hyperintensities

PATHOLOGY

General Features

- Etiology
  - Hypertensive occlusive disease of small penetrating arteries
    - Results in lacunar infarcts, deep white matter lesions
  - Venous collagenosis (controversial)
- Genetics
  - General risk factors for peripheral/cerebral vascular diseases
    - APOE ϵ4 alleles
    - Angiotensinogen gene promoter
  - CADASIL
    - *NOTCH3* mutations
- Associated abnormalities
  - Microangiopathy-related cerebral damage = PVWM hyperintensities, lacunar infarcts
  - PVWM hyperintensities on imaging does not always have pathologic correlate

Staging, Grading, & Classification

- European Task Force on Age-Related White Matter Changes (ARWMC) rating scale for MR and CT (for ill-defined lesions ≥ 5 mm)
  - White matter lesions
    - 0 = no lesions (including symmetrical caps, bands)
    - 1 = focal lesions
    - 2 = beginning confluence of lesions
    - 3 = diffuse involvement, ± U-fibers
  - Basal ganglia lesions
    - 0 = no lesions
    - 1 = 1 focal lesion (≥ 5 mm)
    - 2 = > 1 focal lesion
    - 3 = confluent lesions

Gross Pathologic & Surgical Features

- Prominent sulci, ventricles common
- Periventricular WM spongiosis
- Multifocal lacunes often present

Microscopic Features

- Normal age-related changes
- Imaging PVWM hyperintensities have spectrum of histopathologic correlates
  - Degenerated myelin (myelin "pallor")
  - Axonal loss, increased intra-/extracellular fluid
  - Gliosis, spongiosis
  - Arteriosclerosis, small vessel occlusions
  - Dilated perivascular spaces

CLINICAL ISSUES

Presentation

- Most common signs/symptoms
  - Broad range
    - From normal, minimal cognitive impairment to dementia
- Clinical profile
  - Older patient with cerebrovascular risk factors (hypertension, hypercholesterolemia, diabetes, etc.)

Demographics

- Age
  - PVWM hyperintensities almost universal after 65 years
  - Lacunar infarcts in 1/3 of asymptomatic healthy patients > 65 years
- Gender
  - M = F
- Epidemiology
  - Vascular dementia (VaD): 3rd most common cause of dementia (after Alzheimer disease, Lewy body disease), accounts for 15% of cases
  - VaD is caused by arteriolosclerosis or multiple cortical/subcortical infarcts

Natural History & Prognosis

- Little known

Treatment

- Modification of known cerebrovascular risk factors

DIAGNOSTIC CHECKLIST

Consider

- Use FLAIR, T2* (GRE, SWI) sequences in all elderly patients
- GRE hypointensities suggest chronic hypertension or amyloid
- More peripheral hyperintensities suggest diabetes or amyloid
- Anterior temporal lobe involvement in middle-aged patient suggests CADASIL

Image Interpretation Pearls

- Many causes of PVWMs other than arteriopathy (demyelination, infection, inflammatory, drug related, metabolic)
- Clinical + imaging findings overlap with multi-infarct (vascular) dementia, subcortical arteriosclerotic encephalopathy (Binswanger disease)

SELECTED REFERENCES

1. Kimberly WT et al: Silent ischemic infarcts are associated with hemorrhage burden in cerebral amyloid angiopathy. Neurology. 72(14):1230-5, 2009
2. Vernooij MW et al: Use of antithrombotic drugs and the presence of cerebral microbleeds: the Rotterdam Scan Study. Arch Neurol. 66(6):714-20, 2009
3. Matsusue E et al: White matter changes in elderly people: MR-pathologic correlations. Magn Reson Med Sci. 5(2):99-104, 2006
4. Viswanathan A et al: Cerebral microhemorrhage. Stroke. 37(2):550-5, 2006
5. Yip AG et al: APOE, vascular pathology, and the AD brain. Neurology. 65(2):259-65, 2005
6. Arboix A et al: New concepts in lacunar stroke etiology: the constellation of small-vessel arterial disease. Cerebrovasc Dis. 17 Suppl 1:58-62, 2004

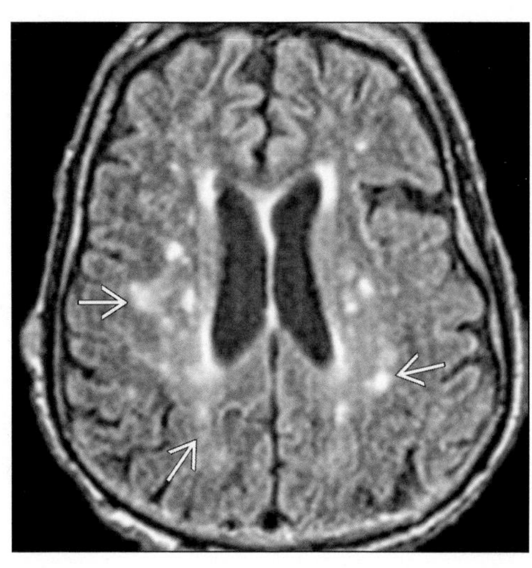

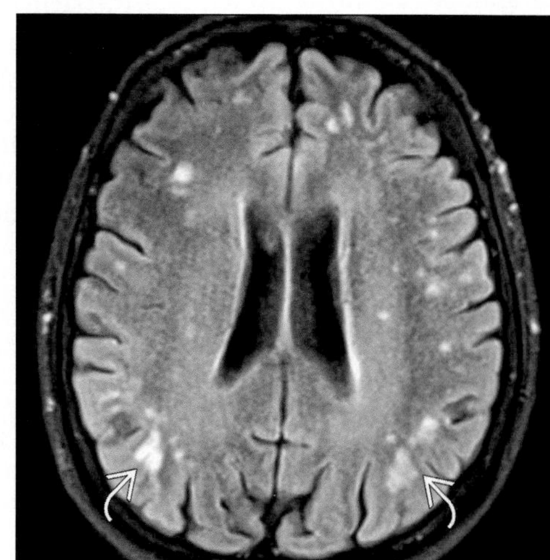

(Left) *Axial FLAIR MR shows multifocal hyperintensities in the central white matter ➔ with lesser involvement of the periventricular WM, a typical distribution in arteriolosclerosis related to diabetes mellitus. FLAIR is superior for periventricular foci of high signal and differentiating perivascular spaces from arteriolosclerosis.* ***(Right)*** *Axial FLAIR MR in a cognitively normal 72-year-old shows numerous nonconfluent WM hyperintensities ➔, findings consistent with age-related microvascular disease.*

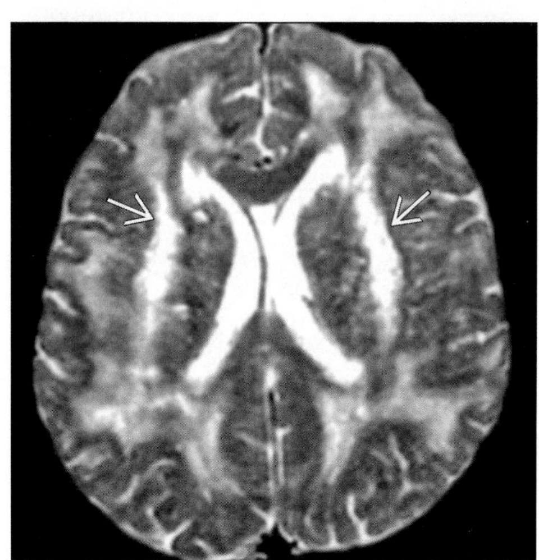

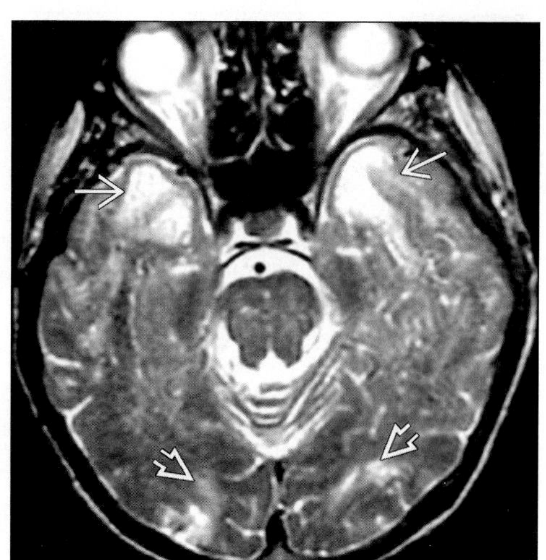

(Left) *Axial T2WI FS MR shows striking confluent hyperintensity throughout the white matter, very prominent in the external capsules ➔, with callosal sparing and minimal atrophy.* ***(Right)*** *Axial T2WI MR in the same patient shows prominent hyperintensity in the subcortical white matter of the anterior temporal lobes ➔, rarely seen in typical arteriolosclerosis, but characteristic of CADASIL. Note also the foci of increased signal in the midbrain & the occipital lobes ➔, which are not specific.*

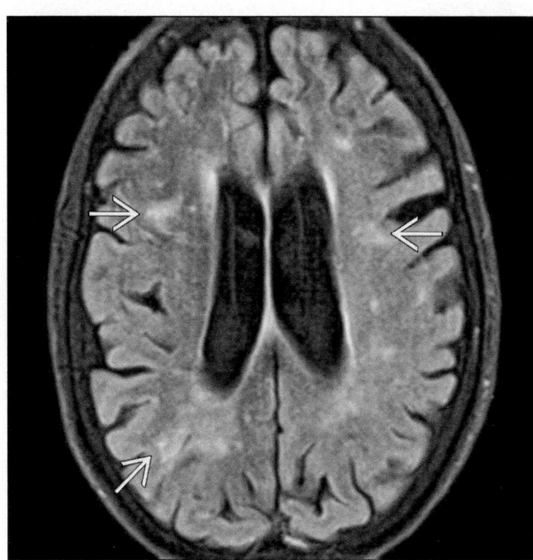

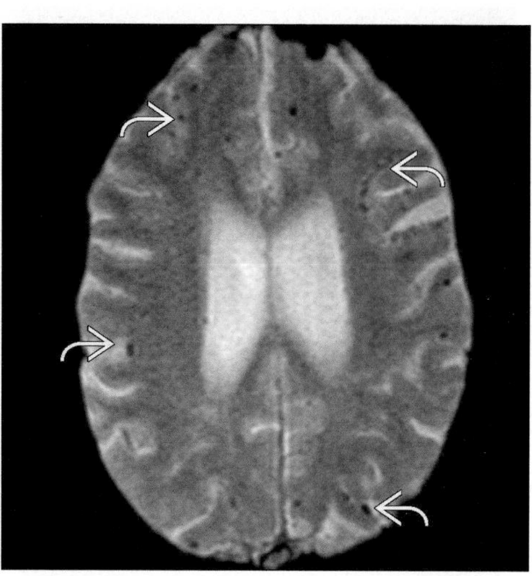

(Left) *Axial FLAIR MR shows moderate diffuse volume loss with enlarged sulci & ventricles and scattered irregular deep & peripheral white matter hyperintensities ➔, a nonspecific finding in this 47-year-old with amyloid angiopathy.* ***(Right)*** *Axial T2* GRE MR in the same patient shows innumerable blooming foci in the cortical & juxtacortical supratentorial parenchyma ➔ with sparing of the basal ganglia, characteristic of amyloid angiopathy. The patient is very young for amyloid; likely familial.*

ABERRANT INTERNAL CAROTID ARTERY

Key Facts

Terminology

- AbICA: Congenital vascular anomaly resulting from failure of formation of extracranial ICA with arterial collateral pathway

Imaging

- Appearance of AbICA on thin-section (< 1 mm) temporal bone CT is diagnostic
- AbICA appears as tubular lesion crossing middle ear posterior to anterior
- Enlarged inferior tympanic canaliculus important observation
- Caveat: Do not mistake AbICA for glomus tympanicum paraganglioma!

Top Differential Diagnoses

- Vascular middle ear lesion
  - Glomus tympanicum paraganglioma
  - Dehiscent jugular bulb
  - Lateralized internal carotid artery

Pathology

- Best explanation: "Alternative blood flow" theory
  - Persistence of pharyngeal artery system means C1 portion of ICA absent
  - Mature arterial collateral system compensates for absent C1 and vertical petrous ICA segments
  - Ascending pharyngeal artery ⇒ inferior tympanic artery ⇒ caroticotympanic artery ⇒ posterolateral aspect of horizontal petrous ICA
- 30% of AbICA have persistent stapedial artery

Clinical Issues

- Discovered at time of routine physical exam, during middle ear surgery, or as incidental imaging finding
- Associated symptoms: Pulsatile tinnitus and conductive hearing loss

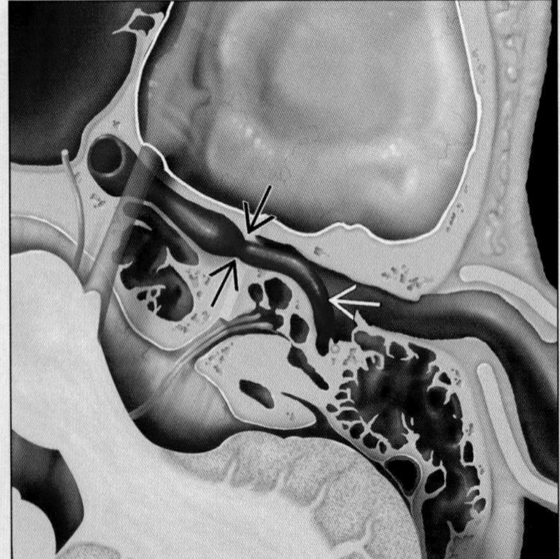

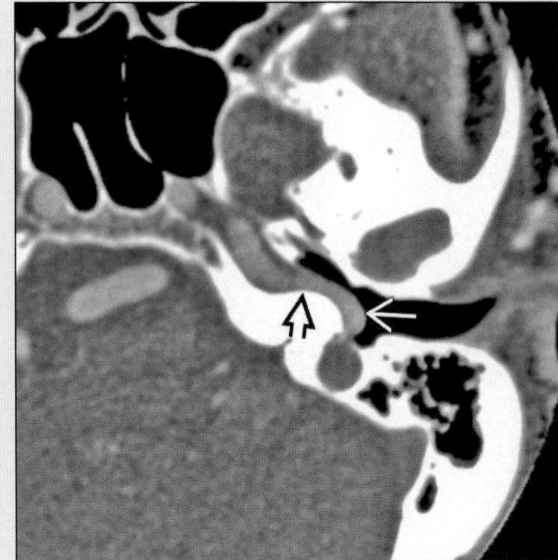

(Left) *Axial graphic of the left temporal bone illustrates a classic AbICA ➔ rising along the posterior cochlear promontory, crossing along the medial middle ear wall to rejoin the horizontal petrous ICA ➔. At the point of reconnection, stenosis is often present.* ***(Right)*** *Axial CTA image through the middle ear shows the looping aberrant internal carotid ➔ on the low cochlear promontory. Note the caliber change ➔ as the AbICA rejoins the normal horizontal segment of the ICA.*

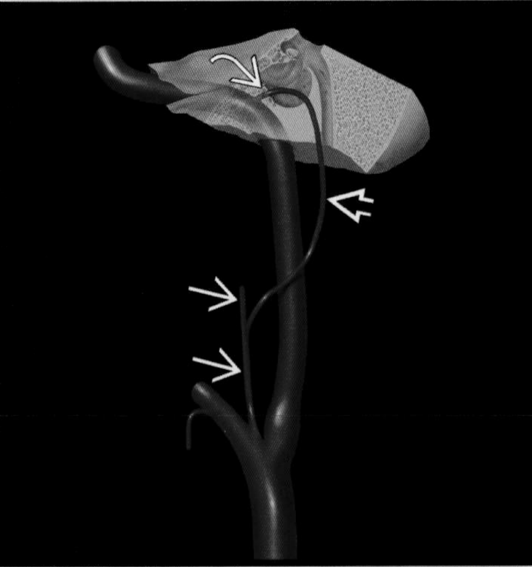

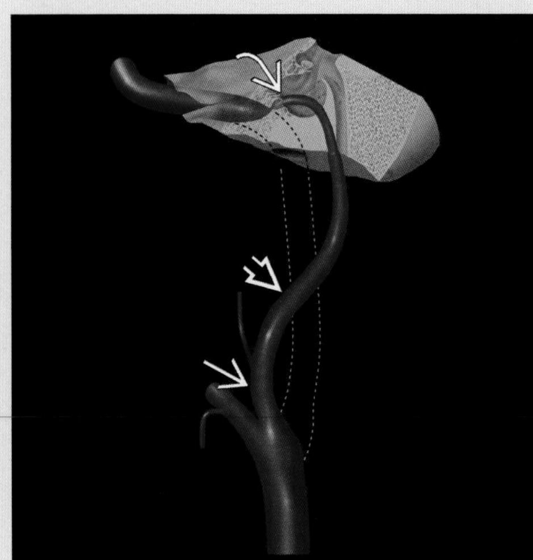

(Left) *Lateral graphic of adult suprahyoid and petrous ICA reveals the inferior tympanic artery ➔ branching off the ascending pharyngeal artery ➔, passing into the T-bone to anastomose with the very small caroticotympanic artery ➔ on the cochlear promontory.* ***(Right)*** *Lateral graphic depicts failure of the cervical ICA to develop (dotted lines) with the ascending pharyngeal ➔, inferior tympanic ➔, and caroticotympanic ➔ arteries providing an alternative collateral arterial channel (AbICA).*

ABERRANT INTERNAL CAROTID ARTERY

TERMINOLOGY

Abbreviations

- Aberrant internal carotid artery (AbICA)

Synonyms

- Lateral internal carotid artery (ICA)
- Aberrant carotid artery

Definitions

- Congenital vascular anomaly resulting from failure of formation of extracranial ICA with arterial collateral pathway

IMAGING

General Features

- Best diagnostic clue
  - Tubular structure running horizontally through middle ear cavity from posterior to anterior
- Location
  - Enters posterior middle ear through enlarged inferior tympanic canaliculus
    - Posterior and lateral to expected site of petrous carotid canal
  - Courses anteriorly across cochlear promontory to join horizontal petrous ICA through dehiscent carotid plate
- Size
  - Smaller than horizontal petrous ICA
- Morphology
  - Tubular morphology is key observation

CT Findings

- CECT
  - Enhancement equivalent to other arteries
    - **Caution**: Glomus tympanicum paraganglioma also enhances
      - Use morphology to differentiate tubular AbICA from ovoid paraganglioma
- Bone CT
  - Appearance of AbICA on thin-section (< 1 mm) temporal bone CT is diagnostic
  - Axial bone CT
    - AbICA appears as tubular lesion crossing middle ear posterior to anterior
    - **Enlarged inferior tympanic canaliculus** important observation
      - Anteromedial to stylomastoid foramen and mastoid segment of facial nerve
    - Smaller AbICA often stenotic at point of reconnection with horizontal petrous ICA
    - Carotid foramen and vertical segment of petrous ICA are absent
  - Coronal bone CT
    - AbICA appears as round, soft tissue lesion on cochlear promontory
      - Single slice looks disturbingly like glomus tympanicum paraganglioma
      - **Caveat**: Do not mistake AbICA for glomus tympanicum paraganglioma!
      - Tubular nature of AbICA is key observation
    - Inferior tympanic canaliculus is vertical tube posterolateral to normal location of vertical segment of petrous ICA
      - Rises at coronal level of round window niche
  - If **persistent stapedial artery** associated
    - Absent foramen spinosum
    - Enlarged anterior tympanic segment of CN7 canal
- CTA
  - Diagnostic for AbICA
  - Usually not necessary as CT alone is diagnostic

MR Findings

- Conventional MR does not reliably identify AbICA
  - Low signal of bone is difficult to distinguish from low signal of arterial flow void
- MRA source and reformatted images show aberrant nature of vessel
  - AbICA enters skull base posterior and lateral, compared to normal contralateral side
  - Frontal reformat: Petrous segment of ICA extends laterally instead of medially
    - In left ear, AbICA looks like "7"
    - In right ear, AbICA looks like "reverse 7"

Angiographic Findings

- Frontal view: Petrous segment of ICA extends laterally instead of medially
- Lateral view: Absent extracranial course of suprabifurcation ICA (C1 segment)
  - Smaller caliber vessels rises from bifurcation posteriorly, looping back to horizontal segment of petrous ICA
    - Stenosis may be present at site of reconnection between AbICA and horizontal petrous ICA
- Conventional angiography no longer necessary to confirm imaging diagnosis
  - CTA or MRA sufficient if uncertainty arises from bone CT images

Imaging Recommendations

- Best imaging tool
  - T-bone CT: Tubular morphology and posterolateral position diagnostic
    - Contrast CT not necessary
- Protocol advice
  - Bone CT: < 1 mm axial and coronal images if possible
  - If MR is used, MRA is critical component

DIFFERENTIAL DIAGNOSIS

Glomus Tympanicum Paraganglioma

- Otoscopy: Rose-colored, pulsatile, retrotympanic mass
- Bone CT: Focal ovoid mass on cochlear promontory
- MR: T1WI C+ enhancing mass

Lateralized Internal Carotid Artery

- Otoscopy: Vague, vascular hue deep behind tympanic membrane
- Bone CT: Dehiscent lateral wall of petrous ICA genu

Aneurysm, Petrous Internal Carotid Artery

- Otoscopy: Negative unless large
- Bone CT: Focal, smooth, petrous ICA canal expansion

- ICA has normal course but focal ovoid, expansile section
- MR: MRA is diagnostic of nonthrombosed aneurysm

Dehiscent Jugular Bulb

- Otoscopy: Gray-blue retrotympanic mass in posteroinferior quadrant
- Bone CT: Focal absence of sigmoid plate
  - "Bud" from superolateral jugular bulb enters middle ear as "mass"

Cholesterol Granuloma, Middle Ear

- Otoscopy: Blue-black retrotympanic mass
- Bone CT: Appears identical to acquired cholesteatoma
- MR: High signal on T1 without contrast suggests diagnosis

PATHOLOGY

General Features

- Etiology
  - Etiology of AbICA is controversial
  - Best explanation: "Alternative blood flow" theory
    - Persistence of pharyngeal artery system means C1 portion of ICA is absent
    - Mature arterial collateral system compensates for absent C1 and vertical petrous ICA segments
      - Ascending pharyngeal artery ⇒ inferior tympanic artery ⇒ caroticotympanic artery ⇒ posterolateral aspect of horizontal petrous ICA
  - Results of absent extracranial ICA C1 segment
    - Ascending pharyngeal, inferior tympanic, and caroticotympanic arteries enlarge
    - Inferior tympanic canaliculus enlarges to accommodate enlarged inferior tympanic artery
    - Bony margin of posterolateral horizontal petrous ICA canal is penetrated at site of caroticotympanic artery origin
- Associated abnormalities
  - 30% of AbICA have **persistent stapedial artery**
    - Enlarged anterior tympanic segment of CN7 canal
    - Absent ipsilateral foramen spinosum

Gross Pathologic & Surgical Features

- Pulsatile aberrant artery is found in middle ear cavity

Microscopic Features

- Histologically normal artery

CLINICAL ISSUES

Presentation

- Most common signs/symptoms
  - Most commonly asymptomatic
    - Discovered at time of routine physical exam, during middle ear surgery, or as incidental imaging finding
  - Associated symptoms
    - Pulsatile tinnitus (PT) (pulse-synchronous sound)
      - May be subjective (only patient hears) or objective (patient and MD hear)
      - Objective PT: When stenosis present at junction of AbICA and normal horizontal petrous ICA
      - Subjective PT: Pulsatile sound may transmit directly through cochlear promontory to basal turn of cochlea
    - Conductive hearing loss
  - Otoscopy: Retrotympanic pink-red mass
    - Inferior aspect of tympanic membrane
    - May mimic paraganglioma

Demographics

- Age
  - Average at presentation: 38 years
- Gender
  - M < F in single study (N = 16)
- Epidemiology
  - Very rare disorder

Natural History & Prognosis

- No long-term sequelae reported with AbICA
- Poor prognosis results only if misdiagnosis ⇒ biopsy
  - Pseudoaneurysm may require endovascular repair
- If tinnitus is loud, AbICA can be debilitating

Treatment

- **No treatment** is best treatment
- Greatest risk is misdiagnosis leading to biopsy

DIAGNOSTIC CHECKLIST

Image Interpretation Pearls

- Radiologist must remain firm on imaging diagnosis despite clinical impression of paraganglioma
  - Biopsy or attempted resection of misdiagnosed AbICA can be disastrous
    - Hemorrhage, stroke, or death may result from vessel injury

Reporting Tips

- Report diagnosis; offer no differential diagnosis
- Equivocal report such as "cannot exclude paraganglioma" may lead to surgical intervention

SELECTED REFERENCES

1. Sauvaget E et al: Aberrant internal carotid artery in the temporal bone: imaging findings and management. Arch Otolaryngol Head Neck Surg. 132(1):86-91, 2006
2. Windfuhr JP: Aberrant internal carotid artery in the middle ear. Ann Otol Rhinol Laryngol Suppl. 192:1-16, 2004
3. Kojima H et al: Aberrant carotid artery in the middle ear: multislice CT imaging aids in diagnosis. Am J Otolaryngol. 24(2): 92-6, 2003
4. Roll JD et al: Bilateral aberrant internal carotid arteries with bilateral persistent stapedial arteries and bilateral duplicated internal carotid arteries. AJNR Am J Neuroradiol. 24(4):762-5, 2003
5. Jain R et al: Management of aberrant internal carotid artery injury: a real emergency. Otolaryngol Head Neck Surg. 127(5): 470-3, 2002
6. Davis WL et al: MR angiography of an aberrant internal carotid artery. AJNR Am J Neuroradiol. 12(6):1225, 1991
7. Lo WW et al: Aberrant carotid artery: radiologic diagnosis with emphasis on high-resolution computed tomography. Radiographics. 5(6):985-93, 1985

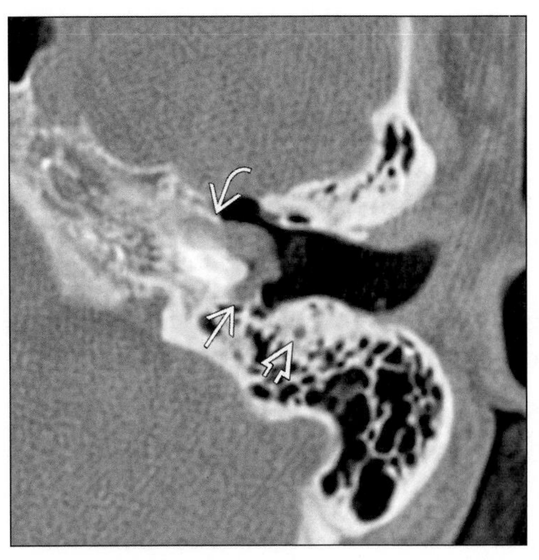

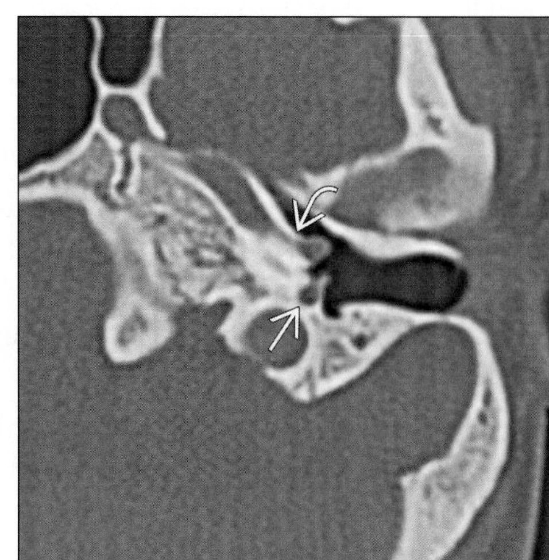

(Left) *Axial bone CT of the left ear shows a larger caliber AbICA entering the posteromedial middle ear cavity ➡, looping anteriorly across the low cochlear promontory to reconnect to the horizontal petrous ICA ➡. CN7 mastoid segment ➡ is posterolateral to AbICA.* ***(Right)*** *Axial bone CT reveals a smaller caliber AbICA entering the middle ear cavity through enlarged inferior tympanic canaliculus ➡, coursing across middle ear on cochlear promontory, and reentering the horizontal petrous ICA ➡.*

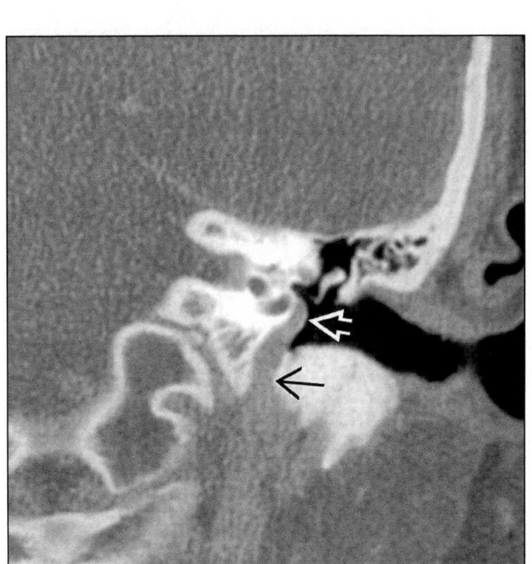

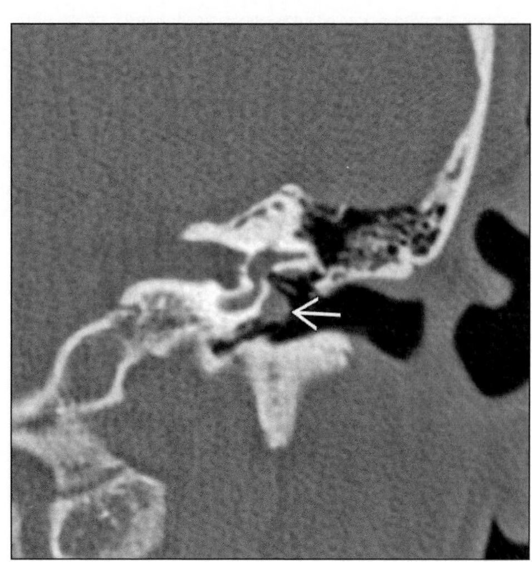

(Left) *Coronal bone CT of the left ear shows the posterior aspect of an AbICA with its enlarged inferior tympanic canaliculus ➡ and looping course ➡ up onto the cochlear promontory. The tubular configuration of the vessel should prevent misdiagnosis.* ***(Right)*** *Coronal left T-bone CT at the level of the oval window shows the AbICA ➡ as a "mass" located on the cochlear promontory resembling a glomus tympanicum paraganglioma. Accidental biopsy of AbICA may have devastating consequences!*

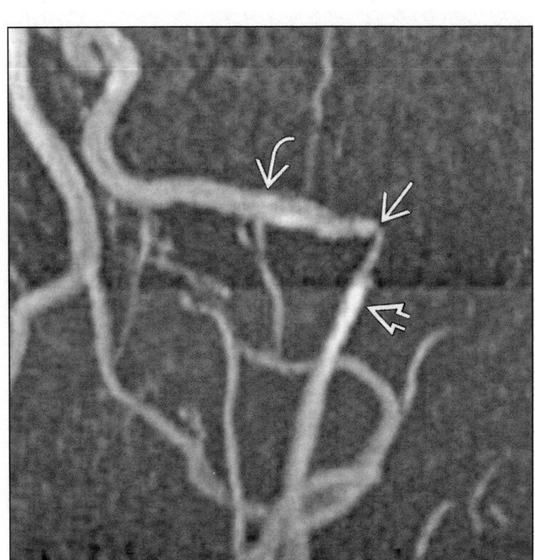

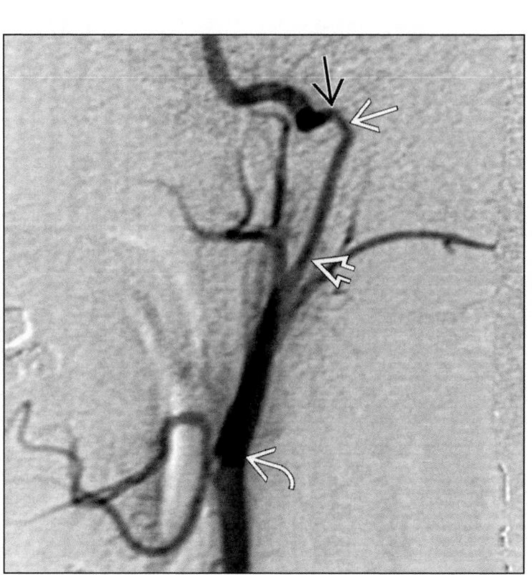

(Left) *Sagittal oblique MRA reveals an AbICA ➡ with significant stenosis ➡ at the junction where the AbICA rejoins the horizontal petrous ICA ➡. Notice the characteristic "7" shape to this left AbICA.* ***(Right)*** *Lateral internal carotid angiography of an AbICA reveals that the normal extracranial ICA is replaced by an enlarged collateral circuit including the ascending pharyngeal ➡, inferior tympanic ➡, and caroticotympanic ➡ arteries. Note the caliber change from AbICA to horizontal petrous ICA ➡.*

PERSISTENT CAROTID BASILAR ANASTOMOSES

Key Facts

Terminology

- Persistent carotid basilar anastomoses (PCBA)
- Vestigial carotid-basilar anastomoses
- Persistence of normally transient embryonic-type arterial supply from carotid to basilar system

Imaging

- Prominent unusual vessel between ICA and basilar artery (BA)
  - Levels distributed from tentorial hiatus to below foramen magnum, presumably at specific nerve levels (CN5, 8, 12; C1)
- Persistent trigeminal artery (PTA); from intracavernous ICA and BA
  - Most common (0.1-0.2%)
- Persistent otic artery (POA); from petrous ICA to BA through internal auditory canal (IAC)
  - Very rare
- Persistent hypoglossal artery (PHA); from cervical ICA (C1-2 level) to BA
  - Rare (0.03-0.26%)
- Proatlantal intersegmental artery (PIA); from cervical ICA (C2-3 level), or rarely ECA to vertebral artery between C1 and occiput
  - 3rd most common

Top Differential Diagnoses

- ICA origin of posterior cerebral artery (PCA)
- Secondary anastomoses

Pathology

- Named according to parallel CN

Clinical Issues

- Asymptomatic; no treatment (unless aneurysms)

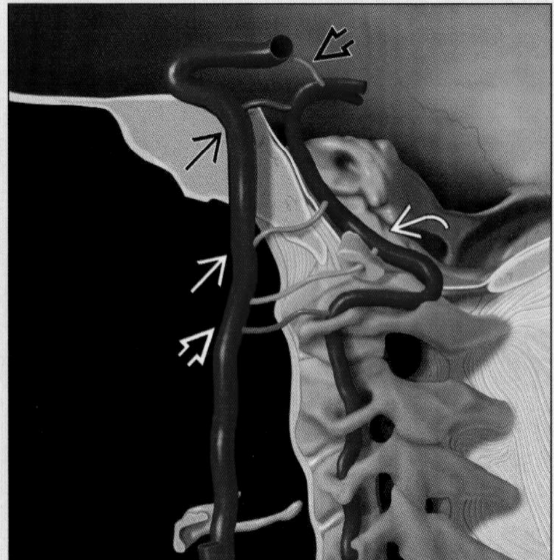

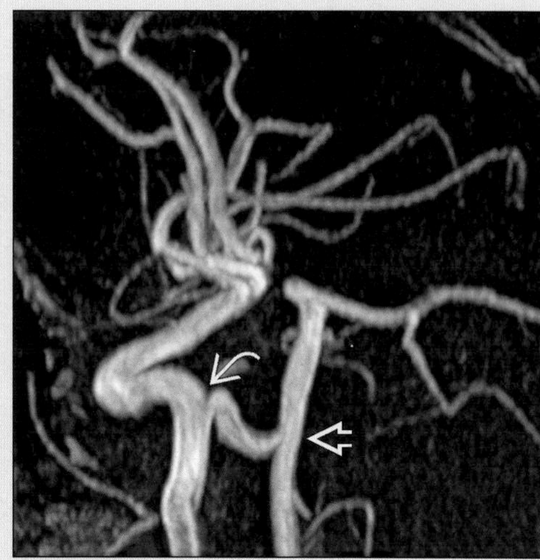

(Left) *Sagittal graphic shows anastomoses between ICA and VA. PCoA ⇨ connects PCA with supraclinoid ICA. The PTA → connects the cavernous ICA and BA. The POA ➡ connects the petrous ICA to the BA through the IAC. The PHA ➡ connects the cervical ICA and the VA through the hypoglossal canal. The proatlantal artery ➡ connects the cervical ICA and the VA through the occipito-atloidal space.* ***(Right)*** *Sagittal MRA shows the PTA connecting the proximal ICA siphon ➡ with the mid-BA ⇨.*

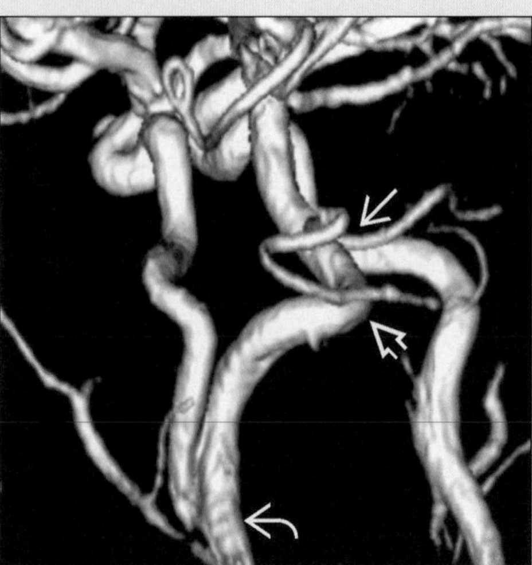

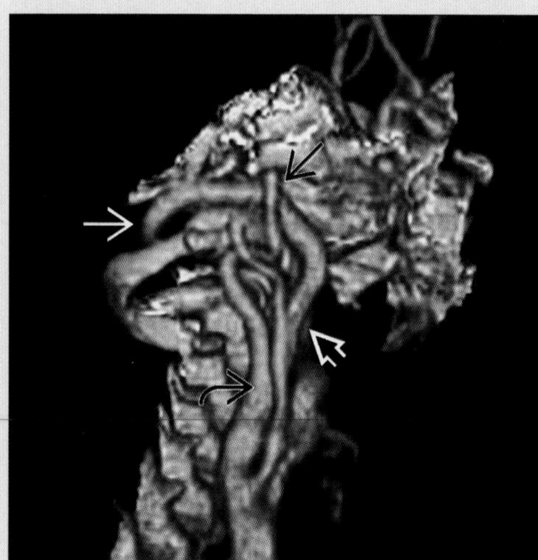

(Left) *Oblique MRA 3D surface rendering shows the PHA originating ➡ from the ICA, running vertically through the hypoglossal canal ➡ and joining the lower end of the BA ➡ like a vertebral artery.* ***(Right)*** *Oblique CTA 3D surface rendering shows PIA ➡ originating from the cervical ICA ⇨ running vertically before turning around the lateral mass of the atlas → to enter the dura in the lateral aspect of the occipitoatloidal space ➡ like a true vertebral artery before joining the BA.*

PERSISTENT CAROTID BASILAR ANASTOMOSES

TERMINOLOGY

Abbreviations

- Persistent carotid basilar anastomoses (PCBA)

Synonyms

- Vestigial carotid-basilar anastomoses

Definitions

- Persistence of normally transient embryonic-type arterial supply from carotid to basilar system

IMAGING

General Features

- Best diagnostic clue
  - Abnormal internal carotid artery (ICA)-basilar artery (BA) connection below level of posterior communicating artery (PCoA)
- Location
  - From sellar to occipito-vertebral level
- Morphology
  - Persistent trigeminal artery (PTA), from intracavernous ICA to BA, most common (0.1-0.2%)
    - Saltzman type 1: PTA supplies distal BA, PCoAs usually absent; proximal BA usually hypoplastic
    - Saltzman type 2: PTA fills superior cerebellar arteries, PCAs supplied via patent PCoAs
  - Persistent otic artery (POA), from petrous ICA to BA through internal auditory canal (IAC)
    - Vertebral arteries (VAs) absent or hypoplastic
  - Persistent hypoglossal artery (PHA), from cervical ICA (C1-2 level) to BA; rare (0.03-0.26%)
    - Parallels CN12 in hypoglossal canal
  - Proatlantal intersegmental artery (PIA); from cervical ICA (C2-3 level), or rarely external carotid (ECA) to VA between C1 and occiput (3rd most common)
    - Most caudal of PCBAs; VAs absent or hypoplastic

CT Findings

- CECT
  - Large caliber vessel between BA and ICA
- CTA
  - Delineates presence and course of vascular anomaly, associated abnormalities (e.g., saccular aneurysm)

MR Findings

- T2WI
  - Prominent unusual vessel between ICA and BA
    - Levels distributed from tentorial hiatus to below foramen magnum, presumably at specific nerve levels (CN5, 8, 12; C1)
- MRA
  - Depicts unusual vessel, its origin, course, and vertebrobasilar connection
  - Associated arterial anomalies (e.g., aneurysm)

Angiographic Findings

- Performed for other reasons (e.g., subarachnoid hemorrhage); shows vestigial artery and arterial flow

Imaging Recommendations

- Best imaging tool: MR and MRA

DIFFERENTIAL DIAGNOSIS

ICA Origin of Posterior Cerebral Artery (PCA)

- Common: Above sella, PCoA prominent, P1 segment of PCA hypoplastic/absent

Secondary Anastomoses

- To feed AV fistula
- To compensate for arterial occlusion/agenesis

PATHOLOGY

General Features

- Etiology
  - Unknown
- Associated abnormalities
  - 25% prevalence of other vascular anomalies
    - Controversial: Aneurysm (15%)
    - Rare: Carotid-cavernous fistula, arteriovenous malformation, arterial fenestration, moyamoya, neurofibromatosis type 1
    - Very rare: Absent CC/ICA, proximal subclavian artery, BA; aorta coarctation
- Embryology
  - Early transient segmental connections from ICA supply BA before intersegmental VAs develop
  - Named by cranial/spinal nerve they parallel
- Anatomy
  - Anatomic change in arterial supply associated with reorganized arterial pattern (hypoplastic/missing arterial segments)

CLINICAL ISSUES

Presentation

- Most common signs/symptoms
  - Incidental finding at imaging or SAH
    - Rarely trigeminal neuralgia or pituitary dysfunction

Natural History & Prognosis

- Asymptomatic; no treatment (unless aneurysms)

SELECTED REFERENCES

1. Vasović L et al: Proatlantal intersegmental artery: a review of normal and pathological features. Childs Nerv Syst. 25(4):411-21, 2009
2. Vasović L et al: Hypoglossal artery: a review of normal and pathological features. Neurosurg Rev. 31(4):385-95; discussion 395-6, 2008
3. Thayer WP et al: Surgical revascularization in the presence of a preserved primitive carotid-basilar communication. J Vasc Surg. 41(6):1066-9, 2005
4. Patel AB et al: Angiographic documentation of a persistent otic artery. AJNR Am J Neuroradiol. 24(1):124-6, 2003
5. Uchino A et al: Persistent trigeminal artery variants detected by MR angiography. Eur Radiol. 10(11):1801-4, 2000

SICKLE CELL DISEASE, BRAIN

Key Facts

Terminology

- Abnormality in hemoglobin (Hgb) → change in shape ("sickling") → ↑ "stickiness" of erythrocytes (RBCs) → capillary occlusions, ischemia, infarctions, premature RBC destruction (hemolytic anemia)

Imaging

- Best diagnostic clue
  - Cerebral infarct(s) in African-American child
  - Moyamoya (MM, secondary)

Top Differential Diagnoses

- Vasculitis
- Other causes of moyamoya (inherited & secondary)

Pathology

- Point mutation hemoglobin β gene, Chr 11p15.5: Glutamate ⇒ valine substitution
- Sickled RBCs adhere to endothelium ⇒ fragmentation of internal elastic lamina, degeneration of muscularis ⇒ large vessel vasculopathy ± aneurysm formation

Clinical Issues

- Stroke
  - 17-26% of all patients with SCD
  - 18x ↑ risk if transcranial Doppler velocities ICA/MCA > 200 cm/s
- 20% of children have WM infarcts on MR but no overt neurologic deficits = "silent infarcts"
  - 14x ↑ risk of stroke
- Regular blood transfusions keep Hgb S < 30%
  - ↓ stroke by up to 75%

Diagnostic Checklist

- Always consider SCD in African-American child with cerebral infarction

*(**Left**) Lateral scout image from a CT examination shows marked diploic thickening ➔ due to red marrow hyperplasia, causing a "hair on end" appearance. (**Right**) Sagittal T1WI MR shows calvarial thickening and ↓ marrow signal intensity ➔ secondary to red marrow hyperplasia caused by chronic anemia. Loss of normal T1 hyperintense fatty marrow is also seen in the cervical spine ➔. Iron deposition from repeat transfusions can also contribute to marrow signal abnormality.*

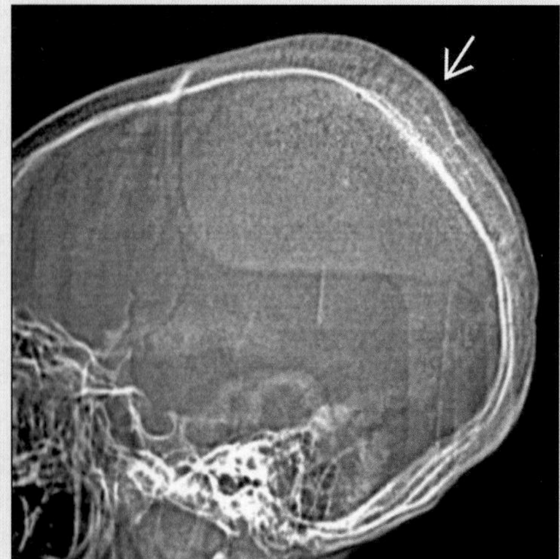

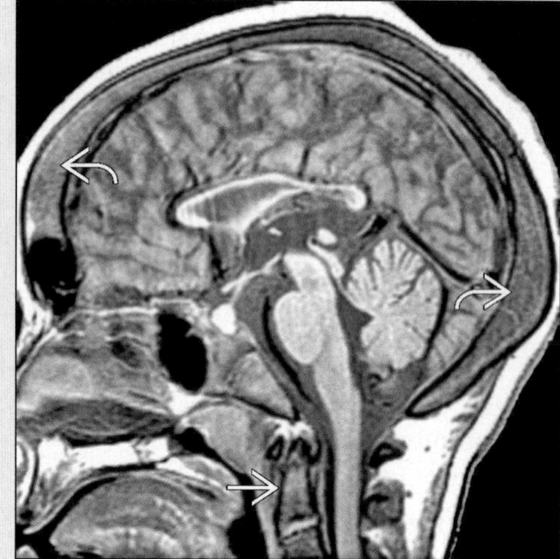

*(**Left**) Axial FLAIR MR shows considerable brain atrophy and signal hyperintensity due to chronic ischemic brain injury. Note the presence of "ivy" sign ➔, branching abnormal hyperintensity in the cerebral sulci. The "ivy" sign is thought to occur secondary to slow collateral flow in engorged pial vessels. (**Right**) Axial MRA in the same patient reveals distal bilateral internal carotid artery (ICA) occlusions ➔. Repetitive injury to the walls of the ICAs has resulted in severe secondary moyamoya.*

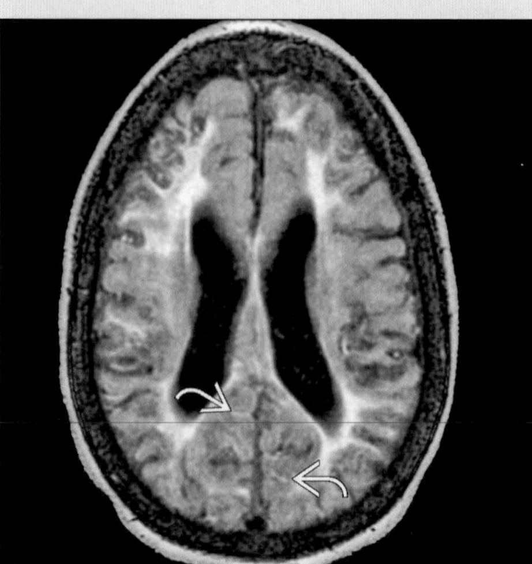

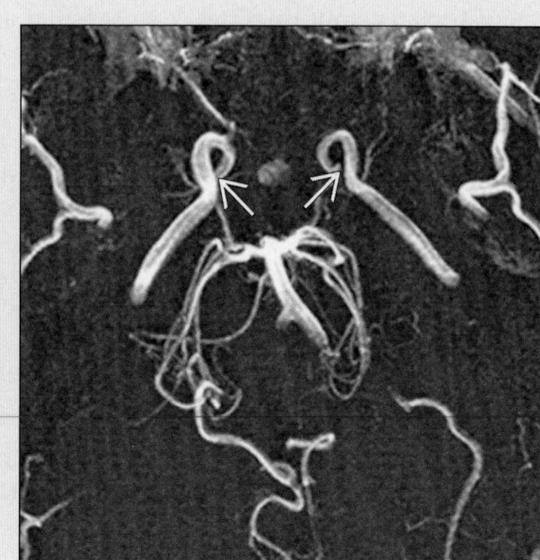

SICKLE CELL DISEASE, BRAIN

TERMINOLOGY

Abbreviations

- Sickle cell disease (SCD)

Definitions

- Abnormality in hemoglobin (Hgb) → change in shape ("sickling") → increased "stickiness" of erythrocytes (RBCs) → capillary occlusions, ischemia, infarctions, premature RBC destruction (hemolytic anemia)

IMAGING

General Features

- Best diagnostic clue
  - Cerebral infarct(s) in African-American child
  - Secondary moyamoya (MM)
    - Narrowing of distal internal carotid arteries or proximal anterior, middle cerebral arteries
    - Lenticulostriate collaterals in basal ganglia (BG)
- Location: ICAs, deep white matter (WM), cortex, bone marrow
- Cognitive impairment does not correlate with imaging findings

Radiographic Findings

- Radiography
  - Thick skull with expanded diploic space
  - Opacified paranasal sinuses

CT Findings

- NECT
  - Hypodense gray or WM infarct(s) → diffuse atrophy
  - Rare: Subarachnoid (SAH) or intraventricular hemorrhage (IVH) from SCD-related aneurysm or MM
- CECT: Punctate enhancement BG from MM collaterals
- CTA: Stenosis of distal ICA, proximal circle of Willis (COW)

MR Findings

- T1WI
  - Hemorrhagic infarcts may be seen
  - Punctate flow voids in BG correspond to MM collaterals
  - Decreased signal, expanded marrow (↑ red marrow)
- T2WI
  - Cortical, deep WM infarcts
    - Often in ACA/MCA watershed distribution
- FLAIR
  - Multifocal hyperintensities ± "ivy" sign of MM
- DWI: Diffusion restriction in acute infarcts
- PWI
  - ↑ cerebral blood flow (CBF) early: Adaptive response to anemia
  - ↓ CBF, ↑ mean transit time (MTT), ↑ time to peak (TTP) with arterial sludging, progressive COW narrowing
- T1WI C+: Vascular stasis and leptomeningeal collaterals in MCA territory with proximal MCA stenosis
- MRA
  - Enlarged, tortuous arteries early
    - Theory: Adaptive response to anemia and ↑ cerebral perfusion
  - Frequent eventual development of MM
  - Aneurysms in atypical locations
- MRS: ↑ lactate, ↓ NAA, ↓ Cho, ↓ Cr in areas of infarction (lactate seen only in acute infarctions)

Ultrasonographic Findings

- Transcranial Doppler (TCD): Hyperdynamic flow distal ICA/MCA secondary to proximal stenosis
  - Time-averaged mean velocities > 200 cm/s → high risk of ischemic stroke
  - Velocities between 170-200 cm/s, conditional

Angiographic Findings

- MM: Stenosis of distal ICA, proximal COW with BG and ECA → ICA collaterals
  - Association between MM with persistent primitive carotid-basilar arterial communications
- Fusiform aneurysms
- Peri-procedural risk of stroke higher than other populations: Hydrate, transfuse before catheter study

Nuclear Medicine Findings

- PET, SPECT: Focal areas of ↓ brain perfusion described

Imaging Recommendations

- Best imaging tool
  - MR/MRA ± DSA
- Protocol advice
  - DWI differentiates acute infarcts from chronic
  - Turbulent dephasing due to anemia, rapid flow can mimic stenosis on "bright blood" MRA: Use lowest possible TE for "bright blood" MRA or "black blood" MRA if stenosis suspected

DIFFERENTIAL DIAGNOSIS

Vasculitis

- Idiopathic, infectious, autoimmune, substance abuse
- Classic imaging findings: Cortical and deep WM infarcts and parenchymal hemorrhage

Moyamoya

- Primary moyamoya
  - Idiopathic, inherited
- Other causes of secondary MM
  - NF1, Down Syndrome, radiation therapy, connective tissue disease, prothrombotic states

Thick Skull with Expanded Diploe

- Other chronic anemias (thalassemia)

PATHOLOGY

General Features

- Etiology
  - Abnormal hemoglobin (Hgb S) becomes "stiff" when deoxygenated → RBCs become sickle-shaped
  - Sickled RBCs loose pliability to traverse capillaries → vascular occlusion ("crisis"), cell destruction (hemolysis)

SICKLE CELL DISEASE, BRAIN

- Sickled RBCs adhere to endothelium → fragments internal elastic lamina, degenerates muscularis → large vessel vasculopathy ± aneurysm formation
- Genetics
  - Point mutation of hemoglobin β gene, Chr 11p15.5: Glutamate ⇒ valine substitution
  - SCD: Autosomal recessive, both β-globin affected
  - Sickle cell trait: 1 β-globin affected → mild disease
    - Carrier
    - ↑ resistance to malaria (hence prevalence)
- Associated abnormalities
  - Anemia, reticulocytosis, granulocytosis
  - Susceptibility to pneumococcal infection (due to malfunctioning spleen)
  - Occasionally causes pseudotumor cerebri

Gross Pathologic & Surgical Features

- Bone, brain, renal, and splenic infarcts; hepatomegaly

Microscopic Features

- Severe anemia with sickled cells on smear
- Vascular occlusions due to masses of sickled RBCs

CLINICAL ISSUES

Presentation

- Most common signs/symptoms
  - Focal neurologic deficit
- Other signs/symptoms
  - Children: Learning difficulties, headache, psychiatric symptoms
- Clinical profile
  - African-American child with stroke
- Stroke
  - 17-26% of all patients with SCD
  - 11% by age 20, 24% by age 45
  - 75% ischemic, 25% hemorrhagic
  - 20% of children have WM infarcts on MR but no overt neurologic deficit = "silent infarcts"
    - TCD usually normal
    - Associated with mild cognitive impairment
    - 14x ↑ risk of stroke consistent with patients with normal MR
  - 18x ↑ risk of stroke if TCD velocity of ICA or MCA > 200 cm/s
- Bone infarcts, avascular necrosis during crisis
- Osteomyelitis, especially *Salmonella*
- Gross hematuria from renal papillary necrosis and ulceration
- Splenic infarction from exposure to high altitude (e.g., flying)
- Infections common, especially *Pneumococcus* after splenic infarction

Demographics

- Age
  - Children = adults
  - Stroke risk highest from 2-5 years of age
- Gender: No predilection
- Ethnicity: Found primarily in African-Americans and their decendents
- Epidemiology
  - Birth prevalence in African-Americans: 1/375
  - Birth prevalence of sickle cell trait: 1/12
  - Primary cause of stroke in African-American children
  - Incidence of cerebral lesions (MR) in patients with sickle cell trait: 10-19%

Natural History & Prognosis

- Unrelenting, severe hemolytic anemia beginning at few months of age after Hgb S replaces Hgb F (fetal)
- Cognitive dysfunction occurs even in absence of cerebral infarctions
- Repeated ischemic events → strokes with worsening motor and intellectual deficits
- Patients usually live to adulthood albeit with complications
- Prognosis poor for SCD without transfusions

Treatment

- Screening TCD
  - Detection ↑ velocity prompts brain MR and treatment with regular blood transfusions
  - Regular blood transfusions keep Hgb S < 30%
    - ↓ incidence of stroke by up to 75%
    - ↓ intimal hyperplasia COW vessels
- Hydroxyurea: ↓ incidence of painful crises and acute chest syndrome; may improve TCD velocities
  - Induces Hgb F, which ↓ vasoocclusion and hemolysis
- Penicillin prophylaxis; pneumococcal vaccine
- Bone marrow transplantation is only curative therapy
  - Available only to few who have HLA-matched donor
- On the horizon: Stem cell-based therapies

DIAGNOSTIC CHECKLIST

Image Interpretation Pearls

- Always consider SCD in African-American child with cerebral infarction

SELECTED REFERENCES

1. Helton KJ et al: Arterial spin-labeled perfusion combined with segmentation techniques to evaluate cerebral blood flow in white and gray matter of children with sickle cell anemia. Pediatr Blood Cancer. 52(1):85-91, 2009
2. Khademian Z et al: Reversible posterior leuko-encephalopathy in children with sickle cell disease. Pediatr Blood Cancer. 52(3):373-5, 2009
3. Dick MC: Standards for the management of sickle cell disease in children. Arch Dis Child Educ Pract Ed. 93(6):169-76, 2008
4. Al-Kandari FA et al: Regional cerebral blood flow in patients with sickle cell disease: study with single photon emission computed tomography. Ann Nucl Med. 21(8):439-45, 2007
5. Alam M et al: Cerebrovascular accident in sickle cell disease. J Coll Physicians Surg Pak. 13(1):55-6, 2003
6. Kral MC et al: Transcranial Doppler ultrasonography and neurocognitive functioning in children with sickle cell disease. Pediatrics. 112(2):324-31, 2003
7. Oguz KK et al: Sickle cell disease: continuous arterial spin-labeling perfusion MR imaging in children. Radiology. 227(2):567-74, 2003

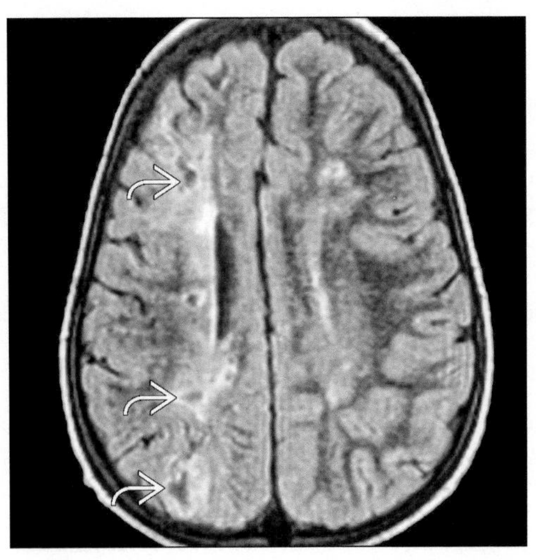

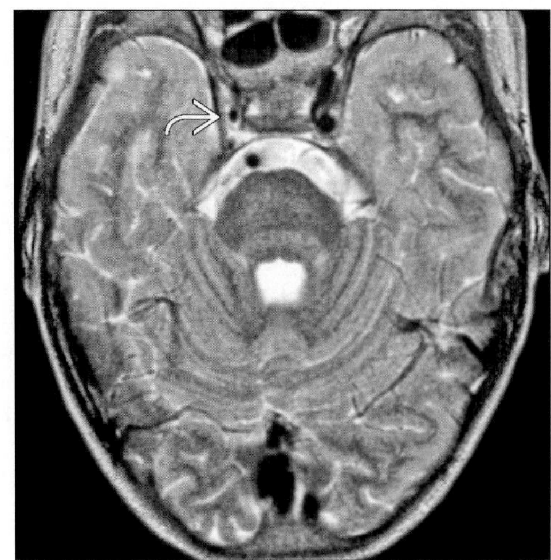

***(Left)** Axial FLAIR MR shows a characteristic appearance of the brain in SCD with bilateral deep white matter and cortical (on right) infarcts with foci of cystic encephalomalacia ➢. The infarcts are linearly arranged in the AP plane, a pattern consistent with watershed infarction. **(Right)** Axial T2WI MR in the same patient shows asymmetry of the internal carotid arteries (ICA) with ↓ caliber on the right ➢, the side with greater brain injury. Vessel narrowing is a result of sickle cell vasculopathy.*

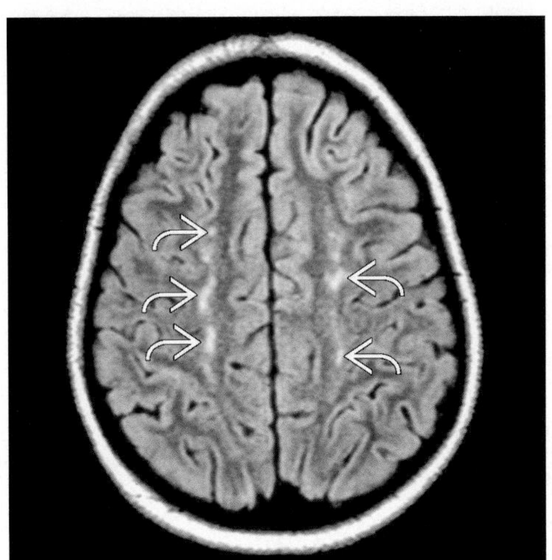

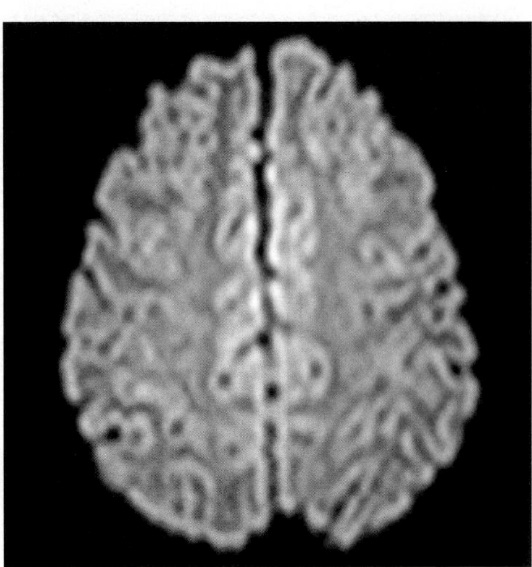

***(Left)** Axial FLAIR MR in an asymptomatic teenager with SCD shows multiple, small foci of increased signal ➢ in the deep white matter watershed. **(Right)** Axial DWI MR in the same patient shows no reduced diffusion to suggest acute infarction; the infarcts are "silent." There is MR evidence of infarct without overt neurologic abnormality and usually normal ICA/MCA velocities on TCD. Such patients often have mild cognitive impairment and are at increased risk of stroke.*

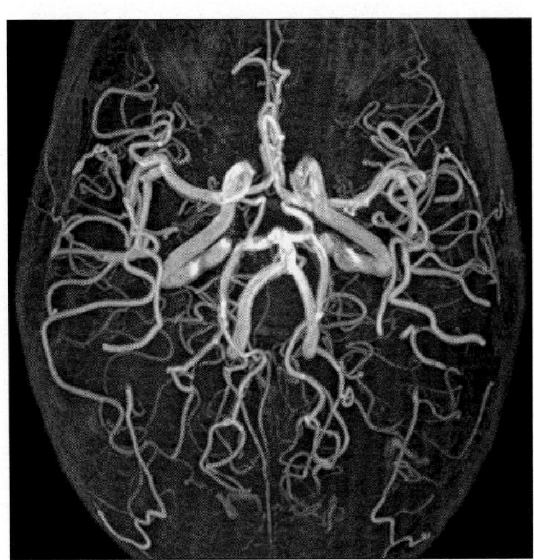

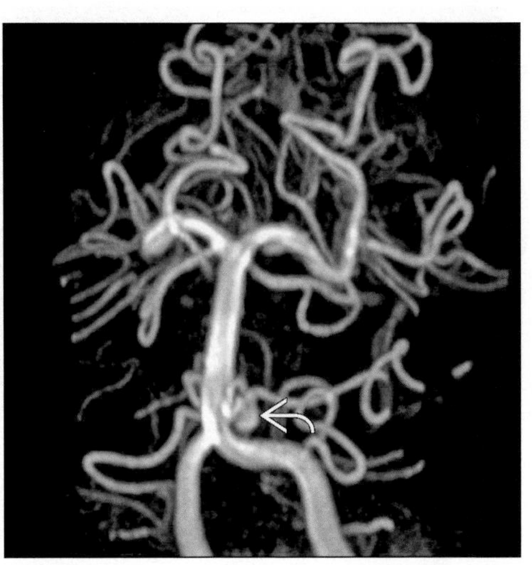

***(Left)** MRA collapsed view does not demonstrate narrowing of the distal ICAs, proximal ACAs, or proximal MCAs. The vessels are mildly enlarged and tortuous, thought to occur as a pathophysiologic response to anemia and ↑ cerebral perfusion. This progressive vasculopathy eventually results in large and small vessel injury. **(Right)** MRA in the same patient shows a proximal basilar artery aneurysm ➢. Patients with SCD are at ↑ risk of aneurysm, often in atypical locations.*

MOYAMOYA

Key Facts

Terminology

- Progressive narrowing of distal ICA and proximal circle of Willis (COW) vessels with secondary to collateralization
- Moyamoya disease = primary (idiopathic) moyamoya
  - More common in Japan, Korea
- Secondary moyamoya occurs in association with other disorders

Imaging

- Best diagnostic clue: Multiple punctate dots (CECT) and flow voids (MR) in basal ganglia (BG)
- "Puff of smoke" (moyamoya in Japanese) = cloud-like lenticulostriate and thalamostriate collaterals on angiography
- Best imaging tool: MR C+/MRA

Pathology

- Moyamoya disease
  - Inherited polygenic or AD with low penetrance
- Secondary moyamoya
  - Syndromes, inflammatory, prothrombotic states, premature aging, congenital mesenchymal defects

Clinical Issues

- Bimodal age peaks: 6 and 35 years
- Most frequent cause of stroke in Asian children
- Presentation (children): TIAs, alternating hemiplegia (exacerbated by crying), headache
- Presentation (adults): TIAs, cerebral infarct, or hemorrhage
- Treatment: Indirect (children) or direct bypass (more common adults)

*(**Left**) Coronal graphic shows severe tapering of both distal internal carotid arteries ➔ and strikingly enlarged lenticulostriate arteries ➔ coursing through basal ganglia. This is the "puff of smoke" (moyamoya) pattern. (**Right**) Axial T1WI MR shows multiple punctate flow voids ➔ representing enlarged lenticulostriate artery collaterals in the basal ganglia. Moyamoya-like collateralization may occur with any progressive vascular occlusive process.*

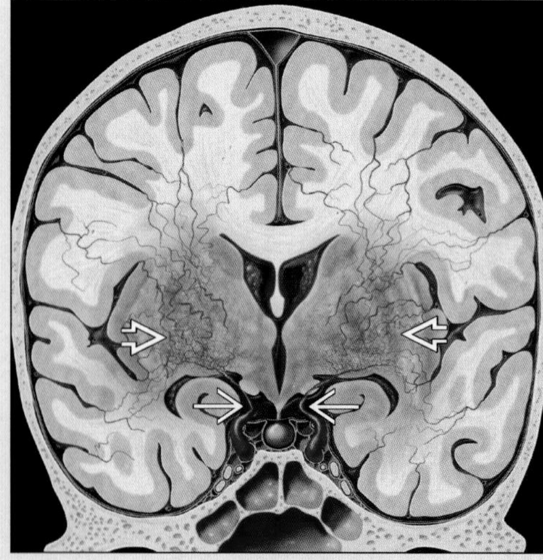

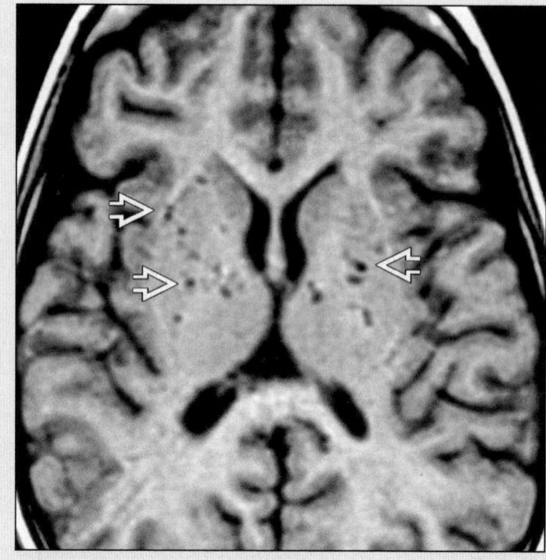

*(**Left**) Axial FLAIR MR shows advanced moyamoya with multifocal ischemic brain injury ➔. Punctate hyperintensities ➔ in the basal ganglia represent slow flow in enlarged lenticulostriate collaterals. Note the bilateral scalp defects ➔ from prior indirect bypass. (**Right**) Collapsed view MRA shows moyamoya on the right, with narrowing of the distal ICA and occlusion of the ACA and MCA. The lenticulostriate ➔ and anterior choroidal ➔ arteries are enlarged with branch extension of the latter.*

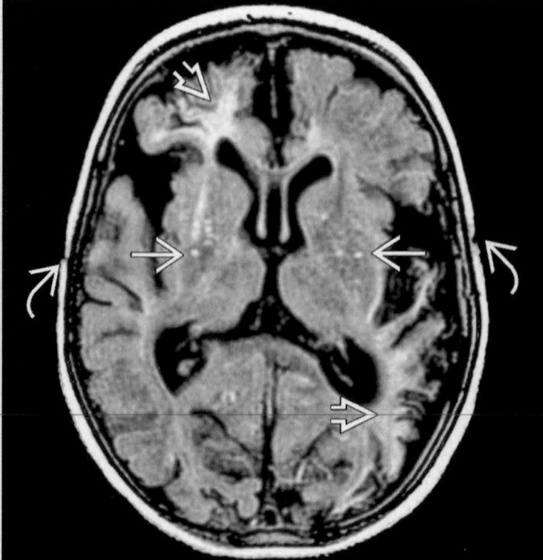

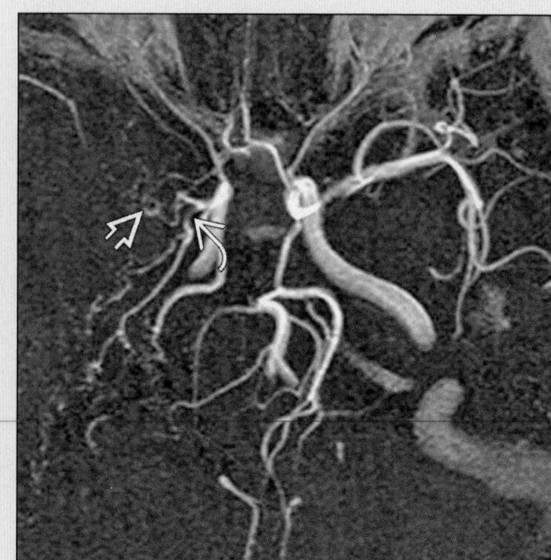

TERMINOLOGY

Synonyms

- Idiopathic progressive arteriopathy of childhood; spontaneous occlusion of circle of Willis

Definitions

- Progressive narrowing of distal internal carotid artery (ICA), proximal circle of Willis (COW) vessels with collateral flow
- Moyamoya disease = primary (idiopathic) moyamoya
  - More common Japan, Korea
- Secondary moyamoya occurs in association with other disorders

IMAGING

General Features

- Best diagnostic clue: Multiple punctate dots (CECT) and flow voids (MR) in basal ganglia (BG)
- Location: COW; anterior > > > posterior circulation
- Size: Large vessel occlusion
- Morphology: "Puff of smoke" (moyamoya in Japanese)
  - Cloud-like lenticulostriate and thalamostriate collaterals on angiography

CT Findings

- NECT
  - Children: 50-60% show anterior > posterior atrophy
  - Adults can present with intracranial hemorrhage
- CECT: Enhancing dots (large lenticulostriates) in BG and abnormal net-like vessels at base of brain
- CTA: Abnormal COW and net-like collaterals
- Xe-133 CT: ↓ cerebral reserve with acetazolamide challenge

MR Findings

- T1WI: Multiple dot-like flow voids in BG
- T2WI
  - ↑ signal small vessel cortical and white matter infarcts
  - Collateral vessels = net-like cisternal filling defects
- FLAIR
  - Bright sulci = leptomeningeal "ivy" sign
    - Slow-flowing engorged pial vessels, thickened arachnoid membranes
    - Correlates with decreased cerebral vascular reserve
- T2* GRE
  - Hemosiderin if prior hemorrhage
  - Asymptomatic microbleeds occasionally seen in adults
- DWI: Very useful for "acute on chronic" disease
- T1WI C+
  - Lenticulostriate collaterals ⇒ enhancing "dots" in BG and net-like thin vessels in cisterns
  - Leptomeningeal enhancement (contrast-enhanced "ivy" sign) ↓ after effective bypass surgery
- MRA: Narrowed distal ICA and proximal COW vessels, ± synangiosis
- MRV: Some vasculopathies may also involve veins
- MRS: Lactate in acutely infarcted tissue
  - NAA/Cr and Cho/Cr ratios frontal white matter improve/increase after revascularization
- PWI: ↓ perfusion in deep hemispheric white matter, relative ↑ perfusion in posterior circulation

Ultrasonographic Findings

- Grayscale: Reduction of ICA lumen size
- Pulsed Doppler
  - Doppler spectral waveforms in ICA show no flow (occluded) or high resistance (stenotic) flow pattern
  - ↑ end-diastolic flow velocity, ↓ vascular resistance in external CA (ECA) collaterals
- Color Doppler: Aliasing suggests stenoses
- Power Doppler: Contrast injection improves visualization of slow-flow stenotic vessels and collaterals

Angiographic Findings

- Conventional
  - Predominantly (not exclusively) anterior circulation
    - Narrow proximal COW and ICA (earliest)
    - Lenticulostriate and thalamoperforator collaterals (intermediate)
    - Transdural and transosseous EC-IC collaterals (late)
  - Dilatation and branch extension of anterior choroidal artery predicts adult hemorrhagic events

Nuclear Medicine Findings

- PET: ↓ hemodynamic reserve capacity
- SPECT I-123-iomazenil: Neuronal density preserved if asymptomatic, ↓ if symptomatic

Imaging Recommendations

- Best imaging tool: MR C+/MRA
- Protocol advice
  - Contrast improves detection: Synangiosis, collaterals
  - Catheter angiography defines anatomy of occlusions prior to bypass
- Diagnostic criteria: MR/MRA or catheter angiography
  - Stenosis/occlusion terminal ICA or proximal ACA and MCA
  - Abnormal vascular network/flow voids in BG
  - Bilateral; unilateral findings presumptive

DIFFERENTIAL DIAGNOSIS

"Ivy" Sign

- Leptomeningeal metastases, subarachnoid hemorrhage (SAH), meningitis, increased inspired oxygen

Punctate Foci in Basal Ganglia

- Cribriform lacunar state: No enhancement

Severely Attenuated Circle of Willis

- SAH, meningitis, tumor encasement

PATHOLOGY

General Features

- Etiology
  - Moyamoya disease
    - Inherited polygenic or AD with low penetrance
    - Gene loci: Chr 3p26-p24.2, Chr 17q25, Chr 8q23

MOYAMOYA

- Increase in growth factors, cytokines, adhesion molecules in CSF implicates inflammation
  - Secondary moyamoya
    - Down syndrome, tuberous sclerosis, sickle cell disease, connective tissue disease, progeria, NF1
      - NF1 + suprasellar tumor + radiation is disastrous
    - Morning glory syndrome; syndromes with aneurysms, cardiac and ocular defects
    - Inflammatory: CNS angiitis (of childhood), basal meningitis, atherosclerosis, H&N infections
    - Vasculopathies and prothrombotic states: XRT, Kawasaki, anticardiolipin antibody, factor V Leiden, polyarteritis nodosa, Behçet, SLE
- Epidemiology: Moyamoya disease
  - Incidence in Japan: 1:100,000
  - Incidence in North America, Europe: 0.1:100,000
  - 10-15% familial

Staging, Grading, & Classification

- Staging criteria (after Suzuki)
  - Stage 1: Narrowing of ICA bifurcation
  - Stage 2: ACA, MCA, PCA dilated
  - Stage 3: Maximal basal collaterals; small ACA/MCA
  - Stage 4: Fewer collaterals (vessels); small PCA
  - Stage 5: Further ↓ collaterals; absent ACA/MCA/PCA
  - Stage 6: Extensive ECA-pial collaterals

Gross Pathologic & Surgical Features

- Increased perforating (early) and ECA-ICA (late) collaterals in atrophic brain
- Hemorrhage (subarachnoid, intraventricular > parenchymal) adults
- Increased saccular aneurysms (especially basilar in adults)

Microscopic Features

- Intimal thickening and hyperplasia
- Excessive infolding, thickening internal elastic lamina
- Periventricular pseudoaneurysms (cause of hemorrhage)

CLINICAL ISSUES

Presentation

- Most common signs/symptoms
  - Children: Transient ischemic attacks (TIAs), alternating hemiplegia (exacerbated by crying), headache
  - Adults: TIAs, cerebral infarct, or hemorrhage
    - Hemorrhagic presentation more common in Asian adults
- Other signs/symptoms
  - Children: Developmental delay, poor feeding, chorea
- Clinical profile
  - Children more likely to have TIAs and to progress, adults more likely to infarct (but slower progression)
  - Children more likely to have ipsilateral anterior plus posterior circulation involvement

Demographics

- Age
  - Bimodal age peaks
    - Japan, Korea: 6 years > 35 years
    - North America, Europe: 35 years > 6 years
- Gender
  - M:F = 1:1.8; in familial cases, M:F = 1:5
- Most frequent cause of stroke in Asian children

Natural History & Prognosis

- Progressive narrowing, collateralization, and ischemia
- Prognosis depends on etiology, ability to form collaterals, age/stage at diagnosis
- Pediatric cases usually advance to stage V within 10 years of onset
  - Infantile moyamoya progresses faster
- Hemorrhagic moyamoya has poorer outcome

Treatment

- Moyamoya disease
  - Indirect bypass: Encephalo-duro-arterio-synangiosis (EDAS) more effective in children
    - 5-year risk of ipsilateral stroke post EDAS = 15%
  - Direct bypass: Superficial temporal artery-middle cerebral artery (STA-MCA) more common in adults
- Anticoagulation; correct/control prothrombotic states and inflammatory etiologies
- Hypertransfusion for sickle cell-related moyamoya
- Perivascular sympathectomy or superior cervical ganglionectomy (adults)

DIAGNOSTIC CHECKLIST

Consider

- Seek secondary causes of moyamoya

Image Interpretation Pearls

- Enhanced asymmetric atrophy found on childhood CT, look for abnormal vascular pattern
- Adult moyamoya can present with IC hemorrhage

Reporting Tips

- Successful revascularization = ↓ basal collaterals, ↑ flow in MCA branches, ↑ caliber of STA (direct bypass)

SELECTED REFERENCES

1. Hayashi T et al: Additional surgery for postoperative ischemic symptoms in patients with moyamoya disease: the effectiveness of occipital artery-posterior cerebral artery bypass with an indirect procedure: technical case report. Neurosurgery. 64(1):E195-6; discussion E196, 2009
2. Narisawa A et al: Efficacy of the revascularization surgery for adult-onset moyamoya disease with the progression of cerebrovascular lesions. Clin Neurol Neurosurg. 111(2):123-6, 2009
3. Kamijo K et al: Dramatic disappearance of moyamoya disease-induced chorea after indirect bypass surgery. Neurol Med Chir (Tokyo). 48(9):390-3, 2008
4. Kraemer M et al: Moyamoya disease in Europeans. Stroke. 39(12):3193-200, 2008
5. Kuroda S et al: Moyamoya disease: current concepts and future perspectives. Lancet Neurol. 7(11):1056-66, 2008
6. Su IC et al: Acute cerebral ischemia following intraventricular hemorrhage in moyamoya disease: early perfusion computed tomography findings. J Neurosurg. 109(6):1049-51, 2008

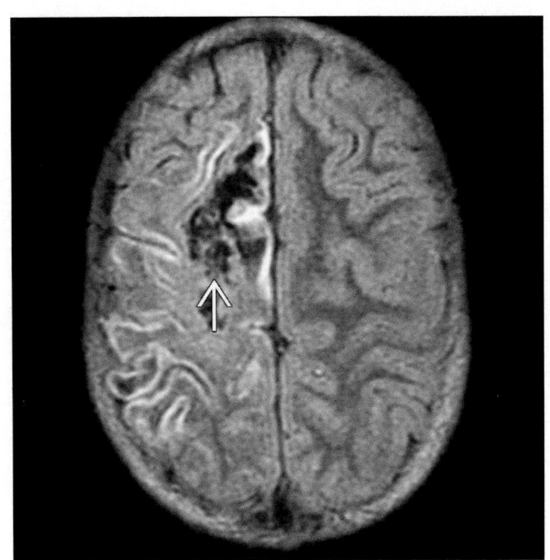

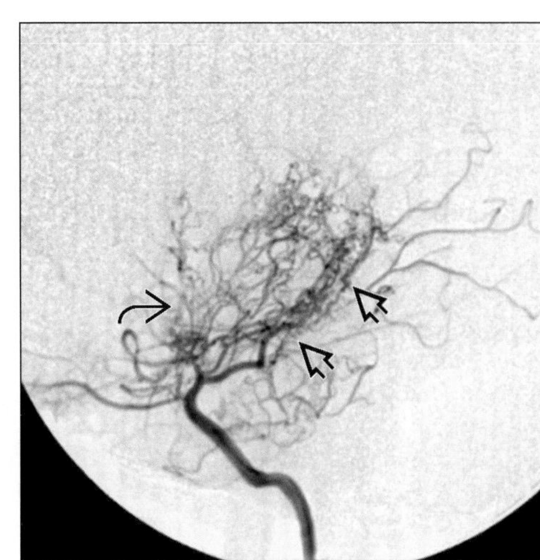

(Left) *Axial FLAIR MR in a 10 year old with Down syndrome shows necrosis in the right frontal-parietal cortex with encephalomalacia → in the deep white matter.* ***(Right)*** *Lateral angiography, right ICA injection in the same patient shows narrowing of the distal ICA & occlusion of the ACA & MCA with the "puff of smoke" appearance → of enlarged lenticulostriate collaterals. Note the additional network of collaterals more posteriorly →, likely thalamoperforators and posterior choroidal branches.*

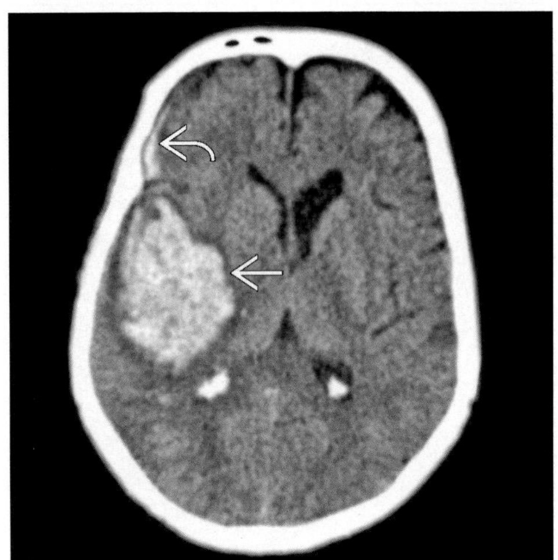

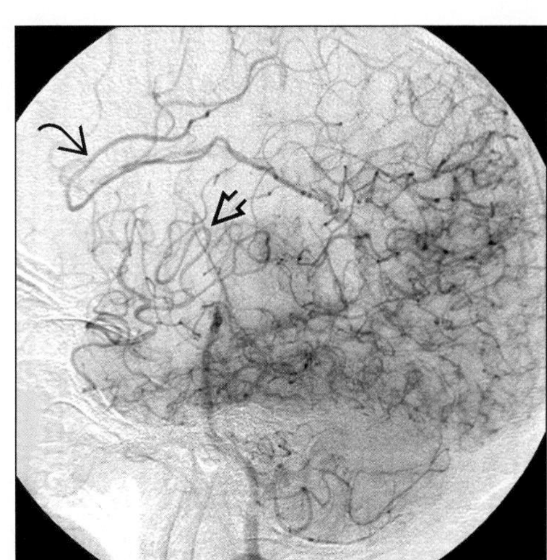

(Left) *Axial NECT in an adult with moyamoya shows intra- → and extraaxial → hemorrhage.* ***(Right)*** *Lateral angiography, delayed vertebral artery injection in the same patient shows extensive slow-flowing pial collateralization from the posterior circulation into the anterior → and middle → cerebral artery branches. This patient had complete occlusion of both proximal ACAs and MCAs. Presentation with intracranial hemorrhage is most common in Asian adults with moyamoya.*

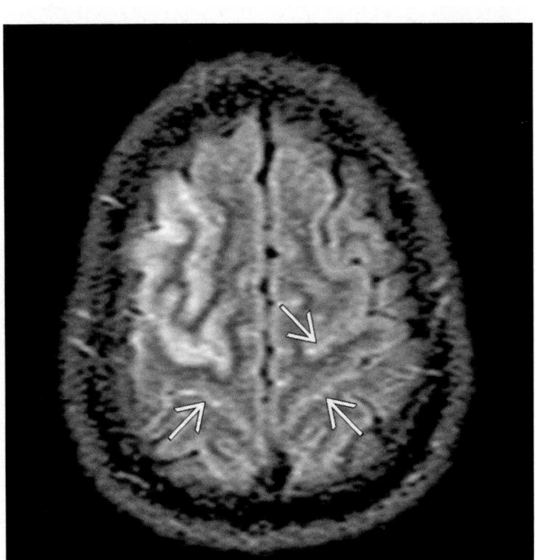

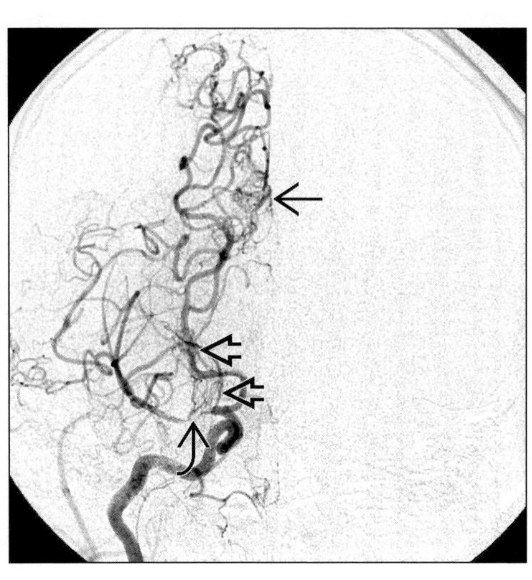

(Left) *Axial FLAIR MR in a 12 year old with sudden left hemiplegia shows an acute right MCA territory infarct. Hyperintense signal in the cerebral sulci → represents the "ivy" sign, caused by slow flow in engorged pial collaterals.* ***(Right)*** *Anteroposterior DSA of right ICA injection in the same patient shows severe focal narrowing of proximal MCA → & occluded ACA. Lenticulostriates and thalamoperforator arteries → are enlarged. Collateral flow from the posterior choroidal artery → is also present.*

PRIMARY ARTERITIS OF THE CNS

Key Facts

Terminology
- Primary arteritis confined to intracranial CNS
- No evidence of secondary (systemic) vasculitis

Imaging
- CT/MR
  - Look for secondary signs of vasculitis (ischemia, infarction)
  - Hypodensities on CT
  - Multifocal hyperintensities (T2WI, FLAIR)
  - Especially basal ganglia, subcortical white matter
- CTA/MRA is useful for screening; spatial resolution may be insufficient for subtle disease
- DSA
  - Imaging "gold standard"
  - Especially useful if high clinical suspicion but lab studies positive and MR/MRA negative
  - Alternating stenoses, dilatations
  - Less common: Long-segment stenoses, pseudoaneurysms, occlusions
  - Peripheral (2nd, 3rd order branches) more commonly affected than circle of Willis

Pathology
- Brain biopsy may be required to confirm diagnosis
  - 75-80% sensitive
  - Negative biopsy does not exclude primary arteritis of CNS
- Leptomeningeal arteries/veins are affected
  - May involve intracranial vessels of any size

Clinical Issues
- Wide age range (mean ~ 42 years)

Diagnostic Checklist
- Older adult with vasculitis-like DSA pattern? Atherosclerosis is much more common than PACNS!

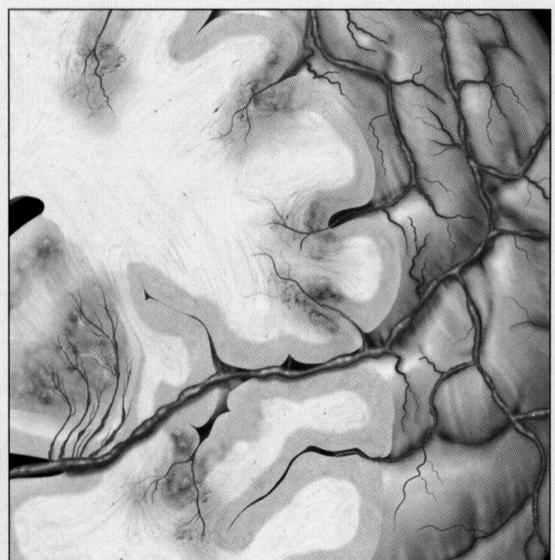
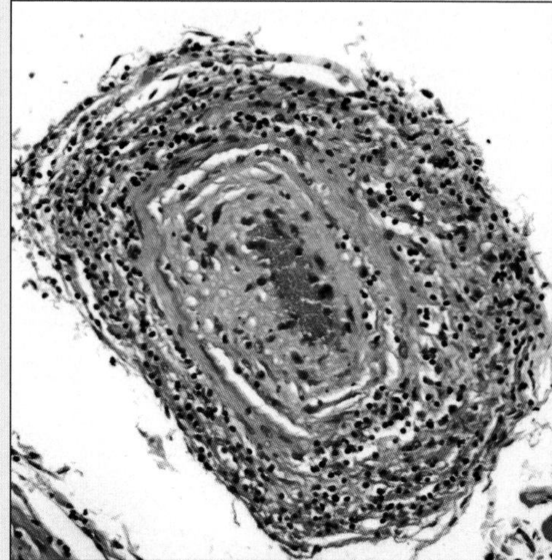

(Left) Coronal oblique graphic illustrates alternating segmental areas of narrowing and dilatation of the opercular and superficial MCA branches, as well as patchy multifocal ischemia within the underlying brain from primary arteritis of the CNS. *(Right)* Micropathology, low-power, H&E from the autopsy of a 71-year-old woman with multifocal T2 and FLAIR brain hyperintensities (not illustrated) shows intimal and adventitial necrosis and inflammatory changes, characteristic for CNS vasculitis.

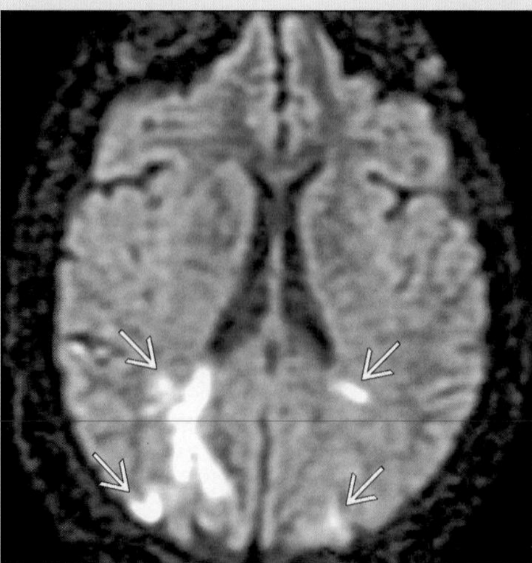
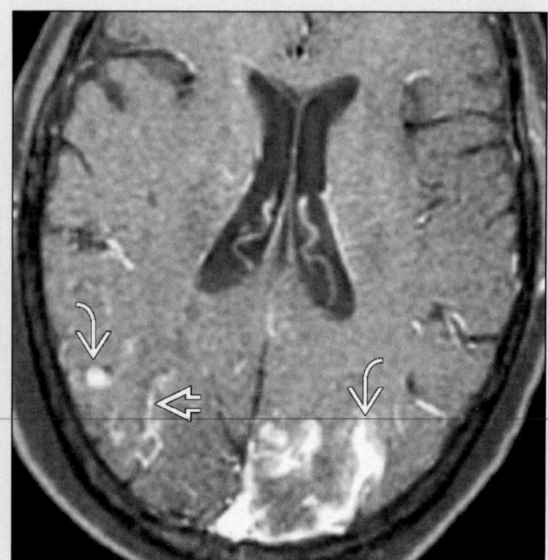

(Left) Axial DWI MR in a 50-year-old man shows diffusion restriction involving the white matter and cortex of both parietal lobes ➔, an atypical pattern for embolic disease. *(Right)* Axial T1WI C+ MR in the same patient shows extensive gyriform and patchy enhancement in the parietal lobes ➔ with subtle linear sulcal enhancement in the larger region of diffusion restriction ➔. This patient was proven to have PACNS with multifocal infarcts. Posterior circulation predominance in this patient is unusual.

PRIMARY ARTERITIS OF THE CNS

TERMINOLOGY

Abbreviations

- Primary arteritis of CNS (PACNS)

Synonyms

- Vasculitis, vasculopathy

Definitions

- Primary arteritis confined to intracranial CNS without any evidence of systemic vasculitis

IMAGING

General Features

- Best diagnostic clue
  - Irregularities, stenoses, and vascular occlusions in atypical pattern for atherosclerotic disease
  - Imaging work-up can be normal; requires clinical/laboratory correlation
- Location
  - Pathologically leptomeningeal arteries & veins are affected, but involves intracranial vessels of any size
  - Brain is primary site but spinal cord can also be involved
- Size
  - Degree of vessel narrowing may range from normal or minimally stenotic to completely occluded
- Morphology
  - Areas of smooth or slightly irregularly shaped stenoses alternating with dilated segments
  - Nonspecific (appearance similar to other vasculitides)

CT Findings

- NECT
  - Relatively insensitive; often normal
  - May see secondary signs, such as ischemia or infarction
    - Multifocal low-density areas especially in basal ganglia, subcortical white matter
  - May see hemorrhage (less typical)
- CECT
  - May see patchy areas of enhancement

MR Findings

- T1WI
  - Multifocal deep gray & subcortical hypointensities
- FLAIR
  - Multifocal deep gray & subcortical hyperintensities
- T2* GRE
  - May show petechial hemorrhage
- DWI
  - Restricted diffusion in acute stages
- T1WI C+
  - May see patchy areas of enhancement
- MRA
  - Relatively insensitive, most often normal
  - May see some classic angiographic signs if larger vessels involved

Ultrasonographic Findings

- Color Doppler
  - Transcranial Doppler may be used to monitor cerebral blood flow velocities and evaluate therapy if large arteries are involved

Angiographic Findings

- Conventional
  - Alternating stenosis with dilatation primarily involving 2nd, 3rd order branches
  - Less common: Long-segment stenoses, pseudoaneurysms, occlusions

Nuclear Medicine Findings

- 11C-(R)-PK11195 PET shows increased binding
  - Specific ligand for peripheral benzodiazepine binding site
  - Particularly abundant on cells of mononuclear phagocyte lineage
  - May be helpful in patients of suspected vasculitis with normal or ambiguous MR findings

Imaging Recommendations

- Best imaging tool
  - Conventional angiography is "gold standard"
  - MR C+; consider MRA
- Protocol advice
  - Conventional angiography if lab studies positive, MR/MRA negative, and high clinical suspicion
  - CTA/MRA is useful for screening; spatial resolution may be insufficient for subtle disease

DIFFERENTIAL DIAGNOSIS

Intracranial Atherosclerotic Vascular Disease (ASVD)

- Advanced patient age
- Typical distribution (carotid siphon, proximal intracranial vessels)

Arterial Vasospasm

- Temporal relationship to subarachnoid hemorrhage
- Involves proximal vasculature

Drug Abuse

- Younger patient population
- Commonly multi-drug users
- DSA appearance indistinguishable from PACNS

Moyamoya

- Sometimes referred to as "idiopathic progressive arteriopathy of childhood"
- Moyamoya is angiographic pattern, not specific disease; may be acquired as well as inherited
- Any slowly progressive occlusion of supraclinoid ICAs may develop moyamoya pattern

Systemic CNS Vasculitis

- Secondary CNS involvement of systemic vasculitis, polyarteritis, SLE are most common
- Systemic disease with characteristic findings and labs
- DSA appearance indistinguishable from PACNS

PRIMARY ARTERITIS OF THE CNS

PATHOLOGY

General Features

- Etiology
  - Unknown
- Brain biopsy may be required to confirm diagnosis
  - Definite diagnosis made from mononuclear inflammation of vessel wall
  - 75-80% sensitive, negative biopsy does not necessarily exclude PACNS
- Diagnosis can be established on clinical grounds, typical findings on DSA, and other investigatory grounds excluding other diseases
- Must be distinguished from other causes of CNS inflammation & noninflammatory vascular disease

Staging, Grading, & Classification

- PACNS: Highly heterogeneous group of vasculitides limited to CNS
  - Spectrum from granulomatous angiitis of CNS (GACNS) to benign angiopathy of central nervous system (BACNS) to reversible vasoconstrictive syndrome (RCVS)
  - BACNS, RCVS has more favorable outcome, all have indistinguishable angiographic appearance
- Clinical manifestations of CNS vasculitides may be identical
  - Acute onset, headache, normal to mildly abnormal CSF findings, female predominance in BACNS, RCVS
  - Focal weakness, seizures, hemorrhage, confusion, memory disorders, altered consciousness can be seen in each
  - Despite "benign" designation in BACNS and RCVS, some patients sustain significant neurological damage
  - Histories of heavy nicotine or caffeine use, OTC cold remedy use, and oral contraceptive or estrogen replacement
  - Precise relationship (if any) of these exposures remains unclear

Gross Pathologic & Surgical Features

- Characterized by ischemic lesions and small petechial hemorrhages
- Vessels of any size can be involved
- May see venulitis with parenchymal hemorrhages

Microscopic Features

- Mononuclear inflammation with necrosis of blood vessel walls is PACNS hallmark
- Variable degree of granulomatous and nongranulomatous angiitis of small vessels
- Typically involves media, adventitia of small leptomeningeal arteries and veins

CLINICAL ISSUES

Presentation

- Most common signs/symptoms
  - Stroke from vascular involvement (stenoses, occlusion, aneurysm)
  - Headache is also common
- Clinical profile
  - Clinical presentation is highly variable: Focal to diffuse manifestations & acute to chronic evolution
  - Subacute presentation over weeks or months is typical (mean = 5 months to diagnosis)
  - Headache & mental status change with focal deficits
  - No evidence of secondary vasculitis or other diseases mentioned in differential diagnosis should arouse suspicion

Demographics

- Age
  - Childhood to adulthood
  - Mean age ~ 42 years; range from age 3 to elderly
  - BACNS, RCVS patients tend to be young women
- Gender
  - Distribution of PACNS is nearly equal between sexes, with perhaps slight male predominance
- Epidemiology
  - Rare

Natural History & Prognosis

- Prognosis greatly improved with early recognition and therapy
- Delay in diagnosis may lead to additional morbidity
- PACNS: More likely to develop symptoms subacutely and remain undiagnosed for months
- BACNS: More likely to have relatively acute presentations and be diagnosed within weeks of onset
- Untreated PACNS: Risk of permanent cognitive dysfunction
- Often diagnosed posthumously; high index of suspicion is necessary to make correct diagnosis in timely basis

Treatment

- Few controlled studies on treatment of vasculitis, with considerable variation among centers on current therapeutic regimens
- Therapy typically comprises aggressive immunosuppressive approach
- High-dose steroid therapy with prolonged course and gradual taper controls disease in most cases
- Close monitoring of patients mandatory
- Without treatment, patients with PACNS tend to have progressively downhill courses often leading to death
- BACNS, RCVS patients may respond to less aggressive corticosteroid and Ca++ channel blocker therapy

DIAGNOSTIC CHECKLIST

Consider

- DSA when clinical suspicion of PACNS is strong, regardless of findings on MR

Image Interpretation Pearls

- Atherosclerosis is by far most common cause of vasculitis-like DSA pattern in older adults, not PACNS

SELECTED REFERENCES

1. Miller DV et al: Biopsy findings in primary angiitis of the central nervous system. Am J Surg Pathol. 33(1):35-43, 2009

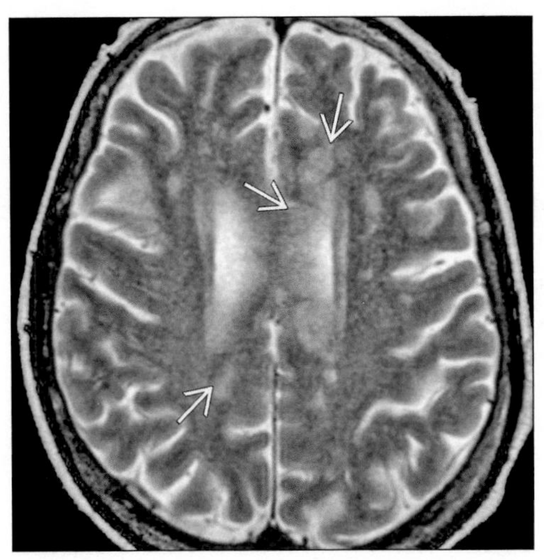

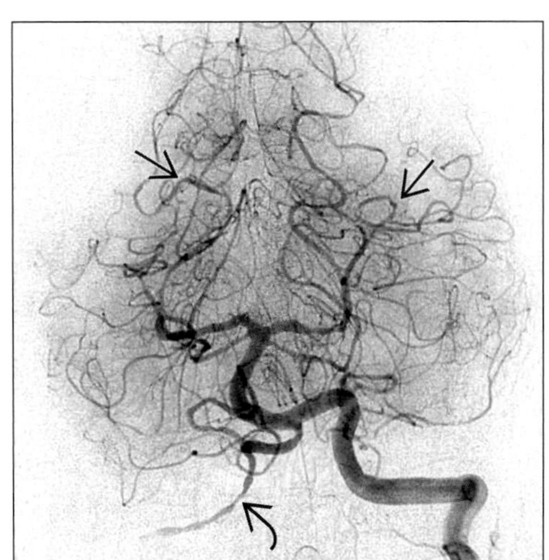

(Left) *Axial T2WI MR shows hyperintensity in the deep white matter that extends along the corpus callosum ➔, which were DWI positive (not shown). Callosal involvement is atypical for embolic or thrombotic infarcts.* ***(Right)*** *Left vertebral DSA in the same patient shows alternating areas of stenosis and irregularity in both PCAs →. Given the appropriate clinical and laboratory findings, vasculitis is the most likely diagnosis. Note extensive involvement of the intracranial right vertebral artery ↪.*

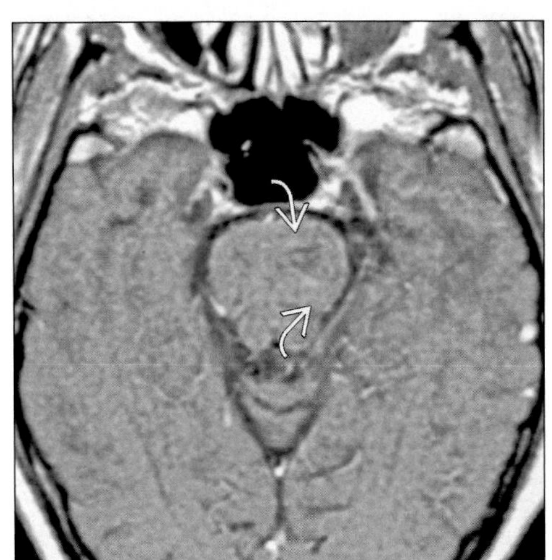

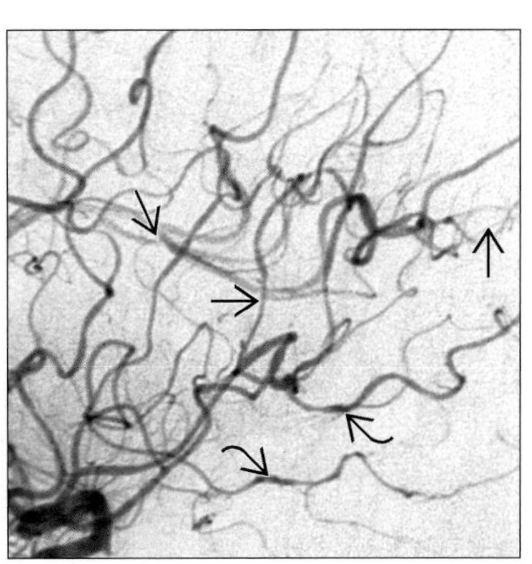

(Left) *Axial T1WI C+ MR in a 40-year-old woman with a headache and mental status changes shows abnormal enhancement in the pons and midbrain ↪. Marked diffusion restriction was present (not shown).* ***(Right)*** *Lateral DSA internal carotid injection in the same patient shows multiple alternating arterial stenoses → with focal fusiform dilatations ↪ typical for PACNS. Conventional DSA, with laboratory, clinical, and pathologic data, remains the "gold standard" for diagnosis.*

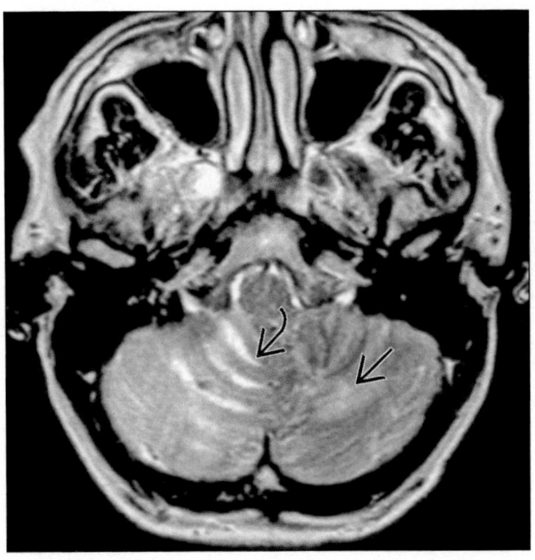

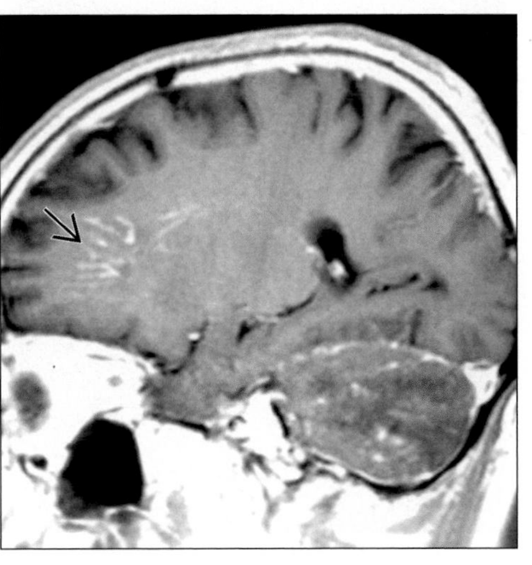

(Left) *Axial T2WI MR shows hyperintensity in the right cerebellum with a small focus of hyperintensity in the left cerebellum →. Linear areas of even greater hyperintensity can be identified involving the folia and sulci ↪.* ***(Right)*** *Sagittal T1WI C+ MR shows nodular and linear enhancement along the pial surface (folia) of the cerebellum and in the deep medullary veins of the frontal lobe →. This has a mixed pattern of arterial and venous involvement in biopsy-proven granulomatous angiitis of the CNS.*

MISCELLANEOUS VASCULITIS

Key Facts

Terminology

- Heterogeneous group of CNS disorders
  - Characterized by nonatheromatous inflammation and necrosis of blood vessel walls
  - Both arteries, veins may be affected

Imaging

- CTA/MRA useful screening; spatial resolution may be insufficient for subtle disease
- CT/MR
  - Look for secondary signs (ischemia/infarction)
  - Multifocal hypodensities/T2 hyperintensities
  - Basal ganglia, cortex, subcortical WM
- DSA
  - Multifocal areas of smooth or slightly irregular-shaped stenoses alternating with dilated segments
  - May occur in intracranial vessels of any size
  - Pattern/distribution atypical for atherosclerotic disease

Pathology

- Vessel wall inflammation, necrosis common to all vasculitides
  - Bacterial, tuberculous meningitis
  - Mycotic, viral, syphilitic, granulomatous arteritis
  - Cell-mediated, collagen-vascular arteritides
  - Drug abuse

Clinical Issues

- Thinking vasculitis?
  - Brain neuroimaging is only beginning
  - Add toxicology screen, lumbar puncture, angiography
  - Only biopsy allows definite diagnosis

*(**Left**) Coronal oblique graphic shows vasculitis with medium vessel changes ⇒ and parenchymal changes seen as multifocal areas of edema, infarction, and scattered hemorrhages within the basal ganglia and at the gray-white junction. (**Right**) Axial FLAIR MR in a 71-year-old patient with TIA-like symptoms shows multifocal peripherally located hyperintensities ➔. Other scans (not shown) demonstrated similar lesions in the cortex and pons.*

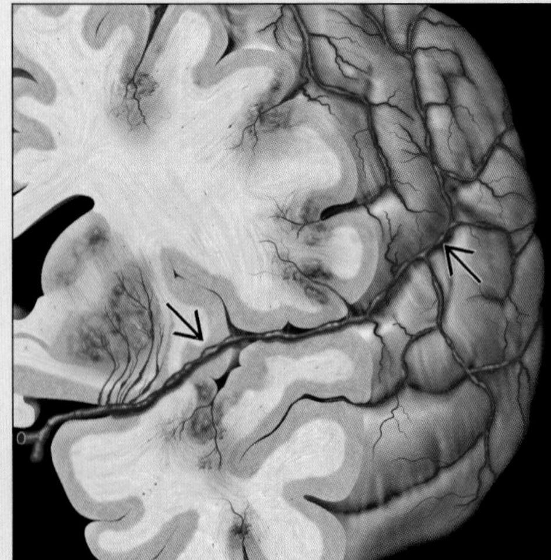

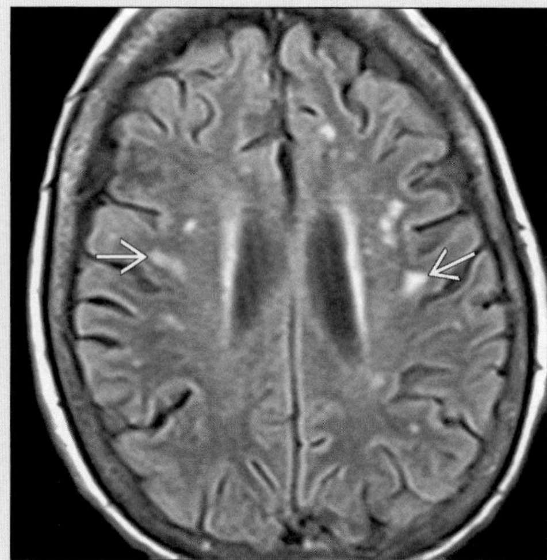

*(**Left**) Axial DWI MR in the same patient shows multiple foci of diffusion restriction ➔ in the cerebral cortex. (**Right**) Anteroposterior DSA in the same patient showed multifocal areas of alternating stenoses and dilatations ⇒. In an older patient, the most common cause of this appearance is atherosclerotic disease. However, laboratory work-up was positive for antinuclear antibodies. The patient died 2 months later from unrelated causes. Brain-only autopsy disclosed giant cell arteritis.*

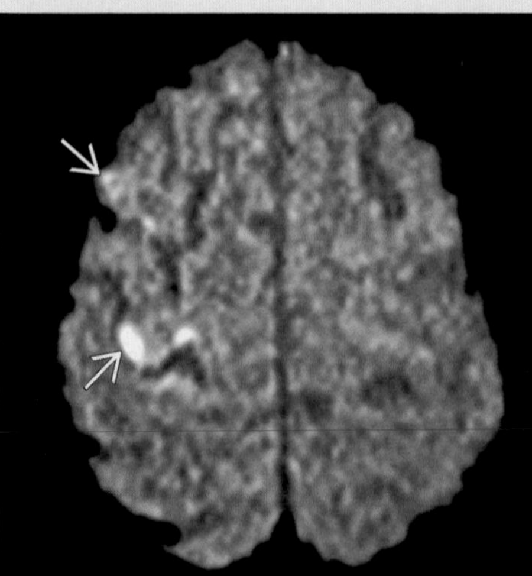

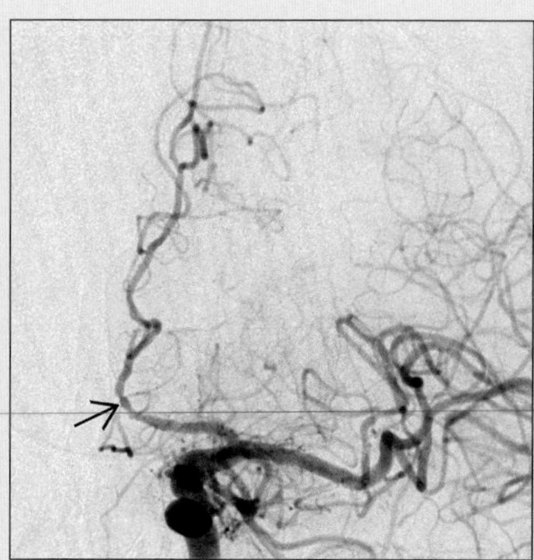

MISCELLANEOUS VASCULITIS

TERMINOLOGY

Synonyms

- Inflammatory vasculopathy (more general term indicating any vascular pathology with inflammation)
- Arteritis (specifies arterial inflammation)
- Angiitis (inflammation of either arteries or veins)

Definitions

- Heterogeneous group of CNS disorders characterized by nonatheromatous inflammation and necrosis of blood vessel walls
- Involves either arteries or veins

IMAGING

General Features

- Best diagnostic clue
  - Irregularities, stenoses, and vascular occlusions in pattern atypical for atherosclerotic disease
  - Imaging work-up can be normal; need clinical/ laboratory correlation
- Location
  - Arteries and veins are affected; occurs in intracranial vessels of any size
- Size
  - Degree of vessel narrowing may range from normal/ minimally stenotic to occluded
- Morphology
  - Classic appearance: Multifocal areas of smooth or slightly irregular-shaped stenosis alternating with dilated segments
  - Variety of angiographic appearances depending on etiology, including vascular irregularities, stenoses, aneurysms, and occlusions

CT Findings

- NECT
  - Relatively insensitive; may be normal
  - May see secondary signs, such as ischemia/ infarction: Multifocal low-density areas in basal ganglia, subcortical white matter
  - May see hemorrhage
- CECT
  - May see patchy areas of enhancement

MR Findings

- T1WI
  - Can be normal early; ± multifocal cortical/ subcortical hypointensities
- T2WI
  - Multifocal hyperintensities
- FLAIR
  - Subcortical, basal ganglia hyperintensities
- T2* GRE
  - May show hemorrhage
- DWI
  - Can see restricted diffusion in acute stage
- T1WI C+
  - May see patchy areas of enhancement
- MRA
  - May see some classic angiographic signs if larger vessels involved/vascular occlusion; may be normal

Ultrasonographic Findings

- Pulsed Doppler
  - Transcranial Doppler may be used to monitor cerebral blood flow velocities if large arteries are involved
  - May also be used to evaluate therapy response if large arteries are involved

Angiographic Findings

- Conventional
  - Alternating stenosis and dilatation primarily involving 2nd, 3rd order branches
  - Less common: Long-segment stenoses, pseudoaneurysms

Imaging Recommendations

- Best imaging tool
  - DSA is cornerstone diagnostic procedure
  - MR findings may be negative in setting of CNS vasculitis confirmed on angiography
- Protocol advice
  - DSA if lab studies positive, MR/MRA negative
  - CTA/MRA useful screening; spatial resolution may be insufficient for subtle disease

DIFFERENTIAL DIAGNOSIS

Intracranial Atherosclerotic Vascular Disease

- Advanced patient age
- Typical distribution (carotid siphon, proximal intracranial vessels); extracranial manifestations of disease

Arterial Vasospasm

- Temporal relationship to subarachnoid hemorrhage (SAH)
- Involves proximal vasculature

PATHOLOGY

General Features

- Etiology
  - Pattern of vessel wall inflammation, necrosis common to all vasculitides
  - Can be primary or secondary, caused by broad spectrum of infectious/inflammatory agents, drugs, etc.
  - Bacterial meningitis
    - Infarction due to vascular involvement seen in 25%
    - *H. influenzae* most common organism; common in children
  - Tuberculous meningitis
    - Vessels at skull base most commonly involved (i.e., supraclinoid ICA and M1-producing occlusions and stenoses)
  - Mycotic arteritis (*Aspergillus*, cocci, etc.)
    - Actinomyces may invade vessel walls leading to hemorrhage
    - Narrowing of basal cerebral or cortical vessels on angiography

MISCELLANEOUS VASCULITIS

- Viral arteritis
  - Herpes simplex most common in North America
  - HIV-associated vasculitis increasing, especially in children
- Syphilis arteritis
  - 2 forms: Syphilitic meningitis and gummatous vasculitis
  - Diffuse vasculitis involves cortical arteries and veins
  - Gummatous vasculitis usually affects proximal MCA branches
- Polyarteritis nodosa
  - Most common systemic vasculitis to involve CNS (though late)
  - Microaneurysms due to necrosis of internal elastic lamina in 75%
- Cell-mediated arteritides
  - Giant cell arteritis (granulomatous infiltration of arterial walls)
  - Takayasu (primarily involves aorta, great vessels, branches)
  - Temporal arteritis (systemic; involves temporal, other extracranial arteries)
- Wegener
  - May cause intracerebral and meningeal granulomas or vasculitis
  - CNS involved in 15-30% due to direct invasion from nose/sinuses
  - Chronic systemic arteritis involving lungs, kidneys, and sinuses
- Sarcoid (CNS involvement in 3-5% of cases)
  - Can extend along perivascular spaces, involve penetrating arteries
  - Meningitis, vasculitis involving vessels at base of brain
- Granulomatous angiitis (PACNS)
  - Primary angiitis isolated to CNS (idiopathic)
  - Manifest as multiple intracranial stenoses
- Collagen vascular disease (SLE, rheumatoid, scleroderma)
  - SLE: Most likely to involve CNS
  - Vasculitis relatively uncommon (variable findings; range from small vessel irregularities/stenoses/ occlusions to fusiform aneurysms)
  - CVA seen in 50% due to cardiac disease or coagulopathy
- Drug abuse vasculitis
  - Drug can injure vessels directly or secondarily (usually hypersensitivity to contaminants)
  - Associated with both legitimate and illegal "street" drugs, including amphetamines, cocaine, heroin, and phenylpropanolamine and ergots
- Radiation
  - Acute arteritis produces transient white matter edema
  - Chronic changes more severe with vessel obliteration and brain necrosis, leukomalacia, mineralizing microangiopathy, and atrophy
  - Effects compounded with concomitant chemotherapy
- Moyamoya disease
  - Sometimes referred to as "idiopathic progressive arteriopathy of childhood"
  - Moyamoya is angiographic pattern, not specific disease; may be acquired or inherited
  - Any slowly progressive occlusion of supraclinoid ICAs may develop moyamoya pattern
  - Pattern has been reported with NF, atherosclerosis, radiation therapy
  - Prognosis depends upon rapidity and extent of vascular occlusions, as well as development of effective collaterals

Gross Pathologic & Surgical Features

- Characterized by ischemic lesions and small petechial hemorrhages
- Vessels of any size can be involved
- May see venulitis with parenchymal hemorrhages

Microscopic Features

- Inflammation and necrosis of blood vessel walls

CLINICAL ISSUES

Presentation

- Most common signs/symptoms
  - Stroke related to manifestations of vascular involvement (stenosis, occlusion, aneurysm)
  - Patients presenting with symptoms suggestive of vasculitis require brain neuroimaging, lumbar puncture, and angiography, but only biopsy allows definite diagnosis

Demographics

- Epidemiology
  - Atherosclerosis is by far most common cause of vasculitis-like angiographic pattern in adults
  - CNS vasculitis occurs in variety of clinical settings, some of which exhibit distinct age preference, others tissue tropism

Natural History & Prognosis

- Varies depending upon etiology; typically progressive if untreated

Treatment

- Most patients with CNS vasculitis should be treated aggressively with combination of immunosuppressive medications

DIAGNOSTIC CHECKLIST

Consider

- Diagnosis is frequently made on basis of clinical presentation, brain MR, and cerebral angiography without pathologic confirmation

SELECTED REFERENCES

1. Birnbaum J et al: Primary angiitis of the central nervous system. Arch Neurol. 66(6):704-9, 2009
2. Melica G et al: Primary vasculitis of the central nervous system in patients infected with HIV-1 in the HAART era. J Med Virol. 81(4):578-81, 2009
3. Yahyavi-Firouz-Abadi N et al: Steroid-responsive large vessel vasculitis: application of whole-brain 320-detector row dynamic volume CT angiography and perfusion. AJNR Am J Neuroradiol. 30(7):1409-11, 2009

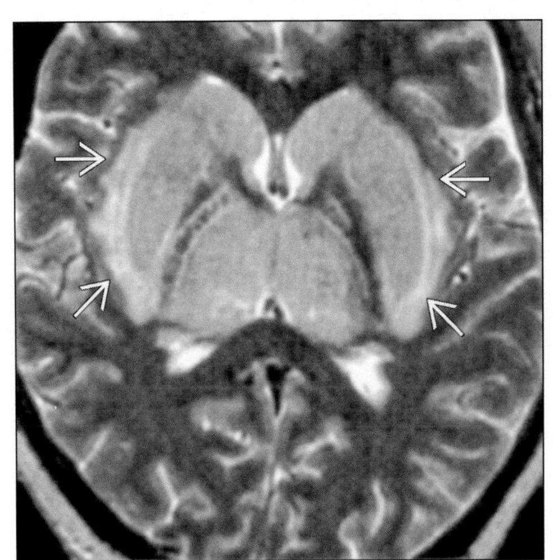

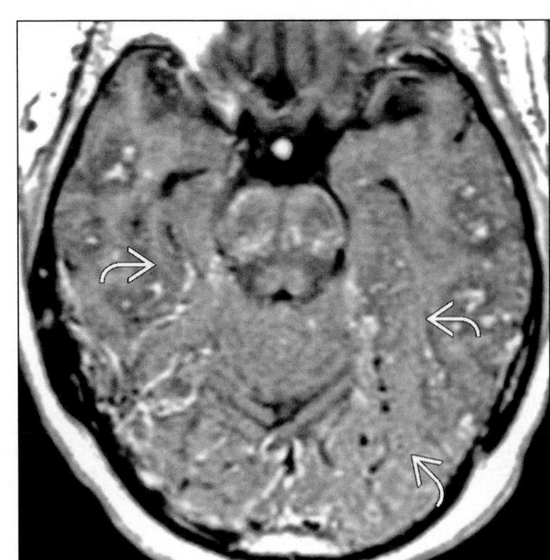

(Left) *Axial T2WI MR in a patient with lupus and no evidence for endocarditis and emboli shows symmetric high signal intensity in the basal ganglia, thalami, and external and extreme capsules ➔.* ***(Right)*** *Axial T1WI C+ MR in a patient with lupus vasculitis shows multifocal linear and punctate enhancing foci in the pons and throughout the juxtacortical white matter ➔. These are 2 common patterns seen with CNS lupus vasculitis.*

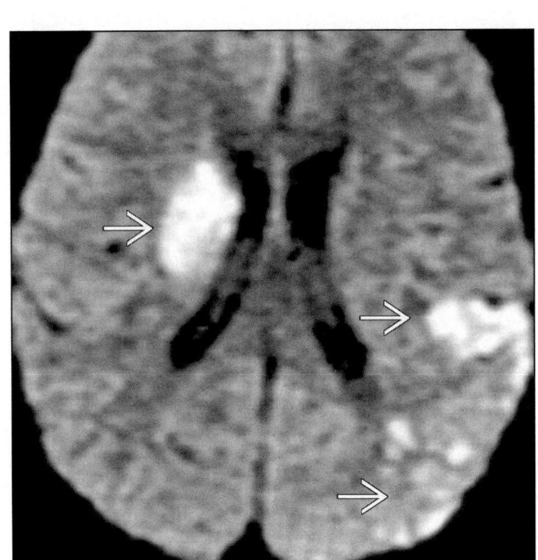

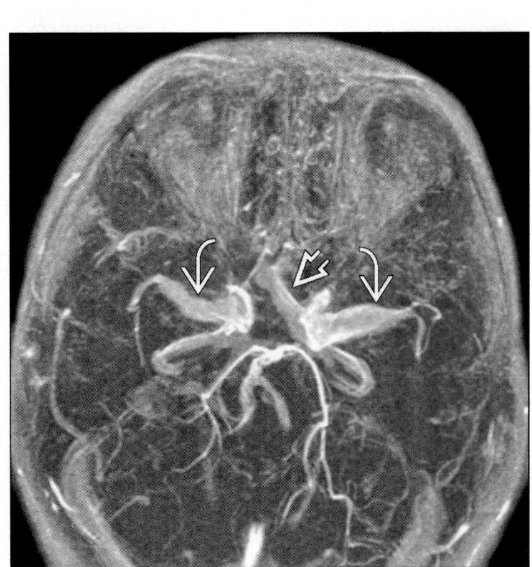

(Left) *Axial DWI MR in a 13 year old shows multifocal hyperintensities in the upper basal ganglia ➔, GM/WM with diffusion restriction due to acute infarcts.* ***(Right)*** *Axial MRA in the same patient shows the fusiform arterial enlargement of the M1 segment of the middle cerebral arteries ➔ as well as the left anterior cerebral artery, A1 segment ➔. Congenital HIV/AIDS is a well-recognized cause of pediatric fusiform arteriopathy, a form of infectious vasculitis.*

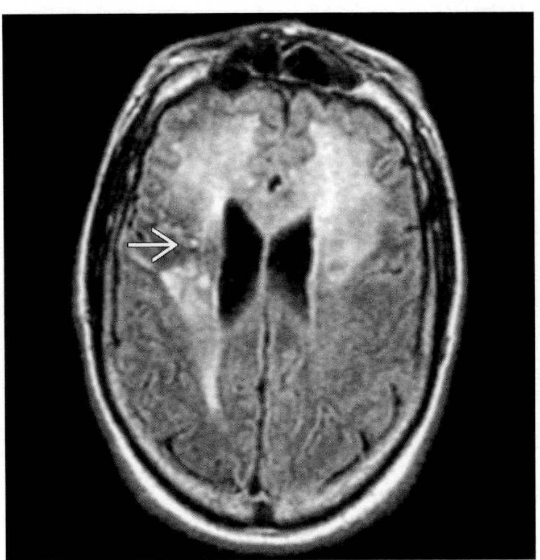

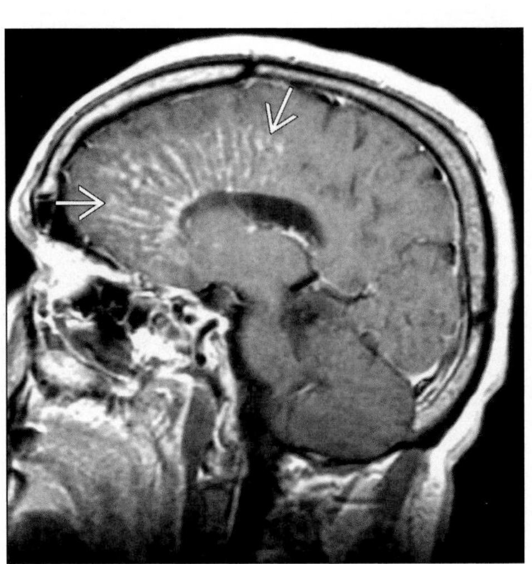

(Left) *Axial FLAIR MR shows confluent white matter hyperintensity primarily affecting the frontal lobes along with old hemorrhage in the right hemisphere ➔.* ***(Right)*** *Sagittal T1WI C+ MR in same patient shows striking multifocal linear enhancement ➔ coursing along deep medullary veins in the same regions as the FLAIR hyperintensities. Imaging diagnosis included sarcoid, amyloid angiopathy, vasculitis, and intravascular (angiocentric) lymphoma. Granulomatous angiitis was found at biopsy.*

REVERSIBLE CEREBRAL VASOCONSTRICTION SYNDROME

Key Facts

Terminology

- Reversible cerebral vasoconstriction syndrome (RCVS)
- Group of disorders characterized by
  - Reversible, multifocal cerebral artery vasoconstrictions
  - Severe headaches ± focal neurological deficits

Imaging

- Acute/recurrent headaches + vasculitic pattern (DSA)
- DSA = crucial for diagnosis (100% sensitive)
  - Involves large, medium-sized arteries
  - Diffuse, multifocal, segmental narrowing
  - Sometimes "string of beads" or "sausage strings"
- NECT often negative
  - Small cortical SAHs (20%) ± parenchymal hemorrhage
- CTA/MRA: May be normal if subtle changes (10%)
  - Diffuse segmental arterial constriction in 90%
- TCD: ↑ arterial velocities in MCA, ICA, ACA

Pathology

- Thought to represent transient disturbance in control of cerebral vascular tone → vasoconstriction → ischemia, stroke, death
- Spontaneous (1/3 of cases) or precipitated by
  - Post-partum state
  - Exposure to vasoactive substances

Clinical Issues

- Symptoms: Severe, acute "thunderclap" headache
  - Often recurrent (95%)
  - Ischemia/stroke (visual disturbance, aphasia, hemiparesis)
- Treatment
  - Discontinuation of vasoactive medications
  - Vasodilators (e.g., Ca++ antagonists)

*(**Left**) Axial NECT in a patient with acute onset severe headache shows limited cortical SAH in the sulci of the right frontal lobe ➔. DSA was performed to exclude aneurysm or vascular malformation (not shown). (**Right**) MR in the same patient was obtained 4 days later when she noticed visual disturbances. FLAIR scan (top) shows multifocal hyperintensities in both occipital lobes ➔. DWI (bottom) shows restricted diffusion ➔, consistent with ischemia or infarction.*

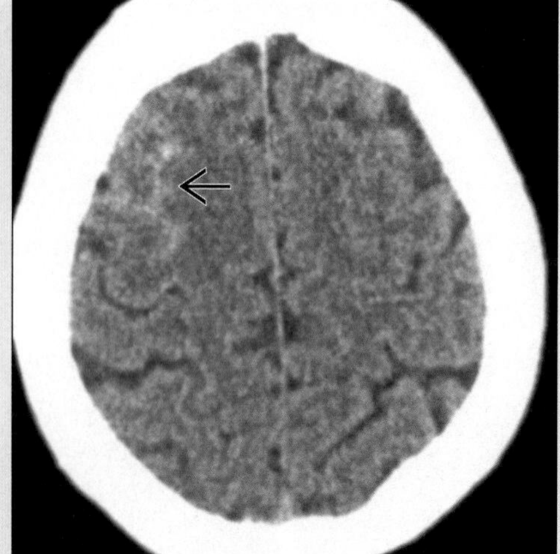

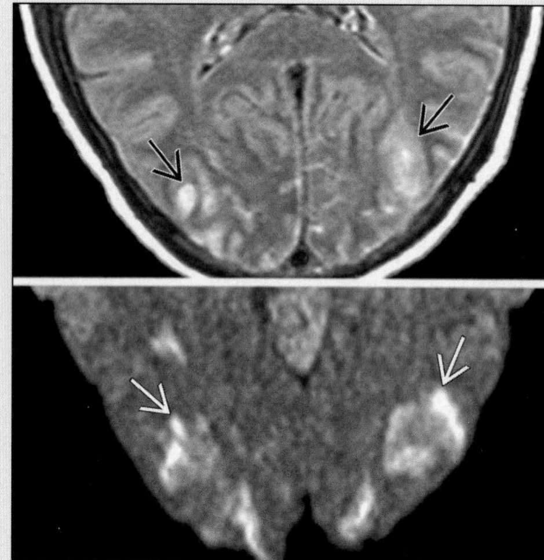

*(**Left**) Anteroposterior right vertebral artery DSA shows diffuse luminal irregularity and focal stenoses involving the basilar artery and posterior cerebral and superior cerebellar arteries ➔. Similar changes were seen in the anterior circulation (not shown). The patient was treated with IA verapamil over the next 10 days. (**Right**) DSA repeated 2 weeks later shows significant interval resolution of the posterior circulation vasospasm. There are a few foci ➔ of mild residual stenoses still evident.*

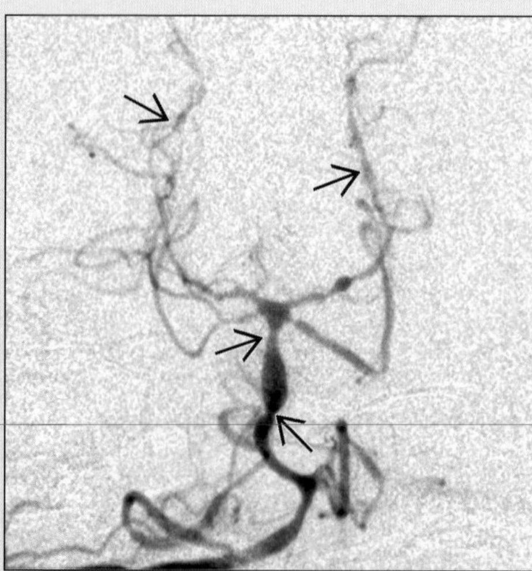

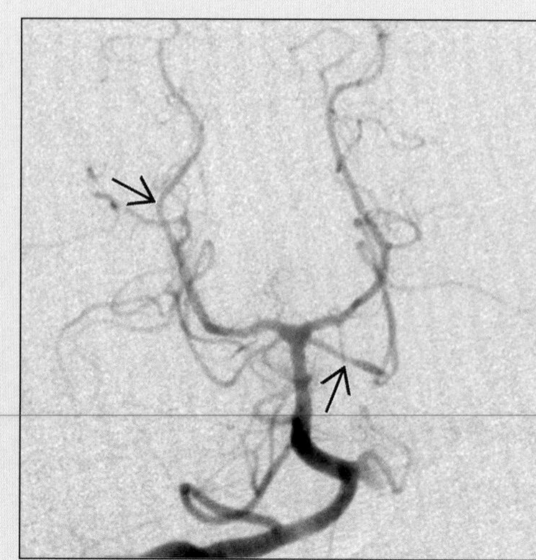

REVERSIBLE CEREBRAL VASOCONSTRICTION SYNDROME

TERMINOLOGY

Abbreviations
- Reversible cerebral vasoconstriction syndrome (RCVS)

Synonyms
- Call-Fleming syndrome

Definitions
- Group of disorders characterized by
  - Reversible, multifocal cerebral artery vasoconstriction
  - Severe headaches ± focal neurological deficits

IMAGING

General Features
- Best diagnostic clue
  - Acute onset, usually recurrent headaches + vasculitic pattern on DSA

CT Findings
- NECT
  - May see small cortical subarachnoid hemorrhage (SAH) in 20% of parenchymal hemorrhages
  - Cortical ± subcortical hypodensity secondary to ischemia/stroke
- CECT
  - Usually normal unless ischemic stroke ensues → gyriform enhancement
- CTA
  - May be normal or can see undulations of large/ medium-sized arteries

MR Findings
- FLAIR
  - May see uni- or bilateral cortical SAH
  - Focal regions of ↑ signal secondary to stroke
- DWI
  - Most sensitive for regions of ischemia/stroke
- MRA
  - May be normal if subtle changes (10%); require DSA for diagnosis
  - Diffuse segmental arterial constriction in 90%

Ultrasonographic Findings
- Transcranial Doppler (TCD): ↑ arterial velocities consistent with vasospasm + ↓ luminal diameter of MCA, ICA, ACA in 70%

Angiographic Findings
- Crucial for diagnosis (100% sensitive)
- Diffuse, multifocal, segmental narrowing of large/ medium-sized arteries
- Occasional dilated segments may appear like "string of beads" or "sausage strings"

DIFFERENTIAL DIAGNOSIS

Cerebral Vasculitis
- Similar angiographic appearance; clinical onset more insidious, CSF abnormalities
- e.g., primary angiitis of central nervous system (PACNS), systemic lupus, infection, sarcoidosis

Nonaneurysmal SAH
- Dural fistula, trauma, arteriovenous malformation

PATHOLOGY

General Features
- Etiology
  - Thought to represent transient disturbance in control of cerebral vascular tone → vasoconstriction → ischemia, stroke, death
- Associated abnormalities
  - Occurs spontaneously (1/3 of cases) or may be precipitated by
    - Postpartum state
    - Exposure to vasoactive substances
      - Cannabis, cocaine, ecstasy, amphetamine derivatives, LSD
      - Selective serotonin reuptake inhibitors (SSRIs)
      - Nasal decongestants, pseudoephedrine
      - Ergotamine tartrate, bromocriptine, sumatriptan
    - Pheochromocytoma, bronchial carcinoid tumor

CLINICAL ISSUES

Presentation
- Most common signs/symptoms
  - Severe, acute-onset ("thunderclap") headache
    - Often recurrent (95%)
    - Mimics SAH secondary to ruptured aneurysm
- Other signs/symptoms
  - Ischemia/stroke may result in visual disturbance, aphasia, hemiparesis
  - Seizures

Natural History & Prognosis
- Stroke occurs in 7-54%
- M:F = 1:2

Treatment
- Discontinuation of vasoactive medications
- Vasodilators (e.g., Ca++ antagonists) PO/IV/IA infusion

DIAGNOSTIC CHECKLIST

Consider
- RCVS in patient with history of thunderclap headache but no SAH or limited cortical SAH

Image Interpretation Pearls
- Interval DSA may show rapid improvement with vasodilator Rx

SELECTED REFERENCES

1. Ducros A et al: The clinical and radiological spectrum of reversible cerebral vasoconstriction syndrome. A prospective series of 67 patients. Brain. 130(Pt 12):3091-101, 2007

VASOSPASM

Key Facts

Terminology

- Reversible stenosis of intracranial arteries
- Caused by exposure to blood breakdown products
  - Contraction of vascular smooth muscle
  - Histological changes in vessel wall

Imaging

- General features (CTA/MRA/DSA)
  - Typically occurs 4-14 days after SAH
  - Smooth, relatively long segmental stenoses
  - Seen as arterial luminal irregularity/undulations
  - Multiple arteries, usually > 1 vascular territory
- CT perfusion
  - ↑ time to peak (TTP), ↑ mean transit time (MTT)
  - ↓ cerebral blood flow (CBF) in areas of hypoperfusion
- Transcranial Doppler (TCD)
  - ↑ mean flow velocity
  - Due to ↓ arterial cross-sectional area

Top Differential Diagnoses

- Non-SAH causes of vasospasm
  - Meningitis
  - Acute hypertensive encephalopathy (PRES)
  - Reversible cerebral vasoconstriction syndrome (RCVS)
  - Migraine headache
- Vasculitis
- Atherosclerosis

Clinical Issues

- Delayed ischemic neurological deficit (DIND)
  - ~ 1 week after SAH is typical
- Management
  - "Triple H" therapy
  - Endovascular (chemical or balloon angioplasty)

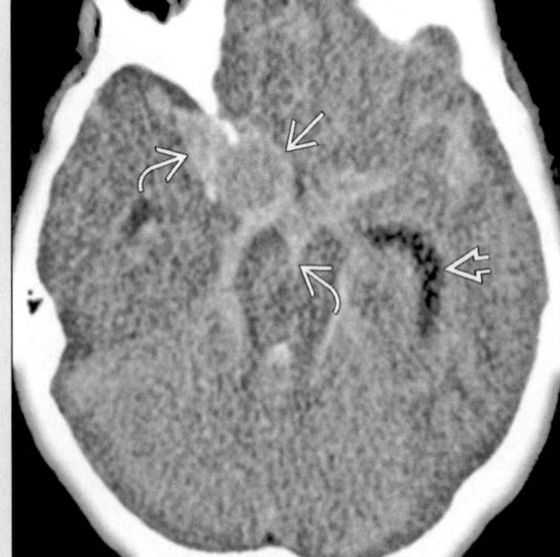

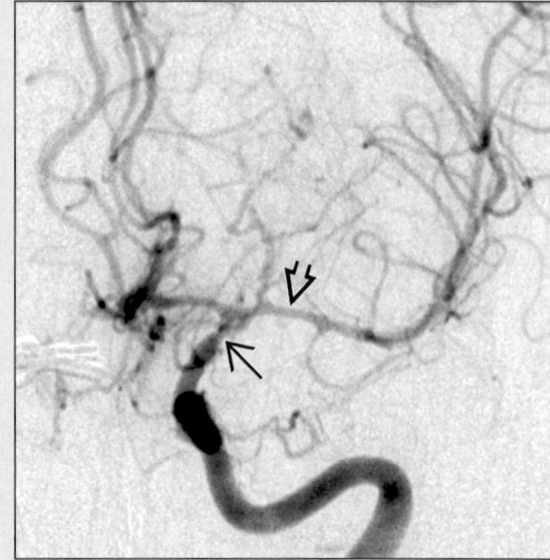

(Left) *Axial NECT in a patient with large SAH due to ruptured PCoA aneurysm. The aneurysm appears as a round filling defect ➡ within the SAH. There are > 1 mm thick layers of SAH present ➦ (Fisher grade 3), predictive of high vasospasm risk. Note hydrocephalus ⇨.* ***(Right)*** *Anteroposterior left ICA DSA in the same patient on day 7 post-SAH shows vasospasm of the M1 segment ⇨ and carotid terminus →. The patient had fluctuating right hemiparesis despite "triple H" therapy and oral nimodipine.*

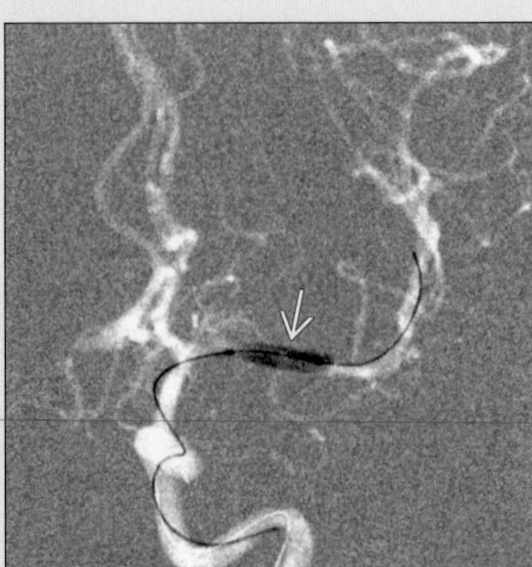

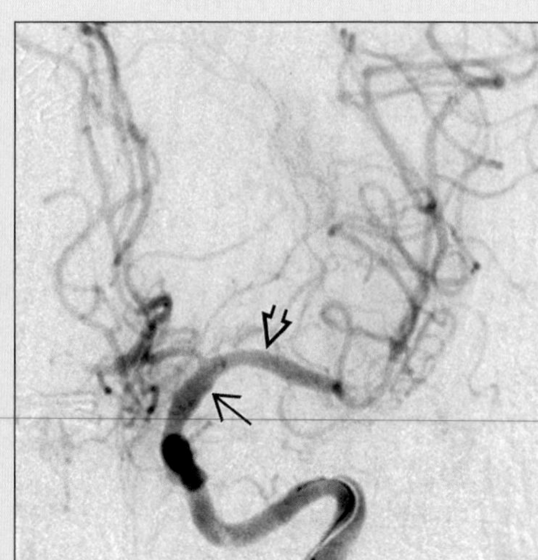

(Left) *Fluoroscopic roadmap image during balloon angioplasty of the left M1 segment shows a compliant balloon inflated within the MCA ➡. The balloon was later retracted into the supraclinoid ICA and inflated during fluoroscopic observation.* ***(Right)*** *Anteroposterior left ICA DSA after balloon angioplasty shows restoration of normal luminal diameter along the supraclinoid ICA → and M1 segment ⇨. The improvement is especially dramatic compared to the pre-angioplasty DSA.*

VASOSPASM

TERMINOLOGY

Synonyms

- Subarachnoid hemorrhage (SAH) vasospasm

Definitions

- Exposure to blood breakdown products → reversible stenosis of intracranial arteries
  - Contraction of vascular smooth muscle
  - Histological changes in vessel wall

IMAGING

General Features

- Best diagnostic clue
  - Segmental stenoses (CTA/MRA/DSA)
    - Typically 4-14 days after SAH
- Location
  - Affects any intradural (subarachnoid) artery
  - Worst vasospasm typically adjacent to site of ruptured aneurysm (highest concentration of SAH)

Imaging Recommendations

- Best imaging tool
  - Gold standard is DSA (100% sensitive but nonspecific)
    - May follow with intraarterial (IA) therapy
  - TCD useful as bedside monitoring/screening tool
- Protocol advice
  - Multi-territorial vascular involvement is typical
  - Visualize both carotids, dominant vertebral artery

CT Findings

- NECT
  - May see residual SAH
  - Otherwise normal (unless ischemia/stroke)
  - Hypodensity in involved vascular territory may herald ischemia/infarction
  - Differentiate from retraction edema
    - Adjacent to surgical clip
    - Not confined to vascular territory
- CTA
  - Screening tool for involvement of large vessels
    - Circle of Willis, M1 segment, basilar artery
  - Attenuation/stenosis of arteries
    - Typically multi-territorial but asymmetric
  - Insensitive for smaller vessels (e.g., M2, distal segments)
- CT perfusion (pCT)
  - Hypoperfusion
    - ↑ time to peak (TTP), ↑ mean transit time (MTT)
    - ↓ cerebral blood flow (CBF)
    - Preservation of cerebral blood volume (CBV) may indicate adequacy of collateral flow
  - May miss distal vasospasm if pCT limited to 2 slices
    - Whole brain pCT recommended

MR Findings

- DWI
  - Most sensitive for vasospasm sequelae
    - If ischemia proceeds to infarction
- MRA
  - Not usually utilized for screening
  - CT more easily performed in patients in ICU S/P SAH
  - Vessel stenosis → signal void on TOF imaging
    - Depends on vasospasm severity

Ultrasonographic Findings

- Transcranial Doppler (TCD)
  - Poiseuille law: ↑ mean flow velocity occurs due to ↓ arterial cross-sectional area from vasospasm/stenosis
  - Low frequency transducer used to evaluate larger arteries at base of brain
  - Transtemporal window absent in 10% patients
  - > 80% accuracy for vasospasm detection if
    - Mean velocity in MCA > 120 cm/s, basilar artery > 70 cm/s
    - Lindegaard ratio (mean MCA velocity to extracranial ICA velocity) > 3
  - Sensitivity ~ 60% (operator dependent)
  - Specificity > 95% (in patients with known SAH)
  - Upward trends in mean velocities may be more indicative of vasospasm than absolute values

Angiographic Findings

- Arterial luminal irregularity/undulations
- Smooth, relatively long-segment stenoses
  - Multiple arteries, > 1 vascular territory typical

DIFFERENTIAL DIAGNOSIS

Meningitis

- Sulcal/cisternal enhancement

Acute Hypertensive Encephalopathy (PRES)

- Posterior > anterior circulation

Reversible Cerebral Vasoconstriction Syndrome (RCVS), Migraine Headaches

- Transient, may look identical

Vasculitis

- Can look identical to vasospasm, RCVS; typically shorter segmental stenoses/"beading" in vasculitis
- Absence of SAH on NECT is typical (SAH secondary to vasculitis is rare)
  - Subacute SAH may be iso-/hypodense on NECT; CSF analysis may help to detect blood breakdown products
- Inflammatory markers in serum, CSF often elevated

Atherosclerosis (ASVD)

- Usually older patients
- Short > long-segment stenoses
- Cavernous/extracranial ICA, vertebral artery often affected

PATHOLOGY

General Features

- Etiology
  - SAH vasospasm most commonly seen after aneurysm rupture
    - Other causes of SAH (e.g., trauma, AVM rupture) may also cause vasospasm

VASOSPASM

- Exact pathophysiology is unknown
  - Causation is likely multifactorial
  - Coating of vessel walls with blood breakdown products (e.g., oxyHgb) → release of free radicals from vessel wall
  - Release of factors, including serotonin, angiotensin, prostaglandins, thromboxane, protein kinase C, phospholipase C and A2
  - Possible role of ↓ nitric oxide activity from endothelium, ↑ endothelin-1 activity

Staging, Grading, & Classification

- Fisher CT score corresponds to risk of vasospasm development
  - 1: No SAH
  - 2: Small SAH, < 1 mm vertical layers
  - 3: Extensive SAH, > 1 mm vertical layers
  - 4: Intraventricular hemorrhage (IVH)

Microscopic Features

- Prolonged exposure of vessel wall to blood components → thickening of tunica media, intimal edema, subintimal cellular proliferation with muscle cells and fibroblasts

CLINICAL ISSUES

Presentation

- Most common signs/symptoms
  - Majority of patients with vasospasm are asymptomatic
  - Vasospasm is significant source of morbidity and mortality in patients with SAH
  - Delayed ischemic neurological deficit (DIND) ~ 1 week after SAH is typical
  - Focal neurological deficit(s): Motor, language, vision
- Other signs/symptoms
  - Altered mental status, ↓ level of consciousness

Demographics

- Age
  - Any age; more common in younger patients
- Epidemiology
  - 30,000 people per year have SAH in USA
  - 70% of patients after aneurysmal SAH develop some degree of vasospasm detectable by DSA; only 30% symptomatic

Natural History & Prognosis

- Approximate time course of vasospasm following SAH
  - D3-4: Vasospasm begins
  - D7-10: Vasospasm peaks
  - D14-21: Vasospasm subsides
- Hyperacute vasospasm occurs in 10% of patients (onset < 48 hours from SAH)
- Aggressive treatment/prophylaxis in SAH patients can prevent stroke, death from ischemic sequela

Treatment

- Medical management
  - "Triple H" therapy = hypertension, hemodilution, hypervolemia
  - Oral or IV Ca++ antagonists (e.g., nimodipine)
  - Magnesium
- Endovascular
  - Chemical angioplasty: IA infusion of Ca++ antagonist has superseded papaverine
    - Less technically demanding than balloon angioplasty; can treat smaller distal vessels
    - Duration of effect may be up to 24 hours; additional IA treatments may be needed
    - Relatively low-risk: Side effect = hypotension, which could exacerbate hypoperfusion
  - Balloon angioplasty
    - Progressive dilatation of larger basal arteries: Intradural ICA and vertebral arteries, basilar artery, MCA (M1 ± M2 segments), ACA (A1 segment), PCA (P1 segment)
    - 1% risk of fatal vessel rupture, thromboembolic stroke, vessel dissection
  - Intracisternal thrombolytic therapy
    - Several clinical trials have shown moderate success; not widely accepted Rx
    - Recombinant tPA infused via ventriculostomy to lyse blood in subarachnoid spaces → ↓ breakdown to oxyHgb → prevent vasospasm

DIAGNOSTIC CHECKLIST

Consider

- Vasospasm as etiology of clinical deterioration, ischemic changes on NECT 4-14 days after aneurysmal SAH

Image Interpretation Pearls

- TCD is insensitive to changes in vessels beyond intradural ICA, M1, A1, and basilar arteries
  - Should proceed to DSA if involvement of more distal vessels suspected (e.g., pericallosal aneurysm rupture, nonaneurysmal SAH)

SELECTED REFERENCES

1. Eddleman CS et al: Endovascular options in the treatment of delayed ischemic neurological deficits due to cerebral vasospasm. Neurosurg Focus. 26(3):E6, 2009
2. Hänggi D et al: Feasibility and safety of intrathecal nimodipine on posthaemorrhagic cerebral vasospasm refractory to medical and endovascular therapy. Clin Neurol Neurosurg. 110(8):784-90, 2008
3. Ionita CC et al: The value of CT angiography and transcranial doppler sonography in triaging suspected cerebral vasospasm in SAH prior to endovascular therapy. Neurocrit Care. 9(1):8-12, 2008
4. Keuskamp J et al: High-dose intraarterial verapamil in the treatment of cerebral vasospasm after aneurysmal subarachnoid hemorrhage. J Neurosurg. 108(3):458-63, 2008
5. Majoie CB et al: Perfusion CT to evaluate the effect of transluminal angioplasty on cerebral perfusion in the treatment of vasospasm after subarachnoid hemorrhage. Neurocrit Care. 6(1):40-4, 2007
6. Tejada JG et al: Safety and feasibility of intra-arterial nicardipine for the treatment of subarachnoid hemorrhage-associated vasospasm: initial clinical experience with high-dose infusions. AJNR Am J Neuroradiol. 28(5):844-8, 2007

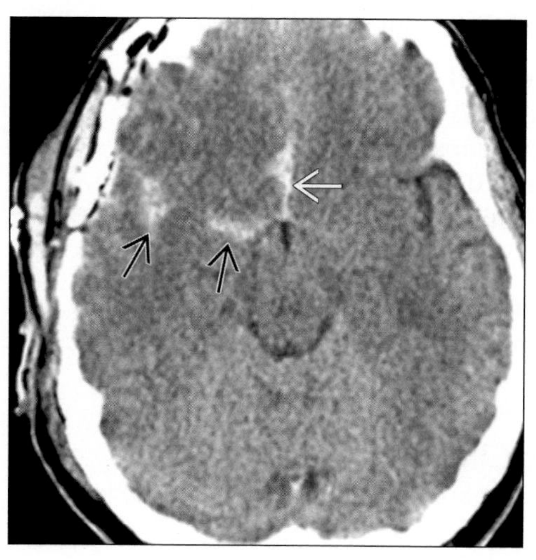

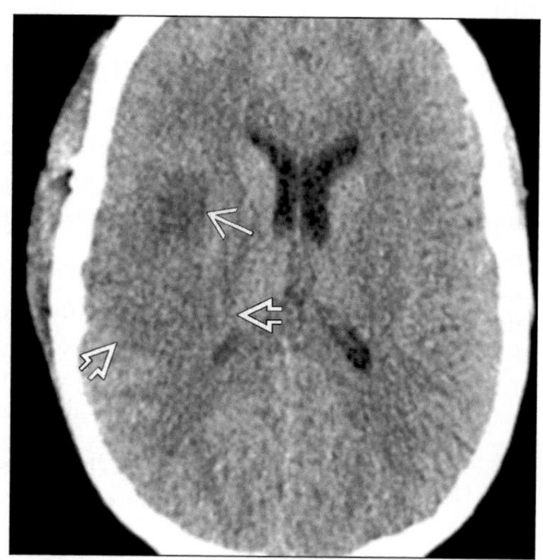

(Left) *Axial NECT in a patient S/P resection of a sphenoidal ridge meningioma complicated by significant intraoperative hemorrhage shows SAH in the right sylvian fissure ⇒ and anterior interhemispheric fissure ➡.* ***(Right)*** *Axial NECT obtained 10 days later when the patient developed hemiparesis shows a focal area of low attenuation in the right frontal lobe ➡, consistent with infarction. There is blurring of both the superficial and deep gray-white interface ➡ adjacent to the infarct.*

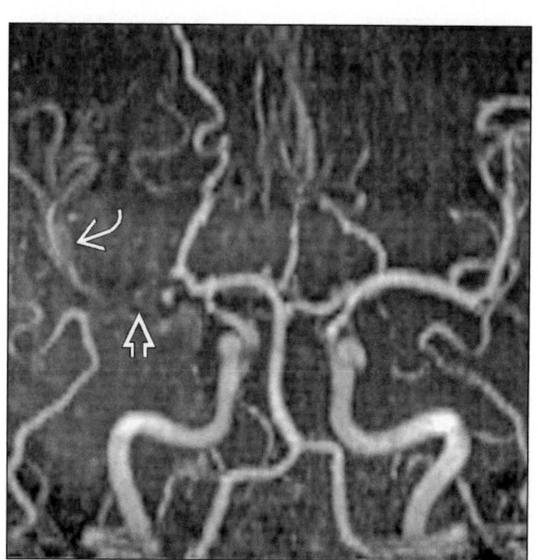

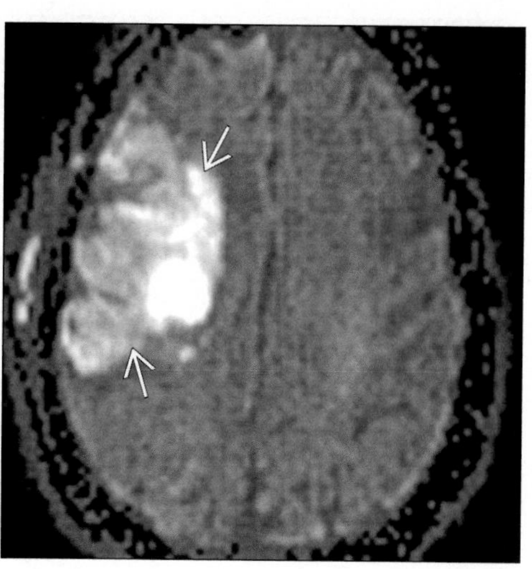

(Left) *Anteroposterior 3D TOF MRA MIP image in the same patient shows no signal from flow-related enhancement along the right M1 segment ➡. The M2 vessels ➡ are attenuated compared with the left side, suggestive of reduced flow.* ***(Right)*** *Axial DTI MR shows a large area of ischemia/ infarction in the right frontal lobe ➡. The constellation of imaging findings along with the delayed clinical deterioration 10 days after documented SAH made vasospasm the most likely etiology.*

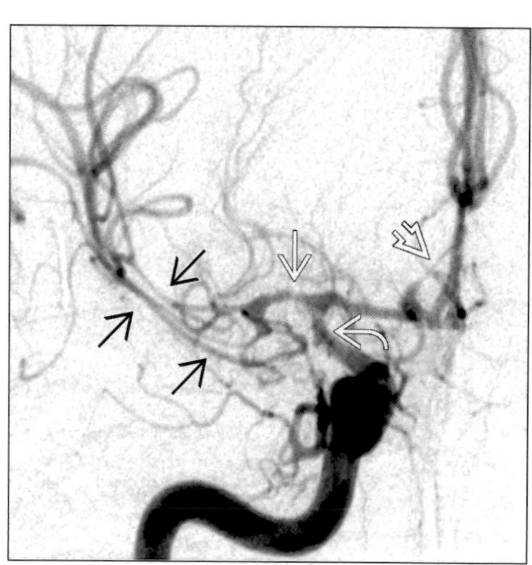

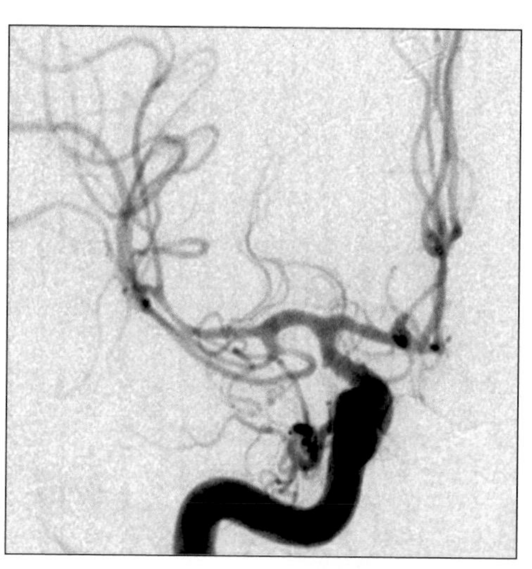

(Left) *AP right ICA DSA confirms the presence of severe vasospasm involving the right M1 ➡ and M2 ⇒ segments, as well as the right A2 segment ➡ and carotid terminus ➡.* ***(Right)*** *DSA after infusion of 25 mg verapamil into the right ICA shows significant increase in caliber of all vasospastic segments. The patient underwent additional IA verapamil treatments in the ensuing days. Recurrence of vasospasm after chemical angioplasty is to be expected whereas balloon angioplasty is more durable.*

SYSTEMIC LUPUS ERYTHEMATOSUS

Key Facts

Terminology

- Systemic lupus erythematosus (SLE), neuropsychiatric SLE (NPSLE)
- Multisystem autoimmune disorder
  - CNS involved in up to 75%

Imaging

- 4 general patterns
  - New infarcts (associated with ↑ anticardiolipin, ↑ lupus anticoagulant antibodies)
  - Focal areas of hyperintensity, primarily in GM
  - Multiple T2WI hyperintensities (microinfarctions)
  - Extensive, reversible WM changes (cerebral edema)
- Most common = multifocal WM microinfarcts, cerebral atrophy
- Mild SLE: PET/SPECT more sensitive than MR
- Restricted diffusion (cytotoxic edema) in ischemia/infarct
- Increased diffusion (vasogenic edema) in vasculopathy
- Acute/active CNS lesions may enhance

Top Differential Diagnoses

- Multiple sclerosis (MS), Susac syndrome
- Lyme encephalopathy
- Microvascular disease (e.g., arteriolosclerosis)
- Other vasculitides (e.g., PACNS)

Pathology

- Antiphospholipid antibodies (APL-Ab)
  - Macro-/microvascular thrombosis, arterial or venous
- Libman-Sacks endocarditis, emboli

Diagnostic Checklist

- Negative brain MR does not exclude cerebral lupus

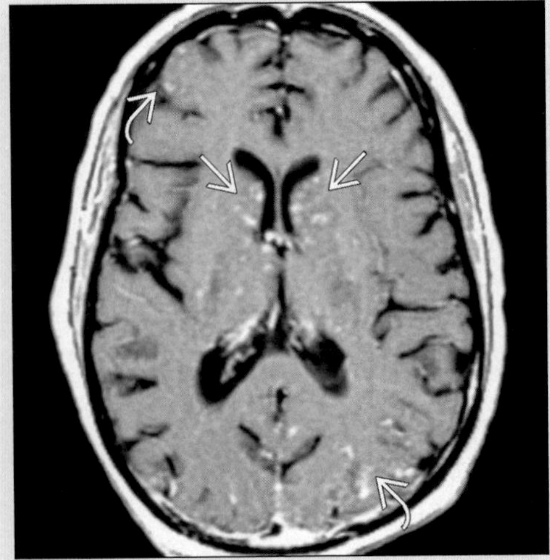
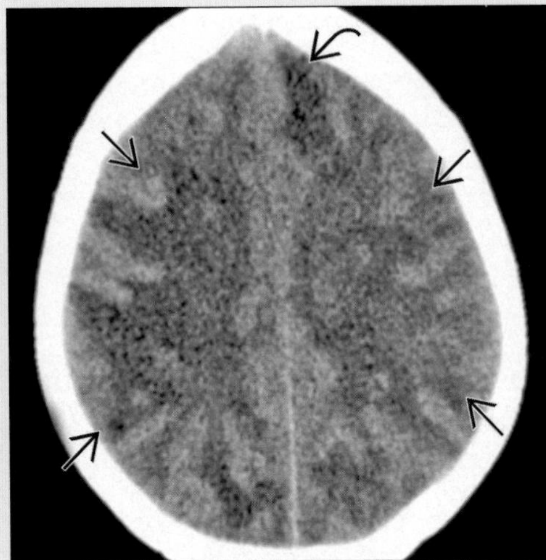

(Left) *Axial T1WI C+ MR shows multifocal linear and punctate enhancing foci in the basal ganglia ➔ and subcortical white matter ➔ due to small infarcts from CNS lupus vasculitis.* ***(Right)*** *Axial NECT shows diffuse confluent low-density areas in the deep and juxtacortical white matter ➔ of both hemispheres with a focal cortical infarct in the left frontal lobe ➔. The diffuse involvement was due to hypertensive encephalopathy secondary to severe renal involvement, a complication of lupus.*

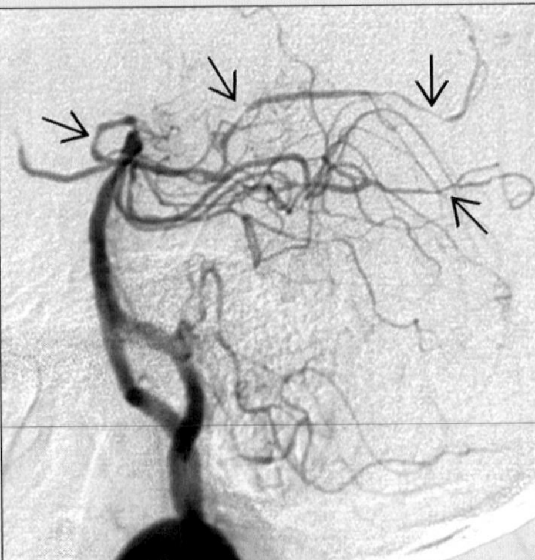
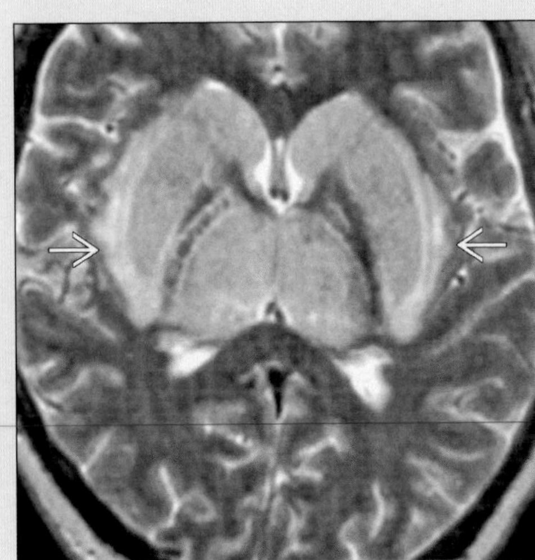

(Left) *Lateral vertebrobasilar DSA shows multifocal stenoses ➔ typical of a nonspecific vasculitis, uncommonly seen with lupus, which is more of a small-vessel vasculitis than other inflammatory vasculitides.* ***(Right)*** *Axial T2WI MR shows extensive hyperintensity in the basal ganglia, which appear somewhat swollen and compress the lateral ventricles. Note the hyperintensity in the external and extreme capsules ➔ due to 1 form of NPSLE, probably a neurotoxic response related to antineuronal antibodies.*

TERMINOLOGY

Abbreviations

- Systemic lupus erythematosus (SLE)
- Neuropsychiatric SLE (NPSLE)

Definitions

- Multisystem autoimmune disorder
  - CNS involved in up to 75%

IMAGING

General Features

- Best diagnostic clue
  - Focal infarcts of various sizes
  - Symptomatic "migratory" edematous areas
- Location
  - White matter (WM), gray matter (GM)
    - Frontal, parietal subcortical WM most common
- Morphology
  - Rounded or patchy lesions

CT Findings

- NECT
  - Other findings
    - Focal infarcts, cerebral calcification
    - Patchy cortical/subcortical hypodensities
  - Extensive, reversible WM changes (cerebral edema)
    - Can be life-threatening
- CECT
  - ↑ sensitivity for acute/subacute lesions
- CTA
  - Often completely normal in NPSLE

MR Findings

- T2WI
  - 4 patterns of involvement
    - Focal infarcts (↑ anticardiolipin, ↑ lupus anticoagulant antibodies)
    - Multiple T2WI hyperintensities (microinfarctions)
    - Focal areas of hyperintensity, primarily in GM
    - Diffuse steroid-responsive subcortical lesions (associated ↑ antineurofilament antibodies)
  - Acute lesions on T2WI suggesting active NPSLE
    - New infarct, discrete GM lesions, diffuse GM hyperintensities, cerebral edema
- FLAIR
  - Multifocal WM hyperintensities
- DWI
  - Restricted diffusion (cytotoxic edema) in ischemia/infarct
  - Increased diffusion (vasogenic edema) in vasculopathy
- T1WI C+
  - Acute/active CNS lesions may enhance
- MRA
  - Look for extra-/intracranial thrombosis
- MRV
  - May show dural venous sinus thrombosis
    - Especially in antiphospholipid syndrome
- MRS
  - ^{1}H-MRS in NPSLE patients
    - ↓ N-acetyl aspartate in lesions, as well as normal-appearing WM/GM
    - ↑ choline related to disease activity, stroke, inflammation, chronic WM disease
    - No ↑ in lactate ⇒ anaerobic metabolism is not fundamental characteristic of NPSLE
  - MRS findings directly correlate with severity of neuropsychiatric symptoms

Angiographic Findings

- CTA/MRA/DSA rarely detects cerebral lupus vasculitis

Nuclear Medicine Findings

- PET
  - Parietooccipital hypometabolism = most conspicuous finding in MR-negative NPSLE
- Tc-99m ethyl cysteinate dimer brain SPECT
  - Sensitive tool for early detection of brain abnormalities in SLE (more sensitive than MR)
  - Relatively nonspecific regional cerebral cortical hypoperfusion
    - Most hypoperfused areas: Parietal, frontal, and temporal lobes (MCA territory)
    - Least hypoperfused area: Cerebellum
  - Positive findings also seen in patients without neuropsychiatric signs/symptoms
    - Secondary to subclinical brain involvement or cerebral atrophy (due to steroid therapy)
    - Occasionally may show transient hyperperfusion

Imaging Recommendations

- Best imaging tool
  - MR more sensitive than CT
- Protocol advice
  - T2WI, FLAIR
  - Consider PET in NPSLE if standard MR normal

DIFFERENTIAL DIAGNOSIS

Multiple Sclerosis (MS)

- Hyperintense WM lesions on T2WI
- Lesions radially oriented along WM tracts
- Periventricular WM (callososeptal interface)
- SLE lesions not confined to periventricular WM, favor gray-white junction or involve cortex/deep nuclei

Antiphospholipid Antibodies (Non-SLE)

- "Antiphospholipid syndrome" in non-SLE patients
  - Early stroke, recurrent arterial + venous thromboses
  - Spontaneous fetal loss, thrombocytopenia
- Infarcts of various sizes and T2 hyperintense WM foci

Lyme Encephalopathy

- Hyperintense periventricular WM lesions on T2WI
- May enhance, resemble MS or ADEM

Small Vessel Cerebrovascular Disease

- Caused by diabetes, HTN, arteriolosclerosis
- T2WI hyperintense lesions within deep GM (basal ganglia, thalamus), centrum semiovale
- Diffuse, confluent regions of periventricular hyperintense WM involvement (leukoaraiosis)

SYSTEMIC LUPUS ERYTHEMATOSUS

Susac Syndrome
- Microangiopathy of unknown etiology
- Triad of HA/encephalopathy, branch retinal artery occlusions, hearing loss
- Deep WM, corpus callosum multifocal hyperintense lesions on T2WI, FLAIR
  - Central CC > callososeptal interface
  - May enhance (acute)
  - Central callosal "holes" in subacute/chronic
- Usually self-limited, fluctuating, monophasic illness
  - Duration 2-4 years (from 6 months up to 5 years)

Other Vasculitides
- Primary angiitis of CNS
- Polyarteritis nodosa (PAN)
- Wegener
- Behçet disease
- Syphilis
- Sjögren syndrome

PATHOLOGY

General Features
- Etiology
  - Pathogenesis of NPSLE is likely multifactorial
  - No pathognomonic brain lesion
  - Diverse nonspecific lesions of varying etiology
  - Diffuse neuropsychiatric symptoms
    - Neuronal dysfunction mediated by antibodies: Anti-neuronal, anti-ribosomal P-protein, and anti-cytokines
  - Focal neurologic symptoms
    - Circulating immune complexes ⇒ vascular injury
    - Endothelial cell activation by cytokines and complement activation ⇒ occlusive vasculopathy
    - Antiphospholipid antibodies (APL-Ab) ⇒ macro- and microvascular thrombosis
  - Late stage SLE: Accelerated atherosclerosis
    - ↑ intravascular complement turnover and APL-Ab
- Genetics
  - Genetic predisposition to SLE
    - HLA-DR2, HLA-DR3, null complement alleles
    - Congenital deficiencies of complement (C4, C2)
- Associated abnormalities
  - Lupus-related myelitis (transverse myelitis)
  - Libman-Sacks endocarditis, emboli

Gross Pathologic & Surgical Features
- Vasculitis ⇒ CNS ischemia or hemorrhage (intraparenchymal/subarachnoid)
- Edema ⇒ reversible leukoencephalopathy
- WM degeneration + myelin vacuolation of spinal cord

CLINICAL ISSUES

Presentation
- Most common signs/symptoms
  - CNS involvement in up to 75% of cases
    - Migraine, seizures, stroke, chorea
    - Transverse myelopathy, cranial neuropathies, aseptic meningitis
    - Psychosis, mood disorders, acute confusional state, cognitive dysfunction
  - Subclinical CNS disease in SLE: Transient event
- Clinical profile
  - Cerebral involvement may precede full-blown SLE picture or may develop during course of disease
    - Most frequently within 1st 3 years
  - Diffuse psychiatric or focal neurologic symptoms
  - Movement disorders (chorea, parkinsonism)

Demographics
- Age
  - All age groups affected; peak incidence in young adulthood (20-45)
- Gender
  - Strong female predominance (as high as 5:1 during childbearing years)
- Ethnicity
  - High prevalence in African-American women
- Epidemiology
  - Incidence of SLE (USA): 14.6-50.8 in 100,000 people
  - NPSLE affects 14-75% of SLE patients

Natural History & Prognosis
- Neurologic complications worsen prognosis of SLE
  - Transient neurologic deficits, chronic brain injury
- SLE patients with APL-Ab have additional risk for neuropsychiatric events
- Mortality rate in NPSLE: 7-40%

Treatment
- Immunosuppressive agents (steroids, cyclophosphamide) for suspected vasculitis
- Lifelong anticoagulation for APL-Ab-mediated thromboembolic events
- Intrathecal methotrexate + dexamethasone in severe cases
- Primary prevention of accelerated ASVD and narrowing of blood vessels: Prophylactic aspirin, lipid-lowering drugs

DIAGNOSTIC CHECKLIST

Consider
- Difficult to differentiate active from old NPSLE lesions
- Obtain MR within 24 hours of neurologic event onset

Image Interpretation Pearls
- Most important role of imaging in NPSLE: Assessment of acute focal (stroke-like) neurologic deficits
  - Lupus-related CNS vasculitis
  - Thromboembolic events due to vasculopathy or endocarditis (Libman-Sacks)
  - APL-Ab-mediated thrombosis
  - Microangiopathy (including thrombotic thrombocytopenic purpura)
  - Accelerated ASVD
- Negative brain MR does not exclude cerebral lupus

SELECTED REFERENCES

1. Baizabal-Carvallo JF et al: Posterior reversible encephalopathy syndrome as a complication of acute lupus activity. Clin Neurol Neurosurg. 111(4):359-63, 2009

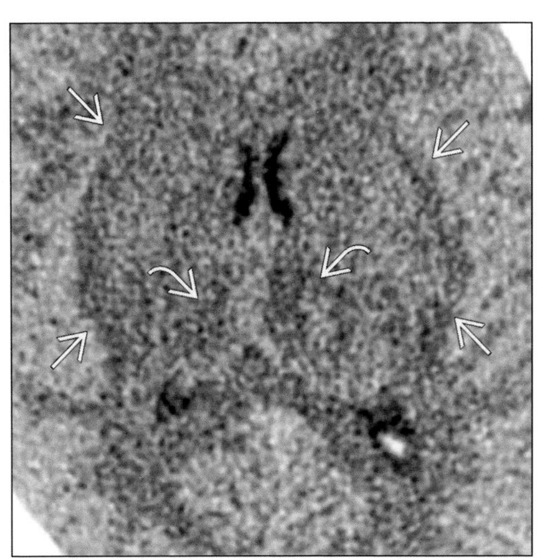

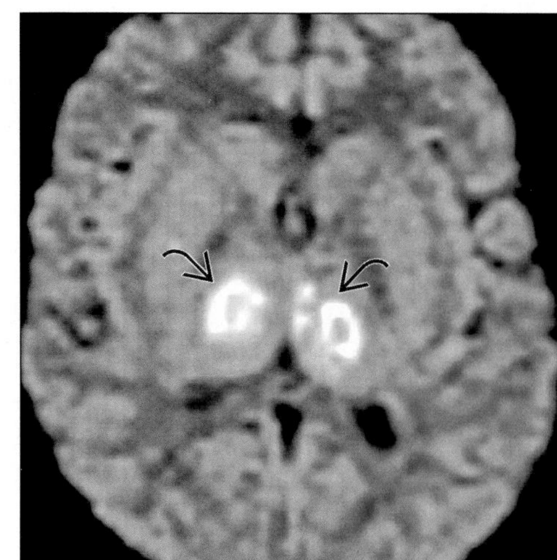

(Left) *Axial NECT in a patient with probable antineuronal antibodies shows bilateral caudate, lentiform, thalamic, and capsular hypodensity* ➔*. Note the more prominent hypodensity in the central thalami* ➦*.* ***(Right)*** *Axial DWI in the same patient 1 week later shows areas of restricted diffusion* ➦ *indicating frank infarction only involving the central thalami, correlating with CT. Although this form of lupus may be reversible and steroid responsive, severe involvement can lead to necrosis.*

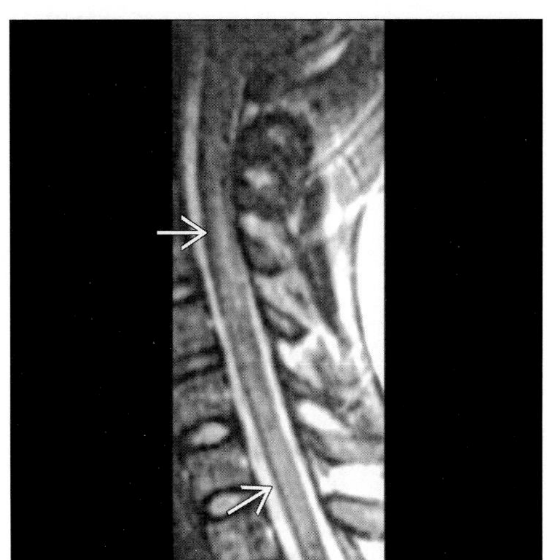

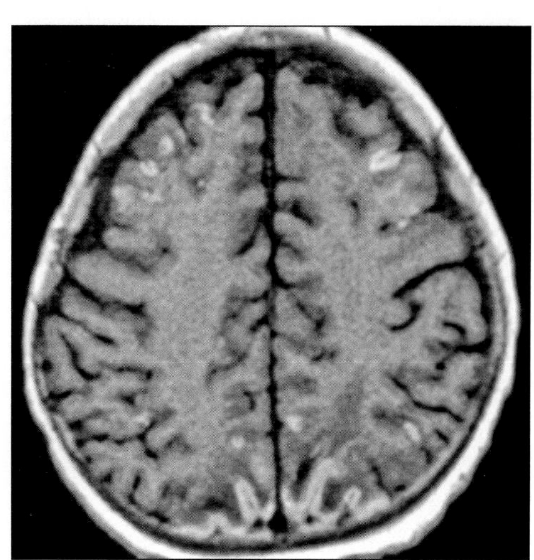

(Left) *Sagittal T2WI MR in the same patient shows multisegmental areas of increased signal intensity in the central gray matter of the spinal cord* ➔*, consistent with lupus myelopathy caused by neuronal toxicity or lupus vasculitis in penetrating spinal arteries.* ***(Right)*** *Axial T1WI MR shows multifocal areas of gyriform hyperintensity in the occipital cortex as well as the frontal gray matter near the anterior watershed zone due to PRES, a secondary complication of systemic renal involvement from lupus.*

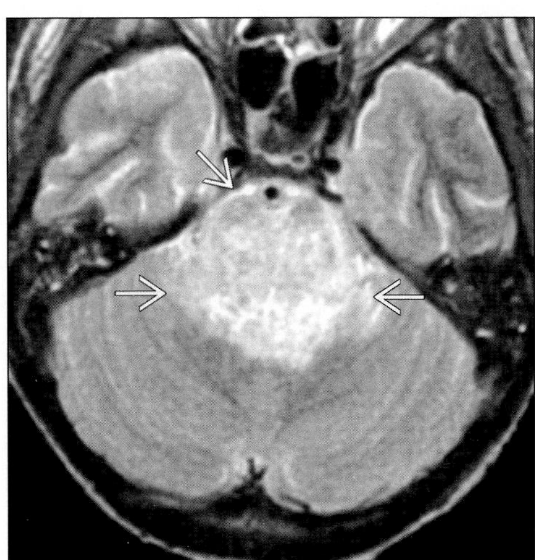

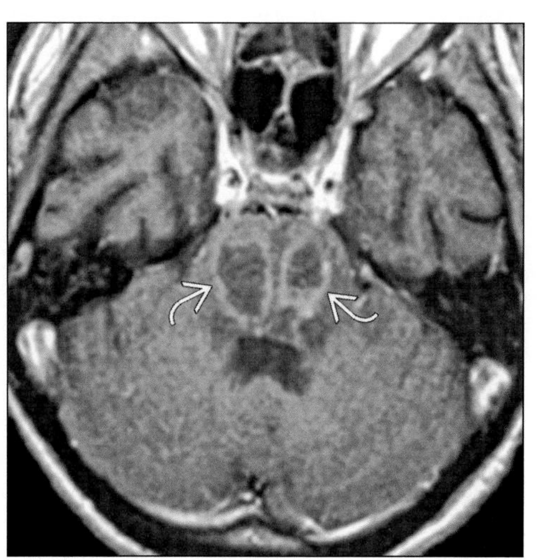

(Left) *Axial T2WI MR shows hyperintensity in the enlarged pons and middle cerebellar peduncles* ➔ *in this unusual variant of lupus vasculitis. Although small vessel vasculitis commonly involves the posterior fossa, it is usually a multifocal peripheral pattern.* ***(Right)*** *Axial T1WI C+ MR in the same patient shows 2 regions of ring enhancement* ➦ *in the central pons due to areas of ischemic necrosis. Lupus vasculitis, which this patient has, is uncommon. Necrotic infarcts in lupus are even less common.*

ANTIPHOSPHOLIPID ANTIBODY SYNDROME

Key Facts

Terminology
- Multisystem disorder characterized by
  - Thromboses, early strokes
  - Cognitive dysfunction
  - Pregnancy loss

Imaging
- More WM hypodensities/hyperintensities than expected for patient's age
- Geographic encephalomalacia from cortical/subcortical infarcts
- Characteristic atrophy pattern in parietal lobes
  - Frontal, temporal lobes relatively spared
- Cardiac valvular abnormalities in 1/3 of patients

Top Differential Diagnoses
- Multi-infarct dementia
- Systemic lupus erythematosus
- Alzheimer disease
- CADASIL
- Multiple sclerosis

Pathology
- Presumed autoimmune; pathophysiology is multifactorial

Clinical Issues
- Pregnancy loss, premature strokes, deep vein thromboses, cardiac valve abnormalities
- Seizures in 13% of APS patients
- Dementia in 10%, more prevalent with ↑ age

Diagnostic Checklist
- Compare parietal to temporal atrophy to distinguish from other dementia patterns

(Left) Axial FLAIR in a 43-year-old man with antiphospholipid antibody syndrome shows subacute ➔ and chronic ➾ infarcts in both PCA distributions ➾, as well as multifocal areas of WM hyperintensity ➦, enlarged sulci, and ventriculomegaly ➔. (Right) Axial FLAIR in the same patient shows subcortical ➦ and centrum semiovale ➔ WM hyperintensities related to advanced microvascular ischemia.

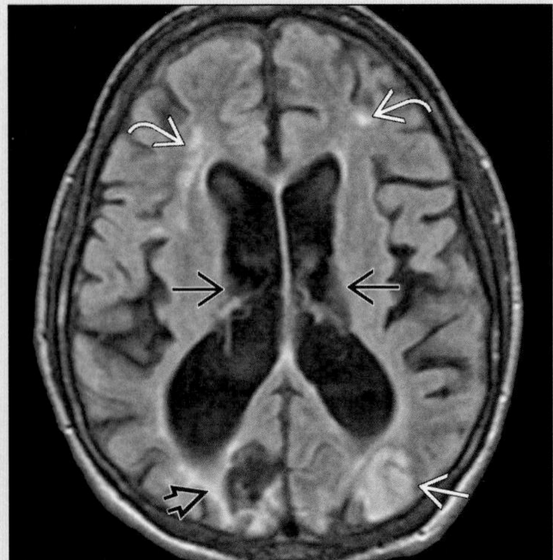

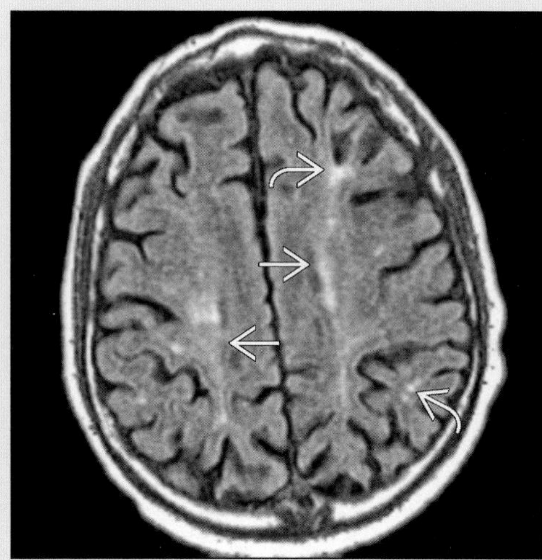

(Left) Axial T2 GRE in another case shows focal perirolandic and post central gyrus atrophy ➔ that is out of proportion to the frontal or temporal atrophy, characteristic for APS. No microhemorrhages or geographic, large-vessel territorial infarcts were present. (Right) Sagittal T1WI MR shows parietal and focal post central gyrus atrophy ➔ with relative sparing of the frontal and temporal lobes in a young patient with antiphospholipid antibody syndrome and dementia.*

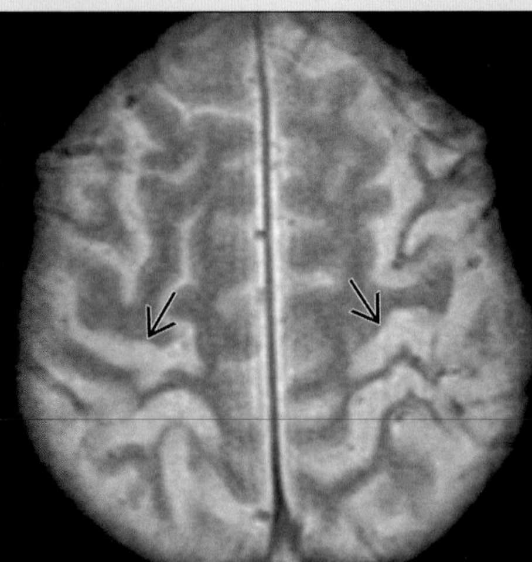

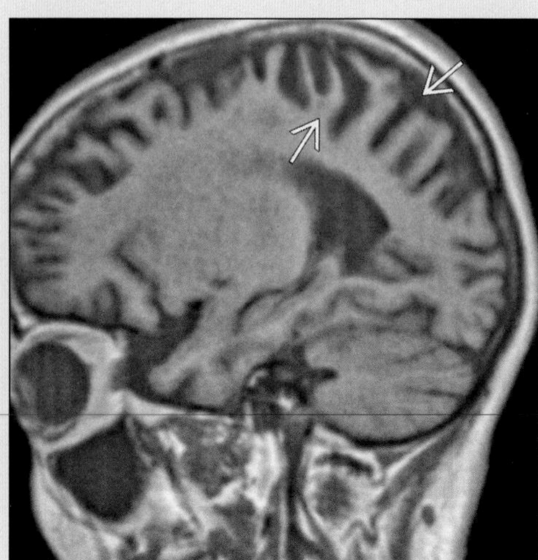

ANTIPHOSPHOLIPID ANTIBODY SYNDROME

TERMINOLOGY

Abbreviations

- Antiphospholipid antibody syndrome (APS)

Definitions

- Multisystem disorder characterized by
  - Thromboses, early strokes
  - Cognitive dysfunction
  - Pregnancy loss

IMAGING

General Features

- Best diagnostic clue
  - Premature strokes, WM hyperintensities
  - Characteristic atrophy pattern in parietal lobes with relative sparing of frontal, temporal lobes

CT Findings

- NECT
  - Multiple cortical/subcortical infarcts
    - More than expected for age
    - Accelerated microvascular ischemic changes

MR Findings

- T1WI
  - Atrophy greatest in parietal lobe (postcentral gyrus)
  - Relative sparing of temporal, frontal lobes
- T2WI
  - Multiple deep WM hyperintensities
  - Geographic encephalomalacia (cortical/subcortical infarcts)
- FLAIR
  - More hyperintensities than expected for patient age
- DWI
  - Acute/early subacute infarcts restrict

Ultrasonographic Findings

- Echocardiography
  - Cardiac valvular abnormalities in 1/3 of patients
    - Mitral valve thickening most common
  - Cardiac US recommended in all APS patients

DIFFERENTIAL DIAGNOSIS

Multi-Infarct Dementia

- May have similar pattern of multiple infarcts and chronic ischemic changes ("Binswanger dementia")
- Typically hemispheric, basal ganglia
- No focal parietal atrophy

Systemic Lupus Erythematosus

- Commonly occurs with APS
- CNS manifestations of vasculitis, infarcts, accelerated T2 hyperintensities

Alzheimer Disease

- Cerebral atrophy more commonly involves temporal and parietal lobes
- Prominent hippocampal atrophy

CADASIL

- May show premature dementia, greater than expected T2 WM hyperintensities
- Characteristic anterior temporal subcortical white matter hyperintensity

Multiple Sclerosis

- T2 lesions more often involve callososeptal margin

PATHOLOGY

General Features

- Etiology
  - Presumed autoimmune; pathophysiology is multifactorial

Staging, Grading, & Classification

- Sapporo criteria (1999) (updated 2006)
  - 1 clinical and 1 laboratory criteria must be met
  - Clinical criteria
    - Vascular thrombosis (arterial or venous, any tissue or organ)
    - Pregnancy morbidity: Normal fetus lost beyond 10th week of gestation, eclampsia, placental insufficiency, 3 or more unexplained spontaneous abortions before 10th week
  - Laboratory criteria
    - Lupus anticoagulant (LA) present in plasma on 2 occasions at least 12 weeks apart
    - Anticardiolipin antibody (aCL) of IgG or IgM in medium or high titer in serum on 2 occasions at least 12 weeks apart
    - Anti-β2-glycoprotein-I antibody in serum on 2 occasions at least 12 weeks apart

CLINICAL ISSUES

Presentation

- Most common signs/symptoms
  - Pregnancy loss, premature cerebral infarcts, deep vein thromboses, cardiac valve abnormalities
- Other signs/symptoms
  - Seizures in 13% of APS patients
  - Dementia in 10%, more prevalent with age

Demographics

- Age
  - With CNS abnormalities
    - Mean = 49 years old, range = 16-79 years old
- Gender
  - M:F = 1:2
  - Female APS patients often diagnosed through pregnancy losses

Treatment

- Anticoagulation, steroids, aspirin, dypiridamole

SELECTED REFERENCES

1. Gómez-Puerta JA et al: Dementia associated with the antiphospholipid syndrome: clinical and radiological characteristics of 30 patients. Rheumatology (Oxford). 44(1):95-9, 2005

THROMBOTIC MICROANGIOPATHIES (HUS/TTP)

Key Facts

Terminology
- Microvascular occlusive disorders characterized by
  - Platelet aggregation, profound thrombocytopenia
  - Vascular occlusions
  - Intravascular hemolysis, hemolytic anemia
- Includes several major disorders
  - Thrombotic thrombocytopenic purpura (TTP)
  - Hemolytic uremic syndrome (HUS)
  - Malignant hypertension (mHTN)
  - Disseminated intravascular coagulopathy (DIC)

Imaging
- General: Multifocal peripheral hemorrhagic infarcts
- CT: Variable cortical hemorrhages, edema
- MR
  - Multifocal peripherally located punctate/gyral hyperintensities on FLAIR
  - "Blooming" foci in cortex on GRE/SWI
  - Multiple foci of diffusion restriction
  - Some patients have PRES-like findings

Top Differential Diagnoses
- Acute hypertensive encephalopathy, PRES
- Multiple acute embolic infarcts
- Antiphospholipid antibody syndrome
- Cortical venous thrombosis

Pathology
- Common pathway may be sepsis/organ failure-related brain microhemorrhages &/or infarcts

Clinical Issues
- Diverse clinical features related to thrombi in multiple organs

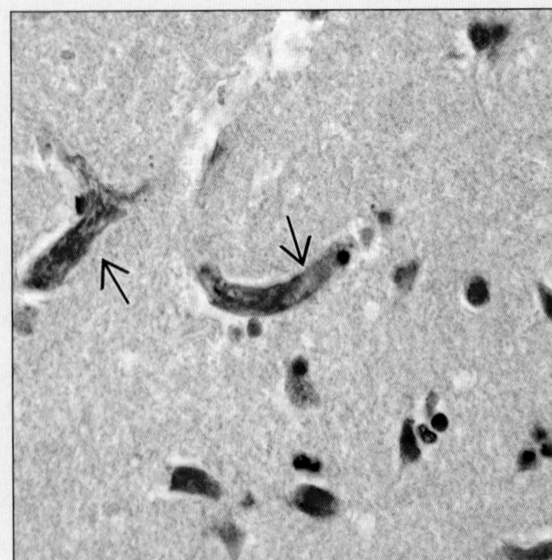
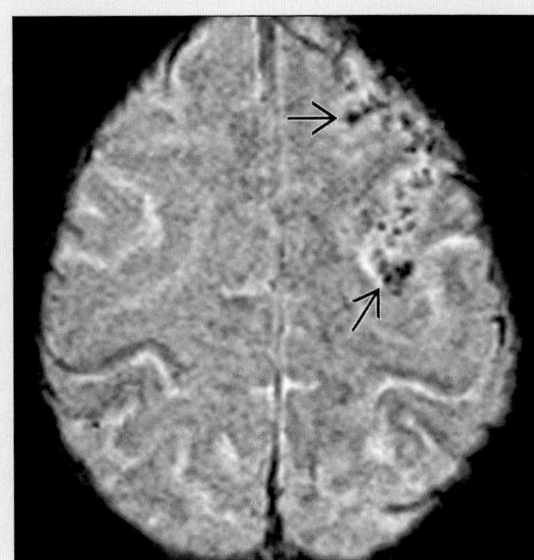

(Left) High-power hematoxylin & eosin stain in a patient with disseminated intravascular coagulopathy shows multiple thrombi in capillaries ➔ causing edema and ischemic changes in the surrounding brain. (Courtesy R. Hewlett, PhD.) (Right) Axial T2 SWI MR in a 40-year-old woman with TTP shows multifocal punctate areas of "blooming" in the left frontal cortex/ subcortical white matter ➔.*

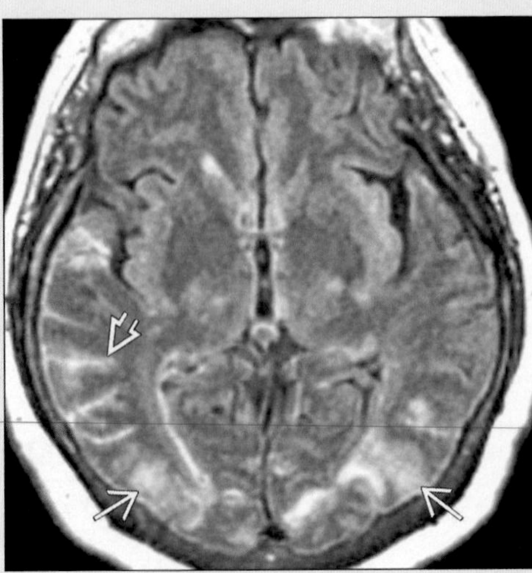
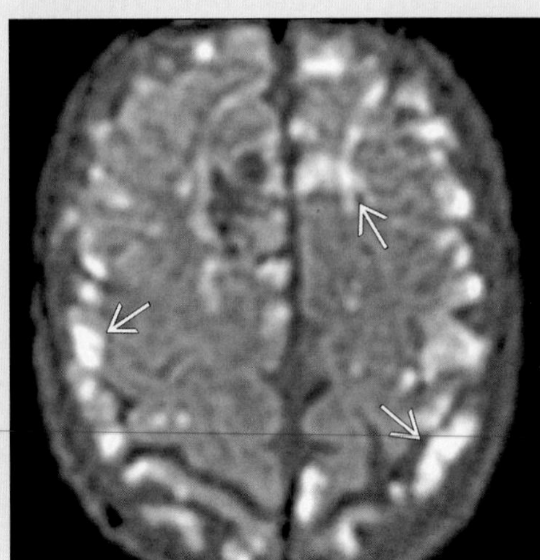

(Left) Axial FLAIR in a 66-year-old woman with mHTN, seizure, anemia with thrombocytopenia, and acute renal failure shows subarachnoid hemorrhage ➔ and occipital hyperintensities ➔. (Right) Axial DWI in a 64-year-old man with altered mental status, β streptococcal pneumonia with sepsis, multi-organ failure, low hematocrit (31%), and low platelets (22,000) shows multifocal cortical foci of restricted diffusion ➔, consistent with DIC-induced small vessel occlusions.

THROMBOTIC MICROANGIOPATHIES (HUS/TTP)

TERMINOLOGY

Abbreviations

- Thrombotic microangiopathies (TMAs)
- Disseminated intravascular coagulation (DIC)
- Thrombocytopenic thrombotic purpura (TTP)
- Hemolytic-uremic syndrome (HUS)

Definitions

- Includes 3 major disorders
  - TTP (± HUS)
  - Disseminated intravascular coagulopathy (DIC)
  - Malignant hypertension (mHTN)

IMAGING

General Features

- Best diagnostic clue
  - Multifocal peripheral hemorrhagic infarcts in patients with HUS/TTP, DIC, or mHTN
- Location
  - Cortex, subcortical white matter

Imaging Recommendations

- Best imaging tool
  - MR with T2* GRE or SWI, DWI

CT Findings

- NECT
  - May be normal early
  - Variable cortical hemorrhages

MR Findings

- T1WI
  - Variable signal depending on hemorrhage age
- T2WI
  - Cortical/subcortical hyperintensities
- FLAIR
  - Multifocal peripherally located punctate/gyral hyperintensities
- T2* GRE
  - Punctate/gyral "blooming" foci in cortex
- DWI
  - Multiple foci of diffusion restriction

DIFFERENTIAL DIAGNOSIS

Acute Hypertensive Encephalopathy, PRES

- HUS/TTP may cause PRES-like imaging pattern with posterior leukoencephalopathy
- May affect only brainstem

Cerebral Infarction, Multiple Embolic

- Air embolism may mimic findings in TMAs

Antiphospholipid Antibody Syndrome (APS)

- HELLP (**h**emolysis, **e**levated **l**iver enzymes, **l**ow **p**latelets) may complicate APS
  - In APS, typically associated with eclampsia/preeclampsia

Cortical Venous Thrombosis

- May occur ± dural sinus occlusion
- Hemorrhages, infarcts in TMA typically more diffuse

PATHOLOGY

General Features

- Etiology
  - Microvascular occlusive disorders characterized by
    - Platelet aggregation with profound thrombocytopenia
    - Variable occlusions in microcirculation
    - Intravascular hemolysis, schistocytosis
    - Microangiopathic hemolytic anemia
  - HUS/TTP may be triggered by enteric infections
  - Common pathway may be sepsis/organ failure-related brain microhemorrhages
  - Some patients have findings similar to posterior reversible encephalopathy syndrome (PRES)
    - Hypertension, renal failure → posterior leukoencephaly
    - Less commonly may occur in absence of HTN
- Associated abnormalities
  - End-organ ischemia/infarctions ± hemorrhage
    - Kidneys most commonly affected

Microscopic Features

- DIC causes segmental vascular damage, necrotizing microvascular hemorrhages
  - ± true intravascular thrombi of platelet-fibrin aggregates
- TTP causes intravascular "plugs" of eosinophilic, somewhat granular thrombi ± surrounding parenchymal injury
- Hypertensive encephalopathy causes "sausage-string" appearance in affected arterioles
  - Segments of fibrinoid necrosis
  - Alternating areas of "blow out" arteriolar dilatations

CLINICAL ISSUES

Presentation

- Most common signs/symptoms
  - Diverse clinical features related to thrombi in multiple organs
    - 50% of patients with TTP have CNS symptoms
      - Seizures
      - Fluctuating focal neurologic deficits
    - Seizures or strokes in patient with mHTN (often eclampsia/pre-eclampsia)
    - Child with abdominal pain, diarrhea (HUS)

Demographics

- Age
  - Adult (mHTN, TTP) vs. child (HUS)
  - DIC in both age groups

SELECTED REFERENCES

1. Zheng XL et al: Pathogenesis of thrombotic microangiopathies. Annu Rev Pathol. 3:249-77, 2008
2. Garewal M et al: MRI changes in thrombotic microangiopathy secondary to malignant hypertension. J Neuroimaging. 17(2):178-80, 2007

CEREBRAL AMYLOID DISEASE

Key Facts

Terminology
- Cerebral amyloid deposition occurs in 3 morphologic varieties
  - Common: Cerebral amyloid angiopathy (CAA)
  - Uncommon: Mass-like lesion ("amyloidoma")
  - Rare: Diffuse (encephalopathic) WM involvement

Imaging
- General findings
  - Normotensive demented patient
  - Lobar hemorrhage(s) of different ages
  - Multifocal "black dots" on T2* MR
- Protocol advice
  - NECT = best initial screening (for acute hemorrhage)
  - MR with T2*

Top Differential Diagnoses
- Multifocal "black dots" on T2/T2* MR
  - Hypertensive microhemorrhages
  - Ischemic stroke with microhemorrhage
  - Multiple cavernous malformations (type 4)
  - Diffuse axonal injury
  - Hemorrhagic metastases
  - CADASIL
  - Posterior reversible encephalopathy syndrome (PRES)

Clinical Issues
- CAA = common cause of "spontaneous" lobar hemorrhage in elderly
  - Causes up to 15-20% of primary intracranial hemorrhage (ICH) in patients > 60 years old
  - Stroke-like clinical presentation with "spontaneous" lobar ICH
  - Incidence of CAA in such patients = 4-10%
  - Chronic: Can cause vascular dementia

*(**Left**) Axial graphic shows acute hematoma ➡ with a fluid level ➝. Multiple microbleeds ➡ and old lobar hemorrhages ⇨ are also typical findings in cerebral amyloid disease. (**Right**) Axial T2WI shows a large right parenchymal hemorrhage. Fluid levels, with dependent T2 hypointense signal ➡, are characteristic of acute hemorrhage. Sagittal images (not shown) confirmed the hemorrhage was centered in the frontal lobe, rather than the basal ganglia. (Basal ganglia bleeds suggest hypertensive etiology.)*

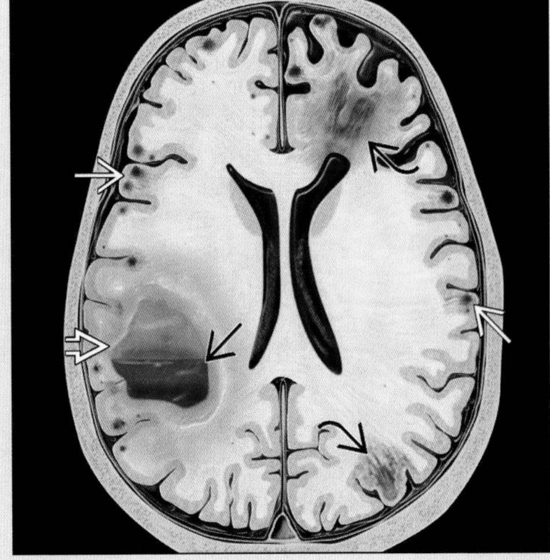

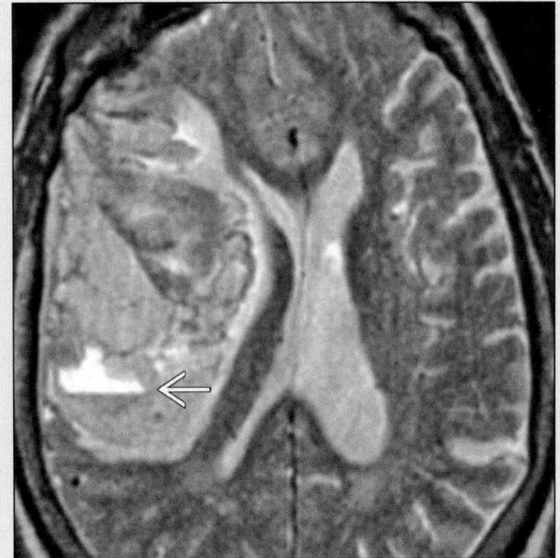

*(**Left**) Axial NECT shows a left posterior, frontal/anterior, parietal acute peripheral lobar hematoma ➡. (**Right**) Axial T2* GRE in the same patient again shows a left hemispheric lobar hematoma with strong susceptibility effect ⇨. Note the multifocal "black dots" ➝, whose peripheral location is suggestive of amyloid. The presence of multiple peripheral microbleeds in an elderly patient in the setting of mild cognitive impairment is highly suspicious for amyloid angiopathy.*

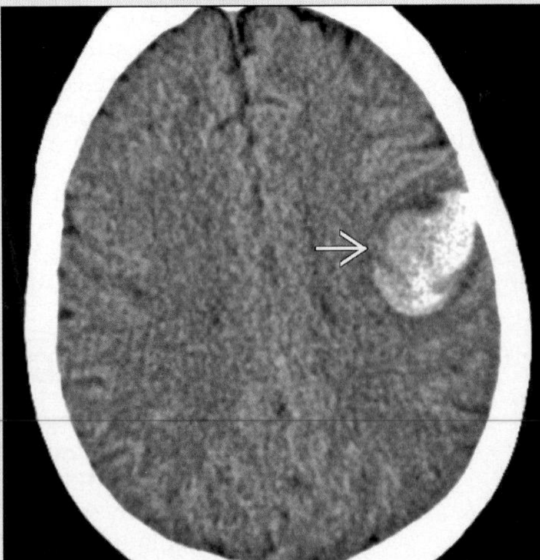

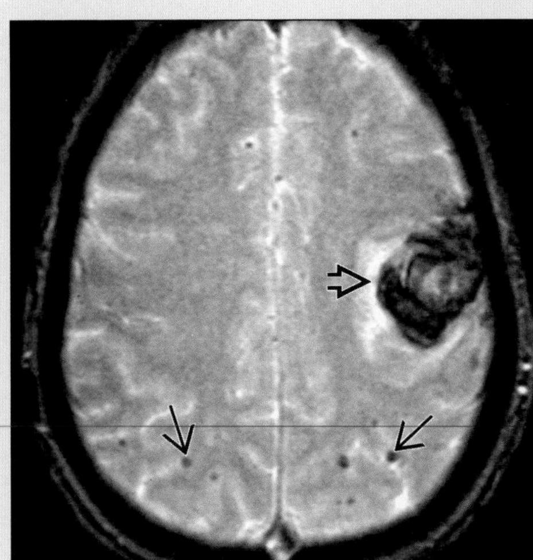

TERMINOLOGY

Abbreviations

- Cerebral amyloid angiopathy (CAA)

Synonyms

- "Congophilic angiopathy," cerebral amyloidosis

Definitions

- Cerebral amyloid deposition occurs in 3 morphologic varieties
  - CAA (common)
  - Amyloidoma (uncommon)
  - Diffuse (encephalopathic) white matter (WM) involvement (rare)
- CAA is common cause of "spontaneous" lobar hemorrhage in elderly

IMAGING

General Features

- Best diagnostic clue
  - Normotensive demented patient with
    - Lobar hemorrhage(s) of different ages
    - Multifocal cortical/subcortical "black dots" on T2*
- Location
  - Subcortical WM (gray-white junction)
  - Parietal + occipital lobes most common at autopsy; also frontal + temporal on imaging
  - Less common in brainstem, deep gray nuclei, cerebellum, hippocampus
- Size
  - Acute lobar hemorrhage tends to be large
  - Hypointense foci on dark T2*/susceptibility sequences (blooming) seen with chronic microbleeds, but not specific for CAA
    - Microbleeds and macrobleeds may represent distinct entities in CAA
    - Increased vessel wall thickness may predispose to microbleed > macrobleed formation
- Morphology
  - Acute hematomas are large, often irregular, with dependent blood sedimentation

CT Findings

- NECT
  - Patchy or confluent cortical/subcortical hematoma with irregular borders, surrounding edema
  - Hemorrhage may extend to subarachnoid space or into ventricles
  - Rare: Gyriform Ca++
  - Generalized atrophy common
- CECT
  - No enhancement, unless amyloidoma (rare)

MR Findings

- T1WI
  - Lobar hematoma (signal varies with age of clot)
- T2WI
  - Acute hematoma iso-/hypointense
    - 1/3 have old hemorrhages (lobar, petechial) seen as multifocal punctate "black dots"
  - Focal or patchy/confluent WM disease associated in nearly 70%
  - Rare form: Nonhemorrhagic diffuse encephalopathy with confluent WM hyperintensities
    - Acute white matter vasogenic edema may be seen in acute inflammatory forms
      - Can mimic posterior reversible encephalopathy syndrome (PRES) on imaging
    - Asymmetric pattern and multiple microbleeds are suggestive
    - Lack typical PRES predisposing factors (e.g., hypertensive crisis, immunosuppressive drugs)
    - Acute inflammatory CAA = steroid responsive
  - Microbleeds: Dark T2 foci variably present; T2* much more sensitive
- T2* GRE
  - Multifocal "black dots" (best sequence to detect chronic microbleeds)
- T1WI C+
  - CAA, lobar hemorrhages usually do not enhance
  - Amyloidoma (focal, nonhemorrhagic mass[es])
    - Mass effect generally minimal/mild
    - May show moderate/striking enhancement, mimic neoplasm
    - Often extends medially to lateral ventricular wall with fine radial enhancing margins
    - Rare: Patchy, infiltrating
- Susceptibility weighted imaging (SWI)
  - Multifocal hypointensities (microbleeds) similar to T2* GRE, but more sensitive

Angiographic Findings

- Conventional: Normal or avascular mass effect

Imaging Recommendations

- Best imaging tool
  - NECT = best initial screening study (for acute hemorrhage)
  - MR with T2* for nonacute evaluation (dementia)
- Protocol advice
  - Include T2*-weighted sequence in all patients > 60 years old

DIFFERENTIAL DIAGNOSIS

Hypertensive Microhemorrhages

- Deep structures (basal ganglia, thalami, cerebellum) > cortex, subcortical WM
- Often coexists with CAA
- Younger patients than CAA (< 65 years old)

Ischemic Stroke with Microhemorrhage

- Multifocal hemosiderin deposits
  - Found in 10-15% of patients with acute ischemic strokes
- Hemorrhagic lacunar infarcts

Multiple Vascular Malformations

- Cavernous malformations
  - Look for "locules" of blood with fluid-fluid levels or multiple ages of hemorrhage
  - Often dense on CT due to calcification
- Capillary telangiectasias
  - Faint, brush-like, or transparent enhancement

- Type seen as multifocal "black dots" on T2* (GRE)
- Brainstem > lobar location

Other Causes of Multifocal "Black Dots"

- Traumatic diffuse axonal injury
  - History of trauma
  - Location in corpus callosum, subcortical/deep white matter, brainstem
- Hemorrhagic metastases
  - Location similar to CAA (gray-white junction)
  - Variable enhancement, edema
- CADASIL
  - Usually nonhemorrhagic
  - Most common site = cortical-subcortical (up to 27% in thalami/brainstem)
- Metallic microemboli from artificial heart valves
- PRES
  - Associated with acute hypertensive crisis or immunosuppressive therapy in most
  - Symmetric lesions more typical

PATHOLOGY

General Features

- Etiology
  - Amyloidosis = rare systemic disease caused by extracellular deposition of β-amyloid
  - 10-20% of cases are localized form, including CNS
  - Can be primary/idiopathic
  - Can be secondary/reactive (e.g., dialysis-related amyloidosis)
- Genetics
  - Sporadic
    - APOE4 allele associated with CAA-related hemorrhage
    - Polymorphisms in presenilin-1 gene
  - Hereditary cerebral hemorrhage with amyloidosis
    - Autosomal dominant inheritance
    - Dutch type = mutated amyloid β precursor protein on chromosome 21
    - Other types include British, Flemish, etc.

Staging, Grading, & Classification

- WHO classification of amyloidoses
  - Primary systemic amyloidosis
  - Secondary amyloidosis
  - Hereditary systemic amyloidosis
  - Hemodialysis-related systemic amyloidosis
  - Medullary thyroid carcinoma
  - Type 2 diabetes

Gross Pathologic & Surgical Features

- Lobar hemorrhage(s)
- Multiple small cortical hemorrhages

Microscopic Features

- Interstitial, vascular/perivascular deposits of amorphous protein
  - Shows apple-green birefringence when stained with Congo red, viewed under polarized light
  - 3 components
    - Fibrillar protein component (varies/defines amyloidosis type)
    - Serum amyloid P
    - Charged glycosaminoglycans (ubiquitous)
- Microaneurysms
- Fibrinoid necrosis
- Hyaline thickening
- 15% have CAA-related perivascular inflammation

CLINICAL ISSUES

Presentation

- Most common signs/symptoms
  - Acute: Stroke-like clinical presentation with "spontaneous" lobar intracranial hemorrhage
    - Incidence of CAA in such patients = 4-10%
  - Chronic: Dementia (CAA)
- Clinical profile
  - CAA common in demented elderly patients
    - 2/3 normotensive, 1/3 hypertensive
    - 40% with subacute dementia/overt Alzheimer (overlap common)

Demographics

- Age
  - Usually older when sporadic (> 60 years old)
  - Inflammatory CAA younger
    - May mimic PRES with acute edema, but steroid responsive
- Gender
  - No gender predilection
- Epidemiology
  - 1% of all strokes
  - Causes up to 15-20% of primary ICH in patients > 60 years old
  - Frequency of CAA in elderly
    - 27-32% of normal elderly (autopsy)
    - 82-88% in patients with Alzheimer disease
    - Common in Down syndrome
  - Other associations: Kuru, Creutzfeldt-Jacob disease, plasmacytoma

Natural History & Prognosis

- Multiple, recurrent hemorrhages
- Progressive cognitive decline

Treatment

- Evacuate focal hematoma if patient < 75 years old, no intraventricular hemorrhage, not parietal
- Consider immunosuppressive therapy in inflammatory CAA
- Adverse prognostic factors: Low Glasgow coma scale scores, APOE4 allele

DIAGNOSTIC CHECKLIST

Consider

- GRE (T2*) &/or SWI in all elderly

SELECTED REFERENCES

1. Alcalay RN et al: MRI showing white matter lesions and multiple lobar microbleeds in a patient with reversible encephalopathy. J Neuroimaging. 19(1):89-91, 2009
2. Greenberg SM et al: Microbleeds versus macrobleeds: evidence for distinct entities. Stroke. 40(7):2382-6, 2009

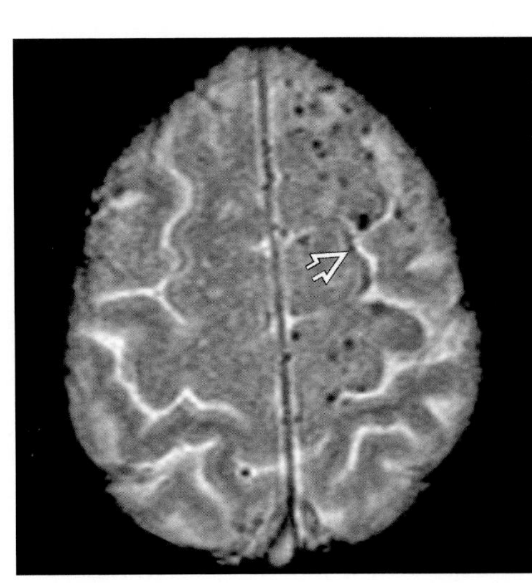

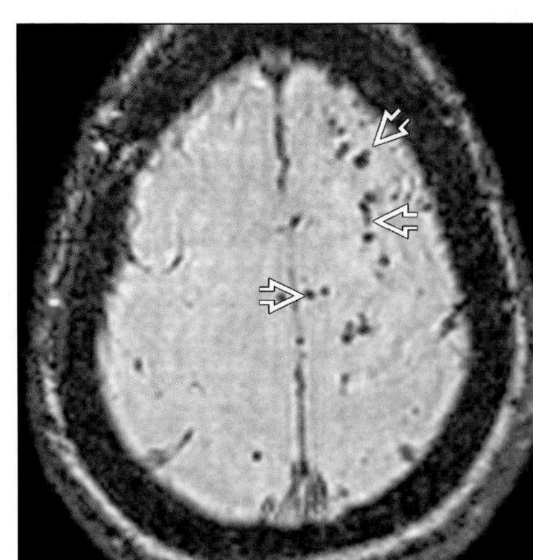

(Left) *Axial T2* GRE MR show large numbers of "black dots" almost exclusively in the cortex and brain surface in this 47 year old. Linear hypointensity along the pial surface ➩ probably represents superficial siderosis.* ***(Right)*** *Axial SWI shows additional hypointensities in the cortex and along the pial surfaces ➩. The findings are those of amyloid angiopathy. Lack of cerebellar and basal ganglia involvement (not shown) argues against hypertensive microbleeds. Indeed, this patient was normotensive.*

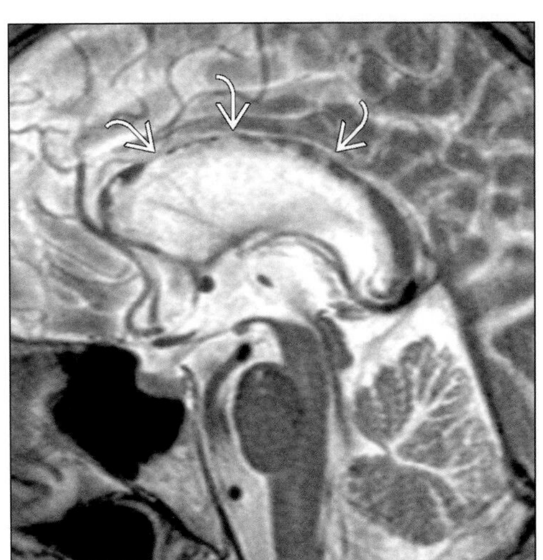

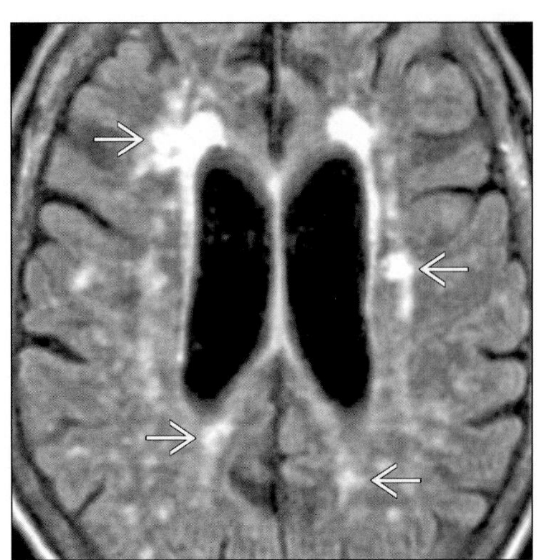

(Left) *Sagittal T2WI in an elderly, demented patient demonstrates severe thinning and multifocal hyperintense foci in the corpus callosum ➦.* ***(Right)*** *Axial FLAIR in the same patient demonstrates multifocal T2 hyperintensities ➔ in the periventricular white matter. The distribution is perivascular but nonspecific. Autopsy disclosed the diffuse leukoencephalopathic variant of amyloidosis. This manifestation of CAA is rare and imaging findings are nonspecific. (Courtesy R. Hewlett, PhD.)*

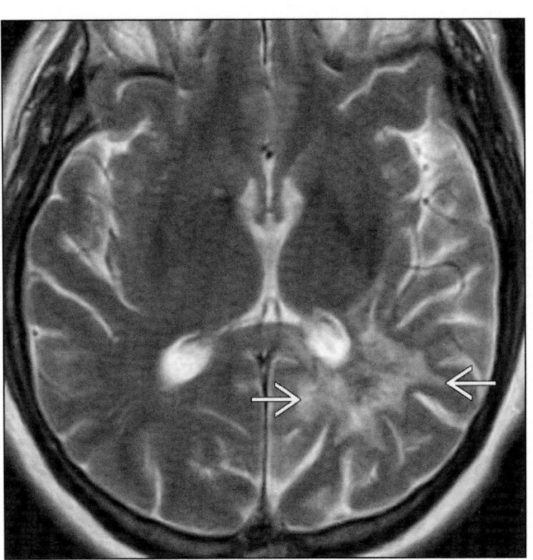

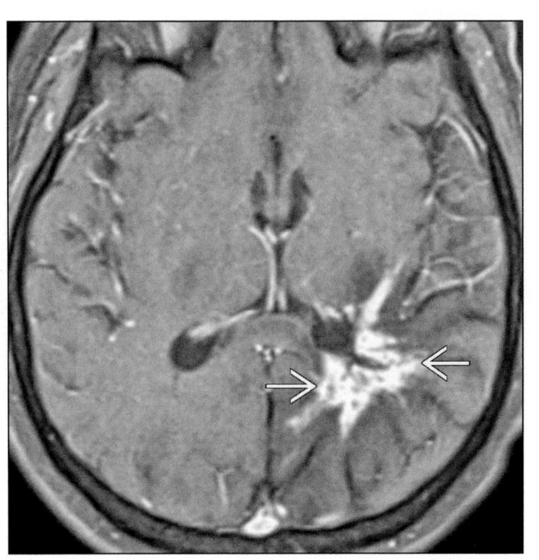

(Left) *Axial T2WI MR shows an area of mixed signal abnormality ➔ in the left periatrial white matter with mild mass effect on the left ventricular atrium.* ***(Right)*** *Axial T1WI C+ FS MR shows stellate enhancement with mild mass effect in the left periatrial white matter ➔ in this patient with biopsy-confirmed amyloidoma. This appearance is not specific, however, and could be seen with other inflammatory and neoplastic etiologies.*

CADASIL

Key Facts

Terminology
- Cerebral autosomal dominant arteriopathy with subcortical infarcts and leukoencephalopathy (CADASIL)
- Hereditary small-vessel disease due to mutations in *NOTCH3* gene on chromosome 19, which causes stroke in young to middle-aged adults

Imaging
- Diffuse WM hyperintensities (WMHs) = leukoaraiosis, early finding
- Discrete hyperintense lacunar infarctions
- Anterior temporal pole and paramedian superior frontal lobe highly sensitive and specific
- Diffusion restriction in acute lacunar infarcts

Top Differential Diagnoses
- Sporadic subcortical arteriosclerotic encephalopathy (sSAE)
- MELAS
- Primary angiitis of CNS

Pathology
- Autosomal dominant disease with mutation in *NOTCH3* results in arteriopathy affecting penetrating cerebral and leptomeningeal arteries

Clinical Issues
- TIA/stroke or migraine with aura often initial presentation
- TIA or stroke most common manifestation of disease (60-85% of all patients)
  - Often absence of traditional risk factors
- Migraines, if present, often precede other findings
- Average onset of stroke slightly earlier for men, but not significantly different (M = 50.7, F = 52.5)
- No specific therapy

*(**Left**) Axial FLAIR MR of a young patient with migraines show focal hyperintensity ➔ in the anterior temporal lobe highly suggestive of CADASIL. (**Right**) Axial FLAIR MR in the same patient shows additional abnormal hyperintensities ➔ in the subcortical and periventricular white matter, advanced for age, in this young adult with CADASIL. These nonspecific white matter changes should raise concern for CADASIL in the appropriate clinical setting (migraines with aura, memory problems, TIA/ stroke-like symptoms).*

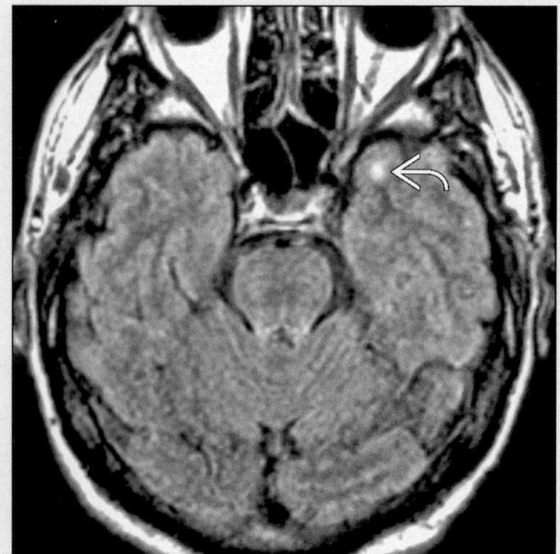

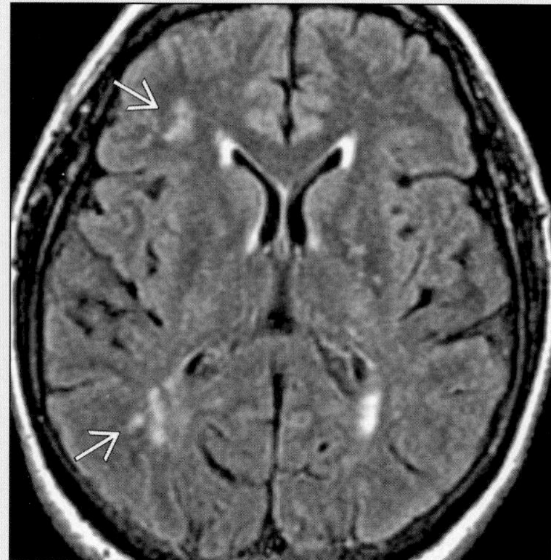

*(**Left**) Axial FLAIR MR shows multiple hyperintense white matter lesions with involvement of the external capsule ➔. External capsule disease is characteristic for CADASIL and rarely seen with ischemic leukoaraiosis. (**Right**) Axial DWI MR in the same patient shows that the lesions are hyperintense, consistent with restricted diffusion due to acute infarction. (Courtesy G. Gibbs, MD, and P. Lindell, MD.)*

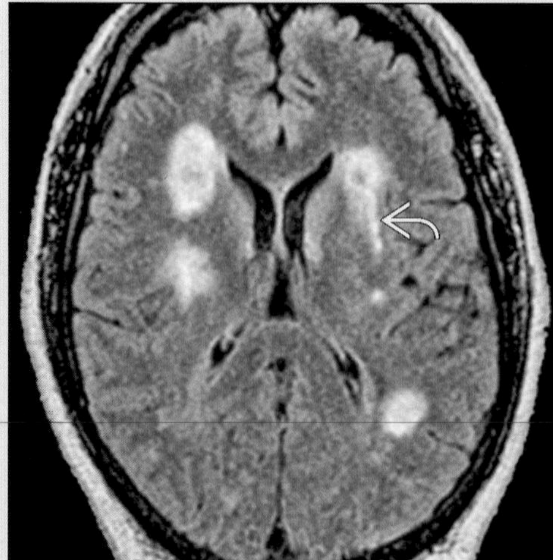

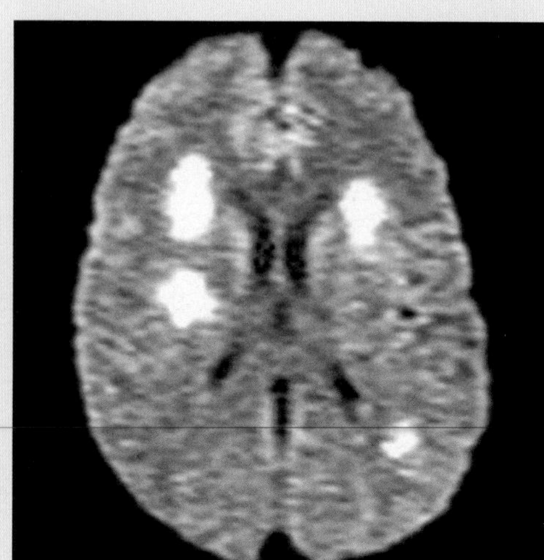

CADASIL

TERMINOLOGY

Abbreviations

- Cerebral autosomal dominant arteriopathy with subcortical infarcts and leukoencephalopathy (CADASIL)

Definitions

- Hereditary small-vessel disease due to mutations in *NOTCH3* gene on chromosome 19, which causes stroke in young to middle-aged adults

IMAGING

General Features

- Best diagnostic clue
  - Characteristic subcortical lacunar infarcts and leukoencephalopathy in young/middle-aged adults
- Location
  - Most common involvement in order of frequency
    - Younger patients: Frontal lobe, parietal lobe, external capsule, anterior temporal lobe
    - Older patients: Additionally posterior temporal and occipital lobes often involved
  - Cerebral cortex is generally spared
  - Lacunar infarcts in basal ganglia (BG) and subcortical location in order of frequency
    - BG > frontal > parietal > anterior temporal lobes
- Size
  - Multiple infarcts of various sizes, typically lacunar
- Morphology
  - Various shapes

CT Findings

- NECT
  - Subcortical and BG hypodense lesions
- CECT
  - No enhancement

MR Findings

- T1WI
  - 2 types of lesions
    - Large, coalescent, isointense WM lesions
    - Small, well-delineated, hypointense lesions that spare cortex
- T2WI
  - Diffuse WM hyperintensities (WMHs) = leukoaraiosis, early finding
  - Discrete hyperintense lacunar infarctions
  - Prominent perivascular spaces may be seen
  - Anterior temporal pole and paramedian superior frontal lobe highly sensitive and specific
- FLAIR
  - Findings akin to T2 findings
- DWI
  - Diffusion restriction in acute lacunar infarcts
- PWI
  - Reduced CBF and CBV in areas of WM signal abnormality without significant MTT changes
    - ↓ CBF may precede WM signal abnormality
  - Decreased hemodynamic reserve after acetazolamide challenge in areas of WM signal abnormality

Angiographic Findings

- Digital subtraction angiogram is normal in CADASIL

Nuclear Medicine Findings

- PET
  - 18F-FDG PET: ↓ cortical and subcortical glucose metabolism

Imaging Recommendations

- Best imaging tool
  - MR imaging
- Protocol advice
  - MR with T2WI and DWI

DIFFERENTIAL DIAGNOSIS

Sporadic Subcortical Arteriosclerotic Encephalopathy (sSAE)

- Associated with hypertension
- Multiple lacunar infarcts in lenticular nuclei, pons, thalamus, internal capsule, and caudate nuclei
- Diffuse, confluent periventricular WM involvement
- Uncommon to have temporopolar WM lesions
- WM lesions typically do not extend into arcuate fibers of temporopolar and paramedian superior frontal lobe

MELAS

- Mitochondrial encephalomyopathy with lactic acidosis and stroke-like episodes
- Bilateral, multifocal, cortical and subcortical hyperintense lesions on FLAIR images
- Normal/↑ ADC values within 48 hours of neurological deficit of abrupt onset should raise possibility of MELAS, especially if conventional MR images show infarct-like lesions
- Lesions disappear with clinical improvement, and ADC returns to normal (tissue recovery)

Primary Angiitis of CNS

- Lumen irregularities in distal cerebral arteries on digital subtraction angiogram

Hypercoagulable States

- Antiphospholipid antibodies, protein S deficiency
  - Stroke in young and middle-aged adults, with high rate of recurrence
- "Antiphospholipid syndrome": Early stroke, recurrent arterial and venous thromboses, spontaneous fetal loss, thrombocytopenia
- Cortical and lacunar infarcts of various sizes
- T2 WMHs, dural sinus thrombosis
- Abnormal angiogram: Vasculitis-like findings and stenoses at origin of great vessels (infrequent in general stroke population)

PATHOLOGY

General Features

- Etiology
  - Autosomal dominant disease with mutation in *NOTCH3* results in arteriopathy affecting penetrating cerebral and leptomeningeal arteries

- Narrowed lumen of affected vessels results in ↓ CBF and metabolism
  - In CADASIL patients with minor WMHs, cerebral vasodilatory capacity preserved but ↓ total CBF
- Genetics
  - Point mutations in *NOTCH3* gene on chromosome 19p13 with autosomal dominant transmission
    - *NOTCH3* codes for large transmembrane receptor physiologically expressed in vascular smooth muscle cell
    - Extracellular domain has 34 epidermal growth factor repeats (EGFR) with 6 cysteine residues
    - More than 150 CADASIL mutations are described
      - Mutations result in odd number of cysteine residues on affected EGFR
  - De novo mutations have been reported
- Associated abnormalities
  - Small vessels of other organs (skin, muscle, liver, spleen) affected, but clinical manifestations are predominantly cerebral
    - 25% of 41 Dutch CADASIL patients had myocardial infarctions

Gross Pathologic & Surgical Features

- Features characteristic of chronic small artery disease
  - Diffuse myelin pallor; periventricular and centrum semiovale WM rarefaction
  - WM and BG lacunar infarcts
  - Dilated perivascular spaces
  - Macroscopic appearance of cortex is usually normal

Microscopic Features

- Specific arteriopathy of small penetrating cerebral and leptomeningeal arteries characterized by
  - Arterial wall thickening (→ luminal stenosis) with normal endothelium
  - Nonamyloid extracellular granular osmiophilic deposits in media extending into adventitia
  - Morphologically altered smooth muscle cells, which can disappear from vessel wall
- Widespread cortical apoptosis, especially of layer 3 and 5

CLINICAL ISSUES

Presentation

- Most common signs/symptoms
  - TIA/stroke or migraine with aura often initial presentation
  - TIA or stroke most common manifestation of disease (60-85% of all patients)
    - Average age of onset 41-49 years, range 20-58 years
    - Often absence of traditional risk factors
    - Most have recurrent strokes
  - Migraine with aura (often atypical) (20-40%)
    - When present often 1st manifestation at younger age than TIA/stroke
  - Cognitive deficits common, increase with age
    - Almost 90% have executive dysfunction, often associated with changes in memory and attention
  - Behavioral disturbances common (75%)
    - Depression (46%), disturbed sleep (45%), irritability/lability (43%), apathy (41%)
  - Seizures (5-10%); may be related to stroke rather than primary manifestation of CADASIL
- Clinical profile
  - Large variations in clinical presentation
  - Young or middle-aged patient often 1st presenting with migraines with aura or TIA/stroke

Demographics

- Age
  - Onset of ischemic symptoms in mid-adulthood
    - MR changes appear at average age of 30 years and precede stroke/TIA by 10-15 years
    - Migraines, if present, often precede other findings
- Gender
  - No gender preference, but prognosis/life expectancy different for females and males
- Epidemiology
  - Prevalence is unknown
    - Over 500 families described worldwide
    - 2% of cases with lacunar infarcts and leukoaraiosis < 65 years and 11% < 50 years in 1 study
    - Small study in Scotland found minimum prevalence of 1.98/100,000
      - Likely underestimates true prevalence due to variety of factors

Natural History & Prognosis

- Average age of stroke onset slightly earlier for men but not significantly different (M = 50.7, F = 52.5 years)
- Disease progression typically more rapid in men with earlier death

Treatment

- No specific therapy

DIAGNOSTIC CHECKLIST

Consider

- Awareness of clinical and radiological features of CADASIL in young and middle-aged adults allows early diagnosis
- Consider CADASIL in acute unexplained encephalopathy

Image Interpretation Pearls

- Radiologic hallmark: Subcortical WMHs and small cystic lesions
- Characteristic WMHs visualized on MR often before onset of symptoms
- Temporal WM involvement = major abnormality differentiating CADASIL from sSAE

SELECTED REFERENCES

1. Chabriat H et al: Cadasil. Lancet Neurol. 8(7):643-53, 2009
2. Liem MK et al: Cerebral autosomal dominant arteriopathy with subcortical infarcts and leukoencephalopathy: progression of MR abnormalities in prospective 7-year follow-up study. Radiology. 249(3):964-71, 2008
3. Singhal S et al: The spatial distribution of MR imaging abnormalities in cerebral autosomal dominant arteriopathy with subcortical infarcts and leukoencephalopathy and their relationship to age and clinical features. AJNR Am J Neuroradiol. 26(10):2481-7, 2005

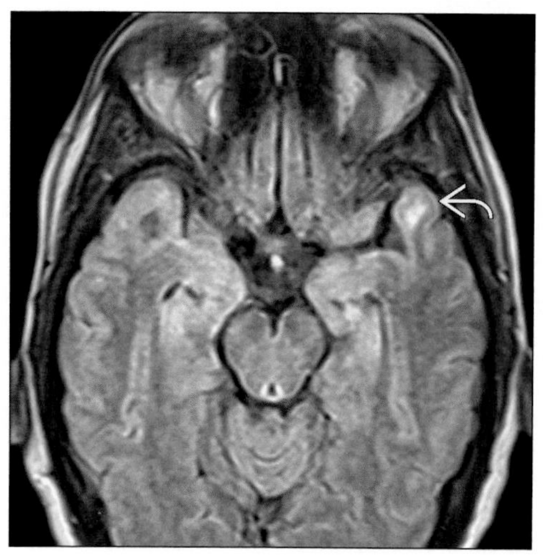

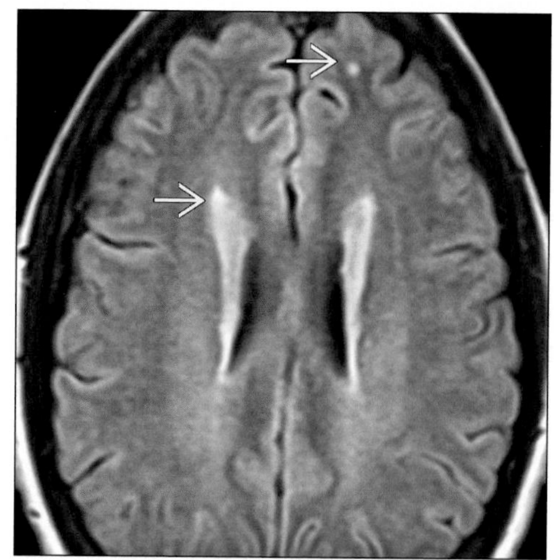

(Left) *Axial FLAIR MR through the temporal lobes shows focal subcortical white matter hyperintensities, very early changes in a 31-year-old patient with genetically proven CADASIL and migraines with visual auras as the only symptom.* **(Right)** *Axial FLAIR MR in the same patient shows nonspecific hyperintensities in the frontal and periventricular white matter. These white matter lesions are often seen before the onset of symptoms.*

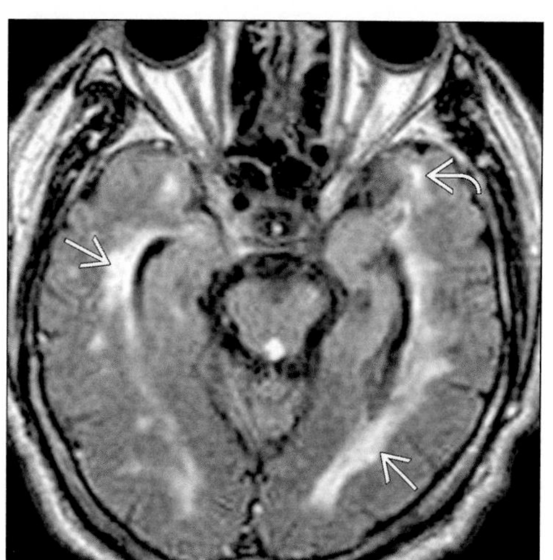

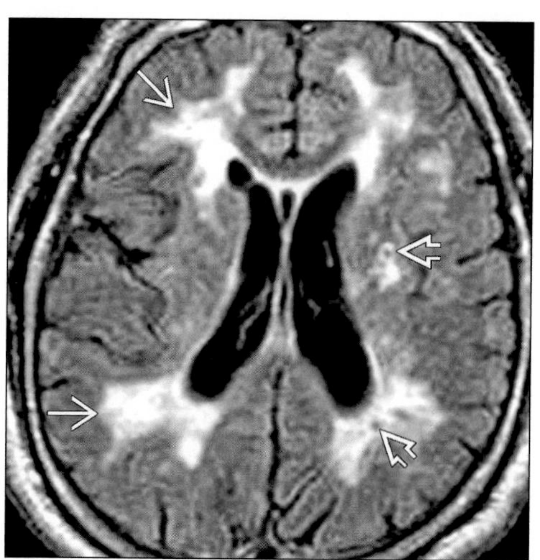

(Left) *Axial FLAIR MR through the temporal lobes shows extensive white matter hyperintensities in the anterior temporal lobe and periventricular white matter in this 32 year old with CADASIL.* **(Right)** *Axial FLAIR MR in the same patient shows confluent white matter disease in the subcortical and periventricular white matter as well as lacunar infarcts. Diffuse white matter disease with associated lacunar infarcts should raise suspicion for CADASIL in a young patient.*

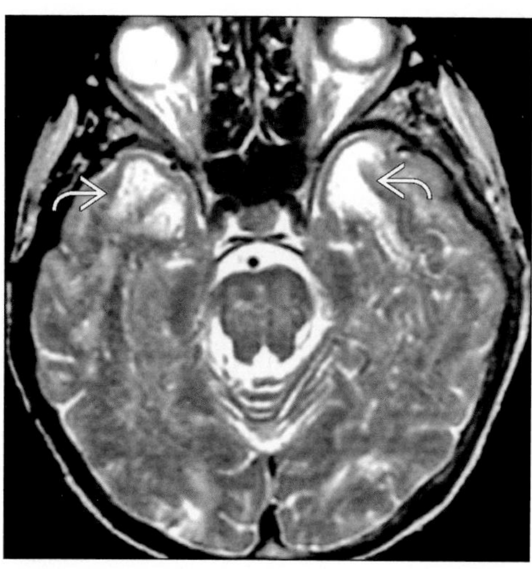

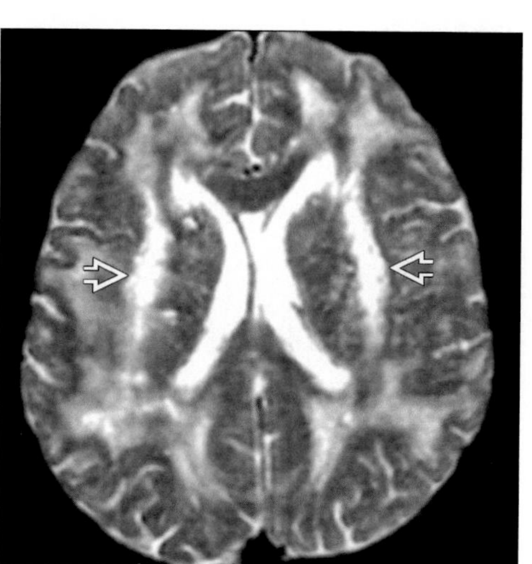

(Left) *Axial T2WI through the temporal lobes shows extensive anterior temporal lobe hyperintensities related to CADASIL.* **(Right)** *Axial T2WI MR in the same patient shows extensive confluent white matter disease involving the subcortical white matter and external capsules. Involvement of the anterior temporal poles, external capsules, and paramedial superior frontal lobes are findings with high specificity for CADASIL.*

BEHCET DISEASE

Key Facts

Terminology

- Chronic, idiopathic relapsing-remitting multisystem vascular-inflammatory disease characterized by recurrent orogenital ulcerations and uveitis
  - CNS involved in up to 20% of patients

Imaging

- Best diagnostic clue: T2 hyperintense brainstem lesion in patient with oral and genital ulcers
  - Midbrain > pons > BG > thalami > white matter
  - Focal or multifocal lesions
  - May see expansion of involved structures acutely
- T2WI: Hyperintense lesions
- T1WI C+: Patchy enhancement typical
- ↓ NAA in acute lesions
  - NAA may normalize when lesions resolve
- May see atrophy of involved structures chronically

Top Differential Diagnoses

- Gliomatosis cerebri
- ADEM
- Primary CNS Lymphoma
- Vasculitis
- Multiple sclerosis

Clinical Issues

- Neurologic deficit (hemiparesis), headache, seizure common presenting features
- Young adults, median age of 40 years

Diagnostic Checklist

- Consider Behçet disease in young adult with brainstem or deep gray nucleus lesion
- Enhancement pattern may help differentiate Behçet disease from other etiologies

*(**Left**) Axial T2WI MR shows abnormal hyperintensity and expansion of the left ventral midbrain in this young adult woman with Behçet disease. Involvement of the cerebral peduncles and associated mild expansion is common. This chronic, idiopathic, relapsing-remitting multisystem vascular-inflammatory disease is also characterized by oral and genital ulcers. (**Right**) Axial T2WI MR in the same patient shows hyperintensity and mild expansion of the left caudate head and anterior putamen.*

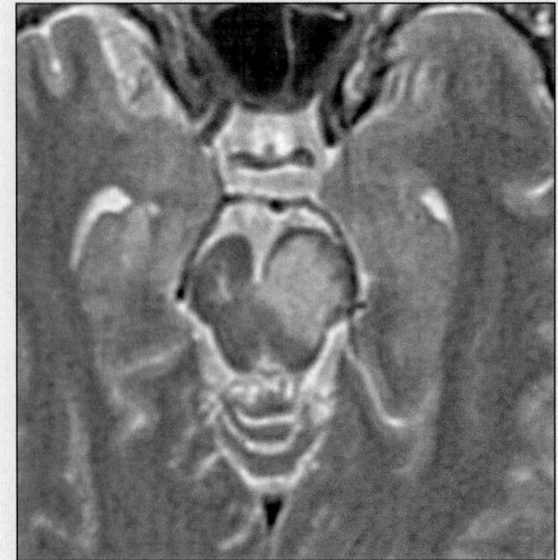

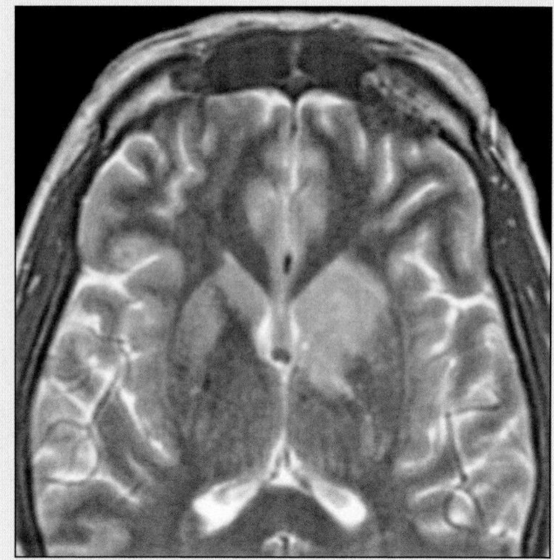

*(**Left**) Axial T1WI C+ MR in the same patient shows patchy enhancement of the brainstem lesion, typical of an acute Behçet lesion. Imaging mimics gliomatosis cerebri and vasculitis in this case. (**Right**) Axial T1WI C+ FS MR shows patchy enhancement of the right basal ganglia ⇨ in a young adult with oral and genital ulcers. Additional T2 hyperintense lesions were present in the midbrain, pons, and medulla. Imaging of Behçet disease often mimics neoplasm, demyelination, and vasculitis.*

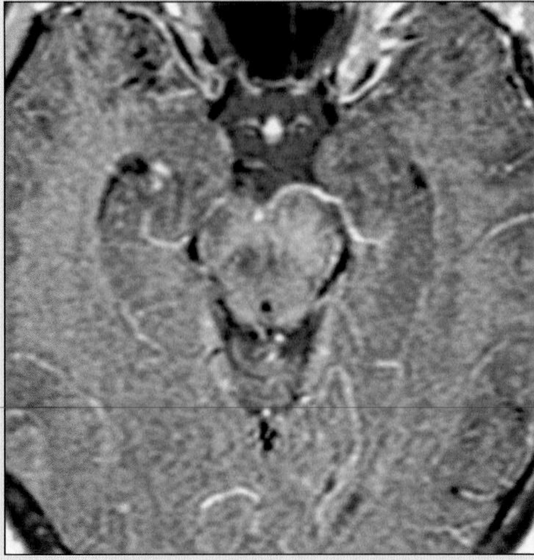

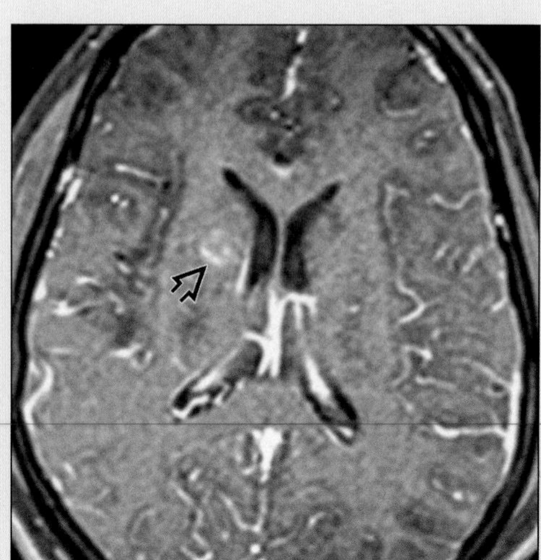

BEHCET DISEASE

TERMINOLOGY

Synonyms

- Behçet disease, neuro-Behçet

Definitions

- Chronic, idiopathic relapsing-remitting multisystem vascular-inflammatory disease characterized by recurrent orogenital ulcerations and uveitis
  - CNS involved in up to 20% of patients

IMAGING

General Features

- Best diagnostic clue
  - T2 hyperintense brainstem lesion in patient with oral and genital ulcers
- Location
  - Brainstem is most common location
    - Ventral midbrain (cerebral peduncles) and pons typically involved
  - Basal ganglia (BG) commonly involved
  - May involve thalami and white matter (WM)
  - Rarely affects spinal cord, mesial temporal lobes
  - Additional form with vessel involvement: Sinus thrombosis, arterial occlusion, aneurysm
- Size
  - Variable
- Morphology
  - May enlarge involved structures acutely
  - Focal or multifocal lesions

Imaging Recommendations

- Best imaging tool
  - Contrast-enhanced MR

CT Findings

- NECT: Often normal
  - May see subtle hypointense lesions

MR Findings

- T1WI: Isointense or hypointense lesions
- T2WI: Hyperintense lesions
  - May see expansion of involved structures
- FLAIR: Hyperintense lesions
- DWI: Variable; acute lesion may show restriction
- T1 C+: Patchy enhancement common
- MRS: ↓ NAA in acute lesions
  - ↑ NAA and ↑ Cho in normal-appearing brain (BG, brainstem)

DIFFERENTIAL DIAGNOSIS

Gliomatosis Cerebri

- T2 hyperintense mass with enlargement of involved structures
- Typically no enhancement

ADEM

- T2 hyperintense lesions in subcortical WM and deep gray nuclei after viral prodrome or vaccination
- Brainstem involvement uncommon

Primary CNS Lymphoma

- Enhancing lesions typically abut ependymal surfaces
- Often T2 hypointense

Vasculitis

- T2 hyperintense lesions, often supratentorial
- Diffusion restriction acutely
- Variable enhancement

Multiple Sclerosis

- Callososeptal interface lesions most common
- Ventral brainstem lesions uncommon

PATHOLOGY

General Features

- Etiology
  - Multi-system, vascular-inflammatory disease of unknown origin
- Associated abnormalities
  - Patients with CNS disease typically have orogenital ulcerations and uveitis

Microscopic Features

- Perivascular infiltration with inflammatory cells ± signs of necrosis

CLINICAL ISSUES

Presentation

- Most common signs/symptoms
  - Neurologic deficit (hemiparesis), headache, seizure
- Clinical profile
  - CSF studies: Pleocytosis and ↑ protein levels

Demographics

- Age
  - Young adults typically; also reported in children
- Gender
  - M > F in neuro-Behçet
- Epidemiology
  - 10-20% of patients with Behçet have CNS involvement

Treatment

- Corticosteroids and immunosuppressive therapy

DIAGNOSTIC CHECKLIST

Consider

- Behçet disease in young adult with brainstem or deep gray nucleus lesion

SELECTED REFERENCES

1. Siva A et al: The spectrum of nervous system involvement in Behçet's syndrome and its differential diagnosis. J Neurol. 256(4):513-29, 2009
2. Heo JH et al: Neuro-Behcet's disease mimicking multiple brain tumors: diffusion-weighted MR study and literature review. J Neurol Sci. 264(1-2):177-81, 2008

FIBROMUSCULAR DYSPLASIA

Key Facts

Terminology

- Fibromuscular dysplasia (FMD)
  - Arterial disease of unknown etiology
  - Overgrowth of smooth muscle, fibrous tissue
  - Affects medium/large arteries

Imaging

- Renal artery is most common overall site
- Cervicocranial FMD
  - ICA (30%) > ECA > vertebral arteries (10%)
  - > 50% of cases are bilateral
  - Intracranial rare (supraclinoid ICA, MCA)
- CTA
  - Arterial luminal irregularity or "beading" ± stenosis or aneurysm (rare)
  - No mural Ca++
- DWI-MR
  - Most sensitive for ischemic sequela of FMD
- DSA
  - Type 1 (85%): Classic "string of beads" = medial fibroplasia
  - Type 2 (10%): Long, tubular stenosis = intimal fibroplasia
  - Type 3 (5%): Asymmetric outpouching from 1 side of artery = periadventitial fibroplasia

Top Differential Diagnoses

- Atherosclerosis
- Standing waves

Clinical Issues

- Symptoms: HTN, stroke
- Treatment
  - Antiplatelet ± anticoagulant Rx to reduce risk of thromboembolic sequela (stroke)
  - Balloon angioplasty
  - Covered stent, arterial reconstruction for aneurysm

(Left) Graphic of the carotid bifurcation shows the principal subtypes of FMD. Type 1 appears as alternating areas of constriction and dilatation ➡, type 2 as tubular stenosis ➡, and type 3 as focal corrugations ± diverticulum ➡. (Right) Coronal oblique CTA shows luminal irregularity and "beaded" appearance of the left ICA ➡, suggestive of FMD. Note the absence of mural calcification along the involved segment compared with the prominent atherosclerotic lesion at the carotid bulb ➡.

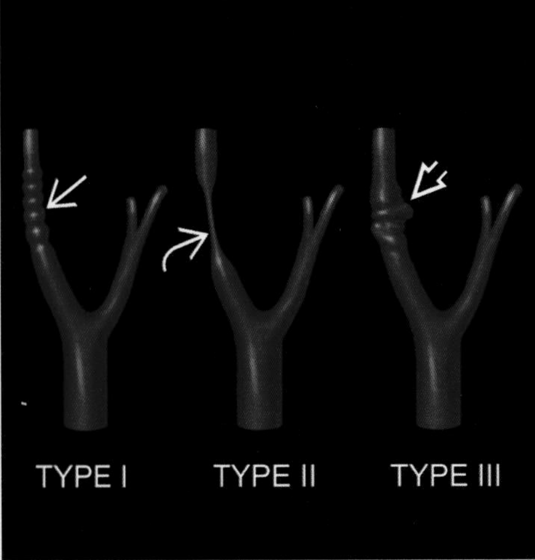

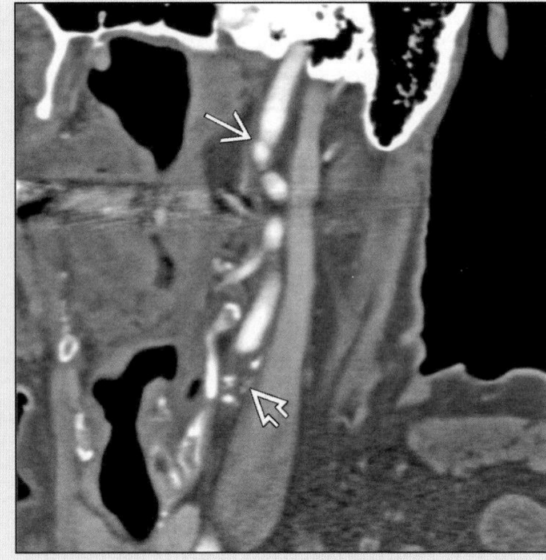

(Left) Oblique DSA of the left carotid artery shows ASVD stenosis of the carotid bulb ➡. Note the mural calcification seen as faint subtraction artifact ➡. Superiorly, the ICA shows luminal irregularity and beading, consistent with FMD ➡. Additional FMD involvement of an ECA branch is evident ➡. (Right) Lateral DSA after carotid stenting across the ASVD stenosis ➡ shows a distal protection device in situ ➡. Note the irregularity of the ICA ➡ and occipital artery ➡ due to FMD.

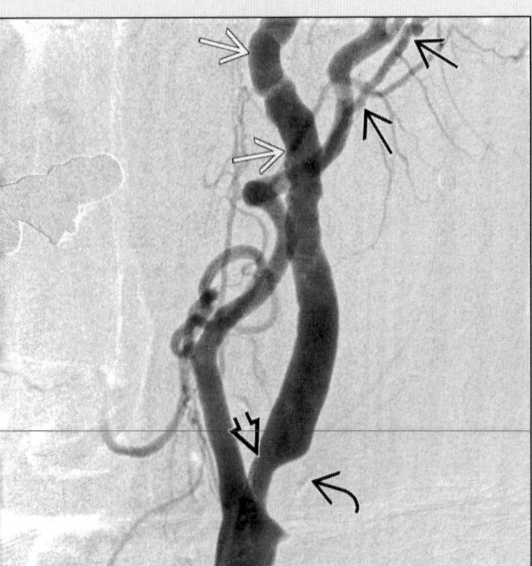

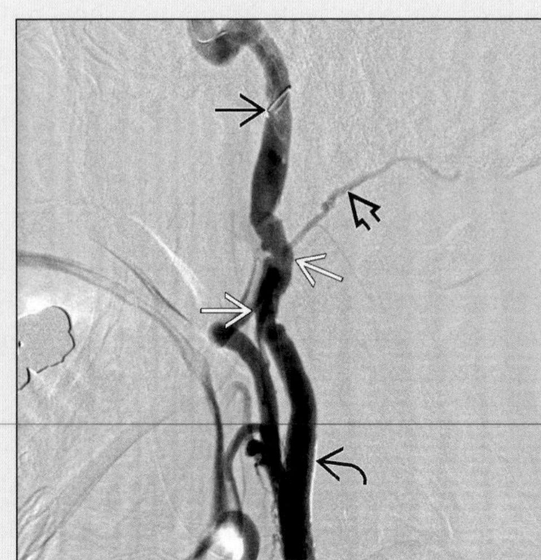

FIBROMUSCULAR DYSPLASIA

TERMINOLOGY

Abbreviations
- Fibromuscular dysplasia (FMD)

Definitions
- Arterial disease of unknown etiology
  - Overgrowth of smooth muscle, fibrous tissue
  - Affects medium/large arteries

IMAGING

General Features
- Best diagnostic clue
  - Luminal irregularity ("beaded") arteries in young/ middle-aged patient
- Location
  - Renal artery = most common site overall
  - Craniocervical arteries
    - ICA (30%) > ECA > vertebral arteries (10%)
    - > 50% of cases have bilateral involvement
  - Intracranial rare (supraclinoid ICA, MCA)
- Morphology
  - Arterial luminal corrugations, classic "string of beads" appearance
    - ± arterial stenosis, aneurysm

CT Findings
- CTA
  - Arterial luminal irregularity or "beading"
    - ± stenosis or aneurysm (rare)
    - Mural Ca++ absent
      - Exception: Dystrophic Ca++ if dissection

MR Findings
- DWI
  - Most sensitive for ischemic sequela of FMD
- MRA
  - May see "string of beads" appearance
    - Differentiate from motion artifact due to swallowing

Ultrasonographic Findings
- Color Doppler
  - Visible ridges or thickening of carotid wall ± stenosis

Angiographic Findings
- 3 subtypes with distinctive appearances on DSA
  - Type 1 (85%): Classic "string of beads" = medial fibroplasia
  - Type 2 (10%): Long, tubular stenosis = intimal fibroplasia
  - Type 3 (5%): Asymmetric outpouching from 1 side of artery = periadventitial fibroplasia

DIFFERENTIAL DIAGNOSIS

Atherosclerosis
- Usually older patients
- Typically short-segment stenosis (not "string of beads"), associated with mural Ca++

Arterial "Standing Waves"
- Unknown etiology
  - Oscillations from normal retrograde flow during cardiac cycle
- Appears as transient "string of beads"
  - Very regular periodicity, smoothness differentiate from FMD

PATHOLOGY

General Features
- Etiology
  - Unknown; thought to be dysplastic rather than degenerative or inflammatory
- Associated abnormalities
  - Intracranial (berry) aneurysms in 10%
  - Spontaneous dissection (20% in ICA)
  - Thromboembolic sequela due to disturbed flow → thrombus formation

Microscopic Features
- Overgrowth of smooth muscle cells and fibrous tissue in arterial wall

CLINICAL ISSUES

Presentation
- Most common signs/symptoms
  - Hypertension due to renal involvement (stenosis)
- Other signs/symptoms
  - Craniocervical FMD
    - Stenosis → TIA/stroke
    - Aneurysm → mass effect on adjacent structures, rupture (rare)

Demographics
- Age
  - Onset of symptoms: 25-50 years old
- Gender
  - M:F = 1:9 (most common subtype)

Natural History & Prognosis
- Slow progression of arterial irregularities ± stenoses

Treatment
- Antiplatelet ± anticoagulant Rx to reduce risk of thromboembolic sequela (stroke)
- Balloon angioplasty of stenoses
- Covered stent, arterial reconstruction for aneurysm

DIAGNOSTIC CHECKLIST

Consider
- FMD in younger patients with HTN, stroke, dissection
- Head CTA/MRA in FMD patients to exclude associated intracranial aneurysm(s)

SELECTED REFERENCES

1. Libman RB: Fibromuscular dysplasia with carotid artery dissection presenting as an isolated hemianopsia. J Stroke Cerebrovasc Dis. 17(5):330, 2008

HYDRANENCEPHALY

Key Facts

Terminology
- In utero cerebral hemispheric destruction

Imaging
- Absent cerebrum with fluid-filled cranial vault
- Thalamus, cerebellum, brainstem, falx intact
- Temporal, occipital lobe remnants common
- Macrocephaly

Top Differential Diagnoses
- Severe hydrocephalus
- Alobar holoprosencephaly (HPE)
- Severe bilateral open-lip schizencephaly
- Cystic encephalomalacia

Pathology
- In utero compromise of anterior cerebral circulation
- Implicated: Anoxia, infection, thrombophilic states, maternal toxin exposure, radiation, genetic factors, twin-twin transfusion

Clinical Issues
- Newborn with macrocephaly, developmental failure, calvarial transillumination
  - Hyperirritability, hyperreflexia, seizures
- Neurological function limited to brainstem
- Prognosis: Death in infancy; prolonged survival rare
- Ventricular shunt treats macrocephaly

Diagnostic Checklist
- Intact falx distinguishes hydranencephaly from alobar HPE
- Thin cortical mantle along inner table distinguishes severe hydrocephalus from hydranencephaly

*(**Left**) Coronal graphic shows classic features of hydranencephaly. The cerebral hemispheres are nearly absent, but the thalami, brainstem, and cerebellum are intact. The falx cerebri ➔ appears to "float" in a CSF-filled rostral cranial vault. (**Right**) Axial NECT shows cerebral hemispheres replaced by CSF with no cortical mantle appreciated except in medial temporal lobes ➔. The posterior fossa and diencephalic structures supplied by the posterior cerebral circulation are intact.*

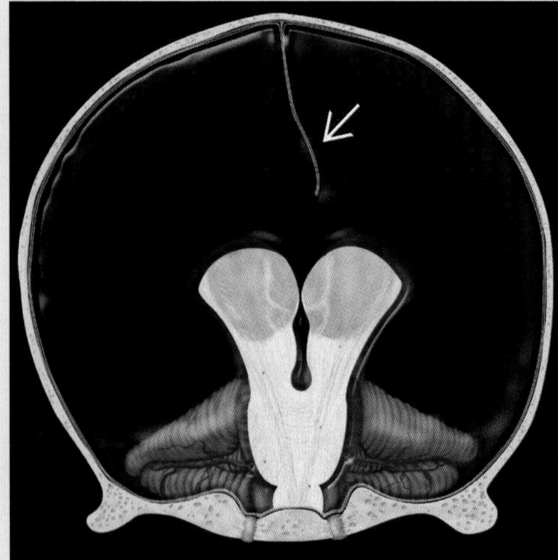

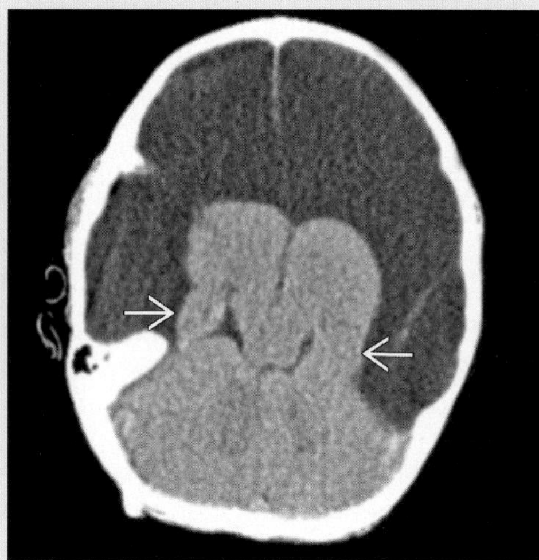

*(**Left**) Axial NECT of the upper head shows a near complete absence of telencephalon with intact falx, medial frontal ➔, and parietal/occipital remnants ➔. Patients with hydranencephaly are often macrocephalic as the choroid plexus continues to secrete CSF. (**Right**) Axial T2WI MR shows the undamaged posterior temporal and occipital cerebral cortex ➔ with nearly normal sulcation, as well as nearly normal appearing thalami ➔ in this otherwise fluid-filled calvarium.*

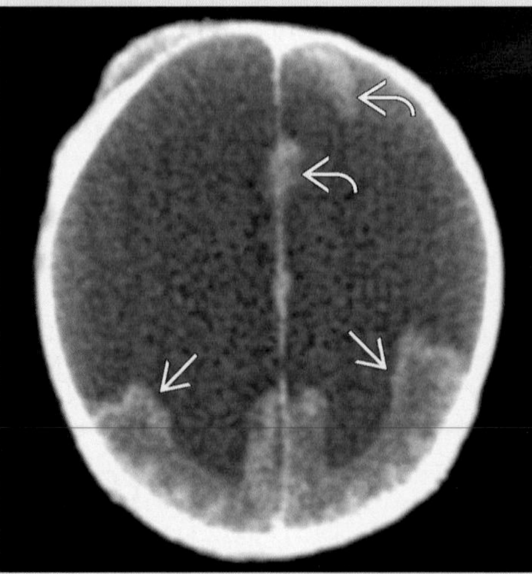

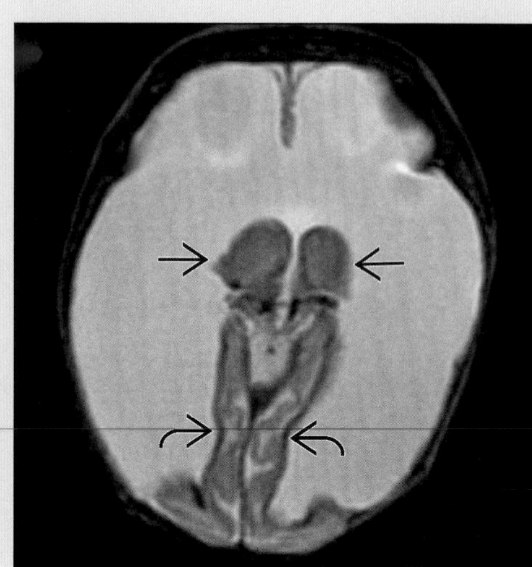

HYDRANENCEPHALY

TERMINOLOGY

Definitions

- In utero cerebral hemispheric destruction
- Hemihydranencephaly: Rare unilateral form

IMAGING

General Features

- Best diagnostic clue
  - Absent cerebrum with fluid-filled cranial vault
  - Falx cerebri and posterior fossa structures intact
- Location
  - Cerebral hemispheres
- Morphology
  - "Water bag brain"
- Thalamus, cerebellum, brainstem, falx intact
- Temporal, occipital lobe remnants common

CT Findings

- Fluid-filled cranial vault
- Macrocephaly

MR Findings

- Absent cerebral mantle
- Falx cerebri partially/completely intact
- No gliosis in remaining brain structures

Ultrasonographic Findings

- Anechoic cranial vault

Other Modality Findings

- CTA, MRA: Atretic, stenotic, occluded, malformed or normal supraclinoid carotids and branch vessels
- Prenatal US/MR: Severe hydrocephalus or hemorrhage may precede hydranencephaly

Imaging Recommendations

- Best imaging tool
  - Prenatal US allows therapeutic intervention
  - Postnatal MR best delineates extent of destruction

DIFFERENTIAL DIAGNOSIS

Severe Hydrocephalus

- Thin cortical mantle compressed against inner table

Alobar Holoprosencephaly (HPE)

- Fused midline structures; absent falx

Severe Bilateral Open-lip Schizencephaly

- Perisylvian transmantle cleft lined by abnormal gray matter

Cystic Encephalomalacia

- Scattered cerebral cavities, gliosis

PATHOLOGY

General Features

- Etiology
  - In utero compromise of anterior cerebral circulation
  - Brain injury results in liquefactive necrosis by 20-27 weeks gestation
  - Implicated: Anoxia, infection, thrombophilic states, maternal toxin exposure, radiation, genetic factors, twin-twin transfusion
- Genetics
  - Sporadic
  - Rare autosomal recessive syndromes
    - Fowler: Hydranencephaly, fetal akinesia, CNS vasculopathy
    - Microhydranencephaly: Hydranencephaly, microcephaly, small body (Chr 16p13.3-12.1)
- Associated abnormalities
  - Few reports: Vascular malformations, renal dysplasia

Gross Pathologic & Surgical Features

- Leptomeningeal-lined, fluid-filled "sacs" in lieu of cerebral hemispheres

Microscopic Features

- Hemosiderin-laden macrophages over remnant brain

CLINICAL ISSUES

Presentation

- Most common signs/symptoms
  - Macrocephaly (intact choroid plexus secretes CSF)
- Other signs/symptoms
  - Hyperirritability, hyperreflexia, seizures
- Clinical profile
  - Newborn with macrocephaly, developmental failure, calvarial transillumination

Demographics

- Age: Diagnosis usually made in 1st few weeks of life
- Epidemiology: < 1:10,000 births; 10x ↑ teenage moms

Natural History & Prognosis

- Neurological function limited to brainstem
- Prognosis: Death in infancy; prolonged survival rare

Treatment

- Ventriculo-peritoneal shunt treats macrocephaly

DIAGNOSTIC CHECKLIST

Image Interpretation Pearls

- Intact falx distinguishes hydranencephaly from alobar HPE
- Thin cortical mantle along inner table distinguishes severe hydrocephalus from hydranencephaly

SELECTED REFERENCES

1. Merker B: Life expectancy in hydranencephaly. Clin Neurol Neurosurg. 110(3):213-4, 2008
2. Tsai JD et al: Hydranencephaly in neonates. Pediatr Neonatol. 49(4):154-7, 2008
3. Counter SA: Preservation of brainstem neurophysiological function in hydranencephaly. J Neurol Sci. 263(1-2):198-207, 2007
4. Sutton LN et al: Hydranencephaly versus maximal hydrocephalus: an important clinical distinction. Neurosurgery. 6(1):34-8, 1980

WHITE MATTER INJURY OF PREMATURITY

Key Facts

Terminology

- WMIP is not the same as germinal matrix hemorrhage (GMH)
  - In WMIP, primary injury is to white matter; in GMH, primary injury is to vessels in germinal matrix
- PVL = WMIP, but term WMIP is used to emphasize that not all white matter injury is periventricular
- Encephalopathy of prematurity = WMIP and associated neuronal/axonal abnormalities

Imaging

- Best early ultrasound (US) clue: Hyperechoic "flare" with loss of normal tissue echo texture
- Most specific US clue: White matter cavitation/cysts (but may not appear for ≥ 1 week)
- Best early MR clue: Decreased diffusion (bright DWI, low ADC) in affected areas
  - Acute DWI abnormality > T1 and T2 abnormality, also acute DWI > chronic injury visible on MR
- Best late MR clue: Gliosis, white matter volume loss, ventriculomegaly

Top Differential Diagnoses

- Normal periventricular halo
- Infection
- Inborn errors of metabolism

Pathology

- Primarily initiating factors: Inflammation (due to maternal infection/postnatal sepsis) and ischemia

Clinical Issues

- Typically silent
- Severity and extent of brain abnormalities = destructive processes + developmental disturbances

*(**Left**) Oblique transfontanelle cranial ultrasound in a 34-week GA infant at age 17 days shows diffusely increased echogenicity throughout the white matter with subtle regions of cavitation ➔, usually called cystic change. (**Right**) Axial T2WI MR in the same 34-week GA infant 1 day later better illustrates the severity and extent of the white matter injury. More extensive white matter cavitation (cystic regions) ➔ are clearly identified.*

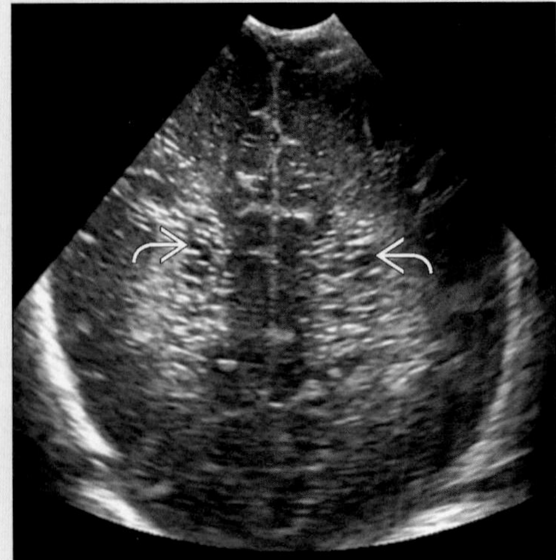

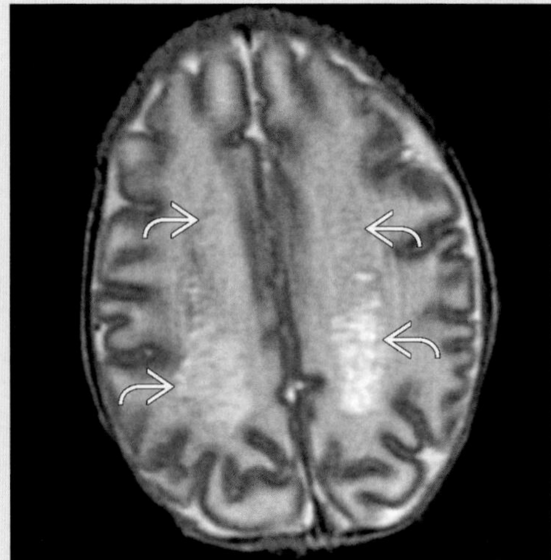

*(**Left**) Axial T1WI MR in the same 34-week GA infant at age 18 days shows cavitary white matter injury in the peritrigonal regions ➔ and, to a lesser degree, adjacent to the left frontal horn ➔. (**Right**) Axial T2WI MR in the same infant at 3 months of age shows almost complete collapse of the cavities, resulting in ex vacuo ventricular enlargement and white matter volume loss. On follow-up at age 2 years, this child has mild spastic diplegia and mild language delay.*

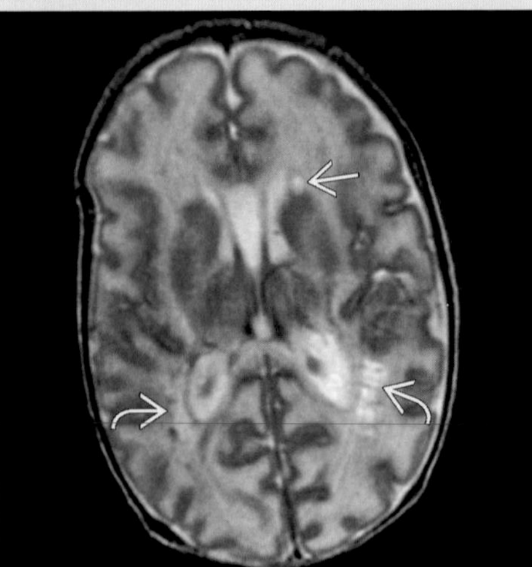

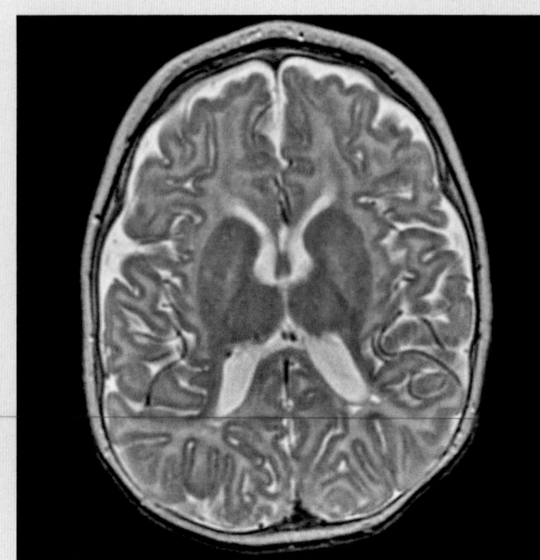

WHITE MATTER INJURY OF PREMATURITY

TERMINOLOGY

Abbreviations

- White matter injury of prematurity (WMIP), hypoxic-ischemic encephalopathy (HIE), hypoxic ischemic injury (HII), periventricular leukomalacia (PVL), very low birthweight (VLBW)

Definitions

- WMIP is not the same as germinal matrix hemorrhage (GMH)
  - In WMIP, primary injury is to white matter; in GMH, primary injury is to vessels in germinal matrix
- PVL = WMIP, but term WMIP is used here to emphasize that not all white matter injury is periventricular
- VLBW = infant ≤ 1,500g (1-5% of all births)
- Encephalopathy of prematurity = WMIP and associated neuronal/axonal abnormalities

IMAGING

General Features

- Best diagnostic clue
  - Best early ultrasound (US) clue: Hyperechoic "flare" with loss of normal tissue echo texture
  - Most specific US clue: White matter cavitation/cysts (but may not appear for ≥ 1 week)
  - Best early MR clue: Decreased diffusion (bright DWI, low ADC) in affected areas
  - Best late MR clue: Gliosis, white matter volume loss, ventriculomegaly
- Location
  - Focal (often but not always adjacent to frontal horns and trigones) or diffuse white matter
  - ± deep gray nuclei
  - ± cerebellar white matter, dentate nucleus, pons
- Size
  - WM cavities 1st detected at 2-3 mm range; larger cysts carry poorer prognosis
- Morphology
  - Chronic: WM volume loss
    - ↓ WM volume (especially corpus callosum [CC])
    - Undulating ventricular borders
    - Secondary ventriculomegaly
    - ± cortical and deep gray volume loss
    - ± pontine and cerebellar volume loss

CT Findings

- NECT
  - Insensitive to nonhemorrhagic WMIP

MR Findings

- T1WI
  - Early
    - May be normal, often underestimates extent of injury
    - WM ↓ T1 signal: Diffuse (edema or ischemia) or focal (cavitation)
    - Focal WM ↑ T1 signal (myelin breakdown products, hemorrhage, or gliosis) ± cavitation
    - ± ↑ T1 signal in dorsal pons, deep gray nuclei
  - Late: Morphological changes as above
- T2WI
  - Early
    - May be normal, often underestimates extent of injury
    - WM ↑ T2 signal: Diffuse (edema or ischemia) or focal (cavitation)
    - Focal WM ↓ T2 signal (myelin breakdown products, hemorrhage, or gliosis)
  - Late: Morphological changes as above, gliosis (if injury occurred > 24-26 weeks GA)
- FLAIR
  - Early: Insensitive to injury
  - Late: Same as T2 but ↑ sensitivity to periventricular gliosis
- T2* GRE
  - Blooming at sites of hemorrhage
- DWI
  - Most sensitive in acute stage
  - ↑ signal and ↓ ADC in areas of recent injury, but time course for DWI and ADC evolution and normalization not known
  - Acute DWI abnormality larger in size than acute or chronic T1 and T2 abnormalities
- MRS
  - ↑ lactate
  - ↓ NAA
  - ↑ excitatory neurotransmitters
  - **Caveat**: Small amounts of lactate are often seen in uninjured premature neonates

Ultrasonographic Findings

- Grayscale ultrasound
  - Early: Focal or diffuse increased echogenicity, most prominent adjacent to frontal horns and trigone
  - Subacute: ± cavitation (may take ~ 7-10 days to appear)
  - Late: Cavities often collapse; WM volume loss, secondary ventriculomegaly

Imaging Recommendations

- Best imaging tool
  - MR with DWI
    - Most sensitive and specific imaging modality
    - Benefits must be balanced with risk of transport to MR
    - ↑ sensitivity and ↑ specificity to type of injury (ischemia, hemorrhage vs. edema) compared to US
  - Head US
    - Still screening tool of choice: Inexpensive and can be performed bedside but ↓ sensitivity and specificity compared to MR
- Protocol advice
  - Current practice parameter recommendations
    - Screening head US in all infants GA < 30 weeks at 7-14 days of age and at 36-40 corrected GA
  - MR
    - When US is abnormal: MR ASAP to clarify scope of injury and aid in prognosticating, include DWI
    - At discharge for "at-risk" VLBW neonates with "normal" screening cranial sonograms

WHITE MATTER INJURY OF PREMATURITY

DIFFERENTIAL DIAGNOSIS

Normal Periventricular Halo

- Normal hyperechoic "blush" posterosuperior to ventricular trigones, seen on parasagittal sonography
- Suspect WMIP if echogenicity is asymmetric, coarse, globular, or more hyperechoic than glomi of choroid plexus

Infection

- Congenital CMV infection: Microcephaly, calcifications, WM edema, ± polymicrogyria, DWI negative
- *Citrobacter*: Frontal lobes
- Neonatal herpes simplex encephalitis

Inborn Errors of Metabolism

- Urea cycle disorders, mitochondrial disorders

PATHOLOGY

General Features

- Etiology
  - Primarily initiating factors: Inflammation (due to maternal infection/postnatal sepsis) and ischemia
  - Unique risk factors of premature brain
    - Intrinsic vulnerability of immature oligodendroglia and subplate neurons to free radicals, excitotoxicity, and cytokines
    - Abundant microglia
    - Impaired cerebrovascular autoregulation → pressure-passive cerebral circulation
    - Periventricular vascular anatomical and physiological factors (arterial end zones)
  - Primary injury to WM ± subplate neurons
  - Currently unclear if more widespread neuronal/ axonal abnormalities primary or secondary to resulting growth disturbances/WM injury
- Associated abnormalities
  - Intraventricular hemorrhage

Staging, Grading, & Classification

- Focal: Localized necrosis in deep white matter with loss of all cellular components
  - Macroscopic: Cysts ≥ 1-2mm (< 5% of VLBW infants, also called cystic PVL)
  - Microscopic: Cysts not resolved by current imaging, evolve to glial scar
- Diffuse: Marked astrogliosis and microgliosis, abnormal promyelinating oligodendrocyte maturation (results in hypomyelination, volume loss)

CLINICAL ISSUES

Presentation

- Most common signs/symptoms
  - Acute: Typically silent, ± perirolandic sharp waves on EEG; need to consider risk and screen
- Clinical profile
  - Mother: Poor antepartum care, preterm premature rupture of membranes, chorioamnionitis, preeclampsia, group B strep
  - Preterm neonate: VLBW, intraventricular hemorrhage, respiratory distress syndrome type 1, hypocarbia, hypotension, sepsis, anemia, apnea

Demographics

- Age
  - Incidence of WMIP in VLBW infants is ≥ 50%
  - Worldwide ~ 5% of preterm infants have WMIP
- Gender
  - M > F
- Epidemiology
  - VLBW ⇒ 45% incidence (higher if associated with intraventricular hemorrhage)
  - Gestational age < 33 weeks ⇒ 38% incidence
  - > 50% of patients with WMIP or grade 3 intraventricular hemorrhage develop cerebral palsy

Natural History & Prognosis

- Severity and extent of brain abnormalities = destructive processes + developmental disturbances
- Spastic diplegia/quadriplegia, seizures, microcephaly, blindness, deafness in severe cases
- Poor outcome if intraventricular hemorrhage + WMIP, WMIP + volume loss, widespread infarction, or seizures
- Spastic diplegia (associated with cystic WMIP)
- Cognitive deficits in absence of motor deficits (associated with noncystic WMIP)
  - Many have impaired working memory and attention deficits
  - Basis of cognitive deficits may be due to thalamic, basal ganglia, cerebellum, as well as cerebral cortical involvement

Treatment

- Prenatal care significantly reduces preterm birth (35% down to 8%)
- Supportive

DIAGNOSTIC CHECKLIST

Image Interpretation Pearls

- Cranial ultrasound underestimates WMIP
- As with HII of term, injuries evolve over time

SELECTED REFERENCES

1. Fu J et al: Studies on the value of diffusion-weighted MR imaging in the early prediction of periventricular leukomalacia. J Neuroimaging. 19(1):13-8, 2009
2. Ligam P et al: Thalamic damage in periventricular leukomalacia: novel pathologic observations relevant to cognitive deficits in survivors of prematurity. Pediatr Res. 65(5):524-9, 2009
3. Volpe JJ: Brain injury in premature infants: a complex amalgam of destructive and developmental disturbances. Lancet Neurol. 8(1):110-24, 2009
4. Kidokoro H et al: Diffusion-weighted magnetic resonance imaging in infants with periventricular leukomalacia. Neuropediatrics. 39(4):233-8, 2008
5. Roelants-van Rijn AM et al: Parenchymal brain injury in the preterm infant: comparison of cranial ultrasound, MRI and neurodevelopmental outcome. Neuropediatrics. 32(2):80-9, 2001

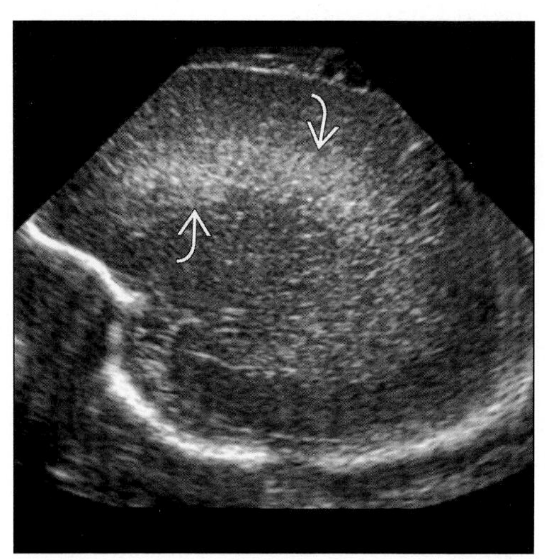

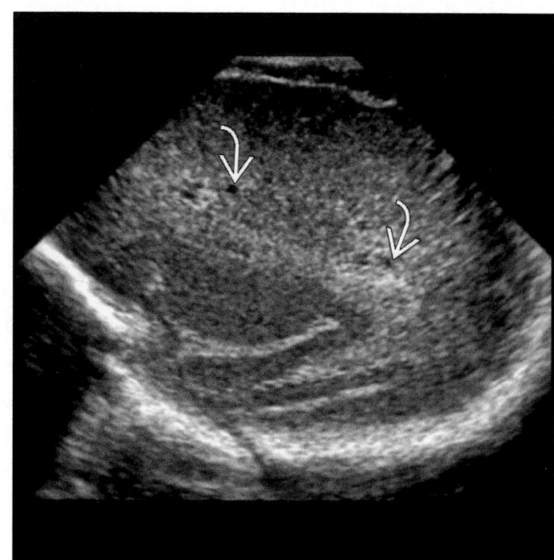

(Left) *Sagittal oblique transfontanelle cranial ultrasound in a 3-day-old premature infant shows hazy increased echogenicity or hyperechoic "flare"* ➦ *throughout the hemispheric white matter.* **(Right)** *Sagittal oblique cranial ultrasound in the same infant a few days later shows development of small cavitations* ➦ *within the hyperechoic white matter. The lesions progressed to large areas of cavitation in the injured white matter during the next week (not shown).*

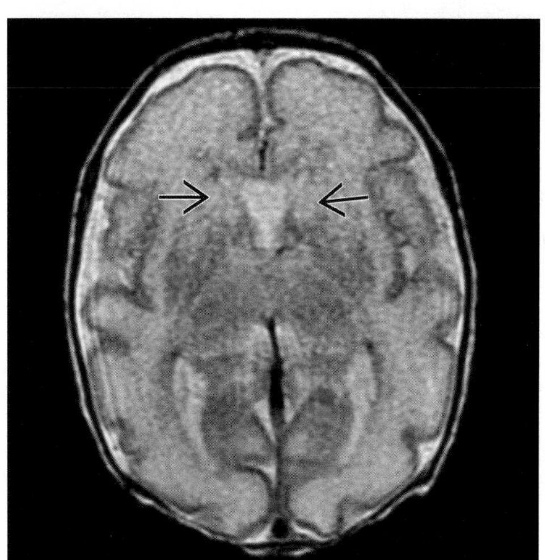

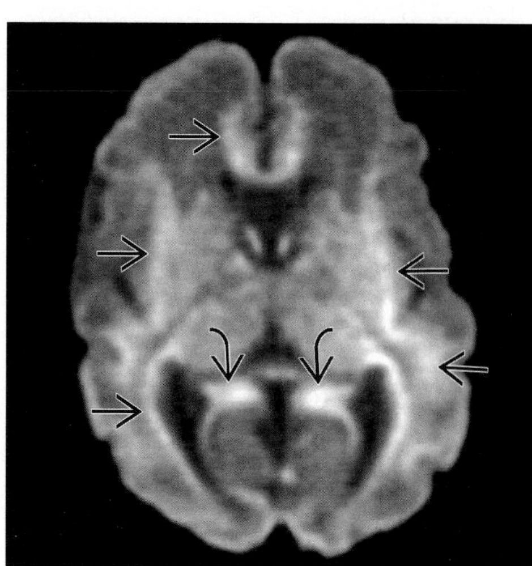

(Left) *Axial T2WI MR in a 30.5-week gestation age infant at age 4 days shows diffusely increased signal* ➔ *throughout the basal ganglia and thalami.* **(Right)** *Axial DWI MR in the same infant at age 4 days shows decreased diffusion throughout the basal ganglia, thalami, and hippocampi* ➦, *as well as more diffusely throughout the white matter* ➔ *where no T2 abnormality was identified. DWI is most sensitive to injury during the 1st week after injury.*

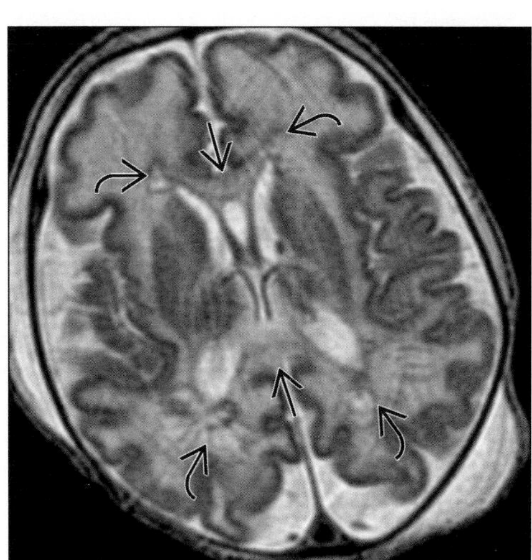

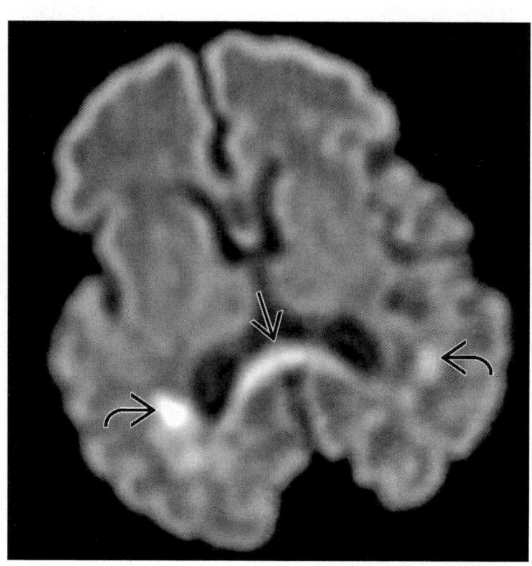

(Left) *Axial T2WI MR at age 10 days in a 35 week gestation age infant, delivered by emergency C-section due to maternal eclampsia and seizures, shows diffusely increased WM signal with cystic changes* ➦ *and edematous corpus callosum* ➔. **(Right)** *Axial DWI MR at 10 days in the same infant shows decreased diffusion in parietal white matter injury* ➦ *and in splenium of the corpus callosum* ➔ *where there was edema. DWI sensitivity starts to decrease after ~ 7-10 days.*

TERM HYPOXIC ISCHEMIC INJURY

Key Facts

Terminology

- HII = imaging pattern of injury due to acquired global arterial hypoperfusion (though many factors can increase vulnerability and potential injury)
- HIE = clinical syndrome defined in term or near-term neonates

Imaging

- Profound HII: Low ADC in VL thalamus ± corticospinal tract (CST) in posterior limb internal capsule (PLIC)
- Partial HII: Ventrolateral thalamus and CST in PLIC spared, cortical injury maximal at depths of sulci
- Bright DWI and ↓ ADC occur early, even when T1WI/T2WI normal
- Injuries evolve over time: DWI and ADC abnormality can ↑ in size and severity over 1st few days due to delayed cell death; DWI and ADC normalize or ↑ around 7-10 days
- US and CT insensitive

Top Differential Diagnoses

- Arterial ischemic stroke
  - Focal arterial vascular ischemic injury
  - Typically not associated with HIE
- Venous injury
  - Edema, hemorrhage, or ischemia in venous distribution
- Hypoglycemia
  - Predominantly posterior distribution, check glucose
- Mitochondrial disorders
- Urea cycle disorders
- Other inborn errors in metabolism
- Kernicterus (accentuated by sepsis, hypoxia)

(Left) Axial ADC map in a 1-day-old neonate with an Apgar score of 0 at 5 min shows marked ADC decrease involving the ventrolateral thalami ➔ and CST in PLIC bilaterally ➚. This case was proven to be profound HII. (Right) Axial ADC in the same neonate at 4 days old shows the ADC decrease to now involve the bilateral caudate ➚ and lentiform nuclei ➔. The delayed appearance of ADC abnormalities suggests that delayed necrosis has occurred in the interval.

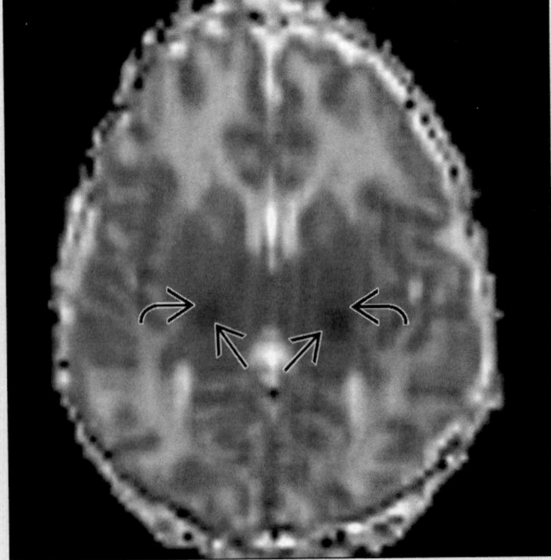

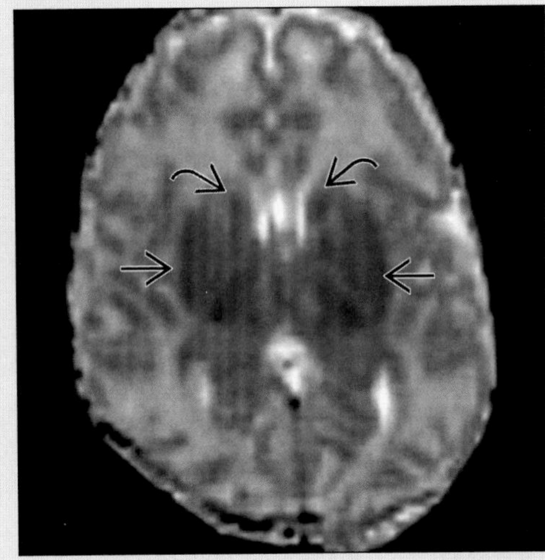

(Left) Axial DWI MR of a 1-day-old neonate presenting with seizures shows scattered small foci of increased signal intensity, primarily at the depths of sulci ➔. This infant was diagnosed with partial HII. (Right) Axial DWI MR in the same neonate at age 3 days shows marked progression of the extent and severity of the DWI abnormality suggesting delayed necrosis. Note the involvement of the depths of sulci ➔, as well as the sparing of ventrolateral thalamus ➔ and CST in PLIC ➚.

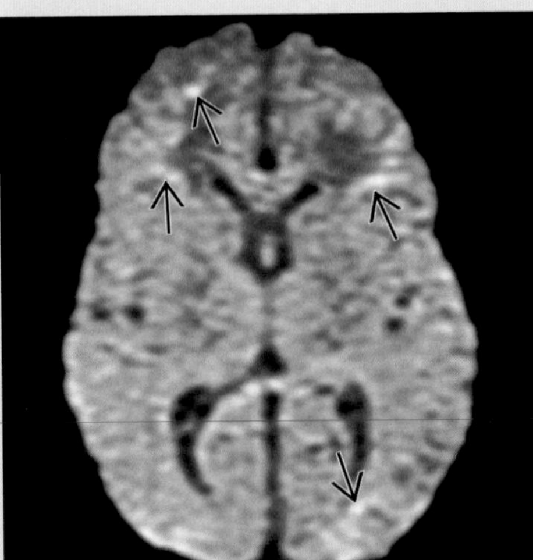

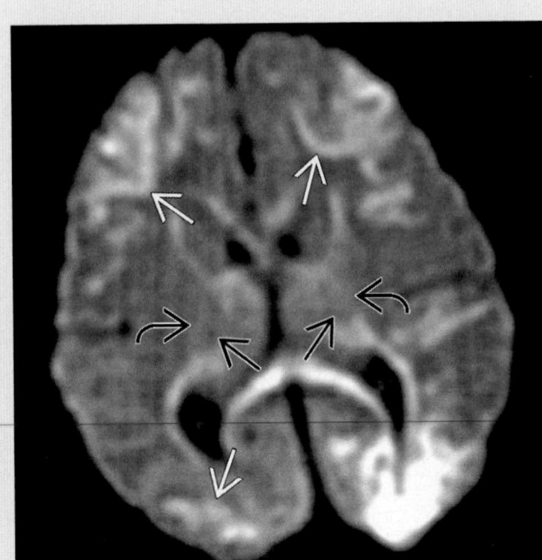

TERM HYPOXIC ISCHEMIC INJURY

TERMINOLOGY

Abbreviations

- Hypoxic ischemic injury (HII), hypoxic ischemic encephalopathy (HIE)

Synonyms

- Hypoxic ischemic insult, perinatal or birth asphyxia, asphyxia neonatorium

Definitions

- HII = imaging pattern of injury due to acquired global arterial hypoperfusion (though many factors can increase vulnerability and potential injury)
  - Not all with HII meet clinical criteria for HIE
- HIE = clinical syndrome defined in term or near-term neonates
  - Not all with HIE have HII on imaging

IMAGING

General Features

- Best diagnostic clue
  - Profound HII: Low ADC in ventrolateral thalamus (VLT) ± corticospinal tract (CST) in posterior limb internal capsule (PLIC)
  - Partial HII: VL thalamus and CST in PLIC spared, cortical injury maximal at depths of sulci
- Location
  - Profound HII
    - VLT + CST in PLIC
    - ± perirolandic cortex, other cortical regions (in cortex depths of sulci more involved than apices of gyri), white matter, hippocampi, midbrain, dorsal brainstem, superior vermis
    - Subacute: Entire thalamus and basal ganglia may become involved
  - Partial HII
    - VLT + CST in PLIC spared
    - Bilateral symmetric or asymmetric involvement of cortex and subcortical white matter usually maximal at sulcal depths
    - Thalamic involvement but not VLT

CT Findings

- NECT
  - Insensitive
  - Profound HII: Deep gray nuclei may be indistinct due to ↓ attenuation
  - Partial HII: Loss of gray-white distinction

MR Findings

- T1WI
  - Profound HII
    - Subacute (beginning ~ 3 days): ↑ signal in VLT, ± posterolateral putamen, ± perirolandic cortex at depths of sulci, loss of normal ↑ signal of CST in PLIC
  - Partial HII
    - Subacute: ↑ signal depths of sulci starting ~ 3 days
- T2WI
  - Profound HII
    - Acute: Blurring of deep gray nuclei ± cortical margins
    - Subacute: ↓ signal in VLT ± posterolateral putamen starting ~ 6 days, ↑ signal in white matter
    - Chronic: ↑ signal ± volume loss in VLT, ± posterolateral putamen, ± other areas of gliosis + volume loss
  - Partial HII
    - Acute: Blurring of cortical margins
    - Subacute: ↑ signal in white matter
    - Chronic: Variable volume loss and gliosis
- T2* GRE
  - Rarely blooming to suggest hemorrhage directly related to HII
- DWI
  - Bright DWI and ↓ ADC occur early, even when T1WI/T2WI normal
  - Injuries evolve over time: DWI and ADC abnormality can ↑ in size and severity over 1st few days due to delayed cell death; DWI normalizes and ADC normalizes or ↑ around 7-10 days
- MRA
  - Typically normal or loss of signal due to turbulent flow in small neonatal arteries
- MRV
  - Typically normal, often focal narrowing in superior sagittal sinus due to moulding
- MRS
  - ↓ NAA correlates with worse prognosis
  - ↑ α-glutamate/glutamine peaks in BG correlate with ↑ severity of injury
  - ↑ lactate correlates with worse prognosis

Ultrasonographic Findings

- Grayscale ultrasound
  - Insensitive, may see ↑ echogenicity in injured areas
- Color Doppler
  - ↓ resistive indices in severe profound HII
  - Good to rule out clot in circle of Willis

Imaging Recommendations

- Best imaging tool
  - DWI: Extremely sensitive for early ischemic necrosis
- Protocol advice
  - In milder injuries, DWI may take 24 hours to become abnormal
    - To ↑ sensitivity to subtle injury, look at ADC as well as DWI and consider ↑ b values

DIFFERENTIAL DIAGNOSIS

Arterial Ischemic Stroke

- Focal arterial vascular ischemic injury
- Typically not associated with HIE
- Not global arterial hypoperfusion = technically not HII

Venous Injury

- Edema, hemorrhage, or ischemia in venous distribution
- Not global arterial hypoperfusion = technically not HII

Hypoglycemia

- Predominantly posterior distribution, check glucose

Mitochondrial Disorders

- Consider if history benign
- Pattern can be identical to HII

Urea Cycle Disorders

- Pattern of BG and thalamus involvement different

Other Inborn Errors in Metabolism

- Many have basal ganglia abnormalities; thalamus uncommon

Kernicterus

- Accentuated by sepsis, hypoxia
- Mimics profound injury, acute on T1WI; has confirmed hyperbilirubinemia
- Globus pallidus (not putamen or thalamus)

PATHOLOGY

General Features

- Etiology
  - Profound HII
    - Sentinel event: Equivalent to cardiorespiratory arrest
    - Severe lack of blood flow & O_2 for min to ~ 1 hour
    - Injury maximal to areas with high metabolic demand
  - Partial HII
    - No sentinel event, therefore less well understood
    - Moderate lack of blood flow and oxygen for hours to days; persistent or intermittent
    - Redistribution of blood flow to areas of high metabolic demand → sparing of these regions
  - Asphyxia triggers cascade of cellular biochemical events → abnormal function, edema, or death of cell
    - Extracellular glutamate accumulates, activates postsynaptic excitatory amino acid receptors
    - Postsynaptic receptor distribution changes with development → different damage patterns at different gestational ages
  - Many chances for cell loss
    - Primary neuronal (death at time of insult)
    - Reactive cell death (reperfusion injury hours or days later)
    - Seizure-related cell injury
- Genetics
  - Seek inborn errors of metabolism if apparent HII with normal Apgar or if > 1 HII child in family
- Associated abnormalities
  - Maternal: Infection, pre-eclampsia, diabetes, cocaine
  - Infant: ↓ gestational age, ↓ Hgb, growth retardation, ↓ Ca++/glucose, sepsis, hyperthermia, seizures, congenital heart disease; ↑ urine S100B protein
  - Ischemia often multi-organ (e.g., cardiac, renal)

Staging, Grading, & Classification

- Sarnat stage (based on clinical and EEG findings)

Gross Pathologic & Surgical Features

- Profound HII: Hippocampal, BG, thalamic, perirolandic atrophy
- Partial HII: Ulegyria, gliosis, and atrophy with sparing perirolandic region

CLINICAL ISSUES

Presentation

- Most common signs/symptoms
  - Sarnat I (mild): Hyperalert/irritable, mydriasis, ↑ HR, EEG normal
  - Sarnat II (mod): Lethargy, hypotonia, miosis, ↓ HR, seizure (SZ)
  - Sarnat III (severe): Stupor, flaccid, reflexes absent, SZ

Demographics

- Age
  - Near or full-term in immediate prenatal, intrapartum, and postnatal period
- Gender
  - M > F
- Epidemiology
  - HIE: Up to 2/1,000 (0.2%) live births

Natural History & Prognosis

- Varies from normal outcome (Sarnat I) to spastic quadriparesis, developmental delay, microcephaly, and SZ (Sarnat III)
- Profound HII (VL thalamus injury): Extrapyramidal cerebral palsy, high mortality, high morbidity
- Partial HII: Spastic quadriparesis

Treatment

- Resuscitation, correct fluid, and electrolyte imbalance
- Treat seizures
- Therapeutic hypothermia

DIAGNOSTIC CHECKLIST

Consider

- Prenatal HII with in utero injury & recovery or inborn errors of metabolism if atypical clinical presentation

Image Interpretation Pearls

- DWI critical, but evolves over time: Can be normal < 1 day, ↑ in severity over days, then normalize ~ 1 week

SELECTED REFERENCES

1. Okereafor A et al: Patterns of brain injury in neonates exposed to perinatal sentinel events. Pediatrics. 121(5):906-14, 2008
2. Vermeulen RJ et al: Diffusion-weighted and conventional MR imaging in neonatal hypoxic ischemia: two-year follow-up study. Radiology. 249(2):631-9, 2008
3. Barkovich AJ et al: MR imaging, MR spectroscopy, and diffusion tensor imaging of sequential studies in neonates with encephalopathy. AJNR Am J Neuroradiol. 27(3):533-47, 2006
4. Ferriero DM: Neonatal brain injury. N Engl J Med. 351(19):1985-95, 2004
5. McKinstry RC et al: A prospective, longitudinal diffusion tensor imaging study of brain injury in newborns. Neurology. 59(6):824-33, 2002
6. Barkovich AJ et al: Proton spectroscopy and diffusion imaging on the first day of life after perinatal asphyxia: preliminary report. AJNR Am J Neuroradiol. 22(9):1786-94, 2001
7. Barkovich AJ et al: Perinatal asphyxia: MR findings in the first 10 days. AJNR Am J Neuroradiol. 16(3):427-38, 1995

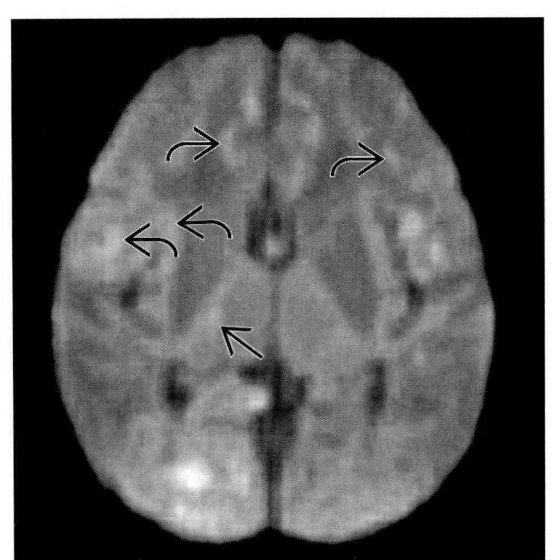

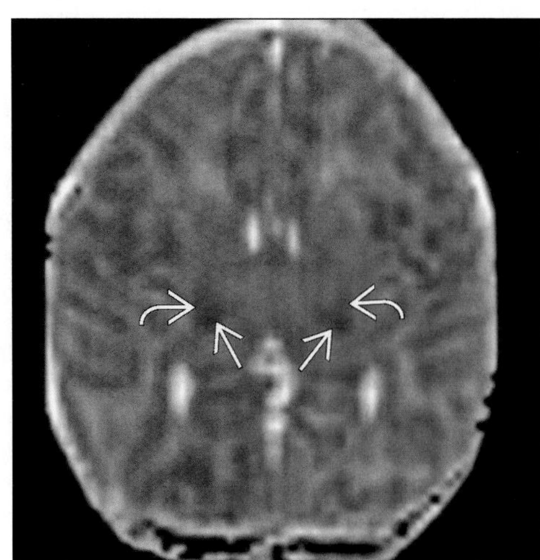

(Left) *Axial DWI MR in a neonate with profound HII shows increased signal in the right VL thalamus/CST region with multiple other foci of cortical/subcortical increased signal. Note the depths of sulci are often preferentially involved in profound HII.* ***(Right)*** *Axial ADC map in the same neonate better demonstrates the low ADC in the VL thalamus and CST with multiple other regions of cortical/subcortical white matter involved. ADC shows neonatal injury better than DWI.*

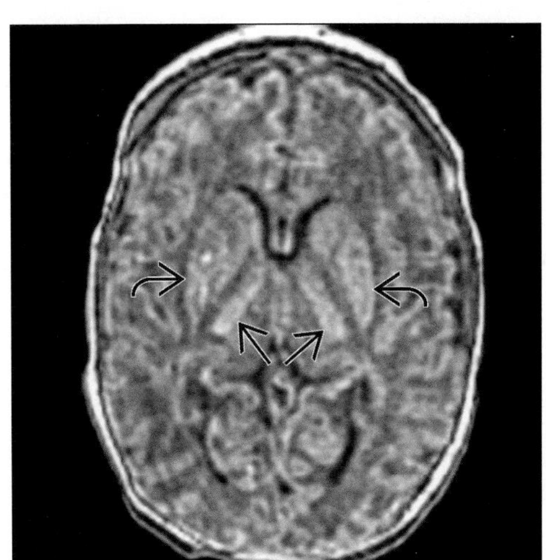

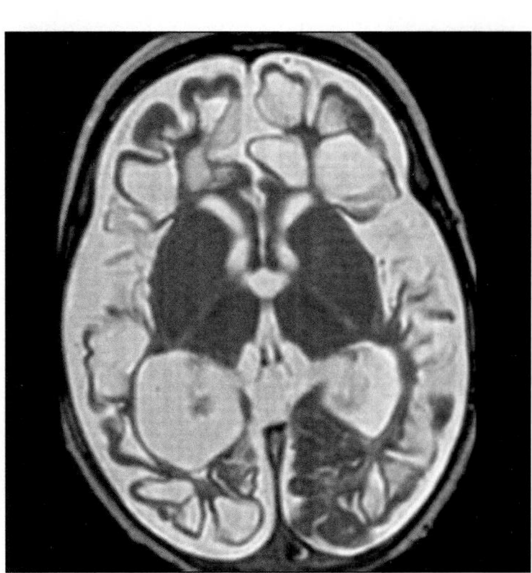

(Left) *Axial T1WI MR of a 9-day-old neonate who suffered birth injury and has profound HII shows increased signal intensity bilaterally in the ventrolateral thalami and putamina.* ***(Right)*** *Axial T2WI MR in the same infant 6 months later. The diffuse cystic encephalomalacia seen here goes beyond the visualized DWI/ADC abnormalities seen on the neonatal MR, suggesting processes of delayed cell death continued after the neonatal period.*

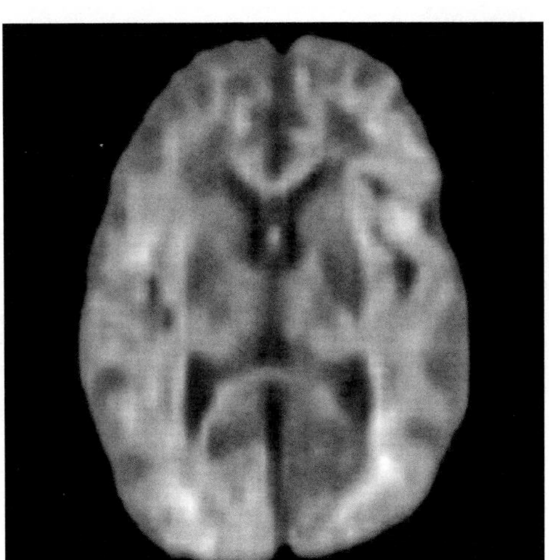

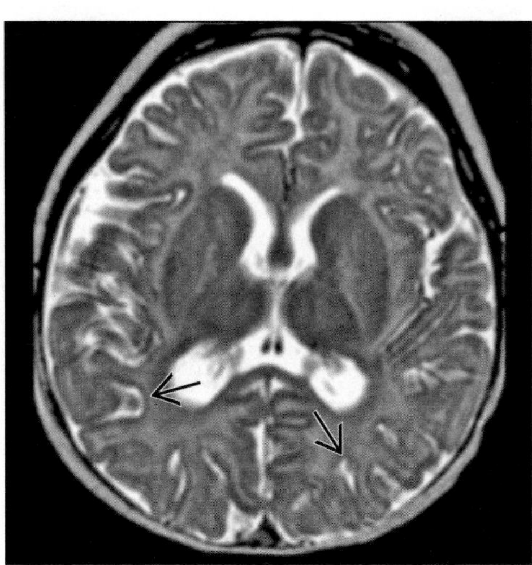

(Left) *Axial DWI MR in an infant with partial HII shows diffuse cortical white matter and deep gray increased signal with sparing of the VL thalamus and CST.* ***(Right)*** *Axial T2WI MR in the same infant at 6 months shows diffuse volume loss with scattered subtle areas of cortical thinning at the depths of sulci, indicating that regions of marked decreased diffusion as seen on the previous image do not always progress to frank cystic encephalomalacia.*

ADULT HYPOXIC ISCHEMIC INJURY

Key Facts

Terminology

- Hypoxic ischemic injury (HII) includes global hypoxic ischemic injury, global anoxic injury, cerebral hypoperfusion injury
  - Etiologies: Cardiac arrest, cerebrovascular disease, drowning, asphyxiation

Imaging

- Injury patterns highly variable depending on brain maturity, severity and length of insult
  - Mild to moderate: Watershed zone infarcts
  - Severe: Gray matter structures (basal ganglia, thalami, cortex, cerebellum, hippocampi)
- MR best to assess overall extent of injury within hours after HII event
  - DWI: 1st modality to be positive (within hours)
  - DWI: Restriction in deep nuclei ± cortex
  - T2/FLAIR: ↑ signal in cerebellum, basal ganglia, cortex
  - Acute changes not reliably identified with T2
- MRS: More sensitive and indicative of severity of injury in 1st 24 hours after HII
  - ↑ lactate, ↑ glutamine-glutamate

Top Differential Diagnoses

- Ischemic territorial infarction
- Traumatic cerebral edema
- Toxic/metabolic disorder
- Acute hypertensive encephalopathy, PRES
- Creutzfeldt-Jakob disease

Pathology

- Common underlying process regardless of cause
  - ↓ CBF and ↓ blood oxygenation
  - Switch from oxidative phosphorylation to anaerobic metabolism
  - Glutamate-related cytotoxic processes

*(**Left**) Axial DWI MR shows symmetrically increased signal in bilateral globi pallidi ➔. DWI is the earliest modality to become positive, within the 1st few hours after a hypoxic-ischemic event. DWI abnormalities may pseudonormalize by the end of the 1st week. (**Right**) Axial T2WI MR in the same patient shows symmetric hyperintensity in the globi pallidi ➔. T2 images typically become positive in the early subacute period (> 24 hours to 2 weeks) with increased signal and swelling of the injured gray matter structures.*

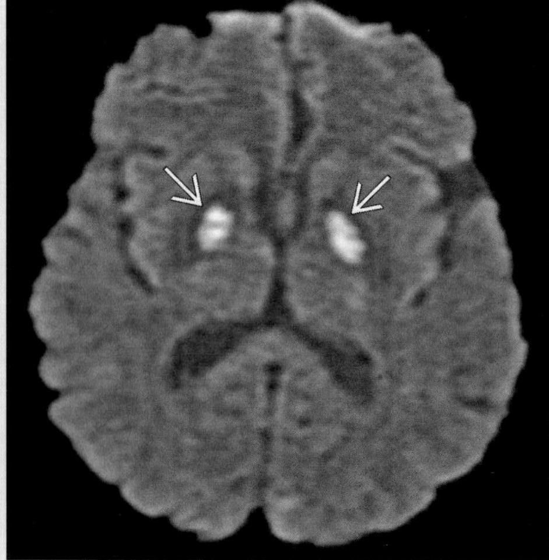

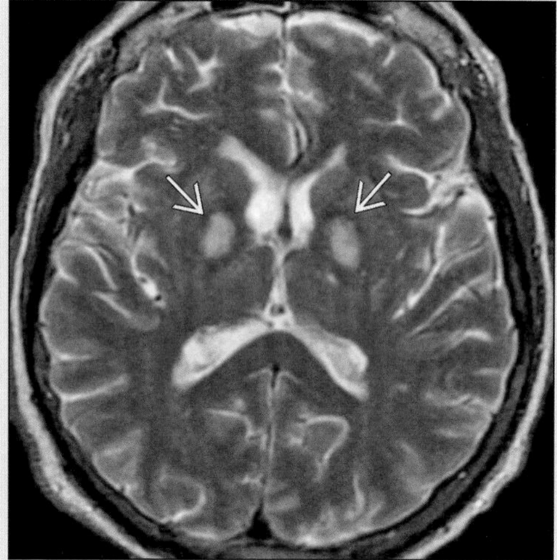

*(**Left**) Axial DWI MR shows symmetric restricted diffusion in the caudate heads, putamina ➔, and cortex in a comatose patient status post cardiac arrest. The cortical involvement is most prominent in the occipital lobes ➔. (**Right**) Axial FLAIR MR shows symmetric hyperintensity in the basal ganglia bilaterally ➔ in a patient with a history of chronic anoxic injury. These deep gray nuclei are also atrophic. Subtle cortical thinning and hyperintensity is also seen in bilateral occipital lobes ➔.*

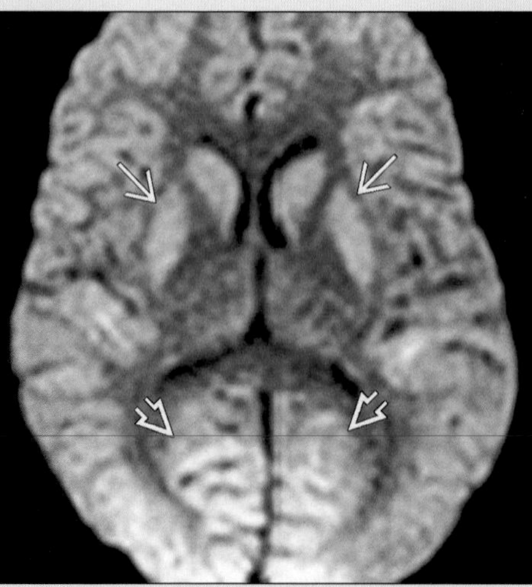

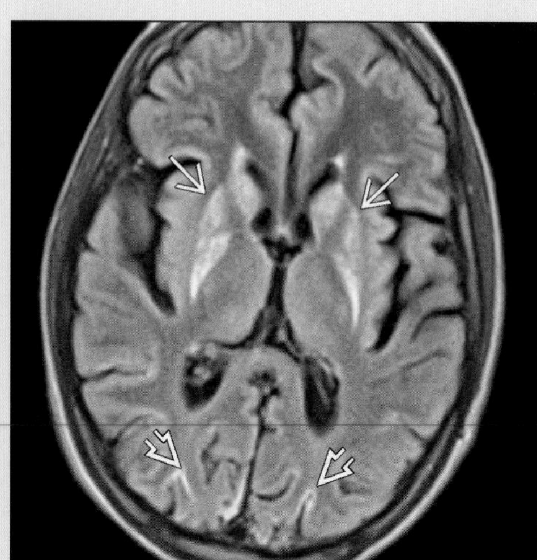

ADULT HYPOXIC ISCHEMIC INJURY

TERMINOLOGY

Synonyms

- Hypoxic ischemic injury (HII), hypoxic ischemic encephalopathy (HIE)

Definitions

- Includes various etiologies of injury: Global hypoxic ischemic injury, global anoxic injury, cerebral hypoperfusion injury

IMAGING

General Features

- Best diagnostic clue
  - Symmetric T2/FLAIR hyperintensity in deep gray nuclei ± cortex
- Location
  - Mild to moderate: Watershed zone infarcts
  - Severe: Gray matter (GM) structures (basal ganglia [BG], thalami, cerebral cortex [sensorimotor and visual], cerebellum, hippocampi)
    - Cerebellar injury tends to be more common in older patients; Purkinje cells are sensitive to ischemia
  - Injury patterns are highly variable depending on brain maturity, severity and length of insult

CT Findings

- NECT
  - Diffuse cerebral edema with effacement of CSF-containing spaces
  - Decreased cortical gray matter attenuation with loss of normal gray-white differentiation
  - Decreased bilateral BG attenuation
  - "Reversal" or "white cerebellum" sign indicates severe injury with poor prognosis

MR Findings

- T1WI
  - Normal to very subtle abnormalities
  - BG may show T1 hyperintensity
  - Gray matter signal abnormalities may persist into end of 2nd week
  - Chronic stages show cortical pseudolaminar necrosis
- T2WI
  - Normal to very subtle abnormalities in 1st 24 hours
  - BG typically show T2 hyperintensity
  - Gray matter signal abnormalities may persist into end of 2nd week
  - Chronic stages show residual BG hyperintensity
- FLAIR
  - Symmetric hyperintensity in deep gray nuclei ± cortex
- DWI
  - 1st imaging modality to become positive, within hours after HII event
    - ↑ signal in cerebellar hemispheres, BG, cerebral cortex
  - DWI abnormalities pseudonormalize by end of 1st week
  - ADC is reduced in hyperacute phase following HII event due to influx of water from extra- to intracellular space
    - ADC values are reduced in severe white matter (WM) and in some severe BG and thalamic injury
    - ADC values may pseudonormalize or even be high initially in some less severe but clinically significant injuries
    - Abnormal ADC values pseudonormalize during 2nd week, whereas fractional anisotropy (FA) values continue to decrease
  - DTI: FA may be abnormal
    - Low FA may reflect breakdown in WM organization
    - Moderate BG/thalamic injury may result in atrophy but not overt infarct due to delayed apoptosis (may account for normal early ADC values)
      - Accompanying low FA within some severe and all moderate gray matter lesions → associated with significant later impairment
- PWI
  - In rat models, luxury perfusion immediately follows resuscitation from HII ⇒ several hours of cortical and striatal mild hypoperfusion followed by hyperemia
- MRS
  - More sensitive and more indicative of injury severity in 1st 24 hours after HII
    - ↑ lactate at 1.3 ppm, ↑ glutamine-glutamate peak at 2.3 ppm
    - ↑ lactate after 24 hours portends poor neurologic outcome
    - NAA is usually normal in acute setting and declines 48 hours after acute injury

Imaging Recommendations

- Best imaging tool
  - MR, particularly DWI/DTI, is most sensitive modality to show abnormalities after ictus
- Protocol advice
  - DTI/DWI are most sensitive
  - Acute ischemic cerebral changes cannot be reliably identified with T2/FLAIR sequences
  - T2*GRE/SWI helpful to detect petechial or subarachnoid hemorrhage

DIFFERENTIAL DIAGNOSIS

Acute Cerebral Ischemia-Infarction

- Wedge-shaped T2 hyperintensity in vascular distribution
- DWI positive acutely

Traumatic Cerebral Edema/Ischemia

- Compressed ventricles and effaced sulci due to combination of vasogenic edema in WM and cytotoxic edema in GM → herniation of brain
- Vascular compression can lead to infarction

Toxic/Metabolic Disorder

- Selective vulnerability of GM to energy depletion
  - Carbon monoxide: T2 hyperintense GP ± subcortical WM

- Methanol: Hyperintense putamen ± hemorrhagic necrosis
- Mitochondrial encephalopathy: Symmetric BG abnormality

Acute Hypertensive Encephalopathy, PRES

- Predominantly vasogenic edema in subcortical WM of bilateral parietooccipital regions

Creutzfeldt-Jakob Disease (CJD)

- Progressive T2 hyperintensity in BG, thalamus, and cerebral cortex
- FLAIR hyperintensity in cortex in sporadic CJD
- DWI: Restriction in deep gray nuclei and cortex; may resolve late in disease

PATHOLOGY

Staging, Grading, & Classification

- Common underlying process regardless of cause of injury
  - Diminished cerebral blood flow and reduced blood oxygenation
  - Brain ischemia due to cardiac arrest or cerebrovascular disease and 2° to hypoxia due to ↓ blood flow
    - Switch from oxidative phosphorylation to anaerobic metabolism: ↓ ATP, ↑ lactate
    - Release of presynaptic glutamate → activation of NMDA receptors → triggers cytotoxic processes
      - Severe energy depletion → cell necrosis; lesser energy depletion → apoptosis
- Sites of brain injury determined by maturity of brain, severity of hypoxic-ischemic insult, and duration
- Selective vulnerability: Patterns of injury reflect dysfunction of selected excitatory neuronal circuits depleted most rapidly
  - Areas with highest concentrations of glutamate or excitatory amino acid receptors (GM) are more susceptible to injury
  - Areas with greatest energy demands become energy deficient
  - Cell death may not be evident until days after initial insult
- Delayed white matter injury: Postanoxic leukoencephalopathy
  - 2-3 weeks after HII in 2-3% of patients
  - Clinical stability followed by acute neurologic decline, most (75%) recover
- Brain-damaging effects of hypoxic-ischemia are age-dependent but do not increase linearly with advancing age and development
  - Immature brain is less resistant to HII than its adult counterpart
  - Intermediate age groups are more tolerant to HII than either very young or more mature ages
- Mechanism behind reduced diffusion during ischemia is thought to be caused by cytotoxic edema, which results from breakdown of cellular membrane Na/K pump system
  - As cytotoxic edema develops → shift of water from extracellular to intracellular space
  - Cell membrane remains intact, no overall ↑ in tissue water; **initially**: ↑ FA, ↓ ADC, normal T2
- Shorter intervals of HII primarily damage cerebral cortex and hippocampus, while longer periods result in more extensive damage and can be associated with cavitary lesions of cerebral hemispheres
  - Cavitary lesions, vertical band-like distribution of noncavitary lesions, mineralization more common in immature brain

CLINICAL ISSUES

Presentation

- Most common signs/symptoms
  - Etiologies: Cardiac arrest, cerebrovascular disease, drowning, asphyxiation
  - Hypoxia in cases of near drowning involves putamen and caudate nucleus

Natural History & Prognosis

- Death or profound long-term neurologic disability
  - Neurological sequela, such as cerebral palsy and epilepsy

Treatment

- Supportive care; however, this does not prevent ongoing injury following causative insult
- Hypothermia
- Excitatory amino acid antagonists

DIAGNOSTIC CHECKLIST

Image Interpretation Pearls

- If MR is negative in 1st 24 hours, repeat exam at 2-4 days to exclude delayed injury

Reporting Tips

- Important to describe extent of cortical and deep gray matter involvement

SELECTED REFERENCES

1. Wu O et al: Comatose patients with cardiac arrest: predicting clinical outcome with diffusion-weighted MR imaging. Radiology. 252(1):173-81, 2009
2. Huang BY et al: Hypoxic-ischemic brain injury: imaging findings from birth to adulthood. Radiographics. 28(2):417-39; quiz 617, 2008
3. Grant PE et al: Acute injury to the immature brain with hypoxia with or without hypoperfusion. Radiol Clin North Am. 44(1):63-77, viii, 2006
4. Schaefer P. Stroke and cerebral ischemia. In Edelman R: Clinical Magnetic Resonance Imaging. 3rd ed. Philadelphia: Saunders Elsevier. 1454-98, 2006
5. van Pul C et al: Selecting the best index for following the temporal evolution of apparent diffusion coefficient and diffusion anisotropy after hypoxic-ischemic white matter injury in neonates. AJNR Am J Neuroradiol. 26(3):469-81, 2005
6. Mutlu H et al: Cranial MR imaging findings of potassium chlorate intoxication. AJNR Am J Neuroradiol. 24(7):1396-8, 2003
7. Dijkhuizen RM et al: Dynamics of cerebral tissue injury and perfusion after temporary hypoxia-ischemia in the rat: evidence for region-specific sensitivity and delayed damage. Stroke. 29(3):695-704, 1998

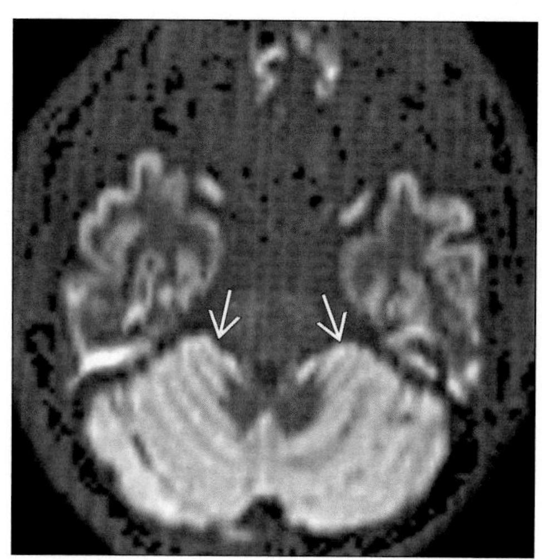

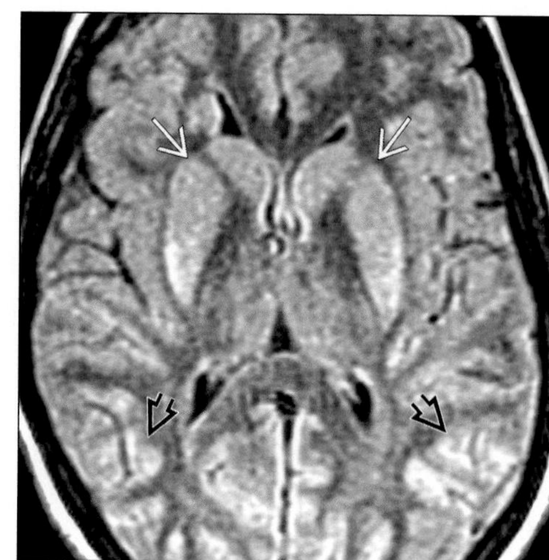

(Left) *Axial DWI demonstrates diffusely increased signal in both cerebellar hemispheres. In adults, severe hypoxic ischemic injury can affect the cerebellum. Purkinje cells are exquisitely sensitive to ischemic damage. Purkinje cell immaturity protects the cerebellar cortex in the neonatal population.* ***(Right)*** *Axial FLAIR MR shows symmetric hyperintensity in the basal ganglia and occipital cortex in this patient with hypoperfusion injury.*

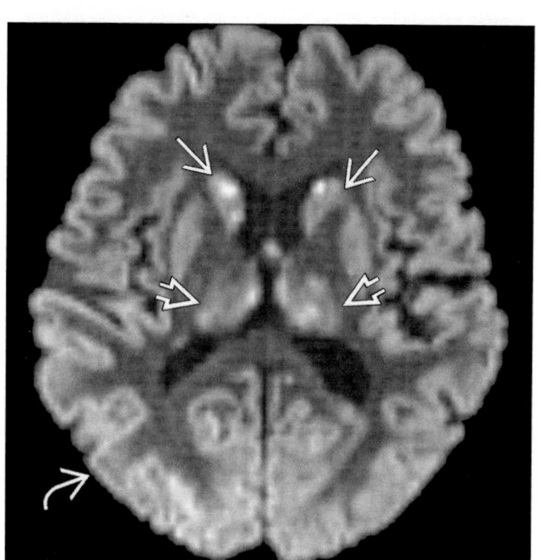

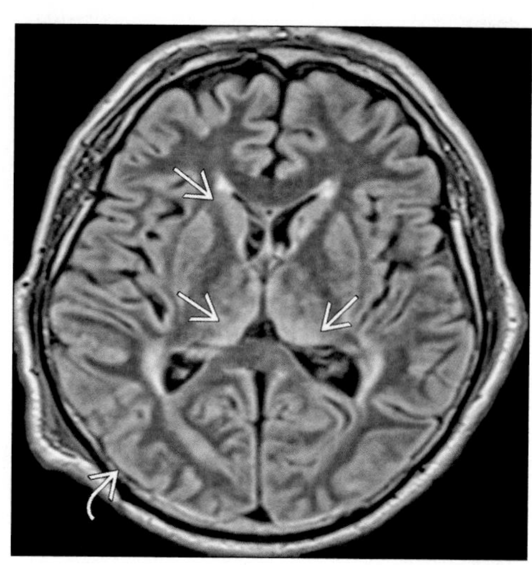

(Left) *Axial DTI TRACE image shows patchy increased signal in bilateral basal ganglia and thalami, as well as in the cerebral cortex diffusely. DTI can be even more sensitive than DWI for the detection of proton movement, indicating acute ischemia.* ***(Right)*** *Axial FLAIR MR in the same patient shows abnormal subtle hyperintensity in the deep gray nuclei and cerebral cortex. Involvement of the visual and sensorimotor cortex is common in hypoxic ischemic injury.*

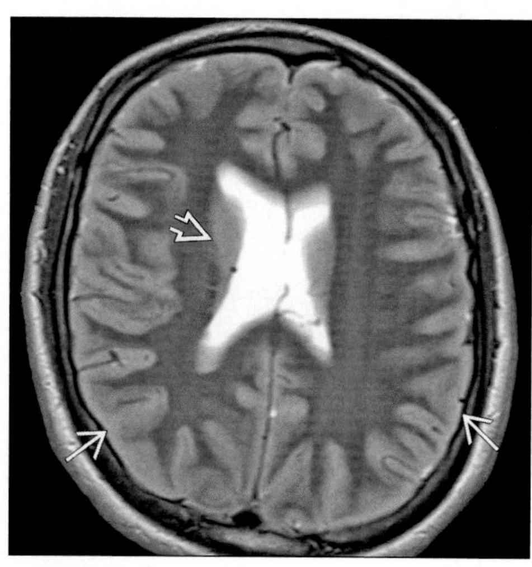

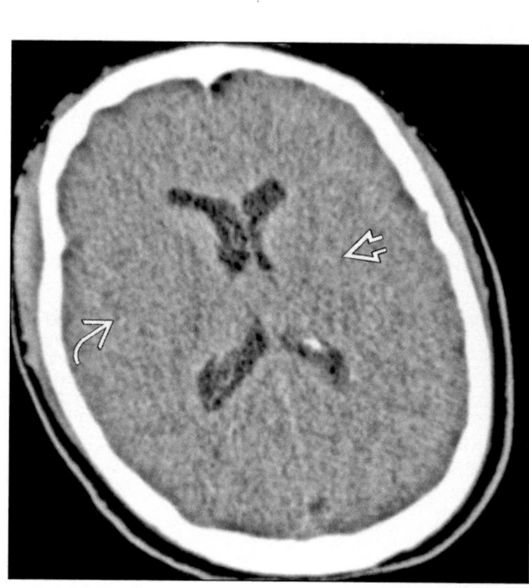

(Left) *Axial T2WI shows diffuse swelling and hyperintensity of the cortex and the caudate bodies. There is a paucity of CSF signal within the sulci due to the gyral swelling.* ***(Right)*** *Axial NECT shows diffuse cerebral parenchymal hypodensity with obscuration of the gray-white interfaces. There is poor delineation of the deep gray nuclei. The sulci and gyri are completely effaced. When hyperdensity of the cerebellum is seen, this indicates severe injury and a poorer prognosis.*

HYPOTENSIVE CEREBRAL INFARCTION

Key Facts

Terminology
- Hypotensive cerebral infarction (HCI)
  - Infarction resulting from insufficient cerebral blood flow to meet metabolic demands (low flow state)
  - "Border zone" or "watershed" infarction

Imaging
- Best imaging tool
  - MR with DWI/ADC ± pMR
- Cortical border zone (between major arterial territories)
  - Typically at gray-white matter junctions
  - Hypodensity between vascular territories
- White matter border zone (between perforating arteries)
  - Typically in deep WM (centrum semiovale)
  - ≥ 3 lesions
  - Linear AP orientation → "string of pearls" appearance
  - If unilateral, look for stenosis of major vessel!
- Imaging recommendations
  - MR + GRE, DWI, MRA (both cervical, intracranial)
  - ± pMR (may show ↓ CBF to affected areas)
  - NECT, pCT, CTA if MR not available
  - CTA/DSA > MRA for determining total vs. near-occlusion of ICA

Top Differential Diagnoses
- Acute embolic cerebral infarction(s)
- Arteriosclerosis ("small vessel disease")
- Posterior reversible encephalopathy (PRES)
- Vasculitis
- Pseudolaminar necrosis (other causes)

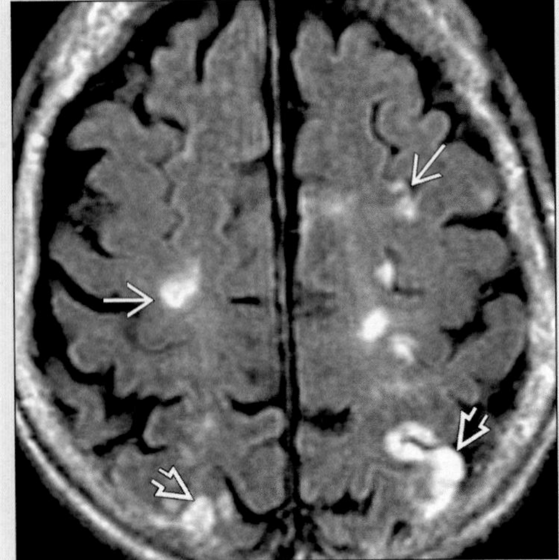

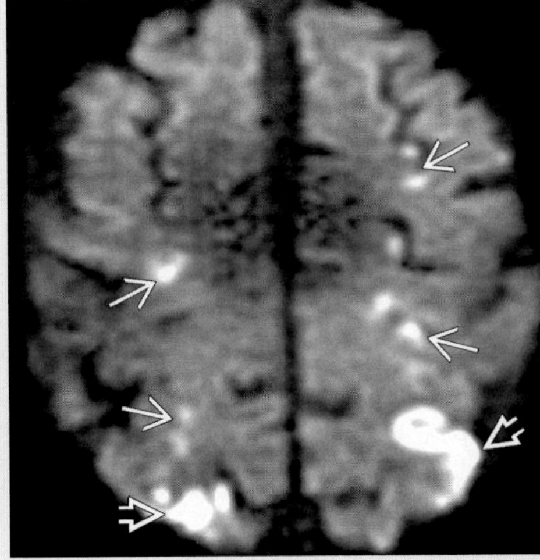

***(Left)** Axial FLAIR MR in a patient with transient global hypoperfusion secondary to a hypotensive episode shows multifocal hyperintensities along the cortical watershed zone ➔. Changes are most severe at the confluence of the ACA, PCA, and MCA cortical vascular territories ➲. **(Right)** DWI in the same patient shows corresponding areas of restricted diffusion in the cortical watershed zones bilaterally ➔, most severe at the trivascular confluence ➲. The diagnosis was hypotensive watershed cerebral infarctions.*

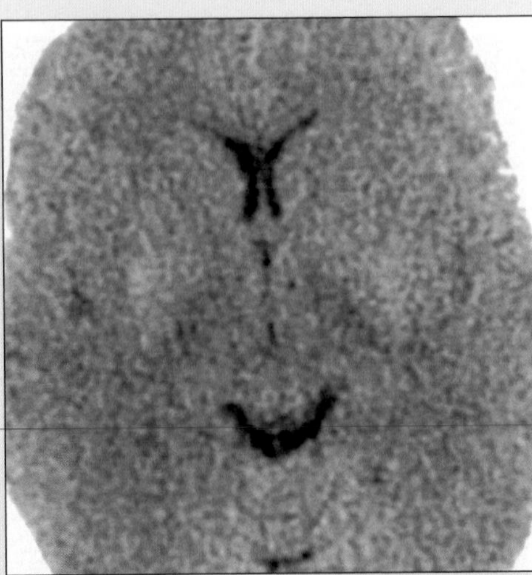

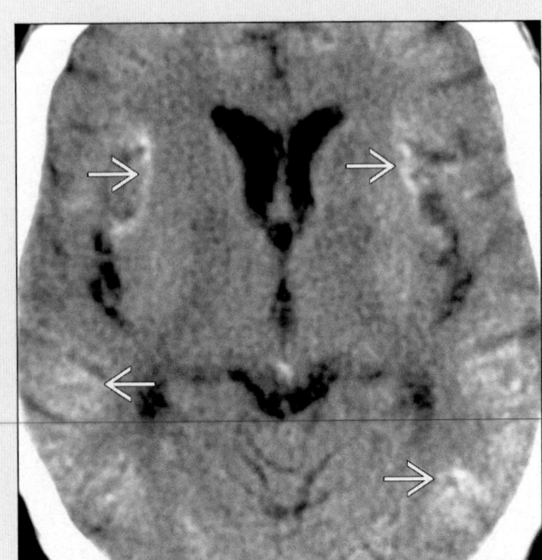

***(Left)** Axial NECT scan obtained a few hours after circulatory arrest and resuscitation shows diffuse cerebral edema with almost complete effacement of all gray-white matter interfaces in both the cortex and basal ganglia. The ventricles appear small, and the sulci are inapparent. **(Right)** Follow-up NECT scan in the same patient shows cortical atrophy and ventricular enlargement. Cortical curvilinear hyperdensities ➔ are typical of pseudolaminar cortical necrosis.*

HYPOTENSIVE CEREBRAL INFARCTION

TERMINOLOGY

Abbreviations

- Hypotensive cerebral infarction (HCI)

Synonyms

- "Border zone" or "watershed" infarction

Definitions

- Infarction resulting from insufficient cerebral blood flow (CBF) to meet metabolic demands (low-flow state)

IMAGING

General Features

- Best diagnostic clue
  - Restricted diffusion on DWI/ADC
- Location
  - 2 types
    - Border zone between major arterial territories
      - Typically at gray-white matter junctions
    - Border zone between perforating arteries
      - Typically in deep white matter
  - Supratentorial structures in severe perinatal asphyxia
  - Bilateral abnormalities in global hypoxic-ischemic (HIE) events (with underlying vascular stenoses + relative hypoperfusion) can lead to unilateral presentations
- Morphology
  - Cortically based wedge-shaped abnormality at border zone between vascular territories
  - Deep white matter (WM) watershed with "rosary" or "string of pearls/beads" appearance
    - Multiple round foci in linear orientation within centrum semiovale
  - Pseudolaminar necrosis = curvilinear, gyriform, cortical T1 shortening
  - Diffuse supratentorial abnormality following severe global asphyxia ("white cerebellar" or "reversal" sign)

CT Findings

- NECT
  - Major arterial border zone infarcts
    - Hypodensity at gray-white matter junction between vascular territories
    - Severe (i.e., global hypoxia-ischemia, HIE)
      - Usually significant hemodynamic compromise (i.e., hypotension)
      - Most all supratentorial gray-white matter junctions effaced
      - Basal ganglia (BG), thalami affected
      - Occasionally isolated to BG ± hippocampus
    - "White cerebellum" ("cerebellar reversal" sign)
      - Cerebellum appears hyperdense compared to supratentorial hypodensity
  - Deep WM watershed infarcts
    - ≥ 3 deep WM lesions within centrum semiovale
    - "String of pearls" appearance
      - Linear orientation in AP (front to back) direction
      - Parallel to lateral ventricle
      - Can resemble multiple emboli
    - Can be unilateral
      - Look for major vessel stenosis on side of infarcts
    - Bilateral if bilateral vessel stenoses ± significant hemodynamic event
- CECT
  - Enhancement in subacute HCI
- CTA
  - Use to determine complete vs. near-complete ICA occlusion
- CT perfusion
  - CBF ↓ in affected areas

MR Findings

- T1WI
  - Acute: Hypointense, swollen gyri ± BG
  - Subacute: Gyriform cortical hyperintensity = pseudolaminar necrosis
    - Usually with global HIE
- T2WI
  - Hyperintensity in involved areas
  - CSF cisterns/sulci compressed if severe
- FLAIR
  - Thrombosed vessels often hyperintense
  - More sensitive to early infarction
- DWI
  - Restricted diffusion (hyperintense on DWI, hypointense ADC)
    - Distinguishes cytotoxic from vasogenic edema
    - Helpful for evaluation following intraoperative anoxia
  - Global HIE may be diffusely hyperintense
    - Creates nearly "pseudonormal" appearance
- T1WI C+
  - Subacute infarcts enhance
    - Gyriform pattern common
    - ± basal ganglia
- MRA
  - Major vessel stenoses predispose to watershed infarction following hypotensive event
- MRS
  - ↑ lactate, ↓ NAA ± lactate doublet (intermediate TE)

Angiographic Findings

- DSA may delineate predisposing conditions for watershed infarct
  - Significant extracranial, major intracranial vessel stenosis

Imaging Recommendations

- Best imaging tool
  - MR + GRE, MRA, DWI
- Protocol advice
  - MR + DWI, MRA (both cervical, intracranial), ± pMR
  - NECT, pCT, CTA if MR unavailable

DIFFERENTIAL DIAGNOSIS

Cerebral Infarction (Acute, Multiple Embolic)

- Often bilateral, multi-territorial
- May also occur at border zones

HYPOTENSIVE CEREBRAL INFARCTION

Arteriosclerosis ("Small Vessel Disease")
- Scattered, multifocal lesions
- No specific predilection for watershed
- Confluent lesions around lateral ventricle atria
  - Common in chronic hypertension

Posterior Reversible Encephalopathy (PRES)
- Usually does not restrict (vasogenic edema)
- Usually cortical/subcortical PCA distribution
- Less commonly can involve watershed zones, BG

Vasculitis
- Often subcortical
- Patchy enhancement in cortex, subcortical WM, BG

Pseudolaminar Necrosis (Other Causes)
- Associations with numerous other entities
  - Reye, lupus, central pontine myelinolysis, immunosuppressive therapy
- Petechial hemorrhage ("hemorrhagic transformation") in subacute thrombolic infarct

PATHOLOGY

General Features
- Etiology
  - Global brain injury due to disruption of perfusion or oxygenation
  - Causes include severe prolonged hypotension, cardiac arrest with resuscitation, profound asphyxia, and carbon monoxide inhalation
  - Major vessel stenoses predispose patient to infarcts at "border zone" between vascular territories during times of hemodynamic compromise
    - Deep WM infarcts ("rosary" pattern) correlate well with clinical hemodynamic compromise
    - Associated with proximal ICA stenosis/occlusion
  - Embolic infarcts also occur at "border zones" and thus complicate clinical and radiographic picture
    - Cortical "border zone" infarcts occur in 3.2% in patients with cardiac embolic sources
      - Compared to 3.6% in those with severe ICA obstruction
    - "Directed embolization" may account for many embolic-type "border zone" infarcts (directional flow at bifurcations occurs from vessel size imbalances in circle of Willis)
- "Border zone" infarction results in encephalomalacic brain, "ulegyria"

Staging, Grading, & Classification
- Pattern classifications
  - Cortical "border zone" infarcts (bi- or unilateral)
  - Deep WM infarcts (penetrating artery "watershed zone")
  - Cortical pseudolaminar necrosis
  - Predominately deep gray nuclei

Gross Pathologic & Surgical Features
- Pale, swollen brain; gray-white matter boundaries "smudged"
- Encephalomalacia (chronic)

Microscopic Features
- After 4 hours: Eosinophilic neurons with pyknotic nuclei
- 15-24 hours: Neutrophils invade, necrotic nuclei look like "eosinophilic ghosts"
- 2-3 days: Blood-derived phagocytes
- 1 week: Reactive astrocytosis, ↑ capillary density
- End result: Fluid-filled cavity lined by astrocytes
- Pseudolaminar necrosis affects 3rd, 5th, 6th cortical layers

CLINICAL ISSUES

Presentation
- Most common signs/symptoms
  - Altered mental status, coma
- Clinical profile
  - Patient with high-grade ICA stenosis, transient hypotension leading to acute cerebral infarction
  - Resuscitated patient with profound asphyxia or prolonged systemic hypotension

Demographics
- Age
  - Any age
- Gender
  - No gender predilection
- Epidemiology
  - Hypotensive infarcts account for 0.7-3.2% of infarcts

Natural History & Prognosis
- Experimental literature suggests isolated hypoxic injury tolerated better than hypoxia complicated by hypotension
- Clinical outcome usually poor, depends on degree of injury
- Diffusion abnormalities restricted to deep nuclei without involvement of cerebral cortex suggest milder injury, and significant neurological recovery can occur

Treatment
- Treatment of underlying conditions
  - Correction of hypotension as rapidly as possible
  - Revascularization of major vessel stenoses

DIAGNOSTIC CHECKLIST

Consider
- MRA, CTA of cervical, intracranial vessels as proximal large vessel disease often present in setting of hypotensive infarction

Image Interpretation Pearls
- "Rosary" or "string of beads" appearance in centrum semiovale highly specific for hemodynamic compromise

SELECTED REFERENCES

1. Moore MJ et al: Reducing the gray zone: imaging spectrum of hypoperfusion and hypoxic brain injury in adults. Emerg Radiol. Epub ahead of print, 2009

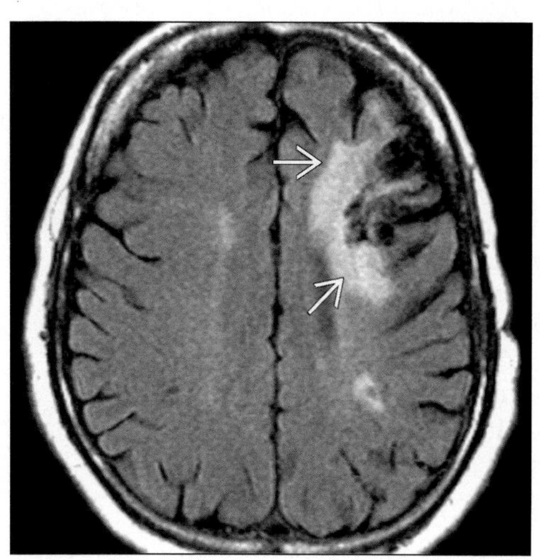

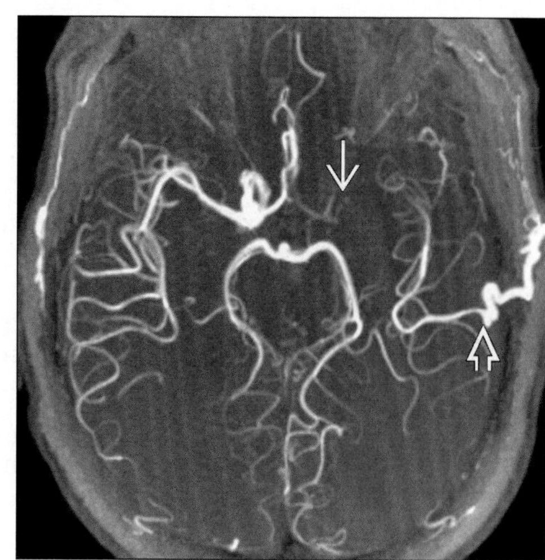

(Left) *Axial FLAIR MR shows a normal right hemisphere and left hemispheric encephalomalacia* ➡ *in the border zone between the ACA and MCA territories, suggesting the infarct may be secondary to hemispheric hypoperfusion.* ***(Right)*** *MIP MRA in the same patient shows an occluded left internal carotid artery* ➡*. This patient had undergone a prior revascularization procedure; note the patent-appearing superficial temporal artery bypass* ➡*, which fills the MCA branches in a retrograde fashion.*

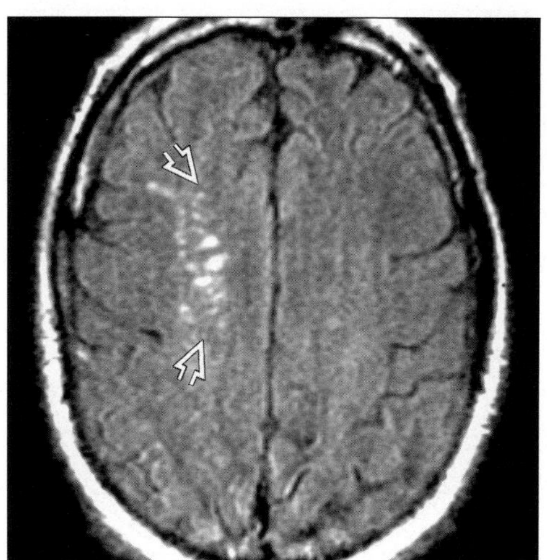

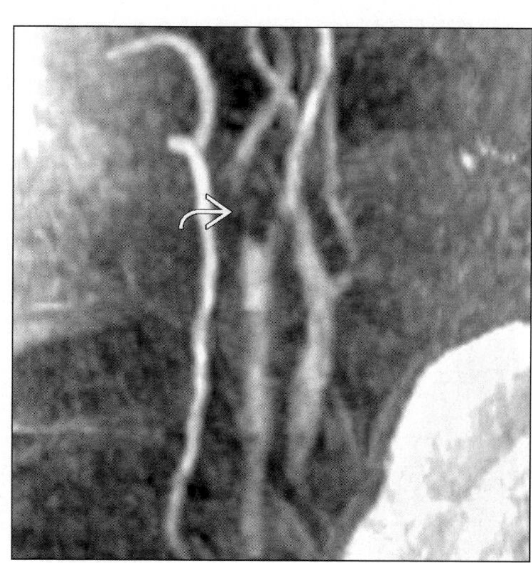

(Left) *Axial FLAIR MR shows hyperintensities in the right centrum semiovale* ➡*, at the deep white matter watershed zone between penetrating arteries. The hyperintensities form a "string of pearls" appearance from front to back.* ***(Right)*** *Cervical MRA in the same patient demonstrates that the underlying predisposing condition leading to infarction was a severe right internal carotid artery stenosis* ➡*. Intracranial MRA (not shown) disclosed a small-caliber right ICA and MCA with poor distal flow.*

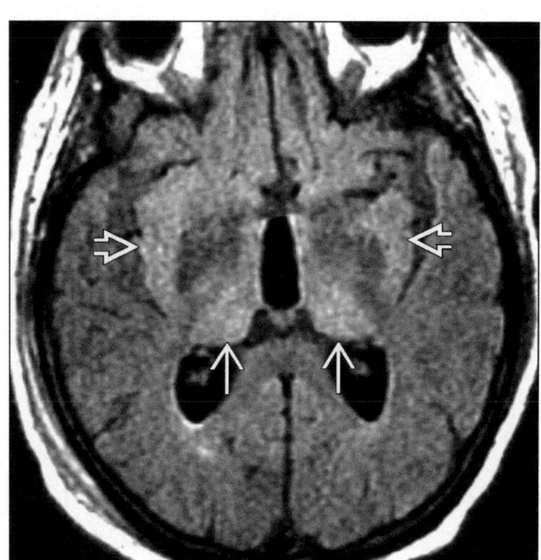

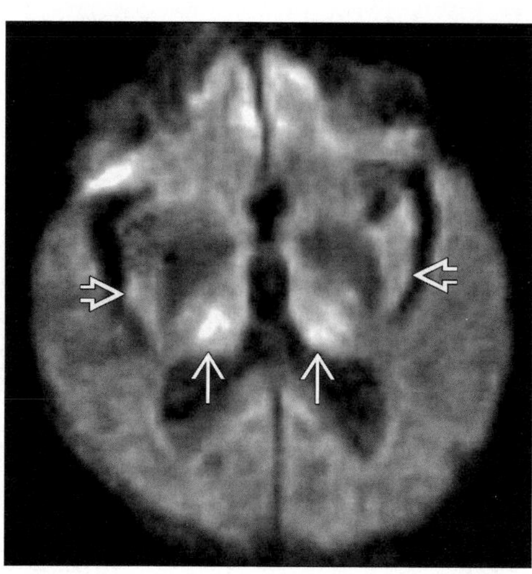

(Left) *This patient with myocardial infarction was resuscitated, then later failed to wake up and lacked response to pain. FLAIR scan obtained several days later shows hyperintense thalami* ➡ *and insular cortex* ➡*, consistent with global ischemic injury.* ***(Right)*** *Axial DWI MR in the same patient shows faint restriction in both thalami* ➡ *and insular cortex* ➡*, less intense than on FLAIR, likely due to the subacute nature of the infarction.*

CHILDHOOD STROKE

Key Facts

Terminology
- Acute alteration of neurologic function due to loss of vascular integrity

Imaging
- "Insular ribbon" sign ⇒ loss of distinction of insular cortex
- "Hyperdense MCA" sign (HMCAS) ⇒ increased density of thrombosed MCA
- Enhancement of infarcted territory typically occurs after 5-7 days
- CTA can show focal vascular abnormalities in acute setting
- DWI is most sensitive imaging sequence for ischemic injury
  - Diffusion restriction seen within 45 minutes of arterial occlusion
- Perfusion studies can identify ischemic penumbra

Pathology
- No underlying cause discovered in > 33% of cases
- Anterior circulation > posterior; left > right

Clinical Issues
- Seizure ⇒ deficit often attributed to post-ictal state (Jacksonian paralysis)
- Under-recognized as significant source of morbidity in pediatric population
- Children with stroke typically present in delayed fashion (> 24 hours)
- 2-3/100,000 per year in USA
- Mortality: 0.6/100,000
- Capacity for recovery much greater than in adults
- Aspirin is mainstay of chronic therapy for fixed vascular lesions and vasculopathies

*(**Left**) Axial T2WI MR shows mature encephalomalacia in the vascular territory of the left MCA in this 4 month old with left hand preference. Handedness should not be apparent before 12-18 months. (**Right**) Axial T1WI C+ MR shows the characteristic "climbing ivy" sign of enhancing sulcal arteries ➔ in a child with moyamoya vasculopathy secondary to sickle cell disease. Slow flow in MCA branches distal to the stenosis allows T1 shortening from contrast to overcome flow void effects.*

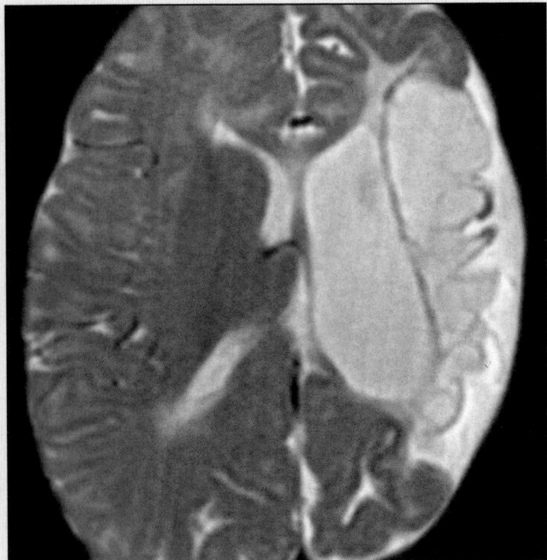

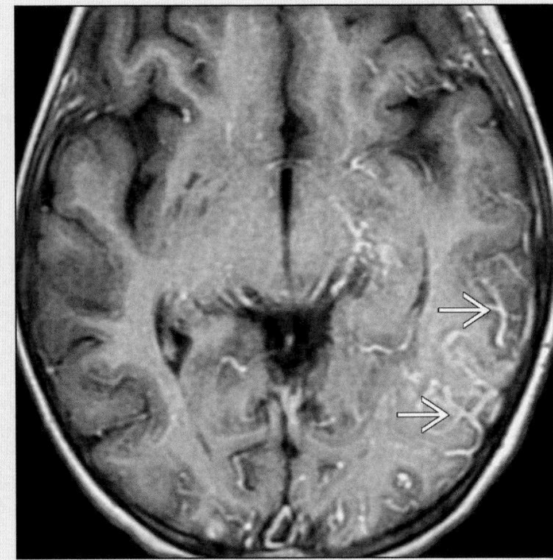

*(**Left**) Axial NECT in 15 year old with difficulty speaking and right hand weakness shows a hyperdense MCA ➔. The patient presented 12 hours after symptom onset and was treated with aspirin only. (**Right**) Axial ADC in the same teenager shows reduced diffusion ➔ in the distal left MCA territory. Encephalomalacia developed, but the patient had a normal neurologic exam 6 months later. Children often have a much greater capacity for neurologic recovery than adults, even with similar imaging findings.*

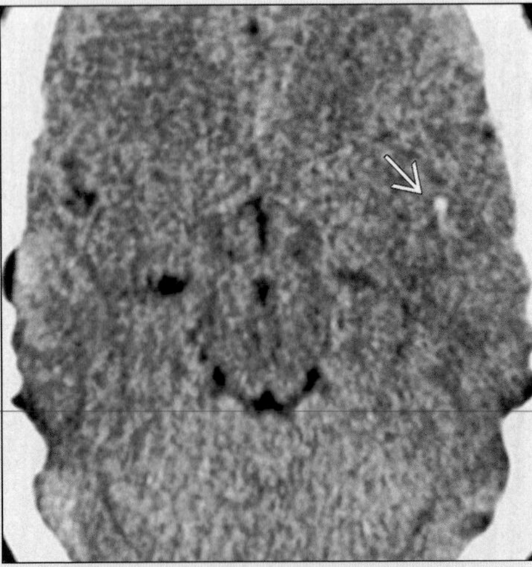

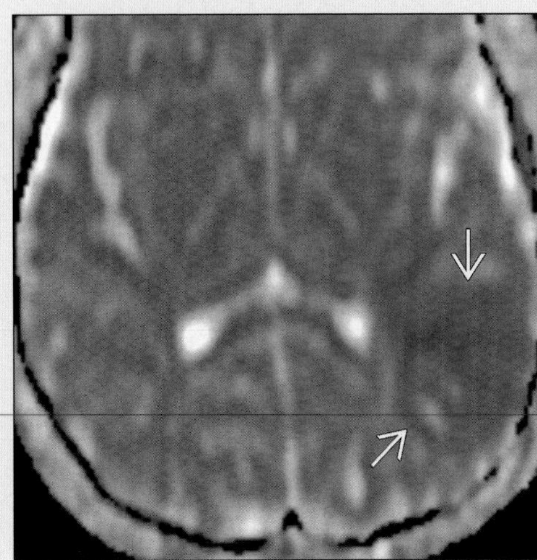

CHILDHOOD STROKE

TERMINOLOGY

Abbreviations

- Cerebrovascular accident (CVA), arterial ischemic stroke (AIS), cerebral venous sinus thrombosis (CVST)

Synonyms

- Cerebral infarct, cerebral ischemia

Definitions

- Acute alteration of neurologic function due to loss of vascular integrity
  - Can be arterial or venous
  - Can be hemorrhagic or nonhemorrhagic

IMAGING

General Features

- Best diagnostic clue
  - Edema, restricted diffusion in affected territory
- Location
  - Proximal and distal middle cerebral artery (MCA) territory most commonly affected
- Morphology
  - Stroke caused by arterial occlusion often conforms to arterial territory
  - Venous territories typically less well recognized

CT Findings

- NECT
  - Decreased attenuation of affected gray matter (GM)
    - "Insular ribbon" sign
      - Loss of distinction of insular cortex
  - "Hyperdense MCA" sign (HMCAS)
    - Increased density of thrombosed MCA
  - Hemorrhagic conversion of stroke
    - Cortical hemorrhage often petechial
    - White matter (WM) or deep nuclear hemorrhage often mass-like
      - Hematoma within infarcted tissue
  - Hyperdense dural sinus in venous thrombosis
    - "Delta" sign
- CECT
  - Enhancement of infarcted territory typically occurs after 5-7 days
  - Enhancement of sagittal sinus wall around nonenhancing clot
    - "Empty delta" sign
- CTA
  - CTA is invaluable for demonstrating focal vascular abnormalities in acute setting
  - Can clearly show arterial occlusion/stenosis
  - Can be used to assess effect of treatment on vessel
    - Restoration of vascular integrity may not correlate with return of neurologic function

MR Findings

- T1WI
  - Gyral swelling and hypointensity in affected territory
  - Loss of normal vascular flow void
    - Entry slice artifact can cause false-positive!
    - Irregular signal can be seen in normal veins due to slow flow
- T1WI FS
  - Use of fat saturation allows confident identification of crescent of mural hematoma in dissected vessel
    - Use in combination with MRA
- T2WI
  - Edema evident in affected territory after 12-24 hours of arterial occlusion
- FLAIR
  - More sensitive than T2WI for ischemia-induced cytotoxic edema
    - Hyperintense after 6-12 hours
  - Also shows loss of normal arterial flow voids
    - "Climbing ivy" sign ⇒ bright vessels in sulci distal to arterial occlusion (slow flow)
      - Same effect is seen with T1WI C+
      - Classically seen in moyamoya
- T2* GRE
  - Sensitive for detection of blood products, especially hemosiderin
    - May impact clinical decision making for acute therapy
- DWI
  - Most sensitive imaging sequence for ischemic injury
  - Diffusion restriction seen within 45 minutes of arterial occlusion
  - Apparent diffusion coefficient (ADC) mapping essential to avoid false-positive from "T2 shine through"
- PWI
  - Can provide valuable information regarding region at risk in setting of acute stroke
  - Ischemic penumbra ⇒ region with diminished perfusion not yet infarcted (perfusion-diffusion mismatch)
  - May define brain salvageable with acute stroke therapy
  - Arterial spin-labeling techniques hold promise for standardized perfusion imaging without contrast administration
- T1WI C+
  - Can provide earliest sign of proximal arterial occlusion ⇒ enhancement of arteries in territory distal to occlusion
    - Collateral flow to distal vascular bed is slower
    - Normal flow void caused by rapid arterial flow is out-weighed by T1 shortening effect of contrast
- MRA
  - Sensitive in detection of arterial occlusion and stenosis in large and medium-sized cerebral vessels
- MRV
  - Can demonstrate focal occlusion, stenosis, or response to treatment
- MRS
  - ↑ lactate hallmark of ischemia/infarct

Ultrasonographic Findings

- Grayscale ultrasound
  - Affected territory hyperechoic in acute/subacute stage
- Color Doppler
  - Direct Doppler evaluation ideal for surveillance of vascular occlusion in neonate with open sutures

- Transcranial Doppler evaluation of circle of Willis through temporal squamosa
  - Increased velocities can predict stenoses detectable by MRA
  - Used as screening tool in children with sickle cell anemia

Angiographic Findings

- Catheter angiography rarely necessary in acute evaluation of childhood stroke
  - Only justified if contemplating endovascular therapy
- Best modality for detailed evaluation of primary arteriopathies

Nuclear Medicine Findings

- Perfusion studies can identify salvageable regions at risk (ischemic penumbra)
- Can evaluate effects of synangiosis surgery in moyamoya

Imaging Recommendations

- Best imaging tool
  - MR with diffusion, perfusion, MRA
    - MRV if MRA negative and DWI positive
- Protocol advice
  - Development of a predetermined stroke imaging protocol can increase efficiency and accuracy

DIFFERENTIAL DIAGNOSIS

Mitochondrial Encephalopathies

- MELAS, MERRF

Encephalitis

- Viral encephalitides, ADEM, cerebritis

Toxins

- Carbon monoxide poisoning, ethylene glycol

PATHOLOGY

General Features

- Etiology
  - No underlying cause discovered in > 33% of cases
- Associated abnormalities
  - Cardiac disease (25-50%), sickle cell (200-400x increased risk), trauma
  - Chemotherapy, sepsis

Gross Pathologic & Surgical Features

- Pathologic findings similar to adults
- Anterior circulation > posterior; left > right

CLINICAL ISSUES

Presentation

- Most common signs/symptoms
  - Focal deficit often masked by lethargy, coma, irritability
  - Seizure ⇒ deficit often attributed to post-ictal state (Jacksonian paralysis)
- Other signs/symptoms
  - Speech difficulties, gait abnormality
  - Preceding transient events occur in 25%
- Under-recognized as significant source of morbidity in pediatric population
  - Children with stroke typically present in delayed fashion (> 24 hours)
    - Poor recognition/understanding of symptoms by child, caregiver, physician

Demographics

- Age
  - Incidence/mortality greatest in infants < 1 year old
- Gender
  - Boys > girls
- Epidemiology
  - 2-3/100,000 per year in USA
  - Mortality: 0.6/100,000
  - "Stroke belt" ⇒ higher incidence in southeastern states

Natural History & Prognosis

- Recurrence (20-40%)
- Capacity for recovery much greater than in adults
  - Fewer concomitant risk factors
  - Better quality of collateral vessels

Treatment

- Clinical window of opportunity/benefit much narrower than in adults
- Aspirin is mainstay of chronic therapy for fixed vascular lesions and vasculopathies
- Transfusion therapy for at-risk children with sickle cell disease
- Thrombolytic therapy has been used in a small number of cases
  - Higher than acceptable risk of hemorrhage
  - Use is mitigated by good outcome with less aggressive therapy in many cases

DIAGNOSTIC CHECKLIST

Consider

- Always consider stroke when evaluating a child with new onset seizure

Reporting Tips

- Be sure to investigate for hemorrhagic complications

SELECTED REFERENCES

1. Amlie-Lefond C et al: Predictors of cerebral arteriopathy in children with arterial ischemic stroke: results of the International Pediatric Stroke Study. Circulation. 119(10):1417-23, 2009
2. Amlie-Lefond C et al: Use of alteplase in childhood arterial ischaemic stroke: a multicentre, observational, cohort study. Lancet Neurol. 8(6):530-6, 2009
3. Kim CT et al: Pediatric stroke recovery: a descriptive analysis. Arch Phys Med Rehabil. 90(4):657-62, 2009
4. Fullerton HJ et al: Pediatric Stroke Belt: geographic variation in stroke mortality in US children. Stroke. 35(7):1570-3, 2004

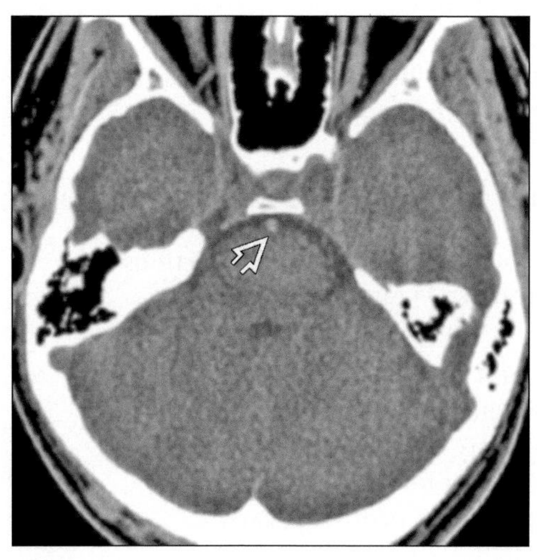

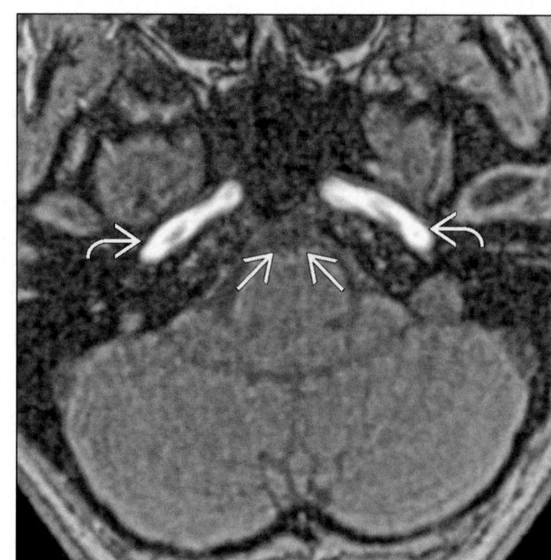

(Left) *Axial NECT in a 12 year old with inflammatory bowel disease and intermittent dysarthria and weakness shows abnormal increased density of the mid-basilar artery, worrisome for thrombosis.* ***(Right)*** *Axial MRA in the same child shows absence of flow in the basilar, with normal flow signal in the carotid arteries. Treatment with intravenous TPA was started within 6 hours and a full recovery was made, despite the lack of contiguous flow through the vessel on follow-up imaging.*

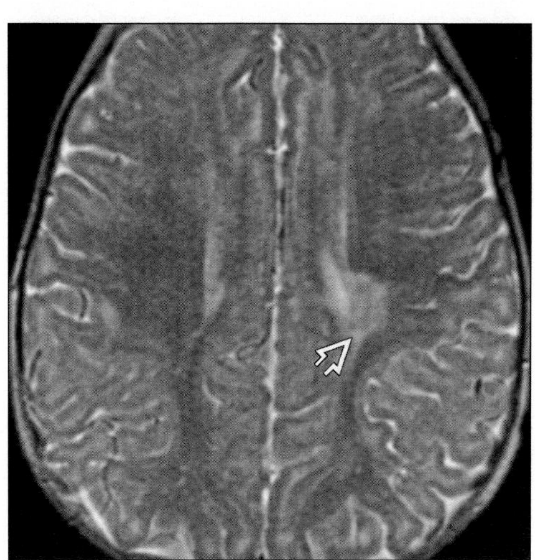

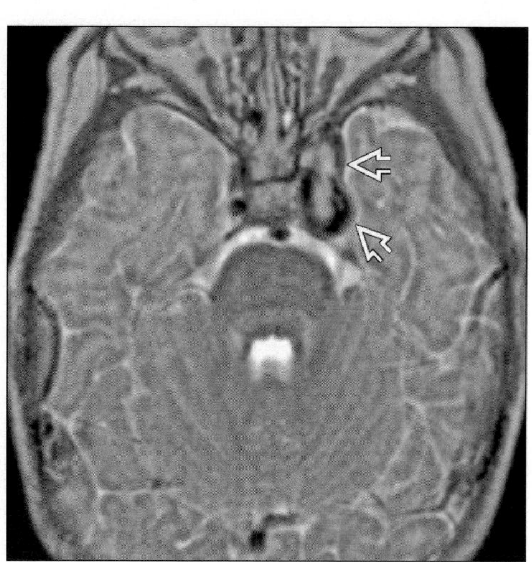

(Left) *Axial T2WI MR in a 7 month old with left hand preference shows focal gliosis in the left periventricular white matter.* ***(Right)*** *Axial T2WI MR through the cavernous sinuses in the same infant shows aneurysm of the left cavernous carotid artery. The aneurysm was coil occluded, and a diagnosis of NF1 was subsequently made. A proximal vascular lesion is not discovered in most cases of perinatal stroke, but it is imperative to exclude the possibility of a treatable lesion.*

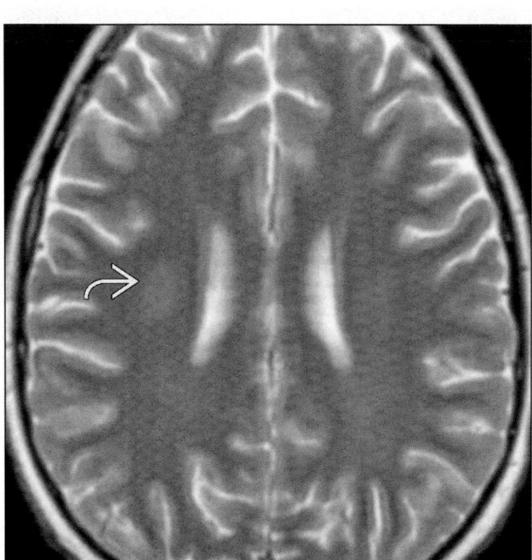

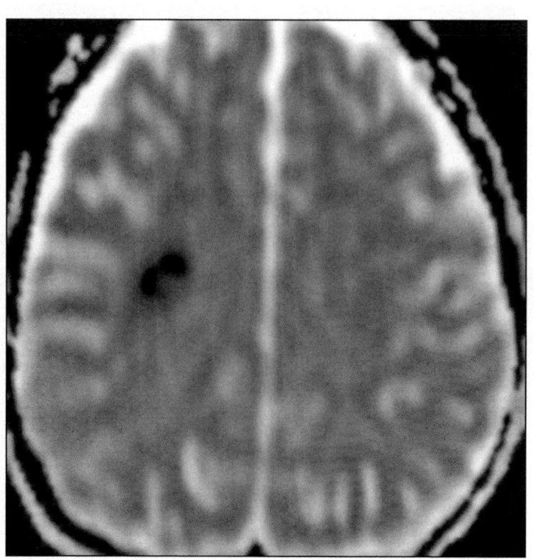

(Left) *Axial T2WI MR in this 12 year old presenting with left-sided weakness shows subtle focal hyperintense signal in the right centrum semiovale. The affected patient had a diagnosis of leukemia and was being treated with L-asparaginase.* ***(Right)*** *Axial ADC map in the same patient confirms the reduced diffusion in the same distribution. Oncologic disease is a significant risk factor for childhood stroke, along with cardiac disease and coagulopathy.*

DYKE-DAVIDOFF-MASSON SYNDROME

Key Facts

Terminology

- Dyke-Davidoff-Masson syndrome (DDMS)
  - a.k.a. cerebral hemiatrophy (CH)

Imaging

- General findings
  - Unilateral cerebral atrophy
  - Ipsilateral paranasal sinuses, mastoids hyperpneumatized
  - Ipsilateral calvarial thickening
- Associated findings
  - Ipsilateral cerebral peduncle, thalamus atrophic (wallerian degeneration)
  - ± crossed cerebellar atrophy/diaschisis
- MR may be helpful for etiology of hemiatrophy
  - Vascular/infectious insult
  - Encephalomalacia/gliosis
  - Corresponding T2/FLAIR hyperintensity

Top Differential Diagnoses

- Large MCA infarction
- Sturge-Weber syndrome
- Rasmussen encephalitis
- Hemimeganencephaly

Pathology

- In utero/early childhood (< 3 yo) hemispheric insult
  - Unilateral
  - Usually vascular, less commonly infectious
  - Lack of ipsilateral brain growth
  - Calvarial diploic spaces, sinuses expand inward

Clinical Issues

- Contralateral hemiplegia/hemiparesis
- Facial asymmetry, mental retardation
- Hemispherectomy for intractable seizures
  - 85% success rate if performed early

*(**Left**) Graphic depicts Dyke-Davidoff-Masson syndrome. The right hemisphere is shrunken and atrophic with a thickened overlying calvarium ➔. If the insult occurs early in development, the falx will be inserted somewhat off-midline ➔. (**Right**) Axial FLAIR in a 13-year-old girl shows right cerebral hemiatrophy with gliotic, hyperintense parenchyma ➔, enlarged lateral ventricle ➔, right frontal sinus ➔, and expansion of the diploic space ➔ compared to the normal left hemisphere. (Courtesy M. Edwards-Brown, MD.)*

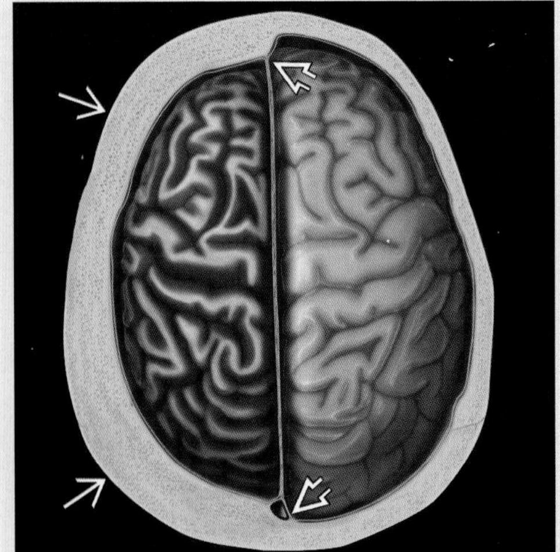

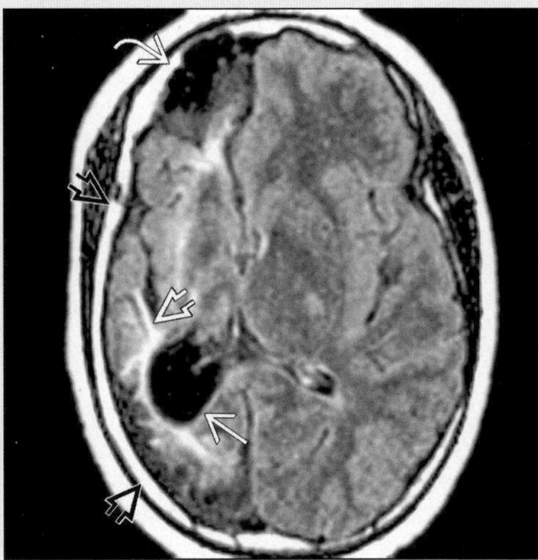

*(**Left**) Coronal T1WI C+ FS MR in the same patient demonstrates the atrophic right hemisphere. The falx ➔ inserts off-midline, and the left temporal bone is expanded and the mastoid ridge is elevated ➔. The calvarium ➔ is thickened compared to the normal left side. (Courtesy M. Edwards-Brown, MD.) (**Right**) Coronal T1WI C+ FS MR in the same patient shows enlargement of the right frontal sinus ➔. (Courtesy M. Edwards-Brown, MD.)*

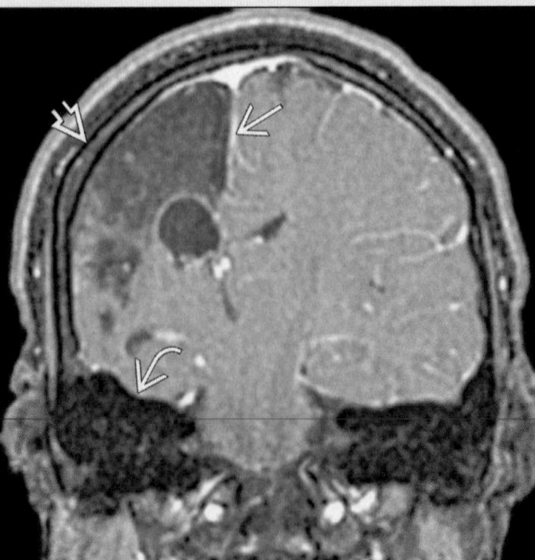

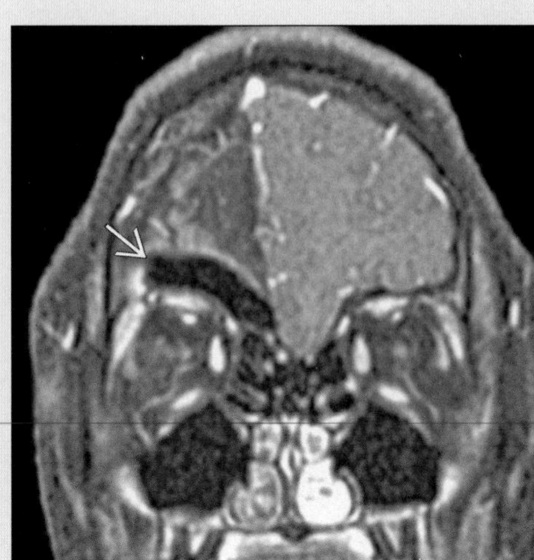

DYKE-DAVIDOFF-MASSON SYNDROME

TERMINOLOGY

Abbreviations

- Dyke-Davidoff-Masson syndrome (DDMS)

Synonyms

- Cerebral hemiatrophy (CH)

Definitions

- Syndrome of hemiplegia, seizures, facial asymmetry, and mental retardation

IMAGING

General Features

- Best diagnostic clue
  - Unilateral cerebral atrophy plus
    - Ipsilateral calvarial thickening
    - Ipsilateral paranasal sinuses, mastoids hyperpneumatized
- Location
  - 70% left hemisphere predominance
  - Right hemisphere ↑ perfusion may be protective in 1st 3 years of life

Imaging Recommendations

- Best imaging tool
  - NECT + bone CT

Radiographic Findings

- Radiography
  - Unilateral calvarial thickening
  - Ipsilateral expansion of paranasal sinuses, mastoid air cells
  - Elevation of ipsilateral greater sphenoid wing, petrous ridge

CT Findings

- NECT
  - Cerebral hemiatrophy
    - Enlarged sulci, CSF spaces
    - Ipsilateral enlarged ventricles
  - Ipsilateral hyperpneumatization
    - Paranasal sinuses
    - Mastoid air cells
  - ± contralateral mild compensatory hemispheric hypertrophy
- Bone CT
  - Ipsilateral calvarium may be thickened

MR Findings

- MR may be helpful for etiology of hemiatrophy
  - Hyperintensity on T2/FLAIR
  - Encephalomalacia, gliosis (vascular or infectious insult)
- Wallerian degeneration
  - Ipsilateral cerebral peduncle, thalamic atrophy

DIFFERENTIAL DIAGNOSIS

Sturge-Weber Syndrome

- Facial port wine stain + ipsilateral atrophy
- Pial angioma + dystrophic cortical Ca++
- Ipsilateral choroid plexus enlarged
- Skull, sinuses, mastoids may resemble DDMS

Rasmussen Encephalitis

- Rare; cause of focal intractable seizures
- Hemiatrophy centered in medial temporal lobe, around sylvian fissure
- No calvarial features of DDMS

Hemimeganencephaly

- Hamartomatous overgrowth of cerebral hemisphere
- Smaller side is normal

Large MCA Infarction

- Atrophy limited to MCA distribution
- Insult after significant calvarial growth has occurred
- Lacks DDMS calvarial changes

PATHOLOGY

General Features

- Etiology
  - In utero/early childhood, unilateral hemispheric insult
    - Usually vascular, less commonly infectious
  - Lack of ipsilateral brain growth
    - Calvarial diploic spaces, sinuses expand inward
- Associated abnormalities
  - Crossed cerebellar atrophy/diaschisis

CLINICAL ISSUES

Presentation

- Most common signs/symptoms
  - Contralateral hemiplegia/hemiparesis
  - Seizures, mental retardation

Demographics

- Age
  - Any age
    - Insult typically in utero or early childhood (< 3 years old)
- Gender
  - Males (70%), females (30%)
  - Males may be functionally more "hemispherically asymmetric"

Treatment

- Hemispherectomy for intractable seizures
  - 85% success rate if performed early

SELECTED REFERENCES

1. Atalar MH et al: Cerebral hemiatrophy (Dyke-Davidoff-Masson syndrome) in childhood: clinicoradiological analysis of 19 cases. Pediatr Int. 49(1):70-5, 2007
2. Unal O et al: Left hemisphere and male sex dominance of cerebral hemiatrophy (Dyke-Davidoff-Masson Syndrome). Clin Imaging. 28(3):163-5, 2004

ACUTE CEREBRAL ISCHEMIA-INFARCTION

Key Facts

Terminology

- Interrupted blood flow to brain resulting in cerebral ischemia/infarction with variable neurologic deficit

Imaging

- Major artery (territorial) infarct
  - Generally wedge-shaped; both GM, WM involved
- Embolic infarcts
  - Often focal/small, at GM-WM interface
- NECT
  - Hyperdense vessel (high specificity, low sensitivity)
  - "Dense MCA" sign: Acute thrombus in artery
  - Loss of GM-WM distinction in 1st 3 hours (50-70%)
  - "Insular ribbon" sign: Loss of gray-white differentiation of insular cortex
- MR
  - Parenchymal ± intraarterial FLAIR hyperintensity
  - ↑ intensity on DWI + corresponding ↓ on ADC
  - ↓ CBF, CBV on perfusion MR (or CT)

Top Differential Diagnoses

- Hyperdense vessel mimics
- Parenchymal hypodensity (nonvascular causes)

Pathology

- Severely ischemic core
  - CBF < $(6\text{-}8\ cm^3)/(100\ g/min)$
- Peripheral "penumbra"
  - CBF between $(10\text{-}20\ cm^3)/(100\ g/min)$

Clinical Issues

- 2nd most common cause of death worldwide
- #1 cause of morbidity in USA
- Treatment
  - IV thrombolysis (< 3 hours of symptom onset)
  - IA thrombolysis (selected acute strokes < 6 hours)

*(**Left**) Coronal graphic illustrates a left M1 occlusion. A proximal occlusion affects the entire MCA territory, including the basal ganglia, which are perfused by lenticulostriate (perforating) arteries ⇒. Acute ischemia is often identified by subtle loss of the gray-white interfaces with blurring of the basal ganglia and an "insular ribbon" sign on the initial CT. (**Right**) Axial NECT demonstrates a hyperdense MCA sign representing acute thrombus ➡ in this patient with acute stroke symptoms.*

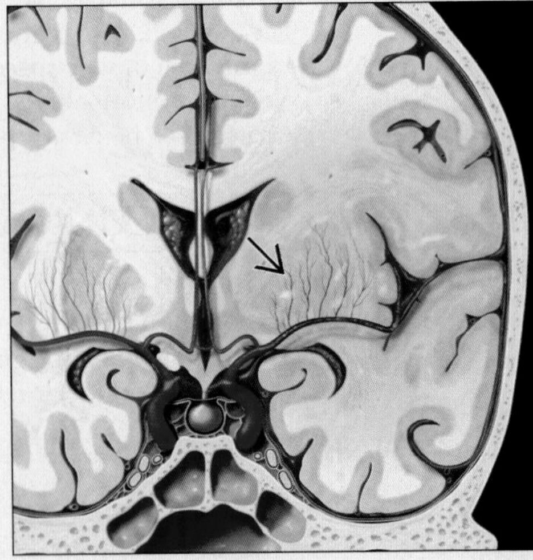

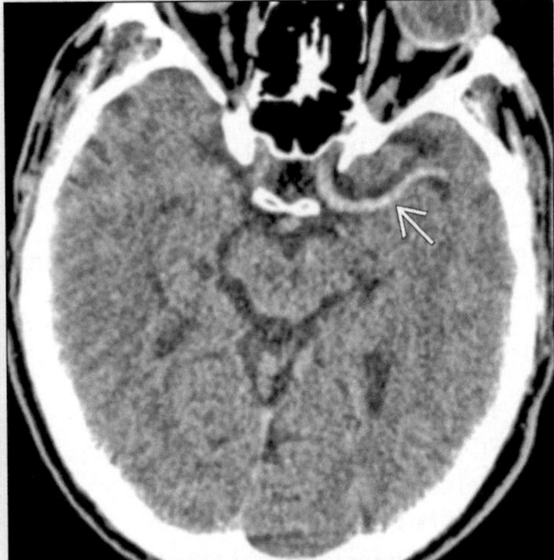

*(**Left**) Axial NECT shows very subtle loss of the right temporal gray-white interfaces ➡ compared to the left, representing an "insular ribbon" sign. (**Right**) Axial pCT (CBF) shows decreased blood flow ⇒ in the right hemisphere related to hyperacute MCA ischemia. The CBF and CBV color maps cephalad to this slice showed a large MCA wedge-shaped defect. There was a similar perfusion abnormality on the TTP maps (not shown). Lack of a mismatch between CBV and TTP maps suggests that no ischemic penumbra is present.*

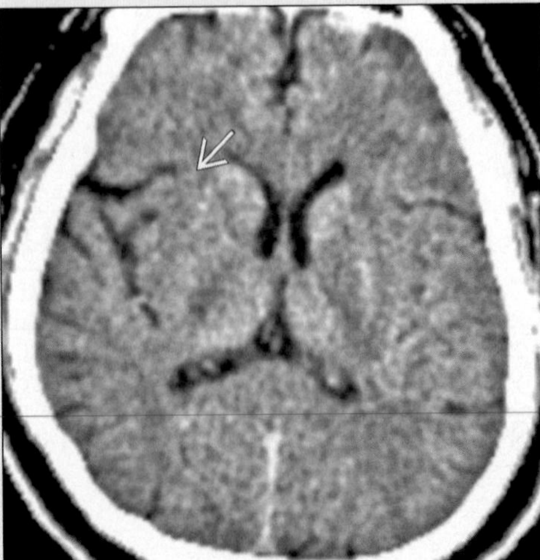

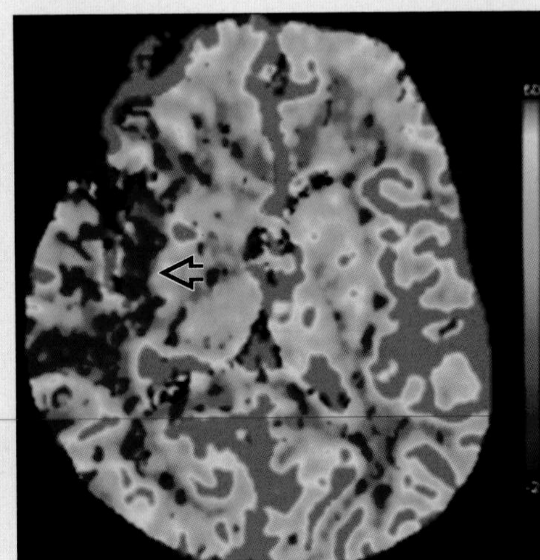

ACUTE CEREBRAL ISCHEMIA-INFARCTION

TERMINOLOGY

Synonyms

- Stroke, cerebrovascular accident (CVA), brain attack

Definitions

- Interrupted blood flow to brain resulting in cerebral ischemia/infarction with variable neurologic deficit

IMAGING

General Features

- Best diagnostic clue
  - High signal on DWI with corresponding low signal on ADC
  - Decreased CBF and CBV on CT or MR perfusion
- Location
  - 1 or more vascular territories or at border-zones ("watershed")
- Size
  - Dependent on degree of compromise and collateral circulation
- Morphology
  - Territorial infarct
    - Conforms to arterial territory
    - Generally wedge-shaped, both gray matter (GM) and white matter (WM) involved
  - Embolic infarcts (often focal, at GM/WM interface)

CT Findings

- NECT
  - Hyperdense vessel (high specificity, low sensitivity)
    - Represents acute thrombus in cerebral vessel(s)
    - Hyperdense M1 MCA in 35-50%
    - "Dot" sign: Occluded MCA branches in sylvian fissure (16-17%)
  - Loss of GM-WM distinction in 1st 3 hours (50-70%)
    - Obscuration of deep gray nuclei
    - Loss of cortical "ribbon"
  - Parenchymal hypodensity
    - If > 1/3 MCA territory initially, larger lesion usually develops later
    - Temporary transition to isodensity (up to 54%) at 2-3 weeks post-ictus (CT "fogging")
  - Gyral swelling, sulcal effacement 12-24 hours
  - "Hemorrhagic transformation" in 15-45%
    - Delayed onset (24-48 hours) most typical
    - Can be gross (parenchymal) or petechial
- CECT
  - Enhancing cortical vessels: Slow flow or collateralization acutely
  - Absent vessels: Occlusion
  - Perfusion CT (pCT): Assess ischemic core vs. penumbra; identify patients who benefit most from revascularization
    - pCT calculates cerebral blood flow (CBF), cerebral blood volume (CBV), time to peak (TTP); deconvolution can give mean transit time (MTT)
  - Cortical/gyral enhancement after 48-72 hours
- CTA: Identify occlusions, dissections, stenoses, status of collaterals

MR Findings

- T1WI
  - Early cortical swelling and hypointensity, loss of GM-WM borders
- T2WI
  - Cortical swelling, hyperintensity develops by 12-24 hours
  - May normalize 2-3 weeks post-ictus (MR "fogging")
- FLAIR
  - Parenchymal hyperintensity appears (6 hours post ictus) while other sequences normal
  - Intraarterial FLAIR hyperintensity is early sign of major vessel occlusion or slow flow
- T2* GRE
  - Detection of acute blood products
  - Arterial "blooming" (thrombosed vessel) from clot susceptibility
- DWI
  - Hyperintense restriction from cytotoxic edema
    - Improves hyperacute stroke detection to 95%
    - Usually correlates to "ischemic core" (final infarct size); some diffusion abnormalities reversible (TIA, migraine)
    - May have reduced sensitivity in brainstem and medulla in 1st 24 hours
    - Restriction typically lasts 7-10 days
      - High signal can persist up to 2 months post ictus
      - After 10 days, T2 effect may predominate over low ADC: T2 "shine-through"
  - Corresponding low signal on ADC maps
    - May normalize after tissue reperfusion
    - Hyper- or isointensity on ADC map (T2 "shine-through") may mimic diffusion restriction
  - Distinguish cytotoxic from vasogenic edema in complicated cases
    - May be helpful to evaluate new deficits after tumor resection
- PWI
  - Dynamic contrast bolus or arterial spin labeled techniques
    - Maximum slope gives relative CBF, CBV
    - Deconvolution gives absolute values
  - Bolus-tracking T2* gadolinium perfusion imaging (PWI) with CBV map
    - ↓ perfusion; 75% larger than DWI abnormality
    - DWI/PWI "mismatch": "Penumbra" or "at-risk" tissue
- T1WI C+
  - Variable enhancement patterns evolve over time
    - Hyperacute: Intravascular enhancement (stasis from slow antegrade or retrograde collateral flow)
    - Acute: Meningeal enhancement (pial collateral flow appears in 24-48 hours, resolves over 3-4 days)
    - Subacute: Parenchymal enhancement (appears after 24-48 hours, can persist for weeks/months)
- MRA: Major vessel occlusions, stenoses, status of collaterals
- MRS: Elevated lactate, decreased NAA
- Conventional MR sequences positive in 70-80%
  - Restricted diffusion improves accuracy to 95%
- Diffusion tensor imaging (DTI)

ACUTE CEREBRAL ISCHEMIA-INFARCTION

- Multidirectional diffusion-weighted images; at least 6 directions can be used to calculate DTI trace and ADC maps
  - Higher spatial resolution
- May be more sensitive for small ischemic foci, emboli, cortical strokes

Angiographic Findings

- Conventional: Vessel occlusion (cut-off, tapered, tram track)
  - Slow antegrade flow, retrograde collateral flow
- Neurointerventional: IA fibrinolytic therapy for treatment of selected acute nonhemorrhagic stroke within 6 hour window
  - IA mechanical clot removal with retriever device

Imaging Recommendations

- Best imaging tool
  - MR + DWI, T2* GRE
- Protocol advice
  - NECT as initial study to exclude hemorrhage/mass
    - CT perfusion and CTA if available
  - MR with DWI, FLAIR, GRE ± MRA, PWI
  - DSA with thrombolysis in selected patients

DIFFERENTIAL DIAGNOSIS

Hyperdense Vessel Mimics

- High hematocrit (polycythemia)
- Microcalcification in vessel wall
- Diffuse cerebral edema makes vessels appear relatively hyperdense
- Normal circulating blood always slightly hyperdense to normal brain

Parenchymal Hypodensity (Nonvascular Causes)

- Infiltrating neoplasm (e.g., astrocytoma)
- Cerebral contusion
- Inflammation (cerebritis, encephalitis)
- Evolving encephalomalacia
- Dural venous thrombosis with parenchymal venous congestion and edema

PATHOLOGY

General Features

- Etiology
  - Many causes (thrombotic vs. embolic, dissection, vasculitis, hypoperfusion)
  - Early: Critical disturbance in CBF
    - Severely ischemic core has CBF < (6-8 cm^3)/(100 g/min) (normal ~ [60 cm^3]/[100 g/min])
    - Oxygen depletion, energy failure, terminal depolarization, ion homeostasis failure
    - Bulk of final infarct → cytotoxic edema, cell death
  - Later: Evolution from ischemia to infarction depends on many factors (e.g., hyperglycemia influences "destiny" of ischemic brain tissue)
  - Ischemic "penumbra" CBF between (10-20 cm^3)/(100 g/min)
    - Theoretically salvageable tissue
    - Target of thrombolysis, neuroprotective agents
- Associated abnormalities
  - Cardiac disease, prothrombotic states
  - Additional stroke risk factors: C-reactive protein, homocysteine

Gross Pathologic & Surgical Features

- Acute thrombosis of major vessel
- Pale, swollen brain; GM-WM boundaries blurred

Microscopic Features

- After 4 hours: Eosinophilic neurons with pyknotic nuclei
- 15-24 hours: Neutrophils invade, necrotic nuclei look like "eosinophilic ghosts"
- 2-3 days: Blood-derived phagocytes
- 1 week: Reactive astrocytosis, ↑ capillary density
- End result: Fluid-filled cavity lined by astrocytes

CLINICAL ISSUES

Presentation

- Most common signs/symptoms
  - Focal acute neurologic deficit
  - Paresis, aphasia, decreased mental status

Demographics

- Age
  - Usually older adults
  - Consider underlying disease (sickle cell, moyamoya, NF1, cardiac, drugs) in children, young adults
- Epidemiology
  - 2nd most common cause of death worldwide
  - #1 cause of morbidity in USA

Natural History & Prognosis

- Clinical diagnosis inaccurate in 15-20% of strokes
- Malignant MCA infarct (coma, death)
  - Up to 10% of all stroke patients
  - Fatal brain swelling with increased ICP

Treatment

- "Time is brain": IV rTPA window < 3 hours
  - IA window < 6 hours
- Patient selection most important factor in outcome
  - Symptom onset < 6 hours
  - No parenchymal hematoma on CT
  - < 1/3 MCA territory hypodensity

DIAGNOSTIC CHECKLIST

Consider

- DWI positive for acute stroke only if ADC correlates
- Rarely, ischemia may mimic tumor or encephalitis

SELECTED REFERENCES

1. Harris AD et al: Diffusion and perfusion MR imaging of acute ischemic stroke. Magn Reson Imaging Clin N Am. 17(2):291-313, 2009
2. Soares BP, Chien JD, Wintermark M. MR and CT monitoring of recanalization, reperfusion, and penumbra salvage: everything that recanalizes does not necessarily reperfuse! Stroke. 40(3 Suppl):S24-7, 2009

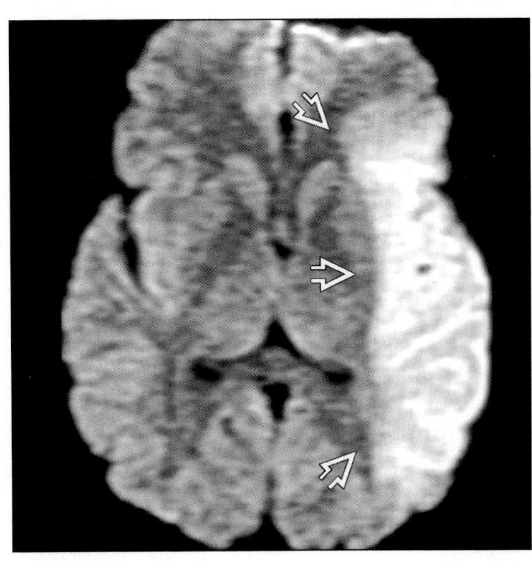

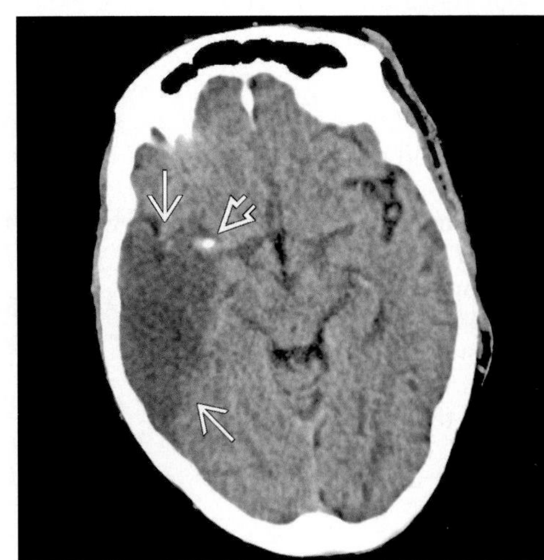

(Left) *Axial DWI MR shows a large wedge-shaped hyperintensity related to restricted diffusion ⇨ representing acute ischemia in a left MCA distribution. There is sparing of the basal ganglia, consistent with distal M1 occlusion.* ***(Right)*** *Axial NECT shows a hypodense wedge-shaped region of acute infarct ➡ with mild mass effect and sulcal effacement related to a right M1 calcified embolus ⇨.*

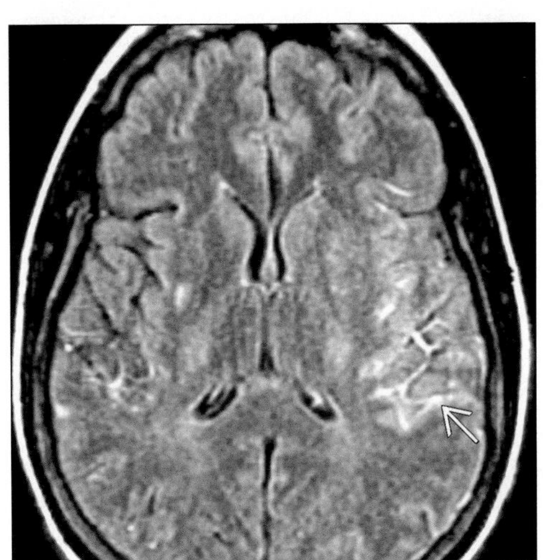

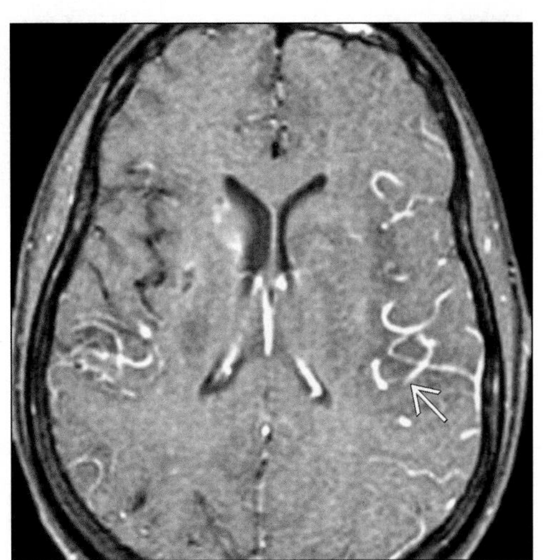

(Left) *Axial FLAIR MR shows hyperintense signal in the left temporal lobe related to acute MCA distribution ischemia. Hyperintensity within the MCA branches ➡ is related to slow flow or occlusion. The MCA territory is the most commonly involved distribution of ischemic stroke.* ***(Right)*** *Axial T1WI C+ FS MR in the same patient shows intravascular enhancement ➡. Meningeal enhancement, related to pial collateral flow, is often seen in the 1st few days (1-4) following acute ischemia.*

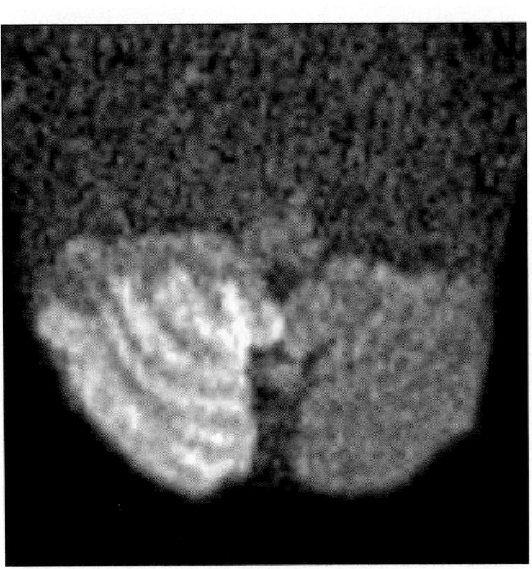

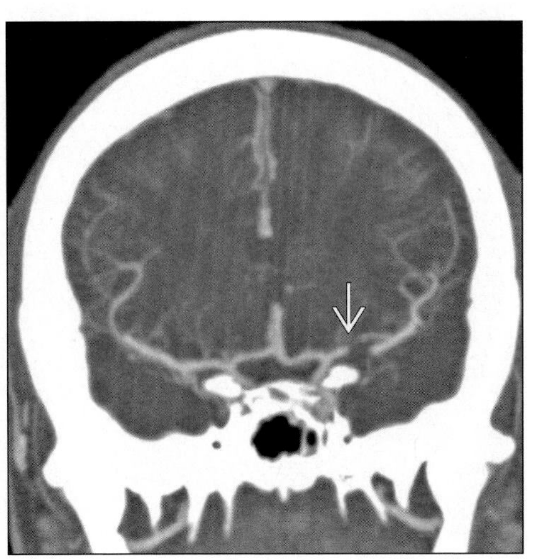

(Left) *Axial DWI MR shows hyperintensity related to restricted diffusion in this patient with vertebrobasilar disease and a posterior inferior cerebellar artery acute infarct. MR is superior to CT in evaluation of a posterior fossa stroke.* ***(Right)*** *Coronal CTA MIP reconstruction shows a focal filling defect within the proximal M1 segment ➡ in a patient with acute MCA ischemia. Intraarterial thrombolysis may be helpful, if the patient presents to the emergency department within 6 hours of symptom onset.*

SUBACUTE CEREBRAL INFARCTION

Key Facts

Terminology

- Subacute stroke ± hemorrhagic transformation (HT)
- Subacute infarction approximately 2-14 days following initial ischemic event

Imaging

- Best diagnostic clue: Gyral edema and enhancement within basal ganglia and cortex
- Typically wedge-shaped abnormality involving gray and white matter within vascular distribution
- HT of initially ischemic infarction occurs in 15-20% of MCA occlusions, usually by 48-72 hours
- "2-2-2" rule = enhancement begins at 2 days, peaks at 2 weeks, disappears by 2 months
- ↑ lactate, ↓ NAA within infarcted tissue

Top Differential Diagnoses

- Neoplasm
- Venous infarction
- Encephalitis/cerebritis

Clinical Issues

- Acute onset focal neurologic deficit
- 1st month after infarction, mortality predominantly from neurologic complications; 1:4 die of recurrent stroke event
- Acute anticoagulation after 1st infarction reduces mortality

Diagnostic Checklist

- Enhancement key to defining subacute stage of cerebral infarction
- Consider
  - Is affected area another space-occupying pathology (i.e., tumor)?
  - Recommend short-term follow-up to ensure expected course of evolution

*(**Left**) Axial NECT obtained 48 hours after presentation demonstrates the classic appearance of a late acute/ early subacute cerebral infarct. Note the wedge-shaped, low-density area involving both the gray and white matter in the left MCA distribution. (**Right**) Axial NECT in the same patient obtained 1 week after ictus demonstrates gyriform areas of slightly increased attenuation ➔ in keeping with hemorrhagic transformation. This typically occurs between 48 and 72 hours after onset.*

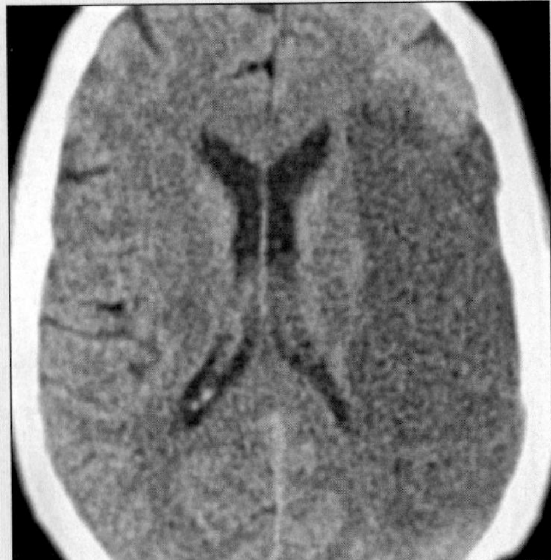

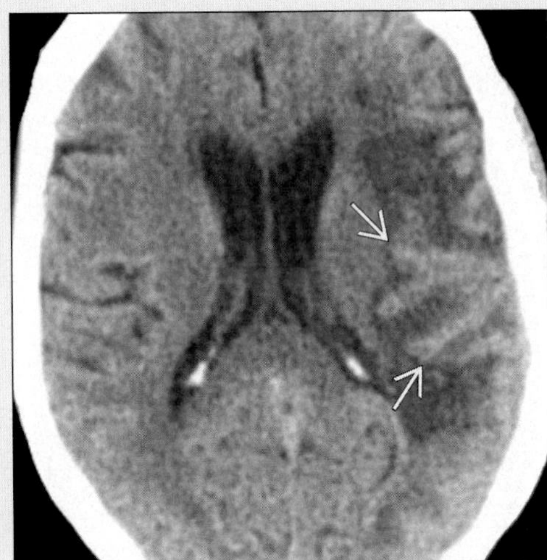

*(**Left**) Axial T1WI C+ MR demonstrates gyriform enhancement ➔ in the right MCA distribution in this late subacute infarct. (**Right**) Sagittal T1 C+ MR in the same patient shows well-defined gyriform enhancement ➔ in the right MCA distribution. Note the lack of significant mass effect in this late subacute infarct.*

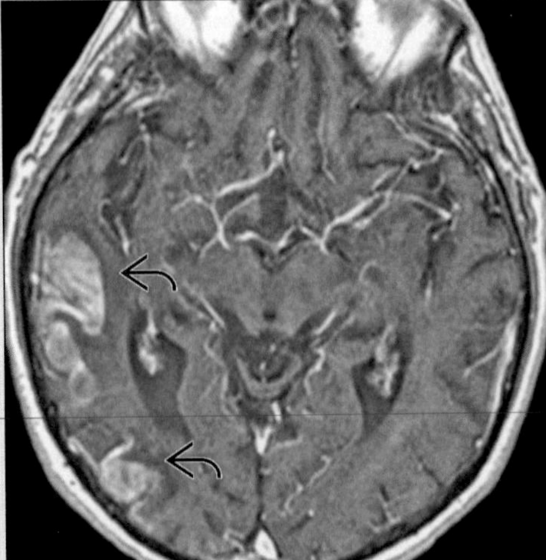

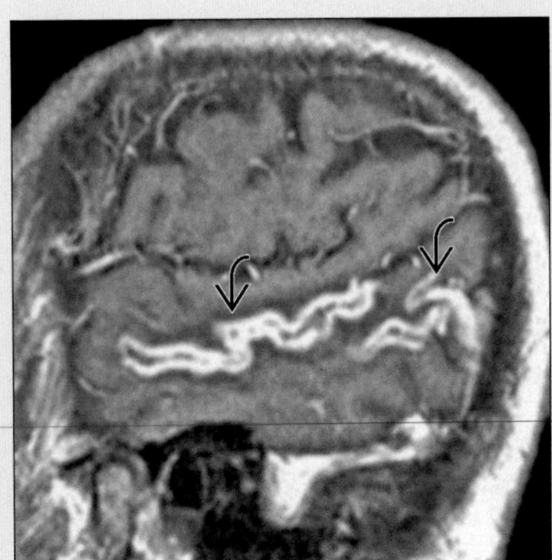

SUBACUTE CEREBRAL INFARCTION

TERMINOLOGY

Abbreviations

- Subacute stroke ± hemorrhagic transformation (HT)

Definitions

- Focal brain necrosis following obstruction of blood flow to localized area of brain
- Subacute infarction ~ 2-14 days following initial ischemic event

IMAGING

General Features

- Best diagnostic clue
  - Gyral edema, enhancement in basal ganglia/cortex
  - Look for HT
- Location
  - Cerebral hemispheres, brainstem, cerebellum in territorial vascular distribution
- Size
  - Extremely variable
  - Ranges from focal ("lacunes") to global (hemispheric)
- Morphology
  - Variable depending on location, size, etiology
  - Typically wedge-shaped, involves both gray and white matter
    - Recognizable vascular distribution

CT Findings

- NECT
  - Wedge-shaped area of ↓ attenuation involving gray and white matter
  - Mass effect initially ↑, then ↓ by 7-10 days; often less than expected given lesion size as acuity resolves
  - HT of initially ischemic infarction occurs in 15-20% of MCA occlusions, usually by 48-72 hours
    - Common locations are basal ganglia and cortex
    - Hemorrhagic foci detected in majority of medium/large subacute infarcts
- CECT
  - Enhancement typically patchy or gyral
  - May appear as early as 2-3 days after ictus, persists up to 8-10 weeks
  - "2-2-2" rule = enhancement begins at 2 days, peaks at 2 weeks, disappears by 2 months
- CTA
  - Evidence of subacute occlusion correlates strongly, independently with poor clinical outcome
    - Significantly worse discharge National Institutes of Health Stroke Scale (NIHSS) score
- CT perfusion
  - More useful in acute > subacute stroke
    - Helpful in predicting tissue outcome
  - Significant difference between infarct and peri-infarct tissue for both rCBF, rCBV

MR Findings

- T1WI
  - Hypointense edema with mass effect
  - HT: Signal changes of hemorrhage
- T2WI
  - Hyperintense edema with mass effect
  - "Fogging" effect = normal T2WI with striking enhancement on T1WI C+ 1-2 weeks following ictus
  - HT: Signal changes of evolving hemorrhage
  - Early wallerian degeneration can occur
    - Look for well-defined hyperintense band in corticospinal tract
- FLAIR
  - Hyperintense edema with mass effect
  - Hyperintensity ("dot" sign) in slow-flowing/occluded vessels
- T2* GRE
  - May see blooming if HT has occurred
- DWI
  - ↑ diffusion restriction, ↓ ADC initially, reversing as it proceeds into/through subacute stage
  - DWI, T1WI C+ complement each other in detecting subacute infarcts
    - Early subacute can be ↑ DWI and ↓ T1 C+
- T1WI C+
  - Intravascular enhancement in initial 48 hours, disappears at 3-4 days as vessels recanalize
  - Parenchymal enhancement (patterns typically patchy or gyral)
    - May appear as early as 2-3 days after ictus
    - Can persist up to 8-10 weeks
- MRA
  - Vessel occlusion (large vessel)
- MRS
  - ↑ lactate, ↓ NAA within infarcted tissue
  - In subacute and chronic infarction, lactate/choline and NAA/choline ratios correlate with outcome
- MR T2* perfusion
  - ↓ rCBV of acute infarct increases in subacute stage, reflecting reperfusion hyperemia
  - Decreases again in chronic stage

Angiographic Findings

- Conventional
  - May see intraluminal thrombus &/or vessel occlusion
  - Slow antegrade flow with delayed arterial emptying
  - Slow retrograde filling through collateral vessels
  - "Bare" areas = regions of nonperfused or slowly perfused brain tissue

Nuclear Medicine Findings

- Diminished/absence of perfusion with SPECT or PET
- HMPAO SPECT may show reflow hyperemia after reperfusion in acute and subacute stages

Imaging Recommendations

- Best imaging tool
  - MR with DWI, T2*, T1WI C+
- Protocol advice
  - CT: Add CT perfusion
  - CT and MR: C+ for assessing subacute age

DIFFERENTIAL DIAGNOSIS

Neoplasm

- DWI: Vasogenic ("tumoral") edema instead of cytotoxic edema

SUBACUTE CEREBRAL INFARCTION

- Enhancing mass instead of patchy, gyral enhancement
- Will not regress on follow-up imaging

Venous Infarction

- Nonarterial distribution
- Venous instead of arterial occlusion, typically major dural sinus
- More commonly hemorrhagic, primarily affecting white matter instead of cortex
- Different clinical presentation/setting (trauma, hypercoagulable states, pregnancy, dehydration)

Encephalitis/Cerebritis

- DWI: Strong restriction
- Nonvascular distribution
- Gyriform, ring-enhancing patterns (late cerebritis)
- Different clinical presentation

PATHOLOGY

General Features

- Etiology
  - Prolonged cerebral ischemia
  - Duration + severity of ischemic insult determines cellular viability
  - Less commonly, may be result of infectious etiologies
    - Sequelae of meningitis (bacterial, mycobacterial, etc.)
  - May also be result of inflammatory diseases, such as vasculopathy, angiitis, etc.
  - Uncontrolled, unilateral, supratentorial expanding lesions can cause descending tentorial herniation → ischemic infarction of occipital lobe
  - Ischemia/infarction involves typical vascular territories or watershed (border-zone) distributions depending on etiology
  - Other factors: Adequacy of collateral blood supply, degree, duration, and distribution of flow reduction
- Genetics
  - Hypercholesterolemia, diabetes, hypertension, and homocysteine increase stroke risk

Gross Pathologic & Surgical Features

- Blurring of gray-white matter demarcation
- Mass effect with narrowing of sulci, displacement of adjacent structures
- Softening of ischemic tissues from water retention

Microscopic Features

- Fragmentation of axons & early disintegration of myelin sheaths; loss of oligodendrocytes, astrocytes
- 48 hours: Neutrophils begin to pass through vessel walls into brain tissue
- 72-96 hours: Macrophages aggregate around vessels
- 2 weeks: Macrophages are predominate reactive cells

CLINICAL ISSUES

Presentation

- Most common signs/symptoms
  - Acute onset focal neurologic deficit
  - ~ 50% of patients with infarction → permanent neurologic deficits have preceding TIAs
- Clinical profile
  - Elderly patient with typical risk factors: Hypertension, diabetes, smoking history, obesity, hypercholesterolemia, etc.

Demographics

- Age
  - Usually > 55 years
  - Women often slightly older than men at presentation
- Gender
  - Females often more disabled after age adjustment
  - Fatality rates similar
- Epidemiology
  - 3rd cause of USA adult mortality
  - Highest cause of USA adult morbidity

Natural History & Prognosis

- 1st month after infarction, mortality predominantly from neurologic complications
  - 1:4 die of recurrent stroke event
- Later mortality from respiratory, cardiovascular causes

Treatment

- To improve long-term survival, aggressive management of pulmonary & cardiac disease is critical
- Acute anticoagulation after 1st infarction reduces mortality
- Current research: Therapeutic hypothermia + gene therapy (antiapoptotic protein BCL-2) during acute stroke event

DIAGNOSTIC CHECKLIST

Consider

- Is affected area another space-occupying pathology (i.e., tumor)?
- Recommend short-term follow-up to ensure expected course of evolution

Image Interpretation Pearls

- Enhancement key to defining subacute stage of cerebral infarction

SELECTED REFERENCES

1. Donnan GA et al: Penumbral selection of patients for trials of acute stroke therapy. Lancet Neurol. 8(3):261-9, 2009
2. Elkind MS: Outcomes after stroke: risk of recurrent ischemic stroke and other events. Am J Med. 122(4 Suppl 2):S7-13, 2009
3. Olivot JM et al: Perfusion MRI (Tmax and MTT) correlation with xenon CT cerebral blood flow in stroke patients. Neurology. 72(13):1140-5, 2009
4. Muñoz Maniega S et al: Changes in NAA and lactate following ischemic stroke: a serial MR spectroscopic imaging study. Neurology. 71(24):1993-9, 2008

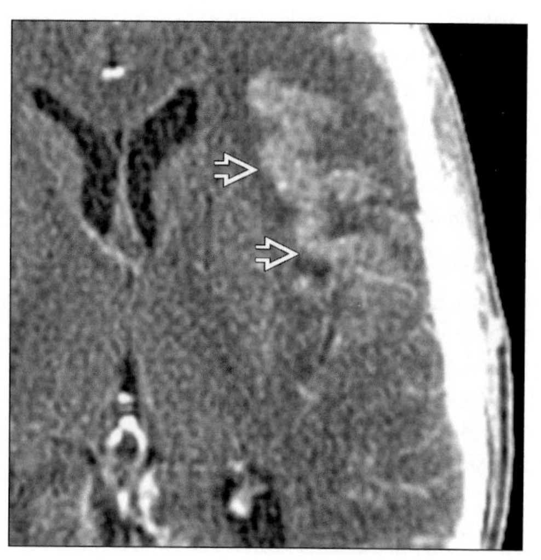

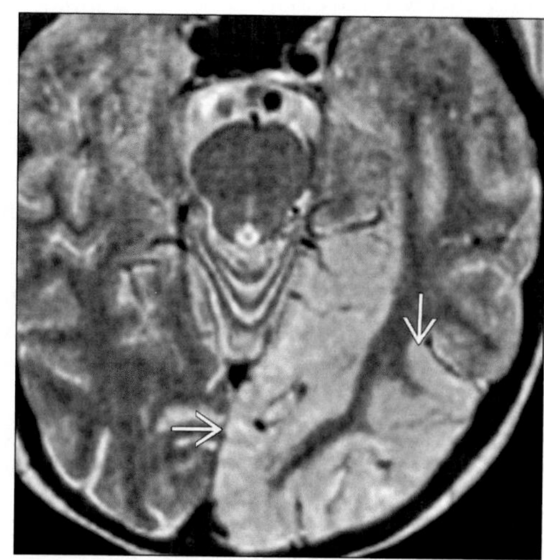

(Left) *Axial CECT demonstrates gyriform enhancement ➲ in the left MCA territory, a finding seen in subacute infarcts.* ***(Right)*** *Axial T2WI MR demonstrates regional gyral effacement and T2 hyperintensity in the left PCA distribution ➔.*

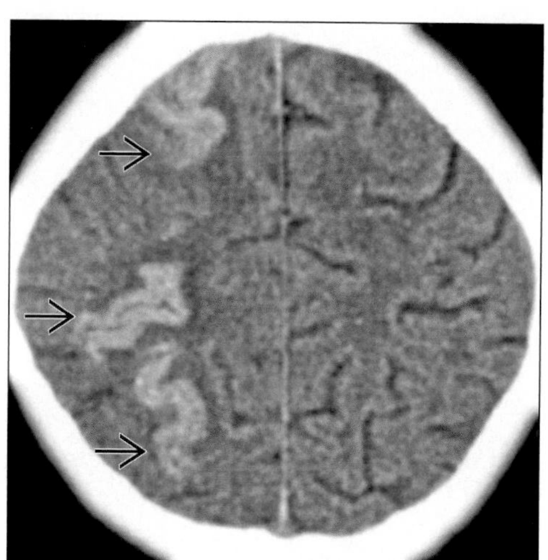

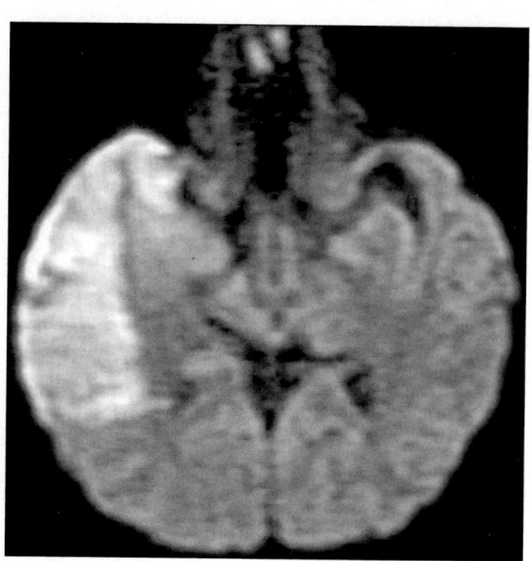

(Left) *Axial NECT demonstrates gyriform hyperdensity ➔ in keeping with cortical laminar necrosis/ hemorrhagic transformation in a right hemispheric watershed infarct.* ***(Right)*** *Axial DWI MR 5 days after a right middle cerebral infarct shows high signal due to restricted diffusion. DWI scans can be hyperintense up to a week following acute stroke onset.*

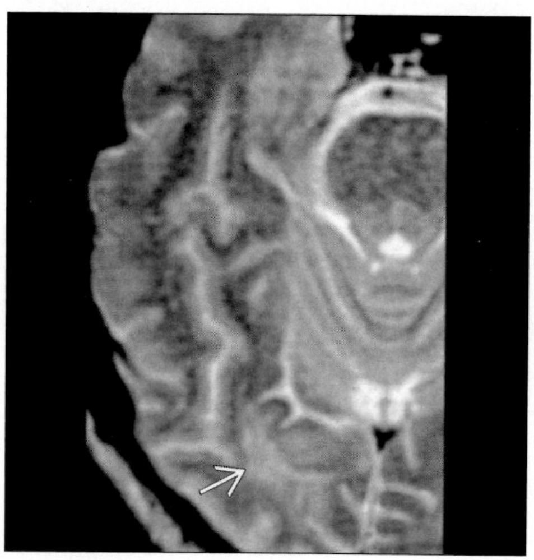

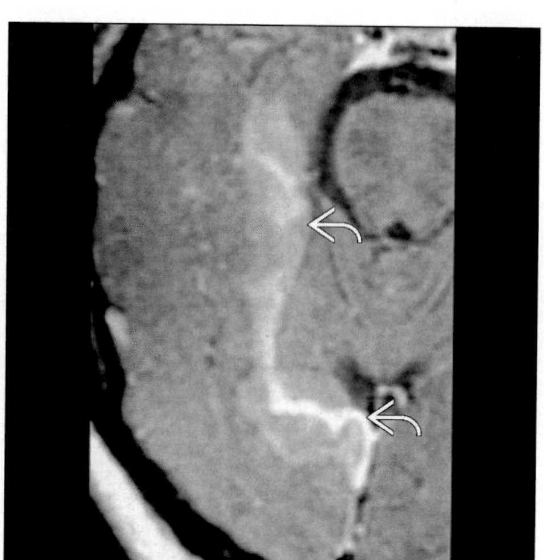

(Left) *Axial T2WI MR shows almost no abnormality except for minimal hyperintensity on the T2WI ➔. Occasionally subacute cerebral infarcts may be difficult to visualize on standard MR scans because of the so-called fogging effect.* ***(Right)*** *Axial T1WI C+ MR in the same patient demonstrates striking gyriform enhancement ➔.*

CHRONIC CEREBRAL INFARCTION

Key Facts

Imaging

- Volume loss with gliosis along affected margins
- Classic: Wedge-shaped area of encephalomalacia
- Territorial infarction
  - Involves brain supplied by major cerebral artery
- Watershed infarction
  - Involves brain **between** main vascular territories
- Lacunar infarction(s)
  - Most common in basal ganglia/thalami, deep WM

Top Differential Diagnoses

- Porencephalic cyst
- Arachnoid cyst
- Postsurgical/post-traumatic encephalomalacia
- Low-attenuating tumors

Pathology

- Volume loss, gliosis are pathological hallmarks

Clinical Issues

- Elderly patient with typical risk factors
- Focal neurologic deficit
  - Varies depending on size, location of CI
- Stroke severity most consistent predictor of 30 day mortality after stroke
- Lacunar stroke most common stroke subtype associated with vascular dementia

Diagnostic Checklist

- Evaluate for associated acute infarcts in same or different vascular territory
- Evaluate for underlying cause
  - CTA/MRA of extra-, intracranial vasculature
  - If negative, consider cardiac source
- Evaluate for risk factors

*(**Left**) Axial gross pathology, sectioned through the mid-ventricular level, shows a chronic left middle cerebral artery infarct with encephalomalacia in the classic MCA vascular distribution ➔. Note the mild compensatory enlargement of the left lateral ventricle. (Courtesy R. Hewlett, PhD.) (**Right**) Axial FLAIR MR in a patient with a chronic left middle cerebral artery infarct shows encephalomalacia ➔ and gliosis ➔ in the classic MCA vascular distribution. The basal ganglia were spared.*

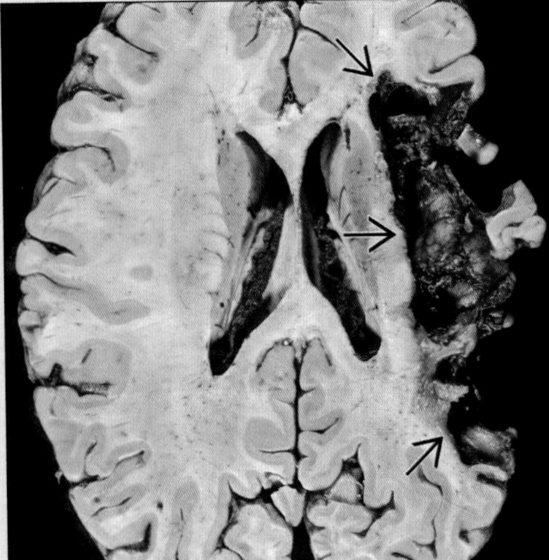

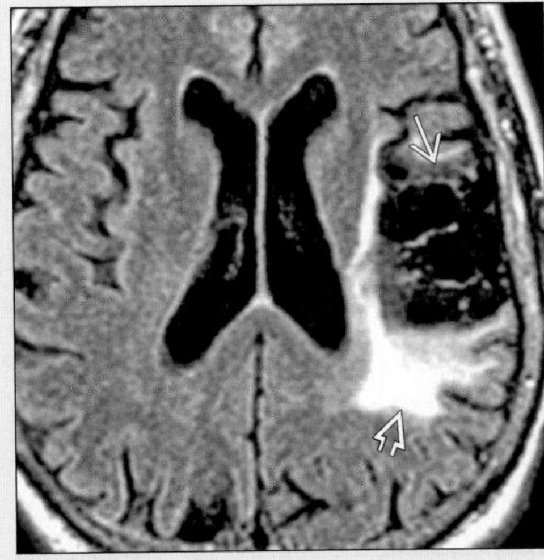

*(**Left**) Axial T2WI MR in a patient injured in a jet ski accident 2 months earlier demonstrates T2 hyperintensity in the left MCA distribution. Findings are consistent with a chronic infarct. Note the mild dilatation of the ipsilateral ventricle secondary to volume loss in the left hemisphere. (**Right**) MRA in the same patient demonstrates absence of flow in the left ICA. T1WI FS MR (not shown) demonstrated hyperintense signal in the wall of a chronically dissected, thrombosed left ICA.*

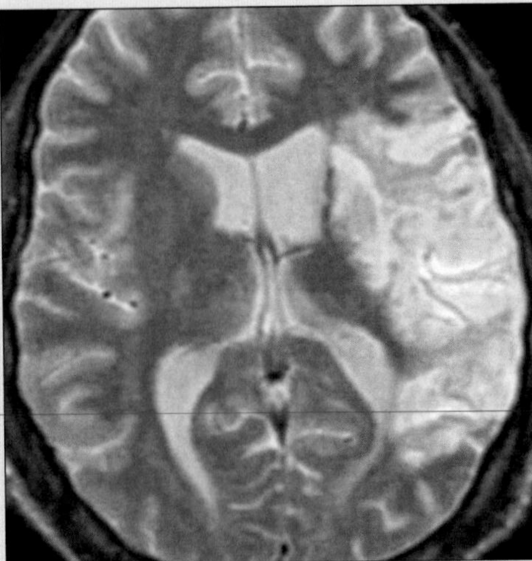

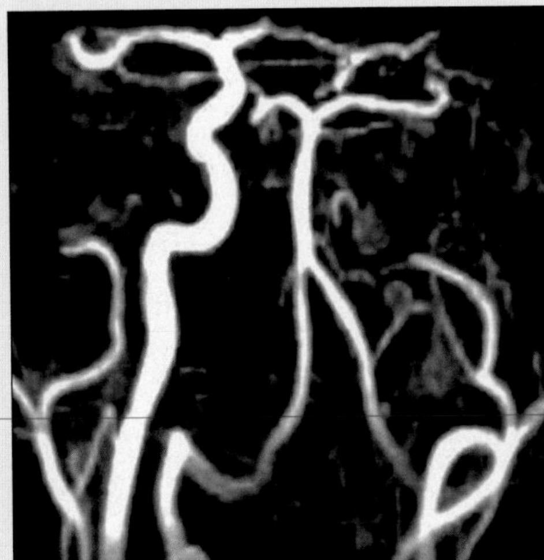

CHRONIC CEREBRAL INFARCTION

TERMINOLOGY

Abbreviations

- Cerebral infarction (CI)

Synonyms

- Old ischemic stroke
- Post-infarction encephalomalacia

Definitions

- End result of prolonged cerebral ischemia

IMAGING

General Features

- Best diagnostic clue
  - Volume loss with gliosis along affected margins
- Location
  - Cerebral hemispheres, brainstem, cerebellum
  - Territorial infarction involves brain tissue supplied by major cerebral artery
    - Common sites
      - Supratentorial: MCA, ACA, PCA distribution
      - Infratentorial: BA, PICA distribution
  - Watershed (border zone) infarction involves brain tissue **between** main vascular territories
  - Lacunar infarctions are small infarcts in deep penetrating artery distributions
    - Typically located in basal ganglia/thalami, white matter (WM)
- Size
  - Extremely variable
    - Ranging from focal ("lacunes") to lobar or global (hemispheric)
- Morphology
  - Extremely variable depending on location, size, etiology of vascular insult
  - Classic: Wedge-shaped area of encephalomalacia

CT Findings

- NECT
  - Focal, well-delineated low-attenuation areas in affected vascular distribution
  - Adjacent sulci become prominent; ipsilateral ventricle enlarges
  - Wallerian degeneration may be present
  - Dystrophic Ca++ may very rarely occur in infarcted brain
- CECT
  - No enhancement
- CTA
  - May see lack of flow in affected vessel

MR Findings

- T1WI
  - Isointense to CSF in affected areas
  - Adjacent sulci become prominent; ipsilateral ventricle enlarges
  - Wallerian degeneration may be present
- T2WI
  - Isointense to CSF in affected areas
  - Borders of infarction may show ↑ signal secondary to gliosis/spongiosis
  - Differentiation of subacute from chronic infarction on standard SE/FSE sequences may be difficult due to prolonged relaxation times in both
- FLAIR
  - Low signal in encephalomalacic area
  - Hyperintense gliotic white matter at margins
- T2* GRE
  - May see hemosiderin staining in gliotic areas or along borders of infarction
- DWI
  - No restriction; increased diffusivity (↑ signal on ADC)
- T1WI C+
  - No enhancement
- MRA
  - May see lack of flow in affected vessel
- MRS
  - Shows loss of NAA peak in affected area

Angiographic Findings

- Conventional
  - May see lack of flow in affected vessel and its vascular territory

Imaging Recommendations

- Best imaging tool
  - CT or MR
- Protocol advice
  - No contrast necessary if imaging typical (i.e., lack of mass effect or volume loss)

DIFFERENTIAL DIAGNOSIS

Porencephalic Cyst

- Congenital cyst typically seen in younger age groups
- Also lined by gliotic white matter

Arachnoid Cyst

- No gliotic margins
- Usually in locations atypical for vascular territory
- Intact gray matter lining brain, displaced by cyst

Postoperative/Post-Traumatic Encephalomalacia

- History and associated findings help to distinguish
- May see leptomeningeal cyst in post-traumatic setting

Low-Attenuation Tumors

- Typically shows mass effect
- Usually slightly hyperdense/intense compared to CSF

PATHOLOGY

General Features

- Etiology
  - Prolonged cerebral ischemia
  - Duration and severity of ischemic insult determines cellular viability
    - Results of CI vary with sensitivity of individual cell types to ischemia

CHRONIC CEREBRAL INFARCTION

- Other factors include adequacy of collateral blood supply, degree, duration, and distribution of flow reduction
  - Most CI caused by territorial, watershed, lacunar infarcts
  - Less commonly result of infectious/inflammatory etiologies
    - Sequelae of meningitis (bacterial, mycobacterial, etc.)
    - Vasculopathy, angiitis, etc.
  - Rare
    - Unilateral descending tentorial herniation
    - May cause secondary ischemic infarction of occipital lobe
- Genetics
  - Hypercholesterolemia, diabetes, hypertension, homocysteine ↑ stroke risk

Gross Pathologic & Surgical Features

- Volume loss and gliosis pathological hallmarks
- Liquefaction resulting in cyst formation
- Cystic areas traversed by trabeculations of blood vessels, surrounded by firm glial tissue
- Typically in main vascular territories or watershed (border zone) distribution depending on etiology

Microscopic Features

- Fibrillary gliosis along margin of infarction
- Macrophages may persist in interstices of infarcts; some may contain hemosiderin

CLINICAL ISSUES

Presentation

- Most common signs/symptoms
  - Focal neurologic deficit with history of acute onset
- Clinical profile
  - Elderly patient with typical risk factors
    - Hypertension, diabetes, smoking history, obesity, hypercholesterolemia, etc.

Demographics

- Age
  - Usually > 55
- Gender
  - Women typically older than men
  - Females often more disabled after age adjustment
  - Fatality rates similar
- Epidemiology
  - 2nd or 3rd leading cause of death in Western world (after noncerebral cardiovascular disease & cancer)
  - Major cause of long-term disability
  - 1 in 5 with 1st stroke will survive to 10 years
  - Estimates in USA range from 760,000-780,000 annually; contributes to ~ 150,000 deaths/year
  - Estimated 5,800,000 stroke survivors in USA

Natural History & Prognosis

- Varies greatly depending on size of CI and degree of neurologic deficit
- Stroke severity most consistent predictor of 30 day mortality after stroke
- Mortality rates in USA declined dramatically in 1970s and 1980s, but plateaued by 1990s
- Stroke mortality in USA predicted to ↑ 3x as fast as general population over next 30 years
- Lacunar stroke most common stroke subtype associated with vascular dementia

Treatment

- Acute anticoagulation after 1st infarction associated with reduced mortality
- To improve long-term survival after CI, aggressive management of pulmonary and cardiac disease critical

DIAGNOSTIC CHECKLIST

Consider

- Could lesion be arachnoid cyst or porencephalic cyst?

Image Interpretation Pearls

- Look for signs of volume loss in vascular territory
- Evaluate for associated acute infarcts in same or different vascular territory

Reporting Tips

- Evaluate for underlying cause
  - Multiple infarcts in different vascular territories
    - Suggests cardioembolic source or vasculitis
  - Bilateral watershed infarcts
    - Hypoperfusion event
  - Unilateral watershed infarct
    - Hypoperfusion event & ipsilateral carotid stenosis
  - Infarct in setting of trauma
    - Evaluate for dissection

SELECTED REFERENCES

1. Danaei G et al: The preventable causes of death in the United States: comparative risk assessment of dietary, lifestyle, and metabolic risk factors. PLoS Med. 6(4):e1000058, 2009
2. Donnan GA et al: Penumbral selection of patients for trials of acute stroke therapy. Lancet Neurol. 8(3):261-9, 2009
3. Elkind MS: Outcomes after stroke: risk of recurrent ischemic stroke and other events. Am J Med. 122(4 Suppl 2):S7-13, 2009
4. Lloyd-Jones D et al: Heart disease and stroke statistics--2009 update: a report from the American Heart Association Statistics Committee and Stroke Statistics Subcommittee. Circulation. 2009 Jan 27;119(3):480-6. Erratum in: Circulation. 119(3):e182, 2009
5. Roberts CS et al: Additional stroke-related and non-stroke-related cardiovascular costs and hospitalizations in managed-care patients after ischemic stroke. Stroke. 40(4):1425-32, 2009
6. Donnan GA et al: Stroke. Lancet. 371(9624):1612-23, 2008
7. Mark VW et al: Poststroke cerebral peduncular atrophy correlates with a measure of corticospinal tract injury in the cerebral hemisphere. AJNR Am J Neuroradiol. 29(2):354-8, 2008
8. Muñoz Maniega S et al: Changes in NAA and lactate following ischemic stroke: a serial MR spectroscopic imaging study. Neurology. 71(24):1993-9, 2008
9. Glodzik-Sobanska L et al: Prefrontal N-acetylaspartate and poststroke recovery: a longitudinal proton spectroscopy study. AJNR Am J Neuroradiol. 28(3):470-4, 2007
10. De Simone T et al: Wallerian degeneration of the pontocerebellar fibers. AJNR Am J Neuroradiol. 26(5):1062-5, 2005

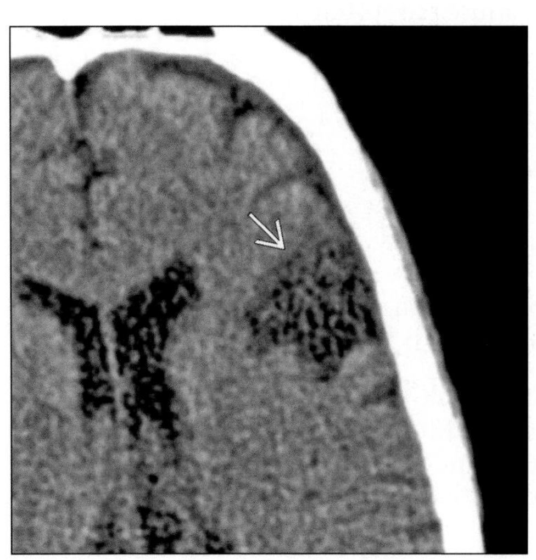

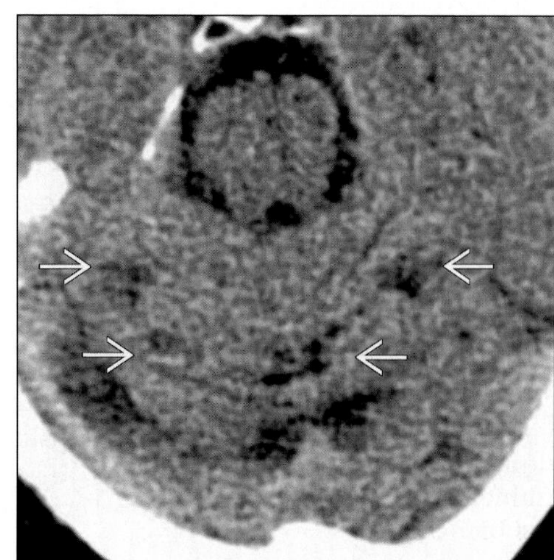

***(Left)** Axial NECT reveals a chronic left MCA infarct (anterior circulation) ➔. **(Right)** Axial NECT in the same patient demonstrates multiple remote cerebellar infarcts ➔ (posterior circulation). Findings are consistent with embolic infarcts in this patient with HHT (Osler-Weber-Rendu disease) who was found to have a pulmonary AV fistula.*

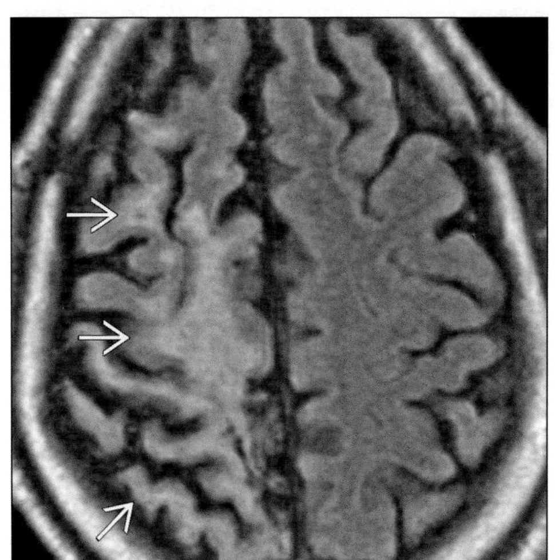

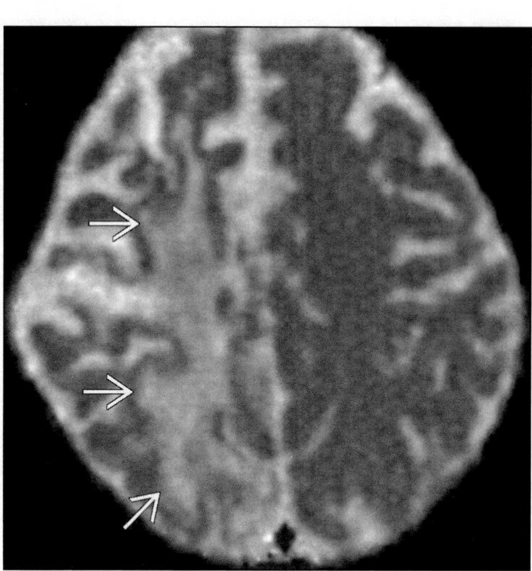

***(Left)** Axial FLAIR MR shows increased signal in a parasagittal distribution on the right ➔ with associated volume loss, in keeping with a remote watershed infarct. **(Right)** Axial ADC map in the same patient shows corresponding increased diffusibility ➔ in the right parasagittal region. No diffusion restriction is present. This patient had an occluded right internal carotid artery with tenuous perfusion to the right hemisphere.*

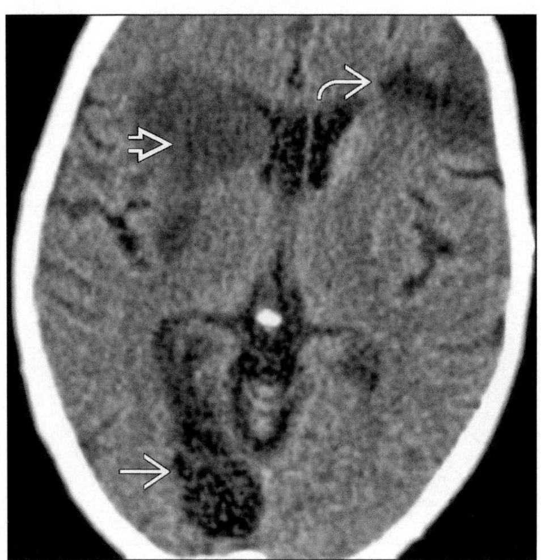

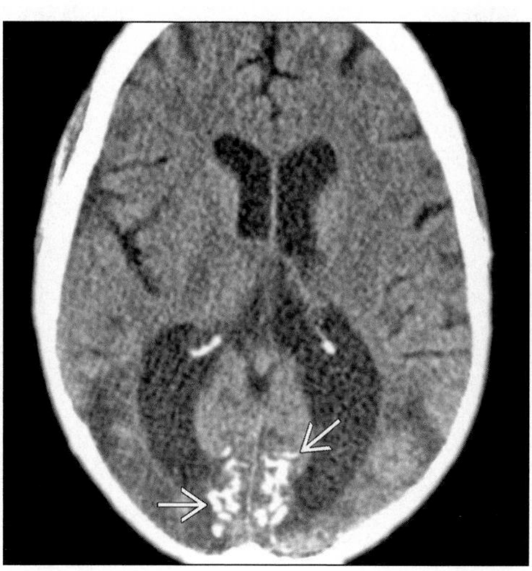

***(Left)** Axial NECT demonstrates remote right PCA ➔ and anterior left MCA ➔ infarcts. An acute deep right MCA infarct ➔ is also present, correlating with new onset left-sided weakness in this patient with cardioembolic disease. **(Right)** Axial NECT shows encephalomalacic changes in both occipital lobes, findings consistent with remote cerebral infarction. The gyriform calcifications in the cortex ➔ are most interesting (and unusual) in this case.*

ACA CEREBRAL INFARCTION

Key Facts

Terminology

- Ischemia/infarct in part or all of ACA vascular territory

Imaging

- CT: Hypodensity/loss of GM/WM differentiation in cortical ACA distribution
  - Hypodensity in caudate head, anteromedial putamen/globus pallidus, anterior limb of internal capsule (lenticulostriate arteries)
  - Perfusion CT shows ↓ CBF/CBV, ↑ TTP in medial cerebral hemisphere
- T2/FLAIR MR: Medial hemisphere hyperintensity
- DTI/DWI: Diffusion restriction acutely
- ACA: A1 segment (ICA bifurcation to ACoA)
  - A2 segment (ACoA to corpus callosum genu)
  - A3 segment (genu to terminal bifurcation)
  - A4 segment (distal cortical branches)

Top Differential Diagnoses

- Low-grade diffuse astrocytoma
- Cerebral edema
- Herpes encephalitis
- Subdural effusion, empyema

Clinical Issues

- Contralateral leg weakness/paraplegia
  - Face, upper extremity spared
- Abulia, motor aphasia, incontinence
- Frontal lobe symptoms, personality changes
- Uncommon, account for < 5% of ischemic strokes

Diagnostic Checklist

- Consider CTA or MRA to evaluate vessels
  - Always evaluate ACoA for aneurysm
- Perfusion CT should include ACA distribution

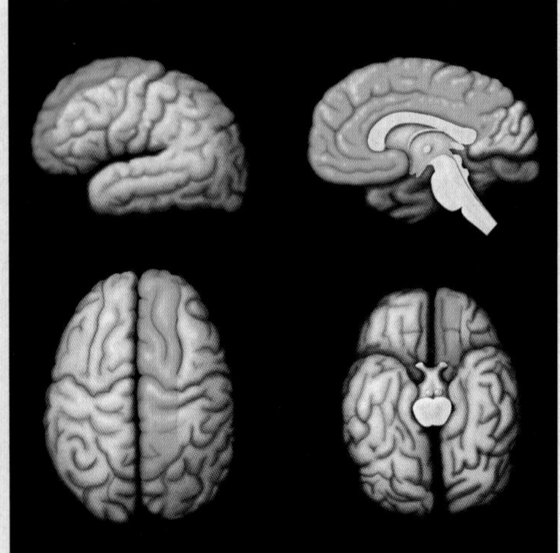

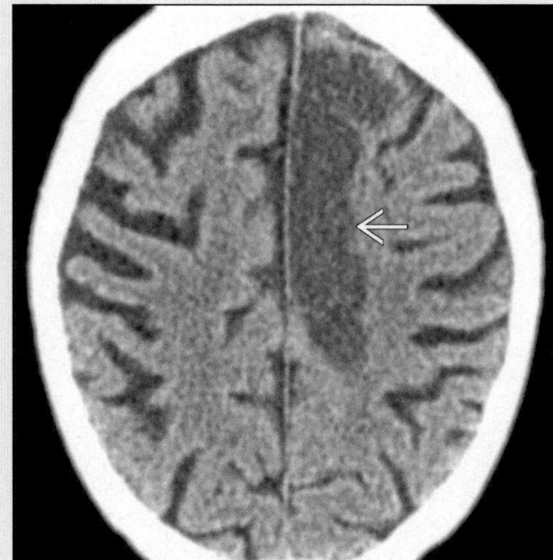

(Left) *Graphic shows the ACA cortical vascular territories in green. The ACA supplies the medial anteroinferior frontal lobe, the anterior 2/3 of the medial hemisphere surface, and a variable amount of territory over the cerebral convexity. The corpus callosum is also typically supplied primarily by the ACA branches: Callosal perforating, pericallosal, and posterior splenial branches.* ***(Right)*** *Axial NECT shows low attenuation within the medial parafalcine left frontal lobe in the ACA territory ➔, related to a subacute stroke.*

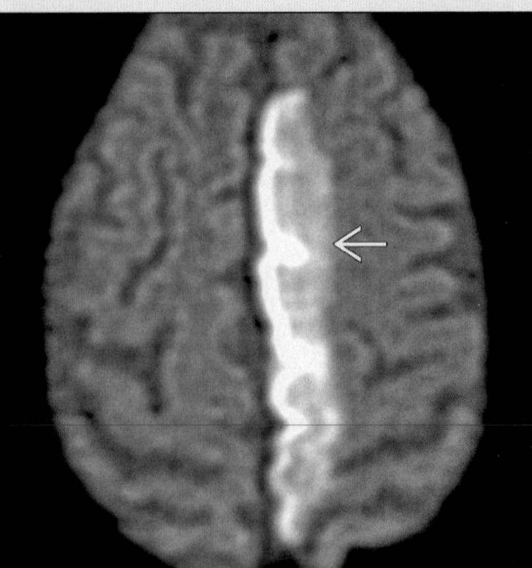

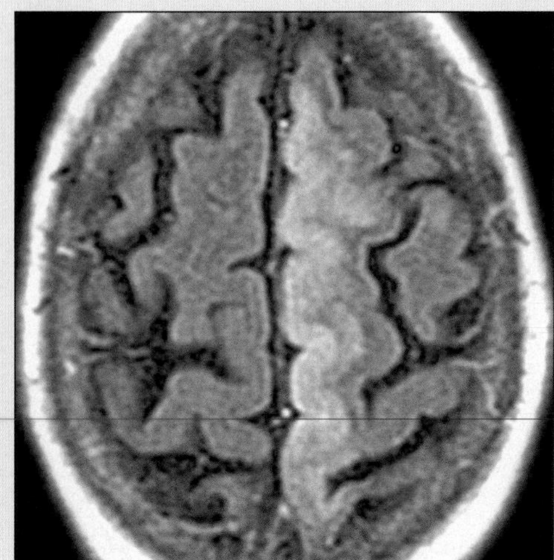

(Left) *Axial DWI MR shows diffusion restriction along the territory of the left ACA ➔. Patients with ACA strokes often present with contralateral leg weakness, abulia, motor aphasia, incontinence, &/ or personality changes.* ***(Right)*** *Axial FLAIR MR shows hyperintensity in the medial left frontal gyri. Note the effacement of sulci and gyral swelling in the classic ACA distribution. This ACA distribution stroke also involved the cingulate gyrus and corpus callosum rostrum (not shown).*

MCA CEREBRAL INFARCTION

Key Facts

Terminology

- Occlusion of middle cerebral artery (MCA) resulting in ischemia and infarct

Imaging

- Best imaging clue: Abnormal perfusion or diffusion in MCA territory
- CT: Hypodensity in frontal, parietal, &/or temporal lobes ± basal ganglia (BG)
- CT perfusion and CTA in acute setting
  - CBF and CBV can help predict ischemic core/ penumbra
  - CTA can identify occlusion
- DWI MR: Restricted diffusion in MCA territory
  - > 95% sensitive for hyperacute stroke detection
- Middle cerebral artery comprised of 4 segments: Horizontal (M1), insular (M2), opercular (M3), cortical (M4) segments
  - Lenticulostriate (perforating) arteries arise from M1 and supply majority of BG

Top Differential Diagnoses

- Low-grade diffuse astrocytoma
- Traumatic cerebral edema
- Herpes encephalitis

Clinical Issues

- Common presentation: Aphasia or motor weakness
- Inferior MCA occlusion: Wernicke aphasia, quadranopsia, hemianopsia, visual neglect
- Superior MCA branch occlusion: Global aphasia, Broca aphasia, visual and parietal neglect, contralateral motor and sensory loss
- Lenticulostriate artery occlusion: Dense hemiplegia
- Treatment: IV thrombolysis within 3 hours, IA thrombolysis within 6 hours

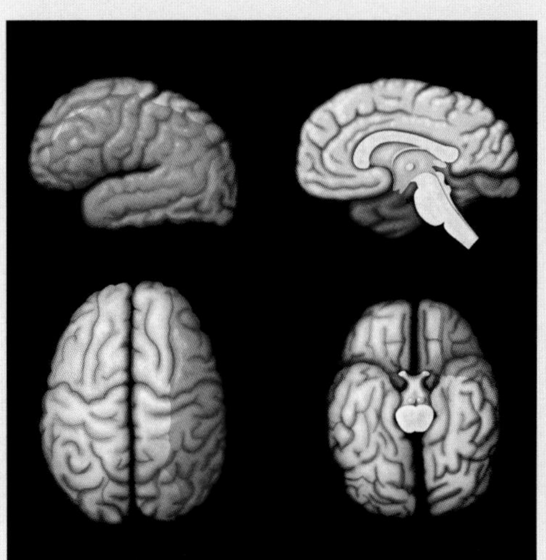

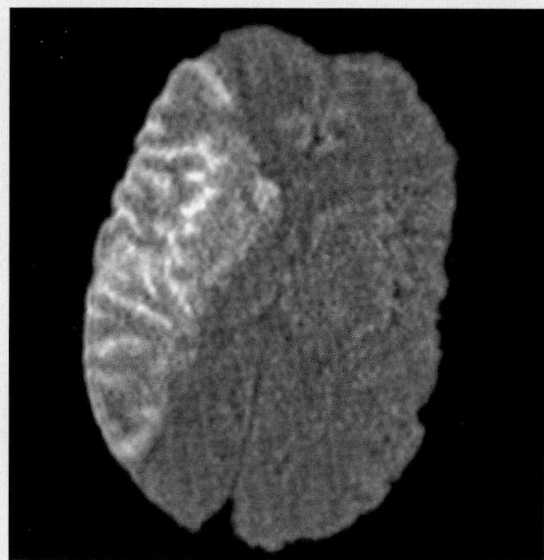

__(Left)__ Graphic shows the cortical MCA distribution in red. MCA distribution typically involves the majority of the lateral surface of the hemisphere, including the frontal, temporal, and parietal lobes. In addition, the majority of the lenticulostriate arteries arise from the M1 segment and supplies the basal ganglia. __(Right)__ Axial DTI trace MR shows diffusion restriction in the MCA distribution. Involvement of the basal ganglia indicates a proximal occlusion with lenticulostriate artery occlusion.

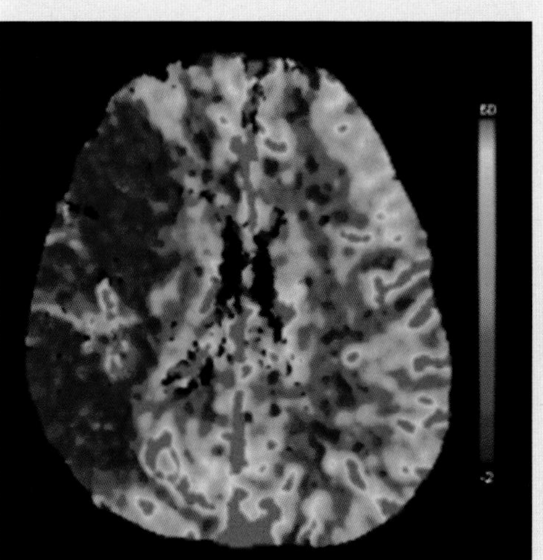

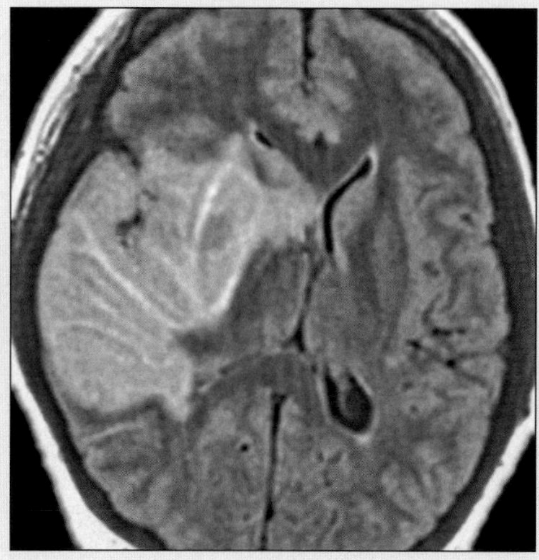

__(Left)__ Axial CT perfusion CBV color map shows significant reduction of cerebral blood volume in the right MCA territory related to hyperacute ischemia. If the patient presents within 3 hours of symptom onset, intravenous thrombolysis is given. If the patient presents within 6 hours of symptom onset, treatment includes intraarterial thrombolysis or mechanical thrombolysis. __(Right)__ Axial FLAIR MR shows marked hyperintensity & edema of the basal ganglia, insula, & temporal lobe, related to an MCA infarct.

PCA CEREBRAL INFARCTION

Key Facts

Imaging

- Best imaging clue: CT hypodensity or DWI/FLAIR/T2 hyperintensity in PCA vascular distribution
  - Occipital or inferior temporal lobes commonly
  - Also includes thalamus, hypothalamus, geniculate bodies, internal capsule posterior limb, upper midbrain, choroid plexus
- Segmental anatomy of PCA
  - P1 (precommunicating segment)
  - P2 (ambient segment)
  - P3 (quadrigeminal segment)
  - P4 (calcarine or cortical segment)
- P1 and P2: Primarily supply inferolateral temporal lobes and occipital lobes
  - Perforators and posterior choroidal arteries also supply thalamus, hypothalamus, internal capsule posterior limb, midbrain, choroid plexus
- P3 and P4: Supply posterior 1/3 of brain along interhemispheric fissure, lower parietal, occipital, and temporal lobes
- PCA ischemia may arise from anterior circulation emboli if PCA of fetal-origin is present

Top Differential Diagnoses

- Herpes encephalitis
- Low-grade diffuse astrocytoma
- Traumatic cerebral edema
- Acute hypertensive encephalopathy, PRES

Clinical Issues

- IV or IA thrombolysis is primary treatment
- Common presentation: Visual changes, including ocular reflexes, eye movement, visual encoding, visual agnosia, or cortical blindness
- Temporal lobe and fornix ischemia impacts memory and visual spatial encoding

__(Left)__ Graphic shows the typical PCA vascular territory, including the occipital lobes, inferior temporal lobes, and medial posterior 1/3 of the interhemispheric brain. Patients with PCA ischemia most commonly present with visual complaints. __(Right)__ Axial NECT shows hypodensity in the medial left occipital lobe ➔ with loss of gray-white differentiation related to an evolving PCA infarct. PCA ischemia is most commonly caused by emboli, typically from a cardiac source or from vertebrobasilar disease.

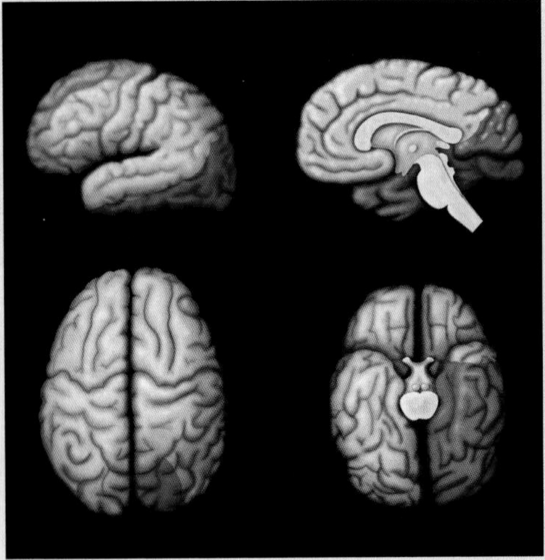

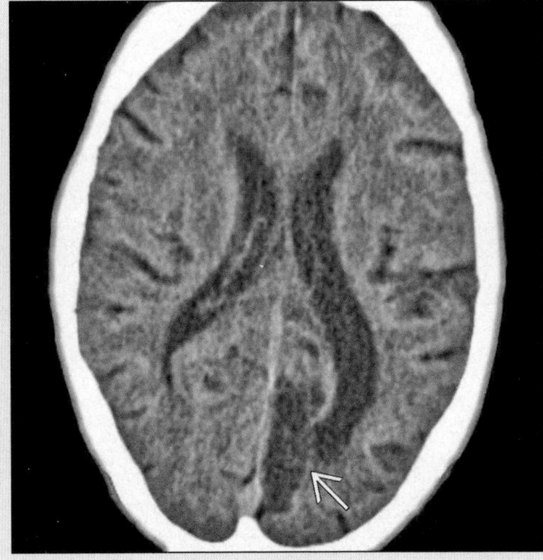

__(Left)__ Axial DWI MR shows diffusion restriction in the right thalamus ➔ and medial occipital lobe related to an acute PCA infarct. The occipital lobe is the region most commonly affected in PCA ischemia; thalamic involvement occurs in 1/3 of PCA territory strokes. __(Right)__ Axial FLAIR MR shows hyperintensity in the medial temporal and occipital lobes related to an acute PCA infarct. Note the involvement of the hippocampus ➯, which typically results in memory impairment.

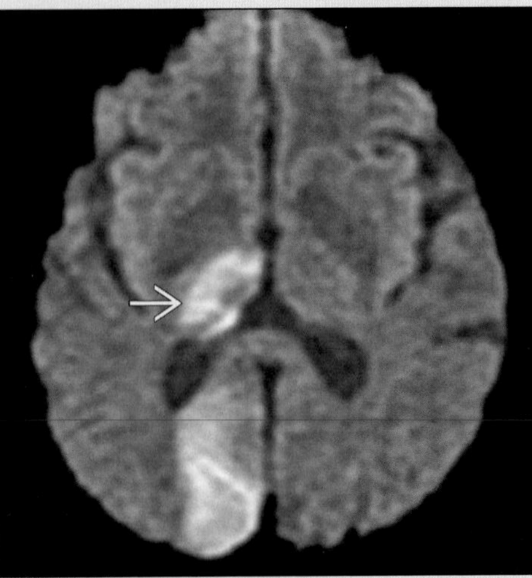

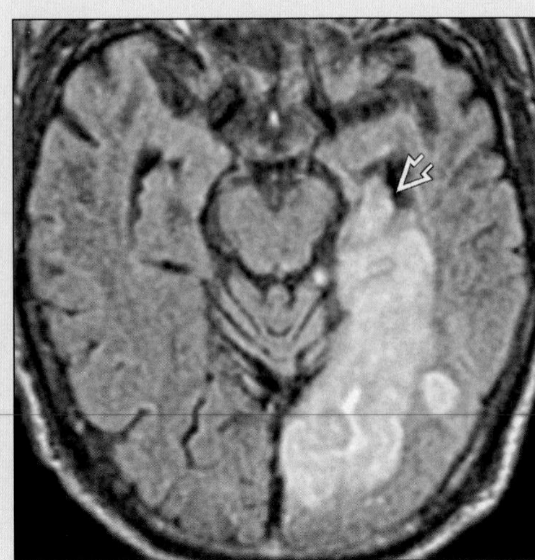

CHOROIDAL ARTERY CEREBRAL INFARCTION

Key Facts

Terminology

- Infarct of anterior choroidal or medial/lateral posterior choroidal arteries

Imaging

- Best diagnostic clue: Acute ischemia in choroidal artery distribution
- NECT: Hypodensity in medial temporal lobe, thalamus, or lateral midbrain
- MR: DWI/T2/FLAIR hyperintensity in choroidal artery territory
- Anterior choroidal artery arises from ICA
  - Supplies optic tract, lateral midbrain, uncus, thalamus, and posterior limb of internal capsule
- Medial/lateral posterior choroidal arteries arise from P2 segment of PCA
  - Supply pulvinar, part of thalamus, medial temporal lobe, splenium, and choroid plexus

Top Differential Diagnoses

- Herpes encephalitis
- Mesial temporal sclerosis
- Low-grade diffuse astrocytoma

Clinical Issues

- Anterior choroidal artery infarct: Triad of hemiparesis, hemianopia, and hemisensory loss
- Posterior choroidal artery infarct: Homonymous hemianopsia, hemisensory loss, memory disturbance

Diagnostic Checklist

- Anterior and posterior choroidal anastomoses allow anterior and posterior circulation disease to affect geniculate, hippocampus, and thalamus

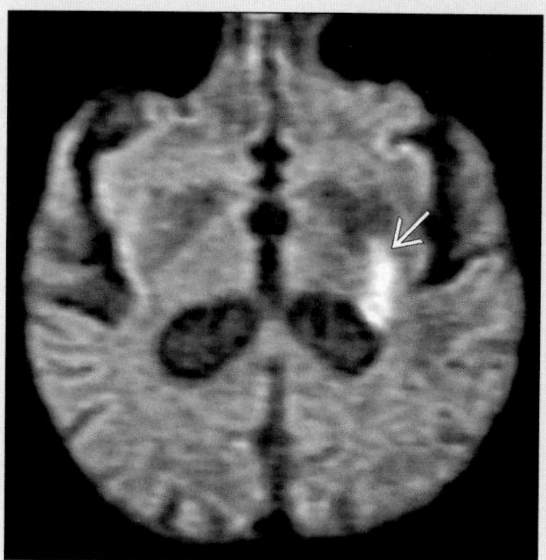

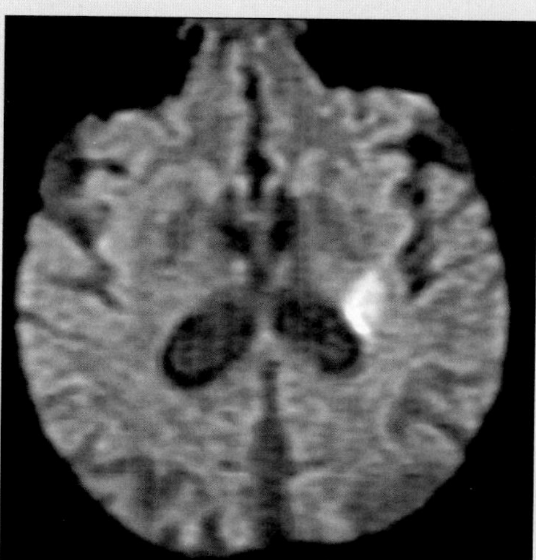

(Left) *Axial DWI MR shows hyperintensity related to acute ischemia in the region of the lateral geniculate nucleus, lateral thalamus, and posterior limb of the internal capsule ➡ in this patient with acute anterior choroidal artery ischemia.* ***(Right)*** *Axial DWI MR in the same patient shows cephalad extension of the ischemia. Patients with anterior choroidal infarcts typically present with a triad of hemiparesis, hemianopia, and hemisensory loss. Embolic disease is the most common etiology.*

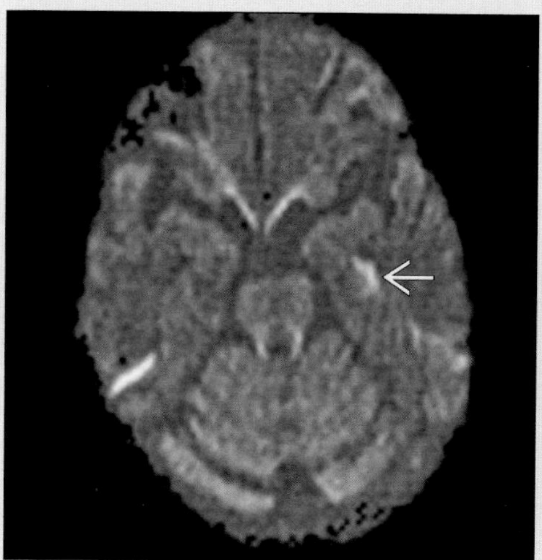

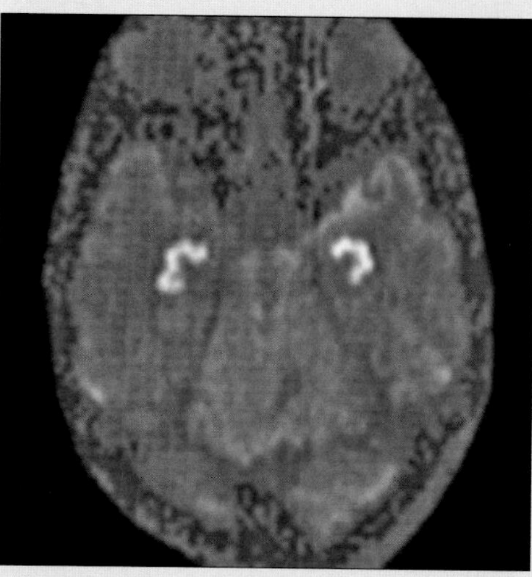

(Left) *Axial DTI trace image shows focal diffusion restriction in the left hippocampus ➡ related to a posterior choroidal artery infarct. The posterior choroidal arteries usually arise from the P2 segment of the PCA.* ***(Right)*** *Axial DTI trace image shows bilateral restriction from acute hippocampal ischemia in this patient with basilar artery embolic stroke. The patient had new onset memory deficit. Posterior choroidal artery infarcts typically result in homonymous hemianopsia, hemisensory loss, or memory disturbance.*

COW PERFORATING ARTERY CEREBRAL INFARCTION

Key Facts

Terminology
- Focal lacunar infarct due to occlusion of small perforators arising from circle of Willis
- Imaging anatomy
  - Small perforating vessels arise from ICA, ACA, ACoA, PCoA, PCA, and basilar artery
  - Anterior choroidal artery: Optic tract, posterior limb of internal capsule, cerebral peduncle, choroid plexus, and medial temporal lobes
  - ACA (medial lenticulostriates): Putamen and globus pallidus; recurrent artery of Huebner supplies caudate head
  - ACoA perforators: Anterior optic chiasm, hypothalamus, fornix
  - PCoA (anterior thalamoperforators): Thalamus, internal capsule posterior limb, optic tracts
  - Basilar and proximal PCA (posterior thalamoperforators): Thalamus and midbrain

Imaging
- Lacunar infarct of basal ganglia (BG), hypothalamus, infundibulum, thalamus, medial temporal lobe, midbrain, or cerebral peduncle
- NECT: Focal hypodensity in perforator territories
- DWI: Restriction in BG, thalamus, midbrain
- MR with DWI or DTI is best imaging tool
  - Consider CTA/MRA to search for aneurysm
- Consider vascular and cardiac evaluation if small lacunar infarcts or emboli

Top Differential Diagnoses
- ADEM
- Enlarged perivascular spaces
- Hippocampal sulcus remnant cysts

Clinical Issues
- Treatment: Supportive; consider IV/IA thrombolysis

(Left) Axial graphic shows the major penetrating artery vascular territories. The pontine and thalamic perforating artery territories are shown in light purple. The medial lenticulostriate arteries, which supply the anterior basal ganglia, are shown in light green, while the lateral lenticulostriate arteries are shown in blue. The anterior choroidal artery territory is shown in magenta. (Right) Axial DTI trace shows thalamic hyperintensity related to thalamoperforator distribution ischemia. Note the additional PCA territory ischemia.

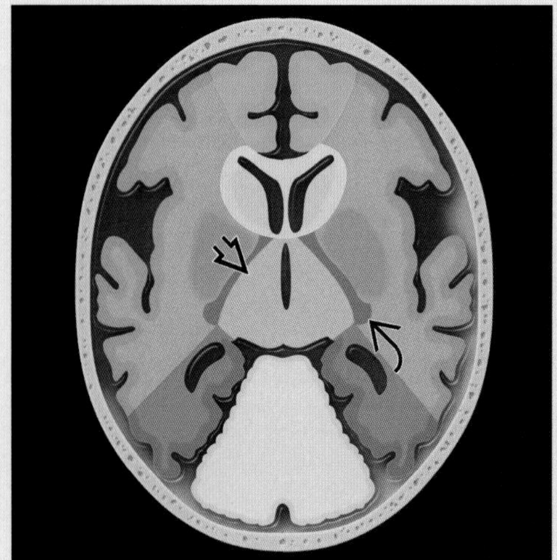

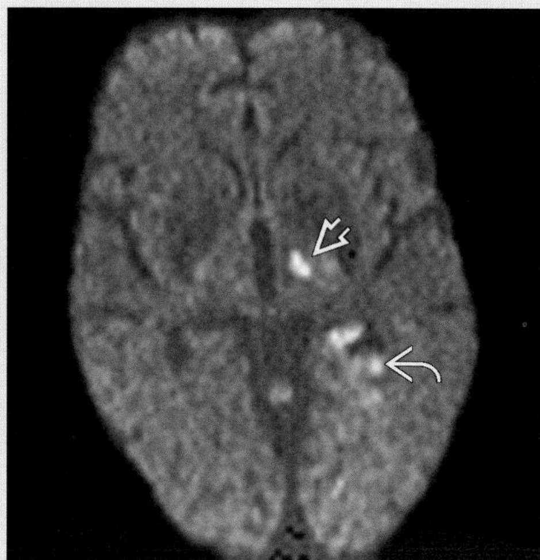

(Left) Axial DWI MR shows diffusion restriction in the left cerebral peduncle related to acute ischemia in the anterior choroidal perforator distribution. (Right) Axial FLAIR MR shows hyperintensity related to ischemia in the medial and lateral lenticulostriate distributions, including the recurrent artery of Huebner (caudate head). The lateral lenticulostriate arteries arise from the M1 segment of the MCA. The majority of perforating artery strokes are present in the deep gray nuclei.

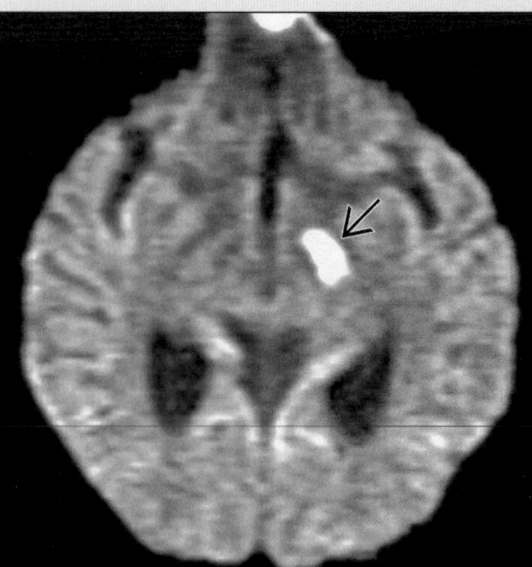

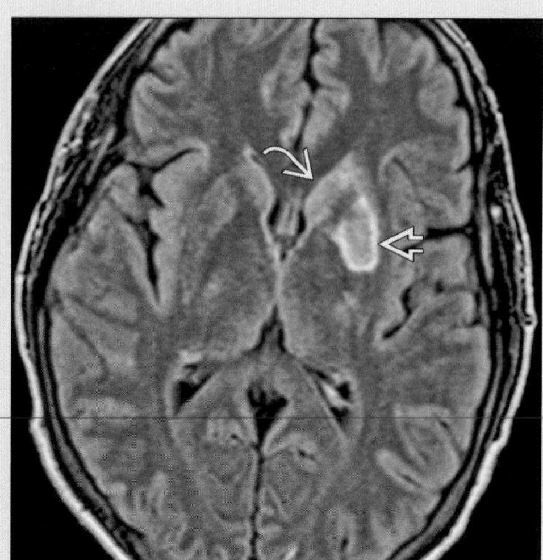

Key Facts

Terminology
- Bilateral paramedian thalamic &/or midbrain infarcts due to occlusion of variant P1 common trunk (Percheron) with bilateral supply

Imaging
- Best imaging clue: T2/FLAIR hyperintensity in bilateral thalami ± midbrain extension
- NECT: Low attenuation in bilateral thalami, may extend into medial midbrain
- DWI: Diffusion restriction in bilateral paramedian thalami ± midbrain
- Imaging anatomy
  - Artery of Percheron can arise from unilateral P1 segment of PCA or rarely tip of basilar
  - Single vessel supplies both paramedian thalami and medial midbrain

Top Differential Diagnoses
- Neoplasm
- "Top of basilar" infarct
- Deep cerebral venous thrombosis
- Wernicke encephalopathy

Clinical Issues
- Obtundation, mental status change, oculomotor and pupillary deficit, vertical gaze palsy, ptosis, lid retraction

Diagnostic Checklist
- CTA or MRA to evaluate posterior circulation, exclude vertebrobasilar source
- Bilateral thalamic infarcts in absence of PCA or SCA findings suggest anatomic variant artery of Percheron infarct

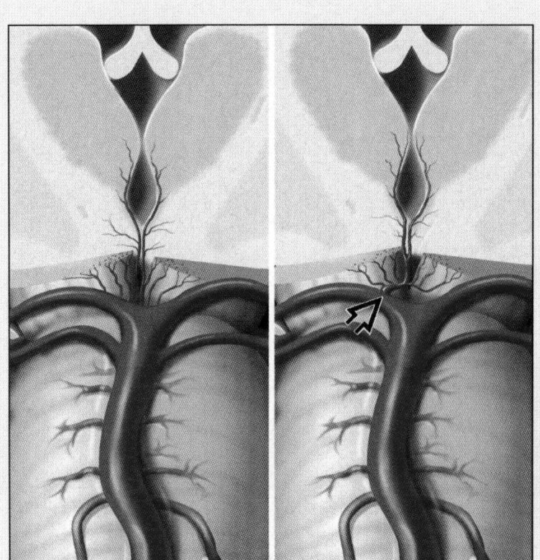

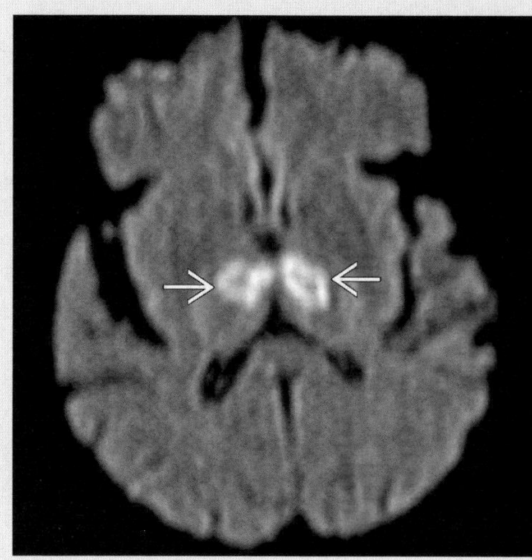

*(**Left**) Coronal oblique graphic of the rostral basilar artery shows (left panel) the typical arterial supply to the medial thalami by multiple PCA and basilar tip perforators. Right panel shows the anatomic variant, artery of Percheron ⇨, in which a single large perforating artery from P1 supplies bilateral thalami and the medial midbrain. (**Right**) Axial DWI MR shows classic diffusion restriction within bilateral medial thalami ➡ in an acute artery of Percheron infarct. Symmetric involvement is typical.*

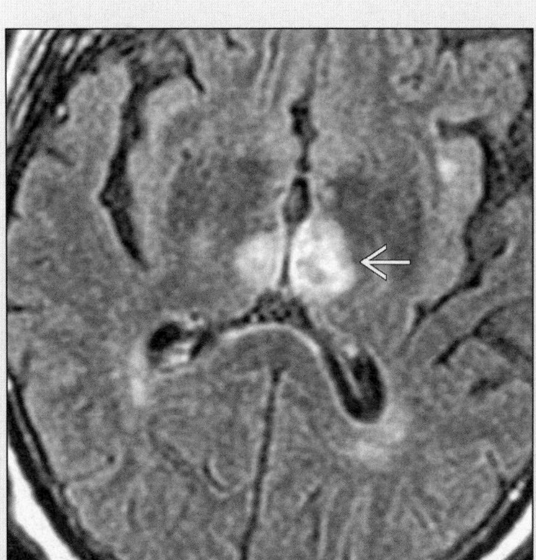

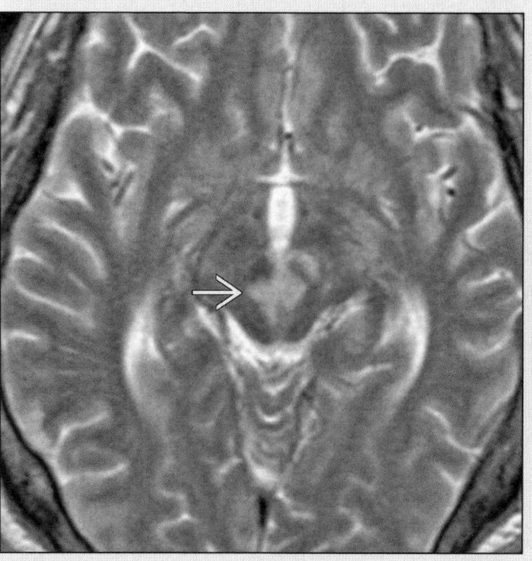

*(**Left**) Axial FLAIR MR shows increased signal in bilateral thalami, asymmetric to the left ➡ related to an acute artery of Percheron infarct. The abnormal signal extended cephalad from the medial cerebral peduncles. When hyperintensity is present only in the thalami, differential considerations include deep venous thrombosis, hypoxic injury, and neoplasm. (**Right**) Axial T2WI MR shows hyperintensity in the medial midbrain ➡ related to an artery of Percheron infarct. Extension to the medial thalami was also present (not shown).*

TOP OF BASILAR CEREBRAL INFARCTION

Key Facts

Terminology

- Infarct of rostral brainstem and cerebral hemispheres supplied by distal basilar artery
- Clinically recognizable syndrome characterized by visual, oculomotor, and behavioral abnormalities

Imaging

- Best diagnostic clue: Diffusion restriction in rostral midbrain, bilateral thalami, and PCA distributions
- CT: Low attenuation of midbrain, bilateral thalami, and PCA territory
  - CT perfusion: ↓ rCBF and rCBV
- MR: T2/FLAIR hyperintensity in midbrain, thalami, occipital and temporal lobes
- Imaging anatomy
  - Distal basilar: Rostral midbrain/pons perforators
  - Distal basilar terminates as PCA branches
  - SCA typically arise just proximal to PCA
- Consider MRA or CTA to evaluate vessels
- Consider MR with DWI/DTI for posterior fossa or visual symptoms

Top Differential Diagnoses

- Acute hypertensive encephalopathy, PRES
- Brainstem glioma
- Osmotic demyelination syndrome
- Miscellaneous vasculitis

Clinical Issues

- Visual and oculomotor deficits, visual agnosia, visual hallucinations
- Somnolence, confusion, or behavioral change
- Relative absence of motor deficit
- Clinical may mimic bilateral thalamic syndromes or artery of Percheron infarct

__(Left)__ Axial FLAIR MR shows hyperintensity in the occipital lobes and left pons ➔ in this patient with visual changes and confusion. Top of the basilar syndrome is most commonly caused by embolic disease, as in this case. __(Right)__ Axial DTI trace shows bilateral rostral midbrain ischemia ➔, which extended into the cerebral peduncles (not shown). This patient presented with oculomotor symptoms. Note the dorsal extension of ischemia ➔ involving the medial longitudinal fasciculus.

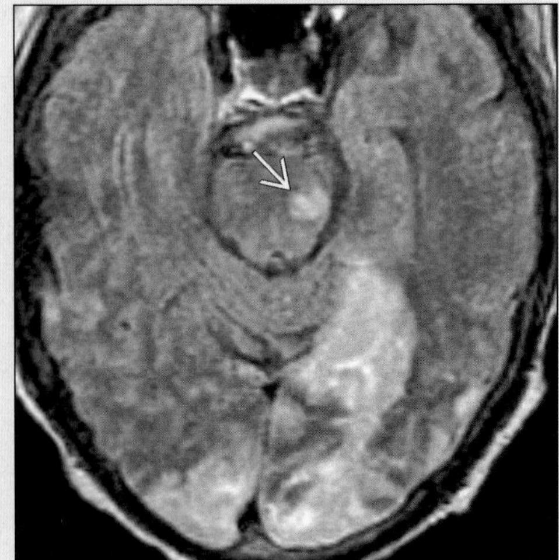

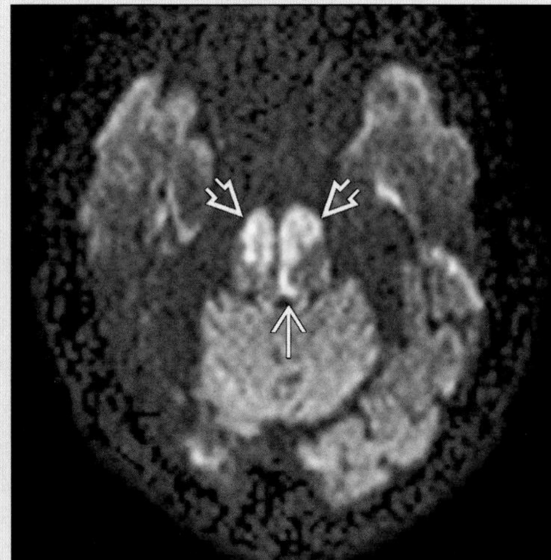

__(Left)__ Axial T2WI MR shows diffuse hyperintensity in the bilateral occipital lobes ➔ and medial temporal lobes. There is involvement of the superior cerebellum ➔ resulting in upward transtentorial herniation and mass effect on the pons. __(Right)__ Axial T2WI MR in the same patient shows additional involvement of the thalami bilaterally ➔ as well as the medial occipital lobes. The top of the basilar syndrome often clinically mimics bilateral thalamic syndromes or artery of Percheron infarcts.

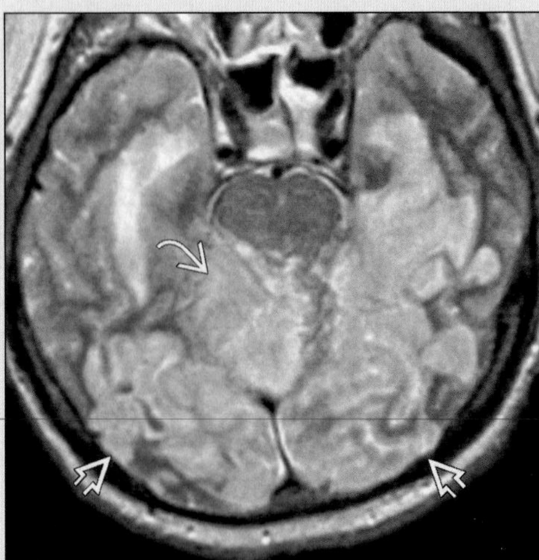

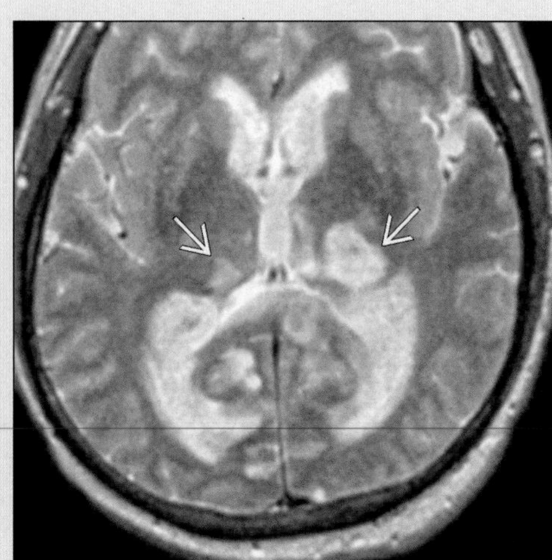

BASILAR THROMBOSIS CEREBRAL INFARCTION

Key Facts

Terminology

- Infarct of pons ± midbrain secondary to basilar artery occlusion; may result in "locked in" syndrome

Imaging

- Best imaging clue: CTA with basilar artery filling defect + hypodensity/hyperintensity of pons
- Basilar artery: Vascular supply to pons, midbrain, mid/upper cerebellum, posteromedial thalami, and posterior limb of internal capsule
- Branches: Paired anterior inferior cerebellar arteries (AICA), superior cerebellar arteries (SCA), posterior cerebral arteries (PCA) + multiple perforators
- CT imaging: May see "hyperdense basilar artery"
  - NECT: Low attenuation in pons, ± hemorrhage
  - CTA: Occlusion, filling defect, dissection, or stenosis of basilar artery
  - CT perfusion: ↓ rCBF, rCBV in pons ± midbrain
- MR imaging
  - T2/FLAIR: Hyperintensity in pons ± midbrain; variable AICA, SCA, PCA involvement
  - DWI or DTI: Diffusion restriction
- Consider MRA or CTA in patients with posterior fossa symptoms, worsening exam, obtundation
- Expedite imaging to neurointervention if basilar occlusion ⇒ IA thrombolysis/thrombectomy

Top Differential Diagnoses

- Brainstem glioma
- Osmotic demyelination syndrome
- Miscellaneous vasculitis

Clinical Issues

- Dizziness, vertigo, ataxia, corticospinal signs, nystagmus, pupillary defect, sensory deficit
- Progressive cranial nerve palsies, corticospinal signs, loss of airway, "locked in" syndrome

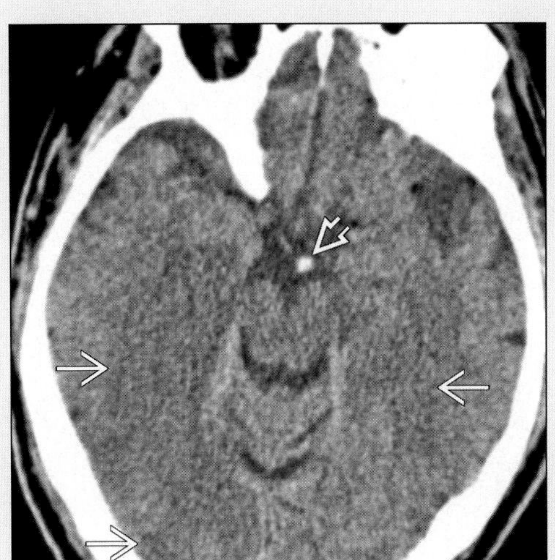

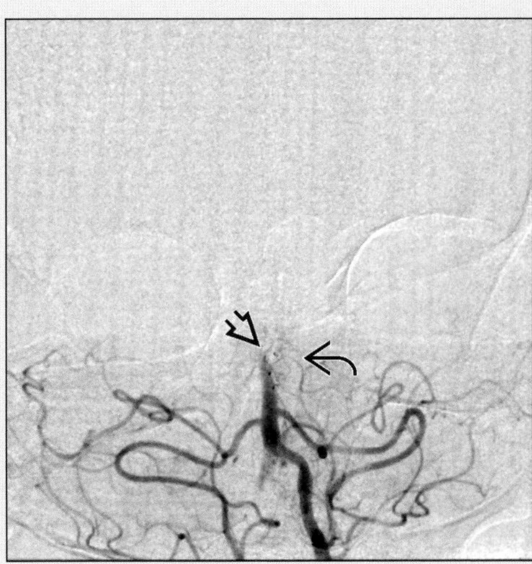

(Left) *Axial NECT shows a "hyperdense basilar artery" ➡ related to atherosclerotic calcification and acute thrombus in this patient with basilar thrombosis. Note the associated inferior temporal and occipital lobe hypodensity ➡ related to PCA ischemia in a patient with absent PCoAs.* ***(Right)*** *AP angiogram of a left vertebral injection shows thrombosis of the distal basilar artery ➡ with lack of filling of the SCA and PCA branches. There is normal opacification of bilateral PICA and AICA. Note the small blush of lower pontine perforator arteries ↪.*

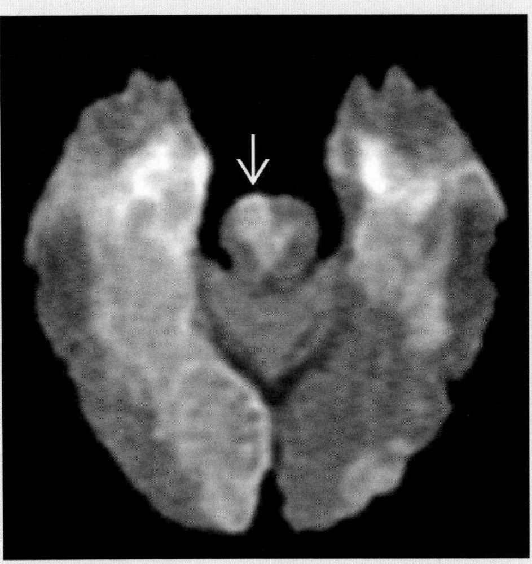

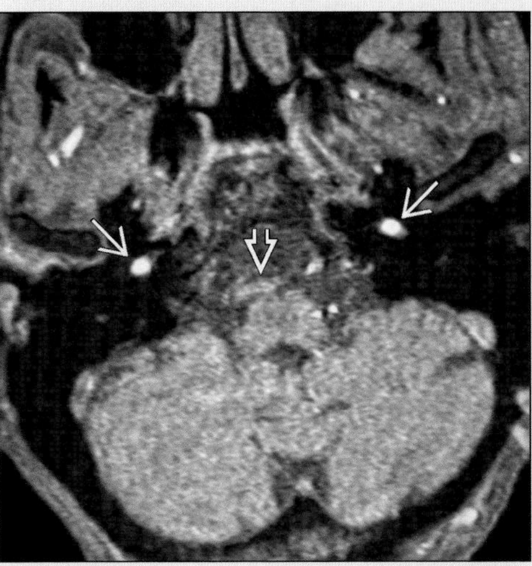

(Left) *Axial DWI MR shows the profound impact of basilar thrombosis in a patient with basilar artery occlusion at the level of the AICA origins. Pontine perforator stroke caused diffusion restriction in the pons ➡ and caudal midbrain. Note the additional involvement of bilateral posterior cerebral artery territories in this patient with absent PCoAs.* ***(Right)*** *Axial MRA source image shows no flow ➡ in the occluded basilar artery. Note the normal signal ➡ in bilateral petrous internal carotid arteries.*

BASILAR PERFORATING ARTERY CEREBRAL INFARCTION

Key Facts

Terminology

- Focal infarct in pons or pontomedullary junction secondary to pontine perforator or basilar branch artery ischemia
- Pontine perforating or basilar branch arteries usually produce unilateral paramedian, lateral pontine, or pontine tegmental infarcts

Imaging

- Best imaging clue: DWI/FLAIR/T2 hyperintensity in pons, typically respects midline
- NECT: Focal hypodensity in medial, paramedian, or lateral pons
- DWI: Focal restriction in paramedian, lateral, or tegmentum of pons or pontomesencephalic junction
- Consider MR with DWI/DTI for posterior fossa symptoms
- Rule out basilar artery occlusion or stenosis with MRA or CTA

Top Differential Diagnoses

- Arteriolosclerosis
- Pontine glioma
- Enlarged perivascular spaces
- Olivopontocerebellar degeneration
- Hypertrophic olivary degeneration

Clinical Issues

- Paramedian pontine infarct causes pure motor hemiparesis, dysarthria, ataxia, "clumsy hand" syndrome
- Basal tegmental infarct causes contralateral hemiparesis, ipsilateral trigeminal sensory deficit, CN6 or gaze paralysis, facial paralysis, loss of position and vibratory sense
- Rarely multiple pontine perforators produce bilateral pontine infarct, mimicking basilar thrombosis

__(Left)__ Axial DTI trace shows punctate diffusion restriction in the right pons ➡ related to acute basilar perforating artery ischemia. The majority of basilar artery ischemia is related to embolic disease from a cardiac source or from vertebrobasilar disease. Note the remote left pontine lacunar infarct ➡. __(Right)__ Axial T1WI C+ FS MR shows irregular enhancement ➡ in the left pons in this patient with a subacute infarct. Imaging may mimic neoplasm if the correct clinical history is unknown.

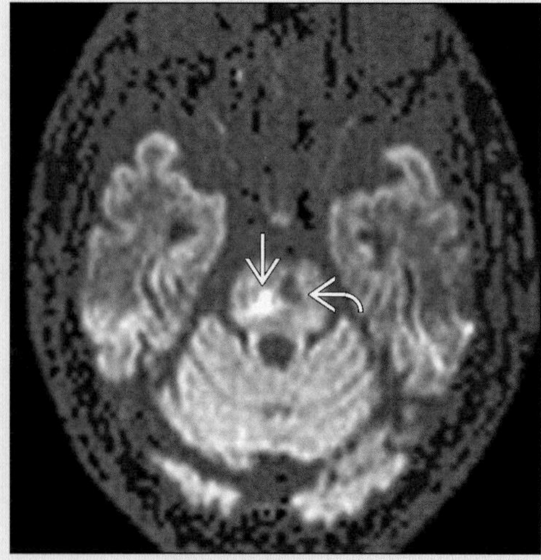

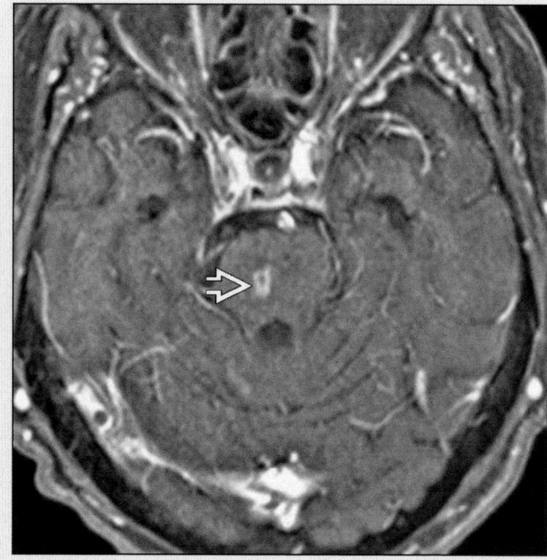

__(Left)__ Axial T2WI MR shows hyperintensity and enlargement of the pons ➡ related to acute ischemia. Note that the lesion respects midline ➡, typical of ischemia. __(Right)__ Axial DWI MR shows restricted diffusion in the left pons ➡ that respects midline in a patient with acute onset of right hemiparesis. Findings are typical of acute ischemia in a basilar perforating artery distribution. Additional acute ischemia is present in the right temporal lobe. (Courtesy N. Fischbein, MD.)

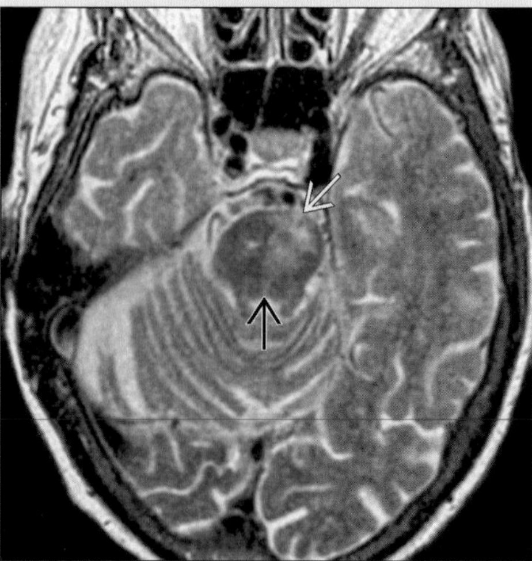

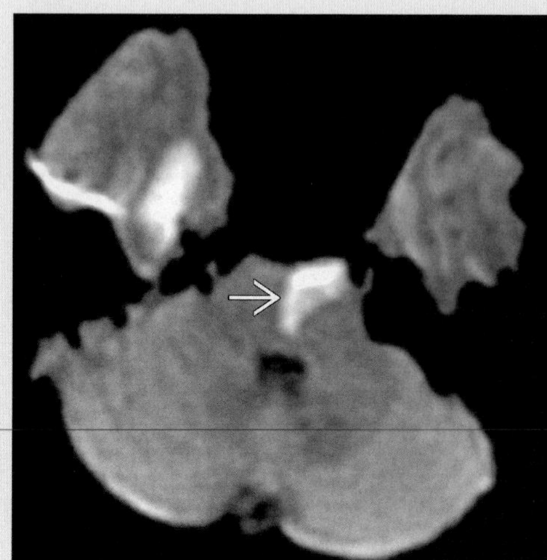

Key Facts

Terminology

- Infarct of superior cerebellum ± upper pons, supplied by superior cerebellar artery (SCA)

Imaging

- Best imaging clue: T2/FLAIR hyperintensity in superior cerebellum ± upper lateral pons
- DWI: Restriction in superior cerebellum ± pons
- Anatomy: SCA bifurcates into medial and lateral SCA
  - Medial SCA: Supplies dorsal and medial superior cerebellum, upper lateral and dorsal pons
  - Lateral SCA: Ventral and lateral superior cerebellum

Top Differential Diagnoses

- Cerebellitis
- Diffuse astrocytoma
- Cerebral contusion/edema

Clinical Issues

- Rostral basilar syndrome
  - Coma, tetraplegia, cerebellovestibular signs
  - Ipsilateral limb ataxia, ipsilateral Horner syndrome, contralateral spinothalamic, contralateral CN4, rarely contralateral deafness
- Lateral superior cerebellar artery syndrome
  - Ataxia, mild truncal and severe extremity ataxia, dysarthria
- Medial superior cerebellar artery syndrome
  - Ataxia, severe truncal and mild extremity, dysarthria
- SCA occlusion can be clinically masked by contralateral MCA stroke
- Pure SCA occlusion is rare in isolation
  - Often associated with rostral basilar infarct of midbrain, dorsal thalamus, occipital lobes

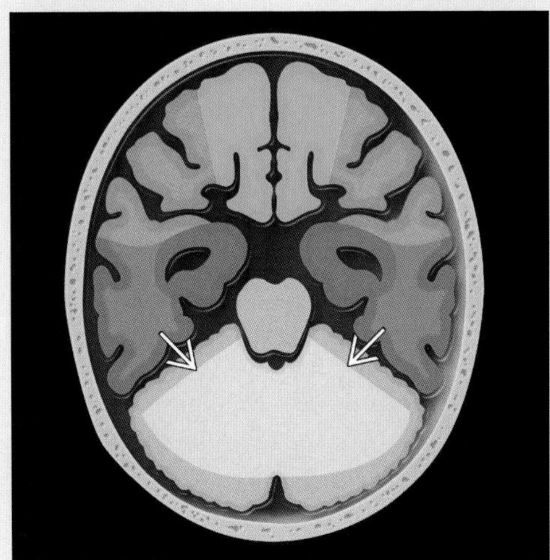

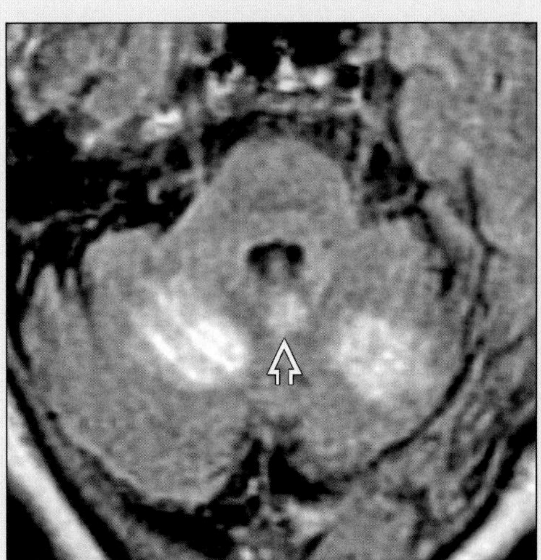

(Left) Graphic displays the territory of the superior cerebellar artery (SCA) in yellow. The superior cerebellar hemispheres and upper lateral and dorsal pons are supplied by the SCA ➡. AICA is shown in blue, and PICA is shown in tan. (Right) Axial FLAIR MR shows hyperintensity in the superior cerebellar hemispheres and the superior cerebellar vermis ⇨ related to acute ischemia. Bilateral SCA infarcts are rare and mimic other etiologies, including cerebellitis. DWI and clinical history help with an accurate diagnosis.

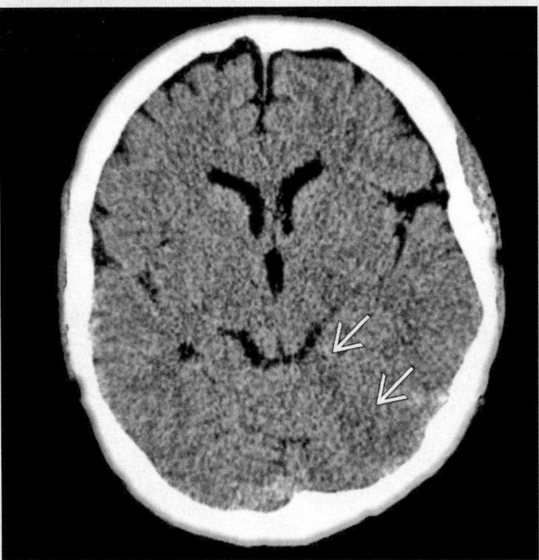

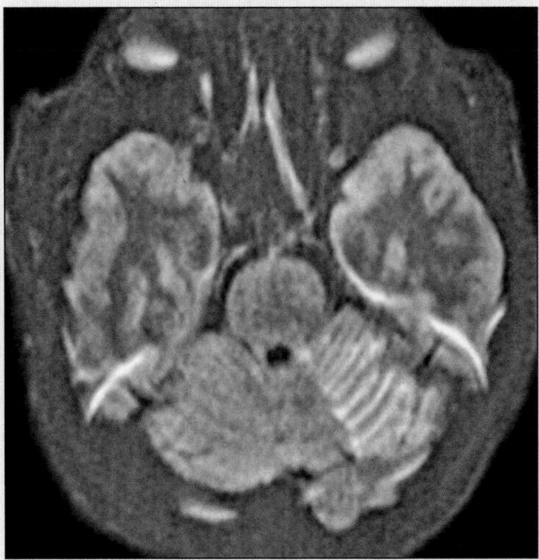

(Left) Axial NECT shows subtle hypodensity and loss of the cerebellar folia definition in the left superior cerebellum ➡. CT evaluation of a posterior fossa stroke is difficult as there is often beam hardening or volume averaging with the tentorium cerebelli, which obscures the lesion. MR can be helpful to further evaluate. (Right) Axial DTI trace image in the same patient shows diffusion restriction in the superior left cerebellum and SCA distribution, related to acute ischemia.

AICA CEREBELLAR INFARCTION

Key Facts

Imaging

- Best diagnostic clue: DWI/T2/FLAIR hyperintensity in anterior inferior cerebellar artery (AICA) territory
  - AICA: Primarily supplies ventral pons and petrosal surface of cerebellar hemispheres
  - Also supplies brachium pontis and foramen of Luschka choroid plexus
  - AICA labyrinthine branch supplies inner ear and CN7 and CN8
  - Variant AICA-PICA trunk may supply inferior cerebellar hemisphere
- NECT findings of early ischemia may be masked by beam hardening artifact in posterior fossa
- MR DWI or DTI is best imaging tool
- Skull base artifacts can obscure subtle findings or give false-positive DWI signal; always compare to ADC

Top Differential Diagnoses

- Cerebellitis
- Traumatic edema
- Demyelination

Clinical Issues

- Brainstem predominant signs: Vertigo, tinnitus, ipsilateral hearing loss, dysarthria, distal facial palsy, Horner syndrome, and ipsilateral limb ataxia
- Auditory symptoms suggest AICA over PICA territory infarct: Labyrinthine artery of AICA supplies inner ear, canalicular facial nerve, vestibular and cochlear apparatus

Diagnostic Checklist

- Variant anatomy (AICA-PICA trunk) may complicate imaging of posterior fossa stroke
- If new ipsilateral hearing loss, carefully evaluate AICA territory

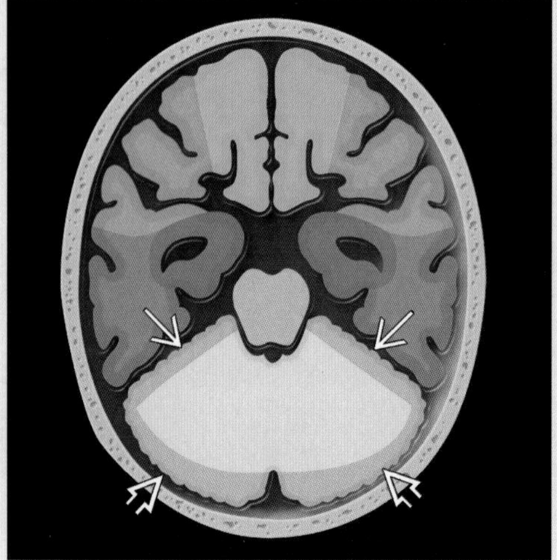

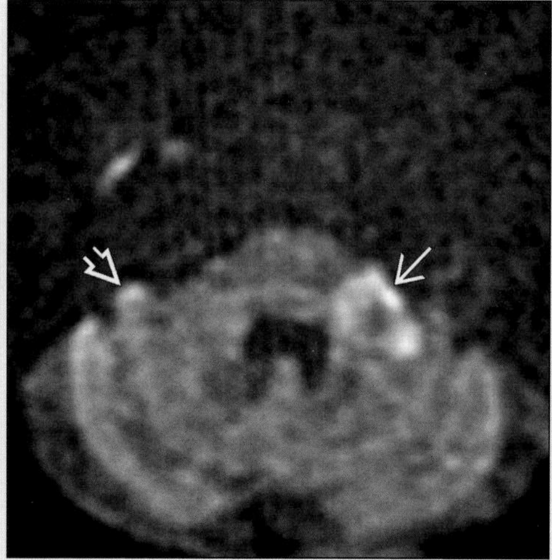

(Left) *Axial graphic shows the primary AICA distribution as the petrosal surface of the cerebellar hemispheres in blue ➡. There can be variable lateral pontine and upper medullary contribution by AICA perforators, including supply of the brachium pontis. PICA-AICA trunk variants can supply both AICA and PICA ⮕ territories. SCA territory is shown in yellow.* ***(Right)*** *Axial DWI MR shows hyperintensity related to acute ischemia in the brachium pontis ➡. The AICA territory includes the cerebellar flocculus ⮕, just lateral to the brachium pontis.*

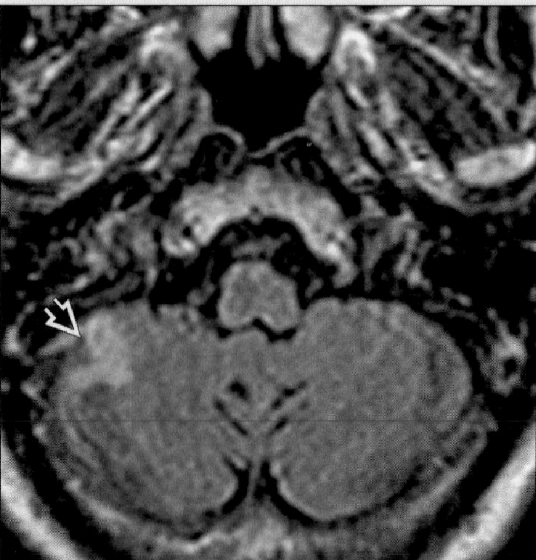

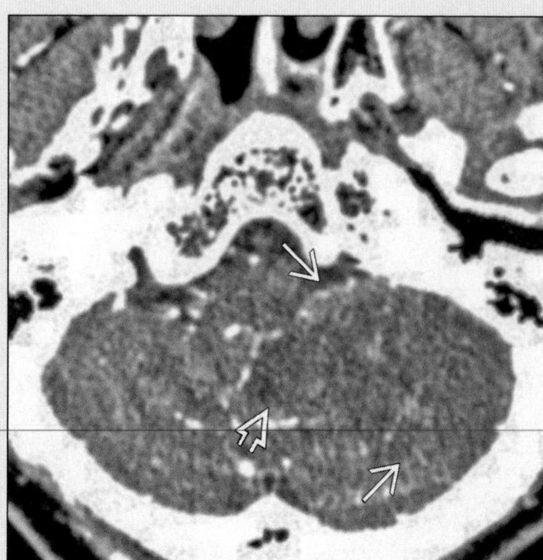

(Left) *Axial FLAIR MR shows hyperintensity related to acute ischemia in the inferolateral cerebellum ⮕, AICA distribution. This elderly woman presented with dizziness, nausea, and vomiting.* ***(Right)*** *Axial CECT shows hypodensity related to an acute infarct in the inferior cerebellum ➡ involving both lateral and medial cerebellum, including the tonsil ⮕, which is typically supplied by PICA. Variable supply is common in the posterior fossa.*

PICA CEREBELLAR INFARCTION

Key Facts

Terminology
- Ischemia in posterior inferior cerebellar artery (PICA) distribution
  - Inferior cerebellar hemispheres, lateral medulla, inferior vermis, tonsils

Imaging
- Best imaging clue: Diffusion restriction of PICA territory, typically lateral medulla and majority of lower cerebellar hemispheres
- PICA: Supplies inferior cerebellar hemispheres, lateral medulla, inferior vermis, tonsils, choroid plexus

Top Differential Diagnoses
- Low-grade diffuse astrocytoma
- Cerebellitis
- Cerebral contusion/edema

Clinical Issues
- Lateral medullary syndrome (Wallenberg syndrome) classic crossed face and body symptoms
  - Ipsilateral Horner (ptosis, anhydrosis, miosis), ipsilateral face loss of pain and temperature, contralateral body loss of pain and temperature
  - Contralateral extremity ataxia
- May have dysphagia, dysarthria, vocal cord paralysis from CN10, nausea, vertigo, hiccups
- Treatment often supportive, IA or IV thrombolysis if associated with additional vertebrobasilar occlusion

Diagnostic Checklist
- If clinical suspicion for posterior fossa stroke, consider MR with DWI or DTI
  - CT findings may be obscured in posterior fossa
- Consider CTA or MRA for vessel evaluation

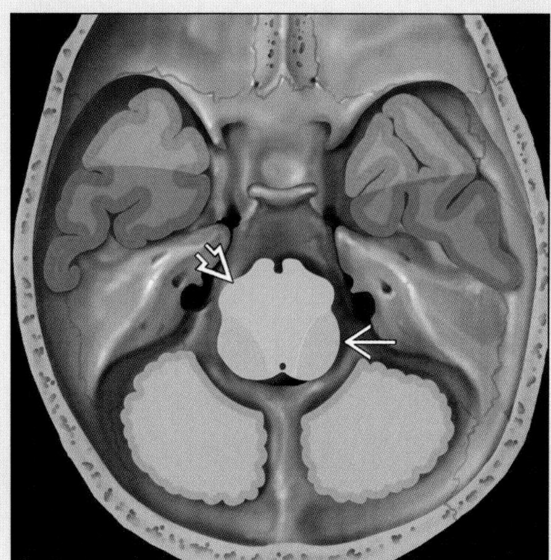

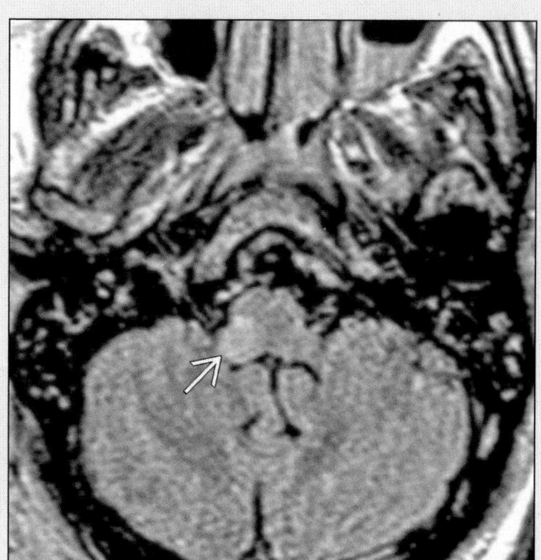

*(**Left**) Axial graphic shows the primary PICA territory of the lateral medulla ➔ and inferior cerebellum in tan. Penetrating arteries from the vertebral and anterior spinal arteries supply the remainder of the medulla ⇨. (**Right**) Axial FLAIR MR shows hyperintensity in the lateral medulla ➔ related to a PICA infarct in this patient with Wallenberg syndrome, including the clinical triad of Horner syndrome, ataxia, and contralateral hemisensory findings. Lateral medullary strokes are typically related to vertebral artery disease, including dissection.*

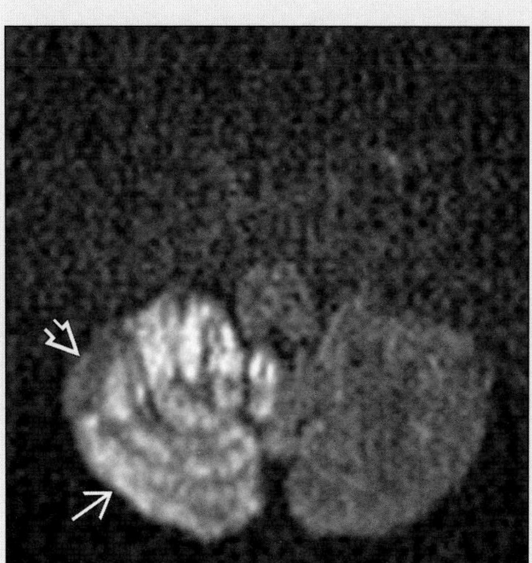

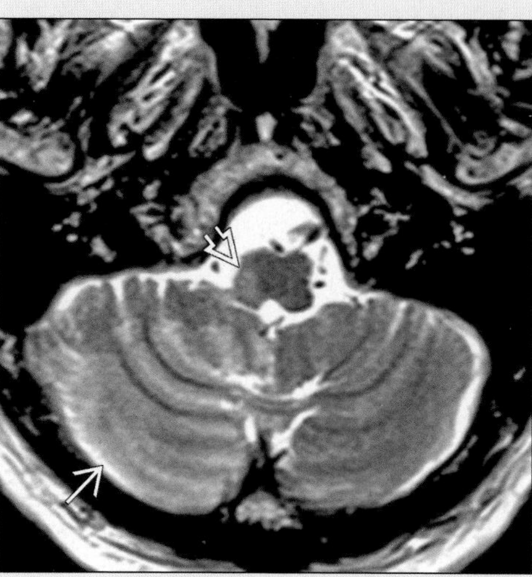

*(**Left**) Axial DTI trace at the level of the upper medulla shows diffusion restriction within the majority of the right cerebellar hemisphere ➔. Note the sparing of the lateral cerebellum ⇨ and AICA distribution. Large PICA distribution infarcts can result in severe posterior fossa mass effect and upward transtentorial herniation. (**Right**) Axial T2WI MR shows high signal with mild edema in the right cerebellar hemisphere ➔ and subtle high signal in the lateral medulla ⇨ due to PICA infarct related to vertebral artery embolus.*

MULTIPLE EMBOLIC CEREBRAL INFARCTIONS

Key Facts

Terminology

- Infarcts in multiple arterial distributions from embolic source, often cardiac origin

Imaging

- Best imaging clue: DWI restriction in multiple vascular distributions
- NECT: Multiple regions of low attenuation, loss of gray-white differentiation
- T2/FLAIR: Multiple supratentorial and infratentorial regions of hyperintensity, often in a vascular distribution
  - May be of different ages
- Embolic infarcts tend to involve terminal cortical branches, producing wedge-shaped infarcts
- Cardiac echocardiography may show valve vegetations, intracardiac filling defect, or atrial or ventricular septal defect
- Best imaging tool: MR with DWI, FLAIR, T1WI C+

Top Differential Diagnoses

- Hypotensive cerebral infarction
- Multiple sclerosis
- Parenchymal metastases

Clinical Issues

- Multiple focal neurologic complaints not conforming to singular vascular distribution
- Peripheral signs of emboli, such as splinter hemorrhages or paradoxical emboli
- Cardiac source most common etiology of multiple embolic infarcts
  - May be septic or benign
- Carotid artery disease may cause multiple embolic infarct, if associated with variant PCA origin
- Cardiac and vascular evaluation ⇒ treat underlying disease

(Left) Axial NECT shows extensive bilateral hypodense infarcts in multiple vascular distributions and varying ages, typical of multiple embolic infarcts. Cardiac evaluation is important in these cases as the etiology is usually cardiac, either bland or septic emboli. (Right) Axial DWI MR shows bilateral areas of restriction ➡ related to acute ischemia in this patient with cardiac valve vegetations. DWI is helpful to determine the age of the infarcts, as they may be of varying ages.

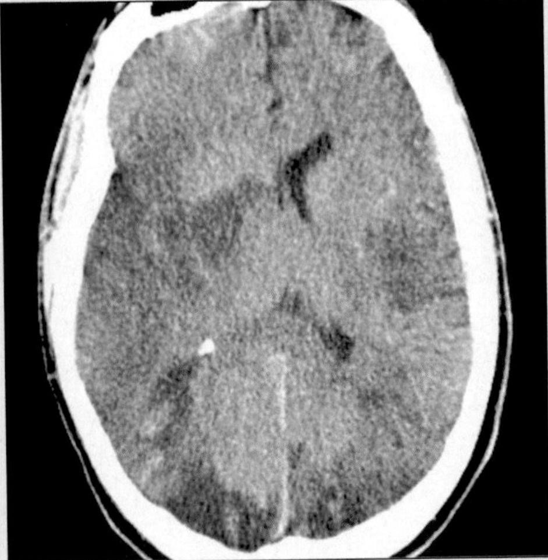

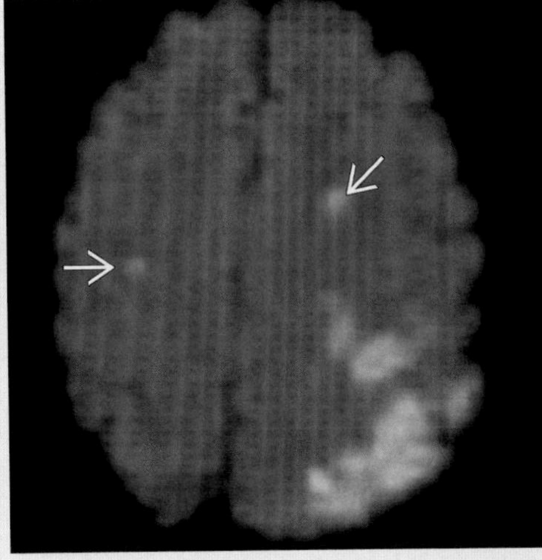

(Left) Axial DTI trace shows diffusion restriction in the left hemisphere in multiple vascular distributions. Note the involvement of the ACA distribution (head of caudate) ➡, as well as the MCA and PCA territories, in this patient with severe internal carotid artery atherosclerotic disease and a fetal origin PCA. (Right) Axial T1WI C+ FS MR shows multiple enhancing lesions in this patient with a history of septic emboli from a cardiac source. Imaging mimics metastatic disease. DWI is often helpful to differentiate infarct from neoplasm.

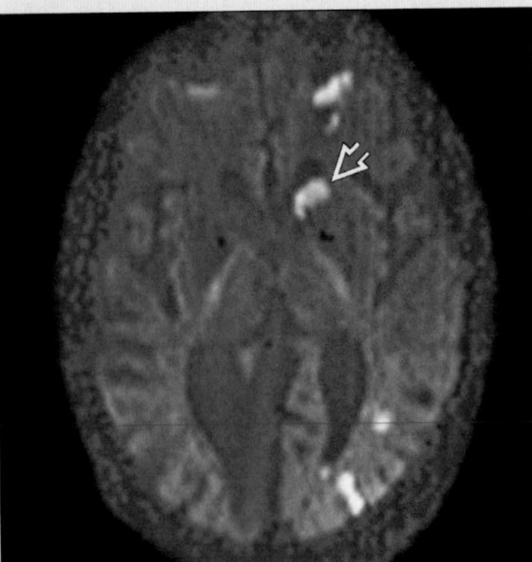

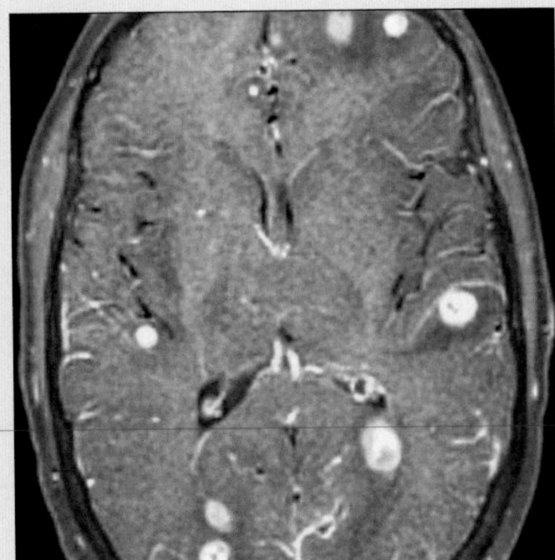

FAT EMBOLI CEREBRAL INFARCTION

Key Facts

Terminology

- Acute stroke related to fat emboli

Imaging

- Acute ischemia with appropriate clinical history
  - Long bone or pelvic fractures, cardiac surgery, joint replacement surgery
- Often mimics thromboembolic stroke
- Commonly affects both gray and white matter (WM)
  - May affect deep and periventricular WM
  - May affect deep gray nuclei
- May involve typical vascular territory
- May mimic "watershed" infarct
- NECT: Typically negative acutely
  - "Hypodense MCA" sign related to fat within MCA
- T2WI: Multiple small, scattered hyperintense foci
- DWI: Acute diffusion restriction

Top Differential Diagnoses

- Acute cerebral ischemia-infarction
- Acute hypertensive encephalopathy, PRES
- Vasculitis

Pathology

- Fat emboli can pass through pulmonary capillaries without shunting lesions and result in systemic embolization (brain, kidneys most commonly)

Clinical Issues

- Fat embolism syndrome: Pulmonary, CNS, and cutaneous manifestations
  - Hypoxia, deteriorating mental status, petechiae
- Neurological dysfunction varies from confusion to encephalopathy with coma and seizures
- Uncommon but potentially life-threatening
- Fat embolism syndrome after fractures: Up to 2.2%

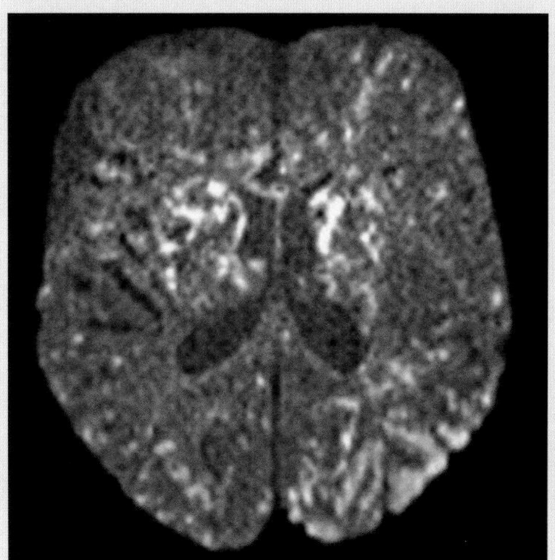

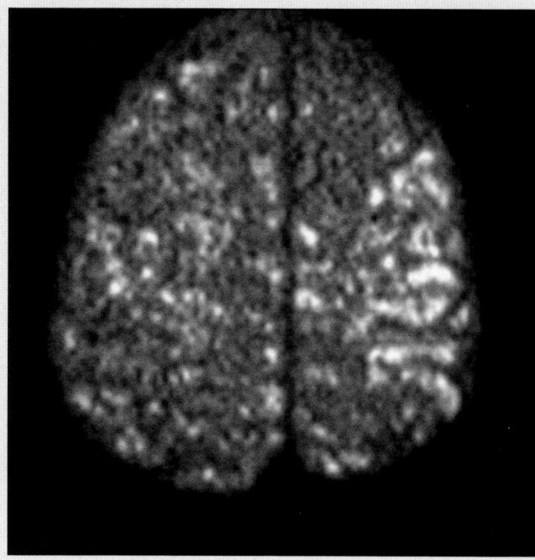

***(Left)** Axial DWI MR shows innumerable punctate foci of restriction throughout the white matter and gray matter of this 68 year old with mental status changes status post hip surgery. Note the extensive involvement of the basal ganglia and thalami. **(Right)** Axial DWI in the same patient shows the extensive foci of restriction related to acute ischemia from the patient's fat emboli. Note the more focal involvement of the left MCA territory with frontal and temporal lobe involvement.*

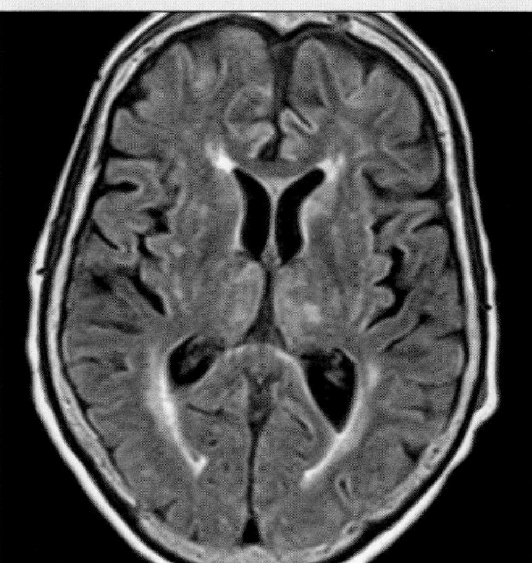

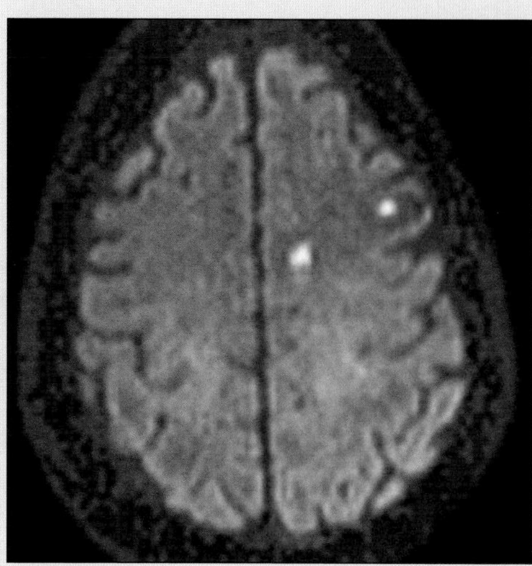

***(Left)** Axial FLAIR MR in the same patient shows minimal abnormal hyperintensities in the deep gray nuclei and periventricular white matter. Diffusion imaging is the most sensitive sequence for acute stroke imaging. **(Right)** Axial DTI trace image shows 2 punctate foci of restriction related to fat emboli in this 39-year-old trauma patient with bilateral acetabular fractures. DTI may be more sensitive than DWI in acute ischemia. Imaging of fat emboli often mimics a typical thromboembolic stroke.*

LACUNAR INFARCTION

Key Facts

Terminology

- Small, deep cerebral infarcts typically located in basal ganglia (BG), thalamus ≤ 15 mm in size

Imaging

- Commonly deep gray nuclei, especially putamen, thalamus, caudate nuclei; internal capsule, pons
  - Other locations include deep and periventricular white matter
- Range in size from microscopic to 15 mm
- Because of small size, most acute lacunar infarcts are not seen on CT scans
- Acute: T2/FLAIR increased signal
- Chronic: FLAIR central low signal with increased peripheral signal
- Restricted diffusion (hyperintense) if acute/subacute
  - May show small lesions otherwise undetectable

Pathology

- Embolic, atheromatous, or thrombotic lesions in long, single penetrating end arterioles supplying deep cerebral gray matter
- Size of lacunar infarct depends on level of occlusion and anatomy of affected vessel
- Most lacunar infarctions are clinically "silent," often subtle neurological deficits that may go unnoticed by patient and physician

Clinical Issues

- Many different presentations, depending on size, location, number
- Typical risk factors for cerebrovascular disease: Hypertension, diabetes, smoking history, obesity, hypercholesterolemia, etc.
- Lacunar infarcts account for 15-20% of all strokes

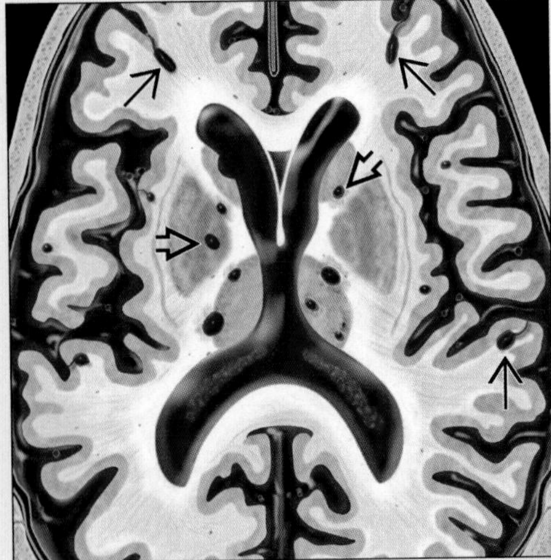

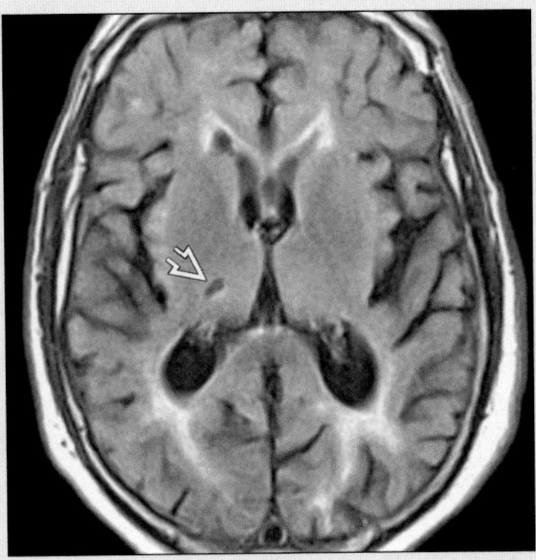

*(**Left**) Axial graphic illustrates numerous bilateral lacunar infarctions within the thalami and basal ganglia ⇨, the most common locations. Also shown are prominent perivascular (Virchow-Robin) spaces →, a common normal variant. (**Right**) Axial FLAIR MR shows a chronic lacunar infarct in the right thalamus ⇨ with central hypointense encephalomalacia and mild peripheral hyperintense gliosis. The surrounding gliosis and typical location can help differentiate a chronic lacunar infarct from a perivascular space.*

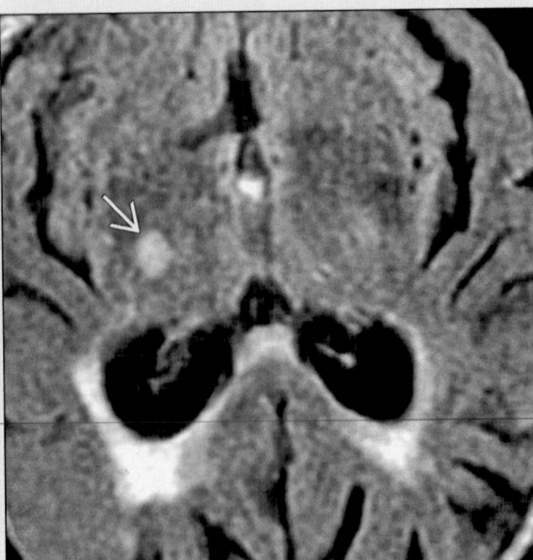

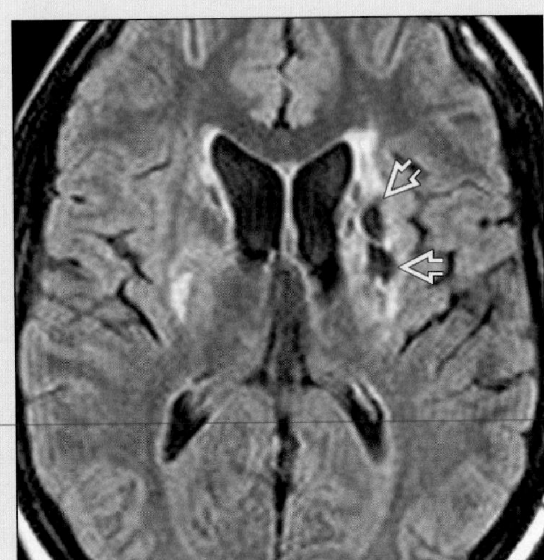

*(**Left**) Axial FLAIR MR shows hyperintensity in the right thalamus ⇨ in a patient with acute sensory symptoms. DWI showed diffusion restriction indicating acute ischemia. Lacunar infarcts are typically less than 1.5 cm in diameter and classically located in the basal ganglia, thalamus, and penetrating artery distributions, including the lenticulostriate arteries and thalamoperforating arteries. (**Right**) Axial FLAIR MR shows multiple chronic left basal ganglia lacunar infarcts ⇨ with surrounding hyperintense gliosis.*

LACUNAR INFARCTION

TERMINOLOGY

Synonyms

- Lacunar infarction (LI)
- "Lacunes"

Definitions

- Small, deep cerebral infarcts typically located in basal ganglia (BG) and thalamus, ≤ 15 mm in size
- From Latin word "lacuna," meaning hole
  - Used to describe small focus of encephalomalacia, mostly in basal ganglia
- "L'état lacunaire" or "lacunar state" = multifocal BG lacunar infarcts with surrounding gliosis

IMAGING

General Features

- Best diagnostic clue
  - Small, well-circumscribed areas of parenchymal abnormality (encephalomalacia) in BG, thalamus
- Location
  - Commonly deep gray nuclei, especially putamen, thalamus, caudate nuclei; internal capsule, pons
  - Can be in other locations
    - Subcortical white matter (WM) in patients > 65 years
    - CADASIL characteristically has subcortical lacunar infarcts
- Size
  - Ranges from microscopic to 15 mm
  - Majority < 8 mm
- Morphology
  - Typically round or ovoid

CT Findings

- NECT
  - Because of small size, most "true" lacunar infarcts are not seen on CT scans
  - Visible lacunes are seen as small, well-circumscribed areas of low (CSF) attenuation
  - Usually seen in setting of more extensive white matter disease; typically multiple
- CECT
  - May enhance if late acute/early subacute

MR Findings

- T1WI
  - Small, well-circumscribed, hypointense foci
- T2WI
  - Small, well-circumscribed, hyperintense foci
- FLAIR
  - Acute: Increased signal
  - Chronic: Central cystic portion suppresses (low signal) with increased peripheral signal
- DWI
  - Restricted diffusion (hyperintense) if acute/subacute
  - May show lesions not seen on standard sequences
- PWI
  - Abnormal PWI seen in 2/3 of cases
- T1WI C+
  - May enhance if late acute/early subacute
- MRA
  - Normal

Imaging Recommendations

- Best imaging tool
  - NECT for chronic lacunes; MR with DWI for acutely symptomatic patient
  - MR better to distinguish lacunar infarcts from perivascular spaces
- Protocol advice
  - MR with DWI if acute

DIFFERENTIAL DIAGNOSIS

Prominent Perivascular Spaces

- Normal variant resulting from accumulation of interstitial fluid within enlarged Virchow-Robin spaces
- Found in all areas but tend to cluster around anterior commissure and in cerebral WM
- Similar to CSF signal on all pulse sequences
- Found in patients of all ages
- Increase in size and frequency with advancing age
- 25% have slight halo of ↑ signal on FLAIR or T2WI
- Can expand, occur in clusters (mimic neoplasm)

Etat Crible

- Multiple enlarged Virchow-Robin spaces most commonly in basal ganglia
- Blood vessels in état criblé are thickened, ectatic, with sclerotic walls
- Perivascular tissues may show reactive astrocytosis and isomorphic gliosis with glial fibers extending along degenerated axons

Neurocysticercosis

- May mimic benign intraparenchymal cysts
- Imaging findings vary with developmental stage of cyst, as well as host response
- Solitary in 20-50%; when multiple, usually small number of cysts
- Inflammatory response around cyst may seal sulcus, making lesions appear intraaxial

PATHOLOGY

General Features

- Etiology
  - Embolic, atheromatous, or thrombotic lesions in long, single penetrating end arterioles supplying deep cerebral gray matter
    - Size of LI depends on level of occlusion and anatomy of affected vessel
  - Some studies suggest chronic endothelial dysfunction in cerebral small vessel disease and LI
    - Subtle white matter blood-brain barrier dysfunction in patients with lacunar infarcts but not with cortical ischemic strokes
  - Endothelial prothrombotic changes may be important in mediating ischemic leukoaraiosis phenotype
- Genetics
  - Usually sporadic

LACUNAR INFARCTION

- May occur secondary to genetic disorder CADASIL (cerebral autosomal dominant arteriopathy with subcortical infarcts and leukoencephalopathy)
- Associated abnormalities
  - Most lacunar infarctions are clinically "silent," often subtle neurological deficits that may go unnoticed by patient and physician
  - Small vessel cerebrovascular disease is an important vascular cause of cognitive impairment

Gross Pathologic & Surgical Features

- Similar to other types of cerebral infarction
- Earliest visible change is slight discoloration and softening of affected area
  - Gray matter structures become blurred, and white matter loses its normal fine-grained appearance
- Within 48-72 hours necrosis is well established, and there is softening, disintegration of ischemic area with circumlesional swelling
- As resolution proceeds, liquefaction results in cyst formation; more apparent in lesions of larger size
- Cysts may be traversed by trabeculations of blood vessels and are surrounded by firm glial tissue

Microscopic Features

- Gliosis along margin of infarction
- Hypertensive hyalinization of supplying arterioles
- Pigmented macrophages can be found in some lacunes, suggesting possible hemorrhagic component

CLINICAL ISSUES

Presentation

- Most common signs/symptoms
  - Many different presentations, depending on size, location, number
  - Variable symptoms, ranging from clinically "silent" to focal neurologic deficit to cognitive impairment to dementia
    - In a study of patients ≥ 65 years 23% had isolated lacunar infarcts
      - 66% of these were single, 89% of them clinically silent
  - Significant correlation between pure motor strokes and presence of lacune in internal capsule
  - About 1/4 of patients with classic lacunar syndrome have nonlacunar infarcts on MR
  - Responsible lacune only seen in about 60% of cases in lacunar syndromes
- Clinical profile
  - Elderly, hypertensive patient
  - Typical risk factors for cerebrovascular disease: Hypertension, diabetes, smoking history, obesity, hypercholesterolemia, etc.

Demographics

- Age
  - Usually > 55 years
  - Prevalence increases with age
  - Patients with coronary artery or peripheral vascular disease are at risk for infarcts at younger age
  - Patients with CADASIL present slightly earlier, with TIA/stroke-like symptoms typically beginning at about 45 years of age; cognitive decline can start as early as age 35 years
- Gender
  - Not gender specific
- Epidemiology
  - Lacunar infarcts account for 15-20% of all strokes
  - Strong association with systemic hypertension
  - Lacunar stroke is most common stroke subtype associated with vascular dementia
  - Statistically significant incidence of isolated ipsilateral carotid stenosis in patients with LI located in carotid territory

Natural History & Prognosis

- Clinically "silent" to focal neurological deficit
- Hypertension and diabetes are significant risk factors for recurrent lacunar infarction
- Many patients with LI have good functional outcomes after 5 years
  - Increased risk of mortality, stroke recurrence, physical and cognitive decline with initial severe strokes and additional vascular risk factors
- **Early** mortality and stroke recurrence less common than nonlacunar infarcts; no difference after 1 month
- Silent infarcts more than double risk of subsequent strokes and dementia
- Presence of multiple LIs may be important prognostic indicator both for functional recovery as well as higher rate of recurrence

Treatment

- Typical treatment is targeted toward underlying etiology of vasculopathy
- More studies on mechanisms, prevention, and treatment are needed to provide specific guidance on long-term management of LI patients
  - Risk-factor modification is likely to play large part in therapeutic interventions targeted at this stroke subtype

DIAGNOSTIC CHECKLIST

Consider

- Are "lacunes" Virchow-Robin spaces?
- Is there a treatable embolic source?

Image Interpretation Pearls

- To be classified as LI, location must be end-artery territory and lesion must be smaller than 15 mm

SELECTED REFERENCES

1. De Reuck J et al: The classic lacunar syndromes: clinical and neuroimaging correlates. Eur J Neurol. 15(7):681-4, 2008
2. Arboix A et al: Recurrent lacunar infarction following a previous lacunar stroke: a clinical study of 122 patients. J Neurol Neurosurg Psychiatry. 78(12):1392-4, 2007
3. Appelros P et al: Lacunar infarcts: functional and cognitive outcomes at five years in relation to MRI findings. Cerebrovasc Dis. 20(1):34-40, 2005
4. Longstreth WT Jr et al: Lacunar infarcts defined by magnetic resonance imaging of 3660 elderly people: the Cardiovascular Health Study. Arch Neurol. 55(9):1217-25, 1998

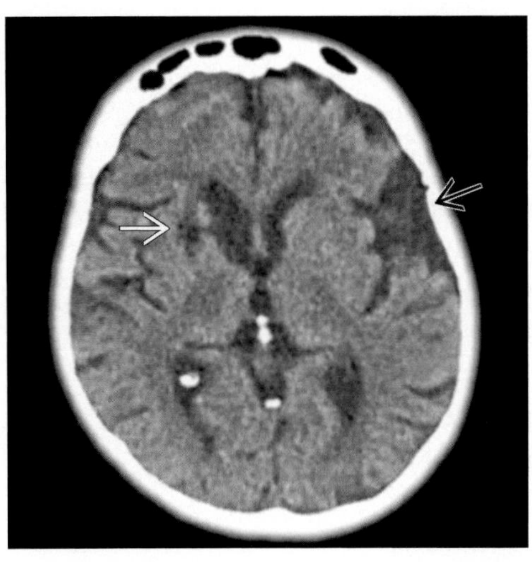

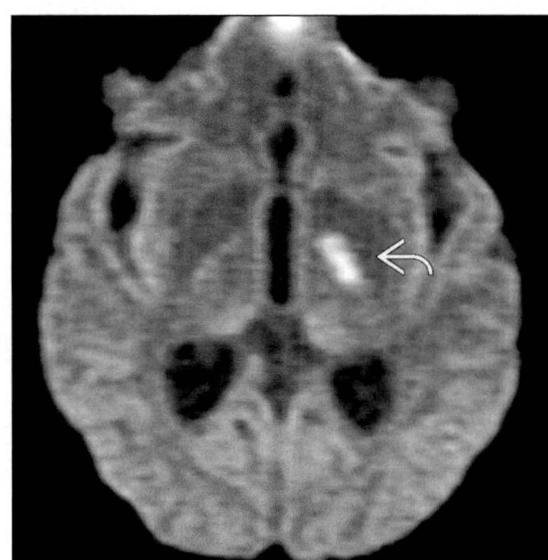

*(**Left**) Axial NECT shows a chronic lacunar infarction in the anterior limb of the right internal capsule ➔. This patient also has a small, chronic left MCA distribution infarct ➔. (**Right**) Axial DWI MR shows hyperintensity related to an acute lacunar infarct ➔ involving the corticospinal tracts in the posterior limb of the internal capsule. Lacunar infarcts in this location have a high association with motor deficits, though the majority are clinically silent. About 20% of all strokes are lacunar infarcts.*

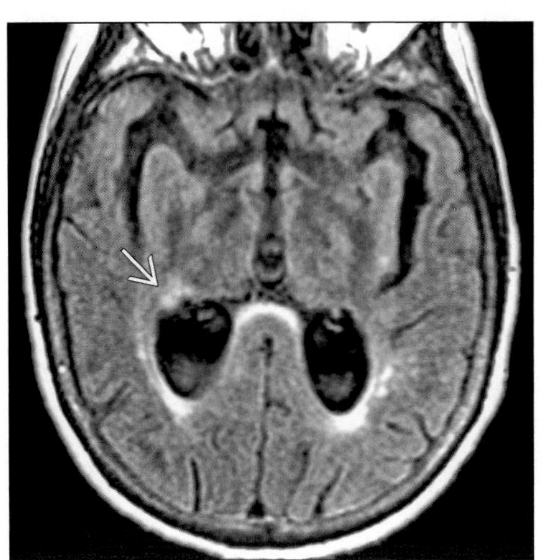

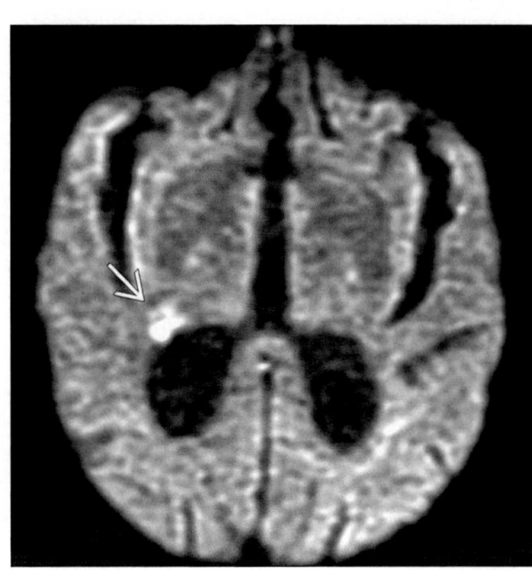

*(**Left**) Axial FLAIR MR shows bilateral periventricular hyperintensity, as well as a focal hyperintensity ➔ along the lateral thalamus related to an acute lacunar infarction. Lacunar infarcts are highly associated with vascular dementia. (**Right**) Axial DWI MR in the same patient shows hyperintensity ➔ related to acute ischemia. Without diffusion weighted imaging, it would be impossible to distinguish this acute lacune from an area of chronic small vessel disease, which commonly coexist.*

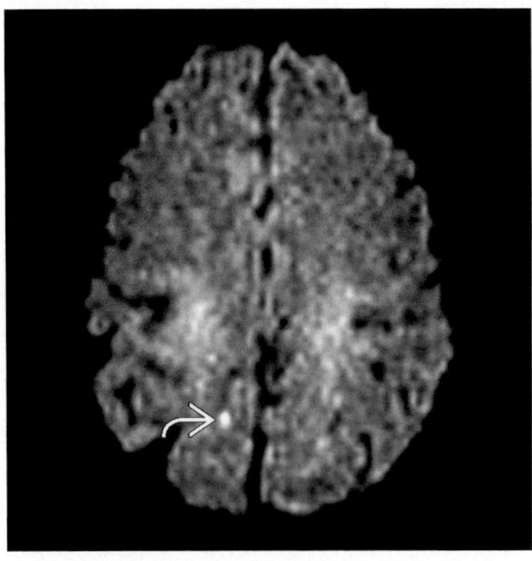

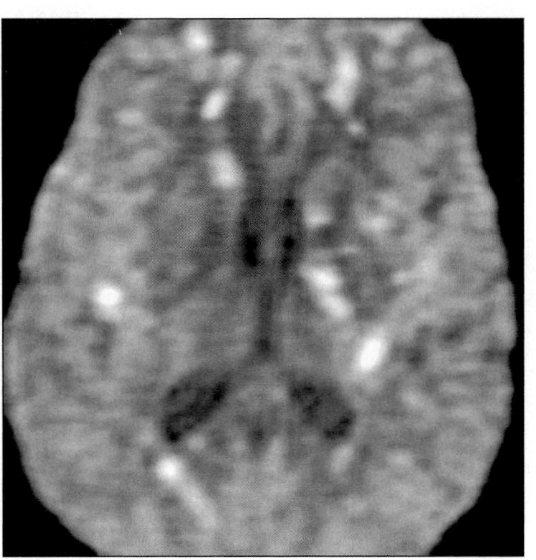

*(**Left**) Axial DWI MR shows a punctate area of diffusion restriction ➔ in a 31-year-old CADASIL patient with history of migraines and an acute presentation of numbness, which had resolved by the time of the exam. The majority of lacunar infarcts are subclinical. (**Right**) Axial DWI MR shows multiple foci of diffusion restriction related to multiple acute lacunar infarcts in this young adult with a drug abuse history. Lacunar infarcts are highly associated with systemic hypertension. (Courtesy N. Fischbein, MD.)*

CEREBRAL HYPERPERFUSION SYNDROME

Key Facts

Terminology

- Rare disorder usually occurring as complication of carotid reperfusion procedure
  - Other settings (e.g., status epilepticus, MELAS) less common
- Major increase in ipsilateral cerebral blood flow (CBF) well above normal metabolic demands

Imaging

- Gyral swelling, sulcal effacement in post-CEA patient
  - ↑ CBF, CBV on pMR
  - MR with DWI, PWI helps in differential diagnosis

Top Differential Diagnoses

- Acute cerebral ischemia-infarction
- Status epilepticus
- MELAS
- Acute hypertensive encephalopathy, PRES
- Hypercapnia

Pathology

- CHS probably caused by maladaptive autoregulatory mechanisms, altered cerebral hemodynamics
  - "Normal perfusion pressure breakthrough"
  - Rapid restoration of normal perfusion following revascularization → hyperperfusion in previously underperfused brain

Clinical Issues

- Unilateral headache, face/eye pain
- Focal neurologic deficit
- 5-10% of post-CEA patients develop mild CHS

Diagnostic Checklist

- Need to distinguish stroke/TIA from CHS!

*(**Left**) Axial NECT in a patient with right-sided weakness after a carotid endarterectomy shows gyral swelling and sulcal effacement ➔ in the left parietooccipital area. (**Right**) Axial CT perfusion shows increased diameter and intravascular enhancement in the vascular distribution of the left internal carotid artery ➔. The time to peak (not shown) was shortened, probably because of hyperperfusion and rapid flow.*

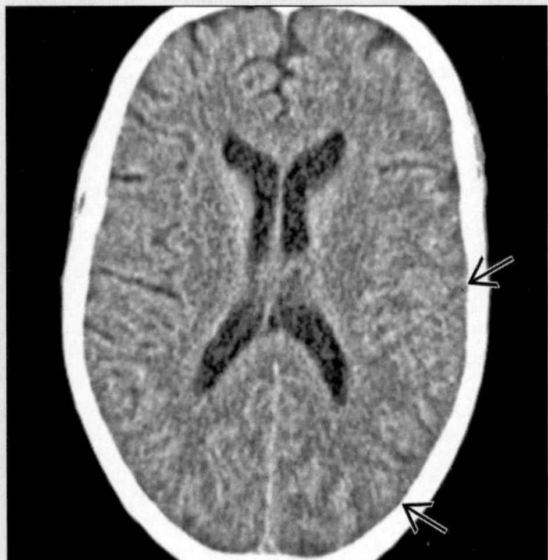

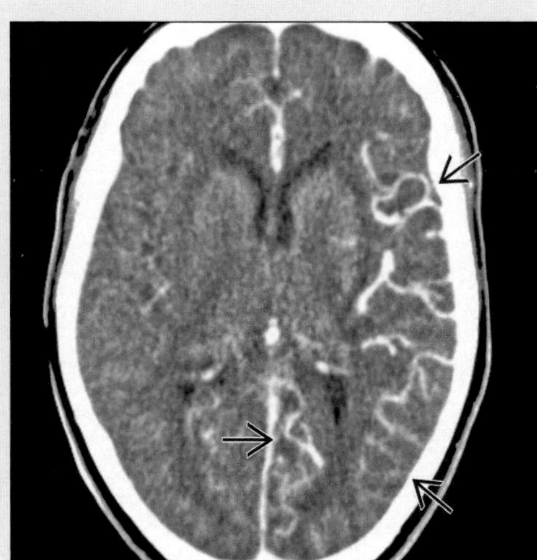

*(**Left**) Axial FLAIR MR in the same patient shows hyperintensity in the cortex ➔ and basal ganglia ➔. (**Right**) Coronal T1WI C+ MR in the same patient reveals contrast extravasation in the left posterior temporal lobe ➔, suggesting damage to the blood-brain barrier.*

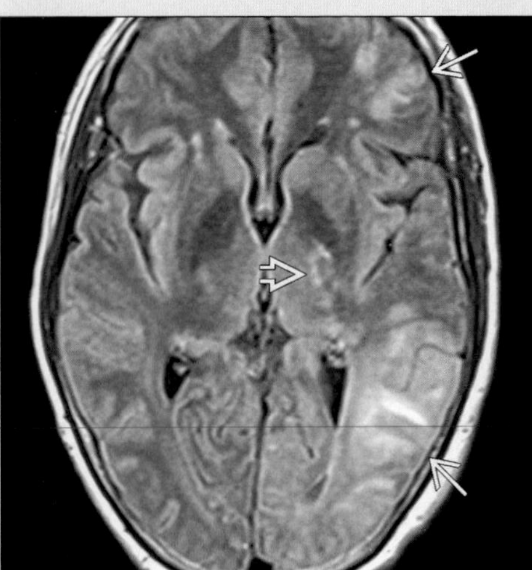

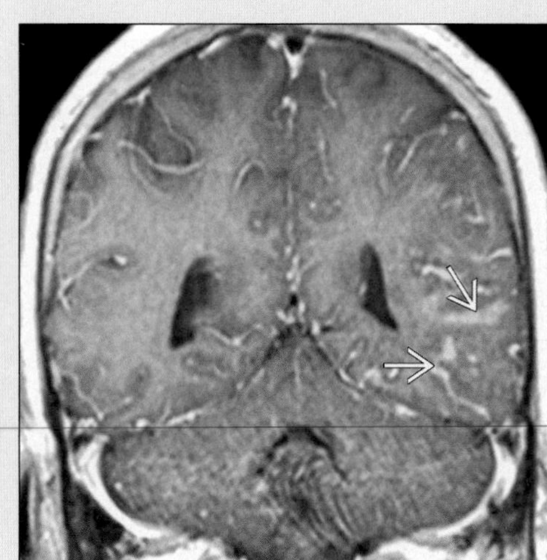

CEREBRAL HYPERPERFUSION SYNDROME

TERMINOLOGY

Abbreviations

- Cerebral hyperperfusion syndrome (CHS)

Synonyms

- Post-carotid endarterectomy hyperperfusion
- Luxury perfusion

Definitions

- Rare (1-3%) but potentially devastating disorder usually occurring as complication of carotid reperfusion procedures
  - Mildly ↑ CBF common after carotid endarterectomy (CEA), typically asymptomatic
  - CHS defined as ≥ 100% increase in rCBF compared to preoperative values
- Major increase in ipsilateral CBF well above normal metabolic demands
  - Usually following carotid revascularization procedure
    - Carotid endarterectomy
    - Angioplasty
    - Stenting
    - Thrombolysis
  - May occur in other settings (e.g., status epilepticus, MELAS)

IMAGING

General Features

- Best diagnostic clue
  - Gyral swelling, sulcal effacement in post-CEA patient
  - ↑ CBF, CBV on perfusion MR (pMR), perfusion CT (pCT)
- Size
  - Variable
- Morphology
  - Follows vascular distribution

Imaging Recommendations

- Best imaging tool
  - MR with DWI, PWI
  - SPECT
- Protocol advice
  - Add T2* (GRE or SWI) to look for hemorrhage

CT Findings

- NECT
  - Gyral swelling
  - Cortical effacement
  - ± hypodensity (may occur without attenuation alterations)
  - Frank hemorrhage in < 1%
- CECT
  - Prominent vessels with ↑ intravascular enhancement
  - May demonstrate contrast extravasation in severe cases (rare)

MR Findings

- T1WI
  - Cortical swelling
  - ± mild hypointensity
  - Sulci effaced
- T2WI
  - Gyral swelling, hyperintensity
- FLAIR
  - Hyperintense cortex
- T2* GRE
  - Frank hemorrhage in < 1%
  - "Blooming" on GRE or SWI
- DWI
  - Usually normal as edema is vasogenic, not cytotoxic
  - Approximately 25% show small foci of restricted diffusion compared to preoperative DWI
- PWI
  - Elevated CBV, CBF
  - Prolonged MTT
    - Side-to-side difference of 3 seconds predictive of CHS
- T1WI C+
  - May be normal
  - May show slightly increased prominence of cerebral vessels
  - Parenchymal enhancement in severe cases
- MRA
  - Preoperative ↓ signal intensity in MCA may identify patients at risk for CHS

Other Modality Findings

- SPECT
  - N-isopropyl-p-I-123-iodoamphetamine or I-123-iomazenil SPECT
    - Shows hyperperfusion in ipsilateral cerebral hemisphere after surgery
    - Can be detected even in asymptomatic patients
    - May be correlated with long-term neuronal damage that CT, MR do not detect
    - May be associated with crossed cerebellar diaschisis

DIFFERENTIAL DIAGNOSIS

Acute Cerebral Ischemia-Infarction

- Time-to-peak/mean transit time prolonged (not decreased)
- Typically shows restriction on DWI (CHS often negative)

Status Epilepticus

- Metabolic hyperperfusion in affected brain
- History of seizure helpful but may not be available

Acute Hypertensive Encephalopathy, PRES

- Failed autoregulation → hyperperfusion → endothelial injury/vasogenic edema
- Predilection for posterior circulation
- Markedly elevated blood pressure (many etiologies)
  - Eclampsia, preeclampsia
  - Chemotherapy
  - Renal failure
  - Hemolytic uremic syndrome/thrombotic thrombocytopenic purpura
  - Drug abuse (especially cocaine)

CEREBRAL HYPERPERFUSION SYNDROME

MELAS

- Acute oxidative phosphorylation defect
- Stroke-like episodes related to vasogenic edema, hyperperfusion, neuronal damage
- Cortical hyperintensity, enhancement
- Perform MRS in unaffected region, look for lactate

Hypercapnia

- Carbon dioxide is potent stimulator of CBF
- Vasodilatory effect on cerebral vasculature

PATHOLOGY

General Features

- Etiology
  - Cognitive impairment after CEA/stenting may result from
    - Cerebral embolization during dissection, stenting
    - Global cerebral hypoperfusion during carotid cross-clamping
    - Cerebral hyperperfusion syndrome
  - CHS probably caused by maladaptive autoregulatory mechanisms, altered cerebral hemodynamics
    - "Normal perfusion pressure breakthrough"
      - Chronic ischemia → impaired autoregulation
      - Loss of normal vasoconstriction
      - "Resistance" vessels become chronically dilated
      - Rapid restoration of normal perfusion following revascularization → hyperperfusion in previously underperfused brain

CLINICAL ISSUES

Presentation

- Characterized by
  - Variable cognitive impairment
  - Focal neurologic deficit
- Other signs/symptoms
  - Unilateral headache
  - Face, eye pain
  - Seizure

Demographics

- Age
  - For post-endarterectomy CHS, generally older patients
  - For other etiologies (e.g., seizure, MELAS), any age
- Epidemiology
  - 5-10% of post-CEA patients develop mild CHS
  - Covariate clinical risk factors
    - Age
    - Hypertension (especially postoperative)
    - Diabetes
    - Bilateral lesions
    - Extent of ICA stenosis
      - High grade > low grade
    - Presence of contralateral carotid occlusion or high-grade stenosis
    - Duration of cross-clamping
    - Diminished carotid reserve
    - Poor collateral blood flow
    - Decreased cerebrovascular reactivity to acetazolamide challenge

Natural History & Prognosis

- Neurologic deficits in CHS without intracranial hemorrhage
  - Usually reversible
  - No major tissue destruction
  - May result in persistent mild cognitive impairment
- 1% of CHS with intracranial hemorrhage
  - Poor prognosis

Treatment

- Prevention
  - Minimize intraoperative cerebral ischemia
  - Consider continuing postoperative anesthesia/ continuous sedation
  - Strict postoperative blood pressure control

DIAGNOSTIC CHECKLIST

Consider

- Post-CEA/carotid artery stenting patient with neurologic deficit? Need to distinguish stroke/ transient ischemic attack from CHS!

SELECTED REFERENCES

1. Brantley HP et al: Hyperperfusion syndrome following carotid artery stenting: the largest single-operator series to date. J Invasive Cardiol. 21(1):27-30, 2009
2. Grunwald IQ et al: Hyperperfusion syndrome after carotid stent angioplasty. Neuroradiology. 51(3):169-74, 2009
3. Kuroda H et al: Prediction of cerebral hyperperfusion after carotid endarterectomy using middle cerebral artery signal intensity in preoperative single-slab 3-dimensional time-of-flight magnetic resonance angiography. Neurosurgery. 64(6):1065-71; discussion 1071-2, 2009
4. Medel R et al: Hyperperfusion syndrome following endovascular cerebral revascularization. Neurosurg Focus. 26(3):E4, 2009
5. Moulakakis KG et al: Hyperperfusion syndrome after carotid revascularization. J Vasc Surg. 49(4):1060-8, 2009
6. Tseng YC et al: Prediction of cerebral hyperperfusion syndrome after carotid stenting: a cerebral perfusion computed tomography study. J Comput Assist Tomogr. 33(4):540-5, 2009
7. Hirooka R et al: Magnetic resonance imaging in patients with cerebral hyperperfusion and cognitive impairment after carotid endarterectomy. J Neurosurg. 108(6):1178-83, 2008
8. Wichert-Ana L et al: Ictal technetium-99 m ethyl cysteinate dimer single-photon emission tomographic findings in epileptic patients with polymicrogyria syndromes: a subtraction of ictal-interictal SPECT coregistered to MRI study. Eur J Nucl Med Mol Imaging. 35(6):1159-70, 2008
9. Fukuda T et al: Prediction of cerebral hyperperfusion after carotid endarterectomy using cerebral blood volume measured by perfusion-weighted MR imaging compared with single-photon emission CT. AJNR Am J Neuroradiol. 28(4):737-42, 2007
10. Muehlschlegel S et al: CT angiography and CT perfusion in post-CEA hyperperfusion syndrome. Neurology. 68(17):1437, 2007

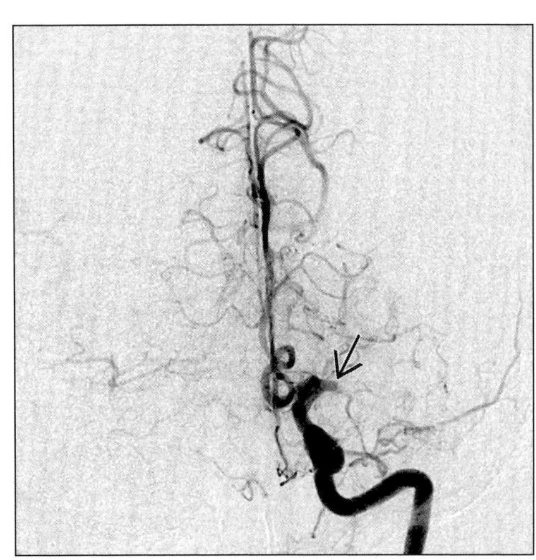

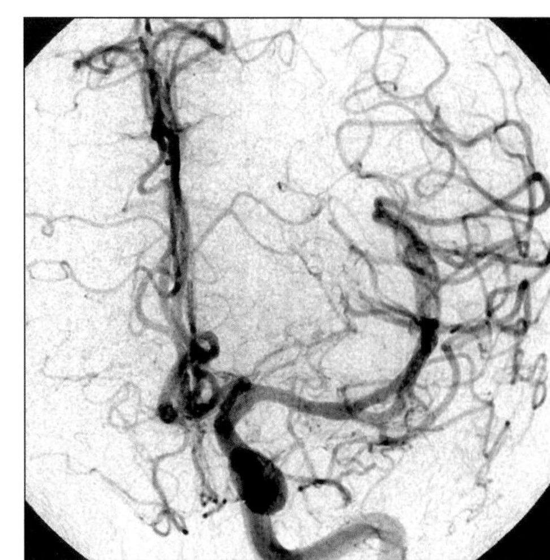

(Left) *Anteroposterior view of DSA shows abrupt occlusion of the left middle cerebral artery just distal to its origin → in a patient with a sudden onset of right-sided weakness and stroke-like symptoms. Little collateral filling of the distal MCA is seen.* ***(Right)*** *After superselective catheterization of the left MCA and infusion of tissue plasminogen activator for 2 hours, normal circulation was restored, as shown on this anteroposterior DSA.*

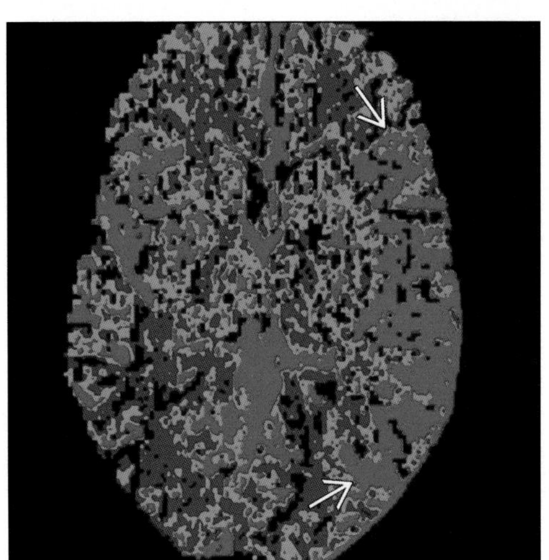

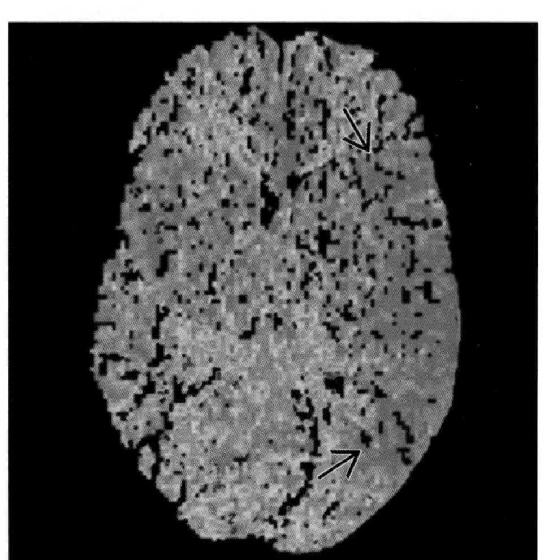

(Left) *Following restoration of normal blood flow in the previously occluded left MCA, the patient experienced worsening right-sided weakness and throbbing headache. This axial MR perfusion study shows elevated (red area →), not decreased, CBF in the left temporal and parietal lobes.* ***(Right)*** *Axial MR perfusion in the same case shows elevated cerebral blood volume →.*

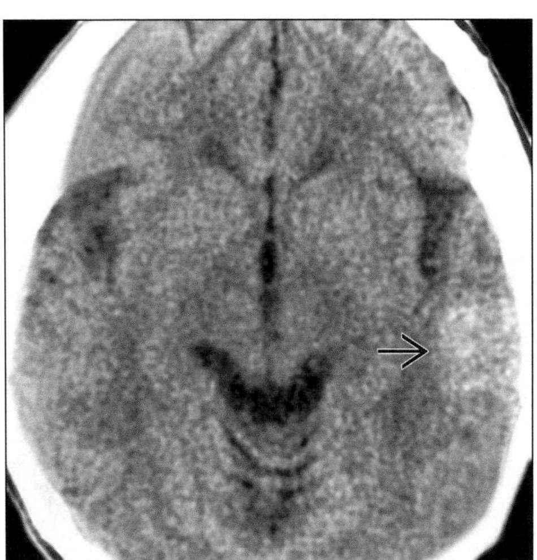

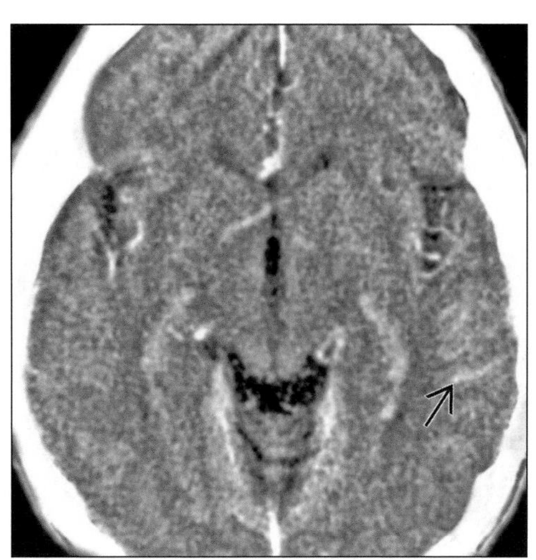

(Left) *Axial NECT in a 30 year old was obtained 36 hours after a prolonged seizure. Note the mildly hyperdense area → that could represent increased cerebral blood volume.* ***(Right)*** *Axial CECT in the same patient shows some enhancement → in the same area, indicating some degree of blood-brain barrier disruption. Cerebral hyperperfusion can be caused by hypermetabolism in the affected cortex following status epilepticus.*

CEREBRAL HYPERPERFUSION SYNDROME

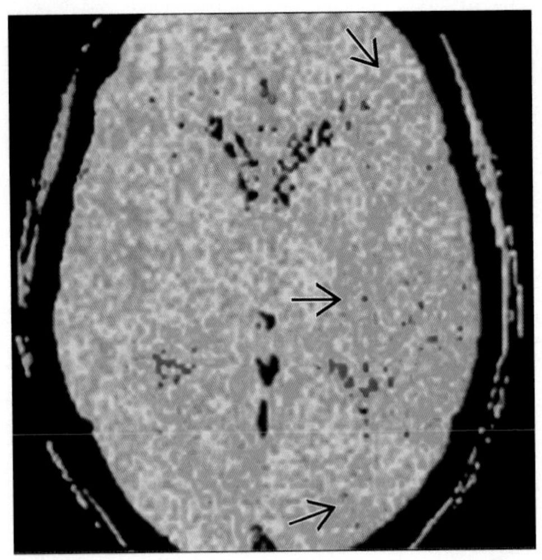

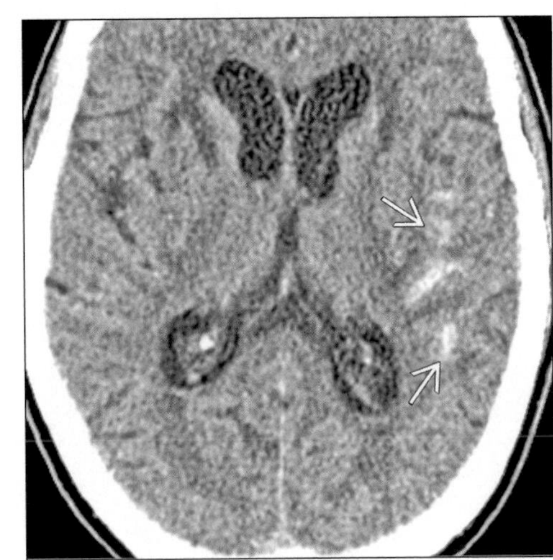

*(**Left**) Axial MR perfusion was obtained prior to angioplasty and stenting in a patient with high-grade left carotid stenosis. Note the decreased perfusion with diminished CBV in the left temporoparietal region ➙. (**Right**) Axial NECT was obtained when the patient developed aphasia and right upper extremity weakness 3 hours after the procedure to "rule out stroke." Note the gyral swelling, sulcal effacement, and high-density foci ➔ suggesting hemorrhage in the left temporal lobe.*

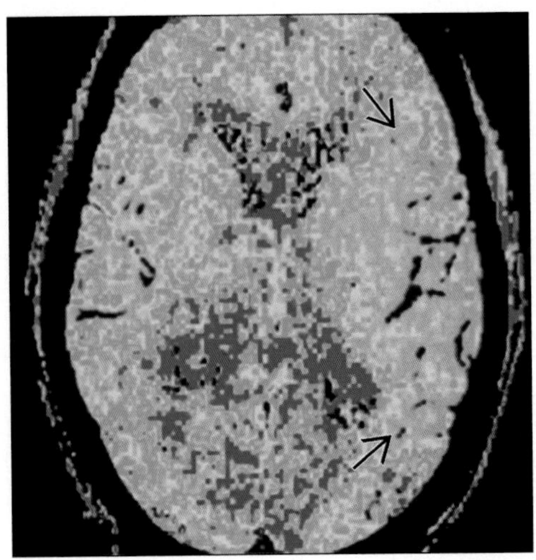

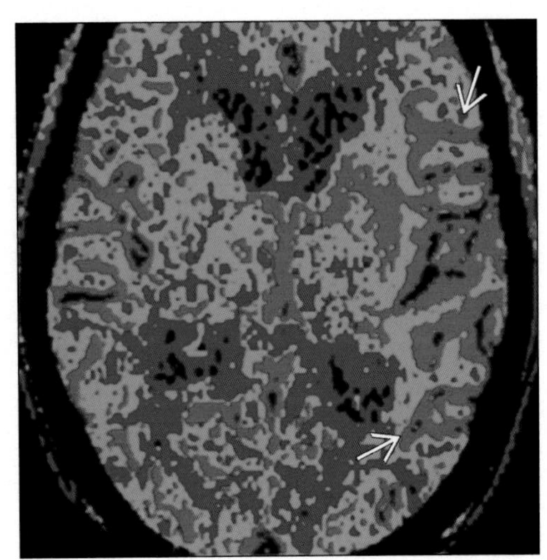

*(**Left**) Repeat axial MR perfusion was then obtained. Even though the color scale of this image appears different, the previously underperfused left temporal lobe and basal ganglia now appear relatively hyperperfused ➙ compared to the contralateral hemisphere. (**Right**) Axial MR perfusion in the same patient shows elevated cerebral blood flow in the left temporal lobe ➔, consistent with cerebral hyperperfusion syndrome.*

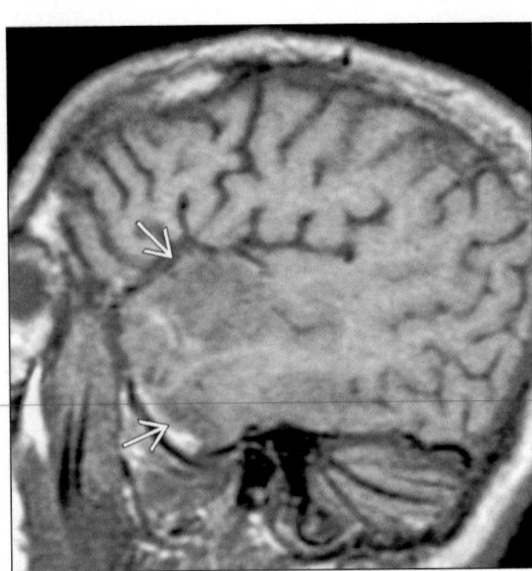

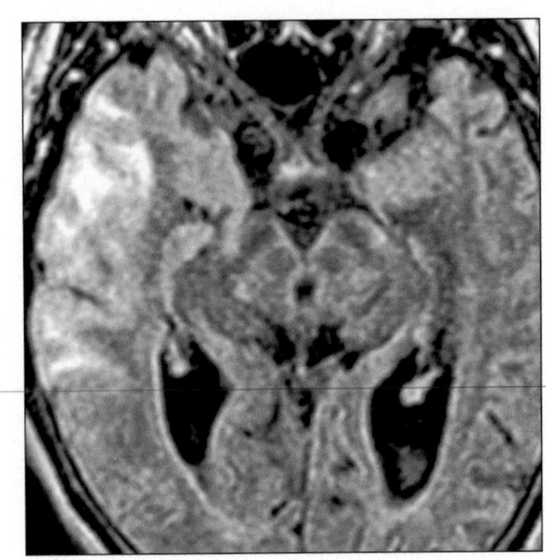

*(**Left**) Sagittal T1WI MR in a 33 year old with acute onset of stroke-like symptoms shows swollen, hypointense gyri in the temporal lobe ➔. (**Right**) Axial FLAIR MR in the same patient shows hyperintensity in the right temporal lobe cortex and subcortical white matter. MRS in the normal unaffected brain showed a lactate peak (not shown), and a subsequent work-up disclosed MELAS.*

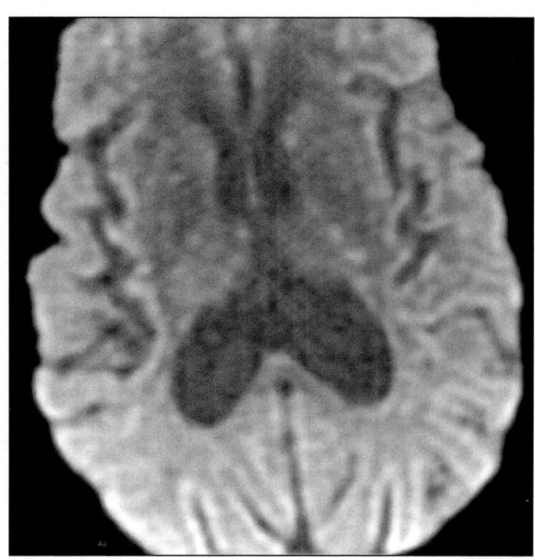

(Left) *This elderly patient with left hemiparesis, who had been "found down," had a normal CT scan. This axial FLAIR MR obtained to "rule out stroke" is also normal.* **(Right)** *Axial DWI MR in the same patient shows no evidence of diffusion restriction that would otherwise suggest cerebral ischemia-infarction.*

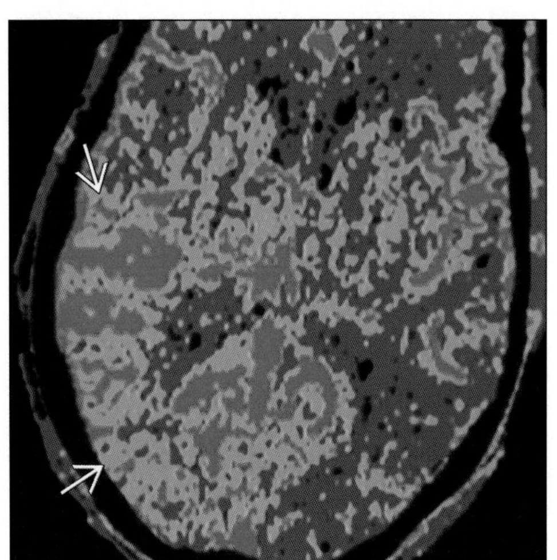

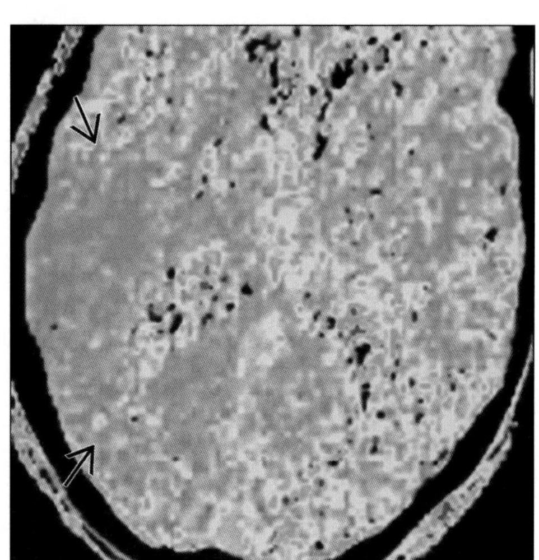

(Left) *Axial MR perfusion in the same patient shows elevated cerebral blood flow ➔.* **(Right)** *Axial MR perfusion again shows markedly increased cerebral blood volume ⇨. The patient's left-sided weakness resolved over the next several hours. It was concluded that the patient had experienced an unobserved seizure with Todd paralysis and that the elevated CBV and CBF were from seizure-induced hyperperfusion.*

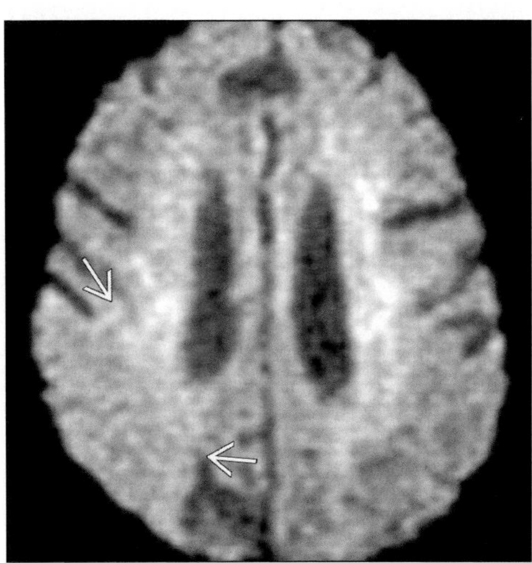

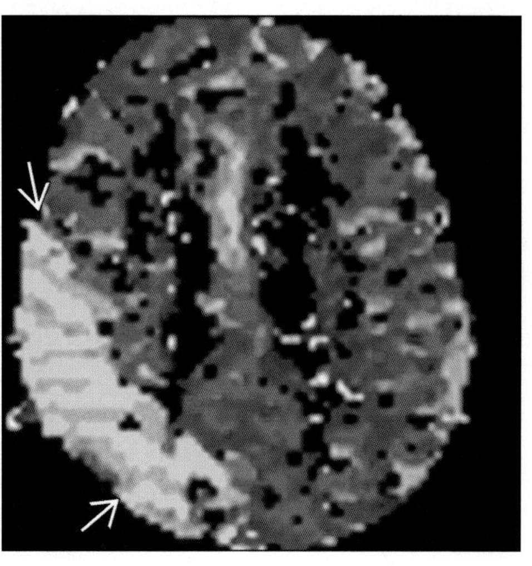

(Left) *Axial DWI MR in a 73-year-old woman who had a history of high blood pressure, elevated cholesterol, and left hemiparesis following seizure shows no definite abnormality although the right parietal lobe ➔ appears very slightly hyperintense.* **(Right)** *Axial PWI MR in the same case shows markedly elevated cerebral blood volume in the right parietal lobe ➔. The hemiparesis (a Todd paralysis) resolved slowly over the next week. Follow-up pMR (not shown) was normal.*

CAVERNOUS SINUS THROMBOSIS/THROMBOPHLEBITIS

Key Facts

Terminology

- Cavernous sinus thrombosis/thrombophlebitis (CST)
- CST = blood clot in CS

Imaging

- Relevant anatomy
  - CSs = trabeculated venous cavities
  - Receive blood from multiple valveless veins
  - Blood flows in any direction (depending on pressure gradient)
- CT findings often subtle or negative in CST
- Look for
  - Enlarged CS with convex margins
  - Filling defects in CS
  - Enlarged superior ophthalmic vein ± clot, proptosis
  - Enlarged extra-ocular muscles

Top Differential Diagnoses

- Cavernous sinus neoplasm
  - Meningioma, lymphoma, metastasis
- Cavernous carotid aneurysm, fistula
- Infection/inflammation
  - Tolosa/Hunt, sarcoid, Wegener

Pathology

- Often complication of sinusitis/midface infection
  - *S. aureus* most common pathogen

Clinical Issues

- Headache most common early symptom
- Orbital pain, ophthalmoplegia, visual loss

Diagnostic Checklist

- Clinical setting + high index of suspicion
- Negative CT ⇒ MR/MRV or CTA

(Left) Axial T1WI MR shows enlargement of the right cavernous sinus ➡ with material isointense to gray matter. There is mild narrowing of the cavernous internal carotid artery ➡. The patient presented with sphenoethmoidal sinusitis, headache, right 6th nerve palsy, and mild right proptosis. *(Right)* Axial T2WI MR shows mild enlargement and a convex margin of the right cavernous sinus with heterogeneous, hyperintense tissue ➡.

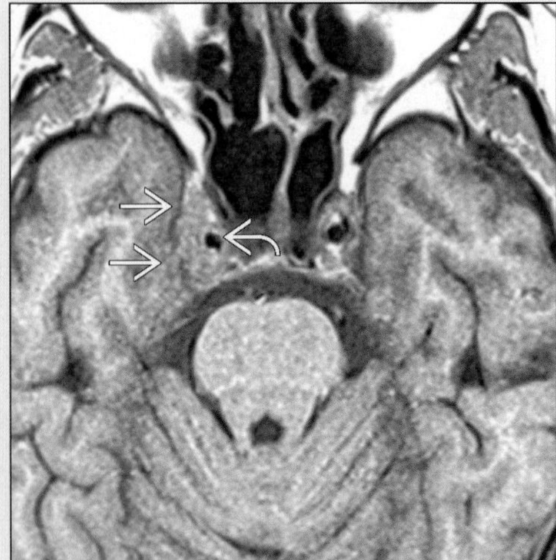

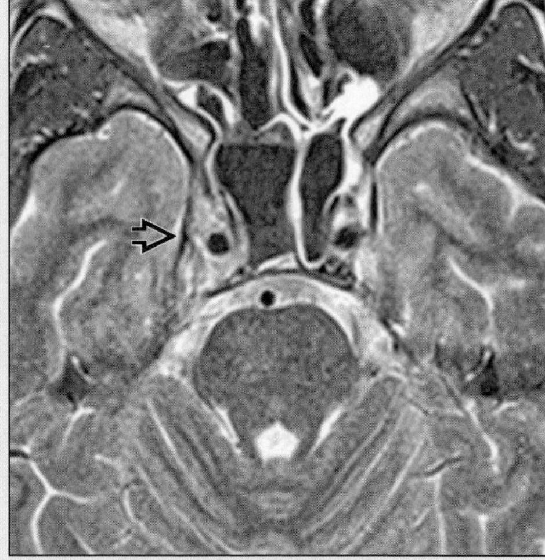

(Left) Axial T1WI C+ MR of bilateral cavernous sinus thrombosis complicating acute pansinusitis. There are filling defects ➡ within the cavernous sinuses consistent with clot. There is prominent enhancement of the lateral dural margins of the CSs ➡ and bilateral proptosis due to venous congestion. *(Right)* Axial DWI MR shows hyperintense clot in the bilateral cavernous sinuses ➡.

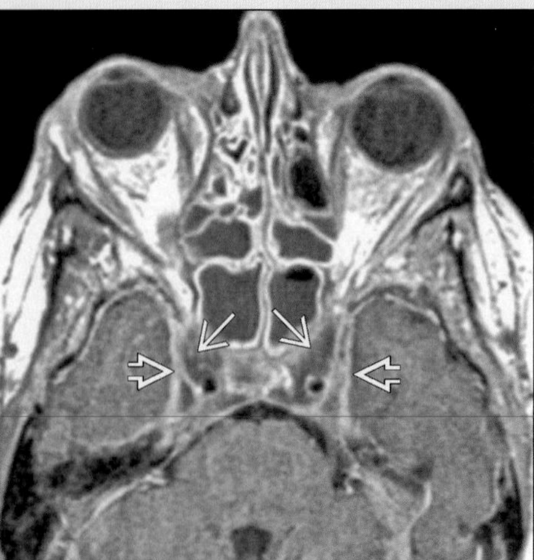

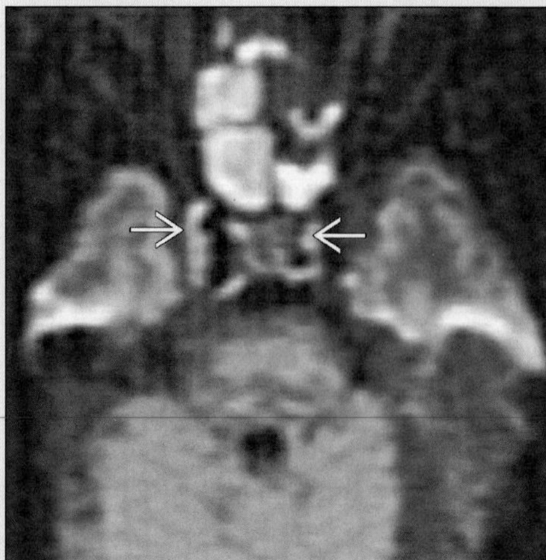

CAVERNOUS SINUS THROMBOSIS/THROMBOPHLEBITIS

TERMINOLOGY

Abbreviations

- Cavernous sinus thrombosis/thrombophlebitis (CST)

Definitions

- CST = blood clot in cavernous sinus (CS)

IMAGING

General Features

- Best diagnostic clue
  - Appropriate clinical setting + high index of suspicion
- Location
  - Relevant anatomy
    - CSs = trabeculated venous cavities (not single pool of blood)
    - Multiple venous interconnections
    - Receive blood from multiple valveless veins
      - Facial veins (via superior ophthalmic vein [SOV], inferior ophthalmic vein [IOV])
      - Sphenoid, deep middle cerebral veins
    - CSs drain into inferior petrosal sinuses ⇒ IJVs
    - Also superior petrosal sinuses ⇒ sigmoid sinuses
    - Blood flows in any direction (depending on pressure gradient)

Imaging Recommendations

- Best imaging tool
  - CTA; MR ± contrast
    - 1-3 mm sections through orbits, CSs

CT Findings

- NECT
  - Findings often subtle or negative
- CECT
  - Filling defects in involved CS
    - CS margins convex, not flat/concave
  - Orbits: SOVs ↑ ± clot
    - Proptosis, enlarged extra-ocular muscles
- CTA/CTV
  - Filling defects in 1 or both CSs

MR Findings

- T1WI
  - Convex, enlarged CS isointense to gray matter
- T2WI
  - Heterogeneous high signal intensity in CS
- DWI
  - May see hyperintense clot in CS
- T1WI C+
  - Variable; classic = filling defects in CS

DIFFERENTIAL DIAGNOSIS

Cavernous Sinus Neoplasm

- Meningioma, schwannoma
- Metastasis, lymphoma, invasive carcinomas

Cavernous Carotid Aneurysm, Fistula

- "Flow voids"

Infection/Inflammation

- Tolosa-Hunt, sarcoid, Wegener

PATHOLOGY

General Features

- Etiology
  - Complication of sinusitis or infection
    - Usually in midface (furuncle), orbits, or tonsils
    - *S. aureus* most common pathogen ± bacteremia
  - Miscellaneous causes: Trauma
    - Otomastoiditis, odontogenic infection
    - Underlying malignancy

CLINICAL ISSUES

Presentation

- Most common signs/symptoms
  - Headache most common early symptom
    - Often localized to regions innervated by V1 and V2
  - Orbital pain, periorbital edema, chemosis
  - Ptosis, ophthalmoplegia, visual loss
- Other signs/symptoms
  - Hypoesthesia or hyperesthesia in V1 and V2 dermatomes
  - Decreased pupillary responses
  - Signs/sx in contralateral eye diagnostic of CST
  - Meningeal signs
  - Systemic signs indicative of sepsis are late findings

Demographics

- Epidemiology
  - *S. aureus* ~ 70% of infections
  - *S. pneumoniae*, gram-rods, anaerobes
  - Fungi (*Aspergillus*, *Rhizopus*) rare

Natural History & Prognosis

- Without therapy, signs appear in contralateral eye in 24-48 hours
  - Spread via communicating veins to contralateral CS
- Can be fatal (death from sepsis or CNS involvement)
- Incidence/fatality significantly ↓ with early antibiotics
- Complete recovery infrequent
  - Permanent visual impairment (15%)
  - Cranial nerve deficits (50%)

Treatment

- Intravenous antibiotics
- Supportive care, hydration, steroids

DIAGNOSTIC CHECKLIST

Image Interpretation Pearls

- Maintain high clinical suspicion
- Negative CT ⇒ MR/MRV or CTA

SELECTED REFERENCES

1. Agayev A et al: Images in clinical medicine. Cavernous sinus thrombosis. N Engl J Med. 359(21):2266, 2008

DURAL SINUS THROMBOSIS

Key Facts

Imaging

- General features
  - "Empty delta" sign on CECT, T1WI C+ MR
- CT
  - Hyperdense sinus on NECT
  - ± hyperdense cortical veins ("cord" sign)
  - CTV: Filling defect (thrombus) in dural sinus
- MR
  - Hypointense thrombus "blooms" on T2* GRE
  - Absence of flow in occluded sinus on 2D TOF MRV
- Protocol recommendations
  - NECT, CECT scans ± CTV as initial screening
  - If CTs negative, MR + MRV (T2*, DWI, T1WI C+)
  - If MRV equivocal, DSA is gold standard

Top Differential Diagnoses

- Normal: Arteries, veins normally slightly hyperdense
- Dural sinus hypoplasia/aplasia
  - No "blooming"; collaterals/venous infarcts absent
- "Giant" arachnoid granulations
  - Round/ovoid, not elongated like thrombus
- Acute subdural hematoma
  - Blood layered on tentorium can mimic transverse sinus (TS) thrombosis

Diagnostic Checklist

- Review MRV source images
  - Exclude pseudo-occlusions (e.g., hypoplastic TS)
- Review T1 images to exclude false-negative MRV
- Review NECT to exclude dense thrombus as false-negative CECT or CTV
- Brain looks normal? Does not exclude CVT!
- DSA helpful if noninvasive imaging inconclusive
- Chronic thrombosis may enhance
  - Recanalization or granulation tissue enhances
  - Can look bizarre, mimic neoplasm

(Left) Sagittal graphic shows thrombosis of the superior sagittal sinus ➡ and straight sinus ⮊. Inset in the upper left reveals a thrombus in the superior sagittal sinus in cross section ("empty delta" sign) ➦ seen on contrast-enhanced imaging. ***(Right)*** *Coronal T1WI C+ MR shows a filling defect ("delta" sign) due to thrombus in the superior sagittal sinus ⮊, consistent with acute thrombosis. Note the left parietal edema ➡ and vascular congestion due to regional cortical vein extension ➦.*

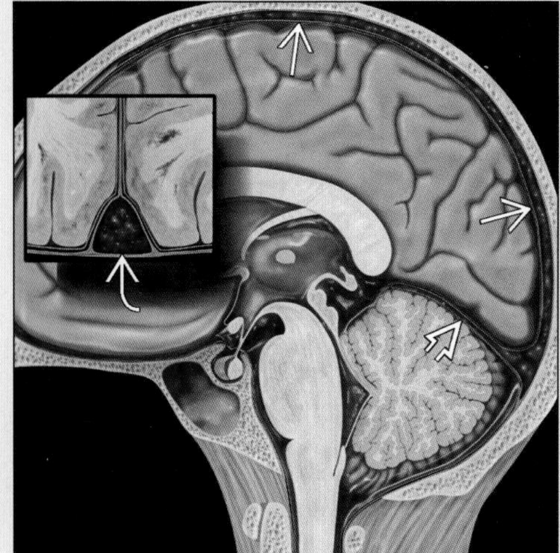

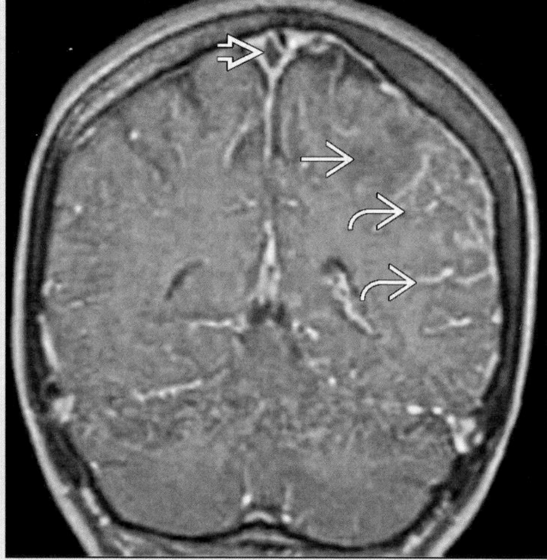

(Left) Axial CTA shows pseudopatent appearance of the deep cerebral veins ➡ and the torcular herophili ⮊ due to inherent high attenuation of clot, a source of potential false-negative CTA/CTV. ***(Right)*** *Axial NECT in the same patient shows high attenuation in the deep cerebral veins ➡ and torcular herophili ⮊, confirming acute venous thrombosis. NECT should always be obtained concurrently with CECT or CTV to avoid potential false-negatives.*

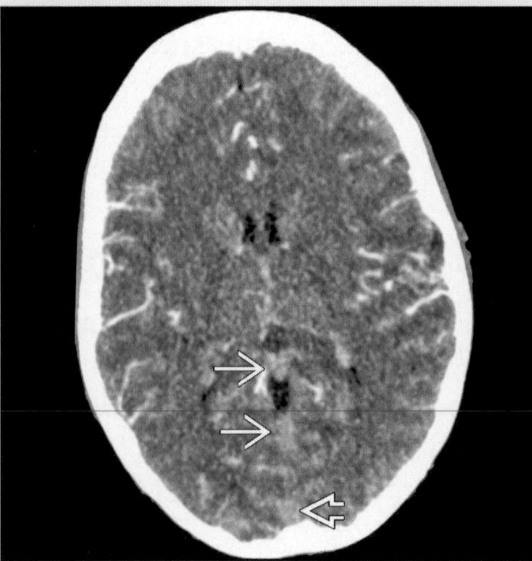

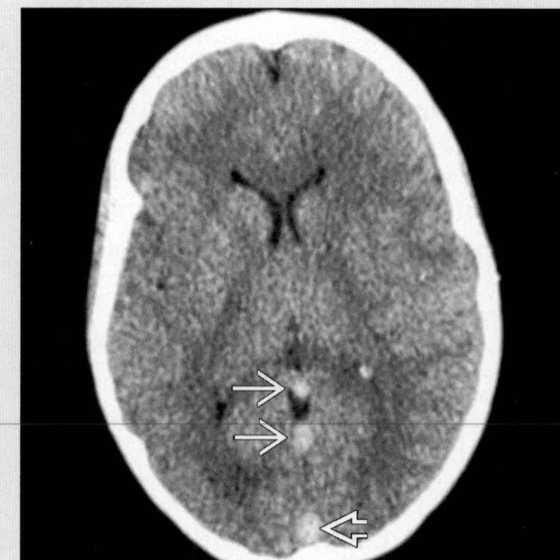

DURAL SINUS THROMBOSIS

TERMINOLOGY

Abbreviations

- Dural sinus thrombosis (DST)
- Cerebral vein thrombosis (CVT)

Definitions

- Thrombotic occlusion of intracranial dural sinuses

IMAGING

General Features

- Best diagnostic clue
  - **"Empty delta" sign** on CECT, T1WI C+ MR
- Location
  - Thrombus in dural sinus ± adjacent cortical vein(s)

CT Findings

- NECT
  - Early imaging findings often subtle
  - Hyperdense sinus (compared to carotid arteries)
  - ± hyperdense cortical veins (**"cord" sign**)
  - ± venous infarct (in 50% of cases)
    - Cortical/subcortical petechial hemorrhages, edema
    - Straight sinus (SS) ± internal cerebral veins (ICV) occlusion
      - Thalami/basal ganglia hypodense, swollen
- CECT
  - **"Empty delta" sign** (25-30%)
    - Enhancing dura surrounds nonenhancing thrombus
  - "Shaggy," enlarged/irregular veins (collateral channels)
- CTA/CTV
  - Filling defect (thrombus) in dural sinus
  - Caution: Acute, hyperdense clot can result in false-negative CECT or CTV
    - Always include NECT for comparison

MR Findings

- T1WI
  - Acute thrombus: Isointense
  - Subacute thrombus: Hyperintense
  - Chronic thrombus: Isointense
  - Normal variations in dural sinus flow may mimic thrombosis; vascular exam (CTV or MRV) more reliable to confirm suspected DST
- T2WI
  - Acute thrombus: Hypointense
    - Pitfall: Hypointense thrombus can mimic normal sinus flow void (potential source of false-negative interpretation)
  - Subacute thrombus: Hyperintense
  - Chronic thrombus: Hyperintense
  - Chronically thrombosed sinus: Fibrotic dural sinus eventually appears isointense
  - Venous infarct: Mass effect with mixed hypo-/ hyperintense signal in adjacent parenchyma
- PD/intermediate
  - Loss of normal flow voids
  - More sensitive than T2WI
- FLAIR
  - Clot signal varies
  - Venous infarcts are hyperintense
- T2* GRE
  - Hypointense thrombus usually "**blooms**"
    - Improves conspicuity of thrombus
  - ± hypointense petechial hemorrhages
- DWI
  - 40% have hyperintense clot in occluded vessel
  - DWI/ADC findings in parenchyma variable, heterogeneous
    - Mixture of vasogenic, cytotoxic edema
      - Cytotoxic edema may precede vasogenic edema
      - Parenchymal abnormalities may be reversible
- T1WI C+
  - Dura enhances around thrombus ("empty delta" sign)
  - Chronic thrombus can enhance
    - Organizing fibrous tissue ± recanalization
    - Potential source of false-negative interpretation
- MRV
  - 2D TOF or contrast MRV
  - Absence of flow in occluded sinus on 2D TOF MRV
    - Frayed or shaggy appearance of venous sinus
    - Abnormal collateral channels (e.g., enlarged medullary veins)
  - T1 hyperintense (subacute) clot can masquerade as flow on MRV; evaluate standard sequences, source images to exclude artifacts
    - Potential cause of false-negative MRV
  - Flow gaps on MIPs must be reviewed on source images to exclude hypoplastic sinus variants, particularly for transverse and sigmoid sinus
    - Potential source of false-positive interpretation on MIPs
  - Contrast-enhanced MRV (CE-MRV) shows thrombus, small vein detail, collaterals much better than 2D TOF
  - Phase contrast MRV not limited by T1 hyperintense thrombus
- SWI not useful since normal veins are hypointense

Angiographic Findings

- Occlusion of involved sinus
- Slow flow in adjacent patent cortical veins
- Collateral venous drainage develops

Imaging Recommendations

- Best imaging tool
  - NECT, CECT scans ± CTV as initial screening
  - MR, MRV (include T2*, DWI, T1WI C+)
- Protocol advice
  - If CT/CECT/CTV negative, MR with MRV
  - If MRV equivocal, cerebral angiography

DIFFERENTIAL DIAGNOSIS

Normal

- Arteries, veins normally slightly hyperdense on NECT
- Common in newborns (unmyelinated low-density brain, physiologic polycythemia)

Dural Sinus Hypoplasia-Aplasia

- Congenital hypoplastic/aplastic transverse sinus

DURAL SINUS THROMBOSIS

- Transverse sinus flow gaps (31%); nondominant sinus
- Right transverse sinus dominant (59%), left dominant (25%), codominant (16%)
- "High-splitting" tentorium

"Giant" Arachnoid Granulations

- Round/ovoid filling defect (clot typically long, linear)
- Cerebrospinal fluid (CSF) density/signal intensity
- Normal in 24% of CECT, 13% of MR
  - Transverse sinus most common location by imaging, left > right
  - Superior sagittal sinus most common location for arachnoid granulations on histopathology (lateral lacunae, not well seen by imaging)

Acute Subdural Hematoma

- Layered blood on tentorium cerebelli may mimic transverse sinus thrombosis

Neoplasm

- Venous infarct can enhance, mimic neoplasm
- Intravascular lymphoma (rare)

PATHOLOGY

General Features

- Etiology
  - Wide spectrum of predisposing causes
    - Trauma, infection, inflammation
    - Pregnancy, oral contraceptives
    - Metabolic (dehydration, thyrotoxicosis, cirrhosis)
    - Hematological (coagulopathy)
    - Collagen-vascular disorders (APLA syndrome)
    - Vasculitis (Behçet)
  - Most common pattern
    - Thrombus forms in dural sinus
    - Clot propagates into cortical veins
    - Venous drainage obstructed, venous pressure elevated
    - Blood-brain barrier breakdown with vasogenic edema, hemorrhage
    - Venous infarct with cytotoxic edema
- Genetics
  - Resistance to activated protein C (typically due to factor 5 Leiden mutation): Most common cause of sporadic CVT
  - Protein S deficiency
  - Prothrombin (factor II) gene mutation (*G20210A*)
- Associated abnormalities
  - Dural AV fistula; venous occlusive disease may be underlying etiologic factor

Staging, Grading, & Classification

- **Venous ischemia grading**
  - Type 1: No abnormality
  - Type 2: Hyperintense on T2/FLAIR; no enhancement
  - Type 3: Hyperintense on T2/FLAIR; enhancement
  - Type 4: Hemorrhage or venous infarction

Gross Pathologic & Surgical Features

- Sinus occluded, distended by acute clot
- Thrombus in adjacent cortical veins
- Edematous adjacent cortex; petechial hemorrhage

Microscopic Features

- Thrombosis of veins, proliferative fibrous tissue in chronic thromboses

CLINICAL ISSUES

Presentation

- Most common signs/symptoms
  - Headache, nausea, vomiting ± neurologic deficit
  - Clinical diagnosis often elusive

Demographics

- Age
  - Any age can be affected
- Gender
  - M < F
- Epidemiology
  - Venous accounts for 1% of acute strokes

Natural History & Prognosis

- Extremely variable: Asymptomatic to coma, death
  - Up to 50% of cases progress to venous infarction
  - Can be fatal if severe brain swelling, herniation

Treatment

- In-patient heparin followed by out-patient warfarin (Coumadin)
- In more severe cases, endovascular mechanical thrombectomy ± local heparin infusion

DIAGNOSTIC CHECKLIST

Consider

- Angiography for patients with suspected chronic DST
- Venous filling defect from arachnoid granulation

Image Interpretation Pearls

- Review MRV source images to exclude pseudo-occlusions
  - Transverse sinus common site for hypoplastic segment variations mimicking occlusion
- Review T1 images to exclude false-negative MRV
- Lack of parenchymal abnormality does not exclude cerebral vein thrombosis
- Review NECT to exclude dense thrombus as false-negative CECT or CTV
- Obtain DSA if noninvasive imaging inconclusive and clinical suspicion remains high
- Chronic thromboses may enhance on any contrast study due to recanalization or granulation tissue

SELECTED REFERENCES

1. Klingebiel R et al: Comparative evaluation of 2D time-of-flight and 3D elliptic centric contrast-enhanced MR venography in patients with presumptive cerebral venous and sinus thrombosis. Eur J Neurol. 14(2):139-43, 2007
2. Leach JL et al: Partially recanalized chronic dural sinus thrombosis: findings on MR imaging, time-of-flight MR venography, and contrast-enhanced MR venography. AJNR Am J Neuroradiol. 28(4):782-9, 2007

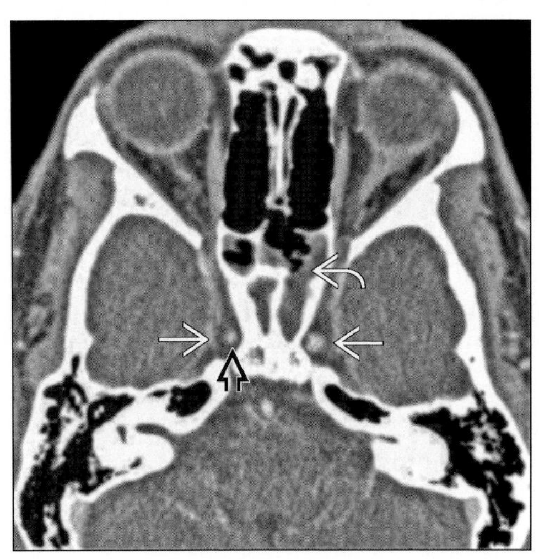

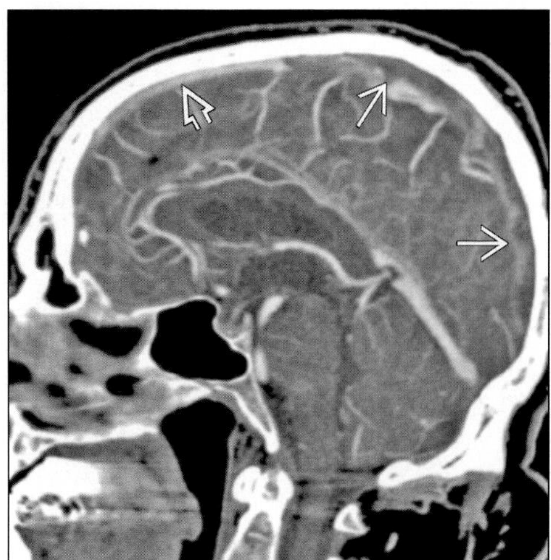

*(**Left**) Axial CTA shows lack of normal enhancement in the bilateral cavernous sinuses ➡, consistent with acute thrombosis, secondary to adjacent sphenoid sinusitis ➡. Inflammatory narrowing of the right internal carotid artery ➡ is characteristic for an infectious/inflammatory etiology. (**Right**) Sagittal CTA shows the anterior 1/3 of the superior sagittal sinus ➡ filling normally with contrast. However, the posterior 2/3 is filled with clot (acute dural sinus thrombosis) and does not enhance ➡.*

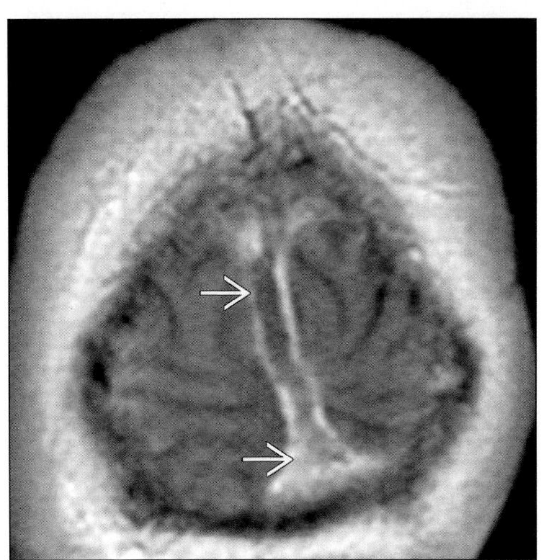

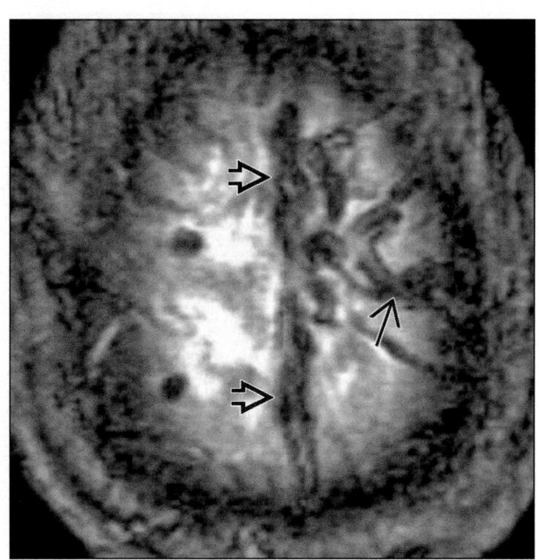

*(**Left**) Coronal T1WI C+ MR in the same patient shows isointense clot ➡ within the intensely enhancing dural leaves of the superior sagittal sinus. (**Right**) Axial T2* GRE MR in the same patient shows blooming clot within the superior sagittal sinus ➡ and left superficial cortical veins ➡. GRE is 1 of the most sensitive conventional MR sequences for sinus thrombosis.*

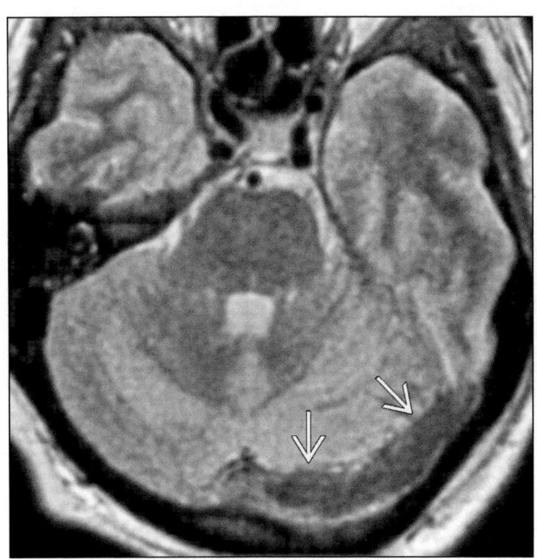

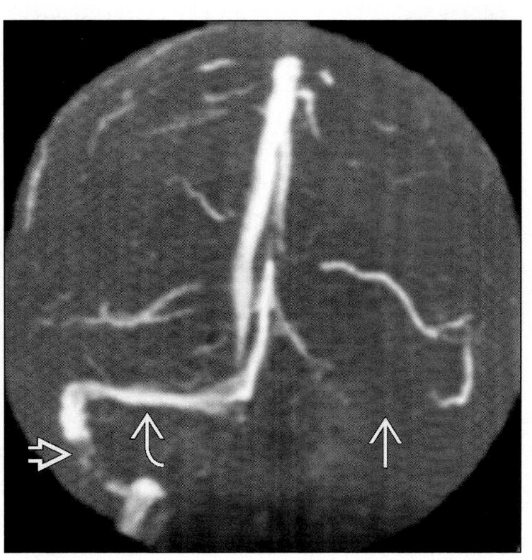

*(**Left**) Axial T2WI MR shows a large irregular left transverse sinus ➡, suspicious for thrombosis. Hypointensity is a potential source of false-negatives; such pseudo flow voids are common and should be confirmed with vascular imaging. (**Right**) Axial MRV in the same patient confirms left transverse sinus occlusion ➡. Note normal flow-related enhancement in the right transverse sinus ➡. A lobulated filling defect was an arachnoid granulation ➡, confirmed on conventional sequences (not shown).*

CORTICAL VENOUS THROMBOSIS

Key Facts

Terminology
- Cortical/cerebral venous thrombosis (CVT)
- Dural sinus thrombosis (DST)
- CVT with DST > isolated CVT without DST

Imaging
- NECT
  - "Cord" sign (hyperdense vein)
  - Involved veins usually enlarged (distended with clot), irregular
  - ± petechial parenchymal hemorrhage, edema
- CECT
  - If DST, "empty delta" sign (25-30% of cases)
  - CTV: Thrombi may be seen as filling defects
- MR
  - Acute thrombus isointense on T1WI
  - Hypointense on T2WI (can mimic flow void)
  - T2* GRE best (clot usually blooms)
- 2D time of flight (TOF) MRV
  - Thrombus seen as sinus discontinuity, loss of vascular flow signal
  - Subacute thrombus T1 hyperintense (mimics patent flow on MIP)
- Imaging recommendations
  - NECT, CECT scans ± CTV
  - If CT negative → MR/MRV with T1WI C+, GRE
  - If MR is equivocal → DSA ("gold standard")

Top Differential Diagnoses
- Normal (circulating blood slightly hyperdense)
- Anatomic variant (hypoplastic segment can mimic DST)

Clinical Issues
- Most common symptom is headache

*(**Left**) Autopsy of superior sagittal sinus thrombosis (not shown) reveals clots extending into multiple superficial cortical veins ➡. Gyral edema, tiny petechial hemorrhages ⇨ without frank venous infarct is seen. (Courtesy E.T. Hedley-Whyte, MD.) (**Right**) Axial MRV shows lack of signal in the expected locations (vein of Labbé ➡, transverse and sigmoid sinuses ➡) consistent with thrombosis in this 69-year-old man recently post surgery, with a history of metastatic carcinoid tumor and new mental status changes.*

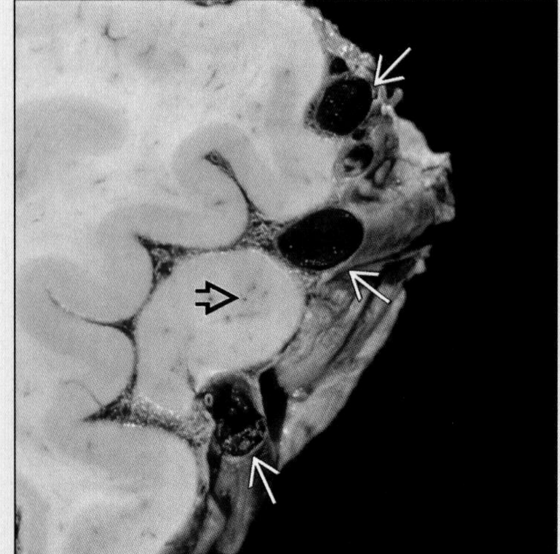

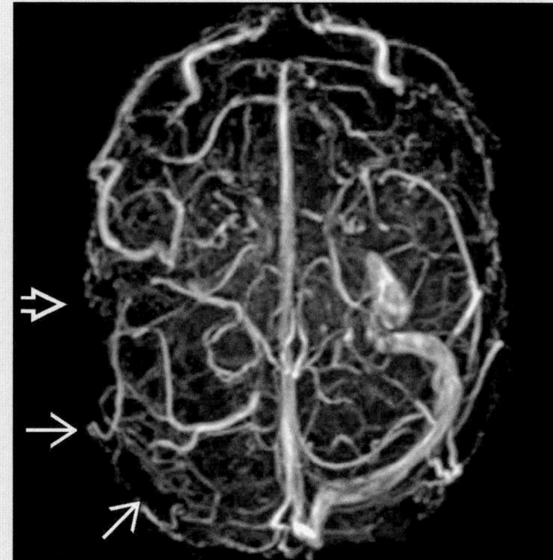

*(**Left**) Axial T2WI MR in the same patient shows extensive vasogenic edema in the right temporal lobe ➡. (**Right**) Axial T1WI C+ MR in the same patient shows gyriform thick cortical enhancement ➡, consistent with late subacute venous ischemia. Enhancement and mass effect may mimic primary CNS neoplasm or infection; however, vascular imaging (such as MRV) confirms the diagnosis of venous thrombosis.*

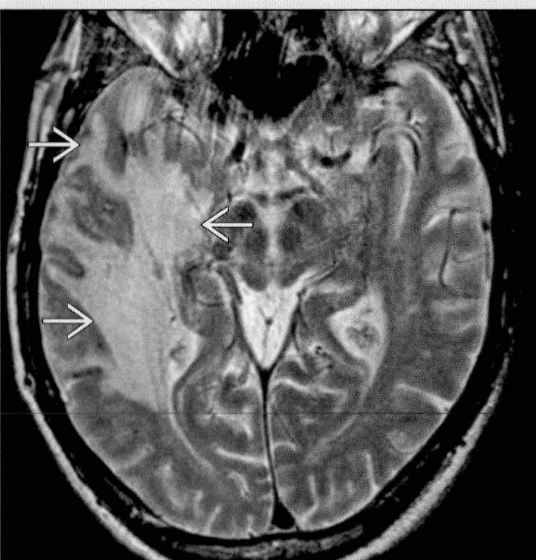

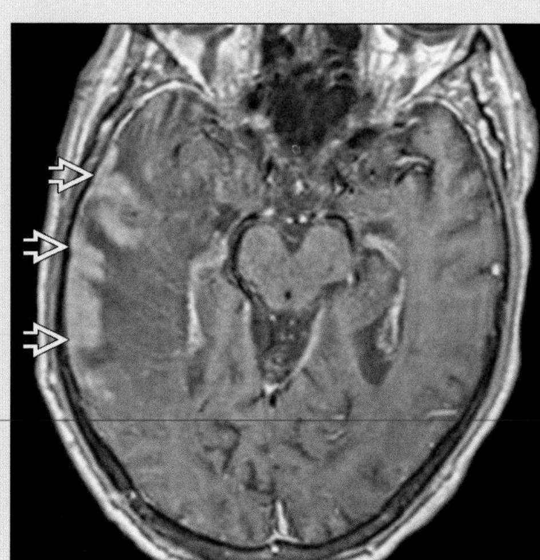

CORTICAL VENOUS THROMBOSIS

TERMINOLOGY

Abbreviations

- Cortical/cerebral venous thrombosis (CVT)
- Dural sinus thrombosis (DST)

Definitions

- Superficial cerebral venous thrombosis
  - Usually with DST but isolated CVT without DST can occur

IMAGING

General Features

- Best diagnostic clue
  - "Cord" sign on NECT, T2* GRE
- Location
  - Cortical veins (unnamed)
    - Anastomotic vein of Labbé
    - Anastomotic vein of Trolard
  - Can be solitary, multiple
- Morphology
  - Veins usually enlarged (distended with clot), irregular
  - Linear, cigar-shaped thrombus

CT Findings

- NECT
  - Hyperdense cortical vein ("cord" sign) ± DST
  - Parenchymal abnormalities common
    - Petechial hemorrhage, edema
    - Hypodensity in affected vascular distribution
  - Need NECT to exclude false-negative CTV
    - Thrombus dense, can mimic enhancement
- CECT
  - If DST present
    - "Empty delta" sign (25-30% of cases)
  - "Shaggy," irregular enhancing veins (collateral channels)
- CTV
  - Thrombus seen as filling defect in cortical veins
  - Abnormal collateral channels (e.g., enlarged medullary veins)
  - Negative CTV does not exclude CVT
    - Limited value for chronic CVT
      - Organizing thrombosis also enhances
    - Limited value for nonocclusive thrombus
    - Optimize technique using thin slice (0.6 mm) MDCT with venous phase enhancement and dedicated sagittal and coronal MPR (1-2 mm)
    - Thick slice (3-5 mm) sliding or overlapping MIPs in sagittal and coronal planes
    - Concurrent NECT important to exclude false-negative CTV due to intrinsically dense thrombus
    - Subacute and chronic thromboses can enhance: Potential false-negative

MR Findings

- T1WI
  - Thrombus is isointense early, hyperintense later
  - ± venous infarct
    - Gyral swelling, edema hypointense
    - Iso- to slightly hyperintense foci if hemorrhagic
- T2WI
  - Thrombus hypointense acutely, hyperintense much later
    - Acute clot can mimic flow void
  - Venous infarct
    - Gyral swelling, edema hyperintense
    - Hypointense foci if hemorrhagic
- FLAIR
  - Thrombus usually hyperintense
  - Parenchymal edema hyperintense
- T2* GRE
  - GRE most sensitive sequence for thrombus
    - Hypointense ("black"), cord-like
  - SWI not as helpful due to intrinsic hypointensity of normal veins
- DWI
  - DWI/ADC varies with ischemia, type of edema, hemorrhage
    - Distinguishes cytotoxic from vasogenic edema
- T1WI C+
  - Thin (1 mm) 3D volume acquisition
  - Acute/early subacute clot: Peripheral enhancement outlines clot
  - Late clot: Thrombus, fibrous tissue often enhances
  - Venous infarct: Patchy enhancement
- MRV
  - 2D time of flight (TOF) MRV depicts thrombus as sinus discontinuity, loss of vascular flow signal
    - May see abnormal collateral channels (e.g., enlarged medullary veins)
    - Occluded veins at time of diagnosis may predict low rate of vessel recanalization 2 or 3 months later
  - Contrast-enhanced MRV (CE-MRV)
    - Faster; better depicts nonenhancing thrombus and small veins than TOF
  - TOF limitations
    - T1 hyperintense thrombus (subacute) may mimic patent flow on MIP (false-negative MRV)
    - Must evaluate source images and conventional MR sequences to exclude potential false-negatives
  - Phase contrast MRV: T1 hyperintense thrombus not misrepresented as flow

Ultrasonographic Findings

- Transcranial Doppler (TCD) ultrasound
  - Monitor venous flow velocities at ICU bedside
  - Follow therapy as decreasing velocities
  - Caveat: Normal venous velocities in serial measurements do not exclude diagnosis of CVT

Angiographic Findings

- Conventional DSA, venous phase
  - More accurate than MR, particularly for isolated cortical vein thrombosis
  - Considered the gold standard
  - Chronic thromboses challenging due to enhancement from recanalization/organizing thrombus
- Interventional: Treatment with thrombolytics &/or mechanical declotting

Imaging Recommendations

- Best imaging tool

- NECT, CECT ± CTV
- MR with T1WI C+, GRE if CTV negative but high suspicion
- DSA is gold standard
- Protocol advice
  - If CT negative → MR with T1WI C+, GRE, MRV
  - If MR, MRV equivocal → DSA

DIFFERENTIAL DIAGNOSIS

Normal

- Circulating blood normally mildly hyperdense on NECT

Anatomic Variant

- Congenital hypoplasia can mimic DST
- Vein of Trolard, Labbé, superficial middle cerebral vein (SMCV) have reciprocal size relationship
  - If 2 are prominent, 3rd usually hypoplastic

"Giant" Arachnoid Granulation

- Can mimic DST
- Round/ovoid filling defect (clot is long, linear)
- CSF density, signal intensity

Cerebral Hemorrhage

- Mimics venous infarct
- Amyloid
- Cerebral contusion
- Hypertensive

PATHOLOGY

General Features

- Etiology
  - No cause identified in 20-25% of cases
  - Wide spectrum of predisposing causes (> 100 identified)
    - Trauma, infection, inflammation, malignancy
    - Pregnancy, oral contraceptives
    - Metabolic (dehydration, thyrotoxicosis, cirrhosis, hyperhomocysteinemia, etc.)
    - Hematological (coagulopathy)
    - Collagen-vascular disorders (e.g., APLA syndrome)
    - Vasculitis (e.g., Behçet)
    - Drugs (androgens, ecstasy)
  - Most common pattern
    - Thrombus initially forms in dural sinus
    - Clot propagates into cortical veins
    - Venous drainage obstructed → ↑ venous pressure
    - Blood-brain barrier breakdown with vasogenic edema, hemorrhage
    - Venous infarct with cytotoxic edema ensues
  - Isolated CVT without DST occurs but is uncommon

Gross Pathologic & Surgical Features

- Sinus occluded, distended by acute clot
- Thrombus in adjacent cortical veins
- Adjacent cortex edematous, usually with petechial hemorrhage

Microscopic Features

- Thrombus in cortical vein(s) and sinus(es)

CLINICAL ISSUES

Presentation

- Most common signs/symptoms
  - Headache (95%)
  - Seizure (47%), paresis (43%), papilledema (41%)
  - Altered consciousness (39%), comatose (15%)
  - Isolated intracranial hypertension (20%)
  - D-dimer is useful in patients with suspected CVT; patients with positive test results should be urgently sent for MR imaging
- Other signs/symptoms
  - Focal neurologic deficits; depend on location

Demographics

- Age
  - Any
- Gender
  - M < F
- Epidemiology
  - 1% of acute strokes

Natural History & Prognosis

- Clinical diagnosis often elusive
- Extremely variable outcome; asymptomatic to death
- Up to 50% of cases progress to venous infarction
- Pulmonary embolism is uncommon but carries poor prognosis
- Poor outcome associated with papilledema, altered consciousness, coma, age > 33 years, diagnostic delay > 10 days, intracerebral hemorrhage, involvement of straight sinus
- Good outcome associated with isolated intracranial hypertension presentation, "delta" sign on CT (leading to earlier diagnosis)
- 1 year following CVT, 40% have lifestyle restrictions, 40% are unable to resume previous level of economic activity, 35% have altered consciousness, 6% are dependent
- Overall mortality = 10%; recurrence as high as 12%

Treatment

- Heparin ± TPA
- Endovascular thrombolysis; thrombolytic &/or mechanical disruption

DIAGNOSTIC CHECKLIST

Consider

- DSA if CT/MR inconclusive, if clinical suspicion is high, or if intervention is planned

Image Interpretation Pearls

- Include T2* GRE sequence on MR/MRV

SELECTED REFERENCES

1. Linn J et al: Noncontrast CT in deep cerebral venous thrombosis and sinus thrombosis: comparison of its diagnostic value for both entities. AJNR Am J Neuroradiol. 30(4):728-35, 2009
2. Idbaih A et al: MRI of clot in cerebral venous thrombosis: high diagnostic value of susceptibility-weighted images. Stroke. 37(4):991-5, 2006

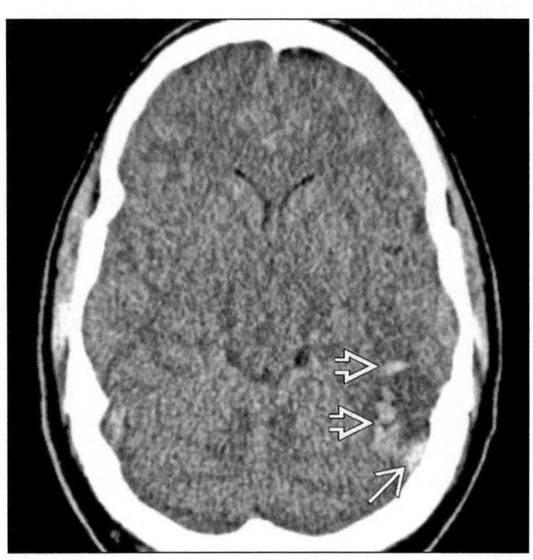

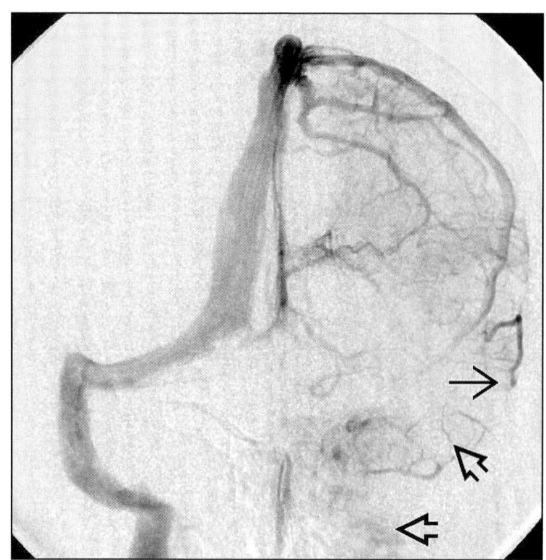

(Left) *Axial NECT shows acute intraparenchymal hemorrhage in the left temporal lobe, in a classic distribution for vein of Labbé thrombosis. Hyperdensity in the left transverse sinus is consistent with acute thrombosis.* ***(Right)*** *Anteroposterior DSA in the same patient during venous phase of a left ICA injection confirms acute thrombosis, with cut-off of the vein of Labbé and nonfilling of the left transverse/sigmoid sinus and internal jugular vein.*

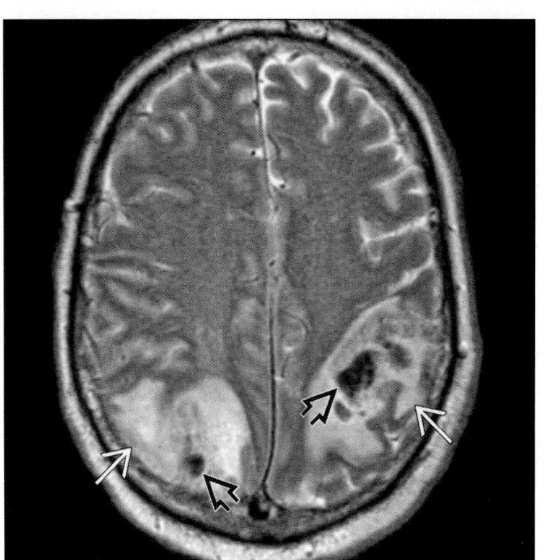

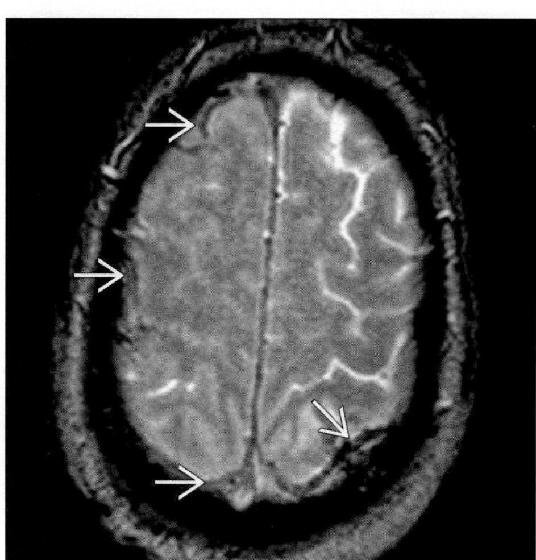

(Left) *Axial T2WI MR shows bilateral juxtacortical areas of vasogenic pattern edema with areas of hemorrhage. This pattern is significant as a classic distribution for multifocal cortical vein thrombosis, prompting vascular imaging.* ***(Right)*** *Axial T2* GRE MR can be 1 of the most sensitive noninvasive techniques for identifying clot within cortical veins. This patient had prior CTV (not shown) which, even in retrospect, was interpreted as negative for vein thrombosis.*

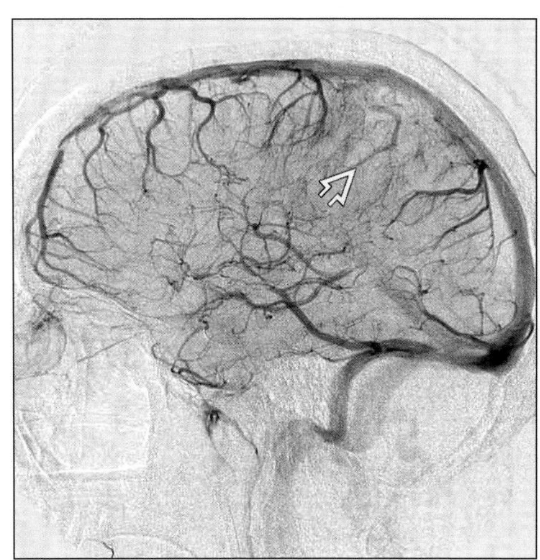

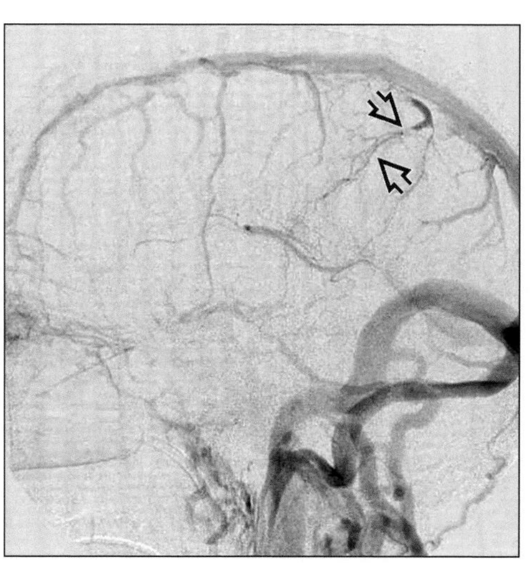

(Left) *Lateral DSA venous phase in the same patient was performed to confirm suspected vein thrombosis. The subacute age of clot likely contributed to difficulty in diagnosis. Despite a nearly normal sagittal sinus, note areas of delayed enhancement and lack of a normal Trolard vein, with collateral venous filling in the left posterior frontal and parietal lobes.* ***(Right)*** *Lateral DSA late venous phase in the same patient shows partial vein of Trolard opacification, with internal filling defects.*

DEEP CEREBRAL VENOUS THROMBOSIS

Key Facts

Terminology

- Thrombotic occlusion of deep cerebral veins
  - Usually affects both internal cerebral vein ± vein of Galen (VOG), straight sinus (SS)
  - May occur in broader setting of widespread deep sinus thrombosis

Imaging

- Best imaging tool
  - NECT/CECT ± CTV venogram
- CT
  - Hyperdense ICV ± bithalamic hypodensity
  - Variable loss of deep gray-white interfaces
  - ± petechial hemorrhages
- Protocol advice
  - If CT/CECT/CTV scans negative → MR with MRV
  - If MRV equivocal → DSA
- MR: Clot hypointense, "blooms" on T2*

Top Differential Diagnoses

- Other bithalamic/basal ganglia lesions
  - Nonvenous ischemia, neoplasm, toxic/metabolic

Clinical Issues

- Venous thrombosis = 1-2% of strokes
- ICV thrombosis = 10% of venous "strokes"

Diagnostic Checklist

- Consider DSA in equivocal cases, intervention
- Image interpretation pearls
  - Early imaging findings subtle, often overlooked
  - Obtain NECT concurrently with CECT/CTV
  - Include T2* sequence on MR
  - 2D TOF MRV should not be interpreted without benefit of standard imaging sequences
  - Nonvisualization of deep venous system on CTA/MRA/DSA always abnormal

*(**Left**) Axial graphic depicts thrombosis of both ICVs and SS ➡ with secondary hemorrhage in the choroid plexus and thalami ⮚. Edema in the thalami, basal ganglia, and deep cerebral white matter are common findings. Linear WM medullary veins ➡ may become engorged and enhance. (**Right**) Axial NECT shows bilateral thalamic low attenuation ➡. Although not a specific finding in this case, a contrast study or MR could confirm suspicion for deep vein thrombosis given the classic venous drainage pattern involved.*

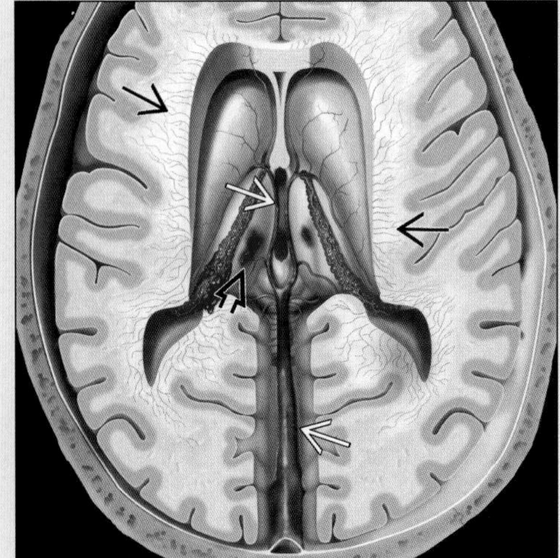

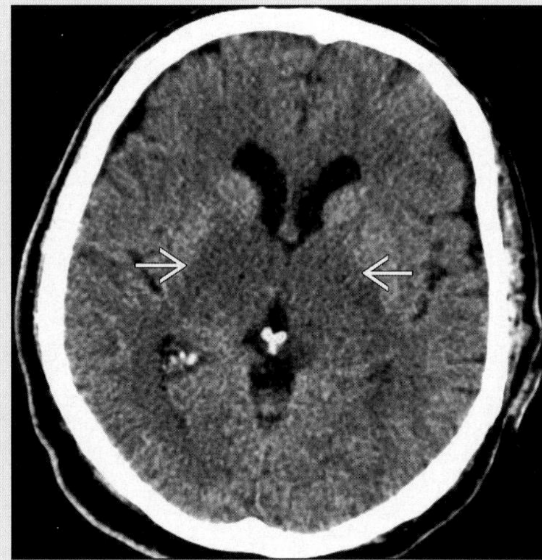

*(**Left**) Axial T2* GRE MR in the same patient confirms abnormal hypointensity ("blooming") in both internal cerebral veins ➡ due to susceptibility. Both thalami are edematous and hyperintense ⮚, a finding confirmed on both FLAIR and T2WI (not shown). (**Right**) Lateral MRV in the same patient shows patent superior sagittal sinus and confirms absence of flow ➡ in the expected location of the deep venous system (ICVs, straight sinus are "missing in action"). Note the prominent deep collateral venous drainage ⮚.*

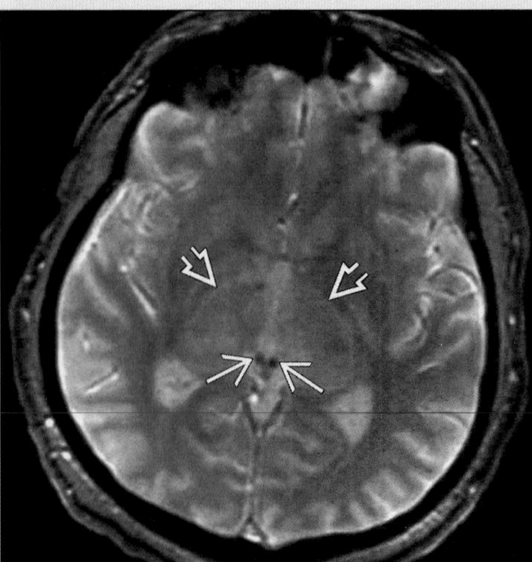

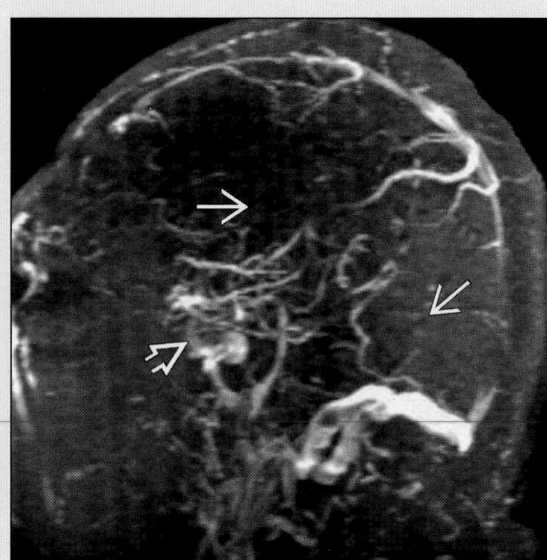

TERMINOLOGY

Abbreviations

- Deep cerebral venous thrombosis (DCVT)
- Internal cerebral vein (ICV) thrombosis

Definitions

- Thrombotic occlusion of deep cerebral veins
  - Usually affects both ICVs ± vein of Galen (VOG), straight sinus (SS)
  - May occur in broader setting of widespread dural sinus thrombosis (DST)

IMAGING

General Features

- Best diagnostic clue
  - Hyperdense ICV on NECT ± bithalamic hypodensity
- Location
  - Clot in ICV ± VOG, SS, basal veins of Rosenthal
  - Bilateral ICV thrombosis >>> unilateral
  - Deep gray nuclei, internal capsule, medullary white matter (WM) typically affected
  - Variable involvement of midbrain, upper cerebellum (VOG, SS territory)

CT Findings

- NECT
  - Hyperdense ICVs ± SS, DST
  - Potential parenchymal abnormalities
    - Hypodense thalami/basal ganglia (BG) hypodense, loss of gray-white matter interfaces
    - ± petechial hemorrhages
- CECT
  - "Empty delta" sign (if DST)
  - "Shaggy," irregular veins (collateral channels) in deep WM, around tentorium
- CTV
  - Loss of ICV enhancement, presence of enlarged collateral channels
  - Limited value in chronic cases as organizing thrombosis also enhances

MR Findings

- T1WI
  - Clot: Early T1 isointense, later hyperintense
  - Venous hypertension: Hypointense swelling of thalami, basal ganglia
  - Venous infarct: Hypointense edema, may be hemorrhagic
- T2WI
  - Clot: Often T2 hypointense mimicking flow void ("pseudo flow void"), much later hyperintense
  - Venous hypertension: Hyperintense swelling of thalami, basal ganglia
    - Corresponds to vasogenic ± cytotoxic edema
  - Venous infarct: Parenchymal swelling, hyperintense edema, may be hemorrhagic
- FLAIR
  - High signal in occluded veins
  - Best demonstrates hyperintense edema
- T2* GRE
  - Clot: Hypointense with blooming on T2*
    - T2* may be most sensitive conventional sequence
  - Venous infarct: More sensitive for hemorrhage, often petechial
- DWI
  - Distinguishes cytotoxic from vasogenic edema
  - DWI/ADC imaging findings heterogeneous
  - May restrict early (hyperintense BG/thalami), normalize later
  - Restriction can be seen in clot proper; occluded veins at time of diagnosis might be predictive of low rate of vessel recanalization 2 or 3 months later
- T1WI C+
  - Acute/early subacute clot: Peripheral enhancement outlines clot
  - Late clot: Thrombus, fibrous tissue often enhances
  - Venous stasis in deep WM (medullary) veins seen as linear enhancing foci radiating outward from ventricles
  - Venous hypertension: No parenchymal enhancement
  - Parenchymal venous infarct: Patchy enhancement
- MRV
  - 2D time of flight (TOF) MRV shows "missing" ICVs, variably absent signal in VOG, SS
    - May see abnormal collateral channels
  - Contrast-enhanced MRV (CE-MRV)
    - Faster; better depicts nonenhancing thrombus and small veins than TOF
  - TOF limitations
    - T1 hyperintense thrombus falsely appears as patent flow on MIP
    - Always evaluate source images and conventional MR sequences
  - Phase contrast MRV: T1 hyperintense thrombus not misrepresented as flow
- SWI not as useful for clot since normal veins are hypointense

Angiographic Findings

- Conventional
  - DSA more accurate than MR
  - Unlike quite variable superficial veins, deep cerebral veins are always present on angiography
    - In DCVT, occluded ICVs do not opacify
    - Collateral venous channels (e.g., pterygoid veins) enlarge
- Interventional: Treatment with thrombolytics &/or mechanical declotting

Imaging Recommendations

- Best imaging tool
  - NECT, CECT scans ± CTV venogram
  - Conventional DSA most sensitive and useful if intervention planned
- Protocol advice
  - If CT/CECT/CTV scans negative → MR with MRV
  - If MRV equivocal → DSA

DIFFERENTIAL DIAGNOSIS

Nonvenous Ischemic Injury

- Arterial occlusion
  - Artery of Percheron cerebral ischemia
  - Top of basilar cerebral infarction

DEEP CEREBRAL VENOUS THROMBOSIS

- Global hypoxia

Primary CNS Lymphoma
- T2 hyperintense, enhancing mass(es)
- Along ependymal surfaces (thalami > basal ganglia)
- Normal venous system

Glioma
- T2 hyperintense mass in deep gray nuclei
- Normal venous system
- Elevated choline, decreased NAA
- Vasogenic not cytotoxic edema

Carbon Monoxide Poisoning
- T2 hyperintense deep gray nuclei, often globus pallidus
- Normal venous system
- Positive carboxyhemoglobin
- Classic cherry red skin is rare

PATHOLOGY

General Features
- Etiology
  - No cause identified in 20-25% of cases
  - Wide spectrum of causes (> 100 identified)
    - Trauma, infection, inflammation
    - Pregnancy, oral contraceptives
    - Metabolic (dehydration, thyrotoxicosis, cirrhosis, etc.)
    - Hematological (coagulopathy)
    - Collagen-vascular disorders (e.g., APLA syndrome)
    - Vasculitis (e.g., Behçet)
    - Drugs (androgens, ecstasy)
  - Most common sequence
    - Thrombus initially forms in dural sinus
    - Clot propagates into cortical veins
    - Venous drainage obstructed, venous pressure elevated
    - Blood-brain barrier breakdown with vasogenic edema, hemorrhage
    - Venous infarct with cytotoxic edema ensues
- Genetics
  - Resistance to activated protein C
    - Factor 5 Leiden mutation is most common cause of sporadic CVT
  - Prothrombin (factor 2) gene mutation (*G20210A*)
  - Protein S deficiency
  - Antithrombin 3 deficiency

Staging, Grading, & Classification
- Venous ischemia
  - Type 1: No abnormality
  - Type 2: High signal on T2WI/FLAIR; no enhancement
  - Type 3: High signal on T2WI/FLAIR; enhancement present
  - Type 4: Hemorrhage or venous infarction

Gross Pathologic & Surgical Features
- ICVs occluded, distended by acute clot
- Venous hypertension ensues
- Adjacent thalami edematous with variable hemorrhage

Microscopic Features
- Thrombus in occluded vessels

CLINICAL ISSUES

Presentation
- Most common signs/symptoms
  - Headache, nausea, vomiting
    - ± neurologic deficit, seizure

Demographics
- Age
  - Any age
    - Especially elderly, debilitated patients
- Gender
  - M < F
- Epidemiology
  - Venous thrombosis causes 1-2% of strokes
  - ICV thrombosis = 10% of venous "strokes"

Natural History & Prognosis
- Clinical diagnosis of CVT often elusive
- Outcome of CVT extremely variable, from asymptomatic to death
  - Majority have no residual deficits at 16 months
  - Subgroup (13%) have poor outcome
  - Predictors of death/dependence
    - Hemorrhage on admission CT
    - DWI demonstration of cytotoxic edema (infarction)

Treatment
- Heparin ± rTPA
- Endovascular thrombolysis

DIAGNOSTIC CHECKLIST

Consider
- DSA in equivocal cases and for intervention

Image Interpretation Pearls
- Early imaging findings subtle, often overlooked
- Obtain NECT concurrently with CECT/CTV
- "Flow voids" on T2 do not rule out DCVT
- 2D TOF MRV should not be interpreted without benefit of standard imaging sequences
- Nonvisualization of deep venous system on CTA/MRA/DSA always abnormal

SELECTED REFERENCES

1. Linn J et al: Noncontrast CT in deep cerebral venous thrombosis and sinus thrombosis: comparison of its diagnostic value for both entities. AJNR Am J Neuroradiol. 30(4):728-35, 2009
2. Rodallec MH et al: Cerebral venous thrombosis and multidetector CT angiography: tips and tricks. Radiographics. 26 Suppl 1:S5-18; discussion S42-3, 2006
3. Favrole P et al: Diffusion-weighted imaging of intravascular clots in cerebral venous thrombosis. Stroke. 35(1):99-103, 2004

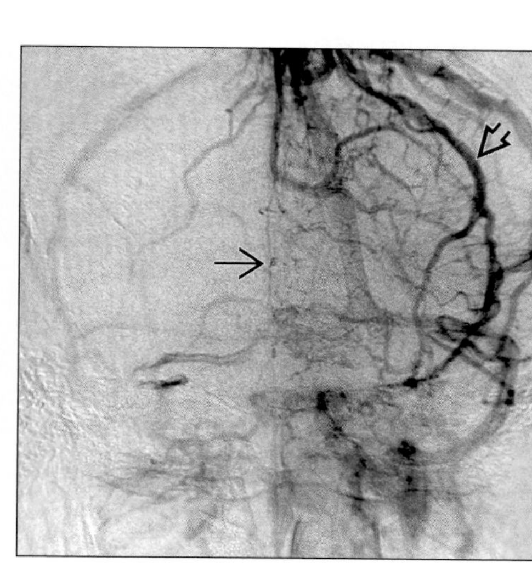

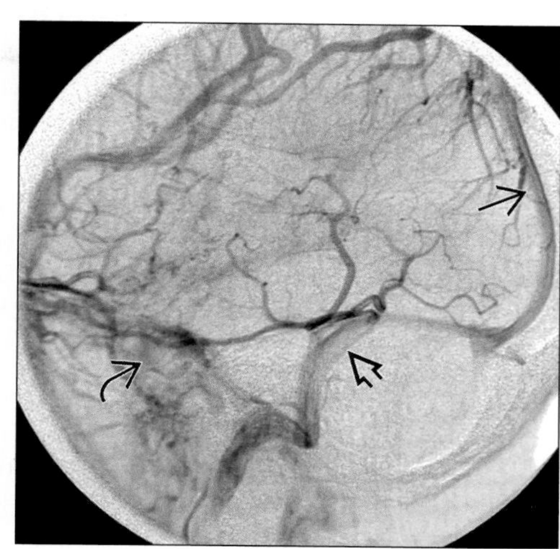

(Left) *AP DSA shows prominent cortical veins ⮚ with no filling of the ICVs →, SS, or VOG.* ***(Right)*** *Lateral DSA venous phase in the same patient shows a normal descending segment of the superior sagittal sinus → and transverse/sigmoid sinuses ⮚. The straight sinus and internal cerebral veins show no filling. There are also very prominent frontal and temporal cortical veins with drainage into the cavernous sinus ↗ and pterygoid venous plexus (immediately below cavernous sinus).*

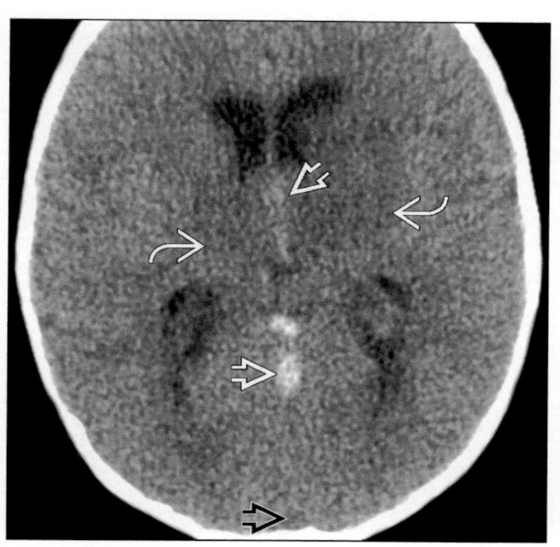

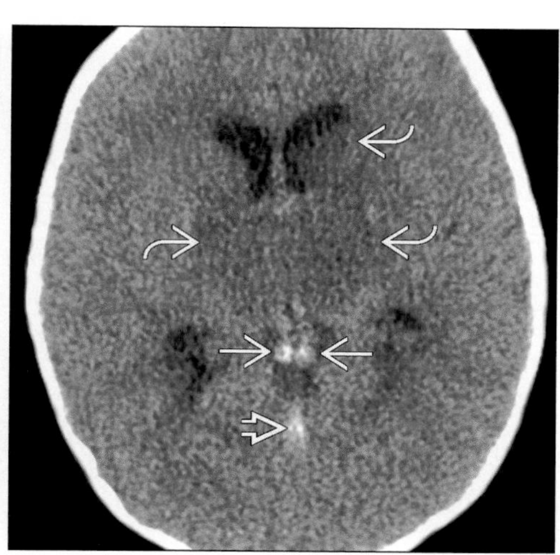

(Left) *Axial NECT demonstrates enlargement/ hyperdensity in the ICVs, VOG, and SS ⮚. Note the normal density in the superior sagittal sinus ⮚ for comparison. There is hypodensity and mild mass effect in both the thalami and basal ganglia ↗.* ***(Right)*** *Axial NECT in the same patient shows definite thrombus in both ICVs → and SS ⮚ and extensive hypodensity in the caudate, thalami, and putamen ↗, consistent with edema secondary to extensive deep cerebral venous occlusion.*

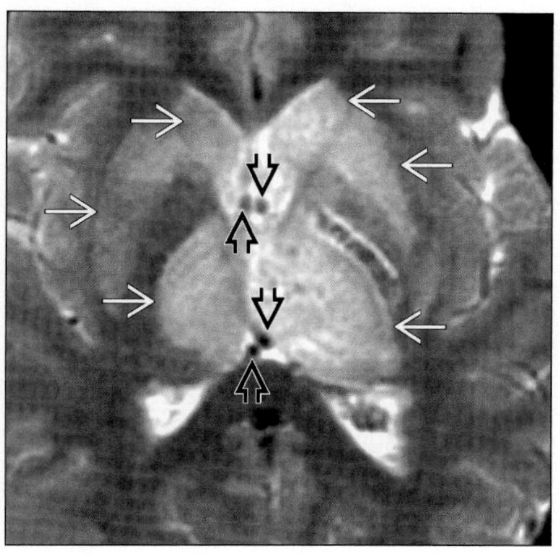

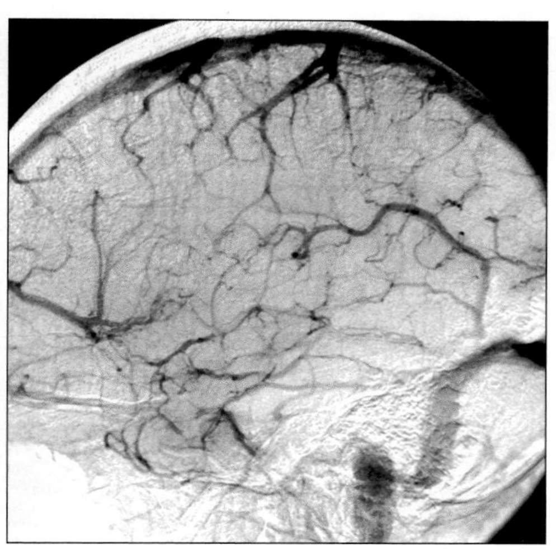

(Left) *Axial T2WI MR demonstrates hyperintense signal and mild mass effect in the bilateral thalami and basal ganglia →. Note the pseudo flow voids in both internal cerebral veins ⮚, an important pitfall and potential source of false-negative interpretation in venous thrombosis.* ***(Right)*** *Lateral DSA venous phase in the same patient shows complete absence of the deep venous system, confirming extensive deep vein thrombosis.*

DURAL SINUS AND ABERRANT ARACHNOID GRANULATIONS

Key Facts

Terminology
- AG: Arachnoid granulation
  - Defined as enlarged arachnoid villi projecting into major dural venous sinus lumen
- AbAG: Aberrant arachnoid granulation
  - Defined as AG that penetrates dura but fails to reach venous sinus, typically in sphenoid bone

Imaging
- Intrasinus AG: Well-circumscribed, discrete, filling defect in venous sinus ± inner calvarial table erosion
  - CECT: Nonenhancing; density like CSF
  - MR: T1/T2 intensity follows CSF; FLAIR often hyperintense
- AbAG: Multiple focal outpouches in sphenoid bone, often greater wing
  - Bone CT: Multiple smooth pits in sphenoid bone
  - MR: T1 and T2 intensity follows CSF
- 5-15 mm range in size

Top Differential Diagnoses
- Dural sinus hypoplasia-aplasia
- Transverse-sigmoid sinus pseudolesion
- Dural sinus thrombosis, skull base
- Dural AV fistula, skull base

Clinical Issues
- Intravenous sinus AG: Asymptomatic with rare exception
  - If pressure gradient across giant AG of venous sinus, venous hypertension with headache possible
- Aberrant AG: Mostly asymptomatic
  - If CSF pulsations enlarge AbAG in sphenoid sinus wall, CSF leak ± meningitis possible
  - If significant cephalocele occurs, seizure possible

(Left) *Graphic shows a giant arachnoid granulation (AG) projecting from subarachnoid space into transverse sinus. CSF core ➡ extends into the AG and is separated by arachnoid cap cells from the venous sinus endothelium ↗. Giant AGs often contain prominent venous channels ⇨ and septations.* ***(Right)*** *Axial CECT shows a giant arachnoid granulation cluster at the transverse-sigmoid venous sinus junction ➡. The 1st imaging interpretation of this finding mistakenly suggested venous sinus thrombosis.*

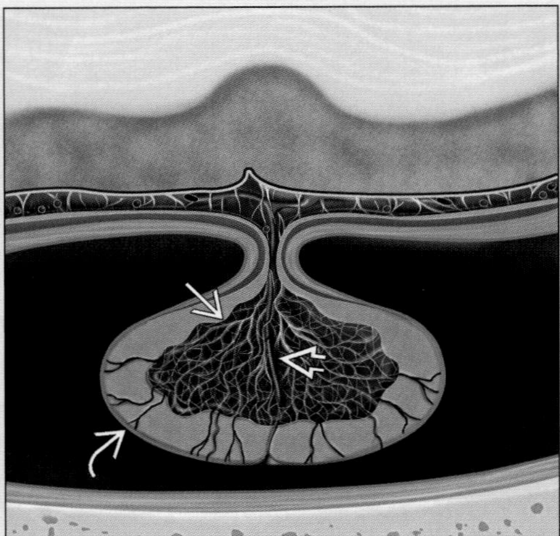

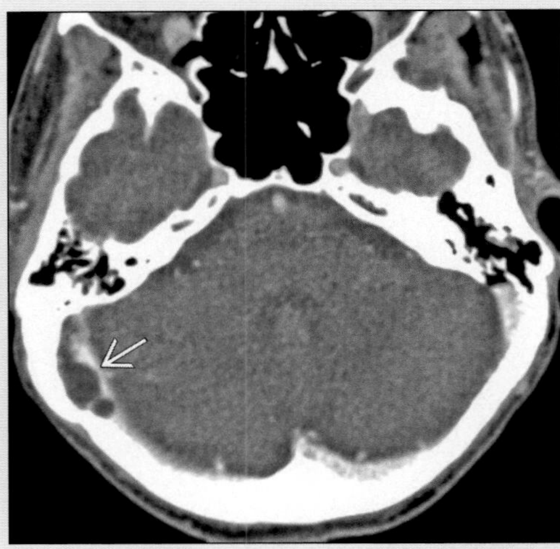

(Left) *Axial T1WI MR in the same patient reveals the multiple giant arachnoid granulations ➡ as low signal within the transverse and proximal sigmoid sinuses. The medial low signal line ⇨ is the dura.* ***(Right)*** *Axial T2WI FS MR in the same patient demonstrates the lesion to be high signal ➡ similar to cerebrospinal fluid in the cerebellopontine angle cistern. The low signal line on the deep surface of arachnoid granulations is the dura ⇨.*

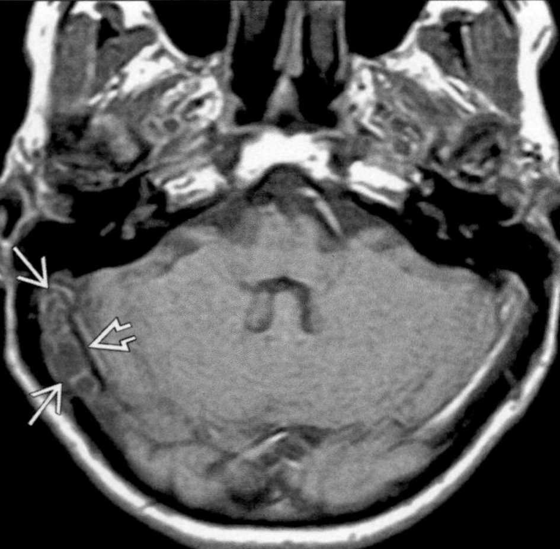

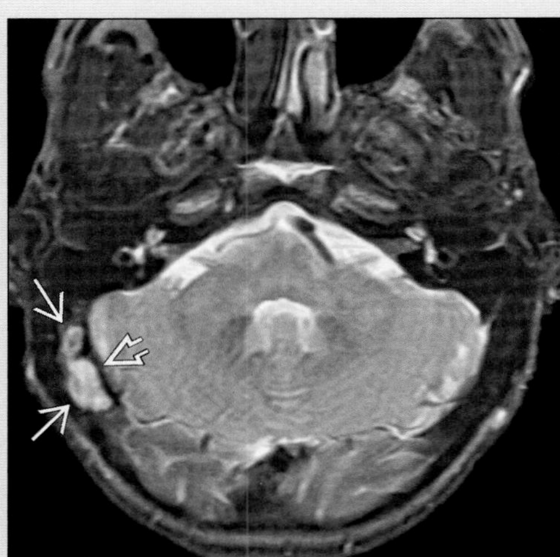

DURAL SINUS AND ABERRANT ARACHNOID GRANULATIONS

TERMINOLOGY

Abbreviations

- Arachnoid granulation (AG)
- Aberrant arachnoid granulation (AbAG)

Synonyms

- Pacchionian depressions, granulations, or bodies
- When large → giant arachnoid granulation
- When in sphenoid bone → AbAG

Definitions

- AG: Enlarged arachnoid villi projecting into major dural venous sinus lumen
- AbAG: AG that penetrated dura but fails to reach venous sinus, typically in sphenoid bone
  - Also referred to as arachnoid pits

IMAGING

General Features

- Best diagnostic clue
  - Intrasinus AG: Discrete filling defect in venous sinus ± inner calvarial table erosion
    - CECT: Nonenhancing; similar density to CSF
    - MR: T1/T2 intensity follows CSF; often hyperintense on FLAIR
  - AbAG: Multiple focal outpouches in sphenoid bone, often greater wing
    - Bone CT: Multiple smooth pits in sphenoid bone
    - MR: T1 and T2 intensity follows CSF
- Location
  - Most common location: Transverse sinus
  - Other locations: Sigmoid, sagittal, straight sinus
  - AbAG location: Sphenoid bone, often greater wing, or lateral sinus wall
- Size
  - 5-15 mm size range
  - If > 15 mm, called "giant AG"
- Morphology
  - Single or multiple ovoid lesions
  - Focal osseous pits in inner table of calvarium

CT Findings

- NECT
  - Intrasinus AG isodense with CSF
  - CSF pulsations may result in erosion or scalloping of inner table
  - AbAG: Focal osseous erosions in sphenoid bone
    - If large, may appear multilocular; mimic cystic bone lesion
- CECT
  - Nonenhancing, ovoid focal filling defect within venous sinus
  - Isodense to CSF
  - AbAG: CSF density with subtle rim (dural) enhancement
- CT venogram
  - Focal filling defect with venous sinus

MR Findings

- T1WI
  - Venous sinus defect isointense to CSF
- T2WI
  - Hyperintense (like CSF)
  - Surrounded by normal flow void of major venous sinus
  - AbAG: High signal outpouching into sphenoid bone
    - If large, may see arachnoid pouch bulging into sphenoid sinus lumen
      - Arachnoid strands seen as low signal lines within pouch
    - Larger lesions may have CSF leak into sphenoid sinus
    - Larger lesions may have cephalocele associated
- T1WI C+
  - Intrasinus AG: Ovoid without enhancement surrounded by enhancing blood in dural sinus
    - Veins, septae may enhance
  - AbAG: Nonenhancing foci in sphenoid bone
- MRV
  - Intrasinus AG
    - Source images show focal signal loss in location of AG
    - MRV reformation shows focal defect in transverse sinus

Imaging Recommendations

- Best imaging tool
  - Intrasinus AG: Enhanced MR with MRV
  - AbAG: Bone CT of skull base
    - Enhanced MR focused to sphenoid bone area

DIFFERENTIAL DIAGNOSIS

Dural Sinus Hypoplasia-Aplasia

- Congenital hypoplastic-aplastic transverse sinus
- "High-splitting" tentorium

Transverse-Sigmoid Sinus Pseudolesion

- Asymmetric complex flow phenomenon in sinus mimics lesions
- Not present on all sequences; MRV sorts out

Dural Sinus Thrombosis, Skull Base

- Long-segment region of ↓ venous sinus flow
- NECT: Hyperdense
- CECT: Nonenhancing clot in venous sinus lumen
- MR: Hyperintense on T1 or lack of flow void on T2

Dural AV Fistula, Skull Base

- MR: Recanalized, irregular transverse-sigmoid sinuses
- Angio: Enlarged, feeding external carotid artery branches

PATHOLOGY

General Features

- Etiology
  - Intrasinus AG: Normal variant enlarged arachnoid villi
    - Arachnoid villi responsible for CSF resorption
  - Aberrant AG: AG that penetrates dura but fails to reach venous sinus in sphenoid bone
    - CSF pulsations suspected in enlarging AbAG causing arachnoid pouch bulging into bone

DURAL SINUS AND ABERRANT ARACHNOID GRANULATIONS

- With enlargement of arachnoid pouch, rupture results in CSF leak into sphenoid sinus
  - Cephalocele may be accompanied by larger AbAG

Gross Pathologic & Surgical Features

- AG: Smooth arachnoid granulation projecting into venous sinus or subarachnoid space
- Aberrant AG: Osteodural defects in lateral sphenoid sinus wall or greater wing of sphenoid

Microscopic Features

- Enlarged arachnoid villi
- Central core of loose, peripheral zone of dense connective tissue
- Projects through dura of venous sinus wall

CLINICAL ISSUES

Presentation

- Most common signs/symptoms
  - Intravenous sinus AG: Asymptomatic with rare exception
    - If pressure gradient across giant AG of venous sinus, venous hypertension with headache is possible
  - Aberrant AG: Mostly asymptomatic
    - If CSF pulsations enlarge AbAG in sphenoid sinus wall, CSF leak ± meningitis possible
    - If significant cephalocele occurs, seizure possible
- Other signs/symptoms
  - Benign intracranial hypertension in obese middle-aged females with empty sella and spontaneous CSF rhinorrhea have been linked to aberrant AG expression

Demographics

- Age
  - ↑ in frequency with ↑ age; ≥ 40 years
- Epidemiology
  - Intravenous sinus AG: 25% CECT or T2WI MR
  - Aberrant AG: Rare; incidence unknown (< 1%)

Natural History & Prognosis

- Intravenous sinus AG: Remains asymptomatic
- Aberrant AG: May remain small or enlarge from CSF pulsations to create CSF leak or cephalocele

Treatment

- Intravenous sinus AG: No treatment required
- Aberrant AG: No treatment needed unless enlarged from CSF pulsation or CSF leak
  - Can follow large, asymptomatic AbAG
  - If CSF leak present into sphenoid sinus, surgical dural repair necessary

DIAGNOSTIC CHECKLIST

Consider

- If intravenous sinus giant AG with history of headache, consider angiogram to look for intrasinus pressure gradient
- If aberrant AG presents in lateral wall sphenoid bone, look for fluid in sphenoid sinus as evidence for CSF leak
  - Also use MR to evaluate for possible associated cephalocele

Image Interpretation Pearls

- Intravenous sinus AG
  - Confirm AG remains CSF density (as seen with CECT or CT angiogram) and intensity (as seen with T1 and T2 MR sequences)
  - Make sure proximal and distal venous sinus is normal from imaging perspective
- Aberrant AG in lateral sphenoid sinus wall
  - If large or multiple, look for evidence of CSF leak (fluid or fluid level in sphenoid sinus)

SELECTED REFERENCES

1. Kiroglu Y et al: Giant arachnoid granulation in a patient with benign intracranial hypertension. Eur Radiol. 18(10):2329-32, 2008
2. La Fata V et al: CSF leaks: correlation of high-resolution CT and multiplanar reformations with intraoperative endoscopic findings. AJNR Am J Neuroradiol. 29(3):536-41, 2008
3. Lloyd KM et al: Imaging of skull base cerebrospinal fluid leaks in adults. Radiology. 248(3):725-36, 2008
4. Schuknecht B et al: Nontraumatic skull base defects with spontaneous CSF rhinorrhea and arachnoid herniation: imaging findings and correlation with endoscopic sinus surgery in 27 patients. AJNR Am J Neuroradiol. 29(3):542-9, 2008
5. Haroun AA et al: Arachnoid granulations in the cerebral dural sinuses as demonstrated by contrast-enhanced 3D magnetic resonance venography. Surg Radiol Anat. 29(4):323-8, 2007
6. Amlashi SF et al: Intracranial hypertension and giant arachnoid granulations. J Neurol Neurosurg Psychiatry. 75(1):172, 2004
7. Liang L et al: Normal structures in the intracranial dural sinuses: delineation with 3D contrast-enhanced magnetization prepared rapid acquisition gradient-echo imaging sequence. AJNR Am J Neuroradiol. 23(10):1739-46, 2002
8. Gacek RR et al: Adult spontaneous cerebrospinal fluid otorrhea: diagnosis and management. Am J Otol. 20(6):770-6, 1999
9. Casey SO et al: Prevalence of arachnoid granulations as detected with CT venography of the dural sinuses. AJNR Am J Neuroradiol. 18(5):993-4, 1997
10. Leach JL et al: Normal appearance of arachnoid granulations on contrast-enhanced CT and MR of the brain: differentiation from dural sinus disease. AJNR Am J Neuroradiol. 17(8):1523-32, 1996
11. Roche J et al: Arachnoid granulations in the transverse and sigmoid sinuses: CT, MR, and MR angiographic appearance of a normal anatomic variation. AJNR Am J Neuroradiol. 17(4):677-83, 1996

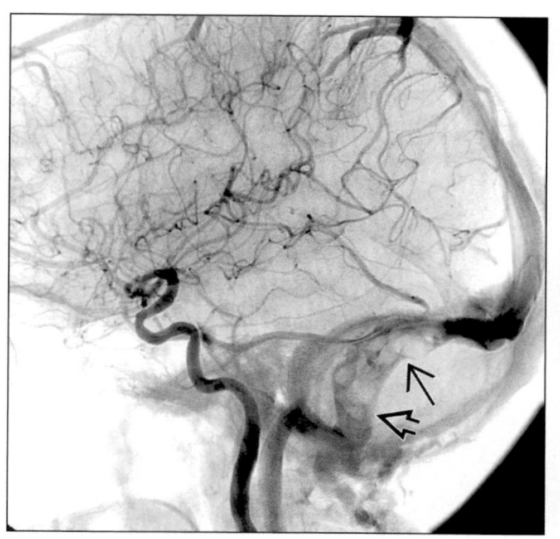

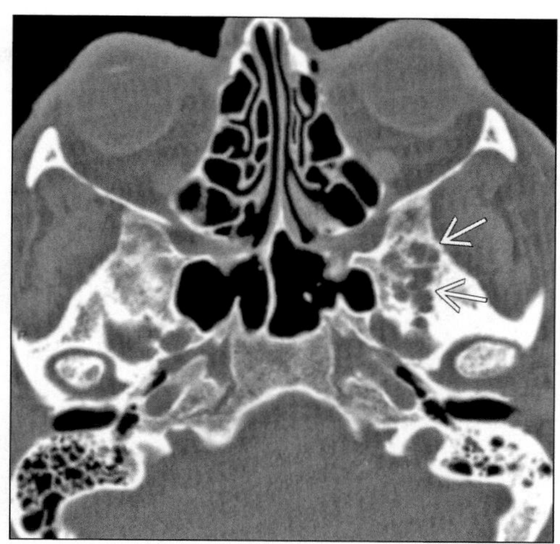

(Left) *Lateral internal carotid artery angiogram clearly depicts multiple giant arachnoid granulations in the transverse ➔ and proximal sigmoid ➲ venous sinuses. No intrasinus pressure gradient was present across the lesion.* ***(Right)*** *Axial bone CT through the mid sphenoid sinus shows multiple ovoid bony defects in the greater wing of sphenoid bone ➔ representing aberrant arachnoid granulations (arachnoid pits). These arachnoid granulations may enlarge from CSF pulsations.*

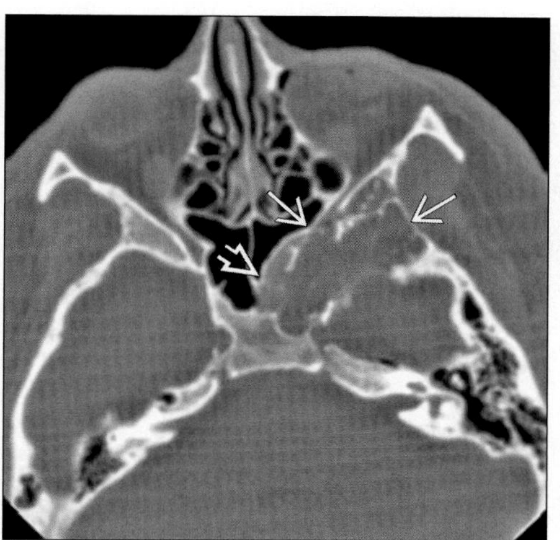

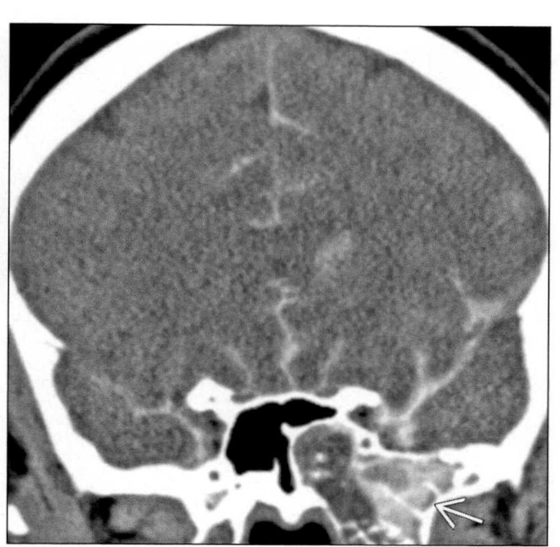

(Left) *Axial bone CT reveals a multilocular lesion in the left greater wing of the sphenoid ➔ and basisphenoid ➲. The most likely etiology of this lesion is CSF pulsations enlarging aberrant arachnoid granulations.* ***(Right)*** *Coronal CT cisternography in the same patient reveals contrast leaking ➔ from the subarachnoid space into the giant aberrant arachnoid granulations.*

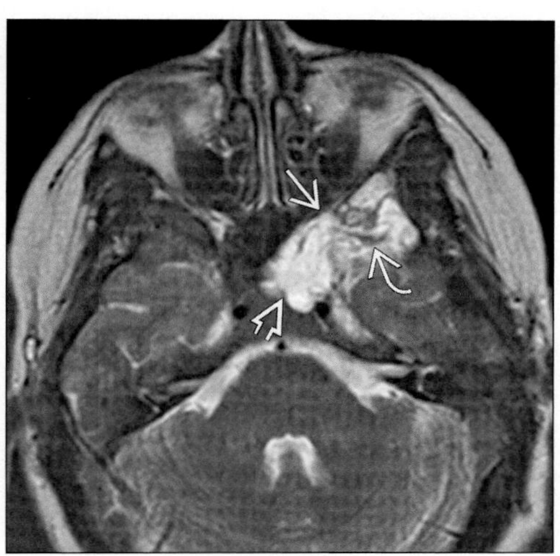

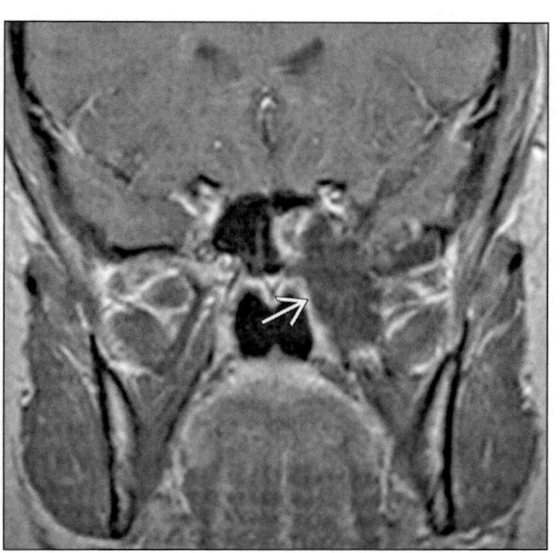

(Left) *Axial T2WI MR in the same patient demonstrates CSF signal within the greater wing of the sphenoid bone ➔ and basi-sphenoid ➲. Arachnoid outpouching with arachnoid stranding ➚ can be seen within the giant aberrant arachnoid granulations.* ***(Right)*** *Coronal T1WI C+ MR in the same patient shows fluid within the expanded pterygoid wing of sphenoid ➔. This represents CSF within an arachnoid pouch filling giant aberrant arachnoid granulations.*

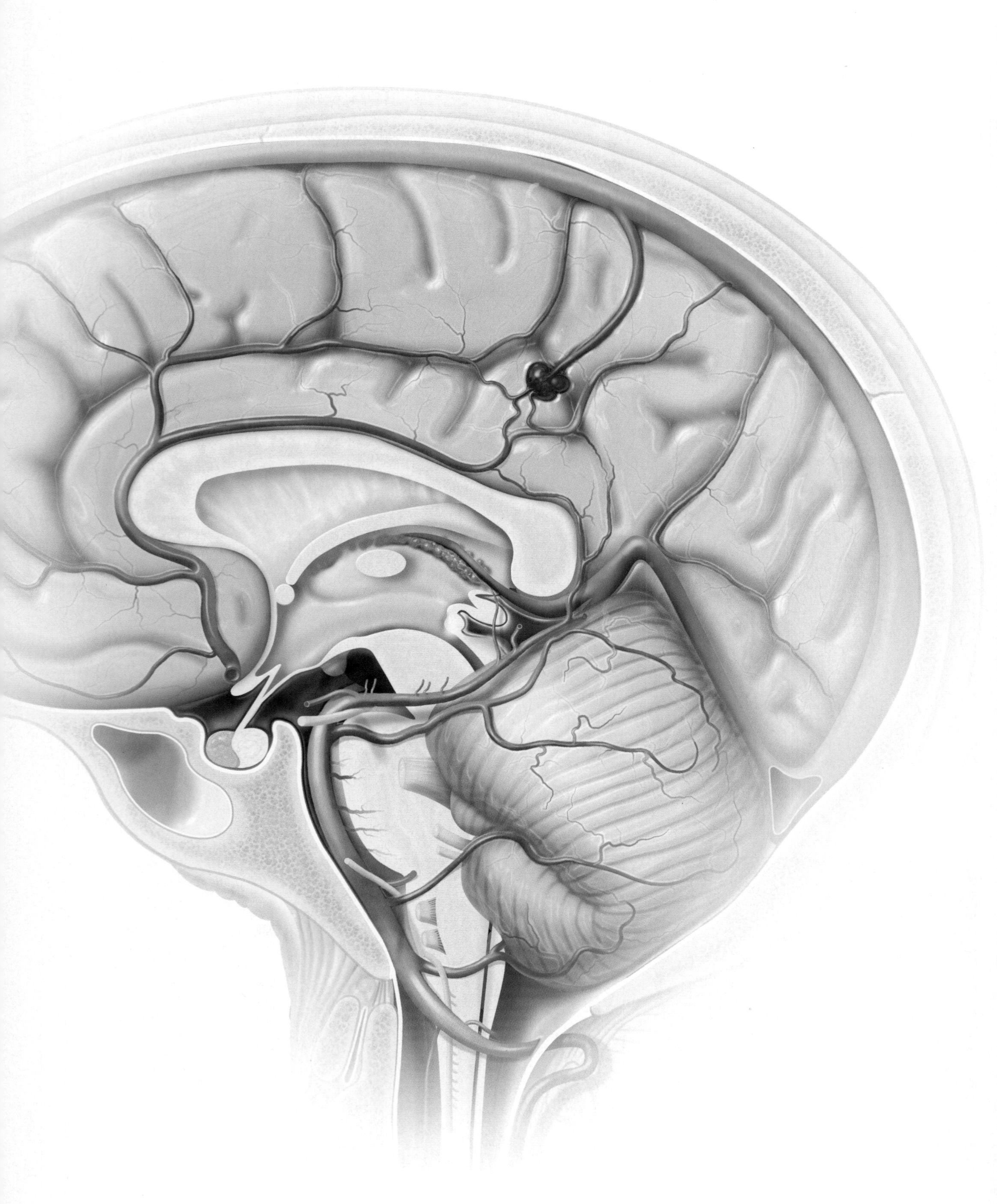

SECTION 5
Vascular Malformations

Introduction and Overview

CVMs with AV Shunting

CVMs without AV Shunting

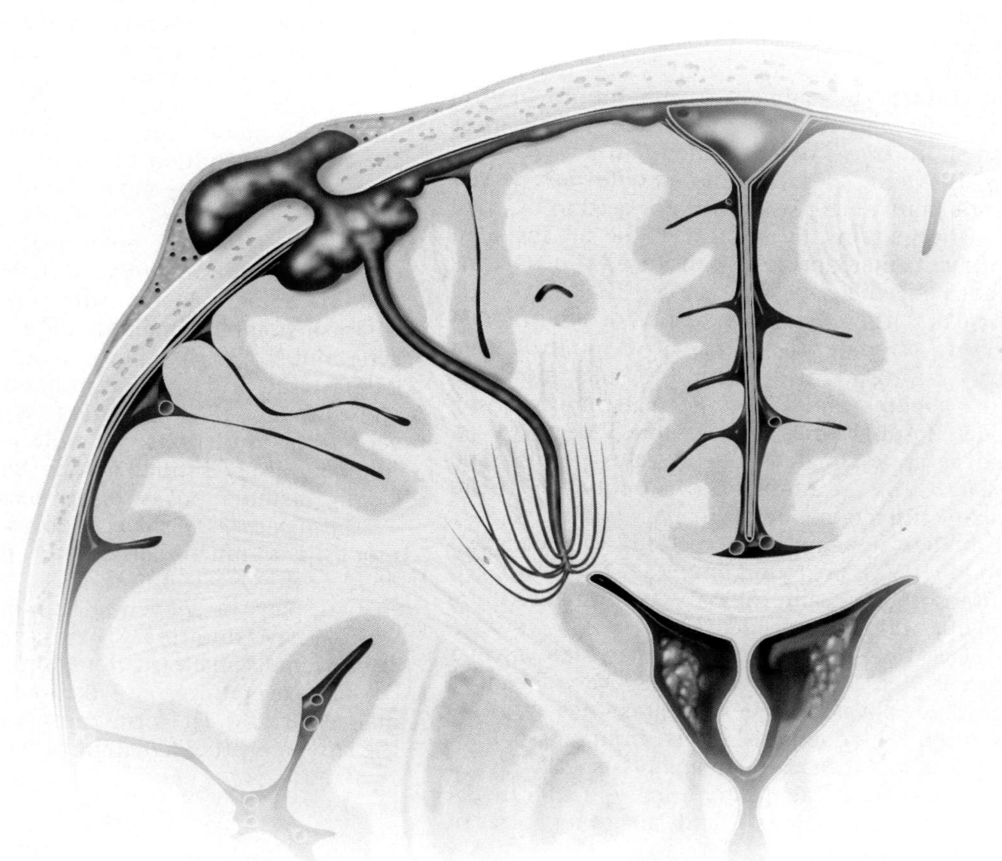

VASCULAR MALFORMATIONS OVERVIEW

General Considerations

Cerebrovascular malformations (CVMs) of the brain are a heterogeneous group of disorders that represent morphogenetic errors affecting arteries, capillaries, veins, or various combinations of vessels.

The presentation, natural history, and management approaches to CVMs depend on their type, location, size, and hemodynamic characteristics. Some CVMs such as venous or capillary malformations are almost always clinically silent and therefore usually identified at imaging or autopsy. Others, such as arteriovenous and cavernous malformations, may hemorrhage unexpectedly and without warning.

Terminology. Without a uniform consensus, there is much confusion regarding the nomenclature of brain CVMs. They have variously been called angiomas, hemangiomas, developmental anomalies, malformations, and hamartomas. For example, venous vascular malformations have been termed venous angiomas, venous anomalies, venous malformations, and developmental venous anomalies (DVAs). Cavernous malformations have been called cavernous angiomas, cavernous hemangiomas, and "cavernomas" in the literature.

Using accurate terminology when discussing brain vascular malformations is important. Two major groups of vascular anomalies are recognized: Vascular malformations and hemangiomas. All cerebrovascular malformations ("angiomas") are malformative lesions. In contrast, "hemangiomas" are true proliferating, vasoformative neoplasms and, in the most recent WHO classification "blue book," are included with the mesenchymal, nonmeningothelial tumors.

Hemangiomas are benign vascular neoplasms, not malformations, and can be capillary or cavernous. Most intracranial hemangiomas are found in the skull, meninges, and dural venous sinuses while most vascular malformations occur in the brain parenchyma. Therefore, the term "hemangioma" should be reserved for vasoproliferative neoplasms and not used to describe vascular malformations. In this text, CVMs are included in this section; hemangiomas are considered as neoplasms and included elsewhere.

Epidemiology. The overall prevalence of brain CVMs is difficult to estimate as accurate epidemiologic data are scarce. Cushing and Bailey found vascular anomalies constituted about 1% of all intracranial tumors. Using ICD-9 codes, hospital admission rates for CVMs have been calculated as approximately 1.5-1.8 cases per 100,000 person-years. CVMs are estimated to cause about 5% of all nontraumatic intracranial hemorrhages.

With modern imaging, and especially with contrast-enhanced MR, CVMs are found in up to 8-10% of imaged patients. Most (venous and capillary malformations) are asymptomatic and found incidentally.

Embryology. Development of the human fetal vascular system occurs via 2 related processes: Vasculogenesis and angiogenesis. Vasculogenesis begins with de novo differentiation of endothelial cells from mesoderm-derived precursors called hemangioblasts. Islands of hemangioblasts form an outer rim of endothelial cell precursors ("angioblasts") and an inner core of hematopoietic stem cells.

Angioblasts form capillary-like tubules that constitute the primitive vascular plexus. This embryonic vascular network is then remodeled by a process of sprouting, progressive anastomosis and retrogressive differentiation. Endothelial cells differentiate into arterial and venous types preceded, and guided by, migrating activated pericytes during definitive organization of the growing vessel wall.

Angiogenesis is regulated by a number of intercell signaling and growth factors. Some of these include Ang-1, Ang-2, Tie2, VEGF, PDGF, and TGF-β1, among others. Mutations in components of the angiogenetic system have been associated with the development of various CVMs.

Classification

In general, CVMs have been traditionally classified by histopathology and, more recently, by embryology and molecular genetics. With the advent of neurovascular interventional procedures, CVMs have also been classified by a practical, more functional approach.

Histopathologic classification. Most neuropathology texts classify CVMs into 4 major types: (1) arteriovenous malformation, (2) venous angioma, (3) capillary telangiectasia, and (4) cavernous malformation. The histopathologic classification is used in this book.

Embryologic classification. Lasjaunias et al. have proposed an embryonic, "metameric" approach to classifying vascular malformations that accounts for the known relationship between some brain and cutaneous vascular malformations. They termed these "cerebral arterial metameric syndromes" or "CAMS." For example, a CAMS1 syndrome links AVMs in the prosencephalon with those of the nose and orbit. Hence a CAMS1 patient may have a neurocutaneous AVM in the nose or retina and a brain parenchymal AVM.

Molecular classification. The identification of underlying causal genes in familial forms of CVMs has allowed the definition of an ever-increasing number of these disorders at the molecular level. Specific mutations in some genes (e.g., *CCM1/KRIT1*, *CCM2/MGC4607*, *CCM3/PDCD10*) cause autosomal dominantly inherited cavernous malformation syndromes (CCM1, CCM2, and CCM3). Some patients with brain AVMs also have cutaneous capillary malformations attributable to *RASA1* gene mutations. Hereditary hemorrhagic telangiectasias (HHT) result from several mutations, among them the endoglin gene (*ENG*) in HHT1. Whether cavernous and venous malformations are "molecularly distinct" or only "phenotypically distinct" lesions that result from the same *CCM* gene mutations is controversial.

Functional classification. Endovascular radiologists have proposed a functional, highly practical system that divides all CVMs into 2 basic categories: (1) CVMs that display arteriovenous shunting and (2) CVMs without AV shunting. The former category includes arteriovenous malformations and fistulae; the latter is basically everything else (venous, capillary, cavernous malformations). The former are amenable to intervention; the latter are either left alone or treated surgically.

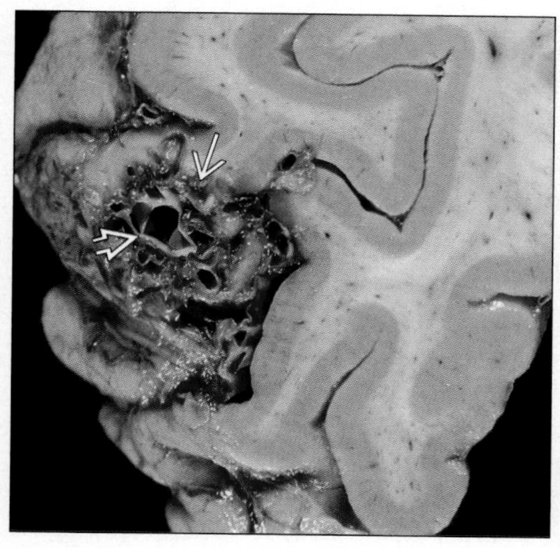

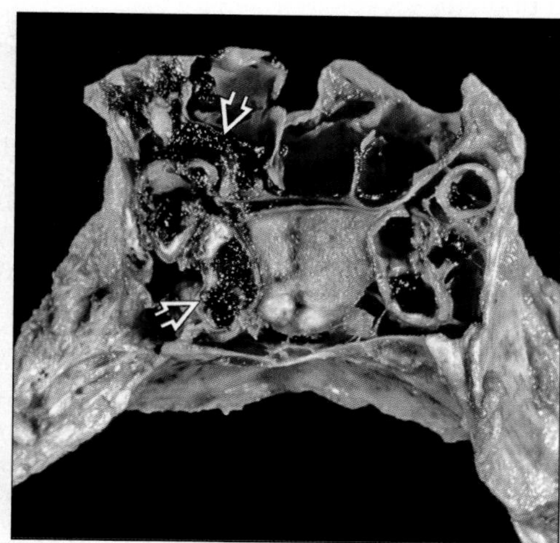

(Left) *Autopsied brain depicts typical findings of an unruptured arteriovenous malformation (AVM), the classic lesion with AV shunting. Multiple thin-walled vessels form the AVM nidus ➔. A larger vessel ➲ may represent an intranidal aneurysm. (Courtesy R. Hewlett, PhD.)* ***(Right)*** *Autopsy of a thrombosed carotid-cavernous fistula, another type of CVM that displays AV shunting, shows multiple enlarged, arterialized venous channels ➲. (Courtesy B. Horten, MD.)*

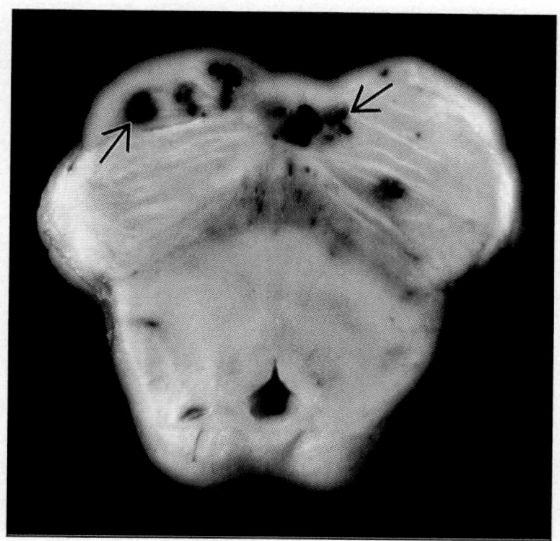

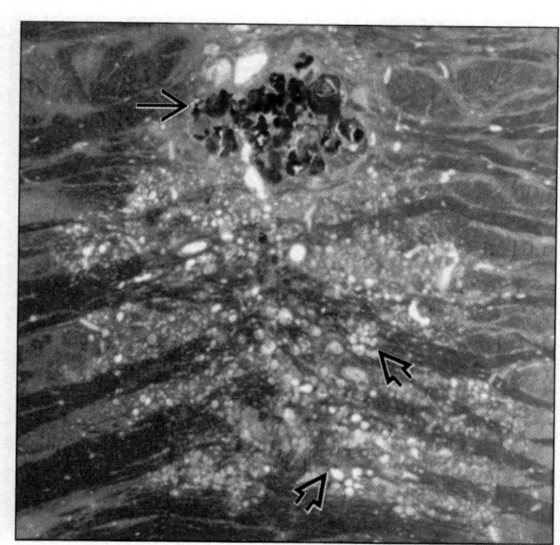

(Left) *Cut section through the upper pons and midbrain in a patient with familial multiple CCM syndrome demonstrates multiple tiny chronic hemorrhages ➔ characteristic of type 4 cavernous malformations. (Courtesy E. Ross, MD.)* ***(Right)*** *Low-power micropathology, Luxol fast blue stain, demonstrates a mixed pontine cavernous-capillary malformation. Normal white matter is interspersed with a cavernous malformation ➔ and multiple tiny thin-walled vessels ➲. (Courtesy AFIP.)*

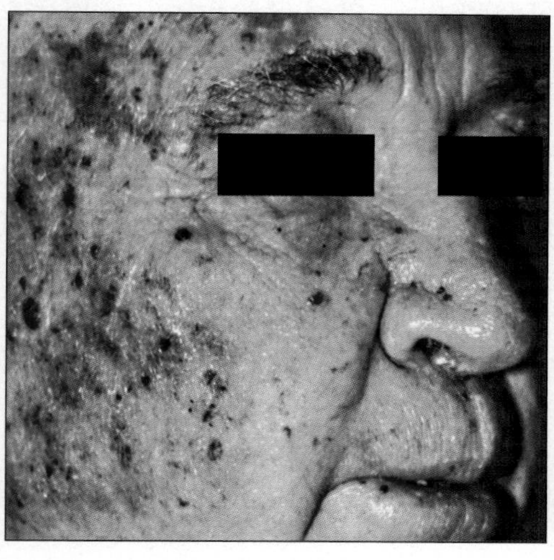

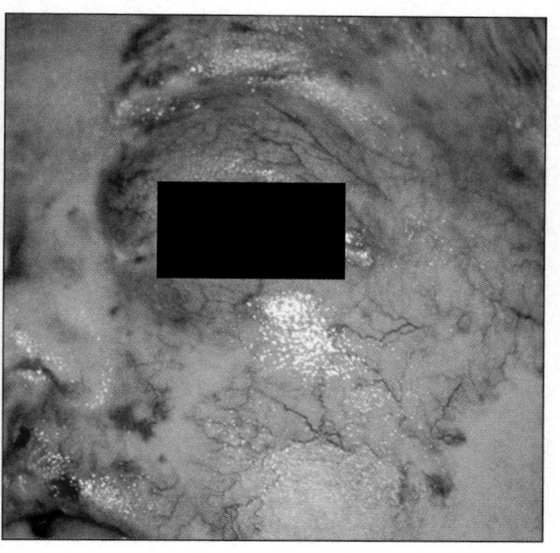

(Left) *Clinical photograph of a patient with hereditary hemorrhagic telangiectasis and multiple episodes of severe epistaxis shows innumerable small capillary telangiectasias of the skin and scalp, nasal and oral mucosa.* ***(Right)*** *Clinical photograph shows a 3-month-old infant with capillary hemangioma of the face. The hemangioma, a true benign vasoformative neoplasm, gradually regressed.*

ARTERIOVENOUS MALFORMATION

Key Facts

Terminology

- Pial vascular malformation of brain
  - Artery → vein (AV) shunting, no intervening capillary bed

Imaging

- General features
  - Supratentorial (85%), posterior fossa (15%)
- CT/CTA
  - Iso-/hyperdense serpentine vessels ± Ca++
  - Arterial feeders, nidus, draining veins enhance
- MR
  - "Bag of worms"/tangle of serpiginous "honeycomb" flow voids
  - No normal brain in between
  - Minimal/no mass effect
  - ± high signal (gliosis) on FLAIR
  - T2* GRE "blooming" if hemorrhage present
- DSA: Best delineates internal angioarchitecture, 3 components of AVM
  - Enlarged feeding arteries
  - Nidus of tightly packed vascular channels
  - Dilated draining veins
- Intranidal "aneurysm" > 50%
- Flow-related aneurysm on feeding artery (10-15%)

Top Differential Diagnoses

- Glioblastoma with AV shunting
- Dural AV fistula

Clinical Issues

- Presentation: Headache with hemorrhage (50%)
- Treatment options
  - Embolization
  - Microsurgical resection
  - Stereotaxic XRT

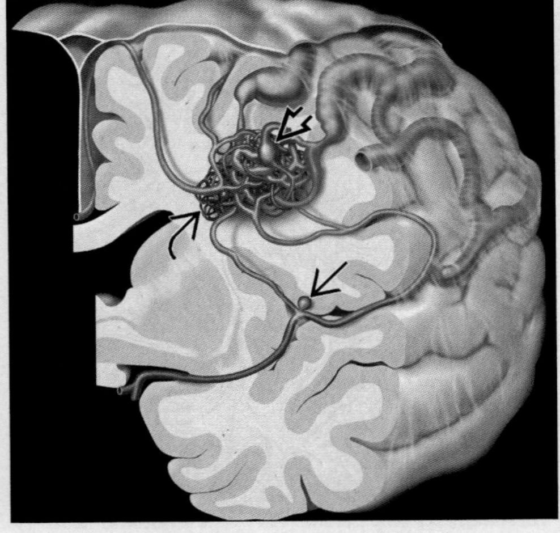

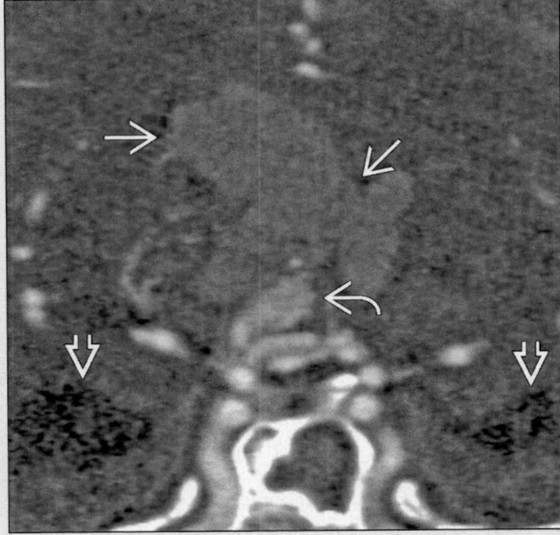

(Left) *Coronal graphic shows a classic cerebral arteriovenous malformation (AVM). Note the nidus with intranidal aneurysm and enlarged feeding arteries with a "pedicle" aneurysm.* ***(Right)*** *Coronal CTA in a young patient with spontaneous intracranial hemorrhage shows parenchymal and intraventricular hemorrhage. Note hydrocephalus with enlarged temporal horns. An ill-defined vascular blush is seen extending to the ventricular surface.*

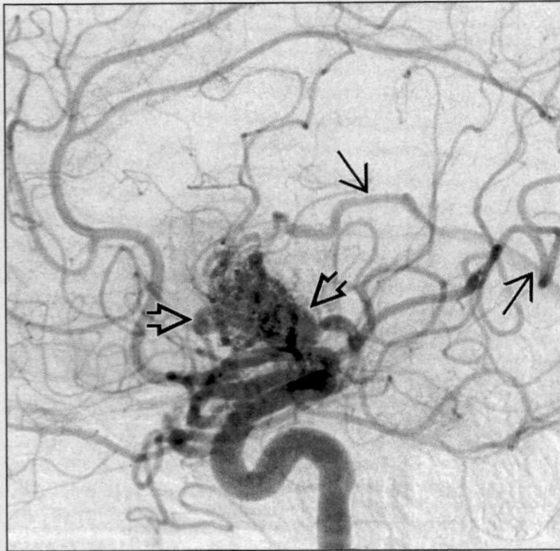

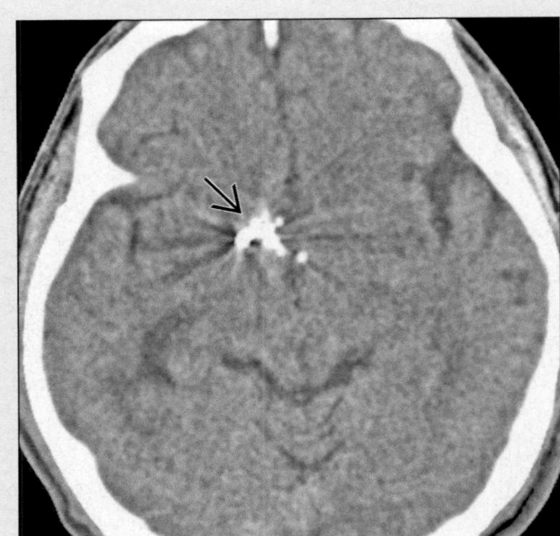

(Left) *Lateral DSA in the same patient shows an AVM nidus superior to the carotid terminus. No intranidal or feeding pedicle aneurysms were identified. Note the early deep venous drainage into the internal cerebral vein and straight sinus.* ***(Right)*** *Axial NECT in the same patient after embolization of 2 arterial feeding pedicles with Onyx shows a hyperdense cast within the nidus. AVMs of this small size do not require staged embolization to prevent normal perfusion pressure breakthrough.*

ARTERIOVENOUS MALFORMATION

TERMINOLOGY

Abbreviations

- Arteriovenous malformation (AVM)

Definitions

- Pial vascular malformation with direct artery → vein (AV) shunting, no intervening capillary bed

IMAGING

General Features

- Best diagnostic clue
  - "Bag of worms" (flow voids) on MR with minimal/ no mass effect
- Location
  - May occur anywhere in brain
    - Supratentorial (85%), posterior fossa (15%)
  - 98% solitary, sporadic
    - Multiple AVMs rare, usually syndromic
- Size
  - Varies from microscopic to giant
  - Most symptomatic AVMs are 3-6 cm
- Morphology
  - 3 components
    - Enlarged feeding arteries
    - Nidus of tightly packed, enlarged vascular channels
    - Dilated draining veins
  - No normal brain in between

CT Findings

- NECT
  - May be normal (if AVM very small)
  - Iso-/hyperdense serpentine vessels
  - Ca++ in 25-30%
  - AVM bleed → parenchymal, intraventricular hemorrhage > > subarachnoid hemorrhage
  - Status post embolization: Liquid embolics appear hyperdense within nidus
- CECT
  - Strong enhancement of arterial feeders, nidus, draining veins
- CTA
  - Depicts enlarged arteries, draining veins

MR Findings

- T1WI
  - Signal varies with flow rate, direction, presence/age of hemorrhage
  - Tightly packed mass: "Honeycomb" of flow voids
- T2WI
  - Tangle of serpiginous, "honeycomb" flow voids
  - Variable hemorrhage
  - Little/no brain inside nidus
    - Some gliotic, high signal tissue may be present
- FLAIR
  - Flow voids ± surrounding high signal (gliosis)
- T2* GRE
  - "Blooming" if hemorrhage present
- T1WI C+
  - Strong enhancement of nidus, draining veins
  - Rapid flow may not enhance ("flow void")
- MRA
  - Helpful for gross depiction of flow, post embo/XRT
  - Does not depict detailed angioarchitecture

Angiographic Findings

- DSA best delineates internal angioarchitecture
- Use high-frame rate, ↑ volume + rate of contrast injection per acquisition
- Depicts 3 components of AVMs
  - Enlarged arteries ± flow-related aneurysm(s)
  - Nidus of tightly packed vessels ± intranidal aneurysm(s)
  - Early draining veins ± venous stenoses due to high-flow venopathy (may ↑ intracranial hemorrhage [ICH] risk)
- 27-32% have "dual" arterial supply (pial, dural)

Imaging Recommendations

- Best imaging tool
  - DSA with high-frame rate acquisitions ± superselective catheterization
- Protocol advice
  - Standard MR (include Gd-MRA, GRE sequences)

DIFFERENTIAL DIAGNOSIS

Glioblastoma with AV Shunting

- GBM enhances (tumor blush on DSA), has mass effect
- Some parenchyma between vessels

Thrombosed ("Cryptic") AVM

- Cavernous angioma
- Calcified neoplasm
- Oligodendroglioma
- Low-grade astrocytoma

Dural AV Fistula (dAVF)

- AV shunts within wall of patent ± partially thrombosed dural venous sinus, parallel venous channel, or adjacent cortical vein
- Most common location = transverse/sigmoid sinuses
- Differentiate from pial AVM by
  - Location: Nidus intimately related to dural venous sinus
  - Predominant blood supply is from dural (meningeal) arteries > > pial artery
    - e.g., middle and posterior meningeal arteries, artery of falx cerebelli, tentorial branches of cavernous ICA, occipital artery, artery of Davidoff and Schechter
  - Some parasitization of pial supply possible with larger dAVFs
  - Flow-related aneurysm are rare

PATHOLOGY

General Features

- Etiology
  - Dysregulated angiogenesis
    - Vascular endothelial growth factors (VEGFs), receptors mediate endothelial proliferation, migration

ARTERIOVENOUS MALFORMATION

  - Cytokine receptors mediate vascular maturation, remodeling
- Genetics
  - Sporadic AVMs have multiple up-/down-regulated genes
    - Homeobox genes, such as *Hox D3* and *B3*, involved in angiogenesis may malfunction
  - Syndromic AVMs (2% of cases)
    - Multiple AVMs in *HHT1* (endoglin gene mutation)
    - Cerebrofacial arteriovenous metameric syndromes (CAMS) have orbit/maxillofacial + intracranial AVMs
- Associated abnormalities
  - Flow-related aneurysm on feeding artery (10-15%)
  - Intranidal "aneurysm" > 50%
  - Vascular "steal" may cause ischemia in adjacent brain
    - PET studies may show hemodynamic impairment

Staging, Grading, & Classification

- Spetzler-Martin scale
  - Sum of following estimates surgical risk, from 1-5
    - Size
      - Small (< 3 cm) = 1
      - Medium (3-6 cm) = 2
      - Large (> 6 cm) = 3
    - Location
      - In "noneloquent" area = 0
      - Involves "eloquent" brain = 1
      - "Eloquent" = sensorimotor cortex, visual cortex, hypothalamus, thalamus, internal capsule, brainstem, cerebellar peduncles, deep nuclei
    - Venous drainage
      - Superficial only = 0
      - Deep = 1

Gross Pathologic & Surgical Features

- Wedge-shaped, compact mass of tangled vessels

Microscopic Features

- Wide phenotypic spectrum
  - Feeding arteries usually enlarged but mature (may have some wall thickening)
  - Enlarged draining veins (may have associated varix, stenosis)
  - Nidus
    - Conglomeration of numerous tiny AV shunts
    - Thin-walled dysplastic vessels (no capillary bed)
    - Disorganized collagen, variable muscularization
    - No intervening normal brain (may have some gliosis)
  - Perinidal capillary network (PDCN)
    - Nidus surrounded by dilated capillaries in brain tissue 1-7 mm outside nidus border
    - Vessels in PDCN 10-25x larger than normal capillaries

CLINICAL ISSUES

Presentation

- Most common signs/symptoms
  - Headache with hemorrhage (50%)
  - Seizure (25%)
  - Focal neurologic deficit (20-25%)
- Clinical profile
  - Young adult with spontaneous (nontraumatic) ICH

Demographics

- Age
  - Peak presentation = 20-40 years (25% by age 15)
- Gender
  - M = F
- Epidemiology
  - Most common symptomatic cerebral vascular malformation (CVM)
  - Prevalence of sporadic AVMs = 0.04-0.52%

Natural History & Prognosis

- All brain AVMs are potentially hazardous
  - Risk of 1st hemorrhage is lifelong, rises with age (2-4% per year, cumulative)
  - Vast majority will become symptomatic during patient's lifetime
- Spontaneous obliteration rare (< 1% of cases)
  - 75% have small lesion (< 3 cm), single draining vein
  - 75% have "spontaneous" ICH

Treatment

- Embolization
  - Staged procedures ↓ risk of normal perfusion pressure breakthrough (→ cerebral edema, ICH)
  - If AVM rupture, aim of embolization = target site of bleed to ↓ recurrence risk (e.g., flow-related or intranidal aneurysms)
  - Often performed as preoperative adjunct to resection
  - Likelihood of complete cure with embolization alone ↑ if small AVM, few feeders, single draining vein, liquid embolics used
- Microneurosurgical resection
- Stereotactic radiosurgery
  - Cure rate ↓ with ↑ nidus size
  - < 3 cm: > 95% cured in 2-3 years
  - Latent period for cure up to 4 years (patient still at risk for ICH until cured)

DIAGNOSTIC CHECKLIST

Consider

- MR of vascular-appearing lesion that has brain parenchyma in between flow voids may be vascular neoplasm, not AVM

Image Interpretation Pearls

- Look carefully for pedicle, intranidal aneurysms
- Look for subtle early draining veins; may be only clue to diagnosis of largely thrombosed AVMs

SELECTED REFERENCES

1. Santos ML et al: Angioarchitecture and clinical presentation of brain arteriovenous malformations. Arq Neuropsiquiatr. 67(2A):316-21, 2009
2. Maruyama K et al: Optimal timing for Gamma Knife surgery after hemorrhage from brain arteriovenous malformations. J Neurosurg. 109 Suppl:73-6, 2008

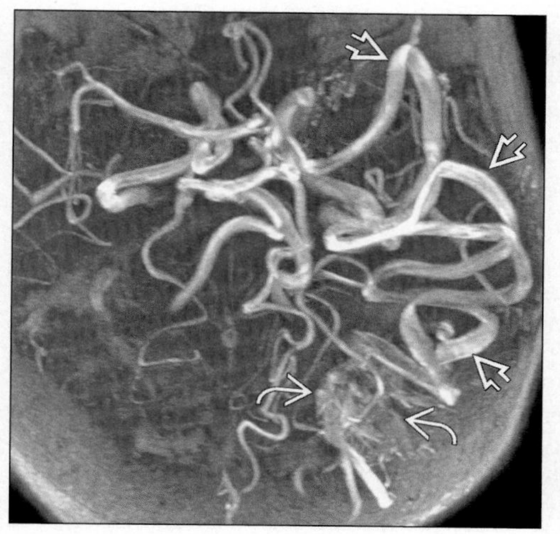

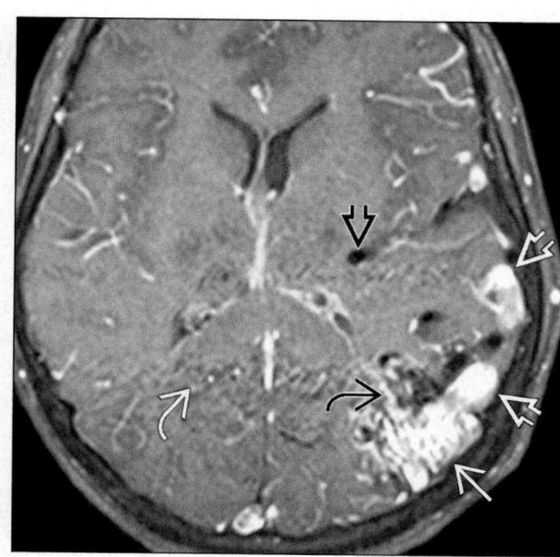

(Left) *Axial TOF MRA MIP in a 38-year-old patient with a worsening headache and visual disturbance shows a left parietooccipital AVM* ➔ *with massively dilated MCA feeding arteries* ➔. ***(Right)*** *Axial T1WI C+ MR in the same patient shows avid enhancement of the nidus* ➔ *and enlarged superficial draining veins* ➔. *Note that a portion of the nidus* ➔ *and feeding arteries* ➔ *appear as flow voids due to the high flow within the vessels. Phase artifact* ➔ *propagation across the image is striking.*

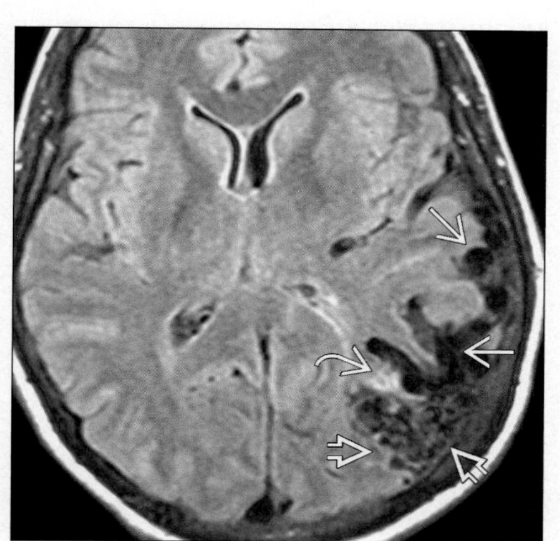

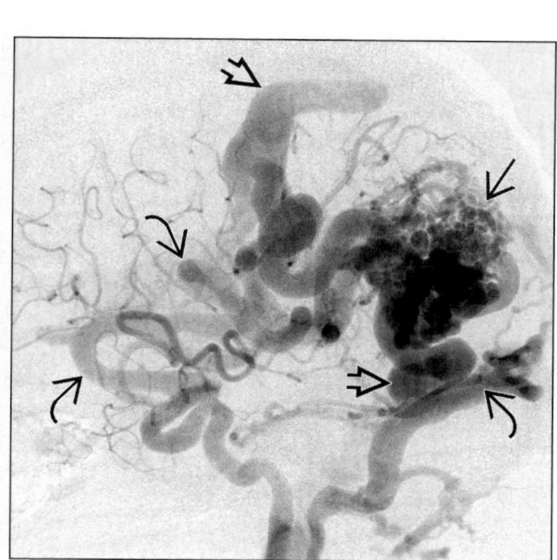

(Left) *Axial FLAIR MR shows "honeycomb" flow voids representing the AVM nidus* ➔. *Large serpentine flow voids anterior to the nidus are MCA feeding arteries ± draining veins* ➔. *Note only mild mass effect on the trigone of the left lateral ventricle relative to the size of the lesion. Some high signal adjacent to the nidus* ➔ *likely represents gliosis.* ***(Right)*** *Lateral ICA DSA in the same patient shows enlarged MCA feeders* ➔, *dilated/ tortuous superficial draining veins* ➔, *and AVM nidus* ➔.

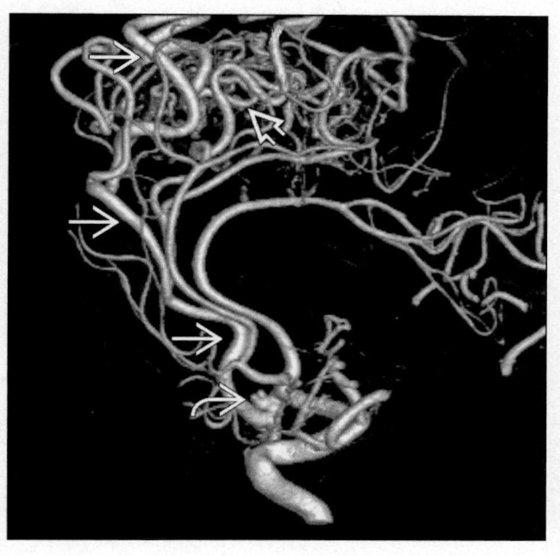

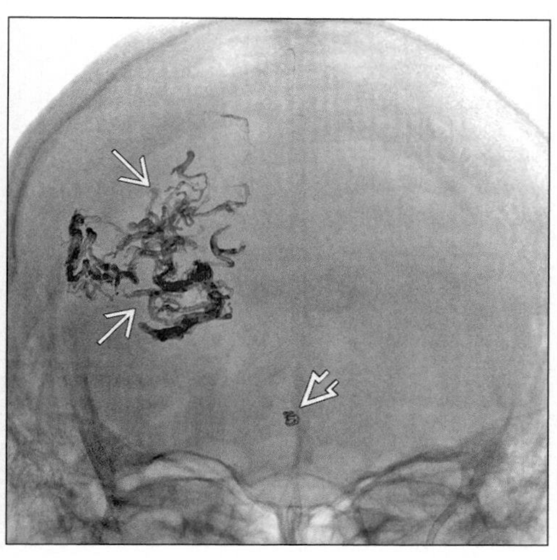

(Left) *Oblique left ICA 3D DSA shows an enlarged right ACA* ➔ *supplying a right frontal lobe AVM* ➔. *Note the flow-related aneurysm of the ACoA* ➔, *which is a potential cause of future subarachnoid hemorrhage.* ***(Right)*** *Posteroanterior unsubtracted image, after 3 sessions of staged embolization of multiple ACA and MCA feeders, shows an Onyx cast within the nidus and adjacent feeding arteries* ➔. *The ACoA flow-related aneurysm was coiled* ➔ *prior to embolization of the ACA feeders.*

DURAL AV FISTULA

Key Facts

Imaging

- General: Network of tiny (crack-like) vessels in wall of thrombosed dural venous sinus
- NECT usually normal
  - Subarachnoid hemorrhage if rupture of dAVF or (rarely) flow-related aneurysm
- CECT
  - Tortuous feeding arteries ± flow-related aneurysms
  - Dilated, tortuous cortical draining veins
- MR
  - Isointense thrombosed sinus ± flow voids on T1/T2WI
  - Thrombosed dural sinus blooms on T2*
  - May show parenchymal hemorrhage in dAVF with cortical venous drainage
  - FLAIR: Isointense thrombosed sinus ± adjacent edema if venous congestion or ischemia present
- DSA: Predominant supply from meningeal arteries
  - Retrograde venous drainage in dural sinus(es) ± cortical veins

Top Differential Diagnoses

- Hypoplastic transverse-sigmoid sinus
- Sigmoid sinus-jugular foramen pseudolesion
- Thrombosed dural sinus

Clinical Issues

- Treatment
  - Conservative (e.g., observation, carotid compression)
  - Endovascular: Embolization of arterial feeders ± venous pouch/sinus
  - Surgical resection: Skeletonization of involved dural venous sinus
  - Stereotaxic radiosurgery: Time delay of 2-3 years for obliteration

*(**Left**) Axial bone CT shows enlargement of the right foramen spinosum ➔, compared with the left side ➔, due to enlargement of the middle meningeal artery, a common arterial supply to dural arteriovenous fistulas (dAVF). (**Right**) Axial T2WI MR shows tiny flow voids (crack-like vessels) ➔ at the junction of the sigmoid and superior petrosal sinuses (SPS). Additional large flow voids are see in the cerebellopontine angle and rostral pons ➔, representing dilated draining veins in this patient with a SPS dAVF.*

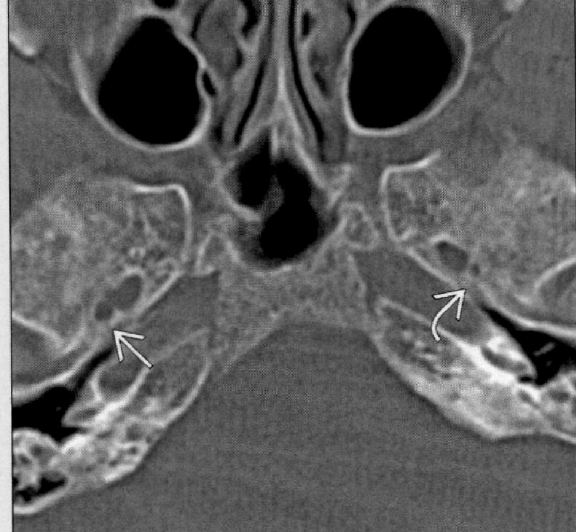

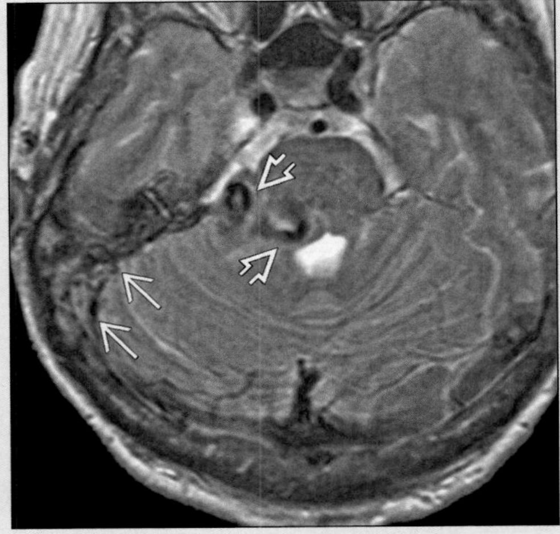

*(**Left**) Lateral DSA of the right external carotid artery shows a high-risk (grade 4) dAVF of the superior petrosal sinus ➔ with dilated, tortuous cortical draining veins ➔. Note the dilated middle meningeal artery ➔ and venous stenosis ➔ from high-flow venopathy. (**Right**) Lateral ECA DSA after embolization and surgical resection of the dAVF shows no residual arteriovenous shunting. A combination of metallic coils and liquid embolics were used preoperatively to reduce flow.*

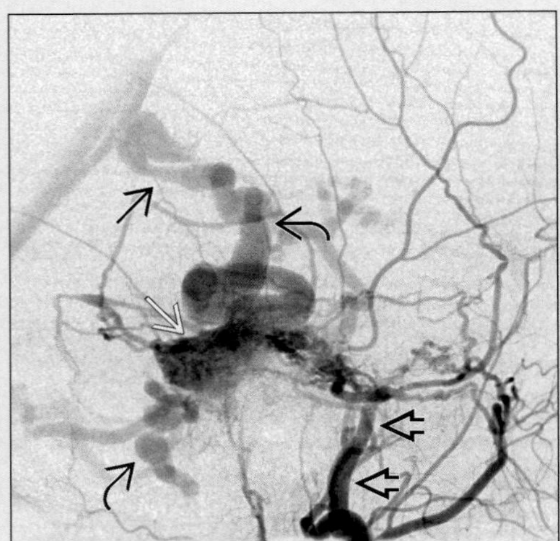

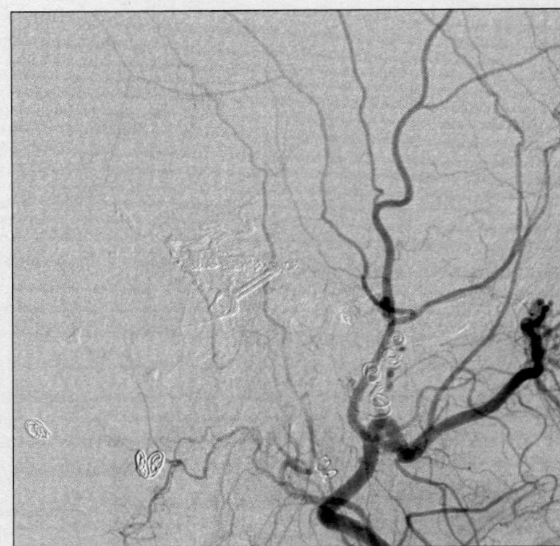

DURAL AV FISTULA

TERMINOLOGY

Abbreviations

- Dural arteriovenous fistula (dAVF)

Synonyms

- Dural arteriovenous malformation (dAVM)

Definitions

- Heterogeneous group of lesions with common angioarchitecture (arteriovenous shunts associated with dural venous sinus wall)

IMAGING

General Features

- Best diagnostic clue
  - MR/CTA: Network of tiny (crack-like) vessels in wall of thrombosed dural venous sinus
  - DSA: Predominant arterial supply from meningeal arteries (compare pial AVMs)
  - Bone CT: Dilated transosseous calvarial vascular channels, enlarged foramen spinosum
- Location
  - Can involve any dural venous sinus
    - Most common (35-40%) = transverse sinus (TS) + sigmoid sinus (SS)
    - Other common sites = cavernous sinus (CS), superior sagittal sinus (SSS), superior petrosal sinus (SPS)

CT Findings

- NECT
  - May see dilated vascular channels in skull from transosseous feeding arteries
  - Ipsilateral enlargement of foramen spinosum
    - Contains middle meningeal artery that commonly supplies dAVFs
  - Look for complications: Subarachnoid hemorrhage, cerebral edema (venous hypertension)
- CECT
  - May see tortuous feeding arteries ± flow-related aneurysms (uncommon), draining veins
  - Involved dural venous sinus usually stenotic/partially thrombosed
- CTA
  - 3D CTA may be useful in static depiction of angioarchitecture

MR Findings

- T1WI
  - Isointense thrombosed dural sinus ± flow voids
- T2WI
  - Isointense thrombosed sinus ± flow voids
  - Focal hyperintensity in adjacent brain = retrograde leptomeningeal venous drainage (RLVD), venous perfusion abnormalities
- FLAIR
  - Isointense thrombosed sinus ± adjacent edema if venous congestion or ischemia present
- T2* GRE
  - May show parenchymal hemorrhage in dAVF with cortical venous drainage
  - Thrombosed dural sinus will bloom
- DWI
  - Normal unless venous infarct or ischemia present
- T1WI C+
  - Chronically thrombosed sinus usually enhances
- MRA
  - Time-resolved contrast-augmented MRA useful for gross depiction of angioarchitecture and dynamics
  - TOF MRA positive in larger dAVF; may be negative with small or slow-flow shunts
- MRV
  - Depicts occluded parent sinus, collateral flow
  - 3D phase contrast MRA with low velocity encoding can identify fistula, feeding arteries, flow reversal in draining veins

Angiographic Findings

- Conventional
  - Multiple arterial feeders are typical
    - Dural/transosseous branches from ECA most common
    - Tentorial/dural branches from ICA, VA
    - Parasitization of pial arteries with larger dAVFs
  - Arterial inflow into parallel venous channel ("recipient pouch") common; can be embolized with preservation of parent sinus
  - Involved dural sinus often thrombosed
  - Flow reversal in dural sinus/cortical veins correlates with progressive symptoms, risk of hemorrhage
  - Tortuous engorged pial veins ("pseudophlebitic" pattern) with venous congestion/hypertension (clinically aggressive)
  - High-flow venopathy → progressive stenosis, outlet occlusion, hemorrhage

Imaging Recommendations

- Best imaging tool
  - DSA ± superselective catheterization of dural, transosseous feeders
- Protocol advice
  - Screening MR, contrast-augmented MRA
  - DSA to delineate vascular supply, venous drainage (assess risk of future intracranial hemorrhage [ICH])

DIFFERENTIAL DIAGNOSIS

Pial AVM

- Congenital vascular lesion with intraaxial nidus and no intervening normal brain parenchyma
- Predominant pial arterial supply, parasitization of dural supply possible (opposite to dAVF)

Sigmoid Sinus-Jugular Foramen Pseudolesion

- Slow or asymmetric flow creates variable signal on MR sequences
- Use MRV with multiple encoding gradients to clarify

Thrombosed Dural Sinus

- Collateral/congested venous drainage can mimic dAVF
- Can be spontaneous, traumatic, infectious (thrombophlebitis)

DURAL AV FISTULA

PATHOLOGY

General Features

- Etiology
  - Adult dAVFs are usually acquired, not congenital
    - Often idiopathic
    - Can occur in response to trauma, venous sinus thrombosis
  - Infant dAVFs are congenital and usually associated with enlargement of dural venous sinuses
  - Pathological activation of neoangiogenesis
    - Proliferating capillaries within granulation tissue in dural sinus obliterated by organized thrombi
    - Budding/proliferation of microvascular network in inner dura connects to plexus of thin-walled venous channels, creating microfistulae
    - High bFGF, VEGF expression in dAVFs
- Associated abnormalities
  - Cortical venous drainage associated with edema, encephalopathy
  - Venous HTN may lead to developmental delay in children
  - Arterialized flow in cortical veins/dural sinuses → high-flow venopathy → cortical vein stenosis, tortuosity, aneurysm + dural venous sinus stenosis, thrombosis → ↑ ICH risk

Staging, Grading, & Classification

- Cognard classification of intracranial dAVFs correlates venous drainage pattern with risk of ICH
  - Grade 1: Located in sinus wall, normal antegrade venous drainage, benign clinical course
  - Grade 2A: Located in main sinus, reflux into sinus but not cortical veins
  - Grade 2B: Reflux (retrograde drainage) into cortical veins, 10-20% hemorrhage rate
  - Grade 3: Direct cortical venous drainage, no venous ectasia, 40% hemorrhage
  - Grade 4: Direct cortical venous drainage, venous ectasia, 65% hemorrhage
  - Grade 5: Spinal perimedullary venous drainage, progressive myelopathy
- Indirect carotid-cavernous fistula (CCF) = 2nd most common dAVF site
  - Barrow classification based on arterial supply
    - Type A: Direct ICA-cavernous sinus high-flow shunt (not dAVF)
    - Type B: Dural ICA branches-cavernous shunt
    - Type C: Dural ECA-cavernous shunt
    - Type D: ECA/ICA dural branches shunt to cavernous sinus

Gross Pathologic & Surgical Features

- Multiple enlarged dural feeders converge on dural sinus, which is often thrombosed
- Enlarged cortical draining veins with stenoses, dilatation, and tortuosity

Microscopic Features

- Arterialized veins with irregular intimal thickening, variable loss of internal elastic lamina

CLINICAL ISSUES

Presentation

- Most common signs/symptoms
  - Varies with site, type of shunt
    - TS-SS = pulsatile tinnitus
    - Cavernous sinus = pulsatile exophthalmos, CN3,4,6 neuropathy
    - Infant dAVF: Developmental delay, ↑ head circumference
  - Uncommon: Encephalopathic symptoms (venous hypertension, ischemia/thrombosis)
    - Progressive dementia
  - Rare: Life-threatening congestive heart failure
    - Usually neonates, infants
- Clinical profile
  - Middle-aged patient with pulse-synchronous tinnitus

Demographics

- Age
  - Adult dAVF usually presents in middle-aged patients
- Epidemiology
  - 10-15% of all cerebrovascular malformations with AV shunting

Natural History & Prognosis

- Prognosis, clinical course depends on location, venous drainage pattern
  - 98% of dAVFs without retrograde venous drainage have benign course
  - dAVFs with retrograde venous drainage have aggressive clinical course

Treatment

- Conservative: Observation ± carotid compression technique
- Treatment options if hemorrhage risk exists
  - Endovascular: Embolization of arterial feeders with particulate or liquid agents, coil embolization of recipient venous pouch/sinus
  - Surgical resection: Skeletonization of involved dural venous sinus
  - Stereotaxic radiosurgery: Time delay of 2-3 years for obliteration

DIAGNOSTIC CHECKLIST

Consider

- DSA for definitive exclusion of dAVF in patient with objective pulsatile tinnitus

Image Interpretation Pearls

- MR + MRA may be normal in small dAVF
- **Always** examine bilateral ICAs, ECAs, and vertebral arteries when performing DSA to exclude dAVF

SELECTED REFERENCES

1. Chew J et al: Arterial Onyx embolisation of intracranial DAVFs with cortical venous drainage. Can J Neurol Sci. 36(2):168-75, 2009

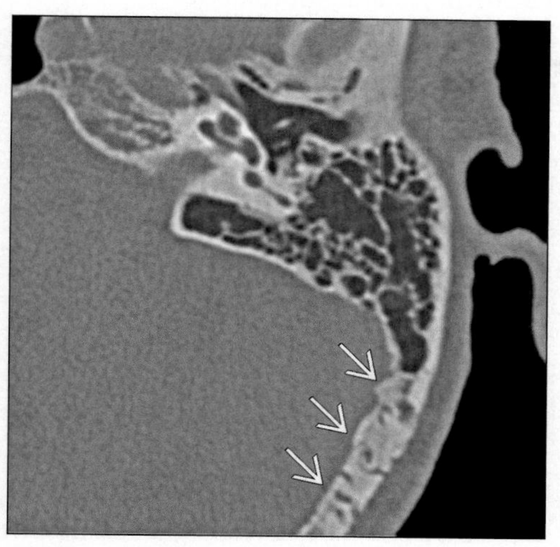

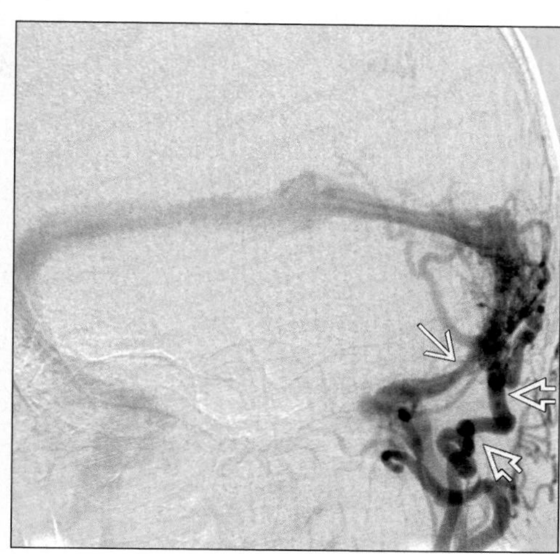

(Left) *Axial left temporal bone CT in a patient with pulsatile tinnitus shows prominent vascular channels in the calvarium, suspicious for underlying dAVF.* ***(Right)*** *Anteroposterior DSA shows a grade 2A dAVF of the left sigmoid sinus (SS). Note the dilated occipital artery supplying the dAVF via innumerable transosseous branches. A stenosis in the distal SS is promoting retrograde flow in the ipsilateral transverse and sigmoid sinuses and across the torcular into the right SS.*

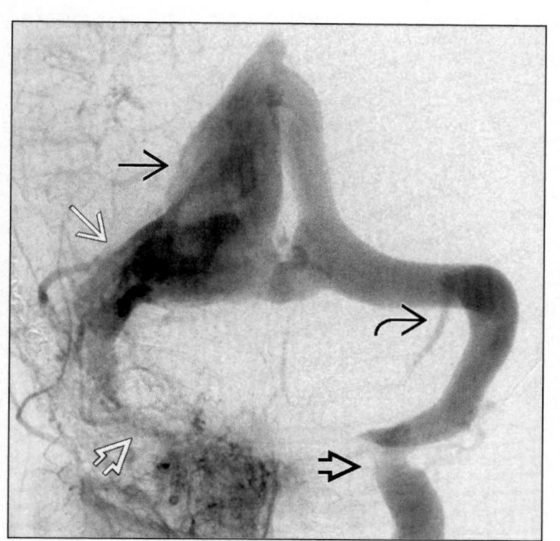

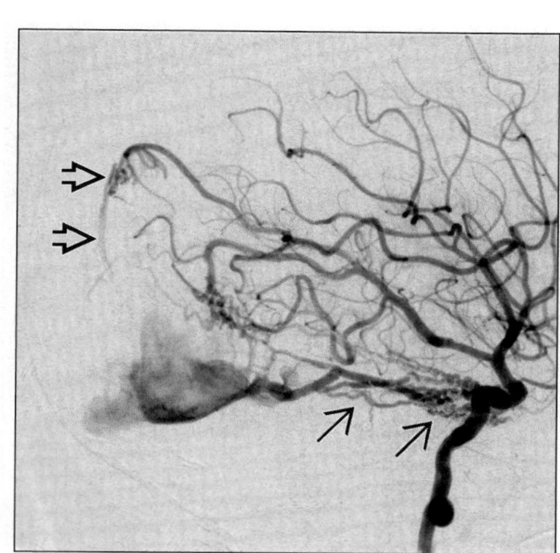

(Left) *Anteroposterior DSA in an infant with extensive dAVF of the right transverse and sigmoid sinuses (TS, SS). The right TS and hemi-torcular are dilated. The ipsilateral SS is occluded with retrograde flow and venous egress via the left TS and SS. A stenosis of the left jugular bulb is present, and some reflux into cortical veins is evident.* ***(Right)*** *Lateral right ICA DSA shows tentorial artery feeders supplying the dAVF. Additional parasitization of pial supply from the PCA is evident.*

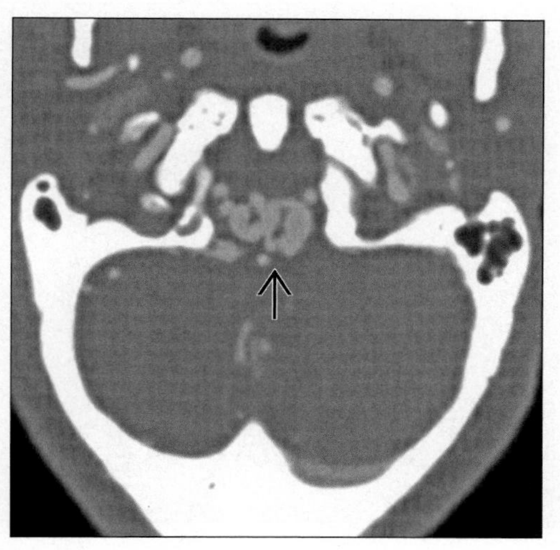

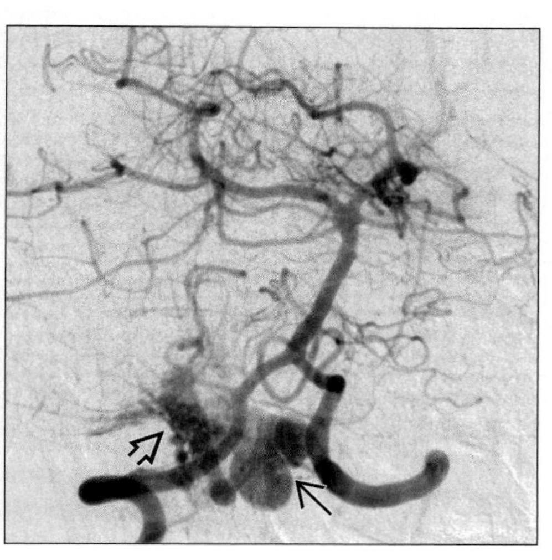

(Left) *Axial CTA in a patient presenting with subarachnoid hemorrhage shows large, enhancing vessels in the vicinity of the foramen magnum, posterior to the medulla oblongata.* ***(Right)*** *Oblique right vertebral artery DSA shows a marginal sinus dAVF supplied predominantly by a posterior meningeal artery arising from the right vertebral artery. There is retrograde venous drainage into dilated, tortuous cortical veins, which increases the risk of intracranial hemorrhage.*

PIAL AV FISTULA

Key Facts

Terminology
- Pial vascular malformation with direct arteriovenous (AV) shunting
  - No intervening capillary bed or nidus
  - May occur anywhere in brain, spinal cord
  - Can lie on surface/within brain or at ependyma

Imaging
- CT: Iso-/hyperdense serpentine vessels ± Ca++
  - Arterial feeder(s), draining veins enhance
- DSA
  - Dilated feeding artery drains directly into enlarged vein
  - ± confluence of arteries just before fistulous connection
  - No intervening nidus

Top Differential Diagnoses
- Arteriovenous malformation (AVM)
- Dural AV fistula
- Vein of Galen aneurysmal malformation

Pathology
- Enlarged mature arteries, variceal draining veins
- Draining veins are "arterialized" with thickened walls
  - May have variceal "aneurysms" ± high-flow venopathy, stenosis

Clinical Issues
- Much higher hemorrhage risk than AVM
- Spontaneous obliteration may be more common, especially in infants
- Embolization curative if draining vein occluded at fistulous site

*(**Left**) Graphic shows a pial AV fistula along the medial cerebral hemisphere. Several slightly enlarged pial ACA branches ➡ connect directly to a dilated cortical draining vein ➡. No nidus is present. A multilobed venous varix ➡ is present at the fistulous site. (**Right**) Axial NECT shows hyperdense, flowing blood density, curvilinear vessels within the right lateral ventricle due to intraventricular varices draining a pAVF ➡. The patient had a small intraventricular hemorrhage (not shown).*

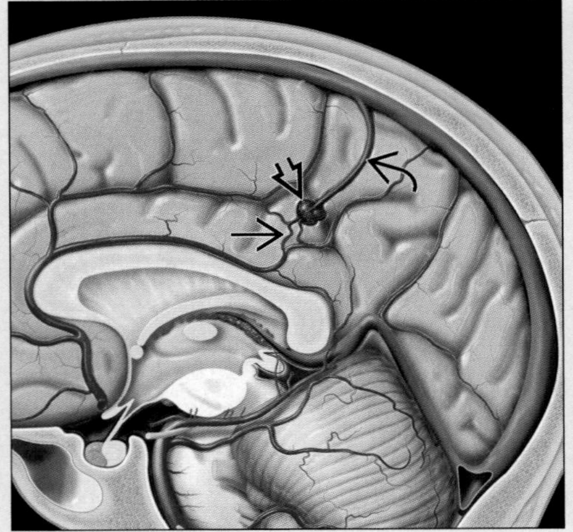

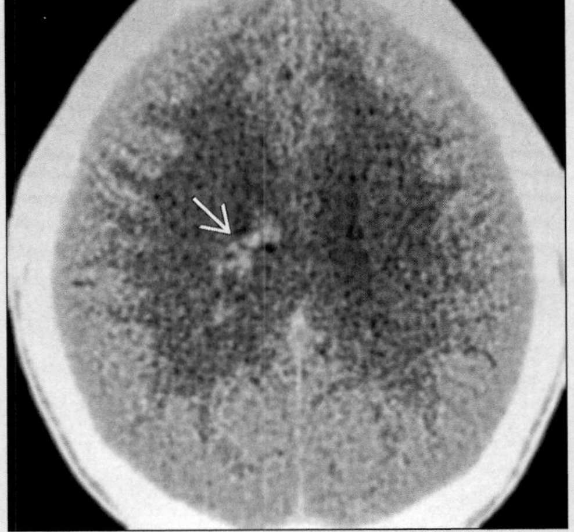

*(**Left**) Axial T2WI MR in the same patient shows serpentine flow voids ➡ and a variceal aneurysm ➡ in the lateral ventricle with no parenchymal or choroidal nidus. An intraventricular location is risky for surgical resection without embolization. (**Right**) Arterial phase frontal DSA in the same patient shows dilated tortuous perforating vessels from an opercular branch of the right MCA ➡, directly filling multiple variceal aneurysms ➡, no intervening nidus, and thalamostriate drainage ➡.*

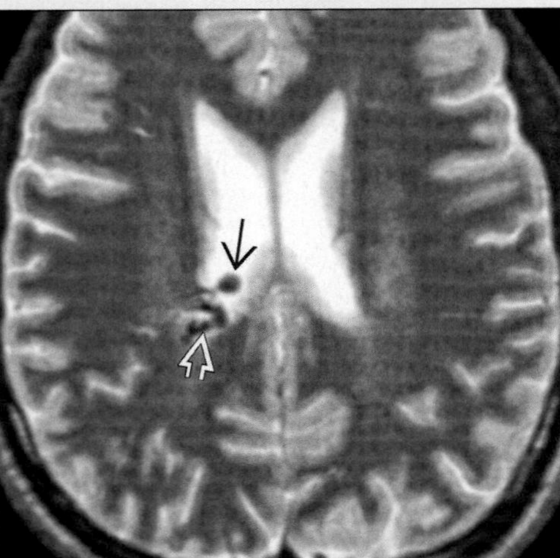

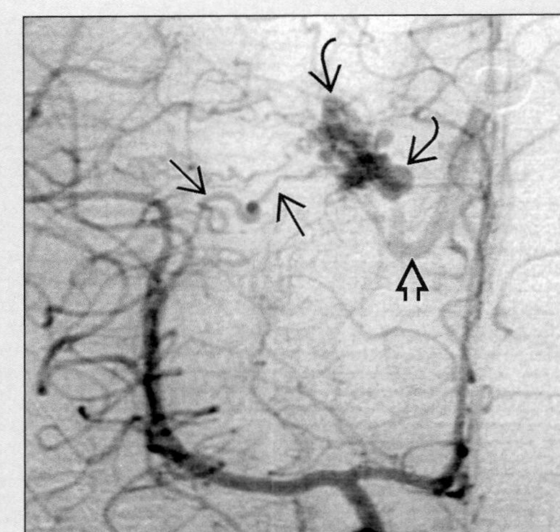

PIAL AV FISTULA

TERMINOLOGY

Abbreviations

- Pial arteriovenous fistula (pAVF)

Definitions

- Pial vascular malformation with direct arteriovenous (AV) shunting
  - No intervening capillary bed or nidus

IMAGING

General Features

- Best diagnostic clue
  - Dilated arteries, veins without focal nidus
- Location
  - Although called "pial," can lie on surface/within brain or at ependyma
  - May occur anywhere in brain, spinal cord
    - Rare in posterior fossa

CT Findings

- NECT
  - Iso-/hyperdense serpentine vessels
  - Variable Ca++ in wall of draining vein(s)
- CTA
  - Shows arterial feeder(s), draining veins

MR Findings

- T2WI
  - Dilated serpiginous flow voids
  - Variable hemorrhage
- T2* GRE
  - ± "blooming" hypointense blood products

Angiographic Findings

- Delineates angioarchitecture
  - Fistula at site of abrupt change in vessel caliber
- Dilated feeding artery
  - Often single
  - Drains directly into enlarged vein
  - No intervening nidus
- ± confluence of arteries just before fistulous connection

Imaging Recommendations

- Best imaging tool
  - DSA best delineates angioarchitecture
- Protocol advice
  - CTA/CE MRA best noninvasive method

DIFFERENTIAL DIAGNOSIS

Arteriovenous Malformation (AVM)

- Has definite nidus composed of microscopic AV shunts
  - Nidus: A few millimeters to several centimeters in size
  - May have large fistulous connections within nidus
  - Angiomatous matrix of small vascular channels on DSA
- Much more common than pAVF

Dural AV Fistula (dAVF)

- AV shunts within wall of patent/partially thrombosed dural venous sinus (DVS)
- Dural sinus drainage or into adjacent pial cortical vein
- Differentiate from pial AVF by
  - Fistulas intimately related to DVS, within DVS wall
  - Predominant blood supply is from dural (meningeal) arteries > > pial artery
    - e.g., anterior, middle, and posterior meningeal arteries, tentorial branches of cavernous ICA, PCA, occipital artery, ascending pharyngeal artery

Vein of Galen Aneurysmal Malformation

- Mural type is pAVF of vein of Galen
- Merely a difference in location
  - Supply from medial posterior choroidal branches to prosencephalic vein
  - Drainage via straight sinus or persistent falcine sinus

PATHOLOGY

General Features

- Etiology
  - Factors of pAVMs: Dysregulated angiogenesis
  - Trauma
- Genetics
  - Sporadic pAVFs, like pAVMs, may have multiple up-/down-regulated genes
  - Syndromic pAVFs associated with *HHT1* (endoglin gene) mutation

Gross Pathologic & Surgical Features

- Draining veins are "arterialized"
  - Thickened walls ± stenosis of high-flow venopathy
  - May have variceal "aneurysms"

CLINICAL ISSUES

Presentation

- Most common signs/symptoms
  - Headache
  - Cranial bruit

Natural History & Prognosis

- ↑ ↑ hemorrhage risk compared to AVM
- Spontaneous obliteration of pAVF
  - May be more common than AVM, especially in infants

Treatment

- Embolization
  - Curative if draining vein occluded at fistulous site
- Surgery rarely necessary unless embolism incomplete

SELECTED REFERENCES

1. Andreou A et al: Transarterial balloon-assisted glue embolization of high-flow arteriovenous fistulas. Neuroradiology. 50(3):267-72, 2008

NONTRAUMATIC CAROTID-CAVERNOUS FISTULA

Key Facts

Terminology
- Nontraumatic AV shunt in cavernous sinus (CS)
  - From CS dAVF (indirect/low-flow CCF)
  - Cavernous ICA aneurysm rupture (high-flow CCF)

Imaging
- General features
  - Asymmetric enlargement/enhancement of SOV, CS
  - Proptosis ± extraocular muscle enlargement
- CTA/MRA/DSA
  - Often associated CS aneurysm present
  - Early filling of CS + outflow pathways
  - SOV, angular, facial veins
  - Inferior, superior petrosal sinuses to internal jugular veins
  - Contralateral CS
  - ± retrograde cortical venous drainage
- If direct CCF from cavernous ICA aneurysm
  - Need very fast acquisition to see aneurysm
- If CS dAVF, supply from dural branches
  - ICA (meningohypophyseal/inferolateral trunks, etc.)
  - ECA (MMA, distal IMA branches)

Top Differential Diagnoses
- Traumatic CCF
  - High-flow CCF, associated skull fracture
- Cavernous sinus thrombosis
  - Dilated SOV, "dirty" fat may be seen, no enhancement of CS

Clinical Issues
- May present days to months after onset
- If severe/rapid vision loss, SAH → emergency
- Treatment: Endovascular
  - Transvenous embolization via various routes
  - Transarterial embolization

*(**Left**) Axial T2WI MR in a middle-aged woman with slowly increasing proptosis and chemosis shows multiple enlarged flow voids ➡ in the left CS, smaller flow voids in the clival dural venous plexus ➡. (**Right**) Lateral MRA in the same patient shows faint flow-related signal in the cavernous sinus ➡ with an unusual-looking vessel at the posterior cavernous segment ➡ of the internal carotid artery. This vessel correlated with the small posterior cavernous sinus pouch on angiography.*

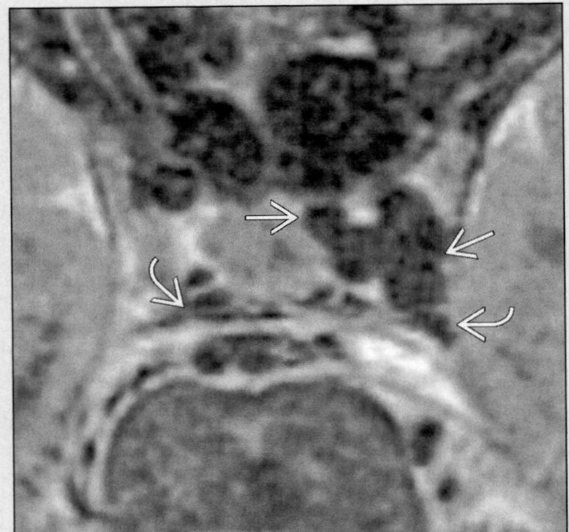

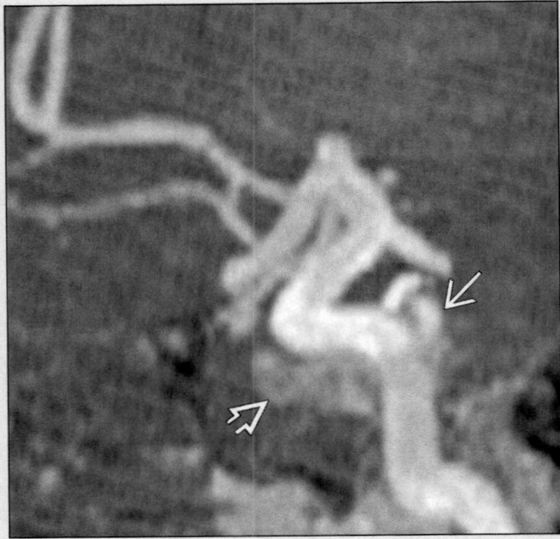

*(**Left**) Lateral DSA, left external carotid artery in the same patient shows enlarged dural branches arising from the maxillary and middle meningeal arteries ➡ have fistulized to the posterior cavernous sinus ➡, which drains into the anterior cavernous sinus and superior ophthalmic vein ➡. (**Right**) Lateral DSA of selective ICA injection in the same patient shows contrast in the CS ➡ and superior ophthalmic vein ➡. Enlarged branches of the inferolateral trunk ➡ supply the low-flow CCF.*

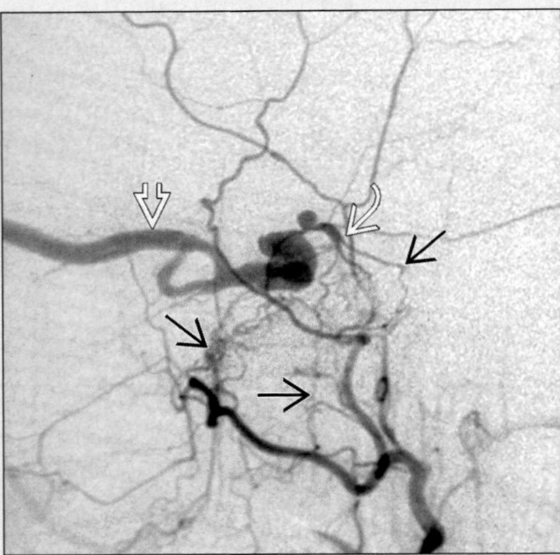

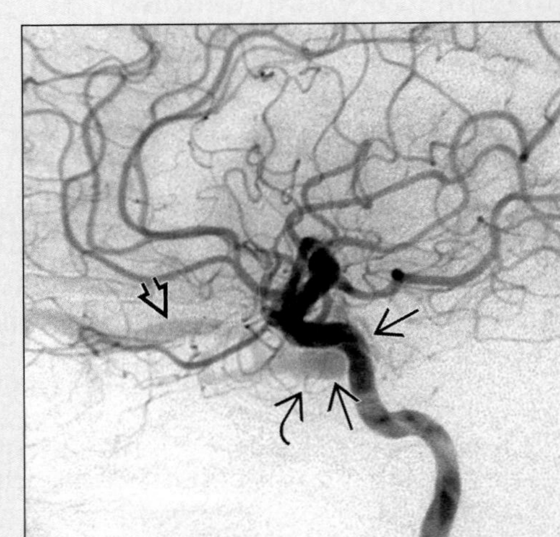

NONTRAUMATIC CAROTID-CAVERNOUS FISTULA

TERMINOLOGY

Abbreviations

- CS dural arteriovenous fistula (dAVF)

Synonyms

- Indirect CCF, low-flow CCF, CS dAVF

Definitions

- Arteriovenous shunt into cavernous sinus due to dural AV fistula or rupture of cavernous ICA aneurysm

IMAGING

General Features

- Best diagnostic clue
  - Proptosis, dilated superior ophthalmic vein (SOV) and CS, extraocular muscle (EOM) enlargement
  - Associated aneurysm located in cavernous sinus in high flow CCF

Imaging Recommendations

- Best imaging tool
  - Conventional angiography definitive
  - CTA/MRA can indicate presence of CCF, DSA necessary for planning and treatment
- Protocol advice
  - DSA: Selective external and internal studies to determine supply, delineate venous drainage

CT Findings

- NECT
  - Proptosis, enlarged SOV, CS, and EOMs
  - Dirty orbital fat secondary to edema
- CECT
  - Dilated SOV and CS
  - ↑ enhancement of EOMs and small orbital vessels
- CTA
  - Early enhancement of CS and SOV compared to other dural sinuses
  - May see dilated middle meningeal and intraorbital arteries

MR Findings

- T2WI
  - Dilated SOV and CS with asymmetric signal due to increased flow voids
- T1WI C+
  - Dilated SOV and CS with asymmetric enhancement
  - May see tortuous collateral with cerebral drainage
- MRA
  - Early enhancement of CS and SOV on CE MRA

Ultrasonographic Findings

- Doppler: Reversal of flow (intracranial to extracranial) in dilated SOV

Angiographic Findings

- Conventional
  - Early filling of CS + outflow pathways including
    - SOV, angular and facial veins
    - Inferior and superior petrosal sinuses to internal jugular vein(s)
    - Contralateral CS
    - Retrograde cortical venous drainage via sphenoparietal sinus or pontine veins
  - Aneurysmal direct CCF: Supply from cavernous ICA aneurysm
    - May need very fast acquisition to see aneurysm
  - CS dAVF: Supply from dural branches
    - ICA: Meningohypophyseal trunk, inferolateral trunk, intraorbital ophthalmic artery
    - ECA: Middle meningeal, distal internal maxillary arterial branches

DIFFERENTIAL DIAGNOSIS

Traumatic CCF

- High-flow CCF, associated skull fracture

Cavernous Sinus Thrombosis

- SOV may be dilated, "dirty" fat may be seen, no CS enhancement on CECT/CTA/CTV/CEMRA/CEMRV

PATHOLOGY

General Features

- Etiology
  - Dural AVF or rupture of cavernous ICA aneurysm
- Associated abnormalities
  - Arterialized flow in CS with retrograde venous hypertension
    - Superior/inferior ophthalmic veins → proptosis, chemosis, ↑ intraocular pressure → ↓ retinal perfusion pressure → blindness
    - Cortical veins → increased SAH or ICH risk

CLINICAL ISSUES

Presentation

- Most common signs/symptoms
  - May present days to months after onset and often treated as inflammatory
  - Bruit, pulsating exophthalmos, orbital edema/erythema, ↓ vision, glaucoma, headache
  - Focal deficits → cranial nerves 3-6
  - Severe/rapid vision loss, SAH → emergency

Treatment

- Endovascular options include
  - Transvenous embolization via various routes
    - Inferior petrosal sinus
    - Superior ophthalmic vein
    - Direct CS puncture via inferolateral orbit
  - Transarterial embolization
    - Usually with particles to facilitate transvenous cure
    - Liquid embolics risk cranial nerve ischemia
    - Aneurysm coiling ± stent with ICA aneurysm

SELECTED REFERENCES

1. Théaudin M et al: Dural carotid-cavernous fistula: relationship between evolution of clinical symptoms and venous drainage changes. Cerebrovasc Dis. 25(4):382-4, 2008

VEIN OF GALEN ANEURYSMAL MALFORMATION

Key Facts

Terminology

- Vein of Galen malformation (VGAM)
- Arteriovenous fistula (AVF) between deep choroidal arteries and embryonic median prosencephalic vein of Markowski (MPV)
- High flow through MPV prevents formation of Vein of Galen → VGAM is misnomer

Imaging

- Best diagnostic clue: Large midline varix (MPV) in neonate/infant
- Embryonic falcine sinus drains MPV in 50%

Top Differential Diagnoses

- Vein of Galen aneurysmal dilatation (VGAD)
- Childhood dural arteriovenous fistula
- Complex developmental venous anomaly (DVA)
- Giant aneurysm

Pathology

- Up to 30% pediatric vascular malformations
- Most common extracardiac cause of high-output cardiac failure in newborn
- Cerebral ischemia/atrophy
- Hydrocephalus

Clinical Issues

- Age: Neonatal presentation most common
- Prognosis related to volume of shunt and timing/success treatment
- Brain damage or multisystem organ failure at presentation are contraindications to treatment
- Initial transarterial embolization (TAE) at 4-5 months
- Frequent neurological and MRI F/U after TAE
- Up to 60% neurologically normal after treatment

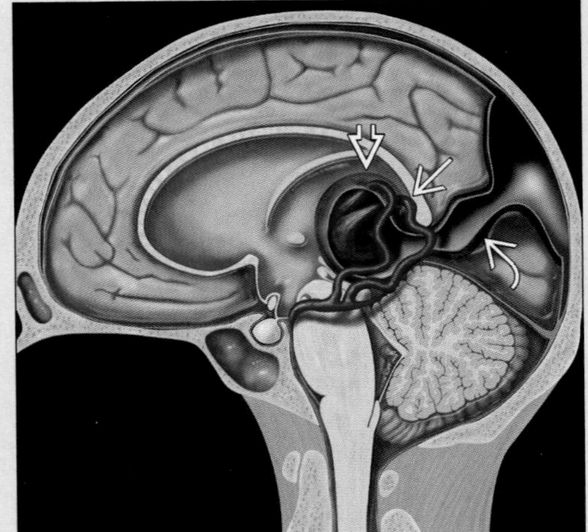

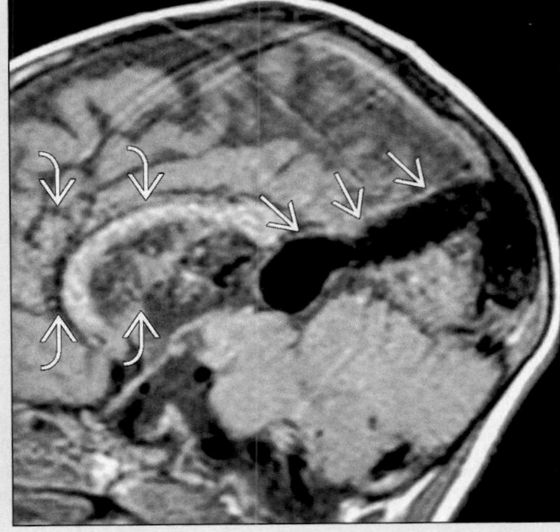

(Left) *Sagittal graphic depicts classic vein of Galen malformation. Enlarged posterior choroidal arteries ➔ drain into a dilated median prosencephalic vein (MPV) of Markowski ⇨. The MPV drains into the superior sagittal sinus via an embryonic falcine sinus ↪; the straight sinus is absent.* ***(Right)*** *Sagittal T1WI MR shows classic VGAM: Large midline falcine sinus ➔ is angled upward toward the sagittal sinus. Phase artifact ↪ from turbulent, high-velocity flow confirms the vascular nature of lesion.*

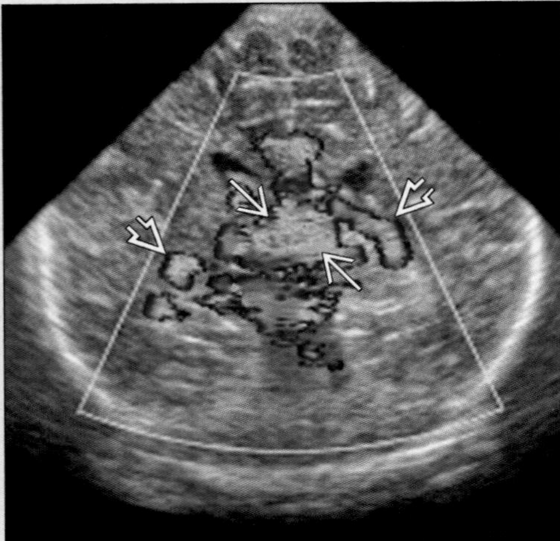

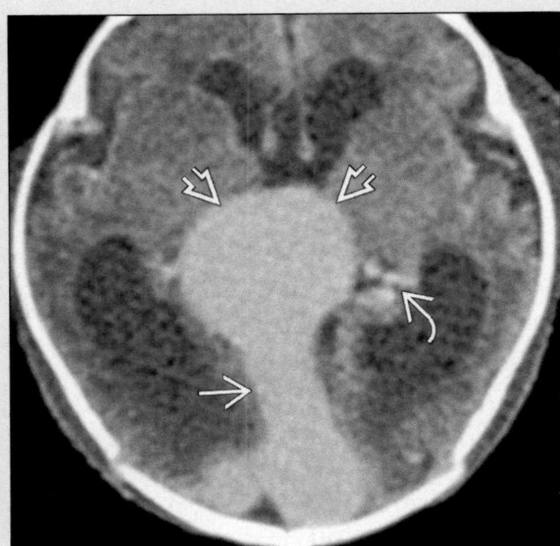

(Left) *Coronal image from neonatal transcranial color Doppler US of a classic VGAM shows the enlarged, midline MPV with both arterial & venous flow ➔. Enlarged vessels with arterial flow (arterial feeders) ⇨ are seen alongside the MPV.* ***(Right)*** *Axial CECT of a classic VGAM shows intense, vascular enhancement in the enlarged, midline MPV ⇨ & adjacent enlarged falcine sinus ➔. Feeding arteries ↪ are seen at the periphery. Hydrocephalus may be mechanical or from increased venous pressure.*

VEIN OF GALEN ANEURYSMAL MALFORMATION

TERMINOLOGY

Abbreviations
- Vein of Galen aneurysmal malformation (VGAM)

Synonyms
- Vein of Galen "aneurysm," Galenic varix

Definitions
- Arteriovenous fistula (AVF) between deep choroidal arteries & embryonic median prosencephalic vein of Markowski (MPV)
- High flow through MPV prevents formation of Vein of Galen; VGAM is misnomer

IMAGING

General Features
- Best diagnostic clue: Large midline varix (MPV) in neonate/infant
- Location: Quadrigeminal plate cistern
- Size: Few to several cm
- Morphology: Tubular > spherical varix

Radiographic Findings
- Chest radiograph: Congestive heart failure (CHF): Cardiomegaly, pulmonary edema

CT Findings
- NECT
  - MPV mildly hyperdense to brain
    - Wall Ca++ in older children or MPV thrombosis
  - Hydrocephalus
  - Subcortical white matter (WM) hypodensity and Ca ++ → chronic venous ischemia
  - Rare intracranial (IC) hemorrhage
- CECT
  - Vascular enhancement feeding arteries, MPV
- CTA
  - Excellent preangiographic delineation of VGAM

MR Findings
- T1WI
  - MPV: Flow void or heterogeneous due to fast or turbulent flow
    - Hyperintense foci: Thrombus
    - Phase artifact from fast, turbulent flow
  - Hyperintense foci within brain: Ca++, ischemia
  - Sag: Tectal compression, tonsillar herniation
- T2WI
  - MPV: Flow void or heterogeneous due to fast or turbulent flow
  - Flow voids from feeding arteries around MPV
  - Ischemic foci poorly seen in unmyelinated infant brain
- DWI: Restriction in acute ischemia/infarction
- MRA: Delineates arterial feeders
- MRA C+: Shows arterial and venous anatomy together
- MRV: Delineates MPV and venous anatomy
- Fetal MR: Can identify brain & other end organ injury
  - Significant antenatal injury is contraindication to aggressive treatment

Ultrasonographic Findings
- Grayscale ultrasound
  - Mildly echogenic midline mass
- Color Doppler
  - Arterialized flow within MPV
- Antenatal US: VGAM identified in 3rd trimester
  - ↑ resistance middle cerebral artery → vascular steal
  - Cardiac dilatation, hydrops fetalis = poor prognosis

Echocardiographic Findings
- Dilatated right heart, superior vena cava (SVC), ascending aorta/great vessels
- 80% left ventricular output diverted to low resistance VGAM
- Poor prognostic indicators
  - Descending aorta diastolic flow reversal
  - Suprasystemic pulmonary artery hypertension
  - PDA with significant right → left shunt

Angiographic Findings
- Common arterial feeders
  - Medial and lateral posterior choroidal arteries
  - Pericallosal arteries
- Venous anatomy
  - Embryonic falcine sinus drains MPV in 50%
    - Associated with absent straight sinus
  - Variable absence, stenoses of other sinuses
  - Reflux into pial venous system ↑ risk IC hemorrhage
    - Requires urgent treatment
  - Venous drainage central brain structures typically not through MPV but superior petrosal and cavernous sinuses

Imaging Recommendations
- Best imaging tool
  - MR with MRA/MRV
  - Catheter angiogram ideally performed with 1st embolization (4-5 months of age)
- Protocol advice
  - MRA C+ may obviate need for MRV

DIFFERENTIAL DIAGNOSIS

Vein of Galen Aneurysmal Dilatation (VGAD)
- Arteriovenous malformation (AVM) with venous drainage into true vein of Galen
- Less common than VGAM
- Does not typically present before 3 years of age

Childhood Dural Arteriovenous Fistula
- High-flow fistulas: Neonatal presentation similar to VGAM
- Frequent giant aneurysms, venous varices
- External carotid artery → torcular, transverse, or superior sagittal sinus
- Spontaneous thrombosis may occur after delivery

Complex Developmental Venous Anomaly
- Dilatation of veins draining normal brain parenchyma
- No nidus or AV shunting
- Associated with blue rubber-bleb nevus syndrome

VEIN OF GALEN ANEURYSMAL MALFORMATION

Giant Aneurysm

- Not associated with venous abnormalities
- "Onion skin" layers in wall

PATHOLOGY

General Features

- Embryology
  - Week 5: Arterial supply to choroid plexus established from meninx primitiva
  - Week 7-8: Choroid plexus drains via single temporary midline vein
  - Week 10: Internal cerebral veins annex drainage of choroid plexus → regression MPV
  - Caudal MPV persists, joins internal cerebral veins (ICVs) to form vein of Galen
- Etiology
  - AVF of choroidal arteries and MPV
  - ↑ flow through fistula prevents normal regression MPV
- Genetics: Sporadic
  - Rare reports of hereditary vascular dysplasia syndromes
- Epidemiology:
  - Rare: < 1% of cerebral vascular malformations
  - Up to 30% of pediatric vascular malformations
  - Most common extracardiac cause of high-output cardiac failure in newborn
- Associated abnormalities
  - Venous occlusion, stenosis
    - Primary atresia vs. occlusion 2° to increased pressure, flow
    - Provides right heart protection
  - Cerebral ischemia/atrophy
    - Arterial steal
    - Chronic venous hypertension
  - Hydrocephalus
    - ↓ CSF resorption 2° to ↑ venous pressure
    - ± Cerebral aqueduct obstruction
  - Atrial septal defects; aortic coarctation

Staging, Grading, & Classification

- "Choroidal" or "mural" classification based on angioarchitecture of VGAM
  - Choroidal: Multiple feeders from pericallosal, choroidal, and thalamoperforating arteries
  - Mural: Single or few feeders from collicular or posterior choroidal arteries

Gross Pathologic & Surgical Features

- Malformations of structures adjacent to MPV
  - Pineal gland, tela choroidea of 3rd ventricle

Microscopic Features

- Thickened wall of MPV, ± Ca++

CLINICAL ISSUES

Presentation

- Most common signs/symptoms
  - Neonate: High-output CHF, cranial bruit
  - Infant: Macrocranium (hydrocephalus)
  - Older child, adult (rare): Headache, IC hemorrhage
- Other signs/symptoms
  - Developmental delay, failure to thrive, seizure, end-organ failure

Demographics

- Age: Neonatal presentation most common
  - Rarely diagnosed after age 3
- Gender: M:F = 2:1

Natural History & Prognosis

- Without treatment, death from intractable heart- and multisystem-failure occurs in neonates
- Prognosis related to volume of shunt and timing/ success treatment
  - Neonatal prognosis worse than infant/child
  - Embolization at 4-5 months associated with improved outcome compared to embolization in newborn period
  - Up to 60% neurologically normal after treatment

Treatment

- Brain damage or multisystem organ failure at presentation are contraindications to treatment
- Medical therapy for CHF until 4-5 months of age
  - Failure therapy warrants earlier neuro-intervention
- Initial transarterial embolization (TAE) at 4-5 months
  - Occlusion arterial side AVF
  - Staged embolizations frequently required
  - Frequent neurological and MR F/U after TAE
    - Evidence of deterioration warrants further therapy
- Transvenous embolization infrequently performed
  - Increased morbidity compared to TAE
  - Complete occlusion MPV contraindicated if contrast seen in choroidal, subependymal veins
- Treatment for hydrocephalus controversial
  - Shunt placement associated with complications
    - Alters venous drainage → exacerbates brain ischemia
    - Risk intraventricular hemorrhage from engorged subependymal veins
    - Ideally, shunt placed only after all TAEs performed

DIAGNOSTIC CHECKLIST

Image Interpretation Pearls

- Imaging appearance diagnostic in appropriate clinical setting

Reporting Tips

- Report progressive brain injury on MRs

SELECTED REFERENCES

1. Alvarez H et al: Vein of galen aneurysmal malformations. Neuroimaging Clin N Am. 17(2):189-206, 2007
2. Gailloud P et al: Diagnosis and management of vein of galen aneurysmal malformations. J Perinatol. 25(8):542-51, 2005
3. Jones BV et al: Vein of Galen aneurysmal malformation: diagnosis and treatment of 13 children with extended clinical follow-up. AJNR Am J Neuroradiol. 23(10):1717-24, 2002

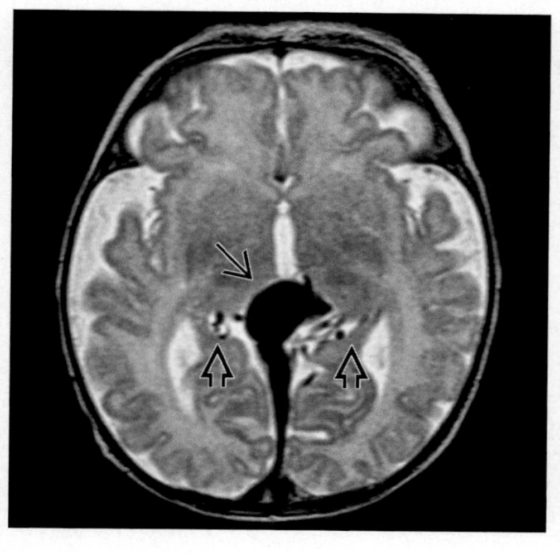

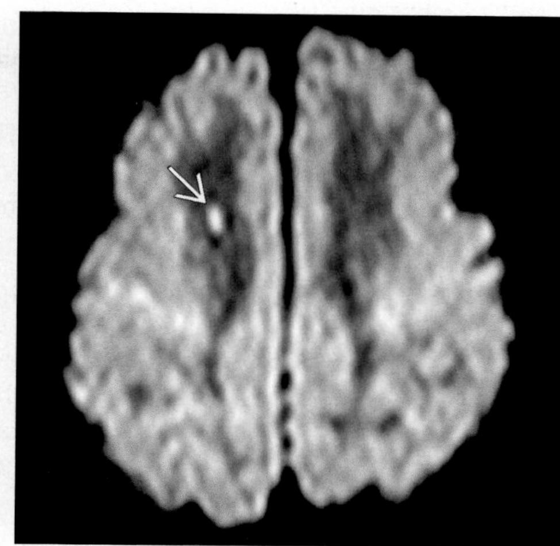

(Left) *Axial T2WI MR in newborn with supraventricular tachycardia shows an enlarged, midline MPV ➙ and large surrounding arterial feeders ➙. Appearance of brain is otherwise normal.* ***(Right)*** *Axial DWI MR in the same patient shows single focus of reduced diffusion (acute ischemia) ➙ in deep white matter. This neonate had small volume shunt with mild cardiac symptoms. He was successfully embolized at 5 months of age with no further brain injury on F/U MR exams.*

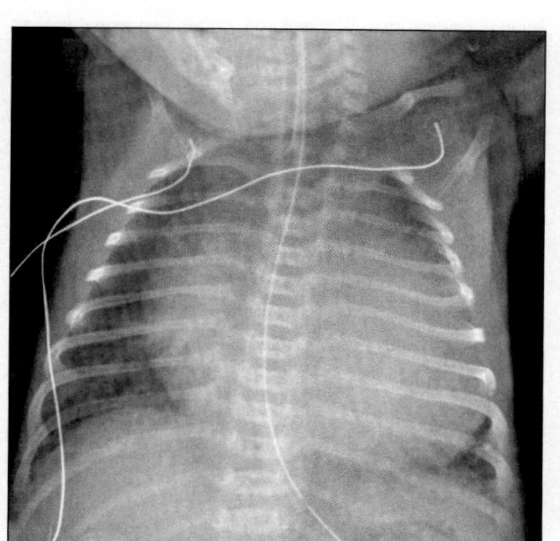

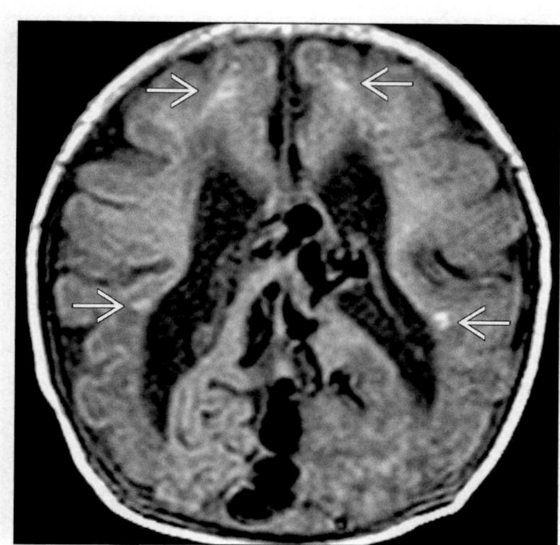

(Left) *AP chest radiograph in a neonate with high-output heart failure shows severe cardiomegaly. Cardiac failure from high-volume shunts may be refractory to medical therapy, requiring VGAM embolization in newborn period, significantly worse prognosis than those embolized at 4-5 months.* ***(Right)*** *Axial T1WI MR in a newborn shows ventriculomegaly and abnormal hyperintense white matter ➙, suggesting injury from increased venous pressure with resultant venous ischemia.*

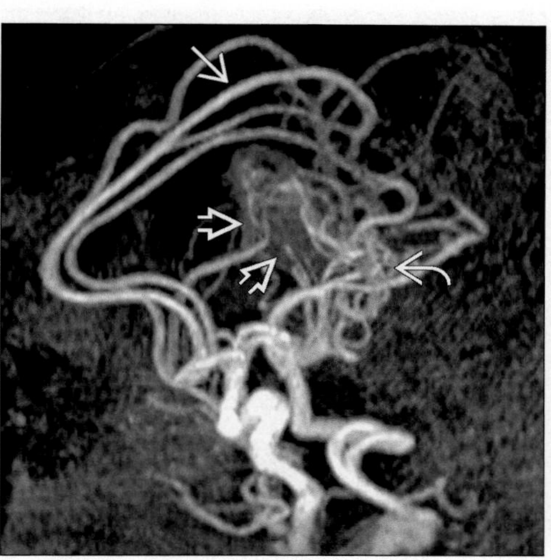

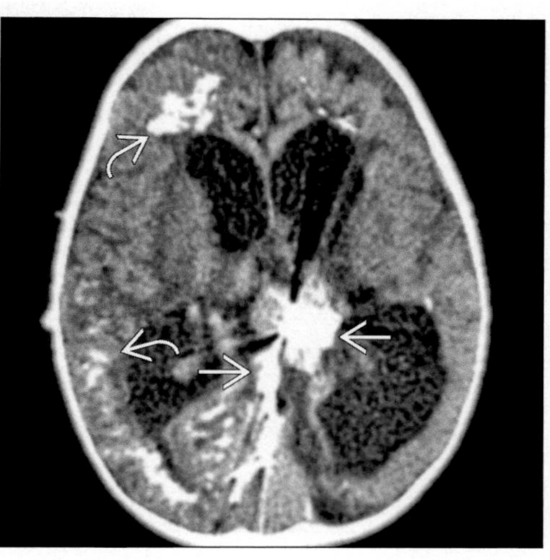

(Left) *Sagittal MRA shows classic VGAM arterial feeders. The pericallosal ➙ and posterior choroidal ➙ arteries are enlarged with branches terminating on a less well-defined midline mass ➙ (the MPV). MRA C+/MRV affords better evaluation of the MPV.* ***(Right)*** *Axial NECT in a toddler who had refractory cardiac failure in the newborn period. Despite multiple embolizations, significant brain atrophy developed, with dystrophic Ca++ ➙ in areas of WM injury. Note the hyperdense embolic material in MPV ➙.*

DEVELOPMENTAL VENOUS ANOMALY

Key Facts

Terminology

- Congenital cerebral vascular malformation with angiogenically mature venous elements

Imaging

- General features
  - Umbrella-like collection of enlarged medullary (white matter) veins ("Medusa head")
  - At angle of ventricle
  - Numerous linear or dot-like enhancing foci
  - Converge on single enlarged "collector" vein
  - "Collector" vein drains into dural sinus/deep ependymal vein
  - Usually solitary, variable size (< 2-3 cm)
  - Hemorrhage may occur if mixed malformation or draining vein thromboses
- CT often normal; enlarged "collector" vein may appear hyperdense
- MR
  - Variable signal depending on size, flow
  - Hypointense on SWI (BOLD effect in draining veins)
  - Strong enhancement

Top Differential Diagnoses

- Mixed vascular malformation (usually cavernous)
- Vascular neoplasm
- Dural sinus thrombosis (chronic)

Pathology

- 15-20% coexisting cavernous &/or capillary malformations
- Blue rubber bleb nevus syndrome (BRBNS)
- Sulcation-gyration disorders (may cause epilepsy)
- Cervicofacial venous or lymphatic malformation (CAMS-3)

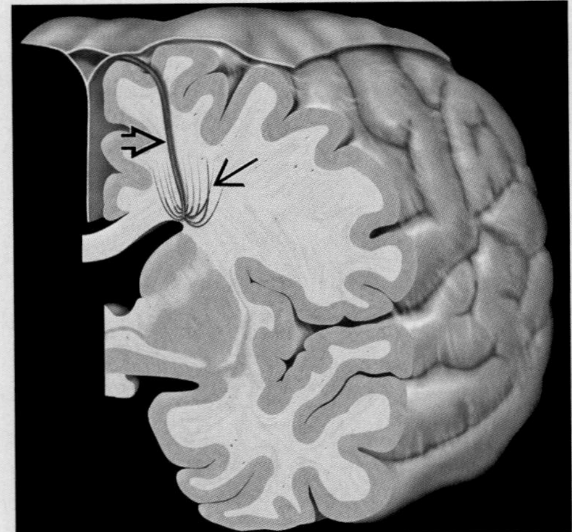

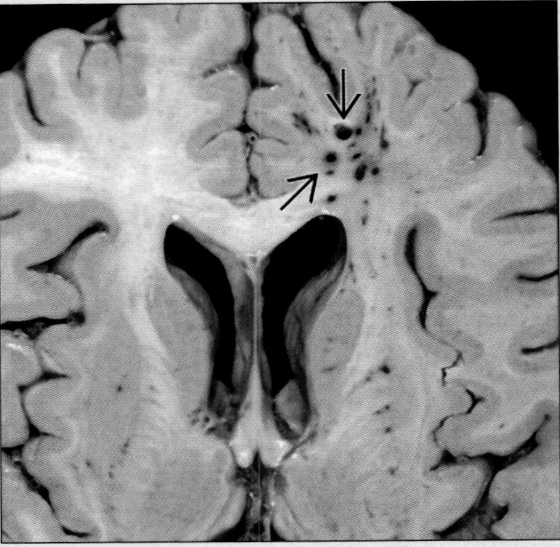

(Left) *Coronal oblique graphic depicts classic DVA with umbrella-like "Medusa head" of enlarged medullary (deep white matter) veins ➔ converging on a dilated transcortical "collector" vein ➲. The "collector" vein drains into the superior sagittal sinus.* ***(Right)*** *Gross pathology shows an incidental finding of DVA, seen here as scattered enlarged venous channels ➔ near the frontal horn of the lateral ventricle. Normal white matter is seen between the venous tributaries. Note the absence of hemorrhage. (Courtesy R. Hewlett, PhD.)*

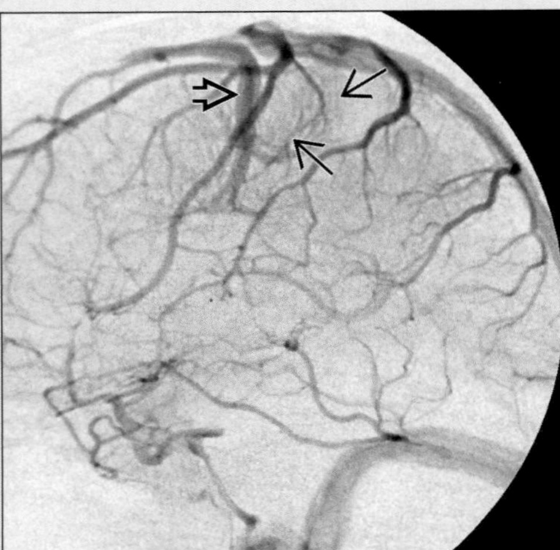

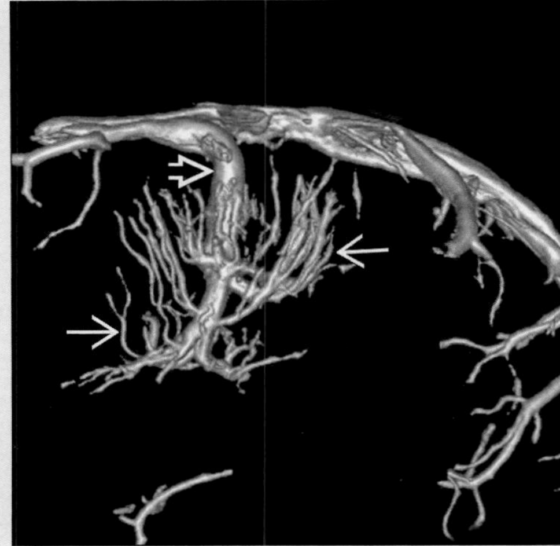

(Left) *Lateral view of internal carotid angiogram, mid-venous phase, shows classic "Medusa head" of DVA. Numerous enlarged medullary veins ➔ converge on an enlarged transcortical "collector" vein ➲.* ***(Right)*** *Lateral DSA with 3D reconstruction in the same patient beautifully demonstrates the DVA with its dilated venous tributaries ➔ and transcortical draining vein ➲. (Courtesy P. Lasjaunias, MD.)*

DEVELOPMENTAL VENOUS ANOMALY

TERMINOLOGY

Abbreviations
- Developmental venous anomaly (DVA)

Synonyms
- Venous angioma

Definitions
- Congenital cerebral vascular malformation with angiogenically mature venous elements
- May represent anatomic variant of otherwise normal venous drainage

IMAGING

General Features
- Best diagnostic clue
  - "Medusa head" (dilated medullary white matter veins)
- Location
  - At angle of ventricle
    - Most common site: Near frontal horn
    - Other: Adjacent to 4th ventricle
- Size
  - Varies (may be extensive) but usually < 3 cm
- Morphology
  - Umbrella-like collection of enlarged medullary (white matter) veins
  - Large "collector" vein drains into dural sinus or deep ependymal vein
  - Usually solitary
    - Can be multiple in blue rubber bleb nevus syndrome

CT Findings
- NECT
  - Usual: Normal; enlarged "collector" vein may appear hyperdense
  - Occasional: Ca++ if mixed cavernous malformation
  - Rare: Acute parenchymal hemorrhage (if draining vein spontaneously thromboses)
- CECT
  - Numerous linear or dot-like enhancing foci
    - Well-circumscribed, round/ovoid, enhancing areas on sequential sections
    - Converge on single enlarged tubular draining vein
    - Occasionally seen as linear structure in single slice

MR Findings
- T1WI
  - Can be normal if DVA is small
  - Variable signal depending on size, flow
    - Flow void
  - Hemorrhage may occur if mixed malformation or draining vein thromboses
- T2WI
  - ± flow void
  - ± blood products
- FLAIR
  - Usually normal; may show hyperintense region if venous ischemia or hemorrhage present
- T2* GRE
  - May be hypointense ("blooms") on GRE if large or if coexisting cavernous malformation (CM) with hemorrhage
  - Hypointense on SWI (BOLD effect in draining veins)
    - If high flow, deoxyhemoglobin reduced; may be isointense
- DWI
  - Usually normal
  - Rare: Acute venous infarct seen as hyperintense area of restricted diffusion
- T1WI C+
  - Strong enhancement
    - Stellate, tubular vessels converge on "collector" vein
    - "Collector" vein drains into dural sinus/ ependymal vein
- MRA
  - Arterial phase usually normal
  - Contrast-enhanced MRA may demonstrate slow-flow DVA
- MRV
  - Delineates "Medusa head" and drainage pattern
- MRS
  - Normal

Angiographic Findings
- DSA
  - Arterial phase normal in > 95% of cases
  - Capillary phase usually normal (rare: Prominent "blush" ± AV shunt)
  - Venous phase: "Medusa head"
  - < 5% atypical (transitional form of venous-arteriovenous malformation with enlarged feeders, AV shunting)

Imaging Recommendations
- Best imaging tool
  - T1 C+ MR plus SWI, MRV
  - 3D VRT of MRV, DSA
- Protocol advice
  - Include T2* sequence (GRE, SWI)
    - Look for BOLD effect (venous tributaries)
    - Hemorrhage (usually mixed malformation)

DIFFERENTIAL DIAGNOSIS

Mixed Vascular Malformation (Usually Cavernous)
- Hemorrhage often associated

Vascular Neoplasm
- Enlarged medullary veins
- Mass effect, usually enhances

Dural Sinus Thrombosis (Chronic)
- Chronic thrombosis → venous stasis
- Medullary veins enlarge as collateral drainage

Sturge-Weber Syndrome
- May develop strikingly enlarged medullary, subependymal, choroid plexus veins
- Coexisting facial angioma

DEVELOPMENTAL VENOUS ANOMALY

Venous Varix (Isolated)
- Occurs but is rare without associated DVA

Demyelinating Disease
- Rare: Active, aggressive demyelination may have prominent medullary veins

PATHOLOGY

General Features
- Etiology
  - Does not express growth factors
  - Expresses structural proteins of mature angiogenesis
  - Mixed malformations may be developmental anomaly of capillary-venous network → transitional vessels, loculated endothelial vascular spaces
- Genetics
  - Mutations in chromosome 9p
    - Encodes for surface cell receptors
    - *TIE-2* mutation results in missense activation
    - Segregates pedigrees with skin, oral and GI mucosa, brain venous malformations
  - Approximately 50% inherited as autosomal dominant
- Associated abnormalities
  - 15-20% of those with DVAs have coexisting cavernous &/or capillary malformations
  - Blue rubber bleb nevus syndrome (BRBNS)
  - Sinus pericranii (cutaneous sign of underlying venous anomaly)
  - Sulcation-gyration disorders (may cause epilepsy)
  - Cervicofacial venous or lymphatic malformation (CAMS-3)
    - Embryology
      - Arrested medullary vein development at time when normal arterial development nearly complete
      - Developmental arrest results in persistence of large primitive embryonic deep white matter veins

Gross Pathologic & Surgical Features
- Radially oriented dilated medullary veins
- Venous radicals are separated by normal brain
- Enlarged transcortical or subependymal draining vein

Microscopic Features
- Dilated thin-walled vessels diffusely distributed in normal white matter (no gliosis)
- Occasional: Thickened, hyalinized vessel walls
- 20% have mixed histology (CM most common), may hemorrhage
- Variant: "Angiographically occult" DVA with malformed, compactly arranged vessels with partly degenerated walls

CLINICAL ISSUES

Presentation
- Most common signs/symptoms
  - Usually asymptomatic
  - Uncommon
    - Headache
    - Seizure (if associated with cortical dysplasia)
    - Hemorrhage with focal neurologic deficit (if associated with cavernous malformation)
- Clinical profile
  - Asymptomatic patient with DVA found incidentally on MR

Demographics
- Age
  - All ages
- Gender
  - M = F
- Ethnicity
  - No known predilection
- Epidemiology
  - Most common cerebral vascular malformation at autopsy
  - 60% of cerebral vascular malformations
  - 2.5-9% prevalence on contrast-enhanced MR scans

Natural History & Prognosis
- Hemorrhage risk: 0.15% per lesion per year
  - Stenosis or thrombosis of draining vein increases hemorrhage risk
  - Coexisting cavernous malformation increases hemorrhage risk

Treatment
- Solitary venous anomaly: None (attempt at removal may cause venous infarction)
- Histologically mixed venous anomaly: Determined by coexisting lesion

DIAGNOSTIC CHECKLIST

Consider
- DVAs contain (and provide main venous drainage for) intervening normal brain!

Image Interpretation Pearls
- If you are not seeing 1 or 2 DVAs per month in usual outpatient setting, you are probably overlooking them
- If you are not doing much contrast-enhanced MR, you are probably missing incidental DVAs

SELECTED REFERENCES

1. Oran I et al: Developmental venous anomaly (DVA) with arterial component: a rare cause of intracranial haemorrhage. Neuroradiology. 51(1):25-32, 2009
2. Abla A et al: Developmental venous anomaly, cavernous malformation, and capillary telangiectasia: spectrum of a single disease. Acta Neurochir (Wien). 150(5):487-9; discussion 489, 2008
3. Fushimi Y et al: A developmental venous anomaly presenting atypical findings on susceptibility-weighted imaging. AJNR Am J Neuroradiol. 29(7):E56, 2008
4. Pozzati E et al: The neurovascular triad: mixed cavernous, capillary, and venous malformations of the brainstem. J Neurosurg. 107(6):1113-9, 2007

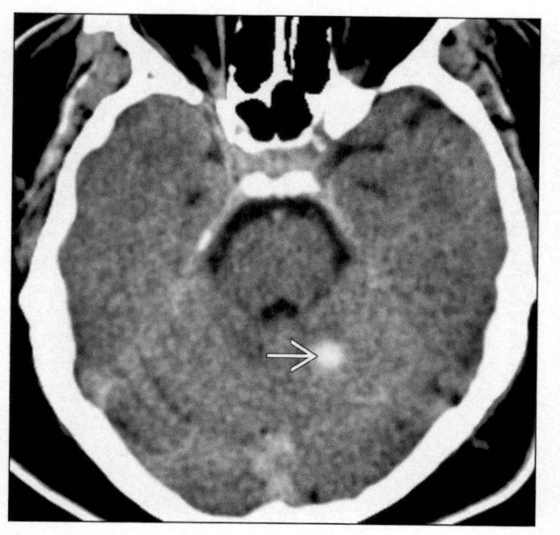

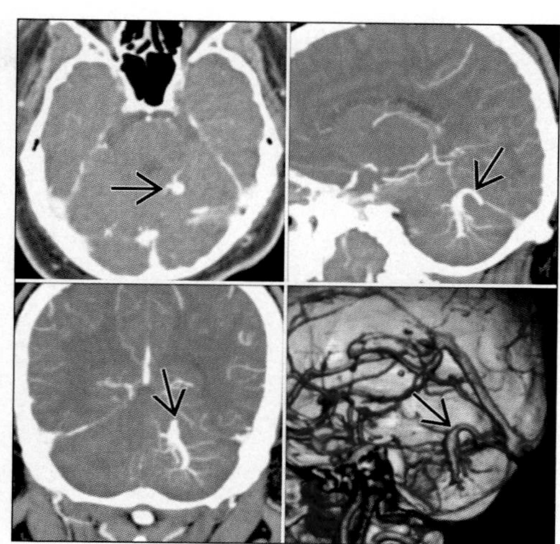

(Left) *Axial NECT shows a well-delineated hyperdensity in the left cerebellar hemisphere ➔.* ***(Right)*** *CTA with axial, sagittal, and coronal views and a 3D reconstruction in the same patient elegantly demonstrates the DVA ➔.*

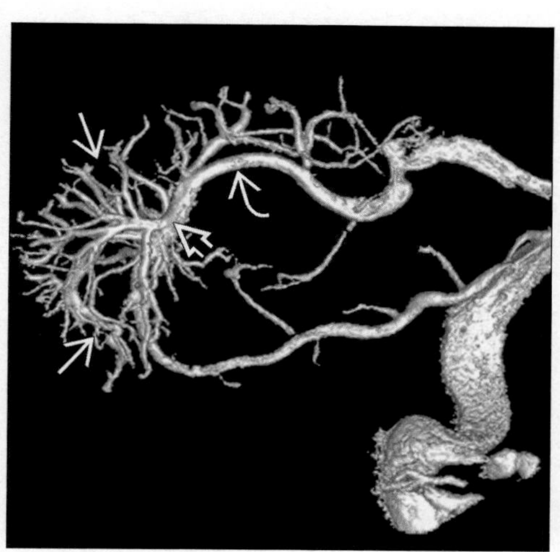

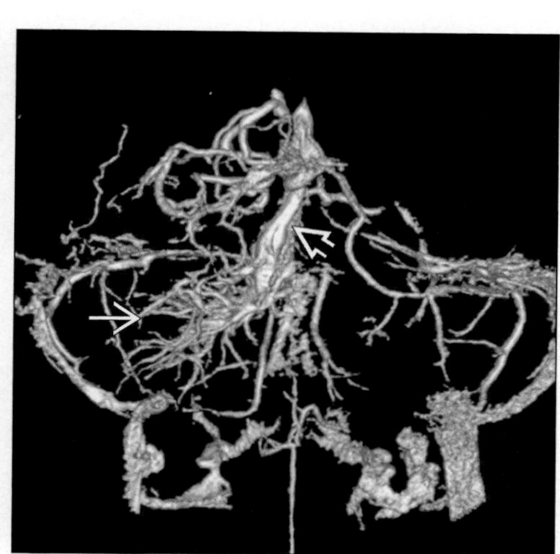

(Left) *Lateral 3D DSA rendered from the late venous phase of an internal carotid angiogram shows a large frontal DVA ➔ that drains into a septal tributary ➔ of the internal cerebral vein ➔. (Courtesy P. Lasjaunias, MD.)* ***(Right)*** *Anteroposterior 3D DSA shows a large right cerebellar DVA ➔ draining into an enlarged precentral cerebellar vein ➔. (Courtesy P. Lasjaunias, MD.)*

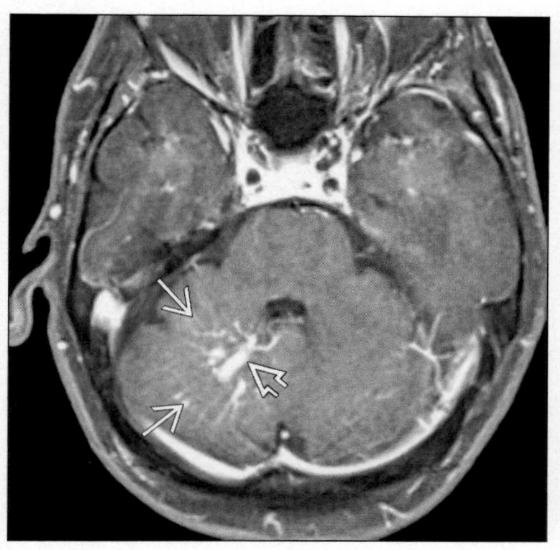

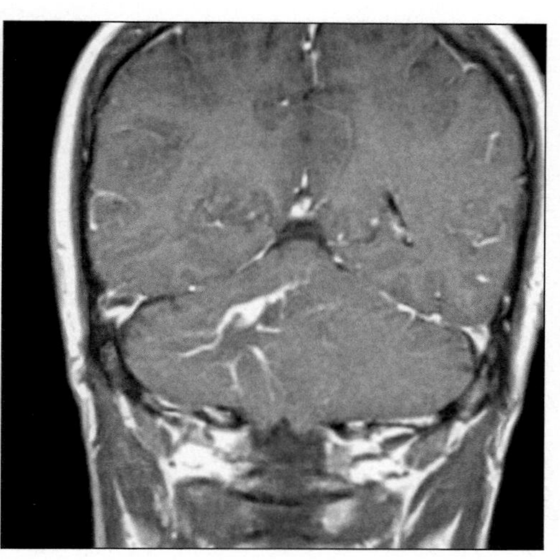

(Left) *Axial T1WI C+ MR shows a classic "Medusa head" of enlarged venous tributaries ➔ draining into a dilated "collector" vein ➔.* ***(Right)*** *Coronal T1WI C+ MR in the same patient shows the DVA occupying much of the deep cerebellar white matter. T2* GRE scans (not shown) demonstrated no evidence for hemorrhage. This DVA was an incidental finding on MR.*

*(**Left**) Axial T1WI C+ MR shows "dots" of enlarged medullary veins, seen "end on" in this patient with a left frontal DVA →. (**Right**) Axial T1WI C+ MR in the same patient shows the enlarged draining "collector" vein → emptying into the anterior superior sagittal sinus →.*

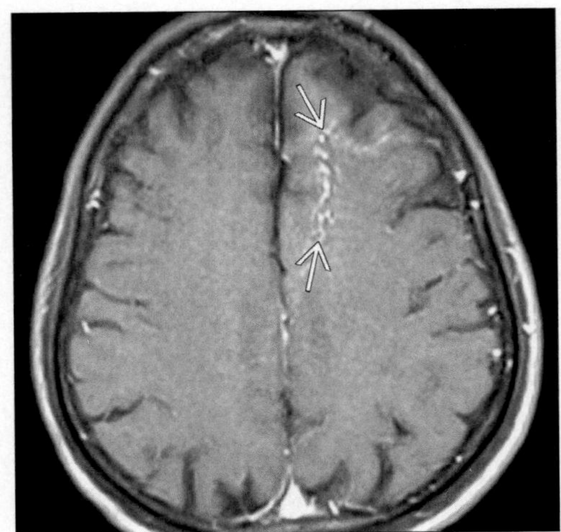

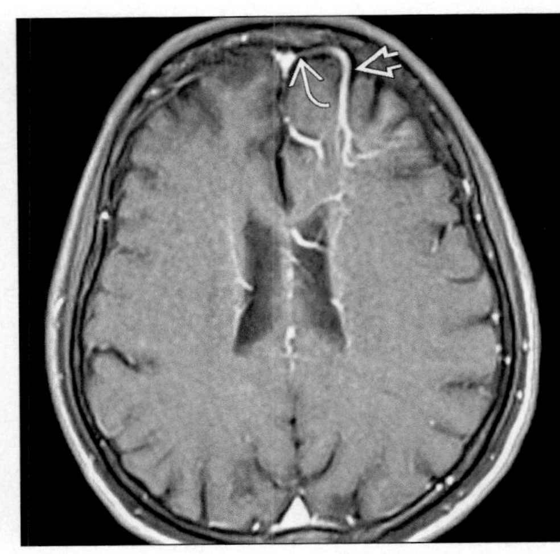

*(**Left**) Axial T2* GRE MR shows "blooming" from a small cavernous malformation in the septum pellucidum →. (**Right**) Axial SWI in the same patient shows hemorrhage in the septum pellucidum → as well as a 2nd, smaller hemorrhagic focus adjacent to the left frontal horn →. Note the prominent DVA → seen especially well on this SWI sequence.*

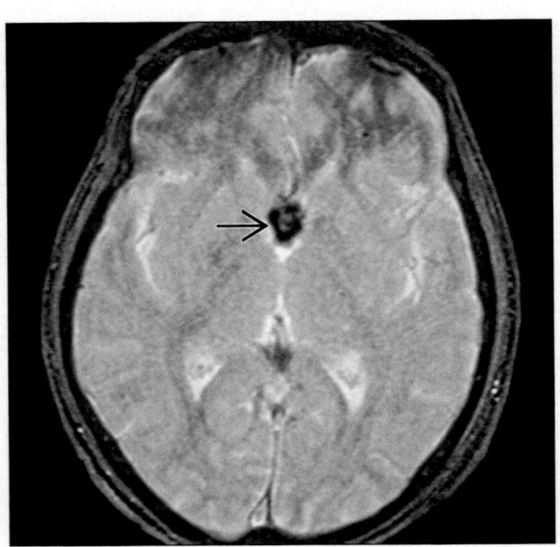

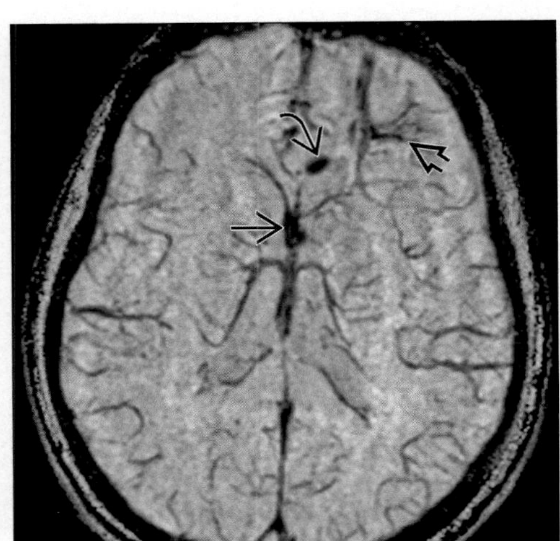

*(**Left**) Axial T2* GRE MR shows brush-like hypointensity in the subcortical white matter extending deep into the centrum semiovale →. (**Right**) Axial T1WI C+ FS MR in the same patient shows brush-like enhancement → with a dilated draining vein → in the center of the lesion. This was an incidental finding, thought to represent a large capillary telangiectasia mixed with a DVA. Large capillary telangiectasias often have a central enlarged draining vein.*

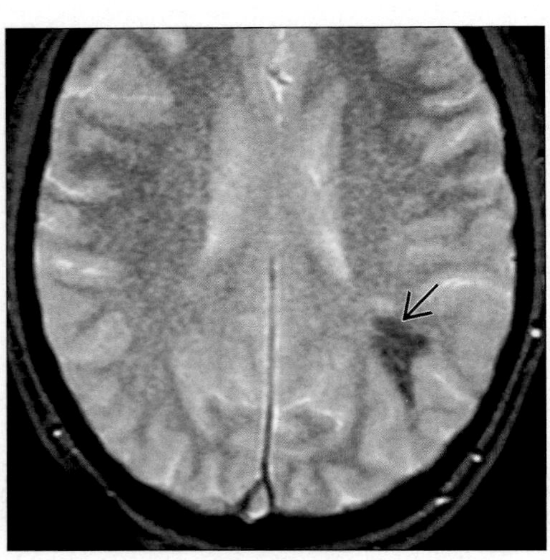

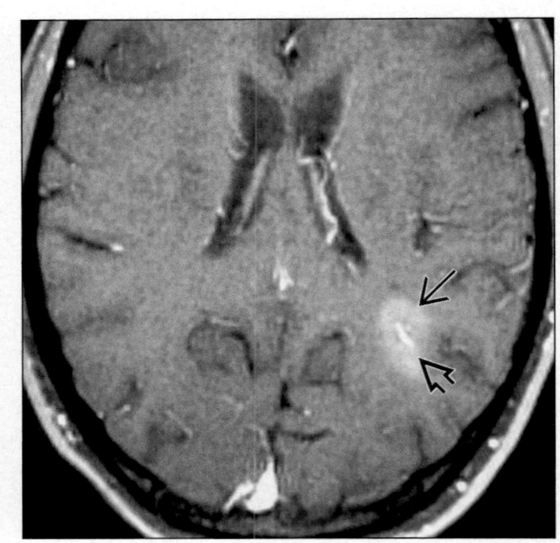

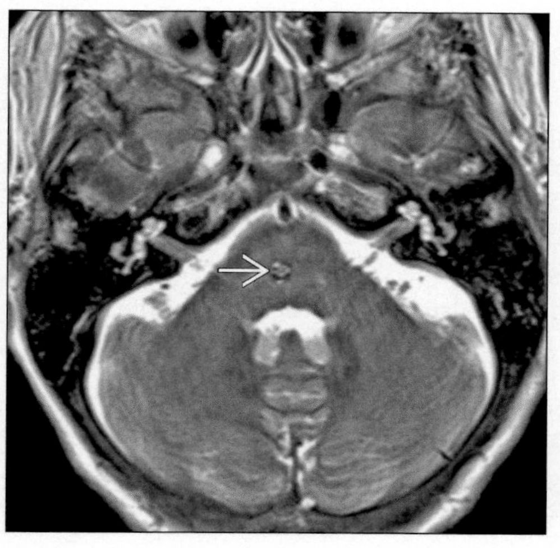

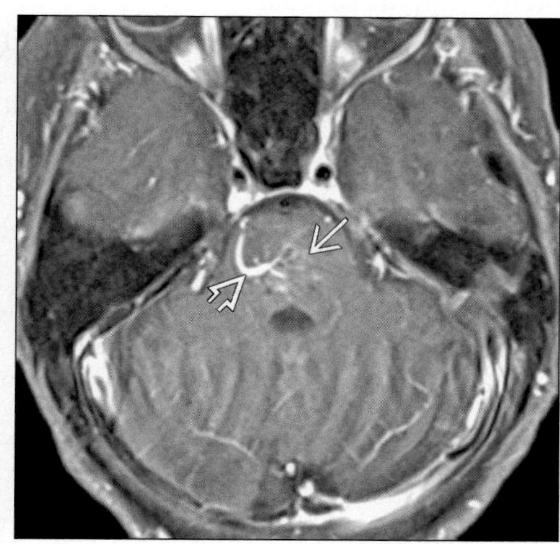

(Left) *Axial T2WI MR shows a small "popcorn" lesion in the central pons ➔ consistent with a cavernous malformation.* ***(Right)*** *Axial T1WI C+ FS MR in the same patient shows the classic "Medusa head" of enlarged veins ➔ draining into a prominent "collector" vein ➲. Mixed cavernous-venous malformations are very common.*

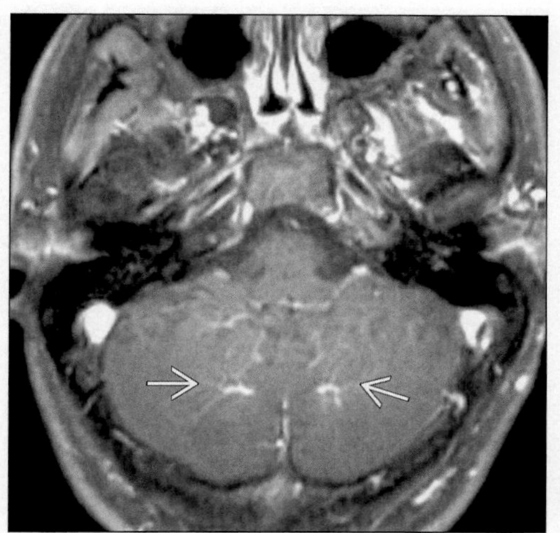

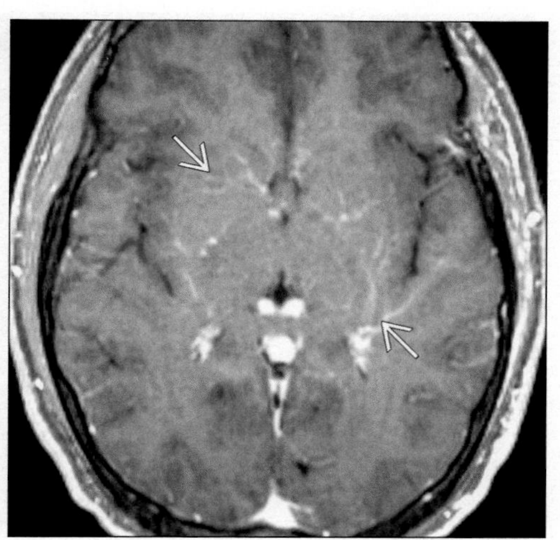

(Left) *Axial T1WI C+ FS MR in a patient with blue rubber bleb nevus syndrome (BRBNS) shows bilateral cerebellar DVAs ➔.* ***(Right)*** *Axial T1WI C+ FS MR in the same patient shows multiple bilateral supratentorial DVAs ➔.*

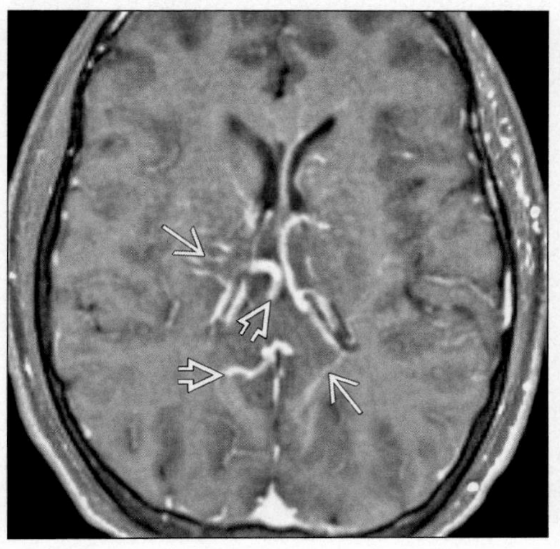

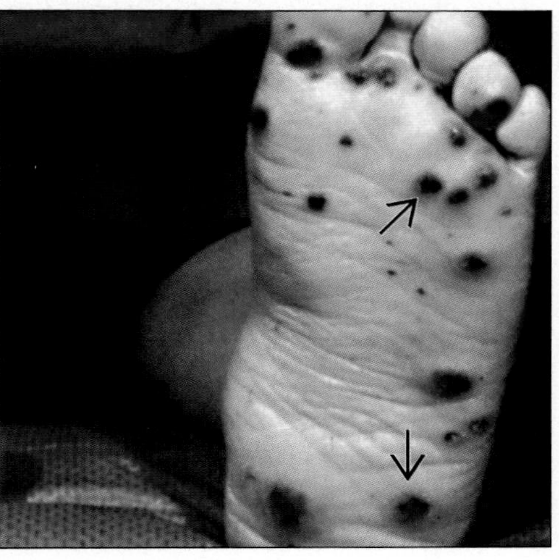

(Left) *Axial T1WI C+ FS MR in the same patient shows DVAs ➔ with multiple enlarged "collector" veins ➲.* ***(Right)*** *Clinical photograph in another patient with blue rubber bleb nevus syndrome shows multiple bluish bleb-like skin lesions → characteristic of this rare neurocutaneous disorder. Angiogram (not shown) demonstrated multiple intracranial DVAs. (Courtesy AFIP.)*

SINUS PERICRANII

Key Facts

Terminology
- Anomalous communication between intracranial (IC) and extracranial venous circulation
- Most common arrangement: Scalp varix communicates with dural venous sinus (DVS) via transosseous emissary vein(s)

Imaging
- Superior sagittal sinus most commonly involved
- CTV, MRV delineates all vascular components of SP
- Bone defect visualized on CT
- Conventional angiography may be required to assess intracranial venous drainage preoperatively

Top Differential Diagnoses
- Encephalocele
- Dermoid cyst
- Hemangioma
- Rhabdomyosarcoma, Langerhans cell histiocytosis, neuroblastoma metastases

Pathology
- Probable anomalous venous development during late embryogenesis, possibly secondary to transient venous hypertension
- Supports association of SPs with other congenital venous anomalies: DVA, DVS hypoplasia/aplasia, persistent embryonic venous sinus, VM

Clinical Issues
- Child with long history of painless, reducible scalp mass
- Prognosis excellent following surgical removal
- Surgery contraindicated if SP serves as major intracranial venous outflow or drains DVA

*(**Left**) Coronal graphic shows a complex lateral SP. This SP is composed of an intracranial varix, cortical vein, & DVA, plus a scalp varix. SPs are typically midline/paramedian scalp varices communicating with the superior sagittal sinus (SSS) via a transosseous vein. Lateral location and association with DVA are uncommon. (**Right**) Coronal CTV reconstruction shows a classic SP. The SSS communicates with a midline scalp varix via a calvarial defect. In this "closed" SP, blood flows from the SSS into the varix & back into the sinus.*

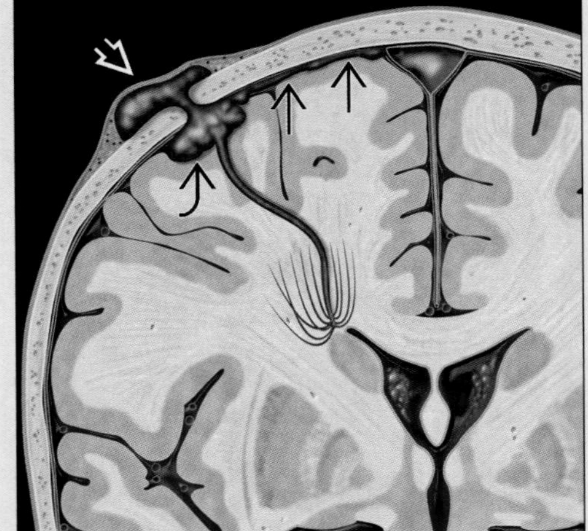

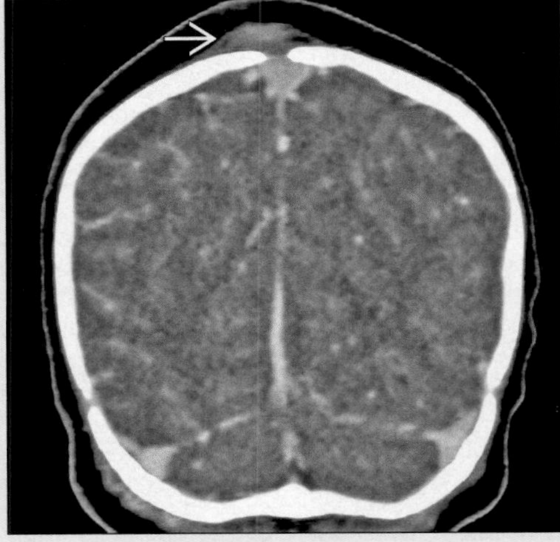

*(**Left**) Sagittal T2WI FS MR shows a small, midline, intermediate signal scalp mass. (**Right**) Sagittal MRV in the same patient reveals a "drainer" SP: A small scalp varix receives venous blood from the underlying SSS via a small transosseous vein and drains into a pericranial scalp vein. This small SP does not contribute significantly to intracranial venous drainage and could be resected. "Drainer" SPs providing major intracranial venous drainage should not be removed.*

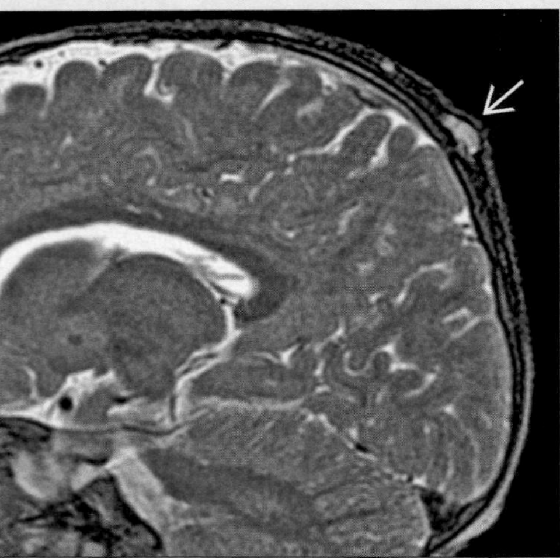

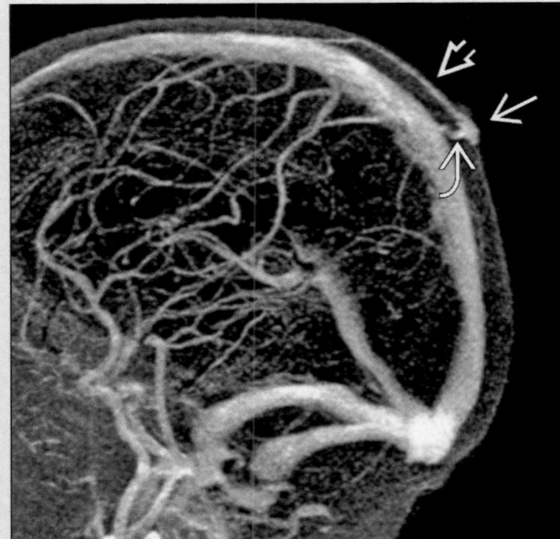

SINUS PERICRANII

TERMINOLOGY

Abbreviations

- Sinus pericranii (SP)

Definitions

- Anomalous communication between intracranial (IC) and extracranial venous circulation
  - Most common arrangement: Scalp varix communicates with dural venous sinus (DVS) via transosseous emissary vein(s)

IMAGING

General Features

- Best diagnostic clue
  - Vascular scalp lesion communicating with underlying DVS
- Location
  - Frontal (40%), parietal (34%), occipital (23%), temporal (4%)
  - Midline or parasagittal; lateral location uncommon
  - Superior sagittal sinus most commonly involved
    - Transverse sinus, torcular distant 2nd
- Size
  - Scalp lesion: 1-13 cm; most 2-6 cm
  - Bone defect: 1-4 mm hole(s); rare large defect
- Morphology
  - Extracranial component
    - Varix, most common
    - Enlarged vein(s) > venous malformation (VM)
    - Arteriovenous malformation (AVM), rare
  - Intracranial component
    - Midline SP: Direct communication with DVS
    - Parasagittal SP: Prominent cortical or scalp vein(s) bridge scalp lesion with DVS
    - Developmental venous anomaly (DVA), uncommon

Radiographic Findings

- Skull radiograph: Normal or focal bone defect(s), thinning, pressure erosion

CT Findings

- NECT
  - Homogeneous soft tissue density scalp mass
  - If VM: Septations, cysts, ± phleboliths
  - Bone algorithm
    - Single/multiple, well-defined bone defect(s)
    - Pressure erosion from overlying varix/VM
- CECT
  - Intense, "vascular" enhancement most common
    - Heterogeneous if thrombus present or VM
- CTV: Delineates all vascular components of SP

MR Findings

- T1WI
  - Most iso-, hypo-, or mixed iso-/hypointense
    - Hyperintense if thrombus present
    - Flow voids if rapidly flowing varix/VM
- T2WI
  - Most hyperintense
    - Mixed signal in large varix/VM secondary to turbulent flow
    - Flow voids in rapidly flowing varix/VM
- T1WI C+
  - Intense, "vascular" enhancement
    - Heterogeneous if thrombus present
    - Peripheral and solid enhancement if VM
- MRV
  - Delineates all vascular components of SP

Ultrasonographic Findings

- Grayscale ultrasound
  - Hypoechoic scalp mass and transosseous feeder(s)
  - Shadowing from skull limits IC evaluation
- Color Doppler
  - Demonstrates direction of flow

Angiographic Findings

- Sinus pericranii identified during venous phase
- "Closed" and "drainer" classification based on venous drainage pattern
  - Closed: Blood flows from and back into DVS
  - Drainer: Blood flows from DVS into scalp lesion and drains into pericranial scalp veins

Nuclear Medicine Findings

- Bone scan
  - ↑ activity in venous and blood pool phases

Other Modality Findings

- Percutaneous venography (PV)
  - Visualization of scalp veins
  - Visualization of transosseous vein, DVS inconstant

Imaging Recommendations

- Best imaging tool
  - C+ MR/MRV or CTV
    - Both modalities suitable for delineation of SP and any associated intracranial venous anomalies
    - Bone defect best visualized on CT
  - US confirms diagnosis; does not define IC component
- Protocol advice
  - Conventional angiography may be required to assess intracranial venous drainage preoperatively

DIFFERENTIAL DIAGNOSIS

Encephalocele

- Herniation of IC contents through skull defect
- No enhancement unless vessels/DVS herniate

Dermoid Cyst

- Well-defined fluid or fat density lesion
- Anterior fontanelle/bregma location classic

Hemangioma

- Intensely enhancing mass with flow voids
- Characteristic evolution

Rhabdomyosarcoma, Langerhans Cell Histiocytosis, Neuroblastoma Metastases

- Enhancing, destructive mass
- Invasion of DVS appears as filling defect

SINUS PERICRANII

PATHOLOGY

General Features

- Etiology
  - Majority congenital
    - Probable anomalous venous development during late embryogenesis, possibly secondary to transient venous hypertension
      - Theory supports association of SPs with other congenital venous anomalies/variants: DVA, DVS hypoplasia/aplasia, persistent embryonic venous sinus, venous malformation
    - Incomplete sutural fusion over prominent/ abundant diploic or emissary veins
    - In utero DVS thrombosis
  - Traumatic
    - Disruption of emissary veins at outer table
    - Laceration or DVS thrombosis
  - Spontaneous
    - Likely secondary to remote, "forgotten" trauma
    - Subclinical, postnatal DVS thrombosis
- Associated abnormalities
  - DVA
  - Systemic venous malformations
  - Blue rubber bleb nevus syndrome
  - Multisutural craniosynostosis
    - SP forms secondary to DVS/internal jugular vein hypoplasia/atresia or IC hypertension
  - Isolated reports of cutis aplasia congenita

Staging, Grading, & Classification

- Classification based on venous drainage pattern
  - Closed: Blood flows from and back into DVS
  - Drainer: Blood flows from DVS into scalp lesion and drains into pericranial scalp veins

Gross Pathologic & Surgical Features

- Scalp varix/VM: Bluish, blood-filled sac or network of sacs beneath > above calvarial periosteum

Microscopic Features

- Scalp varix/VM: Nonmuscular venous channel(s)
  - Endothelial lining = congenital origin
  - Fibrous lining/capsule = traumatic origin
- ± hemosiderin-laden macrophages, thrombus

CLINICAL ISSUES

Presentation

- Most common signs/symptoms
  - Nontender, fluctuant, bluish forehead/scalp mass
    - Reduces in upright position
    - Distends when prone or with Valsalva
  - Rare: Pain, headache, nausea, dizziness
- Clinical profile
  - Child with long history of painless, reducible scalp mass

Demographics

- Age
  - Children, young adults
  - Range: 0-70 years
- Gender
  - M = F (post-traumatic cases: M > F)
- Epidemiology
  - Rare
  - 11% of patients presenting for treatment of craniofacial VMs

Natural History & Prognosis

- Stable or slow enlargement
- Rare spontaneous regression
- Potential lifetime risk hemorrhage, air embolus if sinus pericranii injured
- Prognosis excellent following surgical removal
  - Very rare recurrence

Treatment

- Contraindicated if SP serves as major intracranial venous drainage pathway or drains DVA
- Surgery
  - Preoperative evaluation of entire DVS network necessary to ensure feasibility of SP removal
  - Ligation of transosseous emissary vein(s), removal of scalp lesion, closure of bone hole(s) with bone wax
  - Small risk of significant blood loss
- Endovascular therapy
  - Uncommon, suitable for small drainer SPs
  - Percutaneous injection sclerosants/coils into draining scalp veins
  - Risk of overlying skin necrosis

DIAGNOSTIC CHECKLIST

Consider

- Consider blue rubber bleb nevus syndrome if SP associated with multiple intracranial DVAs

Image Interpretation Pearls

- Assess for associated intracranial venous anomalies (DVA) and congenital venous variants
- Entire DVS network must be evaluated prior to sinus pericranii removal
- Diagnostic imaging appearance characteristic
  - Unless thrombosed, main competing diagnosis is cephalocele with herniated DVS

Reporting Tips

- Describe contribution of SP to IC venous drainage

SELECTED REFERENCES

1. Rozen WM et al: Spontaneous involution of two sinus pericranii - a unique case and review of the literature. J Clin Neurosci. 15(7):833-5, 2008
2. Weinzierl M et al: Off-midline Sinus Pericranii Associated with Ipsilateral Venous Anomaly: Case Report and Therapeutic Considerations. Zentralbl Neurochir. 69(1):40-2, 2008
3. Gandolfo C et al: Sinus pericranii: diagnostic and therapeutic considerations in 15 patients. Neuroradiology. 49(6):505-14, 2007
4. Mitsukawa N et al: Sinus pericranii associated with craniosynostosis. J Craniofac Surg. 18(1):78-84, 2007
5. Nomura S et al: Association of intra- and extradural developmental venous anomalies, so-called venous angioma and sinus pericranii. Childs Nerv Syst. 22(4):428-31, 2006

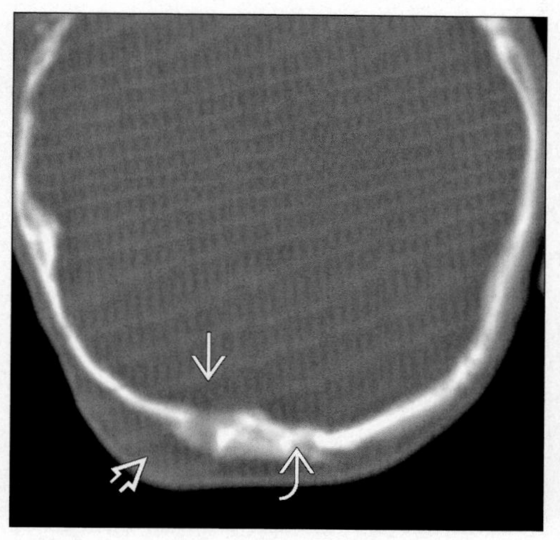

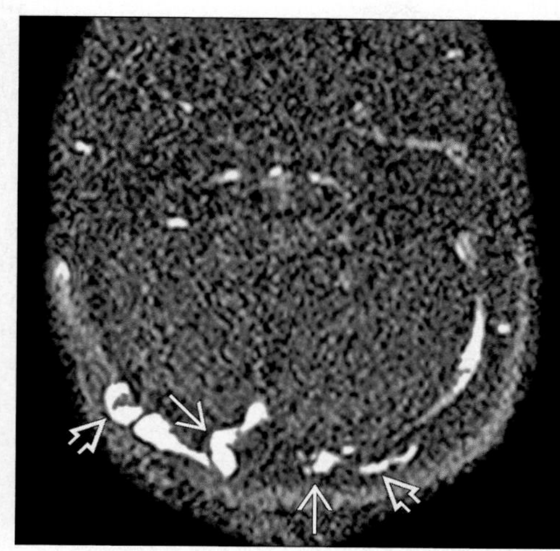

(Left) *Axial NECT demonstrates a large right occipital bone defect ➡ with an overlying scalp mass ➡. A smaller left-sided bone defect can also be seen ➡.* ***(Right)*** *Source images from axial TOF MRV in the same patient demonstrate large, right > left veins extending from the torcular, through the skull ➡ into the scalp ➡. This patient had atretic jugular bulbs with the SPs, accounting for the major venous drainage from the head. Surgery was contraindicated.*

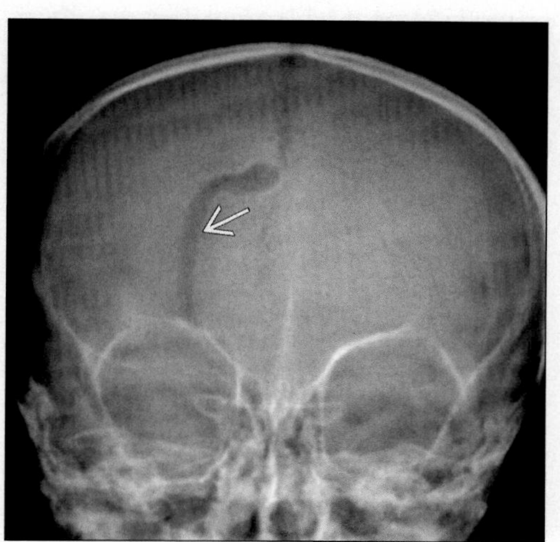

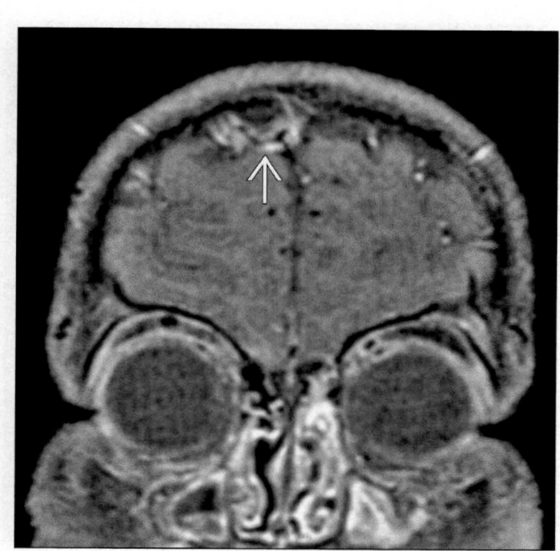

(Left) *Skull radiograph demonstrates an SP variant: A well-defined, vertically oriented calvarial channel extending from the right paramedian frontal bone to the right orbital roof ➡.* ***(Right)*** *Coronal T1WI C+ FS MR in the same patient shows a prominent vein ➡ extending from the superior sagittal sinus into the adjacent calvarium.*

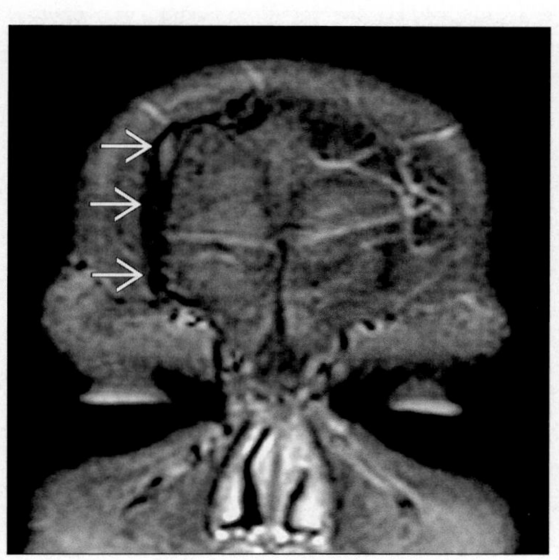

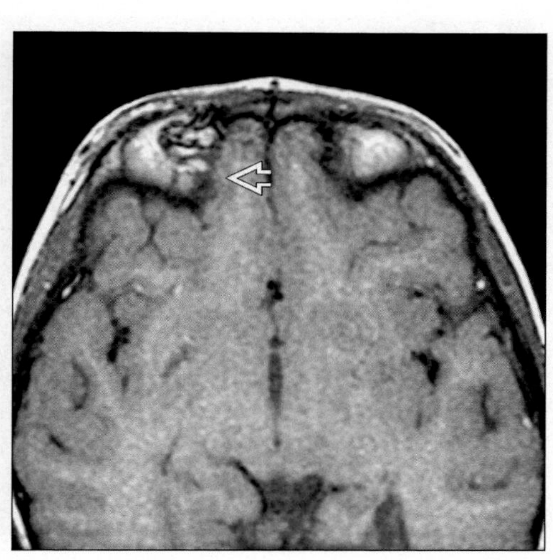

(Left) *Coronal T1 C+ FS MR obtained more anteriorly in the same patient with SP variant shows the transcalvarial vein in the vertically oriented right frontal bone channel extending toward the right orbital roof ➡.* ***(Right)*** *Axial T1WI MR in the same patient shows a mixed signal intensity, lobular mass in the superomedial right orbit ➡. In this patient with SP variant, the extracranial component of the SP is a partially thrombosed orbital varix.*

CAVERNOUS MALFORMATION

Key Facts

Terminology

- Benign vascular hamartoma
  - Contains masses of closely apposed immature blood vessels ("caverns"), no neural tissue
  - Intralesional hemorrhages of different ages
- CMs exhibit range of dynamic behaviors (enlargement, regression, de novo formation)

Imaging

- CMs vary from microscopic to giant (> 6 cm)
- Locules of variable size contain blood products at different stages of evolution
  - Variable appearance depending on hemorrhage/stage
- Zabramski classification of CMs
  - Type 1 = subacute hemorrhage (hyperintense on T1WI; hyper-/hypointense on T2WI)
  - Type 2 = mixed signal intensity on T1, T2WI with degrading hemorrhage of various ages (classic "popcorn ball" lesion)
  - Type 3 = chronic hemorrhage (hypo- to iso on T1, T2WI)
  - Type 4 = punctate microhemorrhages ("black dots"), poorly seen except on T2* sequences
- DSA usually normal ("angiographically occult vascular malformation") **unless** CM is extradural

Top Differential Diagnoses

- Arteriovenous malformation
- Hemorrhagic neoplasm
- Calcified neoplasm
- Hypertensive microbleeds
- Amyloid angiopathy

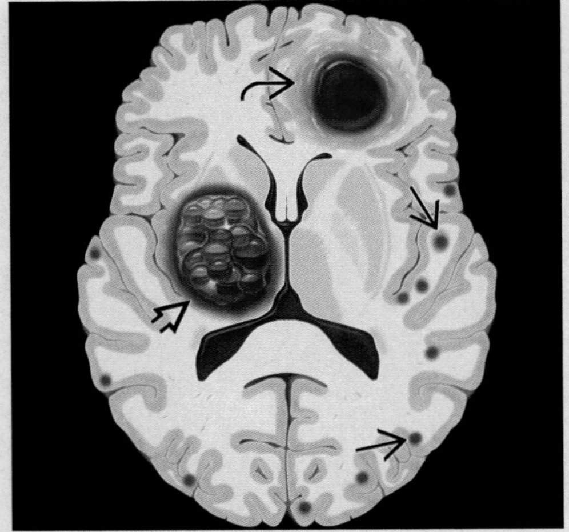

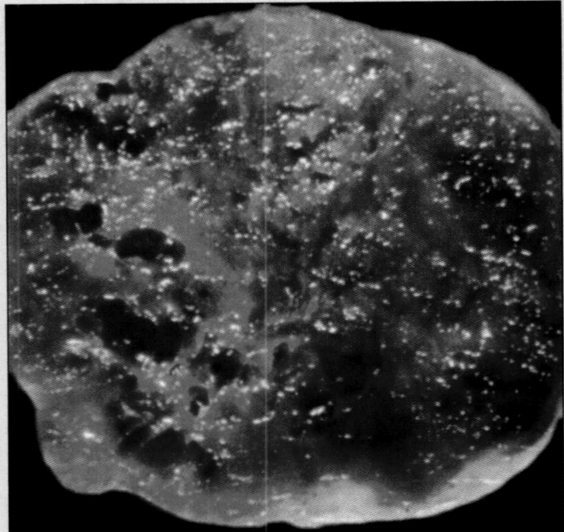

(Left) *Axial graphic depicts multiple cavernous malformations at different stages of evolution. A mixed signal "popcorn ball" (Zabramski type 2) is seen in the right basal ganglia, and subacute hemorrhage with edema (Zabramski type 1) is seen in the left frontal lobe. Multiple old microhemorrhages (Zabramski type 4) are seen as multifocal black dots that bloom on T2*.* ***(Right)*** *Gross pathology section of a cavernous malformation shows multiple locules of blood in various stages of evolution.*

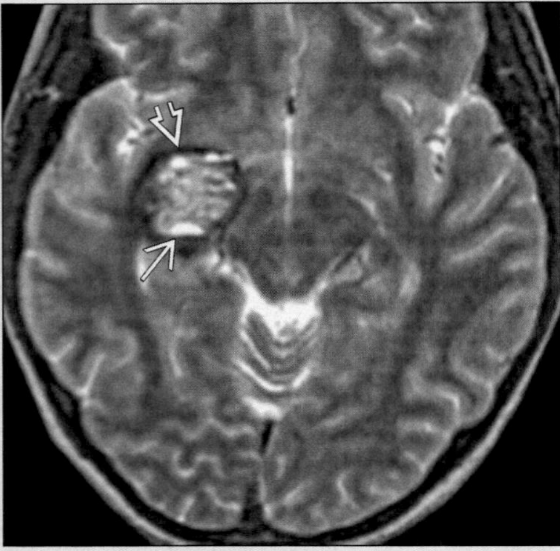

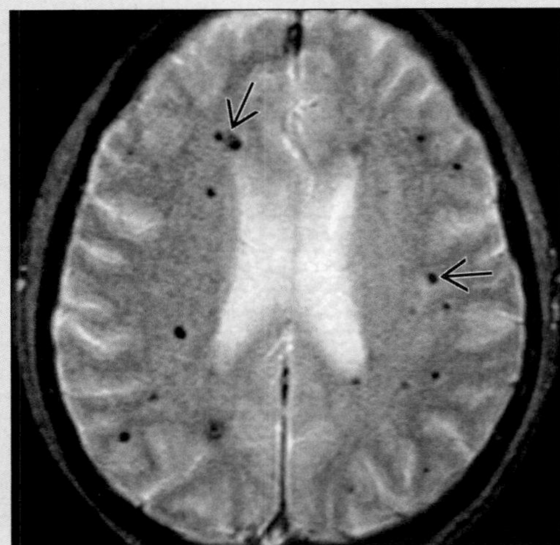

(Left) *Axial T2WI MR shows a classic "popcorn ball" configuration of a Zabramski type 2 cavernous malformation. Note the multiple locules with blood-fluid levels surrounded by a hemosiderin rim.* ***(Right)*** *Axial T2* GRE MR shows multifocal black dots that bloom on susceptibility-weighted imaging. These are Zabramski type 4 cavernous malformations with multiple punctate microhemorrhages.*

CAVERNOUS MALFORMATION

TERMINOLOGY

Abbreviations

- Cavernous malformation (CM)

Synonyms

- "Cavernoma"

Definitions

- Benign vascular hamartoma with intralesional hemorrhages, no neural tissue
  - Contains masses of closely apposed immature blood vessels ("caverns")
  - Intralesional hemorrhages of different ages
- CMs exhibit range of dynamic behaviors (enlargement, regression, de novo formation)

IMAGING

General Features

- Best diagnostic clue
  - "Popcorn ball" appearance with complete hypointense hemosiderin rim on T2WI MR
- Location
  - Occurs throughout CNS
  - Brain parenchymal CMs common
    - Spinal cord rare (more common in patients with multiple CM syndrome)
    - Extraaxial CMs rare
      - Can originate from within any venous sinus
      - Cavernous sinus most common site
      - May attain large size before becoming symptomatic
- Size
  - CMs vary from microscopic to giant (> 6 cm)
  - Majority are 0.5-4 cm
- Morphology
  - Discrete, lobulated mass of interwoven vessels
  - Locules of variable size contain blood products at different stages of evolution
  - Complete hemosiderin rim surrounds lesion

CT Findings

- NECT
  - Negative in 30-50%
  - Well-delineated round/ovoid hyperdense lesion, usually < 3 cm
    - 40-60% Ca++
    - No mass effect unless recent hemorrhage
  - Surrounding brain usually appears normal
- CECT
  - Little/no enhancement unless mixed with other lesion (e.g., developmental venous anomaly [DVA])
- CTA
  - Usually negative

MR Findings

- T1WI
  - Variable, depending on hemorrhage/stage
    - Common: "Popcorn ball" appearance of mixed hyper-, hypointense blood-containing locules
    - Less common: Acute hemorrhage (nonspecific)
  - T1 perilesional hyperintensity common
    - Helps differentiate CM from other hemorrhagic masses
- T2WI
  - Reticulated popcorn-like lesion most typical
    - Mixed signal core, complete hypointense hemosiderin rim
    - Locules of blood with fluid-fluid levels
  - Less common: Hypointense
- FLAIR
  - May show surrounding edema in acute lesions
- T2* GRE
  - Prominent susceptibility effect (hypointense "blooming")
  - Multiple CMs: Numerous punctate hypointense foci ("black dots") on GRE scans most common finding
- DWI
  - Usually normal
- T1WI C+
  - Minimal or no enhancement (may show associated venous malformation)
- MRA
  - Normal (unless mixed malformation present)
- Large acute hemorrhage may obscure more typical features of CM

Angiographic Findings

- Conventional
  - DSA
    - Usually normal ("angiographically occult vascular malformation")
      - Exception: Extradural CM (may be very vascular)
    - Slow intralesional flow without AV shunting
    - Avascular mass effect if large or acute hemorrhage
    - ± associated other malformation (e.g., DVA)
    - Rare: Venous pooling, contrast "blush"

Imaging Recommendations

- Best imaging tool
  - MR
    - Standard T1, T2WI may be negative in small type 4 lesions!
    - Use T2* sequence (SWI > GRE)
- Protocol advice
  - Use T2* GRE sequence with long TE (35 msec)
  - Include T1 C+ to look for associated anomalies (e.g., DVA)

DIFFERENTIAL DIAGNOSIS

"Popcorn Ball" Lesion

- Arteriovenous malformation
- Hemorrhagic neoplasm
- Calcified neoplasm

Multiple "Black Dots"

- Old trauma (DAI, contusions)
- Hypertensive microbleeds
- Amyloid angiopathy
- Capillary telangiectasias

CAVERNOUS MALFORMATION

PATHOLOGY

General Features

- Etiology
  - CMs are angiogenically immature lesions with endothelial proliferation, increased neoangiogenesis
  - VEGF, β-FGF, TGF-α expressed
  - Receptors (e.g., *FLI-1*) upregulated
- Genetics
  - Sporadic CM
    - No *KRIT1* mutation
    - *PTEN* promoter methylation mutation common (also in familial CM syndrome)
  - Multiple (familial) CM syndrome is autosomal dominant, variable penetrance
    - Nonsense, frame-shift, or splice-site mutations consistent with 2-hit model for CM
    - 3 separate loci implicated: *CCM1*, *CCM2*, *CCM3* genes
      - Mutations in these 3 genes account for > 95% of familial CMs
      - Mutations encode truncated KRIT1 protein
      - KRIT1 interacts with endothelial cell microtubules
      - Loss of function leads to inability of endothelial cells to mature, form capillaries
- Associated abnormalities
  - Developmental venous anomaly
  - Superficial siderosis
  - Cutaneous abnormalities
    - Café au lait spots
    - Hyperkeratotic capillary-venous malformations ("cherry angiomas")

Staging, Grading, & Classification

- Zabramski classification of CMs
  - Type 1 = subacute hemorrhage (hyperintense on T1WI; hyper- or hypointense on T2WI)
  - Type 2 = mixed signal intensity on T1, T2WI with degrading hemorrhage of various ages (classic "popcorn ball" lesion)
  - Type 3 = chronic hemorrhage (hypo- to isointense on T1, T2WI)
  - Type 4 = punctate microhemorrhages ("black dots"), poorly seen except on GRE sequences

Gross Pathologic & Surgical Features

- Discrete, lobulated, bluish-purple (mulberry-like) nodule
  - Well-delineated collection of endothelial-lined, hemorrhage-filled vessels without intervening normal brain
  - Pseudocapsule of gliotic, hemosiderin-stained brain

Microscopic Features

- Angioarchitecture
  - "Bland" regions within thin-walled caverns
  - "Honeycombed" regions with notable capillary proliferation
- Thin-walled epithelial-lined spaces
  - Embedded in collagenous matrix
  - Hemorrhage in different stages of evolution
  - ± Ca++
  - Does not contain normal brain tissue
- May be histologically mixed (vascular malformation most common)

CLINICAL ISSUES

Presentation

- Most common signs/symptoms
  - Seizure (50%)
  - Neurologic deficit (25%) (may be progressive)
  - Asymptomatic (20%)

Demographics

- Age
  - Peak presentation: 40-60 years
    - May present in childhood
  - Familial CMs tend to present earlier than sporadic lesions
- Gender
  - M = F
- Ethnicity
  - Multiple (familial) CM syndrome in Hispanic-Americans of Mexican descent
    - Founder mutation in *KRIT1* (Q445X)
    - Positive family history = 90% chance of mutation resulting in CM
  - CMs may occur in any ethnic population
- Epidemiology
  - Most common angiographically "occult" vascular malformation
  - Approximate prevalence 0.5%
  - 2/3 occur as solitary, sporadic lesion
  - 1/3 multiple, familial

Natural History & Prognosis

- Broad range of dynamic behavior (may progress, enlarge, regress)
- De novo lesions may develop
- Propensity for growth via repeated intralesional hemorrhages
  - Sporadic = 0.25-0.7% per year
  - Risk factor for future hemorrhage = previous hemorrhage
  - Rehemorrhage rate high initially, decreases after 2-3 years
- Familial CMs at especially high risk for hemorrhage, forming new lesions
  - Estimated 1% per lesion per year

Treatment

- Total removal via microsurgical resection
  - Caution: If mixed DVA, venous drainage must be preserved

DIAGNOSTIC CHECKLIST

Consider

- Perform T2* scan to look for additional lesions in patients with spontaneous intracranial hemorrhage

Image Interpretation Pearls

- "Giant" CMs can mimic neoplasm

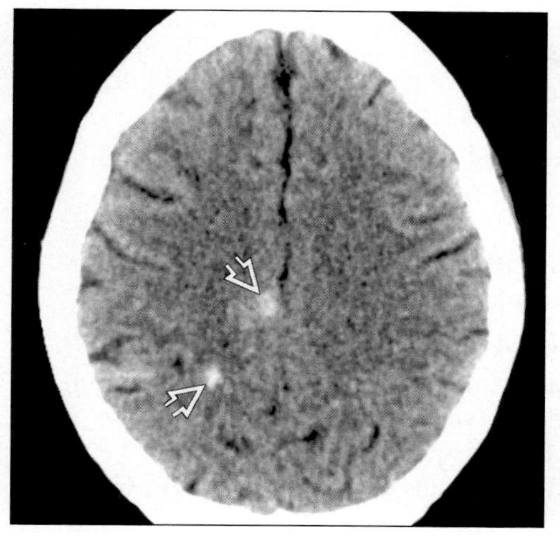

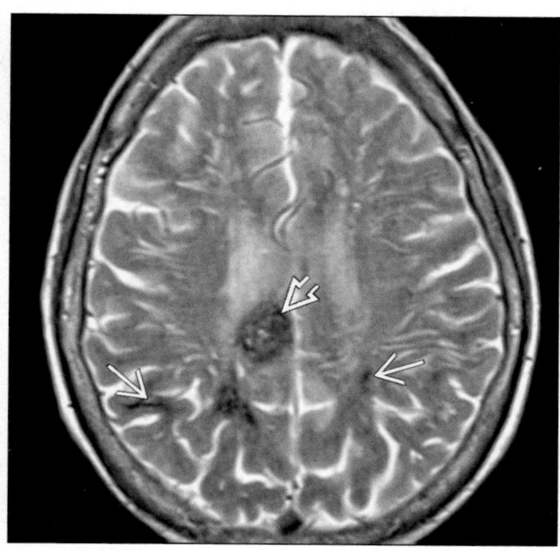

(Left) *Axial NECT shows multiple hyperdense lesions ➲ in this patient with chronic headaches. The lesions appear at least partially calcified.* ***(Right)*** *Axial T2WI MR in a patient with multiple cavernous malformation syndrome shows the classic hypointense lesion of Zabramski type 3 cavernous malformation with chronic hemorrhage ➲. Other lesions are seen as punctate "black dots" and are probably chronic microhemorrhages ➔, Zabramski type 4 cavernous malformations.*

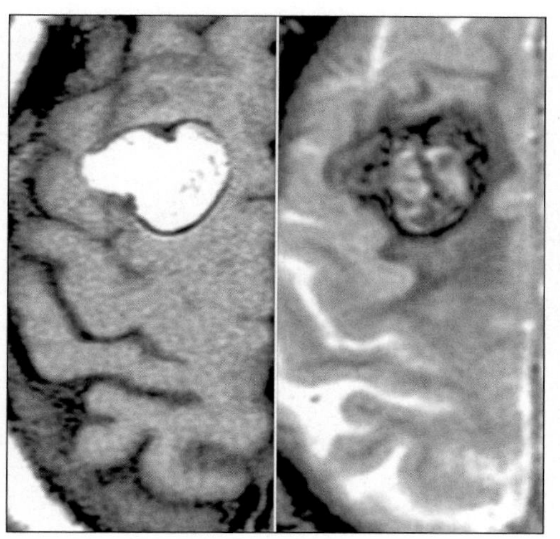

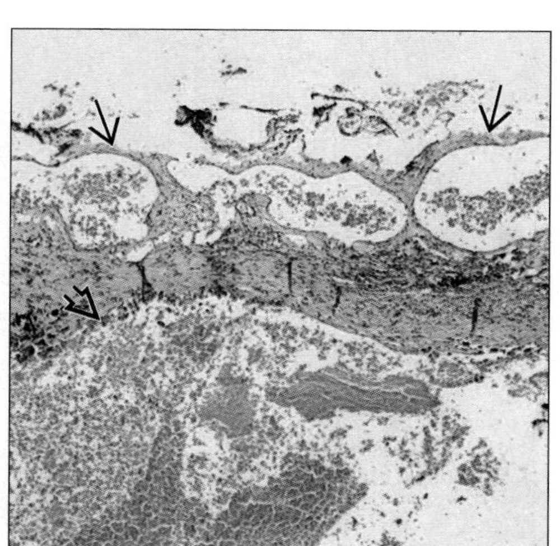

(Left) *Axial T1WI MR (left) and T2* GRE scan (right) in a 49-year-old woman with a 4-month history of convulsions shows a right frontoparietal lesion with subacute hemorrhage.* ***(Right)*** *Micropathology H&E from resected surgical specimen in the same patient shows a cavity filled with clotted blood undergoing patchy organization ➲. The wall consists of thin endothelial-lined vascular channels ➔. Diagnosis was classic cavernous malformation, Zabramski type 1. (Courtesy R. Hewlett, PhD.)*

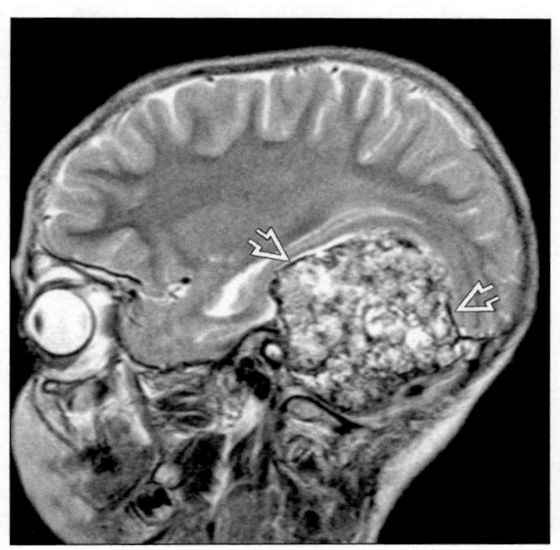

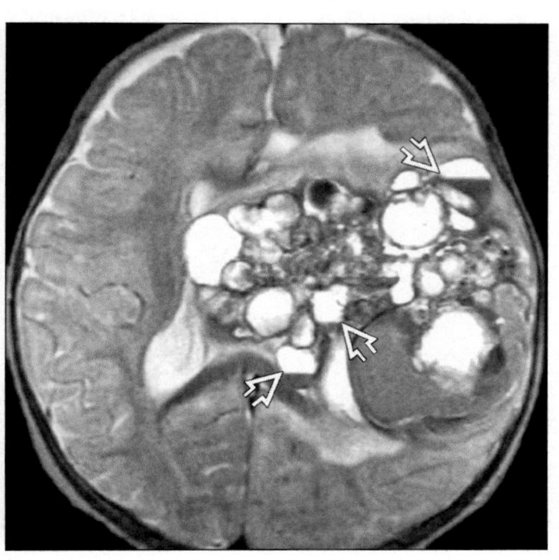

(Left) *Sagittal T2WI MR shows a large popcorn-like posterior fossa mass. Note its extradural location, shown by the displaced thin black line representing dura ➲. CM was found at surgery. CMs arising within dural sinuses are often highly vascular, in contrast to parenchymal CMs, which are typically angiographically occult.* ***(Right)*** *Axial T2WI MR shows a giant cavernous malformation in a child. Note fluid-fluid levels ➲, which confirm proliferating caverns that contain blood-filled "locules."*

CAPILLARY TELANGIECTASIA

Key Facts

Terminology

- Cluster of enlarged, dilated capillaries interspersed with normal brain parenchyma
- BCTs represent 15-20% of all intracranial vascular malformations

Imaging

- General features
  - Common sites: Pons, cerebellum, spinal cord
  - Usually < 1 cm
- CT
  - Usually normal
- MR
  - T1WI usually normal
  - 50% normal on T2WI
  - 50% show faint stippled foci of hyperintensity
  - Large BCTs may show ill-defined FLAIR hyperintensity
  - Moderately hypointense on GRE; profoundly hypointense on SWI
  - T1 C+ shows faint stippled or speckled brush-like enhancement
  - Large BCTs typically contain prominent linear draining vein(s)

Top Differential Diagnoses

- Developmental venous anomaly
- Metastasis
- Cavernous malformation
- Capillary hemangioma

Clinical Issues

- Usually found incidentally at autopsy or imaging
- Rare: Headache, vertigo, tinnitus
- Clinically benign, quiescent
  - Unless histologically mixed (usually with CM)

*(**Left**) Lateral graphic shows a stippled-appearing lesion of the pons with dilated, thin-walled capillaries interspersed with normal brain. Note the absence of mass effect. (**Right**) High-power photomicrography shows typical findings of incidental capillary telangiectasia of the brainstem. Note the enlarged thin-walled vessels ➔ with normal brain interspersed between the dilated capillaries. No hemorrhage is present in the adjacent brain.*

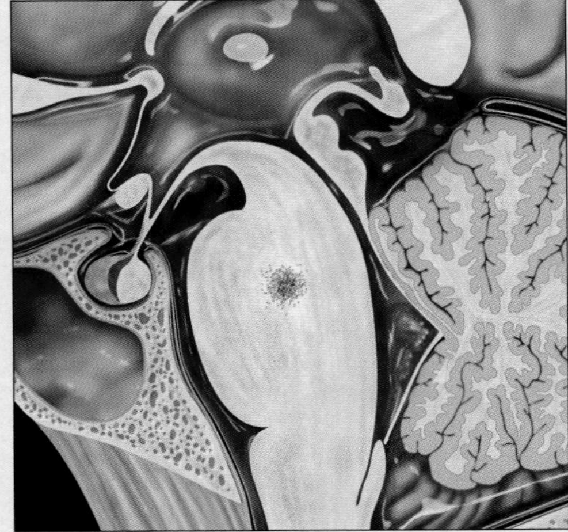

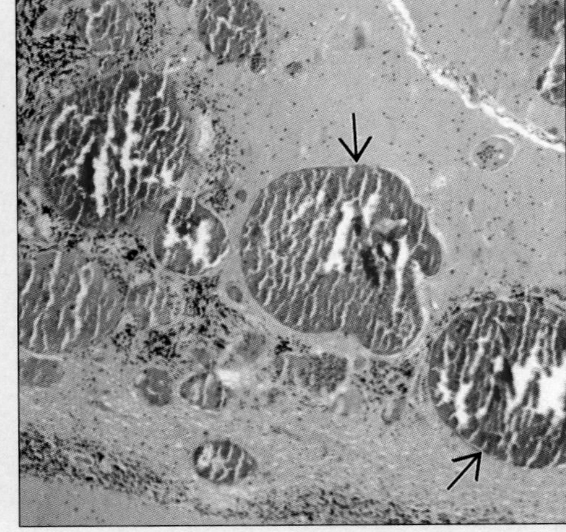

*(**Left**) Axial T2WI MR is normal in an asymptomatic patient with a family history of HHT who underwent a screening MR study. (**Right**) Axial T1WI C+ MR in the same patient shows faint, brush-like enhancement in the pons ➲. This presumed capillary telangiectasia was the only brain lesion in this patient. A T2* (GRE or SWI) sequence was not performed but would show the lesion becoming mildly hypointense because of slow intralesional flow and desaturation from oxy- to deoxyhemoglobin.*

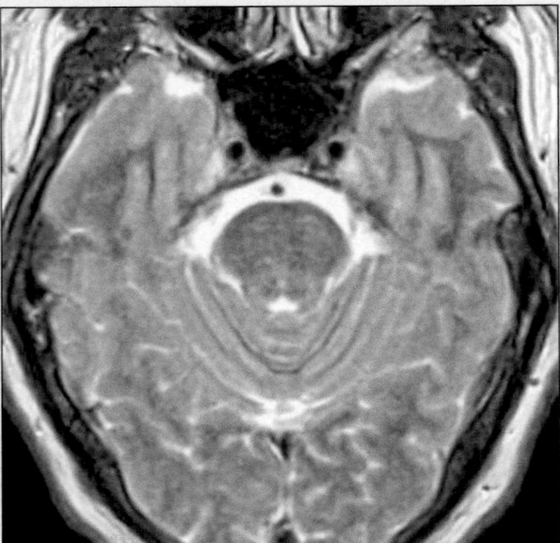

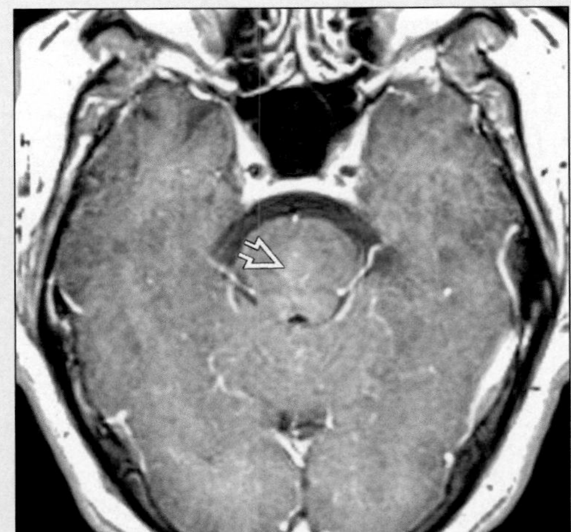

CAPILLARY TELANGIECTASIA

TERMINOLOGY

Abbreviations

- Brain capillary telangiectasia (BCT)
- Cerebrovascular malformation (CVM)

Synonyms

- Capillary malformation
- **Not** capillary "hemangioma"
  - Hemangiomas are true benign vasoformative neoplasms
  - Usually in face, scalp, back, chest, orbit
  - Less common: Dura, venous sinuses
  - Exceptionally rare in brain parenchyma

Definitions

- Cluster of enlarged, dilated capillaries interspersed with normal brain parenchyma

IMAGING

General Features

- Best diagnostic clue
  - Hypointense lesion on T2* with faint brush-like enhancement
- Location
  - Can be found anywhere
  - Most common sites
    - Pons
      - Adjacent to median raphe
      - Adjacent to floor of 4th ventricle
    - Cerebellum
    - Medulla
    - Spinal cord
  - Up to 1/3 in cerebral hemispheres
    - White matter
    - Cortex
- Size
  - Usually < 1 cm
  - Occasionally "giant" (> 1 cm)
  - Solitary > > multiple
- Morphology
  - Small, poorly marginated
  - No mass effect
  - No edema

CT Findings

- NECT
  - Usually normal
  - Occasionally may show Ca++
    - Usually only if mixed histology
      - Cavernous malformation (CM) is most common
- CECT
  - Usually normal

MR Findings

- T1WI
  - Usually normal
  - May be hyperintense or hypo-/hyperintense ("popcorn" appearance) if mixed with CM
- T2WI
  - 50% normal
  - 50% show faint stippled foci of hyperintensity
- FLAIR
  - Usually normal
  - If large, may show ill-defined hyperintensity
  - No mass effect
- T2* GRE
  - GRE
    - Lesion moderately hypointense
    - Slows blood flow with oxy- to deoxyhemoglobin
    - Occasionally multifocal BCTs seen as black or gray "dots," especially if mixed with CMs
  - SWI
    - More sensitive than GRE
    - Lesion may be profoundly hypointense
- DWI
  - Usually normal
- PWI
  - Shows profound drop in signal intensity with relatively rapid recovery to baseline
- T1WI C+
  - Faint stippled or mild speckled brush-like enhancement
    - May have enlarged central draining vein with prominent linear enhancement
  - Large BCTs
    - Usually contain punctate, linear/branching vessel(s)
    - Represent radicles of draining veins
    - Larger "collector" vein often present
    - Mixed BCT, DVA common
- MRV
  - SWI even more sensitive than standard T2*
- DTI
  - BCTs are interspersed with normal WM tracts
  - No alteration of FA
  - No disturbance/displacement of WM tracts

Angiographic Findings

- Conventional
  - Usually normal
  - Faint vascular "stain" ± draining vein
  - Look for associated DVA

Imaging Recommendations

- Best imaging tool
  - MR with T2*, T1 C+ sequences
- Protocol advice
  - Include SWI

DIFFERENTIAL DIAGNOSIS

Developmental Venous Anomaly (DVA)

- Often mixed with BCT

Metastasis

- Strong > > faint enhancement
- Pons/cerebellum rare locations

Cavernous Malformation

- Blood locules with fluid-fluid levels
- Complete hemosiderin rim
- Can be mixed with BCTs, cause hemorrhage

CAPILLARY TELANGIECTASIA

Capillary Hemangioma
- Capillary hemangiomas are vasoformative neoplasms, not congenital CVMs
- Dura, venous sinuses > > > brain parenchyma

PATHOLOGY

General Features
- Etiology
  - Precise etiology of sporadic BCTs unknown
  - May develop as complication of radiation
    - 20% of children after cranial irradiation
- Genetics
  - May be related to mutated *ALK1* ± (same as HHT type 2)
    - ↑ perfusion → upregulated VEGF → ↑ capillary dysplasia
  - Capillary density increases with nonischemic venous hypertension
    - Hypoxia-inducible factor-1-α (HIF-1-α), downstream target VEGF upregulated
- Associated abnormalities
  - Often mixed with other vascular malformations (cavernous, venous)
  - Hereditary hemorrhagic telangiectasia (HHT)
    - a.k.a. Osler-Weber-Rendu disease
    - Autosomal dominant disorder
    - Often complicated by vascular malformations in brain, lung, GI tract, liver
      - Capillary telangiectasias common in nasal mucosa (epistaxis, hemoptysis common, may be life-threatening)
      - Brain parenchymal capillary telangiectasias relatively rare
      - AVMs more common
      - HHT-associated strokes usually secondary to pulmonary AVM/AVF, brain AVM with bleed, SAH with saccular aneurysm
  - Macrocephaly capillary malformation (MCM) syndromes
    - a.k.a. macrocephaly-cutis marmorata telangiectatica congenita (M-CMTC)
      - Facial nevus flammeus, cutis marmorata
    - Rapid brain growth during infancy
      - Megalencephaly, polymicrogyria
      - Tonsillar herniation
      - Ventriculomegaly, dilated dural venous sinuses
      - Prominent PVSs
      - Skin > > brain capillary malformations

Gross Pathologic & Surgical Features
- Readily overlooked at autopsy
- Most BCTs found incidentally
  - Unusually large BCTs may appear pinkish or slightly dusky
  - No hemorrhage unless other vascular malformation (e.g., CM) present

Microscopic Features
- Cluster of dilated but histologically normal capillaries
  - Thin-walled, endothelial-lined vascular channels
  - Largest channels may represent draining veins
- Normal brain interspersed between dilated capillaries
- Uncomplicated BCTs have no surrounding gliosis, hemorrhage, Ca++

CLINICAL ISSUES

Presentation
- Most common signs/symptoms
  - Usually found incidentally at autopsy or imaging
  - Rare: Headache, vertigo, tinnitus
- Clinical profile
  - Asymptomatic middle-aged patient with poorly delineated, enhancing brainstem lesion

Demographics
- Age
  - Any age; 30-40 years most common
  - Rarely identified in children but do occur
- Epidemiology
  - 15-20% of all intracranial vascular malformations

Natural History & Prognosis
- Clinically benign, quiescent unless histologically mixed
- Rare reports of aggressive course

Treatment
- None

DIAGNOSTIC CHECKLIST

Image Interpretation Pearls
- Faintly enhancing pontine lesion that becomes moderately hypointense on T2* is usually BCT

SELECTED REFERENCES

1. Gao P et al: Nonischemic cerebral venous hypertension promotes a pro-angiogenic stage through HIF-1 downstream genes and leukocyte-derived MMP-9. J Cereb Blood Flow Metab. 29(8):1482-90, 2009
2. Govani FS et al: Hereditary haemorrhagic telangiectasia: a clinical and scientific review. Eur J Hum Genet. 17(7):860-71, 2009
3. Gripp KW et al: Significant overlap and possible identity of macrocephaly capillary malformation and megalencephaly polymicrogyria-polydactyly hydrocephalus syndromes. Am J Med Genet A. 149A(5):868-76, 2009
4. Hao Q et al: Increased tissue perfusion promotes capillary dysplasia in the ALK1-deficient mouse brain following VEGF stimulation. Am J Physiol Heart Circ Physiol. 295(6):H2250-6, 2008
5. Pozzati E et al: The neurovascular triad: mixed cavernous, capillary, and venous malformations of the brainstem. J Neurosurg. 107(6):1113-9, 2007
6. Koike S et al: Asymptomatic radiation-induced telangiectasia in children after cranial irradiation: frequency, latency, and dose relation. Radiology. 230(1):93-9, 2004
7. Castillo M et al: MR imaging and histologic features of capillary telangiectasia of the basal ganglia. AJNR Am J Neuroradiol. 22(8):1553-5, 2001

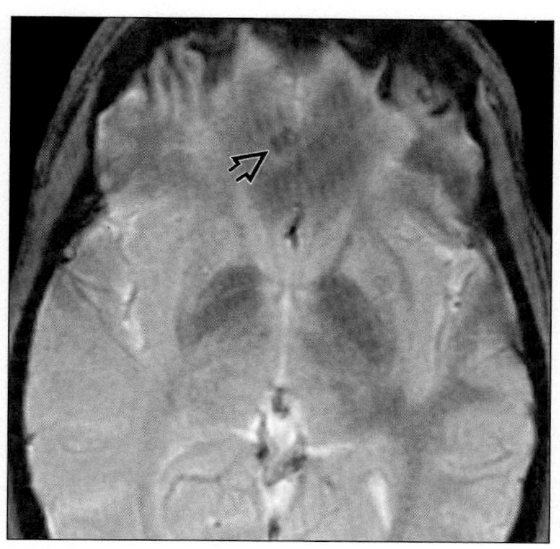

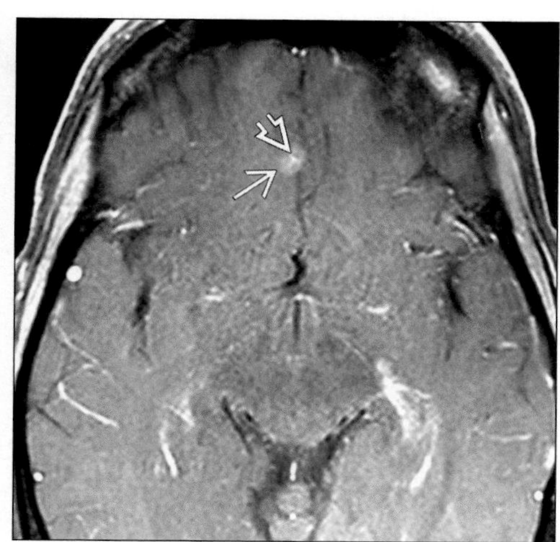

(Left) *Axial T2* GRE MR in a 33-year-old woman with headaches shows small faint hypointensity in the right medial frontal lobe cortex* ➪. *No other abnormalities were identified.* ***(Right)*** *Axial T1WI C+ FS MR in the same case shows mild to moderate enhancement* ➡. *Note the more intensely enhancing linear focus in the center of the lesion* ➪. *Findings are typical for a small capillary telangiectasia with central draining vein. The frontal lobe cortex is a less common location than the pons or cerebellum.*

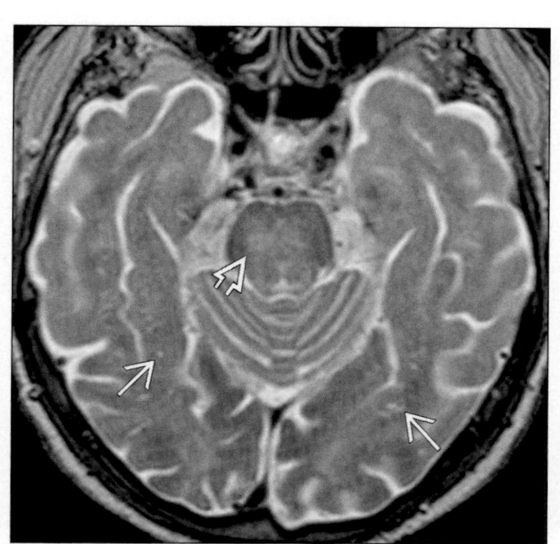

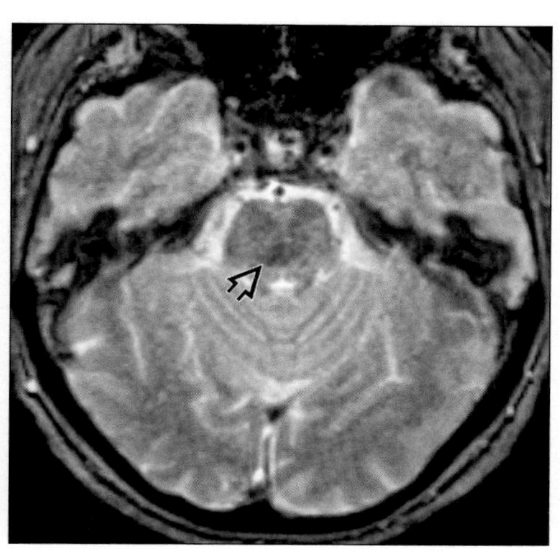

(Left) *Axial T2WI MR in a 71-year-old woman with headaches shows a few scattered hyperintensities in the pons* ➪ *and some prominent perivascular spaces in the temporal lobe white matter* ➡. *The scan appears normal for the patient's age.* ***(Right)*** *Axial T2* GRE MR in the same patient shows a focus of mild central pontine hypointensity* ➪. *The lesion is dark gray, not the black "blooming" typically seen in remote hemorrhage with hemosiderin and ferritin deposition.*

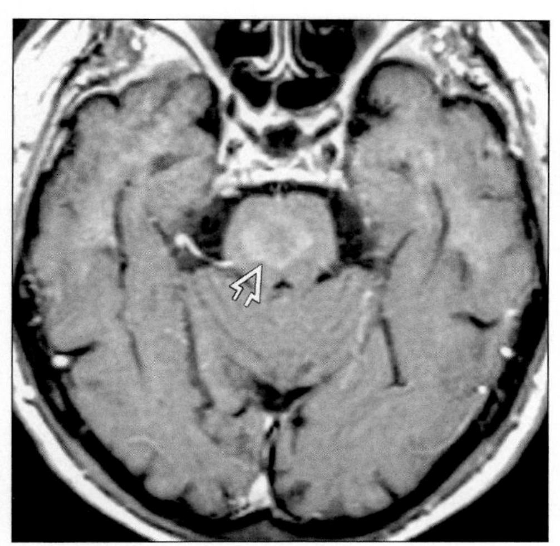

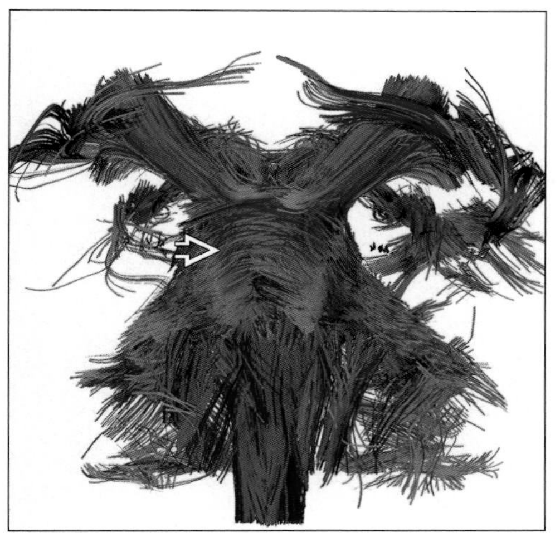

(Left) *Axial T1WI C+ MR in the same patient shows a very large mildly enhancing central pontine lesion* ➪. *Note the absence of mass effect.* ***(Right)*** *Coronal DTI in the same patient shows normal central pontine white matter tracts* ➪. *There is no distortion or alteration of anisotropy to suggest focal mass or tumor infiltration. Findings are those of a classic "giant" capillary telangiectasia of the pons. (Courtesy P. Rodriguez, MD.)*

(Left) Axial T2WI MR in a 37-year-old man with vertigo, obtained to look for demyelinating disease, shows a wedge-shaped, ill-defined hyperintensity present in the left parietal lobe ➔. Note the absence of mass effect on the adjacent ventricle. The overlying gyrus and subcortical white matter appear normal. ***(Right)*** Axial T2* GRE MR in the same patient shows stippled hypointensity in the same area ➔.

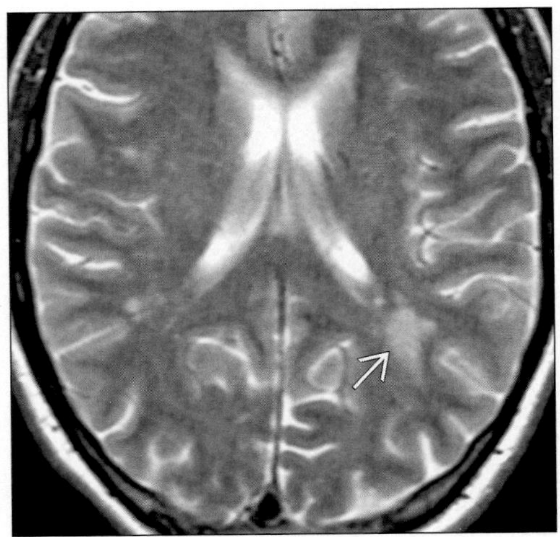

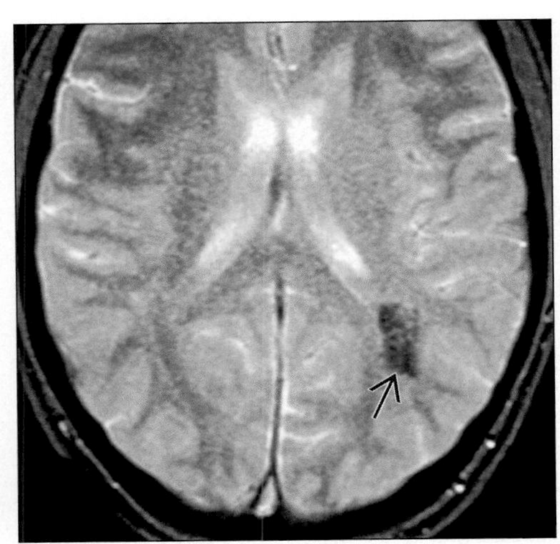

(Left) Axial T1WI C+ FS MR in the same patient shows prominent but poorly marginated enhancement ➔. Note the strongly enhancing linear structure in the lesion's core ➔ with smaller adjacent stippled foci ➔ that probably represent venous radicles draining into a central "collector vein." ***(Right)*** Coronal T1WI C+ MR in the same patient shows that the lesion ➔ extends from the subcortical WM into the centrum semiovale. Note the linear, enhancing "collector vein" ➔, characteristic of "giant" BCT.

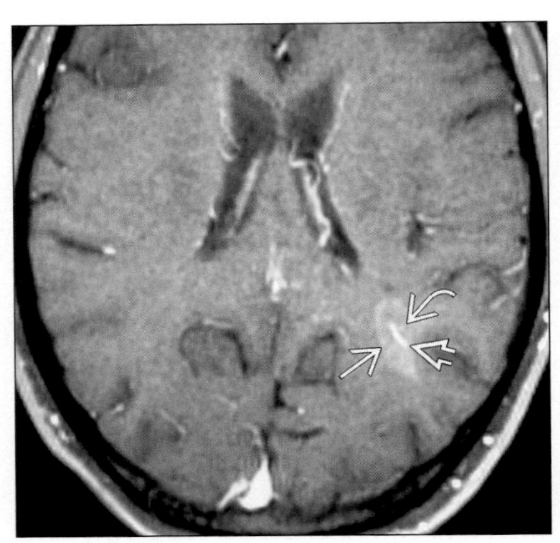

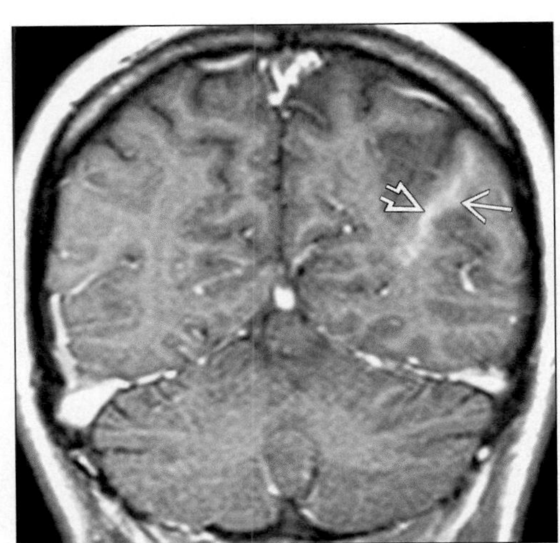

(Left) Axial T2* GRE MR in a 45-year-old, asymptomatic, normotensive patient shows multifocal, moderately hypointense lesions in the left cerebellar hemisphere ➔. ***(Right)*** Axial T2* GRE MR in the same patient shows additional lesions in the cerebellum and pons ➔. No abnormalities were identified in the cerebral hemispheres. Because BCTs rarely hemorrhage, these lesions probably represent either multiple type 4 cavernous malformations or mixed capillary-cavernous malformations.

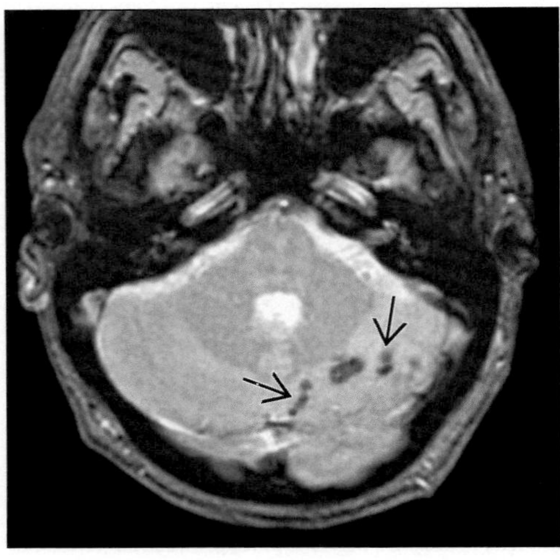

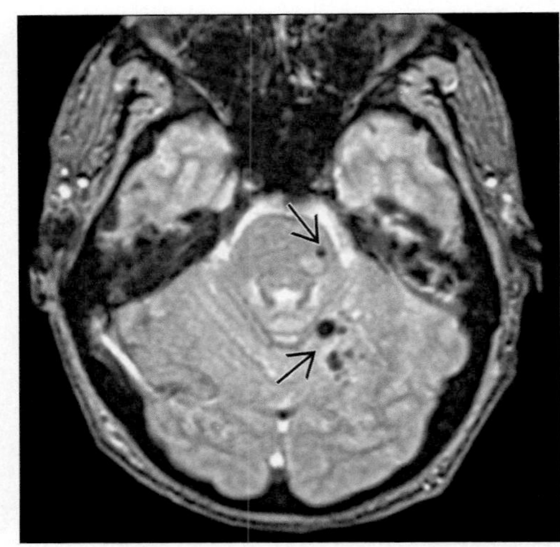

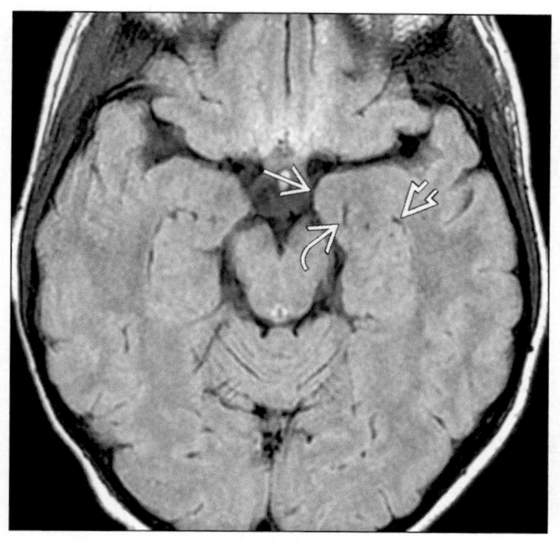

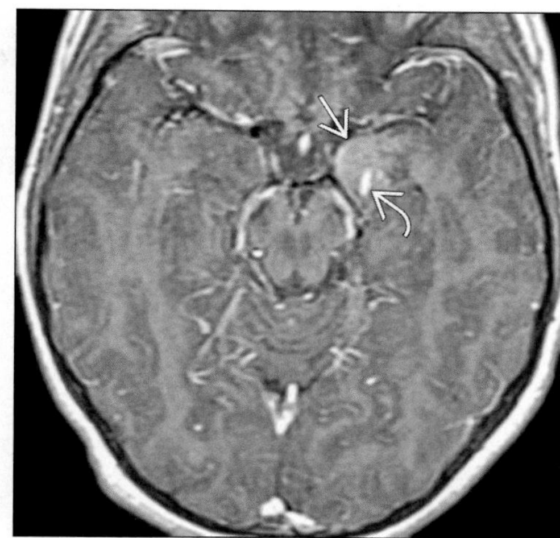

(Left) *Axial FLAIR MR in a 17 year old with headaches, dizziness, "blackouts," and no definite history of seizures. Neurologic examination was normal. Scan shows faint diffuse hyperintensity in the medial temporal lobe ➔. Note the absence of mass effect and normal-appearing temporal horn ➔. A possible linear flow void is present ➔.* ***(Right)*** *Axial T1WI C+ MR in the same patient shows moderate diffuse enhancement ➔ and a prominent draining vein ➔ where the possible flow void was seen on FLAIR.*

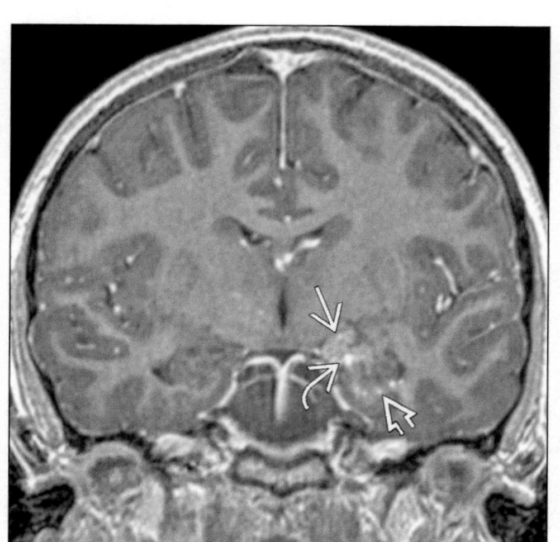

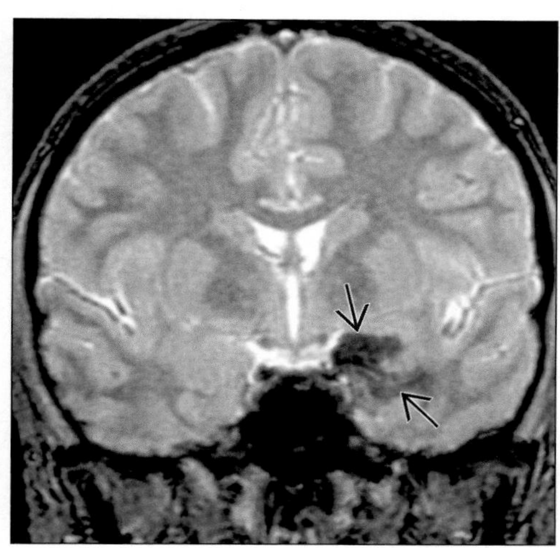

(Left) *Coronal T1 C+ MR shows the diffuse enhancement ➔ and strongly enhancing central draining vein ➔. In addition, several other punctate enhancing foci are identified that may represent venous radicles ➔.* ***(Right)*** *Coronal T2* GRE MR in the same patient shows diffuse hypointensity ➔ within the lesion. The T2WIs (not shown) appeared normal. Note the "giant" capillary telangiectasia with prominent draining veins that may represent a DVA mixed with the BCT. (Courtesy C. Hecht-Leavitt, MD.)*

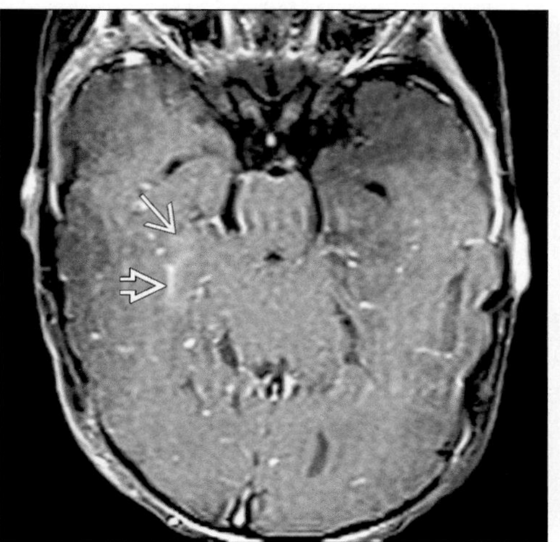

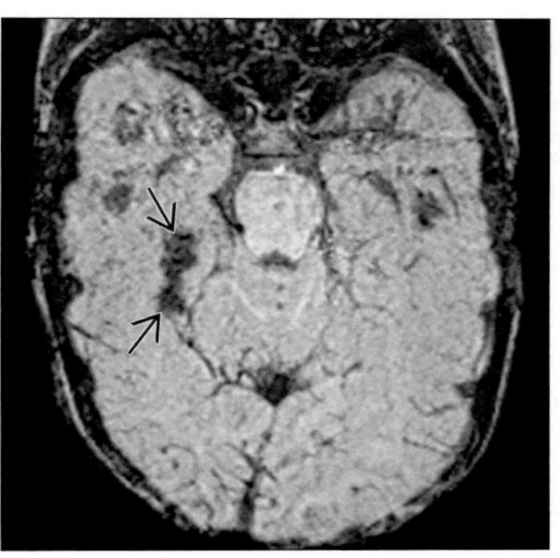

(Left) *Axial T1WI C+ FS MR in a 6-month-old infant with infantile spasms shows faint enhancement in the right medial temporal lobe ➔. A prominent linear enhancing structure ➔ most likely represents a draining vein.* ***(Right)*** *Axial SWI in the same patient shows profound "blooming" ➔ due to the deoxyhemoglobin in the slowly flowing radicles of the presumed capillary telangiectasia. (Courtesy A. Vossough, MD.)*

SECTION 6
Neoplasms

Introduction and Overview

Astrocytic Tumors, Infiltrating

Astrocytic Tumors, Localized

Oligodendroglial and Miscellaneous Tumors

Ependymal Tumors

Choroid Plexus Tumors

Neuronal and Mixed Neuronal-Glial Tumors

Pineal Parenchymal Tumors

Embryonal and Neuroblastic Tumors

Tumors of Cranial/Peripheral Nerves

Blood Vessel and Hemopoietic Tumors

Germ Cell Tumors

Metastatic Tumors and Remote Effects of Cancer

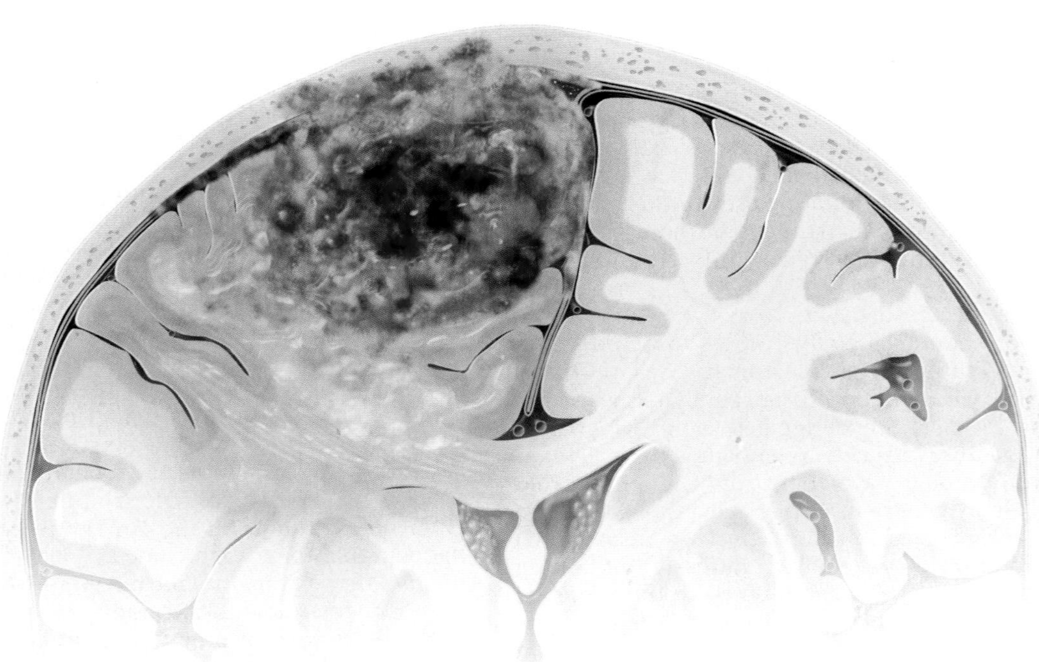

NEOPLASMS OVERVIEW

Introduction

The most widely accepted classification of brain neoplasms is sponsored by the World Health Organization (WHO). A working group of world-renowned neuropathologists is periodically convened for a consensus conference on brain tumor classification and grading. The results are then published, most recently in 2007. The WHO classification follows in this text.

Brain tumors are both classified and graded. Histological grading is a means of predicting the biological behavior of tumors and is an important guide to therapeutic decisions. While many different grading schemas have been proposed, the WHO grading is the most widely accepted and is utilized in this text. Some tumors have been assigned WHO grades, but many others, especially newly defined tumors, remain ungraded.

Classification/Grading of CNS Neoplasms

General Considerations

CNS neoplasms are divided into primary and metastatic tumors. Primary neoplasms are divided into 6 major categories. The largest by far is "tumors of neuroepithelial tissue," followed by tumors of the meninges. Tumors of cranial and spinal nerves, lymphomas and hematopoietic neoplasms, and germ cell tumors are less common but important groupings. The final category of primary neoplasms--tumors of the sellar region--is identified by geographic region rather than histologic type.

Tumors of Neuroepithelial Tissue

This category is huge and therefore divided into several discrete tumor subtypes. The neuropil mostly consists of neurons and glial cells. Glial cells have several subtypes: Astrocytes, oligodendrocytes, ependymal cells, and modified ependymal cells that form the choroid plexus. Each cell type gives rise to a specific type of "glioma." Of all the gliomas, astrocytomas are by far the most common.

Astrocytomas. There are many histologic types and subtypes of astrocytomas. The most common of these are the diffusely infiltrating astrocytomas. Here no distinct border between tumor and normal brain is present (even though the tumor may look discrete on imaging). The lowest grade is simply called "diffuse astrocytoma" and is designated as WHO grade II. Anaplastic astrocytoma (AA) is WHO grade III and glioblastoma (GBM) is a grade IV neoplasm. All diffusely infiltrating astrocytomas have an inherent tendency to malignant progression. Note that there is no such thing as a grade I diffusely infiltrating astrocytoma.

The more benign-behaving astrocytic tumors are less common and generally more localized than the diffusely infiltrating astrocytomas. Two of these, pilocytic astrocytoma (PA) and subependymal giant cell astrocytoma (SGCA), are designated as WHO grade I neoplasms. Neither displays a tendency to malignant progression, although a variant of PA, pilomyxoid astrocytoma, may behave more aggressively.

Patient age has a significant effect on astrocytoma type and location. For example, diffusely infiltrating astrocytomas are most common in the cerebral hemispheres of adults and the pons in children. PAs are tumors of children and young adults. They are common in the cerebellum and around the 3rd ventricle but rarely occur in the hemispheres.

Nonastrocytic gliomas. These tumors include oligodendrogliomas, ependymomas, "mixed" gliomas, and choroid plexus tumors.

Oligodendroglial tumors. These vary from a diffusely infiltrating but relatively well-differentiated WHO grade II neoplasm (oligodendroglioma) to anaplastic oligodendroglioma (WHO grade III). Oligodendrogliomas can be mixed with astrocytic or other elements. Mixed gliomas are graded according to the most anaplastic element, which is usually the astrocytic component.

Ependymal tumors. Ependymomas vary from WHO grade I to III. Subependymoma, a benign-behaving neoplasm of middle-aged and older adults that occurs in the frontal horns and 4th ventricle, is a WHO grade I tumor. So is myxopapillary ependymoma, a tumor of young and middle-aged adults that is almost exclusively found at the conus, cauda equina, and filum terminale of the spinal cord.

Ependymoma, generally a slow-growing tumor of children and young adults, is a WHO grade II neoplasm that may arise anywhere along the ventricular system and in the central canal of the spinal cord. Infratentorial ependymomas, typically arising within the 4th ventricle, predominate in children. Supratentorial ependymomas are more common in the cerebral hemispheres than lateral ventricle and are usually tumors of young children. Anaplastic ependymomas are biologically more aggressive, have poorer prognosis, and are designated as WHO grade III neoplasms.

Choroid plexus tumors. Choroid plexus tumors are papillary intraventricular neoplasms derived from choroid plexus epithelial cells. Almost 80% of choroid plexus tumors are found in children and are 1 of the most common brain tumors in children under the age of 3 years. They have classically been divided into choroid plexus papillomas (CPP), WHO grade I tumors, and choroid plexus carcinomas (CPC), designated as WHO grade III. CPPs are 5-10 times more common than CPCs. Both CPPs and CPCs can spread diffusely through the CSF, so the entire neuraxis should be imaged prior to surgical intervention.

Recently, an intermediate grade of choroid plexus tumor has been recognized. These "atypical choroid plexus papillomas" (aCPPs) are WHO grade II neoplasms.

Other neuroepithelial tumors. These rare neoplasms include astroblastoma, chordoid glioma of the 3rd ventricle, and angiocentric glioma.

Neuronal and mixed neuronal-glial tumors. Neuroepithelial tumors with ganglion-like cells, differentiated neurocytes, or poorly differentiated neuroblastic cells are included in this heterogeneous group. Ganglion cell neoplasms (gangliocytoma, ganglioglioma), DIG/DIA (desmoplastic infantile ganglioglioma or astrocytoma), neurocytoma (central as well as the newly described extraventricular variant), dysembryoplastic neuroepithelial tumor (DNET), papillary glioneuronal tumor, rosette-forming glioneuronal tumor (of the 4th ventricle), and cerebellar liponeuroblastoma are included.

Pineal region tumors. Pineal region neoplasms account for less than 1% of all intracranial neoplasms and can be germ cell tumors or pineal parenchymal tumors. Pineal parenchymal tumors are less common than germ cell tumors. As germ cell neoplasms occur in other intracranial sites as well as the pineal gland, they are considered a separate category.

Pineocytoma is a very slowly growing, well-delineated tumor that is usually found in adults. Pineocytomas are WHO grade I. Pineoblastoma is a highly malignant primitive embryonal tumor mostly found in children. Highly aggressive and associated with early CSF dissemination, pineoblastomas are WHO grade IV neoplasms.

A newly described tumor, pineal parenchymal tumor of intermediate differentiation (PPTID), is intermediate in malignancy, probably WHO grade II or III. Many so-called aggressive pineocytomas would probably be reclassified as PPTIDs. Another newly-described neoplasm, papillary tumor of the pineal region (PTPR), is a rare neuroepitheal tumor of adults. No WHO grade has been assigned.

Embryonal tumors. This group includes medulloblastoma, CNS primitive neuroectodermal tumors (PNETs), and atypical teratoid-rhabdoid tumors (AT/RT). All are highly malignant, invasive tumors. All are WHO grade IV and are mostly tumors of young children.

Meningeal Tumors

Overview. Meningeal tumors are the 2nd largest category of primary CNS neoplasms. They are divided into meningiomas and mesenchymal, nonmeningothelial tumors (i.e., tumors that are not meningiomas). Hemangiopericytomas, hemangioblastomas, and melanocytic lesions are also considered as part of the meningeal tumor grouping.

Meningiomas. Meningiomas arise from meningothelial (arachnoid cap) cells. Most are attached to the dura but can occur in other locations (e.g., choroid plexus of the lateral ventricles). While meningiomas have many histologic subtypes (e.g., meningothelial, fibrous, psammomatous, etc.), the current WHO schema classifies them rather simply. Most meningiomas are benign and correspond to WHO grade I. Atypical meningioma, as well as the chordoid and clear cell variants, are WHO grade II tumors. Anaplastic (malignant) meningiomas correspond to WHO grade III.

Mesenchymal, nonmeningothelial tumors. Both benign and malignant mesenchymal tumors can originate in the CNS. Most correspond to tumors of soft tissue or bone. Generally, both a benign and malignant (sarcomatous) type occur. Lipomas and liposarcomas, chondromas and chondrosarcomas, osteomas and osteosarcomas are examples.

Hemangiopericytoma (HPC) is a highly cellular, vascular mesenchymal tumor that is almost always attached to the dura. HPCs are WHO II or III neoplasms. Hemangioblastoma (HGBL) is a WHO grade I neoplasm consisting of stromal cells and innumerable small blood vessels. It occurs both sporadically and as a part of von Hippel-Lindau (VHL) syndrome. Primary melanocytic neoplasms of the CNS are rare. They arise from leptomeningeal melanocytes and can be diffuse or circumscribed, benign or malignant.

Tumors of Cranial (and Spinal) Nerves

Schwannoma. Schwannomas are benign, encapsulated nerve sheath tumors that consist of well-differentiated Schwann cells. They can be solitary or multiple. Multiple schwannomas are associated with neurofibromatosis type 2 and schwannomatosis, a syndrome characterized by multiple schwannomas but lacking other features of NF2. Intracranial schwannomas are almost always associated with cranial nerves (CN8 is by far the most common) but occasionally occur as a parenchymal lesion. Schwannomas do not undergo malignant degeneration and are designated as WHO grade I neoplasms.

Neurofibroma. Neurofibromas (NFs) are diffusely infiltrating, extraneural tumors that consist of Schwann cells and fibroblasts. Solitary scalp neurofibromas occur. Multiple NFs or plexiform NFs occur as part of neurofibromatosis type 1. Neurofibromas correspond histologically to WHO grade I. Plexiform neurofibromas may degenerate into malignant peripheral nerve sheath tumors (MPNSTs). MPNSTs are graded from WHO II to IV, an approach similar to sarcoma grading.

Lymphomas and Hematopoietic Tumors

Primary CNS lymphoma. As a result of HAART therapy in HIV/AIDS patients, as well as in other immunocompromised individuals, primary CNS lymphomas (PCNSL) are dramatically increasing in prevalence. PCNSL can occur as both focal parenchymal and intravascular (IVL) tumor. PCNSL can be single or multiple and is most commonly seen in the cerebral hemispheres. More than 95% of PCNSLs are diffuse large B-cell lymphomas.

Germ Cell Tumors

Intracranial germ cell tumors (GCTs) are morphologic homologues of germinal neoplasms that arise in the gonads and extragonadal sites. 80-90% occur in adolescents. Most occur in the midline (pineal region, around the 3rd ventricle).

GCT subtypes. Germinomas are the most common intracranial GCT. Teratomas differentiate along ectodermal, endodermal, and mesodermal lines. They can be mature, immature, or occur as teratomas with malignant transformation. Other miscellaneous GCTs include the highly aggressive yolk sac tumor, embryonal carcinoma, and choriocarcinoma.

Sellar Region Tumors

Craniopharyngioma. Craniopharyngioma is a benign (WHO grade I), often partially cystic neoplasm that is the most common nonneuroepithelial intracranial neoplasm in children. It shows a distinct bimodal age distribution, with the cystic adamantinomatous type seen mostly in children and a 2nd, smaller peak in middle-aged adults. The less common papillary type is usually solid and found almost exclusively in adults.

Miscellaneous sellar region tumors. Granular cell tumor of the neurohypophysis, also called "choristoma," is a rare tumor of adults that usually arises from the infundibulum. Pituicytomas are glial neoplasms of adults that also usually arise within the infundibulum. Spindle cell oncocytoma of the adenohypophysis is an oncocytic, nonendocrine neoplasm of the adenohypophysis. All of these rare tumors are WHO grade I. The diagnosis is usually histological, as differentiating these tumors from each other and from other adult tumors, such as macroadenoma, can be problematic.

NEOPLASMS OVERVIEW

Neuroepithelial Tumors

Neoplasm	*Grade*	*Neoplasm*	*Grade*	*Neoplasm*	*Grade*
ASTROCYTIC		**CHOROID PLEXUS**		**NEURONAL, MIXED NEURONAL-GLIAL**	
Pilocytic astrocytoma	I	Choroid plexus papilloma	I	Gangliocytoma	I
Pilomyxoid astrocytoma	II	Atypical choroid plexus papilloma	II	Ganglioglioma	I
Subependymal giant cell astrocytoma	I	Choroid plexus carcinoma	III	DIG/DIA	I
Pleomorphic xanthoastrocytoma	II			DNET	I
Anaplastic astrocytoma	III	**PINEAL REGION**		Central neurocytoma	II
Glioblastoma multiforme	IV	Pineocytoma	I	Extraventricular neurocytoma	II
Gliosarcoma	IV	PPTID	II-III	Cerebellar liponeurocytoma	II
Gliomatosis cerebri	III	Pineoblastoma	IV	Paraganglioma (spinal cord)	I
		PTPR	II-III	Papillary glioneural tumor	I
OLIGODENDROGLIAL				RGNT	I
Oligodendroglioma	II	**EPENDYMAL**			
Anaplastic oligodendroglioma	III	Subependymoma	I	**OTHER NEUROEPITHELIAL**	
Oligoastrocytoma	Variable	Myxopapillary ependymoma	I	Astroblastoma	
		Ependymoma	II	Chordoid glioma of 3rd ventricle	II
EMBRYONAL		Anaplastic ependymoma	III	Angiocentric glioma (ANET)	I
Medulloblastoma	IV				
Primitive neuroectodermal tumor (PNET)	IV				
Atypical teratoid-rhabdoid tumor (AT/RT)	IV				

Meningeal Tumors

Neoplasm	*Grade*	*Neoplasm*	*Grade*	*Neoplasm*	*Grade*
MENINGOTHELIAL		**NONMENINGOTHELIAL MESENCHYMAL**		**PRIMARY MELANOCYTIC**	
Meningioma	I	Lipoma	I	Diffuse melanocytoma	
Atypical meningioma	II	Liposarcoma		Melanocytoma	
Anaplastic/malignant meningioma	III	Chondroma	I	Malignant melanoma	
		Chondrosarcoma		Meningeal melanomatosis	
OTHER RELATED		Osteoma			
Hemangioblastoma	I	Osteosarcoma			
		Osteochondroma			
		Hemangioma	I		
		Hemangiopericytoma	II-III		

Other Tumors

Neoplasm	*Grade*	*Neoplasm*	*Grade*	*Neoplasm*	*Grade*
CRANIAL & SPINAL NERVE TUMORS		**GERM CELL TUMORS**		**SELLAR REGION TUMORS**	
Schwannoma	I	Germinoma		Craniopharyngioma	I
Neurofibroma	I	Embryonal carcinoma		Adamantinomatous	
MPNST	II-IV	Yolk sac tumor		Papillary	
		Mixed germ cell tumor		Granular cell tumor of neurohypophysis	I
LYMPHOMA/HEMATOPOIETIC		Teratoma		Pituicytoma	I
Malignant lymphoma		Mature teratoma		Spindle cell oncocytoma of adenohypophysis	I
Plasmacytoma		Immature teratoma			
Leukemia/granulocytic sarcoma		Teratoma with malignant degeneration			

Tables modified, adapted to conform to 2007 World Health Organization Classification of Tumours of the Central Nervous System.

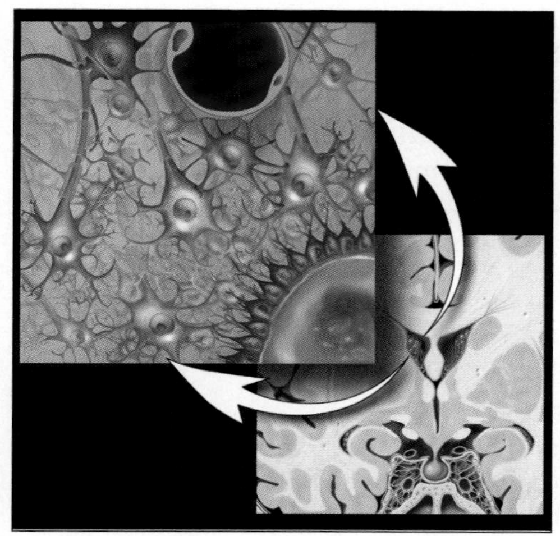

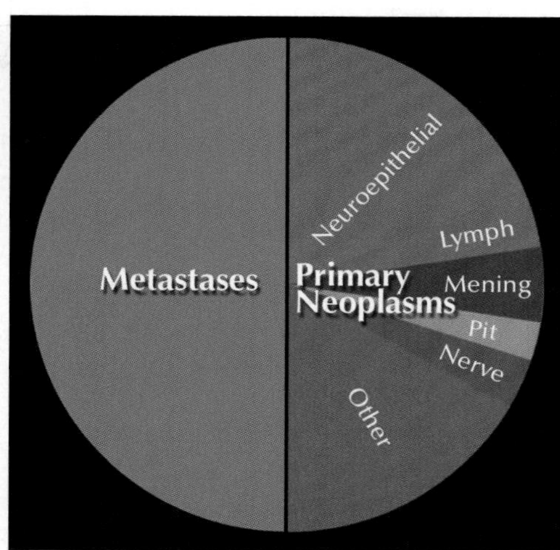

*(**Left**) Graphic depicts cellular constituents of the neuropil. Astrocytes, oligodendrocytes, neurons, microglia, choroid plexus, and ependymal cells are all represented. Any of these can give rise to primary brain neoplasms. In addition, brain tumor stem cells have been found in the subventricular zone that may be involved in tumorigenesis. (**Right**) Graphic depicts the relative prevalence of brain tumors in adults. Nearly half are metastases from systemic cancers; the other half are primary neoplasms.*

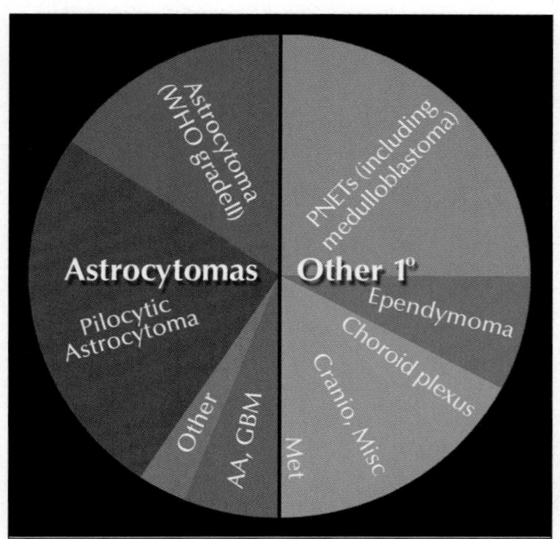

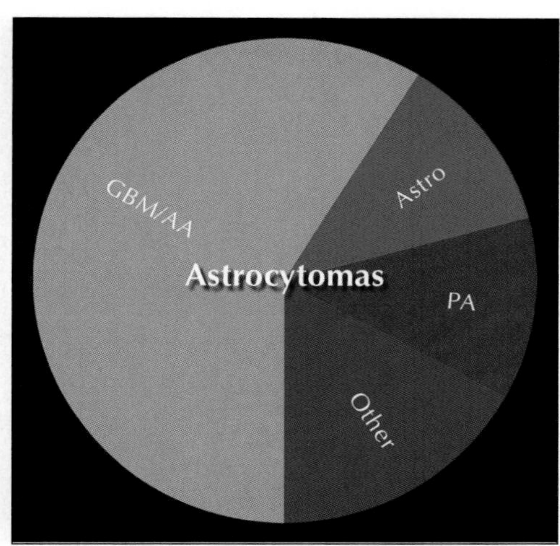

*(**Left**) Graphic depicts brain tumors in children. Metastases, AA, and GBM are rare. Pilocytic astrocytoma and PNETs are more common compared to adults. (**Right**) Overall, astrocytomas comprise the largest single group of primary brain tumors. AA (WHO grade III) and GBM (WHO grade IV) are the most common and account for over half of astrocytomas. Astrocytoma ("low grade," WHO grade II) and pilocytic astrocytoma together account for about 1/3 of all cases.*

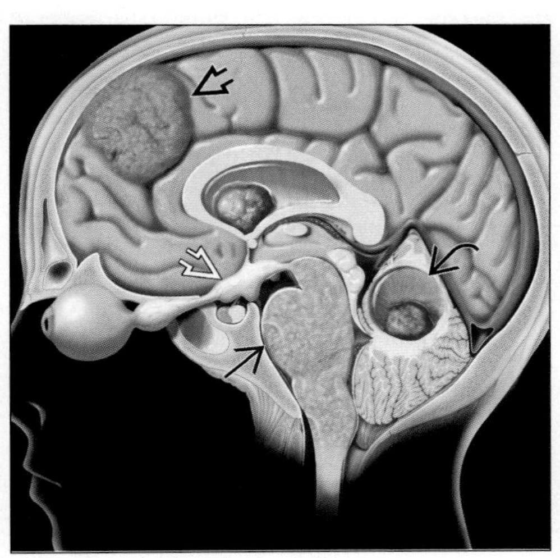

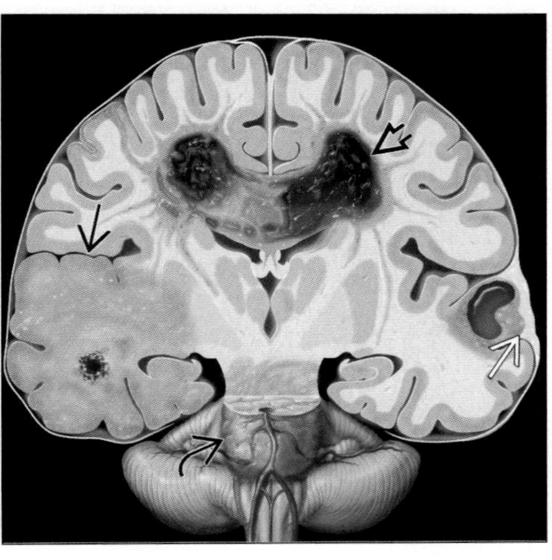

*(**Left**) Graphic depicts astrocytoma locations in children. Posterior fossa brainstem "gliomas" ➔ & pilocytic astrocytoma (PA) ➔ are common. Except for PAs around the 3rd ventricle ➔, supratentorial astrocytomas (WHO II) ➔ are less frequent. (**Right**) Astrocytomas in adults are mostly supratentorial. AA (WHO III) ➔ & GBM ➔ are common. Low-grade astrocytoma occurs in the brainstem ➔ as well as the hemispheres. PXA is a cystic tumor with nodule abutting & thickening meninges ➔.*

LOW-GRADE DIFFUSE ASTROCYTOMA

Key Facts

Terminology

- Well-differentiated but infiltrating neoplasm, slow growth pattern
- Primary brain tumor of astrocytic origin with intrinsic tendency for malignant progression, degeneration into anaplastic astrocytoma (AA)

Imaging

- Focal or diffuse nonenhancing white matter mass
- T2 homogeneously hyperintense mass
- May expand adjacent cortex
- Usually no enhancement
  - Enhancement suggests progression to higher grade
- MRS: High choline, low NAA typical but not specific
- Perfusion: Relatively lower rCBV compared to AA
- Cerebral hemispheres most common location
  - Supratentorial 2/3: Frontal and temporal lobes
- Infratentorial 1/3: Brainstem (50% of brainstem "gliomas" are low-grade astrocytoma)
- May appear circumscribed on imaging, but tumor cells are often found beyond imaged signal abnormality

Top Differential Diagnoses

- Anaplastic astrocytoma (AA)
- Oligodendroglioma
- Ischemia
- Cerebritis

Pathology

- WHO grade II

Clinical Issues

- Seizure is most common presenting feature
- Majority occur between ages of 20-45 years
- Median survival: 6-10 years

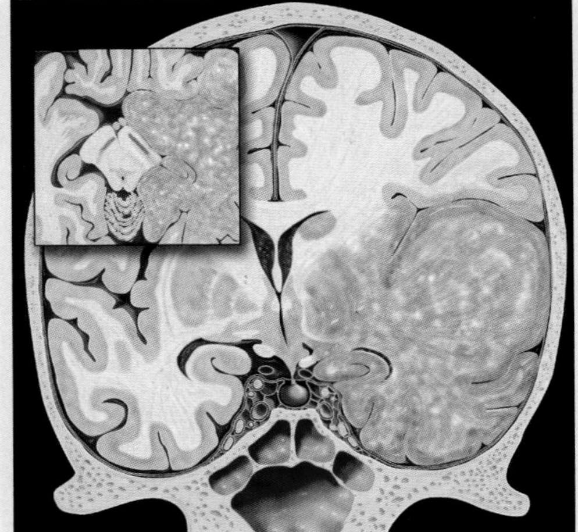

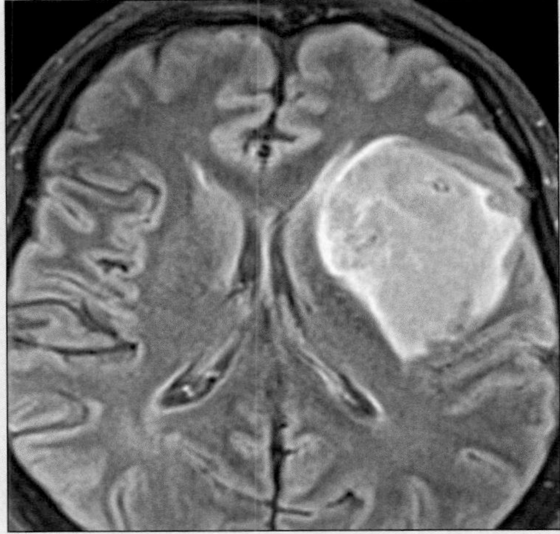

(Left) *Coronal graphic shows an infiltrative mass centered in the white matter expanding the left temporal lobe. Axial insert shows mild mass effect upon the midbrain. Low-grade astrocytomas typically affect young adults.* ***(Right)*** *Axial FLAIR MR shows a relatively homogeneous hyperintense mass with mild local mass effect. No enhancement was seen following contrast, typical of a WHO grade II diffuse astrocytoma. These infiltrative tumors may be focal or diffuse. Fibrillary astrocytoma is the most frequent histologic variant.*

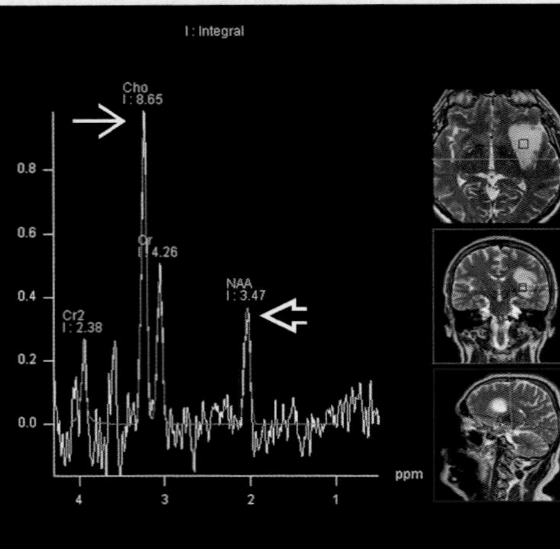

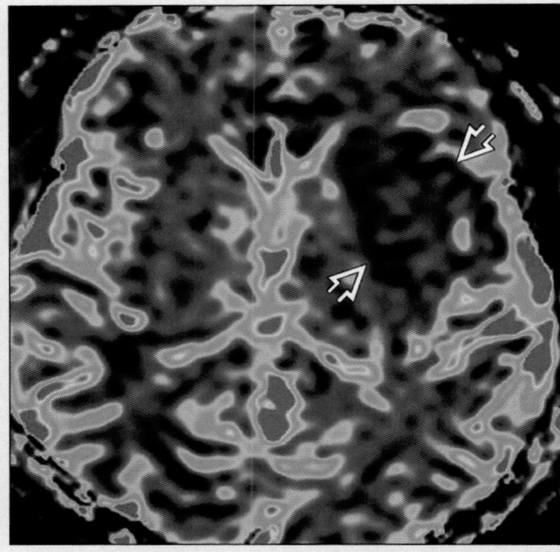

(Left) *MRS in the same patient shows a typical tumor spectrum with a high choline (Cho) peak ➔ and low NAA peak ➔. Note the lack of a lactate doublet at 1.33 ppm. Lactate is often seen in grade IV astrocytomas (GBM).* ***(Right)*** *Axial MR perfusion in the same patient shows a low rCBV ➔ in the frontotemporal mass, suggesting a low-grade tumor. Perfusion MR has been shown to be helpful in preoperative tumor grading, predicting survival, and guiding biopsy.*

LOW-GRADE DIFFUSE ASTROCYTOMA

TERMINOLOGY

Synonyms

- Diffuse astrocytoma, grade II astrocytoma, fibrillary astrocytoma, low-grade astrocytoma

Definitions

- Primary brain tumor of astrocytic origin with intrinsic tendency for malignant progression, degeneration into anaplastic astrocytoma (AA)
- Well-differentiated but infiltrating neoplasm, slow growth pattern

IMAGING

General Features

- Best diagnostic clue
  - Focal or diffuse nonenhancing white matter (WM) mass
- Location
  - Cerebral hemispheres, supratentorial 2/3
    - Frontal lobes 1/3, temporal lobes 1/3
    - Relative sparing of occipital lobes
  - Infratentorial 1/3
    - Brainstem (50% of brainstem "gliomas" are low-grade astrocytoma)
    - Occur in pons and medulla of children/adolescents
    - Cerebellum is uncommon location
  - Tumors of white matter may extend into cortex
    - 20% involve deep gray matter structures: Thalamus and basal ganglia
  - Less commonly occur in spinal cord
- Size
  - Variable
- Morphology
  - Homogeneous mass with enlargement and distortion of affected structures
  - May appear circumscribed on imaging, but tumor cells are often found beyond imaged signal abnormality

CT Findings

- NECT
  - Ill-defined homogeneous hypodense/isodense mass
  - 20% Ca++; cysts are rare
  - Calvarial erosion in cortical masses (rare)
- CECT
  - No enhancement or very minimal
    - Enhancement should raise suspicion of focal malignant degeneration

MR Findings

- T1WI
  - Homogeneous hypointense mass
  - May expand white matter and adjacent cortex
  - Appears circumscribed, but infiltrates adjacent brain
  - Ca++ and cysts (uncommon)
  - Hemorrhage or surrounding edema (rare)
- T2WI
  - Homogeneous hyperintense mass
  - May appear circumscribed, but often infiltrates adjacent brain
  - Ca++ and cysts less common
  - Hemorrhage or surrounding edema are rare
  - May expand adjacent cortex
- FLAIR
  - Homogeneous hyperintense mass
- DWI
  - Typically no diffusion restriction
- T1WI C+
  - Usually no enhancement
  - Enhancement suggests progression to higher grade
- MRS
  - High choline, low NAA typical but not specific
  - High mI/Cr ratio (0.82 ± 0.25)
  - May delineate tumor extent better than conventional MR
- MR perfusion
  - Relatively lower rCBV compared to AA, GBM
  - Lower permeability values than high-grade tumors
  - Increase in rCBV helps predict time to progression

Nuclear Medicine Findings

- PET
  - Low-grade astrocytomas have FDG uptake similar to normal white matter
  - FDG uptake within astrocytoma has good correlation with histologic grade of tumor
  - FDG, 18F-choline, and 11C-choline PET useful for biopsy (most hypermetabolic area)

Imaging Recommendations

- Best imaging tool
  - Newer techniques such as diffusion tensor imaging (DTI) coming into use
- Protocol advice
  - Contrast-enhanced MR
  - MRS and perfusion imaging may be helpful

DIFFERENTIAL DIAGNOSIS

Anaplastic Astrocytoma (AA)

- Hemispheric WM lesion, usually nonenhancing
- Focal or diffuse mass
- May be indistinguishable without biopsy

Oligodendroglioma

- Cortically based mass with variable enhancement
- Ca++ common
- May be indistinguishable

Ischemia

- Vascular territory (MCA, ACA, PCA), acute onset
- Diffusion restriction (acute/early subacute)
- Often wedge-shaped, involves GM and WM

Cerebritis

- Edema, patchy enhancement characteristic
- Usually shows restricted diffusion
- Typically more acute onset

Herpes Encephalitis

- Confined to limbic system, temporal lobes
- Hemorrhage and enhancement common
- Acute onset

LOW-GRADE DIFFUSE ASTROCYTOMA

Status Epilepticus
- Active seizures may cause signal abnormalities and enhancement
- Clinical history of seizures

PATHOLOGY

General Features
- Etiology
  - Arise from differentiated astrocytes or astrocytic precursor cells
  - Astrocytic neoplasm characterized by high degree of cellular differentiation, slow growth, diffuse infiltration of adjacent structures
- Genetics
  - *TP53* mutation > 60%
  - Overexpression of platelet-derived growth factor receptor-α (*PDGFRA*)
  - Chromosomal abnormalities: Gain of 7q; 8q amplification; LOH 10p, 22q; chromosome 6 deletions
- Associated abnormalities
  - Associated with Li-Fraumeni syndrome and inherited multiple enchondromatosis type 1 (Ollier disease)
  - If oligodendroglioma components, oligoastrocytoma

Staging, Grading, & Classification
- WHO grade II

Gross Pathologic & Surgical Features
- Enlargement and distortion of invaded structures
- Diffusely infiltrating mass with blurring of GM/WM interface
- May appear grossly circumscribed but diffusely infiltrates adjacent brain
- Occasional cysts, Ca++

Microscopic Features
- Well-differentiated fibrillary or gemistocytic neoplastic astrocytes
- Background of loosely structured, often microcystic tumor matrix
- Moderately increased cellularity
- Occasional nuclear atypia
- Mitotic activity generally absent or very rare
- No microvascular proliferation or necrosis
- Histologic variants
  - Fibrillary (most frequent)
  - Gemistocytic (most likely to progress to AA, GBM)
  - Protoplasmic (rare)
- MIB-1 (proliferation index) is low (< 4%)
- Immunohistochemistry: GFAP(+)

CLINICAL ISSUES

Presentation
- Most common signs/symptoms
  - Seizures, increased intracranial pressure
  - Other signs/symptoms: Varies with tumor location
    - Seizure, focal neurologic deficit, behavior changes

Demographics
- Age
  - Majority occur between 20-45 years
  - Occur at all ages, mean: 34 years
- Gender
  - Slight male predominance
- Epidemiology
  - Represents 25-30% of gliomas in adults
  - 10-15% of all astrocytomas
  - 2nd most common astrocytoma of childhood (pilocytic is 1st)
  - Approximately 1.4 new cases per 1,000,000/year

Natural History & Prognosis
- Patients rarely succumb to spread of low-grade tumor
- Median survival: 6-10 years
- Inherent tendency for malignant progression to AA and GBM = major cause of mortality
- Recurrent disease associated with malignant degeneration in 50-75% of cases
- Malignant progression tends to occur following mean interval of 4-5 years
- Increased survival: Young age, gross total resection
- Radiation therapy in patients with subtotal resection improves survival
- Prognosis worse for pontine, better for medullary tumors (especially dorsally exophytic)

Treatment
- Surgical resection is primary treatment
- Usually adjuvant chemotherapy and XRT at time of recurrence or progression

DIAGNOSTIC CHECKLIST

Consider
- Low-grade astrocytoma may be indistinguishable from other tumors including AA and oligodendroglioma
- Acute/subacute ischemia may mimic diffuse astrocytoma; DWI, history, and follow-up MR helpful

Image Interpretation Pearls
- Think low-grade astrocytoma if T2 hyperintense expansile mass largely confined to WM

SELECTED REFERENCES

1. Bisdas S et al: Cerebral blood volume measurements by perfusion-weighted MR imaging in gliomas: ready for prime time in predicting short-term outcome and recurrent disease? AJNR Am J Neuroradiol. 30(4):681-8, 2009
2. Cha S: Neuroimaging in neuro-oncology. Neurotherapeutics. 6(3):465-77, 2009
3. Law M et al: Gliomas: predicting time to progression or survival with cerebral blood volume measurements at dynamic susceptibility-weighted contrast-enhanced perfusion MR imaging. Radiology. 247(2):490-8, 2008
4. Chawla S et al: Arterial spin-labeling and MR spectroscopy in the differentiation of gliomas. AJNR Am J Neuroradiol. 28(9):1683-9, 2007
5. Louis DN et al (eds): WHO Classification of Tumours of the Central Nervous System: Diffuse Astrocytoma. Lyon: IARC Press. 25-9, 2007

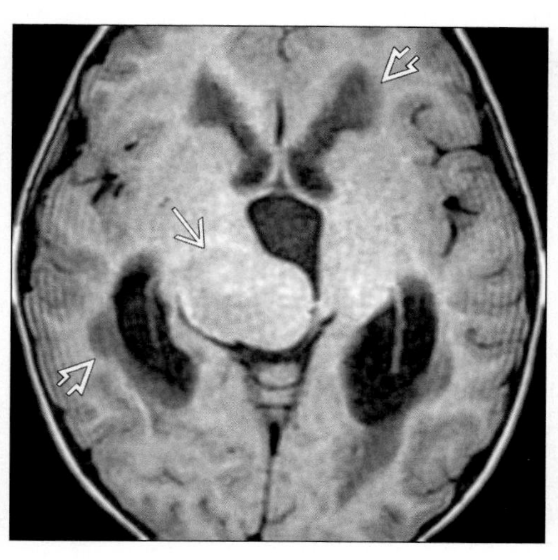

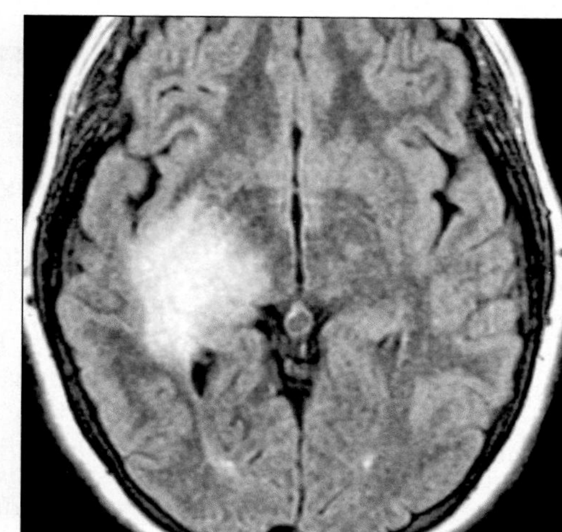

(Left) *Axial T1WI MR shows a large isointense right thalamic mass ➔ with associated severe hydrocephalus. Note the transependymal flow of CSF ➲ seen as a "halo" surrounding the ventricles. Biopsy revealed a diffusely infiltrating fibrillary astrocytoma. Hydrocephalus is a rare complication of diffuse astrocytoma.* ***(Right)*** *Axial FLAIR MR shows a hyperintense infiltrative right temporal mass extending medially into the basal ganglia and thalamus in this patient with WHO grade II fibrillary astrocytoma.*

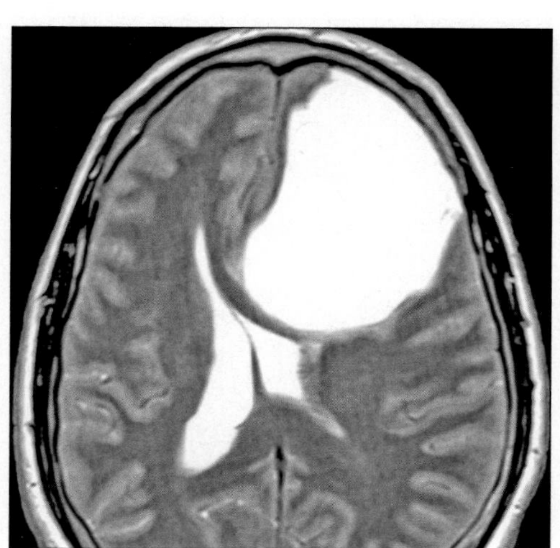

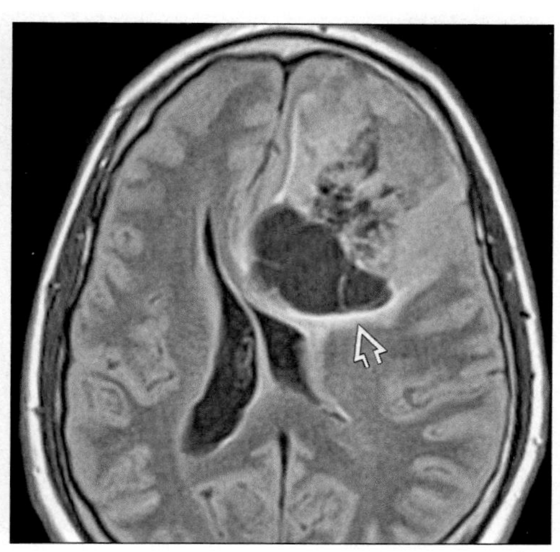

(Left) *Axial T2WI MR shows a large, hyperintense frontal lobe mass with significant mass effect in this young man with seizures. Protoplasmic astrocytoma, WHO grade II was found at resection.* ***(Right)*** *Axial FLAIR MR in the same patient shows the mass to be heterogeneous with minimal surrounding vasogenic edema ➲. Protoplasmic astrocytoma is a rare variant of diffuse astrocytoma. Mucoid degeneration and microcyst formation are common. The frontotemporal region is a classic location.*

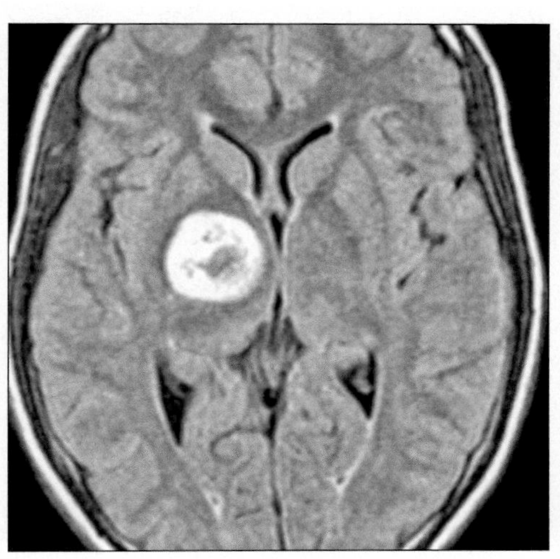

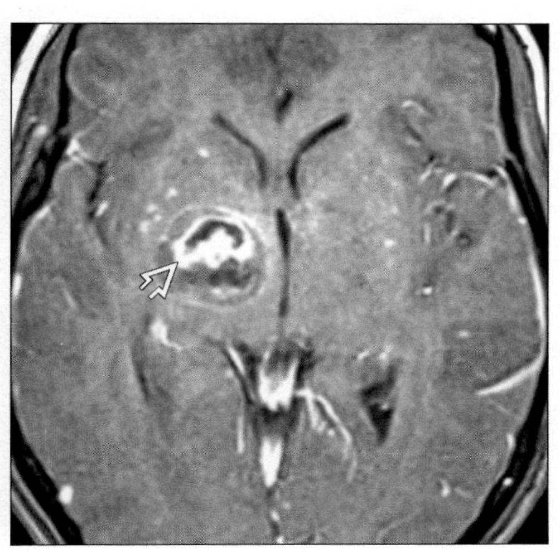

(Left) *Axial FLAIR shows a heterogeneously hyperintense basal ganglia and thalamic mass with discrete margins and a distinct lack of surrounding edema. 20% of low-grade astrocytomas involve the deep gray matter structures.* ***(Right)*** *Axial T1WI C+ MR in the same patient shows heterogeneous enhancement of the mass ➲, atypical for low-grade astrocytoma. Imaging mimics a pilocytic astrocytoma or a higher grade astrocytoma in this young adult. Low-grade, diffuse astrocytoma was found at resection.*

PEDIATRIC BRAINSTEM TUMORS

Key Facts

Imaging

- Brainstem gliomas can be categorized into 2 groups
  - Diffuse pontine gliomas (DPG): Infiltrative fibrillary lesions with poor prognosis
  - Focal gliomas involving mesencephalon, tectum, and lower brainstem, mostly pilocytic with good prognosis
- Borders/margins predictive of prognosis
  - Infiltrative: Symptoms < 6 months; poor prognosis
  - Focal: Long clinical prodrome; good prognosis
- All are variably T2 hyperintense
- Pilocytic: Heterogeneous to intense enhancement
- Diffuse fibrillary does not typically enhance
- DPG: T2 hyperintense mass, typically "engulfs" basilar artery
- Focal gliomas have well-circumscribed borders without significant peritumoral T2 hyperintensity

Top Differential Diagnoses

- Brainstem encephalitis
- ADEM
- Neurofibromatosis type 1
- Osmotic demyelination syndrome
- Pineal region mass

Pathology

- DPG children: Better prognosis with NF1
- DPG adults: Worse prognosis with NF1 than without
- 30-70% DPG: Mutations *p53* (tumor suppressor gene)

Clinical Issues

- Multiple cranial nerve palsies common in diffuse pontine glioma
- Short onset of symptoms prior to diagnosis suggestive of DPG and poor outcome
- Tectal gliomas are distinct, rarely progressive

(Left) Sagittal graphic shows diffuse brainstem enlargement by a diffuse pontine glioma (DPG), the most common pediatric brainstem tumor. Note the characteristic flattening of the pontomedullary junction ➔ and engulfment of the basilar artery by the tumor ➔ (axial insert). (Right) Sagittal T2WI MR demonstrates marked expansion and hyperintensity of the pons by a DPG. Note the marked compression of the 4th ventricle ➔ with a surprising lack of hydrocephalus, which is typical of DPG.

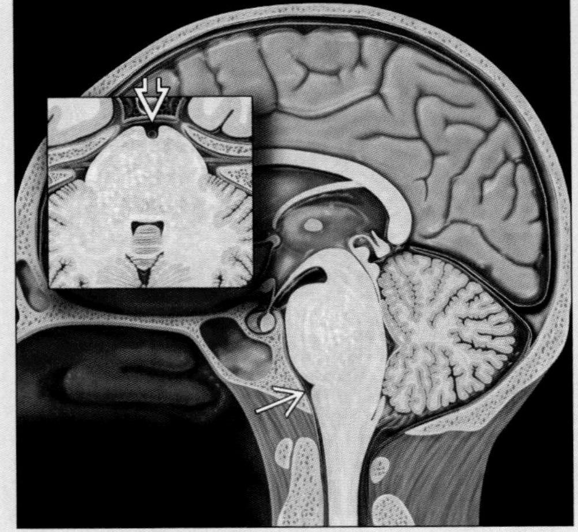

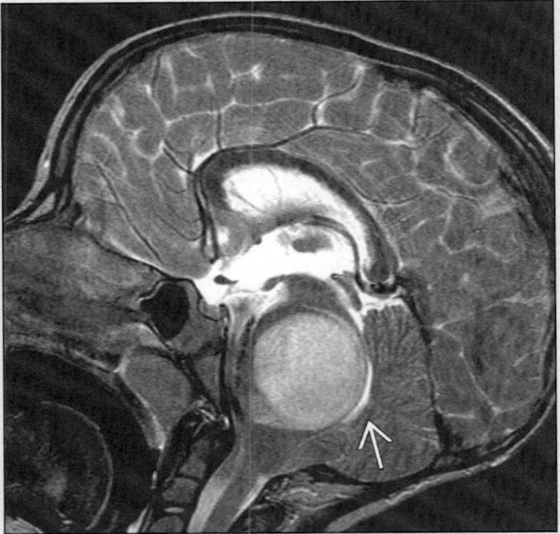

(Left) Axial T2WI MR in the same patient shows marked expansion and hyperintensity of the pons. Note the tumor "wrapping" around the basilar artery ➔, typical of DPGs. DPGs are usually fibrillary and have a poor outcome despite therapy. (Right) Sagittal T1WI C+ MR in the same patient shows no significant enhancement, typical of diffuse pontine glioma. Enhancement and necrosis may occur with higher grade tumors and suggest a worse prognosis. Enhancement may also be seen after therapy.

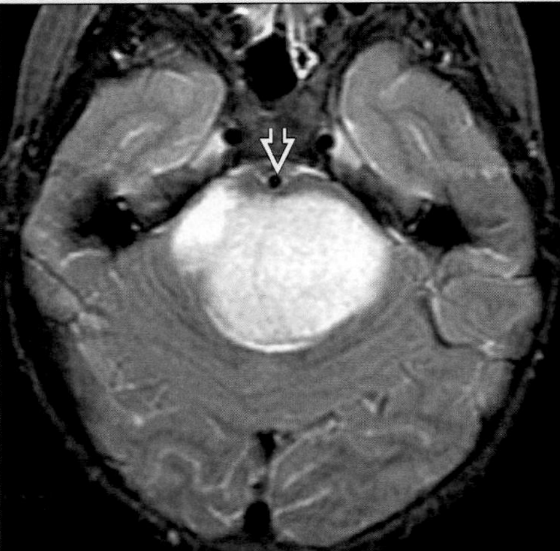

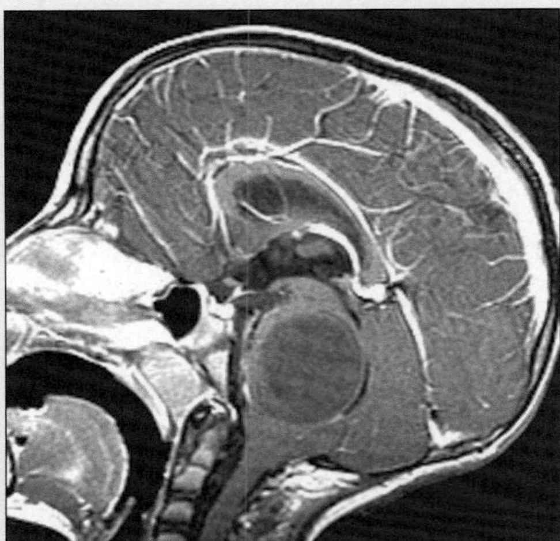

PEDIATRIC BRAINSTEM TUMORS

TERMINOLOGY

Abbreviations

- Brainstem glioma (BSG)
  - Tectal glioma (tectal)
  - Focal tegmental mesencephalic (FTM)
  - Diffuse (intrinsic) pontine glioma (DPG)
  - Pilocytic astrocytoma (PA)
  - Fibrillary astrocytoma (FA)

Definitions

- Heterogeneous group of focal or diffuse gliomas involving mesencephalon, pons, or medulla
- Brainstem gliomas can be categorized into 2 groups
  - Diffuse pontine gliomas: Infiltrative fibrillary lesions with poor prognosis
  - Focal gliomas involving mesencephalon, tectum, and lower brainstem, mostly of pilocytic variety with good prognosis

IMAGING

General Features

- Best diagnostic clue
  - Classic imaging varies with tumor type and location
    - Tectal: T2 hyperintense; variable enhancement
    - FTM: Cyst + mural nodule
    - DPG: T2 hyperintense, expansile mass
- Location
  - All BSGs are not equal! Geography and glioma grading predict prognosis
    - Tectal: Indolent course, most only need CSF diversion
    - FTM: Surgery, radiation, or chemo; do well
    - DPG: Most are infiltrative ⇒ poor survival despite chemotherapy, XRT
    - Focal exophytic (pedunculated) gliomas of medulla-craniocervical junction = better prognosis
- Size
  - Tectal: Even small tectal gliomas will obstruct aqueduct, cause early hydrocephalus
  - DPG: Often large when present, hydrocephalus occurs late
- Morphology
  - Focal or diffusely infiltrative
  - Borders/margins predictive of prognosis
    - Focal: Long clinical prodrome; good prognosis
    - Infiltrative: Symptoms < 6 months; poor prognosis

CT Findings

- NECT
  - Tectal: Hazy increased density over time, ± Ca++; hydrocephalus common
  - FTM and focal brainstem gliomas: Low-attenuation cyst with mural nodule
  - DPG: Decreased density, Ca++ rare, hydrocephalus only 10% at presentation
- CECT
  - Tectal: Variable enhancement
  - FTM and focal brainstem gliomas: Cyst plus brightly enhancing variable-sized nodule, clean margins
  - DPG: Enhancement is uncommon but heterogeneous
    - Increased enhancement/necrosis over time suggests increasing grade or treatment
    - Worse prognosis if enhancement at initial diagnosis

MR Findings

- T1WI
  - Tectal: Iso- to hypointense, may demonstrate T1 hyperintensity with progressive faint calcification
  - FTM and DPG: Hypointense
- T2WI
  - All are variably hyperintense
  - Focal brainstem gliomas have well-circumscribed borders without significant peritumoral T2 hyperintensity
  - Tectal: Hyperintense, expands tectum, causes hydrocephalus early
  - DPG: High signal T2, expands pons, obstructs but does not invade 4th ventricle, engulfs basilar artery, infiltrative without circumscribed borders
- FLAIR: Typically hyperintense
- DWI: No diffusion restriction
- T1WI C+: Variable enhancement
  - Diffuse fibrillary does not typically enhance
  - Pilocytic varieties demonstrate heterogeneous to intense enhancement
- MRS: Pilocytic astrocytomas have ↑ lactate & choline, MRS signature > aggressive than its biological activity
  - NAA preservation may indicate ↓ aggressive course
  - NAA levels higher in DPG with NF1 than without
    - Pediatric NF1 associated with less malignant course

Imaging Recommendations

- Best imaging tool
  - MR with contrast
- Protocol advice
  - Include thin sagittal T2 for tectal, DPG

DIFFERENTIAL DIAGNOSIS

Brainstem Encephalitis

- More acute clinical course; febrile
- *Listeria monocytogenes* often involved
- May be viral: West Nile virus, adenovirus, EBV, herpes

ADEM

- Onset after viral prodrome or vaccination typical
- T2/FLAIR hyperintensities in gray and white matter
  - Supratentorial brain typically involved

Neurofibromatosis Type 1

- Foci areas of signal abnormality (FASI) on T2
  - Typically involve basal ganglia (globus pallidus), brainstem, cerebellum
  - Increase in early childhood and diminish in early adolescence
- May see low-grade BSG associated with NF1

Osmotic Demyelination Syndrome

- Expansile edema of central pons or midbrain, may show restricted diffusion

PEDIATRIC BRAINSTEM TUMORS

- Clinical setting of rapidly corrected hyponatremia

Pineal Region Mass

- Pineoblastoma: Heterogeneous enhancement
- Germinoma
  - Enhancing pineal mass, may infiltrate tectal plate

Langerhans Cell Histiocytosis, Brain

- Often multifocal sites of disease
- May cause T2 hyperintensities of pons and cerebellum

PATHOLOGY

General Features

- Genetics
  - Fibrillary astrocytoma
    - Mutations *p53* (tumor suppressor gene) 30-70%
    - Inactivation *p53* ⇒ Poor outcome with progression to higher grade
    - Loss of heterozygosity chromosomes 10, 17p
  - Tectal and DPG associated with NF1
    - Tectal: Better prognosis with NF1
    - DPG children: Better prognosis with NF1 than without NF1
    - DPG adults: Worse prognosis with NF1 than without NF1
- Associated abnormalities
  - No metastases outside CNS
  - Pilocytic tumors may have leptomeningeal and spinal drop metastases

Staging, Grading, & Classification

- Pilocytic: WHO I
- Fibrillary: WHO II with potential of progression to higher grade (III-IV)

Gross Pathologic & Surgical Features

- Tectal: Grayish, ill-defined mass, same consistency as gliotic white matter
  - Obstructs aqueduct of Sylvius
- FTM: Involves cerebral peduncle between thalamus and upper pons
- DPG: "Hypertrophied," swollen pons
  - Diffuse tumor infiltration ventral pons
  - Caudal/cranial extent along fiber tracts

Microscopic Features

- Pilocytic: Alternating spongy, compact cellular areas
  - Spongy areas: Astrocytes outline microcysts
  - Compact regions: Bipolar cells with Rosenthal fibers
- Fibrillary astrocytoma: ↑ cellularity/mitotic activity
  - Pleomorphism/nuclear atypia
  - ± necrosis, endothelial proliferation

CLINICAL ISSUES

Presentation

- Most common signs/symptoms
  - Tectal: Macrocrania; headache
  - FTM: Hemiparesis
  - DPG: Cranial neuropathies, nausea/vomiting, headache, ataxia

Demographics

- Epidemiology
  - 10% of primary pediatric brain tumors
  - Only 2% of adult gliomas are brainstem tumors
- Age: 3-10 years, mean age 7 years
- Gender: M = F

Natural History & Prognosis

- Focal types: Favorable prognosis with treatment of hydrocephalus
  - If surgical resection possible, may be curative
- DPG: Poor prognosis, CSF dissemination with high-grade progression; caudal/cranial extension
  - Dissemination occurs in 50% prior to death
- Better prognosis in NF1 and dorsally exophytic PA

Treatment

- Focal types
  - Treat hydrocephalus with shunting
  - Surgical resection ± chemotherapy
- DPG: Experimental chemotherapy; XRT
  - Child: Poor, median survival < 1 year despite therapy
  - Adult: Better, median survival 7 years

DIAGNOSTIC CHECKLIST

Consider

- Not all expansile brainstem lesions are neoplasms
- If acute onset of symptoms, consider abscess or demyelination

Image Interpretation Pearls

- Location, location, location!
- Geography and glioma grade predicts prognosis

SELECTED REFERENCES

1. Frazier JL et al: Treatment of diffuse intrinsic brainstem gliomas: failed approaches and future strategies. J Neurosurg Pediatr. 3(4):259-69, 2009
2. Thomale UW et al: Neurological grading, survival, MR imaging, and histological evaluation in the rat brainstem glioma model. Childs Nerv Syst. 25(4):433-41, 2009
3. Ueoka DI et al: Brainstem gliomas--retrospective analysis of 86 patients. J Neurol Sci. 281(1-2):20-3, 2009
4. Massimino M et al: Diffuse pontine gliomas in children: changing strategies, changing results? A mono-institutional 20-year experience. J Neurooncol. 87(3):355-61, 2008
5. Teo C et al: Radical resection of focal brainstem gliomas: is it worth doing? Childs Nerv Syst. 24(11):1307-14, 2008
6. Porto L et al: Proton magnetic resonance spectroscopy in childhood brainstem lesions. Childs Nerv Syst. 23(3):305-14, 2007
7. Recinos PF et al: Brainstem tumors: where are we today? Pediatr Neurosurg. 43(3):192-201, 2007
8. Donaldson SS et al: Advances toward an understanding of brainstem gliomas. J Clin Oncol. 24(8):1266-72, 2006
9. Hargrave D et al: Diffuse brainstem glioma in children: critical review of clinical trials. Lancet Oncol. 7(3):241-8, 2006
10. Fisher PG et al: A clinicopathologic reappraisal of brain stem tumor classification. Identification of pilocystic astrocytoma and fibrillary astrocytoma as distinct entities. Cancer. 89(7):1569-76, 2000

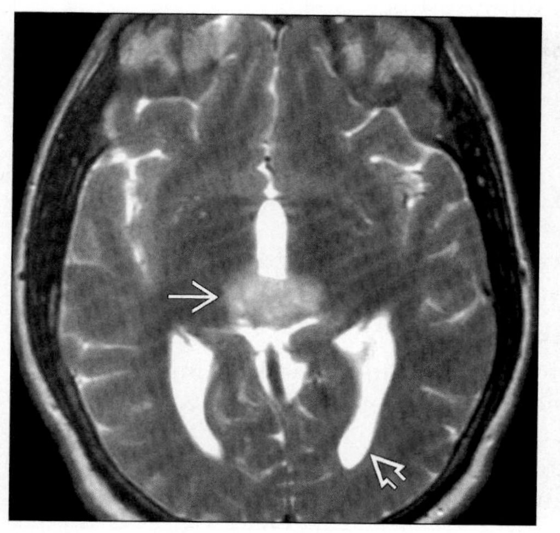

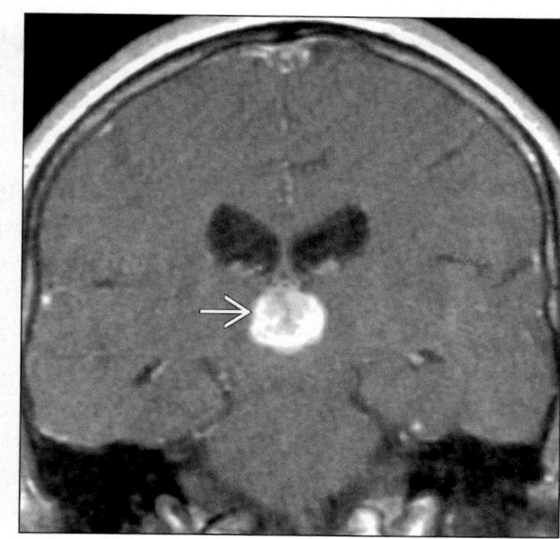

(Left) *Axial T2WI MR shows a focal hyperintense expansile mass ➔ involving the mesencephalon, including the tectum, with extension to the posterior thalami. There is obstruction of the cerebral aqueduct with mild enlargement of the 3rd and lateral ventricles ➔.* ***(Right)*** *Coronal T1WI C+ MR in the same patient shows intense, heterogeneous enhancement of this mesencephalic glioma ➔. Imaging is typical of a pilocytic histology with an indolent course and good prognosis.*

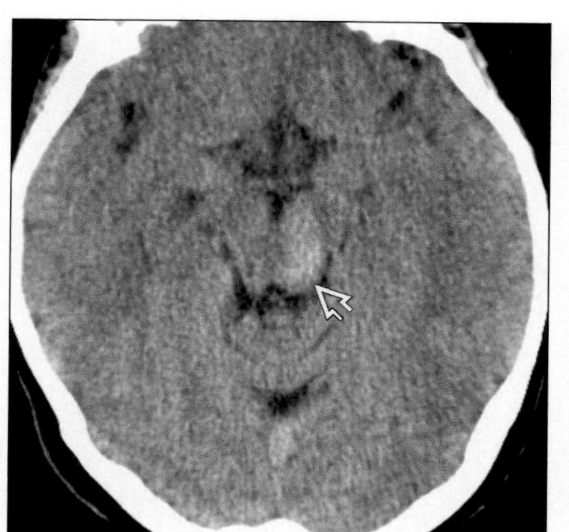

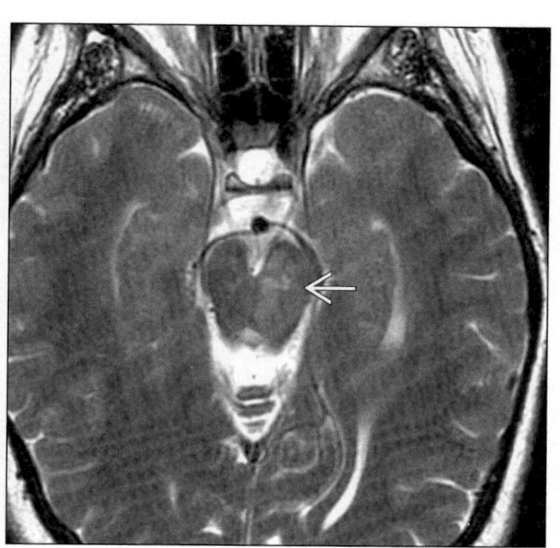

(Left) *Axial CT demonstrates a focal tegmental mesencephalic glioma involving the left midbrain and cerebral peduncle ➔. Note the slight hyperdensity that represents faint calcification.* ***(Right)*** *Axial T2WI MR in the same patient shows a hyperintense, mildly expansile mass of the left midbrain and tectum ➔. These tumors often obstruct the aqueduct early and present with signs and symptoms of hydrocephalus. These tumors often require CSF diversion but have a good prognosis.*

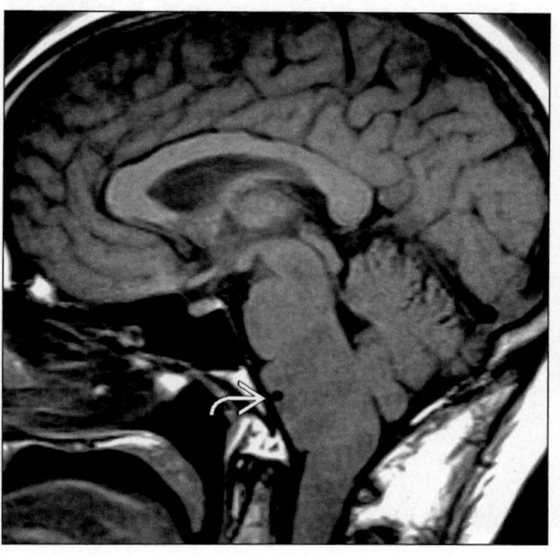

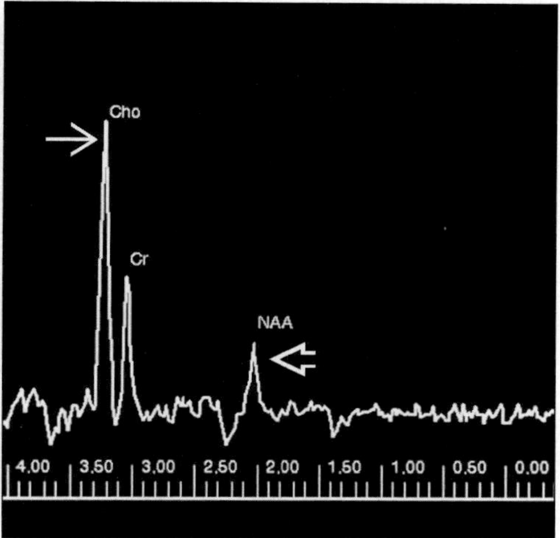

(Left) *Sagittal T1WI MR shows a diffuse brainstem glioma, centered in the medulla. Note expansion of the brainstem by the tumor, resulting in the basilar artery ➔ being engulfed by tumor. These WHO grade II tumors typically do not enhance. Enhancement in this location at presentation implies a worse prognosis.* ***(Right)*** *MRS in the same patient shows a typical tumor spectrum with elevation of choline ➔ and decreased NAA ➔. This tumor spectrum implies a more aggressive tumor.*

ANAPLASTIC ASTROCYTOMA

Key Facts

Terminology
- Diffusely infiltrating malignant astrocytoma with anaplasia and marked proliferative potential

Imaging
- Infiltrating mass that predominately involves white matter with variable enhancement
- T2 heterogeneously hyperintense
- Neoplastic cells almost always found beyond areas of abnormal signal intensity
- May involve and expand overlying cortex
- Usually no enhancement
  - Focal, nodular, homogeneous, patchy enhancement less common
  - Ring enhancement is suspicious for GBM
- Elevated Cho:Cr ratio, decreased NAA
- Elevated maximum rCBV

Top Differential Diagnoses
- Low-grade diffuse astrocytoma
- Glioblastoma multiforme (GBM)
- Oligodendroglioma
- Cerebritis
- Ischemia

Pathology
- WHO grade III
- Usually evolves from low-grade (diffuse) astrocytoma (WHO grade II) (75%)

Clinical Issues
- Most common presentation: Marked clinical deterioration in patient with grade II astrocytoma
- Occurs at all ages, most common 40-50 years
- 1/3 of astrocytomas
- Median survival: 2-3 years

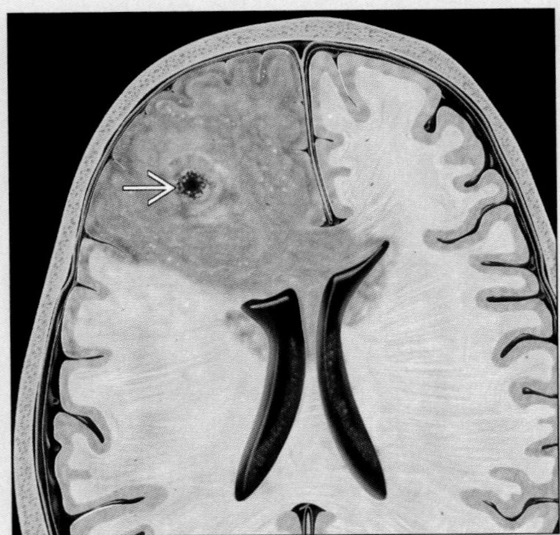

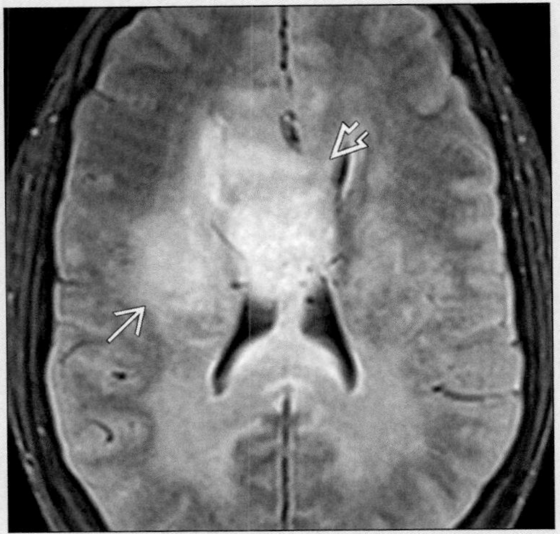

(Left) *Axial graphic shows an infiltrative white matter mass with extension along the corpus callosum, focal hemorrhage →, and local mass effect. White matter extension is typical of anaplastic astrocytoma.* ***(Right)*** *Axial FLAIR MR shows a diffusely infiltrative white matter mass → with extensive involvement of the corpus callosum ⇨, typical of anaplastic astrocytoma. Anaplastic astrocytomas often involve adjacent structures without frank destruction and have a marked tendency to progress to GBM.*

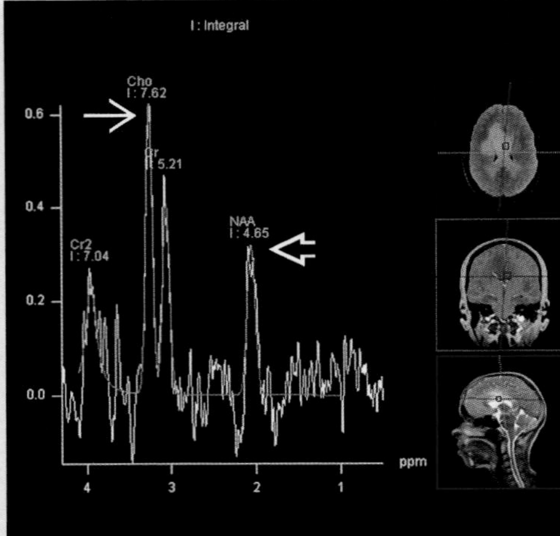

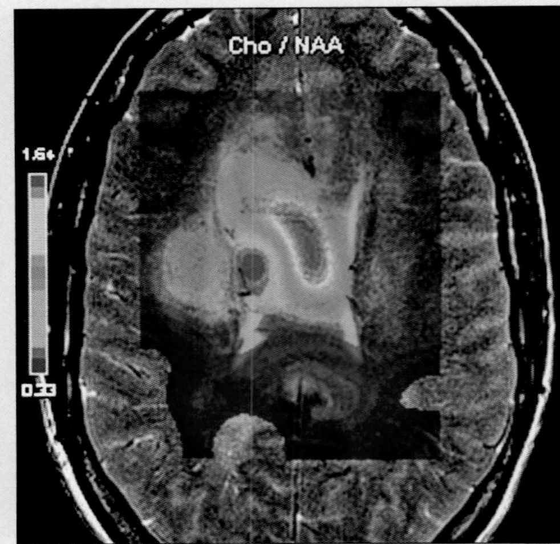

(Left) *MRS from the same patient shows a high choline peak → and a low NAA peak ⇨, characteristic of a malignant glioma.* ***(Right)*** *MRS choline map from the same patient shows the elevated Cho/NAA ratio in striking color. MRS color maps can help guide a biopsy in a patient who is unable to have a complete resection. Correlating a biopsy with MRS or MR perfusion has been shown to improve the diagnostic accuracy of the biopsy by decreasing sampling error.*

ANAPLASTIC ASTROCYTOMA

TERMINOLOGY

Abbreviations
- Anaplastic astrocytoma (AA)

Synonyms
- Grade III astrocytoma, malignant astrocytoma, high-grade astrocytoma

Definitions
- Diffusely infiltrating malignant astrocytoma with focal or diffuse anaplasia and marked proliferative potential

IMAGING

General Features
- Best diagnostic clue
  - Infiltrating mass that predominately involves white matter (WM) with variable enhancement
- Location
  - Hemispheric WM
    - Commonly involves frontal and temporal lobes
  - In children, may involve pons, thalamus
  - Less commonly involves brainstem, spinal cord
- Size
  - Variable
- Morphology
  - Ill-defined hemispheric WM mass typical
  - May appear well circumscribed
  - Neoplastic cells almost always found beyond areas of abnormal signal intensity

CT Findings
- NECT
  - Low-density ill-defined mass
  - Ca++ and hemorrhage rare
- CECT
  - Majority do not enhance
  - Enhancement often focal, patchy, heterogeneous
  - If ring enhancement, consider malignant progression to glioblastoma multiforme (GBM)

MR Findings
- T1WI
  - Mixed isointense to hypointense WM mass
  - May involve and expand overlying cortex
  - Ca++, hemorrhage, cysts rare
- T2WI
  - Heterogeneously hyperintense
  - May appear discrete, but infiltrates adjacent brain
  - May involve and expand overlying cortex
  - Rarely prominent flow voids are present, suggesting progression to GBM
- FLAIR
  - Heterogeneously hyperintense
- DWI
  - No diffusion restriction is typical
- T1WI C+
  - Usually no enhancement
  - Less common: Focal, nodular, homogeneous, patchy enhancement
  - Ring enhancement is suspicious for GBM
- MRS
  - Elevated Cho/Cr ratio, decreased NAA
  - Lower myoinositol (mI)/Cr ratio (0.33 ± 0.16) than low-grade (diffuse) astrocytoma
- Dynamic contrast-enhanced T2-weighted imaging
  - Elevated maximum rCBV compared to low-grade astrocytoma
  - Increased permeability compared to low-grade astrocytoma
- Diffusion tensor imaging (DTI) of white matter tracts may help surgical planning

Nuclear Medicine Findings
- PET
  - Higher metabolism than low-grade astrocytomas
  - FDG shows high-grade gliomas have uptake similar to or exceeding normal gray matter
  - Tumor:WM > 1.5 and tumor:GM > 0.6 suggest high-grade tumors
  - FDG has sensitivity of 81-86%, specificity of 50-94% in differentiation of recurrent tumor from radiation brain injury

Imaging Recommendations
- Protocol advice
  - Contrast-enhanced MR
  - MRS, MR perfusion, and DTI may be helpful

DIFFERENTIAL DIAGNOSIS

Low-Grade Diffuse Astrocytoma
- Focal or diffuse white matter mass
- Typically nonenhancing hemispheric mass
- May be indistinguishable without biopsy

Glioblastoma Multiforme (GBM)
- 95% necrotic core, enhancing rim
- Extensive surrounding T2/FLAIR signal
- Hemorrhage not uncommon

Cerebritis
- T2 hyperintensity and patchy enhancement
- Diffusion restriction typical

Ischemia
- Vascular territory (MCA, ACA, PCA)
- Restricted diffusion if acute/subacute
- Often wedge-shaped, involves GM and WM
- Gyriform enhancement in subacute ischemia

Oligodendroglioma
- Cortical mass with variable enhancement
- Ca++ common
- May be indistinguishable

Status Epilepticus
- Active seizures may cause signal abnormalities and enhancement
- History of seizures
- Follow-up imaging may be necessary

Herpes Encephalitis
- Confined to limbic system, temporal lobes
- Blood products and enhancement common

ANAPLASTIC ASTROCYTOMA

- Typically acute onset

PATHOLOGY

General Features

- Etiology
  - Derived from precursor cells committed to astrocytic differentiation
  - Usually evolves from low-grade (diffuse) astrocytoma (WHO grade II) (approximately 75%)
    - Progression from low-grade (diffuse) astrocytoma to AA is associated with multiple genetic alterations
  - Occasionally arises de novo
- Genetics
  - High frequency of *TP53* mutations (> 70%) and LOH 17p (50-60%)
  - Abnormal cell cycle regulatory genes
  - Loss of heterozygosity: Chromosome 10q, 19q, 22q
  - Deletion of chromosome 6q (30%)
- Biologically aggressive astrocytoma characterized by cytologic atypia and mitotic activity
  - Intrinsic tendency for progression to GBM

Staging, Grading, & Classification

- WHO grade III
- Intermediate between low-grade (diffuse) astrocytoma (WHO grade II) and GBM (grade IV)

Gross Pathologic & Surgical Features

- Infiltrating mass with poorly delineated margins
- Often expands invaded structures without frank destruction
- May appear discrete but tumor always infiltrates adjacent brain
- Cysts, hemorrhage uncommon

Microscopic Features

- Characterized by increased cellularity, marked mitotic activity, distinct nuclear atypia
- High nuclear/cytoplasmic ratio
- Nuclear/cytoplasmic pleomorphism
- No necrosis or microvascular proliferation (presence = grade IV)
- Immunohistochemistry: GFAP(+) common
- KI-67 (MIB-1): 5-10% (proliferation index)
- May have oligodendroglioma components (anaplastic oligoastrocytoma)

CLINICAL ISSUES

Presentation

- Most common signs/symptoms
  - Acceleration in clinical deterioration in patient with low-grade (diffuse) astrocytoma (WHO grade II)
  - Varies with location
    - Seizures, focal neurologic deficit common
    - May have headache, drowsiness
    - Increased intracranial pressure
    - Personality or behavioral changes

Demographics

- Age
  - Occurs at all ages, most common 40-50 years
- Gender
  - M:F = 1.6:1
- Epidemiology
  - 1/3 of astrocytomas
  - 25% of gliomas
  - Diffusely infiltrating gliomas including WHO grades II, III, IV account for > 60% of all primary tumors

Natural History & Prognosis

- Median survival: 2-3 years
- Commonly arise as recurrence after resection of grade II tumor
- Progression to secondary GBM very common
  - 2 years is typical time for progression
- Spreads along white matter tracts commonly
  - May spread along ependyma, leptomeninges, and CSF
- Increased survival: Younger age, high Karnofsky score, gross total resection
- Other factors associated with longer survival
  - Absence of enhancement, proliferation index of 5.1% or lower, oligodendroglial component

Treatment

- Resection with adjuvant radiation therapy and chemotherapy

DIAGNOSTIC CHECKLIST

Consider

- AA may mimic other tumors, particularly diffuse low-grade astrocytomas (grade II)
- Nonneoplastic mimics such as cerebritis may be differentiated with help of clinical history
- AA have histologic and imaging characteristics along spectrum between low-grade astrocytoma and GBM

Image Interpretation Pearls

- AA are typically nonenhancing hemispheric masses
- If new areas of enhancement are seen, malignant degeneration is likely

SELECTED REFERENCES

1. Hirai T et al: Prognostic value of perfusion MR imaging of high-grade astrocytomas: long-term follow-up study. AJNR Am J Neuroradiol. 29(8):1505-10, 2008
2. Louis DN et al (eds): WHO Classification of Tumours of the Central Nervous System: Anaplastic Astrocytoma. Lyon, France: IARC Press. 30-2, 2007
3. Tortosa A et al: Prognostic implication of clinical, radiologic, and pathologic features in patients with anaplastic gliomas. Cancer. 97(4): 1063-71, 2003
4. Provenzale JM et al: Comparison of permeability in high-grade and low-grade brain tumors using dynamic susceptibility contrast MR imaging. AJR Am J Roentgenol. 178(3):711-6, 2002
5. Castillo M et al: Correlation of myo-inositol levels and grading of cerebral astrocytomas. AJNR Am J Neuroradiol. 21(9):1645-9, 2000

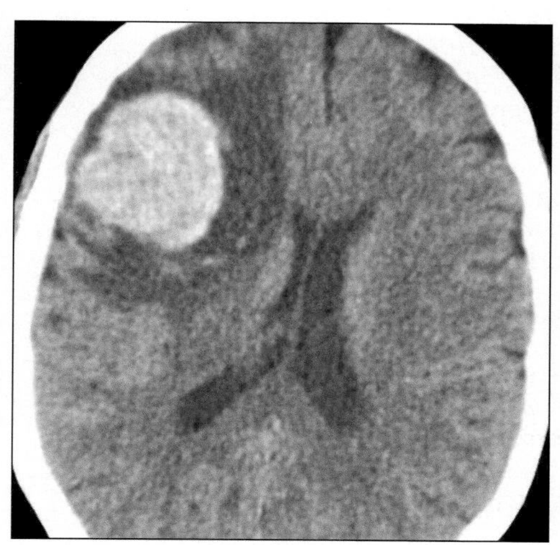

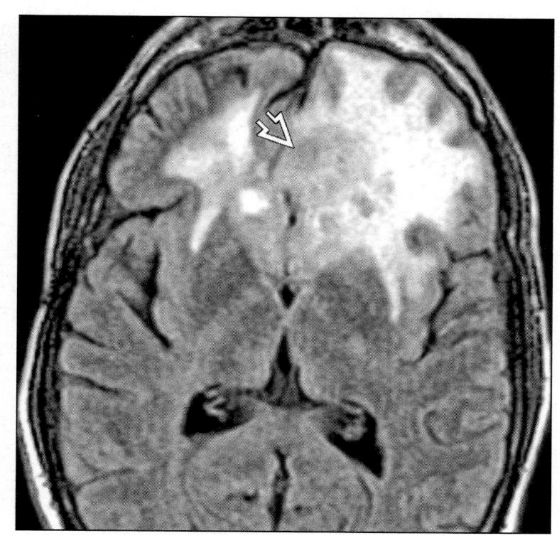

(Left) *Axial NECT shows a hemorrhagic mass in the right frontal lobe with surrounding low density and mass effect. Hemorrhage is more commonly seen in GBM than anaplastic astrocytoma.* ***(Right)*** *Axial FLAIR MR shows an infiltrative left frontal lobe mass ➡ with involvement of the adjacent white matter and extension across the corpus callosum into the right frontal lobe. Note the sparing of the overlying cortex, typical of an infiltrative astrocytoma. Imaging often mimics a grade II astrocytoma.*

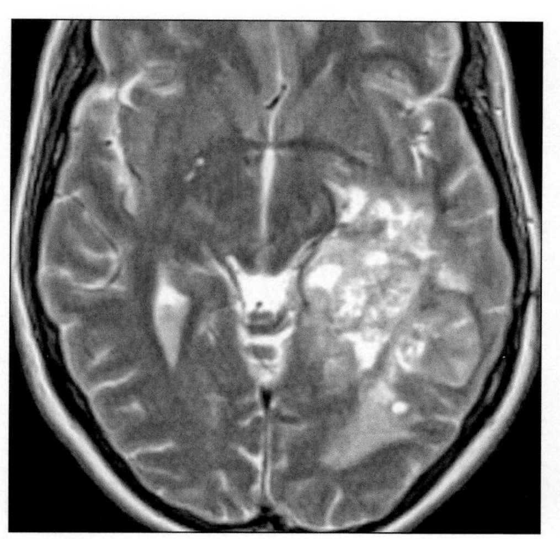

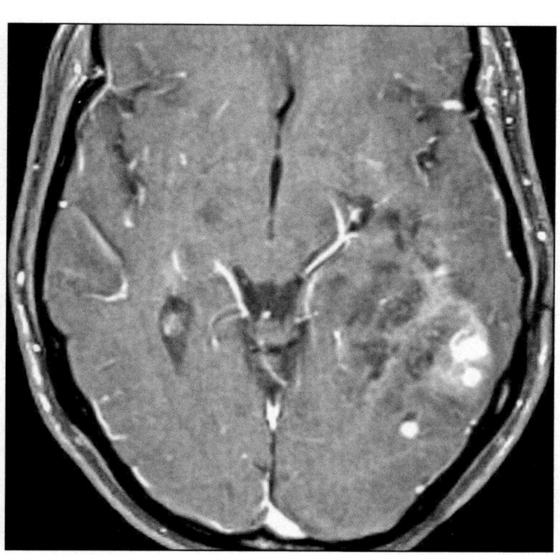

(Left) *Axial T2WI MR shows a heterogeneously hyperintense mass in the left posterior temporal and occipital lobes in a patient with a previously treated low-grade (diffuse) astrocytoma.* ***(Right)*** *Axial T1WI C+ MR in the same patient shows heterogeneous enhancement of the mass, a new finding in this patient with a grade II astrocytoma and clinical deterioration. Repeat biopsy disclosed a grade III astrocytoma. New enhancement always suggests malignant degeneration.*

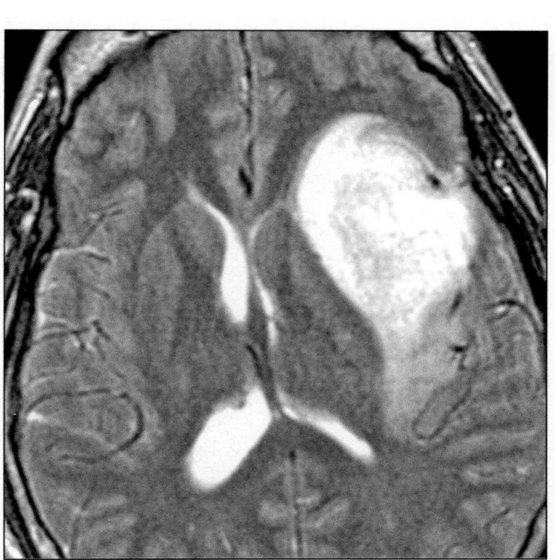

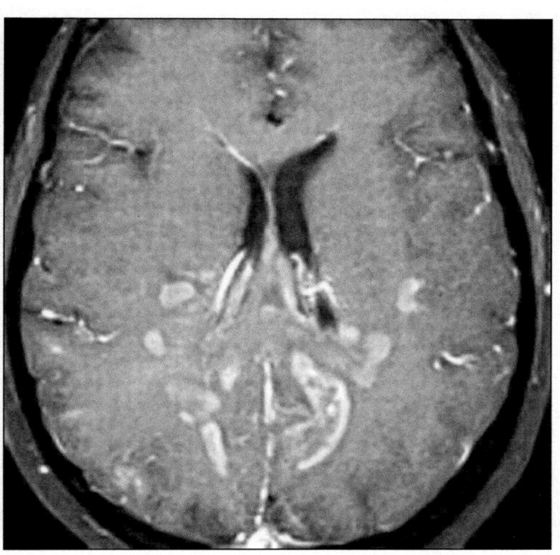

(Left) *Axial T2WI shows a hyperintense white matter mass. Although the mass appears discrete, tumor cells often extend beyond the signal abnormality. No enhancement was seen following contrast, typical of an anaplastic astrocytoma. Imaging mimics a low-grade astrocytoma.* ***(Right)*** *Axial T1 C+ FS MR shows multifocal nodular enhancement involving the parietal and occipital lobes with corpus callosum extension. Enhancement pattern suggests a malignant glioma. AA found at resection.*

GLIOBLASTOMA MULTIFORME

Key Facts

Terminology
- Rapidly enlarging malignant astrocytic tumor characterized by necrosis and neovascularity
- Most common of all primary intracranial neoplasms

Imaging
- Viable tumor extends far beyond signal changes
- Thick, irregularly enhancing rind of neoplastic tissue surrounding necrotic core
- Heterogeneous, hyperintense mass with adjacent tumor infiltration/vasogenic edema
- Necrosis, cysts, hemorrhage, fluid/debris levels, flow voids (neovascularity) may be seen
- Supratentorial white matter most common location
  - Cerebral hemispheres > brainstem > cerebellum

Top Differential Diagnoses
- Abscess
- Metastasis
- Primary CNS lymphoma
- Anaplastic astrocytoma
- "Tumefactive" demyelination
- Subacute ischemia

Pathology
- 2 types: Primary (de novo) and secondary (degeneration from lower grade astrocytoma)
- Necrosis and microvascular proliferation are hallmarks
- WHO grade IV

Clinical Issues
- Varies with location: Seizures, focal neurologic deficits common
- Peak: 45-75 years, but may occur at any age
- Represents 12-15% of all intracranial neoplasms

__(Left)__ Axial graphic shows a centrally necrotic infiltrating mass with extension across the corpus callosum. There is a peripheral rind of tumor surrounding the necrotic core, typical of GBM. __(Right)__ Axial T1WI C+ FS MR in a 60-year-old man with acute onset of seizures shows a heterogeneously enhancing occipital lobe mass with central necrosis and extension across the splenium of the corpus callosum ➔, characteristic of GBM. The frontal and temporal lobes are the most common locations for GBM.

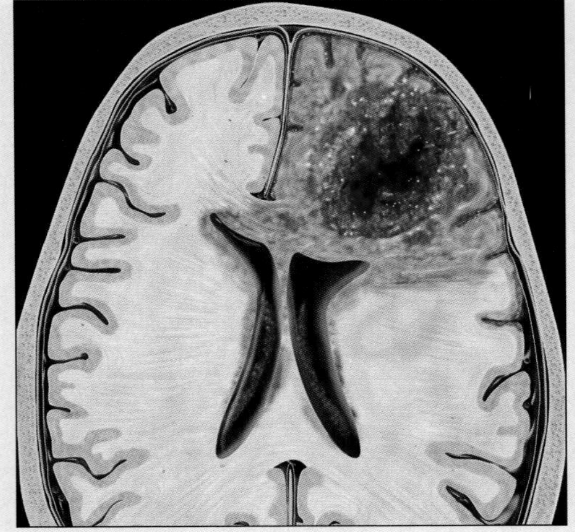

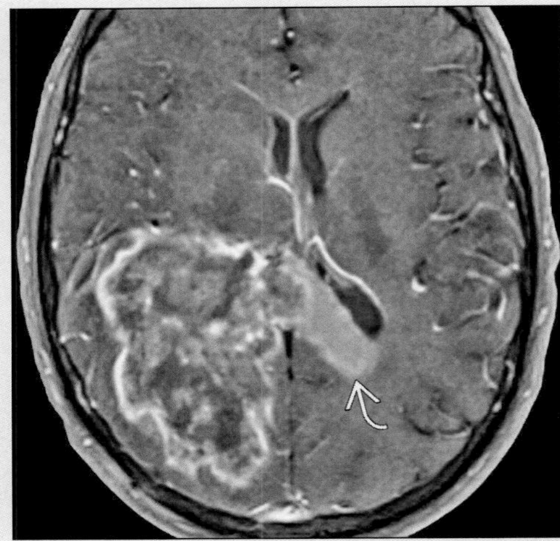

__(Left)__ Axial T2WI MR shows a heterogeneous mass ⇨ with extensive abnormal hyperintensity extending into the temporal and occipital lobes. The areas of low signal ➔ within the mass are related to blood products, a common feature of GBM. __(Right)__ Axial FLAIR MR in the same patient shows abnormal hyperintensity surrounding the mass which represents a combination of tumor spread and vasogenic edema. It is important to remember that tumor cells may extend beyond the area of MR signal abnormality.

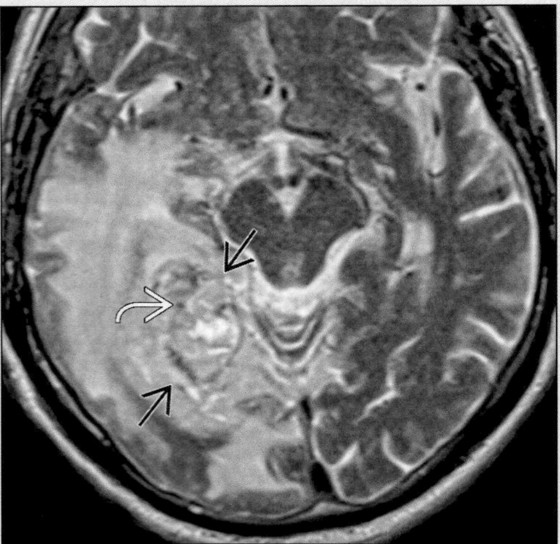

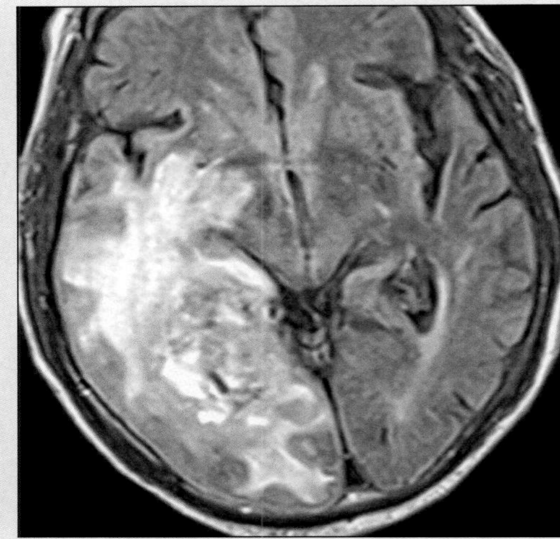

GLIOBLASTOMA MULTIFORME

TERMINOLOGY

Synonyms

- Glioblastoma multiforme (GBM), glioblastoma, grade IV astrocytoma, malignant astrocytoma

Definitions

- Rapidly enlarging malignant astrocytic tumor characterized by necrosis and neovascularity
- Most common of all primary intracranial neoplasms

IMAGING

General Features

- Best diagnostic clue
  - Thick, irregularly enhancing rind of neoplastic tissue surrounding necrotic core
- Location
  - Supratentorial white matter most common
    - Frontal, temporal, parietal > occipital lobes
  - Cerebral hemispheres > brainstem > cerebellum
  - Basal ganglia/thalamus less common
  - Brainstem, cerebellum more common in children
- Morphology
  - Poorly marginated, diffusely infiltrating necrotic hemispheric mass
  - Tumor typically crosses white matter tracts to involve contralateral hemisphere
    - Corpus callosum ("butterfly glioma")
    - Anterior and posterior commissures
  - Rarely may invade meninges
  - Rarely may be multifocal

CT Findings

- NECT
  - Irregular isodense or hypodense mass with central hypodensity representing necrosis
  - Marked mass effect and surrounding edema/tumor infiltration
  - Hemorrhage not uncommon
  - Ca++ rare (related to low-grade tumor degeneration)
- CECT
  - Strong, heterogeneous, irregular rim enhancement

MR Findings

- T1WI
  - Irregular isointense, hypointense white matter mass
  - Necrosis, cysts, and thick irregular margin common
  - May have subacute hemorrhage
- T2WI
  - Heterogeneous, hyperintense mass with adjacent tumor infiltration/vasogenic edema
  - Necrosis, cysts, hemorrhage, fluid/debris levels, flow voids (neovascularity) may be seen
  - Viable tumor extends far beyond signal changes
- FLAIR
  - Heterogeneous, hyperintense mass with adjacent tumor infiltration/vasogenic edema
- T2* GRE
  - Susceptibility artifact related to blood products
- DWI
  - Lower measured ADC than low-grade gliomas
  - No diffusion restriction typical
- T1WI C+
  - Thick, irregular rind of enhancement surrounding central necrosis typical
  - Enhancement may be solid, ring, nodular, or patchy
- MRS
  - Decreased NAA, myoinositol
  - Elevated choline, lactate/lipid peak (1.33 ppm)
- Dynamic contrast-enhanced T2* weighted imaging
  - Elevated maximum rCBV compared to low grade
  - Elevated permeability compared to low grade
- Diffusion tensor imaging (DTI) may help surgical planning

Nuclear Medicine Findings

- PET
  - Malignant tumors have high glucose metabolism and avidly accumulate FDG
  - Tumor:WM > 1.5 and tumor:GM > 0.6 suggests high-grade tumors

Imaging Recommendations

- Best imaging tool
  - Contrast-enhanced MR is most sensitive
  - Newer techniques help improve diagnosis/biopsy accuracy: MRS, perfusion, hypoxia imaging, DTI

DIFFERENTIAL DIAGNOSIS

Abscess

- Ring-enhancement typically thinner than GBM
- T2 hypointense rim, diffusion restriction is typical
- MRS may show succinate, amino acids

Metastasis

- Typically multiple lesions at gray-white junctions
- Round > infiltrating lesion
- Single lesion may be indistinguishable

Primary CNS Lymphoma

- Periventricular enhancing mass
- Often crosses corpus callosum
- Typically isointense/hypointense on T2WI
- Necrosis common in AIDS-related lymphoma

Anaplastic Astrocytoma

- Often nonenhancing white matter mass
- Enhancement may indicate degeneration to GBM
- May be indistinguishable

"Tumefactive" Demyelination

- Often incomplete, horseshoe-shaped enhancement, open towards cortex
- Lesions in typical locations; younger patients

Subacute Ischemia

- Typical vascular territory (MCA, PCA, ACA)
- May have mass effect and enhancement (gyriform)
- Follow-up imaging may be helpful to differentiate

Status Epilepticus

- Active seizures may cause signal abnormality and enhancement
- Enhancement often diffuse, affecting GM and WM

GLIOBLASTOMA MULTIFORME

- Clinical history of seizures

Arteriovenous Malformation (AVM)

- Multiple flow voids with minimal mass effect
- If associated with hemorrhage, may mimic GBM

PATHOLOGY

General Features

- Etiology
  - 2 types: Primary (de novo) and secondary (degeneration from lower grade astrocytoma)
    - Genetically distinct, same appearance
  - Spreads by creating "permissive environment"
  - Rare cases related to irradiation
- Genetics
  - Primary GBM (de novo)
    - Older patients (mean = 62 years), biologically more aggressive
    - Develops de novo (without preexisting lower grade tumor)
    - Amplification, overexpression of *EGFR*, *MDM2*
    - *PTEN* mutation (up to 40% of cases)
    - Chromosome 10p loss of heterozygosity (LOH)
    - Represent > 90% of GBMs
  - Secondary GBM (degeneration from lower grade)
    - Younger patients (mean = 45 years), less aggressive than primary GBM
    - Develops from lower grade astrocytoma (usually 4-5 years of progression)
    - *TP53* mutations
    - *PDGFR* amplification, overexpression
    - Chromosomes 10q, 17p LOH
    - Increased telomerase activity and *hTERT* expression
    - Represent < 10% of GBMs
- Associated abnormalities
  - Occurs sporadically or as part of heritable tumor syndrome
    - NF1, Li-Fraumeni syndrome (*TP53* mutation)
    - Turcot syndrome, Ollier disease, Maffucci syndrome
  - Giant cell glioblastoma, histologic variant of GBM (5%), slightly improved prognosis

Staging, Grading, & Classification

- WHO grade IV

Gross Pathologic & Surgical Features

- Reddish-gray "rind" of tumor surrounds necrotic core
  - Necrosis is hallmark of GBM
- Most GBMs have marked vascularity, ± gross hemorrhage

Microscopic Features

- Necrosis and microvascular proliferation are hallmarks
- Pleomorphic astrocytes, marked nuclear atypia, numerous mitoses
- High MIB-1 (proliferation index): > 10%

CLINICAL ISSUES

Presentation

- Most common signs/symptoms
  - Varies with location: Seizures, focal neurologic deficits common
  - Increased intracranial pressure, mental status change
  - Typically short duration of symptoms (< 3 months)

Demographics

- Age
  - Peak 45-75 years, but may occur at any age
- Gender
  - Male predominance (M:F = 1.3:1)
- Epidemiology
  - Most common primary brain tumor
  - Represents 12-15% of all intracranial neoplasms
  - 60-75% of astrocytomas
  - 3-4:100,000 per year
  - Multifocal in up to 20% (2-5% synchronous independent tumors)

Natural History & Prognosis

- Relentless progression
- Prognosis is dismal (death in 9-12 months)
- Patterns of dissemination
  - Most common: Along white matter tracts
  - Less common: Ependymal/subpial spread, CSF metastases, perivascular spaces
  - Uncommon: Dural/skull invasion
  - Rare: Extraneural spread (lung, liver, nodes, bone)
- Independent predictors of longer survival
  - Age (younger), Karnofsky performance scale (higher), extent of resection (gross total vs. subtotal)
  - Degree of necrosis, enhancement on preoperative MR

Treatment

- Biopsy/tumor debulking followed by XRT, chemotherapy
- Newer antiangiogenesis agents promising

DIAGNOSTIC CHECKLIST

Consider

- Corpus callosum involvement may be seen in GBM, lymphoma, demyelination, or less commonly with metastases

Image Interpretation Pearls

- Viable tumor extends far beyond signal abnormalities

SELECTED REFERENCES

1. Saraswathy S et al: Evaluation of MR markers that predict survival in patients with newly diagnosed GBM prior to adjuvant therapy. J Neurooncol. 91(1):69-81, 2009
2. Louis DN et al: WHO Classification of Tumours of the Central Nervous System: Glioblastoma. Lyon: IARC Press. 33-49, 2007

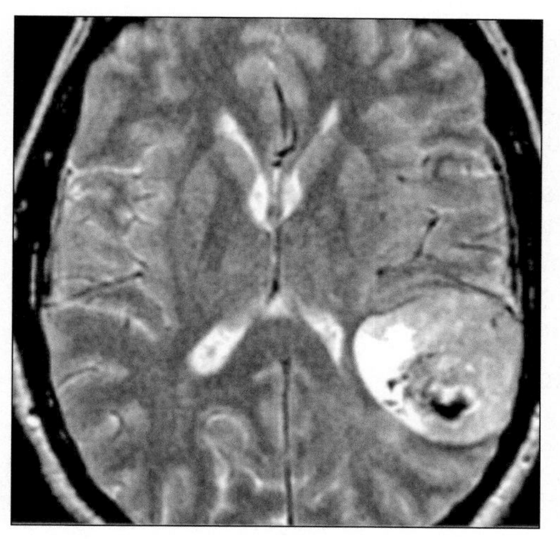

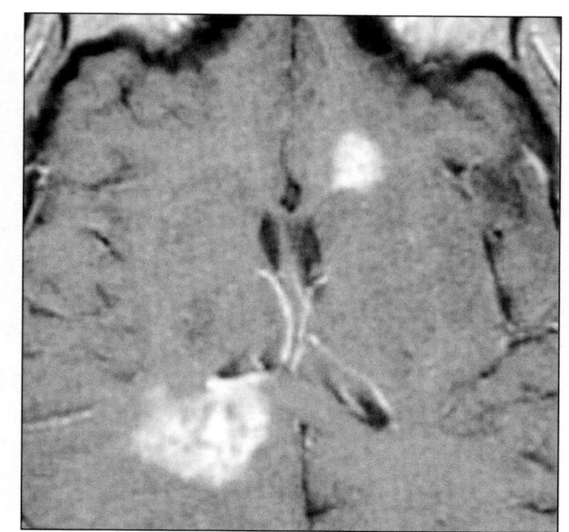

(Left) *Axial T2WI MR shows a heterogeneous, discrete-appearing mass in the posterior temporal region. There is a distinct lack of surrounding T2 signal and mass effect, very unusual for glioblastoma multiforme. Although they may appear discrete, GBMs are always infiltrative and often extend beyond the area of MR signal abnormality.* ***(Right)*** *Axial T1WI C+ MR shows 2 areas of enhancement representing a multifocal GBM. This rare synchronous presentation of GBM occurs in up to 5% of cases.*

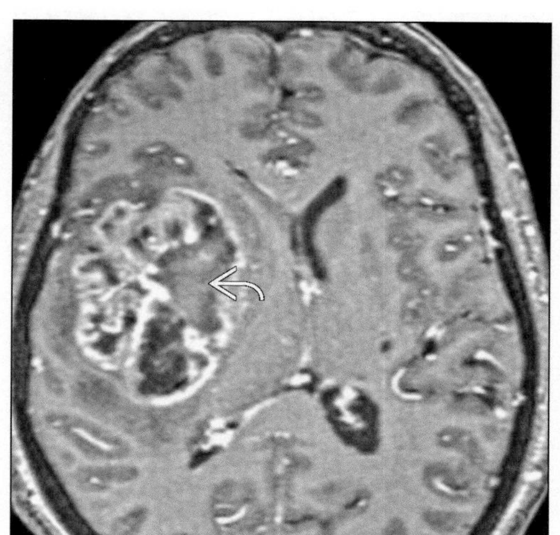

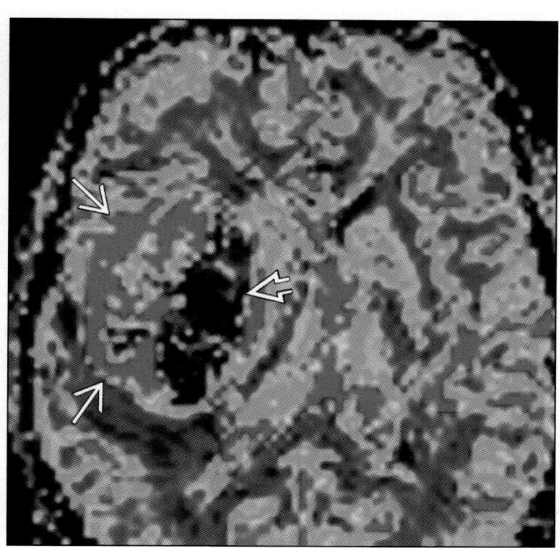

(Left) *Axial T1WI C+ MR shows a heterogeneously enhancing temporal lobe mass with central necrosis, which is characteristic of a GBM.* ***(Right)*** *Axial MR perfusion in the same patient shows an increased rCBV in the solid parts of the tumor and a low rCBV in the necrotic center. Perfusion MR is helpful to provide an accurate preoperative diagnosis. In addition, it is often used to help guide a biopsy if the location of the tumor prevents the patient from undergoing a complete resection.*

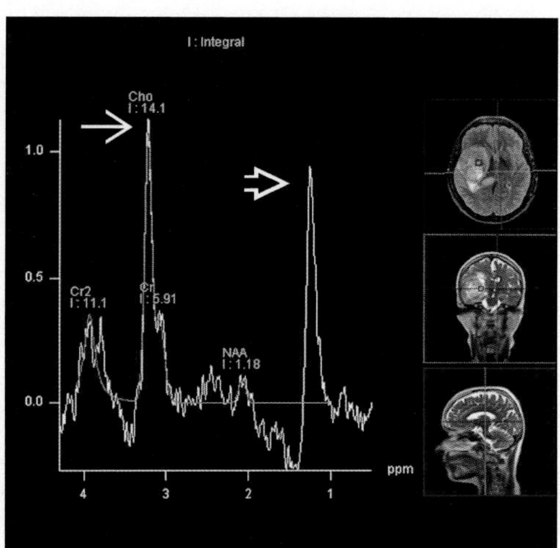

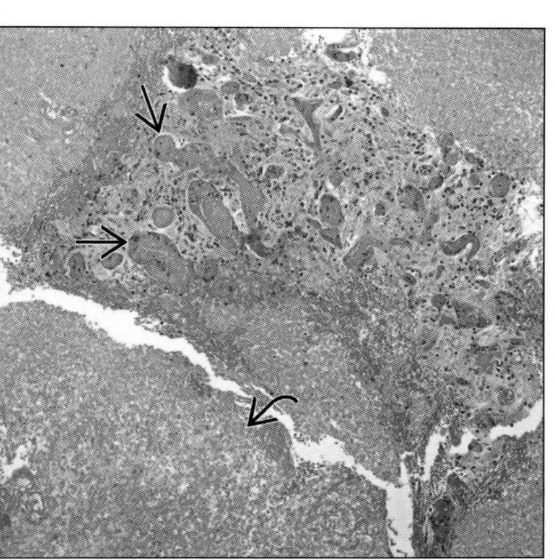

(Left) *MRS in the same patient shows a classic GBM tumor spectrum with a markedly elevated choline (Cho), a low NAA at 2.02 ppm, and lactate peak at 1.33. The lactate peak represents necrosis seen in this WHO grade IV tumor.* ***(Right)*** *Low-power H&E shows neovascularity and necrosis within a hypercellular mass, hallmarks of GBM. High-power views revealed mitotic activity, typical of a grade IV tumor. (Courtesy P. Hildenbrand, MD.)*

GLIOSARCOMA

Key Facts

Terminology
- Rare glioblastoma variant with both glial & mesenchymal elements
- May be primary or secondary (sarcomatous growth in recurrent GBM)

Imaging
- Heterogeneously enhancing mass with dural invasion, ± skull involvement
- May be indistinguishable from GBM
- Temporal > parietal > frontal > occipital lobes
- Heterogeneous mass related to hemorrhage, necrosis
- Heterogeneous, thick irregular enhancement with central necrosis

Top Differential Diagnoses
- Glioblastoma multiforme (GBM)
- Metastasis
- Hemangiopericytoma
- Malignant meningioma

Pathology
- Sarcomatous elements thought to arise from transformed vascular elements within GBM
- WHO grade IV

Clinical Issues
- Increased intracranial pressure: Headache
- Typically 5th to 6th decade
- Poor prognosis, median survival 6-12 months
- Extracranial metastases common (15-30%)

Diagnostic Checklist
- Consider gliosarcoma in event of peripheral mass with dural invasion

*(**Left**) Coronal graphic shows a peripherally located, heterogeneous necrotic mass with an invasion of the dura and adjacent skull, findings typical of gliosarcoma. An infiltrative tumor involves the corpus callosum as well. Dural invasion with or without skull involvement helps distinguish this GBM variant from a typical GBM. (**Right**) Coronal T1WI C+ MR shows a heterogeneously enhancing mass with dural invasion and possible skull involvement ➡. Note the significant mass effect and midline shift.*

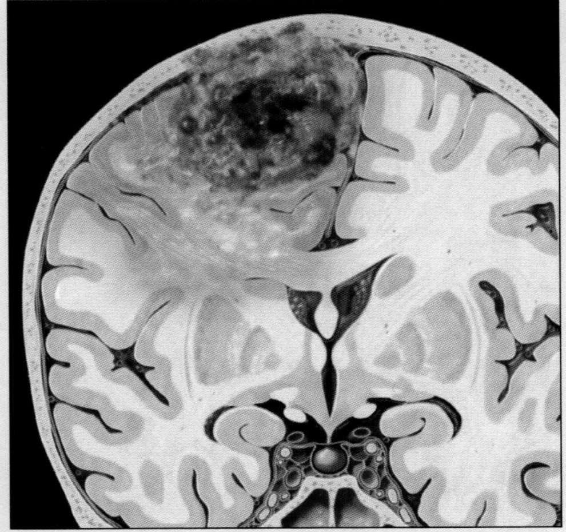

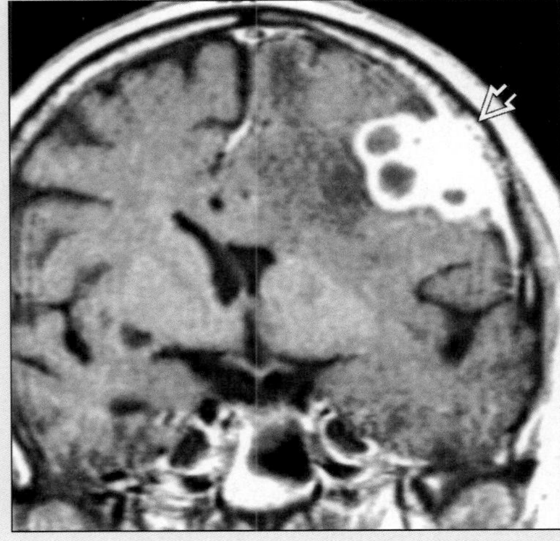

*(**Left**) Axial T1WI C+ MR shows a peripheral frontal lobe mass with dural invasion ➡ and local mass effect, findings typical of gliosarcoma. (**Right**) Axial T1WI C+ FS MR shows heterogeneous enhancement with areas of central low signal related to necrosis. Note the ependymal enhancement of the entrapped occipital horn ➡. When there is no dural involvement, gliosarcoma is indistinguishable from a typical GBM. Both of these WHO grade IV tumors have a poor prognosis.*

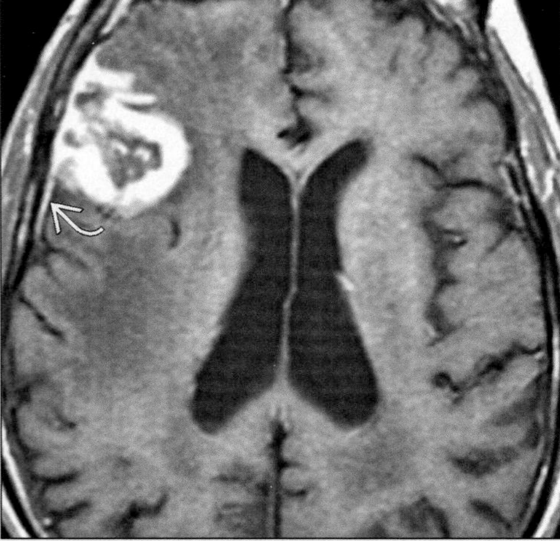

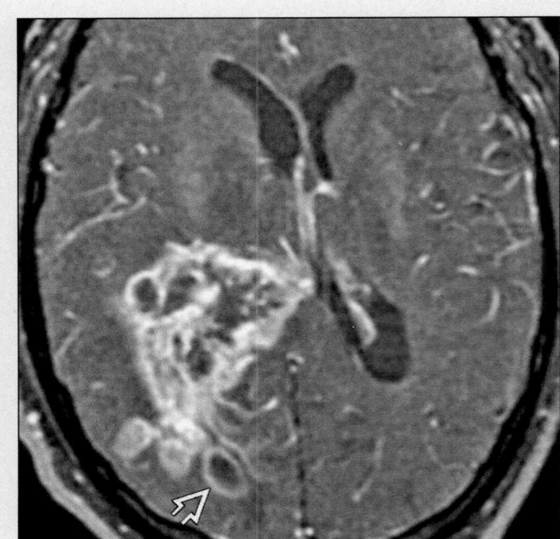

GLIOSARCOMA

TERMINOLOGY

Definitions

- Rare glioblastoma variant with both glial & mesenchymal elements
- May be primary or secondary (sarcomatous growth in recurrent GBM)

IMAGING

General Features

- Best diagnostic clue
  - Heterogeneously enhancing mass with dural invasion, ± skull involvement
  - May be indistinguishable from GBM
- Location
  - Cerebral hemispheres
    - Temporal > parietal > frontal > occipital lobes
  - Rarely posterior fossa
- Size
  - Variable, typically 3-8 cm
- Morphology
  - Infiltrating mass, may have discrete portion

CT Findings

- NECT
  - Heterogeneous mass with surrounding edema
  - Hemorrhage may be seen
- CECT
  - Heterogeneous, thick irregular enhancement
  - May see dural involvement, ± skull involvement

MR Findings

- T1WI
  - Heterogeneous, hypointense mass
- T2WI
  - Heterogeneous mass related to hemorrhage, necrosis
  - Marked surrounding edema
- T1WI C+
  - Heterogeneous, thick, irregular enhancement with central necrosis
  - May see dural involvement, ± skull involvement

DIFFERENTIAL DIAGNOSIS

Glioblastoma Multiforme (GBM)

- Typically indistinguishable
- Heterogeneous mass with hemorrhage, necrosis
- No dural or skull involvement

Metastasis

- Multiple lesions common; primary often known

Hemangiopericytoma

- Extraaxial mass with dural and skull invasion

Malignant Meningioma

- Extraaxial mass with parenchymal invasion

Abscess

- Ring-enhancing lesion with central necrosis
- T2 hyperintense rim and DWI is typical

PATHOLOGY

General Features

- Etiology
  - Sarcomatous elements thought to arise from transformed vascular elements within GBM
  - Reports suggest XRT induces sarcomatous change

Staging, Grading, & Classification

- WHO grade IV

Gross Pathologic & Surgical Features

- May mimic metastasis or meningioma at surgery
- Firm, lobular mass with central necrosis, ± meningeal invasion

Microscopic Features

- Malignant glial and mesenchymal elements

CLINICAL ISSUES

Presentation

- Most common signs/symptoms
  - Increased intracranial pressure: Headache
- Other signs/symptoms
  - Related to location: Seizure, focal neuro deficit

Demographics

- Age
  - Typically 5th to 6th decade
  - Congenital gliosarcoma has been reported (rare)
- Gender
  - M:F = 1.6:1
- Epidemiology
  - Rare, accounts for 2-8% of GBM

Natural History & Prognosis

- Poor prognosis, median survival 6-12 months
- Local recurrence typical
- Extracranial metastases common (15-30%)

Treatment

- Surgery followed by adjuvant XRT, ± chemotherapy

DIAGNOSTIC CHECKLIST

Image Interpretation Pearls

- Consider gliosarcoma in event of peripheral mass with dural invasion
- Gliosarcomas may mimic GBM and metastases

SELECTED REFERENCES

1. Han SJ et al: Secondary gliosarcoma: a review of clinical features and pathological diagnosis. J Neurosurg. Epub ahead of print, 2009
2. Kozak KR et al: Adult gliosarcoma: epidemiology, natural history, and factors associated with outcome. Neuro Oncol. 11(2):183-91, 2009

GLIOMATOSIS CEREBRI

Key Facts

Terminology

- Diffusely infiltrating, frequently bilateral glial tumor involving at least 3 lobes
- Infiltrative extent of tumor is out of proportion to histologic and clinical features

Imaging

- T2 hyperintense infiltrating mass with enlargement of involved structures
- Typically no or minimal enhancement
- Enhancement may indicate malignant progression or focus of malignant glioma
- MRS: Increased choline (Cho), decreased NAA

Top Differential Diagnoses

- Arteriolosclerosis
- Vasculitis
- Anaplastic astrocytoma
- Viral encephalitis
- Demyelination

Pathology

- Usually WHO grade III
- Shares some, but not all, features of diffusely infiltrating astrocytoma
- Rarely oligodendroglioma is predominant cell type
- Diagnosis typically made on basis of histology and imaging

Clinical Issues

- Mental status changes, dementia, headaches, seizures, lethargy
- Peak incidence between 40-50 years
- Relentless progression
- Survival ranges from weeks to years

*(**Left**) Axial graphic shows infiltrating tumor involving frontal lobes, insulae and basal ganglia with preservation of the underlying cerebral architecture. Note the focal malignant degeneration ➔. (**Right**) Axial T2WI MR shows diffuse hyperintensity extending through the white matter of the frontal and temporal lobes, basal ganglia, and splenium of the corpus callosum. No significant enhancement was seen following contrast. Gliomatosis cerebri occasionally mimics a nonneoplastic white matter process.*

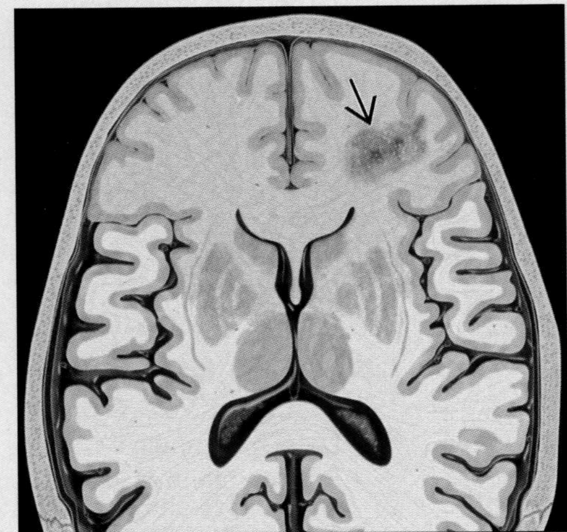

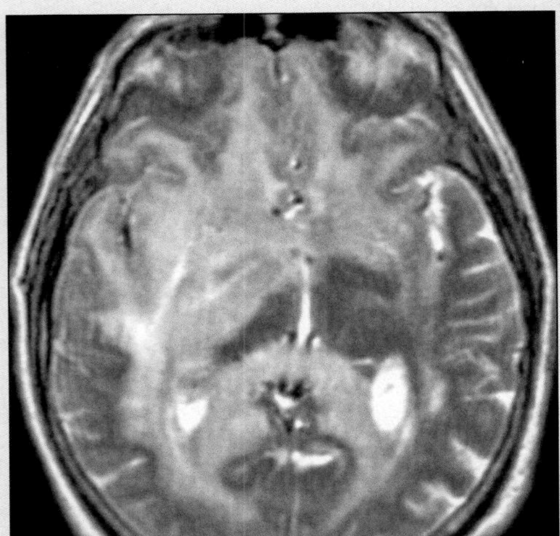

*(**Left**) Axial FLAIR MR shows abnormal hyperintensity in the left brainstem with extension into the temporal lobe. Note the subtle expansion of the involved structures with relative preservation of the underlying architecture, typical of gliomatosis cerebri. (**Right**) Axial FLAIR MR in the same patient shows hyperintensity in the left temporal and parietal lobes, corpus callosum, frontal lobes, & thalamus ➔. Usually a WHO grade III tumor, biopsy revealed a grade IV tumor in this patient.*

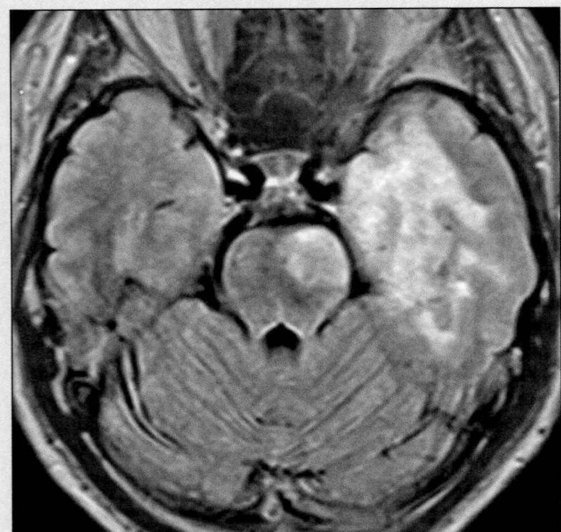

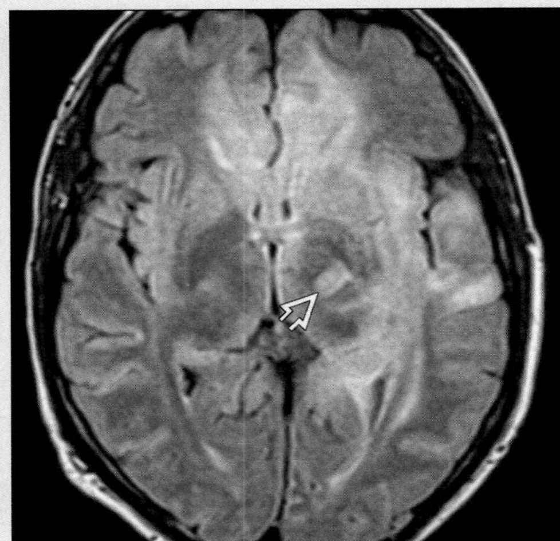

GLIOMATOSIS CEREBRI

TERMINOLOGY

Abbreviations
- Gliomatosis cerebri (GC)

Synonyms
- Gliomatosis, diffuse cerebral gliomatosis

Definitions
- Diffusely infiltrating, frequently bilateral glial tumor involving at least 3 lobes
- Infiltrative extent of tumor is out of proportion to histologic and clinical features

IMAGING

General Features
- Best diagnostic clue
  - T2 hyperintense infiltrating mass with enlargement of involved structures
- Location
  - Typically hemispheric white matter (WM) involvement (76%), may also involve cortex (19%)
  - 3 lobes, diffuse white matter plus
    - Basal ganglia, thalami (75%)
    - Brainstem (52%)
    - Corpus callosum (50%)
    - Cerebellum (29%)
    - Spinal cord (9%)
  - May cross corpus callosum or massa intermedia
- Morphology
  - Infiltrates, enlarges yet preserves underlying brain architecture

CT Findings
- NECT
  - Poorly defined, asymmetric low density (often subtle)
  - Loss of gray-white differentiation with expansion and mild mass effect
- CECT
  - No enhancement typical

MR Findings
- T1WI
  - Isointense or hypointense infiltrating mass
  - Typically homogeneous
- T2WI
  - Homogeneous hyperintense infiltrating mass
  - Mass effect with mild diffuse sulcal and ventricular effacement
  - May cause hydrocephalus (rare)
- FLAIR
  - Homogeneous hyperintense infiltrating mass
- DWI
  - Usually no restriction
- T1WI C+
  - Typically no or minimal enhancement
  - Patchy enhancement rarely
  - Enhancement may indicate malignant progression or focus of malignant glioma
- MRS
  - Marked elevation of myoinositol (mI)
  - Increased choline (Cho)
  - Decreased NAA
  - ± lactate, lipid peaks at 1.33 ppm (suggests decreased survival)
- Dynamic perfusion MR
  - Low rCBV: Correlates with no vascular hyperplasia
  - High rCBV: Suggests higher grade tumor
- Diffusion tensor imaging (DTI)
  - Preservation of nerve fibers in GC compared to other tumors

Nuclear Medicine Findings
- FDG PET shows marked hypometabolism

Imaging Recommendations
- Protocol advice
  - Multiplanar contrast-enhanced MR
  - MRS and perfusion imaging may help further characterize

DIFFERENTIAL DIAGNOSIS

Arteriolosclerosis
- Aging brain, microvascular disease
- No mass effect; spares cortex
- Often associated volume loss
- Some cases may be indistinguishable without biopsy

Vasculitis
- Often multifocal areas of ischemia
- DWI positive acutely
- Patchy, multifocal enhancement may be seen
- May be indistinguishable without biopsy

Anaplastic Astrocytoma
- May appear discrete or infiltrating, often less diffuse
- Variable enhancement

Viral Encephalitis
- More acute presentation, history may distinguish
- ± meningeal involvement
- Herpes involves temporal lobes, limbic system

Demyelination
- Usually multiple lesions in typical locations
- Typically lack significant mass effect
- Often enhances, incomplete ring, open at cortex
- May involve white matter and deep gray nuclei

Progressive Multifocal Leukoencephalopathy
- Asymmetric T2 hyperintensity in periventricular, subcortical white matter
- No or minimal enhancement typical
- Often parietooccipital region, may cross corpus callosum
- Immunosuppressed patients, typically AIDS

Lymphoma
- Periventricular/deep GM enhancing mass in primary CNS lymphoma
  - Corpus callosum involvement classic
  - Isointense/hypointense on T2WI
- Intravascular lymphoma may appear diffusely infiltrating

GLIOMATOSIS CEREBRI

Inherited/Acquired Metabolic Disorder
- Metachromatic leukodystrophy (MLD): Confluent periventricular WM T2 hyperintensity
- Alexander disease: Frontal lobe WM hyperintensity and enhancement

PATHOLOGY

General Features
- Etiology
  - Controversial, classified as neoplasm of unknown histogenesis
  - Shares some, but not all, features of diffusely infiltrating astrocytoma
  - Rarely oligodendroglioma is predominant cell type
- Genetics
  - *TP53* mutation similar to diffuse astrocytoma, lower frequency
  - In oligodendroglioma subtype, chromosome 1p deletion reported

Staging, Grading, & Classification
- Usually WHO grade III (range from grades II-IV)
- Dx typically made on basis of histology and imaging

Gross Pathologic & Surgical Features
- 2 gross pathologic GC types recognized
  - Type 1: Neoplastic overgrowth, expansion of existing structures without circumscribed tumor mass
  - Type 2: Diffuse lesion + focal neoplastic mass with malignant features (may develop from type 1)
- Blurring of gray-white junction borders ± distinct tumor nodule
- Underlying brain architecture preserved
- Diffuse neoplastic overgrowth

Microscopic Features
- Extensive tumor infiltration is disproportionate to histologic features
  - Necrosis and neovascularity typically absent
- Neuroepithelial neoplasm with diffuse invasion of parenchyma with tumor cells
- Elongated glial cells with hyperchromatic nuclei, variable mitoses
- Neoplastic cells often arranged in parallel rows
- Diffuse infiltration along/between myelinated nerve fibers
- Immunohistochemistry: Often GFAP(+), S100(+)
- Ki-67 (proliferation index) = 1-30%

CLINICAL ISSUES

Presentation
- Most common signs/symptoms
  - Mental status changes, dementia, headaches, seizures, lethargy
- Other signs/symptoms
  - Cranial nerve signs, increased intracranial pressure, personality changes
  - Rare: Hydrocephalus

Demographics
- Age
  - Peak incidence between 40-50 years
  - Occurs at all ages, reported in neonates to 83 years
- Gender
  - No gender predominance
- Epidemiology
  - Rare, just over 300 reported cases

Natural History & Prognosis
- Relentless progression
- Poor prognosis
  - 50% mortality by 1 year
  - 75% by 3 years
- Survival ranges from weeks to years
- Karnofsky performance scale ≥ 70 correlates with increased survival
- Ki-67 labeling index may correlate with survival time
- Rarely complicated by hydrocephalus or herniation
- Very rarely GC is complicated by hemorrhage

Treatment
- Stereotaxic biopsy (enhancing nodule, if present)
- Poor response to chemotherapy, radiation therapy
  - Some reports show increased survival with treatment
- Steroids may help as initial treatment
- Surgical decompression, ventricular shunting occasionally required

DIAGNOSTIC CHECKLIST

Consider
- GC = diffusely infiltrating glial tumor that can be mistaken for nonneoplastic WM disease

Image Interpretation Pearls
- Extensive MR findings and tumor infiltration are disproportionate to histologic features
- MR often underestimates extent of disease when correlated with postmortem findings
- 3 or more contiguous lobes of multiregional involvement characterizes GC

SELECTED REFERENCES

1. Park S et al: Gliomatosis cerebri: clinicopathologic study of 33 cases and comparison of mass forming and diffuse types. Clin Neuropathol. 28(2):73-82, 2009
2. Kaloshi G et al: Genetic markers predictive of chemosensitivity and outcome in gliomatosis cerebri. Neurology. 70(8):590-5, 2008
3. Fuller GN et al: WHO Classification of Tumours of the Central Nervous System: Gliomatosis cerebri. Lyon: IARC Press. 50-2, 2007
4. Ware ML et al: Genetic aberrations in gliomatosis cerebri. Neurosurgery. 60(1):150-8; discussion 158, 2007
5. Taillibert S et al: Gliomatosis cerebri: a review of 296 cases from the ANOCEF database and the literature. J Neurooncol. 76(2):201-5, 2006
6. Yang S et al: Dynamic contrast-enhanced T2*-weighted MR imaging of gliomatosis cerebri. AJNR Am J Neuroradiol. 23(3): 350-5, 2002

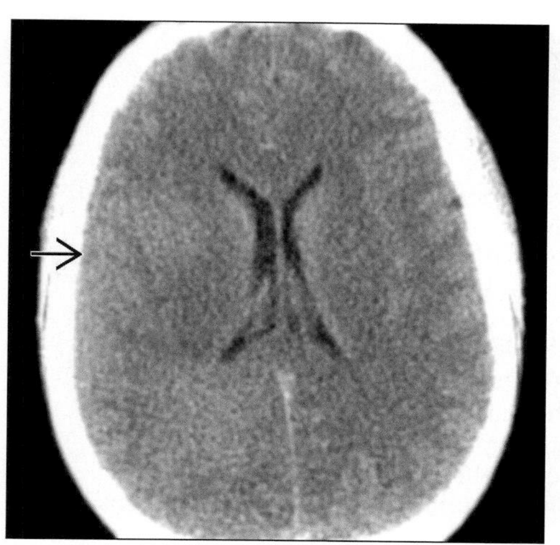

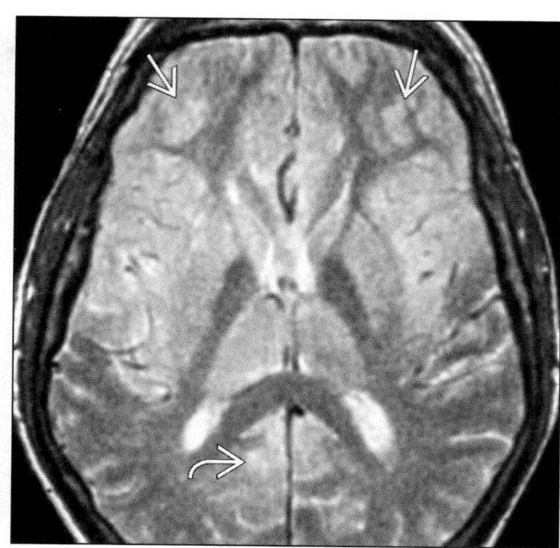

(Left) *Axial NECT shows loss of the normal gray-white interfaces & sulcal effacement →. CT diagnosis of gliomatosis cerebri is difficult as the study may occasionally appear normal.* ***(Right)*** *Axial T2WI MR shows abnormal hyperintensity in the frontal → & temporal lobes & occipital cortex →. The basal ganglia & thalami are also involved in this diffusely infiltrating process. The bilateral, but asymmetric appearance is typical. Biopsy disclosed oligodendroglioma, a rare cause of GC, often with increased survival.*

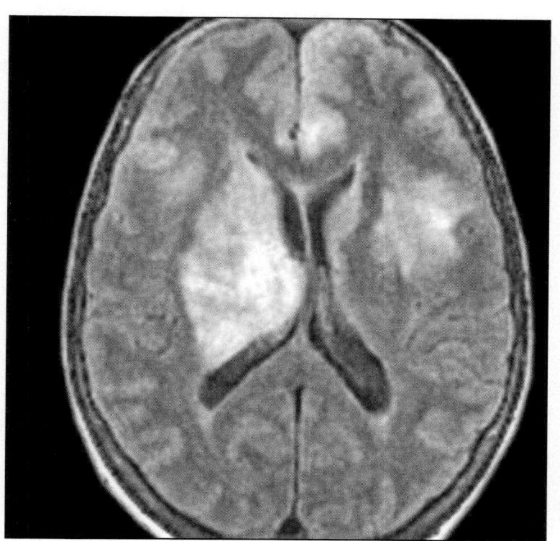

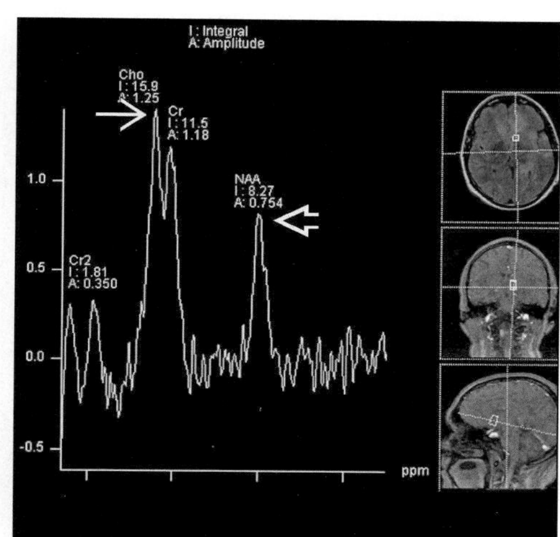

(Left) *Axial FLAIR MR shows multiple hyperintensities in the cortex of both hemispheres, the right basal ganglia, and thalamus. Note the relative lack of mass effect, with a mild right to left shift of the lateral ventricles and slight expansion of the affected structures, typical of GC.* ***(Right)*** *MRS shows a typical tumor spectrum with elevated choline → and decreased NAA → in this GC patient. Degree of choline and the presence of lactate has been show to correlate with decreased survival in GC.*

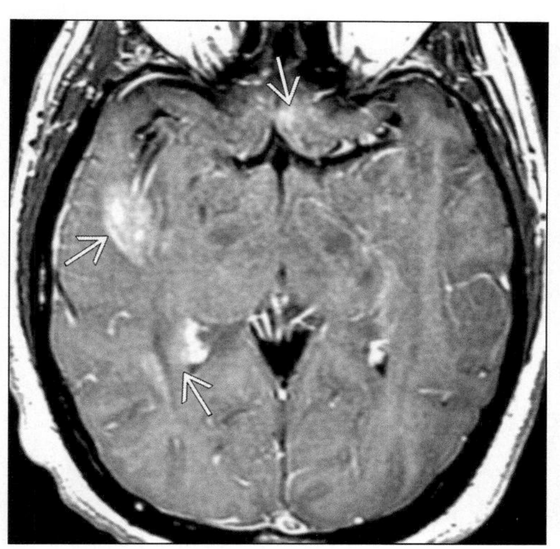

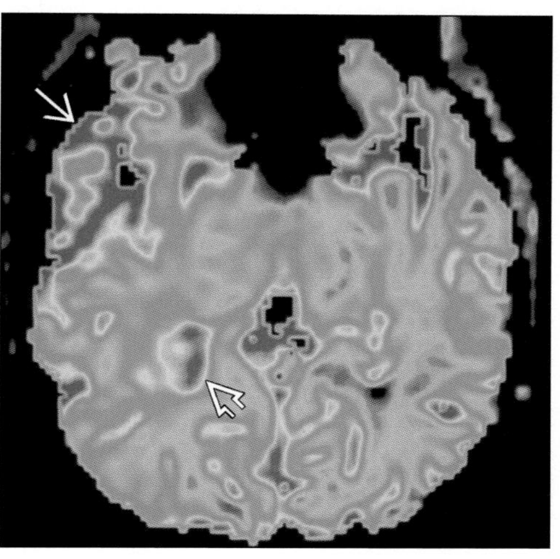

(Left) *Axial T1WI C+ MR shows multifocal areas of enhancement → in this patient with extensive FLAIR hyperintensity. Enhancement is uncommon in GC and may indicate a more malignant focus.* ***(Right)*** *Axial PWI MR in the same patient shows markedly increased cerebral blood volume (rCBV) in the right temporal lobe → and white matter → of the right hemisphere. The increased rCBV correlates to the more malignant portions of the tumor and may help guide biopsy. (Courtesy P. Hildenbrand, MD.)*

PILOCYTIC ASTROCYTOMA

Key Facts

Terminology

- Pilocytic astrocytoma: Well-circumscribed, slow-growing tumor, often with cyst and mural nodule

Imaging

- Cystic cerebellar mass with enhancing mural nodule
  - Arises from cerebellar hemisphere and compresses 4th ventricle
- Enlarged optic nerve/chiasm/tract with variable enhancement
- Cerebellum (60%) > optic nerve/chiasm (25-30%) > adjacent to 3rd ventricle > brainstem
- Well circumscribed with little to no edema
- Aggressive appearance (enhancement and MRS) of tumor is misleading

Top Differential Diagnoses

- Medulloblastoma (PNET-MB)
- Ependymoma
- Ganglioglioma
- Hemangioblastoma
- Demyelination

Pathology

- WHO grade I
- 15% of NF1 patients develop PAs, most commonly in optic pathway
- Up to 1/3 of patients with optic PAs have NF1
- Most common primary brain tumor in children

Clinical Issues

- Clinical presentation varies with location
  - Headache, nausea, vomiting most common
  - Visual loss (optic pathway lesions)
  - Ataxia, cerebellar signs (cerebellar lesions)
- Slowly growing tumor with very good prognosis

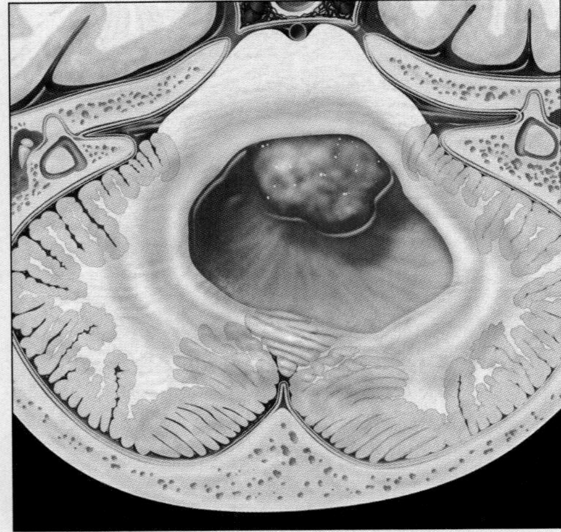

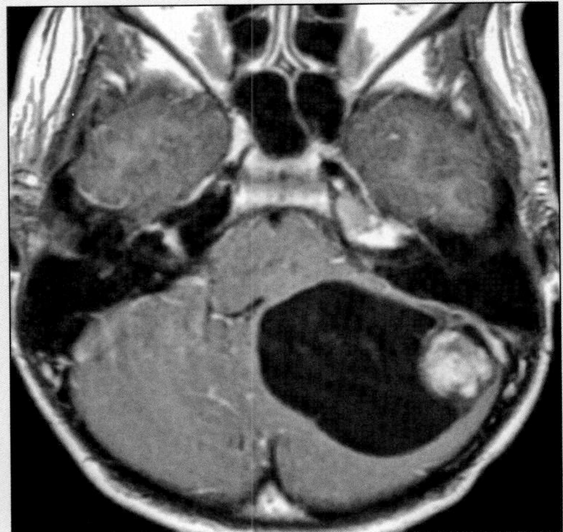

(Left) *Axial graphic shows the characteristic "cyst with mural nodule" appearance of a posterior fossa pilocytic astrocytoma (PA). These WHO grade I tumors most commonly arise in the cerebellar hemispheres and compress the 4th ventricle.* ***(Right)*** *Axial T1WI C+ MR shows a classic "cyst with mural nodule" appearance of a cerebellar PA in a child. Note the typical intense enhancement of the nodule with no enhancement of the cyst wall. Mass effect on the 4th ventricle with associated hydrocephalus is common.*

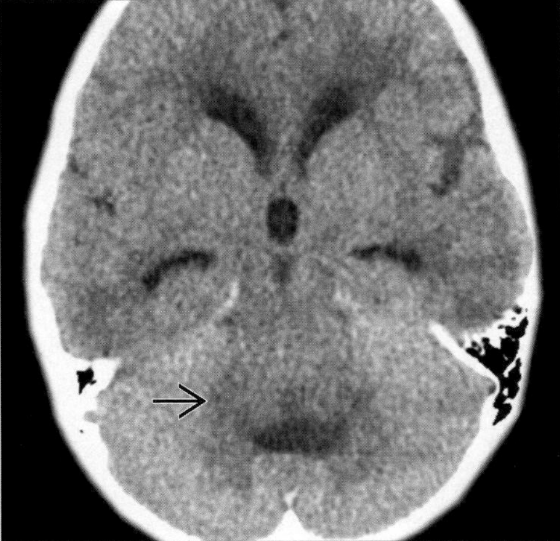

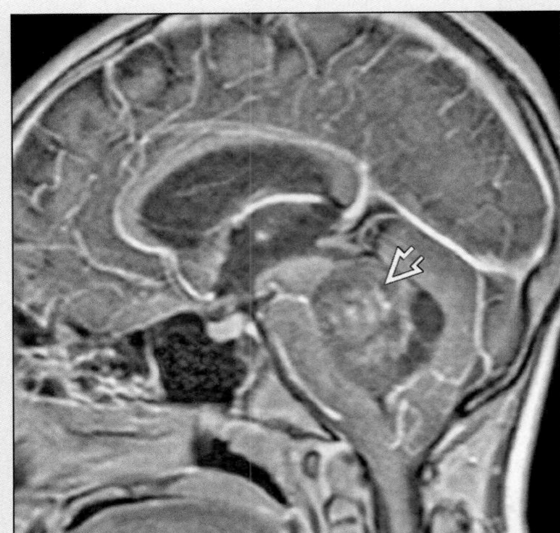

(Left) *Axial NECT shows a cystic and solid isodense mass ➔ extending from the posterior brainstem, causing obstructive hydrocephalus. The lack of increased density helps to differentiate this PA from a medulloblastoma.* ***(Right)*** *Sagittal T1WI C+ MR in the same patient shows mild heterogeneous enhancement ➲ of the solid portion of the mass. PAs most often arise from the cerebellar hemispheres but may be dorsally exophytic from the brainstem. PAs are the most common primary brain tumor in children.*

PILOCYTIC ASTROCYTOMA

TERMINOLOGY

Abbreviations

- Pilocytic astrocytoma (PA), juvenile pilocytic astrocytoma (JPA)

Definitions

- Pilocytic astrocytoma: Well-circumscribed, slow-growing tumor, often with cyst and mural nodule
- Characterized by hair-like cytoplasmic (Rosenthal) fibers &/or eosinophilic granular bodies in stacked bipolar cells

IMAGING

General Features

- Best diagnostic clue
  - Cystic cerebellar mass with enhancing mural nodule
  - Enlarged optic nerve/chiasm/tract with variable enhancement
- Location
  - Cerebellum (60%) > optic nerve/chiasm (25-30%) > adjacent to 3rd ventricle > brainstem
- Size
  - Large lesions in cerebellum, often > 3 cm
  - Optic nerve lesions typically smaller
- Morphology
  - Overall morphology often determined by cystic component
  - Well circumscribed with little to no adjacent T2 prolongation
  - Optic nerve tumors elongate and widen nerve, causing buckling in orbit: "Dotted i" appearance

CT Findings

- NECT
  - Discrete cystic-solid mass
  - May have little or no surrounding edema
  - Solid component hypo- to isodense to gray matter (GM)
  - Ca++ in 20%, hemorrhage uncommon
  - Often causes obstructive hydrocephalus, location dependent
- CECT
  - > 95% enhance (patterns vary)
    - 50% nonenhancing cyst, strongly enhancing mural nodule
    - 40% solid with necrotic center, heterogeneous enhancement
    - 10% solid, homogeneous
    - Cyst may accumulate contrast on delayed images
    - Cyst wall may have some enhancement

MR Findings

- T1WI
  - Solid portions iso-/hypointense to GM
  - Cyst contents iso- to slightly hyperintense to CSF
- T2WI
  - Solid portions hyperintense to GM
  - Cyst contents iso-/hyperintense to CSF
  - Optic pathway: Hyperintense to GM
- FLAIR
  - Solid portions hyperintense to GM
  - Cyst contents do not suppress: Hyperintense to CSF
  - Margins of chiasmatic/hypothalamic tumors in patients with neurofibromatosis type 1 (NF1) difficult to resolve
- DWI
  - Solid tumor has similar diffusivity to GM
- T1WI C+
  - Intense but heterogeneous enhancement of solid portion
  - Cyst wall occasionally enhances
  - Rare: Leptomeningeal metastases
  - Optic pathway: Variable enhancement
- MRS: Aggressive-appearing metabolite pattern
  - ↑ choline, ↓ NAA, ↑ lactate
  - Paradoxical finding: MRS does not accurately reflect clinical behavior of tumor

Ultrasonographic Findings

- Grayscale ultrasound
  - Solid components are hyperechoic relative to brain parenchyma
  - Cysts may contain debris

Angiographic Findings

- Conventional: Avascular mass
  - Occasional neovascularity seen in solid portion

Nuclear Medicine Findings

- PET
  - 18F-fluorodeoxyglucose (FDG) studies show increased tumor metabolism in PAs
  - Paradoxical finding: PET does not accurately reflect histologic behavior of tumor

Imaging Recommendations

- Best imaging tool
  - Contrast-enhanced MR
- Protocol advice
  - Multiplanar or 3D volume post-contrast imaging key to show structure of origin and degree of extension

DIFFERENTIAL DIAGNOSIS

Medulloblastoma (PNET-MB)

- Hyperdense enhancing midline mass fills 4th ventricle
- Solid components T2 isointense to GM; ↓ ADC
- Younger patient age (2-6 years)

Ependymoma

- "Plastic" tumor, extends out 4th ventricle foramina
- Ca++, cysts, hemorrhage common
- Heterogeneous enhancement

Ganglioglioma

- Cortically based cystic and solid enhancing mass
- Ca++ common
- Typically located in temporal or frontal lobes

Hemangioblastoma

- Large cyst with small enhancing mural nodule at periphery of cerebellum, associated with feeding vessel
- Adult tumor!
- Associated with von Hippel-Lindau disease

PILOCYTIC ASTROCYTOMA

Pilomyxoid Astrocytoma

- Chiasmatic/hypothalamic tumor in infants
- Solid and enhancing
- More likely to disseminate, more aggressive

Demyelination/Inflammation

- Optic neuritis in acute multiple sclerosis, ADEM, pseudotumor can mimic optic nerve glioma
- "Tumefactive" MS can mimic hemispheric PA

PATHOLOGY

General Features

- Etiology
  - Astrocytic precursor cell
- Genetics
  - Syndromic: Association with NF1
    - 15% of NF1 patients develop PAs, most commonly in optic pathway
    - Up to 1/3 of patients with optic pathway PAs have NF1
  - Sporadic: No definite loss of tumor suppressor gene
- Associated abnormalities
  - Major source of morbidity in NF1
  - Frequently causes obstructive hydrocephalus
  - Gross appearance and clinical impact varies with location

Staging, Grading, & Classification

- WHO grade I

Gross Pathologic & Surgical Features

- Well-circumscribed, soft, gray mass ± cyst

Microscopic Features

- Classic "biphasic" pattern of 2 astrocyte populations
  - Compacted bipolar cells with Rosenthal fibers
  - Loose-textured multipolar cells with microcysts, eosinophilic granular bodies
- Highly vascular with glomeruloid features
- May have aggressive features, but still grade I tumor
- MIB-1 proliferation index ~ 1%

CLINICAL ISSUES

Presentation

- Most common signs/symptoms
  - Headache, nausea, and vomiting (consequence of hydrocephalus and increased intracranial pressure)
  - Visual loss (optic pathway lesions)
  - Ataxia, cerebellar signs (cerebellar lesions)
- Clinical profile
  - "Middle-aged" child, 5-15 years old
  - Prolonged duration of symptoms on close inquiry: Months to years

Demographics

- Age
  - > 80% under 20 years
  - Peak incidence: 5-15 years of age
    - Older than children with medulloblastoma
- Gender
  - M = F
- Epidemiology
  - 5-10% of all gliomas
  - Most common primary brain tumor in children (up to 25% of total)

Natural History & Prognosis

- Slowly growing, mass effect accommodated
  - Rarely spontaneously involute without treatment or after partial resection or biopsy
- Tumor may spread through subarachnoid space in rare cases (but is still WHO grade I)
- Median survival rates at 20 years > 70%
- Rare reports of malignant features associated with prior radiation therapy

Treatment

- Cerebellar or hemispheric: Resection
  - Adjuvant chemotherapy or radiation only if residual progressive unresectable tumor
- Optic/chiasmatic/hypothalamic: Often none
  - Stable or slowly progressive tumors watched
  - Debulking or palliative surgery considered after vision loss
  - Radiation or chemotherapy for rapidly progressive disease

DIAGNOSTIC CHECKLIST

Consider

- Cerebellar or supratentorial cyst + enhancing nodule in child, most likely PA
- Generally not reasonable diagnostic consideration in adults
- Rarely presents with CSF metastatic disease or as hemorrhagic mass

Image Interpretation Pearls

- Differentiate cerebellar lesions from medulloblastoma
  - PA arises from hemisphere, compresses 4th ventricle, circumscribed, DWI similar to GM
- Aggressive appearance of PA is misleading
  - Enhancing intraaxial tumor with cystic change in child is most likely PA
- MRS pattern of PA is contradictory to clinical behavior

SELECTED REFERENCES

1. Qaddoumi I et al: Pediatric low-grade gliomas and the need for new options for therapy: Why and how? Cancer Biol Ther. 8(1), 2009
2. Fisher PG et al: Outcome analysis of childhood low-grade astrocytomas. Pediatr Blood Cancer. 51(2):245-50, 2008
3. Rozen WM et al: Spontaneous regression of low-grade gliomas in pediatric patients without neurofibromatosis. Pediatr Neurosurg. 44(4):324-8, 2008
4. Burger PC et al: Pilocytic astrocytoma. In Louis DN et al: Tumours of the Central Nervous System. Lyon: IARC Press. 14-21, 2007

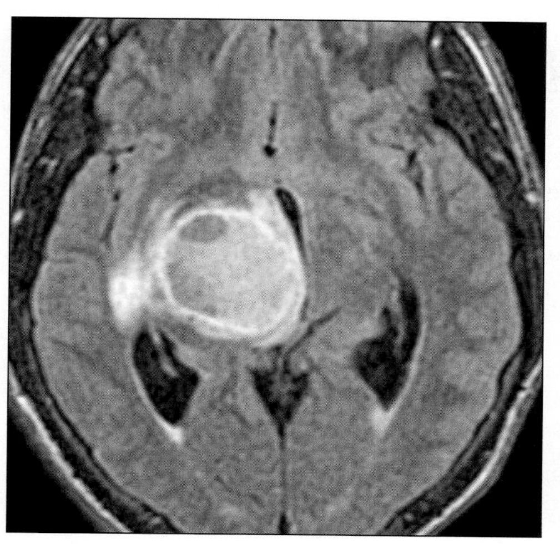

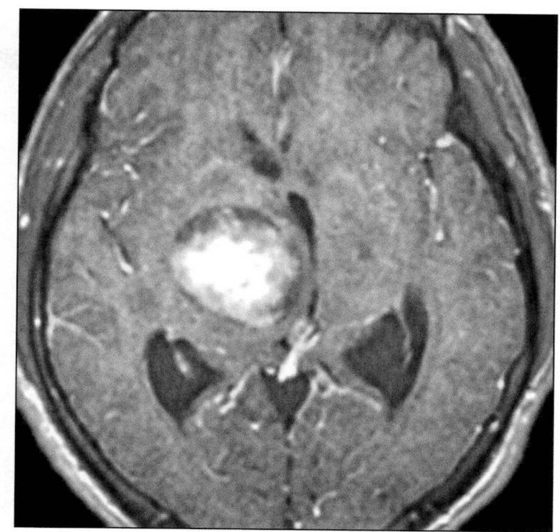

(Left) *Axial FLAIR MR shows a heterogeneously hyperintense thalamic mass with mild peritumoral edema and associated hydrocephalus.* ***(Right)*** *Axial T1WI C+ MR in the same patient shows intense central enhancement of the discrete tumor. PAs are most common in the posterior fossa (60%) and optic nerve/ chiasm (25-30%). Within the supratentorial brain, pilocytic astrocytomas are commonly adjacent to the 3rd ventricle. The cystic and solid appearance is typical of these WHO grade I tumors.*

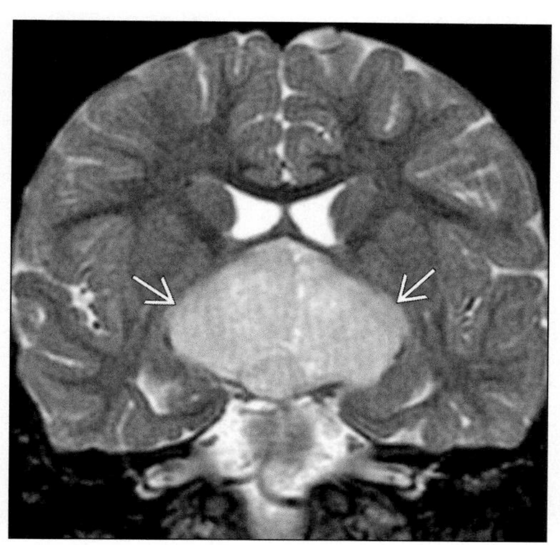

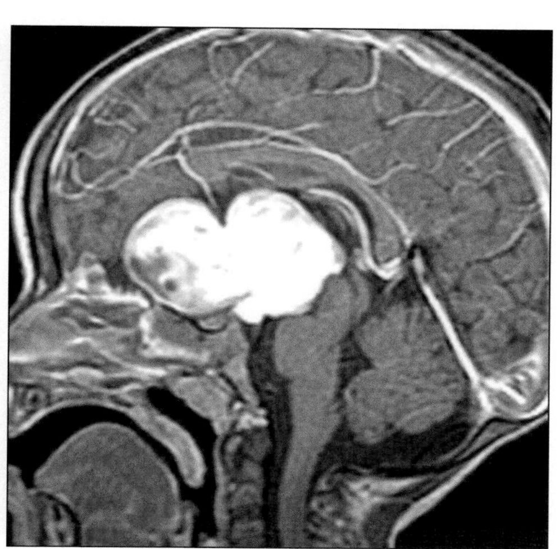

(Left) *Coronal T2WI MR shows a markedly hyperintense hypothalamic/ chiasmatic mass ➔ with no surrounding edema.* ***(Right)*** *Sagittal T1WI C+ MR in the same patient shows intense enhancement of the hypothalamic/chiasmatic PA in this teenager with visual symptoms. Hypothalamic/ chiasmatic tumors have variable enhancement. Optic pathway PAs are highly associated with neurofibromatosis type 1: Up to 1/3 of patients with an optic pathway PA have neurofibromatosis type 1.*

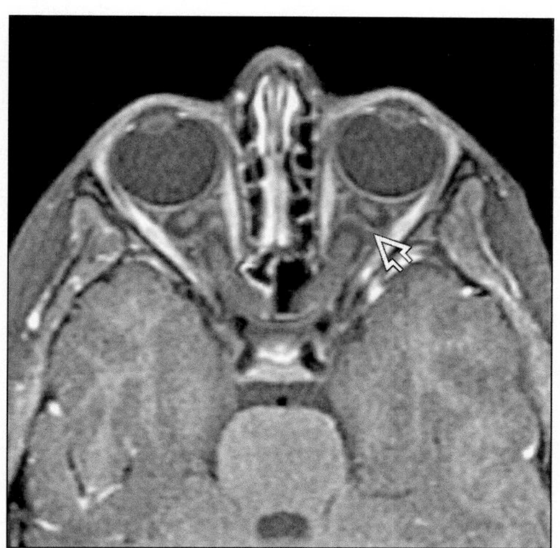

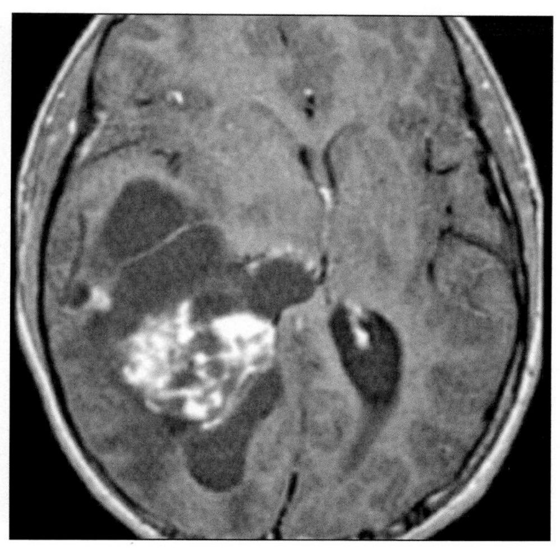

(Left) *Axial T1WI C+ MR with fat saturation in an NF1 patient with bilateral optic nerve gliomas shows the characteristic "dotted i" appearance of the intraorbital optic nerves ➔, caused by buckling of the elongated nerve just proximal to the globe.* ***(Right)*** *Axial T1WI C+ MR shows a large, cystic, and solid mass in a child. Note the associated mass effect. The large size and heterogeneous enhancement might suggest a more aggressive histology. At resection, this proved to be a WHO grade I PA.*

PILOMYXOID ASTROCYTOMA

Key Facts

Terminology

- Pilomyxoid astrocytoma (PMA) = more aggressive, myxoid variant of pilocytic astrocytoma (PA)
  - High risk of local recurrence, CSF dissemination

Imaging

- 60% suprasellar (large, bulky H-shaped mass in hypothalamus/optic chiasm, medial temporal lobes)
- 40% outside diencephalon (hemisphere, ventricles)
- Grossly well circumscribed, little/no edema
- Enhances strongly
- 20% show intratumoral hemorrhage

Top Differential Diagnoses

- Pilocytic astrocytoma
- Low-grade diffuse astrocytoma
- Glioblastoma multiforme

Pathology

- WHO grade II (typical PA is WHO grade I)

Clinical Issues

- Typical: Infants, young children (< 4 years)
- Less common: Older children, young adults
- 5-10% of cases initially diagnosed as PAs may actually be PMAs
  - Especially if tumor is hemorrhagic, presents in very young child, or shows CSF dissemination

Diagnostic Checklist

- PMA if
  - Infant or young child has large/bulky or hemorrhagic H-shaped suprasellar mass
  - Presumed PA in any patient who has atypical imaging (i.e., hemorrhage, metastases)

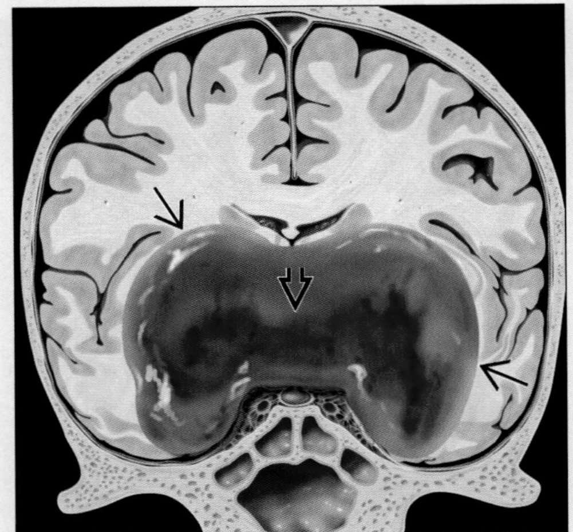
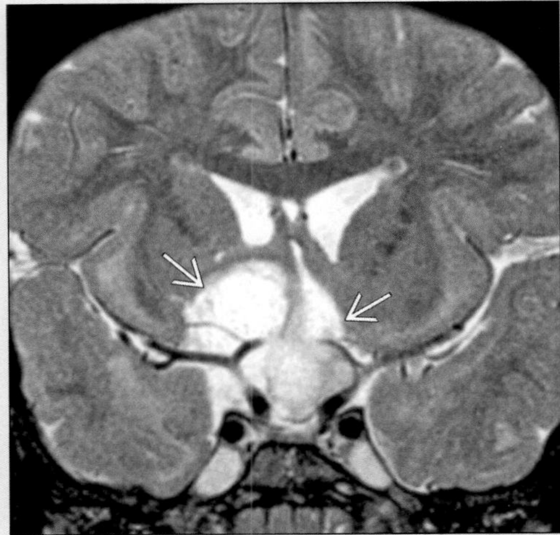

(Left) *Coronal graphic depicts pilomyxoid astrocytoma (PMA). Note the large, bulky H-shaped mass ⇒ centered on the hypothalamic/chiasmatic region & extending into both temporal lobes. The tumor is relatively well circumscribed and shows little/no edema. Glistening myxoid matrix is typical. Hemorrhage ⇒ occurs in about 20% of PMAs but is unusual in classic pilocytic astrocytoma (PA).* ***(Right)*** *Coronal T2WI MR shows well-circumscribed PMA ➡ in an 8 month old. Imaging is indistinguishable from classic PA.*

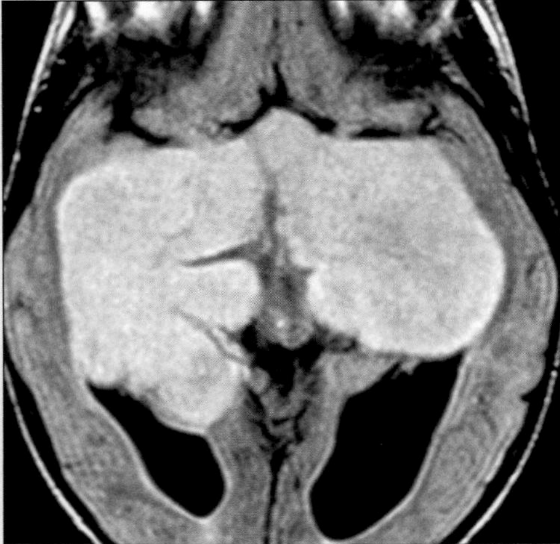
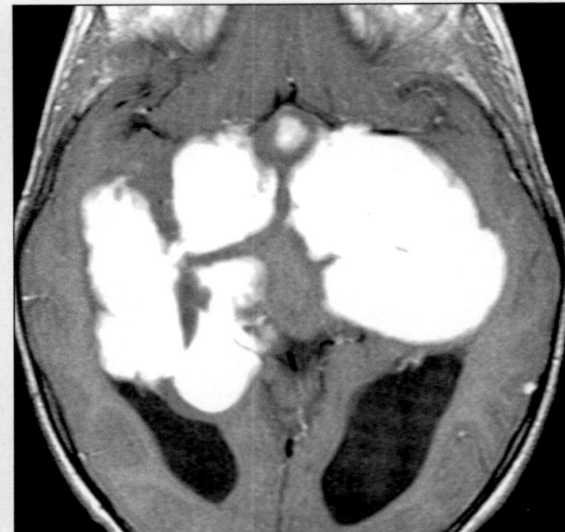

(Left) *Axial FLAIR MR in a 3 year old shows a large H-shaped suprasellar mass with extension into the basal ganglia and both medial temporal lobes. The tumor is quite well delineated despite its size and shows no evidence for surrounding edema.* ***(Right)*** *Axial T1WI C+ MR in the same patient shows intense, uniform enhancement. Biopsy disclosed neoplastic piloid cells in the mucinous matrix, consistent with PMA. MIB-1 was elevated, consistent with this more aggressive variant. (Courtesy R. Hewlett, PhD.)*

PILOMYXOID ASTROCYTOMA

TERMINOLOGY

Abbreviations

- Pilomyxoid astrocytoma (PMA)
- Myxoid variant of pilocytic astrocytoma (PA)

Definitions

- Tumor with monomorphic piloid cells dispersed in mucopolysaccharide-rich matrix
  - More aggressive tumor than PA with high risk of local recurrence, dissemination

IMAGING

General Features

- Best diagnostic clue
  - Infant or young child with large, bulky H-shaped mass in hypothalamus/optic chiasm, medial temporal lobes
- Location
  - 60% suprasellar
    - Optic chiasm, hypothalamus
    - Extension into adjacent structures is common with larger tumors
    - Deep gray nuclei, temporal lobes, adjacent white matter often involved
  - 40% centered **outside** diencephalon!
    - Cerebral hemispheres
      - 2nd most common general location
      - Temporal lobe most common
      - May be purely cortical
    - Less common sites reported
      - Midbrain
      - Cerebellum
      - 4th ventricle
      - Spinal cord
- Size
  - Variable
    - Mean = 4 cm
    - Often large, bulky (up to 12 cm)
- Morphology
  - Grossly well circumscribed

CT Findings

- NECT
  - Uniform hypodensity most common
  - 20% show intratumoral hemorrhage
    - Hyperdense
    - Mixed hypo-/hyperdense
  - Ca++ occurs but uncommon
- CECT
  - Strong but inhomogeneous enhancement
  - Irregular central nonenhancing area in 1/3

MR Findings

- T1WI
  - Typical: Uniformly hypointense (almost 2/3 of cases)
  - Less common: Mixed hypo-/hyperintensity (10-15%)
  - Uncommon: Blood-fluid level
- T2WI
  - 70% uniformly hyperintense
  - 15% inhomogeneously hyperintense
  - 10% hypointense center, hyperintense rim
- FLAIR
  - 50% uniformly hyperintense
  - 33% heterogeneously hyperintense
  - Relatively well-demarcated margins
  - Little or no peritumoral edema
- T2* GRE
  - Intratumoral hemorrhage in 20%
  - May be strikingly hypointense
- DWI
  - Typically does not restrict
- T1WI C+
  - Strong but heterogeneous enhancement
    - 50% heterogeneous (i.e., rim)
    - 40% solid, homogeneous
    - 10% no enhancement
  - Basilar/spinal meningeal enhancement is common and indicates CSF dissemination

Other Modality Findings

- MRS
  - ↑ Cho, ↓ Cr and NAA, ± lactate
  - Some authors report "low metabolite" pattern with ↓ Cho, Cr, NAA
- Angiography
  - Avascular

Imaging Recommendations

- Best imaging tool
  - MR with T1WI C+, DWI, T2* (GRE or SWI), MRS
- Protocol advice
  - Thin-section sagittal, coronal pre- and post-contrast T1WI
  - Whole brain FLAIR
  - Thin-section T2WI through hypothalamus, chiasm
  - GRE or SWI (to look for hemorrhage)
  - Optional: Add DWI, MRS

DIFFERENTIAL DIAGNOSIS

Pilocytic Astrocytoma

- Older children (mean age at diagnosis 6 years)
- In hypothalamus, typically enhances strongly/uniformly
- Occasionally calcified
- Clinically indolent, rarely aggressive
- Rarely hemorrhages
- CSF dissemination uncommon
- ↑ Cho, ↓ Cr and NAA
  - Note: Some PMAs show low metabolite concentrations

Low-Grade Diffuse Astrocytoma

- Peak age 20-45 years
- Cerebral hemispheres, brainstem > diencephalon
- Does not enhance

Glioblastoma Multiforme

- Hemorrhage, necrosis common
- Hypothalamus rare location
- Patients usually older
- May arise from lower grade astrocytoma

PILOMYXOID ASTROCYTOMA

PATHOLOGY

General Features

- Etiology
  - Unknown
  - Some tumors demonstrate synaptophysin reactivity, suggesting PMAs may be of mixed glioneuronal origin
  - May also originate from tanycytic cells
- Genetics
  - Cytogenetics demonstrates chromosome 17 insertion with disruption of *BCR* gene
- Associated abnormalities
  - A few cases associated with neurofibromatosis type 1 have been reported

Staging, Grading, & Classification

- WHO grade II (PA is WHO grade I)
- MIB-1 indices generally 1-2%

Gross Pathologic & Surgical Features

- Large, grossly well-circumscribed mass
- Necrosis, hemorrhage may be present

Microscopic Features

- Lacks classic "biphasic" pattern seen in PAs
  - Alternating solid and loose areas interspersed with microcysts not seen
  - Rosenthal fibers, eosinophilic granular bodies absent
- Consists of monomorphic piloid tumor cells
  - Embedded in myxoid (mucopolysaccharide-rich) matrix
  - GFAP(+), vimentin(+)
- Conspicuous angiocentric growth pattern (perivascular rosettes)
  - Vascular proliferation may be marked
  - Infiltration of tumor cells into adjacent brain common

CLINICAL ISSUES

Presentation

- Most common signs/symptoms
  - Signs of ↑ intracranial pressure
    - Headache
    - Nausea, vomiting
  - Delayed development
  - Failure to thrive (so-called diencephalic syndrome)
  - Visual disturbances
  - Hypothalamic dysfunction
- Other signs/symptoms
  - Seizures
  - Focal neurologic deficit

Demographics

- Age
  - Typical: Infants, young children (< 4 years)
  - Less common: Older children, young adults
  - Rare: Middle-aged adult (up to 46 years)
- Gender
  - Slight male predominance (M:F = 4:3)
- Epidemiology
  - Rare; represent < 1% of astrocytomas
  - 5-10% of cases initially diagnosed as PAs may be PMAs, especially if hemorrhage present or tumor presents in very young child

Natural History & Prognosis

- Higher recurrence rate than PA
- CSF dissemination common

Treatment

- Partial resection + adjuvant therapy may prolong survival

DIAGNOSTIC CHECKLIST

Consider

- Pilomyxoid astrocytoma if
  - Infant or young child has large/bulky or hemorrhagic suprasellar mass
  - Imaging atypical for PA (i.e., hemorrhage)
- "Pilocytic astrocytoma" with repeated recurrences, CSF dissemination? Review histopathology and consider PMA!

Image Interpretation Pearls

- H-shaped suprasellar mass may be PMA

SELECTED REFERENCES

1. Amatya VJ et al: Clinicopathological and immunohistochemical features of three pilomyxoid astrocytomas: comparative study with 11 pilocytic astrocytomas. Pathol Int. 59(2):80-5, 2009
2. Buccoliero AM et al: Occipital pilomyxoid astrocytoma in a 14-year-old girl--case report. Clin Neuropathol. 27(6):373-7, 2008
3. Komotar RJ et al: Magnetic resonance imaging characteristics of pilomyxoid astrocytoma. Neurol Res. 30(9):945-51, 2008
4. Linscott LL et al: Pilomyxoid astrocytoma: expanding the imaging spectrum. AJNR Am J Neuroradiol. 29(10):1861-6, 2008
5. Brat DJ et al: Newly codified glial neoplasms of the 2007 WHO Classification of Tumours of the Central Nervous System: angiocentric glioma, pilomyxoid astrocytoma and pituicytoma. Brain Pathol. 17(3):319-24, 2007
6. Ceppa EP et al: The pilomyxoid astrocytoma and its relationship to pilocytic astrocytoma: report of a case and a critical review of the entity. J Neurooncol. 81(2):191-6, 2007
7. Morales H et al: Magnetic resonance imaging and spectroscopy of pilomyxoid astrocytomas: case reports and comparison with pilocytic astrocytomas. J Comput Assist Tomogr. 31(5):682-7, 2007
8. Komotar RJ et al: Astrocytoma with pilomyxoid features presenting in an adult. Neuropathology. 26(1):89-93, 2006
9. Melendez B et al: BCR gene disruption in a pilomyxoid astrocytoma. Neuropathology. 26(5):442-6, 2006
10. Cirak B et al: Proton magnetic resonance spectroscopic imaging in pediatric pilomyxoid astrocytoma. Childs Nerv Syst. 21(5):404-9, 2005
11. Komotar RJ et al: Pilomyxoid astrocytoma of the spinal cord: report of three cases. Neurosurgery. 56(1):191, 2005
12. Chikai K et al: Clinico-pathological features of pilomyxoid astrocytoma of the optic pathway. Acta Neuropathol (Berl). 108(2):109-14, 2004

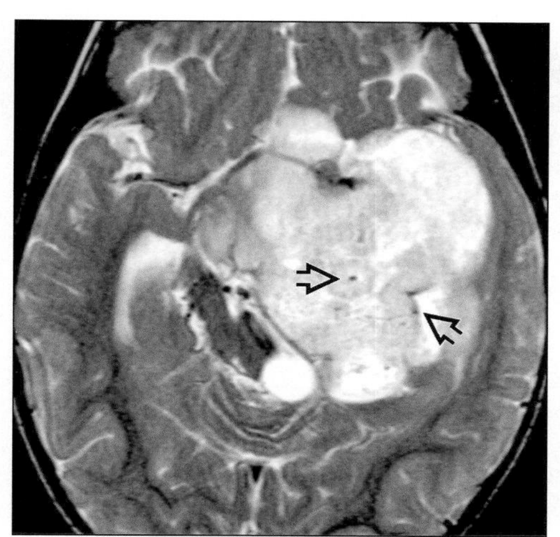

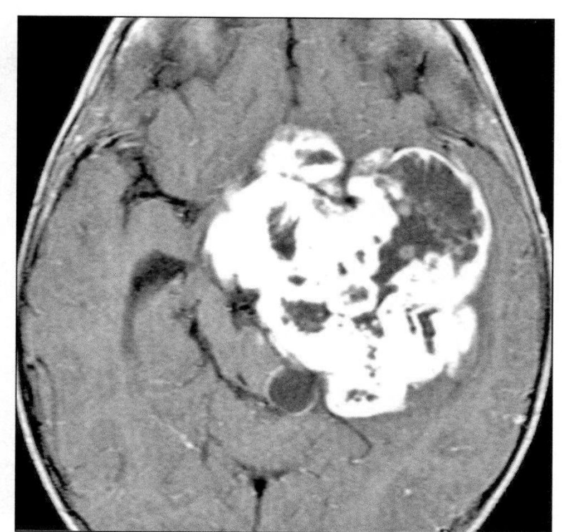

(Left) *Axial T2WI MR in a 20 month old shows a huge bulky suprasellar and medial temporal lobe mass. Scattered foci of T2 shortening within the mass may represent hemorrhage (no T2* imaging was performed.)* ***(Right)*** *Axial T1WI C+ MR in the same patient shows mixed solid and rim enhancement. Biopsy disclosed elongated "piloid" cells in a mucin-rich matrix consistent with PMA. (Courtesy R. Hewlett, PhD.)*

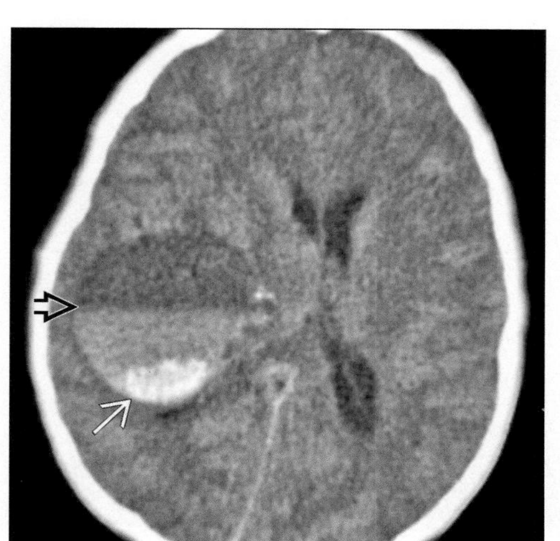

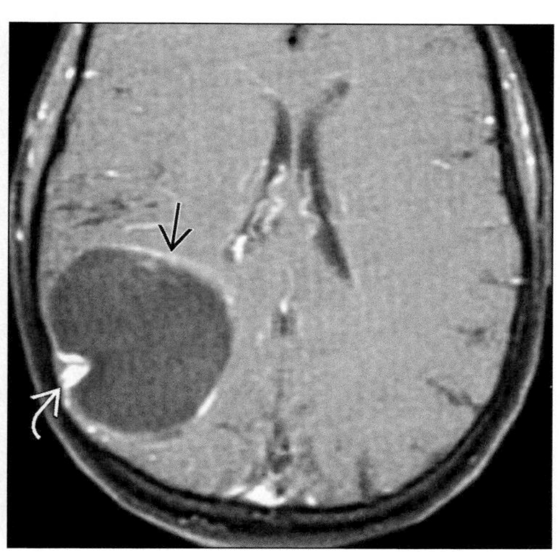

(Left) *Axial NECT in a 24-year-old man shows a right parietal mass with a fluid-fluid level and debris in the dependent portion of this cystic, hemorrhagic mass. PMA was found at histological examination of the surgically resected mass.* ***(Right)*** *Axial T1WI C+ FS MR in a 31-year-old woman with "head-shaking" seizures shows a cystic mass with nodular and rim enhancement. No edema was seen on T2WI or FLAIR. PMA with an elevated MIB-1 index was found at micropathology.*

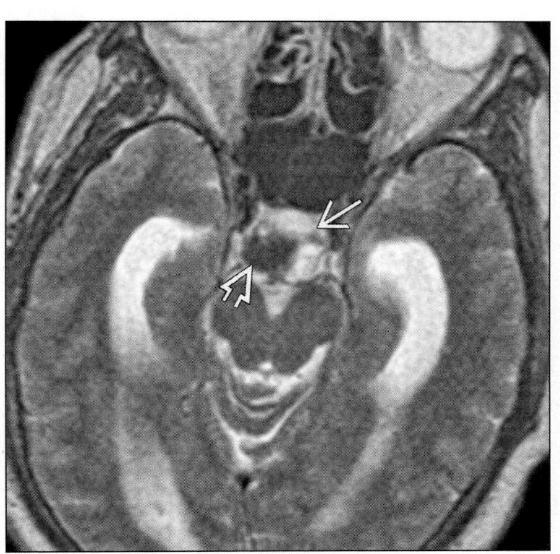

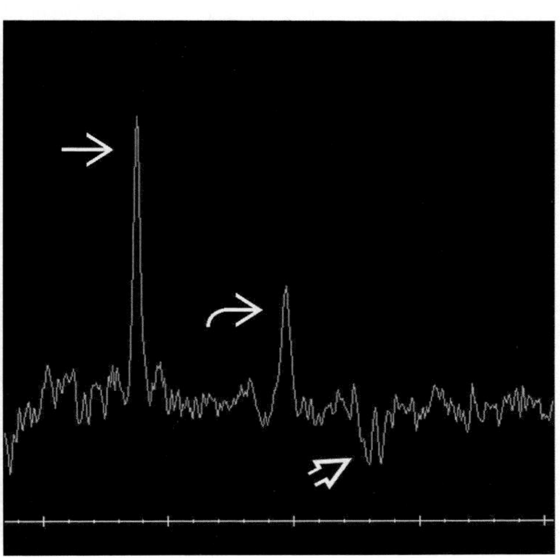

(Left) *Axial T2WI MR in a patient with sudden severe headache shows a mixed signal suprasellar mass with hemorrhage. Moderate obstructive hydrocephalus is present; the preoperative diagnosis was thrombosed aneurysm or pituitary apoplexy; & surgery disclosed a necrotic, hemorrhagic mass arising from the optic pathway. Initial diagnosis was PA; further review disclosed PMA.* ***(Right)*** *MRS (TE 144) from large suprasellar PMA shows elevated Cho, decreased NAA, lactate doublet.*

PLEOMORPHIC XANTHOASTROCYTOMA

Key Facts

Terminology
- Astrocytic neoplasm with generally favorable prognosis in children and young adults

Imaging
- Peripherally located hemispheric mass, often involves cortex and meninges
  - Temporal lobe most common
- Supratentorial cortical mass with adjacent enhancing dural "tail"
  - Cyst and enhancing mural nodule typical
  - Enhancing nodule often abuts pial surface

Top Differential Diagnoses
- Ganglioglioma
- Pilocytic astrocytoma
- Dysembryoplastic neuroepithelial tumor (DNET)
- Oligodendroglioma
- Meningioma

Pathology
- WHO grade II

Clinical Issues
- Majority of patients have longstanding epilepsy, often partial complex seizures (temporal lobe)
  - Rare but important cause of temporal lobe epilepsy
- Tumor of children and young adults, majority < 18 years
- Represent < 1% of all astrocytomas
- Surgical resection is treatment of choice

Diagnostic Checklist
- Cortical mass and meningeal thickening in a young adult with long seizure history? Think PXA!
- Ganglioglioma may mimic PXA clinically and by imaging

*(**Left**) Coronal graphic shows a cystic and solid cortical mass with thickening of the adjacent meninges ➔, characteristic of PXA. The mural nodule often abuts the pial surface and may result in a dural "tail." Thinning of the adjacent calvarium is rare. (**Right**) Coronal T1 C+ MR shows a classic PXA as an enhancing cystic and solid temporal lobe mass in a young seizure patient. Note that the mass touches the dura, and there is a subtle dural "tail" ➔. Surgical resection is the treatment of choice.*

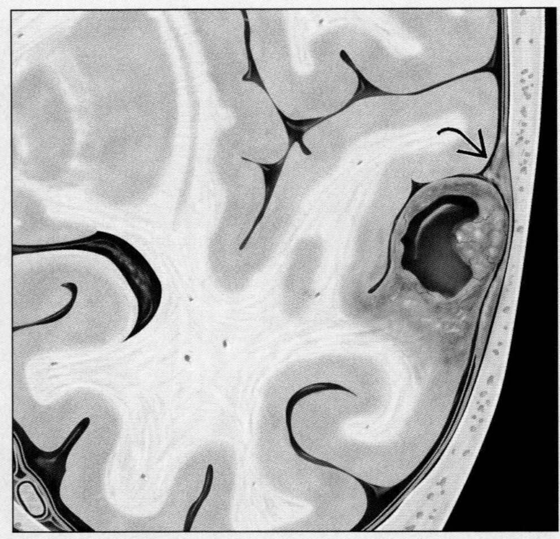

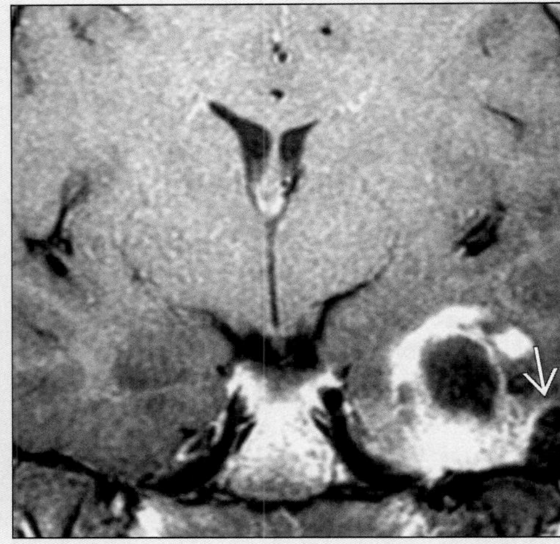

*(**Left**) Axial T2WI MR shows a cystic ➔ and solid ➔ temporal lobe mass in a 6-year-old girl with epilepsy. (**Right**) Axial T1WI C+ MR in the same patient shows marked enhancement ➔ of the solid portions of the mass. Note the relative lack of surrounding edema and mass effect, characteristic of PXA. The imaging differential diagnosis includes ganglioglioma and pilocytic astrocytoma. Enhancement along the meninges helps make an accurate preoperative diagnosis.*

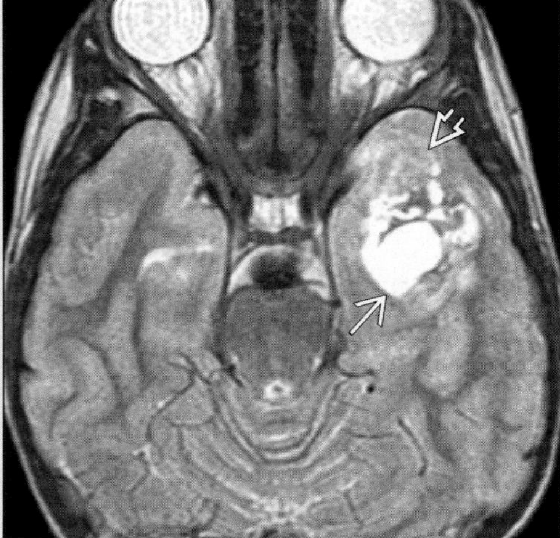

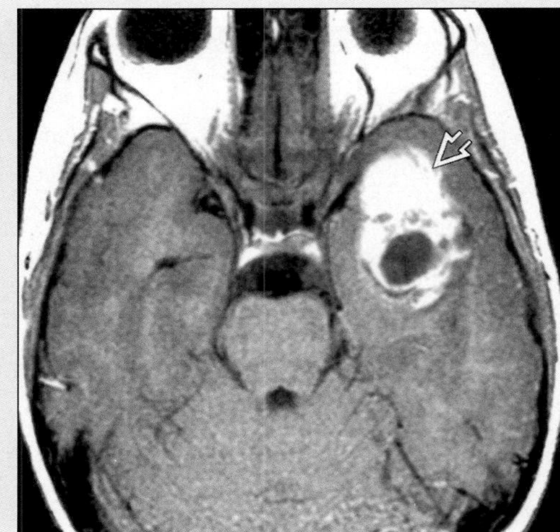

TERMINOLOGY

Abbreviations

- Pleomorphic xanthoastrocytoma (PXA)

Definitions

- Astrocytic neoplasm with generally favorable prognosis in children and young adults
  - Superficial location in cerebral hemispheres with involvement of meninges

IMAGING

General Features

- Best diagnostic clue
  - Supratentorial cortical mass with adjacent enhancing dural "tail"
  - Cyst and enhancing mural nodule typical
- Location
  - Peripherally located hemispheric mass, often involves cortex and meninges
    - 98% supratentorial
  - Temporal lobe most common
    - Parietal > occipital > frontal lobes
  - Rarely found in cerebellum, sella, spinal cord, retina
- Size
  - Variable
- Morphology
  - 50-60% cyst + mural nodule that abuts meninges (may be solid)
  - Discrete round to oval mass typical (may be ill defined)
  - Despite circumscribed appearance, tumor often infiltrates into brain and perivascular spaces

CT Findings

- NECT
  - Cystic/solid mass: Hypodense with mixed density nodule
  - Solid mass: Variable; hypodense, hyperdense, or mixed
  - Minimal or no edema is typical
  - Ca++, hemorrhage, frank skull erosion (rare)
- CECT
  - Strong, sometimes heterogeneous enhancement of tumor nodule

MR Findings

- T1WI
  - Mass is hypo- or isointense to gray matter
  - Mixed signal intensity may be seen
  - Cystic portion isointense to CSF
  - Associated cortical dysplasia may be seen (rare)
- T2WI
  - Hyperintense or mixed signal intensity mass
  - Cystic portion isointense to CSF
  - Surrounding edema (rare)
- FLAIR
  - Hyperintense or mixed signal intensity mass
  - Cystic portion isointense to CSF
- T1WI C+
  - Enhancement usually moderate/strong, well delineated
  - Enhancement of adjacent meninges, dural "tail" common (approximately 70%)
    - Enhancing nodule often abuts pial surface
  - Rare: Deep tumor extension, distant metastases

Angiographic Findings

- Typically avascular
- Vascular blush may indicate necrotic or aggressive PXA

Nuclear Medicine Findings

- PET
  - FDG PET may show hypermetabolic foci even in low-grade PXA

Imaging Recommendations

- Best imaging tool
  - Multiplanar MR is most sensitive
  - CT may be helpful for calvarial changes
- Protocol advice
  - Contrast-enhanced MR including coronal images to better evaluate temporal lobes

DIFFERENTIAL DIAGNOSIS

Ganglioglioma

- Cortically based hemispheric mass, solid/cystic, or solid
- Mural nodule typical, often not adjacent to meninges
- Variable enhancement, no enhancing dural "tail"
- Ca++ is common; may remodel calvarium

Pilocytic Astrocytoma

- Supratentorial location other than hypothalamus/ chiasm is rare
- Typically solid and cystic or solid mass
- Enhancement but no dural "tail"

Dysembryoplastic Neuroepithelial Tumor (DNET)

- Superficial cortical tumor, well demarcated
- Multicystic "bubbly" appearance
- T2 hyperintense mass with rare, mild enhancement
- May remodel calvarium

Oligodendroglioma

- Heterogeneous, Ca++ mass
- Typically larger and more diffuse than PXA
- May remodel/erode calvarium

Meningioma

- Diffusely enhancing dural-based mass with dural "tail"
- Usually older patients

Low-Grade Astrocytoma (Grade II)

- Demarcated but infiltrative white matter mass
- No enhancement

PATHOLOGY

General Features

- Etiology
  - May originate from cortical (subpial) astrocytes

PLEOMORPHIC XANTHOASTROCYTOMA

- May arise from multipotential neuroectodermal precursor cells common to both neurons and astrocytes or from preexisting hamartomatous lesions
- Genetics
  - No definite association with hereditary tumor syndromes
  - Rare reports of PXA in neurofibromatosis type 1 and Sturge-Weber patients
  - PXA with *TP53* mutations reported
- Associated abnormalities
  - PXA may occur with ganglioglioma and oligodendroglioma (rare)
  - PXA reported with DNET and atypical teratoid-rhabdoid tumor
  - Synchronous, multicentric PXA lesions are rare
  - May be associated with cortical dysplasia

Staging, Grading, & Classification

- WHO grade II
- PXA with anaplastic features
  - Significant mitoses (5 or more per 10 HPF) &/or necrosis
  - Has been associated with poorer prognosis
    - Increased recurrence and decreased survival
  - Some classify these PXA as WHO grade III

Gross Pathologic & Surgical Features

- Cystic mass with mural nodule abutting meninges
- May be completely solid
- Leptomeningeal adhesion/attachment is common
- Dural invasion is rare
- Deep margin may show infiltration of parenchyma

Microscopic Features

- Superficial, circumscribed astrocytic tumor noted for cellular pleomorphism and xanthomatous change
- "Pleomorphic" appearance
  - Fibrillary and giant multinucleated neoplastic astrocytes
  - Large xanthomatous (lipid-containing) cells are GFAP positive
  - Dense reticulin network
  - Lymphocytic infiltrates
- Tumor sharply delineated from cortex, but infiltration may be seen
- Some positive for synaptophysin, neurofilament proteins, S100 protein
- CD34 antigen may help differentiate PXA from other tumors
- Necrosis, mitotic figures rare/absent
  - MIB-1 index generally < 1%

CLINICAL ISSUES

Presentation

- Most common signs/symptoms
  - Majority with longstanding epilepsy, often partial complex seizures (temporal lobe)
  - Other signs/symptoms: Headache, focal neurologic deficits

Demographics

- Age
  - Tumor of children and young adults
    - Typically 1st 3 decades
    - 2/3 < 18 years
    - Ranges from 2-82 years, mean 26 years
- Gender
  - No definite gender predominance
- Epidemiology
  - < 1% of all astrocytomas
  - Rare but important cause of temporal lobe epilepsy

Natural History & Prognosis

- Usually circumscribed, slow growing
- Recurrence of tumor is uncommon
- Hemorrhage is rare complication
- Survival 70% at 10 years
- Malignant transformation in 10-25% of cases
- Extent of resection and mitotic index are most significant predictors of outcome
- Aggressive PXA with malignant progression, dissemination occasionally occurs

Treatment

- Surgical resection is treatment of choice
- Repeat resection for recurrent tumors
- Radiation therapy and chemotherapy show mild improvement in outcome in some cases

DIAGNOSTIC CHECKLIST

Consider

- Cortical mass and meningeal thickening in young adult with long seizure history? Think PXA!
- Ganglioglioma may mimic PXA clinically and by imaging

Image Interpretation Pearls

- Meningioma-like lesion in young patient should raise suspicion of PXA

SELECTED REFERENCES

1. Wind JJ et al: Pleomorphic xanthoastrocytoma presenting with life-threatening hemorrhage in a child. J Neurosurg Pediatr. 3(2):157-9, 2009
2. Ng WH et al: Pleomorphic xanthoastrocytoma in elderly patients may portend a poor prognosis. J Clin Neurosci. 15(4):476-8, 2008
3. Ishizawa K et al: A neuroepithelial tumor showing combined histological features of dysembryoplastic neuroepithelial tumor and pleomorphic xanthoastrocytoma--a case report and review of the literature. Clin Neuropathol. 26(4):169-75, 2007
4. Louis DN et al: WHO Classification of Tumours of the Central Nervous System: Pleomorphic xanthoastrocytoma. Lyon: IARC Press. 22-24, 2007
5. Kilickesmez O et al: Coexistence of pleomorphic xanthoastrocytoma with Sturge-Weber syndrome: MRI features. Pediatr Radiol. 35(9):910-3, 2005
6. Koeller KK et al: From the archives of the AFIP: superficial gliomas: radiologic-pathologic correlation. Armed Forces Institute of Pathology. Radiographics. 21(6):1533-56, 2001

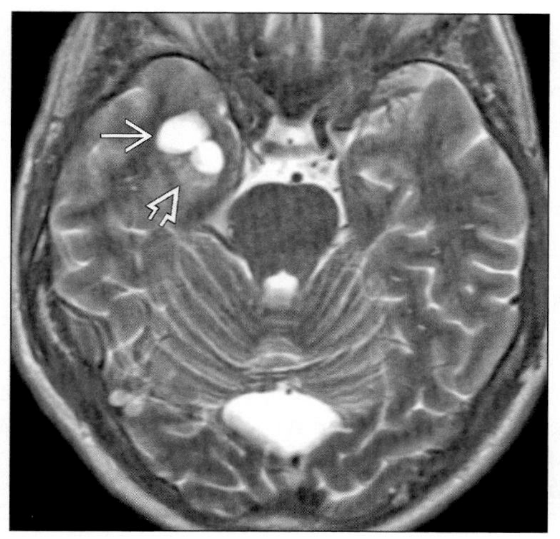

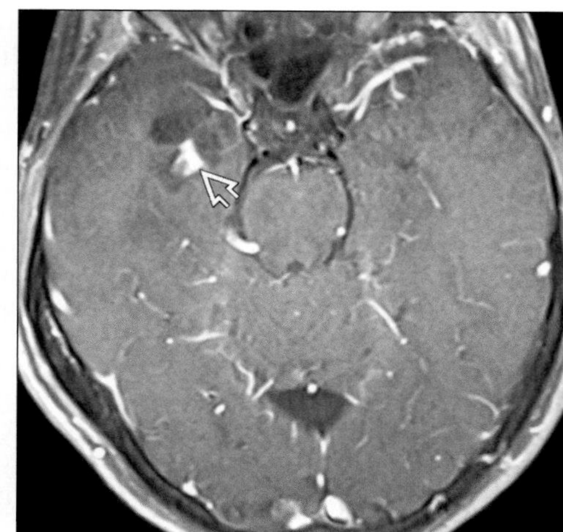

(Left) *Axial T2WI MR in an epilepsy patient shows a cystic & solid temporal lobe mass with no significant mass effect or surrounding edema.* ***(Right)*** *Axial T1 C+ FS MR in the same patient shows minimal nodular enhancement of the mass. Imaging differential diagnosis includes ganglioglioma, pilocytic astrocytoma, PXA, & DNET. However, this proved to be PXA, WHO grade II at resection. Coronal imaging is often helpful to better visualize the presence of meningeal involvement that is typical of PXA.*

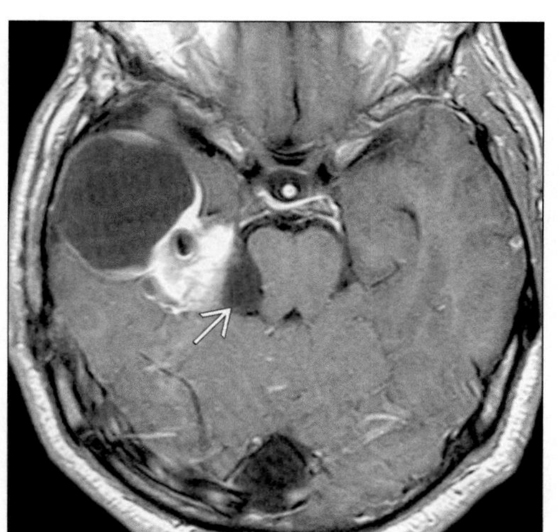

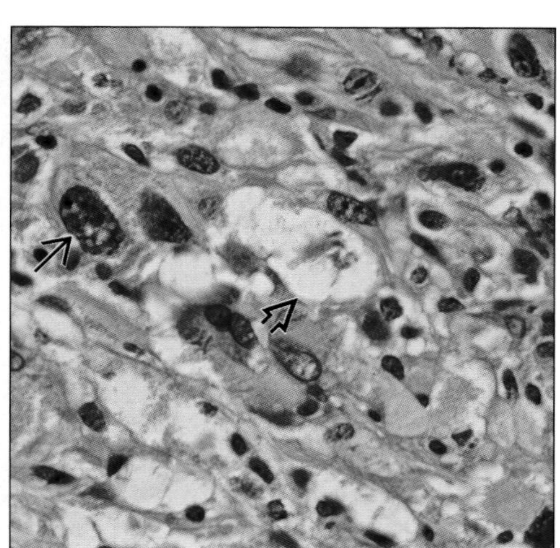

(Left) *Axial T1WI C+ MR shows a solid and cystic temporal lobe mass related to a recurrent PXA. Note the extraaxial portion with mass effect on the adjacent midbrain.* ***(Right)*** *H&E micropathology from the same patient shows conspicuous pleomorphism of the tumor with multinucleated giant cells and vacuolation, characteristic for PXA, WHO grade II. Malignant transformation occurs in 10-25% of cases. (Courtesy R. Hewlett, PhD.)*

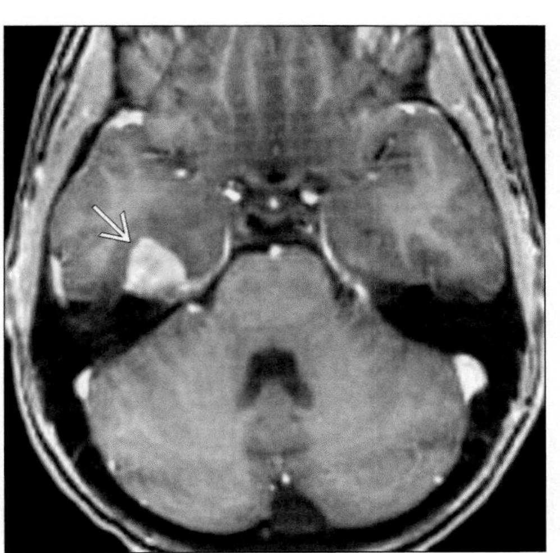

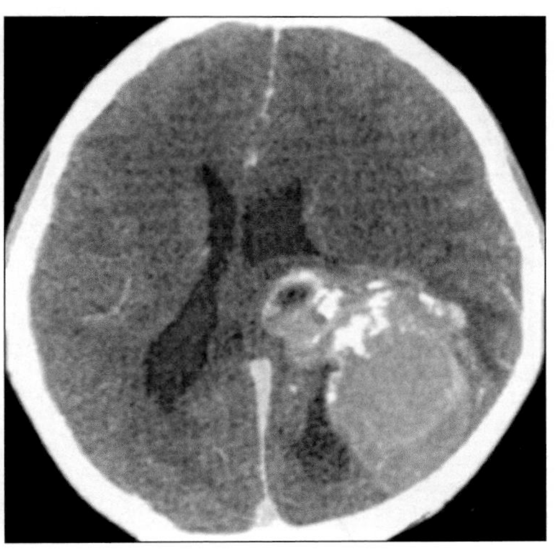

(Left) *Axial T1WI C+ MR shows homogeneous enhancement of a cortically based mass, a PXA at resection. Imaging mimics a ganglioglioma, as solid enhancement of a PXA is uncommon.* ***(Right)*** *Axial CECT shows a large, mixed density, partially calcified, parietooccipital mass with patchy enhancement. This was classified as PXA with anaplastic features, WHO grade III at resection, and the tumor had a high mitotic rate. These anaplastic tumors are uncommon and associated with a poor prognosis.*

SUBEPENDYMAL GIANT CELL ASTROCYTOMA

Key Facts

Terminology

- Subependymal giant cell astrocytoma (SGCA)
- Benign, slow-growing glioneuronal tumor in patient with tuberous sclerosis complex (TSC)
  - Arises near foramen of Monro

Imaging

- General findings
  - Enlarging, enhancing mass near foramen of Monro in patient with TSC
  - Other findings of TS (cortical tubers, SE nodules)

Top Differential Diagnoses

- Choroid plexus tumors
  - Choroid plexus papilloma > atypical choroid plexus papilloma, carcinoma
- Central neurocytoma
  - Body of lateral ventricle
- Astrocytoma
  - Pilocytic astrocytoma, chordoid glioma (rare)
- Subependymoma
  - Middle-aged, older adults
- Supratentorial PNET (rare)
  - Young child without TSC

Pathology

- SGCA probably arises from subependymal nodule in region of germinal matrix
- Likely represents disordered neuronal migration
- WHO grade I, curable with complete resection

Clinical Issues

- Most common CNS neoplasm in TSC
  - SGCA in up to 15% of patients with TSC
  - Rarely (if ever) arises in absence of TSC
- Typically occurs during 1st 2 decades

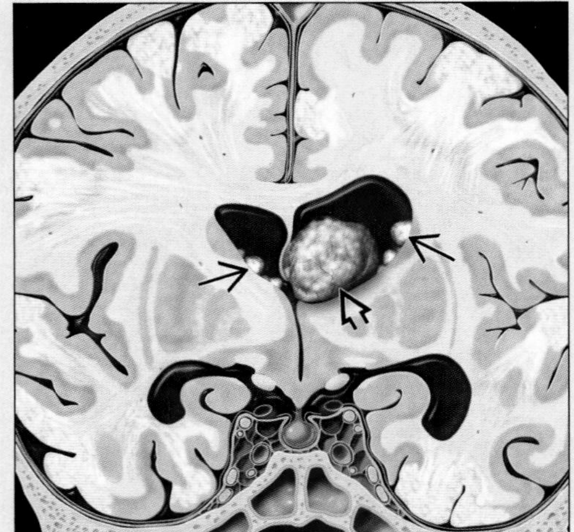

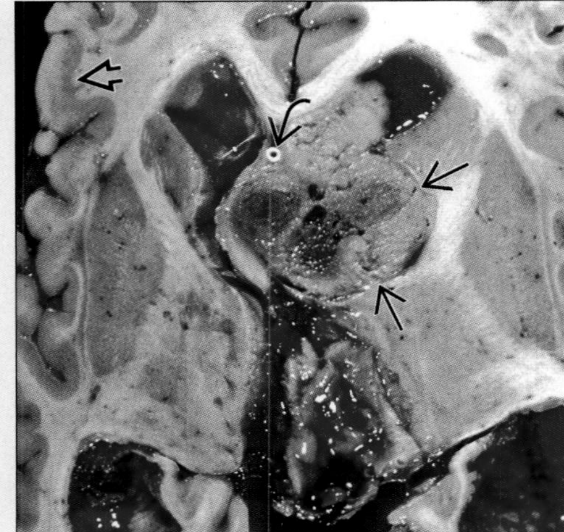

(Left) Coronal graphic demonstrates hydrocephalus secondary to a subependymal giant cell tumor arising near the left foramen of Monro ⇨. Note the subependymal tubers →. (Right) Axial section through the ventricles in a patient with tuberous sclerosis complex shows a large SGCA obstructing the foramen of Monro. Note the well-delineated tumor margins →. A cortical tuber ⇨ is also seen. Despite emergent ventricular shunting ↗, the ventricles were not decompressed successfully. (Courtesy R. Hewlett, PhD.)

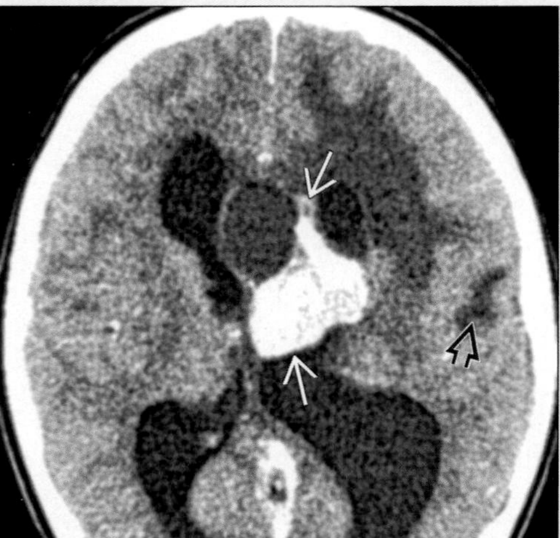

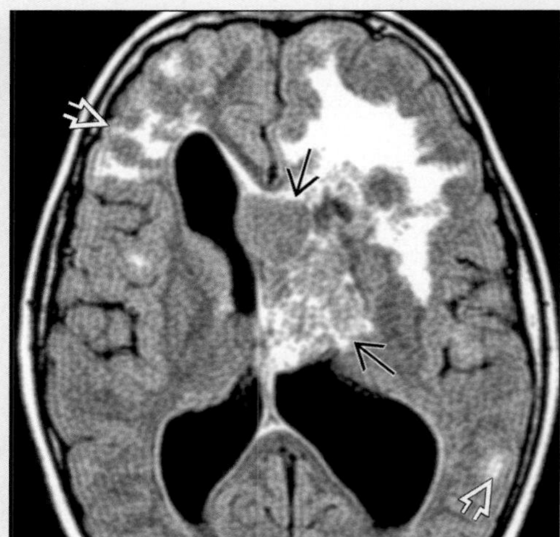

(Left) Axial NECT in a patient with tuberous sclerosis complex shows a large, partially calcified mass → that obstructs the foramen of Monro. Note the hypodense white matter lesion ⇨ underlying a cortical tuber. (Right) Axial FLAIR MR in the same patient shows that the mass is heterogeneously hyperintense →. Note the cortical tubers and subcortical white matter hyperintensities ⇨. Subependymal giant cell astrocytoma was found at surgery.

SUBEPENDYMAL GIANT CELL ASTROCYTOMA

TERMINOLOGY

Abbreviations

- Subependymal giant cell astrocytoma (SGCA)

Synonyms

- Intraventricular astrocytoma of tuberous sclerosis complex (TSC)

Definitions

- Benign, slow-growing glioneuronal tumor arising near foramen of Monro in patient with TSC

IMAGING

General Features

- Best diagnostic clue
  - Enlarging, enhancing foramen of Monro mass in patient with TSC
    - Other imaging findings of TSC (cortical tubers, subependymal nodules)
- Location
  - Almost always near foramen of Monro
- Size
  - Variable, slowly growing
  - Often presents when 2-3 cm, causes obstructive hydrocephalus
- Morphology
  - Well marginated, often lobulated
  - Frond-like margins

CT Findings

- NECT
  - Hypo- to isodense
  - Heterogeneous
  - Ca++ variable
  - Hydrocephalus
- CECT
  - Heterogeneous, strong enhancement
  - Presence of interval growth suggests SGCA
  - Initially tumor typically > 1 cm
- CT Perfusion
  - May be mildly hypervascular

MR Findings

- T1WI
  - Hypointense to isointense to GM
  - ± Ca++ (hyperintense to hypointense)
- T2WI
  - Heterogeneous
    - Isointense to hyperintense
  - Ca++ foci hypointense
  - Hydrocephalus
- PD/intermediate
  - Hyperintense
- FLAIR
  - Heterogeneously hyperintense
  - Periventricular interstitial edema from ventricular obstruction
- T2* GRE
  - Low signal from Ca++
- DWI
  - ADC values less than parenchymal hamartomas of TS
- T1WI C+
  - Robust enhancement
    - Enhancement alone does not allow discrimination from hamartoma
  - Enlarging, enhancing foramen of Monro mass larger than 1.2 cm suggests SGCA
  - CSF dissemination not seen
- MRS
  - Less than expected decrease in NAA due to some neuronal elements in this primarily glial neoplasm

Ultrasonographic Findings

- Intraoperative
  - Hyperechoic intraventricular mass
  - Heterogeneous shadowing foci of Ca++

Angiographic Findings

- Conventional
  - Variable vascularity
  - ± stretched thalamostriate veins (hydrocephalus)

Imaging Recommendations

- Best imaging tool
  - MR demonstrates extent of mass, delineates associated TSC features
- Protocol advice
  - FLAIR MR to detect subtle CNS features of TSC
  - Recommend brain MR with contrast every 1-2 years for SGCA follow-up

DIFFERENTIAL DIAGNOSIS

Choroid Plexus Tumors

- Choroid plexus papilloma
- Choroid plexus carcinoma
  - Vivid enhancement
  - ± CSF seeding
  - Parenchymal invasion and peritumoral edema with choroid plexus carcinoma

Astrocytoma

- Origin: Septum pellucidum fornices or medial basal ganglia
  - Common pediatric intraaxial neoplasm
  - Variable enhancement, Ca++ rare

Germinoma

- Hugs midline, often arises near 3rd ventricle
- May originate from basal ganglia, resemble SGCA
- Early CSF spread

Subependymoma

- Tumor of middle-aged, elderly
- Inferior 4th/frontal horn of lateral ventricle

Central Neurocytoma

- Well-defined, variably vascularized, lobulated mass
- Body of lateral ventricle > foramen of Monro or septum pellucidum
- Necrosis, cyst formation are common
- Seen in young adults

Supratentorial PNET

- May exophytically extend into ventricle
- Lack of peritumoral edema
- Highly cellular tumor, isointense → slightly hyperintense on T2WI

PATHOLOGY

General Features

- Etiology
  - SGCA probably arises from subependymal nodule in region of germinal matrix
  - Likely represents disordered neuronal migration complex
- Genetics
  - 50% of TSC patients have positive family history
    - High rate of de novo mutations
  - In affected kindreds
    - Inheritance: Autosomal dominant
    - High penetrance
    - Considerable phenotypic variability
  - Molecular genetics
    - 2 distinct TSC loci (chromosome 9q on *TSC1* and 16p on *TSC2*)
    - *TSC1* and *TSC2* are likely tumor suppressor genes
- Associated abnormalities
  - Other CNS, extraneural manifestations of TSC

Staging, Grading, & Classification

- WHO grade I

Gross Pathologic & Surgical Features

- Well-marginated mass arising from lateral ventricular wall near foramen of Monro
  - ± cysts, Ca++, and hemorrhage
- Does not seed CSF pathways

Microscopic Features

- Tumor cells of SGCAs show wide spectrum of astroglial phenotypes
  - Giant pyramidal ganglioid astrocytes
  - Perivascular pseudopalisading
- Histology may be indistinguishable from subependymal nodules
  - Diagnosis based on size and growth
- Immunohistochemistry
  - Variable immunoreactivity for GFAP, S100
  - Glial, neuronal antigen expression variable

CLINICAL ISSUES

Presentation

- Most common signs/symptoms
  - Increased intracranial pressure secondary to tumor obstructing foramen of Monro
    - Headache, vomiting, loss of consciousness
  - Other signs/symptoms
    - Worsening epilepsy
    - Massive spontaneous hemorrhage
- Clinical profile
  - Patient with TSC develops signs and symptoms of ventricular obstruction
  - Worsening of epilepsy

Demographics

- Age
  - SGCA typically occurs during 1st 2 decades
  - Mean age = 11 years
- Uncommon reports of congenital cases
- No race or gender predilection
- Epidemiology
  - 1.4% of all pediatric brain tumors
  - Most common CNS neoplasm in TSC
    - Incidence of SGCA: Up to 15% of patients with TSC
    - Rarely (if ever) arises in absence of TSC

Natural History & Prognosis

- Solitary, slow-growing, benign tumor
- Symptoms from ventricular obstruction
- Good outcome and low recurrence rate with complete resection
- Rarely, massive spontaneous hemorrhage

Treatment

- Surgical resection (open vs. endoscopic)
- Massive hemorrhage possible complication

DIAGNOSTIC CHECKLIST

Consider

- SGCA in tuberous sclerosis patient with worsening seizures &/or symptoms of ventricular obstruction

Image Interpretation Pearls

- Enlarging, enhancing, intraventricular mass near foramen of Monro in TSC patient
- Foramen of Monro mass and associated intraventricular hemorrhage

SELECTED REFERENCES

1. Buccoliero AM et al: Subependymal giant cell astrocytoma (SEGA): Is it an astrocytoma? Morphological, immunohistochemical and ultrastructural study. Neuropathology. 29(1):25-30, 2009
2. Khayal IS et al: Characterization of low-grade gliomas using RGB color maps derived from ADC histograms. J Magn Reson Imaging. 30(1):209-13, 2009
3. Voykov B et al: When tuberous sclerosis complex becomes an emergency. Can J Ophthalmol. 44(2):220-1, 2009
4. Jozwiak J et al: Possible mechanisms of disease development in tuberous sclerosis. Lancet Oncol. 9(1):73-9, 2008
5. Phi JH et al: Congenital subependymal giant cell astrocytoma: clinical considerations and expression of radial glial cell markers in giant cells. Childs Nerv Syst. 24(12):1499-503, 2008
6. Ess KC et al: Developmental origin of subependymal giant cell astrocytoma in tuberous sclerosis complex. Neurology. 64(8):1446-9, 2005
7. Koeller KK et al: From the archives of the AFIP. Cerebral intraventricular neoplasms: radiologic-pathologic correlation. Radiographics. 22(6):1473-505, 2002
8. Nishio S et al: Tumours around the foramen of Monro: clinical and neuroimaging features and their differential diagnosis. J Clin Neurosci. 9(2):137-41, 2002

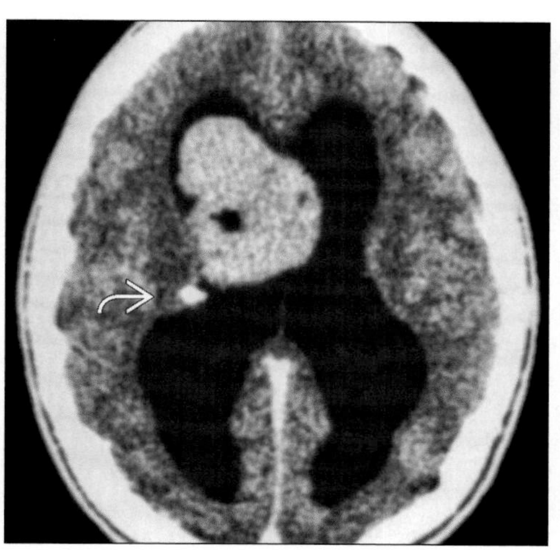

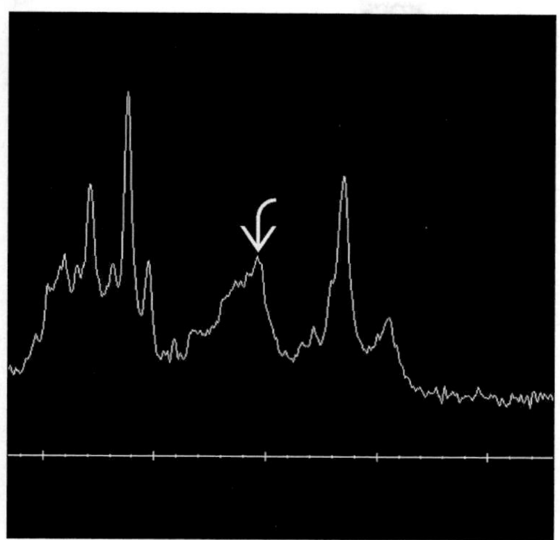

(Left) *Axial CECT shows a moderate subependymal giant cell astrocytoma extending into the right frontal horn. Note the proximal small calcified subependymal nodule ➔, which indicates tuberous sclerosis complex.* ***(Right)*** *MRS in the same patient shows a relative decrease in N-acetyl aspartate (NAA) peak ➔ suggesting a predominantly glial phenotype in this mixed glioneuronal neoplasm.*

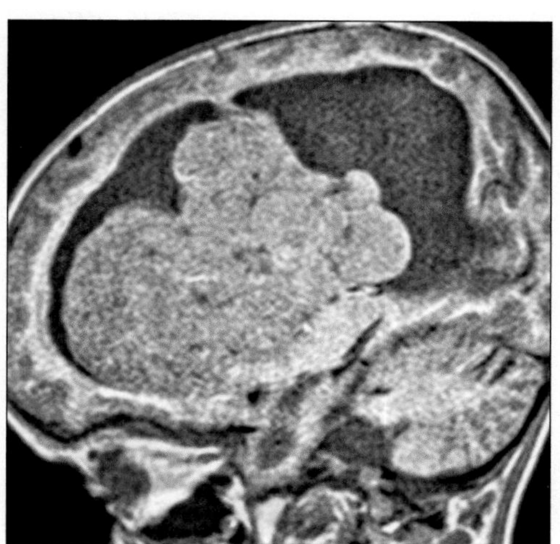

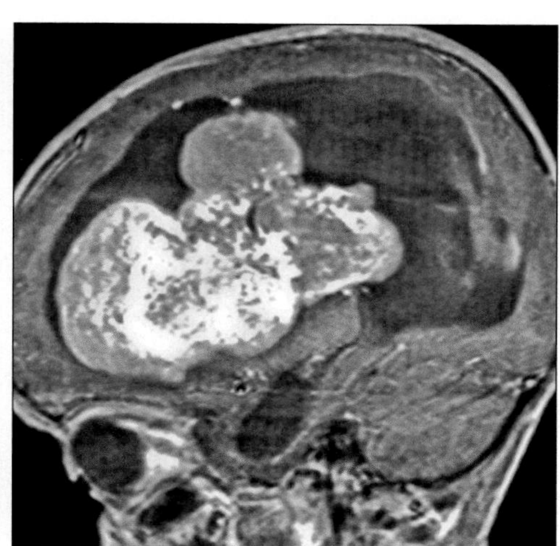

(Left) *Sagittal T1WI MR demonstrates an unusually large subependymal giant cell astrocytoma arising near the right foramen of Monro with marked hydrocephalus and extension into the lateral ventricles.* ***(Right)*** *Post-gadolinium image reveals diffuse but mildly heterogeneous enhancement in this subependymal giant cell astrocytoma, which is more than twice as large as many more typical cases.*

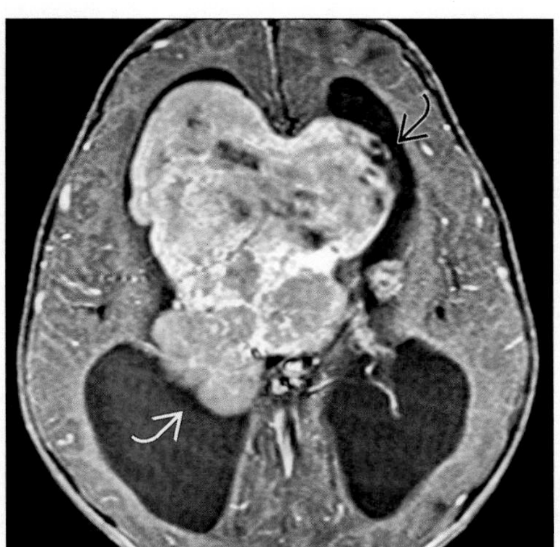

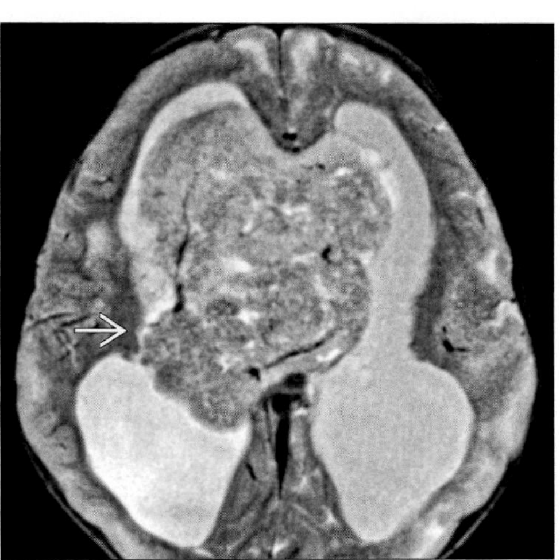

(Left) *Lobularity, heterogeneity, and some areas of nonenhancement are seen in this axial post-contrast image. There is marked hydrocephalus and extension into the contralateral frontal horn ➔, 3rd ventricle, and right more than the left lateral ventricles ➔.* ***(Right)*** *Prominent vascular flow voids and signal heterogeneity are present in this unusually large subependymal giant cell astrocytoma. Note the probable point of origin ➔ on the lateral ventricular. (Courtesy AFIP.)*

OLIGODENDROGLIOMA

Key Facts

Terminology
- Well-differentiated, slowly growing but diffusely infiltrating cortical/subcortical tumor

Imaging
- Most common site is frontal lobe (50-65%)
- Partially Ca++ subcortical/cortical frontal mass in middle-aged adult is best diagnostic clue
  - Typically T2 heterogeneous, hyperintense mass
- Approximately 50% enhance
  - Heterogeneous enhancement is typical

Top Differential Diagnoses
- Anaplastic oligodendroglioma (AO)
- Low-grade diffuse astrocytoma
- Ganglioglioma
- Dysembryoplastic neuroepithelial tumor (DNET)
- Pleomorphic xanthoastrocytoma (PXA)
- Cerebritis
- Cerebral ischemia

Pathology
- WHO grade II
- Loss of heterozygosity for 1p and 19q (50-70%)
- Anaplastic oligodendroglioma = WHO grade III

Clinical Issues
- 5-10% of primary intracranial neoplasms
- Seizures, headaches, focal neurologic deficits most common presentations
- Peak incidence 4th and 5th decades
- Median survival time = 10 years
- Loss of heterozygosity for 1p, 19q is associated with more favorable prognosis & better chemotherapy response

(Left) Axial graphic shows a heterogeneous cystic and solid mass involving the cortex and subcortical white matter, typical of oligodendroglioma. Note the deep infiltrative margin ➔ and calvarial remodeling ⇨. (Right) Axial FLAIR MR shows a hyperintense infiltrative mass expanding the frontal gyri in this young adult who presented with seizures and was diagnosed with grade II oligodendroglioma. The frontal lobe location and involvement of both cortex and subcortical white matter are typical findings.

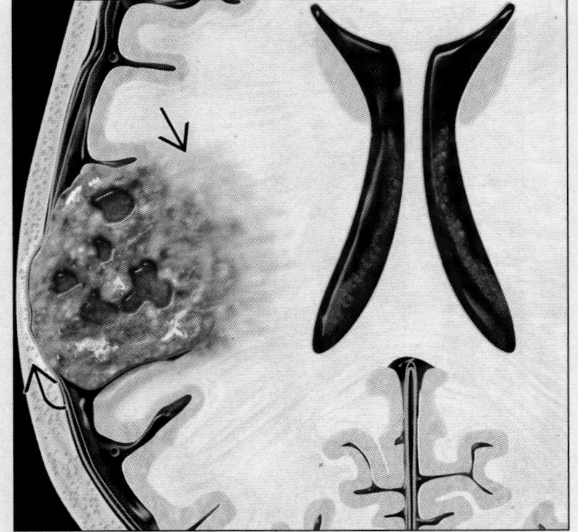

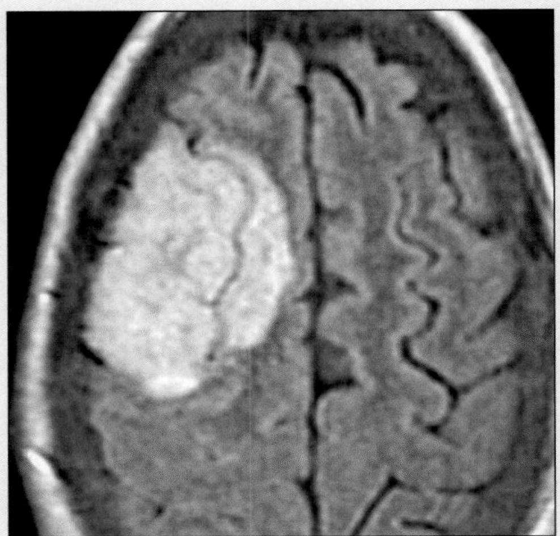

(Left) Axial NECT shows a large, calcified, right frontal lobe mass in a 36-year-old man. The vast majority of oligodendrogliomas (70-90%) show calcification. (Right) Axial T2WI MR in the same patient shows a heterogeneously hyperintense frontal lobe mass with calcification ➔ and cystic change ⇨. Note involvement of the cortex and subcortical white matter, typical of oligodendroglioma. Patients with deletions of 1p and 19q have a more favorable prognosis and better chemotherapy response.

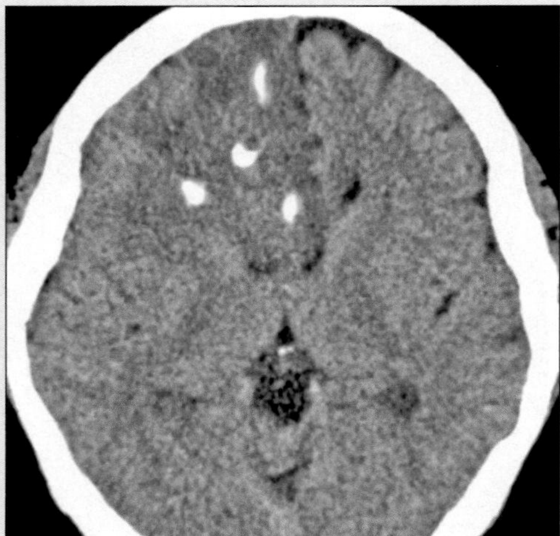

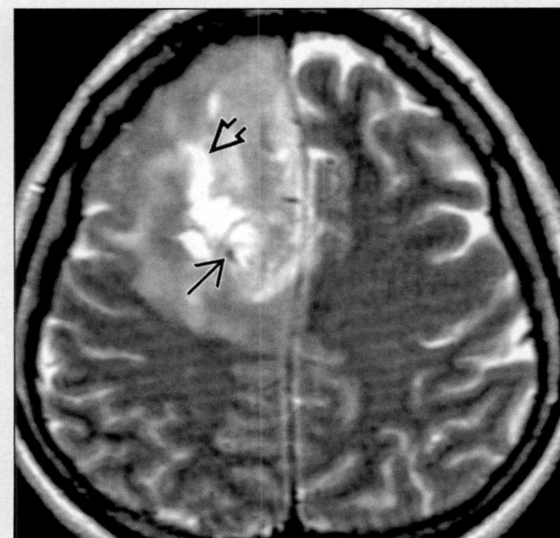

OLIGODENDROGLIOMA

TERMINOLOGY

Abbreviations

- Oligo, low-grade oligodendroglioma

Definitions

- Well-differentiated, slowly growing but diffusely infiltrating cortical/subcortical tumor

IMAGING

General Features

- Best diagnostic clue
  - Partially calcified subcortical/cortical mass in middle-aged adult
- Location
  - Typically involves subcortical white matter (WM) and cortex
  - Majority supratentorial (85%), hemispheric WM
    - Most common site is frontal lobe (50-65%)
    - May involve temporal, parietal, or occipital lobes
    - Rare: Posterior fossa
    - Extremely rare: Intraventricular, brainstem, spinal cord, primary leptomeningeal
- Morphology
  - Infiltrative mass that appears well demarcated

CT Findings

- NECT
  - Mixed density (hypo-/isodense) hemispheric mass that extends to cortex
  - Majority calcify, nodular or clumped Ca++ (70-90%)
  - Cystic degeneration common (20%)
  - Hemorrhage, edema are uncommon
  - May expand, remodel, erode calvarium
- CECT
  - Approximately 50% enhance
  - Enhancement varies from none to striking

MR Findings

- T1WI
  - Hemispheric mass, hypo- to isointense to gray matter
  - Typically heterogeneous
  - Cortical and subcortical with cortical expansion
  - May appear well circumscribed with minimal associated edema
- T2WI
  - Typically heterogeneous, hyperintense mass
    - Heterogeneity related to Ca++, cystic change, less commonly blood products
  - May appear well circumscribed with minimal associated edema
  - Typically expands overlying cortex
  - Hemorrhage, necrosis rare unless anaplastic
  - May expand, erode calvarium
- FLAIR
  - Typically heterogeneous, hyperintense
  - May appear well circumscribed but infiltrative
- T2* GRE
  - Ca++ seen as areas of "blooming"
- DWI
  - No diffusion restriction is typical
- T1WI C+
  - Heterogeneous enhancement is typical
  - Approximately 50% enhance
  - Rarely, leptomeningeal enhancement is seen
- MRS
  - ↑ Cho, ↓ NAA
  - Absence of lipid/lactate peak helps differentiate from anaplastic oligodendroglioma
- Perfusion MR
  - Relative CBV can help differentiate grade II from grade III
  - Foci of elevated rCBV can mimic high-grade tumor!

Nuclear Medicine Findings

- PET
  - FDG uptake similar to normal white matter
  - 11C-methionine studies show marked uptake differences between oligo and anaplastic oligo

Imaging Recommendations

- Best imaging tool
  - MR is most sensitive to delineate tumor
  - CT helpful for identifying Ca++
- Protocol advice
  - Contrast-enhanced MR with T2* GRE or SWI ± MRS, perfusion

DIFFERENTIAL DIAGNOSIS

Anaplastic Oligodendroglioma (AO)

- May require biopsy to distinguish
- MRS, perfusion, or PET may be helpful

Low-Grade Diffuse Astrocytoma

- Calcification less common
- Usually involves white matter, cortex relatively spared
- May be indistinguishable

Ganglioglioma

- Usually temporal lobe, cortical
- Sharply demarcated, cyst with enhancing nodule
- Ca++ common
- Childhood, young adult tumor

Dysembryoplastic Neuroepithelial Tumor (DNET)

- Sharply demarcated cortical neoplasm
- Heterogeneous, "bubbly" appearance
- Variable enhancement
- Childhood, young adult tumor

Pleomorphic Xanthoastrocytoma (PXA)

- Supratentorial cortical mass, dural "tail" common
- Often cyst and mural nodule, may be solid
- Enhancing nodule abuts pial surface
- Childhood, young adult tumor

Cerebritis

- T2 hyperintensity and patchy enhancement
- Diffusion restriction typical

Cerebral Ischemia

- Typical vascular distribution (MCA, ACA, PCA)

OLIGODENDROGLIOMA

- Diffusion restriction if acute/subacute
- Involves gray and white matter, often wedge-shaped
- Cortical, gyriform enhancement if subacute

Arteriovenous Malformation (AVM)

- Typically multiple enlarged flow voids
- Often calcified
- If thrombosed, may be indistinguishable

Herpes Encephalitis

- Confined to limbic system, temporal lobes
- Blood products and enhancement common
- Acute onset is typical

PATHOLOGY

General Features

- Etiology
  - Arises from neoplastic transformation of mature oligodendrocytes or immature glial precursors
- Genetics
  - Loss of heterozygosity for 1p and 19q (50-70%)
  - Familial cases have been reported
- Associated abnormalities
  - Oligoastrocytomas are common
    - Includes neoplastic cell types of both oligodendroglioma and diffuse astrocytoma
  - Majority of "intraventricular oligodendrogliomas" are central neurocytomas
  - Rarely occurs with other tumors, pleomorphic xanthoastrocytoma (PXA)
  - Rarely may be multifocal or multicentric
  - Oligodendroglial gliomatosis cerebri (rare)
  - Primary leptomeningeal oligodendrogliomatosis (extremely rare)

Staging, Grading, & Classification

- WHO grade II
- Anaplastic oligodendroglioma = WHO grade III
  - Mitoses, microvascular proliferation, ± necrosis
- Oligodendrogliomas carry better prognosis than astrocytomas of same grade

Gross Pathologic & Surgical Features

- Solid, infiltrative lesions of cortex/subcortical WM
- Well-defined, grayish-pink, soft, unencapsulated mass
- Ca++ frequent; ± cystic degeneration, hemorrhage

Microscopic Features

- Moderately cellular tumors with occasional mitoses
- Rounded, homogeneous nuclei and clear cytoplasm
  - "Fried egg" and "honeycomb" patterns probably artifactual, perinuclear halos
- May have dense network of branching capillaries
- MIB-1 < 5% (proliferation index)

CLINICAL ISSUES

Presentation

- Most common signs/symptoms
  - Seizures, headaches, focal neurologic deficits
  - Patients have relatively longstanding history of symptoms

Demographics

- Age
  - Peak incidence 4th and 5th decades
- Gender
  - Slight male predominance
- Epidemiology
  - 5-10% of primary intracranial neoplasms
  - 5-25% of all gliomas

Natural History & Prognosis

- More favorable outcome correlated with
  - Younger age
  - Frontal location
  - Lack of enhancement
  - Complete resection
  - Radiation therapy after partial resection
- Worse prognosis correlated with
  - Necrosis, increased cellularity
  - Mitotic activity, nuclear atypia
  - Cellular pleomorphism, microvascular proliferation
- Median survival time = 10 years
- 5-year survival rate 50-75%
- Local recurrence is common
- CSF seeding is uncommon
- Loss of heterozygosity for 1p, 19q associated with more favorable prognosis, better response to chemo

Treatment

- Surgical resection is primary treatment
- Adjuvant radiation therapy + chemotherapy

DIAGNOSTIC CHECKLIST

Consider

- Frontal lobe calcified mass? Think oligodendroglioma!
- Oligos may mimic cortically based masses (i.e., DNET), although these typically occur in younger patients

Image Interpretation Pearls

- Grade II oligos cannot be reliably differentiated from grade III (AO) on conventional imaging
- Oligos are most common intracranial tumor to calcify
- New enhancement in previously nonenhancing oligodendroglioma suggests malignant progression

SELECTED REFERENCES

1. Sepulveda Sanchez JM et al: Classification of oligodendroglial tumors based on histopathology criteria is a significant predictor of survival--clinical, radiological and pathologic long-term follow-up analysis. Clin Neuropathol. 28(1):11-20, 2009
2. Louis DN et al: WHO Classification of Tumours of the Central Nervous System: Oligodendroglioma. Lyon: IARC Press. 54-59, 2007
3. Spampinato MV et al: Cerebral blood volume measurements and proton MR spectroscopy in grading of oligodendroglial tumors. AJR Am J Roentgenol. 188(1):204-12, 2007

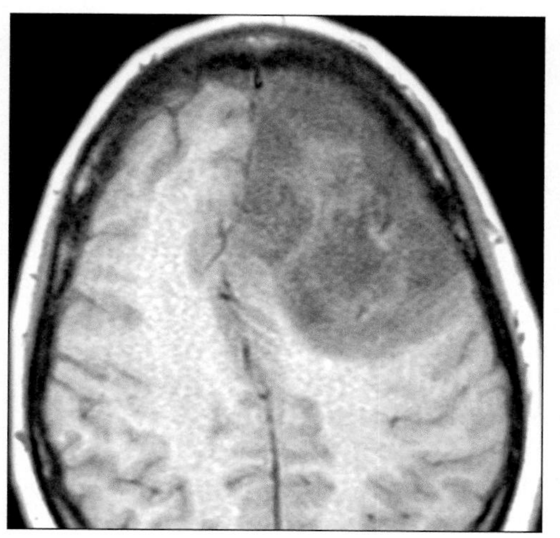

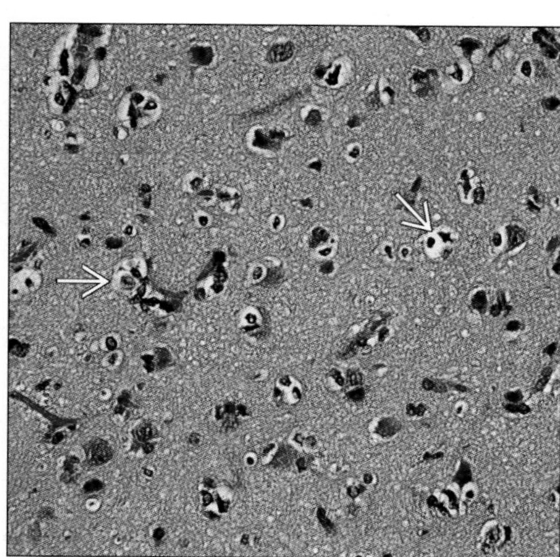

(Left) *Axial T1WI MR shows a hypodense mass involving a large portion of the frontal lobe. Note involvement of the cortex and deep white matter, typical of oligodendroglioma. Minimal enhancement was present along the deep margin of this tumor. About 50% of grade II oligodendrogliomas show enhancement.* ***(Right)*** *High-power micropathology from the same patient shows a classic "fried egg" appearance ➔ related to a perinuclear halo, characteristic for oligodendroglioma.*

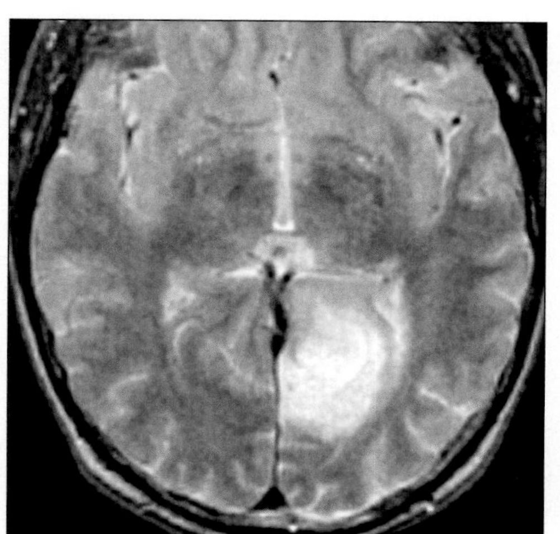

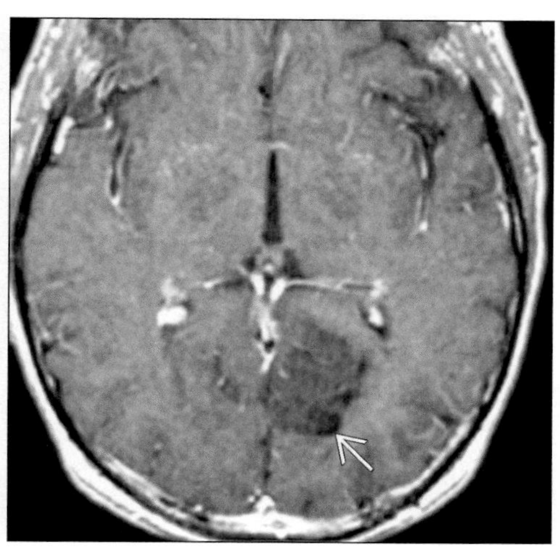

(Left) *Axial T2WI MR in a 43-year-old man with headaches shows a demarcated hyperintense mass with involvement of the cortex and subcortical white matter with mild associated mass effect. The imaging is characteristic of oligodendroglioma, despite the occipital lobe location.* ***(Right)*** *Axial T1WI C+ MR in the same patient shows the occipital mass with cystic change ➔ and no enhancement. Enhancement is variable in oligodendroglioma. New enhancement often indicates malignant progression.*

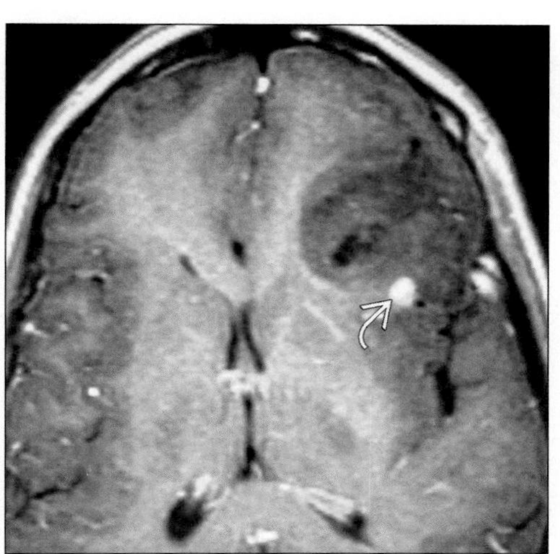

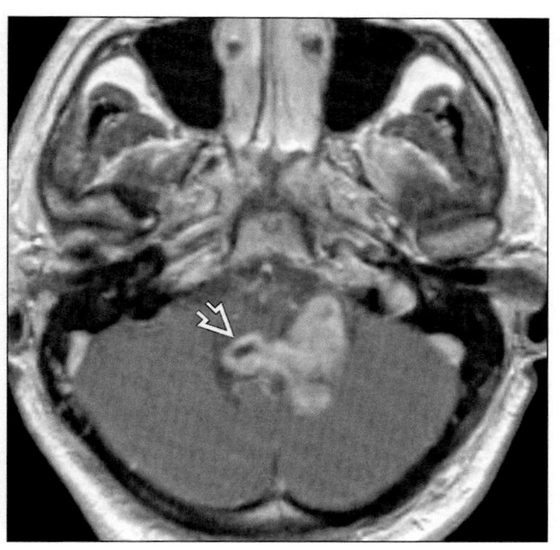

(Left) *Axial T1WI C+ MR shows focal nodular enhancement ➔ in this frontotemporal, grade II oligodendroglioma. Differentiating a grade II from a grade III oligodendroglioma is difficult on conventional imaging. MRS & MR perfusion may help predict the tumor grade preoperatively.* ***(Right)*** *Axial T1WI C+ MR shows a heterogeneously enhancing posterior fossa mass ➔ involving the 4th ventricle. Though imaging mimics an ependymoma, this was a grade II oligodendroglioma at resection.*

ANAPLASTIC OLIGODENDROGLIOMA

Key Facts

Terminology

- Oligodendroglioma with focal or diffuse histologic features of malignancy

Imaging

- Best diagnostic clue: Calcified frontal lobe mass involving cortex and subcortical white matter
  - Frontal lobe most common location, followed by temporal lobe
- Majority have nodular or clumped calcification
- May see hemorrhage or necrosis
- Variable enhancement
  - Anaplastic oligodendroglioma more likely to enhance than low-grade oligo
- Neoplastic cells almost always found beyond areas of abnormal signal intensity
- MRS and MR perfusion may help distinguish grade II from grade III oligos

Top Differential Diagnoses

- Oligodendroglioma
- Anaplastic astrocytoma (AA)
- Glioblastoma multiforme (GBM)
- Cerebritis
- Ischemia

Pathology

- WHO grade III

Clinical Issues

- Headache, seizures most common presentation
- Occurs at all ages; mean is 49 years
- 20-50% of oligodendrogliomas are anaplastic
- Median survival: 4 years
- 5-year survival: 40-45%; 10-year survival: 15%
- 1p and 19q loss of heterozygosity associated with prolonged survival

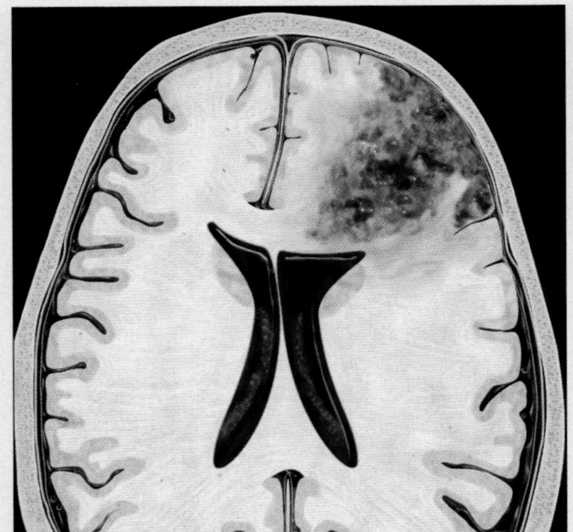

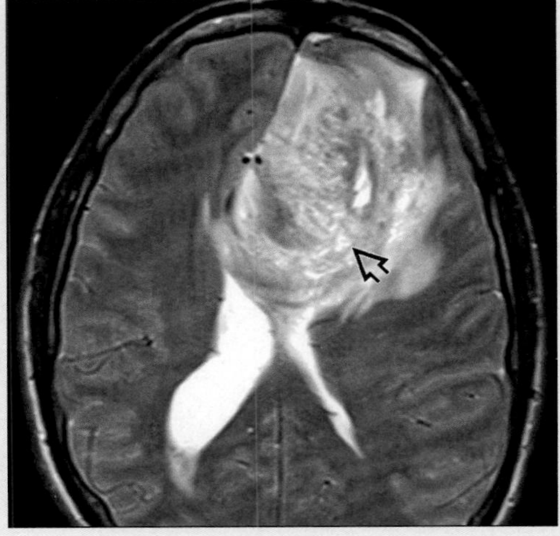

(Left) *Axial graphic shows a heterogeneous frontal cortical and subcortical mass with areas of necrosis and hemorrhage. Note the mass effect and infiltrative margins, typical of anaplastic grade III oligodendroglioma.* ***(Right)*** *Axial T2WI MR in a 31-year-old man with seizures shows a heterogeneously hyperintense frontal lobe mass with significant mass effect and associated hydrocephalus. The T2 heterogeneity is related to cystic change ⮚ and calcification. The calcification is better seen on CT or GRE MR. AO found at resection.*

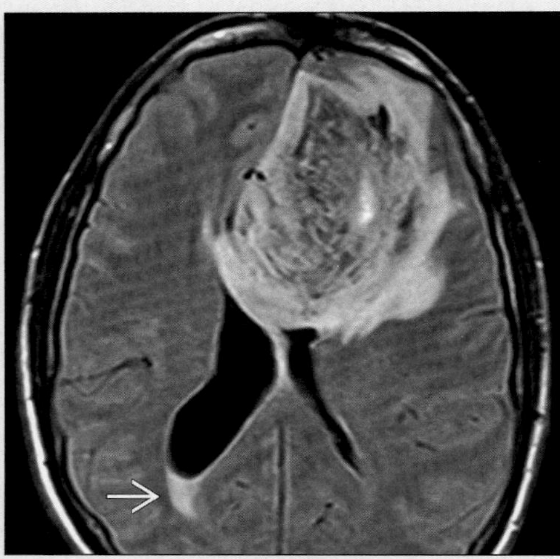

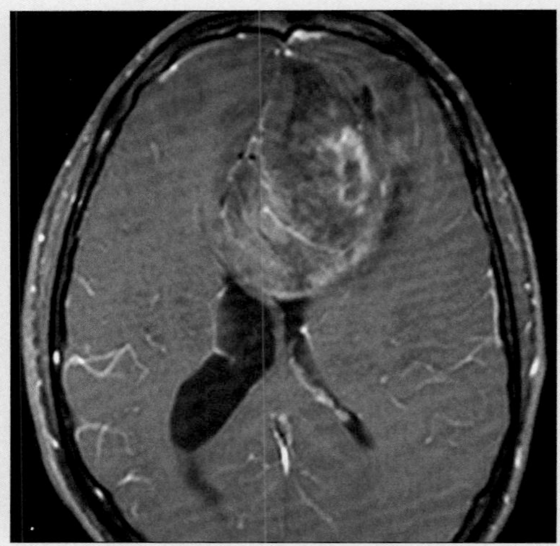

(Left) *Axial FLAIR MR in the same patient shows a heterogeneously hyperintense mass with significant mass effect and associated hydrocephalus. Note the transependymal flow of CSF ➡ and expansion of the overlying cortex.* ***(Right)*** *Axial T1WI C+ FS MR in the same patient shows heterogeneous enhancement of the large mass. Approximately 50% of all oligodendrogliomas enhance. Enhancement does not reliably differentiate between grade II and grade III oligodendrogliomas.*

ANAPLASTIC OLIGODENDROGLIOMA

TERMINOLOGY

Abbreviations

- Anaplastic oligodendroglioma (AO), high-grade oligodendroglioma (oligo)

Definitions

- Highly cellular diffusely infiltrating glioma
- Oligodendroglioma with focal or diffuse histologic features of malignancy

IMAGING

General Features

- Best diagnostic clue
  - Calcified frontal lobe mass involving cortex and subcortical white matter (WM)
- Location
  - Supratentorial hemispheric mass, involves cortex and subcortical WM
  - Frontal lobe most common, followed by temporal
  - May involve parietal or occipital lobes
  - Often expands overlying cortex
- Size
  - Variable
- Morphology
  - Diffusely infiltrative mass
  - May appear discrete, but always infiltrative
  - Neoplastic cells almost always found beyond areas of abnormal signal intensity

CT Findings

- NECT
  - Mixed density (hypodense/isodense) mass
  - Majority calcify, nodular or clumped Ca++
    - May see gyriform Ca++
  - Cystic degeneration common
  - May see hemorrhage or necrosis
  - May expand, remodel, or erode calvarium
- CECT
  - Variable enhancement

MR Findings

- T1WI
  - Heterogeneous hypointense infiltrative mass
  - May appear circumscribed
  - May see blood products, edema, necrosis
  - Cortical expansion may be seen
- T2WI
  - Heterogeneous hyperintense infiltrative mass
    - Heterogeneity related to Ca++, cystic change, blood products
  - Typically expands overlying cortex
  - May see hemorrhage, necrosis
- FLAIR
  - Heterogeneous hyperintense infiltrative mass
  - Typically expands overlying cortex
- T2* GRE
  - Ca++ seen as areas of "blooming"
- DWI
  - No diffusion restriction typical
- T1WI C+
  - Variable enhancement
  - New enhancement suggests malignant progression
  - 50% of all oligodendrogliomas enhance
  - AOs more likely to enhance than low-grade oligo
- MRS
  - ↑ Cho/Cr, ↓ NAA
  - Lipid/lactate peak at 1.33 ppm may be seen
- PWI
  - High rCBV common
  - Helpful to distinguish grade II from grade III
  - May help guide biopsy

Nuclear Medicine Findings

- PET
  - High glucose metabolism, accumulate FDG similar to or exceeding gray matter
  - FDG shows high-grade gliomas have uptake similar to or exceeding normal gray matter
  - Tumor/WM > 1.5 and tumor/GM > 0.6 suggest high-grade tumors
  - 11C-methionine studies show marked uptake differences between oligo, AO

Imaging Recommendations

- Best imaging tool
  - MR to delineate tumor; CT for Ca++
- Protocol advice
  - MR with contrast, GRE ± MRS and PWI

DIFFERENTIAL DIAGNOSIS

Oligodendroglioma

- Calcified mass involving gray and white matter
- May appear more circumscribed
- May be indistinguishable without biopsy
- MRS and perfusion may help preoperative diagnosis

Anaplastic Astrocytoma (AA)

- Infiltrative mass, predominantly involves white matter
- Often nonenhancing
- May be indistinguishable

Glioblastoma Multiforme (GBM)

- 95% necrotic core, enhancing rim
- Extensive surrounding T2/FLAIR signal
- Hemorrhage common

Cerebritis

- T2 hyperintensity and patchy enhancement
- Diffusion restriction is typical
- May appear mass-like
- Acute onset common

Ischemia

- Typical vascular distribution (MCA, ACA, PCA)
- Diffusion restriction if acute/subacute
- Involves GM and WM, often wedge-shaped
- Cortical, gyriform enhancement if subacute

Herpes Encephalitis

- Confined to limbic system, temporal lobes
- Blood products and enhancement common
- Acute onset is typical

ANAPLASTIC OLIGODENDROGLIOMA

Meningioma
- Enhancing extra axial dural-based mass
- Often calcified with broad dural base, dural "tail"
- Hyperostosis and Ca++ is characteristic
- Older patients

PATHOLOGY

General Features
- Etiology
  - Arises from neoplastic transformation of mature oligodendrocytes or immature glial precursors
  - May arise de novo or from malignant progression of preexisting grade II oligo
- Genetics
  - Loss of heterozygosity for 1p and 19q (50-70%)
    - Often occur together, suggesting synergistic effect
  - Average number of chromosomes involved is higher in grade III than grade II oligo
- Associated abnormalities
  - Oligoastrocytoma (mixed tumor with 2 distinct neoplastic cell types) is common (50%)
    - WHO grade II (oligoastrocytoma)
    - WHO grade III (anaplastic oligoastrocytoma)
    - Decreased survival compared with pure oligodendroglioma

Staging, Grading, & Classification
- WHO grade III
- Rarely may be multifocal or multicentric
- Some authors propose dividing AOs into WHO grades III and IV

Gross Pathologic & Surgical Features
- Well-defined, grayish-pink, soft unencapsulated mass
- Located in cortex and subcortical WM
- Ca++ is extremely common
- Cystic degeneration and hemorrhage common
- Necrosis may be present
- Rarely infiltrates overlying leptomeninges

Microscopic Features
- Rounded, homogeneous nuclei and clear cytoplasm
  - Perinuclear halos, "fried egg" and "honeycomb" patterns related to fixation artifact
- Microcalcifications, mucoid/cystic degeneration
- Dense network of branching capillaries
  - "Chicken-wire"
- Increased cellularity, marked atypia
- High mitotic activity
- Microvascular proliferation and necrosis

CLINICAL ISSUES

Presentation
- Most common signs/symptoms
  - Headache, seizures most common
  - Focal neurologic deficits
  - Duration of symptoms shorter than in grade II oligo

Demographics
- Age
  - Peak incidence: 4th through 6th decade
  - Occurs at all ages; mean is 49 years
  - Older on average than WHO grade II patients
- Gender
  - Slight male predominance
- Epidemiology
  - 20-50% of oligodendrogliomas are anaplastic
  - Oligos represent 5-25% of all gliomas

Natural History & Prognosis
- Poor prognosis
- Median survival: 4 years
- 5-year survival: 40-45%; 10-year survival: 15%
- Local tumor recurrence common
- CSF metastasis uncommon
- Systemic metastasis rare
- Leptomeningeal oligodendrogliomatosis, spinal cord metastasis extremely rare
- Positive prognostic factors
  - Age: < 50 years
  - Karnofsky performance status (KPS): 90-100
  - Tumors ≤ 4 cm
  - Complete tumor resection
- *CDKN2A* tumor suppressor gene deletions associated with shorter survival
- 1p and 19q loss of heterozygosity associated with prolonged survival
- Oligos have better prognosis than astrocytomas of same grade

Treatment
- Surgical resection + adjuvant chemo and XRT

DIAGNOSTIC CHECKLIST

Consider
- Many gliomas may mimic AO
- Presence of Ca++, cortical expansion may help distinguish AOs from other gliomas

Image Interpretation Pearls
- AOs cannot be reliably differentiated from grade II oligos on conventional MR
- Neoplastic cells are almost always found beyond areas of abnormal signal intensity
- New enhancement in previously nonenhancing oligo suggests malignant progression

SELECTED REFERENCES

1. Iwamoto FM et al: Clinical relevance of 1p and 19q deletion for patients with WHO grade 2 and 3 gliomas. J Neurooncol. 88(3):293-8, 2008
2. Louis DN et al (eds): WHO Classification of Tumours of the Central Nervous System: Anaplastic Oligodendroglioma. Lyon, France: IARC Press. 60-2, 2007
3. Spampinato MV et al: Cerebral blood volume measurements and proton MR spectroscopy in grading of oligodendroglial tumors. AJR Am J Roentgenol. 188(1):204-12, 2007

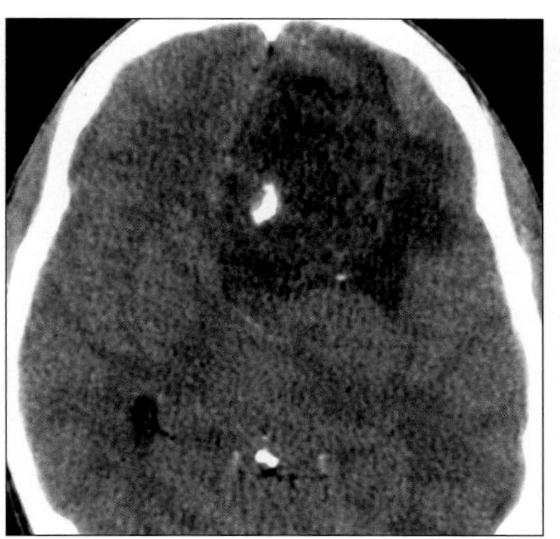

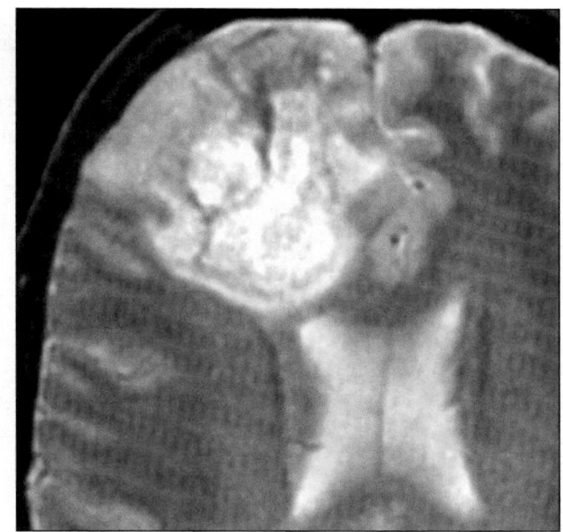

(Left) *Axial NECT shows a large frontal lobe mass with calcification. The calcification suggests the correct diagnosis, oligodendroglioma. CT is also helpful to see hemorrhage which may occur in anaplastic oligodendroglioma, but is more common in GBM. WHO grade III AO at resection.* ***(Right)*** *Axial T2WI MR shows a heterogeneous mass with cortical expansion and mild mass effect. Although it appears discrete, this AO is infiltrative and has a poor prognosis. Imaging mimics a grade II oligodendroglioma.*

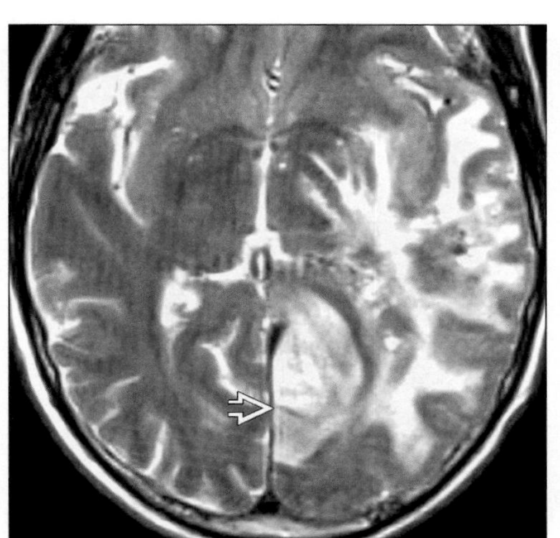

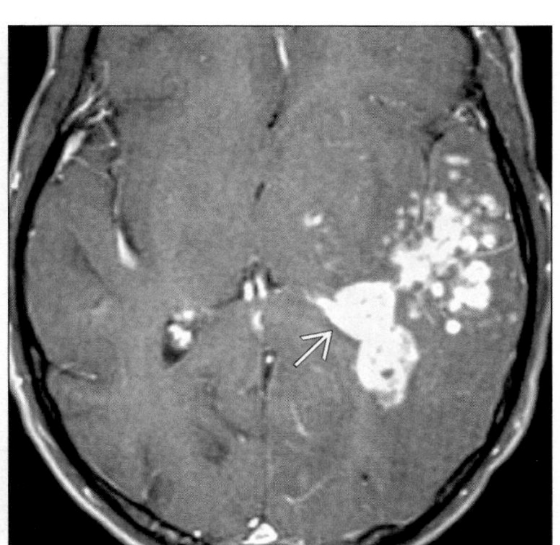

(Left) *Axial T2WI MR shows extensive hyperintensity involving the temporal and parietal lobes in this patient diagnosed with an occipital lobe oligodendroglioma ⇨ 4 years prior.* ***(Right)*** *Axial T1WI C+ FS MR in the same patient with anaplastic oligodendroglioma shows extensive enhancement with ependymal extension → along the ventricles. This enhancement represents malignant degeneration of the grade II tumor. New enhancement of a previously treated tumor suggests malignant degeneration.*

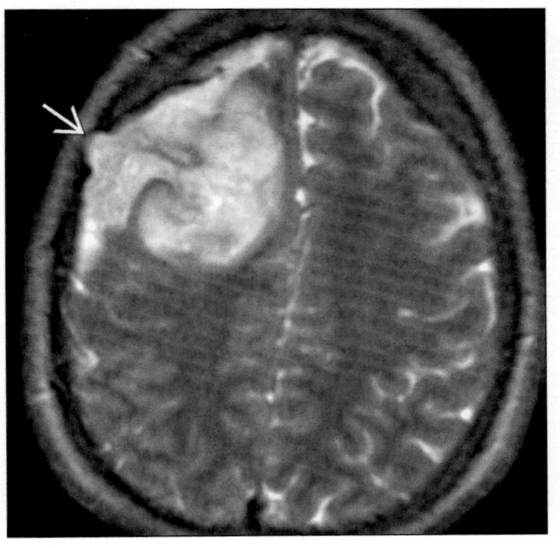

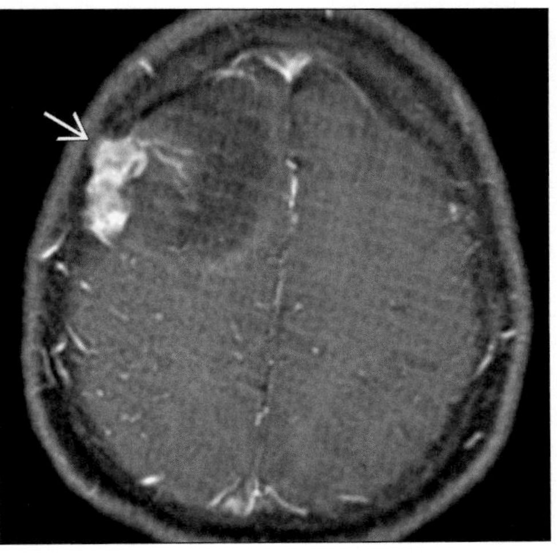

(Left) *Axial T2WI shows a heterogeneously hyperintense frontal lobe mass with skull remodeling →. The tumor appears to have an extraaxial component. However, involvement of the cortex and subcortical white matter is suggestive of oligodendroglioma.* ***(Right)*** *Axial T1WI C+ FS MR in the same patient shows peripheral enhancement →. Grade III oligoastrocytoma was found at resection. Oligoastrocytomas have a better prognosis than pure astrocytomas of the same grade.*

ASTROBLASTOMA

Key Facts

Terminology

- Rare glial neoplasm with perivascular pseudorosettes and variable biological behavior

Imaging

- Well-delineated, mixed solid and cystic hemispheric mass with "bubbly" appearance
- Almost always supratentorial, usually within cerebral hemisphere
- Majority (up to 80%) have calcification
- T2WI: Solid and cystic mass with heterogeneous "bubbly" appearance of solid portion
- GRE/SWI: Hypointensity related to Ca++ or blood products
- Heterogeneous enhancement is typical (75%)
  - Mixed solid, rim-enhancing pattern
- MRS may show ↓ NAA, ↑ choline

Top Differential Diagnoses

- Ependymoma
- Primitive neuroectodermal tumor
- Atypical teratoid-rhabdoid tumor
- Oligodendroglioma
- Pleomorphic xanthoastrocytoma

Pathology

- No WHO grade officially established
  - Low- and high-grade histologic features

Clinical Issues

- Most common presentation: Headache, seizures, focal neurologic deficit
- Occurs at all ages; median is 11 years
- Rare: 0.5-2.8% of primary gliomas
- Low-grade astroblastomas often have good long-term survival

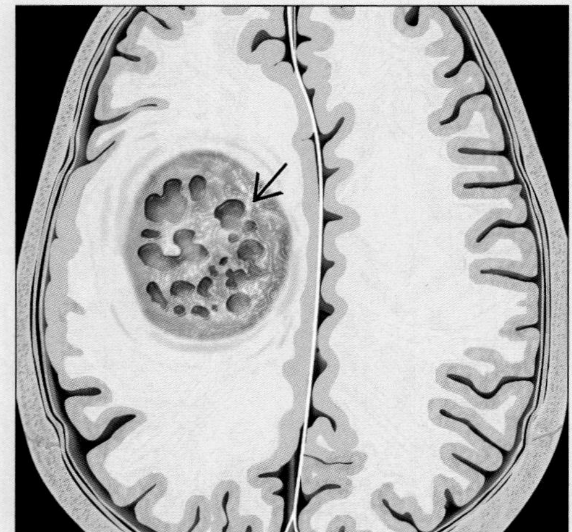

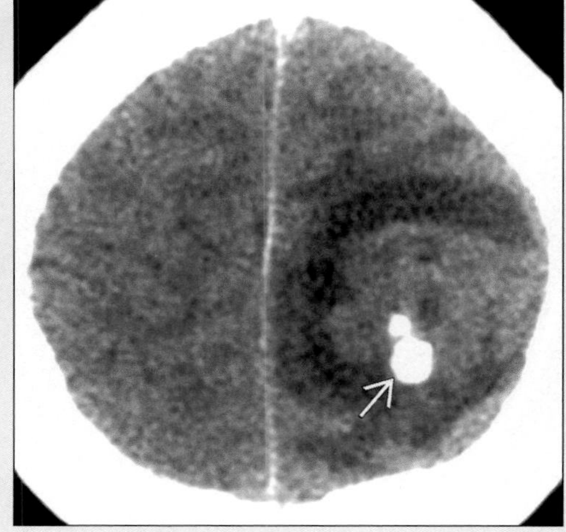

(Left) Axial graphic shows a well-delineated mixed solid and cystic hemispheric mass with calcification ⇒ and a "bubbly" appearance characteristic of astroblastoma. Note the lack of significant mass effect. These rare tumors typically occur in children and young adults. (Right) Axial NECT shows a mixed density hemispheric mass in a 25-year-old patient with seizures. There is globular calcification ⇒, typical of astroblastoma. Note the relative lack of surrounding edema and mass effect.

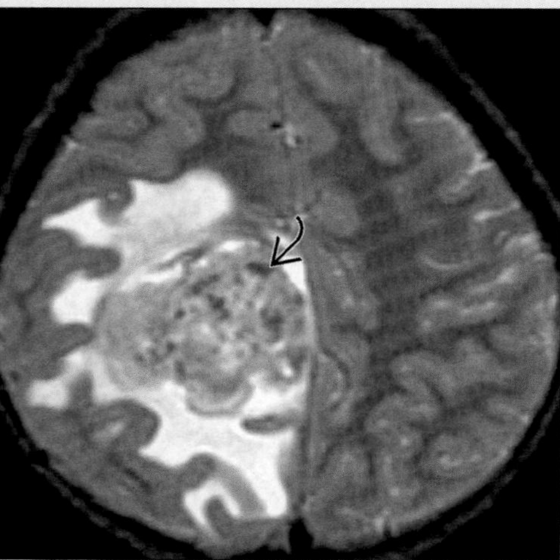

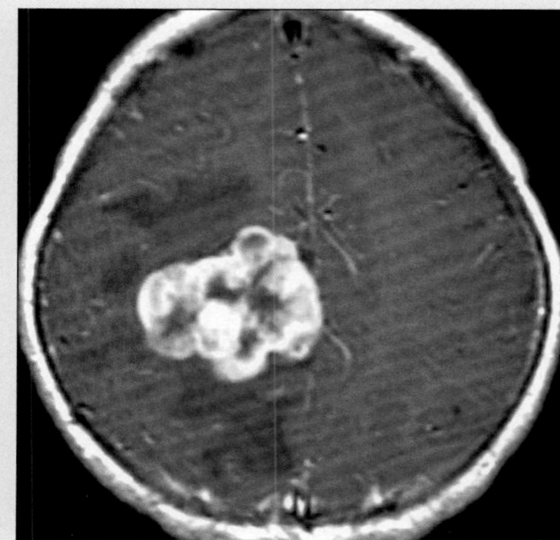

(Left) Axial T2WI MR shows a large heterogeneous hemispheric mass in this 5 year old with seizures. The areas of low signal intensity ⇒ are related to calcifications, better seen on prior CT (not shown). (Right) Axial T1WI C+ MR in the same patient shows strong, heterogeneous enhancement of the mass, typical of an astroblastoma. Histology revealed a well-differentiated astroblastoma. Surgical resection is the primary treatment with adjuvant radiation and chemotherapy reserved for anaplastic tumors.

ASTROBLASTOMA

TERMINOLOGY

Definitions

- Rare glial neoplasm with perivascular pseudorosettes and variable biological behavior

IMAGING

General Features

- Best diagnostic clue
  - Well-delineated mixed solid and cystic hemispheric mass with "bubbly" appearance in child or young adult
- Location
  - Almost always supratentorial, usually within cerebral hemisphere
    - Parietal > frontal lobe
      - Temporal lobe is uncommon site
    - Often superficial, frequently involve cortex
    - Can be extraaxial or even intraventricular
  - Cerebellum and brainstem extremely rare
  - Corpus callosum, optic nerves, cauda equina reported
- Size
  - Range: 1-10 cm
  - Mean: 4 cm
- Morphology
  - Circumscribed, lobular, solid and cystic mass with dominant solid component

CT Findings

- NECT
  - Attenuation variable
    - Mixed areas of hyperdensity, hypodensity, isodensity typical
  - Majority (up to 80%) have calcification (Ca++)
    - Typically dense, globular
    - Can be punctate or psammomatous
- CECT
  - Strong, heterogeneous enhancement of solid portion
    - Rim enhancement may be seen

MR Findings

- T1WI
  - Solid and cystic mass with heterogeneous signal
    - 50% isointense to white matter
    - 40% mixed isointense and hypointense
    - 10% predominately hypointense
- T2WI
  - Solid and cystic mass with heterogeneous "bubbly" appearance of solid portion
  - Hyperintense to white matter (80%)
    - Heterogeneous iso-/hyperintense "bubbly" appearance is typical
    - Mixed isointense and hypointense (10-20%)
    - Intratumoral hemorrhage ± fluid-fluid level may occur
  - 50% lack peritumoral hyperintensity
- FLAIR
  - Hyperintense (80%), isointense (20%)
- T2* GRE
  - Hypointensity related to Ca++ or blood products
- T1WI C+
  - Heterogeneous enhancement (70-75%)
    - Mixed solid, rim-enhancing pattern
  - Solid enhancement (15-20%)
  - < 10% show no enhancement
  - Extraaxial astroblastomas may have enhancing dural "tail"
- MRS
  - Rare reports show decreased NAA, increased choline
    - Additional peaks: Lipids, myoinositol, glycine reported

Imaging Recommendations

- Best imaging tool
  - NECT best to identify calcification
  - Multiplanar contrast-enhanced MR best for tumor evaluation
- Protocol advice
  - Add T2* (GRE or SWI) sequence for Ca++ or blood products

DIFFERENTIAL DIAGNOSIS

Ependymoma

- Supratentorial (1/3): Heterogeneous parenchymal/ periventricular enhancing mass
- Hemorrhage, necrosis, Ca++, and edema common

Primitive Neuroectodermal Tumor (PNET)

- Pediatric tumor, infants and young children
- Peripheral, heterogeneous parenchymal mass
- Hemorrhage, cysts, and Ca++ common

Atypical Teratoid-Rhabdoid Tumor (AT/RT)

- Pediatric tumor, infants and young children
- Heterogeneous solid mass with hemorrhage, necrosis, Ca++, cyst formation

Oligodendroglioma

- Peripheral, cortically based mass ± enhancement
- Ca++ common; minimal surrounding edema

Pleomorphic Xanthoastrocytoma

- Cyst with mural nodule in temporal lobe typical
- Enhancing nodule abuts dura with dural "tail"

Pilocytic Astrocytoma

- Enhancing solid component + cyst common
- Typically in cerebellum

Glioblastoma Multiforme (GBM)

- Thick, irregular enhancing rind with central necrosis
- Rare in children, young adults

Parenchymal Metastases

- Multiple lesions common with marked edema
- Older patients, primary often known

PATHOLOGY

General Features

- Etiology
  - Histogenesis remains controversial

- Putative astrocytic origin
- Some authors propose tanycyte cell origin
- Genetics
  - Gains of chromosomes 19 and 20q reported

Staging, Grading, & Classification

- No WHO grade officially established
- Some pathologists designate well-differentiated (low grade) or anaplastic (high grade) based on histologic features
  - Low grade: Low to moderate mitotic activity, little cellular atypia
  - High grade: Vascular endothelial hyperplasia, high mitotic rates, significant atypia
    - Pseudopalisading necrosis also suggests high grade

Gross Pathologic & Surgical Features

- Circumscribed, well-demarcated mass
- Cysts are common
- Necrosis may be seen in low-grade or high-grade lesions
- Hemorrhage is rare

Microscopic Features

- Perivascular pseudorosettes
  - Broad, nontapering astrocytic cell processes radiate toward central, often hyalinized blood vessel
- Oval to elongated hyperchromatic nuclei; ± Ca++
- GFAP(+), vimentin(+), and S100(+) are characteristic
- Ki-67 proliferation index: 1-18%
- Electron microscopy
  - Intermediate filament-laden cell processes that form parallel or radial arrays terminating on perivascular basement membranes

CLINICAL ISSUES

Presentation

- Most common signs/symptoms
  - Headache, seizures, focal neurologic deficit
- Other signs/symptoms
  - Increased intracranial pressure

Demographics

- Age
  - Occurs at all ages
    - Reported ages range from newborn to 58 years
    - Most commonly seen in children, adolescents, and young adults
    - Median: 11 years
  - Rarely in infants; congenital cases reported
- Gender
  - Striking female predominance noted in recent studies
- Epidemiology
  - Rare, 0.5-2.8% of primary gliomas
  - < 80 cases reported

Natural History & Prognosis

- Gross total resection is associated with favorable outcome
- Low-grade astroblastomas often have good long-term survival
- Anaplastic histology is associated with tumor recurrence and progression
- Metastatic dissemination to CSF and spine is extremely rare

Treatment

- Surgical resection is treatment of choice
- Adjuvant radiation therapy and chemotherapy for high-grade (anaplastic) lesions

DIAGNOSTIC CHECKLIST

Consider

- "Bubbly" hemispheric mass in child or young adult may be astroblastoma

Image Interpretation Pearls

- Astroblastoma often shows lack of significant mass effect for size of lesion

SELECTED REFERENCES

1. Ganapathy S et al: Unusual manifestations of astroblastoma: a radiologic-pathologic analysis. Pediatr Radiol. 39(2):168-71, 2009
2. Kantar M et al: Anaplastic astroblastoma of childhood: aggressive behavior. Childs Nerv Syst. 25(9):1125-9, 2009
3. Denaro L et al: Intraventricular astroblastoma. Case report. J Neurosurg Pediatr. 1(2):152-5, 2008
4. Hirano H et al: Consecutive histological changes in an astroblastoma that disseminated to the spinal cord after repeated intracranial recurrences: a case report. Brain Tumor Pathol. 25(1):25-31, 2008
5. Notarianni C et al: Brainstem astroblastoma: a case report and review of the literature. Surg Neurol. 69(2):201-5, 2008
6. Bannykh SI et al: Malignant astroblastoma with rhabdoid morphology. J Neurooncol. 83(3):277-8, 2007
7. Bell JW et al: Neuroradiologic characteristics of astroblastoma. Neuroradiology. 49(3):203-9, 2007
8. Louis DN et al: WHO Classification of Tumours of the Central Nervous System: Astroblastoma. Lyon: IARC Press. 88-9, 2007
9. Mangano FT et al: Astroblastoma. Case report, review of the literature, and analysis of treatment strategies. J Neurosurg Sci. 51(1):21-7; discussion 27, 2007
10. Tumialán LM et al: An astroblastoma mimicking a cavernous malformation: case report. Neurosurgery. 60(3):E569-70; discussion E570, 2007
11. Hata N et al: An astroblastoma case associated with loss of heterozygosity on chromosome 9p. J Neurooncol. 80(1):69-73, 2006
12. Kubota T et al: Astroblastoma: immunohistochemical and ultrastructural study of distinctive epithelial and probable tanycytic differentiation. Neuropathology. 26(1):72-81, 2006
13. Navarro R et al: Astroblastoma in childhood: pathological and clinical analysis. Childs Nerv Syst. 21(3):211-20, 2005
14. Port JD et al: Astroblastoma: radiologic-pathologic correlation and distinction from ependymoma. AJNR Am J Neuroradiol. 23(2):243-7, 2002
15. Sener RN: Astroblastoma: diffusion MRI, and proton MR spectroscopy. Comput Med Imaging Graph. 26(3):187-91, 2002

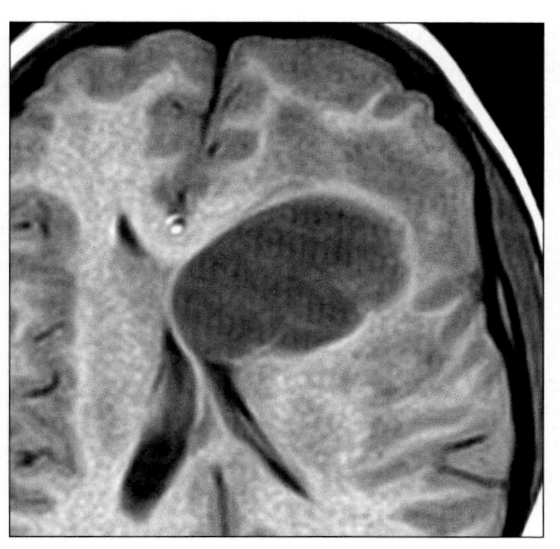

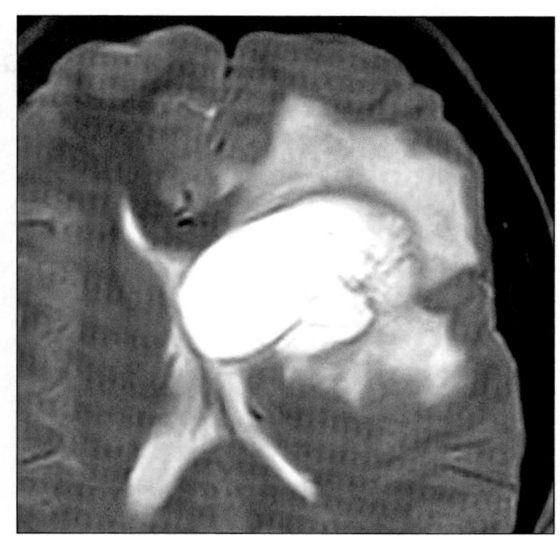

(Left) *Axial T1WI MR in an adolescent girl with headaches shows a predominantly cystic mass in the left frontal lobe with central signal that is mildly hyperintense to CSF in the adjacent ventricle.* ***(Right)*** *Axial T2WI MR in the same patient shows the mass to be predominantly hyperintense with moderate surrounding vasogenic edema. Remember to consider astroblastoma in a child or young adult with a cystic or "bubbly" mass. Astroblastoma found at resection. (Courtesy J. Aufderheide, MD).*

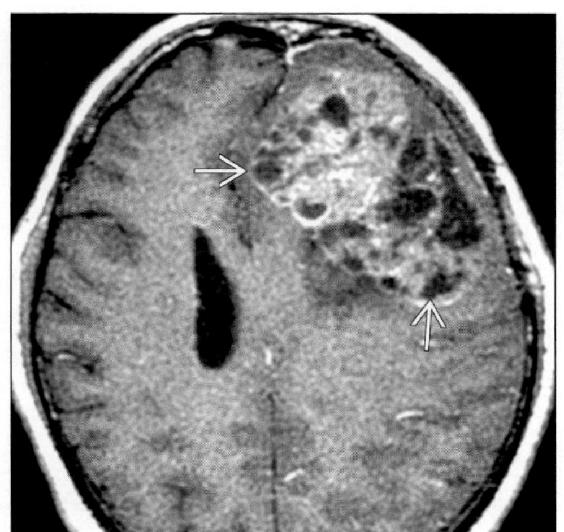

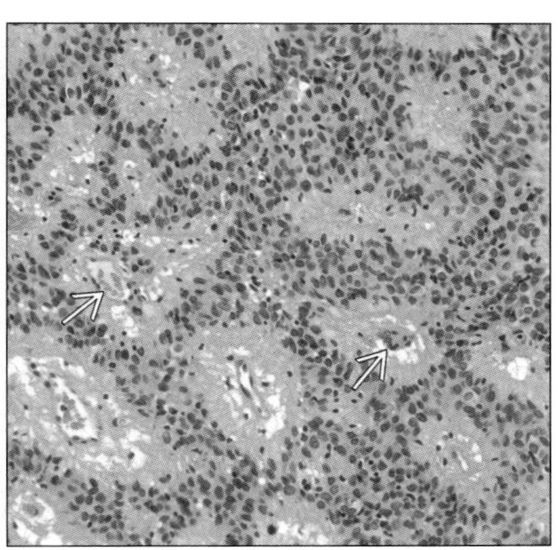

(Left) *Axial T1WI C+ MR shows a large frontal lobe mass with strong, heterogeneous enhancement. Note the multiple cysts ➡ surrounded by rims and solid masses of enhancing tissue. Note the relative lack of surrounding edema and mass effect for the size of the lesion, typical of astroblastoma.* ***(Right)*** *High-power hematoxylin & eosin stain shows a low-grade astroblastoma. Note the small round cells in a typical perivascular "pseudorosette" pattern radiating toward the central blood vessels ➡.*

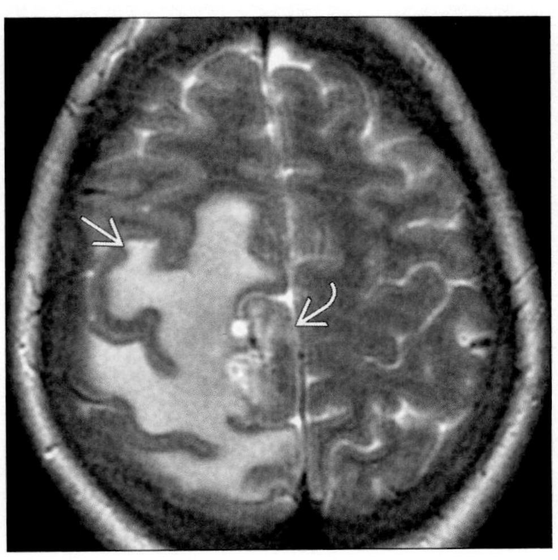

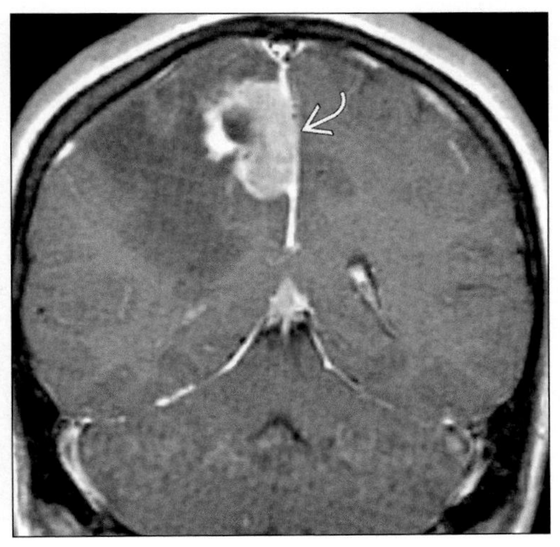

(Left) *Axial T2WI MR shows a heterogeneous dural-based mass ➡ in this young adult with significant surrounding vasogenic edema ➡.* ***(Right)*** *Coronal T1WI C+ MR in the same patient shows strong, heterogeneous enhancement of the dural-based mass ➡. It is difficult to determine if the mass is intra- or extraaxial. Astroblastoma with dural invasion was found at surgery. Imaging mimics an atypical meningioma or a dural metastasis.*

CHORDOID GLIOMA OF THE THIRD VENTRICLE

Key Facts

Terminology
- Rare glioma arising from anterior wall/roof of 3rd V

Imaging
- Adult with well-delineated, T2 hyperintense, homogeneously enhancing 3rd V mass

Top Differential Diagnoses
- Pilocytic astrocytoma
- Craniopharyngioma
- Germinoma
- Choroid plexus papilloma
- Colloid cyst
- Ependymoma

Pathology
- Cords/clusters of oval/polygonal epithelioid cells within mucinous stroma
- WHO grade II
- Likely ependymal origin
  - From ependymal cells in/near lamina terminalis
  - May arise from subcommissural organ

Clinical Issues
- Nonspecific (headache, nausea due to hydrocephalus)
  - Endocrine disturbances (hypothyroidism, diabetes insipidus, amenorrhea)
  - Dysautonomias
  - Visual disturbances

Diagnostic Checklist
- Consider chordoid glioma of 3rd ventricle if adult with T2 hyperintense, enhancing, anterior 3rd V mass

*(**Left**) Sagittal T1WI MR shows a small, round, well-circumscribed mass ➔ arising from the anterior roof of the 3rd ventricle. The lesion is isointense with gray matter and demonstrated strong, uniform enhancement on T1WI C+ (not shown). (**Right**) High-power H&E stain of classic chordoid glioma shows a neoplasm with clusters and cords of epithelioid cells with abundant eosinophilic cytoplasm in a mucinous stroma. GFAP (not shown) was strongly positive.*

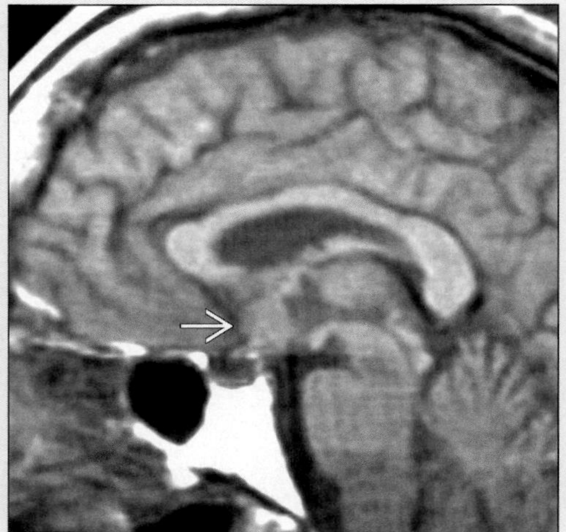

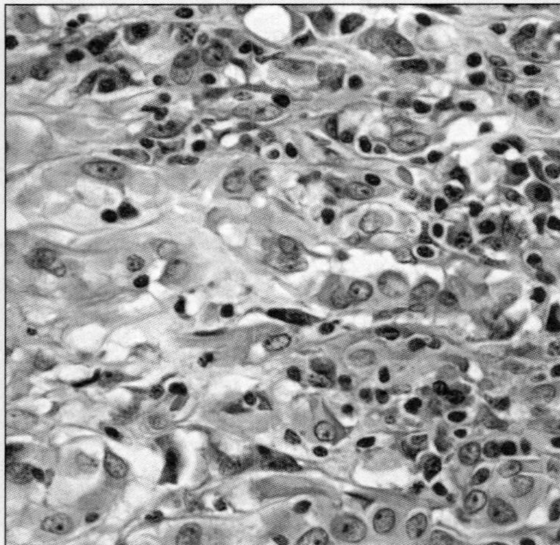

*(**Left**) Coronal T2WI FS MR in this 65-year-old woman, with a 3-year history of weight gain and personality changes, shows a lobulated hyperintense mass ➔ mostly contained within the 3rd ventricle. The optic tract ➔ is displaced inferolaterally. (**Right**) Sagittal T1WI C+ MR in the same patient shows strong, uniform enhancement of the slightly lobulated 3rd ventricle mass ➔. Chordoid glioma was found at histopathology.*

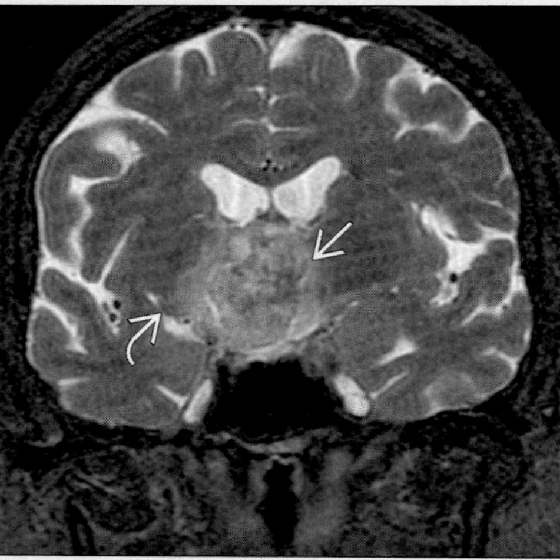

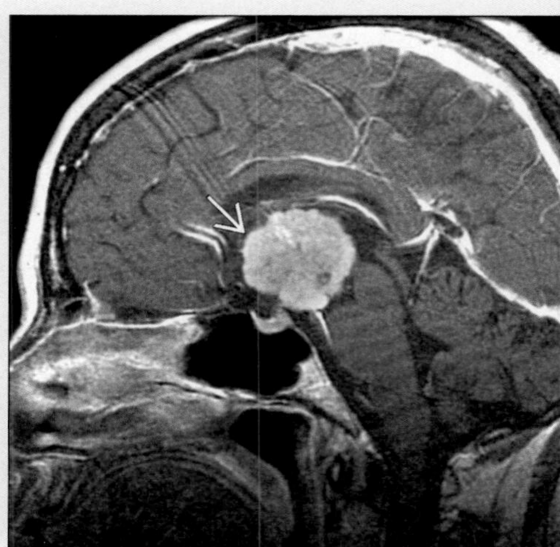

CHORDOID GLIOMA OF THE THIRD VENTRICLE

TERMINOLOGY

Abbreviations

- Chordoid glioma of 3rd ventricle (CGOTV)

Definitions

- Rare glioma arising from anterior wall/roof of 3rd ventricle (V)

IMAGING

General Features

- Best diagnostic clue
  - Well-delineated, T2 hyperintense, homogeneously enhancing 3rd V mass
- Location
  - Suspended from roof/anterior wall of 3rd V
- Size
  - 1-4 cm
- Morphology
  - Rounded or ovoid, well circumscribed

Imaging Recommendations

- Best imaging tool
  - MR
- Protocol advice
  - Pituitary/hypothalamus protocol
    - Thin sagittal, coronal T1WI, T2WI
    - T1WI C+ FS sagittal, coronal

DIFFERENTIAL DIAGNOSIS

Pilocytic Astrocytoma

- Optic tract, hypothalamus, 3rd V floor
- Child, ± neurofibromatosis type 1

Craniopharyngioma

- Heterogeneous, 90% cystic
- Extraventricular, extraaxial
- Child > adult

Germinoma

- Diabetes insipidus common
- Usually involves stalk
- Child, young adult

Choroid Plexus Papilloma

- Rare in 3rd V
- Typically child < 5 years

Colloid Cyst

- At foramen of Monro, wedged between fornices
- Round, nonenhancing

Ependymoma

- Uncommon in 3rd V

PATHOLOGY

General Features

- Etiology
  - Likely ependymal origin
    - From ependymal cells in or around lamina terminalis
    - May arise from subcommissural organ

Staging, Grading, & Classification

- WHO grade II

Gross Pathologic & Surgical Features

- Grossly well circumscribed
- Occasional extension into adjacent hypothalamic tissue
- Variable calcifications, cystic regions; hemorrhage rare

Microscopic Features

- Cords/clusters of oval/polygonal epithelioid cells within mucinous stroma
  - Strongly GFAP(+); vimentin(+)
  - Mitotic figures uncommon
  - ± reactive changes in adjacent tissues
    - Lymphoplasmacytic infiltrates at tumor periphery

CLINICAL ISSUES

Presentation

- Most common signs/symptoms
  - Nonspecific (headache ± nausea due to hydrocephalus)
- Other signs/symptoms
  - Endocrine disturbances
    - Hypothyroidism, diabetes insipidus, amenorrhea
  - Dysautonomias (hyperhidrosis)
  - Visual disturbances

Demographics

- Age: Adults (35-60 years)
- Gender: Female predominance (M:F = 1:1.7)
- Epidemiology: Rare

Natural History & Prognosis

- Slow enlargement

Treatment

- Surgical excision

DIAGNOSTIC CHECKLIST

Consider

- CGOTV if adult with T2 hyperintense, enhancing, anterior 3rd V mass

Image Interpretation Pearls

- Bulky, well-circumscribed 3rd V mass in adult

SELECTED REFERENCES

1. Kawasaki K et al: Chordoid glioma of the third ventricle: a report of two cases, one with ultrastructural findings. Neuropathology. 29(1):85-90, 2009
2. Sangoi AR et al: Distinguishing chordoid meningiomas from their histologic mimics: an immunohistochemical evaluation. Am J Surg Pathol. 33(5):669-81, 2009
3. Vanhauwaert DJ et al: Chordoid glioma of the third ventricle. Acta Neurochir (Wien). 150(11):1183-91, 2008

ANGIOCENTRIC GLIOMA

Key Facts

Terminology

- Angiocentric glioma (AG) includes 2 recently described neoplasms
  - Angiocentric neuroepithelial tumor
  - Monomorphic angiocentric glioma
- Epilepsy-associated, slowly growing, low-grade cortical neoplasm mainly affecting children and young adults

Imaging

- Frontal, temporal lobes most common sites
- Nonenhancing, ill-defined cortical mass
  - Most commonly solid
  - Rarely mixed solid, cystic
  - Rim-like hyperintensity on T1WI
- Hyperintense on T2WI, FLAIR
  - Stalk-like extension toward ventricle common

Pathology

- WHO grade I
  - Angiocentric growth pattern
  - MIB-1 proliferation low (1-5%)
  - No malignant degeneration

Clinical Issues

- Longstanding drug-resistant focal epilepsy
  - Typically starting in childhood
- Complete surgical resection curative

Diagnostic Checklist

- Cortical neoplasm in child/young adult with refractory epilepsy
- Nonenhancing cortical mass with rim-like hyperintensity on T1WI

*(**Left**) Axial T1WI MR in 6-year-old child with refractory epilepsy shows an ill-defined, cortical/subcortical mass. Note the hyperintense ring-like areas ➔, findings typical for an angiocentric glioma. (**Right**) Coronal T2WI MR in the same patient shows high signal intensity of the cortical/subcortical right frontal lobe lesion ➔.*

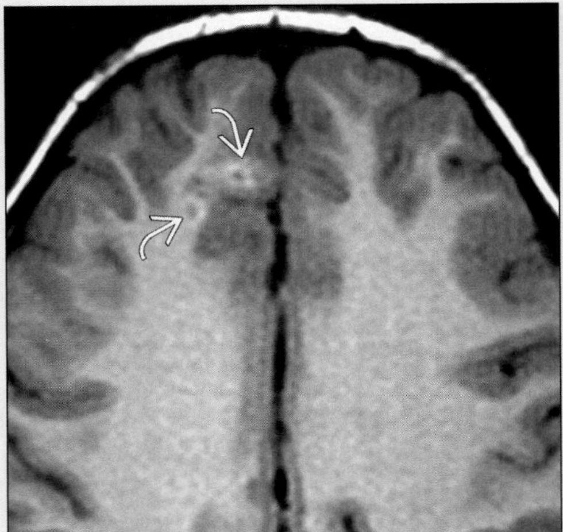

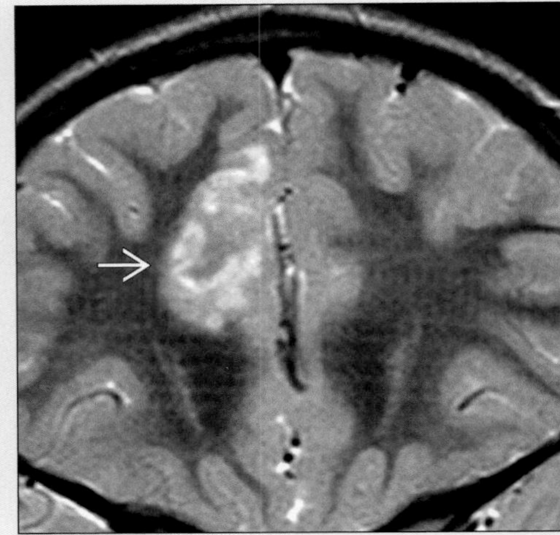

*(**Left**) Axial FLAIR MR in the same patient shows high signal intensity in the mass, which is ill-defined but does not demonstrate surrounding edema. (**Right**) Axial T1WI C+ MR in the same patient shows no enhancement. (Courtesy A. Rossi, MD.)*

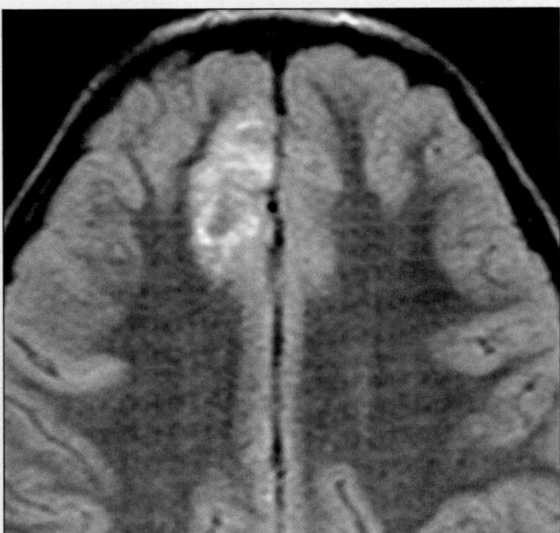

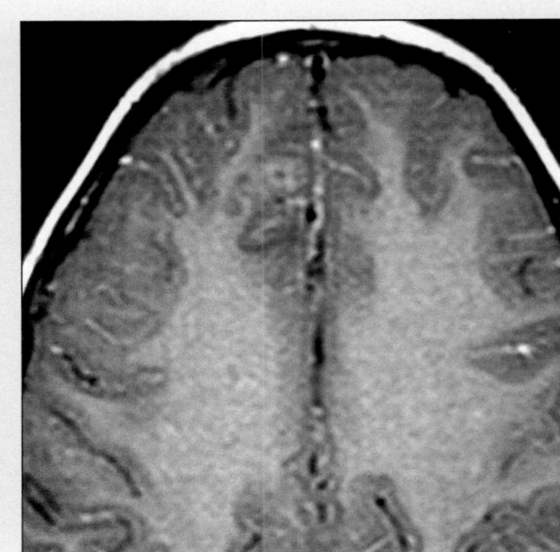

ANGIOCENTRIC GLIOMA

TERMINOLOGY

Abbreviations

- Angiocentric glioma (AG)

Synonyms

- AG spectrum includes 2 recently described tumors
  - Angiocentric neuroepithelial tumor (ANET)
  - Monomorphic angiocentric glioma (MAG)

Definitions

- Epilepsy-associated, slowly growing, low-grade cortical neoplasm mainly affecting children and young adults

IMAGING

General Features

- Best diagnostic clue
  - Nonenhancing, ill-defined cortical mass in child/ young adult with seizures
- Location
  - Cortex or subcortical white matter
  - Frontal, temporal lobes most common sites
- Size
  - 3-4 cm (up to 10 cm)

Imaging Recommendations

- Best imaging tool
  - MR

MR Findings

- T1WI
  - Ill-defined cortical/subcortical mass
  - Most commonly solid
    - Rarely mixed solid, cystic
  - Can be hypo-, iso-, or hyperintense
  - Rim-like hyperintensity!
- T2WI
  - Hyperintense
  - Stalk-like extension toward ventricle common
- FLAIR
  - Hyperintense
  - Stalk-like extension toward ventricle
- T1WI C+
  - Usually no enhancement

DIFFERENTIAL DIAGNOSIS

Ganglioglioma

- Solid cystic appearance

DNET

- Small cysts ("bubbly" appearance) on T2WI

PATHOLOGY

General Features

- Etiology
  - Uncertain origin
  - Dysembryoplastic theory
    - Radial glia suggested cell of origin
- Genetics
  - Loss of chromosomal bands 6q24-q25
  - Gain on 11p11.2 in some cases

Staging, Grading, & Classification

- WHO grade I

Microscopic Features

- Small spindle-/polygonal-shaped tumor cells with ependymal features
- Angiocentric growth pattern
- MIB-1 proliferation low (1-5%)

CLINICAL ISSUES

Presentation

- Most common signs/symptoms
  - Drug-resistant focal epilepsy starting in childhood

Demographics

- Age
  - Children, young adults

Natural History & Prognosis

- Benign course
- No malignant degeneration

Treatment

- Complete surgical resection curative

DIAGNOSTIC CHECKLIST

Consider

- Cortical neoplasm in child/young adult with longstanding seizures

Image Interpretation Pearls

- Ill-defined nonenhancing cortical mass with rim-like hyperintensity on T1WI

SELECTED REFERENCES

1. Arsene D et al: Angiocentric glioma: presentation of two cases with dissimilar histology. Clin Neuropathol. 27(6):391-5, 2008
2. Lum DJ et al: Cortical ependymoma or monomorphous angiocentric glioma? Neuropathology. 28(1):81-6, 2008
3. Sugita Y et al: Brain surface spindle cell glioma in a patient with medically intractable partial epilepsy: a variant of monomorphous angiocentric glioma? Neuropathology. 28(5):516-20, 2008
4. Preusser M et al: Angiocentric glioma: report of clinico-pathologic and genetic findings in 8 cases. Am J Surg Pathol. 31(11):1709-18, 2007
5. Lellouch-Tubiana A et al: Angiocentric neuroepithelial tumor (ANET): a new epilepsy-related clinicopathological entity with distinctive MRI. Brain Pathol. 15(4):281-6, 2005
6. Wang M et al: Monomorphous angiocentric glioma: a distinctive epileptogenic neoplasm with features of infiltrating astrocytoma and ependymoma. J Neuropathol Exp Neurol. 64(10):875-81, 2005
7. Shakur SF et al: Angiocentric glioma: a case series. J Neurosurg Pediatr. 2009 Mar;3(3):197-202. PubMed PMID: 19338465.

INFRATENTORIAL EPENDYMOMA

Key Facts

Terminology

- Infratentorial ependymoma (ITE)
  - Subtypes: Cellular, papillary, clear cell, tanycytic
- Slow-growing tumor of ependymal cells

Imaging

- 2/3 of all ependymomas are infratentorial
  - Most in 4th ventricle
  - Soft or "plastic" tumor
  - Squeezes through 4th ventricle foramina
  - Extends into CPA/cisterna magna
- Ca++ common (50%)
- ± cysts, hemorrhage
- Variable enhancement, hydrocephalus
- Low cellularity → high ADC
- NAA:Cho ratio higher than in PNET-MB

Top Differential Diagnoses

- Medulloblastoma (PNET-MB)
- Cerebellar pilocytic astrocytoma (PA)
- Brainstem glioma
- Atypical teratoid-rhabdoid tumor (AT/RT)
- Choroid plexus papilloma
- Oligodendroglioma

Clinical Issues

- Signs of increased intracranial pressure
- 3-17% CSF dissemination

Diagnostic Checklist

- Much less common than PNET-MB or PA
- Indistinct interface
  - With **floor** of 4th ventricle = ependymoma
  - With **roof** of 4th ventricle = PNET-MB

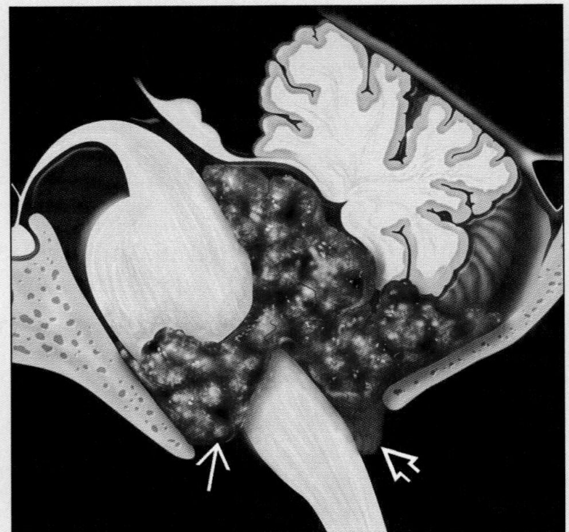

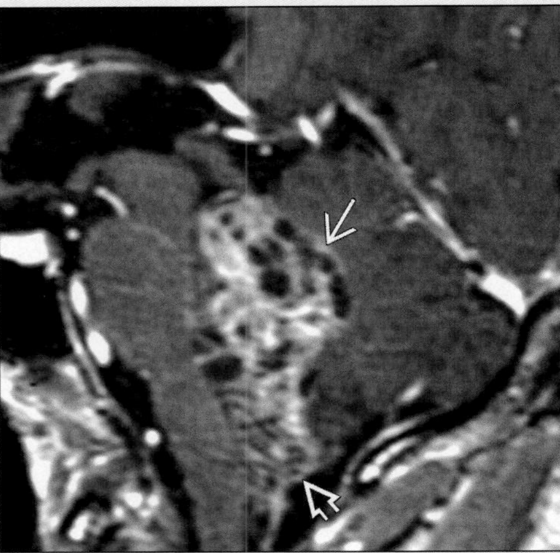

(Left) *Sagittal graphic shows a posterior fossa ependymoma extending through the 4th ventricle outlet foramina into the cisterna magna and CPA cistern. This "plastic" pattern of growth is typical of ependymoma in this location and increases the difficulty of surgical resection.* ***(Right)*** *Sagittal T1WI C+ FS MR shows a classic ependymoma extending from the 4th ventricle into the cisterna magna. The appearance of cystic areas intermixed with enhancing solid tumor is typical.*

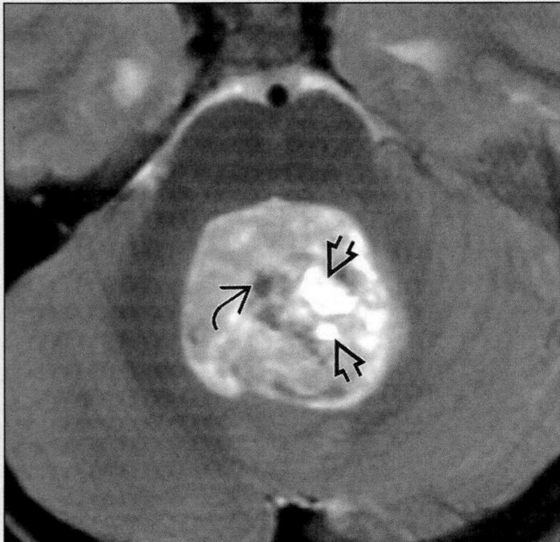

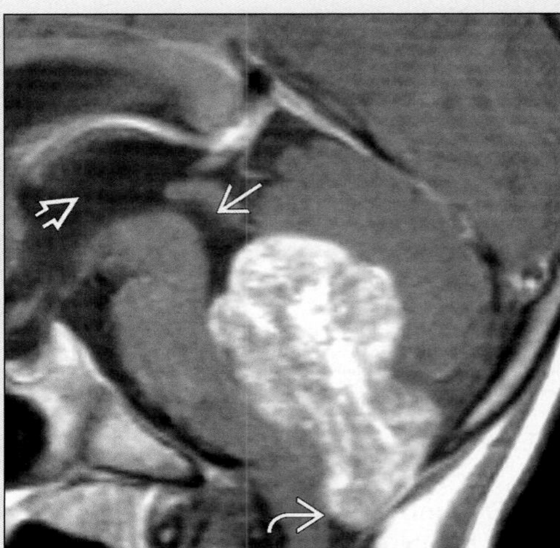

(Left) *Axial T2WI MR in a 9-year-old boy reveals a midline mass with heterogeneous internal features. The focal regions of hyperintensity corresponded to focal necrosis and the hypointense regions correlated with calcifications on NECT.* ***(Right)*** *Sagittal T1WI C+ MR in the same patient shows strong tumor enhancement. Note the "upstream" ventricular obstruction with an enlarged cerebral aqueduct, dilated 3rd ventricle, and tumor extruding through the foramen of Magendie into the cisterna magna.*

INFRATENTORIAL EPENDYMOMA

TERMINOLOGY

Definitions

- Infratentorial ependymoma (ITE)
  - Slow-growing tumor of ependymal cells
  - Subtypes: Cellular, papillary, clear cell, tanycytic

IMAGING

General Features

- Best diagnostic clue
  - Heterogeneous signal
  - Soft or "plastic" tumor squeezes out through 4th ventricle foramina into cisterns
  - Indistinct interface with floor of 4th ventricle
- Location
  - 2/3 infratentorial (most in 4th ventricle)
    - "Midfloor" type: Arises from inferior 1/2 of 4th ventricle
    - "Roof" type: Arises from inferior medullary velum
    - Lateral (off-midline) ependymomas = worse prognosis
  - 1/3 supratentorial
    - Majority outside ventricles, in periventricular white matter (WM)
- Size
  - 2-4 cm
- Morphology
  - Irregular shape in posterior fossa
    - Accommodates to shape of ventricle or cisterns

CT Findings

- NECT
  - 4th ventricle mass extending into CPA/cisterna magna
  - Ca++ common (50%); ± cysts, hemorrhage
  - Hydrocephalus common
- CECT
  - Variable heterogeneous enhancement

MR Findings

- T1WI
  - Heterogeneous, usually iso- to hypointense
  - Cystic foci slightly hyperintense to CSF
  - Hyperintense foci (Ca++, blood products) common
- T2WI
  - Heterogeneous, usually iso- to hyperintense
  - Hyperintense cystic foci
  - Hypointense foci (Ca++, blood products)
- FLAIR
  - Can show sharp interface between tumor, CSF
  - Tumor cysts very hyperintense to CSF
- T2* GRE
  - "Blooming" of hypointense Ca++ foci
- DWI
  - Relatively low cellularity → high ADC
- T1WI C+
  - Enhancement varies from none to mild/moderate
    - Typically heterogeneous
- MRS
  - ↓ NAA, ↑ Cho
    - NAA/Cho ratio higher than in PNET-MB
  - ↑ lactate
  - MR spectroscopy alone does not reliably differentiate ependymoma from astrocytoma or PNET-MB

Angiographic Findings

- Findings vary from avascular to hypervascular with arteriovenous shunting

Nonvascular Interventions

- Myelography
  - May be helpful in showing "drop" metastases

Nuclear Medicine Findings

- Increased FDG uptake on PET

Imaging Recommendations

- Best imaging tool
  - NECT + MR with contrast, MRS
- Protocol advice
  - Image entire neuraxis before surgery
  - Need combination of imaging, clinical findings to distinguish from PNET-MB
  - High-quality sagittal imaging can distinguish point of origin as floor vs. roof of 4th ventricle

DIFFERENTIAL DIAGNOSIS

Medulloblastoma (PNET-MB)

- Hyperdense on NECT
- Homogeneous mass
- Arises from roof of 4th ventricle
- More distinct interface with floor
- Low ADC, high cellularity

Cerebellar Pilocytic Astrocytoma (PA)

- Heterogeneous tumor of cerebellar hemisphere
- Cyst with mural nodule
- Solid portion enhances vigorously

Brainstem Glioma

- Infiltrating mass expanding brainstem
- Homogeneous signal on MR
- May project into 4th ventricle

Atypical Teratoid-Rhabdoid Tumor (AT/RT)

- Large mass with cyst or necrosis
- Variable enhancement pattern

Choroid Plexus Papilloma

- Vigorously enhancing intraventricular tumor
- 4th ventricle location more common in adults

Oligodendroglioma

- Heterogeneous supratentorial mass in young adults
- Frontal lobe lesion with Ca++

Glioblastoma Multiforme

- Older adults; rare in posterior fossa
- Heterogeneous malignant supratentorial mass
- Necrosis, hemorrhage common

INFRATENTORIAL EPENDYMOMA

PATHOLOGY

General Features

- Etiology
  - Arise from ependymal cells or ependymal rests
    - Periventricular ependymal rests account for supratentorial tumors
  - Possible link with simian virus 40 (SV40)
    - Large percentage express SV40 DNA sequences
    - SV40 can induce ependymoma when injected in rodents
- Genetics
  - Intracranial tumors associated with aberrations on chromosomes 1q, 6q, 9, 13, 16, 17, 19, 20, 22
    - Gain of 1q, loss on 9 associated with anaplastic tumors

Staging, Grading, & Classification

- WHO grade II (low grade, well differentiated)
- WHO grade III (high grade, anaplastic)

Gross Pathologic & Surgical Features

- Well demarcated
- Soft, lobulated, grayish-red mass
- ± cysts, necrosis, hemorrhage
- Extrudes through 4th ventricle outlet foramina → "plastic development"
- Typically displaces rather than invades adjacent brain parenchyma

CLINICAL ISSUES

Presentation

- Most common signs/symptoms
  - ↑ intracranial pressure: Headache, nausea, vomiting
- Clinical profile
  - Age 1-5 years; headache, vomiting
- Other
  - Ataxia, hemiparesis, visual disturbances, neck pain, torticollis, dizziness
  - Infants: Irritability, lethargy, developmental delay, vomiting, macrocephaly

Demographics

- Age
  - Bimodal age distribution
    - Major peak: 1-5 years
    - 2nd smaller peak: Mid 30s
- Gender
  - Slight male predominance
- Epidemiology
  - 3-5% of all intracranial tumors
  - 15% of posterior fossa tumors in children
    - 3rd most common posterior fossa tumor in children
      - Most common are PA and PNET-MB

Natural History & Prognosis

- 3-17% CSF dissemination
- Generally poor prognosis
  - 5-year overall survival: 50-60%
  - Progression-free survival: 30-50%
- Tumor expression of metalloproteinase MMP2 and MMP14 → better prognosis

Treatment

- Surgical resection ± chemo, radiation therapy (XRT)
  - Gross total resection + XRT correlates with improved survival
  - 5-year survival after recurrence: 15%
- Surgical resection often difficult due to adherence and infiltrating nature of tumor

DIAGNOSTIC CHECKLIST

Consider

- Much less common than PNET-MB or PA
- Gross total resection has greater impact on survival than in PNET-MB or PA
- Surveillance imaging to detect asymptomatic recurrence can increase survival

Image Interpretation Pearls

- Indistinct interface
  - With **floor** of 4th ventricle = ependymoma
  - With **roof** of 4th ventricle = PNET-MB

SELECTED REFERENCES

1. Merchant TE et al: Conformal radiotherapy after surgery for paediatric ependymoma: a prospective study. Lancet Oncol. 10(3):258-66, 2009
2. Puget S et al: Candidate genes on chromosome 9q33-34 involved in the progression of childhood ependymomas. J Clin Oncol. 27(11):1884-92, 2009
3. Yuh EL et al: Imaging of ependymomas: MRI and CT. Childs Nerv Syst. 25(10):1203-13, 2009
4. Schneider JF et al: Multiparametric differentiation of posterior fossa tumors in children using diffusion-weighted imaging and short echo-time 1H-MR spectroscopy. J Magn Reson Imaging. 26(6):1390-8, 2007
5. Korshunov A et al: The histologic grade is a main prognostic factor for patients with intracranial ependymomas treated in the microneurosurgical era: an analysis of 258 patients. Cancer. 100(6):1230-7, 2004
6. Fouladi M et al: Clear cell ependymoma: a clinicopathologic and radiographic analysis of 10 patients. Cancer. 98(10):2232-44, 2003
7. Korshunov A et al: Gene expression patterns in ependymomas correlate with tumor location, grade, and patient age. Am J Pathol. 163(5):1721-7, 2003
8. Dyer S et al: Genomic imbalances in pediatric intracranial ependymomas define clinically relevant groups. Am J Pathol. 161(6):2133-41, 2002
9. Good CD et al: Surveillance neuroimaging in childhood intracranial ependymoma: how effective, how often, and for how long? J Neurosurg. 94(1):27-32, 2001
10. Hirose Y et al: Chromosomal abnormalities subdivide ependymal tumors into clinically relevant groups. Am J Pathol. 158(3):1137-43, 2001
11. Figarella-Branger D et al: Prognostic factors in intracranial ependymomas in children. J Neurosurg. 93(4):605-13, 2000

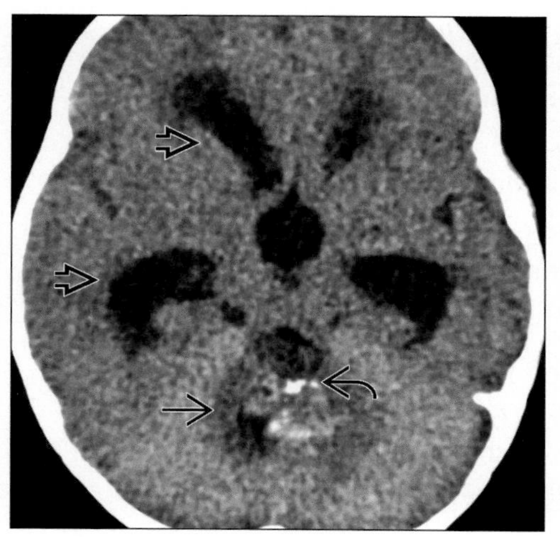

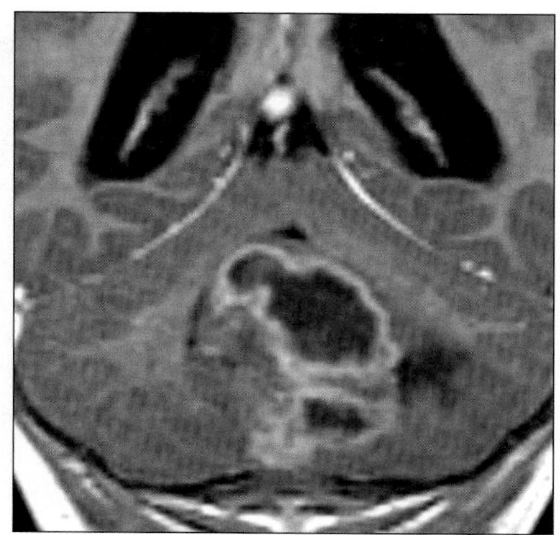

(Left) *Axial NECT in a 2-year-old girl presenting with nausea and vomiting shows a partially calcified midline mass causing obstructive hydrocephalus.* ***(Right)*** *Coronal T1WI C+ MR in the same patient shows inhomogeneous peripheral enhancement of the tumor. At surgery anaplastic ependymoma (WHO grade III) was found.*

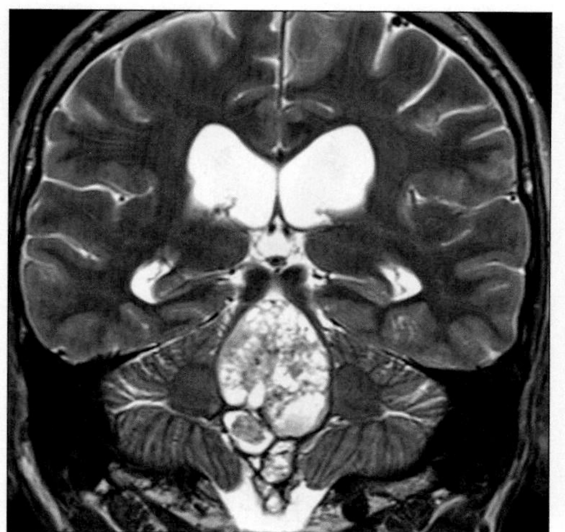

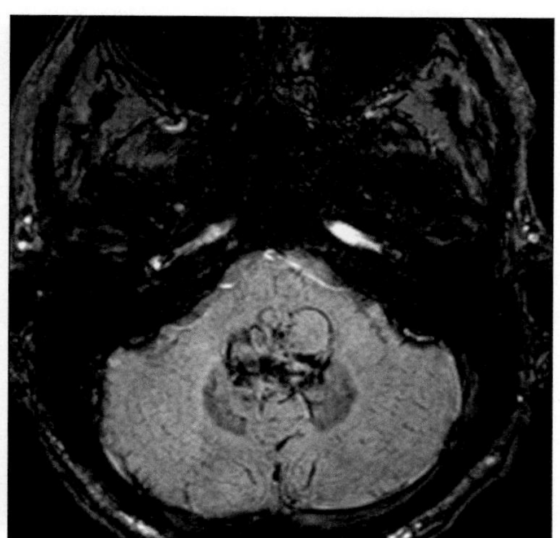

(Left) *Coronal T2WI MR in a 29-year-old man shows a typical infratentorial ependymoma in the region of the 4th ventricle. The tumor shows inhomogeneous high signal with multiple foci of low signal intensity.* ***(Right)*** *Axial T2* SWI MR in the same patient demonstrates intratumoral, low signal areas, most probably representing calcification and hemorrhagic components.*

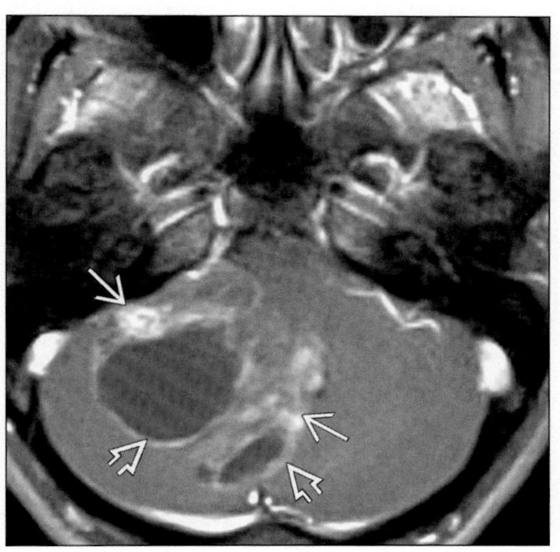

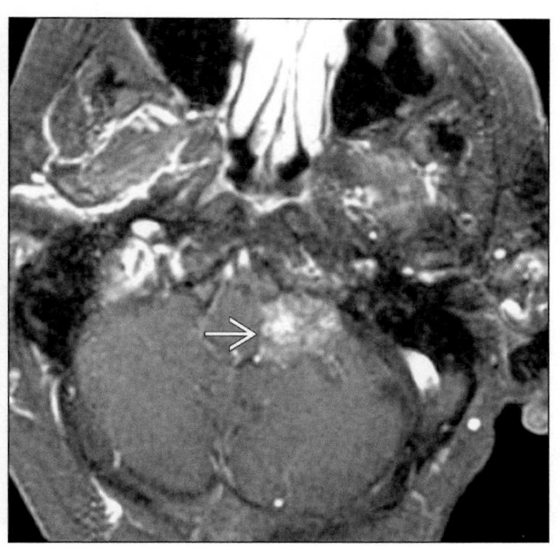

(Left) *Axial T1WI C+ MR in a 12-year-old boy shows an off-midline mass. Note the heterogeneous enhancement of the solid tumor components with marginal enhancement in the cyst walls. Surgery disclosed ependymoma. "Lateral ependymomas" have a worse prognosis.* ***(Right)*** *Axial T1WI C+ MR in a middle-aged woman with headaches shows a lobulated mass in the inferior left CPA cistern. Preoperative diagnosis was choroid plexus papilloma; at surgery, cellular ependymoma was found.*

SUPRATENTORIAL EPENDYMOMA

Key Facts

Imaging

- General location of ependymomas
  - 2/3 infratentorial, 1/3 supratentorial
  - 45-65% of supratentorial ependymomas (STEs) are **extraventricular**
  - Common locations of STEs: Cerebral hemisphere > 3rd > lateral ventricle
- General features
  - Cystic + mural nodule > solid mass
  - Calcification common
  - Variable intratumoral hemorrhage
  - Moderate but inhomogeneous enhancement

Top Differential Diagnoses

- Glioblastoma multiforme
- Ganglioglioma
- Angiocentric glioma
- Astroblastoma
- Papillary glioneuronal tumor
- Oligodendroglioma
- Anaplastic oligodendroglioma
- Pilocytic astrocytoma
- Ependymoblastoma

Pathology

- Majority of adult STE are WHO grade III tumors

Clinical Issues

- Older children, adults
  - Seizures
- Most important prognostic factor: Location
- Children < 3 years have poor outcome

Diagnostic Checklist

- Large mixed solid-cystic, calcified hemispheric/ cortical mass in older children or adult

(Left) Axial FLAIR MR in a 47-year-old man with anaplastic (grade III) hemispheric supratentorial ependymoma (STE) shows an inhomogeneous extraventricular mass in the left frontal lobe ⇨ with perifocal edema ➡. ***(Right)*** Axial T2* GRE MR in the same patient demonstrates a rim of peripheral low signal intensity → indicating hemorrhage. STEs commonly demonstrate intratumoral hemorrhage.

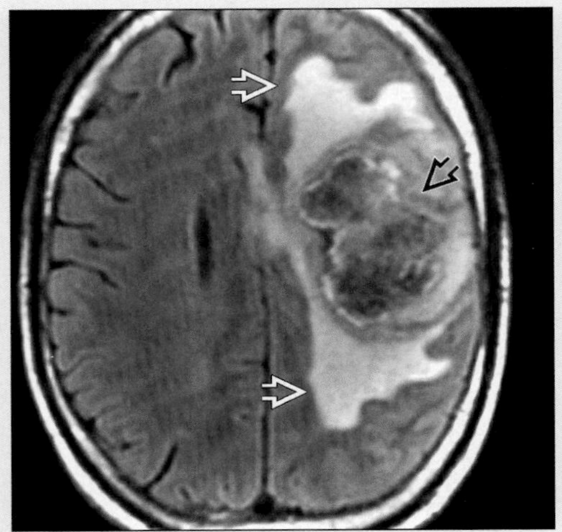

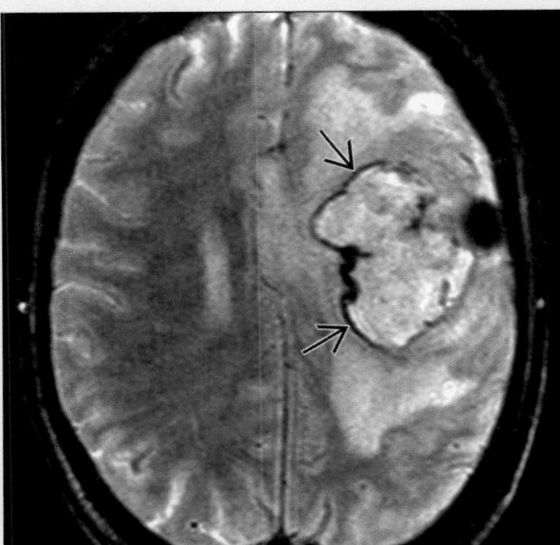

(Left) Axial DWI MR in the same patient reveals inhomogeneous high signal of the tumor representing areas of elevated diffusion (dark) and areas of restricted diffusion due to hemorrhage (hyperintense). ***(Right)*** Coronal T1WI C+ MR in the same patient shows a peripherally enhancing tumor with central necrosis, compression of the left ventricle, and midline shift. Note the contiguity with the ventricular system ➡.

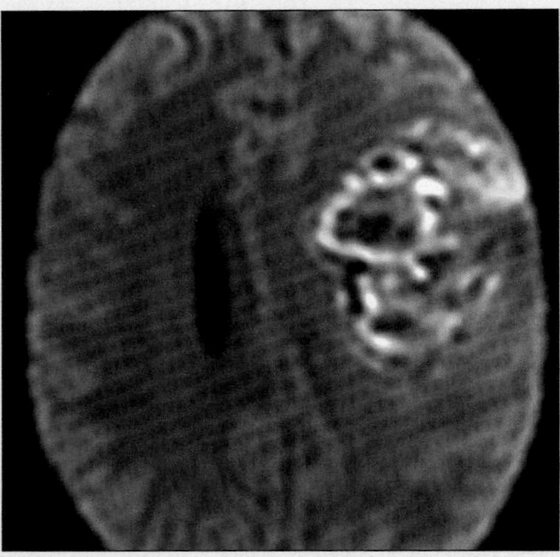

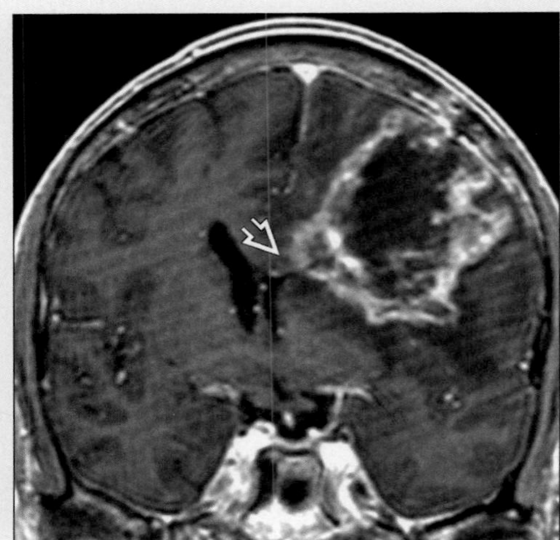

SUPRATENTORIAL EPENDYMOMA

TERMINOLOGY

Abbreviations

- Supratentorial ependymoma (STE)

Synonyms

- Hemispheric STE (a.k.a. "brain surface ependymoma")
- Supratentorial ectopic cortical ependymoma
- Cortical ependymoma

Definitions

- Ependymoma in supratentorial location

IMAGING

General Features

- Best diagnostic clue
  - Cystic-mural nodule mass in older children or adults, either brain hemispheres or 3rd ventricle
- Location
  - General location of ependymomas
    - 2/3 infratentorial (ITE)
    - 1/3 supratentorial (STE)
  - 45-65% of STEs are **extraventricular**
    - Hemispheric white matter or cortex
      - Frontal lobe most common location of cortical STEs
      - In cortex or infiltrating cortex from white matter
    - Rare: Suprasellar region
  - Less common location = intraventricular
    - 3rd ventricle > lateral ventricle
- Size
  - Larger size at presentation than ITE
  - > 4 cm (95%)

CT Findings

- NECT
  - Mixed iso-/hypodense
    - Hyperdense = solid portion
    - Hypodense = cystic component
    - Calcifications (44%)
      - Can be small scattered foci or very extensive
  - May show bone destruction (tumor invades meninges, dura, and bone)

MR Findings

- T1WI
  - Iso-/hypointense
  - Cysts follow CSF
- T2WI
  - Variable morphological features
    - Cystic with mural nodule
    - Solid mass
    - Huge, partially necrotic mass
  - Variable signal
    - Hyper-/hypointense (high cellularity, calcifications)
    - Cysts hyperintense (CSF)
- T2* GRE
  - Low signal indicates hemorrhage or calcifications
- DWI
  - High signal with low ADC in hypercellular solid portions
- T1WI C+
  - Moderately intense enhancing tumor (solid parts) with necrotic foci
  - Rarely nonenhancing
  - Pattern
    - Cystic + mural nodule appearance (often in hemispheric location)
      - Mural nodule moderate or intense enhancing
      - Nonenhancing or rim-enhancing cysts
  - Continuity with ventricle may be present
  - Continuity with surface present in cortical STE

Imaging Recommendations

- Best imaging tool
  - MR ± contrast
  - T2* (hemorrhage, calcification)

DIFFERENTIAL DIAGNOSIS

Glioblastoma Multiforme

- If STE presents as huge partially necrotic mass
- Less common: Low-grade anaplastic astrocytoma

Ganglioglioma

- Most common in temporal lobe

Angiocentric Glioma

- Children, young adults
- Nonenhancing cortical mass
- Rim-like hyperintensity on T1WI
- Epilepsy since childhood

Astroblastoma

- Older children and young adults
- Solid cystic mass
- Supratentorial location
- Calcifications

Papillary Glioneuronal Tumor

- Cortical mass, often with connection to ventricle
- Calcifications
- May be cystic or have nodule-cystic appearance

Oligodendroglioma (and Anaplastic Oligodendroglioma)

- Cerebral hemispheres
- Cortical and subcortical locations
- Calcifications
- Scalloping of inner table of skull

Pilocytic Astrocytoma

- Rarely hemispheric when supratentorial
- Most often around 3rd ventricle, hypothalamus, optic chiasm

Ependymoblastoma

- Usually supratentorial
- Children < 5 years of age
- Clearly separated from ventricle
- Rare embryonal tumor (PNET features + ependymal rosettes)

SUPRATENTORIAL EPENDYMOMA

- Histology: Should be distinguished from anaplastic ependymoma = different prognosis

PATHOLOGY

General Features

- Etiology
  - General: Ependymoma is glial-based neoplasm arising from ependymal lining of ventricular system
  - Extraventricular STE arise either from
    - Fetal rests of ependymal cells located at angle of ventricles
    - Random distribution of fetal ependymal rests located periventricularly
- Genetics
  - Gains of 1q (associated with aggressive clinical behavior), 12q, 7q, 8, 9
  - Perinuclear LRIG3 proteins more highly expressed in STE than ITE
  - Complete and partial losses of chromosomes 22, 22q, 10q, 3, 6q, 9q
    - 9q contains P16 *INK4A* gene often seen in STE
  - Upregulation of components of EphB-ephrin and Notch signaling pathways in STE
  - New entity: **Trisomy 19 ependymoma**
    - WHO grade III
    - Occurs in 9% of ependymomas

Staging, Grading, & Classification

- WHO grade I includes subependymoma & myxopapillary ependymoma
- WHO grade II ependymoma
  - 4 variants: Cellular, papillary, clear cell, & tanycytic
- WHO grade III anaplastic ependymoma
  - Majority of adult STE are WHO grade III tumors
  - Defined by presence of any 2 of 4 + factors
    - 4 mitoses per 10 high-power fields (brisk mitotic activity)
    - Hypercellularity
    - Endothelial proliferation
    - Necrosis (pseudopalisading necrosis)

Gross Pathologic & Surgical Features

- Well-delineated tumors
- Lobulated mass, grayish-red surface, hemorrhagic and calcified parts

Microscopic Features

- Histological hallmarks
  - Perivascular rosettes
  - Ependymal rosettes
  - GFAP(+)
- Nonrosetting angiocentric growth pattern
- Variable amount of solid tumor growth
- Low proliferative index
- Infiltrating brain parenchyma
  - Infiltration along axonal tracts, perineuronal satellitosis, subpial mounding

CLINICAL ISSUES

Presentation

- Most common signs/symptoms
  - Seizures most common symptom
  - Focal motor or sensory deficit, headache

Demographics

- Age
  - STEs found in older children, adults
- Gender
  - M > F
- Epidemiology
  - Ependymomas = 1.2-7.8% of all intracranial tumors
  - 3rd most common intracranial neoplasm in children

Natural History & Prognosis

- 5-year survival for supratentorial ependymomas (57.8%)
- Higher recurrence rate for 3rd ventricular tumors (compared to hemispheric tumors)
- Most important prognostic factor: Location
- Children < 3 years have poor outcome

Treatment

- Gross total resection with adjuvant radiotherapy

DIAGNOSTIC CHECKLIST

Consider

- Large solid-cystic, calcified mass in ventricular or cortical location in older children or adults

SELECTED REFERENCES

1. Niazi TN et al: WHO Grade II and III supratentorial hemispheric ependymomas in adults: case series and review of treatment options. J Neurooncol. 91(3):323-8, 2009
2. Yi W et al: Expression of leucine-rich repeats and immunoglobulin-like domains (LRIG) proteins in human ependymoma relates to tumor location, WHO grade, and patient age. Clin Neuropathol. 28(1):21-7, 2009
3. Lehman NL: Central nervous system tumors with ependymal features: a broadened spectrum of primarily ependymal differentiation? J Neuropathol Exp Neurol. 67(3):177-88, 2008
4. Lehman NL: Patterns of brain infiltration and secondary structure formation in supratentorial ependymal tumors. J Neuropathol Exp Neurol. 67(9):900-10, 2008
5. Miyazawa T et al: Supratentorial ectopic cortical ependymoma occurring with intratumoral hemorrhage. Brain Tumor Pathol. 24(1):35-40, 2007
6. Rousseau E et al: Trisomy 19 ependymoma, a newly recognized genetico-histological association, including clear cell ependymoma. Mol Cancer. 6:47, 2007
7. Vinchon M et al: Supratentorial ependymoma in children. Pediatr Neurosurg. 34(2):77-87, 2001
8. Schwartz TH et al: Supratentorial ependymomas in adult patients. Neurosurgery. 44(4):721-31, 1999
9. Spoto GP et al: Intracranial ependymoma and subependymoma: MR manifestations. AJR Am J Roentgenol. 154(4):837-45, 1990

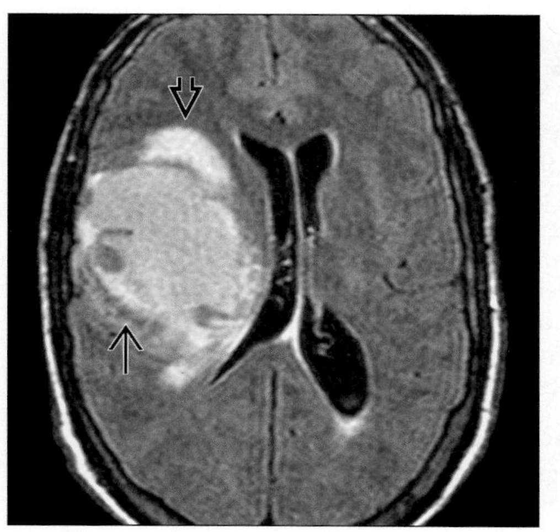

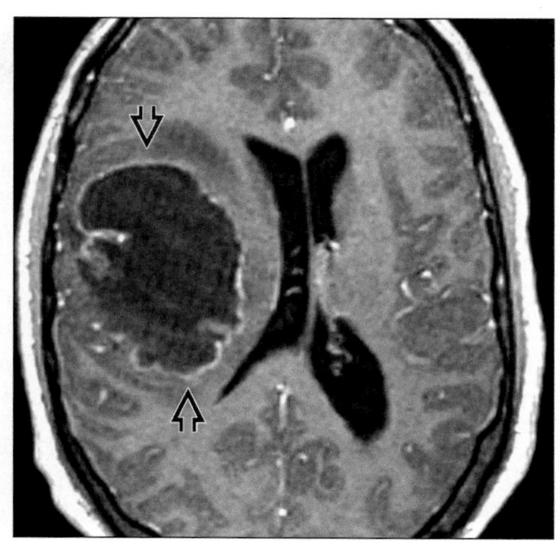

(Left) *Axial FLAIR MR shows a large cystic mass ➡ in the right hemisphere with perifocal edema ⇨ and compression of the right ventricle with minimal midline shift.* ***(Right)*** *Axial T1WI C+ MR in the same patient shows peripheral enhancement around a nonenhancing cystic component ⇨. STE was found at surgery. This STE does not show any contiguity with the ventricular system.*

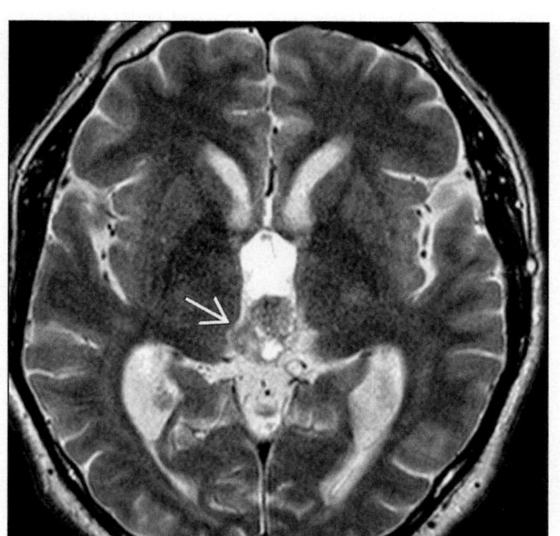

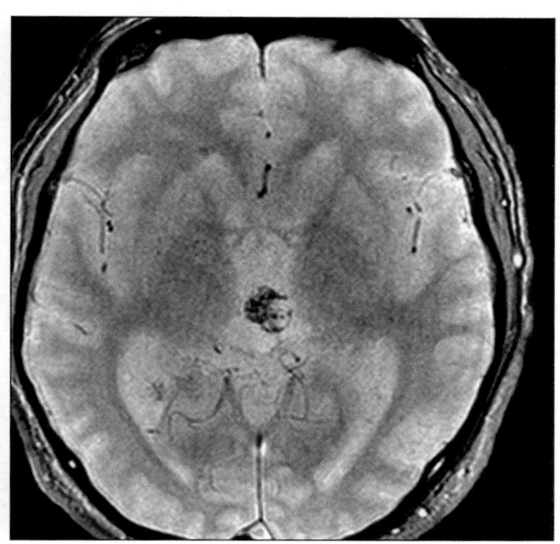

(Left) *Axial T2WI MR in a patient with supratentorial intraventricular ependymoma (STE) shows an inhomogeneous mass in the 3rd ventricle ➡. Note the relatively low signal, small intratumoral cysts.* ***(Right)*** *Axial T2* GRE MR in the same case shows blooming, hypointense foci indicating calcification or hemorrhage.*

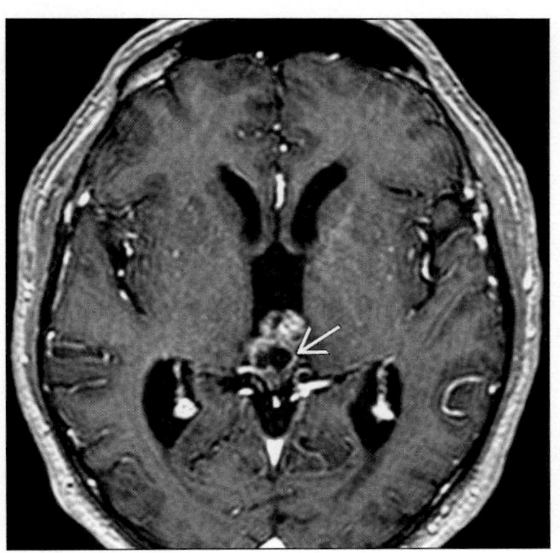

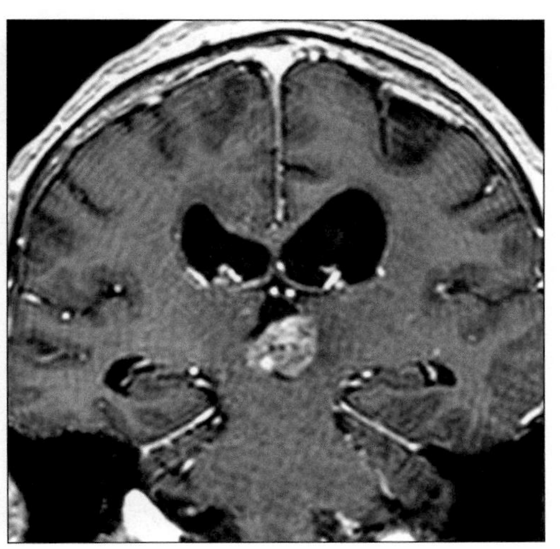

(Left) *Axial T1WI C+ MR in the same patient demonstrates marked but inhomogeneous enhancement. Note the solid portions, intratumoral cysts of various sizes, and a larger cyst with rim enhancement ➡.* ***(Right)*** *Coronal T1WI C+ MR in the same patient demonstrates an inhomogeneously enhancing nodular mass within the 3rd ventricle.*

SUBEPENDYMOMA

Key Facts

Terminology
- Rare, benign well-differentiated intraventricular ependymal tumor, typically attached to ventricular wall

Imaging
- Intraventricular, inferior 4th ventricle typical (60%)
- Other locations: Lateral > 3rd ventricle > spinal cord
- T2/FLAIR hyperintense intraventricular mass
  - Heterogeneity related to cystic changes; blood products or Ca++ may be seen in larger lesions
- Variable enhancement, typically none to mild

Top Differential Diagnoses
- Ependymoma
- Central neurocytoma
- Subependymal giant cell astrocytoma
- Choroid plexus papilloma (CPP)
- Hemangioblastoma
- Metastases

Pathology
- WHO grade I

Clinical Issues
- 40% become symptomatic, often supratentorial
  - Related to increased intracranial pressure, hydrocephalus
- Present in middle-aged/elderly adult (typically 5th-6th decades)
- Excellent prognosis for supratentorial lesions
  - Recurrence is extremely rare
- Surgical resection is curative in most cases

Diagnostic Checklist
- 4th or lateral ventricular hyperintense mass in an elderly man? Think subependymoma!

(Left) Sagittal graphic shows a solid, well-circumscribed mass arising from the floor of the 4th ventricle with mild mass effect ⇒. Note the lack of hydrocephalus, typical of subependymoma. (Right) Sagittal T2WI MR shows a solid, hyperintense mass along the inferior 4th ventricle ➡ in a 43-year-old man with headaches and trigeminal neuralgia. Subependymoma was found at resection. These 4th ventricular tumors are often asymptomatic. T2 and FLAIR are typically the most sensitive sequences for this tumor.

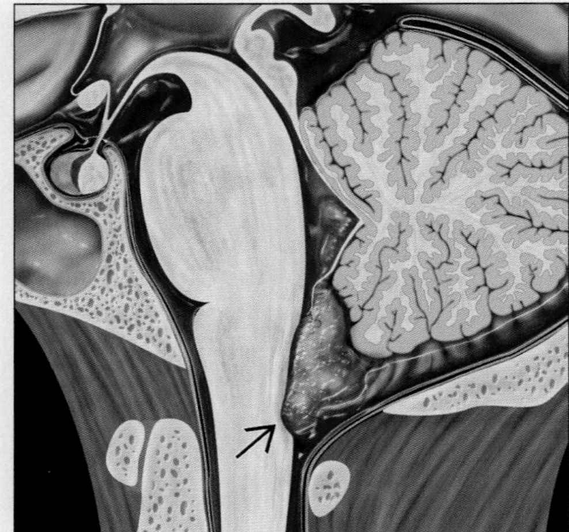

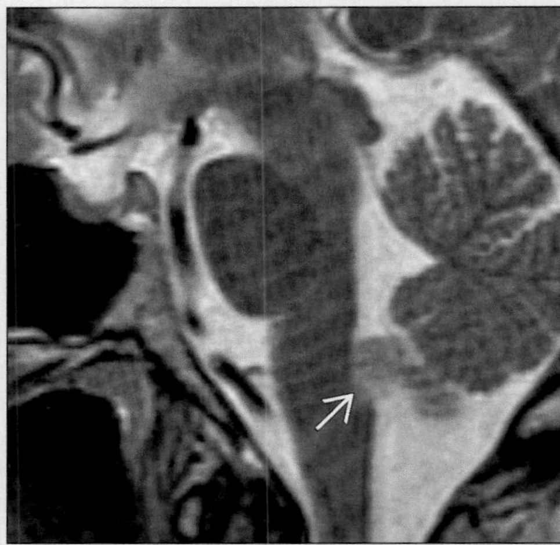

(Left) Axial T2WI MR shows a hyperintense mass ➡ along the inferior 4th ventricle at the level of the medulla. (Right) Sagittal T1WI C+ MR in the same patient shows mild enhancement of the mass ➡ found incidentally. Subependymomas are most commonly found in the inferior 4th ventricle (50-60%); the lateral ventricle is the next most common location (30-40%). These WHO grade I tumors are primarily treated with surgical resection, which is typically curative.

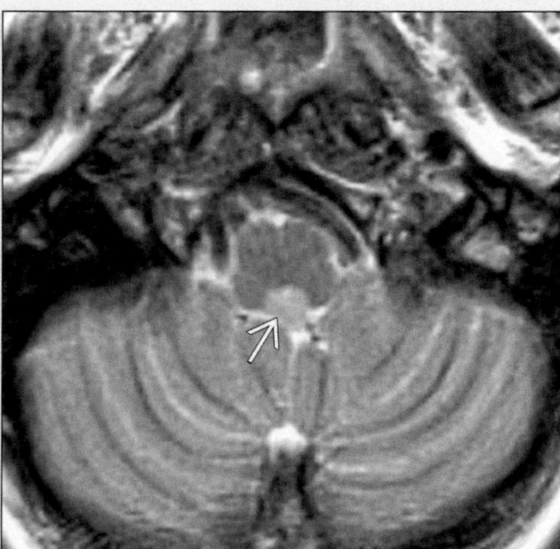

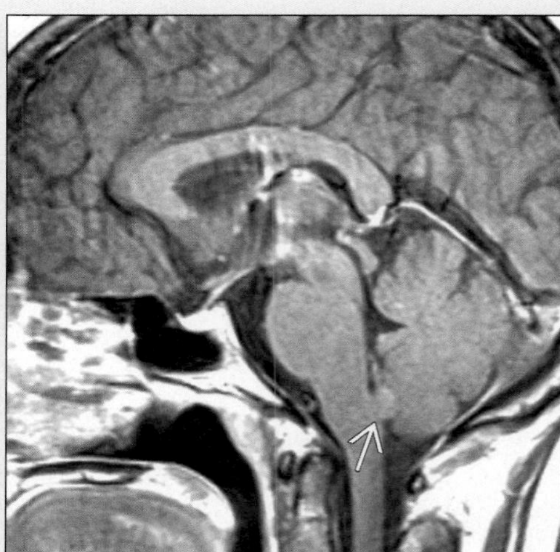

TERMINOLOGY

Synonyms

- Older literature: Subependymal glomerulate astrocytoma, subependymal astrocytoma, subependymal mixed glioma

Definitions

- Rare, benign, well-differentiated, intraventricular ependymal tumor, often attached to ventricular wall

IMAGING

General Features

- Best diagnostic clue
  - T2-hyperintense, lobular, nonenhancing, intraventricular mass
- Location
  - Typical: Intraventricular, inferior 4th ventricle (60%)
    - Often protrudes through foramen of Magendie
  - Other locations: Lateral > 3rd ventricle > spinal cord (cervical or cervicothoracic)
    - Lateral ventricle: Attached to septum pellucidum or lateral wall
  - Rare: Periventricular
- Size
  - Typically small, 1-2 cm
  - May become large, > 5 cm
    - When large, more commonly symptomatic
- Morphology
  - Well-defined, solid, lobular mass
  - When large, may see cysts, hemorrhage, Ca++

CT Findings

- NECT
  - Iso- to hypodense intraventricular mass
  - Cysts or Ca++ may be seen in larger lesions
  - Rarely hemorrhage
- CECT
  - No or mild enhancement typical
  - Heterogeneous enhancement may be seen

MR Findings

- T1WI
  - Intraventricular mass, hypo- or isointense to white matter
  - Typically homogeneous solid mass
  - Heterogeneity may be seen in larger lesions
- T2WI
  - Hyperintense intraventricular mass
  - Heterogeneity related to cystic changes; blood products or Ca++ may be seen in larger lesions
  - No edema seen in adjacent brain parenchyma
- FLAIR
  - Hyperintense intraventricular mass
  - No edema seen in adjacent brain parenchyma
- T2* GRE
  - May see Ca++ "bloom" in larger lesions and 4th ventricle location
- T1WI C+
  - Variable enhancement, typically none to mild
  - Marked enhancement may be seen: More common in 4th than lateral ventricular subependymomas

Nuclear Medicine Findings

- PET
  - Rare reports show exceedingly low rates of glucose metabolism and kinetic constants
    - Hypometabolism indicates low cellular density and slow growth

Imaging Recommendations

- Best imaging tool
  - MR is most sensitive
  - CT may be useful for calcification
- Protocol advice
  - Multiplanar contrast-enhanced MR including T2WI, FLAIR

DIFFERENTIAL DIAGNOSIS

Ependymoma

- Younger patients
- Heterogeneous, enhancing mass with edema
- Typically 4th ventricular mass with hydrocephalus
- Often parenchymal when supratentorial

Central Neurocytoma

- Typical "bubbly" appearance, Ca++ common
- Lateral ventricle, attached to septum pellucidum
- Moderate to strong enhancement

Subependymal Giant Cell Astrocytoma

- Enhancing mass at foramen of Monro
- Ca++ common
- Tuberous sclerosis patients: Subependymal nodules, cortical tubers, white matter lesions

Choroid Plexus Papilloma (CPP)

- Typically pediatric tumors, lateral ventricle
- In adults, 4th ventricle
- Enhancing papillary mass, hydrocephalus common

Hemangioblastoma

- Cystic mass with enhancing mural nodule
- Typically cerebellar hemispheres, often at pial surface
- Rarely intraventricular

Metastases

- Primary tumor often known
- Often multiple lesions at gray-white junctions
- Typically involve choroid plexus if intraventricular

Cavernous Malformation

- Rarely intraventricular, 2.5-11% of cases
- Ca++ and T2 hypointense hemosiderin rim common
- Enhancement variable

PATHOLOGY

General Features

- Etiology
  - Proposed cells of origin: Subependymal glia, astrocytes of subependymal plate, ependymal cells

SUBEPENDYMOMA

    - Development from subependymal glial precursors appears likely
- Genetics
  - Most are sporadic
  - Rare familial cases have been reported
- Associated abnormalities
  - Contains both astrocytes and ependymal elements
  - Occasionally coexists with cellular ependymomas
  - Rare: Multiple lesions

Staging, Grading, & Classification

- WHO grade I

Gross Pathologic & Surgical Features

- Solid, well-delineated, white to grayish, avascular mass
- Firmly attached to site of origin
  - 4th ventricle: Floor typical
  - Lateral ventricle: Septum pellucidum or lateral wall
- Larger lesions are lobulated, more often Ca++; hemorrhage, cyst formation common
- 4th ventricular lesions often protrude out of foramen of Magendie

Microscopic Features

- Highly fibrillar, low cellularity with nuclei clustering
- Microcystic change common in tumors near foramen of Monro
- Ca++ is commonly seen in 4th ventricle tumors
- Mitoses are rare or absent, MIB < 1%
- Hemorrhage is rare
- Immunohistochemistry: Strongly GFAP(+)
- Electron microscopy: Closely packed cell processes filled with glial intermediate filaments

CLINICAL ISSUES

Presentation

- Most common signs/symptoms
  - Most asymptomatic
  - 40% become symptomatic, often supratentorial
    - Related to increased intracranial pressure, hydrocephalus
      - Headache, gait ataxia, visual disturbance, cranial neuropathy, nystagmus, vertigo, nausea, vomiting

Demographics

- Age
  - Middle-aged/elderly adult (typically 5th-6th decades)
    - Asymptomatic patients: Mean age = 60 years
    - Symptomatic patients: Mean age = 40 years
  - Rare in children
- Gender
  - Male predominance
- Epidemiology
  - Reported in 0.4% of 1,000 consecutive autopsies
  - Account for 0.7% of intracranial neoplasms
  - Represent ~ 8% of ependymal tumors

Natural History & Prognosis

- Excellent prognosis for supratentorial lesions
- Recurrence is extremely rare
- Complications include hydrocephalus and rarely hemorrhage

Treatment

- Surgical resection is curative in most cases
  - Lateral ventricle lesions: Complete resection
  - 4th ventricle lesions: Subtotal resection more common
- Perioperative mortality low but increased by attachment of tumor to adjacent structures
- If hydrocephalus, CSF diversion may be required
- Adjuvant radiation therapy is controversial, likely of no benefit
- Conservative management with serial imaging if asymptomatic

DIAGNOSTIC CHECKLIST

Consider

- Other intraventricular tumors tend to enhance more prominently
- May be indistinguishable from ependymoma or central neurocytoma

Image Interpretation Pearls

- 4th or lateral ventricular hyperintense mass in an elderly man? Think subependymoma!
- T2WI and FLAIR are often most sensitive

SELECTED REFERENCES

1. Louis DN et al: WHO Classification of Tumours of the Central Nervous System: Subependymoma. Lyon: IARC Press. 70-71, 2007
2. Rushing EJ et al: Subependymoma revisited: clinicopathological evaluation of 83 cases. J Neurooncol. 85(3):297-305, 2007
3. Ragel BT et al: Subependymomas: an analysis of clinical and imaging features. Neurosurgery. 58(5):881-90; discussion 881-90, 2006
4. Rath TJ et al: Massive symptomatic subependymoma of the lateral ventricles: case report and review of the literature. Neuroradiology. 47(3):183-8, 2005
5. Shuangshoti S et al: Supratentorial extraventricular ependymal neoplasms: a clinicopathologic study of 32 patients. Cancer. 103(12):2598-605, 2005
6. Kim HC et al: Subependymoma in the third ventricle in a child. Clin Imaging. 28(5):381-4, 2004
7. Im SH et al: Clinicopathological study of seven cases of symptomatic supratentorial subependymoma. J Neurooncol. 61(1):57-67, 2003
8. Maiuri F et al: Symptomatic subependymomas of the lateral ventricles. Report of eight cases. Clin Neurol Neurosurg. 99(1):17-22, 1997
9. Mineura K et al: Subependymoma of the septum pellucidum: characterization by PET. J Neurooncol. 32(2):143-7, 1997
10. Jallo GI et al: Intramedullary subependymoma of the spinal cord. Neurosurgery. 38(2):251-7, 1996
11. Chiechi MV et al: Intracranial subependymomas: CT and MR imaging features in 24 cases. AJR Am J Roentgenol. 165(5):1245-50, 1995
12. Hoeffel C et al: MR manifestations of subependymomas. AJNR Am J Neuroradiol. 16(10):2121-9, 1995
13. Iqbal Z et al: Subependymoma of the lateral ventricle: case report and literature review. Br J Neurosurg. 8(1):83-5, 1994

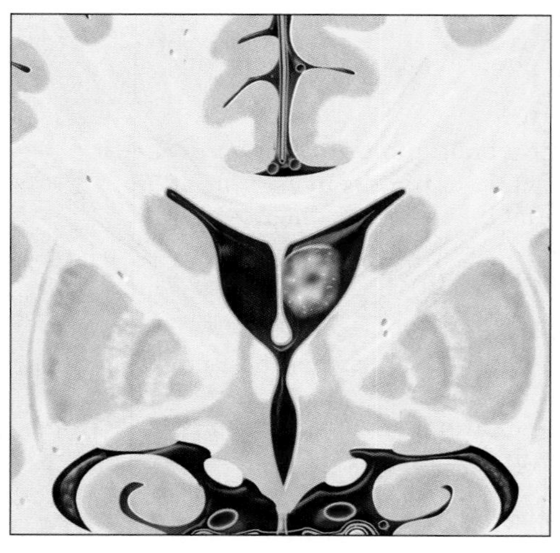

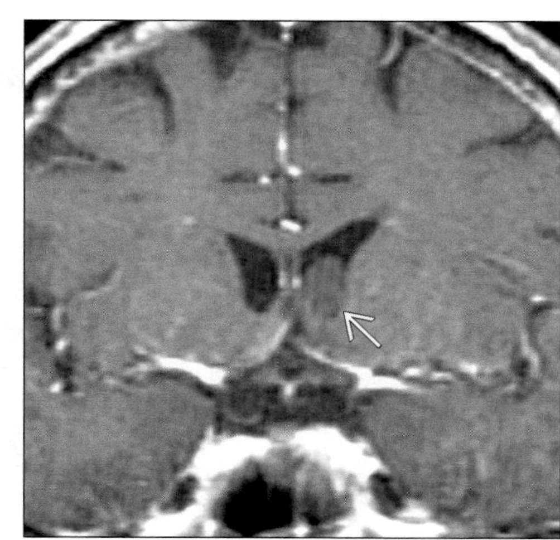

(Left) *Coronal graphic shows a solid, well-circumscribed, intraventricular mass attached to the septum pellucidum with neither mass effect nor hydrocephalus. Subependymomas are typically asymptomatic, but they may cause hydrocephalus and increased intracranial pressure.* ***(Right)*** *Coronal T1WI C+ MR shows a small nonenhancing mass in the left lateral ventricle ➔. There is no evidence of obstructive hydrocephalus. The location and imaging findings are classic for subependymoma.*

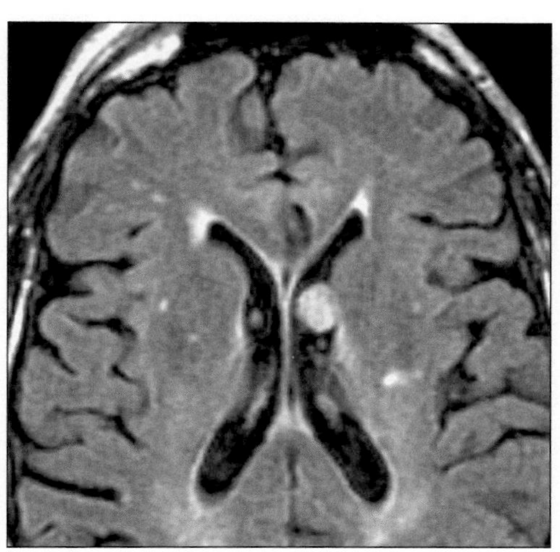

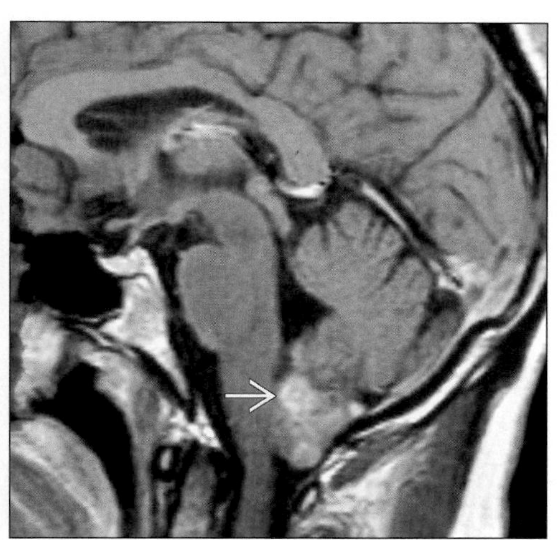

(Left) *Axial FLAIR MR shows a hyperintense lateral ventricle mass at the level of the septum pellucidum. Subependymomas are often best visualized on T2 and FLAIR MR. When in the lateral ventricle, they are typically attached to the septum pellucidum or lateral wall.* ***(Right)*** *Sagittal T1 C+ MR shows a circumscribed, enhancing mass in the region of the 4th ventricular outflow tract ➔ and cisterna magna. Subependymomas often protrude through the foramen of Magendie. The moderate enhancement is uncommon.*

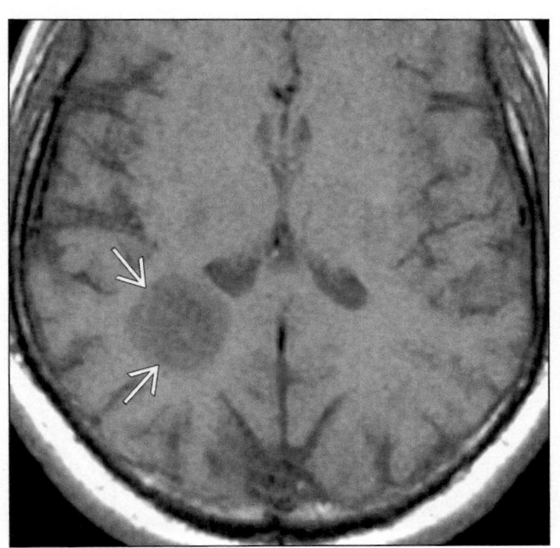

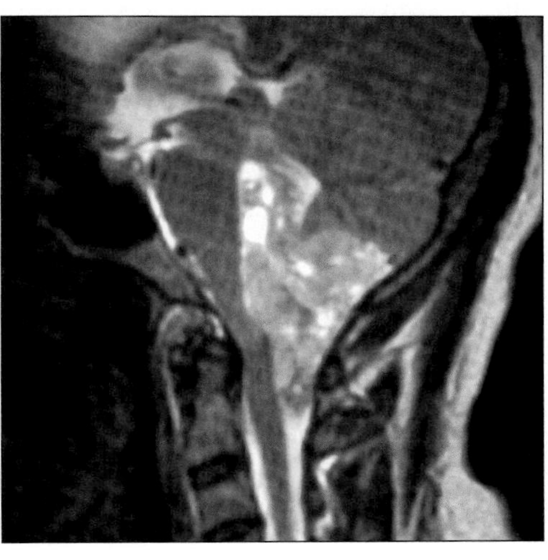

(Left) *Axial T1WI MR shows a circumscribed hypointense mass ➔ in the right periatrial region. Note the mass effect upon the adjacent lateral ventricle. Subependymomas rarely occur in the periventricular location.* ***(Right)*** *Sagittal T2WI MR shows a heterogeneous mass filling the 4th ventricle with inferior extension. Enhancement was present on contrast images of this WHO grade I subependymoma. Cysts, blood, and calcification may be seen in larger lesions. Imaging mimics ependymoma and hemangioblastoma.*

TYPICAL CHOROID PLEXUS PAPILLOMA

Key Facts

Terminology

- Intraventricular, papillary neoplasm derived from choroid plexus epithelium (WHO grade I)

Imaging

- Child with strongly enhancing, lobulated intraventricular mass
- CPPs occur in proportion to amount of normally present choroid plexus
  - 50% ⇒ lateral ventricle
  - 40% ⇒ 4th ventricle and foramina of Luschka
  - 5% ⇒ 3rd ventricle (roof)
- Choroidal artery enlargement for lateral ventricular (trigonal) CPPs
- Hydrocephalus common

Top Differential Diagnoses

- Choroid plexus carcinoma
- Medulloblastoma
- Infratentorial ependymoma
- Intraventricular metastasis
- Meningioma
- Physiologic choroid plexus enlargement

Clinical Issues

- Most common brain tumor in children < 1 year
  - 13.1% of all brain tumors in 1st year of life
  - 7.9% of fetal brain tumors diagnosed by ultrasound
- Rarely seed CSF pathways

Diagnostic Checklist

- Consider CPP if intraventricular mass in child under 2 years
- Imaging alone cannot reliably distinguish CPP from choroid plexus carcinoma

*(**Left**) Axial graphic shows a choroid plexus papilloma (CPP) arising from the glomus of the left lateral ventricular trigone. Note the characteristic frond-like surface projections. CPP are most common in the lateral ventricles of a child. (**Right**) Axial T1WI MR shows a lobular, isointense, left lateral ventricular mass in an 18-month-old child, typical of CPP. Note the associated hydrocephalus, which is often related to overproduction of CSF by the tumor.*

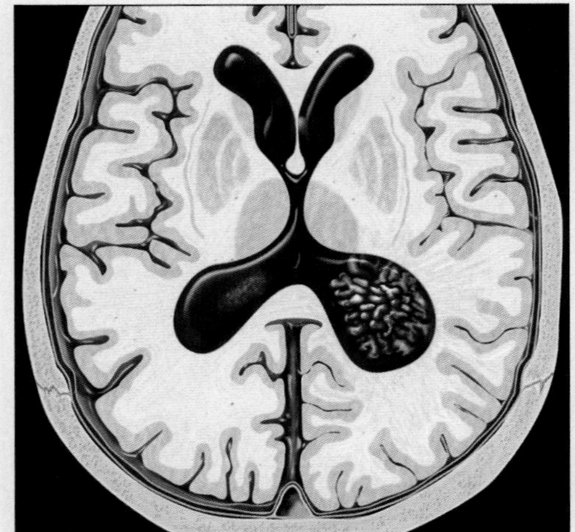

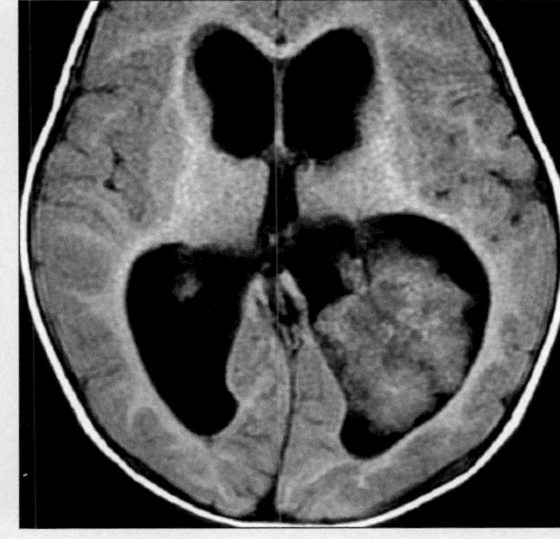

*(**Left**) Axial T2WI MR in the same patient shows a heterogeneously hyperintense lateral ventricle mass with scattered hypointense flow voids →, indicating high vascularity. No significant T2 hyperintensity is present in the adjacent parenchyma to suggest local invasion. (**Right**) Axial T1WI C+ MR shows marked enhancement of the lobular mass with frond-like projections, characteristic of CPP. CPP cannot be reliably differentiated from carcinoma by conventional imaging alone.*

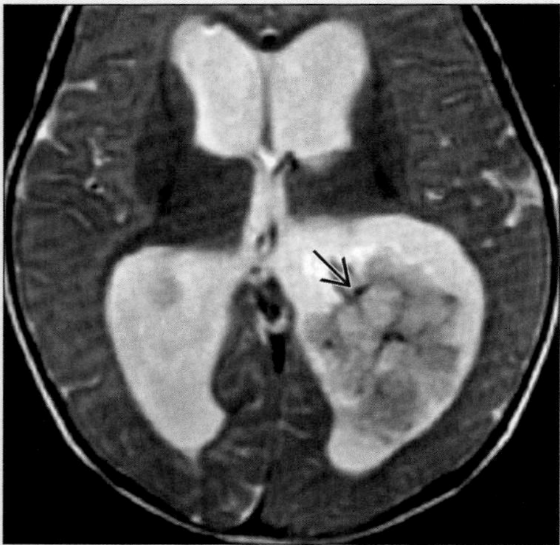

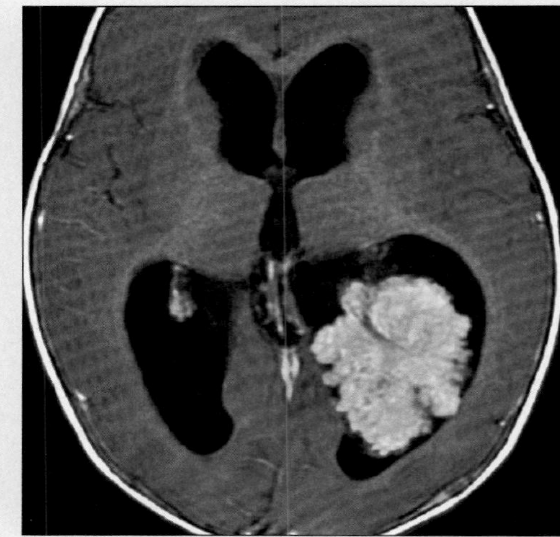

TYPICAL CHOROID PLEXUS PAPILLOMA

TERMINOLOGY

Abbreviations

- Choroid plexus tumor (CPT)
  - Choroid plexus papilloma (CPP) or choroid plexus carcinoma (CPCa)

Definitions

- Intraventricular, papillary neoplasm derived from choroid plexus epithelium (WHO grade I)

IMAGING

General Features

- Best diagnostic clue
  - Child with strongly enhancing, lobulated, intraventricular mass
- Location
  - CPPs occur in proportion to amount of normally present choroid plexus
    - 50% ⇒ atrium of lateral ventricle, left > right
    - 40% ⇒ 4th ventricle (posterior medullary velum) and foramina of Luschka
    - 5% ⇒ 3rd ventricle (roof)
    - 5% ⇒ multiple sites
    - Rare: Cerebellopontine angle, suprasellar, intraparenchymal
- Size
  - Often of remarkable size at diagnosis
- Morphology
  - Cauliflower-like mass

CT Findings

- NECT
  - Intraventricular lobular mass
  - 75% iso- or hyperattenuating
  - Ca++ in 25%
  - Hydrocephalus
    - Often related to overproduction of CSF by tumor
- CECT
  - Intense, homogeneous enhancement
    - Heterogeneous enhancement suggests choroid plexus carcinoma (CPCa)
  - Occasionally, minimal parenchymal invasion
  - Rarely, vascular pedicle twists leading to CPP infarction and dense Ca++ ("brain stone")
- CTA: Choroidal artery enlargement for lateral ventricular (trigonal) CPPs

MR Findings

- T1WI
  - Well-delineated iso- to hypointense lobular mass
- T2WI
  - Iso- to hyperintense mass
  - ± internal linear and branching vascular flow voids
  - Large CPP may bury itself within brain parenchyma
    - Extensive invasion suggests CPCa
  - Hydrocephalus common
- FLAIR
  - Bright periventricular signal
    - Transependymal interstitial edema due to ventricular obstruction
    - Asymmetric ipsilateral T2 hyperintensity may suggest invasion and CPCa
- T2* GRE
  - ± foci of diminished signal if Ca++ &/or blood products are present
- T1WI C+
  - Robust homogeneous enhancement
  - Occasional cysts and small foci of necrosis
  - ± CSF seeding lesions
- MRA
  - Flow-related signal within mass
  - Enlarged choroidal artery (trigonal mass)
- MRS
  - NAA absent, mild ↑ choline, lactate if necrotic
  - Myoinositol (mI) elevation in CPP may help to distinguish from CPCa

Ultrasonographic Findings

- Grayscale ultrasound
  - Hyperechoic mass with frond-like projections
  - Mass echogenicity similar to normal choroid plexus
  - Hydrocephalus
- Pulsed Doppler
  - Vascular pedicle and internal sampling of mass
    - Bidirectional flow through diastole
    - Arterial tracing shows low impedance
- Color Doppler
  - Hypervascular mass with bidirectional flow

Angiographic Findings

- Conventional
  - Enlarged anterior or posterior choroidal artery
  - Prolonged vascular stain
  - Arteriovenous shunting

Nuclear Medicine Findings

- PET
  - 11C-methionine → high tumor/normal brain ratios in CPP compared to gliomas
  - FDG → unable to distinguish between CPP and glioma

Imaging Recommendations

- Best imaging tool
  - MR with contrast
- Protocol advice
  - Perform contrast-enhanced MR of entire neuraxis before surgery

DIFFERENTIAL DIAGNOSIS

Choroid Plexus Carcinoma

- Difficult to distinguish from CPP by imaging
- More likely to invade brain
- May see heterogeneous enhancement

Medulloblastoma

- Hyperdense 4th ventricular mass in child
- More spherical than CPP

Infratentorial Ependymoma

- More common in 4th ventricle in children
- Heterogeneous enhancing mass

TYPICAL CHOROID PLEXUS PAPILLOMA

Intraventricular Metastasis
- Known history of primary tumor
- Rare in children

Meningioma
- Enhancing, circumscribed, intraventricular mass
- Consider neurofibromatosis type 2
- Older adults

Physiologic Choroid Plexus Enlargement
- Collateral venous drainage (Sturge-Weber)
- Enlargement of choroid following hemispherectomy

Subependymoma
- Nonenhancing intraventricular mass

Villous Hypertrophy (VH)
- Many presumed VH cases may be bilateral CPPs
- Proliferation index (MIB-1) is useful to distinguish

PATHOLOGY

General Features
- Genetics
  - DNA sequences from simian virus 40 (SV40) have been found in CPTs
  - High expression of *TWIST1*, a transcription factor that inhibits p53
  - Association with Aicardi and Li-Fraumeni syndromes
  - Duplication of short arm of chromosome 9 reported
- Associated abnormalities
  - Diffuse hydrocephalus from
    - CSF overproduction
    - Mechanical obstruction
    - Impaired CSF resorption (due to hemorrhage)

Staging, Grading, & Classification
- WHO grade I

Gross Pathologic & Surgical Features
- Well-circumscribed, lobulated, intraventricular mass
- ± cysts, necrosis, and hemorrhage

Microscopic Features
- Fibrovascular connective tissue fronds, covered by cuboidal or columnar epithelium
- Mitotic activity, necrosis, and brain invasion typically absent
- Resembles nonneoplastic choroid plexus (CP)
- Immunohistochemistry
  - Transthyretin may help distinguish from normal CP
  - GFAP reactivity can distinguish from normal CP
  - Kir7.1 and stanniocalcin-1 reactivity differentiates normal CP and CPT from other cell origins

CLINICAL ISSUES

Presentation
- Most common signs/symptoms
  - Macrocrania, bulging fontanelle, vomiting, headache, ataxia, seizure
- Clinical profile
  - Child < 2 years with signs and symptoms of elevated intracranial pressure

Demographics
- Age
  - Lateral ventricular CPPs: 80% < 20 years
  - 4th ventricular CPPs: More common in adults
- Gender
  - Lateral ventricle: M:F = 1:1
  - 4th ventricle: M:F = 3:2
- Epidemiology
  - 0.5% of all adult brain tumors
  - 2-3% of all pediatric brain tumors
  - Most common brain tumor in children < 1 year
    - 50% manifest in 1st decade
    - 86% present by 5 years
    - 13.1% of all brain tumors in 1st year of life
    - 7.9% of fetal brain tumors diagnosed by ultrasound

Natural History & Prognosis
- Benign, slowly growing
  - Rarely seed CSF pathways
- 5-year survival ~ 100%

Treatment
- Total surgical resection: Recurrence rare

DIAGNOSTIC CHECKLIST

Consider
- CPP if intraventricular mass in child under 2 years

Image Interpretation Pearls
- Imaging alone cannot reliably distinguish CPP from CPCa
  - Final diagnosis is histologic
- Lobulated intraventricular mass with strong enhancement in young child most likely represents choroid plexus tumor

SELECTED REFERENCES

1. Hasselblatt M et al: TWIST-1 is overexpressed in neoplastic choroid plexus epithelial cells and promotes proliferation and invasion. Cancer Res. 69(6):2219-23, 2009
2. Naeini RM et al: Spectrum of choroid plexus lesions in children. AJR Am J Roentgenol. 192(1):32-40, 2009
3. Buckle C et al: Choroid plexus papilloma of the third ventricle. Pediatr Radiol. 37(7):725, 2007
4. Frye RE et al: Choroid plexus papilloma expansion over 7 years in Aicardi syndrome. J Child Neurol. 22(4):484-7, 2007
5. Jeibmann A et al: Malignant progression in choroid plexus papillomas. J Neurosurg. 107(3 Suppl):199-202, 2007
6. Jinhu Y et al: Metastasis of a histologically benign choroid plexus papilloma: case report and review of the literature. J Neurooncol. 83(1):47-52, 2007
7. Kaptanoglu E et al: Spinal drop metastasis of choroid plexus papilloma. J Clin Neurosci. 14(4):381-3, 2007
8. Hasselblatt M et al: Identification of novel diagnostic markers for choroid plexus tumors: a microarray-based approach. Am J Surg Pathol. 30(1):66-74, 2006

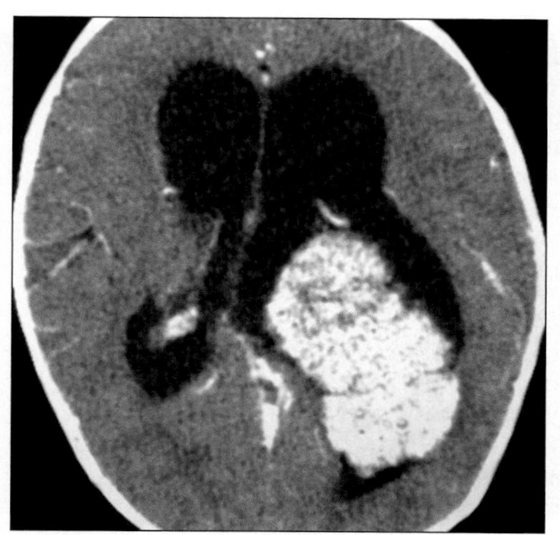

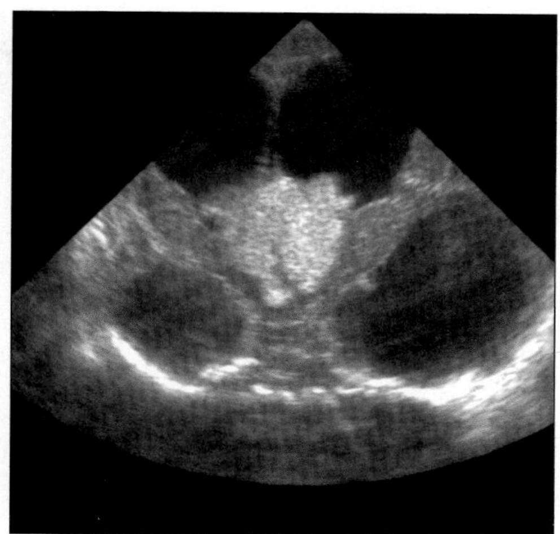

(Left) *Axial CECT shows a vividly enhancing lobular mass arising from the left lateral ventricle trigone, typical of CPP. Note the normal contralateral choroid plexus. The associated hydrocephalus is more commonly related to overproduction of CSF rather than mechanical obstruction or poor resorption.* ***(Right)*** *Coronal ultrasound shows a markedly hyperechoic mass with frond-like projections in the superior 3rd ventricle. Note the marked associated hydrocephalus in this infant with a grade I CPP.*

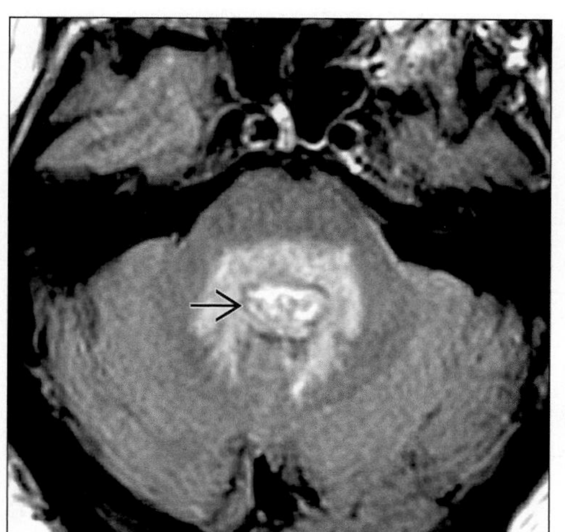

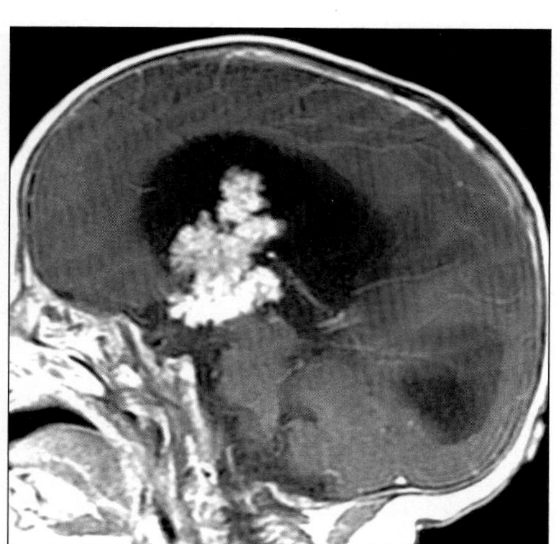

(Left) *Axial FLAIR MR in a 52 year old with headaches and vomiting shows a hyperintense 4th ventricular mass ⇒ with marked edema in the surrounding brain, an atypical feature of WHO grade I CPP. The imaging mimics an atypical CPP or choroid plexus carcinoma. (Courtesy P. Hildenbrand, MD.)* ***(Right)*** *Sagittal T1WI C+ MR shows a lobular, markedly enhancing, 3rd ventricle mass with frond-like projections, an uncommon location for choroid plexus tumors. Note the associated hydrocephalus.*

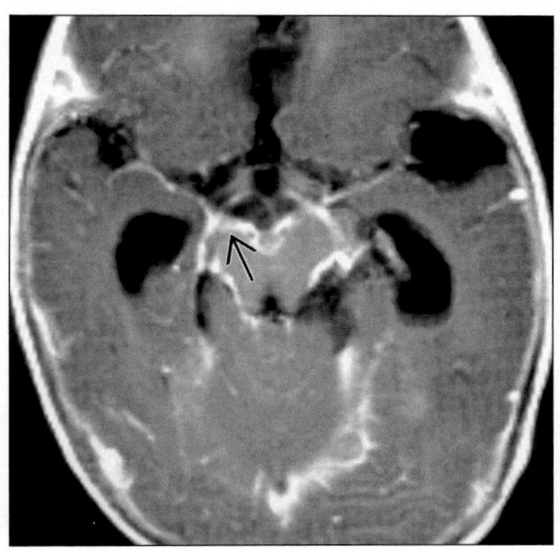

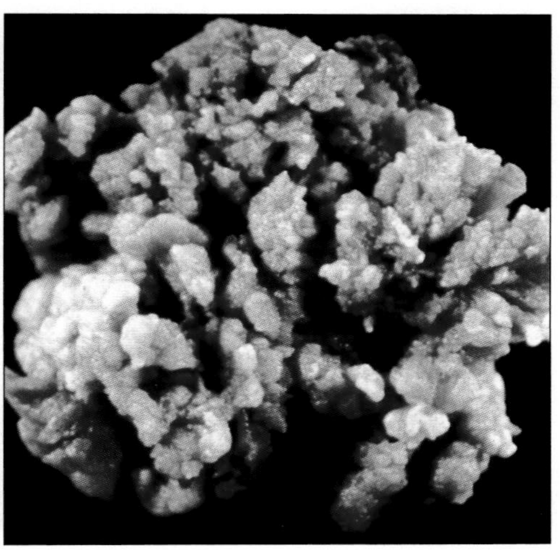

(Left) *Axial T1WI C+ MR shows diffuse basal cistern tumor seeding from a CPP ⇒, WHO grade I. Although CSF seeding may occur with all choroid plexus tumors, it is much more common in choroid plexus carcinomas, WHO grade III.* ***(Right)*** *Coronal gross pathology shows a typical CPP with a cauliflower-like appearance and multiple frond-like projections. These benign tumors rarely cause CSF seeding and may mimic a more aggressive choroid plexus tumor. (Courtesy AFIP.)*

ATYPICAL CHOROID PLEXUS PAPILLOMA

Key Facts

Terminology
- Choroid plexus papilloma (CPP) with increased mitotic activity and higher likelihood of recurrence (WHO grade II)

Imaging
- Child with lobulated, strongly enhancing intraventricular mass
  - May see hemorrhage and necrosis
  - Internal vascular flow voids common
  - Hydrocephalus common
- Not reliably distinguished from choroid plexus papilloma (CPP) or carcinoma (CPCa) on imaging

Top Differential Diagnoses
- CPP and CPCa
- Ependymoma
- Medulloblastoma
- Atypical teratoid-rhabdoid tumor

Pathology
- ≥ 2 mitoses per 10 high-power fields
  - Single microscopic criteria to distinguish aCPP (WHO grade II) from CPP (WHO grade I)
  - Most significant factor related to ↑ recurrence
- ↑ likelihood of atypical features: Hypercellularity, nuclear pleomorphism, necrosis, solid growth
- May demonstrate higher Ki-67 and MIB-1 proliferation indices

Clinical Issues
- Macrocephaly and vomiting most common presentation
- Complete surgical resection is generally curative
- Atypical CPP has 4.9x recurrence rate compared to WHO grade I CPP
- 5-year survival approaches 100%

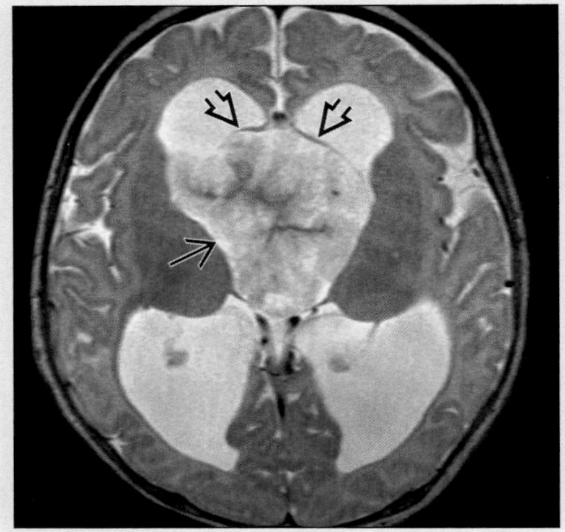
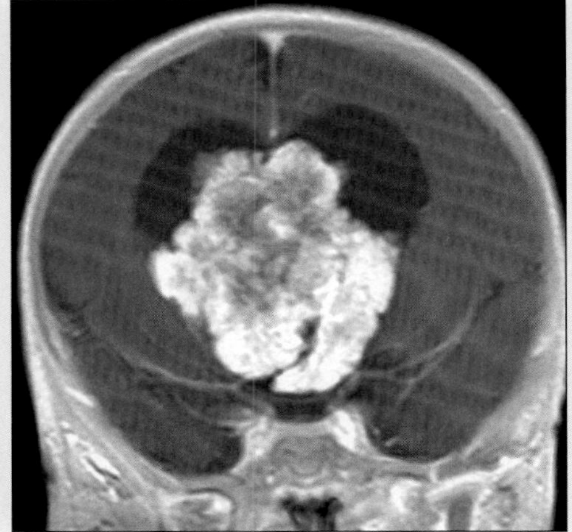

(Left) *Axial T2WI MR shows a heterogeneous, hyperintense 3rd ventricular mass → extending upward through the foramen of Monro into the lateral ventricles. Note the splaying of the pillars of the fornices anterosuperiorly ⇨, confirming the 3rd ventricular origin of the tumor. Note also the marked ventriculomegaly.* ***(Right)*** *Coronal T1WI C+ MR in the same patient shows a lobular, intensely enhancing mass, typical of a choroid plexus tumor. WHO grade II was found at resection. (Courtesy M. Castillo, MD.)*

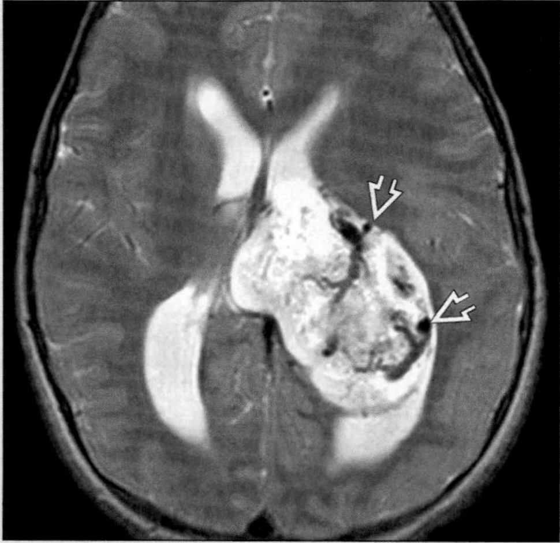
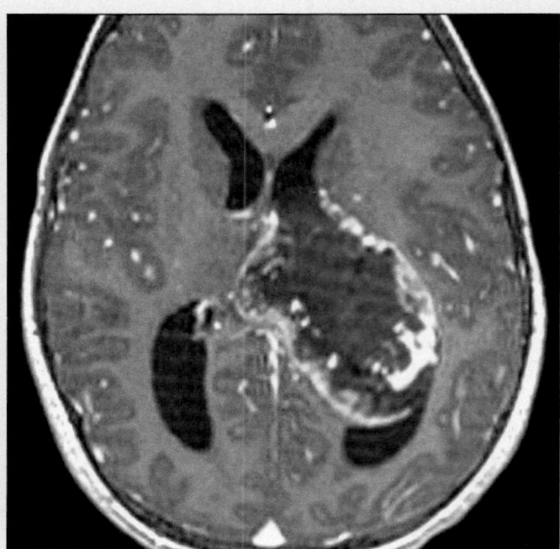

(Left) *Axial T2WI MR in a 15 year old with headaches and papilledema shows a hyperintense intraventricular mass with prominent vascular flow voids ⇨ and associated hydrocephalus.* ***(Right)*** *Axial T1WI C+ MR in the same patient shows peripheral enhancement of the mass with central lack of enhancement suggesting necrosis. WHO grade II, atypical CPP found at resection. These rare tumors may mimic a typical grade I CPP or have atypical imaging features, as in this case.*

TERMINOLOGY

Abbreviations

- Atypical choroid plexus papilloma (aCPP)

Definitions

- Choroid plexus papilloma (CPP) with increased mitotic activity and higher likelihood of recurrence (WHO grade II)

IMAGING

General Features

- Best diagnostic clue
  - Child with lobulated, strongly enhancing intraventricular mass
    - May see hemorrhage and necrosis
  - Not reliably distinguished from CPP or choroid plexus carcinoma (CPCa) on imaging
- Location
  - Follows CPP in location
  - Lateral > 4th > 3rd ventricle
- Size
  - Often large at diagnosis
- Morphology
  - Cauliflower-like mass

Imaging Recommendations

- Best imaging tool
  - MR with contrast
- Protocol advice
  - Evaluate entire neuraxis for CSF seeding

CT Findings

- Intraventricular, strongly enhancing lobulated mass
- Hydrocephalus common

MR Findings

- T2WI: Hyperintense lobular mass + hydrocephalus
  - Internal vascular flow voids common
  - May see necrosis, hemorrhage, &/or calcification
  - Periventricular focal edema may suggest invasion
- T1WI C+: Strongly enhancing

DIFFERENTIAL DIAGNOSIS

CPP and CPCa

- Lobular, strongly enhancing ventricular mass
- Cannot be reliably distinguished on imaging
- CPP may have less necrosis or hemorrhage
- CPCa may show ependymal invasion

Ependymoma

- Strongly enhancing heterogeneous tumor
- Commonly in 4th ventricle in children
- Supraventricular cases often periventricular

Medulloblastoma

- Hyperdense 4th ventricular mass in child
- Enhancing mass arises from 4th ventricle roof (superior medullary velum)
- CSF dissemination common

Atypical Teratoid-Rhabdoid Tumor

- Heterogeneous, strongly enhancing mass in young child (often < 3 years old)
- Cerebellopontine angle, cerebellum, hemispheric

PATHOLOGY

General Features

- Genetics
  - Simian virus 40 (SV40) DNA sequences reported
  - High expression of TWIST-1, a transcription factor that inhibits p53
  - Li-Fraumeni and Aicardi syndromes associated

Staging, Grading, & Classification

- WHO grade II

Gross Pathologic & Surgical Features

- Lobulated intraventricular mass
- ± cysts, necrosis, and hemorrhage

Microscopic Features

- ≥ 2 mitoses per 10 high-power fields
  - Single microscopic criteria to distinguish from CPP
  - Most significant factor related to ↑ recurrence
- ↑ likelihood of atypical features: Hypercellularity, nuclear pleomorphism, necrosis, solid growth
- May show high Ki-67 and MIB-1 proliferation indices

CLINICAL ISSUES

Presentation

- Macrocephaly and vomiting most common

Demographics

- Age: Infants, children, and young adults

Natural History & Prognosis

- Slow growing
- Atypical CPP has 4.9x recurrence rate compared to WHO grade I CPP
- 5-year survival approaches 100%
- Complete surgical resection is often curative

DIAGNOSTIC CHECKLIST

Consider

- Atypical CPP with intraventricular mass with atypical features in child/young adult

SELECTED REFERENCES

1. Jeibmann A et al: Malignant progression in choroid plexus papillomas. J Neurosurg. 107(3 Suppl):199-202, 2007
2. Louis DN et al: The 2007 WHO classification of tumours of the central nervous system. Acta Neuropathol. 2007 Aug;114(2):97-109. Epub 2007 Jul 6. Review. Erratum in: Acta Neuropathol. 114(5):547, 2007
3. Hasselblatt M et al: Identification of novel diagnostic markers for choroid plexus tumors: a microarray-based approach. Am J Surg Pathol. 30(1):66-74, 2006

CHOROID PLEXUS CARCINOMA

Key Facts

Terminology
- Malignant tumor originating from epithelium of choroid plexus (WHO grade III)

Imaging
- Best imaging clue: Child < 5 years with enhancing intraventricular mass and ependymal invasion, ± prominent flow voids
  - Asymmetric periventricular white matter edema suggests invasion
- MR may not distinguish papilloma from carcinoma
  - Heterogeneity, brain invasion, CSF spread favors CPCa
- Important to image spine prior to surgery

Top Differential Diagnoses
- Choroid plexus papilloma (CPP)
- Ependymoma
- Subependymal giant cell astrocytoma

Pathology
- Microscopic features: Hypercellularity, pleomorphism, increased mitotic activity
  - Cysts, necrosis, hemorrhage, microcalcifications
  - Brain invasion common
- Increased incidence in Li-Fraumeni and Aicardi syndromes

Clinical Issues
- Occurs in infants and young children
  - 70% occur before 2 years of age
- Nausea, vomiting, headache, obtundation are most common presenting features
- CPCa represent 20-40% of all choroid plexus tumors
- Grows rapidly, 30-50% 5-year survival
- Poor outcome with brain invasion or CSF seeding

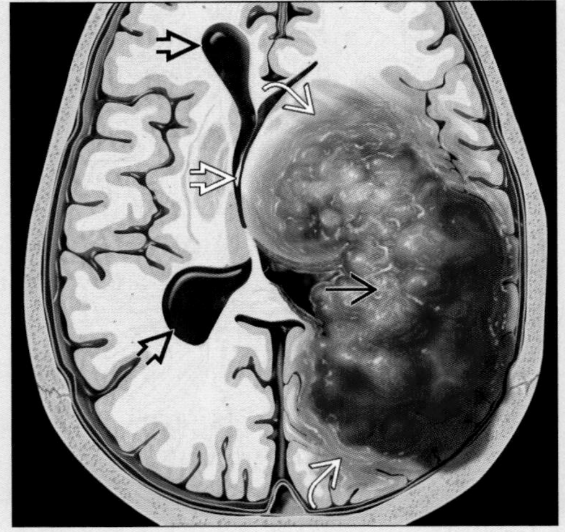

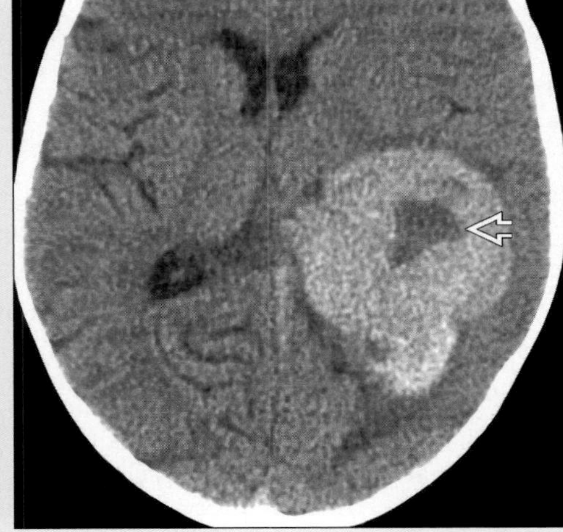

(Left) *Axial graphic demonstrates a lobular mass centered in the atria of the left lateral ventricle. Note the invasion and expansion of the surrounding parenchyma, more characteristic of a choroid plexus carcinoma. There is associated midline shift and entrapment of the right lateral ventricle.* ***(Right)*** *Axial NECT in a 2-year-old with altered mental status shows a hyperdense mass with areas of necrosis in the atrium of the left lateral ventricle.*

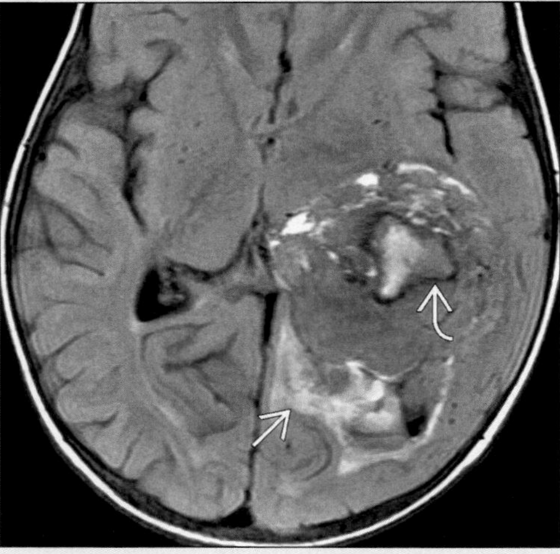

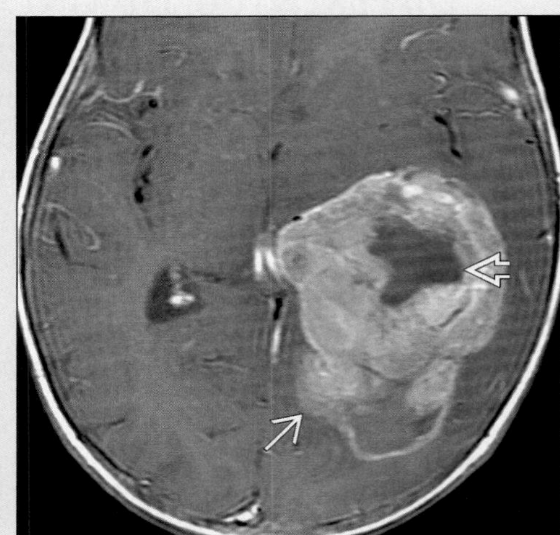

(Left) *Axial FLAIR MR in the same patient shows a heterogeneous mass centered in the left lateral ventricle atrium. Hyperintensity in the adjacent brain parenchyma is suspicious for brain invasion. Note the areas of hypointensity related to blood products.* ***(Right)*** *Axial T1WI C+ MR in the same patient shows intense enhancement of the intraventricular mass with central necrosis. Note the enhancement of the adjacent occipital lobe, confirming tumor invasion. CPCa was found at resection.*

CHOROID PLEXUS CARCINOMA

TERMINOLOGY

Abbreviations
- Choroid plexus carcinoma (CPCa)
- Choroid plexus tumor (CPT)

Definitions
- Malignant tumor originating from epithelium of choroid plexus

IMAGING

General Features
- Best diagnostic clue
  - Child (< 5 years) with enhancing intraventricular mass and ependymal invasion
  - Differentiation from choroid plexus papilloma (CPP) is histologic, not radiologic
- Location
  - Almost always arise in lateral ventricle
- Size
  - Variable
- Morphology
  - Cauliflower-like mass
  - Necrosis, cysts, and hemorrhage are common

CT Findings
- NECT
  - Iso- to hyperattenuating mass with irregular contours
  - Necrosis, cysts, and hemorrhage common
  - Hydrocephalus common
  - Calcification (Ca++) in 20-25%
- CECT
  - Heterogeneous, strong enhancement
  - Peritumoral edema
  - ± CSF tumor seeding

MR Findings
- T1WI
  - Iso- to hypointense intraventricular mass
  - Lobulated or irregularly marginated, papillary appearance
  - Heterogeneous (necrosis, cysts, hemorrhage)
- T2WI
  - Mixed signal mass, hypo-/iso-/hyperintense
  - Heterogeneous related to necrosis, cysts, hemorrhage, Ca++)
  - ± prominent flow voids
  - Many invade brain and cause edema
- PD/intermediate
  - Heterogeneous mass with vascular flow voids
- FLAIR
  - Heterogeneous intraventricular mass
  - Periventricular white matter edema suggests invasion
  - Transependymal CSF flow from hydrocephalus
- T2* GRE
  - Low signal from hemorrhage or calcification
- DWI
  - Low ADC values in solid portions of tumor
- T1WI C+
  - Heterogeneous enhancement, ± CSF seeding
- MRS
  - NAA absent; ↑ choline ± ↑ lactate

Ultrasonographic Findings
- Grayscale ultrasound
  - Hyperechoic intraventricular mass
- Pulsed Doppler
  - Bidirectional flow through diastole
- Color Doppler
  - Hypervascular mass

Angiographic Findings
- Conventional
  - Enlarged choroidal artery and vascular stain

Nuclear Medicine Findings
- PET
  - 11C-methionine ⇒ ↑ tumor/normal brain ratios
- Tc-99m sestamibi ⇒ ↑ in CPTs

Imaging Recommendations
- Best imaging tool
  - Contrast-enhanced MR of brain and spine
- Protocol advice
  - Enhanced MR of entire neuraxis prior to surgery

DIFFERENTIAL DIAGNOSIS

Choroid Plexus Papilloma (CPP)
- MR may not distinguish papilloma from carcinoma
- Aggressive CPP may seed through CSF pathways
- CPP rarely shows minimal brain invasion

Ependymoma
- Heterogeneous 4th ventricular mass
- Classically squeezes out 4th ventricular foramina into cisterns
- Supratentorial ependymoma often extraventricular

Subependymal Giant Cell Astrocytoma
- Associated CNS findings of tuberous sclerosis
- Characteristic location near foramen of Monro
- Rarely cause edema

Astrocytic Tumors
- May arise from periventricular tissues (septum pellucidum, thalamus)
- Smooth or lobular masses, no papillary margins
- High-grade tumor may cause periventricular edema

Medulloblastoma
- Hyperdense, round 4th ventricular mass
- Arises from roof of 4th ventricle (superior medullary velum)

Central Neurocytoma
- "Bubbly" intraventricular mass in adult
- Often attached to septum pellucidum

Meningioma
- Delineated, oval enhancing mass
- Uncommon in children, associated with neurofibromatosis type 2

Primitive Neuroectodermal Tumor (PNET)
- Heterogeneous tumor can be lobulated within lateral ventricle
- May arise deep in hemisphere
- Peritumoral edema often minimal

Atypical Teratoid-Rhabdoid Tumor (AT/RT)
- Heterogeneous tumor with cysts or hemorrhage
- Common in posterior fossa, may occur in lateral ventricle, often intraaxial
- Typically present in patients < 2 years of age
- INI1 protein negative on immunohistochemistry
  - Most CPCa are positive

Vascular Lesions
- AVM
- Cavernous malformation

Metastases
- History of previous tumor often known
- Multiple lesions common
- Rare in children

PATHOLOGY

General Features
- Etiology
  - SV40 virus DNA sequences in 50% of CPTs
- Genetics
  - Increased incidence in Li-Fraumeni and Aicardi syndromes
    - Li-Fraumeni *p53* mutation/deletion
      - Autosomal dominant tumor predisposition syndrome
  - Overlap with rhabdoid tumors and *SNF5/INI1* mutation
- Associated abnormalities
  - Diffuse hydrocephalus ⇒ mechanical obstruction, increased CSF production, decreased resorption

Staging, Grading, & Classification
- WHO grade III

Gross Pathologic & Surgical Features
- Well-circumscribed lobulated intraventricular mass
- Ependymal invasion

Microscopic Features
- Hypercellular, pleomorphic, increased mitotic activity
- Cysts, necrosis, hemorrhage, microcalcifications
- Brain invasion common
- May have CSF seeding
- Ki-67(MIB-1) proliferation indices high (~ 14-20%)

Immunochemistry expression
- Kir7.1 and Stanniocalcin-1 may distinguish choroid plexus origin from other tumors
- CPC express cytokeratins
- Transthyretin, S100(+) (less than CPP)

CLINICAL ISSUES

Presentation
- Most common signs/symptoms
  - Nausea, vomiting, headache, obtundation
  - Focal neurologic signs and symptoms
- Clinical profile
  - Infant or child with elevated ICP and focal neuro deficits

Demographics
- Age
  - Infants and young children (typically < 5 years)
  - Median: 26-32 months
- Gender
  - M = F
- Epidemiology
  - 80% arise in children
  - 70% before 2 years of age
  - 20-40% of all CPTs
  - ~ 5% of supratentorial tumors in children
  - < 1% of all pediatric intracranial tumors

Natural History & Prognosis
- Small percentage may be malignant progression from WHO grade I and II papillomas
- Grows rapidly, 30-50% 5-year survival
- Poor outcome with brain invasion, CSF seeding

Treatment
- Total resection has best prognosis
- Chemoradiation demonstrates some increased survival

DIAGNOSTIC CHECKLIST

Consider
- CPCa in child with invasive intraventricular mass and focal neurologic signs

Image Interpretation Pearls
- MR may not distinguish papilloma from carcinoma
- Heterogeneity, brain invasion, CSF spread favors CPCa
- Image spine prior to surgery

SELECTED REFERENCES

1. Gonzalez KD et al: Beyond Li Fraumeni Syndrome: clinical characteristics of families with p53 germline mutations. J Clin Oncol. 27(8):1250-6, 2009
2. Gopal P et al: Choroid plexus carcinoma. Arch Pathol Lab Med. 132(8):1350-4, 2008
3. Wrede B et al: Chemotherapy improves the survival of patients with choroid plexus carcinoma: a meta-analysis of individual cases with choroid plexus tumors. J Neurooncol. 85(3):345-51, 2007
4. Levy ML et al: Choroid plexus tumors in children: significance of stromal invasion. Neurosurgery. 48(2):303-9, 2001
5. Malkin D et al: Tissue-specific expression of SV40 in tumors associated with the Li-Fraumeni syndrome. Oncogene. 20(33):4441-9, 2001

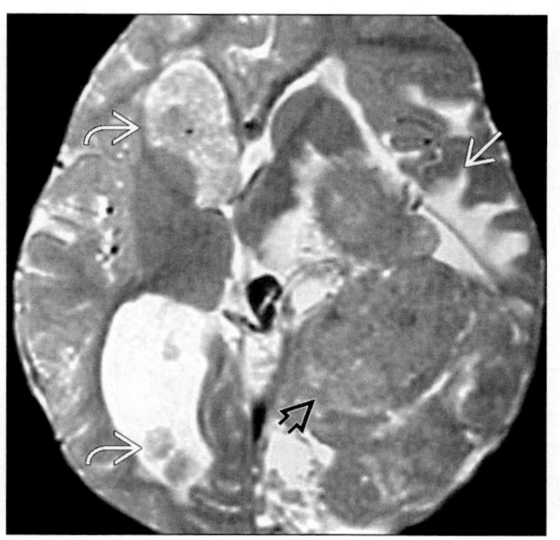

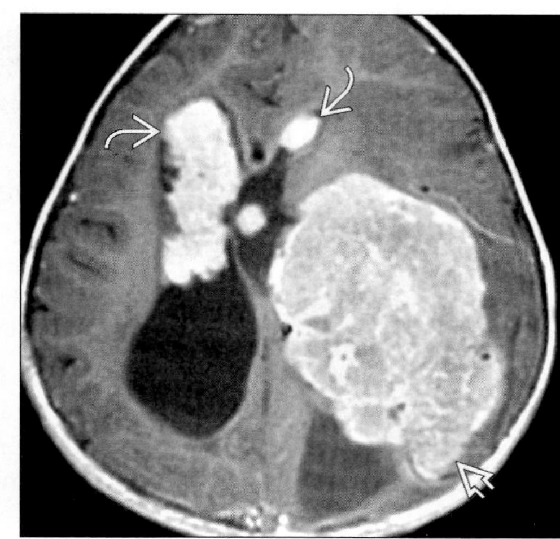

(Left) *Axial T2WI MR shows a massive left lateral ventricle choroid plexus carcinoma with multiple nodules of metastatic CSF spread. Note the asymmetric periventricular T2 hyperintensity related to brain invasion.* ***(Right)*** *Axial T1WI C+ MR in the same patient shows marked enhancement of the lateral ventricle choroid plexus carcinoma with ependymal invasion and multiple nodules of metastatic CSF spread. CSF spread and brain invasion is associated with a poor prognosis.*

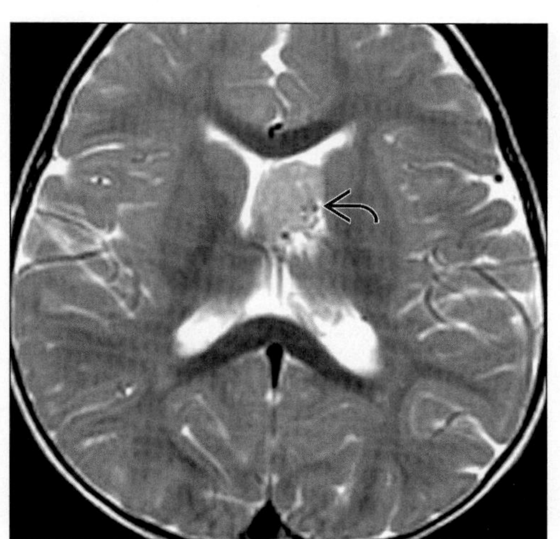

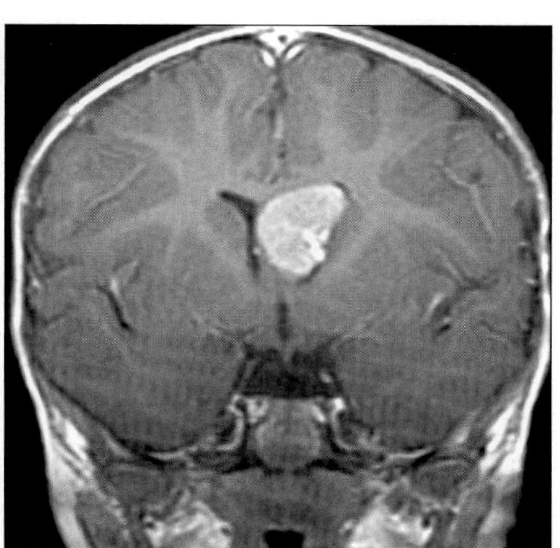

(Left) *Axial T2WI MR in a patient with Li-Fraumeni syndrome and a known adrenocortical carcinoma shows a lobulated, isointense mass in the lateral ventricle body, extending to the foramen of Monro with prominent vascular flow voids.* ***(Right)*** *Coronal T1WI C+ MR in the same patient shows strong, uniform enhancement of the mass. Imaging suggests either a choroid plexus papilloma or carcinoma. There is no evidence of brain invasion or CSF seeding. CPCa was found at surgery.*

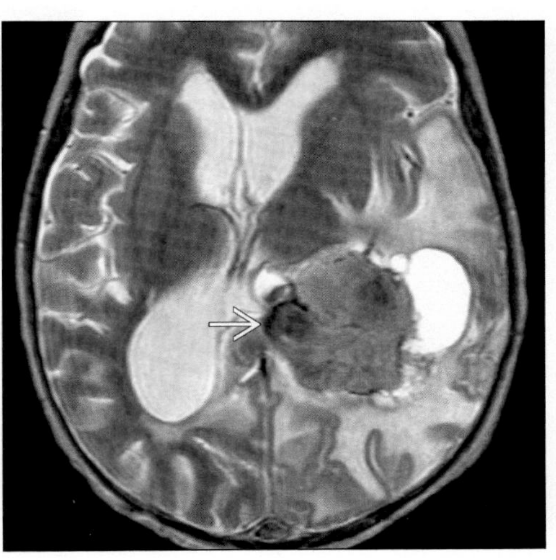

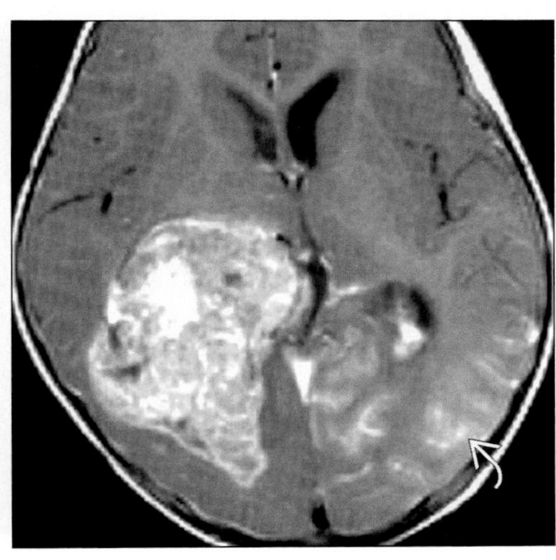

(Left) *Axial T2WI MR shows a heterogeneous left lateral ventricle trigone mass with prominent flow voids and areas of hypointensity related to blood products. The marked periventricular edema is indicative of brain invasion.* ***(Right)*** *Axial T1WI C+ MR shows a markedly enhancing lateral ventricular trigone mass with extensive leptomeningeal tumor spread. Choroid plexus papillomas are much more common than carcinomas, with a ratio of at least 4-5:1. CSF seeding and brain invasion favor carcinoma.*

GANGLIOGLIOMA

Key Facts

Terminology

- Well-differentiated, slowly growing neuroepithelial tumor composed of neoplastic ganglion cells and neoplastic glial cells
- Most common cause of temporal lobe epilepsy (TLE)

Imaging

- Partially cystic, enhancing, cortically based mass in child/young adult with TLE
- Can occur anywhere, but most commonly superficial hemispheres, temporal lobe (> 75%)
- Circumscribed cyst + mural nodule most common
- Calcification is common (up to 50%)
- Superficial lesions may expand cortex, remodel bone
- Approximately 50% enhance
- May see associated cortical dysplasia

Top Differential Diagnoses

- Pleomorphic xanthoastrocytoma (PXA)
- Dysembryoplastic neuroepithelial tumor (DNET)
- Astrocytoma
- Oligodendroglioma
- Neurocysticercosis

Pathology

- WHO grade I or II (80% grade I)
- Uncommon: Anaplastic ganglioglioma (WHO III)
- Rare: Malignant with GBM-like glial component (WHO IV)

Clinical Issues

- Occurs at all ages, peak: 10-20 years
- Most common mixed neuronal-glial tumor
- Excellent prognosis if surgical resection complete

*(**Left**) Coronal graphic shows a discrete cystic and solid temporal lobe mass expanding the overlying cortex. Calvarial remodeling is seen, typical of a superficially located ganglioglioma. Gangliogliomas are the most common tumors to cause temporal lobe epilepsy. (**Right**) Coronal T1WI C+ MR in a young adult with temporal lobe epilepsy shows a circumscribed, cystic and solid temporal lobe mass with intense enhancement of the mural nodule ➡. This is the classic enhancement pattern of a ganglioglioma.*

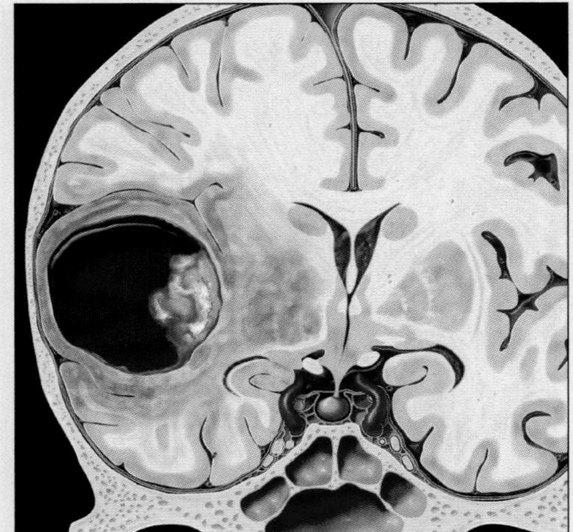

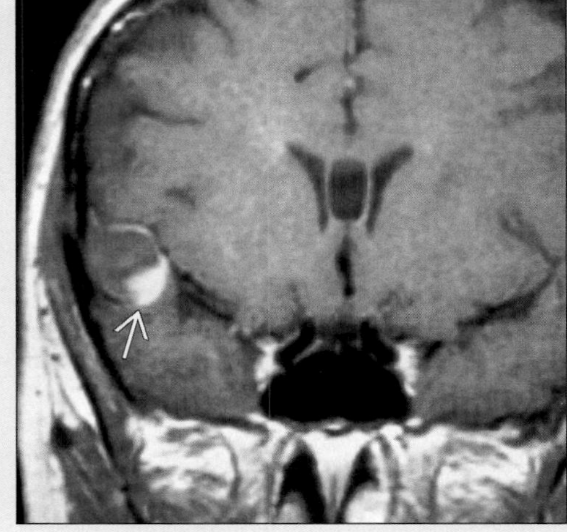

*(**Left**) Axial T1WI C+ MR shows a solidly enhancing frontal lobe mass ➡. The lack of surrounding edema and superficial location is typical for ganglioglioma. The temporal lobe is the most common location (> 75%) followed by the frontal and parietal lobes. (**Right**) Coronal T1WI C+ MR shows subtle enhancement ➡ within a right temporal lobe ganglioglioma in a female patient with seizures. The differential diagnosis for this lesion includes DNET, astrocytoma, PXA, and oligodendroglioma.*

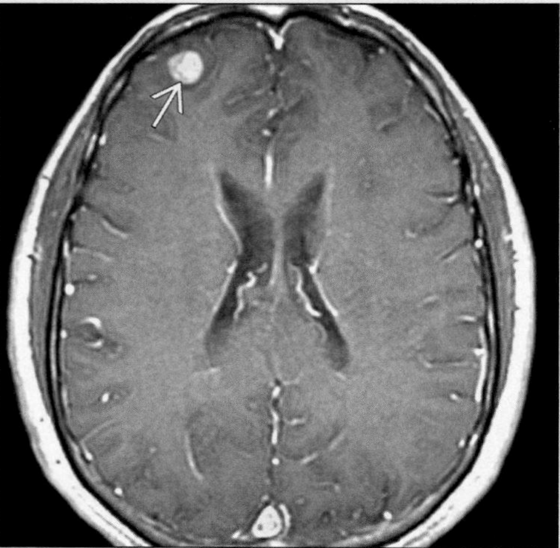

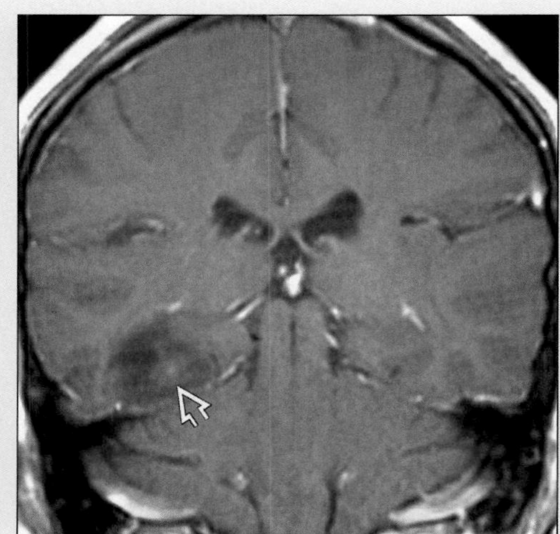

GANGLIOGLIOMA

TERMINOLOGY

Abbreviations
- Ganglioglioma (GG)

Definitions
- Well-differentiated, slowly growing neuroepithelial tumor composed of neoplastic ganglion cells and neoplastic glial cells
- Most common cause of temporal lobe epilepsy (TLE)

IMAGING

General Features
- Best diagnostic clue
  - Partially cystic, enhancing, cortically based mass in child/young adult with TLE
- Location
  - Can occur anywhere, but most commonly superficial hemispheres, temporal lobe (> 75%)
    - Frontal and parietal lobes next most common
  - Rare locations: Brainstem, cerebellum, pineal region, optic nerve/chiasm, intraventricular, pituitary axis, spinal cord, cranial nerves
- Size
  - Variable, typically 2-3 cm in adults
  - Larger in children, typically > 4 cm
  - Up to 6 cm reported
- Morphology
  - 3 patterns
    - Most common: Circumscribed cyst + mural nodule
    - Solid tumor (often thickens, expands gyri)
    - Uncommon: Infiltrating, poorly delineated mass
  - Calcification is common (up to 50%)
  - In younger patients (< 10 years), gangliogliomas are larger and more cystic

CT Findings
- NECT
  - Variable density
    - 40% hypodense
    - 30% mixed hypodense (cyst), isodense (nodule)
    - 15% isodense or hyperdense
  - Ca++ common (35-50%)
  - Superficial lesions may expand cortex, remodel bone
- CECT
  - Approximately 50% enhance
    - Varies from moderate, uniform to heterogeneous
    - Can be solid, rim, or nodular
    - Often shows cyst with enhancing nodule

MR Findings
- T1WI
  - Mass is hypointense to isointense to gray matter
    - Rarely hyperintense
  - Ca++ has variable signal intensity
  - May see associated cortical dysplasia
- T2WI
  - Hyperintense mass typical
  - May be heterogeneous
  - No surrounding edema
- T2* GRE
  - May show Ca++ as areas of "blooming"
- T1WI C+
  - Variable enhancement, usually moderate but heterogeneous
    - May be minimal, ring-like, homogeneous
  - Meningeal enhancement rarely seen
- MRS
  - Elevated Cho has been described

Nuclear Medicine Findings
- PET
  - Typically decreased activity with FDG PET indicating tumor hypometabolism
  - May have some hypermetabolic foci
- 201Tl-SPECT: Increased activity in high-grade gangliogliomas (grade III, IV)
  - Typical gangliogliomas have decreased or normal SPECT activity

Imaging Recommendations
- Best imaging tool
  - Multiplanar MR
- Protocol advice
  - Contrast-enhanced MR to include coronal T2 images for better evaluation of temporal lobes

DIFFERENTIAL DIAGNOSIS

Pleomorphic Xanthoastrocytoma (PXA)
- Supratentorial cortical mass, dural "tail" common
- Often cyst and mural nodule, may be solid
- Enhancing nodule abuts pial surface
- Temporal lobe most common location

Dysembryoplastic Neuroepithelial Tumor (DNET)
- Superficial cortical tumor, well demarcated
- Multicystic "bubbly" appearance
- T2 hyperintense mass with rare, mild enhancement
- May remodel calvarium

Pilocytic Astrocytoma
- Supratentorial location other than hypothalamus/chiasm rare
- Typically solid and cystic or solid mass
- Enhancement typical

Low-Grade Astrocytoma (Grade II)
- Circumscribed but infiltrative white matter mass
- No enhancement

Oligodendroglioma
- Calcified, heterogeneous mass
- Typically more diffuse than ganglioglioma
- May remodel/erode calvarium

Neurocysticercosis
- Cyst with "dot" inside
- Often calcified
- Multiple lesions common
- Imaging varies with pathologic stage, host response

GANGLIOGLIOMA

PATHOLOGY

General Features

- Etiology
  - 2 theories
    - Origin from dysplastic, malformative glioneuronal precursor lesion with glial element neoplastic transformation
    - Neoplastic transformation of glial hamartoma or subpial granule cells
- Genetics
  - Gain of chromosome 7 reported
  - Sporadic
    - *Tp53* mutations found in malignant degeneration
  - Syndromic
    - GG has been reported in Turcot syndrome, NF1, and NF2
- Associated abnormalities
  - Gangliogliomas have been found in association with oligodendroglioma, DNET, tanycytic ependymoma
  - Malignant transformation into GBM, neuroblastoma has been reported
  - Cortical dysplasia is commonly associated

Staging, Grading, & Classification

- WHO grade I or II (80% WHO grade I)
- Uncommon: Anaplastic ganglioglioma (WHO grade III)
- Rare: Malignant with GBM-like glial component (WHO grade IV)

Gross Pathologic & Surgical Features

- Solid or cystic mass with mural nodule
- Firm, well-circumscribed mass, often expands cortex

Microscopic Features

- Mix of mature but neoplastic ganglion cells and neoplastic glial cells (usually astrocytes)
- Dysmorphic, occasionally binucleate neurons
  - Immunohistochemistry of neuronal cells
    - Synaptophysin and neurofilament protein are positive
    - Majority exhibit CD34 immunoreactivity (70-80% of gangliogliomas)
- Electron microscopy shows dense core granules, variable synapses
- Neoplastic glial cells are GFAP(+)
- Mitoses rare (75% have Ki-67 < 1%, low MIB)

CLINICAL ISSUES

Presentation

- Most common signs/symptoms
  - Chronic temporal lobe epilepsy (approximately 90%)
    - Often partial complex seizures
  - Other signs/symptoms: Headache and signs of increased intracranial pressure

Demographics

- Age
  - Tumor of children, young adults
  - 80% of patients < 30 years
  - Occurs at all ages, peak: 10-20 years
- Gender
  - Slight male predominance
- Epidemiology
  - 1% of primary intracranial neoplasms
  - Most common mixed neuronal-glial tumor
  - Represents 1-4% of pediatric CNS neoplasms
  - Most common tumor to cause TLE (> 45%)
    - Ganglioglioma > DNET > pilocytic astrocytoma > low-grade astrocytoma > oligodendroglioma > PXA

Natural History & Prognosis

- Excellent prognosis if surgical resection complete
- 94% have 7.5-year recurrence-free survival
- Vast majority of patients seizure-free after surgery (80%)
- Well-differentiated tumor with slow growth pattern
- Malignant degeneration is rare (approximately 5-10% glial component)

Treatment

- Surgical resection is treatment of choice
- Radiation therapy &/or chemotherapy for aggressive or unresectable tumors

DIAGNOSTIC CHECKLIST

Consider

- Ganglioglioma in young patient with history of temporal lobe epilepsy
- In children under 10 years old, gangliogliomas are larger and more cystic

Image Interpretation Pearls

- Cyst with enhancing mural nodule is classic, but not specific for ganglioglioma

SELECTED REFERENCES

1. Allende DS et al: The expanding family of glioneuronal tumors. Adv Anat Pathol. 16(1):33-9, 2009
2. Karremann M et al: Anaplastic ganglioglioma in children. J Neurooncol. 92(2):157-63, 2009
3. Adachi Y et al: Gangliogliomas: Characteristic imaging findings and role in the temporal lobe epilepsy. Neuroradiology. 50(10):829-34, 2008
4. Brat DJ et al: Surgical neuropathology update: a review of changes introduced by the WHO classification of tumours of the central nervous system, 4th edition. Arch Pathol Lab Med. 132(6):993-1007, 2008
5. Hauck EF et al: Intraventricular ganglioglioma. J Clin Neurosci. 15(11):1291-3, 2008
6. Park YS et al: Factors contributing to resectability and seizure outcomes in 44 patients with ganglioglioma. Clin Neurol Neurosurg. 110(7):667-73, 2008
7. Louis DN et al: Ganglioma and gangliocytoma. WHO Classification of Tumours of the Central Nervous System. Lyon: IARC Press. 103-105, 2007
8. Koeller KK et al: From the archives of the AFIP: superficial gliomas: radiologic-pathologic correlation. Armed Forces Institute of Pathology. Radiographics. 21(6):1533-56, 2001

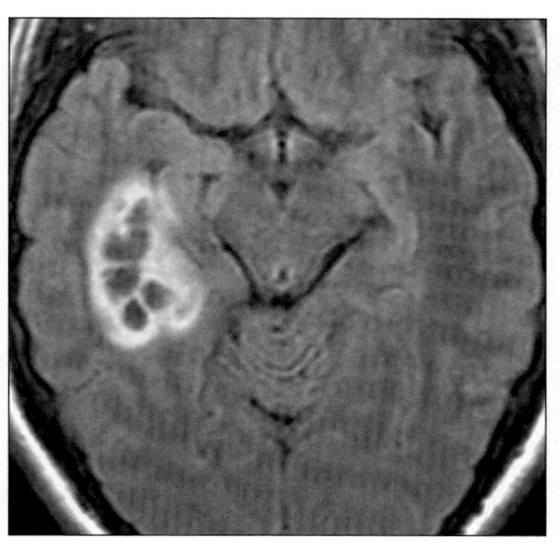

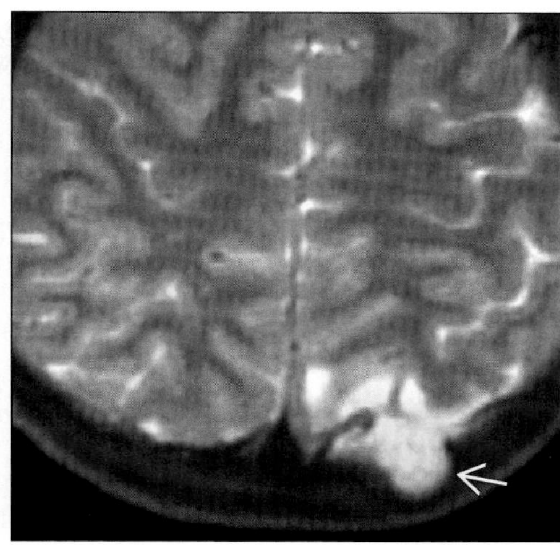

*(**Left**) Axial FLAIR MR shows a discrete, multiseptated temporal lobe mass. The lack of surrounding edema and lack of significant mass effect is typical of ganglioglioma. This WHO grade I tumor has a very good prognosis with resection. (**Right**) Axial T2WI MR shows a hyperintense, cystic parietal lobe mass ➔ with remodeling of the overlying calvarium. This mass showed a cyst with an enhancing mural nodule, classic for ganglioglioma. Superficial tumors often have associated bone remodeling.*

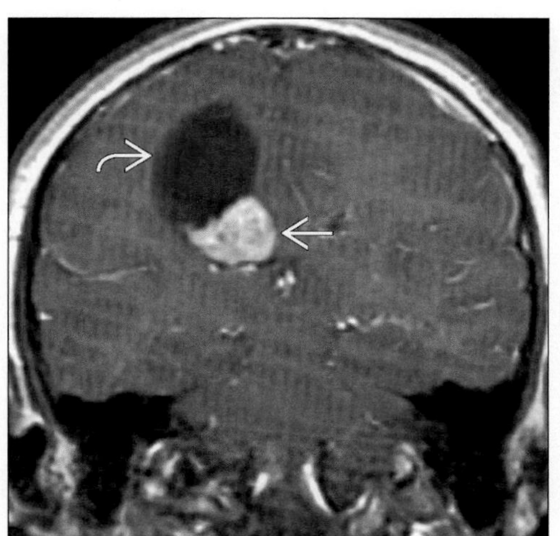

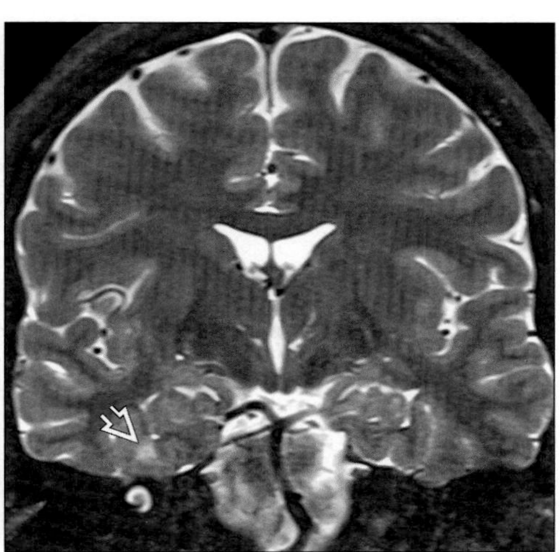

*(**Left**) Coronal T1WI C+ MR shows a well-circumscribed frontal lobe mass with a sharply demarcated cystic portion ➔ and an enhancing deep soft tissue nodule ➔ that indents the ventricle. This deep white matter location is atypical of ganglioglioma. (**Right**) Coronal T2WI MR shows a discrete hyperintense mass ➔ in this temporal lobe epilepsy patient. Thin section T2 imaging is very helpful for evaluation of patients with temporal lobe epilepsy. This case proved to be ganglioglioma at resection.*

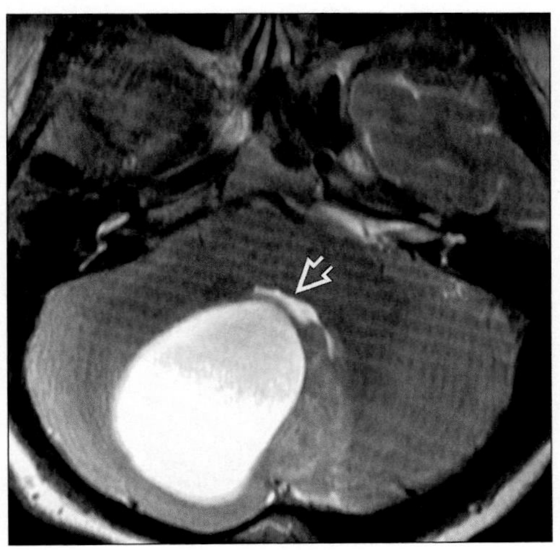

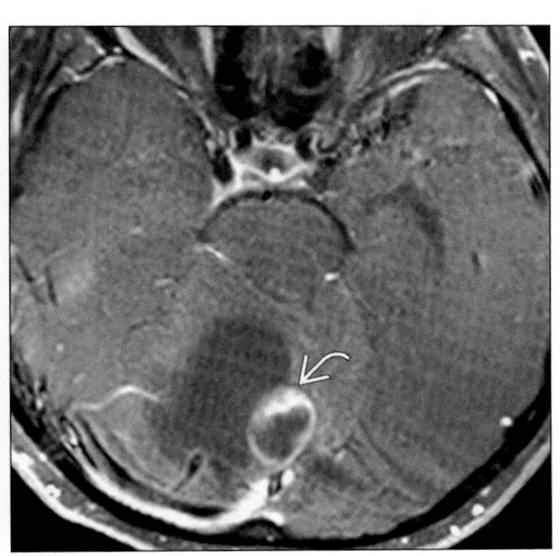

*(**Left**) Axial T2WI MR shows a well-circumscribed cystic mass in the posterior fossa with mass effect on the 4th ventricle ➔. (**Right**) Axial T1WI C+ FS MR in the same patient shows an enhancing cyst and mural nodule along the medial border of the large cystic mass ➔. The posterior fossa is an uncommon location for this mixed neuronal-glial tumor. Differential considerations would include hemangioblastoma and pilocytic astrocytoma in this young adult.*

DESMOPLASTIC INFANTILE ASTROCYTOMA AND GANGLIOGLIOMA

Key Facts

Terminology

- Large cystic tumors of infants involving superficial cerebral cortex and leptomeninges
- Desmoplastic infantile ganglioglioma (DIG/DIGG)
  - Prominent desmoplastic stroma + neoplastic astrocytes, variable neuronal component
- Desmoplastic infantile astrocytoma (DIA)
  - Desmoplastic stroma + neoplastic astrocytes

Imaging

- Best diagnostic clue: Peripheral supratentorial tumor with cyst and nodule in infant < 2 years
  - Large cyst + cortical-based tumor nodule
  - Enhancement of adjacent meninges
  - T2 hypointense solid portion
- Frontal and parietal > temporal > occipital
- Cysts may be very large, cause macrocephaly and bulging fontanelles in infants

Top Differential Diagnoses

- Primitive neuroectodermal tumor (PNET)
- Supratentorial ependymoma
- Pleomorphic xanthoastrocytoma (PXA)
- Hemangioblastoma
- Ganglioglioma
- Pilocytic astrocytoma

Pathology

- WHO grade 1
- Areas of cellular proliferation, mitoses, and necrosis may cause misdiagnosis as higher grade tumor

Clinical Issues

- Most are found at 1-24 months (peak: 3-6 months)
- 16% of intracranial tumors in 1st year of life
- Median survival rate is > 75% at 15 years
- Surgical resection typically curative

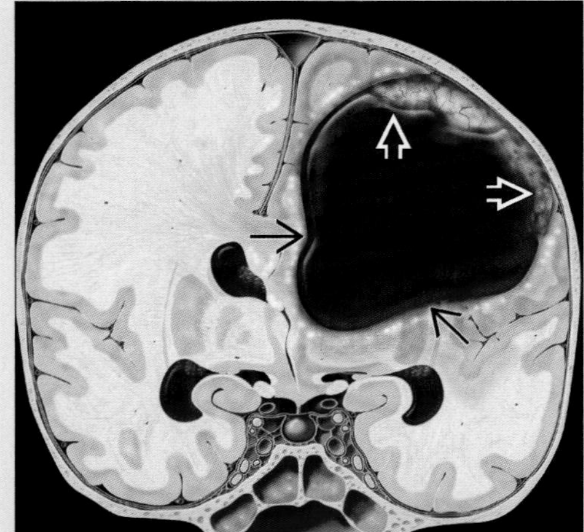

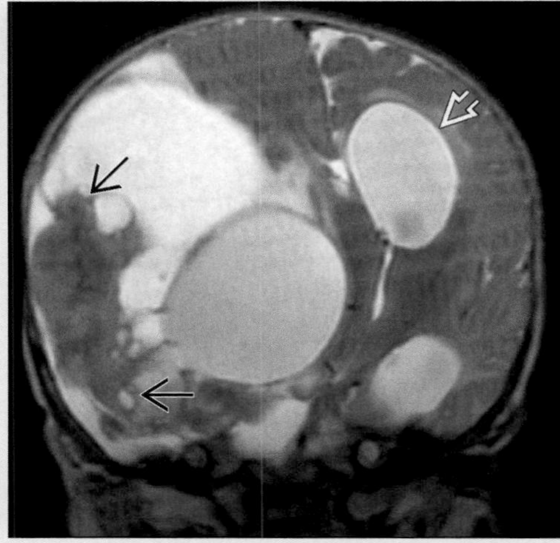

(Left) *Coronal graphic shows an infant with an enlarged head caused by DIG/DIA. Note the dominant cystic component → with a dural-based plaque of desmoplastic stroma ➡. Mild surrounding edema and hydrocephalus is present.* ***(Right)*** *Coronal T2WI MR shows a large cystic and solid mass with a T2 hypointense, peripheral plaque-like solid component →, characteristic of desmoplastic infantile ganglioglioma and astrocytoma. Note the significant associated mass effect and hydrocephalus ➡.*

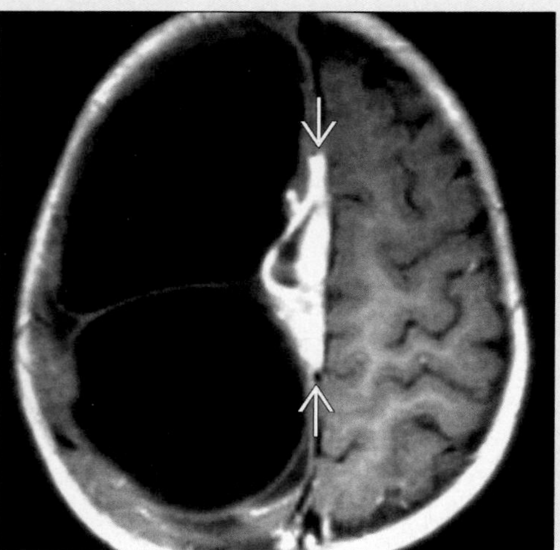

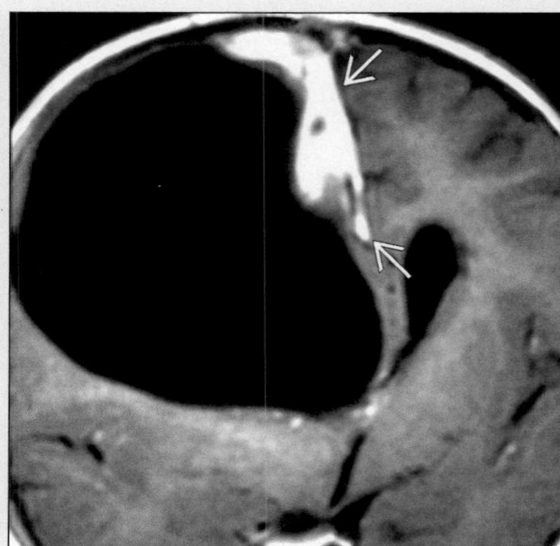

(Left) *Axial T1WI C+ MR shows a large cystic and solid mass with a markedly enhancing solid component along the falx ➡.* ***(Right)*** *Coronal T1WI C+ MR in the same patient shows the large cystic and solid mass with a dural-based enhancing solid portion ➡, characteristic of DIG/DIA. Involvement of the adjacent dura is typical. DIG/DIA should be considered in supratentorial tumors demonstrating cysts and peripheral nodules in the 1st year of life. (Courtesy M. Sage, MD.)*

DESMOPLASTIC INFANTILE ASTROCYTOMA AND GANGLIOGLIOMA

TERMINOLOGY

Abbreviations
- Desmoplastic infantile ganglioglioma (DIG/DIGG)
- Desmoplastic infantile astrocytoma (DIA)

Synonyms
- Desmoplastic supratentorial neuroepithelial tumors of infancy
- Superficial cerebral astrocytoma ± neuronal elements attached to dura

Definitions
- Large cystic tumors of infants involving superficial cerebral cortex and leptomeninges, often attached to dura
- DIG: Prominent desmoplastic stroma + neoplastic astrocytes, variable neuronal component
- DIA: Desmoplastic stroma + neoplastic astrocytes

IMAGING

General Features
- Best diagnostic clue
  - Large cyst + cortical-based enhancing tumor nodule/plaque in infant < 2 years
  - Enhancement of adjacent pia PLUS reactive dural thickening
  - T2 hypointense solid portion
- Location
  - Supratentorial: Frontal/parietal > temporal > occipital
- Size
  - Cysts may be very large, cause macrocephaly and bulging fontanelles in infants
- Morphology
  - Solid and cystic mass usually with dural attachment

CT Findings
- NECT
  - Large heterogeneous solid and cystic mass
  - Well-demarcated hypodense cyst (isodense to CSF)
  - Solid tumor nodule(s) isodense/slightly hyperdense to GM
  - Calcification extremely rare
- CECT
  - Cyst → no enhancement
  - Nodule → marked enhancement
- CTA
  - Hypovascular; supply from intra- and extraparenchymal vessels
  - Vessels markedly stretched around large cyst

MR Findings
- T1WI
  - Cyst: Hypointense, often multilobulated
    - May contain septae
  - Solid portion: Nodule or plaque-like areas → heterogeneous
- T2WI
  - Cyst is hyperintense
  - Lobular, solid tumor nodule is hypointense
  - Degree of surrounding edema dependent upon local ventricular obstruction
- FLAIR
  - Cysts are isointense to CSF
  - Solid portions usually isointense to GM
- T2* GRE
  - No hemorrhage or calcification
- DWI
  - Reduced diffusivity in solid portion
- T1WI C+
  - Solid tumor nodule(s) enhance markedly
  - Enhancement of leptomeninges, dura adjacent to solid tumor is typical
  - Cyst typically more central than enhancing solid nodule, ± wall enhancement
- MRS
  - ↓ NAA, ↑ choline

Ultrasonographic Findings
- Grayscale ultrasound
  - Large, multicystic mass
  - Hypoechoic tumor nodule, if identified

Imaging Recommendations
- Best imaging tool
  - Multiplanar contrast-enhanced MR

DIFFERENTIAL DIAGNOSIS

Primitive Neuroectodermal Tumor (PNET)
- Solid tumor is hyperdense on CT, iso- to GM on T2, contains cysts, Ca++, edema
- Large heterogeneously enhancing hemispheric mass
- Large cyst less common than in DIG/DIA

Supratentorial Ependymoma
- Nonspecific imaging findings but commonly contains Ca++
- Solid portion usually less peripherally located than DIG/DIA
- Cysts are often less complex than DIG/DIA

Pleomorphic Xanthoastrocytoma (PXA)
- May appear identical to DIG
- Occurs in older patients, children, and young adults
- Temporal lobe most common location

Hemangioblastoma
- Cyst with mural nodule appearance in posterior fossa
- Solid nodule is vascular, flow void may be seen
- Older patients
- Imaging features similar to DIG but rare above tentorium

Ganglioglioma
- Similar appearance to DIG but generally smaller in size
- Ca++ is common
- Older patients, children, and young adults
- Temporal lobe most common location

Pilocytic Astrocytoma
- Rare in infancy
- Uncommon in cerebral hemispheres

- Cyst is usually smaller; nodule hyperintense on T1WI

PATHOLOGY

General Features

- Etiology
  - Possibly related to progenitor cells in subcortical zone along with mature subpial astrocytes
- Genetics
  - No consistent chromosomal alterations

Staging, Grading, & Classification

- WHO grade I

Gross Pathologic & Surgical Features

- 2 distinct components
  - Cortical-based solid tumor nodule with adjacent dural thickening
  - Large associated cyst compresses adjacent ventricular system
- Large cyst(s) containing xanthochromic fluid
- Firm attachment to dura and brain parenchyma
- No necrosis within solid component of tumor, no hemorrhage

Microscopic Features

- DIA: Astrocytes are sole tumor cell
- DIG: Astrocytes + neoplastic neurons
  - Intense desmoplasia with mixture of astroglial and neuronal cells
  - Immature neuronal component and neoplastic astrocytes
- Spindle cells in collagenous stroma forming whorled patterns
- Areas of cellular proliferation, mitoses, and necrosis may cause misdiagnosis as higher grade tumors
- Mitoses are rare
- Ki-67 (MIB-1) proliferation indices < 2-5%

Immunohistochemistry

- GFAP and vimentin positive
- Synaptophysin(+) if neuronal elements (DIG)

CLINICAL ISSUES

Presentation

- Most common signs/symptoms
  - ↑ head size, bulging fontanelles, paresis, and seizures
  - Older children: Seizures and focal neurologic signs/ symptoms
- Clinical profile
  - Infant with rapidly progressive macrocephaly

Demographics

- Age
  - Most are found at 1-24 months (peak: 3-6 months)
  - Children, < 24 months, usually ≤ 12 months; occasionally older patients (5-17 years)
- Gender
  - Slightly more common in males (M:F = 2:1)
- Epidemiology
  - 1.25% of intracranial tumors in childhood
  - 16% of intracranial tumors in 1st year of life

Natural History & Prognosis

- Median survival rate is > 75% at 15 years after diagnosis
- Spontaneous disappearance rare
- Anaplasia is very rare
- Leptomeningeal metastasis rare

Treatment

- Surgical resection curative, no recurrence with complete resection
- Chemotherapy if brain invasion or recurrence

DIAGNOSTIC CHECKLIST

Consider

- Large cystic mass in infant with plaque-like or nodular component along meninges, think DIG/DIA
- Important to mention DIG/DIA in report as pathologists may initially misinterpret as highly malignant tumor

Image Interpretation Pearls

- Solid portion is peripheral involving cortex, often invades adjacent meninges
- Solid portion is T2 hypointense

SELECTED REFERENCES

1. Balaji R et al: Imaging of desmoplastic infantile ganglioglioma: a spectroscopic viewpoint. Childs Nerv Syst. 25(4):497-501, 2009
2. Hoving EW et al: Desmoplastic infantile ganglioglioma with a malignant course. J Neurosurg Pediatr. 1(1):95-8, 2008
3. Brat DJ et al: Desmoplastic infantile astrocytoma and ganglioglioma. In Louis DN et al: Tumours of the Central Nervous System. Lyon: IARC Press. 96-8, 2007
4. Darwish B et al: Desmoplastic infantile ganglioglioma/ astrocytoma with cerebrospinal metastasis. J Clin Neurosci. 14(5):498-501, 2007
5. Lönnrot K et al: Desmoplastic infantile ganglioglioma: novel aspects in clinical presentation and genetics. Surg Neurol. 68(3):304-8; discussion 308, 2007
6. Bhardwaj M et al: Desmoplastic infantile ganglioglioma with calcification. Neuropathology. 26(4):318-22, 2006
7. Cerdá-Nicolás M et al: Desmoplastic infantile ganglioglioma. Morphological, immunohistochemical and genetic features. Histopathology. 48(5):617-21, 2006
8. Bächli H et al: Therapeutic strategies and management of desmoplastic infantile ganglioglioma: two case reports and literature overview. Childs Nerv Syst. 19(5-6):359-66, 2003
9. Tamburrini G et al: Desmoplastic infantile ganglioglioma. Childs Nerv Syst. 19(5-6):292-7, 2003
10. Shin JH et al: Neuronal tumors of the central nervous system: radiologic findings and pathologic correlation. Radiographics. 22(5):1177-89, 2002

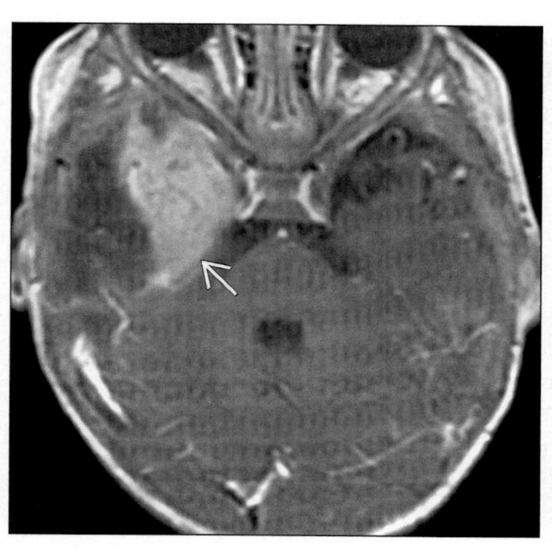

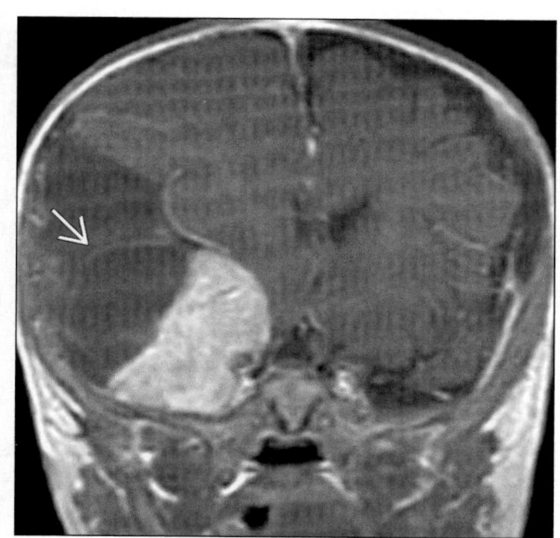

***(Left)** Axial T1WI C+ MR shows a cystic and solid mass in the temporal lobe with intense enhancement of the solid portion ➡. **(Right)** Coronal T1WI C+ MR in the same patient shows the cystic and solid mass with internal septations ➡ present in the cystic portion of the tumor. There is mild associated mass effect. DIA/DIA are often very large at presentation. Enhancement of the cortically based solid portion with involvement of the adjacent pia and dura is characteristic of these rare tumors.*

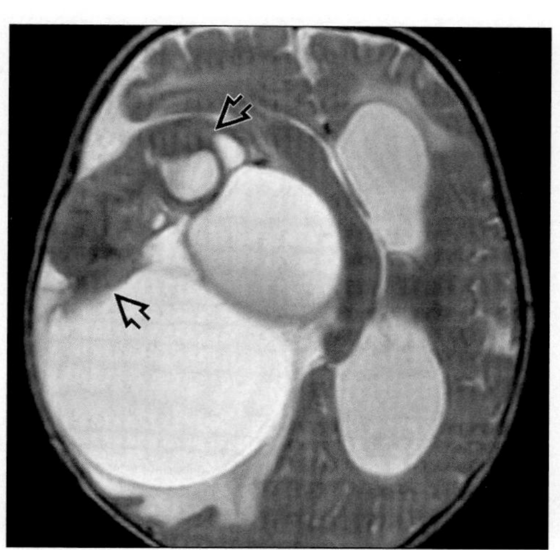

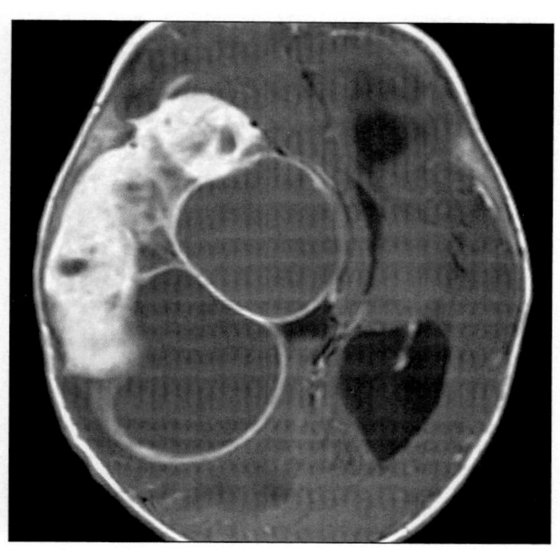

***(Left)** Axial T2WI MR shows a large multicystic and solid mass of the right hemisphere. The cortically based T2 hypointense solid portion ➡ is typical of DIG/DIA. **(Right)** Axial T1WI C+ MR in the same patient shows marked enhancement of the solid elements with mild cyst wall enhancement. Desmoplastic infantile astrocytoma and ganglioglioma presents in infants as large tumors, often approaching 13 cm. Macrocephaly with seizures are the most common presenting features.*

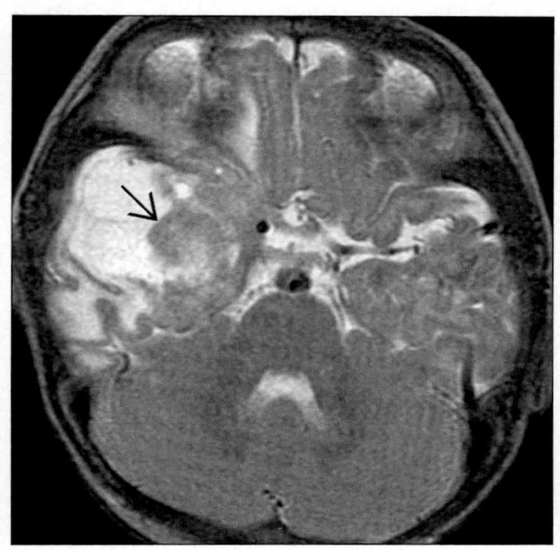

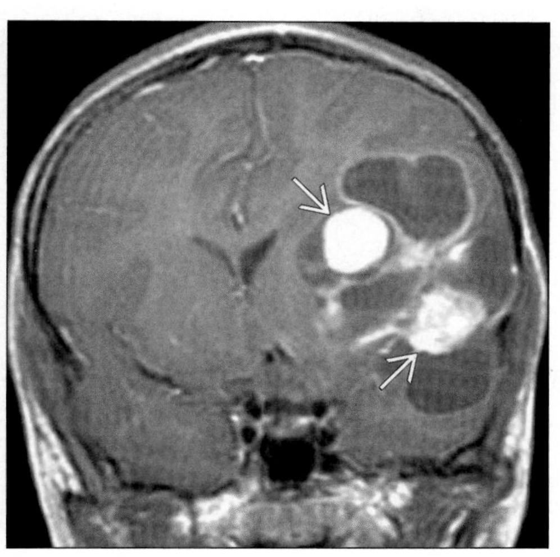

***(Left)** Axial T2WI MR shows a heterogeneous cystic and solid mass with a hypointense cortically based ➡ medial solid portion. Diagnosis was DIA/DIG. **(Right)** Coronal T1WI C+ MR shows a heterogeneous cystic and solid frontal mass with marked enhancement of the multiple solid nodules ➡. Typically, the solid portion is peripheral and dural-based in DIA/DIG. These WHO grade I tumors are important to recognize, as the initial pathology may suggest a more malignant tumor.*

DNET

Key Facts

Terminology

- Dysembryoplastic neuroepithelial tumor (DNET)
  - Benign mixed glial-neuronal neoplasm
  - Frequently associated with cortical dysplasia

Imaging

- May occur in any region of supratentorial cortex
  - Mesial temporal lobe most common
  - Mass frequently "points" towards ventricle
- Sharply demarcated, wedge-shaped
  - Cystic ("bubbly ") intracortical mass
  - Minimal/no mass effect
  - No surrounding edema
- Slow growth over years
- Usually does not enhance
- Faint focal punctate or ring enhancement in 20-30%
  - Higher rate of recurrence if enhancement

Top Differential Diagnoses

- Taylor dysplasia
- Neuroepithelial cyst
- Ganglioglioma
- Pleomorphic xanthoastrocytoma (PXA)
- Angiocentric glioma (a.k.a. ANET)

Pathology

- WHO grade I
- Hallmark = "specific glioneuronal element" (SGNE)

Clinical Issues

- Longstanding drug-resistant partial complex seizures in child/young adult
- Surgical resection usually curative
- Histology usually remains benign even if tumor recurs, enhances

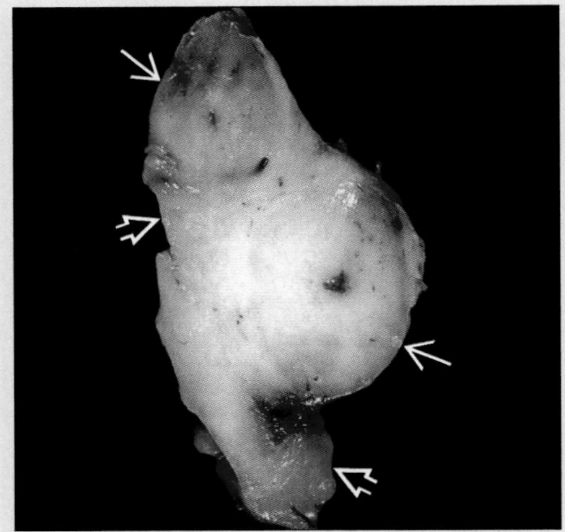

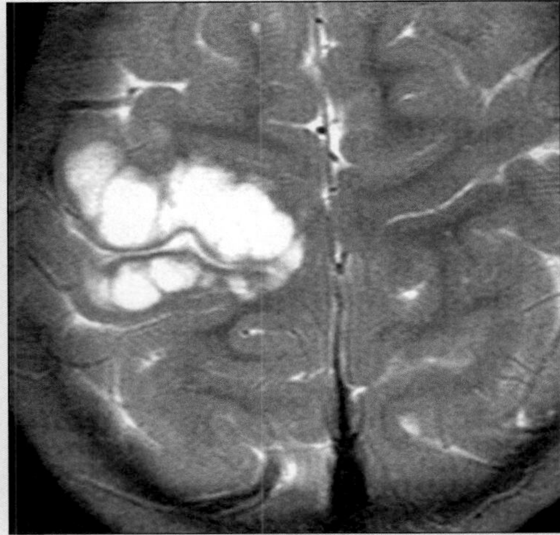

(Left) *Surgical specimen shows the typical nodular pattern of a DNET. The glioneuronal components are somewhat viscous areas ➡ intermixed with single or multiple firmer nodules ➡. Cut sections through surgical specimens like this often reflect the complex histoarchitecture of DNETs. (Courtesy R. Hewlett, PhD.)* ***(Right)*** *Axial T2WI MR shows a multilobular, wedge-shaped cystic cortically based mass in the right frontal lobe. Note the lack of edema and mass effect given the size of the tumor.*

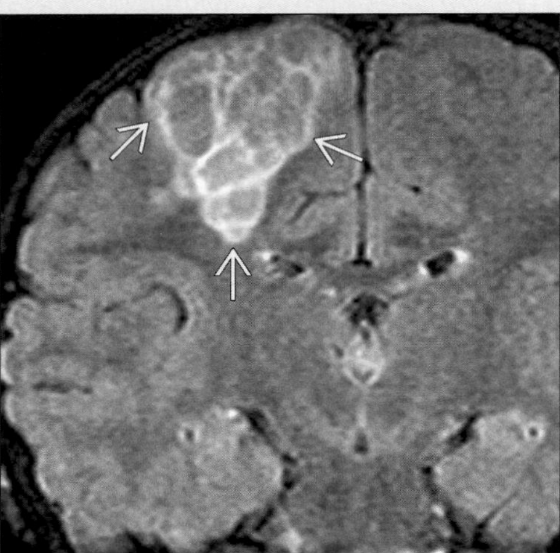

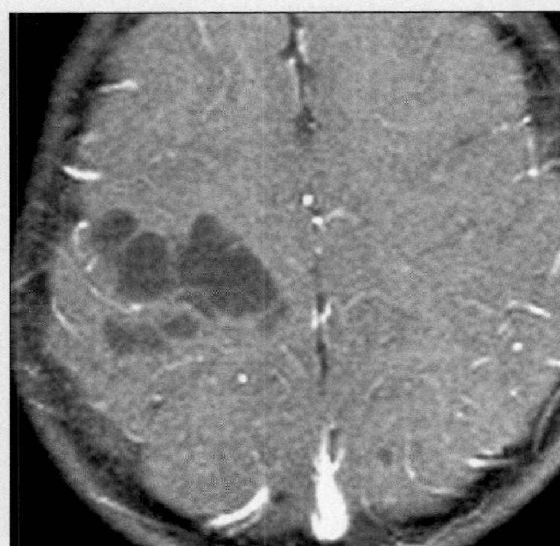

(Left) *Axial FLAIR MR in the same patient shows the characteristic appearance of a DNET. Note the cortically based, sharply demarcated, wedge-shaped mass with a hyperintense "rim" ➡. The tumor points towards the ventricle, and there is no surrounding edema.* ***(Right)*** *Axial T1WI C+ MR shows the cystic nature of the mass with a multiloculated appearance. There is no solid enhancement.*

DNET

TERMINOLOGY

Abbreviations
- Dysembryoplastic neuroepithelial tumor (DNET)

Synonyms
- Mixed glial-neuronal neoplasm

Definitions
- Benign tumor frequently associated with cortical dysplasia

IMAGING

General Features
- Best diagnostic clue
  - Demarcated, wedge-shaped cystic cortical mass in young patient with longstanding partial complex seizures
- Location
  - May occur in any region of supratentorial cortex
    - Mesial temporal lobe most common (68%)
      - Often amygdala/hippocampus
    - Caudate nucleus, septum pellucidum less frequent sites
  - Cortical mass frequently "points" towards ventricle
- Size
  - Variable: Small (involving part of gyrus)
  - Large (several cm lesions involving large portion of lobe have been reported)
- Morphology
  - Circumscribed, wedge-shaped, cystic
  - Minimal or no mass effect relative to size of lesion
  - No associated surrounding edema
  - Slow growth over many years
    - May remodel overlying bone

CT Findings
- NECT
  - Wedge-shaped
    - Cortical/subcortical
    - Scalloped inner table in 44-60%
  - Low density
    - May resemble stroke on initial CT
      - BUT no temporal evolution to atrophy
  - Calcification in 20-36%
- CECT
  - Usually nonenhancing
  - Faint nodular or patchy enhancement in 20%
    - Higher incidence of recurrence if enhancement
- CTA
  - Avascular CTA, MRA, conventional angiography

MR Findings
- T1WI
  - Multilobular, hypointense "bubbly" mass
    - Cortex ± extension into subcortical WM
- T2WI
  - Multilobular or septated appearance
  - Very hyperintense on T2
  - "Pseudocystic" or multicystic appearance
    - True cysts uncommon
- PD/intermediate
  - Hyperintense rim
- FLAIR
  - Variable
    - Mixed hypo/isointense signal
    - Well-defined, complete or incomplete, hyperintense ring(s) surrounding mass
  - No peritumoral edema
- T2* GRE
  - Bleeding into DNET uncommon but does occur
    - Possibly in association with microvascular abnormalities
    - May simulate cavernoma
- DWI
  - Usually lacks restricted diffusion
- T1WI C+
  - Usually does not enhance
  - Focal punctate or ring enhancement in up to 30%
- MRS
  - Nonspecific, but lactate present in some
  - Often spectroscopy normal

Nuclear Medicine Findings
- PET
  - 18F-FDG PET demonstrates glucose hypometabolism
  - Lower 11C-methionine (MET) uptake in DNET than in ganglioglioma or gliomas
- Tc-99m-HMPAO SPECT
  - Ictal may show hyperperfusion
  - Interictal hypoperfusion typical

Imaging Recommendations
- Best imaging tool
  - MR with T1WI C+, FLAIR ± MRS

DIFFERENTIAL DIAGNOSIS

Taylor Dysplasia
- Single tuberous sclerosis lesion
- Expands single gyrus
- Looks like tuber, nonenhancing

Neuroepithelial Cyst
- Nonenhancing single or complex cystic structure
- No bright rim on FLAIR

Ganglioglioma
- Ca++ common
- Frequently solid and cystic components
- Solid components avidly enhance

Pleomorphic Xanthoastrocytoma (PXA)
- Enhancing nodule abuts pia
- May have pial enhancement
- Look for dural "tail"

Angiocentric Glioma
- a.k.a. "angiocentric neuroepithelial tumor" (ANET)
- Rare superficial cortical lesion, usually frontoparietal
- Child/young adult with longstanding epilepsy

DNET

PATHOLOGY

General Features

- Etiology
  - Embryology: Dysplastic cells in germinal matrix
  - Extend along migratory path of neurons towards cortex
  - Associated with cortical dysplasia
  - Ring-like, slightly hyperintense rim on T1WI
- Genetics
  - Sporadic
  - Nonneoplastic focal cortical dysplasias may be syndrome related
  - Reported cases with NF1

Staging, Grading, & Classification

- WHO grade I

Gross Pathologic & Surgical Features

- Neocortical lesion
- Thick gyrus
- Glioneuronal component of tumor is viscous in consistency
- Firm nodules represent more stromal components

Microscopic Features

- Hallmark = "specific glioneuronal element" (SGNE)
  - Characterized by columns of bundled axons oriented perpendicular to cortex
  - Columns lined by oligodendroglia-like cells
  - Other cells show astrocytic, neuronal differentiation
- Several histological types
  - Complex form
    - Multinodular architecture
    - Mixed cellular composition
    - Foci of cortical disorganization
    - SGNE
  - Simple form with SGNE only
  - 3rd "nonspecific" form has no SGNE
    - But has same neuroimaging characteristics as complex form
- Microcystic degeneration
  - Neurons "float" in pale, eosinophilic mucoid matrix
- Calcification and leptomeningeal involvement common
- Adjacent cortical dysplasia common
- Low proliferative potential with variable MIB-1 index

CLINICAL ISSUES

Presentation

- Most common signs/symptoms
  - Partial complex seizures
- Clinical profile
  - Longstanding frequently drug-resistant partial complex seizures in child or young adult

Demographics

- Age
  - Children and young adults
    - 2nd to 3rd decades
    - Majority present by 20 years
- Gender
  - Slight male predominance
- Epidemiology
  - < 1% of all primary brain tumors
  - Approximately 1% of primary neuroepithelial brain tumors in patients < 20 years
  - Represents 0.2% of neuroepithelial tumors in patients > 20 years
  - Reported in 5-80% of epilepsy specimens

Natural History & Prognosis

- Benign lesions
- No or very slow increase in size over time
- Rare recurrence
  - Beware of atypical features (enhancement) on preoperative imaging
  - Malignant transformation extremely rare
    - Imaging may look alarming (e.g., new ring-enhancing mass)
    - Histology usually remains benign

Treatment

- Seizures may become intractable
  - Glutamate receptors shown within tumor and margins may explain typical difficult-to-control seizures
- Surgical resection of epileptogenic foci (may include cortical dysplasia)
- Surgical resection usually curative

DIAGNOSTIC CHECKLIST

Consider

- DNET if "bubbly" cortical mass in child/young adult with longstanding epilepsy

Image Interpretation Pearls

- Beware of enhancing lesions; they may represent more ominous lesion than DNET

SELECTED REFERENCES

1. Alexiou GA et al: Benign lesions accompanied by intractable epilepsy in children. J Child Neurol. 24(6):697-700, 2009
2. Bilginer B et al: Surgery for epilepsy in children with dysembryoplastic neuroepithelial tumor: clinical spectrum, seizure outcome, neuroradiology, and pathology. Childs Nerv Syst. 25(4):485-91, 2009
3. Ray WZ et al: Clinicopathologic features of recurrent dysembryoplastic neuroepithelial tumor and rare malignant transformation: a report of 5 cases and review of the literature. J Neurooncol. Epub ahead of print, 2009
4. Lee J et al: Dysembryoplastic neuroepithelial tumors in pediatric patients. Brain Dev. Epub ahead of print, 2008

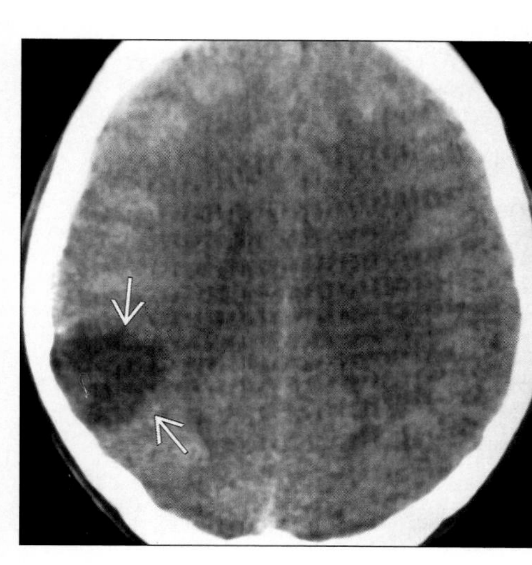

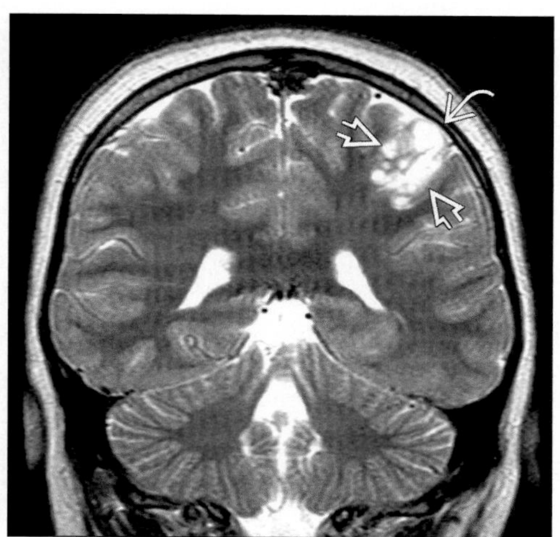

(Left) *Axial NECT in a 16 year old with longstanding seizures shows a low-density, cortically based mass in the right parietal lobe* ➡*. DNET was found at surgery.* ***(Right)*** *Coronal T2WI MR in a 10-year-old boy with longstanding seizures shows a cortically based mass with the classic "bubbly" appearance of a DNET* ➡*. The overlying cortex is slightly thinned* ➡*.*

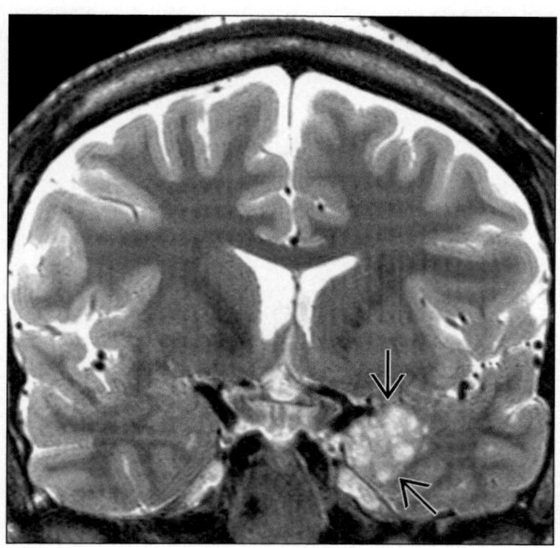

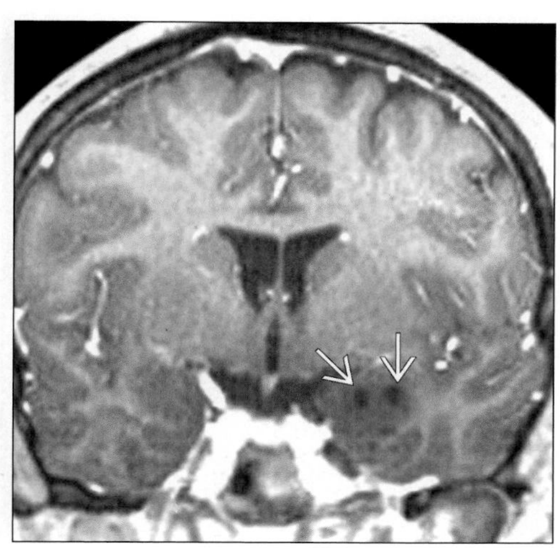

(Left) *Coronal T2WI MR shows a demarcated, "bubbly" mass* ➡ *in the medial left temporal lobe. The tumor is heterogeneous with both cystic and more solid areas. There is no associated surrounding edema.* ***(Right)*** *Coronal FLAIR C+ MR in the same patient shows the cortically based mass with cystic areas* ➡*. There is no enhancement of the solid portion of the tumor.*

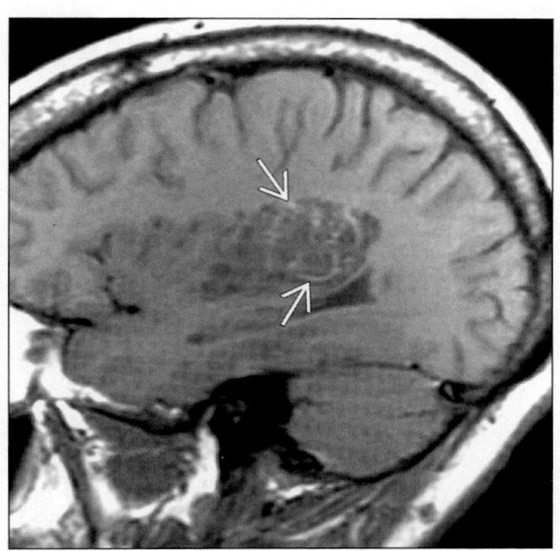

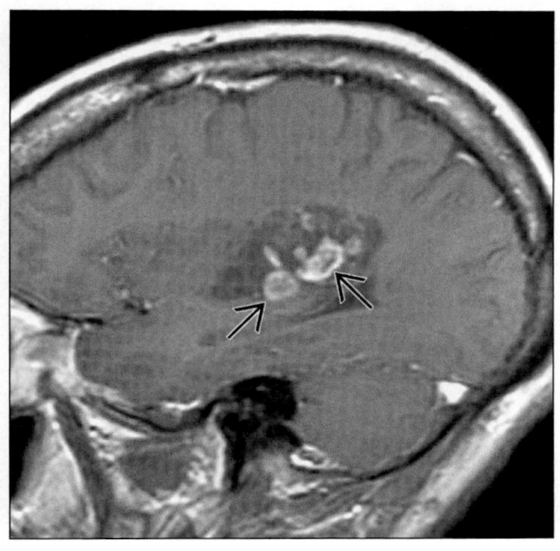

(Left) *Sagittal T1WI MR in a patient with DNET and multiple resections shows a "bubbly," cortically based temporal lobe mass, mostly hypointense, and with a few scattered areas of T1 shortening* ➡*.* ***(Right)*** *Sagittal T1WI C+ MR in the same patient shows foci of inhomogeneous but avid enhancement* ➡*, mostly around the cystic-appearing components. DNETs with "atypical" features may behave more aggressively. This tumor continued to show benign histology despite multiple recurrences.*

CENTRAL NEUROCYTOMA

Key Facts

Terminology

- Intraventricular neuroepithelial tumor with neuronal differentiation, typically in young adult

Imaging

- Best diagnostic clue: "Bubbly" mass in frontal horn or body of lateral ventricle
  - May involve 3rd ventricle
- CT: Usually mixed solid and cystic mass with calcification
  - Hydrocephalus common
  - Rarely complicated by hemorrhage
- MR: Heterogeneous, T2 hyperintense, "bubbly" appearance
  - Moderate to strong heterogeneous enhancement
- MRS: ↑ Cho, ↓ NAA
  - Glycine peak at 3.55 ppm

Top Differential Diagnoses

- Subependymoma
- Subependymal giant cell astrocytoma
- Intraventricular metastasis
- Ependymoma
- Choroid plexus papilloma

Clinical Issues

- Usually benign, local recurrence is uncommon
  - Surgical resection is typically curative
- 5-year survival rate: 90%
- MIB-1 > 2-3% associated with poorer prognosis

Diagnostic Checklist

- Think central neurocytoma if "bubbly" or "feathery" intraventricular mass near foramen of Monro in young adult

*(**Left**) Axial graphic shows a circumscribed, lobular, "bubbly" mass attached to the septum pellucidum. Ventricular dilatation is related to foramen of Monro obstruction. This is the classic appearance of a central neurocytoma. Complete surgical resection is often curative for these WHO grade II tumors. (**Right**) Axial FLAIR MR shows a heterogeneously hyperintense, "bubbly" mass in the lateral ventricles attached to the septum pellucidum. Associated hydrocephalus and transependymal flow of CSF are well seen ➔.*

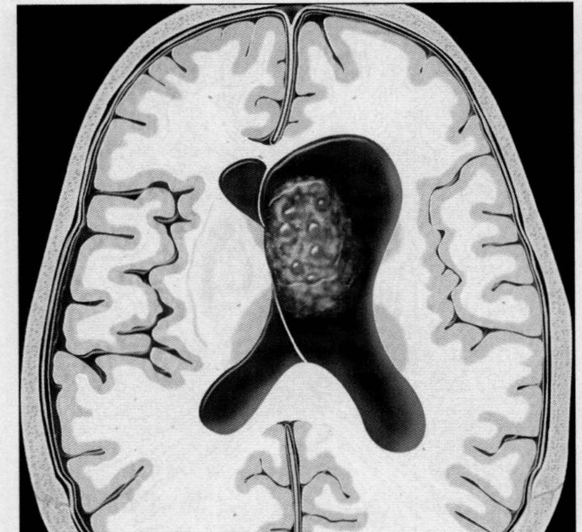

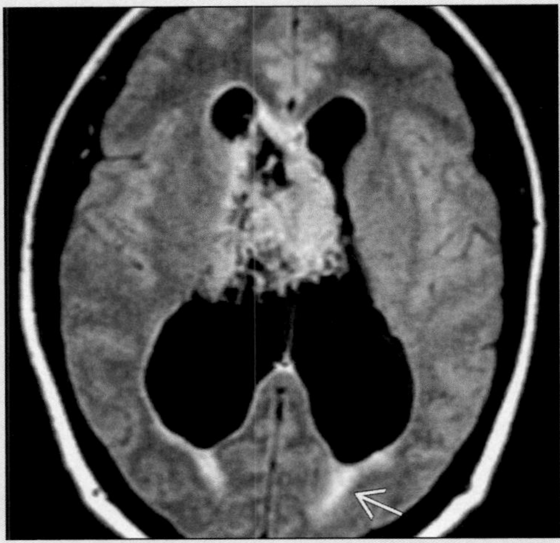

*(**Left**) Axial T2WI MR shows a heterogeneous "bubbly" and cystic lateral ventricular mass with attachment to the septum pellucidum ➔ and hydrocephalus, typical for central neurocytoma. (**Right**) Axial T1WI C+ MR in the same patient shows marked enhancement of the lobular mass with a large cyst filling the frontal horn. Central neurocytoma was found at resection. The imaging features of subependymoma and subependymal giant cell astrocytoma may mimic a central neurocytoma; clinical features can help differentiate.*

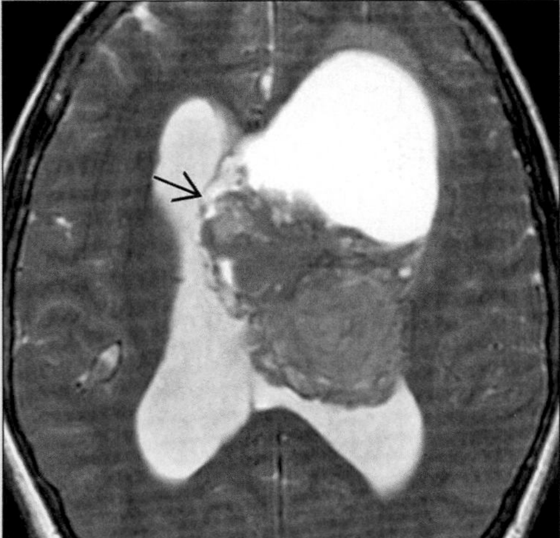

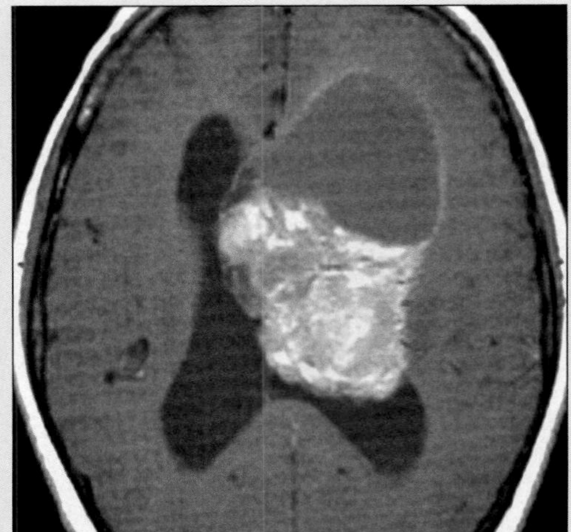

CENTRAL NEUROCYTOMA

TERMINOLOGY

Abbreviations

- Central neurocytoma (CN)

Synonyms

- Neurocytoma

Definitions

- Intraventricular neuroepithelial tumor with neuronal differentiation
- Well-demarcated, intraventricular, neurocytic neoplasm located in foramen of Monro region

IMAGING

General Features

- Best diagnostic clue
  - "Bubbly" mass in frontal horn or body of lateral ventricle
- Location
  - Typically supratentorial, intraventricular
  - Intraventricular mass attached to septum pellucidum
    - > 50% in frontal horn/body of lateral ventricle, near foramen of Monro
    - 15% extend into 3rd ventricle
  - Both lateral ventricles: 13%
  - 3rd ventricle only: 3%
  - 4th ventricle: Extremely rare
  - Rare extraventricular tumors with neurocytoma features ("extraventricular neurocytoma")
    - Brain parenchyma, cerebellum, spinal cord
- Morphology
  - Circumscribed, lobulated mass with intratumoral "cysts"
  - Characteristic "bubbly" appearance on imaging studies
  - May be predominantly solid

CT Findings

- NECT
  - Usually mixed solid and cystic (iso-/hyperdense)
  - Ca++ common (50-70%)
  - Hydrocephalus common
  - Rarely complicated by hemorrhage
- CECT
  - Moderate heterogeneous enhancement

MR Findings

- T1WI
  - Heterogeneous, mostly isointense to gray matter
  - Cysts are hypointense
  - Prominent flow voids may be seen
  - Hemorrhage is rare
- T2WI
  - Heterogeneous, hyperintense "bubbly" appearance
  - Associated hydrocephalus is common
  - Ca++ often hypointense
  - Prominent flow voids may be seen
- FLAIR
  - Heterogeneous, predominantly hyperintense mass
- T2* GRE
  - Ca++ seen as areas of "blooming"
- T1WI C+
  - Moderate to strong heterogeneous enhancement
- MRS
  - Elevated Cho peak, decreased NAA typical
  - Glycine peak at 3.55 ppm typical
  - Alanine peak may be seen

Angiographic Findings

- DSA: Variable appearance
  - Avascular mass to marked vascularity

Nuclear Medicine Findings

- PET
  - Typically characterized by decreased metabolism on FDG PET
  - Hypermetabolic activity has been described in atypical central neurocytoma

Imaging Recommendations

- Protocol advice
  - Multiplanar contrast-enhanced MR

DIFFERENTIAL DIAGNOSIS

Subependymoma

- May be indistinguishable
- Older patients
- Usually faint or no enhancement
- 4th > lateral ventricle

Subependymal Giant Cell Astrocytoma

- Mass at foramen of Monro, Ca++ common
- Look for stigmata of tuberous sclerosis
  - Subependymal nodules, cortical tubers, white matter lesions

Intraventricular Metastasis

- Uncommon, usually older patients
- Primary often known

Ependymoma

- Supratentorial ependymomas rarely intraventricular
- Heterogeneous enhancing mass with edema
- Aggressive features

Choroid Plexus Papilloma

- Typically younger patients, lateral ventricle
- In adults, 4th ventricle
- Intensely enhancing papillary mass, hydrocephalus common

Meningioma

- Circumscribed, intensely enhancing mass
- Typically at trigone of lateral ventricle
- Older patients

Cavernous Malformation

- Rarely intraventricular (2.5-11%)
- Ca++, T2-hypointense hemosiderin rim common

Oligodendroglioma

- Typically cortical mass with variable enhancement
- Main histologic differential

CENTRAL NEUROCYTOMA

PATHOLOGY

General Features

- Etiology
  - Likely arise from neuroglial or bipotential progenitor cells
- Genetics
  - Chromosomal abnormalities on 7, 2p, 10q, 18q, 13q reported
- Associated abnormalities
  - "Central neurocytoma" describes typical intraventricular tumors
    - Parenchymal invasion is rare, found in more aggressive tumors
  - Central neurocytoma rarely found in association with medulloblastoma

Staging, Grading, & Classification

- WHO grade II
- "Atypical central neurocytoma" (aggressive variant)
  - MIB-1 index > 2%
  - Vascular proliferation

Gross Pathologic & Surgical Features

- Grayish, friable, circumscribed, intraventricular mass
- Moderately vascular; may calcify; hemorrhage rare
- Typically attached to septum pellucidum or lateral ventricular wall

Microscopic Features

- Resembles oligodendroglioma
  - Many central neurocytomas misdiagnosed in past
- Uniform round cells with neuronal differentiation
  - Stippled nuclei, perinuclear halos
- Various architectural patterns (can resemble other neoplasms)
  - Monotonous sheets of cells
  - Perivascular pseudorosettes (ependymoma)
  - Honeycomb appearance (oligodendroglioma)
  - Large fibrillary areas (pineocytoma)
- Benign (low proliferation rate, mitoses rare)
  - MIB-1 usually low (< 2%)
- Anaplasia, necrosis rare
  - May have brisk mitotic activity, MIB-1 > 2-3%
  - Microvascular proliferation
- Synaptophysin and neuron-specific enolase positive; rarely GFAP positive
- Electron microscopy: Finely speckled chromatin, small distinct nucleolus, cell processes with neuritic features (microtubules)

CLINICAL ISSUES

Presentation

- Most common signs/symptoms
  - Headache, increased intracranial pressure, mental status changes, seizure
- Other signs/symptoms
  - Hydrocephalus secondary to foramen of Monro obstruction
  - Tumors of septum, 3rd ventricle, hypothalamus may have visual disturbances, hormonal dysfunction
  - Acute ventricular obstruction and death reported
  - Rarely asymptomatic

Demographics

- Age
  - Young adults, commonly 20-40 years (70%)
  - Range: 1-67 years; mean: 29 years
- Gender
  - No gender predominance
- Epidemiology
  - < 1% of all primary intracranial neoplasms
  - Approximately 10% of intraventricular neoplasms
  - Represents 50% of intraventricular tumors in patients 20-40 years

Natural History & Prognosis

- Usually benign, local recurrence is uncommon
  - Surgical resection is typically curative
- Rarely complicated by hemorrhage
- 5-year survival rate: 90%
- MIB-1 > 2-3% associated with poorer prognosis
- Craniospinal dissemination extremely rare (< 10 cases reported)
- Tumors with extraventricular extension have poorer clinical outcome

Treatment

- Complete surgical resection is treatment of choice
- If incomplete resection, radiation therapy, chemotherapy, &/or radiosurgery may be helpful
- Gamma knife radiosurgery may improve local control rates and increase survival

DIAGNOSTIC CHECKLIST

Consider

- Subependymoma and giant cell astrocytoma mimic central neurocytoma, clinical information may help
- May mimic other tumors pathologically, so imaging correlation is important

Image Interpretation Pearls

- Think central neurocytoma if "bubbly" or "feathery" intraventricular mass near foramen of Monro in young adult
- Central neurocytoma is typically attached to septum pellucidum

SELECTED REFERENCES

1. Kocaoglu M et al: Central neurocytoma: proton MR spectroscopy and diffusion weighted MR imaging findings. Magn Reson Imaging. 27(3):434-40, 2009
2. Chen CM et al: Central neurocytoma: 9 case series and review. Surg Neurol. 70(2):204-9, 2008
3. Paek SH et al: Long-term outcome of conventional radiation therapy for central neurocytoma. J Neurooncol. 90(1):25-30, 2008
4. Louis DN et al: WHO Classification of Tumours of the Central Nervous System:Central neurocytoma and extraventricular neurocytoma. Lyon: IARC Press. 106-109, 2007

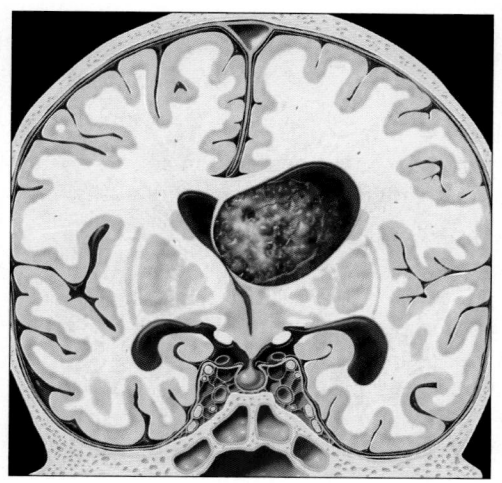

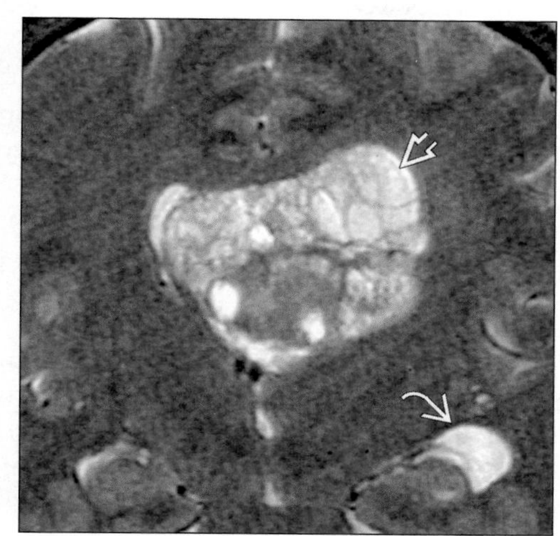

(Left) *Coronal graphic shows a "bubbly," lobular, intraventricular mass attached to the septum pellucidum with associated ventricular dilatation, typical of central neurocytoma.* ***(Right)*** *Coronal T2WI MR shows the characteristic "bubbly" or "soap bubble" appearance of this lateral ventricular central neurocytoma ➔ with bowing of the septum pellucidum and temporal horn dilatation ➔. Strong heterogeneous enhancement is typical. These tumors typically present in young adults between 20 and 40 years old.*

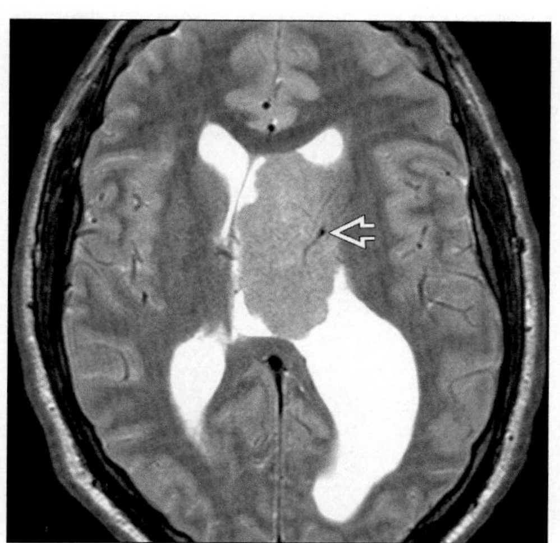

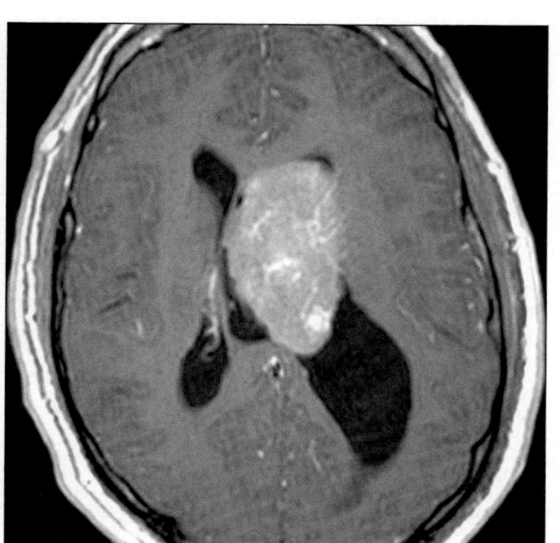

(Left) *Axial T2WI MR in a 20 year old with headaches shows a predominantly solid ventricular mass in the body of the left lateral ventricle with prominent scattered flow voids ➔. Flow voids are best seen on T2 and PD MR.* ***(Right)*** *In the same patient with central neurocytoma, axial T1WI C+ MR shows diffuse enhancement of the mass. Imaging differential considerations include subependymal giant cell astrocytoma, subependymoma, and meningioma. (Courtesy S. van der Westhuizen, MD.)*

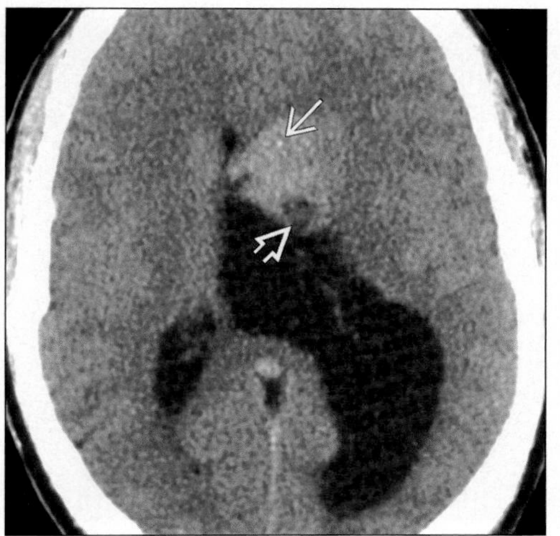

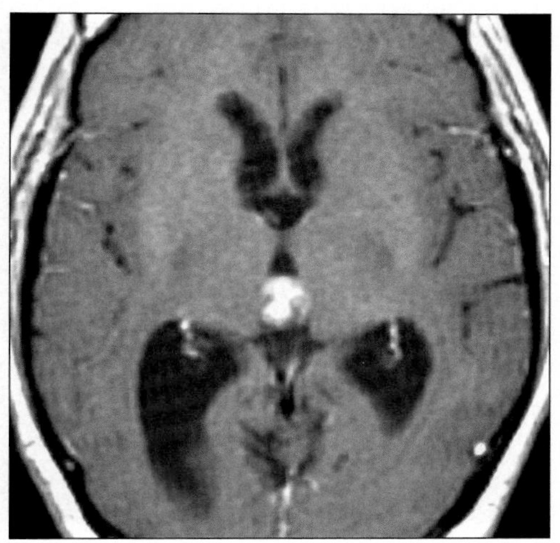

(Left) *Axial NECT shows a mildly hyperdense mass at the foramen of Monro with a focal calcification ➔ and a small cystic component ➔. The predominantly solid appearance of this central neurocytoma is unusual; Ca++ is seen in 50-70% of central neurocytomas.* ***(Right)*** *Axial T1WI C+ MR shows an enhancing mass in the posterior 3rd ventricle, suggesting a pineal mass. Calcification was present on CT. Central neurocytoma was found at resection. Less than 5% of central neurocytomas occur in the 3rd ventricle.*

EXTRAVENTRICULAR NEUROCYTOMA

Key Facts

Terminology
- Neuroepithelial tumor located outside ventricular system, commonly in brain parenchyma

Imaging
- Best diagnostic clue: Well-circumscribed, enhancing, cystic-solid parenchymal mass in young adult
- Majority are supratentorial involving cerebral hemispheres
  - Frontal and parietal lobes most common
  - Deep gray nuclei less common
- T2 MR: Heterogeneously hyperintense mass
- T2* GRE: May show "blooming" related to blood products or Ca++
- T1WI C+: Variable enhancement of solid portions
  - May have cyst with mural nodule appearance

Top Differential Diagnoses
- Oligodendroglioma
- Pilocytic astrocytoma
- Ganglioglioma
- DNET
- Glioblastoma multiforme

Pathology
- WHO grade II
- May be identical to central neurocytoma
  - Often contain ganglion cells or ganglioid cells

Clinical Issues
- Seizures, hemiparesis are most common presenting features
- Occur in children & young adults (median: 34 years)
- Rare: < 0.5% of primary CNS tumors
- Surgical resection is typically curative
- Subtotal resection, atypical histologic features, and high cell proliferation rates correlate with recurrence

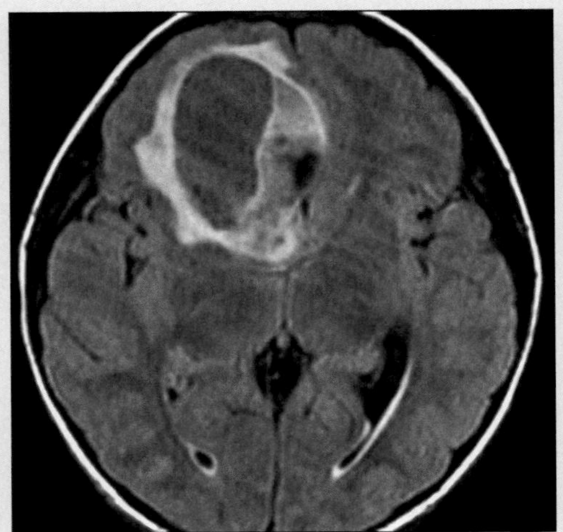

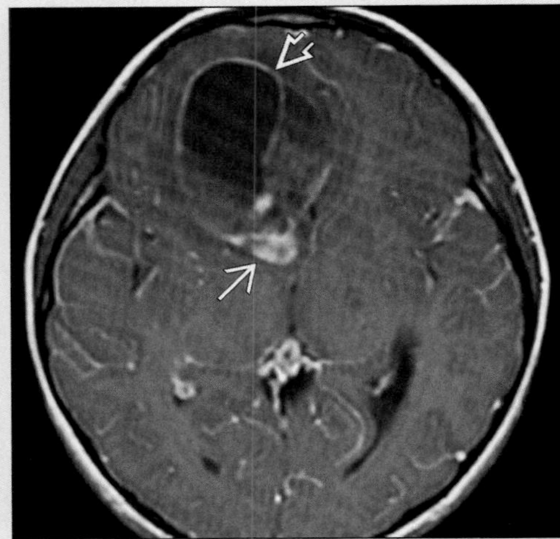

(Left) *Axial FLAIR MR shows a cystic and solid mass in the frontal lobe with mild surrounding vasogenic edema. (Courtesy N. Fischbein, MD.)* ***(Right)*** *Axial T1WI C+ MR in the same patient shows heterogeneous enhancement of the solid portion* ➔ *and rim enhancement of the cystic portion* ⇨*. The lack of significant vasogenic edema is typical for extraventricular neurocytoma. Imaging differential considerations include oligodendroglioma, astrocytoma, and ganglioglioma. (Courtesy N. Fischbein, MD.)*

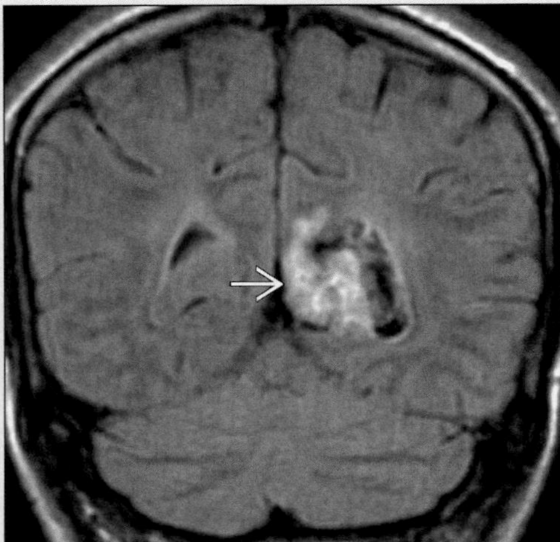

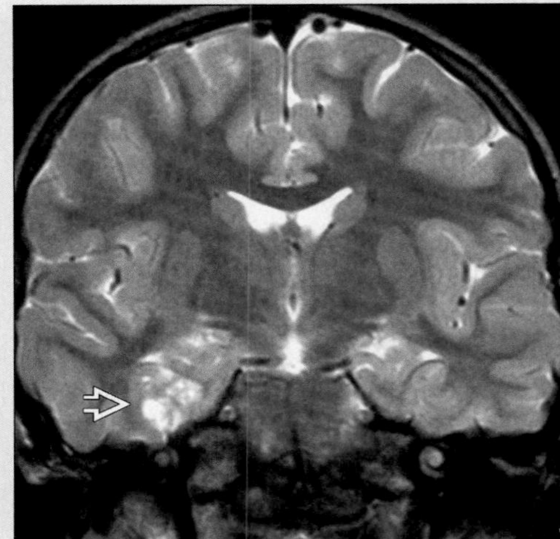

(Left) *Coronal FLAIR MR shows a heterogeneously hyperintense mass* ➔ *within the medial occipital lobe parenchyma. Note the lack of surrounding vasogenic edema, typical for extraventricular neurocytoma. The occipital lobe is an uncommon location.* ***(Right)*** *Coronal T2WI MR shows a heterogeneously hyperintense superficial temporal lobe mass* ⇨*. The "bubbly" appearance mimics a DNET, but this proved to be an extraventricular neurocytoma. (Courtesy A. Rossi, MD.)*

EXTRAVENTRICULAR NEUROCYTOMA

TERMINOLOGY

Abbreviations
- Extraventricular neurocytoma (EVN)

Definitions
- Neuroepithelial tumor located outside of ventricular system, commonly in brain parenchyma

IMAGING

General Features
- Best diagnostic clue
  - Well-circumscribed, enhancing, cystic and solid parenchymal mass in young adult
- Location
  - Majority are supratentorial involving cerebral hemispheres
    - Frontal and parietal lobes most common
    - Deep grey nuclei less common
  - Cerebellum and brainstem rare
  - Sella, pineal region, spinal cord reported
- Morphology
  - Cystic and solid masses
  - May have cyst with mural nodule appearance

Imaging Recommendations
- Protocol advice
  - Contrast enhanced MR with GRE, ± MRS

CT Findings
- NECT
  - Circumscribed, complex, cystic and solid mass
  - Ca++ in 10-15%
  - Vasogenic edema variable

MR Findings
- T1WI: Cystic, heterogeneously solid mass
  - Usually involve deep WM, may involve cortex
- T2WI: Heterogeneously hyperintense mass
  - Mild vasogenic edema typical
- T2* GRE: May show "blooming" related to blood products or Ca++
- T1WI C+: Variable enhancement of solid portions
  - May see cyst and mural nodule
- MRS: ↓ NAA and ↑ choline (Cho)

DIFFERENTIAL DIAGNOSIS

Oligodendroglioma
- Calcified, heterogeneous mass
- Variable enhancement

Pilocytic Astrocytoma
- Solid-cystic or solid enhancing mass
- Typically posterior fossa or chiasmatic/hypothalamic

Ganglioglioma
- Enhancing cystic and solid cortically based mass in child or young adult
- Temporal lobe commonly > parietal, frontal

DNET
- Cortical "bubbly" mass in young adult

Glioblastoma Multiforme
- Heterogeneous mass with central necrosis
- Typically older patients

PATHOLOGY

General Features
- Etiology
  - May arise from neuroglial precursor cells
- Associated abnormalities
  - Single case reported in patient with neurofibromatosis type 1

Staging, Grading, & Classification
- WHO grade II

Gross Pathologic & Surgical Features
- Cysts, necrosis, Ca++ may be seen
- Hemorrhage rare

Microscopic Features
- May be identical to central neurocytoma
  - Densely cellular, cytologically monomorphous
- Often contain ganglion cells or ganglioid cells
- Hyalinized vessels and dense Ca++ common
- Synaptophysin positive, often GFAP positive

CLINICAL ISSUES

Presentation
- Most common signs: Seizures, hemiparesis

Demographics
- Age
  - Typically children, young adults (median: 34 years)
- Gender
  - No gender predominance
- Epidemiology
  - Rare: < 0.5% of primary CNS tumors

Natural History & Prognosis
- Surgical resection is typically curative
- Subtotal resection, atypical histologic features, and high cell proliferation rates correlate with recurrence

Treatment
- Surgical resection ± adjuvant therapy
- Radiation therapy in recurrent tumors

SELECTED REFERENCES

1. Mpairamidis E et al: Extraventricular neurocytoma in a child: case report and review of the literature. J Child Neurol. 24(4):491-4, 2009
2. Yang GF et al: Imaging findings of extraventricular neurocytoma: report of 3 cases and review of the literature. AJNR Am J Neuroradiol. 30(3):581-5, 2009
3. Sharma MC et al: Neurocytoma: a comprehensive review. Neurosurg Rev. 29(4):270-85; discussion 285, 2006

CEREBELLAR LIPONEUROCYTOMA

Key Facts

Terminology

- Cerebellar liponeurocytoma (CLN)
- Rare cerebellar parenchymal neoplasm of adults
  - Consistent neuronal, variable astrocytic and lipomatous elements

Imaging

- CT
  - Hypodense (fat density)
- MR
  - Hyperintense on T1WI
  - Inhomogeneously hyperintense on T2WI
  - Lipomatous component suppresses with FS
  - Inhomogeneous enhancement

Top Differential Diagnoses

- Teratoma
- Medulloblastoma with lipidized cells
- Anaplastic oligodendroglioma
- Ependymoma

Pathology

- *Tp53* missense mutations
- WHO grade II
- Moderate to low mitotic index
  - MIB-1 mean: 2.5%

Clinical Issues

- Headache
  - More focal cerebellar symptoms depending on location
- Age range: 24-77 years; mean: 50 years
- Approximately 2/3 recur after resection within 1-12 years
  - 5-year survival: 48%

*(**Left**) Precontrast T1WI MR shows irregular areas of high signal intensity ➔ within a left cerebellar mass due to areas of fatty tissue that cause T1 shortening. The majority of the mass is isointense with nearly indistinguishable borders ➔. (Courtesy AFIP.) (**Right**) Sagittal T1WI C+ MR in the same patient shows minimal/ no enhancement. Most of the high signal was seen previously due to fatty components of this tumor. Images are degraded slightly by pulsation artifact from the carotid arteries. (Courtesy AFIP.)*

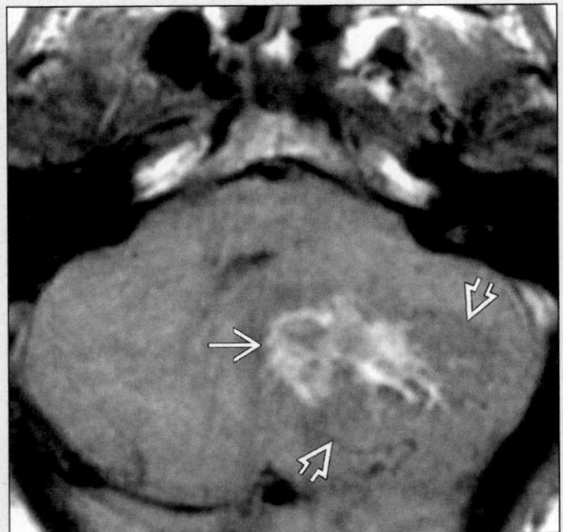

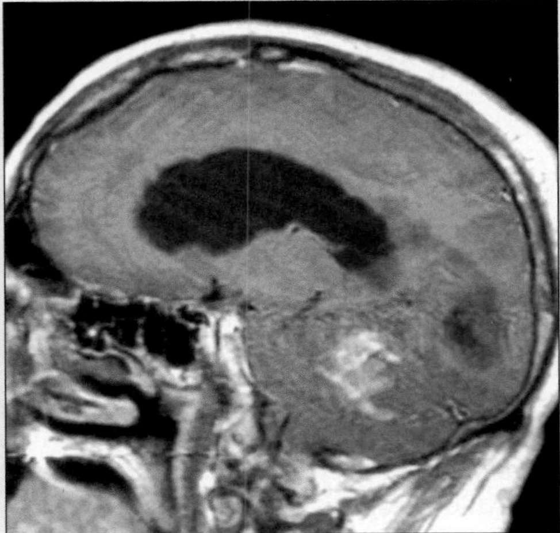

*(**Left**) The left cerebellar mass is more clearly delineated on T2 images, which show the fatty component ➔ as slightly hypointense compared to the larger, more cellular non-fatty, hyperintense componets ➔ surrounding the fatty elements. (Courtesy AFIP.) (**Right**) The mass effect from the tumor significantly effaces the inferior 4th ventricle ➔, resulting in the supratentorial hydrocephalus seen on the sagittal T1WI C+ MR. (Courtesy AFIP.)*

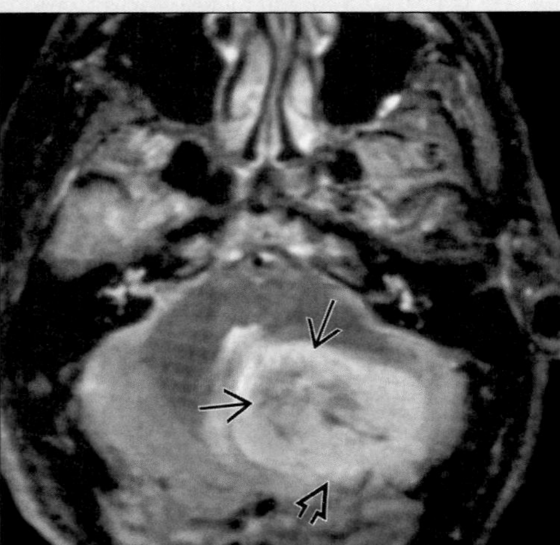

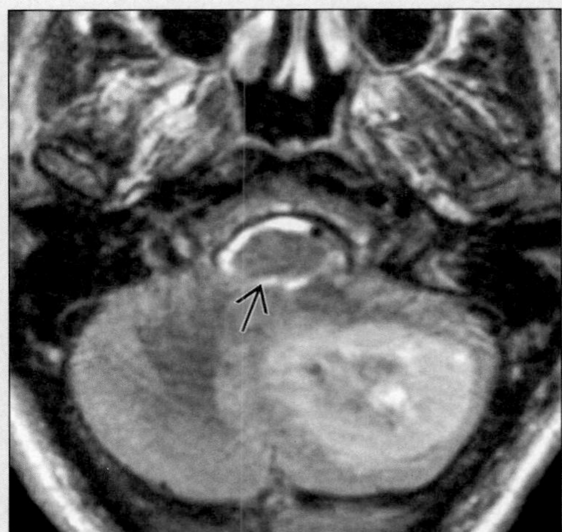

Key Facts

Terminology

- Indolent glioneuronal tumor
  - Previously considered ganglioglioma subtype
  - Also described as pseudopapillary neurocytoma with glial differentiation

Imaging

- General features
  - Cerebral hemispheres most common site
  - Parenchymal mass with solid, cystic, or cyst-mural nodule architecture
- CT
  - Partially calcified mass ± cystic regions
- MR
  - Isointense ± hypointense cysts on T1WI
  - Inhomogeneously hyperintense on T2WI
  - Inhomogeneously hyperintense nodule on FLAIR (cyst may suppress)
  - Strong, heterogeneous enhancement on T1WI C+

Top Differential Diagnoses

- Ganglioglioma
- Oligodendroglioma
- Ependymoma
- Chronic inflammatory lesion (e.g., neurocysticercosis)

Pathology

- "Biphasic" neurocytic, glial components
- WHO grade I with low MIB-1 index (1-2%)

Clinical Issues

- Seizures, headache most common symptoms
- Affects children, young adults (range 4-75 years)
- Potentially curable with complete resection
- Generally indolent course although aggressive papillary glioneuronal tumors reported

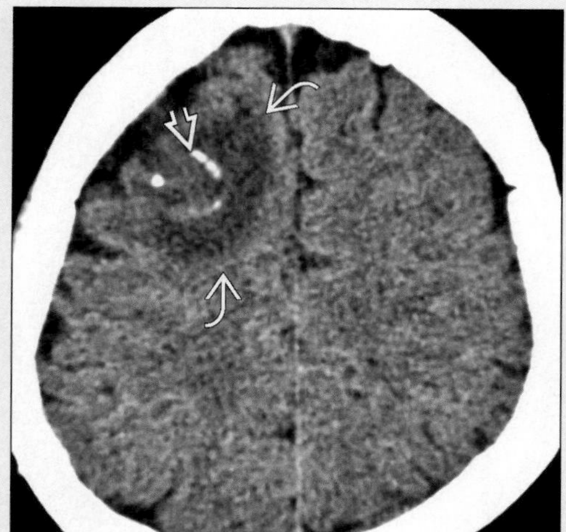

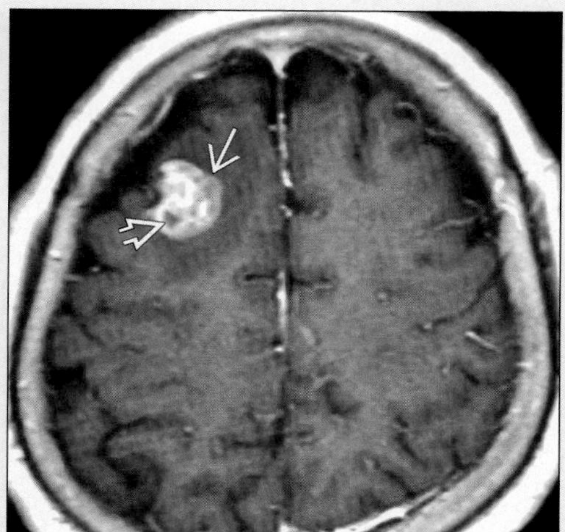

(Left) *Axial NECT in a recently arrived immigrant with seizures shows a right frontal mass with incomplete ring calcification ➡ and moderate perilesional edema ↗. Parasitic infection was considered.* ***(Right)*** *Axial T1WI C+ MR in the same patient shows an intensely but inhomogeneously enhancing component ➡. Note the small intratumoral cysts ➡. Lower images (not shown) demonstrated a larger cystic area with rim enhancement. Ultrasound-guided stereotaxic biopsy disclosed papillary glioneuronal tumor.*

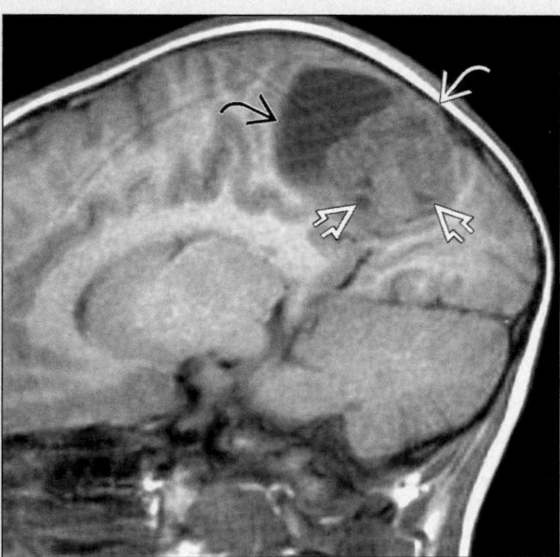

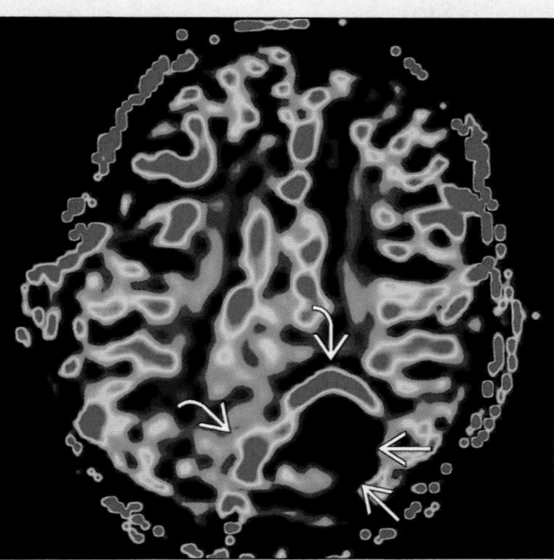

(Left) *Sagittal T1WI in an 8-year-old boy with seizures shows a solid ➡ and cystic ↗ parietal lobe mass. The solid component shows lobulations with some intratumoral cystic-appearing spaces ➡. (Courtesy M. Castillo, MD.)* ***(Right)*** *Axial perfusion MR in the same patient shows a parietal lobe mass with relatively decreased perfusion ➡ surrounded by a rim of relatively increased perfusion ↗. Papillary glioneuronal tumor was found at surgery. (Courtesy M. Castillo, MD.)*

ROSETTE-FORMING GLIONEURONAL TUMOR

Key Facts

Terminology
- Rosette-forming glioneuronal tumor (RGNT)
- Rare, slowly growing benign tumor of young adults
  - 4th ventricle most common site
  - Rarely in pineal region, cerebellopontine angle, brain hemispheres

Imaging
- Midline cerebellar neoplasm
  - Mixed solid-cystic appearance
  - Variable Ca++, hemorrhage
  - Hyperintense on T2WI
- Enhancement usually absent
  - When present, usually mild
  - Peripheral, nodular, or inhomogeneous

Top Differential Diagnoses
- Ependymoma
- Medulloblastoma (PNET-MB)
- Pilocytic astrocytoma

Pathology
- WHO grade I
- 2 components
  - "Neurocytic": Neurocytes forming neurocytic/ perivascular pseudorosette
  - "Astrocytic": Resembles pilocytic astrocytoma

Clinical Issues
- Headache (60% associated hydrocephalus)
- Benign, no malignant transformation

Diagnostic Checklist
- Suspect RGNT when young adult presents with well-circumscribed 4th ventricle mass with combined cystic-nodule appearance, no edema

*(**Left**) Axial T2* GRE MR in a patient with headaches and papilledema on physical examination demonstrates a large multicystic midline mass in the posterior fossa. Note fluid-fluid levels ➡ and regions of low signal intensities ⇨ representing calcifications. (**Right**) Axial T1WI C+ in the same patient shows mild inhomogeneous enhancement ➡. Note the dilated optic nerve sheaths and elevated optic discs ➡ from papilledema. A RGNT was found at surgery.*

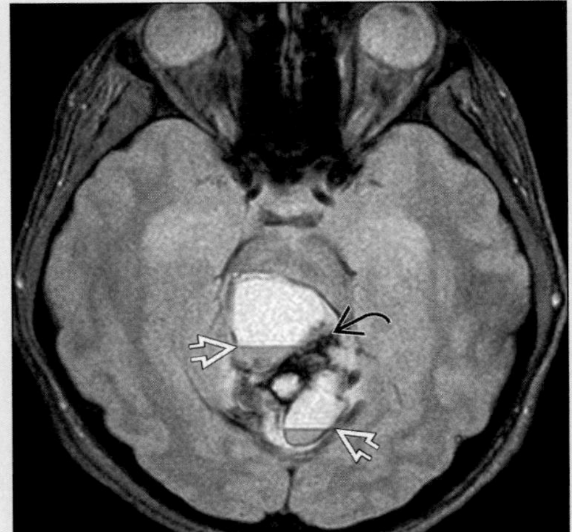

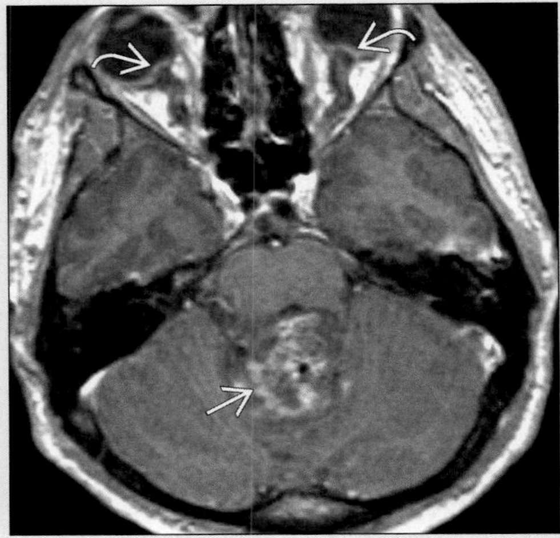

*(**Left**) Sagittal T1WI MR in a young adult with headaches shows a mixed signal intensity mass ⇨ filling the 4th ventricle. Foci of T1 shortening represent hemorrhage. No enhancement was seen on T1WI C+ scans. Pathology showed a RGNT. (**Right**) Sagittal T1WI C+ MR in a teenager with headaches shows a nonenhancing hypointense pineal region mass ➡. The lesion involves the tectum as well as the pineal gland. Histology disclosed a RGNT, which are often found in locations other than the 4th ventricle.*

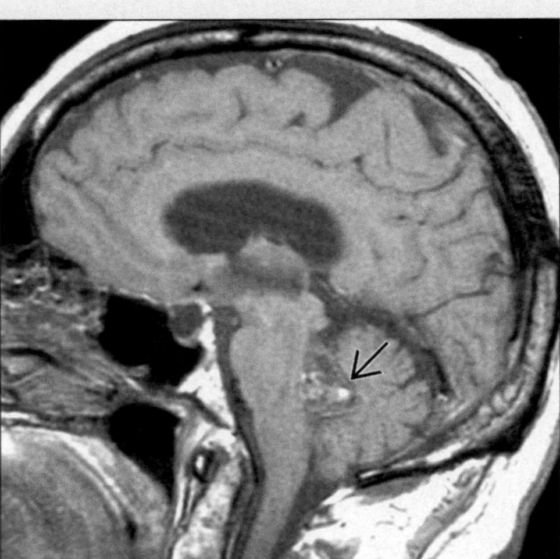

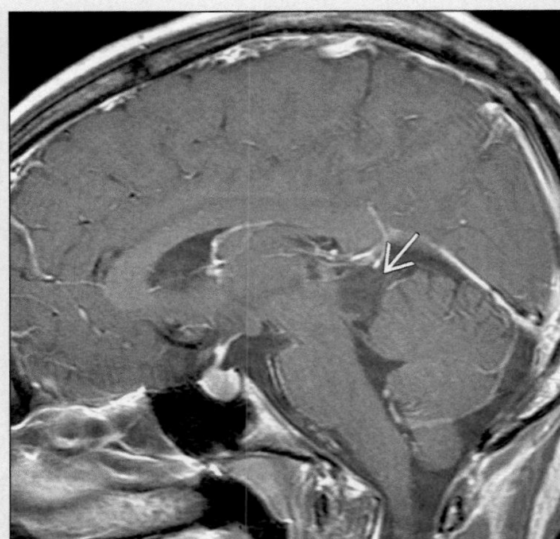

ROSETTE-FORMING GLIONEURONAL TUMOR

TERMINOLOGY

Abbreviations

- Rosette-forming glioneuronal tumor (RGNT)

Synonyms

- 1st described as dysembryoplastic neuroepithelial tumor (DNT) of cerebellum
- Also formerly called cerebellar DNT

Definitions

- Rare, slowly growing benign tumor
  - 4th ventricle most common (sometimes called RGNT of 4th ventricle)

IMAGING

General Features

- Best diagnostic clue
  - Cerebellar-based neoplasm with solid-cystic appearance without edema in young/middle-aged adults
- Location
  - Majority in cerebellar midline around 4th ventricle
  - Rarely in pineal region, cerebellopontine angle, brain hemispheres
- Size
  - Varies between 1.5 and 10 cm

Imaging Recommendations

- Best imaging tool
  - MR with T1WI C+, T2* (hemorrhage, Ca++)

CT Findings

- NECT
  - Midline posterior fossa cystic/solid mass
  - Variable Ca++, hemorrhage

MR Findings

- T1WI
  - Iso-/hypointense
- T2WI
  - Hyperintense
- T2* GRE
  - Hemorrhage common
- T1WI C+
  - Usually absent
    - Usually mild when present ; may be peripheral, nodular, or inhomogeneous

DIFFERENTIAL DIAGNOSIS

Ependymoma

- Usually tumor of childhood
- "Squeezes" out through lateral recesses
- Strong but heterogeneous enhancement

Medulloblastoma (PNET-MB)

- Children > adults
- Usually (not always) enhances strongly
- Gross hemorrhage, cyst formation less common

Pilocytic Astrocytoma (PA)

- Children > adults
- Cyst with nodule appearance
  - Nodule enhances strongly
  - If cyst wall enhances, may resemble RGNT

PATHOLOGY

General Features

- Etiology
  - Derives from pluripotential cells of subependymal plate

Staging, Grading, & Classification

- WHO grade I

Gross Pathologic & Surgical Features

- Cystic/nodular appearance

Microscopic Features

- 2 components
  - "Neurocytic": Neurocytes forming neurocytic/ perivascular pseudorosette
  - "Astrocytic": Resembles pilocytic astrocytoma

CLINICAL ISSUES

Presentation

- Most common signs/symptoms
  - Headache
- Other signs/symptoms
  - Nausea, vertigo, ataxia
  - 60% of patients present with obstructive hydrocephalus

Demographics

- Age
  - Young/middle-aged adults
    - Mean age ~ 30 years old
- Gender
  - M:F = 1:2

Natural History & Prognosis

- Benign; no malignant transformation

Treatment

- Surgical removal

DIAGNOSTIC CHECKLIST

Consider

- Suspect RGNT when young adult presents with well-circumscribed 4th ventricle mass with combined cystic-nodule appearance, no edema

SELECTED REFERENCES

1. Marhold F et al: Clinicoradiological features of rosette-forming glioneuronal tumor (RGNT) of the fourth ventricle: report of four cases and literature review. J Neurooncol. 90(3):301-8, 2008

PINEOCYTOMA

Key Facts

Terminology

- Pineocytoma (PC), pineal parenchymal tumor (PPT)
- PCs are composed of small, uniform, mature cells
  - Cells resemble pineocytes

Imaging

- General features
  - Typically less than 3 cm
  - Rarely extends into 3rd ventricle
  - Rarely invasive
  - May compress adjacent structures
  - Can compress aqueduct → hydrocephalus
  - Occasionally hemorrhages
- CT
  - Circumscribed iso-/hypodense pineal region mass on NECT
  - Peripheral ("exploded") Ca++ common
  - Enhances (solid, ring, nodular) on CECT
- MR (most sensitive)
  - Cystic change may be present
  - Enhancement may be solid or peripheral

Top Differential Diagnoses

- Nonneoplastic pineal cyst
- Pineal parenchymal tumor of intermediate differentiation
- Pineoblastoma
- Germinoma, other germ cell tumors

Clinical Issues

- Headache, Parinaud syndrome
- Increased intracranial pressure, ataxia, hydrocephalus, mental status changes
- Germ cell markers (α-fetoprotein, hCG) absent
- Peak incidence 10-20 years, mean age = 35 years
- Stable- or slow-growing tumor

*(**Left**) Sagittal graphic shows a cystic pineal gland mass with a fluid-fluid level and a nodular tumor along the periphery of the mass, typical of pineocytoma. No significant mass effect is present. (**Right**) Axial NECT shows a classic example of a pineocytoma. Note the "exploded" peripheral calcification ➔ in this small mass that arises from the pineal region. The tumor is just over 1 cm in size. There is no hydrocephalus.*

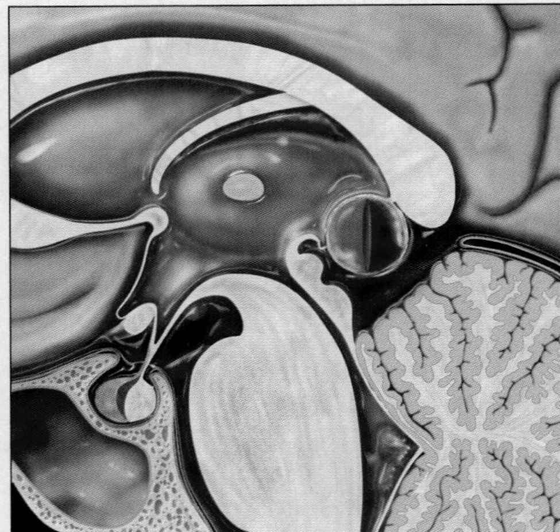

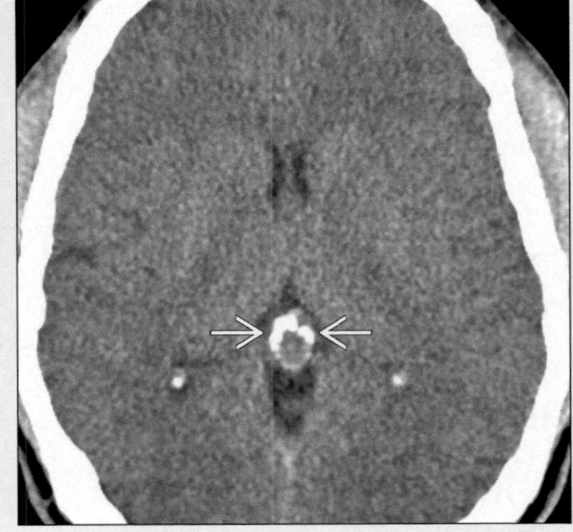

*(**Left**) Sagittal T1WI MR in the same patient shows a demarcated mass of the pineal gland that is isointense to the brain parenchyma ➔. It exerts mild mass effect on the tectum, but the aqueduct is patent ➔ and there is no hydrocephalus. The pineal tumor sits underneath the internal cerebral veins ➔ and splenium of the corpus callosum. (**Right**) Sagittal T1WI C+ MR shows the demarcated, but heterogeneously enhancing nature of the tumor, with avid enhancement of the superior nodular component ➔.*

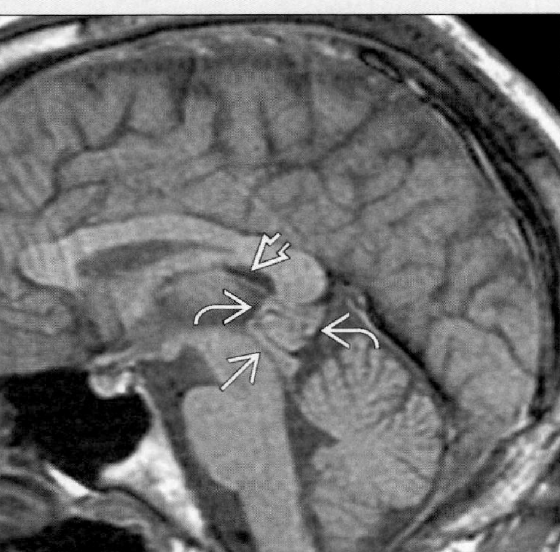

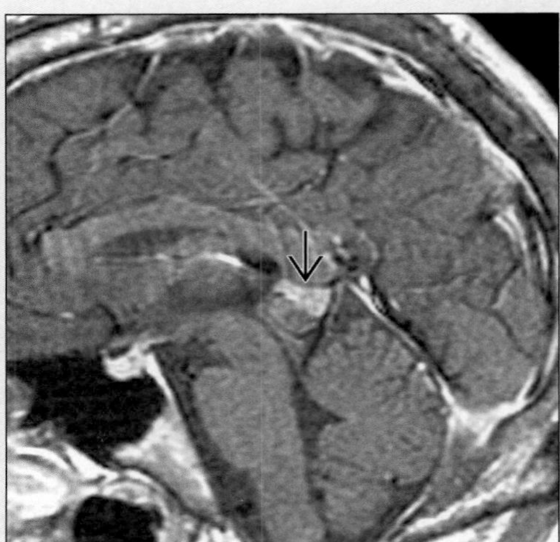

PINEOCYTOMA

TERMINOLOGY

Abbreviations
- Pineocytoma (PC)

Definitions
- Slow-growing pineal parenchymal tumor (PPT) of young adults
  - Composed of small, uniform, mature cells resembling pineocytes

IMAGING

General Features
- Best diagnostic clue
  - Circumscribed pineal mass that "explodes" pineal calcification peripherally
  - May mimic pineal cyst, pineal parenchymal tumor of intermediate differentiation (PPTID)
- Location
  - Pineal region
  - Rarely extends into 3rd ventricle
  - Rarely invasive
  - May compress adjacent structures
    - Rarely, associated hydrocephalus if aqueduct compression
- Size
  - Typically less than 3 cm
- Morphology
  - Demarcated round or lobular mass

CT Findings
- NECT
  - Iso-/hypodense mass
  - Peripheral ("exploded") Ca++
  - Cystic change may be present
- CECT
  - Enhancement present, often heterogeneous

MR Findings
- T1WI
  - Iso- to hypointense round or lobular mass
- T2WI
  - Hyperintense round or lobular mass
- FLAIR
  - Hyperintense round or lobular pineal mass
- T2* GRE
  - May see Ca++
    - Areas of "blooming" at periphery/within mass
  - May hemorrhage (less common)
- T1WI C+
  - Avid enhancement is typical
  - Enhancement may be solid or peripheral

Imaging Recommendations
- Best imaging tool
  - MR imaging most sensitive
  - CT helpful to confirm Ca++
- Protocol advice
  - Include post-contrast coronal and sagittal images

DIFFERENTIAL DIAGNOSIS

Nonneoplastic Pineal Cyst
- Round, smooth, cystic mass
- Typically < 1 cm, may be up to 2 cm
- Variable calcification and cyst fluid
- No/minimal rim enhancement
  - Compressed enhancing gland often seen posteriorly
- May be indistinguishable from PC on imaging

Pineal Parenchymal Tumor of Intermediate Differentiation (PPTID)
- Often middle-aged, older patients
- PPTIDs more aggressive appearance than PC
  - Intermediate between PC, pineoblastoma
  - WHO grade II or III

Pineoblastoma
- Younger patients
- Large, lobulated, heterogeneous
- Mass effect, parenchymal invasion, CSF spread
- May be seen in patients with retinoblastoma ("trilateral retinoblastoma")

Germinoma
- "Engulfs" calcified pineal gland
- Intensely enhancing, often homogeneous
- CSF spread often present at diagnosis
- Hyperdense on CT
- Typically young male patients

Papillary Tumor of Pineal Region
- Rare
- May be indistinguishable from PC, PPTID on imaging

Astrocytoma
- Infiltrative, T2 hyperintense mass
- Significant mass effect
- Variable enhancement

Other Germ Cell Tumors (GCT)
- Teratoma
- Choriocarcinoma, endodermal sinus (yolk sac) tumor, embryonal carcinoma, mixed GCT
- May have fat, hemorrhage, cystic change
- Lab studies may help, i.e., α-fetoprotein, hCG

Meningioma
- Avidly enhancing, homogeneous mass
- Middle-aged, older female patients

PATHOLOGY

General Features
- Etiology
  - Derived from pineal parenchymal cells ("pineocytes") or their embryonic precursors
  - Pineocytes have photosensory and neuroendocrine function
- Genetics
  - No *Tp53* mutations

- Inconsistent reports of chromosomal gains/ deletions

Staging, Grading, & Classification

- WHO grade I
- Grading system for PPTs
  - Based on mitoses, neurofilament (NF) protein staining
    - Grade 1: Classic PC with no mitoses, NF(+)
    - Grade 2: < 6 mitoses/10 high-power fields, NF(+) (PPTID)
    - Grade 3: < 6 mitoses, NF(-) or ≥ 6 mitoses, NF(+) (PPTID)
    - Grade 4: Variable mitoses ± NF (pineoblastoma)

Gross Pathologic & Surgical Features

- Well-circumscribed, gray-tan mass
  - Homogeneous or granular cut surface
- Cysts, small hemorrhagic foci may be present
- Compresses, does not invade adjacent structures
- Rarely extends into 3rd ventricle

Microscopic Features

- Well-differentiated tumor
  - Small, uniform, mature cells
    - Resemble pineocytes
  - Sheets/lobules of tumor
  - Separated by mesenchymal septae
  - Variable neuronal, ganglionic, astrocytic differentiation
- Large fibrillary "pineocytomatous rosettes" characteristic
  - Large rosettes surround a fine network of processes
- Mitoses, necrosis absent
- Immunohistochemistry
  - Synaptophysin strongly positive
  - Neuron-specific enolase (NSE) strongly positive
- Electron microscopy
  - Microtubules
  - Clear-core or dense-core vesicles
  - Synapses
- Pleomorphic subset (probably PPTID)
  - Mixed/intermediate differentiation, mitoses
  - Occasional areas of necrosis, endothelial hyperplasia

CLINICAL ISSUES

Presentation

- Most common signs/symptoms
  - Headache
  - Parinaud syndrome (paralysis of upward gaze)
- Other signs/symptoms
  - ↑ intracranial pressure, hydrocephalus
  - Ataxia
  - Mental status changes
- Clinical profile
  - Germ cell markers
    - α-fetoprotein, hCG absent

Demographics

- Age
  - May occur at any age, including children
  - Mean = 35-40 years
- Gender
  - M = F
- Epidemiology
  - < 1% of primary brain tumors
  - Pineocytoma, pineoblastomas = 15% of all pineal region neoplasms
    - Germinoma > > PPTs
  - Pineocytomas = 45% of PPTs

Natural History & Prognosis

- Stable or slow-growing tumor
- Overall 5-year survival 86%
  - 90% (grade II) to 100% (grade I) 5-year survival
- Rarely complicated by hemorrhage

Treatment

- Surgical excision or stereotactic biopsy
- CSF diversion may be necessary
- Postoperative radiation therapy is controversial
- Early reports suggest stereotactic radiosurgery may be used as primary therapy

DIAGNOSTIC CHECKLIST

Consider

- Pineocytoma may be cystic, mimic pineal cyst
- May appear aggressive, mimic pineoblastoma
- Germ cell tumors often have positive serum markers
- Clinical information often helpful to differentiate pineal region masses

Image Interpretation Pearls

- Pineocytomas have peripheral Ca++
  - Germinomas "engulf" gland Ca++
- Enhancement often solid, may be peripheral

SELECTED REFERENCES

1. Kano H et al: Role of stereotactic radiosurgery in the management of pineal parenchymal tumors. Prog Neurol Surg. 23:44-58, 2009
2. Boco T et al: Papillary tumor of the pineal region. Neuropathology. 28(1):87-92, 2008
3. Fakhran S et al: Pineocytoma mimicking a pineal cyst on imaging: true diagnostic dilemma or a case of incomplete imaging? AJNR Am J Neuroradiol. 29(1):159-63, 2008
4. Reis F et al: Neuroimaging in pineal tumors. J Neuroimaging. 16(1):52-8, 2006
5. Deshmukh VR et al: Diagnosis and management of pineocytomas. Neurosurgery. 55(2):349-55; discussion 355-7, 2004
6. Hirato J et al: Pathology of pineal region tumors. J Neurooncol. 54(3):239-49, 2001
7. Rickert CH et al: Comparative genomic hybridization in pineal parenchymal tumors. Genes Chromosomes Cancer. 30(1):99-104, 2001
8. Jouvet A et al: Pineal parenchymal tumors: a correlation of histological features with prognosis in 66 cases. Brain Pathol. 10(1):49-60, 2000
9. Nakamura M et al: Neuroradiological characteristics of pineocytoma and pineoblastoma. Neuroradiology. 42(7):509-14, 2000

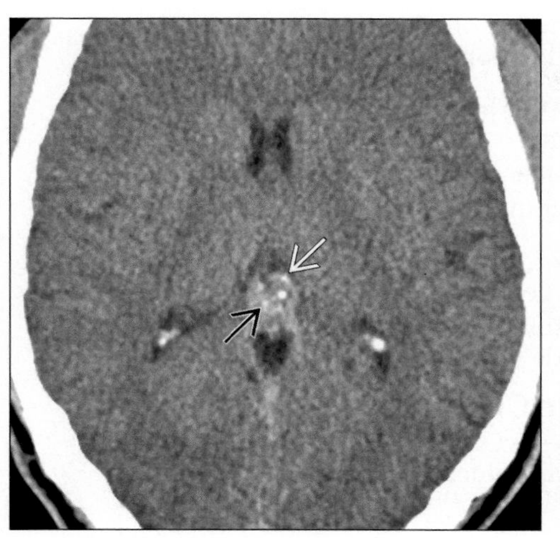

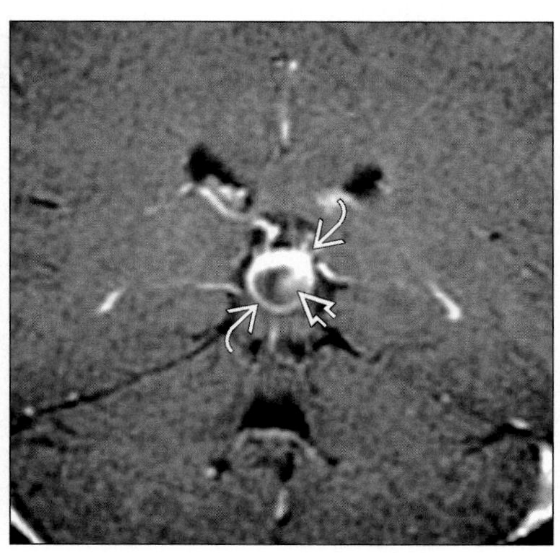

(Left) *Axial NECT shows a small, mildly hyperdense pineal tumor. In this variant case, there are a few punctate calcifications that are peripheral ➔ and central ➔. There is no hydrocephalus.* ***(Right)*** *Coronal T1WI C+ MR in a patient with pineocytoma shows both peripheral and more solid enhancement of a cystic pineal mass ➔. A small central "target" of enhancement is also present ➔.*

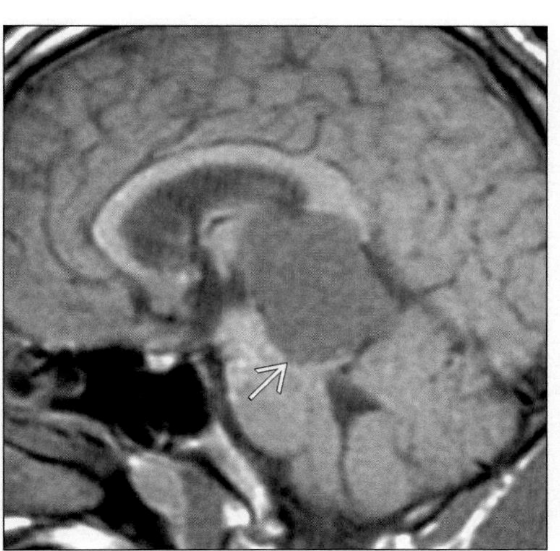

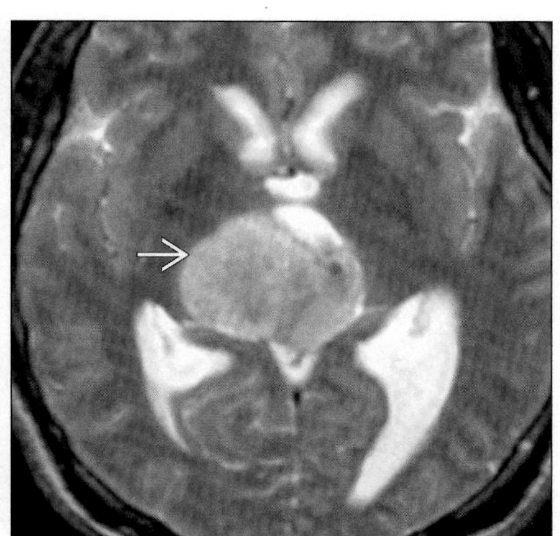

(Left) *Sagittal T1WI MR shows a variant appearance of a pineocytoma. There is a large, lobular, circumscribed tumor that causes obstructive hydrocephalus due to compression of the aqueduct of Sylvius ➔. The tumor is slightly hyperintense relative to CSF and mildly hypointense relative to the brain.* ***(Right)*** *Axial T2WI MR in the same patient shows that the tumor ➔ is hyperintense to brain. There is hydrocephalus. The tumor is more than 3 cm in diameter and extends into the 3rd ventricle.*

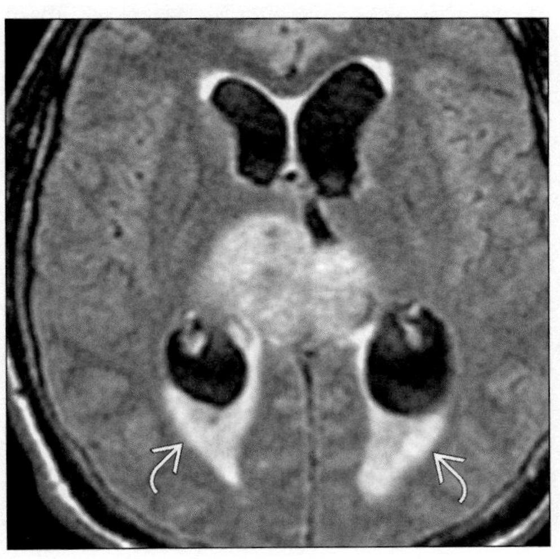

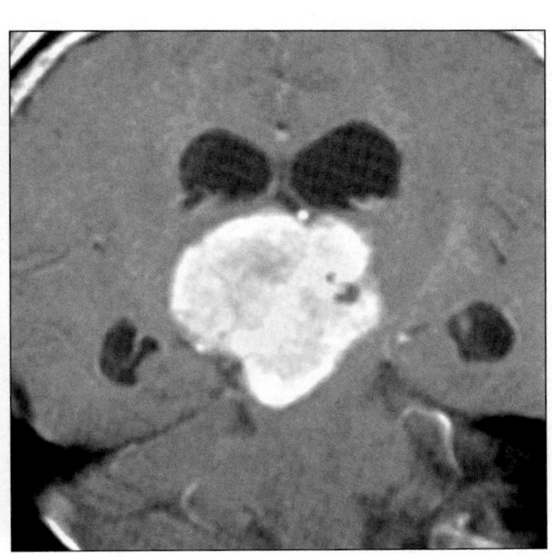

(Left) *Axial FLAIR MR in the same patient shows the tumor is hyperintense relative to brain. There is hydrocephalus with periventricular transependymal flow of CSF ➔.* ***(Right)*** *Coronal T1WI C+ MR shows avid enhancement of the tumor with mild heterogeneity. The demarcation between tumor and normal brain is well delineated. "Variant" cases of presumed pineocytoma must be distinguished from pineal parenchymal tumor of intermediate differentiation, a more aggressive tumor.*

PINEAL PARENCHYMAL TUMOR OF INTERMEDIATE DIFFERENTIATION

Key Facts

Terminology

- Primary parenchymal neoplasm of pineal gland
  - Intermediate in malignancy between pineoblastoma and pineocytoma

Imaging

- General features
  - Aggressive-looking pineal mass in adult
  - Extension into adjacent structures (ventricles, thalami) is common
  - Lobulated, moderately vascular
  - Size varies from small (< 1 cm) to huge
- CT
  - Hyperdense mass centered in pineal region
  - Engulfs pineal gland Ca++
- MR
  - Mixed iso-, hypointense on T1WI
  - Isointense with gray matter on T2WI
  - Small hyperintense cystic-appearing foci is common on T2WI
  - Hyperintense on FLAIR
  - Strong, heterogeneous enhancement

Top Differential Diagnoses

- Germinoma
- Pineocytoma
- Pineoblastoma

Pathology

- Neuroepithelial neoplasm
  - Arises from pineocytes or their precursors
- WHO grade II or III proposed

Diagnostic Checklist

- Odd/aggressive-looking pineal region tumor in middle-aged, older adult? Consider PPTID

*(**Left**) Sagittal T1WI MR in a 57-year-old woman with headaches and "visual problems" and an outside MR interpreted as germinoma. Repeat imaging shows a slightly hypointense pineal mass → that compresses and invades the tectal plate ⇨. (**Right**) Axial T2WI MR in the same patient shows an inhomogeneously iso-/mildly hyperintense pineal mass → that contains some cystic foci ⇨. The mass appears lobulated and relatively well demarcated but may focally invade the right thalamus.*

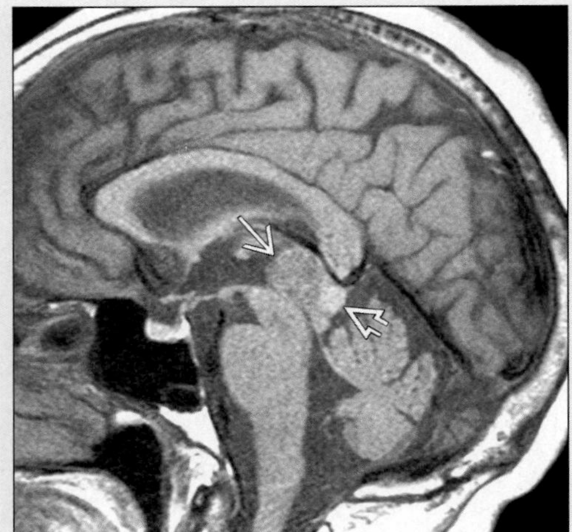

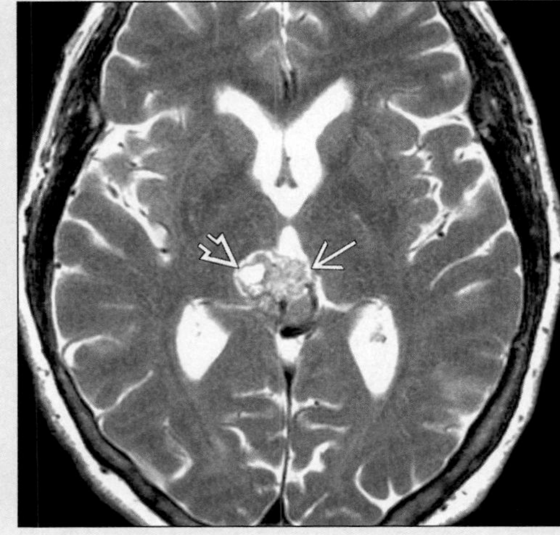

*(**Left**) Axial T1WI C+ MR in the same patient shows strong but heterogeneous enhancement. (**Right**) MRS in the same patient shows elevated choline, decreased NAA, and a lactate doublet. Imaging does not fit pineocytoma. Germinomas are rare in middle-aged females. By process of elimination, this is most likely a PPTID, although a papillary tumor of the pineal region would be a possible diagnosis. The lesion was biopsied stereotaxically and resected. PPTID was confirmed at histologic examination.*

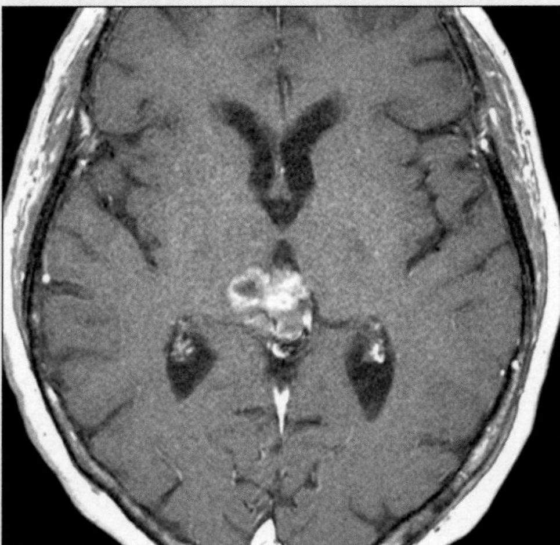

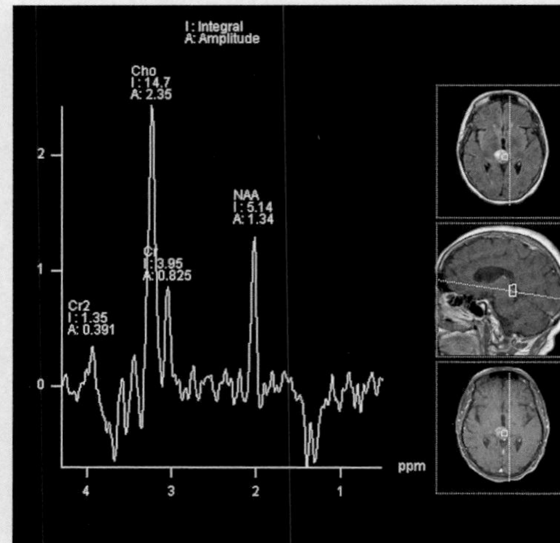

PINEAL PARENCHYMAL TUMOR OF INTERMEDIATE DIFFERENTIATION

TERMINOLOGY

Abbreviations

- Pineal parenchymal tumors (PPT)
- Pineal parenchymal tumor of intermediate differentiation (PPTID)

Synonyms

- "Atypical pineocytoma" (old)

Definitions

- Primary parenchymal neoplasm of pineal gland
  - Intermediate in malignancy between pineocytoma and pineoblastoma
    - Pineocytoma = slow-growing neoplasm with small mature cells that resemble pineocytes
      - Adults predominate
      - Well-differentiated histology with large "pineocytomatous rosettes"
      - Indolent course (imaging may remain stable for years)
      - Generally good prognosis
    - Pineoblastoma = highly malignant primitive embryonal tumor of pineal gland
      - Occurs primarily (but not exclusively) in children
      - Poorly differentiated
      - Aggressive behavior
      - Poor prognosis

IMAGING

General Features

- Best diagnostic clue
  - Aggressive-looking pineal mass in adult
- Location
  - Pineal gland
  - Extension into adjacent structures common
    - Ventricles
    - Tectum
    - Thalamus
  - CSF dissemination (rare)
- Size
  - Varies from small (< 1 cm) to huge
- Morphology
  - Lobulated, moderately vascular

CT Findings

- NECT
  - Hyperdense mass centered in pineal region
  - Engulfs pineal gland Ca++
  - Gross hemorrhage, cysts (rare)
  - Hydrocephalus (common)
- CECT
  - Strong, generally uniform enhancement

MR Findings

- T1WI
  - Mixed iso-, hypointense
- T2WI
  - Isointense with gray matter
  - Small, intratumor, hyperintense, cystic-appearing foci common
- FLAIR
  - Hyperintense
- T2* GRE
  - May show foci of "blooming"
    - Ca++ common
    - Gross hemorrhage (rare)
- T1WI C+
  - Strong, heterogeneous enhancement
- MRS
  - Elevated Cho
  - Decreased NAA
  - Variable lactate

Imaging Recommendations

- Best imaging tool
  - MR
- Protocol advice
  - Pre-, post-contrast sagittal/axial/coronal T1WI
    - T2WI, FLAIR
    - T2* (GRE, SWI)
    - DWI
    - Multivoxel MRS
  - Perform complete imaging of entire neuraxis prior to surgery to look for CSF dissemination
    - CSF spread to spine does occur but is uncommon

DIFFERENTIAL DIAGNOSIS

Germinoma

- Most common pineal neoplasm
- 80-90% of patients < 25 years old
  - Rare in middle-aged, older adults
- M > > F
- Engulfs pineal gland Ca++
- Intraventricular, distant CSF spread is common

Pineocytoma

- Most common pineal parenchymal neoplasm
- Generally tumor of adults (mean = 35-40 years)
- "Explodes" pineal gland Ca++
- Solid or partially solid and cystic
- Solid portion enhances strongly, mostly uniformly
- CSF spread is very rare

Pineoblastoma

- Most common in children but can occur at any age
- M = F
- May require biopsy to distinguish from large PPTID
- CSF spread common, early

Papillary Tumor of Pineal Region (PTPR)

- Rare neuroepithelial tumor with papillary architecture
- All ages except very young children reported
- Indistinguishable on imaging, gross pathology from PPTID, pineocytoma

Metastases

- Metastases to pineal gland is rare
- Solitary metastasis is even less common
- Usually known primary neoplasm elsewhere

PINEAL PARENCHYMAL TUMOR OF INTERMEDIATE DIFFERENTIATION

PATHOLOGY

General Features

- Etiology
  - Neuroepithelial neoplasm
    - Probably arises from pineocytes or their precursors
  - Many reported chromosomal abnormalities but none consistent
    - Pineoblastomas may occur in patients with *RB1* mutation
    - PPTID chromosomal imbalances common but variable
  - No known familial predilection
    - Pineoblastomas occur in bi-, trilateral retinoblastoma syndrome
- Historical background
  - PPTID not generally recognized as distinct entity until 2007
  - Neoplasms diagnosed as "pineocytoma vs. pineoblastoma" or "atypical pineocytoma" prior to 2007 may be PPTIDs

Staging, Grading, & Classification

- Definitive WHO not established
- WHO grade II or III proposed

Gross Pathologic & Surgical Features

- Circumscribed, soft tumor without gross hemorrhage or necrosis
- Focal invasion of adjacent structures may be present

Microscopic Features

- Diffuse sheets of relatively uniform small cells
- Moderate to high cellularity
- Mild to moderate nuclear atypia
- Wide range of reported mitotic activity
  - Generally low to moderate
  - MIB-1 index usually in 1-5% range
  - Some reports of PPTID dedifferentiation to pineoblastoma
    - MIB-1 markedly elevated
    - Tumor dissemination
- GFAP(+)
- Immunohistochemistry helpful
  - Neuronal markers positive
    - Synaptophysin strongly positive
    - Variable neurofilament protein, chromogranin, β-tubulin positivity
    - Diffuse staining for neuron-specific enolase (NSE)

CLINICAL ISSUES

Presentation

- Most common signs/symptoms
  - Diplopia
  - Parinaud syndrome
- Other signs/symptoms
  - Signs of elevated intracranial pressure
  - Ataxia

Demographics

- Pineal region tumors uncommon as a group
  - 1% of all intracranial neoplasms
- Histologically heterogeneous
  - Germinomas > > pineal parenchymal neoplasms
  - PPTIDs probably represent at least 20% of pineal parenchymal tumors

Natural History & Prognosis

- Limited number of reported cases
- Still being defined
- Highly variable behavior
  - Local recurrence is common
  - Dissemination rare
- Survival even with subtotal resection is common
  - May be years
  - Slowly progressive
  - Clinical course can be relatively benign despite histologic pleomorphism

Treatment

- Stereotaxic biopsy, surgical resection
- Role of chemo-, radiation therapy unknown

DIAGNOSTIC CHECKLIST

Consider

- Aggressive-looking pineal region tumor in middle-aged, older adult? Consider PPTID
- Patient with long history of atypical-appearing "pineocytoma"? Consider PPTID
- Review histopathology of atypical pineal region tumors diagnosed prior to 2007

Image Interpretation Pearls

- Odd-looking pineal region mass in adult? May be a PPTID!

Reporting Tips

- Ask for review of histopathology in patients with follow-up imaging and history of "atypical" pineocytoma

SELECTED REFERENCES

1. Kim BS et al: Pineal parenchymal tumor of intermediate differentiation showing malignant progression at relapse. Neuropathology. Epub ahead of print, 2009
2. Sato K et al: Pathology of pineal parenchymal tumors. Prog Neurol Surg. 23:12-25, 2009
3. Fèvre-Montange M et al: Pineocytoma and pineal parenchymal tumors of intermediate differentiation presenting cytologic pleomorphism: a multicenter study. Brain Pathol. 18(3):354-9, 2008
4. Rousseau A et al: The 2007 WHO classification of tumors of the central nervous system - what has changed? Curr Opin Neurol. 21(6):720-7, 2008
5. Senft C et al: Pineal parenchymal tumor of intermediate differentiation: diagnostic pitfalls and discussion of treatment options of a rare tumor entity. Neurosurg Rev. 31(2):231-6, 2008
6. Nakazato Y et al: Pineal parenchymal tumour of intermediate differentiation. In DN Louis et al: WHO Classification of Tumours of the Central Nervous System. Lyon: IARC Press. 124-5, 2007

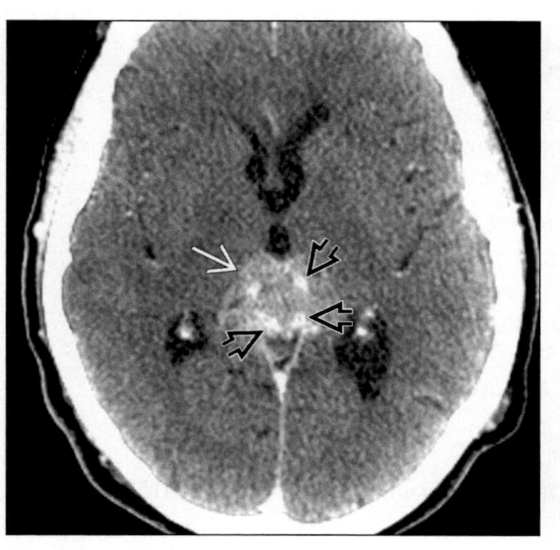

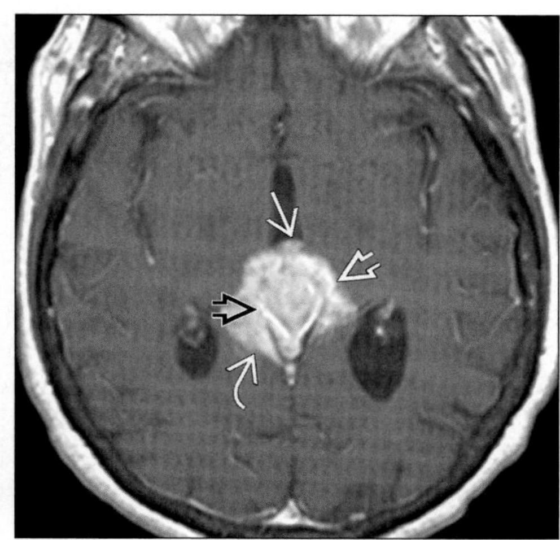

(Left) *Axial CECT shows classic "exploded" calcifications ➡. characteristic of PPTs. The strongly enhancing mass ➡ extends into the posterior 3rd ventricle.* ***(Right)*** *Axial T1WI C+ MR in the same patient shows the strongly enhancing lobulated mass extending into the 3rd ventricle ➡, thalami ➡, and forceps major of the corpus callosum ➡. Note splaying apart of the internal cerebral veins ➡. Other scans (not shown) disclosed tumor spread into the 4th ventricle and spinal canal. This proved to be PPTID.*

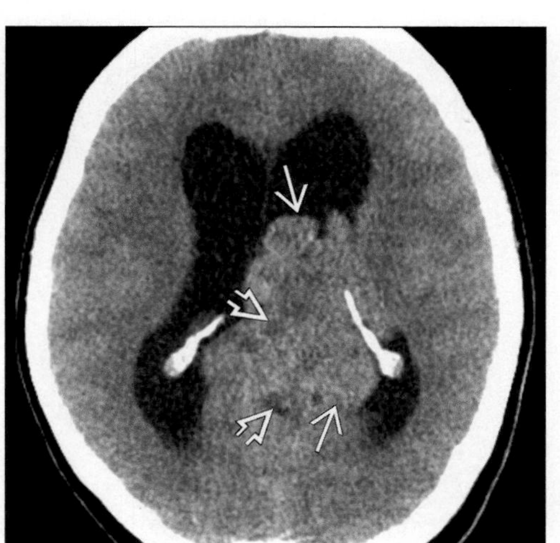

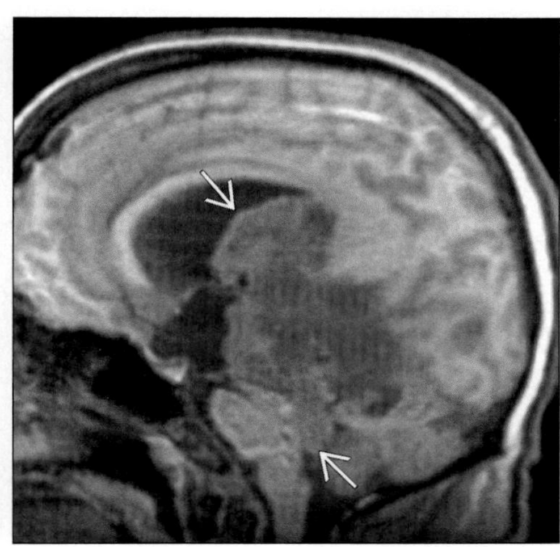

(Left) *Axial NECT in a 50-year-old woman with progressive headaches & incontinence shows a large, bulky, lobulated, midline mass ➡ with some small focal hypodensities that suggest cysts ➡. The precise origin of the mass (i.e., ventricles vs. pineal gland vs. corpus callosum) is difficult to determine on this study, so MR was obtained.* ***(Right)*** *Sagittal T1WI MR in the same patient shows a huge hypointense mass extending into the ventricles & posterior fossa ➡. The epicenter of the mass is the pineal gland.*

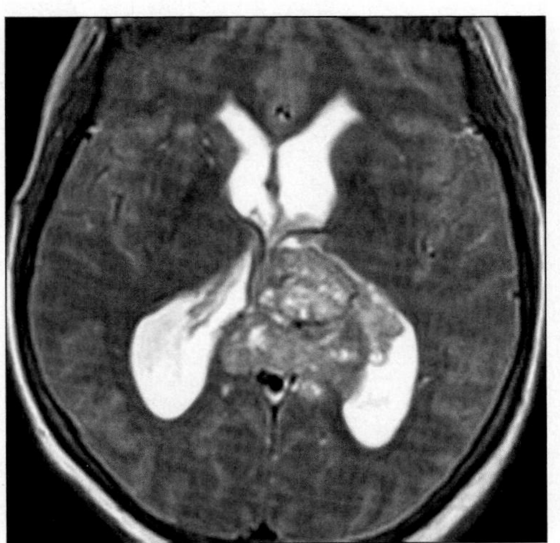

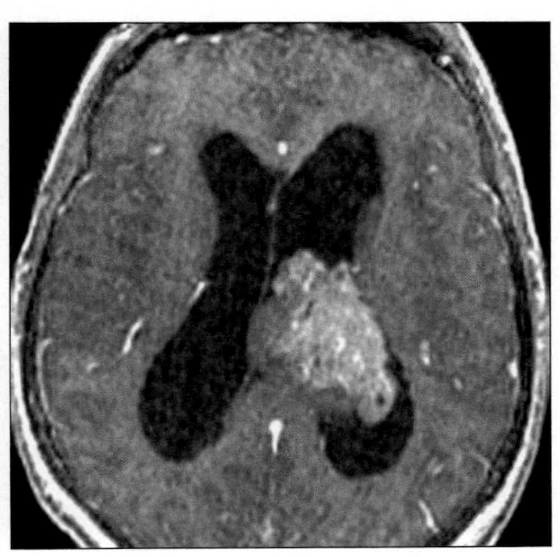

(Left) *Axial T2WI MR in the same patient shows that the mass is mostly iso- to mildly hyperintense compared to the adjacent white matter. Numerous small hyperintense cysts are present within the tumor. Moderate obstructive hydrocephalus is present.* ***(Right)*** *Contrast-enhanced T1 study shows strong but heterogeneous enhancement. The mass was biopsied and subtotally resected. PPTID was found at histologic examination.*

PINEOBLASTOMA

Key Facts

Terminology

- Pineoblastoma (PB)
  - Highly malignant, primitive embryonal tumor (PNET)

Imaging

- General features
  - Large, heterogeneous pineal mass
  - Lobulated with poorly delineated margins
  - Nearly 100% have obstructive hydrocephalus
- Frequent invasion into adjacent brain
  - Corpus callosum, thalamus, midbrain, vermis
- Solid portion frequently
  - Hyperdense with peripheral Ca++
  - Iso- to hypointense on T2WI compared to cortex
  - Often shows restricted diffusion
  - Variable heterogeneous enhancement
- Image entire neuraxis preoperatively!
  - 15-45% CSF dissemination on MR or CSF

Pathology

- WHO grade IV
- Derived from embryonic precursors of pineal parenchymal cells ("pinealocytes")
- Common phylogenetic origin of retina and pineal gland as light-sensing organs

Clinical Issues

- ↑ intracranial pressure (hydrocephalus)
  - Headache, nausea, vomiting, lethargy
  - Papilledema, abducens nerve palsy
- Parinaud syndrome, ataxia
- Mean age at diagnosis in children = 3 years
- M:F = 1:2
- Treatment
  - Resection plus cranial/spinal XRT, chemotherapy

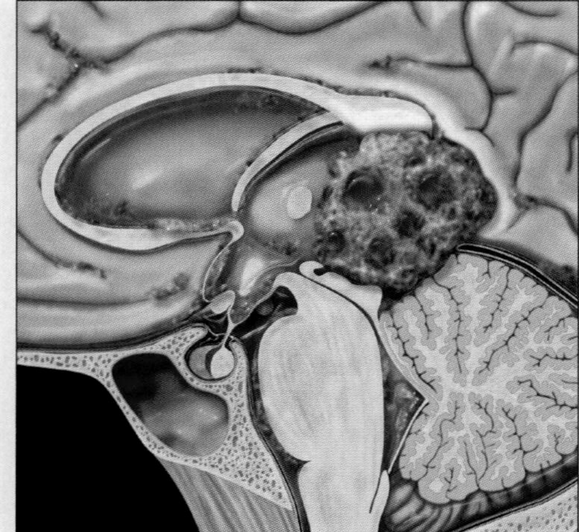

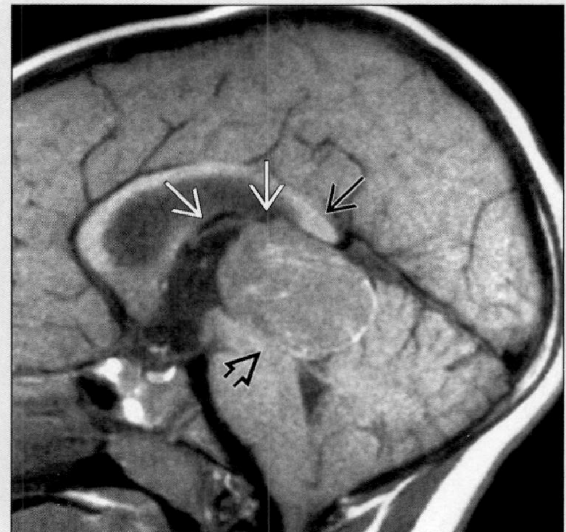

(Left) *Sagittal graphic shows a large, heterogeneous pineal mass with areas of hemorrhage and necrosis. Note the compression of adjacent structures, hydrocephalus, and diffuse CSF seeding, which is typical of pineoblastoma.* ***(Right)*** *Sagittal T1WI MR of a pineal region retinoblastoma shows the classic findings indicative of a pineal region mass, including its position underneath the splenium →, elevation of the internal cerebral veins ➡, and compression of the tectal plate ⇨. There is hydrocephalus.*

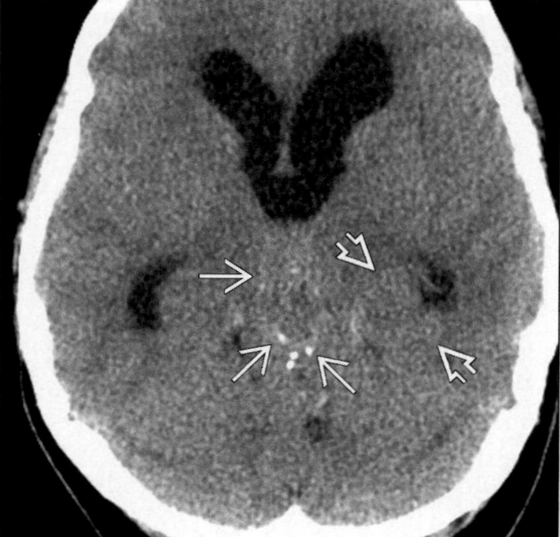

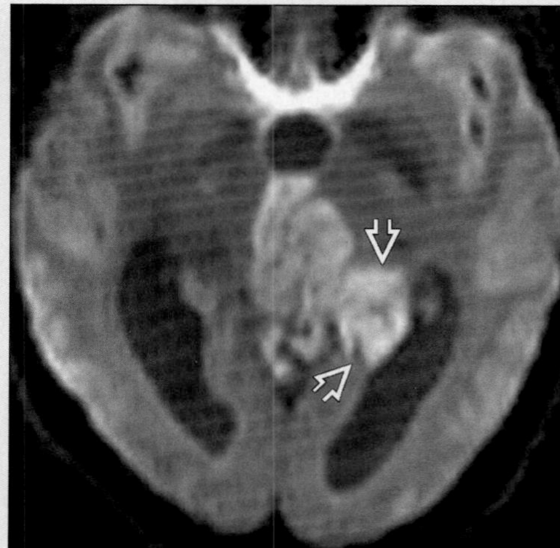

(Left) *Axial NECT shows a poorly demarcated, infiltrative, mildly hyperdense mass centered in the pineal region. Classic peripheral calcifications are present →. On close evaluation there is invasion of the adjacent brain parenchyma ⇨. There is compression of the aqueduct of Sylvius and resultant hydrocephalus.* ***(Right)*** *Axial DWI MR shows restricted diffusion in the solid mass and better delineates the neoplasm and the invasion of the adjacent brain parenchyma ⇨.*

PINEOBLASTOMA

TERMINOLOGY

Abbreviations

- Pinealoblastoma (PB)

Synonyms

- Primitive neuroectodermal tumor (PNET) of pineal gland

Definitions

- Highly malignant primitive embryonal tumor of pineal gland

IMAGING

General Features

- Best diagnostic clue
  - Child with large, heterogeneous pineal mass with peripheral Ca++
    - Pineal region masses elevate internal cerebral veins
    - Lie below splenium
  - Solid portion hyperdense on CT, iso-/hypointense on T2WI compared to cortex
- Location
  - Pineal region
  - Frequent invasion of adjacent brain
    - Corpus callosum, thalamus, midbrain, vermis
- Size
  - Large (most ≥ 3 cm)
- Morphology
  - Irregular, lobulated mass with poorly delineated margins

CT Findings

- NECT
  - Mixed density; solid portion frequently hyperdense
  - Ca++ classic
  - Nearly 100% have obstructive hydrocephalus
- CECT
  - Weak to avid but heterogeneous enhancement

MR Findings

- T1WI
  - Heterogeneous; solid portion iso-/hypointense
- T2WI
  - Heterogeneous
    - Solid portion iso-/hypointense > minimally hyperintense to cortex
    - Frequent necrosis/hemorrhage
  - Mild peritumoral edema characteristic
- T2* GRE
  - Ca++ and hemorrhage may "bloom"
- DWI
  - Solid portion frequently restricts
- T1WI C+
  - Heterogeneous enhancement
- MRS
  - ↑ Cho, ↓ NAA
  - Prominent glutamate and taurine peak (~ 3.4 ppm) described at TE 20 msec

Angiographic Findings

- Conventional

Nuclear Medicine Findings

- PET
  - Increased 18F-FDG

Other Modality Findings

- No elevation of serum tumor markers

Imaging Recommendations

- Best imaging tool
  - MR with T1WI C+
- Protocol advice
  - Image entire neuraxis preoperatively
    - 15-45% present with CSF dissemination!
  - Sagittal images ideal for pineal region anatomy

DIFFERENTIAL DIAGNOSIS

Germ Cell Tumors (GCTs)

- 1% of CNS tumors in Western population; 4% of CNS tumors in Asia
- M > F; 2nd decade most common
- Germinoma
- Mature teratoma
  - 2nd most common GCT and pineal region tumor
  - Heterogeneous, multicystic mass with foci of Ca++ and fat
- Choriocarcinoma, endodermal sinus tumor, embryonal cell carcinoma
  - Uncommon, highly malignant
  - Characteristic elevation of serum tumor markers
    - Choriocarcinoma: β-hCG
    - Endodermal sinus tumor: α-fetoprotein (AFP)
    - Embryonal cell carcinoma: β-hCG and AFP
- 10% of GCTs are mixed histology (mixed GCT)

Astrocytoma

- Rarely arise from pineal gland
- More commonly from thalamus or midbrain tectum
- Pilocytic astrocytoma (WHO grade I) most common
- Tectal astrocytoma
  - Nonenhancing, well-defined, expansile tectal mass
- Thalamic astrocytoma
  - T2 hyperintense, paramedian mass or cyst with enhancing mural nodule

Meningioma

- Females (5th-7th decades)
- Well-defined, round, dural-based mass isointense to cortex on all sequences with intense, homogeneous enhancement
- Pineal region meningiomas arises from tentorium cerebelli, falx
- Dural "tail" (35-80%)

Pineocytoma (PC)

- Differentiated tumor arising from pineal gland parenchymal cell
- Older age group compared to pineoblastomas
- Well-defined, round, homogeneous mass with uniform homogeneous enhancement

Metastases

- Pineal gland metastases uncommon
- Adenocarcinoma reported

PATHOLOGY

General Features

- Etiology
  - Derived from embryonic precursors of pineal parenchymal cells ("pinealocytes")
  - Pinealocytes have photosensory and neuroendocrine function
  - Common phylogenetic origin of retina and pineal gland as light-sensing organs
- Genetics
  - No *Tp53* mutations
  - Some reports of chromosome 11 deletions
  - "Trilateral retinoblastoma" has bilateral retinoblastomas, pineal PNET-like pineoblastoma

Staging, Grading, & Classification

- WHO grade IV
- New prognostic grading system for PPTs
  - Grade 1 = pineocytoma
  - Grade 2 and 3 = PPTs with intermediate differentiation
    - Grade 2 if < 6 mitoses and (+) immunolabeling for neurofilaments
    - Grade 3 if ≥ 6 mitoses or < 6 mitoses but (-) immunolabeling for neurofilaments
  - Grade 4 = pineoblastoma

Gross Pathologic & Surgical Features

- Soft, friable, poorly marginated, infiltrative
- Compresses/invades cerebral aqueduct leading to hydrocephalus
- CSF dissemination at autopsy frequent

Microscopic Features

- Highly cellular tumor
  - Sheets of packed, small undifferentiated cells
  - Carrot-shaped hyperchromatic nuclei, scant cytoplasm
    - High nuclear cytoplasmic ratio in solid portion accounts for hyperdensity on CT and hypointensity on MR
  - Occasional Homer-Wright or Flexner-Wintersteiner rosettes
  - Variable (+) immunolabeling for synaptophysin, neuronal specific enolase, neurofilaments, and chromogranin A , but < than PCs, mixed PB/PCs
  - Necrosis and hemorrhage common
  - Mitoses common, MIB-1 elevated

CLINICAL ISSUES

Presentation

- Most common signs/symptoms
  - ↑ intracranial pressure (hydrocephalus)
    - Headache, nausea, vomiting, lethargy
    - Papilledema, abducens nerve palsy
- Other signs/symptoms
  - Parinaud syndrome, ataxia
- Clinical profile
  - Toddler with Parinaud syndrome, signs/symptoms of ↑ intracranial pressure

Demographics

- Age
  - Children > young adults
  - Mean age at diagnosis in children = 3 years
- Gender
  - M:F = 1:2
- Epidemiology
  - PPTs comprise 0.5-1% of primary brain tumors and 15% of pineal region neoplasms
  - PBs comprise 30-45% of PPTs

Natural History & Prognosis

- CSF seeding common
  - Up to 45% of patients present with spinal dissemination on MR &/or CSF analysis
- Rare reports of hematogenous metastases to bone
- Dismal; median survival 16-25 months from presentation

Treatment

- Surgical resection plus cranial/spinal radiation and chemotherapy

DIAGNOSTIC CHECKLIST

Consider

- Could pineal region mass be GCT? (more common than PPTs)
  - Does patient have elevated serum tumor markers?
  - Is patient male?
  - Is there a coexistent suprasellar mass (germinoma)?

Image Interpretation Pearls

- Both PBs and germinomas frequently hyperdense on CT (hypointense on T2WI) and prone to CSF dissemination
- Peripheral "exploded" Ca++ in PB and central "engulfed" Ca++ in classic germinoma but not always identified

Clinical Pearl

- Pineal region astrocytomas typically do not present with Parinaud syndrome

SELECTED REFERENCES

1. Papaioannou G et al: Imaging of the unusual pediatric 'blastomas'. Cancer Imaging. 9:1-11, 2009
2. Gasparetto EL et al: Diffusion-weighted MR images and pineoblastoma: diagnosis and follow-up. Arq Neuropsiquiatr. 66(1):64-8, 2008
3. Senft C et al: Pineal parenchymal tumor of intermediate differentiation: diagnostic pitfalls and discussion of treatment options of a rare tumor entity. Neurosurg Rev. 31(2):231-6, 2008
4. Cuccia V et al: Pinealoblastomas in children. Childs Nerv Syst. 22(6):577-85, 2006
5. Korogi Y et al: MRI of pineal region tumors. J Neurooncol. 54(3): 251-61, 2001

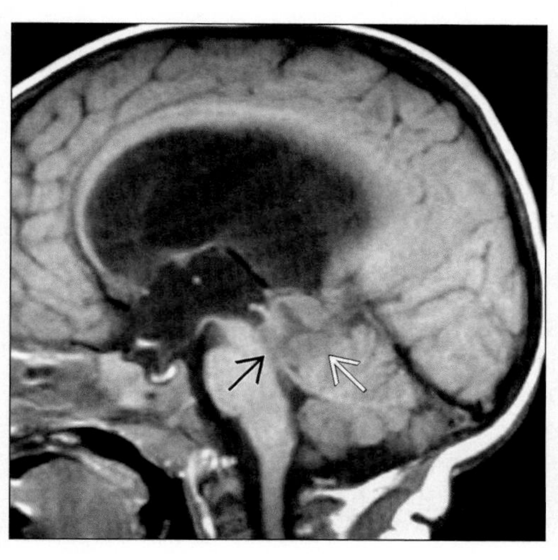

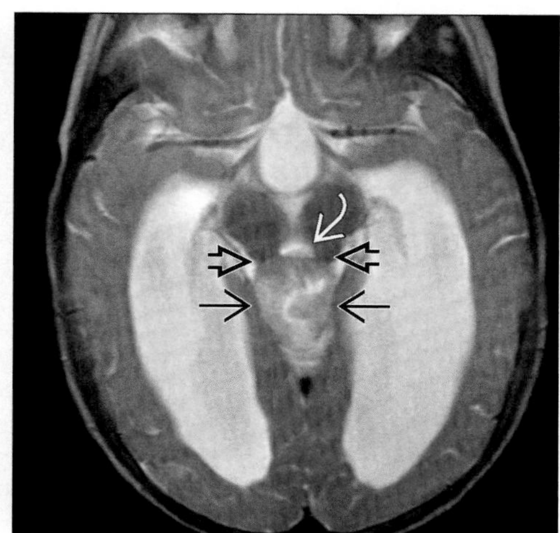

(Left) *Sagittal T1WI MR shows a heterogeneous pineal region tumor →. There is compression and invasion of the distal aqueduct →, resulting in massive hydrocephalus.* ***(Right)*** *Axial T2WI MR in the same patient shows the heterogeneous mass → with mild central necrosis and solid tumor peripherally that is isointense to brain. There is compression of the tectum and posterior midbrain shown here →, as well as dilatation of the proximal aqueduct → with massive hydrocephalus.*

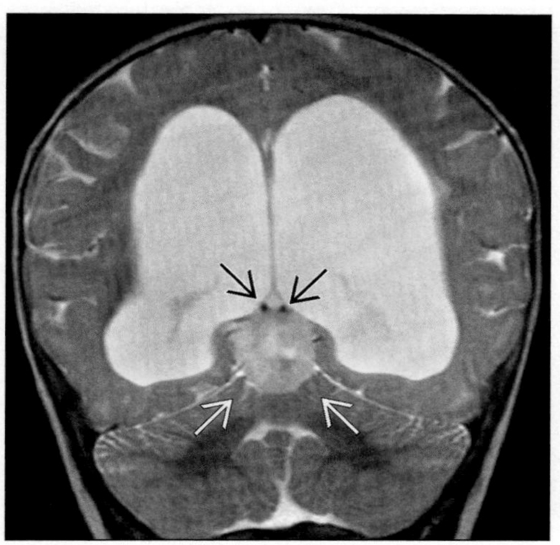

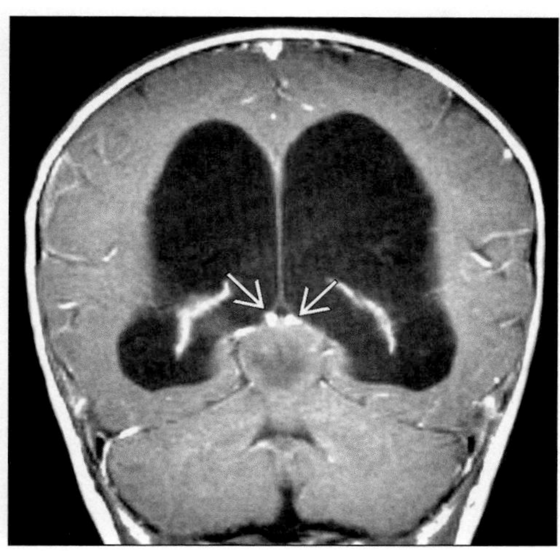

(Left) *Coronal T2WI MR again shows the demarcated solid mass in the pineal region with mild central necrosis. Note the compression of the cerebellar vermis → and elevation of the bilateral internal cerebral veins →.* ***(Right)*** *Coronal T1WI C+ MR shows solid peripheral enhancement of the tumor, hydrocephalus, and elevation of the internal cerebral veins →.*

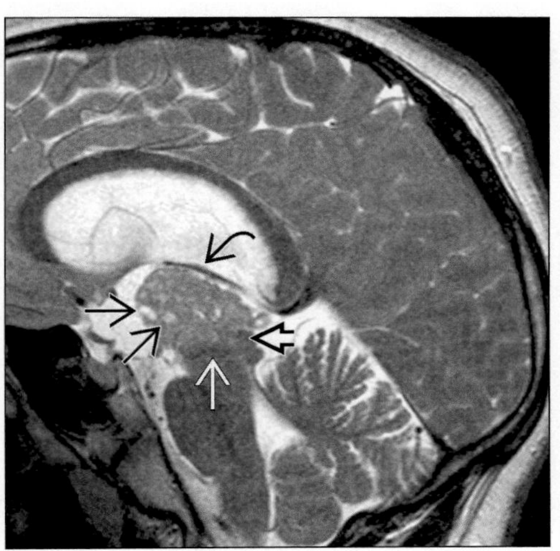

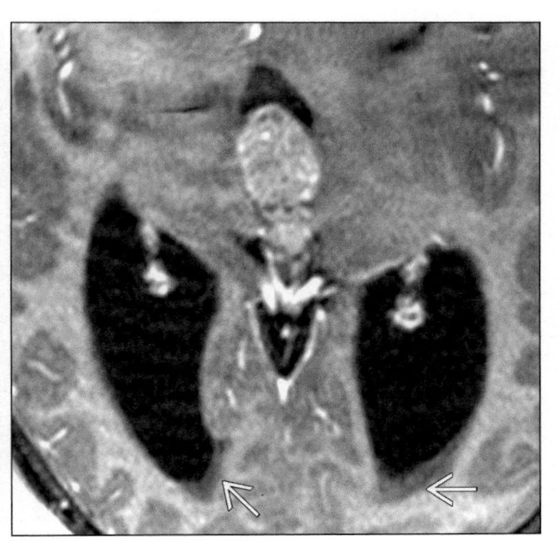

(Left) *Sagittal T2WI MR shows a solid mass isointense to cortex with small areas of cystic change/necrosis →. Note the compression of midbrain →, superior tectum →, & aqueduct with hydrocephalus. The mass fills the posterior 3rd ventricle, & tumor is below internal cerebral veins →.* ***(Right)*** *Axial T1WI C+ MR in the same patient shows avid enhancement with tiny regions of cystic change/necrosis. The tumor fills 3rd ventricle. Note hydrocephalus and mild transependymal flow of CSF →.*

PAPILLARY TUMOR OF THE PINEAL REGION

Key Facts

Terminology
- Papillary tumor of pineal region (PTPR)

Imaging
- Enhancing pineal mass
- Well circumscribed
- Cystic regions common

Top Differential Diagnoses
- Pineocytoma
  - Arises from pineal gland
  - "Explodes" pineal gland Ca++
- Pineal parenchymal tumor of intermediate differentiation (PPTID)
  - Imaging can be indistinguishable
  - Histologic diagnosis
- Germinoma
  - Adolescent males > middle-aged, older adults
- Teratoma
  - Suppresses with FS sequences

Pathology
- May derive from specialized ependymocytes of subcommissural organ
- WHO grade II-III
- Epithelial tumor
  - Papillary regions with large cuboidal/columnar cells
  - Cytokeratin(+), EMA(-)

Clinical Issues
- Nonspecific headache
- Reported in ages 5-66 but primarily tumor of adults
- > 5 mitoses per 10 high-power fields correlates with decreased survival and increased likelihood of recurrence

*(**Left**) Axial T2WI in a 66-year-old man with headaches shows a small irregular mass in the pineal region ➔ that displays complex mixed signal intensity. The mass is mostly inhomogeneously isointense with the brain but contains a small, more focal, cystic-like area ➔. Note hydrocephalus with transependymal CSF flow, seen here as "blurred" ventricular margins ➔. (Courtesy AFIP.) (**Right**) FLAIR image in the same patient confirms the mass ➔ is inhomogeneously hyperintense. (Courtesy AFIP.)*

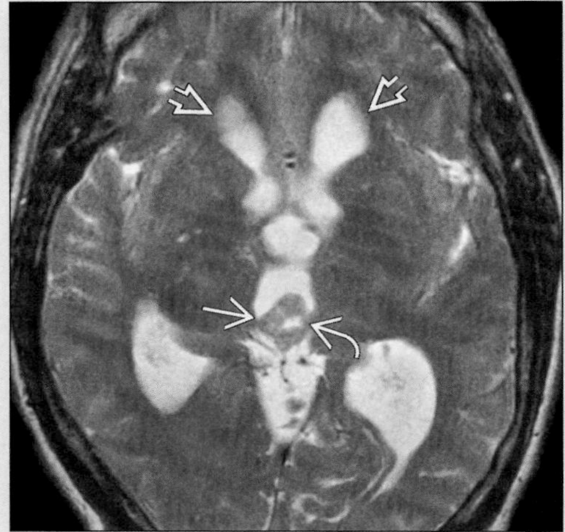

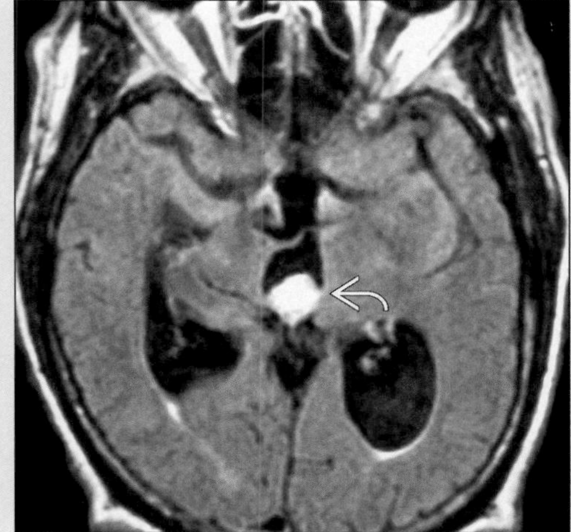

*(**Left**) Sagittal T1WI C+ MR in the same patient shows the small, slightly irregular pineal region mass ➔ enhances somewhat heterogeneously. The mass arises separately from both the tectum and the tegmentum of the midbrain and obstructs the superior meatus of the aqueduct of Sylvius, causing moderate hydrocephalus. (Courtesy AFIP.) (**Right**) In the same patient, axial T1WI C+ MR shows the pineal region mass ➔ enhances diffusely but somewhat heterogeneously. (Courtesy AFIP.)*

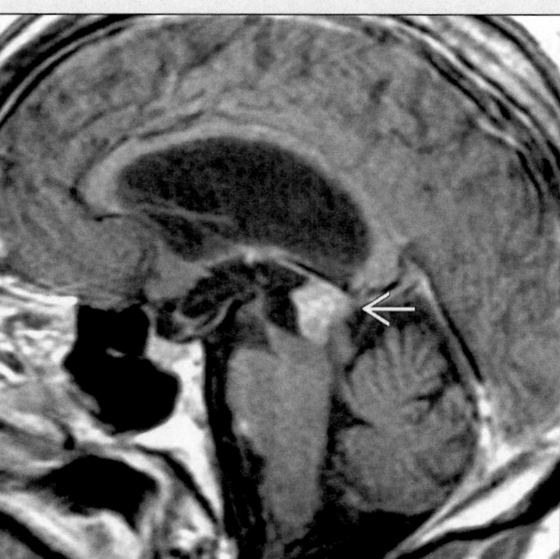

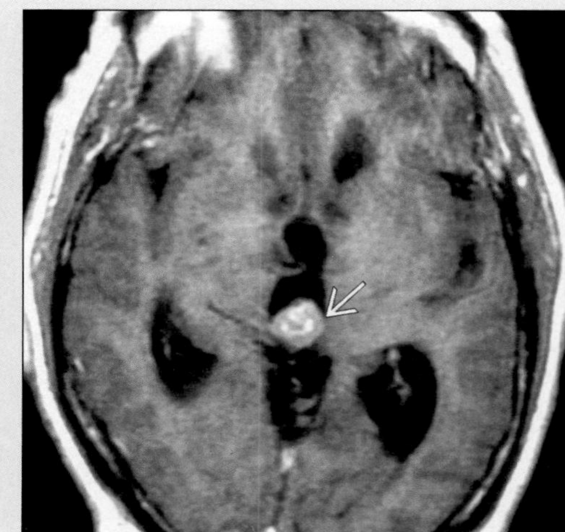

PAPILLARY TUMOR OF THE PINEAL REGION

TERMINOLOGY

Abbreviations

- Papillary tumor of pineal region (PTPR)

IMAGING

General Features

- Best diagnostic clue
  - Enhancing pineal mass in adult
- Size
  - Varies; usually moderate
- Morphology
  - Well circumscribed, ± cystic regions

Imaging Recommendations

- Best imaging tool
  - MR ± gadolinium
- Protocol advice
  - Pre-, post-contrast thin section sagittal T1WIs

MR Findings

- T1WI
  - Variable but can be heterogeneously hyperintense
- T2WI
  - Heterogeneously iso-/hyperintense
- FLAIR
  - Hyperintense
- T1WI C+
  - Moderate heterogeneous enhancement

DIFFERENTIAL DIAGNOSIS

Pineocytoma

- Arises from pineal gland; "explodes" pineal gland Ca++

Pineal Parenchymal Tumor of Intermediate Differentiation

- Can be indistinguishable
- Histologic diagnosis

Germinoma

- Adolescent males > middle-aged adults

Teratoma

- Suppresses with FS sequences

PATHOLOGY

General Features

- Etiology
  - May derive from specialized ependymocytes of subcommissural organ
  - May be related to ependymal cells in pineal recess
- Genetics
  - Most show losses on chromosomes 10 and 22q
  - Gains on chromosomes 4, 8, 9, and 12
- Associated abnormalities
  - No other anomalies or syndromal associations

Staging, Grading, & Classification

- WHO grade II-III

Gross Pathologic & Surgical Features

- Moderate to large well-circumscribed mass

Microscopic Features

- Epithelial tumor with characteristic papillary regions with large cuboidal or columnar cells or, less commonly, smaller cells
- Some ependymal-type rosettes and tubular regions as well as perivascular pseudorosettes
- Immunohistochemistry
  - Strongly positive for cytokeratin, S100, NSE, vimentin
  - Weak or nonreactive to GFAP
- Occasional areas of necrosis, variable mitotic figures

CLINICAL ISSUES

Presentation

- Most common signs/symptoms
  - Nonspecific CNS symptoms, headache

Demographics

- Age
  - Reported in ages 5-66 but primarily tumor of adults

Natural History & Prognosis

- Variable: 5-year survival (73%); progression free (27%)
- > 5 mitoses per 10 high-power fields correlates with decreased survival and increased likelihood of recurrence

Treatment

- Complete resection affords highest chance of cure

SELECTED REFERENCES

1. Cerase A et al: Neuroradiological follow-up of the growth of papillary tumor of the pineal region: a case report. J Neurooncol. Epub ahead of print, 2009
2. Sato TS et al: Papillary tumor of the pineal region: report of a rapidly progressive tumor with possible multicentric origin. Pediatr Radiol. 39(2):188-90, 2009
3. Boco T et al: Papillary tumor of the pineal region. Neuropathology. 28(1):87-92, 2008
4. Chang AH et al: MR imaging of papillary tumor of the pineal region. AJNR Am J Neuroradiol. 29(1):187-9, 2008
5. Fèvre-Montange M et al: Bcl-2 expression in a papillary tumor of the pineal region. Neuropathology. 28(6):660-3, 2008
6. Inoue T et al: Papillary tumor of the pineal region: a case report. Brain Tumor Pathol. 25(2):85-90, 2008
7. Lehman NL: Central nervous system tumors with ependymal features: a broadened spectrum of primarily ependymal differentiation? J Neuropathol Exp Neurol. 67(3):177-88, 2008
8. Louis DN et al: The 2007 WHO classification of tumours of the central nervous system. Acta Neuropathol. 2007 Aug;114(2):97-109. Epub 2007 Jul 6. Review. Erratum in: Acta Neuropathol. 114(5):547, 2007
9. Roncaroli F et al: Papillary tumor of the pineal region and spindle cell oncocytoma of the pituitary: new tumor entities in the 2007 WHO Classification. Brain Pathol. 17(3):314-8, 2007

MEDULLOBLASTOMA

Key Facts

Terminology
- Medulloblastoma (MB), posterior fossa PNET
- Malignant highly cellular embryonal tumor

Imaging
- 4th ventricle tumor
  - Arises from roof (superior medullary velum)
  - Lateral origin (cerebellar hemisphere) more common in older children/adults
- Spherical, pushes brain away on all sides
- 90% hyperdense on NECT
- Small intratumoral cysts/necrosis in 40-50%
- Hydrocephalus common (95%)
- > 90% enhance
- Restricted diffusion, low ADC
- Up to 1/3 have subarachnoid metastatic disease at presentation

Top Differential Diagnoses
- Cerebellar pilocytic astrocytoma (PA)
- Ependymoma
- Choroid plexus papilloma (CPP)
- Atypical teratoid/rhabdoid tumor (AT/RT)

Pathology
- WHO grade IV

Clinical Issues
- 30-40% of childhood posterior fossa tumors
- Rare in adults
- Rapid growth, early subarachnoid spread
- Children < 3 years of age have inferior survival

Diagnostic Checklist
- Thinking of MB in childhood posterior fossa tumor? Include AT/RT!

(Left) Axial graphic shows a spherical tumor centered in the 4th ventricle, typical of medulloblastoma. (Right) Axial FLAIR MR shows an inhomogeneous, high signal intensity mass with well-defined borders in the region of the 4th ventricle ➔. Note the multiple intratumoral cysts ➔. Classic medulloblastoma was found at surgery.

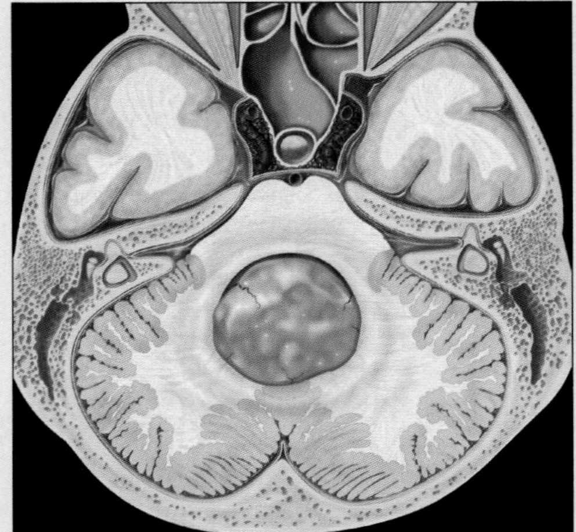

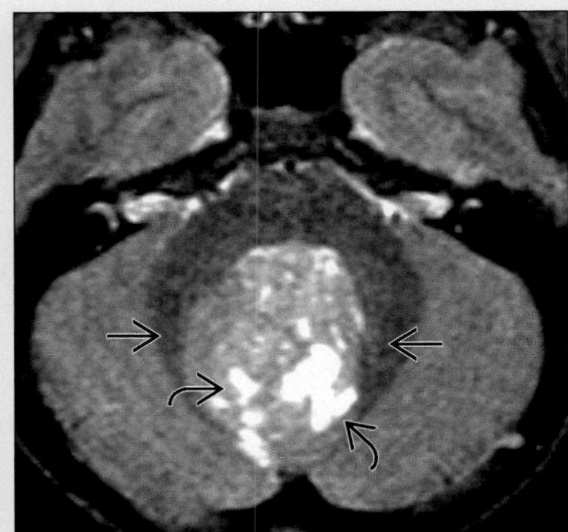

(Left) Axial T2WI MR demonstrates a large, inhomogeneously hyperintense mass in the posterior fossa ➔ (originating from the 4th ventricle) with extension to the right CPA and internal auditory canal ➔. The mass has multiple cystic foci. (Right) Axial T1WI C+ MR shows subtle enhancement of this large medulloblastoma.

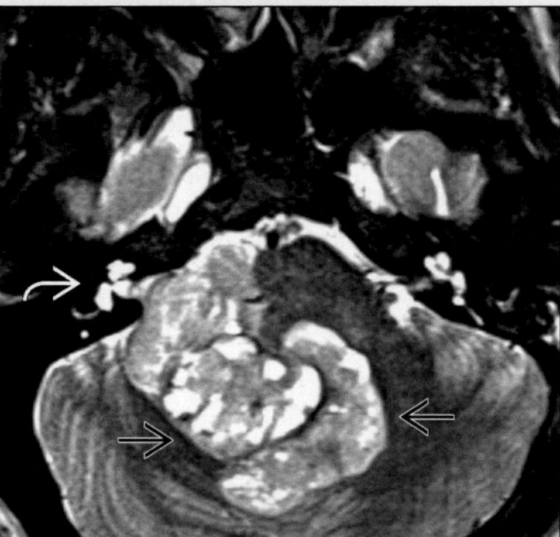

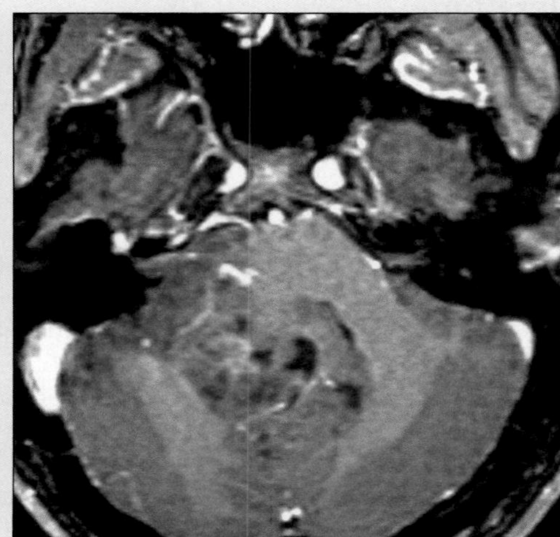

MEDULLOBLASTOMA

TERMINOLOGY

Abbreviations
- Medulloblastoma (MB)
- Medulloblastoma with extensive nodularity (MBEN)

Synonyms
- Posterior fossa PNET, PNET-MB

Definitions
- Malignant, invasive, highly cellular embryonal tumor

IMAGING

General Features
- Best diagnostic clue
  - Round, dense 4th ventricle mass
- Location
  - 4th ventricle tumor
    - Arises from roof (superior medullary velum)
    - Distinguished from ependymoma which arises from floor of 4th ventricle
  - Lateral origin (cerebellar hemisphere) more common in older children/adults (50-89%)
  - May grow into CPA
- Size
  - 1-3 cm
- Morphology
  - Spherical, pushes brain away on all sides

Radiographic Findings
- Radiography
  - Hyperdense bone metastases may occur late in disease course (rare)

CT Findings
- NECT
  - Solid mass in 4th ventricle
    - 90% hyperdense
    - Ca++ in up to 20%; hemorrhage rare
    - Small intratumoral cysts/necrosis in 40-50%
  - Hydrocephalus common (95%)
- CECT
  - > 90% enhance
    - Relatively homogeneous
    - Occasionally patchy (may fill in slowly)

MR Findings
- T1WI
  - Hypointense to gray matter (GM)
- T2WI
  - Near GM intensity, or slightly hyperintense to GM
- FLAIR
  - Hyperintense to brain
  - Good differentiation of tumor from CSF in 4th ventricle
- DWI
  - Restricted diffusion, low ADC
- T1WI C+
  - > 90% enhance
  - Often heterogeneous
  - Contrast essential to detect CSF dissemination
    - Linear icing-like enhancement over brain surface: "Zuckerguss"
    - Extensive grape-like tumor nodules common in desmoplastic or MBEN
    - May have dural tail and resemble meningioma (cerebellar hemispheres)
  - Contrast-enhanced MR of spine (entire neuraxis)
    - Up to 1/3 have subarachnoid metastatic disease at presentation
    - Image preoperatively to avoid postoperative false positive: Blood in spinal canal may mimic or mask metastases
- MRS
  - ↓↓ NAA
  - ↑↑ choline
  - Lactate usually present
  - Elevation in Tau (short TE)
  - Cr/Cho < 0.75 and mI/NAA < 2.1 indicative for MB (DD ependymoma)

Angiographic Findings
- Conventional
  - Avascular or hypovascular posterior fossa mass

Nonvascular Interventions
- Myelography
  - May be helpful in identifying "drop" mets
  - Largely replaced by spinal MR with contrast

Imaging Recommendations
- Best imaging tool
  - Contrast-enhanced MR
- Protocol advice
  - Pre- and post-contrast sagittal images to show site of origin (roof vs. floor)
  - Quality of spine MR better if performed as separate exam

DIFFERENTIAL DIAGNOSIS

Cerebellar Pilocytic Astrocytoma (PA)
- Older children
- Hemispheric lesion
- Cyst with enhancing nodule

Ependymoma
- Older children
- More heterogeneous, Ca++ and hemorrhage more common
- Extension through 4th ventricle foramina/foramen magnum: "Plastic tumor"
- Higher ADC values (less cellular)

Choroid Plexus Papilloma (CPP)
- Much less common in 4th ventricle
- Vigorous and homogeneous enhancement
- Less mass effect

Atypical Teratoid/Rhabdoid Tumor (AT/RT)
- Indistinguishable by imaging
  - ↑ percentage of hemorrhage compared with MB
  - CPA involvement more common in AT/RT
- Younger children

MEDULLOBLASTOMA

Dorsally Exophytic Brainstem Glioma
- MR to show origin from brainstem

PATHOLOGY

General Features
- Etiology
  - 2 cell lines suspected as source
    - Cell rests of posterior medullary velum (roof of 4th ventricle)
    - External granular layer of cerebellum
- Associated abnormalities
  - Association with familial cancer syndromes
    - Gorlin (nevoid basal cell carcinoma) syndrome
    - Li-Fraumeni syndrome
    - Turcot syndrome
    - Gardner syndrome
    - Cowden syndrome
  - Associated with Taybi & Coffin-Siris syndromes

Staging, Grading, & Classification
- WHO grade IV

Gross Pathologic & Surgical Features
- Firm/discrete to soft/less well defined
  - Tumor outside of 4th ventricle more likely to be desmoplastic variant

Microscopic Features
- Densely packed hyperchromatic cells with scanty cytoplasm
- Frequent mitoses
- Anaplasia 24%

CLINICAL ISSUES

Presentation
- Most common signs/symptoms
  - Ataxia, signs of increased intracranial pressure
  - Macrocephaly in infants with open sutures
- Clinical profile
  - Relatively short (< 1 month) of symptoms
  - Symptoms reflect local mass effect &/or ↑ ICP
    - Nausea and vomiting, ataxia
    - Cranial nerve palsies (less common than in brainstem astrocytomas)
  - Gastrointestinal workup for N & V may precede diagnostic neuroimaging

Demographics
- Age
  - 75% < 10 years
  - Most diagnosed by 5 years
- Gender
  - M:F = 2-4:1
- Epidemiology
  - 15-20% of all pediatric brain tumors
  - 30-40% of posterior fossa tumors in children
  - Rare in adults

Natural History & Prognosis
- Rapid growth with early subarachnoid spread
- Initial positive response to treatment reflects high mitotic activity
- "Standard risk" clinical profile
  - No metastases or gross residual tumor s/p resection
  - With ERBB-2 tumor protein negative = high 5-year survival rate (100%)
  - With ERBB-2 tumor protein positive = low 5-year survival rate (54%)
- "High risk" clinical profile
  - 5-year survival rate ≈ 20%
  - Gross residual tumor after surgery
  - Documented metastatic disease
  - Children < 3 years of age have inferior survival
- Adult presentation has slightly better outcome (may reflect greater resectability of lateral lesions, desmoplastic variant)
  - Late relapse common in adults

Treatment
- Surgical excision, adjuvant chemotherapy
- Craniospinal irradiation if > 3 years

DIAGNOSTIC CHECKLIST

Consider
- AT/RT in patients under 3 years
- Preoperative evaluation of entire neuraxis and postoperative evaluation of surgical bed are key to prognosis

Image Interpretation Pearls
- 4th ventricle tumor arising from roof = PNET-MB
- 4th ventricle tumor arising from floor = ependymoma
- Thinking of MB in childhood posterior fossa tumor? Include AT/RT!

SELECTED REFERENCES

1. Papaioannou G et al: Imaging of the unusual pediatric 'blastomas'. Cancer Imaging. 9:1-11, 2009
2. Riffaud L et al: Survival and prognostic factors in a series of adults with medulloblastomas. J Neurosurg. Epub ahead of print, 2009
3. Yamashita Y et al: Minimum apparent diffusion coefficient is significantly correlated with cellularity in medulloblastomas. Neurol Res. Epub ahead of print, 2009
4. Davies NP et al: Identification and characterisation of childhood cerebellar tumours by in vivo proton MRS. NMR Biomed. 21(8):908-18, 2008
5. Holthouse DJ et al: Classic and desmoplastic medulloblastoma: Complete case reports and characterizations of two new cell lines. Neuropathology. Epub ahead of print, 2008
6. Koral K et al: Imaging characteristics of atypical teratoid-rhabdoid tumor in children compared with medulloblastoma. AJR Am J Roentgenol. 190(3):809-14, 2008
7. Harris LM et al: The use of short-echo-time 1H MRS for childhood cerebellar tumours prior to histopathological diagnosis. Pediatr Radiol. 37(11):1101-9, 2007
8. Peet AC et al: Magnetic resonance spectroscopy suggests key differences in the metastatic behaviour of medulloblastoma. Eur J Cancer. 43(6):1037-44, 2007
9. Rumboldt Z et al: coefficients for differentiation of cerebellar tumors in children. AJNR Am J Neuroradiol. 27(6):1362-9, 2006

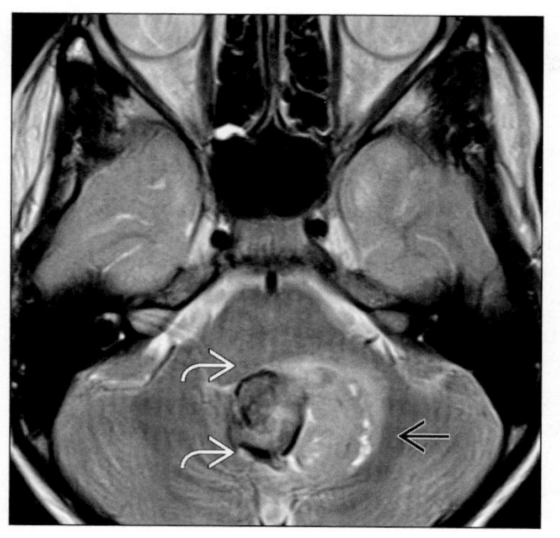

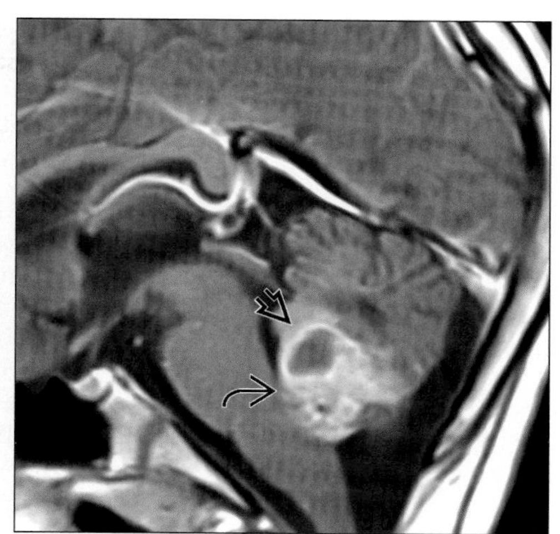

(Left) *Axial T2WI MR in an 11-year-old girl presenting with clumsiness, vomiting, and weight loss shows isointense cortex and an inhomogeneous mass in the 4th ventricle ➔ with low signal areas representing hemorrhage ➔. Neurological examination revealed ataxia, nystagmus, and right facial palsy.* ***(Right)*** *Sagittal T1WI C+ MR shows marked enhancement ➔ of the tumor with nonenhancing necrotic parts ➔.*

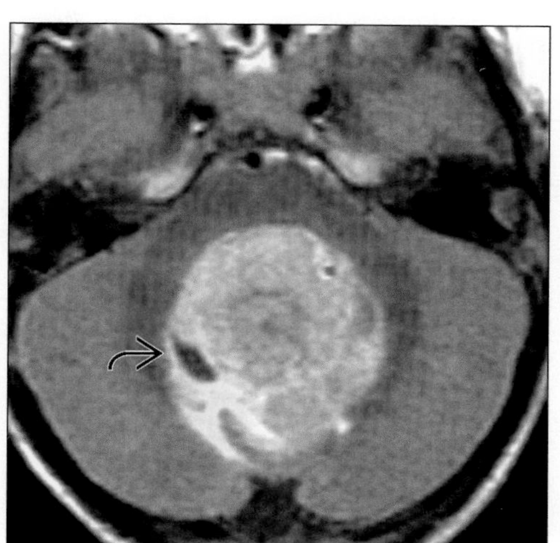

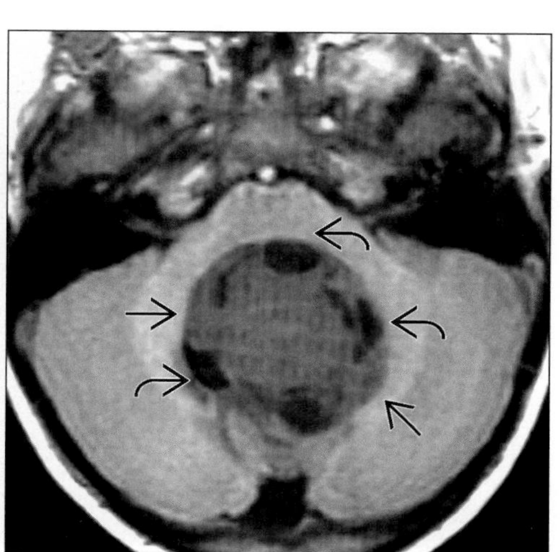

(Left) *Axial FLAIR MR shows classic medulloblastoma with high signal, well-defined borders, and small cystic parts ➔ in the region of the 4th ventricle.* ***(Right)*** *Axial T1WI MR demonstrates a low signal intensity mass in the 4th ventricle ➔ with cystic elements ➔.*

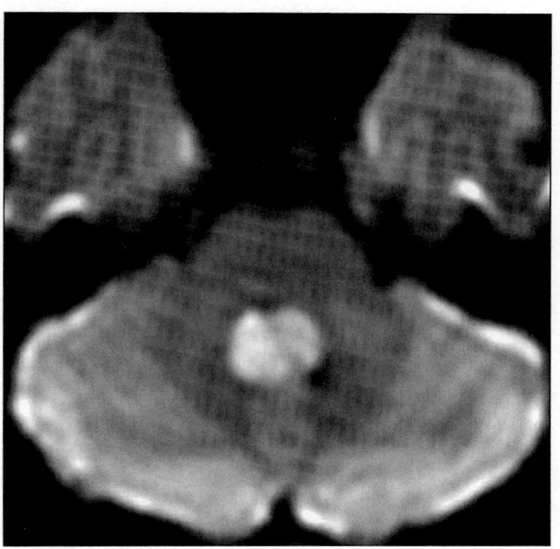

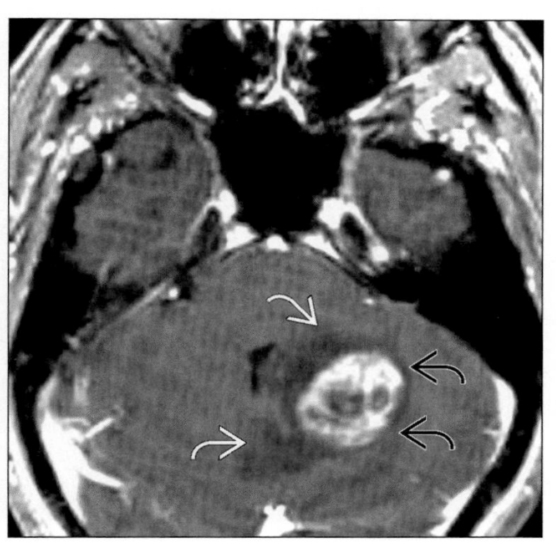

(Left) *Axial DWI MR shows a high signal, classic medulloblastoma located in the 4th ventricle suggesting restricted diffusion in a high cellularity tumor. This feature is frequently seen in medulloblastoma, whereas ependymomas will show low signal on DWI and high ADC values.* ***(Right)*** *Axial T1WI C+ MR in a 50-year-old female patient demonstrates enhancing mass ➔ with perifocal edema ➔ in the left cerebellar hemisphere. Classic medulloblastoma was found at surgery.*

VARIANT MEDULLOBLASTOMA

Key Facts

Terminology

- Medulloblastoma variants (MB-V)
  - Anaplastic and large cell medulloblastoma (LCA)
  - Medulloblastoma with extensive nodularity (MBEN)
  - Desmoplastic/nodular medulloblastoma
- Malignant "small blue cell" tumors

Imaging

- Hyperdense posterior fossa tumor in child
- Marked, inhomogeneous enhancement of solid tumor portions
- Grape-like appearance with solid and cystic parts in MBEN
- Multiple coalescing nodules in MBEN
- Elevated choline, low NAA

Top Differential Diagnoses

- Ependymoma
- Pilocytic astrocytoma
- AT/RT

Pathology

- WHO grade IV

Clinical Issues

- MBEN strongly associated with cancer predisposition syndrome (Gorlin syndrome)
- MBEN, desmoplastic/nodular medulloblastoma occur in children ≤ 5 years
- Anaplastic/large-cell MB
  - CSF dissemination common at presentation
- Desmoplastic medulloblastoma, MBEN better prognosis than LCA
- Obstructive hydrocephalus common

__(Left)__ Axial autopsy section through the mid-cerebellum shows a rather firm, laterally located cerebellar hemispheric mass ➡, a desmoplastic medulloblastoma. (Courtesy R. Hewlett, PhD.) __(Right)__ Axial T1WI C+ MR in a 66-year-old man demonstrates inhomogeneous but marked enhancement of a poorly marginated, lateral cerebellar hemispheric mass ➡. Venous structures in the posterior fossa are not invaded ➡. Histological analysis after surgical resection revealed anaplastic medulloblastoma.

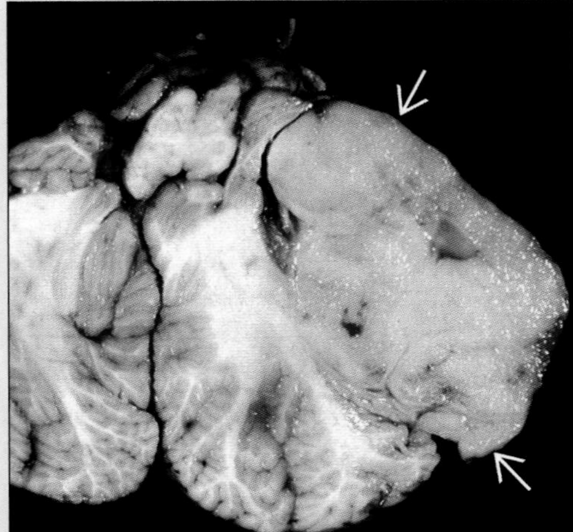

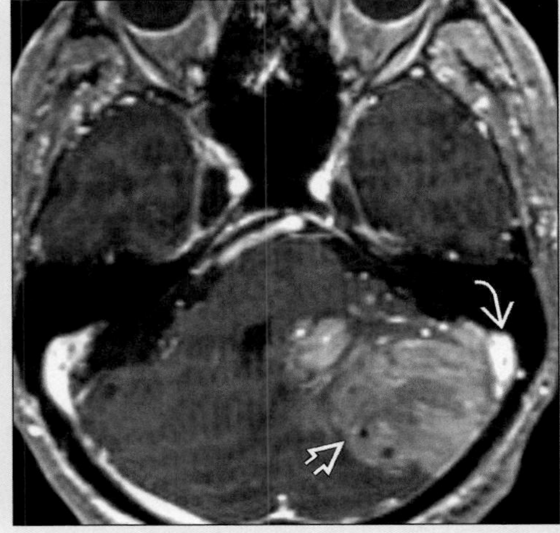

__(Left)__ Axial FLAIR MR in a 1-year-old boy shows a multilobulated, low signal intensity mass in the right cerebellum ➡. __(Right)__ Coronal T1WI C+ MR in the same patient shows marked enhancement of the solid tumor portions ➡ with a scar-like central part ➡. Biopsy revealed a medulloblastoma with extensive nodularity (MBEN).

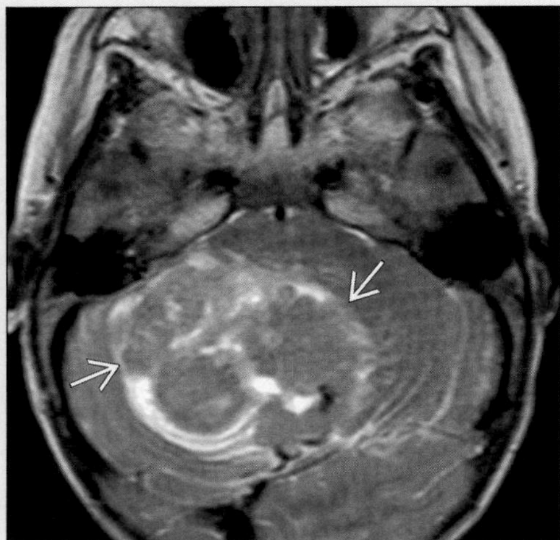

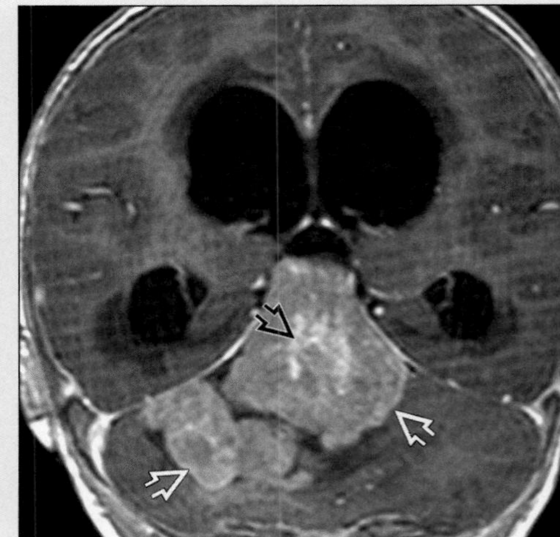

VARIANT MEDULLOBLASTOMA

TERMINOLOGY

Abbreviations

- Medulloblastoma (MB) variants (MB-V)

Synonyms

- MB variants
  - Anaplastic and large cell medulloblastoma (LCA)
  - Medulloblastoma with extensive nodularity (MBEN)
    - Sometimes called "cerebellar neuroblastoma"
  - Desmoplastic/nodular medulloblastoma

Definitions

- Malignant posterior fossa tumor in children
- "Small blue cell" tumors

IMAGING

General Features

- Best diagnostic clue
  - Child with highly cellular, posterior fossa tumor
- Location
  - Posterior fossa
    - Midline or lateral (cerebellar hemispheres)
- Morphology
  - Inhomogeneous mass with solid, cystic parts

Imaging Recommendations

- Best imaging tool
  - MR with T1WI C+, DWI
- Protocol advice
  - DWI (high signal + low ADC indicates high cellularity)
    - Differentiates from ependymoma, pilocytic astrocytoma

CT Findings

- NECT
  - Hyperdense or hypodense nodular mass in MBEN

MR Findings

- T1WI
  - Iso-/hypointense
- T2WI
  - Low signal in solid parts (high cellularity), high signal in cystic parts
- DWI
  - High signal on DWI, low ADC values (cutoff < 0.9 x 103 mm²/s)
- T1WI C+
  - Marked, inhomogeneous enhancement of solid tumor portions
    - Grape-like appearance, multiple coalescing nodules in MBEN
- MRS
  - Elevated choline, low NAA

DIFFERENTIAL DIAGNOSIS

Ependymoma

- ADC = 1.0-1.3 x 10^3 mm²/s

Pilocytic Astrocytoma

- ADC cutoff > 1.4 x 10^3 mm²/s

Atypical Teratoid-Rhabdoid Tumor

- Heterogeneous intracranial tumor in infant

PATHOLOGY

General Features

- Etiology
  - Arises from primitive cells of external granular layer of cerebellum

Staging, Grading, & Classification

- All medulloblastoma variants are WHO grade IV tumors

CLINICAL ISSUES

Presentation

- Other signs/symptoms
  - LCA: CSF dissemination is common finding at presentation
  - Obstructive hydrocephalus common

Demographics

- Age
  - MBEN and desmoplastic medulloblastoma occur in children ≤ 5 years
- Epidemiology
  - MBEN is strongly associated with cancer predisposition syndrome (Gorlin syndrome)
  - Large cell/anaplastic represent 10-22% of MB
    - 2-4% of MB are large cell
  - Nodular/desmoplastic and MBEN represent 7-13%

Natural History & Prognosis

- Desmoplastic medulloblastoma and MBEN have better prognosis than LCA
- Overall 5-year survival of desmoplastic and MBEN is 95%
  - Overall 5-year survival of classic MB is only 41%

Treatment

- Surgery followed by radio- and chemotherapy

SELECTED REFERENCES

1. Garrè ML et al: Medulloblastoma variants: age-dependent occurrence and relation to Gorlin syndrome--a new clinical perspective. Clin Cancer Res. 15(7):2463-71, 2009
2. Gulino A et al: Pathological and molecular heterogeneity of medulloblastoma. Curr Opin Oncol. 20(6):668-75, 2008
3. Louis DN et al: The 2007 WHO classification of tumours of the central nervous system. Acta Neuropathol. 2007 Aug;114(2):97-109. Epub 2007 Jul 6. Review. Erratum in: Acta Neuropathol. 114(5):547, 2007
4. McManamy CS et al: Nodule formation and desmoplasia in medulloblastomas-defining the nodular/desmoplastic variant and its biological behavior. Brain Pathol. 17(2):151-64, 2007
5. Giangaspero F et al: Medulloblastoma with extensive nodularity: a variant with favorable prognosis. J Neurosurg. 91(6):971-7, 1999

SUPRATENTORIAL PNET

Key Facts

Terminology

- Supratentorial primitive neuroectodermal tumor (S-PNET)
  - Cerebral embryonal tumor composed of undifferentiated neuroepithelial cells

Imaging

- Large, complex-appearing hemispheric mass with minimal peritumoral edema in infant/young child
- Variable size, based on location
  - Cerebral hemispheric PNETs larger (mean diameter = 5 cm)
  - Suprasellar, pineal PNETs smaller (earlier symptoms from mass effect on adjacent structures)
- Sharply delineated to diffusely infiltrative
- Calcification (50-70%)
- Heterogeneous enhancement
- Restricted diffusion common
- Prone to subarachnoid tumor seeding
- Do enhanced MR of entire neuraxis before surgery!
  - Enhanced FLAIR detects subarachnoid seeding

Top Differential Diagnoses

- Astrocytoma
- Ependymoma
- Atypical teratoid-rhabdoid tumor

Pathology

- WHO grade IV
- Histology similar to medulloblastoma (PNET-MB)

Clinical Issues

- Most common in younger children
- M:F = 2:1

Diagnostic Checklist

- Large bulky hemispheric mass, sparse edema

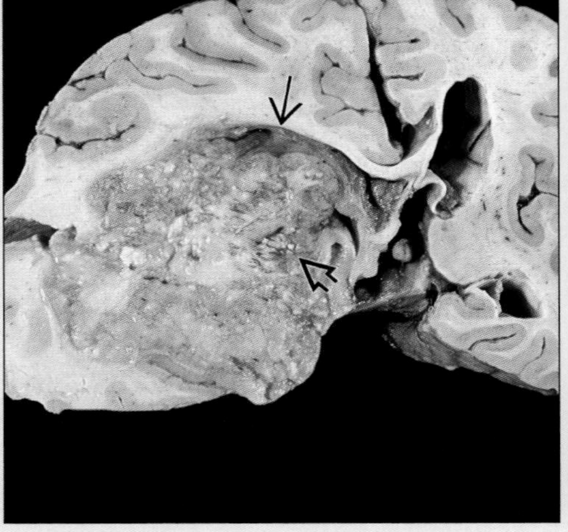

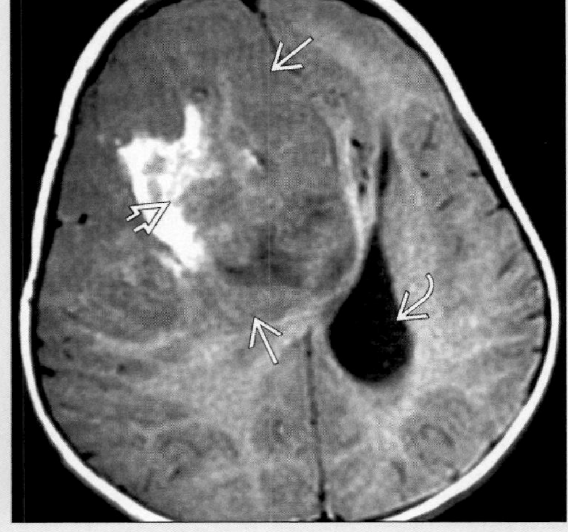

(Left) Coronal gross pathology shows a cerebral PNET as a large, bulky hemispheric mass →. Note the heterogeneous appearance, foci of hemorrhage, and necrosis ⇒. (Courtesy Rubinstein Collection, AFIP.) (Right) Axial T1WI MR shows a typical, very large, solid, intraaxial mass → with distinctive lack of peritumoral edema. The mass is overall mildly hypointense relative to gray matter, though regions of hemorrhage are hyperintense ⇒. Ventricular obstruction with dilatation ↪ results from subfalcine herniation.

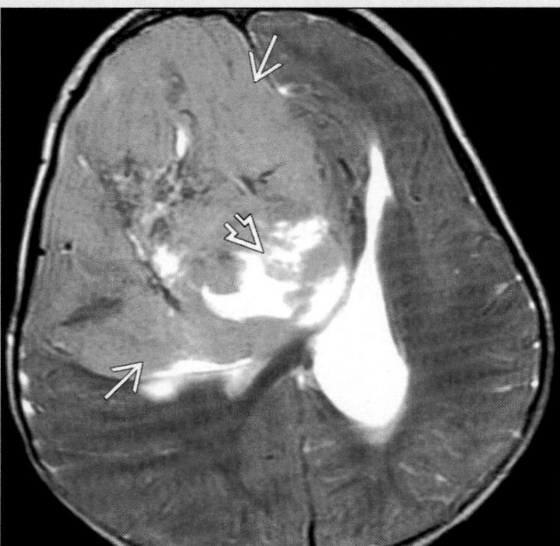

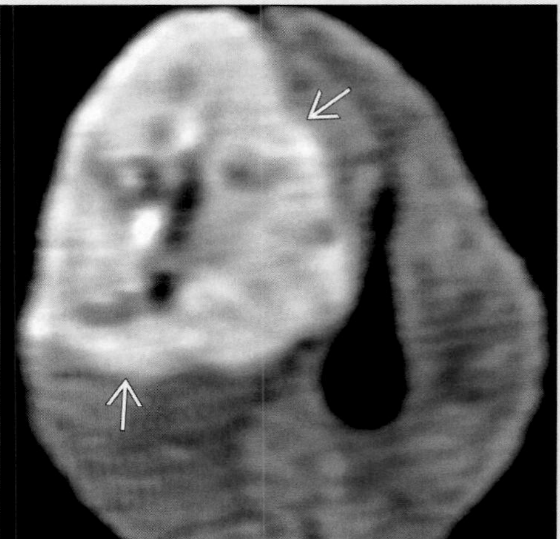

(Left) Axial T2WI MR shows a large, mildly hyperintense, right frontal lobe mass →. Note that the signal intensity is just slightly greater than gray matter. Also note the lack of peritumoral edema. Central and medial tumoral heterogeneity and hyperintensity represent necrosis ⇒. (Right) Axial DWI MR image shows restricted diffusion within this highly cellular mass →. Restricted diffusion was confirmed on corresponding ADC maps (not shown).

TERMINOLOGY

Abbreviations

- Supratentorial primitive neuroectodermal tumor (S-PNET)

Synonyms

- Supratentorial primitive neuroepithelial tumor
- Primary cerebral neuroblastoma
- Cerebral ganglioneuroblastoma

Definitions

- Primitive cerebral embryonal tumor
  - Composed of undifferentiated neuroepithelial cells
  - Broad capacity for divergent differentiation
    - Astrocytic, ependymal, neuronal, muscular, melanotic elements

IMAGING

General Features

- Best diagnostic clue
  - Large, complex-appearing hemispheric mass with minimal peritumoral edema in infant/young child
- Location
  - Cerebral hemisphere
    - Cortical/subcortical
    - Thalamic
  - Suprasellar
  - Pineal
- Size
  - Variable, based on location
    - Cerebral hemispheric PNETs are larger at diagnosis, mean diameter ~ 5 cm
      - Hemispheric lesions in infants often huge
    - Suprasellar PNETs tend to be smaller
      - Earlier symptoms (e.g., neuroendocrine and visual disturbances) due to mass effect on adjacent structures
    - Pineal PNETs cause hydrocephalus and gaze/ convergence difficulties
- Morphology
  - Sharply delineated to diffusely infiltrative

Radiographic Findings

- Radiography
  - Macrocephaly and widened sutures (neonate and infant)

CT Findings

- NECT
  - Iso- to hyperattenuating
  - Calcification (50-70%)
  - Hemorrhage and necrosis common
- CECT
  - Heterogeneous enhancement
  - Prone to subarachnoid tumor seeding

MR Findings

- T1WI
  - Hypo- to isointense to gray matter
  - Homogeneous to heterogeneous
- T2WI
  - Solid elements isointense to slightly hyperintense to gray matter
  - No or minimal peritumoral edema
  - Ca++ → hypointense foci
  - Blood products → mixed signal intensity
- PD/intermediate
  - Slightly hyperintense
- FLAIR
  - Solid components hyperintense
  - Little peritumoral edema
  - Post-contrast-enhancement FLAIR detects leptomeningeal metastases
- T2* GRE
  - Dephasing from blood products
- DWI
  - Restricted diffusion common
- T1WI C+
  - Heterogeneous enhancement
  - Subarachnoid seeding common
  - Subtraction imaging helpful with hemorrhagic masses
- MRS
  - ↓ ↓ NAA, ↓ creatine, ↑ ↑ choline, + lipid and lactate

Ultrasonographic Findings

- Congenital S-PNET (antenatal sonography)
  - Large hyperechoic hemispheric mass
  - Hydrocephalus

Imaging Recommendations

- Best imaging tool
  - MR with T1WI C+, FLAIR, DWI, MRS
- Protocol advice
  - Do T1WI C+ MR of entire neuraxis before surgery!
  - Adding post-contrast-enhancement FLAIR aids in detecting leptomeningeal metastases

DIFFERENTIAL DIAGNOSIS

Astrocytoma (AA, GBM)

- Extensive vasogenic edema
- Ca++

Ependymoma

- When supratentorial (30%), usually intraaxial
  - Only 15-25% arise within 3rd or lateral ventricle
- Necrosis and hemorrhage not uncommon

Oligodendroglioma

- Predilection for frontotemporal region
- Peripheral location
- Coarse Ca++ common

Atypical Teratoid-Rhabdoid Tumor

- Posterior fossa > 50%, supratentorial 39%
- Necrosis, cysts, and vasogenic edema common
- Subarachnoid seeding common

Choroid Plexus Carcinoma

- Parenchymal invasion can be dramatic
- Extensive vasogenic edema
- Avid enhancement

Giant Cavernoma
- Can be huge in newborn, infant
- Mimics hemorrhagic tumor

PATHOLOGY

General Features
- Etiology
  - Tumor suppressor gene aberrations may play role
- Genetics
  - Unlike medulloblastoma (PNET-MB), chromosome 17 aberrations (rare)
  - Somatic mutations in tumor suppressor genes
    - *HASH1*
    - *hSNF5* on chromosome 22
  - Other chromosome anomalies in S-PNETs
    - Aberrations of short arm of chromosome 11
    - Trisomies of chromosomes 9,13,1q, and 18p telomere maintenance
- Associated abnormalities
  - Hereditary syndromes
    - Gorlin syndrome
    - Turcot syndrome
    - Hereditary retinoblastoma and risk for secondary malignancies
    - Rubinstein-Taybi syndrome

Staging, Grading, & Classification
- WHO grade IV

Gross Pathologic & Surgical Features
- Variable consistency
  - Solid and homogeneous → cystic, necrotic, hemorrhagic, and partially calcified
  - Solid portions and soft pink-red coloration, unless prominent desmoplasia
  - Demarcation between tumor and brain may range from indistinct to sharp

Microscopic Features
- Similar to medulloblastoma (PNET-MB)

CLINICAL ISSUES

Presentation
- Most common signs/symptoms
  - Vary with site of origin and size of tumor
    - Hemispheric → seizures, altered mental status, motor deficit, elevated intracranial pressure
    - Suprasellar → visual disturbance, endocrine dysfunction
    - Pineal → hydrocephalus, Parinaud syndrome
- Other signs/symptoms
  - Cranial neuropathies due to herniation or diffuse CSF metastases
- Clinical profile
  - Infant presenting with macrocephaly, seizures, and large hemispheric mass

Demographics
- Age
  - Most common in younger children
    - Median age at diagnosis: 35 months
- Gender
  - M:F = 2:1
- Ethnicity
  - No ethnic predilection
- Epidemiology
  - S-PNETs constitute 1% of pediatric brain tumors
  - Of all CNS PNETs, 5-6% are supratentorial

Natural History & Prognosis
- Compared to posterior fossa PNET (PNET-MB), S-PNETs have poorer survival
  - S-PNET → 5-year survival (30-35%)
  - PNET-MB → 5-year survival (80-85%)
- Critical survival factors include
  - Complete surgical resection
  - Absence of metastases
  - Patient age > 2 years
  - Small, solid tumor (necrosis is unfavorable)
  - Immunohistochemical labeling indices (Ki-67 index > 10%, unfavorable)
  - M stage of tumor
- Heavily calcified S-PNETs have slightly better prognosis

Treatment
- Aggressive surgical resection, chemotherapy, craniospinal radiation

DIAGNOSTIC CHECKLIST

Consider
- S-PNET in newborn, infant, or young child with
  - Hemispheric tumor lacking edema
  - Suprasellar or pineal mass

Image Interpretation Pearls
- Large hemispheric mass with sparse peritumoral edema

SELECTED REFERENCES

1. Biswas S et al: Non-pineal supratentorial primitive neuro-ectodermal tumors (sPNET) in teenagers and young adults: Time to reconsider cisplatin based chemotherapy after cranio-spinal irradiation? Pediatr Blood Cancer. 52(7):796-803, 2009
2. Brandes AA et al: Adult neuroectodermal tumors of posterior fossa (medulloblastoma) and of supratentorial sites (stPNET). Crit Rev Oncol Hematol. 71(2):165-79, 2009
3. Johnston DL et al: Supratentorial primitive neuroectodermal tumors: a Canadian pediatric brain tumor consortium report. J Neurooncol. 86(1):101-8, 2008
4. Smee RI et al: Medulloblastomas-primitive neuroectodermal tumours in the adult population. J Med Imaging Radiat Oncol. 52(1):72-6, 2008
5. Chawla A et al: Paediatric PNET: pre-surgical MRI features. Clin Radiol. 62(1):43-52, 2007
6. Yamada T et al: Prenatal imaging of congenital cerebral primitive neuroectodermal tumor. Fetal Diagn Ther. 18(3):137-9, 2003
7. Poussaint TY: Magnetic resonance imaging of pediatric brain tumors: state of the art. Top Magn Reson Imaging. 12(6):411-33, 2001

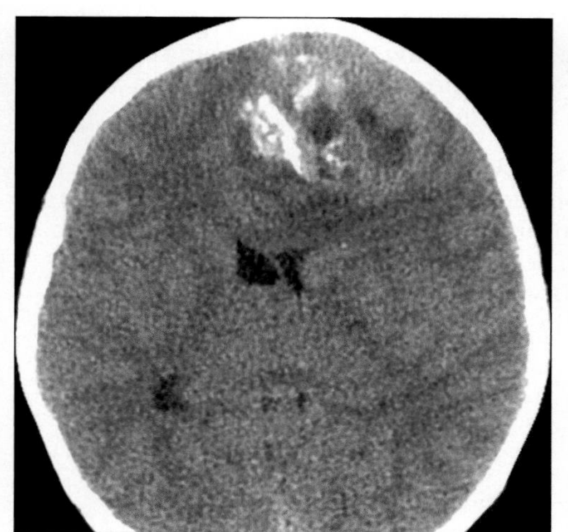

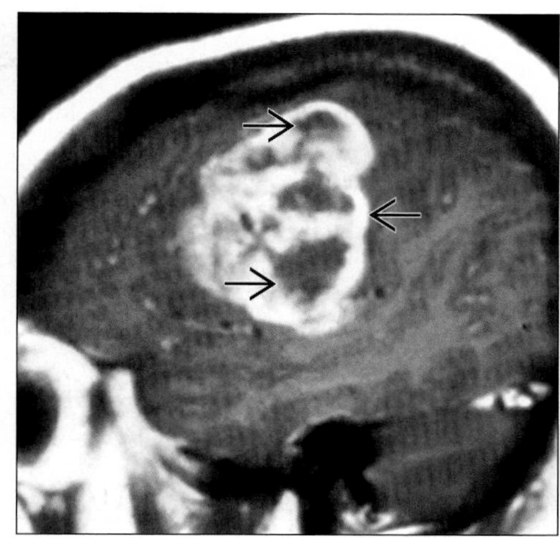

*(**Left**) Axial NECT shows a typical, intraaxial, frontal lobe cerebral PNET with heterogeneity, features of high cellularity and little or no peritumoral edema. The tumor is largely hyperattenuating with scattered calcifications. (**Right**) Sagittal T1WI C+ MR in a different supratentorial PNET shows a demarcated, lobular mass with heterogeneous enhancement due to areas of necrosis and hemorrhage ➔.*

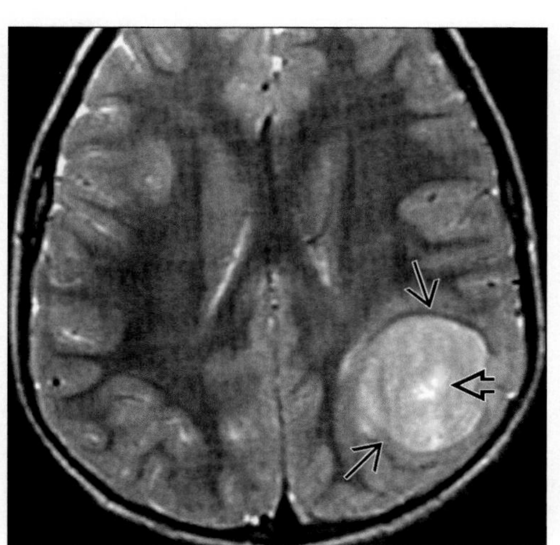

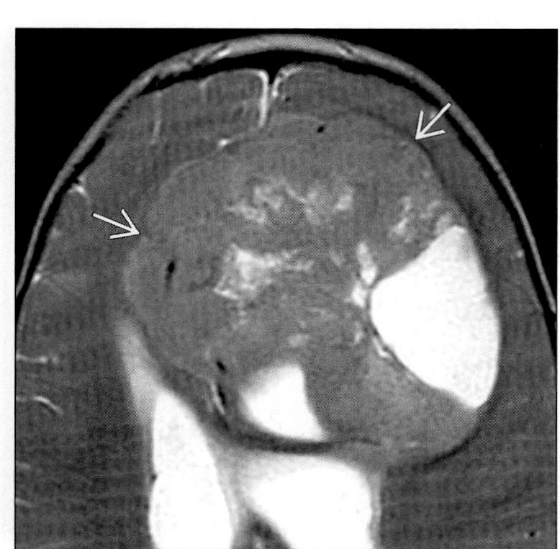

*(**Left**) Axial T2WI MR shows a demarcated mass ➔ in the left cerebrum with central necrosis ➔. Note the minimal edema in the surrounding brain. (**Right**) Axial T2WI MR in a 13-month-old child shows a large bifrontal mass ➔. Its solid components are only slightly hyperintense to the adjacent gray matter, characteristic of a highly cellular tumor. Heterogeneous hyperintense foci correspond to regions of necrosis. Supratentorial PNET was found at surgery.*

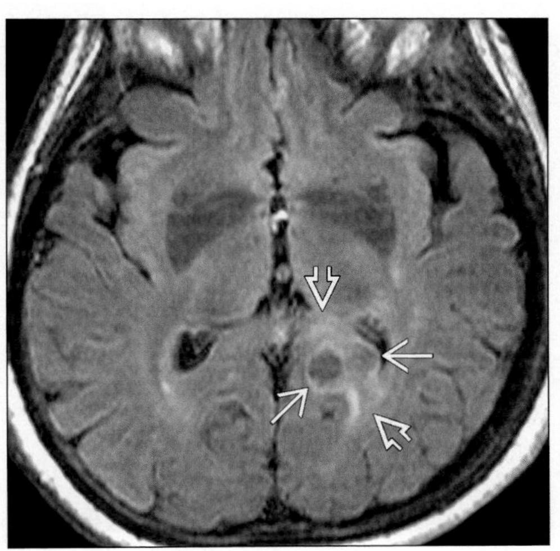

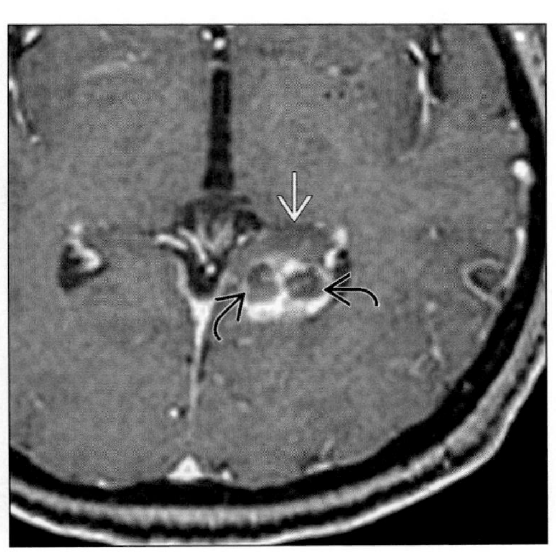

*(**Left**) Axial FLAIR MR shows a lobular, heterogeneous mass ➔ medial to the trigone of the left lateral ventricle at the parietooccipital junction. More subtle areas of hyperintensity in the surrounding white matter ➔ proved to be an infiltrating tumor at surgery and pathologic evaluation. (**Right**) Axial T1 C+ MR in the same patient shows heterogeneous enhancement of the lobular portion with regions of central necrosis ➔. The infiltrating portions do not enhance ➔. Supratentorial PNET was concluded.*

ATYPICAL TERATOID-RHABDOID TUMOR

Key Facts

Imaging

- Heterogeneous intracranial mass in infant
- Hyperattenuating mass on CT
- Commonly contains cysts or hemorrhage
- Relatively little edema for size of tumor
- Heterogeneous enhancement
- Leptomeningeal spread common
- May restrict on DWI, show ↓ ADC

Pathology

- WHO grade IV
- Extreme morphological, immunophenotypic heterogeneity
- Divergent differentiation accounts for "teratoid" label
  - Sheets of nonspecific primitive small cells interrupted by fibrovascular septa
  - Rhabdoid cells resemble those in malignant rhabdoid tumor of kidney
- Monosomy of chromosome 22 or deletion of band 22q11
  - Band 22q11 is site of *hSNF5/INI1* gene
- Lack of immunostaining for INI1 protein correlates with *hSNF5/INI1* mutation
  - Reliable for diagnosing AT/RT

Diagnostic Checklist

- Always consider AT/RT when large tumor found in child younger than 3 years
- Include AT/RT whenever medulloblastoma (PNET-MB) is diagnostic consideration
  - May be impossible to distinguish by imaging

*(**Left**) Coronal graphic shows an AT/RT. A foci of central necrosis can coalesce, as in this example, forming a thick nodular enhancing tumor rind around the central cavity. (**Right**) Axial NECT demonstrates typical findings of AT/RT with an off-midline, heterogeneous, hyperdense tumor ➡ with calcifications ⮚. Although PNET-medulloblastoma is much more common than AT/RT in the posterior fossa of a child, AT/RT should be considered when the tumor is off midline.*

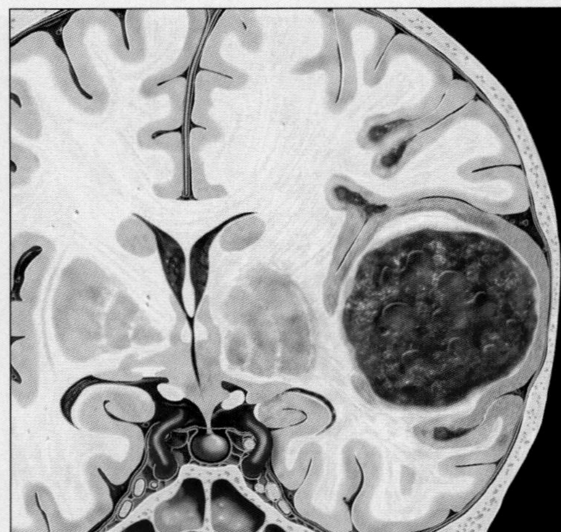

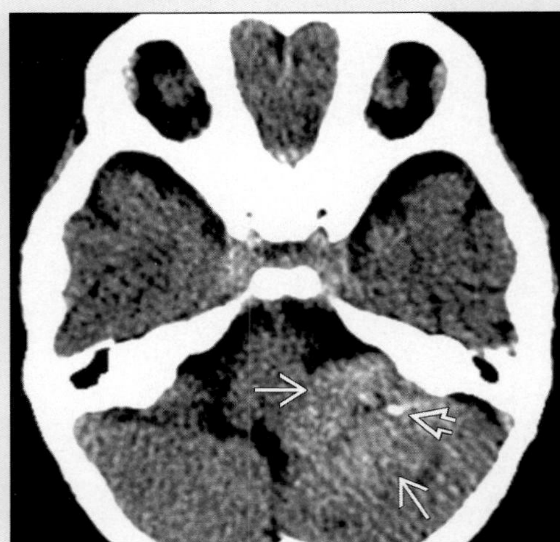

*(**Left**) Axial T1WI MR in the same patient demonstrates heterogeneous enhancement ➡ of the cerebellar pontine angle mass. (**Right**) Axial DWI MR demonstrates mild restricted diffusion ➡ with central hemorrhagic products. Restricted diffusion is typical of central necrosis or highly cellular tumors. This is seen in both PNET-MB and AT/RT.*

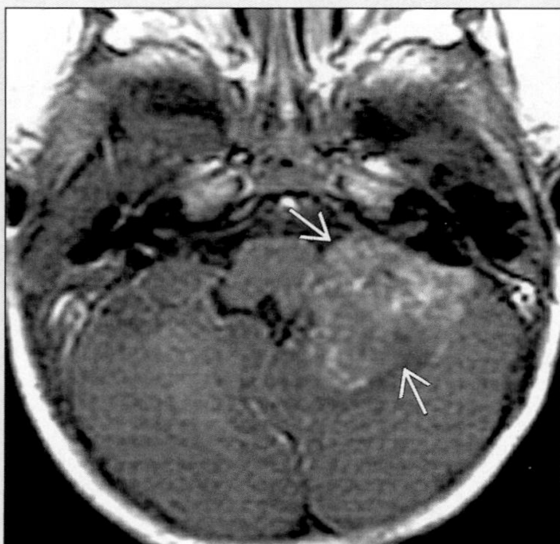

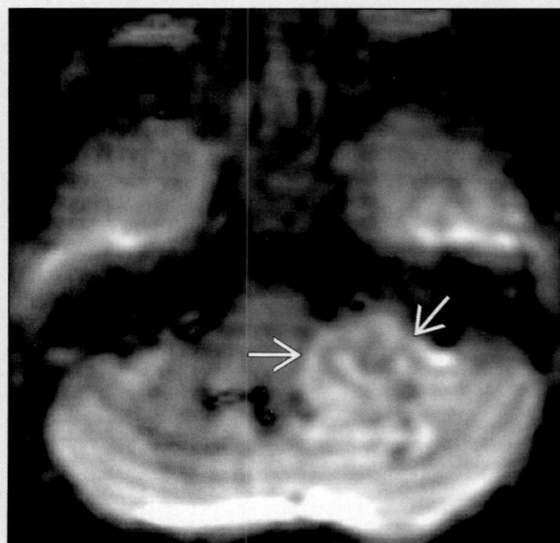

ATYPICAL TERATOID-RHABDOID TUMOR

TERMINOLOGY

Abbreviations
- Atypical teratoid-rhabdoid tumor (AT/RT)

Synonyms
- Malignant rhabdoid tumor of brain
- Cranial rhabdoid tumor

Definitions
- Rare, highly malignant aggressive tumor of early childhood
  - Composed of rhabdoid cells
  - Often contains primitive neuroectodermal cells that resemble PNET
  - Divergent differentiation along mesenchymal, neuronal, glial, or epithelial lines

IMAGING

General Features
- Best diagnostic clue
  - Heterogeneous mass in infant/young child
  - Moderately large, bulky tumor with mixed solid cystic components
- Location
  - Infratentorial (47%)
    - Most off-midline
    - Cerebellopontine angle (CPA)
    - Cerebellum &/or brainstem
  - Supratentorial (41%)
    - Hemispheric or suprasellar
  - Both infra- and supratentorial (12%)
  - 15-20% present with disseminated tumor at time of initial diagnosis
- Size
  - Most 1-3 cm at presentation (can be very large)
- Morphology
  - Roughly spherical, irregular/lobulated

CT Findings
- NECT
  - Hyperattenuating mass
  - Commonly contains cysts &/or hemorrhage
  - May contain Ca++
  - Obstructive hydrocephalus common
- CECT
  - Strong but heterogeneous enhancement typical

MR Findings
- T1WI
  - Heterogeneous
    - Isointense to brain
    - ± hyperintense hemorrhagic foci
    - Cysts slightly hyperintense to CSF
- T2WI
  - Heterogeneous
    - Hypointense foci (hemorrhage)
    - Hyperintense foci (cysts)
- FLAIR
  - Solid tumor isointense to hyperintense
  - Cysts hyperintense to CSF
  - Transependymal edema from hydrocephalus
  - Relatively little edema for size of tumor
- T2* GRE
  - Hypointense "blooming" of hemorrhagic foci
- DWI
  - May restrict because of cellularity
  - Decreased apparent diffusion coefficient (ADC)
- T1WI C+
  - Heterogeneous enhancement
  - Leptomeningeal spread common (15-20%)
    - Diffuse linear
    - Multiple nodular
  - "Brain-to-brain" parenchymal metastases
- MRA
  - May show narrowing of encased vessels
- MRS
  - Aggressive metabolite pattern
    - Elevated choline
    - Low or absent N-acetylaspartate (NAA), creatine
    - Lipid/lactate peak common

Imaging Recommendations
- Best imaging tool
  - MR with contrast
- Protocol advice
  - Entire CNS must be imaged at presentation to identify subarachnoid spread of tumor

DIFFERENTIAL DIAGNOSIS

Medulloblastoma (PNET-MB)
- Posterior fossa tumor
- AT/RT more likely to have cysts than PNET-MB
- Heterogeneous CPA tumors statistically more likely to be PNET-MB but more typical of AT/RT

Ependymoma
- "Plastic" tumor, extends out 4th ventricle foramina
- Ca++, cysts, hemorrhage common
- Strong, heterogeneous enhancement

Choroid Plexus Papilloma
- Intraventricular mass
- Homogeneous enhancement

Glioblastoma/Sarcoma
- High-grade glioma
- Exophytic from brainstem

Teratoma
- More often pineal or parasellar in location
- Heterogeneous on imaging due to Ca++, hemorrhage

PATHOLOGY

General Features
- Etiology
  - Unknown, may arise from neural crest cells
  - Combination of primitive neuroectodermal, peripheral epithelial, mesenchymal elements
  - Rhabdoid cells resemble those in malignant rhabdoid tumor of kidney

- Divergent differentiation accounts for "teratoid" label
  - Diverse immunohistological staining suggests multiple cell lines
  - Unlike teratoma, cells do not develop beyond primitive stage
- Genetics
  - Monosomy of chromosome 22 or deletion of band 22q11
    - Inactivating mutation of *hSNF5/INI1* gene on chromosome 22
    - Choroid plexus neoplasms have same mutation
    - Choroid plexus carcinomas occur in families with "rhabdoid predisposition syndrome"

Staging, Grading, & Classification

- WHO grade IV

Gross Pathologic & Surgical Features

- Frequently unresectable at presentation
- Poorly defined tumor margins
- Infiltration into parenchyma

Microscopic Features

- Extreme morphological, immunophenotypic heterogeneity
- Sheets of nonspecific primitive small cells interrupted by fibrovascular septa
- Rhabdoid cells
  - Large, pale, bland cells with moderate eosinophilic cytoplasm
- Embracing cells
  - Sickle-shaped cells that "embrace" rhabdoid cells
- Frequent positive immunoreactivity
  - Vimentin (VIM)
  - Epithelial membrane antigen (EMA)
  - Neuron-specific enolase (NSE)
  - Glial fibrillary acidic protein (GFAP)
  - Claudine 6 (CLDN6)
    - Key component of tight junctions
    - Moderate/high expressivity in AT/RTs
    - Little to none in other neoplasms including medulloblastoma, PNETs
- Lack of immunostaining for INI1 protein correlates with *hSNF5/INI1* mutation
  - Reliable for diagnosing AT/RT

CLINICAL ISSUES

Presentation

- Most common signs/symptoms
  - Signs of increased intracranial pressure
    - Lethargy
    - Vomiting
    - Increased head circumference
  - Other signs/symptoms
    - Torticollis
    - Seizure
    - Regression of skills
- Clinical profile
  - Child < 3 years with increasing head size, vomiting, and lethargy

Demographics

- Age
  - < 3 years
- Gender
  - M = F
- Epidemiology
  - Rare > 3 years
  - Up to 20% of primitive CNS tumors in children younger than 3
  - No gender predominance

Natural History & Prognosis

- Median survival = 16 months with leptomeningeal disease, 149 months without
- Death rate = 64%

Treatment

- Aggressive resection and chemoradiation have increased survival times but still remains poor
- Radiation has shown to ↑ survival time, especially in older children
  - Controversial in younger children due to damage to developing brain
- Chemotherapy regimens designed for PNET-MB largely ineffectual

DIAGNOSTIC CHECKLIST

Consider

- Always consider AT/RT when large tumor found in child younger than 3 years
- Include AT/RT whenever medulloblastoma (PNET-MB) is diagnostic consideration

Image Interpretation Pearls

- Imaging appearance is nonspecific
- More likely to be heterogeneous or supratentorial than PNET-MB

SELECTED REFERENCES

1. Birks DK et al: Claudin 6 Is a Positive Marker for Atypical Teratoid/Rhabdoid Tumors. Brain Pathol. Epub ahead of print, 2009
2. Chi SN et al: Intensive multimodality treatment for children with newly diagnosed CNS atypical teratoid rhabdoid tumor. J Clin Oncol. 27(3):385-9, 2009
3. Koral K et al: Imaging characteristics of atypical teratoid-rhabdoid tumor in children compared with medulloblastoma. AJR Am J Roentgenol. 190(3):809-14, 2008
4. Warmuth-Metz M et al: CT and MR imaging in atypical teratoid/rhabdoid tumors of the central nervous system. Neuroradiology. 50(5):447-52, 2008
5. Squire SE et al: Atypical teratoid/rhabdoid tumor: the controversy behind radiation therapy. J Neurooncol. 81(1):97-111, 2007
6. Meyers SP et al: Primary intracranial atypical teratoid/rhabdoid tumors of infancy and childhood: MRI features and patient outcomes. AJNR Am J Neuroradiol. 27(5):962-71, 2006
7. Parmar H et al: Imaging findings in primary intracranial atypical teratoid/rhabdoid tumors. Pediatr Radiol. 36(2):126-32, 2006

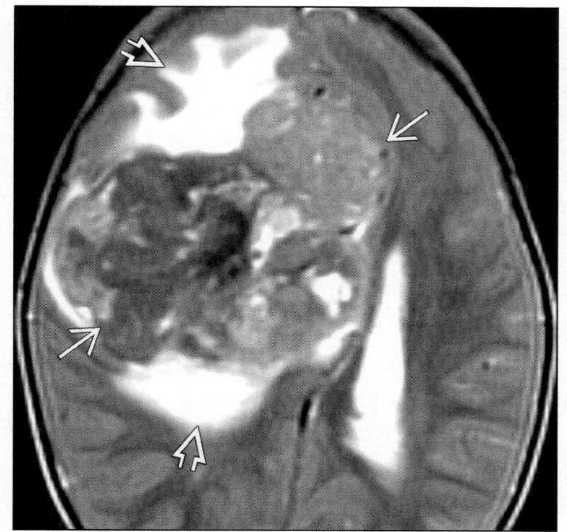

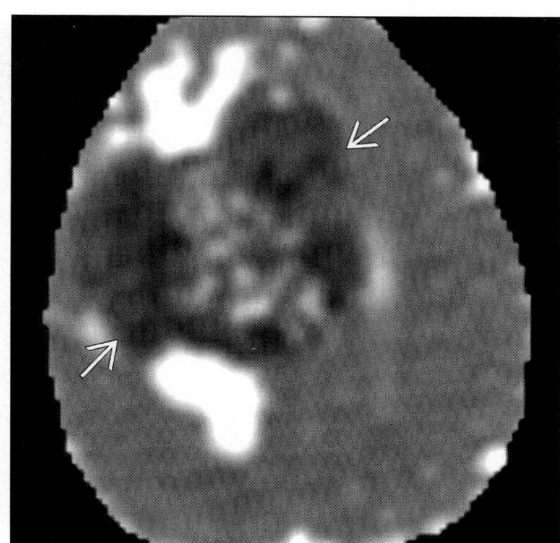

(Left) *Axial T2WI MR shows a large, bulky, supratentorial, heterogeneous tumor ➔ with central hemorrhage and mass effect. Although some edema is present ⇨, it is less than expected given the size of the tumor.* ***(Right)*** *Axial ADC in the same case shows decreased attenuated diffusion coefficient ➔ compatible with the hypercellular nature of the tumor.*

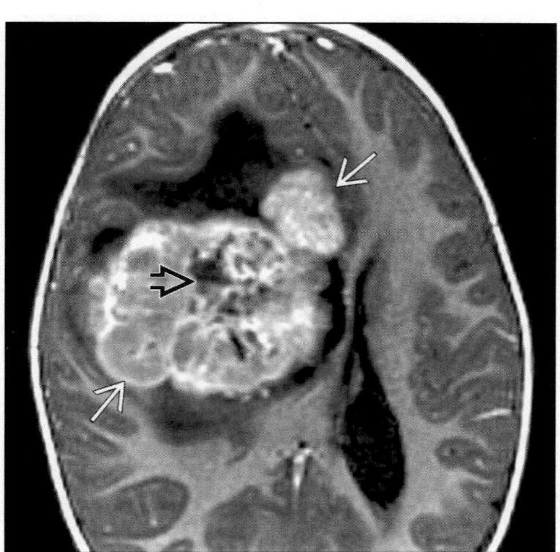

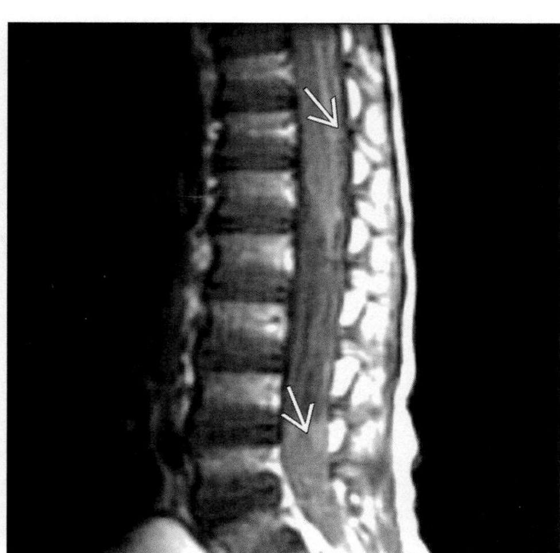

(Left) *Axial T1WI C+ MR in the same patient shows strong but rather heterogeneous enhancement ➔. Some central areas of necrosis ⇨ can be seen within the generally solid mass.* ***(Right)*** *Sagittal T1WI C+ MR demonstrates "drop" metastases ➔. Preoperative contrast-enhanced scans of the entire neuraxis should be obtained in all cases of posterior fossa neoplasms in children to rule out subarachnoid metastases, as in this example.*

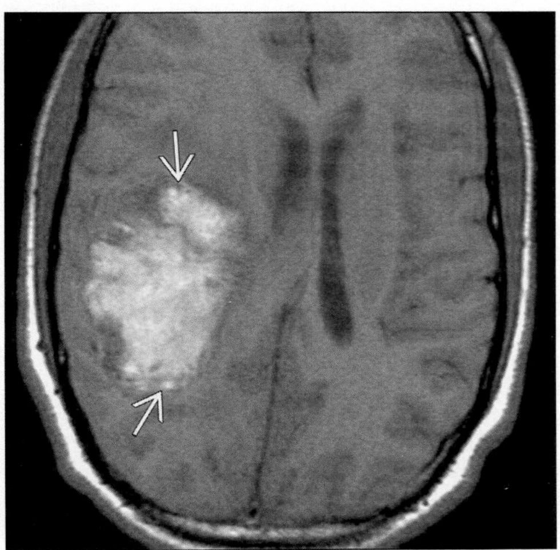

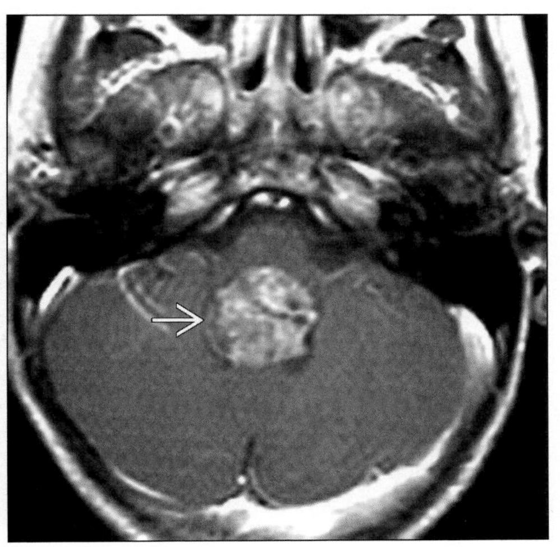

(Left) *Axial T1WI without contrast shows a T1 hyperintense right parietal mass ➔. This was confirmed as hemorrhage on gradient echo imaging. Surgical resection resulted in aggregates of highly pleomorphic cells strongly suggestive of AT/RT.* ***(Right)*** *Axial T1 C+ MR demonstrates a heterogeneously enhancing midline tumor ➔ in the 4th ventricle, which was pathologically proven to be AT/RT. Imaging findings are indistinguishable from those of medulloblastoma (PNET-MB).*

METASTATIC NEUROBLASTOMA

Key Facts

Terminology

- Malignant tumor of sympathetic nervous system arising from embryonal neural crest cell derivatives

Imaging

- Best diagnostic clue: Spiculated periorbital bone mass causing proptosis in child with "raccoon eyes"
- Often from bone marrow of bony orbit, typically roof or lateral wall/sphenoid wings
- Cranial metastases nearly always extradural, calvarial-based mass
  - Vigorously enhances but may be heterogeneous
- Classic imaging appearance: "Hair on end" spiculated periostitis of orbits and skull ± bone destruction
- Bone scan essential for differentiating stage IV disease from stage IV-S in children < 1 year

Top Differential Diagnoses

- Leukemia
- Langerhans cell histiocytosis (LCH)
- Extraaxial hematoma
- Ewing sarcoma

Pathology

- Calvarial metastases indicate stage IV disease
- Stage 4: < 1 year 60-75% survival; > 1 year 15% survival despite aggressive treatment
- Calvarial metastases indicate stage IV disease

Clinical Issues

- Most common tumor < 1 month (congenital)
- Median age at diagnosis = 22 months
- Ophthalmic manifestation in 20-55% at presentation
- Most common solid extracranial tumor < 5 years
- Metastasis to bone most common, 2/3 of patients at diagnosis

__(Left)__ Coronal NECT of a child with an abdominal mass reveals orbital, facial bone, and calvarial spiculated periostitis giving rise to a "hair on end" appearance ➔ with associated large soft tissue masses. Note bilateral disease ⇨. Metastatic stage IV neuroblastoma typically involves the skull and bony orbits. __(Right)__ Axial NECT in the same patient shows the "hair on end" appearance. Involvement of the orbits often gives rise to proptosis and ecchymosis "raccoon eyes," which may be mistaken for abuse.

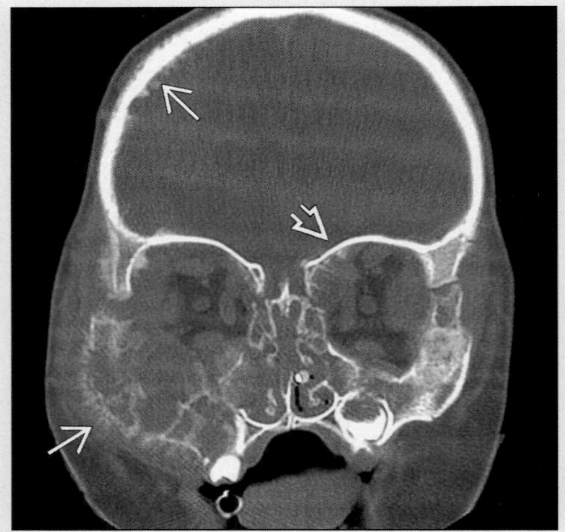

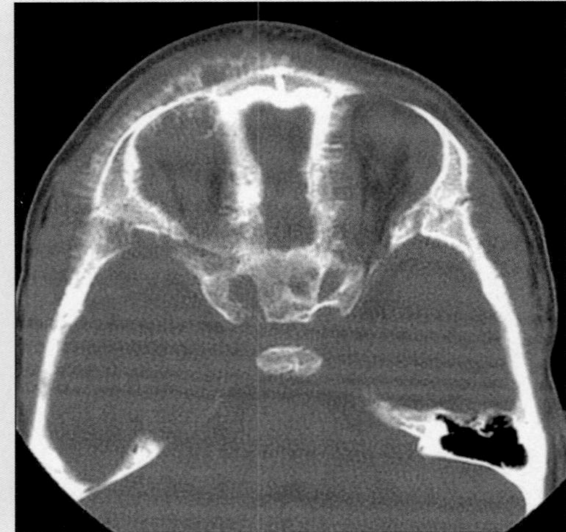

__(Left)__ Axial CECT shows strong, heterogeneously enhancing epidural masses ➔ with mass effect and edema in the frontal lobe. Intracranial involvement is typically from adjacent calvarial metastases with dural invasion. Brain parenchymal metastases are rare. __(Right)__ Axial T1WI C+ FS MR shows bilateral, orbital, enhancing soft tissue masses centered on the sphenoid bones. There is marked distortion of the right globe and proptosis. Note the intracranial dural extension ⇨.

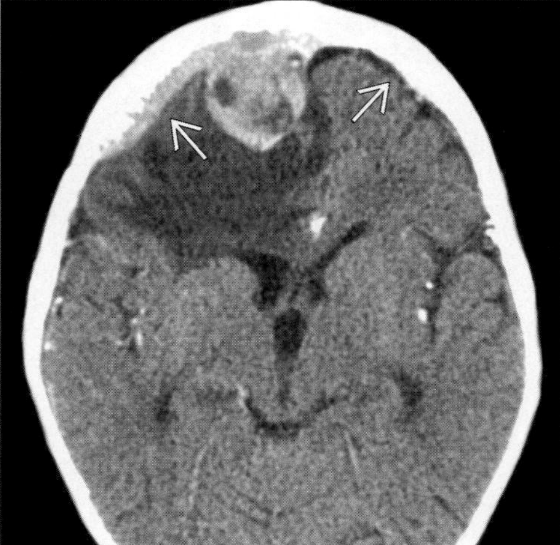

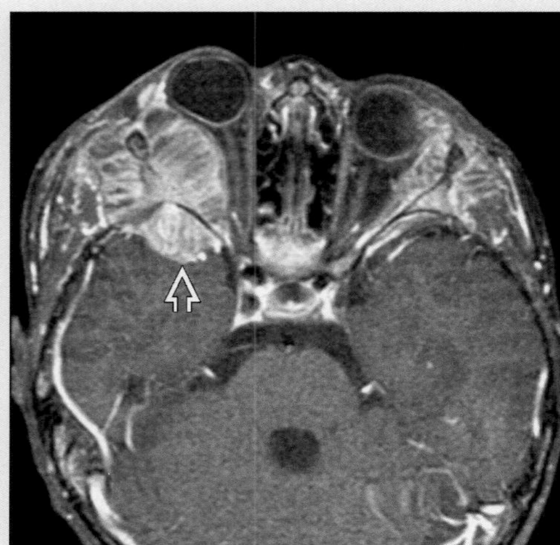

METASTATIC NEUROBLASTOMA

TERMINOLOGY

Abbreviations

- Neuroblastoma (NB), neuroblastic tumors (NBT)

Definitions

- Malignant tumor of sympathetic nervous system arising from embryonal neural crest cell derivatives

IMAGING

General Features

- Best diagnostic clue
  - Spiculated periorbital bone mass causing proptosis in child with "raccoon eyes"
- Location
  - Cranial metastases nearly always extradural calvarial-based masses
  - Often around bony orbit (roof/lateral wall) and sphenoid wings
  - Intraaxial lesions rare
- Morphology
  - Crescentic or lenticular, following contour of bone
  - Typically poorly defined
- Classic imaging appearance: "Hair on end" spiculated periostitis of orbits and skull, ± bony destruction

Radiographic Findings

- Radiography: Coronal suture widening and periosteal new bone

CT Findings

- NECT
  - NECT best for showing fine spicules of periosteal bone projecting off skull or sphenoid wings
  - Soft tissue mass typically iso- to hyperdense to brain
    - May mimic epidural or subdural hematoma
  - Mass projects into orbit (extraconal), with extension to surrounding spaces, not preseptal space
  - May project through inner and outer tables of skull
  - May be bilateral
- CECT
  - Enhancing dural metastasis if intracranial
  - Rare ring-enhancing brain parenchymal metastasis

MR Findings

- T1WI
  - Slightly heterogeneous
  - Hypointense to muscle
- T2WI
  - Heterogeneous
  - Hypointense to brain
  - Slightly hyperintense to muscle
- FLAIR: Heterogeneous; hyperintense to muscle
- T2* GRE: Hypointense
- T1WI C+: Vigorously enhances, may be heterogeneous
- MRV: May narrow or invade adjacent dural sinuses

Nuclear Medicine Findings

- Bone scan
  - MIBG (meta-iodobenzylguanidine)
    - Catecholamine analog
    - Labeled with iodine-131 or iodine-123
    - Avid uptake by neural crest tumors
      - NB, ganglioneuroblastoma, ganglioneuroma, carcinoid, medullary thyroid carcinoma
    - 99% specific for NBT
    - Caveat: Up to 30% of NB are not MIBG positive
      - Misses 50% of recurrent tumors
    - Cannot distinguish marrow disease from bone disease
  - Tc-99m-MDP (methylene diphosphonate)
    - Increased uptake from calcium metabolism of tumor not specific to neural crest tissue
    - 74% sensitivity for bony metastases
    - May distinguish marrow from bone disease
    - Bone scan essential for differentiating stage IV disease from stage IV-S in children < 1 year
  - In111 pentetreotide
    - Somatostatin analog
    - Not specific to NBT; not superior to MIBG
- PET
  - FDG PET has shown high sensitivity and specificity for recurrent tumor in small numbers of cases
  - FDG PET may identify recurrence when MIBG is negative due to dedifferentiation

Imaging Recommendations

- Best imaging tool
  - CT/MR to evaluate primary tumor
  - Nuclear medicine MIBG & Tc-99m-MDP bone scan
  - Brain/orbit CT if scintigraphy indicates metastases
- Protocol advice
  - MR C+ and fat saturation complementary to CT

DIFFERENTIAL DIAGNOSIS

Leukemia

- Dural- or calvarial-based masses
- More frequent parenchymal masses
- Less heterogeneous on MR

Langerhans Cell Histiocytosis (LCH)

- Lytic bone lesions without periosteal new bone
- Often associated with diabetes insipidus

Extraaxial Hematoma

- Subdural or epidural hematoma
- Bleeding disorder or child abuse to be considered

Ewing Sarcoma

- < 1% of cases involve skull
- Aggressive bone destruction
- Spiculated periosteal reaction

Osteosarcoma

- Rarely primary in calvarium

Rhabdomyosarcoma

- Most common soft tissue malignancy of pediatric orbit
- Less likely bilateral; may invade preseptal space

Beta Thalassemia Major

- Classic "hair on end" calvarial expansion
- Not focal or destructive like neuroblastoma

METASTATIC NEUROBLASTOMA

PATHOLOGY

General Features

- Etiology
  - Arises from pathologically maturing neural crest progenitor cells
  - Primary tumors arise at sites of sympathetic ganglia
  - No known causative factor
- Genetics
  - Multiple gene loci associated with NB 1p, 4p, 2p, 12p, 16p, 17q
    - Myc-N oncogene (chromosome 2) important marker
    - 35% have chromosome 1 short arm deletion
  - 1-2% of cases inherited
- Associated abnormalities
  - Rarely associated with Beckwith-Wiedemann syndrome, neurofibromatosis type 1
  - Some association with neurocristopathy syndromes
    - Hirschsprung disease, congenital central hypoventilation, DiGeorge syndrome

Staging, Grading, & Classification

- Calvarial metastases indicate stage IV disease
- International Neuroblastoma Staging System
  - Stage I: Confined to primary organ
  - Stage IIA: Unilateral tumor, no positive lymph nodes (LN)
  - Stage IIB: Unilateral tumor, unilateral positive LN
  - Stage III: Contralateral involvement
  - Stage IV: Distal metastases
  - Stage IV-S: < 1 year at diagnosis, stage I or II + metastatic disease confined to skin, liver, or bone marrow

Gross Pathologic & Surgical Features

- Grayish-tan soft nodules
- Infiltrating or circumscribed without capsule
- Necrosis, hemorrhage, and calcifications variable

Microscopic Features

- Undifferentiated round blue cells with scant cytoplasm, hyperchromatic nuclei
- May form Homer-Wright rosettes
- Ganglioneuroblastoma has interspersed mature ganglion cells
  - Different regions of same tumor may have ganglioneuroblastoma or NB

CLINICAL ISSUES

Presentation

- Most common signs/symptoms
  - "Raccoon eyes" (periorbital ecchymosis)
  - Palpable calvarial masses
- Other signs/symptoms
  - Palpable abdominal or paraspinal mass
  - Cranial metastatic disease rarely occurs in isolation
- Clinical profile
  - Ophthalmic manifestation in 20-55% at presentation
    - Proptosis and "raccoon eyes," 50% bilateral
    - Horner syndrome
    - Opsoclonus, myoclonus, and ataxia
      - Myoclonic encephalopathy of infancy
      - Paraneoplastic syndrome (not metastatic)
      - Up to 2-4% of NB patients; more favorable prognosis
  - Elevated vasoactive intestinal peptides (VIP)
    - Up to 7% of NBT patients
    - Diarrhea, hypokalemia, achlorhydria
  - Elevated homovanillic acid and vanillylmandelic acid in urine (> 90%)

Demographics

- Age
  - Median at diagnosis = 22 months
  - 40% diagnosed by 1 year
  - 35% between 1-2 years
  - 25% > 2 years
  - 89% by 5 years
- Gender
  - M:F = 1.2:1
- Epidemiology
  - Most common solid extracranial tumor < 5 years
  - 8-10% of all childhood cancer
  - Most common tumor in patients < 1 month (congenital)
  - Bony metastasis most common, 2/3 of patients at diagnosis
  - 1-2% spontaneously regress in 6-12 months, mostly stage IV-S
  - NB is most common and aggressive of NBT

Natural History & Prognosis

- Stage I, II, and IV-S have 3-year event free survival (EFS) of 75-90%
- Stage III: < 1 years old (80-90%) 1 year EFS; > 1 years old (50%) 3-year EFS
- Stage IV: < 1 years old (60-75%) 1 year EFS; > 1 years old (15%) 3-year EFS
- Poor prognostic indicators: Deletion of 1p, translocation of 17q, Myc-N amplification
- Good prognostic indicators: Localized disease, stage IV-S, decreased Myc-N amplification

Treatment

- Surgical resection + chemotherapy, radiation
- Bone marrow transplant
- Stage IV-S may spontaneously regress

DIAGNOSTIC CHECKLIST

Consider

- Abdominal imaging to identify primary tumor site

Image Interpretation Pearls

- CT without contrast can help identify bone spicules, eliminating LCH from differential

SELECTED REFERENCES

1. Heck JE et al: The epidemiology of neuroblastoma: a review. Paediatr Perinat Epidemiol. 23(2):125-43, 2009
2. Rothenberg AB et al: The association between neuroblastoma and opsoclonus-myoclonus syndrome: a historical review. Pediatr Radiol. 39(7):723-6, 2009

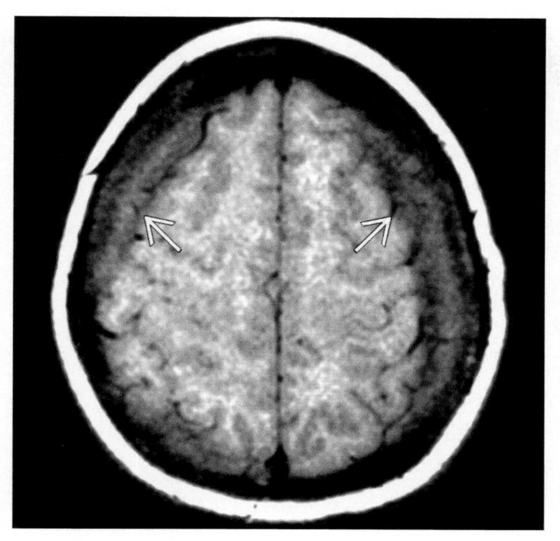

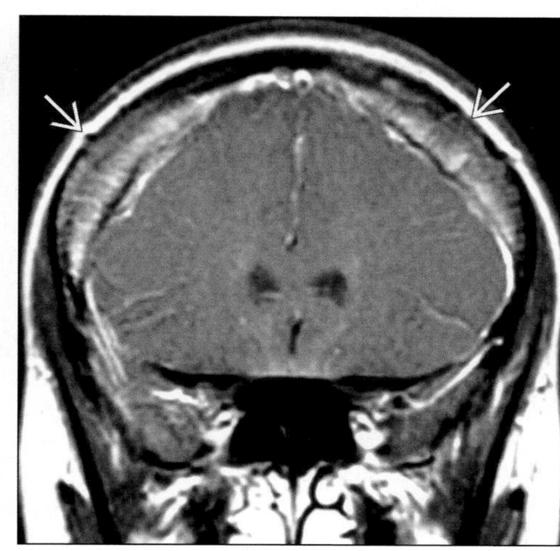

(Left) *Axial T1WI MR shows diffuse skull and dural thickening ➔ with no significant signal abnormality of the underlying parenchyma.* ***(Right)*** *Coronal T1WI C+ MR in the same patient shows enhancement of the skull and dura. Note the "hair on end" pattern ➔, typical for metastatic neuroblastoma. Stage IV neuroblastoma has a good prognosis when diagnosed in patients younger than 1 year. In patients older than 1 year, the 3-year survival rate drops below 15% despite aggressive treatment.*

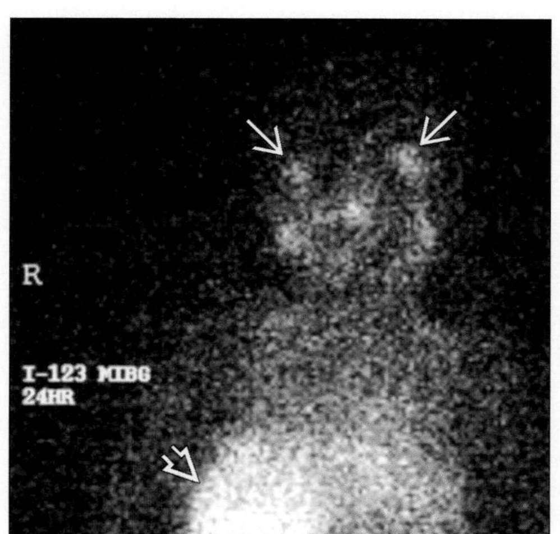

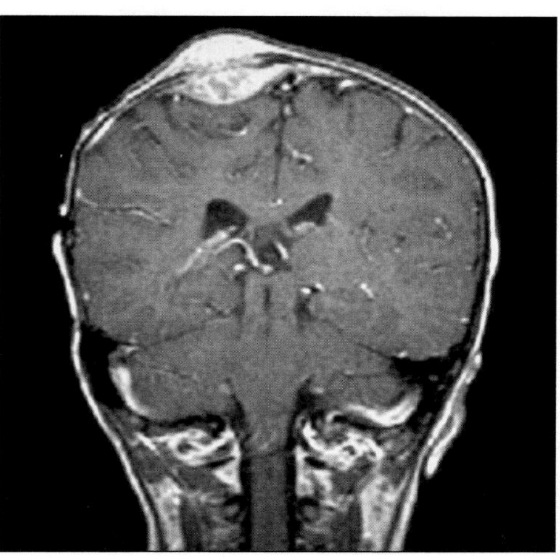

(Left) *Coronal I-123-labeled MIBG shows areas of increased uptake in the orbits ➔ related to neuroblastoma metastases. Note the large area of uptake in the right abdomen from the primary tumor ➔. Although MIBG scanning is highly specific for neuroblastic tumors, up to 30% of primary and 50% of recurrent neuroblastomas do not take up MIBG.* ***(Right)*** *Coronal T1WI C+ MR shows an enhancing convexity mass centered at the diploic space with subperiosteal and epidural components in a child with neuroblastoma.*

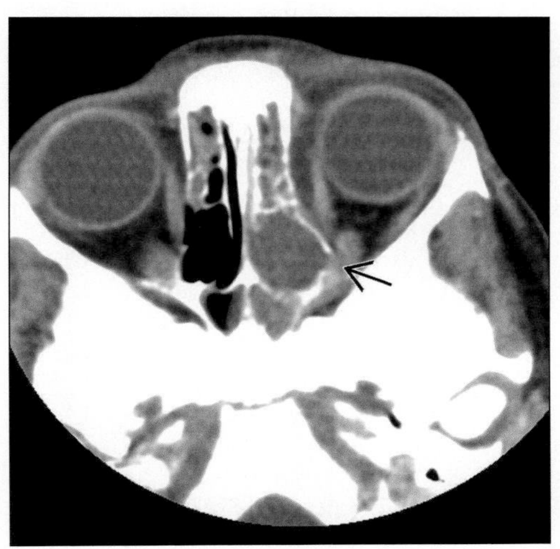

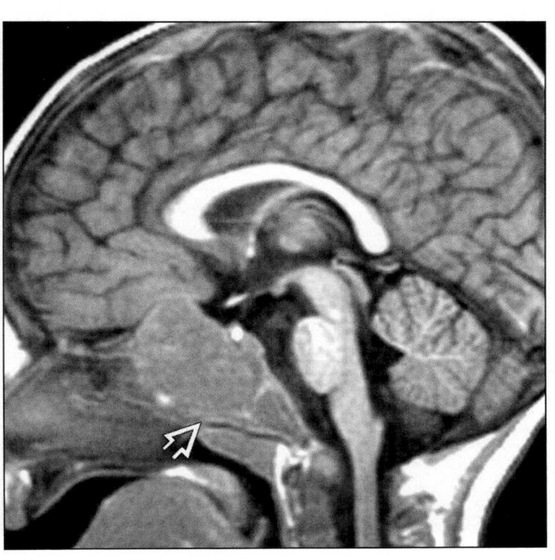

(Left) *Axial NECT in a child with neuroblastoma shows an ethmoid mass. There is a small focus of bony erosion ➔ suggesting the correct diagnosis of neuroblastoma metastasis.* ***(Right)*** *Sagittal T1WI MR shows a mildly heterogeneous, large, central skull base mass ➔ with marked expansion of the clivus in this 2 year old with stage IV neuroblastoma. Imaging mimics other malignancies. Neuroblastoma metastases most commonly involve the calvarium or orbital region.*

NONVESTIBULAR SCHWANNOMA

Key Facts

Terminology

- Benign encapsulated nerve sheath tumor composed of differentiated neoplastic Schwann cells
  - 99% of all schwannomas associated with cranial nerves
  - 95% involve CN8
  - < 1% of all intracranial schwannomas are intraparenchymal

Imaging

- CT
  - Iso- to slightly hyperdense compared to brain
  - Adjacent bone, foramina may show smooth, scalloped enlargement
  - Strong, sometimes heterogeneous enhancement
- MR
  - Heterogeneously hyperintense on T2WI, FLAIR
  - 100% enhance (strongly, heterogeneously)

Top Differential Diagnoses

- CN schwannoma (enlarged, enhancing cranial nerve[s])
  - Metastases
  - Lymphoma
  - Multiple sclerosis
  - Neurofibromatosis type 2
- Parenchymal schwannoma (rare)
  - Ganglioglioma
  - Pleomorphic xanthoastrocytoma
  - Pilocytic astrocytoma

Pathology

- Spindle-shaped neoplastic Schwann cells
- 2 basic tissue types seen
  - Compact, elongated cells (Antoni A pattern)
  - Less cellular, loosely textured ± lipidization (Antoni B pattern)

*(**Left**) Autopsy specimen sectioned through the 3rd ventricle and mammillary bodies shows a markedly enlarged left 3rd nerve ➔ compared to the normal-sized right oculomotor nerve ➔. Schwannoma of CN3 in a patient without evidence of NF2. (Courtesy E.T. Hedley-Whyte, MD.) (**Right**) Sagittal T1WI C+ MR shows an avidly enhancing olfactory schwannoma extending through the cribriform plate ➔. CSF collection ➔ behind the schwannoma leads to a deep frontal nonneoplastic tumor-associated cyst ➔.*

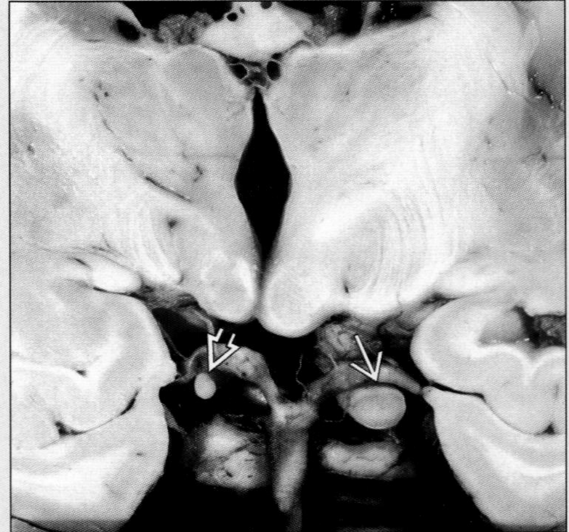

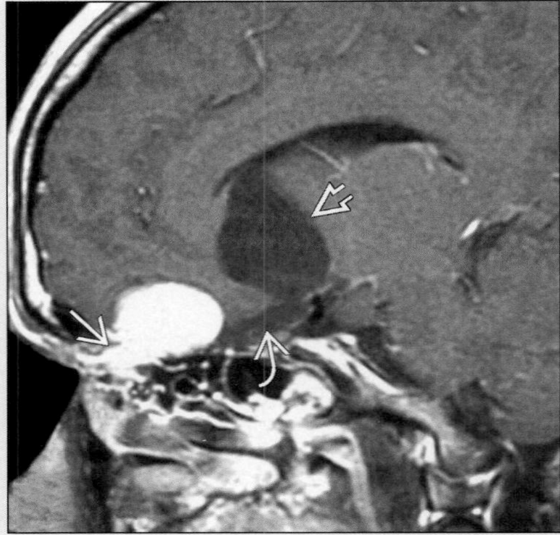

*(**Left**) Sagittal T2WI MR shows a giant trigeminal schwannoma that extends posteriorly from the Meckel cave ➔, eroding the clivus and abutting the pons ➔. (Courtesy M. Hartel, MD.) (**Right**) Axial T2WI MR in the same patient shows the classic "dumbbell" shape of a trigeminal schwannoma ➔. The lesion is inhomogeneously hyperintense. Note the indentation of the pons ➔ and enlargement of the ipsilateral CPA cistern ➔. (Courtesy M. Hartel, MD.)*

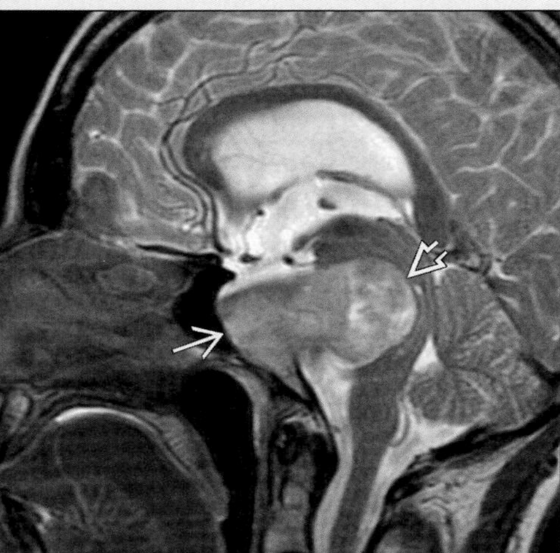

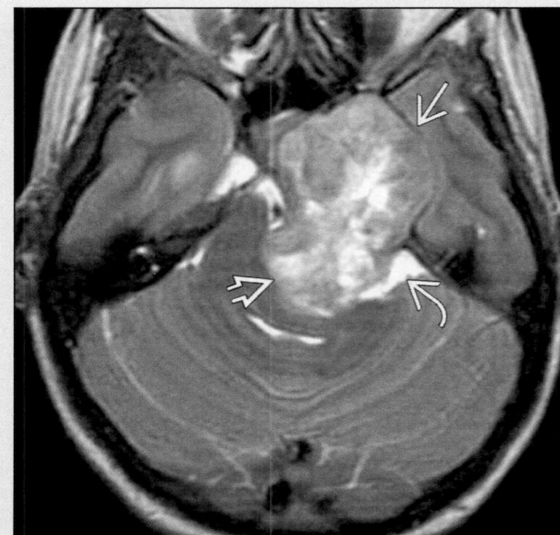

NONVESTIBULAR SCHWANNOMA

TERMINOLOGY

Abbreviations

- Nonvestibular schwannoma (nVS)

Synonyms

- Neurilemoma, neurinoma

Definitions

- Benign encapsulated nerve sheath tumor composed of differentiated neoplastic Schwann cells

IMAGING

General Features

- Best diagnostic clue
  - T2 hyperintense, strongly but heterogeneously enhancing cranial nerve mass
- Location
  - Extraaxial
    - 99% of all intracranial schwannomas are extraaxial
      - Arise from a cranial nerve
    - 95% associated with CN8 (vestibular schwannoma [VS])
      - VS = 2nd most common extraaxial tumor in adults (meningioma is most common)
      - VS accounts for ~ 90% of all CPA-IAC masses
    - Between 1-5% of intracranial schwannomas are nonvestibular schwannomas
    - Relative incidence of nVSs
      - Trigeminal nerve (CN5) 2nd most common schwannoma
      - Schwannomas of all other CNs are uncommon
      - 9 > 10 > 7 > 11 > 12
      - Nonvestibular schwannomas of CN3, 4, 6 rare in absence of neurofibromatosis type 2
  - Intraparenchymal
    - < 1% of all intracranial schwannomas
  - Schwannomas can be solitary or multiple
    - Solitary (sporadic) schwannoma
    - Multiple schwannomas
      - Neurofibromatosis type 2
      - Multiple schwannomatosis syndrome
- Size
  - Varies from tiny to enormous
    - Small schwannomas along oculomotor CNs (3, 4, 6)
    - Largest along CN8, 5
- Morphology
  - Smooth, well-demarcated, often lobulated

CT Findings

- NECT
  - Iso- to slightly hyperdense compared to brain
  - Look for effect on adjacent bone, foramina
    - **Smooth enlargement**
    - Thin, sclerotic but well-demarcated margins
    - CN5 schwannoma often extends into (or originates from) Meckel cave
    - Extracranial extension of nVS (e.g., CN5, 9) more common than with VS
  - Nonneoplastic tumor-associated cyst between tumor, brain in ~ 5%
  - Ca++, gross hemorrhage uncommon
- CECT
  - Strong, sometimes heterogeneous enhancement

MR Findings

- T1WI
  - Isointense to brain
  - Tumor-associated cyst hypointense
- T2WI
  - Inhomogeneously hyperintense
  - Tumor-associated cyst very hyperintense
- FLAIR
  - Both nodule, tumor-associated cyst may be hyperintense
- T2* GRE
  - May show small "blooming" hemorrhagic foci
- DWI
  - No restriction
- T1WI C+
  - 100% enhance
    - Strong, often heterogeneous
    - 10-15% have intramural cysts (nonenhancing)
    - Nonneoplastic tumor-associated cysts do not enhance

Imaging Recommendations

- Best imaging tool
  - Precontrast T1-, T2WIs; whole brain FLAIR with axial, coronal T1WI C+ FS
- Protocol advice
  - For suspected cranial nerve schwannoma
    - Add thin-section high-resolution T2 or CISS

DIFFERENTIAL DIAGNOSIS

CN Schwannoma

- Enlarged, enhancing cranial nerve(s)
  - Metastases
  - Lymphoma
  - Multiple sclerosis
  - Neurofibromatosis type 2
  - Neurosarcoid
  - Chronic inflammatory demyelinating polyneuropathy (CIDP)

Parenchymal Schwannoma (Rare)

- Ganglioglioma
- Pleomorphic xanthoastrocytoma
- Pilocytic astrocytoma
- Hemangioblastoma

PATHOLOGY

General Features

- Etiology
  - Benign cranial nerve tumor
    - Arises from glial-Schwann cell junction
    - Distance from brain to glial-Schwann cell junction varies according to CN

NONVESTIBULAR SCHWANNOMA

- Parenchymal schwannoma may arise from dedifferentiated neural crest cells
- Genetics
  - Inactivating mutations of neurofibromatosis type 2 tumor suppressor gene in 60% of sporadic schwannomas
    - Loss of remaining wild-type allele on chromosome 22q
    - Encodes Merlin (schwannomin) protein

Staging, Grading, & Classification

- WHO grade I

Gross Pathologic & Surgical Features

- Yellowish tan, rubbery
  - Round/ovoid
  - Encapsulated, well delineated
- Arises eccentrically from cranial nerve
  - Nerve often appears "splayed" over schwannoma
- 15-20% have associated fluid-filled cysts
  - Most are small, intratumoral
  - Occasionally large, nonneoplastic, fluid-containing collections form between tumor and brain
- Hemorrhage
  - Small hemorrhagic foci occur but are uncommon
  - Gross hemorrhage rare (< 1%)

Microscopic Features

- Spindle-shaped neoplastic Schwann cells
- 2 basic tissue types seen
  - Compact, elongated cells with occasional nuclear palisading (Antoni A pattern)
    - "Verocay" bodies = foci of prominent nuclear palisades separated by anuclear area
  - Less cellular, loosely textured cells with variable lipidization (Antoni B pattern)
- Immunohistochemistry
  - S100 protein strongly expressed
  - Vimentin variably expressed
  - Usually GFAP negative
- Rare variant = melanotic schwannoma

CLINICAL ISSUES

Presentation

- Most common signs/symptoms
  - Cranial nerve schwannoma
    - Vestibular schwannoma
      - Unilateral sensorineural hearing loss
      - Small VS: Tinnitus, disequilibrium common
      - Large VS: Trigeminal ± facial neuropathy
    - Symptoms of nVS vary depending on which nerve is affected
  - Parenchymal schwannoma
    - Much less common
    - Seizure
    - Headache
    - Focal neurologic deficit uncommon

Demographics

- Age
  - Adult (unless neurofibromatosis type 2)
    - Age range = 30-70 years
    - Peak = 40-60 years
- Epidemiology
  - Schwannomas account for 8% of all intracranial tumors
  - Vestibular schwannoma accounts for 90% of all CPA masses
  - 90% of schwannomas are solitary
  - 5% associated with neurofibromatosis type 2
  - 5% associated with multiple schwannomatosis syndrome

Natural History & Prognosis

- Benign, slowly growing
- Malignant change extremely rare

Treatment

- Vestibular schwannoma
  - Resection
  - Fractionated/stereotaxic neurosurgery
- Other (nonvestibular schwannoma)
  - Varies with location

DIAGNOSTIC CHECKLIST

Consider

- Patient may have NF2 if
  - nVS in unusual location
  - > 1 schwannoma
  - Coexisting meningioma identified

SELECTED REFERENCES

1. Ambekar S et al: Frontal intraparenchymal Schwannoma--case report and review of literature. Br J Neurosurg. 23(1):86-9, 2009
2. Asthagiri AR et al: Neurofibromatosis type 2. Lancet. 373(9679):1974-86, 2009
3. Ito E et al: Factors predicting growth of vestibular schwannoma in neurofibromatosis type 2. Neurosurg Rev. 32(4):425-33, 2009
4. James MF et al: NF2/merlin is a novel negative regulator of mTOR complex 1, and activation of mTORC1 is associated with meningioma and schwannoma growth. Mol Cell Biol. 29(15):4250-61, 2009
5. Kano H et al: Stereotactic radiosurgery for trigeminal schwannoma: tumor control and functional preservation Clinical article. J Neurosurg. 110(3):553-8, 2009
6. Marzo SJ et al: Facial nerve schwannoma. Curr Opin Otolaryngol Head Neck Surg. Epub ahead of print, 2009
7. Mathiesen T et al: Hypoglossal schwannoma-successful reinnervation and functional recovery of the tongue following tumour removal and nerve grafting. Acta Neurochir (Wien). 151(7):837-41; discussion 841, 2009
8. Menkü A et al: Atypical intracerebral schwannoma mimicking glial tumor: case report. Turk Neurosurg. 19(1):82-5, 2009
9. Mukherjee J et al: Human schwannomas express activated platelet-derived growth factor receptors and c-kit and are growth inhibited by Gleevec (Imatinib Mesylate). Cancer Res. 69(12):5099-107, 2009
10. Sughrue ME et al: The natural history of untreated sporadic vestibular schwannomas: a comprehensive review of hearing outcomes. J Neurosurg. Epub ahead of print, 2009

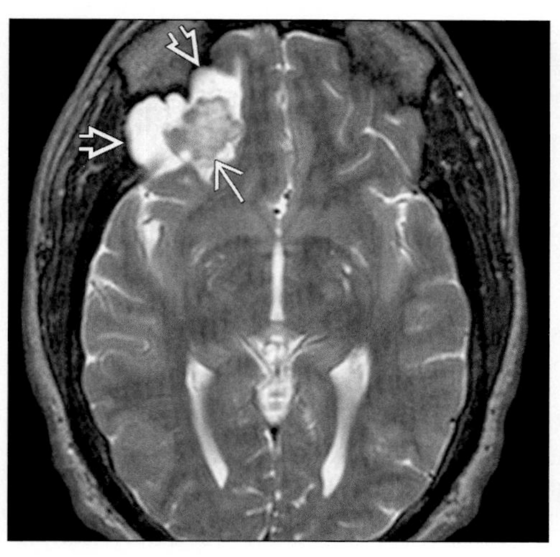

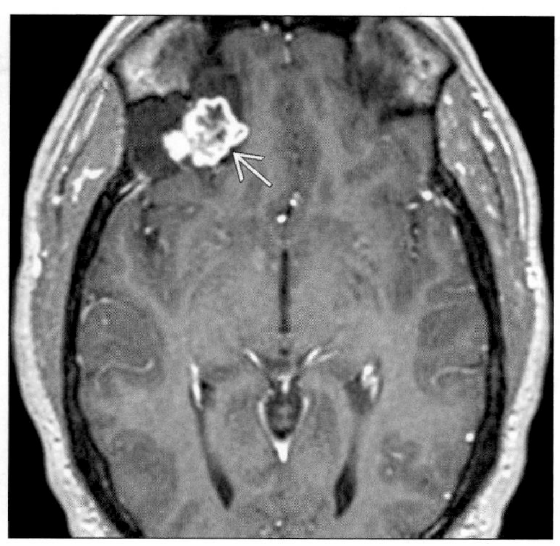

(Left) *Axial T2WI MR demonstrates a cystic mass with a mural nodule in the right inferior frontal lobe. Note the remodeling/scalloping of the adjacent calvarium, characterizing this as a slow-growing mass.* ***(Right)*** *Axial T1WI C+ MR in the same patient shows that the mural nodule enhances inhomogeneously. Most intracranial schwannomas are extraaxial, associated with cranial nerves. Parenchymal schwannomas are rare (< 1% of schwannomas). Most are seen as a cyst with a mural nodule.*

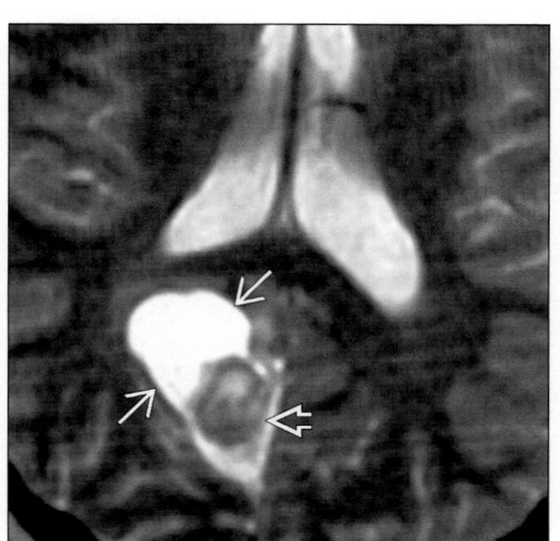

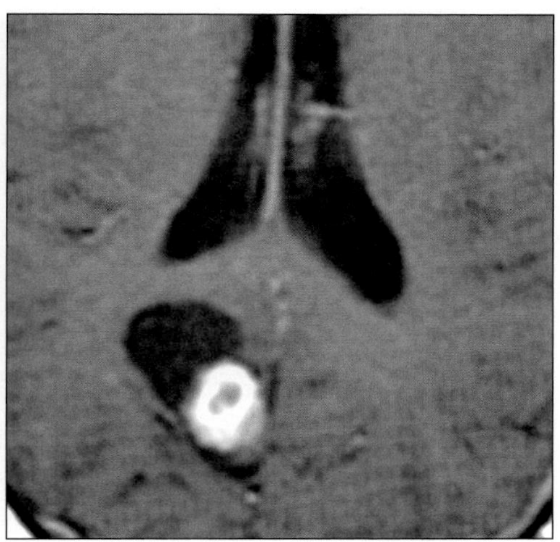

(Left) *Axial T2WI MR in a young adult with epilepsy shows a cystic occipital mass with a superficial mural nodule that abuts the interhemispheric fissure.* ***(Right)*** *Axial T1WI C+ MR in the same patient shows that the nodule enhances strongly but heterogeneously. The preoperative diagnosis was ganglioglioma; intraparenchymal schwannoma was found at surgery.*

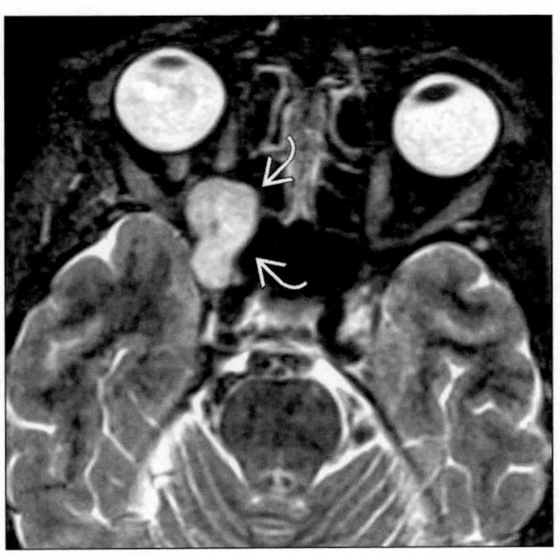

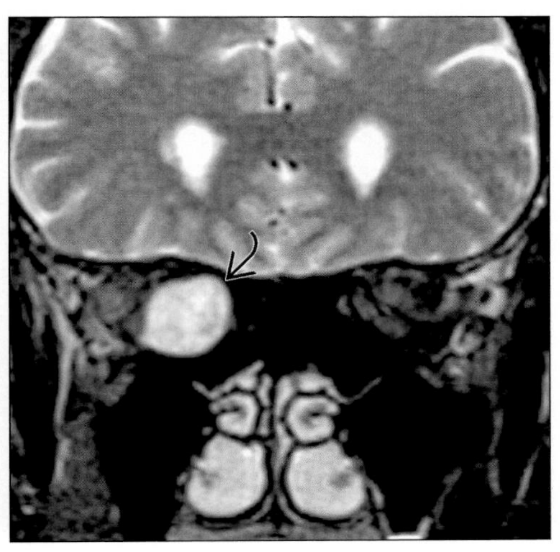

(Left) *Axial T2WI MR shows a lobulated, densely enhancing mass at the right orbital apex proven to be a ciliary schwannoma.* ***(Right)*** *Coronal T2WI MR shows the hyperintense ciliary schwannoma displacing orbital structures laterally.*

NEUROFIBROMA

Key Facts

Terminology
- PNF: Infiltrative extraneural tumor
  - Occurs exclusively in NF1
- SNF: Round/ovoid subcutaneous mass
  - Usually solitary
  - Not associated with NF1

Imaging
- General features
  - PNF: NF1 patient with poorly delineated, infiltrating, worm-like, soft tissue mass
  - PNF: Orbit (CNV1), scalp, parotid
  - SNF: Well-circumscribed round/oval scalp mass
  - SNF: Skin, spinal, or peripheral nerve roots (rarely, if ever, involves CNs)
- CT
  - PNF infiltrates CNV1, may enlarge superior orbital fissure
  - May extend intracranially into cavernous sinus
- MR
  - Isointense, infiltrating on T1WI
  - Hyperintense on T2WI
  - Strong, somewhat heterogeneous enhancement

Top Differential Diagnoses
- Schwannoma
- Metastasis
- Malignant peripheral nerve sheath tumor (MPNST)
- Sarcoma

Clinical Issues
- 2-12% of PNFs degenerate into MPNST

Diagnostic Checklist
- Look for other imaging stigmata of NF1 (WM lesions, sphenoid aplasia, etc.)

*(**Left**) Axial graphic shows extensive plexiform neurofibroma of the right face and orbit, resulting in proptosis. (**Right**) Axial T2WI FS MR shows a large, multilobulated, right cavernous sinus mass → with extension through markedly enlarged superior orbital fissure into the retrobulbar space →. Note the right temporal scalp involvement →. Plexiform neurofibromas in and around the orbit and scalp rarely have this degree of intracranial involvement.*

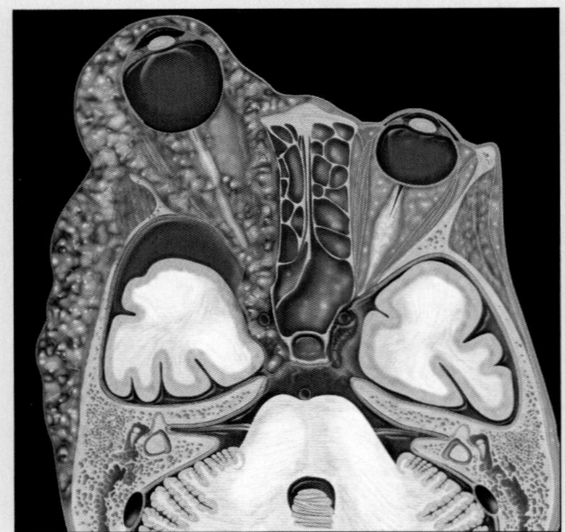

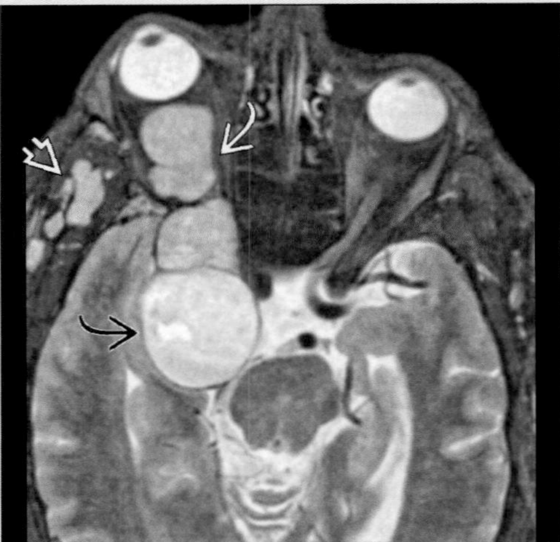

*(**Left**) Sagittal T1WI MR in a 17 year old with a longstanding history of a "lump on my head" shows a well-delineated, focal enhancing scalp mass →. The lesion abuts but does not invade the skull. (**Right**) In the same patient, axial T1WI C+ FS MR shows that the well-delineated mass enhances strongly and uniformly →. No other subcutaneous lesions were identified, and the brain appeared normal. This was diagnosed as a solitary neurofibroma in a patient without neurofibromatosis type 1.*

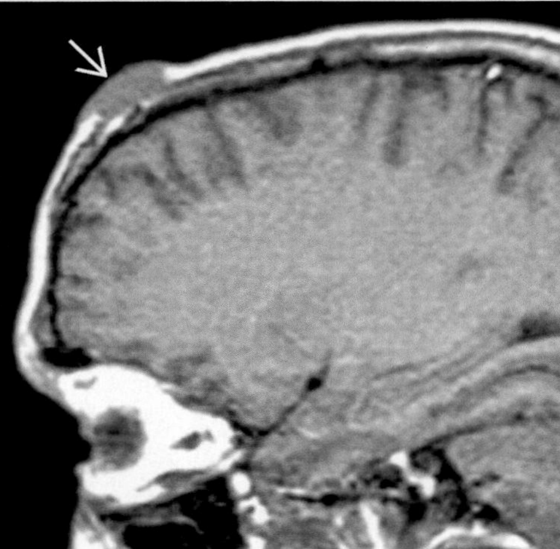

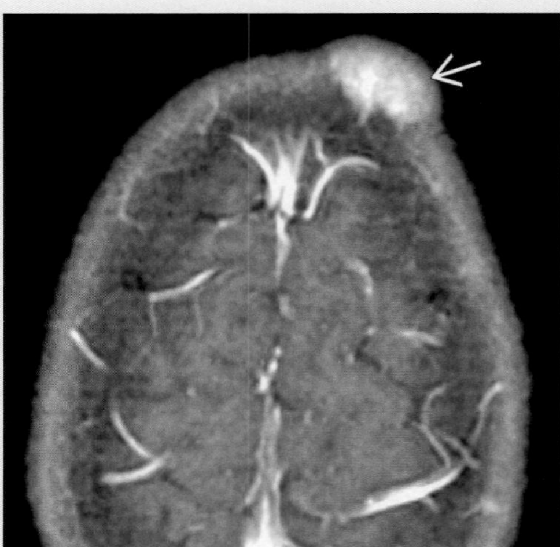

NEUROFIBROMA

TERMINOLOGY

Abbreviations
- Neurofibroma (NF)
- Plexiform neurofibroma (PNF)
- Solitary neurofibroma (SNF)

Definitions
- PNF: Infiltrative extraneural tumor
  - Occurs exclusively in patients with neurofibromatosis type 1 (NF1)
- SNF: Round/ovoid subcutaneous mass
  - Not associated with NF1

IMAGING

General Features
- Best diagnostic clue
  - PNF: NF1 patient with poorly delineated, worm-like, soft tissue mass infiltrating scalp, orbit, or parotid
  - SNF: Well-circumscribed round/oval scalp mass
- Location
  - PNF: Orbit (CNV1) most common head/neck site
    - Scalp, parotid gland (CN7)
    - Spinal, peripheral nerve roots
  - SNF: Skin, spinal, or peripheral nerve roots
    - Rarely (if ever) involves cranial nerves
- Morphology
  - Can be small or large; well demarcated (SNF) or diffusely infiltrating (PNF)

CT Findings
- NECT
  - Plexiform NF
    - Mass infiltrates CNV1
    - PNFs may enlarge orbital fissure
      - May extend into cavernous sinus (almost never posterior to Meckel cave)
    - Other sites: Scalp, skull base (e.g., parotid gland, pterygopalatine fossa)
- CECT
  - Moderate/strong enhancement

MR Findings
- T1WI
  - Plexiform NF = isointense infiltrating mass
- T2WI
  - Hyperintense
- T1WI C+
  - Enhances strongly, sometimes heterogeneously

Imaging Recommendations
- Best imaging tool
  - MR ± contrast
- Protocol advice
  - PNF: Scan entire neuraxis to detect other manifestations of NF1

DIFFERENTIAL DIAGNOSIS

Schwannoma
- Usually solitary, well circumscribed
- May involve CNs, spinal nerve roots (rare in scalp)

Metastasis
- Scalp lesions rare without underlying bone/dura involvement

Malignant Peripheral Nerve Sheath Tumor
- Infiltrative, invasive

Sarcoma of Skull/Scalp
- Kaposi sarcoma (usually in AIDS patients)
- Ewing sarcoma (metastatic)

Lymphoma
- Skull, dura often involved

Vascular Malformation of Scalp
- Can be seen in patients with NF1

PATHOLOGY

General Features
- Genetics
  - Germline *NF1* mutation + loss of remaining wild-type allele
- Associated abnormalities
  - PNFs = other stigmata of NF1

Staging, Grading, & Classification
- NF = WHO grade I

Gross Pathologic & Surgical Features
- Plexiform NF may look like infiltrating "bag of worms"
- Solitary NF is ovoid/fusiform circumscribed nodule

Microscopic Features
- Neoplastic Schwann cells + fibroblasts
- Matrix of collagen fibers, mucoid substances

CLINICAL ISSUES

Presentation
- Most common signs/symptoms
  - Painless scalp or skin mass

Natural History & Prognosis
- Slow growth
- 2-12% of PNFs and NFs of major nerves degenerate into malignant peripheral nerve sheath tumor

Treatment
- ± surgical resection (PNFs have high recurrence rate)

DIAGNOSTIC CHECKLIST

Consider
- Look for other stigmata of NF1 (café au lait spots, axillary freckling, Lisch nodules, etc.)

SELECTED REFERENCES

1. Canelas MM et al: Lipomatous neurofibroma associated with segmental neurofibromatosis. J Cutan Pathol. Epub ahead of print, 2009

HEMANGIOBLASTOMA

Key Facts

Terminology
- Highly vascular tumor of adults most commonly found in cerebellum, brainstem, spinal cord
  - 25-40% of HGBLs occur in patients with VHL

Imaging
- General features
  - Adult with intraaxial posterior fossa mass
  - 60% cyst + "mural" nodule
  - 90-95% in posterior fossa
  - 5-10% supratentorial (around optic pathways, hemispheres; usually in VHL)

Top Differential Diagnoses
- von Hippel-Lindau syndrome (VHL)
- Metastasis
- Pilocytic astrocytoma
- Cavernous malformation (CM)
- Hereditary hemorrhagic telangiectasia (HHT)

Pathology
- Red or yellowish, well-circumscribed, unencapsulated, highly vascular mass that abuts leptomeninges
- Histology shows stromal cells, innumerable small vessels
- WHO grade I

Clinical Issues
- Primary therapy = en bloc surgical resection; piecemeal may result in catastrophic hemorrhage

Diagnostic Checklist
- Most common posterior fossa intraaxial mass in middle-aged/older adult is metastasis, not HGBL!
- Most common posterior fossa primary tumor in middle-aged/older adult is HGBL

__(Left)__ Coronal graphic shows a classic cerebellar hemangioblastoma, seen here as a largely cystic mass ➔ with a very vascular tumor nodule ➔ that is abutting the pia. __(Right)__ Coronal gross pathology shows a solitary hemangioblastoma of the cerebellar hemisphere. The well-delineated, very vascular-appearing tumor nodule ➔ abuts the pia, a classic finding of hemangioblastomas. Note the lack of edema and invasion of adjacent tissue. (Courtesy E. Ross, MD.)

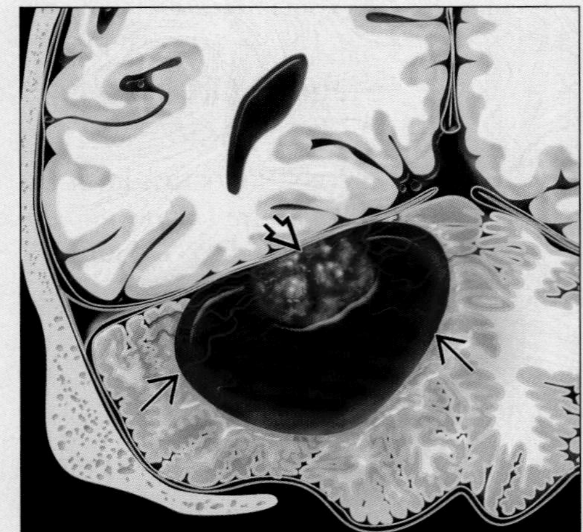

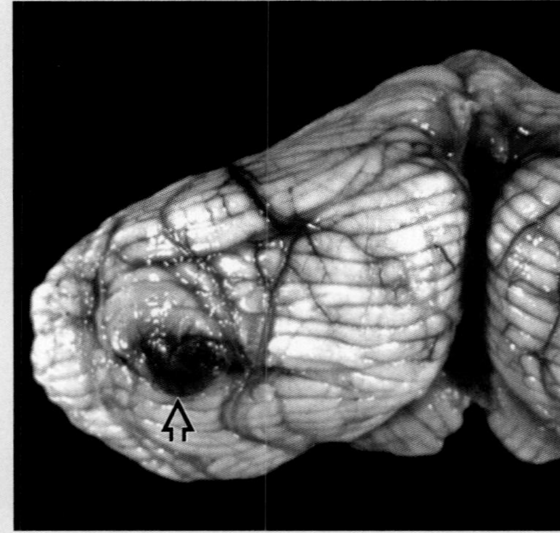

__(Left)__ Axial T1WI C+ MR shows a mixed cystic ➔ and solid enhancing ➔ tumor of the right cerebellar hemisphere. The solid enhancing nodule abuts the pia and projects into the right cerebellopontine angle cistern. Note the lack of enhancement of the cyst wall, which consists of compressed but normal cerebellum. __(Right)__ Coronal T1WI C+ MR shows a typical hemangioblastoma with a benign, nonenhancing cyst wall ➔ and a strongly enhancing tumor nodule ➔ abutting the pial surface of the cerebellum.

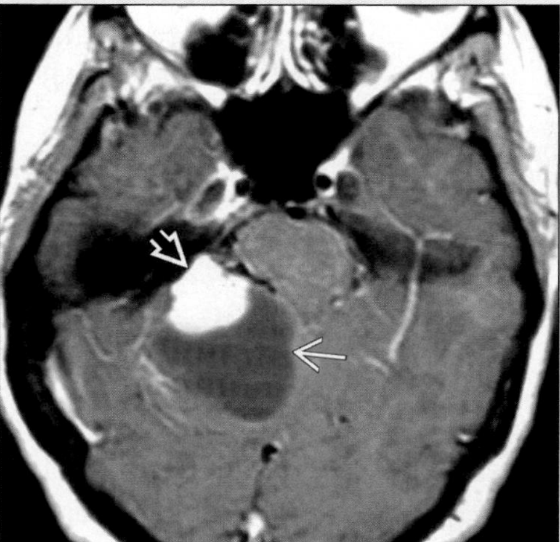

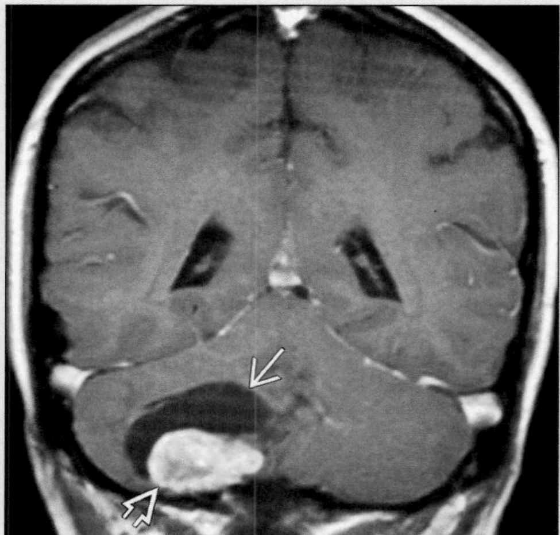

HEMANGIOBLASTOMA

TERMINOLOGY

Abbreviations

- Hemangioblastoma (HGBL)

Synonyms

- Capillary hemangioblastoma

Definitions

- Slow-growing, highly vascular tumor of adults most commonly found in cerebellum, brainstem, spinal cord

IMAGING

General Features

- Best diagnostic clue
  - Adult with intraaxial posterior fossa mass with cyst, enhancing mural nodule abutting pia (classic)
- Location
  - Posterior fossa (90-95%)
    - Cerebellar hemispheres (80%)
    - Vermis (15%), other, e.g., medulla, 4th ventricle (5%)
  - Supratentorial (5-10%) (around optic pathways, hemispheres; usually in von Hippel-Lindau)
  - Rarely extraaxial dural-based mass
    - May also rarely be extramedullary in spine
- Size
  - Size varies from tiny to several cms
- Morphology
  - 60% cyst + "mural" nodule; 40% solid

CT Findings

- NECT
  - Low-density cyst + isodense nodule
- CECT
  - Nodule enhances intensely, relatively uniformly
  - Cyst wall usually does not enhance
- CTA
  - May demonstrate arterial feeders

MR Findings

- T1WI
  - Nodule isointense with brain ± flow voids
  - Cyst slightly/moderately hyperintense compared to CSF
- T2WI
  - Both nodule, cyst are hyperintense
  - Prominent flow voids in some cases
- FLAIR
  - Both cyst and nodule hyperintense
- T2* GRE
  - May "bloom" if blood products present
- DWI
  - Cyst slightly or markedly low signal
- T1WI C+
  - Common: Nodule enhances strongly, intensely
  - Less common: Solid tumor enhancement
  - Rare: Ring-enhancing mass

Angiographic Findings

- Rarely performed as diagnosis is established by MR and preoperative embolization not generally used
  - Large avascular mass (cyst)
  - Highly vascular nodule
    - Prolonged blush
    - ± arteriovenous shunting (early draining vein)

Nuclear Medicine Findings

- Thallium-201 SPECT shows fast washout

Imaging Recommendations

- Best imaging tool
  - Contrast-enhanced MR (sensitivity > > CT for small HGBLs)
- Protocol advice
  - Begin MR screening of patients from von Hippel-Lindau families after 10 years of age
  - Screen complete spine, as cord lesions are common

DIFFERENTIAL DIAGNOSIS

von Hippel-Lindau Syndrome (VHL)

- 25-40% of HGBLs occur in VHL
- Multiple HGBLs are rule in VHL
- Other markers (visceral cysts, renal clear cell carcinoma), + family history

Metastasis

- Solitary posterior fossa metastasis uncommon
  - **But** most common parenchymal posterior fossa mass in middle-aged, older adults is metastasis!
- May be very vascular
- Solid > cystic
- Multiple > single
- Vascular mets (renal cell carcinoma) do not express inhibin A or GLUT1; HGBL does

Astrocytoma

- Pilocytic astrocytoma (PA)
  - Usually in children
- Glioblastoma
  - Adults with irregular ring-enhancing mass
  - Posterior fossa uncommon location

Vascular Neurocutaneous Syndromes

- Hereditary hemorrhagic telangiectasia (HHT)
- Wyburn-Mason
- Multiple intracranial AVMs may mimic HGBLs

Cavernous Malformation (CM)

- Gross intratumoral hemorrhage rare in HGBL
- Complete hemosiderin rim typical in CMs

Clear Cell Ependymoma

- Rare; younger patients

PATHOLOGY

General Features

- Etiology
  - Precise histogenesis unknown

HEMANGIOBLASTOMA

- Presence of 2 cell types suggests undifferentiated precursor cell with angiogenic and stromal potential
- Alternative theory: Stromal cells are neoplastic and vascular cells are nonneoplastic response to stromal VEGF

- Genetics
  - Familial HGBL (von Hippel-Lindau disease)
    - Autosomal dominant
    - Chromosome 3p mutation
    - Suppressor gene product (VHL protein) causes neoplastic transformation
    - VEGF highly expressed in stromal cells
    - Other *VHL* gene mutations common
  - Sporadic HGBL
    - Upregulation of erythropoietin common in both sporadic, VHL-related HGBL
- Associated abnormalities
  - Secondary polycythemia (may elaborate erythropoietin)
  - 25-40% of patients with HGBL have VHL

Staging, Grading, & Classification

- WHO grade I
- Low MIB-1 index (mean 0.8%)
- No difference between sporadic, VHL-associated HGBLs

Gross Pathologic & Surgical Features

- Red or yellowish, well-circumscribed, unencapsulated, highly vascular mass that abuts leptomeninges
- ± cyst with yellow-brown fluid

Microscopic Features

- Nodule
  - Large vacuolated stromal cells
    - Neoplastic component
    - Lipid-containing vacuoles ("clear cell" morphology)
  - Immunohistochemistry
    - Negative for cytokeratin, EMA
    - Positive for inhibin A, GLUT1
    - Overexpress VEGF protein
  - Rich capillary network
- Cyst wall
  - Usually compressed brain (not neoplasm)
  - Variable intratumoral hemorrhage

CLINICAL ISSUES

Presentation

- Most common signs/symptoms
  - Sporadic HGBL
    - Headache (85%), dysequilibrium, dizziness
  - Familial
    - Retinal HGBL: Ocular hemorrhage often 1st manifestation of VHL
    - Other: Symptoms due to renal cell carcinoma, polycythemia, endolymphatic sac tumor

Demographics

- Age
  - Sporadic HGBL
    - Peak 40-60 years
    - Rare in children
  - Familial
    - VHL-associated HGBLs occur at younger age (rare < 15 years)
    - Retinal HGBL: Mean onset 25 years
- Gender
  - Slight male predominance
- Epidemiology
  - VHL seen in 1:36-40,000
  - Less than half (25-40%) HGBLs associated with VHL
  - 1-2% of primary intracranial tumors
    - 7-10% of posterior fossa tumors
  - 3-13% of spinal cord tumors

Natural History & Prognosis

- Usually benign tumor with slow growth pattern
  - Symptoms usually associated with cyst expansion (may occur rapidly)
  - Rare: Leptomeningeal tumor dissemination, leptomeningeal hemangioblastomatosis
- 2/3 with a single VHL-associated HGBL develop additional lesions
  - Average: 1 new lesion every 2 years
  - Require periodic screening, lifelong follow-up
  - Periods of intermixed growth, relative quiescence common with VHL-associated HGBL
  - Median life expectancy in patients with VHL: 49 years

Treatment

- En bloc surgical resection (piecemeal may result in catastrophic hemorrhage)
  - 10-year survival rate: 85%
  - Recurrence rate: 15-20%
- Preoperative embolization: Limited efficacy and usage
- Expectant management without surgery may occasionally be considered if lesion is stable and nonsymptomatic
- Evolving medical and gene target therapies

DIAGNOSTIC CHECKLIST

Consider

- Screen entire neuraxis for other HGBLs

Image Interpretation Pearls

- Most common posterior fossa intraaxial mass in middle-aged/older adult is metastasis, not HGBL!
- Most common posterior fossa primary tumor in middle-aged/older adult is HGBL

Reporting Tips

- Degree of mass effect
- Presence of hemorrhage
- Extent of additional screening needed

SELECTED REFERENCES

1. Courcoutsakis NA et al: Aggressive leptomeningeal hemangioblastomatosis of the central nervous system in a patient with von Hippel-Lindau disease. AJNR Am J Neuroradiol. 30(4):758-60, 2009
2. Parker F et al: Results of microsurgical treatment of medulla oblongata and spinal cord hemangioblastomas: a comparison of two distinct clinical patient groups. J Neurooncol. 93(1):133-7, 2009

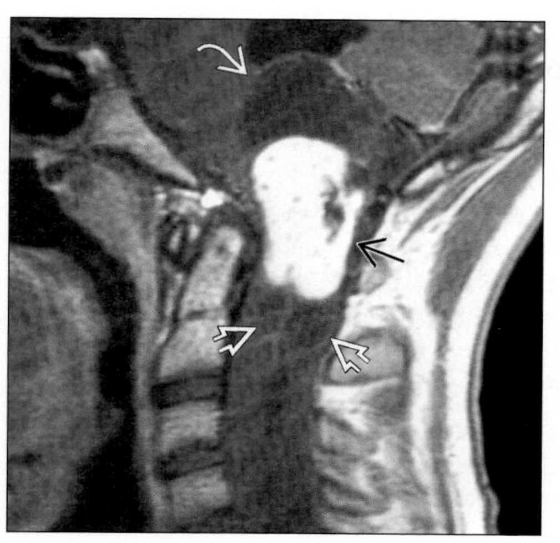

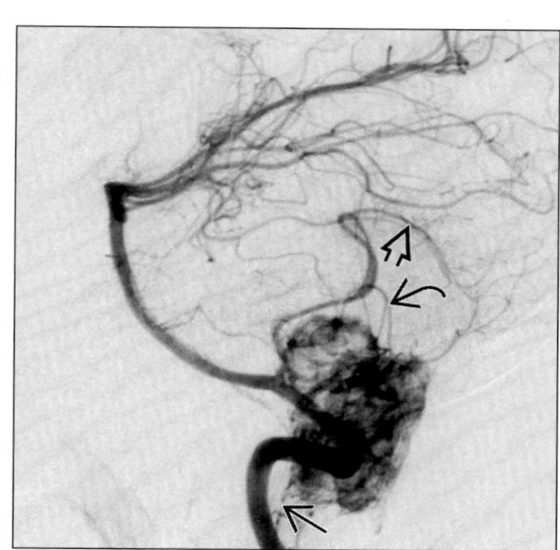

(Left) *A strongly enhancing intramedullary tumor ➔ with a superior cystic component ➔ extends into the upper cervical spinal cord. Other cystic components ➔ are present in the cord inferior to the enhancing tumor nodule.* ***(Right)*** *Lateral DSA in the same patient shows a highly vascular tumor nodule supplied by PICA ➔ and branches of the vertebral and anterior spinal arteries ➔. Avascular mass effect caused by the large associated cyst displaces the hemispheric branches superiorly ➔. (Courtesy AFIP.)*

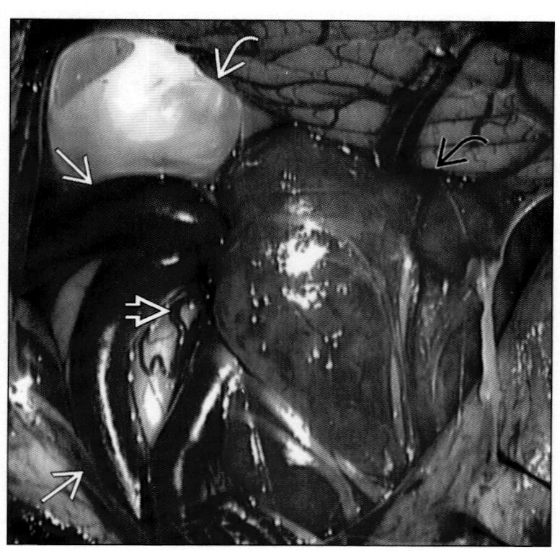

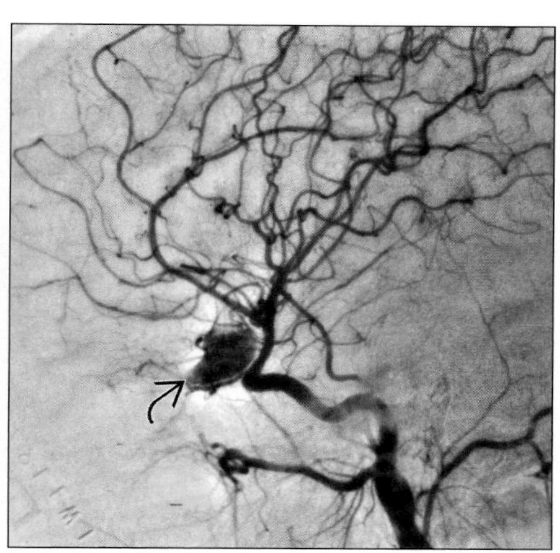

(Left) *Lateral surgical photograph of the same lesion shows the solid, highly vascular tumor nodule ➔, the cystic component with yellowish fluid ➔, and a markedly enlarged PICA ➔ with prominent dilated feeding vessels ➔. (Courtesy AFIP.)* ***(Right)*** *Lateral DSA of an orbital hemangioblastoma shows a highly vascular suprasellar mass ➔ fed by branches of the ophthalmic artery.*

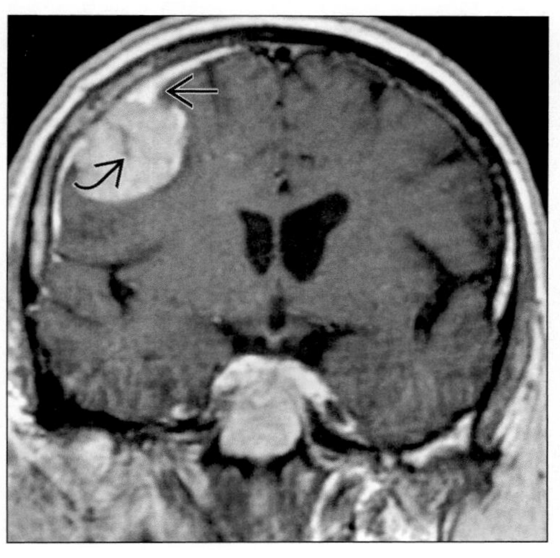

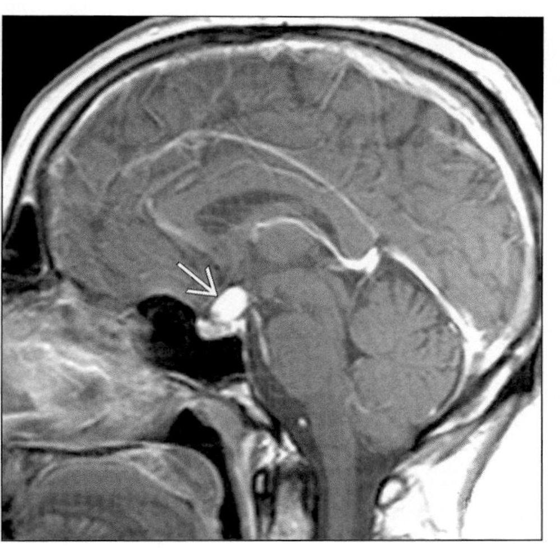

(Left) *Rare extraaxial dural-based hemangioblastoma shows diffuse enhancement with a visible central flow void ➔. A slight enhancing dural tail is present ➔. Imaging findings in this variant case mimic meningioma. Most supratentorial hemangioblastomas cluster around the optic nerves and chiasm. (Courtesy AFIP.)* ***(Right)*** *Sagittal T1WI C+ MR in a 37-year-old man shows a solid enhancing suprasellar mass ➔. Surgery disclosed a hemangioblastoma. (Courtesy R. Bert, MD).*

HEMANGIOPERICYTOMA

Key Facts

Terminology

- Highly cellular and vascularized mesenchymal tumor, nearly always attached to dura

Imaging

- Lobular enhancing extraaxial mass with dural attachment, ± skull erosion
  - Mimics meningioma, but no Ca++ or hyperostosis
- Typically supratentorial heterogeneous, extraaxial mass; occipital region most common
- Commonly involve falx, tentorium, or dural sinuses
- Marked enhancement, often heterogeneous
- Dural "tail" seen in approximately 50%

Top Differential Diagnoses

- Meningioma
- Dural metastases
- Lymphoma

Pathology

- WHO grade II and WHO grade III (anaplastic)
- HPC: Distinctive mesenchymal neoplasm unrelated to meningioma
  - Arises from primitive mesenchymal cells throughout body

Clinical Issues

- Headache is most common presenting feature
- Commonly occur in 4th-6th decades, mean: 43 years
- Represents < 1% of primary CNS tumors
- Surgical resection with radiation therapy or radiosurgery is treatment of choice
- Local recurrence common (50-90%)

Diagnostic Checklist

- Think HPC when "meningioma" has atypical features (frank bone erosion, multiple flow voids)

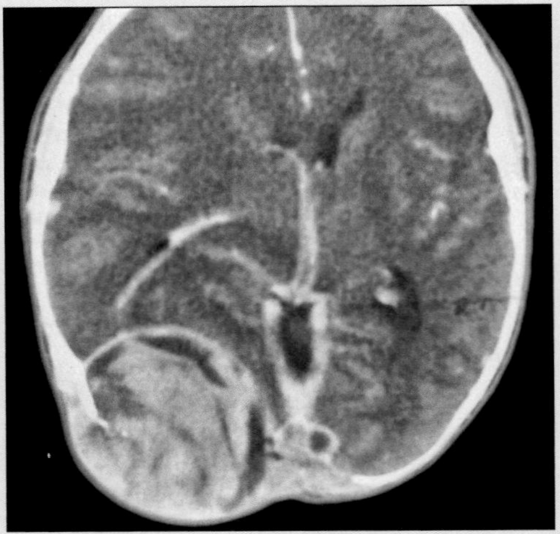

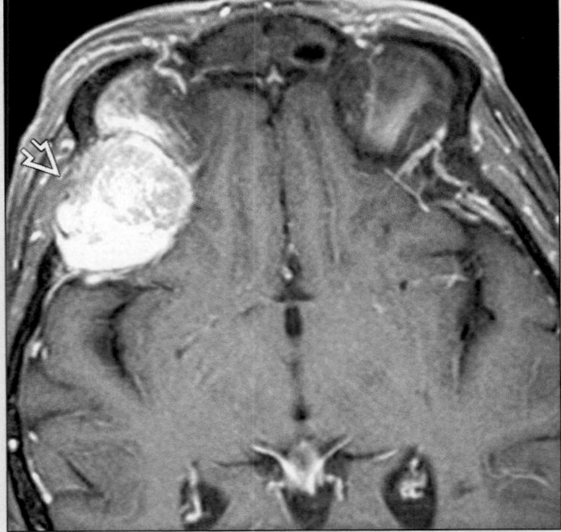

(Left) *Axial CECT shows a heterogeneously enhancing mass in the occipital region with extensive bone erosion. Note the surrounding edema and mass effect. Location and appearance are typical of hemangiopericytoma.* ***(Right)*** *Axial T1WI C+ FS MR shows an enhancing extraaxial mass along the greater sphenoid wing that extends into the right orbit. Although this mimics a meningioma, the associated bone erosion, not hyperostosis, helps correctly diagnose this as the more aggressive hemangiopericytoma.*

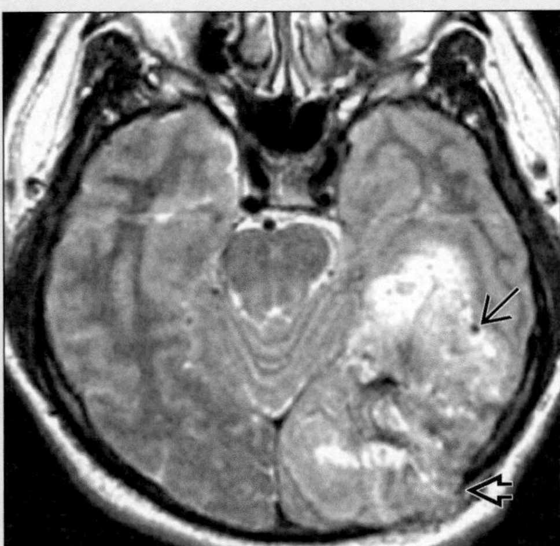

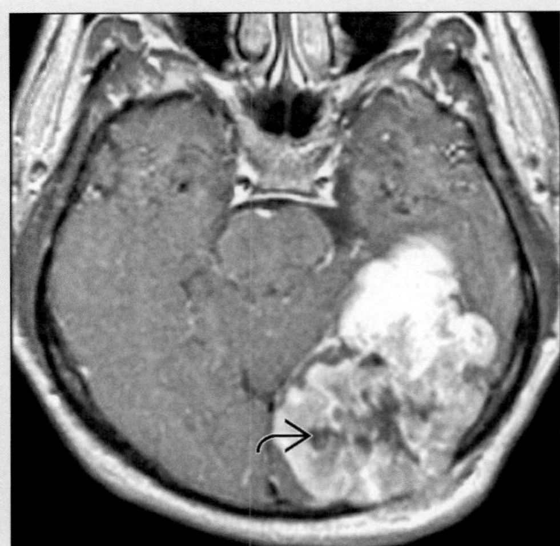

(Left) *Axial T2WI MR shows a large, heterogeneous occipital mass with flow voids and calvarial erosion, characteristic of hemangiopericytoma.* ***(Right)*** *Axial T1WI C+ MR in the same patient shows a lobular, heterogeneously enhancing extraaxial mass with central low signal, likely related to necrosis. Hemangiopericytomas are typically attached to the falx, tentorium, or dural sinuses. These rare tumors have a high rate of recurrence and often metastasize outside the CNS.*

HEMANGIOPERICYTOMA

TERMINOLOGY

Abbreviations

- Hemangiopericytoma (HPC), meningeal hemangiopericytoma

Synonyms

- In older literature called "angioblastic meningioma," hemangiopericytic type

Definitions

- Highly cellular and vascularized mesenchymal tumor, nearly always attached to dura
- Sarcoma related to neoplastic transformation of pericytes, contractile cells about capillaries
  - Occur in any region of body where capillaries are found

IMAGING

General Features

- Best diagnostic clue
  - Lobular enhancing extraaxial mass with dural attachment, ± skull erosion
  - May mimic meningioma, but without Ca++ or hyperostosis
- Location
  - Supratentorial: Occipital region most common
  - Typically involve falx, tentorium, or dural sinuses
  - Rare reports of intraparenchymal, skull base, cranial nerve, intraventricular involvement
- Size
  - Variable; 2-9 cm, often > 4 cm
- Morphology
  - Lobular dural-based extraaxial mass
    - Dural attachment may be narrow pedicle or broad based
  - Dural "tail" commonly seen, approximately 50%
  - Rarely may appear intraaxial

CT Findings

- NECT
  - Hyperdense extraaxial mass with surrounding edema
    - Low-density cystic or necrotic areas are common
  - Calvarial erosion may be seen
  - No Ca++ or hyperostosis
- CECT
  - Strong, heterogeneous enhancement

MR Findings

- T1WI
  - Heterogeneous mass, isointense to gray matter
  - Flow voids may be seen
- T2WI
  - Heterogeneous isointense mass
  - Prominent flow voids are common
  - Surrounding edema, mass effect typical
  - Hydrocephalus may be seen
- T1WI C+
  - Marked enhancement, often heterogeneous
  - Dural "tail" seen in approximately 50%
  - Central necrosis may be seen
- MRV
  - May show occlusion of dural sinuses
- MRS
  - Early reports have shown elevated myoinositol (3.56 ppm) using short TE (20 m/sec) may help differentiate HPC from meningioma

Angiographic Findings

- Hypervascular mass with irregular tumor vessels and prolonged, dense tumor stain
- Extensive arteriovenous shunting
- Mixed dural-pial vascular supply typical
- Preoperative embolization has been shown helpful

Nuclear Medicine Findings

- Bone scan
  - Helpful to detect extracranial metastases
- PET
  - Early FDG studies show lower metabolic rate in HPC than gray matter

Imaging Recommendations

- Best imaging tool
  - CT helpful to evaluate bone erosion
  - Multiplanar MR is most sensitive
- Protocol advice
  - Multiplanar contrast-enhanced MR, ± MRS
  - Bone scan useful in patient follow-up as extracranial metastases are common

DIFFERENTIAL DIAGNOSIS

Meningioma

- May be indistinguishable
- Enhancing extraaxial dural based mass
- Often calcified with broad dural base, dural "tail"
- Hyperostosis and Ca++ is characteristic

Dural Metastases

- Dural metastases with calvarial invasion may be indistinguishable
- Typically multiple lesions
- Primary tumor often known
  - Breast and prostate cancer most common

Lymphoma

- Dural involvement by lymphoma may mimic HPC
  - Diffusely enhancing dural mass, often multifocal
  - T2 low signal related to hypercellularity
- Calvarial involvement uncommon
- Flow voids usually absent

Neurosarcoidosis

- Dural-based masses can occur, often multifocal
- No calvarial involvement
- Typically leptomeningeal enhancement

Gliosarcoma

- Rare glial tumor often with dural involvement
- Heterogeneously enhancing parenchymal mass

Solitary Fibrous Tumor

- Circumscribed enhancing dural-based mass

- May have associated hyperostosis
- Extremely rare, < 20 reported cases

PATHOLOGY

General Features

- Etiology
  - Distinctive mesenchymal neoplasm unrelated to meningioma
  - Uncertain histogenesis
    - May form morphological continuum with solitary fibrous tumor
  - Arises from primitive mesenchymal cells throughout body
    - Most commonly involves soft tissues of lower extremities, pelvis, and retroperitoneum
    - Approximately 15% occur in head and neck region (scalp, face, neck, sinonasal)
- Genetics
  - No consistent chromosomal losses or gains
  - Reports of abnormalities of chromosomes 12 and 3

Staging, Grading, & Classification

- WHO grade II
- WHO grade III (anaplastic)

Gross Pathologic & Surgical Features

- Extremely vascular with tendency to bleed at surgery
- Well-circumscribed, encapsulated firm mass with dural attachment
- Cut surface is gray to red-brown with visible vascular spaces

Microscopic Features

- Highly cellular, monotonous tumor with randomly oriented plump cells in dense reticulin network
- "Staghorn" vascular pattern characteristic
  - Lobules of tumor cells surrounding wide, branching capillaries
- Immunohistochemistry: Antibodies to factor XIIIa, Leu-7, and CD34 may help differentiate from other tumors
  - Vimentin positive
  - Epithelial membrane antigen (EMA) negative, S100 negative
- Prominent mitotic activity, median Ki-67 index (MIB-1) of 5-10%
- Histologic features are not predictive of outcome

CLINICAL ISSUES

Presentation

- Most common signs/symptoms
  - Headache
- Other signs/symptoms
  - Related to tumor location: Focal neurologic deficit, seizure

Demographics

- Age
  - Most common 4th to 6th decade, mean = 43 years
  - Occur at all ages, uncommon in children
- Gender
  - Slight male predominance
- Epidemiology
  - Represents < 1% of primary CNS tumors, approximately 0.4%
  - Represents 2-4% of all meningeal tumors
  - HPC to meningioma ratio = 1:50

Natural History & Prognosis

- Local recurrence common (50-90%)
  - Recurrence usually within 40-70 months
- Extracranial metastases common (up to 30%)
  - Commonly liver, lungs, lymph nodes, bones
  - Mean survival after metastases: 2 years
- Complications
  - Invasion of dural sinuses, bone, and cranial nerves
  - Hemorrhage (rare)
- May cause oncogenic osteomalacia
  - Rare paraneoplastic syndrome associated with mesenchymal tumors
- 5-year survival rate has improved (up to 93%)

Treatment

- Preoperative embolization may be helpful, tumors are highly vascular
- Surgical resection with radiation therapy or radiosurgery is treatment of choice
  - Reduces risk of local recurrence
- Radiosurgery may be effective alternative to repeated surgical resection in recurrent tumors
- Chemotherapy shows some improved survival in recurrent tumors in recent reports
- Careful long-term follow-up is mandatory
  - Potential for local recurrence and metastases many years after initial diagnosis

DIAGNOSTIC CHECKLIST

Consider

- Bone erosion is most commonly seen in metastatic disease, but can suggest HPC
- Dural "tail" is nonspecific and is much more common in meningioma

Image Interpretation Pearls

- Think HPC when "meningioma" has atypical features (frank bone erosion, multiple flow voids)

SELECTED REFERENCES

1. Park MS et al: New insights into the hemangiopericytoma/solitary fibrous tumor spectrum of tumors. Curr Opin Oncol. 21(4):327-31, 2009
2. Chamberlain MC et al: Sequential salvage chemotherapy for recurrent intracranial hemangiopericytoma. Neurosurgery. 63(4):720-6; author reply 726-7, 2008
3. Louis DN et al: WHO Classification of Tumours of the CNS: Haemangiopericytoma. Lyon: IARC Press. 178-80, 2007
4. Sibtain NA et al: Imaging features of central nervous system haemangiopericytomas. Eur Radiol. 17(7):1685-93, 2007
5. Fountas KN et al: Management of intracranial meningeal hemangiopericytomas: outcome and experience. Neurosurg Rev. 29(2):145-53, 2006

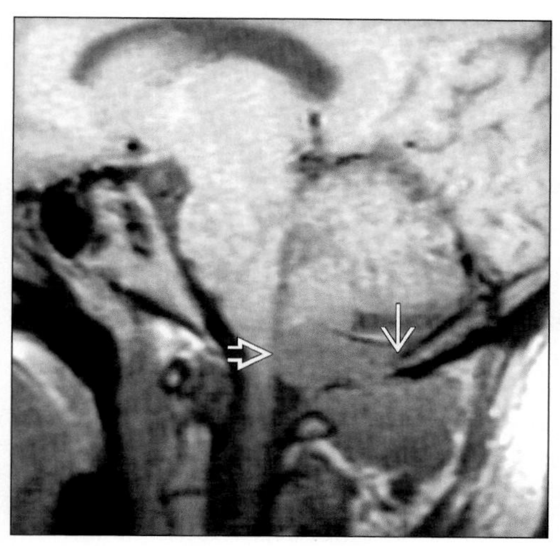

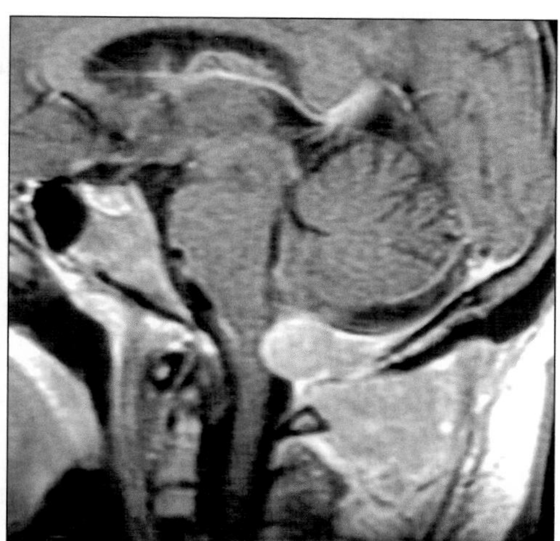

(Left) *Sagittal T1WI MR shows a mildly heterogeneous posterior fossa extraaxial mass with displacement of the cerebellum and erosion of the opisthion. There is extracranial extension of tumor into the cervical region.* ***(Right)*** *Sagittal T1WI C+ MR in the same patient shows diffuse, mildly heterogeneous enhancement. Hemangiopericytomas are most commonly supratentorial tumors, often involving the occipital region, These rare mesenchymal tumors represent < 1% of all primary CNS tumors.*

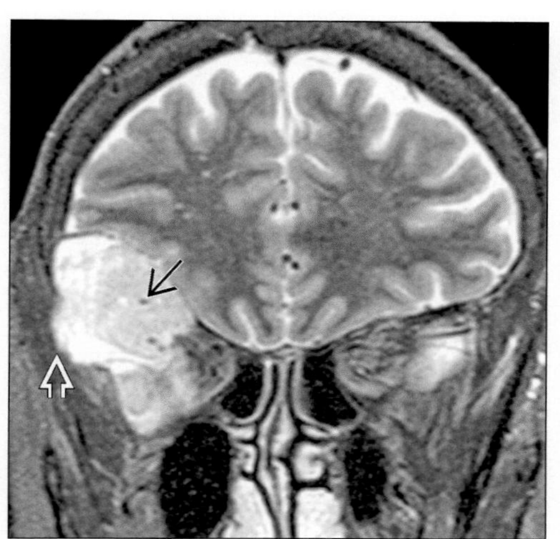

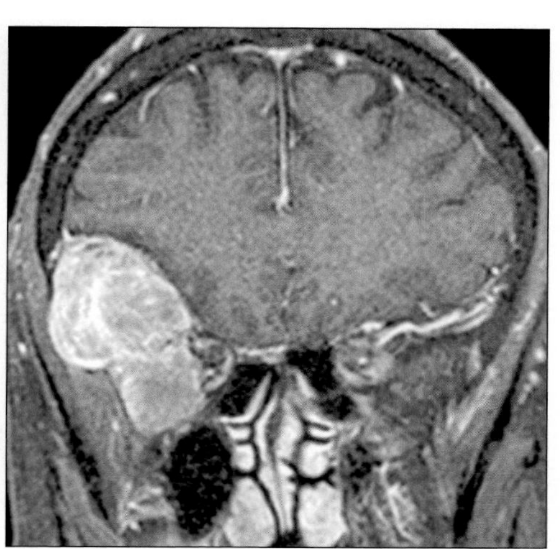

(Left) *Coronal T2WI FS MR shows a heterogeneous hyperintense mass in the inferior frontal region with central flow voids and bone erosion, characteristic of hemangiopericytoma.* ***(Right)*** *Coronal T1WI C+ FS MR in the same patient shows diffuse enhancement of the lobular mass. Imaging mimics a meningioma. CT can be helpful to further define bone erosion. Other imaging differential considerations would include a dural metastasis and lymphoma.*

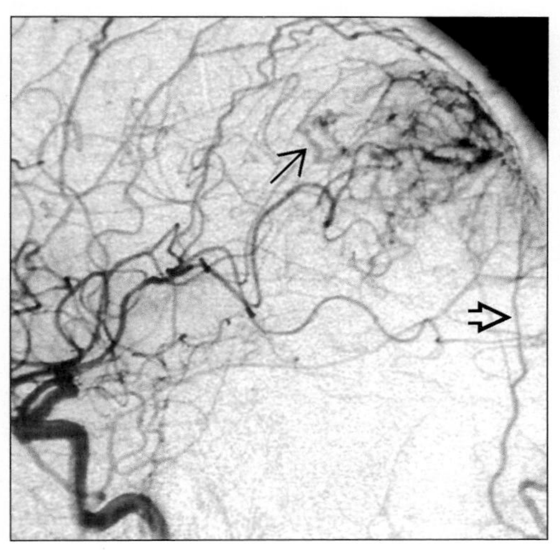

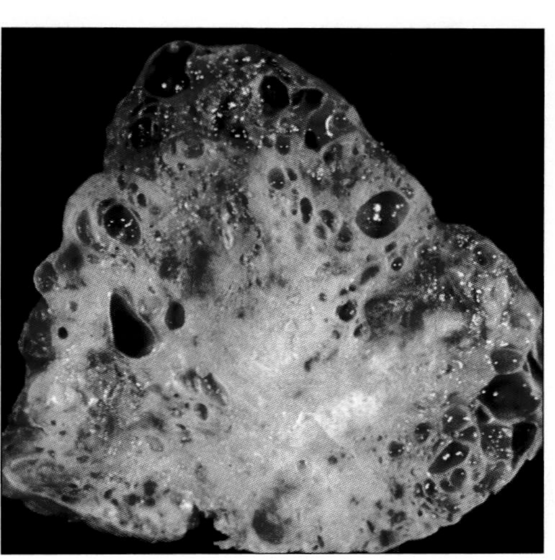

(Left) *Lateral ICA injection DSA shows arteriovenous shunting with early draining veins. An additional dural feeding vessel, a branch of the occipital artery, is also seen. A mixed dural-pial vascular supply is typical of hemangiopericytoma. Preoperative embolization is often helpful.* ***(Right)*** *Gross pathology cut section shows a lobulated, circumscribed vascular mass with multiple enlarged vascular channels characteristic of hemangiopericytoma. (Courtesy R. Hewlett, PhD.)*

PRIMARY CNS LYMPHOMA

Key Facts

Terminology

- Malignant primary CNS neoplasm primarily composed of B lymphocytes

Imaging

- Best diagnostic clue: Enhancing lesion(s) within basal ganglia &/or periventricular white matter
- 60-80% supratentorial
  - Often involve, cross corpus callosum
  - Frequently abut, extend along ependymal surfaces
- Classically hyperdense on CT (helpful for diagnosis)
- Diffusely enhancing periventricular mass in immunocompetent
- May see hemorrhage or necrosis in immunocompromised
- DWI: Low ADC values
- PWI: Low rCBV ratios
- Periventricular location and subependymal involvement is characteristic of PCNSL

Top Differential Diagnoses

- Acquired toxoplasmosis
- Glioblastoma multiforme (GBM)
- Abscess
- Progressive multifocal leukoencephalopathy (PML)

Pathology

- 98% diffuse large B-cell, non-Hodgkin lymphoma

Clinical Issues

- Imaging and prognosis varies with immune status
- 6.6% of primary brain tumors, incidence rising
- Poor prognosis
- Stereotactic biopsy, followed by XRT and chemotherapy is treatment of choice

*(**Left**) Axial graphic shows multiple periventricular lesions with involvement of the basal ganglia, thalamus, and corpus callosum, typical of primary CNS lymphoma (PCNSL). Note the extensive subependymal spread of disease ⇒; indeed, PCNSL typically extends along ependymal surfaces. (**Right**) Axial NECT shows multiple hyperdense lesions ➡ along the ventricular margins. CT hyperdensity is characteristic of PCNSL and is helpful for an accurate preoperative diagnosis. (Courtesy N. Fischbein, MD.)*

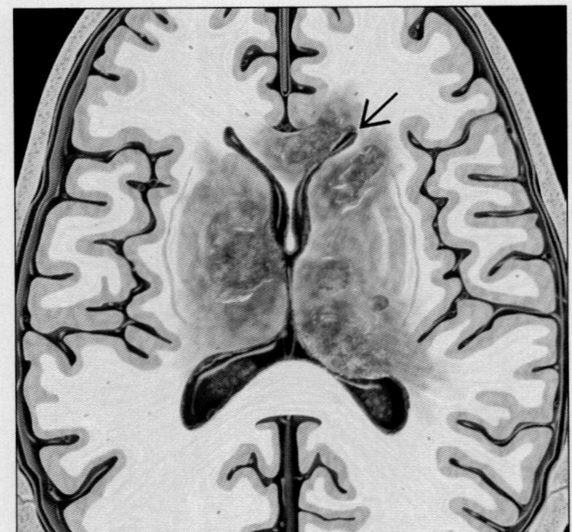

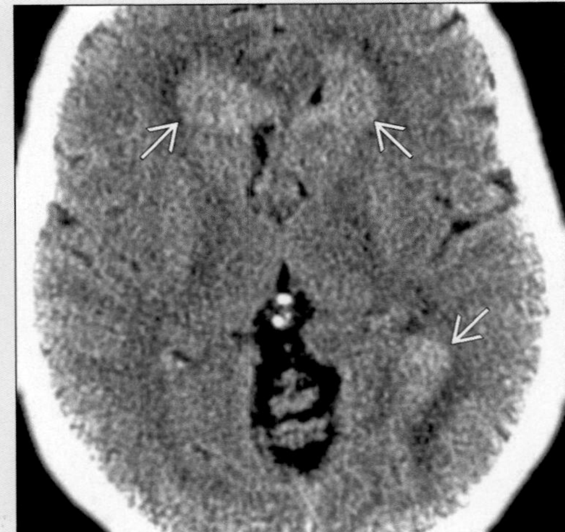

*(**Left**) Coronal T1WI C+ MR shows a homogeneously enhancing mass crossing the corpus callosum and an additional periventricular lesion ➡, typical of PCNSL, in this 72-year-old man with a headache. (**Right**) Axial T1WI C+ MR in an AIDS patient shows a ring-enhancing mass with a "target" sign ➡, suggestive of toxoplasmosis. The ependymal enhancement ➡ along the lateral ventricles is key to the correct diagnosis of PCNSL. Hemorrhage, necrosis, and ring-enhancing lesions are typical of PCNSL in AIDS patients.*

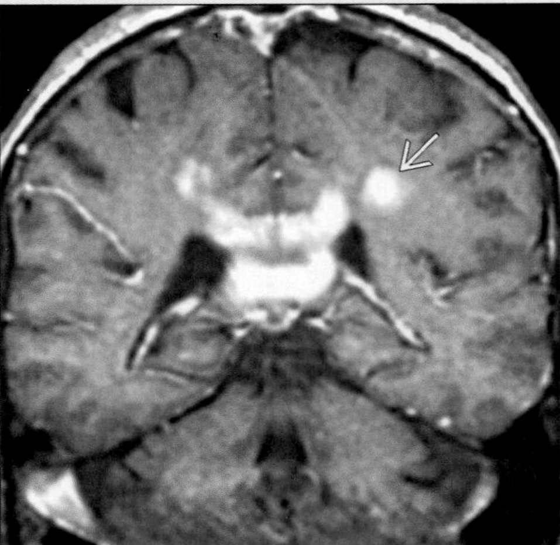

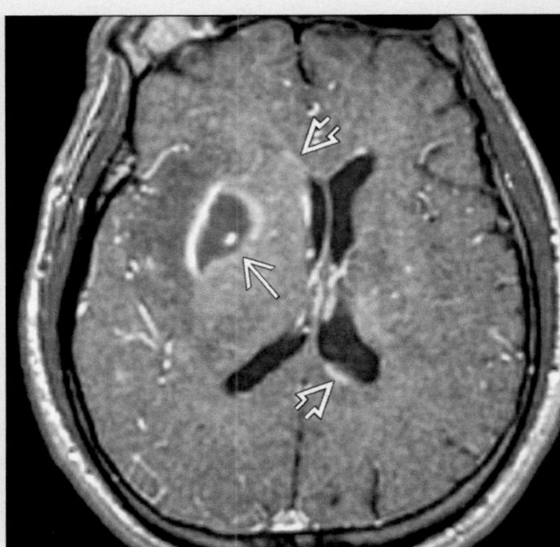

TERMINOLOGY

Abbreviations

- Primary central nervous system lymphoma (PCNSL)

Definitions

- Extranodal malignant lymphoma arising in CNS in absence of systemic lymphoma

IMAGING

General Features

- Best diagnostic clue
  - Enhancing lesion(s) within basal ganglia, periventricular white matter (WM)
- Location
  - 60-80% supratentorial
    - Frontal, temporal, and parietal lobes most common
  - Deep gray nuclei commonly affected (10%)
  - Lesions cluster around ventricles, gray-white matter junction
  - Often involve, cross corpus callosum (5-10%)
  - Frequently abut, extend along ependymal surfaces
  - Posterior fossa, sella, pineal region uncommon
  - Spine involvement rare (1%)
  - May involve leptomeninges or dura (more common in secondary lymphoma)
- Morphology
  - Solitary mass or multiple lesions
  - May be circumscribed or infiltrative

CT Findings

- NECT
  - Classically hyperdense; may be isodense
  - ± hemorrhage, necrosis (immunocompromised)
- CECT
  - Common: Moderate, uniform (immunocompetent)
  - Less common: Ring (immunocompromised)
  - Rare: Nonenhancing (infiltrative)

MR Findings

- T1WI
  - Immunocompetent: Homogeneously iso-/hypointense to cortex
  - Immunocompromised: Iso-/hypointense
    - May be heterogeneous from hemorrhage, necrosis
- T2WI
  - Immunocompetent: Homogeneously iso-/hypointense to cortex
    - Hypointensity related to high nuclear to cytoplasmic ratio
  - Immunocompromised: Iso-/hypointense
    - May be heterogeneous from hemorrhage, necrosis
    - Ca++ may rarely be seen, usually after therapy
  - Mild surrounding edema is typical
- FLAIR
  - Homogeneously iso-/hypointense
  - Immunocompromised: Iso-/hypointense
  - May be hyperintense
- T2* GRE
  - May see blood products or calcium as areas of "blooming" (immunocompromised)
- DWI
  - May show restricted diffusion
  - Low ADC values compared to malignant glioma
    - Minimal ADC = 0.51± 0.09 in 1 study, lower than glioblastoma multiforme (0.79 ± 0.21)
- PWI
  - Relative CBV ratios are lower than malignant glioma
    - Relative CBV = 2.33 ± 0.68 in 1 study, much lower than glioblastoma multiforme (6.33 ± 2.03)
- T1WI C+
  - Immunocompetent: Strong homogeneous enhancement
  - Immunocompromised: Peripheral enhancement with central necrosis or homogeneous enhancement
  - Nonenhancement extremely rare
- MRS
  - NAA ↓, Cho ↑
  - Lipid and lactate peaks reported
- Diffusion tensor imaging (DTI)
  - Low fractional anisotropy (FA) and ADC
    - FA & ADC of PCNSL significantly lower than GBM

Nuclear Medicine Findings

- FDG PET and Tl-201 SPECT: Hypermetabolic

Imaging Recommendations

- Protocol advice
  - Contrast-enhanced MR ± DWI, PWI, DTI
  - PET or Tl-201 SPECT may be helpful when toxoplasmosis is considered

DIFFERENTIAL DIAGNOSIS

Acquired Toxoplasmosis

- Involves basal ganglia, corticomedullary junction
- Enhancing lesions, "eccentric target" sign
- No ependymal spread
- Often indistinguishable on standard MR
  - DWI, DTI, perfusion may be helpful
  - SPECT, PET helpful (iso-/hypometabolic)

Glioblastoma Multiforme (GBM)

- "Butterfly glioma" involving corpus callosum
- Hemorrhage common
- Enhancement typically heterogeneous
- Necrosis with ring enhancement in 95%

Abscess

- T2 hypointense rim, diffusion restriction typical
- Peripheral enhancement with central necrosis
- Enhancement often thinner on ventricular side
- MRS: Elevated amino acids in cystic cavity (low TE)

Progressive Multifocal Leukoencephalopathy

- White matter T2 hyperintensity, nonenhancing
- Involves subcortical U-fibers and corpus callosum

Demyelination

- May involve corpus callosum
- Often incomplete, horseshoe-shaped enhancement, open toward cortex
- Other lesions in characteristic locations
- Younger patients

PRIMARY CNS LYMPHOMA

Metastases
- Multiple lesions common
- Significant associated vasogenic edema

Neurosarcoidosis
- "Lacy" leptomeningeal enhancement typical
- Dural, leptomeningeal > > parenchymal disease
- Most patients have systemic disease

Secondary CNS Lymphoma
- Lymphomatous meningitis or dural disease common
- Can have single/multiple deep, periventricular lesions

PATHOLOGY

General Features
- Etiology
  - Site of origin controversial as CNS does not have lymphoid tissue or lymphatic circulation
  - Inherited or acquired immunodeficiency predisposes
- Genetics
  - Clonal abnormalities in chromosomes 1, 6, 7, & 14
  - Translocations reported in (1;14), (6;14), (13;18), & (14;21)
- Associated abnormalities
  - Epstein-Barr virus (EBV) plays major role in immunocompromised (95%)
  - 8% of PCNSL patients have had prior malignancy, commonly leukemia or adenocarcinoma
  - Rarely PCNSL is preceded by demyelinating lesions

Staging, Grading, & Classification
- Majority are diffuse large B-cell, non-Hodgkin lymphoma

Gross Pathologic & Surgical Features
- Single or multiple mass(es) in cerebral hemispheres
- Well-circumscribed > infiltrative mass
- Central necrosis, hemorrhage in HIV-positive patients

Microscopic Features
- Cells surround, infiltrate vessels and perivascular spaces
- High nuclear to cytoplasmic ratio (high electron density)
- MIB-1, proliferation index, usually high (50-70%)

CLINICAL ISSUES

Presentation
- Most common signs/symptoms
  - Altered mental status, focal neurologic deficits
- Other signs/symptoms
  - Cognitive, neuropsychiatric disturbance
  - Headache, increased intracranial pressure, seizure
- Clinical profile
  - Cytology positive in 5-30% of PCNSL

Demographics
- Age
  - Immunocompetent: 6th-7th decades, mean 60 years
  - Immunocompromised
    - AIDS: Mean age 39 years
    - Transplant recipients: Mean age 37 years
    - Inherited immunodeficiency: Mean age 10 years
- Gender: Male predominance
- Epidemiology
  - 6.6% of primary brain tumors
  - Represents ~ 1% of lymphomas
  - PCNSL is present in 0.4% of AIDS patients
    - PCNSL is AIDS-defining condition
    - Highly effective antiviral therapy (HAART) has reduced occurrence of all NHL in AIDS patients
  - In post-transplant lymphoma, CNS involvement occurs in 22%

Natural History & Prognosis
- Poor prognosis
- Median survival
  - 50 months in immunocompetent
  - 36 months in AIDS patients
    - Marked improvement with HAART and XRT
- Favorable prognostic factors
  - Single lesion
  - Absence of meningeal or periventricular disease
  - Immunocompetent patient
  - Age < 60 years
    - Patients < 61 years: 5-year survival 75%
- Dramatic but short-lived response to steroids and XRT
- Rarely, PCNSL is complicated by systemic disease

Treatment
- Stereotactic biopsy, followed by XRT and chemotherapy
- Treatment with enhanced chemotherapy delivery with blood-brain barrier disruption may be helpful

DIAGNOSTIC CHECKLIST

Consider
- Corpus callosum involvement may be seen with PCNSL, GBM and rarely metastases, demyelination
- Steroids may dramatically ↓ ↓ mass, enhancement; mask biopsy results
- Occult systemic disease present in up to 8% of PCNSL, systemic staging helpful

Image Interpretation Pearls
- Imaging and prognosis varies with immune status
- PCNSL is characteristically hyperdense on NECT
- Periventricular location and subependymal involvement is characteristic of PCNSL

SELECTED REFERENCES

1. Liao W et al: Differentiation of primary central nervous system lymphoma and high-grade glioma with dynamic susceptibility contrast-enhanced perfusion magnetic resonance imaging. Acta Radiol. 50(2):217-25, 2009
2. Toh CH et al: Primary cerebral lymphoma and glioblastoma multiforme: differences in diffusion characteristics evaluated with diffusion tensor imaging. AJNR Am J Neuroradiol. 29(3):471-5, 2008
3. Louis DN et al: WHO Classification of Tumours of the Central Nervous System: Malignant lymphomas. Lyon: IARC Press. 188-92, 2007

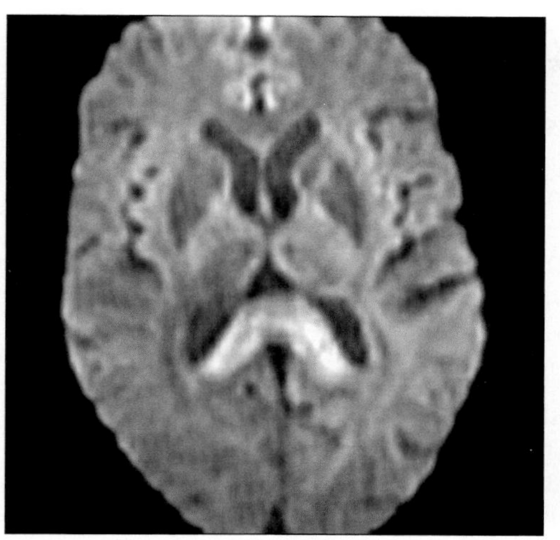

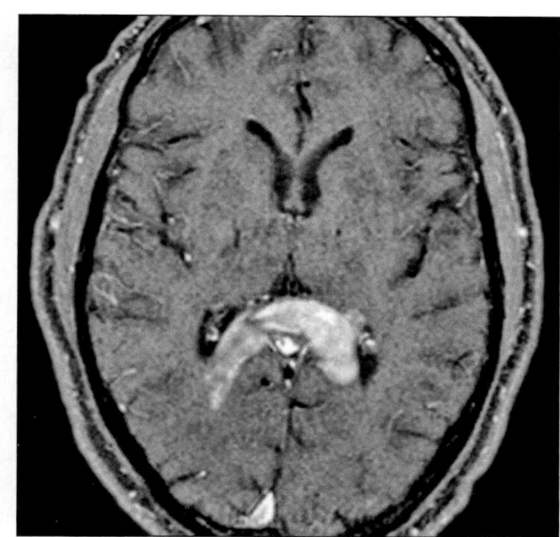

(Left) *Axial DWI MR in a 58-year-old man with confusion shows diffusion restriction along the splenium of the corpus callosum. DWI and DTI are often helpful to differentiate PCNSL from glioblastoma multiforme, which also classically crosses the corpus callosum.* ***(Right)*** *Axial T1WI C+ FS MR in the same patient shows homogeneous enhancement of the tumor. It is important to recognize PCNSL as the preoperative diagnosis, as a biopsy rather than a resection is the initial treatment of choice.*

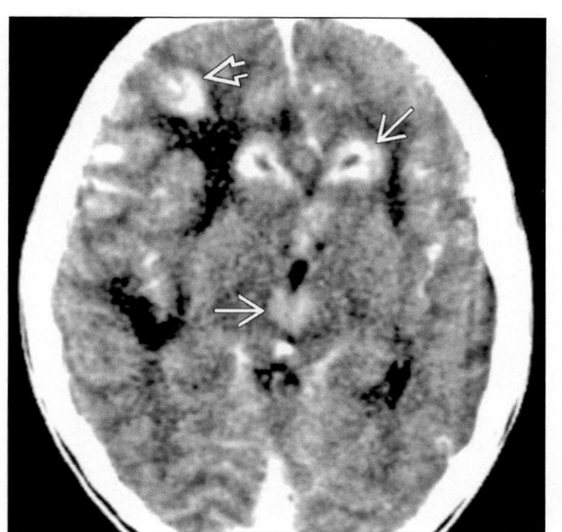

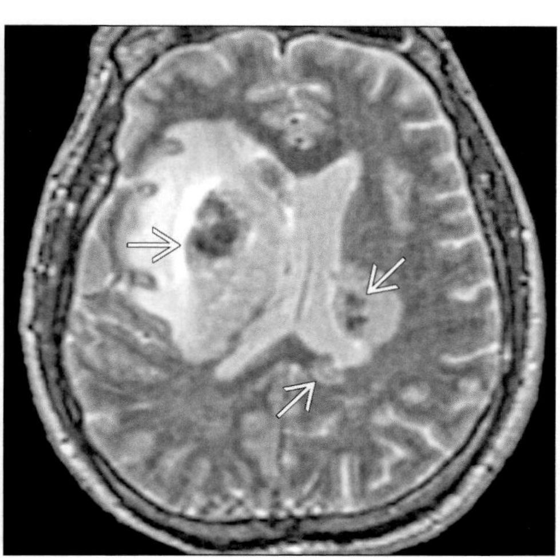

(Left) *Axial CECT shows extensive ependymal enhancement ➔ along the frontal horns of the lateral and 3rd ventricles. An additional frontal mass is present ➲ in this immunocompromised teen with PCNSL.* ***(Right)*** *Axial T2WI MR shows multifocal, heterogeneously hypointense lesions ➔ in the basal ganglia and periventricular region with surrounding edema in this AIDS patient. PCNSL is often T2 hypointense due to hemorrhage and necrosis within the tumor in AIDS patients.*

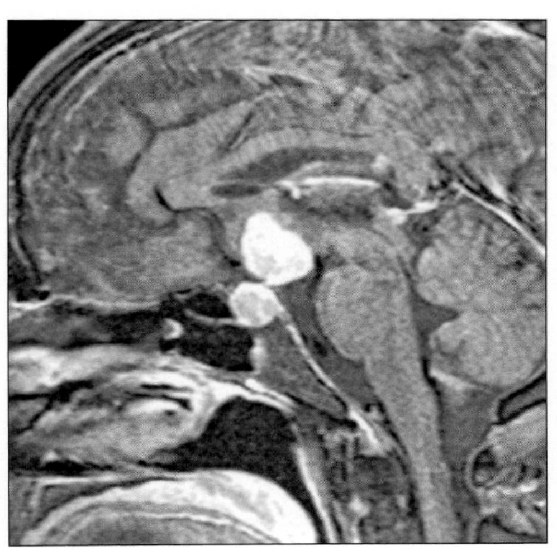

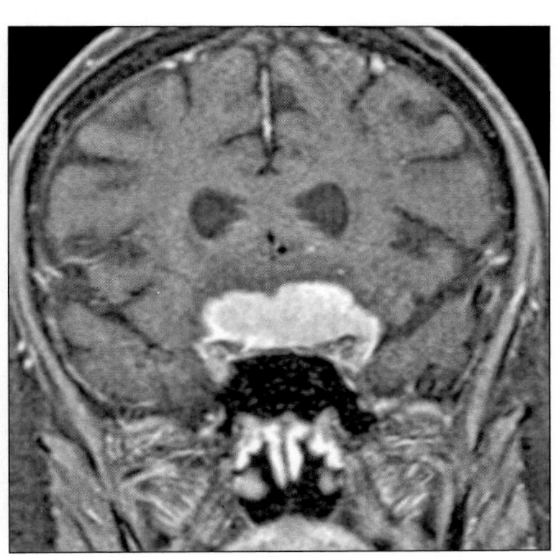

(Left) *Sagittal T1WI C+ FS MR shows an enhancing suprasellar mass involving the optic chiasm, hypothalamus, and anterior 3rd ventricle. Primary involvement of the sellar and suprasellar regions is a fairly uncommon manifestation of PCNSL.* ***(Right)*** *Coronal T1 C+ FS MR shows a dural-based mass along the anterior cranial fossa in an elderly woman with optic neuropathy. Imaging mimics a meningioma, but PCNSL was found at biopsy. Dural involvement is more common in secondary CNS lymphoma.*

INTRAVASCULAR (ANGIOCENTRIC) LYMPHOMA

Key Facts

Terminology
- Rare malignancy characterized by intravascular proliferation of lymphoid cells with predilection for CNS and skin

Imaging
- T2/FLAIR multifocal hyperintensities in deep white matter, cortex, and basal ganglia
  - May mimic infarct
- Diffusion restriction common
- Linear and punctate enhancement typical
  - May see meningeal &/or dural enhancement
- Often mimics vasculitis

Top Differential Diagnoses
- Vasculitis
- Multi-infarct dementia
- Primary CNS lymphoma (PCNSL)
- Neurosarcoid

Pathology
- Malignant lymphoid cells occlude and distend small arteries, veins, and capillaries

Clinical Issues
- Dementia is most common presenting feature
- Presents in 5th through 7th decade; mean: 63 years
- Diagnosis may be made by skin or brain biopsy
- Rare, but underdiagnosed
  - CNS involved in > 30% of cases
- Mean survival: 7-13 months
- Mortality rate: > 80%

Diagnostic Checklist
- Imaging of IVL is nonspecific, but IVL should be considered in patients with dementia, multifocal lesions, and enhancement

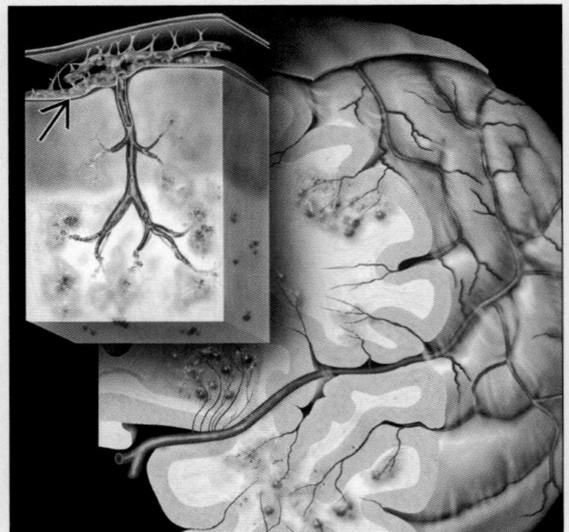

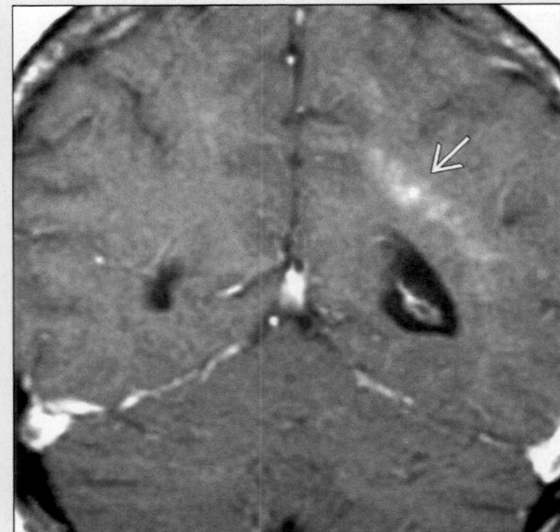

***(Left)** Graphic shows malignant lymphoid cells occluding and distending small arteries, veins, and capillaries, resulting in ischemic regions. Note also meningeal involvement →, typical of intravascular lymphoma (IVL). **(Right)** Coronal T1WI C+ MR shows a classic multifocal linear and patchy enhancement pattern in the deep white matter ➡ related to IVL in this patient with dementia. The enhancement occurs in regions of T2/FLAIR hyperintensity and is often the key to a correct preoperative diagnosis.*

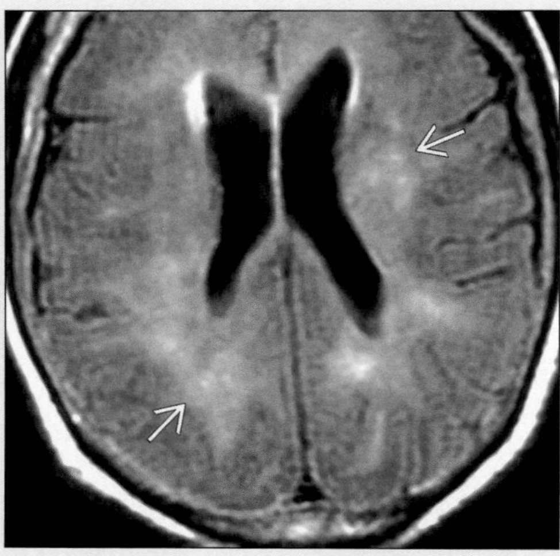

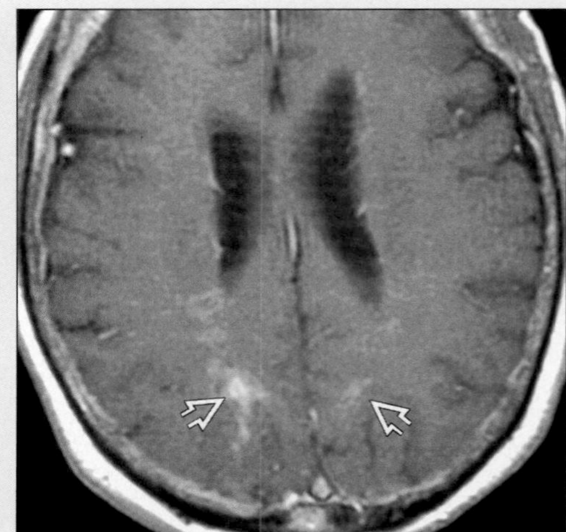

***(Left)** Axial FLAIR MR shows confluent areas of hyperintensity in the periventricular white matter ➡ in this 76-year-old patient. The FLAIR hyperintensities seen in IVL are nonspecific and mimic other disease processes, including chronic small vessel ischemia. Cortical lesions are also commonly seen. **(Right)** Axial T1WI C+ MR in the same patient shows multifocal linear and nodular enhancement ⇨ in the periventricular and subcortical white matter, typical of IVL. (Courtesy B. Sekar, MD.)*

INTRAVASCULAR (ANGIOCENTRIC) LYMPHOMA

TERMINOLOGY

Abbreviations

- Intravascular (angiocentric) lymphoma (IVL)

Synonyms

- Intravascular malignant lymphomatosis
- Malignant angioendotheliomatosis
- Angiotropic large-cell lymphoma
- Intravascular B-cell lymphoma

Definitions

- Rare malignancy characterized by intravascular proliferation of lymphoid cells with predilection for CNS and skin
- Form of non-Hodgkin lymphoma (NHL) characterized by angiotropic growth

IMAGING

General Features

- Best diagnostic clue
  - Multifocal abnormal T2 hyperintensities in deep white matter (WM), cortex, or basal ganglia + enhancement
  - Linear and nodular enhancement commonly
- Location
  - Supratentorial
    - Periventricular/deep WM, gray-white junction
  - May involve basal ganglia, brainstem, cerebellum
  - Spinal cord involvement reported

CT Findings

- NECT
  - Often normal or nonspecific
  - Focal, bilateral, asymmetric, low-density lesions in WM, cortex, or basal ganglia
- CECT
  - Variable enhancement
    - None to moderate

MR Findings

- T1WI
  - Multifocal hypointense lesions
  - May see blood products
- T2WI
  - Majority show hyperintensities in deep WM
    - e.g., edema, gliosis
  - May see cortex hyperintensity, infarct-like lesions (1/3 of cases)
  - Hyperintense basal ganglia lesions common
  - May see hemorrhagic transformation
- T2* GRE
  - May see blood products "blooming"
- DWI
  - Diffusion restriction common
  - Often mimics acute stroke or vasculitis
- T1WI C+
  - Variable enhancement
    - Linear, punctate, patchy, nodular, ring-like, gyriform, homogeneous
  - Meningeal &/or dural enhancement

Angiographic Findings

- Often mimics vasculitis
  - Alternating stenoses and dilatation, "beading," primarily involving 2nd and 3rd order branches

Imaging Recommendations

- Best imaging tool
  - Multiplanar MR
- Protocol advice
  - Contrast-enhanced MR with DWI

Nuclear Medicine Findings

- PET
  - FDG PET helpful in diagnosing IVL in bone marrow and kidneys

DIFFERENTIAL DIAGNOSIS

Vasculitis

- Multifocal subcortical ischemia, ± enhancement
- DWI positive in acute setting
- DSA suggests diagnosis (IVL may mimic)
- Enhancement pattern may mimic IVL (particularly granulomatous angiitis)

Multi-Infarct Dementia

- Large and small infarcts, WM disease
- Deep gray nuclei typically involved
- Clinical diagnosis can mimic IVL

Primary CNS Lymphoma (PCNSL)

- Enhancing lesions in basal ganglia, periventricular WM
- Corpus callosum often involved
- Ependymal involvement characteristic

Neurosarcoid

- Dural or leptomeningeal enhancement
- Brain parenchyma typically spared
- Patients often have systemic disease

PATHOLOGY

General Features

- Etiology
  - Aggressive B-cell non-Hodgkin lymphoma, angiotropic
    - May arise from T cells or rarely NK cells
  - IVL typically affects CNS and skin
    - May affect any organ
      - Reported in kidneys, bone marrow, breast, uterus, testes, lungs, larynx, adrenal gland
- Associated abnormalities
  - Possible association with Epstein-Barr virus (EBV)
    - NK-IVL is typically Epstein-Barr virus positive

Gross Pathologic & Surgical Features

- Small infarcts of varying ages throughout cortex and subcortical WM
  - May be hemorrhagic
- May cause cerebral masses

INTRAVASCULAR (ANGIOCENTRIC) LYMPHOMA

Microscopic Features

- Accumulations of large B cells typical
- Malignant lymphoid cells occlude and distend small arteries, veins, and capillaries
- Minimal perivascular extension into adjacent brain parenchyma

CLINICAL ISSUES

Presentation

- Most common signs/symptoms
  - Dementia, confusion, memory loss
- Other signs/symptoms
  - Cognitive failure, focal deficits, seizure, fever
  - Myelopathy reported with spinal cord involvement
- Clinical profile
  - Skin changes
    - Raised plaques or nodules over abdomen and thighs (50%)
  - CSF studies may show elevated protein
  - No malignant cells in peripheral blood smear or bone marrow
  - Laboratory studies often inconclusive

Demographics

- Age
  - 5th through 7th decade; mean: 63 years
- Gender
  - Slight male predominance
- Epidemiology
  - Rare, but underdiagnosed
  - CNS involved in > 30% of cases

Natural History & Prognosis

- Mean survival: 7-13 months
  - Mildly improved survival in recent reports
- Mortality rate: > 80%
- Rarely, spontaneous regression of symptoms occurs
- Diagnosis often made postmortem

Treatment

- Diagnosis may be made by skin or brain biopsy
- Treatment primarily includes steroids and chemotherapy
- Variable results with radiation therapy

DIAGNOSTIC CHECKLIST

Consider

- In evaluation of patients with dementia, contrast-enhanced MR may be helpful
- IVL often mimics vasculitis and vascular dementia clinically and by imaging

Image Interpretation Pearls

- Imaging of IVL is nonspecific, but IVL should be considered in patients with dementia, multifocal lesions, and enhancement
- Linear enhancement along perivascular spaces suggests diagnosis of IVL

SELECTED REFERENCES

1. Liu H et al: Spinal cord infarct as the initial clinical presentation of intravascular malignant lymphomatosis. J Clin Neurosci. 16(4):570-3, 2009
2. Pusch G et al: Intravascular lymphoma presenting with neurological signs but diagnosed by prostate biopsy: suspicion as a key to early diagnosis. Eur J Neurol. 16(3):e39-41, 2009
3. Sumer M et al: Intravascular lymphoma masquerading as multiembolic stroke developing after coronary artery by-pass surgery. Neurologist. 15(2):98-101, 2009
4. Anda T et al: Ruptured distal middle cerebral artery aneurysm filled with tumor cells in a patient with intravascular large B-cell lymphoma. J Neurosurg. 109(3):492-6, 2008
5. Cerroni L et al: Intravascular large T-cell or NK-cell lymphoma: a rare variant of intravascular large cell lymphoma with frequent cytotoxic phenotype and association with Epstein-Barr virus infection. Am J Surg Pathol. 32(6):891-8, 2008
6. Grove CS et al: Intravascular lymphoma presenting as progressive paraparesis. J Clin Neurosci. 15(9):1056-8, 2008
7. Matsue K et al: A clinicopathological study of 13 cases of intravascular lymphoma: experience in a single institution over a 9-yr period. Eur J Haematol. 80(3):236-44, 2008
8. Savard M et al: Intravascular lymphoma with conus medullaris syndrome followed by encephalopathy. Can J Neurol Sci. 35(3):366-71, 2008
9. Szots M et al: Intravascular lymphomatosis of the nervous system. J Neurol. 255(10):1590-2, 2008
10. Ganguly S: Acute intracerebral hemorrhage in intravascular lymphoma: a serious infusion related adverse event of rituximab. Am J Clin Oncol. 30(2):211-2, 2007
11. Holmøy T et al: Intravascular large B-cell lymphoma presenting as cerebellar and cerebral infarction. Arch Neurol. 64(5):754-5, 2007
12. Louis DN et al: WHO Classification of Tumours of the Central Nervous System: Malignant lymphomas. Lyon: IARC Press. 188-192, 2007
13. Song DE et al: Intravascular large cell lymphoma of the natural killer cell type. J Clin Oncol. 25(10):1279-82, 2007
14. Gaul C et al: Intravascular lymphomatosis mimicking disseminated encephalomyelitis and encephalomyelopathy. Clin Neurol Neurosurg. 108(5):486-9, 2006
15. Zuckerman D et al: Intravascular lymphoma: the oncologist's "great imitator". Oncologist. 11(5):496-502, 2006
16. Kinoshita T et al: Intravascular malignant lymphomatosis: diffusion-weighted magnetic resonance imaging characteristics. Acta Radiol. 46(3):246-9, 2005
17. Burger PC et al: Surgical pathology of the nervous system and its coverings: The Brain: Tumors. 4th ed. Philadelphia: Churchill Livingstone. 323-4, 2002
18. Martin-Duverneuil N et al: Intravascular malignant lymphomatosis. Neuroradiology. 44(9):749-54, 2002
19. Williams RL et al: Cerebral MR imaging in intravascular lymphomatosis. AJNR Am J Neuroradiol. 19(3):427-31, 1998

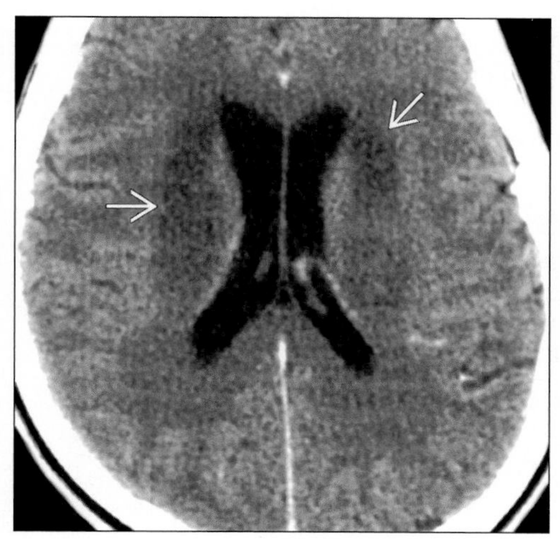

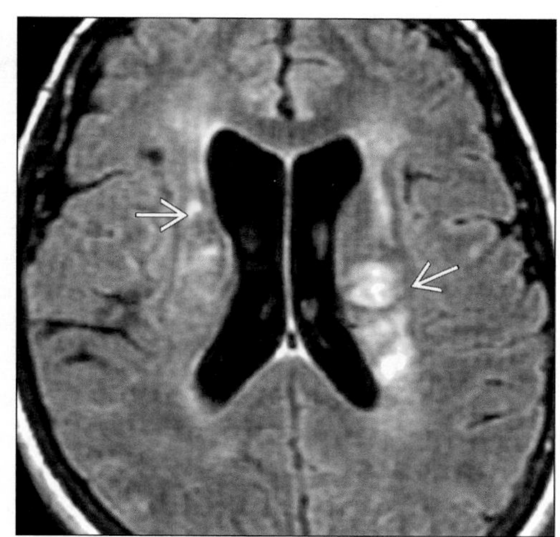

(Left) *Axial CECT shows multifocal, nonenhancing, low-density areas in the basal ganglia and deep cerebral white matter ➔. CT is often normal or nonspecific in patients with intravascular lymphoma, as in this case.* ***(Right)*** *Axial FLAIR MR in the same patient shows confluent areas of increased signal intensity ➔. No diffusion restriction was present on DWI sequences. Without contrast, the imaging is nonspecific, and this patient may have been diagnosed with chronic small vessel ischemia.*

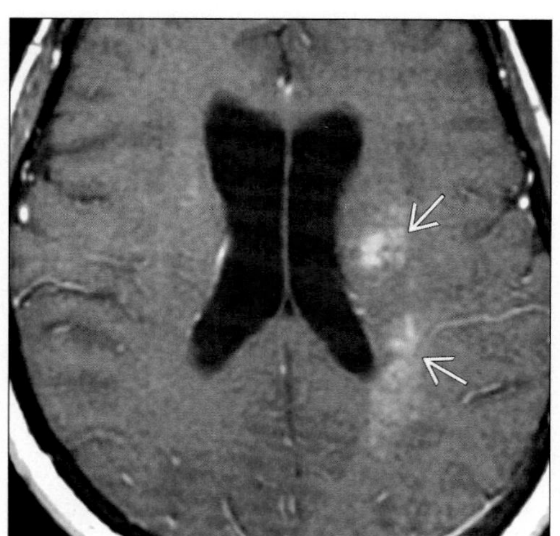

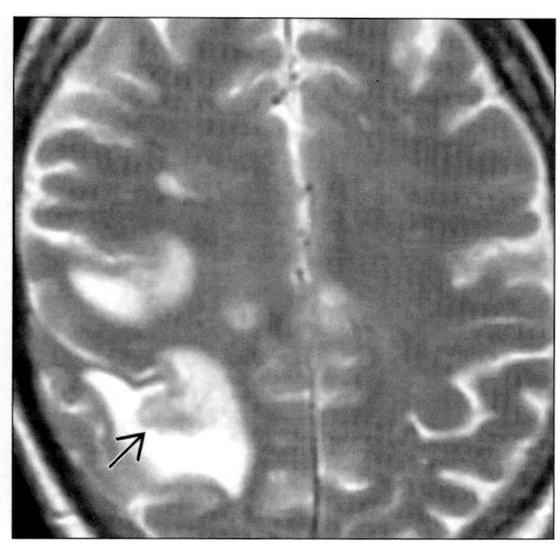

(Left) *Axial T1WI C+ MR in the same patient shows numerous foci of punctate and linear enhancement ➔ within the areas of FLAIR signal abnormality. The enhancement pattern suggests the correct diagnosis of intravascular lymphoma in this patient with dementia.* ***(Right)*** *Axial T2WI MR shows multifocal areas of abnormal hyperintensity involving the subcortical and deep white matter with mild cortical involvement ➔. Cortical involvement is often seen in intravascular lymphoma and may mimic an infarct.*

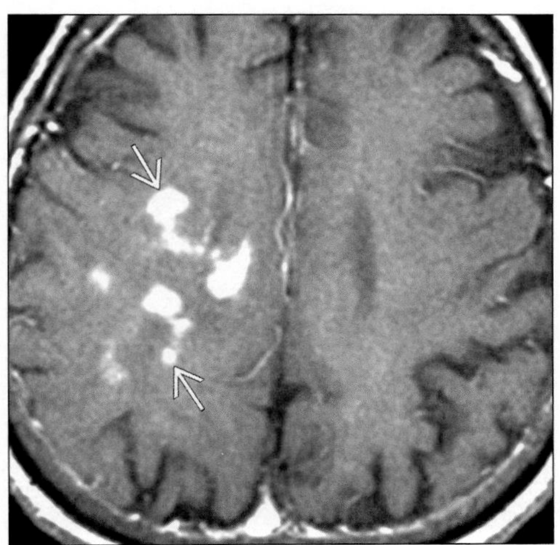

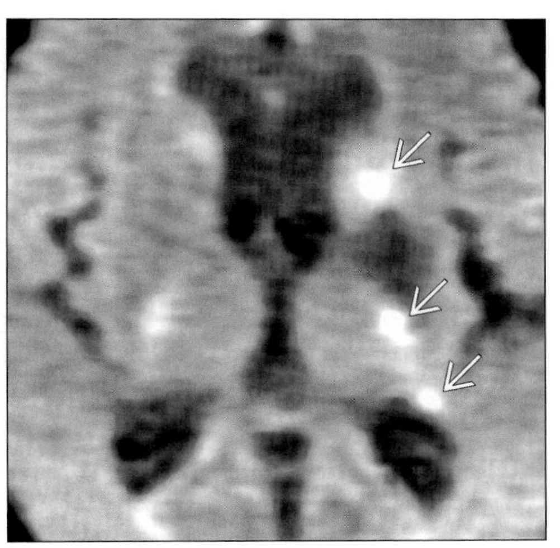

(Left) *Axial T1WI C+ MR shows multifocal areas of nodular & linear enhancement in the right periventricular & subcortical white matter ➔ in this IVL patient. Enhancement patterns of IVL are variable and may be linear, punctate, patchy, nodular, ring-like, gyriform, or homogeneous. Meningeal &/or dural enhancement has also been described.* ***(Right)*** *Axial DWI MR shows multifocal areas of restriction in the basal ganglia and periventricular regions ➔. Imaging of IVL may mimic vasculitis.*

LEUKEMIA

Key Facts

Terminology

- Granulocytic sarcoma, chloroma, extramedullary leukemic tumors (EML)
- Multiple other intracranial manifestations, complications of leukemia/treatment
  - PRES, invasive fungal infection
  - Late development of cavernous angiomas after radiation therapy
  - PTLD after bone marrow transplantation
  - Venous thrombosis associated with chemotherapy

Imaging

- Homogeneous enhancing tumor(s) in patients with known or suspected myeloproliferative disorder
- May present with/mimic hematoma
- Meningeal (dural-based or pial) > intraparenchymal lesions

Top Differential Diagnoses

- Metastatic neuroblastoma (NBT)
- Meningioma
- Extraaxial hematoma
- Extramedullary hematopoiesis
- Langerhans cell histiocytosis (LCH)

Pathology

- CNS leukemia presents in 3 forms
  - Meningeal disease (usually with ALL)
  - Intravascular aggregates (leukostasis): Can rupture, hemorrhage with markedly ↑ leukocyte counts
  - Tumor masses (chloroma)

Diagnostic Checklist

- Hemorrhagic lesions in children with AML can be chloroma **or** complication of therapy

*(**Left**) Coronal graphic shows multiple foci of leukemic infiltrates in the skull base/paranasal sinuses ➡, hypothalamus/infundibulum ➡, basal ganglia ➡, and dura ➡. Green color observed at pathology results in the name "chloroma." The accepted term is "granulocytic sarcoma." (**Right**) Coronal T1WI C+ MR shows an enhancing dural-based granulocytic sarcoma ➡ with an enhancing dural "tail" ➡.*

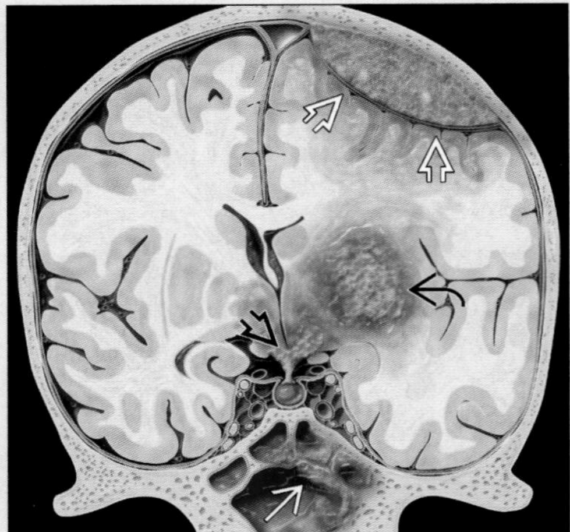

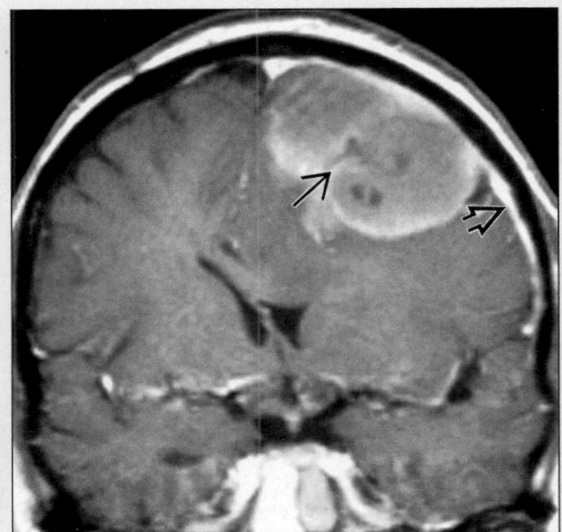

*(**Left**) Axial NECT demonstrates a hyperdense frontoparietal mass ➡ surrounded by a collar of edema ➡. The presentation of cerebral granulocytic sarcomas have been most commonly reported in the context of AML relapse. (**Right**) Axial T1WI C+ MR in a patient with ALL shows enhancement in both Meckel caves which are expanded and filled with leukemic infiltrates ➡. Both trigeminal nerves are markedly enlarged in their cisternal segments ➡. Other scans showed multiple, enhancing cranial nerves.*

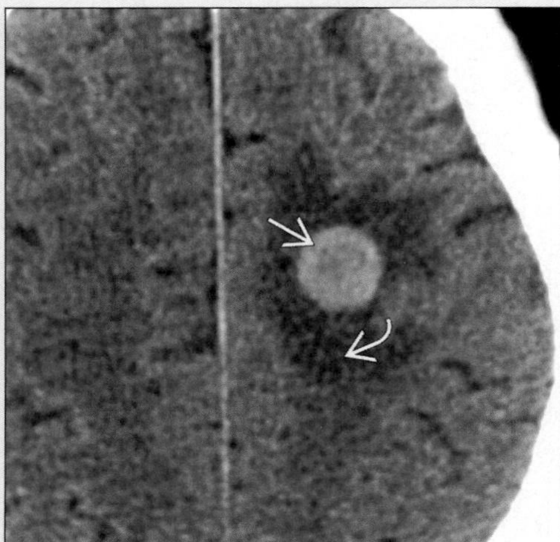

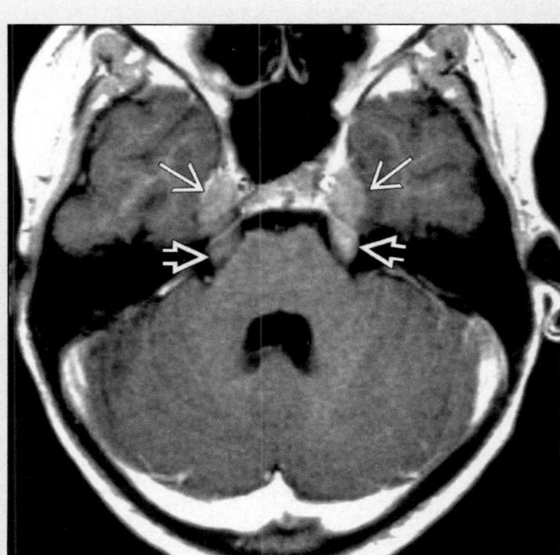

TERMINOLOGY

Abbreviations
- Extramedullary leukemic tumors (EML)
- Extramedullary myeloblastoma, extramedullary myeloid cell tumors (EmMCT)

Synonyms
- Granulocytic sarcoma, chloroma

Definitions
- Solid tumor of myeloblasts/myelocytes/promyelocytes
  - In patients with myeloproliferative disorder
- Multiple other intracranial manifestations of leukemia/treatment complications
  - Posterior reversible encephalopathy syndrome (PRES)
  - Invasive fungal infection
  - Late development of cavernous angiomas after radiation therapy
  - Post-transplantation lymphoproliferative disease (PTLD) after bone marrow transplantation
  - Venous thrombosis associated with chemotherapy (L-asparaginase)
  - Vasculitis
    - Primary manifestation of leukemia
    - Secondary to treatment (transretinoic acid)
    - Secondary to infection (e.g., *Aspergillus*)

IMAGING

General Features
- Best diagnostic clue
  - Homogeneous enhancing tumor(s) in patients with known or suspected myeloproliferative disorder
  - Most often complication of acute myelogenous leukemia (AML)
- Location
  - Meningeal (dural-based or pial) > intraparenchymal lesions

CT Findings
- NECT
  - Iso-/hyperdense to brain
    - May rapidly become hypodense (necrosis, liquefaction)
  - May present with (or mimic) hematoma
  - Look for skull base/paranasal sinus involvement
- CECT
  - Homogeneous enhancement
    - Hyperdensity or presence of hemorrhage may mask enhancement
  - May have rim enhancement, mimic abscess

MR Findings
- T1WI
  - Hypo-/isointense to brain
  - Can distinguish between acute hematoma, nonhemorrhagic mass
- T2WI
  - Heterogeneously hyper- to isointense
  - Pial disease may extend into perivascular spaces, appear as patchy WM hyperintensities
- FLAIR
  - More sensitive than T2WI for leptomeningeal disease
- T2* GRE
  - Helpful for identifying cavernous angiomas as very late complication of leukemia treatment
- DWI
  - May restrict (hyperintense on DWI, hypointense on ADC)
  - Helps distinguish ischemic complications from PRES
- T1WI C+
  - Homogeneous enhancement
    - May become heterogeneous with necrosis/ liquefaction
  - Leptomeningeal or perivascular space enhancement
  - Fat-saturation technique essential for assessment of skull base disease
- MRA
  - May show vasospasm in cases of PRES
  - May identify medium-vessel vasculitis
- MRV
  - Essential in evaluation of hemorrhagic lesions
  - Identify presence or extent of venous thrombosis

Nuclear Medicine Findings
- Bone scan
  - Tc-99m MDP commonly used for bone disease in leukemia
  - Soft tissue uptake typically reflects hypercalcemia, not chloroma
- PET
  - Avid uptake on FDG PET exams

Imaging Recommendations
- Best imaging tool
  - MR with contrast
  - NECT provides additional information in hemorrhagic lesions
- Protocol advice
  - Use T1WI C+ FS

DIFFERENTIAL DIAGNOSIS

Metastatic Neuroblastoma (NBT)
- Rarely occurs without extracranial disease
- Characteristic "raccoon eyes" clinical presentation
- Spiculated periostitis

Meningioma
- May be very difficult to distinguish
- Dural "tail" may be more common in meningioma

Extraaxial Hematoma
- Extracranial soft tissue swelling or skull fracture
- If no appropriate history, consider possibility of child abuse

Extramedullary Hematopoiesis
- Markedly hypointense on T2WI
- Same at-risk patient population

Langerhans Cell Histiocytosis (LCH)
- Destruction of adjacent bone without periosteal reaction

- Diabetes insipidus

Ewing Sarcoma

- Aggressive pattern of growth
- Destruction of adjacent bone

Neurosarcoidosis

- Mimic of leptomeningeal disease
- Less commonly presents as dural-based masses

PATHOLOGY

General Features

- Etiology
  - Some association with exposures
    - Ionizing radiation, hydrocarbons, benzene, alkylating agents
- Genetics
  - Children with CNS leukemic infiltrates in AML have ↑ chromosome 11 abnormalities compared to those without CNS disease
  - Chromosomal 8, 21 translocations reported in cases of AML with chloroma
  - AML has higher incidence in some genetic syndromes
    - Down, Bloom, Fanconi syndromes
- Associated abnormalities
  - Less common in non-AML myeloproliferative disorders
    - Myeloid metaplasia
    - Hypereosinophilic syndrome
    - Polycythemia vera
- CNS leukemia presents in 3 forms
  - Meningeal disease
    - Usually with acute lymphoblastic leukemia (ALL)
  - Intravascular aggregates (leukostasis)
    - May rupture, hemorrhage (with markedly high leukocyte counts)
  - Focal tumor masses (chloroma)
- Chloroma
  - Leukemic masses 1st described in 1811
  - "Chloroma" coined in 1853
  - Renamed granulocytic sarcoma in 1966

Gross Pathologic & Surgical Features

- Called "chloroma" because of green color in 70% of cases
  - Caused by high levels of myeloperoxidase

Microscopic Features

- Moderate to large cells
- Pleomorphic nuclei
- Multiple mitoses give "starry sky" appearance

CLINICAL ISSUES

Presentation

- Most common signs/symptoms
  - May precede marrow diagnosis of leukemia
  - 50% of cases diagnosed only at autopsy
  - CNS lesions more likely symptomatic
  - Focal signs from local mass effect
  - Headache from hemorrhage
- Clinical profile
  - Child with AML develops new neurological signs or symptoms

Demographics

- Age
  - 60% of patients < 15 years
- Gender
  - M:F = 1.38:1
- Ethnicity
  - Hispanic children < 19 years have highest rates of leukemia
  - Incidence in Americans of European descent > African descent
- Epidemiology
  - 11% of patients with AML
  - 1-2% of patients with chronic myelogenous leukemia (CML)

Natural History & Prognosis

- Overall survival rates for AML (40-50%)
- Chloroma in setting of other myeloproliferative syndrome
  - Implies blastic transformation
  - Poor prognostic sign

Treatment

- Chemotherapy for induction
  - Cytarabine (Ara-C)
  - Anthracycline
- Bone marrow transplant for consolidation

DIAGNOSTIC CHECKLIST

Consider

- Extramedullary hematopoiesis can present in same patient population with similar appearance
- Hemorrhagic lesions in children with AML can be manifestation of chloroma or complication of therapy

Image Interpretation Pearls

- Multiple lesions at multiple sites suggestive of diagnosis
- Chloromas with enhancing rim (rare) can mimic abscess

SELECTED REFERENCES

1. Dicuonzo F et al: Posterior Reversible Encephalopathy Syndrome Associated With Methotrexate Neurotoxicity: Conventional Magnetic Resonance and Diffusion-Weighted Imaging Findings. J Child Neurol. Epub ahead of print, 2009
2. Koenig MK et al: Central nervous system complications of blastic hyperleukocytosis in childhood acute lymphoblastic leukemia: diagnostic and prognostic implications. J Child Neurol. 23(11):1347-52, 2008

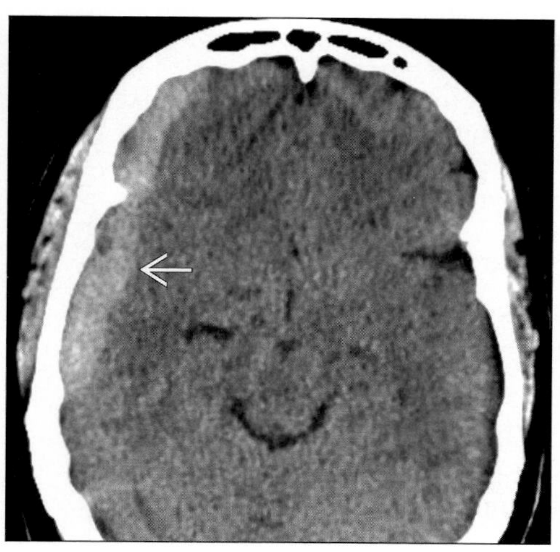

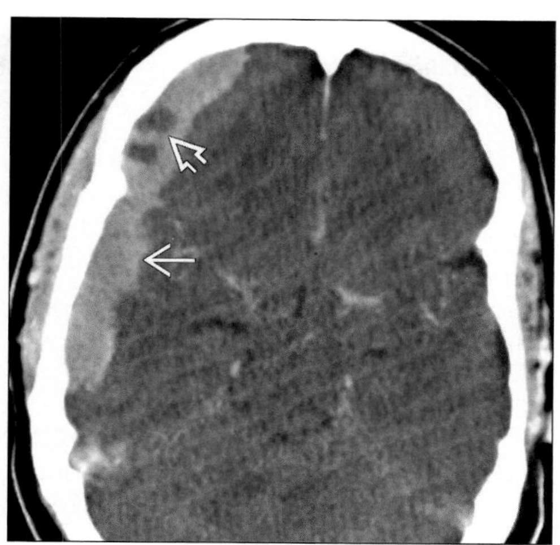

(Left) *Axial NECT demonstrates a hyperdense dural-based mass mimicking a subdural hematoma in a patient with acute myelocytic leukemia ➡.* ***(Right)*** *Axial CECT shows homogeneous enhancement in the dural-based mass ➡, thus excluding simple hemorrhage. Small areas of nonenhancement ➡ are due to necrosis/liquefaction rather than rapid bleeding. These are typical findings in dural-based leukemic infiltrates in patients with AML.*

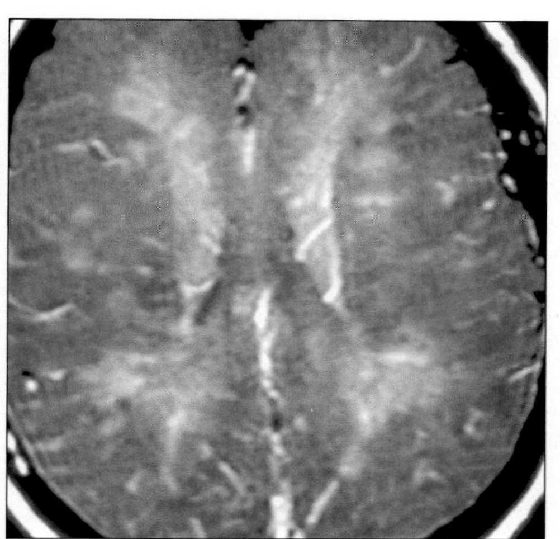

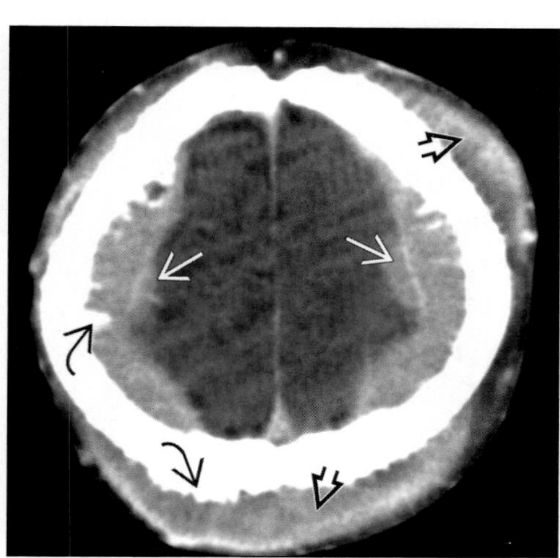

(Left) *Axial T1WI C+ MR in a patient with leukemia and progressive encephalopathy shows multiple, enhancing intra- and perivascular infiltrates. "Carcinomatous encephalitis" is a rare complication of leukemia.* ***(Right)*** *Axial CECT in a patient with leukemic disease & skull involvement shows large, bilateral, convexity epidural leukemic masses ➡. Note the subperiosteal accumulations of tumor ➡. The spiculated appearance of the outer and inner calvarium ➡ speaks to the extensive marrow involvement.*

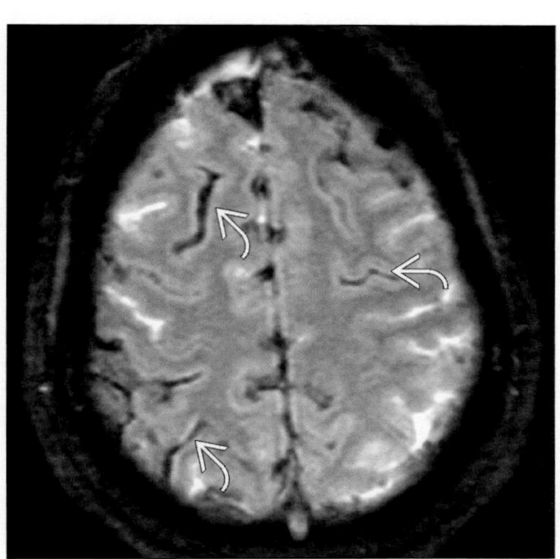

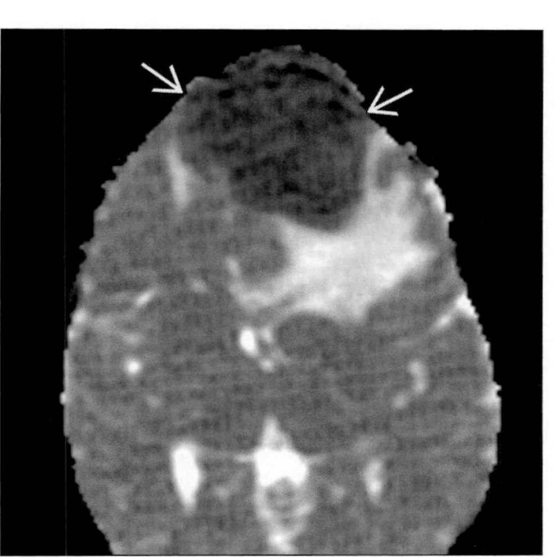

(Left) *Axial T2* GRE MR shows leptomeningeal low signal ➡ in a patient with AML and blast crisis. CSF analysis showed hemorrhage and leukemic cell infiltrates.* ***(Right)*** *Axial ADC in a 13-year-old girl with sinusitis and scalp swelling shows a restricting, profoundly hypointense mass ➡ that was hyperdense on CT and hyperintense and strongly enhancing on DWI (not shown). Biopsy and blood studies showed high-risk ALL.*

GERMINOMA

Key Facts

Terminology

- Synonyms: Dysgerminoma, extragonadal seminoma (formerly called atypical teratoma)
- Basal ganglia, internal capsule, thalamic germinoma = "off-midline" or "ectopic" germinoma

Imaging

- 80-90% of CNS germinomas in midline near 3rd ventricle
  - Pineal region mass ("engulfs" Ca++ pineal gland)
  - Pituitary/stalk/hypothalamus mass
  - Pineal + suprasellar germinomas ("double midline atypical teratoma" or bifocal germinoma)
  - Basal ganglia/thalami ~ 5-10% (uni-/bilateral)
- Strong, homogeneous enhancement, ± CSF seeding, ± brain invasion
- Show restricted diffusion (high cellularity)

Top Differential Diagnoses

- Other benign/malignant pineal region GCTs
  - Malignant mixed germ cell, yolk sac, choriocarcinoma, embryonal Ca
  - Immature teratoma, mature teratoma, mixed mature/immature
- Pineoblastoma
- Pineal parenchymal tumor of intermediate differentiation
- Histiocytosis, sarcoid

Clinical Issues

- 90% of patients < 20 years
- M:F ≈ 10:1

Diagnostic Checklist

- Young patient presents with diabetes insipidus? Think germinoma or LCH!

*(**Left**) Sagittal graphic shows synchronous germinomas in the suprasellar and pineal regions. Note the CSF spread of tumor in the lateral, 3rd, and 4th ventricles ➔. (**Right**) Sagittal T1WI C+ MR in a 14-year-old female with sleep disturbances, behavioral problems, and personality change demonstrates homogeneously, intensely enhancing suprasellar germinoma ➲. β-HCG/AFP were normal.*

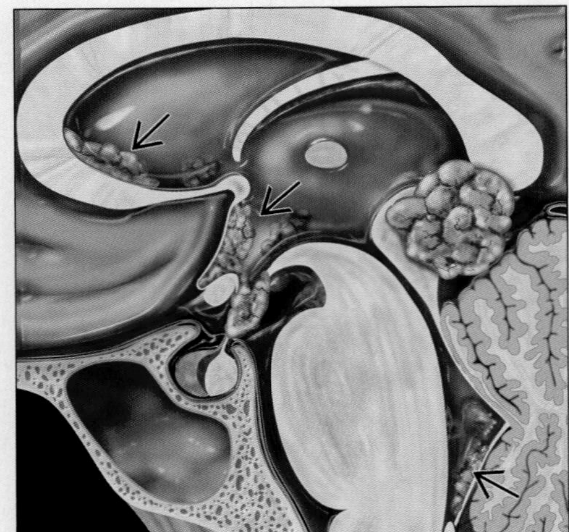

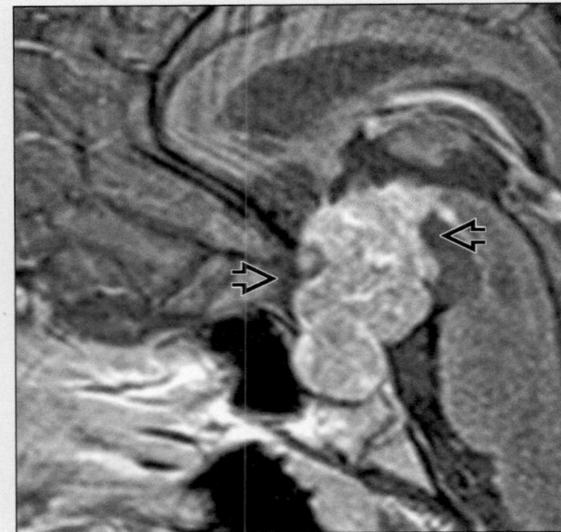

*(**Left**) Axial T1WI C+ MR shows an inhomogeneously enhancing midline mass of the pineal region ➲ in a boy who presented with double vision, nausea, vomiting, & headache in the frontal region. After surgical removal, histological analysis revealed a pineal germinoma. (**Right**) Axial NECT in an 18-year-old male with treated suprasellar germinoma presenting with a worsening headache. Note the thick rind of hyperdense tumor ➔ surrounding the lateral ventricles & infiltrating the corpus callosum & caudate nuclei.*

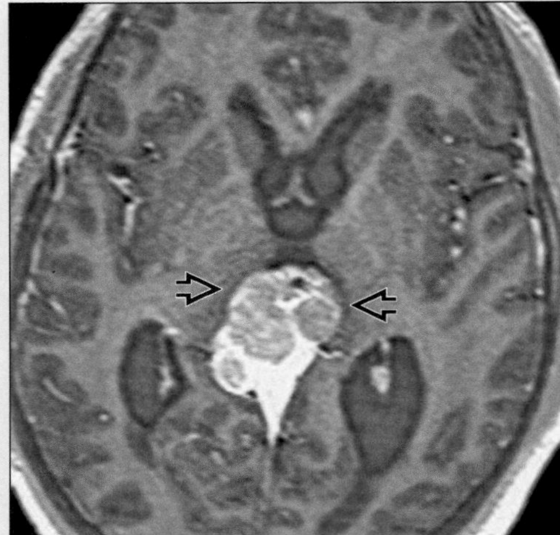

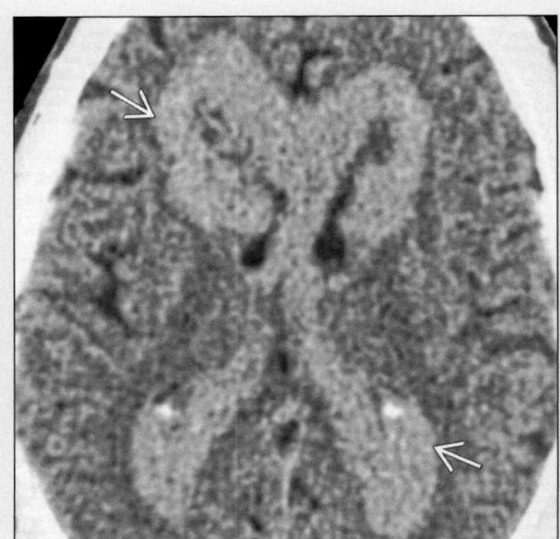

GERMINOMA

TERMINOLOGY

Synonyms

- Dysgerminoma, extragonadal seminoma
  - Formerly called atypical teratoma
- Off-midline or "ectopic" germinoma
  - Germinoma originating in basal ganglia (BG), internal capsule, thalami

Definitions

- Morphologic homologues of germinal neoplasms arising in gonads, extragonadal sites

IMAGING

General Features

- Best diagnostic clue
  - Pineal region mass that "engulfs" pineal gland
  - Suprasellar mass with diabetes insipidus (DI)
  - Bilateral BG lesions with ipsilateral hemiatrophy
- Location
  - CNS germinomas have propensity to hug midline near 3rd ventricle ~ 80-90%
    - Pineal region ~ 50-65%
    - Suprasellar ~ 25-35%
    - Basal ganglia/thalami ~ 5-10% (uni-/bilateral)
  - Other sites: Intraventricular (3rd), intrasellar, bulbar, intramedullary, midbrain, hemispheric
  - Simultaneous pineal & suprasellar in 21% of germinomas → "double midline atypical teratoma" or bifocal germinoma
  - Simultaneous midline + off-midline germinomas reported
- Size
  - Location dictates size at presentation
    - Suprasellar germinoma: Early presentation with DI, mass may be small
    - Pineal region germinoma: Due to tectal compression, ± invasion, mass may be small

CT Findings

- NECT
  - Sharply circumscribed dense mass (hyperdense to GM)
    - Pineal: Mass drapes around posterior 3rd ventricle or "engulfs" Ca++ pineal gland
    - Suprasellar: Retrochiasmatic, noncystic, noncalcified
    - Basal ganglia: Often no abnormality in early stage, later iso-/hyperdense lesions without mass effect
      - Single calcified spot may be seen on NECT in early stage
  - ± hydrocephalus
- CECT
  - Strong uniform enhancement, ± CSF seeding
    - Pineal region: Look for posterior 3rd ventricular wall infiltration
    - Suprasellar: Look for thick stalk, infiltration of 3rd ventricular floor, lateral walls, and anterior columns of fornices
  - Cystic/necrotic/hemorrhagic components not uncommon with larger germinomas (especially in basal ganglia)

MR Findings

- T1WI
  - Iso-/hyperintense to GM
  - Early → may only see absent posterior pituitary bright spot
  - Basal ganglia/thalami: 20-33% associated ipsilateral hemiatrophy
- T2WI
  - Iso- to hyperintense to GM (high nuclear to cytoplasmic ratio)
    - Cystic/necrotic foci (high T2 signal)
      - Multiple cysts common in germinoma and all GCTs (up to 44%)
    - Less common: Hypointense foci (hemorrhage)
- FLAIR
  - Slightly hyperintense to GM
- T2* GRE
  - Calcification, hemorrhage (rare)
- DWI
  - Restricted diffusion due to high cellularity
- T1WI C+
  - Strong, homogeneous enhancement, ± CSF seeding, ± brain invasion
  - BG & thalami: Ill-defined enhancement
    - Later cystic changes (due to previous hemorrhage and tumor progression)
- MRS
  - ↑ choline, ↓ NAA, ± lactate

Imaging Recommendations

- Best imaging tool
  - Enhanced MR of brain and spine
- Protocol advice
  - MR evaluation of entire neuraxis before surgery

DIFFERENTIAL DIAGNOSIS

Other Pineal GCTs

- Malignant mixed germ cell, yolk sac, choriocarcinoma, embryonal carcinoma
- Immature teratoma, mature teratoma, mixed mature/immature

Pineoblastoma

- Large, heterogeneous pineal mass; peripheral Ca++
- Obstructive hydrocephalus

Pineocytoma

- Mass "explodes" rather than "engulfs" pineal Ca++

Pineal Parenchymal Tumor of Intermediate Differentiation

- Pineal mass with histopath between pineocytoma and pineoblastoma

Pineal Cyst (Atypical)

- Often > 15 mm, rim-enhancing, variable signal of cyst contents, ± tectal compression

Craniopharyngioma

- Cystic, solid, and Ca++ components

Hypothalamic/Chiasmatic Astrocytoma
- Homogeneous enhancement, rarely associated with DI

Other Pineal Region Masses
- Astrocytoma
- Metastasis
- Meningioma
- Retinoblastoma
  - Trilateral → evaluate orbits and suprasellar regions

Other Suprasellar Region Lesions
- PNET
- Hamartoma (isointense with GM, nonenhancing)
- Suprasellar arachnoid cyst (CSF density/intensity; no enhancement)
- Langerhans cell histiocytosis (LCH)
- Sarcoid
- Metastases

PATHOLOGY

General Features
- Etiology
  - Toti-/pluripotential stem cells native to all 3 embryonic layers
  - BG & thalami: Ectopic totipotential cells that deviate from midline during very early stage of rostral neural tube development
- Associated abnormalities
  - Klinefelter syndrome (47XXY)
  - Down syndrome
  - Neurofibromatosis type 1
  - Laboratory derangements
    - Elevated placental alkaline phosphatase (PLAP)
    - ± elevation of serum and CSF β-HCG

Staging, Grading, & Classification
- Multiple site involvement (pineal, suprasellar, BG, thalamus) considered metastatic in USA, synchronous in Canada and Europe
- Pure germinoma: WHO grade II
- Germinoma with syncytiotrophoblastic giant cells (STGCs): WHO grade II-III

Gross Pathologic & Surgical Features
- Soft and friable, tan-white mass, ± necrosis

Microscopic Features
- Sheets of large polygonal primitive germ cells
- Lymphocytic infiltrates along fibrovascular septa

CLINICAL ISSUES

Presentation
- Most common signs/symptoms
  - Pineal region germinoma
    - Parinaud syndrome (upward gaze paralysis and altered convergence)
    - Headache due to tectal compression or invasion (hydrocephalus)
  - Suprasellar germinoma
    - Diabetes insipidus (DI)
    - Visual loss
    - Hypothalamic-pituitary dysfunction (↓ growth, precocious puberty)
  - Off-midline germinoma
    - Slow progressive hemiparesis (due to involvement of internal capsule and subsequent Wallerian degeneration)
    - Progressive mental deterioration, personality change, fever of unknown origin
    - Precocity, diabetes insipidus, hemianopsia, speech disturbance
    - Choreoathetoid movements

Demographics
- Age
  - CNS GCTs primarily seen in young patients (90% of patients < 20 years)
    - Peak: 10-12 years
- Gender
  - Pineal region germinoma: M:F ≈ 10:1
  - Suprasellar germinoma: More common in females
  - For all CNS germinomas: M:F = 1.5-2:1
- Ethnicity
  - CNS GCTs far more prevalent in Asia (9-15% of all CNS tumors in Japan)
- Epidemiology
  - Germinomas → 1-2% of all CNS tumors
    - 2-4% of pediatric CNS tumors (9-15% of CNS tumors in Japanese children)

Natural History & Prognosis
- Pure germinoma has favorable prognosis
  - Moderate elevation of β-HCG (< 50 IU/l) → favorable
- CSF dissemination and invasion of adjacent brain common

Treatment
- Biopsy to confirm histology, "pure" germinomas have best outcome
- Reduced dose and volume of XRT ± adjuvant chemotherapy

SELECTED REFERENCES

1. Lee J et al: Atypical basal ganglia germinoma presenting as cerebral hemiatrophy: diagnosis and follow-up with 11C-methionine positron emission tomography. Childs Nerv Syst. 25(1):29-37, 2009
2. Guerrero-Vázquez S et al: [Simultaneous suprasellar and pineal germinoma: a case report] Rev Neurol. 46(7):411-5, 2008
3. Rossi A et al: Bilateral germinoma of the basal ganglia. Pediatr Blood Cancer. 50(1):177-9, 2008
4. Villani A et al: Inherent diagnostic and treatment challenges in germinoma of the basal ganglia: a case report and review of the literature. J Neurooncol. 88(3):309-14, 2008
5. Sartori S et al: Germinoma with synchronous involvement of midline and off-midline structures associated with progressive hemiparesis and hemiatrophy in a young adult. Childs Nerv Syst. 23(11):1341-5, 2007
6. Ueno T et al: Spectrum of germ cell tumors: from head to toe. Radiographics. 24(2):387-404, 2004

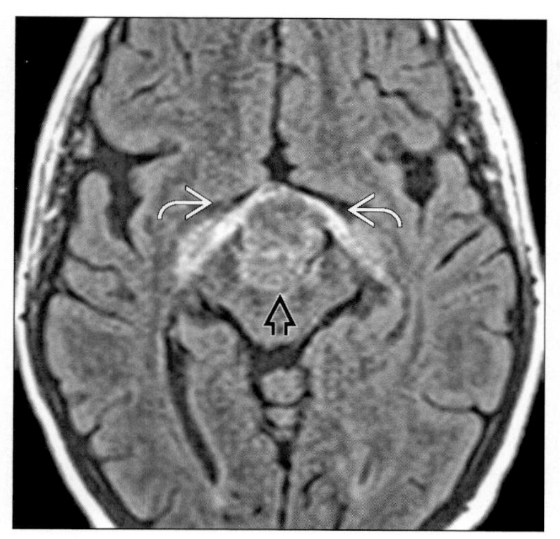

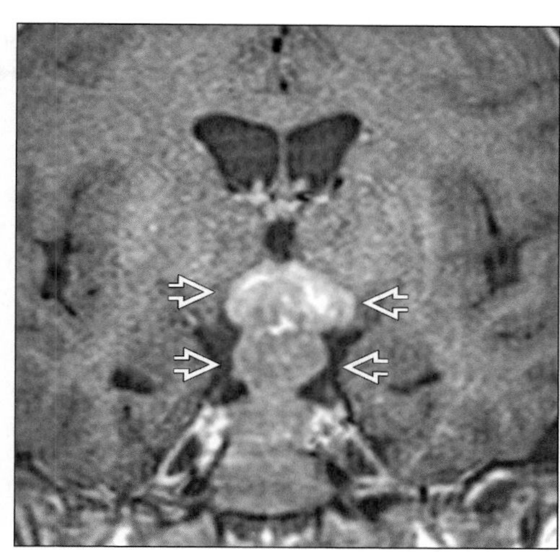

(Left) *Axial FLAIR MR demonstrates a well-defined mass in the suprasellar region ⇨ with elevation of the optic chiasm ➡. Optic chiasm hyperintensity is secondary to compression, not tumor infiltration.* ***(Right)*** *Coronal T1WI C+ MR in the same patient reveals a suprasellar, homogeneously enhancing mass ➡ with well-defined borders. Histological diagnosis was germinoma.*

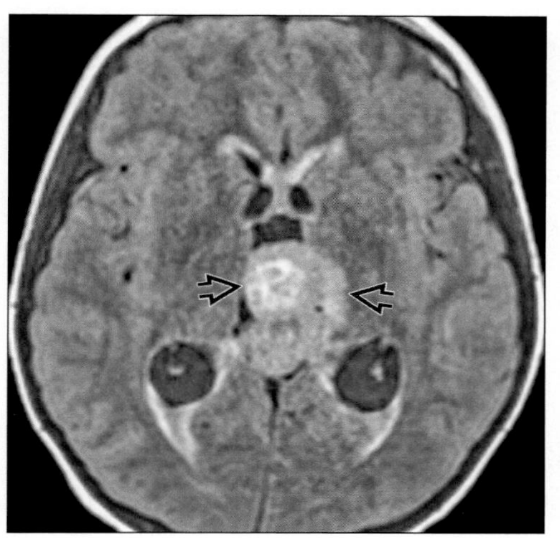

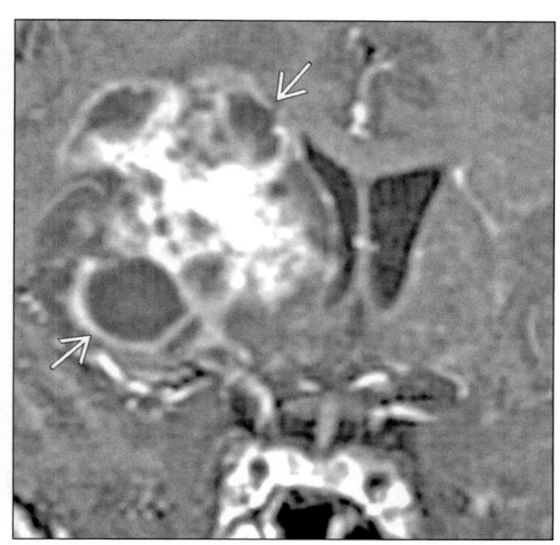

(Left) *Axial FLAIR MR in a 15-year-old boy with pineal germinoma, presenting with headache and papilledema, demonstrates an inhomogeneous, multilobulated midline mass in the pineal region ⇨. Note the absence of perifocal edema.* ***(Right)*** *Coronal T1WI C+ MR in 6-year-old boy with left-sided weakness and headaches shows a mixed solid/multicystic right basal ganglia mass ➡. Approximately 5-10% of intracranial germinomas arise within the basal ganglia.*

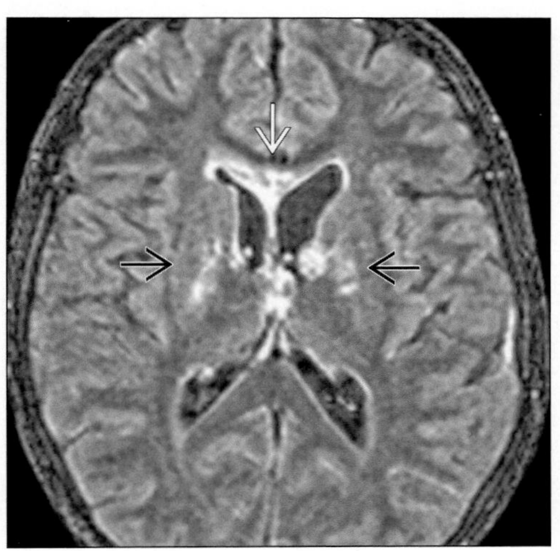

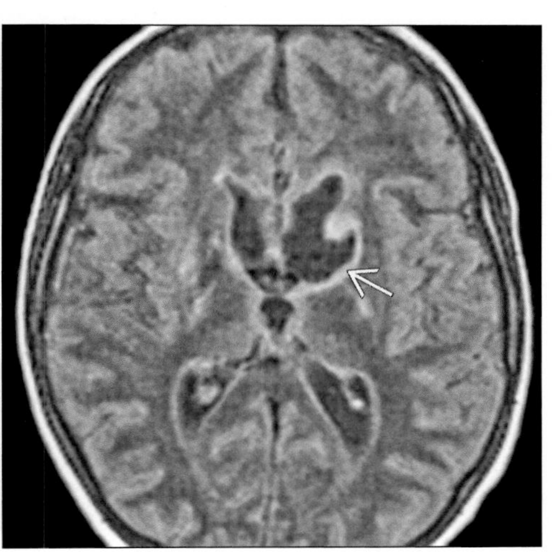

(Left) *Axial FLAIR MR in a 15-year-old girl with bilateral germinoma of the BG, presenting with dystonia, diabetes insipidus, and personality change, shows hyperintensities in the BG region on both sides →, as well as in the corpus callosum ➡. Note the missing mass effect.* ***(Right)*** *Axial FLAIR MR in the same patient 1 year later shows progression of the disease with cavitations in the BG ➡. Mild elevation of β-HCG was found in the CSF, consistent with germinoma.*

TERATOMA

Key Facts

Terminology

- Intracranial teratoma
- Intracranial germ cell tumor (ICGCT)

Imaging

- Midline mass containing Ca++, soft tissue, cysts, and fat
- Soft tissue components iso- to hyperintense, enhancing
- CT: ↑ signal from fat, variable signal from Ca++
- T2WI: ↓ signal from Ca++
- Restricted diffusion in solid (high cellular) parts
- Anatomic location can not be determined in 50%
  - Lost anatomic landmarks in large masses
- Huge holocranial mass in newborns or fetus

Top Differential Diagnoses

- Craniopharyngioma
- Dermoid
- Nongerminoma germ cell tumor
- Pineoblastoma, PNET

Clinical Issues

- Detected in utero or as neonate
- M > F
- Leading perinatal brain tumor (42%)
- Lowest survival rate of all fetal brain tumors
- Fetal US: Macrocephaly and hydrocephaly
- More common among Asians

Diagnostic Checklist

- Midline tumor
  - Predominantly in sellar, pineal region
  - Contents: Fat, soft tissue, Ca++
- Newborn with holocranial tumor? Think teratoma!

*(**Left**) Sagittal graphic shows a heterogeneous pineal teratoma with a solid, calcific ⇨, and fatty → composition. (**Right**) Sagittal gross pathology section shows a pineal teratoma ➡ with obstructive hydrocephalus. (Courtesy B. Alvord, MD.)*

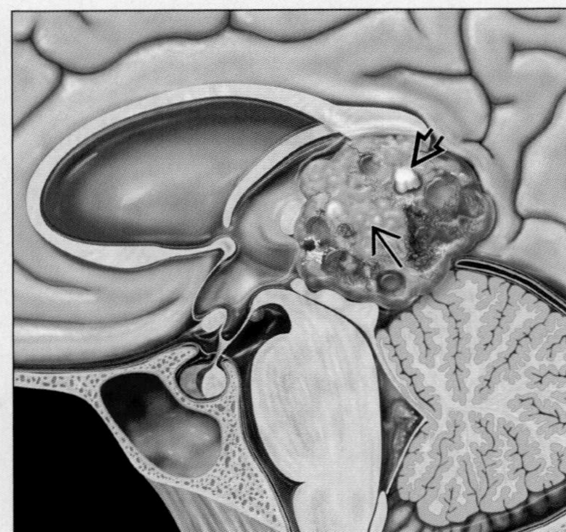

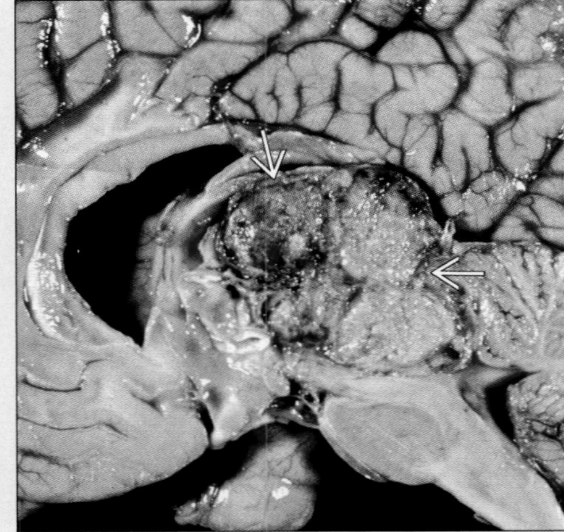

*(**Left**) Axial T1WI MR demonstrates a heterogeneous pineal region teratoma with soft tissue, calcific, and fatty → elements. (**Right**) Coronal T2WI MR in a 1-year-old child with a large hemispheric tumor shows inhomogeneous, predominantly low signal intensity in the solid portion of the mass ⇨ with cystic parts located on the periphery of the tumor ➡.*

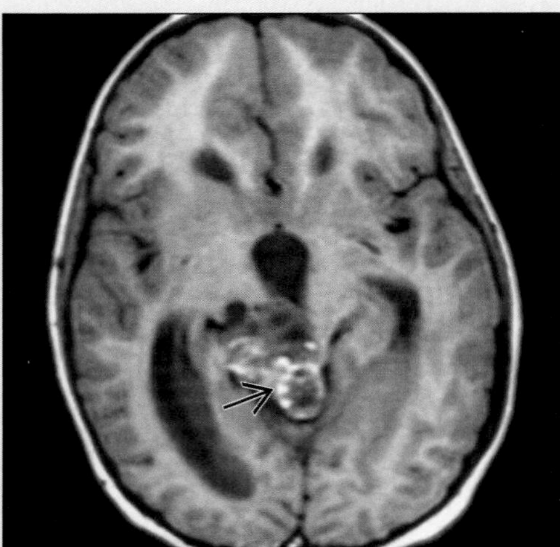

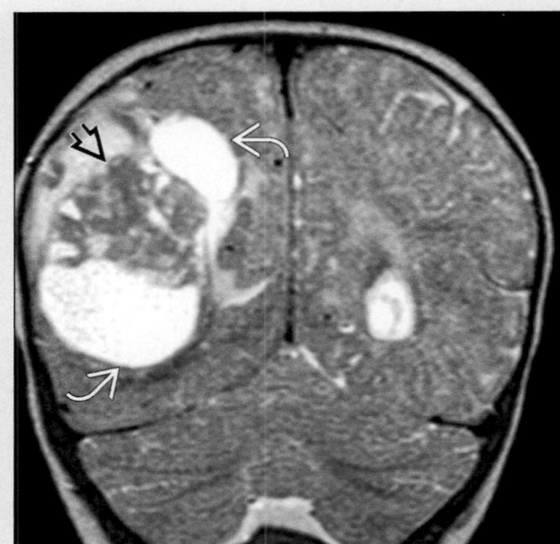

TERATOMA

TERMINOLOGY

Abbreviations

- Intracranial teratoma
- Intracranial germ cell tumor (ICGCT)

Definitions

- Tridermal mass originating from
  - Displaced embryonic tissue that is misenfolded
  - Embryonic stem cells
  - Parthenogenetic → "blighted twins"
- Types
  - Mature teratoma
  - Immature teratoma
  - Teratoma with malignant transformation

IMAGING

General Features

- Best diagnostic clue
  - Midline mass containing Ca++, soft tissue, cysts, fat
  - Huge holocranial mass in newborn or fetus
- Location
  - Hugs midline
    - Suprasellar
      - Hypothalamus, optic chiasm
    - Pineal gland ± involvement of mesencephalic tectum
      - Tectum commonly involved
  - Rare locations
    - Brain hemispheres
    - Ventricles
    - Cavernous sinus
  - Almost 50% are so large that precise anatomic origin cannot be determined
- Size
  - Variable
  - Holocranial teratomas are huge!

CT Findings

- NECT
  - Fat, soft tissue, Ca++
  - Cystic components common
- CECT
  - Soft tissue components enhance
- Bone CT
  - Skull erosions may be seen in huge tumors

MR Findings

- T1WI
  - Increased signal from fat
  - Variable signal from Ca++
- T2WI
  - Soft tissue components iso- to hyperintense
  - Perifocal edema
    - Usually minimal or absent (mature teratoma)
    - Common in immature (malignant) teratoma
- FLAIR
  - ↓ signal from cysts, ↑ signal from solid tissue
- T2* GRE
  - Decreased signal from Ca++
- DWI
  - Restricted diffusion in solid (high cellular) parts
- T1WI C+
  - Soft tissue enhancement

Ultrasonographic Findings

- Heterogeneous mass with internal shadowing (Ca++)
- In utero ultrasound
  - Intracranial mass (often huge)
  - Hydrocephalus, polyhydramnios

Imaging Recommendations

- Best imaging tool
  - CT to demonstrate soft tissue, fat, Ca++
  - MR best characterizes relationship of teratoma to midline structures
- Protocol advice
  - Fat-suppressed MR

DIFFERENTIAL DIAGNOSIS

Craniopharyngioma

- Cystic and solid, calcifications

Dermoid

- Minimal/no enhancement
- Look for rupture with fat "droplets"

Other Nongerminomatous Germ Cell Tumor

- Heterogeneous suprasellar or pineal mass
- Includes embryonal carcinoma, yolk sac tumor, choriocarcinoma, mixed germ cell tumor

Pineoblastoma

- Large pineal mass with "exploded" Ca++
- Hydrocephalus present in 100%

Supratentorial PNET

- Ca++, hemorrhage, necrosis common
- Does not contain fat

Astrocytoma

- Calcifications rare

PATHOLOGY

General Features

- Etiology
  - Originates during 3rd or 4th week of fetal development
  - Anomalous development of primitive streak or its derivatives
- Genetics
  - Gains of hypomethylated, active X chromosomes occur in all ICGCTs
- Associated abnormalities
  - Increased serum carcinoembryonic antigen (CEA)
  - Increased α-fetoprotein if tumor contains enteric glandular elements (yolk sac cells)

Staging, Grading, & Classification

- WHO classification
  - Mature teratoma
  - Immature

- Teratoma with malignant transformation (TMT)

Gross Pathologic & Surgical Features

- Mature teratomas → fully differentiated tissue
  - Cystic component frequent in mature teratoma
- Immature or malignant teratoma → resembles fetal tissues

Microscopic Features

- Contain elements representing 3 germinal layers
  - Ectoderm
  - Mesoderm
  - Endoderm

CLINICAL ISSUES

Presentation

- Most common signs/symptoms
  - Macrocephaly → congenital teratoma
  - Parinaud syndrome → pineal lesions
- Other signs/symptoms
  - Increased serum carcinoembryonic antigen (CEA)
- Clinical profile
  - In utero demonstration of hydrocephalus, macrocephaly, and heterogeneous mass
  - Congenital teratomas
    - Diffuse intracranial form: Large tumors replacing intracranial content
    - Small tumors causing hydrocephalus
    - Massive form: Extension in orbits, pharynx, neck

Demographics

- Age
  - Detected in utero or as neonate
- Gender
  - M > F
- Ethnicity
  - More common among Asians
- Epidemiology
  - 2-4% of intracranial tumors in children
  - Leading perinatal brain tumor (42%)

Natural History & Prognosis

- 5-year survival for malignant teratomas: 18%
- Congenital teratoma
  - Majority stillborn or die 1st week of life
- Lowest survival rate of all fetal brain tumors
- Pineal mature teratomas have good prognosis
- CSF metastases common in malignant (immature) teratoma

Treatment

- Surgical removal
  - Operative mortality in 1st year: 20%

DIAGNOSTIC CHECKLIST

Consider

- Think teratoma in newborn with holocranial tumor
- Young age, male predominance, pineal preferential location = teratoma

Image Interpretation Pearls

- Midline tumor predominantly in sellar and pineal region containing fat, soft tissue, and Ca++

SELECTED REFERENCES

1. Isaacs H: Fetal brain tumors: a review of 154 cases. Am J Perinatol. 26(6):453-66, 2009
2. Sato K et al: Pathology of intracranial germ cell tumors. Prog Neurol Surg. 23:59-75, 2009
3. Berhouma M et al: Transcortical approach to a huge pineal mature teratoma. Pediatr Neurosurg. 44(1):52-4, 2008
4. Köken G et al: Prenatal diagnosis of a fetal intracranial immature teratoma. Fetal Diagn Ther. 24(4):368-71, 2008
5. Noudel R et al: Intracranial teratomas in children: the role and timing of surgical removal. J Neurosurg Pediatr. 2(5):331-8, 2008
6. Arslan E et al: Massive congenital intracranial immature teratoma of the lateral ventricle with retro-orbital extension: a case report and review of the literature. Pediatr Neurosurg. 43(4):338-42, 2007
7. Baykaner MK et al: A mature cystic teratoma in pineal region mimicking parietal encephalocele in a newborn. Childs Nerv Syst. 23(5):573-6, 2007
8. Shim KW et al: Congenital cavernous sinus cystic teratoma. Yonsei Med J. 48(4):704-10, 2007
9. Erman T et al: Congenital intracranial immature teratoma of the lateral ventricle: a case report and review of the literature. Neurol Res. 27(1):53-6, 2005
10. Cavalheiro S et al: Fetal brain tumors. Childs Nerv Syst. 19(7-8):529-36, 2003
11. Im SH et al: Congenital intracranial teratoma: prenatal diagnosis and postnatal successful resection. Med Pediatr Oncol. 40(1):57-61, 2003
12. Jaing TH et al: Intracranial germ cell tumors: a retrospective study of 44 children. Pediatr Neurol. 26(5):369-73, 2002
13. Liang L et al: MRI of intracranial germ-cell tumours. Neuroradiology. 44(5):382-8, 2002
14. Okada Y et al: Hypomethylated X chromosome gain and rare isochromosome 12p in diverse intracranial germ cell tumors. J Neuropathol Exp Neurol. 61(6):531-8, 2002

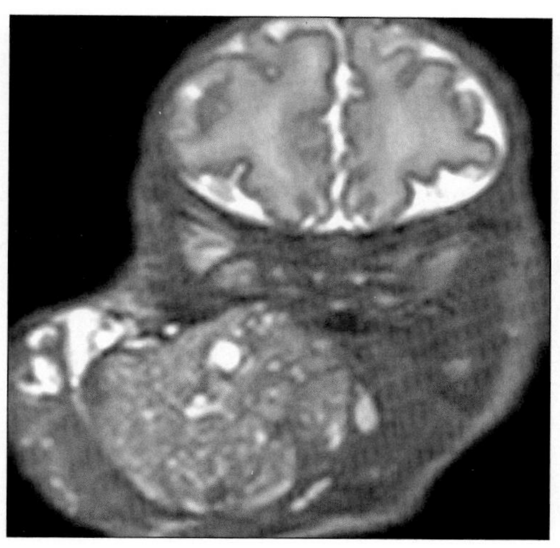

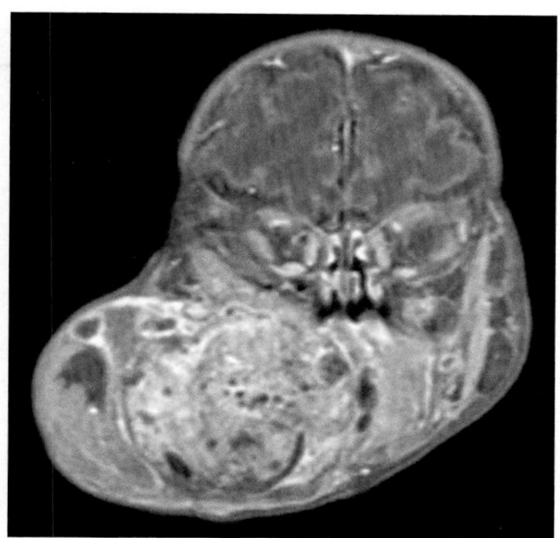

(Left) *Coronal T2WI MR shows a huge neck mass with relatively low signal intensity (indicating high cellularity) without extension into the brain. Immature (malignant) teratoma was found at surgery.* ***(Right)*** *Coronal T1WI C+ FS MR shows a huge, inhomogeneously enhancing neck mass.*

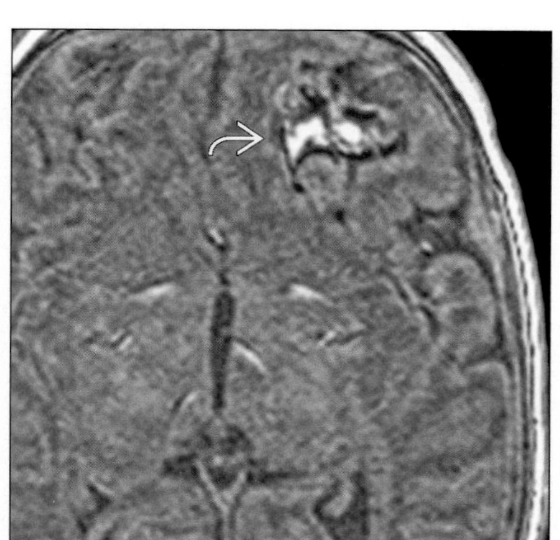

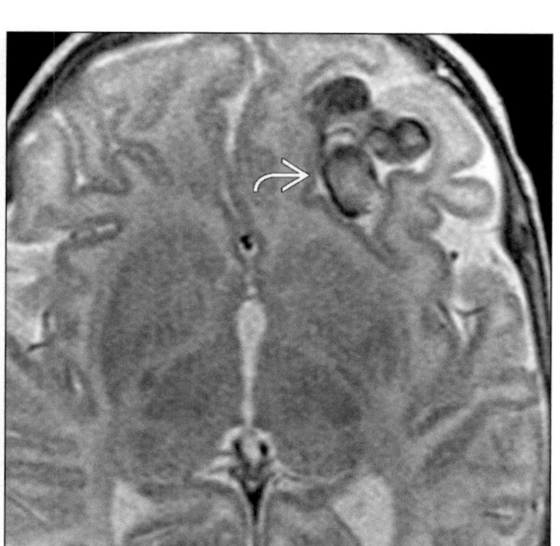

(Left) *Axial T1WI MR demonstrates an inhomogeneous mass in the left frontal lobe ➔ in a male newborn.* ***(Right)*** *Axial T2WI MR shows a hypointense lesion with relatively well-defined margins ➔. The perifocal edema is missing.*

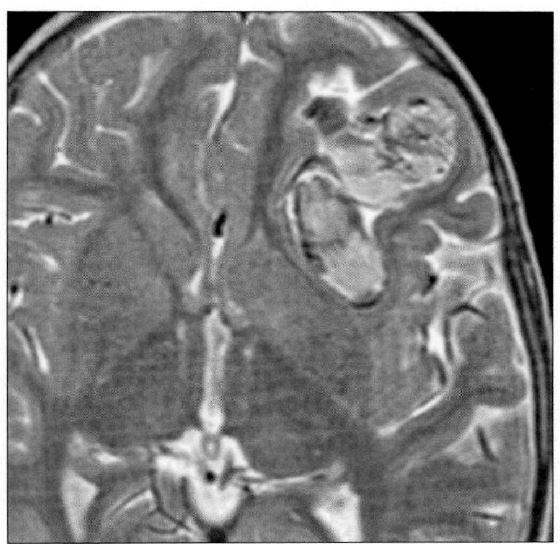

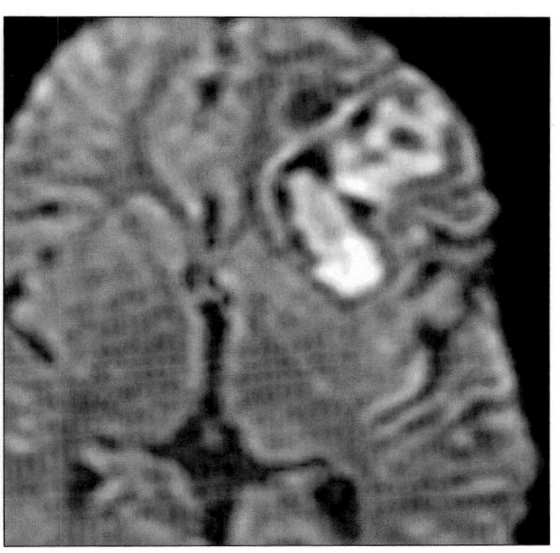

(Left) *Axial T2WI MR in the same patient 6 years later shows a significant interval increase in the size of the lesion.* ***(Right)*** *On axial DWI MR, the left frontal mass appears hyperintense, indicating high cellularity. At surgery mature teratoma was found.*

MISCELLANEOUS MALIGNANT GERM CELL NEOPLASMS

Key Facts

Terminology
- 2 major types of GCTs
  - Most common = germinoma (50-70%)
  - Nongerminomatous GCTs
- Nongerminomatous malignant GCTs
  - Teratoma with malignant transformation
  - Embryonal carcinoma
  - Yolk sac tumor
  - Choriocarcinoma

Imaging
- Location
  - Propensity to hug midline
  - Pineal + suprasellar lesions common
- MR features
  - Hypo-/isointense to gray matter
  - T1 shortening common (protein, blood, or fat)
  - Heterogeneous enhancement, ± CSF spread

Top Differential Diagnoses
- Supratentorial PNET
- Astrocytoma
- Dermoid
- Choroid plexus tumors of 3rd ventricle

Clinical Issues
- Peripubertal patients (rare < 4 years)
- M:F = 14:1 (purely pineal tumors)
- Visual/endocrine symptoms, Parinaud syndrome
- Signs of hypothalamic/pituitary dysfunction

Diagnostic Checklist
- Difficult to differentiate from other CNS GCTs on imaging alone

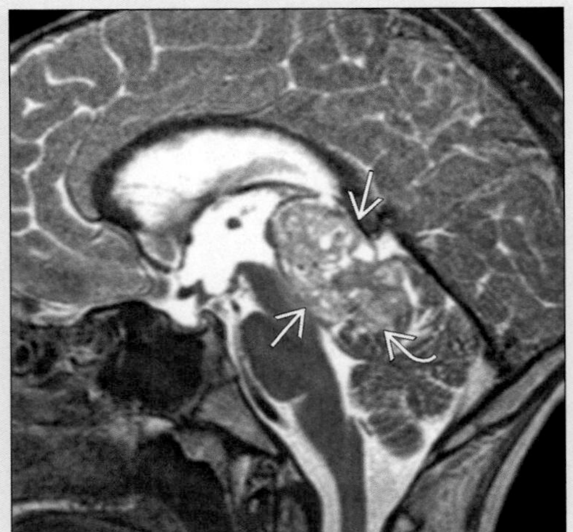
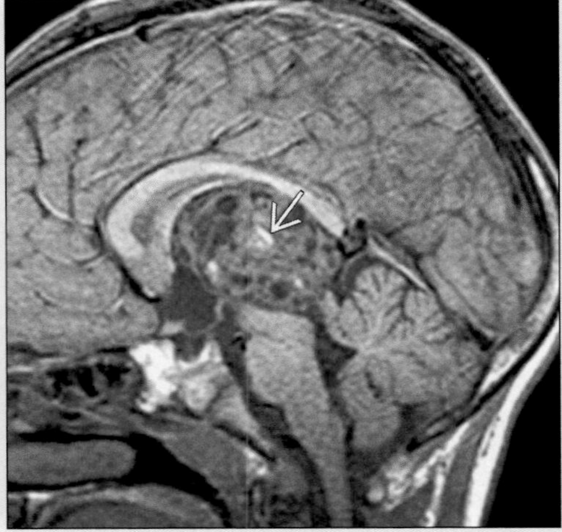

(Left) *Sagittal T2WI FS MR in a 13-year-old boy shows a mixed GCT presenting as a lobulated mixed solid-cystic pineal region mass ➡ with focal invasion of the vermis ➡.* ***(Right)*** *Sagittal T1WI MR in an 8-year-old boy with Parinaud syndrome and embryonal carcinoma shows a heterogeneous mass with foci of T1 shortening that represent hemorrhage ➡. This tumor, like other intracranial GCTs, tends to hug the midline and typically occurs as a component of a histologically mixed germ cell tumor.*

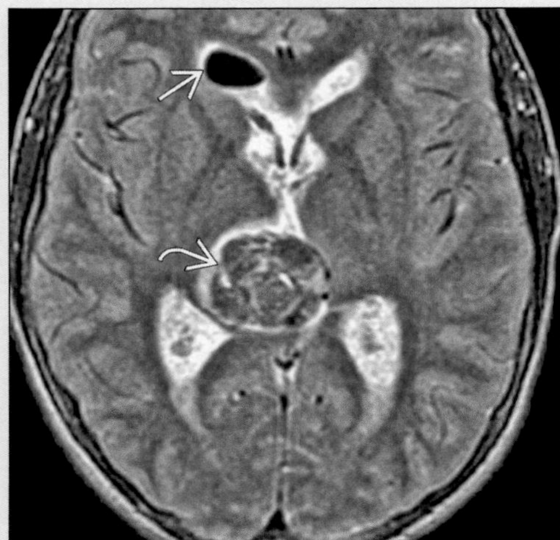
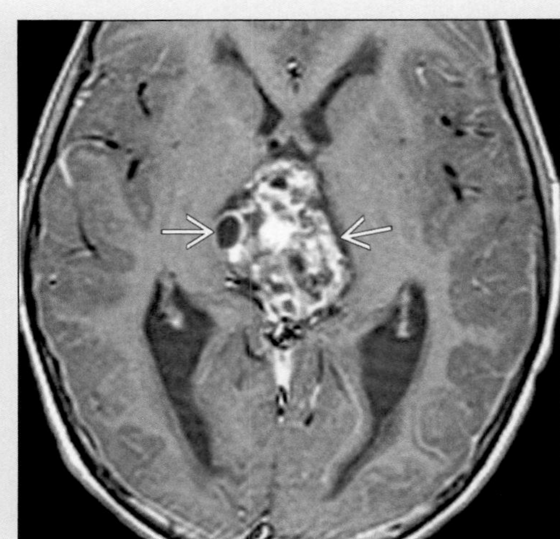

(Left) *Axial T2WI MR of a patient with embryonal carcinoma shows a heterogeneous, predominantly iso- to hypointense, pineal region mass ➡. Relatively low signal intensity is due to the high nuclear to cytoplasmic ratio in the cells of this highly malignant neoplasm. Also note the air within the right frontal horn following ventricular catheter placement ➡.* ***(Right)*** *Axial T1WI C+ MR shows heterogeneous enhancement within a pineal embryonal carcinoma ➡.*

MISCELLANEOUS MALIGNANT GERM CELL NEOPLASMS

TERMINOLOGY

Synonyms

- Malignant germ cell tumor (GCT)
- Primary germ cell tumor (PGCT)
- Primary intracranial choriocarcinoma (PICCC)
- Intracranial germ cell tumor (ICGCT)

Definitions

- Malignant tumor composed of undifferentiated epithelial cells
- Morphological, immunophenotypic homologues of gonadal/extraneuraxial GCTs but in CNS
- 2 major types of GCTs
  - Germinoma (50-70%)
  - Nongerminomatous GCTs (NGGCTs)
    - Embryonal carcinoma
    - Yolk sac tumor (YST)
    - Choriocarcinoma
    - Teratoma
    - Mixed germ cell tumors

IMAGING

General Features

- Best diagnostic clue
  - Heterogeneous pineal or suprasellar mass in adolescent
- Location
  - Hugs midline as do other CNS GCTs
    - Bifocal germinoma (tumors in both pineal and suprasellar regions)
  - Brainstem GCT (rare)
- Size
  - Suprasellar, pineal region GCTs usually smaller than hemispheric tumors
- Morphology
  - Typically lobulated, well circumscribed

CT Findings

- NECT
  - Heterogeneous (mixed iso- to hyperdense)
- CECT
  - Enhancing, ± cysts, hemorrhage

MR Findings

- T1WI
  - Hypo- to isointense to gray matter
  - Short T1 due to protein, blood, or fat
- T2WI
  - Iso- to slightly hyperintense to gray matter
- FLAIR
  - Hyperintense solid elements
  - ± hydrocephalus
- T2* GRE
  - Dephasing from hemorrhagic foci
- DWI
  - ± restriction within solid components
- T1WI C+
  - Heterogeneous enhancement
  - Variable CSF spread
- MRS
  - ↑ choline, lipid, and lactate
  - ↓ NAA

Angiographic Findings

- Variable (can be very vascular)

Imaging Recommendations

- Best imaging tool
  - MR of entire neuraxis
  - ± contrast
- Protocol advice
  - Preoperative MR of **entire** neuraxis

DIFFERENTIAL DIAGNOSIS

Intracranial Germ Cell Tumors

- Various histologies
  - Germinoma
  - Mixed malignant germ cell tumor, yolk sac tumor
  - Choriocarcinoma
  - Teratoma (immature, malignant)
- May have similar imaging; age, histology help differentiate

Supratentorial PNET

- Minimal peritumoral edema

Other Suprasellar, Pineal Tumors

- Astrocytoma
- Dermoid
- Choroid plexus tumors of 3rd ventricle

PATHOLOGY

General Features

- Etiology
  - Aberrations in
    - Histogenesis
    - Germ cell migration
    - Stem cells
  - 2 possible theories
    - "Germ cell" theory
      - GCTs arise from primordial germ cells that have migrated aberrantly during embryonic development with subsequent malignant transformation
    - "Embryonic cell" theory
      - Mismigrational pluripotent embryonic cells give rise to GCTs
- Genetics
  - Reports of near triploid complex karyotypes
  - *p14* and *C-Kit* gene alterations in germinomas
  - Homozygous deletion or frameshift mutation of *INK4a/ARF* (71% of ICGCTs)
  - Overexpression of *p21*(*WAF1/Cip1*)
    - Associated with poor prognosis in intracranial GCTs
- Associated abnormalities
  - Klinefelter syndrome (47,XXY)
  - Down syndrome

Staging, Grading, & Classification

- Malignant GCTs often histologically mixed

MISCELLANEOUS MALIGNANT GERM CELL NEOPLASMS

- May exist with both germinomatous, other nongerminomatous GCTs
- Prognosis correlated with most malignant component
  - PICCC, YST, embryonal carcinoma elements have worst prognosis

Gross Pathologic & Surgical Features

- Soft, often friable mass

Microscopic Features

- Undifferentiated epithelial cells
- YST: Tubulo-papillary structures with vacuolated cuboidal cells, colloid-like matrix, Schiller-Duval bodies
- PICCC: Extraembryonic differentiation
- Teratoma and germinoma: Pure tumor types
- Other GCTs usually mixed

Special Immunohistochemical Markers

- Human chorionic gonadotropin (hCG)
- Fetoprotein
- Human placental alkaline phosphatase
- Cytokeratin
- C-Kit (CD117)
- OCT4 (POU5F1)

CLINICAL ISSUES

Presentation

- Most common signs/symptoms
  - Signs of hypothalamic/pituitary dysfunction
  - ↑ intracranial pressure from suprasellar or pineal region mass
  - Other signs/symptoms
    - Visual, endocrine symptoms
    - Parinaud syndrome
  - Brainstem GCT: Pulmonary complaints, cranial neuropathies
- Other signs/symptoms
  - PICCC: High serum and CSF hCG
- Clinical profile
  - Adolescent with obstructing midline mass in vicinity of 3rd ventricle, ± focal neuro deficits

Demographics

- Age
  - Strong predilection for peripubertal patients
    - Peak incidence 10-15 years
    - Rare < 4 years
- Gender
  - Males show slight increased incidence for pineal region
    - When purely pineal tumors, M:F = 14:1
  - Female predominance in suprasellar cases
- Ethnicity
  - More common in Asians
    - In Japan 1.8-3% of all primary brain tumors are GCT (in patients < 15 years, 15%)
- Epidemiology
  - Rare (0.3 -3.4% of all CNS tumors)
  - Teratoma is leading perinatal brain tumor
    - Accounts for 42% of fetal brain tumors

Natural History & Prognosis

- Locally invasive with metastatic potential
- Follow-up: PLAP, cytokeratin markers
- YST
  - Median survival < 2 years
  - 5-year survival rate < 25%
- PICCC is most malignant intracranial GCT
  - High risk of hemorrhage
  - Extraneural/CSF dissemination

Treatment

- Surgical resection → chemotherapy → neuraxis radiation
- Combination of pre- and post-irradiation chemotherapy: Improved survival

DIAGNOSTIC CHECKLIST

Consider

- Embryonal carcinoma if heterogeneous pineal region or suprasellar mass in adolescent
- Metastasis of embryonal carcinoma from testicular source
- Metastasis of choriocarcinoma from other source in patients with cerebral hemorrhage and multiple pseudoaneurysms

Image Interpretation Pearls

- Difficult to differentiate from other CNS GCTs on imaging alone

SELECTED REFERENCES

1. Isaacs H: Fetal brain tumors: a review of 154 cases. Am J Perinatol. 26(6):453-66, 2009
2. Sato K et al: Pathology of intracranial germ cell tumors. Prog Neurol Surg. 23:59-75, 2009
3. Echevarría ME et al: Pediatric central nervous system germ cell tumors: a review. Oncologist. 13(6):690-9, 2008
4. Vuillermet P et al: Simultaneous suprasellar and pineal germ cell tumors in five late stage adolescents: endocrinological studies and prolonged follow-up. J Pediatr Endocrinol Metab. 21(12):1169-78, 2008
5. Kageji T et al: Successful neoadjuvant synchronous chemo- and radiotherapy for disseminated primary intracranial choriocarcinoma: case report. J Neurooncol. 83(2):199-204, 2007
6. Cuccia V et al: Pure pineal germinomas: analysis of gender incidence. Acta Neurochir (Wien). 148(8):865-71; discussion 871, 2006
7. Kamakura Y et al: C-kit gene mutation: common and widely distributed in intracranial germinomas. J Neurosurg. 104(3 Suppl):173-80, 2006
8. Sawamura Y et al: Germ cell tumours of the central nervous system: treatment consideration based on 111 cases and their long-term clinical outcomes. Eur J Cancer. 34(1):104-10, 1998
9. Salzman KL et al: Primary intracranial germ cell tumors: clinicopathologic review of 32 cases. Pediatr Pathol Lab Med. 17(5):713-27, 1997
10. Fujimaki T et al: CT and MRI features of intracranial germ cell tumors. J Neurooncol. 19(3):217-26, 1994
11. Smirniotopoulos JG et al: Pineal region masses: differential diagnosis. Radiographics. 12(3):577-96, 1992

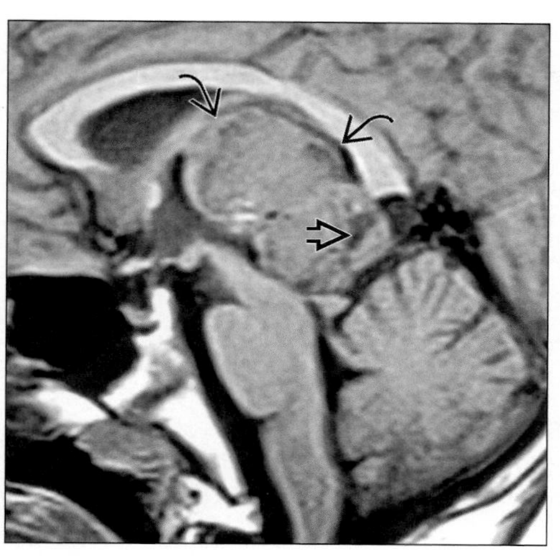

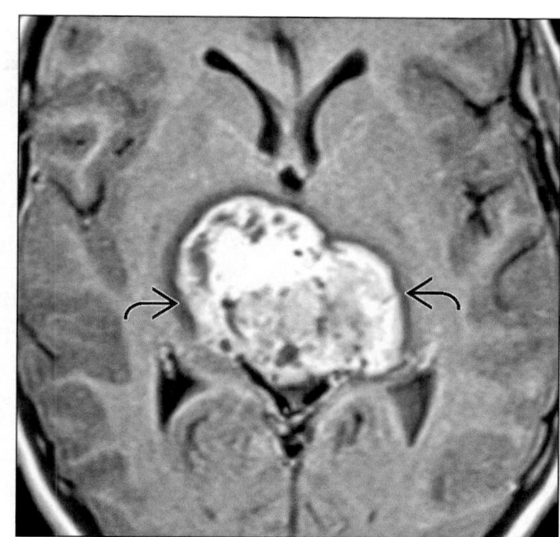

(Left) *Sagittal T1WI MR in a 5-year-old boy shows a well-circumscribed, lobulated, low signal intensity, midline, pineal region mass with a small cystic component. (Courtesy A. Rossi, MD.)* ***(Right)*** *Axial T1WI C+ MR in the same patient shows intense but slightly inhomogeneous enhancement of the mass. No evidence of CSF dissemination was identified on preoperative evaluation of the entire neuraxis. Histopathology revealed a yolk sac tumor. (Courtesy A. Rossi, MD.)*

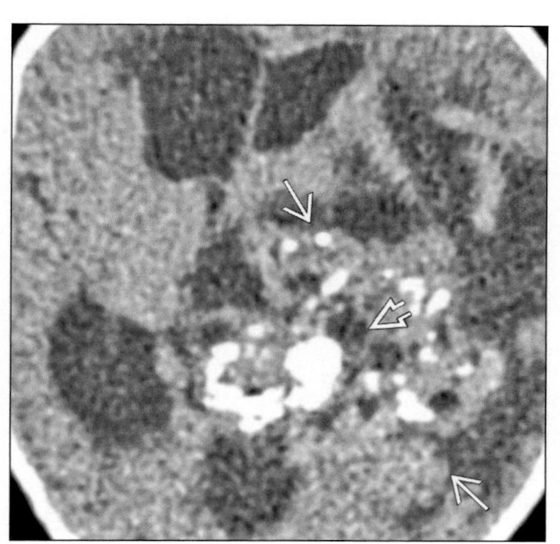

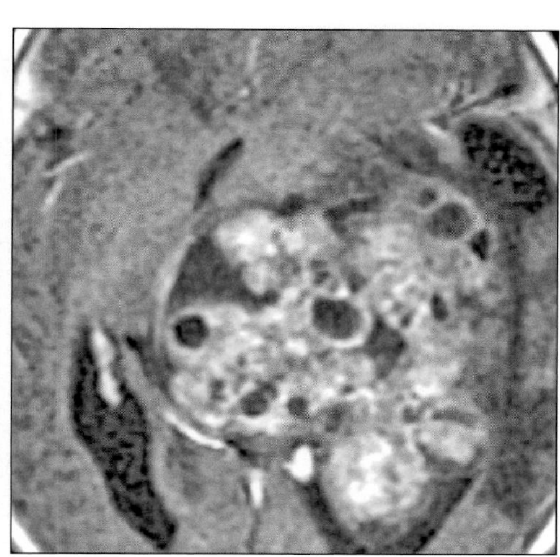

(Left) *Axial NECT shows a lobulated heterogeneous mass centered in the left hypothalamus and causing obstructive hydrocephalus. Note the multiple calcifications, intratumoral cysts, and surrounding edema.* ***(Right)*** *Axial T1WI MR in the same patient nicely demonstrates the very heterogeneous nature of the mass. Foci of enhancing solid tumor intermixed with cysts characterize this neoplasm. An immature teratoma was found at histopathological examination.*

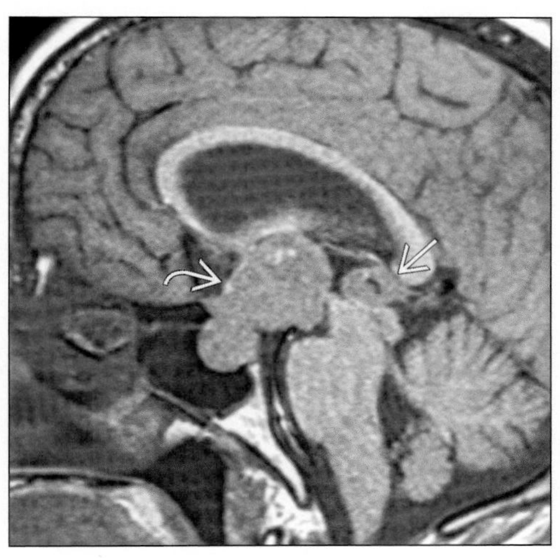

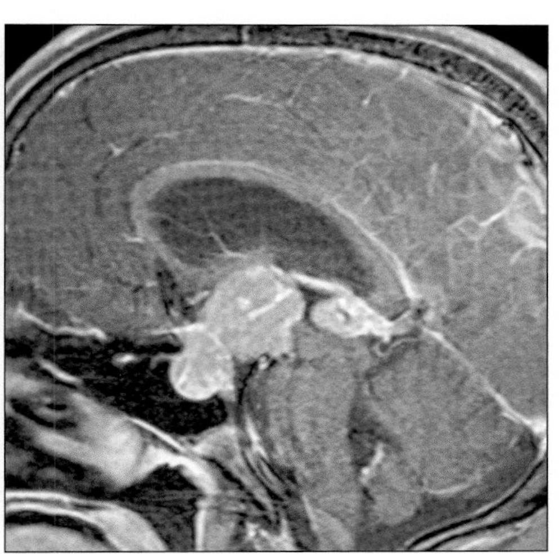

(Left) *Sagittal T1WI MR in a 22-year-old man with headaches, diabetes insipidus, and a hyperdense suprasellar mass on NECT (not shown) reveals a "double midline" mass with a small pineal lesion and a larger intra-/suprasellar mass.* ***(Right)*** *Sagittal T1WI C+ FS MR in the same patient shows intense but heterogeneous enhancement. Preoperative diagnosis was germinoma. Biopsy disclosed embryonal carcinoma.*

PARENCHYMAL METASTASES

Key Facts

Terminology

- Secondary brain tumors (metastases) arise from
  - Tumors outside CNS spreading to CNS (usually via hematogenous dissemination)
  - Primary CNS neoplasms spreading from 1 site to another (usually geographic extension, i.e., along WM tracts)

Imaging

- General features
  - Round enhancing lesion(s) at gray-white interface (arterial border zones)
  - Most mets are circumscribed/discrete > > infiltrating, spherical > > linear
  - 50% are solitary; 20% have 2 metastases
  - 30% of patients have 3 or more
- MR signal intensity varies with
  - Cellularity, nuclear to cytoplasmic ratio
  - Presence/absence of hemorrhage
- Usually no restriction on DWI
  - Exception: Densely cellular metastases may restrict!

Top Differential Diagnoses

- Abscess (solitary or multiple)
- Glioblastoma multiforme
- Cerebral infarction (multiple embolic)
- Demyelinating disease (e.g., "tumefactive" MS)

Pathology

- Mets represent at least 50% of all brain tumors
- In 10% of cases, brain is only site

Clinical Issues

- Progressive increase in size and numbers is typical
- Median survival with whole brain XRT = 3-6 months

(Left) Axial graphic shows parenchymal metastases ⇨ with surrounding edema ⇨. The gray-white matter junction is the most common location. Most metastases are round, not diffusely infiltrating. ***(Right)*** *Close-up view of an axial section through an autopsied brain shows a classic metastasis ⇨ in the classic location, the gray-white matter junction. Note the round shape, central necrosis, and relative lack of edema. Diffuse leptomeningeal metastatic spread ⇨ is also present.*

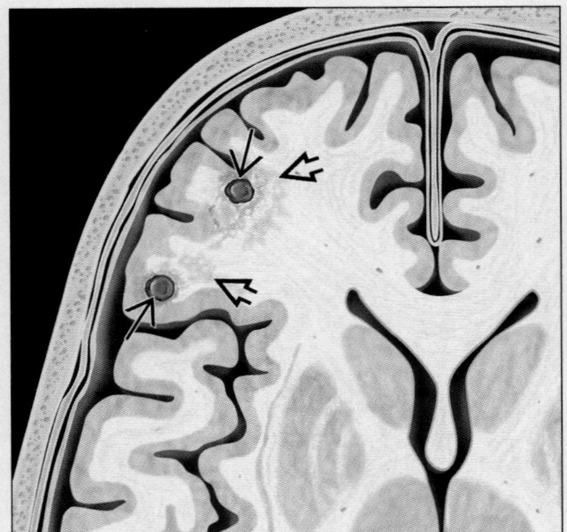

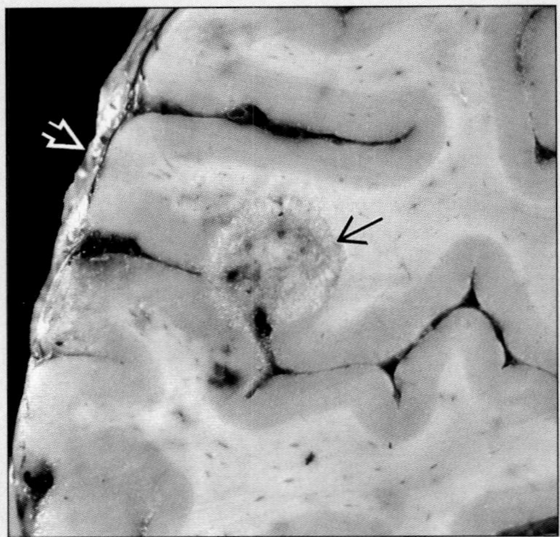

(Left) *Axial T1WI MR in a patient with multiple hemorrhagic metastases ➡ from renal cell carcinoma shows multiple round lesions at the gray-white matter junction with intrinsically short T1.* ***(Right)*** *Axial CECT in a patient with carcinoma of the breast shows multiple enhancing masses ➡ at the gray-white matter junction. Lesions vary in size from tiny to large. The large lesions have moderate surrounding edema ⇨.*

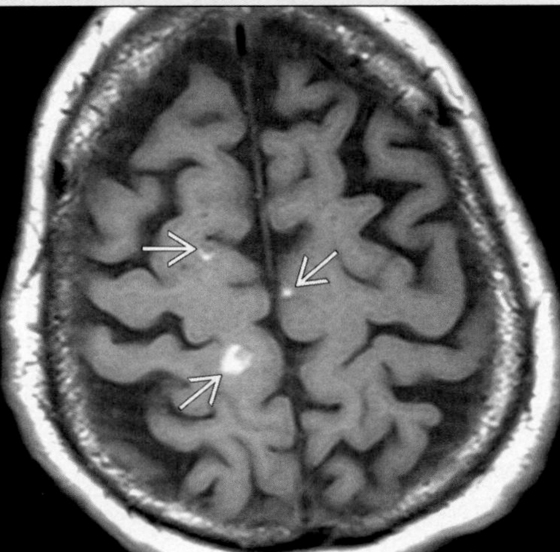

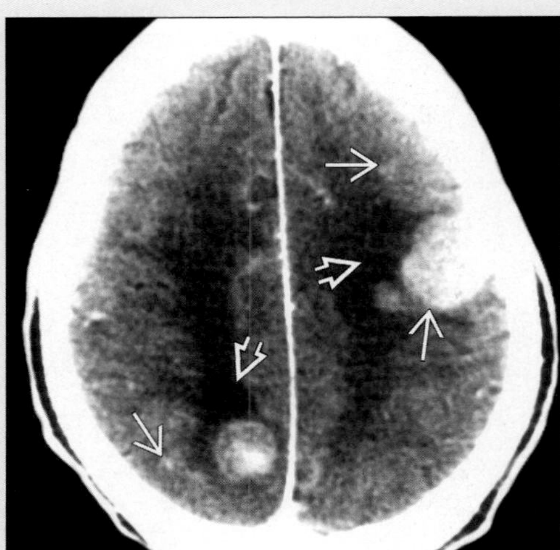

TERMINOLOGY

Abbreviations

- Parenchymal metastases (mets)

Synonyms

- Secondary brain tumors
- Body-to-brain metastases
- Brain-to-brain metastases

Definitions

- Secondary brain tumors (metastases) arise from
  - Tumors outside CNS that spread to CNS (usually via hematogenous dissemination)
  - Primary CNS neoplasms that spread from 1 site to another (usually geographic spread, i.e., along white matter [WM] tracts)

IMAGING

General Features

- Best diagnostic clue
  - Discrete enhancing lesion(s) at gray-white interface
- Location
  - Common: At arterial border zones/gray-white matter (GM-WM) junctions
    - 80% hemispheres
    - 15% cerebellum
    - 3% basal ganglia
    - < 1% midbrain, pons, medulla
  - Uncommon: Diffusely infiltrating tumors ("carcinomatous encephalitis")
    - Perivascular (e.g., intravascular lymphoma)
    - Perineural (e.g., adenocystic carcinoma along CN5 to pons)
- Size
  - Varies from microscopic to several cm
- Morphology
  - Most mets are circumscribed/discrete > > infiltrating, spherical > > linear
  - 50% of metastases are solitary
  - 20% 2 metastases
  - 30% 3 or more

CT Findings

- NECT
  - Iso-/hypodense mass(es) at GM-WM interface
  - Variable peritumoral edema (none to striking)
  - Variable intracranial hemorrhage (ICH)
    - Mets may cause "spontaneous" ICH in elderly
- CECT
  - Intense, punctate, nodular, or ring enhancement
  - Conspicuity, number, volume of tumors may increase on delayed scans

MR Findings

- T1WI
  - Most common: Iso-/hypointense
  - Less common: Hyperintense
    - Some nonhemorrhagic mets (e.g., melanoma) have intrinsically short T1
    - Hemorrhagic metastases
      - Disordered/bizarre appearance, evolution (compared to nonneoplastic ICH)
- T2WI
  - Signal varies depending on
    - Cellularity, nuclear to cytoplasmic ratio
    - Presence/absence of hemorrhage
  - Multifocal hyperintense mets mimic vascular WM disease
- FLAIR
  - Usually moderately hyperintense with strikingly hyperintense adjacent edema
- T2* GRE
  - "Blooms" if hemorrhage present
- DWI
  - Usually no restriction on DWI
    - Exception: Densely cellular mets may restrict!
- T1WI C+
  - Almost all mets enhance
    - Enhancement usually strong
    - Patterns variable
      - Solid, uniform
      - Nodular
      - Ring-like
  - Dynamic susceptibility contrast-enhanced MR
    - May show elevated rCBV
    - Can be difficult to distinguish metastasis from high-grade gliomas
- MRS
  - Elevated Cho
  - Lipid or lipid/lac peak often present
  - 80-85% lack Cr peak
- DTI
  - Fractional anisotropy helpful in distinguishing met from glioblastoma multiforme (GBM)
  - Tractography may help detect WM tract invasion

Angiographic Findings

- Occasionally very hypervascular
  - Intense prolonged "blush" ± AV shunting
  - Can mimic hemangioblastoma, AVM

Nuclear Medicine Findings

- PET/CT
  - Helpful for systemic mets
  - Not as sensitive as MR for brain lesions

Imaging Recommendations

- Best imaging tool
  - MR with DWI, T2*, T1WI C+
- Protocol advice
  - T1WI C+ with FS enhances lesion conspicuity
  - 3D MP-RAGE sequence may improve detection
  - Delayed sequences at 20-30 minutes often show additional lesions
  - Double- or triple-contrast dose increases sensitivity but of questionable value on routine basis

DIFFERENTIAL DIAGNOSIS

Abscess

- Usually restricts on DWI
- MRS: Elevated amino acids, lactate in cystic component; no Cho elevation

PARENCHYMAL METASTASES

Glioblastoma Multiforme

- Tends to be infiltrating, deep location (rather than discrete gray-white junction masses)
- Solitary > multifocal
  - Solitary met can mimic GBM

Multiple Embolic Cerebral Infarction

- Arterial border-zone location common
- Ring-enhancing pattern uncommon
- Multiple acute embolic strokes usually show restricted diffusion
- Chronic-appearing hyperintensities
  - If they do not enhance, they are not metastases!

Multiple Sclerosis

- Periventricular > gray-white junction
- Incomplete ring, horseshoe-shaped enhancement
- Younger patients

PATHOLOGY

General Features

- Etiology
  - Hematogenous spread from systemic primary neoplasm
    - Lung, breast, melanoma most common primary malignancies
    - 10% unknown source
  - Brain-to-brain spread from primary CNS neoplasm (e.g., glioblastoma multiforme)
    - Along compact WM tracts (e.g., corpus callosum, internal capsule), ependyma
    - CSF dissemination to pia may then spread to parenchyma via perivascular spaces
- Genetics
  - Metastasis formation is complex, often genetically mediated event
    - Inactivation of tumor suppressor genes
    - Activation of protooncogenes
  - Organ-specific metastasis formation
    - Specific receptors mediate attachment, infiltration of circulating tumor cells into CNS
    - Chromosome 17q (*RHO* gene family), 8q (*c-Myc*) gains
    - Overexpression, amplification of *EGFR* gene common
  - Some tumor-specific patterns of disease spread
    - ER(+), PR(+) breast cancers: Osseous > brain mets
    - ER(-), PR(-) breast cancers: Brain > osseous mets
- Associated abnormalities
  - Other organs often involved
  - In 10% of cases, brain is only site
  - Limbic encephalitis
    - Paraneoplastic syndrome (remote effect of cancer)
    - Resembles herpes encephalitis (subacute clinical presentation)

Gross Pathologic & Surgical Features

- Round/confluent, relatively discrete, tan or grayish-white mass
- Edema, mass effect varies from little to striking
- Hemorrhage common with some mets (melanoma, choriocarcinoma, lung/renal cell carcinomas)

Microscopic Features

- Usually similar to primary neoplasm
- Metastases usually displace rather than infiltrate tissue
- Necrosis, neovascularity common
- Marked mitoses; labeling index may be greater than primary

CLINICAL ISSUES

Presentation

- Most common signs/symptoms
  - Seizure, focal neurologic deficit
- Clinical profile
  - Middle-aged/elderly patient with known systemic cancer, new onset of neurological symptoms

Demographics

- Age
  - Incidence increases with age
    - Rare in children (skull/dura more common site than parenchyma)
    - Peak prevalence over 65 years
- Gender
  - Slight male predominance
- Epidemiology
  - With better treatment, patients with systemic cancers are surviving longer
  - Result
    - Prevalence of metastases vs. primary CNS neoplasms increasing
    - Now account for up to 50% of all brain tumors
    - Brain involvement is found in 25% of systemic cancer patients at autopsy

Natural History & Prognosis

- Progressive increase in size and numbers is typical
- Median survival with whole brain XRT = 3-6 months
  - Younger age, high Karnofsky performance status associated with longer survival

Treatment

- Varies with number, location of metastases
- Resection of solitary metastasis may improve survival

DIAGNOSTIC CHECKLIST

Consider

- "Spontaneous" ICH or new onset seizures in elderly patient may be caused by metastasis

Image Interpretation Pearls

- White matter disease ("UBOs") in elderly patient can be caused by multifocal metastases
- Consider T1WI C+ in patients with "WM disease," unexplained mental decline

SELECTED REFERENCES

1. Wang W et al: Diffusion tensor imaging in glioblastoma multiforme and brain metastases: the role of p, q, L, and fractional anisotropy. AJNR Am J Neuroradiol. 30(1):203-8, 2009

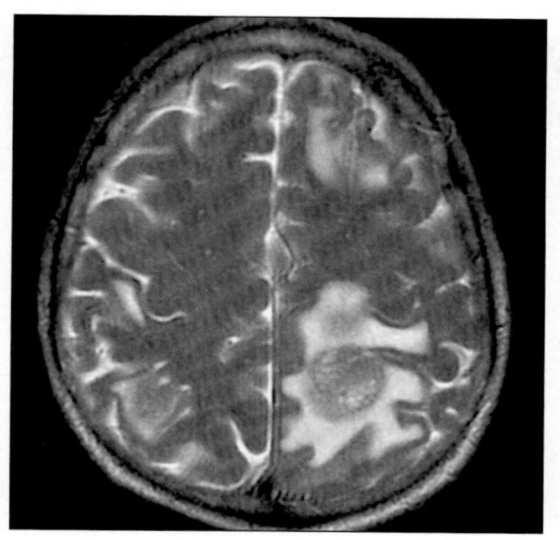

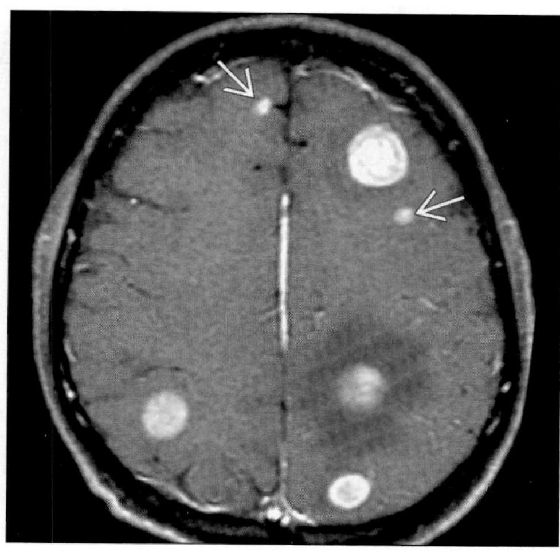

(Left) *Axial T2WI MR in a patient with known colon carcinoma demonstrates that multiple metastases at the gray-white junction are mostly isointense with brain, surrounded by variable edema.* ***(Right)*** *Axial T1 C+ FS MR in the same patient shows multiple large and enhancing foci at the gray-white matter junctions ➔. Innumerable other lesions were present on other images.*

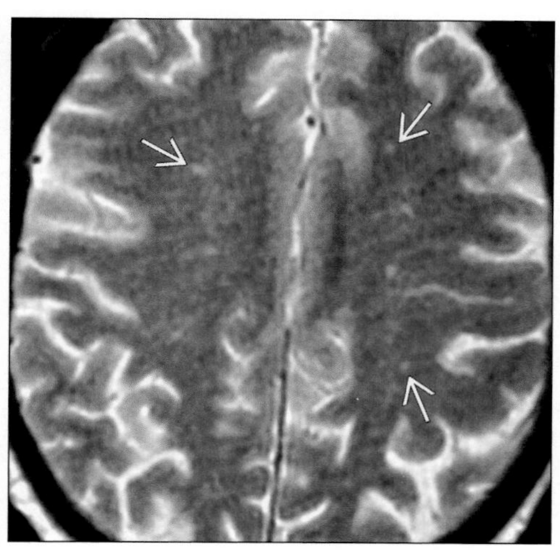

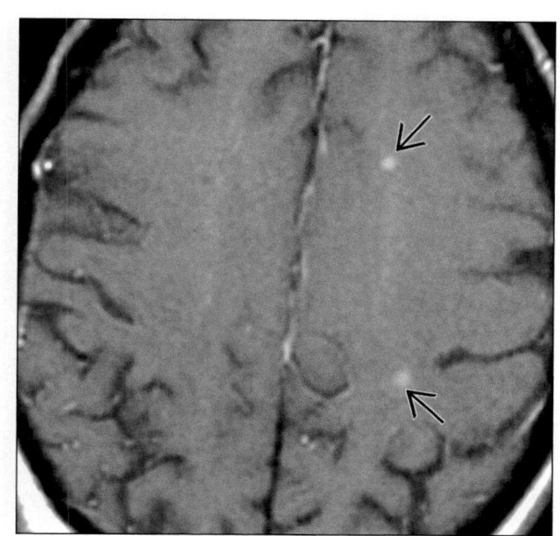

(Left) *Axial T2WI MR in a middle-aged patient with unexplained mental decline and normal neurologic examination shows multifocal white matter hyperintensities (WMHs) ➔. These are indistinguishable from the usual WMHs of small vessel disease, most commonly arteriolosclerosis.* ***(Right)*** *Axial T1WI C+ MR in the same patient demonstrates that several of the WMHs enhance ➔. Other images (not shown) revealed several subependymal enhancing foci. Further evaluation revealed breast carcinoma.*

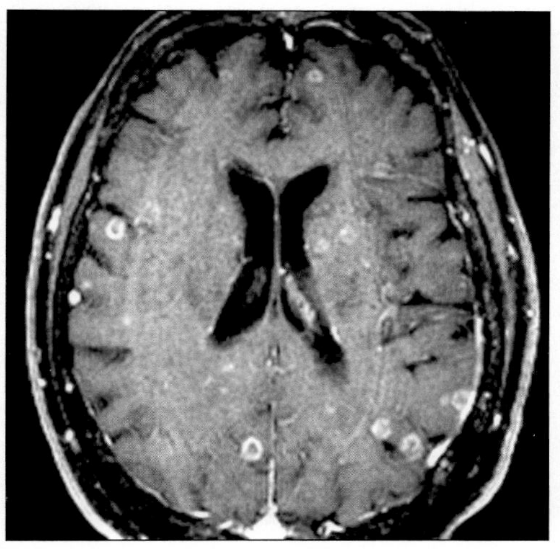

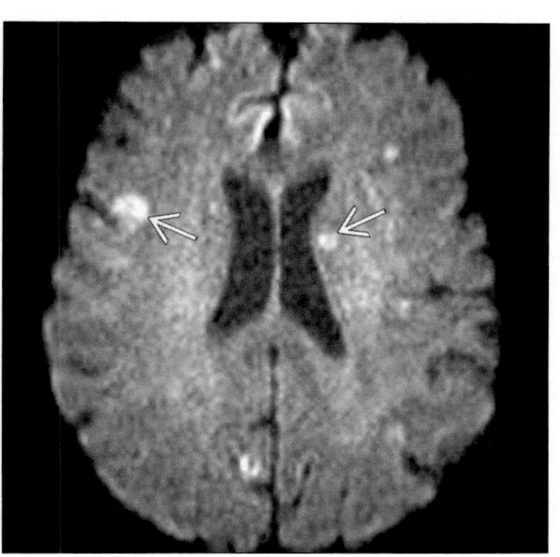

(Left) *Axial T1WI C+ FS MR in a 70-year-old woman with breast cancer shows multiple punctate and ring-enhancing lesions.* ***(Right)*** *Axial DWI MR in the same patient shows several foci of restricted diffusion ➔ that were hypointense on ADC (not shown). Most neoplasms do not restrict, but metastases often have a high nuclear to cytoplasm ratio and sometimes show restricted diffusion.*

MISCELLANEOUS INTRACRANIAL METASTASES

Key Facts

Terminology
- Brain metastases in locations other than skull/ meninges or parenchyma

Imaging
- General features
  - > 95% of brain metastases are parenchymal
  - Only 1-2% in ventricles, pituitary gland, etc.
  - Sites are generally very vascular
  - Extraventricular metastases more diffuse, infiltrative than parenchymal mets (usually round)
- Location
  - Choroid plexus ± ventricular ependyma
  - Pituitary gland infundibulum
  - Eye (choroid)
  - Cranial nerves
  - Pineal gland
  - Preexisting neoplasm ("collision tumor")
- Best imaging tool = MR with T1WI C+ FS
  - Metastases almost always enhance

Top Differential Diagnoses
- Varies with location
- Choroid plexus, ventricle = meningioma
- Pituitary gland, infundibular stalk
  - Pituitary macroadenoma
  - Lymphocytic hypophysitis
  - Lymphoma
- Cranial nerves = NF2, lymphoma
- Eye (globe)
  - Ocular melanoma
  - Retinal or choroidal detachment
  - Choroidal hemangioma

Diagnostic Checklist
- Look for "secret sites" outside parenchyma when imaging brain for possible metastatic disease

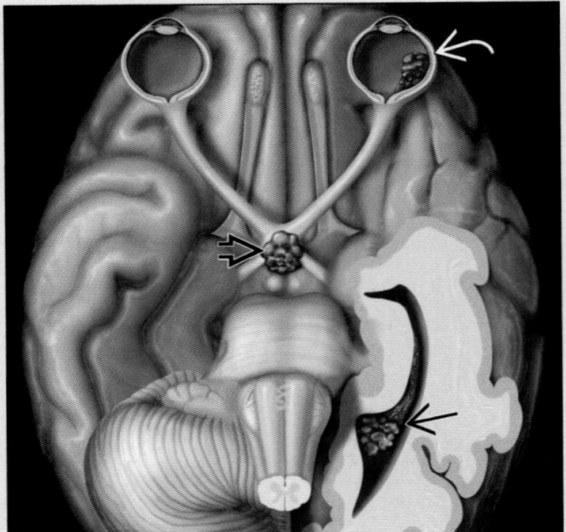

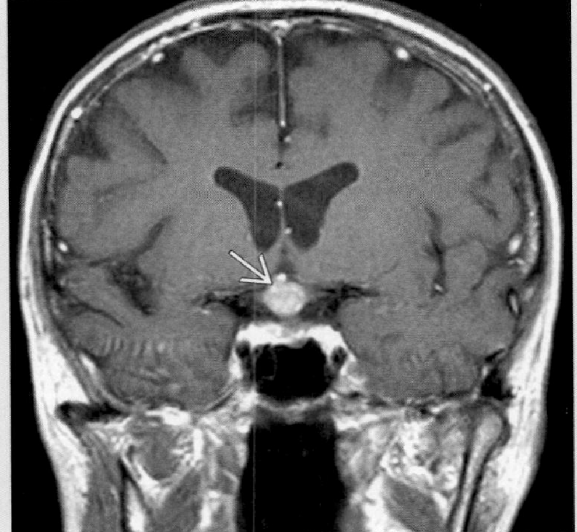

***(Left)** Submentovertex graphic shows the typical sites for miscellaneous nonparenchymal CNS metastases. These include the choroid plexus and ventricles ➔, pituitary gland, infundibular stalk ➔, & eye (choroid of the retina) ➔. **(Right)** Coronal T1WI C+ MR in an elderly woman with known breast carcinoma shows a thickened, enhancing infundibular stalk ➔. This was the only intracranial metastasis identified in this patient.*

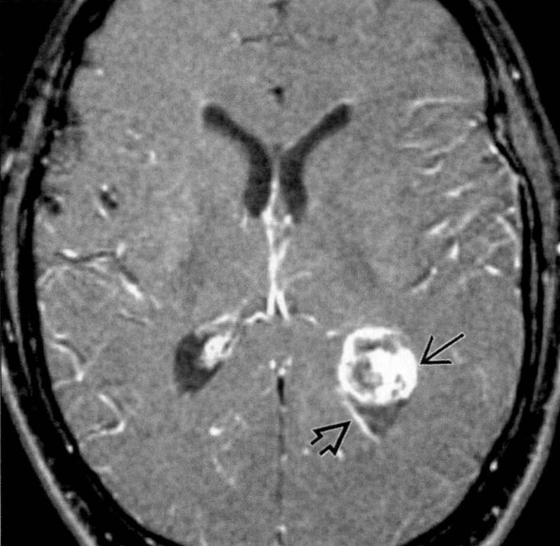

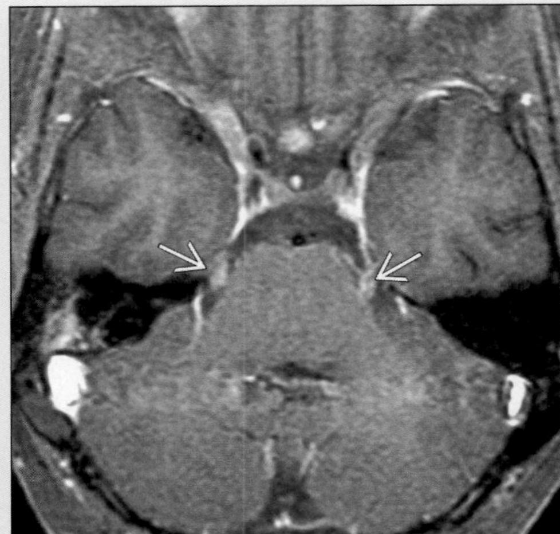

***(Left)** Axial T1WI C+ FS MR shows a metastasis to the choroid plexus glomus ➔. Note the subtle abnormal ependymal enhancement ➔ adjacent to the choroid plexus metastasis. This was the only intracranial lesion identified in this patient with known renal cell carcinoma. **(Right)** Axial T1WI C+ FS MR in a patient with known systemic lymphoma and multiple cranial neuropathies shows enlarged, enhancing trigeminal nerves ➔. Other scans (not shown) disclosed the involvement of several other nerves.*

TERMINOLOGY

Definitions

- Brain metastases in locations other than skull/ meninges, parenchyma

IMAGING

General Features

- Best diagnostic clue
  - "Unusual" mass in patient with known systemic primary neoplasm
- Location
  - In general, sites very vascular
  - Choroid plexus ± ventricular ependyma
  - Pituitary gland, infundibulum
  - Cranial nerves
  - Eye
    - Posterior segment (uvea)
    - Biconvex mass along choroid
  - Pineal gland
  - Preexisting neoplasm ("collision tumor")
    - 2 unique tumor types within single lesion
    - Metastasis to meningioma most common
- Size
  - Usually small
- Morphology
  - Often more diffuse, infiltrative than parenchymal metastases (round > > infiltrating)

Imaging Recommendations

- Best imaging tool
  - MR with T1WI C+ FS (metastases almost always enhance regardless of location)

DIFFERENTIAL DIAGNOSIS

Choroid Plexus, Ventricle

- Meningioma
- Choroid plexus cyst (xanthogranuloma)
- Ventriculitis/choroid plexitis

Pituitary Gland, Infundibular Stalk

- Pituitary macroadenoma
- Lymphocytic hypophysitis
- Lymphoma

Cranial Nerves (Multiple Enhancing)

- Lymphoma
  - May be indistinguishable from other metastases
  - CNs, brain surface often coated
- Neurofibromatosis type 2
  - Multiple schwannomas, meningiomas
- Lyme disease
  - Nerves enhance; usually not enlarged
- Chronic inflammatory demyelinating polyneuropathy
  - Spinal nerves > > CNs
  - Multiple enlarged mildly enhancing CNs
  - Parenchymal/skull/meningeal lesions absent

Eye (Globe)

- Ocular melanoma
  - Most ocular melanomas are choroidal
  - Ciliary body, iris lesions less common
  - Usually T1 hyperintense, T2 hypointense
  - Associated hemorrhage, choroidal detachment common
- Retinal or choroidal detachment
  - Retina is V-shaped
  - Choroid is ovoid, parallel to choroidal plane
  - Often hyperintense on T1WI
- Choroidal hemangioma
  - Congenital vascular hamartoma
  - Middle-aged/elderly patients
  - Lenticular mass in juxtapapillary or macular region
  - Can be solitary or diffuse
  - T1, T2 hyperintense
  - Avid enhancement (> metastasis, melanoma)
  - Ocular ultrasound helpful

PATHOLOGY

General Features

- Etiology
  - Extracranial primary sources
    - Breast carcinoma most common
    - Others include lung, kidney, colon
  - Intracranial sources of "brain-to-brain" metastases
    - Glioblastoma multiforme, anaplastic astrocytoma most common
      - White matter > extraparenchymal sites
- Associated abnormalities
  - Other CNS metastases (often multifocal)
    - Parenchyma
    - Pia-subarachnoid space
    - Skull, meninges
  - Systemic metastases
    - Often multiorgan
    - In 10% of cases, brain is only metastatic site

CLINICAL ISSUES

Presentation

- Most common signs/symptoms
  - Varies with location

Demographics

- Age
  - Middle-aged, older patients
- Epidemiology
  - > 95% of brain metastases are parenchymal
  - Only 1-2% found in ventricles, pituitary gland, etc.

DIAGNOSTIC CHECKLIST

Consider

- Metastasis in middle-aged or older patient with intraventricular or intraocular mass

Image Interpretation Pearls

- Look for "secret sites" outside parenchyma when imaging brain for possible metastatic disease

METASTATIC INTRACRANIAL LYMPHOMA

Key Facts

Terminology
- Secondary involvement of CNS in patients with systemic lymphoma

Imaging
- Secondary CNS lymphoma typically involves dura or leptomeninges, but it may cause parenchymal mass
- Best diagnostic clue: Diffusely enhancing dural mass ± bone involvement
  - May see leptomeningeal enhancement or nonsupression of CSF on FLAIR
- Lower rCBV than other tumors

Top Differential Diagnoses
- Meningioma
- Meningeal metastases
- Primary CNS lymphoma
- Leptomeningeal disease
- Hemangiopericytoma

Clinical Issues
- Prognostic markers suggestive of CNS relapse
  - Elevated serum lactate dehydrogenase (LDH) levels
  - Presence of B symptoms
  - Extranodal involvement at more than 1 site
  - Advanced stage
- Aggressive histologic features increase risk for SCNSL
- Involvement of liver, bladder, testis, or adrenals increases risk of CNS spread
- CNS involvement of lymphoma almost always fatal

Diagnostic Checklist
- Occult lymphoma found in 8% of patients presenting with CNS lymphoma
- SCNSL commonly mimics meningioma or other metastatic disease

(Left) Axial T1WI C+ MR shows 2 homogeneously enhancing dural-based posterior fossa masses ➡ in this patient with systemic lymphoma. An associated dural tail is present ⇨. Imaging of secondary CNS lymphoma may mimic a meningioma. (Right) Axial T1WI C+ FS MR shows enhancement along the maxillary division (V2) of CN5 ➡, extending from the cavernous sinus into the pterygopalatine fossa ⇨, in this patient with systemic lymphoma and new facial paresthesias.

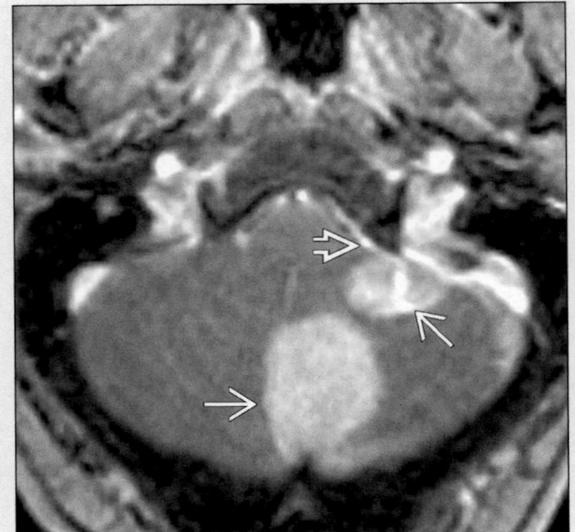

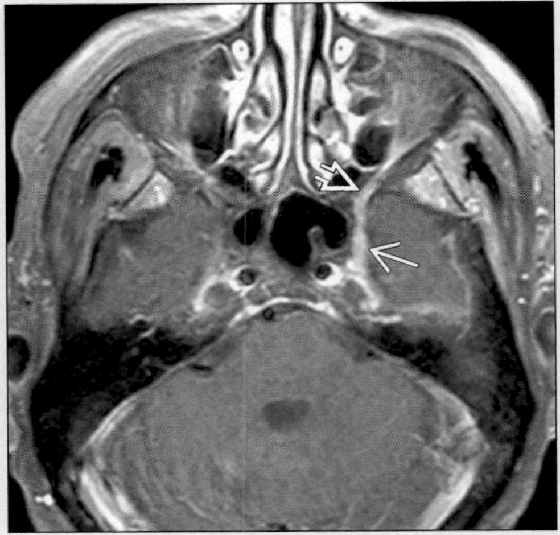

(Left) Axial CECT in a lymphoma patient with new onset seizures shows extensive leptomeningeal enhancement. Lymphomatous meningitis mimics other leptomeningeal disease, including infectious and carcinomatous meningitis. CSF studies are the key to diagnosis. (Right) Sagittal T1WI C+ FS MR shows a destructive enhancing central skull base mass with a retroclival dural tail ⇨. The clivus is often involved by metastatic disease, particularly breast cancer and lymphoma. Myeloma may a have similar appearance.

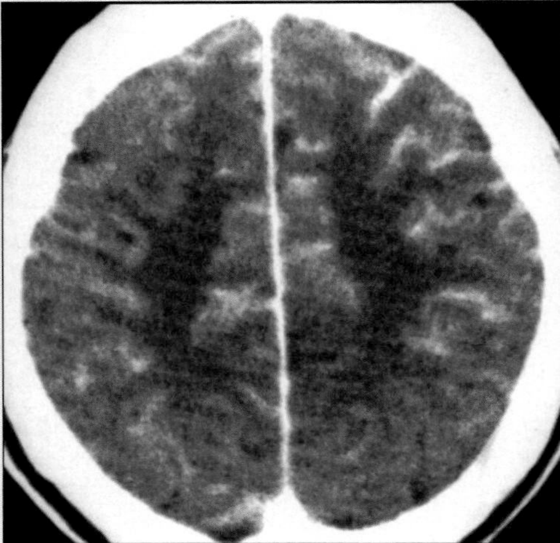

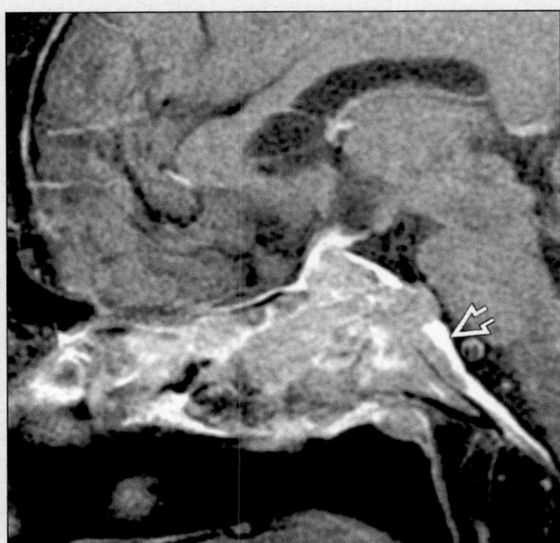

METASTATIC INTRACRANIAL LYMPHOMA

TERMINOLOGY

Synonyms
- Secondary CNS lymphoma (SCNSL)

Definitions
- Secondary involvement of CNS in patients with systemic lymphoma

IMAGING

General Features
- Best diagnostic clue
  - Enhancing dural mass ± bone involvement
- Location
  - Typically involves dura or leptomeninges
  - Parenchymal lesions may occur
  - Peripheral nerve = neurolymphomatosis
- Morphology
  - Solitary mass or multiple lesions
  - May be circumscribed or infiltrative

Imaging Recommendations
- Protocol advice
  - Contrast-enhanced MR

MR Findings
- T1WI
  - Single or multiple iso- or hypointense mass(es)
- T2WI
  - Homogeneously iso- or hypointense to cortex
- FLAIR
  - Leptomeningeal: Nonsuppression of CSF in sulci
- PWI
  - Lower rCBV than other tumors
- T1WI C+
  - Diffusely enhancing dural mass ± bone changes
  - May see leptomeningeal enhancement

DIFFERENTIAL DIAGNOSIS

Meningioma
- Enhancing mass with dural tail in older female
- May be indistinguishable

Meningeal Metastases
- Prostate and breast primaries may cause dural metastases
- Calvarial erosion may be seen

Primary CNS Lymphoma
- Periventricular or basal ganglia enhancing mass
- May rarely present as dural mass

Leptomeningeal Disease
- Infectious meningitis usually diagnosed clinically
- Carcinomatous meningitis indistinguishable

Hemangiopericytoma
- Lobular extraaxial mass ± skull erosion
- Heterogeneous enhancement typical

PATHOLOGY

General Features
- Etiology
  - Secondary involvement of CNS in patient with systemic lymphoma
  - CNS involvement occurs in 22% of post-transplantation lymphomas

Staging, Grading, & Classification
- Highly aggressive lymphomas (i.e., lymphoblastic and Burkitt) carry high risk of CNS relapse
- Intermediately aggressive subtypes (i.e., diffuse large B-cell lymphoma) carry lower risk of CNS relapse
- Hodgkin disease uncommon

Gross Pathologic & Surgical Features
- Typically firm dural mass
- Parenchymal mass less common

CLINICAL ISSUES

Presentation
- Most common signs/symptoms
  - Headache, altered mental status
- Clinical profile
  - Polymerase chain reaction (PCR) and flow cytometry assays of CSF useful for correct diagnosis

Demographics
- Age
  - Typically 6th-7th decade

Natural History & Prognosis
- Prognostic markers suggestive of CNS relapse of lymphoma
  - Elevated serum lactate dehydrogenase (LDH) levels
  - Presence of B symptoms
    - Fever, night sweats, weight loss
  - Extranodal involvement at more than 1 site
  - Advanced stage
- Aggressive histologic features increase risk for SCNSL
- Involvement of liver, bladder, testis, or adrenals increases risk of CNS spread
- CNS involvement is almost always fatal

Treatment
- Prophylactic CNS chemotherapy for patients considered at high risk of CNS recurrence

DIAGNOSTIC CHECKLIST

Consider
- Occult systemic lymphoma found in 8% of patients presenting with CNS lymphoma

SELECTED REFERENCES

1. Lee IH et al: Analysis of perfusion weighted image of CNS lymphoma. Eur J Radiol. Epub ahead of print, 2009
2. van Besien K et al: Secondary lymphomas of the central nervous system: risk, prophylaxis and treatment. Leuk Lymphoma. 49 Suppl 1:52-8, 2008

PARANEOPLASTIC SYNDROMES

Key Facts

Terminology

- Remote neurological effects of cancer, associated with extra-CNS tumors
  - Most common tumor: Small cell lung carcinoma
- Limbic encephalitis (LE) is most common clinical paraneoplastic syndrome

Imaging

- Limbic encephalitis: Hyperintensity in mesial temporal lobes, limbic system
  - Mimics herpes encephalitis but subacute/chronic
- Paraneoplastic cerebellar degeneration (PCD): Cerebellar atrophy
- Brainstem encephalitis: T2 hyperintensity in midbrain, pons, cerebellar peduncles, basal ganglia
- Most paraneoplastic syndromes do not have associated imaging findings

Top Differential Diagnoses

- Herpes encephalitis
- Low-grade (grade II) diffuse astrocytoma
- Status epilepticus
- Gliomatosis cerebri

Clinical Issues

- < 1% of patients with systemic cancers develop paraneoplastic syndrome
- Immune-mediated by autoantibodies or cytotoxic T-cell-related mechanisms
  - 60% have circulating serum autoantibodies
- LE: Memory loss, cognitive dysfunction, dementia, psychological features, seizures
- PCD: Ataxia, incoordination, dysarthria, nystagmus
- Brainstem encephalitis: Brainstem dysfunction including cranial nerve palsies, visual changes
- Treatment of primary tumor may improve symptoms

__(Left)__ Axial FLAIR MR shows abnormal hyperintensity in the medial temporal lobes bilaterally, characteristic of limbic encephalitis, the most common paraneoplastic syndrome. Bilateral involvement is typical of limbic encephalitis. __(Right)__ Axial T1WI C+ MR in the same patient shows patchy enhancement ⮚ of the medial temporal lobes. Limbic encephalitis is the only paraneoplastic syndrome with defined imaging features. The patient's symptoms often improve after treatment of the primary tumor.

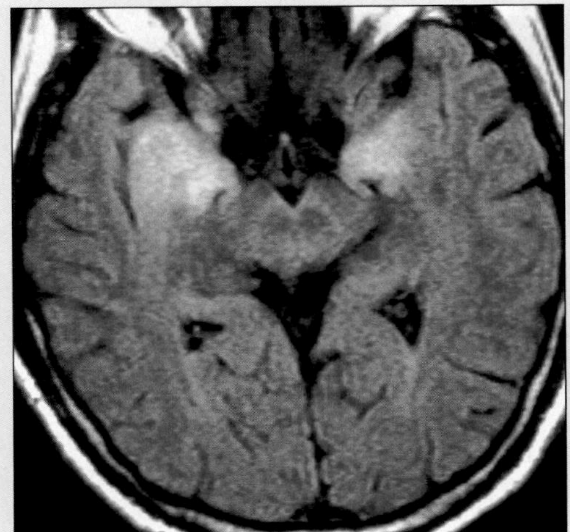

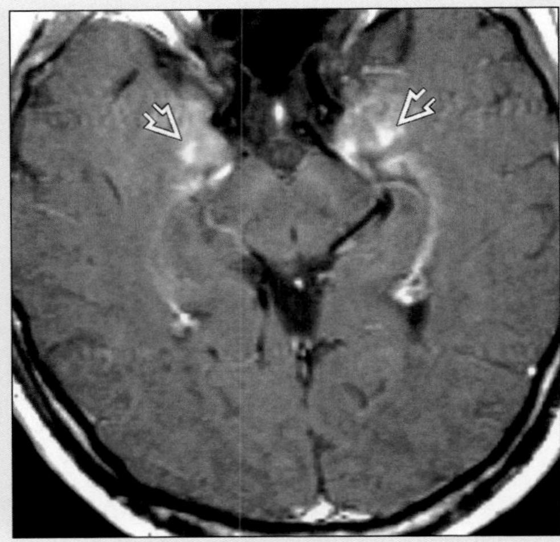

__(Left)__ Axial FLAIR MR in an older adult with small cell lung cancer and subacute dementia shows striking hyperintensity in the right insula ⮚. __(Right)__ Coronal T2WI in the same patient shows abnormal hyperintensity in both medial temporal lobes ➔ and right insular cortex ⮚. Imaging of limbic encephalitis mimics that of herpes encephalitis; however, patients with limbic encephalitis have a subacute presentation. Hemorrhage suggests herpes rather than limbic encephalitis.

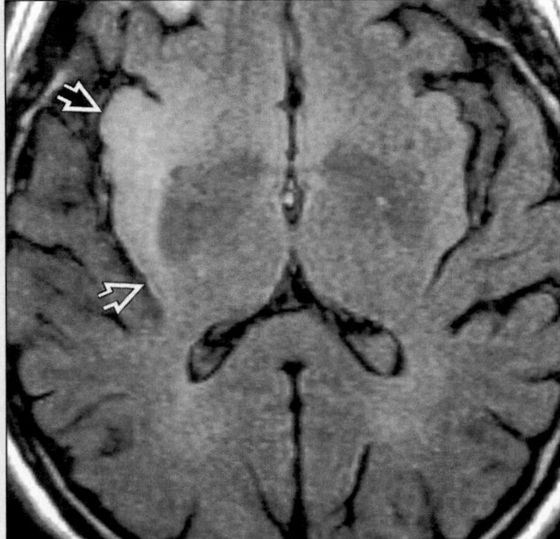

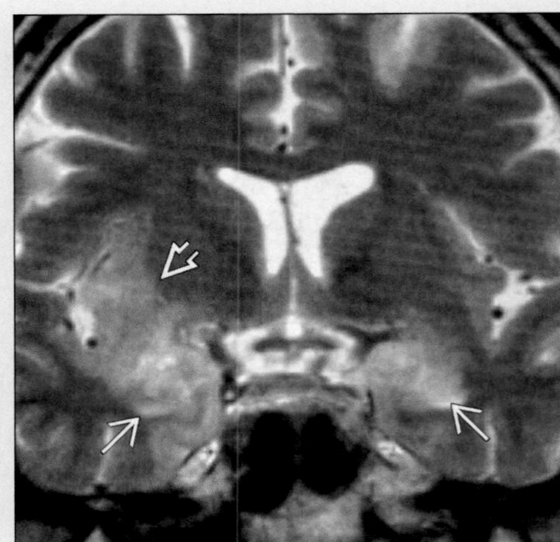

PARANEOPLASTIC SYNDROMES

TERMINOLOGY

Synonyms

- Paraneoplastic syndromes (PSs), paraneoplastic disease

Definitions

- Remote neurological effects of cancer, associated with extra-CNS tumors
  - Most common tumor: Small cell lung carcinoma
- Limbic encephalitis (LE) is most common clinical paraneoplastic syndrome
  - Only PS with clearly defined imaging features

IMAGING

General Features

- Best diagnostic clue
  - Limbic encephalitis: Hyperintensity in mesial temporal lobes, limbic system
    - Looks like herpes encephalitis but different clinical course (subacute vs. chronic)
  - Initial study normal in 20-40%
- Location of LE: Hippocampus, amygdala, cingulate gyrus, pyriform cortex, subfrontal cortex, insula

CT Findings

- NECT: Initial CT scan normal in > 95%
  - Rare: Low density within mesial temporal lobes
- CECT: Usually no visible enhancement

MR Findings

- T1WI
  - Hypointensity in mesial temporal lobes (hippocampus, amygdala), insula, cingulate gyrus, subfrontal cortex, inferior frontal white matter (WM)
  - May see minimal mass effect
  - May see atrophy in chronic cases
  - No hemorrhage
- T2WI: Hyperintensity in mesial temporal lobes (hippocampus, amygdala), insula, cingulate gyrus, subfrontal cortex, inferior frontal WM
  - May see minimal mass effect
- FLAIR: Hyperintensity in temporal lobes, insula, cingulate gyrus, subfrontal cortex, inferior frontal WM
- T2* GRE: No hemorrhage
  - If blood products seen, consider herpes encephalitis
- T1WI C+: Patchy enhancement common
- Rare case reports show MR findings in other PSs
  - Paraneoplastic cerebellar degeneration (PCD)
    - Cerebellar atrophy
  - Brainstem encephalitis: T2 hyperintensity in midbrain, pons, cerebellar peduncles, basal ganglia

Nuclear Medicine Findings

- FDG PET: Increased glucose metabolism in medial temporal lobes in LE patients

Imaging Recommendations

- Protocol advice
  - Contrast-enhanced MR with coronal T2 or FLAIR
  - Consider repeat MR if initial scan normal + high clinical suspicion

DIFFERENTIAL DIAGNOSIS

Herpes Encephalitis

- T2 hyperintensity in temporal lobes, limbic system
- Mass effect common; restricted DWI common
- Rapid onset, febrile illness
- HSV titers (CSF, serum) may be negative early
- Late acute/subacute may hemorrhage
- May be indistinguishable from limbic encephalitis

Low-Grade (Grade II) Diffuse Astrocytoma

- Unilateral T2 hyperintense mass
- May involve medial temporal lobe
- No enhancement typical

Status Epilepticus

- Seizures may cause abnormal T2/FLAIR of mesial temporal lobes
- Cortical enhancement is typical
- Clinical history of seizures

Gliomatosis Cerebri

- Diffuse process, no predilection for limbic system
- T2 hyperintensity in multiple contiguous lobes
- Enlarges affected area

Parenchymal Metastases

- Typically multifocal enhancing lesions
- Primary tumor often known

PATHOLOGY

General Features

- Etiology
  - Immune-mediated by autoantibodies or cytotoxic T-cell-related mechanisms
  - 60% of patients have circulating serum autoantibodies
    - Anti-Hu (lung cancer): Limbic encephalitis
    - Anti-Ta (testicular germ cell tumors): Limbic encephalitis, brainstem encephalitis
    - Anti-Yo (breast and ovarian): Paraneoplastic cerebellar degeneration
    - Anti-Tr (Hodgkin disease): Paraneoplastic cerebellar degeneration
    - Anti-Ri (lung, breast, ovarian): Opsoclonus-myoclonus
  - Reversible extralimbic paraneoplastic encephalopathy
    - Associated with breast cancer and lung cancer
    - Reversible when primary tumors controlled
  - New cell surface antigens reported: Voltage-gated potassium channels (VGKC) and N-methyl-D-aspartate receptor (NMDAR)
    - Associated with other tumors (thymoma, teratoma, Hodgkin lymphoma)
    - Appear to be antibody-mediated and respond better to immunotherapy (90%)
    - Patients may present with limbic encephalitis; more frequently manifest severe psychiatric symptoms, seizures, dyskinesias, autonomic instability, or hypoventilation

Staging, Grading, & Classification

- PSs divided into disorders of CNS, peripheral NS, CNS/PNS, neuromuscular junction
  - CNS: Paraneoplastic cerebellar degeneration (PCD), opsoclonus-myoclonus, retinopathy
  - Peripheral NS: Sensory-motor neuropathy, autonomic neuropathy
  - Both CNS/PNS: Encephalomyelitis (limbic encephalitis, brainstem encephalitis, myelitis, motor neuron disease)
  - Neuromuscular junction: Lambert-Eaton myasthenic syndrome
- Limbic encephalitis most common PS
  - Nonparaneoplastic limbic encephalitis reported
- PCD is 2nd most common PS
- Multiple PSs may occur in same patient

Gross Pathologic & Surgical Features

- LE: Ill-defined softening, discoloration of GM
  - Hippocampus, cingulate gyrus, pyriform cortex, frontal orbital surface of temporal lobe, insula, amygdala; typically bilateral
- PCD: Cerebellar atrophy, gyral thinning
- Brainstem encephalitis: Brainstem softening

Microscopic Features

- Limbic encephalitis
  - Neuronal loss, reactive gliosis, perivascular infiltration of lymphocytes, microglial nodules
  - No neoplasm and no viral inclusions
- PCD: Purkinje cell loss, microglial proliferation, Bergmann glia hyperplasia, decrease in granule cells
- Brainstem encephalitis: Perivascular inflammatory infiltrates, glial nodules, neuronophagia

CLINICAL ISSUES

Presentation

- Most common signs/symptoms
  - LE: Memory loss, cognitive dysfunction, dementia, psychological features (anxiety, depression, hallucinations), seizures; subacute presentation
  - PCD: Ataxia, incoordination, dysarthria, nystagmus
    - In patients > 50 years, cerebellar degeneration is paraneoplastic in 50% of cases, often precedes remote malignancy
  - Brainstem encephalitis: Brainstem dysfunction including cranial nerve palsies, visual changes
  - In patients with known primary tumor, must exclude other complications
    - Metastases, infection, metabolic disorder, chemotherapy effects
- Clinical profile
  - Up to 60% have no known primary tumor at presentation, many have no tumor found at work-up
  - Identification of antineuronal antibodies in serum or CSF facilitates diagnosis of PS and primary cancer
  - Primary neoplasms
    - Limbic encephalitis
      - Most common: Small cell lung carcinoma
      - Other = GI, GU (ovary > renal > uterus), Hodgkin lymphoma, breast, testicular, thymus, neuroblastoma (pediatric)
      - 90% have positive CSF (pleocytosis, ↑ protein, oligoclonal bands)
      - EEG reveals involvement of temporal lobes
    - Paraneoplastic cerebellar degeneration
      - GU (ovary), breast, lung, lymphoma
    - Opsoclonus-myoclonus
      - Neuroblastoma, lung cancer
    - Lambert-Eaton myasthenic syndrome
      - Small cell lung cancer

Demographics

- Age: Occurs at all ages, most commonly adults
- Epidemiology: < 1% of patients with systemic cancers develop paraneoplastic syndrome

Natural History & Prognosis

- Relates to primary neoplasm
- Some reports suggest patients with PSs have more indolent primary tumor growth than those without
- Relates to type of paraneoplastic syndrome
  - Slow long-term cognitive decline (LE)
  - Progressive ataxia, weakness (PCD, spinal cord degeneration)

Treatment

- Treatment of primary malignancy may improve neurologic symptoms of PSs (25-45%)
- Primary neoplasm resected, ± chemoradiation
- Treatment of paraneoplastic syndromes is variable
  - Treatment of primary tumor is best therapy
  - ± steroids, immunoglobulins, plasmapheresis

DIAGNOSTIC CHECKLIST

Consider

- LE is only PS with defined imaging features
- Paraneoplastic syndromes are often clinically evident before diagnosis of primary tumor
- Repeat MR if initial scan normal and high clinical suspicion, as initial MR often normal in LE

Image Interpretation Pearls

- Herpes encephalitis mimics LE on imaging but has an acute presentation
  - Patients often initially treated with antiviral therapy until HSV titers final
- Hemorrhage suggests herpes rather than limbic encephalitis

SELECTED REFERENCES

1. Khan NL et al: Histopathology of VGKC antibody-associated limbic encephalitis. Neurology. 72(19):1703-5, 2009
2. McKeon A et al: Reversible extralimbic paraneoplastic encephalopathies with large abnormalities on magnetic resonance images. Arch Neurol. 66(2):268-71, 2009
3. Darnell RB et al: Paraneoplastic syndromes affecting the nervous system. Semin Oncol. 33(3):270-98, 2006
4. Dalmau J et al: Paraneoplastic neurologic syndromes: pathogenesis and physiopathology. Brain Pathol. 9(2):275-84, 1999

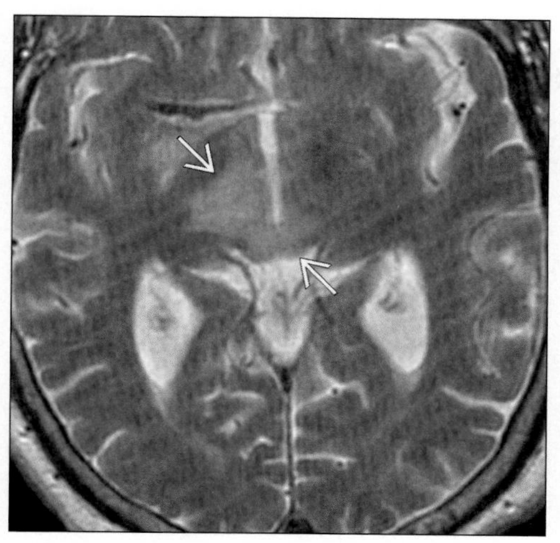

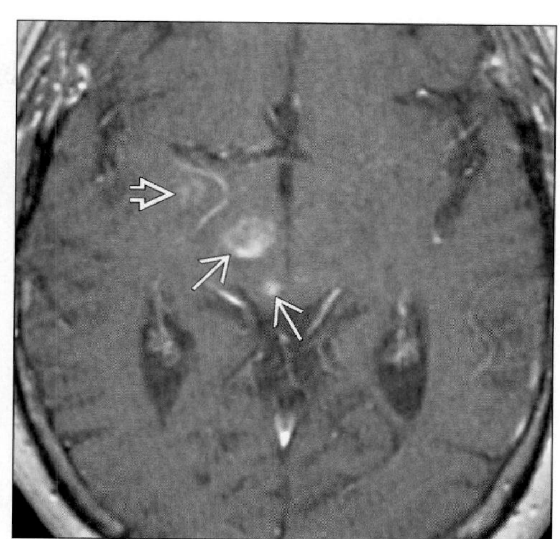

(Left) *Axial T2WI MR shows midbrain hyperintensity ➔ related to brainstem encephalitis, which is characterized by hyperintensity in the midbrain, pons, cerebellar peduncle, and basal ganglia.* ***(Right)*** *Axial T1WI C+ MR in the same patient shows patchy enhancement of the midbrain lesions ➔ and of the medial temporal lobe ➲. This patient was diagnosed with limbic encephalitis with new brainstem symptoms. Multiple paraneoplastic syndromes may occur in the same patient.*

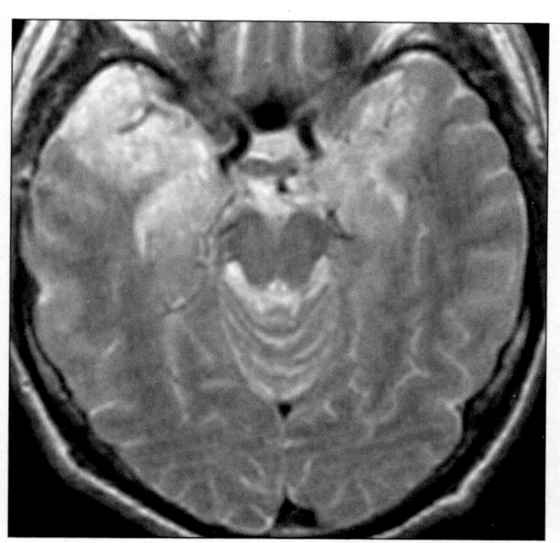

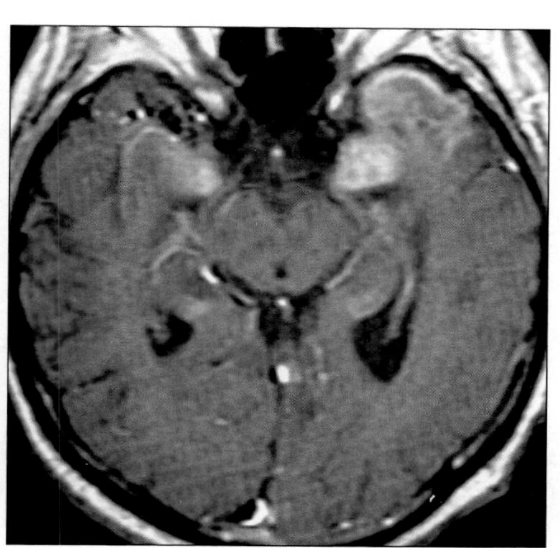

(Left) *Axial T2WI MR shows abnormal hyperintensity within the medial temporal lobes bilaterally related to limbic encephalitis. Less than 1% of patients with systemic cancers develop a paraneoplastic syndrome.* ***(Right)*** *Axial T1WI C+ MR shows enhancement in the medial temporal lobes and left anterior temporal lobe related to limbic encephalitis. As imaging mimics herpes encephalitis, most patients are initially treated with antiviral therapy until HSV titers are found to be negative.*

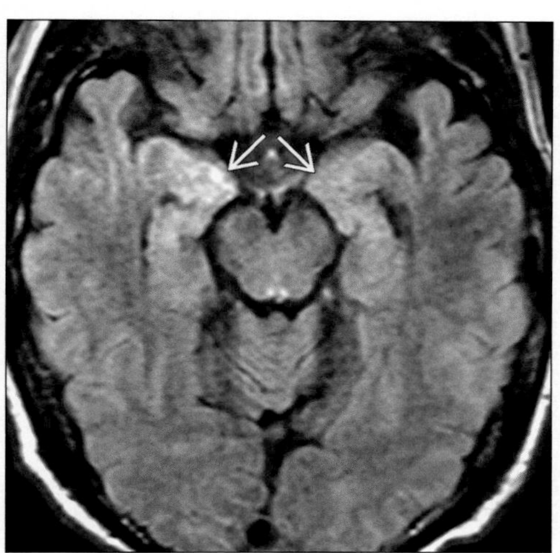

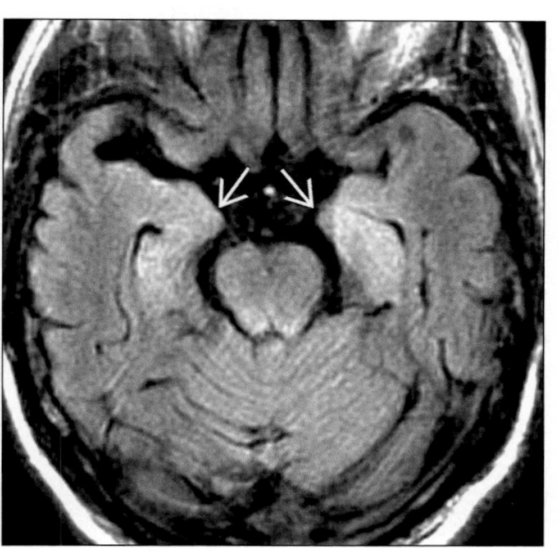

(Left) *Axial FLAIR MR shows subtle asymmetric hyperintensity of the hippocampi ➔ in this young patient with melanoma and subacute dementia.* ***(Right)*** *Axial FLAIR MR shows hyperintensity in both medial temporal lobes ➔ in this patient with subacute dementia and voltage-gated potassium channel (VGKC) autoimmunity. VGKC may occur without a primary neoplasm or may present as a paraneoplastic syndrome and mimic limbic encephalitis. VGKC responds well to immunotherapy.*

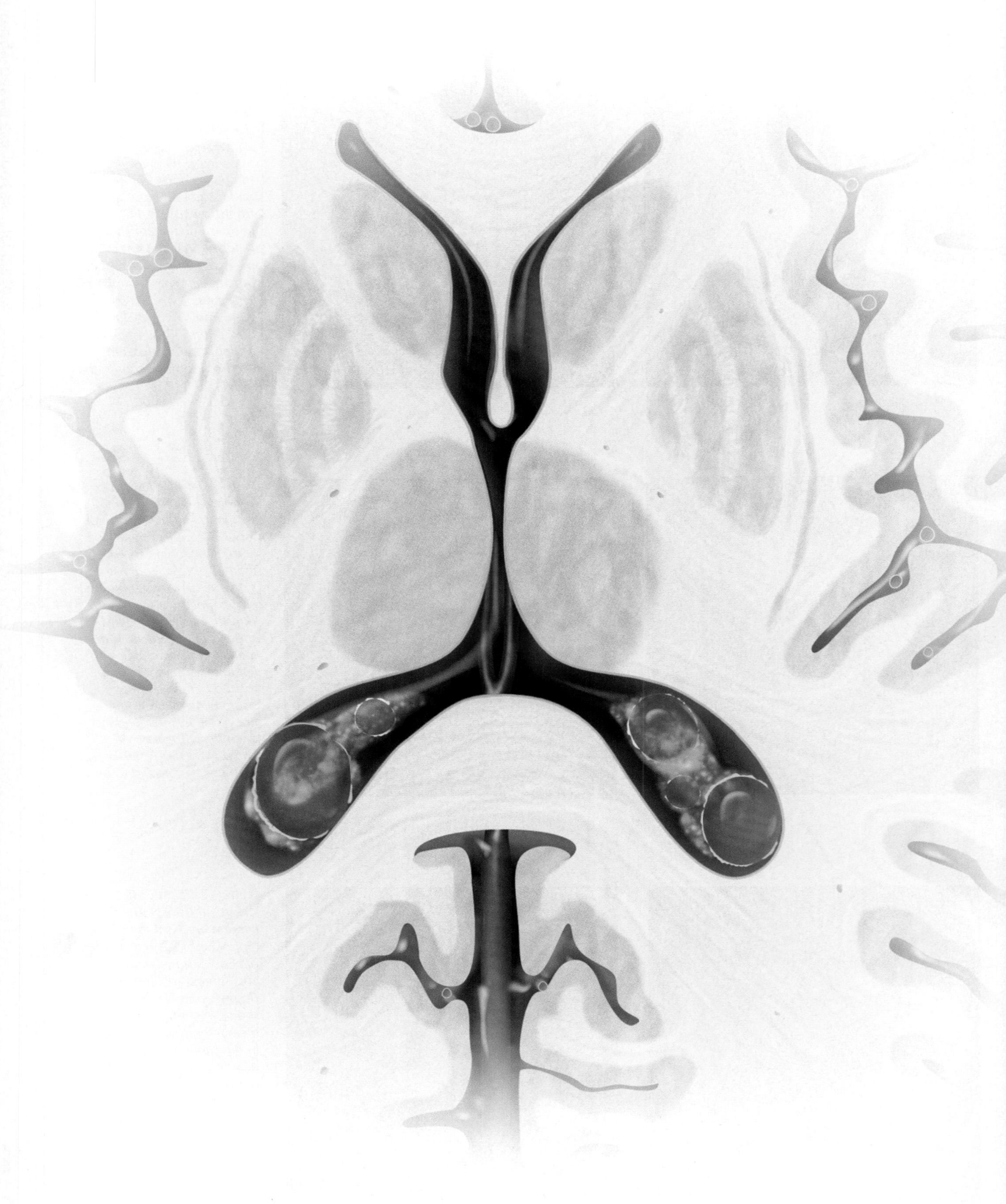

SECTION 7
Primary Nonneoplastic Cysts

Introduction and Overview

Primary Nonneoplastic Cysts

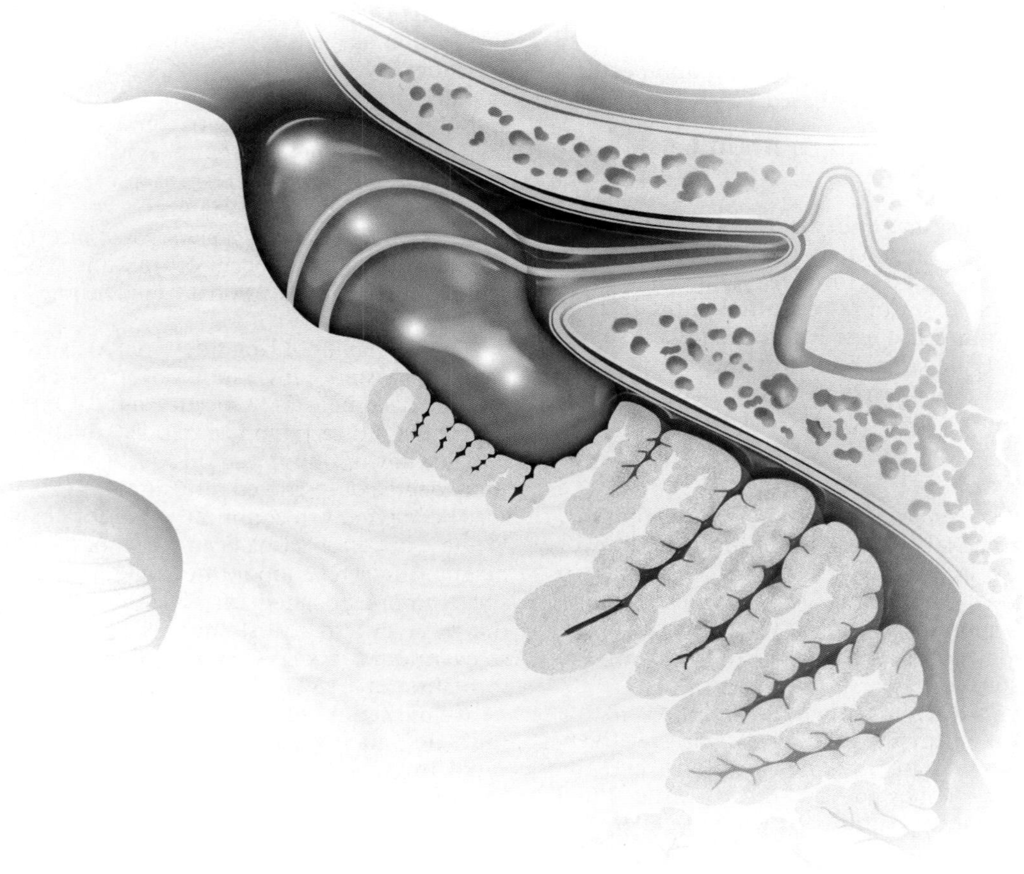

General Approach to Brain Cysts

General Considerations

Overview. Cysts are common findings on MR and CT brain scans. There are many types of intracranial cysts, some significant, some incidental. In this section we exclude cystic neoplasms (such as pilocytic astrocytoma and hemangioblastoma), solid neoplasms that commonly have intratumoral cysts (such as ependymoma), and tumors that often display central necrosis (e.g., glioblastoma multiforme).

We also exclude parasitic cysts (neurocysticercosis, hydatid disease) and cystic brain malformations (Dandy-Walker spectrum) from the discussion. Thus the focus of this particular section is primary nonneoplastic cysts.

Because the etiology, pathology, and clinical importance of nonneoplastic cysts is so varied, classifying them presents a real challenge. Some neuropathologists typically classify cysts according to the histology of the cyst wall. Others group them according to putative origin or pathogenesis.

In a schema based on pathogenesis, cysts may occur as normal anatomic variants (e.g., enlarged perivascular [Virchow-Robin] spaces), congenital inclusion cysts (e.g., dermoid and epidermoid cysts), or lesions derived from embryonic ecto-/endoderm (colloid and neurenteric cysts). Of course, there is a group of miscellaneous cysts (such as choroid plexus cysts and nonneoplastic tumor-associated cysts) that does not fit nicely into any category.

Neuroimagers face a very real dilemma: A cystic-appearing lesion is identified on MR or CT. What is it? What else could it be? Histopathology of the cyst wall isn't a practical consideration. What **is** readily apparent is (1) the anatomic location of the cyst; (2) its imaging characteristics (density/signal intensity, presence or absence of calcification, enhancement, etc.); and (3) the patient's age. The recommended initial approach to analyzing brain cysts is anatomy-based.

Anatomy-Based Approach to Brain Cysts

General Considerations

Key features. Four features help the diagnostic approach to cystic-appearing intracranial lesions. The 1st step is to determine if the cyst is intra- or extraaxial. If it is extraaxial, is the cyst supra- or infratentorial? Is it midline or off-midline? If a cyst is intraaxial, is it supra- or infratentorial? Is it parenchymal or intraventricular? While many intracranial cysts certainly may occur in more than 1 location, some sites are "preferred" by certain cysts.

Extraaxial Cysts

Supratentorial extraaxial cysts. Nonneoplastic, noninfectious extraaxial cysts can occur in the midline or off-midline. Pineal and Rathke cleft cysts occur only in the midline. While dermoid cysts seem to prefer a midline location like the suprasellar cistern, they also occur off-midline. Look for rupture with fatty "droplets" in the subarachnoid cisterns.

Arachnoid cysts (AC) are usually off-midline. In the supratentorial compartment, midline ACs are relatively rare. The most frequent midline locations are the suprasellar cistern, followed by the quadrigeminal cistern and velum interpositum. Large suprasellar ACs usually present in children and may cause obstructive hydrocephalus.

The most common off-midline extraaxial supratentorial cyst is an arachnoid cyst. While these can occur virtually anywhere, the middle cranial fossa is the location of at least 50% of all ACs. Occasionally ACs occur over the cerebral convexities, most commonly over the parietal lobe. ACs follow CSF on all sequences and are differentiated from epidermoid cysts using FLAIR and DWI. ACs suppress completely on FLAIR and do not show diffusion restriction.

Extraaxial tumors such as meningioma, schwannoma, pituitary macroadenoma and craniopharyngioma may be associated with prominent extratumoral cysts. These nonneoplastic tumor-associated cysts (TACs) occur in both the supra- and infratentorial compartments.

TACs are benign collections of fluid that vary from clear and CSF-like to proteinaceous. TACs are typically positioned between at the tumor-brain interface, between the mass and adjacent cortex. Whether TACs are true arachnoid cysts, obstructed PVSs, or fluid collections mostly lined by gliotic brain is debatable.

Scalp and skull cysts are less common than intracranial cysts. Sebaceous cysts (more accurately termed trichilemmal cysts [TCs]) are a common scalp mass in middle-aged and older patients. Most are identified incidentally on MR and CT scans. TCs can be solitary or multiple, are well-delineated, and vary in size from a few millimeters to several centimeters. The classic finding is a subepidermal scalp tumor in a female over the age of 60 years.

Leptomeningeal cysts, also known as "growing fractures," are a rare but important extraaxial cyst that is most commonly found in the parietal bone. An enlarging calvarial fracture adjacent to post-traumatic encephalomalacia is typical. The vast majority of patients are under 3 years of age. They present with an enlarging, palpable soft tissue mass. Fluid and encephalomalacic brain extrude through torn dura and arachnoid and then through the enlarging linear calvarial fracture. Leptomeningeal cysts are seen as linear lucent skull lesions with rounded, scalloped margins.

Infratentorial extraaxial cysts. Most nonneoplastic cysts in the posterior fossa occur off-midline. The 2 major cyst types found in this location are epidermoid and arachnoid cysts.

The cerebellopontine angle (CPA) is by far the most common posterior fossa sublocation of an epidermoid cyst (EC). Occasionally an EC occurs in the 4th ventricle. A 4th ventricular EC can mimic a trapped, dilated 4th ventricle, but ECs do not suppress on FLAIR and usually exhibit some degree of restricted diffusion.

The next most common posterior fossa cyst is AC. While ACs can also occur in the midline cisterna magna, the cerebellopontine angle is the most common site. Tumor-associated cysts (TACs) sometimes occur in the CPA cistern. Most are associated with vestibular schwannoma, but a CPA meningioma may also cause formation of a TAC.

Neurenteric cysts (NE) are congenital endodermal cysts that are much more commonly found in the spinal canal. Intracranial NE cysts occur in the cerebromedullary cistern and are usually midline or slightly off-midline, lying just anterior to the pontomedullary junction. Sometimes NE cysts occur off-midline, in the lower CPA (cerebromedullary) cistern. Bony skull defects can occur but are rare.

An anatomic variant that can be confused with a posterior fossa NE cyst is retroclival ecchordosis physaliphora (EP), found in about 2% of autopsies. EP is a gelatinous notochordal remnant that can occur anywhere from the dorsum sellae to the sacrococcygeal region. Intracranial EPs typically occur in the prepontine cistern and are attached to a defect in the dorsal clivus by a thin, stalk-like pedicle. NE cysts and EPs are both hyperintense on T2WI. Chordomas are the malignant counterparts of ecchordosis.

Intraaxial Cysts

Supratentorial intraaxial cysts. Here anatomic sublocation is key to the differential diagnosis. Parenchymal cysts represent a completely different group than intraventricular cysts. The most common parenchymal cysts in the brain are enlarged perivascular (Virchow-Robin) spaces (PVSs). PVSs have a distinct predilection for the basal ganglia, where they tend to cluster around the anterior commissure. The midbrain is another common site. When they occur here, enlarged PVSs may cause obstructive hydrocephalus. Prominent PVSs also occur in the subcortical and deep white matter. They are pial-lined, interstitial fluid-containing structures that tend to occur in clusters of variably-sized cysts. Most PVSs suppress completely; 75% are surrounded by normal-appearing brain, which helps distinguish them from porencephalic cysts.

Hippocampal sulcus remnant cysts are common normal variants, seen as a "string" of small CSF-like cysts lying in the hippocampus just medial to the temporal horn of the lateral ventricle. They are caused by defective or incomplete fusion of the embryonic cornu ammonis and dentate gyrus and are of no clinical significance.

Porencephalic cysts are the 3rd most common supratentorial parenchymal cysts. They may communicate with the ventricles and are typically lined by gliotic white matter, not ependyma, and are caused by brain destruction (e.g., peri- or antenatal insult). The brain surrounding a porencephalic cyst is typically hyperintense on T2WI and FLAIR.

Periventricular cysts of newborns encompasses a wide, overlapping variety of periventricular cystic lesions that ranges from cystic periventricular leukomalacia to connatal and germinolytic cysts. This somewhat confusing and controversial topic is covered in its own separate chapter.

Neuroglial cysts, sometimes called neuroepithelial cysts, are benign glial-lined cavities buried within the cerebral white matter. While they can occur anywhere, the frontal lobe is the most common site. They tend to be solitary whereas PVSs are usually collections of multiple cysts of different sizes. A choroid fissure cyst is a neuroglial cyst that occurs anywhere along the infolded choroid fissure. Most are found medial to the temporal horn of the lateral ventricle. Hippocampal sulcus remnant cysts (HSRCs) occur when there is incomplete fusion of the cornu ammonis and the dentate gyrus. HSRCs are often multiple, appearing like a string of small CSF-containing cysts along the lateral margin of the hippocampus.

Supratentorial intraventricular cysts are most often found in the atria of the lateral ventricles and foramen of Monro. Choroid plexus cysts (CPCs) are the most common of all intracranial neuroepithelial cysts, occurring in up to 50% of autopsies. Most CPCs are actually xanthogranulomas. Lipid accumulates in the choroid plexus from degenerating &/or desquamating choroid epithelium. CPCs are common incidental imaging findings in middle-aged and older adults. They are usually bilateral and are often multicystic. Most CPCs are small, measuring 2-8 mm in diameter. They typically do not suppress completely on FLAIR and may show moderately high signal intensity on DWI.

Ependymal cysts (EC) are rare, benign, ependymal-lined cysts of the lateral ventricles. Most ECs, even large ones, are asymptomatic and incidental. EC patients presenting with headache, seizure, &/or obstructive hydrocephalus have been reported in the literature. They contain clear serous CSF-like fluid secreted from ependymal cells. ECs typically follow CSF on all sequences and suppress completely on FLAIR.

Colloid cysts (CCs) occur almost exclusively in the foramen of Monro, attached to the anterosuperior portion of the 3rd ventricular roof. They are wedged into the foramen and are typically straddled by the fornices. CCs are endodermal in origin and contain viscous gelatinous material consisting of mostly mucin. CCs may also contain blood degradation products, foamy cells and cholesterol crystals. Even relatively small CCs may suddenly obstruct the foramen of Monro, causing acute hydrocephalus. Occasionally brain herniation with rapid clinical deterioration ensues. The imaging appearance of a well-delineated hyperdense mass at the foramen of Monro on NECT is virtually pathognomonic of a CC.

Infratentorial intraaxial cysts. Parenchymal infratentorial cysts are rare; most are PVSs. The only common site is in and around the dentate nuclei. Most are asymptomatic. Occasionally large PVSs occur in the pons and can be a rare cause of cranial neuropathy.

Nonneoplastic, nonparasitic cysts in the 4th ventricle are uncommon. The most common cause is not a true cyst but an enlarged, "encysted" 4th ventricle. Infection or aneurysmal subarachnoid hemorrhage may cause outlet foraminal obstruction. When combined with superior obstruction near the aqueduct, the 4th ventricle can become completely encysted. Choroid plexus continues to produce CSF. With egress blocked, the 4th ventricle enlarges. Epidermoid cysts can arise in the 4th ventricle, a much less common posterior fossa location than the CPA. Some ECs are so similar to CSF that only FLAIR and DWI permit distinction of an EC from CSF in an enlarged but otherwise normal-appearing 4th ventricle.

References

1. Tseng J et al: Peripheral cysts: a distinguishing feature of esthesioneuroblastoma with intracranial extension. Ear Nose Throat J. 88(6):E14, 2009
2. Yurt A et al: Magnetic resonance spectroscopic imaging associated with analysis of fluid in cystic brain tumors. Neurol Res. Epub ahead of print, 2009
3. Osborn AG et al: Intracranial cysts: radiologic-pathologic correlation and imaging approach. Radiology. 239(3):650-64, 2006

PRIMARY NONNEOPLASTIC CYSTS OVERVIEW

INTRACRANIAL CYSTIC-APPEARING LESIONS

Extraaxial	*Intraaxial*
Supratentorial	Supratentorial
Midline	Parenchymal
Pineal cyst	Enlarged perivascular spaces (PVSs)
Dermoid cyst	Neuroglial cyst
Rathke cleft cyst	Porencephalic cyst
Arachnoid cyst (suprasellar)	Connatal, germinolytic cysts
	Hippocampal sulcus remnants
Off-midline	Intraventricular
Arachnoid cyst (middle cranial fossa, convexity)	Choroid plexus cysts
Epidermoid cyst	Ependymal cyst
TACs (macroadenoma, meningioma)	Colloid cyst
Sebaceous cyst (scalp)	
Leptomeningeal cyst ("growing fracture")	
Infratentorial	Infratentorial
Midline	Parenchymal
Neurenteric cyst	Enlarged PVSs (dentate nuclei)
Arachnoid cyst	
Off-midline	Intraventricular
Epidermoid (CPA)	Epidermoid (4th ventricle, cisterna magna)
Arachnoid cyst (CPA)	Cystic ("trapped") 4th ventricle
TACs (schwannoma, meningioma)	

Nonneoplastic, noninfectious cystic brain lesions classified by common anatomic locations. The 1st division is extra- vs. intraaxial, then supra- vs. infratentorial. Extraaxial cysts are further subdivided into midline and off-midline lesions. Intraaxial cysts are subdivided into parenchymal and intraventricular. Cerebellopontine angle (CPA), perivascular (Virchow-Robin) spaces (PVSs), tumor-associated cysts (TACs).

INTRACRANIAL CYSTS BY TYPE, MOST COMMON LOCATION(S)

Cyst Type	*Common Location(s)*
Arachnoid cyst	Middle cranial fossa; cerebellopontine angle (CPA); suprasellar cistern
Choroid fissure cyst	Choroid fissure, between temporal horn and suprasellar cistern
Choroid plexus cyst	Choroid plexus glomus
Colloid cyst	Interventricular foramen/anterosuperior 3rd ventricle
Connatal cyst(s)	Peri- or intraventricular, adjacent to frontal horn, body of lateral ventricle
Dermoid cyst	Suprasellar, frontonasal (anteroinferior interhemispheric fissure)
Enlarged perivascular spaces (PVSs)	Basal ganglia, midbrain, cerebral white matter, dentate nuclei
Epidermoid cyst	Cerebellopontine angle (CPA)
Ependymal cyst	Lateral ventricle (atrium most common)
Germinolytic pseudocyst(s)	Periventricular, subependymal along caudothalamic groove
Hippocampal sulcus remnants	Hippocampus, just medial to lateral ventricle
Leptomeningeal cyst ("growing fracture")	Parietal bone
Neurenteric cyst	Prepontine at pontomedullary junction
Neuroglial cyst	Frontal/temporal subcortical WM, choroid fissure
Pineal cyst	Pineal gland
Porencephalic cyst	Cerebral hemispheres, adjacent to lateral ventricles
Rathke cleft cyst	Suprasellar, intrasellar
Sebaceous (trichilemmal) cyst	Scalp (dermis or subcutaneous tissues)
Tumor-associated cyst	Between schwannoma, meningioma, macroadenoma, and brain

Nonneoplastic, noninfectious cysts of the brain, as well as the skull and scalp, are listed alphabetically, with most common location(s) noted.

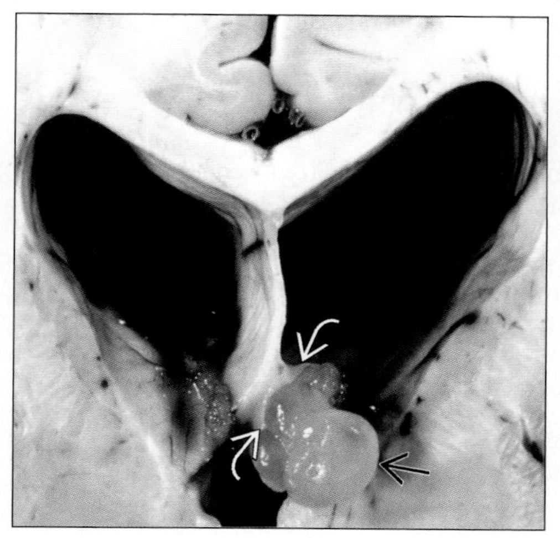

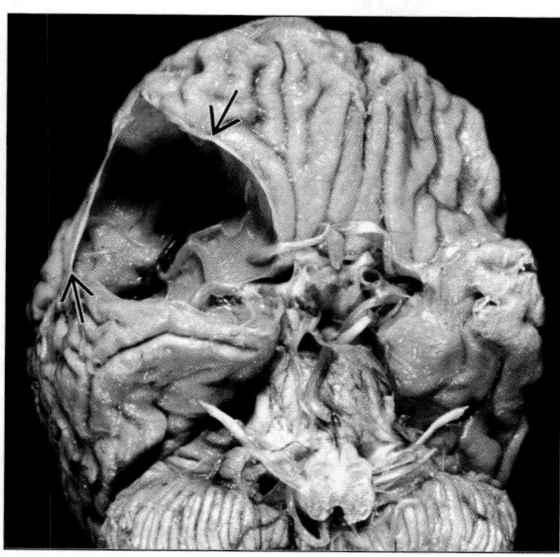

(Left) *Gross pathology shows an autopsied case of a colloid cyst, sectioned in the coronal plane through the foramen of Monro. Note the gelatinous-appearing lobulated cyst* → *with the fornices* ➔ *straddling the cyst. This patient died of sudden obstructive hydrocephalus. (Courtesy J. Townsend, MD.)* ***(Right)*** *Gross pathology of an autopsied brain, seen from below, shows a large arachnoid cyst of the middle cranial fossa. The cyst contained CSF within split layers of arachnoid* →*. (Courtesy J. Townsend, MD.)*

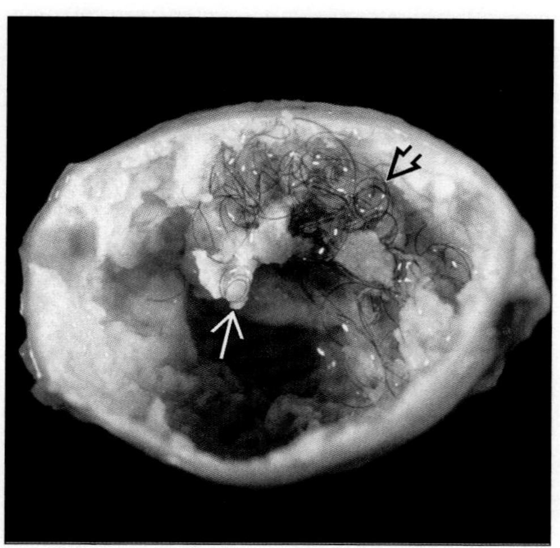

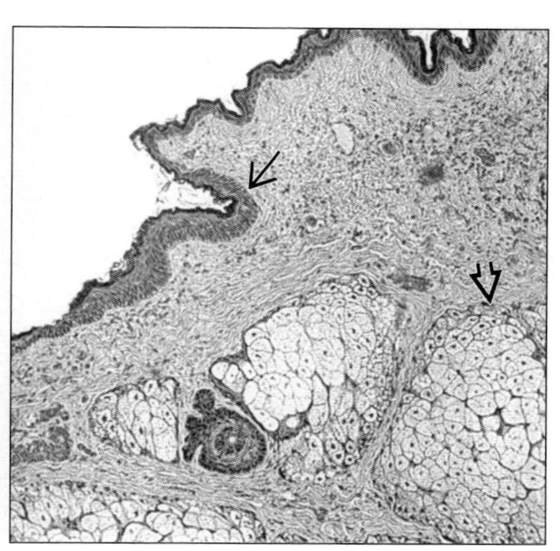

(Left) *Gross surgical specimen of a sectioned dermoid cyst shows the characteristic lining of stratified squamous epithelium plus intracystic keratin debris* ➔*. Matted, tangled hairs* ⇒ *are present within the cyst which contained thick, greasy sebaceous material when sectioned. (Courtesy R. Hewlett, PhD.)* ***(Right)*** *Microscopy of a typical dermoid cyst shows squamous epithelium* → *and sebaceous glands* ⇒ *lining a cavity that contains desquamated keratinaceous debris.*

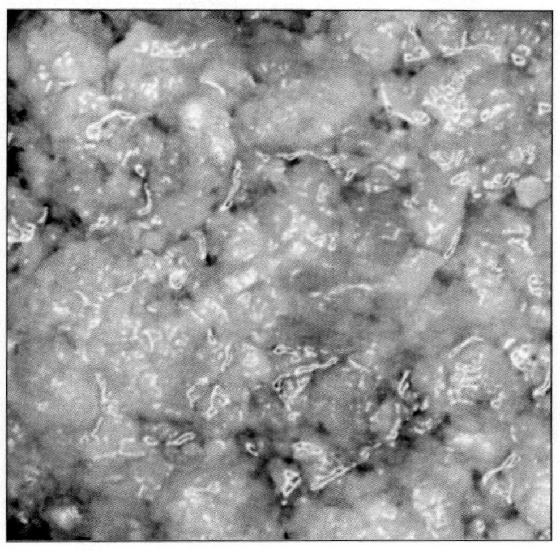

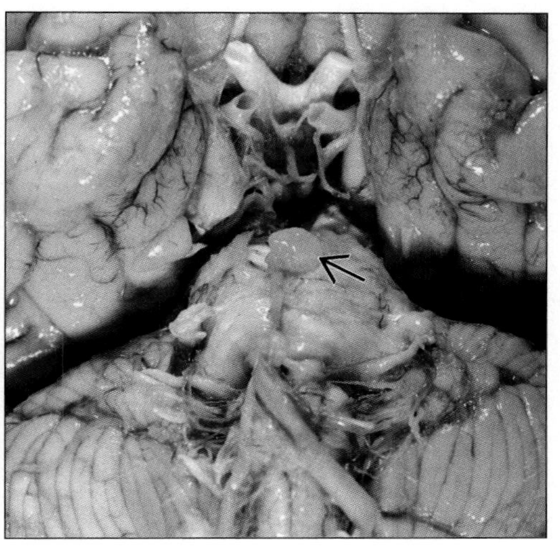

(Left) *Close-up view of an epidermoid cyst shows the cauliflower-like cyst surface that is composed of nodular masses of squamous epithelium and pearly white keratin.* ***(Right)*** *Autopsy specimen shows a small gelatinous-appearing nodule* → *just anterior to the pons. Ecchordosis physaliphora, a notochordal remnant, grossly appears similar to neurenteric cyst. (Courtesy R. Hewlett, PhD.)*

ARACHNOID CYST

Key Facts

Terminology

- Intraarachnoid CSF-filled sac that does not communicate with ventricular system

Imaging

- General findings
  - Sharply demarcated round/ovoid extraaxial cyst
  - Isodense/isointense with CSF
- Location
  - Middle cranial fossa (50-60%)
  - Cerebellopontine angle (10%)
  - Suprasellar (10%)
  - Miscellaneous (10%) (convexity, quadrigeminal)
- MR
  - Isointense with CSF on all sequences
  - Suppresses completely with FLAIR
  - No restriction on DWI
  - CISS, FIESTA: Use to delineate cyst wall, adjacent structures
  - 2D cine PC: Use to detect communication between AC, adjacent subarachnoid space

Top Differential Diagnoses

- Epidermoid cyst
- Other nonneoplastic cysts (e.g., porencephalic)
- Chronic subdural hematoma

Clinical Issues

- Most common congenital intracranial cystic abnormality
- 1% of all intracranial masses
- Can be found at any age (75% in children)

Diagnostic Checklist

- FLAIR, DWI best for AC vs. epidermoid

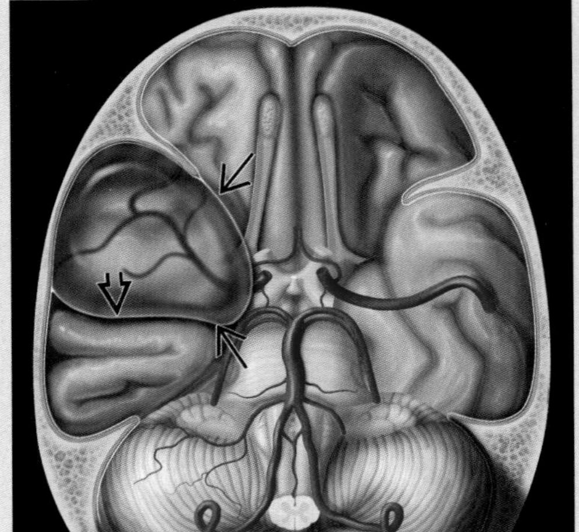

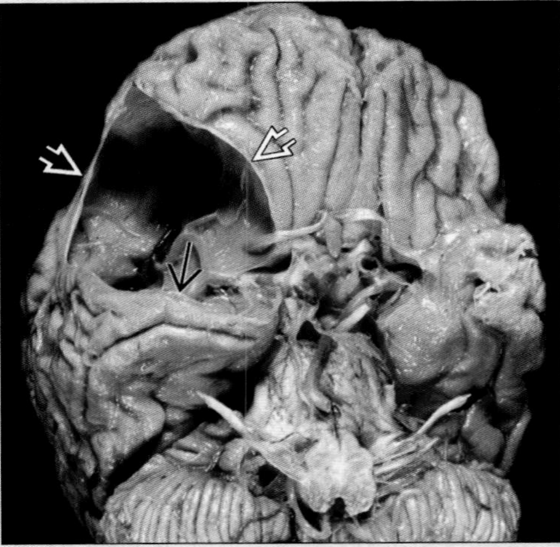

(Left) Graphic depicts the middle cranial fossa AC. Note the arachnoid → splits and encloses CSF. The middle fossa is expanded, and the overlying bone is thinned. Note the temporal lobe → is displaced posteriorly. (Right) Submentovertex view of autopsied brain with incidental finding of middle cranial fossa AC. Note "splitting" of arachnoid → containing a large CSF collection (drained during removal). The temporal lobe is displaced posteriorly →, and the middle fossa is expanded. (Courtesy J. Townsend, MD.)

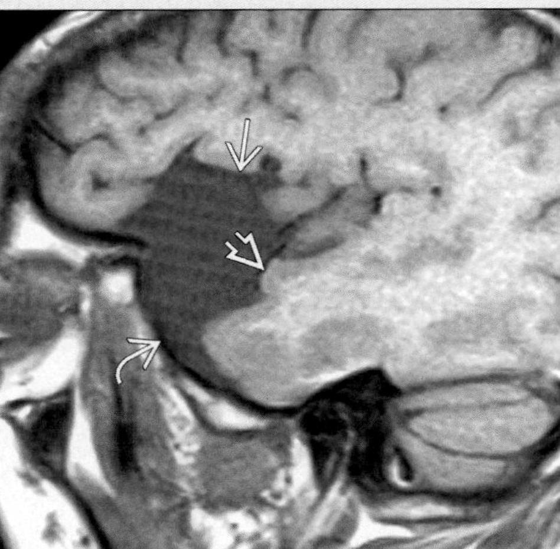

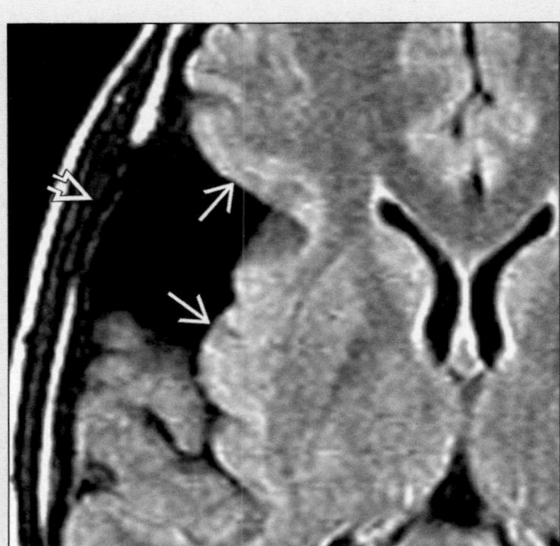

(Left) Sagittal T1WI MR shows a classic middle fossa arachnoid cyst →. Note the expansion of the greater sphenoid wing → and posteriorly displaced temporal lobe →. (Right) Axial FLAIR MR in the same patient shows the classic "scalloped" appearance of the arachnoid cyst, with smooth, sharply demarcated edges that displace the adjacent cortex →. Note the thinning of the overlying calvarium →.

ARACHNOID CYST

TERMINOLOGY

Abbreviations
- Arachnoid cyst (AC)
- Middle cranial fossa AC (MCF AC)

Definitions
- Intraarachnoid CSF-filled sac that does not communicate with ventricular system

IMAGING

General Features
- Best diagnostic clue
  - Sharply demarcated round/ovoid extraaxial cyst that follows CSF attenuation/signal
- Location
  - Middle cranial fossa (50-60%)
  - Cerebellopontine angle (CPA) (10%)
  - Suprasellar arachnoid cyst (SSAC), variable types (10%)
    - Noncommunicating = cyst of membrane of Liliequist
    - Communicating = cystic dilation of interpeduncular cistern
  - 10% miscellaneous (convexity, quadrigeminal)
- Size
  - Varies from a few mm to giant
- Morphology
  - Sharply delineated translucent cyst
  - Displays features of extraaxial mass
    - Displaces cortex
    - "Buckles" gray-white interface

CT Findings
- NECT
  - Usually CSF density
    - Hyperdense if intracyst hemorrhage present (rare)
  - May expand, thin/remodel bone
- CECT
  - Does not enhance
- CTA
  - Posterior displacement of MCA in MCF ACs
- CT: Cisternography may demonstrate communication with subarachnoid space

MR Findings
- T1WI
  - Sharply marginated extraaxial fluid collection isointense with CSF
- T2WI
  - Isointense with CSF
- PD/intermediate
  - Isointense with CSF
- FLAIR
  - Suppresses completely
- T2* GRE
  - No "blooming" unless hemorrhage present (rare)
- DWI
  - No restriction
- T1WI C+
  - Does not enhance
- MRA
  - Cortical vessels displaced away from calvarium
- MRV
  - Can demonstrate anomalies of venous drainage
- MRS
  - Can predict pathology in > 90% of similar-appearing intracranial cystic lesions

Ultrasonographic Findings
- Grayscale ultrasound
  - Useful for demonstrating sonolucent ACs in infants < 1 year

Angiographic Findings
- MCA, sylvian triangle displaced posteriorly in MCF ACs

Nuclear Medicine Findings
- SPECT
  - May show hypoperfusion in brain adjacent to cyst

Imaging Recommendations
- Best imaging tool
  - MR with FLAIR, DWI
- Protocol advice
  - Consider adding
    - Magnetic resonance cisternography
      - CISS, FIESTA (high-resolution sequences to delineate cyst wall, adjacent anatomic structures)
      - Can help distinguish AC from enlarged subarachnoid space
    - MR CSF flow imaging, quantification
      - 2D cine PC (to look for communication between AC, adjacent subarachnoid space)

DIFFERENTIAL DIAGNOSIS

Epidermoid Cyst
- Scalloped margins
- Insinuating growth pattern
  - Creeps along into CSF cisterns
  - Surrounds, engulfs vessels/nerves
    - ACs displace but usually do not engulf vessels, cranial nerves
- Does not suppress on FLAIR
- Restricted diffusion (bright) on DWI

Chronic Subdural Hematoma
- Signal not identical to CSF
- Often bilateral, lentiform-shaped
- ± enhancing membrane
- Look for foci of "blooming" on T2*
  - < 5% of ACs hemorrhage

Subdural Hygroma
- Often bilateral
- Crescentic or flat configuration

Other Nonneoplastic Cysts
- Porencephalic cyst
  - Surrounded by gliotic brain, not compressed cortex
  - History of trauma, stroke common
- Neurenteric cyst

ARACHNOID CYST

  - Rare; spine, posterior fossa = most common locations
  - Often proteinaceous fluid
- Neuroglial (glioependymal) cyst
  - Rare
  - Usually intraaxial

PATHOLOGY

General Features

- Etiology
  - Old concept = "splitting" or diverticulum of developing arachnoid
  - New concept (middle fossa ACs)
    - Frontal, temporal embryonic meninges (endomeninx) fail to merge as Sylvian fissure forms
    - Remain separate, forming "duplicated" arachnoid
  - Possible mechanisms
    - Active fluid secretion by cyst wall
    - Slow distention by CSF pulsations
    - CSF accumulates by 1-way (ball-valve) flow
  - Rare: ACs may form as shunt complication
- Genetics
  - Usually sporadic, nonsyndromic, rarely familial
  - Inherited disorders of metabolism
    - "Sticky" leptomeninges: Mucopolysaccharidoses
- Associated abnormalities
  - Temporal lobe may appear (or be) hypoplastic (MCF ACs)
  - Subdural hematoma
    - 5% in middle fossa ACs
  - Syndromic ACs
    - Acrocallosal (cysts in 1/3), Aicardi, Pallister-Hall syndromes
  - Periventricular giant ACs may cause hydrocephalus, may be associated with
    - Foramen of Monro stenosis
    - Aqueductal stenosis/occlusion

Staging, Grading, & Classification

- Galassi classification for middle fossa ACs: Increases with ↑ size/mass effect and ↓ communication with basal cisterns
  - Type 1: Small, spindle-shaped; limited to anterior MCF
  - Type 2: Superior extent along Sylvian fissure; temporal lobe displaced
  - Type 3: Huge, fills entire MCF; frontal/temporal/ parietal displacement

Gross Pathologic & Surgical Features

- Fluid-containing cyst with translucent membrane
- Arachnoid layers bulge around, contain CSF collection

Microscopic Features

- Wall consists of flattened but normal arachnoid cells
- No inflammation, neoplastic change

CLINICAL ISSUES

Presentation

- Most common signs/symptoms
  - Often asymptomatic, found incidentally
  - Symptoms vary with size and location of cyst
    - Headache, dizziness, sensorineural hearing loss, hemifacial spasm/tic
    - SSACs may cause obstructive hydrocephalus

Demographics

- Age
  - ACs can be found at any age
  - 75% in children (symptom onset, if any, may be delayed)
- Gender
  - M:F = 3-5:1; especially middle cranial fossa
- Ethnicity
  - None reported
- Epidemiology
  - Most common congenital intracranial cystic abnormality
  - 1% of all intracranial masses
  - 2% incidental finding on imaging for seizure

Natural History & Prognosis

- May (but usually do not) slowly enlarge
- Occasionally decompress spontaneously

Treatment

- Treatment: Often none
- Resection (may be endoscopic)
- Fenestration/marsupialization
- Shunt (cystoperitoneal is common option)

DIAGNOSTIC CHECKLIST

Image Interpretation Pearls

- FLAIR, DWI best sequences for distinguishing etiology of cystic-appearing intracranial masses

SELECTED REFERENCES

1. Rangel-Castilla L et al: Coexistent intraventricular abnormalities in periventricular giant arachnoid cysts. J Neurosurg Pediatr. 3(3):225-31, 2009
2. Russo N et al: Spontaneous reduction of intracranial arachnoid cysts: a complete review. Br J Neurosurg. 22(5):626-9, 2008
3. Tsitsopoulos P et al: Intracranial arachnoid cyst associated with traumatic intracystic hemorrhage and subdural haematoma. Hippokratia. 12(1):53-5, 2008
4. Wester K et al: How often do chronic extra-cerebral haematomas occur in patients with intracranial arachnoid cysts? J Neurol Neurosurg Psychiatry. 79(1):72-5, 2008
5. Awaji M et al: Magnetic resonance cisternography for preoperative evaluation of arachnoid cysts. Neuroradiology. 49(9):721-6, 2007
6. Yildiz H et al: Evaluation of CSF flow patterns of posterior fossa cystic malformations using CSF flow MR imaging. Neuroradiology. 48(9):595-605, 2006

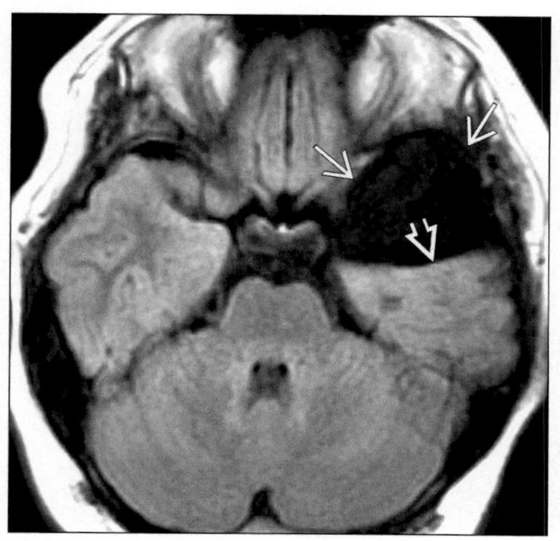

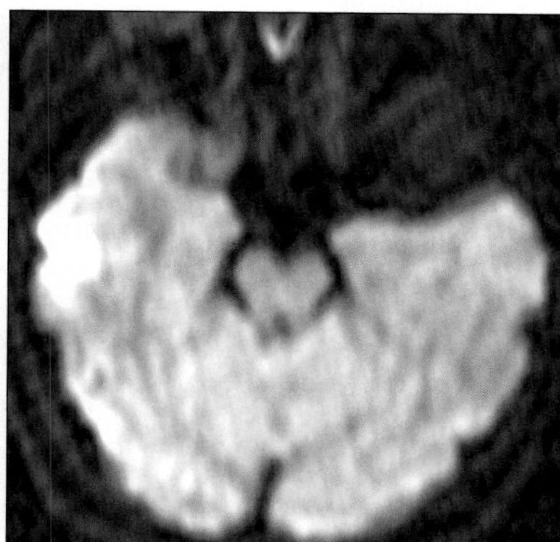

(Left) *Axial FLAIR MR in a 9 year old with seizures shows a large CSF-like mass ➡ that slightly expands the middle cranial fossa and displaces the temporal lobe posteriorly ➡.* ***(Right)*** *Axial DWI MR in the same patient shows that the cystic mass does not restrict. Typical ACs follow CSF on all sequences, suppress completely on FLAIR, and show no restriction on DWI.*

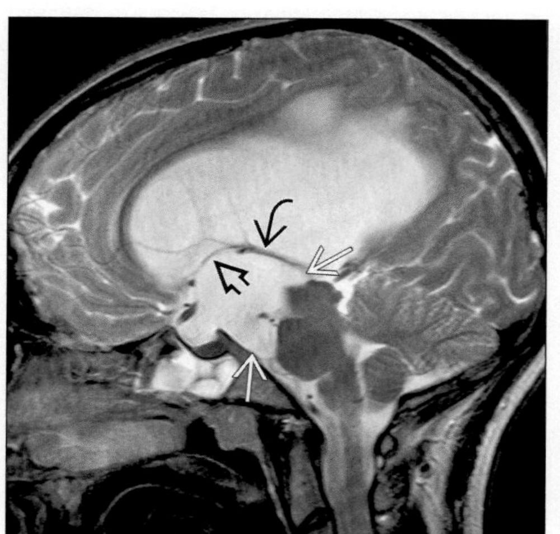

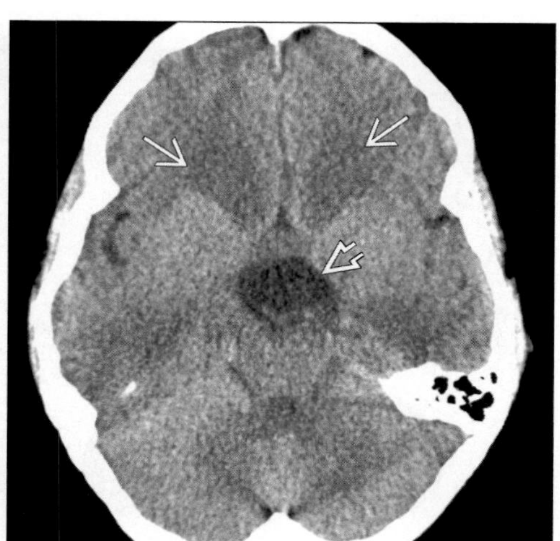

(Left) *Sagittal T2WI FS MR in an 18-year-old female with longstanding headaches shows a large CSF-like suprasellar mass ➡ with obstructive hydrocephalus seen here as an enlarged lateral ventricle flattening the fornix ➡. The floor of the 3rd ventricle ➡ is thinned and elevated over the cyst.* ***(Right)*** *Axial NECT in the same case after instillation of dilute contrast into the lateral ventricles shows moderate opacification ➡. The suprasellar cyst ➡ is unopacified and does not communicate.*

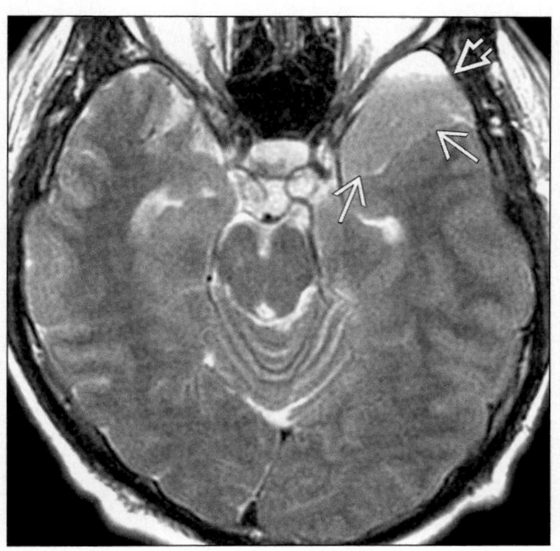

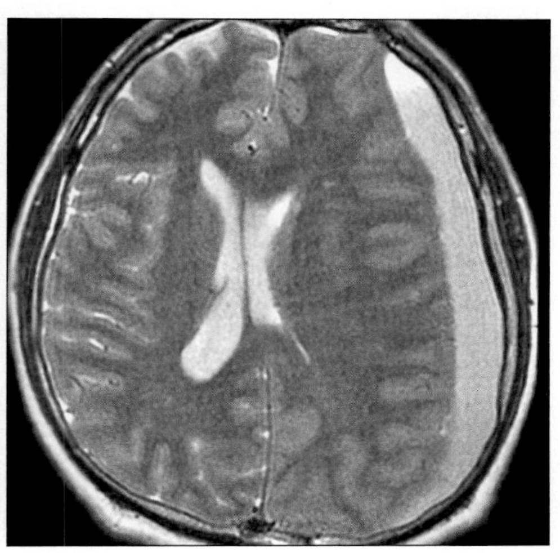

(Left) *A patient with head trauma had a middle fossa arachnoid cyst on initial imaging (not shown). Repeat MR obtained a few days later, after the patient became drowsy & developed progressive right-sided weakness, shows hemorrhage into the cyst ➡. Note fluid-fluid level ➡ between acute blood & the CSF in the AC.* ***(Right)*** *Axial T2WI cephalad image in the same case shows a subdural hematoma that had developed. Patients with ACs are at increased risk for developing SDHs. Intracyst hemorrhage is uncommon.*

COLLOID CYST

Key Facts

Terminology
- Unilocular mucin-containing 3rd ventricular cyst

Imaging
- > 99% are wedged into foramen of Monro
  - Pillars of fornix straddle, drape around cyst
  - Majority are hyperdense on NECT
  - Density correlates inversely with hydration state
- MR signal more variable
  - Generally reflects water content
  - Majority isointense to brain on T2WI (small cysts may be difficult to see)
  - 25% mixed hypo/hyper ("black hole" effect)
  - May show mild rim enhancement (rare)

Top Differential Diagnoses
- Neurocysticercosis
- CSF flow artifact (MR "pseudocyst")
- Vertebrobasilar dolichoectasia (VBD)/aneurysm
- Subependymoma
- Craniopharyngioma

Pathology
- From embryonic endoderm, not neuroectoderm
- Similar to other foregut-derived cysts (neurenteric, Rathke)

Clinical Issues
- 40-50% asymptomatic, discovered incidentally
- Headache (50-60%)
  - Acute foramen of Monro obstruction may lead to rapid onset hydrocephalus, herniation, death
- Peak age = 3rd to 4th decade (rare in children)

Diagnostic Checklist
- Could possible CC be flow artifact?

*(**Left**) Axial graphic shows a classic CC at the foramen of Monro causing mild/moderate obstructive hydrocephalus. Note that the fornices and choroid plexus are elevated and stretched over the cyst ⇨. (**Right**) Axial gross pathology in a patient who suddenly and inexplicably died shows a large colloid cyst ⇨ causing moderate obstructive hydrocephalus. A small cavum septi pellucidi is present. Fornices ➔ are draped over the cyst. (Courtesy R. Hewlett, PhD.)*

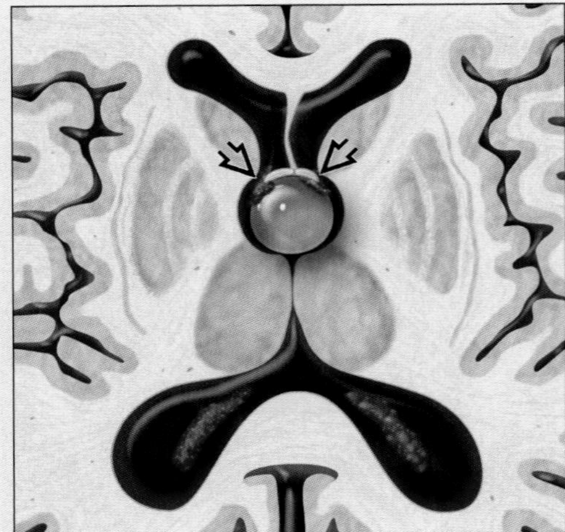

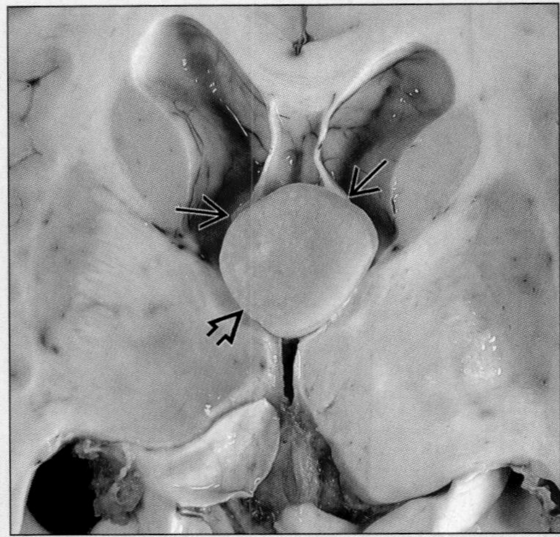

*(**Left**) Axial NECT in a 65-year-old man with "thunderclap" headache, obtained to look for a subarachnoid hemorrhage, shows a classic colloid cyst, seen here as a hyperdense mass ➔ wedged into the foramen of Monro and upper 3rd ventricle. (**Right**) Sagittal T2WI MR in the same case shows the mass ➔ to be very hypodense, indicating inspissated proteinaceous contents. Note the markedly enlarged lateral ventricle with a normal-sized 3rd ventricle. The colloid cyst was removed emergently.*

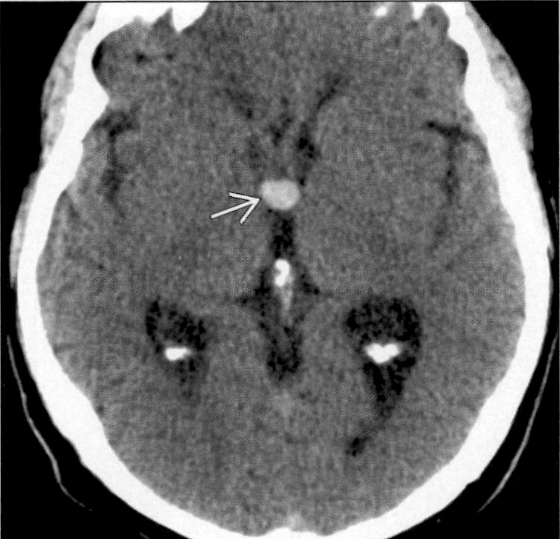

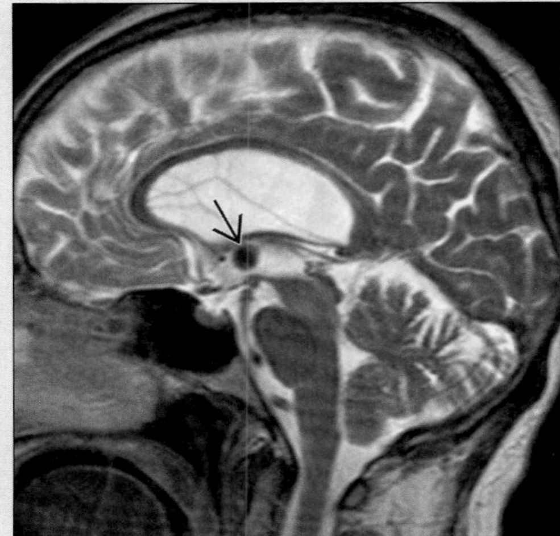

COLLOID CYST

TERMINOLOGY

Abbreviations

- Colloid cyst (CC)

Synonyms

- Paraphyseal cyst, endodermal cyst

Definitions

- Unilocular, mucin-containing 3rd ventricular cyst

IMAGING

General Features

- Best diagnostic clue
  - Hyperdense foramen of Monro mass on NECT
- Location
  - > 99% are wedged into foramen of Monro
    - Attached to anterosuperior 3rd ventricular roof
    - Pillars of fornix straddle, drape around cyst
    - Posterior part of frontal horns splayed laterally around cyst
  - < 1% found at other sites
    - Lateral, 4th ventricles
    - Extraventricular CCs (very rare)
      - Parenchyma (cerebellum)
      - Extraaxial (prepontine, meninges, olfactory groove)
- Size
  - Variable (few mm to 3 cm)
  - Mean: 15 mm
- Morphology
  - Well-demarcated round > ovoid/lobulated mass

CT Findings

- NECT
  - Density correlates inversely with hydration state
    - 2/3 hyperdense
    - 1/3 iso-/hypodense
  - ± hydrocephalus
  - Rare
    - Hypodense
    - Change in density/size
    - Hemorrhage (cyst "apoplexy"), Ca++
- CECT
  - Usually does not enhance
  - Rim enhancement (rare)

MR Findings

- T1WI
  - Signal correlates with cholesterol concentration
    - 2/3 hyperintense on T1WI
    - 1/3 isointense
      - Small CCs may be difficult to see
  - May have associated ventriculomegaly
- T2WI
  - Signal more variable
    - Generally reflects water content
    - Majority isointense to brain on T2WI
      - Small CCs may be difficult to see
  - Less common findings
    - 25% mixed hypo/hyper ("black hole" effect)
    - Fluid-fluid level
- FLAIR
  - Does not suppress
- DWI
  - Does not restrict
- T1WI C+
  - Usually no enhancement
  - Rare: May show peripheral (rim) enhancement
- MRS
  - Normal brain metabolites absent

Imaging Recommendations

- Protocol advice
  - NECT + contrast-enhanced MR
  - ± serial imaging for asymptomatic cysts < 1 cm, no hydrocephalus

DIFFERENTIAL DIAGNOSIS

Neurocysticercosis

- Multiple lesions within parenchyma and cisterns
- Associated ependymitis or basilar meningitis common
- Ca++ common
- Look for scolex

CSF Flow Artifact (MR "Pseudocyst")

- Multiplanar technique confirms artifact
- Look for phase artifact

Vertebrobasilar Dolichoectasia (VBD)/ Aneurysm

- Extreme VBD can cause hyperdense foramen of Monro mass
- Look for flow void, phase artifact on MR

Neoplasm

- Subependymoma
  - Frontal horn of lateral ventricle
  - Attached to septum pellucidum
  - Patchy/solid enhancement
- Craniopharyngioma
  - 3rd ventricle rare location
  - Usually not wedged into foramen of Monro, fornix
  - Ca++, rim/nodular enhancement common
- Pituitary adenoma
  - Rare in 3rd ventricle
  - Enhances (usually strongly, uniformly)

Choroid Plexus Mass

- Choroid plexus papilloma
  - Rare in 3rd ventricle
  - Tumor of early childhood
- Xanthogranuloma
  - Rare in 3rd ventricle
  - Ovoid > round
  - Can be hyper- or hypodense ± Ca++
  - Can obstruct foramen of Monro
  - Can be indistinguishable on imaging studies
- Choroid plexus cyst
  - Usually found in infants
  - Anechoic at ultrasound

COLLOID CYST

PATHOLOGY

General Features

- Etiology
  - From embryonic endoderm, not neuroectoderm
    - Similar to other foregut-derived cysts (neurenteric, Rathke)
    - Ectopic endodermal elements migrate into embryonic diencephalic roof
  - Contents accumulate from mucinous secretions, desquamated epithelial cells
- Genetics
  - None known
- Associated abnormalities
  - Variable hydrocephalus

Gross Pathologic & Surgical Features

- Smooth, spherical/ovoid well-delineated cyst
  - Thick gelatinous center, variable viscosity (mucinous or desiccated)
  - Rare = evidence for recent/remote hemorrhage
- Gross appearance, location virtually pathognomonic

Microscopic Features

- Outer wall = thin fibrous capsule
- Inner lining
  - Simple or pseudostratified epithelium
  - Interspersed goblet cells, scattered ciliated cells
  - Rests on thin connective tissue layer
- Cyst contents
  - PAS + gelatinous ("colloid") material
  - Variable viscosity
  - ± necrotic leukocytes, cholesterol clefts
- Immunohistochemistry
  - ± epithelial antigen reactivity (cytokeratins, EMA)
  - Neuroepithelial markers negative
- Electron microscopy
  - Resembles mature respiratory epithelium
  - Nonciliated or tall columnar cells
  - Basal cells contain dense core vesicles

CLINICAL ISSUES

Presentation

- Most common signs/symptoms
  - Headache (50-60%)
  - Less common = nausea, vomiting, memory loss, altered personality, gait disturbance, visual changes
  - Acute foramen of Monro obstruction may lead to rapid onset hydrocephalus, herniation, death
  - 40-50% asymptomatic, discovered incidentally
    - 3-, 5-, and 10-year incidence of developing cyst-related symptoms = 0, 0, and 8%, respectively
- Clinical profile
  - Adult with headache

Demographics

- Age
  - 3rd to 4th decade
    - Peak: 40
    - Rare in children (only 8% < 15 at diagnosis)
- Gender
  - M = F
- Epidemiology
  - 0.5-1.0% primary brain tumors
  - 15-20% intraventricular masses
  - Few familial cases reported

Natural History & Prognosis

- Varies with presence/rate of growth, development of CSF obstruction
- 90% stable or stop enlarging
  - Older age
  - Small cyst
  - No hydrocephalus
  - Hyperdense on NECT, hypointense on T2-weighted MR
- 10% enlarge
  - Younger patients
  - Larger cyst, hydrocephalus
  - Iso-/hypodense on NECT, often hyperintense on T2WI
  - May enlarge rapidly, cause coma/death
- Prognosis excellent when CCs diagnosed early and excised

Treatment

- Most common = complete surgical resection
  - Neuronavigation-guided endoscopic approach increasingly common
  - 50% experience short-term memory disturbance (usually resolves)
  - Recurrence rare if resection complete
- Options
  - Precoronal, paramedian minicraniotomy
  - Stereotactic aspiration (difficult with extremely viscous/solid cysts)
  - Imaging features that may predict difficulty with percutaneous therapy
    - Hyperdensity on CT/hypointensity on T2WI suggest high viscosity
  - Ventricular shunting
  - Observation (rare; not recommended as sudden obstruction can occur with even small CCs)

DIAGNOSTIC CHECKLIST

Consider

- Consider CT or MR in patient with longstanding history of intermittent headaches
- Notify referring MD immediately if CC identified (especially if hydrocephalus is present)

Image Interpretation Pearls

- Could possible CC be flow artifact?

SELECTED REFERENCES

1. Demirci S et al: Sudden death due to a colloid cyst of the third ventricle: report of three cases with a special sign at autopsy. Forensic Sci Int. 189(1-3):e33-6, 2009
2. Majós C et al: In vivo proton magnetic resonance spectroscopy of intraventricular tumours of the brain. Eur Radiol. 19(8):2049-59, 2009

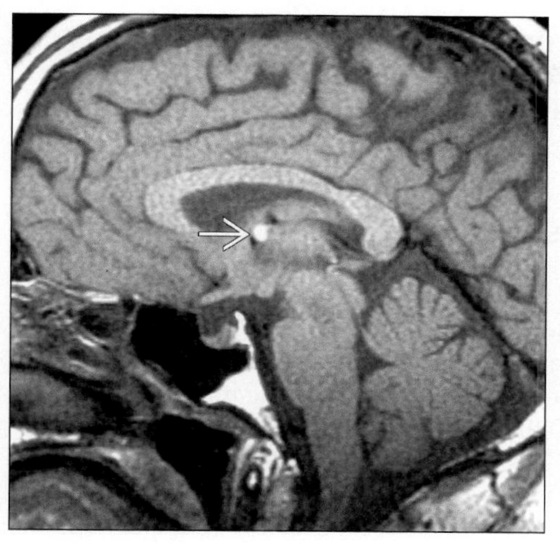

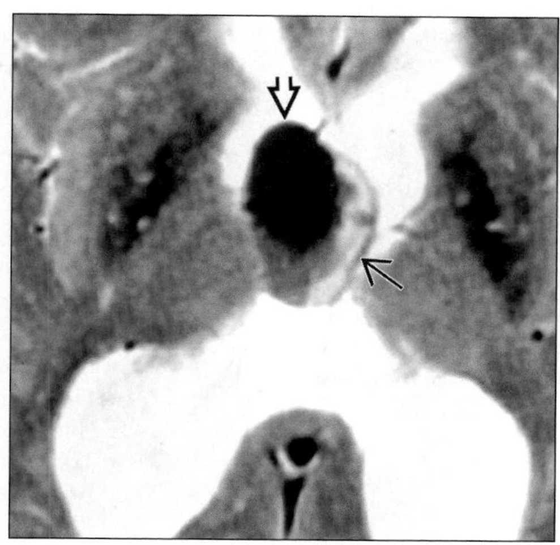

(Left) *Sagittal T1WI MR shows a tiny colloid cyst ➔ discovered incidentally in this asymptomatic patient.* ***(Right)*** *Axial T2WI MR in a patient with a large colloid cyst shows the "black hole" effect ➔, a focus of profound hypointensity within the larger lesion ➔ caused by inspissated, dessicated proteinaceous contents. These cysts are difficult to aspirate and generally must be surgically removed.*

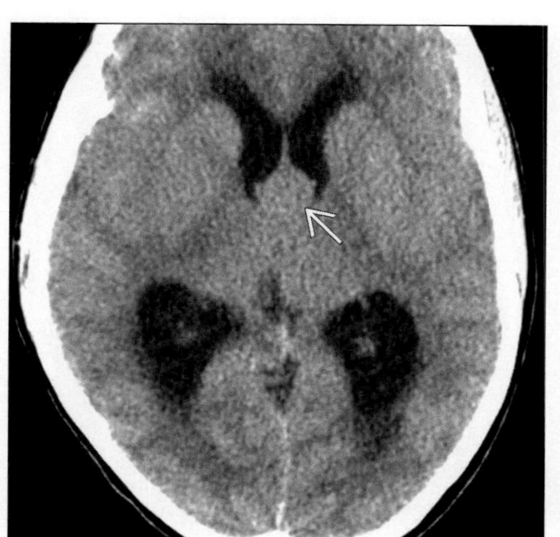

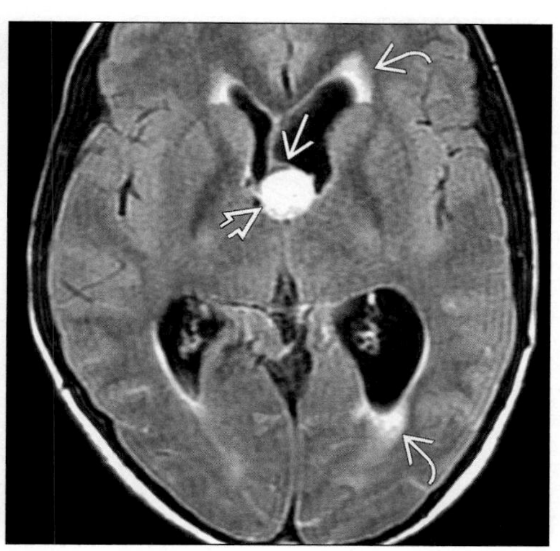

(Left) *Axial NECT in a 16-year-old boy, who presented in the ER with severe headaches and papilledema, shows severe obstructive hydrocephalus with dilated lateral ventricles & complete effacement of all superficial sulci. An isodense mass ➔ is present at the foramen of Monro.* ***(Right)*** *Axial FLAIR MR in the same patient shows the lesion ➔ to be very hyperintense & straddled by the fornix ➔. Ventricles are dilated and transependymal CSF flow ➔ is present. The colloid cyst was removed at surgery.*

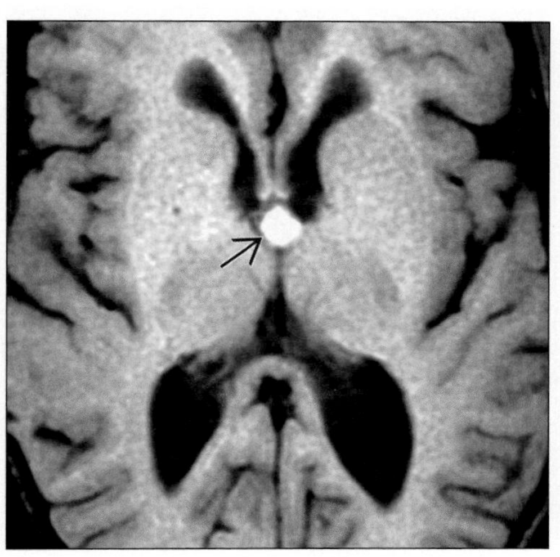

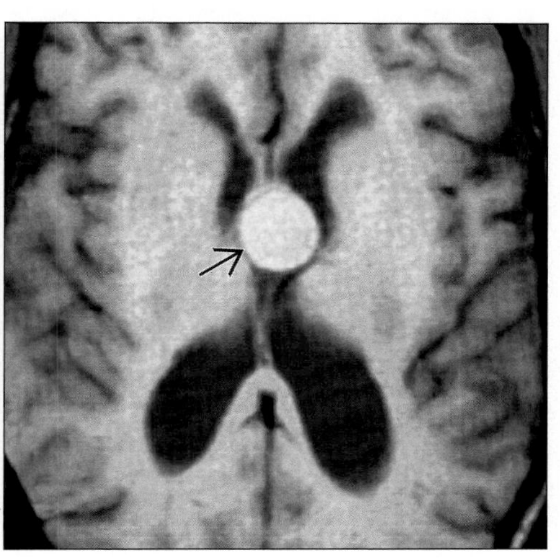

(Left) *Axial T1WI MR in this patient with only mild headaches shows a small CC ➔ at the foramen of Monro. The patient declined surgery. Occasionally colloid cysts may increase in size over a relatively short period of time.* ***(Right)*** *Axial T1WI MR in the same case, performed after the patient developed sudden, dramatic increase in headaches a few months later. The cyst ➔ enlarged & is now causing moderate obstructive hydrocephalus. A classic colloid cyst without evidence for hemorrhage was found.*

DERMOID CYST

Key Facts

Terminology

- Benign, ectopic, squamous epithelial cyst containing dermal elements, including hair follicles, sebaceous and sweat glands

Imaging

- Midline unilocular cystic lesion with fat
  - Subarachnoid fatty droplets if ruptured
- Suprasellar or posterior fossa most common intracranial sites
- Extracranial sites = spine, orbit
  - May have fistulous connections to skin (dermal sinus tract)
- CT hypodensity and negative Hounsfield units (fat)
  - 20% capsular Ca++
- MR: T1 hyperintense
  - Fat-suppression sequence confirms lipid elements
  - Fat-fluid level in cyst and in ventricles (if ruptured)
- With rupture: Extensive leptomeningeal enhancement possible from chemical meningitis

Top Differential Diagnoses

- Epidermoid cyst
- Craniopharyngioma
- Teratoma
- Lipoma

Clinical Issues

- Rare: < 0.5% of primary intracranial tumors
- Intradural dermoid cysts 4-9x less common than epidermoid cysts
- Rupture can cause significant morbidity/mortality
- Dermoid + dermal sinus may cause meningitis, hydrocephalus
- Treatment: Complete surgical excision ± shunt for hydrocephalus

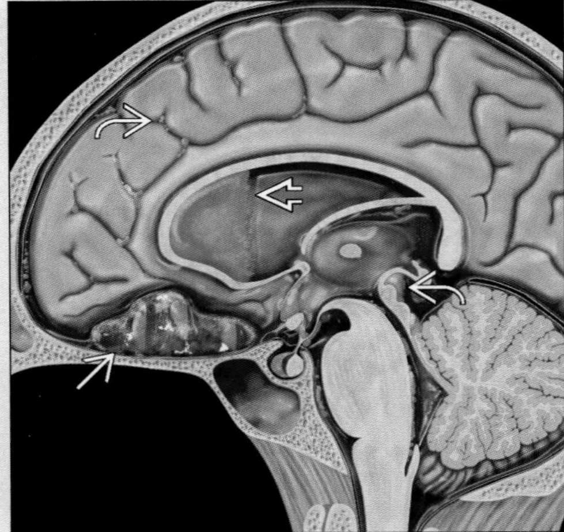

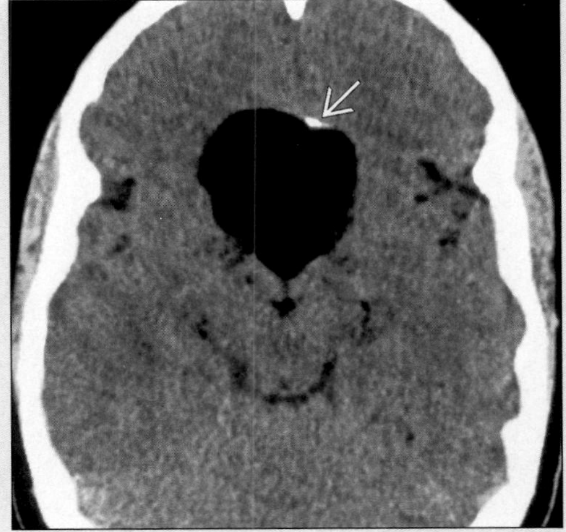

(Left) *Sagittal graphic of an inferior frontal dermoid ➔ shows a discrete, heterogeneous fat-containing mass with squamous epithelium and dermal appendages. There is a ventricular fat-fluid level ➔ and fat within the subarachnoid spaces ➔ related to the rupture.* ***(Right)*** *Axial NECT shows a midline fatty mass with focal calcification ➔. Dermoid cysts are typically midline in the sellar, parasellar, and frontonasal region, with only 20% having capsular calcification.*

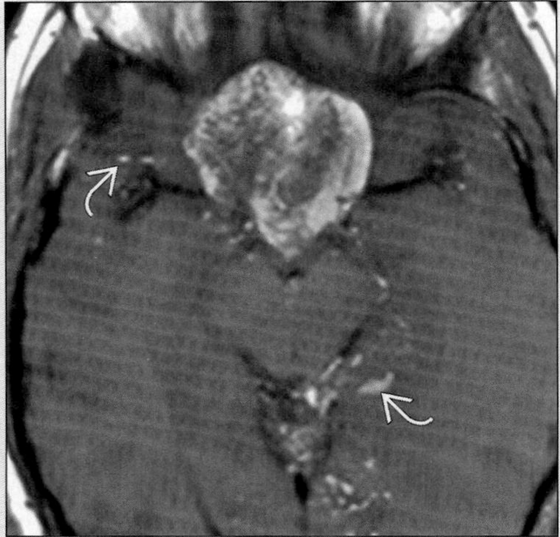

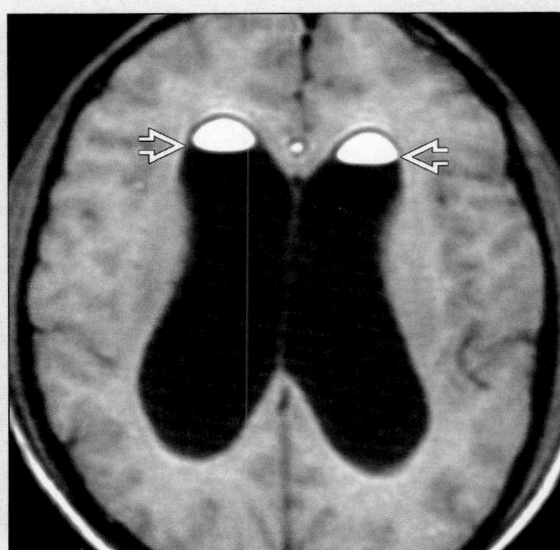

(Left) *Axial T1WI MR shows a heterogeneously hyperintense mass with scattered hyperintense fat droplets throughout the subarachnoid space ➔, indicating rupture of the dermoid cyst. Fat droplets in the cisterns, sulci, and ventricles are pathognomonic for a ruptured dermoid cyst. Chemical meningitis and hydrocephalus may be associated with cyst rupture.* ***(Right)*** *Axial T1 MR shows a fat-fluid level ➔ in the lateral ventricles related to a ruptured dermoid cyst obstructing the 3rd ventricle.*

DERMOID CYST

TERMINOLOGY

Synonyms

- Dermoid inclusion cyst, ectodermal inclusion cyst

Definitions

- Benign, ectopic, squamous epithelial cyst containing dermal elements, including hair follicles, sebaceous and sweat glands

IMAGING

General Features

- Best diagnostic clue
  - Midline nonenhancing unilocular cystic lesion with fat
    - Subarachnoid fatty droplets if ruptured
- Location
  - Suprasellar, parasellar
  - Less common is posterior fossa: Cisterna magna, 4th ventricle, and basal cisterns
  - Extracranial sites = spine, orbit
    - May have fistulous connections to skin (dermal sinus tract)
    - Orbit: Dermolipoma at zygomatico-frontal suture
  - Ruptured: Subarachnoid/intraventricular spread of contents
- Size
  - Variable
- Morphology
  - Well-circumscribed, lipid-containing mass

CT Findings

- NECT
  - Round/lobulated, well-delineated, unilocular cystic mass
  - Hypodensity and negative Hounsfield units from fat
  - Capsular Ca++ (20%)
  - With rupture, droplets of fat disseminate in cisterns, may cause fat-fluid level within ventricles
  - Skull/scalp dermoid expands diploe
  - Frontonasal dermoid sinus tract: Bifid crista galli, large foramen cecum + sinus tract
  - Rare "dense" dermoid: Hyperattenuating on CT
- CECT
  - Generally no enhancement

MR Findings

- T1WI
  - Unruptured: Hyperintense on
  - Ruptured: Droplets very hyperintense
    - Fat-suppression sequence confirms lipid elements
    - Fat-fluid level in cyst; if ruptured, in ventricles as well
  - Rare "dense" dermoid: Very hyperintense
- T2WI
  - Unruptured: Heterogeneous, hypo- to hyperintense
    - Chemical shift artifact in frequency encoding direction with long TR
  - Ruptured: Typically hyperintense droplets
  - Rare "dense" dermoid: Very hypointense
  - With hair: Fine curvilinear hypointense elements
- T1WI C+
  - ± mild enhancement of capsule without central enhancement
  - With rupture: Extensive leptomeningeal enhancement possible from chemical meningitis
- MRS
  - Elevated lipid peak from 0.9-1.3 ppm

Angiographic Findings

- Vasospasm with chemical meningitis from rupture
  - May relieve vasospasm with angioplasty
- Dermoid-encased vessels may have ↑ rupture risk

Imaging Recommendations

- Best imaging tool
  - MR with fat saturation
- Protocol advice
  - Use fat-suppression sequence to confirm diagnosis
  - Chemical shift-selective sequence useful to detect tiny droplets

DIFFERENTIAL DIAGNOSIS

Epidermoid Cyst

- Most epidermoid cysts resemble CSF, no fat
- Restricted diffusion on DWI classic
- Cyst lined with squamous epithelium without dermal elements
- 4-9x more common than dermoid
- Off-midline > midline: In CPA (40-50%), parasellar/middle fossa (10-15%), diploic (10%)

Craniopharyngioma

- Also suprasellar/midline, often with intrasellar component
- CT: Multilocular with solid enhancing tissue (> 90%), nodular Ca++ in majority
- MR: Commonly T1WI hypointense, T2WI hyperintense, enhances strongly
- More common than dermoid (3-5% of primary intracranial tumors)

Teratoma

- Location similar but usually pineal region
- 90% have all 3 embryologic layers: Ectoderm, mesoderm, endoderm
- Often multicystic/multiloculated
- Heterogeneous appearance containing calcification, CSF, lipid, and soft tissue components
- Does not have fat fluid level

Lipoma

- Homogeneous midline fat
- Dermoids more likely heterogeneous
- Ca++ less frequent than in dermoid

PATHOLOGY

General Features

- Etiology
  - Embryology (2 theories)
    - Sequestration of surface ectoderm at lines of epithelial fusion/along course of normal embryonic invaginations

DERMOID CYST

- Inclusion of cutaneous ectoderm at time of neural tube closure; 3rd to 5th week of embryogenesis
  - Can also arise at any age from traumatic implantation (i.e., lumbar puncture)
  - Similar etiology with epidermoid, which is thought to be later in development and off midline
- Genetics
  - Usually sporadic
  - Association with Goldenhar syndrome
  - Possible association with Klippel-Feil syndrome
- Associated abnormalities
  - Occipital/nasofrontal dermal sinus may be present; 89% of dermal sinuses associated with inclusion cysts
  - Goldenhar syndrome (a.k.a. oculoauriculovertebral dysplasia); congenital condition includes
    - Cranial lipomas and dermoids
    - Ocular dermoids
    - Anomalies of 1st and 2nd branchial arch derivatives
    - Cardiovascular, facial, oral, auricular, visceral, and spinal defects

Gross Pathologic & Surgical Features

- Unilocular cyst with thick wall
- Contents = lipid and cholesterol elements from sebaceous secretions floating on proteinaceous material

Microscopic Features

- Outer wall of squamous epithelium
- Inner lining contains dermal elements of hair follicles, sebaceous and apocrine glands
- Rare squamous cell carcinoma (SCCa) degeneration
  - Squamous cell predominance with some glandular differentiation
  - Suggestive of poorly differentiated squamous cell carcinoma with adenomatous component

CLINICAL ISSUES

Presentation

- Most common signs/symptoms
  - Uncomplicated dermoid: Headache (32%), seizure (30%) are most common symptoms
    - Large cyst can cause obstructive hydrocephalus
    - Less commonly hypopituitarism, diabetes insipidus, or cranial nerve (CN) defects
    - Suprasellar may present with visual symptoms
  - Cyst rupture causes chemical meningitis (6.9%)

Demographics

- Age
  - 2nd to 3rd decade
- Gender
  - Slight male predilection
- Epidemiology
  - Rare: < 0.5% of primary intracranial tumors
  - Intradural dermoid cysts 4-9x less common than epidermoid cysts

Natural History & Prognosis

- Benign, slow growing
- Larger lesions associated with higher rupture rate
- Rupture can cause significant morbidity/mortality
  - Relatively rare and typically spontaneous
  - Seizure, coma, vasospasm, infarction, death
- Dermoid + dermal sinus may cause meningitis, hydrocephalus
- Rare malignant transformation into SCCa
  - Postulated prolonged or reparative process from foreign material leads to cellular atypia and neoplasia
  - May occur years after surgical resection

Treatment

- Treatment: Complete surgical excision
  - Residual capsule may lead to recurrence
  - Rare SCCa degeneration within surgical remnants
- Subarachnoid dissemination of contents may occur during operative/postoperative course
  - Cause aseptic meningitis or other complications (hydrocephalus, seizures, CN deficits)
    - May require shunt placement for hydrocephalus
  - Alternatively, disseminated fat particles can remain silent without radiological/neurological change
    - Justifies "wait-and-see" approach
    - Regular MR and clinical exams are necessary to avoid complications

DIAGNOSTIC CHECKLIST

Image Interpretation Pearls

- Follows fat characteristics on NECT and T1WI fat-suppressed MR

SELECTED REFERENCES

1. Turgut M: Klippel-Feil syndrome in association with posterior fossa dermoid tumour. Acta Neurochir (Wien). 151(3):269-76, 2009
2. Liu JK et al: Ruptured intracranial dermoid cysts: clinical, radiographic, and surgical features. Neurosurgery. 62(2):377-84; discussion 384, 2008
3. Orakcioglu B et al: Intracranial dermoid cysts: variations of radiological and clinical features. Acta Neurochir (Wien). 150(12):1227-34; discussion 1234, 2008
4. Ecker RD et al: Delayed ischemic deficit after resection of a large intracranial dermoid: case report and review of the literature. Neurosurgery. 52(3):706-10; discussion 709-10, 2003
5. Manfre L et al: Absence of the common crus in Goldenhar syndrome. AJNR Am J Neuroradiol. 18(4):773-5, 1997
6. Higashi S et al: Occipital dermal sinus associated with dermoid cyst in the fourth ventricle. AJNR Am J Neuroradiol. 16(4 Suppl):945-8, 1995
7. Nishio S et al: Primary intracranial squamous cell carcinomas: report of two cases. Neurosurgery. 37(2):329-32, 1995
8. Poptani H et al: Characterization of intracranial mass lesions with in vivo proton MR spectroscopy. AJNR Am J Neuroradiol. 16(8):1593-603, 1995
9. Smirniotopoulos JG et al: Teratomas, dermoids, and epidermoids of the head and neck. Radiographics. 15(6):1437-55, 1995

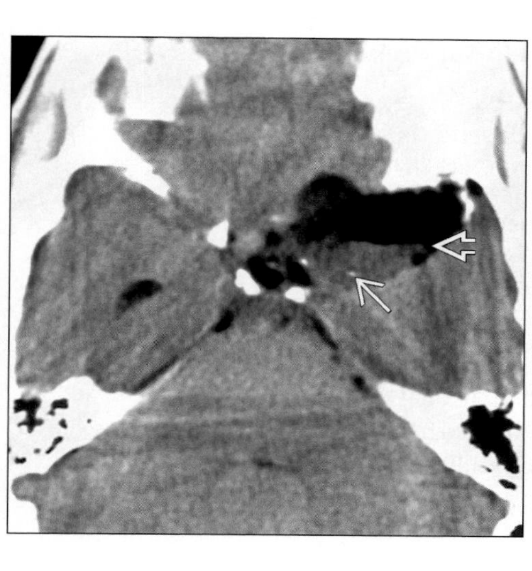

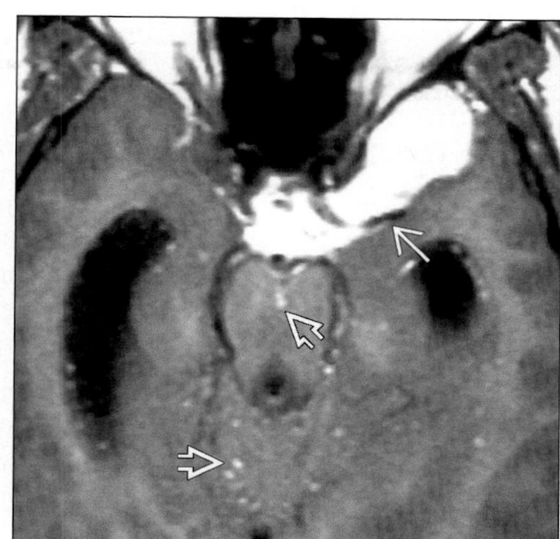

(Left) *Axial NECT shows a large, heterogeneous fatty mass in the left parasellar region. Note the typical fat-fluid level ➪ within the dermoid cyst and minimal calcification ➡.* ***(Right)*** *Axial T1WI MR in the same patient shows a hyperintense mass ➡ with scattered foci of hyperintensity throughout the subarachnoid space ➪. Chemical meningitis from a ruptured dermoid, while uncommon, can cause significant morbidity from seizures, vasospasm, infarction, and even death.*

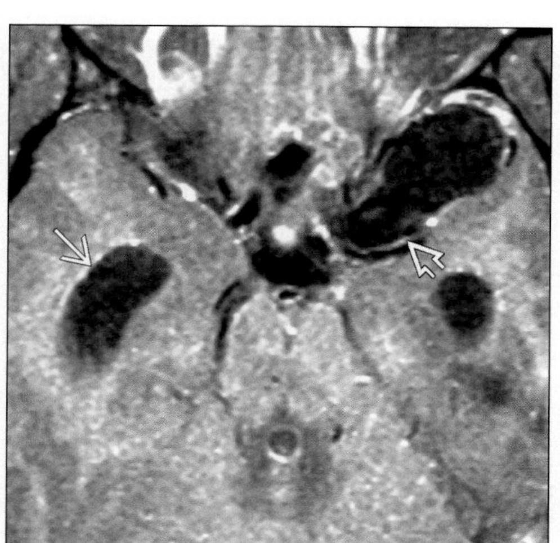

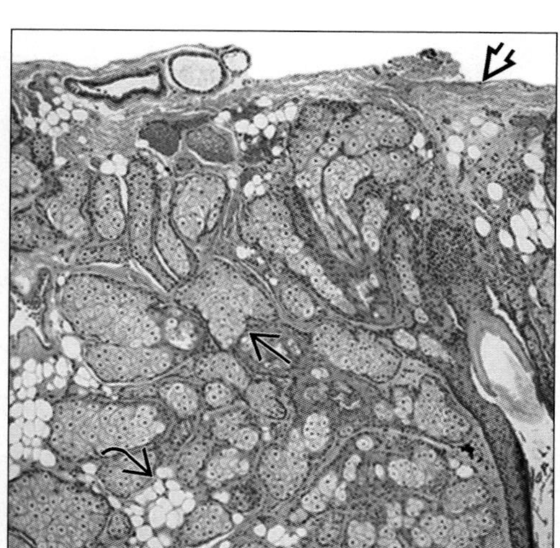

(Left) *Axial T1WI C+ FS MR in the same patient shows complete suppression of the fatty mass with minimal capsular enhancement ➪. The severe communicating hydrocephalus is caused by a chemical meningitis ➡. Patients with a ruptured dermoid are typically treated with resection of the cyst and ventricular decompression.* ***(Right)*** *High-power micropathology shows typical dermoid cyst features with keratin lining ➪, multiple sebaceous glands ➡, and fat ➡.*

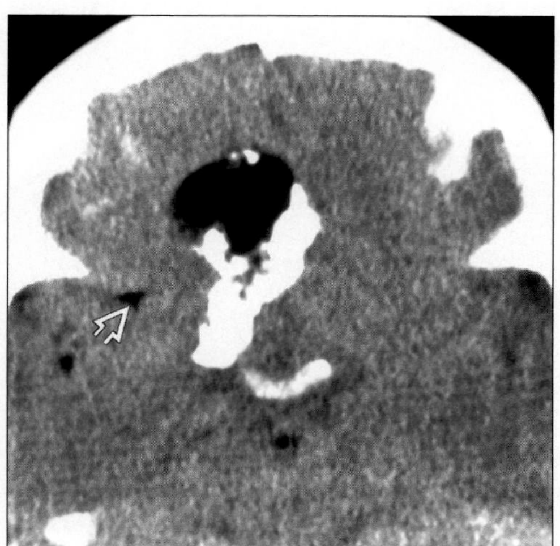

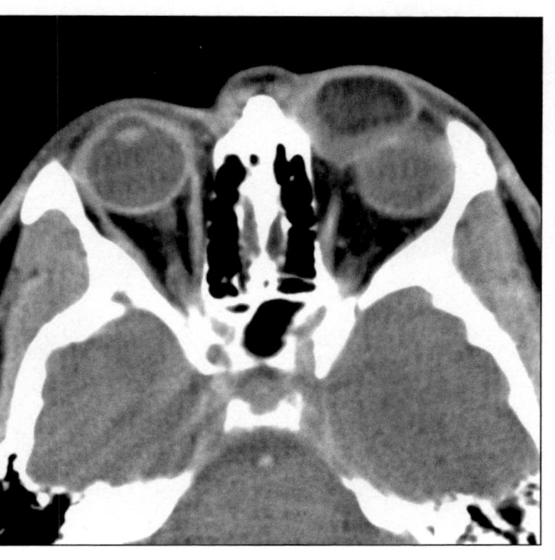

(Left) *Axial NECT shows a large mixed fatty and calcified suprasellar and subfrontal mass. Low-density "fat droplets" ➪ are seen in the adjacent sylvian fissure, related to dermoid rupture. Headaches and seizures are the most common presenting features of these cysts. Rupture may cause a chemical meningitis.* ***(Right)*** *Axial CECT shows a fat-containing orbital mass in a young adult. Dermoids of the orbit are most commonly "dermolipomas" and are associated with the zygomatico-frontal suture.*

EPIDERMOID CYST

Key Facts

Terminology
- Intracranial epidermoids: Congenital inclusion cysts

Imaging
- CSF-like mass that insinuates cisterns and encases neurovascular structures
- Morphology: Lobulated, irregular, cauliflower-like mass with "fronds"
- FLAIR: Usually does not completely null
- DWI: Diffusion hyperintensity definitively distinguishes from arachnoid cyst

Top Differential Diagnoses
- Arachnoid cyst
- Inflammatory cyst (i.e., neurocysticercosis)
- Cystic neoplasm
- Dermoid cyst

Pathology
- Arise from ectodermal inclusions during neural tube closure, 3rd to 5th week embryogenesis

Clinical Issues
- Symptoms depend on location and affect on adjacent neurovascular structures
  - Most common symptom: Headache
  - Cranial nerve 5, 7, 8 neuropathy common
- 0.2-1.8% of all primary intracranial tumors
- Rare malignant degeneration into squamous cell Ca
- Treatment: Microsurgical resection
  - Recurrence common if incompletely removed

Diagnostic Checklist
- Insinuates and surrounds rather than displaces
- Incomplete nulling on FLAIR; DWI hyperintense

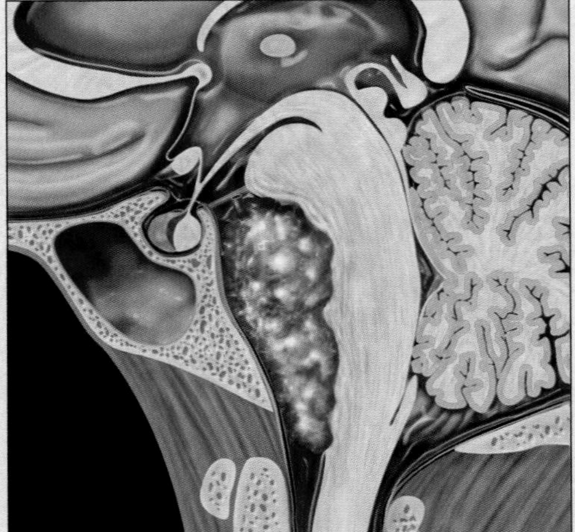

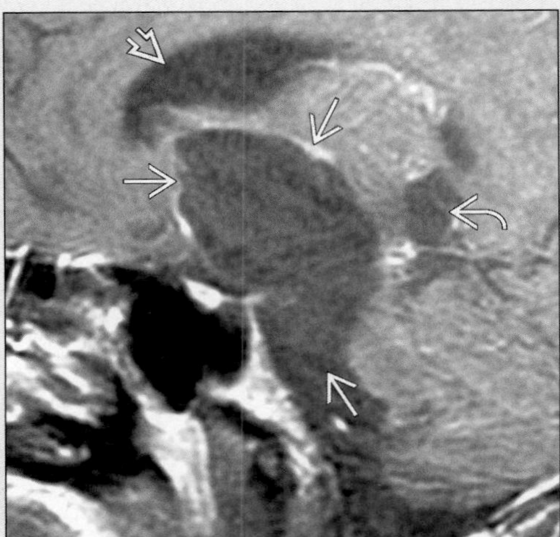

(Left) *Sagittal graphic illustrates a multilobulated epidermoid, primarily within the prepontine cistern. Significant mass effect displaces the pons, cervicomedullary junction, and upper cervical spine.* ***(Right)*** *Sagittal T1WI C+ MR shows a nonenhancing epidermoid ➔ arising from the prepontine cistern with extensive mass effect upon the pons, midbrain, and hypothalamus. Its intensity is slightly greater than normal CSF ⇨, and it has insinuated itself around the pons into the ambient cistern ↪.*

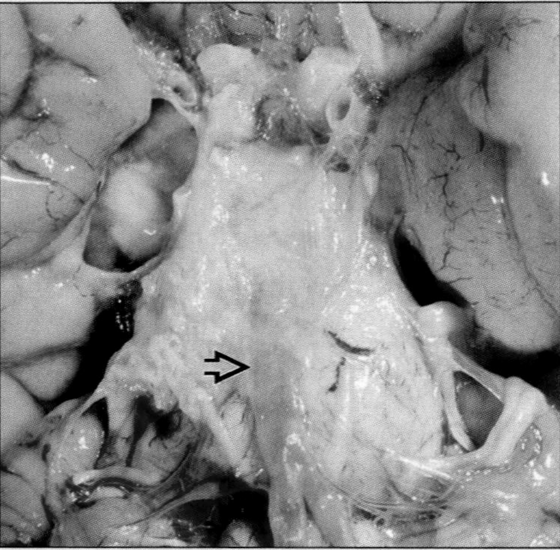

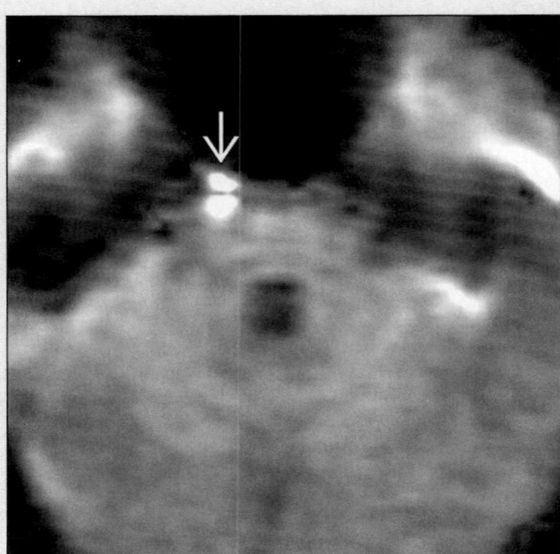

(Left) *Gross pathology shows an epidermoid cyst extending anterosuperiorly from the CPA cistern, insinuating within the prepontine cistern and encasing the basilar artery ⇨. Note its typical "pearly" appearance. (Courtesy E. Hedley-Whyte, MD.)* ***(Right)*** *Axial DWI MR following epidermoid resection reveals a very small focus of residual tumor ➔ that was not visible on other sequences. DWI may play a more important role postoperatively when assessing for small foci of residual tumor.*

EPIDERMOID CYST

TERMINOLOGY

Synonyms

- Ectodermal inclusion cyst

Definitions

- Intracranial epidermoids: Congenital inclusion cysts

IMAGING

General Features

- Best diagnostic clue
  - CSF-like mass that insinuates cisterns and encases neurovascular structures
- Location
  - Intradural (90%), primarily in basal cisterns
    - Cerebellopontine angle (CPA) (40-50%)
    - 4th ventricle (17%)
    - Parasellar/middle cranial fossa (10-15%)
    - Cerebral hemispheres (rare) (1.5%)
    - Brain stem location exceedingly rare
    - Intraventricular within tela choroidea of temporal horn, 3rd or 4th ventricles
  - Extradural (10%): Skull (intradiploic within frontal, parietal, occipital, sphenoid skull) as well as spine
- Morphology
  - Lobulated, irregular, cauliflower-like mass with "fronds"
  - Insinuates without mass effect unless large

Radiographic Findings

- Radiography
  - Diploic space epidermoids
    - May alter scalp, outer/inner skull tables, and epidural space appearance
    - Typically round or lobulated
    - Well delineated with sclerotic rim

CT Findings

- NECT
  - Round/lobulated mass
  - > 95% hypodense, resembling CSF
  - 10-25% contain calcifications
  - Rare variant = "dense" epidermoid
    - 3% of intracranial epidermoids
    - Secondary to hemorrhage, high protein, saponification of cyst debris to calcium soaps or iron-containing pigment
- CECT
  - Usually none, though margin of cyst may show minimal enhancement
- Bone CT
  - May have bony erosion; sharply corticated margins when intradiploic

MR Findings

- T1WI
  - Often (~ 75%) slightly hyperintense to CSF
  - Lobulated periphery may be slightly more hyperintense than center
  - Uncommonly hyperintense to brain ("white epidermoid") due to high triglycerides and unsaturated fatty acids
  - Uncommonly hypointense to CSF ("black epidermoid")
    - Presence of solid crystal cholesterol & keratin
    - Lack of triglycerides & unsaturated fatty acids
- T2WI
  - Often isointense (65%) to slightly hyperintense (35%) to CSF
  - Very rarely hypointense due to calcification, ↓ hydration, viscous secretions, & iron pigments
- FLAIR
  - Usually does not completely null
- DWI
  - Characteristic hyperintensity
    - High fractional anisotropy due to diffusion along 2D geometric plane
      - Attributed to microstructure of parallel-layered keratin filaments and flakes
    - In comparison to white matter, which also shows high fractional anisotropy, due to diffusion along single direction
  - ADC = brain parenchyma
- T1WI C+
  - Usually none, though margin of cyst may show minimal enhancement (25%)
  - Enhancing tumor is sign of malignant degeneration
- MRS
  - Resonances from lactate
  - No NAA, choline, or lipid

Angiographic Findings

- Conventional
  - Depending on location and size, may show avascular mass effect

Nonvascular Interventions

- Myelography
  - Cisternography contrast delineates irregular lobulated tumor borders, extends into interstices

Imaging Recommendations

- Best imaging tool
  - MR
- Protocol advice
  - FLAIR will often distinguish whereas conventional sequences may not
  - Diffusion hyperintensity definitively distinguishes from arachnoid cyst

DIFFERENTIAL DIAGNOSIS

Arachnoid Cyst

- Usually isointense to CSF on all standard sequences
  - Completely nulls on FLAIR
  - Hypointense diffusion: Contains highly mobile CSF, ADC = stationary water
- Rather than insinuate and engulf local structures, arachnoid cysts displace them
- Smooth surface, unlike lobulations of epidermoids

Inflammatory Cyst

- i.e., neurocysticercosis
- Often enhances
- Density/signal intensity usually not precisely like CSF

- Adjacent edema, gliosis common

Cystic Neoplasm
- Attenuation/signal intensity not that of CSF
- Often enhances

Dermoid Cyst
- Usually at or near midline
- Resembles fat, not CSF, and contains dermal appendages; often ruptured

PATHOLOGY

General Features
- Etiology
  - Congenital: Embryology
    - Arise from ectodermal inclusions during neural tube closure, 3rd to 5th week embryogenesis
    - Congenital intradural CPA epidermoids derived from cells of 1st branchial groove
  - Acquired: Develop as result of trauma
    - Uncommon etiology for intracranial tumors
    - More common as spine etiology following LP
- Genetics
  - Sporadic
- Associated abnormalities
  - May have occipital/nasofrontal dermal sinus tract

Gross Pathologic & Surgical Features
- Outer surface often has shiny, glistening "mother of pearl" appearance ("beautiful tumor")
- Soft and pliable, conforms to shape of adjacent local structures/spaces
- Lobulated excrescences, may invaginate into brain
- Insinuating growth pattern, extends through cisterns, surrounds and encases vessels/nerves
- Cyst filled with soft, waxy, creamy, or flaky material

Microscopic Features
- Cyst wall = internal layer of simple stratified cuboidal squamous epithelium covered by fibrous capsule
- Cyst contents = solid crystalline cholesterol, keratinaceous debris; no dermal appendages
- Grows by progressive desquamation with conversion to keratin/cholesterol crystals, forming concentric lamellae

CLINICAL ISSUES

Presentation
- Most common signs/symptoms
  - Symptoms depend on location and affect on adjacent neurovascular structures
    - Most common symptom: Headache
    - Cranial nerve 5, 7, 8 neuropathy common
    - 4th ventricular cerebellar signs common, yet increased intracranial pressure rare
    - Less commonly hypopituitarism, diabetes insipidus
    - Seizures if in sylvian fissure/temporal lobe
  - May remain clinically silent for many years

Demographics
- Age
  - Presents between 20-60 years with peak at 40 years
- Gender
  - M = F
    - CT hyperdense variant lesions have female predominance (M:F = 1:2.5)
- Epidemiology
  - 0.2-1.8% of all primary intracranial tumors
  - 4-9x more common than dermoid
  - Most common congenital intracranial tumor
  - 3rd most common CPA/IAC mass, after vestibular schwannoma and meningioma

Natural History & Prognosis
- Grows slowly: Epithelial component growth rate commensurate to that of normal epithelium
- Chemical meningitis possible from content leakage
- Rare malignant degeneration into squamous cell carcinoma (SCCa) reported
  - Postulated prolonged or reparative process from foreign material leads to cellular atypia and neoplasia
  - Often predated by frequent recurrences
  - May occur years after surgical resection
  - Mean age at presentation: 52 years with male preponderance

Treatment
- Treatment: Microsurgical resection
  - Complicated by investment of local structures
  - Recurrence common if incompletely removed
  - Subarachnoid dissemination of contents may occur during operative/postoperative course
    - May cause chemical meningitis
    - CSF seeding and implantation reported
- Rare malignant degeneration of resection bed into SCCa reported

DIAGNOSTIC CHECKLIST

Consider
- Epidermoid if insinuates and surrounds rather than displaces

Image Interpretation Pearls
- Resembles CSF on imaging studies, except usually incomplete nulling on FLAIR
- DWI hyperintensity is diagnostic

SELECTED REFERENCES

1. Guttal KS et al: Trigeminal neuralgia secondary to epidermoid cyst at the cerebellopontine angle: case report and brief overview. Odontology. 97(1):54-6, 2009
2. Jolapara M et al: Diffusion tensor mode in imaging of intracranial epidermoid cysts: one step ahead of fractional anisotropy. Neuroradiology. 51(2):123-9, 2009
3. Praveen KS et al: Calcified epidermoid cyst of the anterior interhemispheric fissure. Br J Neurosurg. 23(1):90-1, 2009
4. Li F et al: Hyperdense intracranial epidermoid cysts: a study of 15 cases. Acta Neurochir (Wien). 149(1):31-9; discussion 39, 2007

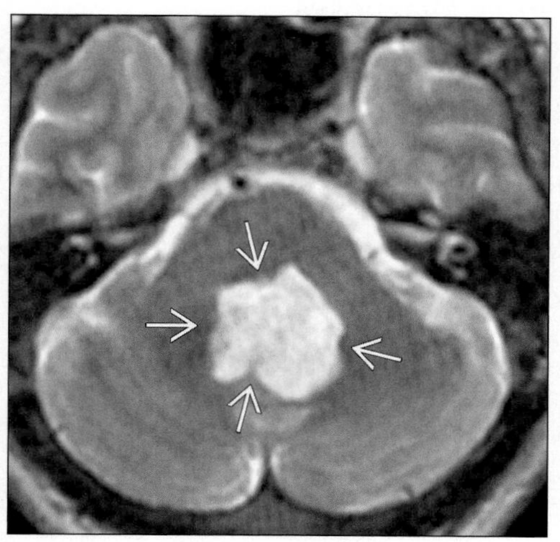

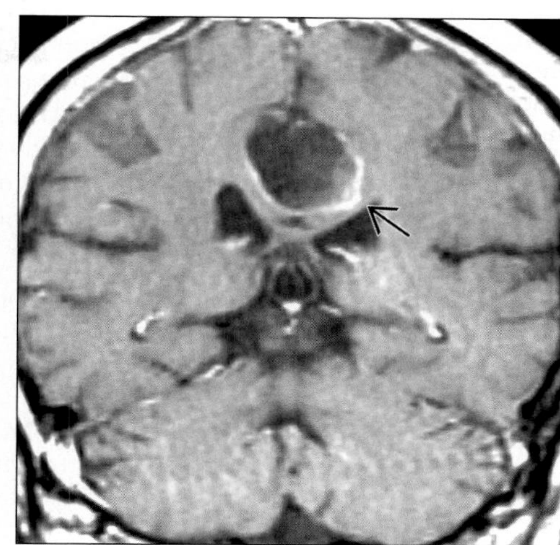

(Left) *Axial T2WI MR demonstrates "scalloped" expansion of an epidermoid within the 4th ventricle ➔. This is the 2nd most common location for epidermoids yet is statistically uncommon at only 17%.* ***(Right)*** *Coronal T1WI C+ MR demonstrates the typical appearance of an epidermoid in an atypical interhemispheric location. Note the slight marginal enhancement ➔.*

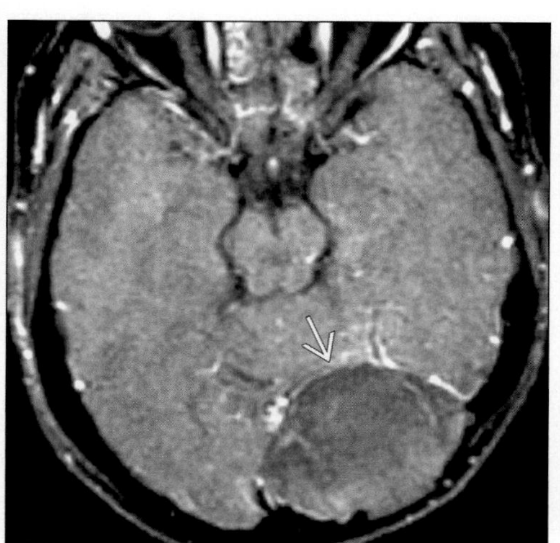

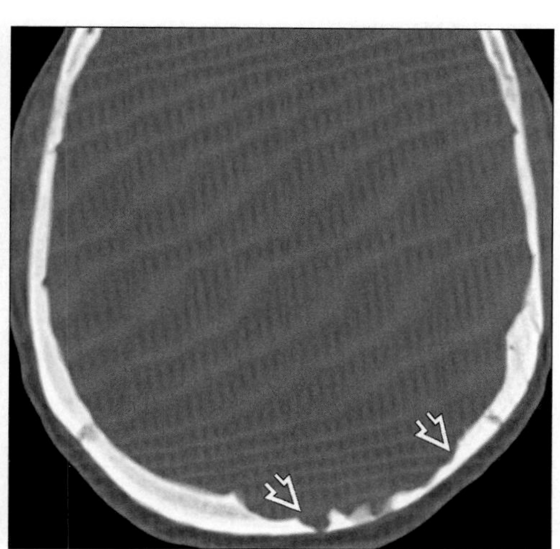

(Left) *Axial T1WI C+ FS MR shows an extraaxial mass in the left occipital region that is hyperintense to CSF and does not enhance ➔. DWI (not shown) clinched the diagnosis as an epidermoid cyst. This is an atypical location for epidermoid.* ***(Right)*** *Axial bone CT in the same patient reveals significant yet benign-appearing remodeling and scalloping of the inner calvarial table ➔.*

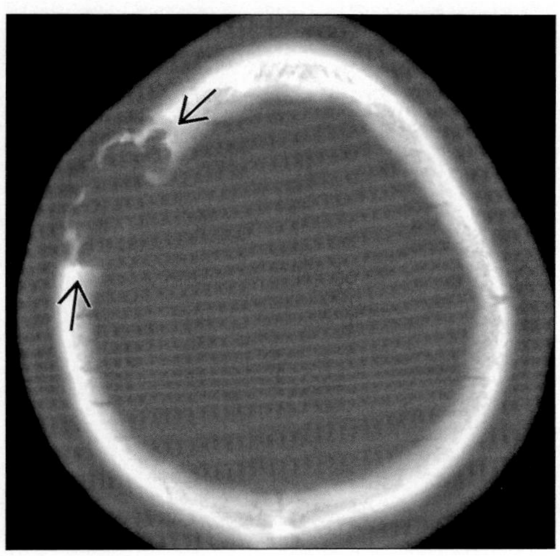

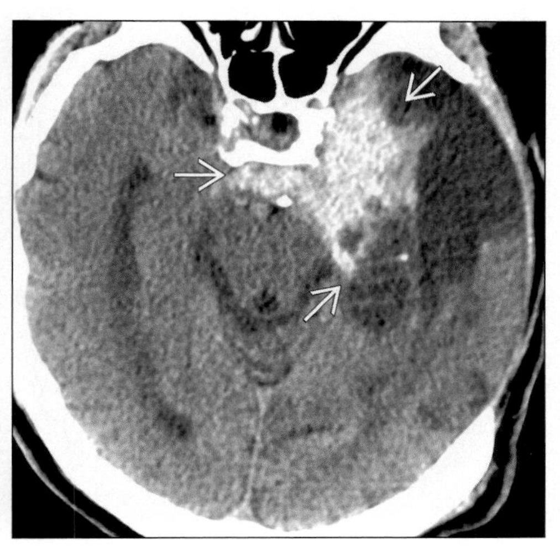

(Left) *Axial bone CT demonstrates the typical appearance of an intradiploic epidermoid as an expansile lesion with sharply corticated margins ➔.* ***(Right)*** *Axial NECT nicely shows a rare "dense" epidermoid ➔ that had been previously debulked at another institution. Only 3% of intracranial epidermoids have a "dense" CT appearance, which is thought to be secondary to hemorrhage, high protein, saponification of cyst debris to calcium soaps, or iron-containing pigment.*

NEUROGLIAL CYST

Key Facts

Terminology

- Neuroglial cyst (NGC), a.k.a. glioependymal cyst
- Benign, glial-lined, fluid-containing cavity buried within cerebral white matter
  - May occur anywhere throughout neuraxis
  - Frontal lobe most common site
  - Size varies from a few mm up to several cm

Imaging

- CT
  - Well-delineated, low-density, unilocular parenchymal cyst
  - No Ca++ or enhancement
- MR
  - T1 hypo-/T2 hyperintense (resembles CSF)
  - Usually suppresses on FLAIR
  - Does not restrict on DWI
  - No enhancement
  - Minimal/no surrounding signal abnormality

Top Differential Diagnoses

- Porencephalic cyst
- Enlarged perivascular spaces (PVSs)
- Arachnoid cyst
- Ependymal cyst
- Epidermoid cyst
- Infectious cyst (e.g., neurocysticercosis, echinococcosis)

Diagnostic Checklist

- Parenchymal cysts that do not communicate with ventricular system and have minimal/no surrounding gliosis may be NGC
- Use FLAIR, DWI to help distinguish between different types of intracranial cysts

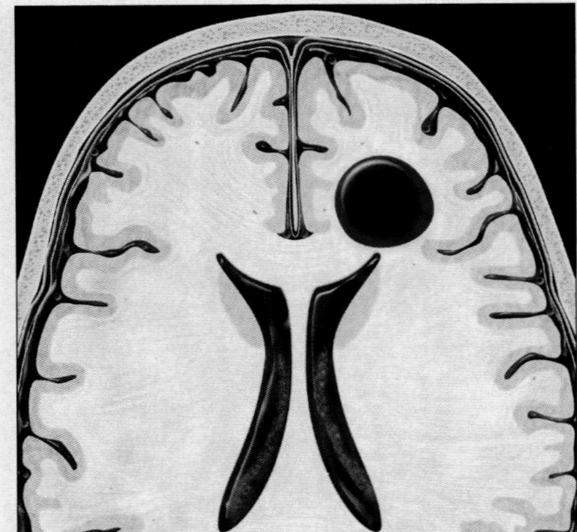

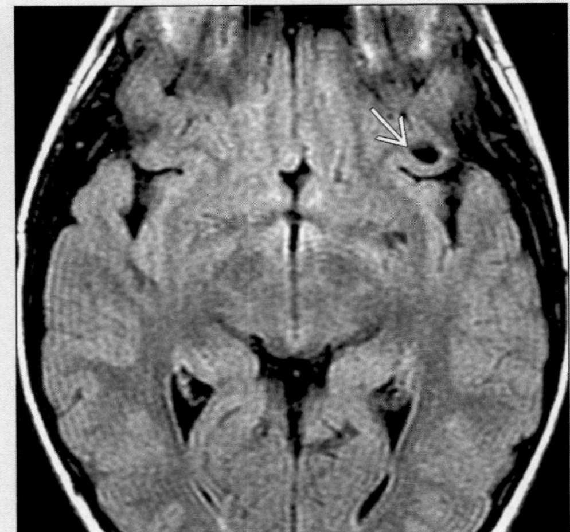

(Left) *Axial graphic shows a classic neuroglial cyst. This well-delineated unilocular lesion does not communicate with the ventricles and contains clear fluid. The surrounding brain is normal. Neuroglial cysts are lined with glial cells, astrocytes, and rarely ependymal cells.* ***(Right)*** *Axial FLAIR MR in a child shows incidental finding of a benign-appearing cyst in the left frontal subcortical white matter ➡. The cyst followed CSF on all sequences and did not enhance.*

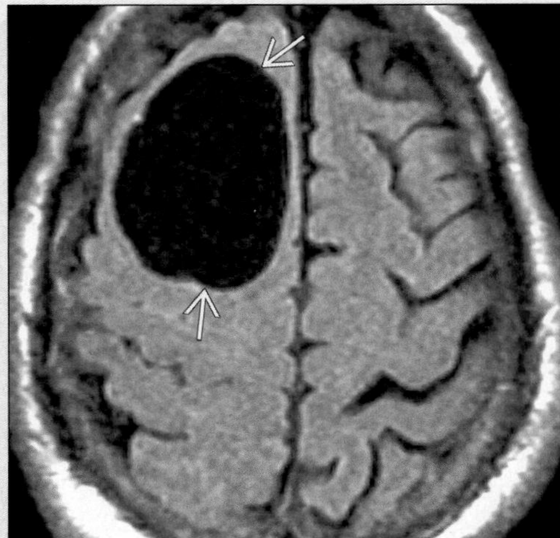

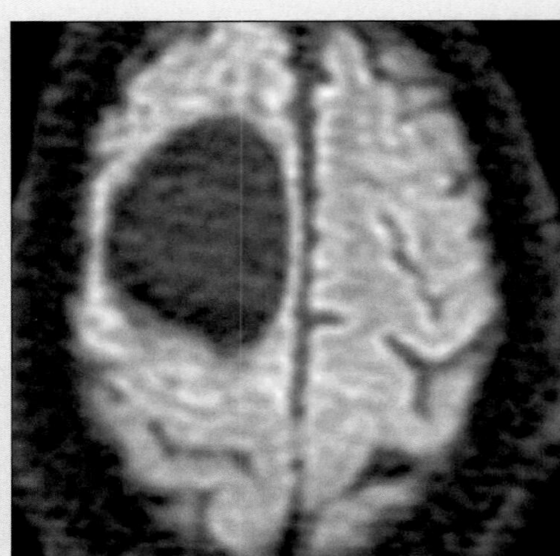

(Left) *Axial FLAIR MR in a young adult with headaches shows a large right frontal CSF-like cyst ➡.* ***(Right)*** *Axial DWI MR in the same patient shows no restriction. The cyst was biopsied and drained. Histological examination showed the cyst lining was glial tissue with no evidence for epithelial elements.*

NEUROGLIAL CYST

TERMINOLOGY

Abbreviations
- Neuroglial cyst (NGC)

Synonyms
- Glioependymal cyst

Definitions
- Benign, glial-lined, fluid-containing cavity buried within cerebral white matter

IMAGING

General Features
- Best diagnostic clue
  - Nonenhancing CSF-like parenchymal cyst with minimal/no surrounding signal abnormality
- Location
  - May occur anywhere throughout neuraxis
    - Frontal lobe most common site
    - Intraparenchymal > extraparenchymal
- Size
  - Varies from a few mm up to several cm
- Morphology
  - Smooth, rounded, unilocular, benign-appearing cyst

CT Findings
- NECT
  - Well-delineated, low-density cyst
    - Unilocular; no Ca++
- CECT
  - Wall does not enhance

MR Findings
- T1WI
  - Usually hypointense, resembles CSF
- T2WI
  - Hyperintense
- PD/intermediate
  - May be slightly hyperintense to CSF
- FLAIR
  - Usually suppresses
- DWI
  - Typically no diffusion restriction
- T1WI C+
  - No enhancement

Imaging Recommendations
- Best imaging tool
  - MR with T1WI C+, FLAIR, DWI

DIFFERENTIAL DIAGNOSIS

Porencephalic Cyst
- Communicates with ventricles
- Adjacent brain usually shows gliosis, spongiosis

Enlarged Perivascular Spaces (PVSs)
- Clusters of variable-sized cysts > single, unilocular cyst

Arachnoid Cyst
- Extraaxial

Ependymal Cyst
- Intraventricular

Epidermoid Cyst
- Does not suppress on FLAIR, restricts on DWI

Infectious Cyst
- e.g., neurocysticercosis, echinococcosis

PATHOLOGY

Gross Pathologic & Surgical Features
- Rounded, smooth, unilocular cyst usually containing clear fluid resembling CSF

Microscopic Features
- Varies from columnar (ependymal type) epithelium to low cuboidal cells resembling choroid plexus
  - Variable expression of GFAP
  - Cytokeratin, EMA expression absent

CLINICAL ISSUES

Presentation
- Most common signs/symptoms
  - Headache
- Other signs/symptoms
  - Seizures
  - Neurologic deficit (depends on cyst size, location)

Demographics
- Age
  - Any age; adults > children
- Gender
  - M = F
- Epidemiology
  - Uncommon (< 1% of intracranial cysts)

Natural History & Prognosis
- Varies with cyst size, location
- May be stable over many years

Treatment
- Observation vs. fenestration/drainage of cyst

DIAGNOSTIC CHECKLIST

Consider
- Parenchymal cysts that do not communicate with ventricular system and have minimal/no surrounding gliosis may be NGC

Image Interpretation Pearls
- Use FLAIR, DWI to help distinguish between different types of intracranial cysts

SELECTED REFERENCES

1. Osborn AG et al: Intracranial cysts: radiologic-pathologic correlation and imaging approach. Radiology. 239(3):650-64, 2006

PERIVENTRICULAR CYST

Key Facts

Terminology

- Periventricular cysts of newborn
  - Encompasses wide variety of periventricular cystic lesions

Imaging

- Anterior choroid plexus cysts (ACPC)
  - Posterior to caudothalamic groove, within choroid plexus or protruding into lateral ventricle
- Subependymal pseudocysts (SEPC)
  - Nonhemorrhagic: Anterior to caudothalamic groove
  - Posthemorrhagic: Commonly in caudothalamic notch
- Connatal (CS)
  - At or just below superolateral angles of frontal horns &/or body of lateral ventricles
- Cystic periventricular leukomalacia (cPVL)
  - At or above superolateral angle of frontal horn
  - Along margins of lateral ventricles

Clinical Issues

- Bilateral ACPC or SEPC → look for systemic disease
  - Inborn error of metabolism, TORCH, cocaine, etc.
- Cystic periventricular leukomalacia: More common in association with cytokine damage
  - Neonatal enterovirus
  - Maternal chorioamniitis
  - Sepsis
- SEPC &/or ACPC detected in up to 5% of neonates
  - Frequently involute over time

Diagnostic Checklist

- May be extremely difficult/impossible to differentiate SEPC from ACPC

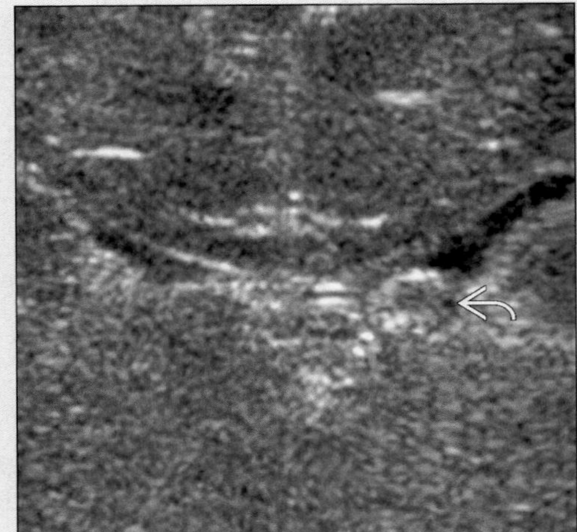

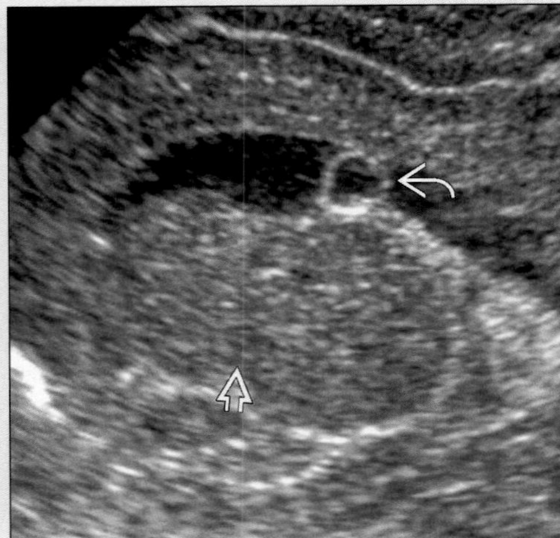

(Left) *Coronal ultrasound in a newborn with intrauterine growth retardation demonstrates a round cyst ➔ in the anterior horn of the left lateral ventricle.* ***(Right)*** *Longitudinal ultrasound in the same infant shows the cyst ➔ behind the caudothalamic groove ➔. The cyst may "bounce" on ultrasound.*

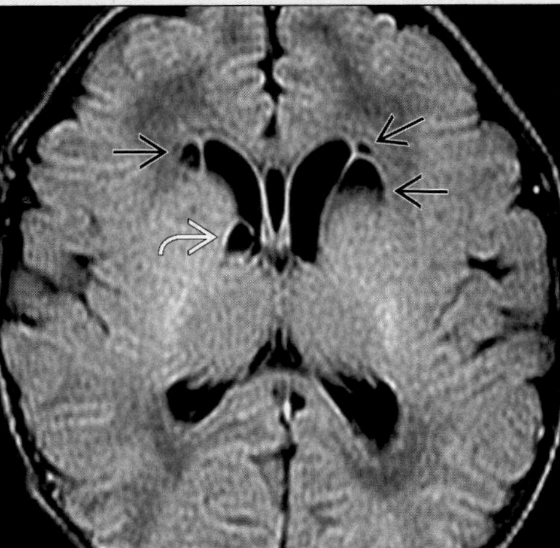

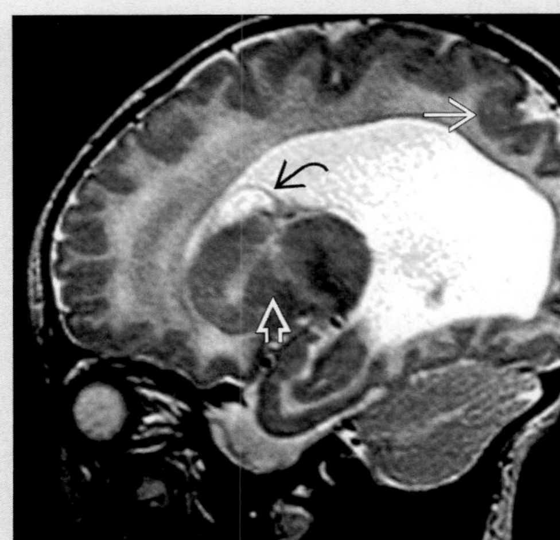

(Left) *Axial FLAIR MR in newborn with mitochondrial depletion syndrome and lactic acidosis demonstrates multiple periventricular cysts. Large paraventricular cysts (cPVL) ➔ adjacent to the frontal horns were noted in utero. Additionally, a subependymal cyst ➔ is anterior to the caudothalamic groove.* ***(Right)*** *Sagittal T2WI MR in a newborn with Zellweger syndrome reveals ventriculomegaly, focal cortical dysplasia ➔, and a large subependymal cyst ➔ anterior to the caudothalamic groove ➔.*

PERIVENTRICULAR CYST

TERMINOLOGY

Abbreviations

- Neonatal periventricular cysts (PCs)
  - Anterior choroid plexus cyst (ACPC)
  - Subependymal pseudocyst (SEPC)
  - Germinolytic cyst (GC)
  - Connatal cyst (CS)
  - Cystic periventricular leukomalacia (cPVL), previously known as paraventricular cysts

Definitions

- Periventricular cysts of newborn: Encompasses wide variety of periventricular cystic lesions
  - Anterior choroid plexus cyst
    - Cyst of anterior portion of choroid plexus in body of lateral ventricles
  - Subependymal pseudocyst
    - Subependymal cyst in region of caudate nucleus; may be congenital (germinolytic) or acquired (posthemorrhagic)
  - Connatal cyst, a.k.a. coarctation of anterior horns
    - Controversial, some authors consider connatal cysts to be germinolytic cysts
  - Cystic periventricular leukomalacia
- Considerable overlap and confusion in literature

IMAGING

General Features

- Best diagnostic clue
  - Anterior choroid plexus cyst
    - Spherical, thick or double walled
    - On US, look for "bouncing" of ACPC with pulsation to confirm location within choroid plexus
  - Subependymal pseudocyst
    - Teardrop-shaped, thin walled
    - Nonhemorrhagic
      - Anterior to caudothalamic groove
    - Hemorrhagic
      - In caudothalamic groove, blood products identifiable during acute phase
  - Cystic periventricular leukomalacia
    - Local loss of brain volume
- Location
  - Anterior choroid plexus cyst
    - Posterior to caudothalamic groove
    - Within choroid plexus or protruding into lateral ventricle
  - Subependymal pseudocyst
    - Nonhemorrhagic
      - Anterior to caudothalamic groove
    - Posthemorrhagic
      - Commonly in caudothalamic notch
    - Slightly more common on left side
  - Connatal cyst
    - At or just below superolateral angles of frontal horns &/or body of lateral ventricles
    - Anterior to foramina of Monro
  - Cystic periventricular leukomalacia
    - At or above superolateral angle of frontal horn
    - Along margins of lateral ventricles, anterior to posterior
    - Cysts may communicate with ventricles (porencephaly) or be separated from ventricles by ependyma
- Size
  - SEPC: 2-11 mm
  - Cysts in cystic periventricular leukomalacia are most variable in size, may be several centimeters in diameter
- Morphology
  - ACPC: Spherical, may exhibit double wall, nonseptate
  - SEPC: Teardrop-shaped, thin walled

CT Findings

- NECT: Hemorrhage within cysts may give clue to etiology

Ultrasonographic Findings

- ACPC: Double wall, may "bounce" with pulsation

Imaging Recommendations

- Best imaging tool
  - High-resolution sonography/linear array
- Protocol advice
  - Include gradient sequences with MR to exclude or confirm hemorrhagic etiology

DIFFERENTIAL DIAGNOSIS

Arachnoid Cyst

- Giant arachnoid cysts of foramen of Monro
- Distinguished by location
  - Not along caudothalamic groove
  - Not at superolateral frontal horn
  - Not along ventricular margins

Choroid Plexus Papilloma

- Rarely, choroid plexus papillomas can be purely cystic
- Intra- rather than periventricular

Hippocampal Sulcus Remnant Cysts

- Cornu ammonis, dentate gyrus normally fuse
- Defects leave remnant cysts within primitive hippocampal fissure
- Seen medial to temporal horn of lateral ventricle
- CSF-like "string of pearls" along hippocampus

PATHOLOGY

General Features

- Etiology
  - SEPC: Subependymal germinal matrix of neuronal and glial proliferation
    - Metabolically active and richly vascular
    - Insult (infection, hemorrhage, genetic) → lysis of cells

Gross Pathologic & Surgical Features

- Subependymal cyst
  - Cystic cavity bounded by pseudocapsule

- Pseudocapsule consists of aggregates of germinal cells and glial tissue, not epithelium
- ± hemorrhage or reactive astrocytes, cystic necrosis
- Connatal cysts: Ependymal lined
- cPVL: Cavitary white matter necrosis

CLINICAL ISSUES

Presentation

- Most common signs/symptoms
  - SEPC vs. ACPC
    - SEPC somewhat more likely than ACPC to be associated with anomalies or systemic disease
    - Unilateral ACPC or SEPC
      - Low likelihood of associated anomalies
    - Bilateral ACPC or SEPC
      - Look for systemic disease
- Other signs/symptoms
  - ACPC very occasionally causes obstruction at foramina of Monro

Natural History & Prognosis

- SEPC &/or ACPC detected in up to 5% of neonates, frequently involute over time
- Postnatal acquired SEPC (hemorrhagic) in very low-birth-weight infants = risk factor for impaired motor development
- cPVL prognosis dependent upon amount of destroyed tissue, become incorporated into ventricle over time

Treatment

- None unless obstruction of lateral ventricles occurs

DIAGNOSTIC CHECKLIST

Consider

- Bilateral SEPCs are markers for systemic disease
  - Aneuploidy and multiple congenital anomaly syndromes
  - Growth disorders: Intrauterine growth restriction, large for gestational dates, Soto syndrome
  - TORCH: CMV, rubella
  - Intrauterine exposure to cocaine
  - Inborn error of metabolism
    - Peroxisomal biogenesis disorders (Zellweger)
    - Congenital lactic acidoses, PDH deficiency
    - Holocarboxylase synthetase deficiency
    - D-2OH and L-2OH glutaric aciduria

Image Interpretation Pearls

- CT or gradient sequences may aid in differentiation

Reporting Tips

- May be extremely difficult or even impossible to differentiate SEPC and ACPC

SELECTED REFERENCES

1. Fernandez Alvarez JR et al: Diagnostic value of subependymal and choroid plexus cysts on neonatal cerebral ultrasound: a meta-analysis. Arch Dis Child Fetal Neonatal Ed. Epub ahead of print, 2009
2. van Baalen A et al: From fossil to fetus: nonhemorrhagic germinal matrix echodensity caused by mineralizing vasculitis--hypothesis of fossilizing germinolysis and gliosis. J Child Neurol. 24(1):36-44, 2009
3. Soares-Fernandes JP et al: Neonatal pyruvate dehydrogenase deficiency due to a R302H mutation in the PDHA1 gene: MRI findings. Pediatr Radiol. 38(5):559-62, 2008
4. van Baalen A et al: Anterior choroid plexus cysts: distinction from germinolysis by high-resolution sonography. Pediatr Int. 50(1):57-61, 2008
5. Chuang YC et al: Neurodevelopment in very low birth weight premature infants with postnatal subependymal cysts. J Child Neurol. 22(4):402-5, 2007
6. van Baalen A et al: [Non-haemorrhagic subependymal pseudocysts: ultrasonographic, histological and pathogenetic variability.] Ultraschall Med. 28(3):296-300, 2007
7. Epelman M et al: Differential diagnosis of intracranial cystic lesions at head US: correlation with CT and MR imaging. Radiographics. 26(1):173-96, 2006
8. Finsterer J et al: Adult unilateral periventricular pseudocysts with ipsilateral headache. Clin Neurol Neurosurg. 108(1):73-6, 2005
9. Read MH et al: Clinical, biochemical, magnetic resonance imaging (MRI) and proton magnetic resonance spectroscopy (1H MRS) findings in a fourth case of combined D- and L-2 hydroxyglutaric aciduria. J Inherit Metab Dis. 28(6):1149-50, 2005
10. Wilson CJ et al: Severe holocarboxylase synthetase deficiency with incomplete biotin responsiveness resulting in antenatal insult in samoan neonates. J Pediatr. 147(1):115-8, 2005
11. Cuillier F et al: [Subependymal pseudocysts in the fetal brain revealing Zellweger syndrome.] J Gynecol Obstet Biol Reprod (Paris). 33(4):325-9, 2004
12. Habek D et al: Fetal biophysical profile and cerebro-umbilical ratio in assessment of brain damage in growth restricted fetuses. Eur J Obstet Gynecol Reprod Biol. 114(1):29-34, 2004
13. Qian JH et al: [Prospective study on prognosis of infants with neonatal subependymal cysts.] Zhonghua Er Ke Za Zhi. 42(12):913-6, 2004
14. Herini E et al: Clinical features of infants with subependymal germinolysis and choroid plexus cysts. Pediatr Int. 45(6):692-6, 2003
15. Pal BR et al: Frontal horn thin walled cysts in preterm neonates are benign. Arch Dis Child Fetal Neonatal Ed. 85(3):F187-93, 2001
16. van der Knaap MS et al: D-2-hydroxyglutaric aciduria: further clinical delineation. J Inherit Metab Dis. 22(4):404-13, 1999
17. Rosenfeld DL et al: Coarctation of the lateral ventricles: an alternative explanation for subependymal pseudocysts. Pediatr Radiol. 27(12):895-7, 1997
18. Shackelford GD et al: Cysts of the subependymal germinal matrix: sonographic demonstration with pathologic correlation. Radiology. 149(1):117-21, 1983
19. Takashima S et al: Old subependymal necrosis and hemorrhage in the prematurely born infants. Brain Dev. 1(4):299-304, 1979
20. De León GA et al: Cystic degeneration of the telencephalic subependymal germinal layer in newborn infants. J Neurol Neurosurg Psychiatry. 38(3):265-71, 1975

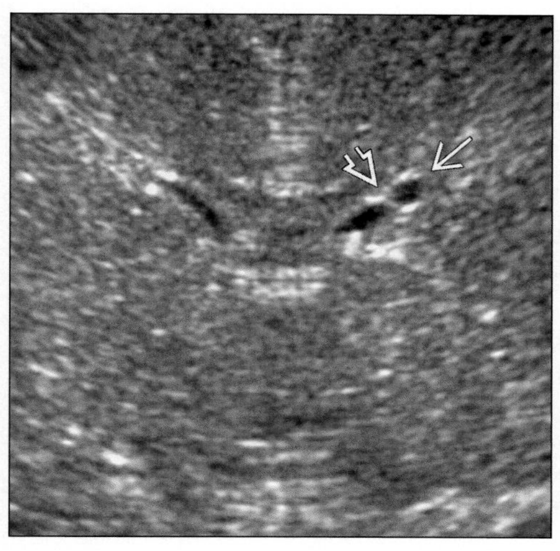

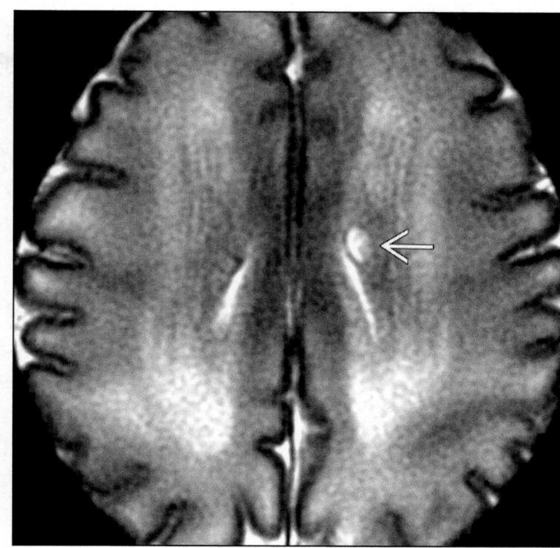

(Left) *Coronal ultrasound 1 day after birth in a 31-week gestational infant demonstrates a cyst ➡ adjacent to the lateral corner of the anterior horn. It is formed by a web-like adhesion ⇨ or coarction of the anterior horn, representing a connatal cyst.* ***(Right)*** *Axial T2WI MR in the same infant shows the connatal cyst ➡. As is typical, the cyst was not present on follow-up ultrasound or MR.*

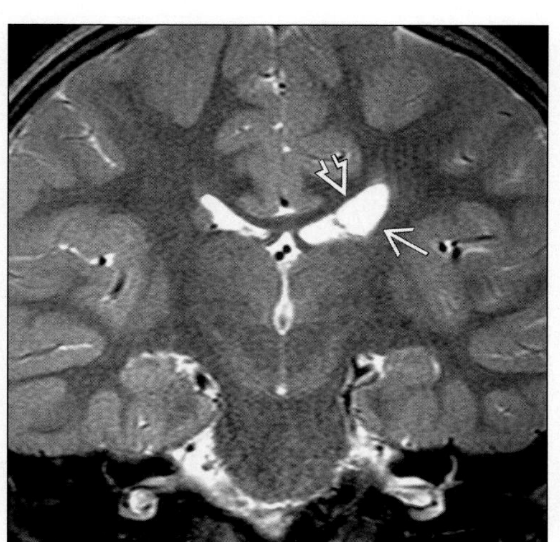

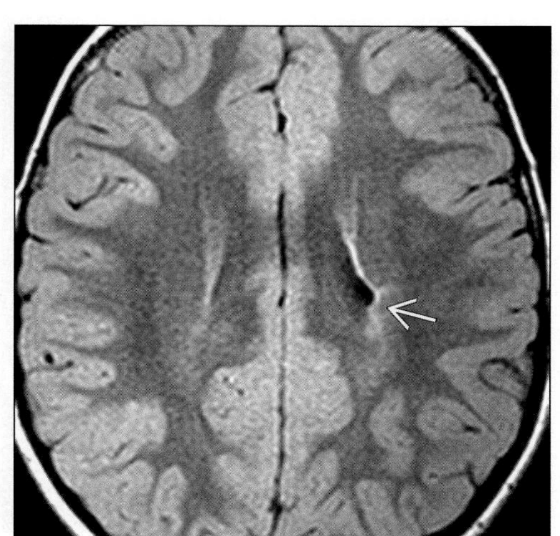

(Left) *Coronal T2WI MR in a toddler with a history of congenital hemiparesis demonstrates an apparent cyst of the anterior horn ⇨. However, note the loss of the body of the caudate nucleus ➡ in this child with a paraventricular volume loss following neonatal ischemia.* ***(Right)*** *Axial FLAIR MR in the same child reveals focal atrophy in the body of the caudate nucleus and surrounding white matter gliosis ➡.*

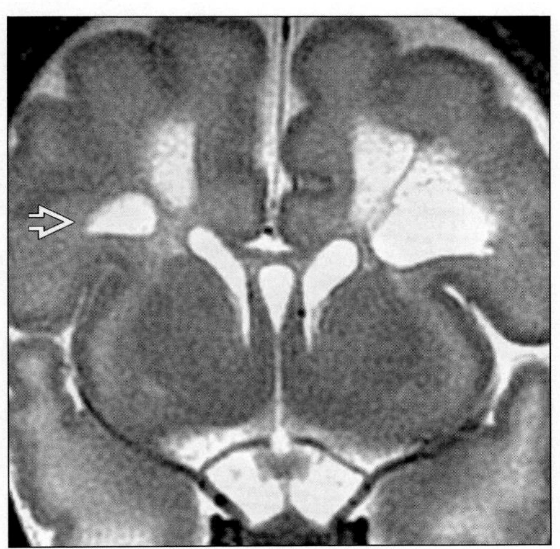

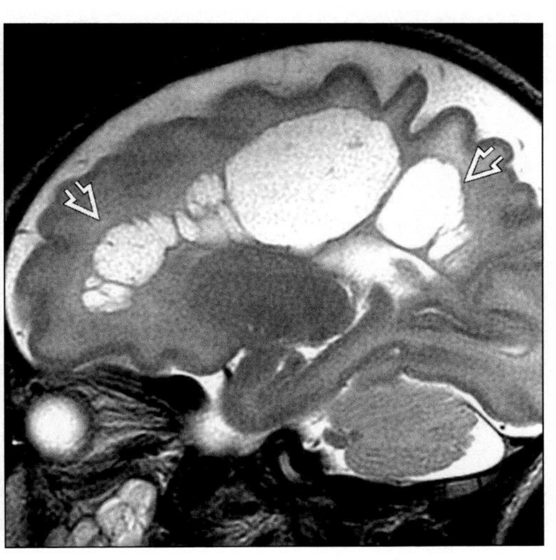

(Left) *Coronal T2WI MR in a pre-term infant with a history of maternal chorioamnionitis reveals large "paraventricular" cysts ⇨. This pattern is more commonly called extensive cystic periventricular leukomalacia (cPVL).* ***(Right)*** *Sagittal T2WI MR again reveals extensive cystic white matter damage ⇨. Lesions do not communicate with the ventricles, an appearance reported in term and pre-term infants who present with neonatal enterovirus or who have had exposure to maternal chorioamnionitis.*

CHOROID FISSURE CYST

Key Facts

Terminology

- Extraaxial neuroepithelial cyst arising in or near choroid fissure

Imaging

- Best imaging clue: Cystic lesion following CSF involving medial temporal lobe, choroid fissure
  - Well-circumscribed round or oval cyst
- NECT: Hypodense lesion of medial temporal lobe
  - May cause mass effect on hippocampus
- MR: Follows CSF on all sequences
  - FLAIR: Complete suppression
  - DWI: No restricted diffusion
  - T1 C+: No enhancement
- Sagittal MR shows typical "spindle" shape
- Coronal T2 shows relationship to choroid fissure

Top Differential Diagnoses

- Arachnoid cyst
- Epidermoid cyst
- Dermoid cyst
- Cystic tumor

Pathology

- Choroid fissure: CSF space between fimbria of hippocampus and diencephalon

Clinical Issues

- Incidental benign finding
- Most commonly asymptomatic
- Rare association with complex partial seizures
  - Questionable epileptogenic focus
- Some authors advocate surgical resection if significant mass effect or documented medically refractory epileptogenic focus

*(**Left**) Sagittal T1WI MR shows a large choroidal fissure cyst ➔ with mass effect on the adjacent hippocampus. While these are most commonly incidental, there are case reports suggesting an association with complex partial seizures. (**Right**) Axial FLAIR MR in the same patient shows the isointense choroid fissure cyst ➔ just posterior to the uncus. The cyst displaces the temporal horn and distorts the normal hippocampus. Choroid fissure cysts follow CSF on all sequences.*

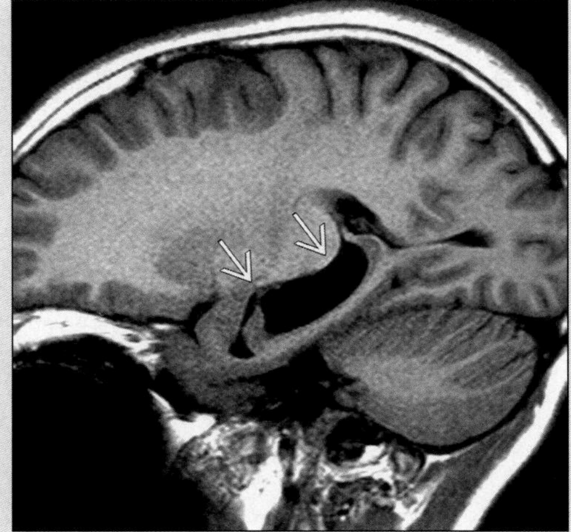

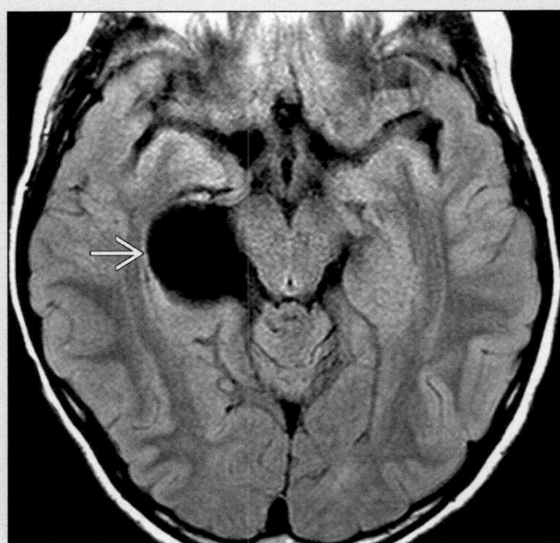

*(**Left**) Coronal T2WI MR shows a choroid fissure cyst displacing the temporal horn and causing hippocampal and parahippocampal gyrus flattening and distortion ⇨. (**Right**) Axial FLAIR MR shows an incidental choroid fissure cyst ➔, medial to the temporal horn, in a young adult with headaches. These benign cysts follow CSF signal intensity on all sequences, including DWI, and do not enhance. These cysts usually require no treatment unless associated with medically refractory epilepsy.*

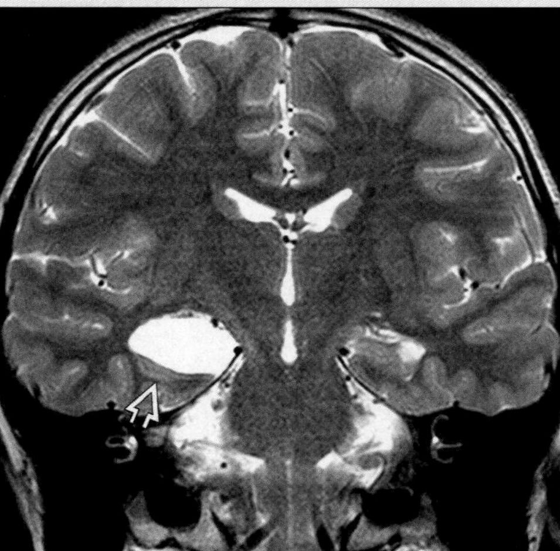

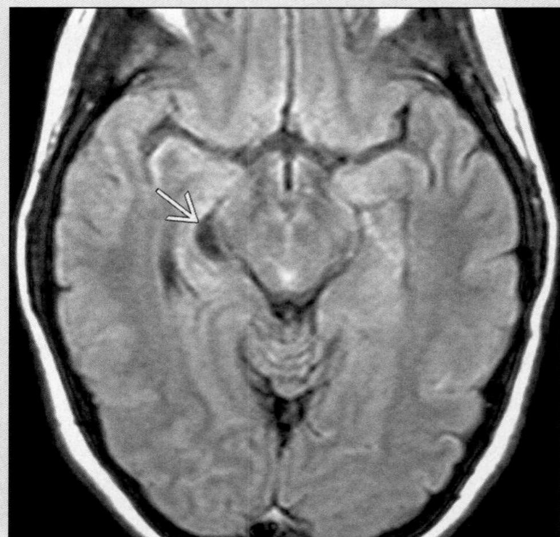

HIPPOCAMPAL SULCUS REMNANT CYSTS

Key Facts

Terminology

- Synonyms: Hippocampal remnant cyst, hippocampal sulcal cavities
- Cyst or string of cysts along residual cavity of primitive hippocampal sulcus

Imaging

- String of cysts along lateral margin of hippocampus
- Cysts follow CSF signal on all MR sequences
  - T2: Hyperintense
  - FLAIR: Complete suppression
  - T1WI C+: No enhancement

Top Differential Diagnoses

- Mesial temporal sclerosis
- Choroid fissure cyst
- Arachnoid cyst
- DNET

Pathology

- Represent partially unfused hippocampal sulcus
- Embryology
  - Primitive hippocampal fissure is formed as cornu ammonis and dentate gyrus fold on each other to form cleft
  - Cornu ammonis and dentate gyrus then fuse, leaving shallow hippocampal sulcus
  - Defects in this fusion cause remnant cysts within primitive sulcus

Clinical Issues

- Incidental finding, not associated with pathology
- Often observed on high-resolution imaging for evaluation of seizure patients (10-15%)
- Have been noted to enlarge with temporal lobe atrophy in Alzheimer disease

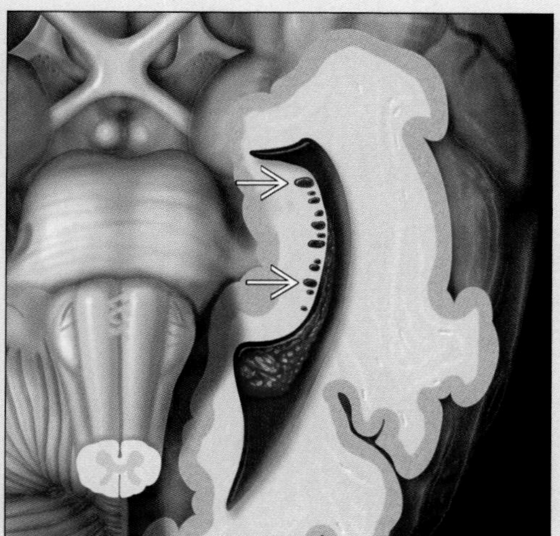

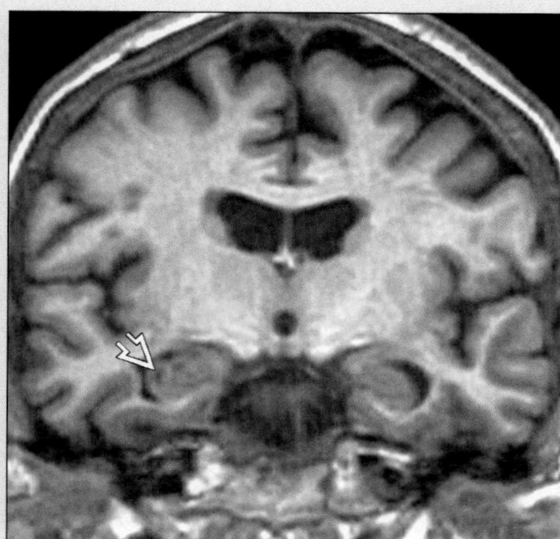

(Left) *Axial graphic of the normal temporal lobe shows a string of cysts within the lateral hippocampus, along the residual cavity of the primitive hippocampal sulcus ➔, representing hippocampal sulcus remnant cysts. These incidental findings have a characteristic appearance.* ***(Right)*** *Coronal T1WI MR shows small hypointense cysts ➔ in the lateral hippocampus, which follow CSF signal on all sequences. These normal variants are related to a partially unfused hippocampal sulcus and require no treatment.*

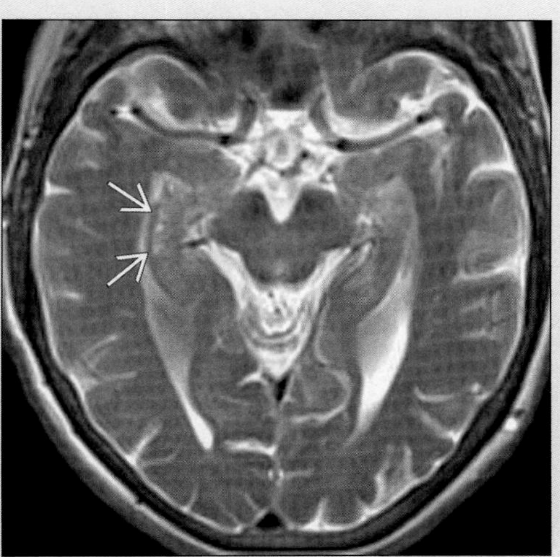

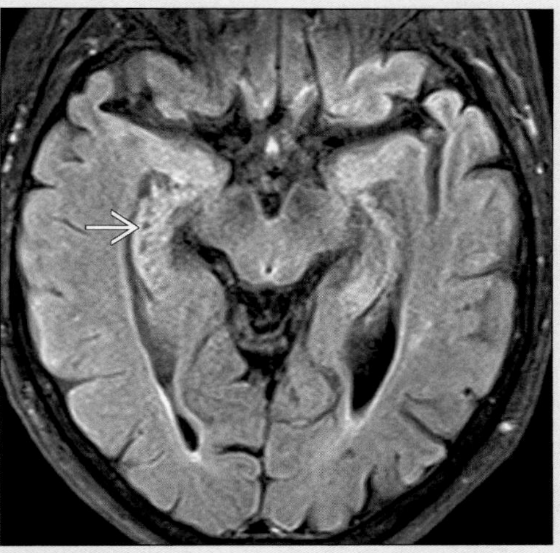

(Left) *Axial T2WI MR shows small hyperintense cysts in the hippocampus ➔. These unfused remnants of the embryonic hippocampal sulcus present as CSF-like cysts, appearing as a "string of beads" coursing through the hippocampus.* ***(Right)*** *Axial FLAIR MR in the same patient shows complete suppression of the hippocampal sulcus remnant cysts ➔. The "string of beads" appearance is typical of these common normal variants. They have been found to enlarge in patients with temporal lobe atrophy.*

ENLARGED PERIVASCULAR SPACES

Key Facts

Terminology
- Pial-lined interstitial fluid (ISF)-filled structures
  - Accompany penetrating arteries
  - Do not communicate with subarachnoid space

Imaging
- Clusters of variable-sized, well-delineated nonenhancing cysts
- PVSs occur in all locations, at all ages; easily seen in most patients on 3T imaging
- Most common site for normal PVSs = basal ganglia (clustered around anterior commissure)
  - Midbrain, thalami
  - Deep white matter (including corpus callosum, subinsular cortex, extreme capsule)
  - Almost never involve cortex (PVSs expand within subcortical white matter)
- PVSs usually 5 mm or less
  - Occasionally expand, attain large size
  - Most common location for expanded ("giant" or "tumefactive") PVSs = midbrain
  - May cause mass effect, obstructive hydrocephalus
- Isodense/isointense with CSF

Top Differential Diagnoses
- Lacunar infarcts
- Cystic neoplasm (e.g., DNET, cystic astrocytoma)
- Infectious/inflammatory cysts

Clinical Issues
- Should not be mistaken for serious disease
- Usually remain stable in size over years

Diagnostic Checklist
- Prominent but normal PVSs are identified in nearly all patients, in virtually every location at 3T imaging

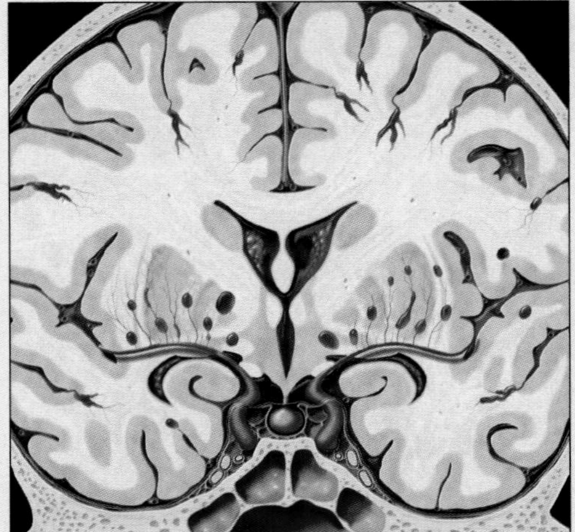
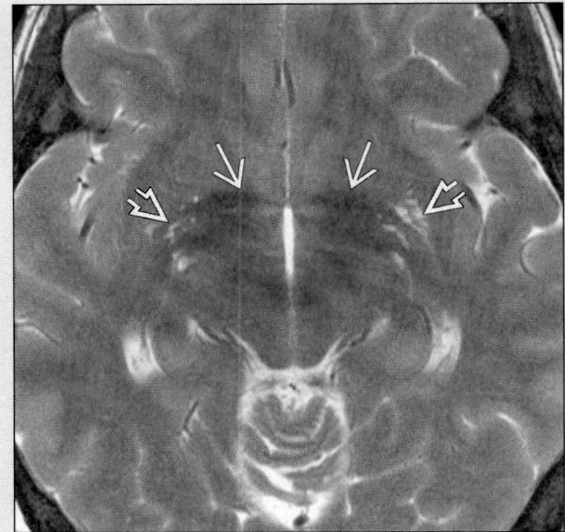

(Left) *Coronal graphic shows normal PVSs as they accompany penetrating arteries into the basal ganglia and subcortical white matter. Normal PVSs cluster around the anterior commissure but occur in all areas.* ***(Right)*** *Axial T2WI 3T MR with thin sections shows multiple small perivascular spaces ⇨ clustered around the anterior commissure ➡ in the inferior 3rd of the basal ganglia. These are normal findings.*

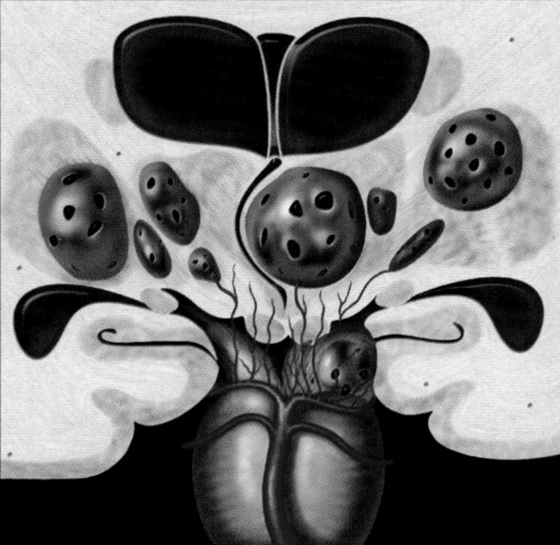
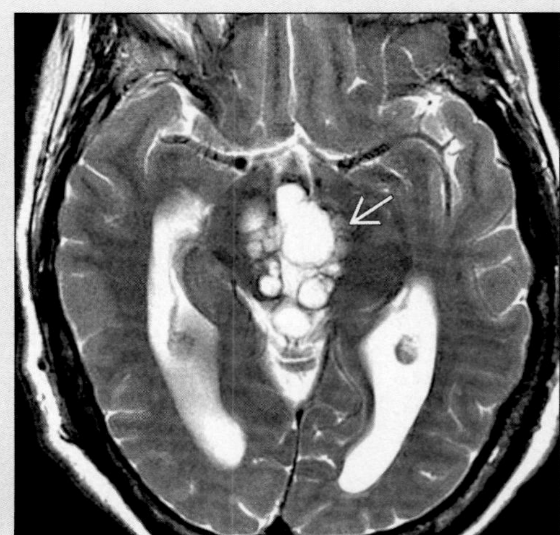

(Left) *Coronal graphic shows enlarged perivascular spaces in the midbrain and thalami causing mass effect on the 3rd ventricle and aqueduct with resulting hydrocephalus.* ***(Right)*** *Axial T2WI MR shows multiple variable-sized, CSF-like cysts in the midbrain ➡ causing obstructive hydrocephalus. The lateral ventricles were shunted.*

ENLARGED PERIVASCULAR SPACES

TERMINOLOGY

Abbreviations
- Perivascular spaces (PVSs)

Synonyms
- Virchow-Robin spaces

Definitions
- Pial-lined interstitial fluid (ISF)-filled structures that accompany penetrating arteries but do not communicate directly with subarachnoid space

IMAGING

General Features
- Best diagnostic clue
  - Clusters of variable-sized fluid-filled spaces resembling CSF
    - Surround/accompany penetrating arteries
    - Found in virtually all locations, in patients of all ages
- Location
  - Most common site for normal PVSs = basal ganglia (clustered around anterior commissure)
  - Other common locations
    - Midbrain
    - Deep white matter
    - Subinsular cortex, extreme capsule
  - Less common sites
    - Thalami
    - Dentate nuclei
    - Corpus callosum, cingulate gyrus
  - Most common location for expanded ("giant" or "tumefactive") PVSs = midbrain
    - Can be found almost anywhere
    - Almost never involve cortex (PVSs expand within subcortical white matter)
- Size
  - PVSs usually 5 mm or less
    - Occasionally expand, attain large size (up to several cm)
    - May cause focal mass effect, hydrocephalus
    - Widespread dilatation of PVSs may look very bizarre
- Morphology
  - Clusters of well-demarcated, variable-sized parenchymal cysts
  - Multiple > solitary cysts

CT Findings
- NECT
  - Clusters of round/ovoid/linear/punctate cyst-like lesions
    - Low density (attenuation = CSF)
    - No Ca++
- CECT
  - Do not enhance

MR Findings
- T1WI
  - Multiple well-delineated cysts isointense with CSF
  - Focal mass effect common
    - Expand overlying gyri
    - Midbrain enlarged PVSs may compress aqueduct/3rd ventricle, cause hydrocephalus
- T2WI
  - Appear isointense with CSF
    - Signal intensity within PVSs actually measures slightly < CSF
  - No edema in adjacent brain; may have ↑ SI
- PD/intermediate
  - Isointense with CSF
- FLAIR
  - Suppress completely
  - 25% have minimal increased signal in brain surrounding enlarged PVSs
- T2* GRE
  - No "blooming"
- DWI
  - No restricted diffusion
- T1WI C+
  - No enhancement
  - ± visualization of penetrating arteries with contrast
- MRS
  - Spectra in adjacent brain typically normal

Angiographic Findings
- Conventional
  - High-resolution DSA may depict penetrating arteries in area of enlarged PVSs

Nuclear Medicine Findings
- Tc-99m HMPAO SPECT normal, shows no ischemic changes

Imaging Recommendations
- Best imaging tool
  - Routine MR + FLAIR, DWI
- Protocol advice
  - Contrast optional

DIFFERENTIAL DIAGNOSIS

Lacunar Infarcts
- Older patients
- Common in basal ganglia, white matter
- Adjacent parenchymal hyperintensity

Cystic Neoplasm
- Usually in pons, cerebellum, thalamus/hypothalamus
- Single > multiple cysts
- Signal not quite like CSF
- Parenchymal signal abnormalities common
- May enhance

Infectious/Inflammatory Cysts
- Neurocysticercosis
  - Cysts often have scolex
  - Most are < 1 cm
  - Can be multiple but do not typically occur in clusters
  - Cyst walls often enhance
  - Surrounding edema often present
- Other parasites

ENLARGED PERIVASCULAR SPACES

- Hydatid cysts often unilocular, almost all in children
- Multilocular parasitic cysts typically enhance, mimic neoplasm more than PVSs

PATHOLOGY

General Features

- Etiology
  - Theory: ISF accumulates between penetrating vessel, pia
  - Egress of ISF blocked, causing cystic enlargement of PVS
    - Enlarged cystic-appearing spaces
    - Actually contain interstitial fluid, not CSF
- Genetics
  - Usually normal unless PVSs expanded by undergraded mucopolysaccharides (Hurler, Hunter disease)
  - PVSs expand in some congenital muscular dystrophies
- Associated abnormalities
  - Hydrocephalus (midbrain expanding PVSs can obstruct aqueduct)
  - "Cysts" caused by enlarged/obstructed PVSs reported with pituitary adenomas, large aneurysms
  - PVSs provide entry site into CNS in inflammatory, neoplastic disorders
    - Transmigration across capillaries, venules into PVSs
    - Progress across glia limitans into parenchyma

Gross Pathologic & Surgical Features

- Smoothly demarcated, fluid-filled cyst(s)

Microscopic Features

- Single or double layer of invaginated pia
- Pia becomes fenestrated, disappears at capillary level
- PVSs usually very small in cortex, often enlarge in subcortical white matter
- Surrounding brain usually lacks gliosis, amyloid deposition

CLINICAL ISSUES

Presentation

- Most common signs/symptoms
  - Usually normal, discovered incidentally at imaging/ autopsy
  - Nonspecific symptoms (e.g., headache)
- Clinical profile
  - Patient with nonspecific, nonlocalizing symptoms and bizarre, alarming multicystic-appearing brain mass initially diagnosed as "cystic neoplasm"

Demographics

- Age
  - Occur in all locations, at all ages
    - Easily seen on 3T imaging
  - Present in 25-30% of children (benign normal variant)
  - Enlarged PVSs
    - Mean age = mid 40s
    - May occur in children
- Gender
  - Giant PVSs: M:F = 1.8:1
- Epidemiology
  - Common nonneoplastic brain "cyst"
  - Common cause of multifocal hyperintensities on T2WI

Natural History & Prognosis

- Usually remain stable in size
- Occasionally continue to expand

Treatment

- "Leave me alone" lesion that should not be mistaken for serious disease
- Shunt ventricles if midbrain lesions cause obstructive hydrocephalus

DIAGNOSTIC CHECKLIST

Consider

- Could multicystic, nonenhancing mass on MR or CT be cluster of enlarged PVSs?

Image Interpretation Pearls

- Prominent but normal PVSs are identified in nearly all patients, in virtually every location at 3T imaging

SELECTED REFERENCES

1. Caner B et al: Dilatation of Virchow-Robin perivascular spaces: report of 3 cases with different localizations. Minim Invasive Neurosurg. 51(1):11-4, 2008
2. Carare RO et al: Solutes, but not cells, drain from the brain parenchyma along basement membranes of capillaries and arteries: significance for cerebral amyloid angiopathy and neuroimmunology. Neuropathol Appl Neurobiol. 34(2):131-44, 2008
3. Kara S et al: Dilated perivascular spaces: an informative radiologic finding in Sanfilippo syndrome type A. Pediatr Neurol. 38(5):363-6, 2008
4. Leclerc X et al: [Case No. 4. Giant perivascular spaces (Virchow Robin).] J Radiol. 89(7-8 Pt 1):936-7, 2008
5. Owens T et al: Perivascular spaces and the two steps to neuroinflammation. J Neuropathol Exp Neurol. 67(12):1113-21, 2008
6. Stephens T et al: Giant tumefactive perivascular spaces. J Neurol Sci. 266(1-2):171-3, 2008
7. Wuerfel J et al: Perivascular spaces--MRI marker of inflammatory activity in the brain?. Brain. 131(Pt 9):2332-40, 2008
8. Salzman KL et al: Giant tumefactive perivascular spaces. AJNR Am J Neuroradiol. 26(2):298-305, 2005
9. Papayannis CE et al: Expanding Virchow Robin spaces in the midbrain causing hydrocephalus. AJNR Am J Neuroradiol. 24(7):1399-403, 2003
10. Ozturk MH et al: Comparison of MR signal intensities of cerebral perivascular (Virchow-Robin) and subarachnoid spaces. J Comput Assist Tomogr. 26(6):902-4, 2002
11. Song CJ et al: MR imaging and histologic features of subinsular bright spots on T2-weighted MR images: Virchow-Robin spaces of the extreme capsule and insular cortex. Radiology. 214(3):671-7, 2000
12. Adachi M et al: Dilated Virchow-Robin spaces: MRI pathological study. Neuroradiology. 40(1):27-31, 1998

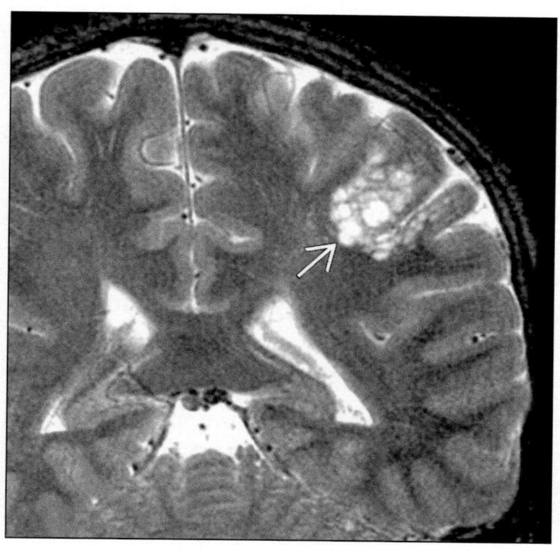

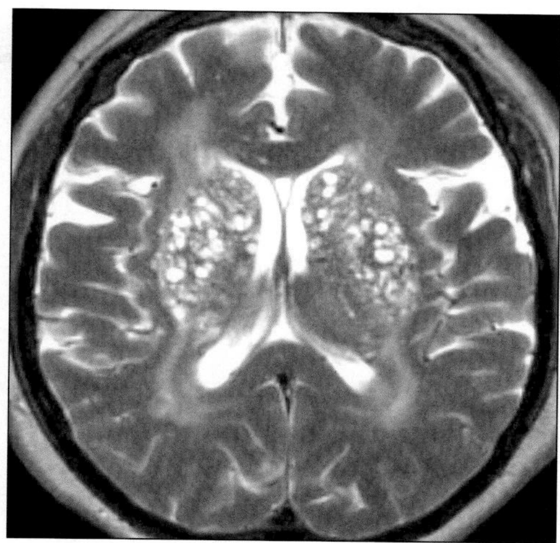

(Left) *Coronal T2WI MR in a 15-year-old boy with headaches shows a cluster of variable-sized cysts ➡ in the parietal subcortical white matter. Note the sparing of the overlying gray matter, which distinguishes this condition from DNET.* ***(Right)*** *Axial T2WI MR in a 56-year-old woman shows multiple bilateral hyperintensities in the basal ganglia. Multiple dilated PVSs in this location are also called "état criblé."*

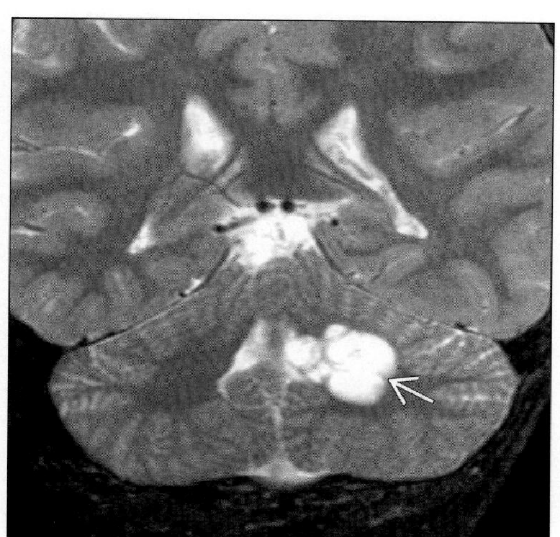

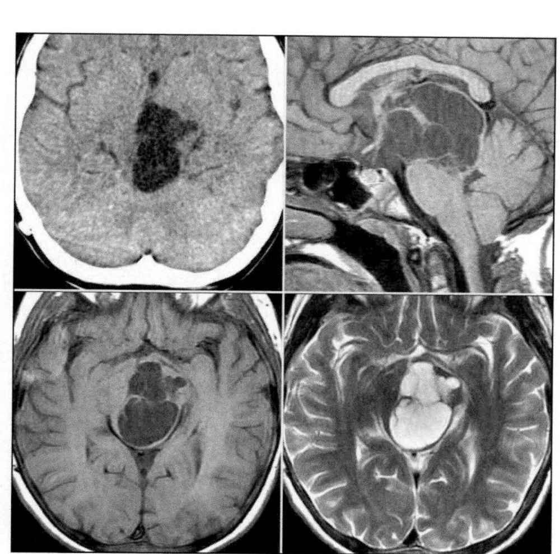

(Left) *This coronal T2WI MR of a child with headaches who was referred for overread with a diagnosis of "cystic brain tumor" shows dilated PVSs in the left dentate nucleus ➡.* ***(Right)*** *Composite imaging in a 15-year-old boy with longstanding shunted hydrocephalus caused by "cystic brain mass." These are multiple enlarged PVSs that expand the midbrain, causing hydrocephalus. The PVSs are of variable size and follow CSF on all sequences.*

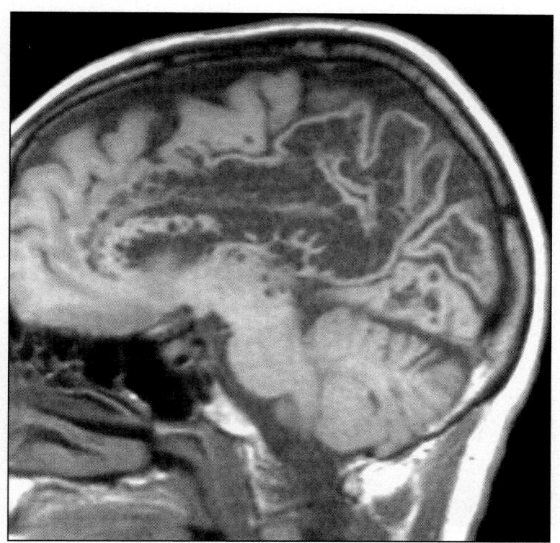

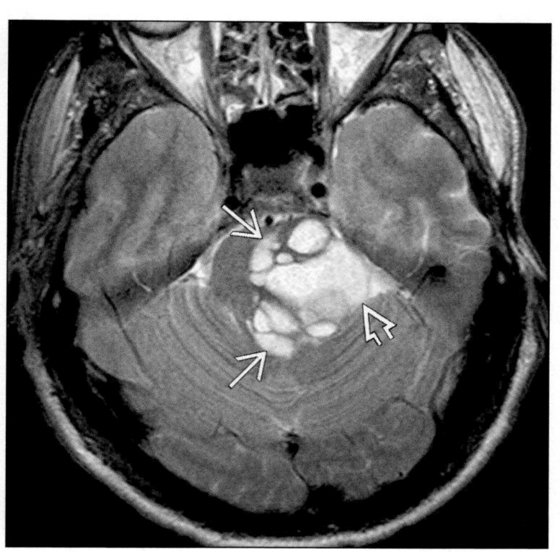

(Left) *Sagittal T1WI MR shows CSF-like cysts in the corpus callosum, cingulate gyrus, and occipital lobe. Note the mass effect with gyral expansion but striking sparing of the overlying gray matter. (Courtesy L. Valanne, MD.)* ***(Right)*** *Axial T2WI MR in a 27 year old with left-sided facial numbness and sensorineural hearing loss shows variable-sized cysts ➡ with a large cyst ➡ expanding into the CPA and probably compressing the 7th and 8th cranial nerves. No enhancement was seen on T1WI C+ MR.*

PINEAL CYST

Key Facts

Terminology

- Nonneoplastic intrapineal glial-lined cyst

Imaging

- CT
  - Sharply demarcated, smooth cyst behind 3rd ventricle
  - 80% < 10 mm (can be large, reported up to 4.5 cm)
  - Fluid iso-/slightly hyperdense to CSF
  - 25% Ca++ in cyst wall
- MR
  - Slightly hyperintense to CSF (55-60%)
  - Isointense (40%)
  - 1-2% hemorrhage (heterogeneous signal intensity)
  - Does not suppress on FLAIR

Top Differential Diagnoses

- Normal pineal gland
- Pineocytoma
- Epidermoid cyst
- Arachnoid cyst

Clinical Issues

- Vast majority clinically silent, discovered incidentally
  - Occur at all ages (older adults > children)
  - Found in 1-5% of normal MRs
- Presentation: Headache (less common), "pineal apoplexy" (rare)
  - Intracystic hemorrhage, acute hydrocephalus, sudden death

Diagnostic Checklist

- Cannot distinguish benign PC from neoplasm (pineocytoma) on basis of imaging studies alone
- Heterogeneous, nodular, or ring-like enhancing pineal mass may be benign cyst, not neoplasm

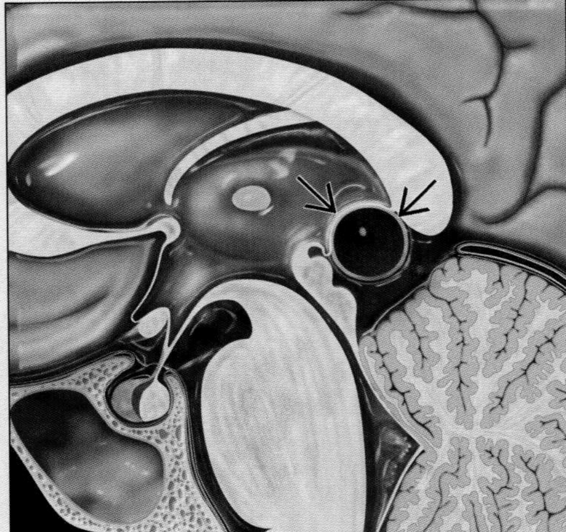

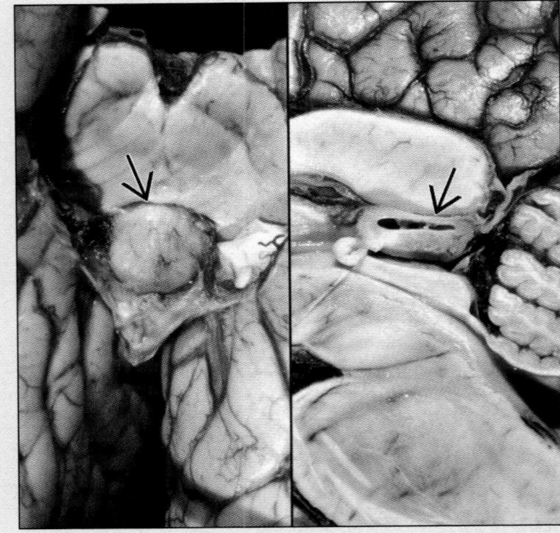

(Left) *Sagittal graphic shows a small cystic lesion within the pineal gland →. Small benign pineal cysts (PCs) are often found incidentally at autopsy or imaging.* ***(Right)*** *Submentovertex (left) and sagittal midline section (right) show a benign, nonneoplastic pineal gland cyst found incidentally at autopsy. The cyst → is very well delineated and has a moderately thick wall surrounding the cystic cavity. (Courtesy E. Tessa Hedley-Whyte, MD.)*

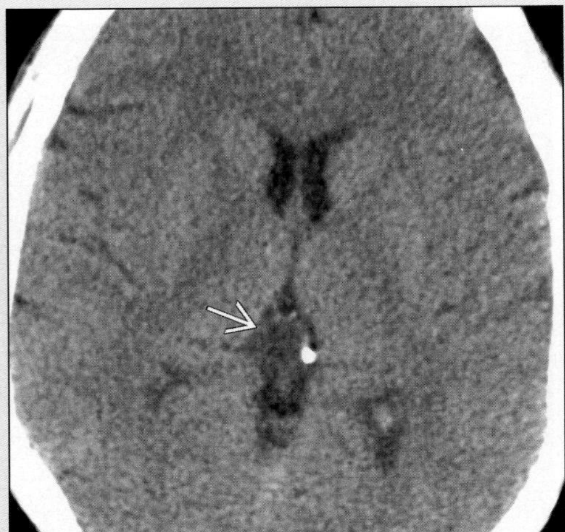

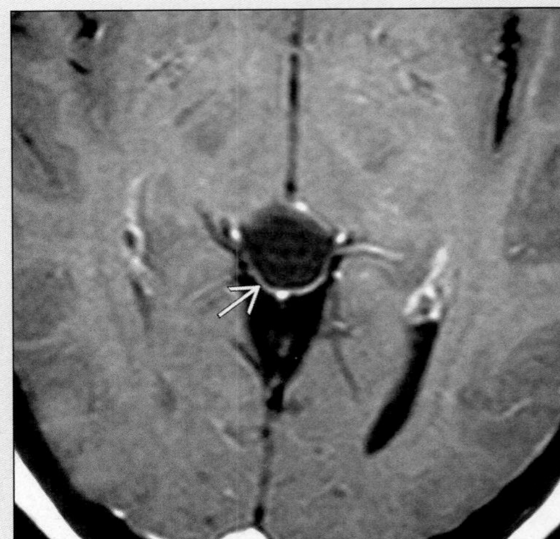

(Left) *Axial NECT shows a 15 mm partially calcified pineal gland cyst →. No surgery was performed. Approximately 25% of pineal cysts show a rim or nodular calcification.* ***(Right)*** *Axial T1 C+ MR shows smooth, thin rim enhancement around a pineal gland cyst →. The cyst fluid was slightly hyperintense to CSF on the precontrast study (not shown). This was an incidental finding in an asymptomatic patient.*

PINEAL CYST

TERMINOLOGY

Abbreviations

- Pineal cyst (PC)

Synonyms

- Glial cyst of pineal gland

Definitions

- Nonneoplastic intrapineal glial-lined cyst

IMAGING

General Features

- Best diagnostic clue
  - Fluid-filled pineal region mass
- Location
  - Above, clearly distinct from tectum
  - Below velum interpositum, internal cerebral veins (ICVs)
- Size
  - Most are small (< 1 cm)
  - Occasionally up to 2 cm or more
- Morphology
  - Round/ovoid, relatively thin-walled cyst
    - 95% minimal/no compression of tectum, aqueduct
    - 5% flatten tectum, occasionally compress aqueduct
    - Variable hydrocephalus (with large cysts or cyst apoplexy)
      - Enlarged 3rd, lateral ventricles
      - Normal 4th ventricle

CT Findings

- NECT
  - Sharply demarcated, smooth cyst behind 3rd ventricle
    - Fluid iso-/slightly hyperdense to CSF
    - Ca++ in cyst wall (25%)
    - Rare: Hyperdense cyst
      - Acute hemorrhage ("pineal apoplexy")
- CECT
  - Rim or nodular enhancement

MR Findings

- T1WI
  - Slightly hyperintense to CSF (55-60%)
  - Isointense (40%)
  - Hemorrhagic (heterogeneous signal intensity) (1-2%)
- T2WI
  - Iso-/slightly hyperintense to CSF
  - Multicystic/septated (20-25%)
- PD/intermediate
  - Hyperintense to CSF (85-90%)
- FLAIR
  - Does not suppress
  - Moderately hyperintense
- T2* GRE
  - Usually normal
  - Uncommon: Blooming (old or recent hemorrhage)
- DWI
  - Typically shows no restriction
- T1WI C+
  - ~ 90% enhance
    - Most common: Thin rim (≤ 2 mm)
      - Can be partial, eccentric, incomplete
    - Less common: Nodular, irregular enhancement
    - Cystic areas may fill in on delayed scans, resemble solid tumor
- MRV
  - Internal cerebral veins (ICVs) may be elevated by large lesions
- MRS
  - Neuronal markers absent

Angiographic Findings

- Arterial phase almost always normal
- Venous phase
  - May show elevation, displacement of ICVs if large PC present
  - Thalamostriate veins splayed, bowed if hydrocephalus present

Imaging Recommendations

- Best imaging tool
  - MR ± contrast
    - DWI, T2*, MRS may be helpful
- Protocol advice
  - Use thin sections (3 mm or less) for detecting, defining lesions in this anatomically complex region

DIFFERENTIAL DIAGNOSIS

Normal Pineal Gland

- Can be cystic
- 3 anatomic appearances on contrast-enhanced imaging
  - Nodule (52%)
  - Crescent (26%)
  - Ring-like (22%)

Pineocytoma

- Usually solid or partially solid/cystic
- Purely cystic pineocytoma much less common
  - May be indistinguishable on imaging studies
  - Require histology for definitive diagnosis
- Both pineal cyst, indolent pineocytoma may not change on serial imaging

Epidermoid Cyst

- Quadrigeminal cistern relatively rare location
- "Cauliflower" configuration
- Mild/moderate restriction on DWI

Arachnoid Cyst

- No Ca++, enhancement
- Follows CSF attenuation, signal intensity

PATHOLOGY

General Features

- Etiology
  - Etiology/pathogenesis: 3 major theories

PINEAL CYST

- Enlargement of embryonic pineal cavity
- Ischemic glial degeneration ± hemorrhagic expansion
- Small preexisting cysts enlarge with hormonal influences
- Genetics
  - None known
- Associated abnormalities
  - Hydrocephalus (uncommon)
  - Embryology
    - Primitive pineal diverticulum divides into pineal recess, cavum pineal
    - Cavum pineal usually obliterated by glial fibers
    - Incomplete obliteration may leave residual cavity

Gross Pathologic & Surgical Features

- Smooth, soft, tan to yellow cyst wall
  - Cavity can be uni- or multilocular
  - Fluid contents vary
    - Clear yellow (most common) to hemorrhagic
- 80% < 10 mm
- Can be large (reported up to 4.5 cm)

Microscopic Features

- Delicate (usually incomplete) outer leptomeningeal layer
- Middle layer of attenuated pineal parenchyma
  - ± Ca++
- Inner layer of dense fibrillar glial tissue with
  - Variable granular bodies
  - ± hemosiderin-laden macrophages
- Compare with pineocytoma
  - Pseudolobular arrangement of small, round cells with pleomorphic nuclei
  - "Pinocytic" rosettes
  - Neuronal differentiation
    - NSE, synaptophysin positive cells

CLINICAL ISSUES

Presentation

- Most common signs/symptoms
  - Vast majority clinically silent
    - Discovered incidentally at imaging/autopsy
  - Large cysts (> 1 cm) may become symptomatic
    - 50% headache (aqueduct compression, hydrocephalus)
    - 10% Parinaud syndrome (tectal compression)
  - Rare: "Pineal apoplexy"
    - Severe headache (can be "thunderclap," mimic aneurysmal subarachnoid hemorrhage)
    - Intracystic hemorrhage, acute hydrocephalus, sudden death
- Clinical profile
  - Young female with nonfocal headache

Demographics

- Age
  - Can occur at **any** age
    - Older adults > children
  - Incidence among women between 21-30 years significantly higher than any other group
    - Incidence in women decreases with age
    - No change in males
- Gender
  - F:M = 3:1
- Ethnicity
  - None known
- Epidemiology
  - 1-5% of normal MRs
    - 2% in children, young adults
  - 25-40% of microscopic cysts within pineal gland found at autopsy

Natural History & Prognosis

- Size generally remains unchanged in males
- Cystic expansion of pineal in some females begins in adolescence, decreases with aging
- Rare: Sudden expansion, hemorrhage ("pineal apoplexy")

Treatment

- Usually none
- Atypical/symptomatic lesions may require stereotactic aspiration or biopsy/resection
  - Preferred approach = infratentorial supracerebellar

DIAGNOSTIC CHECKLIST

Consider

- PCs often asymptomatic, incidental MR finding
- MR appearance of PCs varies
  - Uncomplicated cystic mass
  - Mass with hemorrhage, enhancement, or hydrocephalus
- Heterogeneous, nodular, or ring-like enhancing pineal mass **may be benign cyst, not neoplasm**

Image Interpretation Pearls

- Cannot distinguish benign PC from neoplasm (pineocytoma) on basis of imaging studies alone
- Histopathology required for definitive diagnosis
  - May be complicated by tissue fragmentation, cyst collapse, reactive changes in adjacent tissue

SELECTED REFERENCES

1. Al-Holou W et al: Prevalence of pineal cysts in children and young adults. J Neurosurg Pediatrics. 4(3): 230-236, 2009
2. Cauley KA et al: Serial follow-up MRI of indeterminate cystic lesions of the pineal region: experience at a rural tertiary care referral center. AJR Am J Roentgenol. 193(2):533-7, 2009
3. Costa F et al: Symptomatic pineal cyst: case report and review of the literature. Minim Invasive Neurosurg. 51(4):231-3, 2008
4. Fakhran S et al: Pineocytoma mimicking a pineal cyst on imaging: true diagnostic dilemma or a case of incomplete imaging? AJNR Am J Neuroradiol. 29(1):159-63, 2008
5. Taraszewska A et al: Asymptomatic and symptomatic glial cysts of the pineal gland. Folia Neuropathol. 46(3):186-95, 2008
6. Michielsen G et al: Symptomatic pineal cysts: clinical manifestations and management. Acta Neurochir (Wien). 144(3):233-42; discussion 242, 2002
7. Korogi Y et al: MRI of pineal region tumors. J Neurooncol. 54(3):251-61, 2001

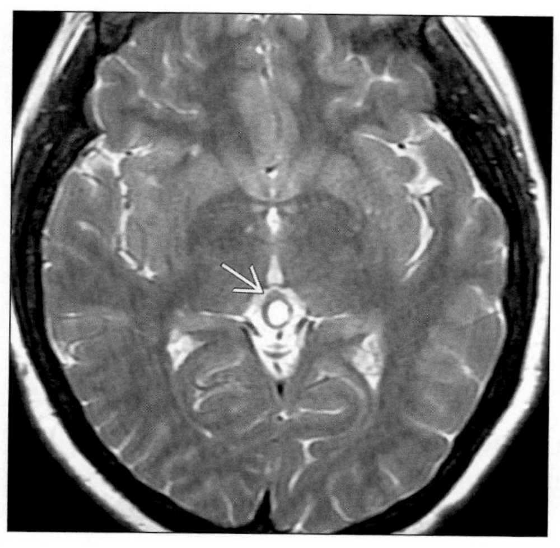

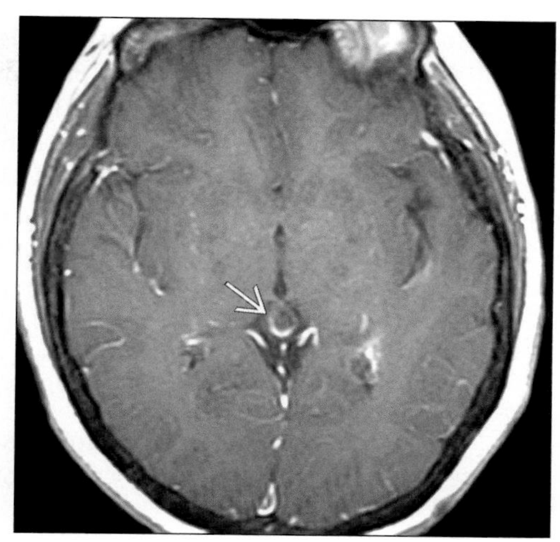

(Left) *Axial T2WI MR in a 42-year-old man shows a thick-walled, slightly nodular pineal cyst ➡. Cyst fluid was hyperintense to CSF on FLAIR (not shown) and did not restrict on DWI.* ***(Right)*** *Axial T1WI C+ MR in the same case shows asymmetric rim enhancement of the cyst wall ➡. This was an incidental finding on normal brain MR.*

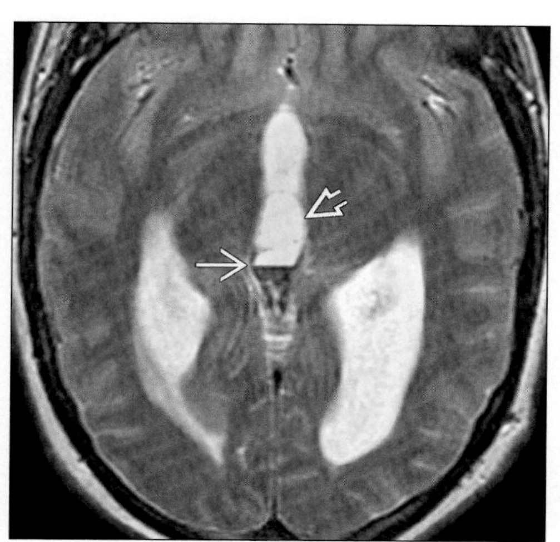

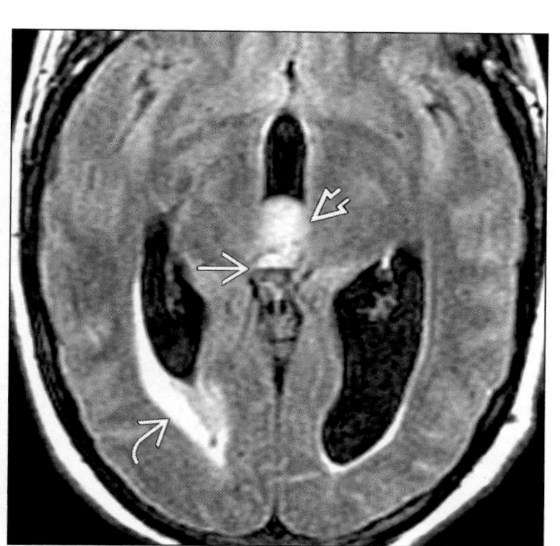

(Left) *Axial T2WI in a 29-year-old pregnant woman, with a 1-month history of daily occipital headache that increased with blurred vision on bending forward, shows a large bilobed pineal cyst ⇨ projecting into the 3rd ventricle. Fluid-fluid level ➡ suggests acute hemorrhage.* ***(Right)*** *Axial FLAIR in the same patient shows blood-fluid level ➡ in the hyperintense pineal cyst ⇨. Note the transependymal CSF flow ↗. A "pineal apoplexy," benign, nonneoplastic hemorrhagic cyst was found at surgery.*

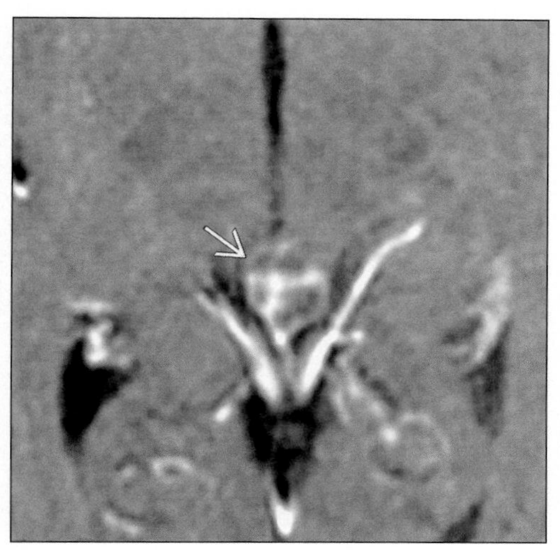

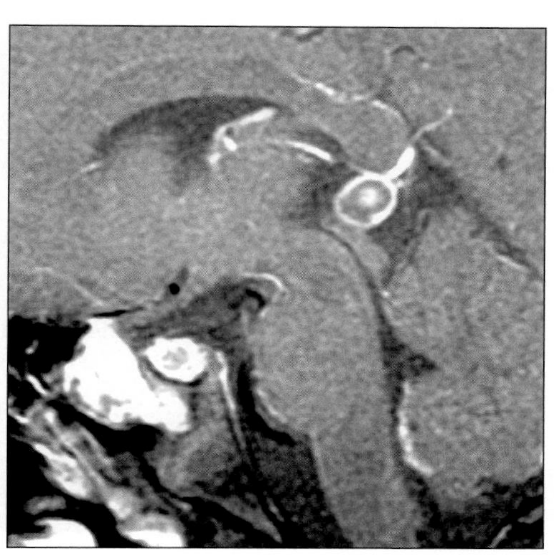

(Left) *Axial T1WI C+ MR shows a multicystic pineal gland ➡ with rim and septal enhancement, a less common appearance of pineal cyst.* ***(Right)*** *Sagittal T1WI C+ MR shows an enlarged pineal gland with rim enhancement and a central enhancing nodule. "Target" appearance is atypical for a pineal cyst. A benign nonneoplastic glial cyst of the pineal gland was found at surgery. Pineal cysts, especially variants like this, can be clinically and radiologically indistinguishable from cystic neoplasms.*

CHOROID PLEXUS CYST

Key Facts

Terminology
- Nonneoplastic, noninflammatory cysts
  - Contained within choroid plexus
  - Lined by compressed connective tissue

Imaging
- General
  - Usually small (2-8 mm)
  - Rare: Large cysts (> 2 cm)
  - Usually multiple, often bilateral
- CT
  - Isodense or slightly hyperdense to CSF
  - Irregular, peripheral Ca++ common in adults
- MR
  - Isointense or slightly hyperintense compared to CSF on T1WI
  - 2/3 isointense, 1/3 hypointense on FLAIR
  - 60-80% show restricted diffusion
  - Enhancement (ring, nodular, solid) varies from none to strong

Top Differential Diagnoses
- Ependymal cyst
- Neurocysticercosis
- Epidermoid cyst
- Choroid plexus papilloma
  - Purely cystic CPP very rare

Clinical Issues
- Found at both ends of age spectrum
  - Common in fetus, infants, older adults
  - Less common in children, young adults
- Clinically silent, discovered incidentally

Diagnostic Checklist
- Most common choroid plexus mass in adults = CPC

*(**Left**) Axial graphic shows multiple cystic masses in the choroid plexus glomi ⇨, often seen incidentally on scans of middle-aged and older adults. Most are degenerative xanthogranulomas. (**Right**) Axial NECT obtained in an elderly adult with minor head trauma and normal neurological examination shows dense peripheral calcifications ➡ around cystic masses in the atria of both lateral ventricles. This was an incidental finding with no clinical significance.*

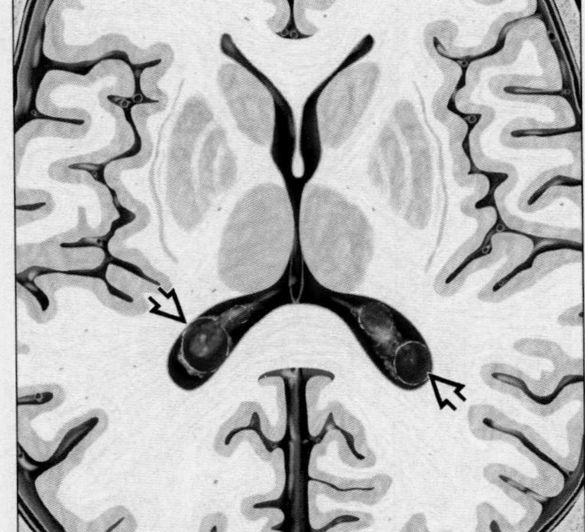

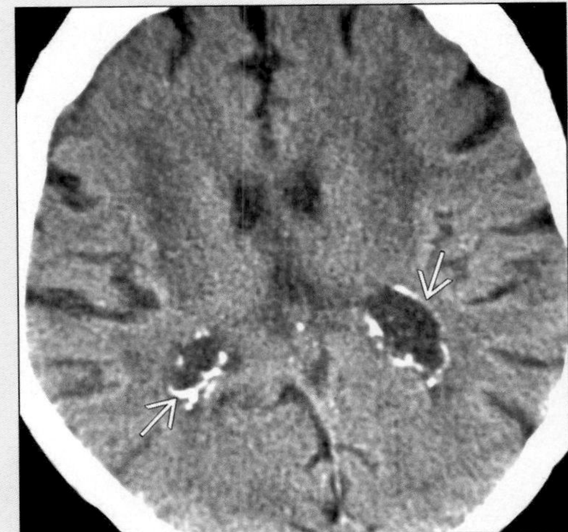

*(**Left**) Axial T1WI C+ FS MR in a 52-year-old man with headaches and no neurological abnormalities shows multiple mixed solid and ring-enhancing cysts in the atria of both lateral ventricles ➡. (**Right**) Coronal T1WI C+ MR in the same patient shows multiple small to medium-sized, ring-enhancing cysts filling the atria of both lateral ventricles ➡.*

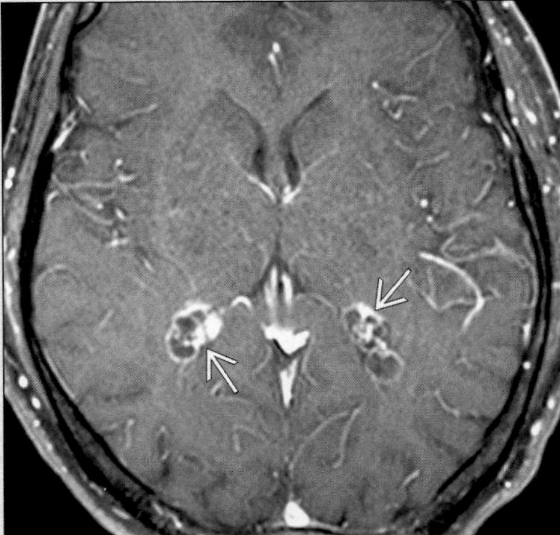

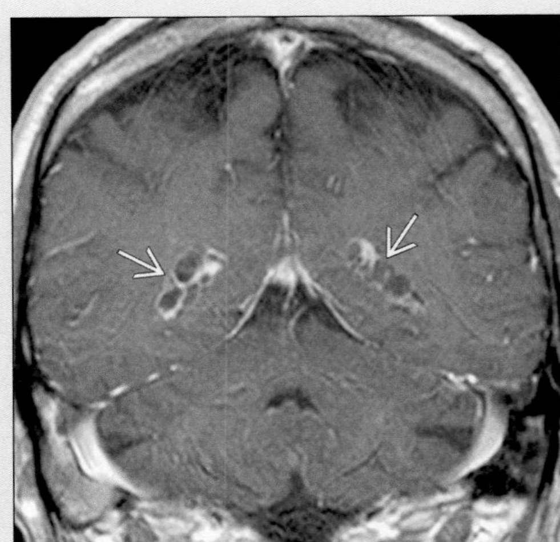

CHOROID PLEXUS CYST

TERMINOLOGY

Abbreviations

- Choroid plexus cyst (CPC)
- Choroid plexus xanthogranuloma (CPX)

Definitions

- Nonneoplastic, noninflammatory cysts of choroid plexus
  - Lined by compressed connective tissue
  - Adult: CPC is common incidental finding on imaging studies in older patients (~ 40% prevalence)
  - Fetus: CPCs seen in 1% of 2nd trimester pregnancies

IMAGING

General Features

- Best diagnostic clue
  - Older patient with "bright" choroid plexi on T2WI
  - Fetus or newborn with large (> 2 mm) choroid plexus cyst(s) on US
- Location
  - Most common: Atria of lateral ventricles
    - Attached to or within choroid plexus
    - > 2/3 bilateral
  - Less common: 3rd and 4th ventricles
- Size
  - Variable
    - Usually small (2-8 mm)
    - Often multiple
    - Rare: Large cysts (> 2 cm)
- Morphology
  - Cystic or nodular/partially cystic mass(es) in choroid plexus glomi

CT Findings

- NECT
  - Iso-/slightly hyperdense to CSF
  - Irregular, peripheral Ca++ in majority of adult cases
- CECT
  - Varies from none to rim of solid enhancement

MR Findings

- T1WI
  - Isointense or slightly hyperintense compared to CSF
- T2WI
  - Hyperintense compared to CSF
- PD/intermediate
  - Hyperintense
- FLAIR
  - 2/3 isointense, 1/3 hypointense
- T2* GRE
  - Foci of "blooming" common
    - Ca++ (intracystic hemorrhage rare)
- DWI
  - 60-80% show restricted diffusion (high signal)
- T1WI C+
  - Enhancement varies from none to strong
  - Variable pattern (solid, ring, nodular)
  - Delayed scans may show filling in of contrast within cysts

Ultrasonographic Findings

- Grayscale ultrasound
  - Prenatal US
    - Cyst > 2 mm surrounded by echogenic choroid
    - In absence of other abnormalities, low risk for chromosomal abnormalities

Imaging Recommendations

- Best imaging tool
  - Adults: MR ± contrast
  - Fetus, newborn
    - Antenatal: Maternal US or MR
    - Postnatal: US of infant with anterior, posterior, mastoid fontanelles as acoustic windows
- Protocol advice
  - MR with contrast, FLAIR, DWI
  - US transverse view of lateral ventricle at atrial level

DIFFERENTIAL DIAGNOSIS

Ependymal Cyst

- Does not enhance
- Usually unilateral
- Attenuation, signal more like CSF
- Immunohistochemistry differentiates

Neurocysticercosis (NCC)

- Multiple cysts common (subarachnoid space, parenchyma ventricles)
- Not associated with choroid plexus
- Look for scolex, other signs of NCC (e.g., parenchymal Ca++)
- May be migratory

Epidermoid Cyst

- Intraventricular location rare (4th > > lateral ventricle)
- "Cauliflower," insinuating pattern

Choroid Plexus Papilloma (CPP)

- Children < 5 years
- Strong, relatively uniform enhancement
- Purely cystic CPP very rare

Villous Hyperplasia of Choroid Plexus

- Very rare
- Often overproduces CSF
- Causes hydrocephalus

Ultrasound "Pseudolesion"

- Tiny anechoic areas in fetal choroid are normal, not CPC
- Normal fluid-filled atria can be confused with CPC on transverse view
- "Split" or "truncated" choroid can mimic CPC

Neoplasm

- Meningioma (usually solid)
- Metastasis (rarely cystic)
- Cystic astrocytoma (rare in older patients)

Sturge-Weber Syndrome

- Enlarged "angiomatous" choroid plexus ipsilateral to malformation

CHOROID PLEXUS CYST

Choroid plexus Infarct

- Usually seen in choroid artery infarct
- May cause ↑ intraventricular signal on DWI

PATHOLOGY

General Features

- Etiology
  - CPCs
    - Lipid from desquamating, degenerating choroid epithelium accumulates in choroid plexus
    - Lipid provokes xanthomatous response
- Genetics
  - Large fetal choroid plexus cysts associated with trisomy 21 or 18 in only 6% of cases
  - Presence of additional malformations increases risk factors for aneuploidy
- Associated abnormalities
  - Fetal CPC
    - Trisomy 18 (mildly increased risk < 2x baseline risk)
    - Trisomy 21 (only if other markers present)
  - Adult CPC: May cause obstructive hydrocephalus (rare)
  - Aicardi syndrome: Usually associated with choroid plexus papillomas but may occur with choroid plexus cysts

Gross Pathologic & Surgical Features

- CPC commonly found at autopsy in middle-aged, older adults
  - Nodular, partly cystic, yellowish-gray masses in choroid plexus glomus
  - Contents often gelatinous, highly proteinaceous
  - Rare: Hemorrhage

Microscopic Features

- Neuroepithelial microcysts
- Trapped choroid plexus epithelium often associated
- Cysts contain nests of foamy, lipid-laden histiocytes
- Foreign body giant cells
- Chronic inflammatory infiltrates (lymphocytes, plasma cells)
- Cholesterol clefts, hemosiderin
- Peripheral psammomatous Ca++ common
- Immunohistochemistry positive for prealbumin, cytokeratins, GFAP, EMA, S100

CLINICAL ISSUES

Presentation

- Most common signs/symptoms
  - Adult CPC
    - Typical: Clinically silent, discovered incidentally at autopsy/imaging
    - Rare: Headache

Demographics

- Age
  - Found at both ends of age spectrum
    - Adult CPC: Prevalence increases with age
    - Fetal CPC: Prevalence decreases with age
- Gender
  - No known prevalence
- Ethnicity
  - No known prevalence
- Epidemiology
  - Most common type of neuroepithelial cyst
    - 1% of all pregnancies on routine US
    - 50% of fetuses with T18
    - Small asymptomatic CPCs found incidentally in more than 1/3 of all autopsied adults

Natural History & Prognosis

- Fetal CPCs
  - Transient finding; typically resolve in 3rd trimester regardless of whether isolated or with associated anomalies
  - CPC + minor markers = 20% risk for chromosome abnormality
  - CPC + major markers = 50% risk for chromosome abnormality
- Adult CPCs
  - Usually remain asymptomatic, nonprogressive

Treatment

- Adult CPC: Usually none
  - Rare: Shunt for obstructive hydrocephalus
- Fetal CPC
  - In absence of other markers, none
  - With other markers, amniocentesis warranted

DIAGNOSTIC CHECKLIST

Consider

- Amniocentesis with karyotyping if CPCs + other anomalies (e.g., cardiac anomaly, clenched hands with overlapping fingers, clubfeet) present on fetal US

Image Interpretation Pearls

- Benign degenerative cyst (xanthogranuloma): Most common cause of choroid plexus mass in adults

SELECTED REFERENCES

1. Naeini RM et al: Spectrum of choroid plexus lesions in children. AJR Am J Roentgenol. 192(1):32-40, 2009
2. Herman TE et al: Aicardi syndrome choroid plexus cysts. J Perinatol. 27(5):323-4, 2007
3. Kinoshita T et al: Clinically silent choroid plexus cyst: evaluation by diffusion-weighted MRI. Neuroradiology. 47(4):251-5, 2005
4. Boockvar JA et al: Symptomatic lateral ventricular ependymal cysts: criteria for distinguishing these rare cysts from other symptomatic cysts of the ventricles: case report. Neurosurgery. 46(5):1229-32; discussion 1232-3, 2000
5. Muenchau A et al: Xanthogranuloma and xanthoma of the choroid plexus: evidence for different etiology and pathogenesis. Clin Neuropathol. 16(2):72-6, 1997

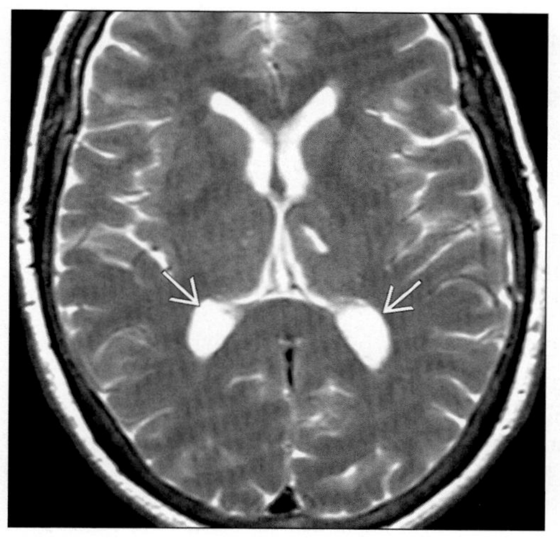

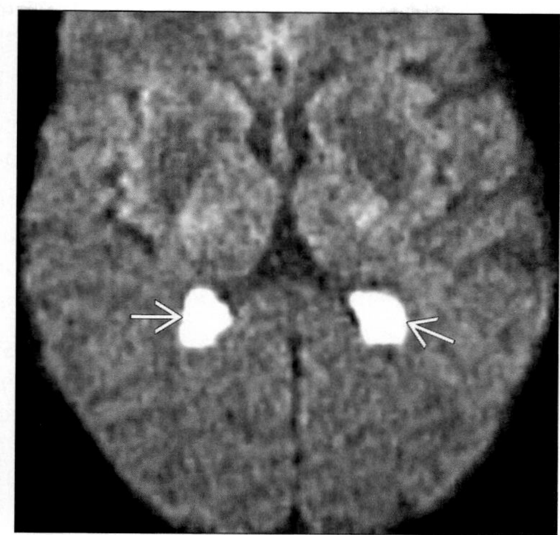

(Left) *Axial T2WI MR in an asymptomatic patient with an old left thalamic infarct shows hyperintense lesions in the atria of both lateral ventricles ➔ that are difficult to see because they are isointense with CSF.* ***(Right)*** *Axial DWI MR shows restriction in the choroid plexus lesions ➔. Choroid plexus cysts often restrict on diffusion-weighted imaging.*

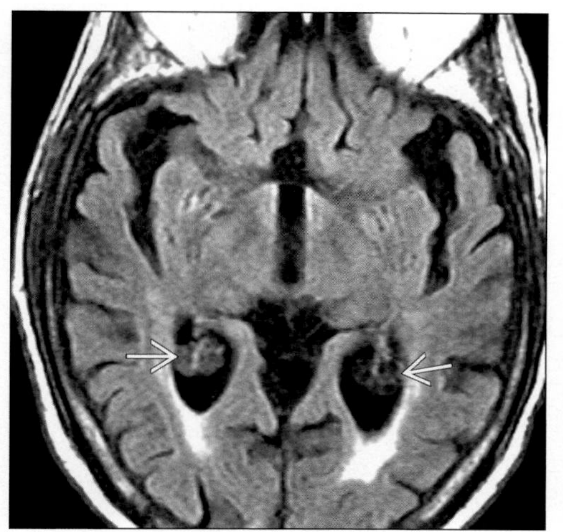

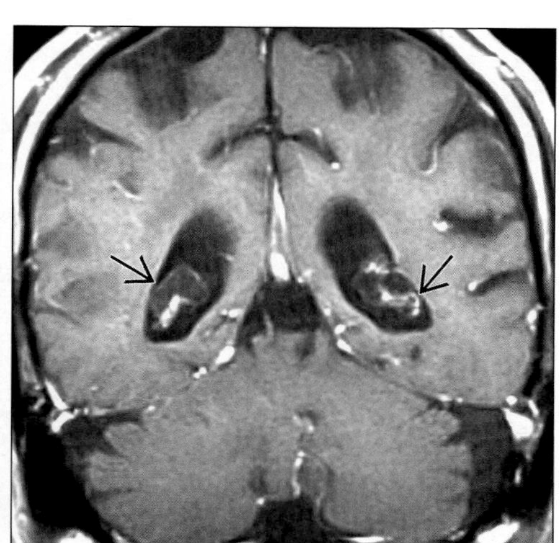

(Left) *Axial FLAIR MR in an elderly hypertensive patient scanned for memory problems shows diffuse atrophy, especially in the temporal lobes. Periventricular hyperintensity is seen around both atria and occipital horns. Note the intraventricular cysts that seem to be "dangling" from the choroid plexus glomi ➔.* ***(Right)*** *Coronal T1WI C+ MR in the same patient shows enhancement around the cyst margins ➔, findings typical for choroid plexus cysts.*

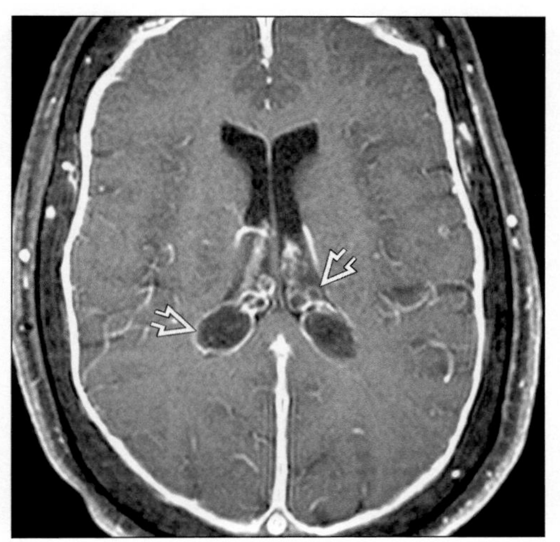

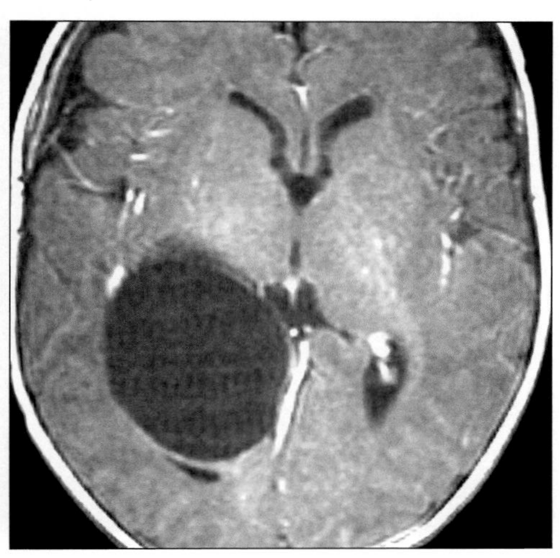

(Left) *Axial T1 C+ FS MR in a patient with a remote history of childhood meningitis shows rim-enhancing cysts in the choroid plexus of both lateral ventricles ➔. The largest cysts are in the atria, but other smaller cysts follow the body of the choroid plexus anteriorly.* ***(Right)*** *Axial T1WI C+ MR in an infant with multiple congenital anomalies shows a huge unilocular choroid plexus cyst in the right lateral ventricle. Scan obtained 5 years later (not shown) demonstrated significant decrease in cyst size.*

EPENDYMAL CYST

Key Facts

Terminology
- Congenital, benign, ependymal-lined cyst of brain

Imaging
- Nonenhancing thin-walled cyst
  - CSF density/intensity
- Most common location = intraventricular (lateral; 3rd rare)
  - Less common: Parenchyma, subarachnoid space

Top Differential Diagnoses
- Asymmetric lateral ventricles (normal variant)
- Choroid plexus cyst
- Arachnoid cyst
- Epidermoid cyst
- Neurenteric cyst
- Porencephalic cyst
- Neurocysticercosis

Pathology
- Thin-walled cyst filled with clear serous liquid
- Fluid-filled space lined by columnar or cuboidal cells

Clinical Issues
- Typically asymptomatic
- Headache, seizure, gait disturbance, dementia
- Symptoms related to CSF obstruction/↑ ICP
- Young adults (typically < 40 years old)
- Interval follow-up typically shows no clinical or imaging changes in asymptomatic lesions

Diagnostic Checklist
- Ependymal cysts may be indistinguishable from other benign intracranial cysts
- Ependymal cysts follow CSF on all MR sequences, including DWI; no enhancement

*(**Left**) Axial graphic depicts a typical ependymal cyst of the lateral ventricle →, seen here as a CSF-containing simple cyst that displaces the choroid plexus around it. Ependymal cysts typically follow CSF signal on all sequences. (**Right**) Axial T2WI MR in a 25-year-old woman with daily headaches shows a thin-walled ependymal cyst → in the atrium of the lateral ventricle. The lateral ventricle is not obstructed, and the relationship of the cyst to the patient's symptoms is unclear.*

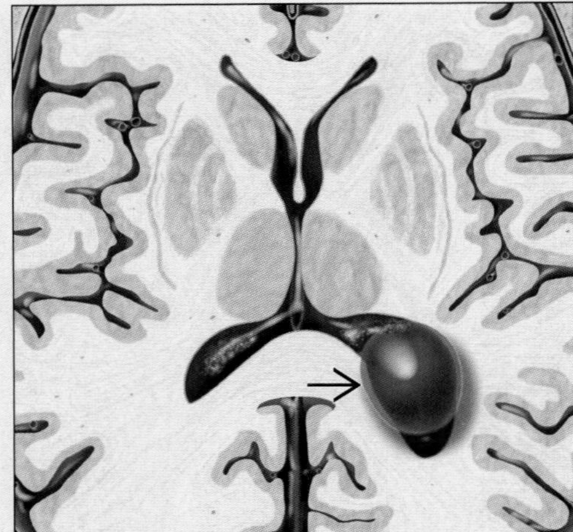

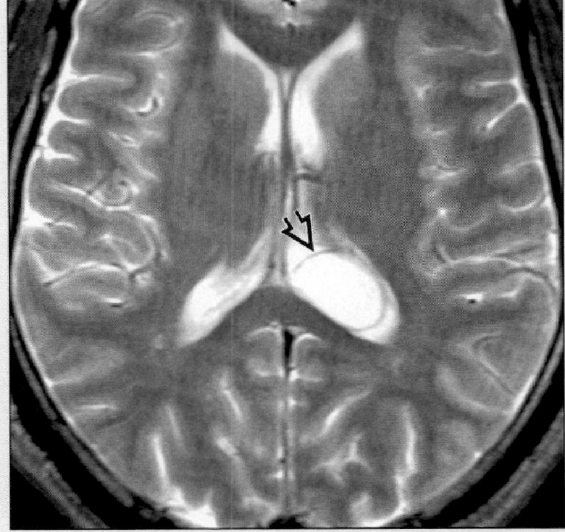

*(**Left**) Axial T2WI MR in a 25-year-old woman with headaches shows an enlarged, trapped temporal horn → that is expanded and obstructed by a thin-walled CSF-containing ependymal cyst →. (**Right**) Sagittal T2WI MR in a 2 year old with failure to thrive and severe papilledema on physical examination shows a CSF cyst within the 3rd ventricle that thins and depresses the hypothalamus → and elevates the ICVs →. An ependymal cyst of the 3rd ventricle was found at surgery and fenestrated.*

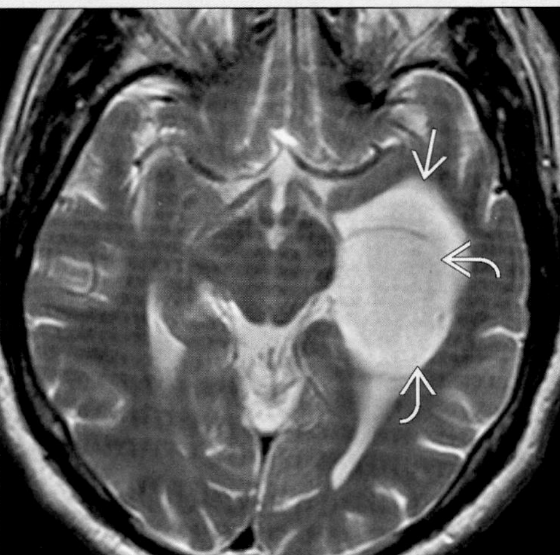

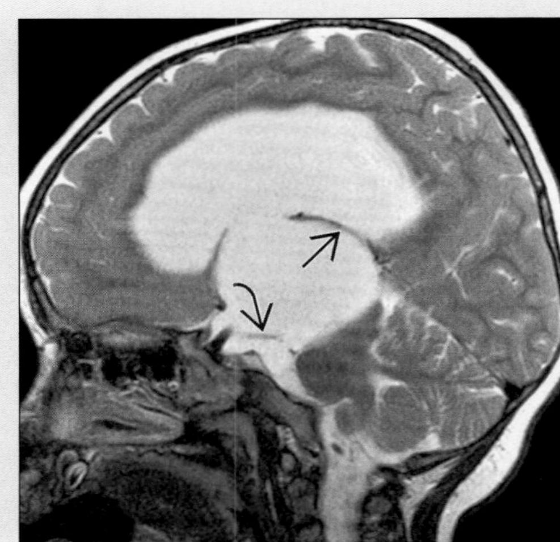

EPENDYMAL CYST

TERMINOLOGY

Abbreviations

- Ependymal cyst (EC)

Synonyms

- Neuroepithelial cyst, glioependymal cyst

Definitions

- Congenital, benign, ependymal-lined cyst of brain

IMAGING

General Features

- Best diagnostic clue
  - Nonenhancing, thin-walled, CSF density/intensity
- Location
  - Most common: Intraventricular (lateral > 3rd, 4th)
  - Less common: Cerebral parenchyma
  - Rare: Subarachnoid space
- Size
  - Typically small (2-3 mm) but up to 8-9 cm reported
- Morphology
  - Smooth, thin-walled cyst

CT Findings

- NECT
  - Cyst is isodense to CSF; Ca++ extremely rare
- CECT
  - No enhancement

MR Findings

- T1WI
  - Isointense to CSF, cyst wall may be seen
- T2WI
  - Isointense to hyperintense to CSF (protein content)
- FLAIR
  - Isointense to CSF (suppresses)
- DWI
  - No diffusion restriction
- T1WI C+
  - No enhancement

Imaging Recommendations

- Best imaging tool
  - Multiplanar MR with T1WI C+, DWI

DIFFERENTIAL DIAGNOSIS

Asymmetric Ventricles

- Lateral ventricle asymmetry, normal variant

Choroid Plexus Cyst

- Typically bilateral, arises in choroid plexus glomus

Neurocysticercosis

- Scolex present; does not suppress on FLAIR

Arachnoid Cyst

- May be indistinguishable; CSF intensity

Epidermoid Cyst

- Subarachnoid space > ventricles (4th most common)
- Heterogeneous on FLAIR, DWI positive

Neurenteric Cyst

- Extraaxial (typically posterior fossa) > parenchyma

PATHOLOGY

Gross Pathologic & Surgical Features

- Thin-walled cyst filled with clear serous liquid

Microscopic Features

- Fluid-filled space lined by columnar or cuboidal cells

CLINICAL ISSUES

Presentation

- Most common signs/symptoms
  - Typically asymptomatic
- Other signs/symptoms
  - Headache, seizure, gait disturbance, dementia
  - Symptoms related to CSF obstruction/↑ ICP

Demographics

- Age
  - Young adults (typically < 40 years old)
- Gender
  - Male predominance

Natural History & Prognosis

- Uncommon so natural history unknown
- Interval follow-up typically shows no clinical or imaging changes in asymptomatic lesions
- Recurrence after surgical intervention uncommon

Treatment

- If asymptomatic, conservative management
- If symptomatic, surgical excision or decompression

DIAGNOSTIC CHECKLIST

Consider

- Ependymal cysts may be indistinguishable from other benign intracranial cysts

Image Interpretation Pearls

- Ependymal cysts follow CSF on all MR sequences, including DWI; no enhancement

SELECTED REFERENCES

1. Utsunomiya H et al: Midline cystic malformations of the brain: imaging diagnosis and classification based on embryologic analysis. Radiat Med. 24(6):471-81, 2006
2. Yano S et al: Third ventricular ependymal cyst presenting with acute hydrocephalus. Pediatr Neurosurg. 42(4):245-8, 2006
3. Pawar SJ et al: Giant ependymal cyst of the temporal horn -- an unusual presentation. Case report with review of the literature. Pediatr Neurosurg. 34(6):306-10, 2001

PORENCEPHALIC CYST

Key Facts

Terminology

- CSF-filled parenchymal cavity
  - Deep, unilateral/bilateral cavity/excavation
  - Usually communicates with ventricle &/or subarachnoid space
  - Lined by reactive gliosis/astrocytic proliferation
- Congenital (perinatal brain destruction) or acquired (trauma, infection, etc)

Imaging

- Best diagnostic clue: CSF-filled cavities with enlarged adjacent ventricle
- MR: Smooth-walled cavity; CSF isointense; lined by gliotic white matter

Top Differential Diagnoses

- Consider arachnoid, ependymal, neoplastic, or inflammatory cyst
- Agenesis of corpus callosum
- Encephalomalacia
- Schizencephaly
- Dandy-Walker malformation
- Hydranencephaly

Pathology

- Congenital: In utero destructive process caused by cerebral vascular events or infectious injury (CMV)
- Acquired: Injury later in life, following head trauma, surgery, vascular occlusion, or infection
- Genetics: Rare, autosomal dominant familial porencephaly → procollagen defect

Clinical Issues

- Spastic hemiplegia most common symptom
- Indications for therapy: Mass effect, localized/generalized refractory symptoms

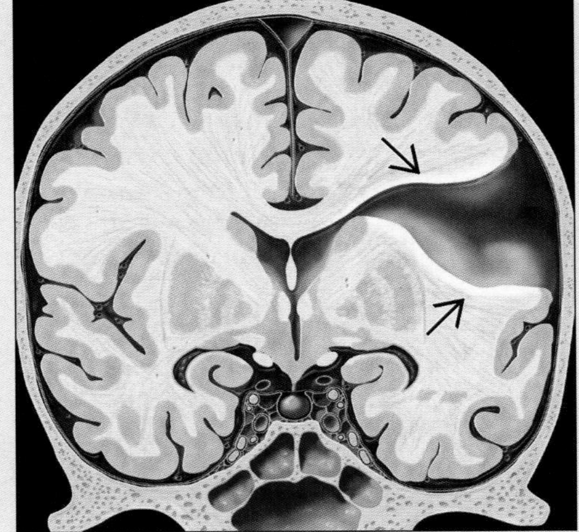

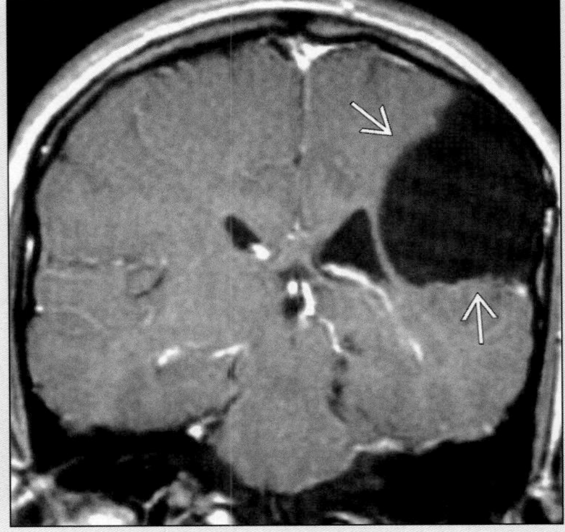

(Left) *Coronal graphic illustrates an intraparenchymal CSF-filled cavity that communicates with the left lateral ventricle and subarachnoid space. Note the classic porencephalic cyst is lined with gliotic white matter ➙.* ***(Right)*** *Coronal T1WI C+ MR shows a large CSF-filled space in the left parietal lobe ➙. This classic porencephalic cyst does not enhance and appears to be lined with white matter. Adjacent slices demonstrated direct communication with an enlarged lateral ventricle (not shown).*

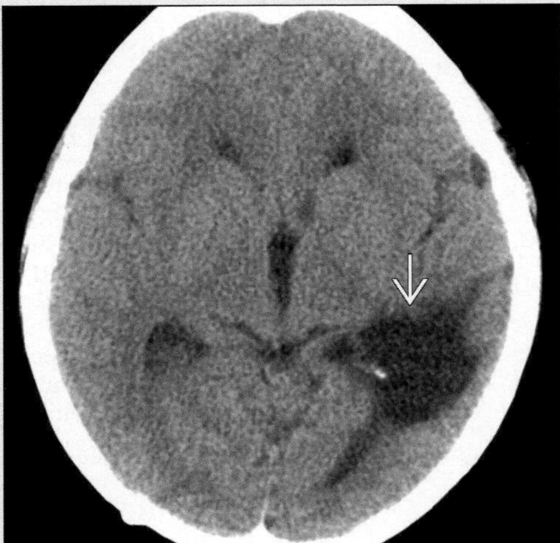

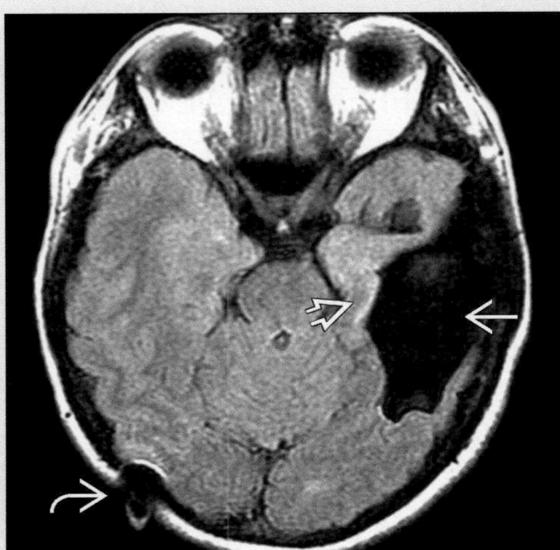

(Left) *Axial NECT demonstrates a CSF-density parenchymal defect ➙ communicating with the atrium of the left lateral ventricle, accompanied by slight dilatation of the occipital horn.* ***(Right)*** *Axial FLAIR reveals a CSF intensity parenchymal defect, which was isointense to CSF on all sequences, including FLAIR nulling ➙. Also note the small amount of associated white matter gliosis ➙. Susceptibility artifact is secondary to a ventriculostomy shunt ➙.*

PORENCEPHALIC CYST

TERMINOLOGY

Synonyms

- Porencephaly

Definitions

- Various definitions of porencephaly
  - Congenital/acquired CSF-filled cavity that usually communicates with ventricular system
    - Deep, unilateral/bilateral cavities or excavations
    - Lined by reactive gliosis/astrocytic proliferation
  - Presence of cysts/cavities in brain parenchyma
    - Communicating by "pore" with arachnoid space
  - Cavities arising in fetal life or early infancy
    - Brain destruction during perinatal period
    - Frequently communicate with subarachnoid space &/or lateral ventricles

IMAGING

General Features

- Best diagnostic clue
  - CSF-filled cavities; enlarged adjacent ventricle
- Location
  - Often corresponds to territories supplied by cerebral arteries (ischemic injury in mid-gestation)
  - Cortical/subcortical cavity, unilateral/bilateral
  - Usually connected with a lateral ventricle
- Size
  - Varies from small to enormous

CT Findings

- NECT
  - Intraparenchymal smooth-walled cavity
    - Isodense with CSF
  - Directly communicates with ventricle
  - May see thin membrane separating cavity from ventricle
- CECT
  - No contrast enhancement of fluid-filled cavity
- Bone CT
  - Skull remodeling from chronic CSF pulsation
- CTA
  - Absence of vessels at site of porencephaly

MR Findings

- T1WI
  - Smooth-walled cavity; CSF isointense; lined by WM
- T2WI
  - Brain atrophy, gliosis common; CSF isointense; lined by white matter
- FLAIR
  - Accurately depicts CSF content of cyst and gliosis
- T1WI C+
  - Nonenhancing cyst

Ultrasonographic Findings

- Prenatal ultrasound for congenital porencephaly
  - Solitary or multiple echo-spared lesions(s)
  - Some cortical tissue may be preserved

Nonvascular Interventions

- Myelography
  - Contrast material injected into lumbar region may fill cystic space

Nuclear Medicine Findings

- PET
  - Area of absent glucose metabolism

Imaging Recommendations

- Best imaging tool
  - MR
- Protocol advice
  - FLAIR

DIFFERENTIAL DIAGNOSIS

Arachnoid Cyst

- CSF-isointense extraaxial cyst that exerts variable degrees of mass effect
- Unlike porencephalic cyst, extraaxial and displaces brain tissue away from adjacent skull

Ependymal Cyst

- Intraventricular; brain usually normal

Neoplastic Cyst

- Any cystic appearance of neoplastic processes

Inflammatory Cyst

- Mass effect, contrast enhancement if neoplastic

Agenesis of Corpus Callosum

- CSF-filled space extending cephalad from 3rd ventricle
- Parallel appearance of lateral ventricles
- Colpocephaly: Dilatation of occipital horns and posterior portions of temporal horns

Encephalomalacia

- Late gestational, perinatal, or postnatal injuries (thrombotic/embolic infarction, asphyxia, infection)
- May be slightly hyperdense/hyperintense to CSF (T1, T2, FLAIR)
- Cavity typically does not communicate with ventricle
  - Often contains septations and is lined by astrocytic proliferation

Schizencephaly

- Intraparenchymal cavity lined by gray matter, extending from ventricular surface to brain surface

Dandy-Walker Malformation

- Large median posterior fossa cyst widely communicating with 4th ventricle
- Rotated, raised, and small cerebellar vermis in contact with tentorium
- Upward displacement of tentorium and lateral sinuses

Hydranencephaly

- Early destructive process of developing brain caused by toxoplasmosis, CMV, or arterial occlusion
- Cortex and white matter destroyed and replaced by thin-walled CSF-filled sacs of leptomeninges

PORENCEPHALIC CYST

PATHOLOGY

General Features

- Etiology
  - Congenital: In utero destructive process caused by cerebral vascular events or infectious injury (CMV)
    - May be induced by antenatal trauma, even when mild or not directed at uterine wall
  - Acquired: Injury later in life, following head trauma, surgery, vascular occlusion, or infection
- Genetics
  - Most cases are sporadic
  - Inherited cases often result from bleeding
    - Rare, autosomal dominant familial porencephaly
      - Chromosome 13qter → mutation of collagen *4A1* gene encoding procollagen type IV α1
      - Encodes a basement membrane protein expressed in all tissues
      - ↑ intracerebral hemorrhage risk for life
    - Inherited thrombophilia, most often heterozygosity for factor V Leiden mutation (gene *F5*)
- Associated abnormalities
  - Amygdala-hippocampal atrophy often coexists with congenital porencephaly (95% in some reports)
    - May be bilateral despite unilateral cysts
  - Syndromes: Septo-optic dysplasia, oro-facio-digital syndrome type I, encephalocraniocutaneous lipomatosis, Proteus syndrome, Delleman syndrome, DK-focomelia
  - Alloimmune thrombocytopenia
  - Coagulopathies, e.g., von Willebrand disease, factor V or X deficiency, maternal warfarin use
  - Multiple gestation associated with vascular disruption defects: Large intestinal atresia, transverse limb deficiency, porencephaly, and renal agenesis

Gross Pathologic & Surgical Features

- CSF-filled cavity with smooth walls
  - Lined by gliotic or spongiotic white matter
- Overlying skull
  - May be remodeled due to long-term transmission of CSF pulsations
  - May be thickened when intervening brain tissue precludes transmission of CSF pulsations

Microscopic Features

- Congenital porencephalic cyst
  - Gray and white matter necrosis
  - Fluid-filled, focal cavity with smooth walls and minimal surrounding glial reaction
- Acquired porencephalic cyst
  - Mature brain reacts to injury by significant astrocytic proliferation
  - Resulting cavity often has septations and irregular wall composed primarily of reactive astrocytes

CLINICAL ISSUES

Presentation

- Most common signs/symptoms
  - Spastic hemiplegia most common feature
  - May be associated with severe neurological deficits
    - Mental retardation, medically intractable epilepsy
- Clinical profile
  - Cerebellar symptoms; ophthalmological signs
  - Various forms of cerebral paralysis
  - Seizures, psychomotor retardation

Demographics

- Age
  - Pediatric age most common; also occurs in adults
- Gender
  - Male > female infants, especially with mothers < 20 years
- Epidemiology
  - 2.5% incidence of porencephalic cysts among 1,000 congenital and acquired brain lesions
  - 0.035% prevalence per 10,000 live births

Natural History & Prognosis

- Narrow communication with ventricular system may ↑ pressure in cyst ⇒ mass effect
- Children with neonatal intraparenchymal echodensities and porencephaly have much worse long-term neurodevelopmental outcome

Treatment

- Usually no treatment required
- Indications for therapy: Mass effect, localized/generalized refractory symptoms
  - Cystoperitoneal shunt (preferred)
  - If no communication with ventricular system: Fenestration or partial resection of cyst wall
  - Children with intractable seizures benefit from uncapping and cyst fenestration to lateral ventricle
- Congenital porencephaly should prompt collagen *4A1* genetic screening

DIAGNOSTIC CHECKLIST

Consider

- Arachnoid cyst simulating porencephalic cyst

Image Interpretation Pearls

- Assess hippocampus in setting of seizures

SELECTED REFERENCES

1. de Vries LS et al: COL4A1 mutation in two preterm siblings with antenatal onset of parenchymal hemorrhage. Ann Neurol. 65(1):12-8, 2009

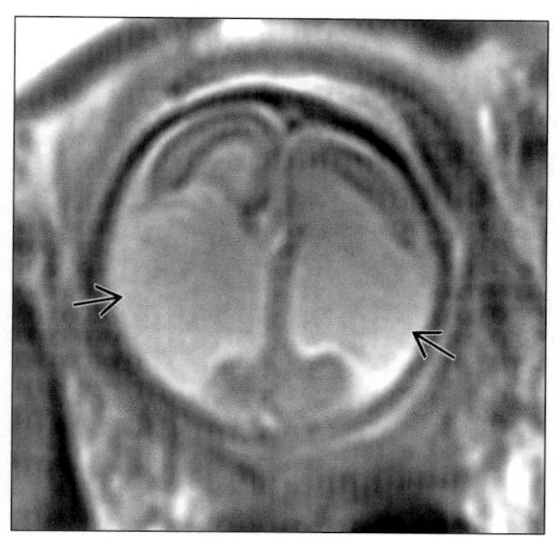

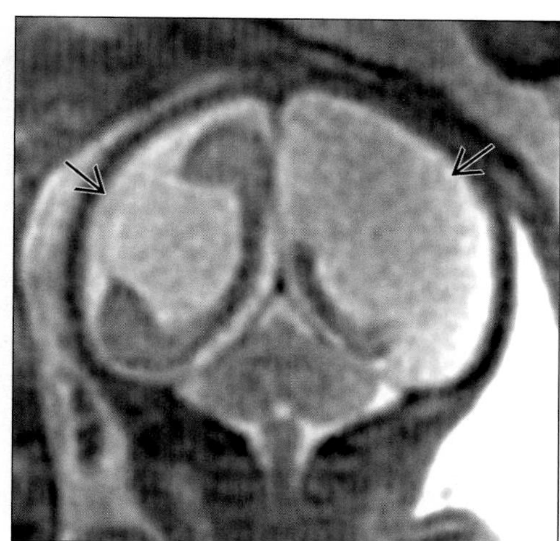

(Left) *Axial T2WI fetal MR technique demonstrates bilateral supratentorial porencephalic cysts* ➙ *as CSF isointense lesions communicating with dilated lateral ventricles.* ***(Right)*** *Coronal T2WI fetal MR in the same patient nicely shows bilateral supratentorial porencephalic cysts* ➙ *with normal posterior fossa contents. Congenital porencephalic cysts are the result of an in utero destructive process, usually cerebral vascular events or infectious injury.*

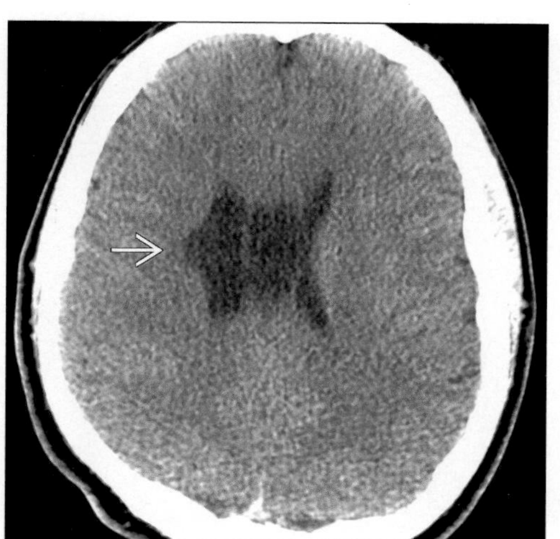

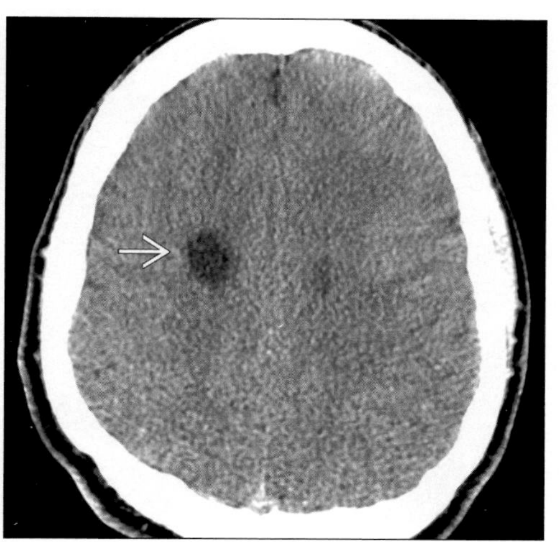

(Left) *Axial NECT reveals porencephalic dilatation of the right lateral ventricle* ➙ *as a smooth-walled extension from the lateral ventricular wall which appears CSF-isodense.* ***(Right)*** *Axial NECT in the same fetal patient shows how the lesion extends into the parenchyma and appears as a deep, smooth-walled, unilateral cavity* ➙*. Note that the overlying brain has a normal morphology.*

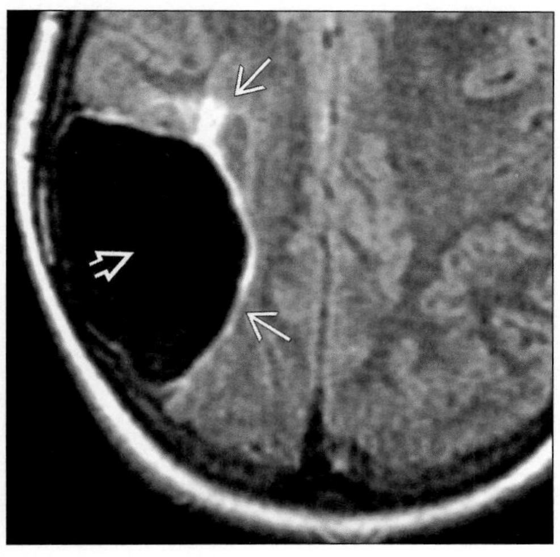

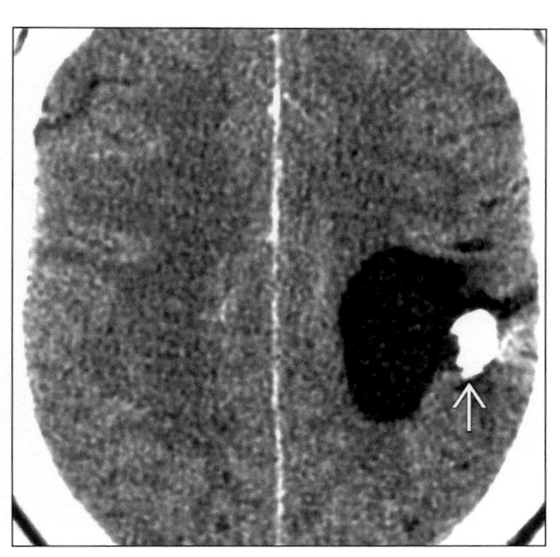

(Left) *Axial FLAIR MR shows the fluid within a right parietal lesion suppressing completely* ➙*. Note how this classic porencephalic cyst is lined by hyperintense gliotic white matter* ➙*.* ***(Right)*** *Axial CECT demonstrates a well-delineated, nonenhancing CSF-density mass containing globular calcification* ➙*. Surgery disclosed a benign, CSF-filled cyst lined with gliotic brain. This is a very unusual case, as porencephalic cysts rarely calcify.*

NEURENTERIC CYST

Key Facts

Terminology

- Congenital endodermal cyst
  - Like Rathke cleft, colloid cysts

Imaging

- General
  - Oblong nonenhancing, slightly hyperintense (to CSF) mass in front of medulla
- Location
  - More common in spine than brain (3:1)
  - 70-75% of intracranial NECs infratentorial, extraaxial
  - Anterior/lateral to pontomedullary junction
  - 25-30% supratentorial (suprasellar, cerebral hemispheres)
- CT
  - Hypo-/iso-/hyperdense, no Ca++
  - Bony anomalies usually absent
- MR
  - Almost always iso-/hyperintense to CSF on T1WI
  - 90% hyperintense to CSF, 10% hypointense on T2WI
  - Usually does not restrict on DWI
  - Usually no enhancement (mild rim in some)

Top Differential Diagnoses

- Epidermoid cyst
- Dermoid cyst
- Arachnoid cyst
- Schwannoma
- Other endodermal cysts (e.g., Rathke cleft, colloid)
- Ecchordosis physaliphora

Diagnostic Checklist

- Mass in front of brainstem, hyperdense/hyperintense to CSF may be neurenteric cyst

*(**Left**) Sagittal graphic shows a classic neurenteric cyst ⇨. Intracranial NECs are most often found near the midline, anterior to the brainstem. (**Right**) Sagittal T1WI MR shows a subtle lobulated mass ➔ anterior to the pontomedullary junction. The lesion is isointense with the brain on this sequence and was very hyperintense on T2WI. It did not suppress on FLAIR, did not restrict on DWI, and showed no enhancement. A neurenteric cyst was found at surgery.*

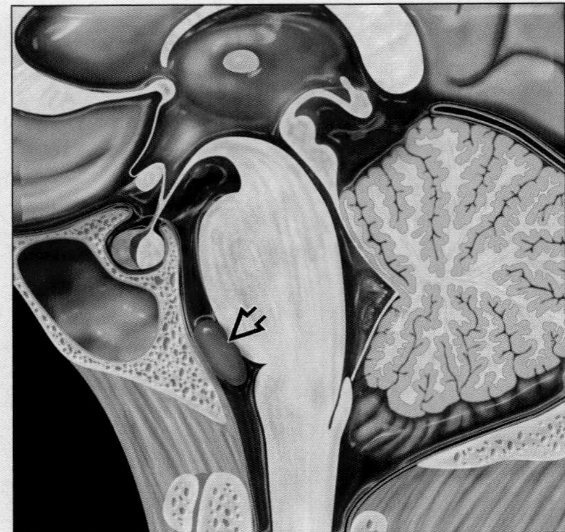

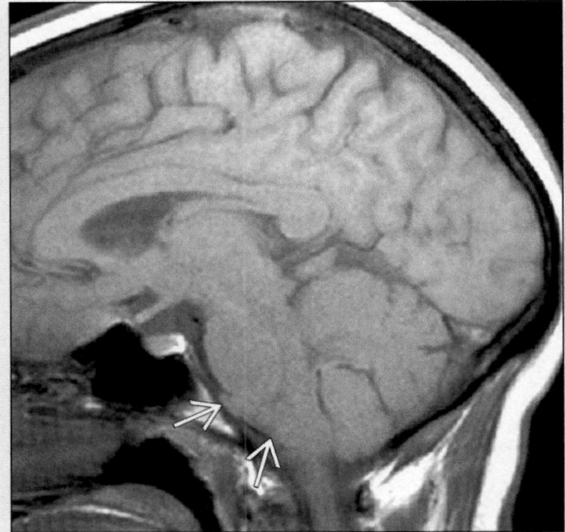

*(**Left**) shows a slightly hyperintense lobulated mass at the pontomedullary junction ➔. The lesion extended laterally on axial images, was hyperintense to brain on T2WI, and did not enhance following contrast administration. Classic posterior fossa neurenteric cyst. (**Right**) Axial T2WI MR shows a large left hemispheric cyst. It is difficult to tell whether the mass is extra- or intraaxial. It did not suppress on FLAIR. An intraaxial neurenteric cyst was found at surgery.*

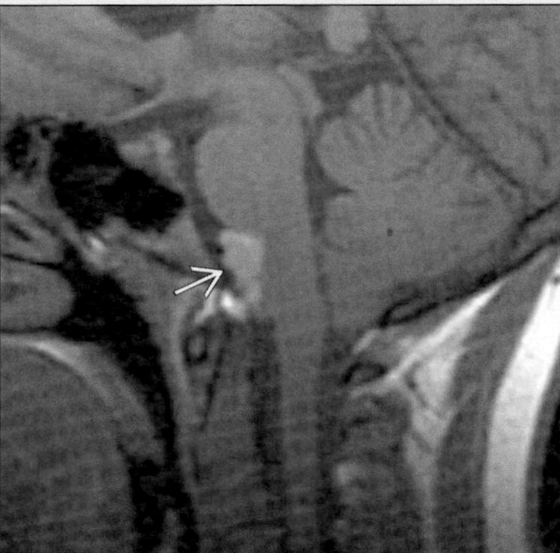

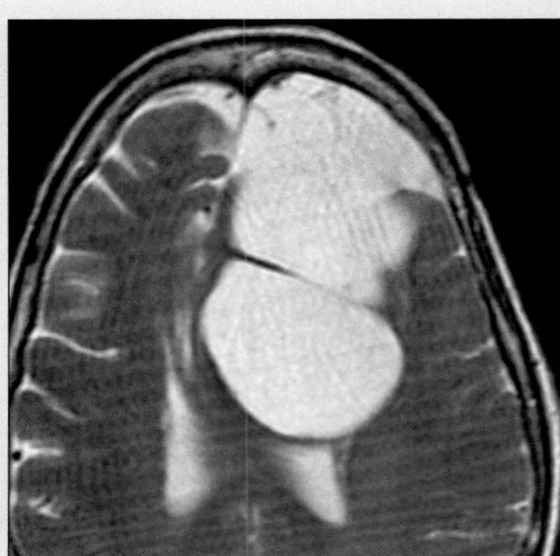

NEURENTERIC CYST

TERMINOLOGY

Abbreviations

- Neurenteric cyst (NEC)

Synonyms

- Enterogenous cyst, enteric cyst

Definitions

- Rare benign malformative endodermal CNS cyst

IMAGING

General Features

- Best diagnostic clue
  - Oblong nonenhancing, slightly T1/T2 hyperintense mass in front of medulla
- Location
  - More common in spine than brain (3:1)
  - 70-75% of intracranial NECs found in posterior fossa
    - > 95% extraaxial
    - Anterior/lateral to pontomedullary junction
    - 70% extend to midline
  - 25-30% supratentorial
    - Suprasellar, quadrigeminal cisterns
    - Cerebral hemispheres (frontal most common)
- Size
  - Posterior fossa usually < 2 cm; supratentorial often large
- Morphology
  - Smooth, lobulated, well demarcated

CT Findings

- NECT
  - Hypo-/iso-/hyperdense mass, no Ca++
  - Bony anomalies usually absent
- CECT
  - No enhancement

MR Findings

- T1WI
  - Almost always iso-/hyperintense to CSF
- T2WI
  - 90% hyperintense to CSF, 10% hypointense
- FLAIR
  - Hyperintense to CSF
- DWI
  - Usually none, but may show mild restriction
- T1WI C+
  - Usually none; occasionally mild rim

Imaging Recommendations

- Best imaging tool
  - MR with T1 C+, FLAIR, DWI

DIFFERENTIAL DIAGNOSIS

Epidermoid Cyst

- Usually restricts on DWI

Dermoid Cyst

- Like fat; often Ca++

Arachnoid Cyst

- Like CSF on all sequences

Schwannoma

- Enhances strongly; usually not midline

Other Endodermal Cysts

- Rathke cleft, colloid cysts
- Excluded by location

Ecchordosis Physaliphora

- Notochordal remnant
- Often involves clivus

PATHOLOGY

General Features

- Etiology
  - Congenital endodermal cyst
  - Probably arises from persistent neurenteric canal

Gross Pathologic & Surgical Features

- Transparent, thin-walled, smooth, round/lobulated cyst
- Contents vary from clear, colorless fluid (like CSF) to thicker, more viscous/mucoid

CLINICAL ISSUES

Presentation

- Most common signs/symptoms
  - Brain = asymptomatic or headache

Demographics

- Age
  - Any age
- Gender
  - M:F = 1:3
- Epidemiology
  - Rare (only 75 intracranial cases reported)

Natural History & Prognosis

- May be stable or enlarge slowly

Treatment

- Observation vs. total surgical excision

DIAGNOSTIC CHECKLIST

Consider

- Mass in front of brainstem, hyperdense/hyperintense to CSF may be NEC

SELECTED REFERENCES

1. Preece MT et al: Intracranial neurenteric cysts: imaging and pathology spectrum. AJNR Am J Neuroradiol. 27(6):1211-6, 2006

NONNEOPLASTIC TUMOR-ASSOCIATED CYSTS

Key Facts

Terminology
- Nonneoplastic tumor-associated cysts (TACs)
- Benign fluid-containing cyst
  - Directly adjacent to, but not within neoplasm

Imaging
- General features of TAC
  - Smooth, well demarcated
  - Can be single, multiple, multiloculated
  - Abuts tumor directly
  - Usually lies between tumor, brain
  - Extraaxial > > intraaxial TACs
  - Size varies from small to very large
  - Neoplasms that cause TACs are typically large
- CT
  - Hypodense fluid collection adjacent to mass
  - No Ca++, hemorrhage
  - No enhancement
- MR
  - Variable signal (depending on protein content)
  - Often hyperintense to CSF
  - May suppress on FLAIR
  - Usually no restriction on DWI
  - Enhancement absent/minimal

Top Differential Diagnoses
- Arachnoid cyst
- Enlarged perivascular spaces
- Cystic neoplasms

Pathology
- Considered tumor "epiphenomenon"
- Most likely represent trapped, encysted pools of CSF adjacent to large extraaxial neoplasm
- As tumor grows, traps CSF between itself and adjacent brain

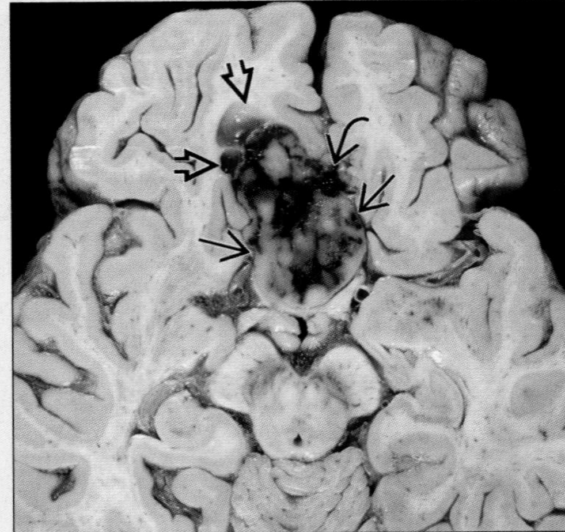

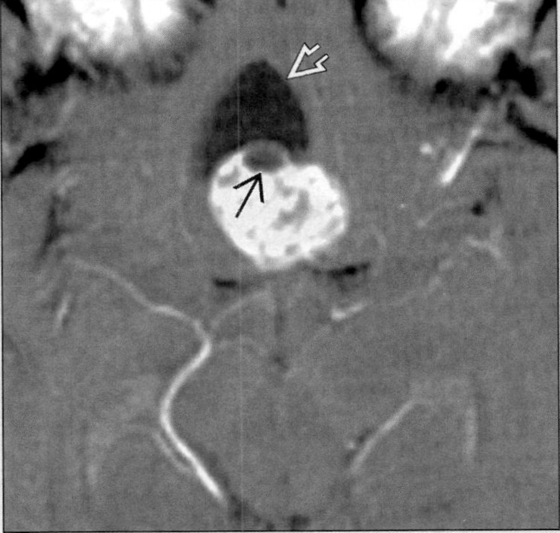

(Left) *Gross pathology shows a large hemorrhagic pituitary macroadenoma → with an intratumoral cyst containing blood products ↗. Note the 2 small nonneoplastic tumor-associated cysts ⇨ immediately adjacent to the mass. (Courtesy R. Hewlett, PhD.)* ***(Right)*** *Axial T1 C+ MR shows a strongly but heterogeneously enhancing pituitary macroadenoma with an intratumoral cyst →. Note the nonenhancing CSF-like cyst ➡ that directly abuts the tumor, though clearly not part of the neoplasm itself.*

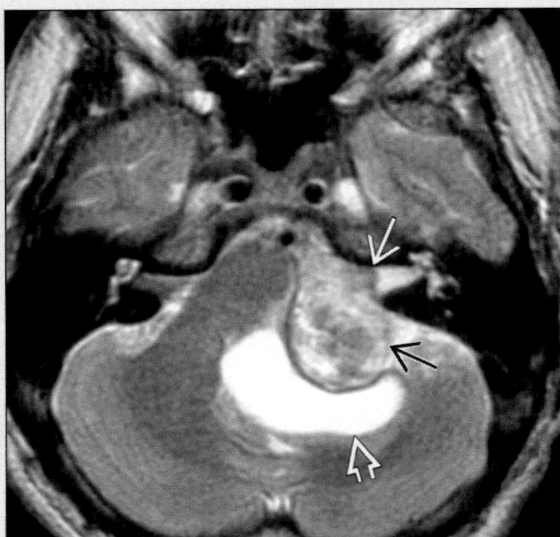

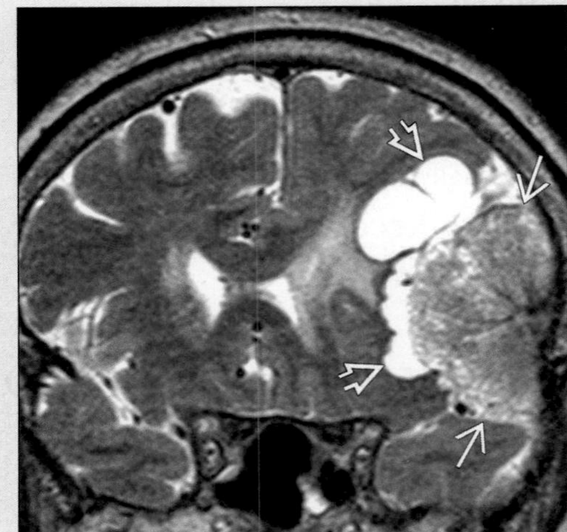

(Left) *Axial T2WI MR in a 33-year-old man with gradually increasing left-sided hearing loss shows a large, mixed signal intensity, CPA mass → that extends into the proximal IAC ➡. Note the large cyst ⇨, hyperintense to CSF, associated with the tumor. Vestibular schwannoma.* ***(Right)*** *Coronal T2WI MR shows a classic meningioma ➡ with several large tumor-associated cysts ⇨. The neoplasm enhanced strongly but heterogeneously after contrast administration; the cysts showed no enhancement.*

NONNEOPLASTIC TUMOR-ASSOCIATED CYSTS

TERMINOLOGY

Abbreviations

- Nonneoplastic tumor-associated cysts (TACs)
- Arachnoid cyst (AC)
- Perivascular spaces (PVSs)

Synonyms

- Peritumoral cyst
- "Herald" cyst (at surgery, may "herald" immediately adjacent mass)
- Tumor-associated arachnoid cyst
- Tumor-associated enlarged PVSs

Definitions

- Benign fluid-containing cyst adjacent to, but not within, neoplasm

IMAGING

General Features

- Best diagnostic clue
  - Nonenhancing cyst immediately adjacent to neoplasm
- Location
  - Adjacent to tumor
    - Extraaxial TACs much more common than intraaxial
    - TACs generally between tumor, brain
- Size
  - TACs vary from small to very large
  - Neoplasms that cause TACs are typically large
- Morphology
  - Smooth, well demarcated
  - Can be single, multiple, multiloculated

Imaging Recommendations

- Best imaging tool
  - Contrast-enhanced MR
- Protocol advice
  - Include FLAIR, DWI

CT Findings

- NECT
  - Hypodense
  - No Ca++, hemorrhage
- CECT
  - No enhancement

MR Findings

- T1WI
  - Variable depending on protein content
    - Hypointense to brain
    - Iso- to hyperintense to CSF
- T2WI
  - Hyperintense
- FLAIR
  - May suppress
- DWI
  - Usually no restriction
  - May show mildly increased diffusivity
- T1WI C+
  - Usually none
  - Minimal/mild peripheral enhancement may occur
    - Secondary to reactive inflammatory changes, not neoplastic cells in cyst wall

DIFFERENTIAL DIAGNOSIS

Arachnoid Cyst

- Non-tumor-associated arachnoid cysts more common than TACs
- Typically behave **exactly** like CSF
  - Suppress on FLAIR
  - Does not restrict/show increased diffusivity on DWI

Enlarged Perivascular Spaces

- Intraparenchymal, not extraaxial
- Clustered variably-sized cysts > > solitary lesion
- Contain interstitial fluid but behave like CSF

Cystic Neoplasms

- Pilocytic astrocytoma
- Hemangioblastoma
- Schwannoma

PATHOLOGY

General Features

- Etiology
  - Precise etiology unknown
  - Considered tumor "epiphenomenon"
  - Most likely represent trapped, encysted pools of CSF adjacent to large extraaxial neoplasm
    - As tumor grows, traps CSF between itself and adjacent brain
  - Trapped PVSs less likely etiology
  - Some TACs may be true arachnoid cysts

Gross Pathologic & Surgical Features

- Thin cyst wall
- Fluid varies from clear to turbid, proteinaceous

Microscopic Features

- TAC cyst wall is generally gliotic brain ± reactive astrocytes, lymphocytes
- No tumor cells

CLINICAL ISSUES

Presentation

- Most common signs/symptoms
  - Usually related to neoplasm itself, not TAC

DIAGNOSTIC CHECKLIST

Consider

- TAC if large CSF collection adjacent to large extraaxial mass

SELECTED REFERENCES

1. Osborn AG et al: Intracranial cysts: radiologic-pathologic correlation and imaging approach. Radiology. 239(3):650-64, 2006

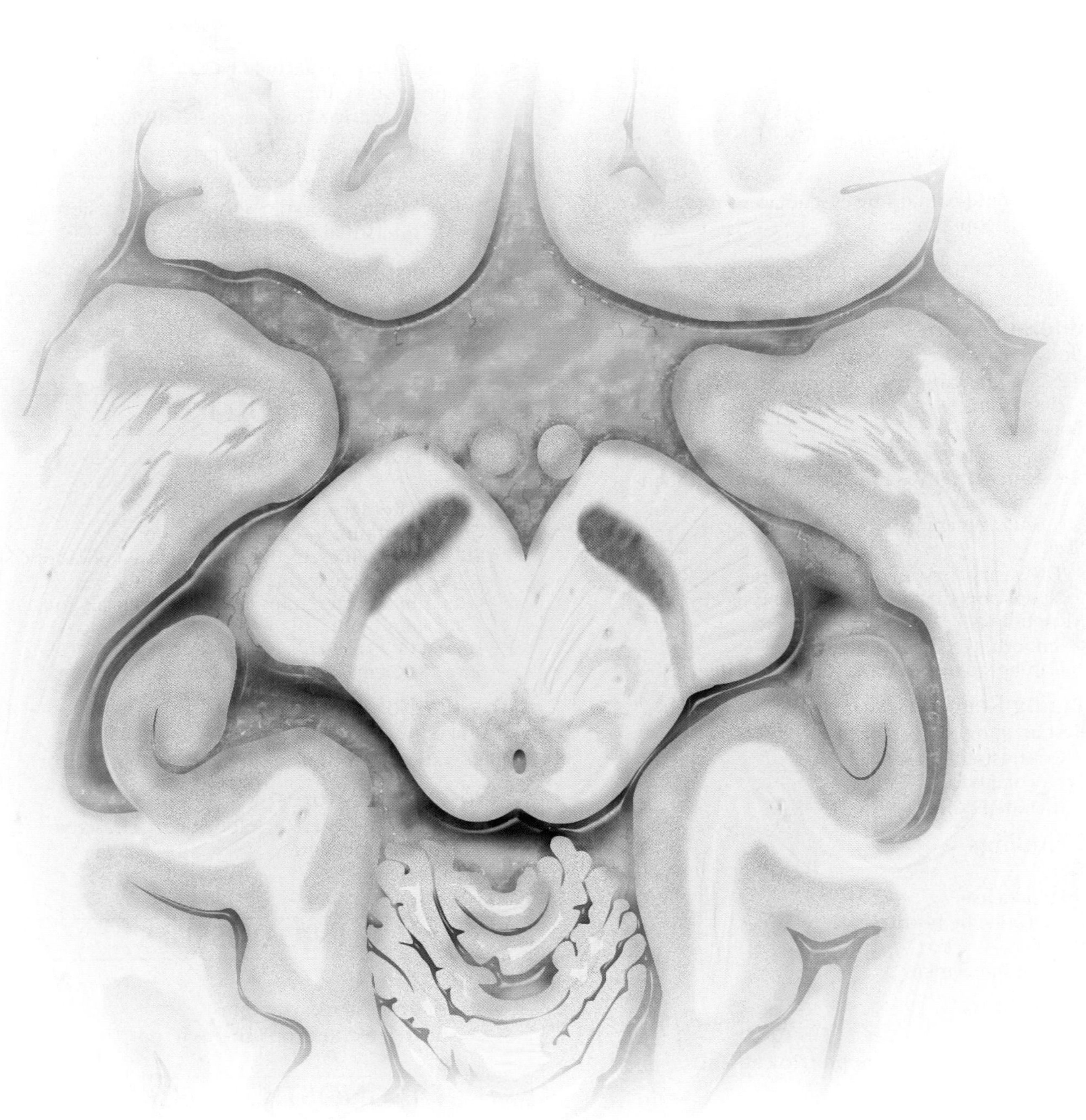

SECTION 8
Infectious and Demyelinating Disease

Introduction and Overview

Congenital/Neonatal Infections

Acquired Infections

Demyelinating Disease

Overview of CNS Infections

General Considerations

Classification. Infectious diseases can be classified into congenital/neonatal and acquired infections. They can be further subdivided by etiology, i.e., bacterial, viral, granulomatous, parasitic, and rickettsial diseases.

Infectious/inflammatory diseases can also have different manifestations depending on disease acuity. Some diseases like herpes encephalitis are typically acute and fulminant. Others are subacute or chronic (e.g., subacute sclerosing panencephalitis (SSPE) and Rasmussen encephalitis). Some, such as HIV/AIDS, look very different in the acute stage in patients who are coinfected with tuberculosis versus in patients who have been on prolonged antiretroviral therapy (HAART).

Congenital/Neonatal Infections

General Considerations

Terminology. Congenital brain infections are often grouped together and simply called TORCH infections (for **to**xoplasmosis, rubella, Cytomegalovirus, and **h**erpes). If congenital syphilis is included, the grouping is called TORCH(S) or (S)TORCH.

Other congenital infections include human immunodeficiency virus (HIV) and lymphocytic choriomeningitis (LCM). HIV is an increasingly common congenital infection in certain parts of the world. It is estimated that almost 30% of pregnancies in HIV(+) women will result in transmission to the developing fetus unless HAART is administered.

Etiology. With 1 exception, neonatal herpes encephalitis, most congenital infections are secondary to transplacental passage of the infectious agent and are acquired antenatally. With 2 exceptions, toxoplasmosis and syphilis, most are viral. All are relatively rare with the possible exceptions of cytomegalovirus (CMV) and herpes encephalitis.

Pathology. Transplacental transmission of various pathogens results in a spectrum of findings depending on both the agent and timing of infection. When infections occur early in fetal development (e.g., the 1st trimester), they tend to result in miscarriage or birth defects. Malformations, such as migrational defects and schizencephaly, are seen in surviving neonates. When infections occur later, encephaloclastic manifestations predominate. Microcephaly with frank brain destruction and widespread encephalomalacia occur. Dystrophic parenchymal calcifications are characteristic of CMV, toxoplasmosis, HIV, and congenital rubella infections.

Acquired Infectious/Inflammatory Diseases

Bacterial Infections

Meningitis. Purulent exudates, predominately in the basal cisterns, are the common pathologic feature of meningitis, regardless of the specific infectious agent. The pia is congested, thickened, and inflamed. Exudates may fill the cisterns and subarachnoid spaces.

Pia-subarachnoid enhancement is the most common imaging finding. The brain may be swollen and edematous. Complications, such as hydrocephalus, empyema, and vasculitis, with or without cerebral infarction, are common.

Abscess. Abscesses develop in 4 general stages: Early and late cerebritis and early and late capsule. In early cerebritis, infection is focal but not yet localized. An unencapsulated mass of inflammatory cells, edema, necrotic foci, and petechial hemorrhage forms. In late cerebritis, the infection coalesces. Central necrosis with a poorly delineated rim of inflammatory cells, granulation tissue, and fibroblasts is seen.

The early capsule stage follows late cerebritis. A well-defined collagenous capsule with a liquified necrotic core forms 2-4 weeks after the initial infection. Eventually the abscess cavity shrinks and collapses. This "late capsule" stage can last for months, with imaging findings still present long after symptoms resolve.

Ventriculitis. An abscess rim is thinnest on the paraventricular side. If the abscess ruptures into the ventricle, it causes ventriculitis ("pyocephalus") and choroid plexitis. Intraventricular abscess rupture is often fatal.

Viral Infections

Acute viral infections. Herpes simplex encephalitis (HSE) is the most common nonepidemic viral encephalitis. Over 95% are caused by HSV-1 (oral herpes virus). Currently the most common epidemic viral encephalitis is the West Nile virus.

Subacute and chronic viral infections. Many viruses have a slow incubation period and are characterized by symptoms that progress over months or even years. Subacute sclerosing panencephalitis (SSPE) is an example. Progressive multifocal leukoencephalopathy (PML), caused by JC virus (a ubiquitous polyomavirus), is another.

Miscellaneous Infections

Tuberculosis. With 8-10 million new cases each year and rising prevalence in developing countries, TB is a special public health concern. The emergence of multi-drug resistant TB (MDR TB) and extremely drug-resistant TB (XDR TB) make early recognition and urgent treatment of TB even more important. The "deadly intersection" between HIV and TB, with each disease amplifying the lethality of the other, is of special concern.

Parasites. Neurocysticercosis (NCC) has become the most common CNS parasitic infection in the world and the most common worldwide cause of epilepsy. Although most parasites rarely infect the brain, CNS lesions eventually develop in most patients infected with NCC.

Fungal and rickettsial diseases. Fungi are ubiquitous organisms and endemic in many areas of the world. Most, such as *Aspergillus*, infect humans infrequently, usually through inhalation or puncture wounds. When fungal infections occur in immunocompetent patients, lung disease is more common than brain infection.

CNS and disseminated systemic fungal infections typically occur in immunocompromised patients. HIV/AIDS and immunosuppressive drugs are factors that increasingly predispose patients to opportunistic infections.

Rickettsial diseases, such as Rocky Mountain and Mediterranean spotted fever, usually have associated skin rashes. CNS infection is uncommon. When it occurs, *Rickettsiae* have a distinct predilection for the perivascular spaces and cause infarct-like lesions in the basal ganglia.

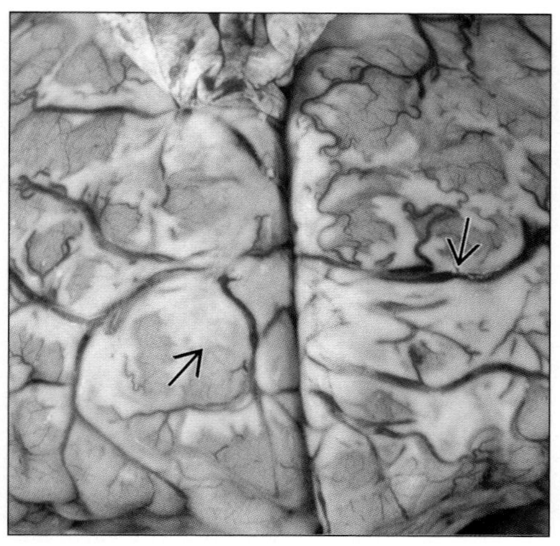

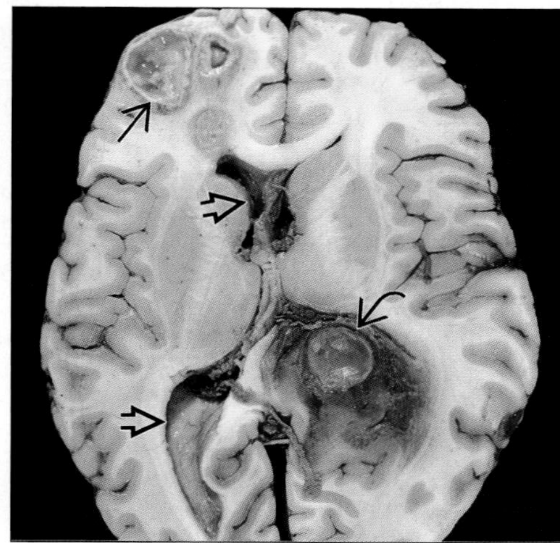

(Left) *Close-up view of the autopsied brain in a patient who died from acute bacterial meningitis. Note thick purulent exudate filling the sulci* ➔*. The underlying gyri are edematous and diffusely swollen. The pia is inflamed and congested, with prominent cortical vessels. (Courtesy R. Hewlett, PhD.)* ***(Right)*** *Autopsy case shows multiple pyogenic abscesses* ➔*. A large abscess in the deep white matter* ➔ *has ruptured into the ventricles, causing ventriculitis* ➔*. (Courtesy R. Hewlett, PhD.)*

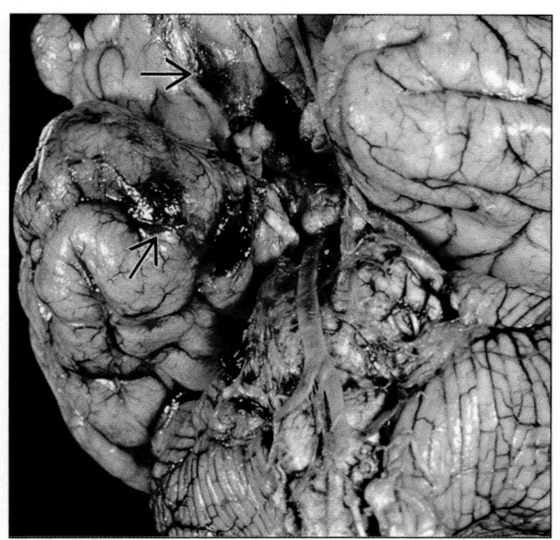

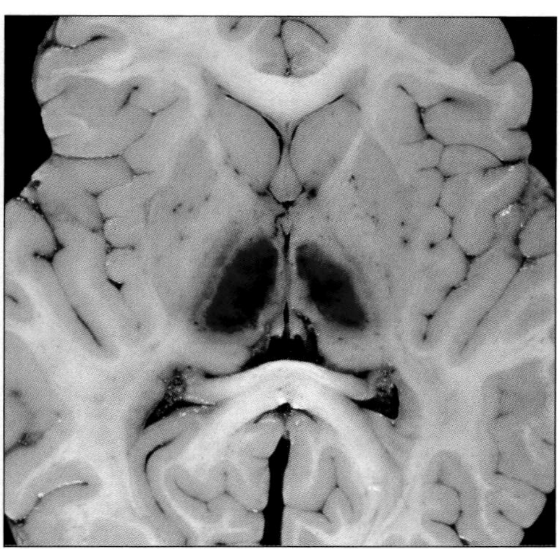

(Left) *Autopsied brain shows classic findings of acute herpes encephalitis. Note the predilection for the limbic system, seen here as hemorrhagic necrosis in the temporal lobe and subfrontal cortex* ➔*. (Courtesy R. Hewlett, PhD.)* ***(Right)*** *Autopsy case of acute hemorrhagic, necrotizing encephalitis, probably viral. Many nonepidemic viral encephalidites have a predilection for the basal ganglia, thalami, midbrain, and pons. (Courtesy R. Hewlett, PhD.)*

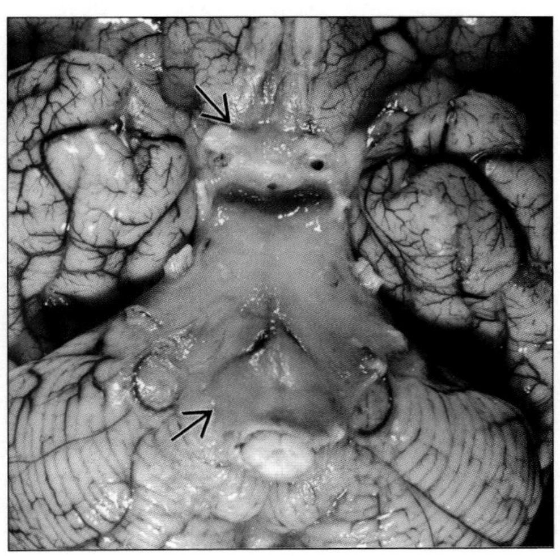

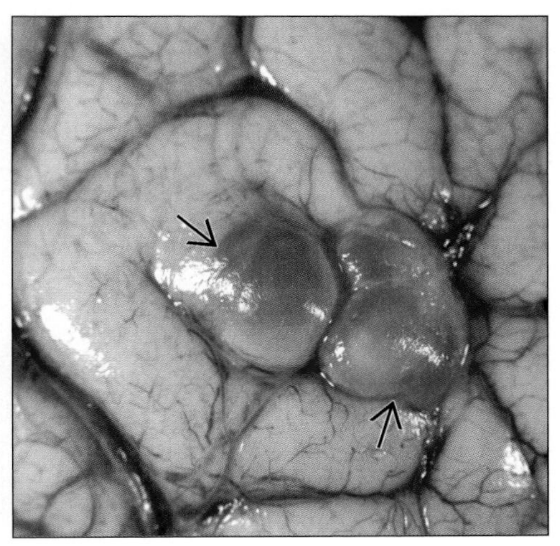

(Left) *Autopsy case demonstrates tuberculous meningitis (TBM). TBM* ➔ *typically causes thick, purulent-appearing exudates with a predilection for the basal cisterns. The imaging and pathologic appearance of meningitis is generally similar, regardless of the etiology. (Courtesy R. Hewlett, PhD.)* ***(Right)*** *Autopsy case shows 2 neurocysticercosis (NCC) cysts* ➔ *lodged within the superficial sulci. The subarachnoid spaces are the most common location for NCC cysts in the brain. (Courtesy R. Hewlett, PhD.)*

Key Facts

Terminology

- Acronym for congenital infections caused by transplacental transmission of pathogens
- TORCH(S), (S)TORCH, congenital infections, intrauterine infection, TORCH infections

Imaging

- CMV, Toxo, lymphocytic choriomeningitis, HIV, and rubella all have parenchymal calcifications (Ca++)
- CMV ⇒ periventricular Ca++ ± cysts, cortical clefts, cortical dysplasia, WM abnormalities, and cerebellar hypoplasia
- Sonography for neonatal screening, MR for comprehensive evaluation, NECT to detect or confirm Ca++

Top Differential Diagnoses

- Pseudo-TORCH syndromes ⇒ basal ganglia Ca++, progressive demyelination
- Congenital lymphocytic choriomeningitis ⇒ micro- or macrocephaly, Ca++ precise mimic of CMV

Pathology

- CMV ⇒ most common cause of intrauterine infection, DNA herpes virus

Clinical Issues

- CMV can present at birth (10%) with micrencephaly, hepatosplenomegaly, petechial rash

Diagnostic Checklist

- CMV ⇒ microcephaly, cortical dysplasia, periventricular Ca++ and ± cysts, WM disease, and cerebellar hypoplasia

*(**Left**) Axial graphic shows periventricular parenchymal calcifications ⇗, damaged white matter ⇨, and dysplastic cortex →, all characteristic of an in utero cytomegalovirus infection. (**Right**) Axial NECT in a microcephalic infant with cytomegalovirus shows extensive parenchymal Ca++ →. Note the open sylvian cisterns ⇗. MR (not shown) confirmed bilateral perisylvian polymicrogyria. Bilateral frontal white matter hypodensity ⇨ corresponded to regions of demyelination.*

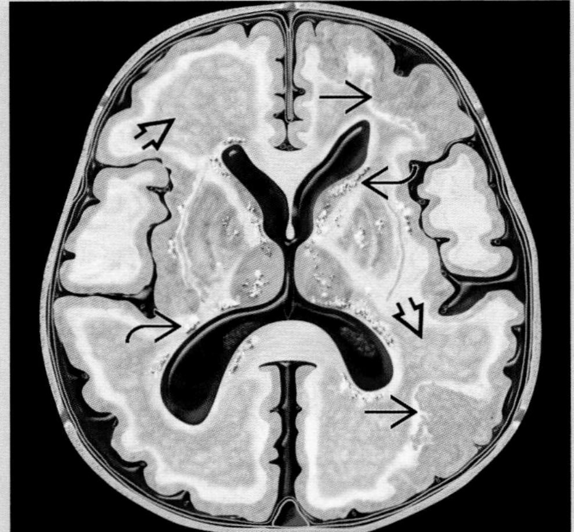

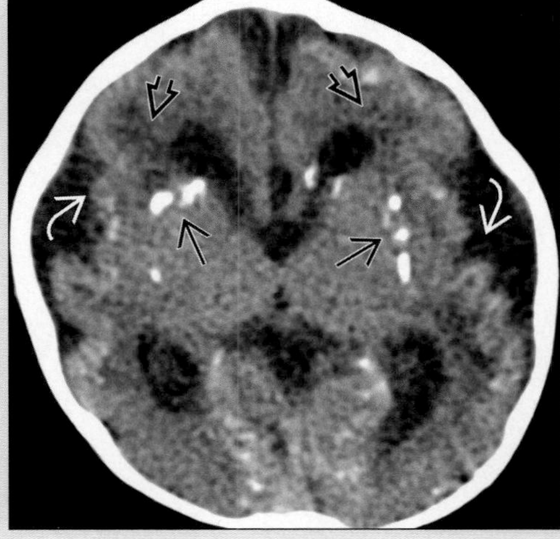

*(**Left**) Periventricular foci of hyperechogenicity ➡ correspond to Ca++ on a NECT in this patient with congenital CMV. Ultrasound may also detect cysts, clefts, and schizencephaly, all associated with congenital CMV. (**Right**) Coronal T2WI FSE MR in an infant with a congenital CMV infection shows periventricular germinolytic cysts ➡. These CMV-related cysts may also be seen anterior to the temporal horns and may be associated with white matter signal abnormalities.*

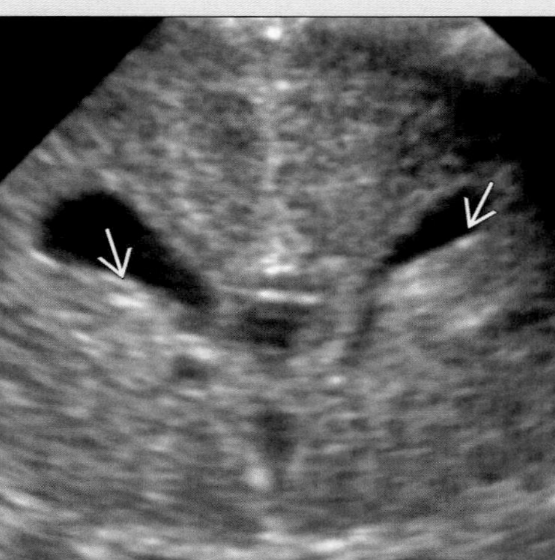

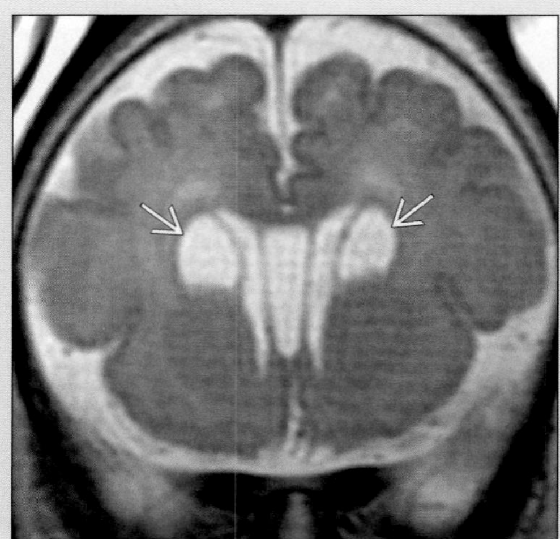

TERMINOLOGY

Synonyms

- TORCH(S), (S)TORCH, congenital infections, intrauterine infection, TORCH infections

Definitions

- Congenital infections caused by transplacental transmission of pathogens
  - Toxoplasmosis (toxo) ⇒ *Toxoplasma gondii*
  - Rubella ⇒ rubella virus
  - Cytomegalovirus (CMV) ⇒ most common TORCH infection
  - Herpes ⇒ herpes simplex virus 2 (HSV-2)
  - Other ⇒ human immunodeficiency virus (HIV), lymphocytic choriomeningitis (LCM), syphilis

IMAGING

General Features

- Best diagnostic clue
  - Toxo, CMV, HIV, and rubella all cause parenchymal calcifications (Ca++)
  - CMV causes periventricular cysts, clefts, schizencephaly, and migrational defects
  - Rubella and HSV cause lobar destruction/ encephalomalacia
  - Syphilis causes basilar meningitis

CT Findings

- NECT
  - Cytomegalovirus
    - ~ 50% of patients have parenchymal &/or periventricular Ca++
    - Focal regions of white matter (WM) low attenuation, ± cysts
    - Migrational defects, cortical clefts, schizencephaly
    - Ventricular dilatation, cerebral volume loss, cerebellar hypoplasia
  - Toxoplasmosis
    - Parenchymal and periventricular Ca++ ⇒ usually less extensive than CMV, scattered
  - Herpes simplex virus
    - Large regions of decreased attenuation, ± high attenuation foci of hemorrhage
  - HIV
    - Combination of volume loss, basal ganglia, and subcortical Ca++
- CECT
  - Lesions with meningeal inflammatory components (syphilis, HSV) may show enhancement

MR Findings

- T1WI
  - Cytomegalovirus
    - Periventricular subependymal foci of T1 shortening due to Ca++, hypoattenuating WM
  - Herpes simplex virus
    - Hemorrhagic regions may be hyperintense
- T2WI
  - Cytomegalovirus
    - Cortical abnormalities (polymicrogyria, clefts), hippocampal dysplasia (vertical orientation)
  - Herpes simplex virus
    - Obliterated normal "dark cortex" on T2WI, diffusion restriction, ± hemorrhagic foci
- FLAIR
  - Cytomegalovirus
    - Focal, patchy, or confluent regions of increased signal due to gliosis and demyelination
- T2* GRE
  - Hypointense signal due to Ca++ in CMV, toxo, and HIV
  - Blooming blood in HSV and rubella
- T1WI C+
  - Thickened and enhancing basal meninges in syphilis
  - Patchy mild parenchymal enhancement in HSV
- MRS
  - Active lesions: ↑ myoinositol and excitatory amino acids
  - Chronic disease: ↓ N-acetylaspartate (NAA)

Ultrasonographic Findings

- Grayscale ultrasound
  - Echogenic periventricular foci (Ca++) in CMV, toxo
  - Branching basal ganglia and thalamic echoes ⇒ "mineralizing vasculopathy"
    - Associated with CMV, toxo, syphilis, rubella, and trisomies
  - Periventricular pseudocysts and ventricular adhesions

Imaging Recommendations

- Best imaging tool
  - Cranial sonography for neonatal screening
  - MR brain to completely characterize abnormalities
- Protocol advice
  - T2* GRE &/or NECT to detect periventricular Ca++ or hemorrhage

DIFFERENTIAL DIAGNOSIS

Tuberous Sclerosis

- Subependymal Ca++ characteristic
- Peripheral tubers will mimic migrational abnormalities
- WM lesions can mimic gliosis in TORCH infections

Congenital Lymphocytic Choriomeningitis

- Produces necrotizing ependymitis → aqueductal obstruction; microcephaly (43%), microcephaly (13%)
- NECT may perfectly mimic CMV

Pseudo-TORCH Syndromes

- Baraitser-Reardon, Aicardi-Goutières (cerebrospinal fluid [CSF] pleocytosis, ↑ CSF α interferon)
  - Progressive cerebral and cerebellar demyelination
  - Basal ganglia Ca++, ± periventricular Ca++

PATHOLOGY

General Features

- Etiology
  - Cytomegalovirus
    - Ubiquitous DNA virus of herpes virus family
    - Most common cause of intrauterine infection

- Mother has primary or reactivation infection during pregnancy
  - Herpes encephalitis
    - HSV-2
    - Active genital infection during delivery; transplacental infection less common
  - Rubella
    - Togaviridae family of viruses, very rare in USA
    - High risk of miscarriage and birth defects with 1st trimester maternal infection
  - Toxoplasmosis
    - Cats are definitive hosts for protozoan parasite
    - 50% of toxoplasmosis infections in USA are from contaminated meat
    - Active infection in pregnancy ⇒ 20-50% congenital infection
  - HIV
    - Transmitted by transcervical route
    - 30% of pregnancies in HIV(+) women will result in transmission unless preventative measures taken
  - Syphilis
    - Caused by spirochetal bacterium *Treponema pallidum*

Gross Pathologic & Surgical Features

- Microcephaly, schizencephaly, polymicrogyria in CMV
- Inflammation/destruction in toxo, rubella, HSV

Microscopic Features

- May find encysted parasites in toxo
- Ischemic necrosis in rubella
- Microglial nodules and cytomegalic cells in CMV

CLINICAL ISSUES

Presentation

- Most common signs/symptoms
  - CMV can present at birth (10%) with micrencephaly, hepatosplenomegaly, petechial rash
    - 55% with systemic disease have central nervous system (CNS) involvement
  - Congenital toxoplasmosis is usually inapparent at birth, presenting at 2-3 months
    - Leukokoria (chorioretinitis)
  - HSV acquired during delivery typically presents at 3-15 days with seizures, lethargy
    - HSV acquired in utero (5%) typically presents at birth with hydranencephaly and growth retardation
  - HIV typically diagnosed at 6-12 months with developmental delay
  - Rubella presents with petechial rash, low birth weight, and leukokoria (cataracts)
  - Syphilis ⇒ failure to thrive and irritability in newborn, bone pain in infant

Demographics

- Epidemiology
  - CMV affects ~ 1% of all newborns
  - More than 20% of USA population is seropositive for *Toxoplasma gondii*; high risk for illness during pregnancy
  - 20-25% of pregnant women in USA have genital herpes
  - ~ 750,000 HIV(+) people in USA
  - 20,000 new syphilis cases in USA each year

Natural History & Prognosis

- Up to 95% of newborns with neurological symptoms from CMV have major neurodevelopmental sequelae

Treatment

- Ganciclovir may benefit CMV-infected infants
- No treatment for rubella
- Antiretroviral treatment in 2nd and 3rd trimesters and during labor can prevent transmission of HIV
- Pyrimethamine and sulfadiazine are used to treat neonatal toxo ⇒ improved outcomes compared to untreated infants
- HSV is treated with acyclovir
- All forms of syphilis are treated with penicillin

DIAGNOSTIC CHECKLIST

Consider

- TORCH infection in newborn and infant with microcephaly, ocular abnormalities, and intrauterine growth restriction

Image Interpretation Pearls

- Congenital CMV encephalitis should be considered when imaging shows
  - Microcephaly, polymicrogyria, periventricular Ca++ and cysts, cortical clefts, WM disease, and cerebellar hypoplasia

SELECTED REFERENCES

1. Abdel-Salam GM et al: Microcephaly, malformation of brain development and intracranial calcification in sibs: pseudo-TORCH or a new syndrome. Am J Med Genet A. 146A(22):2929-36, 2008
2. Briggs TA et al: Band-like intracranial calcification with simplified gyration and polymicrogyria: a distinct "pseudo-TORCH" phenotype. Am J Med Genet A. 146A(24):3173-80, 2008
3. Kang SS et al: Lymphocytic choriomeningitis infection of the central nervous system. Front Biosci. 13:4529-43, 2008
4. Bale JF et al: Herpes Simplex Virus Infections of the Newborn. Curr Treat Options Neurol. 7(2):151-156, 2005
5. Sanchis A et al: Genetic syndromes mimic congenital infections. J Pediatr. 146(5):701-5, 2005
6. de Vries LS et al: The spectrum of cranial ultrasound and magnetic resonance imaging abnormalities in congenital cytomegalovirus infection. Neuropediatrics. 35(2):113-9, 2004
7. Jones J et al: Congenital toxoplasmosis. Am Fam Physician. 67(10):2131-8, 2003
8. Bale JF Jr: Congenital infections. Neurol Clin. 20(4):1039-60, vii, 2002
9. Vivarelli R et al: Pseudo-TORCH syndrome or Baraitser-Reardon syndrome: diagnostic criteria. Brain Dev. 23(1):18-23, 2001

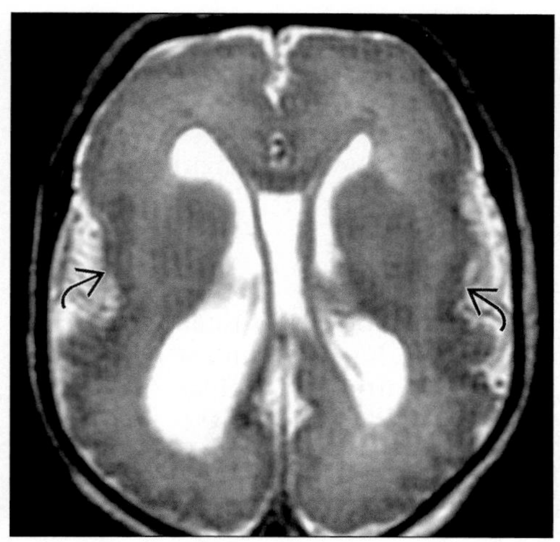

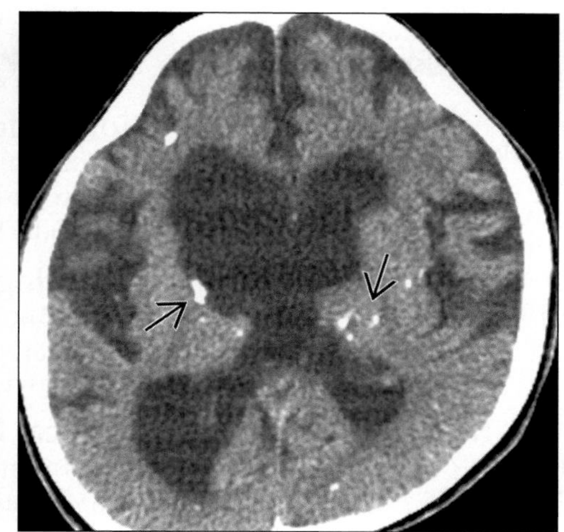

(Left) *Axial T2WI FSE MR in an infant with congenital CMV shows primitive, broad, sylvian cisterns due to extensive bi-hemispheric perisylvian polymicrogyria →. Sparse periventricular calcifications and cysts were detected on NECT (not shown).* ***(Right)*** *Axial NECT in a patient with toxoplasmosis shows multiple scattered cerebral calcifications →. Note the ventricular dilation and cerebral hemispheric volume loss. The infection is caused by the protozoan Toxoplasma gondii.*

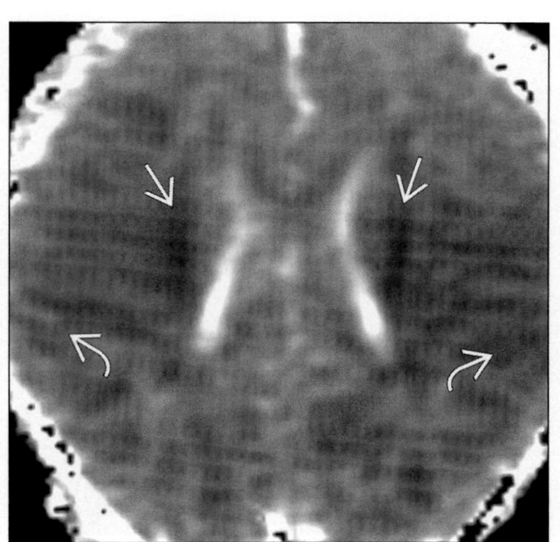

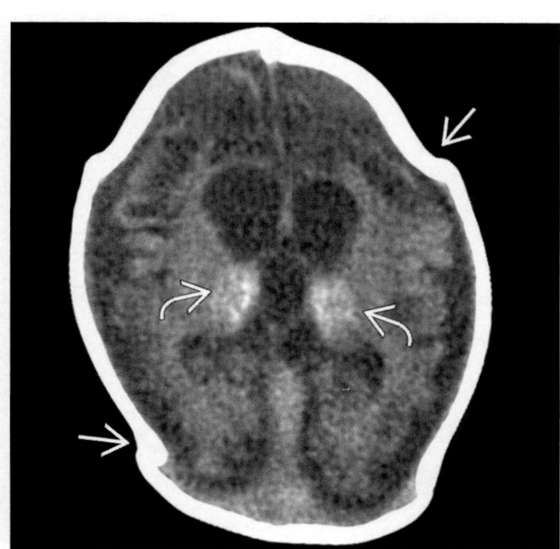

(Left) *Axial ADC of an acutely infected, seizing neonate with herpes simplex virus type 2 sepsis shows widespread low diffusivity (hypointensity) within the periventricular white matter →, cortex, and subcortical white matter →.* ***(Right)*** *Axial NECT in an infant with congenital rubella and cataracts shows atrophy of the cerebral hemispheres. There is overlap of the cranial sutures →, secondary to volume loss. Note the central basal ganglia calcification →.*

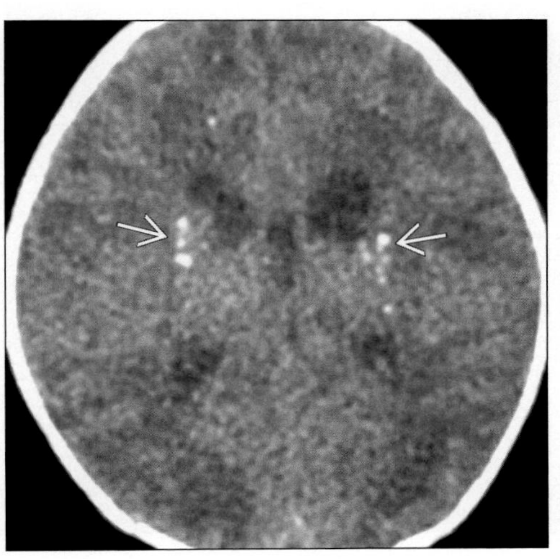

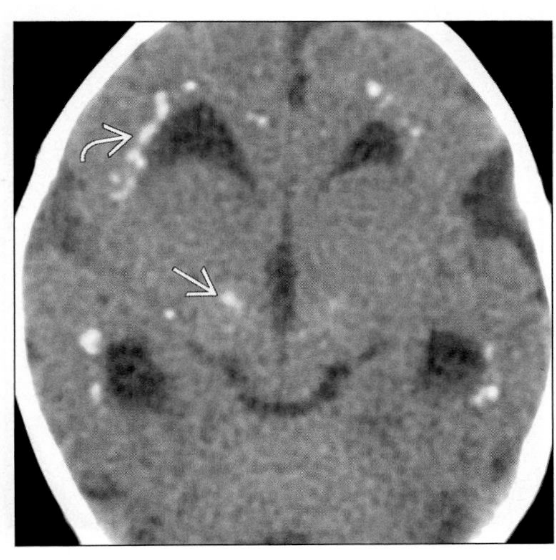

(Left) *Axial NECT in a microcephalic infant with a lymphocytic choriomeningitis virus infection shows scattered basal ganglia calcifications →. The clinical and imaging features of this disorder may precisely mimic congenital cytomegalovirus infection.* ***(Right)*** *Axial NECT in pseudo-TORCH shows basal ganglia calcification → and periventricular calcification →. Pseudo-TORCH states are autosomal recessive disorders showing mineralization and progressive demyelination.*

CONGENITAL CMV

Key Facts

Terminology

- Human Cytomegalovirus (HCMV)
- Most common cause of intrauterine infection in USA

Imaging

- Microcephaly: Spectrum and severity of brain injury depends on timing of fetal infection
- Cranial sonography
  - Periventricular hyperechoic foci
  - Branching basal ganglia hyperechogenicities (lenticulostriate vasculopathy)
  - Ring-like regions of periventricular lucency may precede subependymal Ca++
- NECT when CMV is clinically suspected &/or to complement brain MR
  - Intracranial Ca++ (40-70%): Periventricular (subependymal) (germinolytic zones)
- MR brain to completely characterize abnormalities
  - Agyria ↔ pachygyria ↔ diffuse polymicrogyria ↔ focal cortical dysplasia ↔ schizencephalic clefting
  - WM abnormalities: Periventricular germinolytic cysts, demyelination, gliosis
  - Cerebellar hypoplasia

Top Differential Diagnoses

- Congenital lymphocytic choriomeningitis (LCM)
- Toxoplasmosis
- Pseudo-TORCH syndromes

Pathology

- Ubiquitous DNA virus of herpes virus family
- Hematogenously seeds choroid plexus, replicates in ependyma, germinal matrix, and capillary endothelia

Clinical Issues

- Most infected newborns appear normal
- 55% with systemic disease have CNS involvement

*(**Left**) Axial graphic shows numerous periventricular ➔ and basal ganglia ➔ calcifications. Note regions of cortical dysplasia (polymicrogyria) ➔. Ventricular dilation reflects adjacent white matter (WM) volume loss. The yellowish white matter abnormalities reflect regions of edema, demyelination, &/or gliosis. (**Right**) Axial NECT shows extensive periventricular and parenchymal calcification ➔. Note the open sylvian fissures and simplified perisylvian cortex ➔. MR confirmed polymicrogyria.*

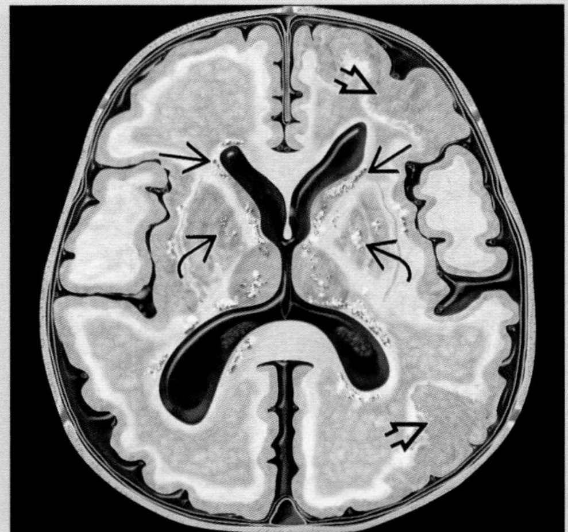

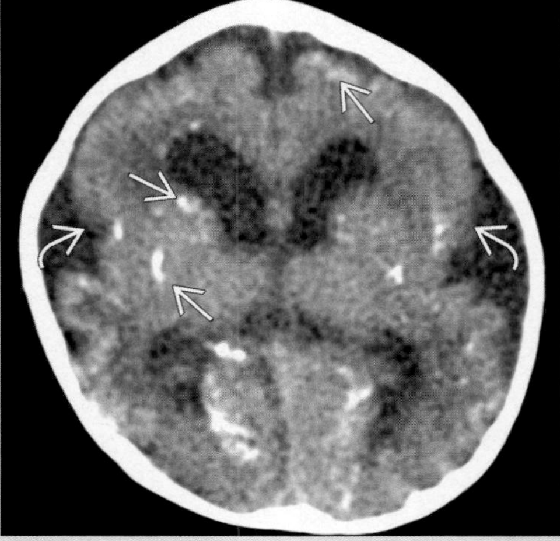

*(**Left**) Axial NECT demonstrates sparse intracranial Ca++ ➔ in an infant with congenital CMV infection. Cerebral periventricular/parenchymal Ca++ is observed in about 40-70% of infected patients. (**Right**) Longitudinal ultrasound in a microcephalic newborn with congenital CMV infection demonstrates focal periventricular hyperechogenicities ➔, shown as Ca++ on NECT. Sonography may also demonstrate germinolytic cysts and ventriculomegaly.*

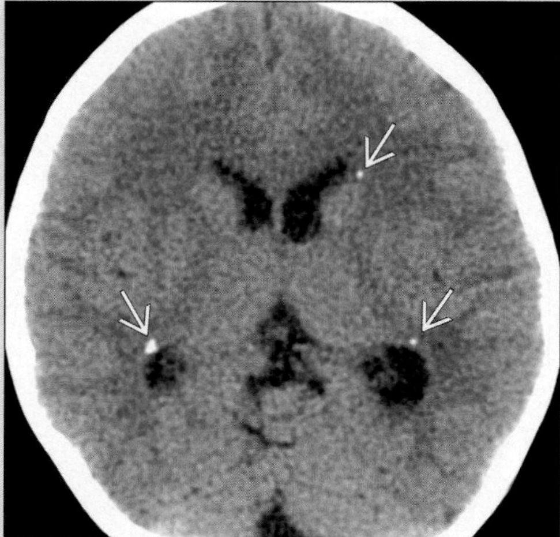

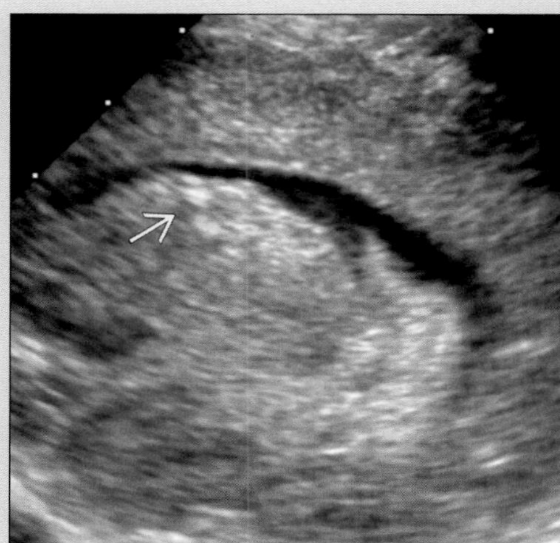

TERMINOLOGY

Abbreviations
- Congenital Cytomegalovirus (CMV) encephalitis

Synonyms
- Human Cytomegalovirus (HCMV)

Definitions
- Congenital infection caused by transplacental transmission of human herpes virus
  - Most common source of intrauterine infection in USA

IMAGING

General Features
- Best diagnostic clue
  - Microcephaly, spectrum of brain injury depending on timing of fetal infection
  - Cerebral calcification (40-70%); periventricular (subependymal germinal matrix zones)
  - Cortical abnormalities: Agyria ↔ pachygyria ↔ polymicrogyria ↔ schizencephalic clefting
  - Cerebellar hypoplasia
  - Myelin delay or destruction
- Gestational age at time of infection determines pattern of CNS injury
  - Prior to 18 weeks → reduction in neurons and glia, lissencephaly, small cerebellum, ventriculomegaly
  - 18-24 weeks → cortical gyral abnormalities, frontal > temporal
  - 3rd trimester → myelin delay or destruction, periventricular cysts
  - Perinatal infection → delay in myelin maturation, focal white matter injury (astrogliosis)

Radiographic Findings
- Radiography
  - ↓ cranial-to-facial ratio

CT Findings
- NECT
  - Intracranial Ca++ (40-70%): Periventricular (subependymal) (germinolytic zones)
  - White matter (WM) volume loss, WM low attenuation, ± germinolytic periventricular cysts, ventriculomegaly
  - Cortical gyral abnormalities
  - Cerebellar hypoplasia

MR Findings
- T1WI
  - Periventricular subependymal foci of T1 shortening secondary to Ca++
  - Ventricular dilatation and periventricular WM volume loss, ± germinolytic cysts
  - Cerebellar hypoplasia
- T2WI
  - Cortical abnormalities ranging from: Agyria ↔ diffuse &/or focal cortical dysplasia
  - Myelination delay or destruction, ± germinolytic periventricular cysts (temporal tip cysts)
  - Focal WM lesions with ↑ T2 intensity (gliosis/demyelination) predominantly in parietal deep WM
  - Hippocampal dysplasia (vertical orientation)
- FLAIR
  - Focal, patchy, or confluent regions of increased signal due to gliosis, ± germinolytic hypointense cysts
- T2* GRE
  - Periventricular ↓ signal due to Ca++
- MRS
  - ↓ NAA/Cr ratio due to loss of neuronal elements, ↑ myoinositol (gliosis)

Ultrasonographic Findings
- Grayscale ultrasound
  - Ring-like regions of periventricular lucency may precede subependymal Ca++
  - Branching basal ganglia and thalamic echoes (lenticulostriate vasculopathy)
  - Periventricular pseudocysts and ventricular adhesions
  - Cerebellar hypoplasia

Imaging Recommendations
- Best imaging tool
  - Cranial sonography for neonatal screening
  - NECT when CMV clinically suspected or to complement MR findings
  - Brain MR to completely characterize abnormalities
- Protocol advice
  - NECT for detecting periventricular Ca++
  - T2* GRE to detect subtle calcification or hemorrhage

DIFFERENTIAL DIAGNOSIS

Congenital Lymphocytic Choriomeningitis
- Rodent-borne arenavirus: Carried by feral house mouse and hamster
- Necrotizing ependymitis leading to aqueductal obstruction (macrocephaly 43%, microcephaly 13%)
- Appearance on NECT may perfectly mimic CMV

Toxoplasmosis
- Protozoan parasite
  - Maternal risk factors include
    - Exposure to cat excreta during pregnancy
    - Eating raw or undercooked meat
- 1/10 as common as CMV, macrocrania > microcrania, cortical dysplasia less common, random cerebral Ca++

Pseudo-TORCH Syndromes
- Baraister-Reardon, Aicardi-Goutières (CSF pleocytosis, ↑ CSF α interferon)
  - Autosomal recessive, progressive cerebral and cerebellar demyelination and degeneration
  - Basal ganglia and brainstem Ca++, periventricular Ca++ less common

PATHOLOGY

General Features
- Etiology
  - CMV is ubiquitous DNA virus of herpes virus family

CONGENITAL CMV

- Hematogenously seeds choroid plexus; replicates in ependyma, germinal matrix, and capillary endothelia
- Capillary involvement leads to thrombosis and ischemia
- Chronic ischemia from placentitis leading to secondary perfusion insufficiency

- Most common cause of intrauterine infection
- Mechanisms of infection
  - Mechanism of fetal infection
    - Mother with primary infection during pregnancy vs. mother with reactivation of latent infection
  - Mechanism of neonatal infection
    - Mother infected at delivery ↔ transmission of virus in breast milk ↔ blood transfusion

Staging, Grading, & Classification

- Timing of gestational infection determines insult
  - Neuronal formation between 8-20 weeks
  - Neuron migration until 24-26 weeks
  - Astrocyte generation begins near end of neuronal production
  - Maximal size of germinal zones at 26 weeks
  - Oligodendrocytes produced during 1st half of 3rd trimester

Gross Pathologic & Surgical Features

- Micrencephaly
- Early gestational infection
  - Germinal zone necrosis, diminished number of glia and neurons, WM volume loss

Microscopic Features

- Hallmark of CMV infection→ cytomegaly with viral nuclear and cytoplasmic inclusions
- Patchy and focal cellular necrosis (particularly germinal matrix cells)
- Vascular inflammation and thrombosis, vascular and subependymal dystrophic Ca++

CLINICAL ISSUES

Presentation

- Most common signs/symptoms
  - Most infected newborns appear normal
  - 10% have systemic signs of disease
    - Hepatosplenomegaly, petechiae, chorioretinitis, jaundice, intrauterine growth retardation
  - 55% with systemic disease have CNS involvement
    - Microcephaly, seizures, hypotonia or hypertonia, sensorineural hearing loss (SNHL)
- Clinical profile
  - Seronegative women are at greatest risk for vertical transmission
- Methods of diagnosis
  - Shell-vial assay for CMV (urine)
  - Late diagnosis with PCR for CMV-DNA from neonatal Guthrie card

Demographics

- Epidemiology
  - Affects ~ 1% of all newborns (10% of whom have CNS or systemic signs and symptoms)
  - 40% of mothers who acquire infection during pregnancy transmit virus to fetus

Natural History & Prognosis

- 3 prognostic groups
  - Newborns with CNS manifestations (microcephaly, periventricular Ca++)
    - Up to 95% have major neurodevelopmental sequelae
  - Newborns with only systemic manifestations (hepatosplenomegaly, petechiae, jaundice)
    - Have better prognosis but still significantly affected
  - Infected newborns with neither CNS nor systemic manifestations
    - Best prognosis, yet still at risk for developmental delays, motor deficits, and SNHL
  - Overall mortality ~ 5%

Treatment

- Ganciclovir may benefit infected infants

DIAGNOSTIC CHECKLIST

Consider

- Congenital CMV in developmentally delayed, microcephalic infant with SNHL

Image Interpretation Pearls

- Congenital CMV encephalitis should be considered when MR shows
  - Microcephaly, cortical dysplasia, germinolytic cysts, WM abnormalities, and cerebellar hypoplasia
- When NECT is classic for CMV encephalitis but work-up for (S)TORCH infection is negative, consider
  - Lymphocytic choriomeningitis (LCM) and pseudo-TORCH syndromes

SELECTED REFERENCES

1. Briggs TA et al: Band-like intracranial calcification with simplified gyration and polymicrogyria: a distinct "pseudo-TORCH" phenotype. Am J Med Genet A. 146A(24):3173-80, 2008
2. Picone O et al: Comparison between ultrasound and magnetic resonance imaging in assessment of fetal cytomegalovirus infection. Prenat Diagn. 28(8):753-8, 2008
3. Malm G et al: Congenital cytomegalovirus infections. Semin Fetal Neonatal Med. 12(3):154-9, 2007
4. Wright R et al: Congenital lymphocytic choriomeningitis virus syndrome: a disease that mimics congenital toxoplasmosis or Cytomegalovirus infection. Pediatrics. 100(1):E9, 1997
5. Barkovich AJ et al: Congenital cytomegalovirus infection of the brain: imaging analysis and embryologic considerations. AJNR Am J Neuroradiol. 15(4):703-15, 1994

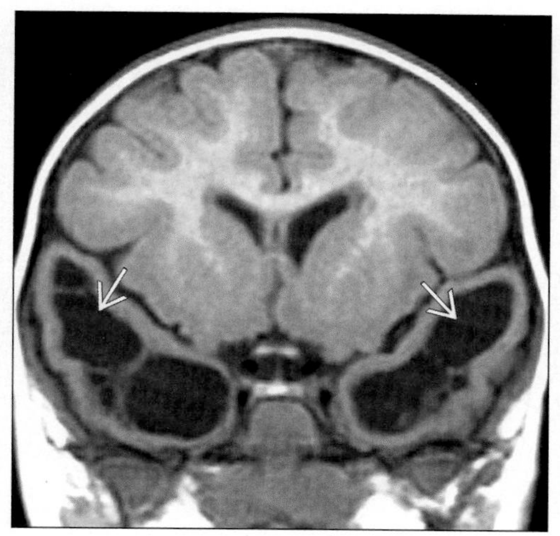

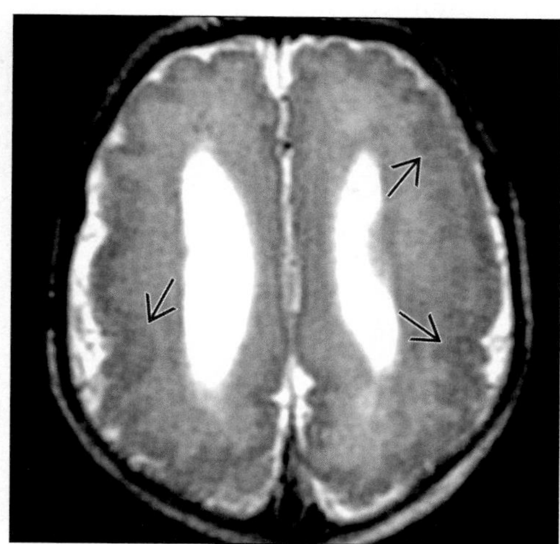

(Left) *Coronal T1WI MR in a microcephalic infant shows numerous periventricular cavitary germinolytic cysts* → *. Detecting these cysts on US, CT, or MR imaging should prompt the consideration of possible congenital CMV infection.* ***(Right)*** *Axial T2WI MR in a newborn shows bihemispheric polymicrogyria* → *. The ventricular dilation is a reflection of WM volume loss. Early cranial US showed periventricular germinolytic cysts.*

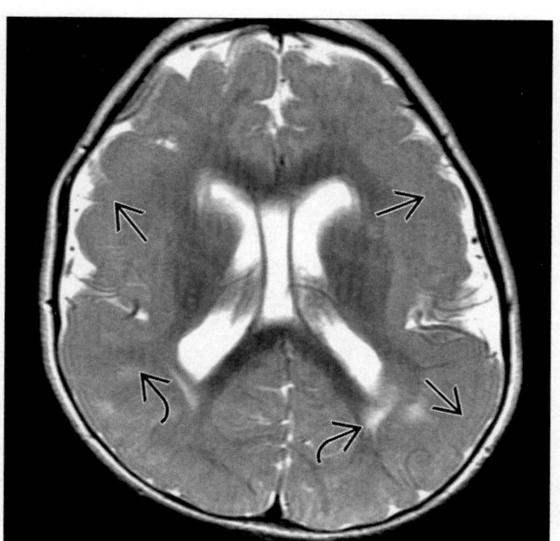

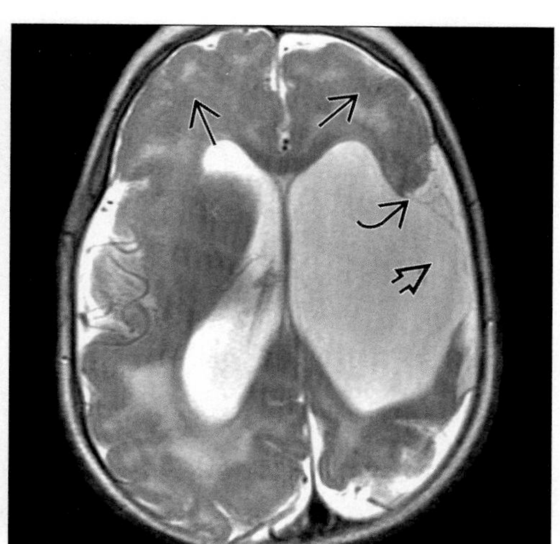

(Left) *Axial T2WI MR in an infant shows an extensive perisylvian dysplastic cortex* → *(likely polymicrogyria) and regions of abnormal WM signal* ↷*, likely gliosis &/or demyelination. Ventricular dilation is secondary to WM volume loss.* ***(Right)*** *Axial T2WI MR shows a left hemispheric "open-lip" schizencephaly* ⇨ *lined by polymicrogyric cortex* ↷*. Note the extensive bifrontal polymicrogyria* →*. Patchy central WM hyperintensity reflects regions of demyelination or gliosis.*

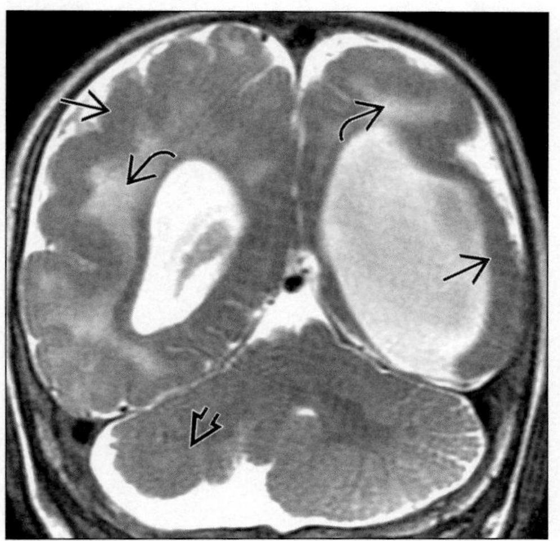

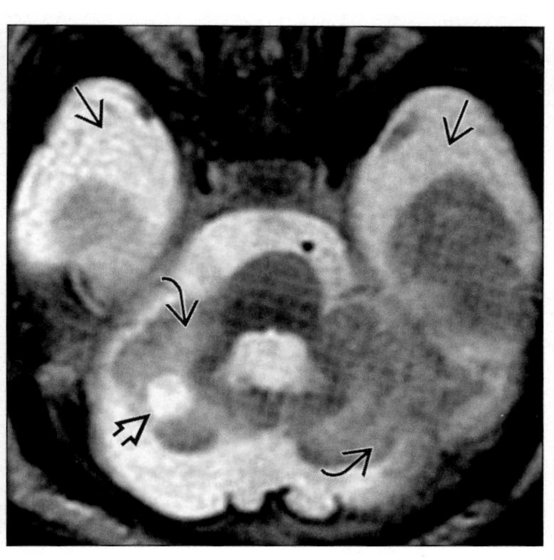

(Left) *Coronal T2WI MR shows ventriculomegaly secondary to central WM volume loss; WM hyperintensities reflecting edema, gliosis, or demyelination* ↷*; and polymicrogyria* →*. Also note the hypoplastic right cerebellar hemisphere* ⇨*.* ***(Right)*** *Axial T2WI MR in a neonate demonstrates cerebellar hypoplasia* ↷ *and focal cystic injury of the cerebellum* ⇨*. Expansion of the middle cranial fossa subarachnoid spaces* → *is indicative of temporal lobe atrophy.*

CONGENITAL HIV

Key Facts

Terminology

- Congenital AIDS, maternally transmitted AIDS

Imaging

- Basal ganglia (BG) Ca++, cerebral atrophy
- Atrophy (57-86%), frontal > BG > diffuse
- Mineralizing microangiopathy: BG Ca++ (30-85%) > frontal WM > cerebellum
- Atrophy, ± T1 shortening within BG due to Ca++
- ± high signal in frontal subcortical WM
- Fusiform vasculopathy (late)
- Include MRA with baseline NECT/MR in symptomatic patients

Top Differential Diagnoses

- Cytomegalovirus: Periventricular Ca++, microcephaly, cortical dysplasia
- Toxoplasmosis: Scattered Ca++, ± hydrocephalus
- Pseudo-TORCH: Basal ganglia, brainstem, and parenchymal Ca++, neurodegeneration

Clinical Issues

- Developmental delay, progressive encephalopathy, ↓ motor milestones, stroke
- Pediatric HIV: HIV cases in USA (2%), worldwide (5-25%); 90% are vertically transmitted (90%)
- Most acquired at birth, 3rd trimester, or via breast feeding

Diagnostic Checklist

- Consider congenital HIV with bilateral symmetrical BG Ca++ in children > 2 months
- Consider congenital HIV when fusiform arteriopathy is detected

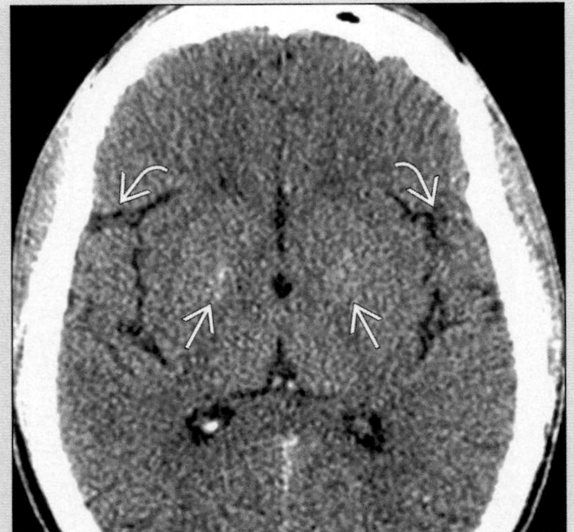

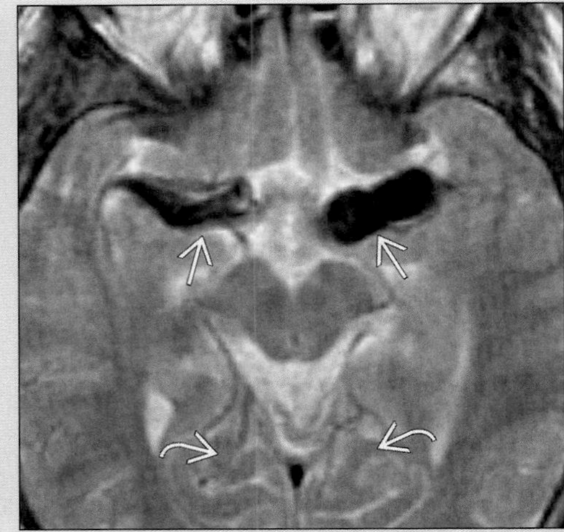

(Left) *Axial NECT in a 5-year-old girl with vertically transmitted HIV infection shows mild to moderate atrophy, most notable at the sylvian cisterns ↪. Note the focal calcification involving the globus pallidus ➔.* ***(Right)*** *Axial T2WI MR in a 12-year-old boy with a history of previous strokes and congenital HIV infection demonstrates fusiform aneurysmal dilation of the arteries of the circle of Willis ➔. There is evidence of early atrophy involving the occipital lobes ↪.*

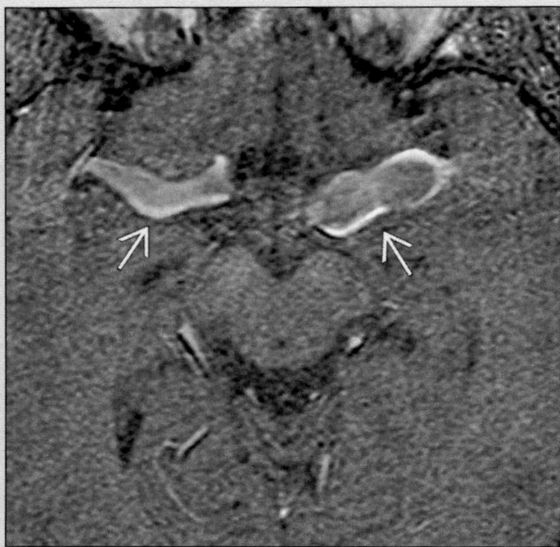

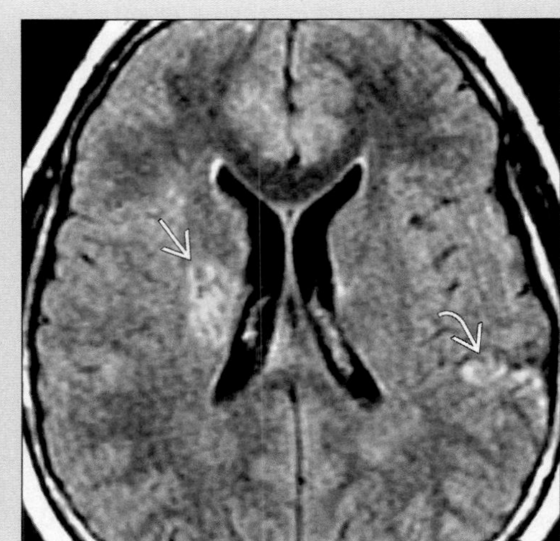

(Left) *Axial MRA without contrast in the same patient demonstrates flow-related enhancement within the fusiform, aneurysmally dilated M1 segments of the middle cerebral arteries ➔.* ***(Right)*** *Axial FLAIR MR in same patient with HIV-associated cerebral aneurysms and previous strokes demonstrates encephalomalacia and gliosis involving the right corona radiata ➔ and posterior left angular gyrus ↪. Stroke &/ or subarachnoid hemorrhage may herald the diagnosis of congenital HIV.*

CONGENITAL HIV

IMAGING

General Features

- Best diagnostic clue
  - Basal ganglia (BG) Ca++
  - Cerebral atrophy

CT Findings

- NECT
  - Atrophy (57-86%), frontal > BG > diffuse
  - Mineralizing microangiopathy: BG Ca++ (30-85%) > frontal white matter (WM) > cerebellum

MR Findings

- T1WI
  - Atrophy, ± T1 shortening within BG due to Ca++
- T2WI
  - ± high signal in frontal subcortical WM
- T2* GRE
  - May accentuate Ca++
- DWI
  - ± restricted diffusion for patients presenting with stroke
- T1WI C+
  - ± faint BG enhancement initially
- MRA
  - Fusiform vasculopathy (late)
- MRS
  - ↓ NAA, ↑ Cho/Cr, presence of excitatory neurotransmitters

Angiographic Findings

- DSA: Ectasia &/or fusiform aneurysmal dilation of intracranial arteries

Imaging Recommendations

- Best imaging tool
  - NECT
- Protocol advice
  - Include MRA with baseline NECT/MR in symptomatic patients

DIFFERENTIAL DIAGNOSIS

Cytomegalovirus

- Periventricular Ca++, microcephaly, cortical dysplasia

Toxoplasmosis

- Scattered Ca++, ± hydrocephalus

PATHOLOGY

General Features

- Etiology
  - HIV in microglial cells and macrophages
- Genetics
  - Co-receptors allow virus into cell, mutations in receptor gene ⇒ immunity in small percent

Gross Pathologic & Surgical Features

- Cerebrovascular disease found in 25% at autopsy (less than 3% on imaging)
- Fibrosing and calcific vasculopathy, aneurysms, strokes, demyelination, ± hemorrhage

Microscopic Features

- Microglial nodules, multinucleated giant cells, mononuclear cells, Ca++ vasculopathy, myelin loss

CLINICAL ISSUES

Presentation

- Most common signs/symptoms
  - Developmental delay
  - Encephalopathy
  - ↓ motor milestones
  - Stroke
  - Microcephaly

Demographics

- Age
  - Symptoms begin at 12 weeks of life; some asymptomatic until 10 years
- Epidemiology
  - Pediatric HIV: HIV cases in USA (2%), worldwide (5-25%); 90% are vertically transmitted
    - Most acquired at birth, 3rd trimester, or via breast feeding

Natural History & Prognosis

- If symptomatic in 1st year of life → 20% die in infancy
- Opportunistic infections less common than in adult HIV

Treatment

- Confirm diagnosis with polymerase chain reaction, HIV blood culture, p24-antigen assay
- Retroviral therapy improves survival (50% rebound in 1st year)

DIAGNOSTIC CHECKLIST

Image Interpretation Pearls

- Consider congenital HIV with bilateral symmetrical BG Ca++ in children > 2 months
- Consider HIV when fusiform arteriopathy is detected

SELECTED REFERENCES

1. Modi G et al: Human immunodeficiency virus associated intracranial aneurysms: report of three adult patients with an overview of the literature. J Neurol Neurosurg Psychiatry. 79(1):44-6, 2008
2. Tardieu M et al: Cerebral MR imaging in uninfected children born to HIV-seropositive mothers and perinatally exposed to zidovudine. AJNR Am J Neuroradiol. 26(4):695-701, 2005
3. Meleski ME et al: HIV exposure: neonatal considerations. J Obstet Gynecol Neonatal Nurs. 32(1):109-16, 2003
4. Mitchell W: Neurological and developmental effects of HIV and AIDS in children and adolescents. Ment Retard Dev Disabil Res Rev. 7(3):211-6, 2001
5. Tovo PA et al: Brain atrophy with intracranial calcification following congenital HIV infection. Acta Paediatr Scand. 77(5):776-9, 1988

NEONATAL HERPES ENCEPHALITIS

Key Facts

Terminology

- Neonatal herpes simplex encephalitis, HSV-2, neonatal HSV

Imaging

- Early: Edema, DWI abnormality ↔ late: Atrophy, cysts, ventriculomegaly, Ca++
- Variable brain involvement, early DWI abnormality
- Variable: WM, GM (cortical, BG), temporal lobe, brainstem, cerebellum, ± watershed
- Early: CT normal (27%); variable distribution, low attenuation
- Early: Swelling, T1 prolongation in affected regions
- Early: T2 prolongation (edema, neuronal necrosis), BG involved ~ 57%
- Hemorrhage less common than with HSV-1

Top Differential Diagnoses

- Peripartum &/or postnatal infection
- Stroke/ischemia, arterial or venous
- Vertically transmitted infection, TORCH
  - CMV → microcephaly, Ca++, cortical clefting or malformation
  - Toxoplasmosis → scattered Ca++, hydrocephalus

Pathology

- Transmission: Peripartum (85%), postnatal (10%), in utero (5%)

Diagnostic Checklist

- Suspect HSV-2 in neonates with unexplained DWI abnormality

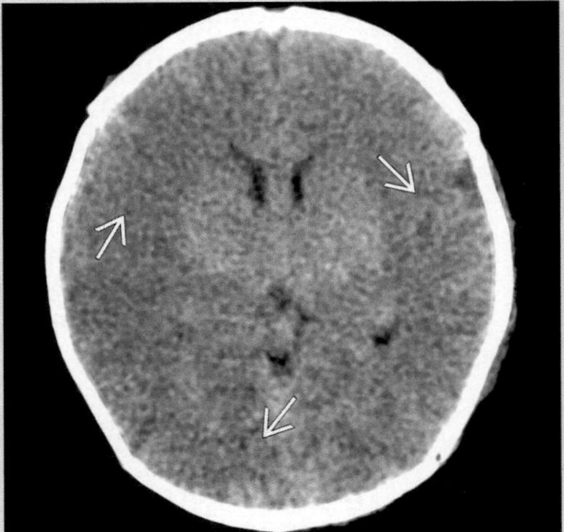

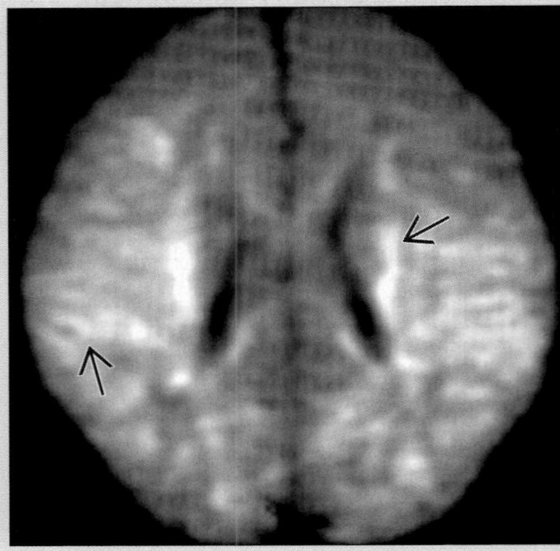

(Left) *Axial NECT in a neonate with HSV-2 encephalitis demonstrates widespread regions of gray and white matter hypoattenuation ➔. The initial NECT will be negative in up to 27% of infected neonates.* ***(Right)*** *Axial DWI MR in a 2-week-old with seizures & bulging fontanelle demonstrates extensive bihemispheric reduced diffusion ➔ involving gray and white matter structures in a random widespread manner. Increased IgM & positive PCR against HSV were detected. DWI is essential for early detection.*

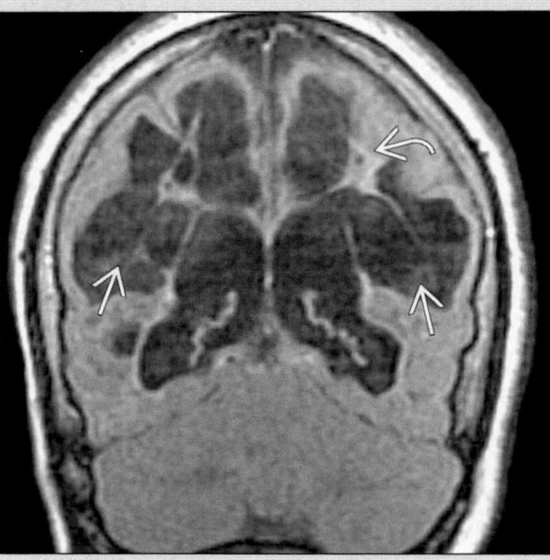

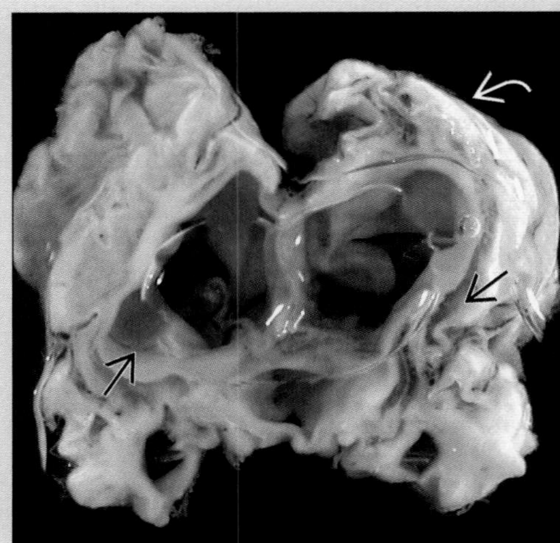

(Left) *Coronal FLAIR MR in a microcephalic infant who had HSV-2 peripartum encephalitis demonstrates extensive bihemispheric cystic encephalomalacia ➔. Note the adjacent regions of FLAIR hyperintensity ➔ representing gliosis.* ***(Right)*** *Coronal gross pathology section of a neonatal brain with changes of vertically transmitted HSV-2 infection, including ventricular dilation, cystic encephalomalacia ➔, and lack of normal cortical sulcation ➔. About 5% of neonatal HSV-2 is acquired in utero.*

NEONATAL HERPES ENCEPHALITIS

TERMINOLOGY

Abbreviations

- Neonatal HSV, HSV-2

IMAGING

General Features

- Best diagnostic clue
  - Variable brain involvement, early DWI abnormality
- Location
  - Variable: White matter (WM), gray matter (GM) (cortical, basal ganglia [BG]), temporal lobe, brainstem, cerebellum, ± watershed

CT Findings

- NECT
  - Early: Normal (27%), variable distribution, low attenuation
  - Late: Hydrocephalus, cysts, Ca++ (BG, thalami, cortex, or WM)

MR Findings

- T1WI
  - Early: Swelling, T1 prolongation in affected regions
  - Late: Atrophy, cysts, ventriculomegaly, ± T1 shortening (Ca++)
- T2WI
  - Early: T2 prolongation (edema, neuronal necrosis), BG involved ~ 57%
  - Late: Cystic encephalomalacia, atrophy, WM hyperintensity
- T2* GRE
  - Hemorrhage less common than with HSV-1
- DWI
  - Reduced diffusion in affected regions
- T1WI C+
  - Patchy enhancement in affected regions, ± meningeal enhancement
- MRS
  - Acute: ↑ Cho, Glx, glutamine, ± lipid lactate, ↓ NAA
  - Chronic: All metabolites ↓

Ultrasonographic Findings

- Early: Linear echoes in BG ↔ late; multicystic encephalomalacia, ± Ca++

Imaging Recommendations

- Protocol advice
  - NECT, MR

DIFFERENTIAL DIAGNOSIS

Peripartum &/or Postnatal Infection

- Stroke/ischemia: Arterial or venous

Vertically Transmitted Infection, TORCH

- CMV → microcephaly, Ca++, cortical clefting or malformation
- Toxoplasmosis → scattered Ca++, hydrocephalus

PATHOLOGY

General Features

- Etiology
  - Transmission: Peripartum (85%), postnatal (10%), in utero (5%)

Gross Pathologic & Surgical Features

- Early: Meningoencephalitis, necrosis, ± hemorrhage, microglial proliferation
- Late: Atrophy, cysts, Ca++, ± hydranencephaly

CLINICAL ISSUES

Presentation

- Most common signs/symptoms
  - Postnatal: Lethargy, apnea, poor feeding, ± seizures, bulging fontanelle
  - In utero: Low birth weight, microcephaly, microphthalmia, ± mucous membrane ulceration
- Clinical profile
  - CSF: Pleocytosis (mononuclear cells), ↑ protein
  - EEG: Nonspecific

Demographics

- Age
  - Onset for peripartum infection → 2-4 weeks
- Epidemiology
  - Newborns of African-American, low-income mothers with multiple sexual partners → 1:2,500 births → 40-45% are premature → 2% of mothers become HSV(+) during pregnancy

Natural History & Prognosis

- Death in ~ 50% of neonates with CNS disease and 85% with disseminated disease

Treatment

- C-section if active maternal infection ↔ intravenous acyclovir

DIAGNOSTIC CHECKLIST

Consider

- HSV-2 in neonates with unexplained MR diffusion abnormalities

Image Interpretation Pearls

- Postnatal: Varied distribution, + DWI, ± hemorrhage
- In utero: Atrophy, scattered brain Ca++, cystic encephalomalacia, ventriculomegaly

SELECTED REFERENCES

1. Vossough A et al: Imaging findings of neonatal herpes simplex virus type 2 encephalitis. Neuroradiology. 50(4):355-66, 2008
2. Pelligra G et al: Brainstem involvement in neonatal herpes simplex virus type 2 encephalitis. Pediatrics. 120(2):e442-6, 2007

GROUP B STREPTOCOCCAL MENINGITIS

Key Facts

Terminology

- GBS meningitis, group B β-hemolytic streptococcal meningitis
- Leading cause of newborn meningitis in developed countries

Imaging

- Acute manifestations: Meningitis, cerebritis, vasculitis, ventriculitis, subdural effusion, empyema, arterial and venous infarction
- Arterial distributions often affected
- Variable: Dural, leptomeningeal, and parenchymal enhancement
- Ependymal enhancement and ventricular debris = ventriculitis
- Blurring/loss of gray-white matter junction ⇒ ± BG, thalamic, WM hyperintensities
- FLAIR hyperintensity in cortex, SAS, and subdural, cisternal, and ventricular spaces
- Diffusion restriction within infarcts and empyema
- Rim enhancement with subdural effusion (thinner) and empyema (thicker)
- Dural venous sinus/cortical vein thrombosis ~ 30%

Top Differential Diagnoses

- Enteric, gram-negative meningitis
- *E. coli*: Along with GBS meningitis, major cause of newborn meningitis in developed countries
- Listeria monocytogenes: Gram-positive rod
- *Enterobacter*: Most common cause of meningitis in 1st few months of life

Diagnostic Checklist

- No imaging features distinguish GBS meningitis from other neonatal meningitides

*(**Left**) Axial CECT in an infant with group B streptococcal meningitis shows cortical enhancement ➡ and leptomeningeal enhancement ⇨. Note the dilation of the frontal horns and 3rd ventricle ↪ reflecting impeded CSF circulation. (**Right**) Axial T1 C+ MR of the same patient, performed for evaluation of status epilepticus 24 hours following CECT, more clearly shows the peripheral frontal cortical ➡ and leptomeningeal enhancement ⇨. CSF Gram stain showed gram-positive diplococci.*

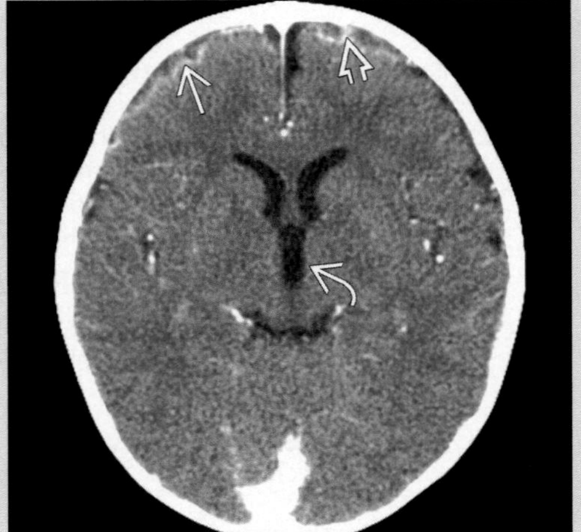

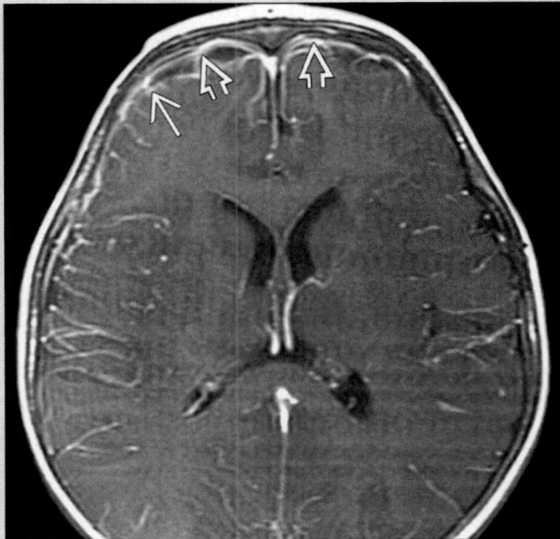

*(**Left**) Axial FLAIR MR is a sensitive tool to detect early complicated extraaxial fluid collections. FLAIR hyperintensity is seen in the right frontal cortex ➡ and within the right frontal temporal subarachnoid spaces ⇨. Note the early involvement of the left frontal subarachnoid space ↪. (**Right**) Axial DWI MR in the same patient with meningitis can help to differentiate subdural effusions from subdural empyemas. These bifrontal hyperintense subdural collections ➡ showed low ADC values.*

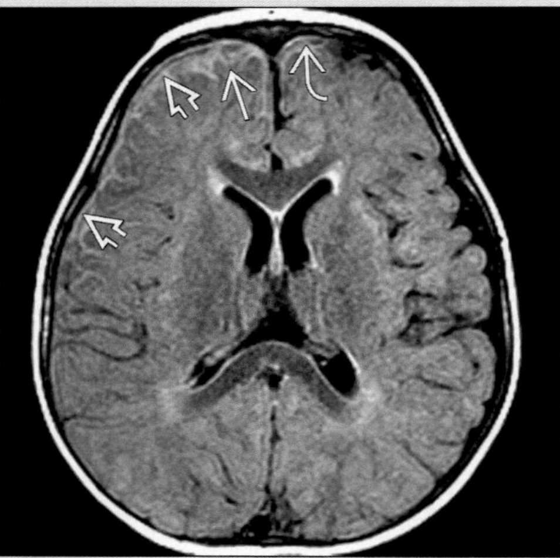

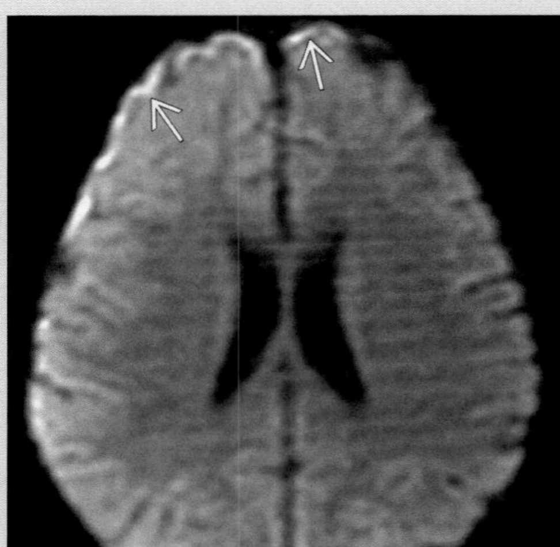

GROUP B STREPTOCOCCAL MENINGITIS

TERMINOLOGY

Abbreviations
- Group B streptococcal (GBS) meningitis

Synonyms
- Group B β-hemolytic streptococcal meningitis

Definitions
- Leading cause of newborn meningitis in developed countries
  - Early-onset disease (EOD): GBS sepsis presenting in 1st week of life
  - Late-onset disease (LOD): GBS sepsis presenting between 1-4 weeks of life

IMAGING

General Features
- Best diagnostic clue
  - Meningoencephalitis in newborn
- Location
  - Cerebral hemispheres and deep gray matter
- Size
  - Extensive panlobar involvement typical
- Morphology
  - Multifocal involvement
  - Arterial distributions often affected, particularly BG and thalami
- Acute manifestations: Meningitis, cerebritis, vasculitis, ventriculitis, subdural effusion, empyema, arterial and venous infarction
- Chronic sequelae: Loculated hydrocephalus, cystic encephalomalacia

CT Findings
- NECT
  - Hydrocephalus ± dependent debris in ventricles
  - Occasional hyperdense foci = hemorrhagic venous infarcts, laminar necrosis
  - Hypodense subdural collections (effusion vs. empyema)
- CECT
  - Variable: Dural, leptomeningeal, and parenchymal enhancement
    - Rim enhancement around subdural effusions and empyemas
  - Ependymal enhancement/ventricular debris

MR Findings
- T1WI
  - Hypo- and hyperintense foci common
    - Multifocal hypointensities = edema, ischemia, infarction
    - Hyperintense foci cortex, BG, and WM = laminar necrosis, hemorrhagic venous infarction
- T2WI
  - Blurring/loss of gray-white matter junction, ± BG, thalamic and WM hyperintensity
- FLAIR
  - Hyperintensity in cortex and subarachnoid, subdural, cisternal, and ventricular spaces
- T2* GRE
  - Blooming of hemorrhagic foci
- DWI
  - Diffusion reduced in infarcts, pus collections
- T1WI C+
  - Variable: Dural, leptomeningeal, parenchymal, and ependymal enhancement
  - Rim enhancement with subdural effusion (thinner) and empyema (thicker)
- MRA
  - Arterial narrowing, ± occlusions
- MRV
  - Dural venous sinus/cortical vein thrombosis (in up to 30%)
- MRS
  - ↑ choline, ↓ NAA; positive lactate in areas of ischemia/infarction

Ultrasonographic Findings
- Grayscale ultrasound
  - ↑ echogenicity of sulci and parenchyma ⇒ hydrocephalus ⇒ ventricular debris

Imaging Recommendations
- Best imaging tool
  - MR with IV contrast, DWI, MRA, and MRV
- Protocol advice
  - CECT for rapid, initial assessment of hemodynamically unstable neonate

DIFFERENTIAL DIAGNOSIS

Other Neonatal Meningitides
- Enteric, gram-negative meningitis
  - Account for majority of early onset meningitis in developing countries
  - Higher mortality than GBS meningitis
  - Specific pathogens
    - *E. coli*: Major cause of newborn meningitis in developed countries (along with GBS meningitis)
    - *Enterobacter*: Most common cause of meningitis in 1st few months of life
    - *Citrobacter*: Rare; high morbidity/mortality secondary to frequent abscess formation
- Other meningitides
  - Listeria monocytogenes: Gram-positive rod

Congenital Infections (TORCH)
- CMV, toxoplasmosis, rubella: Infection occurs in utero with chronic sequelae present in neonate/infant
  - CMV: Periventricular Ca++, microcephaly, migrational abnormalities, encephalomalacia, cerebellar hypoplasia
  - Toxoplasmosis: Parenchymal Ca++, encephalomalacia, microphthalmia
- Herpes simplex virus type 2 (HSV-2): Infection acquired during vaginal birth; presents in 1st 2-4 weeks of life
  - Meningoencephalitis with extensive edema, necrosis, cystic encephalomalacia

Hypoxic Ischemic Encephalopathy
- Preterm: Injury to periventricular WM (mild) or thalami, basal ganglia, brainstem (severe)

- Term: Injury to mature vascular watershed (mild) or areas of early myelination/metabolic activity (severe)

PATHOLOGY

General Features

- Etiology
  - EOD: Aspiration of infected amniotic fluid or birth canal secretions
  - LOD: As EOD or postnatal maternal contact, breast milk, nosocomial
  - Bacteremia facilitated by immature neonatal immune system
  - Development of meningitis related to magnitude/duration of bacteremia
  - Production of β-hemolysin facilitates access of GBS across blood-brain barrier
- GBS agalactiae serotype 3 responsible for majority of GBS meningitis
- Embryology/anatomy
  - GBS is potent activator of neonatal immune/inflammatory response

Gross Pathologic & Surgical Features

- Debris, exudates within subarachnoid spaces and ventricles
- Parenchymal infarction/encephalomalacia; luminal narrowing of vessels

Microscopic Features

- Inflammation of adventitia and vaso vasorum = vasculitis

CLINICAL ISSUES

Presentation

- Most common signs/symptoms
  - Lethargy, poor feeding, irritability
  - Seizures (40%) and bulging fontanelle are typically late findings
- Clinical profile
  - Newborn with sepsis
  - Typical signs/symptoms of meningitis subtle or absent in neonate
- CSF analysis: ↑ WBCs, ↑ protein ↓ glucose
- CSF/blood Gram stain: Gram-positive diplococci
- Maternal risk factors for EOD: GBS colonization, GBS chorioamnionitis/bacteruria, membrane rupture > 18 hours, intrapartum fever ≥ 38°C, previous newborn with EOD, delivery at < 37 weeks gestation

Demographics

- Age
  - 90% of newborns with GBS EOD present within 1st 24 hours of life
  - GBS LOD presents between 1 to 4 weeks after birth; occasionally up to 6 months
- Gender
  - Male, preterm infants (< 37 weeks) most at risk for EOD
- Ethnicity
  - Maternal GBS colonization rates highest in African-American women
- Epidemiology
  - 10-30% of pregnant women have asymptomatic GBS colonization of genital/GI tract
    - Actual < 1% of newborns born to colonized women develop EOD
  - EOD incidence: 0.5/1,000 live births
    - Incidence decreased by > 50% as result of maternal screening and intrapartum chemoprophylaxis
    - ↓ incidence of GBS EOD accompanied by ↑ incidence of neonatal gram-negative sepsis
    - Term infants account for 50% of GBS EOD secondary to preterm intrapartum chemoprophylaxis

Natural History & Prognosis

- Prognosis
  - Mortality of early-onset disease
    - Full-term newborns (2%), 34-36 weeks gestational age (10%), < 33 weeks gestational age (30%)
  - Morbidity meningitis: Neurological sequelae (12-30%) (cortical blindness, spasticity, global mental retardation)

Treatment

- Maternal
  - GBS screen: Rectovaginal swab at 35-37 weeks gestation
  - Positive maternal GBS screen or presence of other risk factors: Intrapartum IV penicillin
  - Future strategies
    - GBS PCR assay and rapid strep screen at onset of labor
    - GBS vaccine: Ideal prevention strategy; would prevent development of antibiotic-resistant pathogens
- Neonatal meningitis
  - High-dose IV penicillin ⇒ ± antiepileptics ⇒ CSF diversion may be required for complicated hydrocephalus

DIAGNOSTIC CHECKLIST

Image Interpretation Pearls

- No imaging features distinguish GBS meningitis from other neonatal meningitides

SELECTED REFERENCES

1. Centers for Disease Control and Prevention (CDC): Trends in perinatal group B streptococcal disease - United States, 2000-2006. MMWR Morb Mortal Wkly Rep. 58(5):109-12, 2009
2. Yikilmaz A et al: Sonographic findings in bacterial meningitis in neonates and young infants. Pediatr Radiol. 38(2):129-37, 2008
3. Heath PT et al: Perinatal group B streptococcal disease. Best Pract Res Clin Obstet Gynaecol. 21(3):411-24, 2007
4. Smirniotopoulos JG et al: Patterns of contrast enhancement in the brain and meninges. Radiographics. 27(2):525-51, 2007
5. Miyairi I et al: Group B streptococcal ventriculitis: a report of three cases and literature review. Pediatr Neurol. 34(5):395-9, 2006

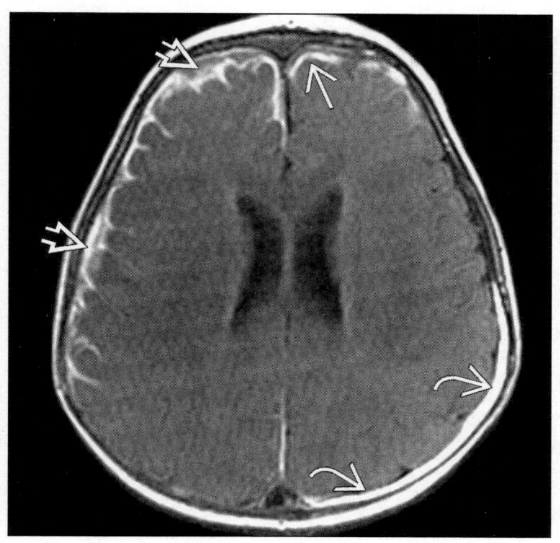

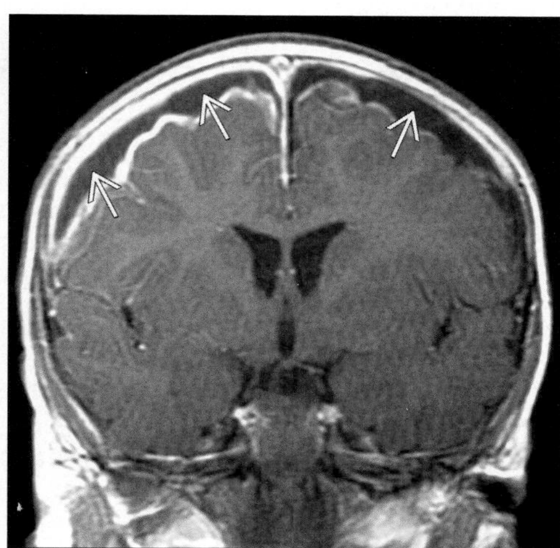

(Left) *Axial FLAIR MR with IV contrast in a neonate with group B streptococcal meningitis shows asymmetric hyperintensity in supratentorial subarachnoid spaces → and cortical hyperintensity →. Note the hyperintense subdural collection → that had reduced diffusion on DWI (empyema).* ***(Right)*** *Coronal T1WI C+ MR shows bilateral frontal convexity subdural effusions → that had restricted diffusion on DWI. Effusions typically regress with appropriate IV therapy.*

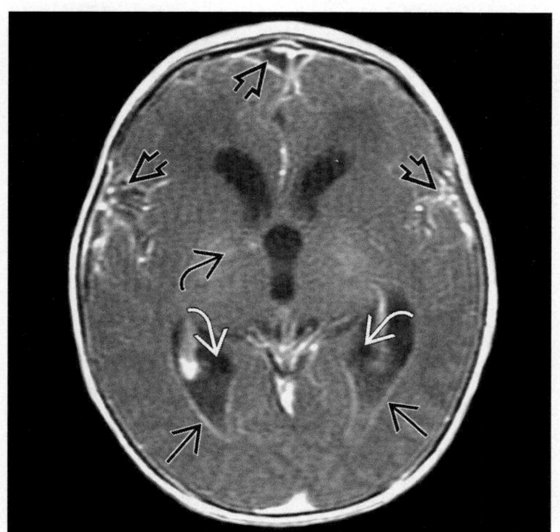

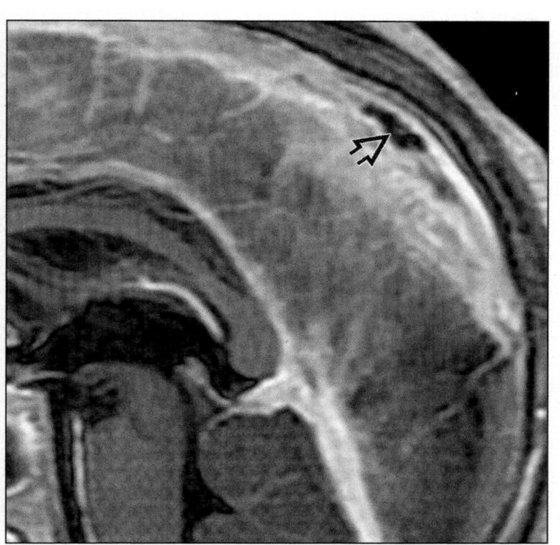

(Left) *Axial T1WI C+ MR shows extensive leptomeningeal enhancement →. Note the ventricular ependymal enhancement →, dependent ventricular debris → (ventriculitis), and basal ganglia enhancement → due to perivascular space inflammation/arteritis. Ventricular dilation reflects early hydrocephalus.* ***(Right)*** *Sagittal MRV with contrast shows a hypointense clot → within the sagittal sinus, creating a partial occlusion. Small clots were also detected in the transverse sinuses.*

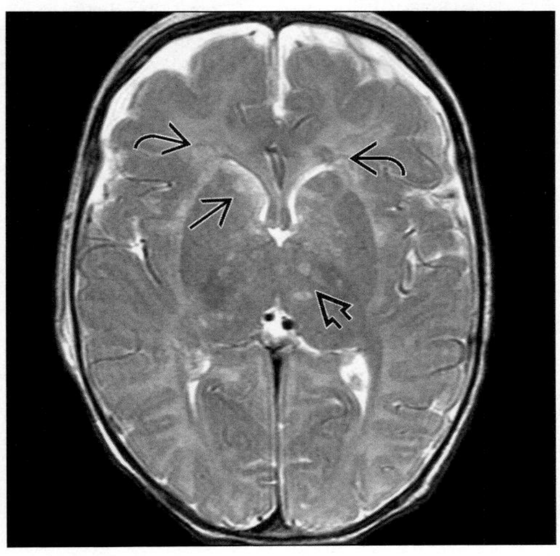

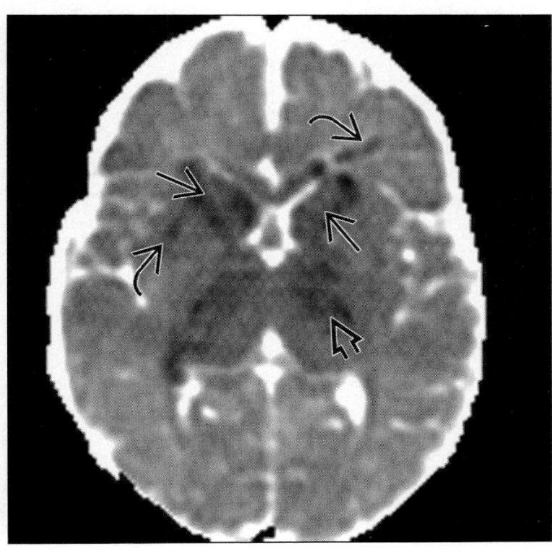

(Left) *Axial T2WI MR demonstrates focal basal ganglia →, thalamic →, and white matter → hyperintensities, reflecting infarction secondary to perivascular space inflammatory involvement/ arteritis.* ***(Right)*** *Axial ADC in the same patient shows multiple basal ganglia → and thalamic → infarctions. Note the scattered white matter infarctions →. Early detection of infarction is best achieved with diffusion imaging, which shows abnormality when T2 and FLAIR images may be "normal."*

CITROBACTER MENINGITIS

Key Facts

Imaging

- Multiple, large, cystic white matter (WM) lesions
- ± diffuse pneumocephalus (due to gas production)
- Square morphology of abscesses
- Rim or dot-like septal enhancement
- Best imaging tool: MR with contrast

Top Differential Diagnoses

- Other bacterial brain infections
- Periventricular white matter injury
- Cystic encephalomalacia
- White matter lacerations in nonaccidental head injury

Pathology

- Infection acquired: Horizontally (nosocomial) or vertically (maternal)
- Colonization (skin, umbilicus stump) → bacteremia → meningitis

Clinical Issues

- Immunocompromised patients at higher risk
- Neonates & sick preterms are immunocompromised
- Preterm newborns are most susceptible
- 5% of neonatal (gram-negative) meningitis → 80% of neonatal brain abscesses
- Abscesses may only appear near completion of therapy
- 80% of neonates with *Citrobacter* meningitis develop brain abscesses

Diagnostic Checklist

- Square WM abscesses with rim or dot-like septal enhancement

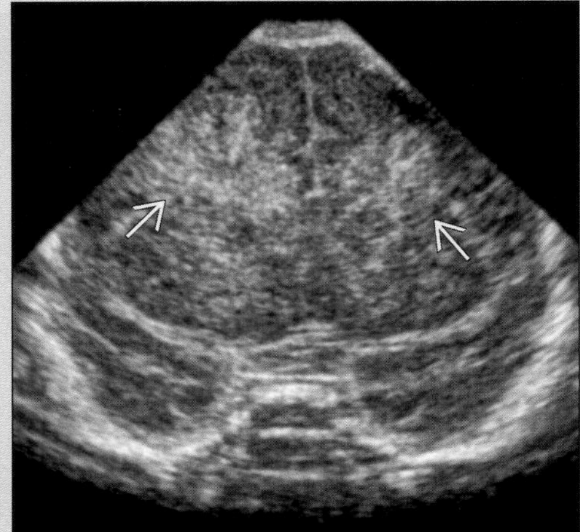

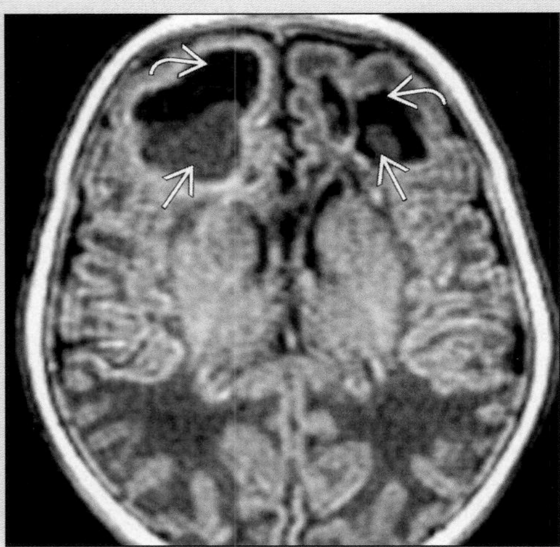

(Left) *Coronal cranial ultrasound in a newborn with Citrobacter sepsis shows bilateral frontal lobe white matter hyperechogenicity ➔ corresponding to regions of cerebritis on earlier MR (not shown). (Courtesy C. Glasier, MD.)* ***(Right)*** *Axial T1WI MR in a newborn with peripartum Citrobacter sepsis shows bifrontal "square" cavitary white matter abscesses ➔. These cavitary lesions progressed from foci of cerebritis. Note the necrotic debris ➔ within the cavities. (Courtesy C. Glasier, MD.)*

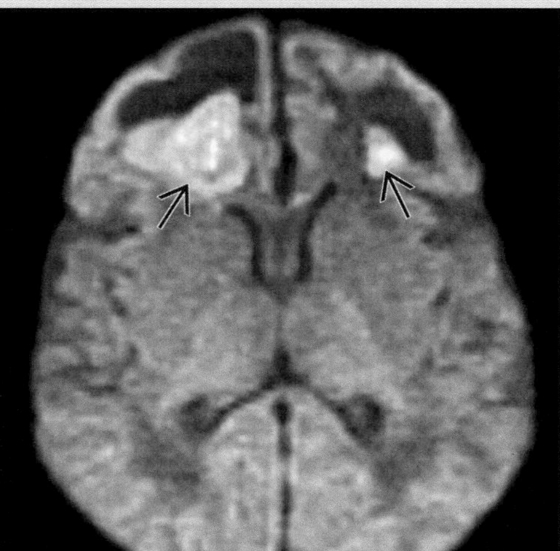

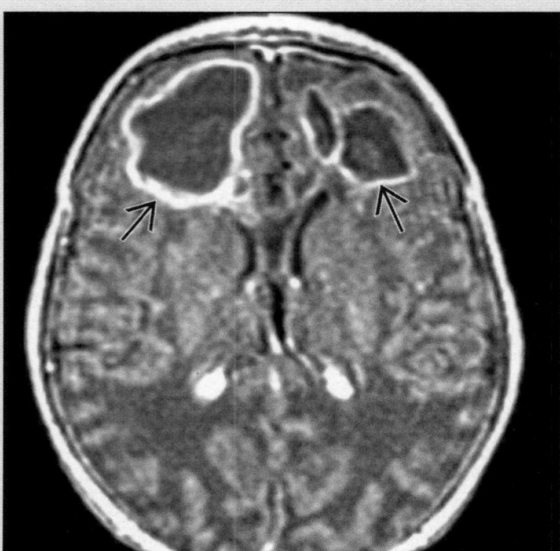

(Left) *Axial DWI MR in the same patient demonstrates reduced diffusivity (increased signal intensity) within the dependent infected debris ➔. (Courtesy C. Glasier, MD.)* ***(Right)*** *Axial T1 C+ MR in the same patient shows rim enhancement ➔ of the abscesses. Dot-like septal enhancement within the abscesses is another finding that may be seen on CECT or T1WI C+ MR. (Courtesy C. Glasier, MD.)*

CITROBACTER MENINGITIS

TERMINOLOGY

Synonyms

- *Citrobacter* cerebritis

Definitions

- Gram-negative (Gm-) enteric bacterium
  - Predilection for very young, very old patients
    - Newborns (NB) → sepsis, meningitis, and cerebral abscesses
    - Elderly → causes urinary, upper respiratory tract infections

IMAGING

General Features

- Best diagnostic clue
  - Multiple, large, cystic ("square") white matter (WM) lesions
    - Replace (not displace) white matter
  - "Square" abscesses
    - Square abscess that "rounds" more likely to have infected contents
    - Increasing mass effect/edema more likely to have infected contents
- Location
  - Predilection for lobar white matter
- Size
  - Multiple large WM cysts
- Morphology
  - Square abscesses

CT Findings

- NECT
  - Early (cerebritis)
    - Patchy, multilobar WM lesions
    - Low attenuation compared to unmyelinated brain
    - ± diffuse pneumocephalus (due to gas production)
  - Late (abscess)
    - Lobar WM cavities with septations
    - Square morphology of abscesses
    - Dot-like focus of septal Ca++
- CECT
  - Early (cerebritis)
    - Variable, often subtle parenchymal enhancement
  - Late (abscess)
    - Rim or dot-like septal enhancement
    - Multiple large cavities (± septations), replace WM

MR Findings

- T1WI
  - Early (cerebritis)
    - Patchy multilobar areas of diminished T1 signal
  - Late (abscess)
    - Multiple large cysts
    - Square morphology
    - Septations
    - T1 WM signal abnormality diminishes
- T2WI
  - Early (cerebritis)
    - Patchy multilobar T2 prolongation
  - Late (abscess)
    - Multiple, often septated cavities
    - Usually bilateral
    - T2 prolongation within WM
    - Variable edema, mass effect
    - Eventually, cavities may contract, causing profound WM loss
- FLAIR
  - Increased signal within lobar WM
- T2* GRE
  - Dot-like Ca++ within septal walls shows diminished signal
- T1WI C+
  - Early (cerebritis)
    - Subtle patchy WM enhancement
  - Late (abscess)
    - Patchy WM enhancement
    - Rim or septal wall enhancement
    - Dot-like focus of septal enhancement
- MRS
  - Products of fermentation
    - Lactate, acetate, and succinate
  - Proteolysis end-products released from neutrophils
    - Valine and leucine

Ultrasonographic Findings

- Grayscale ultrasound
  - Early (meningitis/cerebritis)
    - Sulcal thickening and increased sulcal echogenicity
    - Regions of WM hyperechogenicity
    - Loss of normal WM echo architecture
  - Late (abscess)
    - Multiple, septated, WM, anechoic or hypoechoic cavities
- Color Doppler
  - Subtle flow within abscess septal walls

Imaging Recommendations

- Best imaging tool
  - MR with contrast best depicts extent of involvement
- Protocol advice
  - MR with contrast
    - Shows early parenchymal enhancement of cerebritis
    - Reveals dot-like foci of septal enhancement of "squared" abscesses
    - Detects complications of brain infection (vascular, extraaxial purulent collections)

DIFFERENTIAL DIAGNOSIS

Other Bacterial Brain Infections

- Usually with greater surrounding edema and mass effect
- Possible sinus, mastoid, or embolic/hematogenous sources of infection

Periventricular Leukomalacia

- Perifrontal and peritrigonal locations of WM cysts
- Nonprogressive cystic change
- No rim or septal "dot" enhancement

Cystic Encephalomalacia

- Cortical and deep gray matter involved

- Thalamic and basal ganglia Ca++
- Cysts replaces WM
- Passive ventricular dilatation

White Matter Lacerations in Nonaccidental Head Injury (NAHI)

- Frontal lobe WM
- Fluid level may be seen dependently within laceration
- Associated intracranial manifestations of NAHI
  - Parafalcine/convexity subdural hematoma, subarachnoid hemorrhage

PATHOLOGY

General Features

- Etiology
  - Neurovirulence factors of *Citrobacter* species
    - Unique 32-kD outer membrane protein
    - Resistance to phagocytosis
  - *Citrobacter* invades/transcytoses microvascular endothelial cells
    - Leads to hemorrhagic necrosis and abscess
  - Intracellular replication of *Citrobacter* in microvascular endothelial cells
    - Contributes to persistence of brain infection
- Genetics
  - No particular genetic predisposition known
- Associated abnormalities
  - Infection acquired: Horizontally (nosocomial) or vertically (maternal)
  - Colonization (skin, umbilicus stump) → bacteremia → meningitis
  - *Citrobacter* is facultative anaerobe
    - Hydrolyzes urea and ferments glucose → produces gas

Gross Pathologic & Surgical Features

- Opaque leptomeninges, purulent exudate
- Diffuse ependymitis

Microscopic Features

- No well-formed fibrotic capsule
- Organisms in walls of congested vessels
- Neutrophils plus necrotic cell debris

CLINICAL ISSUES

Presentation

- Most common signs/symptoms
  - Septic newborn or preterm infant: Bulging fontanelle, apnea, seizures
- Clinical profile
  - In very premature neonates
    - Sepsis, irritability, poor feeding, bulging fontanelle
- Immunocompromised patients at higher risk
  - Neonates, sick preterms are immunocompromised

Demographics

- Age
  - Mean age of sepsis onset = 5 days
  - Preterm newborns are most susceptible
  - *Citrobacter* CNS infection beyond 1 month of age is rare
- Epidemiology
  - Epidemiology of *Citrobacter* infection
    - 5% of neonatal (gram-negative) meningitis → 80% of neonatal brain abscesses
    - Abscesses may only appear near completion of therapy
  - *Citrobacter* CNS infection
    - Most cases considered sporadic ↔ neonatal ICU outbreaks do occur

Natural History & Prognosis

- 30% of neonates and infants with *Citrobacter* CNS infection die
- 80% of neonates with *Citrobacter* meningitis develop brain abscesses
- 50% of *Citrobacter* meningitis/abscess survivors have significant CNS damage

Treatment

- Antibiotics are mainstay of therapy
- 2 drug therapy is standard
  - Late abscesses occur, and prolonged IV therapy is rule
- Adjunctive surgical drainage of abscesses
  - For enlarging cysts on optimized IV therapy
  - Poorly responsive to initial antibiotic therapy

DIAGNOSTIC CHECKLIST

Image Interpretation Pearls

- Minimal edema surrounding abscesses
- Square abscesses with focal septal enhancement
- Not all rim-enhancing cavities are abscesses
  - Some are WM necrosis and liquefaction
- *Citrobacter* species and *Enterobacter sakazakii* have similar imaging

SELECTED REFERENCES

1. Samonis G et al: Citrobacter infections in a general hospital: characteristics and outcomes. Eur J Clin Microbiol Infect Dis. 28(1):61-8, 2009
2. Benca J et al: Nosocomial meningitis caused by Enterobacteriaceae: risk factors and outcome in 18 cases in 1992-2007. Neuro Endocrinol Lett. 28 Suppl 2:27-9, 2007
3. Alviedo JN et al: Diffuse pneumocephalus in neonatal Citrobacter meningitis. Pediatrics. 118(5):e1576-9, 2006
4. Agrawal D et al: Vertically acquired neonatal citrobacter brain abscess - case report and review of the literature. J Clin Neurosci. 12(2):188-90, 2005
5. Pooboni SK et al: Pneumocephalus in neonatal meningitis: diffuse, necrotizing meningo-encephalitis in Citrobacter meningitis presenting with pneumatosis oculi and pneumocephalus. Pediatr Crit Care Med. 5(4):393-5, 2004
6. Doran TI: The role of Citrobacter in clinical disease of children: review. Clin Infect Dis. 28(2):384-94, 1999
7. Meier A et al: Neonatal citrobacter meningitis: neurosonographic observations. J Ultrasound Med. 17(6):399-401, 1998

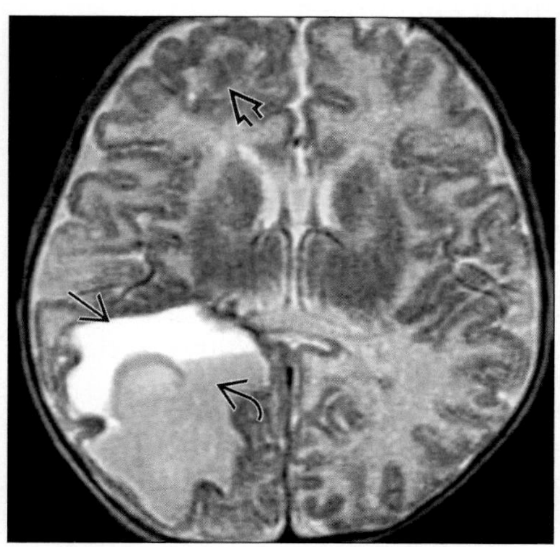

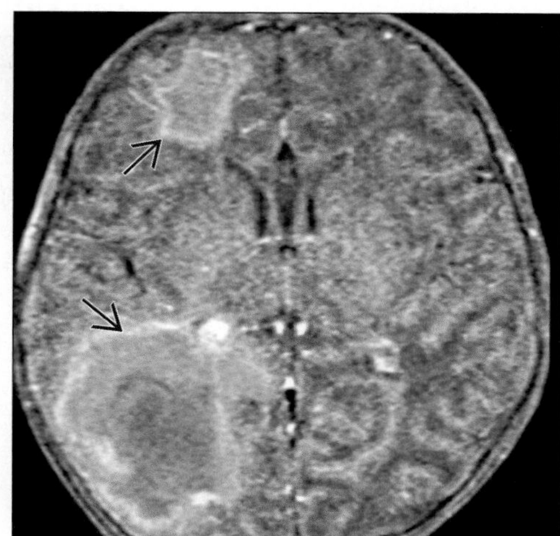

(Left) *Axial T2WI MR in a 1 month old with neonatal Citrobacter sepsis demonstrates a large cavitary right parietooccipital abscess* ➔ *with dependent debris* ➔. *Note the developing small right frontal lobe abscess* ➔, *which is just starting to cavitate. (Courtesy L. Lowe, MD.)* ***(Right)*** *Rim enhancement* ➔ *of a more mature parietooccipital and less mature frontal abscess is seen. Progression from meningitis to cerebritis to abscess is common (~ 80%). (Courtesy L. Lowe, MD.)*

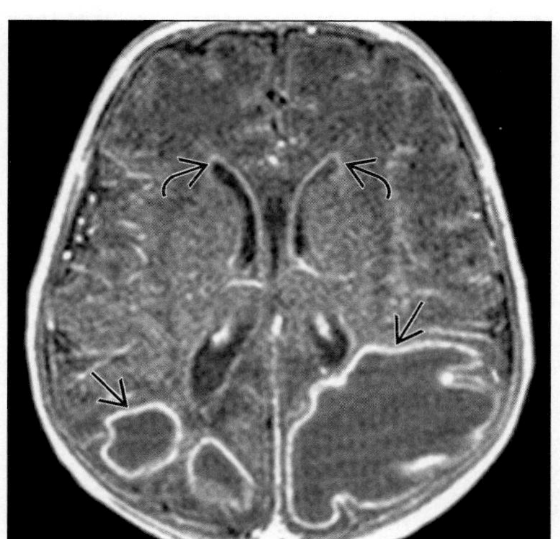

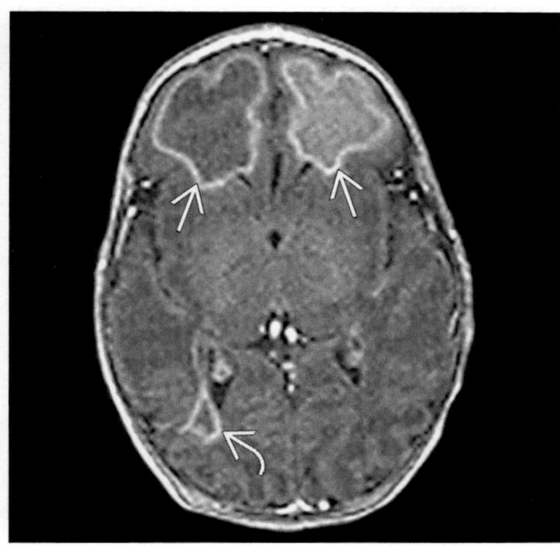

(Left) *Axial T1WI C+ MR in an infant with "treated" Citrobacter meningitis demonstrates large bilateral parietooccipital rim-enhancing abscesses* ➔. *Note the associated ependymal thickening and enhancement reflecting ventriculitis* ➔. *(Courtesy T. Booth, MD.)* ***(Right)*** *In this newborn with "treated" Citrobacter meningitis, bilateral frontal* ➔ *and right peritrigonal* ➔ *rim-enhancing abscesses are seen. Long-term IV therapy is the rule in such cases. (Courtesy T. Feygin, MD.)*

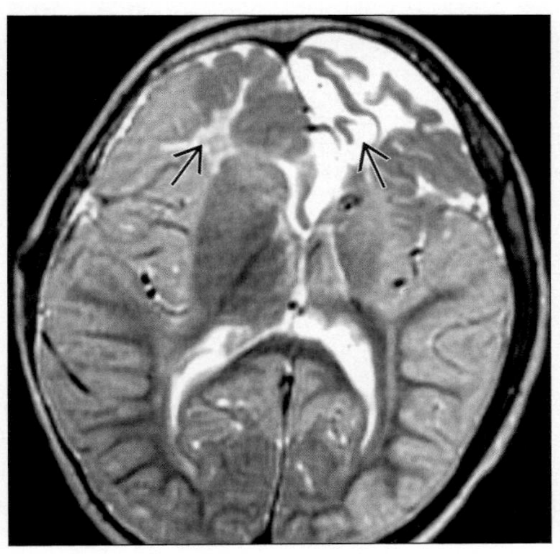

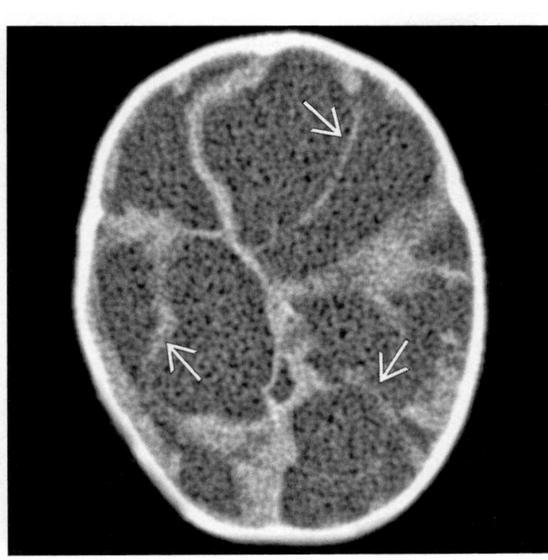

(Left) *Axial T2WI MR in a 1 year old with refractory seizures remote from long-term IV therapy for Citrobacter brain abscesses shows bilateral frontal retraction cavities, gliosis, and atrophy* ➔. *(Courtesy C. Glasier, MD.)* ***(Right)*** *Axial NECT in an infant originally diagnosed with Citrobacter sepsis and meningitis shows that the meningitis has progressed. Note the multifocal cerebral abscesses lead to macrocystic encephalomalacia and multiple septated cavities* ➔. *(Courtesy S. Gorges, MD.)*

MENINGITIS

Key Facts

Terminology

- Acute or chronic inflammatory infiltration of pia, arachnoid, and CSF
- Classified as acute pyogenic (bacterial), lymphocytic (viral), chronic (tuberculosis or granulomatous)

Imaging

- Imaging best delineates complications: Empyema, ischemia, hydrocephalus, cerebritis/abscess
- FLAIR MR: Hyperintense signal in sulci, cisterns
- T1WI C+: Exudate and brain surface (pia) enhance
- Delayed C+ FLAIR most sensitive sequence for leptomeningeal disease
- DWI: Invaluable for detecting complications
- Basilar meningitis typical of pyogenic infections, TB, cryptococcosis, neurosyphilis, sarcoid, lymphoma
- Meningitis is clinical/laboratory diagnosis, not imaging diagnosis
    - Can occur in presence of normal imaging

Top Differential Diagnoses

- Carcinomatous meningitis
- Neurosarcoidosis
- Increased FLAIR signal in CSF (SAH, high inspired oxygen, artifact, venous congestion from stroke)

Pathology

- Hematogenous spread from remote infection (i.e., heart, teeth) is most common etiology

Clinical Issues

- Adults: Headache, fever, nuchal rigidity, ± altered mental status
- Children: Fever, irritability, nuchal rigidity
- Infants: Fever, lethargy, irritability
- Intravenous antibiotics are mainstay of therapy

*(**Left**) Axial graphic shows diffuse inflammatory exudate that involves the leptomeninges and fills the basal cisterns and sulci. This typically results in increased density on CT or T1 signal intensity on MR. It is important to remember that meningitis is a clinical/laboratory diagnosis, not an imaging diagnosis. (**Right**) Axial T1WI C+ MR shows the classic findings of meningitis, with striking sulcal and cisternal enhancement, as well as hydrocephalus. This basilar pattern of enhancement is typical of TB meningitis.*

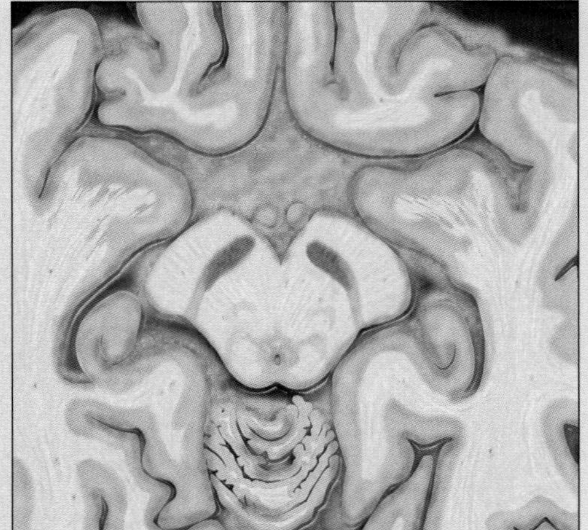

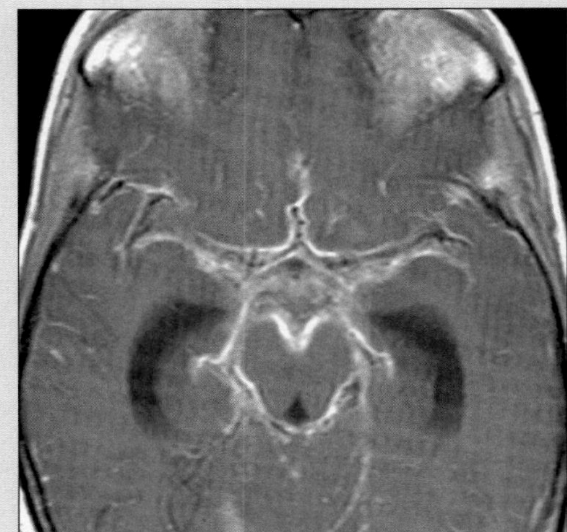

*(**Left**) Axial FLAIR MR shows diffusely abnormal signal throughout the sulci and pial surface of the brain ➔ caused by pyogenic meningitis. (**Right**) Axial T1WI C+ MR shows extensive enhancement of the basal cisterns with an enlarged cerebral aqueduct related to coccidioidomycosis meningitis. Causes of infectious basilar meningitis include bacterial infection, TB, cryptococcosis, and neurosyphilis. Sarcoidosis and lymphoma also have a predilection for the basal meninges. (Courtesy T. Swallow, MD.)*

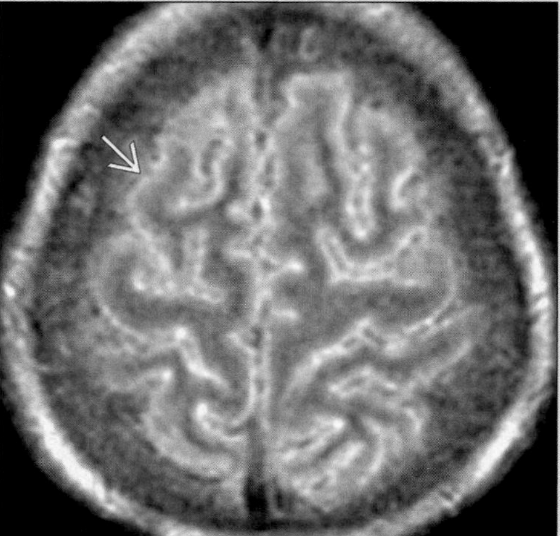

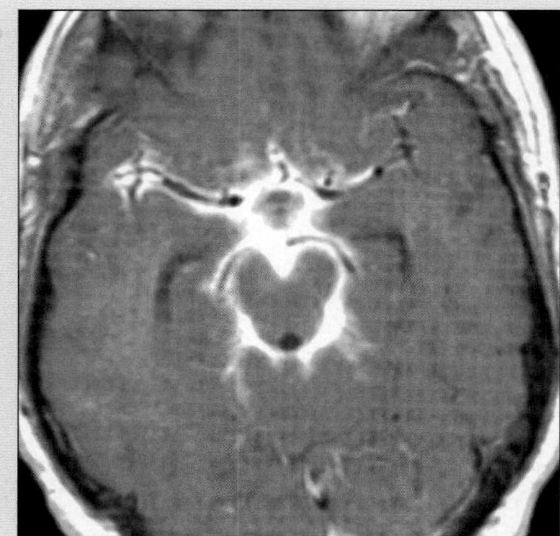

MENINGITIS

TERMINOLOGY

Synonyms

- Leptomeningitis; infectious meningitis

Definitions

- Acute or chronic inflammatory infiltration of pia, arachnoid, and CSF
- Classified as acute pyogenic (bacterial), lymphocytic (viral), or chronic (tubercular or granulomatous)

IMAGING

General Features

- Best diagnostic clue
  - Positive CSF by lumbar puncture
- Location
  - Pia, arachnoid, and subarachnoid space of brain and spine
- Morphology
  - Typically smooth ± thick, intense sulcal-cisternal enhancement
  - Tuberculosis (TB), fungal meningitis often basilar/ confluent; may be nodular
- Imaging may be normal early
- Imaging best delineates complications
  - Hydrocephalus (often early complication)
  - Cerebritis/abscess
  - Empyema
- Imaging findings often nonspecific

CT Findings

- NECT
  - Most common = normal
  - Mild ventricular enlargement common
  - Sulci, basal cisterns may appear effaced
  - May see increased density in basilar cisterns or sylvian fissures related to inflammatory debris
  - ± subdural effusion in pediatric patients
- CECT
  - Enhancing exudate in sulci, cisterns
  - Low-density areas related to ischemic complications
- CTA
  - Arterial narrowing, occlusion may be seen

MR Findings

- T1WI: Isointense exudate
- T2WI: Hyperintense exudate
- FLAIR: Hyperintense signal in sulci, cisterns (nonspecific)
  - May see hydrocephalus
- DWI: Useful to detect vascular complications, empyema, abscess
- T1WI C+: Exudate and brain surface (pia) enhance
  - Characterizes complications
- MRA: May see arterial narrowing or occlusion
- MRV: May see venous thrombosis
- MRS: Helpful for evaluation of complications
  - e.g., cerebritis, abscess, infarct

Ultrasonographic Findings

- Sulcal enlargement, echogenic deposits in subarachnoid space in infants
- Ventricular dilatation and subdural collections

Imaging Recommendations

- Protocol advice
  - MR with FLAIR, DWI, T1WI C+
  - Delayed enhanced FLAIR most sensitive sequence for leptomeningeal disease

DIFFERENTIAL DIAGNOSIS

Carcinomatous Meningitis

- Primary tumor often known (exception = lymphoma)
- Breast, lung most common extracranial sources
- Primary CNS tumors: GBM, medulloblastoma, pineal/ choroid plexus tumors, PNET, ATRT, ependymoma

Neurosarcoidosis

- Lacy leptomeningeal enhancement
- May have ventricular or dural-based enhancing masses

Increased FLAIR Signal in CSF

- Nonspecific; many causes
  - Subarachnoid hemorrhage (SAH)
  - High inspired oxygen
  - Artifact
  - Acute stroke (parenchymal edema, vascular congestion)
  - Retained gadolinium in CSF
    - Dialysis-dependent patient with end-stage renal disease

PATHOLOGY

General Features

- Etiology
  - Hematogenous (most common)
    - Spread from remote infection (heart, teeth, etc.)
    - Some may enter CNS via choroid plexus (lacks blood-brain barrier)
  - Direct extension
    - Less common
    - Sinusitis, otitis media, orbital infection
    - Skull base fracture
  - Penetrating injury (least common)
  - Basilar meningitis typical of pyogenic infections, TB, cryptococcosis, neurosyphilis, sarcoid, lymphoma
- Associated abnormalities
  - Complications
    - Extraventricular obstructive hydrocephalus (EVOH)
    - Ventriculitis, choroid plexitis
    - Cerebritis, abscess
    - Subdural fluid collections (empyema, effusion)
  - Cerebrovascular complications
    - Venous and arterial thrombosis
    - Ischemia/infarct

Gross Pathologic & Surgical Features

- Gross pathology generally same regardless of agent
- Cisterns, sulci filled with cloudy CSF, then purulent exudate
- Pia-arachnoid congested, may mimic SAH
- Cortex may be edematous

MENINGITIS

Microscopic Features

- Meningeal exudate: PMNs, fibrin, bacteria
- Vessels within exudate may show fibrinoid necrosis, thrombosis
- Infection may extend into perivascular spaces (PVSs), ventricles
  - PVSs may act as conduit for infection to reach brain parenchyma
- May spread by direct invasion of pia
- Subpial, microglial, astrocytic proliferation

CLINICAL ISSUES

Presentation

- Most common signs/symptoms
  - Adults: Headache, fever, nuchal rigidity, ± altered mental status
    - Brudzinski sign: Hips and knees flex involuntarily when neck is flexed
    - Kernig sign: Flex hips and knees, try to extend knees; pain in hamstrings, patient resistance
  - Children: Fever, irritability, nuchal rigidity
  - Infants: Fever, lethargy, irritability
  - Seizures in 30%
  - Meningitis is clinical/laboratory diagnosis, not imaging diagnosis
- Clinical profile
  - CSF shows increased white blood cells (leukocytosis)
    - Elevated CSF protein, decreased glucose typical of infectious meningitis
  - Purpuric rash may develop in *N. meningitidis* (meningococcal) meningitis, highly morbid

Demographics

- Epidemiology
  - Bacterial meningitis increase in last 30 years related to nosocomial infection
    - Approximately 3/100,000 in USA
  - Meningitis is most common form of CNS infection in children
  - Incidence of bacteria based on age
    - Elderly: *Listeria monocytogenes*, *Streptococcus pneumoniae*, *Neisseria meningitidis*, gram-negative bacilli
    - Adults: *S. pneumoniae*, *N. meningitidis*, group B *Streptococcus*
    - Children: *N. meningitidis*
    - Infants: *S. pneumoniae*, *N. meningitidis*
    - Neonates: Group B *Streptococcus*, *Escherichia coli*, *Enterobacter*
  - Vaccine has markedly decreased incidence of *Haemophilus influenzae* meningitis
  - Viral meningitis: Enteroviruses most common
  - Chronic meningitis
    - TB most common
    - High morbidity, mortality despite treatment
  - Fungal meningitis: *Cryptococcus neoformans* (AIDS) and *Coccidioides immitis* most common

Natural History & Prognosis

- Effective antimicrobial agents have reduced but not eliminated mortality, morbidity
- Impaired CSF resorption may cause hydrocephalus
- Elevated intracranial pressure, cerebral perfusion alterations can be early complications
- Complications occur in 50% of adult patients
  - Infectious: Cerebritis/abscess, ventriculitis, empyema, effusion
  - Vascular: Ischemia related to arterial spasm or infectious arteritis, dural venous thrombosis
  - Labyrinthine ossificans is uncommon complication
    - Infection of labyrinth via cochlear aqueduct from subarachnoid space
    - Typically results in bilateral hearing loss
- Mortality up to 20-25%

Treatment

- Intravenous antibiotics
  - Empiric therapy based on age
    - < 1 month: Ampicillin and cefotaxime
    - > 1 month: Ceftriaxone or cefotaxime + vancomycin + dexamethasone
  - Specific therapy based on culture and sensitivity
  - Most bacterial meningitides: Ceftriaxone or cefotaxime ± vancomycin is treatment of choice
  - Fungal meningitis: Amphotericin B ± fluconazole or flucytosine
  - TB meningitis requires combination therapy: Isoniazid, pyrazinamide, rifampin
  - Viral meningitis: Supportive care, except for herpes meningitis (acyclovir)
- Surgery for complications (hydrocephalus, empyema)

DIAGNOSTIC CHECKLIST

Consider

- Imaging may be normal, most useful for complications

Image Interpretation Pearls

- Meningitis is clinical/laboratory diagnosis, not imaging diagnosis
  - Can occur in presence of normal imaging
- T1WI C+, FLAIR often complementary in diagnosis
- Delayed contrast-enhanced FLAIR best for subtle disease
- DWI invaluable for detecting complications of meningitis

SELECTED REFERENCES

1. Helbok R et al: Chronic meningitis. J Neurol. 256(2):168-75, 2009
2. Lee BE et al: Aseptic meningitis. Curr Opin Infect Dis. 20(3):272-7, 2007
3. Lepur D et al: Community-acquired bacterial meningitis in adults: antibiotic timing in disease course and outcome. Infection. 35(4):225-31, 2007
4. Smirniotopoulos JG et al: Patterns of contrast enhancement in the brain and meninges. Radiographics. 27(2):525-51, 2007
5. Kremer S et al: Accuracy of delayed post-contrast FLAIR MR imaging for the diagnosis of leptomeningeal infectious or tumoral diseases. J Neuroradiol. 33(5):285-91, 2006
6. Meyer S et al: Tuberculous meningitis. Lancet. 367(9523):1682, 2006

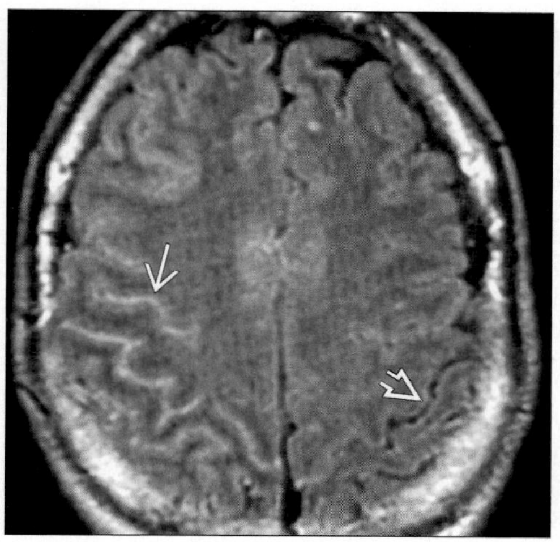

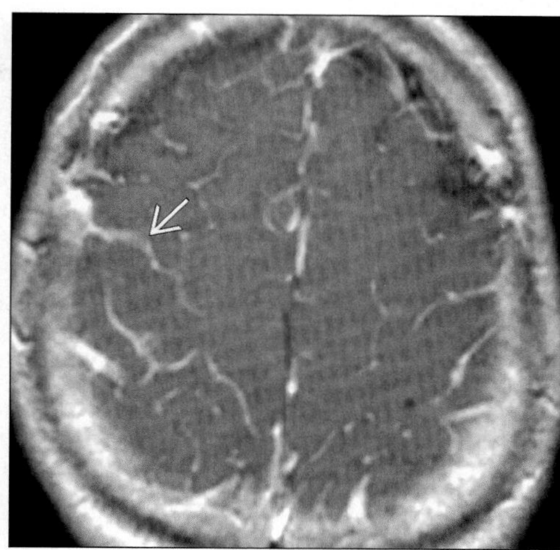

(Left) *Axial FLAIR MR shows hyperintensity in the right frontal and parietal sulci ➔ compared to the nearly normal hypointense CSF on the left ➲, findings related to meningeal infiltration by inflammatory cells.* ***(Right)*** *Axial T1WI C+ MR in the same patient shows striking enhancement in the right sulci ➔. Diagnosis was Streptococcus pneumoniae meningitis. MR is particularly helpful in identifying the complications of meningitis, including hydrocephalus, cerebritis, abscess, empyema, and ischemia.*

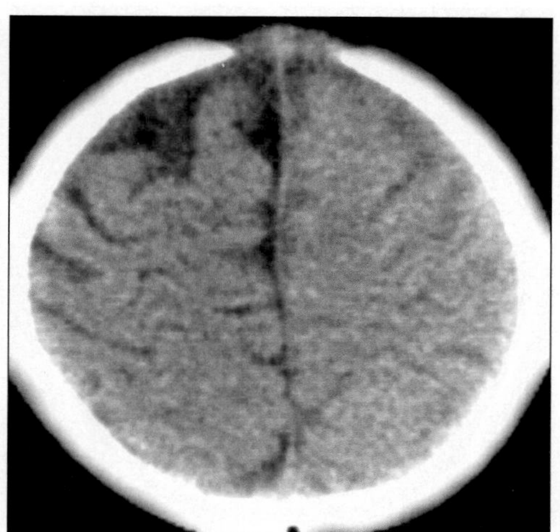

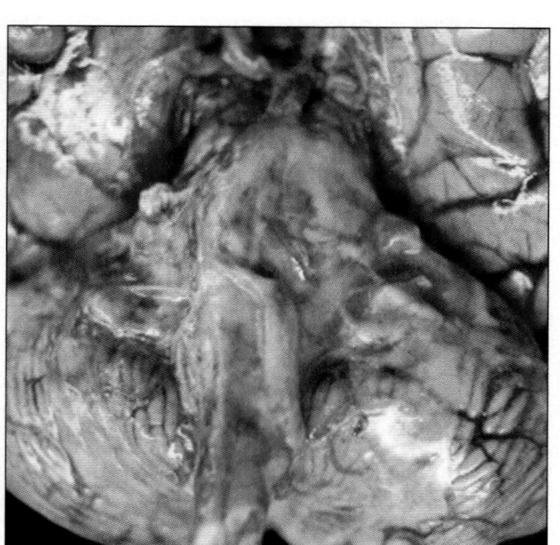

(Left) *Axial NECT in an infant shows poor visualization of the left convexity sulci related to an inflammatory exudate due to bacterial meningitis. There has been a markedly decreased incidence of Haemophilus influenzae meningitis since the development of vaccination programs.* ***(Right)*** *Gross pathology from a patient with E. coli meningitis shows extensive purulent exudate coating the base of the brain, involving the leptomeninges. The sulci and cisterns were also involved. (Courtesy J. Townsend, MD.)*

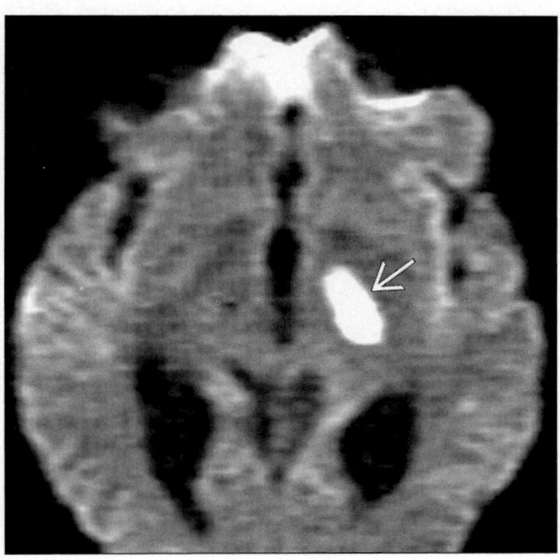

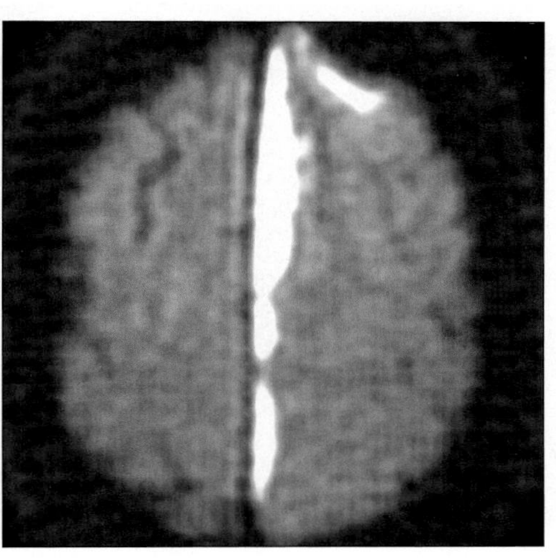

(Left) *Axial DWI MR shows focal high signal in the left posterior limb of the internal capsule ➔, as well as moderately enlarged ventricles, in this patient with bacterial meningitis complicated by ischemia & hydrocephalus. Ischemia may be the result of arterial spasm/occlusion or true arteritis.* ***(Right)*** *Axial DWI MR shows a hyperintense subdural collection in a patient with sinusitis complicated by meningitis, cerebritis, & empyema. DWI is invaluable in the evaluation of meningitis complications.*

Key Facts

Terminology
- Focal pyogenic infection of brain parenchyma, typically bacterial; fungal or parasitic less common
- 4 pathologic stages: Early cerebritis, late cerebritis, early capsule, late capsule

Imaging
- Ring-enhancing lesion with T2 hypointense rim and diffusion restriction characteristic
- Typically supratentorial in frontal and parietal lobes
- Imaging varies with stage of abscess development
  - Early cerebritis: Ill-defined T2 hyperintense mass
- Findings with contrast enhancement
  - Early cerebritis: Patchy enhancement
  - Late cerebritis: Intense, irregular rim enhancement
  - Early capsule: Well-defined, thin-walled, enhancing rim
  - Late capsule: Cavity collapses, capsule thickens
- MRS: Central necrotic area may show acetate, lactate, alanine, succinate, pyruvate, amino acids

Top Differential Diagnoses
- Glioblastoma multiforme
- Parenchymal metastases
- Demyelinating disease
- Resolving intracerebral hematoma
- Subacute cerebral infarction

Clinical Issues
- Headache is most common presentation; may have seizures, altered mental status, focal deficits
- Most common 20-40 years; 25% in patients < 15 years
- Potentially fatal but treatable lesion
- Lumbar puncture hazardous; pathogen often cannot be determined from CSF unless related to meningitis

*(**Left**) Axial graphic shows early cerebritis, the initial phase of abscess formation, in the frontal lobe. There is a focal unencapsulated mass of petechial hemorrhage, inflammatory cells, and edema. (**Right**) Axial T1WI C+ MR shows a low signal lesion with patchy central enhancement ⮚ in this young adult with early cerebritis. Imaging varies with the stage of abscess development and may mimic a neoplasm, demyelination, or subacute infarct, as in this case. DWI is often helpful to distinguish cerebritis from its mimics.*

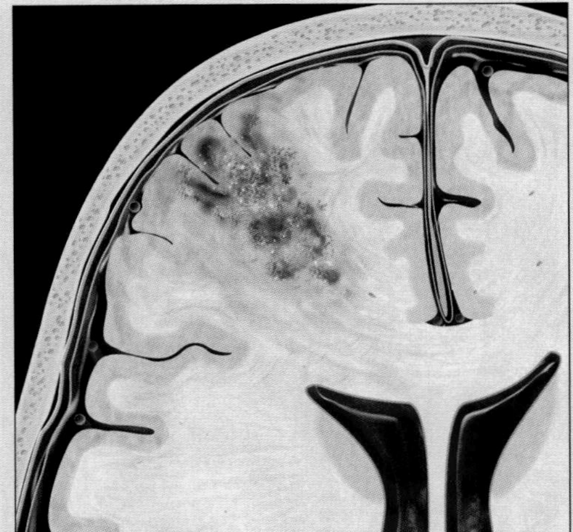

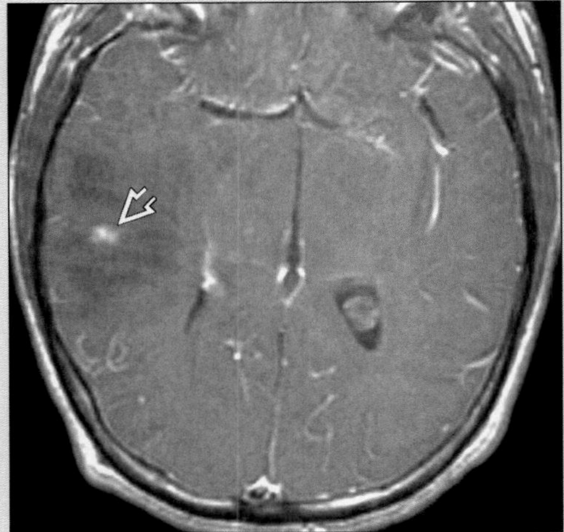

*(**Left**) Axial graphic shows the early capsule formation of an abscess with central liquified necrosis and inflammatory debris. Collagen and reticulin form the well-defined abscess wall. Note the surrounding edema. (**Right**) Axial T1WI C+ FS MR in a teenager shows a ring-enhancing mass with central necrosis and surrounding edema. A T2 hypointense rim and diffusion restriction can differentiate this abscess from a brain tumor. MRS and perfusion MR may also help determine the correct preoperative diagnosis.*

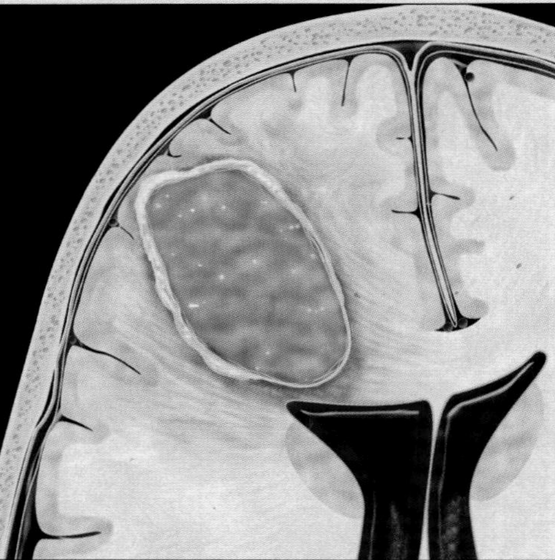

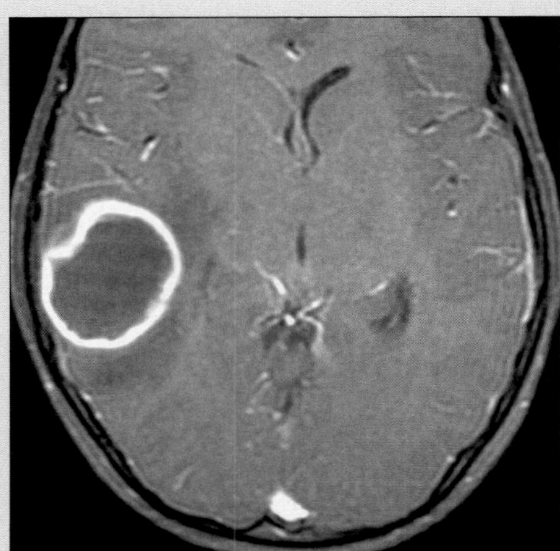

TERMINOLOGY

Definitions

- Focal pyogenic infection of brain parenchyma, typically bacterial; fungal or parasitic less common
- 4 pathologic stages: Early cerebritis, late cerebritis, early capsule, late capsule

IMAGING

General Features

- Best diagnostic clue
  - Imaging varies with stage of abscess development
  - Early capsule: Well-defined, thin-walled enhancing rim
    - Ring-enhancing lesion: DWI high signal, low ADC
    - T2 hypointense rim with surrounding edema
- Location
  - Typically supratentorial; up to 14% infratentorial
  - Frontal, parietal lobes most common
  - Usually at gray-white junction (hematogenous)
  - Multiple lesions may represent septic emboli
- Size
  - 5 mm up to several cm
- Morphology
  - Thin-walled, well-delineated, ring-enhancing, cystic-appearing mass

CT Findings

- NECT
  - Early cerebritis: Ill-defined, hypodense subcortical lesion with mass effect; may be normal early
  - Late cerebritis: Central low-density area; peripheral edema, increased mass effect
  - Early capsule: Hypodense mass with moderate vasogenic edema and mass effect
  - Late capsule: Edema, mass effect diminish
  - Gas-containing abscess rare
- CECT
  - Early cerebritis: ± mild patchy enhancement
  - Late cerebritis: Irregular rim enhancement
  - Early capsule: Low-density center with thin, distinct enhancing rim
    - Deep part of capsule thinnest; thickest near cortex
  - Late capsule: Cavity shrinks, capsule thickens
    - May have "daughter" abscesses

MR Findings

- T1WI
  - Early cerebritis: Poorly marginated, mixed hypo-/isointense mass
  - Late cerebritis: Hypointense center, iso-/mildly hyperintense rim
  - Early capsule: Rim iso-/hyperintense to white matter (WM); center hyperintense to CSF
  - Late capsule: Cavity shrinks, capsule thickens
- T2WI
  - Early cerebritis: Ill-defined hyperintense mass
  - Late cerebritis: Hyperintense center, hypointense rim; hyperintense edema
  - Early capsule: Hypointense rim (due to collagen, hemorrhage, or paramagnetic free radicals)
  - Late capsule: Edema and mass effect diminish
- DWI
  - Increased signal intensity in cerebritis and abscess
  - ADC map: Markedly decreased signal centrally within abscess
- T1WI C+
  - Early cerebritis: Patchy enhancement
  - Late cerebritis: Intense, irregular rim enhancement
  - Early capsule: Well-defined, thin-walled enhancing rim
  - Late capsule: Cavity collapses, capsule thickens
    - Capsule thinnest on ventricular side
- MRS
  - Central necrotic area may show presence of acetate, lactate, alanine, succinate, pyruvate, amino acids
- PWI: Low rCBV ratio in capsule
  - rCBV 0.76 ± 0.12 reported
- Resolving abscess: T2 hypointense rim resolves, central ADC increases, enhancement resolves last
  - Small ring/punctate enhancing focus may persist for months

Nuclear Medicine Findings

- PET: FDG and carbon-11-methionine show increased uptake in brain abscess

Imaging Recommendations

- Best imaging tool
  - Contrast-enhanced MR
- Protocol advice
  - Multiplanar MR ± contrast, DWI, ± MRS, PWI

DIFFERENTIAL DIAGNOSIS

Glioblastoma Multiforme

- Thick, nodular > thin wall
- Low signal on DWI (rarely high, mimics abscess)
- Hemorrhage common
- Other cystic primary neoplasms can also mimic abscess

Parenchymal Metastases

- Thick-walled, centrally necrotic mass
- Often multiple with marked edema
- May be solitary ring-enhancing lesion
- DWI typically negative (rarely positive and mimics abscess)

Demyelinating Disease

- Multiple sclerosis, ADEM
- Ring enhancement often incomplete ("horseshoe")
- Characteristic lesions elsewhere in brain
- Mass effect small for size of lesion

Resolving Intracerebral Hematoma

- History of trauma or vascular lesion
- Blood products present on MR

Subacute Cerebral Infarction

- History of stroke
- Vascular distribution
- Gyriform > > ring enhancement (rare)

PATHOLOGY

General Features

- Etiology
  - Hematogenous from extracranial location (pulmonary infection, endocarditis, urinary tract infections)
  - Direct extension from calvarial or meningeal infection
    - Paranasal sinus, middle ear, teeth infections (via valveless emissary veins)
  - Penetrating trauma (bone fragments > metal)
  - Postoperative
  - Right-to-left shunts (congenital cardiac malformations, pulmonary arteriovenous fistulas)
  - Neonatal: 2/3 associated with meningitis
  - 20-30% have no identifiable source (cryptogenic)
    - Often polymicrobial (*Streptococci*, *Staphylococci*, anaerobes)
- Cerebritis: Unencapsulated zone of vessels, inflammatory cells, edema; necrotic foci coalesce
- Capsule: Well-defined capsule develops around necrotic core; edema/mass effect decreases as matures

Gross Pathologic & Surgical Features

- Early cerebritis (3-5 days)
  - Infection focal but not localized
  - Unencapsulated mass of PMNs, edema, scattered foci of necrosis, petechial hemorrhage
- Late cerebritis (4-5 days to 2 weeks)
  - Necrotic foci coalesce
  - Rim of inflammatory cells, macrophages, granulation tissue, fibroblasts surrounds central necrotic core
  - Vascular proliferation, surrounding vasogenic edema
- Early capsule (begins about 2 weeks)
  - Well-delineated collagenous capsule
  - Liquified necrotic core, peripheral gliosis
- Late capsule (weeks to months)
  - Central cavity shrinks
  - Thick wall (collagen, granulation tissue, macrophages, gliosis)

Microscopic Features

- Early cerebritis: Hyperemic tissue with PMNs, necrotic blood vessels, microorganisms
- Late cerebritis: Progressive necrosis of neuropil, PMN destruction, and inflammatory cells
- Early capsule: Granulation tissue proliferation around necrotic core
- Late capsule: Multiple layers of collagen & fibroblasts

CLINICAL ISSUES

Presentation

- Most common signs/symptoms
  - Headache (up to 90%); may have seizures, altered mental status, focal deficits
  - Fever in only 50%
- Other signs/symptoms
  - Increased ESR (75%), elevated WBC count (50%)

Demographics

- Age
  - Most common during 3rd and 4th decades, but 25% occur in patients < 15 years
- Gender
  - M:F = 2:1
- Epidemiology
  - Uncommon; approximately 2,500 cases/year in USA
  - Bacterial: *Staph*, *Strep*, *Pneumococcus*
  - Diabetic: *Klebsiella pneumoniae*
  - Post-transplant: *Nocardia*, *Aspergillus*, *Candida*
  - AIDS: *Toxoplasmosis*, *Mycobacterium tuberculosis*
  - Neonates: *Citrobacter*, *Proteus*, *Pseudomonas*, *Serratia*, *Staphylococcus aureus* (meningitis related)

Natural History & Prognosis

- Potentially fatal but treatable lesion
  - Stereotactic surgery + medical therapy have greatly reduced mortality
- Complications of inadequately or untreated abscesses
  - Meningitis, "daughter" lesions
  - Mass effect, herniation
  - Intraventricular rupture, ventriculitis
    - May be fatal (80%)
    - Ventricular debris with irregular fluid level
    - Hydrocephalus and ependymal enhancement
- Factors affecting prognosis: Size, location, virulence of infecting organism(s), and systemic conditions
- Mortality variable: 0-30%
- Epilepsy: Common complication in pediatric patients

Treatment

- Primary therapy: Surgical drainage &/or excision
- If < 2.5 cm or early phase cerebritis: Antibiotics only
- Steroids to treat edema and mass effect
- Lumbar puncture hazardous; pathogen often cannot be determined from CSF unless related to meningitis

DIAGNOSTIC CHECKLIST

Consider

- DWI, MRS helpful to distinguish abscess from mimics

Image Interpretation Pearls

- Search for local cause (sinusitis, otitis media, mastoiditis)
- T2 hypointense abscess rim resolves before enhancement in successfully treated patients

SELECTED REFERENCES

1. Nath K et al: Role of diffusion tensor imaging metrics and in vivo proton magnetic resonance spectroscopy in the differential diagnosis of cystic intracranial mass lesions. Magn Reson Imaging. 27(2):198-206, 2009
2. Menon S et al: Current epidemiology of intracranial abscesses: a prospective 5 year study. J Med Microbiol. 57(Pt 10):1259-68, 2008
3. Lai PH et al: Proton magnetic resonance spectroscopy and diffusion-weighted imaging in intracranial cystic mass lesions. Surg Neurol. 68 Suppl 1:S25-36, 2007

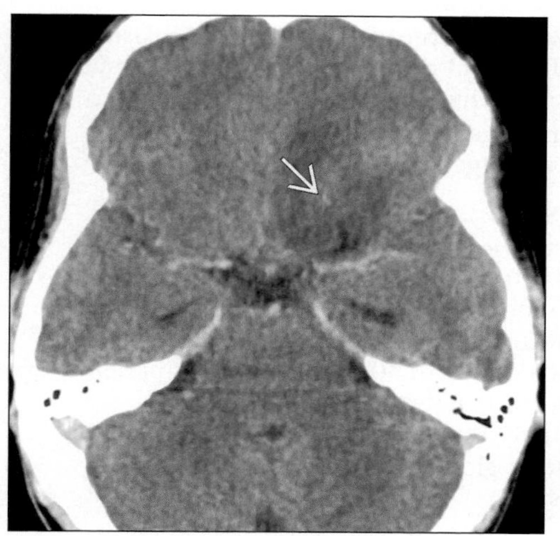

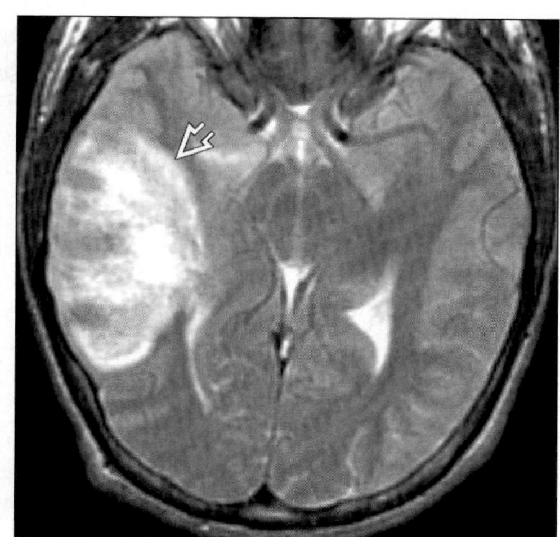

(Left) *Axial CECT shows left inferior frontal lobe cerebritis in a 24 year old with sinusitis and meningitis. Faint enhancement is noted centrally. (Courtesy R. Hewlett, PhD.)* ***(Right)*** *Axial T2WI MR shows a heterogeneous temporal lobe lesion related to early cerebritis in this young adult. DWI can help confirm the diagnosis of cerebritis. Although brain abscesses are potentially fatal, with a mortality up to 40%, they are treatable lesions. It is thus important to suggest infection in such cases.*

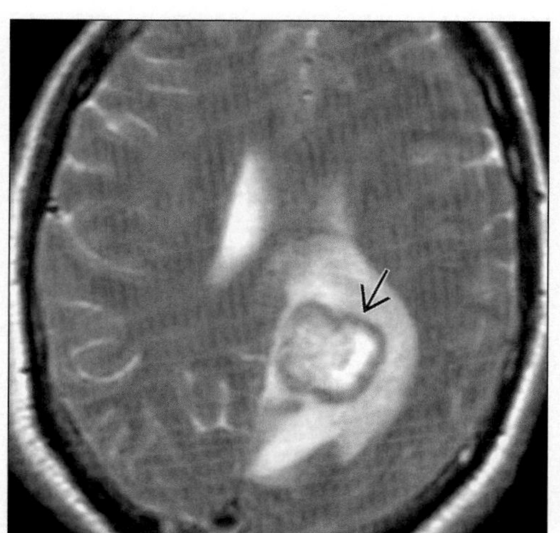

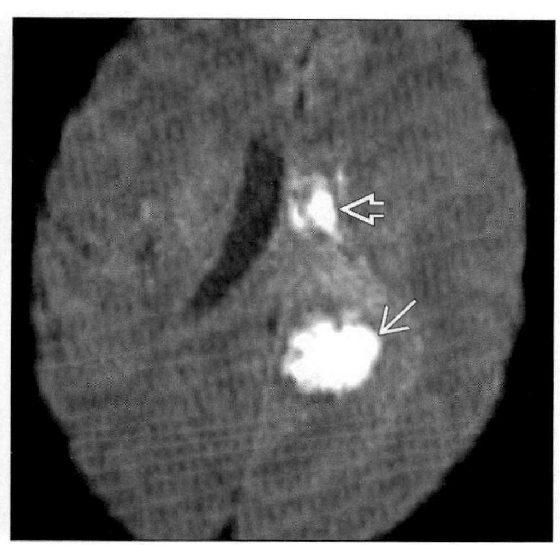

(Left) *Axial T2WI MR shows the characteristic hypointense rim related to collagen, blood products, or paramagnetic free radicles in this patient with an abscess due to meningitis.* ***(Right)*** *Axial DWI MR in the same patient shows diffusion restriction characteristic of abscess within the parenchymal mass. DWI restriction within the ventricle is related to ventriculitis. Intraventricular rupture of a brain abscess is a potentially fatal complication, with mortality rates up to 80%.*

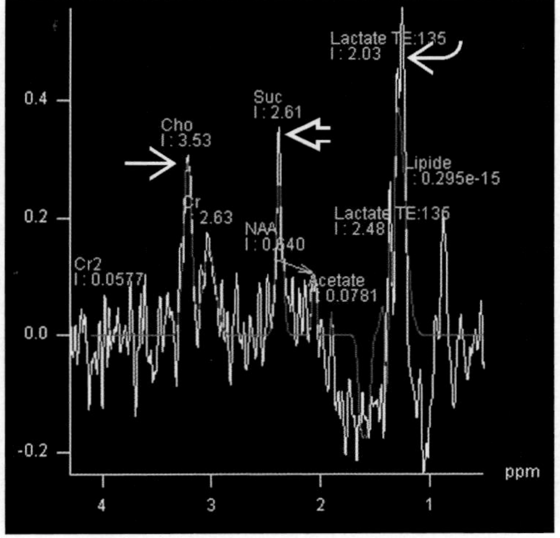

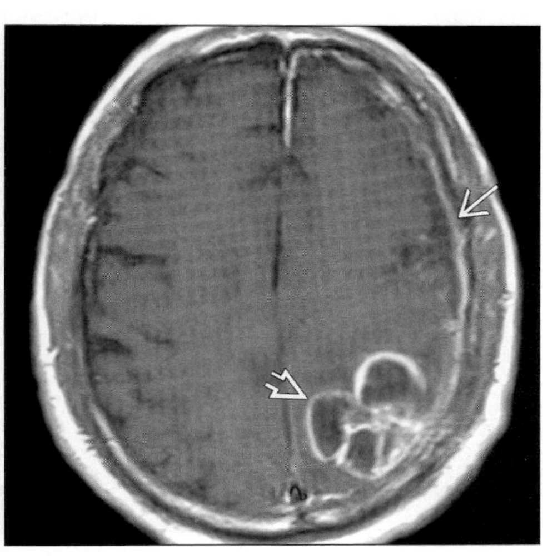

(Left) *MRS (CSI) shows the typical spectrum for a bacterial brain abscess. There is elevated choline with decreased NAA and high lactate-lipid complex. Succinate and acetate peaks are typically seen in abscess but not neoplasm.* ***(Right)*** *Axial T1WI C+ MR in this patient with a pyogenic abscess and subdural empyema shows a multiloculated, rim-enhancing lesion with associated dural enhancement over the left hemisphere and extending into the interhemispheric fissure.*

VENTRICULITIS

Key Facts

Terminology

- Ventricular ependyma infection related to meningitis, ruptured brain abscess, or ventricular catheter

Imaging

- Best imaging clue: Ventriculomegaly with debris level, abnormal ependyma, periventricular T2/FLAIR hyperintensity
- DWI: Restriction of layering debris with low ADC is characteristic
- T1WI C+: Marked ependymal enhancement with ventriculomegaly
- Ultrasound: Ventriculomegaly with echogenic ependyma and debris in infant
  - Can play important role in detection of postinfectious hydrocephalus

Top Differential Diagnoses

- Primary CNS lymphoma
- Ependymal tumor spread (GBM, medulloblastoma, pineal and choroid plexus tumors, ependymoma)
- Intraventricular hemorrhage
- Prominent ependymal veins (e.g., AVM, DVA, cavernoma, Sturge-Weber)

Clinical Issues

- Bacterial ventriculitis may occur in healthy individuals after trauma or neurosurgical procedure
- Fungal or viral ventriculitis occurs most commonly in immunosuppressed patients
- Ventriculitis occurs in 30% of meningitis patients; up to 80-90% in neonates/infants
- High mortality rate: 40-80%
- Treatment: Surgical irrigation, drainage, &/or antibiotics

__(Left)__ Axial graphic shows a right frontal abscess that has ruptured into the ventricular system, resulting in ventriculitis. Note the characteristic debris level within the ventricles and the inflammation along the ventricular margins →. __(Right)__ Axial FLAIR MR shows striking hyperintensity along the ventricular ependyma ⇨ with hyperintense debris filling the atria of the lateral ventricles →. FLAIR and DWI are the most sensitive sequences to identify ventriculitis. Note the right basal ganglia abscess.

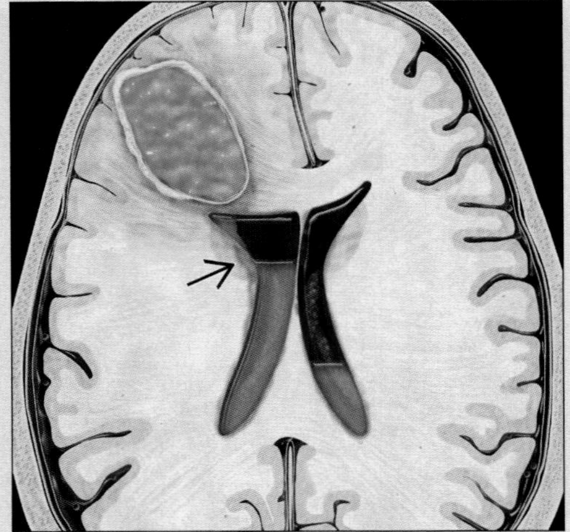

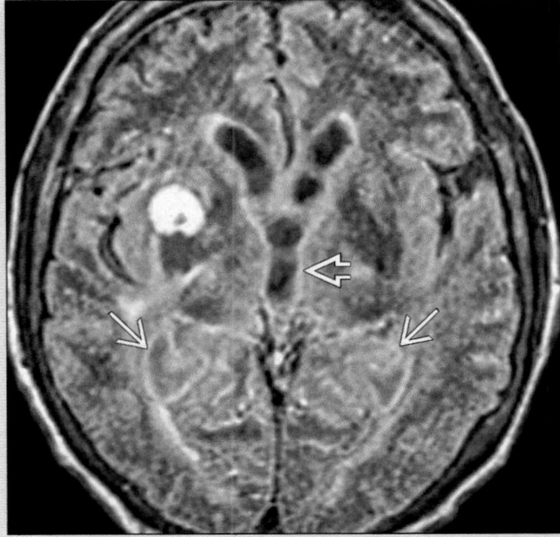

__(Left)__ Axial CECT shows marked ventriculomegaly with a debris level → and ependymal enhancement ⇨, characteristic of ventriculitis. Note the subtle periventricular hypodensity ⇨ in this patient with a temporal lobe abscess rupture. (Courtesy T. Swallow, MD.) __(Right)__ Axial DWI MR shows diffusion restriction of the lateral ventricular debris and temporal lobe abscess in this patient with multiple abscesses and ventriculitis related to a tooth abscess. DWI is invaluable in the diagnosis of ventriculitis.

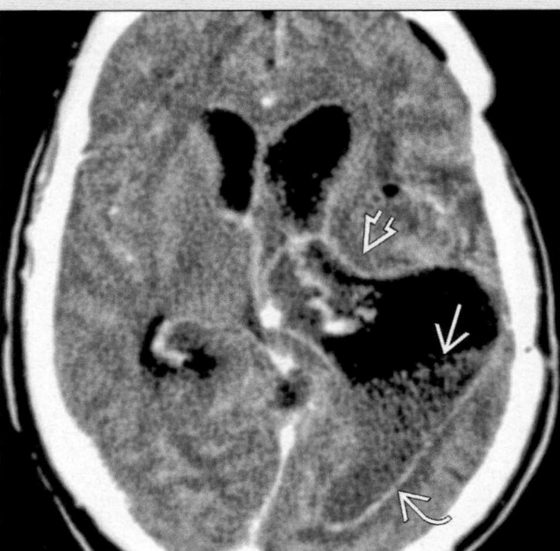

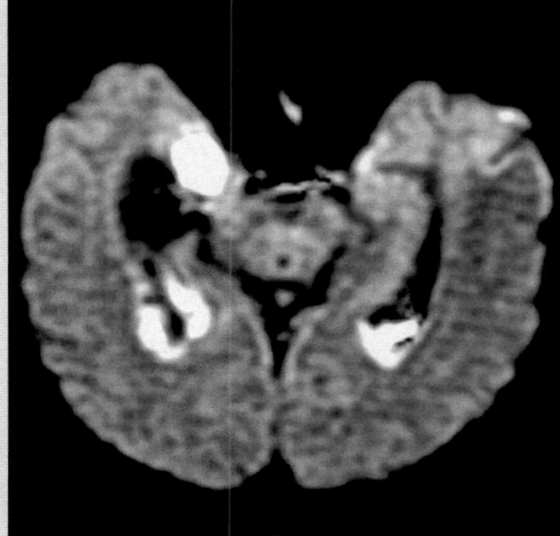

VENTRICULITIS

TERMINOLOGY

Synonyms

- Ependymitis, ventricular abscess, pyocephalus

Definitions

- Ventricular ependyma infection related to meningitis, ruptured brain abscess, or ventricular catheter

IMAGING

General Features

- Best diagnostic clue
  - Ventriculomegaly with debris level, abnormal ependyma, periventricular T2 hyperintensity

CT Findings

- NECT
  - Ventriculomegaly with dependent debris level
  - Subtle low density along ventricular margins
- CECT
  - Enhancement of ventricular walls

MR Findings

- T1WI
  - Ventriculomegaly with hyperintense debris
  - Subtle periventricular hypointensity
- T2WI
  - Hyperintensity along ventricular margins
- FLAIR
  - Hyperintensity along ventricular margins
  - Hyperintense debris layering dependently
- DWI
  - Diffusion restriction of layering debris, low ADC
- T1WI C+
  - Marked ependymal enhancement
  - Inflammatory septations and loculations (chronic)

Ultrasonographic Findings

- Ventriculomegaly with echogenic debris and echogenic ependyma, increased periventricular echogenicity, poor definition of choroid plexus in infant

Imaging Recommendations

- Best imaging tool
  - MR in adults, ultrasound in infants
- Protocol advice
  - Multiplanar MR with contrast, DWI, FLAIR

DIFFERENTIAL DIAGNOSIS

Primary CNS Lymphoma

- Ependymal enhancement, typically nodular
- Parenchymal disease usually present

Ependymal Tumor Spread

- Primary brain tumors: Glioblastoma multiforme, medulloblastoma, pineal tumors, ependymoma, choroid plexus tumors
- Metastatic tumor from extracranial primary

Intraventricular Hemorrhage

- History of trauma; other sequelae seen
- Ventricles typically not enlarged acutely

Prominent Ependymal Veins

- Vascular malformations: Arteriovenous malformation, developmental venous anomaly, cavernoma
- Abnormal venous drainage (i.e., Sturge-Weber)

PATHOLOGY

General Features

- Etiology
  - Complication of meningitis or cerebral abscess that ruptures into ventricular system
  - Complication of neurosurgical procedure, most commonly intraventricular catheter
  - Pathogens include bacteria, fungus, virus, parasites
    - Common bacterial organisms: *Staphylococcus*, *Streptococcus*, *Enterobacter*
- Associated abnormalities
  - Associated choroid plexitis is rare

Gross Pathologic & Surgical Features

- Intraventricular sedimentation levels with inflammation and proteinaceous debris

Microscopic Features

- Ependymal and subependymal inflammation with macrophages, lymphocytes

CLINICAL ISSUES

Presentation

- Most common signs/symptoms
  - Dependent on etiology; often indolent
- Clinical profile
  - CSF cytology, cultures may be normal

Demographics

- Gender
  - M > F
- Epidemiology
  - Bacterial ventriculitis may occur in healthy individuals after trauma or neurosurgical procedure
  - Fungal or viral ventriculitis occurs most commonly in immunosuppressed patients
  - Ventriculitis occurs in 30% of meningitis patients; up to 80-90% in neonates/infants
  - Intrathecal chemotherapy, rarely associated

Natural History & Prognosis

- Mortality rate: 40-80%

Treatment

- Surgical irrigation, drainage, &/or antibiotics

SELECTED REFERENCES

1. Hong JT et al: Significance of diffusion-weighted imaging and apparent diffusion coefficient maps for the evaluation of pyogenic ventriculitis. Clin Neurol Neurosurg. 110(2):137-44, 2008

EMPYEMA

Key Facts

Terminology

- Collection of pus in subdural or epidural space, or both (15%); subdural much more common
- Subdural empyema (SDE), epidural empyema (EDE)

Imaging

- Best diagnostic clue: Extraaxial collection with enhancing rim, DWI positive
- Supratentorial typical
  - EDE: Often adjacent to frontal sinus
  - SDE: Convexity in > 50%, parafalcine in 20%
- Infratentorial (up to 10%); related to mastoiditis
- T2 MR: Inwardly displaced dura seen as hypointense line between fluid and brain
- T1 C+: Prominent enhancement at margin related to granulomatous tissue and inflammation
- MR with DWI best to demonstrate presence, nature, extent, and complications

Top Differential Diagnoses

- Chronic subdural hematoma
- Subdural effusion, subdural hygroma

Pathology

- Infants, young children: Complication of bacterial meningitis
- Older children, adults: Related to paranasal sinus disease (> 2/3)

Clinical Issues

- Sinus or ear infection in > 75% of cases
- EDE, SDE rare, yet highly lethal
- Complications common: Cerebritis, abscess, venous thrombosis, ischemia, hydrocephalus
- Mortality: 10-15%
- Surgical drainage is primary treatment
- Sinus drainage + antibiotics: Small sinus-related EDE

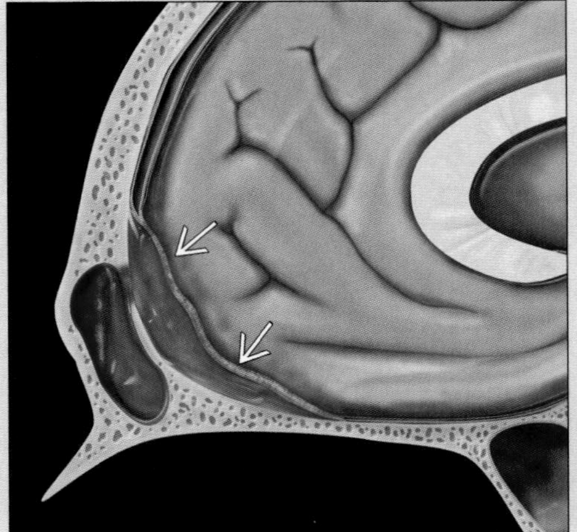

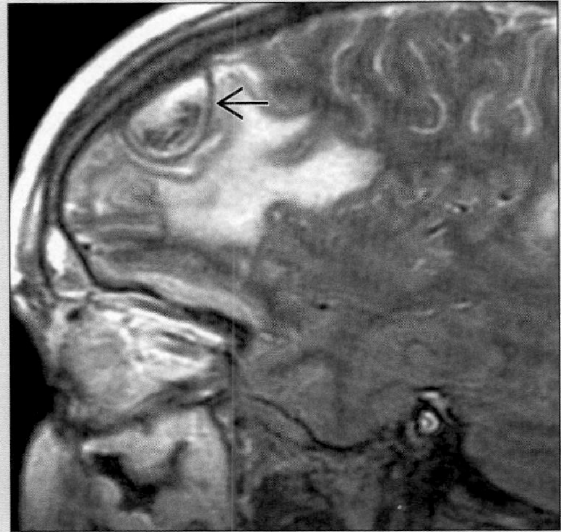

(Left) *Sagittal graphic shows frontal sinus purulence and direct extension into the epidural space, resulting in an epidural empyema (EDE). Note the displaced dura ➔ and inflammation in the adjacent frontal lobe. EDE is often located adjacent to the frontal sinus.* ***(Right)*** *Sagittal T2WI MR shows an EDE with abnormal signal in the adjacent brain related to cerebritis. Note the inwardly displaced dura ➔, seen as a hypointense line between the EDE and the brain, in this child with sinusitis.*

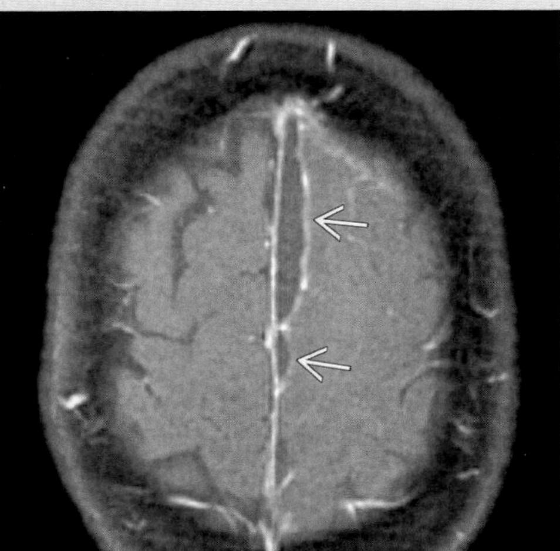

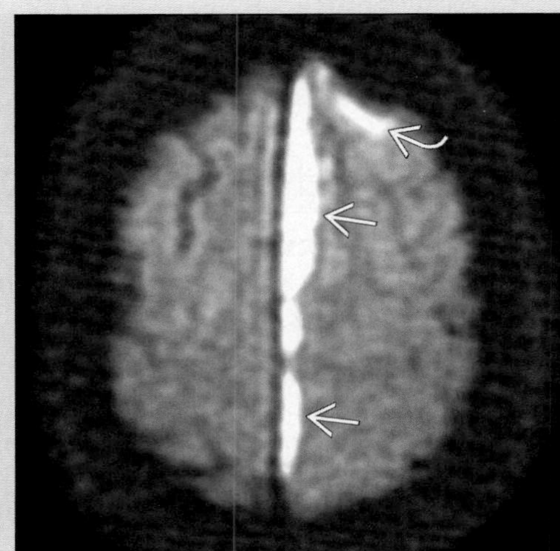

(Left) *Axial T1WI C+ FS MR in a patient with frontal sinusitis shows a rim-enhancing parafalcine collection related to a subdural empyema ➔.* ***(Right)*** *Axial DWI MR in the same patient shows bright diffusion restriction throughout the parafalcine ➔ and left frontal ➔ SDE. DWI is very important to demonstrate the presence, extent, and complications of a subdural or epidural empyema. In older children and adults, a sinus or ear infection is present in more than 75% of empyema cases.*

EMPYEMA

TERMINOLOGY

Abbreviations

- Subdural empyema (SDE), epidural empyema (EDE)

Synonyms

- Epidural empyema = epidural abscess

Definitions

- Collection of pus in subdural or epidural space, or both; subdural much more common

IMAGING

General Features

- Best diagnostic clue
  - Extraaxial collection with enhancing rim
- Location
  - Supratentorial typical
    - SDE: Convexity in > 50%, parafalcine in 20%
    - EDE: Often adjacent to frontal sinus
  - Infratentorial (up to 10%)
    - Often associated with mastoiditis
    - > 90% associated with hydrocephalus
- Morphology
  - SDE: Crescentic typical; may be lens-shaped (lentiform) on coronal images
  - EDE: Biconvex, lentiform

CT Findings

- NECT
  - Extraaxial collection, iso- to hyperdense to CSF
  - SDE: Crescentic iso- to hyperdense collection, confined by falx
    - Frequently bilateral
    - Warning: Can be small, easily overlooked
  - EDE: Biconvex low-density collection between dura, calvarium; contained by cranial sutures
    - Often continuous across midline
  - Posterior fossa EDE
    - Typically at sinodural angle
    - Tegmen tympani ± sigmoid plate eroded
    - Pus may extend into cerebellopontine angle
- CECT
  - Strong peripheral rim enhancement
  - Posterior fossa EDE: Look for venous thrombosis
- Bone CT
  - **Sinusitis** common in **supratentorial** SDE-EDE
  - **Otomastoiditis** common in **infratentorial** SDE-EDE

MR Findings

- T1WI
  - Extraaxial collection, hyperintense to CSF
  - SDE: Crescentic extraaxial collection
  - EDE: Lentiform bifrontal or convexity collection
    - Inwardly displaced dura seen as **hypointense line** between fluid and brain
    - May cross midline in frontal region
- T2WI
  - Iso- to hyperintense to CSF
  - SDE: Crescentic collection, underlying brain may be hyperintense
  - EDE: Lentiform bifrontal or convexity collection
    - Inwardly displaced dura seen as **hypointense line** between fluid and brain
    - Underlying brain usually spared
- FLAIR
  - Hyperintense to CSF
  - SDE: Crescentic collection, underlying brain may be hyperintense
  - EDE: Lentiform bifrontal or convexity collection
    - Underlying brain rarely hyperintense
- DWI
  - SDE: **Restricted diffusion** (↑ signal intensity) typical
  - EDE: Variable signal with hyperintense components
- T1WI C+
  - Prominent enhancement at margin related to granulomatous tissue and inflammation
  - SDE: Encapsulating membranes enhance strongly, may be loculated with internal fibrous strands
  - EDE: Strong enhancement of collection margins
  - May see enhancement of adjacent brain parenchyma (cerebritis/abscess)
  - Subgaleal phlegmon or abscess ("Pott puffy tumor")
- MRV: Venous thrombosis may be seen as lack of flow

Ultrasonographic Findings

- Useful in infants
- Heterogeneous echogenic convexity collection with mass effect
  - Hyperechoic fibrous strands
  - Thick hyperechoic inner membrane
  - Increased echogenicity of pia-arachnoid and exudates in subarachnoid space

Imaging Recommendations

- Best imaging tool
  - **MR with DWI** best to demonstrate presence, nature, extent, and complications
- Protocol advice
  - Contrast-enhanced multiplanar MR with DWI
  - **DWI** helpful to evaluate extent and complications

DIFFERENTIAL DIAGNOSIS

Chronic Subdural Hematoma

- MR shows blood products; may be loculated
- Often enhances along edge; usually thinner than SDE
- May be indistinguishable; history may help

Subdural Effusion

- Sterile, CSF-like collection associated with meningitis
- Follows CSF on all MR sequences
- Usually nonenhancing; may enhance mildly
- Frontal and temporal regions common, often bilateral

Subdural Hygroma

- Nonenhancing CSF collection, often trauma history

Dural Metastasis

- Primary tumor often known, typically breast, prostate
- Often diffuse, nodular enhancement
- May have associated bone metastases

EMPYEMA

PATHOLOGY

General Features

- Etiology
  - Infants, young children: Complication of **bacterial meningitis**
  - Older children, adults: Related to **paranasal sinus disease** (> 2/3)
    - Direct spread via posterior wall of frontal sinus
    - Retrograde spread through **valveless bridging emissary veins** of extra-, intracranial spaces
  - **Mastoiditis** (± cholesteatoma) in 20%
  - Complication of head trauma or neurosurgical procedure (rare)
  - Complication of meningitis in adults (very rare)
  - Causative organism: *Streptococci, H. influenzae, S. aureus, S. epidermidis* most common
  - Anaerobic or microaerophilic organisms (strep, bacteroides) common
- SDE much more common than EDE
- SDE more commonly complicated by abscess and venous thrombosis (> 10%)
- 15% of cases have both EDE and SDE

Gross Pathologic & Surgical Features

- Encapsulated, yellowish, purulent collection
- Spreads widely but may be loculated
- Osteitis in 35%

Microscopic Features

- Inflammatory infiltrate-granulomatous tissue

CLINICAL ISSUES

Presentation

- Most common signs/symptoms
  - Majority have fever, headaches
  - Meningismus common, may mimic meningitis
  - Sinusitis often present
  - Cerebritis-brain abscess causes neurologic signs
- Clinical profile
  - Sinus or ear infection in > 75% of cases
  - Frontal subgaleal abscess ("Pott puffy tumor") in up to 1/3; typically adolescent males
  - Periorbital swelling may be seen
  - Confused with meningitis; delayed diagnosis
  - EDE, SDE rare, yet highly lethal

Demographics

- Age
  - Can occur at any age
- Epidemiology
  - Uncommon; occur 25-50% as often as abscess
  - SDE and EDE account for ~ 30% of intracranial infections
  - SDE: Sinusitis (67%), mastoiditis (10%)

Natural History & Prognosis

- Progresses rapidly, **neurosurgical emergency**
- Rapidly evolving, fulminant course
- EDE may occasionally have indolent course, as dura mater functions as barrier between infection and brain
  - Much better prognosis than SDE
- Can be fatal unless recognized and treated
  - **Lumbar puncture** can be **fatal**
  - CSF can be normal
- Complications common
  - Cerebritis and brain abscess: ~ 5%
  - Cortical vein, dural sinus thrombosis (ischemia)
  - Cerebral edema
  - Hydrocephalus (> 90% of infratentorial SDE)
- **Mortality: 10-15%**

Treatment

- Surgical drainage via wide craniotomy is gold standard
- Intravenous antibiotics
- Sinus drainage + antibiotics possible in small sinus-related EDE

DIAGNOSTIC CHECKLIST

Consider

- Chronic subdural hematoma may be difficult to differentiate from SDE; history may help
- Look for empyema in patient with sinusitis and neurologic symptoms
- If SDE or EDE discovered, look also for sinusitis, otomastoiditis, dural sinus thrombosis, brain abscess

Image Interpretation Pearls

- MR with contrast and **DWI** is most sensitive; CT may miss small collections
- DWI differentiates SDE from subdural effusions
- MR with DWI may be used to monitor treatment response

SELECTED REFERENCES

1. Legrand M et al: Paediatric intracranial empyema: differences according to age. Eur J Pediatr. 168(10):1235-41, 2009
2. Karaman E et al: Pott's puffy tumor. J Craniofac Surg. 19(6):1694-7, 2008
3. Ziai WC et al: Update in the diagnosis and management of central nervous system infections. Neurol Clin. 26(2):427-68, viii, 2008
4. Foerster BR et al: Intracranial infections: clinical and imaging characteristics. Acta Radiol. 48(8):875-93, 2007
5. Osborn MK et al: Subdural empyema and other suppurative complications of paranasal sinusitis. Lancet Infect Dis. 7(1):62-7, 2007
6. Fanning NF et al: Serial diffusion-weighted MRI correlates with clinical course and treatment response in children with intracranial pus collections. Pediatr Radiol. 36(1):26-37, 2006
7. Venkatesh MS et al: Pediatric infratentorial subdural empyema: analysis of 14 cases. J Neurosurg. 105(5 Suppl):370-7, 2006
8. Wong AM et al: Diffusion-weighted MR imaging of subdural empyemas in children. AJNR Am J Neuroradiol. 25(6):1016-21, 2004
9. Heran NS et al: Conservative neurosurgical management of intracranial epidural abscesses in children. Neurosurgery. 53(4):893-7; discussion 897-8, 2003
10. Tsai YD et al: Intracranial suppuration: a clinical comparison of subdural empyemas and epidural abscesses. Surg Neurol. 59(3):191-6; discussion 196, 2003

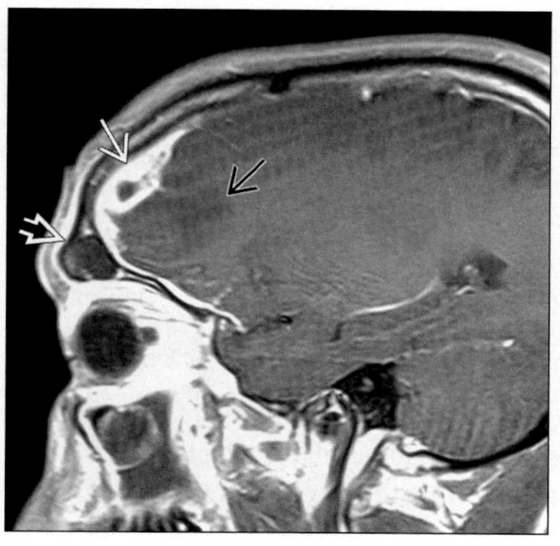

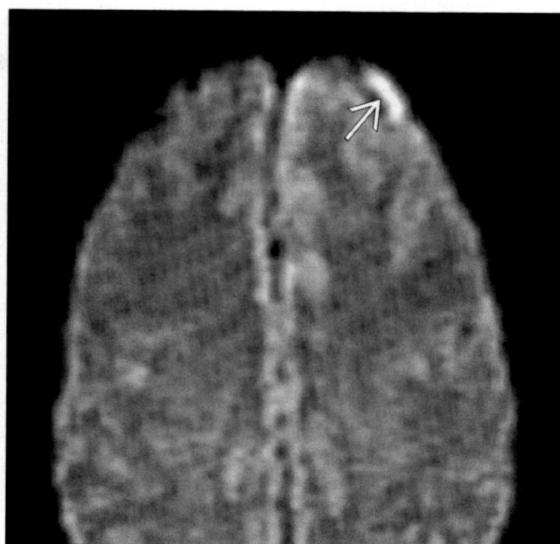

(Left) *Sagittal T1WI C+ FS MR shows a rim-enhancing extraaxial collection ➔ and frontal sinusitis ➔. This subdural empyema extends inferiorly along the frontal lobe. There is low signal within the brain parenchyma ➔ related to cerebritis.* ***(Right)*** *Axial DWI MR in the same patient shows diffusion restriction within the subdural empyema ➔. DWI may help differentiate empyemas from other subdural collections, including chronic subdural hematoma, subdural effusion, and hygroma.*

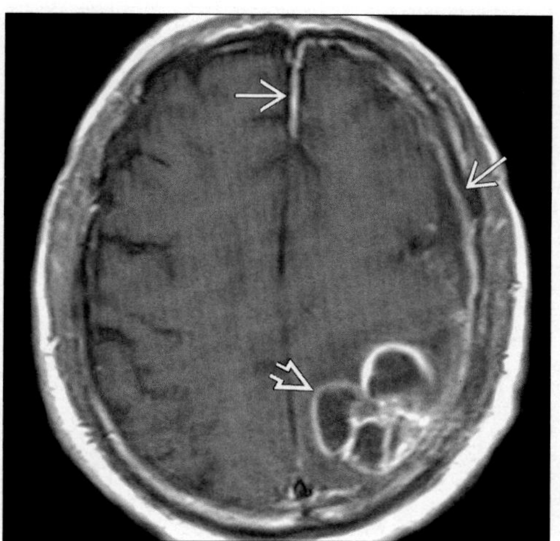

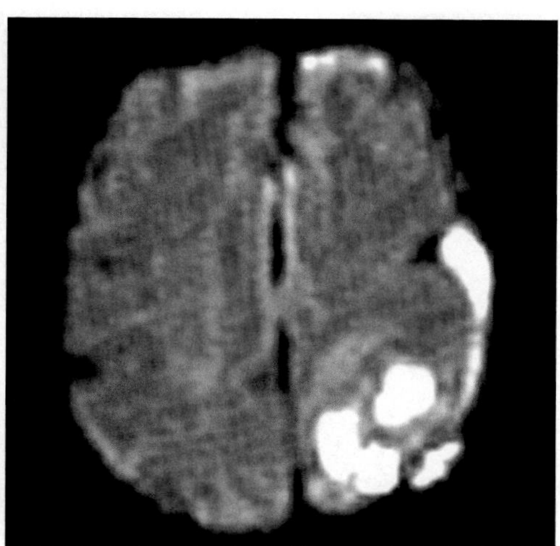

(Left) *Axial T1WI C+ MR in this 67-year-old patient with weakness shows a multiloculated, rim-enhancing parietal "mass" ➔ and thick dural enhancement over the hemisphere extending into the interhemispheric fissure ➔.* ***(Right)*** *Axial DWI MR in the same patient shows diffusion restriction in the "mass" as well as in the subdural collection, confirming the diagnosis of empyema and brain abscess. Subdural and epidural empyemas are rare, yet highly lethal. (Courtesy C. Sutton, MD.)*

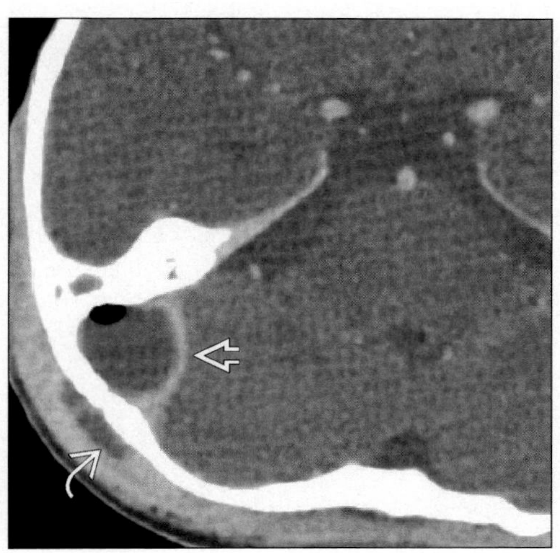

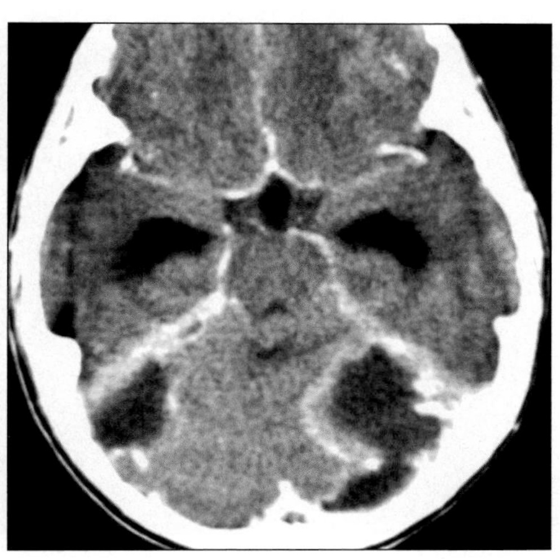

(Left) *Axial CECT shows a large epidural empyema ➔ related to acute otomastoiditis. Note the associated soft tissue abscess ➔. Infratentorial epidural empyema is commonly associated with otomastoiditis.* ***(Right)*** *Axial CECT shows bilateral posterior fossa subdural empyemas with irregularly enhancing margins in this patient with mastoiditis further complicated by hydrocephalus and venous thrombosis. Hydrocephalus is a common complication of subdural empyemas.*

HERPES ENCEPHALITIS

Key Facts

Terminology

- Brain parenchyma infection caused by herpes simplex virus type 1 (HSV-1)
- Typically reactivation in immunocompetent patients

Imaging

- Best imaging clue: T2/FLAIR hyperintensity of limbic system (medial temporal and inferior frontal cortex) with DWI restriction
  - Typically bilateral disease, but asymmetric
  - Deep gray nuclei usually spared
- CT often normal early
- MR with DWI most sensitive for early diagnosis
- T2/FLAIR: Cortical, subcortical hyperintensity with relative white matter sparing
- GRE: If hemorrhagic, hypointensity "blooms" within edematous brain
- DWI: Restricted diffusion in limbic system
- T1WI C+: May see mild, patchy enhancement early
  - Gyriform enhancement usually seen 1 week after initial symptoms

Top Differential Diagnoses

- Acute cerebral ischemia-infarction
- Status epilepticus
- Limbic encephalitis
- Infiltrating neoplasm

Clinical Issues

- Common presentation: Fever, headache, seizures, ± viral prodrome
- Children often present with nonspecific symptoms
- Polymerase chain reaction (PCR) of CSF most accurate diagnosis
- HSV-1 causes 95% of all herpetic encephalitis
- Start IV acyclovir immediately if HSE suspected

__(Left)__ Coronal graphic shows the classic features of herpes encephalitis with bilateral but asymmetric involvement of the limbic system. There is inflammation involving the temporal lobes, cingulate gyri, and insular cortices. __(Right)__ Coronal T1WI C+ MR shows bilateral but asymmetric gyriform enhancement of the temporal lobes, insular cortices ➲, and minimally the cingulate gyri ➡. Gyriform enhancement is usually a subacute feature, seen 1 week after the initial onset of patient symptoms.

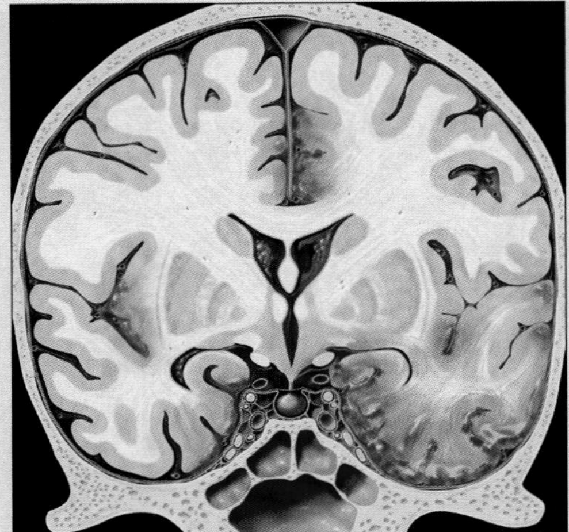

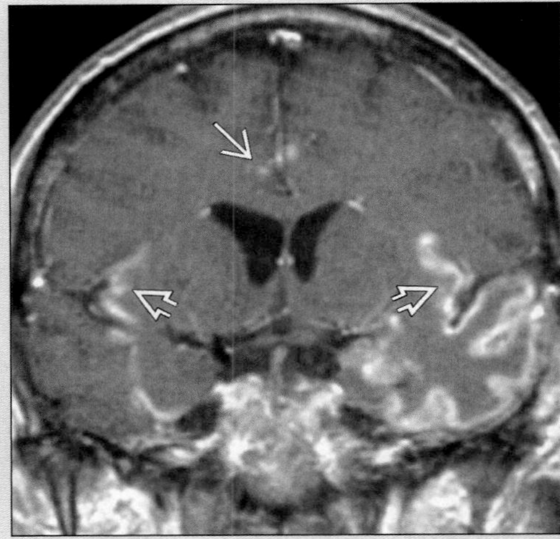

__(Left)__ Axial FLAIR MR shows classic bilateral but asymmetric abnormal hyperintense signal in the medial temporal lobes of this patient with herpes encephalitis. Note involvement of the hippocampi ➡. __(Right)__ Axial DWI MR in the same patient shows diffusion restriction as bright signal in the medial temporal lobes ➲ and hippocampi ➡. DWI and FLAIR are the most sensitive sequences for detection of encephalitis. CT is often normal early in the course of herpes encephalitis.

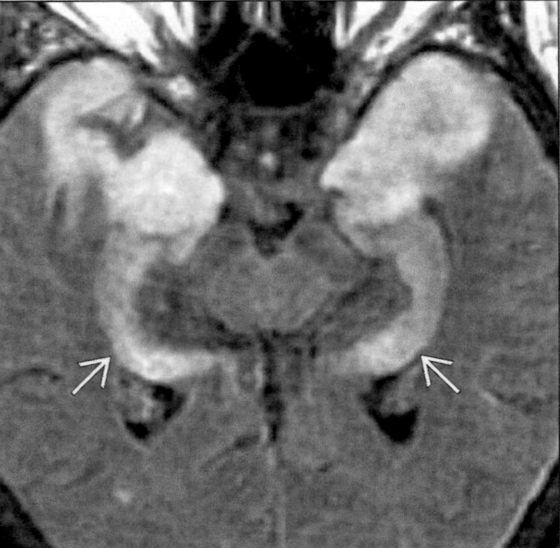

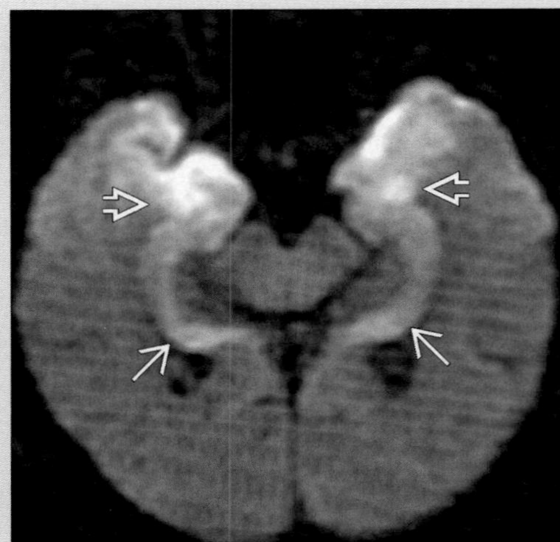

HERPES ENCEPHALITIS

TERMINOLOGY

Abbreviations

- Herpes simplex encephalitis (HSE)

Definitions

- Brain parenchyma infection caused by herpes simplex virus type 1 (HSV-1)
- Typically reactivation in immunocompetent patients

IMAGING

General Features

- Best diagnostic clue
  - Abnormal signal of medial temporal and inferior frontal cortex with DWI restriction
  - Involvement of cingulate gyrus, contralateral temporal lobe highly suggestive
- Location
  - Limbic system: Temporal lobes, insula, subfrontal area, cingulate gyri typical
  - Cerebral convexity, posterior occipital cortex may become involved
  - Typically bilateral disease, but asymmetric
  - Basal ganglia usually spared
  - Atypical patterns seen in infants, children (may be caused by HSV-1 or HSV-2)
    - May primarily affect cerebral hemispheres
  - Rarely affects midbrain and pons (mesenrhombencephalitis)

CT Findings

- NECT
  - CT often normal early
    - Low attenuation, mild mass effect in medial temporal lobes, insula
    - Hemorrhage typically late feature
  - Predilection for limbic system; basal ganglia spared
  - Earliest CT findings at 3 days after symptom onset
- CECT
  - Patchy or gyriform enhancement of temporal lobes (late acute/subacute feature)

MR Findings

- T1WI
  - Cortical swelling with loss of gray-white junction, mass effect
  - May see subacute hemorrhage as increased signal within edematous brain
  - Atrophy, encephalomalacia in late subacute/chronic cases
- T2WI
  - Cortical and subcortical hyperintensity with relative white matter sparing
  - May see subacute hemorrhage as increased signal within edematous brain
- PD/intermediate
  - Increased signal in affected areas
- FLAIR
  - Cortical and subcortical hyperintensity with relative white matter sparing
  - Often see changes earlier than on T2WI
- T2* GRE
  - If hemorrhagic, hypointensity "blooms" within edematous brain
- DWI
  - Restricted diffusion in limbic system
  - Look for bilateral disease
  - DWI findings may precede T2/FLAIR changes
- T1WI C+
  - May see mild, patchy enhancement early
  - Gyriform enhancement usually seen 1 week after initial symptoms
  - Meningeal enhancement occasionally seen
  - Enhancement seen in temporal lobes, insular cortex, subfrontal area, cingulate gyrus

Imaging Recommendations

- Best imaging tool
  - MR (positive 24-48 hours earlier than CT)
- Protocol advice
  - Multiplanar MR with coronal T2 &/or FLAIR, DWI, T2* GRE, contrast

DIFFERENTIAL DIAGNOSIS

Acute Cerebral Ischemia-Infarction

- Typical vascular distribution (MCA, ACA, PCA)
- Hyperacute symptoms vs. 2-3 day history of flu-like illness
- DWI positive in acute infarct
- ACA distribution ischemia may mimic HSE

Status Epilepticus

- Active seizures may disrupt blood-brain barrier, cause signal abnormalities and enhancement
- Temporal lobe epilepsy hyperperfusion may mimic HSE
- No hemorrhage in status epilepticus

Limbic Encephalitis

- Rare paraneoplastic syndrome associated with primary tumor, often lung
- Predilection for limbic system, often bilateral
- Hemorrhage not present
- Imaging may be indistinguishable
- Symptom onset weeks to months (vs. acute in HSE)

Infiltrating Neoplasm

- Low-grade gliomas often involve medial temporal lobe and cause epilepsy
- Gliomatosis cerebri may involve frontal and temporal lobes, may be bilateral
- Onset usually indolent

Other Encephalitides

- Limbic system not typically involved
- Neurosyphilis can affect medial temporal lobes and mimic HSE
  - May involve meninges, blood vessels (obliterative endarteritis)
- West Nile can mimic HSE clinically, but typically involves basal ganglia &/or thalami

HERPES ENCEPHALITIS

PATHOLOGY

General Features

- Etiology
  - Initial HSV-1 infection usually occurs in oronasopharynx via contact with infected secretions
  - HSV-1 invades along cranial nerves (via lingual nerve, division of trigeminal nerve) to ganglia
  - HSV-1 remains dormant in trigeminal ganglion
  - HSV-1 reactivation may occur spontaneously or be precipitated by various factors
    - Local trauma, immunosuppression, hormonal fluctuations, emotional stress
  - HSV-1 causes acute hemorrhagic, necrotizing encephalitis (primarily involving limbic system)

Staging, Grading, & Classification

- Herpes viruses include HSV-1, HSV-2, Epstein-Barr virus (EBV), cytomegalovirus (CMV), varicella-zoster virus (VZV), B virus, HSV-6, HSV-7
- HSV-1 in adults, children
- HSV-2 is more common in neonates
- HSV-1 and HSV-2 are DNA viruses
- Viruses are obligate intracellular pathogens

Gross Pathologic & Surgical Features

- Hemorrhagic, necrotizing encephalitis
  - Severe edema, massive tissue necrosis with hemorrhage typical
  - Involvement of temporal lobes, insular cortex, orbital surface of frontal lobes
  - Less frequent involvement of cingulate gyrus and occipital cortex

Microscopic Features

- Intense perivascular cuffing, interstitial lymphocytic inflammation
- Intranuclear inclusion bodies in infected cells (neurons, glia, endothelial cells)
  - Typically eosinophilic Cowdry A nuclear inclusions
- Immunohistochemistry shows viral antigens, antibodies to HSV-1
- Chronic cases, microglial nodules form

CLINICAL ISSUES

Presentation

- Most common signs/symptoms
  - Fever, headache, seizures, ± viral prodrome
  - Children often present with nonspecific symptoms
    - Behavioral changes, fever, headaches, seizures
  - Patients typically immunocompetent
    - HSV-1 uncommon in AIDS patients
- Other signs/symptoms
  - Altered mental status
  - Focal or diffuse neurologic deficit (< 30%)
- Clinical profile
  - CSF studies show lymphocytic pleocytosis, ↑ protein
  - Polymerase chain reaction (PCR) of CSF most accurate diagnosis
    - Sensitivity/specificity nearly 95-100%
    - False-negatives can occur early after disease onset
  - EEG shows temporal lobe activity
  - Brain biopsy may be required for diagnosis

Demographics

- Age
  - May occur at any age
  - Highest incidence in adolescents and young adults
  - Approximately 1/3 of all patients < 20 years old
- Gender
  - No gender predominance
- Epidemiology
  - HSV-1 causes 95% of all HSE
  - Most common cause of fatal sporadic encephalitis
  - Most common nonepidemic cause of viral meningoencephalitis
  - In adults, typically related to viral reactivation
  - In neonates, related to maternal infection
  - Incidence: 1-3/1,000,000

Natural History & Prognosis

- May progress to coma and death
  - 50-70% mortality rate
  - Rapid diagnosis, early treatment with antiviral agents can decrease mortality, may improve outcome
- Nearly 2/3 of survivors have significant neurological deficits, despite acyclovir therapy
- Survival complicated by memory difficulties, hearing loss, intractable epilepsy, personality changes

Treatment

- Antiviral therapy with intravenous acyclovir

DIAGNOSTIC CHECKLIST

Consider

- Start IV acyclovir immediately if HSE suspected
- Unilateral disease may mimic stroke or tumor; history often helpful
- Limbic encephalitis if all clinical HSE tests negative and subacute onset of symptoms
- Acute onset of HSE helps differentiate from other etiologies

Image Interpretation Pearls

- MR with FLAIR/DWI most sensitive for early diagnosis
- Imaging often key in diagnosis

SELECTED REFERENCES

1. Akyldz BN et al: Diffusion-weighted magnetic resonance is better than polymerase chain reaction for early diagnosis of herpes simplex encephalitis: a case report. Pediatr Emerg Care. 24(6):377-9, 2008
2. Baringer JR: Herpes simplex infections of the nervous system. Neurol Clin. 26(3):657-74, viii, 2008
3. Hatipoglu HG et al: Magnetic resonance and diffusion-weighted imaging findings of herpes simplex encephalitis. Herpes. 15(1):13-7, 2008
4. McCabe K et al: Diffusion-weighted MRI abnormalities as a clue to the diagnosis of herpes simplex encephalitis. Neurology. 61(7):1015-6, 2003
5. Sämann PG et al: Serial proton MR spectroscopy and diffusion imaging findings in HIV-related herpes simplex encephalitis. AJNR Am J Neuroradiol. 24(10):2015-9, 2003

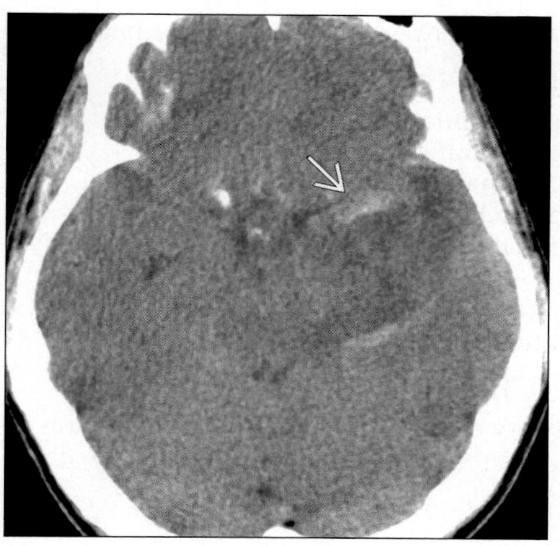

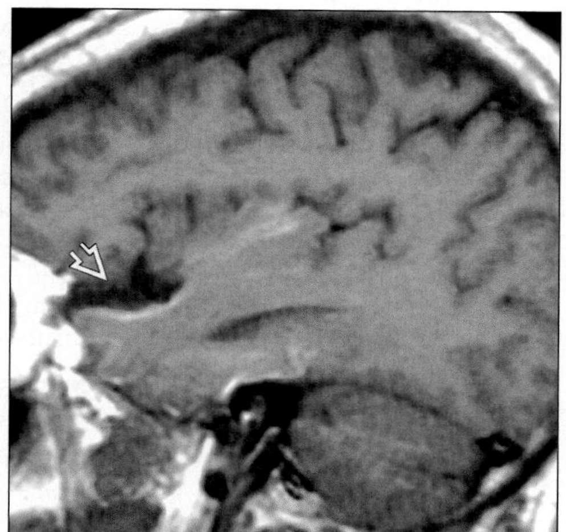

(Left) *Axial NECT shows edema and hemorrhage ➡ in the left temporal lobe in this young adult with altered mental status. Despite early acyclovir therapy, the patient succumbed to his disease. Mortality ranges from 50-70% of HSE patients.* ***(Right)*** *Sagittal T1WI in a patient 2 weeks after the initial presentation of herpes encephalitis. There is volume loss in the temporal lobe ➡ and linear gyriform T1 shortening within the temporal lobe cortex, characteristic of subacute cortical hemorrhage.*

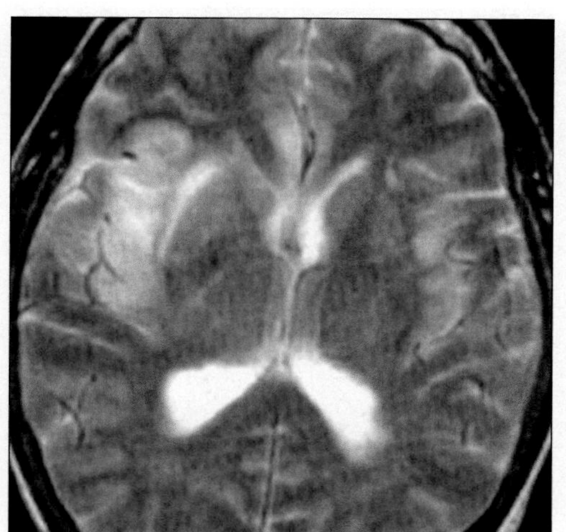

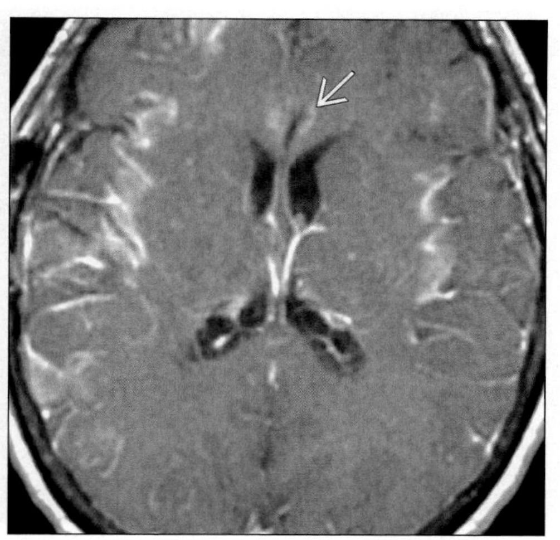

(Left) *Axial T2WI MR shows the classic appearance of herpes encephalitis with bilateral but asymmetric hyperintensity involving the cortex and subcortical white matter of the temporal lobes. Note the typical sparing of the deep gray nuclei. FLAIR may show subtle changes of HSE earlier than T2WI.* ***(Right)*** *Axial T1 C+ MR in the same patient shows bilateral, asymmetric enhancement of the medial temporal lobes and insular cortex. Subtle enhancement of the cingulate gyri ➡ is also noted.*

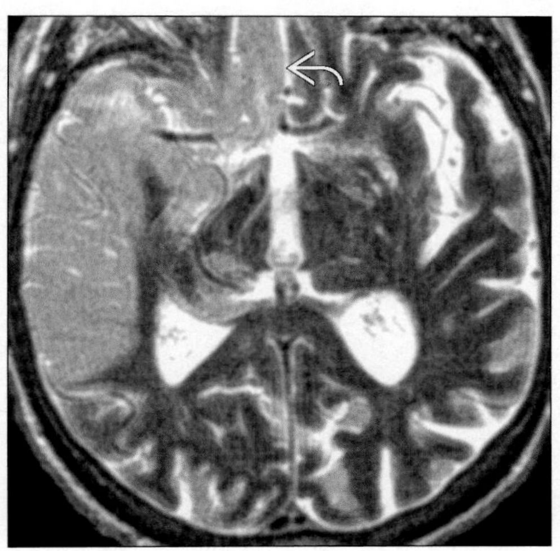

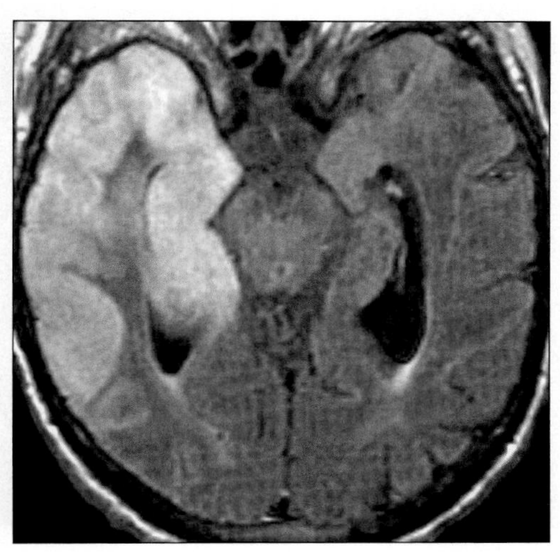

(Left) *Axial T2WI MR in an older adult with fever and confusion shows diffuse swelling and hyperintensity in the right temporal lobe and orbito frontal gyrus ➡.* ***(Right)*** *Axial FLAIR MR in the same patient shows marked edema and hyperintensity in the right temporal lobe cortex with relative sparing of the subcortical white matter. This unilateral involvement by herpes encephalitis is atypical and may mimic a stroke. Clinical history is often helpful.*

MISCELLANEOUS ENCEPHALITIS

Key Facts

Terminology
- Diffuse brain parenchymal inflammation caused by variety of pathogens, most commonly viruses
- Location dependent on etiology

Imaging
- Abnormal T2 hyperintensity of gray matter ± white matter or deep gray nuclei
- Large, poorly delineated areas of involvement common, ± patchy hemorrhage
- Imaging is often nonspecific, mimics other etiologies

Top Differential Diagnoses
- Acute ischemia
- Infiltrating neoplasm
- Herpes encephalitis
- Status epilepticus
- Toxic/metabolic lesions

Pathology
- Most (but not all) are caused by viruses
- Spread of virus to CNS is hematogenous or neural

Clinical Issues
- Herpes: Most common cause of sporadic (nonepidemic) viral encephalitis
- Japanese encephalitis: Most common endemic encephalitis in Asia
- Many encephalitides have high morbidity, mortality
- Rapid diagnosis and early treatment with antiviral or antibacterial agents can decrease mortality, may improve outcome

Diagnostic Checklist
- Clinical history often helpful for accurate diagnosis
- DWI may detect lesions earlier than conventional MR

*(**Left**) Axial FLAIR MR shows hyperintense signal primarily in the left posterior frontal lobe ➔ in an immunosuppressed patient with CMV meningoencephalitis. CMV typically involves the periventricular white matter. (**Right**) Axial DWI MR in the same patient shows restricted diffusion in the left posterior frontal lobe ➔ with involvement of the gray and white matter. DWI is often positive in encephalitis and may be the most sensitive MR sequence.*

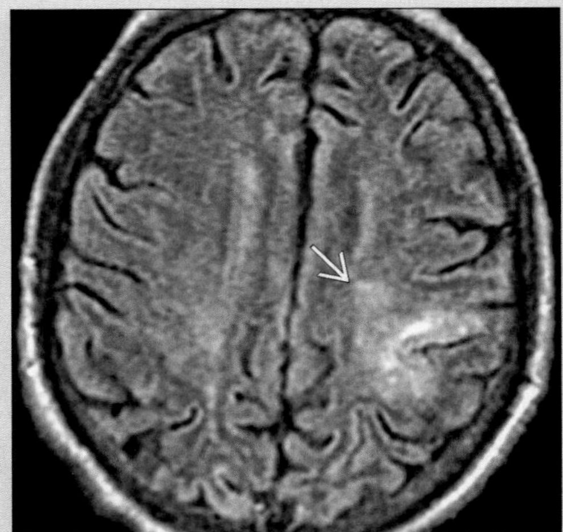

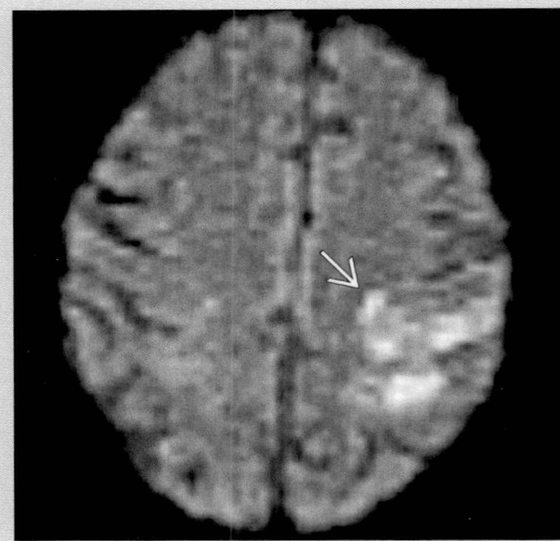

*(**Left**) Axial FLAIR MR shows symmetric abnormal hyperintensity in the basal ganglia ➲ and thalami in this patient with West Nile virus encephalitis. The symmetric appearance of deep gray nuclei involvement mimics toxic and metabolic etiologies, as well as hypoxic-ischemic encephalopathy. (**Right**) Axial T2WI MR shows bilateral hyperintensity ➔ of the cerebellar hemispheres in this 10-year-old patient with headache, vertigo, and emesis. Cerebellitis is often seen in pediatric patients.*

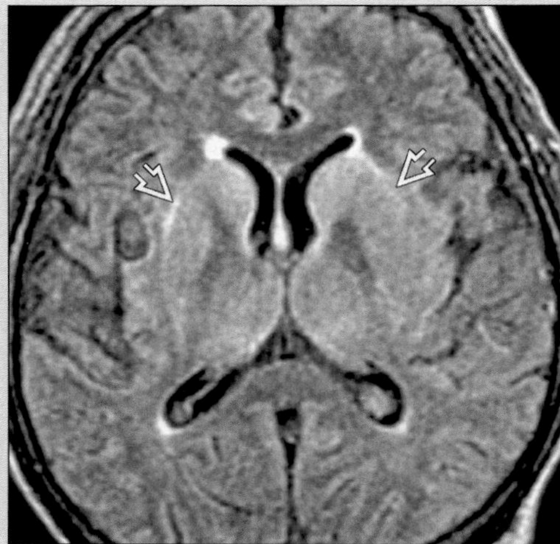

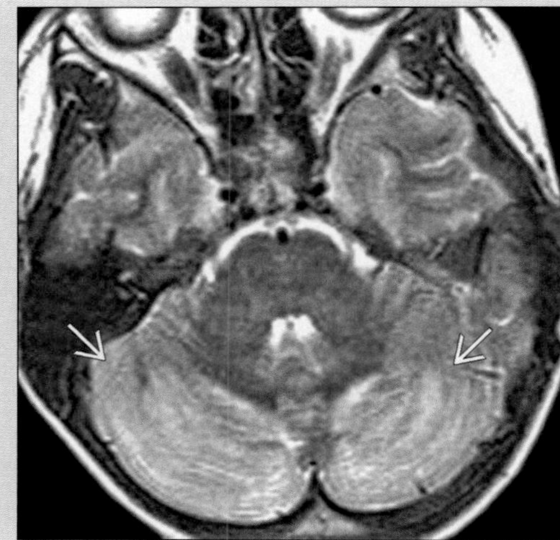

MISCELLANEOUS ENCEPHALITIS

TERMINOLOGY

Definitions

- Diffuse brain parenchymal inflammation caused by variety of pathogens, most commonly viruses
- Location dependent on etiology

IMAGING

General Features

- Best diagnostic clue
  - Abnormal T2 hyperintensity of gray matter (GM) ± white matter (WM) or deep gray nuclei
  - Large, poorly delineated areas of involvement common, ± patchy hemorrhage
  - Imaging is often nonspecific
- Location
  - Herpes simplex virus type 1 (**HSV-1**): Limbic system
  - Cytomegalovirus (**CMV**): Periventricular WM
  - Epstein-Barr virus (**EBV**): Symmetric basal ganglia (BG), thalami, cortex, or brainstem
  - Varicella-zoster virus (**VZV**)
    - Varicella: May affect multifocal areas of cortex
    - Zoster: Brainstem/cortical GM, cranial nerves
  - **Cerebellitis**: Bilateral cerebellar hemispheres
  - Eastern equine encephalitis (**EEE**): BG and thalami
  - **Enteroviral** encephalomyelitis
    - **Enterovirus (EV) 71**: Posterior medulla, pons, midbrain, dentate nuclei, spinal cord
    - **Polio, coxsackie**: Midbrain, anterior spinal cord
  - **Hantavirus**: Pituitary gland hemorrhage
  - **HIV-1**: Cerebral WM, brainstem, thalamus, BG
  - **Japanese encephalitis**: Bilateral thalami, brainstem, cerebellum, spinal cord, cerebral cortex
  - Murray Valley encephalitis (**MVE**): Bilateral thalami; may affect midbrain, cervical spinal cord
  - **Nipah viral encephalitis**: Multifocal WM
  - **Rabies encephalitis**: Brainstem, hippocampi, hypothalamus, WM, GM
  - **Rhombencephalitis**: Brainstem and cerebellum
  - **St. Louis encephalitis**: Substantia nigra
  - West Nile virus (**WNV**): BG &/or thalami; may affect brainstem, cerebral WM, substantia nigra, cerebellum, spinal cord

CT Findings

- NECT: Initial CT negative in vast majority of patients
  - Japanese encephalitis: May see thalamic hemorrhage

MR Findings

- T1WI
  - **Japanese encephalitis**: Low signal foci in WM, brainstem, BG, thalami bilaterally
  - **Rabies encephalitis**: Hyperintense bilateral BG (rare)
- T2WI
  - **CMV**: Periventricular WM patchy increased signal
  - **EBV**: Hyperintensity in BG, thalamus, cortex
  - **Varicella**: Multifocal increased cortical signal
  - **Zoster**: Increased signal in brainstem, cortex
  - **Cerebellitis**: Hyperintense cerebellar signal
  - **EEE**: Increased signal in BG and thalami; may involve brainstem, cortex, periventricular WM
  - Enteroviral encephalomyelitis (**EV71**): Hyperintense lesions in posterior medulla, pons, midbrain, dentate nuclei of cerebellum
    - Less common: Cervical cord, thalamus, putamen
  - **Japanese encephalitis**: High signal foci in WM, brainstem, BG, thalami bilaterally
  - **MVE**: Hyperintensity in bilateral thalami; may involve midbrain, cerebral peduncles
  - **Nipah viral encephalitis**: Multifocal WM hyperintensities; may affect GM
  - **Rabies encephalitis**: Ill-defined mild hyperintensity in brainstem, hippocampi, thalami, WM, BG
    - Paralytic rabies: Medulla and spinal cord hyperintensity
  - **Rhombencephalitis**: Patchy hyperintensity in pons, medulla, midbrain
  - **St. Louis encephalitis**: May see hyperintensity of substantia nigra, often normal
  - **WNV**: Hyperintensity in deep gray nuclei ± cerebral WM
- FLAIR
  - **Nipah encephalitis**: Discrete high signal lesions in subcortical, deep WM ± GM
    - Confluent cortical involvement in relapsed and late-onset encephalitis
- DWI: Diffusion restriction is commonly seen
- T1 C+: Variable enhancement, none to intense
  - Meningeal enhancement can be seen
  - Herpes zoster oticus (Ramsay Hunt syndrome): Enhancing CN7, 8, membranous labyrinth
- MRS: May help distinguish encephalitis from infarct

Imaging Recommendations

- Protocol advice
  - Multiplanar MR with FLAIR, DWI, and contrast

DIFFERENTIAL DIAGNOSIS

Acute Ischemia

- Typical vascular distribution, DWI positive

Infiltrating Neoplasm

- Often unilateral disease with subacute onset

Herpes Encephalitis

- Limbic system and temporal lobe involvement

Status Epilepticus

- Active seizures with cerebral hyperperfusion, BBB disruption causes abnormal signal and enhancement

Toxic/Metabolic Lesions

- Symmetric BG or thalamic involvement common

PATHOLOGY

General Features

- Etiology
  - Most (but not all) are caused by viruses
    - Viruses are obligate intracellular parasites
  - Arboviruses are transmitted by mosquitoes and ticks
  - Replicate in skin or mucous membranes of respiratory, GI tracts

MISCELLANEOUS ENCEPHALITIS

- Spread of virus to CNS is hematogenous or neural
- Some invade along CNs (i.e., HSV-1 via lingual nerve to trigeminal ganglia)
  - Latent infections may reactivate, spread along meningeal branches
- Zoster: Latent virus in ganglia of CN (often 5 and 7) can reactivate, spread to brainstem
- Nipah encephalitis: Inflammation of small blood vessels with thrombosis and microinfarction
- Rabies: Reaches CNS by retrograde axoplasmic flow

Staging, Grading, & Classification

- Herpes viruses include HSV-1, HSV-2, CMV, EBV, VZV, B virus, HSV-6, HSV-7
- HSV-2 is major cause of neonatal encephalitis
- **Varicella**: Meningoencephalitis, cerebellar ataxia, and aseptic meningitis (< 1% of patients)
- **Zoster** infection: Encephalitis, neuritis, myelitis, or herpes ophthalmicus
  - Immunocompetent patients: Cranial and peripheral nerve palsies
  - Immunosuppressed patients: Diffuse encephalitis
  - Herpes zoster ophthalmicus can cause ICA necrotizing angiitis
- **EBV**: Agent in infectious mononucleosis
  - Diffuse encephalitis seen in < 1% of patients
  - Associated with meningoencephalitis, Guillain-Barré syndrome, transverse myelitis
- **Enteroviruses** include Coxsackie viruses A and B, poliovirus, echoviruses, enteroviruses 68 to 71
- **Arboviruses** (arthropod-borne viruses) include Eastern, Western, and Venezuelan equine encephalitis, St. Louis encephalitis, Japanese B encephalitis, California encephalitis, tick-borne encephalitis
- **Nipah encephalitis**: Paramyxovirus related to close contact with infected pigs
- **Rhombencephalitis**: Viruses most commonly (i.e., HSV), *Listeria monocytogenes*, Legionnaire disease, mycoplasma, Lyme disease, TB

Gross Pathologic & Surgical Features

- Vascular congestion, generalized or local edema, ± hemorrhage, necrosis

Microscopic Features

- Infiltration by polymorphonuclear cells (PMNs), lymphocytes, plasma cells, and mononuclear cells
- Perivascular cuffing characteristic
- May see inclusion bodies (i.e., Negri bodies in rabies)

CLINICAL ISSUES

Presentation

- Most common signs/symptoms
  - Varies widely: Slight meningeal to severe encephalitic symptoms, ± fever, prodrome
  - Varicella and herpes zoster: Different clinical manifestations of infection by same virus (VZV)
    - **Varicella encephalitis**: Fever, headache, vomiting, seizures, altered mental status days to weeks after onset of (chicken pox) rash
    - **Zoster**: Immunocompetent, CN and peripheral nerve palsies in dermatomes involved by skin lesions
      - CN5, ophthalmic branch most affected (herpes zoster ophthalmicus)
      - Rare complication: Contralateral hemiplegia related to cerebral angiitis and mycotic aneurysms
  - **Zoster**: Immunosuppressed patient with fever, meningismus, altered mental status
  - **Cerebellitis**: Sudden onset of limb &/or gait ataxia after infectious prodrome
  - Enterovirus encephalitis (**EV 71**)
    - Hand-foot-and-mouth disease (HFMD): Fever, vesicles on hands, feet, elbows, knees, lips
    - Herpangina: Ulcers of palate and pharynx
    - Cranial neuropathies, ocular disturbance, dyspnea, tachycardia if brainstem involved
  - **Nipah virus**: Fever, headache, dizziness, vomiting; segmental myoclonus, areflexia, hypotonia, hypertension, tachycardia
  - **MVE**: Fever, headache, confusion, tremors; may progress to paralysis, coma, respiratory failure
  - **Rabies** (encephalitic): Fever, malaise, altered mental status, limbic dysfunction, autonomic stimulation
    - Paralytic: Weakness of all extremities
  - **Rhombencephalitis**: Areflexia, ataxia, ophthalmoplegia
  - **St. Louis encephalitis**: Tremors, fevers

Demographics

- Epidemiology
  - Herpes: Most common cause of sporadic (nonepidemic) viral encephalitis
  - Japanese encephalitis: Most common endemic encephalitis in Asia
  - CNS involvement in EBV is uncommon (< 10% of cases)
  - VZV: < 1% have CNS involvement
  - Marked seasonal variation in USA

Natural History & Prognosis

- Many encephalitides have high morbidity, mortality
- Rapid diagnosis, early treatment with antiviral or antibacterial agents can decrease mortality, may improve outcome

DIAGNOSTIC CHECKLIST

Consider

- Imaging often nonspecific, mimics other etiologies
- Clinical and travel history often helpful

Image Interpretation Pearls

- DWI may detect lesions earlier than conventional MR

SELECTED REFERENCES

1. Nagel MA et al: The varicella zoster virus vasculopathies: clinical, CSF, imaging, and virologic features. Neurology. 70(11):853-60, 2008
2. Rumboldt Z: Imaging of topographic viral CNS infections. Neuroimaging Clin N Am. 18(1):85-92; viii, 2008
3. Baskin HJ et al: Neuroimaging of herpesvirus infections in children. Pediatr Radiol. 37(10):949-63, 2007
4. Kennedy PG: Viral encephalitis: causes, differential diagnosis, and management. J Neurol Neurosurg Psychiatry. 75 Suppl 1:i10-5, 2004

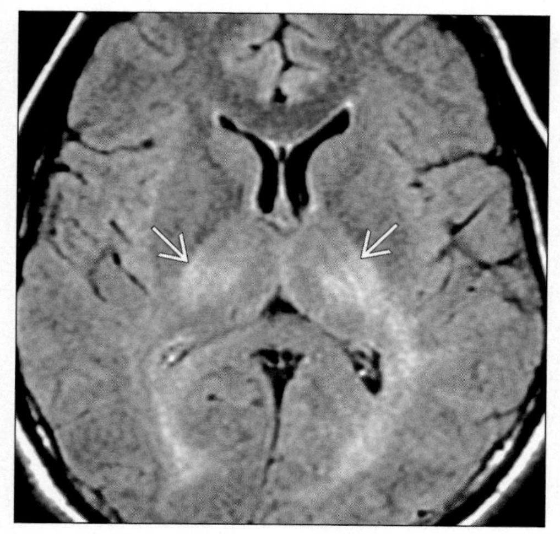

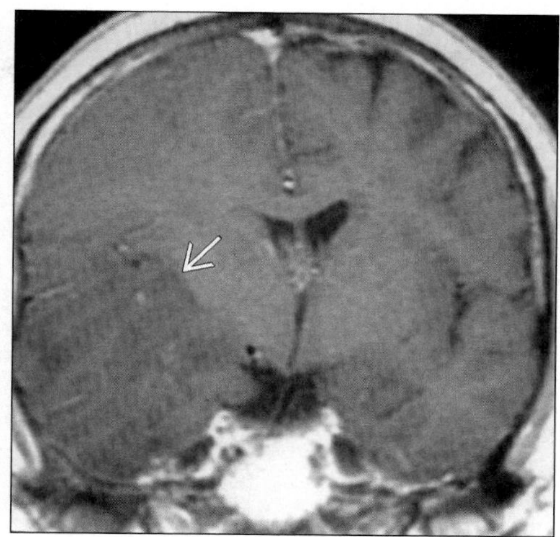

(Left) *Axial FLAIR MR shows symmetric hyperintense signal in the thalami ➡ in this patient with a history of infectious mononucleosis. EBV commonly involves the basal ganglia, thalami, cortex, &/or brainstem. Imaging of encephalitis is often nonspecific and commonly mimics other disease processes.* ***(Right)*** *Coronal T1WI C+ MR shows a nonenhancing right temporal lobe "mass" ➡ in this patient with viral encephalitis. Enhancement is variable in the encephalitides. (Courtesy C. Sutton, MD.)*

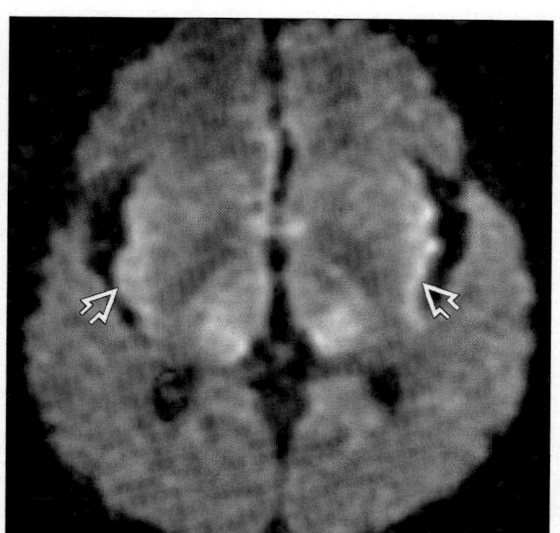

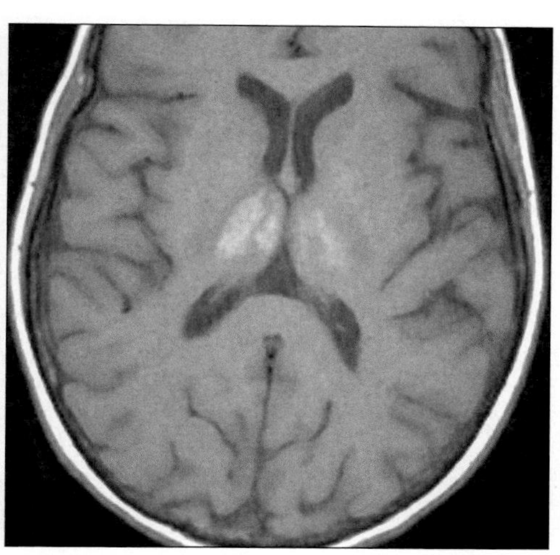

(Left) *Axial DWI MR shows symmetric diffusion restriction in the thalami and insular cortex ➡ in this patient with West Nile virus encephalitis. Basal ganglia and thalamic involvement is classic for West Nile virus encephalitis. DWI may help detect lesions earlier than conventional MR imaging.* ***(Right)*** *Axial T1WI MR shows T1 shortening in the thalami bilaterally in this patient with West Nile virus encephalitis. T1 shortening is suggestive of blood products and is atypical of West Nile virus.*

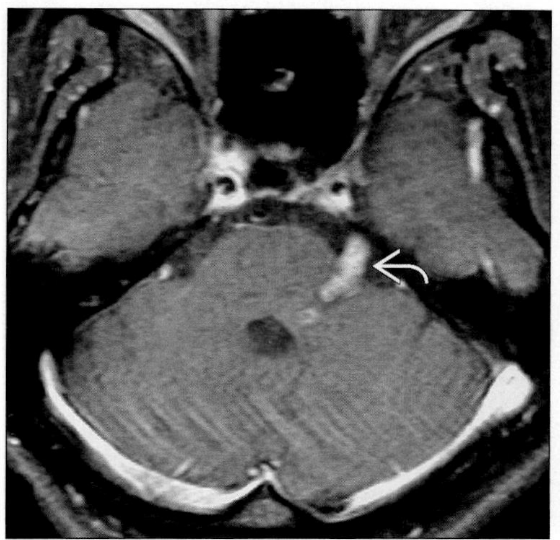

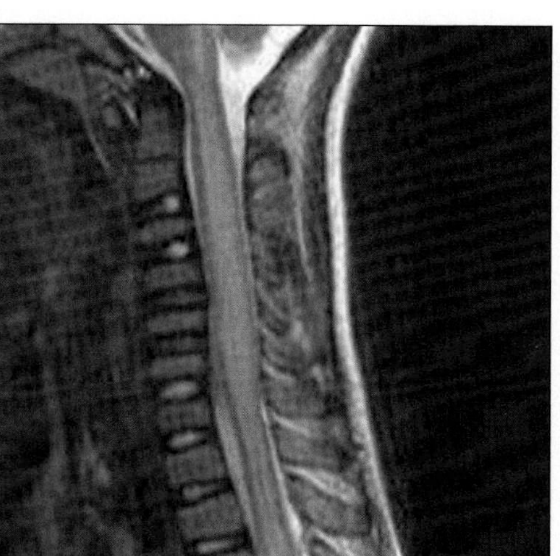

(Left) *Axial T1WI C+ MR shows enhancement of CN5, cisternal segment ➡, root entry zone, and brachium pontis in this patient with trigeminal neuralgia. The ophthalmic branch (V1) is most affected in herpes zoster. Zoster commonly affects cranial nerves in immunocompetent patients. VZV encephalitis is rare.* ***(Right)*** *Sagittal T2WI MR shows diffuse enlargement and hyperintensity of the cervical spinal cord in this paralytic rabies patient. Paralytic rabies often affects the medulla and spinal cord.*

WEST NILE VIRUS ENCEPHALITIS

Key Facts

Terminology

- West Nile virus (WNV); West Nile fever (WNF); West Nile neuroinvasive disease (WNND)
- Mosquito-transmitted acute meningoencephalitis

Imaging

- Head CT usually normal
- MR with DWI, T1 C+
  - Classic: Bilateral basal ganglia, thalamic hyperintensity
  - Patchy, poorly demarcated hyperintense foci in cerebral WM on T2WI/FLAIR
  - Enhancement usually absent (has been reported)
  - DWI may show restricted diffusion
- Other sites of involvement
  - Midbrain
  - Corpus callosum splenium
  - Mesial temporal lobes
  - Cerebellum
  - Spinal cord, cauda equina

Clinical Issues

- Approximately 1/140 patients infected with WNV develop CNS symptoms
  - Incubation period: 2-14 days
- ~ 80% of infected individuals asymptomatic
  - Mild febrile syndrome (West Nile fever) in 20%
  - Meningoencephalitis in < 1%
  - Rare: Anterior myelitis
- CNS symptoms more common in diabetics, immunocompromised
- Treatment is supportive; hydration, antipyretics, airway and seizure management as indicated
- No human vaccine
  - Best way to prevent infection? Fight the bite!

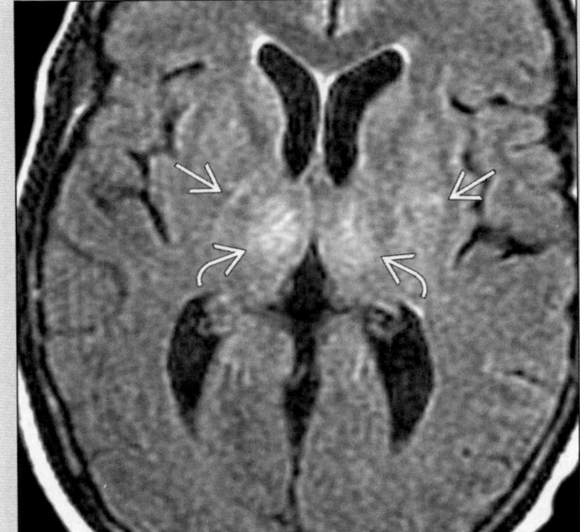

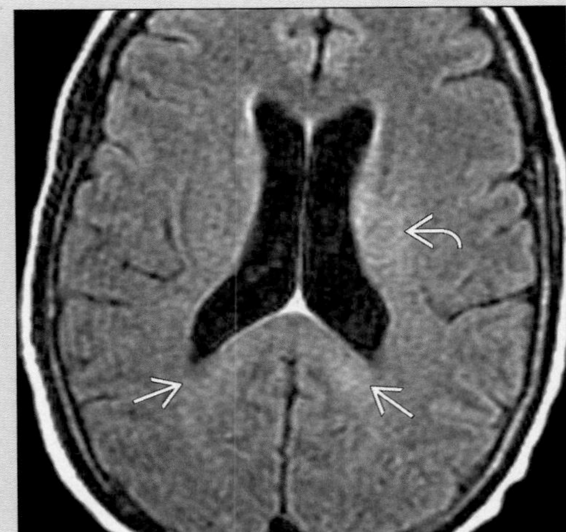

(Left) *Axial FLAIR MR in patient with West Nile virus meningoencephalitis shows bilaterally symmetric high signal intensity in the thalami ➔. There is subtle hyperintensity in the basal ganglia and right internal capsule ➔.* ***(Right)*** *Axial FLAIR MR in the same patient shows mild hyperintensity in the splenium of the corpus callosum ➔ and in the left corona radiata ➔.*

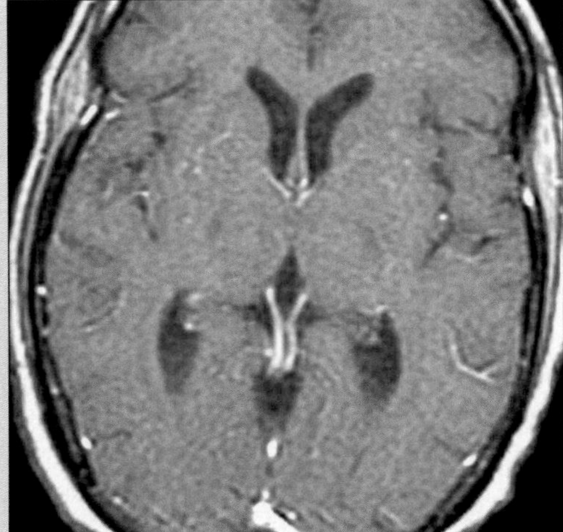

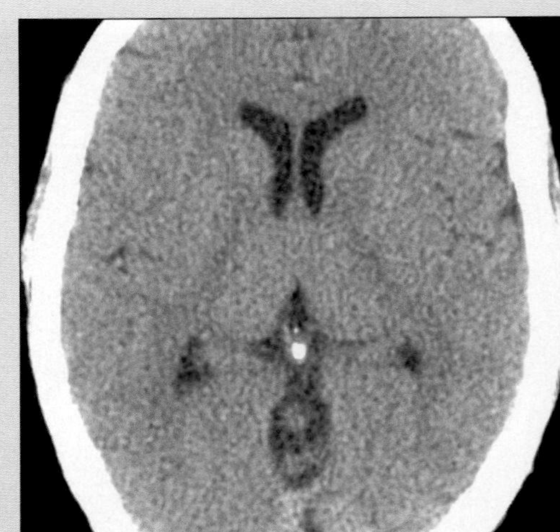

(Left) *Axial T1WI C+ MR in the same patient shows that the thalamic lesions do not enhance. The remainder of the study showed no evidence for abnormal enhancement elsewhere.* ***(Right)*** *Axial NECT in the same patient performed 6 hours prior to the MR exam is normal. No edema is seen in the thalami or white matter. Indeed, early in the disease course, CT scans are frequently unremarkable.*

WEST NILE VIRUS ENCEPHALITIS

TERMINOLOGY

Abbreviations

- West Nile virus (WNV); West Nile fever (WNF); West Nile neuroinvasive disease (WNND)

Definitions

- Mosquito-transmitted acute meningoencephalitis caused by West Nile arbovirus

IMAGING

General Features

- Best diagnostic clue
  - Bilateral basal ganglia &/or thalamic lesions
- Location
  - Classic: Bilateral basal ganglia, thalami
  - Cerebral white matter
  - Other
    - Midbrain
    - Corpus callosum splenium
    - Mesial temporal lobes
    - Cerebellum
    - Spinal cord, cauda equina

Imaging Recommendations

- Best imaging tool
  - Standard MR; include T1 C+, DWI

CT Findings

- Frequently normal

MR Findings

- Patchy, poorly demarcated foci of T2 signal in cerebral white matter on T2 and FLAIR sequences
- Bilateral, frequently symmetric T2 hyperintense signal in basal ganglia, thalami, and brainstem
- DWI may show restricted diffusion
- Enhancement usually absent (though has been reported)

DIFFERENTIAL DIAGNOSIS

Encephalitis (Other Infectious Etiologies)

- Herpes usually affects mesial temporal lobe(s)

Demyelinating Diseases

- e.g., ADEM, multiple sclerosis, Susac
- ADEM often (but not always) spares deep gray matter

PATHOLOGY

General Features

- Etiology
  - WNV: Flavivirus (like Japanese encephalitis)
    - Arthropod-transmitted (mosquito)
      - *Culex pipiens* is vector in eastern USA
      - *Culex quinquefasciatus* species in southeastern USA
      - *Culex tarsalis* species in western, midwestern USA
    - Mosquitos infect birds ("amplifying hosts")
      - Birds transmit infection to other biting mosquitos
      - Uncommonly infects humans/other mammals
    - Human-to-human transmission rare but reported
      - Blood transfusions, transplant recipients
      - Intrauterine exposure, conjunctival exposure
      - Breast feeding, occupational exposure
- Genetics
  - Increased susceptibility to WNV disease in carriers with 2 mutated copies of gene *CCR5*

CLINICAL ISSUES

Presentation

- Most common signs/symptoms
  - ~ 80% of infected individuals asymptomatic
  - Mild febrile syndrome (WNF) in 20%
    - Fever, headache, fatigue, lymphadenopathy, arthralgia typical
    - May develop GI symptoms including nausea, vomiting, and diarrhea
    - Occasional truncal maculopapular rash
    - Incubation period: 2-14 days
  - Meningoencephalitis (WNND) in < 1%
    - Symptoms of mild febrile syndrome plus
      - Seizures, altered mental status, coma
      - Extrapyramidal signs (brisk followed by ↓ DTRs)
- Other signs/symptoms
  - Rare associations
    - Anterior myelitis ± encephalitis
      - Guillain-Barré syndrome
    - Multifocal chorioretinitis
    - Nephritis, hepatitis, myocarditis

Demographics

- Age
  - WNND more common in elderly
- Epidemiology
  - Approximately 1/140 patients infected with WNV develop CNS symptoms
  - CNS symptoms more common in diabetics, immunocompromised

Natural History & Prognosis

- Prolonged convalescent period with fatigue common
- Mortality rate of neuroinvasive infection < 4%

Treatment

- No human vaccine
- Best way to prevent infection? Fight the bite!
  - Wear light clothing that covers extremities
  - Use insect repellents
- Treatment is supportive
  - Hydration, antipyretics, airway and seizure management as indicated

SELECTED REFERENCES

1. Kramer LD et al: West Nile virus. Lancet Neurol. 6(2):171-81, 2007
2. Ali M et al: West Nile virus infection: MR imaging findings in the nervous system. AJNR Am J Neuroradiol. 26(2):289-97, 2005

HHV-6 ENCEPHALITIS

Key Facts

Terminology
- Encephalitis caused by human herpes virus 6 (HHV-6)

Imaging
- Immunocompromised patient with abnormal signal medial temporal lobe(s)
  - Limbic system: Hippocampus, amygdala, parahippocampal gyrus
  - Insular region, frontal white matter, corona radiata may be involved
  - Atypical pattern in infants/children (basal ganglia, thalami, cerebellum, brainstem)
- Best imaging: MR (coronal T2/FLAIR, DWI, T1 C+)

Top Differential Diagnoses
- Herpes simplex virus (HSV) encephalitis
- Paraneoplastic limbic encephalitis
- Status epilepticus

Pathology
- HHV-6: DNA virus belongs to herpes virus family
- 2 variants: HHV-6A and HHV-6B

Clinical Issues
- Mental status changes, fever, seizure, headache
- Reactivation in immunocompromised
- Post hemopoietic stem cell transplant, lung/liver transplant
- Antiviral drugs: Ganciclovir and foscarnet
- Mortality of HHV-6 encephalitis > 50%

Diagnostic Checklist
- Consider HHV-6 encephalitis in immunocompromised patients with CNS symptoms + unilateral/bilateral medial temporal lobe signal changes

*(**Left**) Coronal T2WI MR in a 37-year-old man with immunosuppression, a fever, and seizures shows hyperintense signal in the medial temporal lobes, basal ganglia, and subinsular white matter. (**Right**) Axial T2WI MR in the same patient shows asymmetric hyperintense signal in the subinsular white matter. Extrahippocampal involvement in HHV-6 encephalitis has been commonly reported.*

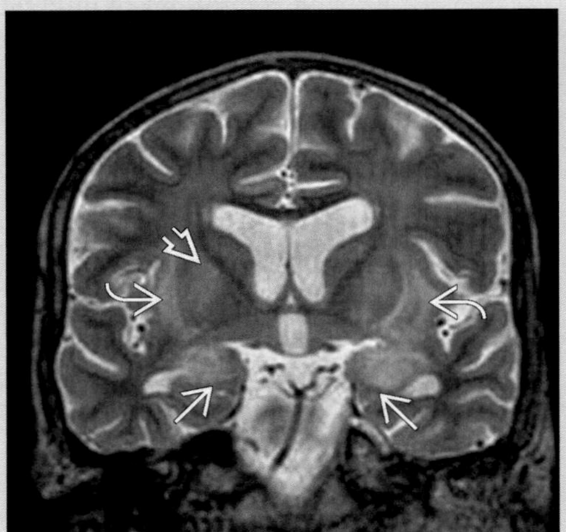

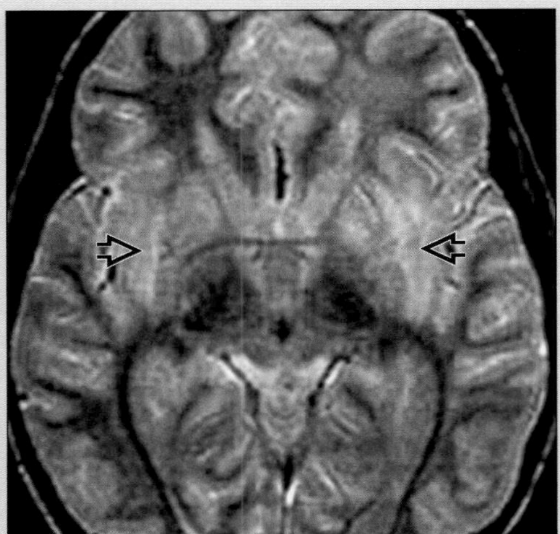

*(**Left**) Axial PWI MR shows asymmetric hyperintense signal in the medial temporal lobes in this immunosuppressed patient with HHV-6 encephalitis. (**Right**) Axial DWI MR shows bright signal consistent with restricted diffusion within both amygdalae and hippocampi in a 10-year-old boy with immunosuppression. ADC map (not shown) confirmed restricted diffusion.*

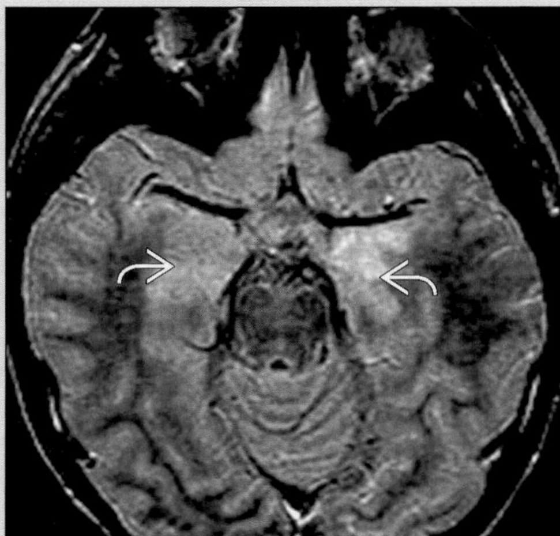

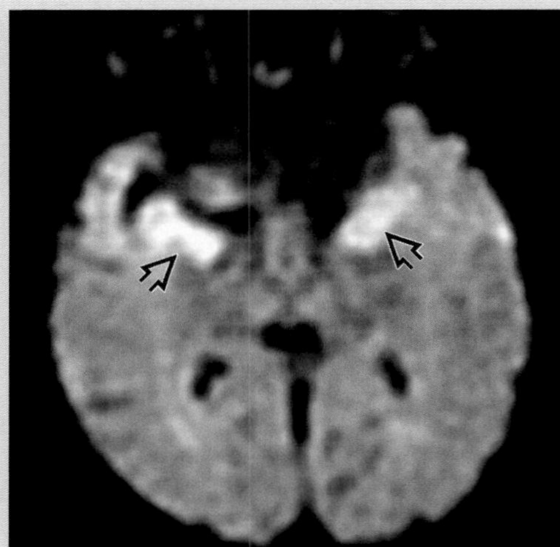

Key Facts

Terminology
- Acute cerebellitis

Imaging
- Bilateral, often confluent cerebellar hemispheric gray matter and white matter low attenuation (NECT), T1 and T2 prolongation (MR)
- DWI/ADC → affected regions typically show increased diffusivity

Top Differential Diagnoses
- Acute disseminated encephalomyelitis
- Infiltrating cerebellar neoplasm

Pathology
- Infectious
  - Enteroviruses, Epstein-Barr, varicella, Coxsackie, influenza A and B, mumps and measles viruses
- Other
  - Acute disseminated encephalomyelitis, vasculitis, lead intoxication, cyanide and methadone poisoning

Clinical Issues
- Nausea, vomiting, ± bradycardia, truncal ataxia, abnormal eye movements
- Most symptoms and signs resolve completely over weeks to months

Diagnostic Checklist
- Idiopathic acute cerebellitis is diagnosis of exclusion
- DWI and ADC maps usually show increased diffusivity

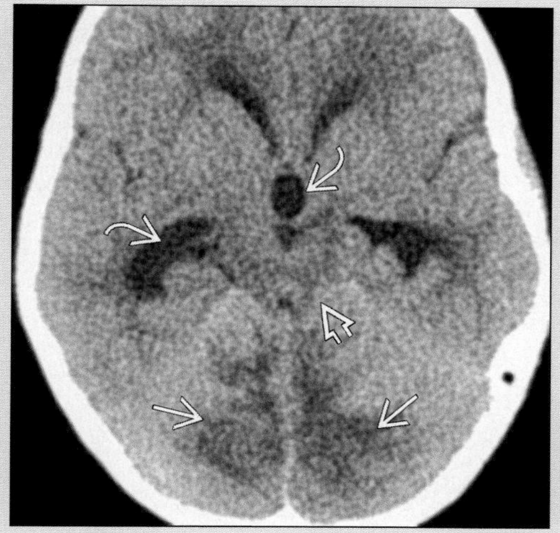

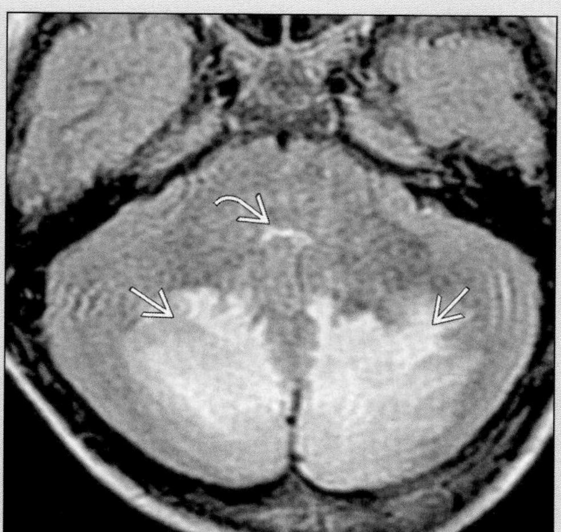

*(**Left**) Axial NECT in a 4-year-old girl with proven influenza A infection shows cerebellar hemispheric edema (low attenuation) ➡ involving both gray and white matter. The edema causes upward cerebellar herniation and effacement of the quadrigeminal plate cistern ➡. The resultant aqueductal compression causes hydrocephalus ➡. (**Right**) Axial T2WI MR demonstrates cerebellar edema (T2 hyperintensity) involving both gray and white matter ➡. Note the compressed 4th ventricle ➡.*

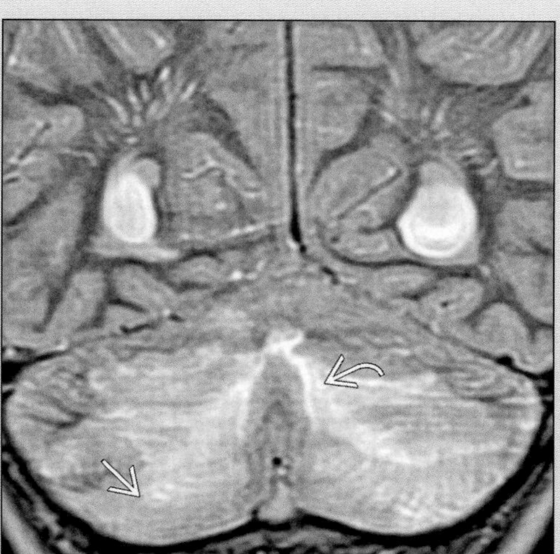

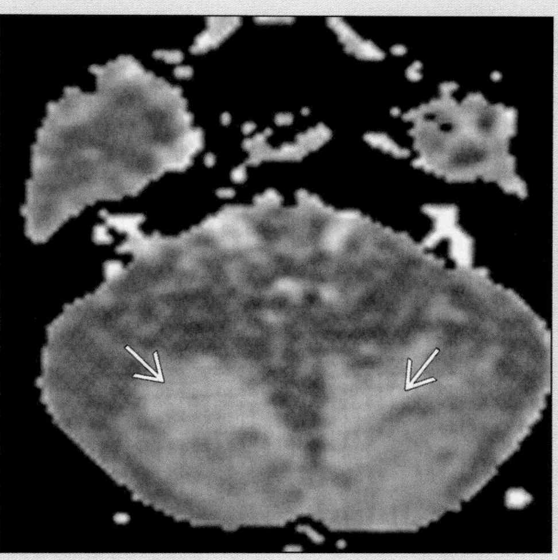

*(**Left**) Coronal T2WI MR in a patient with acute onset of bradycardia, ataxia, and abnormal eye movements shows confluent bilateral cerebellar hemispheric regions of T2 prolongation, involving both gray ➡ and white ➡ matter. In acute cerebellitis, involvement is typically bilateral. (**Right**) Axial ADC map in a patient with influenza A cerebellitis demonstrates confluent regions of increased diffusivity ➡ corresponding to areas of T2 prolongation and FLAIR hyperintensity on spin echo MR (not shown).*

RASMUSSEN ENCEPHALITIS

Key Facts

Terminology

- Chronic focal (localized) encephalitis
- Chronic, progressive, unilateral brain inflammation of uncertain etiology

Imaging

- Unilateral progressive cortical atrophy
- CT/MR often normal initially
- Early cortical swelling, then atrophy ensues
- Usually unilateral, predominantly frontal and parietal
- Best Imaging tools: MR with contrast, ± PET (FDG)

Top Differential Diagnoses

- Sturge-Weber syndrome
- **M**itochondrial **e**ncephalopathy, **l**actic **a**cidosis, and **s**troke-like episodes (MELAS)
- Hemispheric infarction (Dyke-Davidoff-Masson)

Pathology

- Hemispheric cortical atrophy

Clinical Issues

- Intractable epilepsy, clonic movements
  - Other: Visual and sensory deficits, dysarthria, dysphasia, personality changes
- Partial complex seizures that increase in frequency → 20% present in status epilepticus

Diagnostic Checklist

- Consider Rasmussen encephalitis when/if
  - ↑ frequency of partial complex seizures, postictal deficit in patients (1-15 years) with initial "normal" imaging
  - Intractable epilepsy with progressive atrophy of 1 hemisphere showing high T2 signal

*(**Left**) Coronal T2WI MR in a 6-year-old girl with worsening partial complex seizures and progressive right hemiplegia demonstrates marked left hemispheric atrophy. Note the profound hippocampal volume loss ➙. (**Right**) Axial T2WI MR demonstrates diffuse atrophy of the left hemisphere in a child with progressive seizures refractory to medical therapy. Note the atrophy of the insular region ➙, typically involved early in Rasmussen encephalitis, and the right frontal lobe ➙.*

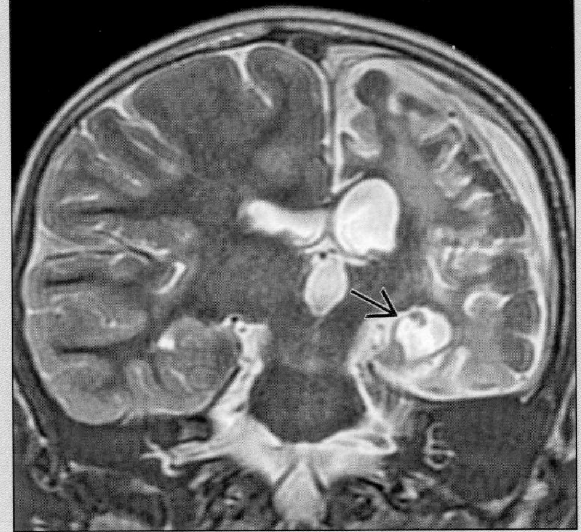

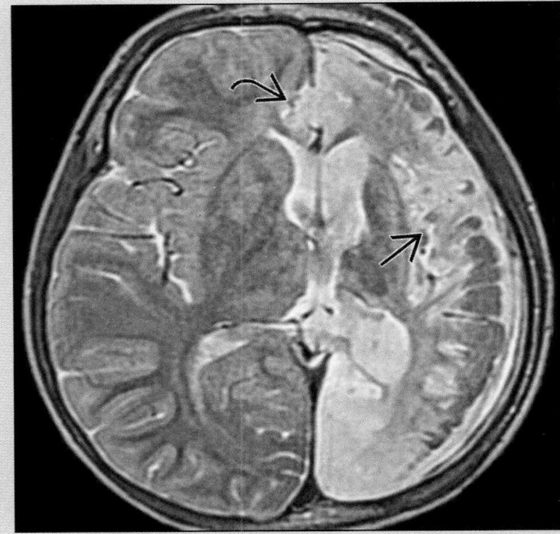

*(**Left**) Axial FLAIR MR shows atrophy of the left hemisphere. Gliosis is manifest as FLAIR hyperintensity ➙. Note the insular cortical and subcortical atrophy ➙ and the involvement of the right frontal cortex ➙. (**Right**) Coronal T1WI C+ MR shows extensive atrophy of the left hemisphere. Note the profound left hippocampal volume loss ➙. Rasmussen encephalitis is distinguished on T1WI C+ MR from Sturge-Weber syndrome by the lack of enhancing leptomeningeal angiomatosis.*

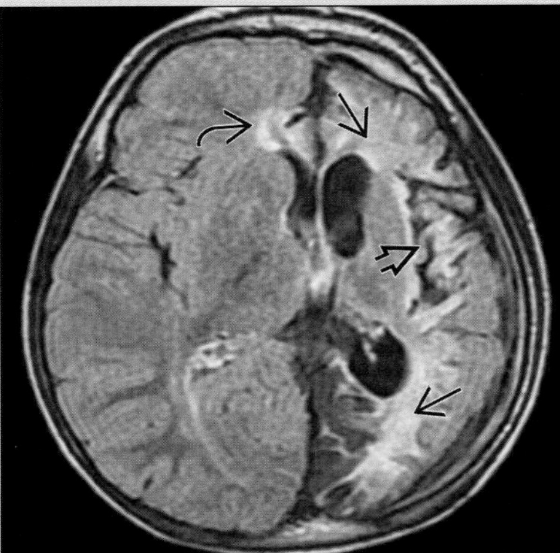

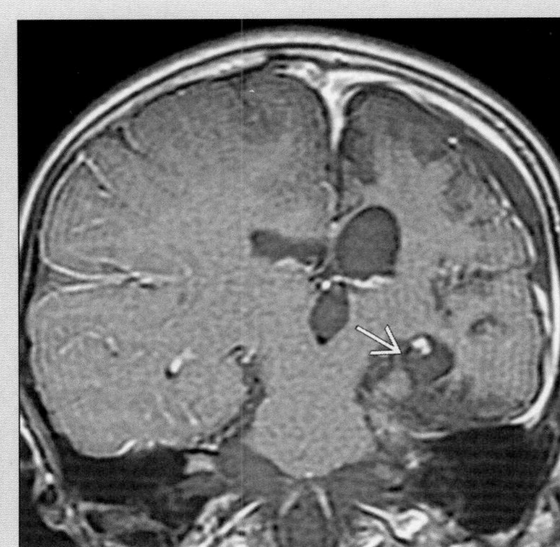

TERMINOLOGY

Abbreviations

- Rasmussen syndrome (RS)

Synonyms

- Chronic focal (localized) encephalitis

Definitions

- Chronic, progressive, unilateral brain inflammation of uncertain etiology
- Characterized by hemispheric volume loss and difficulty controlling focal seizure activity

IMAGING

General Features

- Best diagnostic clue
  - Unilateral progressive cortical atrophy
  - CT/MR often normal initially
    - Early cortical swelling, then atrophy ensues
    - Most cerebral damage occurs in 1st 12 months after clinical onset of disease
- Location
  - Cerebral hemisphere
  - Usually unilateral, predominantly frontal and parietal
    - Precentral, inferior frontal atrophy
      - Contralateral cerebellar volume loss (crossed cerebellar diaschisis)
- Size
  - Variable, usually lobar, occasionally entire hemisphere affected
- Morphology
  - Focal abnormality, "spreads across hemisphere"
  - Becomes progressively more diffuse

CT Findings

- NECT
  - Initially normal → atrophy
- CECT
  - Usually no enhancement
  - **Rare** transient pial &/or cortical enhancement

MR Findings

- T1WI
  - Sulcal effacement due to early swelling
- T2WI
  - Early focal swelling of gyri
    - Gray-white matter (GM-WM) "blurring" and T2 prolongation
    - ± basal ganglia, hippocampi involvement
  - Late: Atrophy of involved cerebral hemisphere or lobe
- PD/intermediate
  - Same as T2WI
- FLAIR
  - Cortical and subcortical areas of hyperintensity that progressively increase over time
  - Late: Atrophy, encephalomalacia/gliosis
- T2* GRE
  - Typically normal
  - Nonhemorrhagic
- DWI
  - Subtle high signal on trace images; ↑ diffusivity
- T1WI C+
  - Usually does not enhance
    - Occasionally, subtle pial &/or cortical enhancement
- MRS
  - ↓ N-acetyl-aspartate (NAA) and choline; ↑ myoinositol, ↑ glutamine/glutamate

Nuclear Medicine Findings

- Tc-99m-HMPAO scintigraphy: ↓ perfusion even if normal MR
- PET and SPECT
  - ↓ cerebral perfusion/metabolism
  - Crossed cerebellar diaschisis
  - Transient hypermetabolism may be related to recent seizures (rare)
    - C-11-methionine shows increased multifocal uptake

Imaging Recommendations

- Best imaging tool
  - MR + clinical signs/symptoms + appropriate EEG findings
- Protocol advice
  - MR with contrast, ± PET (FDG)

DIFFERENTIAL DIAGNOSIS

Sturge-Weber Syndrome

- Port wine facial nevus and enhancement of pial angioma
- Progressive hemispheric atrophy
- Cortical Ca++

Mitochondrial Encephalopathy, Lactic Acidosis, and Stroke-Like Episodes (MELAS)

- Acute: May cause cortical hyperintensity (parietooccipital most common) → + DWI/ADC
- Chronic: Cortical atrophy, lacunes (basal ganglia, thalami)

Prenatal/Neonatal Hemispheric Infarction (Dyke-Davidoff-Masson)

- Unilateral brain atrophy
- Compensatory calvarial thickening
- Elevation of petrous ridge and hyperaeration of paranasal sinuses
- Following in utero or perinatal infarct

PATHOLOGY

General Features

- Etiology
  - Autoimmune theory (1 theory)
    - Glutamate is excitatory neurotransmitter
    - Glutamate antibodies cross damaged blood-brain barrier
    - Antibodies bind and activate glutamate receptors (GluR3)
    - Nerve cells stimulated → seizures induced

RASMUSSEN ENCEPHALITIS

- Genetics
  - Possibly viral trigger of genetic predisposition to immunodysfunction
- Associated abnormalities
  - 3 potentially overlapping factors may initiate or perpetuate events leading to injury
    - Viral infection
    - Autoimmune antibodies
    - Autoimmune cytotoxic T lymphocytes

Staging, Grading, & Classification

- Classification and staging: MR (T2WI)
  - Stage 1: Swelling/hyperintense signal
  - Stage 2: Normal volume/hyperintense signal
  - Stage 3: Atrophy/hyperintense signal
  - Stage 4: Progressive atrophy and normal signal

Gross Pathologic & Surgical Features

- Hemispheric cortical atrophy

Microscopic Features

- Robitaille classification
  - Group 1 (pathologically active): Ongoing inflammatory process
    - Microglial nodules, ± neuronophagia, perivascular round cells
  - Group 2 (active and remote disease): Acute on chronic
    - Above plus at least 1 gyral segment of complete necrosis and cavitation including full-thickness cortex
  - Group 3 (less active "remote" disease)
    - Neuronal loss/gliosis and fewer microglial nodules
  - Group 4 (burnt out)
    - Nonspecific scarring with little active inflammation

CLINICAL ISSUES

Presentation

- Most common signs/symptoms
  - Intractable epilepsy, clonic movements
  - Progresses to epilepsia partialis continua
  - Other: Visual and sensory deficits, dysarthria, dysphasia, personality changes
- Clinical profile
  - Young child with progressive partial epilepsy unresponsive to medical therapy
- Clinical course
  - Partial complex seizures that increase in frequency
  - 20% present in status epilepticus
  - Followed by
    - Worsening seizures, progressive hemiparesis, cognitive deterioration, death
- EEG: Slow focal activity (early); epilepsia partialis continua (late)
- CSF: ± oligoclonal bands
- Other: GluR3 antibodies found in ~ 50%; but not specific

Demographics

- Age
  - Usually begins in childhood (6-8 years)
- Gender
  - M = F
- Ethnicity
  - No predilection
- Epidemiology
  - Preceded by inflammatory episode (50%)
    - Tonsillitis, upper respiratory infection, otitis media

Natural History & Prognosis

- Hemiplegia and cognitive deterioration in most cases
- Older patients have longer prodromal stage and protracted course
- Prognosis is poor
- Hemiplegia is inevitable ± treatment

Treatment

- Refractory to antiepileptic medications
- ± transient improvement with plasma exchange, ganciclovir, steroids, immunoadsorption
- Surgical options
  - Hemispherectomy
  - Functional hemispherectomy/central disconnection

DIAGNOSTIC CHECKLIST

Image Interpretation Pearls

- Consider Rasmussen encephalitis
  - ↑ frequency of partial complex seizures + postictal deficit in patients (1-15 years) with initial "normal" imaging
  - Intractable epilepsy with progressive atrophy of 1 hemisphere showing high T2 signal

SELECTED REFERENCES

1. Cauley KA et al: Diffusion tensor imaging and tractography of Rasmussen encephalitis. Pediatr Radiol. 39(7):727-30, 2009
2. Faingold R et al: MRI appearance of Rasmussen encephalitis. Pediatr Radiol. Epub ahead of print, 2009
3. Terra-Bustamante VC et al: Rasmussen encephalitis: long-term outcome after surgery. Childs Nerv Syst. 25(5):583-9, 2009
4. Misra UK et al: The prognostic role of magnetic resonance imaging and single-photon emission computed tomography in viral encephalitis. Acta Radiol. 49(7):827-32, 2008
5. Tessonnier L et al: Perfusion SPECT Findings in a Suspected Case of Rasmussen Encephalitis. J Neuroimaging. Epub ahead of print, 2008
6. Cook SW et al: Cerebral hemispherectomy in pediatric patients with epilepsy: comparison of three techniques by pathological substrate in 115 patients. J Neurosurg. 100(2 Suppl Pediatrics):125-41, 2004
7. Bien CG et al: Diagnosis and staging of Rasmussen's encephalitis by serial MRI and histopathology. Neurology. 58(2):250-7, 2002
8. Kim SJ et al: A longitudinal MRI study in children with Rasmussen syndrome. Pediatr Neurol. 27(4):282-8, 2002

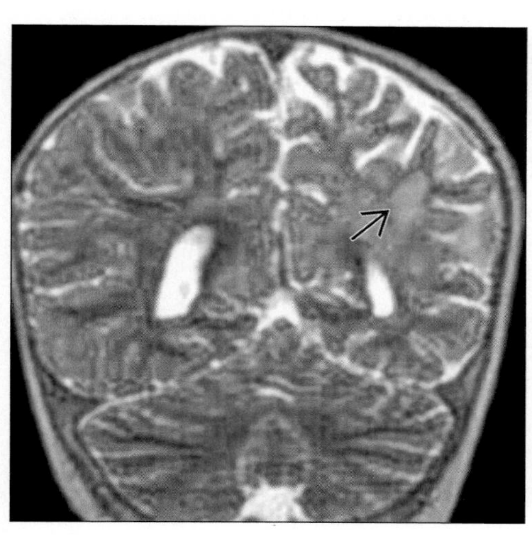

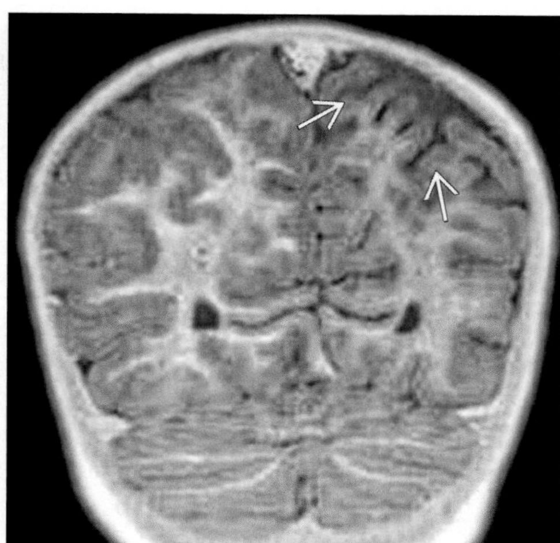

(Left) *Coronal T2WI MR in a 7-year-old girl with epilepsia partialis continua and cognitive decline shows left parietal atrophy. Note the subcortical white matter T2 hyperintensity reflecting gliosis ➡. (Courtesy A. Gupta, MD.)* ***(Right)*** *Coronal T1WI MR in the same patient shows left parietal cortical and subcortical atrophy ➡. The frontal and parietal lobes are commonly the 1st regions of the cerebral hemisphere to show changes on MR. (Courtesy A. Gupta, MD.)*

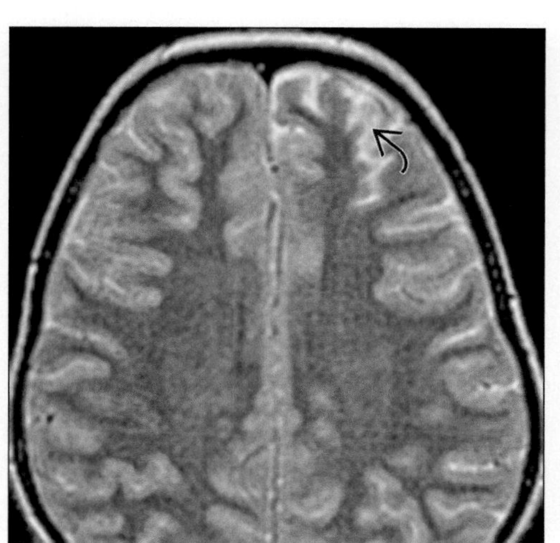

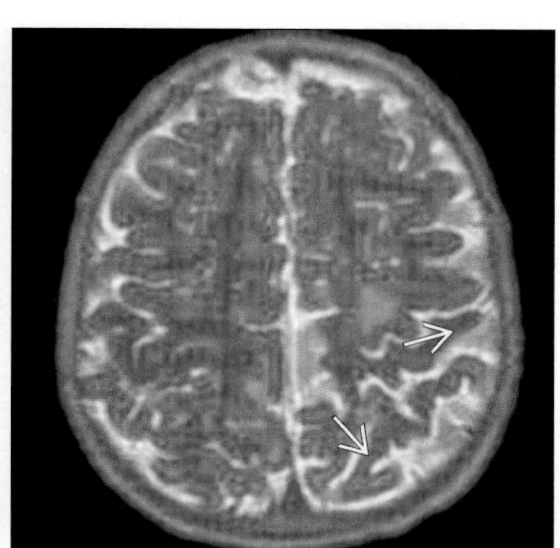

(Left) *Axial T2WI MR in a 5-year-old boy with progressive cognitive decline and seizures demonstrates left frontal atrophy predominately affecting the cortex ➡. The atrophy in Rasmussen encephalitis is progressive with cortical and subcortical involvement.* ***(Right)*** *Axial T2WI MR in a patient with an escalating frequency of partial complex seizures and right hemiparesis shows moderate left cerebral hemispheric atrophy most severely affecting the parietal lobe ➡. (Courtesy A. Gupta, MD.)*

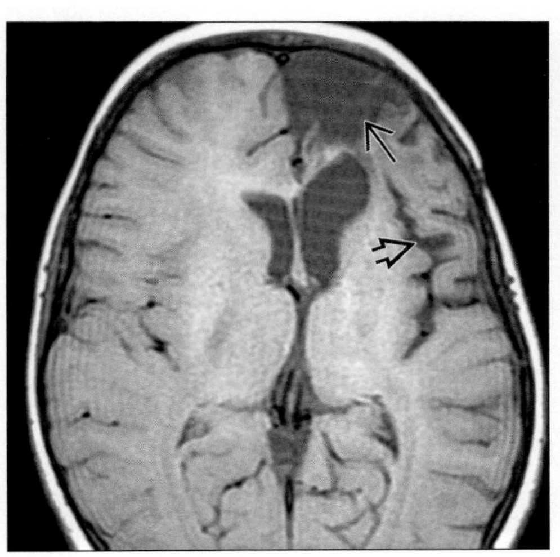

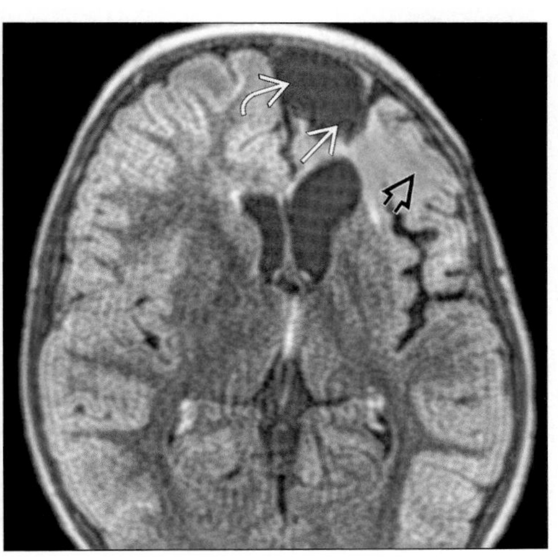

(Left) *Axial T1WI MR in a 4-year-old girl with chronic localized Rasmussen encephalitis demonstrates marked atrophy of the frontal lobe ➡. Note the ex vacuo dilation of the left frontal horn and the enlargement of the circular sulcus ➡ reflecting insular volume loss.* ***(Right)*** *Axial FLAIR MR in the same patient shows atrophy of the superior frontal ➡ and middle frontal gyrus ➡. Atrophy and subcortical gliosis extends into the left inferior frontal gyrus ➡.*

SUBACUTE SCLEROSING PANENCEPHALITIS

Key Facts

Terminology
- Definition: Rare, progressive measles virus-mediated encephalitis

Imaging
- CT: Imaging often initially normal → cortical swelling → cortical/subcortical hypoattenuation
- MR: Ill-defined T2 hyperintensities in periventricular or subcortical white matter (WM)
  - Frontal > parietal > occipital, no mass effect
- MRS: Increased choline and myoinositol; decreased NAA (may precede MR abnormalities)

Top Differential Diagnoses
- Acute disseminated encephalomyelitis (ADEM)
- Tumefactive multiple sclerosis (MS)
- Human immunodeficiency virus (HIV)

Pathology
- Measles virus (mutant or defective form), aberrant response to measles infection

Clinical Issues
- Progressive mental deterioration, motor impairment, myoclonus, emotional instability
- Begins insidiously → subacute course → death (duration generally 1-6 months)
- Positive CSF, plasma complement fixation test for measles; CSF plus oligoclonal bands

Diagnostic Checklist
- Consider SSPE in immigrant child with behavior changes and multifocal white matter disease

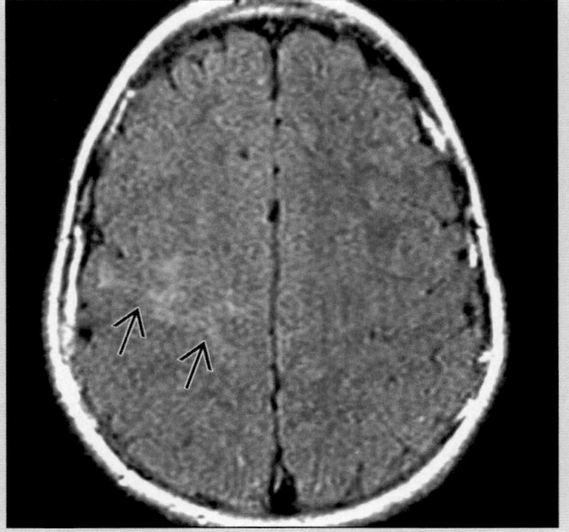

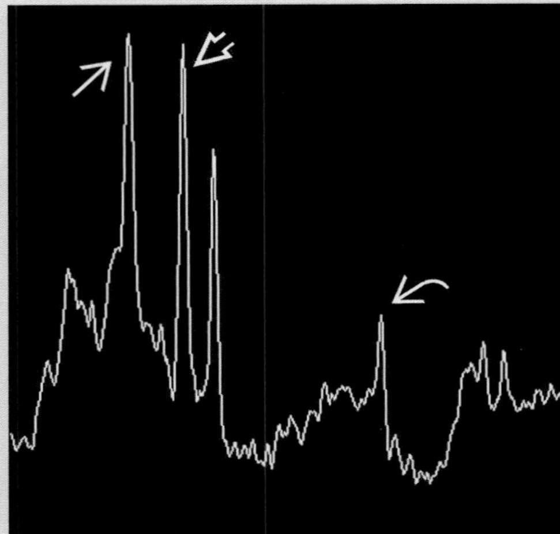

(Left) *Axial FLAIR MR in a 7-year-old boy with worsening gait disturbance and myoclonic jerks. Note the subtle right posterior frontal lobe cortical and subcortical white matter FLAIR hyperintensity ➔.* ***(Right)*** *Single voxel proton MRS (TE = 35 msec) from the right parietal subcortical white matter in the same patient shows increased choline ➔ and myoinositol ➔ and a marked decrease in NAA ➔. These metabolic changes were present with only subtle FLAIR and T2 signal abnormality.*

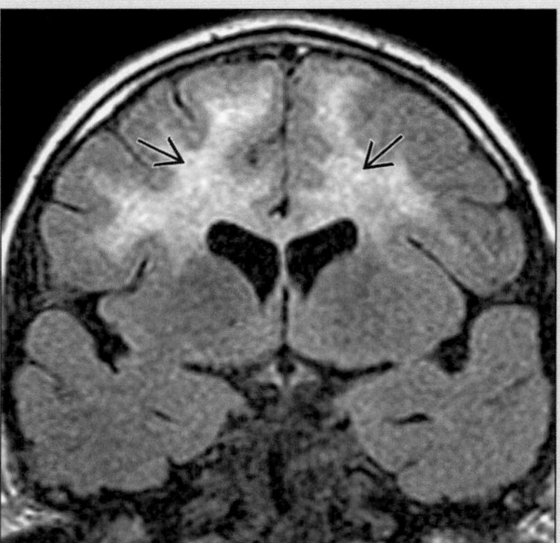

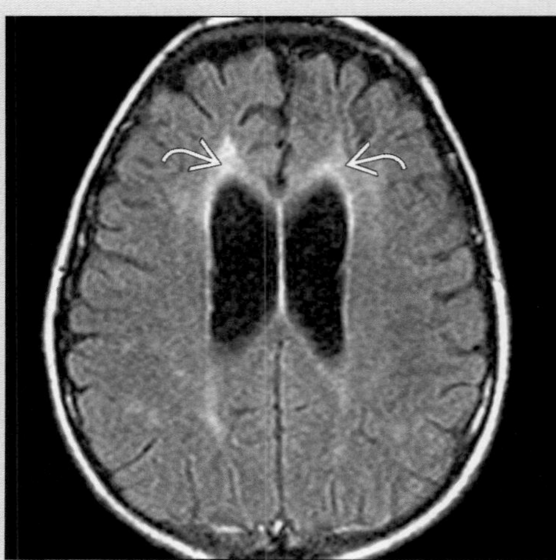

(Left) *Coronal FLAIR MR in a 7-year-old boy 6 months after initial presentation, following confirmatory CSF complement fixation test for measles, demonstrates progressive frontal lobe white matter FLAIR hyperintensity ➔.* ***(Right)*** *Axial FLAIR MR in the same patient, 10 months after initial clinical presentation with progressive cognitive deterioration and worsening myoclonus, shows bilateral frontal lobe WM volume loss and FLAIR hyperintensity ➔ (demyelination and gliosis).*

SUBACUTE SCLEROSING PANENCEPHALITIS

TERMINOLOGY

Abbreviations

- Subacute sclerosing panencephalitis (SSPE), Dawson encephalitis

Definitions

- Progressive measles virus-mediated encephalitis

IMAGING

General Features

- Best diagnostic clue
  - T2 hyperintensities in periventricular or subcortical white matter (WM)
- Location
  - Frontal > parietal > occipital lobes

CT Findings

- NECT
  - CT: Imaging often initially normal → cortical swelling → cortical/subcortical hypoattenuation

MR Findings

- T1WI
  - Areas of ↓ signal in WM, corpus callosum
- T2WI
  - Increased signal in WM, frontal > parietal > occipital, generally symmetric and eventually leading to diffuse atrophy
- T1WI C+
  - No enhancement
- MRS
  - Increased choline and myoinositol; decreased NAA (may precede MR abnormalities)

Imaging Recommendations

- Best imaging tool
  - MR
- Protocol advice
  - MR + IV contrast + MRS

DIFFERENTIAL DIAGNOSIS

Acute Disseminated Encephalomyelitis (ADEM)

- Prior viral illness, peripheral areas of ↑ T2 signal

Tumefactive Multiple Sclerosis (MS)

- Mass-like lesions in periventricular WM, perimeter enhancement

Human Immunodeficiency Virus (HIV)

- Atrophy, ill-defined areas of increased T2 signal in WM, increased attenuation of basal ganglia (NECT)

PATHOLOGY

General Features

- Etiology
  - Measles virus (mutant form), aberrant response to measles infection

Gross Pathologic & Surgical Features

- Swelling → cortical petechial hemorrhage → subcortical encephaloclastic lesions

Microscopic Features

- Widespread myelin loss, gliosis, macrophage infiltration, increased microglial (Hortega) cells
- Perivascular lymphocytic cuffing → diffuse neuronal loss, Alzheimer-type neurofibrillary tangles

CLINICAL ISSUES

Presentation

- Most common signs/symptoms
  - Progressive mental deterioration, motor impairment, myoclonus, emotional instability
- Clinical profile
  - Positive CSF, plasma complement fixation test for measles; CSF plus oligoclonal bands
  - EEG: Periodic complexes with generalized polyspike, high voltage slow waves

Demographics

- Age
  - Childhood, early adolescence; rare in adults
- Epidemiology
  - History of measles before age 2 in most patients → 16x risk of developing SSPE

Natural History & Prognosis

- Begins insidiously → subacute course → death (duration generally 1-6 months)

Treatment

- No treatment → some benefits from intraventricular interferon α and ribavirin

DIAGNOSTIC CHECKLIST

Consider

- SSPE in immigrant child with behavior changes and multifocal white matter disease

Image Interpretation Pearls

- MR findings correlate poorly with clinical stage

SELECTED REFERENCES

1. Aydin K et al: Reduced gray matter volume in the frontotemporal cortex of patients with early subacute sclerosing panencephalitis. AJNR Am J Neuroradiol. 30(2):271-5, 2009
2. Oguz KK et al: MR imaging, diffusion-weighted imaging and MR spectroscopy findings in acute rapidly progressive subacute sclerosing panencephalitis. Brain Dev. 29(5):306-11, 2007

TUBERCULOSIS

Key Facts

Terminology
- Typically causes tuberculous meningitis (TBM) &/or localized CNS infection, tuberculoma

Imaging
- Basilar meningitis + extracerebral TB (pulmonary)
- Meningitis + parenchymal lesions highly suggestive
- Tuberculomas
  - Supratentorial parenchyma most common
  - Usually T2 hypointense
  - Enhances strongly (solid or ring-enhancing)

Top Differential Diagnoses
- Meningitis
- Neurosarcoidosis
- Abscess
- Neoplasm

Pathology
- CNS TB almost always secondary (often pulmonary source)
- Meningitis = most frequent manifestation of CNS TB
  - More common in children

Clinical Issues
- Varies from mild meningitis with no neurologic deficit to coma
- Long-term morbidity up to 80%: Mental retardation, paralysis, seizures, rigidity, speech or visual deficits
- Mortality in 25-30% of patients; higher in AIDS patients
- Reemerging disease (immigration from endemic areas, AIDS, drug-resistant strains)

Diagnostic Checklist
- TB often mimics other diseases, such as neoplasm

*(**Left**) Coronal graphic shows basilar TB meningitis and tuberculomas ⇒, which often coexist. Note the vessel irregularity and early basal ganglia ischemia related to arteritis. (**Right**) Axial gross pathology section shows numerous features of CNS TB. Exudates with meningitis in the basilar cisterns ⇒, tuberculoma ⇒, and vasculitic changes ⇒ are all present in this autopsy specimen. (Courtesy R. Hewlett, PhD.)*

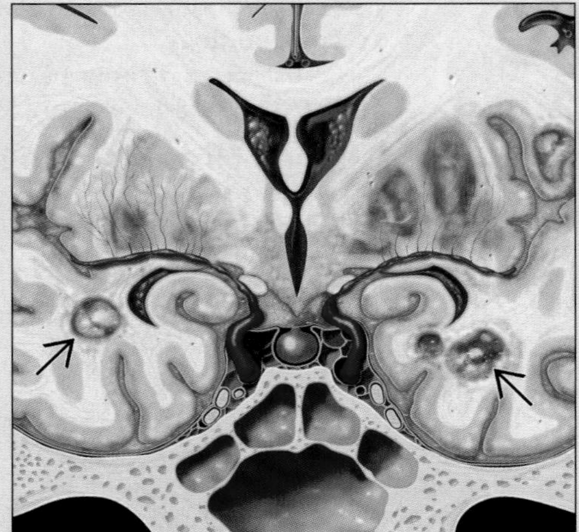

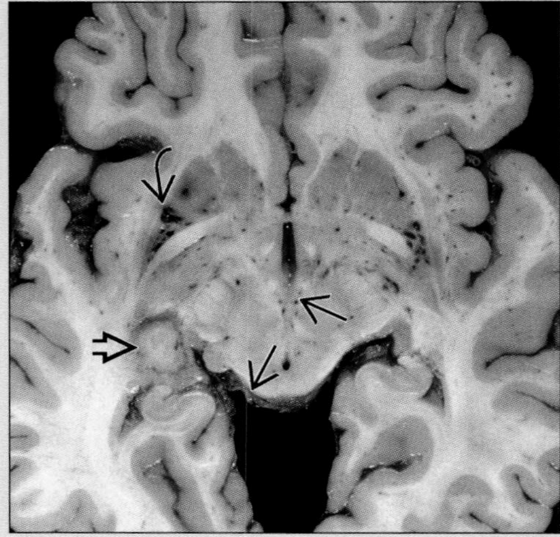

*(**Left**) Axial T1WI C+ MR in a child with documented tuberculous meningitis shows thick, linear enhancement along the midbrain and temporal lobes ⇒. Note the enlarged lateral ventricles and cerebral aqueduct. (**Right**) Axial T2WI MR in a patient with tuberculoma shows a large, mostly hypointense left parietal lesion ⇒ with edema affecting almost the entire hemisphere. Note the extension into the subcortical U-fibers with sparing of the overlying cortex.*

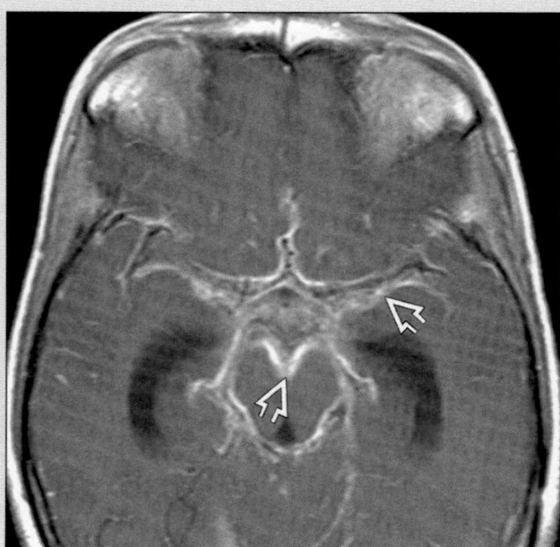

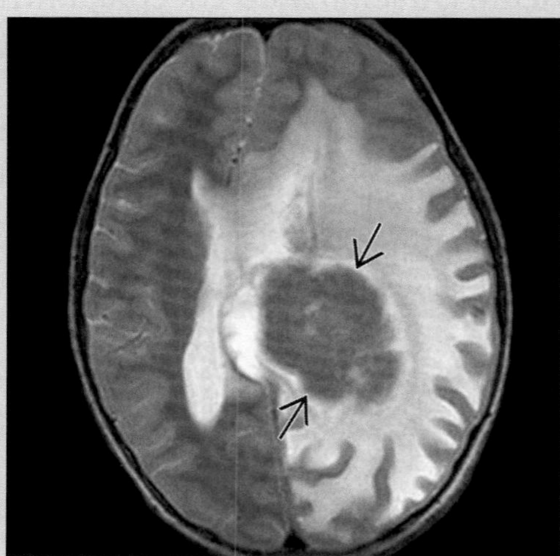

TERMINOLOGY

Definitions

- Infection by acid-fast bacillus *Mycobacterium tuberculosis* (TB)
- CNS TB almost always secondary to hematogenous spread (often pulmonary)
  - Manifestations include tuberculous meningitis (TBM)
  - Localized parenchymal infection (tuberculoma) (common); TB abscess (rare)

IMAGING

General Features

- Best diagnostic clue
  - Basilar meningitis + extracerebral TB (pulmonary)
  - Meningitis + parenchymal lesions highly suggestive
- Location
  - Meningitis (basal cisterns > superficial sulci)
  - Tuberculomas
    - Typically parenchymal
      - Supratentorial most common
      - Infratentorial lesions less common, rare brainstem involvement
    - Dural tuberculomas may occur
- Size
  - Tuberculomas range from 1 mm to 6 cm
- Morphology
  - TBM: Thick basilar exudate
  - Tuberculoma: Round or oval mass
    - Solitary or multiple (more common)
- Associated findings
  - Less common sites: Calvarium (± dura), otomastoid
  - TB cervical adenitis
    - Child/young adult with pulmonary disease, conglomerate nodal neck mass

CT Findings

- NECT
  - TBM: May be normal early (10-15%)
    - Isodense to hyperdense exudate effaces CSF spaces, fills basal cisterns, sulci
  - Tuberculoma
    - Hypodense to hyperdense round or lobulated nodule/mass with moderate to marked edema
    - Ca++ uncommon (approximately 20%)
- CECT
  - TBM: Intense basilar meningeal enhancement
  - Tuberculoma: Solid or ring-enhancing
    - "Target" sign: Central Ca++ or enhancement surrounded by enhancing rim
      - Not pathognomonic for TB

MR Findings

- T1WI
  - TBM: Exudate isointense or hyperintense to CSF
  - Tuberculoma
    - Noncaseating granuloma: Hypointense to brain
    - Caseating granuloma
      - Solid center: Hypointense or isointense
      - Necrotic center: Central hypointensity
      - May have hyperintense rim (paramagnetic material)
- T2WI
  - TBM: Exudate is isointense or hyperintense to CSF; may see low-signal nodules (rare)
  - Tuberculoma
    - Noncaseating granuloma: Hyperintense to brain
    - Caseating granuloma: Hypointense rim
      - Solid center: Usually hypointense
      - Necrotic center: Hyperintense
    - Surrounding edema common
- FLAIR
  - TBM: Increased intensity in basal cisterns, sulci
  - Tuberculoma: Similar to T2 characteristics
- DWI
  - May show hyperintense center of tuberculoma
  - Helpful for detecting complications (stroke, cerebritis)
- T1WI C+
  - TBM: Marked meningeal enhancement, basilar prominence; may be nodular
    - Punctate/linear basal ganglia enhancement = vasculitis
    - Rare: Ventriculitis, choroid plexitis
    - Rare: Pachymeningitis with dural thickening, enhancement (may mimic meningioma)
  - Tuberculomas
    - Noncaseating granuloma: Nodular, homogeneous enhancement
    - Caseating granuloma: Peripheral rim enhancement
      - Necrotic center will show low signal
- MRA
  - May see vessel narrowing, irregularity, occlusion
- MRS
  - TB abscess has prominent lipid, lactate but no amino acid resonances
    - Lipids at 0.9 ppm, 1.3 ppm, 2.0 ppm, 2.8 ppm
- Complications: Hydrocephalus, ischemia
- Chronic changes: Atrophy, Ca++, chronic ischemia

Angiographic Findings

- Narrowing of major arteries
  - Supraclinoid ICA, M1, A1
- Narrowing/occlusion of small &/or medium arteries

Imaging Recommendations

- Best imaging tool
  - MR with FLAIR, DWI, T1 C+, ± MRA, MRS

DIFFERENTIAL DIAGNOSIS

Meningitis

- Infectious meningitis (bacterial, fungal, viral, parasitic)
  - Coccidioidomycosis, cryptococcosis often basilar
- Carcinomatous meningitis (CNS or systemic primary) or lymphoma

Neurosarcoidosis

- Typically leptomeningeal &/or dural enhancement
- Rarely causes parenchymal nodules

TUBERCULOSIS

Abscess
- Other granuloma, parasite (neurocysticerosis), bacteria
- Pyogenic abscess often has more edema
- Classically T2 hypointense rim and DWI(+)

Neoplasm
- Primary or metastatic tumors may be indistinguishable
- Thick, nodular enhancing wall and DWI(-) are typical
- Typically more indolent onset, history may help

PATHOLOGY

General Features
- Etiology
  - CNS TB almost always secondary to hematogenous spread (often pulmonary; rarely GI or GU tract)
    - Hyperemia, inflammation extend to meninges
    - May involve perivascular spaces, cause vasculitis
  - TBM pathophysiology
    - Penetration of meningeal vessel walls by hematogenous spread
    - Rupture of subependymal or subpial granulomata into CSF
  - Tuberculoma pathophysiology
    - Hematogenous spread (gray-white matter junction lesions)
    - Extension of meningitis into parenchyma via cortical veins or small penetrating arteries
  - Arteries directly involved by basilar exudate or indirectly by reactive arteritis (up to 40% of patients)
    - Infection causes arterial spasm resulting in thrombosis and infarct
    - Lenticulostriate arteries, MCA, thalamoperforators most often affected
    - Infarcts most common in basal ganglia, cerebral cortex, pons, cerebellum
    - Arteritis: More common in children, HIV(+)

Gross Pathologic & Surgical Features
- TBM: Thick, gelatinous, cisternal exudate
- Tuberculoma: Noncaseating, caseating with solid center, or caseating with necrotic center
  - Rarely progresses to TB abscess
    - Lobulated mass with thick rim, occurs in parenchyma, subarachnoid space, dura

Microscopic Features
- TBM: Inflammatory cells, fragile neocapillaries
  - Caseous necrosis, chronic granulomas, endarteritis, perivascular inflammatory changes
- Tuberculoma
  - Early capsule: Peripheral fibroblasts, epithelioid cells, Langerhans giant cells, lymphocytes
  - Late capsule: Thick collagen layer, central liquefied caseating material in mature tuberculoma

CLINICAL ISSUES

Presentation
- Most common signs/symptoms
  - Varies from mild meningitis with no neurologic deficit to coma
  - TBM: Fevers, confusion, headache, lethargy, meningismus
  - Tuberculoma: Seizures, increased intracranial pressure, papilledema
- Clinical profile
  - LP: Increased protein, pleocytosis (lymphocytes), low glucose, negative for organisms
    - CSF positive on initial LP in < 40%
    - *Mycobacteria* grow slowly, culture 4-8 weeks
    - PCR for TB may help confirm diagnosis earlier
  - TB skin test may be negative, particularly early
  - Elevated erythrocyte sedimentation rate common

Demographics
- Age
  - Occurs at all ages, more often in 1st 3 decades
- Gender
  - No gender predilection
- Epidemiology
  - Worldwide: 8,000,000-10,000,000 cases annually
  - Reemerging disease (immigration from endemic areas, AIDS, drug-resistant strains)

Natural History & Prognosis
- Long-term morbidity up to 80%: Mental retardation, paralysis, seizures, rigidity, speech or visual deficits
- Mortality in 25-30% of patients; higher in AIDS patients
- Complications: Hydrocephalus (70%), stroke (up to 40%), cranial neuropathies (3, 4, 6 common), syrinx
- Tuberculomas may take months to years to resolve
  - Size of lesion determines healing time

Treatment
- Untreated TBM can be fatal in 4-8 weeks
- Multidrug therapy required: Isoniazid, rifampin, pyrazinamide, ± ethambutol or streptomycin
- Despite therapy, lesions may develop or increase
- Hydrocephalus typically requires CSF diversion

DIAGNOSTIC CHECKLIST

Consider
- TB often mimics other diseases, such as neoplasm

Image Interpretation Pearls
- Combination of meningitis and parenchymal lesions suggests TB

SELECTED REFERENCES

1. Be NA et al: Pathogenesis of central nervous system tuberculosis. Curr Mol Med. 9(2):94-9, 2009
2. van Well GT et al: Twenty years of pediatric tuberculous meningitis: a retrospective cohort study in the western cape of South Africa. Pediatrics. 123(1):e1-8, 2009

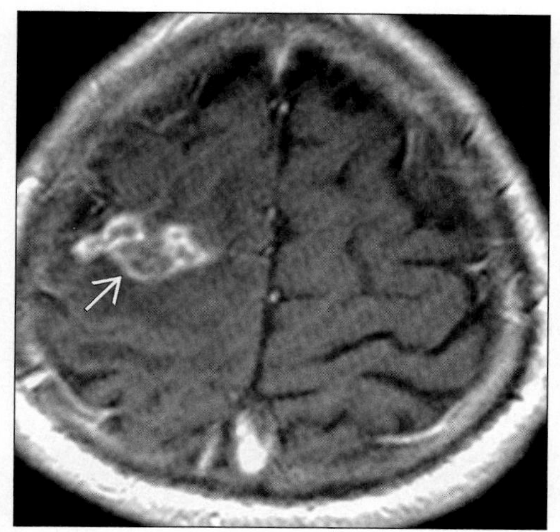

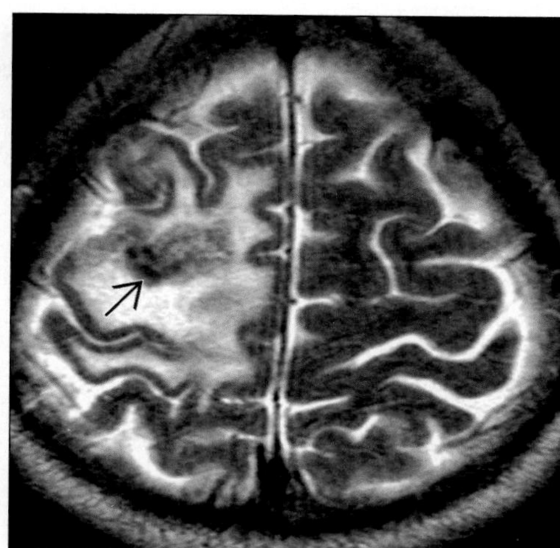

***(Left)** Axial T1WI C+ MR demonstrates a cluster of ring-enhancing granulomas → in the right frontal lobe. **(Right)** Axial T2WI MR in the same patient reveals low signal intensity related to the granulomas → as well as surrounding vasogenic edema.*

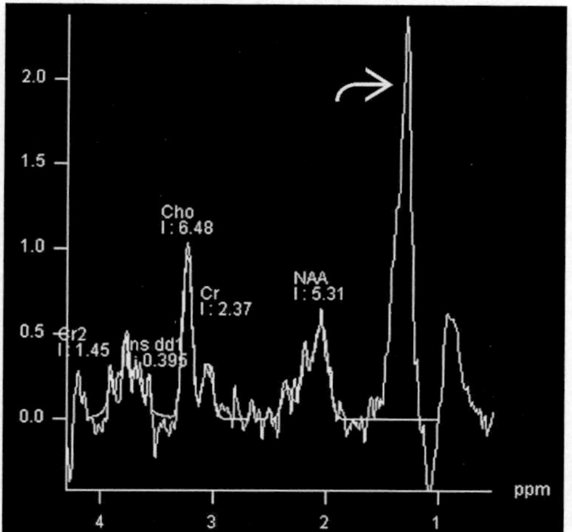

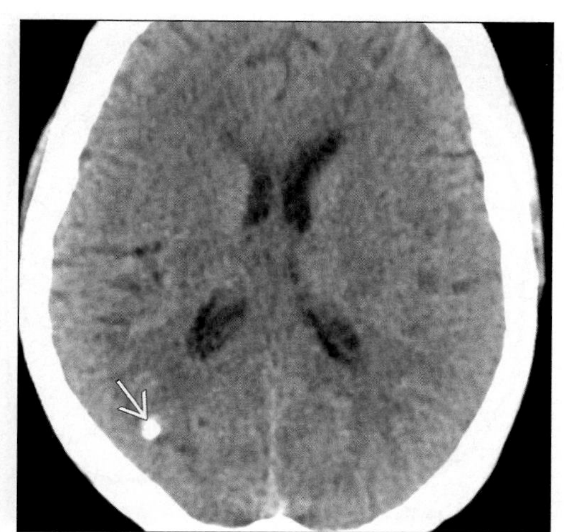

***(Left)** MRS (PRESS, intermediate echo) in the same patient shows dimunition in NAA and a large lipid peak →, a common finding in tuberculosis. **(Right)** Axial NECT shows a calcified, healed tuberculous granuloma →.*

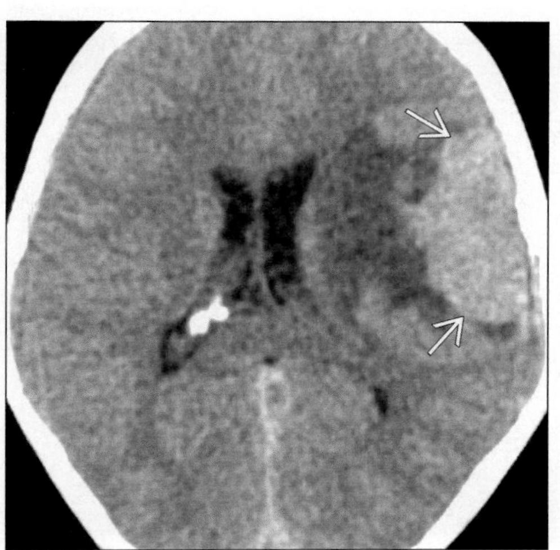

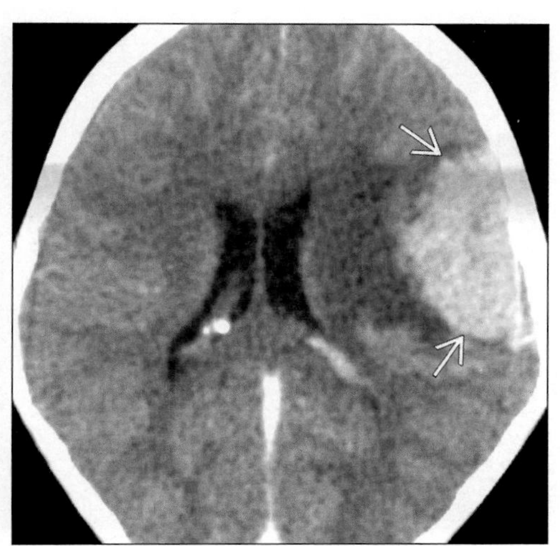

***(Left)** Axial NECT shows a predominantly hyperdense dural-based mass →. (Courtesy R. Ramakantan, MD.) **(Right)** Axial CECT in the same patient demonstrates the moderately strong enhancement of this lesion →. This extraaxial mass looks like a meningioma. Dural tuberculoma was found at surgery. (Courtesy R. Ramakantan, MD.)*

NEUROCYSTICERCOSIS

Key Facts

Terminology

- Intracranial parasitic infection caused by the pork tapeworm *Taenia solium*
  - 4 pathologic stages: Vesicular, colloidal vesicular, granular nodular, and nodular calcified

Imaging

- Best diagnostic clue: Cyst with "dot" inside
- Convexity subarachnoid spaces most common location
  - Inflammatory response around cyst may seal sulcus, making lesions appear intraaxial
- May involve cisterns > parenchyma > ventricles
- Intraventricular cysts are often isolated
- Basal cistern cysts may be racemose (grape-like)
- Imaging varies with development stage and host response
- Lesions may be at different stages in same patient
- FLAIR and T1 MR helpful to identify scolex and intraventricular lesions

Top Differential Diagnoses

- Abscess
- Tuberculosis
- Neoplasm
- Arachnoid cyst

Clinical Issues

- Seizure, headaches, hydrocephalus common
  - NCC asymptomatic until larvae degenerate
- Cysticercosis is most common parasitic infection worldwide
  - CNS involved in 60-90% of cysticercosis cases
- Most common cause of epilepsy in endemic areas
- Increased travel, immigration have spread disease
- Diagnosis confirmed by ELISA of serum or CSF

__(Left)__ Coronal graphic shows subarachnoid and ventricular cysts. The convexity cysts have a scolex and surrounding inflammation. Note that the inflammation around the largest cyst "seals" the sulcus ➔ and makes it appear parenchymal. Racemose cysts ⇨ are seen in the basal cisterns. These multilocular cysts are nonviable and typically lack a scolex. __(Right)__ Axial FLAIR MR shows a right frontal "mass" in a young adult with new focal seizures. The NCC cyst follows CSF signal ➔. Note the surrounding edema.

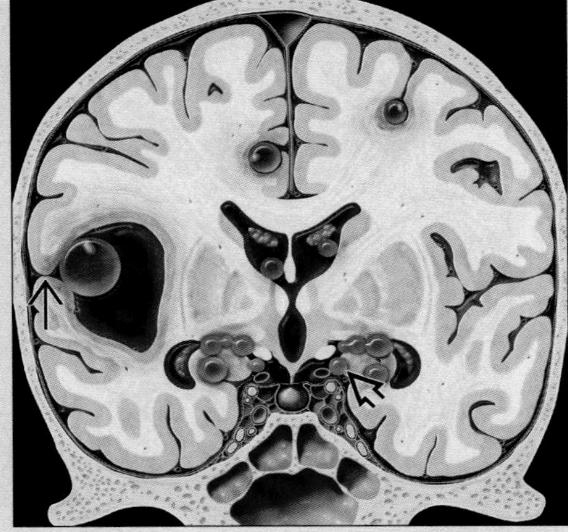

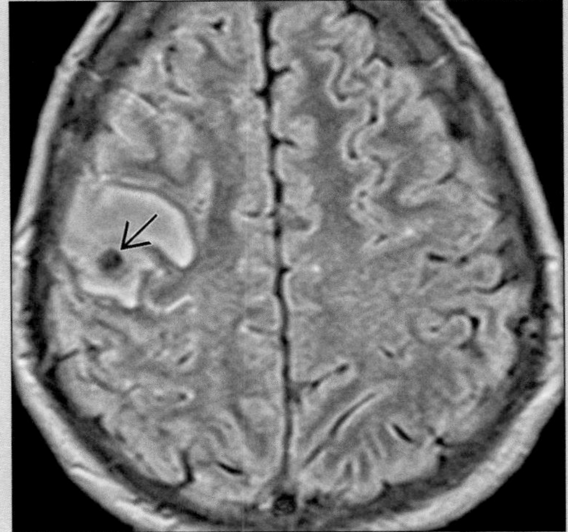

__(Left)__ Axial T1WI C+ MR in the same patient shows peripheral enhancement of the cyst wall ⇨ with a central "dot" representing the scolex. The surrounding inflammation has caused the overlying sulcus to seal, making the lesion appear intraaxial. Occasionally, linear enhancement may be seen extending from the lesion, representing inflammation along the pial surface of the sulcus. __(Right)__ Coronal T1WI C+ MR in the same patient shows peripheral enhancement of the NCC cyst (colloidal vesicular stage).

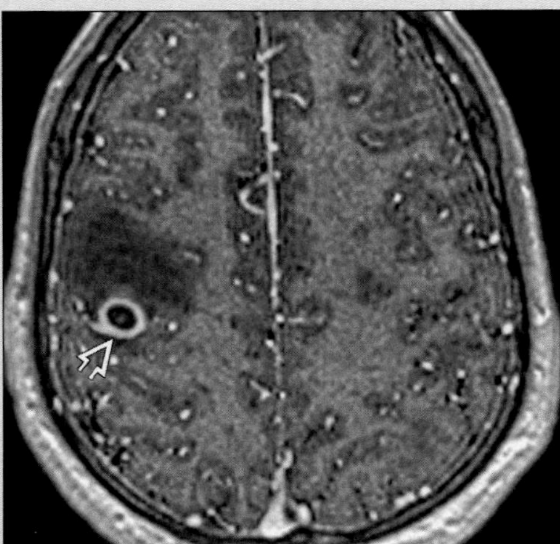

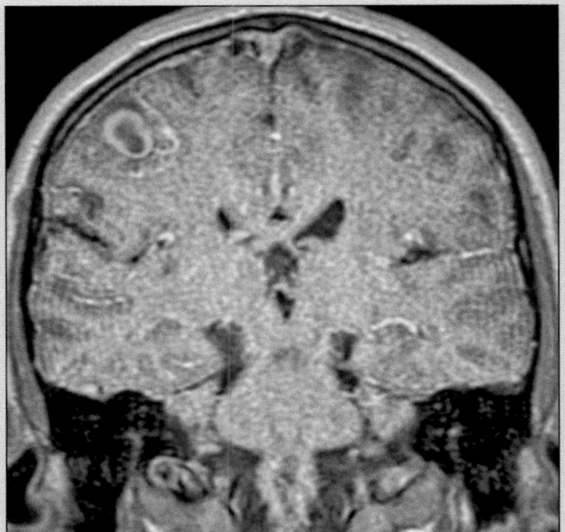

NEUROCYSTICERCOSIS

TERMINOLOGY

Abbreviations

- Neurocysticercosis (NCC)

Synonyms

- Cysticercosis

Definitions

- Intracranial parasitic infection caused by pork tapeworm *Taenia solium*
  - 4 pathologic stages: Vesicular, colloidal vesicular, granular nodular, and nodular calcified

IMAGING

General Features

- Best diagnostic clue
  - Cyst with "dot" inside
- Location
  - Convexity subarachnoid spaces most common
  - May involve cisterns > parenchyma > ventricles
  - Parenchymal cysts often hemispheric, at gray-white junction
  - Intraventricular cysts are often isolated
    - 4th ventricle is most common
  - Basal cistern cysts may be racemose (grape-like)
  - Rare CNS locations: Sella, orbit, spinal cord
- Size
  - Cysts variable, typically 1 cm, range from 5-20 mm; contain scolex (1-4 mm)
  - Parenchymal cysts ≤ 1 cm
  - Subarachnoid cysts may be larger; up to 9 cm reported
- Morphology
  - Round or ovoid cyst, solitary in 20-50%
  - When multiple, usually small number of cysts
  - Disseminated form (a.k.a. miliary NCC): Rare
- Imaging varies with development stage and host response
- Lesions may be at different stages in same patient
- Inflammatory response around cyst may seal sulcus, making lesions appear intraaxial

CT Findings

- NECT
  - **Vesicular** stage (viable larva): Smooth, thin-walled cyst, isodense to CSF, no edema
    - Hyperdense "dot" within cyst = protoscolex
  - **Colloidal vesicular** stage (degenerating larva): Hyperdense cyst fluid with surrounding edema
  - **Granular nodular** stage (healing): Mild edema
  - **Nodular calcified** stage (healed): Small, calcified nodule
- CECT
  - **Vesicular** stage: No (or mild) wall enhancement
  - **Colloidal vesicular** stage: Thicker ring-enhancing fibrous capsule
  - **Granular nodular** stage: Involuting, enhancing nodule
  - **Nodular calcified** stage: Shrunken, Ca++ nodule
- Subarachnoid lesions: Multiple isodense cysts without scolex; may cause meningitis, vasculitis, or hydrocephalus
- Intraventricular cysts not well seen on CT, may see hydrocephalus

MR Findings

- T1WI
  - **Vesicular** stage: Cystic lesion isointense to CSF
    - May see discrete, eccentric scolex (hyperintense)
  - **Colloidal vesicular** stage: Cyst is mildly hyperintense to CSF
  - **Granular nodular** stage: Thickened, retracted cyst wall; edema decreases
  - **Nodular calcified** stage: Shrunken, Ca++ lesion
  - Useful to detect intraventricular cysts
- T2WI
  - **Vesicular** stage: Cystic lesion isointense to CSF
    - May see discrete, eccentric scolex
    - No surrounding edema
  - **Colloidal vesicular** stage: Cyst is hyperintense
    - Surrounding edema, mild to marked
  - **Granular nodular** stage: Thickened, retracted cyst wall; edema decreases
  - **Nodular calcified** stage: Shrunken, Ca++ lesion
- FLAIR
  - **Vesicular** stage: Cystic lesion isointense to CSF
    - May see discrete, eccentric scolex (hyperintense to CSF); no edema
  - **Colloidal vesicular** stage: Cyst is hyperintense
    - Surrounding edema, mild to marked
  - Useful to detect intraventricular cysts (hyperintense)
  - 100% inspired oxygen increases conspicuity
- T2* GRE
  - Useful to demonstrate calcified scolex
  - May show "multiple black dot" appearance
- T1WI C+
  - **Vesicular** stage: No enhancement typical, may see mild enhancement
    - May see discrete, eccentric scolex enhancement
  - **Colloidal vesicular** stage: Thick cyst wall enhances
    - Enhancing marginal nodule (scolex)
  - **Granular nodular** stage: Thickened, retracted cyst wall; may have nodular or ring-like enhancement
  - **Nodular calcified** stage: Small calcified lesion, rare minimal enhancement
- MRS: Few reports show ↑ lactate, alanine, succinate, choline; ↓ NAA and Cr
- DWI: Cystic lesion typically isointense to CSF
- In children, may see "encephalitic cysticercosis" with multiple small enhancing lesions and diffuse edema
- Intraventricular cysts may cause ventriculitis &/or hydrocephalus
- **Cisternal** NCC may appear **racemose** (multilobulated, grape-like), typically lacks scolex

Imaging Recommendations

- Best imaging tool
  - MR is most sensitive
  - Calcified lesions may be better seen on CT
- Protocol advice
  - MR with T1, T2, FLAIR, GRE, contrast

NEUROCYSTICERCOSIS

DIFFERENTIAL DIAGNOSIS

Abscess
- Typically T2 hypointense rim and DWI positive
- Multiple lesions may occur related to septic emboli

Tuberculosis
- Tuberculomas often occur with meningitis
- Typically not cystic

Neoplasm
- Primary or metastatic (primary often known)
- Thick, irregular margin enhancement typical
- May have cyst and mural nodule (e.g., pilocytic astrocytoma, hemangioblastoma)

Arachnoid Cyst
- Solitary lesion with CSF density/intensity
- No enhancement

Enlarged Perivascular Spaces
- Follow CSF on all MR sequences
- No enhancement

Other Parasitic Infection
- May be cystic, but no scolex seen

PATHOLOGY

General Features
- Etiology
  - Caused by larval form of pork tapeworm *Taenia solium*
  - Man is intermediate host in life cycle of tapeworm
    - Fecal-oral most common route of infection
    - Ingestion of eggs from contaminated water, food
    - From GI tract, primary larvae (oncospheres) disseminate into CNS and skeletal muscle
    - Once intracranial, primary develop into secondary larvae, cysticerci
  - Man may also be definitive host (infected with tapeworm)
    - Typically from uncooked pork
    - Viable larvae ingested, attach in GI tract

Staging, Grading, & Classification
- 4 pathologic stages
  - Vesicular, colloidal vesicular, granular nodular, and nodular calcified
- **Vesicular** stage: Larva is small marginal nodule projecting into small cyst with clear fluid
  - Viable parasite with little or no inflammation
  - May remain in this stage for years or degenerate
- **Colloidal vesicular** stage: Larva begins to degenerate
  - Scolex shows hyaline degeneration, slowly shrinks
  - Cyst fluid becomes turbid, and capsule thickens
  - Surrounding edema and inflammation
- **Granular nodular** stage: Cyst wall thickens and scolex is mineralized granule; surrounding edema regresses
- **Nodular calcified** stage: Lesion is completely mineralized and small; no edema

Gross Pathologic & Surgical Features
- Usually small translucent cyst with invaginated scolex

Microscopic Features
- Cyst wall has 3 distinct layers: Outer (cuticular) layer, middle cellular (pseudoepithelial) layer, inner reticular (fibrillary) layer
- Scolex has rostellum with hooklets, muscular suckers

CLINICAL ISSUES

Presentation
- Most common signs/symptoms
  - Seizure, headaches, hydrocephalus
  - Varies with organism development stage, host immune response
  - NCC asymptomatic until larvae degenerate
  - Other signs/symptoms: Syncope, dementia, visual changes, focal neurologic deficits, stroke
- Clinical profile
  - Diagnosis confirmed by ELISA of serum or CSF

Demographics
- Epidemiology
  - Cysticercosis is most common parasitic infection
  - CNS infection in 60-90% of cysticercosis cases
  - Endemic in many countries (Latin America, parts of Asia, India, Africa, eastern Europe)
    - USA: Incidence rising in CA, AZ, NM, TX
  - Increased travel, immigration have spread disease
- Age: Any age; commonly young, middle-aged adults
- Ethnicity: In USA, Latin American patients common

Natural History & Prognosis
- Most common cause of epilepsy in endemic areas
- Variable time from initial infection until symptoms: 6 months to 30 years; typically 2-5 years
- Variable time to progress through pathologic stages: 1-9 years; mean 5 years
- Subarachnoid disease may be complicated by meningitis, vasculitis, and hydrocephalus
- Intraventricular NCC has increased morbidity and mortality (↑ morbidity related to acute hydrocephalus)

Treatment
- Oral albendazole (reduces parasitic burden, seizures)
  - Steroids often required to decrease edema
- Consider excision or drainage of parenchymal lesions
- Consider endoscopic resection of ventricular lesions
- CSF diversion often required to treat hydrocephalus

DIAGNOSTIC CHECKLIST

Consider
- Complex parasitic cysts may mimic brain tumor

Image Interpretation Pearls
- FLAIR and T1WI helpful to identify scolex and intraventricular lesions
- GRE helpful in young adults presenting with seizures

SELECTED REFERENCES

1. Sinha S et al: Neurocysticercosis: a review of current status and management. J Clin Neurosci. 16(7):867-76, 2009

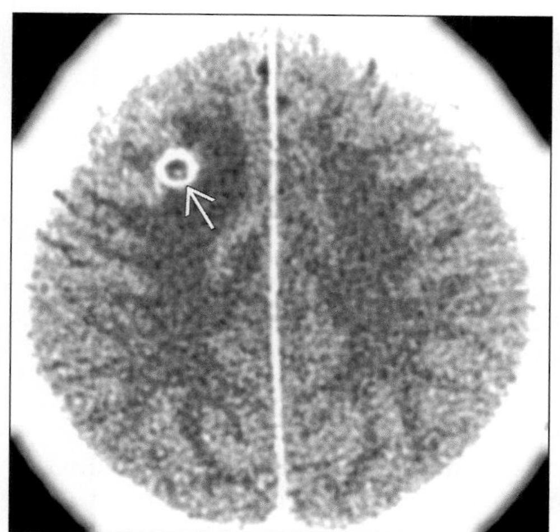

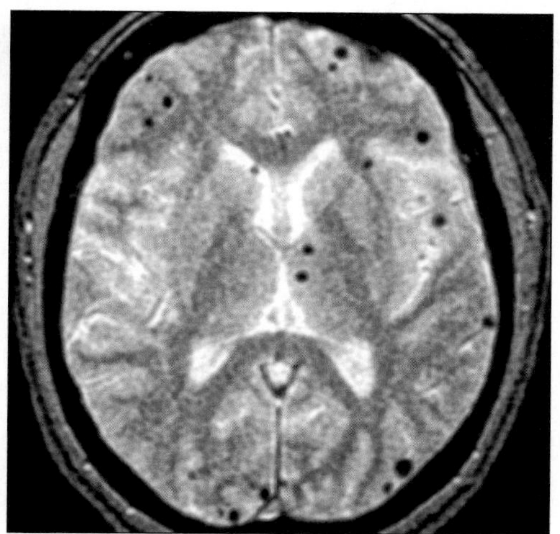

*(**Left**) Axial CECT shows a ring-enhancing frontal lobe lesion with a central "dot" ➔ and surrounding edema in this patient with colloidal vesicular NCC. CT often shows calcified lesions to better advantage than MR. (**Right**) Axial T2* GRE MR in this seizure patient shows multifocal "black dots" in the sulci, parenchyma, and right frontal horn related to the nodular calcified stage of NCC. It is important to remember that different lesions may be at different stages in the same patient.*

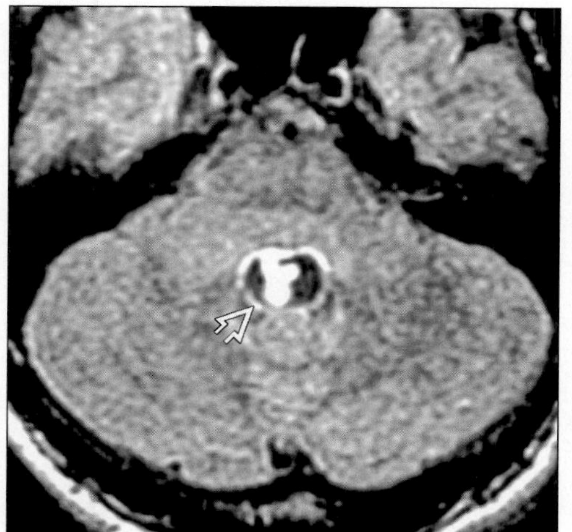

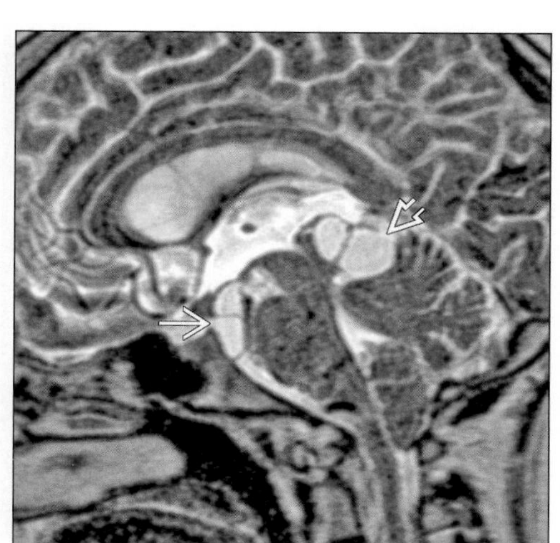

*(**Left**) Axial FLAIR MR shows a 4th ventricular lesion ➔ related to NCC (colloidal vesicular stage). Note the eccentric scolex. FLAIR and T1 are the best MR sequences to identify intraventricular lesions, which are often complicated by acute hydrocephalus. (**Right**) Sagittal STIR MR shows multiple hyperintense cysts in the quadrigeminal cistern ➔ and basal subarachnoid spaces ➔ related to racemose NCC. Note the typical lack of a scolex. (Courtesy E. Bravo, MD.)*

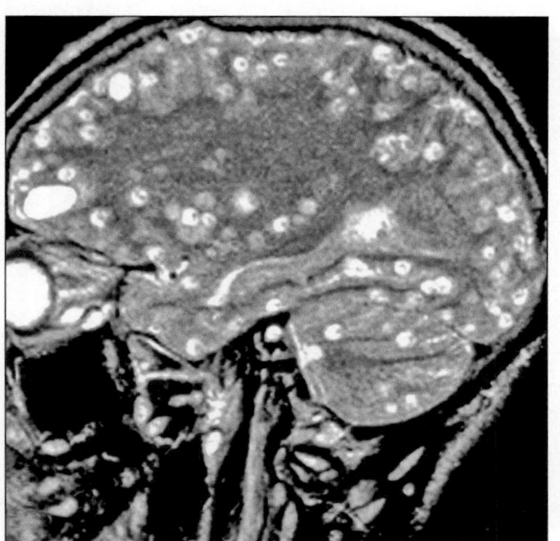

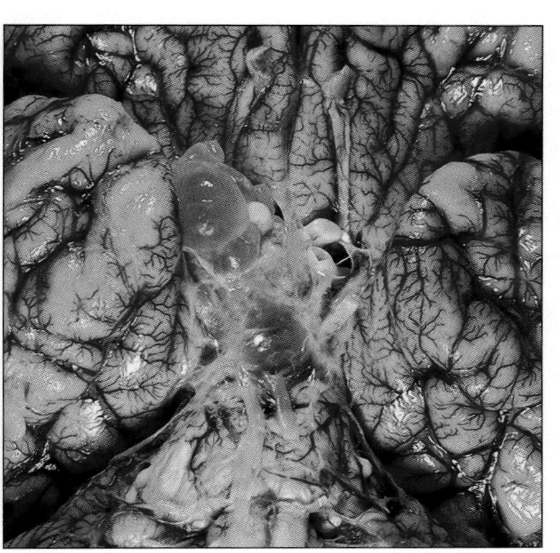

*(**Left**) Sagittal T2WI MR shows a rare case of disseminated or miliary NCC. Note the innumerable cysts, each with a hypointense central "dot" representing the scolex. Note the lack of edema, typical of the vesicular stage. Disseminated NCC is generally only seen in patients from endemic areas. (**Right**) Inferior view of the brain at autopsy shows multiple racemose NCC cysts. Basal cistern cysts are commonly complicated by meningitis, hydrocephalus, and vasculitis. (Courtesy R. Hewlett, PhD.)*

HYDATID DISEASE

Key Facts

Terminology
- Hydatid disease (HD), hydatid cyst (HC)
- *Echinococcus granulosus* (EG)
- *Echinococcus multilocularis/alveolaris* (EM/EA)

Imaging
- General: Child/young adult with large supratentorial unilocular thin-walled cyst
  - No Ca++ or surrounding edema
  - CSF density/intensity
- MR
  - EG: Well-defined T2 hypointense rim, no enhancement
  - EM/EA: Small irregular cysts with nodular/ring enhancement, edema
  - Lactate, alanine, acetate, pyruvate (at 2.4 ppm)

Top Differential Diagnoses
- Arachnoid cyst
- Epidermoid cyst
- Neuroglial cyst
- Porencephalic cyst

Pathology
- Parasitic infection by *Echinococcus* tapeworms
  - Definitive host = dog (or other carnivore)
  - Intermediate host = sheep (most commonly)
  - Humans may become intermediate hosts
- CNS involvement: 1-2% in EG, 3-5% EM/EA
- HC has 3 layers: Outer pericyst, middle laminated membrane, inner germinal layer

Clinical Issues
- Treatment: Surgical removal (caution: HC germinal tissue, protoscolices are viable, transplantable)

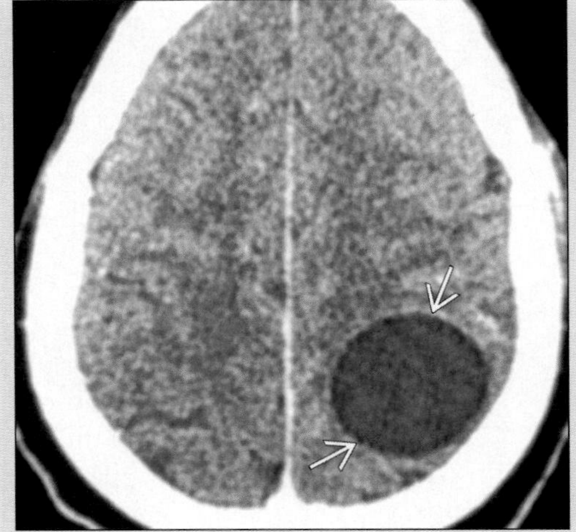

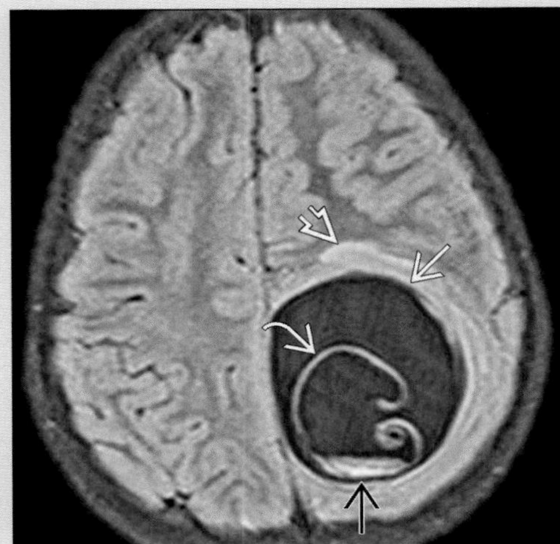

(Left) *Axial CECT shows a nonenhancing unilocular fluid-containing cyst in the left parietal lobe ➡. Note the complete lack of edema surrounding the lesion. Surgery disclosed typical Echinococcus cyst (hydatid disease). (Courtesy S. Nagi, MD.)* ***(Right)*** *Axial FLAIR MR demonstrates a large left parietal hydatid cyst ➡ with an internal membrane representing the detached germinal membrane ↪ and dependent hyperintense "hydatid sand" ⇨. There is very mild surrounding pericystic edema ⇨.*

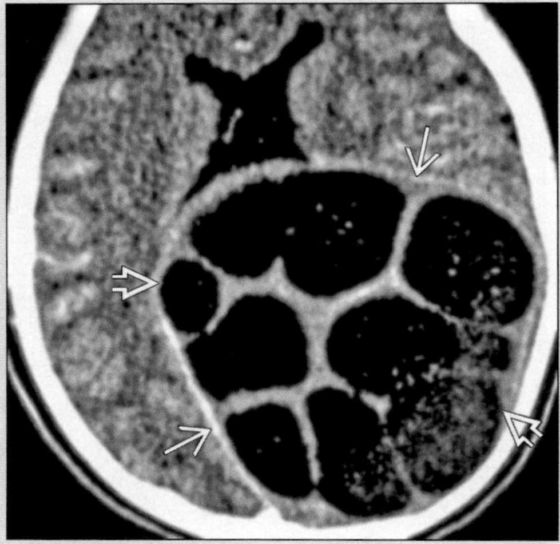

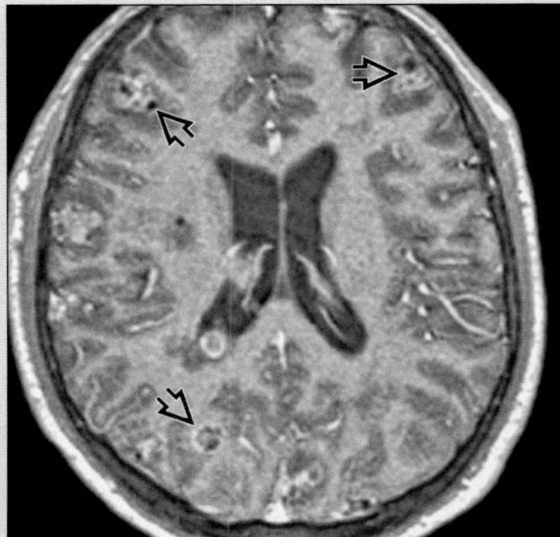

(Left) *Axial CECT shows a variant manifestation of hydatid disease. Multiple "daughter" cysts ⇨ are present within a very large unilocular cyst ➡. (Courtesy S. Nagi, MD.)* ***(Right)*** *Axial T1WI C+ MR demonstrates clusters of small cysts with peripheral ring enhancement ⇨. Alveolar echinococcosis (AE) with CNS involvement was finally diagnosed. AE is composed of numerous irregular cysts (between 1 and 20 mm in diameter), not sharply demarcated. Necrosis with liquefaction causes the cystic central areas.*

HYDATID DISEASE

TERMINOLOGY

Abbreviations

- Hydatid disease (HD), hydatid cyst (HC)
- *Echinococcus granulosus* (EG)
- *Echinococcus multilocularis/alveolaris* (EM/EA)

Synonyms

- Echinococcosis, hydatid cyst

IMAGING

General Features

- Best diagnostic clue
  - Large unilocular thin-walled cyst
    - No Ca++ or surrounding edema
    - CSF density/intensity
- Location
  - Majority of HCs occur in liver, lungs
  - CNS involvement: 1-2% of EG, 3-5% of EM/EA
    - Most commonly supratentorial (MCA territory)
      - Parietal lobe most frequently involved
- Size
  - EG: Large cysts
  - EM/EA: Smaller, partially solid/cystic (1-20 mm)
- Morphology
  - EG: Generally solitary; may be multiple if ruptures present
  - Multivesicular cysts uncommon in brain

CT Findings

- NECT
  - EG: Unilocular cyst isodense to CSF
    - Ca++ < 1% (more common with EM/EA)
- CECT
  - Normally no enhancement

MR Findings

- T1WI
  - EG: Unilocular cyst, isointense to CSF
- T2WI
  - EG: Cyst with well-defined hypointense rim
  - EM/EA: Small irregular cysts with edema
- T1WI C+
  - EG: None (rim only if superinfected)
  - EM/EA: Nodular/ring-like enhancement
- MRS
  - Lactate, alanine, acetate, pyruvate (at 2.4 ppm)

DIFFERENTIAL DIAGNOSIS

Arachnoid Cyst

- Extraaxial cysts follow CSF signal/attenuation

Epidermoid Cyst

- Does not suppress on FLAIR, ↑ DWI

Neuroglial Cyst

- Difficult to differentiate (travel history helps for EG)

Porencephalic Cyst

- Cystic space with adjacent enlarged ventricle

PATHOLOGY

General Features

- Etiology
  - Parasitic infection by *Echinococcus* tapeworm
    - Usually caused by EG, less frequently EM/EA
  - Life cycle
    - Definitive host = dog (or other carnivore)
    - Intermediate host = sheep (most commonly)
  - Humans may become intermediate hosts via
    - Contact with definitive host
    - Ingestion of contaminated water/vegetables

Gross Pathologic & Surgical Features

- Vesicles resemble "bunch of grapes"

Microscopic Features

- HC has 3 layers
  - Outer pericyst: Modified host cells form dense, fibrous protective zone
  - Middle laminated membrane: A-cellular (allows passage of nutrients)
  - Inner germinal layer: Scolices (larval stage of parasite), laminated membrane are produced

CLINICAL ISSUES

Presentation

- Most common signs/symptoms
  - Headache, nausea, vomiting, papilledema (↑ ICP)

Demographics

- Age
  - Usually child, young adult
- Epidemiology
  - EG: Endemic in Australia, New Zealand, Middle East, Mediterranean, South America
  - EM/EA: Endemic in North America, central Europe, Russia, China, Turkey

Natural History & Prognosis

- Rupture, infection: Important complications of HC

Treatment

- Surgical excision = treatment of choice
  - Caution: HC germinal tissue, protoscolices are viable, transplantable
- Antihelmintic therapy (praziquantel, albendazole)

DIAGNOSTIC CHECKLIST

Consider

- HC if large unilocular noncalcified parietal cyst without edema, enhancement
  - Residence in or travel to endemic regions

SELECTED REFERENCES

1. Izci Y et al: Cerebral hydatid cysts: technique and pitfalls of surgical management. Neurosurg Focus. 24(6):E15, 2008

AMEBIC DISEASE

Key Facts

Terminology
- Parasitic infection caused by free-living amebae
  - *Entamoeba histolytica* (EH), *Naegleria fowleri* (NF), *Acanthamoeba* (Ac)
  - Primary amebic meningoencephalitis (PAM)
  - Granulomatous amebic encephalitis (GAE)

Imaging
- EH: Ring-enhancing lesion(s)
- NF: (PAM) enhancing leptomeninges, cisterns (most prominent around olfactory bulbs)
- Ac: (GAE) ring-enhancing lesions, gyriform enhancement

Top Differential Diagnoses
- Pyogenic abscess
- Other encephalitides

Pathology
- *E. histolytica*, *N. fowleri*, *Acanthamoeba* frequent
  - *N. fowleri* causes PAM
  - *Acanthamoeba* causes GAE

Clinical Issues
- Endemic to southern USA, South America, Latin America, Southeast Asia, Africa
  - GAE: Patients often debilitated, immunocompromised
  - Ac: Insidious (headache, low-grade fever, seizures)
- Symptoms: Headache, nausea, vomiting, lethargy, seizures

Diagnostic Checklist
- "Odd-looking" lesion(s); can mimic neoplasm
- Consider amebic infection in setting of meningoencephalitis with travel to endemic areas

(Left) Axial FLAIR MR shows a mixed hypo-/hyperintense right posterior frontal mass ➡. Smaller lesions are also seen in the parietooccipital regions ➡. (Right) Axial T2 GRE MR in the same patient shows "blooming "artifact ➡ due to hemorrhage. Some enhancement was present on T1 C+ study (not shown). Initial diagnosis proved possible metastases from unknown primary. The frontal lobe mass was biopsied, and amebic infestation was identified. The patient had recently traveled to Africa.*

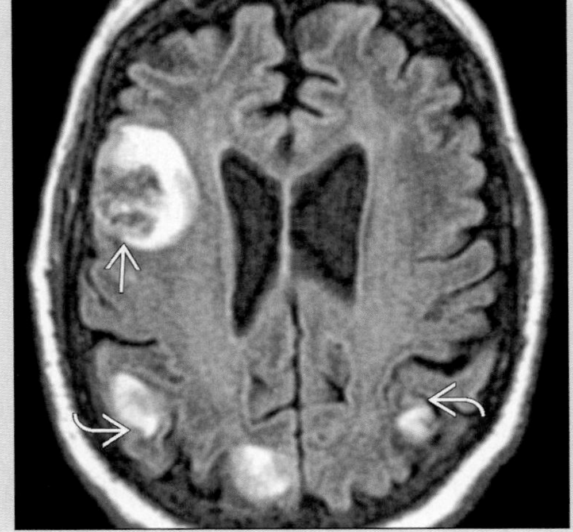

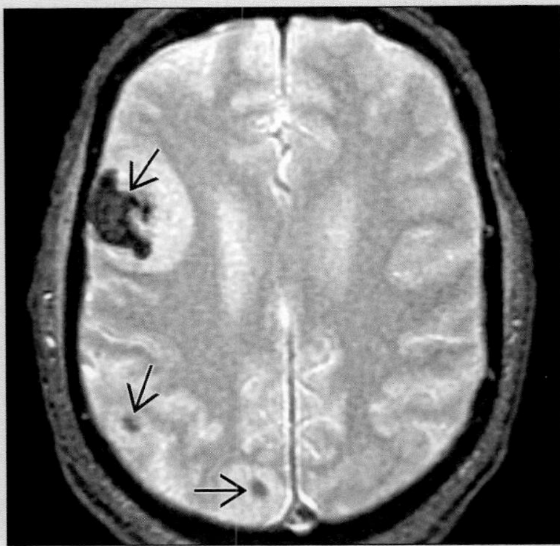

(Left) Axial T1WI C+ MR shows inhomogeneous ring-like enhancement in a right thalamic mass ➡. Note the leptomeningeal enhancement, consistent with meningoencephalitis ➡. (Right) Hematoxylin & eosin micropathology obtained from biopsy in this case shows an ameba ➡ surrounded by inflammatory cells ➡. Note the complex nucleolus with an eosinophilic rim, pyknotic core. This proves necrotizing amebic meningoencephalitis is caused by free-living forms of Acanthamoeba. (Courtesy R. Hewlett, PhD.)

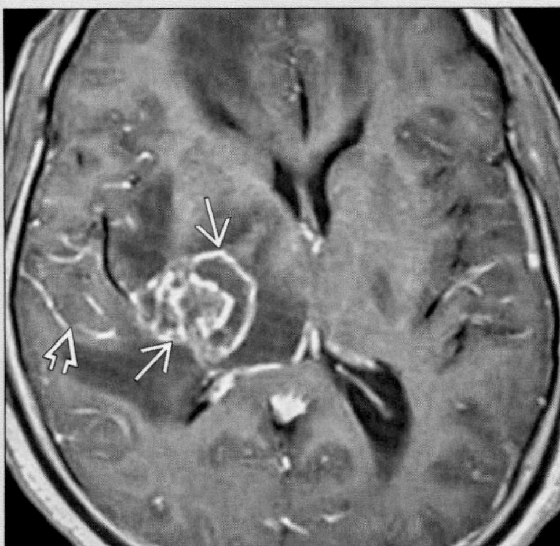

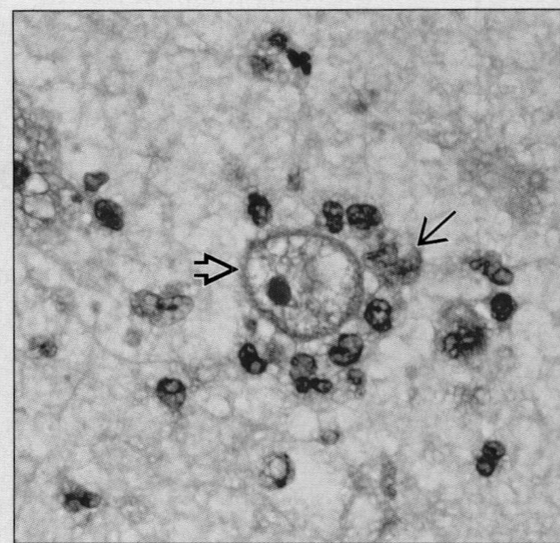

AMEBIC DISEASE

TERMINOLOGY

Abbreviations

- *Entamoeba histolytica* (EH), *Naegleria fowleri* (NF), *Acanthamoeba* (Ac)
- Primary amebic meningoencephalitis (PAM)
- Granulomatous amebic encephalitis (GAE)

Synonyms

- Central nervous system amebiasis

Definitions

- Parasitic infection caused by free-living amebic organisms

IMAGING

General Features

- Best diagnostic clue
  - Meningoencephalitis, ring-enhancing lesion(s) in patients who traveled to endemic areas
- Location
  - EH: Meninges, cortical/deep gray matter
  - NF: (PAM) meninges in region of olfactory bulb, frontal/temporal lobes
  - Ac: (GAE) meninges, brain parenchyma

CT Findings

- NECT
  - Hypodense lesion(s) with surrounding edema
    - Cortical, deep gray matter
- CECT
  - Single/multiple ring-enhancing lesions
  - Gyriform, leptomeningeal enhancement (PAM)

MR Findings

- T1WI
  - Hypointense edema, focal lesions
- T2WI
  - EH: Hyperintense lesions with edema
  - PAM: Ill-defined areas of ↑ T2 signal, mass effect
- FLAIR
  - Meningitis may cause ↑ signal in CSF
- T2* GRE
  - Lesions may show ↓ signal due to hemorrhage
- T1WI C+
  - EH: Ring-enhancing lesion(s)
  - NF: (PAM) enhancing leptomeninges, cisterns (most prominent around olfactory bulbs)
  - Ac: (GAE) Ring, gyriform enhancement

Imaging Recommendations

- Best imaging tool
  - Multiplanar MR with T2, FLAIR, DWI, T1 C+

DIFFERENTIAL DIAGNOSIS

Pyogenic Abscess

- High signal on DWI, low ADC

Other Encephalitides

- Difficult to differentiate

PATHOLOGY

General Features

- Etiology
  - Caused by free-living amebae
  - *E. histolytica, N. fowleri,* & *Acanthamoeba* frequent
    - *N. fowleri* causes PAM
    - *Acanthamoeba* causes GAE
- Most are transmitted by fecal-oral contamination
  - Enter CNS by hematogenous dissemination
- NF: Organisms in stagnant freshwater
  - Nasal mucosa → olfactory neuroepithelium → CNS

Gross Pathologic & Surgical Features

- EH: Single/multiple, 2-60 mm in size, central necrosis
- NF: Purulent exudate, hyperemic meninges (region of olfactory bulbs), necrosis frontal/temporal lobes
- Ac: Multifocal hemorrhagic necrosis, edema, abscess

CLINICAL ISSUES

Presentation

- Most common signs/symptoms
  - Headache, nausea, vomiting, lethargy, seizures
  - Ac: Insidious, headache, low-grade fever, seizures

Demographics

- Age
  - EH: 20-40 years; NF in children
- Gender
  - M > F
- Epidemiology
  - Endemic to southern USA, South America, Latin America, southeast Asia, Africa
  - GAE in debilitated/immunocompromised patients

Natural History & Prognosis

- PAM: Rapid progression (fatal if untreated)
- GAE: More insidious, prolonged duration

Treatment

- Surgical intervention, drugs (miconazole, metronidazole, amphotericin B, clotrimazole)

DIAGNOSTIC CHECKLIST

Consider

- Amebic infection in clinical setting of meningoencephalitis with travel to endemic areas

Image Interpretation Pearls

- "Odd-looking" lesion(s); can mimic neoplasm

SELECTED REFERENCES

1. Fukuma T: [Amebic meningoencephalitis.] Brain Nerve. 61(2):115-21, 2009
2. Kaushal V et al: Primary amoebic meningoencephalitis due to Naegleria fowleri. J Assoc Physicians India. 56:459-62, 2008

CEREBRAL MALARIA

Key Facts

Terminology
- Cerebral malaria (CM)
- *Plasmodium*-infected RBCs sequester in cerebral microvasculature → multiple infarcts
  - Only 2% of infected patients develop CM
  - **But** CM most common cause of death from parasitic infection

Imaging
- Multiple cortical, thalamic infarcts ± hemorrhages
  - Cortex, deep WM, basal ganglia (thalami) > cerebellum
  - May show restriction on DWI
  - Hemorrhages "bloom" on T2* (GRE/SWI)

Top Differential Diagnoses
- Multiple cerebral emboli/infarction
- Acute infantile bilateral striatal necrosis

Pathology
- Malaria caused by 4 species of *Plasmodium*
  - > 95% *P. falciparum, P. vivax*
- Infected erythrocytes sequestered in microvasculature
  - Vascular occlusions → infarcts ± hemorrhages

Clinical Issues
- Usually young children/adults visiting endemic areas
- Incubation period 1-3 weeks
  - Fever, headache
  - Altered sensorium
  - Seizures
- 15-20% mortality despite appropriate therapy
- Sickle cell trait confers some protection

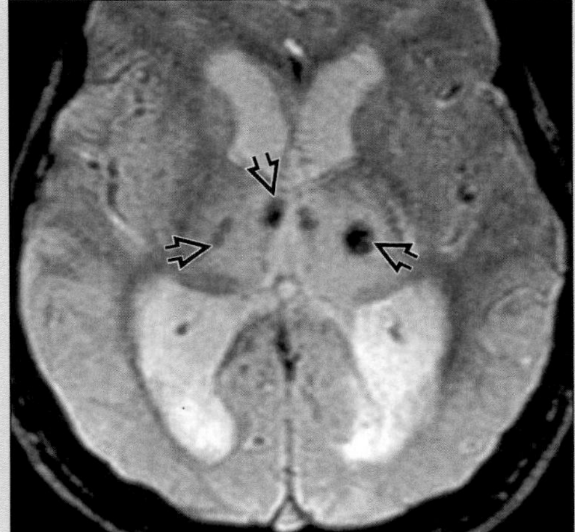
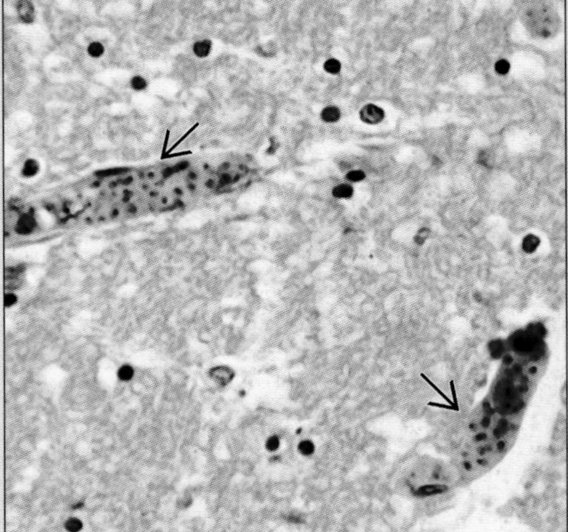

(Left) *Axial T2* GRE MR in a child with known malaria who had altered sensorium, then lapsed into coma. Note the hyperintensity in both thalami with numerous hemorrhagic foci ⇨. DWI and ADC (not shown) disclosed multiple areas of restriction consistent with infarcts. Autopsy showed bithalamic infarcts. (Courtesy R. Ramakantan, MD.)* ***(Right)*** *Hematoxylin & eosin in the same patient shows pale-staining ischemic parenchyma and capillary plugging → from RBCs containing innumerable parasites. (Courtesy R. Ramakantan, MD.)*

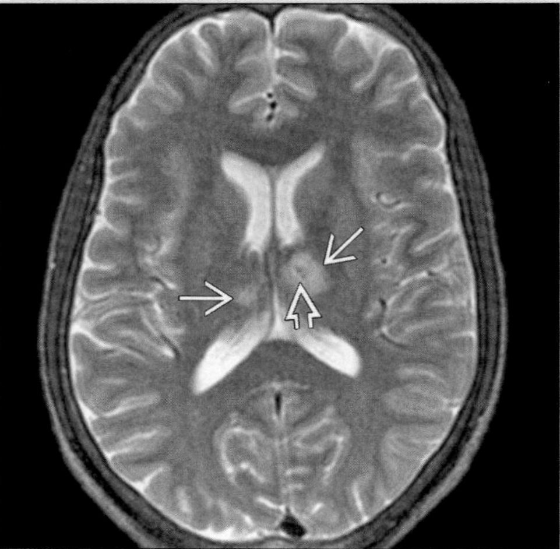
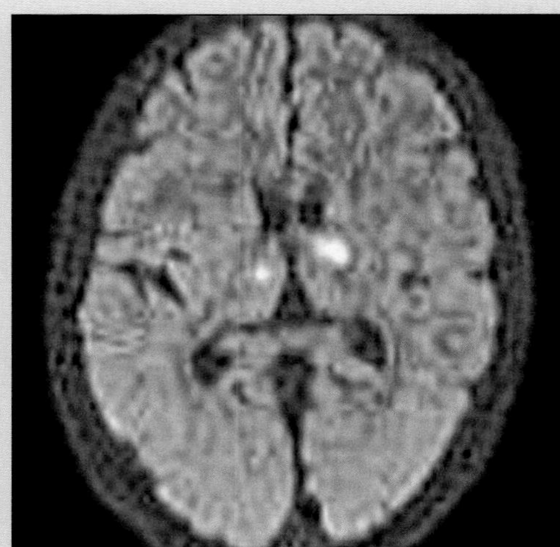

(Left) *Axial T2WI MR in a patient with cerebral malaria and altered sensorium shows bilateral medial thalamic hyperintensities → with a faint area of hypointensity in the left thalamus ⇨ suggesting hemorrhage. T2* GRE (not shown) confirmed hemorrhage. (Courtesy R. Ramakantan, MD.)* ***(Right)*** *Axial DWI MR in the same patient shows bilateral foci of diffusion restriction indicating acute basal ganglionic and thalamic infarcts. (Courtesy R. Ramakantan, MD.)*

CEREBRAL MALARIA

TERMINOLOGY

Abbreviations

- Cerebral malaria (CM)

Definitions

- *Plasmodium*-infected RBCs sequester in cerebral microvasculature → multiple infarcts

IMAGING

General Features

- Best diagnostic clue
  - Multiple cortical, thalamic infarcts ± hemorrhages in patient with known *Plasmodium* infection
- Location
  - Cortex, deep white matter (WM), basal ganglia (thalami)

CT Findings

- NECT
  - Findings vary from normal to striking
    - Diffuse edema ± obstructive hydrocephalus
    - Focal infarcts, often multiple
      - Cortex, basal ganglia (especially thalami)
      - White matter, cerebellum
    - Gross hemorrhage uncommon

MR Findings

- T1WI
  - Variable hypointensity
- T2WI
  - Focal hyperintensities
    - Bilateral thalami
    - Periventricular WM including corpus callosum splenium
- FLAIR
  - Multifocal hyperintensities in WM, thalami
- T2* GRE
  - Hemorrhages "bloom"
- DWI
  - Variable; may show restriction
- T1WI C+
  - Generally none

Imaging Recommendations

- Best imaging tool
  - MR with FLAIR, T2* (GRE/SWI), DWI

DIFFERENTIAL DIAGNOSIS

Multiple Cerebral Emboli/Infarction

- Peripheral (gray-white junction) > > basal ganglia

Acute Infantile Bilateral Striatal Necrosis

- Usually follows respiratory illness, influenza
- Also associated with HHV-6, rotavirus gastroenteritis

PATHOLOGY

General Features

- Etiology
  - Malaria caused by 4 species of *Plasmodium*
    - > 95% *P. falciparum, P. vivax*
    - Less common: *P. malariae, P. ovale*
  - Carrier is *Anopheles* mosquito
  - Infected erythrocytes sequestered in microvasculature
    - Vascular occlusions → infarcts ± hemorrhages

Gross Pathologic & Surgical Features

- Grossly swollen brain

Microscopic Features

- Parasitized RBCs may become ghost-like, contain malaria parasites

CLINICAL ISSUES

Presentation

- Most common signs/symptoms
  - Incubation period 1-3 weeks
    - Fever, headache
    - Altered sensorium
    - Seizures
    - Decreased consciousness
    - Coma
- Other signs/symptoms
  - Backache
  - Photophobia
  - Nausea, vomiting

Demographics

- Age
  - Usually young children
  - Foreign visitors to endemic areas
- Ethnicity
  - Sickle cell trait confers some protection
- Epidemiology
  - Only 2% of patients infected by *Plasmodium falciparum* develop CM
  - CM most common cause of death from parasitic infection

Natural History & Prognosis

- 15-20% mortality despite appropriate therapy

DIAGNOSTIC CHECKLIST

Consider

- Malaria in adult with travel to endemic area

SELECTED REFERENCES

1. Nickerson JP et al: Imaging cerebral malaria with a susceptibility-weighted MR sequence. AJNR Am J Neuroradiol. 30(6):e85-6, 2009
2. Potchen MJ et al: Neuroimaging findings in children with retinopathy-confirmed cerebral malaria. Eur J Radiol. Epub ahead of print, 2009
3. Yadav P et al: Magnetic resonance features of cerebral malaria. Acta Radiol. 49(5):566-9, 2008
4. Sakai O et al: Diffusion-weighted imaging of cerebral malaria. J Neuroimaging. 15(3):278-80, 2005

Key Facts

Imaging

- **Paragonimiasis**: Acutely may cause hemorrhage or infarct followed by granuloma formation
  - Conglomerated, multiple ring-enhancing lesions
- **Schistosomiasis**: Granulomatous encephalitis, hyperintense mass, enhancing dots along linear area
  - Central linear enhancement surrounded by multiple punctate nodules, arborized appearance
- **Sparganosis**: Conglomerate, multicystic hemispheric mass with surrounding edema
  - May cause "tunnel" sign (worm migration)
  - Conglomerate ring enhancement
- **Trichinosis**: Eosinophilic meningoencephalitis, vascular thrombi, infarcts
- **Trypanosomiasis**: Meningoencephalitis, organisms in PVS → edema, congestion, petechial hemorrhages
- Patient travel history is often key to diagnosis!

Top Differential Diagnoses

- Neoplasms (glioblastoma multiforme, metastases)
- Abscess
- Neurocysticercosis
- Neurosarcoid

Pathology

- **Paragonimiasis**: Ingestion of undercooked fresh water crabs or crayfish contaminated with *Paragonimus westermani* flukes (lung fluke)
- **Schistosomiasis**: Infestation from trematode worms
- **Sparganosis**: Ingestion of contaminated water or food (snake, frogs)
- **Trichinosis**: Ingestion of uncooked meat containing infective encysted larvae
- **Trypanosomiasis**: African (tsetse fly) and American (Chagas disease, reduviid bugs)

__(Left)__ Axial T2WI MR shows a heterogeneous lesion in the right frontal lobe with mass effect and surrounding edema in this patient from east Asia. Note the hypointense rim ➔ typical of paragonimiasis. __(Right)__ Coronal T1 C+ MR in the same patient shows conglomerated, ring-enhancing lesions with marked surrounding edema. Paragonimiasis may acutely cause hemorrhage or infarct followed by granuloma formation. Imaging mimics a neoplasm. Chronically, calcifications and atrophy will develop.

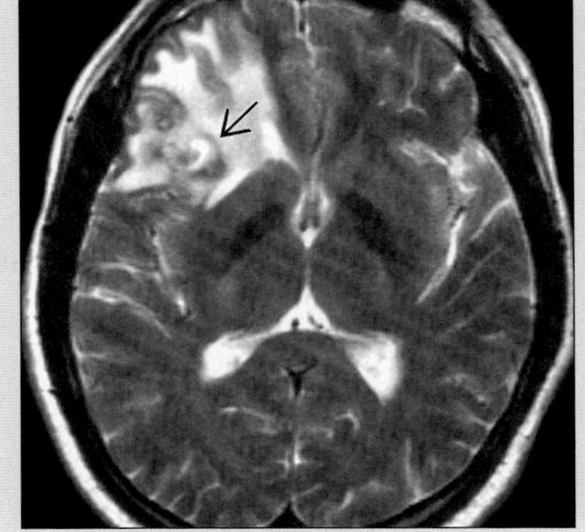

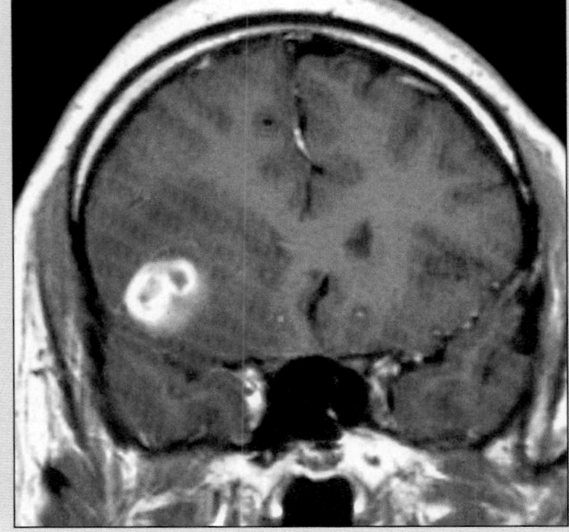

__(Left)__ Axial CECT shows diffuse brain atrophy with ventriculomegaly and basal ganglia hyperdensity ➔ in this patient with a remote history of paragonimiasis. Acutely, these parasites may cause brain infarction. __(Right)__ Axial T1WI C+ MR shows patchy, nodular enhancement in the left temporal lobe. The enhancement has a mildly arborized appearance, characteristic of schistosomiasis. This parasite often causes a granulomatous encephalitis and presents as encephalopathy or seizures.

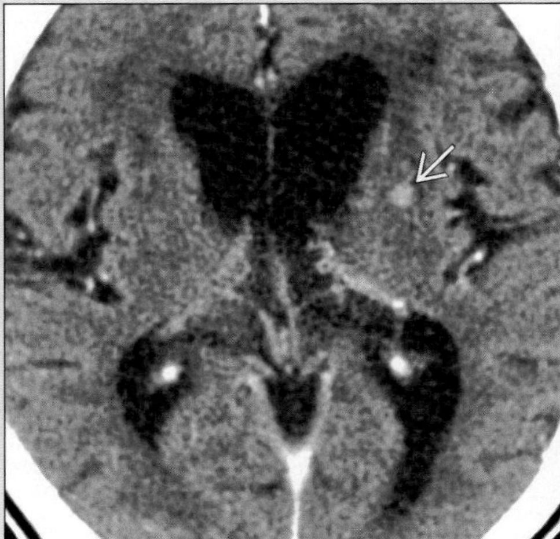

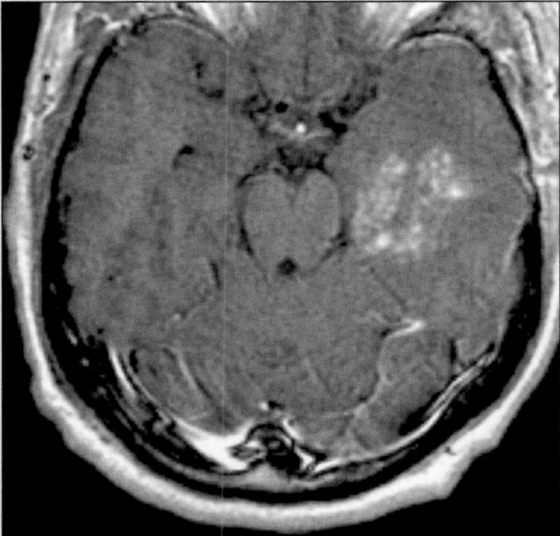

TERMINOLOGY

Definitions

- Rare parasitic infection affecting CNS
- Includes paragonimiasis, schistosomiasis, sparganosis, trichinosis, trypanosomiasis

IMAGING

General Features

- Best diagnostic clue
  - Enhancing supratentorial mass, may be multiloculated
- Location
  - Majority of parasitic infections are supratentorial
  - **Paragonimiasis**: Hemispheric, commonly posterior
  - **Schistosomiasis**: Hemispheric and cerebellar
  - **Sparganosis**: Hemispheric
  - **Trichinosis:** Cerebral cortex and white matter (WM)
- Morphology
  - **Paragonimiasis**: Acutely may cause hemorrhage or infarct followed by granuloma formation
    - In chronic stage, round and ovoid Ca++ in mass
  - **Schistosomiasis**: Granulomatous encephalitis, hyperintense mass, enhancing dots along linear area
  - **Sparganosis**: Conglomerate, multicystic mass with surrounding edema
    - May cause "tunnel" sign related to worm migration
  - **Trichinosis**: Eosinophilic meningoencephalitis, vascular thrombi, infarcts
  - **Trypanosomiasis**: Meningoencephalitis, organisms in perivascular spaces (PVSs) cause brain edema, congestion, petechial hemorrhages

CT Findings

- NECT
  - **Paragonimiasis**: Multiple conglomerated granulomas, ± hemorrhage
    - Multiple round or oval calcifications, surrounding low density, cortical atrophy, ventriculomegaly
  - **Schistosomiasis**: Single or multiple hyperdense lesion(s) with edema, mass effect
  - **Sparganosis**: Conglomerate, multicystic mass with surrounding edema; ± Ca++
    - Typically unilateral, hemispheric
    - Atrophy, ventricular dilatation in chronic cases
  - **Trichinosis**: Hypodense white matter lesions, cortical infarcts
  - **Trypanosomiasis**: Edema with scattered petechial hemorrhage
- CECT
  - **Paragonimiasis**: Ring enhancement
  - **Trichinosis**: Ring-enhancing lesions

MR Findings

- T2WI
  - **Paragonimiasis**: Heterogeneous mass with surrounding edema, ± hemorrhage
    - May have isointense or hypointense rim
  - **Schistosomiasis**: Hyperintense mass with surrounding edema
  - **Sparganosis**: Conglomerate, multicystic mass with surrounding edema, ± hemorrhage
    - May see mixed-signal lesion, central low signal and peripheral high signal
    - Unilateral white matter degeneration, cortical atrophy in chronic cases
- T1WI C+
  - **Paragonimiasis**: Conglomerated multiple ring-enhancing lesions
    - Chronic: Atrophy and calcification
  - **Schistosomiasis**: Central linear enhancement surrounded by multiple punctate nodules, **arborized** appearance
  - **Sparganosis**: Variable; pattern may change on follow-up related to worm migration
    - **"Tunnel" sign**: Peripherally enhancing hollow tube
    - May see conglomerate ring enhancement with multiple rings (bead appearance)

Imaging Recommendations

- Best imaging tool
  - Contrast MR is most sensitive for detection
  - CT may be helpful to identify associated Ca++
- Protocol advice
  - Contrast-enhanced MR

DIFFERENTIAL DIAGNOSIS

Glioblastoma Multiforme

- Thick, irregular margin enhancement with central necrosis typical
- Often involves corpus callosum
- Typically in older adult

Parenchymal Metastases

- Enhancing mass at corticomedullary junctions
- Multiple lesions common
- Primary tumor often known

Abscess

- T2 hypointense rim and DWI(+) typical
- Ring enhancement, thinner on ventricular margin

Neurocysticercosis

- Cyst with marginal scolex
- Multiple lesions common

Neurosarcoid

- Enhancing lesions involving dura, leptomeninges, and subarachnoid space
- Rarely affects brain parenchyma
  - Hypothalamus > brainstem > cerebral hemispheres > cerebellar hemispheres

Porencephalic Cyst

- Encephalomalacia ± surrounding gliosis
- Typically communicates with ventricle

Arachnoid Cyst

- Nonenhancing solitary lesion with CSF density/ intensity
- Anterior middle cranial fossa most commonly

PATHOLOGY

General Features

- Etiology
  - **Paragonimiasis**: Ingestion of undercooked fresh water crabs or crayfish contaminated with *Paragonimus westermani* flukes (lung fluke)
    - Worms penetrate skull base foramina and meninges and directly invade brain parenchyma
  - **Schistosomiasis**: Infestation from trematode (fluke) worms
    - Host is freshwater snail
    - Humans affected through skin
    - Migrate to lungs and liver, reach venous system
  - **Sparganosis**: Ingestion of contaminated water or food (snake, frogs)
  - **Trichinosis**: Ingestion of uncooked meat containing infective encysted larvae
  - **Trypanosomiasis**: African (sleeping sickness) and American (Chagas disease)
    - African: Transmitted to humans by tsetse fly; invade meninges, subarachnoid, PVSs
    - American: Transmitted by reduviid bugs

Gross Pathologic & Surgical Features

- **Paragonimiasis**: Cystic lesions elaborate toxins that result in infarction, meningitis, adhesions
- **Schistosomiasis**: Granulomatous encephalitis, eggs seen at microscopy
- **Sparganosis**: Live worm or degenerated worm with surrounding granuloma found at surgery
- **Trichinosis**: Eosinophilic meningoencephalitis, ischemic lesions, petechial hemorrhage, necrosis
- **Trypanosomiasis**: Edema, congestion, hemorrhage

CLINICAL ISSUES

Presentation

- Most common signs/symptoms
  - **Paragonimiasis**: Headache, seizure, visual changes
  - **Schistosomiasis**: Encephalopathy, seizures, paresis, headache, visual changes
  - **Sparganosis**: Headache, seizure, neurologic signs
  - **Trichinosis**: Fever, headache, delirium, seizures, focal neurologic deficits
  - **African trypanosomiasis**: Behavior change, indifference, daytime somnolence
  - **American trypanosomiasis**: Acute (fever, swollen face, conjunctivitis), chronic (neurologic)
- Clinical profile
  - Varies with organism, development stage, host immune response
  - ELISA studies can be helpful in some diseases

Demographics

- Age
  - Most parasitic infections occur at all ages but commonly affect children and young adults
- Gender
  - Most parasitic infections have male predominance
- Epidemiology
  - Neurocysticercosis most common parasitic infection worldwide
  - Increased travel, immigration have spread diseases
  - **Paragonimiasis**: Brain involvement in 2-27% of cases
  - **Schistosomiasis**: 2% of cases have CNS complications
  - **Sparganosis**: Extremely rare
  - **Trichinosis**: CNS involvement in 10-24% of cases

Natural History & Prognosis

- Some parasitic infections (e.g., echinococcosis) develop slowly over many years
- **Trichinosis**: Mortality in 5-10% of affected individuals
- **American trypanosomiasis**: Mortality 2-10% of meningoencephalitis patients

Treatment

- Variable, ranges from oral therapy to lesion resection

DIAGNOSTIC CHECKLIST

Consider

- Complex conglomerated parasitic cysts of any etiology may mimic brain tumor!
- Patient travel history is often key to diagnosis

SELECTED REFERENCES

1. George J et al: Cerebral schistosomiasis--an unusual presentation of an intracranial mass lesion. Can J Neurol Sci. 36(2):244-7, 2009
2. Shu K et al: Surgical treatment of cerebellar schistosomiasis. Neurosurgery. 64(5):941-3; discussion 943-4, 2009
3. Chen Z et al: Acute cerebral paragonimiasis presenting as hemorrhagic stroke in a child. Pediatr Neurol. 39(2):133-6, 2008
4. Devine MJ et al: Neuroschistosomiasis presenting as brainstem encephalitis. Neurology. 70(23):2262-4, 2008
5. Ferrari TC et al: Immune response and pathogenesis of neuroschistosomiasis mansoni. Acta Trop. 108(2-3):83-8, 2008
6. Rengarajan S et al: Cerebral sparganosis: a diagnostic challenge. Br J Neurosurg. 22(6):784-6, 2008
7. Kim IY et al: Contralateral migration of cerebral sparganosis through the splenium. Clin Neurol Neurosurg. 109(8):720-4, 2007
8. Silva JC et al: Schistosomiasis mansoni presenting as a cerebellar tumor: case report. Arq Neuropsiquiatr. 65(3B):845-7, 2007
9. Song T et al: CT and MR characteristics of cerebral sparganosis. AJNR Am J Neuroradiol. 28(9):1700-5, 2007
10. Bo G et al: Neuroimaging and pathological findings in a child with cerebral sparganosis. Case report. J Neurosurg. 105(6 Suppl):470-2, 2006
11. Liu HQ et al: Characteristic magnetic resonance enhancement pattern in cerebral schistosomiasis. Chin Med Sci J. 21(4):223-7, 2006
12. Roberts M et al: Cerebral schistosomiasis. Lancet Infect Dis. 6(12):820, 2006
13. Zhang JS et al: MRI features of pediatric cerebral paragonimiasis in the active stage. J Magn Reson Imaging. 23(4):569-73, 2006
14. Gelal F et al: Diffusion-weighted and conventional MR imaging in neurotrichinosis. Acta Radiol. 46(2):196-9, 2005
15. Im JG et al: Current diagnostic imaging of pulmonary and cerebral paragonimiasis, with pathological correlation. Semin Roentgenol. 32(4):301-24, 1997

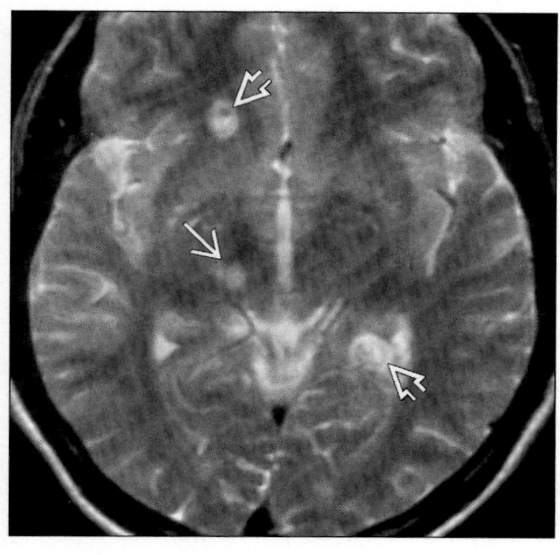

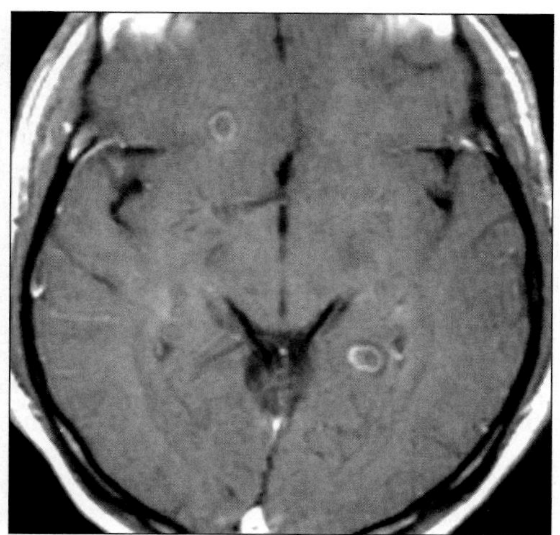

(Left) *Axial T2WI MR shows multiple round lesions scattered in the hemispheres and right brainstem ➔. Some of the lesions have mixed signal with hypointense foci or a hypointense rim ➲.* ***(Right)*** *Axial T1WI C+ MR in the same patient with sparganosis shows ring enhancement of the lesions. Imaging mimics other parasites, including the much more common neurocysticercosis. Sparganosis is extremely rare and is related to ingestion of contaminated water or food. (Courtesy M. Castillo, MD.)*

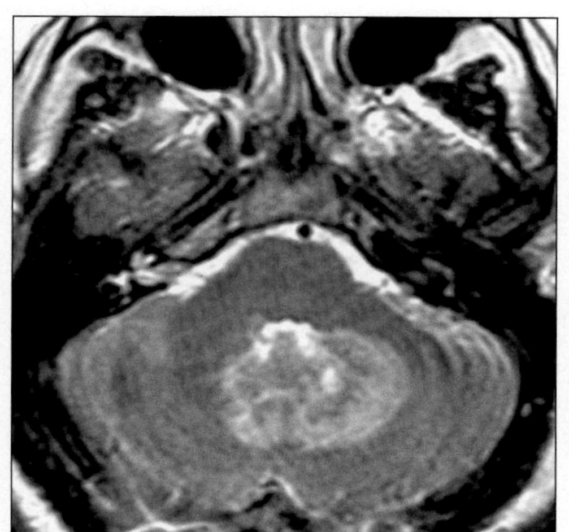

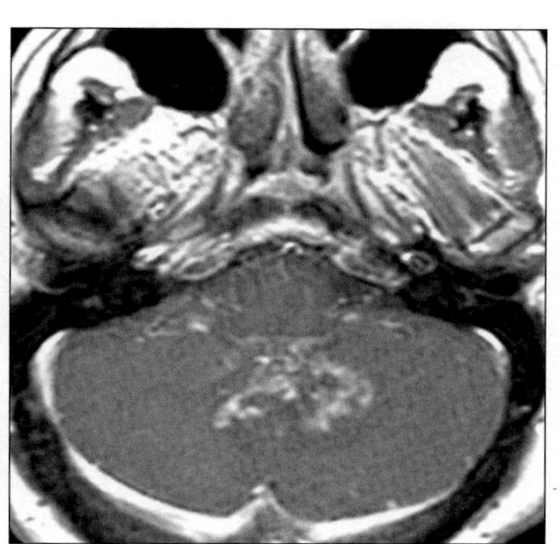

(Left) *Axial T2WI MR shows hyperintensity in the cerebellum related to edema in this young adult male with schistosomiasis.* ***(Right)*** *Axial T1WI C+ MR in the same patient shows patchy, mildly nodular enhancement in the cerebellum with surrounding edema. Imaging mimics granulomatous disease or neoplasm. Schistosomiasis often has central linear enhancement surrounded by multiple punctate nodules, causing an arborized appearance.*

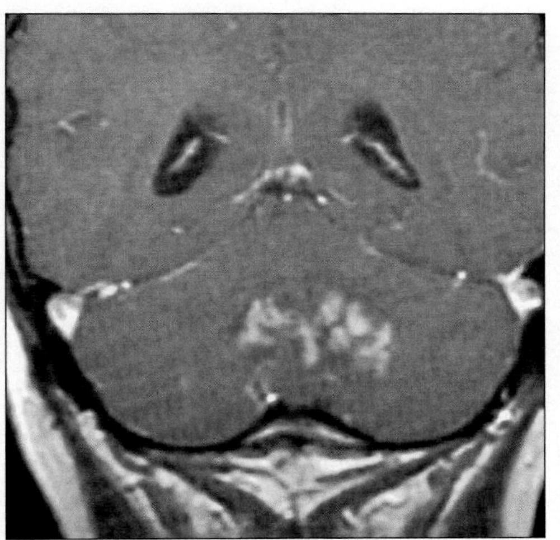

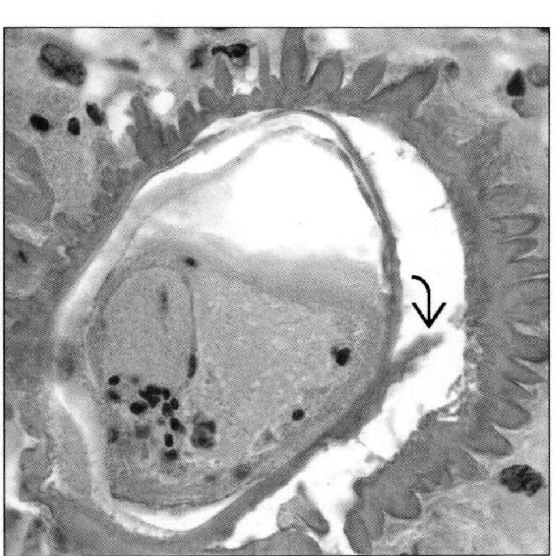

(Left) *Coronal T1WI C+ MR shows irregular punctate and nodular enhancement in the posterior fossa related to schistosomiasis. Schistosomiasis most commonly affects the cerebral hemispheres or the cerebellum.* ***(Right)*** *Microscopic pathology in the same patient shows a Schistosomiasis mansoni egg with a characteristic lateral spine ⮫. Schistosomiasis infection is related to infestation from a trematode (fluke) worm and is very uncommon. (Courtesy D. Kremens, S. Galetta, MD.)*

FUNGAL DISEASES

Key Facts

Terminology
- Coccidioidomycosis, histoplasmosis (common)
- Invasive fungal infection (immunocompromised)
  - Candidiasis (common)
  - Aspergillus, mucormycosis are angioinvasive

Imaging
- General features
  - Meningeal enhancement
  - Ring-enhancing brain lesions
  - Infarctions (both lacunar, territorial)
  - Diffuse brain edema, herniation, hydrocephalus
  - Hemorrhage(s)
  - Vasculitis, occlusions, mycotic aneurysms

Top Differential Diagnoses
- Invasive skull base neoplasm (e.g., SCCa)
  - Fungus often angioinvasive → ICA occlusion
  - Vessel occlusion rare in SCCa
- Ring-enhancing lesions (immunocompetent)
  - Metastases, pyogenic abscesses, septic emboli
- Ring-enhancing lesions (immunocompromised)
  - TB, toxoplasmosis, lymphoma

Pathology
- General
  - Congested meninges, swollen brain
  - Focal granulomas, abscesses
- Angioinvasive fungi
  - Vasculitis, infarcts
  - Hemorrhages, mycotic aneurysm

Diagnostic Checklist
- Consider fungus in immunocompromised when
  - Acute neurologic deficit
  - Multiple brain lesions
  - Stroke, vascular occlusion

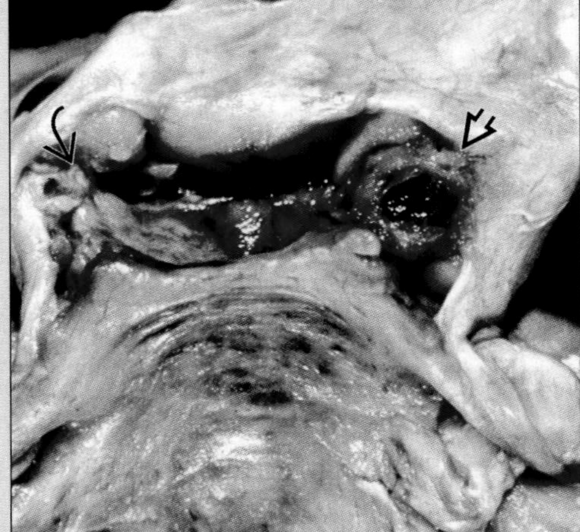

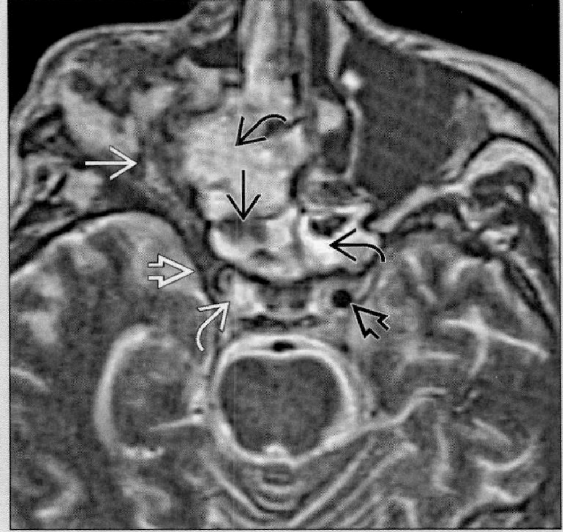

(Left) *Autopsy specimen shows aspergillosis invading the paranasal sinuses and skull base. One internal carotid artery is encased by fungus while the other has been occluded. (Courtesy R. Hewlett, PhD.)* ***(Right)*** *Axial T2WI MR shows the typical sequela of invasive rhinocerebral mucormycosis: Sinonasal opacification, hypointense fungus, orbital invasion, cavernous sinus extension, and occlusion of the right internal carotid artery. The left internal carotid artery is normal.*

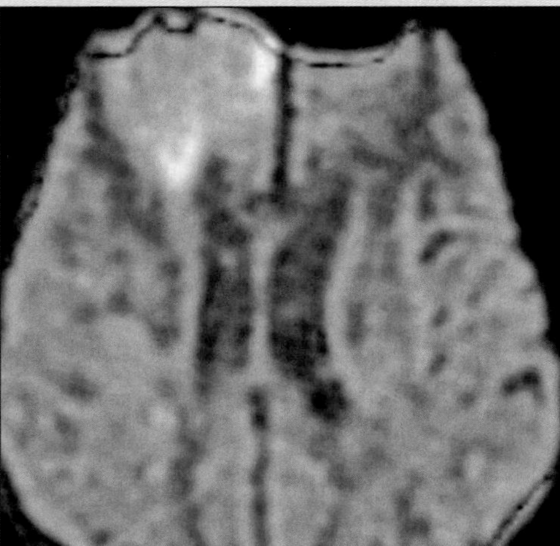

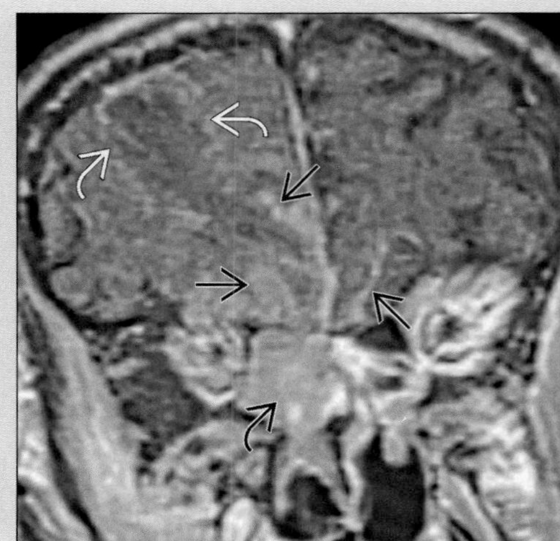

(Left) *Axial DWI MR shows acute infarcts in the right anterior and middle cerebral artery territories related to fungal invasion and occlusion of the right internal carotid artery.* ***(Right)*** *Coronal T1WI C+ MR shows extensive meningeal involvement with mucormycosis, as well as direct cerebral invasion. An area of nonenhancing abnormality in the right frontal lobe is secondary to acute cerebral infarction from invasive fungal occlusion of the internal carotid artery. Note the sphenoid sinus fungal infection.*

FUNGAL DISEASES

TERMINOLOGY

Definitions

- Coccidioidomycosis
  - Sporadic, relatively common
- Histoplasmosis
  - Common
- Blastomycosis
  - Rare, sporadic, generally affects lungs/skin
- Invasive CNS fungal infections
  - Patients usually immunocompromised
  - Agents
    - Hyphae: Aspergillosis, mucormycosis
    - Pseudo-hyphae/yeast: Candidiasis

IMAGING

General Features

- Best diagnostic clue
  - Meningeal enhancement, enhancing lesions in brain in immunosuppressed patient
- Location
  - Meninges, brain, spinal cord
- Size
  - Variable (mm to cm)
- Morphology
  - Many lesions are ring-like

CT Findings

- NECT
  - Areas of low density = infection, lacunar infarctions, territorial infarcts
  - Diffuse brain edema, herniation, hydrocephalus
  - Hemorrhages
- CECT
  - Foci of enhancement, some ring-like

MR Findings

- T1WI
  - Ill-defined areas of low signal intensity
- T2WI
  - Focal or diffuse areas of high signal intensity
  - May have peripheral hypointense rim
- T2* GRE
  - Blooming of Ca++ and blood products
- DWI
  - May have restricted diffusion
- T1WI C+
  - Thick meningeal enhancement
  - Cerebral enhancement may be ring-like, solitary to miliary
- MRA
  - Vasculitis, occlusions, mycotic aneurysms
- MRS
  - Mildly ↑ Cho, ↓ NAA, ↑ lactate

Angiographic Findings

- Vasculitis, mycotic aneurysms

Nuclear Medicine Findings

- PET
  - ↓ metabolism and ↓ blood flow to lesions

Imaging Recommendations

- Best imaging tool
  - MR
- Protocol advice
  - Contrast-enhanced MR essential
  - MRS (infection vs. neoplasm)

DIFFERENTIAL DIAGNOSIS

Locally Invasive Skull Base Neoplasm

- e.g., SCCa
- Look for soft tissue mass in nasopharynx
- Fungal infection often angioinvasive with ICA occlusion (extremely rare in SCCa)

Multiple Ring-Enhancing Brain Lesions

- Immunocompetent patients
  - Metastases
  - Pyogenic abscesses
  - Parasites (e.g., neurocysticercosis)
  - Septic emboli
- Immunocompromised patients
  - Tuberculosis
  - Toxoplasmosis
  - Primary CNS lymphoma

PATHOLOGY

General Features

- Etiology
  - Blastomycosis: *B. dermatitidis*
    - Inhalation, may be acquired by pet bites
  - Coccidioidomycosis: *C. immitis*
    - Inhalation, then hematogenous spread
  - Histoplasmosis: *H. capsulatum*
    - Inhalation, then hematogenous spread
  - Candidiasis: *C. albicans*
    - Initially involves gastrointestinal &/or respiratory systems
    - Then spreads hematogenously
  - Aspergillosis: *A. fumigatus*
    - Inhalation of spores, hypersensitivity reaction
    - Hematogenous dissemination in immunosuppressed
    - Angioinvasive
  - Mucormycosis: Phycomycetes (*Mucor*, *Rhizopus*)
    - Enter via nasopharynx
    - Can be inhaled into lungs
    - Can have rhinocerebral extension
    - Angioinvasive
- Associated abnormalities
  - Histoplasmosis
    - Calcified/cavitating lung lesions
    - Mediastinal nodes
  - Coccidioidomycosis
    - Generally affects lungs

Gross Pathologic & Surgical Features

- All: Congested meninges, swollen brain, focal granulomas, abscesses
- Coccidioidomycosis
  - Involvement of CNS in 30%

FUNGAL DISEASES

- Meningitis most common
- Vasculitis (40%), infarcts, hemorrhages
- Candidiasis
  - Hemorrhagic infarcts
  - Abscess, granulomas (may be miliary)

Microscopic Features

- Granulomas or small abscesses
  - Caseous necrosis, giant cells, neutrophils, lymphocytes
- Identification of specific organism needed for diagnosis
- Fibropurulent meningitis → meningeal fibrosis

CLINICAL ISSUES

Presentation

- Most common signs/symptoms
  - Initially for all
    - Weight loss, fever, malaise, fatigue
  - Meningitis
    - Acute focal neurological deficits from stroke/ hemorrhage
- Clinical profile
  - Many fungal infections have associated lung lesions (granulomas, airspace disease) in immunocompetent patients
  - CSF usually shows pleocytosis, ↓ glucose, ↑ protein

Demographics

- Age
  - More common in young and older individuals
  - Seen at any age if immunocompromised
- Gender
  - M > F (more outdoor activities)
- Ethnicity
  - No predilection
- Epidemiology
  - Blastomycosis
    - Fungus lives in damp places, rotting wood
    - Endemic in Africa, USA (Mississippi, Arkansas, Kentucky, Tennessee, Wisconsin)
  - Coccidioidomycosis
    - Fungus lives in damp places, rotting wood
    - Southwestern USA, northern Mexico, South America
    - 60,000-80,000 new cases/year in USA
  - Histoplasmosis
    - Fungus in chicken, pigeon, bat feces
    - Worldwide distribution
    - Approximately 25% of USA population infected
    - Disseminated disease usually seen in infancy/ childhood, immunosuppression
  - Candidiasis
    - Worldwide distribution
    - Most common nosocomial fungal infection
    - Higher incidence in diabetics, immunocompromised
    - Occasionally seen in immunocompetent individuals
  - Mucormycosis
    - Ubiquitous; found in organic matter, soil
    - Mostly affects immunocompromised
  - Aspergillosis
    - Ubiquitous; found in damp places
    - Mostly affects immunocompromised
    - Occasionally becomes invasive in immunocompetent

Natural History & Prognosis

- Delay in diagnosis and treatment → poor prognosis

Treatment

- Options, risks, complications
  - Survival depends on early diagnosis, prompt initiation of antifungal therapy
    - Amphotericin B in immunocompromised, life-threatening cases
  - Survival depends on management of underlying disease process

DIAGNOSTIC CHECKLIST

Consider

- Consider fungal infection when acute neurologic deficit in immunocompromised patient

Image Interpretation Pearls

- Consider fungal infection with multiple brain lesions in immunocompromised patient
- Consider fungal infection with associated stroke, vascular occlusion

SELECTED REFERENCES

1. Berkeley JL et al: Fatal immune reconstitution inflammatory syndrome with human immunodeficiency virus infection and Candida meningitis: case report and review of the literature. J Neurovirol. 14(3):267-76, 2008
2. Luthra G et al: Comparative evaluation of fungal, tubercular, and pyogenic brain abscesses with conventional and diffusion MR imaging and proton MR spectroscopy. AJNR Am J Neuroradiol. 28(7):1332-8, 2007
3. Redmond A et al: Fungal infections of the central nervous system: A review of fungal pathogens and treatment. Neurol India. 55(3):251-9, 2007
4. Zivković S: Neuroimaging and neurologic complications after organ transplantation. J Neuroimaging. 17(2):110-23, 2007
5. Sundaram C et al: Pathology of fungal infections of the central nervous system: 17 years' experience from Southern India. Histopathology. 49(4):396-405, 2006
6. da Rocha AJ et al: Granulomatous diseases of the central nervous system. Top Magn Reson Imaging. 16(2):155-87, 2005
7. Gaviani P et al: Diffusion-weighted imaging of fungal cerebral infection. AJNR Am J Neuroradiol. 26(5):1115-21, 2005

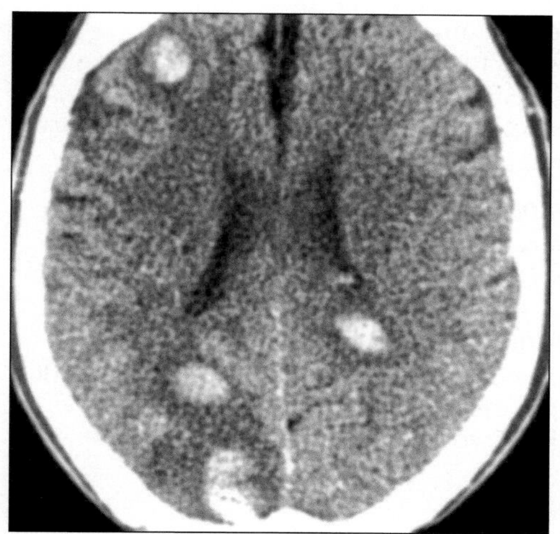

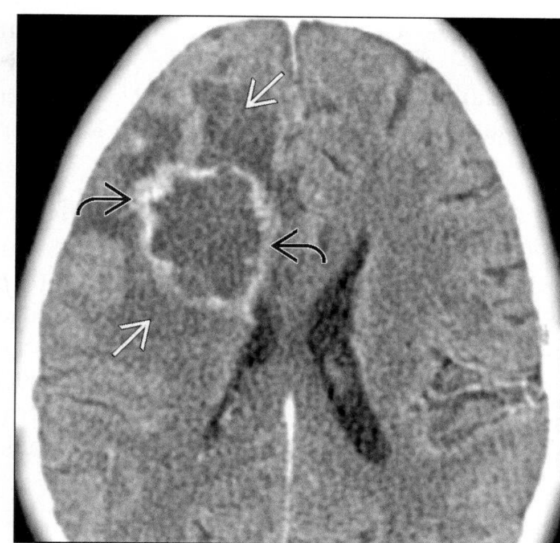

(Left) *Axial NECT shows multiple round and ovoid foci of increased attenuation at the gray-white matter interface with surrounding edema. Hemorrhagic mycetomas from aspergillosis with angioinvasion were documented at surgery.* ***(Right)*** *Axial CECT in a different patient shows a large, low-density mass in the right frontal lobe and deep basal ganglia with irregular rim enhancement → and surrounding edema → with local mass effect. Aspergilloma abscess was found at surgery.*

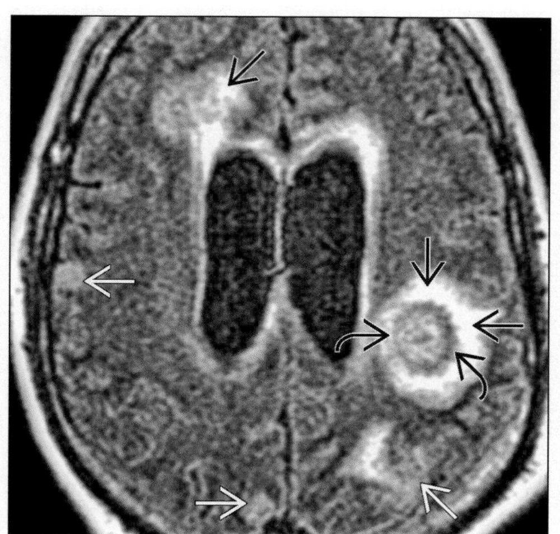

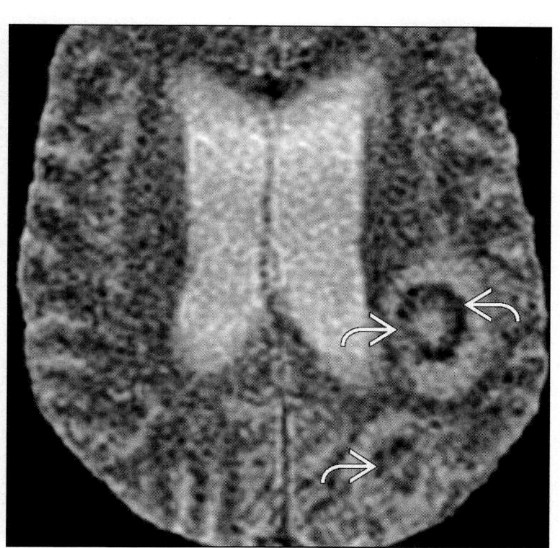

(Left) *Axial FLAIR MR in this immunocompromised patient with Aspergillus infection shows multiple cerebral masses at the gray-white matter interface →. Larger lesions are associated with surrounding hyperintense vasogenic edema →. Note the hypointense rim → around a left cerebral lesion.* ***(Right)*** *Axial T2* GRE MR shows blooming of the hypointense rims → associated with some of the larger cerebral lesions. The hypointense rim may be due to iron needed for hyphae growth.*

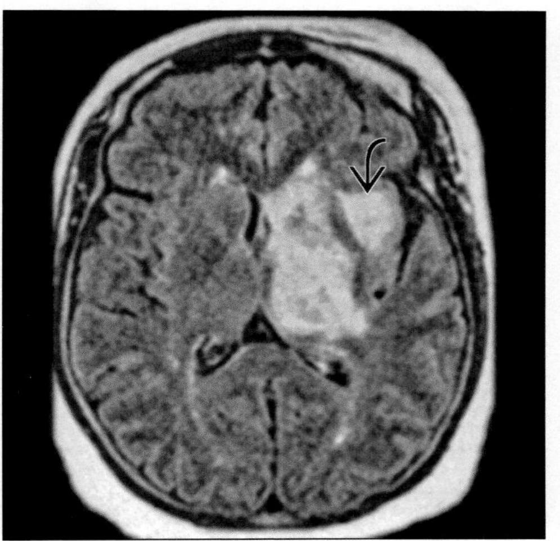

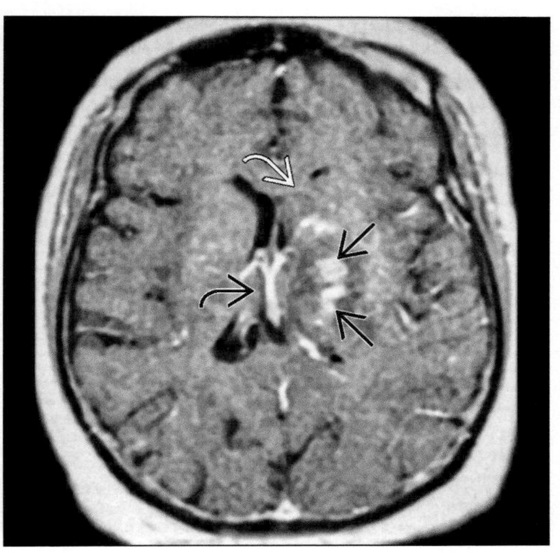

(Left) *Axial FLAIR MR in patient with HIV and cryptococcal infection shows extensive hyperintensity in the deep gray matter of the left basal ganglia and thalamus, as well as in the subinsular white matter →. There is mass effect upon the 3rd ventricle and the left frontal horn.* ***(Right)*** *Axial T1WI C+ MR shows enhancement in the basal ganglia along the perivascular spaces →. There is mild left-to-right shift of the internal cerebral veins → and mass effect on the left frontal horn →.*

RICKETTSIAL DISEASES

Key Facts

Terminology

- Rocky Mountain spotted (RMS) fever, Q fever, typhus, Mediterranean spotted fever, African tick bite fever
- Zoonotic infections of squirrels and other animals → ticks carrying *Rickettsia* → humans

Imaging

- ~ 20% of patients with RMS have abnormal imaging
  - End artery infarct-like lesions (especially BG)
  - Ill-defined hypodensities on CT
  - T2 hyperintensities in perivascular spaces, deep gray nuclei
  - ± diffuse brain swelling
  - Perivascular lesions, meninges may enhance
- Cauda equina, low spinal cord may be abnormal

Pathology

- Caused by *Rickettsia rickettsii* species of bacterium, transmitted to humans via ixodid ticks
- 2 major vectors for *R. rickettsii* in USA
  - Dog tick, Rocky Mountain wood tick
- RMS is most common, most lethal rickettsial disease
  - 800 cases reported per year in USA

Clinical Issues

- RMS: Sudden onset fever, myalgias, headache
  - Petechial rash then develops (palms, soles, then spreads to trunk in 90%)
- RMS can be difficult to diagnose in early stages
- RMS: 90% die if untreated; 20% of patients with MR abnormalities die regardless of treatment
- Normal MR is favorable prognostic sign

*(**Left**) Axial NECT in a patient with headaches and severe joint pain caused by dengue fever shows low density in the basal ganglia bilaterally, with areas of petechial hemorrhage ➔. (**Right**) Axial CECT in a patient with Rocky Mountain spotted fever shows pial enhancement, especially striking along the left insula ➔. Some faint enhancement in the basal ganglia is present ➔.*

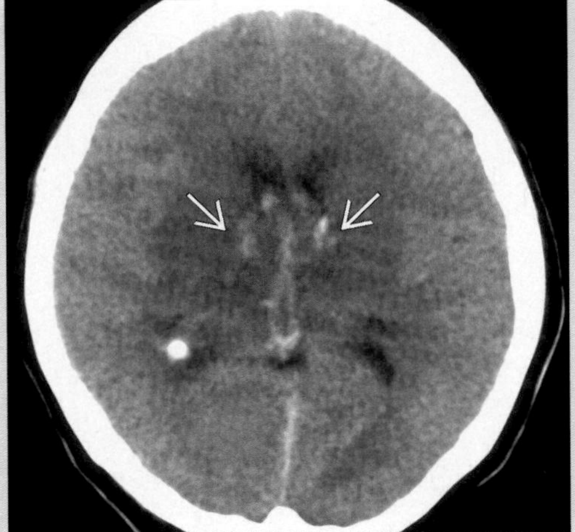

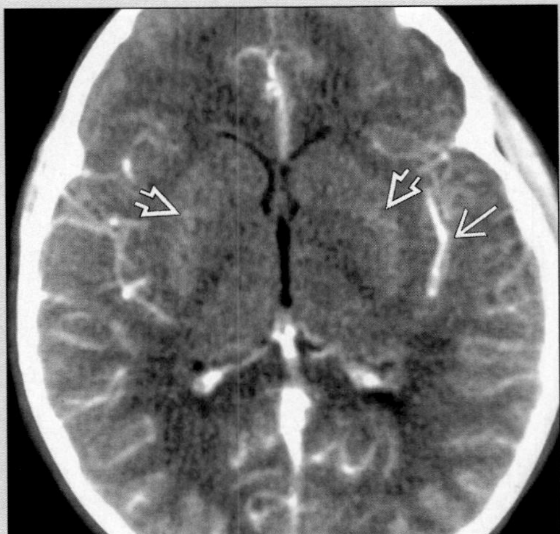

*(**Left**) Axial T2WI MR in the same patient shows punctate areas of increased signal intensity in the basal ganglia and subinsular white matter ➔. (**Right**) Axial T1WI C+ MR in the same patient shows some enhancement in both basal ganglia ➔. (Courtesy C. Bonowitz, MD.)*

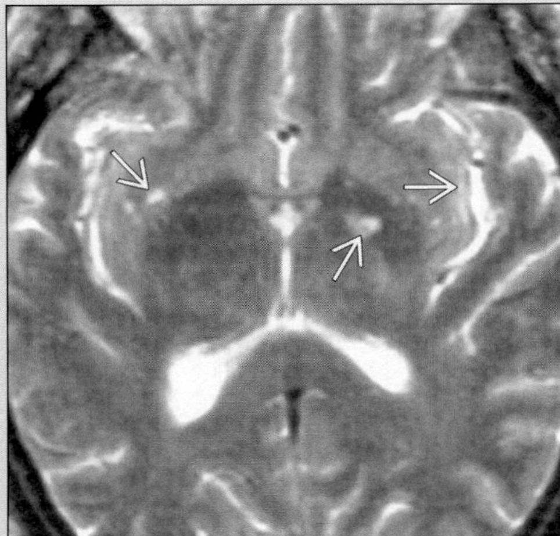

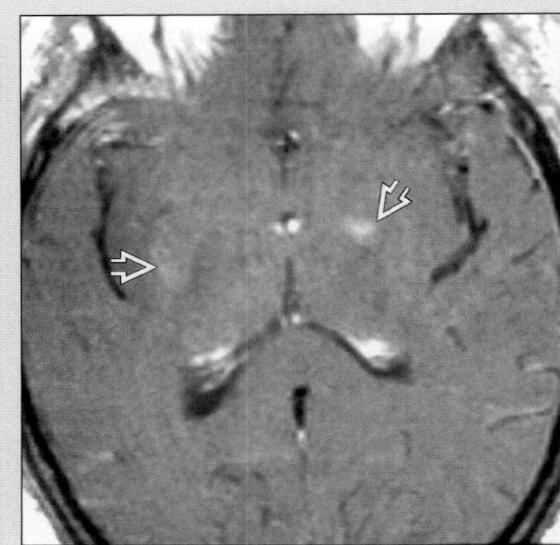

RICKETTSIAL DISEASES

TERMINOLOGY

Abbreviations

- Rocky Mountain spotted (RMS) fever, Q fever, typhus, Mediterranean spotted fever (MSF)

Synonyms

- Tick typhus, Tobia fever (Colombia), Febre maculosa (Brazil), fiebre manchada (Mexico)

Definitions

- Zoonotic infections of squirrels and other animals → ticks carrying *Rickettsia* → humans

IMAGING

General Features

- Best diagnostic clue
  - Ill-defined areas of low density on CT, high signal on T2WI along perivascular spaces and deep gray matter
  - Associated skin rash
- Location
  - Perivascular spaces, deep gray matter nuclei, cauda equina, low spinal cord
- Morphology
  - End artery infarct-like lesions

CT Findings

- NECT
  - Small ill-defined WM low-density foci
  - Infarct-like lesions in deep gray matter
  - Lesions may have small focal hemorrhages

MR Findings

- T2WI
  - Hyperintense lesions in distribution of perivascular spaces, deep gray nuclei, pons
  - Diffuse brain swelling
- DWI
  - Some lesions show restricted diffusion
- T1WI C+
  - Some lesions and meninges enhance
  - Enhancement in cauda equina nerve roots and lower thoracic spinal cord

Imaging Recommendations

- Best imaging tool
  - MR (only 20% of patients have abnormal MR)
- Protocol advice
  - Brain MR with DWI, T1 C+

DIFFERENTIAL DIAGNOSIS

Cryptococcosis and Lyme Disease

- No associated rash

Vasculitis

- Segmental arterial narrowing on DSA
- Multiple infarcts of different ages on DWI

Sarcoidosis

- Suprasellar region, orbit also frequently involved

PATHOLOGY

General Features

- Etiology
  - Caused by *Rickettsia rickettsii* species of bacterium, transmitted to humans via ixodid ticks
    - 2 major vectors for *R. rickettsii* in United States
      - Dog tick, Rocky Mountain wood tick
    - RMS is most common/most lethal rickettsial disease
      - 800 cases reported per year in USA

Microscopic Features

- RMS: Diagnosis → identification of *Rickettsia* on direct or indirect (> 1:64) immunofluorescence
- RMS: Destructive systemic thrombovasculitis
- Confirmation of RMS by histologic examination of skin biopsy

CLINICAL ISSUES

Presentation

- Most common signs/symptoms
  - RMS: Sudden onset fever, myalgias, headache
    - Petechial rash (90% in palms, soles) develops later
  - Can be difficult to diagnose in early stages
  - Often fatal without prompt treatment
- Clinical profile
  - RMS: Anemia, thrombocytopenia, coagulopathy, abnormal liver function tests, ↑ BUN

Demographics

- Epidemiology
  - Increased incidence in Oklahoma, North Carolina, South Carolina, Tennessee, Arkansas

Natural History & Prognosis

- RMS: Early antibiotics → effective
  - If not treated → rapidly progressive
- RMS: 90% die if untreated; 20% of patients with MR abnormalities die regardless of treatment
- RMS: Complications in ~ 1/2 of patients

Treatment

- RMS: Doxycycline, chloramphenicol

DIAGNOSTIC CHECKLIST

Consider

- Normal MR does not exclude diagnosis but is favorable prognostic sign

SELECTED REFERENCES

1. Aliaga L et al: Mediterranean spotted fever with encephalitis. J Med Microbiol. 58(Pt 4):521-5, 2009
2. Singh-Behl D et al: Tick-borne infections. Dermatol Clin. 21(2):237-44, v, 2003
3. Bonawitz C et al: Comparison of CT and MR features with clinical outcome in patients with Rocky Mountain spotted fever. AJNR Am J Neuroradiol. 18(3):459-64, 1997

LYME DISEASE

Key Facts

Terminology

- Lyme disease (LD), Lyme neuroborreliosis (LNB)
- Multisystem inflammatory disease
  - Caused by spirochete *Borrelia burgdorferi* (USA)
  - Transmitted by *Ixodes* tick bite
  - Reservoirs = white tail deer/field mouse

Imaging

- MS-like WM lesions (may enhance)
  - 2-8 mm (large "tumefactive" lesions rare)
- ± multiple enhancing cranial nerves
- ± cauda equina, meningeal enhancement

Top Differential Diagnoses

- Demyelinating disease
- Vasculitis
- Sarcoidosis
- Chronic fatigue syndrome

Clinical Issues

- Most common tick-borne disease in USA
  - Round, "bull's-eye" skin rash
  - ± flu-like symptoms
  - Meningopolyneuritis, radiculitis common
- Confirm with ELISA, PCR
- Peak incidence: May through August
- Incubation period varies from days to weeks
- Progressive debilitating disorder if not treated early
- 10-15% of untreated patients develop neurologic manifestations

Diagnostic Checklist

- Consider geography, recreational/travel history, season
- Consider LNB if MS-like lesions in patient with erythema migrans
  - ± enhancing CNs, cauda equina

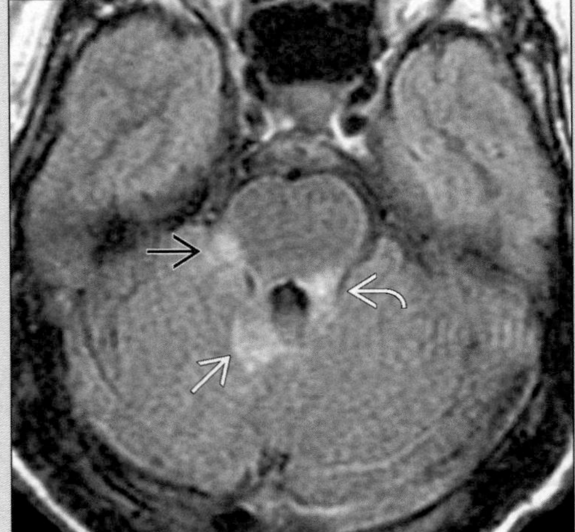

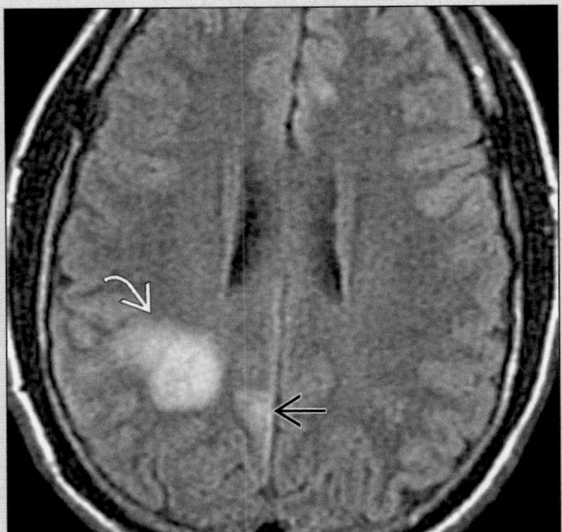

(Left) *Axial FLAIR MR in a patient with serologically documented Lyme disease shows multiple hyperintense foci in the left superior cerebellar peduncle ➔, right lateral pons ➔, and cerebellum ➔.* ***(Right)*** *Axial FLAIR MR in the same patient shows a large focus of signal abnormality in the deep right cerebral white matter ➔. There is also a small region of abnormality in the medial right parietooccipital lobe junction ➔.*

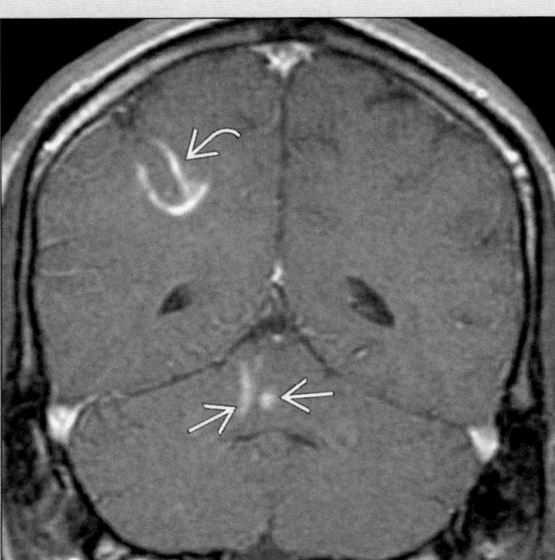

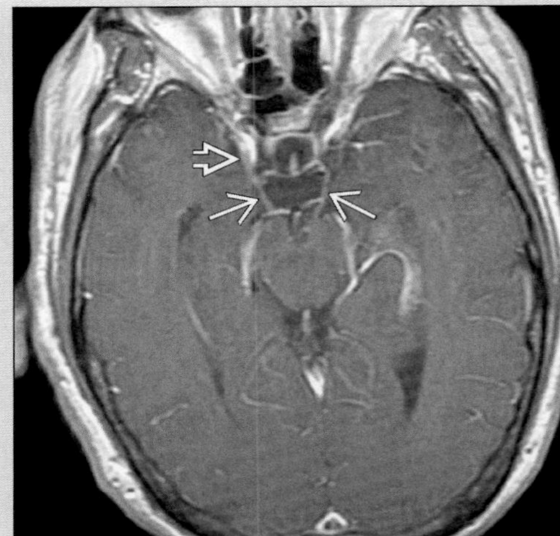

(Left) *Coronal T1WI C+ MR in the same patient shows enhancement of the right cerebral white matter lesion ➔, as well as posterior fossa lesions ➔.* ***(Right)*** *Axial T1WI C+ MR in a patient with headache, diplopia, and left facial droop shows enhancement of the cisternal segment of both oculomotor nerves ➔ as well as enhancement in the right cavernous segment ➔. The patient was subsequently found to have Lyme disease (serologically documented).*

TERMINOLOGY

Abbreviations

- Lyme disease (LD), Lyme neuroborreliosis (LNB)

Definitions

- Multisystem inflammatory disease
  - Caused by spirochete *Borrelia burgdorferi* (different subspecies in Europe)
  - Transmitted by hard-bodied tick bite

IMAGING

General Features

- Best diagnostic clue
  - MS-like lesions + cranial neuritis
  - Meningoradiculoneuritis (Bannwarth syndrome) in Europe
- Location
  - Periventricular white matter (WM)
  - Cranial nerves (CN7 > CN3 and CN5)
  - Cauda equina, leptomeninges
- Size
  - 2-8 mm (large "tumefactive" lesions rare)

CT Findings

- NECT
  - Usually normal

MR Findings

- T2WI
  - Hyperintensities in periventricular WM, spinal cord
- DWI
  - Some lesions may show restriction
- T1WI C+
  - Variable enhancement
    - WM lesions/meninges/cauda equina
    - ± CN enhancement (including CN7 root exit zone, fundal tuft)

Imaging Recommendations

- Protocol advice
  - Brain MR (include T1 C+, DWI)

DIFFERENTIAL DIAGNOSIS

Demyelinating Disease

- WM lesions; lesions in optic nerve, spinal cord, callosal-septal interface more common in MS

Vasculitis

- T2 lesions ± arterial narrowing (DSA)

Sarcoidosis

- Meningeal, perivascular spaces, infundibulum

PATHOLOGY

General Features

- Etiology
  - Spirochete *Borrelia burgdorferi* (USA)
  - Transmitted by hard-bodied ticks of genus *Ixodid*

Microscopic Features

- Perivascular lymphocyte/plasma cell infiltrates
  - Endo-/peri-/epineurial blood vessels
  - Causes endarteritis obliterans
- Axonal degeneration
- Lymphocytes, plasma cells accumulate in autonomic ganglia

CLINICAL ISSUES

Presentation

- Most common signs/symptoms
  - Early local: Round, outwardly expanding rash ("bull's-eye")
    - ± flu-like symptoms
  - Early disseminated: Erythema migrans (may develop at sites different from tick bite)
    - Neurologic symptoms: Facial nerve palsy, meningitis, mild encephalitis, memory loss
  - Late: Brain, nerves, eyes, joints, heart
    - Knee most common joint involved
- Clinical profile
  - Confirmation of diagnosis: ELISA, PCR

Demographics

- Epidemiology
  - Most common tick-borne disease in USA (also occurs in Europe)
    - Approximately 10,000 new cases in USA per year
    - > 90% in Midatlantic states, Michigan, Minnesota
    - Peak incidence: May through August
  - White tail deer/white-footed mouse most important reservoirs

Natural History & Prognosis

- Progressive debilitating disorder if not treated early
- 10-15% of untreated patients develop neurologic manifestations
- Most recover with minimal or no residual deficits

Treatment

- Doxycycline, tetracycline, chloramphenicol; amoxicillin (children)
- Ketolides (new, experimental)

DIAGNOSTIC CHECKLIST

Consider

- Lyme neuroborreliosis if MS-like lesions in patient with erythema migrans
  - ± enhancing CNs, cauda equina
- Geography, recreational/travel history, season of year

SELECTED REFERENCES

1. Hildenbrand P et al: Lyme neuroborreliosis: manifestations of a rapidly emerging zoonosis. AJNR Am J Neuroradiol. 30(6):1079-87, 2009
2. Kalina P et al: Lyme disease of the brainstem. Neuroradiology. 47(12):903-7, 2005

ACQUIRED HIV ENCEPHALITIS

Key Facts

Terminology

- HIV-1 encephalitis/HIV-1 encephalopathy (HIVE)
- HIV-associated neurocognitive disorders (HAND)
- Moderate cognitive impairment common despite good virologic response to therapy
- Cause = direct effect of HIV brain infection itself
  - Opportunistic infections absent
  - Cognitive, behavioral, motor abnormalities in 25-70%
  - Most frequent neurological manifestation of HIV infection

Imaging

- CT
  - Atrophy
  - Bilateral periventricular/diffuse WM hypointensities
  - Basal ganglia, cerebellum, brainstem hypodensity
- MR
  - Diffuse "hazy" hyperintense WM on T2/FLAIR
  - Nonenhancing (if present consider PML, IRIS)
  - MRS may detect ↓ metabolites during asymptomatic stage
  - Nonenhancing (if present, consider opportunistic infections, IRIS)

Pathology

- HIV has ability to cause neurologic disease
  - Does not replicate within neural/glial cells
  - Microglial nodules with multinucleated giant cells
- WM pallor early, neocortical infection/atrophy late

Diagnostic Checklist

- Evidence of "cerebral atrophy" by CT/MR does not indicate AIDS dementia complex in HIV(+) patient
- Consider reversible causes 1st (dehydration, malnutrition, protein depletion, alcoholism)

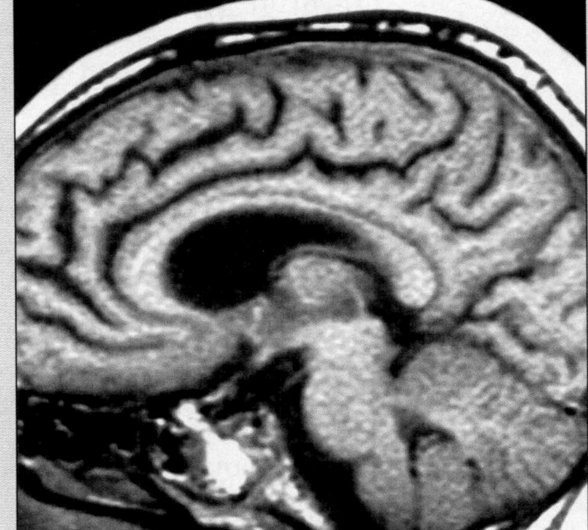

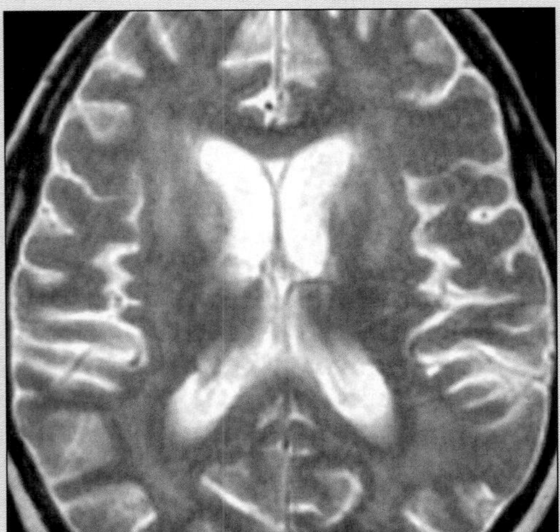

(Left) *Sagittal T1WI MR in an 11-year-old HIV-positive patient shows generalized atrophy, diffusely enlarged sulci, and thinned corpus callosum.* ***(Right)*** *Axial T2WI in the same patient shows diffuse, symmetric periventricular white matter hyperintense signal abnormality, highly suggestive of HIV encephalopathy (HIVE). This symmetrical pattern would not be expected in progressive multifocal leukoencephalopathy, another white matter disease that affects HIV-positive patients.*

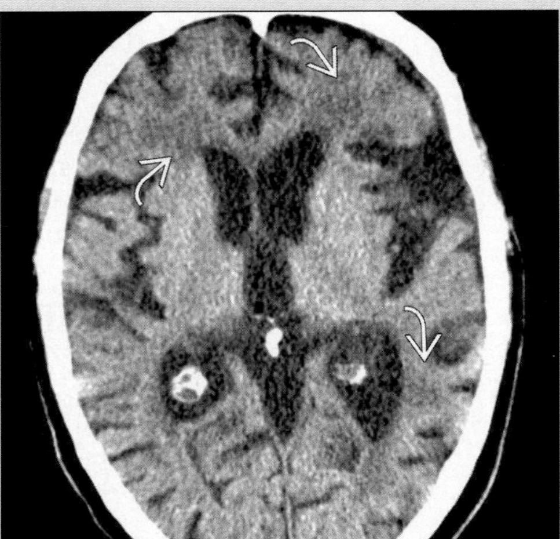

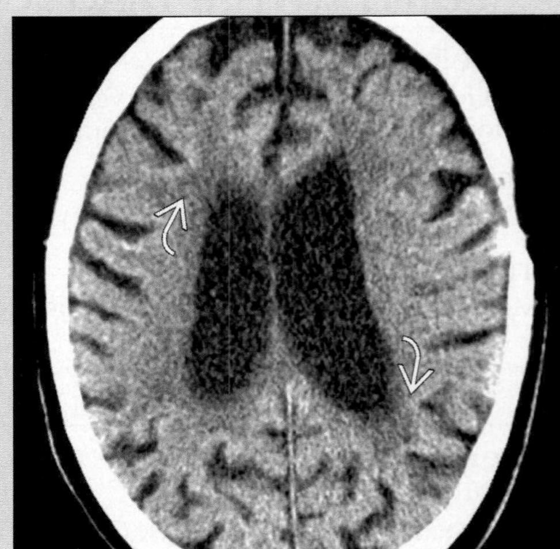

(Left) *Axial NECT in a 38-year-old man with longstanding HIV/AIDS, who was receiving HAART, was obtained for decreasing cognitive function. Note the gross atrophy and low density ➔ within the subcortical white matter.* ***(Right)*** *Axial NECT in the same patient shows characteristic low density in the periventricular white matter ➔ along with diffusely enlarged sulci and lateral ventricles.*

ACQUIRED HIV ENCEPHALITIS

TERMINOLOGY

Definitions

- HIV-1 encephalitis/encephalopathy (HIVE)
- Cause = direct effect of HIV infection itself on brain
  - Opportunistic infections absent
  - Cognitive, behavioral, motor abnormalities in 25-70%
  - HIV-associated neurocognitive disorders (HAND) = most frequent neurological manifestations of HIV infection
- Moderate cognitive impairment common despite good virologic response to therapy

IMAGING

General Features

- Best diagnostic clue
  - Atrophy + bilateral diffuse white matter (WM) abnormalities
    - Pathology/imaging varies with patient age, acuity of onset
- Location
  - Bilateral periventricular/centrum semiovale WM, basal ganglia, cerebellum, brainstem
- Size
  - Variable, often diffuse
- Morphology
  - Extends to gray-white matter junction

CT Findings

- NECT
  - Children: Atrophy and diffuse WM hypodensity
    - In utero HIV infection: Characteristic bilateral and symmetrical calcifications in basal ganglia and frontal WM with eventual contrast enhancement
  - Adults: Normal or mild atrophy, WM hypodensity
  - No mass effect
- CECT
  - Usually no contrast enhancement

MR Findings

- T1WI
  - WM abnormality may not be evident
- T2WI
  - 2 imaging patterns
    - Focal abnormalities of high signal intensity
    - Diffuse moderate-high signal WM changes
  - Distribution and extent of WM lesions does not always correlate with clinical picture
- FLAIR
  - Same imaging patterns as T2WI
  - Allows early detection of small (< 2 cm) lesions in cortical/subcortical and deep WM locations
  - Greater overall lesion conspicuity (when compared to T2-weighted fast spin-echo imaging)
- T1WI C+
  - No enhancement in involved regions
- MRS
  - AIDS patients with CD4(+) < 200/mm³, neurologic evidence of AIDS dementia complex, and atrophy
    - ^{1}H-MRS in subcortical region shows ↓ N-acetyl aspartate (neuronal loss) and ↑ choline in WM (astrocytosis or microglial proliferation)
  - Asymptomatic patients with normal cognition
    - ^{1}H-MRS in subcortical region shows only ↑ choline
- 2 major consequences of brain tissue HIV infection
  - Atrophy of brain parenchyma due to neuronal death
  - Alterations of deep WM (usually periventricular regions) → high signal intensity on T2WI
- Magnetization transfer ratio (MTR)
  - MTR allows differentiation of HIVE from progressive multifocal leukoencephalopathy (PML)
    - Dramatic ↓ in MTR for PML lesions (as compared to HIVE lesions) likely due to demyelination
  - Diffusion tensor imaging
    - May show early ↓ fractional anisotropy in HIV-associated cognitive impairment

Imaging Recommendations

- Best imaging tool
  - MR better than CT for WM lesion detection
  - MRS may detect changes in WM even during asymptomatic stage (in patients with laboratory evidence of immunosuppression)
- Protocol advice
  - CT scan should be performed when
    - New seizure, new onset of headache, depressed, or altered orientation
  - MR scan should be performed when
    - CT shows focal mass

DIFFERENTIAL DIAGNOSIS

Progressive Multifocal Leukoencephalopathy (PML)

- Patchy WM lesions
  - May be unilateral but more often bilateral, asymmetric
  - Parietooccipital locations most common
  - Subcortical U-fibers affected (unlike HIV or CMV)
- No enhancement; if present, consider immune reconstitution inflammatory syndrome (IRIS)

CMV-Associated CNS Disease

- Encephalitis (diffuse WM hyperintensities)
- Ventriculitis (ependymal enhancement)

Herpes Virus Encephalitis

- Herpes simplex virus (HSV), human herpes virus 6 (HHV-6): Initially hippocampal and medial temporal lesions

Toxoplasmosis

- Ring-enhancing mass(es)
- Hyperintense lesions on T2WI/FLAIR, DWI

Primary CNS Lymphoma

- Solitary/multifocal lesions, deep > subcortical lesions
- Marked predilection for basal ganglia, cerebellar hemispheres, thalamus, brain stem, corpus callosum, and subependymal region
- CECT: Usually rim enhancement in HIV(+) patients

- Positive thallium-201 SPECT

Cryptococcosis

- "Gelatinous" pseudocysts within perivascular spaces
- Meningoencephalitis ± vasculitis, infarction

PATHOLOGY

General Features

- Etiology
  - During primary infection, HIV is transported into brain by monocyte/macrophage system
  - HIV has ability to cause neurologic disease but does not replicate within neural/glial cells
  - Myelin destruction is not typical; T2WI WM hyperintensities may be due to ↑ water content
  - Inflammatory (T-cell) reaction with vasculitis, leptomeningitis
- Genetics
  - HIV genomic → more neurovirulent strains
  - Dementia affects only some patients depending on whether critical mutations occur in HIV strain
- Associated abnormalities
  - HIVE can occur in conjunction with other AIDS-related abnormalities (e.g., other infections)
  - Progressive encephalopathy in children is frequently associated with myelopathy
- Hallmark of HIVE: Microglial nodules with multinucleated giant cells (MGCs)
- Reactive gliosis, focal necrosis, and demyelination
- Mild neuronal loss; minor inflammatory changes
- Viral entry into brain occurs very early after systemic infection

Staging, Grading, & Classification

- 3 types of neuropathological findings
  - Finding 1: HIV encephalitis
    - Multiple disseminated foci of microglia, macrophages, and MGCs; if no MGCs found, HIV antigen/nucleic acids required
  - Finding 2: HIV leukoencephalopathy
    - Diffuse and symmetric WM damage (myelin loss, reactive astrogliosis, macrophages, and MGCs); if no MGCs found, HIV antigen/nucleic acids required
  - Finding 3: HIV giant cells
    - PAS(+) mono- or multinuclear macrophages
- Mild HIVE: Finding 1 without MGCs
- Moderate HIVE: Finding 1, 2, or 3
- Severe HIVE: Cerebral atrophy with finding 1 or 2

Gross Pathologic & Surgical Features

- Early: WM pallor
- Late: Neocortical infection, atrophy

Microscopic Features

- HIVE
  - Infected cells: Mostly macrophages and microglia; few astroglia; rarely oligodendrocytes
  - Neurons undergo secondary damage
  - Minor inflammatory changes: Perivascular macrophage infiltrates and microglial nodules
- Progressive encephalopathy in pediatric AIDS population
  - Inflammatory infiltrates with MGCs
  - Extensive calcific vasculopathy primarily in small vessels of basal ganglia, also cerebral WM and pons
  - Atrophy from impaired development of myelin or myelin loss

CLINICAL ISSUES

Presentation

- Most common signs/symptoms
  - Subcortical dementia with cognitive, motor, and behavioral deficits
- Clinical profile
  - HIV cognitive syndrome: Minor or major (dementia)
  - Deficits of central motor function
  - Behavioral: Pseudodementia (depression), delirium, and confusion
  - Pediatric: Microcephaly, cognitive defects, weakness, pyramidal signs, ataxia, and seizures

Demographics

- Age
  - Both pediatric and adult HIV(+) patients
- Gender
  - No gender preference; gender distribution of HIVE reflects that of HIV infection
- Epidemiology
  - 33-67% of adult AIDS patients and 30-50% of pediatric AIDS patients are affected by HIVE
  - HIVE occurs before opportunistic infections and neoplasms; prevalence unrelated to disease stage

Natural History & Prognosis

- Cognitive decline occurs once patients become immunocompromised
- Slowly progressive impairment of fine motor control, verbal fluency, and short-term memory
- After few months: Severe deterioration and subcortical dementia with near vegetative state as final stage

Treatment

- Highly active antiretroviral therapy (HAART) cannot prevent occurrence of HIVE but ↓ HIVE severity
  - HAART era: ↓ frequency of severe HIVE, but ↑ frequency of mild-moderate HIVE

DIAGNOSTIC CHECKLIST

Consider

- Evidence of "cerebral atrophy" by CT/MR does not indicate AIDS dementia complex in HIV(+) patient
  - Consider reversible causes 1st (dehydration, malnutrition, protein depletion, alcoholism)

Image Interpretation Pearls

- Characteristic parenchymal changes often missed by CT, but detected by MR (T2, FLAIR)

SELECTED REFERENCES

1. Letendre SL et al: Neurologic complications of HIV disease and their treatment. Top HIV Med. 17(2):46-56, 2009

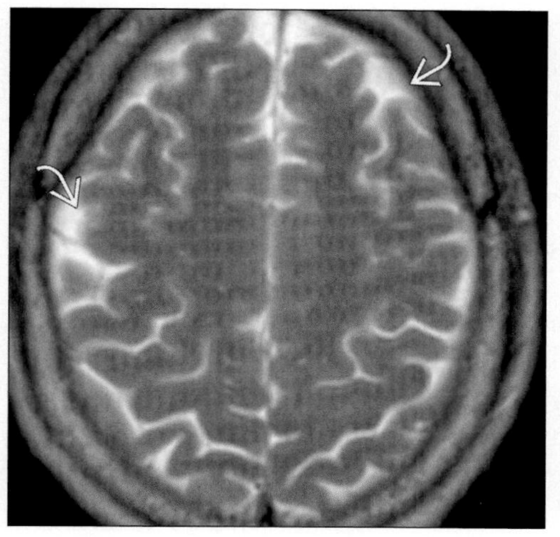

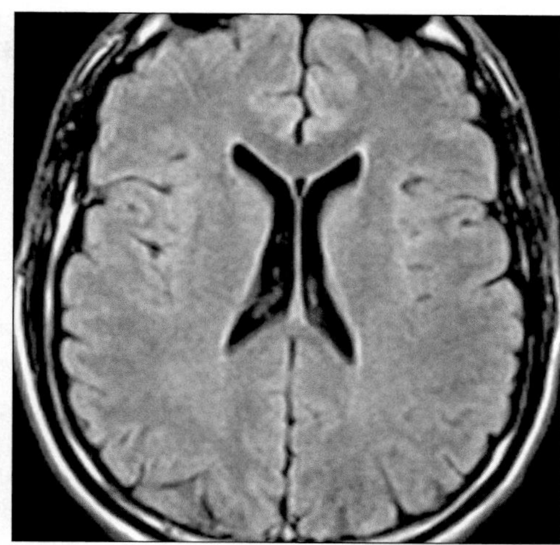

(Left) *Axial T2WI in an HIV-positive patient with early signs of subcortical dementia shows a variant appearance. Atrophy is obvious near the vertex with an increase in the CSF spaces around the brain ⮫. HIV encephalitis most commonly presents on imaging as diffuse "hazy" white matter abnormality in association with atrophy. However, occasionally atrophy may be the dominant feature, as in this case.* ***(Right)*** *FLAIR image in the same patient reveals mild atrophy without significant white matter disease.*

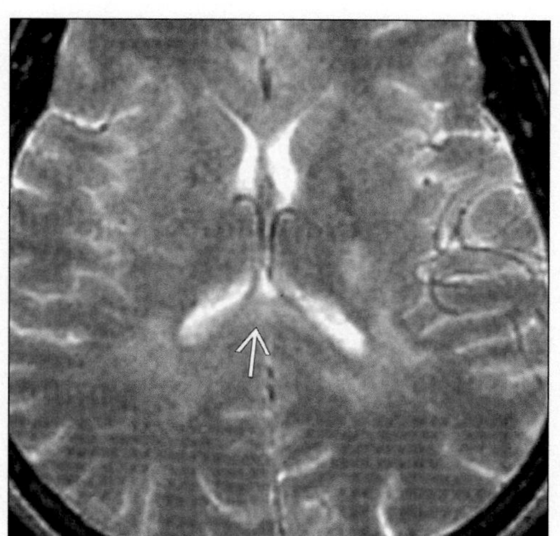

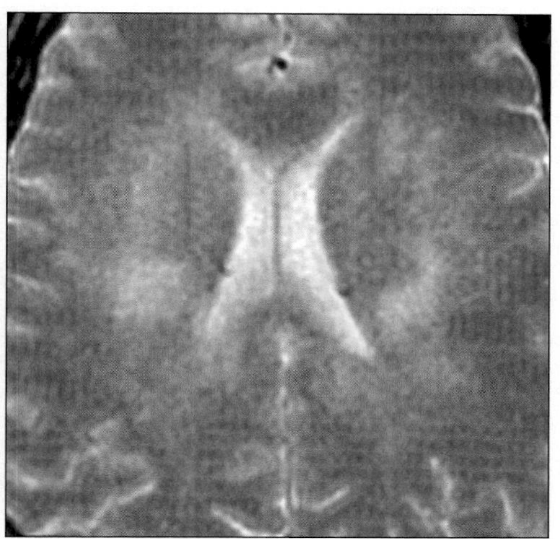

(Left) *White matter changes may appear in the brains of HIV/AIDS patients before atrophy and dementia ensue, as happened in this 34-year-old HIV-positive man with headaches. The ventricles appear normal, but bilateral "hazy" white matter hyperintensity is present, including abnormality in the corpus callosum ➡.* ***(Right)*** *Axial T2WI in the same patient shows ill-defined, multifocal, bilateral, asymmetric, "hazy," hyperintense white matter signal intensity.*

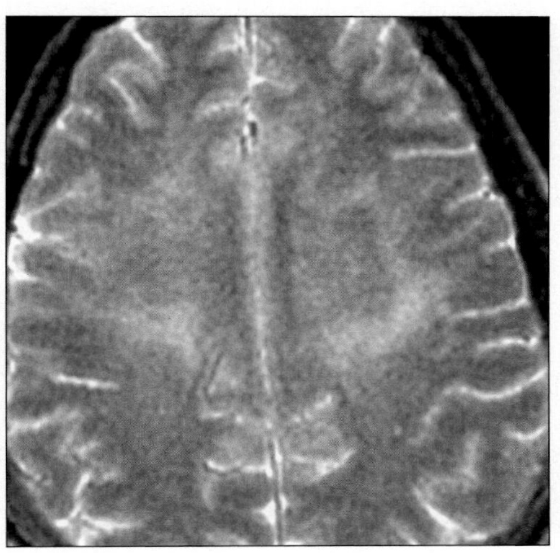

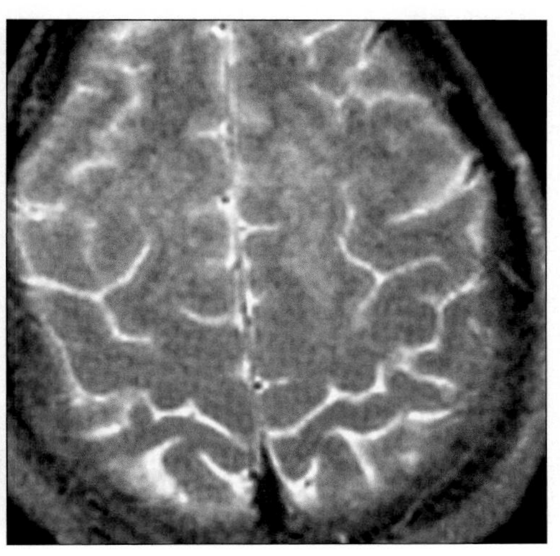

(Left) *Axial T2WI in the same patient shows ill-defined regions of hyperintense signal in the centrum semiovale bilaterally. These findings could potentially represent the effects of PML. However, PML is usually more asymmetric than HIV encephalitis.* ***(Right)*** *Axial T2WI shows "hazy," bilateral but somewhat asymmetrical, confluent areas of increased signal intensity in the white matter of the cerebral hemispheres. These findings are classic for HIV encephalitis.*

ACQUIRED TOXOPLASMOSIS

Key Facts

Terminology

- Opportunistic infection
  - Caused by parasite *Toxoplasma gondii*
- Most common CNS infection in AIDS patients

Imaging

- CT
  - Ill-defined hypodense lesions + edema
  - Basal ganglia, corticomedullary junction, thalamus, cerebellum
  - Rim, nodular, "target" enhancement
- MR
  - T2 hypointense
  - T1 C+ "target" sign highly suggestive

Top Differential Diagnoses

- Lymphoma
  - Solitary mass in patient with HIV/AIDS? Lymphoma > toxoplasmosis
- Other opportunistic infections
  - Cryptococcosis, PML (usually does not enhance)

Pathology

- Usually reactivation of latent infection
  - 20-70% of population seropositive for *T. gondii* in USA

Clinical Issues

- TE = most common mass lesion in AIDS patients
- Fever, malaise, headache
  - Personality change, seizures later

Diagnostic Checklist

- Multiple "target" lesions on T1WI C+ that are dark on T2WI? Consider TE
- TE lesions usually resolve in 2-4 weeks

*(**Left**) Axial gross pathology specimen sectioned through the ventricles in a patient with HIV/AIDS shows a toxoplasmosis abscess in the right lentiform nucleus →. The lesion is necrotic and poorly demarcated. (Courtesy R. Hewlett, PhD.) (**Right**) Axial T1WI C+ MR shows several ring-enhancing lesions in the thalami and left occipital lobe ⇨. Note the large lesion showing a classic "target" appearance ➡. These lesions were hypointense on T2WI.*

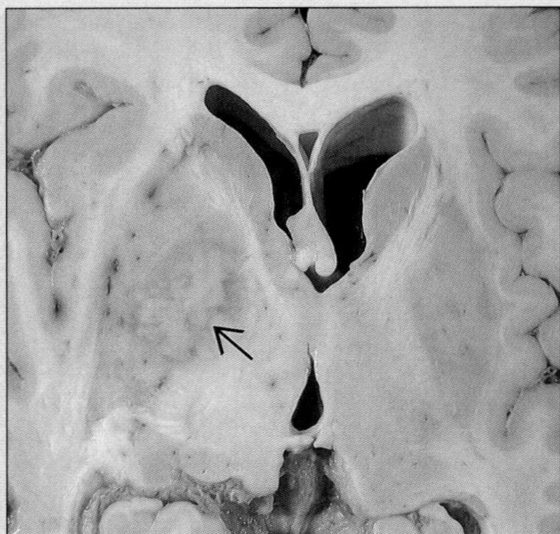

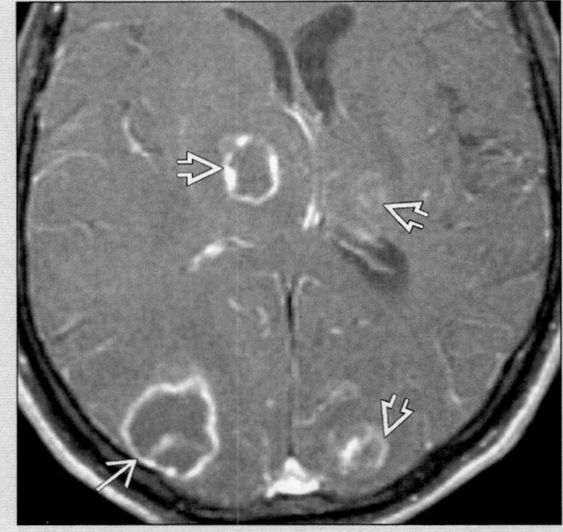

*(**Left**) Axial FLAIR MR in a 30-year-old man with HIV/AIDS shows multifocal parenchymal lesions, 1 of which has a very hypointense rim → with a hyperintense necrotic center ⇨. Lesions showed rim and "target" enhancement on T1WI C+. The key differential consideration is toxoplasmosis vs. lymphoma. (**Right**) Axial MR perfusion in the same patient shows very low CBV ⇨, suggesting toxoplasmosis rather than lymphoma. Antitoxoplasmosis therapy was instituted; the lesions regressed in size and enhancement on follow-up studies.*

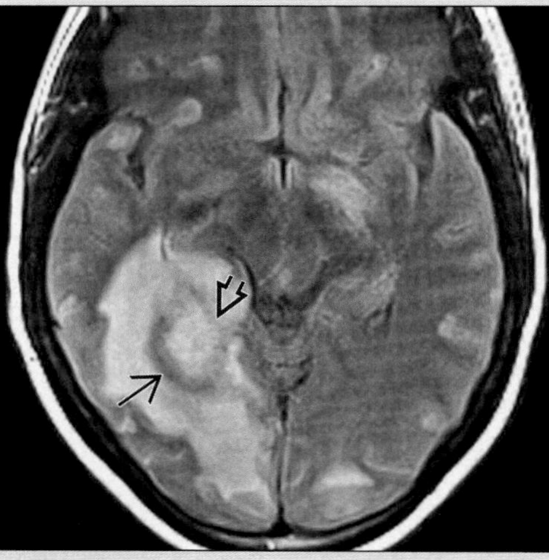

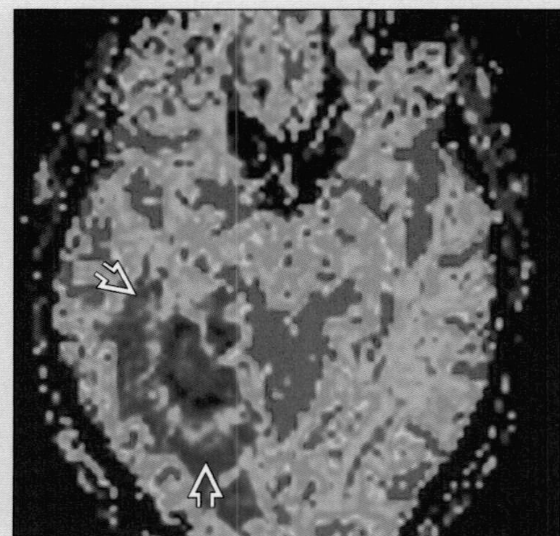

ACQUIRED TOXOPLASMOSIS

TERMINOLOGY

Abbreviations

- Toxoplasmosis encephalitis (TE)

Definitions

- Opportunistic parasitic infection caused by *Toxoplasma gondii*
- Most common opportunistic CNS infection, mass lesion in patients with AIDS

IMAGING

General Features

- Best diagnostic clue
  - T2 hypointense lesion with peripheral nodular enhancement
- Location
  - Basal ganglia, corticomedullary junction, thalamus, cerebellum most common sites
- Size
  - Variable but generally 2-3 cm in diameter
- Morphology
  - Round or oval

Imaging Recommendations

- Best imaging tool
  - MR for sensitivity; thallium-201-SPECT for specificity
- Protocol advice
  - MR with T2WI, FLAIR, T1 C+ plus DWI, MRS

CT Findings

- NECT
  - Ill-defined hypodense lesions with edema
- CECT
  - Multiple rim-/nodular-enhancing masses

MR Findings

- T1WI
  - Ill-defined hypointense lesions
  - Occasionally lesions are hyperintense
    - Not due to hemorrhage or calcification
    - May be coagulative necrosis/proteins
- T2WI
  - Hypointense + hyperintense peripheral edema
- FLAIR
  - May see "target" sign
- DWI
  - Increased diffusivity in necrotic centers
- PWI
  - Extremely hypovascular
- T1WI C+
  - Rim, nodular, punctate enhancement
  - "Target" sign highly suggestive of TE
    - Enhancing nodule within enhancing rim
- MRS
  - Prominent lipid peak

DIFFERENTIAL DIAGNOSIS

Lymphoma

- Solitary mass in patient with HIV/AIDS?
  - Lymphoma > toxoplasmosis

Other Opportunistic Infections

- Cryptococcosis, PML (usually does not enhance)

PATHOLOGY

General Features

- Etiology
  - Usually reactivation of latent infection
    - 20-70% of USA population seropositive for *T. gondii*
  - Definitive host = cat
    - Any mammal can be carrier (intermediate host)
      - Parasites invade cells, forming bradyzoites
      - Cell rupture releases tachyzoites

CLINICAL ISSUES

Presentation

- Most common signs/symptoms
  - Fever, malaise, headache
  - Later: Personality change, seizures

Demographics

- Epidemiology
  - CNS TE occurs in 3-10% of AIDS patients in USA
    - 35-50% of AIDS patients in Europe and Africa
  - More common when CD4(+) counts are < 200 cells/μL

Natural History & Prognosis

- In resource-poor socioeconomic environments, median survival is 28 months

Treatment

- Pyrimethamine plus sulfadiazine; trimethoprim sulfamethoxazole is acceptable alternative
- TE lesions usually resolve in 2-4 weeks; lack of resolution suggests another etiology

DIAGNOSTIC CHECKLIST

Consider

- Primary CNS lymphoma

Image Interpretation Pearls

- Multiple "target" lesions on T1WI C+; dark on T2WI

Reporting Tips

- Know whether therapy has been administered; if poor response, suggest alternative diagnosis

SELECTED REFERENCES

1. Masamed R et al: Cerebral toxoplasmosis: case review and description of a new imaging sign. Clin Radiol. 64(5):560-3, 2009

ACQUIRED CMV

Key Facts

Terminology

- Acquired CNS cytomegalovirus infections: Meningitis, encephalitis, ventriculitis, transverse myelitis, radiculomyelitis, chorioretinitis
- Immunocompromised (AIDS, organ transplant) patients are at risk ⇒ reactivation of previously silent infection

Imaging

- Best diagnostic clue: Ventriculitis with fluid-debris level with ependymal enhancement in immunocompromised patient
- Encephalitis: T2 hyperintense mass, variable enhancement
- May mimic HIV encephalitis with patchy nonspecific T2 hyperintense lesions
- Contrast should be used for imaging of all immunocompromised patients

Top Differential Diagnoses

- HIV encephalitis
- PML
- Toxoplasmosis

Clinical Issues

- Primary CMV infection is generally asymptomatic
- Infection may occur 2° to reactivation of latent viral infection or newly acquired via organ or bone marrow transplant from seropositive donor
  - CMV disseminates to CNS in late stages of HIV infection, low CD4(+) count
  - Clinically may mimic HIV encephalitis
- M > > > F
- Disease manifestations vary in severity depending on degree of host immunosuppression
- HAART: Markedly ↓ incidence of CMV disease in AIDS; ↑ immunocompetence against CMV

*(**Left**) Axial FLAIR MR shows mild ventriculomegaly and periventricular hyperintensities ➔ related to ventriculo-encephalitis. (**Right**) Axial T1WI C+ MR in the same patient shows ependymal ➔ and periventricular ➔ enhancement. This patient was immunocompromised, with ventriculitis and associated encephalitis. CMV encephalitis is commonly a ventriculo-encephalitis, involving the periventricular white matter. However, CMV may also cause hemorrhagic or necrotic lesions or micronodular encephalitis.*

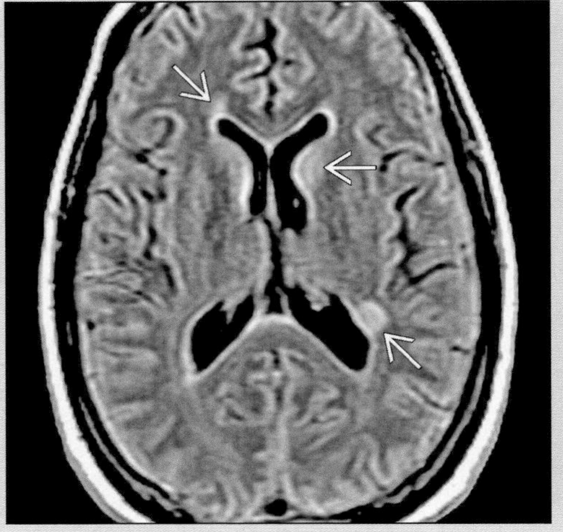

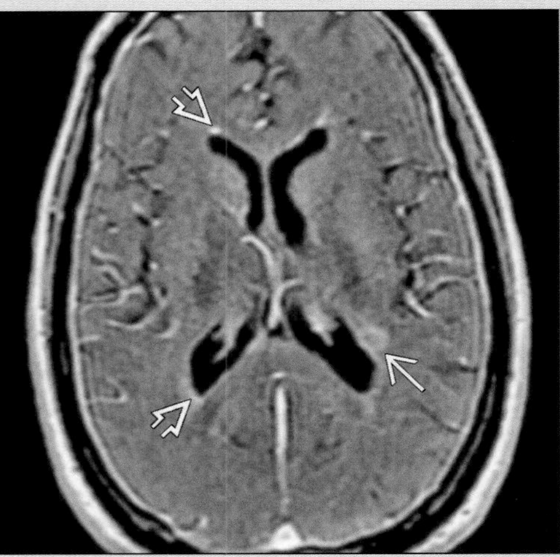

*(**Left**) Coronal T1WI C+ MR shows diffuse ependymal enhancement ➔ and mild ventriculomegaly in this AIDS patient with CMV ventriculitis. Ventriculitis in an AIDS patient is most commonly caused by CMV. (**Right**) Coronal T1WI C+ MR in the same patient shows marked ependymal enhancement of the temporal horns and right basal ganglia enhancing masses ➔ related to ventriculitis and encephalitis. The basal ganglia lesions cannot be reliably differentiated from toxoplasmosis encephalitis.*

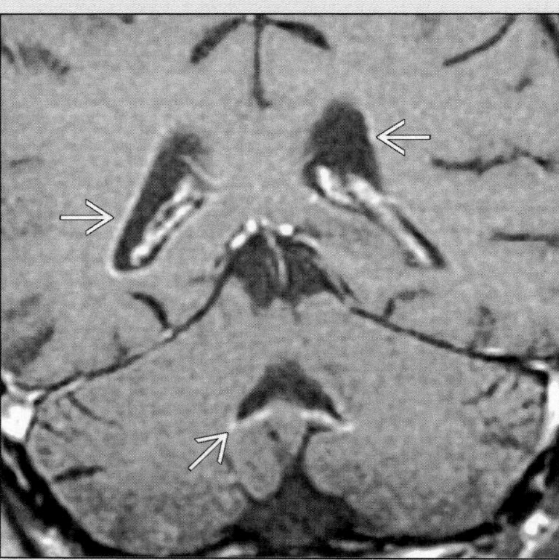

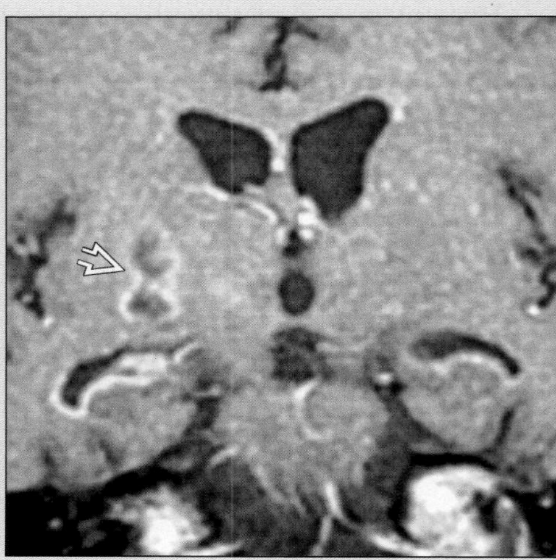

ACQUIRED CMV

TERMINOLOGY

Abbreviations

- Cytomegalovirus (CMV) infection

Definitions

- Acquired CNS infections: Meningitis, encephalitis, ventriculitis, retinitis, polyradiculopathy, myelitis
- Primary CMV infection: Generally no symptoms in healthy adults
- Immunocompromised (AIDS, organ transplant) patients at risk ⇒ reactivation of previously silent infection

IMAGING

General Features

- Best diagnostic clue
  - Ventriculitis in immunocompromised patient
    - Enlarged ventricles with ependymal enhancement
  - Absent periventricular Ca++ (in congenital CMV)
  - Encephalitis may occur, commonly periventricular
- Location
  - Ventricles (ependymal and subependymal)
  - Periventricular white matter (WM)
- Morphology: Encephalitis may cause "mass" lesion

Imaging Recommendations

- Best imaging tool: MR with contrast

MR Findings

- T1WI
  - Encephalitis: Hypointense mass
  - Ventriculitis: Enlarged ventricles with debris level
- T2WI
  - Encephalitis: Hyperintense periventricular mass
  - Ventriculitis: Enlarged ventricles with surrounding hyperintensity
- FLAIR
  - Encephalitis: Hyperintense mass
  - Ventriculitis: Enlarged ventricles with surrounding hyperintensity
  - May cause nonspecific, multifocal, periventricular WM hyperintensity
- T1WI C+
  - Encephalitis: No significant enhancement typically
    - May become necrotizing, with enhancement
  - Ventriculitis: Ependymal and periventricular enhancement
- MRS: Necrotizing encephalitis may show ↑ Cho, ↑ Lac
- PWI: Lower rCBV than tumor

DIFFERENTIAL DIAGNOSIS

HIV Encephalitis

- Periventricular patchy WM T2 hyperintensity with atrophy; no enhancement

PML

- T2 hyperintense WM lesions involving subcortical U-fibers; often frontal/parietooccipital
- Subcortical U-fibers > periventricular WM > gray matter

Toxoplasmosis

- Multiple ring-enhancing lesions
- Deep gray nuclei and cerebral hemispheres

ADEM

- Patchy periventricular WM T2 hyperintensities, with enhancement; 10-14 days after infection/vaccination

PATHOLOGY

General Features

- Etiology
  - Vast majority of adults are infected with CMV
  - Transmission of CMV chiefly via contact with infected secretions
  - CNS disease primarily in immunodepressed host
    - Reaches brain hematogenously
- Associated abnormalities
  - HHV-6 reactivation associated with CMV infection in post liver transplant patients
  - JC virus may be transactivated by CMV

Microscopic Features

- Cytomegalic inclusion cell: Enlarged cells with intranuclear inclusions, histologic "owl's eyes"

CLINICAL ISSUES

Presentation

- Most common signs/symptoms
  - CMV encephalitis: Confusion, gait disturbance, cranial neuropathies, hyperreflexia

Demographics

- Epidemiology
  - Most children acquire CMV infection early in life, with adult seroprevalence approaching 100%
  - CMV disseminates to CNS in late stages of HIV infection, low CD4(+) count
  - Prior to advent of highly active antiretroviral therapy (HAART) for HIV, CMV retinitis was most common cause of blindness in AIDS (> 90%)

Natural History & Prognosis

- Primary infection is generally asymptomatic; acute febrile illness rare, termed CMV mononucleosis
- Infection may occur 2° to reactivation of latent viral infection or be newly acquired via organ or bone marrow transplant (BMT) from seropositive donor

Treatment

- Ganciclovir and other antiviral drugs for severe disease
- HAART: ↓ incidence of CMV disease in AIDS

SELECTED REFERENCES

1. Pirskanen-Matell R et al: Impairment of short-term memory and Korsakoff syndrome are common in AIDS patients with cytomegalovirus encephalitis. Eur J Neurol. 16(1):48-53, 2009
2. Miller RF et al: Comparison of magnetic resonance imaging with neuropathological findings in the diagnosis of HIV and CMV associated CNS disease in AIDS. J Neurol Neurosurg Psychiatry. 62(4):346-51, 1997

CRYPTOCOCCOSIS

Key Facts

Terminology

- *Cryptococcus neoformans* infection
- Opportunistic fungal infection that typically affects HIV and other immunosuppressed patients
- Cryptococci spread along PVS to deep brain: Basal ganglia (BG), thalamus, brainstem, cerebellum, dentate nucleus, periventricular white matter (WM)

Imaging

- Dilated perivascular spaces in deep gray nuclei of AIDS patient, often no enhancement
  - Degree of enhancement depends on cell-mediated immunity of host
- May see miliary or leptomeningeal enhancing nodules + gelatinous pseudocysts
- Cryptococcoma: Ring-like or solid enhancement
- Dilated PVS in AIDS patients ⇒ consider cryptococcus infection
- 4 imaging patterns: Miliary enhancing parenchymal nodules, leptomeningeal-cisternal nodules, cryptococcoma, gelatinous pseudocysts

Top Differential Diagnoses

- Acquired toxoplasmosis
- Tuberculosis
- Primary CNS lymphoma

Clinical Issues

- CNS infection related to hematogenous dissemination from lungs
- Headache most common symptom
- Most common fungal infection in AIDS patients
- 3rd most common infection seen in AIDS patients (HIV > toxoplasmosis > crypto)
- Indian ink test: Highly specific
  - Antigen titers correspond to severity of illness

(Left) Coronal graphic shows multiple dilated perivascular (Virchow-Robin) spaces ⇒, filled with fungi and mucoid material, resulting in gelatinous pseudocysts. Gelatinous pseudocysts are characteristic of cryptococcal infection in AIDS. (Right) Axial T2WI MR shows multiple dilated perivascular spaces ⇒ in this immunocompromised patient with cryptococcal meningitis. Gelatinous pseudocysts are most commonly located in the basal ganglia and thalami but may be seen in the brainstem, cerebellum, and cerebral hemispheres.

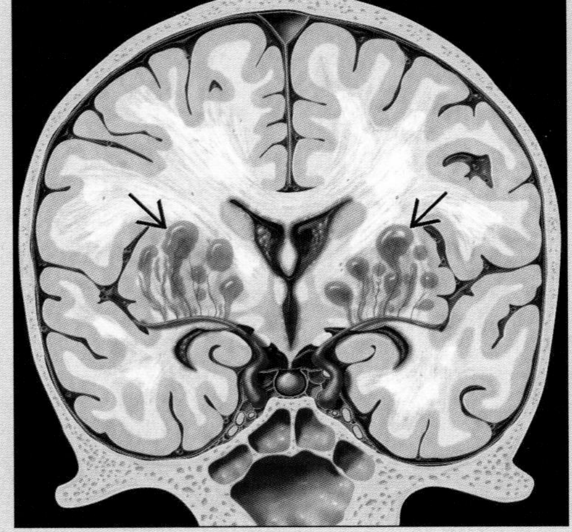

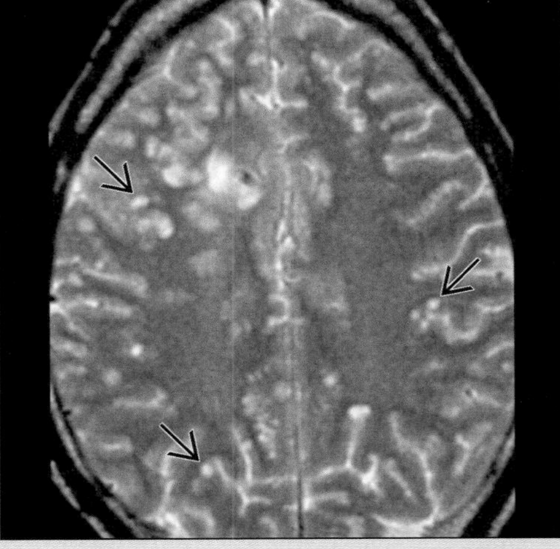

(Left) Axial FLAIR MR shows bilateral dilated perivascular spaces ➡ with hyperintense rims in this AIDS patient with Cryptococcus meningitis. Hydrocephalus is a common complication of this infection. (Right) Axial T1WI C+ MR in the same patient shows subependymal enhancement ➡ along the frontal horns of the lateral ventricles as well as nodular leptomeningeal enhancement ➡. Enhancement in Cryptococcus infection is dependent on the cell-mediated immunity of the host.

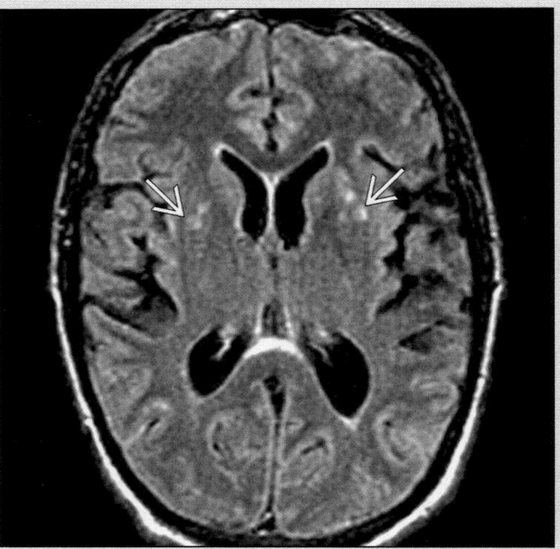

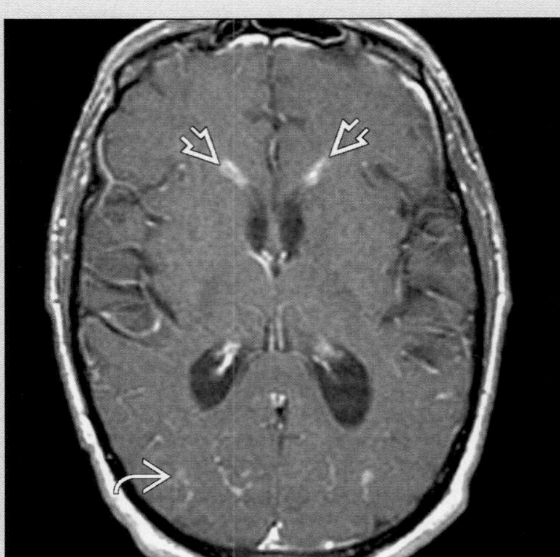

TERMINOLOGY

Definitions

- *Cryptococcus neoformans* infection
- Opportunistic fungal infection that typically affects HIV and other immunocompromised patients
- Pulmonary infection with subsequent transfer of circulating *Cryptococci* into subarachnoid spaces, perivascular spaces ⇒ leptomeningitis

IMAGING

General Features

- Best diagnostic clue
  - Dilated perivascular spaces in deep gray nuclei of AIDS patient, no enhancement
  - Degree of enhancement depends on cell-mediated immunity of host
    - Immunocompromised: Typically no C+
  - May see miliary or leptomeningeal enhancing nodules or cryptococcomas
- Location
  - Perivascular spaces (PVS)
  - Cryptococci spread along PVS to deep brain: Basal ganglia (BG), thalamus, brainstem, cerebellum, dentate nucleus, white matter (WM)
- Size: 2-3 mm nodules, up to 3-4 cm
- Morphology: Small round or oval-shaped lesions
  - May become confluent and form gelatinous pseudocysts or "soap bubbles"

Imaging Recommendations

- Best imaging tool: Contrast-enhanced MR

CT Findings

- CECT: Often normal
  - Subtle meningeal or miliary enhancement rare

MR Findings

- T2WI: PVS filled with fungi, isointense to CSF
- FLAIR: Multiple bilateral, small, cystic lesions
  - Follow CSF, may see small hyperintense rim
  - May form gelatinous pseudocysts
    - BG, thalamus, brainstem, cerebellum, periventricular and subcortical WM
  - Cryptococcoma: Hyperintense lesion
- T1 C+: Enhancement depends on host immune status
  - No enhancement is typical
    - May see leptomeningeal enhancement
  - Cryptococcoma: Ring-like or solid enhancement
  - Rare: Miliary or leptomeningeal enhancing nodules

DIFFERENTIAL DIAGNOSIS

Acquired Toxoplasmosis

- Multiple ring-enhancing masses + surrounding edema
- Typically BG and cerebral hemispheres

Tuberculosis

- Basal meningitis + parenchymal lesions (tuberculoma)
- Tuberculomas may be T2 hypointense

Primary CNS Lymphoma

- Enhancing lesion(s), often along ependymal surface
- T2 hypointense tumor

Neurosarcoid

- Leptomeningeal enhancement ± dural lesions

Enlarged Perivascular Spaces

- Typical locations, near anterior commissure
- Follow CSF on all MR sequences

PATHOLOGY

General Features

- Etiology
  - *Cryptococcus* is found in mammal and bird feces
  - In AIDS, CNS infection related to hematogenous dissemination from lungs

Gross Pathologic & Surgical Features

- Gelatinous mucoid material (pseudocysts) in or near prominent PVS in BG, midbrain, WM

Microscopic Features

- Large polysaccharide capsules stain with Indian ink

CLINICAL ISSUES

Presentation

- Most common signs/symptoms
  - Headache most common
- Other signs/symptoms
  - Seizure, blurred vision, focal neuro deficits (rare)
- Clinical profile
  - Lumbar puncture: ↑ CSF pressure, ↓ glucose, ↑ protein, mild to moderate leucocytosis

Demographics

- Epidemiology
  - 3rd most common infection seen in AIDS patients (HIV > toxoplasmosis > crypto)
    - 10% of AIDS patients have Cryptococcus infection

Treatment

- Antifungal treatment (i.e. amphotericin B)

DIAGNOSTIC CHECKLIST

Consider

- In AIDS patients with dilated PVS

SELECTED REFERENCES

1. Thurnher MM et al: Neuroimaging in the brain in HIV-1-infected patients. Neuroimaging Clin N Am. 18(1):93-117; viii, 2008
2. Saigal G et al: Unusual presentation of central nervous system cryptococcal infection in an immunocompetent patient. AJNR Am J Neuroradiol. 26(10):2522-6, 2005
3. Berkefeld J et al: Cryptococcus meningoencephalitis in AIDS: parenchymal and meningeal forms. Neuroradiology. 41(2):129-33, 1999

PROGRESSIVE MULTIFOCAL LEUKOENCEPHALOPATHY (PML)

Key Facts

Terminology

- Progressive multifocal leukoencephalopathy (PML)
- JC polyomavirus infects oligodendrocytes, causes demyelination in immunocompromised patients
- Associated with immunosuppression, often AIDS
  - Organ transplant, cancer, chemotherapy, myeloproliferative disease, and steroid treatment
  - Recently reported in treatment for multiple sclerosis (MS) and in rheumatic diseases

Imaging

- Multifocal T2 hyperintense demyelinating plaques involve subcortical white matter (WM), extend to deep WM; gray matter often spared until late stage
- Characteristic involvement of **subcortical U-fibers**
- Generally no contrast enhancement or mass effect
- Late: Confluent WM disease, cystic changes
- Propensity for frontal and parietooccipital region, thalamus, and basal ganglia
  - May involve brainstem and cerebellum
- May be solitary, multifocal, or widespread confluent

Top Differential Diagnoses

- HIV encephalitis
- ADEM
- Acquired CMV
- Immune reconstitution inflammatory syndrome

Clinical Issues

- Highly active antiretrovirus therapy (HAART) reported to improve survival

Diagnostic Checklist

- If multifocal subcortical white matter lesions without mass effect or enhancement in AIDS patients, consider PML over HIV encephalopathy

*(**Left**) Axial FLAIR MR in an AIDS patient shows bilateral, asymmetric hyperintensity in the frontal lobe white matter with involvement of the subcortical U-fibers, characteristic of PML. Note the lack of mass effect and involvement of the corpus callosum. (**Right**) Axial FLAIR MR shows white matter hyperintensity involving the right more than left temporal white matter and right cerebral peduncle ➔ related to PML in this immunocompromised patient. PML most commonly involves the frontal and parietooccipital regions.*

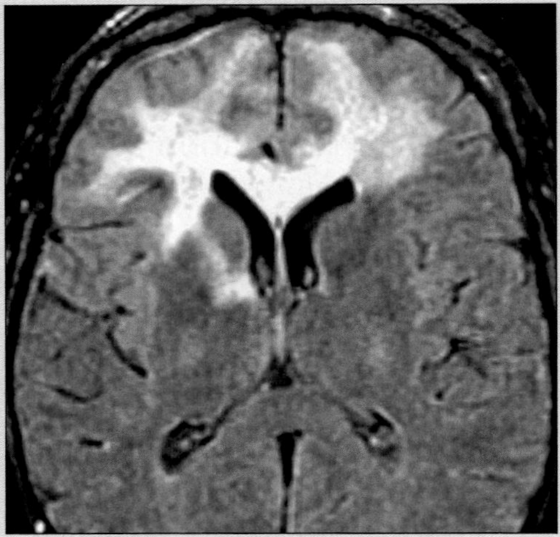

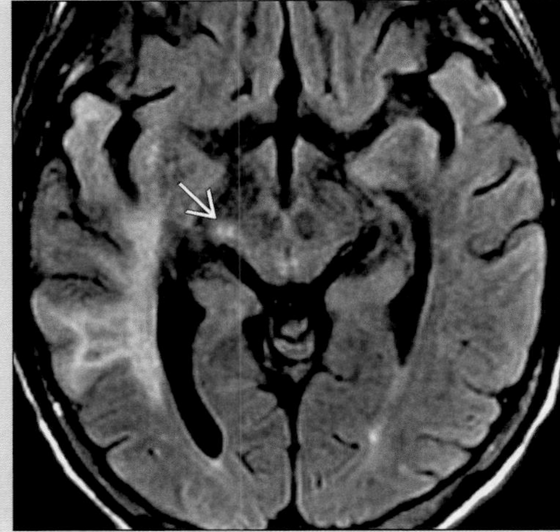

*(**Left**) Axial T2WI MR reveals extensive confluent white matter hyperintensity involving the left cerebral hemisphere without significant mass effect. There is involvement of the subcortical U-fibers, left basal ganglia, and bilateral thalami. Note the classic scalloped appearance ➲ at the gray-white interface. No enhancement is typical. (**Right**) Axial T2WI MR in the same patient shows confluent T2 hyperintensity with cavitary changes ➲ in the left cerebral white matter. Biopsy confirmed PML in this AIDS patient.*

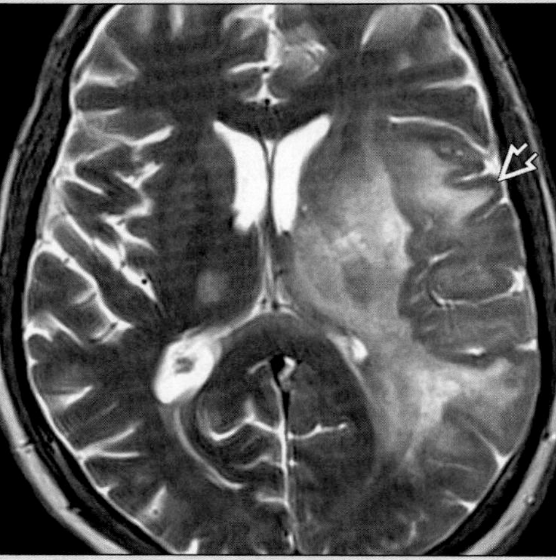

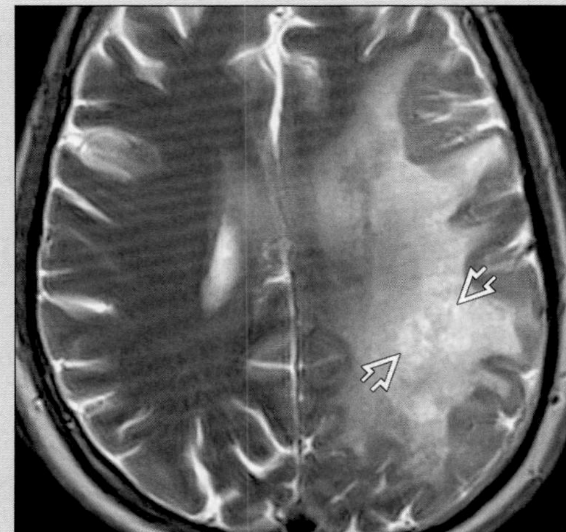

PROGRESSIVE MULTIFOCAL LEUKOENCEPHALOPATHY (PML)

TERMINOLOGY

Abbreviations

- Progressive multifocal leukoencephalopathy (PML)

Definitions

- JC polyomavirus infecting oligodendrocytes, causing demyelination in immunocompromised patients

IMAGING

General Features

- Best diagnostic clue
  - T2 hyperintense, multifocal, demyelinating plaques involve subcortical white matter (WM), extend to deep WM; gray matter often spared until late stage
  - Typically bilateral, but asymmetric; no mass effect or contrast enhancement
  - Late stage: Confluent WM lesions with cavitary changes
- Location
  - Propensity for parietooccipital region, thalamus, and basal ganglia (BG)
  - Rarely, lesions are only in posterior fossa
- Size
  - Variable, small subcortical lesions to confluent hemispheric lesions
- Morphology
  - May be solitary, multifocal, or widespread hemispheric WM lesions

Imaging Recommendations

- Best imaging tool
  - MR with contrast

MR Findings

- T1WI: Hypointense lesions → aggressive forms and burnt out PML lesions
- T2WI: Hyperintensity predominantly in subcortical and periventricular WM
  - Involves **subcortical U-fibers → scalloped** appearance
- FLAIR: Hyperintensity in subcortical and periventricular WM
- DWI: Newer lesion has slightly restricted diffusion; older lesion is unrestricted
- T1WI C+: Typically no enhancement
  - Faint peripheral enhancement may rarely be seen, typically in patients with long-term survival
- MRS: ↓ NAA; ↑ lactate, Cho, lipids
- Magnetization transfer: ↓ ratio compared to HIV encephalitis

DIFFERENTIAL DIAGNOSIS

HIV Encephalitis

- Atrophy and symmetric periventricular or diffuse WM disease; affects subinsular and peritrigonal WM

Acquired CMV

- May see ventriculitis, encephalitis, retinitis, or polyradiculopathy

Immune Reconstitution Inflammatory Syndrome (IRIS)

- Most often caused by PML (JC virus)

ADEM

- Post-infection/vaccination immune-mediated inflammatory demyelination

PATHOLOGY

General Features

- Etiology
  - JC polyomavirus infects oligodendroglia, causes demyelination
  - ~ 4-10% of adult AIDS patients develop PML
    - Rare in children
- Associated abnormalities
  - Commonly associated with AIDS, organ transplantation, cancer, chemotherapy, or any immunosuppression
  - Recently reported in multiple sclerosis patients treated with biologic drug therapy (natalizumab) and in patients with rheumatic diseases

Microscopic Features

- Numerous macrophages and bizarre transformed astrocytes, hyperchromatic oligodendrocytes with intranuclear inclusion bodies

CLINICAL ISSUES

Presentation

- Most common signs/symptoms
  - Altered mental status, progressive neurological symptoms, headache, lethargy

Demographics

- Epidemiology
  - AIDS, organ transplantation, cancer patients undergoing chemotherapy

Natural History & Prognosis

- Fatal disease, death in 6-8 months

Treatment

- Highly active antiretrovirus therapy (HAART) reported to improve survival

DIAGNOSTIC CHECKLIST

Image Interpretation Pearls

- If multifocal subcortical WM lesions without mass effect or enhancement in AIDS patients, consider PML over HIV encephalitis

SELECTED REFERENCES

1. Carson KR et al: Monoclonal antibody-associated progressive multifocal leucoencephalopathy in patients treated with rituximab, natalizumab, and efalizumab: a Review from the Research on Adverse Drug Events and Reports (RADAR) Project. Lancet Oncol. 10(8):816-24, 2009

IMMUNE RECONSTITUTION INFLAMMATORY SYNDROME (IRIS)

Key Facts

Terminology

- Immune reconstitution inflammatory syndrome (IRIS)
  - Atypical/worsening opportunistic infection
  - HIV/AIDS patients following commencement of HAART
  - Patients with MS, immunomodulatory therapy

Imaging

- PML-IRIS
  - WM hypodensities with ↑ mass
  - Patchy atypical enhancement
- TB-IRIS
  - ↑ leptomeningeal enhancement
  - ↑ size of ring-/nodular-enhancing tuberculomas
- Crypto-IRIS
  - ↑ nodular meningeal/subependymal enhancement
  - ↑ in size of "gelatinous" pseudocysts

Top Differential Diagnoses

- Diffuse/patchy WM abnormalities in AIDS
  - HIV encephalitis, PML, CMV infection
- Focal/multifocal brain lesions in AIDS
  - Lymphoma, toxo, tuberculoma, cryptococcosis

Pathology

- Reconstitution of immunity → abnormal immune response to infectious/noninfectious antigens

Clinical Issues

- 1/4 to 1/3 HIV-infected patients develop IRIS
- PML, TB common IRIS-associated pathogens

Diagnostic Checklist

- IRIS if worsening/enhancing lesions in
  - HIV patient + recently started HAART
  - MS patient on immunomodulatory therapy

__(Left)__ Axial T1WI C+ MR does not show any abnormal enhancement. FLAIR images (not shown) demonstrated multifocal confluent white matter hyperintensities, and a diagnosis of PML was suspected. __(Right)__ An axial T1WI C+ follow-up MR was obtained after the patient developed significant worsening of symptoms after HAART. Note the patchy nodular and linear foci of enhancement ⇒. Biopsy showed PML with IRIS. PCR demonstrated presence of JC virus DNA. (Courtesy T. Hutchins, MD.)

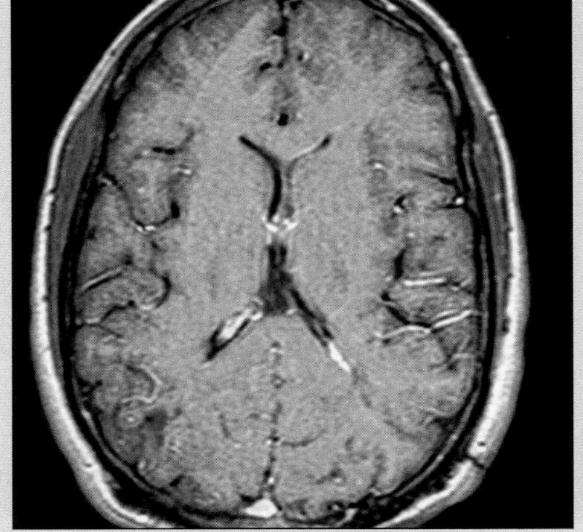

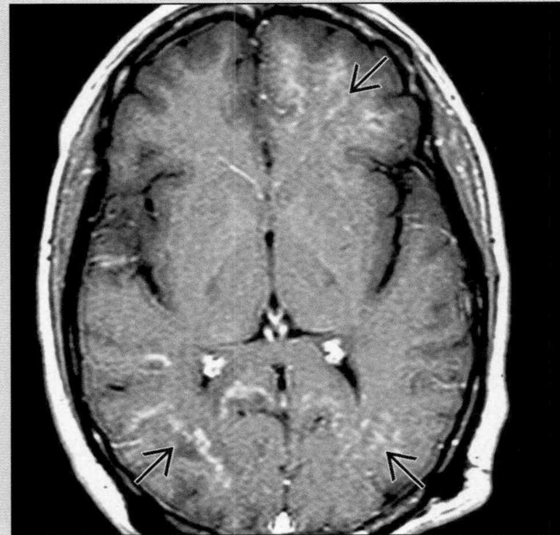

__(Left)__ Axial T1WI C+ MR demonstrates meningeal enhancement in the left sylvian fissure ➡ in an HIV-positive patient with tuberculous meningitis. __(Right)__ Axial T1WI C+ MR shows worsening of imaging appearance after placement on HAART. There is an increase in enhancement, which appears more nodular in the left sylvian fissure ➡, and there is development of surrounding edema ➡. This worsening of disease could be due to drug resistance; however, the time course after starting HAART makes IRIS most likely.

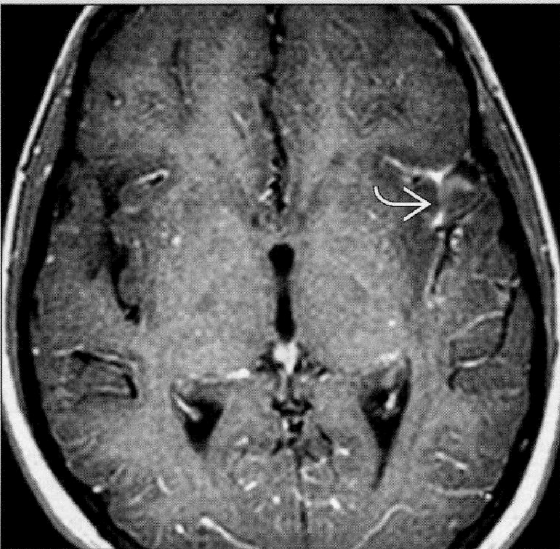

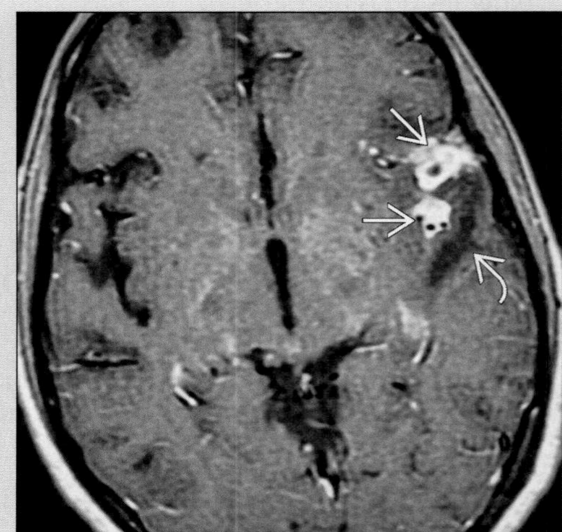

IMMUNE RECONSTITUTION INFLAMMATORY SYNDROME (IRIS)

TERMINOLOGY

Abbreviations

- Immune reconstitution inflammatory syndrome (IRIS)

Synonyms

- Immune restoration disease (IRD)
- Immune restitution syndrome (IRS)

Definitions

- Paradoxical worsening of opportunistic infection
  - After starting highly active antiretroviral therapy (HAART)
  - Patients with MS, immunomodulatory therapy

IMAGING

General Features

- Best diagnostic clue
  - Atypical/worsening imaging appearance of infection in HIV/AIDS following commencement of HAART
  - Other: Patient on immunomodulation therapy
    - MS with monoclonal antibody therapy
- Location
  - PML: Frontal/parietooccipital lobes most common
    - Less common: Posterior fossa
  - TB: Meninges, brain parenchyma
  - Cryptococcosis: Virchow-Robin spaces (VRSs), meninges

CT Findings

- NECT
  - PML-IRIS: White matter (WM) hypodensities with ↑ mass
- CECT
  - PML-IRIS: Atypical heterogeneous enhancement
  - TB-IRIS: Increased size of tuberculomas

MR Findings

- T1WI
  - PML-IRIS: Hypointense lesions become confluent
- T2WI
  - PML-IRIS: Hyperintense WM lesions ↑
    - Enlarge, become confluent, exert mass effect
  - TB-IRIS: ↑ edema around tuberculomas
- T1WI C+
  - PML-IRIS: Patchy atypical enhancement
  - TB-IRIS: ↑ pial enhancement
    - ↑ size of ring-/nodular-enhancing tuberculomas
  - Crypto-IRIS: ↑ nodular meningeal/subependymal enhancement, ↑ in size of "gelatinous" pseudocysts

Imaging Recommendations

- Best imaging tool
  - MR with T1 C+, T2WI, FLAIR

DIFFERENTIAL DIAGNOSIS

Diffuse/Patchy WM Abnormalities in AIDS

- HIV encephalitis, PML, CMV infection

Focal/Multifocal Brain Lesions in AIDS

- Lymphoma, toxo, TB, cryptococcosis

PATHOLOGY

General Features

- Etiology
  - Reconstitution of immunity → abnormal immune response to infectious/noninfectious antigens
  - Typical in 1st 2-12 weeks after starting HAART
  - Unmasking of preexisting disease can occur
  - Pathogens: TB, CMV, crypto, JC virus (PML), and others
  - Can occur in non-HIV immunocompromised
    - MS patient on monoclonal antibody therapy

Gross Pathologic & Surgical Features

- PML-IRIS: Multifocal discoloration of WM
- TB-IRIS: Granulomas, basal exudates

Microscopic Features

- ↑ CD8(+) T cells: Parenchymal and perivascular lymphocytic inflammatory infiltrates

CLINICAL ISSUES

Presentation

- Most common signs/symptoms
  - PML-IRIS: Headache, visual disturbance, dementia
  - TB-IRIS: Fever, lymphadenopathy, seizures

Demographics

- Age
  - Young
- Epidemiology
  - IRIS risk factors at HAART initiation
    - Lower CD4 cell count/cell %, ↓ CD4:CD8 ratio
    - Higher HIV RNA
  - TB common reported copathogen associated with IRIS

Natural History & Prognosis

- May progress to death in severe cases

Treatment

- Continue primary therapy for opportunistic infection
- Continue HAART + anti-inflammatory agents

DIAGNOSTIC CHECKLIST

Consider

- IRIS: HIV + recently started HAART + worsening/unmasking of preexisting opportunist infection

SELECTED REFERENCES

1. Elston JW et al: Immune reconstitution inflammatory syndrome. Int J STD AIDS. 20(4):221-4, 2009
2. Major EO: Progressive multifocal leukoencephalopathy in patients on immunomodulatory therapies. Annu Rev Med. Epub ahead of print, 2009
3. McCombe JA et al: Neurologic immune reconstitution inflammatory syndrome in HIV/AIDS: outcome and epidemiology. Neurology. 72(9):835-41, 2009

HIV/AIDS, MISCELLANEOUS MANIFESTATIONS

Key Facts

Terminology

- Primary CNS lymphoma (PCNSL)
- Kaposi sarcoma (KS)
- Bacterial abscesses (BA)
- Aspergillosis (As)
- Neurosyphilis (NS)
- Benign lymphoepithelial lesions of HIV (BLL-HIV)
- HIV/AIDS-related opportunistic infections and neoplasms

Imaging

- Findings
  - PCNSL: Enhancing lesions, often hemorrhagic/ necrotic within basal ganglia, periventricular WM
  - KS: Intense enhancing soft tissue mass in scalp
  - BA: Ring-enhancing lesion with ↑ signal on DWI
  - As: Multiple ring-enhancing lesions
  - NS: Cortical/subcortical infarcts, granulomas, leptomeningeal enhancement
  - BLL-HIV: Multiple cystic masses enlarging both parotid glands
- MR is most sensitive
- PET or thallium-201-SPECT helpful to differentiate from toxoplasmosis

Top Differential Diagnoses

- Toxoplasmosis
- Metastases
- Tuberculosis

Diagnostic Checklist

- Consider using DWI, MRS, PET/SPECT to differentiate opportunistic infections from malignant lesions
- Bacterial abscess, aspergillosis, neurosyphilis may need surgical biopsy for diagnosis

*(**Left**) Axial graphic through the suprahyoid neck shows lymphoepithelial lesions of HIV in both parotids. Notice that there are both cystic and solid elements. Adenoidal hypertrophy ➔ is also seen. (**Right**) Axial T1WI C+ MR in an HIV patient demonstrates primary CNS lymphoma that mimics toxoplasmosis. There is a peripherally enhancing mass ➔ with central necrosis. There is also an eccentric enhancing nodule ➔ suggesting an "eccentric target" sign, which is typically seen in toxoplasmosis.*

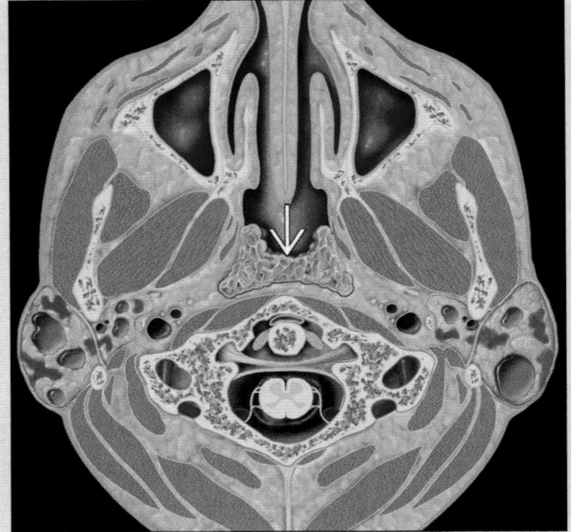

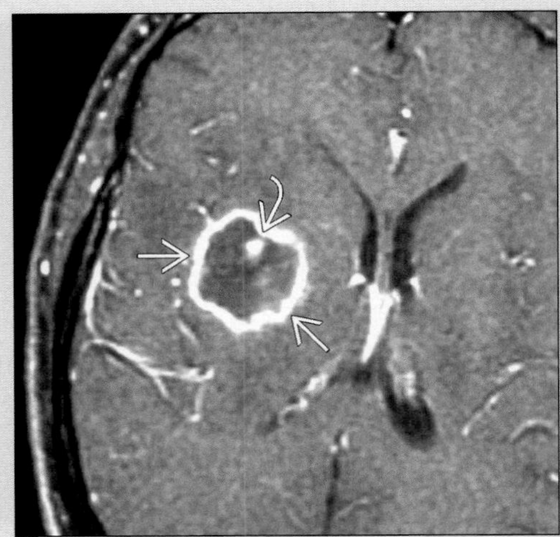

*(**Left**) Axial T1WI MR shows bilateral but asymmetrical, inhomogeneously hyperintense lesions in the basal ganglia, suggesting subacute hemorrhage in primary CNS lymphoma ➔. Hemorrhage and necrosis are not uncommon in patients with HIV/AIDS. (**Right**) Coronal T1WI C+ MR demonstrates a left frontal cortical lesion ➔ involving the adjacent dura ➔ in a patient with tertiary syphilis. The presence of a cortical lesion with adjacent meningeal enhancement should suggest this diagnosis.*

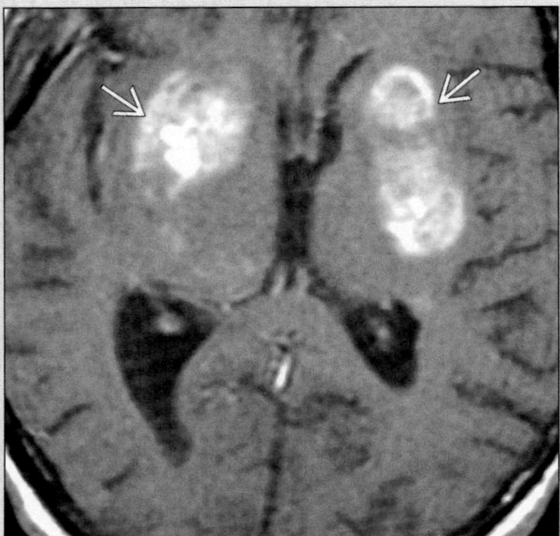

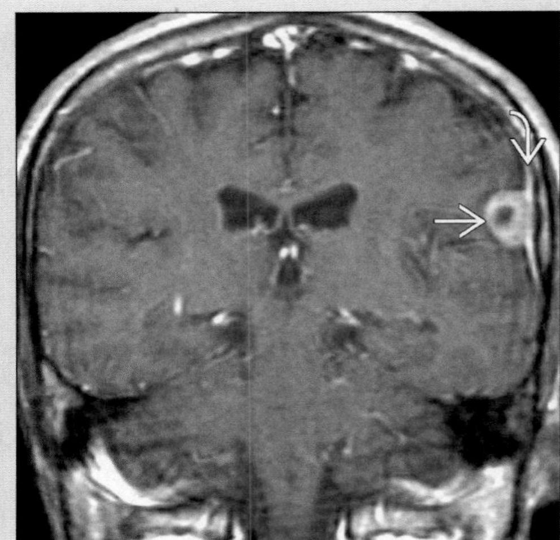

TERMINOLOGY

Abbreviations

- Primary CNS lymphoma (PCNSL)
- Kaposi sarcoma (KS)
- Bacterial abscesses (BA)
- Aspergillosis (As)
- Neurosyphilis (NS)
- Benign lymphoepithelial lesions of HIV (BLL-HIV)

Definitions

- HIV/AIDS-related opportunistic infections, neoplasms

IMAGING

General Features

- Best diagnostic clue
  - PCNSL: Enhancing lesions, often hemorrhagic/necrotic within basal ganglia, periventricular white matter (WM)
  - KS: Intense enhancing soft tissue mass in scalp
  - BA: Ring-enhancing lesion with ↑ signal on DWI
  - As: Multiple ring-enhancing lesions
  - NS: Cortical/subcortical infarcts, granulomas, leptomeningeal enhancement
  - BLL-HIV: Multiple cystic masses enlarging both parotid glands
- Location
  - PCNSL: 90% supratentorial; deep gray nuclei, periventricular white matter commonly affected
  - KS: Face, scalp, and skin of neck
  - BA: Typically supratentorial, frontal, and parietal
  - As: Distribution of MCA, cortical/subcortical, basal ganglia/thalami perforating arteries
  - NS: Cortical/subcortical, meninges
  - BLL-HIV: Parotid glands
- Morphology
  - PCNSL: Solitary mass or multiple lesions
  - KS: Infiltrating soft tissue mass
  - BA: Smooth, ring-enhancing lesion
  - As: Multiple lesions, often in distribution of MCA

CT Findings

- NECT
  - PCNSL: Hypodense or hyperdense, ± hemorrhage, necrosis
  - KS: Soft tissue thickening in scalp, face
  - BA: Hypodense mass with edema and mass effect
  - As: Multiple cortical/subcortical, low-attenuation lesions; may be associated with hemorrhage
  - NS: Peripherally located lesions isointense to cortex
  - BLL-HIV: Multiple bilateral, well-circumscribed, cystic masses within enlarged parotid glands
- CECT
  - PCNSL: Ring enhancement in HIV patients
  - KS: Marked enhancing scalp soft tissue mass
  - BA: Thin ring enhancement
  - As: Multiple ring-enhancing lesions
    - Enhancement may be subtle or well defined related to immune status
  - NS: Enhancing cortical lesions ± dural thickening
  - BLL-HIV: Thin rim enhancement of cystic lesions

MR Findings

- T1WI
  - PCNSL: Iso-/hypointense to cortex
  - KS: Localized thickening scalp isointense to muscle
  - BA: Early poorly marginated hypo-/isointense mass, late hypointense center
  - As: Hypointense masses
    - Hemorrhage ↑ T1 signal
  - NS: Isointense to gray matter
- T2WI
  - PCNSL: Iso-/hypointense to cortex, mild surrounding edema
    - May be heterogeneous due to hemorrhage, necrosis
  - KS: Scalp mass hyperintense to muscle
  - BA: Capsule with hypointense rim
  - As: Heterogeneous if hemorrhage present
  - NS: Hyperintense lesions, infarcts
- DWI
  - PCNSL: Variable restricted diffusion
  - BA: ↑ signal DWI, low ADC
  - As: Restricted diffusion in wall of abscess
- T1WI C+
  - PCNSL: Peripheral enhancement with central necrosis more common in HIV patients than homogeneous enhancement
  - KS: Intensely enhancing soft tissue mass in scalp
  - BA: Early patchy enhancement, late capsule with well-defined, thin rim enhancement
  - As: Multiple ring-enhancing lesions
  - NS: Lesions enhance; overlying leptomeningeal/dural enhancement also seen
  - BLL-HIV: Well-defined, rim-enhancing, cystic lesions in parotid glands
- MRS
  - PCNSL: ↓ NAA, ↑ choline
  - BA: Central necrotic area may show acetate, lactate, alanine, succinate, pyruvate, and amino acids

Imaging Recommendations

- Best imaging tool
  - MR is most sensitive
- Protocol advice
  - PCNSL: Contrast-enhanced MR
    - PET or Tl-201 SPECT helpful to differentiate from toxoplasmosis
  - BA: MR C+, DWI, MRS

Nuclear Medicine Findings

- PCNSL: FDG PET/Tl-201 SPECT hypermetabolic

DIFFERENTIAL DIAGNOSIS

Toxoplasmosis

- Enhancing lesions, "eccentric target" sign
- PET, SPECT helpful to differentiate from PCNSL

Metastases

- Multiple lesions common, significant vasogenic edema, primary tumor often known

HIV/AIDS, MISCELLANEOUS MANIFESTATIONS

Tuberculosis
- Ring/nodular enhancing lesions in cortex, gray-white junction; Ca++ in chronic cases

PATHOLOGY

General Features
- Etiology
  - PCNSL: Typically diffuse, large B-cell non-Hodgkin lymphoma
    - Associated with CD4(+) counts < 100 cells/mm³
    - EBV plays major role in immunosuppressed
  - KS: Caused by herpes virus HHV-8
    - Classified as AIDS-defining cancers (ADCs)
    - Develop as result of combination of factors: HHV-8, altered immunity, and inflammatory/angiogenic milieu
  - BA: *Staphylococcus* and *Streptococcus* most common causative organisms
  - As: *Aspergillus* species = hyaline septate molds
    - *Aspergillus fumigatus* most common agent
    - Hematogenous spread from pulmonary focus or direct extension via sinus
    - Infectious vasculopathy: Acute infarction, hemorrhage, infectious cerebritis/abscess
  - NS: Sexually transmitted disease results from infection with spirochete *Treponema pallidum*

Gross Pathologic & Surgical Features
- PCNSL: Single multiple masses in cerebral hemispheres, central necrosis/hemorrhage in HIV
- BA: Depends on stage; necrotic foci, rim of inflammatory cells, granulation tissue, surrounding vasogenic edema
- As: Hemorrhagic infarcts with variable inflammation
- NS: Syphilitic gummas; well-circumscribed necrotic masses of granulation tissue (avascular)

Microscopic Features
- PCNSL: Small, noncleaved, and large immunoblastic type
  - High nuclear-to-cytoplasmic ratio
  - Angiocentric: Surrounds, infiltrates vessels, perivascular spaces
- KS: Diffuse positivity for vimentin; pedunculated, ulcerated, or both
- BA: Granulation tissue about necrotic core
- As: Septate hyphae branch at acute angles
  - Invade blood vessels, spread along internal elastica and lamina
- NS: Leptomeningitis, multifocal arteritis
  - Cerebral gummas; infiltration of meninges and brain by lymphocytes and plasma cells

CLINICAL ISSUES

Presentation
- Most common signs/symptoms
  - PCNSL: Lethargy, confusion, headache, seizures, focal weakness
  - KS: Usually asymptomatic; symptoms may appear when lesions ulcerate or produce local mass effect
  - BA: Headache most common symptom
    - Seizures, focal neurologic deficits
  - As: Seizures, altered mental status, focal deficits
  - NS: Often asymptomatic
    - Headaches, seizures, personality changes, confusion
  - BLL-HIV: Bilateral parotid space masses
- Clinical profile
  - PCNSL: CD4(+) < 100 cells/mm³
    - CSF: Pleocytosis, ↑ proteins, cytology (+) for monoclonal, malignant-appearing lymphocytes
    - PCR amplification of EBV DNA in CSF
  - KS: Low CD4 count (i.e., < 150-200 cells/mm³)
  - NS: CSF ↑ WBC count, reactive CSF VDRL &/or positive CSF *T. pallidum* antibody index

Demographics
- Epidemiology
  - PCNSL: 2nd most common mass lesion after toxoplasmosis in patients with AIDS
    - 2-6% of AIDS patients
  - KS: Prevalence of AIDS-related KS has ↓, presumably due to use of HAART
  - BA: Relatively uncommon in AIDS patients
  - NS: Affects approximately 1.5% of AIDS population
  - BLL-HIV: 5% of HIV(+) patients

Treatment
- PCNSL: Definitive diagnosis requires stereotactic brain biopsy
  - HAART with radiation
- KS: Biopsy still required to confirm diagnosis
  - Radiotherapy is primary therapy
- BA: Surgical drainage, antibiotics
- As: Surgery, antifungals
- NS: Penicillin ± steroids
- BLL-HIV: HAART therapy tends to completely or partially treat

DIAGNOSTIC CHECKLIST

Consider
- Consider using DWI, MRS, PET/SPECT to differentiate opportunistic infections from malignant lesions

Image Interpretation Pearls
- In HIV patients, difficult to differentiate between PCNSL and toxoplasmosis
  - PET/SPECT studies may be helpful
- Bacterial abscess, aspergillosis, neurosyphilis may need surgical biopsy for diagnosis

SELECTED REFERENCES

1. Crum-Cianflone N et al: Cutaneous malignancies among HIV-infected persons. Arch Intern Med. 169(12):1130-8, 2009
2. Smith AB et al: From the archives of the AFIP: central nervous system infections associated with human immunodeficiency virus infection: radiologic-pathologic correlation. Radiographics. 2008 Nov-Dec;28(7):2033-58. Review. Erratum in: Radiographics. 29(2):638, 2009
3. Descamps M et al: Neuroimaging of CNS involvement in HIV. J HIV Ther. 13(3):48-54, 2008

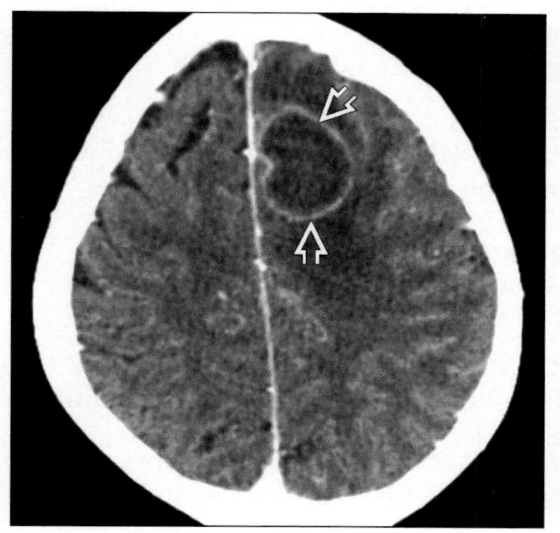

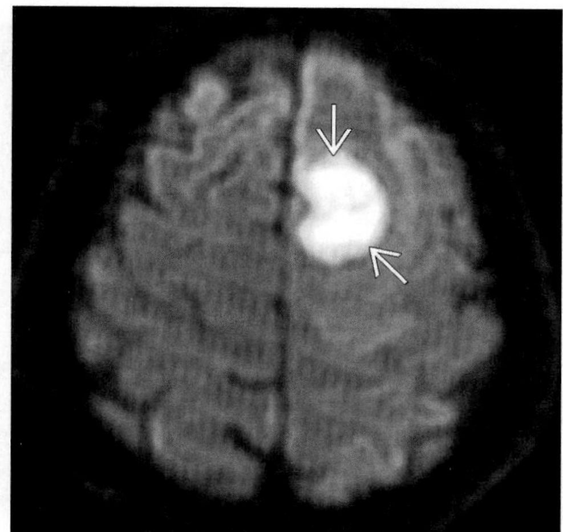

(Left) *Axial CECT shows a well-defined ring-enhancing lesion ➨ with surrounding vasogenic edema in an HIV-positive patient who presented with seizures. On surgery, purulent material was drained and proved positive for enterococci.* ***(Right)*** *Axial DWI MR in the same patient demonstrates homogeneous high signal ➡, which was low on ADC (not shown). These findings are consistent with a bacterial abscess. Purulent material drained at surgery was positive for enterococci.*

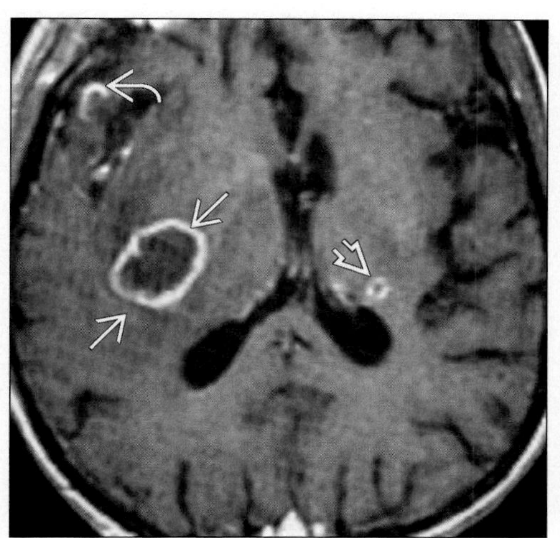

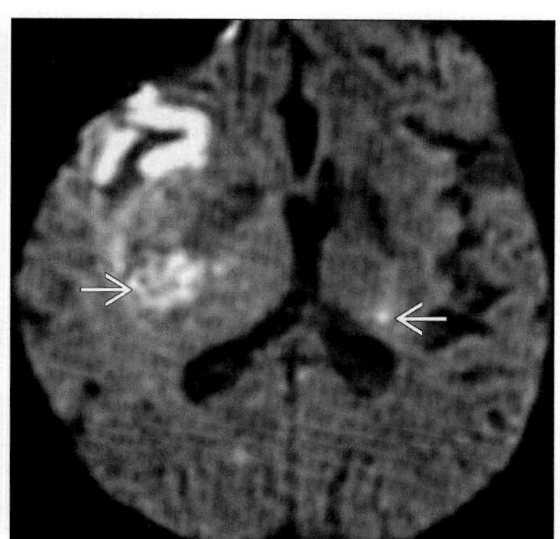

(Left) *Axial T1WI C+ MR shows a ring-enhancing lesion in the right basal ganglia ➡ and a smaller lesion in the left thalamus ➨. The basal ganglia lesion at surgery was due to Aspergillus infection. Note the subtle gyral enhancement in right perisylvian region ↪.* ***(Right)*** *Axial DWI MR in the same patient shows restricted diffusion in the lesion within the basal ganglia and thalamus ➡. There is also restricted diffusion in the right sylvian cortical infarct, presumably due to associated vasculitis.*

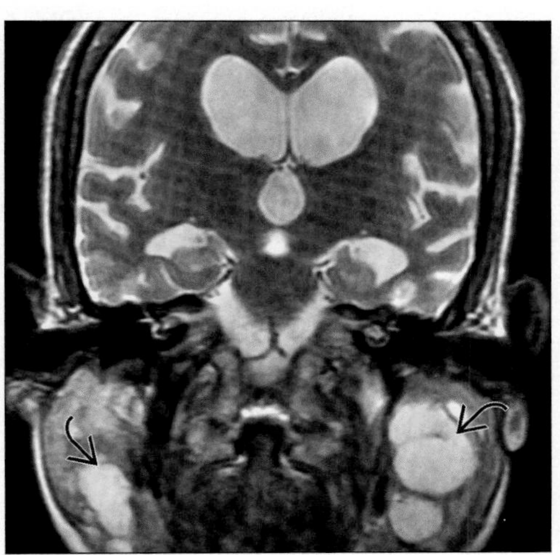

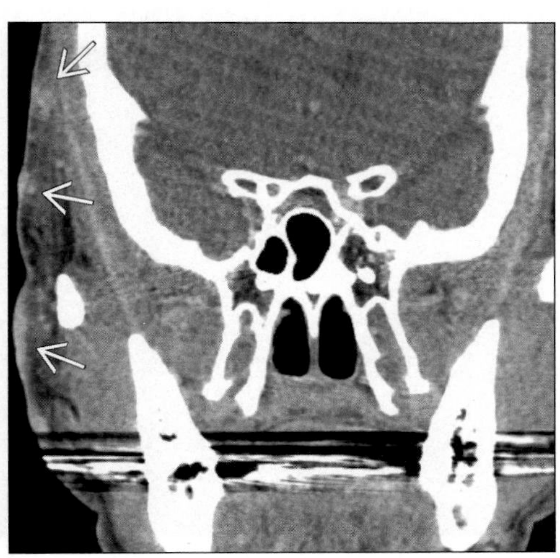

(Left) *Coronal T2WI MR in a young HIV patient demonstrates diffuse cerebral volume loss. Note the multiple cystic lesions ↪ in the parotid glands, findings consistent with benign lymphoepithelial cysts.* ***(Right)*** *Coronal CECT in an immunocompromised patient shows multiple infiltrating soft tissue nodules in the skin and subcutaneous areas ➡ due to Kaposi sarcoma.*

MULTIPLE SCLEROSIS

Key Facts

Imaging

- Multiple perpendicular callososeptal T2 hyperintensities characteristic of MS
  - Perivenular extension: "Dawson fingers"
- Bilateral, asymmetric linear/ovoid FLAIR hyperintensities
  - > 85% periventricular/perivenular
  - 50-90% callososeptal interface
  - May also commonly involve subcortical U-fibers, brachium pontis, brainstem, spinal cord common
- Transient enhancement during active demyelination
  - > 90% disappear within 6 months
- Rare: Large tumefactive enhancing rings
- T1: Hyperintense lesions suggest worse prognosis
  - Correlate with disability, atrophy, progressive disease
- Advanced imaging techniques show disease in normal-appearing white matter

Top Differential Diagnoses

- Acute disseminated encephalomyelitis (ADEM)
- Neuromyelitis optica
- Autoimmune-mediated vasculitis

Clinical Issues

- Estimated 2,500,000 people in world have MS
- Most common disabling CNS disease of young adults; 1:1,000 in Western world
- Age: 20-40 years
  - Peak onset = 30; 3-5% < 15, 9% > 50
- Adults: M:F = 1:2; adolescents: M:F = 1:3-5

Diagnostic Checklist

- Requires dissemination in time and space in central nervous system for diagnosis
- McDonald criteria: Consensus statement for diagnostic criteria, last revised in 2005

(Left) Sagittal graphic illustrates multiple sclerosis plaques involving the corpus callosum, pons, and spinal cord. Note the characteristic perpendicular orientation of the lesions ➔ at the callososeptal interface along penetrating venules. (Right) Axial T1WI C+ MR shows numerous enhancing MS plaques that were present throughout the infratentorial and supratentorial brain. Lesions may show homogeneous enhancement but may also exhibit ring or an incomplete ring pattern of enhancement.

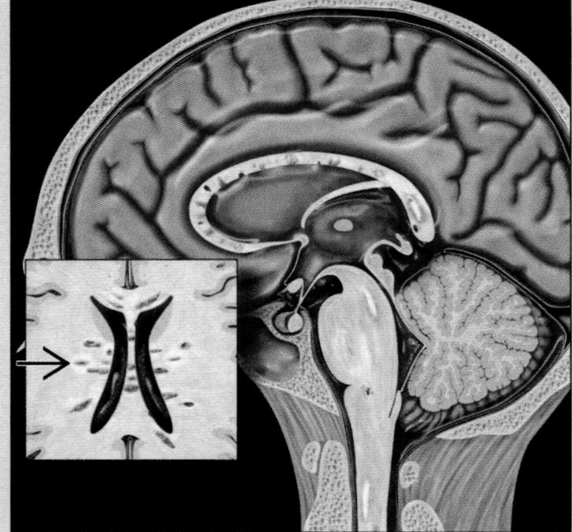

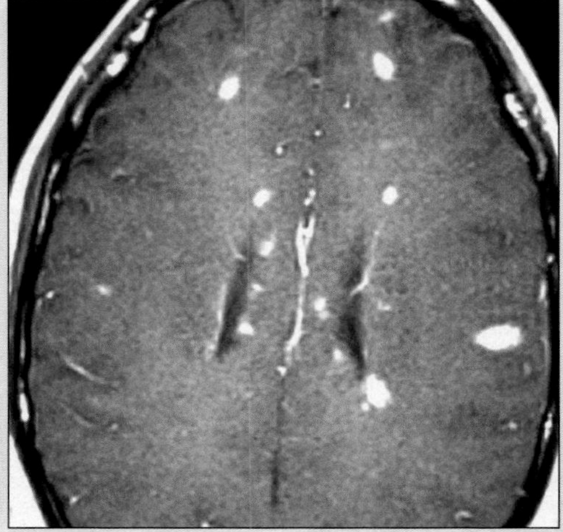

(Left) Sagittal FLAIR shows callososeptal hyperintensities radiating from the lateral ventricles with a typical perpendicular orientation, characteristic of multiple sclerosis. (Right) Axial FLAIR MR 3T shows multiple nonenhancing, periventricular, hyperintense MS lesions oriented perpendicular to the callosomarginal interface. These lesions are perivenular, along the path of the deep medullary veins, and represent Dawson fingers. Confluent lesions are also seen along the right periventricular margin.

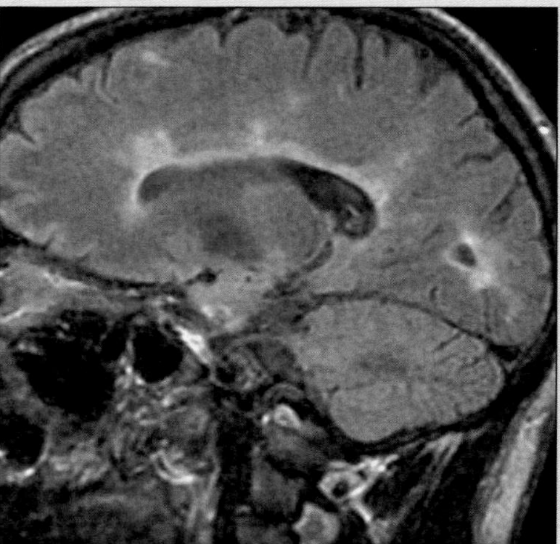

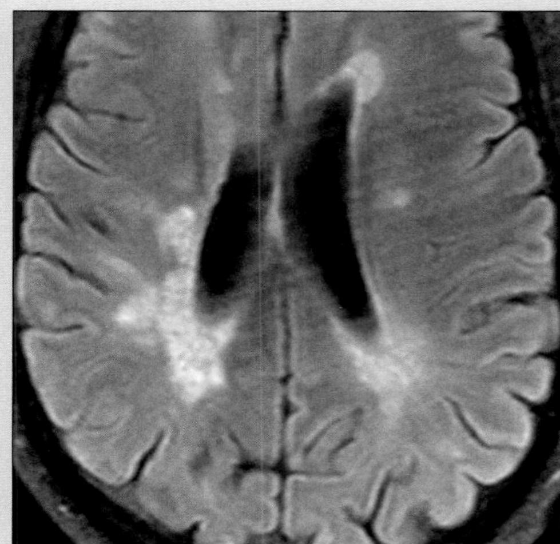

MULTIPLE SCLEROSIS

TERMINOLOGY

Abbreviations

- Multiple sclerosis (MS)

Definitions

- Probable autoimmune-mediated demyelination in genetically susceptible individuals

IMAGING

General Features

- Best diagnostic clue
  - Multiple perpendicular callososeptal T2 hyperintensities
- Location
  - > 85% periventricular/perivenular
  - 50-90% callososeptal interface
  - Subcortical U-fibers, brachium pontis, brainstem, spinal cord common
  - Infratentorial (10% adults, ↑ in children)
- Size
  - Small 5-10 mm, tumefactive lesions several cm
- Morphology
  - Linear, round, or ovoid; beveled, target, lesion-in-a-lesion appearance

CT Findings

- CECT
  - Iso-/hypodense ± mild/moderate enhancement
  - Both solid and ring enhancement patterns

MR Findings

- T1WI
  - Typically hypo- or isointense
  - Hypointensity correlates with axonal destruction ("black holes")
  - Hyperintense lesions suggest worse prognosis
    - Correlated with disability, atrophy, progressive disease
  - Hyperintense dentate nuclei seen in secondary progressive form
- T2WI
  - Hyperintense, linear foci radiating from ventricles
  - Also prevalent in subcortical U-fibers, brachium pontis, brainstem, and spinal cord
  - High cortical disease burden can be predictor of primary progressive MS
  - Hypointense basal ganglia 10-20% of chronic MS
- FLAIR
  - Bilateral, asymmetric, linear/ovoid hyperintensities
  - Perivenular extension; "Dawson fingers"
    - Along path of deep medullary veins
  - Hyperintensities become confluent with severity
- DWI
  - Acute lesions
    - Concentric ring pattern with hyperintense rim
    - Plaque rims: Variable ADC/anisotropic values, not statistically different from normal-appearing white matter (NAWM)
    - Plaque centers: ↑ ADC, ↓ ↓ anisotropy (cf. rim, NAWM, chronic plaques)
  - Subacute/chronic lesions: Intermediate ↑ ADC, moderate ↓ anisotropy (cf. NAWM)
  - ADC/anisotropy abnormal in all WM, worse in periplaque regions
  - ADC positive correlates with expanded disability status scale (EDSS)/disease duration
- T1WI C+
  - Transient enhancement during active demyelination (> 90% disappear within 6 months)
    - Nodular (68%) or ring (23%)
    - Semilunar, incomplete, horseshoe-shaped (9%)
    - Rare: Large tumefactive enhancing rings
- MRS
  - ↓ NAA (NAA/Cr), ↑ choline (Cho/Cr), ↑ myoinositol
  - MRS abnormalities found in NAWM
  - Only secondary progressive MS shows ↓ NAA in normal-appearing gray matter (NAGM)
    - May allow early distinction between relapsing-remitting and secondary-progressive
- Perfusion MR (contrast-enhanced T2*): Low rCBV
  - Can separate tumefactive MS from neoplasm
- Magnetization transfer (MT)
  - ↓ MT ratio (MTR) in lesions/NAWM
- Functional connectivity MR (fcMR)
  - ↓ functional connectivity between right/left hemisphere primary visual and motor cortices
- 3.0 T vs. 1.5 T: 21% ↑ number of contrast-enhancing lesions, 30% ↑ enhancing lesion volume, 10% ↑ total lesion volume

Nuclear Medicine Findings

- PET
  - ↑ glucose utilization correlates with ↓ NAA in lesions and NAWM

Imaging Recommendations

- Protocol advice
  - Contrast-enhanced MR with sagittal FLAIR
  - Fat saturation to assess for optic neuritis

DIFFERENTIAL DIAGNOSIS

Acute Disseminated Encephalomyelitis (ADEM)

- Viral prodrome, monophasic illness
- Can mimic MS; gray matter often involved

Neuromyelitis Optica

- Optic neuritis and spinal cord lesions, sparing of brain

Autoimmune-Mediated Vasculitis

- Enhancing lesions spare callososeptal interface
- "Beaded" angiogram appearance

CADASIL

- Premature dementia and recurrent strokes with *NOTCH3* mutations

Lyme Disease

- Can be identical to MS (skin rash common)

Susac Syndrome

- Classic triad: Encephalopathy, branch retinal artery occlusions, hearing loss

MULTIPLE SCLEROSIS

McDonald Criteria (2005 Revisions) for Diagnosis of MS

Dissemination in space by MR (at least 3 required)	*Dissemination in time by MR (at least 1 required)*
1. Gadolinium-enhancing lesion or 9 T2 lesions	1. Gadolinium-enhancing lesion 3 months after clinical onset
2. At least 3 periventricular T2 lesions	2. New T2 lesion at least 30 days after reference scan
3. At least 1 infratentorial or spinal cord T2 lesion	
4. At least 1 juxtacortical T2 lesion	

PATHOLOGY

General Features

- Etiology
  - Unknown; probably virus &/or autoimmune-mediated in genetically susceptible individuals
  - Activated T cells attack myelinated axons
  - Cox-2, iNOS may cause excitotoxic death of oligodendrocytes
- Genetics
  - Multifactorial; ↑ incidence in 1st-order relatives

Staging, Grading, & Classification

- Major clinical subtypes
  - **Relapsing-remitting** (RR) (85% initial presentation)
  - **Secondary-progressive** (SP), a.k.a. relapsing progressive
    - By 10 years 50%, and by 25 years 90% of RR patients enter SP phase
  - **Primary-progressive** (PP), a.k.a. chronic progressive
    - 5-10% of MS population progressive from start
  - **Progressive-relapsing** (PR)
    - Rare; defined as progressive disease with clear acute relapses ± full recovery
    - Periods between relapses characterized by continuing disease progression
- MS variants/subtypes
  - **Malignant**: Younger patients, febrile prodrome, clinically fulminant, death in months
  - **Schilder** type ("diffuse sclerosis"): Extensive, confluent, asymmetric demyelination in bilateral supra-/infratentorial parenchyma
  - **Balo** type ("concentric sclerosis"): Large lesions with alternating zones of demyelinated/myelinated WM

Gross Pathologic & Surgical Features

- Acute: Poorly delineated, yellowish-white, periventricular plaques
- Chronic: Gray, granular, well-demarcated plaques ± generalized volume loss

Microscopic Features

- Perivenous demyelination, oligodendrocyte loss
  - Active: Foamy macrophages with myelin fragments, lipids; reactive astrocytes + perivascular inflammation; some hypercellular with atypical reactive astrocytes, mitoses (mimic tumor)
  - Chronic: Marked loss of myelin, oligodendrocytes; dense astrogliosis; minimal/no perivascular inflammation
- Axonal transection
- CSF positive for oligoclonal bands

CLINICAL ISSUES

Presentation

- Most common signs/symptoms
  - Variable; initially impaired/double vision of acute optic neuritis (50% with positive MR develop MS)
  - Weakness, numbness, tingling, gait disturbances
  - ↓ sphincter control, blindness, paralysis, dementia
  - Cranial nerve palsy; usually multiple, 1-5% isolated (CN5, 6 most common)
  - Spinal cord symptoms in 80%

Demographics

- Age
  - 20-40; peak onset is 30; 3-5% < 15, 9% > 50
- Gender
  - Adults: M:F = 1:2
  - Adolescents: M:F = 1:3-5
- Ethnicity
  - All groups, but Caucasian most common
  - Most often occurs in temperate zones
- Epidemiology
  - Estimated 2,500,000 people in world have MS
  - Most common disabling CNS disease of young adults; 1:1,000 in Western world

Natural History & Prognosis

- 45% patients not severely affected, nearly normal
- > 80% with "probable" MS, positive MR progress to clinically definite MS
- Majority: Protracted course with progression of deficits
- Late: Severe disability, cognitive impairment

Treatment

- Immunomodulators &/or immunosuppressants

DIAGNOSTIC CHECKLIST

Image Interpretation Pearls

- 95% with clinically definite MS have positive MR

SELECTED REFERENCES

1. Calabrese M et al: Cortical lesions in primary progressive multiple sclerosis: a 2-year longitudinal MR study. Neurology. 72(15):1330-6, 2009
2. Filippi M et al: Conventional MRI in multiple sclerosis. J Neuroimaging. 17 Suppl 1:3S-9S, 2007
3. Polman CH et al: Diagnostic criteria for multiple sclerosis: 2005 revisions to the "McDonald Criteria". Ann Neurol. 58(6):840-6, 2005

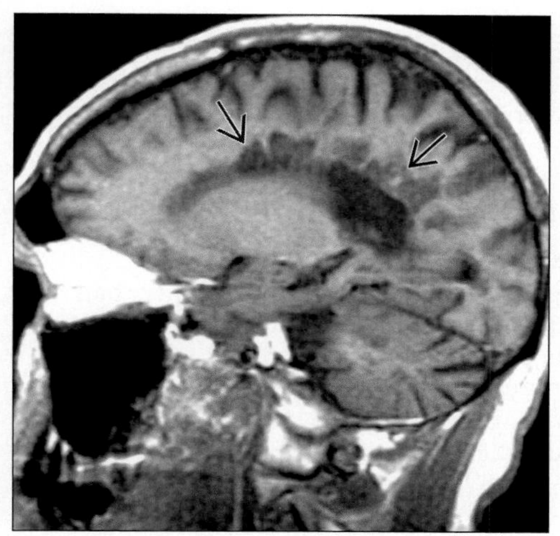

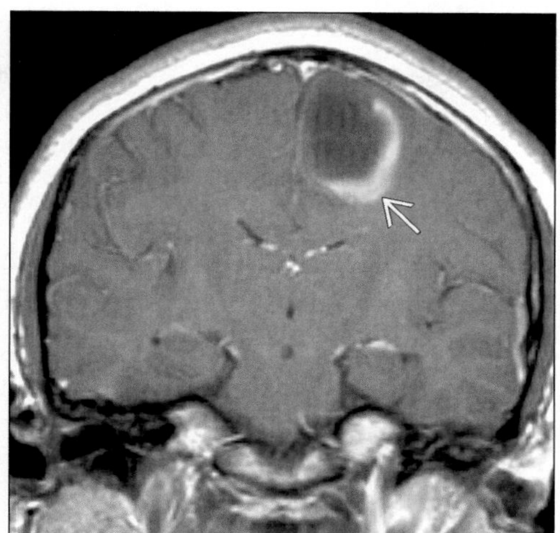

(Left) *Sagittal T1WI MR shows multiple hypointense lesions ("black holes") in the deep white matter* → *related to axonal destruction. Note the associated moderate ventricular and sulcal enlargement.* ***(Right)*** *Coronal T1WI C+ MR shows a hypointense mass in the left posterior frontal region with a peripheral crescent of incomplete or "horseshoe" enhancement* →*. This enhancement pattern is classic for tumefactive demyelinating disease, most commonly MS.*

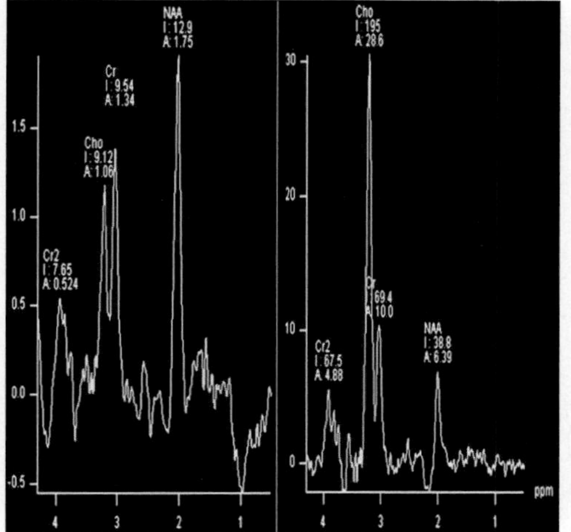

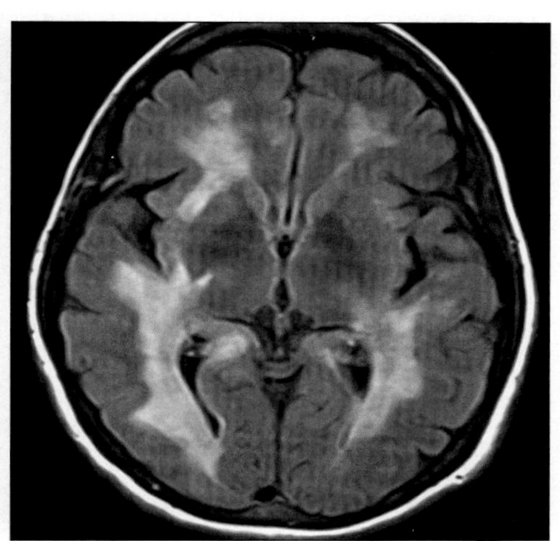

(Left) *MRS (TE = 135) of normal-appearing white matter (left) shows mildly decreased NAA, typical of MS. The tumefactive lesion in the opposite hemisphere (right) shows marked decrease in NAA and increase in choline. The tumor was biopsy-proven glioblastoma in an MS patient.* ***(Right)*** *Axial FLAIR MR shows confluent periventricular white matter hyperintensity typical of advanced, longstanding MS with loss of discrete, linear, periventricular lesions.*

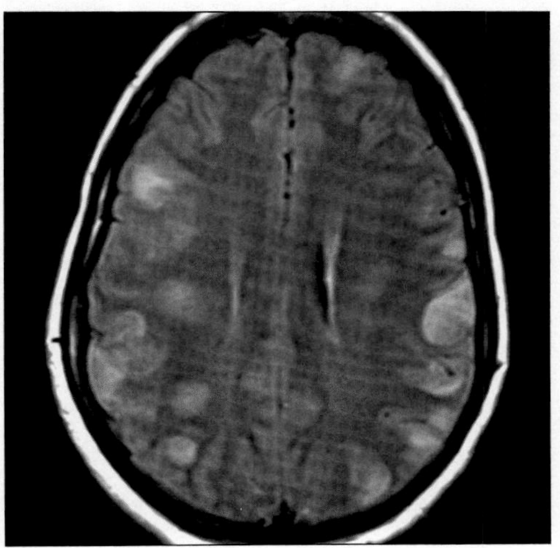

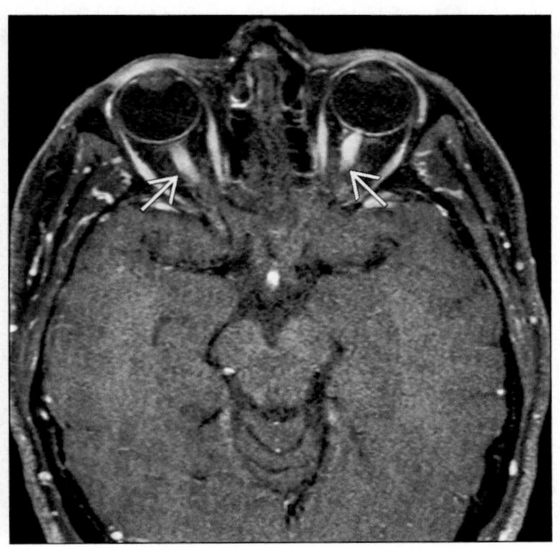

(Left) *Axial FLAIR MR shows numerous peripheral white matter and cortical lesions that exhibited robust contrast enhancement in an 18-year-old female with malignant (Marburg) MS. The patient presented with a 2-week history of behavioral changes and leg pain and died 3 weeks after presentation. Autopsy showed typical demyelinating pathology.* ***(Right)*** *Axial T1WI C+ FS shows bright enhancement of the optic nerves* →*, similar to the extraocular muscles, in an MS patient with acute bilateral optic neuritis.*

NEUROMYELITIS OPTICA

Key Facts

Terminology

- Idiopathic, severe, demyelinating disease that preferentially affects optic nerve and spinal cord

Imaging

- Optic neuritis and myelitis with relative sparing of brain WM
  - 60% will have some nonspecific brain lesions, does not exclude diagnosis
- Expansile, hyperintense T2 cord signal, ≥ 3 segments
- DTI: Higher cord diffusivity, lower fractional anisotropy than MS patients or controls
- T1WI C+: Acute spinal cord and optic nerve lesions typically enhance

Top Differential Diagnoses

- Multiple sclerosis
- Optic neuritis
- Transverse myelitis
- Syringomyelia
- Spinal cord neoplasm

Pathology

- Serum marker: NMO-IgG, targets water channel aquaporin-4
  - Seen in 60% of NMO patients, 99% specificity
- NMO-IgG predicts recurrence in transverse myelitis

Clinical Issues

- Worse prognosis with more severe disability than MS despite lack of brain involvement
  - Relapsing course in 90% of patients
- Systemic immunosuppression to prevent relapses
- Rituximab treatment found to decrease frequency of attacks and reduce disability

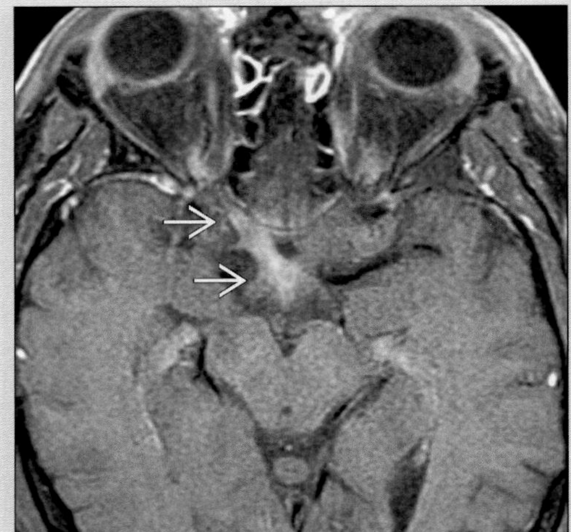

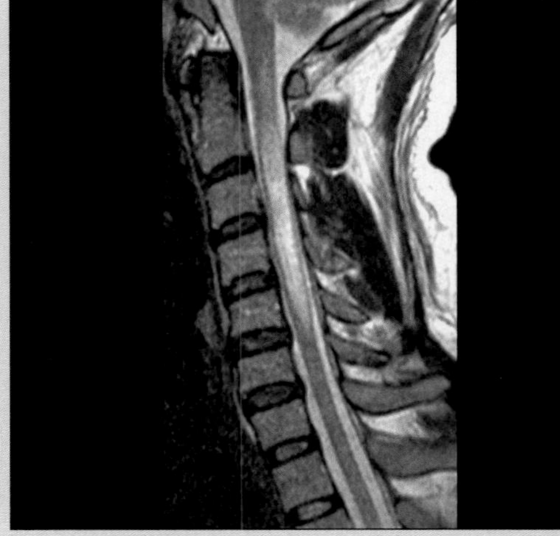

(Left) *Axial T1WI C+ FS MR shows a markedly enhancing prechiasmatic right optic nerve and chiasm ➔, consistent with acute optic neuritis.* ***(Right)*** *Sagittal PD FSE MR in the same patient shows a long segment of cord enlargement with hyperintensity. Ill-defined enhancement was also present in the cervical cord in this patient with myelopathy and vision loss. Patients with NMO have a worse prognosis with more severe disability than multiple sclerosis, despite lack of brain involvement.*

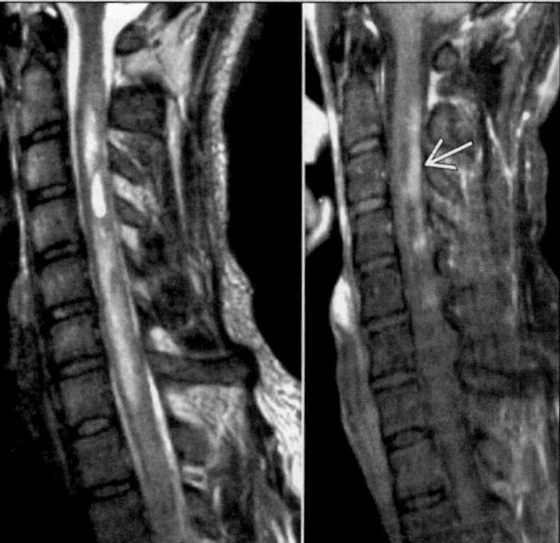

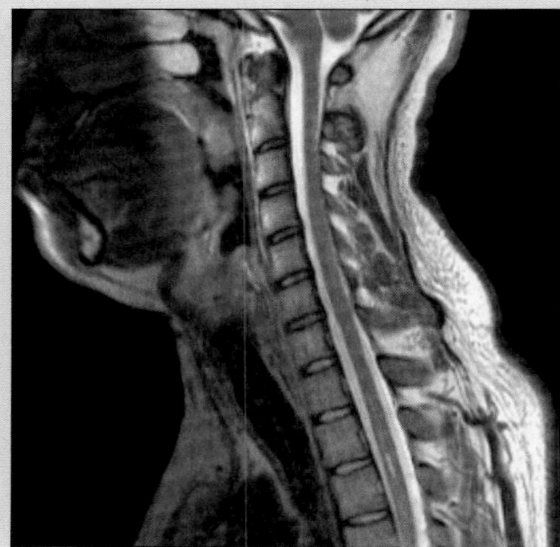

(Left) *Sagittal T2 (left) and T1WI C+ FS (right) images show multilevel T2 hyperintensity with irregular posterior enhancement ➔ in the cervical cord in a patient with a previous history of optic neuritis.* ***(Right)*** *Sagittal T2WI MR in the same patient 1 year after treatment shows near complete resolution of the T2 signal abnormality. Enhancement was no longer seen in the cervical cord. The cord lesions seen in NMO typically extend over 3 or more segments.*

NEUROMYELITIS OPTICA

TERMINOLOGY

Abbreviations

- Neuromyelitis optica (NMO)

Synonyms

- Devic syndrome

Definitions

- Idiopathic, severe, demyelinating disease that preferentially affects optic nerve and spinal cord

IMAGING

General Features

- Best diagnostic clue
  - Optic neuritis and myelitis with relative sparing of brain white matter (WM)
- Location
  - Most common in cervical spinal cord, optic nerves
  - 60% will have some nonspecific brain lesions → does not exclude diagnosis
- Size
  - Spinal lesions typically expansile, multisegment

MR Findings

- T2WI
  - Hyperintense, mildly enlarged optic nerves
  - Expansile, hyperintense cord signal, ≥ 3 segments
    - May have heterogeneous areas of brighter (fluid) T2 signal
- STIR: Hyperintense optic nerve and spinal cord
- DWI: Higher diffusivity, lower fractional anisotropy than multiple sclerosis (MS) patients or controls
- T1WI C+ FS: Acute lesions typically show enhancement

Imaging Recommendations

- Best imaging tool
  - Contrast-enhanced MR of spine and orbits
- Protocol advice
  - Orbits: Axial or coronal STIR or T2 FS & T1 C+ FS
  - Spine: Sagittal T2, T1WI C+

DIFFERENTIAL DIAGNOSIS

Multiple Sclerosis

- Brain more extensively involved
- Optic neuritis and spinal involvement may be seen
- Multisegment, expansile cord lesion more common in neuromyelitis optica

Optic Neuritis

- 1 component of NMO
- Consider NMO-IgG in case of 1st optic neuritis but otherwise normal brain MR

Transverse Myelitis

- 1 component of NMO
- Idiopathic inflammatory or postinfectious myelitis

Syringomyelia

- Enlargement and T2 hyperintensity of spinal cord
- May appear similar to NMO

Spinal Cord Neoplasm

- Astrocytoma or ependymoma can show similar multisegment cord T2 hyperintensity & enhancement

PATHOLOGY

Staging, Grading, & Classification

- Diagnostic criteria
  - Optic neuritis
  - Transverse myelitis
  - At least 2 of following
    - Spinal cord MR with T2 hyperintensity extending over ≥ 3 consecutive segments
    - Seropositive NMO-IgG
    - Brain MR does not meet criteria for MS

Gross Pathologic & Surgical Features

- Cavitation of spinal cord

Microscopic Features

- Serum marker: **NMO-IgG**, targets water channel aquaporin-4
  - Seen in 60% of NMO patients, **99% specificity**
- Aquaporin-4 likely involved in pathogenesis
- NMO-IgG predicts recurrence in transverse myelitis

CLINICAL ISSUES

Natural History & Prognosis

- Relapsing course in 90% of patients
- Worse prognosis with more severe disability than MS despite lack of brain involvement
- Secondary progressive form is rare; disability associated with relapses

Treatment

- Systemic immunosuppression required to prevent relapses
- At least 5 years immunosuppression recommended in NMO-IgG seropositive patient with 1st attack of myelitis
- Rituximab treatment found to decrease frequency of attacks and reduce disability
- Rescue plasmapheresis has shown benefit

DIAGNOSTIC CHECKLIST

Consider

- Neuromyelitis optica in patient with optic neuritis with normal brain MR

SELECTED REFERENCES

1. Jacob A et al: Treatment of neuromyelitis optica with rituximab: retrospective analysis of 25 patients. Arch Neurol. 65(11):1443-8, 2008
2. Jarius S et al: NMO-IgG in the diagnosis of neuromyelitis optica. Neurology. 68(13):1076-7, 2007
3. Matiello M et al: Neuromyelitis optica. Curr Opin Neurol. 20(3):255-60, 2007
4. Pittock SJ et al: Brain abnormalities in neuromyelitis optica. Arch Neurol. 63(3):390-6, 2006

ADEM

Key Facts

Imaging

- Best diagnostic clue: Multifocal WM and deep grey lesions 1-2 weeks following infection/vaccination
  - 93% within 3 weeks of infection, range 2 days to 4 weeks
- Can involve brainstem and posterior fossa
  - Do not usually involve callososeptal interface
- Tumefactive, mass-like lesions possible
- Spinal cord involvement in up to 30%
- C+ MR: Punctate, ring, incomplete ring, peripheral enhancement
- Tc-99m-HMPAO SPECT shows more extensive hypoperfusion than MR lesions
- DWI: Variably hyperintense lesions
  - Diffusion restriction may portend worse prognosis
- MRS: ↓ NAA within lesions; may see ↑ Cho, ↑ lactate

Top Differential Diagnoses

- Multiple sclerosis (MS)
- Autoimmune-mediated vasculitis
- Acute hypertensive encephalopathy, PRES
- Fabry disease
- Behçet disease

Pathology

- Over 30 different infectious agents and immunizations reported

Clinical Issues

- Mean age is 5-8 years, but can occur at any age
- Male predominance (M:F = 1:0.6-0.8), unlike MS
- Usually monophasic, self-limited
- Complete recovery within 1 month: 50-60%
- Mortality: 10-30%

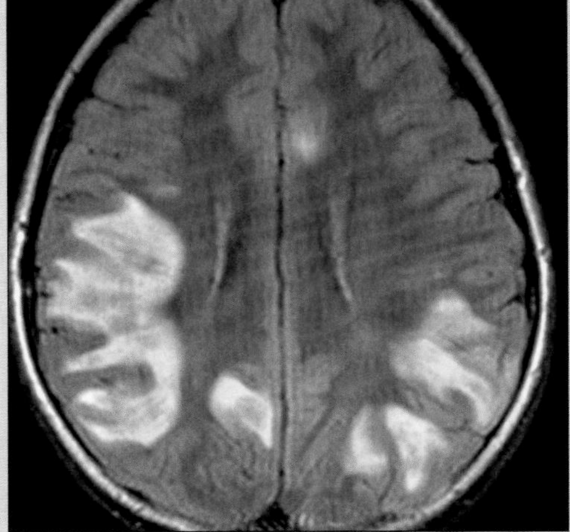
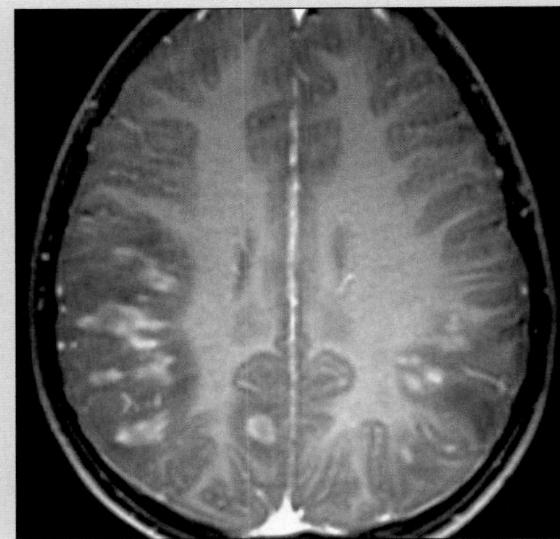

(Left) *Axial FLAIR MR shows peripheral, confluent areas of hyperintensity predominantly involving the subcortical white matter in this child with ADEM. The bilateral but asymmetric pattern is typical of ADEM.* ***(Right)*** *Axial T1WI C+ MR in the same patient shows marked, irregular enhancement of nearly all of the lesions. As ADEM is a monophasic illness, enhancement of the majority of lesions is typical, as the lesions all have a similar time course. Enhancement of MS lesions is more variable.*

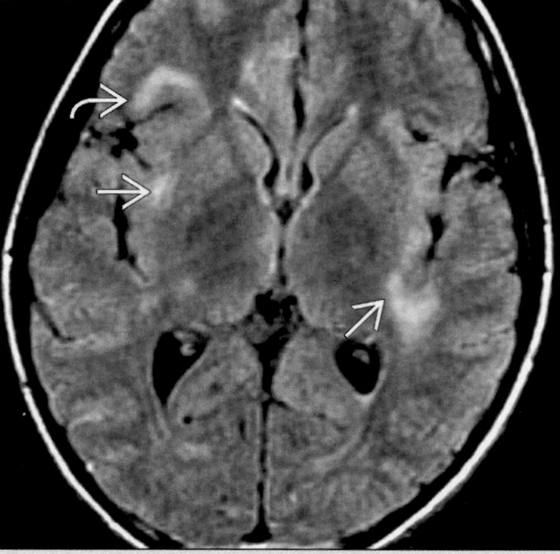
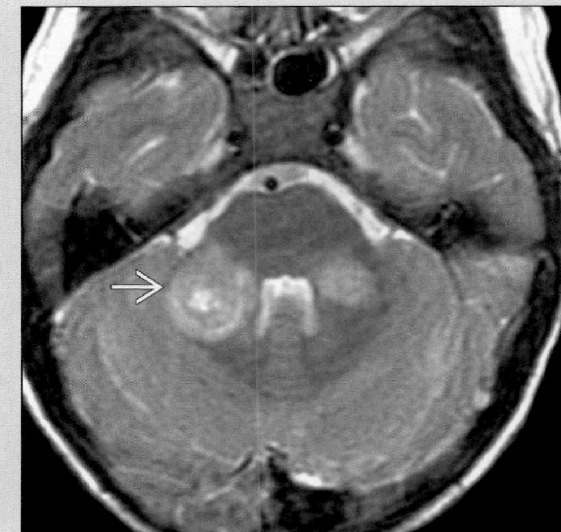

(Left) *Axial FLAIR MR shows typical findings of ADEM with peripheral, subcortical hyperintense foci ➔. Bilateral insular involvement is seen ➔. Periventricular and callososeptal lesions, which are typical of multiple sclerosis, are not commonly seen in ADEM.* ***(Right)*** *Axial T2WI MR shows hyperintense lesions in the brachium pontis bilaterally, typical for demyelination. The right-sided lesion shows a targetoid ➔ appearance. Enhancement of several of the lesions was present on post-contrast T1 images (not shown).*

TERMINOLOGY

Abbreviations

- Acute disseminated encephalomyelitis (ADEM)

Definitions

- Autoimmune-mediated white matter (WM) demyelination of brain &/or spinal cord, usually with remyelination

IMAGING

General Features

- Best diagnostic clue
  - Multifocal WM/basal ganglia lesions 2 days to 4 weeks following infection/vaccination
    - 93% within 3 weeks of infection, 5% within 1 month of vaccination
- Location
  - May involve both brain and spinal cord; predominantly WM but also gray matter (GM)
    - Deep gray nuclei involved in 50%
    - Spinal cord involvement in 11-28%
- Size
  - Tumefactive lesions may be large, but with less mass effect than expected from tumor size
- Morphology
  - Punctate to "flocculent"
  - Tumefactive, mass-like lesions possible

CT Findings

- NECT
  - Initial CT normal in 40%
- CECT
  - Multifocal punctate or ring-enhancing lesions

MR Findings

- T2WI
  - Hyperintensities may be better visualized in brainstem and posterior fossa on T2
- FLAIR
  - Multifocal punctate to large flocculent FLAIR hyperintensities
    - Bilateral but asymmetric
  - Involve peripheral white-gray matter junction subcortical WM
  - Can involve brainstem and posterior fossa
  - Do not usually involve callososeptal interface
- DWI
  - Variably hyperintense lesions on DWI (trace) images
  - Apparent diffusion coefficient (ADC) may be increased or decreased
    - Most lesions show increased signal (T2* "shine through")
    - Diffusion restriction uncommon, suggests worse prognosis
    - Diffusivity normal within normal-appearing white matter (NAWM), unlike MS
- T1WI C+
  - Punctate, ring, incomplete ring, peripheral enhancement
  - Cranial nerve(s) may enhance
  - Absence does not exclude diagnosis
- MRS
  - NAA low within lesions, lactate may be elevated
  - Other metabolites usually normal
  - NAA normalizes with resolution of symptoms/MR abnormalities
- Magnetization transfer ratio (MTR)
  - ADEM MTR normal within NAWM, unlike MS

Imaging Recommendations

- Best imaging tool
  - Contrast-enhanced MR
    - Initial imaging often normal but more sensitive than CT
    - May appear identical to MS; repeat MR necessary to distinguish with certainty
- Protocol advice
  - Limited rapid interval follow-up may be provided by FLAIR alone

Nuclear Medicine Findings

- Tc-99m-HMPAO SPECT shows more extensive hypoperfusion than T2 lesions

DIFFERENTIAL DIAGNOSIS

Multiple Sclerosis (MS)

- Predilection for periventricular WM (callososeptal interface), involves subcortical U-fibers, commonly in posterior fossa
- Lesions often more symmetric than ADEM
- Relapsing-remitting course common

Autoimmune-Mediated Vasculitis

- Multifocal GM-WM lesions
  - Bilateral, usually cortical/subcortical, basal ganglia/thalami
  - Ring-enhancing lesions may mimic infection

Acute Hypertensive Encephalopathy, PRES

- T2 hyperintense edema induced by hypertension
- Typically posterior circulation in cortex/subcortical WM
- May affect deep gray nuclei

Aging Brain with Hyperintense WM Lesions

- Atherosclerotic brain changes in 50% patients > 50 years old
- Found in normotensive patients; more common in hypertensives
- Present in 10-30% of cognitively normal elderly patients
- MR: Scattered, asymmetric WM lesions, without enhancement
  - Often periatrial; posterior fossa uncommon
  - Spares callososeptal interface, subcortical U-fibers

Fabry Disease

- MR: Scattered, asymmetric WM lesions, without enhancement
  - May involve brainstem and posterior fossa
  - Spares callososeptal interface and subcortical U-fibers
  - Cranial MR sensitive to identify neurologic involvement in asymptomatic patients

- Present with renal failure/heart disease

Behcet Disease

- MR: Scattered, asymmetric, subcortical WM lesions without cortical involvement
  - Nodular enhancement in acute phase
  - Predilection for midbrain
- ADC ↑, similar to ADEM
- Classic triad: Oral and genital ulcerations with uveitis

PATHOLOGY

General Features

- Etiology
  - Autoimmune-mediated severe acute demyelination
  - Following nonspecific upper respiratory tract infection, often viral
    - Over 30 different infectious agents and immunizations reported
  - After specific viral illness: Epstein-Barr, influenza A, mumps, coronavirus
  - Especially after exanthematous diseases of childhood (chickenpox, measles)
  - After vaccination: Diphtheria, influenza, rabies, smallpox, tetanus, typhoid
  - Spontaneously (no known cause)
- Genetics
  - ADEM associated with DRB1*01 and DRB1*017(03) in Russian population
- Associated abnormalities
  - Acute hemorrhagic leukoencephalopathy variant associated with ulcerative colitis and asthma

Gross Pathologic & Surgical Features

- None, unless hemorrhage (rare) or tumefactive edema

Microscopic Features

- Acute myelin breakdown
- Perivenous inflammation; lymphocytic infiltrates
- Relative axonal preservation; atypical astrogliosis
- Virus generally not found, unlike viral encephalitides
- Similar to experimental allergic encephalomyelitis, supporting autoimmune-related etiology

CLINICAL ISSUES

Presentation

- Most common signs/symptoms
  - Usually preceded by prodromal phase: Fever, malaise, myalgia
  - Multifocal neurological symptoms, 2 days to 4 weeks after viral illness/immunization
    - Initial symptoms: Headache, fever, drowsiness
    - Cranial nerve palsies, seizures, hemiparesis
    - Decreased consciousness (from lethargy to coma)
    - Behavioral changes
- Other signs/symptoms
  - Seizures in 10-35%
- Clinical profile
  - CSF often abnormal (leukocytosis, elevated protein)
    - Usually lacks CSF oligoclonal bands

Demographics

- Age
  - Children > adults
  - Mean age is 5-8 years but can occur at any age
- Gender
  - Male predominance (M:F = 1.0:0.6-0.8), unlike MS
- Epidemiology
  - Rare, yet most common para-/post-infectious disorder
  - Most common in winter and spring
  - Exact epidemiology unknown, but increasingly reported

Natural History & Prognosis

- Usually monophasic, self-limited
- Variable prognosis
  - Complete recovery within 1 month (50-60%)
  - Neurologic sequelae (most commonly seizures) (20-30%)
  - Mortality (10-30%)
  - Relapses are rare
    - "Relapsing disseminated encephalomyelitis"
    - May not be separate entity from relapsing-remitting MS
- Typically delay between symptom onset and imaging findings
- Varicella and rubella ADEM have preferential patterns
  - Varicella ADEM characterized by cerebellar ataxia and mild pyramidal dysfunction
  - Rubella ADEM characterized by acute explosive onset, seizures, coma, and moderate pyramidal signs
- Rare manifestations of ADEM
  - Acute hemorrhagic leukoencephalopathy (2%)
    - Young patients with abrupt symptom onset
    - Fulminant, often ending in death
  - Bilateral striatal necrosis (usually in infants, may be reversible)

Treatment

- Immunosuppressive/immunomodulatory therapy
  - MR may show prompt improvement after therapy
- Plasma exchange therapy
  - 40% of patients failing steroid treatment may show marked improvement

DIAGNOSTIC CHECKLIST

Image Interpretation Pearls

- Imaging findings often lag behind symptom onset, resolution

SELECTED REFERENCES

1. Callen DJ et al: Role of MRI in the differentiation of ADEM from MS in children. Neurology. 72(11):968-73, 2009
2. Noorbakhsh F et al: Acute disseminated encephalomyelitis: clinical and pathogenesis features. Neurol Clin. 26(3):759-80, ix, 2008
3. Rossi A: Imaging of acute disseminated encephalomyelitis. Neuroimaging Clin N Am. 18(1):149-61; ix, 2008
4. Tenembaum S et al: Acute disseminated encephalomyelitis. Neurology. 68(16 Suppl 2):S23-36, 2007
5. Menge T et al: Acute disseminated encephalomyelitis: an update. Arch Neurol. 62(11):1673-80, 2005

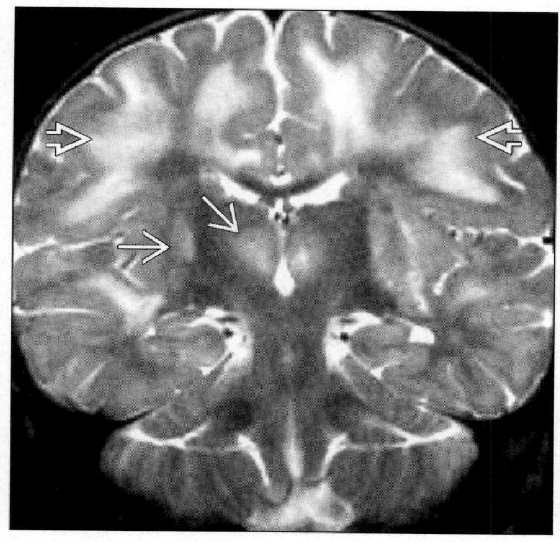

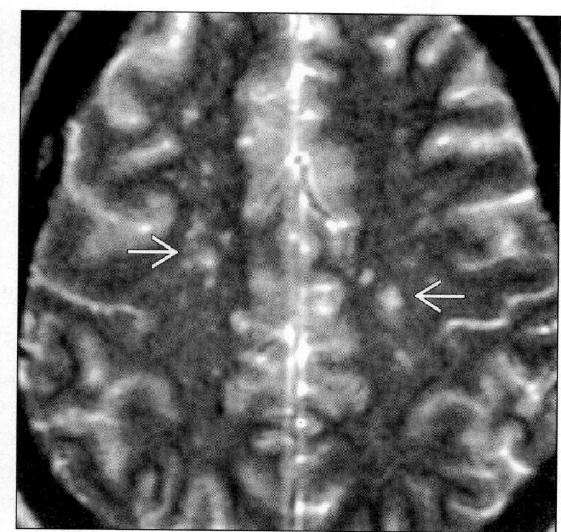

(Left) *Coronal T2WI MR shows large confluent regions of hyperintense signal in the hemispheric white matter ⇨ and deep gray nuclei ➔ of a child with ADEM. Although ADEM predominantly involves white matter, gray matter is often affected.* ***(Right)*** *Axial T2WI MR shows multiple bilateral, but asymmetric, T2 hyperintense foci ➔. None of the lesions demonstrates significant mass effect in this adult patient with ADEM. Imaging mimics multiple sclerosis, vasculitis, and microvascular ischemia.*

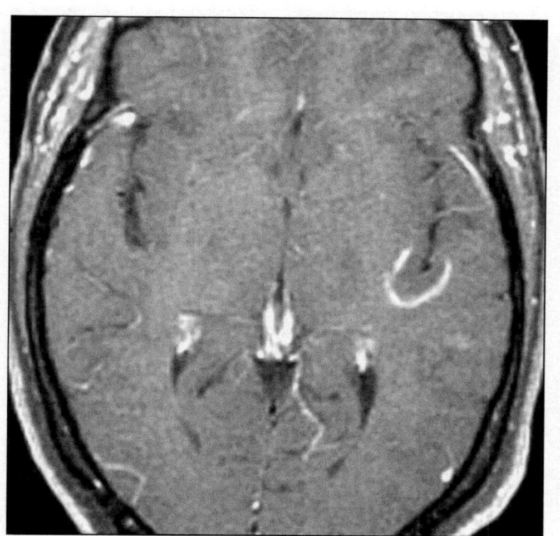

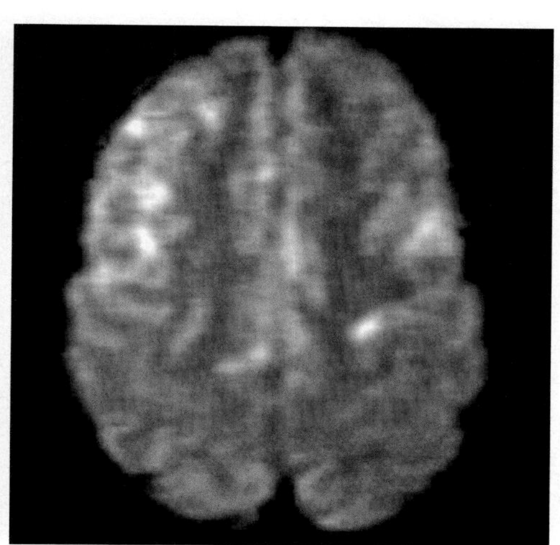

(Left) *Axial T1WI C+ MR shows an incomplete ring of peripheral enhancement, typical of a demyelinating process. Other contrast enhancement patterns include ovoid or punctate homogeneous enhancement.* ***(Right)*** *Axial DWI MR shows increased signal in areas of FLAIR hyperintensity. The foci were hypointense on ADC images, indicating diffusion restriction. Both white and gray matter involvement is present. Diffusion restriction is an uncommon imaging finding and is associated with a worse prognosis.*

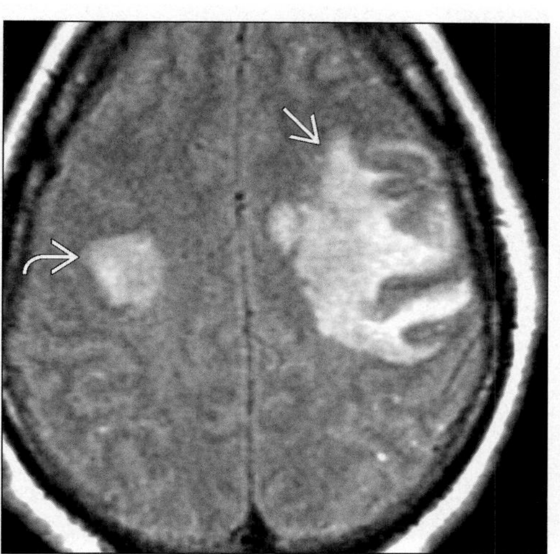

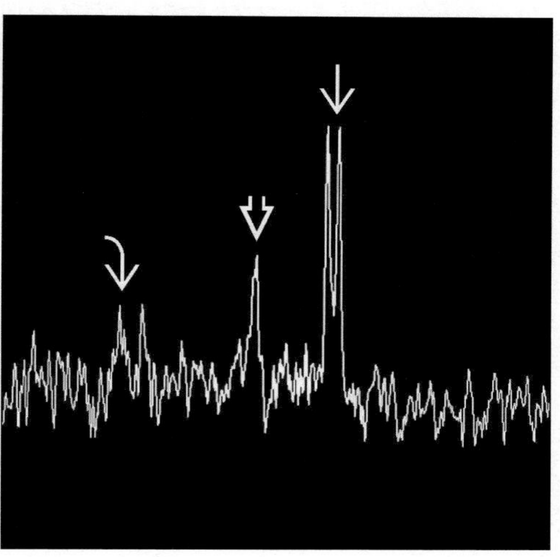

(Left) *Axial FLAIR image shows a large, tumefactive, hyperintense ADEM lesion ➔ with mass effect less than expected for the size of the lesion. Another clue to its nonneoplastic nature is the right-sided lesion ↪.* ***(Right)*** *MRS at a long TE in the same patient shows the tumefactive lesion has a depressed choline ↪ and NAA ⇨ metabolites in the presence of a large lactate doublet ➔. This MRS helps distinguish this lesion from a neoplasm. MRS of ADEM may show elevated choline acutely.*

SUSAC SYNDROME

Key Facts

Terminology
- Microangiopathy of brain, retina, and cochlea

Imaging
- T2 hyperintense corpus callosum (CC) lesions in patient with clinical triad
  - Encephalopathy, bilateral hearing loss, and branch retinal artery occlusions
- Multifocal T2 hyperintensities similar to MS
  - More often round, mid-callosal rather than callosal septal location
- May involve brainstem, basal ganglia, thalamus, subcortical white matter, centrum semiovale
- Callosal lesions may show acute diffusion restriction
- Variable enhancement of lesions and leptomeninges

Top Differential Diagnoses
- Multiple sclerosis
- ADEM
- Systemic lupus erythematosus

Pathology
- Microinfarctions in cerebral cortex that are generally not seen on imaging
- No demyelination seen on pathology

Clinical Issues
- 20-40 years old
- Usually self-limited (2-4 years) but may lead to permanent deafness or blindness

Diagnostic Checklist
- Most patients do not exhibit entire triad (up to 97% at time of presentation)
- Complete triad seen after 2 weeks or after 2 years
- Consider Susac syndrome in patients with corpus callosum lesions and clinical triad

__(Left)__ Axial FLAIR MR image shows multiple hyperintensities ➔ in the middle of the corpus callosum in this patient with Susac syndrome. The classic clinical triad includes encephalopathy, bilateral hearing loss, and branch retinal artery occlusions. __(Right)__ Sagittal PD image shows hyperintense lesions in the anterior corpus callosum body ➔ and thalamus ➔. Note the predilection for the middle layers of the corpus callosum rather than the callososeptal interface, as is typically seen in multiple sclerosis.

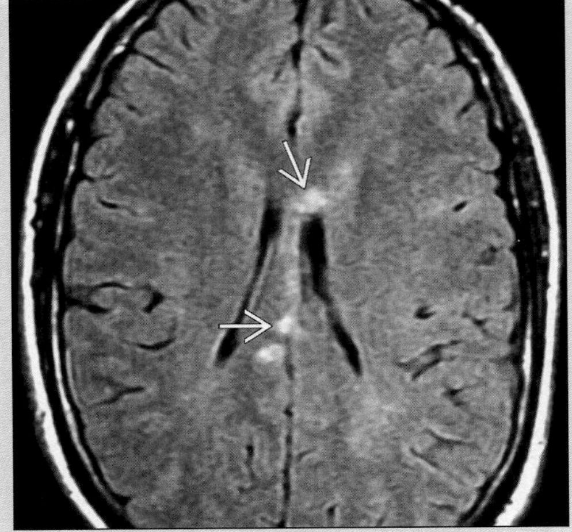

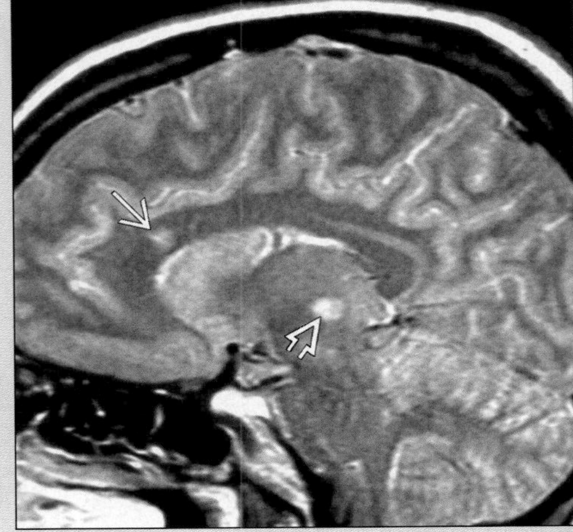

__(Left)__ Axial T1WI C+ MR in the same patient shows homogeneous enhancement of the left thalamic lesion ➔. Enhancement may be seen in white matter lesions and the leptomeninges. __(Right)__ Funduscopic examination shows multiple retinal artery branch occlusions and irregularities ➔, classic for Susac syndrome. Susac syndrome is often mistaken for multiple sclerosis on imaging studies. Its etiology is uncertain but most likely represents a vasculitis, not a demyelinating disorder.

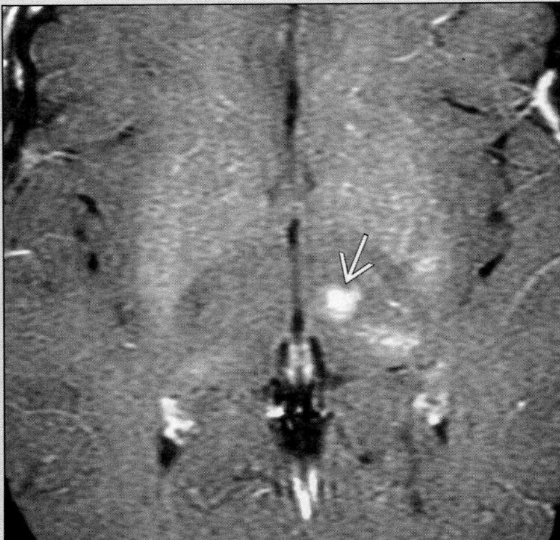

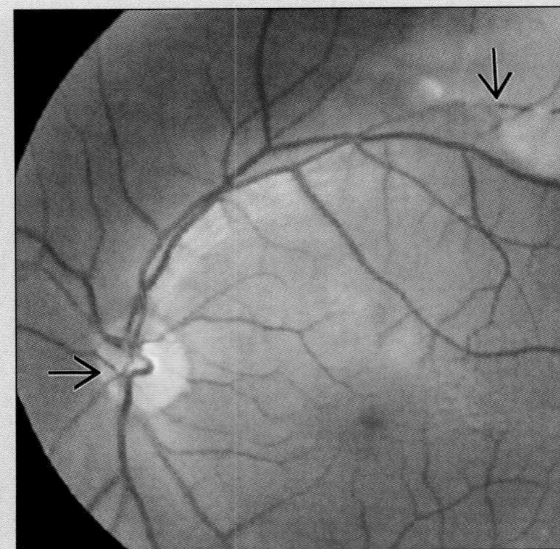

SUSAC SYNDROME

TERMINOLOGY

Synonyms

- RED-M, SICRET syndrome, retinocochleocerebral vasculopathy

Definitions

- Microangiopathy of brain, retina, and cochlea

IMAGING

General Features

- Best diagnostic clue
  - T2 hyperintense corpus callosum (CC) lesions in patient with clinical triad
  - Encephalopathy, bilateral hearing loss, and branch retinal artery occlusions
- Location
  - Body and splenium of CC, middle layers, classically
  - May involve brainstem, basal ganglia (BG), thalamus, subcortical white matter (WM), centrum semiovale

Imaging Recommendations

- Best imaging tool
  - Contrast-enhanced MR

CT Findings

- NECT
  - Often normal
  - May exclude other causes of hearing loss

MR Findings

- T2WI
  - Multifocal T2 hyperintensities similar to those seen in multiple sclerosis (MS)
    - More often round, mid-callosal rather than located at callososeptal interface
  - May see lesions in brainstem, BG, thalamus, subcortical WM, centrum semiovale
- FLAIR
  - Round, punched out, hyperintense callosal lesions
- DWI
  - Callosal lesions may show diffusion restriction acutely (microinfarcts), unlike MS
- T1WI C+
  - Variable enhancement of WM lesions
  - Variable leptomeningeal enhancement
- DTI: Decreased fractional anisotropy (FA) in WM tracts, particularly CC

DIFFERENTIAL DIAGNOSIS

Multiple Sclerosis

- Most common misdiagnosis, with similar appearance of callosal T2 WM lesions
- Typically periventricular and callososeptal interface location

ADEM

- Viral prodrome or post vaccination, monophasic
- T2 hyperintense lesions in BG and WM

Systemic Lupus Erythematosus

- Multifocal WM T2 hyperintensities, vasculitic features

PATHOLOGY

Microscopic Features

- No demyelination seen on pathology
- Normal axon density, reactive glial changes
- Microinfarctions in cerebral cortex, generally not seen on imaging

CLINICAL ISSUES

Presentation

- Most common signs/symptoms
  - Bilateral hearing loss (cochlear)
    - May be unilateral or asymmetric
    - May be associated with tinnitus, vertigo, unsteady gait, nausea, vomiting, and nystagmus
  - Encephalopathy (headaches most common, often severe or migrainous)
  - Branch retinal artery occlusions
- Other signs/symptoms
  - Memory impairment, confusion, behavioral disturbances, ataxia, dysarthria, paranoid psychosis, occasional mutism
  - CSF: High protein and lymphocytic pleocytosis
- Clinical differential diagnosis: Migraine headaches, Ménière disease (bilateral sensorineural hearing loss)

Demographics

- Age: 20-40 years old
- Gender: M < < F

Natural History & Prognosis

- Usually self-limited (2-4 years) but may lead to permanent deafness or blindness

Treatment

- Immunosuppressants and antithrombotics

DIAGNOSTIC CHECKLIST

Consider

- Most patients do not exhibit entire triad (up to 97% at time of presentation)
- Complete triad may be seen after 2 weeks or after 2 years

Image Interpretation Pearls

- Consider Susac syndrome in patients with corpus callosum lesions and clinical triad

SELECTED REFERENCES

1. Kleffner I et al: Diffusion tensor imaging demonstrates fiber impairment in Susac syndrome. Neurology. 70(19 Pt 2):1867-9, 2008
2. Susac JO et al: Susac's syndrome: 1975-2005 microangiopathy/autoimmune endotheliopathy. J Neurol Sci. 257(1-2):270-2, 2007

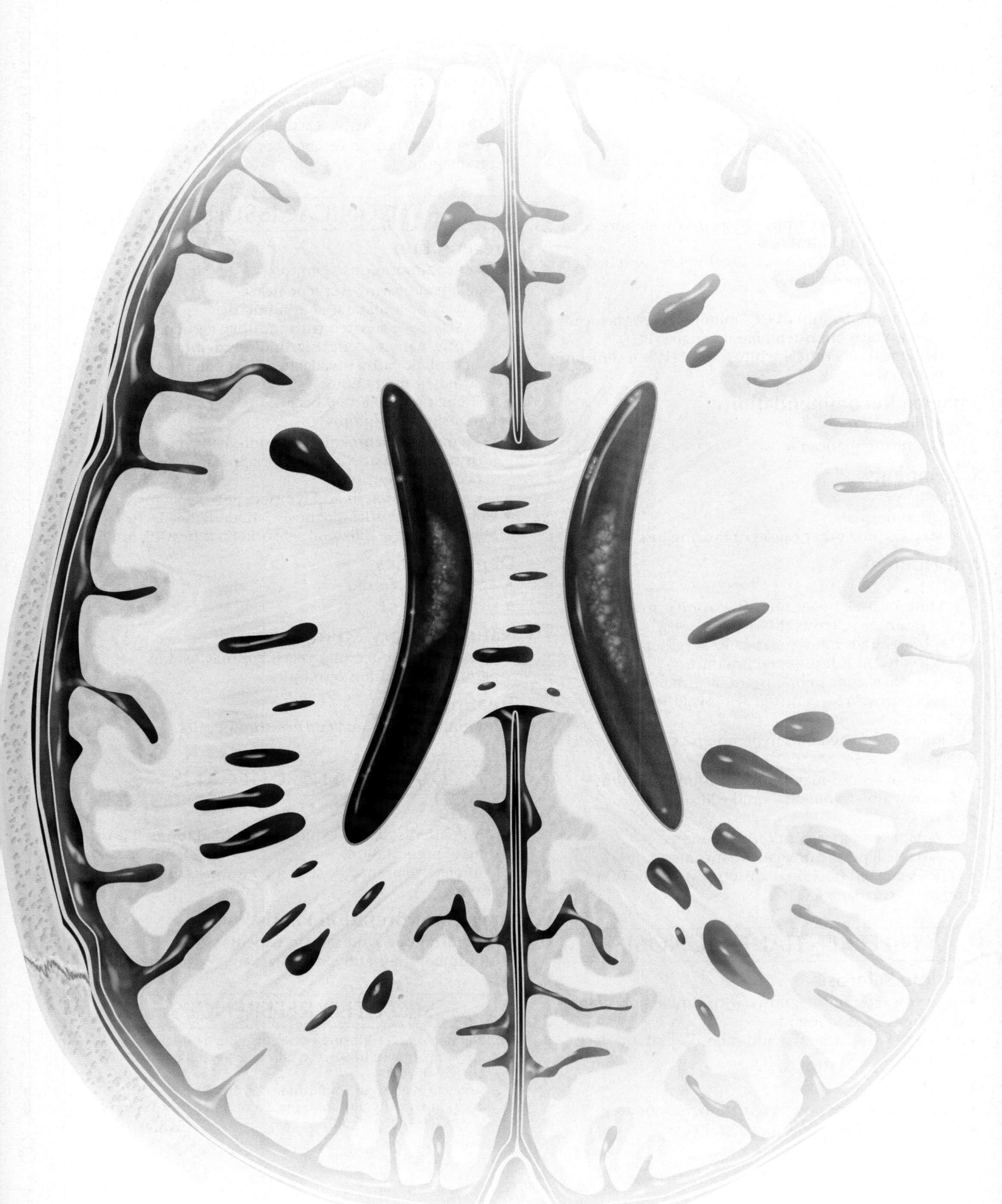

SECTION 9
Inherited Metabolic/Degenerative Disorders

Introduction and Overview

Normal Variants

Mitochondrial Disorders

Lysosomal Disorders

Peroxisomal Disorders

Organic and Aminoacidopathies

Miscellaneous

Overview

Inherited metabolic disorders (IMD) are very difficult to diagnose: Affected patients can present at any age; symptoms vary depending upon age of onset and severity of the biochemical defect. Completely different parts of the brain may be involved in less severely affected patients as compared to more severely affected patients. The same enzyme may perform different functions, in different parts of the brain, as the person matures from infancy to childhood to adulthood. Clearly, patients will have different symptoms if different parts of the brain are involved!

Adding to the confusion, IMDs have been classified in many different ways: Biochemical characteristics, the biochemical pathway that is affected, the cellular organelle in which the affected protein or affected biochemical pathway is located, characteristics of clinical presentation, and the gene that is affected. None of these classifications have been very successful. The imaging features of inherited metabolic disorders can be equally confusing, particularly if not approached methodically.

The imaging appearances of many disorders overlap and often vary with the stage and the variant of the disease. Imaging is most helpful early in the course of the disease. From a neuroimaging perspective, it is most useful to classify disorders based on the pattern of brain involvement on MR early the the course of the disease. This pattern can be supplemented by the use of metabolic data (obtained from proton MR spectroscopy), diffusion data (obtained from diffusion tensor imaging), and occasionally, magnetization transfer.

First Analysis: White vs. Gray Matter

The 1st important determination is whether the disease involves primarily gray matter, primarily white matter, or both gray and white matter.

If the gray matter is primarily involved, scrutinize both the cortex and deep nuclei to determine whether involvement is primarily cortical, primarily deep nuclear, or both. Sometimes disorders that primarily affect cortical gray matter will show cortical swelling with effaced sulci early in the course of the disease; more commonly, cortical thinning is found, with prominent cortical sulci. In later stages, cortical thinning is the rule in all such disorders. The cerebral white matter will often have an abnormal appearance in patients with primary cortical disorders, as Wallerian degeneration of axons causes diminished white matter volume and sometimes mild hyperintensity on FLAIR and T2-weighted images. This appearance should be differentiated from that of primary white matter disorders if the study is performed early in the course of the disease; primarily affected white matter will typically be edematous and, therefore, brighter and more voluminous (causing compressed, smaller sulci) than the white matter that has undergone secondary degeneration. In the acute phase, disorders primarily affecting deep gray matter will typically show edema (FLAIR hyperintensity and prolonged T1 and T2 relaxation times) in the involved structures; in the chronic phase, volume loss with gliosis (resulting in T2 hyperintensity) is more typical.

Disorders primarily affecting white matter cause marked signal abnormality before any volume loss is apparent. Some white matter disorders cause spongiform changes, result in intramyelinic edema, or have an inflammatory component in the early stages. These conditions cause edema with accompanying mass effect upon adjacent structures. (Diffusion weighted images can add specificity as spongiform changes typically cause increased diffusivity, while intramyelinic edema and inflammation cause reduced diffusivity.) Alternatively, many white matter disorders, such as X-linked adrenoleukodystrophy and fibrinoid leukodystrophy (Alexander disease), start locally and expand to involve adjacent areas. Neither of these appearances is seen in the white matter of gray matter disorders. White matter diseases can result in necrosis and cavitation of the affected regions and subsequent ex vacuo dilation of the ventricles, whereas the abnormal white matter in gray matter disorders appears less severely damaged.

Gray Matter Disorders

Gray matter disorders need to be further analyzed to determine whether the disorder primarily involves the cerebral cortex or the deep gray matter nuclei. If the pattern of the imaging study indicates that the metabolic disorder is primarily one of cortical involvement (cortical thinning with enlarged cortical sulci), consideration should be given to disorders such as the neuronal ceroid lipofuscinoses, the mucolipidoses, glycogen storage diseases, or GM1 gangliosidosis.

When only deep gray matter is involved, it is important to identify the specific structures that are affected and their signal intensities. Involvement of the striatum (caudate and putamen) is typically seen in mitochondrial disorders (primarily Leigh syndrome, mitochondrial encephalopathy with lactic acidosis and stroke-like symptoms [MELAS], and the glutaric acidurias) propionic acidemia, Wilson disease, juvenile Huntington disease, molybdenum cofactor deficiency, asphyxia, and childhood or adult hypoglycemia.

Associated white matter or cortical injury may be present in many disorders. If globi pallidi show isolated T2 prolongation, succinate semialdehyde dehydrogenase deficiency, methylmalonic acidemia, guanidinoacetate methyltransferase deficiency (a creatine synthesis disorder), isovaleric acidemia, pyruvate dehydrogenase deficiency (due to mutation of the dihydrolipoamide acetyltransferase [E2] component), carbon monoxide poisoning, or the chronic phase of kernicterus should be considered. If T2 or FLAIR hyperintensity of the globi pallidi is associated with subcortical white matter demyelination, sparing of the periventricular white matter, and involvement of the cerebellar dentate nuclei, L-2-hydroxyglutaric aciduria and Kearns-Sayre syndrome should be considered. When the MR shows atrophy of the dorsal brain stem and cerebellar nuclei, one should consider Leigh syndrome secondary to *SURF1* mutation. If T1 hyperintensity of the globi pallidi is associated with normal T2 signal, and the patient is not receiving hyperalimentation, consider chronic hepatic disease. If both T1 and T2 hyperintensity are seen in a neonate or young infant, consider acute hyperbilirubinemia of infancy, systemic lupus erythematosus, and hemolytic-uremic syndrome; in the presence of edema involving the external and extreme capsules and the claustrum, hemolytic-uremic syndrome is the most likely. If the globi pallidi, the insula, and perirolandic cortex are all hyperintense on T2-weighted or FLAIR images, the diagnosis of hyperammonemia (and a urea cycle disorder) should be suggested. If the involvement of the globus pallidus is manifested on MR as T2 hypointensity with central T2 hyperintensity, the diagnosis of pantothenate kinase-associated neuropathy (formerly called Hallervorden-Spatz disease) can be made with some confidence.

White Matter Disorders

White matter disorders can be divided into disorders in which white matter never myelinates completely (hypomyelination) and disorders in which myelin forms and breaks down (demyelination) with or without cavitation of white matter. The pattern of a lack of myelination, or **hypomyelination**, is seen in very few disorders, called the hypomyelinating leukoencephalopathies. The appearance of the brain in these disorders is that of a normal, much more immature brain. For example, the MR of a 5-year-old child with hypomyelination might be mistaken for that of a 5-month-old infant; diffusivity is normal, while magnetization transfer is reduced. Such disorders include: Pelizaeus-Merzbacher and like diseases, leukodystrophies with trichothiodystrophy and photosensitivity, Tay syndrome, 18q- syndrome (deletion of a large portion of the long arm of chromosome 18), sialic acidemia (Salla disease), hypomyelination with atrophy of basal ganglia and cerebellum, and hypomyelination with congenital cataracts.

When myelin develops but is subsequently damaged, the condition is called **demyelination** to differentiate it from breakdown of abnormal myelin, sometimes called dysmyelination. By the use of diffusion tensor imaging, it may eventually be possible to differentiate these 2 entities, but the differentiation cannot currently be made. Myelin destruction can, however, be differentiated from white matter cavitation (cystic degeneration). Cystic degeneration has much lower signal on FLAIR sequences, significantly less magnetization transfer, and greater diffusivity than areas of myelin destruction without cavitation. In disorders where inflammation is associated with demyelination (typically peroxisomal disorders), the inflammatory infiltrate causes reduced diffusivity and blood-brain barrier breakdown (resulting in contrast enhancement). When myelin breakdown occurs, the white matter becomes more hypointense on T1-weighted images and more hyperintense on T2-weighted images. In these situations, analyze the brain to determine whether the region primarily affected is the periventricular white matter, the deep white matter, or the subcortical white matter.

Disorders Affecting Gray and White Matter

Disorders involving both gray and white matter are 1st separated by the type of gray matter involvement: Those involving only the cerebral cortex and those involving deep gray matter (with or without cortical involvement).

Disorders involving only cortical gray matter can be subdivided depending on the involvement of long bones and the spinal column. If the long bones are normal, the cortex should be analyzed for malformations of cortical development (MCD). If an MCD is present in addition to a lack of myelination, the differential diagnosis includes the generalized peroxisomal disorders, congenital cytomegalovirus disease, and the so-called cobblestone cortical malformations. If no MCD is found, differential considerations include Alpers disease and Menkes disease, both of which cause considerable cerebral cortical destruction. If the bones are abnormal, the differential diagnoses include primarily storage diseases, such as the mucopolysaccharidoses and lipid storage disorders.

If deep gray matter is involved, determine precisely which nuclei are affected. If thalami are involved, differential considerations include Krabbe disease and the GM1 and GM2 gangliosidoses; the thalami in these disorders display high attenuation on CT and short T1 and T2 relaxation times (hyperintense on T1-weighted images and hypointense on T2-weighted images) on MR. Krabbe disease is distinguished by the presence of abnormal T2 hyperintensity along the corticospinal tracts and in the cerebellar dentate nuclei.

Another disorder with thalamic involvement is profound neonatal hypoxic-ischemic injury, which typically involves the ventrolateral thalami, posterior putamina, and perirolandic cortex; a characteristic history of perinatal distress and neonatal encephalopathy simplifies the diagnosis. Another consideration when thalamic involvement is identified is autosomal dominant acute necrotizing encephalitis, particularly if T2 hyperintensity is also seen in the dorsal brain stem. Thalami may also be affected in mitochondrial disorders, Wilson disease, and Canavan disease; typically other deep gray matter nuclei will be affected as well (e.g., putamina in mitochondrial disorders and Wilson disease, globi pallidi in Canavan disease). Globus pallidus involvement in association with diffuse white matter disease including the subcortical, deep, and periventricular regions suggests a diagnosis of Canavan disease. Association of globus pallidus involvement with affected subcortical white matter but sparing of periventricular white matter suggests a later phase of Kearns-Sayre syndrome or L-2-hydroxyglutaric aciduria; the latter will often show involvement of the cerebellar dentate nuclei.

Globus pallidus injury with sparing of subcortical white matter in early stages suggests methylmalonic acidemia, maple syrup urine disease, carbon monoxide toxicity, or cyanide toxicity. MR of maple syrup urine disease during the acute neonatal phase of the disease shows involvement of the centrum semiovale, internal capsules, cerebral peduncles, dorsal pons, and cerebellar white matter, reduced diffusivity in the affected regions, and a peak at 0.9 ppm on proton MR spectroscopy. Carbon monoxide and cyanide toxicity typically involve the cerebral cortex, globi pallidi, and cerebellum. White matter disease associated with striatal involvement suggests Leigh syndrome, MELAS, propionic acidemia, glutaric aciduria type 1, molybdenum cofactor deficiency, isolated sulfite oxidase deficiency, hypomyelination with atrophy of the basal ganglia and cerebellum, toxic exposure, later infantile or childhood profound hypoxic-ischemic injury, or childhood hypoglycemia. Proper analysis of the MR scans using this pattern system can facilitate the work-up of patients with inborn errors of metabolism.

INHERITED METABOLIC DISORDERS OVERVIEW

Imaging Patterns

Metabolic Disorders with ...

T2 or FLAIR Hyperintensity of the Corpus Striatum

- Leigh syndrome (includes pyruvate dehydrogenase deficiency, respiratory complex I and complex II disorders)
- Wilson disease
- Glutaric aciduria type 1
- Juvenile Huntington disease
- Molybdenum cofactor deficiency
- Propionic acidemia

T2 or FLAIR Hyperintensity of the Globi Pallidi

- Methylmalonic acidemia
- Succinic semialdehyde dehydrogenase deficiency
- Urea cycle disorders
- Guanidinoacetate methyltransferase deficiency
- Pyruvate dehydrogenase (E2) deficiency
- Systemic lupus erythematosus
- Hemolytic-uremic syndrome
- Bilirubin toxicity
- Isovaleric acidemia
- Carbon monoxide toxicity
- Cyanide toxicity

Early Involvement of Subcortical White Matter

- Alexander disease
- Kearns-Sayre syndrome
- Megalencephalic leukoencephalopathy with subcortical cysts
- Galactosemia
- Mitochondrial disorders

Early Involvement of Periventricular and Deep White Matter with Sparing of Subcortical White Matter

- X-linked adrenoleukodystrophy
- Krabbe disease (globoid cell leukodystrophy)
- Metachromatic leukodystrophy
- GM2 gangliosidoses
- Childhood ataxia with CNS hypomyelination (vanishing white matter disease)
- Lowe syndrome (oculocerebrorenal syndrome)
- Mucolipidosis type 4
- Merosin deficient congenital muscular dystrophy
- Damage from radiation or chemotherapy

Globus Pallidus and White Matter Involvement

- Canavan disease
- Methylmalonic acidemia
- Kearns-Sayre syndrome
- L-2-hydroxyglutaric aciduria
- Maple syrup urine disease
- Carbon monoxide poisoning
- Cyanide toxicity

Striatal (Caudate and Putaminal) and White Matter Involvement

- Leigh syndrome
- Mitochondrial encephalopathy with lactic acidosis and stroke-like symptoms (MELAS)
- Other mitochondrial leukoencephalopathies
- Propionic acidemia
- Glutaric acidemia type 1
- Isolated sulfite oxidase deficiency
- Late infantile/childhood profound hypoxic-ischemic injury
- Childhood hypoglycemia

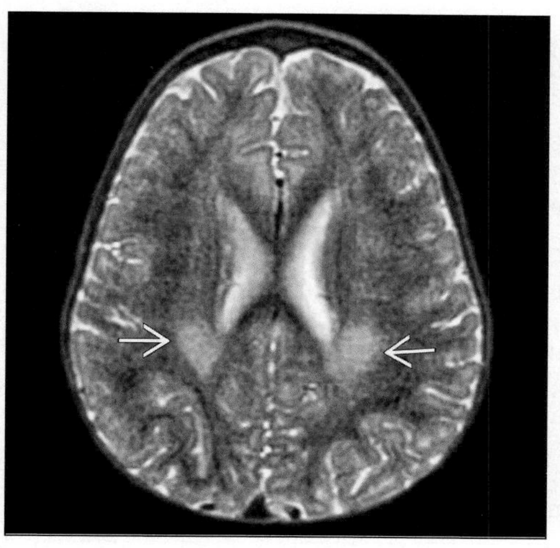

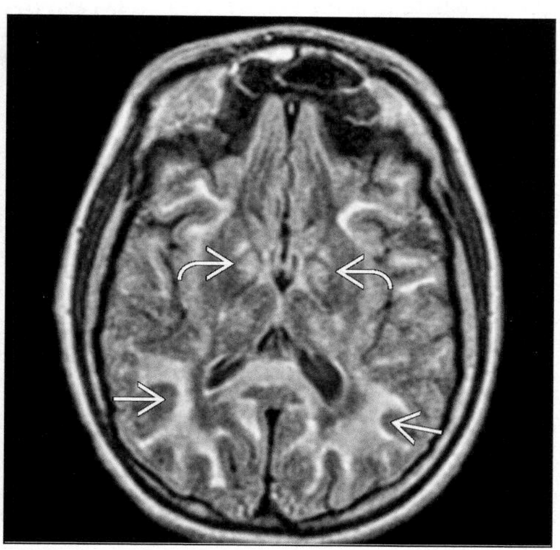

*(**Left**) Axial T2WI MR in a patient with Krabbe disease shows T2 hyperintensity ➡ of the deep and periventricular white matter with sparing of subcortical white matter. Involvement in Krabbe disease typically starts along the corticospinal tracts. (**Right**) Axial FLAIR MR in a patient with Kearns-Sayre syndrome shows involvement ➡ of subcortical and deep white matter with sparing of periventricular regions. Note also bilateral globus pallidus hyperintensity ↷.*

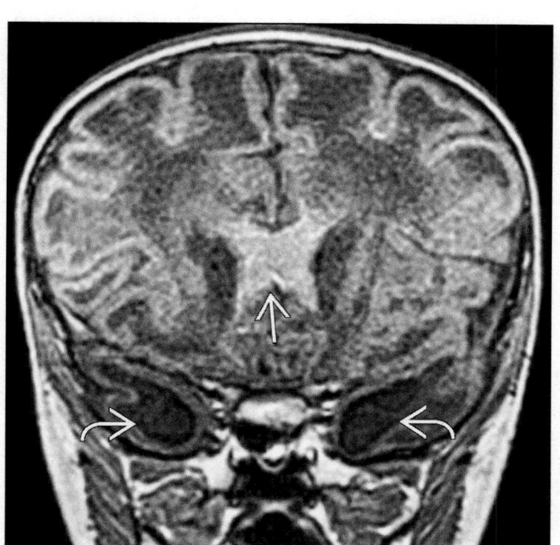

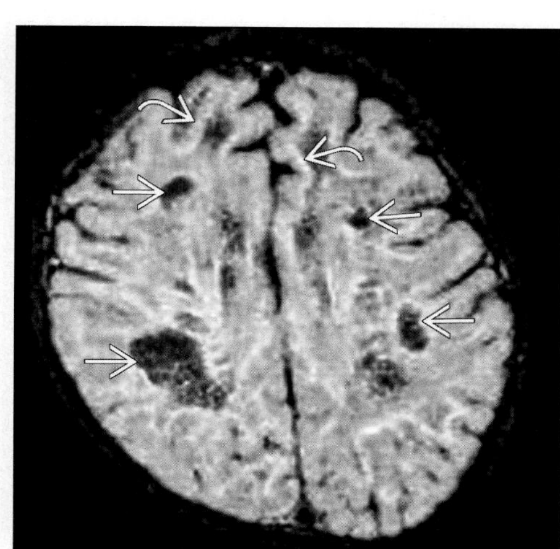

*(**Left**) Coronal T1WI MR in an infant with megalencephaly with leukoencephalopathy and cysts shows complete lack of myelination other than in the genu of the corpus callosum ➡. An important clue to this diagnosis is the subcortical cysts ↷ in the anterior temporal lobes. (**Right**) Axial FLAIR MR shows multiple areas of hypointense cavitation ➡ in the cerebral white matter in this patient with vanishing white matter disease. The less affected subcortical white matter ↷ is hyperintense.*

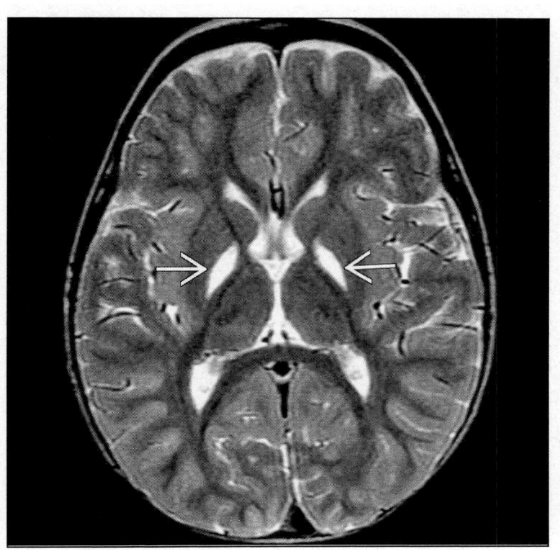

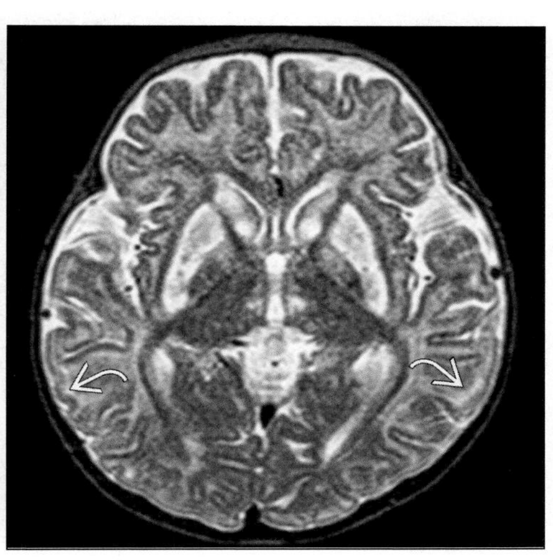

*(**Left**) Axial T2WI MR in a child with methylmalonic acidemia shows abnormal hyperintensity ➡ of the bilateral globi pallidi. The white matter is unaffected in this patient. (**Right**) Axial T2WI MR in an infant with Leigh syndrome due to pyruvate dehydrogenase disease with a typical pattern. Note that there is abnormal hyperintensity of the caudate heads, putamina, and medial thalami. The white matter shows a few areas of subcortical hyperintensity ↷.*

HYPOMYELINATION

Key Facts

Terminology

- Diminished or absent degree of white matter (WM) myelination for age
- May be primary hypomyelination syndrome or secondary to other pathology

Imaging

- T1 shortening reflects presence of mature oligodendrocytes with proteolipid protein
  - Myelination on T1WI is complete by 1 year of age
- T2 shortening reflects displacement of interstitial water by myelin wrapping on axons
  - Myelination on T2WI is complete by 3 years of age, usually by 2 years of age

Top Differential Diagnoses

- Pelizaeus-Merzbacher disease, 18q-syndrome
- Mucopolysaccharidoses, mitochondrial encephalopathies
- Leukodystrophies, trichothiodystrophy

Pathology

- Hypomyelination often reflects abnormalities of proteolipid protein (PLP) or myelin basic protein (MBP)
  - Defects in PLP prevent normal myelin compaction
  - MBP is thought to stabilize myelin spiral at major dense line

Diagnostic Checklist

- It may not be possible to distinguish hypomyelination, dysmyelination, and demyelination
- Define degree of myelination by age at which it would be appropriate → "degree of myelination appropriate for x months of age"
  - Assess myelination prior to learning chronologic age of patient

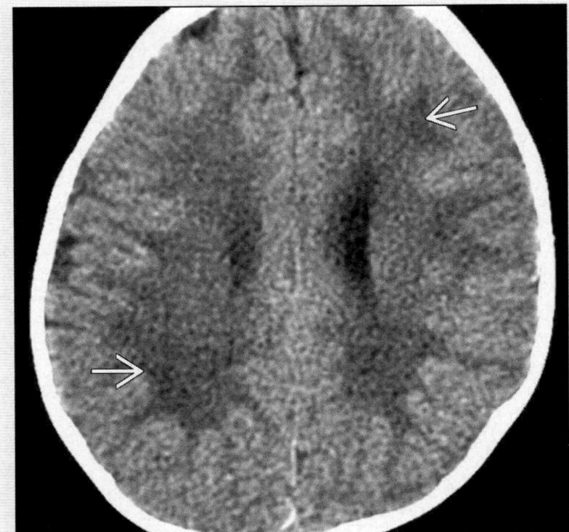

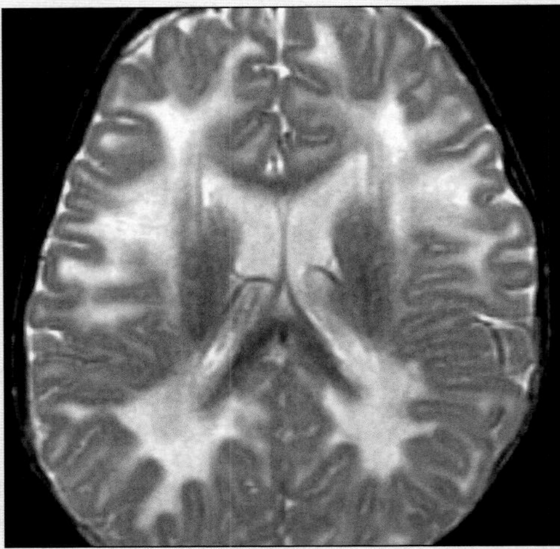

(Left) *Axial NECT in a 1 year old with Jacobsen syndrome (11q-chromosomal deletion) shows irregular hypoattenuation that is most severe in the subcortical cerebral white matter ➔.* ***(Right)*** *Axial T2WI MR in the same patient confirms that the decreased attenuation on CT correlates with marked and diffuse hypomyelination. Hypomyelination has been described in numerous chromosomal deletion syndromes, although the prevalence is difficult to gauge.*

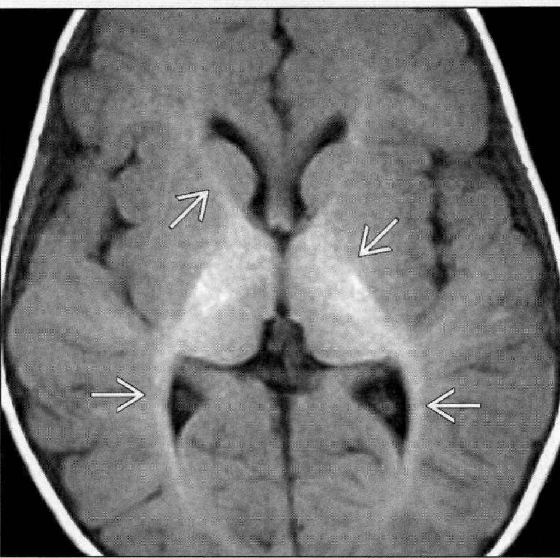

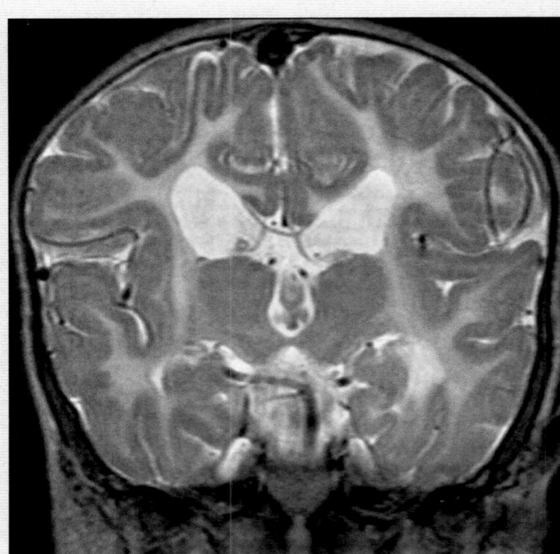

(Left) *Axial T1WI MR in a 9 month old with 18q-syndrome shows only faint T1 shortening that is limited to the internal capsules and optic radiations ➔. At 9 months, only the most distal rami of white matter should be without bright signal on T1WI.* ***(Right)*** *Coronal T2WI MR in a 14 year old with hypomyelination and atrophy of the basal ganglia and cerebellum (H-ABC). Note absence of visible caudate nuclei and corpus callosum, in addition to the abnormal hyperintense signal of unmyelinated white matter.*

HYPOMYELINATION

TERMINOLOGY

Synonyms

- Delayed myelin maturation, undermyelination

Definitions

- Diminished or absent degree of white matter (WM) myelination for age
- Myelin "milestones" not achieved
- May be primary hypomyelination syndrome or secondary to other pathology

IMAGING

General Features

- Best diagnostic clue
  - Poor gray-white differentiation on T1WI in children > 1 year
  - Poor gray-white differentiation on T2WI in children > 2 years
- Location
  - Key areas to assess are internal capsule, pyramidal tracts, and peripheral frontal lobe WM rami
- Size
  - Hypomyelination will result in reduced brain volume
    - Thin corpus callosum evident on sagittal images
- Morphology
  - Typically normal

CT Findings

- NECT
  - Lack of myelin generally too subtle to identify on CT

MR Findings

- T1WI
  - Myelinated WM is hyperintense on T1WI
    - T1 shortening reflects presence of mature oligodendrocytes with proteolipid protein
  - WM structures become hyperintense in stereotypical order
  - Myelination on T1WI is complete by 1 year of age
- T2WI
  - Myelinated WM is hypointense on T2WI
    - T2 shortening reflects displacement of interstitial water by myelin wrapping on axons
  - Hypointensity on T2WI lags hyperintensity on T1WI by 4-8 months
  - Myelination on T2WI is complete by 3 years of age (usually by 2 years of age)
  - "Terminal zones"
    - Regions of persistent hyperintense signal on T2WI in otherwise normal brains
    - Typically around trigones of lateral ventricles
    - Likely due to concentration of interstitial water migrating to ventricles in these areas
    - Must be distinguished from periventricular leukomalacia or perivascular spaces
- PD/intermediate
  - Key for distinguishing gliosis from undermyelination
    - Gliosis is more hyperintense
- FLAIR
  - Not recommended in children < 2 years
    - Heterogeneous signal makes assessment of myelination and distinction of pathology more difficult
- DWI
  - ADC values predate T1- and T2-weighted signal changes
    - ADC drops as WM diffusivity decreases
  - Fractional anisotropy increases with brain maturation
- T1WI C+
  - Some leukodystrophies have abnormal enhancement
    - Not strictly hypomyelination
- MRS
  - Choline decreases as myelination progresses
  - Relative increases in myoinositol, choline, and lipid resonances with hypomyelination
  - Significant increases in choline may indicate demyelination or dysmyelination

Imaging Recommendations

- Best imaging tool
  - MR
- Protocol advice
  - T1WI most helpful in children < 10 months
  - T2WI most helpful in children > 10 months

DIFFERENTIAL DIAGNOSIS

Primary Hypomyelination Syndromes

- Pelizaeus-Merzbacher disease (PMD)
- Spastic paraplegia type 2 (SPG2)
- 18q-syndrome
- Hypomyelination with atrophy of basal ganglia and cerebellum (H-ABC)

Prematurity

- Use of normal milestones assumes full-term gestation
- Adjust chronologic age for degree of prematurity

External Stresses

- Chronic debilitating conditions in infancy
  - Congenital vascular malformations (AVF)
  - Malnutrition
- Treatments for diseases in neonate
  - Organ transplantation
  - Chemotherapy
- Myelination typically rebounds with treatment of primary illness

Syndromes with Hypomyelination and Other Findings

- Typically cause dysmyelination, not hypomyelination
- Mucopolysaccharidoses
  - Hunter, Hurler
  - Mitochondrial encephalopathies
    - Electron transport chain (ETC) defects
    - Mitochondrial membrane abnormalities
- Leukodystrophies
  - Metachromatic leukodystrophy
  - Globoid leukodystrophy (Krabbe)

- Trichothiodystrophy
  - Group of disorders of DNA repair
  - Osteosclerosis of axial skeleton
  - "Tiger-band hair" under polarized light

PATHOLOGY

General Features

- Etiology
  - Hypomyelination often reflects abnormalities of proteolipid protein (PLP) or myelin basic protein (MBP)
  - Defects in PLP prevent normal myelin compaction
    - Compaction displaces water and accounts for T2 hypointensity
  - MBP is thought to stabilize myelin spiral at major dense line
- Genetics
  - 10-30% of PMD and SPG2 caused by defects in proteolipid protein (*PLP*) gene (Xq21-q22)
  - 18q-syndrome causes hemizygous deletion (1 copy of gene missing) of *MBP* gene
- Associated abnormalities
  - Craniofacial-facial malformations associated with 18q-syndrome
  - PMD and 18q-syndrome are prototypes of hypomyelination

Microscopic Features

- Pelizaeus-Merzbacher disease
  - Patchy myelin deficiency; no sparing of subcortical U-fibers
  - Islands of persistent perivascular myelin result in classic "tigroid" appearance
  - Absent or deficient compact myelin sheaths, "redundant myelin balls"

CLINICAL ISSUES

Presentation

- Most common signs/symptoms
  - Developmental delay, hypotonia
- Other signs/symptoms
  - Classic PMD: Head titubation, hypotonia, only 50% able to sit
  - 18q-syndrome: Developmental delays, short stature, delayed bone age, limb anomalies
  - Trichothiodystrophy: Short stature, osteosclerosis

Demographics

- Age
  - Primary hypomyelination syndromes typically present in infancy
- Gender
  - Classic PMD is X-linked recessive and thus exclusive to males
  - Other forms of PMD are autosomal recessive and equally distributed

Natural History & Prognosis

- Late progression of symptoms may occur in some

Treatment

- No treatment yet for heritable disorders of hypomyelination

DIAGNOSTIC CHECKLIST

Consider

- It may not be possible to distinguish hypomyelination, dysmyelination, and demyelination
- Remember to adjust chronologic age for degree of prematurity

Image Interpretation Pearls

- Assess myelination prior to learning chronologic age of patient
  - Avoid predetermination bias
- Correlate imaging findings with clinical history and neurological exam to narrow scope of differential

Reporting Tips

- Define degree of myelination by age at which it would be appropriate → "degree of myelination appropriate for x months of age"

SELECTED REFERENCES

1. Schiffmann R et al: Invited article: an MRI-based approach to the diagnosis of white matter disorders. Neurology. 72(8):750-9, 2009
2. Rossi A et al: Hypomyelination and congenital cataract: neuroimaging features of a novel inherited white matter disorder. AJNR Am J Neuroradiol. 29(2):301-5, 2008
3. Barkovich AJ: Myelin mishaps. Ann Neurol. 62(2):107-9, 2007
4. van der Knaap MS et al: Hypomyelination with atrophy of the basal ganglia and cerebellum: follow-up and pathology. Neurology. 69(2):166-71, 2007
5. van der Voorn JP et al: Childhood white matter disorders: quantitative MR imaging and spectroscopy. Radiology. 241(2):510-7, 2006
6. Hudson LD: Pelizaeus-Merzbacher disease and spastic paraplegia type 2: two faces of myelin loss from mutations in the same gene. J Child Neurol. 18(9):616-24, 2003
7. Linnankivi TT et al: 18q-syndrome: brain MRI shows poor differentiation of gray and white matter on T2-weighted images. J Magn Reson Imaging. 18(4):414-9, 2003
8. Pizzini F et al: Proton MR spectroscopic imaging in Pelizaeus-Merzbacher disease. AJNR Am J Neuroradiol. 24(8):1683-9, 2003
9. Engelbrecht V et al: Diffusion-weighted MR imaging in the brain in children: findings in the normal brain and in the brain with white matter diseases. Radiology. 222(2):410-8, 2002
10. Koeppen AH et al: Pelizaeus-Merzbacher disease. J Neuropathol Exp Neurol. 61(9):747-59, 2002
11. Takanashi J et al: Brain N-acetylaspartate is elevated in Pelizaeus-Merzbacher disease with PLP1 duplication. Neurology. 58(2):237-41, 2002
12. Cecil KM et al: Magnetic resonance spectroscopy of the pediatric brain. Top Magn Reson Imaging. 12(6):435-52, 2001
13. Woodward K et al: CNS myelination and PLP gene dosage. Pharmacogenomics. 2(3):263-72, 2001
14. Barkovich AJ: Concepts of myelin and myelination in neuroradiology. AJNR Am J Neuroradiol. 21(6):1099-109, 2000

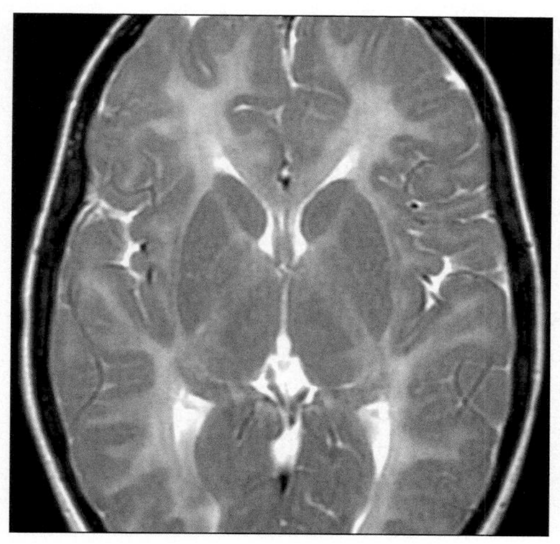

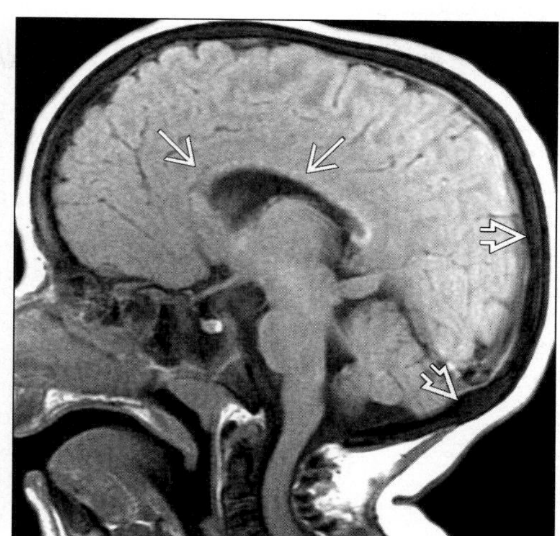

(Left) *Axial T2WI MR in this 12 year old with trichothiodystrophy shows essentially complete absence of myelination throughout the brain. Examination of the hair under polarized light demonstrated characteristic "tiger-tail" bands, and radiographs showed central osteosclerosis.* ***(Right)*** *Sagittal T1WI MR in the same child shows absence of myelin deposition throughout the brain, making the corpus callosum ➔ difficult to define on this midline image. Note the thickened skull posteriorly ➩.*

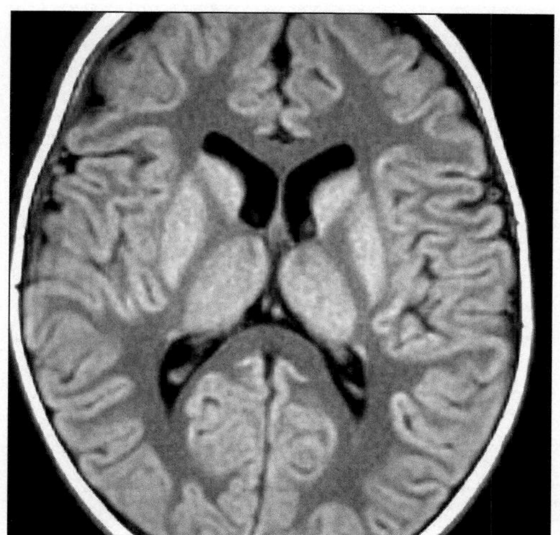

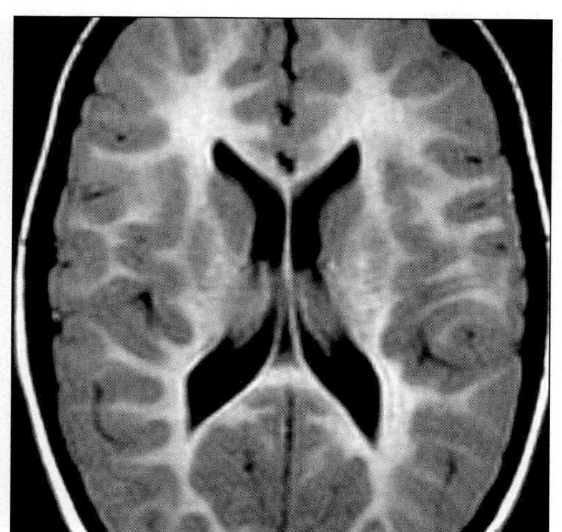

(Left) *Axial T1WI MR in a 26-month-old child with nystagmus and head titubation, diagnosed with Pelizaeus-Merzbacher disease. The homogeneous absence of myelin deposition causes the appearance to mimic a normal FLAIR image in a mature brain.* ***(Right)*** *Conversely, this axial FLAIR image in a 6 year old with Pelizaeus-Merzbacher disease resembles a normal T1WI, with hyperintense signal of the white matter relative to gray matter throughout.*

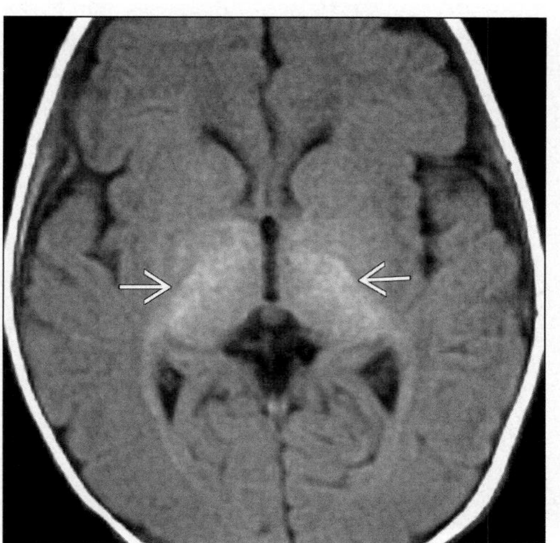

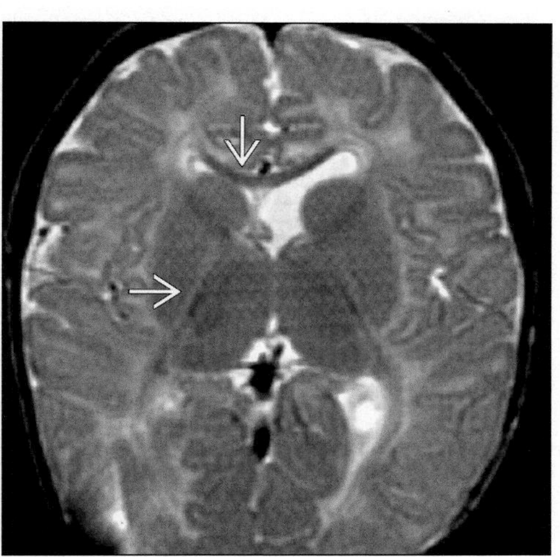

(Left) *Axial T1WI MR in a 2 year old with nystagmus shows minimal T1 shortening in the PLIC ➔; myelination should appear complete on T1WI at this age. Chromosomal analysis showed a mutation of PLP, confirming a diagnosis of Pelizaeus-Merzbacher disease.* ***(Right)*** *Axial T2WI MR in a 14 month old with an arteriovenous fistula shows hypointense signal of myelin maturation in the genu and internal capsules only ➔. Concomitant illness is a common cause of delayed myelin maturation.*

LEIGH SYNDROME

Key Facts

Terminology

- Genetically heterogeneous mitochondrial disorder characterized by progressive neurodegeneration

Imaging

- Bilateral, symmetric ↑ T2/FLAIR corpora striata (putamen > caudate) > globi pallidi (GP), periaqueductal gray matter (PAG), substantia nigra/subthalamic nuclei, dorsal pons, cerebellar nuclei
- Reduced diffusion in regions of acute disease
- Lactate peak often present; may be large
- Best imaging: MR with DWI/MRS
- Uncommon appearance: Predominant WM disease (simulates leukodystrophy)

Top Differential Diagnoses

- Profound perinatal asphyxia
- Mitochondrial encephalopathy, lactic acidosis, stroke-like episodes (MELAS)
- Glutaric aciduria type 1 (GA-1)
- Wilson disease

Pathology

- Bioenergetic failure (ATP loss) and production of reactive oxygen species likely key factors in mitochondria-mediated cell apoptosis
- 50-75% patients with LS have detectable biochemical or molecular abnormality

Clinical Issues

- Presentation: Psychomotor delay/regression, hypotonia
- Prenatal diagnosis: Chorionic villus sampling (mutations and biochemical defects)
- Majority present by age 2 years

(Left) Axial FLAIR MR shows swelling and abnormal hyperintensity in the caudate heads and putamina ➔. Foci of hyperintensity are also present in the medial thalami ➔, a typical location of involvement in Leigh syndrome. *(Right)* Single voxel proton MR spectroscopy (TE = 26 msec) of the same patient shows a large lactate doublet ➔ at 1.3 ppm. The identification of a lactate peak supports the diagnosis of mitochondrial disease, but is variably present.

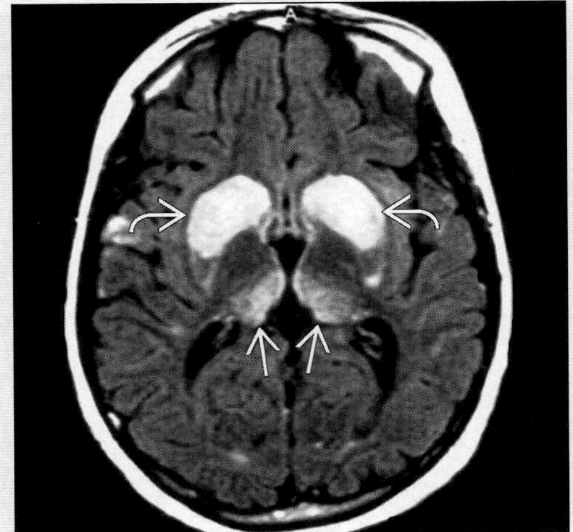

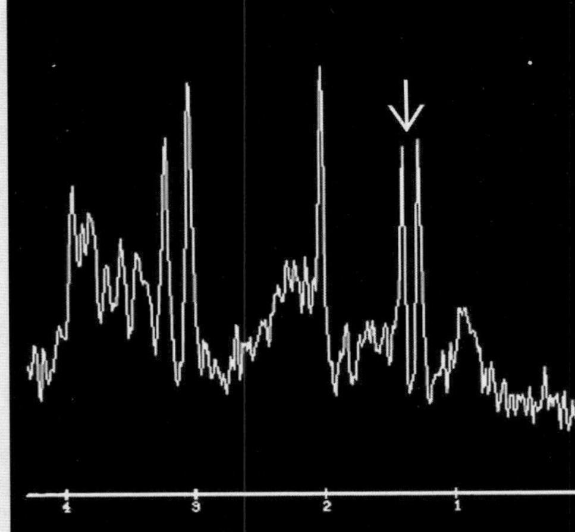

(Left) Axial T2WI MR shows T2 hyperintensity and some swelling of the lentiform nuclei ➔ bilaterally. In addition, the genu ➔ and splenium ➔ of the corpus callosum are affected. Note that foci of unaffected tissue ➔ are present in the putamina; heterogeneous involvement is common. *(Right)* Axial T2WI MR in the same patient shows T2 hyperintensity of the cerebral peduncles ➔. This is another common site of involvement in Leigh syndrome.

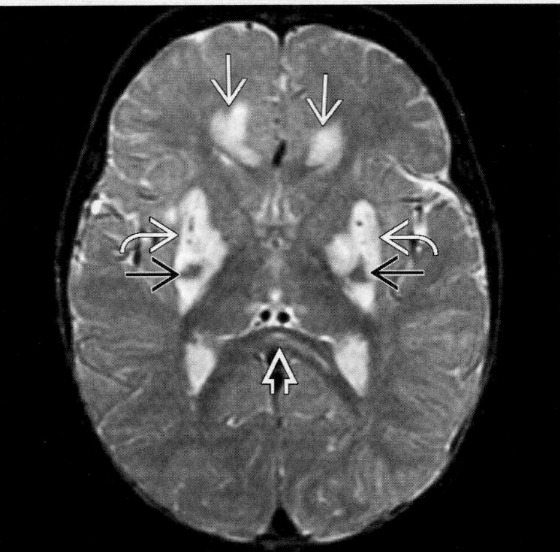

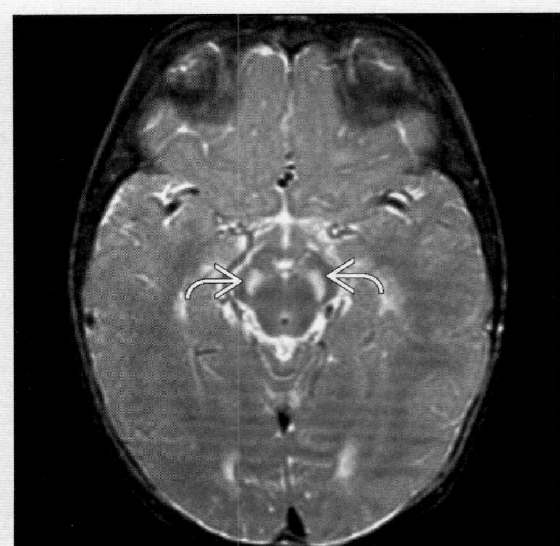

LEIGH SYNDROME

TERMINOLOGY

Abbreviations

- Leigh syndrome (LS)

Synonyms

- Subacute necrotizing encephalomyelopathy

Definitions

- Genetically heterogeneous mitochondrial disorder characterized by progressive neurodegeneration

IMAGING

General Features

- Best diagnostic clue
  - Bilateral, symmetric, ↑ T2/FLAIR putamina and peri-aqueductal gray matter (PAG)
- Location
  - Common
    - Basal ganglia (BG): Corpora striata (putamina > caudate heads) > globi pallidi (GP)
    - Brain stem (BS): PAG, substantia nigra/ subthalamic nuclei, pons, medulla
    - Thalami, dentate nuclei
  - Infrequent: White matter (WM) (cerebral > cerebellar, may be cavitary), spine, cortical gray matter
- Size
  - BS: Small, discrete foci (< 1 cm)
    - Involvement of central WM tracts typical
  - BG: Involvement of posterior putamina classic but variable; may affect entire lentiform nuclei
  - Thalami: Focal involvement of dorsomedial nuclei classic but variable
- Morphology
  - Except WM, lesions are bilaterally symmetric
  - Edema, expansion characteristic of early disease; volume loss characteristic of late disease
    - PAG edema may cause hydrocephalus
  - Involvement of lower BS (pons, medulla) and lack of BG involvement characteristic of LS secondary to *SURF1* mutation
  - Uncommon appearance
    - Predominant WM disease (simulates leukodystrophy)

CT Findings

- NECT
  - Hypodense; occasionally normal
- CECT
  - Enhancement uncommon

MR Findings

- T1WI
  - Hypointense
    - Variable foci hyperintensity = blood or necrosis
- T2WI
  - Hyperintense
- FLAIR
  - Hyperintense
    - Resolution of signal abnormality or cystic encephalomalacia (hypointense) may be seen in chronic disease
- DWI
  - Reduced diffusion in regions of acute disease
- MRS
  - ↑ choline, ↓ NAA
  - Lactate peak often present; may be large

Ultrasonographic Findings

- Hyperechoic deep gray structures, WM

Imaging Recommendations

- Best imaging tool
  - MR with DWI/MRS

DIFFERENTIAL DIAGNOSIS

Profound Perinatal Asphyxia

- ↑ T2 & T1 dorsolateral putamina, lateral thalami, dorsal BS, perirolandic cortex
  - T2 hyperintensity difficult to identify in unmyelinated brain
  - T1 hyperintensity seen subacutely (3-10 days)
- History of perinatal asphyxia

Mitochondrial Encephalopathy, Lactic Acidosis, Stroke-Like Episodes (MELAS)

- ↑ T2/FLAIR putamina (Ca++ in chronic disease)
  - May be asymmetric or unilateral
- Stroke-like signal abnormality parietooccipital lobes
  - Nonvascular distribution and (-) DWI typical

Glutaric Aciduria Type 1 (GA-1)

- ↑ T2/FLAIR corpora striata, GP, ± WM disease
- Characteristic opercular widening

Wilson Disease

- ↑ T2/FLAIR putamina, GP, midbrain, thalami
  - T2 changes evident in older children, teens
- T1 hyperintense GP 2° to hepatic failure

PATHOLOGY

General Features

- Etiology
  - Exact mechanistic relationship between mitochondrial dysfunction and neurodegeneration unknown
  - Bioenergetic failure (ATP loss) and production of reactive oxygen species likely key factors in mitochondria-mediated cell apoptosis
  - Coenzyme Q10 deficiency and mitochondrial depletion also implicated in LS
- Genetics
  - LS characterized by extreme genetic heterogeneity
  - Autosomal recessive (AR), X-linked, and maternal inheritance of mutated proteins involved in mitochondrial energy production
    - Mutations frequently involve electron transport chain complexes (COs) I-V

LEIGH SYNDROME

- AR: Mutation of *SURF1* gene (9q34) is most frequent cause of LS due to CO IV (cytochrome C oxidase, COX) deficiency
- Other AR mutations: *NDUFV1/NDUFS8* (11q13), *NDUFS4* (5q11.1), *NDUFS7* genes ⇒ CO I deficiency; *NDUFS3* gene ⇒ NADH dehydrogenase deficiency; *SDHA* gene (5p15) ⇒ CO II deficiency; *BCS1L* gene (2q33) ⇒ CO III deficiency, and non-*SURF1* mutations ⇒ COX deficiency
- X-linked: *PDHA1* gene (Xp22.2-p22.1) ⇒ pyruvate dehydrogenase CO deficiency
- Maternally inherited (mtDNA mutations): *MTATP6* gene ⇒ CO V deficiency (causes LS if mutation load > 90%), NARP (neuropathy, ataxia, retinitis pigmentosa) if load 70-90%); *MTND5*, *MTND6* genes ⇒ CO I deficiency; *MTCO3* gene ⇒ COX deficiency; *MTTK*, *MTTV* tRNA genes

- Associated abnormalities
  - 50-75% of patients with LS have detectable biochemical or molecular abnormality
  - Embryology-anatomy
    - Main role mitochondria = production ATP via oxidative phosphorylation
    - Mitochondria contain own DNA (mtDNA, average of 5 mtDNA per mitochondrion)
    - mtDNA contribution to zygote exclusively from oocyte (maternal inheritance)
    - Mitochondria/mtDNA randomly distributed among daughter cells
    - mtDNA & nuclear DNA (nDNA) encode subunits of electron transport chain complexes (COs) I, III-V; nDNA encodes subunits CO II
  - Brain & striated muscle highly dependent on oxidative phosphorylation ⇒ most severely affected in mitochondrial disorders
  - Variable number of mitochondria/cell, random distribution of mitochondria/mtDNA into daughter cells ⇒ phenotypic heterogeneity typical of all mitochondrial disorders

Gross Pathologic & Surgical Features

- Brownish-gray, gelatinous or cavitary foci in corpora striata, GP, BS, dentate nuclei, thalami, spinal cord, white matter

Microscopic Features

- Spongiform degeneration, gliosis, neuronal loss, demyelination, capillary proliferation

CLINICAL ISSUES

Presentation

- Most common signs/symptoms
  - Presentation: Psychomotor delay/regression, hypotonia
  - Other signs/symptoms
    - Progressive BS & BG dysfunction
      - Ataxia, ophthalmoplegia, ptosis, vomiting, swallowing and respiratory difficulties, dystonia
  - Early presentation, BS dysfunction, peripheral neuropathy, & rapid neurologic deterioration typical of LS 2° *SURF1* mutation
  - Metabolic stressors (e.g., infection) may unmask disease or cause deterioration
  - Elevated CSF, serum, urine lactate classic but not invariable
  - Clinical diagnosis
    - Progressive neurodegeneration
    - Signs/symptoms of BS & BG dysfunction
    - ↑ lactate in blood + CSF
    - Biochemical defect identified by mitochondrial analysis of muscle biopsy or cultured skin fibroblasts
    - MR → characteristic BG or BS lesions
  - Prenatal diagnosis: Chorionic villus sampling (mutations and biochemical defects)
- Clinical profile
  - Infant with psychomotor regression, hypotonia

Demographics

- Age
  - Majority present by age 2
  - Childhood & adult presentations uncommon
- Gender
  - No gender predilection
- Ethnicity
  - No ethnic predilection
- Epidemiology
  - Mitochondrial disorders = 1:8,500
  - LS in children < 6 years = 1:32,000 (most common mitochondrial disease in this age group)

Natural History & Prognosis

- Natural history: Progressive neurodegeneration leading to respiratory failure and death in childhood
- Prognosis: Dismal (particularly *SURF1*); childhood/adult LS more slowly progressive

Treatment

- No curative treatment
- Potential role of antioxidants and inhibitors in mtDNA replication

DIAGNOSTIC CHECKLIST

Image Interpretation Pearls

- Putaminal involvement classic but variable
- Thalamic and PAG involvement simulates Wernicke encephalopathy; however, mamillary bodies spared in Leigh syndrome
- Only brain stem involvement in *SURF1* mutations

SELECTED REFERENCES

1. Lee HF et al: Leigh syndrome: clinical and neuroimaging follow-up. Pediatr Neurol. 40(2):88-93, 2009
2. Finsterer J: Leigh and Leigh-like syndrome in children and adults. Pediatr Neurol. 39(4):223-35, 2008
3. Okumura A et al: Subacute encephalopathy: clinical features, laboratory data, neuroimaging, and outcomes. Pediatr Neurol. 38(2):111-7, 2008
4. Saneto RP et al: Neuroimaging of mitochondrial disease. Mitochondrion. 8(5-6):396-413, 2008
5. Horváth R et al: Leigh syndrome caused by mutations in the flavoprotein (Fp) subunit of succinate dehydrogenase (SDHA). J Neurol Neurosurg Psychiatry. 77(1):74-6, 2006

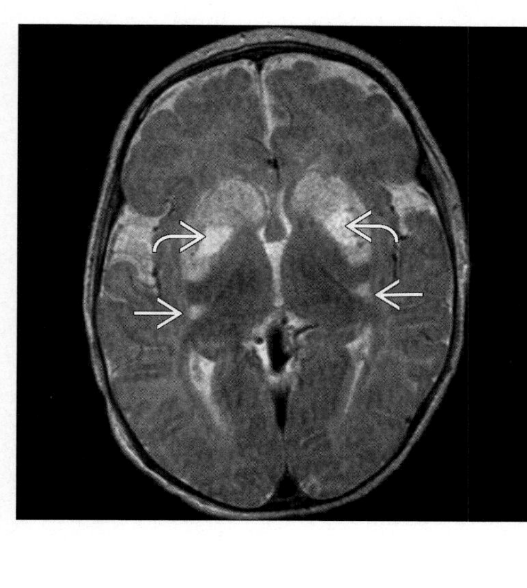

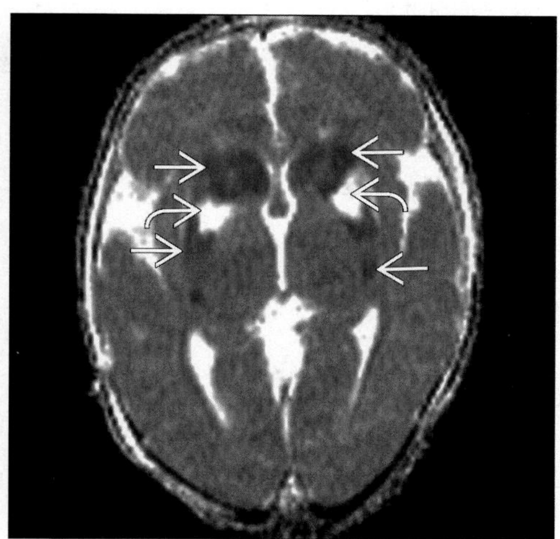

(Left) *Axial T2WI FSE MR in an infant with hypotonia and encephalopathy shows hyperintensity of caudate heads and putamina. Note involvement of most posterior putamina ➡. Central putamina ↪ have increased hyperintensity.* ***(Right)*** *Axial ADC map in the same patient shows that the caudate heads and most of the affected putamina ➡ have reduced diffusivity, whereas the central putamina ↪ have increased diffusivity, indicating prior injury with cavitation.*

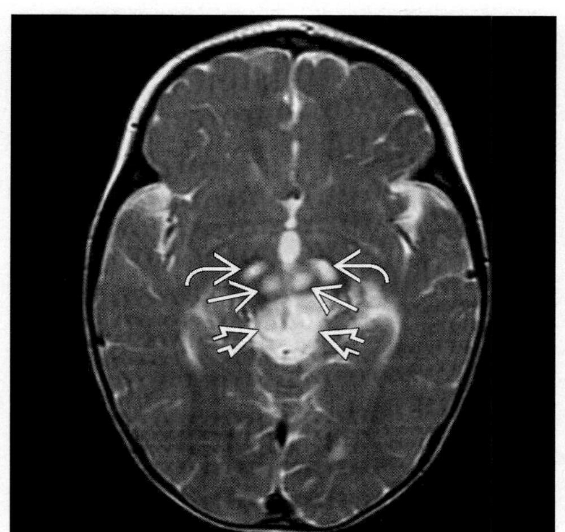

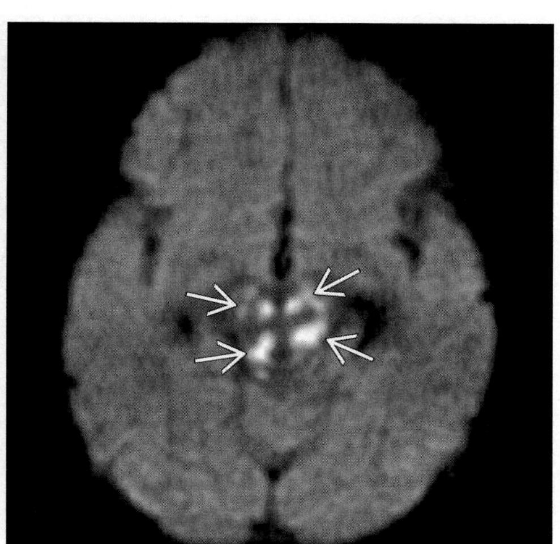

(Left) *Axial T2WI MR shows hyperintensity of cerebral peduncles ↪, red nuclei ➡, and midbrain tegmentum ⇨ (including periaqueductal gray matter). These are common locations of brain stem involvement in Leigh syndrome.* ***(Right)*** *Axial DWI MR shows reduced diffusivity (hyperintense areas ➡) in portions of the affected midbrain. The reduced diffusivity indicates acute injury, while normal or increased diffusivity indicates more chronic injury.*

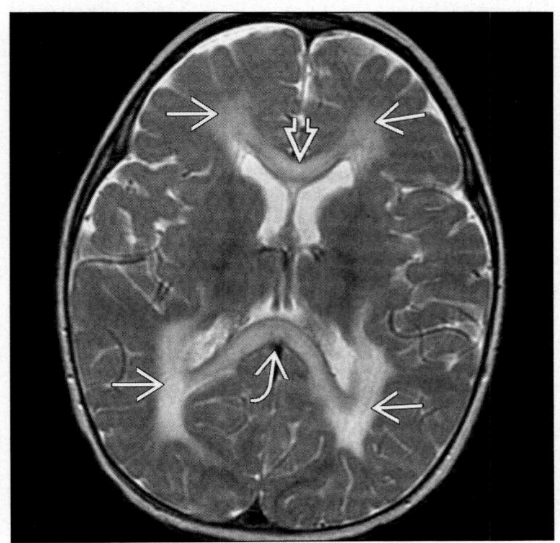

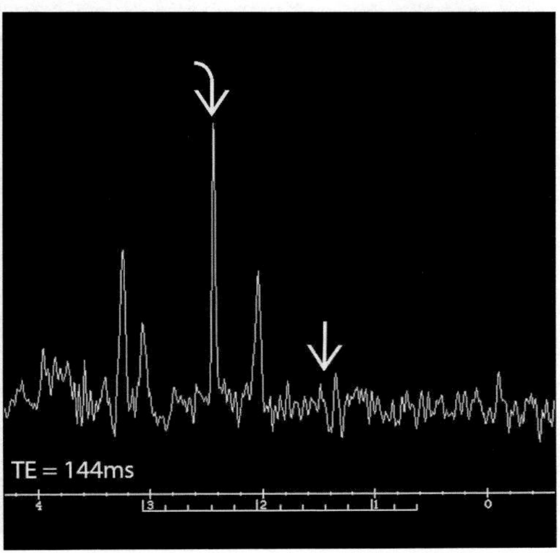

(Left) *Axial T2WI MR shows hyperintensity in the callosal genu ⇨ and splenium ↪, which extends into the periventricular and deep white matter ➡, as well as the posterior limbs of the internal capsules.* ***(Right)*** *Single voxel proton MRS (TE = 144 msec) in the same patient shows minimal lactate ➡ at 1.33 ppm and an abnormal peak ↪ at 2.4 ppm, which corresponds to succinate. The diagnosis was succinate dehydrogenase deficiency from SDHA mutation.*

MELAS

Key Facts

Terminology

- Mitochondrial myopathy, encephalopathy, lactic acidosis, and stroke-like episodes (MELAS)
- Inherited disorder of intracellular energy production caused by point mutation in mtDNA

Imaging

- Stroke-like cortical lesions crossing vascular territories
  - Posterior location most common
- "Shifting spread" (appearance, disappearance, reappearance elsewhere) is classic
- Lactate (Lac) "doublet" at 1.3 ppm in 60-65%
  - Elevated lactate in CSF, "normal" brain on MRS
- Basal ganglia (BG) lesions and calcifications

Pathology

- mtDNA contribution to zygote exclusively maternal inheritance
- Caution: Relationship of phenotype to genotype complex, variable
- Mutations may present as MELAS, but also as other phenotypes

Clinical Issues

- Classic MELAS triad: Lactic acidosis, seizures, stroke-like episodes
  - Onset of stroke-like episodes usually occurs in childhood/early adulthood
- Also: Sensorineural hearing loss, diabetes, short stature
- Heteroplasmy and random mitotic mtDNA segregation, tissue-to-tissue variability ⇒ phenotypic heterogeneity and "overlap" with other mitochondrial syndromes
- Carrier prevalence of *m.3243A > G* mutation 0.6% or 60 per 100,000 individuals

*(**Left**) Axial NECT in an 8-year-old girl with short stature and new onset stroke-like symptoms reveals bilateral basal ganglia calcifications ➡ and prominence of supratentorial sulci ➡ and enlarged sulci of the cerebellar vermis ➡. (**Right**) Axial FLAIR MR in the same child reveals a focus of abnormally increased signal intensity in the right thalamus ➡ and extensive hyperintensity and abnormal thickening of the cerebral cortex ➡ in the right occipital lobe.*

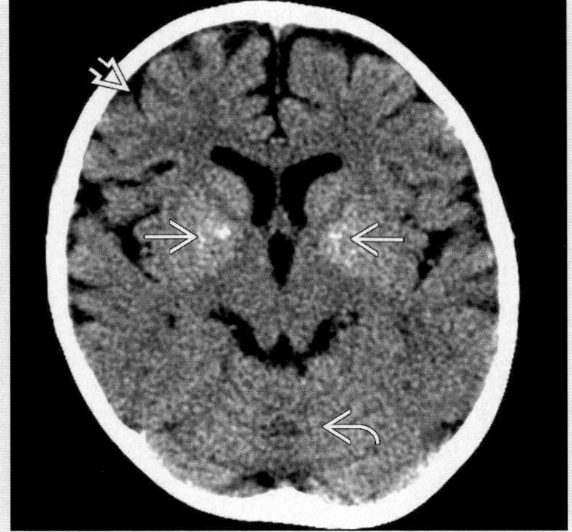

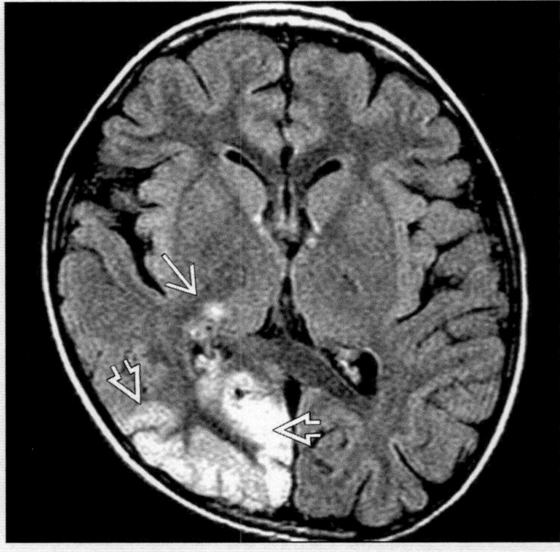

*(**Left**) Axial T2WI MR in the same 8 year old with short stature and new stroke-like symptoms shows similar abnormal signal hyperintensity lesions in the same thalamic focus of signal increase ➡ and in the edematous right occipital cortex ➡. Note the prominent subarachnoid spaces, which may result from malnutrition, medications, or the disease process itself. (**Right**) Axial DWI MR demonstrates reduced diffusion in the affected regions of brain ➡, confirming acuity of the lesion.*

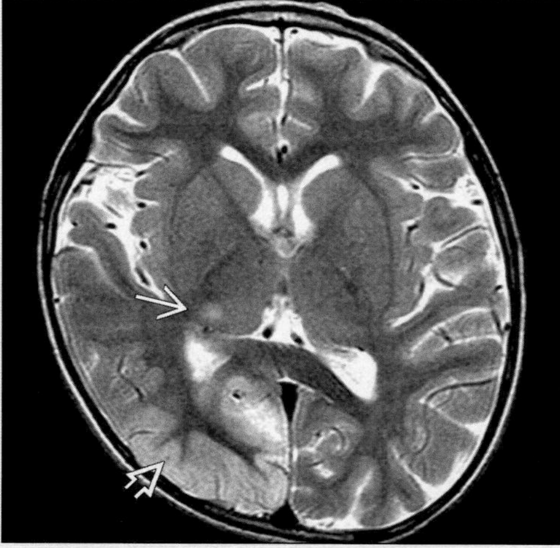

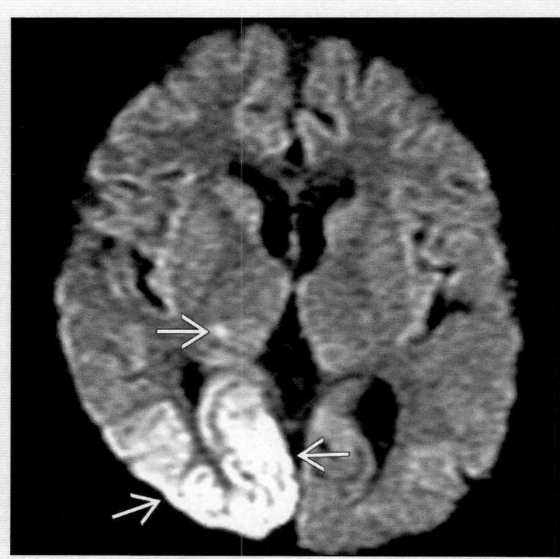

MELAS

TERMINOLOGY

Abbreviations

- Mitochondrial myopathy, encephalopathy, lactic acidosis, and stroke-like episodes (MELAS)
- Mitochondrial DNA (mtDNA), nuclear DNA (nDNA)

Definitions

- Inherited disorder of intracellular energy production caused by point mutations in mtDNA

IMAGING

General Features

- Best diagnostic clue
  - Acute: Stroke-like cortical lesions
    - "Shifting spread" (appearance, disappearance, reappearance elsewhere) is classic
    - Lesions cross typical vascular territories
- Location
  - Stroke-like: Parietooccipital > temporoparietal
  - Calcifications: Basal ganglia (BG)
- Size
  - Variable, progressive, multifocal
- Morphology
  - Acute: Gyral swelling
  - Chronic: Supra- and infratentorial atrophy, deep white matter (WM), & BG lacunar infarcts

CT Findings

- NECT
  - Symmetric BG calcification
- CECT
  - Variable gyral enhancement

MR Findings

- T1WI
  - Acute: Swollen gyri, compressed sulci
  - Subacute: Band of cortical hyperintensity consistent with laminar necrosis
  - Chronic: Progressive atrophy of BG, temporal-parietal-occipital cortex with preservation of hippocampal, entorhinal structures
- T2WI
  - Acute: Hyperintense cortex/subcortical WM
  - Chronic: Multifocal BG, deep WM hyperintensities
- FLAIR
  - Infarct-like swelling and mass effect
- T2* GRE
  - No hemorrhage
- DWI
  - Acute: DWI positive, ADC variable
- T1WI C+
  - Acute: Gyral enhancement
- MRA
  - Normal without major vessel occlusion
- MRS
  - Lactate (Lac) "doublet" at 1.3 ppm in 60-65%
  - Caution: Lac presence variable
    - Lac may be elevated in CSF but not brain (measure ventricular Lac)
    - Lac not always elevated and may precede imaging changes of brain
    - Other causes of elevated CNS Lac (e.g., hypoxia, ischemia, neoplasm, infection) must be excluded

Angiographic Findings

- Conventional
  - Acute: Dilated cortical arteries, prominent capillary blush without arterial occlusion

Nuclear Medicine Findings

- SPECT
  - Acute: Tc-99m-HMPAO SPECT shows striking increase in tracer accumulation

Other Modality Findings

- Xenon CT shows focal hyperperfusion during acute stroke-like episode, hypoperfusion later
- Electromyographic findings consistent with myopathy found in majority of cases
- EEG may show focal periodic epileptiform discharges

Imaging Recommendations

- Best imaging tool
  - MR with multivoxel MRS
- Protocol advice
  - Confirm lactate in normal regions of brain

DIFFERENTIAL DIAGNOSIS

Myoclonic Epilepsy with Ragged-Red Fibers (MERRF)

- Propensity for BG, caudate nuclei
- Watershed ischemia/infarcts common

Leigh Disease

- Mutations commonly involve electron transport chain complexes (COs) I-V
- Subacute necrotizing encephalomyopathy
- *SURF1* gene mutation
  - Involvement of lower brainstem (pons/medulla) characteristic

Kearns-Sayre Syndrome (KSS)

- Ataxia, ophthalmoplegia, retinitis pigmentosa
- Diffuse symmetric Ca++ in BG, caudate nuclei, subcortical WM
- Hyperintense BG on T1 & T2WI; cerebellar WM, posterior columns of medulla often involved

Status Epilepticus

- May cause transient gyral swelling, enhancement
- No Lac elevation in normal unaffected brain, CSF

Maternally Inherited Diabetes and Deafness (MIDD)

- Also *A3243G* mutation of mitochondrial DNA
- Diabetes mellitus, sensorineural hearing loss, short stature, ± spontaneous abortion
- No stroke-like episodes
- NECT: Diffuse atrophy and BG calcification

PATHOLOGY

General Features

- Etiology
  - Pathophysiology remains unclear
    - Impaired oxidative cerebral metabolism
    - Mitochondrial angiopathy of small cerebral arteries, arterioles, capillaries
  - May also be hyperperfusion, vasogenic edema with blood-brain barrier disruption during acute stroke-like episodes
- Genetics
  - mtDNA contribution to zygote exclusively maternal inheritance
  - Caution: Relationship of phenotype to genotype complex, variable
    - Mutations may present as MELAS, but also as other phenotypes
      - MTT1: A-to-G translation at nucleotide 3243 of mtDNA most common
    - Polygenetic: *MTTQ, MTTH, MTTK, MTTS1, MTND1, MTND5, MTND6, MTTS2*
- Associated abnormalities
  - Some cortical malformations associated with *A3243G* mutations

Gross Pathologic & Surgical Features

- Diffuse generalized atrophy
- Multiple focal cortical, deep WM/BG infarcts
- Prominent mineralization of BG
  - Pericapillary and small vessel Ca++

Microscopic Features

- Trichrome stain shows increased numbers of ragged-red fibers in skeletal/cardiac muscle
- Perivascular Ca++ in both gray matter (GM), WM may occur
- Immunohistochemistry: COX(+) ragged-red fibers (may help distinguish from MERRF)
- EM: Swelling, increase in number of dysfunctional mitochondria in smooth muscle, endothelial cells of small arteries, and pial arterioles

CLINICAL ISSUES

Presentation

- Most common signs/symptoms
  - Triad: Lactic acidosis, seizures, stroke-like episodes
  - Common: Sensorineural hearing loss, diabetes, short stature
  - Cognitive deficits, depression, psychosis, dementia
  - Ataxia, muscle weakness (myopathy), peripheral neuropathy
  - Acute onset headache, migraines, episodic vomiting, intermittent dystonia, alternating hemiplegia
- Other signs/symptoms
  - Heteroplasmy and random mitotic mtDNA segregation, tissue-to-tissue variability ⇒ phenotypic heterogeneity and "overlap" with other mitochondrial syndromes
    - Cardiac: Cardiomyopathy, cardiac conduction defects
    - Ocular findings: Scotomata, hemianopsia, ophthalmoplegia, maculopathy (progressive macular retinal pigment epithelial atrophy)
    - Renal dysfunction (including Fanconi syndrome and focal segmental glomerular sclerosis)
    - GI dysmotility, gastroparesis, intestinal pseudo-obstruction
- Clinical profile
  - Older child or young adult with muscle weakness and epilepsy or acute stroke-like syndrome

Demographics

- Age
  - Onset of stroke-like episodes usually occurs in childhood/early adulthood
    - Mean age onset = 15 years
    - 90% symptomatic by 40 years
- Epidemiology
  - Uncommon but important cause of stroke in pediatric cases
  - Carrier prevalence of *m.3243A > G* mutation 0.6% or 60 per 100,000 individuals
  - Incidence (Finland): *3243A > G* =18.4 per 100,000 individuals

Natural History & Prognosis

- Recurrent stroke-like events with either permanent or reversible neurologic deficits
- Progressive course with periodic acute exacerbation

Treatment

- Cofactor and supplement therapy

DIAGNOSTIC CHECKLIST

Consider

- Think MELAS in patient with acute "stroke-like" cortical lesion that crosses usual vascular territories

Image Interpretation Pearls

- Obtain MRS in CSF, "uninvolved" brain

SELECTED REFERENCES

1. Abe K et al: Comparison of conventional and diffusion-weighted MRI and proton MR spectroscopy in patients with mitochondrial encephalomyopathy, lactic acidosis, and stroke-like events. Neuroradiology. 46(2):113-7, 2004
2. Iizuka T et al: Slowly progressive spread of the stroke-like lesions in MELAS. Neurology. 61(9):1238-44, 2003
3. Sparaco M et al: MELAS: clinical phenotype and morphological brain abnormalities. Acta Neuropathol (Berl). 106(3):202-12, 2003
4. Wang XY et al: Serial diffusion-weighted imaging in a patient with MELAS and presumed cytotoxic oedema. Neuroradiology. 45(9):640-3, 2003
5. Sue CM et al: Neuroradiological features of six kindreds with MELAS tRNA(Leu) A2343G point mutation: implications for pathogenesis. J Neurol Neurosurg Psychiatry. 65(2):233-40, 1998
6. Hamazaki S et al: Mitochondrial myopathy, encephalopathy, lactic acidosis, and stroke-like episodes. Report of an autopsy. Acta Pathol Jpn. 39(9):599-606, 1989

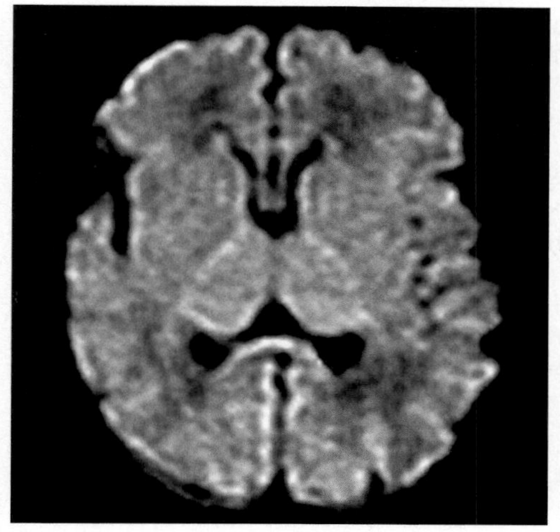

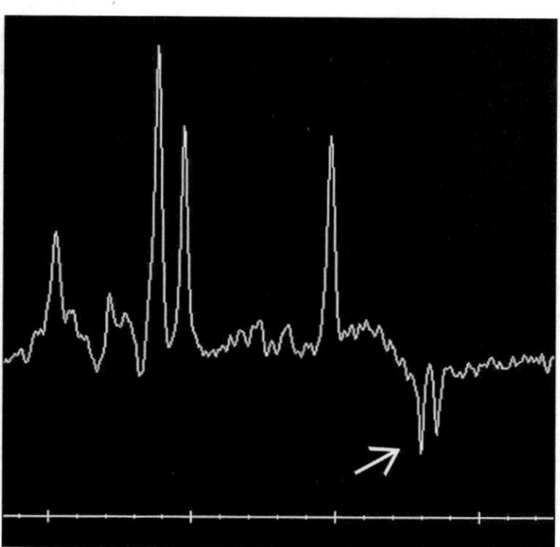

***(Left)** Axial DWI MR in a 22-day-old girl with microcephaly and lactic acidosis is essentially normal; it fails to reveal any areas of reduced diffusion. **(Right)** Proton MRS with an echo time of 144 msec localized to the basal ganglia of the same newborn with lactic acidosis confirms a lactate doublet ➔ at 1.3 ppm. Note that the lactate peak is inverted at an echo time of 135-144 msec. Proton MRS with this echo time can be a useful finding to distinguish lactate from lipid.*

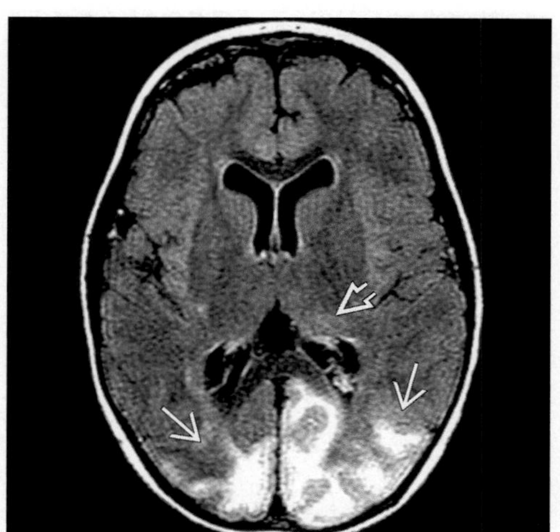

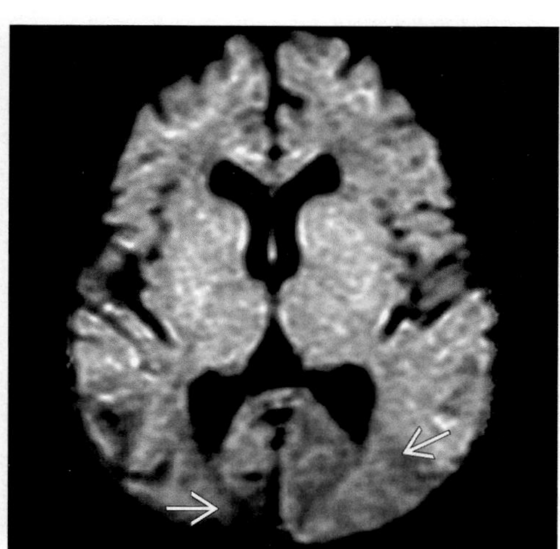

***(Left)** Follow-up axial FLAIR MR in the same child that had microcephaly and lactic acidosis at birth, now 3 and a 1/2 years old, demonstrates a new subtle signal increase in the left thalamus ➔ as well as extensive new bilateral occipital cortical/subcortical hyperintensity and swelling ➔. **(Right)** Axial DWI MR shows hypointensity ➔ in the affected regions, indicating that the lesions are subacute. Proton MRS (not shown) showed the presence of lactate, often seen in the subacute phase.*

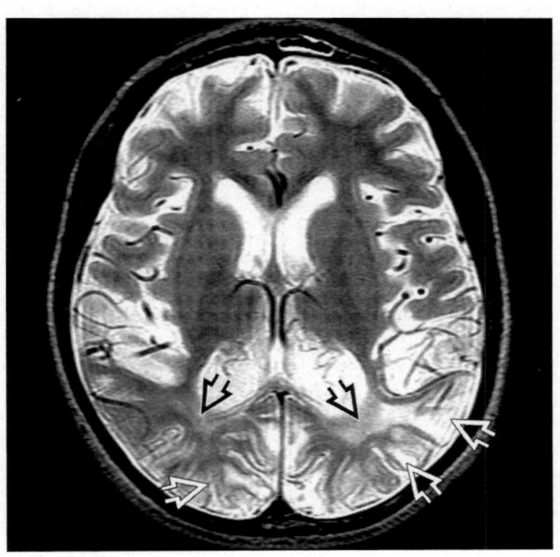

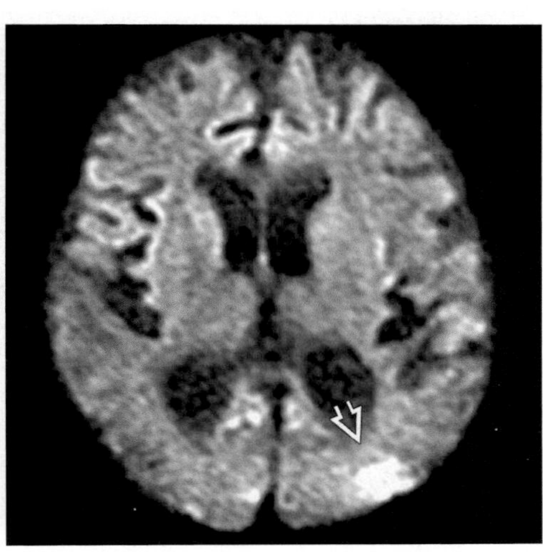

***(Left)** Axial T2WI MR in a 12-year-old girl with longstanding diagnosis of MELAS reveals extensive volume loss in the cerebral cortex and subcortical white matter, in addition to increased signal intensity of peritrigonal white matter ➔ and of the parietooccipital subcortical white matter/ cortex ➔. **(Right)** Axial DWI MR in the same 12 year old demonstrates reduced diffusivity ➔ in the left occipital pole, indicating an acute exacerbation in superimposed upon chronic changes.*

KEARNS-SAYRE SYNDROME

Key Facts

Terminology

- Kearns-Sayre syndrome (KSS)
- Mitochondrial encephalomyopathy presenting with ophthalmoplegia, ataxia, retinitis pigmentosa, heart block

Imaging

- Diffuse symmetric Ca++ in BG on NECT
- ↑ T2 signal in peripheral subcortical WM, U-fibers, cerebellar WM, corpus callosum, globi pallidi, substantia nigra, posterior brainstem
- Early sparing of periventricular WM
- Occasional radial stripes in hyperintense WM

Top Differential Diagnoses

- Other mitochondrial (mtDNA) deletion syndromes

Pathology

- Polygenetic: Caused by various mtDNA rearrangements
- Status spongiosus, spongy myelinopathy
- Cerebellar atrophy
- Ragged-red fibers on muscle biopsy

Clinical Issues

- Common symptoms: Ophthalmoplegia, ataxia, retinitis pigmentosa, heart block present before 20 years old
- Additional symptoms: Dementia, sensorineural hearing loss, muscle weakness, short stature, diabetes
- Age of onset usually before 20 years
- Cardiac conduction problems may manifest during anesthetic care

(Left) Axial T2WI MR in a teenager with symptomatic Kearns-Sayre syndrome demonstrates abnormal increased signal intensity bilaterally in the brachium pontis ➡ and the dorsal pons ➡. Widening of the interfoliate sulci results from mild cerebellar atrophy. (Right) Axial T2WI MR in the same teenager demonstrates foci of abnormal signal bilaterally within the globi pallidi ➡ and the corticospinal tracts ➡. Note the subtle loss of myelin arborization into the subcortical U-fibers ➡.

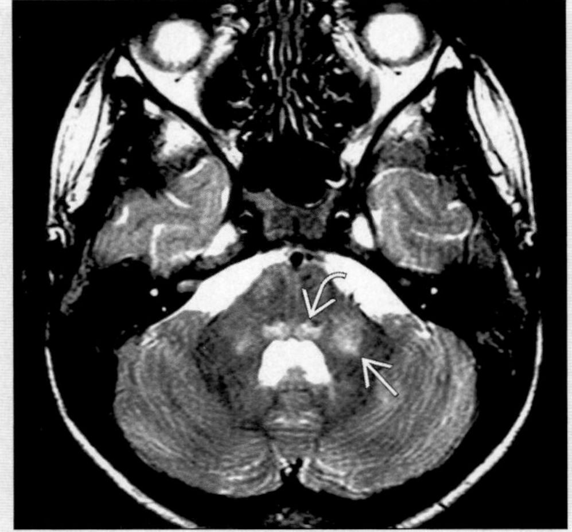

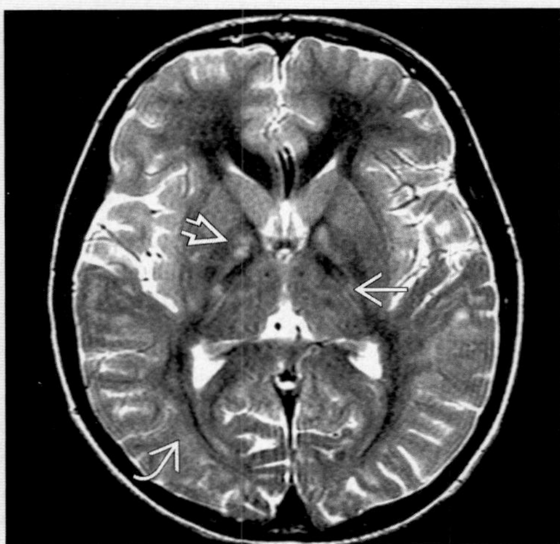

(Left) Axial T2WI MR in the same teenager with symptomatic Kearns-Sayre syndrome reveals linear hyperintense white matter "stripes" in the corona radiata ➡ and multifocal areas of abnormal hyperintense subcortical U-fibers ➡. No lactate was identified on proton MRS (not shown) obtained at the same time as the routine MR imaging. (Right) Coronal FLAIR MR in the same patient shows abnormal hyperintense signal in corticospinal tracts ➡, subcortical U-fibers ➡, and thalami ➡.

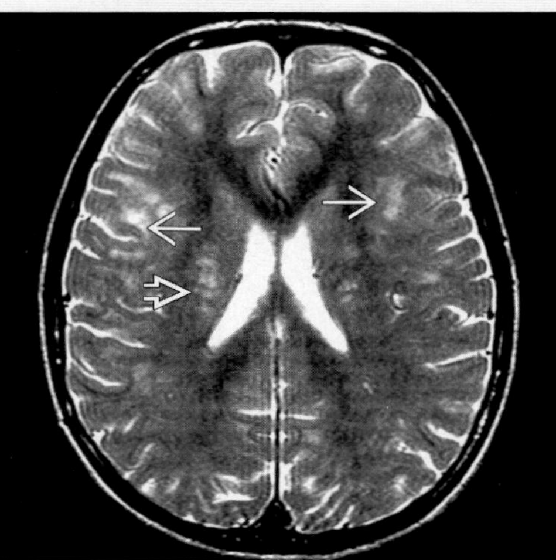

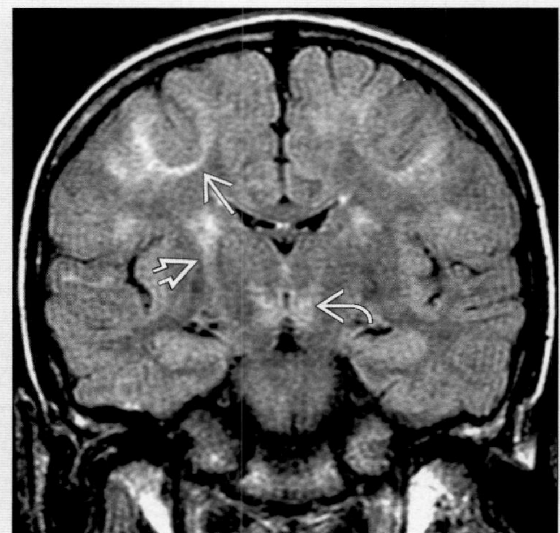

KEARNS-SAYRE SYNDROME

TERMINOLOGY

Abbreviations

- Kearns-Sayre syndrome (KSS)

Synonyms

- Kearns-Sayre ophthalmoplegic syndrome

Definitions

- Mitochondrial encephalomyopathy presenting with ophthalmoplegia, ataxia, retinitis pigmentosa, heart block

IMAGING

General Features

- Best diagnostic clue
  - Diffuse symmetric Ca++ BG
  - Hyperintense GP on T1 & T2WI
  - WM signal increase on T2/FLAIR involves subcortical WM
- Morphology
  - Spongy myelinopathy

CT Findings

- NECT
  - Basal ganglia calcifications

MR Findings

- T2WI
  - Occasional radial stripes in hyperintense WM
  - ↑ signal in peripheral subcortical WM, U-fibers, cerebellar WM, corpus callosum, globi pallidi, substantia nigra, posterior brainstem
  - Early sparing of periventricular WM
- DWI
  - Abnormal white matter (T2-DWI match) has reduced diffusion
  - DTI demonstrates brainstem white matter alterations

DIFFERENTIAL DIAGNOSIS

Other Mitochondrial (mtDNA) Deletion Syndromes

- MELAS
  - Stroke-like episodes (posterior distribution)
  - Lactic acidosis
  - Seizures
- Chronic progressive external ophthalmoplegia (CPEO)
  - Upper eyelid ptosis
  - Progressive weakness of extraocular muscles
  - Normal imaging or atrophy common, lactate uncommon
    - Severe phenotype: Pyramidal tract T2/FLAIR hyperintensity
- Pearson marrow-pancreas syndrome
  - Refractory anemia, vacuolization of bone marrow cells, exocrine pancreatic dysfunction
  - Mild phenotype or progression to KSS

PATHOLOGY

General Features

- Genetics
  - Polygenetic: Caused by multiple mtDNA rearrangements
  - Identical mutations reported in KSS, MELAS, Pearson, and CPEO; however, mutant mtDNA tissue distribution is different in these disorders

Gross Pathologic & Surgical Features

- Status spongiosus, spongy myelinopathy
  - Spongy degeneration and vacuolization
- Cerebellar atrophy
- Ragged-red fibers on muscle biopsy

CLINICAL ISSUES

Presentation

- Most common signs/symptoms
  - Ophthalmoplegia, ataxia, retinitis pigmentosa, heart block
- Other signs/symptoms
  - Dementia, sensorineural hearing loss
  - Short stature, diabetes
  - Proximal muscle weakness, fatigue
  - ↑ CSF protein, ± ↑ lactate

Natural History & Prognosis

- Age of onset usually before 20 years
- Cardiac conduction problems may manifest during anesthetic care

Treatment

- Vitamins and cofactors
- Pacemaker or cochlear implant may be required

DIAGNOSTIC CHECKLIST

Image Interpretation Pearls

- White matter involvement spares periventricular WM, involves "subcortical U-fibers"

SELECTED REFERENCES

1. Duning T et al: Diffusion tensor imaging in a case of Kearns-Sayre syndrome: striking brainstem involvement as a possible cause of oculomotor symptoms. J Neurol Sci. 281(1-2):110-2, 2009
2. Wabbels B et al: [Chronic progressive external ophthalmoplegia and Kearns-Sayre syndrome : interdisciplinary diagnosis and therapy.] Ophthalmologe. 105(6):550-6, 2008
3. Yamashita S et al: Genotype and phenotype analyses in 136 patients with single large-scale mitochondrial DNA deletions. J Hum Genet. 53(7):598-606, 2008
4. Heidenreich JO et al: Chronic progressive external ophthalmoplegia: MR spectroscopy and MR diffusion studies in the brain. AJR Am J Roentgenol. 187(3):820-4, 2006
5. Hourani RG et al: Atypical MRI findings in Kearns-Sayre syndrome: T2 radial stripes. Neuropediatrics. 37(2):110-3, 2006

MUCOPOLYSACCHARIDOSES

Key Facts

Terminology

- Mucopolysaccharidoses (MPS): MPS 1-9
- Prognosis depends upon specific enzyme deficiency
- Prototype: MPS 1H (Hurler)
- Inherited disorder of metabolism characterized by inability to break down glycosaminoglycan (GAG) → accumulation of toxic intracellular substrate
- GAG accumulates in most organs/ligaments

Imaging

- Perivascular spaces (PVS) dilated by accumulated GAG
- Favored sites of dilated VRS in MPS: Corpus callosum (CC), peritrigonal white matter (WM)
  - Can occur in other lobes
- Range: 1 to too-many-to-count
- Dysostosis multiplex, broad ribs, trident hands
- Progressive odontoid dysplasia → risk atlantoaxial subluxation; some correction follows BMT

Clinical Issues

- Rate of deterioration depends upon specific deficiency
- Treatment: BMT or IV recombinant human enzyme (e.g., MPS 1H: α-L-iduronidase)
- Significant correlation exists between WM alterations and mental retardation

Diagnostic Checklist

- Always visualize foramen magnum on any CNS study to seek CVJ compression
- Airway: Major sedation and anesthesia risk
- Not all MPS have typical facial features, dilated VRS may still signal 1 of less common MPS

*(**Left**) Axial graphic of a prototype mucopolysaccharidosis shows multiple dilated perivascular spaces that are radially oriented in the white matter of the brain. Note the posterior predominance and involvement of the corpus callosum ➡. (**Right**) Axial T1WI MR in a toddler with MPS 1H demonstrates prominent perivascular spaces involving the white matter, including the corpus callosum ➡. Note the posterior predominance of involvement, which is typical in MPS.*

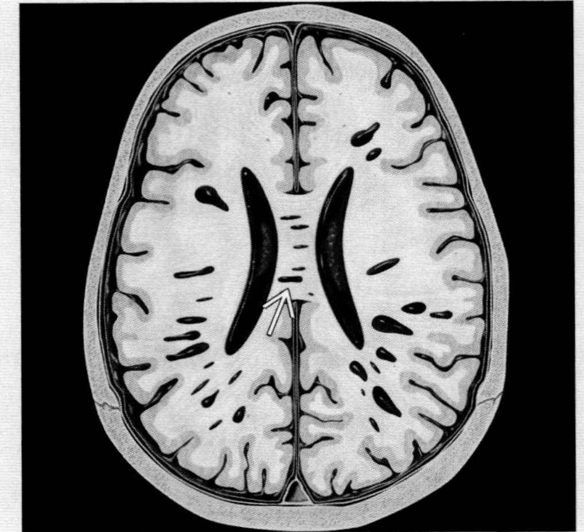

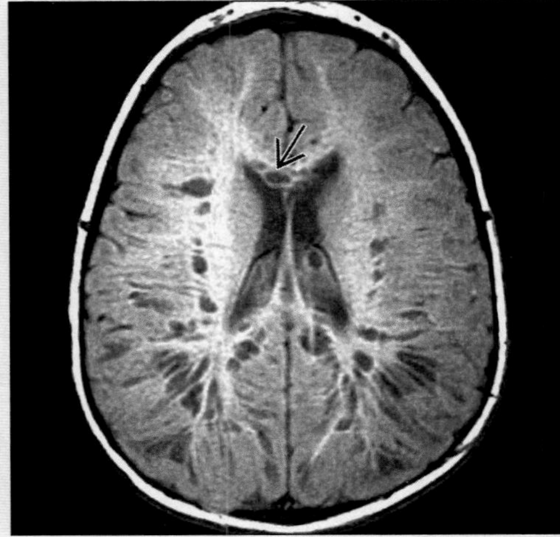

*(**Left**) Axial FLAIR MR in a male child with MPS 2 reveals a few dilated perivascular spaces ➡ surrounded by gliotic white matter ➡. Note the unilateral subdural hematoma ➡. Extraaxial bleeds, while uncommon, have been reported in MPS with vasculopathy, trauma, or large subdural effusions. (**Right**) Axial FLAIR MR in a different school-aged male with MPS 2 demonstrates dilated perivascular spaces ➡, hyperintense white matter ➡, and hydrocephalus. Note the typical anterior beaking ➡.*

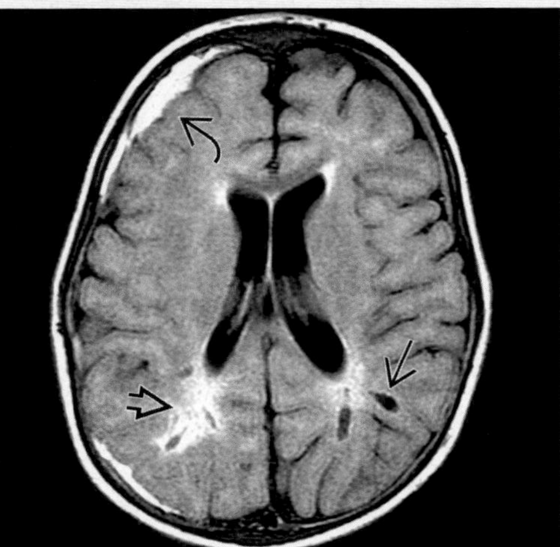

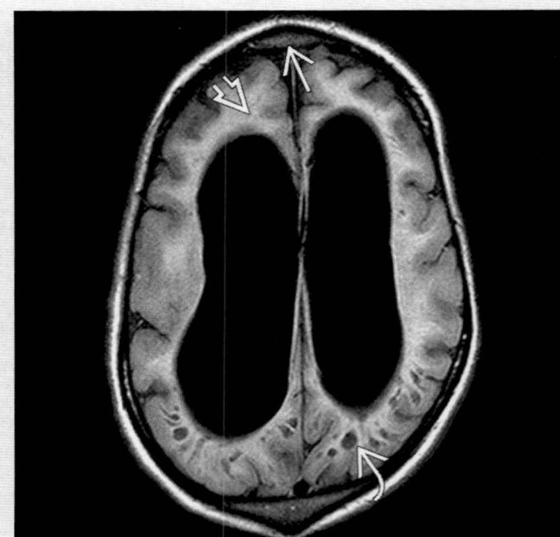

MUCOPOLYSACCHARIDOSES

TERMINOLOGY

Abbreviations

- Mucopolysaccharidoses (MPS)
  - Prototype: MPS 1H (Hurler)

Synonyms

- Old term "gargoylism"

Definitions

- Inherited disorder of metabolism characterized by enzyme deficiency
  - Inability to break down glycosaminoglycan (GAG) → accumulation of toxic intracellular substrate

IMAGING

General Features

- Best diagnostic clue
  - Perivascular spaces (PVS), a.k.a. Virchow-Robin spaces (VRS), dilated by accumulated GAG
- Location
  - Favored sites of dilated VRS in MPS: Corpus callosum (CC), peritrigonal white matter (WM)
    - Can occur in other lobes
- Size
  - Variably sized dilated VRS, usually under 5 mm; occasional large obstructed VRS occur
  - Range in number: 1 to too-many-to-count
- Morphology
  - Round, oval, spindle, parallel to veins

Radiographic Findings

- Radiography
  - Dysostosis multiplex, broad ribs, trident hands, J-shaped sella, "rosette" formation of multiple impacted teeth in single follicle

CT Findings

- NECT
  - Metopic beaking despite macrocrania
  - Macrocrania, ↓ density WM, dilated VRS are rarely visible on CT
  - Progressive hydrocephalus **and** atrophy
    - MPS 1: Hydrocephalus is early finding in 25%
    - MPS 3B: Severe atrophy
- CECT
  - Enhancing pannus associated with ligaments and dura at craniocervical junction (CVJ)

MR Findings

- T1WI
  - Cribriform appearance WM, CC, basal ganglia (BG)
    - Dilated VRS filled with GAG: "Hurler holes"
    - Especially in severe MPS (MPS 1H, 2 > > other MPS types)
    - Except MPS 4 (Morquio): CNS spared
  - Occasional arachnoid cysts (meningeal GAG deposition)
- T2WI
  - ↑ signal of WM surrounding dilated VRS: Gliosis, edema, de- or dysmyelination
  - ± additional patchy WM signal
- FLAIR
  - VRS isointense with CSF
  - ↑ signal surrounds VRS
- T1WI C+
  - CV junction pannus enhances
- MRS
  - ↓ NAA, ↑ Cho/Cr ratio; ↑ peak at 3.7 ppm contains signals from MPS
    - Improvement in presumptive MPS peaks following bone marrow transplant (BMT)
- Spinal MR
  - Compression CVJ in majority MPS
    - C2 meningeal hypertrophy
    - Progressive odontoid dysplasia → risk atlantoaxial subluxation; some correction reported following BMT
    - Short C1 posterior arch
  - ↑ T2 signal cord in 50% of CVJ compression
  - Upper lumbar gibbus
    - MPS 1H (Hurler): Inferior beaking
    - MPS 4 (Morquio): Middle beaking

Imaging Recommendations

- Best imaging tool
  - MR brain
- Protocol advice
  - Baseline MR/MRS
  - Follow-up: Complications (CVJ compression, hydrocephalus), therapeutic response to BMT
  - Always visualize foramen magnum on any CNS study to seek CVJ compression

DIFFERENTIAL DIAGNOSIS

Velocardiofacial Syndrome (22q11DS)

- Dilated VR spaces and plaques, typical frontal predominance
- Deviated carotid arteries in pharynx is clue

Macrocephaly with Dilated VRS

- Lacks typical beaked metopic suture and foramen magnum compression

Hypomelanosis of Ito

- Periventricular signal change (brighter and more persistent than MPS) with large VRS
- May also have hemimegalencephaly
- Typical whorled skin lesions
- Lack "beaked" metopic suture present in MPS

Perinatal Hypoxic Ischemic Encephalopathy

- Transient phase of cystic change following hypoxic ischemic encephalopathy → atrophy

Normal VR Spaces

- Vary in number and prominence

PATHOLOGY

General Features

- Etiology
  - Ganglioside accumulation (toxic to neurons)
- Genetics

- Autosomal recessive (exception: X-linked MPS 2)
- Associated abnormalities
  - Dermal melanocytosis (mongolian-like spots)
    - Extensive, blue skin pigmentation differs from typical mongolian spots in persistence or progression
  - GAG accumulates in most organs/ligaments
    - Hepatosplenomegaly (HSM), umbilical hernia
    - Skeletal dysostosis multiplex, joint contractures
    - Arterial wall (mid-aortic stenosis) and cardiac valve thickening
    - Thick dura (cord compressed at foramen magnum)
    - Coarse facies (formerly "gargoylism")
    - Upper airway obstruction (38%): Submucosal deposition → small, abnormally shaped trachea (difficult intubation); abnormal configuration vocal cords
  - Embryology-anatomy
    - Dilated VR spaces may be seen in utero

Staging, Grading, & Classification

- Diagnosis depends on specific enzyme deficiency
  - MPS 1H, 1HS (Hurler/Hurler-Scheie): α-L-iduronidase (4p16.3)
  - MPS 2 (Hunter): Iduronate 2-sulfatase (Xq28)
  - MPS 3A (Sanfilippo): Heparin N-sulfatase (17q25.3)
  - MPS 4A (Morquio): Galactose 6-sulfatase (16q24.3)
  - MPS 6 (Maroteaux-Lamy): Arylsulfatase B (5q11-q13)

Gross Pathologic & Surgical Features

- Thick meninges
- Cribriform appearance to cut surface of brain

Microscopic Features

- MPS: Glycosaminoglycans accumulate in leptomeninges and VR spaces

CLINICAL ISSUES

Presentation

- Most common signs/symptoms
  - Typical coarse facies develop (mild in MPS 3, 6, 7)
    - Macroglossia, bushy eyebrows, flat nasal bridge
- Clinical profile
  - Prototype MPS 1H, appear normal at birth
    - Corneal clouding (except MPS 2): Proteoglycans in keratocytes
    - Mental retardation (except MPS 2b, 4, 1HS)
    - Joint contractures, dysostosis multiplex, short stubby fingers, carpal tunnel syndrome
    - Loss of walking skills: Spinal claudication/ myelopathy C1-2 and vascular claudication from mid-aortic stenosis
    - Recurrent upper respiratory infection, nasal discharge, ear infections, sleep apnea, sensorineural deafness
    - Middle ear effusions (73%), otolaryngologist notes this prediagnosis MPS
    - Cardiac valvular disease: Mitral > aortic
    - Skin blistering in MPS 3
  - MPS 7 may present with fetal nuchal translucency, hydrops fetalis, or isolated ascites

Demographics

- Age
  - MPS 1H presents in infancy
- Gender
  - MPS 2 (Hunter) is X-linked: Male
- Ethnicity
  - Geographic variability in prevalence of specific MPS disorders
- Epidemiology
  - 1:29,000 live births (series from Australia)
    - MPS 1H = 1:107,000 live births
    - MPS 2 = 1:165,000 male live births
    - MPS 3 = 1:58,000 live births
    - MPS 4A = 1:640,000 live births
    - MPS 6 = 1:320,000 live births

Natural History & Prognosis

- Significant correlation exists between WM alterations and mental retardation
- Rate of deterioration depends upon specific deficiency
  - MPS 1H death by 10 years, without therapy
  - MPS 2A death in late teens (cardiac)
  - Others variable

Treatment

- BMT or IV recombinant human enzyme (e.g., MPS 1H: α-L-iduronidase)
  - ↓ visceral accumulation MPS; ameliorate some manifestations

DIAGNOSTIC CHECKLIST

Consider

- Airway: Major sedation and anesthesia risk

Image Interpretation Pearls

- Not all MPS have typical facial features; dilated VRS may still signal 1 of less common MPS
- Not all dilated VRS are MPS
- Always look for CVJ compression
  - Treatable cause of morbidity in MPS
  - Lack of CVJ compression suggests there may be different etiology of dilated VRS than MPS

SELECTED REFERENCES

1. Yeung AH et al: Airway management in children with mucopolysaccharidoses. Arch Otolaryngol Head Neck Surg. 135(1):73-9, 2009
2. Kara S et al: Dilated perivascular spaces: an informative radiologic finding in Sanfilippo syndrome type A. Pediatr Neurol. 38(5):363-6, 2008
3. Gabrielli O et al: Correlation between cerebral MRI abnormalities and mental retardation in patients with mucopolysaccharidoses. Am J Med Genet. 125A(3):224-31, 2004
4. Takahashi Y et al: Evaluation of accumulated mucopolysaccharides in the brain of patients with mucopolysaccharidoses by (1)H-magnetic resonance spectroscopy before and after bone marrow transplantation. Pediatr Res. 49(3):349-55, 2001

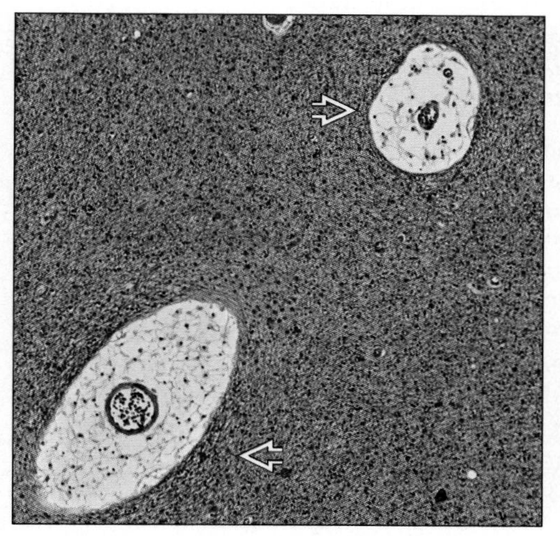

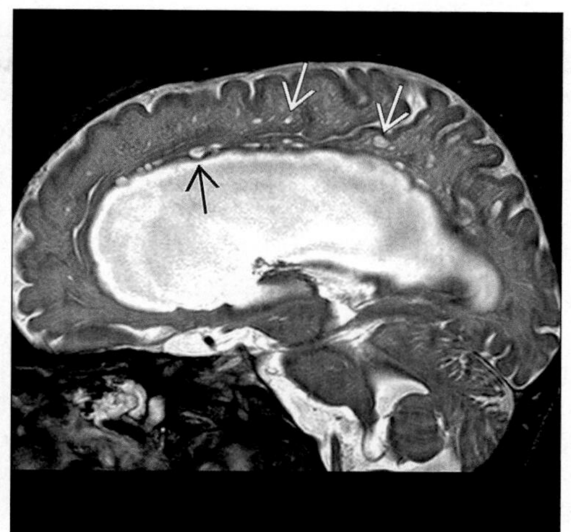

(Left) *Axial micropathology with Luxol fast blue stain in a teenager with MPS 1HS reveals dilated perivascular spaces ➡ filled by mucopolysaccharide. (Courtesy P. Shannon, MD.)* ***(Right)*** *Sagittal T2WI MR in a 10-year-old boy with MPS 2 demonstrates ventriculomegaly due to hydrocephalus, scaphocephaly, and numerous dilated perivascular spaces ➡. Characteristic involvement of the corpus callosum by the perivascular spaces ➡ can be seen.*

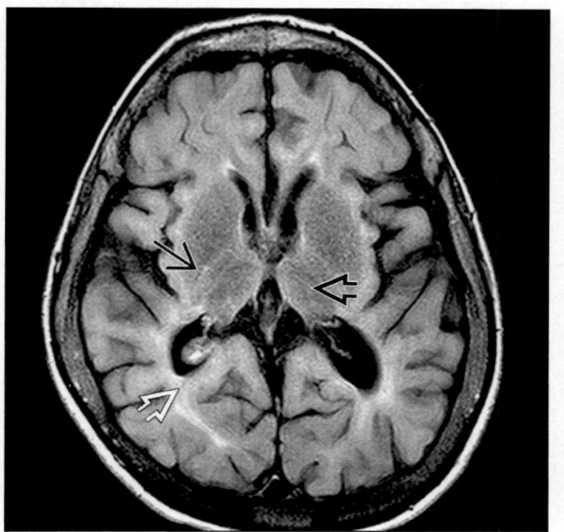

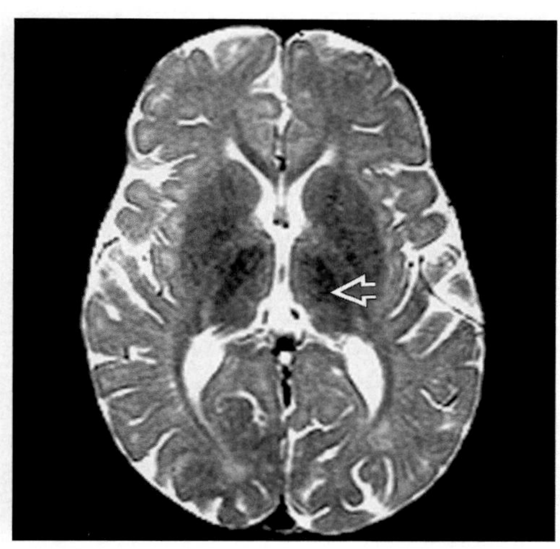

(Left) *Axial FLAIR MR in a child with MPS 3 reveals increased signal in the abnormal myelin of the peritrigonal white matter ➡ and the internal capsules ➡. The thalami are dark and small ➡. Thalamic findings are uncommon in the other MPS disorders but can be seen in MPS 3 and other lysosomal disorders.* ***(Right)*** *Axial T2WI MR in another child with MPS 3 reveals similar thalamic findings ➡. Again, there is abnormal white matter due to hypomyelination.*

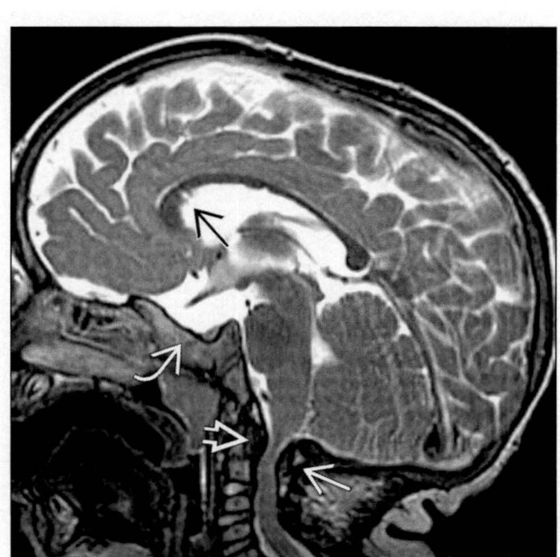

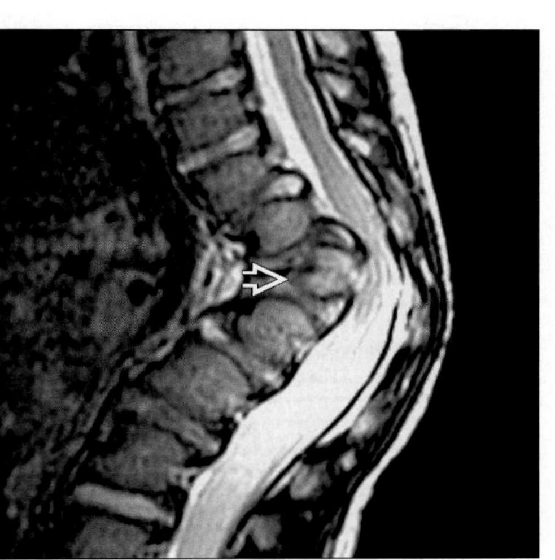

(Left) *Sagittal T2WI MR in a child with MPS 6 demonstrates dilated perivascular spaces ➡ in the corpus callosum (a typical location), scaphocephaly, and an abnormal sella turcica ➡. The upper cervical spinal cord is significantly compressed by prominent pannus dorsal to the odontoid ➡ and by a short posterior arch of C1 ➡.* ***(Right)*** *Sagittal T2WI MR in MPS 1 demonstrates severe acute thoracolumbar kyphosis due to abnormal thoracic vertebra ➡. Note the compression of the conus medullaris.*

GANGLIOSIDOSIS (GM2)

Key Facts

Terminology

- Tay-Sachs disease (TS), Sandhoff disease (SD)
- Inherited lysosomal storage disorder characterized by GM2 ganglioside accumulation in brain
- TS & SD exist in infantile, juvenile, and adult forms

Imaging

- Infantile: T2 hypointense, T1 hyperintense (CT hyperdense) thalami
- Juvenile/adult: Cerebellar atrophy

Top Differential Diagnoses

- Status marmoratus
- Neuronal ceroid lipofuscinosis
- Krabbe disease
- Juvenile GM1 gangliosidosis

Pathology

- Autosomal recessive inheritance
- Accumulation of GM2 ganglioside in neuronal lysosomes causes neuronal degradation, apoptosis with secondary hypo-/demyelination

Clinical Issues

- TS: 1:30 carrier frequency in Ashkenazi Jewish and French Canadians
- SD, GM2 variant AB, juvenile/adult GM2 = pan-ethnic (↑ in small gene pools)
- Presentation
  - Infant: Psychomotor retardation/regression
  - Juvenile/adult: Atypical spinocerebellar ataxia
- Prognosis for infantile: Death by 4 years of age
- Treatment: Supportive, seizure control; promising new therapies on horizon

*(**Left**) Axial NECT shows classic hyperdense thalami ⇨ in this developmentally delayed 1 year old with infantile Tay-Sachs disease. The basal ganglia appear small and were hypodense on lower images (not shown). (**Right**) Axial T2WI MR in a patient with infantile Tay-Sachs disease shows thalamic hypointensity limited to the ventral nuclei ➡, findings in contrast to those in patients with Sandhoff disease. The dorsal thalamus (not shown) is often mildly hyperintense.*

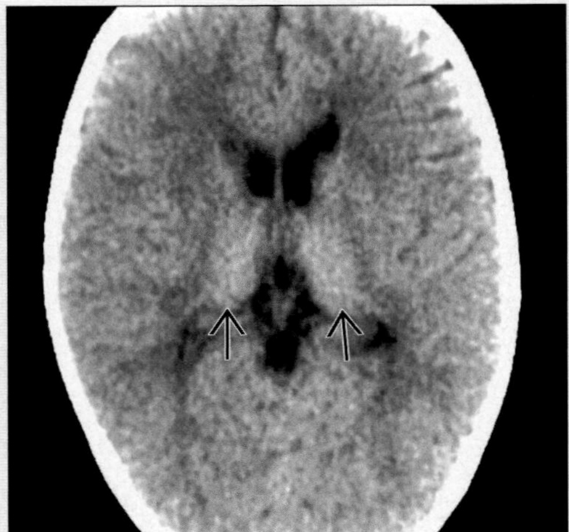

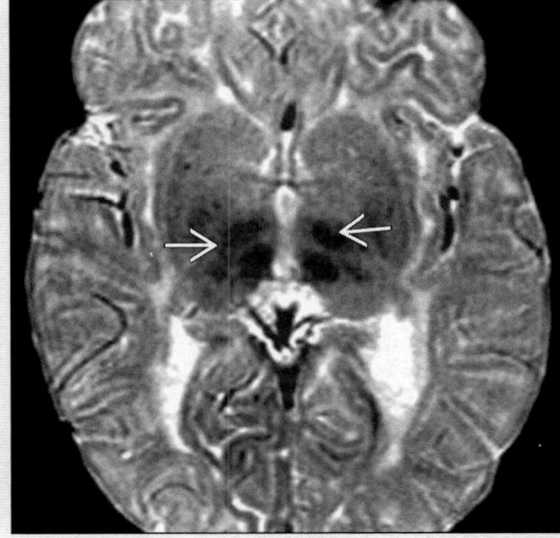

*(**Left**) Sagittal T1WI MR in an older child with psychosis and extrapyramidal symptoms shows enlarged vermian fissures, indicating volume loss. Cerebellar atrophy is the main finding in patients with juvenile or adult onset GM2. (**Right**) Coronal T2WI MR in a 15 year old with juvenile onset GM2 shows cerebellar atrophy. The supratentorial brain is normal. The cerebral WM is variably affected in juvenile/adult GM2. Rarely deep gray structure and mass-like brainstem involvement can occur.*

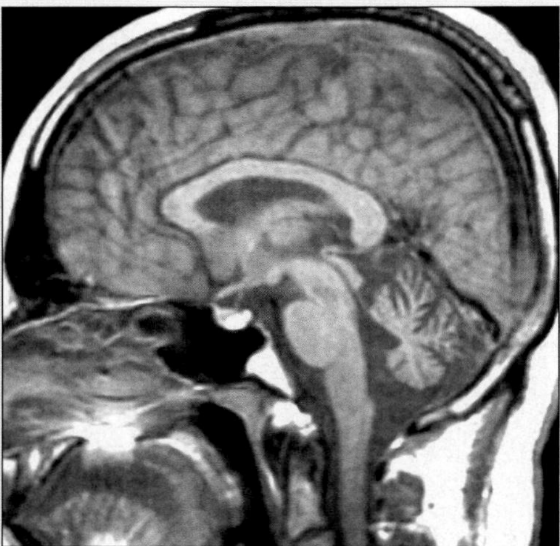

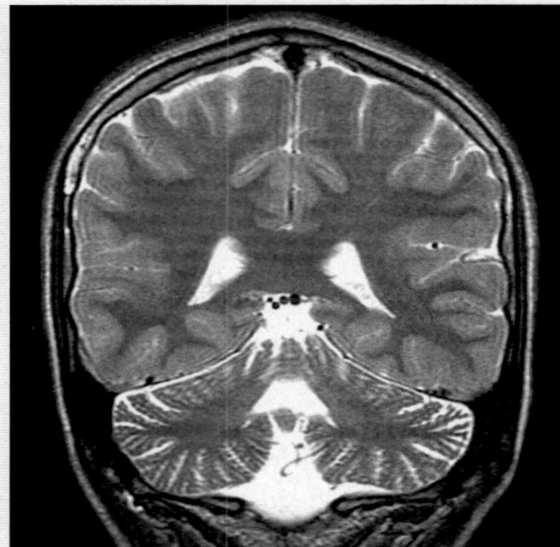

GANGLIOSIDOSIS (GM2)

TERMINOLOGY

Abbreviations

- Gangliosidosis (GM2)

Synonyms

- Tay-Sachs disease, Sandhoff disease

Definitions

- Inherited lysosomal storage disorder characterized by GM2 ganglioside accumulation in brain
- 3 major biochemically distinct, but clinically indistinguishable types
  - Tay-Sachs disease (TS)
  - Sandhoff disease (SD)
  - GM2 variant AB (rare)
- TS and SD exist in infantile, juvenile, and adult forms
- GM2 variant AB exists in infantile form only

IMAGING

General Features

- Best diagnostic clue
  - Infantile
    - T2 hypointense, T1 hyperintense (CT hyperdense) thalami
    - Mild T2 hyperintensity striatum
  - Juvenile/adult
    - Cerebellar atrophy
- Location
  - Infantile: Thalami, striatum, cerebral > > cerebellar white matter (WM)
    - Corpus callosum (CC) spared
  - Juvenile/adult: Cerebellum, cerebral WM
    - Rare striatal and mass-like brainstem involvement
- Morphology
  - Symmetric involvement of deep gray structures
  - Late: Atrophy

CT Findings

- NECT
  - Infantile
    - Hyperdense thalami (classic but variable)
    - Hypodense striatum, WM
  - Juvenile/adult
    - Cerebellar atrophy
    - ± cerebral WM hypodensity
- CECT
  - No abnormal enhancement

MR Findings

- T1WI
  - Hyperintense thalami
  - Striatal intensity variable
  - Hypointense cerebral WM
- T2WI
  - TS: **Hypo**intense ventral thalami, **hyper**intense dorsal thalami
  - SD: Thalami diffusely hypointense
  - Mild striatal and cerebral WM hyperintensity
- DWI
  - Variably ↓ diffusivity ventral thalami (TS)
- T1WI C+
  - No abnormal enhancement
- MRS
  - Infantile: ↓ NAA, ↑ choline, ↑ myoinositol
  - Juvenile/adult: ↓ NAA; normal-appearing thalami, cerebral WM reported

Ultrasonographic Findings

- Infantile: Echogenic thalami

Imaging Recommendations

- MR (CT may confirm thalamic abnormality)

DIFFERENTIAL DIAGNOSIS

Status Marmoratus

- Hyperdense, atrophic thalami
- Atrophy putamina, perirolandic region
- History of profound perinatal ischemia

Neuronal Ceroid Lipofuscinosis

- Thalami, globi pallidi hyperdense, T2 hypointense
- Cerebral, cerebellar atrophy

Krabbe Disease

- Hyperdense thalami, caudate and dentate nuclei
- T2 hyperintense cerebral, cerebellar WM
- CC involved

Juvenile GM1 Gangliosidosis

- Imaging findings identical to SD
- GM1 ganglioside accumulates in brain & viscera

PATHOLOGY

General Features

- General pathology comments
  - Neuronal accumulation of GM2 ganglioside caused by deficient lysosomal enzyme, β-hexosaminidase A
- Embryology-anatomy
  - GM2 ganglioside resides in neuronal membranes; plays role in cell-cell recognition, synaptogenesis
  - β-hexosaminidase A (HexA) and GM2 activator protein (GMAP) required for lysosomal GM2 ganglioside catabolism
  - HexA is 1 of 3 isoenzymes of β-hexosaminidase formed by dimerization α and β subunits
    - HexA = αβ dimer, HexB = ββ, HexS = αα
  - HexA and HexB are major forms; HexS is minor form with unclear physiologic function
  - *HEXA*, chr 15q23-24, encodes α subunit
  - *HEXB*, chr 5q13, encodes β subunit
  - *GM2A*, chr 5q31.3-q33.1, encodes GMAP
- Genetics
  - Autosomal recessive inheritance
  - > 100 different mutations *HEXA* cause TS
  - > 30 different mutations *HEXB* cause SD
  - ~ 4 mutations *GM2A* cause GM2 variant AB
  - Mutations allowing residual HexA activity (0.5-4% normal activity) account for milder juvenile/adult phenotypes
- Etiology

GANGLIOSIDOSIS (GM2)

- ○ Accumulation of GM2 ganglioside in neuronal lysosomes causes neuronal degradation, apoptosis with secondary hypo-/demyelination
    - ▪ GM2 ganglioside accumulation in myelin membrane may also contribute to demyelination
- ○ Exact mechanism by which GM2 ganglioside accumulation → neuronal apoptosis is unknown
    - ▪ Activation microglia, macrophages, and astrocytes suggest inflammatory component
    - ▪ Identification of autoantibodies in mouse models of SD suggests autoimmune component

Gross Pathologic & Surgical Features

- Infantile: Early megalencephaly, late atrophy
    - ○ Gelatinous, hemispheric WM, ± cavitation
- Juvenile/adult: Cerebellar atrophy

Microscopic Features

- GM2 ganglioside accumulation in cerebral neurons
- Less severe GM2 ganglioside accumulation in glial, Purkinje, anterior horn, and retinal ganglion cells
- EM: GM2 ganglioside contained in membranous cytoplasmic bodies (MCBs) in neuronal cytoplasm, proximal nerve processes, axons
    - ○ MCBs in cytoplasm cause distortion and ballooning
    - ○ MCBs in proximal nerve processes form meganeurites
- Hypomyelination, demyelination, wallerian degeneration
- Juvenile/adult GM2: Ganglioside accumulation in anterior horn cells, cerebellar neurons, basal ganglia, brainstem
    - ○ MCBs occasionally absent
- SD: Additional storage of GM2 (and globoside) in viscera

CLINICAL ISSUES

Presentation

- Most common signs/symptoms
    - ○ Infantile: Psychomotor retardation/regression
    - ○ Juvenile/adult: Atypical spinocerebellar ataxia
    - ○ Other signs/symptoms
        - ▪ Infantile: Macrocranium, hypotonia, seizures, blindness (90% with cherry-red spot macula), exaggerated startle response to noise
        - ▪ Juvenile/adult: Dysarthria, extrapyramidal and pyramidal dysfunction, peripheral neuropathy, stuttering, psychosis/depression (late, 30%)
- Clinical profile
    - ○ Diagnosis: Documentation HexA deficiency in serum leukocytes, cultured skin fibroblasts, amniotic fluid, or chorionic villus sample
    - ○ Abnormal results should be followed by DNA analysis to detect mutation &/or exclude pseudodeficiency allele

Demographics

- Age
    - ○ Infantile: Symptom onset in 1st year
    - ○ Juvenile: Symptom onset by 2-6 years old
    - ○ Adult: Symptom onset in 1st-3rd decades
- Gender
    - ○ No predilection
- Epidemiology
    - ○ TS
        - ▪ 1:30 carrier frequency in Ashkenazi Jewish and French Canadians
        - ▪ 1:300 carrier frequency in Sephardic, Oriental, Jewish and non-Jewish
        - ▪ ↑ incidence in Cajuns and Druze
    - ○ SD, GM2 variant AB, juvenile/adult GM2 = pan-ethnic (↑ in small gene pools)
        - ▪ 1:1,000 Jewish, 1:600 non-Jewish
        - ▪ 1:16-29 Creole population of Cordoba, Argentina
        - ▪ 1:7 Maronite Christian Cypriots
    - ○ Incidence of TS in USA and Canada has decreased by > 90% since 1970 due to carrier screening and prenatal diagnosis

Natural History & Prognosis

- Infantile: Rapidly progressive psychomotor regression culminating in paralysis, blindness, deafness; death typically by 4 years of age
- Juvenile: More slowly progressive with death between 5-15 years of age
    - ○ Death often 2° to respiratory infection; preceded by several years of decerebrate rigidity in vegetative state
- Adult: Prolonged survival to age 60-80 can occur

Treatment

- Supportive therapy, seizure control
- Promising new therapies: Substrate deprivation, enzyme replacement, bone marrow transplantation, gene therapy, pharmacologic chaperone therapy

SELECTED REFERENCES

1. Lee SM et al: Newly observed thalamic involvement and mutations of the HEXA gene in a Korean patient with juvenile GM2 gangliosidosis. Metab Brain Dis. 23(3):235-42, 2008
2. Mu TW et al: Chemical and biological approaches synergize to ameliorate protein-folding diseases. Cell. 134(5):769-81, 2008
3. Sharma S et al: Thalamic changes in Tay-Sachs' disease. Arch Neurol. 65(12):1669, 2008
4. Wang SZ et al: A novel HEXB mutation and its structural effects in juvenile Sandhoff disease. Mol Genet Metab. 95(4):236-8, 2008
5. Akeboshi H et al: Production of recombinant beta-hexosaminidase A, a potential enzyme for replacement therapy for Tay-Sachs and Sandhoff diseases, in the methylotrophic yeast Ogataea minuta. Appl Environ Microbiol. 73(15):4805-12, 2007
6. Jeyakumar M et al: Central nervous system inflammation is a hallmark of pathogenesis in mouse models of GM1 and GM2 gangliosidosis. Brain. 126(Pt 4):974-87, 2003
7. Yuksel A et al: Neuroimaging findings of four patients with Sandhoff disease. Pediatr Neurol. 21(2):562-5, 1999
8. Myerowitz R: Tay-Sachs disease-causing mutations and neutral polymorphisms in the Hex A gene. Hum Mutat. 9(3):195-208, 1997
9. Brismar J et al: Increased density of the thalamus on CT scans in patients with GM2 gangliosidoses. AJNR Am J Neuroradiol. 11(1):125-30, 1990

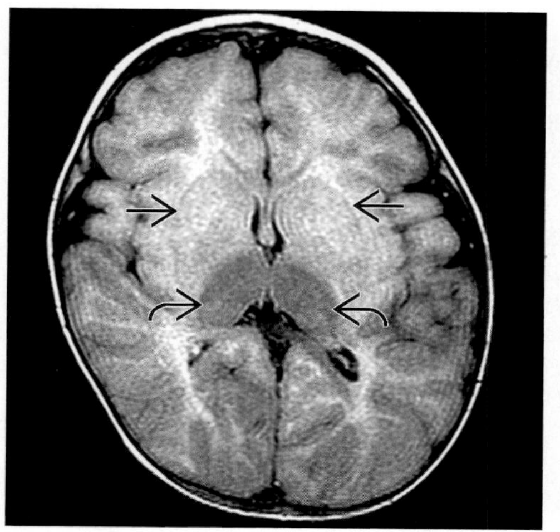

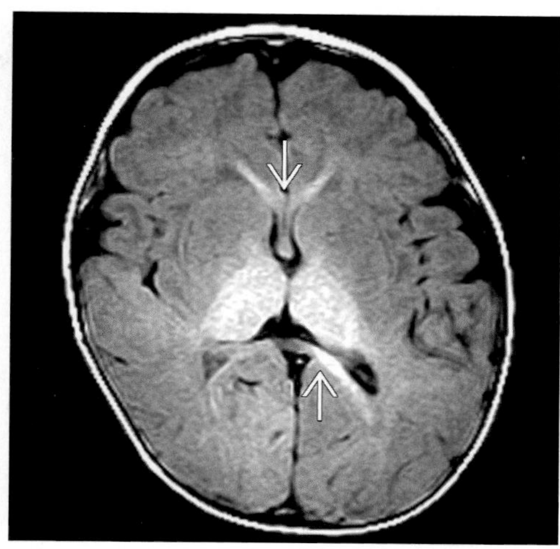

*(**Left**) Axial FLAIR MR in a 1 year old with infantile Sandhoff disease shows ⇒ diffusely hypointense thalami. The striatum ⇒ is diffusely hyperintense. Evaluation of the cerebral WM on FLAIR MR is difficult at this age. (**Right**) Axial T1WI MR in the same patient shows symmetric thalamic hyperintensity and diffusely hypointense (hypo-/demyelinated) cerebral WM. White matter should appear completely myelinated on T1WI at this age. Note the spared (hyperintense) corpus callosum ➡.*

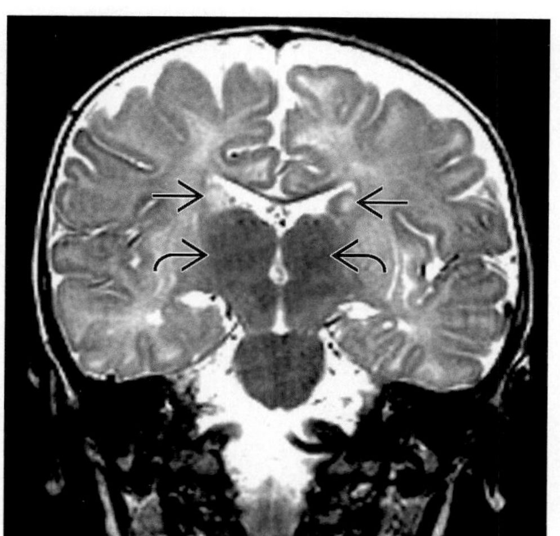

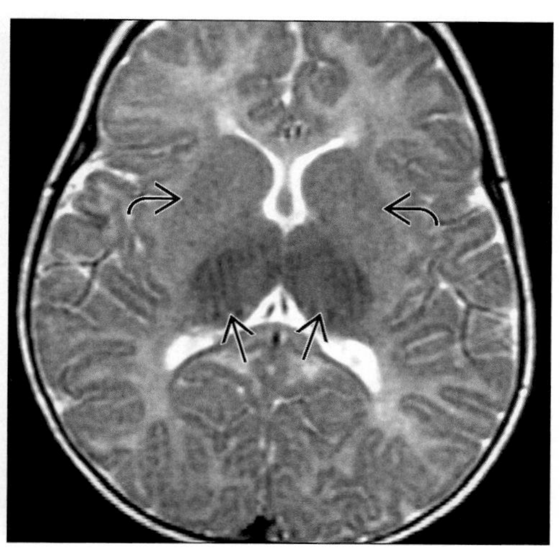

*(**Left**) Coronal T2WI MR in a 1 year old with infantile Sandhoff disease shows diffusely hypointense thalami ⇒. The striatum is abnormally hyperintense, particularly the caudate nuclei ⇒. The cerebral white matter is also mildly hyperintense. (**Right**) Axial T2WI MR shows symmetric hypointense thalami ⇒ in this 7 month old with infantile Sandhoff disease. The putamina ⇒ are mildly hyperintense, more so posteriorly than anteriorly. Myelination appears within a normal range.*

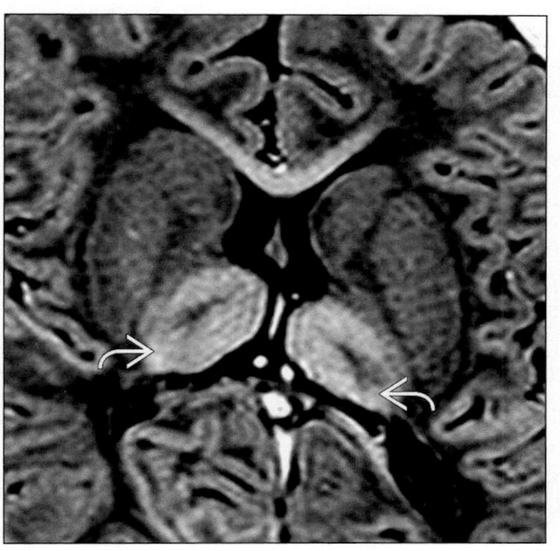

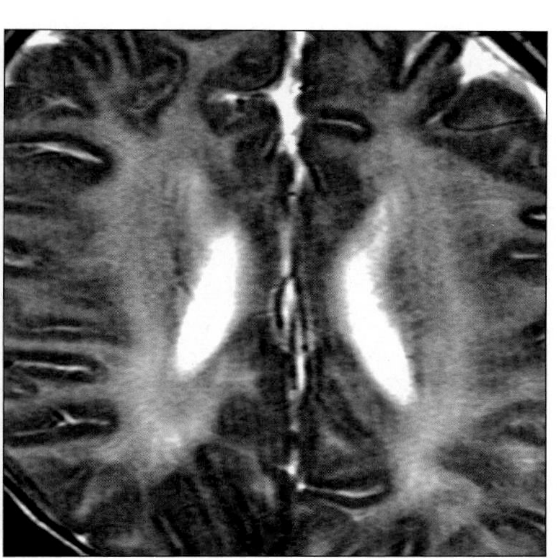

*(**Left**) Axial T1WI MR in a 2 year old with infantile Sandhoff disease shows symmetric thalamic hyperintensity ➡. The central hypointense foci are atypical. The cerebral WM is grossly hypointense, with sparing of the corpus callosum. (**Right**) Axial T2WI MR in the same patient shows diffuse white matter hyperintensity, confirming extensive hypo-/demyelination. The cerebral cortex has a normal appearance.*

METACHROMATIC LEUKODYSTROPHY (MLD)

Key Facts

Terminology

- Lysosomal storage disorder caused by ↓ arylsulfatase A (ARSA) resulting in central (CNS) and peripheral (PNS) nervous system demyelination
- 3 clinical forms: Late infantile (most common), juvenile, adult

Imaging

- Best diagnostic clue: Confluent butterfly-shaped ↑ T2 signal deep cerebral hemispheric white matter
  - Early: Spares subcortical U-fibers
  - Late: Involves subcortical U-fibers
- Sparing of perivenular myelin = "tigroid" or "leopard" pattern
- No WM enhancement
  - Reports cranial nerve, cauda equina enhancement

Top Differential Diagnoses

- Pelizaeus-Merzbacher disease
- TORCH
- Pseudo-TORCH
- Periventricular leukomalacia
- Sneddon syndrome (arylsulfatase A pseudodeficiency)
- Krabbe disease
- Megalencephaly with leukoencephalopathy and cysts

Clinical Issues

- Clinical profile: Toddler with visuomotor impairment and abdominal pain
- Treatment: Supportive
  - Possible future role for retroviral-vector-mediated *ARSA* gene transfer

*(**Left**) Axial T2WI MR shows the typical butterfly-shaped pattern of white matter involvement in MLD. Note the sparing of internal/external capsules and subcortical U-fibers ➡, typical of early disease. (**Right**) Axial T2WI MR shows confluent, symmetric, hyperintense signal in the white matter. Multiple hypointense lines and dots within the white matter ➡ create the characteristic "tigroid" or "leopard" pattern of MLD. The sparing of perivenular myelin is thought to account for this appearance.*

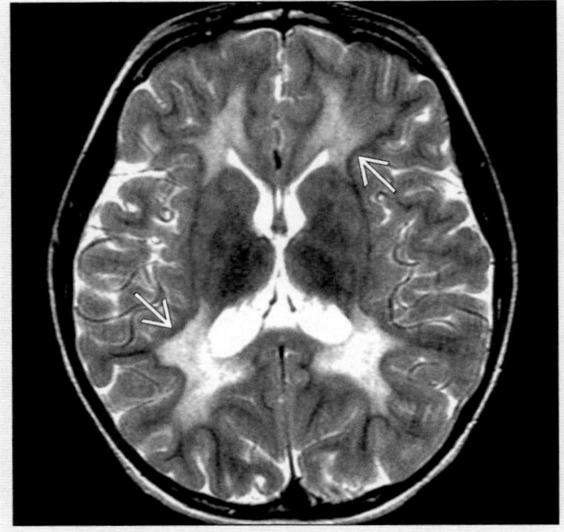

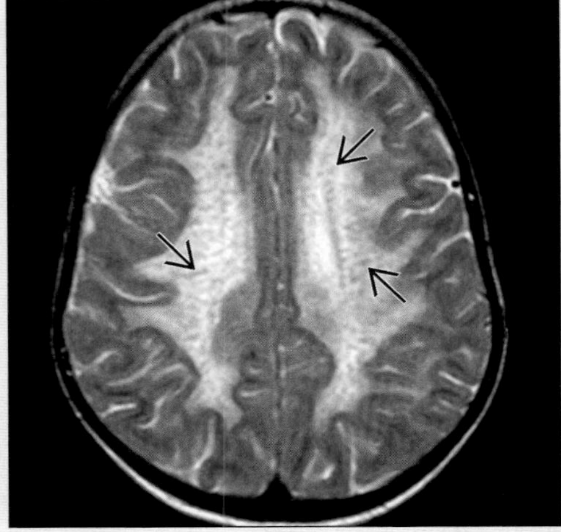

*(**Left**) Axial FLAIR MR demonstrates the characteristic confluent, symmetric, central white matter involvement of MLD. The "tigroid" or "leopard" pattern of lines ➡ and dots within the cerebral hemispheric white matter is evident. (**Right**) Axial ADC map in the same patient shows high signal intensity within the affected white matter, consistent with increased diffusivity and probable interstitial edema. Reduced diffusivity (cytotoxic edema) is sometimes seen in areas of active demyelination.*

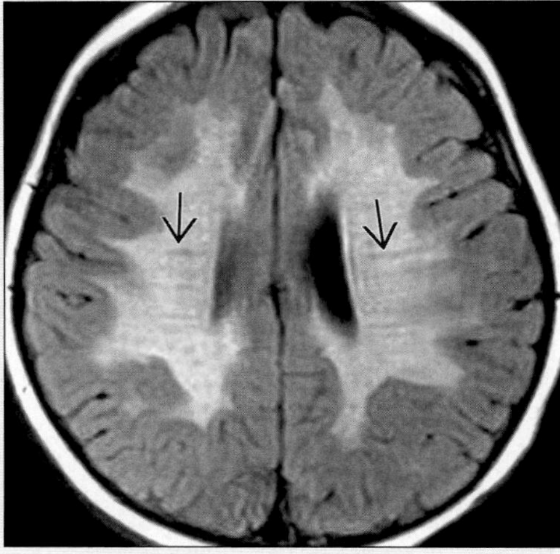

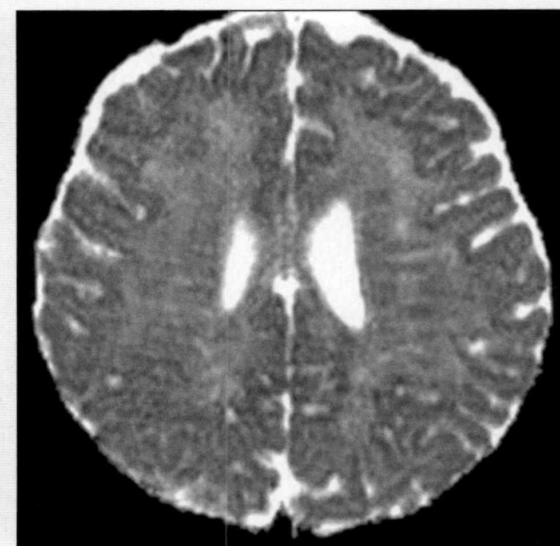

METACHROMATIC LEUKODYSTROPHY (MLD)

TERMINOLOGY

Abbreviations
- Metachromatic leukodystrophy (MLD)

Synonyms
- Sulfatide lipoidosis

Definitions
- Lysosomal storage disorder caused by ↓ arylsulfatase A (ARSA) resulting in central (CNS) and peripheral (PNS) nervous system demyelination
- 3 clinical forms: Late infantile (most common), juvenile, adult

IMAGING

General Features
- Best diagnostic clue: Confluent butterfly-shaped ↑ T2 signal deep cerebral hemispheric white matter (WM)
- Location: Deep cerebral hemispheric white matter
  - Early: Spares subcortical U-fibers
  - Late: Involves subcortical U-fibers
- Morphology: Symmetric, confluent periventricular (PV) and deep WM high T2 signal

CT Findings
- NECT: Symmetric ↓ attenuation central cerebral hemispheric white matter (WM); late atrophy
- CECT: No enhancement (lacks inflammation)
- CT perfusion: ↓ perfusion hemispheric WM

MR Findings
- T1WI
  - Early: ↓ T1 signal within PV/deep WM
  - Late: Atrophy
- T2WI
  - Early
    - Confluent periventricular hyperintensity (butterfly-shaped)
    - Sparing of perivenular myelin = "tigroid" or "leopard" pattern
    - Sparing of subcortical U-fibers
  - Late
    - Progressive subcortical WM extension
    - Involvement of U-fibers, corpus callosum, descending pyramidal tracts, internal capsules
    - Atrophy
- PD/Intermediate: ↑ signal within PV/deep WM
- FLAIR: Butterfly-shaped periventricular hyperintensity
- T2* GRE: No petechial hemorrhage
- DWI: Reduced diffusivity in areas of active demyelination
- T1WI C+: No WM enhancement
  - Reports cranial nerve, cauda equina enhancement
- MRS: ↑ choline, ± ↑ myoinositol

Ultrasonographic Findings
- Thick gallbladder wall, ± sludge, polypoid growths

Nuclear Medicine Findings
- PET: I-123-IMP shows cerebral hypoperfusion

Imaging Recommendations
- Best imaging tool
  - Early MR & MRS in presymptomatic enzyme-deficient siblings
- Protocol advice
  - MR: Include FLAIR
  - MRS: Sample central hemispheric WM

DIFFERENTIAL DIAGNOSIS

Pelizaeus-Merzbacher Disease
- Usually manifests in neonates and infants
- Lack of myelination without myelin destruction
- Cerebellum may be markedly atrophic

TORCH
- Variable WM hyperintensity (demyelination & gliosis)
- Not progressive
- Varied patterns of Ca++ depending on etiology

Pseudo-TORCH
- Progressive cerebral and cerebellar demyelination
- Brainstem, basal ganglia, and periventricular Ca++
- Elevated CSF neurotransmitters

Periventricular Leukomalacia
- Usually symmetric periventricular bright T2 signal
- Periventricular volume loss (nonprogressive)
- Static spastic diplegia or quadriplegia

Sneddon Syndrome (Arylsulfatase A Pseudodeficiency)
- Demyelination
  - May be precipitated by hypoxic event
- Periventricular WM bright T2 signal
- Confirmed by skin biopsy

Krabbe Disease
- Early involvement of cerebellar WM
- CT shows ↑ attenuation of thalami

Megalencephaly with Leukoencephalopathy and Cysts
- Slowly progressive, sparing of cognition, macrocephaly

PATHOLOGY

General Features
- General path comments
  - ↓ ARSA results in systemic storage of sulfatide
    - Symptomatic storage: CNS, PNS, gallbladder
    - Asymptomatic: Kidneys, adrenals, pancreas, liver
  - Diagnosis confirmed by
    - Excess urine sulfatide
    - Absent or deficient ARSA activity in fibroblasts &/ or leukocytes
- Genetics: Autosomal recessive
  - *ARSA* gene located at 22q13.31-qter
  - > 110 different mutations

METACHROMATIC LEUKODYSTROPHY (MLD)

- Late infantile form caused by mutations resulting in extremely low levels ARSA
- Juvenile/adult forms associated with residual ARSA activity
- Etiology
  - Absent or ↓ ARSA ⇒ increased lysosomal storage sulfatide ⇒ lethal demyelination
- Associated abnormalities: Gallbladder disease

Gross Pathologic & Surgical Features

- Early
  - Enlarged brain and demyelination
  - Lack of inflammatory component to WM
- Late
  - Progressive cerebral hemispheric demyelination
  - Cerebral atrophy

Microscopic Features

- Central nervous system
  - PAS(+) metachromatic material accumulates in glial cells, neurons, Schwann cells, macrophages
  - Sulfatide deposition within plasma membranes
  - Sulfatide membrane-bound inclusions at inner layer of myelin sheaths
  - Demyelination may be extensive, yet inflammatory component is lacking
  - Sulfatide content in WM is considerably higher in late infantile form

CLINICAL ISSUES

Presentation

- Most common signs/symptoms
  - Late infantile
    - Insidious onset 2nd year of life
    - Strabismus, gait disturbance, ataxia, weakness, hypotonia
    - ± cherry-red macular spot
    - Bulbar signs ⇒ progressive hypotonia ⇒ decerebrate posturing ⇒ optic atrophy
    - Death frequently within 4 years of diagnosis
  - Juvenile
    - Appears between 5 and 10 years of age
    - Impaired school performance (nonverbal learning disability)
    - Spastic gait, ataxia, intellectual impairment
    - Brisk deep tendon reflexes
    - Progressive spasticity ⇒ progressive dementia ⇒ decerebrate posturing ⇒ seizures
    - Rare to survive longer than 20 years
  - Adult form
    - May present as MS
    - Dementia between 3rd and 4th decades
    - Some adults present with schizophrenia
    - Progressive: Corticobulbar, corticospinal, and cerebellar changes
- Clinical profile: Toddler with visuomotor impairment and abdominal pain

Demographics

- Age: Variable depending on clinical form
- Gender: No gender predilection
- Epidemiology of all forms in USA: 1:100,000
  - ↑ in Habbanite Jewish (1:75 live births)
  - ↑ In Navajo Indians (1:2,500 live births)

Natural History & Prognosis

- Variable depending on clinical form

Treatment

- Supportive
- Bone marrow and umbilical cord blood transplant
  - May arrest motor and intellectual deterioration
  - Questionable effectiveness
    - Considered only in presymptomatic late infantile and early juvenile/adult forms
- Attempts to promote ARSA enzymatic activity have shown poor results
- Future role for retroviral-vector-mediated *ARSA* gene transfer

DIAGNOSTIC CHECKLIST

Consider

- If WM involvement appears as "worst case MLD," involving internal capsule and brainstem ⇒ MLD look-alike, consider
  - Pseudo-TORCH
  - Megalencephaly with leukoencephalopathy and cysts

Image Interpretation Pearls

- "Butterfly" pattern of cerebral hemispheric WM
- "Tigroid" or "leopard" pattern on T2WI
- Early sparing of subcortical U-fibers
- Lack of WM enhancement

SELECTED REFERENCES

1. Haberlandt E et al: Peripheral neuropathy as the sole initial finding in three children with infantile metachromatic leukodystrophy. Eur J Paediatr Neurol. 13(3):257-60, 2009
2. Singh RK et al: Isolated cranial nerve enhancement in metachromatic leukodystrophy. Pediatr Neurol. 40(5):380-2, 2009
3. Pierson TM et al: Umbilical cord blood transplantation for juvenile metachromatic leukodystrophy. Ann Neurol. 64(5):583-7, 2008
4. Görg M et al: Stabilization of juvenile metachromatic leukodystrophy after bone marrow transplantation: a 13-year follow-up. J Child Neurol. 22(9):1139-42, 2007
5. Maia AC Jr et al: Multiple cranial nerve enhancement: a new MR imaging finding in metachromatic leukodystrophy. AJNR Am J Neuroradiol. 28(6):999, 2007
6. Patay Z: Diffusion-weighted MR imaging in leukodystrophies. Eur Radiol. 15(11):2284-303, 2005
7. van der Voorn JP et al: Histopathologic correlates of radial stripes on MR images in lysosomal storage disorders. AJNR Am J Neuroradiol. 26(3):442-6, 2005
8. Sener RN: Metachromatic leukodystrophy: diffusion MRI findings. AJNR Am J Neuroradiol. 23(8):1424-6, 2002
9. Weber Byars AM et al: Metachromatic leukodystrophy and nonverbal learning disability: neuropsychological and neuroradiological findings in heterozygous carriers. Child Neuropsychol. 7(1):54-8, 2001
10. Kim TS et al: MR of childhood metachromatic leukodystrophy. AJNR Am J Neuroradiol. 18(4):733-8, 1997

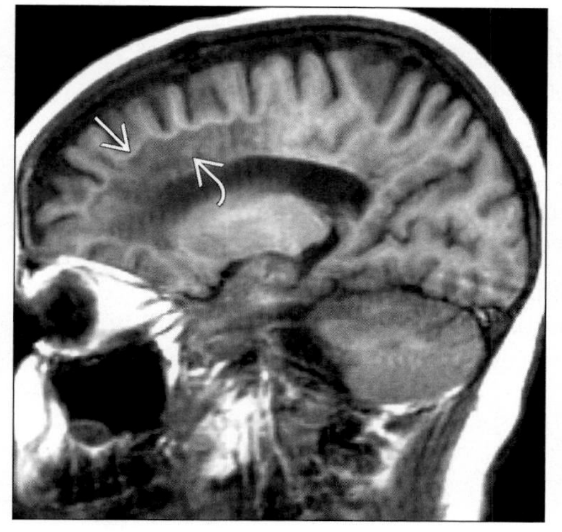

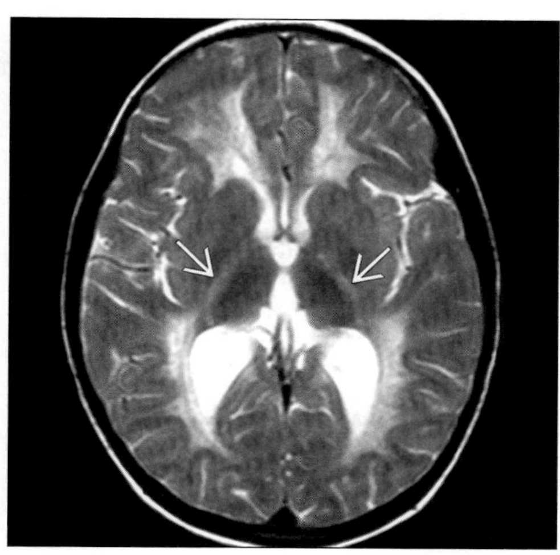

(Left) *Sagittal T1WI MR shows confluent hypointense signal in the periventricular and deep white matter, with sparing of the subcortical U-fibers ➔. Although less well evaluated in the sagittal plane, dot-like areas of spared perivenular myelin can be identified ➔.* ***(Right)*** *Axial T2WI MR shows the butterfly-shaped pattern of white matter involvement typical in more advanced MLD. Although the subcortical U-fibers remain spared, the posterior limbs of the internal capsules ➔ are involved.*

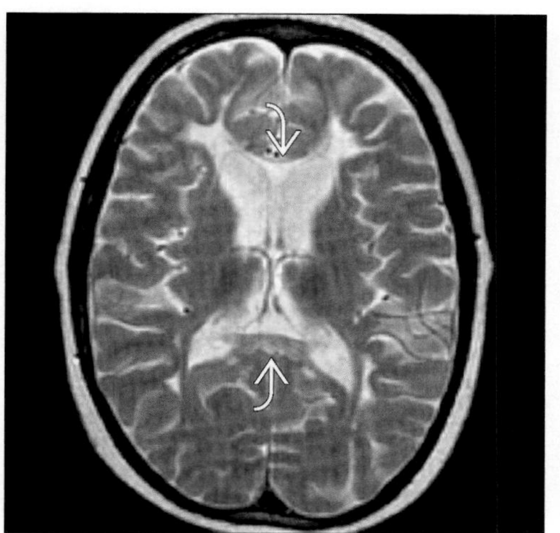

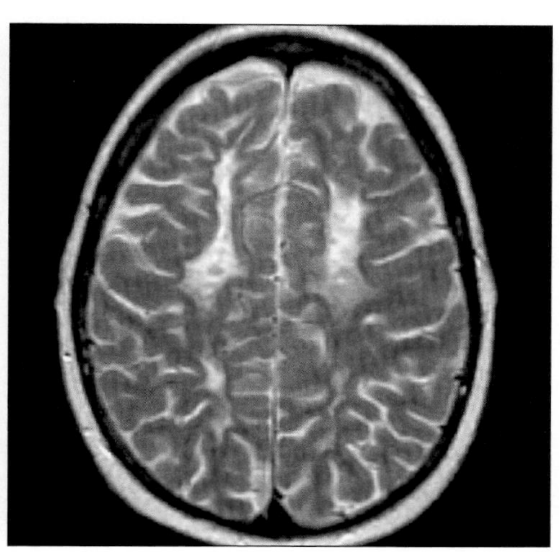

(Left) *In this axial T2WI MR in a patient with late MLD, the characteristic butterfly-shaped pattern of disease can be recognized despite severe loss of white matter volume. Lateral ventricles are enlarged (ex-vacuo), and the basal ganglia are atrophic. Hyperintense signal is present in the corpus callosum ➔.* ***(Right)*** *Axial T2WI MR in the same patient shows confluent hyperintense signal and severe volume loss of the WM. Although spared in this patient, the subcortical U-fibers are often affected in late disease.*

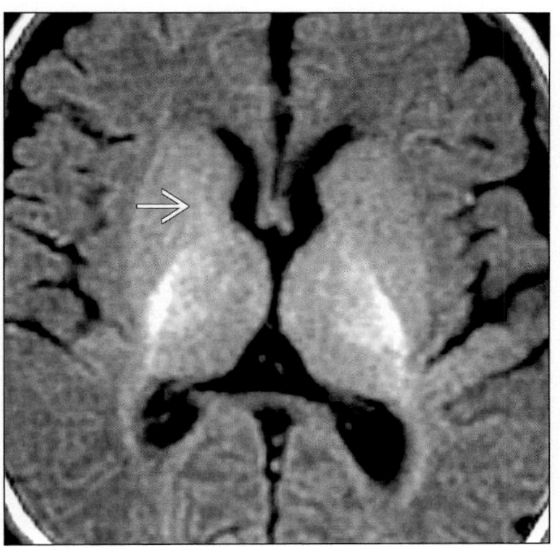

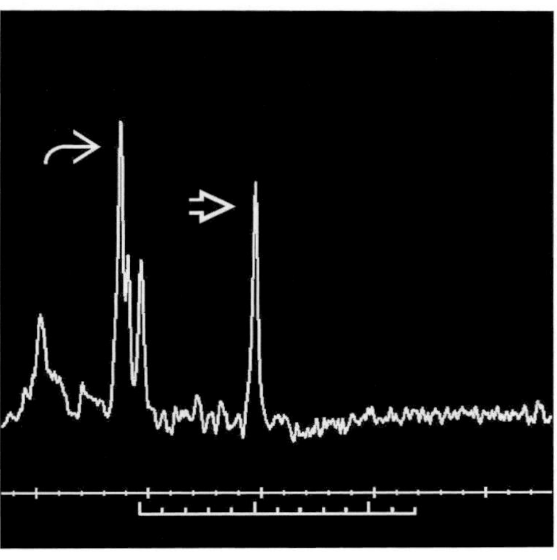

(Left) *Axial T1WI MR in a 4-month-old infant with affected older siblings status post bone marrow transplant (BMT). Excepting mild myelin maturation delay in the anterior limbs of the internal capsule ➔, the conventional images were normal.* ***(Right)*** *Single voxel MRS (TE = 288 msec) obtained from the periventricular white matter of the same patient shows increase in the choline peak ➔. The NAA peak ➔ should be the dominant peak at this age.*

KRABBE

Key Facts

Terminology

- Progressive autosomal-recessive degenerative leukodystrophy of CNS and PNS

Imaging

- Symmetric hyperdensity in thalami, basal ganglia on CT
- Enlargement of optic nerves and cranial nerves
- Confluent symmetric deep periventricular white matter (WM) hyperintensity
- Cerebellar WM hyperintense signal on T2WI
  - Ring-like appearance around dentate nuclei
- Fractional anisotropy values in corticospinal tracts are low compared to controls
- Enhancement of lumbar nerve roots
- MRS: Pronounced ↑ choline, myoinositol; moderate NAA reduction; mild lactate accumulation

Pathology

- Deficiency of lysosomal galactocerebroside β-galactosidase (GALC)
  - Accumulation of psychosine 100x normal concentrations
  - Psychosine is toxic to brain
- Infantile form is most common and most severe
- "Globoid" cells = macrophages containing PAS(+) galactocerebrosides
  - Identified in enlarged optic nerves

Clinical Issues

- Most common symptom is extreme irritability
- Neonatal screening has been instituted in New York, Illinois
- Stem cell transplant can halt disease progression

__(Left)__ Axial NECT in a 6 month old with irritability and feeding difficulties shows abnormal increased attenuation in the thalami ➾. __(Right)__ The hyperdensities are more punctate ➔ in this axial NECT from an 18 month old with Krabbé disease. Infantile Krabbé is 1 of the few leukodystrophies in which CT features may be apparent before MR findings; however, DTI shows promise in detecting decreased fractional anisotropy in the corticospinal tracts in presymptomatic neonates.

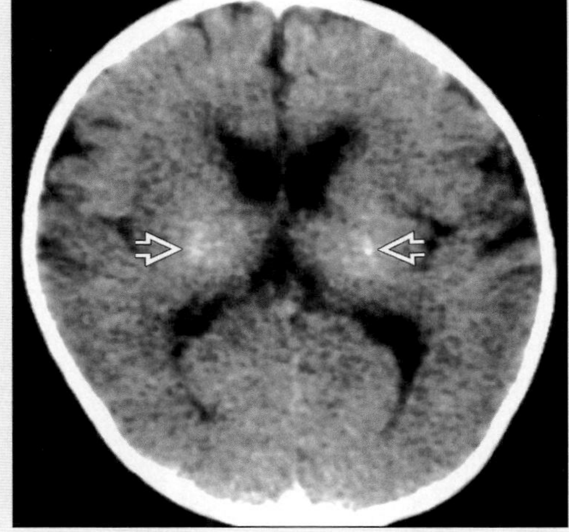

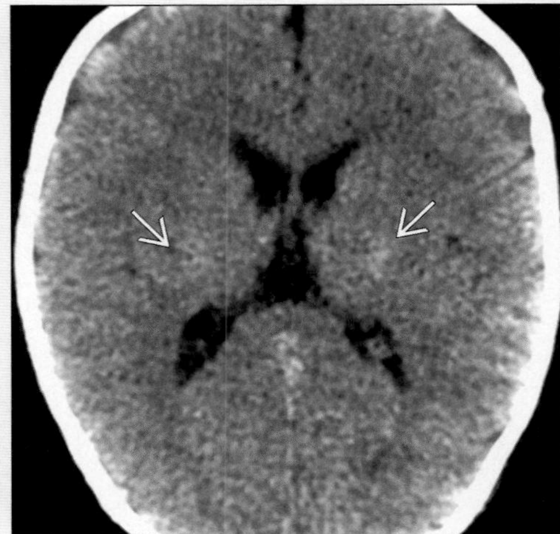

__(Left)__ Axial T1WI MR in an 8-month-old male child with Krabbé shows abnormal hypointensity ➔ in the hila of the cerebellar nuclei bilaterally. Regions of increased density on CT often have hyperintense signal on T1WI. __(Right)__ Axial T2WI MR in the same patient shows correlating alternating hyper- (edema in hila ➔), hypo- (nuclei ➾), and hyperintense (cerebellar white matter ➾) signal around the cerebellar nuclei. Krabbé is 1 of the few leukodystrophies that has early cerebellar imaging findings.

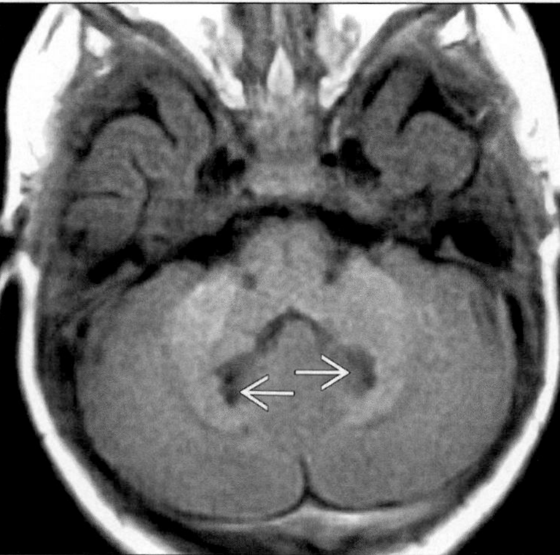

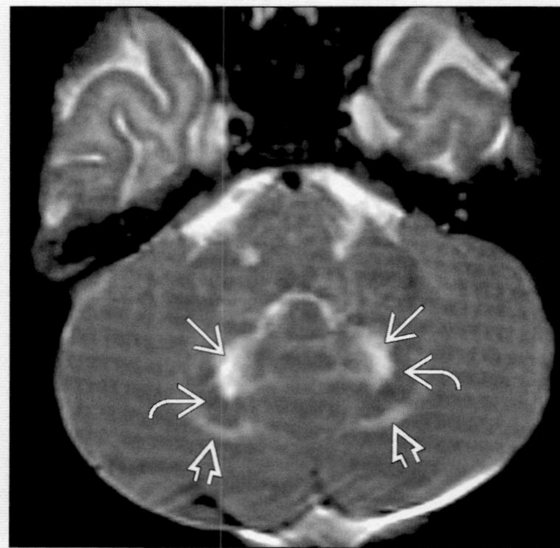

KRABBE

TERMINOLOGY

Synonyms

- Globoid cell leukodystrophy (GLD)

Definitions

- Progressive autosomal-recessive degenerative leukodystrophy of central (CNS) and peripheral (PNS) nervous systems

IMAGING

General Features

- Best diagnostic clue
  - Hyperdensity on CT in thalami, corona radiata, and body of caudate nuclei in irritable infant
- Location
  - Thalami, basal ganglia (BG), white matter (WM), corticospinal and pyramidal tracts, PNS

CT Findings

- NECT
  - Symmetric hyperdensity in thalami, BG, corona radiata, cerebellum
    - Globoid cell accumulation with calcifications
    - Fades over time
  - Deep, periventricular WM hypodensity
  - Atrophy develops → microcephaly

MR Findings

- T1WI
  - Deep, periventricular WM hypointensity
  - Faint hyperintensity in thalami and basal ganglia
  - Enlargement of optic nerves and cranial nerves
- T2WI
  - Confluent symmetric deep periventricular WM hyperintensity
    - Spares subcortical U-fibers
    - Becomes diffuse with time
  - Cerebellar WM hyperintense signal
    - Ring-like appearance around dentate nuclei
  - Corpus callosum frequently involved in adult onset disease
- FLAIR
  - Better delineates WM hyperintensities in older children
- DWI
  - Fractional anisotropy (FA) values in corticospinal tracts are significantly lower in neonates with Krabbé disease than in controls
  - Diffusion tensor-derived anisotropy maps → loss of diffusion anisotropy
    - Relative anisotropy (RA) differences found in BG, middle cerebellar peduncles, internal capsule, corpus callosum, periventricular WM
    - After stem cell transplantation, mean RA between RA of untreated patients and control subjects
- T1WI C+
  - Enhancement of lumbar nerve roots
- MRS
  - Infantile: Pronounced ↑ choline, myoinositol; moderate NAA reduction; mild lactate accumulation
  - Late infantile-juvenile: ↑ choline, myoinositol; mild NAA reduction
  - Adult: Mild ↑ choline and myoinositol, may be close to normal

Imaging Recommendations

- Best imaging tool
  - MR + contrast and DTI
- Protocol advice
  - Pay attention to cranial nerves!
  - Consider NECT to look for hyperintensity

DIFFERENTIAL DIAGNOSIS

Neuronal Ceroid Lipofuscinosis

- Batten disease
- Hyperdense thalami on CT
- Progressive cerebral atrophy

GM2 Gangliosidoses

- e.g., Tay-Sachs
- Lysosomal lipid storage disorders caused by mutations in at least 1 of 3 recessive genes: *HEXA*, *HEXB*, *GM2A*
- Hypointense/hyperdense thalami; patchy hyperintense WM

Neurofibromatosis Type 1

- Optic nerve enlargement (optic nerve glioma)
- Patchy WM signal abnormalities
- Not progressive, does not present with irritability in infant

Metachromatic Leukodystrophy (MLD)

- Progressive WM hyperintensity on T2WI
- Initial sparing of subcortical U-fibers

PATHOLOGY

General Features

- Etiology
  - Gene defects result in deficiency of lysosomal galactocerebroside β-galactosidase (GALC)
    - Normally aids in cleavage of galactose from psychosine and galactosylceramide, leaving sphingosine and ceramide respectively
      - Galactosylceramidase 2 & 3 can catalyze galactosylceramide but not psychosine
    - Results in accumulation of psychosine 100x normal concentrations
      - Psychosine is toxic to brain, especially oligodendroglia → destruction of oligodendrocytes
    - Accumulation of psychosine causes
      - Up-regulation of AP-1 (pro-apoptotic pathway)
      - Down-regulation of NF-κ-B pathway (antiapoptotic pathway)
  - Sulfotransferase may also be deficient → suggests galactosylceramide degradation may be complex
- Genetics
  - Autosomal recessive lysosomal disorder
  - Gene mapped to chromosome 14 (14q24.3 to 14q32.1) and has been cloned

- Different mutations associated with differing severity for both age of onset and progression
- 65 mutations & polymorphic changes described

Staging, Grading, & Classification

- Infantile: Before age 2
  - Most common and most severe
- Late infantile-juvenile: After age 2
- Adult: After age 10
  - Corticospinal, pyramidal tract symptoms
  - Mimics peripheral neuropathy
  - Often undiagnosed for many years

Gross Pathologic & Surgical Features

- Small, atrophic brain

Microscopic Features

- Myelin loss with astrogliosis and dysmyelination
  - Severe oligodendrocyte loss
- Perivascular large multinucleated "globoid" and mononuclear epithelioid cells in demyelinated zones
  - "Globoid" cells = macrophages containing PAS(+) galactocerebrosides
- Demyelination is marked within cerebrum, cerebellum, brainstem, spinal cord with segmental involvement of peripheral nerves
- "Globoid" cells identified in enlarged optic nerves
- "Globoid" cell inclusions in sweat gland epithelial cells

CLINICAL ISSUES

Presentation

- Most common signs/symptoms
  - Neonatal: Most common symptom is extreme irritability
    - Seizures result in medical attention
    - Hypersensitivity to sensory stimuli (e.g., hyperacusis), fevers, feeding problems, failure to thrive, optic atrophy, cortical blindness
  - Infantile-juvenile
    - Visual failure, cerebellar ataxia, spasticity, polyneuropathy, dementia, psychosis
  - Adult
    - Hemiparesis, spastic paraparesis, cerebellar ataxia, intellectual impairment, visual failure, peripheral polyneuropathy, talipes cavus
- Clinical profile
  - Diagnosis made from leukocyte or skin fibroblast β-galactosidase assay
  - Molecular assay available for genetic counseling, prenatal testing
  - Universal neonatal screening has been instituted in New York, Illinois

Demographics

- Gender
  - M = F
- Ethnicity
  - Most reported patients have European ancestry but can affect all
- Epidemiology
  - 1:100,000 USA and Europe
  - 1:25-50,000 in Sweden
  - 6:1,000 in Druze community in Israel

Natural History & Prognosis

- Neonatal: Rapidly progressive, few live more than 2 years
  - Motor deterioration → quadriparesis, decerebrate
  - Hypertonicity becomes flaccidity as PNS involved
  - Blindness
- Infantile-juvenile: More protracted course, slower rate of progression
- Adult: Heterogeneous, progresses more slowly
  - MR may remain normal for many years, even in presence of symptoms
- Sequelae (e.g., infection) cause most deaths

Treatment

- Hematopoietic stem cell transplantation
  - Halts disease progression in mild forms of Krabbé
  - Both clinical and radiologic manifestations may reverse or retard

DIAGNOSTIC CHECKLIST

Consider

- Use contrast on MR when considering leukodystrophies
- Think of Krabbé when dealing with hyperirritable infant

Image Interpretation Pearls

- Look for faint hyperdensity on CT in deep nuclei

SELECTED REFERENCES

1. Duffner PK et al: Newborn screening for Krabbe disease: the New York State model. Pediatr Neurol. 40(4):245-52; discussion 253-5, 2009
2. Beslow LA et al: Thickening and enhancement of multiple cranial nerves in conjunction with cystic white matter lesions in early infantile Krabbe disease. Pediatr Radiol. 38(6):694-6, 2008
3. Patel B et al: Optic nerve and chiasm enlargement in a case of infantile Krabbe disease: quantitative comparison with 26 age-matched controls. Pediatr Radiol. 38(6):697-9, 2008
4. Wang C et al: The earliest MR imaging and proton MR spectroscopy abnormalities in adult-onset Krabbe disease. Acta Neurol Scand. 116(4):268-72, 2007
5. McGraw P et al: Krabbe disease treated with hematopoietic stem cell transplantation: serial assessment of anisotropy measurements--initial experience. Radiology. 236(1):221-30, 2005
6. Brockmann K et al: Proton MRS profile of cerebral metabolic abnormalities in Krabbe disease. Neurology. 60(5):819-25, 2003
7. Suzuki K: Globoid cell leukodystrophy (Krabbe's disease): update. J Child Neurol. 18(9):595-603, 2003
8. Guo AC et al: Evaluation of white matter anisotropy in Krabbe disease with diffusion tensor MR imaging: initial experience. Radiology. 218(3):809-15, 2001
9. Farina L et al: MR imaging and proton MR spectroscopy in adult Krabbe disease. AJNR Am J Neuroradiol. 21(8):1478-82, 2000
10. Jones BV et al: Optic nerve enlargement in Krabbe's disease. AJNR Am J Neuroradiol. 20(7):1228-31, 1999
11. Zafeiriou DI et al: Early infantile Krabbe disease: deceptively normal magnetic resonance imaging and serial neurophysiological studies. Brain Dev. 19(7):488-91, 1997

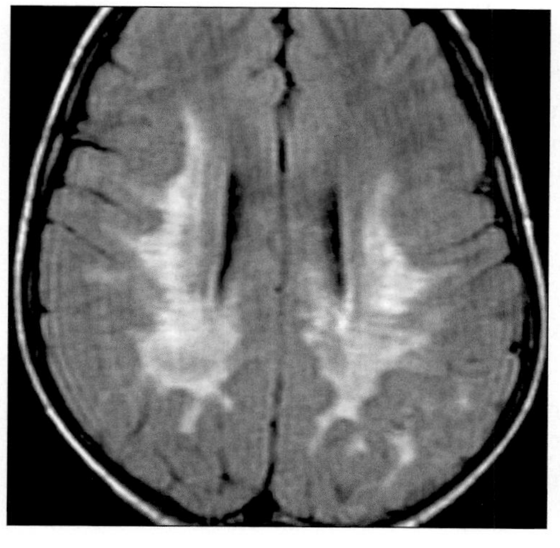

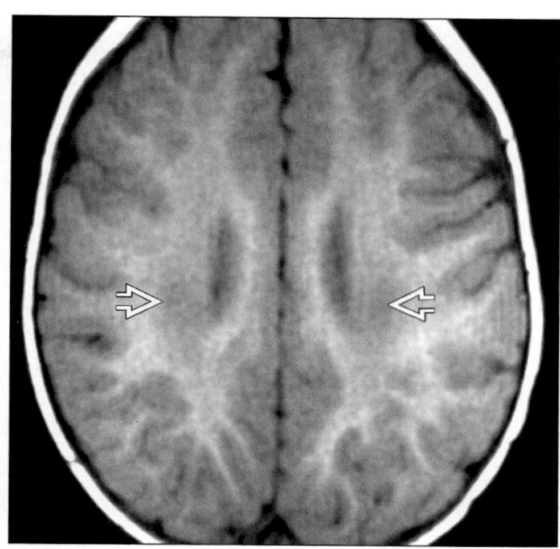

(Left) *Axial FLAIR MR in a 4 year old with Krabbé disease treated with stem cell transplantation shows confluent abnormal hyperintense signal in the periventricular white matter, primarily affecting the posterior frontal and parietal lobes.* ***(Right)*** *Axial T1WI MR in the same child shows subtle hypointense signal ➪ that appears less extensive but is in the same distribution. These findings did not progress after the stem cell transplant.*

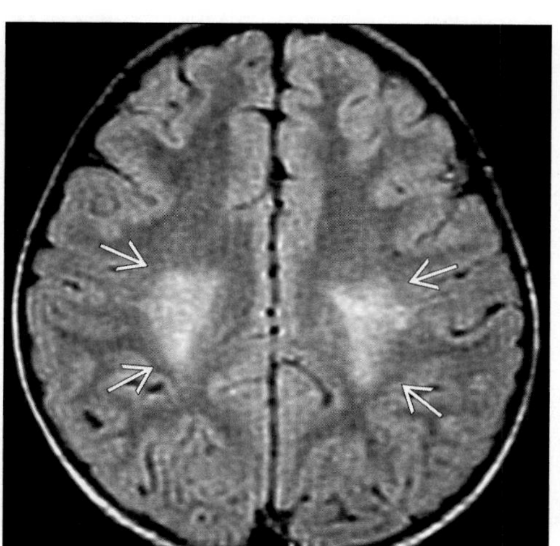

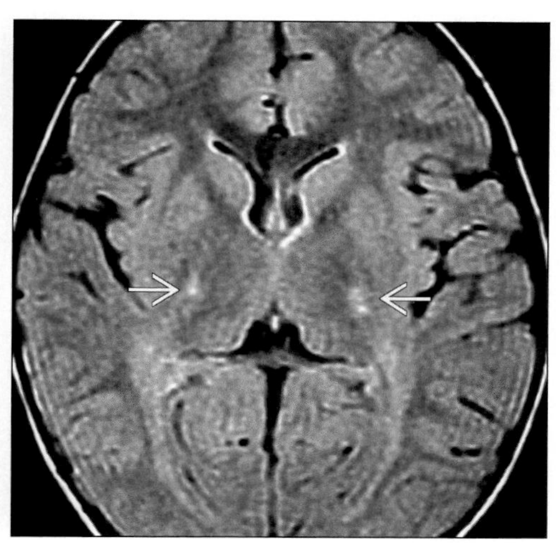

(Left) *Axial FLAIR MR in a 30 year old with juvenile-onset Krabbé disease demonstrates abnormal hyperintense signal ➔ in the corona radiata on each side. Symmetric corticospinal tract involvement is a hallmark of globoid cell leukodystrophy.* ***(Right)*** *Axial FLAIR MR in the same patient shows focal symmetric hyperintensity in the capsular portion of the corticospinal tracts ➔. The infantile juvenile onset form is characterized by a more protracted course with a slower rate of progression.*

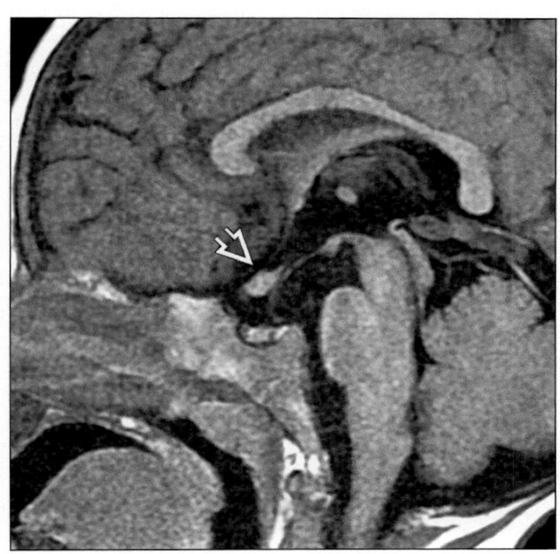

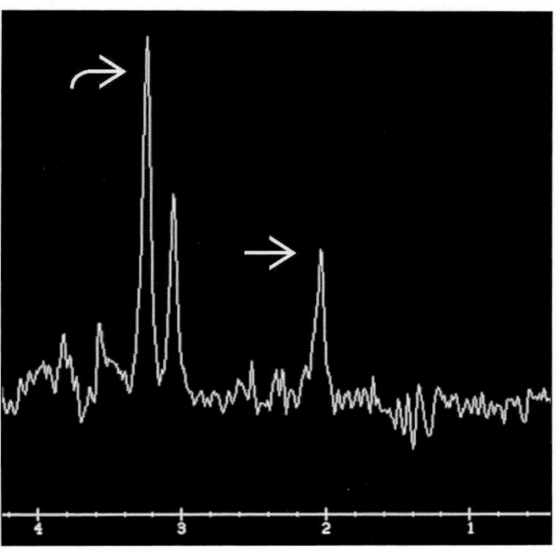

(Left) *Sagittal T1WI MR clearly shows focal enlargement of the optic chiasm ➪ in this child with Krabbé disease. A unique feature of this leukodystrophy is the occasional enlargement of optic nerves, described by Krabbé in his original paper on the condition.* ***(Right)*** *Axial MRS in the affected WM of a child with Krabbé shows elevated choline ➚ and diminished NAA ➔. Although nonspecific, this pattern is typical of Krabbé disease, and these alterations will worsen without treatment.*

FABRY DISEASE

Key Facts

Terminology
- Fabry disease (FD)

Imaging
- NECT
  - Ca++ in lateral pulvinar, globus pallidus, putamen, substantia nigra, dentate nuclei
- MR may show earlier changes
  - ↑ T1 signal in deep gray nuclei
  - T1 lateral pulvinar hyperintensity considered pathognomonic of FD
  - T2/FLAIR hyperintensities in periventricular WM, deep gray matter

Top Differential Diagnoses
- Endocrinologic disorders
  - Hyperparathyroidism, hypoparathyroidism, pseudohypoparathyroidism, hypothyroidism
- HIV-associated mineralizing calcific microangiopathy
- Fahr disease

Pathology
- X-linked disorder of glycosphingolipid metabolism
- Deficient activity of α-galactosidase A
- Endothelial accumulation of glycosphingolipids
  - Compromises vessel lumen size
  - Leads to vascular events (myocardial ischemia, strokes)

Clinical Issues
- Neurologic complications in 4th/5th decades
- Enzyme replacement therapy may help

Diagnostic Checklist
- Consider FD in young males with white matter disease, basal ganglia/pulvinar calcification

*(**Left**) Axial T1WI MR in a patient with Fabry disease shows bilateral hyperintense lesions in the lateral putamina → and lateral aspects of both pulvinars ↷. T1 hyperintensity in the lateral pulvinar is considered a virtually pathognomonic sign of Fabry disease. (**Right**) Axial NECT in the same patient shows calcifications in the right caudate →, both putamina ↷, and lateral pulvinars ⇨, corresponding to the T1 hyperintensities seen on the previous MR scan.*

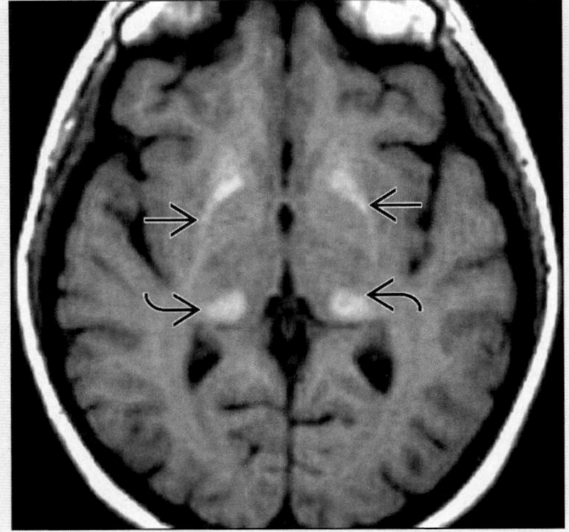

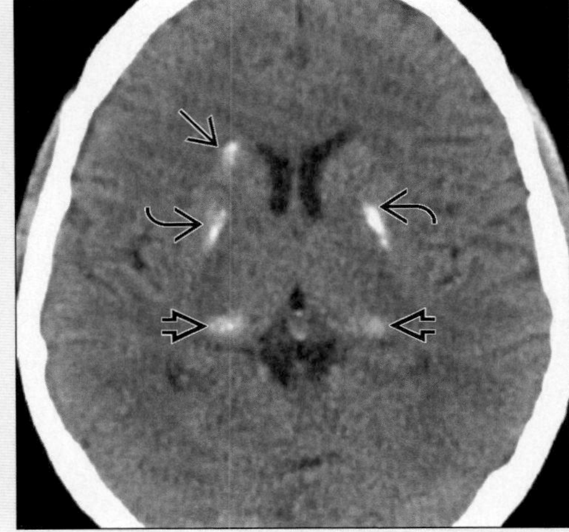

*(**Left**) Axial T2WI MR in a 50-year-old man with Fabry disease shows multifocal lacunar infarcts in the basal ganglia → and thalami ↷, as well as confluent hyperintensities in the deep periventricular white matter ⇨. (**Right**) Axial T2WI MR in the same patient shows multifocal, discrete, and confluent white matter hyperintensities in the deep cerebral white matter →. Deep white matter and basal ganglia infarcts are due to large and small vessel involvement in Fabry disease.*

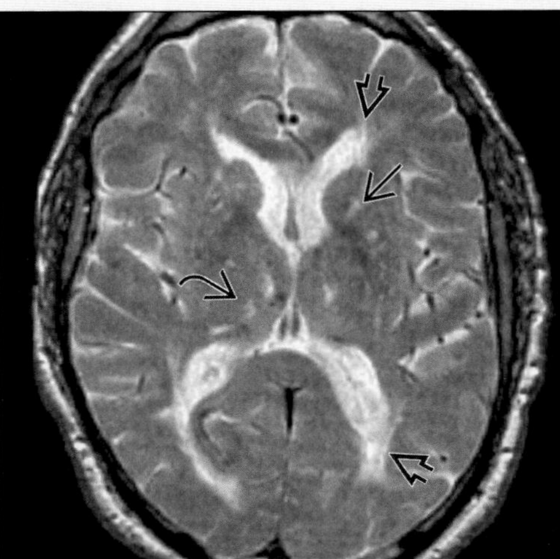

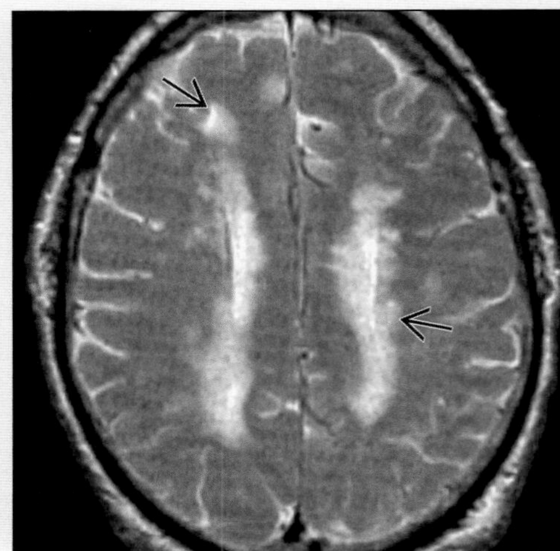

FABRY DISEASE

TERMINOLOGY

Abbreviations

- Fabry disease (FD)

Synonyms

- Anderson-Fabry disease

Definitions

- X-linked disorder of glycosphingolipid metabolism
- Deficient activity of α-galactosidase A

IMAGING

General Features

- Best diagnostic clue
  - Lateral pulvinar ↑ T1 signal (MR), Ca++ (CT)
- Location
  - Typical: Lateral pulvinar, globus pallidus, putamen
  - Other: Substantia nigra, dentate nuclei

Imaging Recommendations

- Best imaging tool
  - CT: Sensitive for small quantities of calcification
  - MR may show earlier changes, T1 hyperintensity
- Protocol advice
  - NECT + MR (T1-, T2WI; FLAIR best)

CT Findings

- NECT
  - Bilateral deep gray nuclei Ca++
  - Deep white matter (WM) hypodensities

MR Findings

- T1WI
  - Increased T1 signal in deep gray nuclei
    - Lateral pulvinar ↑ T1 signal considered pathognomonic
  - T1 hyperintensity varies
    - Depends on stage, volume of Ca++
- T2WI
  - ↑ T2 areas in periventricular WM, deep gray matter
    - ↑ in intensity, coalesce over time
  - Later: Large cortical, deep gray matter infarcts
- T2* GRE
  - Pulvinar hypointensity only in severe disease

DIFFERENTIAL DIAGNOSIS

Endocrinologic Disorders

- Hyperparathyroidism, hypoparathyroidism, pseudohypoparathyroidism, hypothyroidism
- Ca++ distribution similar
  - Thalamus involvement more diffuse
- Serum Ca, PTH, T3/T4, TSH levels helpful

HIV-Associated Mineralizing Calcific Microangiopathy

- Ca++ in basal ganglia (BG) and cerebral atrophy

Fahr Disease

- Bilateral dense, thick Ca++ in BG/thalami
- Cortical atrophy

PATHOLOGY

General Features

- Etiology
  - Disorder of glycosphingolipid metabolism
  - α-galactosidase A deficient activity
    - Causes progressive accumulation of glycosphingolipids (ceramide trihexoside)
      - Vascular endothelium and smooth muscle cells affected
      - Endothelial accumulation causes ↓ vessel lumen
      - Parenchymal cells in kidney, heart, and brain affected
    - Leads to myocardial ischemia and stroke
- Genetics
  - X-linked inheritance, abnormality in *GLA* gene
- Associated abnormalities
  - Left ventricular hypertrophy, short PR interval, AV block
  - Renal cysts (subcapsular predilection)

Microscopic Features

- Glycosphingolipid deposits in neurons
  - Basal ganglia, brain stem, amygdala, hypothalamus

CLINICAL ISSUES

Presentation

- Most common signs/symptoms
  - Acroparesthesias, neuropathic pain
  - Corneal inclusions, cataracts
  - Cutaneous angiokeratomas
- Other signs/symptoms
  - Strokes, angina, heart block, renal failure

Demographics

- Age
  - Neurologic complications in 4th/5th decades
  - Hemizygous men: Onset in adolescence
- Gender
  - Heterozygous females are normally healthy carriers but may develop symptoms of FD

DIAGNOSTIC CHECKLIST

Consider

- FD in young males with white matter disease, basal ganglia/pulvinar calcification

Image Interpretation Pearls

- T1 hyperintensity in pulvinar is pathognomonic

SELECTED REFERENCES

1. Buechner S et al: Central nervous system involvement in Anderson-Fabry disease: a clinical and MRI retrospective study. J Neurol Neurosurg Psychiatry. 79(11):1249-54, 2008
2. Burlina AP et al: The pulvinar sign: frequency and clinical correlations in Fabry disease. J Neurol. 255(5):738-44, 2008

ZELLWEGER SYNDROME SPECTRUM

Key Facts

Terminology

- Zellweger syndrome: Cerebrohepatorenal syndrome
- Zellweger syndrome spectrum (ZSS): ZS + neonatal adrenoleukodystrophy + infantile Refsum disease
- Peroxisome biogenesis disorders: ZSS (80%) + rhizomelic chondrodysplasia punctata

Imaging

- Microgyria, pachygria, hypomyelination, germinolytic cysts
  - Microgyria most severe in perisylvian region
  - Pachygyria most common frontoparietal
- Central volume loss common
- MRS: ↓ NAA, ↑ Cho
- Short TE MRS: Mobile lipid peaks at 0.9 and 1.33 ppm
- Diffuse hypomyelination, cerebellum, and brainstem may be involved especially if present > 1 year

Top Differential Diagnoses

- Congenital CMV
- Pseudo-TORCH
- Single peroxisomal enzyme deficiencies

Pathology

- Defect in biogenesis of peroxisomes
- Autosomal-recessive phenotype resulting from defect in any of at least 12 *PEX* genes

Clinical Issues

- Severe hypotonia, seizures, poor sucking
- Elevated liver enzymes, hepatomegaly
- Cataract, nystagmus, retinitis pigmentosa, or optic atrophy
- Large fontanelle + sutures, high forehead, broad nasal bridge, hypertelorism

*(**Left**) Coronal T2WI MR of a fetus at 32 weeks gestation age shows right ventricular enlargement (30 mm), a subtle germinolytic cyst → in the left frontal horn, diffuse microgyria ➔, and abnormal variation of white matter signal intensity. (**Right**) Coronal T2WI MR in the same patient 2 days after term delivery shows right ventricular enlargement, a germinolytic cyst → in the right frontal horn, diffuse cerebral and cerebellar microgyria ➔, and abnormally increased signal in the deep white matter.*

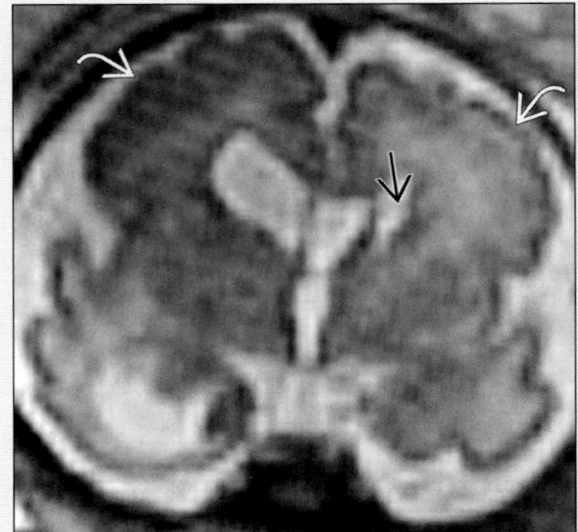

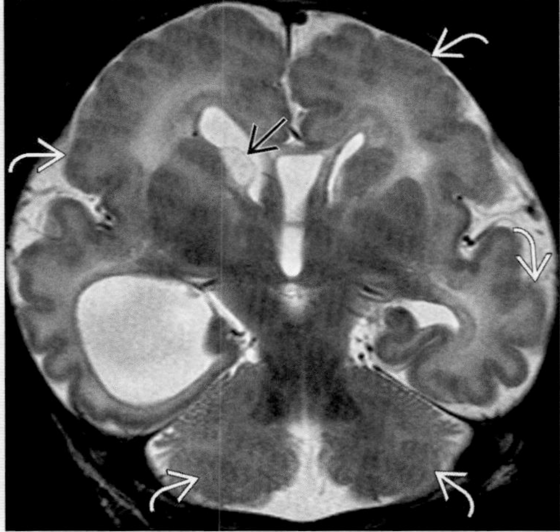

*(**Left**) Axial T2WI MR of the same 32-week gestational age fetus shows diffusely abnormal signal intensity in the cerebral hemispheric white matter, in addition to extensive cerebral microgyria ➔. (**Right**) Axial T2WI MR in the same patient 2 days after term delivery. Note the presence of diffuse cerebral cortical microgyria → along with areas of decreased sulcation ➔, in addition to abnormally increased signal in the white matter ➔.*

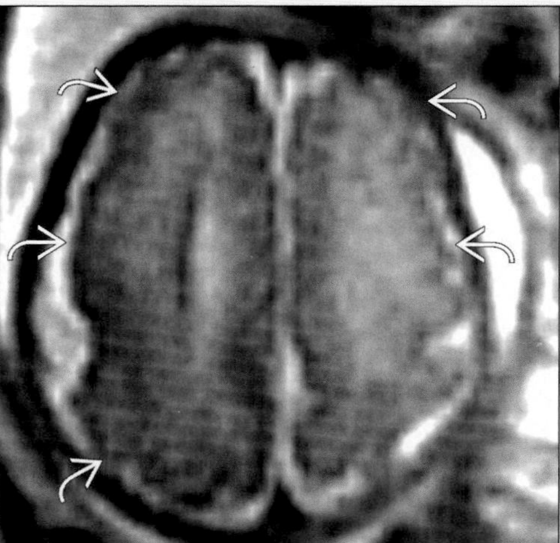

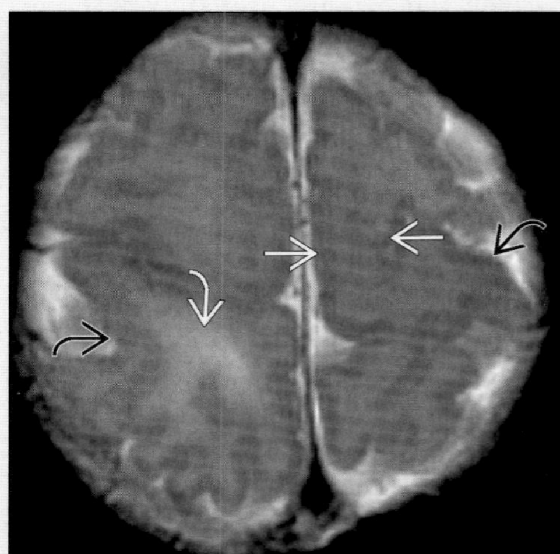

ZELLWEGER SYNDROME SPECTRUM

TERMINOLOGY

Abbreviations

- Zellweger syndrome spectrum (ZSS)

Synonyms

- Cerebrohepatorenal syndrome
- Zellweger syndrome (ZS)

Definitions

- ZSS: ZS + neonatal adrenoleukodystrophy + infantile Refsum disease
- Peroxisome biogenesis disorders: ZSS (80%) + rhizomelic chondrodysplasia punctata (RCDP)

IMAGING

General Features

- Best diagnostic clue
  - Microgyria, pachygria, hypomyelination, germinolytic cysts
  - Leukoencephalopathy; volume loss > 1 year
- Location
  - Microgyria most severe in perisylvian region
  - Pachygyria most common frontoparietal
  - Diffuse hypomyelination; cerebellum and brainstem may be involved especially if present > 1 year
- Size
  - Central volume loss common
- Morphology
  - ± heterotopia (periventricular or subcortical)

MR Findings

- T1WI
  - Microgyria, pachygyria, germinolytic cysts, ↓ white matter (WM) signal
  - ± ↑ globus pallidus signal from hyperbilirubinemia
- T2WI
  - Microgyria, pachygyria, germinolytic cysts, ↑ WM signal
- MRS
  - Use short TE: ↓ NAA; ↑ Cho; lipid peaks at 0.9 and 1.33 ppm

Imaging Recommendations

- Best imaging tool
  - MR + MRS
- Protocol advice
  - Volumetric T1/FLAIR for cysts, TE = 20-30 ms for MRS

DIFFERENTIAL DIAGNOSIS

Congenital CMV

- Ca++, periventricular cysts usually not caudothalamic

Pseudo-TORCH

- Basal ganglia, thalamic, and periventricular Ca++

Single Peroxisomal Enzyme Deficiencies

- Brain MR may be similar; biochemistry different

PATHOLOGY

General Features

- Etiology
  - Defect in biogenesis of peroxisomes
    - Defective transport of proteins into peroxisomal matrix → accumulation of very long chain fatty acids
- Genetics
  - AR defect in any of at least 12 *PEX* genes
- Associated abnormalities
  - Eye: Brushfield spots, retinal pigment degeneration
  - Hepatomegaly, renal cortical cysts
  - Skeletal: Stippled chondral calcification

Gross Pathologic & Surgical Features

- Leukoencephalopathy, germinolytic cysts, cortical and cerebellar malformations
- Subcortical heterotopia, cerebellar hypoplasia

Microscopic Features

- Pachygyria, polymicrogyria, or microgyria
- Sudanophilic leukodystrophy

CLINICAL ISSUES

Presentation

- Most common signs/symptoms
  - Severe hypotonia, seizures, poor sucking
  - Large fontanelle + sutures, high forehead, broad nasal bridge, hypertelorism
- Other signs/symptoms
  - Elevated liver enzymes, hepatomegaly
  - Cataract, nystagmus, retinitis pigmentosa, or optic atrophy
- Clinical profile
  - Low Apgar scores; very floppy, dysmorphic facies

Demographics

- Age
  - Severe at birth, milder at < 6 months, rare adult

Natural History & Prognosis

- Most severely affected die < 3 months, milder may live > 20 years

Treatment

- Supportive, no proven therapy

SELECTED REFERENCES

1. Krause C et al: Rational diagnostic strategy for Zellweger syndrome spectrum patients. Eur J Hum Genet. 17(6):741-8, 2009
2. Weller S et al: Cerebral MRI as a valuable diagnostic tool in Zellweger spectrum patients. J Inherit Metab Dis. Epub ahead of print, 2008
3. Groenendaal F et al: Proton magnetic resonance spectroscopy (1H-MRS) of the cerebrum in two young infants with Zellweger syndrome. Neuropediatrics. 32(1):23-7, 2001
4. Barkovich AJ et al: MR of Zellweger syndrome. AJNR Am J Neuroradiol. 18(6):1163-70, 1997

X-LINKED ADRENOLEUKODYSTROPHY

Key Facts

Terminology

- X-linked adrenoleukodystrophy (X-ALD): Severe progressive form usually affects pre-teen males
- At least 6 variants other than childhood cerebral X-ALD (CCALD) exist: Presymptomatic X-ALD, adolescent (AdolCALD), adult (ACALD), AMN, Addison only, symptomatic female carriers
- Inherited disorder of peroxisome metabolism → impaired β-oxidation of very long chain fatty acids (VLCFA)

Imaging

- CCALD: Enhancing (CT or MR) peritrigonal demyelination
- Usually symmetrical, confluent, posterior involvement; rare frontal pattern (~ 10%)

Pathology

- Clinical heterogeneity attributed to specific mutations, modifying factors
- Phenotypic variability: CCALD, AMN → presymptomatic presentations even within same family

Clinical Issues

- Lorenzo oil delays symptoms in presymptomatic ALD
- X-ALD and variants = 1:16,800 North American births

Diagnostic Checklist

- X-ALD presenting at atypical ages → atypical appearances (lacks enhancement, may have frontal rather than posterior "gradient")
- Always enhance unknown leukodystrophy!

*(**Left**) Axial graphic demonstrates multiple layers of demyelination. The layers correspond to 3 zones histopathologically. The outer layer ➢ consists of active destruction, the middle layer ➢ of active inflammation. Note that the central area → is burnt out. (**Right**) Axial T1WI C+ MR reveals marked rim enhancement ➡ surrounding the most severely damaged parietal white matter ➡ and the splenium of the corpus callosum ➢ in a pre-teen male with typical CCALD (Loes pattern 1).*

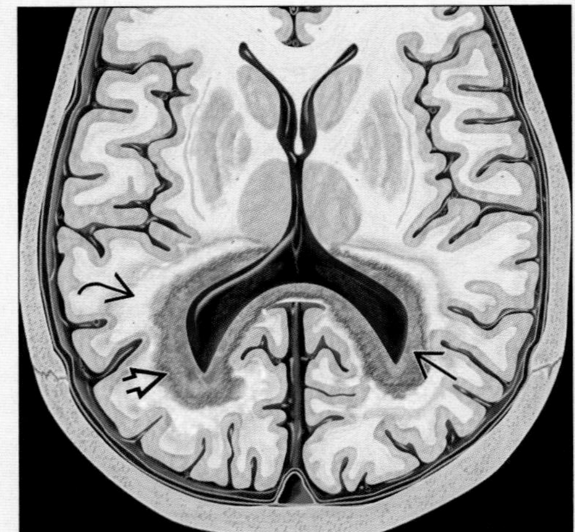

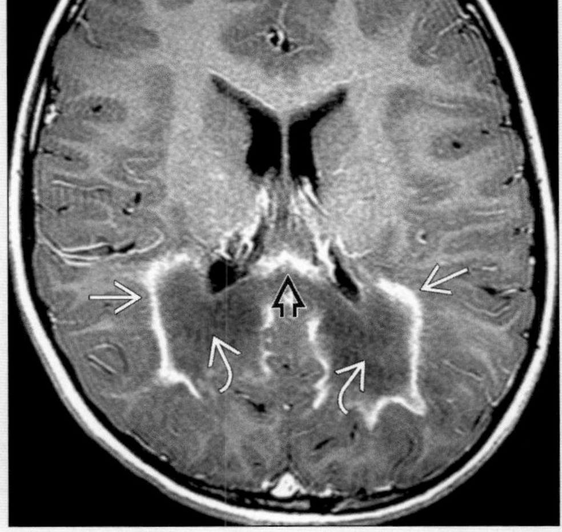

*(**Left**) Axial T2WI MR distinguishes the active inflammation of the outer zone ➡ from the innermost "burnt-out" zone of white matter destruction ➢ in this pre-teen male who presented with well-developed brain involvement. (**Right**) Axial tractograph of the corpus callosum from a DTI sequence demonstrates significant loss of white matter tracts crossing the splenium of the corpus callosum ➢ and forceps major in another pre-teen symptomatic male with CCALD.*

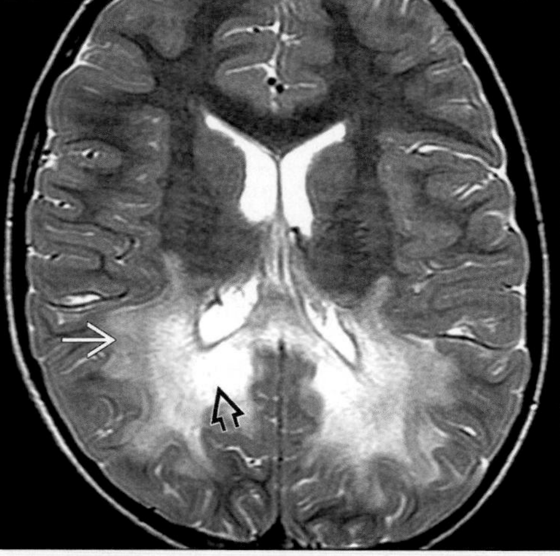

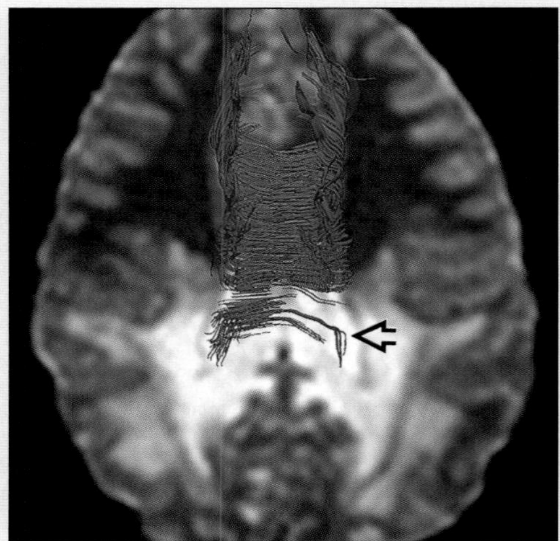

X-LINKED ADRENOLEUKODYSTROPHY

TERMINOLOGY

Synonyms

- Bronze Schilder disease

Definitions

- Inherited disorder of peroxisome metabolism → impaired β-oxidation (β-ox) of very long chain fatty acids (VLCFA)
  - X-linked adrenoleukodystrophy (X-ALD): Severe progressive form usually affects pre-teen males
  - Adrenomyeloneuropathy (AMN): "Mild" adult (spinocerebellar) form, cerebral involvement in up to 50%
  - At least 6 variants other than childhood cerebral X-ALD (CCALD) exist: Presymptomatic X-ALD, adolescent (AdolCALD), adult (ACALD), AMN, Addison only, symptomatic female carriers
  - X-ALD and AMN account for 80% of cases

IMAGING

General Features

- Best diagnostic clue
  - CCALD: Enhancing peritrigonal demyelination
- Location
  - Classic CCALD: Peritrigonal white matter (WM)
    - Pattern: Splenium → peritrigonal WM → corticospinal tracts/fornix/commisural fibers/ visual and auditory pathways
    - Typically spares subcortical U-fibers
- Morphology
  - Usually symmetrical, confluent, posterior involvement; rare frontal pattern occurs
  - Central (splenium) to peripheral gradient is usual

CT Findings

- NECT
  - ↓ density splenium/posterior WM
  - ± Ca++ of involved WM
- CECT
  - CCALD: Linear enhancement of intermediate zone

MR Findings

- T1WI
  - ↓ T1 signal of involved WM
- T2WI
  - ↑ T2 signal of involved WM
    - CCALD: Splenium → peritrigonal WM → corticospinal tracts/fornix/commisural fibers/ visual and auditory pathways
    - AMN: Cerebellum, spinal cord; most common intracranial feature is corticospinal involvement but may resemble CCALD
- FLAIR
  - Same as T2WI
- DWI
  - Restricted diffusion in involved WM
  - DTI: Reduced brain "connectivity," ↑ isotropic diffusion and loss of fractional anisotropy in obvious WM change **and** in presymptomatic WM
- T1WI C+
  - Leading edge (intermediate zone) enhances
    - Enhancement strongly linked to progression
- MRS
  - Peaks between 0.9 and 2.4 ppm probably represent VLCFA macromolecules
  - X-ALD: ↓ NAA even in normal-appearing WM predicts progression; ↑ Cho, myoinositol, lactate
- Spinal MR: Spinal atrophy in AMN

Nuclear Medicine Findings

- PET
  - Hypometabolism of occipital lobes
- Tc-99m-HMPAO SPECT: ↑ regional cerebral blood flow in enhancing zone (decreased elsewhere)

Imaging Recommendations

- Best imaging tool
  - MR + contrast
- Protocol advice
  - DWI/DTI and MRS may predict onset of presymptomatic disease

DIFFERENTIAL DIAGNOSIS

Neonatal Hypoglycemia (Acute & Follow-Up)

- May involve splenium, calcar avis, and posterior peritrigonal WM but does not enhance

White Matter Disease with Lactate (WML)

- Involves splenium, peritrigonal WM, and corticospinal tracts but does not enhance

Alexander Disease

- Enhances, but frontal not peritrigonal WM

PATHOLOGY

General Features

- Etiology
  - Peroxisomes: Ubiquitous organelles involved in catabolic pathways
    - Involved with myelin formation/stabilization
    - Defect in VLCFA importer → impaired β-ox of VLCFA
    - VLCFA accumulate in WM → brittle myelin
- Genetics
  - X-ALD: X-linked recessive
    - Mutations of *ABCD1* gene at Xq28 (> 300 described!)
    - ABCD1 is ATPase transporter protein: "Traffic" ATPase
    - Required for transport hydrophilic molecules across peroxisomal membrane
  - Phenotypic variability: CCALD, AMN, or presymptomatic presentations even within same family
  - Clinical heterogeneity attributed (in part) to specific mutations, modifying factors
    - Insertion allele of CBS c.844_845ins68 protects against CNS demyelination
    - G allele of Tc2 c.776C > G more common in demyelinating forms (CCALD)
- Associated abnormalities

X-LINKED ADRENOLEUKODYSTROPHY

- VLCFA accumulates in all tissues of body
- Symptomatic accumulation: CNS myelin, adrenal cortex, Leydig cell testes
  - Adrenal failure: Skin bronzing
  - Testes: Early androgenetic alopecia in adults

Staging, Grading, & Classification

- Loes MR scoring system: Severity score based upon location, extent of disease, and atrophy
  - Pattern 1: Parietooccipital WM (rapid progression if contrast-enhancement present and very young)
  - Pattern 2: Frontal WM (same as pattern 1)
  - Pattern 3: Corticospinal tract (adults, slower progression)
  - Pattern 4: Corticospinal tract and cerebellar WM (adolescents, slower progression)
  - Pattern 5: Concomitant parietooccipital and frontal WM (mainly childhood, extremely rapid)

Gross Pathologic & Surgical Features

- Atrophy, WM softened

Microscopic Features

- Complete myelin loss (U-fibers preserved), astrogliosis
- Zone specific features
  - Innermost zone of necrosis, gliosis ± Ca++
  - Intermediate zone of active demyelination and inflammation
  - Peripheral zone of demyelination without inflammation

CLINICAL ISSUES

Presentation

- Most common signs/symptoms
  - Skin bronzing, behavioral difficulties, hearing problems
- Clinical profile
  - Phenotypes unpredictable (even intrafamilial)
- Classic childhood cerebral X-ALD (CCALD): 35-50%, but percentage ↓ as new forms diagnosed
  - Pre-teen male (3-10 years): Behavioral, learning, gait, hearing, vision difficulties
  - Addison/adrenal insufficiency (skin bronzing, nausea and vomiting, fatigue) may predate X-ALD diagnosis
- Adrenomyeloneuropathy (AMN) (25%)
  - 14-60 years
  - Spinal involvement > > brain involvement; peripheral nerve involvement
  - Brain inflammatory reaction eventually in 50%; variable demyelination/enhancement
- Presymptomatic ALD (12%)
  - Abnormal genetic testing (due to known symptomatic brother or maternal uncle)
- 20-50% female carriers show AMN-like symptoms (milder, late onset)
- Other presentations less common
  - AdolCALD: 10-20 years, symptoms and course similar to CCALD
  - ACALD: May be misdiagnosed as psychiatric disorder; very rapid progression; diffuse rather than posterior pattern

Demographics

- Age
  - CCALD: Pre-teen males
- Gender
  - Males in classic X-ALD
  - Female carriers may show AMN-like symptoms
- Ethnicity
  - CCALD predominates in North America and France
  - AMN predominates in Netherlands
- Epidemiology
  - X-ALD & variants = 1:16,800 North American births

Natural History & Prognosis

- CCALD: Progresses to spastic quadriparesis, blindness, deafness, vegetative state
- AMN: Spastic, weak legs; sphincter/sexual dysfunction

Treatment

- CCALD: Vegetative state, death in 2-5 years without bone marrow transplant (BMT)
  - Lorenzo oil delays symptoms in presymptomatic ALD
  - Early BMT stabilizes demyelination: RARE reversal demyelination

DIAGNOSTIC CHECKLIST

Consider

- X-ALD presenting at atypical ages → atypical appearances (may lack enhancement or have frontal rather than posterior "gradient")

Image Interpretation Pearls

- Always enhance unknown leukodystrophy!

Reporting Tips

- Loes scoring aids pattern analysis

SELECTED REFERENCES

1. Semmler A et al: Genetic variants of methionine metabolism and X-ALD phenotype generation: results of a new study sample. J Neurol. 256(8):1277-80, 2009
2. Shukla P et al: Three novel variants in X-linked adrenoleukodystrophy. J Child Neurol. 24(7):857-60, 2009
3. Ratai E et al: Seven-Tesla proton magnetic resonance spectroscopic imaging in adult X-linked adrenoleukodystrophy. Arch Neurol. 65(11):1488-94, 2008
4. Mo YH et al: Adrenomyeloneuropathy, a dynamic progressive disorder: brain magnetic resonance imaging of two cases. Neuroradiology, 2004
5. Loes DJ et al: Analysis of MRI patterns aids prediction of progression in X-linked adrenoleukodystrophy. Neurology. 61(3):369-74, 2003
6. Schneider JF et al: Diffusion tensor imaging in cases of adrenoleukodystrophy: preliminary experience as a marker for early demyelination? AJNR Am J Neuroradiol. 24(5):819-24, 2003
7. Melhem ER et al: X-linked adrenoleukodystrophy: the role of contrast-enhanced MR imaging in predicting disease progression. AJNR Am J Neuroradiol. 21(5):839-44, 2000

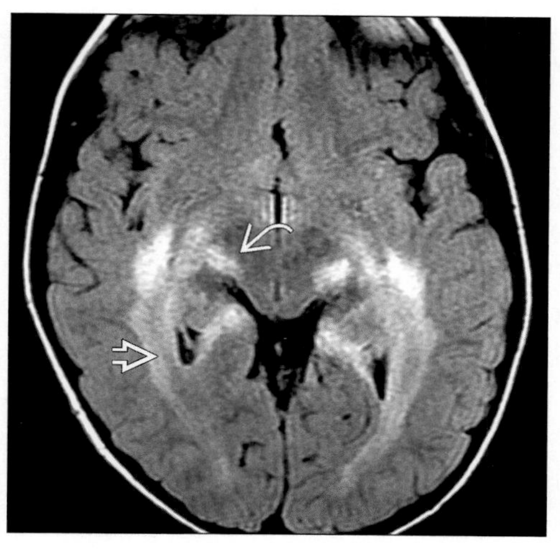

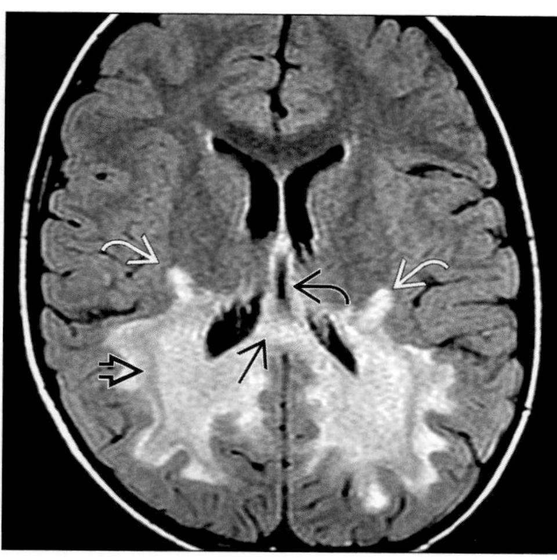

(Left) *Axial FLAIR MR in CCALD (ALD pattern 1) demonstrates hyperintensity of the medial geniculate body along with the periventricular and deep white matter of the temporal and occipital lobes.* ***(Right)*** *Axial FLAIR MR in the same child with CCALD reveals hyperintensity of the posterior columns of the fornices, the splenium of the corpus callosum, and multilayered involvement in the peritrigonal white matter and external/extreme capsules.*

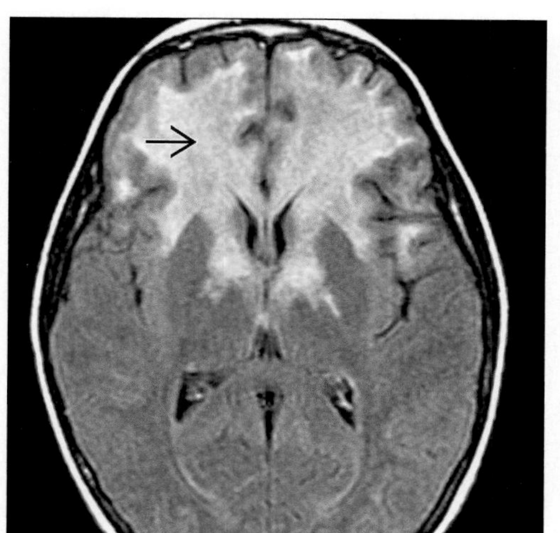

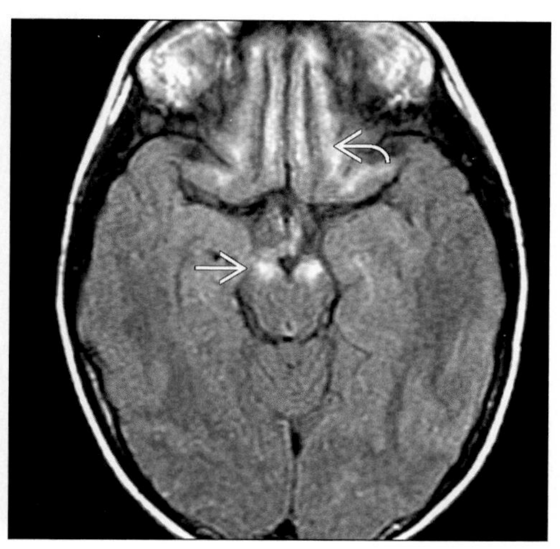

(Left) *Axial FLAIR shows confluent bifrontal white matter hyperintensity. Abnormal signal extends into the caudate heads, globi pallidi, and anterior limbs of internal capsules in this frontal variant case (Loes pattern 2) of proven X-ALD in a school-aged male.* ***(Right)*** *Axial FLAIR in the same patient shows symmetrical white matter hyperintensities in the internal capsules as they extend into the cerebral peduncles and in the juxtacortical frontal white matter.*

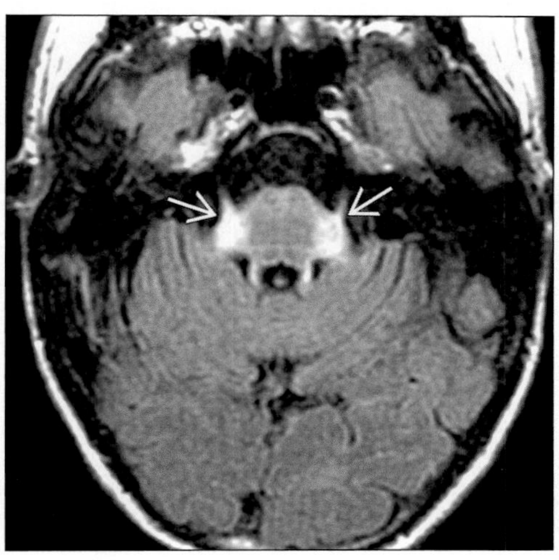

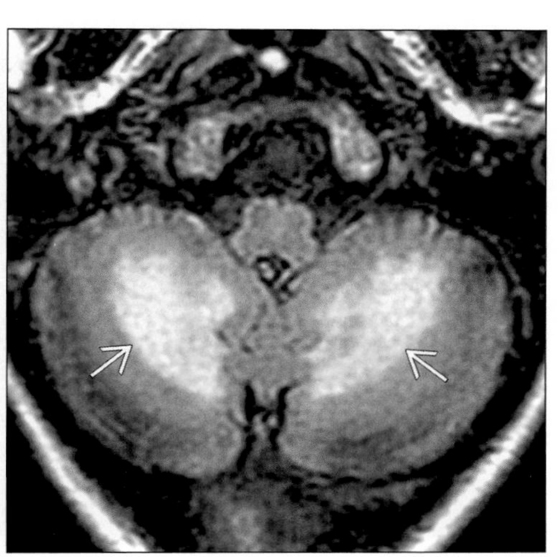

(Left) *Axial FLAIR MR through the mid-pons shows striking demyelination in the lateral pons/root entry zones and both CN5s in an adult with Loes pattern 4.* ***(Right)*** *Axial FLAIR MR at the level of the medulla and lower cerebellum in the same adult with trigeminal nerve involvement shows symmetric hyperintensity in the cerebellar white matter (Loes pattern 4 of ALD).*

OTHER PEROXISOMAL DISORDERS

Key Facts

Terminology

- Peroxisomal disorders; peroxisomal biogenesis or assembly disorders (PBD); single peroxisomal enzyme (transporter) deficiencies (PED)
- PBD: Zellweger syndrome (ZS), neonatal adrenoleukodystrophy (NALD), infantile Refsum disease (IRD), rhizomelic chondrodysplasia punctata (RCDP) type 1
- PED comprised of ≥ 16 disorders with gene mutation affecting single protein in peroxisomal function
- Peroxisomes: Membrane-bound subcellular organelles involved in catabolic and anabolic pathways
- *PEX* genes encode peroxins (proteins required for peroxisome biosynthesis)

Imaging

- ZSD continuum: ZS most severe, NALD intermediate, IRD least severe
- D-BP & Acyl-CoA oxidase deficiencies: ZS-like
  - Look for WM disease in corticospinal tracts
- RCDP: ↑ intensity periventricular WM, centrum semiovale, delayed occipital myelination

Pathology

- Intact peroxisomal function required for normal brain formation, deficiency ⇒ neocortical dysgenesis
- Peroxisomes normally located near developing myelin sheaths in oligodendroglial cells at peak of myelin formation

Diagnostic Checklist

- Use MR with DWI, MRS

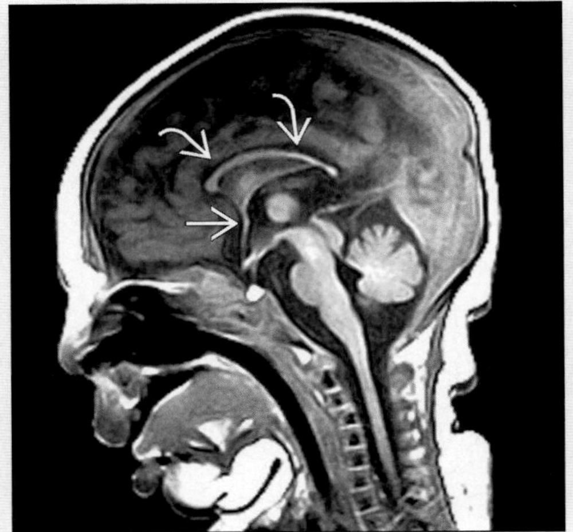

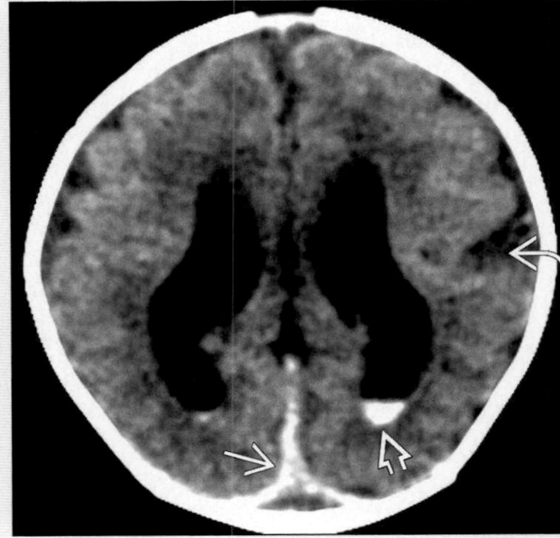

(Left) *Sagittal T1WI MR in a 28 day old with non-Zellweger peroxisomal biogenesis disorder and facial dysmorphism reveals flat face, significant retrognathia, microcephaly, thin corpus callosum ➔, and small anterior commissure ➔.* ***(Right)*** *Axial NECT in a 5 day old with non-Zellweger peroxisomal biogenesis disorder and hepatic dysfunction reveals primitive sylvian fissures ➔, small subdural collection ➔, and blood layering ➔ within the posterior horns of the lateral ventricles.*

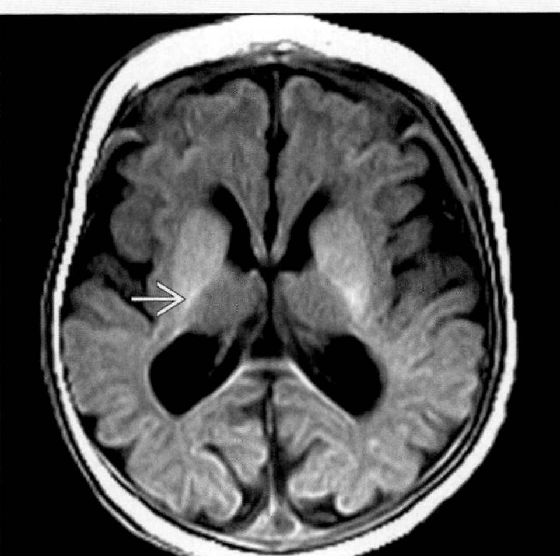

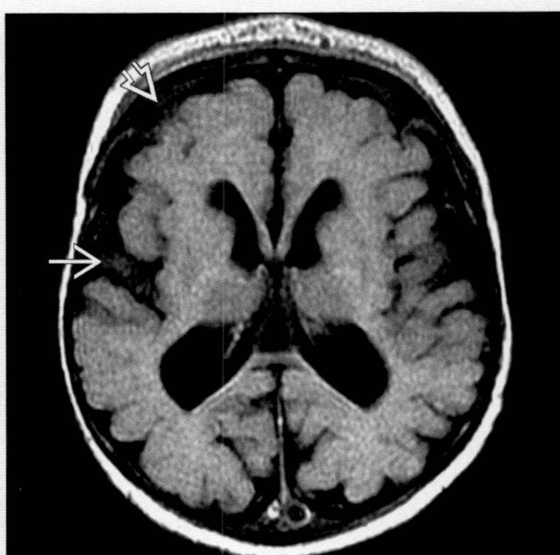

(Left) *Axial T1WI MR in a full-term infant with non-Zellweger peroxisomal biogenesis disorder demonstrates mild ventriculomegaly, enlarged subarachnoid spaces, and failure of myelin maturation within the posterior limb of the internal capsule ➔. Lentiform nuclei are abnormally hyperintense.* ***(Right)*** *Axial FLAIR MR in the same microcephalic infant demonstrates prominent pericerebral fluid spaces ➔ and underoperculized sylvian fissures ➔.*

OTHER PEROXISOMAL DISORDERS

TERMINOLOGY

Abbreviations

- Peroxisomal biogenesis or assembly disorders (PBD)
- Single peroxisomal enzyme (transporter) deficiencies (PED)
- PBD: Zellweger syndrome (ZS), neonatal adrenoleukodystrophy (NALD), infantile Refsum disease (IRD), rhizomelic chondrodysplasia punctata (RCDP) type 1, other nonspecific phenotypes
  - Zellweger spectrum disorders (ZSD): Triad of ZS, NALD, IRD (but not RCDP) phenotypes
  - RCDP type 1: Normal β-oxidation of very long chain fatty acids (VLCFA), therefore different profile
- PED comprised of ≥ 16 disorders with gene mutation affecting single protein in peroxisomal function
  - Peroxisomal fatty acid β-oxidation
    - X-ALD; deficiencies of alkyl-DHAP-synthase (RCDP type 3); Acyl-CoA oxidase, D-bifunctional protein (D-BP), sterol carrier protein X (SCPx), and 2-methylacyl CoA racemase (AMACR)
  - Ether phospholipid biosynthesis (especially plasmalogens)
    - DHAP-alkyl transferase (DHAPAT; RCDP type 2)
  - Phytanic acid α-oxidation: Adult Refsum disease (ARD)
  - Glyoxylate detox: Primary hyperoxaluria type 1
  - Hydrogen peroxide metabolism: Acatalasemia

Definitions

- Peroxisomes: Membrane-bound subcellular organelles involved in catabolic and anabolic pathways, collaborate with other organelles
- *PEX* genes encode peroxins (proteins required for peroxisome biosynthesis)

IMAGING

General Features

- Best diagnostic clue
  - PBD: Abnormal myelin in corticospinal tracts ± dentate nuclei, ± cortical dysplasia
- Location
  - Corticospinal tracts ± dentate nuclei

Radiographic Findings

- Radiography
  - ZS and RCDP: Rhizomelia, stippled epiphyses
  - RCDP and DHAP deficiencies: Coronal vertebral clefts
  - ARD: Short metacarpals/metatarsals (30%)

CT Findings

- NECT
  - X-ALD: Occasional punctate WM calcifications

MR Findings

- T2WI
  - ZSD continuum: ZS most severe, NALD intermediate, IRD least severe
    - ZS: ↑ intensity WM/myelin delay, neocortical dysplasia/PMG, atrophy, late cerebral and cerebellar demyelination
    - NALD: PMG, progressive WM disease
    - IRD: No neuronal migration anomalies, WM nonprogressive ± improvement
  - D-BP & Acyl-CoA oxidase deficiencies: ZS-like
    - D-BP: Occasional thalami & globus pallidus involvement (unlike PBD)
  - RCDP: ↑ intensity periventricular WM, centrum semiovale, delayed occipital myelination
  - SCPx: Thalamic, pons, occipital ↑ intensity
  - AMACR: Deep WM ↑ intensity
- DWI
  - X-ALD: Intermediate zone ↓ ADC
  - PBD: ↑ ADC values
- T1WI C+
  - X-ALD: Leading edge enhancement
  - Acyl-CoA oxidase deficiency: Enhancing centrum semiovale lesions

Ultrasonographic Findings

- ZS: Renal cysts
- ZSD & D-BP: Hepatomegaly

Imaging Recommendations

- Best imaging tool
  - MR
- Protocol advice
  - MR, DWI, MRS, C+

DIFFERENTIAL DIAGNOSIS

ZSD Mimics

- Bilateral perisylvian polymicrogyria

RCDP 1 Mimics

- X-linked dominant chondrodysplasia punctata: Conradi-Hünermann-Happle syndrome
- Warfarin embryopathy

PATHOLOGY

General Features

- Etiology
  - VLCFA and phytanic acid incorporated into cell membranes ⇒ cell dysfunction, atrophy, and death
- Genetics
  - Phenotype severity varies with nature of mutation
    - *PEX1*: G843D does not abolish peroxisomal protein import completely ⇒ mild (NALD, IRD); while c.2097-2098insT mutation abolishes import completely ⇒ severe (ZS)
    - *PEX7*: L292X ⇒ classical, severe RCDP phenotype, while A218V ⇒ milder RCDP
  - PED may clinically resemble PBD
    - D-BP & Acyl-CoA oxidase deficiencies: ZS-like
    - Defects involving 1st 2 steps of plasmalogens (DHAP-alkyl transferase, DHAP-synthase deficiencies): RCDP/*PEX7*-like
- PBD: Organelle fails to form, multiple peroxisomal functions defective
- PBD have *PEX* gene mutations
  - *PEX 1, 6, 12, 26*: ZS, NALD, IRD
  - *PEX 2*: ZS, IRD
  - *PEX 5, 10, 13*: ZS, NALD
  - *PEX 3, 14, 16, 19*: ZS

OTHER PEROXISOMAL DISORDERS

- *PEX 7*: RCDP 1
- PED: Single peroxisomal enzyme deficiency
  - ARD: Phytanoyl-CoA hydroxylase
  - X-ALD: *ABCD1* gene mutation
  - Acyl-CoA oxidase: ZS-like phenotype (less severe)
  - D-BP: ZS-like phenotype (severe)
  - SCPx: Sterol carrier protein X, single family
  - PH1: *AGXT* gene mutation, glyoxylate aminotransferase 1 (AGT) deficient (catalyzes transamination of glyoxylate to glycine) ⇒ ↑ glyoxylate oxidation to oxalate ⇒ renal stones ± systemic hyperoxaluria
  - Acatalasemia: Impaired hydrogen peroxide detoxification ⇒ ↑ risk of diabetes

Staging, Grading, & Classification

- Marked genetic heterogeneity complicates genotype-phenotype correlation

Gross Pathologic & Surgical Features

- Intact peroxisomal function required for normal brain formation, deficiency ⇒ neocortical dysgenesis
- Peroxisomes located near developing myelin sheaths in oligodendroglial cells at peak of myelin formation
  - Deficiency ⇒ defect in central WM formation/ maintenance and myelin lipid reduction

Microscopic Features

- Neuropathologic lesions
  - Abnormalities in neuronal differentiation/migration
  - Inflammatory dysmyelination or noninflammatory demyelination
- Postdevelopmental neuronal degeneration
  - Adrenomyeloneuropathy (AMN): Spinal cord axonopathy
  - IRD, RCDP: Cerebellar atrophy
- PH1: Rare reports of oxalate crystals in brain
- ZS: Additional olivary dysplasia

CLINICAL ISSUES

Presentation

- Most common signs/symptoms
  - CNS involvement manifests during development &/ or later in life
- Other signs/symptoms
  - BPD
    - ZSD: Frontal bossing, marked hypotonia, hepatomegaly, perinatal apnea, seizures, jaundice, cataracts, retinopathy, deafness
    - RCDP: Rhizomelia, dwarfism/short stature, broad nasal bridge (koala bear face), epicanthus, microcephaly, mental retardation, cataracts
  - PED
    - D-BP & Acyl-CoA oxidase deficiencies: ZS-like
    - ARD: Classic tetrad of peripheral polyneuropathy, cerebellar ataxia, ↑ CSF protein, retinitis pigmentosa; also ichthyosis, psychiatric disorders, cardiac arrhythmias, anosmia, deafness
    - X-ALD: Behavioral, learning, and hearing difficulties, skin bronzing
    - SCPx: Dystonia, azoospermia/hypogonadism, hyposmia
    - AMACR: Rare, variable findings (tremor, pyramidal signs, seizures, sensory motor neuropathy)
    - PH1: Renal stones or renal failure with systemic oxalosis (bone pain, fractures, myocarditis, embolic stroke, retinopathy)

Demographics

- Age
  - Most: Neonatal
  - X-ALD, classic Refsum: Childhood or adult onset
- Epidemiology
  - Peroxisomal disorders in 1:5,000 births

Natural History & Prognosis

- PBD: Variable neurodevelopmental delays, retinopathy, deafness, liver disease
  - ZSD & look-alikes share imaging and clinical phenotype; most fail to gain milestones, severe phenotypes die within 1st year of life
  - RCDP & look-alikes: Severe and mild phenotypes
- PED: Variable
  - X-ALD: Progression to vegetative state if untreated
  - PH1: Progression to systemic oxalosis (myocardium, bone marrow, eyes, peripheral nerves); rapidly progressive (death in 1st year) and mild phenotypes

Treatment

- PBD: Limited by multiple malformations and metabolic defects originating in utero
- PED: X-ALD (cholesterol lowering drugs, VLCFA restriction, bone marrow transplant); ARD (phytanic acid restriction); PH1 (pyridoxin ⇒ ↓ production oxalate; alkalinize urine to ↑ oxalate solubility

DIAGNOSTIC CHECKLIST

Consider

- Plasma biochemical abnormalities may be absent
- Analysis of cultured skin fibroblasts indicated if strong imaging and clinical suspicion

SELECTED REFERENCES

1. Brites P et al: Plasmalogens participate in very-long-chain fatty acid-induced pathology. Brain. 132(Pt 2):482-92, 2009
2. Carrozzo R et al: Peroxisomal acyl-CoA-oxidase deficiency: two new cases. Am J Med Genet A. 146A(13):1676-81, 2008
3. Saitoh M et al: Changes in the amounts of myelin lipids and molecular species of plasmalogen PE in the brain of an autopsy case with D-bifunctional protein deficiency. Neurosci Lett. 442(1):4-9, 2008
4. Weller S et al: Cerebral MRI as a valuable diagnostic tool in Zellweger spectrum patients. J Inherit Metab Dis. Epub ahead of print, 2008
5. Ferdinandusse S et al: Clinical and biochemical spectrum of D-bifunctional protein deficiency. Ann Neurol. 59(1):92-104, 2006
6. Wanders RJ et al: Peroxisomal disorders: The single peroxisomal enzyme deficiencies. Biochim Biophys Acta. 1763(12):1707-20, 2006

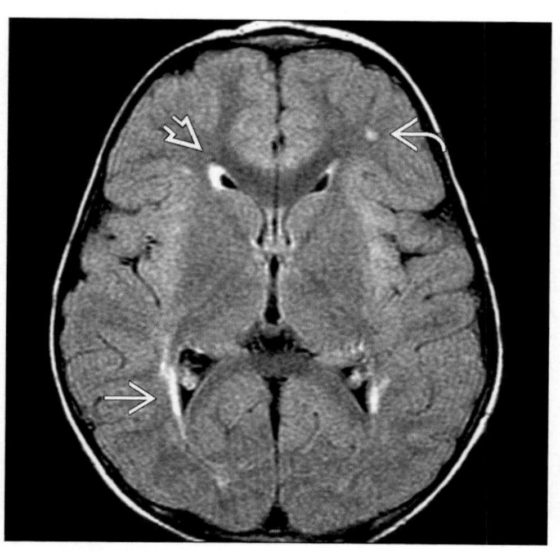

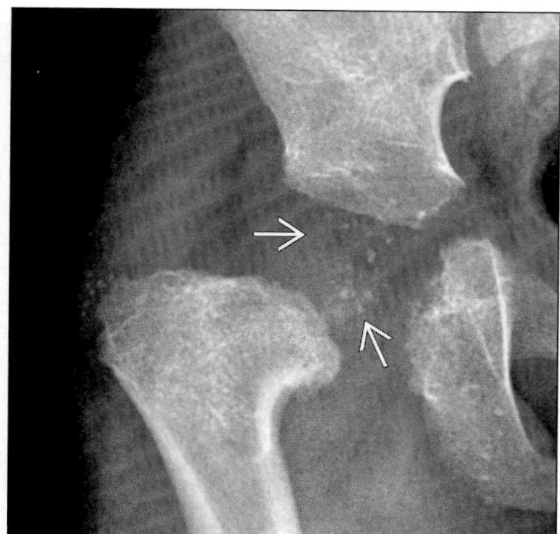

(Left) *Axial FLAIR MR in a 3 year old with peroxisomal chondrodysplasia punctata demonstrates increased signal intensity in the peritrigonal white matter ➔ and periventricular white matter of the right frontal horn ➔, as well as scattered foci of abnormal increased signal ➔.* ***(Right)*** *Anteroposterior radiograph in a 2 year old with peroxisomal chondrodysplasia punctata demonstrates coxa vara with stippling of the triradiate cartilage ➔. Bone radiographs can help to specify diagnosis.*

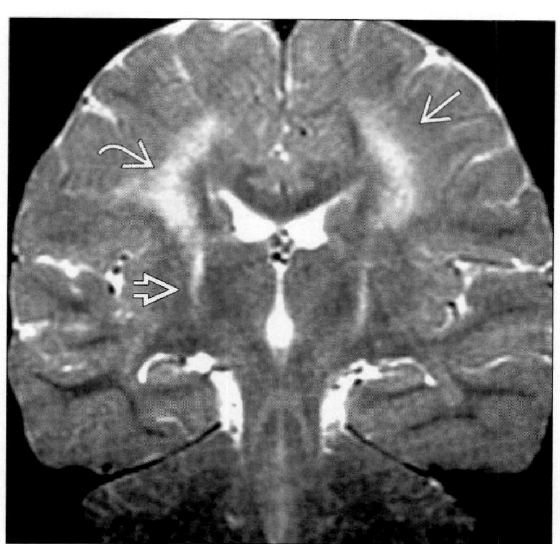

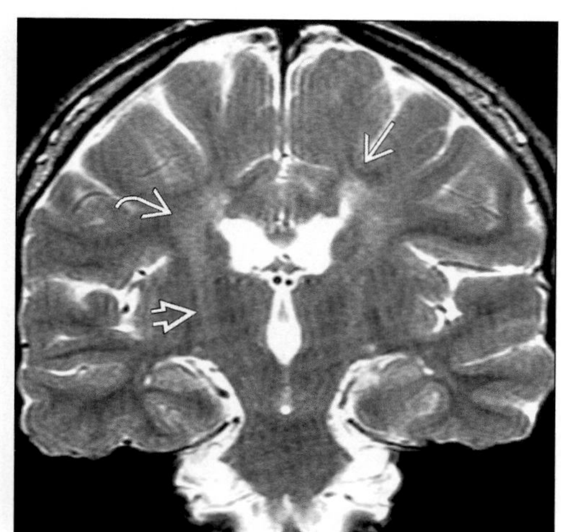

(Left) *Coronal T2WI MR in a 4 year old with infantile Refsum demonstrates abnormal signal intensity within the corticospinal tracts ➔ and periventricular white matter ➔. Note the poor myelin maturation in the subcortical U-fibers ➔.* ***(Right)*** *Follow-up coronal T2WI MR in the same patient at age 16 shows partial resolution of findings. Note progressive myelin maturation of the subcortical U-fibers ➔ & (incomplete) improvement of periventricular white matter ➔ & corticospinal tracts ➔.*

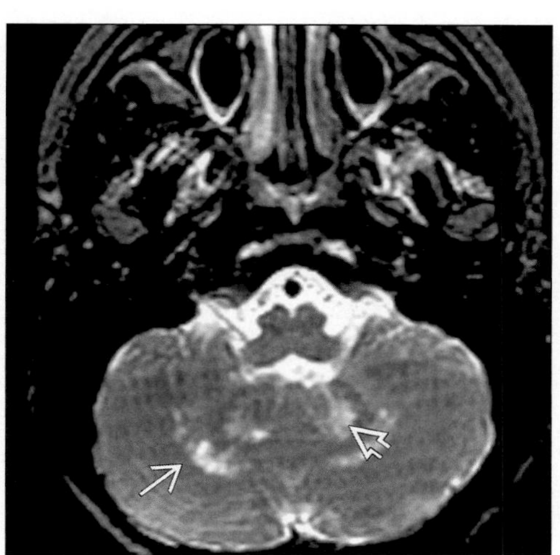

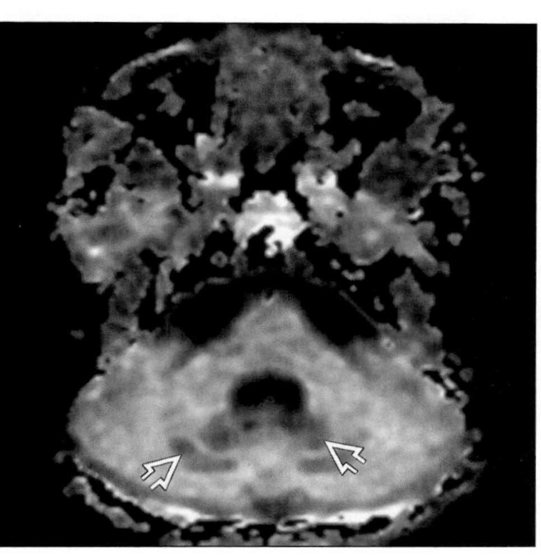

(Left) *Axial T2WI MR in the same patient demonstrates persistent and typical abnormal signal intensity in the cerebellar white matter ➔ and hila of the deep cerebellar nuclei ➔. The brain stem appears normal.* ***(Right)*** *Axial DWI MR in the same patient fails to demonstrate any evidence of reduced diffusion in the abnormal foci ➔, suggesting that the injury is subacute or chronic.*

MAPLE SYRUP URINE DISEASE

Key Facts

Terminology

- Maple syrup urine disease (MSUD)
- Inherited disorder of branched chain amino acid metabolism
- Typically presents at 4-10 days of age with neurologic deterioration, ketoacidosis, hyperammonemia

Imaging

- MR with DWI best, but CT can make diagnosis in critically ill infant
- Classic MSUD edema/restriction pattern
  - Cerebellar white matter, dorsal brainstem, cerebral peduncles, thalami, globi pallidi
  - Pyramidal and tegmental tracts
  - Infratentorial > > supratentorial edema
- Broad peak at chemical shift of 0.9 ppm

Pathology

- MSUD: ↓ activity BCKD → accumulation of branched-chain L-amino (BCAA) and metabolites (neuro- and leukotoxic)

Clinical Issues

- Initial symptoms of classic MSUD: Poor feeding, vomiting, poor weight gain, increasing lethargy, encephalopathy, seizures
- Patients in crisis often (but not always) smell like maple syrup (or burnt sugar)
- 1:850,000 in general population but as frequent as 1:170 in population isolates
- MSUD has potentially favorable outcome with strict dietary control and aggressive treatment of metabolic crises
- Response to therapy; however, can be variable

*(**Left**) Axial NECT in a seizing newborn who returned to the hospital at 10 days of age demonstrates classic MSUD edema pattern. Note hypodensity in cerebellar white matter ⇨, dorsal pons, and 4 foci in the anterior and middle pons, which are paired pyramidal → and tegmental tracts ↩. (**Right**) Axial T1WI MR in a different infant with lethargy and feeding difficulty shows the same MSUD pattern: Hypointensity in the cerebellar white matter ⇨ and paired pyramidal → and tegmental tracts ↩.*

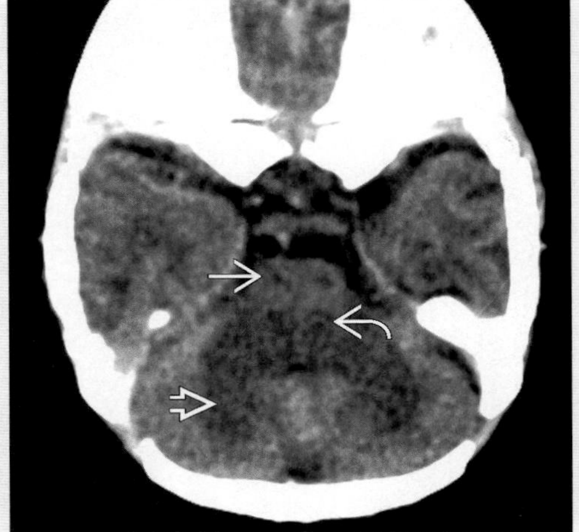

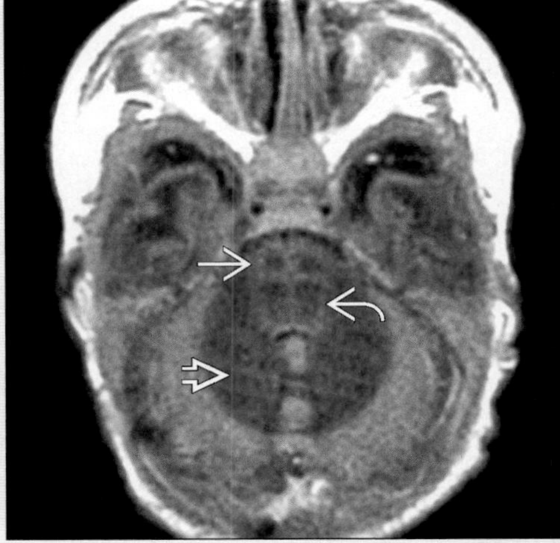

*(**Left**) Axial T2WI MR demonstrates crisp margins of the signal abnormality of the cerebellar white matter. Again seen are the paired tracts (4 bright pontine foci) superimposed on signal abnormality in the pons. The dentate nuclei ⇨ stand out against the abnormal MSUD edema. (**Right**) Axial DWI MR confirms intramyelinic edema in a MSUD pattern, showing reduced diffusivity (hyperintensity). DWI is extremely useful in the acute and subacute phase of MSUD.*

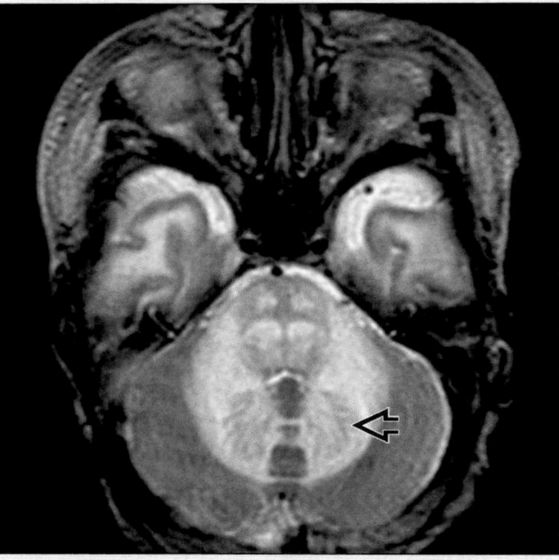

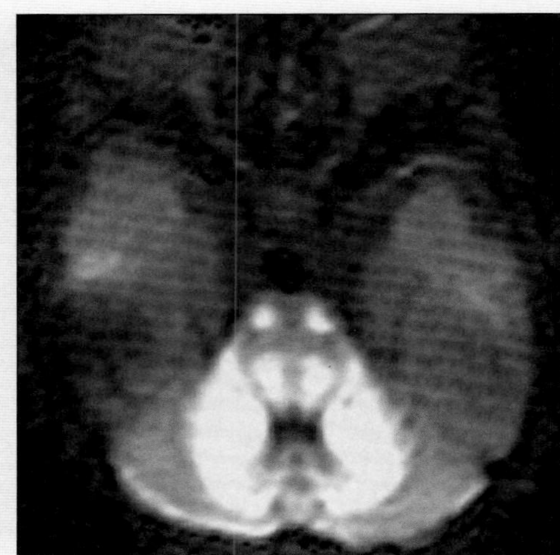

MAPLE SYRUP URINE DISEASE

TERMINOLOGY

Abbreviations

- Maple syrup urine disease (MSUD)
- Leucine encephalopathy

Definitions

- Inherited disorder of branched chain amino acid metabolism presenting in newborns with neurologic deterioration, ketoacidosis, and hyperammonemia

IMAGING

General Features

- Best diagnostic clue
  - Radiologist may be 1st to suggest diagnosis based on classic-appearing MSUD edema
    - Cerebellar white matter, brain stem, thalamus, globus pallidus
    - Pyramidal and tegmental tracts
- Location
  - Cerebellar and brainstem edema > > > supratentorial hemispheres
  - Edema of corticospinal tracts

CT Findings

- NECT
  - Early: Diffuse edema **not** sparing brainstem and cerebellum
    - Recognize here for best neurocognitive outcome
  - Subacute: Rapid formation of typical (classic) MSUD edema pattern
    - Cerebellar white matter, dorsal brainstem, cerebral peduncles, thalami, pyramidal, and tegmental tracts > supratentorial hemispheres
    - Margins become sharp during subacute phase

MR Findings

- T1WI
  - ↓ signal intensity, margins may be sharp
- T2WI
  - Late: Generalized and MSUD edema disappear
    - Resolve to "pallor" and volume loss
- FLAIR
  - Insensitive to fluid shifts in newborns
- DWI
  - Marked restriction (↑ intensity) and ↓ ADC (MSUD edema = cytotoxic/intramyelinic)
  - DTI: ↓ anisotropy
- MRS
  - Broad peak at chemical shift of 0.9 ppm

Ultrasonographic Findings

- Grayscale ultrasound
  - ↑ echogenicity of globi pallidi, periventricular white matter, brainstem, cerebellar white matter

Imaging Recommendations

- Best imaging tool
  - DWI during hyperacute and acute phases
- Protocol advice
  - MR with diffusion weighted imaging best, but CT can make diagnosis in critically ill infant

DIFFERENTIAL DIAGNOSIS

Disorders Causing Brainstem and Cerebellar Swelling

- Mitochondrial *SURF1* mutations: Lactate may be seen in this **and** in MSUD during crisis
- Alexander disease: Abnormal signal and enhancement of brainstem and aqueduct
- Vanishing white matter: Findings are persistent

Hypoxic-Ischemic Encephalopathy

- No symptom-free interval, usually positive history
- Cerebellum, brainstem relatively spared (MSUD involves these areas)

Marchiafava-Bignami

- Myelin splitting disorder of adult red wine drinkers
- Splits corpus callosum

PATHOLOGY

General Features

- Etiology
  - MSUD: ↓ activity branched chain α-keto acid dehydrogenase complex (BCKD) → accumulation of branched chain L-amino (BCAA) and metabolites (neuro- and leukotoxic)
  - ↑ brain leucine displaces other essential amino → neurotransmitter depletion, disrupted brain growth and development
  - Branched-chain ketoacid accumulation → thought to disrupt Krebs cycle
- Genetics
  - > 50 different mutations in genes governing enzyme components of BCKD
    - For example, E1α (33%), E1β (38%), E2 (19%)
  - Autosomal recessive
- Associated abnormalities
  - ↑ plasma isoleucine associated with maple syrup odor
  - Maternal ingestion of fenugreek during labor gives false impression of MSUD
    - Shares component and smell with MSUD urine

Staging, Grading, & Classification

- Classical, intermediate, and intermittent forms of MSUD; thiamine-responsive MSUD

Gross Pathologic & Surgical Features

- Brainstem edema
- Spongy degeneration: White matter, basal ganglia

Microscopic Features

- ↓ oligodendrocytes and astrocytes
- Alterations in neuronal migration, maturation
  - Aberrant orientation of neurons
  - Abnormal dendrites/dendritic spines

CLINICAL ISSUES

Presentation

- Most common signs/symptoms

MAPLE SYRUP URINE DISEASE

- Initial symptoms of classic MSUD: Poor feeding, vomiting, poor weight gain, increasing lethargy
  - In neonates, develops within 4-7 days
- Patients in crisis often (but not always) smell like maple syrup (or burnt sugar)
  - Resuscitation with non-protein-containing oral or IV hydrating fluids may "clear" odor
  - Maple syrup odor may be difficult to identify in 1st days of life unless urine soaked diaper allowed to dry
  - Maple syrup odor of cerumen "more predictable"
- Neonates in communities with known high MSUD risk diagnosed within hours of blood sampling
  - If tested **and** receive immediate results **and** therapy is instituted → may have excellent outcome
  - Tandem mass spectrometry of whole blood filter paper shortens diagnosis time
  - Guthrie test insensitive before 24 hours, requires incubation period and has high false-positive rate

- Clinical profile
  - Normal at birth
  - Presents after disease-free interval, usually within the 1st 48 hours to 2 weeks of life
  - Mimic of sepsis: Acute encephalopathy, vomiting, seizures, neurological distress, lethargy, coma, leukopenia/thrombopenia
    - Additionally free water retention, renal salt wasting and hyponatremia, dehydration
  - Plasma detection of alloisoleucine diagnostic
    - May not appear until 6th day of life
  - Ketosis or ketoacidosis and hyperammonemia
  - Typical EEG: Comb-like rhythms
  - Prenatal diagnosis can be performed on cultured amniocytes or chorion villus cells

Demographics

- Age
  - May be diagnosed on day 1 of life if MSUD suspected
- Ethnicity
  - 1/170 live births in certain population isolates (founder effect in old order Mennonites)
  - High carrier rate in Middle East and Ashkenazi Jewish decendents
- Epidemiology
  - 1:850,000 in general population but as frequent as 1:170 in population isolates

Natural History & Prognosis

- Breast feeding may delay onset of symptoms to 2nd week of life
- MSUD has potentially favorable outcome with strict dietary control and aggressive treatment of metabolic crises
  - Response to therapy; however, can be variable
  - Exposure to high levels, branched chain amino acids (BCAA) and their metabolites neurotoxic
  - Uncontrolled BCAA levels → profound cognitive impairment/death
  - Pretreatment plasma leucine > 40 mg/100 mL **or** encephalopathy > days associated with poor cognitive outcome
- May survive to adulthood if well controlled
  - Metabolic "intoxication" **at any age** may be provoked by infection, injury, stress, fasting, or even pregnancy
- Reports of late (adulthood) development of peripheral neuropathy
- Exfoliative skin and corneal lesions from inadequate amino-acid intake

Treatment

- Acute "metabolic rescue" to reverse cerebral edema
- May require hemodialysis during acute crisis to limit neurotoxicity/damage
- Metabolically appropriate diet (protein-modified) minimizes severity
  - Inhibit endogenous protein catabolism while sustaining protein synthesis
  - Prevent deficiencies of essential amino acids
  - Maintain normal serum osmolarity
  - Commercially available formulas, foods are available without branched chain amino acids or with reduced levels of branched chain amino acids
  - Dietary therapy must be lifelong
- Neonatal screening (tandem mass spectrometry) can diagnose
- Orthotopic liver transplantation increases availability of BCKD (rarely used)
- Gene therapy experimental

DIAGNOSTIC CHECKLIST

Consider

- Neonatal testing for MSUD is **not** universal
- Not all MSUD occurs in population isolates
- Even if testing performed, results may be available only after 1-2 weeks in nonendemic areas

Image Interpretation Pearls

- Neonatal brain edema which includes posterior fossa and brainstem is highly suggestive of MSUD

SELECTED REFERENCES

1. Zinnanti WJ et al: Dual mechanism of brain injury and novel treatment strategy in maple syrup urine disease. Brain. 132(Pt 4):903-18, 2009
2. Silao CL et al: Early diagnosis of maple syrup urine disease using polymerase chain reaction-based mutation detection. Pediatr Int. 50(3):312-4, 2008
3. Parmar H et al: Maple syrup urine disease: diffusion-weighted and diffusion-tensor magnetic resonance imaging findings. J Comput Assist Tomogr. 28(1):93-7, 2004
4. Henneke M et al: Identification of twelve novel mutations in patients with classic and variant forms of maple syrup urine disease. Hum Mutat. 22(5):417, 2003
5. Morton DH et al: Diagnosis and treatment of maple syrup disease: a study of 36 patients. Pediatrics. 109(6):999-1008, 2002

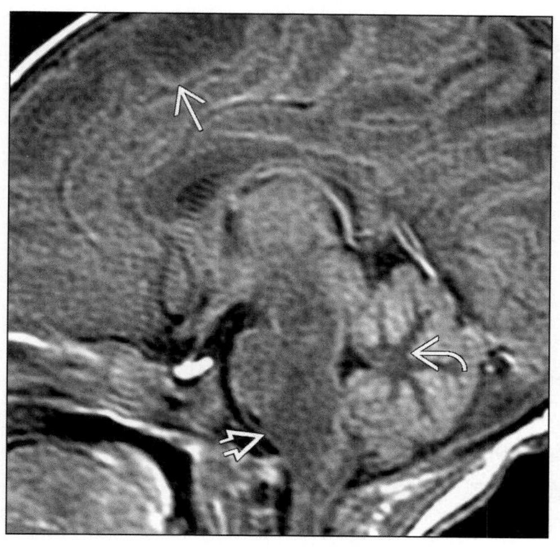

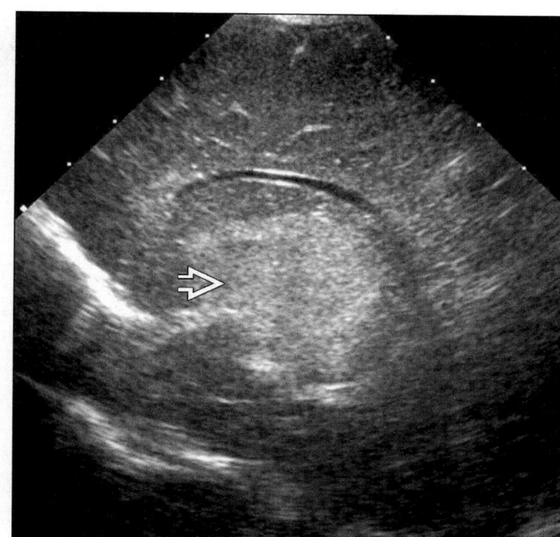

(Left) *Sagittal T1WI MR in an encephalopathic newborn reveals marked swelling of the entire brainstem. Low signal of the involved brainstem* ➪*, cerebellar white matter* ➪*, and subcortical cerebral white matter* ➪ *is also present.* ***(Right)*** *Parasagittal ultrasound in another symptomatic newborn with MSUD demonstrates markedly increased echogenicity* ➪ *of the thalami due to the severe edema.*

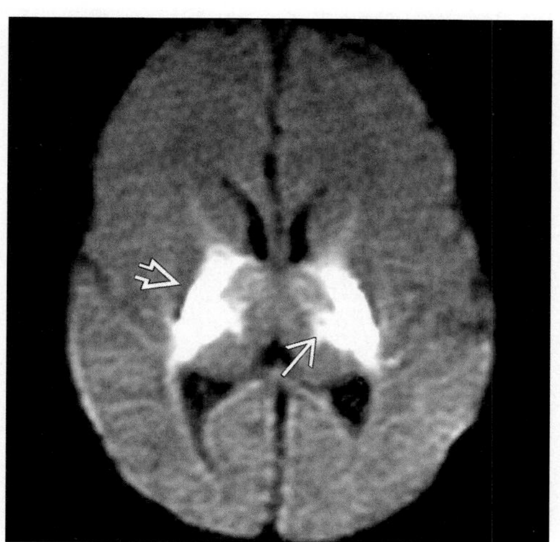

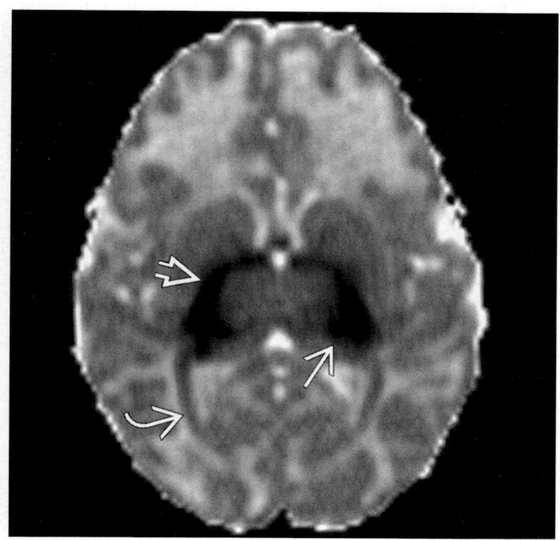

(Left) *Axial DWI MR shows markedly reduced diffusivity (hyperintensity) of the posterior limbs of the internal capsules* ➪ *and of the internal medullary lamina* ➪ *of the thalami during the acute phase of MSUD.* ***(Right)*** *Axial diffusivity (ADC) map in the same infant confirms reduced diffusivity of the posterior limbs of the internal capsules* ➪ *and of the internal medullary lamina* ➪ *of the thalami, as well as the optic tracts* ➪*.*

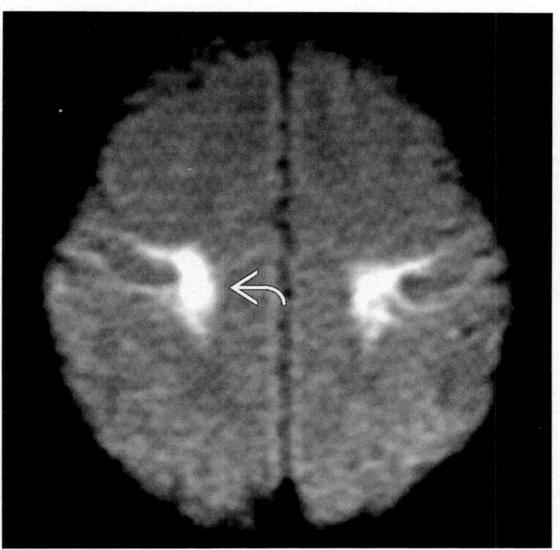

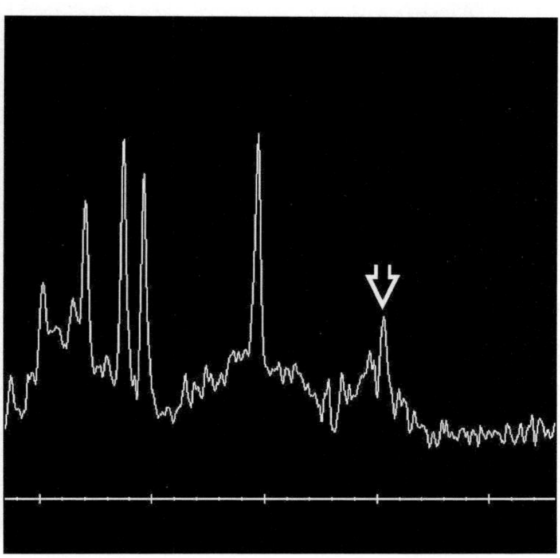

(Left) *Axial DWI MR demonstrates extension of intramyelinic edema (manifest as reduced diffusivity) in the corticospinal tracts as they extend upward to the perirolandic cortex* ➪*.* ***(Right)*** *Peaks at 0.9 -1.0 ppm* ➪ *on MRS with a TE of 30 milliseconds represent branched chain α-keto acids peaks, which can be seen during acute metabolic decompensation in maple syrup urine disease. They are also seen at longer echo times, a finding that helps to confirm the diagnosis.*

UREA CYCLE DISORDERS

Key Facts

Terminology

- 6 disorders of urea cycle
  - Ornithine transcarbamylase deficiency (OTCD)
  - Carbamoyl phosphate synthetase 1 deficiency
  - Citrullinemia or argininosuccinate synthetase deficiency
  - Argininosuccinate aciduria or argininosuccinate lyase deficiency
  - Argininemia or arginase deficiency (AD)
  - N-acetylglutamate synthase deficiency

Imaging

- Neonates: Deep gray nuclei, depths of sulci in frontal, parietal, and insular > temporal cortex
- Older: As above or asymmetric cortical/subcortical white matter mimicking stroke
- Posterior fossa spared
- Acute/subacute: ↑ T2 signal, swelling areas involved
- Acute/subacute: Iso/↑ DWI signal, iso/↓ ADC
- Acute/subacute: ↓ MI, ↑ Glx, ↑ lipids/lactate

Top Differential Diagnoses

- Hypoxic-ischemic encephalopathy
- Mitochondrial disorders
- Arterial ischemic stroke
- Nonketotic hyperglycinemia
- Organic acidemias

Pathology

- Urea cycle incorporates nitrogen → urea → urine, prevents accumulation of toxic nitrogen products
- ↑ ammonia → ↑ glutamate → ↑ glutamine in astrocytes → swelling + dysfunction

Clinical Issues

- Triad of hyperammonemia, encephalopathy, respiratory alkalosis

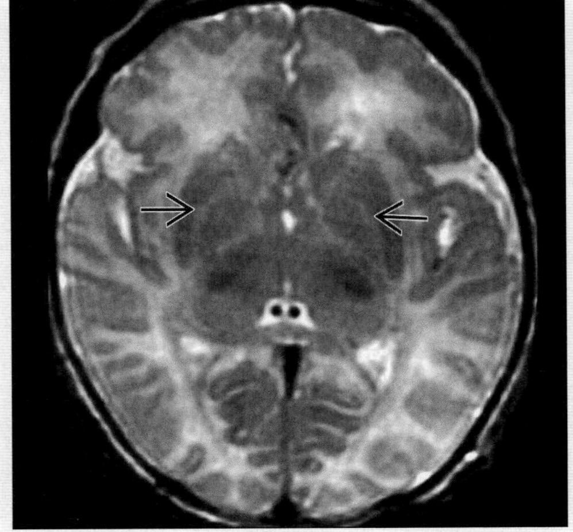

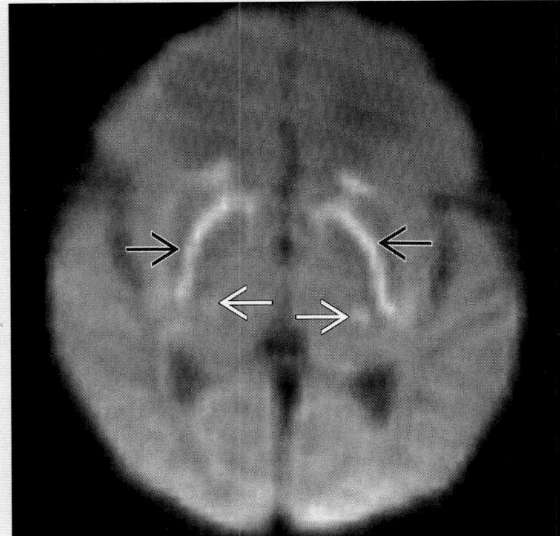

(Left) *Axial T2WI MR shows abnormally increased signal ⇒ between lateral nuclei of the globi pallidi and the putamina in 2-day-old male neonate presenting acutely with ornithine transcarbamylase deficiency.* ***(Right)*** *Axial DWI MR in the same patient shows reduced diffusivity (abnormally increased signal ⇒) in the same location between the globi pallidi and putamina, extending into the caudates; this corresponded to decreased ADC. More subtle thalamic hyperintensity ➡ (and low ADC) is also seen.*

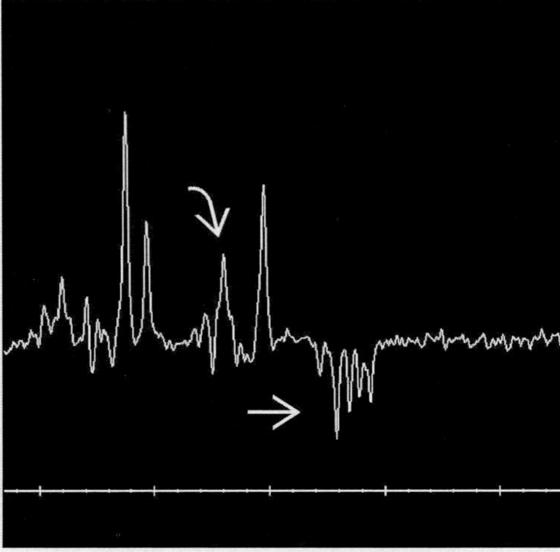

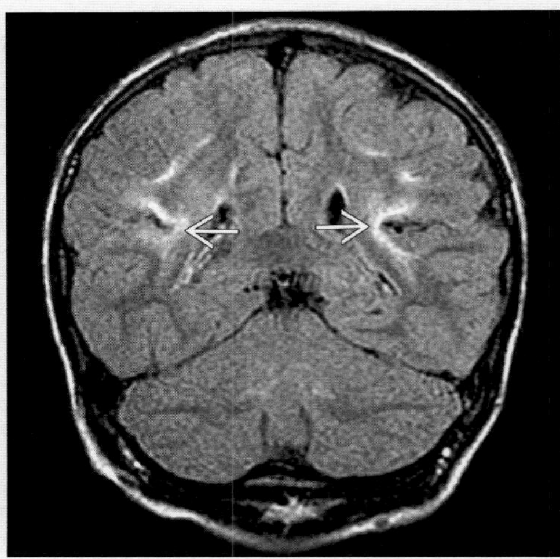

(Left) *Axial proton MRS (TE = 144 msec) in a neonate presenting acutely demonstrates 2 inverted doublets ➡ of lactate (at 1.33 ppm) and 1,2-propene-diol (found in anticonvulsants, at 1.1 ppm). Also noted is a large glutamine-glutamate (glx) peak ➡ at 2.1-1.4 ppm.* ***(Right)*** *Coronal FLAIR MR in the chronic stage of another child with OTCD shows cortical and subcortical posterior insular and temporoparietal increased signal ➡ that is most marked at the depths of the sulci.*

UREA CYCLE DISORDERS

TERMINOLOGY

Definitions

- 6 disorders of urea cycle
  - Ornithine transcarbamylase deficiency (OTCD)
  - Carbamoyl phosphate synthetase 1 deficiency
  - Citrullinemia or argininosuccinate synthetase deficiency
  - Argininosuccinate aciduria or argininosuccinate lyase deficiency
  - Argininemia or arginase deficiency (AD)
  - N-acetylglutamate synthase deficiency

IMAGING

General Features

- Best diagnostic clue
  - Neonate presenting 24-48 hours with basal ganglia (BG) and cortical ↑ DWI signal
- Location
  - Neonates: Deep gray nuclei, depths of sulci in frontal, parietal, and insular > temporal cortex
  - Older: As above or asymmetric cortical/subcortical white matter (WM) mimicking stroke
  - Posterior fossa spared

CT Findings

- NECT
  - ↓ attenuation deep gray nuclei, WM + cortex with swelling → atrophy when chronic

MR Findings

- T1WI
  - Subacute/chronic: ↑ signal cortical, deep gray nuclei areas involved
- T2WI
  - Acute/subacute: ↑ signal, swelling areas involved
  - Chronic: Volume loss, gliosis ± cystic change
- DWI
  - Acute/subacute: Iso/↑ DWI signal, iso/↓ ADC
- MRS
  - Acute/subacute: ↓ myoinositol, ↑ glutamine-glutamate, ↑ lipids/lactate

Imaging Recommendations

- Best imaging tool: MR
- Protocol advice: T1WI, T2WI, DWI, MRS

DIFFERENTIAL DIAGNOSIS

Hypoxic Ischemic Encephalopathy

- Lateral putamen and ventrolateral thalamus involved; difficult to differentiate in chronic state

Arterial Ischemic Stroke

- Vascular distribution

Metabolic Disorders

- Mitochondrial disorders
- Organic acidemias: Globi pallidi but not cortex; metabolic acidosis/ketosis
- Nonketotic hyperglycinemia: No BG involvement

PATHOLOGY

General Features

- Etiology
  - Urea cycle incorporates nitrogen → urea → urine; prevents accumulation of toxic nitrogen products
  - ↑ ammonia → ↑ glutamate → ↑ glutamine in astrocytes → swelling + dysfunction
- Genetics
  - All autosomal recessive except OTCD (X-linked)

Gross Pathologic & Surgical Features

- Brain swelling in acute; atrophy + ulegyria in chronic

Microscopic Features

- GM Alzheimer type 2 astrocytes; GM, WM spongiosis

CLINICAL ISSUES

Presentation

- Most common signs/symptoms
  - Triad of hyperammonemia, encephalopathy, respiratory alkalosis
  - Progressive lethargy, hypothermia, vomiting, apnea
  - Neonates develop encephalopathy > 24-48 hours
  - Episodic in older patients (often when ↑ protein intake or ↑ catabolism)
- Clinical profile
  - ↑ ammonium blood levels (except AD)
  - Diagnosis: Liver cell enzyme assessment/DNA

Demographics

- Age
  - Neonate if severe, older if less severe
- Epidemiology
  - Whites > African-Americans
  - OTCD most common

Natural History & Prognosis

- Improved with treatment but most mentally retarded
- Neonates: Worst prognosis with high mortality

Treatment

- Hemodialysis in acute crisis
- Liver transplant in severe
- ↓ protein intake, adequate caloric intake, supplements
- Sodium benzoate/phenylbutyrate/phenylacetate
- Valproate contraindicated; can cause death

SELECTED REFERENCES

1. Summar ML et al: Diagnosis, symptoms, frequency and mortality of 260 patients with urea cycle disorders from a 21-year, multicentre study of acute hyperammonaemic episodes. Acta Paediatr. 97(10):1420-5, 2008
2. Choi JH et al: Two cases of citrullinaemia presenting with stroke. J Inherit Metab Dis. 29(1):182-3, 2006
3. Takanashi J et al: Brain MR imaging in neonatal hyperammonemic encephalopathy resulting from proximal urea cycle disorders. AJNR Am J Neuroradiol. 24(6):1184-7, 2003

GLUTARIC ACIDURIA TYPE 1

Key Facts

Terminology

- GA 1: Glutaric acidemia type 1 (GA 1), mitochondrial glutaryl-coenzyme A dehydrogenase deficiency
- Inborn error of metabolism characterized by encephalopathic crises and resultant severe dystonic-dyskinetic movement disorder

Imaging

- Wide opercula and bright basal ganglia
  - Common: ↑ signal caudate/putamina > globus pallidus
  - Occasional: Pallidal and dentate signal change may occur even in absence of crisis
  - Severe: White matter, thalami, dentate nuclei may be involved
- Child abuse mimic: Easily torn bridging veins within enlarged cerebrospinal fluid spaces → subdural hematomas

Pathology

- Accumulated substances toxic to striate cells and white matter
- Multiple mutations govern varied clinical presentation

Clinical Issues

- Episodic crises follow trigger (infection, immunization, surgery)
- Generally manifests during 1st year of life
- 10% carrier rate in old order Amish

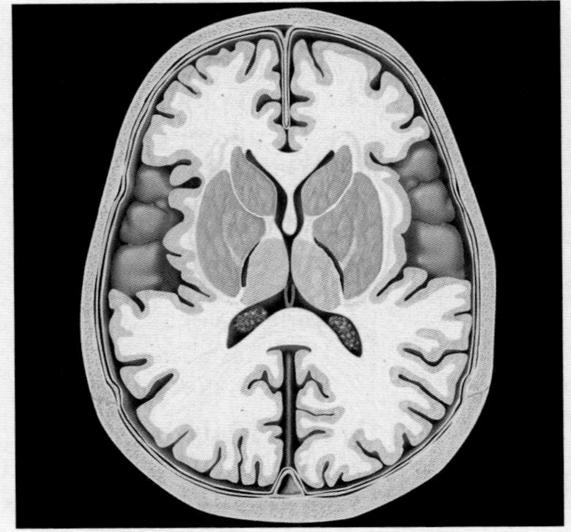

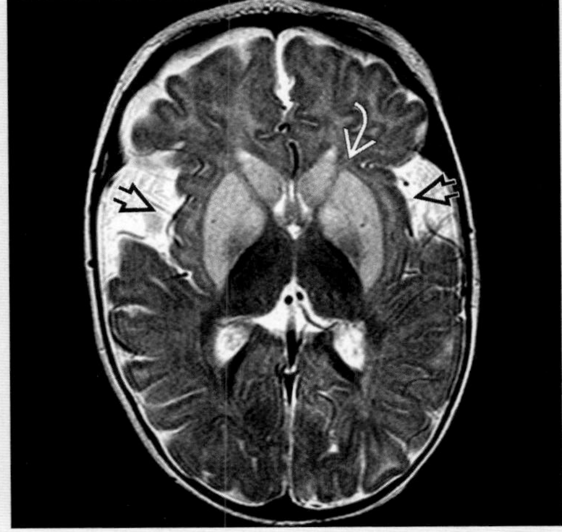

(Left) *Axial graphic demonstrates the pattern of involvement in GA 1. The sylvian fissures are enlarged, and the basal ganglia are diffusely and symmetrically abnormal in signal.* ***(Right)*** *Axial T2WI in a 7 month old reveals enlarged sylvian fissures ➢. Note the swelling and abnormally increased signal intensity of the basal ganglia ➔, including the heads of caudate nuclei, the putamina, and the globi pallidi bilaterally. Myelination is delayed.*

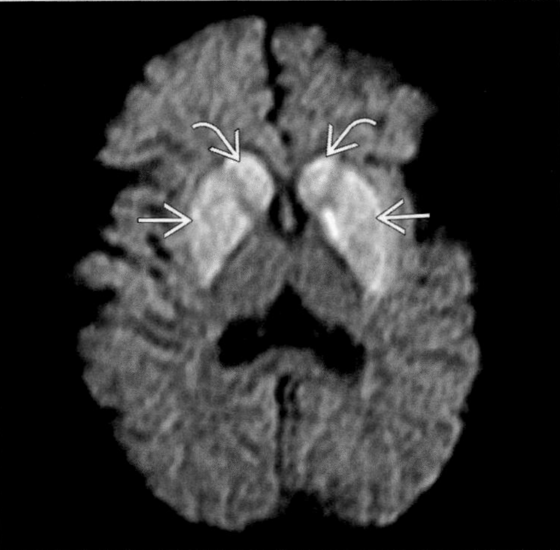

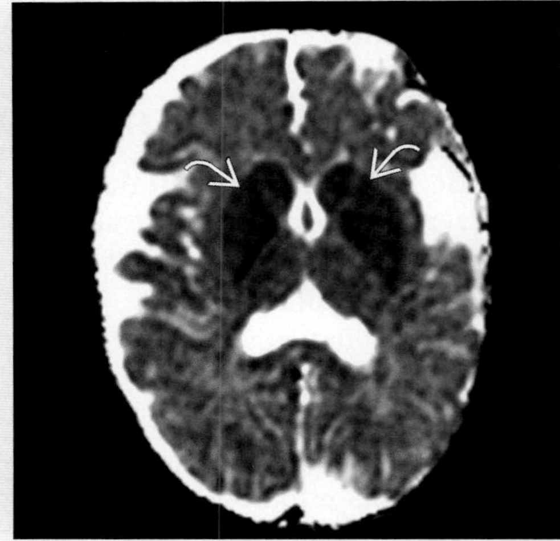

(Left) *Axial diffusion weighted MR of an infant in the midst of a severe metabolic crisis shows hyperintense signal resulting from reduced diffusion within the heads of the caudate nuclei ➔ and putamina ➔ bilaterally.* ***(Right)*** *ADC map shows hypointensity ➔ in the same areas, the caudates and putamina, confirming the presence of acute brain injury with resultant reduced diffusivity, rather than T2 shine-through.*

GLUTARIC ACIDURIA TYPE 1

TERMINOLOGY

Abbreviations

- Glutaric acidemia type 1 (GA 1)
- Mitochondrial glutaryl-coenzyme A dehydrogenase (GCDH) deficiency

Definitions

- Inborn error of metabolism characterized by encephalopathic crises and resultant severe dystonic-dyskinetic movement disorder

IMAGING

General Features

- Best diagnostic clue
  - Wide opercula and bright basal ganglia (BG)
- Location
  - Sylvian fissures, basal ganglia
- Size
  - Enlarged sylvian fissures
- Morphology
  - Wide opercula (frontotemporal hypoplasia) = "bat-wing" dilatation of sylvian fissures

CT Findings

- NECT
  - > 95% cyst-like middle cranial fossa cerebrospinal fluid (CSF) spaces, opercular extension
    - Sylvian fissure widening (93%), mesencephalic cistern widening (86%)
  - Striatal hypodensity
  - Early macrocephaly, late atrophy (mostly ventricular enlargement)
  - Subdural hematoma with minimal trauma
- CECT
  - No enhancement

MR Findings

- T1WI
  - Sylvian fissure cyst-like spaces isointense to CSF
    - May decrease in size over time
  - Subependymal pseudocysts (disappear by 6 months)
  - Frontotemporal atrophy
  - Delayed myelination
  - Occasional mild immature-appearing gyral pattern
- T2WI
  - Common: ↑ signal caudate/putamina > globus pallidus
  - Occasional: Pallidal and dentate signal change may occur even in absence of crisis
    - May predate involvement of caudate & putamina
  - Striatal atrophy over time
  - If severe: White matter (WM), thalami, dentate nuclei may be involved
- FLAIR
  - Same as T2WI
- DWI
  - Acute phase: Reduced diffusion in BG and selected WM tracts; may show more extensive disease than apparent on either CT or MR
- T1WI C+
  - No enhancement
- MRS
  - ↑ Cho/Cr ratio, ↓ NAA
  - During crisis: ± increased lactate

Imaging Recommendations

- Best imaging tool
  - MR
- Protocol advice
  - MRS, DWI

DIFFERENTIAL DIAGNOSIS

Nonaccidental Injury

- a.k.a. child abuse
- GA 1 does not cause fractures
- Subdural hematoma (SDH) in GA 1 from torn-bridging veins in presence of large CSF, atrophy
- SDH in GA 1 do not occur without enlarged CSF spaces
- Head trauma = most common cause of death
  - SDH most common finding, often interhemispheric
  - Skull fracture subarachnoid, epidural hemorrhage
  - Cerebral edema, contusion(s), shear injuries

Other Disorders with Bilateral Middle Cranial Fossa Cyst-like Spaces

- Mucopolysaccharidoses
  - Types 1-4: Hurler, Hunter, Sanfilippo, Scheie, Maroteaux-Lamy, Sly
  - CSF-like mucopolysaccharide pachymeningeal deposition in all but Morquio type 4
- "Idiopathic" middle cranial fossae arachnoid cysts
  - 5% may be bilateral, usually asymptomatic
  - CSF intensity; may be slightly different on FLAIR
  - No DWI restriction

Causes of Macrocephaly

- Hydrocephalus
  - Congenital, post-traumatic, or obstructive
  - Ventricular prominence out of proportion to sulci
  - Enlarged temporal horns, rounded frontal horns, transependymal CSF flow
- Idiopathic enlargement of subarachnoid spaces (SAS) during 1st year of life
- Benign familial macrocephaly: Family tendency toward large head size

PATHOLOGY

General Features

- Etiology
  - GCDH required for metabolism of lysine, hydroxylysine, and tryptophan
  - ↓ GCDH → accumulation glutaric, glutaconic, and 3-OH-glutaric acid
  - Accumulated substances toxic to striate cells and white matter
- Genetics
  - Autosomal recessive
  - *GCDH* gene mutations (Chr 19p13.2) result in amino acid substitutions

GLUTARIC ACIDURIA TYPE 1

- Multiple mutations govern varied clinical presentation
  - European variant (most common): Arg402-to-trp
  - Amish variant, riboflavin sensitive: Ala421-to-val
  - Severe, 1% residual enzyme, symptoms despite treatment (Tx): Glu365-to-lys
- Rare adult onset: Compound heterozygosity with deletion and novel missense mutation
- Associated abnormalities
  - Embryology: Toxic effects in utero impede operculization during 3rd trimester
  - Mild hepatocellular dysfunction during crisis

Staging, Grading, & Classification

- Symptomatic: Frontotemporal atrophy, BG signal changes
- Presymptomatic: Symptom-free, lack BG changes, but CSF spaces still enlarged

Gross Pathologic & Surgical Features

- Macrocrania, frontotemporal atrophy/hypoplasia; ↑ CSF spaces ± SDH
- Hypo- and de-myelination

Microscopic Features

- Myelin vacuolation and splitting, excess intramyelinic fluid
- Spongiform changes, neuronal loss basal ganglia

CLINICAL ISSUES

Presentation

- Most common signs/symptoms
  - Initially normal development
  - Acute encephalopathy, seizures, dystonia, choreoathetosis, mental retardation
- Acute onset group: Majority
  - Episodic crises follow trigger (infection, immunization, surgery)
    - Acute Reye-like encephalopathy, ketoacidosis, ↑ NH4, vomiting
    - Dystonia, opisthotonus, seizures, excessive sweating
    - Follow-up: Alert child (intellect preserved > > motor); rapid infantile head growth → frontal bossing; severe dystonia
- Insidious onset (25%): Dystonia without crisis
- Presymptomatic may remain asymptomatic: Diagnose, treat, avoid catabolic stress
- Rare asymptomatic without treatment: Still frontotemporal atrophy but normal BG
- Diagnosis: Frequent long interval between presentation and diagnosis
  - Tandem mass spectrometry of newborn filter-paper blood specimens
    - Chromatography of mass; spectroscopy of urine
  - Deficient or absent GCDH activity in fibroblasts
  - Laboratory (may be relatively normal between crises)
    - Metabolic acidosis/ketosis, hypoglycemia, ↓ carnitine
    - Urinary organic acids: ↑ glutaric, glutaconic, and 3-OH-glutaric acid

Demographics

- Age
  - Generally manifests during 1st year of life
- Gender
  - No predilection
- Ethnicity
  - 10% carrier rate in old order Amish
- Epidemiology
  - 1:30,000 newborns

Natural History & Prognosis

- Symptomatic: Most severely handicapped, 20% die before 5 years
- Presymptomatic: Many (not all) remain asymptomatic with diagnosis and therapy
- Treat before 1st encephalopathic crisis; avoid catabolic crises
- Prognosis poor if has already presented with encephalopathic crisis

Treatment

- Intrauterine diagnosis available
  - DNA analysis: Cultured amniotic fluid cells and chorionic villi biopsy
  - Fetal sonography and MR: Dilated perisylvian CSF in 3rd trimester
- Early treatment may prevent or ameliorate symptoms and imaging
  - Low-protein diet (reduced tryptophan and lysine), synthetic protein drink
  - Riboflavin (vit B2) to ensure cofactor supply for GCDH
  - Oral carnitine replacement; gamma aminobutyric acid (GABA), analog (baclofen)

DIAGNOSTIC CHECKLIST

Image Interpretation Pearls

- Consider GA in young children with bilateral "cysts" in sylvian fissures and abnormal basal ganglia
- Pallidal and dentate signal change may occur even in absence of crisis; may predate involvement of caudate and putamina

SELECTED REFERENCES

1. Harting I et al: Dynamic changes of striatal and extrastriatal abnormalities in glutaric aciduria type I. Brain. Epub ahead of print, 2009
2. Mellerio C et al: Prenatal cerebral ultrasound and MRI findings in glutaric aciduria Type 1: a de novo case. Ultrasound Obstet Gynecol. 31(6):712-4, 2008
3. Elster AW: Glutaric aciduria type I: value of diffusion-weighted magnetic resonance imaging for diagnosing acute striatal necrosis. J Comput Assist Tomogr. 28(1):98-100, 2004
4. Strauss KA et al: Type I glutaric aciduria, part 1: natural history of 77 patients. Am J Med Genet. 121C(1):38-52, 2003
5. Strauss KA et al: Type I glutaric aciduria, part 2: a model of acute striatal necrosis. Am J Med Genet. 121C(1):53-70, 2003
6. Twomey EL et al: Neuroimaging findings in glutaric aciduria type 1. Pediatr Radiol. 33(12):823-30, 2003

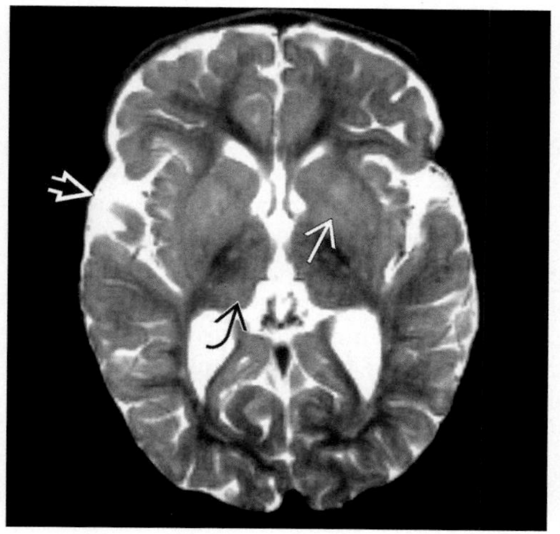

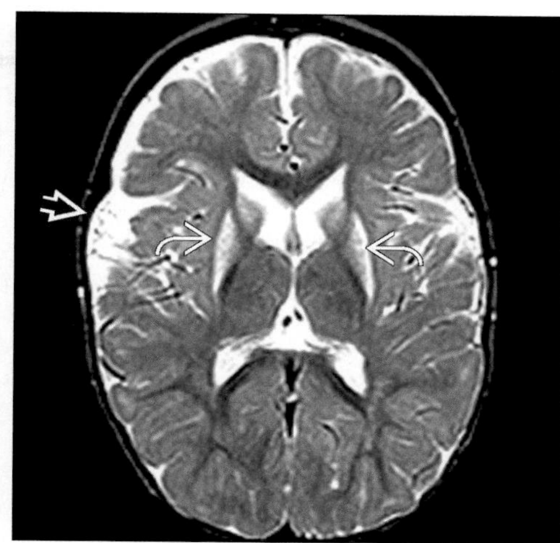

(Left) *Axial T2WI MR shows mild prominence of the sylvian fissures ➡ and mottled, early signal abnormalities in the basal ganglia ➡ and thalami ➡. The presence of macrocrania is an additional clue when imaging findings are subtle in cases of GA 1.* ***(Right)*** *Axial T2WI MR in another child 21 months of age, long after resolution of metabolic crisis, reveals slit-like atrophy, gliosis of the basal ganglia ➡, and persistence of the sylvian fissure enlargement ➡.*

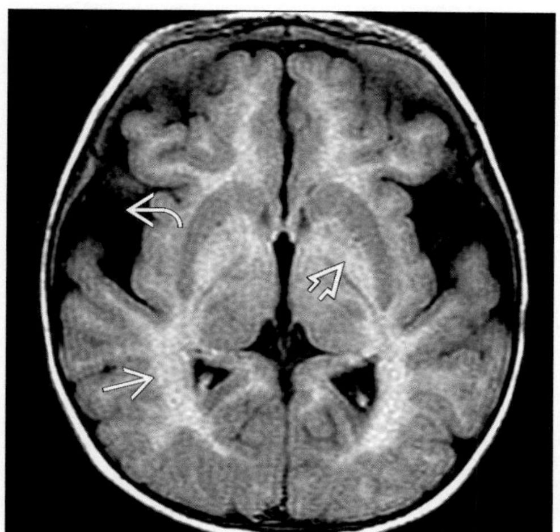

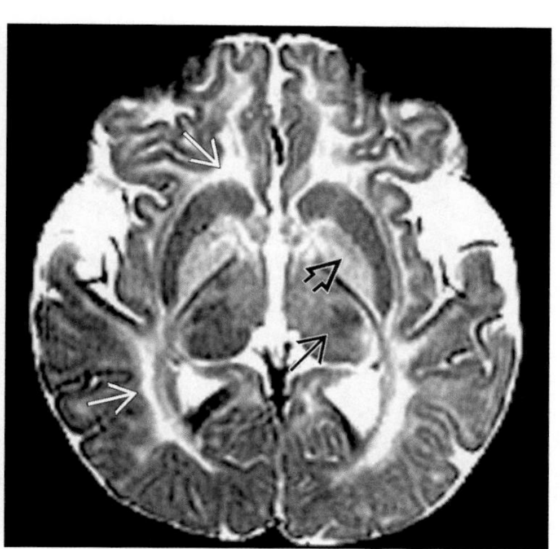

(Left) *Axial FLAIR MR demonstrates typical enlargement of the sylvian fissures ➡ in a 7-month-old child. Abnormal signal is identified within the globi pallidi ➡ as expected and in cerebral white matter ➡. The latter finding is unusual and is felt to reflect the combination of GA 1 and DHPR deficiency in this child.* ***(Right)*** *T2WI MR in the same child shows diffusely abnormal white matter ➡, abnormal signal within the globi pallidi ➡, and thalami ➡.*

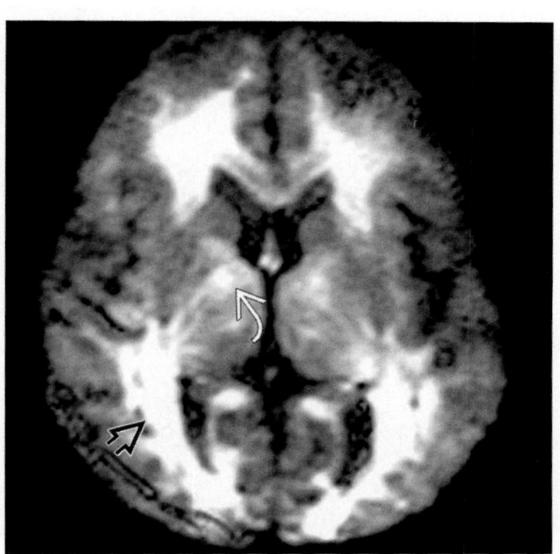

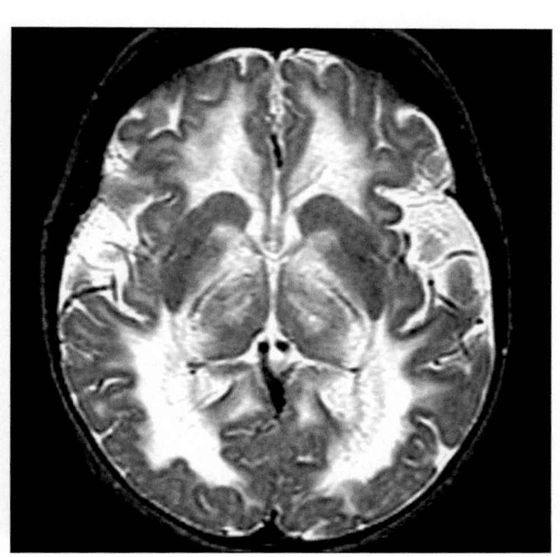

(Left) *Follow-up DWI MR in the same child at nearly 2 years of age shows reduced diffusivity, which confirms active disease and marked progression of disease, particularly within the white matter ➡. There is also reduced diffusivity within the involved globi pallidi ➡.* ***(Right)*** *T2WI MR at the same time as the DWI shows marked progression of white matter abnormality. White matter is now isointense to CSF. The prominent sylvian fissures remain a strong clue to the diagnosis of GA 1.*

CANAVAN DISEASE

Key Facts

Terminology
- Progressive autosomal-recessive spongiform leukodystrophy

Imaging
- WM (involves subcortical U-fibers), sparing internal capsule, and corpus callosum
- Thalami, globi pallidi (GP), ± dentate nuclei, sparing caudate, and putamen
- ↑ T2 + DWI signal, normal to ↓ ADC in involved areas
- ↑ NAA/Cr, ↓ Ch/Cr

Top Differential Diagnoses
- Maple syrup urine disease
- Pelizaeus-Merzbacher disease
- Merosin-deficient congential muscular dystrophy
- Alexander disease

Pathology
- Spongiform degeneration of white matter; GP and thalami with swollen astrocytes
- Deficiency of aspartoacyclase → N-acetyl aspartic acid ↑ in brain and urine

Clinical Issues
- ↑ risk for Ashkenazi Jewish (1 in 40 carriers)
- Early severe hypotonia and macrocephaly
- No proven treatment (gene therapy and acetate supplementation under evaluation)
- Evident by 4 months
- Relentless, progressive neurodegenerative disorder: Chronic vegetative state with autonomic crises → death by end of 1st decade

*(**Left**) Axial T2WI MR in a 6-month-old boy shows diffusely increased signal in the cerebral white matter, thalami ⇨, and right globus pallidus ➡ with relative sparing of the internal capsule, corpus callosum, caudate, and putamen. (**Right**) Axial T1WI MR in the same 6-month-old boy shows diffusely decreased signal in the white matter, thalami ⇨, and globi pallidi ➡. Normal signal intensity is present within the internal capsule, corpus callosum, caudates, and putamina.*

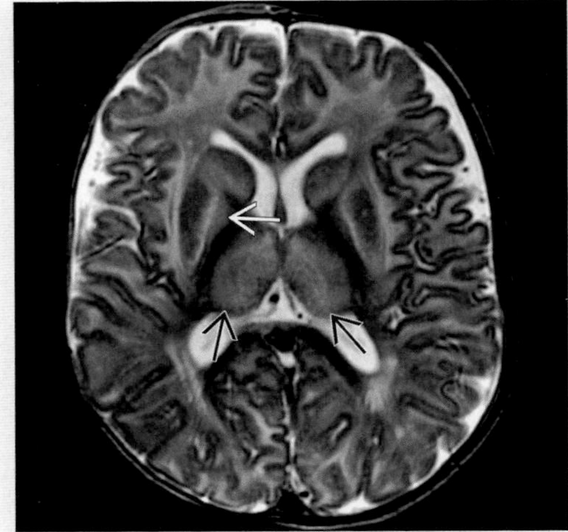

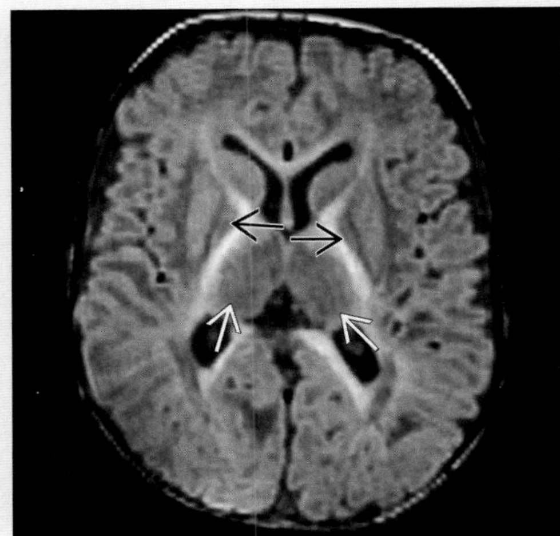

*(**Left**) Axial DWI MR in the same 6-month-old boy shows diffusely increased signal (reduced diffusivity) in the cerebral white matter and globi pallidi ➡. Normal diffusivity is seen in the myelinated internal capsule and corpus callosum. Caudates and putamina appear unaffected. (**Right**) Axial long echo (TE = 144 msec) proton MRS acquired in the centrum semiovale at 1.5T shows a marked relative increase in NAA ➡ and decrease in choline ➡ relative to Cr for age.*

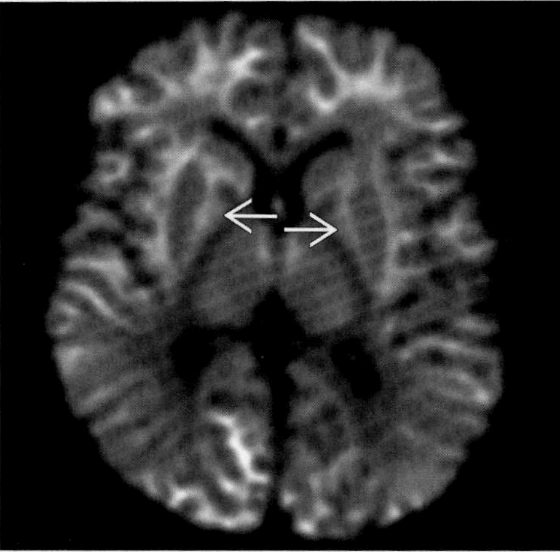

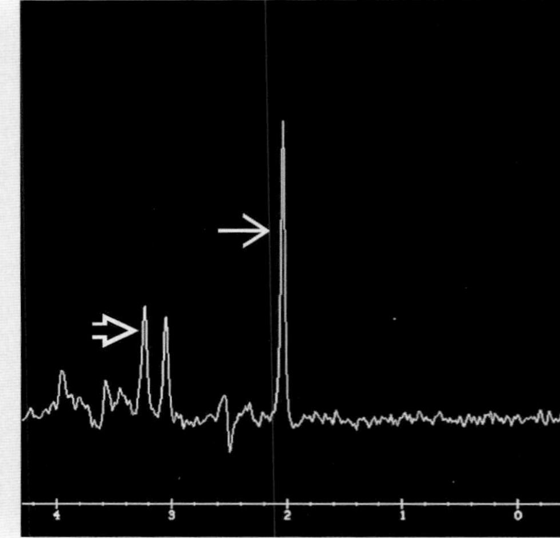

CANAVAN DISEASE

TERMINOLOGY

Synonyms

- Spongiform leukodystrophy, spongy degeneration of CNS, Canavan-van Bogaert-Bertrand disease, aspartoacylase deficiency, *ASPA* deficiency, *ASP* deficiency, aminoacylase 2 deficiency, *ACY2* deficiency

Definitions

- Progressive autosomal-recessive spongiform leukodystrophy

IMAGING

General Features

- Best diagnostic clue
  - Megalencephaly with diffuse ↑ white matter T2 and DWI signal and ↑ NAA
- Location
  - White matter (WM): Involves subcortical U-fibers, sparing internal capsule, and corpus callosum
  - Thalami, globi pallidi (GP), ± dentate nuclei, sparing caudate, and putamen

CT Findings

- NECT
  - Diffuse ↓ attenuation in involved areas

MR Findings

- T1WI
  - Hypointense in involved areas
- T2WI
  - Hyperintense in involved areas
- DWI
  - Bright DWI signal, normal to ↓ ADC in involved areas
- T1WI C+
  - No enhancement
- MRS
  - ↑ NAA/Cr, ↓ Ch/Cr

Imaging Recommendations

- Best imaging tool
  - MR
- Protocol advice
  - T2WI, DWI, and MRS

DIFFERENTIAL DIAGNOSIS

Maple Syrup Urine Disease

- ↑ branched chain AA + ketoacids

Pelizaeus-Merzbacher Disease

- ↑ ADC, spares GP and thalami

Merosin-Deficient Congential Muscular Dystrophy

- ↑ ADC, spares GP and thalami

Alexander Disease

- Predilection for frontal WM, enhances

PATHOLOGY

General Features

- Etiology
  - Deficiency of aspartoacylase → N-acetyl aspartic acid ↑ in brain and urine
- Genetics
  - Autosomal recessive → *ASPA* gene = long arm chromosome 17

Staging, Grading, & Classification

- Earlier onset → more rapid progression

Gross Pathologic & Surgical Features

- Swollen brain

Microscopic Features

- Spongiform degeneration of white matter; GP and thalami with swollen astrocytes

CLINICAL ISSUES

Presentation

- Most common signs/symptoms
  - 3 clinical variants
    - Congenital (1st few days of life)
      - Hypotonia, rapid death
    - Infantile (3-6 months); most common form
      - Hypotonia, head lag, macrocephaly → seizures, spasticity, visual loss
    - Juvenile
      - Onset at 4-5 years; slower progression
- Clinical profile
  - Early severe hypotonia and macrocephaly

Demographics

- Age
  - Evident by 4 months
- Gender
  - No sex predilection
- Ethnicity
  - ↑ risk for Ashkenazi Jewish (1 in 40 carriers)

Natural History & Prognosis

- Relentless, progressive neurodegenerative disorder: Chronic vegetative state with autonomic crises → death by end of 1st decade

Treatment

- No proven treatment (gene therapy and acetate supplementation under evaluation)

DIAGNOSTIC CHECKLIST

Image Interpretation Pearls

- Swollen brain with ↑ T2, ↑ DWI signal in white matter, involvement of GP and thalami

SELECTED REFERENCES

1. van der Knaap MS et al: Defining and categorizing leukoencephalopathies of unknown origin: MR imaging approach. Radiology. 213(1):121-33, 1999

ALEXANDER DISEASE

Key Facts

Terminology

- Rare leukoencephalopathy characterized by Rosenthal fibers (RFs), intracytoplasmic astrocytic inclusions
- 3 clinical forms: Infantile (most common), juvenile, adult
- 1 of few metabolic disorders that enhances

Imaging

- Infantile: Symmetric, ↑ T2 signal bifrontal WM
- Juvenile/adult: ↑ T2 signal brainstem, cerebellum, cervical cord
- Other findings: ↓ T2, ↑ T1 enhancing nodular periventricular rim

Top Differential Diagnoses

- Canavan disease
- Megaloencephalic leukoencephalopathy with subcortical cysts (MLC)
- Glutaric aciduria type 1 (GA-1)
- Mucopolysaccharidoses (MPS)

Pathology

- Dominant mutations *GFAP* (17q21) (> 95% of cases)

Clinical Issues

- Clinical profile: Infant with macrocephaly, seizures
- Natural history: Variable rate of progression ultimately leading to death in all forms
- Treatment: Supportive

Diagnostic Checklist

- Enhancing, symmetric bifrontal WM disease in macrocephalic infant highly characteristic of AD
- Consider adult AD if ↑ T2 signal, atrophy in medulla & cervical cord

***(Left)** Axial NECT shows the typical appearance of infantile Alexander disease (AD). The striatum and periventricular rim ➔ are hyperdense. Note the symmetric, frontal predominant, white matter (WM) hypodensity. **(Right)** Axial T2WI MR shows a nodular, hypointense, periventricular rim ➔ with symmetric, mild hyperintensity in the striata and thalami →. The cerebral WM is diffusely hyperintense, greatest in the frontal lobes, where it extends from the ventricular margin to the subcortical U-fibers.*

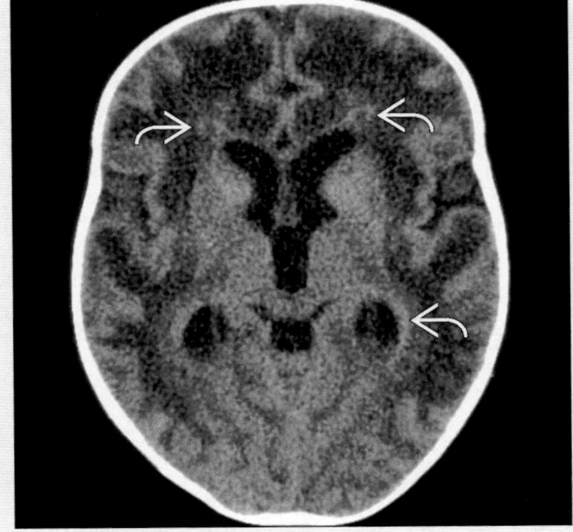

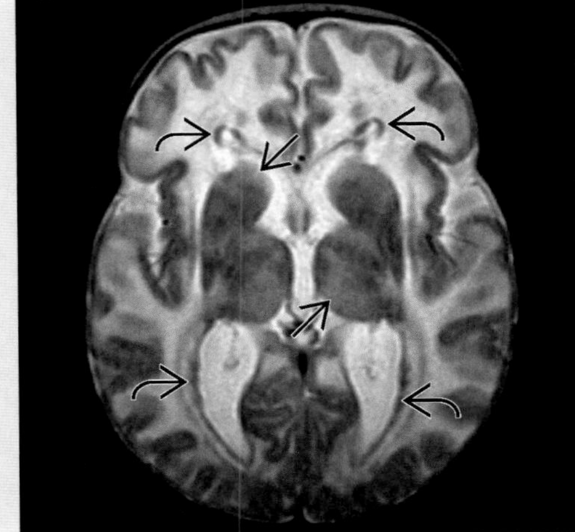

***(Left)** Axial T1WI MR shows diffusely hypointense, swollen-appearing WM with a frontal-to-occipital gradient. Only the occipital WM appears myelinated. The nodular periventricular rim ➔ is hyperintense. The lateral ventricles are abnormally enlarged. **(Right)** Axial T1WI C+ MR shows enhancement of the periventricular rim, the caudate heads, and the putamina bilaterally. The nodular, "rabbit ear" appearance of the frontal periventricular rim ➔ is typical of Alexander disease.*

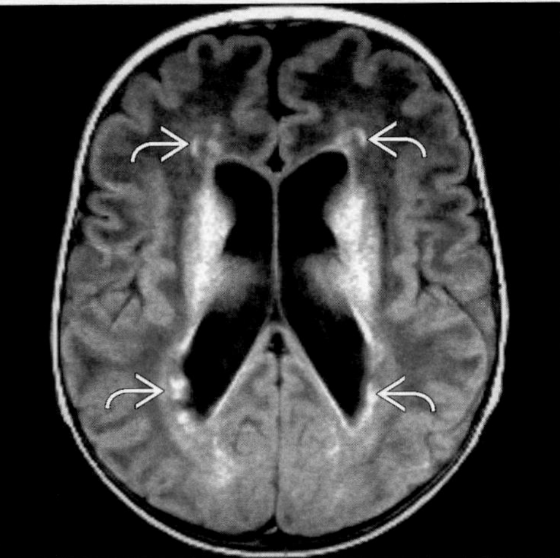

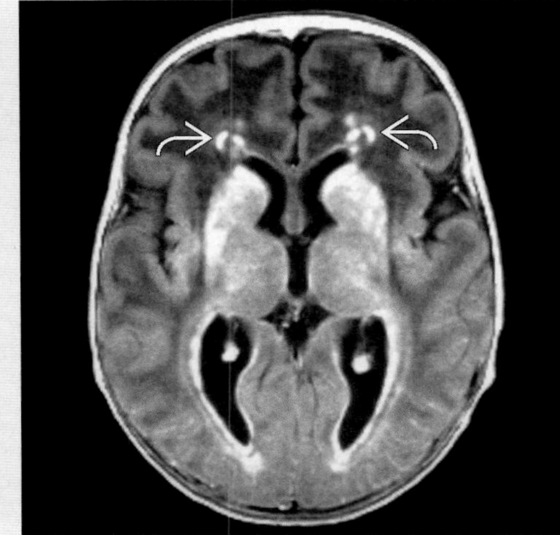

ALEXANDER DISEASE

TERMINOLOGY

Abbreviations
- Alexander disease (AD)

Synonyms
- Fibrinoid leukodystrophy

Definitions
- Rare leukoencephalopathy characterized by Rosenthal fibers (RFs), intracytoplasmic astrocytic inclusions
- 3 clinical forms: Infantile (most common), juvenile, adult
- 1 of the few metabolic disorders that enhance

IMAGING

General Features
- Best diagnostic clue
  - Macrocephalic infant with
    - Symmetric, ↑ T2 signal bifrontal white matter (WM)
    - ↓ T2, ↑ T1, enhancing, nodular periventricular rim
  - Juvenile: Enhancing, ↑ T2 signal brainstem (BS), cerebellum
  - Adult: ↑ T2 signal, atrophy medulla, cervical cord
- Other findings
  - Infantile
    - ↑ T2 signal, enhancement striatum
    - Variable ↑ T2 signal, enhancement in BS (especially periaqueductal), dentate nuclei, optic chiasm, fornix
    - ± hydrocephalus (periaqueductal disease)
  - Juvenile/adult
    - Characterized by BS, cerebellar, spinal cord involvement
    - Involvement cerebral WM, periventricular rim, striatum variable (usually mild)
  - Enhancement, swelling early (infantile AD)
  - Atrophy, cystic encephalomalacia (infantile) late
- Location
  - White matter
    - Frontal: Periventricular → subcortical
    - External/extreme capsules, ± callosal genu
  - Periventricular rim
  - Basal ganglia (BG), thalami, BS, cerebellum, fornix, optic chiasm, spinal cord
- Morphology
  - Posterior extension WM changes frequent with disease progression
  - Rostral caudal gradient less pronounced in juvenile/adult disease

CT Findings
- NECT
  - Hypodense frontal WM
  - Dense periventricular rim, caudate heads
- CECT: Intense enhancement typical of early disease

MR Findings
- T1WI
  - Hypointense frontal WM
  - Hyperintense periventricular rim, ± basal ganglia
- T2WI
  - Hyperintense frontal WM, caudate heads
  - Hypointense periventricular rim
  - Juvenile/adult: Hypertense foci BS, ± cervical cord
- FLAIR
  - Cystic encephalomalacia frontal WM (late infantile)
- DWI: Normal to increased diffusivity
- T1WI C+: Intense enhancement typical of early disease
  - Infantile: Frontal periventricular WM, striatum, periventricular rim; rare BS, fornix, optic chiasm
  - Juvenile/adult: BS and cerebellar enhancement may mimic tumor
- MRS: ↓ NAA, ↑ myoinositol; ± ↑ choline, lactate

Nuclear Medicine Findings
- 18F-fluorodeoxyglucose (FDG) PET
  - Hypometabolism in affected frontal white matter
  - Preserved overlying normal glucose metabolism

Imaging Recommendations
- Best imaging tool: MR C+/MRS
- Protocol advice: Enhance all "unknown" cases of hydrocephalus and abnormal WM
- Proposed MR criteria for infantile AD (4/5 required)
  - Extensive cerebral WM change with frontal predominance
  - ↓ T2, ↑ T1 periventricular rim
  - Abnormal signal basal ganglia, thalami
  - Abnormal signal BS
  - Enhancement of frontal WM, periventricular rim, BG, thalami, BS, dentate nuclei, cerebellum, optic chiasm, or fornix

DIFFERENTIAL DIAGNOSIS

Canavan Disease
- WM: Diffuse; subcortical U-fibers involved early
- Deep gray matter: Globi pallidi, thalami
- No enhancement
- Characteristic ↑↑ NAA peak on MRS

Megalencephaly with Leukoencephalopathy and Cysts (MLC)
- WM: Diffuse with subcortical U-fiber involvement
- No involvement deep gray structures
- No enhancement
- Characteristic temporal, frontoparietal, subcortical cysts

Glutaric Aciduria Type 1
- WM: Periventricular WM involved in severe disease
- Deep gray: Symmetric basal ganglia
- No enhancement
- Characteristic widened opercula

Mucopolysaccharidoses
- WM: Mild periventricular
- No involvement of deep gray structures
- Characteristic cribriform WM, corpus callosum

ALEXANDER DISEASE

PATHOLOGY

General Features

- General pathology comments
  - AD characterized by accumulation of Rosenthal fibers (RFs) in astrocytes and hypo-/demyelination
- Embryology and anatomy
  - Astrocytes play role in myelin formation by oligodendrocytes
  - Astrocytic end-feet form part of blood-brain barrier
  - Glial fibrillary acidic protein (GFAP): Major intermediate filament protein in astrocytes
- Genetics
  - Dominant mutations *GFAP* (17q21) (> 95% of cases)
    - > 65 different mutations identified
    - Same mutation may be seen in all clinical forms ⇒ additional epigenetic or environmental factors influence phenotype
    - Majority of mutations arise de novo; familial cases seen in adult AD
    - Mutations cause gain in function
- Etiology
  - RFs: Abnormal intracellular protein aggregates containing GFAP, αβ-crystalline, hsp27, & ubiquitin
  - Mechanism by which *GFAP* mutation induces RF formation uncertain
  - Mechanism by which RF accumulation leads to hypo-/demyelination uncertain
    - Theory: RF accumulation causes cell dysfunction
      - Includes blood-brain barrier disruption and loss of normal cell-cell interaction with oligodendrocytes
  - RFs also seen in astrocytomas, hamartomas, gliosis

Gross Pathologic & Surgical Features

- Megaloencephalic, heavy brain with large ventricles
- Swollen, gelatinous WM with cortical thinning
- Frontal WM cavitation
- BG swelling early; atrophy and cystic change late

Microscopic Features

- RFs: Eosinophilic, electron-dense, cytoplasmic inclusions in fibrous astrocytes
  - Greatest concentration in subependymal, subpial, and perivascular astrocytic end-feet areas of enhancement
- Hypomyelination/myelin loss frontal lobes > caudal brain, ± cerebellar WM, dentate nucleus, brainstem
- Generalized astrocytosis ± neuraxonal degeneration
- Abnormalities of muscle mitochondria reported

CLINICAL ISSUES

Presentation

- Most common signs/symptoms
  - Infantile: Macrocephaly, seizures, developmental delay/arrest, spasticity
  - Juvenile: Developmental regression, bulbar/pseudobulbar signs, ataxia, spasticity
  - Adult: Bulbar/pseudobulbar signs, ataxia
    - Palatal myoclonus (40%) ⇒ highly suggestive
- Other signs/symptoms in juvenile/adult
  - Bowel/bladder dysfunction, sleep disturbance, dysautonomia
- Clinical profile: Infant with macrocephaly, seizures
- CSF: Variable ↑ protein, αβ-crystalline, hsp27, lactate
- Diagnosis: MR findings & *GFAP* gene blood analysis

Demographics

- Age
  - Infantile: Birth to 2 years
  - Juvenile: 2-12 years
  - Adult: > 12 years old
- Gender: Slight male predominance in infantile AD
- Epidemiology: Rare; incidence unknown
  - Adult AD more common than previously thought

Natural History & Prognosis

- Natural History
  - Variable rate of progression ultimately leading to death in all forms
    - Neonatal variant of infantile form is most rapidly fatal; infantile form is next most severe
    - Juvenile form is more slowly progressive
    - Adult form is mildest
- Prognosis
  - Infantile: Average survival 3 years after disease onset
  - Juvenile: Average survival 8 years after disease onset
  - Adult: Average survival 15 years after disease onset

Treatment

- Supportive; hydrocephalus may respond to shunting
- Potential future therapeutic role for agents causing down-regulation of *GFAP* expression

DIAGNOSTIC CHECKLIST

Consider

- Adult AD if ↑ T2 signal, atrophy in medulla & cervical cord

Image Interpretation Pearls

- Enhancing, symmetric bifrontal WM disease in macrocephalic infant highly characteristic of AD

SELECTED REFERENCES

1. Mignot C et al: Tumor-like enlargement of the optic chiasm in an infant with Alexander disease. Brain Dev. 31(3):244-7, 2009
2. Farina L et al: Can MR imaging diagnose adult-onset Alexander disease?. AJNR Am J Neuroradiol. 29(6):1190-6, 2008
3. Matarese CA et al: Magnetic resonance imaging findings in Alexander disease. Pediatr Neurol. 38(5):373-4, 2008
4. Pareyson D et al: Adult-onset Alexander disease: a series of eleven unrelated cases with review of the literature. Brain. 131(Pt 9):2321-31, 2008
5. Quinlan RA et al: GFAP and its role in Alexander disease. Exp Cell Res. 313(10):2077-87, 2007
6. Dinopoulos A et al: Discrepancy between neuroimaging findings and clinical phenotype in Alexander disease. AJNR Am J Neuroradiol. 27(10):2088-92, 2006
7. van der Knaap MS et al: Alexander disease: diagnosis with MR imaging. AJNR Am J Neuroradiol. 22(3):541-52, 2001

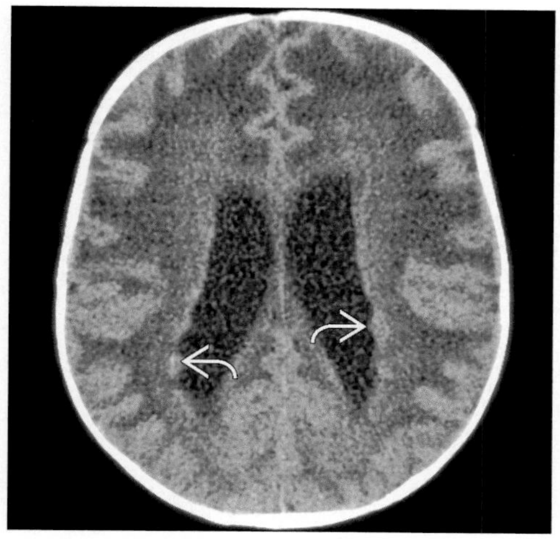

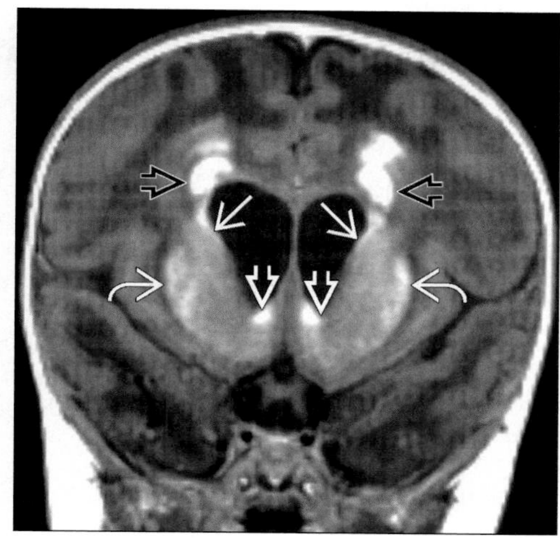

(Left) *Axial NECT shows swollen, hypodense, cerebral WM with frontal predominance. The hyperdense, nodular periventricular rim* ➔ *is made more conspicuous by the adjacent hypodense WM.* ***(Right)*** *Coronal T1WI C+ MR shows intense enhancement in the frontal periventricular rims* ➔ *and adjacent frontal WM. Enhancement is also present over the surface of the caudate heads* ➔ *and in the putamina* ➔ *and fornix* ➔*. Note the symmetric, hypointense, swollen frontal and temporal lobe WM.*

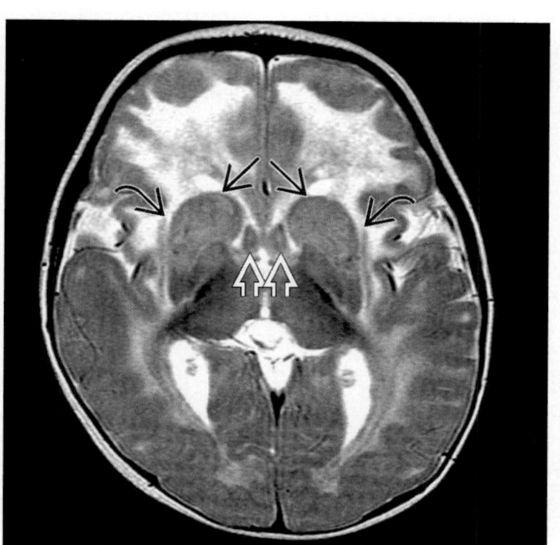

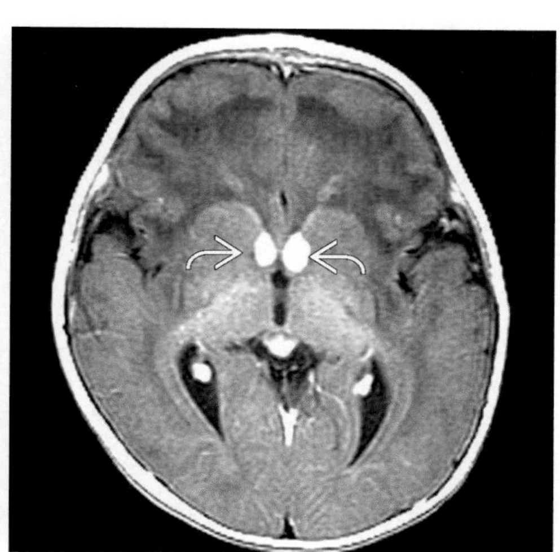

(Left) *Axial T2WI MR in this more advanced case shows symmetric, hyperintense cerebral WM and deep gray structures with greatest hyperintensity in the frontal WM and striata. Note the swollen caudate heads* ➔ *and fornices* ➔*. WM hyperintensity extends into the external and extreme capsules, causing the claustra to stand out* ➔*.* ***(Right)*** *Axial T1WI C+ MR in the same patient shows intense enhancement of the fornices* ➔ *and mild enhancement over the surface of the caudate heads.*

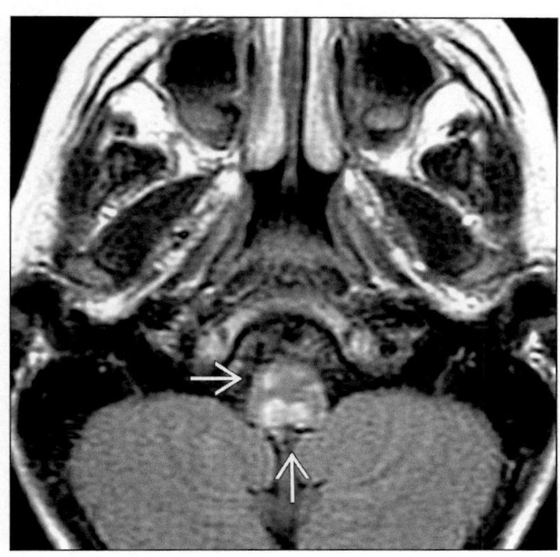

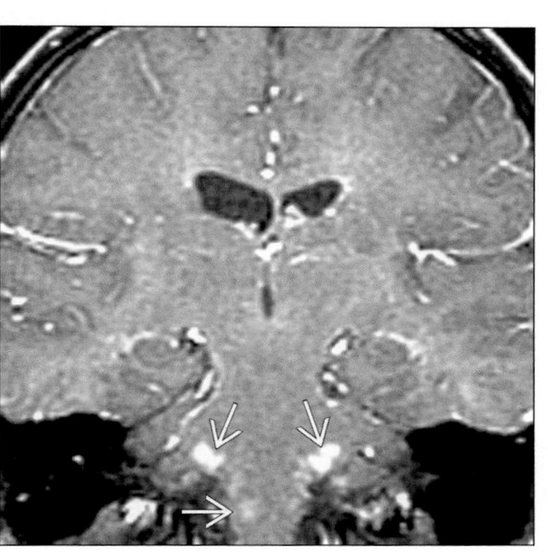

(Left) *Axial FLAIR MR in an older child shows multiple foci of hyperintense signal* ➔ *within the medulla.* ***(Right)*** *Coronal T1WI C+ MR in the same patient shows focal areas of enhancement in the medulla and middle cerebellar peduncles* ➔*. Note the normal appearance of the cerebral WM. Juvenile and adult AD are characterized by the involvement of the brainstem (especially medulla), cerebellum, and cervical cord (particularly adults), with little to no involvement of the supratentorial structures.*

MISCELLANEOUS ORGANIC/AMINOACIDOPATHIES

Key Facts

Terminology

- Phenylketonuria (PKU): Most common inborn error of amino-acid metabolism
  - Caused by mutations in phenylalanine hydroxylase (*PAH*) gene resulting in ↑ phenylalanine (Phe)
- Hyperhomocysteinemia (HHcy): Multiple disorders resulting in ↑ plasma homocysteine (Hcy) > 12 μmol/L
  - Causes: Inborn errors of homocysteine, folate, vitamin B12 metabolism; ↓ vitamin B12/folate intake; renal failure
  - Known risk factor for arteriosclerotic disease > venous thrombosis
  - Most recognized metabolic causes: Cystathionine β-synthase deficiency (CBSD), 5,10 methylenetetrahydrofolate reductase deficiency (MTHFRD), disorders Vit B12 metabolism (Cbl-C), methionine adenosyltransferase deficiency (MAT I/IIID)

Imaging

- PKU, HHcy: ↑ T2 periventricular/deep cerebral WM
- CBSD, MTHFRD, late-onset Cbl-C: Arterial > venous infarcts

Clinical Issues

- PKU: Severe mental retardation if untreated; sublet cognitive impairment in early-treated disease
- HHcy: Variable phenotype; CBSD: Thromboembolic events, mental retardation; others: Varying neurologic impairment/strokes infancy to adulthood
- Diagnosis: PKU, CBSD, MAT I/IIID = newborn screen
- PKU treatment: Phe-free diet starts 1st month of life

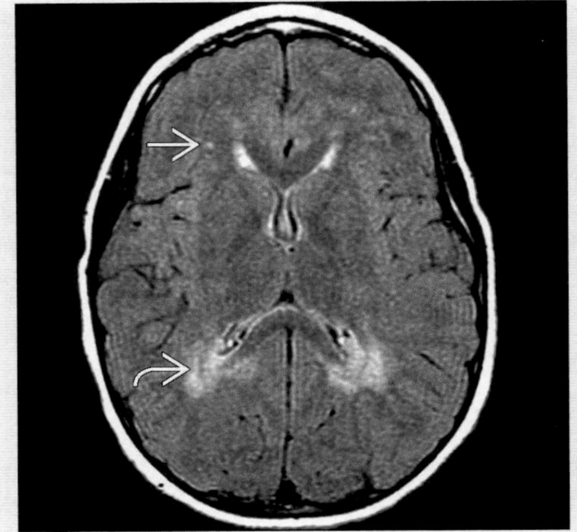

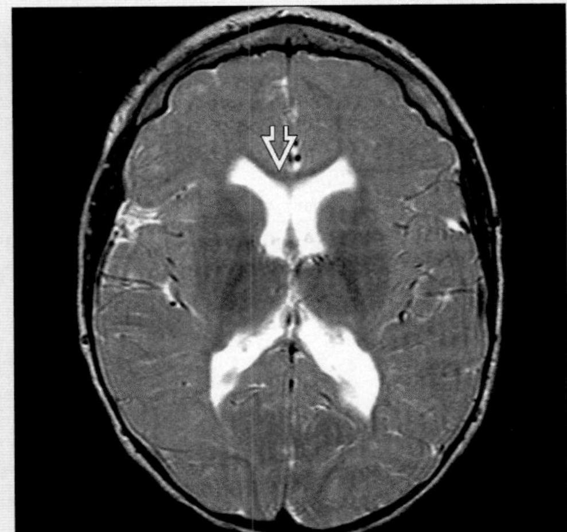

(Left) *Axial FLAIR MR in a 10 year old with PKU. Note the increased signal in the peritrigonal ➔ and frontal ➔ white matter. As is typical of PKU, the parietal white matter lesions are more pronounced than those in the frontal or temporal lobes.* ***(Right)*** *Axial T2WI MR in a 4 year old with MTHFRD. There is marked central white matter volume loss with associated ex vacuo ventricular enlargement and callosal thinning ➔. Note the white matter is hypomyelinated for age.*

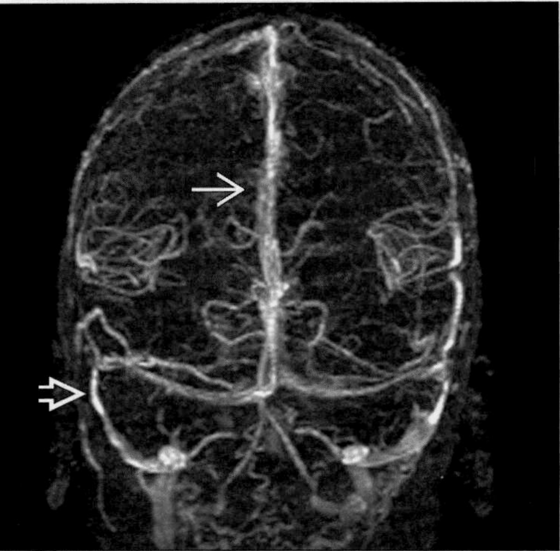

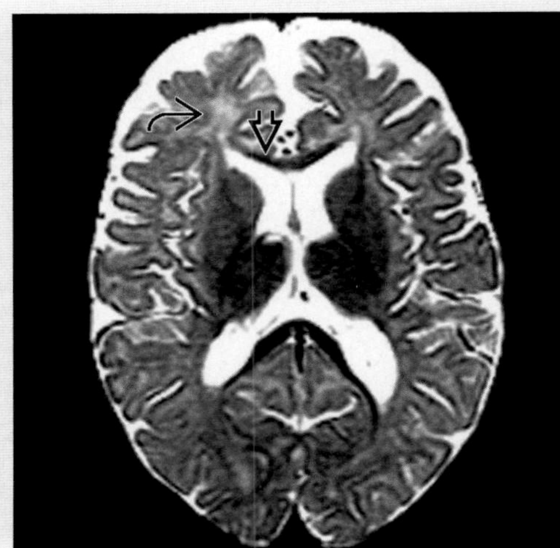

(Left) *Coronal maximum intensity projection from MR venogram in 4 year old with MTHFRD demonstrates irregular, recanalized sigmoid sinus ➔ and superior sagittal sinus ➔ several years following acute sinovenous thrombosis.* ***(Right)*** *Axial T2WI MR in an 8 month old with Cbl-C shows diffusely diminished white matter volume with increased signal in the periventricular and deep frontal white matter ➔. Note mild ex vacuo ventricular enlargement and callosal thinning ➔.*

MISCELLANEOUS ORGANIC/AMINOACIDOPATHIES

TERMINOLOGY

Abbreviations

- Phenylketonuria (PKU)
- Hyperhomocysteinemia (HHcy)
- Cystathionine β-synthase deficiency (CBSD)
- 5,10 methylenetetrahydrofolate reductase deficiency (MTHFRD)
- Methionine adenosyltransferase deficiency (MAT I/IIID)
- Cobalamin C (Cbl-C), disorder vitamin B12 metabolism

Definitions

- PKU: Most common inborn error of amino acid metabolism resulting in ↑ phenylalanine (Phe)
- Hyperhomocysteinemia: Multiple disorders resulting in ↑ plasma homocysteine (Hcy) > 12 μmol/L
  - ↑ risk arteriosclerotic disease > venous thrombosis
  - Caused by inborn errors of Hcy, folate, or vitamin B12 metabolism; ↓ vitamin B12/folate intake; renal failure
  - 4 most recognized metabolic disorders: CBSD, MTHFRD, Cbl-C, MAT I/IIID
  - Variable phenotype among & within each disorder

IMAGING

General Features

- PKU: ↑ T2 periventricular white matter (PVWM)
  - Posterior > anterior PVWM
  - Subcortical WM, corpus callosum late
- CBSD: Small foci ↑ T2 cerebral WM > cortical infarct > sinovenous thrombosis (SVT)
- MTHFRD: ↑ T2 PV/deep WM > arterial infarct, SVT
- Early onset Cbl-C: Swollen, ↑ T2 cerebral WM; ± hydrocephalus, ↑ T2 basal ganglia; Late: WM atrophy
- Late-onset Cbl-C: ↑ T2 PV/deep WM, atrophy > arterial infarct; ± ↑ T2 posterior spinal cord columns
- MAT I/IIID: Reversible ↑ T2 PV/deep WM, dorsal pons during severe hypermethioninemia (also with CBSD)
- PKU & HHcy: Imaging may be normal

CT Findings

- NECT
  - ↓ density cerebral WM, infarct

MR Findings

- T1WI: Variable ↓ signal cerebral WM
- T2WI/FLAIR: ↑ signal affected structures
- DWI: ↓ ADC PVWM reported PKU, HHcy
  - HHcy: ↓ ADC acute infarct, dorsal pons MAT I/IIID
- MRS: PKU: Phe peak 7.37 ppm; Cbl-C: (+) lactate

Imaging Recommendations

- PKU: MR/MRS; HHcy: MR/MRS/MRA

DIFFERENTIAL DIAGNOSIS

Metachromatic Leukodystrophy

- ↑ T2 central cerebral WM with "tigroid" appearance

Periventricular Leukomalacia

- ↑ T2 signal, volume loss PVWM, and positive hypoxia-ischemia history

PATHOLOGY

General Features

- General pathology comments
  - PKU: ↓ phenylalanine hydroxylase (PAH) ⇒ ↑ Phe
    - ↑ Phe toxic to developing brain
  - HHcy: ↑ Hcy ⇒ oxidative stress, ↓ methylation, vascular endothelial damage
- Genetics: Autosomal recessive
  - PKU: > 450 mutations *PAH* gene 12q24.1
  - CBSD: > 100 mutations *CBS* gene 21q22.3
  - MTHFRD: > 50 mutations *MTHFR* gene 1p36.3
  - MAT I/IIID: > 27 mutations *MAT1A* gene 10q22
- Associated abnormalities
  - CBSD: Ectopia lentis, marfanoid, ↓ bone density

CLINICAL ISSUES

Presentation

- Signs/symptoms
  - Untreated PKU: Severe mental retardation
    - Early treated: Subtle cognitive impairments
  - Late-treated CBSD: Mental retardation, thrombosis
  - MTHFRD: Developmental delay, gait difficulties, seizures, psychiatric symptoms > thrombotic events
  - Early-onset Cbl-C (infant): Neurologic, hematologic, renal, GI impairments
    - Late onset: Neurologic deterioration as adult
  - MAT I/IIID: Most normal, rare neurologic signs
- Diagnosis: PKU, CBSD, MAT I/IIID = newborn screen

Demographics

- Epidemiology
  - PKU: 1:8,000 Caucasians in USA (↓ African-Americans)
  - 5-7% population have ↑ Hcy (from all causes)
  - 5-15% Caucasians homozygous *MTHFR* C667T allele

Natural History & Prognosis

- PKU: Strict diet during childhood improves outcome
- Untreated CBSD: 12-27% have thromboembolic event by age 15; 4-23% die by age 30
- MTHFRD/Cbl-C: Significant neurologic impairment, early death if late diagnosis/poor therapy compliance
- MAT I/IIID: Most have normal development

Treatment

- PKU: Phe-free diet begins 1st month of life
- CBSD/MTHFRD: Vit B6, folate, betaine; Cbl-C: IM/IV Vit B12; MAT I/IIID: None typically necessary

SELECTED REFERENCES

1. Castro R et al: Homocysteine metabolism, hyperhomocysteinaemia and vascular disease: an overview. J Inherit Metab Dis. 29(1):3-20, 2006

MEGALENCEPHALY WITH LEUKOENCEPHALOPATHY AND CYSTS (MLC)

Key Facts

Terminology
- Megaloencephalic leukoencephalopathy with subcortical cysts (MLC)
- Inherited leukodystrophy

Imaging
- Swollen white matter
  - Early white matter swelling decreases over time; atrophy ensues
- Subcortical temporal and frontoparietal cysts
- Cysts increase in size and number over time
- No contrast enhancement or reduced diffusion

Pathology
- Genetics
  - Autosomal recessive; gene localized on Chr 22q(tel); 50 different mutations of *MLC1* gene
  - Mutations mostly private mutations
  - Founder effect occurs in population subisolates

Clinical Issues
- Macrocephaly
- Seizures common
- Delayed onset of slow motor deterioration (despite very abnormal MR)
- Even slower cognitive decline
- Cerebellar ataxia
- Pyramidal tract involvement
- Rare disorder, but carrier rate in some communities with high levels of consanguinity as high as 1/40
- Prenatal diagnosis is option in families with known mutations

Diagnostic Checklist
- Consider 1 of "new" leukodystrophies, such as MLC, when imaging features are more severe than metachromatic leukodystrophy

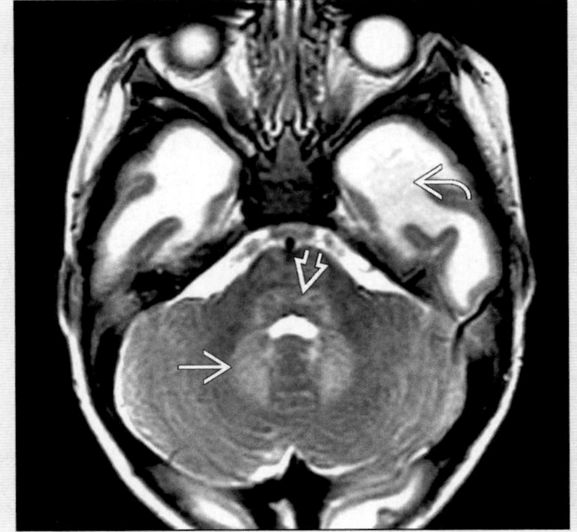

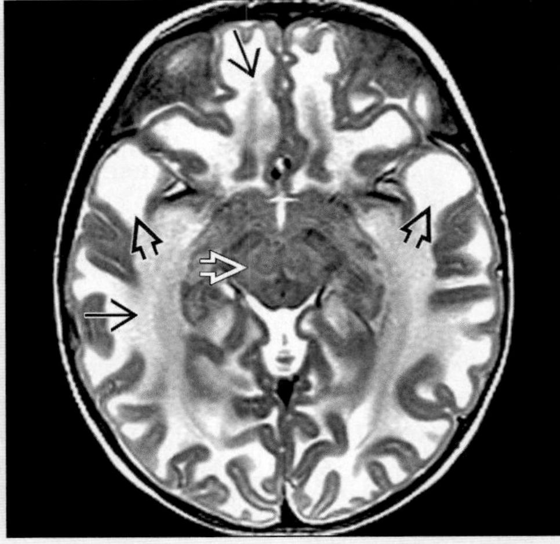

***(Left)** Axial T2WI MR in a 10-month-old infant, with increasing head circumference but normal development, reveals abnormally increased signal intensity of the cerebellar white matter ➡, the dorsal brainstem ➡, and the anterior temporal lobes ➡. **(Right)** Axial T2WI MR in the same infant confirms extensive swelling and increased signal of white matter of the cerebrum ➡ and the white matter tracts ➡ surrounding the red nuclei in the midbrain. Note the anterior temporal lobe cysts ➡.*

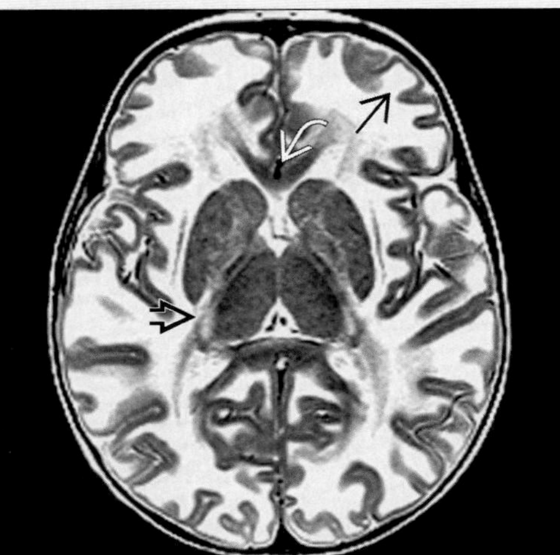

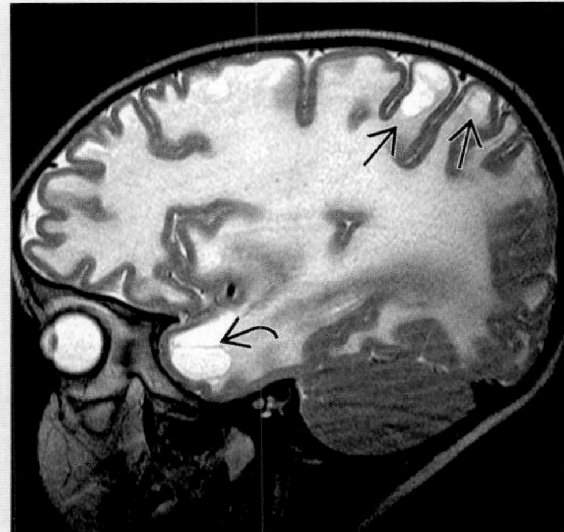

***(Left)** Axial T2WI MR of the same 10-month-old infant reveals sparing (normal myelination) of the corpus callosum ➡, diminished myelination of portions of the posterior limb of the internal capsule ➡, and definitely impaired myelination of the subcortical U-fibers throughout the cerebral hemispheres ➡. **(Right)** Sagittal T2WI MR in the same infant nicely confirms the presence of temporal ➡ and frontoparietal ➡ cysts, as well as extensive hypomyelination.*

MEGALENCEPHALY WITH LEUKOENCEPHALOPATHY AND CYSTS (MLC)

TERMINOLOGY

Abbreviations

- Megaloencephalic leukoencephalopathy with subcortical cysts (MLC)

Synonyms

- Formerly
  - Vacuolating megaloencephalic leukoencephalopathy with benign, slowly progressive course
  - Infantile-onset leukoencephalopathy with swelling and discrepantly mild course
  - van der Knaap disease
    - 1 of many disorders eponymously named after that author
  - Indian Agarwal megaloencephalic leukodystrophy

Definitions

- Inherited leukodystrophy with megalencephaly and large subcortical cysts

IMAGING

General Features

- Best diagnostic clue
  - Swollen white matter (WM)
  - Subcortical cysts
- Location
  - Diffuse WM, includes subcortical U-fibers
    - Subcortical cysts
      - Anterotemporal most common
      - Frontoparietal also common
    - ± involvement of posterior internal capsules, basal ganglia (BG), thalami
    - Cerebellar WM involvement subtle
- Size
  - Cysts increase in size and number over time

CT Findings

- NECT
  - Involved WM ↓ attenuation
- CECT
  - No contrast enhancement

MR Findings

- T1WI
  - Involved WM ↓ signal on T1WI
- T2WI
  - Involved WM ↑ signal on T2WI
    - Cerebral white matter
      - Relative sparing of corpus callosum
    - Posterior 1/3 of posterior limb of internal capsule ± involvement
    - White matter tracts of brainstem ± involvement in very young
- FLAIR
  - Involved WM ↑ signal on FLAIR
  - Subcortical cysts
    - Anterotemporal and frontoparietal most common
    - Cysts approximate CSF signal
- DWI
  - DTI shows ↓ anisotropy, ↑ ADC values
    - Suggests ↓ cell density, ↑ extracellular space
- T1WI C+
  - No contrast enhancement
  - Probably not necessary
- MRS
  - All metabolites ↓ in cystic regions
  - ↓ NAA in WM
  - Normal myoinositol
  - ± lactate signal

Imaging Recommendations

- Best imaging tool
  - MR with MRS
    - ± contrast administration (to exclude enhancing leukodystrophies)

DIFFERENTIAL DIAGNOSIS

Other Leukodystrophies, Nonenhancing

- Metachromatic leukodystrophy (MLD)
  - Look for WM "stripes" on T2WI
- Hypomyelination
- Canavan
  - Subcortical U-fibers involved early
  - Markedly elevated NAA on MRS
- Cree leukoencephalopathy
  - Involvement of WM
  - Deep structures
    - Involves globus pallidus, thalami, medulla
    - Spares olives, red nuclei, and caudate nuclei

Other Leukodystrophies, Enhancing

- Alexander disease
  - Abnormal signal + enhancement of frontal WM and ependymal surfaces
  - Basal nuclei involved
- X-linked adrenoleukodystrophy
  - Abnormal signal and enhancement of peritrigonal WM and splenium

PATHOLOGY

General Features

- Etiology
  - Inborn genetic errors
- Genetics
  - Autosomal recessive; gene localized on Chr 22q(tel)
    - 50 different mutations of *MLC1* gene
    - Mutations distributed along whole gene, types include
      - Splice-site mutations
      - Nonsense mutations
      - Missense mutations
      - Deletions and insertions
    - Mutations identified in 80%; 2nd locus suspected
    - Mutations mostly private mutations
    - Founder effect occurs in population subisolates
- Associated abnormalities
  - *MLC1* in CNS expressed in astrocytic end-feet at blood-brain and CSF-brain barriers
  - *MLC1* also expressed in peripheral white blood cells, spleen

- But no systemic or other organ involvement

Gross Pathologic & Surgical Features

- Spongiform leukoencephalopathy
  - Vacuolization in subcortical white matter

Microscopic Features

- Myelin splitting at intraperiod line
- Vacuolization of outermost lamellae of myelin sheaths

CLINICAL ISSUES

Presentation

- Most common signs/symptoms
  - Macrocephaly at birth or within 1st year of life
  - Delayed onset of slow motor deterioration (even slower cognitive decline) despite very abnormal MR
- Other signs/symptoms
  - Rare early presentation with developmental delay
  - Rare transient coma following minor head trauma
- Clinical profile
  - Macrocephaly
  - Very slow cognitive decline
    - Although learning problems in 50%
  - Cerebellar ataxia and pyramidal tract involvement
  - Motor deterioration
    - Late loss of ability to walk
    - Occasional delayed autonomous walking
  - Seizures common

Demographics

- Age
  - Macrocephaly before 1 year of age
- Ethnicity
  - Increased in population isolates
    - Common *MLC* mutations in
      - Specific Indian community (Agarwal)
      - Libyan Jewish community
      - Turkish community
      - Some Japanese families due to founder effect
    - Agarwal community mutation
      - Insertion (c.135_136insC) usual, phenotypic variation occurs
- Epidemiology
  - Rare
  - Carrier rate in some communities with high levels of consanguinity as high as 1/40

Natural History & Prognosis

- Early white matter swelling
  - Swelling decreases over time
  - Atrophy ensues
- Clinical features progress slowly

Treatment

- Treat symptoms (seizures, spasticity)
- Prenatal diagnosis is option in families with known mutations

DIAGNOSTIC CHECKLIST

Consider

- 1 of "new" leukodystrophies when imaging involvement more severe than metachromatic leukodystrophy

Image Interpretation Pearls

- Always enhance unknown leukoencephalopathy

Reporting Tips

- Differentiation from MLD
  - Involvement of subcortical U-fibers
  - Subcortical cysts
- Differentiate from Canavan
  - No basal ganglia involvement in MLC
  - Normal NAA in MLC

SELECTED REFERENCES

1. Duarri A et al: Molecular pathogenesis of megalencephalic leukoencephalopathy with subcortical cysts: mutations in MLC1 cause folding defects. Hum Mol Genet. 17(23):3728-39, 2008
2. Miles L et al: Megalencephalic Leukoencephalopathy with Subcortical Cysts (MLC): a third confirmed case with literature review. Pediatr Dev Pathol. Epub ahead of print, 2008
3. Shukla P et al: Prenatal diagnosis of megalencephalic leukodystrophy. Prenat Diagn. 28(4):357-9, 2008
4. Boor I et al: MLC1 is associated with the dystrophin-glycoprotein complex at astrocytic endfeet. Acta Neuropathol. 114(4):403-10, 2007
5. Kiriyama T et al: SPECT revealed cortical dysfunction in a patient who had genetically definite megalencephalic leukoencephalopathy with subcortical cysts. Clin Neurol Neurosurg. 109(6):526-30, 2007
6. Teijido O et al: Expression patterns of MLC1 protein in the central and peripheral nervous systems. Neurobiol Dis. 26(3):532-45, 2007
7. Ilja Boor PK et al: Megalencephalic leukoencephalopathy with subcortical cysts: an update and extended mutation analysis of MLC1. Hum Mutat. 27(6):505-12, 2006
8. Morita H et al: MR imaging and 1H-MR spectroscopy of a case of van der Knaap disease. Brain Dev. 28(7):466-9, 2006
9. Schiffmann R et al: The latest on leukodystrophies. Curr Opin Neurol. 17(2):187-92, 2004
10. Brockmann K et al: Megalencephalic leukoencephalopathy with subcortical cysts in an adult: quantitative proton MR spectroscopy and diffusion tensor MRI. Neuroradiology. 45(3):137-42, 2003
11. De Stefano N et al: Severe metabolic abnormalities in the white matter of patients with vacuolating megalencephalic leukoencephalopathy with subcortical cysts. A proton MR spectroscopic imaging study. J Neurol. 248(5):403-9, 2001
12. Leegwater PA et al: Mutations of MLC1 (KIAA0027), encoding a putative membrane protein, cause megalencephalic leukoencephalopathy with subcortical cysts. Am J Hum Genet. 68(4):831-8, 2001
13. van der Knaap MS et al: Defining and categorizing leukoencephalopathies of unknown origin: MR imaging approach. Radiology. 213(1):121-33, 1999
14. van der Knaap MS et al: Histopathology of an infantile-onset spongiform leukoencephalopathy with a discrepantly mild clinical course. Acta Neuropathol. 92(2):206-12, 1996

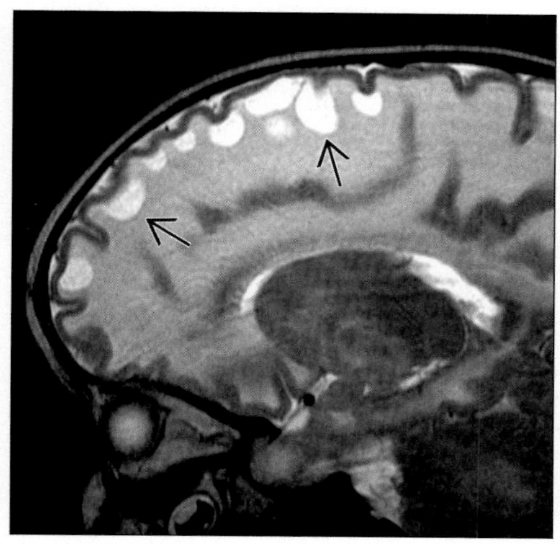

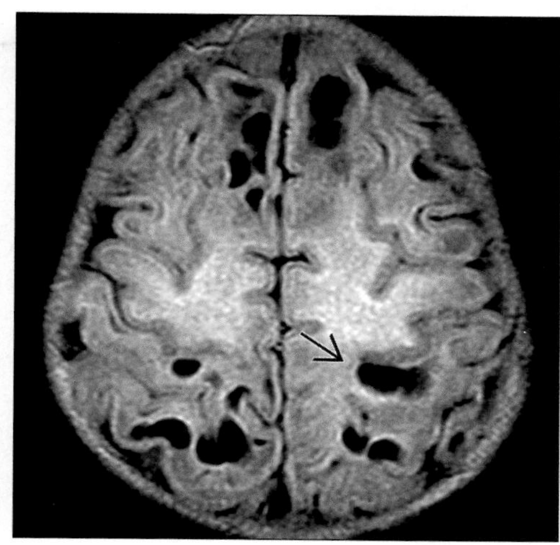

(Left) *Sagittal T2WI MR in a 2-year-old patient with megalencephaly and slowing of acquisition of developmental milestones shows swollen white matter, as well as fairly extensive subcortical cysts → involving the frontal lobe.* ***(Right)*** *Axial FLAIR MR in the same 2-year-old patient shows white matter with abnormally high signal intensity due to hypomyelination, as well as extensive, bilateral, frontal and frontoparietal subcortical cysts →.*

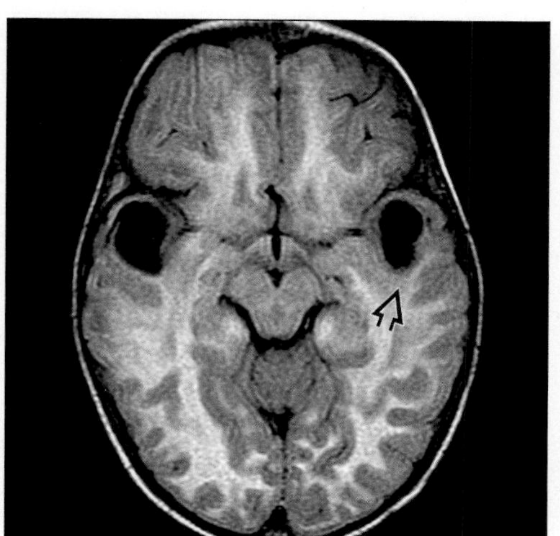

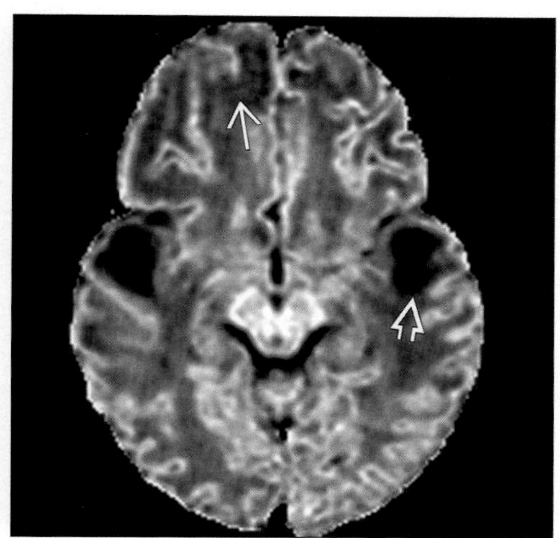

(Left) *Axial FLAIR MR in a 22-month-old child with macrocephaly and decreasing acquisition of developmental milestones shows large, bilateral temporal lobe cysts ⇨, typical of MLC, on a background of swollen, abnormally hyperintense white matter.* ***(Right)*** *Axial DWI MR in the same 22-month-old infant confirms markedly increased diffusivity in the cysts ⇨ and, less dramatically, in the subcortical white matter →.*

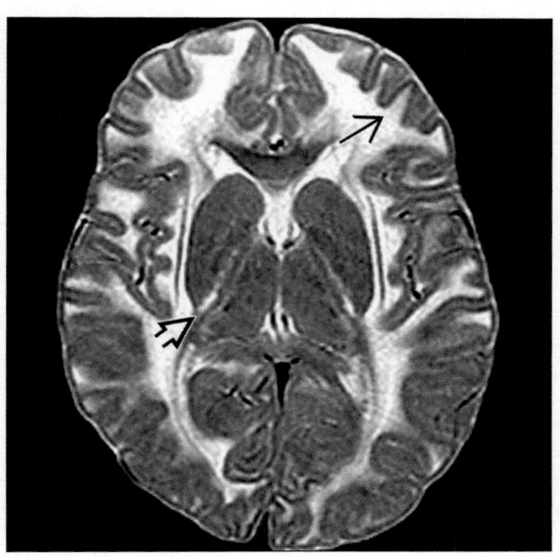

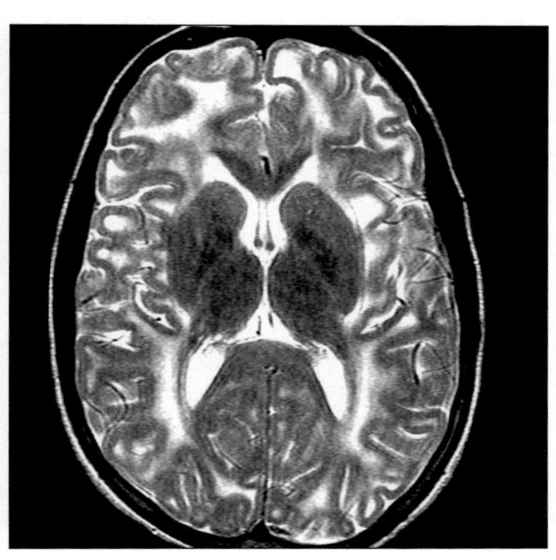

(Left) *Axial T2WI MR in a 6-year-old child with MLC shows less pronounced white matter swelling, although the posterior limbs of the internal capsules ⇨ and subcortical U-fibers → show persistence of abnormal signal hyperintensity.* ***(Right)*** *Axial T2WI MR in a 14-year-old patient with MLC demonstrates sulcal widening due to atrophy, a common finding as the disease progresses. Note the persistent hyperintensity of the cerebral white matter with involvement of the subcortical U-fibers.*

NEURODEGENERATION WITH BRAIN IRON ACCUMULATION (NBIA)

Key Facts

Terminology
- Group of extrapyramidal neurodegenerative disorders with brain iron accumulation
  - PKAN (*PANK2* mutation)
  - INAD (*PLA2G6* mutation)
  - Neuroferritinopathy (*FTL* mutation)
  - Aceruloplasminemia (*CP* mutation)
  - Idiopathic NBIA (mutation unknown)

Imaging
- Consider MR with T2* (gradient echo) or susceptibility weighted imaging (SWI)
- Globus pallidus T2 hypointensity with central hyperintensity of GP: "Eye of the tiger" sign
  - Specific to classic PKAN (*PANK2* mutations)
  - May also be seen in neuroferritinopathy
- GP ± SN, DN, cortex, striatum, & thalamus T2 dark without "eye of the tiger" = other NBIA
- Globus pallidus normally hypointense on T2 at 3T or above!

Pathology
- Iron directly causes or facilitates cellular injury, or is a consequence of axonal disruption

Clinical Issues
- PKAN: Classic < 6 years, atypical during teenage years
- INAD: Classic < 2 years, atypical at 4-6 years
- Aceruloplasminemia and neuroferritinopathy: Mean age 40 years

Diagnostic Checklist
- T2 hypointensity of globus pallidus in patient with movement disorder

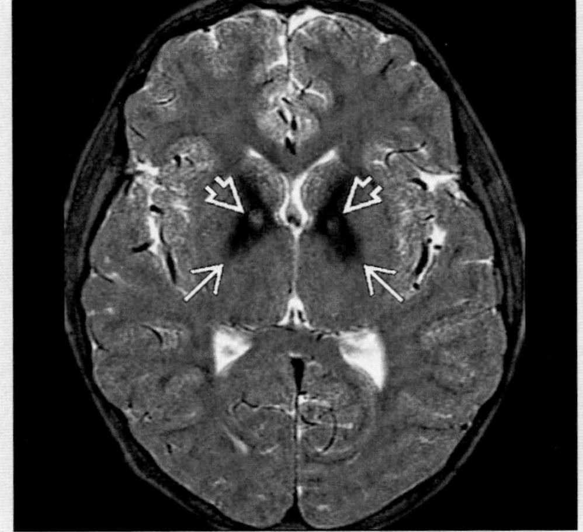
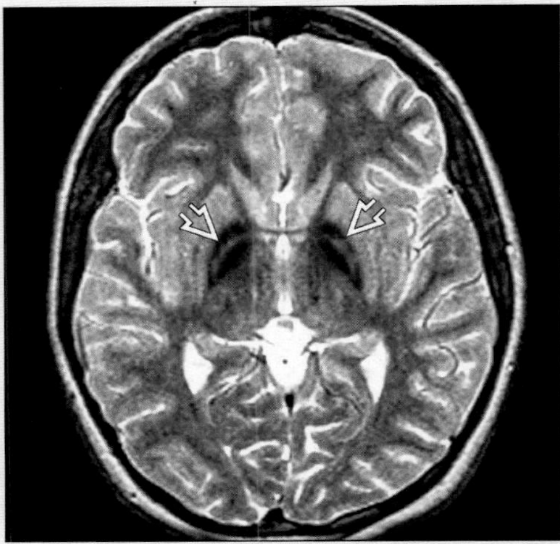

(Left) *Axial T2WI FS MR shows classic imaging of PKAN (Hallervorden-Spatz syndrome), which is within the spectrum of NBIA. Note the globus pallidi hypointensity ➔ related to iron deposition with central hyperintensity ➔, consistent with the "eye of the tiger" sign, highly specific for the PANK2 mutation.* ***(Right)*** *Axial T2WI MR shows symmetric hypointensity within the globus pallidi ➔. The "eye of the tiger" sign is absent; therefore, this is not PKAN. These findings are characteristic of NBIA.*

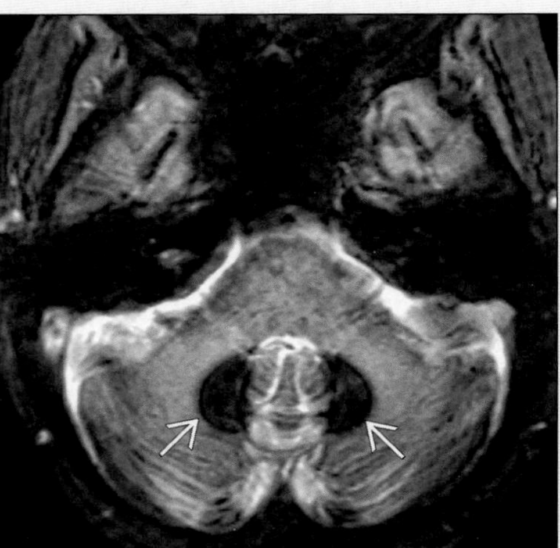
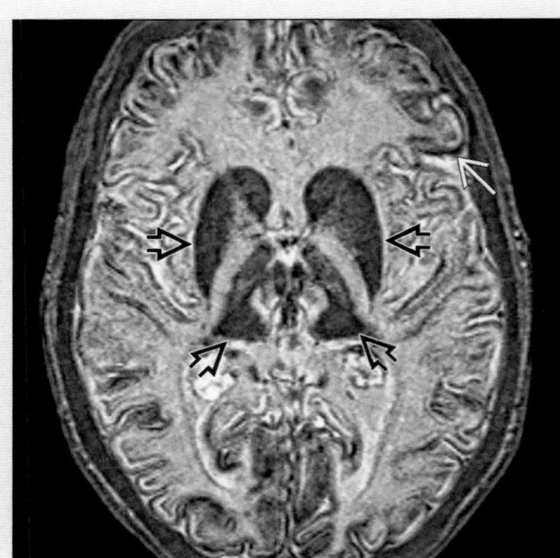

(Left) *Axial T2* GRE MR shows marked hypointensity related to iron deposition in the dentate nuclei ➔ of the cerebellum in this patient with aceruloplasminemia. Aceruloplasminemia and neuroferritinopathy occur in adults and have a similar imaging appearance.* ***(Right)*** *Axial T2* SWI MR in the same patient shows diffuse linear hypointensity in the cortex ➔ with marked "blooming" in the basal ganglia and thalami ➔ related to iron deposition. Substantia nigra involvement is also typical.*

NEURODEGENERATION WITH BRAIN IRON ACCUMULATION (NBIA)

TERMINOLOGY

Abbreviations

- Pantothenate kinase-associated neurodegeneration (PKAN)
- Infantile neuroaxonal dystrophy (INAD)
- Neurodegeneration with brain iron accumulation (NBIA)

Synonyms

- Formerly known as Hallervorden-Spatz disease

Definitions

- Group of extrapyramidal neurodegenerative disorders
  - All characterized by abnormal brain Fe accumulation
  - Includes PKAN, INAD, aceruloplasminemia, etc.

IMAGING

General Features

- Best diagnostic clue
  - T2 hypointensity in globus pallidus (GP)
- Location
  - PKAN and INAD
    - GP, substantia nigra (SN), ± dentate nuclei (DN)
  - Neuroferritinopathy and aceruloplasminemia
    - GP, SN, DN, cortex, striatum, and thalamus

Imaging Recommendations

- Best imaging tool
  - MR with T2* (gradient echo) or susceptibility weighted imaging (SWI)

CT Findings

- NECT
  - Cerebral and cerebellar atrophy in non-*PANK2* NBIA

MR Findings

- T2WI
  - GP hypointensity with central hyperintensity of GP interna: "Eye of the tiger" sign
    - Specific to classic PKAN (*PANK2* mutations)
    - Can see only T2 hyperintensity early in disease
    - May also be seen in neuroferritinopathy
  - GP, ± SN, DN, cortex, striatum, and thalamus dark without "eye of the tiger" = other NBIA
  - GP normally hypointense on T2 at 3T or above!
- T2* GRE
  - Accentuation of hypointense T2 findings
- Imaging findings do not always correlate with clinical symptoms

DIFFERENTIAL DIAGNOSIS

Normal Iron Deposition

- Imaging at 3T
- Seen in normal aging process

Parkinson and Alzheimer Diseases

- No "eye of the tiger"; older patients

Multiple Sclerosis

- Iron accumulation in basal ganglia associated with MS
- Should have other classic demyelinating lesions

Superficial Siderosis

- Iron overload from transfusions or recurrent CNS hemorrhage

Hemochromatosis

- Liver and spleen usually affected before CNS

PATHOLOGY

General Features

- Genetics
  - Autosomal recessive *PANK2*, *PLA2G6*, and *CP*
  - Autosomal dominant *FTL* mutation

Gross Pathologic & Surgical Features

- Iron accumulation, rust brown pigmentation

Microscopic Features

- Iron accumulation in GP and SN, neuronal loss, axonal swellings ("spheroids")
- "Eye of the tiger " may represent cystic degeneration
- Neurofibrillary tangles and Lewy bodies suggest shared pathway with Alzheimer and Parkinson diseases

CLINICAL ISSUES

Presentation

- Most common signs/symptoms
  - Ataxia, dysarthria, dystonia
  - Retinal degeneration and optic atrophy
- Other signs/symptoms
  - Aceruloplasminemia: Adult onset triad of diabetes, retinal degeneration, and movement disorder
  - Neuroferritinopathy: Adult onset chorea or dystonia

Demographics

- Age
  - PKAN: Classic < 6 years, teenage atypical
  - INAD: Classic < 2 years, 4-6 years atypical
  - Adult onset NBIA: Mean age = 40 years

Natural History & Prognosis

- PKAN & INAD: Death is variable, usually from secondary causes such as malnutrition & aspiration
- Adult onset NBIA: Progressive motor decline

Treatment

- Symptom palliation: Medications and deep brain stimulator
- Aceruloplasminemia: Iron chelation with desferrioxamine and ceruloplasmin from fresh frozen plasma

SELECTED REFERENCES

1. Gregory A et al: Clinical and genetic delineation of neurodegeneration with brain iron accumulation. J Med Genet. 46(2):73-80, 2009

PKAN

Key Facts

Terminology

- Pantothenate kinase-associated neurodegeneration (PKAN)
  - Most common form of neurodegeneration with brain iron accumulation (NBIA)
  - Caused by mutation pantothenate kinase 2 gene (*PANK2*)

Imaging

- Best diagnostic clue: "Eye of the tiger" sign = diffuse pallidal T2 hypointensity with medial foci ↑ T2 signal
  - Highly suggestive of PKAN

Top Differential Diagnoses

- Disorders with ↑ T2 signal globus pallidus
  - Metabolic: Methylmalonic acidemia, Kearns-Sayre, L-2-Hydroxyglutaric aciduria, Canavan, neuroferritinopathy
  - Ischemic/toxic: Anoxic encephalopathy, carbon monoxide/cyanide poisoning, kernicterus

Clinical Issues

- Classic PKAN: Dystonia, dysarthria, rigidity, choreoathetosis in young child
- Atypical PKAN: Psychiatric, speech, pyramidal/extrapyramidal disturbances in older child/teenager
- Epidemiology: Rare; incidence unknown
- Prognosis
  - Classic PKAN: Fatal; mean disease duration after symptom onset is 11 years
  - Atypical PKAN: Eventual severe impairment/death
- No curative treatment

__(Left)__ Axial T2WI MR in a 5 year old with a diagnosis of "cerebral palsy" demonstrates an "eye of the tiger" sign typical of PKAN: Symmetric areas of high T2 signal ➔ within the medial globus pallidus with surrounding pallidal hypointensity. __(Right)__ Four years later, dystonia prompted repeat MR imaging in the same patient. Axial T2WI MR shows that the "eyes" have diminished in size and intensity with greater surrounding pallidal hypointensity. Volume loss is now evident, particularly frontal.

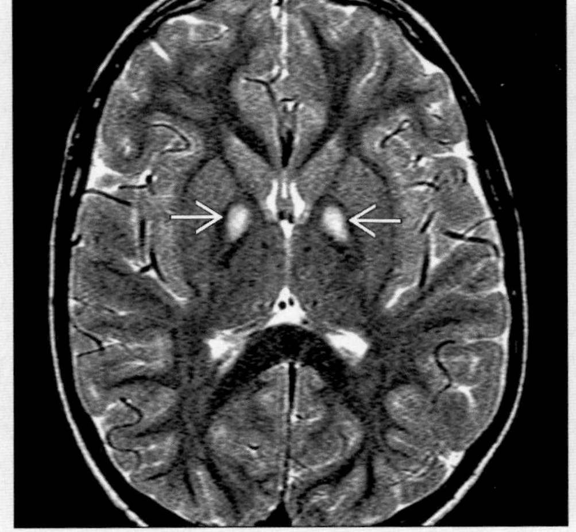

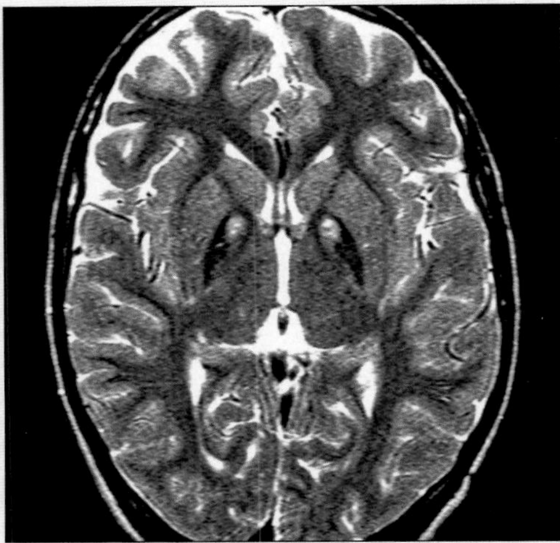

__(Left)__ Coronal T2WI MR of same patient at 9 years old shows abnormal hypointense signal in the globus pallidus ➔ and substantia nigra ➔. __(Right)__ Axial T2 GRE MR in same patient at 9 years old shows "blooming" of hypointense signal in the globus pallidus secondary to the paramagnetic effect of iron. The findings in this patient are typical of the evolution of classic PKAN: Diminishing caliber of the "eye," increasing surrounding pallidal hypointensity, and progressive volume loss.*

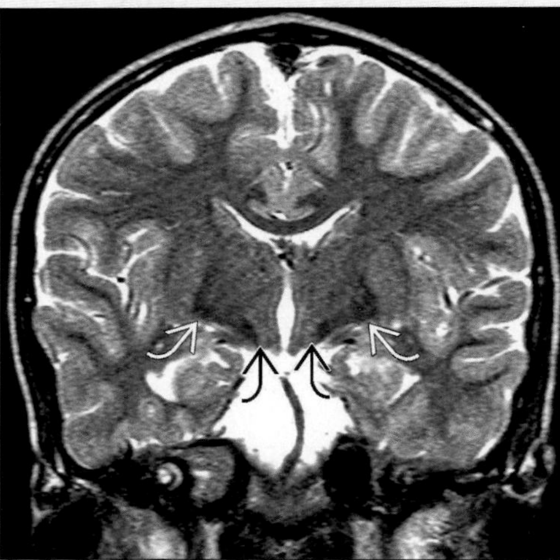

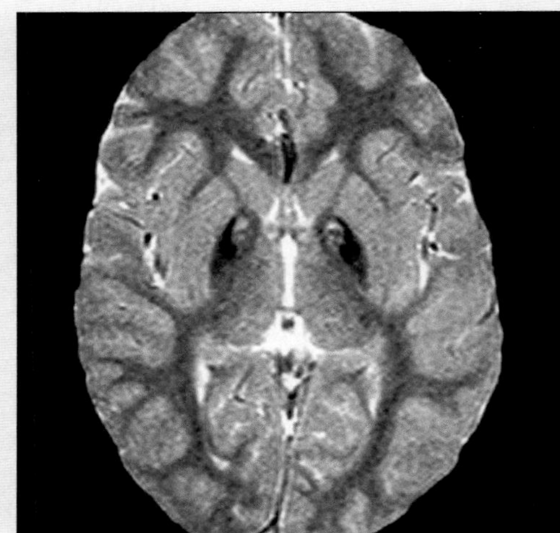

TERMINOLOGY

Abbreviations

- Pantothenate kinase-associated neurodegeneration (PKAN)

Synonyms

- Neurodegeneration with brain iron accumulation type 1 (NBIA-1)
- Hallervorden-Spatz syndrome
  - PKAN and NBIA-1 preferred terms

Definitions

- Neurodegeneration with brain iron accumulation (NBIA) = umbrella term for neurodegenerative disorders characterized by brain iron accumulation
  - Known causes include PKAN (most common), aceruloplasminemia, neuroferritinopathy, and infantile neuroaxonal dystrophy
- PKAN caused by mutation pantothenate kinase 2 gene (*PANK2*)

IMAGING

General Features

- Best diagnostic clue: "Eye of the tiger" sign = diffuse pallidal T2 hypointensity with medial foci ↑ T2 signal
  - Highly suggestive of PKAN
  - Hyperintense "eye" may predate surrounding pallidal hypointensity
  - "Eye" caliber & intensity ↓ as disease progresses
  - Pallidal hypointensity increases as disease progresses
  - "Eye of the tiger" sign has been described in neuroferritinopathy
- Variable ↓ T2 signal substantia nigra > > dentate nuclei
- Atrophy in advanced diseases
- Location: Globus pallidus (GP), substantia nigra (SN), dentate nuclei (DN)
- Morphology: Signal alteration of globus pallidus resembles tiger eyes
- Iron deposition (ferritin-bound) responsible for T2 hypointense imaging appearance

CT Findings

- NECT: Variable; hypodense, hyperdense, normal GP
- CECT: No abnormal enhancement

MR Findings

- T1WI: Variable (ferritin-bound iron has > T1 shortening than hemosiderin-bound)
- T2WI
  - "Eye of the tiger" sign = diffuse pallidal hypointensity with medial foci ↑ signal
  - Variable ↓ signal SN; more common in older patients
- FLAIR: "Eye" persists
- T2* GRE: ↓ T2 signal GP, SN "blooms" due to paramagnetic effect iron
- Susceptibility weighted imaging (SWI): Greater "blooming" artifact than T2* GRE
- T1WI C+: No abnormal enhancement
- MRS: ↓ NAA GP (neuronal loss)

Nuclear Medicine Findings

- Tc-99m SPECT: ↑ activity in medial GP
  - Possible chelation Tc-99m by pallidal cysteine

Imaging Recommendations

- Best imaging tool
  - MR
- Protocol advice
  - Consider SWI or T2* GRE sequence for mineralization
  - T2 hypointensity more conspicuous on spin-echo (vs. fast spin-echo) and high field strength magnets

DIFFERENTIAL DIAGNOSIS

Disorders with ↑ T2 Signal Globus Pallidus

- Metabolic
  - Methylmalonic acidemia (MMA): ↑ T2 signal GP ± periventricular white matter (WM)
  - Kearns-Sayre/L-2-Hydroxyglutaric aciduria: ↑ T2 GP (> than other deep gray) and peripheral WM
  - Canavan: ↑ T2 GP (> than other deep gray) and subcortical WM; macrocephaly; ↑ ↑ NAA
  - Neuroferritinopathy: Variable-sized foci ↑ T2 signal GP, putamen, caudate heads with ↓ T2 SN, DN; disease of adults
- Ischemic/toxic
  - Anoxic encephalopathy: ↑ T2 GP (and other deep gray) and cortex
  - Carbon monoxide poisoning: ↑ T2 GP (± other deep gray, cortex, WM)
  - Cyanide poisoning: ↑ T2 basal ganglia followed by hemorrhagic necrosis
  - Kernicterus: ↑ T2/T1 globus pallidus in neonate

PATHOLOGY

General Features

- Iron accumulation likely secondary phenomenon in PKAN
  - Serial MRs in PKAN patients show hyperintense foci in GP predating surrounding hypointensity
- Embryology, anatomy
  - Progressive, physiologic brain iron accumulation occurs in GP, SN > red and dentate nuclei
  - ↓ T2 signal GP identified in majority of normal patients by age ≥ 25, but never before age 10
- Genetics
  - Autosomal recessive (50% sporadic)
  - > 100 *PANK2* mutations chr 20p12.3-p13 identified
    - MR "eye of the tiger" sign highly correlative with *PANK2* mutation
    - *PANK2* gene encodes mitochondrial-targeted pantothenate kinase 2, key enzyme in biosynthesis of coenzyme A (CoA)
      - CoA essential to energy and fatty acid metabolism, among other functions
    - Null mutations are more common in early onset, rapidly progressive disease
    - Missense mutations more common in late onset, more slowly progressive disease

- Suggests residual pantothenate kinase 2 activity in late onset (less severe) disease
  - HARP: **H**ypoprebetalipoproteinemia, **a**canthocytosis, **r**etinitis pigmentosa, and **p**allidal degeneration
    - Allelic with PKAN
    - Prominent orofacial dystonia; early onset parkinsonism
- Etiology
  - Leading theory
    - *PANK2* mutation → CoA deficiency → energy and lipid dyshomeostasis → production of oxygen free radicals → phospholipid membrane destruction
    - Basal ganglia and retina vulnerable to oxidative damage secondary to high metabolic demand
  - Additional factors
    - Cysteine accumulation in GP secondary to ↓ phosphopantothenate causes iron chelation and peroxidative cell membrane damage
    - Axonal spheroids further compromise glial and neuronal function

Gross Pathologic & Surgical Features

- Symmetric, rust-brown pigmentation GP (interna > externa), and pars reticulata SN
  - In addition to iron, intra-/extraneuronal ceroid lipofuscin and melanin contribute to pigmentation
- Variable atrophy

Microscopic Features

- Classic features
  - ↑ ↑ iron GP interna and pars reticulata SN
    - Iron located in astrocytes, microglial cells, neurons, and around vessels
  - Neuronal loss, gliosis, and glial inclusions primarily involving GP interna and pars reticulata SN
  - Round or oval, non-nucleated, axonal swellings ("spheroids") in GP, SN, cortex, and brainstem
- "Loose" tissue (consisting of reactive astrocytes, dystrophic axons, and vacuoles in anteromedial GP) corresponds to "eye" in "eye of the tiger" sign on MR
- Variably present acanthocytes (on blood smear)

CLINICAL ISSUES

Presentation

- Clinical classification into classic and atypical disease
  - Classic PKAN: Early onset; more rapidly progressive disease; uniform phenotype
  - Atypical PKAN: Late onset; more slowly progressive disease; heterogeneous phenotype
- Most common signs/symptoms
  - Classic PKAN: Dystonia
    - Other extrapyramidal signs/symptoms: Dysarthria, rigidity, choreoathetosis
    - Upper motor neuron signs/symptoms and cognitive decline are frequent
    - Pigmentary retinopathy (66%)
  - Atypical PKAN: Psychiatric and speech disturbances
    - Other signs/symptoms: Pyramidal/extrapyramidal disturbances (including freezing), dementia
- Clinical profile
  - Classic PKAN: Young child with gait, postural deficits
  - Atypical PKAN: Teenager with speech, psychiatric disturbance
- Normal serum and CSF iron levels
- Confirmatory *PANK2* mutation analysis should be performed in all suspected cases of PKAN

Demographics

- Age
  - Classic PKAN: Majority present before 6 years of age
  - Atypical PKAN: Mean age at presentation is 13 years
- Epidemiology: Rare; incidence unknown

Natural History & Prognosis

- Natural History
  - Classic PKAN: Rapid, nonuniform progression with periods of deterioration interspersed with stability, leading to early adulthood death
  - Atypical PKAN: More slowly progressive with loss of ambulation 15-40 years after disease onset
- Prognosis
  - Classic PKAN: Fatal; mean disease duration after symptom onset is 11 years
  - Atypical PKAN: Eventual severe impairment, ± death, adulthood

Treatment

- No curative treatment; iron chelation ineffective
- Palliative therapy
  - Baclofen, trihexyphenidyl frequently ineffective
  - Stereotactic pallidotomy
  - Promising initial results with pallidal deep brain stimulation

DIAGNOSTIC CHECKLIST

Image Interpretation Pearls

- "Eye of the tiger" sign highly suggestive of PKAN
- Physiologic GP hypointensity difficult to distinguish from pathologic hypointensity in teenager/adult

SELECTED REFERENCES

1. Gregory A et al: Clinical and genetic delineation of neurodegeneration with brain iron accumulation. J Med Genet. 46(2):73-80, 2009
2. Mikati MA et al: Deep brain stimulation as a mode of treatment of early onset pantothenate kinase-associated neurodegeneration. Eur J Paediatr Neurol. 13(1):61-4, 2009
3. McNeill A et al: T2* and FSE MRI distinguishes four subtypes of neurodegeneration with brain iron accumulation. Neurology. 70(18):1614-9, 2008
4. Hayflick SJ et al: Brain MRI in neurodegeneration with brain iron accumulation with and without PANK2 mutations. AJNR Am J Neuroradiol. 27(6):1230-3, 2006
5. Hayflick SJ. Related Articles et al: Unraveling the Hallervorden-Spatz syndrome: pantothenate kinase-associated neurodegeneration is the name. Curr Opin Pediatr. 15(6):572-7, 2003
6. Dooling EC et al: Hallervorden-Spatz syndrome. Arch Neurol. 30(1):70-83, 1974

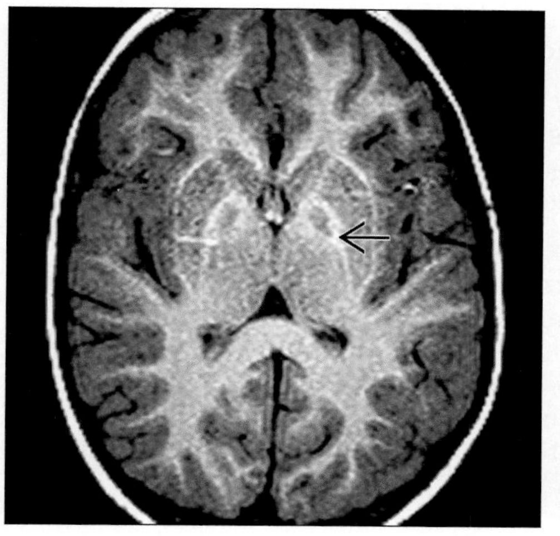

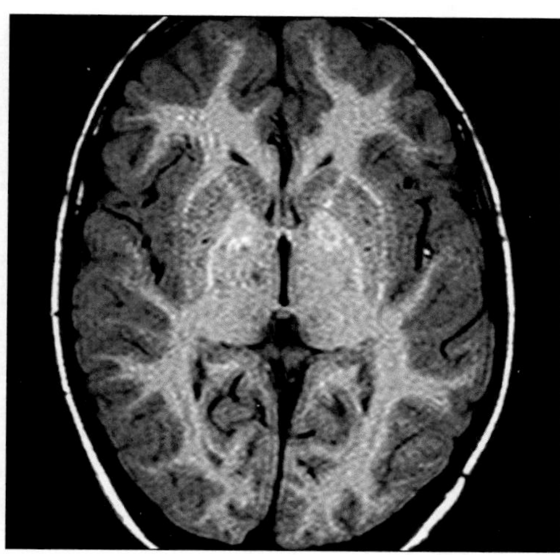

(Left) *Axial T1WI MR in a 5 year old with classic PKAN. The "eye" in the "eye of the tiger" is hypointense with few punctate areas of surrounding hyperintensity ➔.* ***(Right)*** *Axial T1WI MR in the same patient at 9 years of age shows that the "eye" has become mostly hyperintense. The appearance of the "eye" in "eye of the tiger" is variable depending on the stage of the disease. Progressive iron deposition within the globus pallidus likely accounts for greater T1 shortening seen in later disease.*

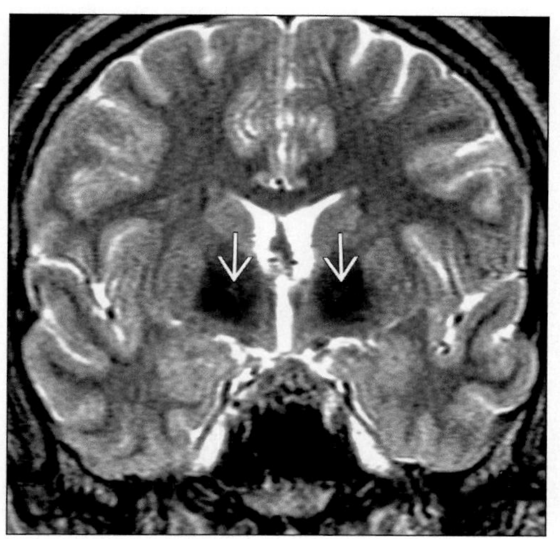

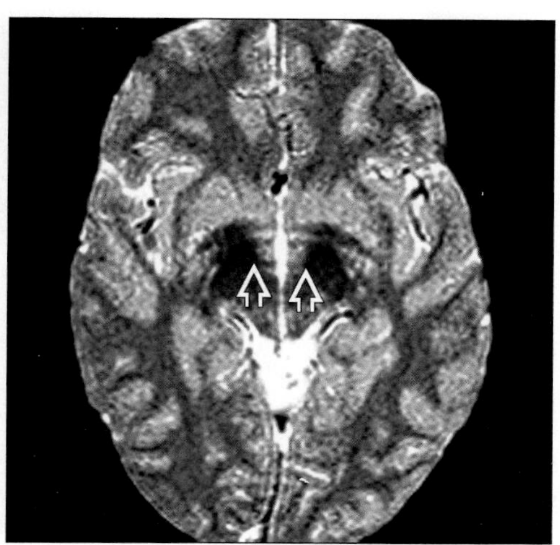

(Left) *Coronal T2WI MR in a patient with classic PKAN shows the classic "eye of the tiger" sign with small foci of increased T2 signal in the medial globi pallidi ➔ surrounded by abnormal pallidal hypointensity.* ***(Right)*** *Axial T2* GRE MR in a patient with classic PKAN shows "blooming" of hypointense signal in the inferior globus pallidus and substantia nigra ➔. Abnormal iron accumulation within the substantia nigra is more conspicuous on imaging as the disease progresses.*

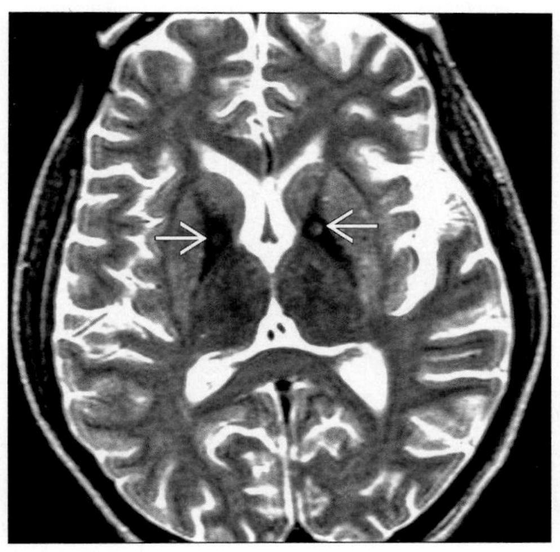

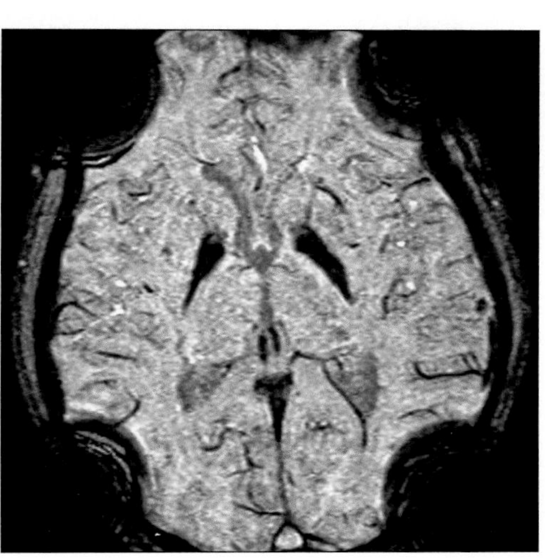

(Left) *Axial T2WI MR in a 12 year old with advanced classic PKAN undergoing preoperative imaging for pallidotomies. Globi pallidi are hypointense and atrophic with subtle "eye of the tiger" signs ➔. Note also the diffuse volume loss.* ***(Right)*** *Axial SWI in the same patient shows "blooming" of hypointense signal within the globi pallidi. The "eyes of the tiger" are no longer seen, obscured by the "blooming" effect. SWI is more sensitive than T2* GRE due to magnetic susceptibility effects.*

HUNTINGTON DISEASE

Key Facts

Terminology

- Autosomal dominant neurodegenerative disease
  - Loss of GABAergic neurons of basal ganglia (BG)

Imaging

- Diffuse cerebral atrophy
- Atrophy of caudate nucleus → frontal horns enlarged
- ↑ CC/IT ratio (bicaudate ratio)
  - Shrinkage of CN and ↑ CC
  - Increased intercaudate distance (CC) between medial aspects of CN
  - Most specific & sensitive measure for HD
- Hyperintense signal in CN, putamina in juvenile HD
- ↓ FDG uptake in BG before any detectable atrophy
- ± frontal lobe hypometabolism

Top Differential Diagnoses

- Leigh disease
- Wilson disease
- Pantothenate kinase-associated neurodegeneration (formerly called Hallervorden-Spatz)
- Carbon monoxide poisoning

Pathology

- Autosomal dominant with complete penetrance
- CAG trinucleotide repeat disease affecting HD gene on chromosome 4p16.3

Diagnostic Checklist

- Rule out reversible dementias, movement disorders
- Caudate atrophy is main radiologic feature of HD
- ↑ bicaudate diameter: Sensitive for CN atrophy
- Decline in size of GP, putamen correlates with disease progression
- Consider HD in child with ↑ signal in CN/putamina on PD-/T2WI

*(**Left**) Axial graphic shows the convex margins of the frontal horns ➡ due to atrophy of the heads of the caudate nuclei. (**Right**) Axial T2WI MR in a patient with juvenile Huntington disease shows generalized volume loss and striking atrophy and hyperintensity ➡ of both caudate nuclei. The frontal horns of the lateral ventricles are enlarged, and there is atrophy and hyperintensity in the putamina ↪.*

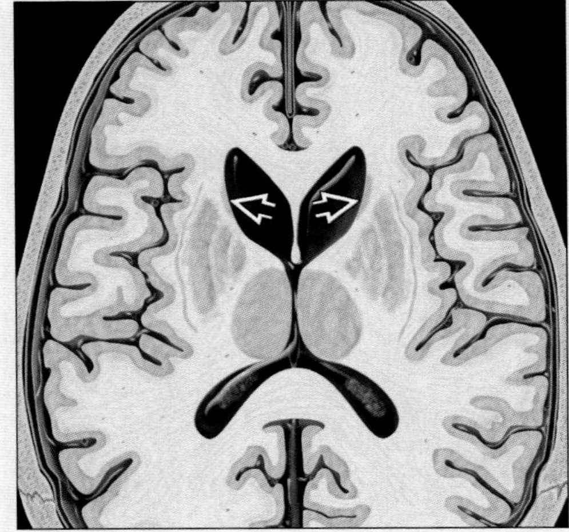

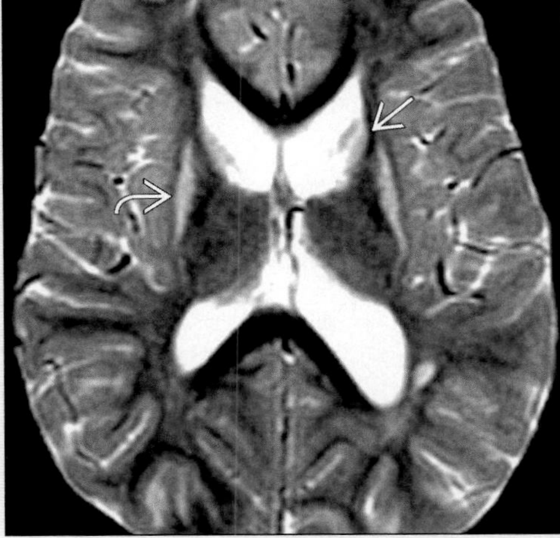

*(**Left**) Autopsy specimen sectioned in the coronal plane shows enlarged lateral ventricles ➡ and basal cisterns ↪. Both caudate nuclei → appear thinned and atrophic. (**Right**) Coronal CECT, cut in same plane to correspond to the autopsy specimen in the previous image, shows straightening of the lateral borders of the lateral ventricles due to caudate atrophy and increased intercaudate (CC) distance ➡, which are characteristic findings of Huntington disease.*

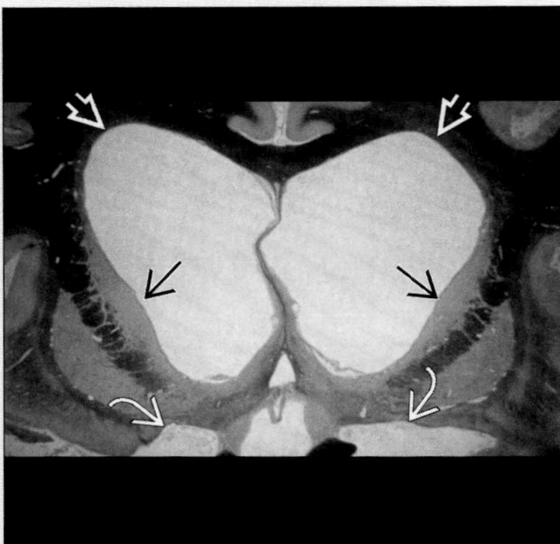

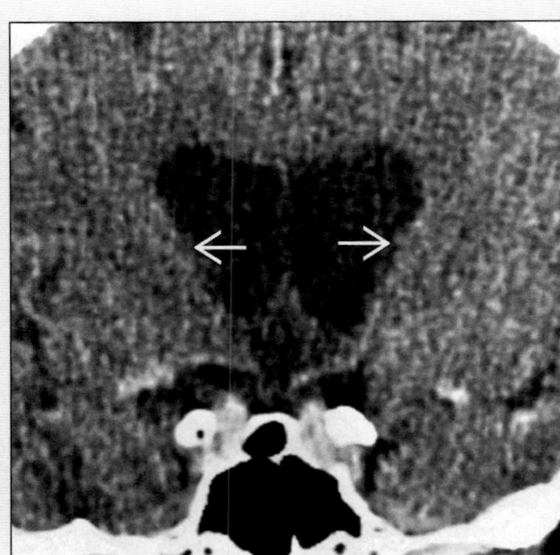

HUNTINGTON DISEASE

TERMINOLOGY

Abbreviations
- Huntington disease (HD)

Synonyms
- Huntington chorea

Definitions
- Autosomal dominant neurodegenerative disease
  - Loss of GABAergic neurons of basal ganglia (BG)
- Clinical triad: Early onset dementia, choreoathetosis, psychosis

IMAGING

General Features
- Best diagnostic clue
  - Atrophy of caudate nucleus (CN) → frontal horns enlarged
- Location
  - Primarily striatum (especially CN, putamen)
  - Cerebral cortex, globus pallidus (GP), thalamus
  - Substantia nigra (SN), brainstem
- Size
  - Decreased caudate nucleus size
- Morphology
  - Loss of convex surface of caudate head

CT Findings
- NECT
  - Atrophy of CN, putamen, and (lesser degree) GP
  - Compensatory enlargement of frontal horns of lateral ventricles
  - Diffuse cerebral atrophy (reported to be predominantly frontal in some studies)
  - CN atrophy is measured on axial images at level of 3rd ventricle
    - Increased intercaudate distance (CC) between medial aspects of CN
    - CC can be compared with distance between inner tables (IT) of skull (CC to IT ratio)
    - In HD, CC is typically > 20 mm & often > 25 mm (compared to 10-14 mm in normal individuals)
    - CC to IT (bicaudate) ratio ↑ in HD; considered most specific & sensitive HD measurement
    - In HD, CC to IT ratio usually ranges from 0.175-0.185 compared to approximately 0.12 in normal individuals
    - CC compared with distance across lateral margins of frontal horns (FH) provides FH to CC ratio
    - In HD, FH to CC ratio typically ranges from 1.3-1.8 compared to 2.3-2.8 in normal individuals
- CECT
  - No contrast enhancement of affected structures

MR Findings
- T1WI
  - Shrinkage of CN and increased CC
  - MR measurements: ↓ volume in all BG structures
    - Reported even in presymptomatic stage of HD
  - Diffuse cerebral atrophy
- T2WI
  - Hyperintense signal in CN, putamina in juvenile HD
    - Related to gliosis
  - Shrinkage of CN; ↑ CC
  - Striatum may have ↓ signal due to iron deposition
- MRS
  - ↑ lactate concentration in occipital cortex of symptomatic HD, also in BG in some patients
  - ↓ N-acetylaspartate to creatine ratio in BG (neuronal loss)
  - ↑ ↑ choline to creatine ratio in BG due to gliosis

Ultrasonographic Findings
- Transcranial real time sonography (TCS)
  - Hyperechogenic lesions primarily in SN and CN
- Functional transcranial Doppler ultrasonography
  - ↓ vasoreactivity in anterior cerebral artery during motor activation in early stage HD

Nuclear Medicine Findings
- PET
  - ↓ FDG uptake in BG precedes detectable atrophy
  - ± frontal lobe hypometabolism
- SPECT: Perfusion defects in motor cortex, prefrontal cortex, and BG correlate with clinical disease

Imaging Recommendations
- Best imaging tool
  - MR
- Protocol advice
  - T2WI

DIFFERENTIAL DIAGNOSIS

Leigh Disease
- Subacute necrotizing encephalomyelopathy
- Onset usually < 2 years old, but juvenile/adult forms also exist
- Changes in putamen, CN, and tegmentum
  - T1 hypointensities, T2 hyperintensities (infarcts)
  - No atrophy of CN and putamina
- Focal involvement of white matter, thalamus, brain stem, and cerebellum

Wilson Disease
- Rigidity, tremor, dystonia, gait difficulty, dysarthria
- T2WI: Symmetrical signal hyperintensity in CN, putamen, midbrain, and pons (gliosis and edema)
  - Asymmetrical hypointensity in frontal white matter
  - Characteristic irregular areas of hypointensity in CN and putamen
- Atrophy of CN and brainstem on CT, MR

Pantothenate Kinase-Associated Neurodegeneration
- Neurodegeneration with brain iron accumulation (formerly called Hallervorden-Spatz)
- Involuntary movements (choreoathetosis), spasticity
- Progressive dementia in young adults
- Characteristic iron deposition in GP, red nuclei, SN
  - "Eye of the tiger" sign: Central spot of high signal in medial GP on T2WI
- GP atrophy, ± cortical, CN atrophy

Carbon Monoxide Poisoning

- Bilateral CT hypodensity, T2 hyperintensity in GP

PATHOLOGY

General Features

- Etiology
  - Polyglutamine expansion → Huntington accumulates in nucleus and cytoplasm → cytoplasmic Huntington aggregates in axonal terminals
- Genetics
  - Autosomal dominant with complete penetrance
  - CAG trinucleotide repeat disease affecting HD gene on chromosome 4p16.3
  - Genetic anticipation: ↑ severity or ↓ age of onset in successive generations
    - More commonly in paternal transmission of mutated allele
  - Homozygosity for HD mutation (very rare)
    - Associated with more severe clinical course

Staging, Grading, & Classification

- Based on gross striatal pathology, neuronal loss, gliosis
- Grade 0: Normal gross, histologic examination
- Grade 1: No gross striatal atrophy (only histologic changes)
- Grade 2: Striatal atrophy, convex CN
- Grade 3: More severe striatal atrophy, flat CN
- Grade 4: Most severe striatal atrophy, concave CN

Gross Pathologic & Surgical Features

- Diffuse cerebral atrophy (marked in CN, putamen)
- Juvenile HD: Involvement of GP, cerebellum (typically not involved in adults)

Microscopic Features

- Neuropathological hallmarks of HD
  - Intranuclear inclusions containing Huntington protein
  - Perinuclear aggregates in cortex, striatum

CLINICAL ISSUES

Presentation

- Most common signs/symptoms
  - Classic triad
    - Movement disorder (choreoathetosis)
    - Dementia of subcortical type
    - Behavioral changes/psychosis
- Other signs/symptoms
  - Dysarthria, dysphagia, abnormal eye movements
- Clinical profile
  - Pathognomonic feature of HD: Movement disorder
    - Chorea: Often facial twitching or writhing and twitching of distal extremities; ballism later on
    - Progressive cytoplasmic → impaired gait ("dancing" gait)
    - Rigidity and dystonia in later stages (adult HD)
  - Juvenile HD: Rigidity > chorea
    - Rigidity & dystonia may occur as initial symptoms
    - Cerebellar signs, dyslalia, rapid cognitive decline
    - Seizures, parkinsonism, dystonia, long-tract signs

Demographics

- Age
  - Mean at onset: 35-44 years in adult-onset HD
  - Juvenile HD (5-10% of cases): Onset at < 20 years
- Gender
  - M = F; gender-related factor affecting disease onset
    - Earlier onset, faster progression of HD in offspring of male patients
    - 70% of juvenile cases have affected father
- Ethnicity
  - Less common in African/Asian populations
- Epidemiology
  - Worldwide prevalence: 5-10/100,000 people
  - 3-7/100,000 in populations of W. European descent

Natural History & Prognosis

- Early symptoms: Personality changes and subtle movement disturbances
- Progression to choreoathetosis and dementia
- Behavioral disorganization, depression, suicidal behavior, psychotic features (visual hallucinations)
- Adult HD: Progressive deterioration until death 15-20 years after onset
- Higher degree of volume loss ↔ earlier age of onset
- Juvenile HD: More progressive clinical course

Treatment

- Antidepressants, high-potency antipsychotics
- Tetrabenazine (Dopamine depleters)
- Antiglutamatergic drugs (amantadine, memantine, riluzole)
- Ubiquinone (coenzyme Q10) → normalization of lactate levels in cortex and striatum
- Bilateral neural transplantation
- Experimental: Grafting of trophic factor-producing cell lines

DIAGNOSTIC CHECKLIST

Consider

- Reversible dementias & movement disorders

Image Interpretation Pearls

- Caudate atrophy is main radiologic feature of HD
  - Bicaudate diameter: Sensitive for CN atrophy
- Consider HD in child with ↑ signal in CN/putamina on PD-/T2WI

SELECTED REFERENCES

1. Adam OR et al: Symptomatic treatment of Huntington disease. Neurotherapeutics. 5(2):181-97, 2008
2. Imarisio S et al: Huntington's disease: from pathology and genetics to potential therapies. Biochem J. 412(2):191-209, 2008
3. Schapiro M et al: MR imaging and spectroscopy in juvenile Huntington disease. Pediatr Radiol. 34(8):640-3, 2004
4. Aylward EH et al: Bicaudate ratio as a measure of caudate volume on MR images. AJNR Am J Neuroradiol. 12(6):1217-22, 1991
5. Stober T et al: Bicaudate diameter--the most specific and simple CT parameter in the diagnosis of Huntington's disease. Neuroradiology. 26(1):25-8, 1984

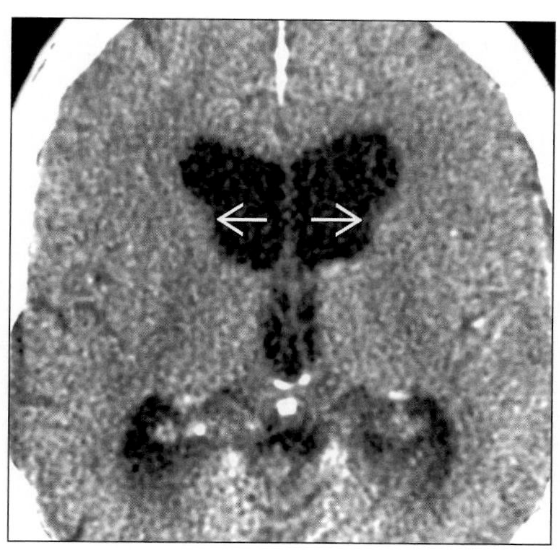

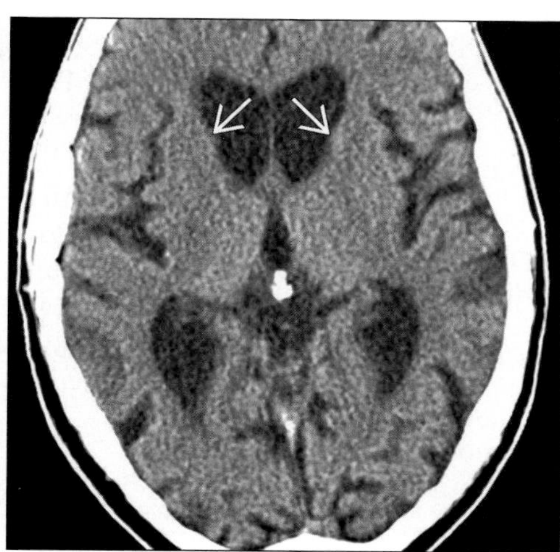

(Left) *Axial CECT shows classic CT findings of Huntington disease involving the caudate nuclei, including caudate atrophy and increased CC distance ➔.* ***(Right)*** *Axial NECT in a patient with Huntington disease shows generalized atrophy. The frontal horns of the lateral ventricles are disproportionately enlarged and flattened, with a loss of normal concavity ➔ caused by marked caudate head atrophy.*

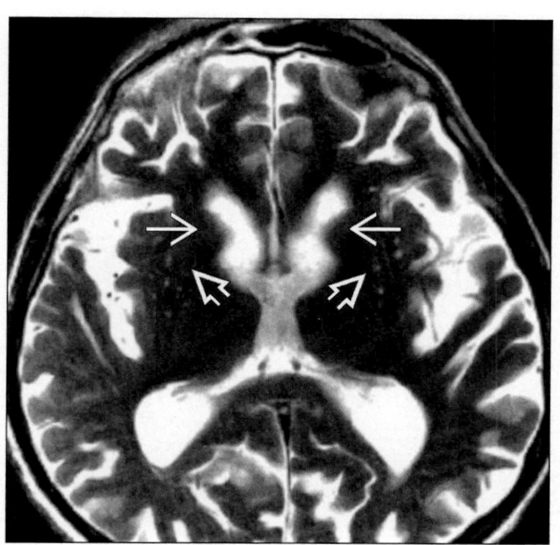

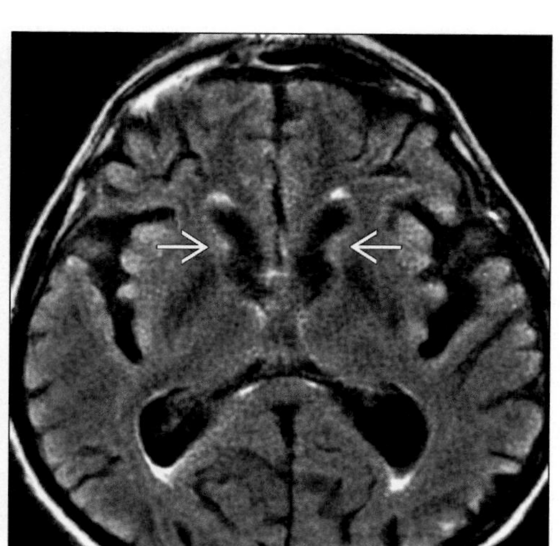

(Left) *Axial T2WI MR in a patient with Huntington disease shows atrophy in the bilateral caudate nuclei ➔ and putamina ➔. Also note the generalized brain atrophy with dilatation of the lateral ventricles and cortical sulci.* ***(Right)*** *Axial FLAIR MR in the same patient shows a slight increase in signal intensity of both caudate ➔ nuclei in addition to atrophy.*

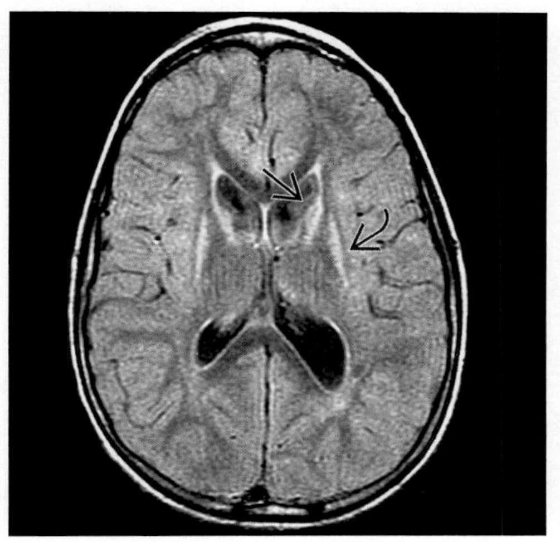

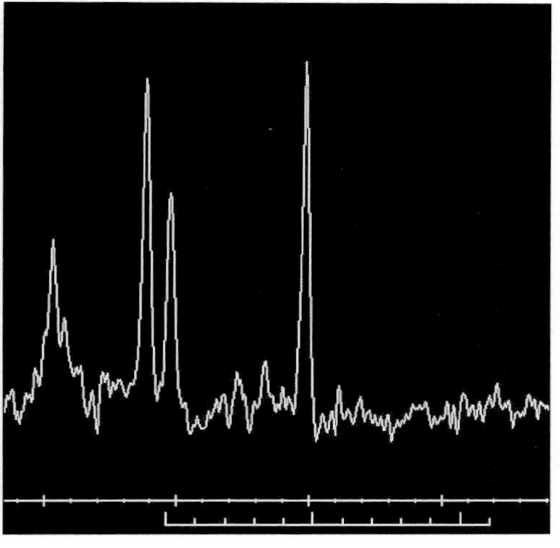

(Left) *Axial FLAIR MR in an 8 year old with dysarthria, rigidity, and a family history of HD demonstrates a combination of volume loss and ↑ signal intensity of the caudate heads ➔ & putamina ➔.* ***(Right)*** *MRS (TR of 144) in the same patient demonstrates abnormal choline to creatine peak and low NAA. Differential diagnosis would include mitochondrial disorders such as Leigh syndrome. No lactate doublet & a family history of Huntington favors Huntington disease over Leigh syndrome.*

WILSON DISEASE

Key Facts

Terminology

- Wilson disease (WD), hepatolenticular degeneration
- Autosomal recessive inherited copper metabolism disorder characterized by
  - Abnormal accumulation of copper in various tissues
  - Particularly in liver and brain (basal ganglia)

Imaging

- Usually normal MR in presymptomatic patients
- SI improvement correlated with clinical response to copper-chelating therapy
- Symmetrical T2 hyperintensity or mixed intensity in putamina (with hyperintense peripheral putaminal rim), caudate nuclei, thalami, and globus pallidi (GP)
- Characteristic "face of giant panda" sign on axial sections at midbrain level

Top Differential Diagnoses

- Leigh disease
- Creutzfeldt-Jakob disease
- Japanese encephalitis
- Organic aciduria
- Hypoxic ischemic encephalopathy

Clinical Issues

- Kayser-Fleischer ring in cornea
- Neurologic: Asymmetric tremor, ataxia, dyskinesia, dysarthria, dystonia (mainly face), incoordination

Diagnostic Checklist

- MR improvement correlated with clinical recovery

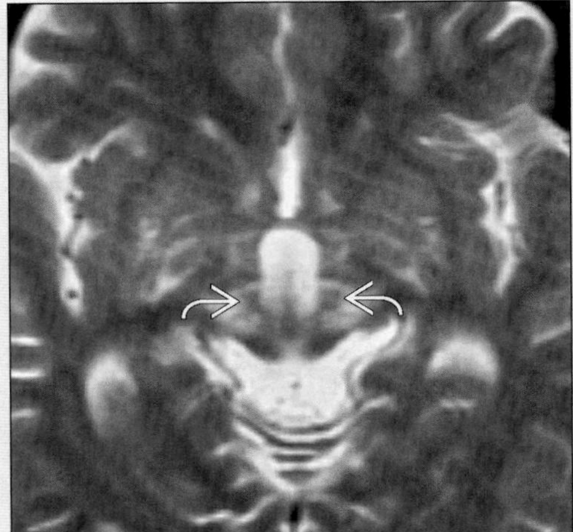

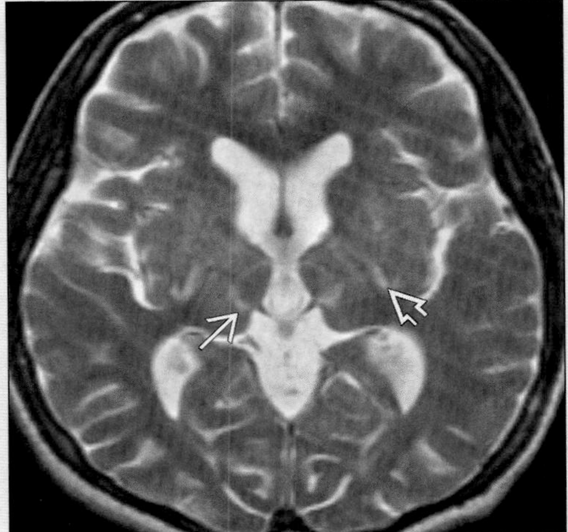

(Left) *Axial T2WI MR at midbrain level shows the "face of giant panda" sign with a normal red nucleus ➔ against the background of high signal in the tegmentum, which is characteristic of Wilson disease.* ***(Right)*** *Axial T2WI MR shows bilateral symmetric hyperintensity in the putamen, globus pallidus, posterior limb of internal capsule ➔, and thalamus ➔. Bilateral symmetric involvement of these structures is characteristic of Wilson disease.*

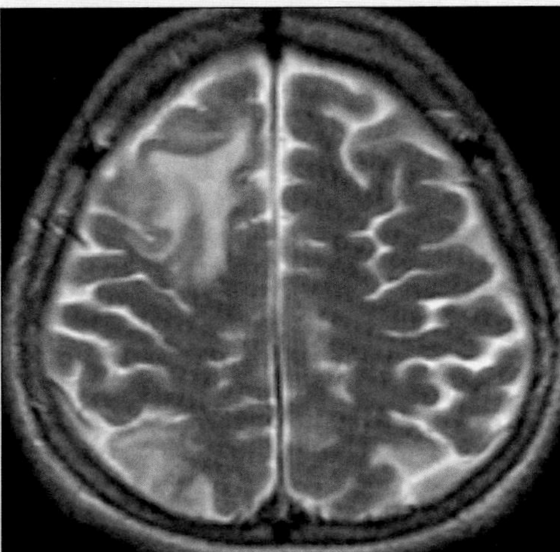

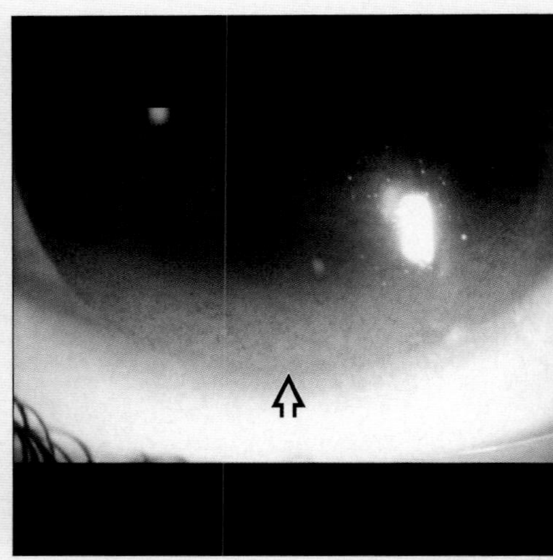

(Left) *Axial T2WI MR demonstrates bilateral, but asymmetric, cortical and subcortical hyperintense signal in the frontoparietal regions. Involvement of cortex and cortical white matter by Wilson disease is usually asymmetric.* ***(Right)*** *Slit lamp examination shows Kayser-Fleischer ring of cornea ➔, an important marker in Wilson disease that is almost always present in patients with neurological involvement.*

WILSON DISEASE

TERMINOLOGY

Abbreviations

- Wilson disease (WD)

Synonyms

- Progressive hepatolenticular degeneration

Definitions

- Autosomal recessive inherited copper metabolism disorder characterized by abnormal accumulation of copper in various tissues

IMAGING

General Features

- Best diagnostic clue
  - Symmetrical T2 hyperintensity or mixed intensity in putamina, caudate nuclei, thalami, and globus pallidi (GP)
- Location
  - Most common: Putamen (predilection for outer rim)
  - Caudate nuclei, GP, thalami (ventrolateral nuclei)
  - Midbrain, pons, cerebellum (vermis and dentate nucleus)
  - Cortical and subcortical lesions (mostly frontal lobe)
- Size
  - Initially ↑ (swelling of basal ganglia), then ↓ (atrophy)
- Morphology
  - No change in shape of affected structures

CT Findings

- NECT
  - Widening of frontal horns of lateral ventricles; diffuse brain atrophy
  - ± hypodensity in lentiform nuclei and thalami
- CECT
  - Lesions do not contrast enhance

MR Findings

- T1WI
  - T1 signal generally reduced in basal ganglia (BG)
  - Signal intensity may ↑ in affected BG (paramagnetic effects of copper)
- T2WI
  - Usually normal MR in presymptomatic patients
  - Hyper-/hypo-/mixed intensity in putamen, GP, caudate, thalamus
    - Bilateral symmetric concentric-laminar T2 putaminal hyperintensity
    - BG can be hypointense due to ↑ iron content
  - Characteristic "face of giant panda" sign; normal signal intensity in red nucleus against background of hyperintense signal in tegmentum
  - ± hyperintensity in periaqueductal gray matter, pontine tegmentum, medulla oblongata, dentate nucleus, and cerebral and cerebellar white matter, especially frontal lobe
  - Clinical response to copper-chelating therapy correlates with improvement in signal abnormalities
  - In adults, BG lesions may differ from those in children
    - Putaminal lesions may be absent; GP and substantia nigra may be hypointense on T2WI
- PD/intermediate
  - Symmetrical high signal intensity in affected BG
- DWI
  - Abnormally low ADC values immediately after onset of neurologic symptoms; subsequently high ADC values (necrosis, spongiform degeneration)
- T1WI C+
  - No contrast enhancement is typically seen
- MRS
  - ↓ N-acetyl aspartate to creatine ratio (neuronal loss) in basal ganglia, parietooccipital cortex, frontal white matter
  - ↓ myoinositol to creatine ratio in basal ganglia and ↓ choline:creatine ratio in GP
  - ↓ myoinositol to creatine ratio in WD with portosystemic shunting (pattern of hepatic encephalopathy)

Nuclear Medicine Findings

- PET
  - ↓ ↓ glucose metabolism in cerebellum, striatum, and, to lesser extent, in cortex and thalamus
  - ↓↓ dopa-decarboxylase activity (impaired nigrostriatal dopaminergic pathway)
- SPECT
  - (I-123)2β-carbomethoxy-3β-(4(I-123)iodophenyl)tropane binds to presynaptic striatal dopamine carriers
  - (I-123)iodobenzamide binds to postsynaptic striatal dopamine D2R
  - In symptomatic WD patients
    - ↓ ↓ striatal binding ratios of both tracers
  - In all WD patients, highly correlated binding ratios of both tracers corresponding to severity of neurologic features

Imaging Recommendations

- Best imaging tool
  - MR more sensitive than CT for detection of early lesions
- Protocol advice
  - T2WI, FLAIR, DWI

DIFFERENTIAL DIAGNOSIS

Leigh Disease

- Subacute necrotizing encephalomyelopathy
- Symmetrical spongiform brain lesions with onset in infancy/early childhood
- Lesions predominantly bilateral and symmetrical, in brainstem, BG (particularly putamen), and cerebral white matter (WM)

Creutzfeldt-Jakob Disease

- Progressively hyperintense changes in BG, thalamus, and cerebral cortices on T2WI

Japanese Encephalitis (JE)

- Homogeneous T2 hyperintensities in BG and posteromedial thalami (very characteristic of JE, spared in WD)

Organic Aciduria
- Symmetrical diffuse WM changes, wide CSF spaces
- BG changes (↑ T2 signal ± volume loss in caudate &/or lentiform nuclei)

Hypoxic Ischemic Encephalopathy
- Bilateral symmetric hyperintense lesions with restricted diffusion in putamen, caudate, thalamus, and cortex

Methanol Poisoning
- Bilateral symmetric T2 hyperintensity in putamen, caudate ± WM

Osmotic Demyelination Syndrome
- Involvement of pons (central median raphe), basal ganglia, and, rarely, midbrain

PATHOLOGY

General Features
- Etiology
  - Defective incorporation of copper into ceruloplasmin and impaired biliary copper excretion
  - Brain lesions caused by accumulation of copper, chronic ischemia, vasculopathy, or demyelination
- Genetics
  - Autosomal recessive: ATPase copper transporting β-polypeptide (*ATP7B*) gene on chromosome 13q14.3-q21.1
- General comments
  - Excess copper throughout brain (lesions often bilateral and symmetrical), with unexplained tendency for extensive BG damage

Staging, Grading, & Classification
- Stage 1: Initial period of accumulation of copper by hepatic binding sites
- Stage 2: Acute redistribution of copper within liver and release into circulation
- Stage 3: Chronic accumulation of copper in brain and other extrahepatic tissues

Gross Pathologic & Surgical Features
- Ventricular enlargement, sulcal widening

Microscopic Features
- Edema, necrosis, and spongiform degeneration of BG; gliosis and demyelination in WM
- Opalski cells = PAS(+) altered glial cells
- Deep pyramidal cell layers of cerebral cortex involved

CLINICAL ISSUES

Presentation
- Most common signs/symptoms
  - Neurologic: Asymmetric tremor, ataxia, incoordination, dyskinesia, dysarthria, dystonia (mainly facial)
    - Parkinsonian symptoms: Rigidity, bradykinesia
  - Psychiatric: Hyperkinetic behavior, irritability, emotional lability, difficulty in concentration, depression, psychosis, mania, personality change
  - Acute hepatitis
  - Kayser-Fleischer ring in cornea due to abnormal copper accumulation in Descemet membrane
- Clinical profile
  - 40-50% of patients present with liver disease
  - 40-50% present with neurological or psychiatric symptoms (corneal rings almost always present)
  - ↓ ceruloplasmin and total serum copper levels, ↑ 24-hour urinary copper excretion, and ↑ ↑ hepatic copper content

Demographics
- Age
  - Onset of liver disease usually at age 8-16 years
  - Neurological symptoms often 1st recognized in 2nd-3rd decade (rarely age < 12 years)
- Gender
  - Generally M = F, but M:F = 1:4 for fulminant WD, i.e., liver failure, encephalopathy, coagulopathy
- Epidemiology
  - Prevalence: 1 in 30,000-40,000 people
  - Carrier frequency in USA: 1 in 90 individuals

Natural History & Prognosis
- Children: Liver disease most common presentation
- Older individuals: Neuropsychiatric symptoms
  - ↑ symptom severity with ↑ brain copper deposition
- Once symptomatic, WD is fatal if untreated; 70% mortality for patients with fulminant liver failure
- Good prognosis with early chelation treatment
- Best prognosis: Treated asymptomatic siblings

Treatment
- Restriction of food abundant in copper (e.g., chocolate, liver, nuts, mushrooms, shellfish)
- Penicillamine (side effect of initial neurological deterioration in 20-50%)
- Other treatments: Trientine (better alternative chelator), ammonium tetrathiomolybdate, zinc (especially for presymptomatic and asymptomatic patients)
- Liver transplant (for severe hepatic decompensation)

DIAGNOSTIC CHECKLIST

Image Interpretation Pearls
- T2 hyperintensity in striatum with neurologic dysfunction
- T1 hyperintensity in basal ganglia with hepatic dysfunction
- MR improvement correlated with clinical recovery

SELECTED REFERENCES

1. Ala A et al: Wilson's disease. Lancet. 369(9559):397-408, 2007
2. Kim TJ et al: MR imaging of the brain in Wilson disease of childhood: findings before and after treatment with clinical correlation. AJNR Am J Neuroradiol. 27(6):1373-8, 2006
3. Sinha S et al: Wilson's disease: cranial MRI observations and clinical correlation. Neuroradiology. 48(9):613-21, 2006

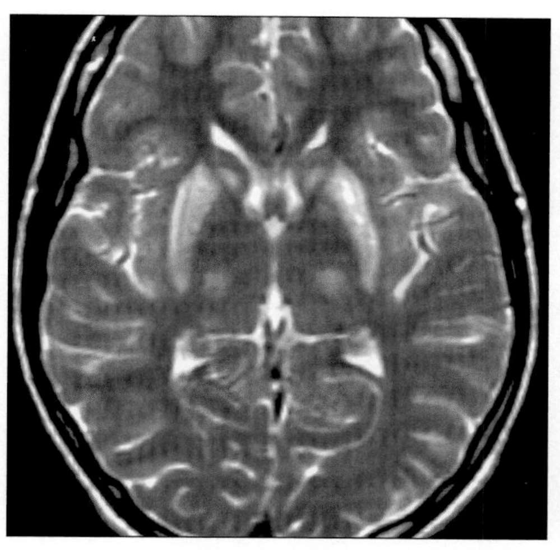

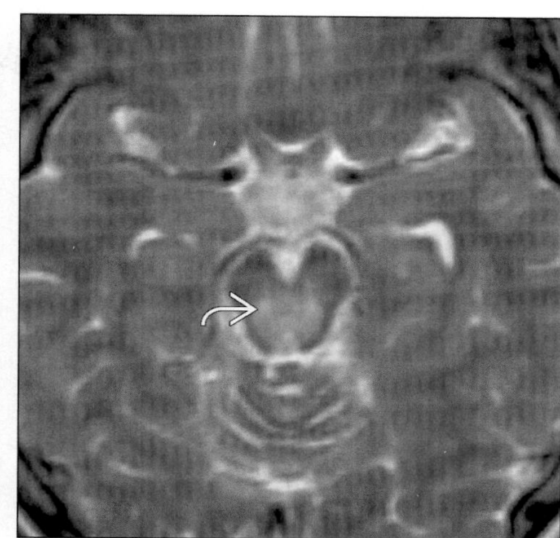

(Left) *Axial T2WI MR in a 13-year-old boy shows typical bilateral symmetric increased signal intensity in the putamen, head of caudate nuclei, and thalamus.* ***(Right)*** *Axial T2WI MR in the same patient shows typical areas of hyperintense signal without mass effect, primarily involving the dorsal part of midbrain →.*

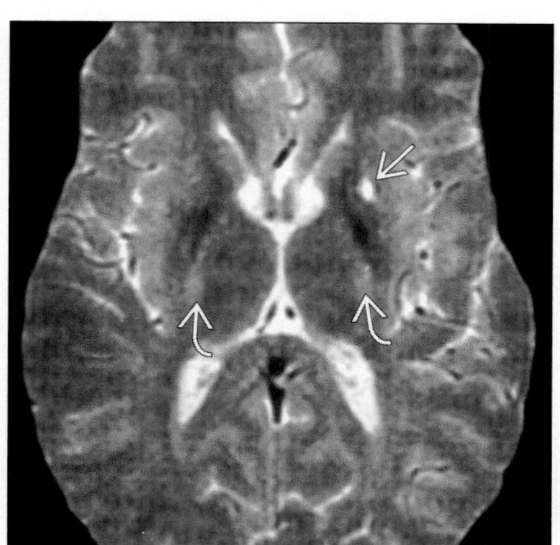

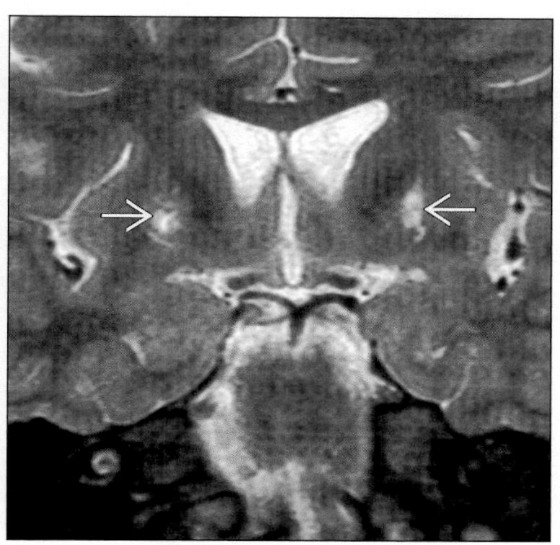

(Left) *Axial T2WI MR in a 19-year-old male shows laminar hyperintense signal in the anterior putamen → and within the corticospinal tracts → in the posterior limbs of the internal capsule.* ***(Right)*** *Coronal T2WI MR in the same patient shows hyperintense lesions in the putamina →.*

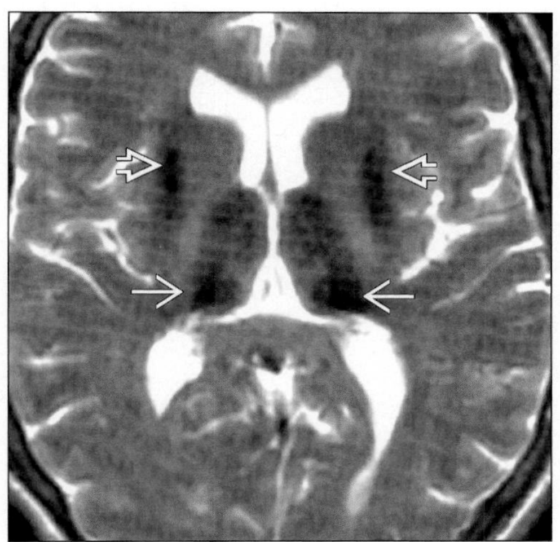

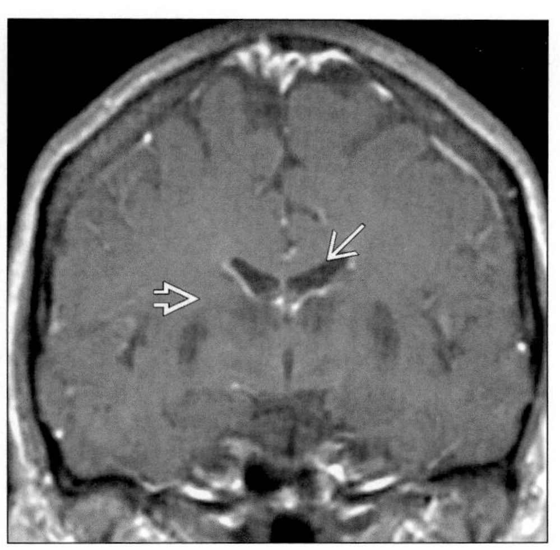

(Left) *Axial T2WI MR in a patient with Wilson disease shows hypointense signal within the thalami → and basal ganglia →.* ***(Right)*** *Coronal T1WI C+ MR in the same patient shows symmetric, hypointense, nonenhancing lesions in both putamina → and caudate nuclei →.*

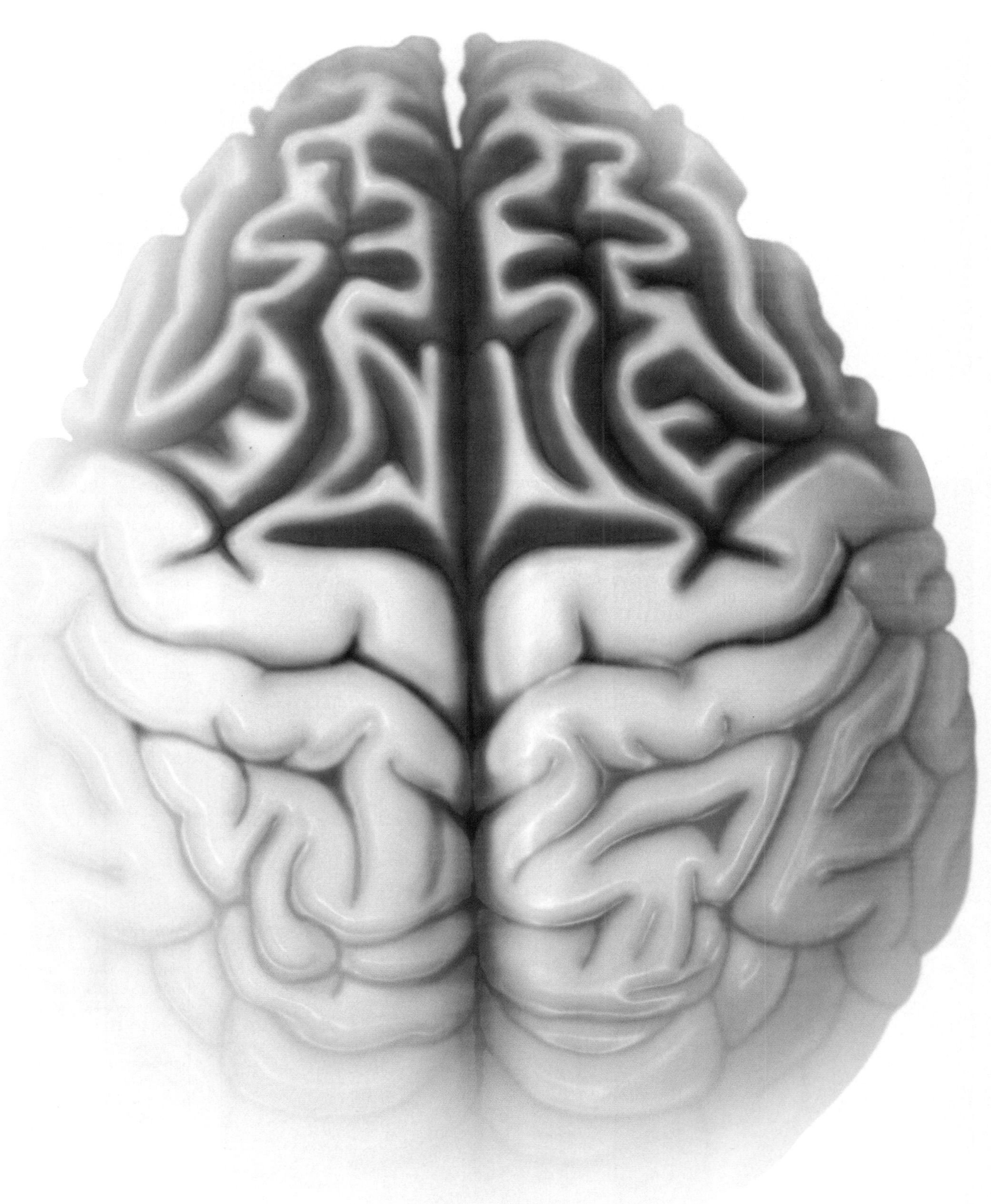

SECTION 10
Acquired Toxic/Metabolic/Degenerative Disorders

Introduction and Overview

Toxic, Metabolic, Nutritional, Systemic Diseases with CNS Manifestations

Dementias and Degenerative Disorders

Approach to Toxic and Metabolic Disorders

Acquired toxic and metabolic disorders of the brain result from a wide variety of agents, including toxic exposures, substance abuse, radiation, and chemotherapy, as well as metabolic alterations, including hypertension, hepatic failure, hypoglycemia, and osmotic demyelination. The vast majority of toxic and metabolic disorders of the brain involve the deep gray nuclei (basal ganglia and thalamus) or the cerebral white matter. Typically, there is symmetric abnormality of the involved structures, which can provide a clue to the correct diagnosis. Most of the toxic and metabolic disorders are best identified on MR. DWI and FLAIR are often extremely valuable in differentiating among the various pathologies in this group and can help the radiologist arrive at a correct diagnosis. Of course, clinical history of possible exposure or substance abuse is often the key to the patient's diagnosis.

Imaging Anatomy

Basal Ganglia

The basal ganglia (BG) are paired nuclei in the inferior hemispheres that are involved in motivation and controlling movement. They are comprised of the caudate nucleus, putamen, and globus pallidus (GP). The caudate nucleus is a C-shaped nucleus with a large head, tapered body, and down-curving tail. The head forms the floor and lateral wall of the anterior horn of the lateral ventricle. The caudate body parallels the lateral ventricles. The anterior limb of the internal capsule separates the caudate head from the putamen and GP. The putamen is located lateral to the GP and is separated by the lateral or external medullary lamina. The GP has 2 segments, lateral (external) and medial (internal). The posterior limb of the internal capsule separates the BG from the thalamus.

Thalamus

The thalamus is comprised of paired ovoid nuclear complexes that act as relay stations for most of the sensory pathways. The thalami extend from the foramen of Monro to the quadrigeminal plate of the midbrain. The medial aspect of the thalami form the 3rd ventricle lateral walls. The posterior limb of the internal capsule forms the lateral border of the thalami. The thalamus is subdivided into several nuclear groups, the anterior, medial, lateral, medial geniculate nuclei, lateral geniculate nuclei, and pulvinar. These nuclear groups are further subdivided into 10 additional nuclei. The pulvinar is easily identified as it is the most posterior of the thalamic nuclei and overhangs the superior colliculus. The subthalamic nucleus is small, lens-shaped, lies superolateral to the red nucleus, and is rarely involved in toxic or metabolic disorders.

Pathologic Issues

The mechanisms for various toxic and metabolic lesions of the brain are complex and often represent a combination of various pathways. Since the deep gray nuclei are highly metabolically active and require significant oxygenation, they are commonly affected by toxins, metabolic abnormalities, and hypoxic-ischemic injury. Often, as in CO poisoning and cyanide, there is a component of hypoxic injury that helps explain the predilection for involvement of the GP, which is extremely sensitive to hypoxia. Selective vulnerability of the deep gray nuclei is also related to dysfunction of selected excitatory neuronal circuits, inhibition of mitochondrial function, and selective loss of dopaminergic neurons.

Differential Diagnosis

Most of the pathologies that affect the brain have a characteristic location, which helps the radiologist arrive at a correct diagnosis. The following differential diagnosis considerations will provide clues to the common toxic and metabolic processes that affect the deep gray nuclei and white matter.

Basal Ganglia Calcification

Basal ganglia calcification is the end result of many toxic, metabolic, inflammatory, and infectious insults. Fahr disease is a rare neurodegenerative disorder that results in extensive bilateral BG calcifications. The GP is most commonly involved, followed by the putamen, caudate, and thalamus. Additionally, there may be involvement of the cerebellum, particularly the dentate nuclei and cerebral white matter.

Other endocrinologic disorders, including hypothyroidism and hypoparathyroidism, may cause calcification, particularly involving the GP and putamen, dentate nuclei, thalami, and subcortical white matter. Radiation and chemotherapy may result in mineralizing microangiopathy that commonly causes BG and subcortical white matter calcification and atrophy. Physiologic calcification as part of the normal aging brain typically occurs in the GP more than the putamen.

T1 Hyperintense Basal Ganglia

Basal ganglia T1 hyperintensity is usually symmetric, related to calcification or other mineralization. T1 hyperintensity is often seen in the GP and substantia nigra in patients with a history of liver disease or hyperalimentation related to abnormal manganese metabolism. Kernicterus, related to toxic unconjugated bilirubin in a newborn, results in increased T1 signal in the GP, as well as the substantia nigra, hippocampus, and dentate nucleus.

Many endocrine disorders that result in BG calcification will also cause T1 hyperintensity. These include hypothyroidism, hyperparathyroidism, hypoparathyroidism, and pseudohypoparathyroidism. Fahr disease also results in T1 hyperintensity, particularly in the GP.

T2 Hyperintense Basal Ganglia

T2 hyperintensity within the BG is typically symmetric in toxic and metabolic disorders. Often DWI helps to differentiate the various lesions of the BG. Carbon monoxide (CO) poisoning classically causes symmetric GP hyperintensity but occasionally also involves the putamen, thalamus, and white matter. DWI may be positive acutely. Methanol toxicity typically results in putaminal necrosis and may be hemorrhagic. Drug abuse is another cause for abnormalities of the basal ganglia, often in young adults. Often, drug abuse results in strokes or vasculitis. Heroin and MDMA (ecstasy) often result in GP ischemia. Drug abuse may be asymmetric and often results in associated hemorrhage. Osmotic demyelination syndrome is acute demyelination caused by rapid shifts in serum osmolality, often in the setting of rapid correction of hyponatremia. Extrapontine myelinolysis commonly affects the caudate and putamen as well as the white matter.

Wilson disease causes symmetric hyperintensity in the putamen, GP, caudate, and thalami. It also results in a "face of the giant panda" sign at the midbrain level with T2 hyperintense white matter tracts. Acute hypertensive encephalopathy (PRES) is a caused by hypertension and may be related to chemotherapy. PRES typically affects the cortex and subcortical white matter of the posterior circulation. However, involvement of the BG may occur. The main considerations besides toxic and metabolic insults that may cause T2 hyperintense BG are hypoxic-ischemic encephalopathy, deep venous occlusion, and infectious etiologies.

Globus Pallidus Lesions

Lesions that often only involve the GP include CO poisoning, cyanide poisoning, heroin and MDMA (ecstasy) abuse, kernicterus, neurodegeneration with brain iron accumulation (NBIA), pantothenate kinase-associated neurodegeneration (PKAN), hyperalimentation, hepatic encephalopathy, and methylmalonic acidemia. NBIA is a group of progressive neurodegenerative disorders with extrapyramidal motor impairment and brain iron accumulation, resulting in GP T2 hypointensity. PKAN, also known as Hallervorden-Spatz syndrome or NBIA-1, has a classic "eye-of-the-tiger" appearance with bilateral, symmetric GP T2 hyperintensity surrounded by hypointensity.

Other disorders that commonly affect the GP more prominently than the other BG nuclei include Fahr disease, hypothyroidism, and Wilson disease. As with other lesions of the BG, hypoxic-ischemic encephalopathy should also be considered.

Bilateral Thalamic Lesions

Thalamic lesions are most commonly caused by arterial or venous ischemia or hypoxic-ischemic encephalopathy. However, they are also involved in many toxic and metabolic processes. Alcoholic encephalopathy, particularly Wernicke encephalopathy, typically results in T2 hyperintense medial thalami, mamillary bodies, hypothalamus, and periaqueductal gray matter. Wernicke encephalopathy results from a vitamin B1 deficiency and is frequently associated with alcohol abuse. T1 hyperintensity in the pulvinar is a common and sensitive finding for Fabry disease and is considered by many as the T1 "pulvinar" sign. Fabry disease is a rare multisystem X-linked disorder that includes renal and cardiac dysfunction and strokes. Although Fahr disease most commonly causes extensive bilateral calcification of the BG, the thalami are frequently affected.

Other diseases that affect the thalami include PRES, vasculitis, osmotic demyelination, and acute disseminated encephalomyelitis. Additionally, many of the encephalitides affect the thalami, including Ebstein-Barr virus, Japanese encephalitis, and West Nile Virus. Creutzfeldt-Jakob disease (CJD) often affects the basal ganglia and thalami symmetrically.

Diffuse White Matter Abnormality

Toxic and metabolic disorders often cause a confluent T2 hyperintense leukoencephalopathy. Radiation and chemotherapy classically causes a leukoencephalopathy with T2 hyperintensity throughout the cerebral white matter. Sparing of the subcortical U-fibers is typical. A diffuse necrotizing leukoencephalopathy may also result, commonly from a combination of radiation and chemotherapy, which causes white matter necrosis in addition to leukoencephalopathy. Heroin vapor inhalation, a.k.a. "chasing the dragon" syndrome, causes a toxic leukoencephalopathy that results in T2 hyperintense cerebellar white matter and the posterior limb of the internal capsule showing involvement of the posterior cerebral white matter, with relative sparing of the subcortical white matter.

Hypothyroidism related to Hashimoto thyroiditis may result in a diffuse confluent white matter encephalopathy that typically affects the anterior cerebral white matter. There is involvement of the subcortical U-fibers but relative sparing of the posterior hemispheres. Acute liver failure may also result in diffuse edema with T2 hyperintensity in the periventricular and subcortical white matter. Cortex involvement is typical. PRES typically involves the cortex and subcortical white matter in a posterior circulation. Alcoholic encephalopathy may rarely result in diffuse white matter T2 hyperintensity related to acute demyelination.

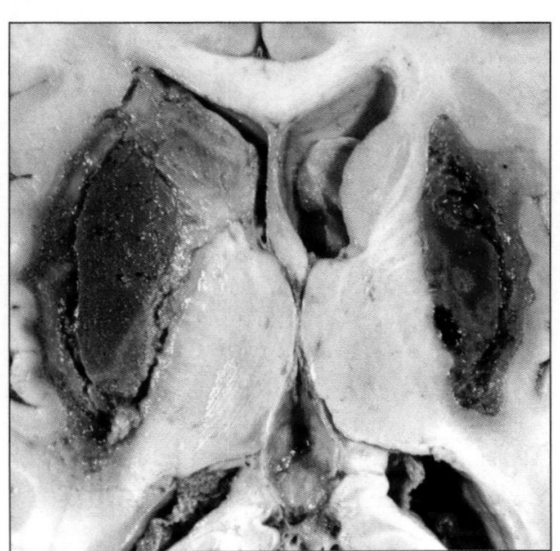

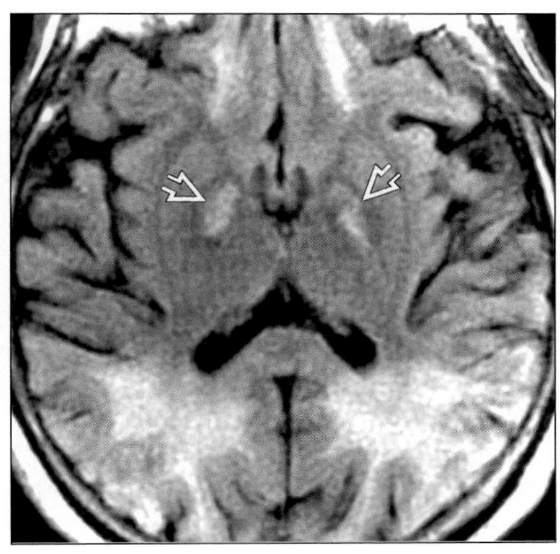

(Left) *Axial gross pathology section shows bilateral hemorrhagic necrosis in the putamen, characteristic of methanol injury to the brain. The right-sided injury extends to involve the globus pallidus and caudate head. (Courtesy R. Hewlett, PhD.)* ***(Right)*** *Axial FLAIR MR shows acute CO poisoning with symmetric hyperintensity in the globi pallidi ➡ and cerebral white matter. CO poisoning commonly involves only the globi pallidi, but may also affect the putamen, thalami, and white matter.*

(Left) *Axial NECT shows bilateral basal ganglia and subcortical white matter calcification related to hypothyroidism. Imaging is similar in other endocrinologic disorders and Fahr disease.* ***(Right)*** *Axial NECT shows extensive subcortical white matter, cerebellar, and basal ganglia calcification in this patient with a history of radiation and chemotherapy for a posterior fossa medulloblastoma. Mineralizing microangiopathy typically occurs 2 or more years after treatment.*

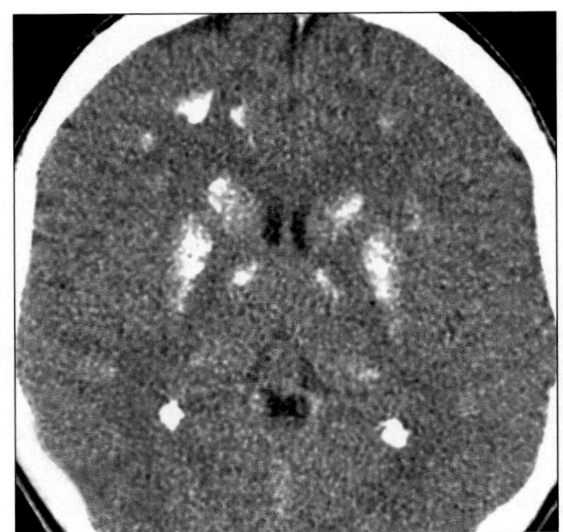

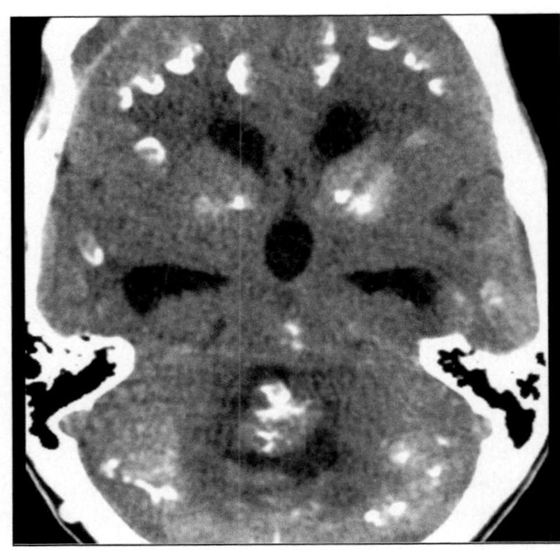

(Left) *Axial T2WI MR shows symmetric hyperintensity in the globi pallidi ➔ related to cyanide poisoning. Cyanide also typically affects the subthalamic nuclei, substantia nigra, and cerebellum.* ***(Right)*** *Axial FLAIR MR shows symmetric hyperintensity in both posteromedial thalami ⇨ and in the region of the mamillary bodies related to Wernicke encephalopathy. DWI is often positive acutely. Wernicke encephalopathy is related to a thiamine deficiency and is often related to alcohol abuse.*

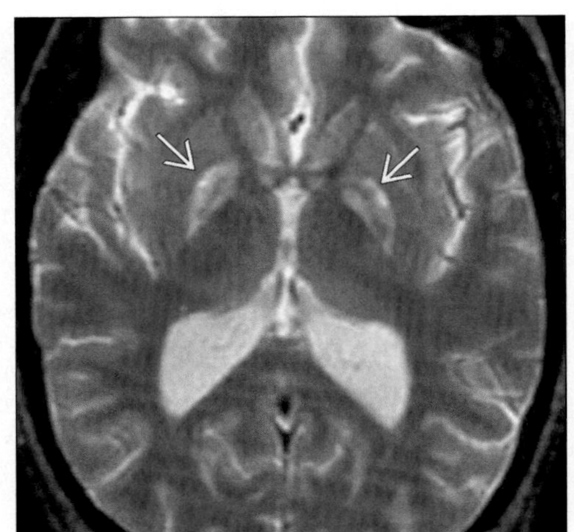

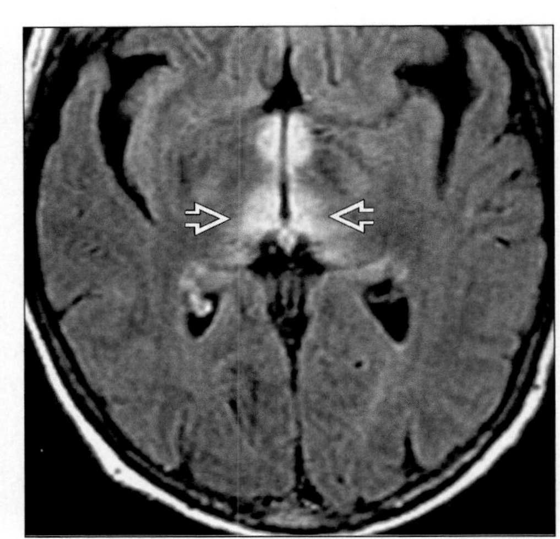

(Left) *Axial FLAIR MR shows symmetric hyperintensity in the caudate and putamen in this patient with both extrapontine and central pontine myelinolysis. Osmotic demyelination is often DWI positive and is typically related to a rapid correction of hyponatremia. Cerebral white matter demyelination may also occur.* ***(Right)*** *Axial gross pathology section shows bilateral necrosis of the putamen and globus pallidus ⇨ with areas of cavitation related to neurotoxicity. (Courtesy R. Hewlett, PhD.)*

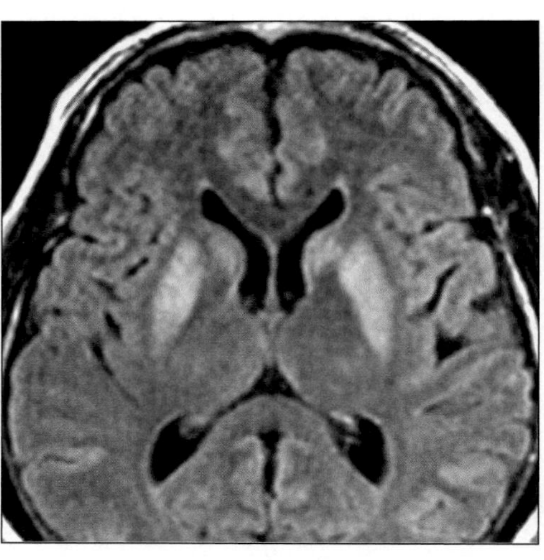

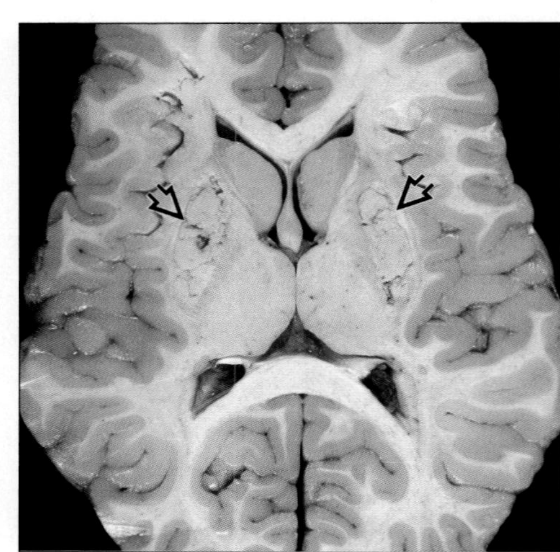

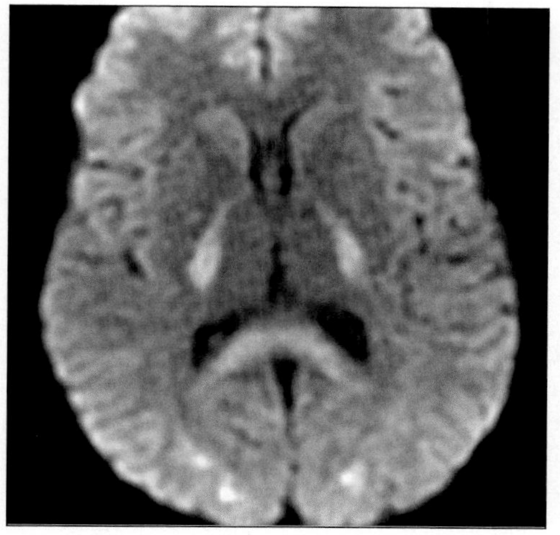

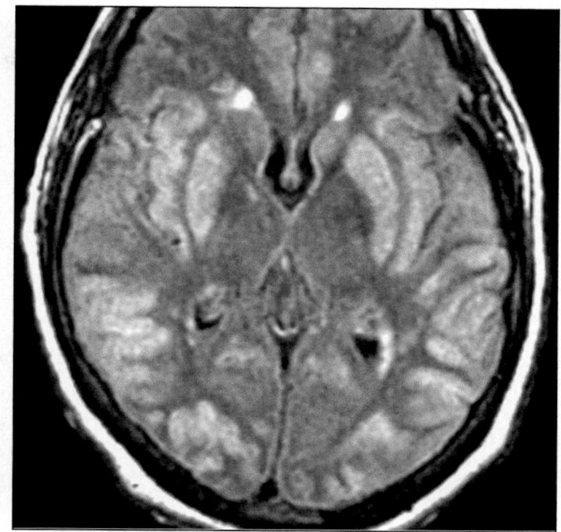

(Left) *Axial DWI MR shows hyperintensity in the internal capsule posterior limbs, corpus callosum splenium, and occipital white matter related to heroin-induced leukoencephalopathy, a.k.a. "chasing the dragon" syndrome. Extensive white matter involvement is seen in severe cases.* ***(Right)*** *Axial FLAIR MR shows extensive, symmetric hyperintensity in the basal ganglia, cortex, and subcortical white matter related to profound hypoglycemia. Predilection for the parietal and occipital lobes is typical.*

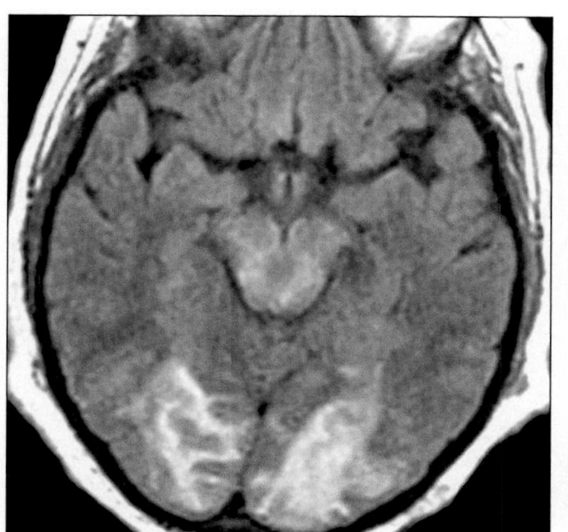

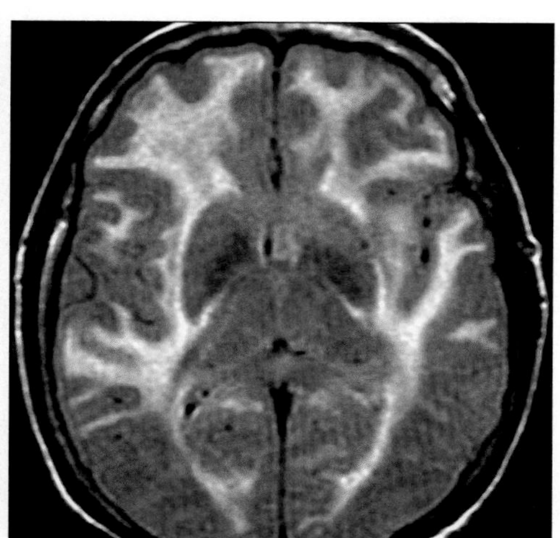

(Left) *Axial FLAIR MR shows bilateral hyperintensity in the occipital lobes related to acute hypertensive encephalopathy or PRES. This encephalopathy is often related to hypertension and is typically reversible.* ***(Right)*** *Coronal FLAIR MR shows diffuse, symmetric white matter hyperintensity with involvement of the subcortical U-fibers. There is relative sparing of the occipital lobes, typical of Hashimoto encephalopathy, a rare complication of Hashimoto thyroiditis.*

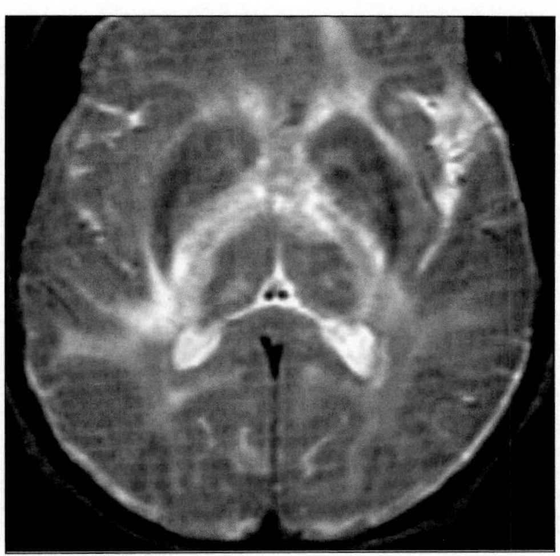

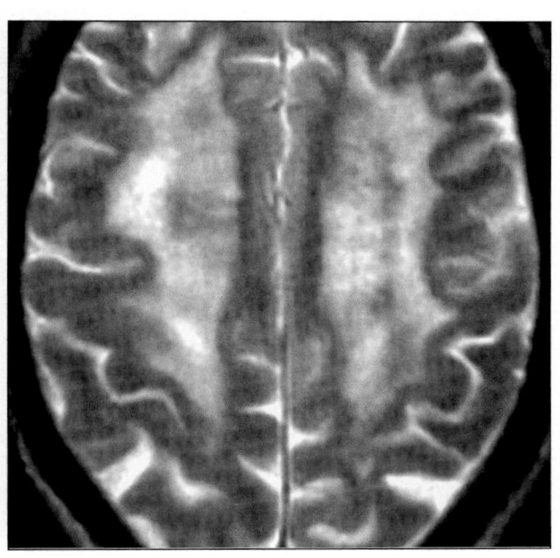

(Left) *Axial T2WI MR shows diffuse white matter hyperintensity related to severe alcohol poisoning from binge drinking and acute demyelination.* ***(Right)*** *Axial T2WI MR shows extensive hyperintensity throughout the white matter and sparing of the subcortical U-fibers, typical of treatment related leukoencephalopathy. This patient has a history of whole brain radiation therapy. Radiation and chemotherapy cause a variety of toxic injuries to the brain, with leukoencephalopathy being the most common.*

PEDIATRIC HYPOGLYCEMIA

Key Facts

Imaging

- Consider if bilateral occipital/parietal bright DWI signal in neonate with seizures
- Occipital > parietal > frontal, temporal lobe
- ± basal ganglia, thalamus, brainstem involvement
- White matter injury common, may be predominantly periventricular in premature
- As few as 29% may have posterior predominance if no DWI and MR performed in subacute phase
- Increased DWI signal corresponds to normal to low ADC acutely, DWI normalizes after 1st week
- Normal to low NAA, ± lactate

Top Differential Diagnoses

- Term hypoxic-ischemic injury
- Preterm hypoxic-ischemic injury
- Inborn error of metabolism

Pathology

- Upper cortical layers involved, not intermediate and deep layers as in hypoxic-ischemic injury
- No selective involvement of watershed areas

Clinical Issues

- Stupor, jitteriness, seizures, apnea, irritability, hypotonia
- Usually presents within 1st 3 days of life
- Threshold for injury unknown but likely a factor of severity and duration as well as associated insults
- M > F

Diagnostic Checklist

- Do not equate DWI abnormalities with infarcts (pannecrosis) as acute DWI abnormalities may result in only mild volume loss, especially if ADC not decreased

(Left) *Axial CECT in a 3 day old with severe hypoglycemia shows decreased attenuation in the posterior cerebrum → involving the occipital, parietal (not shown), and posterior temporal lobes bilaterally with loss of gray-white differentiation.* ***(Right)*** *Axial T2WI MR in the same patient 1 day later shows posterior T2 cortical and subcortical hyperintensity → involving occipital, parietal (not shown), and posterior temporal lobes bilaterally. Note the loss of gray-white differentiation.*

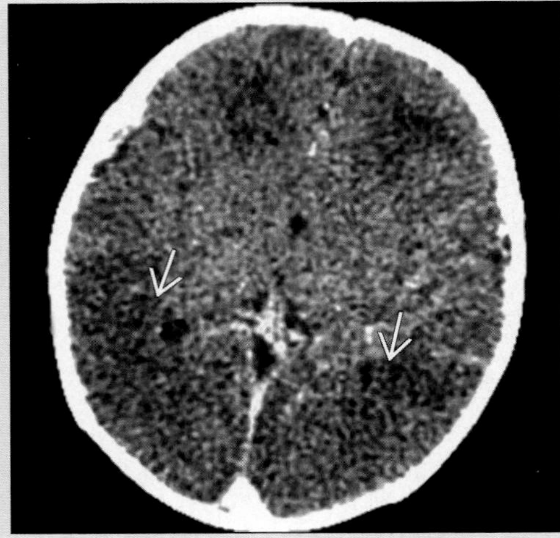

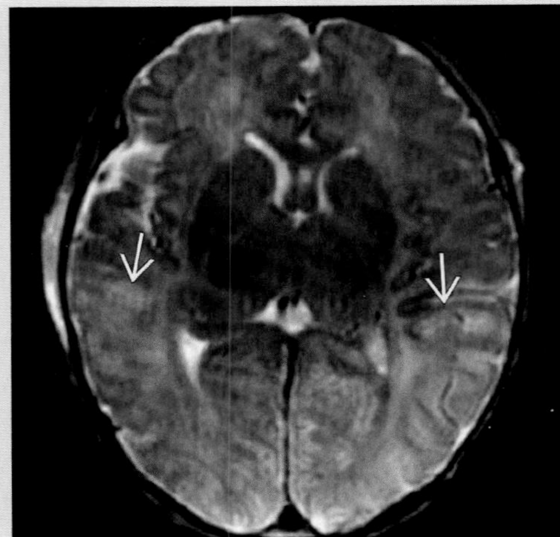

(Left) *Axial DWI MR in the same patient shows increased signal → in the occipital, parietal (not shown), and posterior temporal lobe bilaterally, with less severe right frontal lobe → and insular cortex involvement.* ***(Right)*** *Axial ADC in the same patient shows markedly decreased signal intensity in the posterior regions of the cerebral hemispheres →. The right frontal lobe → is actually reduced diffusivity and not a result of T2 effects "shining through."*

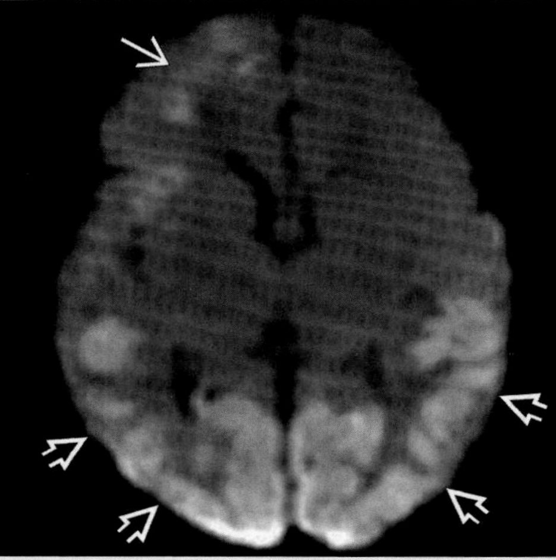

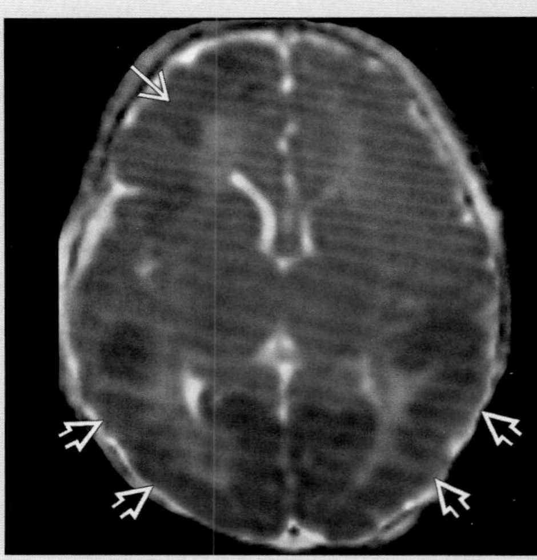

PEDIATRIC HYPOGLYCEMIA

TERMINOLOGY

Definitions

- Significant hypoglycemia
  - < 35 mg/dL (0-3 hours), < 40 mg/dL (3-24 hours), < 45 mg/dL (> 24 hours) in term infant plasma
  - < 25 mg/dL in preterm infant plasma

IMAGING

General Features

- Best diagnostic clue
  - Bilateral occipital/parietal bright DWI in neonate with seizures
- Location
  - Occipital > parietal > frontal, temporal lobes
  - ± basal ganglia, thalamus, brainstem involvement
  - White matter injury common, may be predominantly periventricular in premature
  - As few as 29% may have posterior predominance if no DWI and MR performed in subacute phase

CT Findings

- NECT
  - Decreased attenuation with loss of gray-white differentiation in acute and subacute phase
  - Cortical Ca++ in chronic phase

MR Findings

- T1WI
  - Cortical ± deep gray hyperintensity in subacute phase
  - ± foci of increased T1 signal in white matter
- T2WI
  - Increased signal in gray and white matter with loss of gray-white distinction in acute phase
  - Increased signal in gray and white matter with variable cortical low signal in subacute phase
  - Volume loss ± gliosis that may be subtle to cystic encephalomalacia in chronic phase
- DWI
  - Increased DWI signal corresponds to low ADC acutely, DWI normalizes after 1st week
- MRS
  - Normal to low NAA, ± lactate

Ultrasonographic Findings

- Grayscale ultrasound
  - Increased echogenicity

Imaging Recommendations

- Best imaging tool
  - MR with DWI
- Protocol advice
  - Higher b values (b = 1,000-1,500 s/mm²) make areas of decreased diffusion more conspicuous

DIFFERENTIAL DIAGNOSIS

Term Hypoxic-Ischemic Injury

- Hypoglycemia potentiates hypoxic-ischemic injury (HII)
- HII causes hypoglycemia
- MR with DWI in partial HII may be indistinguishable from hypoglycemic brain injury

Preterm Hypoxic-Ischemic Injury

- Hypoglycemia potentiates periventricular leukomalacia

Inborn Error of Metabolism

- Consider if marked elevation in lactate or if no history of hypoglycemia

Status Epilepticus

- Seizures are typical response of newborn brain to injury
  - DWI abnormalities in newborns more likely to be cause (not consequence) of seizures
- Vicious cycle may develop where cerebral injury is exacerbated by seizures

Venous Infarct

- Often associated hemorrhage and edema; MRV to rule out

Acute Hypertensive Encephalopathy (PRES)

- Predominantly increased ADC, older patients

PATHOLOGY

General Features

- Etiology
  - Inadequate substrate availability/reserve: IUGR, preeclampsia, maternal hypoglycemia, prolonged fasting, prematurity
  - ↑ glucose utilization: Hypoxia, stress
  - Hyperinsulinemia
    - Uncontrolled maternal diabetes
    - Hyperinsulinemic hypoglycemia, familial, 1 or 2 (HHF1 or HHF2)
    - Beckwith-Wiedemann syndrome (BWS)
  - Other endocrine abnormalities: Panhypopituitarism, hypothyroidism, adrenal insufficiency
  - Other: Polycythemia, congenital heart disease
  - Excitatory amino acids (glutamate) and oxidative stress are thought to play central role in neuronal death
- Glucose metabolism
  - Glucose primary metabolic fuel for brain
  - Brain is major determinant of hepatic glucose production
  - Neonates have disproportionally high glucose production relative to body size due to disproportionately large neonatal brain
  - Immature brain more resilient to hypoglycemia than adult
    - Lower absolute demand
    - Increased ability to increase cerebral blood flow
    - Utilization of other substrates (i.e., lactate)
    - Resistance of neonatal heart to hypoglycemia

Staging, Grading, & Classification

- Clinical categories
  - Transitional adaptive hypoglycemia
    - Very early onset; mild, brief hypoglycemia
    - Responds rapidly to treatment

- Diabetic mothers, erythroblastosis, difficulty transitioning to extrauterine life
- Secondary associated hypoglycemia
  - Early 1st day; mild, short-duration hypoglycemia
  - Responds rapidly to treatment
  - Associated CNS disorder (hypoxic-ischemic injury, intracranial hemorrhage, sepsis)
- Classic transient hypoglycemia
  - End of 1st day; moderate to severe, often prolonged hypoglycemia
  - Requires large amounts of glucose
  - IUGR, ↓ substrate/impaired gluconeogenesis
- Severe recurrent hypoglycemia
  - Variable onset; severe, prolonged hypoglycemia
  - May persist despite treatment
  - Most have primary disorder of glucose metabolism
    - e.g., BWS, HHF1 or HHF2/persistent hyperinsulinemia hypoglycemia of infancy (PHHI)/nesidioblastosis, β-cell hyperplasia, endocrine deficiencies, inborn errors in metabolism

Gross Pathologic & Surgical Features

- Pale, edematous brain; blurred gray-white junction

Microscopic Features

- Widespread injury to cerebral cortex, hippocampus, basal ganglia, thalamus, brainstem, spinal cord
- Upper cortical layers involved, not intermediate and deep layers as in hypoxic-ischemic injury
- No selective involvement of watershed areas
- Severe degeneration of glial cells
- Periventricular white matter injury may be prominent

CLINICAL ISSUES

Presentation

- Most common signs/symptoms
  - Stupor, jitteriness, seizures, apnea, irritability, hypotonia
  - May have no symptoms
- Clinical profile
  - Small or large neonates

Demographics

- Age
  - Usually presents within 1st 3 days of life
- Gender
  - M > F

Natural History & Prognosis

- Cerebral glucose metabolism probably flow limited, so dependent on CBF
- Threshold for injury unknown but likely a factor of severity and duration as well as associated insults
- < 50 mg/dL may have deleterious long-term effects even if no neonatal signs
- Epilepsy (may have intractable seizures), developmental delay, motor delay, learning and behavior problems, hyperactivity and attention difficulties, autistic features, microcephaly, cortical blindness
- DWI abnormalities associated with later deficits (occipital lobe low ADC associated with later cortical visual loss)
- Regions of bright DWI and minimal ADC decrease may have minimal to no volume loss on follow-up

Treatment

- Glucose level to treat controversial, consider if 45-50 mg/dL
- Glucose infusion to restore normal glucose levels, often even if asymptomatic
- PHHI → frequent feeds, increased caloric density, continuous NG feeds ± cornstarch, continuous IV dextrose, hydrocortisone, diazoxide, octreotide, glucagon, Ca++ channel blocker, partial pancreatectomy

Prevention

- Control maternal diabetes, preeclampsia/eclampsia, nutrition, prevention/rapid treatment of perinatal asphyxia
- Identify high-risk infant, temperature control, oral feeds in 1st hours of life, glucose test when indicated

DIAGNOSTIC CHECKLIST

Reporting Tips

- Do not equate DWI abnormalities with infarcts (pan-necrosis), as acute DWI abnormalities may result in only mild volume loss, especially if ADC not decreased

SELECTED REFERENCES

1. Musson RE et al: Diffusion-weighted imaging and magnetic resonance spectroscopy findings in a case of neonatal hypoglycaemia. Dev Med Child Neurol. 51(8):653-4, 2009
2. Burns CM et al: Patterns of cerebral injury and neurodevelopmental outcomes after symptomatic neonatal hypoglycemia. Pediatrics. 122(1):65-74, 2008
3. Per H et al: Neurologic sequelae of neonatal hypoglycemia in Kayseri, Turkey. J Child Neurol. 23(12):1406-12, 2008
4. Tam EW et al: Occipital lobe injury and cortical visual outcomes after neonatal hypoglycemia. Pediatrics. 122(3):507-12, 2008
5. Volpe JJ: Neurology of the Newborn. 5th ed. Philadelphia: Saunders. 2008
6. Yalnizoglu D et al: Neurologic outcome in patients with MRI pattern of damage typical for neonatal hypoglycemia. Brain Dev. 29(5):285-92, 2007
7. Kim SY et al: Neonatal hypoglycaemic encephalopathy: diffusion-weighted imaging and proton MR spectroscopy. Pediatr Radiol. 36(2):144-8, 2006
8. Alkalay AL et al: Brain imaging findings in neonatal hypoglycemia: case report and review of 23 cases. Clin Pediatr (Phila). 44(9):783-90, 2005
9. Vannucci RC et al: Hypoglycemic brain injury. Semin Neonatol. 6(2):147-55, 2001
10. Cornblath M et al: Hypoglycemia in the neonate. Semin Perinatol. 24(2):136-49, 2000
11. Hawdon JM et al: Clinical features of neonates with hyperinsulinism. N Engl J Med. 341(9):701-2, 1999
12. Barkovich AJ et al: Imaging patterns of neonatal hypoglycemia. AJNR Am J Neuroradiol. 19(3):523-8, 1998

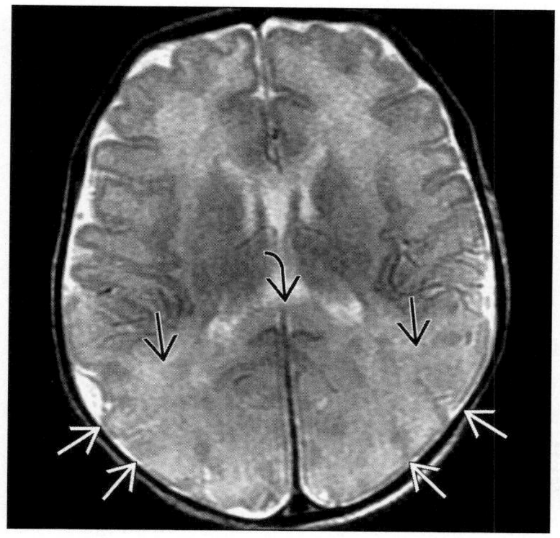

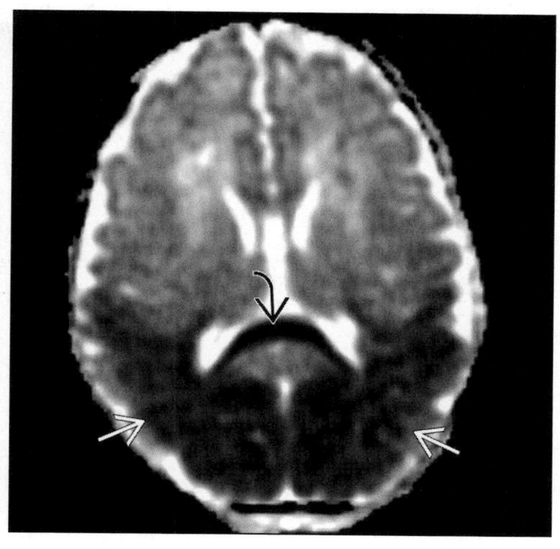

(Left) Axial T2WI MR in a 5-day-old hypoglycemic infant shows increased signal in the parietal cortex ➔ and underlying parietal white matter ➔ with loss of gray-white distinction. Note the extension of hyperintensity ➔, probably representing interstitial edema, into the splenium of the corpus callosum. **(Right)** Axial ADC in the same infant shows reduced diffusivity in the parietal cortex and white matter ➔, as well as in the posterior corpus callosum ➔.

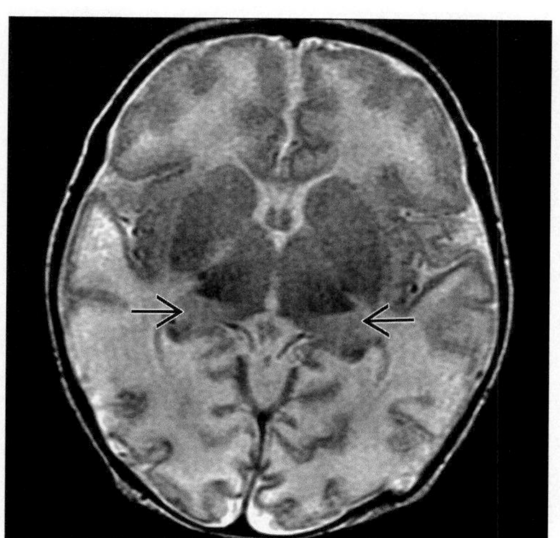

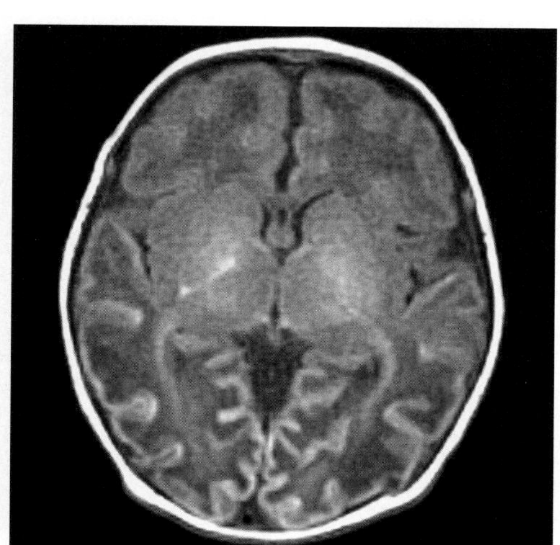

(Left) Axial T2WI MR in the same patient at 7 days shows the evolution of hypoglycemic injury, with increased signal in the posterior white matter, including posterior limb of the internal capsules and pulvinar thalamus ➔. The overlying cortex shows patchy increased and decreased signal. **(Right)** Axial T1WI MR at 7 days shows evolving injury: Decreased signal in the posterior white matter and pulvinar thalamus, increased signal in the overlying cortex and posterior limb internal capsule.

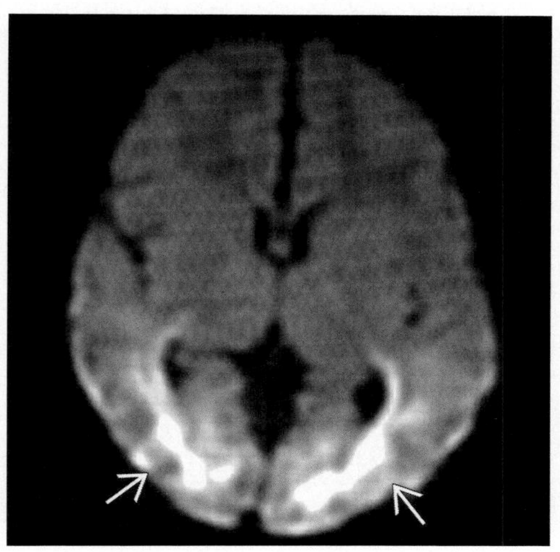

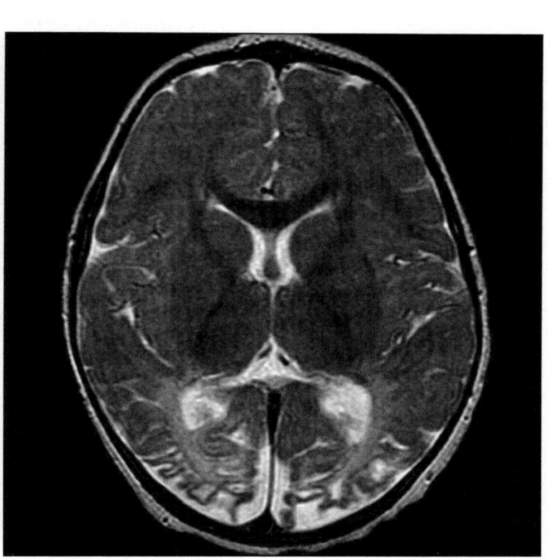

(Left) Axial DWI MR at 7 days in the same patient with hypoglycemic injury shows increased signal ➔ in the posterior white matter and overlying cortex. At this stage, diffusivity is pseudonormalizing, so the increased signal is likely a result of T2 "shine through." **(Right)** Axial T2WI MR in the same patient at 1 year old shows chronic injury with marked volume loss and gliosis involving the cortex and white matter of the posterior temporal lobes, parietal lobes (not shown), and occipital lobes.

ADULT HYPOGLYCEMIA

Key Facts

Terminology
- Adult hypoglycemic encephalopathy (AHE)
- Imbalance between glucose supply, utilization → brain injury

Imaging
- General features
  - Stroke or coma in adult diabetic on insulin
  - Parietal/occipital lobes ± hippocampi, amygdalae
  - ± globus pallidus, striatum
  - Thalami, white matter (WM) usually spared
- MR
  - Parietal/occipital gyral swelling, sulci effaced
  - Restricted diffusion, ↓ ADC (may be transient)
  - Later: T1 gyral hyperintensity (laminar necrosis)

Top Differential Diagnoses
- Acute cerebral ischemia/infarction
- Hypoxia, hypoperfusion
- Acute hypertensive encephalopathy (PRES)

Pathology
- Caused by IRT either without adequate glucose intake or excessive glucose utilization
- Ingestion of oral hypoglycemic medication, either accidental or intentional
- Accumulation/release of excitatory neurotransmitters increases glucose utilization
- Patchy or diffuse laminar necrosis
  - Varying severity, WM generally spared

Clinical Issues
- Often elderly diabetic, altered dietary glucose intake
  - Due to deprivation or other factors (e.g., EtOH)
- Coma, depressed level of consciousness
- May be preceded by seizures

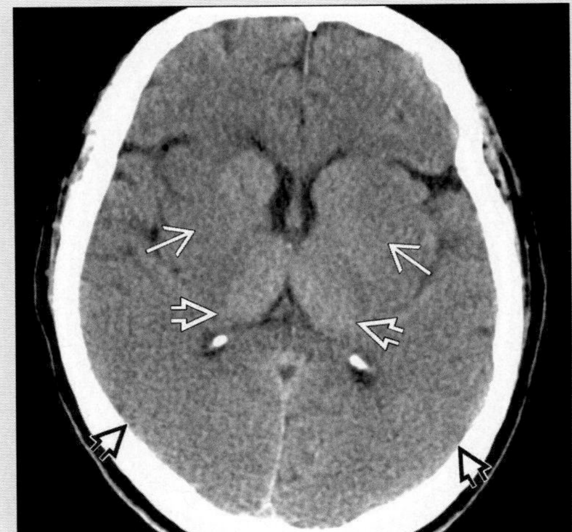

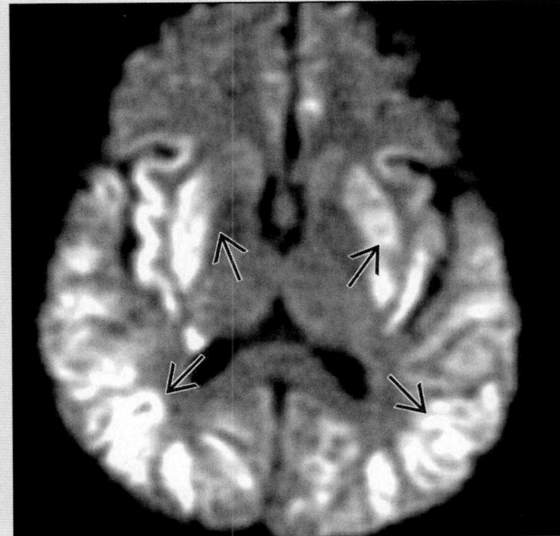

(Left) *Axial NECT in a diabetic with stupor and seizures shows profound parietooccipital gyral swelling with complete effacement of the gray-white interfaces ⇨. Both basal ganglia → (especially the putamina) are edematous. Note the thalamic sparing ⇨.* ***(Right)*** *Axial DWI MR in the same patient shows diffusion restriction → in regions matching the NECT abnormalities. Note the sparing of thalami and deep white matter, with the most severe abnormalities in the putamina and parietooccipital cortex.*

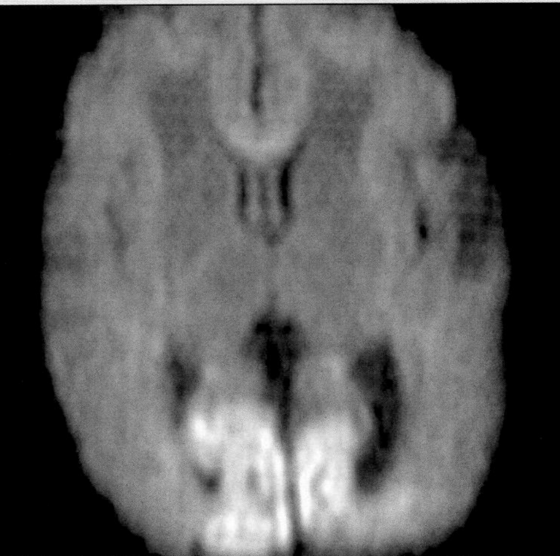

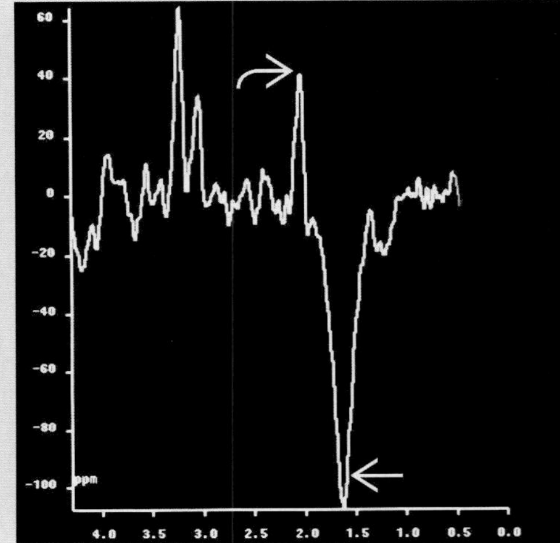

(Left) *Axial DWI MR demonstrates restricted diffusion (hyperintensity) in the occipital lobes of a hypoglycemic patient, indicating irreversible cellular injury. Note the sparing of the basal ganglia and thalami.* ***(Right)*** *Intermediate TE MR spectroscopy in the same patient shows a relatively low NAA peak →, as well as a prominent lactate peak →.*

ADULT HYPOGLYCEMIA

TERMINOLOGY

Abbreviations

- Adult hypoglycemic encephalopathy (AHE)

Synonyms

- Hypoglycemic brain injury
- Diabetic coma (nonspecific; term may include AHE)

Definitions

- Imbalance between glucose supply, utilization → brain injury

IMAGING

General Features

- Best diagnostic clue
  - Stroke/coma in adult diabetic on insulin replacement therapy (IRT)
- Location
  - Common: Parietal/temporal/occipital lobes ± hippocampi, amygdalae
  - Severe: Globus pallidus, striatum (thalami usually spared)

CT Findings

- NECT
  - Hypodense parietal, occipital lobes
    - Superimposed on diffuse edema

MR Findings

- T1WI
  - Early: Gyral swelling, sulcal effacement
  - Later: Gyral hyperintensity (laminar necrosis)
- T2WI
  - Infarcts (parietal/occipital cortex ± basal ganglia)
  - Generally spares white matter (WM) (unlike neonatal hypoglycemic brain injury)
- DWI
  - Restricted diffusion, ↓ ADC (may be transient)
- MRS
  - ↓ NAA, ↑ lactate

Imaging Recommendations

- Best imaging tool
  - MR + DWI

DIFFERENTIAL DIAGNOSIS

Acute Cerebral Ischemia/Infarction

- Wedge-shaped, vascular distribution (MCA > PCA)
- Both cortex, underlying WM involved
- Patchy focal hemorrhage common
  - Uncommon in AHE

Hypoxia, Hypoperfusion

- Post cardiac arrest, global hypoperfusion

Acute Hypertensive Encephalopathy (PRES)

- Uncontrolled HTN or immunosuppressive medication
- Usually no restriction on DWI

PATHOLOGY

General Features

- Etiology
  - Cellular glucose needs, supply imbalance
    - IRT without adequate dietary intake
    - Accidental/intentional ingestion of oral hypoglycemic agents
    - β-cell hypertrophy (nesidioblastosis)
      - Post gastric bypass similar to persistent hyperinsulinemic hypoglycemia of infancy (PHHI)
      - May require subtotal pancreatectomy
  - Accumulation/release of excitatory neurotransmitters
    - ↑ glucose utilization, may ↑ severity of injury

Gross Pathologic & Surgical Features

- Pale/edematous brain, blurred GM-WM boundary
- Cortical ± basal ganglia injury

Microscopic Features

- Variable patchy/diffuse laminar necrosis
- WM generally spared

CLINICAL ISSUES

Presentation

- Most common signs/symptoms
  - Coma, depressed level of consciousness
  - May be preceded by seizures
- Clinical profile
  - Elderly diabetic with altered dietary intake
    - Due to deprivation or other factors (e.g., EtOH)

Natural History & Prognosis

- Prognosis varies with extent of brain injury
- Correlates with basal ganglia (BG) injury
  - If BG significantly involved, meaningful neurologic recovery diminished
  - If no/minimal BG injury, residual deficits are determined by extent and severity of cortical injury

Treatment

- Intravenous glucose, monitoring, supportive care

DIAGNOSTIC CHECKLIST

Image Interpretation Pearls

- WM sparing, lack of hemorrhage help differentiate from hypoxic-ischemic injury
- Bilateral thalamic injury more typical of hypoperfusion/hypoxia

SELECTED REFERENCES

1. Guseva N et al: Successful Treatment of Adult Persistent Hyperinsulinemic Hypoglycemia with Nifedipine. Endocr Pract. Epub ahead of print, 2009
2. Ma JH et al: MR imaging of hypoglycemic encephalopathy: lesion distribution and prognosis prediction by diffusion-weighted imaging. Neuroradiology. 51(10):641-9, 2009

KERNICTERUS

Key Facts

Imaging
- Acute: ↑ T1 signal in globus pallidus (GP), subthalamic nuclei (STN), hippocampi, substantia nigra (SN)
- Chronic: ↑ T2 signal GP, hippocampi
- MRS: ↑ Tau/Cr, ↑ glx/Cr, ↑ mI/Cr, ↓ Cho/Cr

Top Differential Diagnoses
- Hyperalimentation, liver failure: ↑ T1 signal GP, SN
- Toxic: CO poisoning
- Metabolic: Methyl-malonic acidemia, creatine deficiency, succinic semialdehyde dehydrogenase deficiency, L2-hydroxyglutaric aciduria
- Term hypoxic-ischemic injury

Pathology
- Encephalopathy due to ↑ unconjugated bilirubin crossing immature blood-brain barrier (BBB)
- Neurons > glia, neuropil spongiosis
- Yellow staining > MR abnormality

Clinical Issues
- Stupor, hypotonia, poor suckling, high-pitched cry
- Incidence ↑ with early discharge, ↑ breast feeding
- Specific damage to brainstem auditory nuclei → ± deafness or abnormal auditory processing (most common)
- Athetosis, gaze abnormal in most; intellectual deficits in few

Diagnostic Checklist
- Normal MR does not rule out long-term sequelae
- ↑ T1 signal in GP can be normal in neonate, look for other areas of involvement
- Findings may resolve with therapy

__(Left)__ Axial T1WI MR in a neonate with hyperbilirubinemia, stupor, hypotonia, and increased irritability shows increased signal within the globi pallidi ⇒ and hippocampal tails ↪ bilaterally. __(Right)__ Axial T1WI MR in the same kernicteric neonate again shows abnormally increased signal within the substantia nigra ⇒ and hippocampus ↪ bilaterally. The cerebral cortex and the underlying white matter have a normal appearance.

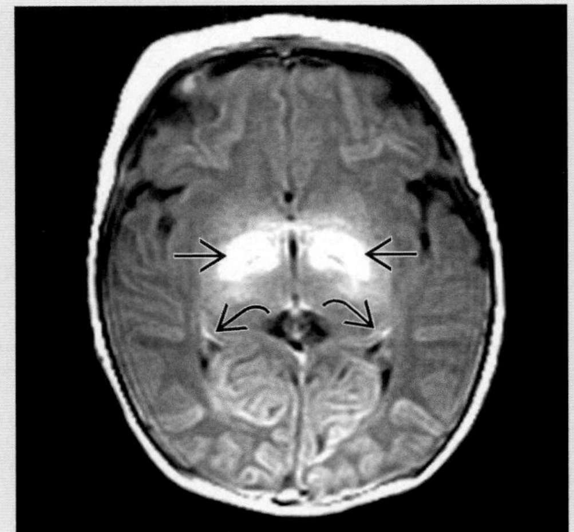

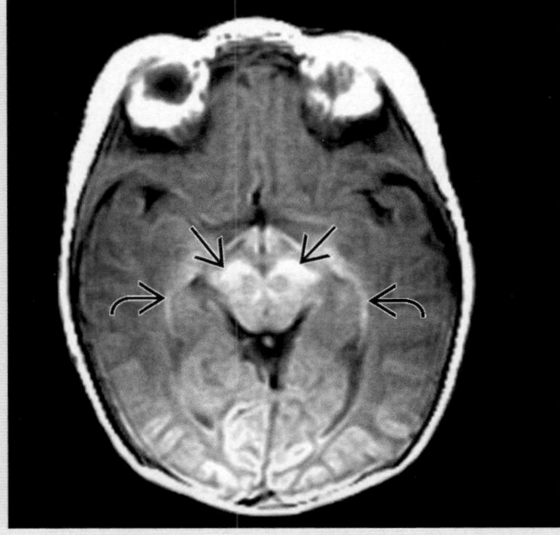

__(Left)__ Axial T2WI MR of the same infant at the age of 6 months shows high T2 signal intensity and volume loss in globus pallidus bilaterally ➡. The volume of the cerebral white matter is somewhat diminished. __(Right)__ Coronal T2WI MR in a young child who had severe neonatal hyperbilirubinemia shows increased T2 signal and volume loss in the bilateral globi pallidi ➡, as well as in the hippocampal heads ↪ bilaterally.

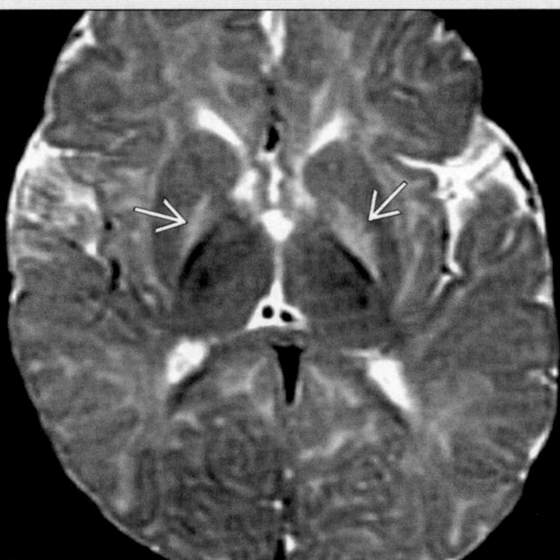

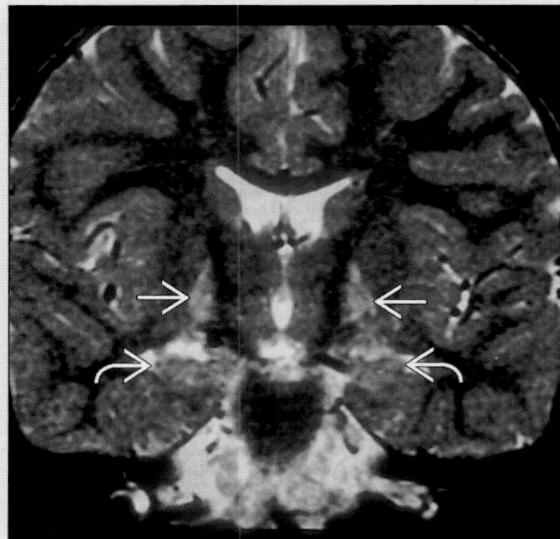

KERNICTERUS

TERMINOLOGY

Synonyms

- Bilirubin (BR) or posticteric encephalopathy

IMAGING

General Features

- Best diagnostic clue
  - Acute: ↑ T1 signal in globus pallidus (GP), subthalamic nuclei (STN), hippocampi, substantia nigra (SN)
  - Chronic: ↑ T2 signal in GP, hippocampi

MR Findings

- T1WI
  - Acute: ↑ T1 signal in GP > STN > hippocampi > SN
    - Deposition of unconjugated BR (UBR) or ↑ manganese (Mn)
- T2WI
  - Chronic: ↑ T2 signal/volume loss in GP, hippocampi, ± SN
- MRS
  - ↑ Tau/Cr, Glx/Cr, mI/Cr, ↓ Cho/Cr

Imaging Recommendations

- Best imaging tool
  - MR

DIFFERENTIAL DIAGNOSIS

T1 Hyperintense Globus Pallidus

- Hyperalimentation, liver failure: ↑ T1 signal GP, SN

T2 Hyperintense Globus Pallidus

- Toxic: CO poisoning
- Metabolic: Methyl-malonic acidemia, creatine deficiency, succinic semialdehyde dehydrogenase deficiency, L2-hydroxyglutaric aciduria

Term Hypoxic-Ischemic Injury

- Acute: ↑ T2 signal; subacute/chronic: ↑ T1 signal in ventrolateral thalamus, corticospinal tract

PATHOLOGY

General Features

- Etiology
  - Encephalopathy due to ↑ UBR crossing immature blood-brain barrier (BBB)
  - Risk factors for ↑ BR
    - Hemolytic disorders (especially erythroblastosis fetalis), breast feeding, > 10% loss of birth weight, polycythemia, dehydration
  - Risk factors for ↑ susceptibility to brain damage at approximately normal BR levels
    - Drugs compete for albumin binding of bilirubin
    - Sulphonamides, ceftriaxone, salicylates, Na-benzoate, hormones
    - Renal hypoalbuminemia, hepatic failure, ↓ thyroidism
    - Prematurity, asphyxia, sepsis
    - ↑ cerebral blood flow; abnormal BBB
- Genetics
  - Some 2q37 (Crigler-Najjar syndrome, etc.)

Gross Pathologic & Surgical Features

- Yellow staining > MR abnormality
  - GP, SN, STN, hippocampi > thalamus, striatum, cranial nerve nuclei (3, 8), dentate nuclei, reticular formation, spinal cord
  - Also Purkinje cells (premies)

Microscopic Features

- Neurons > glia, neuropil spongiosis

CLINICAL ISSUES

Presentation

- Most common signs/symptoms
  - Stupor, hypotonia, poor suckling, high-pitched cry
  - Over days may develop stupor, irritability, ↑ tone
  - May have no or equivocal neurological signs

Demographics

- Age
  - Preterm > term; 1st days of life
- Gender
  - M > F
- Ethnicity
  - More prevalent in Asians, Hispanics
- Epidemiology
  - Incidence ↑ with early discharge, ↑ breast feeding

Natural History & Prognosis

- Specific damage to brainstem auditory nuclei → ± deafness or abnormal auditory processing (common)
- Athetosis, gaze abnormality; intellectual deficits in few

Treatment

- Maternal screen, anti-Rh; fetal blood transfusion
- Hydration, phototherapy for moderate + exchange transfusion for severe
- Other, such as heme oxygenase inhibitors

DIAGNOSTIC CHECKLIST

Consider

- Normal MR does not rule out long-term sequelae

Image Interpretation Pearls

- ↑ T1 signal in GP can be normal in neonates; look for other areas; findings may resolve with therapy

SELECTED REFERENCES

1. Okumura A et al: Kernicterus in preterm infants. Pediatrics. 123(6):e1052-8, 2009
2. Gkoltsiou K et al: Serial brain MRI and ultrasound findings: relation to gestational age, bilirubin level, neonatal neurologic status and neurodevelopmental outcome in infants at risk of kernicterus. Early Hum Dev. 84(12):829-38, 2008
3. Katar S et al: Clinical and cranial magnetic resonance imaging (MRI) findings of 21 patients with serious hyperbilirubinemia. J Child Neurol. 23(4):415-7, 2008

THYROID DISORDERS

Key Facts

Terminology
- Hashimoto thyroiditis (HT), encephalopathy (HE)

Imaging
- Symmetrical pituitary enlargement reversible with thyroid hormone replacement therapy
- BG variably hyperintense (Ca++)
- Hashimoto encephalopathy: Diffuse/focal cortical, subcortical WM T2 hyperintensity with relative sparing of occipital lobes

Top Differential Diagnoses
- Pituitary macroadenoma
- Physiologic pituitary hyperplasia
- Lymphocytic hypophysitis

Pathology
- Diffuse hyperplasia of anterior pituitary responds to treatment
- HT is associated with other autoimmune diseases
  - Encephalopathy associated with HT (rare)
  - Circulating antithyroid peroxidase antibodies in 70-95% of patients with HT

Clinical Issues
- Hypothyroidism: Poor memory, psychomotor slowing, depression, reversible dementia
- HE: Seizures, stroke-like symptoms, neuropsychiatric episodes, cognitive decline
  - HE: Responsive to steroids suggests autoimmune mechanism
- In congenital hypothyroidism, thyroid hormone replacement ASAP (< 13 days)
- ↑ in brain size and ↓ in ventricular size with treatment correlate with changes in levels of circulating thyroid hormones

*(**Left**) Sagittal T1WI C+ MR shows an enlarged homogeneously enhancing pituitary gland ➔ with infundibular thickening ➔ related to hypothyroid-induced pituitary hyperplasia. The hyperplasia resolves with thyroid replacement therapy. (**Right**) Axial T1WI MR shows a focal T1 hyperintensity related to hypothyroidism, involving the caudate heads and globus pallidus bilaterally. These changes are related to mineralization of the basal ganglia, which are hyperdense on CT.*

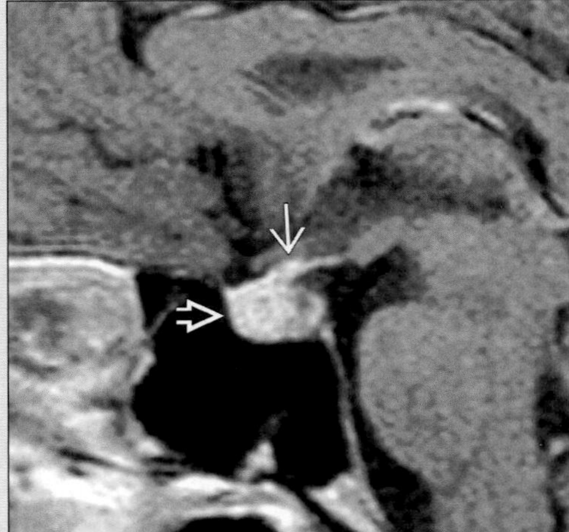

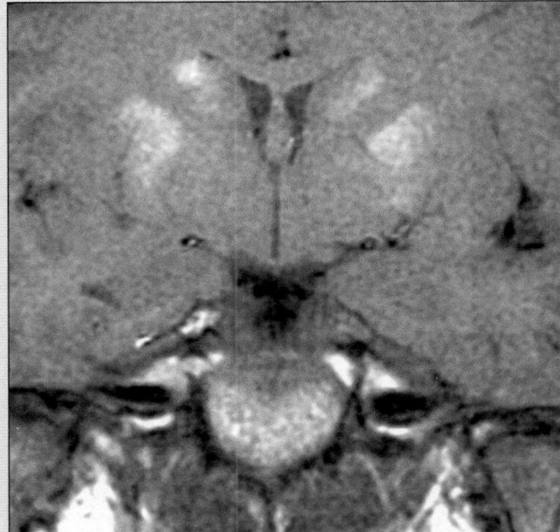

*(**Left**) Axial FLAIR MR shows extensive hyperintensity throughout the anterior temporal white matter and dorsal pons related to leukoencephalopathy in a hypothyroid patient with Hashimoto encephalopathy. (**Right**) Axial FLAIR MR of the same patient shows extensive involvement of the white matter with relative sparing of the posterior cerebral hemispheres. Involvement of the subcortical U-fibers is typical of Hashimoto encephalopathy. This leukoencephalopathy usually progresses to cerebral atrophy.*

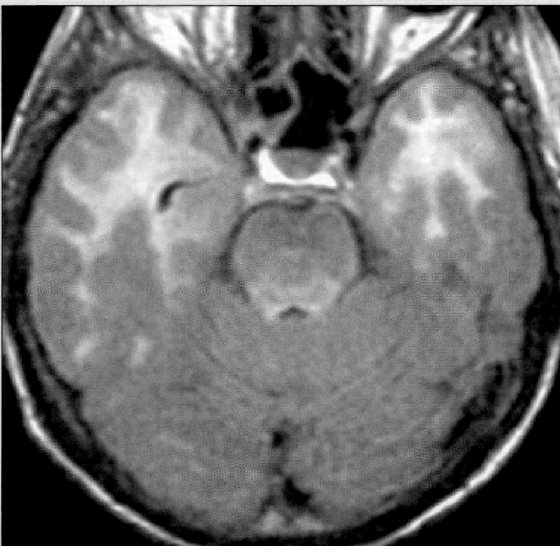

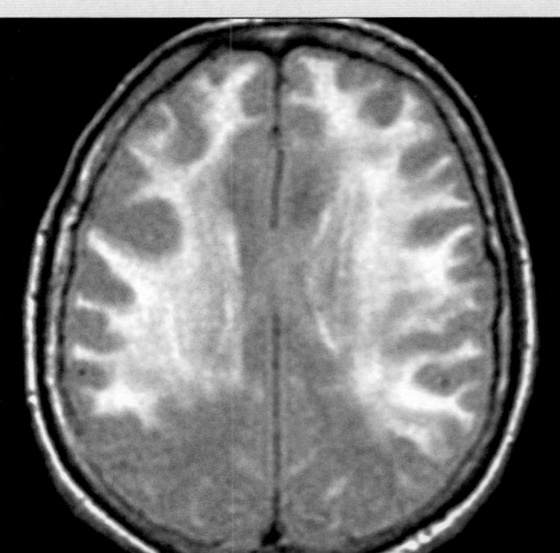

THYROID DISORDERS

TERMINOLOGY

Abbreviations

- Hashimoto thyroiditis (HT), encephalopathy (HE)

Synonyms

- Corticosteroid-responsive encephalopathy associated with autoimmune thyroiditis

Definitions

- Thyroid hormone deficiency affecting multiorgan systems

IMAGING

General Features

- Best diagnostic clue
  - Symmetrical pituitary enlargement that is reversible with thyroid hormone replacement therapy (THRT)
- Location
  - Pituitary enlarged, variable suprasellar extension/ mass effect
- Size
  - Correlates with circulating thyrotropin levels, ↑ with hyperthyroid and ↓ with hypothyroid
- Morphology
  - Hyperplasia of anterior pituitary

CT Findings

- NECT
  - Sellar mass ± suprasellar extension
  - Basal ganglia (BG), variable cerebellar Ca++
- CECT
  - Enhancing intra-/suprasellar mass

MR Findings

- T1WI
  - Enlarged pituitary isointense to cerebral white matter (WM)
  - With THRT: Brain size ↑, ventricular size ↓
  - BG variably hyperintense (Ca++)
  - In endemic neurological cretinism
    - Bilateral globi pallidi, substantia nigra hyperintensity
    - Mild generalized atrophy
    - Enlargement of sylvian fissures
- T2WI
  - Homogeneous diffuse enlargement of pituitary gland, ± suprasellar extension, ± partial or complete obliteration of infundibulum, ± compression of optic chiasm
  - Enlarged pituitary gland is isointense to cerebral white matter
  - In patients with HT-associated ataxia
    - Cerebellar vermis or olivopontocerebellar atrophy
  - Hashimoto encephalopathy
    - HE: Diffuse/focal cortical, subcortical WM T2 hyperintensity with relative sparing of occipital lobes
  - In endemic neurological cretinism
    - Hypointensity in area of globus pallidus and substantia nigra bilaterally
    - Mild generalized atrophy and enlarged sylvian fissures with hypothyroidism
- T1WI C+
  - Enlarged pituitary enhances homogeneously, intensely, ~ cavernous sinuses
  - No focal hypointensity (suggestive of adenoma)
- MRS
  - ↑ Cho in untreated congenital hypothyroidism reflecting blocked myelin maturation

Nuclear Medicine Findings

- PET
  - Severe hypothyroidism (short duration): Generalized ↓ regional CBF, glucose metabolism

Other Modality Findings

- Tc-99m HMPAO SPECT: Reversible cerebral hypoperfusion (25% ↓ mean CBF) in reversible dementia caused by hypothyroidism

Imaging Recommendations

- Best imaging tool
  - MR
- Protocol advice
  - Coronal T1WI C+, axial T2 for white matter

DIFFERENTIAL DIAGNOSIS

Pituitary Macroadenoma

- Difficult to differentiate adenoma from pituitary hyperplasia
- T1WI
  - Adenomas may be homogeneous or heterogeneous, typically with lower signal than normal pituitary gland
  - Isointense signal if hemorrhage or necrosis within adenoma
- T1WI C+: Focal hypointensity suggests macro- or microadenoma

Physiologic Pituitary Hyperplasia

- Puberty, pregnancy, postpartum (1st week)
- Can be indistinguishable on imaging studies

Lymphocytic Hypophysitis

- Thick/bulbous stalk ± enlarged pituitary
- Intense uniform enhancement

Enlargement of Pituitary Gland with Spontaneous Intracranial Hypotension

- Look for diffuse dural thickening, "slumping midbrain," tonsillar herniation

PATHOLOGY

General Features

- Etiology
  - Primary hypothyroidism
    - HT (most common cause in North America): Autoimmune disease
    - Iatrogenic hypothyroidism (2nd most common): Post-thyroidectomy, post-radioactive I-131 therapy

THYROID DISORDERS

  - Congenital hypothyroidism: Aplasia/hypoplasia or ectopic gland, enzymatic defects in thyroid hormone synthesis
  - Goitrous hypothyroidism: Endemic iodine deficiency; extinct in USA, but major cause of mental deficiency worldwide
- ○ Secondary hypothyroidism: Uncommon cause
  - Hypothalamic-pituitary axis failure (↓ thyroid releasing hormone [TRH]/thyroid stimulating hormone [TSH])
- ○ Lack of inhibition of hypothalamic TRH, pituitary TSH caused by insufficient quantity of thyroid hormones
- ○ High TRH levels increase mainly TSH release but also prolactin release from pituitary
- ○ 2 mechanisms of cerebellar dysfunction in hypothyroidism
  - Endocrine disorder, reversible with THRT
  - Autoimmune-mediated HT, not reversed by THRT
- ○ Encephalopathy associated with HT
  - Likely autoimmune pathogenesis
  - Possible underlying cerebral vasculitis

- Associated abnormalities
  - ○ HT is associated with other autoimmune diseases
    - Rheumatoid arthritis, SLE, insulin-dependent diabetes mellitus, ulcerative colitis, myasthenia gravis, MS, pernicious anemia
  - ○ Circulating antithyroid peroxidase antibodies in 70-95% of patients with HT
  - ○ Encephalopathy associated with subclinical HT with high titers of antithyroid antibodies
  - ○ Diffuse hyperplasia of anterior pituitary
  - ○ Cretinism
    - Malformed convolution, poor differentiation of cortical layers, reduction in quantity of white matter, delayed myelination

Gross Pathologic & Surgical Features

- Diffuse enlargement of pituitary gland
- HT with cerebellar dysfunction: Atrophy of anterosuperior vermis

Microscopic Features

- Hyperplasia of thyrotrophs (thyrotropin-producing cells), ± lactotrophs (prolactin-producing cells) in anterior lobe of otherwise normal pituitary gland
- HT with cerebellar dysfunction: Loss of Purkinje cells
  - ○ ± gliosis of ventral pons

CLINICAL ISSUES

Presentation

- Most common signs/symptoms
  - ○ Hypothyroidism: Poor memory, psychomotor slowing, depression, reversible dementia
  - ○ Acquired cerebellar ataxia
  - ○ HE: Seizures, stroke-like symptoms, neuropsychiatric episodes, cognitive decline
  - ○ Other: Headache, visual impairment (bitemporal hemianopsia) if enlarged pituitary

Demographics

- Age
  - ○ In acquired hypothyroidism, prevalence ↑ with age
  - ○ HE reported in pediatric and adult patients
- Gender
  - ○ Females commonly affected in acquired hypothyroidism
- Epidemiology
  - ○ Acquired hypothyroidism affects 8-9 million Americans
  - ○ Congenital hypothyroidism: Caucasian infants (1:4,000) affected more than African-American infants (1:30,000)

Natural History & Prognosis

- Rapid progression (3 weeks) of hyperplasia of anterior pituitary proven in acute development of hypothyroidism
- In congenital hypothyroidism: Main developmental delay originates during 1st 3 months after birth

Treatment

- Prompt regression of pituitary enlargement with THRT
- ↑ in brain size and ↓ in ventricular size with treatment correlate with changes in levels of circulating thyroid hormones
- In congenital hypothyroidism, thyroid hormone replacement ASAP (< 13 days)
  - ○ Patients with early treated congenital hypothyroidism often develop subnormally and display subtle neurological defects
- Endemic cretinism is determined in utero, irreversible by postnatal treatment
- Acquired cerebellar ataxia is typically reversible with THRT
  - ○ In few patients: Ataxia persists despite THRT
- HE: Responsive to corticosteroid suggestive of autoimmune mechanism

DIAGNOSTIC CHECKLIST

Consider

- Urgent thyroid function tests should be performed in all patients with pituitary enlargement prior to surgery to exclude hypothyroid-induced pituitary swelling
- Consider hypothyroidism in child (especially male) with diagnosis of "pituitary adenoma!"
- HE: Exclude other toxic metabolic or infectious etiologies, high antithyroid peroxidase antibody

SELECTED REFERENCES

1. Eom KS et al: Primary hypothyroidism mimicking a pituitary macroadenoma: regression after thyroid hormone replacement therapy. Pediatr Radiol. 39(2):164-7, 2009
2. Alves C et al: Primary hypothyroidism in a child simulating a prolactin-secreting adenoma. Childs Nerv Syst. 24(12):1505-8, 2008
3. Oatridge A et al: Changes in brain size with treatment in patients with hyper- or hypothyroidism. AJNR Am J Neuroradiol. 23(9):1539-44, 2002
4. Selim M et al: Ataxia associated with Hashimoto's disease: progressive non-familial adult onset cerebellar degeneration with autoimmune thyroiditis. J Neurol Neurosurg Psychiatry. 71(1):81-7, 2001
5. Shimono T et al: Rapid progression of pituitary hyperplasia in humans with primary hypothyroidism: demonstration with MR imaging. Radiology. 213(2):383-8, 1999

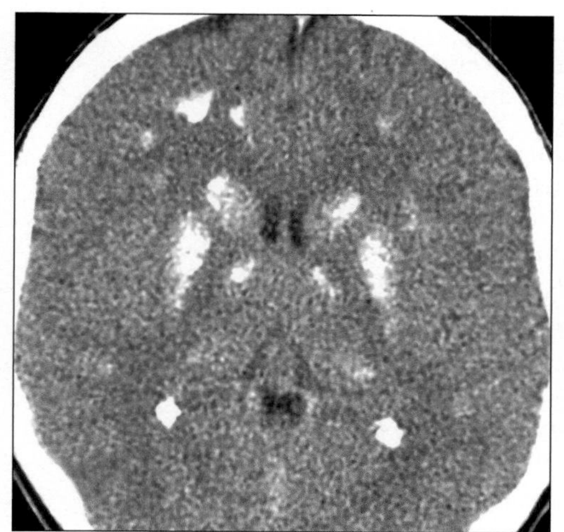

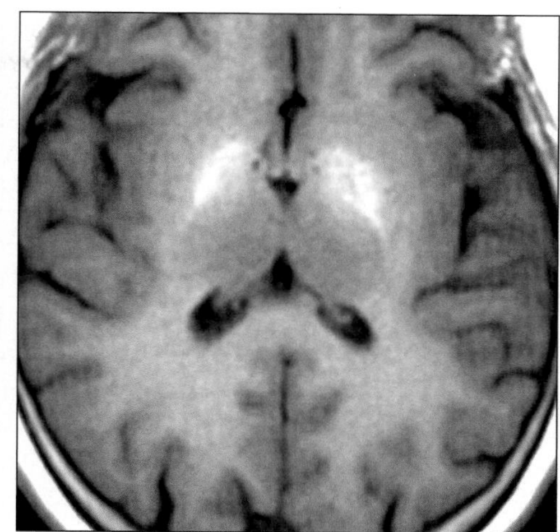

(Left) *Axial NECT shows diffuse calcifications within the basal ganglia and subcortical white matter in a patient with hypothyroidism. Imaging mimics that of other thyroid and parathyroid disorders.* ***(Right)*** *Axial T1WI MR shows focal hyperintensity in both globi pallidi related to longstanding hypothyroidism. NECT scan (not shown) disclosed dense calcifications in the basal ganglia, especially in the globi pallidi, typical of hypothyroidism.*

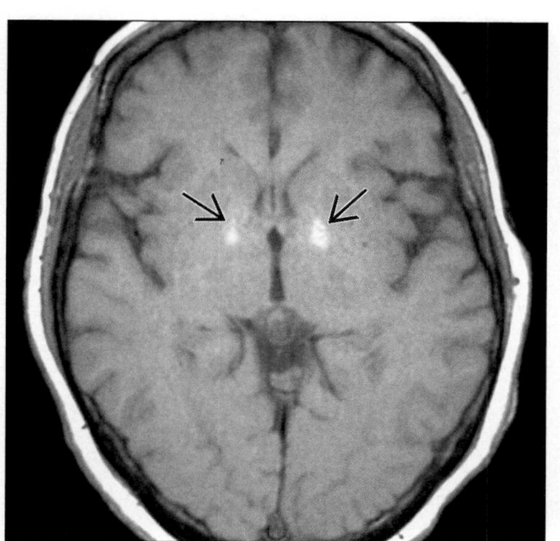

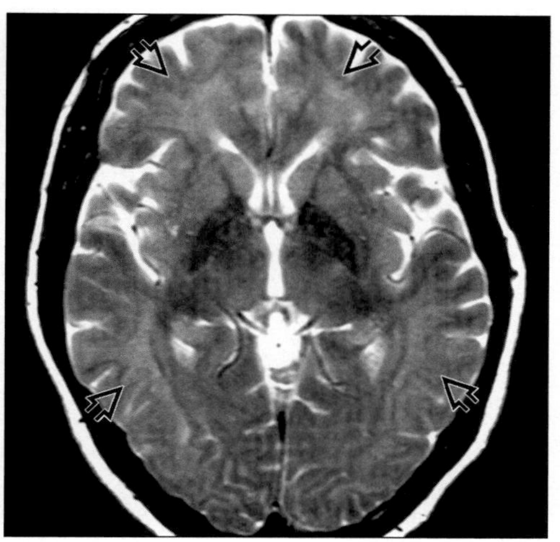

(Left) *Axial T1WI shows bilateral hyperintensities in the medial globi pallidi ⇒ in a patient who is status post thyroidectomy.* ***(Right)*** *Axial T2WI MR shows striking confluent, symmetric hyperintensity throughout the white matter ⇒ with involvement of the subcortical U-fibers. This diffuse white matter hyperintensity is a very rare but recognized manifestation of hypothyroidism. Sometimes called "myxedema madness," it is also known as Hashimoto encephalopathy.*

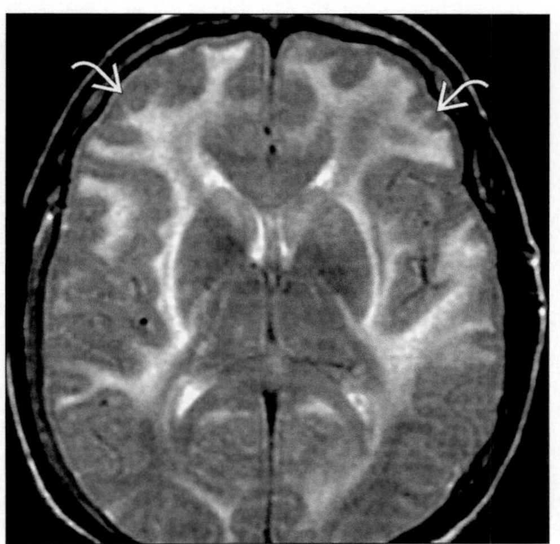

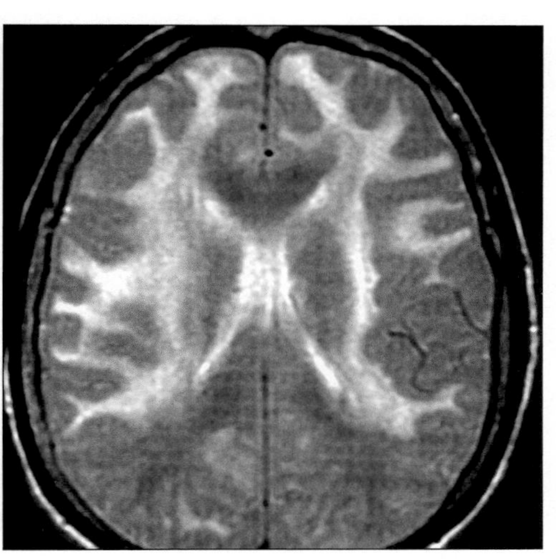

(Left) *Axial FLAIR MR shows diffuse confluent white matter hyperintensity with relative sparing of the occipital lobes ➡. This diffuse white matter hyperintensity with involvement of the subcortical U-fibers with relative sparing of the occipital lobes is characteristic for Hashimoto encephalopathy.* ***(Right)*** *Axial FLAIR MR in the same patient shows diffuse white matter hyperintensity extending to involve the subcortical U-fibers. Note the relative sparing of the occipital lobes and corpus callosum.*

Key Facts

Terminology

- CNS manifestations related to parathyroid hormone (PTH) metabolic abnormalities

Imaging

- Best imaging clue: Ca++ in basal ganglia, thalamus, subcortical white matter (WM), dentate nucleus
  - May see dural Ca++
- Best imaging tools: CT and MR (T2WI and T2* GRE)

Top Differential Diagnoses

- Toxic-metabolic disorders
- Fahr disease
- Physiologic calcification
- Congenital HIV
- Hypoxic-ischemic encephalopathy

Pathology

- 1° hyperPT: Parathyroid adenoma (80-90%), rarely carcinoma (1-5%)
- 2° hyperPT: Chronic renal failure, kidney fails to convert vitamin D to active form and excrete phophate
- 1° hypoPT: Parathyroids are absent or atrophied; genetic autoimmune syndrome or DiGeorge syndrome (total absence of PT glands at birth)
- PseudohypoPT: Insensitivity of end-organ to PTH, rather than decreased production of PTH

Clinical Issues

- HyperPT: ↑ Ca++ affects transsynaptic nerve conduction, fatigue, pain, nausea, osteoporosis
- HypoPT: Muscle cramp, convulsion, seizure, parkinsonism, dystonia, ataxia, dysarthria

*(**Left**) Axial NECT shows symmetric bilateral calcification of the globus pallidi ➡ and caudate nucleus. The patient has known secondary hyperparathyroidism from chronic renal failure. (**Right**) Axial NECT in the same patient shows subcortical white matter calcification ⮞. A small subdural hematoma is also present in the right frontal region ⮫. Imaging mimics other toxic-metabolic disorders and Fahr disease.*

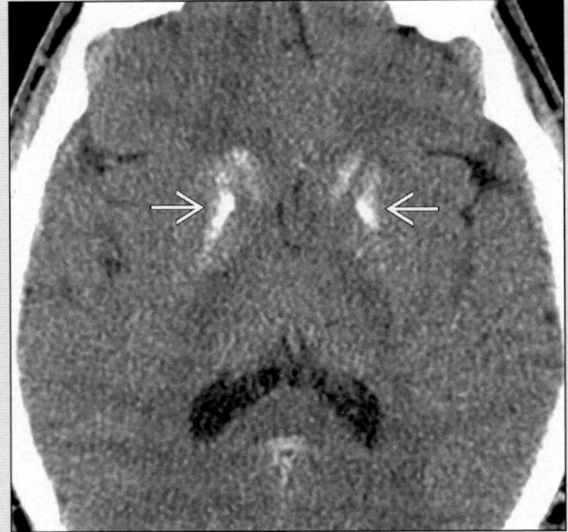

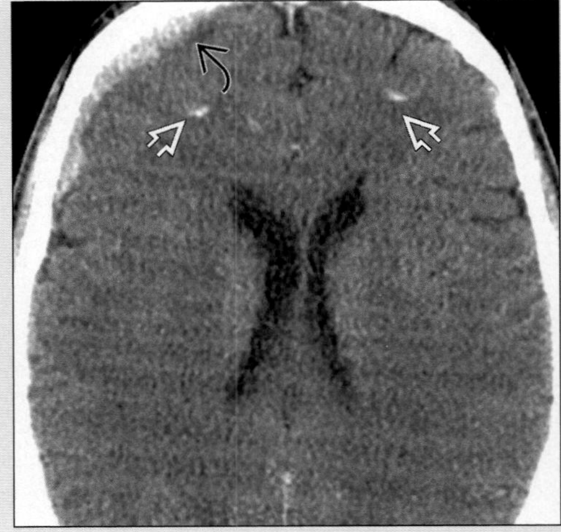

*(**Left**) Axial NECT shows extensive calcification along the tentorium ⮞ in a patient with a long history of dialysis for chronic renal failure. Chronic renal failure is a common cause of secondary hyperparathyroidism which often results in ectopic dural calcification. Secondary hyperparathyroidism may also be caused by parathyroid hyperplasia. (**Right**) Axial NECT in the same patient shows extensive tentorial calcifications ⮞. Dural calcifications may also be seen in basal cell nevus syndrome, a rare phacomatosis.*

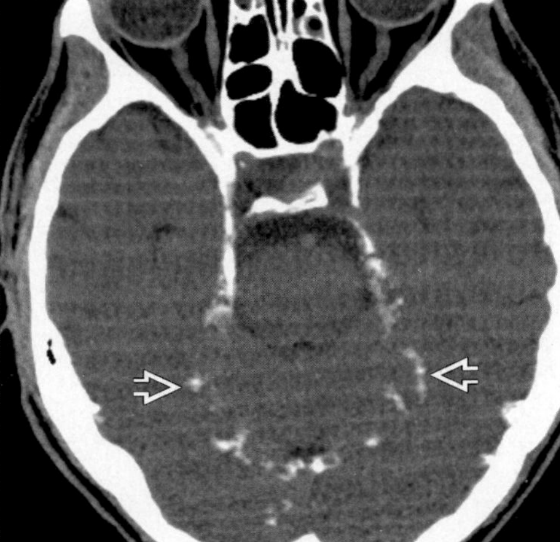

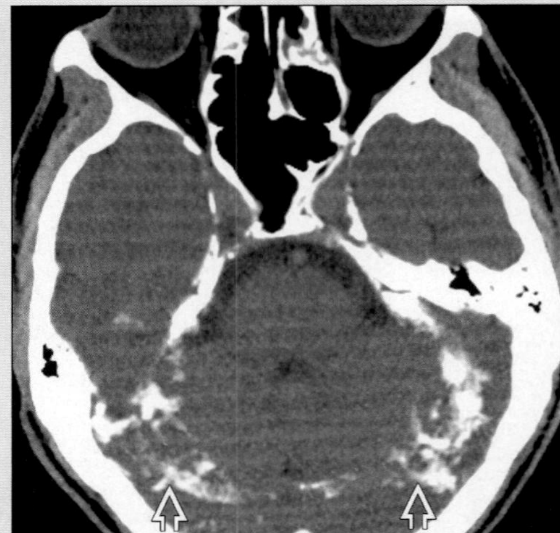

PARATHYROID DISORDERS

TERMINOLOGY

Definitions

- CNS manifestations related to parathyroid hormone (PTH) metabolic abnormalities
  - 1° and 2° hyperparathyroidism (hyperPT)
  - 1° and 2° hypoparathyroidism (hypoPT)
  - pseudohypoparathyroidism (pseudohypoPT)
  - pseudo-pseudohypoparathyroidism (pseudo-pseudohypoPT)
  - Albright hereditary osteodystrophy (AHO)

IMAGING

General Features

- Best diagnostic clue
  - Calcium (Ca++) deposition in basal ganglia (BG)
- Location
  - Ca++ in globus pallidi (GP), putamen, caudate, thalamus, subcortical WM, dentate nucleus

Imaging Recommendations

- Best imaging tool: CT and MR (T2WI and T2* GRE)

CT Findings

- NECT
  - Bilateral Ca++ of BG
  - May see dural heterotopic Ca++

MR Findings

- T1WI: BG hyperintensity
- T2WI: Hypointensity involving BG, cerebral cortex, or dentate nucleus due to Ca++ deposition
- T2* GRE: "Blooming" artifact related to Ca++

DIFFERENTIAL DIAGNOSIS

Toxic-Metabolic Disorders

- Multiple etiologies result in abnormal Ca++
- Hepatic encephalopathy: Ammonia accumulation
- Carbon monoxide (CO) poisoning, MDMA exposure: GP ischemia
- Hyperalimentation: Manganese deposition
- Wilson disease: Abnormal ceruloplasmin metabolism
- Nonketonic hyperglycemia

Fahr Disease

- Symmetric Ca++ in BG, thalamus, and dentate nucleus

Physiologic Calcification

- Almost always GP, ↑ incidence with age

Congenital HIV

- Microangiopathy and infarction → Ca++ and atrophy

Hypoxic-Ischemic Encephalopathy

- GP, thalamus, and brainstem Ca++

PATHOLOGY

General Features

- Etiology
  - 1° hyperPT: Parathyroid adenoma (80-90%) and rarely carcinoma (1-5%), ↑ PTH, ↑ Ca++
  - 2° hyperPT: Chronic renal failure commonly → kidneys fail to convert vitamin D to active form & excrete phophate (P): ↑ PTH, normal or ↓ Ca++, ↑↑ P
    - Parathyroid hyperplasia less common
  - 1° hypoPT: Parathyroid glands are absent or atrophied; surgically removed; genetic autoimmune syndrome or DiGeorge syndrome (total absence of parathyroid glands at birth)
  - PseudohypoPT: Insensitivity of end-organ to PTH, rather than ↓ production of PTH; dysfunction of G protein (Gs alpha subunit): ↓ Ca++, ↑ P, ↑↑ PTH
- Genetics
  - AHO: Rare inherited metabolic disorder, short stature, brachydactyly, round face, and mild mental retardation, can be pseudohypoPT (type 1a) or pseudo-pseudohypoPT (AHO with normal response to PTH)
- Associated abnormalities
  - Dialysis-associated encephalopathy: Dementia (aluminum accumulation), renal osteodystrophy, brown tumor
  - HypoPT could be due to hemochromatosis or magnesium deficiency

CLINICAL ISSUES

Presentation

- Most common signs/symptoms
  - HyperPT: ↑ Ca++ affects transsynaptic nerve conduction; fatigue, pain, nausea, osteoporosis
  - HypoPT: Muscle cramp, convulsion, seizure, parkinsonism, dystonia, ataxia, dysarthria
- Other signs/symptoms
  - HyperPT: Excessive secretion of PTH: ↑ Ca++ (1° hyperPT) or response to low Ca++ level (2° hyperPT)
  - HypoPT: Dry, puffy, coarse skin, brittle nails, cataract, ↓ Ca++

Treatment

- Primary hyperPT: Remove parathyroid adenoma
- Secondary hyperPT: Calcimimetics → mimics Ca++ in body, reduce PTH secretion, lowering Ca++
- HypoPT: Intravenous calcium with vitamin D3

DIAGNOSTIC CHECKLIST

Consider

- Excessive Ca++ in BG or heterotopic Ca++, consider PTH abnormality and other toxic-metabolic disorders

SELECTED REFERENCES

1. Kung B et al: Parathyroid carcinoma: a rare cause of primary hyperparathyroidism. Ear Nose Throat J. 88(9):E10-3, 2009
2. Dorenbeck U et al: Tentorial and dural calcification with tertiary hyperparathyroidism: a rare entity in chronic renal failure. Eur Radiol. 12 Suppl 3:S11-3, 2002

FAHR DISEASE

Key Facts

Terminology
- Fahr disease (FD)
  - Also known as cerebrovascular ferrocalcinosis
- Rare degenerative neurological disorder
  - Extensive bilateral basal ganglia (BG) calcifications (Ca++)
  - ± progressive dystonia, parkinsonism, neuropsychiatric manifestations

Imaging
- Best diagnostic clue: Bilateral symmetric BG Ca++ on NECT

Top Differential Diagnoses
- Normal (physiologic)
  - Symmetrical BG Ca++ in middle-aged, elderly
- Pathologic BG Ca++ (e.g., endocrinological)

Pathology
- FD is often familial, yet heterogeneous
- Characteristic feature: Diffuse neurofibrillary tangles with calcification (a.k.a. Fahr-type calcification)

Clinical Issues
- Most common signs/symptoms
  - Neuropsychiatric disturbance
  - Cognitive impairment (subcortical dementia)
  - Extrapyramidal movement disorders
- Ca++/P metabolism, PTH levels normal
- Bimodal pattern of clinical onset
  - Early adulthood (schizophrenic-like psychosis)
  - 6th decade (extrapyramidal syndrome, subcortical dementia)

Diagnostic Checklist
- BG Ca++ if < 50 years old merits investigation

(Left) *Axial NECT shows the bilateral, slightly asymmetric, hyperdense calcifications of the basal ganglia and thalami that are characteristic of Fahr disease ➡. The dentate nuclei (not shown) were also calcified.* ***(Right)*** *Axial T1WI MR in the same patient shows the lesions as hyperintense foci ➡. T1 shortening is typical and is secondary to the presence of Fahr-type calcification.*

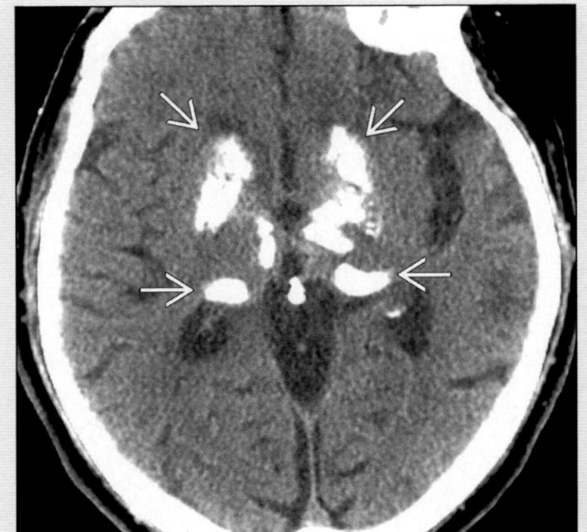

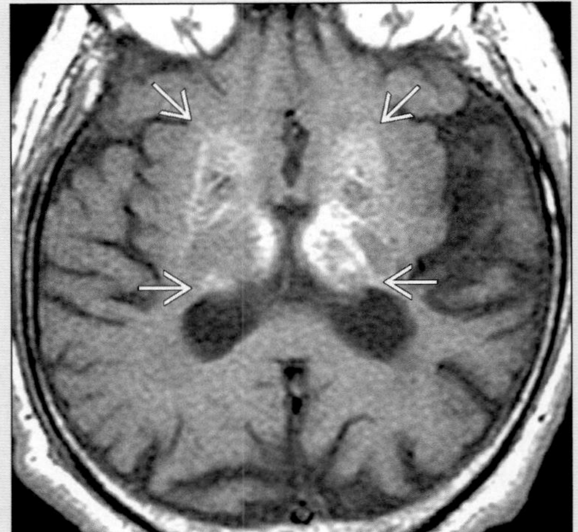

(Left) *Axial T2* GRE MR in the same patient reveals susceptibility within the lesions ➡, which is less prominent than the hyperdensity seen on NECT and the T1 shortening seen on MR. This gradient "blooming" appearance is secondary to iron deposition.* ***(Right)*** *Axial T2WI MR in the same patient, obtained slightly more cephalad, shows the typical concomitant changes of chronic microvascular disease, most prominent around the atria ➡.*

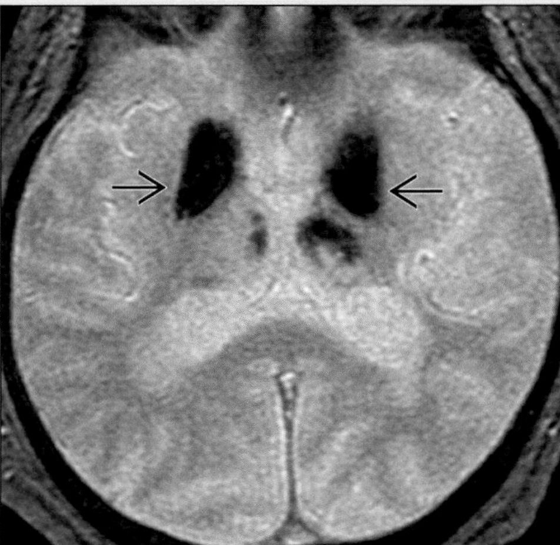

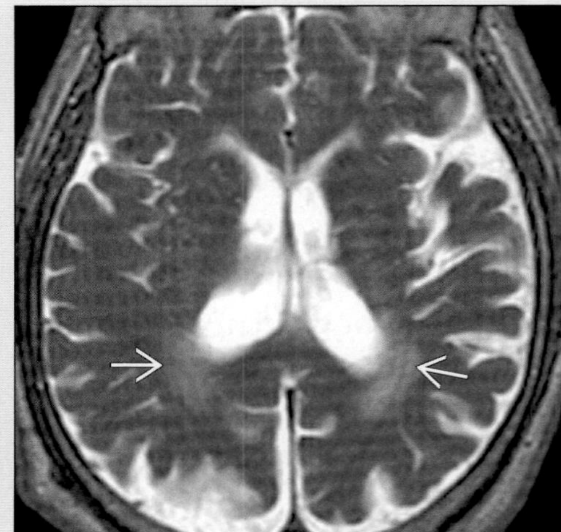

TERMINOLOGY

Abbreviations

- Fahr disease (FD)

Synonyms

- Idiopathic basal ganglia calcification (IBGC), cerebrovascular ferrocalcinosis, bilateral striopallidodentate calcinosis

Definitions

- Rare degenerative neurological disorder
  - Extensive bilateral basal ganglia (BG) calcifications (Ca++)
  - Can lead to progressive dystonia, parkinsonism, neuropsychiatric manifestations

IMAGING

General Features

- Best diagnostic clue
  - Bilateral symmetric BG Ca++ on CT
- Location
  - Globus pallidus = most common site of Ca++
    - Lateral pallidum > medial pallidum
  - Also putamen, caudate, thalami, cerebellum (especially dentate), internal capsule, cerebral white matter
- Morphology
  - Variable extent
  - Dense Ca++ often conforms to outline of BG

CT Findings

- NECT
  - Bilateral symmetric Ca++ in typical locations
- CECT
  - No enhancement

MR Findings

- T1WI
  - Varying signal intensities related to
    - Stage of disease, volume of calcium deposit
    - Differences in calcium metabolism
  - Ca++ usually hyperintense on T1WI
- T2WI
  - Dense Ca++ can appear hypo-/hyperintense
  - T2 hyperintense areas in white matter
    - Do not correspond to any calcification
    - May reflect metabolic or inflammatory brain process, which subsequently becomes calcified
    - Entire centrum semiovale may appear hyperintense in patients with dementia
    - Focal internal capsule hyperintense foci may correlate with contralateral hemiparesis
- FLAIR
  - Same as T2WI
- SWI
  - Marked hypointensity
  - SWI may prove to be more sensitive than CT

Nuclear Medicine Findings

- PET
  - May show ↓ bilateral FDG uptake in BG
    - Also seen in frontal and temporoparietal cortices and hippocampal area
  - Functional abnormalities may precede morphological changes in FD process
- SPECT with Tc-99-ethyl-cysteinate-dimer (ECD)
  - ↓ perfusion to calcified lesions
    - Especially in setting of dementia
    - Not associated with volume of calcium deposits
  - May see ↑ perfusion if acquired during symptomatology
    - Especially temporal lobes with auditory hallucinations

Imaging Recommendations

- Best imaging tool
  - NECT
- Protocol advice
  - MR SWI may prove to be superior

DIFFERENTIAL DIAGNOSIS

Normal

- Symmetrical BG Ca++ in middle-aged, elderly
- Localized in globus pallidus
- Usually punctate but can be quite heavy
- Detected on CT scan, no clinical significance
- Extremely common finding in older age group
- If accompanied by other calcifications, consider pathologic condition

Inherited, Acquired BG Ca++

- In children/young adults
- Associated with Down syndrome
- Trisomy 5
- Mitochondrial encephalopathies
  - Kearns-Sayre, MELAS, MERRF
  - T2 hyperintense lesions in BG
  - BG Ca++ can occur but not prominent feature
- Aicardi-Goutières syndrome
  - Autosomal recessive
  - Encephalopathy after birth → developmental arrest
- HIV encephalitis
  - BG Ca++ and cerebral atrophy
- Cockayne syndrome
  - Autosomal recessive disorder of DNA repair
  - CT: Cortico-subcortical atrophy, BG and dentate nuclei Ca++
  - T2WI: Hyperintensity of periventricular white matter and subcortical U-fibers
  - T2WI hypointense putamina and caudate nuclei
  - Atrophy of cerebellar vermis and brainstem
  - Dwarfism, microcephaly, mental retardation
  - Photosensitivity, ocular abnormalities
  - Gait disturbance, progeroid appearance
- Long-term complications of radiation for childhood brain tumors and intrathecal chemotherapy
  - Bilateral BG Ca++, leukoencephalopathy
- Phakomatoses: Tuberous sclerosis and neurofibromatosis

Pathologic BG Ca++

- Endocrinologic disorders

- Hyperparathyroidism, hypoparathyroidism, pseudohypoparathyroidism, pseudopseudohypoparathyroidism, post-thyroidectomy
- Similar distribution of calcifications to FD
- Hypoparathyroidism: ↑ ionic calcium in interstitial tissues with ↓ levels of circulating calcium
- Calcification in primary hypoparathyroidism is more diffuse than in other etiologies of calcification
- Post-thyroidectomy hypoparathyroidism calcifications are more focal

- Neuropsychiatric (e.g., lupus, motor neuron disease)
- Postinfectious (e.g., TB, toxoplasmosis, cysticercosis)
- Toxic (e.g., carbon monoxide, lead intoxication)

PATHOLOGY

General Features

- Etiology
  - CNS Ca++ in FD could represent
    - Metastatic deposition secondary to local blood-brain barrier disruption
    - Disorder of neuronal calcium metabolism
  - Defective iron transport and free radicals → tissue damage → calcification
- Genetics
  - Autosomal dominant in most families with FD
    - Occasionally autosomal recessive
  - FD is often familial, yet heterogeneous
    - Variable expressivity and reduced penetrance can be found in same family, but most patients are symptomatic
    - "Genetic anticipation" = age of onset ↓ with each transmission in multigenerational family
    - In some kindreds, most individuals are largely asymptomatic
  - 1st locus identified: IBGC1 on chromosome 14q
    - IBGC1 region contains over 100 known genes, expressed sequence tags, and predicted genes
    - Now known not to be the main locus

Staging, Grading, & Classification

- Fahr disease = idiopathic calcifications with cognitive and neurobehavioral manifestations
  - Diagnosis of exclusion; requires normal calcium, phosphorous, and parathyroid hormone levels
- Fahr syndrome = same appearance as FD but secondary to underlying disorder (e.g., hypoparathyroidism)

Microscopic Features

- Characteristic feature: Diffuse neurofibrillary tangles with calcification (a.k.a. Fahr-type calcification)
  - Neurofibrillary tangles comprised of tau and phosphorylated-tau protein
- Predominant element is calcium
  - Other elements (Zn, P, Fe, Mg, Al, K) also present
- Ca++ in extracellular, extravascular space, often surrounding capillaries
  - Ca++ of medial walls and adventitia
  - Ca++ in areas of demyelination, lipid deposition
  - Ca++ incorporated into proteins or bound to polysaccharides

CLINICAL ISSUES

Presentation

- Most common signs/symptoms
  - Neuropsychiatric disturbance
  - Cognitive impairment (subcortical dementia)
  - Extrapyramidal movement disorders
- Clinical profile
  - Calcium-phosphorus metabolism and parathyroid hormone levels are normal
  - Usually asymptomatic in 1st 2 decades of life, despite presence of multiple brain calcifications
  - Neurological manifestations vary, but movement disorders are most common
    - Parkinsonism most common, usually permanent and progressive
    - Childhood transient parkinsonism also reported
    - Paroxysmal dystonic choreoathetosis

Demographics

- Age
  - Onset of clinical symptoms is typically 30-60 years
  - Infantile form also described
  - Bimodal pattern of clinical onset
    - Early adulthood (schizophrenic-like psychosis)
    - 6th decade (extrapyramidal syndrome, subcortical dementia)
- Gender
  - No gender predominance
- Epidemiology
  - Rare

Natural History & Prognosis

- Characterized by very slow progression
- Mental deterioration and loss of motor skills
  - Degenerative rather than developmental disorder
- Adult-onset FD: Calcium deposition begins in 3rd decade, with neurological deterioration 2 decades later
- Symmetrical spastic paralysis and sometimes athetosis appear, progressing to decerebrate state
- Commonly develop neuropsychiatric disturbances
- Proposed disruption in thalamo-cortico-striatal circuit leads to disconnection syndrome, termed "cognitive dysmetria," producing symptoms of schizophrenia

DIAGNOSTIC CHECKLIST

Consider

- FD in parkinsonian patients with dementia and cerebellar signs
- Discovery of BG Ca++ if < 50 years old merits investigation

Image Interpretation Pearls

- Symmetric BG Ca++ in middle-aged/older adults?
  - Common, of no clinical significance

SELECTED REFERENCES

1. Shirahama M et al: A young woman with visual hallucinations, delusions of persecution and a history of performing arson with possible three-generation Fahr disease. Acta Psychiatr Scand. Epub ahead of print, 2009

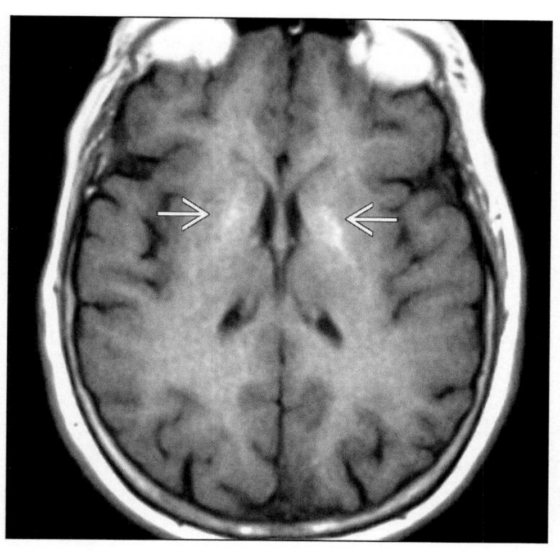

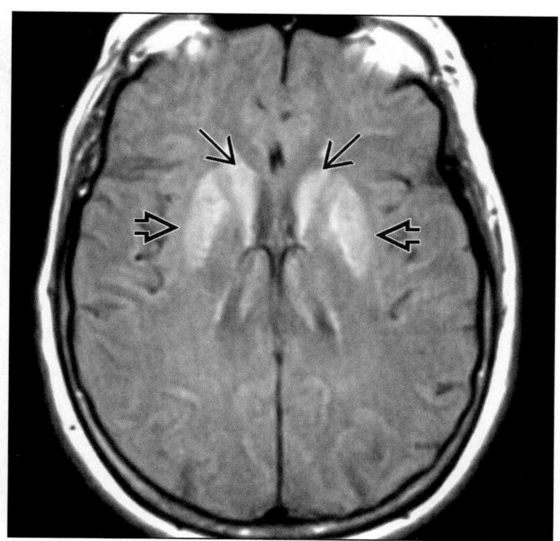

(Left) *Axial T1WI MR demonstrates the typical MR appearance of Fahr disease with T1 hyperintense basal ganglia calcifications →. These calcifications were also documented on head CT (not shown).* ***(Right)*** *Axial PD/intermediate MR in the same patient reveals the typical pattern of basal ganglia calcifications as T1 hyperintensity within a larger region of T2 hyperintense abnormality →. Note that the T2 technique reveals that the caudate nuclei are also involved →.*

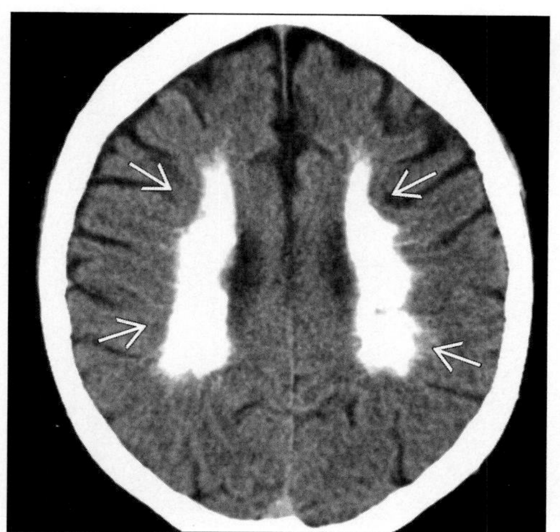

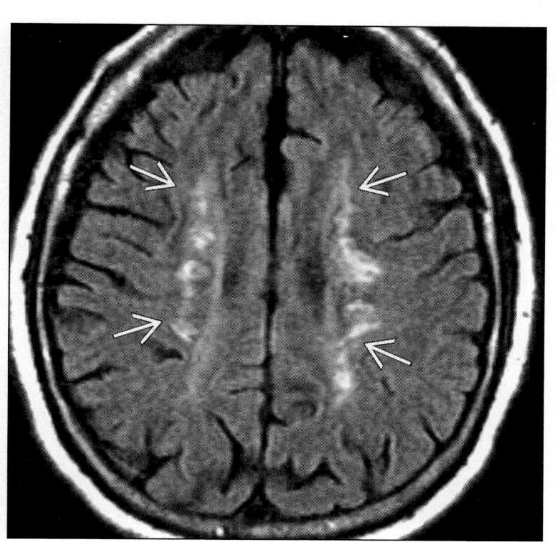

(Left) *Axial NECT of a patient with Fahr disease shows extensive calcifications involving the periventricular deep white matter →. Patients with extensively affected centrum semiovale are more likely to present with dementia.* ***(Right)*** *Axial FLAIR MR in the same patient shows T2 hyperintensity within the areas of calcification →. In advanced cases, hyperintense abnormality may affect the entire centrum semiovale.*

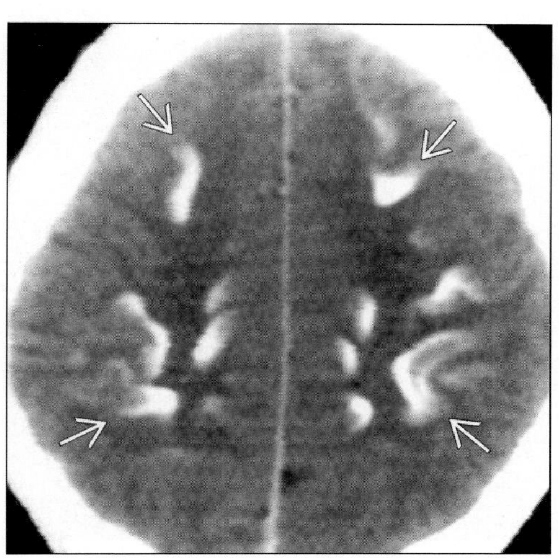

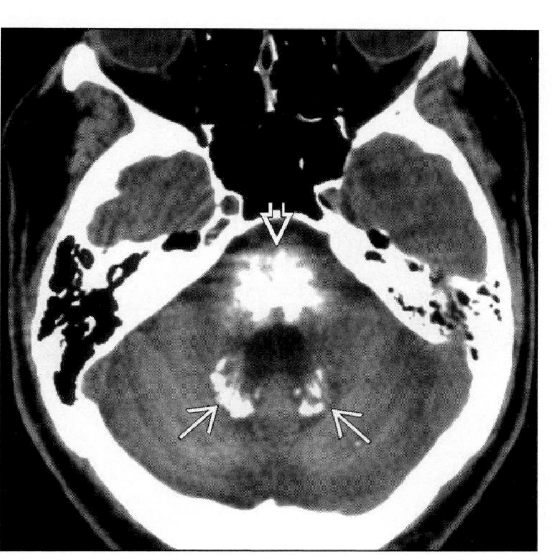

(Left) *Axial NECT demonstrates extensive Fahr-type calcifications at subcortical gray-white junctions →.* ***(Right)*** *Axial NECT illustrates both the typical dentate → as well as atypical and extremely dense midbrain → calcifications of Fahr disease, which is often familial, as in this case.*

ALCOHOLIC ENCEPHALOPATHY

Key Facts

Terminology
- Acute/subacute/chronic toxic effects of EtOH on CNS

Imaging
- EtOH
  - Superior vermian atrophy
  - Enlargement of lateral ventricles, sulci with chronic EtOH
- WE: Mamillary body, medial thalamus, hypothalamus, periaqueductal gray abnormal signal/ enhancement/diffusion restriction
- Corpus callosum (Marchiafava-Bignami disease)
- Diffuse toxic demyelination, rare
- Protocol advice: Contrast-enhanced MR + DWI

Top Differential Diagnoses
- Nonalcoholic atrophy
- Diffuse demyelination
  - Toxic demyelination
  - Acquired/inherited metabolic disorders
- Corpus callosal hyperintensity
  - Status epilepticus
  - Drug toxicity
  - Encephalitis
  - Hypoglycemia

Pathology
- EtOH
  - Causes both direct/indirect neurotoxicity
- WE
  - Thiamine deficiency
- WE can be alcoholic or nonalcoholic

Diagnostic Checklist
- 50% of WE cases occur in nonalcoholics, including children!

*(**Left**) Sagittal graphic shows generalized and superior vermian atrophy, necrosis in the corpus callosum related to alcoholic toxicity. Mammillary body, periaqueductal gray necrosis is seen with Wernicke encephalopathy. (**Right**) Coronal T2WI MR demonstrates pronounced cerebellar atrophy.*

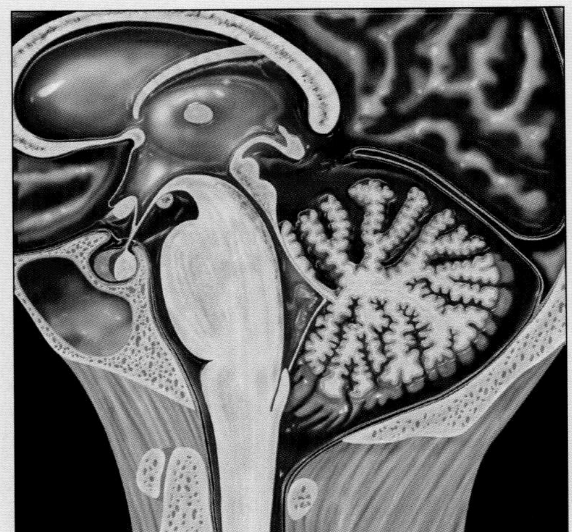

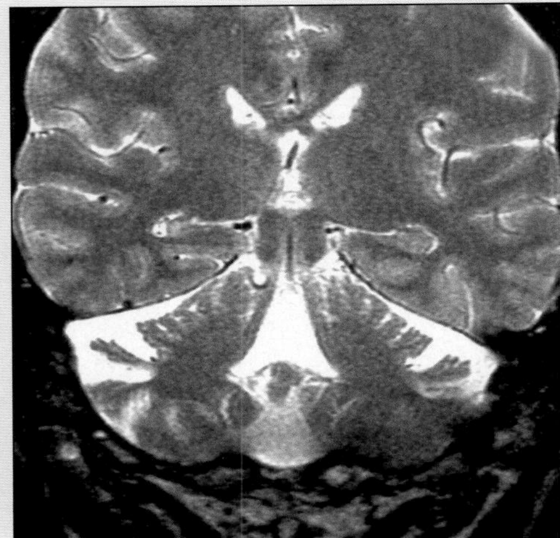

*(**Left**) Sagittal T1WI MR shows a classic finding for Marchiafava-Bignami disease with thinned corpus callosum and hypointensity in middle layers ⇒. Note that the genu, body, and splenium are all involved. (Courtesy A. Datir, MD.) (**Right**) Axial DWI MR shows restricted diffusion in the mammillary bodies ➡ in this patient with acute Wernicke encephalopathy.*

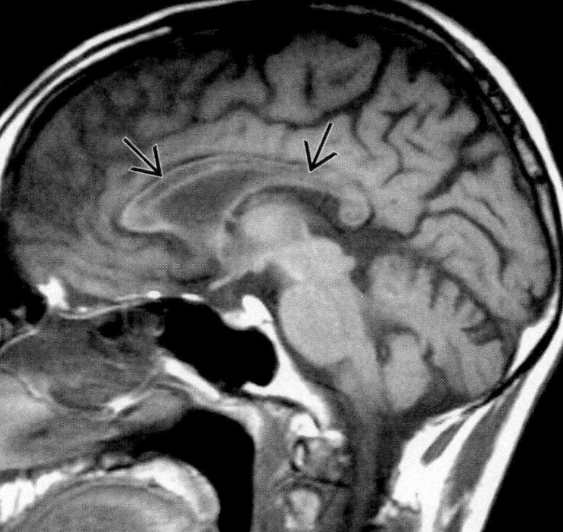

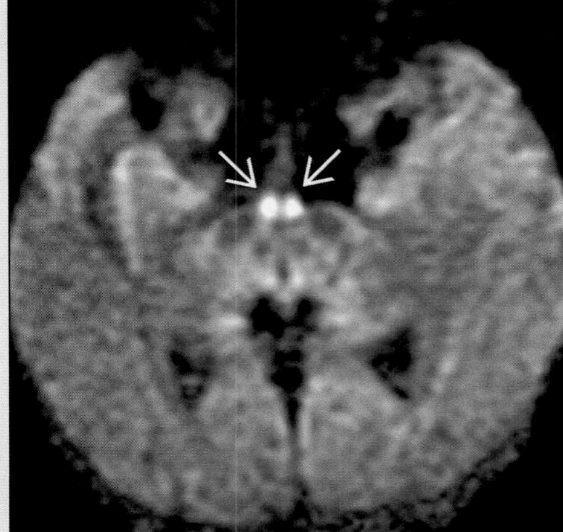

ALCOHOLIC ENCEPHALOPATHY

TERMINOLOGY

Abbreviations

- Alcoholic (EtOH) encephalopathy
- Wernicke encephalopathy (WE)

Definitions

- Acute, subacute, or chronic toxic effects of EtOH on CNS
- Can be primary (direct) or secondary (indirect)
  - Primary (direct) effects of EtOH = neurotoxicity
    - Cortical/cerebellar degeneration, peripheral polyneuropathy
  - Secondary (indirect) effects
    - Trauma, malnutrition, coagulopathy
- Rare treatable complication = WE

IMAGING

General Features

- Best diagnostic clue
  - EtOH: Disproportionate superior vermian atrophy
  - WE: Mamillary body, medial thalamus, hypothalamus, periaqueductal gray abnormal signal/enhancement
- Location
  - EtOH
    - Cerebral hemispheres, especially frontal lobes
    - Cerebellum, superior vermis
    - Corpus callosum (Marchiafava-Bignami disease) ± lateral extension into adjacent white matter
    - Diffuse toxic demyelination = unusual manifestation of alcoholic encephalopathy
    - Basal ganglia (associated liver disease)
  - WE
    - Mamillary bodies, periaqueductal gray matter, hypothalamus
    - Thalami (adjacent to 3rd ventricle)

CT Findings

- NECT
  - EtOH: Generalized atrophy; superior vermis atrophy
  - Marchiafava-Bignami disease: Hypodensity in corpus callosum
  - WE (acute): Often normal
    - May see hypodensity in periaqueductal gray matter, mamillary bodies, and medial thalamus
- CECT
  - Acute alcohol-induced demyelination may enhance

MR Findings

- T1WI
  - EtOH
    - Symmetric enlargement of lateral ventricles, sulci with chronic EtOH
    - ↑ size of cerebral sulci, interhemispheric/sylvian fissures
    - ± hyperintensity in basal ganglia (liver dysfunction)
    - Marchiafava-Bignami disease: Linear or punctate hypointensity in middle layers of corpus callosum
  - WE
    - May see hypointensity in periaqueductal gray matter, mamillary bodies, hypothalamus, and medial thalamus
    - Chronic: Atrophic mamillary bodies (sagittal scan) and 3rd ventricular enlargement
- T2WI
  - EtOH
    - Nonspecific multifocal white matter hyperintensities
    - Less common: Diffuse white matter hyperintensity from toxic demyelination
    - Marchiafava-Bignami disease: Hyperintense corpus callosum (middle layers) virtually pathognomonic
  - WE
    - Hyperintensity around 3rd ventricle, mamillary bodies, hypothalamus, medial thalamus, midbrain (tectal plate and periaqueductal gray)
    - Atypical findings: Hyperintensity in cerebellum, cranial nerve nuclei, red nuclei, dentate nuclei, splenium, and cerebral cortex
- FLAIR
  - Lesions all typically hyperintense
- DWI
  - WE: Restriction in/around 3rd ventricle, midbrain
- T1WI C+
  - WE: Enhancement of mamillary bodies, periaqueductal gray, medial thalamus
- MRS
  - EtOH: NAA/Cr, Cho/Cr decreased in frontal lobes, cerebellum; recover after detoxification
- FMRI
  - EtOH-induced motor inefficiency, alterations of cortical-cerebellar circuits

Nuclear Medicine Findings

- PET
  - EtOH
    - 18F-FDG PET: Significant decrease in whole-brain metabolism with chronic EtOH
  - WE: 18F-FDG PET: Diencephalic, medial temporal, limbic, and retrosplenial hypometabolism

Imaging Recommendations

- Best imaging tool
  - NECT for complications, such as subdural hematoma, related to trauma/coagulopathy
  - MR for possible Wernicke encephalopathy
    - NB: Lack of imaging abnormalities does not exclude WE
- Protocol advice
  - Contrast-enhanced MR + DWI

DIFFERENTIAL DIAGNOSIS

Nonalcoholic Atrophy

- Alzheimer dementia (AD) = hippocampal, temporal atrophy, hypometabolism
- Multi-infarct dementia pattern = focal infarcts ± generalized atrophy
- Malnutrition, eating disorders = generalized
- Remote trauma = atrophy + cortical/axonal hemorrhages common

ALCOHOLIC ENCEPHALOPATHY

- Inherited cerebellar degeneration syndromes (Marie ataxia, olivopontocerebellar degeneration, etc.)
- Longstanding phenytoin (Dilantin) use = cerebellar atrophy + thick skull

Diffuse Demyelination

- Toxic demyelination, including chemotherapy, CO poisoning, and inhaled heroin ("chasing the dragon")
- Acquired/inherited metabolic disorders
  - Osmotic demyelination syndrome = pontine > putamen, cortical involvement
  - Inherited metabolic disorders

Corpus Callosal Hyperintensity

- Status epilepticus
- Drug toxicity
- Encephalitis
- Hypoglycemia

PATHOLOGY

General Features

- Etiology
  - EtOH
    - Alcohol readily crosses blood-brain barrier
    - Causes both direct/indirect neurotoxicity
  - WE
    - Thiamine (vitamin B_1) deficiency impairs dependent enzymes, results in glutamate accumulation/cell damage
    - WE can be alcoholic or nonalcoholic
    - **Alcoholic WE**: Chronic thiamine deficiency due to associated malnourishment
    - **Nonalcoholic WE**: Same pathophysiology but different etiology
      - Malabsorption secondary to GI neoplasm/ surgery
      - Hyperemesis (hyperemesis gravidarum, chemotherapy)
      - Malnutrition (starvation, anorexia nervosa)
      - Prolonged hyperalimentation
- Associated abnormalities
  - EtOH
    - May ↑ stroke risk (especially in putamen, ACA)
    - Hepatic encephalopathy
  - Chronic EtOH
    - Brain shrinkage, cortical atrophy reflect lifetime consumption
    - EtOH modulates GABAergic neurotransmission

Gross Pathologic & Surgical Features

- EtOH
  - Atrophy (especially frontal), ↑ ventricles, sulci
  - Callosal necrosis, atrophy (Marchiafava-Bignami disease)
- WE
  - Mamillary bodies; periventricular midbrain/ brainstem
    - Petechial hemorrhage (acute)
    - Mamillary body atrophy (chronic)
  - Dorsal medial thalamic nuclei (may cause Korsakoff psychosis)

Microscopic Features

- Axonal degeneration, demyelination (alcoholic polyneuropathy)
- Purkinje cell loss (alcoholic cerebellar degeneration)
- WE: Demyelination, neuronal loss in affected areas

CLINICAL ISSUES

Presentation

- Most common signs/symptoms
  - Chronic EtOH
    - Cognitive problems, impaired memory
    - Most common neurologic abnormality = polyneuropathy
    - Gait abnormalities, nystagmus (cerebellar degeneration)
  - WE = triad of ataxia, oculomotor abnormalities, confusion
    - 80% have polyneuropathy
    - 50% nonalcoholic
    - Korsakoff psychosis (amnestic syndrome) may complicate WE
  - Marchiafava-Bignami disease = sudden onset of altered mental status, seizures, dysarthria, ataxia, hypertonia, pyramidal signs

Demographics

- Age
  - Any age (NB: WE can occur in children)
- Epidemiology
  - EtOH, brain atrophy = dose dependent, independent of gender/ethnicity

Natural History & Prognosis

- EtOH: Ventricular, sulcal enlargement often reversible
- WE: Ocular palsies respond 1st to thiamine; ataxia, apathy, and confusion clear more slowly
  - High mortality if untreated
  - Only 25% of Korsakoff patients achieve full recovery

Treatment

- EtOH: Cessation, establishment of adequate nutrition
- WE: Immediate administration of IV thiamine → quick response

DIAGNOSTIC CHECKLIST

Consider

- 50% of WE cases occur in nonalcoholics, including children!

SELECTED REFERENCES

1. Wobrock T et al: Effects of abstinence on brain morphology in alcoholism: A MRI study. Eur Arch Psychiatry Clin Neurosci. 259(3):143-50, 2009
2. Zuccoli G et al: MR imaging findings in 56 patients with Wernicke encephalopathy: nonalcoholics may differ from alcoholics. AJNR Am J Neuroradiol. 30(1):171-6, 2009

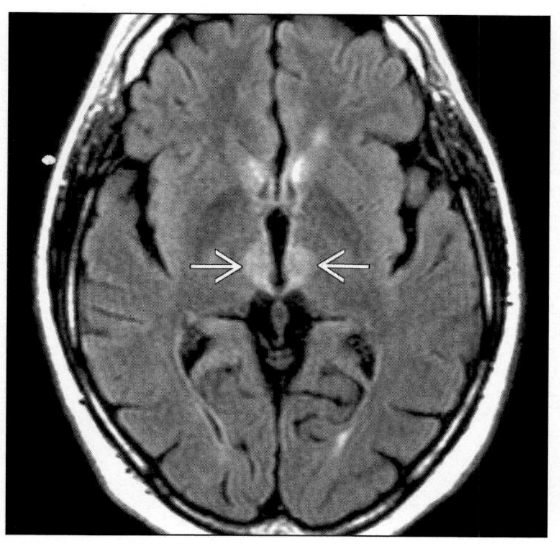

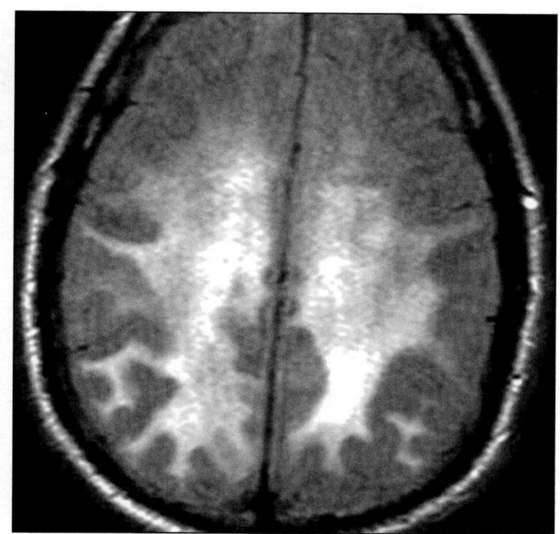

(Left) *Axial FLAIR shows hyperintensity in the medial thalami* ➔*, a common finding in Wernicke encephalopathy.* ***(Right)*** *Axial FLAIR MR shows confluent hyperintensity in the hemispheric white matter in this patient with alcoholic demyelination.*

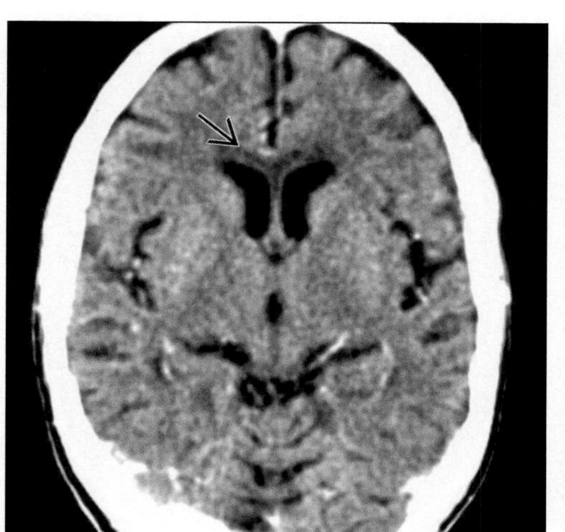

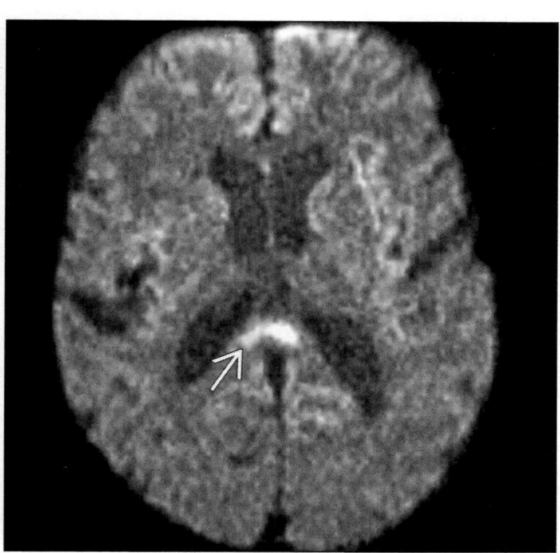

(Left) *Axial CECT scan shows prominent sulci and ventricles for the patient's age. Note the striking linear hypodensity in the corpus callosum genu* ➔ *in this patient with Marchiafava-Bignami disease. (Courtesy A. Datir, MD.)* ***(Right)*** *Axial DWI MR shows diffusion restriction limited to the corpus callosum splenium* ➔*. Acute alcoholic encephalopathy is 1 of the reported causes of hyperintense splenium lesion.*

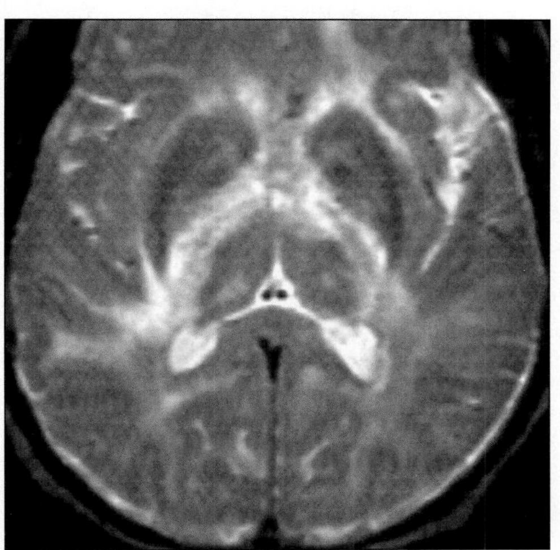

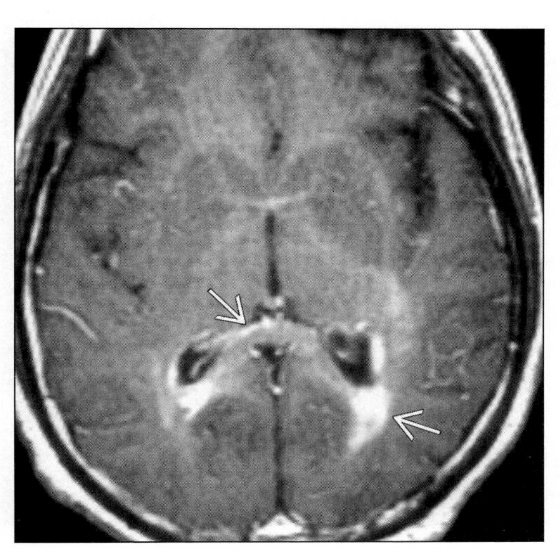

(Left) *Axial T2WI MR in a patient with acute alcohol poisoning caused by binge drinking shows symmetric, confluent, white matter hyperintensity in the internal capsules, corpus callosum, and hemispheric white matter. Acute alcohol toxicity may induce striking demyelination, as occurred in this case.* ***(Right)*** *Axial T1WI C+ MR in the same patient with acute alcohol-induced demyelination shows enhancement in the corpus callosum splenium and forceps major* ➔*.*

HEPATIC ENCEPHALOPATHY

Key Facts

Terminology

- Functional, potentially reversible clinical syndrome during acute or chronic liver disease
- Characterized by psychiatric, cognitive, and motor components

Imaging

- Chronic hepatic encephalopathy (HE)
  - Bilateral T1WI hyperintensity in basal ganglia (BG), particularly globus pallidus (GP)
  - ↑ signal intensity in pituitary gland, hypothalamus, mesencephalon
- Acute HE
  - High signal in most of cerebral cortex
  - Perirolandic/occipital regions relatively spared
  - ↓ mI/Cr and Cho/Cr ratios and ↑ Glx/Cr ratios

Top Differential Diagnoses

- Cholestatic diseases
- Liver copper overload
- Hyperalimentation
- Other causes of T1 hyperintense BG
  - Hypoxic-ischemic encephalopathy
  - Fahr disease (idiopathic calcification of BG)
  - Carbon monoxide poisoning
  - Neurofibromatosis type 1
  - Langerhans cell histiocytosis

Diagnostic Checklist

- After liver transplantation
  - MRS, clinical response improve first
  - Reversal of T1 hyperintense BG sign is delayed 3-6 months
  - BG return to normal intensity within 1 year

*(**Left**) Axial T1WI MR demonstrates findings of both chronic and acute hepatic encephalopathy (HE). Note the hyperintensity in the basal ganglia, especially the globi pallidi ➡. Blurring of gray-white junctions in the insula and cortex are characteristic of acute HE. (**Right**) Axial FLAIR MR in the same patient shows diffuse cortical hyperintensity with relative sparing of the occipital poles.*

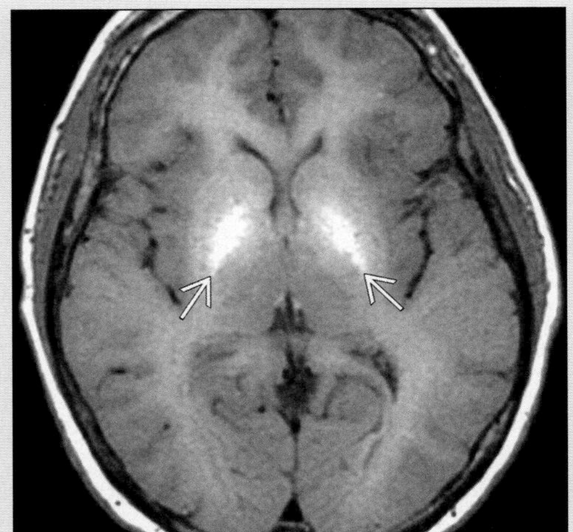

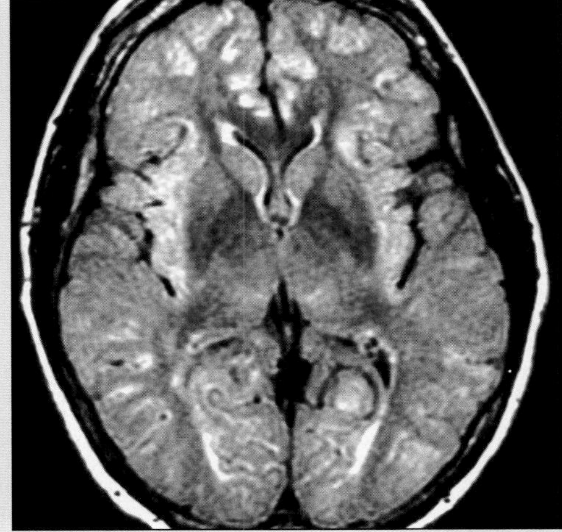

*(**Left**) Sagittal T1WI MR shows hyperintense changes in the lentiform nucleus ➡ and also extension into the midbrain ➡, characteristic findings in chronic HE. (**Right**) Sagittal T1WI MR in a 50-year-old man with cirrhosis, encephalopathy, and gait disorder shows increased signal intensity in the anterior pituitary gland ➡ in addition to normal bright posterior pituitary ➡. "White" pituitary gland can be seen in severe cases of chronic hepatic encephalopathy. (Courtesy P. Hildenbrand, MD.)*

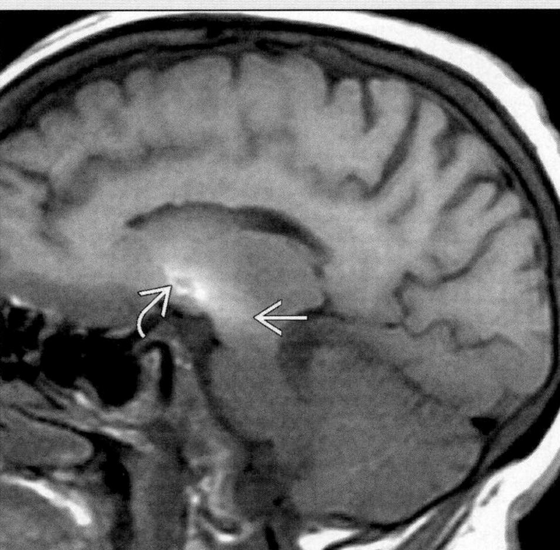

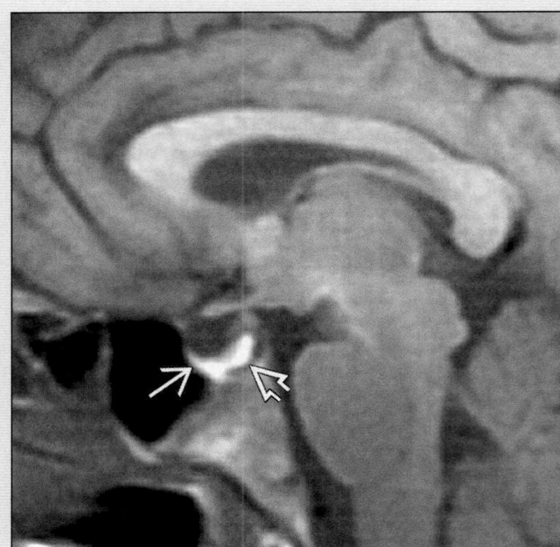

HEPATIC ENCEPHALOPATHY

TERMINOLOGY

Abbreviations

- Hepatic encephalopathy (HE)

Synonyms

- Hepatic coma

Definitions

- Functional, potentially reversible clinical syndrome during acute or chronic liver disease
- Characterized by psychiatric, cognitive, and motor components

IMAGING

General Features

- Best diagnostic clue
  - Bilateral T1WI hyperintensity in basal ganglia (BG), particularly globus pallidus (GP)
- Location
  - BG, particularly GP
- Morphology
  - Generally similar in shape to outline of lentiform nuclei

CT Findings

- NECT
  - Acute HE: Severe diffuse cerebral edema
  - Chronic HE: Cerebral atrophy, mild brain edema
- CECT
  - No enhancement of affected BG

MR Findings

- T1WI
  - Bilateral hyperintensity in BG, particularly GP
    - Reported in 80-90% of chronic liver failure patients
    - Probably caused by manganese accumulation
      - Blood-brain barrier permeability to manganese may be selectively increased in chronic condition
  - ↑ T1WI signal intensity in pituitary gland, hypothalamus, and mesencephalon surrounding red nuclei
    - Occasionally ↑ signal in pituitary gland only
  - Atrophy, especially affecting cerebellum
  - Acute HE: Blurring of gray-white matter junction
- T2WI
  - Acute HE: High T2WI signal in most of cerebral cortex, sparing perirolandic and occipital regions
  - Dentate nucleus, periventricular WM hyperintensity
- FLAIR
  - Fast-FLAIR sequences: ↑ signal along hemispheric WM in/around corticospinal tract
- DWI
  - ↑ mean diffusivity in hemispheric white matter, normal fractional anisotropy; ↓ mean diffusivity in fulminant hepatic failure due to cytotoxic edema
- T1WI C+
  - No contrast enhancement
- MRS
  - ↓ myoinositol (mI), ↑ glutamine/glutamate (Glx), ↓ choline (Cho)
    - Brain glutamine concentrations ↑ in direct correlation with severity of HE in patients with chronic liver failure
    - Brain ammonia removal relies primarily on formation of glutamine
  - ↓ mI/Cr and Cho/Cr ratios and ↑ Glx/Cr ratios
    - After correction of hepatic dysfunction, these ratios normalize or may reverse
    - mI/Cr: Most sensitive (80-85%) indicator of HE
  - May play role in monitoring lactulose therapy

Ultrasonographic Findings

- Transcranial Doppler ultrasonography
  - Cerebral pulsatility and resistive indices
    - Elevated in cirrhotic patients with HE and correlated with severity

Nuclear Medicine Findings

- PET
  - NH_3-13-PET in chronic liver failure with mild HE
    - ↑ cerebral metabolic rate for ammonia
    - ↑ "permeability-surface area" product (measure of blood-brain barrier permeability to ammonia)
  - Redistribution of cerebral blood flow from cortical to subcortical areas (including BG)

Imaging Recommendations

- Best imaging tool
  - Multiplanar MR

DIFFERENTIAL DIAGNOSIS

Liver Copper Overload

- Wilson disease
  - Symmetrical hyperintensity in putamina, GP, caudate nuclei, and thalami on T2WI
  - Hyperintensity in dentatorubrothalamic, pontocerebellar, and corticospinal tracts on T2WI
  - Lesions appear hypointense (occasionally hyperintense) on T1WI, without enhancement
- Cholestatic disease
- Inefficient biliary excretion of copper in newborn

Hyperalimentation

- Bilateral hyperintense signal in GP and subthalamic nuclei on T1WI, without contrast
  - Caused by manganese deposition, astrogliotic reaction to such deposition, or both
- No corresponding abnormalities on T2WI or CT

Other Causes of T1 Hyperintense BG

- Microangiopathy and infarcts in AIDS patients
- Chorea-ballism associated with hyperglycemia
  - T1 hyperintense putamen, caudate nucleus, or both
  - No significant T2 signal alteration, no mass effect, no gadolinium enhancement
- Endocrine disorders leading to BG calcifications
  - Hyperparathyroidism, hypothyroidism
  - Hypoparathyroidism, pseudohypoparathyroidism, pseudo-pseudohypoparathyroidism
- Fahr disease (idiopathic calcification of BG)
- Hypoxic-ischemic encephalopathy

- BG, parasagittal cortical areas most frequently involved
  - Hyperintense BG lesions on T1/T2WI
  - Diffuse laminar cortical hyperintensity on T1WI in subacute stage
  - Laminar cortical, BG enhancement
- Carbon monoxide poisoning
  - Most specific findings: GP hypodensity on CT and hyperintensity on T2WI
- Langerhans cell histiocytosis
- Neurofibromatosis type 1
  - Hyperintensities in BG (usually GP), internal capsule bilaterally on T1WI
  - Smaller foci of hyperintensity in brainstem, cerebellar WM, dentate nucleus, BG, and periventricular WM on T2WI

PATHOLOGY

General Features

- Etiology
  - Underlying cirrhosis, acute fulminant viral hepatitis
  - Drugs and toxins
  - Shock &/or sepsis
  - Childhood hepatic diseases associated with bright hypothalamus and pituitary gland
  - Portosystemic shunting through collateral vessels
  - Brain accumulation of neurotoxic &/or neuroactive substances
    - Ammonia, manganese, aromatic amino acids
  - Alterations in neurotransmission, blood-brain barrier permeability, and energy metabolism
  - Proinflammatory cytokines (TNF α, interleukin 1α) may affect brain by production of nitric oxide in endothelial or neural cells after crossing defective blood-brain barrier
  - HE precipitated by ammoniagenic situations
- Associated abnormalities
  - Parkinsonian signs especially with midbrain involvement
  - Hepatic myelopathy in chronic liver disease with extensive shunts

Gross Pathologic & Surgical Features

- Laminar and pseudolaminar necrosis of cerebral cortex
- Polymicrocavitation at gray-white matter junction

Microscopic Features

- Acute HE: Severe cytotoxic edema in astrocytes with anoxic neuronal damage
- HE in chronic liver failure
  - Astrocytosis: Alzheimer type 2 astrocytes
  - Neuronal degeneration

CLINICAL ISSUES

Presentation

- Most common signs/symptoms
  - Altered mental status leading to stupor and coma
  - Motor abnormalities: Tremor, bradykinesia, asterixis, ataxia, apraxia, hyperreflexia
  - Seizures: Rare manifestation of HE
- Clinical profile
  - HE classified into 3 main groups
    - Episodic/acute: Use neuroimaging to exclude other diseases
    - Chronic HE
      - Relapsing HE: Similar to episodic with completely normal neurocognition between attacks
      - Persistent HE: No reversal of manifestations despite treatment
    - Minimal HE (a.k.a. latent or subclinical HE)
      - Abnormalities that cannot be detected by standard examination

Demographics

- Age
  - Both pediatric and adult patients with severe hepatic dysfunction
- Gender
  - No gender preference
- Epidemiology
  - Occurs in > 50% of all cirrhosis cases

Natural History & Prognosis

- Acute HE: Severe brain edema may ↑ intracranial pressure → cerebral herniation → death
- Neuropsychologic signs of HE follow ^{1}H-MRS rather than MR changes

Treatment

- Identify and remove/treat precipitating factors
- Nonabsorbable disaccharides (lactulose, lactitol)
- Antibiotics (neomycin) with oto-/nephrotoxicity
- L-ornithine-L-aspartate
- Molecular adsorbents recirculating system (MARS) albumin dialysis: Improves encephalopathy grade

DIAGNOSTIC CHECKLIST

Image Interpretation Pearls

- After therapy, clinical features and MRS abnormalities improve first, followed 3-6 months later by normalization of BG signal
- BG signal abnormality typically normalizes within 1 year of liver transplantation

SELECTED REFERENCES

1. Pinarbasi B et al: Are acquired hepatocerebral degeneration and hepatic myelopathy reversible? J Clin Gastroenterol. 43(2):176-81, 2009
2. Rovira A et al: MR imaging findings in hepatic encephalopathy. AJNR Am J Neuroradiol. 29(9):1612-21, 2008
3. Saksena S et al: Cerebral diffusion tensor imaging and in vivo proton magnetic resonance spectroscopy in patients with fulminant hepatic failure. J Gastroenterol Hepatol. 23(7 Pt 2):e111-9, 2008
4. Sugimoto R et al: Value of the apparent diffusion coefficient for quantification of low-grade hepatic encephalopathy. Am J Gastroenterol. 103(6):1413-20, 2008

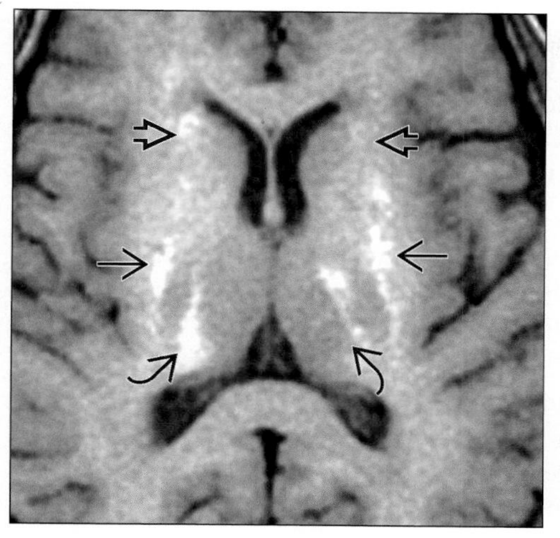

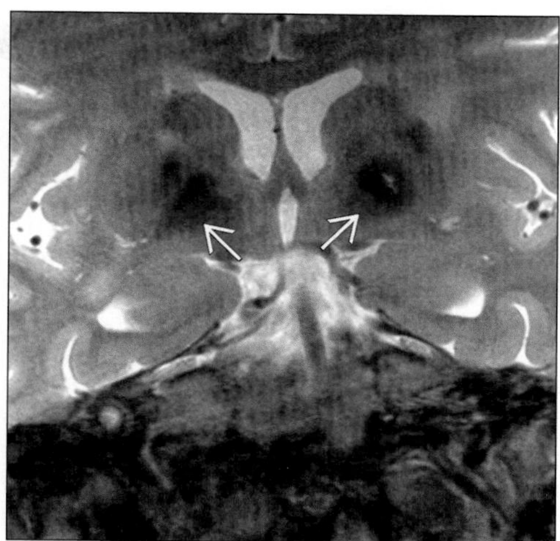

(Left) *Axial T1WI MR exhibits severe increased signal within the white matter ⇨, basal ganglia →, and thalami ↷ in this patient with advanced chronic HE.* ***(Right)*** *Coronal T2WI MR shows the typical T2 hypointense appearance of basal ganglia → in a patient with chronic hepatic encephalopathy.*

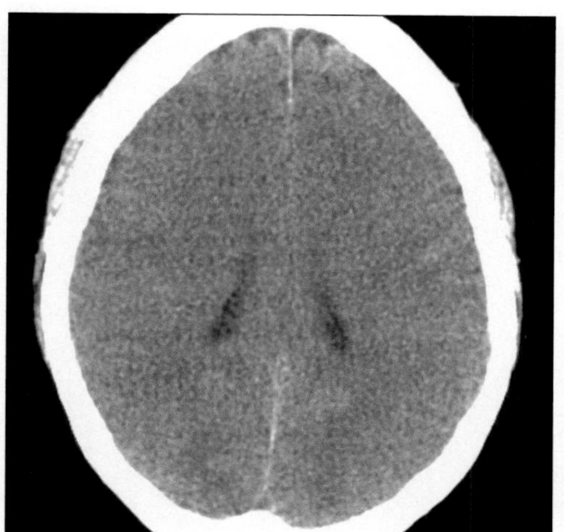

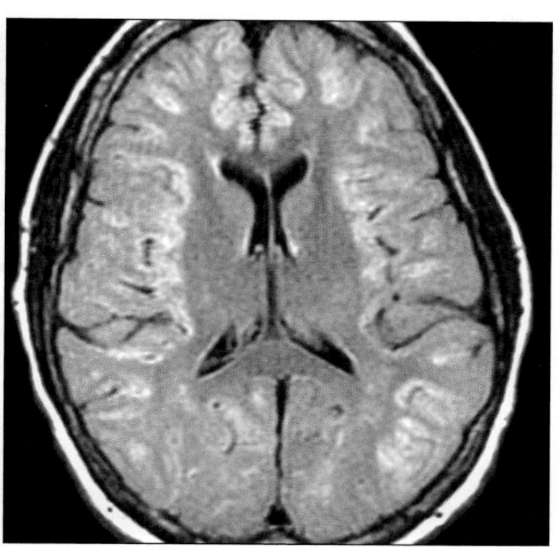

(Left) *Axial NECT shows diffuse cerebral edema in a patient with acute hepatic encephalopathy manifested by loss of gray-white matter distinction and obliteration of the sulci.* ***(Right)*** *Axial FLAIR MR in a patient with acute hepatic encephalopathy shows diffuse cortical hyperintensity with relative sparing of the occipital regions.*

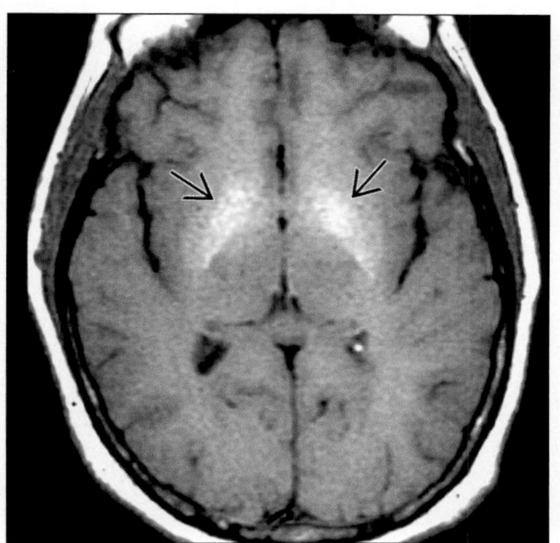

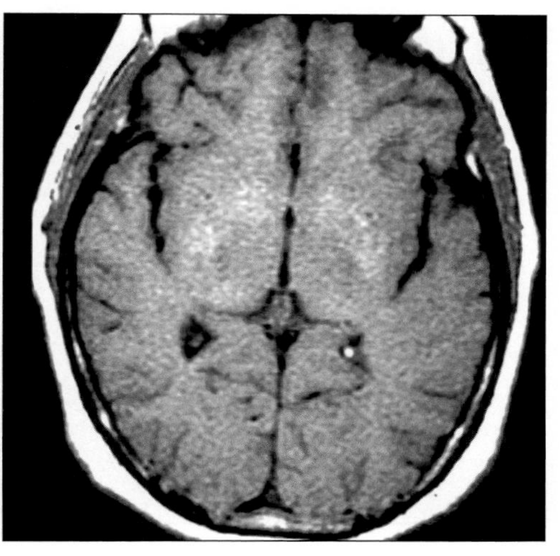

(Left) *Axial T1WI MR obtained prior to liver transplant shows bilateral symmetric hyperintensity in the globi pallidi →, typical findings for chronic hepatic encephalopathy.* ***(Right)*** *Axial T1WI MR in the same patient obtained 14 months after transplant shows nearly complete interval resolution of the hyperintensity. The patient's movement disorder also resolved. Both clinical and imaging findings of hepatocerebral degeneration are potentially reversible. (Courtesy P. Hildenbrand, MD.)*

ACUTE HYPERTENSIVE ENCEPHALOPATHY, PRES

Key Facts

Terminology
- Cerebrovascular autoregulatory disorder
- Many etiologies with HTN as common component
  - Preeclampsia, eclampsia
  - Drug toxicity (e.g., chemotherapy)
  - Uremic encephalopathies

Imaging
- General
  - Predilection for posterior circulation
  - Occipital lobes, cortical watershed zones
- CT
  - Bilateral nonconfluent hypodense foci
  - ± symmetric lesions in basal ganglia
- MR
  - Parietooccipital T2/FLAIR hyperintensities in 95%
  - ± basal ganglia, pontine, cerebellar involvement
  - "Blooming" on T2* if hemorrhagic (uncommon)
  - Generally no restriction on DWI
  - Variable patchy enhancement

Top Differential Diagnoses
- Acute cerebral ischemia-infarction
- Status epilepticus
- Hypoglycemia
- Thrombotic microangiopathies (DIC, TTP, mHTN)

Pathology
- Acute HTN damages vascular endothelium
- Breakthrough of autoregulation causes hyperperfusion, blood-brain barrier disruption
- Result = vasogenic (not cytotoxic) edema

Clinical Issues
- Headache, seizure, ↓ mental status, visual symptoms
- Caution: Some patients, especially children, may be normotensive/minimally elevated BP!

__(Left)__ Axial graphic shows the classic posterior circulation cortical/subcortical vasogenic edema characteristic of PRES. Petechial hemorrhage occurs in some cases but is unusual. __(Right)__ Gross pathology of a patient with complicated PRES demonstrates diffuse cerebral edema with swollen gyri. Multifocal petechial microhemorrhages are present in the occipital cortex ⊳ together with several areas of focal encephalomalacia secondary to infarction →. (Courtesy R. Hewlett, PhD.)

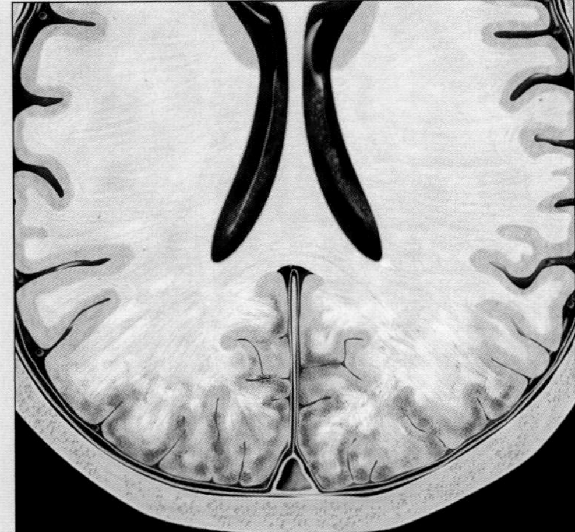

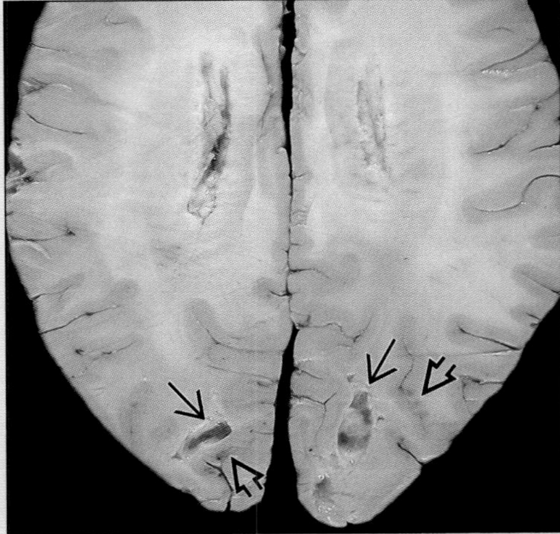

__(Left)__ Axial NECT scan in a 26-year-old pregnant patient with eclampsia was initially read as normal; however, it shows subtle but definite hypodensities ⊳ in the cortex and subcortical white matter of both occipital lobes. __(Right)__ Axial T2WI MR in the same patient shows hyperintensities in both occipital lobes ⊳ corresponding to the hypodensities noted on NECT. DWI (not shown) was normal. If clinical suspicion of PRES is high and NECT is scan normal/ subtly abnormal, MR with T2WI, FLAIR, and DWI is helpful.

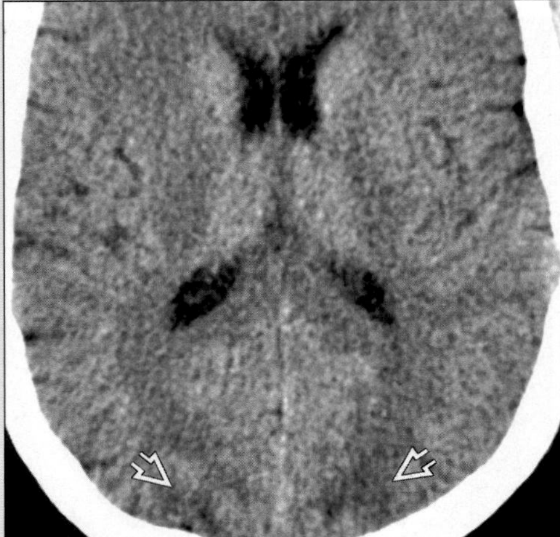

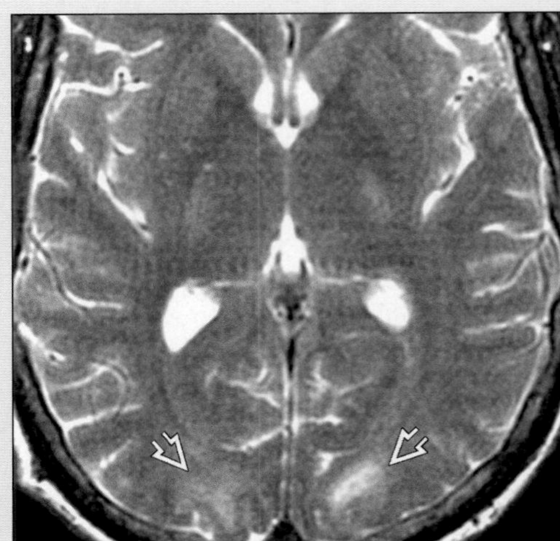

ACUTE HYPERTENSIVE ENCEPHALOPATHY, PRES

TERMINOLOGY

Abbreviations

- Posterior reversible encephalopathy syndrome (PRES)

Synonyms

- Hypertensive encephalopathy
- Reversible posterior leukoencephalopathy syndrome (RPLS)

Definitions

- Variant of hypertensive encephalopathy characterized by headache, visual disturbances, altered mental function
- Cerebrovascular autoregulatory disorder
  - Multiple etiologies
  - Most caused by acute hypertension (HTN)

IMAGING

General Features

- Best diagnostic clue
  - Patchy cortical/subcortical PCA territory lesions in patient with severe acute/subacute HTN
- Location
  - Most common: Cortex, subcortical white matter
    - Predilection for posterior circulation (parietal, occipital lobes, cerebellum)
    - At junctions of vascular watershed zones
    - Usually bilateral, often somewhat asymmetric
  - Less common: Basal ganglia
  - Rare: Predominant/exclusive brainstem involvement
- Size
  - Extent of abnormalities highly variable
- Morphology
  - Patchy > confluent

CT Findings

- NECT
  - May be normal or subtly abnormal
    - If PRES suspected, do MR to confirm!
  - Common: Bilateral nonconfluent hypodense foci
    - Posterior parietal, occipital lobes
    - Cortical watershed zones
  - Less common: Petechial cortical/subcortical or basal ganglionic hemorrhages
  - Uncommon: Thalamic, basal ganglia, brainstem, cerebellar hypodensities
- CECT
  - Usually no enhancement
  - Occasionally mild patchy/punctate enhancement
- CTA
  - Usually normal
  - Rare: Vasospasm with multifocal areas of arterial narrowing

MR Findings

- T1WI
  - Hypointense cortical/subcortical lesions
- T2WI
  - Hyperintense cortical/subcortical lesions
    - Occipital lobes, cortical watershed zones
  - Less common
    - Basal ganglia involvement
    - Extensive brain stem, cerebellar hyperintensity
    - Generalized white matter edema
- FLAIR
  - Parietooccipital hyperintense cortical lesions in 95%
  - ± symmetric lesions in basal ganglia
  - Variable pontine, cerebellar involvement
  - "Leaky" blood-brain barrier may cause gadolinium accumulation in CSF, FLAIR hyperintensity
- T2* GRE
  - Blooms if hemorrhage present
- DWI
  - Most common: No restriction
  - Less common: Hyperintense on DWI with "pseudonormalized" ADC
    - May indicate irreversible infarction
  - ADC map: Markedly elevated (bright areas)
- PWI
  - May show increased CBF
- T1WI C+
  - Variable patchy enhancement
- MRS
  - May show widespread metabolic abnormalities
    - ↑ Cho, Cr
    - Mildly ↓ NAA
    - Usually return to normal within 2 months
- DTI
  - Shows foci of increased diffusion representing anisotropy loss
  - Vasogenic edema due to cerebrovascular autoregulatory dysfunction

Nuclear Medicine Findings

- SPECT
  - Variable findings reported; some show hyper-, others hypoperfusion in affected areas

Imaging Recommendations

- Best imaging tool
  - Contrast-enhanced MR + DWI
- Protocol advice
  - Repeat scan after blood pressure normalized

DIFFERENTIAL DIAGNOSIS

Acute Cerebral Ischemia-Infarction

- MCA distribution > > PCA
- Infarcts restrict on DWI; PRES usually does not

Status Epilepticus

- May cause transient gyral edema, enhancement
- Can mimic PRES, stroke, infiltrating neoplasm
- Unilateral (PRES often bilateral)

Hypoglycemia

- Severe parietooccipital edema
- Can resemble PRES, so history important

Thrombotic Microangiopathies

- Malignant hypertension, DIC, HUS, TTP
- Significant overlap as PRES is common imaging manifestation

ACUTE HYPERTENSIVE ENCEPHALOPATHY, PRES

Cerebral Hyperperfusion Syndrome

- Postcarotid endarterectomy, angioplasty, or stenting
  - Hyperperfusion syndrome occurs in 5-9% of cases
  - Perfusion MR or CT scans show elevated rCBF
  - Aggressive control of blood pressure associated with clinical, radiological improvement

Gliomatosis Cerebri

- Entire lobe(s) involved rather than patchy cortical/subcortical
- Occipital lobe involvement less common
- Can mimic brainstem PRES

PATHOLOGY

General Features

- Etiology
  - Diverse causes and clinical entities with HTN as common component
  - Acute HTN damages vascular endothelium
  - Breakthrough of autoregulation causes blood-brain barrier disruption
  - Result = vasogenic (not cytotoxic) edema
    - Arteriolar dilatation with cerebral hyperperfusion
    - Hydrostatic leakage (extravasation, transudation of fluid/macromolecules through arteriolar walls)
    - Interstitial fluid accumulates in cortex, subcortical white matter
    - Posterior circulation sparsely innervated by sympathetic nerves
      - Predilection for parietal, occipital lobes
  - Frank infarction with cytotoxic edema rare in PRES
- Associated abnormalities
  - Acute/subacute systemic HTN
  - Preeclampsia, eclampsia
    - Typically occurs after 20 weeks gestation
    - Rare: Headache, seizures up to several weeks postpartum
  - Drug toxicity ± tumor lysis syndrome
    - Chemotherapeutic agents
      - e.g., cyclosporine, cisplatin
  - Thrombotic microangiopathies (DIC, TTP, malignant hypertension)
  - Uremic encephalopathies
    - Acute glomerulonephritis, lupus nephropathy, etc.
  - Severe infection
    - 25% of septic patients in shock develop PRES
    - Blood pressure can be normal or elevated

Gross Pathologic & Surgical Features

- Common
  - Cortical/subcortical edema
  - ± petechial hemorrhage in parietal, occipital lobes
- Less common: Basal ganglia, cerebellum, brain stem, anterior frontal lobes
- Rare: Gross hemorrhage, frank infarction

Microscopic Features

- Autopsy in severe cases shows microvascular fibrinoid necrosis, ischemic microinfarcts, variable hemorrhage
- Chronic HTN associated with mural thickening, deposition of collagen, laminin, fibronectin in cerebral arterioles

CLINICAL ISSUES

Presentation

- Most common signs/symptoms
  - Headache, seizure, ↓ mental status, visual disturbances
  - Caution: Some patients, especially children, may be normotensive/minimally elevated BP!
- Clinical profile
  - Pregnant female with acute systemic HTN, headache ± seizure
  - Middle-aged, older adult on chemotherapy
  - Child with kidney disease or transplant

Demographics

- Age
  - Any age but young > old
- Gender
  - M < F
- Epidemiology
  - Preeclampsia in 5% of pregnancies
  - Eclampsia lower rate (< 1%)

Natural History & Prognosis

- Usually no residual abnormalities after HTN corrected
  - Reversibility related to blood pressure normalization
  - Brainstem, deep white matter lesions less reversible than cortical/subcortical
  - Eclampsia more reversible than drug-related PRES
- In rare cases may be life threatening
- Permanent infarction rare
- 4% of patients develop recurrent PRES

Treatment

- Control blood pressure, remove precipitating factors
- Delayed diagnosis/therapy can result in chronic neurologic sequelae

DIAGNOSTIC CHECKLIST

Consider

- Patchy bilateral occipital lobe hypodensities may be earliest NECT manifestation of PRES

Image Interpretation Pearls

- Major DDx of PRES is cerebral ischemia; DWI is positive in latter, usually negative in former

SELECTED REFERENCES

1. Burrus TM et al: Brain lesions are most often reversible in acute thrombotic thrombocytopenic purpura. Neurology. 73(1):66-70, 2009
2. Hamilton BE et al: Delayed CSF enhancement in posterior reversible encephalopathy syndrome. AJNR Am J Neuroradiol. 29(3):456-7, 2008
3. Ishikura K et al: Posterior reversible encephalopathy syndrome in children: its high prevalence and more extensive imaging findings. Am J Kidney Dis. 48(2):231-8, 2006

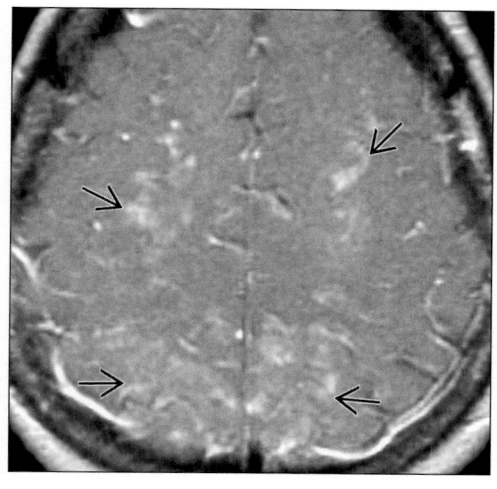

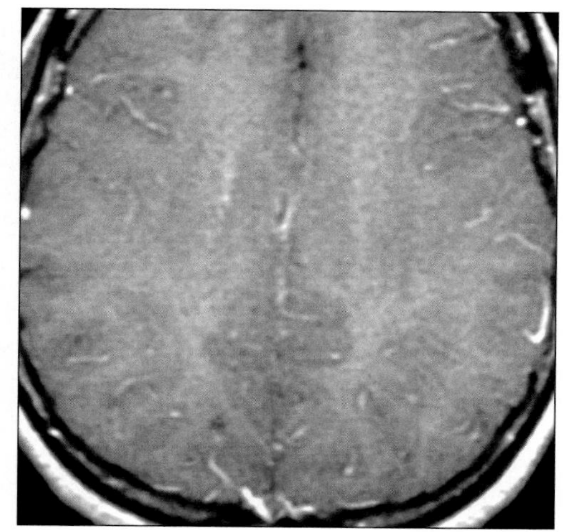

(Left) *Axial T1WI C+ MR in a patient with eclampsia shows numerous patchy cortical and subcortical enhancing foci → in both occipital lobes and along the watershed zones. T2WIs (not shown) demonstrated hyperintensities in the same areas.* ***(Right)*** *Repeat scan was obtained 2 days after delivery and normalization of blood pressure. MR is normal with the disappearance of the enhancing foci previously seen. Even florid MR changes of PRES usually resolve without clinical or imaging residua.*

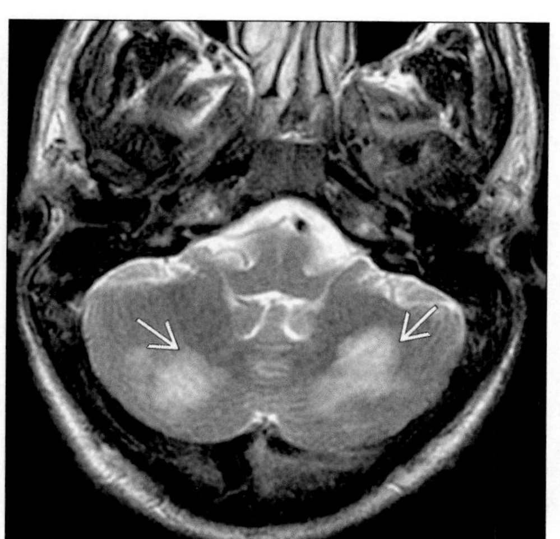

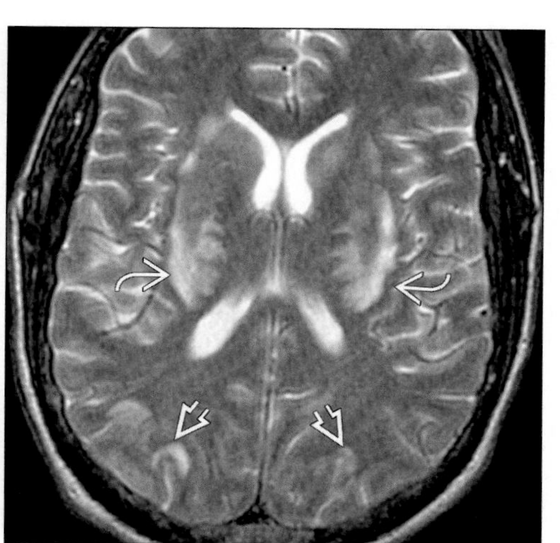

(Left) *Axial T2WI MR in a patient on cyclosporine who developed acute onset of extreme hypertension shows symmetric hyperintensities in both cerebellar hemispheres →.* ***(Right)*** *Axial T2WI MR in the same patient shows striking hyperintensity in both basal ganglia → with relatively subtle findings in the occipital poles →.*

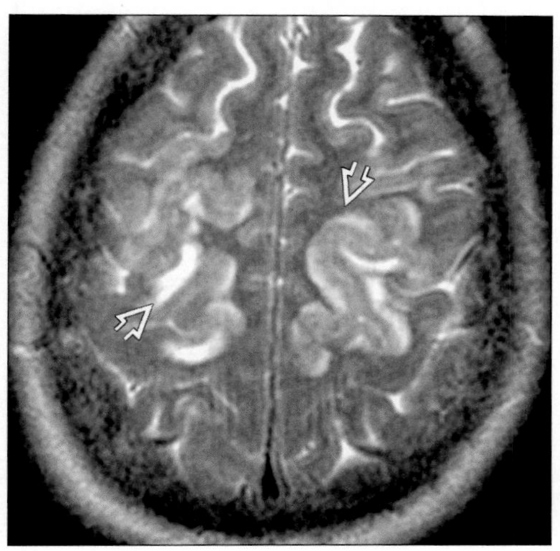

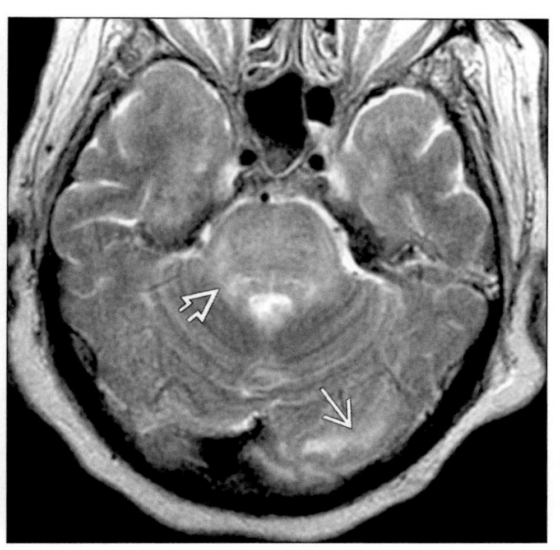

(Left) *Axial T2WI MR in the same patient shows florid changes in the cortical watershed zones →. DWI showed no restriction, which is typical even in severe cases of PRES. All findings resolved when the patient was taken off chemotherapy and blood pressure normalized.* ***(Right)*** *Axial T2WI MR in a patient with PRES shows pontine-predominant pattern → with only subtle change in the occipital lobe →. Sometimes pontine or cerebellar abnormalities can be found without other imaging evidence of PRES.*

CHRONIC HYPERTENSIVE ENCEPHALOPATHY

Key Facts

Terminology
- Chronic hypertensive encephalopathy (CHE)
- Subcortical arteriosclerotic encephalopathy

Imaging
- General features
  - Lacunae (lenticular nuclei, pons, thalamus, internal capsule, caudate)
  - Cerebral hemorrhage (basal ganglia/external capsule, thalamus)
  - Confluent WM disease (centrum semiovale, corona radiata)
- CT
  - Diffuse WM hypodensity on CT
  - Lacunar infarcts (BG, thalamus/brainstem)
- MR
  - Multifocal hyperintensities (T2/FLAIR)
  - Multiple microhemorrhages (GRE, SWI)

Top Differential Diagnoses
- Amyloid angiopathy
- CADASIL
- Dementing disorders
  - Alzheimer dementia
  - Multi-infarct dementia
- Antiphospholipid antibody syndrome
- Neuropsychiatric systemic lupus erythematosus
- Vasculitis

Clinical Issues
- Stepwise/gradual mental deterioration
- Acute strokes, lacunar syndrome
- Subacute pseudobulbar, extrapyramidal signs

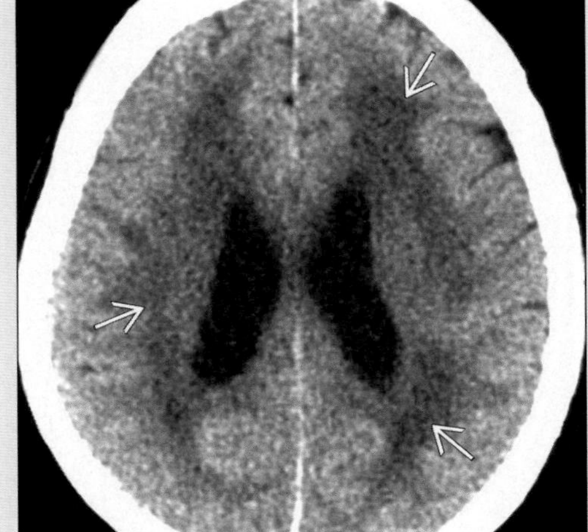
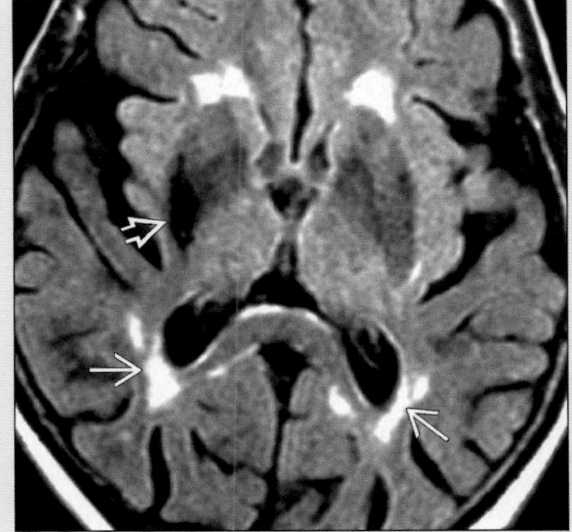

*(**Left**) Axial NECT shows the typical appearance of chronic hypertensive encephalopathy, seen here as diffuse confluent periventricular white matter hypodensity ➔. (**Right**) Axial FLAIR in a 72-year-old woman with longstanding systemic HTN demonstrates multifocal discrete and confluent hyperintensities scattered throughout the deep periventricular white matter, especially near the atria and occipital horns ➔. Note the old, hypertensive, basal ganglionic hemorrhage ➔.*

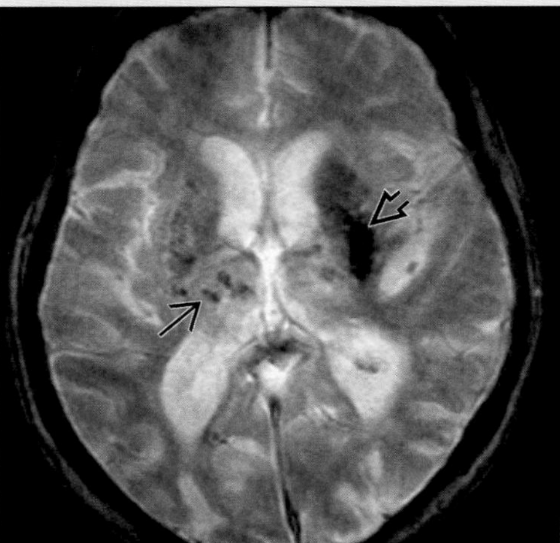
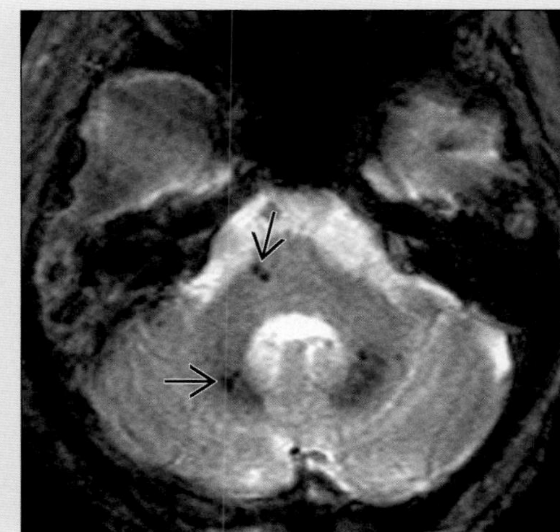

*(**Left**) Axial T2* GRE MR in a patient with remote history of hypertensive basal ganglionic hemorrhage shows residua of the old hemorrhage ➔ with multiple microhemorrhages in the basal ganglia and thalami ➔. (**Right**) Axial T2* GRE MR in the same patient shows multiple brainstem and cerebellar "microbleeds," seen here as multifocal "black dots" ➔. Microbleeds from amyloid angiopathy are less common in the posterior fossa, a helpful distinguishing feature.*

CHRONIC HYPERTENSIVE ENCEPHALOPATHY

TERMINOLOGY

Abbreviations

- Chronic hypertensive encephalopathy (CHE)

Synonyms

- Subcortical arteriosclerotic encephalopathy
  - a.k.a. Binswanger disease
- Hypertension-related microvascular disease

Definitions

- Brain parenchymal changes due to longstanding effects of untreated or poorly treated systemic hypertension (HTN)
  - CHE is most common cause of leukoaraiosis (diffuse rarefaction of white matter)
    - Others include diabetes, chronic vascular disease (arteriolosclerosis, lipohyalinosis)
- CHE: Important cause of cognitive deficits caused by vascular disease (i.e., vascular dementia)

IMAGING

General Features

- Best diagnostic clue
  - 2 major features
    - Diffuse white matter (WM) lesions (hypodense on CT, hyperintense on T2WI)
    - Microhemorrhages ("bloom" on T2*)
- Location
  - WM lesions
    - Centrum semiovale, corona radiata
    - Brainstem, cerebellum
  - Gray matter lesions
    - Basal ganglia (BG), thalami, brainstem
  - Microhemorrhages
    - Cerebellum, subcortical WM, basal ganglia/thalami

CT Findings

- NECT
  - Focal hypodensities (usually multiple)
    - BG, thalamus, brainstem
    - Often due to lacunar infarcts
  - Diffuse periventricular hypodensity
  - ± hyperdense lesions
    - Focal/confluent petechial hemorrhages

MR Findings

- T1WI
  - Lesions usually hypointense
    - Less conspicuous than on T2WI or FLAIR
- T2WI
  - Hyperintense lesions within corona radiata, centrum semiovale, basal ganglia
- FLAIR
  - Hyperintense or central hypointensities + peripheral hyperintensity
- T2* GRE
  - Multifocal hypointense lesions (microhemorrhages)
    - Predilection for BG/thalami, cerebellum
    - Subcortical WM (especially posterior brain regions)
- DWI
  - Acute WM lesions may restrict
  - ADC lower (acute) or higher (chronic)
- PWI
  - ↓ perfusion measurements in patients with confluent lesions
- T1WI C+
  - Generally no enhancement
- MRS
  - Older HTN patients have ↑ myoinositol to creatine ratio
    - Similar to patients with Alzheimer disease (AD)
  - Lower NAA levels in chronic hypertension
- DTI
  - ↑ mean diffusivity (MD), ↓ fractional anisotropy (FA)
    - Seen in both T2WI hyperintensities, normal-appearing WM

Nuclear Medicine Findings

- Frontal lobe (cingulate, superior frontal gyri) predominantly affected
- Regional CBF Tc-99m-HMPAO SPECT
  - Mild CHE: Reduced frontal CBF
  - Severe CHE: diffuse cerebral hypoperfusion

Imaging Recommendations

- Best imaging tool
  - FLAIR (WM lesions) + T2* (GRE, SWI) for microhemorrhages

DIFFERENTIAL DIAGNOSIS

Amyloid Angiopathy

- Amyloid deposition in small/medium arteries of cerebral leptomeninges, cerebral cortex
- Recurrent cerebral hemorrhages, most common in frontal and parietal lobes, involving cortex and subcortical WM
- Rarely cerebellar, putaminal, thalamic, or brainstem

CADASIL

- Nonarteriosclerotic, amyloid-negative hereditary angiopathy primarily affecting leptomeningeal and long perforating arteries
- Characteristic subcortical lacunar infarcts and leukoencephalopathy in young adults
- Anterior temporal WM and external capsule lesions are highly suggestive of CADASIL

Various Dementias

- Alzheimer disease
  - Parietal and temporal cortical atrophy, volume loss in hippocampi, entorhinal cortex
  - Often coexisting microvascular disease, WM hyperintensities
- Multi-infarct dementia
  - Hyperintense lesions on T2WI and focal atrophy suggestive of chronic infarcts

Antiphospholipid Antibody Syndrome

- Early stroke, recurrent arterial and venous thromboses, spontaneous fetal loss, thrombocytopenia

Systemic Lupus Erythematosus (SLE)

- Most common: Small multifocal WM lesions; usually diagnosed in 3rd or 4th decade (earlier than in CHE)
- Periventricular or more diffuse WM changes

Other Vasculitides

- Primary angiitis of CNS
- Granulomatous angiitis
- Polyarteritis nodosa, Behçet disease

Pseudoxanthoma Elasticum

- Systemic HTN, subcortical leukoencephalopathy, multiple strokes, and dementia in 3rd and 4th decade (younger than CHE patients)

PATHOLOGY

General Features

- Etiology
  - Chronic HTN is associated with hyaline deposition within small arteries (so-called lipohyalinosis)
  - 2 major mechanisms postulated for leukoaraiosis related to lipohyalinosis
    - Increased permeability of blood vessels may allow leakage of plasma contents
  - Chronic HTN impairs dilatation of collateral vessels in cerebral circulation
    - Impaired cerebral autoregulation and decreased vasodilatory capacity; ↑ susceptibility to cerebral infarction
- Associated abnormalities
  - Over time, lesions continue to accumulate, principally within subcortical WM
  - Various genetic factors, including DNA sequence variations occurring within single nucleotide (single-nucleotide polymorphisms), appear to place some patients at increased risk
  - Patients with HTN may also develop large parenchymal hemorrhages

Staging, Grading, & Classification

- No well-defined staging or grading scale exists

Gross Pathologic & Surgical Features

- Demyelination of periventricular and central WM
- Multiple lacunae and infarctions
- Tortuosity of small arteries and small artery occlusions

Microscopic Features

- Multiple petechial microhemorrhages
- Leukoaraiosis: Partial loss of myelin, axons, oligodendroglia, glial cells
- Alterations of small penetrating arteries leading to luminal stenosis

CLINICAL ISSUES

Presentation

- Most common signs/symptoms
  - Usually seen in middle-aged or elderly
    - Memory loss, depression, various features of dementia
  - Long tract findings, pseudobulbar syndrome
- Clinical profile
  - Stepwise or gradual progression of mental deterioration
  - Acute strokes, lacunar syndrome
  - Subacute onset of focal, pseudobulbar, and extrapyramidal signs

Demographics

- Age
  - Incidence increases with age
- Gender
  - HTN more prevalent in men than women
- Ethnicity
  - HTN more prevalent in African-Americans
- Epidemiology
  - In addition to HTN, higher prevalence in patients with diabetes mellitus and peritoneal dialysis for renal failure

Natural History & Prognosis

- Arteriolosclerosis associated with systemic HTN and increasing age
  - Small vessel occlusive changes are primary factor in pathogenesis of hyperintense WM lesions on T2WI in elderly
- Periventricular hyperintense WM lesions
  - Increased in patients with untreated systemic HTN
- Age, smoking, and HTN are independent predictors of hyperintense lesions on T2WI
- Untreated or poorly controlled systemic HTN ⇒ intracranial hemorrhages usually involving BG, thalamus, brainstem, or dentate nucleus of cerebellum
- CHE eventually causes vascular-type dementia

DIAGNOSTIC CHECKLIST

Consider

- Is history of chronic hypertension present?
  - Many disease states have imaging findings like CHE

Image Interpretation Pearls

- T2* GRE or SWI superior sensitivity for chronic microhemorrhages

SELECTED REFERENCES

1. Bastos-Leite AJ et al: Cerebral blood flow by using pulsed arterial spin-labeling in elderly subjects with white matter hyperintensities. AJNR Am J Neuroradiol. 29(7):1296-301, 2008
2. Della Nave R et al: Whole-brain histogram and voxel-based analyses of diffusion tensor imaging in patients with leukoaraiosis: correlation with motor and cognitive impairment. AJNR Am J Neuroradiol. 28(7):1313-9, 2007
3. O'Sullivan M et al: Diffusion tensor MRI correlates with executive dysfunction in patients with ischaemic leukoaraiosis. J Neurol Neurosurg Psychiatry. 75(3):441-7, 2004
4. Wardlaw JM et al: Is breakdown of the blood-brain barrier responsible for lacunar stroke, leukoaraiosis, and dementia? Stroke. 34(3):806-12, 2003

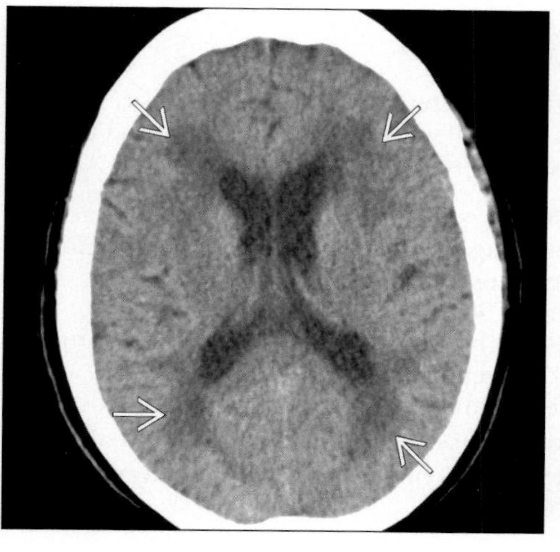

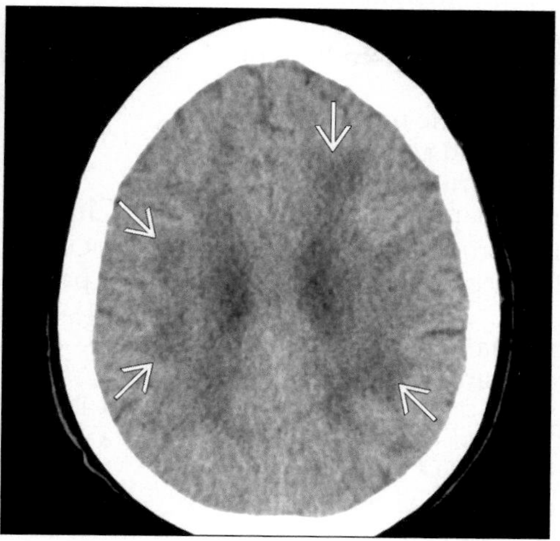

(Left) *Axial NECT demonstrates frontal and parietal periventricular confluent white matter hypodensities ➡ in a patient with chronic hypertensive encephalopathy and clinical Binswanger disease.* ***(Right)*** *Axial NECT slice through corona radiata in the same patient shows bilateral confluent hypodense lesions ➡. These findings are sometimes termed "subcortical arteriosclerotic encephalopathy."*

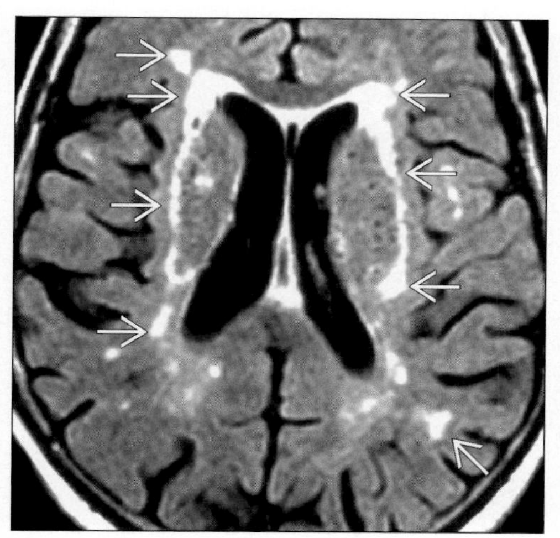

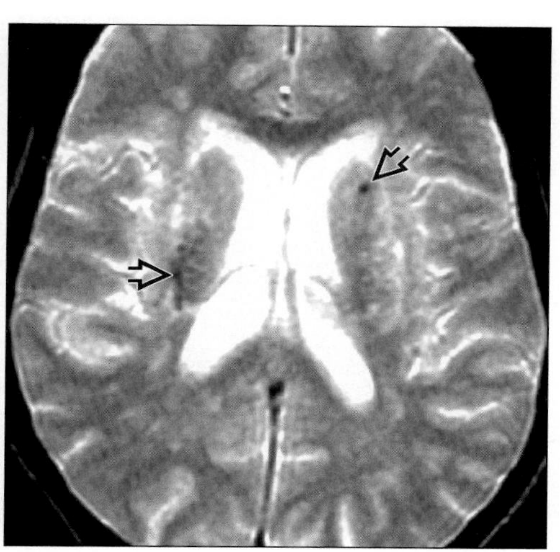

(Left) *Axial FLAIR MR demonstrates hyperintense abnormality scattered throughout the white matter ➡.* ***(Right)*** *Axial T2* GRE MR in the same patient shows punctate hemorrhages ⇨.*

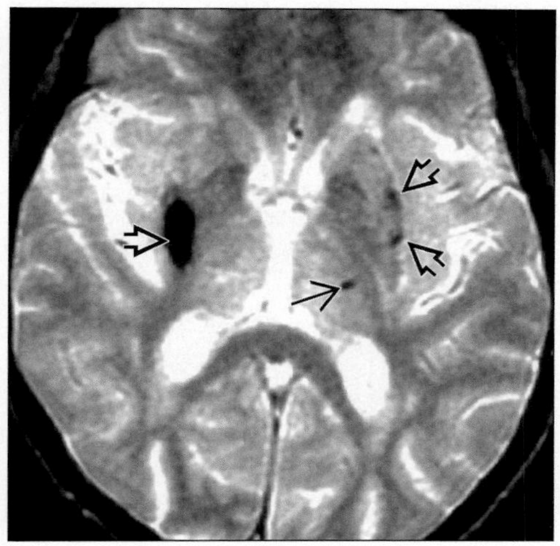

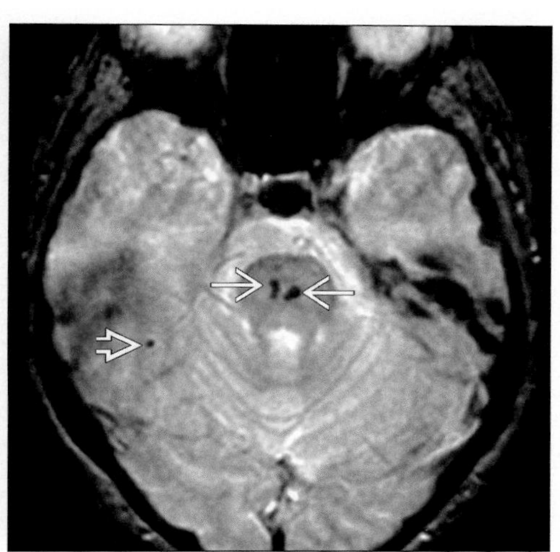

(Left) *Axial T2* GRE MR shows multiple hypointense lesions within the basal ganglia ⇨ bilaterally and left thalamus →, secondary to hemosiderin deposition from past microhemorrhages.* ***(Right)*** *Axial T2* GRE MR shows 2 foci of chronic microhemorrhage in the central pons ➡. Note a dot-like chronic microhemorrhage seen in the right temporooccipital white matter ⮕.*

IDIOPATHIC INTRACRANIAL HYPERTENSION

Key Facts

Imaging

- Best imaging clue: Partial empty sella, dilation/ tortuosity of optic nerve sheath, flattening of posterior sclera in patient with clinical findings of intracranial hypertension
- T2 MR: Increased fluid around optic nerves ± bulbous dilation of sheath behind globes
  - Optic nerve papilla may "protrude" into globe
- T1WI C+: Enhancement of prelaminar optic nerve
- MRV to exclude dural sinus thrombosis/stenosis
- Best imaging tool: MR with fat-saturated T1WI C+ of orbits and whole brain
- Must exclude causes of intracranial hypertension: Venous thrombosis, space-occupying lesion

Top Differential Diagnoses

- Secondary pseudotumor syndromes
- Idiopathic or post-inflammatory (i.e., multiple sclerosis) optic nerve atrophy
- Idiopathic empty sella (normal variant)

Pathology

- Modified Dandy criteria must be met (e.g., symptoms of ↑ ICP with > 25 cm H_2O, normal CT/ MR without DST, mass, etc.)

Clinical Issues

- Obese woman age 20-44 years with headache and papilledema most common presentation
  - Headache in 90-95%
  - Papilledema (bilateral optic nerve head swelling) virtually universal
- Progressive visual loss ± CN6 paresis, diplopia
- Chief hazard: Vision loss from chronic papilledema
- Treatment: Medical or surgical (LP, optic nerve fenestration)

*(**Left**) Axial T2WI MR shows dilated CSF spaces around the optic nerves ➡ and protrusion of the optic nerve papilla into the posterior globes ➡. Opening CSF pressure in this 32-year-old woman was 45 cm of H_2O. Prominent CSF space in the suprasellar cistern represents an empty sella ➡. Note the tortuosity of the left optic nerve. (**Right**) Sagittal T1WI MR in the same patient shows a partially empty sella ➡, suggesting high CSF pressure in this young obese woman with headaches.*

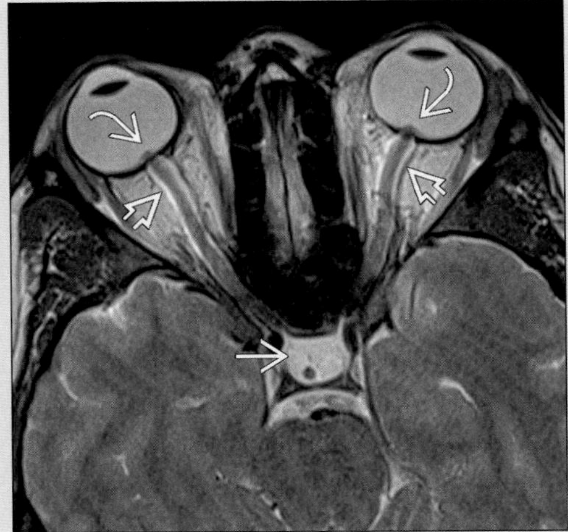

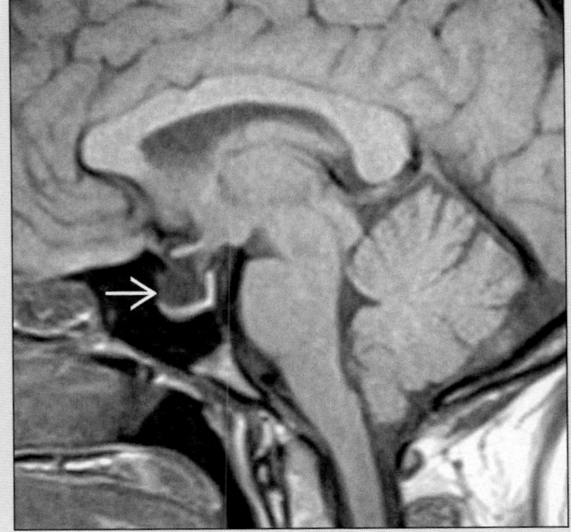

*(**Left**) Axial T1WI C+ MR in the same patient demonstrates enhancement, as well as protrusion of prelaminar optic nerves bilaterally ➡. Mild diffuse optic nerve sheath enhancement is also present. (**Right**) Coronal T1WI C+ FS MR in the same patient shows diffuse enhancement of the optic nerve sheaths ➡ associated with prominent subarachnoid spaces along the optic nerves. Treatment for pseudotumor cerebri includes weight loss and medications, as well as lumbar punctures, shunt, and optic nerve fenestration.*

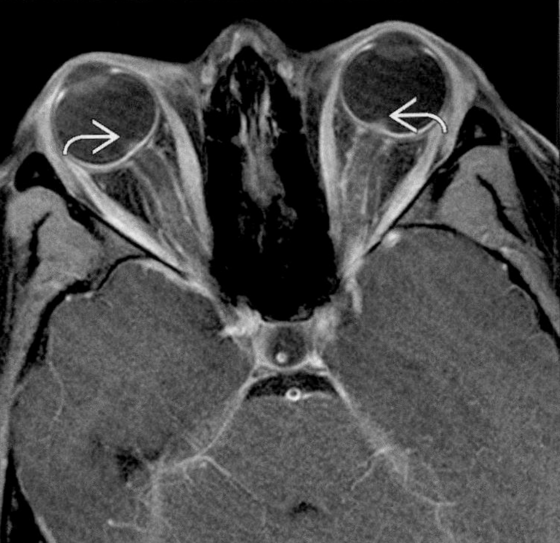

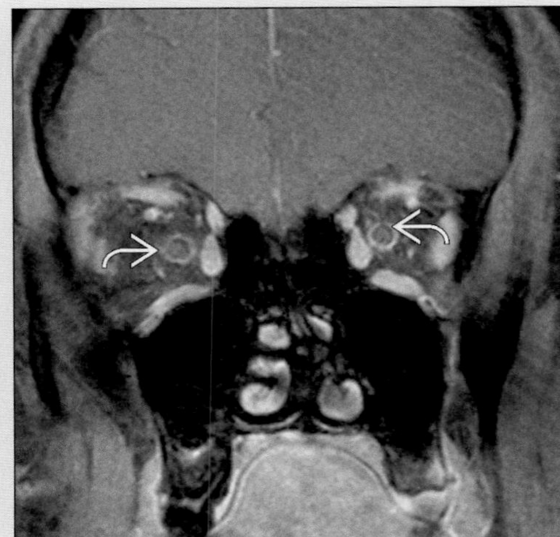

IDIOPATHIC INTRACRANIAL HYPERTENSION

TERMINOLOGY

Synonyms

- Idiopathic intracranial hypertension (IIH)
- Pseudotumor cerebri

Definitions

- ↑ intracranial pressure without obvious underlying brain pathological condition
- Multiple potential causes of intracranial hypertension (e.g., dural sinus thrombosis) must be excluded
- Association of any medication or condition with IIH better termed "secondary pseudotumor syndrome"

IMAGING

General Features

- Best diagnostic clue
  - Partial empty sella, dilation/tortuosity of optic nerve sheath, flattening of posterior sclera in patient with clinical findings of IIH

CT Findings

- NECT
  - Usually normal; enlarged optic nerve sheaths ± empty sella (40-50%)
  - Less common: Slit ventricles (10%)

MR Findings

- T1WI
  - Partially empty sella turcica
  - Enlarged/tortuous optic nerve sheaths, posterior sclera flattened
  - Small "pinched" ventricles
- T2WI
  - Increased fluid around optic nerves ± bulbous dilation of sheath behind globes
  - Optic nerve papilla may "protrude" into globe in severe cases
- DWI: Normal brain water diffusion
  - Suggests diffuse brain edema **not** associated with IIH
- T1WI C+: Enhancement of prelaminar optic nerve
- MRV: Use to exclude dural sinus thrombosis/stenosis

Imaging Recommendations

- Best imaging tool
  - MR with fat-saturated T1WI C+ of orbits, whole brain

DIFFERENTIAL DIAGNOSIS

Secondary Pseudotumor Syndromes

- Dural sinus stenosis/thrombosis
- Medications, such as vitamin A or its derivatives, some antibiotics (e.g., tetracycline), steroid withdrawal, hormones, lithium
- Post Chiari 1 malformation decompression surgery
- Systemic lupus erythematosus associated

Idiopathic or Post-Inflammatory Optic Nerve Atrophy

- Small optic nerves without scleral flattening

Idiopathic Empty Sella

- Normal variant; normal optic nerve sheaths

PATHOLOGY

General Features

- Etiology
  - ↑ intracranial pressure of unknown etiology

Staging, Grading, & Classification

- Modified Dandy criteria must be met (e.g., symptoms of ↑ ICP with > 25 cm H_2O, normal CT/MR without dural sinus thrombosis, mass, etc.)

Gross Pathologic & Surgical Features

- Bilateral papilledema

Microscopic Features

- Normal CSF cytology, chemistry

CLINICAL ISSUES

Presentation

- Most common signs/symptoms
  - Headache in 90-95%
    - Generalized, episodic, throbbing, aggravated by Valsalva
  - Papilledema (bilateral optic nerve head swelling) virtually universal
  - Progressive visual loss ± CN6 paresis, diplopia
  - Uncommon: Vertigo, tinnitus, occasional pituitary disfunction
  - In children: Irritability, "sunset" sign, bulging anterior fontanelle
- Clinical profile
  - Obese, young to middle-aged woman with headache, papilledema

Natural History & Prognosis

- Chief hazard: Vision loss from chronic papilledema

Treatment

- Goal: Prevent visual loss, improve associated symptoms
- Options
  - Medical (e.g., weight loss, carbonic anhydrase inhibitors)
  - Surgical (e.g., LP, shunt, optic nerve sheath fenestration)

DIAGNOSTIC CHECKLIST

Image Interpretation Pearls

- Must exclude venous stenosis/space-occupying lesion

SELECTED REFERENCES

1. Randhawa S et al: Idiopathic intracranial hypertension (pseudotumor cerebri). Curr Opin Ophthalmol. 19(6):445-53, 2008
2. Binder DK et al: Idiopathic intracranial hypertension. Neurosurgery. 54(3):538-51; discussion 551-2, 2004

CARBON MONOXIDE POISONING

Key Facts

Terminology

- Anoxic-ischemic encephalopathy, usually with bilateral lesions, caused by inhalation of CO gas

Imaging

- Best diagnostic clue: GP T2/FLAIR hyperintensity
- T1 MR: Both hypointensity in GP (likely necrosis) & hyperintensity in GP (likely hemorrhage) reported
- T2 MR: Ischemia/infarct of GP
  - Cerebral hemispheric WM: Bilateral confluent hyperintense WM (periventricular, centrum semiovale)
  - Cortical hyperintensity (commonly temporal lobe)
  - Medial temporal lobe hyperintensity (uncommon despite frequent pathologic findings)
- DWI MR: Acute restriction is common
- MRS: Progressively ↓ NAA/Cr with time; ↑ Cho/Cr
  - Progressively ↑ Lac/Cr with time

Top Differential Diagnoses

- Wilson disease
- Japanese encephalitis (JE)
- Creutzfeldt-Jakob disease (CJD)

Pathology

- Impairs the ability of erythrocytes to transport oxygen, causing hypoxia and reducing cellular oxygen metabolism
- CO-induced parkinsonism
- Demyelination, edema, and hemorrhagic necrosis

Clinical Issues

- Acute toxicity: Nausea, vomiting, headache
- Neuropsychological sequelae
- Hyperbaric oxygen (HBO) therapy: Treatment of choice in acute COP (within 6 hours for best effect)
- Delayed neurologic sequelae (10-30% of victims)

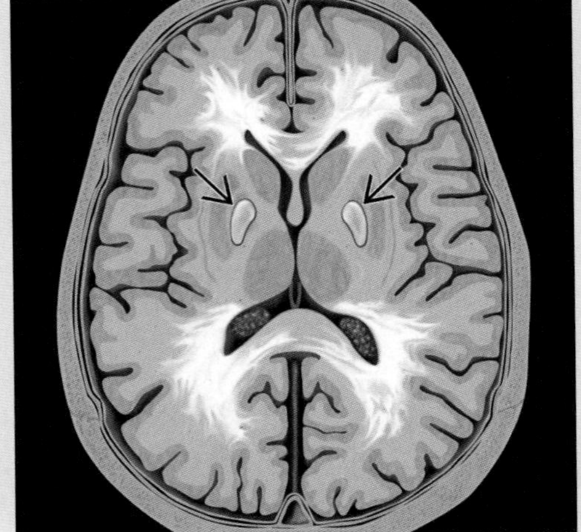

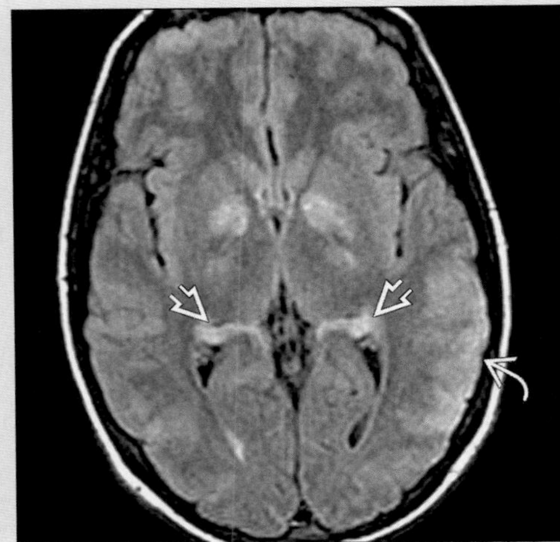

(Left) Axial graphic shows the typical involvement of the brain by CO poisoning. The globi pallidi (GP) ➔ are most affected, followed by the cerebral white matter. Pathologically, there is necrosis of the GP with variable areas of necrosis and demyelination in the white matter. (Right) Axial FLAIR MR in this patient with acute CO poisoning shows the classic appearance with symmetric GP hyperintensity. Note the additional involvement of the posterior temporal cortex ➔ and hippocampi ➔, a less common finding.

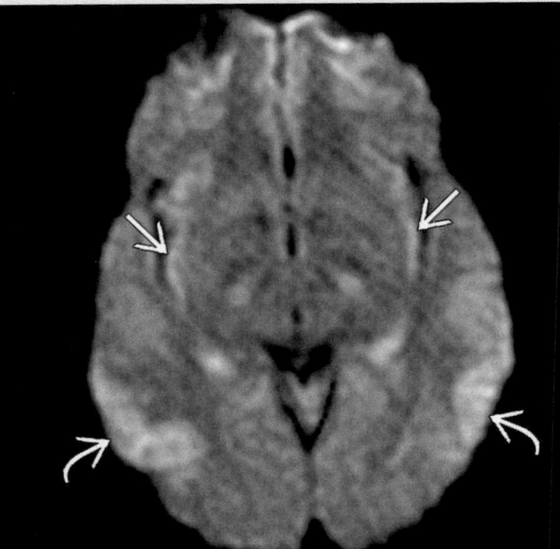

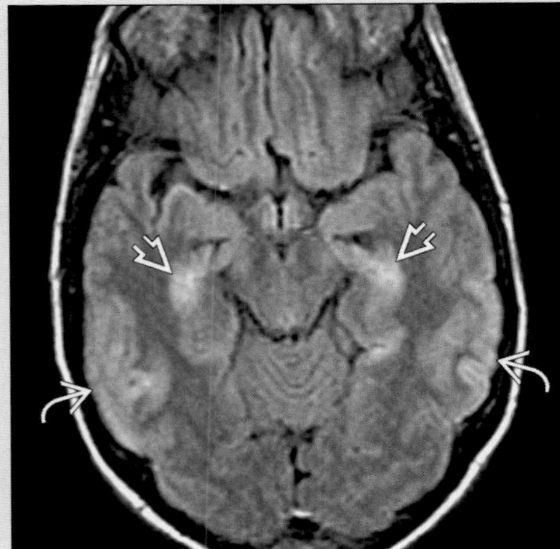

(Left) Axial DWI MR in the same patient shows areas of restricted diffusion involving the posterior temporal cortex ➔, hippocampal tail, and insular cortex ➔ bilaterally. DWI often shows the affected areas more readily than corresponding T2 or FLAIR MR images. (Right) Axial FLAIR MR in the same patient shows symmetric hyperintensity involving the bilateral hippocampi ➔ and posterior temporal cortex ➔.

CARBON MONOXIDE POISONING

TERMINOLOGY

Abbreviations

- Carbon monoxide (CO) poisoning (COP)

Definitions

- Anoxic-ischemic encephalopathy, usually with bilateral lesions, caused by inhalation of CO gas

IMAGING

General Features

- Best diagnostic clue
  - Globi pallidi (GP) hyperintensity on T2WI or hypodensity on CT
- Location
  - GP: Most common site of abnormality
  - Cerebral white matter (WM): 2nd most common
  - Putamen, caudate nucleus, thalamus, substantia nigra, corpus callosum, fornix, hippocampus: Less common
- Morphology
  - Typically oval lesions confined to GP
  - Severe changes show loss of gray-white differentiation due to diffuse edema

CT Findings

- NECT
  - Symmetric hypodensity in GP and symmetric diffuse hypodensity in cerebral WM

MR Findings

- T1WI
  - In GP, both T1 hypointensity (likely due to necrosis) and T1 hyperintensity (likely due to hemorrhage) reported
- T2WI
  - Ischemia/infarct of GP
    - Bilateral T2 hyperintensities of GP surrounded by hypointense rim (likely due to hemosiderin)
    - Caudate nucleus and putamen may be affected, either alone or in addition to GP abnormality
  - Cerebral hemispheric WM: Bilateral, confluent, T2 hyperintense WM (periventricular, centrum semiovale)
    - Reflects diffuse demyelination
  - Abnormal signal in cerebral cortex (less frequent)
    - Cortical hyperintensity: Most common pattern, with predilection for temporal lobe
    - Abnormalities in perisylvian cortex, anterior temporal lobe, and insular cortex
    - Asymmetrical, diffuse cortical hyperintensity affecting parietal and occipital lobes also possible
  - Medial temporal lobe in region of hippocampus may show signal abnormality
    - Uncommon despite frequent pathological findings
  - Diffuse, bilateral high signal within cerebellar hemispheres, affecting cortex and WM
    - Not seen in acute setting; develops later
  - Delayed encephalopathy 2-3 weeks after recovery
    - Additional high intensity in corpus callosum, subcortical U-fibers, internal and external capsules
    - Associated with low intensity in thalamus and putamen (due to iron deposition)
- FLAIR
  - Same as T2WI
  - Additional periventricular high signal in acute COP
    - May not be visible on conventional T2 FSE
- DWI
  - Early (acute) stage of COP
    - Diffuse symmetric DWI hyperintensity in subcortical hemispheric WM (restricted diffusion due to cytotoxic edema)
      - WM may appear normal on FLAIR, particularly in low-dose exposure
    - Corresponding ADC maps: Low signal intensity and low ADC values in same regions
  - Delayed stage of COP (weeks post exposure)
    - High signal area in cerebral WM
    - ± abnormal WM findings on T2WI
    - Low ADC values persist at this stage
  - Chronic stage of COP
    - Gradual increase in ADC values, consistent with macrocystic encephalomalacia
    - Hyperintense WM areas on T2WI and symmetric bright lesions in GP
  - Diffusion tensor imaging (DTI): FA values decreased in corpus callosum, orbitofrontal WM, high frontal WM, parietal WM, and temporal lobes
    - High correlation between FA and Mini-Mental State Exam (MMSE)
- T1WI C+
  - Variable enhancement in GP, often in patients with acute COP
- MRS
  - Serial ^{1}H-MRS scans performed after appearance of delayed sequelae in COP, disturbances of neuronal function, membrane metabolism, and anaerobic energy metabolism
    - Persistently ↑ Cho/Cr at DWI abnormal WM site
    - Progressively ↓ NAA/Cr with time
      - ↓ NAA suggests neuron and axon degeneration
    - Progressively ↑ Lac/Cr with time, often seen in high-dose exposure cases

Nuclear Medicine Findings

- SPECT studies show cerebral hypoperfusion deficits
  - ↓ regional cerebral blood flow in frontal and temporal cortices and diffuse hypoperfusion defects have been reported

Imaging Recommendations

- Best imaging tool
  - DWI best for lesion detection in acute stage of COP
    - ADC value decreases progressively and persists much longer than acute cerebral infarction
- Protocol advice
  - Multiplanar MR including DWI, T2WI

DIFFERENTIAL DIAGNOSIS

Wilson Disease

- WM/GM lesions, involving BG, dentate nucleus, pons, mesencephalon
- T1 hypointense (occasionally hyperintense) lesions

- Variably T2 hyperintense/hypointense

Japanese Encephalitis (JE)

- Homogeneous T2 hyperintensities in BG & thalami
- Most characteristic finding in JE
  - Bilateral thalamic hyperintensities ± hemorrhage
- JE is meningoencephalitis → meningeal enhancement

Creutzfeldt-Jakob Disease (CJD)

- Progressively symmetric hyperintense changes in BG, thalami, cerebral cortex
- DWI and FLAIR most sensitive

Leigh Syndrome

- Symmetrical spongiform brain lesions with onset in infancy/early childhood
- Lesions predominantly in brainstem, BG (particularly putamen), and cerebral WM
- Focal, bilateral, and symmetric T2 hyperintense lesions

PATHOLOGY

General Features

- Etiology
  - CO: Colorless, odorless, tasteless gas, has 210x higher affinity to Hgb than for O_2; brain and heart damage once CO-Hgb level exceeds 20%
  - Mechanisms of brain injury
    - Impairs ability of erythrocytes to transport oxygen, causing hypoxia and reducing cellular oxygen metabolism
    - Lipid peroxidation leading to oxidative injury
    - Damage to vascular endothelium due to deposition of peroxynitrite
    - Excitotoxicity, apoptosis
- Associated abnormalities
  - CO-induced parkinsonism
    - GP lesions after COP or periventricular and deep WM hyperintensities without BG lesions
    - Extrapyramidal syndrome may be due to lesions of WM areas containing BG output &/or input
    - Improvement usually accompanied by ↓ extent and signal intensity of WM abnormalities, especially in frontoparietal centrum semiovale

Staging, Grading, & Classification

- 4 main pathological types
  - GP lesions: Variable degree of necrosis
  - WM lesions: Scattered/focal areas of necrosis or confluent areas of demyelination
  - Cortical lesions: Spongy changes, intense capillary proliferation, degeneration, and loss of neurons
  - Hippocampal lesions: Coagulation necrosis

Gross Pathologic & Surgical Features

- GP necrosis, WM pallor

Microscopic Features

- Demyelination, edema, and hemorrhagic necrosis
  - Necrotic lesions in GP, other BG, hippocampus, cortex, and cerebellum
  - WM lesions: Foci of necrosis or demyelination

CLINICAL ISSUES

Presentation

- Most common signs/symptoms
  - Nonspecific symptoms; controversial association of specific symptoms with known CO-Hgb levels
  - Acute toxicity: Nausea, vomiting, headache
    - Confusion, cognitive impairment, loss of consciousness, seizures, coma, death
  - Neuropsychological sequelae
    - Dementia, memory deficits, decreased attention, irritability, mood and personality disturbance
    - Gait disturbance, parkinsonian-like symptoms, apraxia, convulsive disorders, visual-spatial and speech impairment
- Clinical profile
  - Depends on duration and intensity of exposure

Demographics

- Age
  - Equivalent age-specific fatality rates in adults, death rates from COP: ↑ in patients > 65 years
- Epidemiology
  - Most common cause of accidental poisoning in Europe and North America
  - Causes 2-6,000 deaths/year in USA, from both accidental and nonaccidental overdoses

Natural History & Prognosis

- Persistent neurologic sequelae: Occur immediately following COP and persist over time
- Delayed neurologic sequelae (10-30% of victims)
  - Occur weeks after initial recovery from acute COP
- 2 categories with regard to outcome
  - Normal/mild functional impairment: No or minimal abnormality on brain MR
  - Death/severe functional impairment (coma): Diffuse brain damage on MR

Treatment

- Hyperbaric oxygen (HBO) therapy: Treatment of choice in acute COP (within 6 hours for best effect)
- Early administration of 100% oxygen or HBO may prevent long-term neuropsychiatric sequelae

DIAGNOSTIC CHECKLIST

Consider

- MR to monitor progression/resolution of lesions

SELECTED REFERENCES

1. Kondziella D et al: 1H MR spectroscopy of gray and white matter in carbon monoxide poisoning. J Neurol. 256(6):970-9, 2009
2. Lin WC et al: White matter damage in carbon monoxide intoxication assessed in vivo using diffusion tensor MR imaging. AJNR Am J Neuroradiol. 30(6):1248-55, 2009
3. Prockop LD et al: Carbon monoxide intoxication: an updated review. J Neurol Sci. 262(1-2):122-30, 2007
4. Sener RN: Acute carbon monoxide poisoning: diffusion MR imaging findings. AJNR Am J Neuroradiol. 24(7):1475-7, 2003

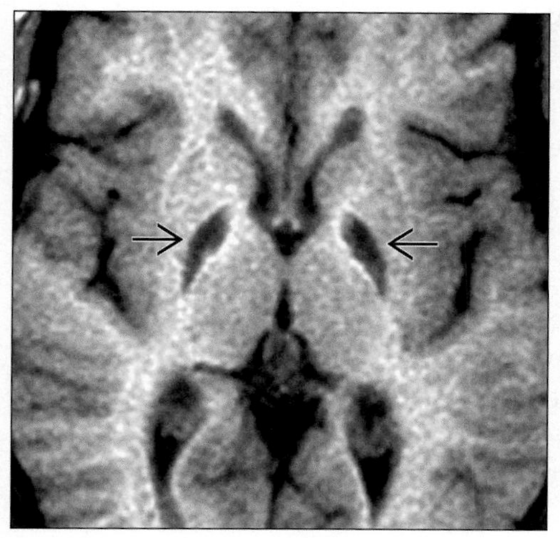

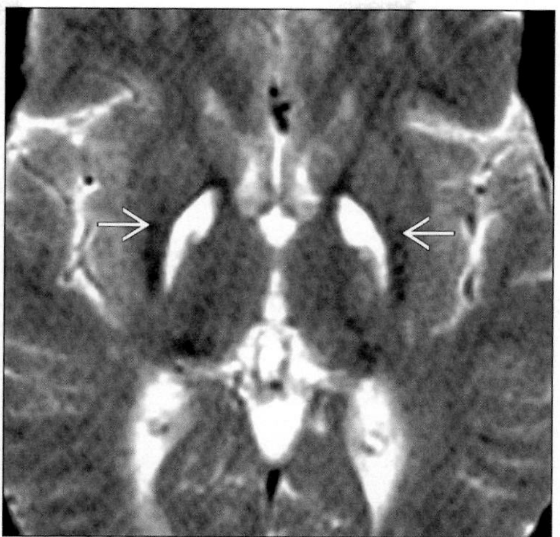

(Left) *Axial T1WI MR shows the appearance of chronic CO poisoning involving the basal ganglia. There are bilateral, nonenhancing, CSF intensity lesions present within the globi pallidi* →. ***(Right)*** *Axial T2WI MR in the same patient shows symmetric, bilateral, CSF intensity lesions within the globi pallidi* ➡. *Often, there is a rim of hypointensity related to hemosiderin surrounding the injured deep gray nuclei. Up to 30% of patients with CO poisoning have delayed neurologic sequelae.*

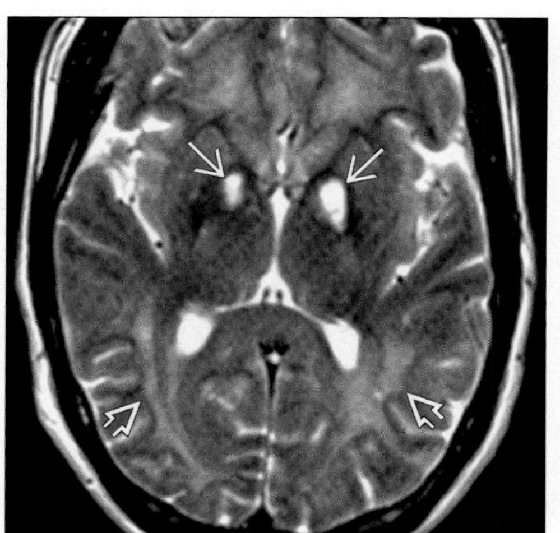

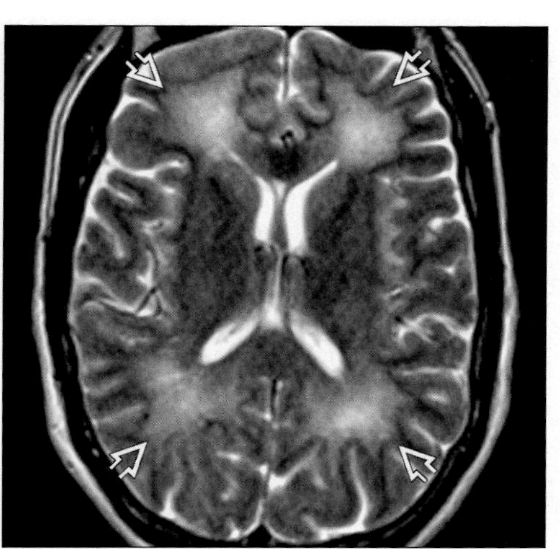

(Left) *Axial T2WI MR shows symmetric, bilateral, globus pallidus hyperintensities* ➡ *and diffuse hyperintensity throughout the white matter* ➡ *with sparing of the subcortical U-fibers.* ***(Right)*** *Axial T2WI MR in the same patient shows bilateral diffuse hyperintensity throughout the white matter* ➡ *with typical sparing of the subcortical U-fibers. The white matter hyperintensity is related primarily to demyelination with variable amounts of necrosis. The hyperintensity typically shows diffusion restriction.*

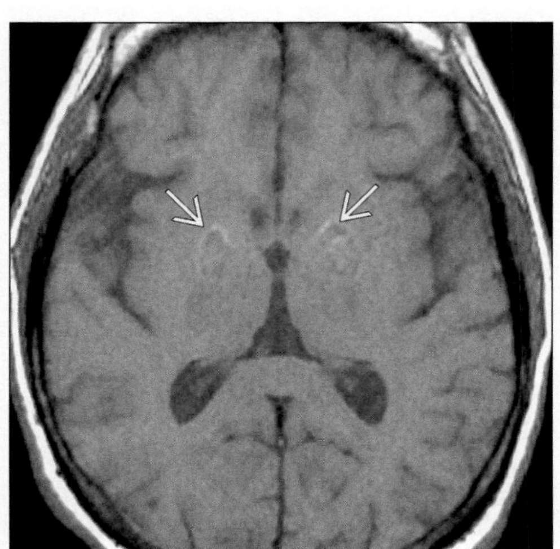

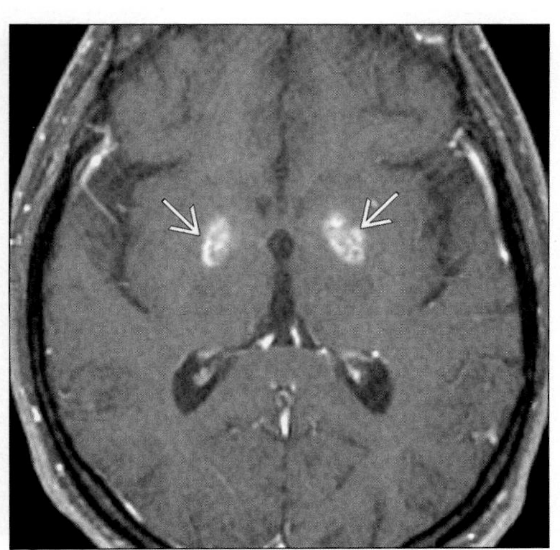

(Left) *Axial T1WI MR of a patient with acute CO poisoning shows heterogeneous signal in the globus pallidus bilaterally with areas of central hypointensity with a surrounding rim of hyperintensity* ➡. *The hyperintensity is likely related to blood products.* ***(Right)*** *Axial T1WI C+ FS MR in the same patient shows heterogeneous enhancement of the globus pallidus bilaterally* ➡. *Enhancement is variably seen in CO poisoning.*

DRUG ABUSE

Key Facts

Terminology

- Many drugs (prescription, illicit, or "street") have adverse CNS effects
  - Illicit drug use often causes cerebrovascular disease
  - Polydrug abuse common, including EtOH
- Nitrous oxide (NO_2) abuse → inactivates vitamin B12 → subacute combined degeneration
- Chronic EtOH abuse → thiamine deficiency → Wernicke encephalopathy

Imaging

- Best imaging clue: Young/middle-aged adult with ischemic or hemorrhagic stroke in close temporal proximity to drug administration
  - Hemorrhage: Intracranial (ICH), subarachnoid (SAH), intraventricular (IVH)
  - Nonhemorrhagic ischemic stroke: MCA territory most common
- Heroin, MDMA: Globus pallidus (GP) ischemia
- Amphetamines: Hemorrhage, vasculitis, pseudoaneurysm, infarcts
- NECT for suspected hemorrhage → if CT reveals hemorrhage, consider CTA/MRA/DSA
- Consider drug abuse or dissection in young or middle-aged patient with stroke

Top Differential Diagnoses

- Intracranial hemorrhage in young adults
  - Vascular malformations
  - Dural sinus thrombosis with hemorrhagic infarct
  - Severe posterior reversible encephalopathy syndrome with secondary hemorrhage

Clinical Issues

- 4% of all strokes occur in patients < 45 years old
- 30% of strokes in patients < 45 years old are drug-related

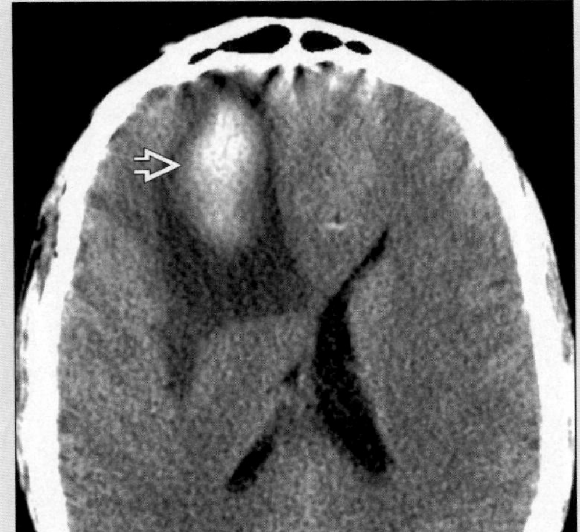

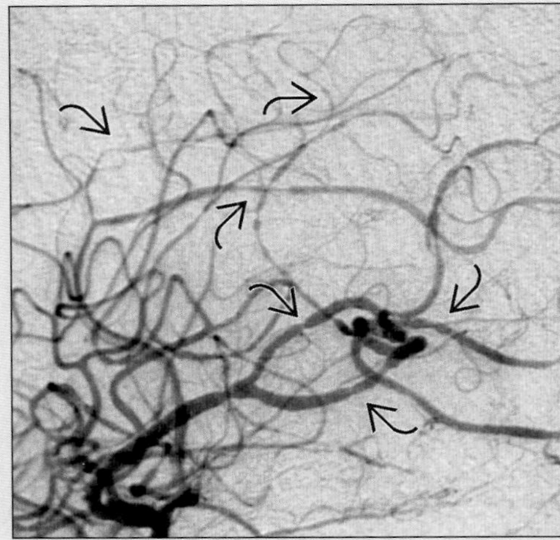

(Left) *Axial NECT in a 42-year-old man who presented with a history of recurrent severe headache and a longstanding history of amphetamine abuse shows hyperdensity related to lobar hemorrhage with surrounding edema in the right frontal lobe.* ***(Right)*** *Lateral DSA of a right internal carotid artery injection shows irregularity and a beaded appearance of the medium to small-sized vessels in the MCA and ACA distributions. Findings are consistent with drug-induced vasculitis in this young adult.*

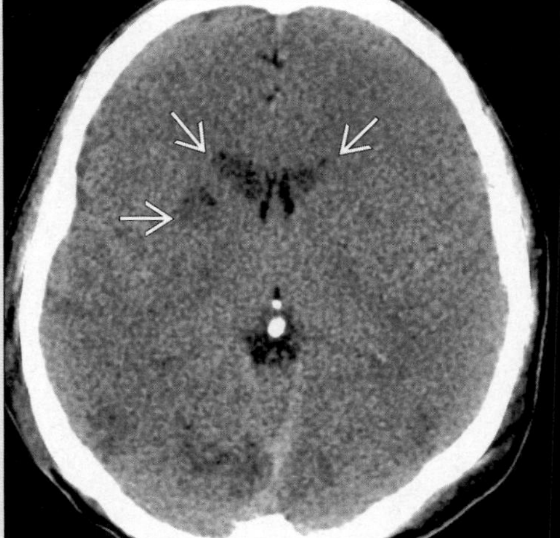

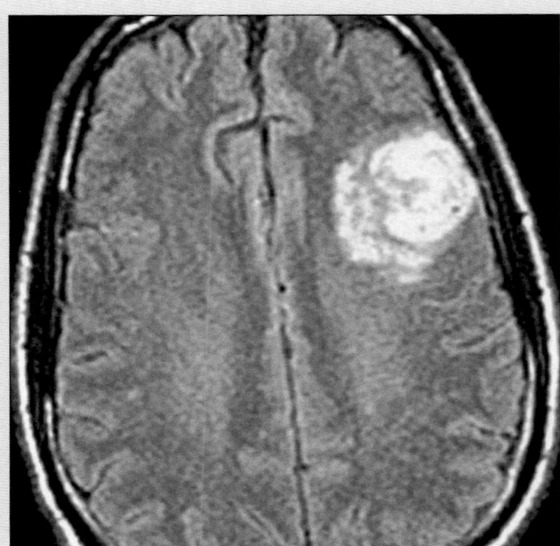

(Left) *Axial NECT in a comatose patient after cocaine abuse shows focal hypodensities in the basal ganglia related to ischemia. Note also the diffuse loss of the corticomedullary differentiation due to severe anoxia.* ***(Right)*** *Axial FLAIR MR in a 22-year-old patient with a history of cocaine abuse shows a rounded hyperintense "mass" in the left frontal lobe. The lesion demonstrated acute restriction on DWI and represents a drug-related cortical infarct in this young adult.*

TERMINOLOGY

Definitions
- Many drugs (prescription, illicit, or "street") have adverse CNS effects
  - Major pathology generally vascular or metabolic
  - Polydrug abuse (including EtOH) is common
- Cerebrovascular disease caused by illicit drug use
  - Cocaine: Intranasal, intravenous (IV), intramuscular, smoked, transplacental transfer
    - Cocaine hydrochloride (HCl) not smokable
    - Alkaloid form ("freebase," "crack") smokable
  - Amphetamines: Oral, intranasal, parenteral use
    - 3-, 4-methylenedioxymethamphetamine (MDMA, "ecstasy")
  - Heroin: IV use, inhaled ("chasing the dragon")
  - EtOH abuse: Interference with normal clotting increases risk of spontaneous hemorrhage and extent of hemorrhage due to primary pathology
    - Traumatic brain injury
    - Hypertensive cerebral vascular disease
- May interfere with critical metabolic pathways
  - Nitrous oxide (NO_2) abuse → inactivates vitamin B12 → subacute combined degeneration
- May lead to nutritional deficiencies
  - Chronic EtOH abuse → thiamine deficiency → Wernicke encephalopathy
- Organ damage from chronic drug abuse
  - EtOH → liver failure → manganese deposition in basal ganglia (BG)

IMAGING

General Features
- Best diagnostic clue
  - Young/middle-aged adult with ischemic or hemorrhagic stroke in close temporal proximity to drug administration
- Location
  - Hemorrhage: Intracranial (ICH), subarachnoid (SAH), intraventricular (IVH)
  - Nonhemorrhagic ischemic stroke: MCA territory most common
  - Cocaine: Infarctions in cerebrum, thalamus, brainstem, cerebellum, retina
  - Heroin, MDMA: Globus pallidus (GP) ischemia
  - Amphetamines: Hemorrhage, vasculitis, pseudoaneurysm, infarcts
  - Wernicke: Bilateral posterior thalamus, mammillary bodies, posterior mesencephalon
  - Liver failure: BG
  - NO_2: Posterior columns, spinal cord

CT Findings
- NECT
  - Cocaine: ICH, SAH, IVH
  - Heroin inhalation: Symmetric hypodensity in cerebellar and posterior cerebral WM, posterior limb of internal capsule, GP

MR Findings
- T1WI
  - Heroin vapor inhalation: Leukoencephalopathy
  - Hepatic encephalopathy: Hyperintense BG
- T2WI
  - Cocaine: May have severe T2 hyperintense lesions
    - Cerebral, insular subcortex WM lesions, transient arterial occlusion in MCA territory: Small infarctions
  - Heroin vapor inhalation
    - Hyperintense cerebral, cerebellar tracts
    - WM cerebellum, posterior cerebral, posterior limb of internal capsule, sparing of subcortical WM and dentate nuclei
  - Wernicke encephalopathy
    - Hyperintensity in medial thalami, tectum, periaqueductal gray matter (GM), mammillary bodies, rarely cortex
  - Subacute combined degeneration
    - Hyperintensity in posterior spinal cord (cervical and thoracic)
- T2* GRE
  - Hemorrhagic lesions have decreased signal
- DWI
  - Restricted diffusion in acute ischemic and metabolic lesions
- MRA
  - Arterial spasm &/or vasculitis
    - Vasculitis difficult to diagnose on MRA unless high quality; 3T MRA > 1.5T MRA

Other Modality Findings
- Cerebral angiography may show irregularity of medium-sized intracranial vessels consistent with amphetamine-induced vasculitis

Imaging Recommendations
- Protocol advice
  - NECT for suspected hemorrhage
    - If CT reveals hemorrhage, consider CTA/MRA/DSA
  - MR: Include DWI, GRE, T1WI C+

DIFFERENTIAL DIAGNOSIS

Spontaneous ICH in Young Adults
- Hypertension (HTN): BG hemorrhages
- Vascular malformations
  - Cavernous angiomas
  - Arteriovenous malformations (AVMs)
- Intratumoral hemorrhage
  - Seen in ~ 1% of brain tumors, usually malignant
    - Incomplete hemosiderin rings, enhancing nodule, persistent mass effect
- Dural sinus thrombosis with hemorrhagic infarct
  - Underlying coagulable state often present with hemorrhagic venous infarct
- Severe posterior reversible encephalopathy syndrome (PRES) with secondary hemorrhage
- Mycotic aneurysm with parenchymal hemorrhage
  - Often related to infectious endocarditis

Vasculitis
- Inflammation and necrosis of vessel walls
- Multiple etiologies: Infectious, granulomatous, autoimmune, collagen vascular disease
- Drug-induced differentiated by history

DRUG ABUSE

PATHOLOGY

General Features

- Etiology
  - Cocaine, amphetamines
    - Systemic vasoconstriction ⇒ acute arterial HTN ⇒ hemorrhagic stroke (rupture of preexisting aneurysms, bleeding from AVM)
    - Cerebral vasoconstriction, vasculitis ⇒ infarction
  - Parenteral drugs
    - Infective endocarditis (IE) ⇒ emboli ⇒ cerebral infarction, hemorrhage, abscess, mycotic aneurysm
    - Bacteremia in absence of IE: Brain abscess
    - Hepatitis: Bleeding diathesis
  - Cocaine
    - ↑ platelet aggregation with thrombosis
    - Heart disease: Source of emboli
  - MDMA abuse: Loss of serotoninergic neurons
  - Heroin: Toxic leukoencephalopathy, hypoxic brain injury, ischemic stroke, brain abscess
    - Generalized hypoxia and hypotension
    - Possible immunologic-mediated vasculitis
    - Nephropathy ⇒ severe HTN
  - Wernicke encephalopathy: ↓ thiamine affects membrane function → failure to maintain osmotic gradients
  - Subacute combined degeneration
    - NO_2 inactivates B12 so serum B12 levels normal; may obscure diagnosis
  - Concomitant alcohol use may potentiate illicit drug effects (↓ hepatic metabolism)
- Associated abnormalities
  - Drug-related ICH frequently related to underlying vascular malformation (cerebral aneurysm, AVM)
  - Drug-induced IE, vasculitis
  - Cocaine HCl: Hemorrhagic (80%) > ischemic stroke
  - Alkaloidal cocaine: Hemorrhagic = ischemic stroke
  - Amphetamines: Hemorrhagic > ischemic stroke
  - Heroin: Cerebral infarctions (MCA area, not watershed distribution), toxic leukoencephalopathy

Gross Pathologic & Surgical Features

- Amphetamine, cocaine: Arterial spasm/vasculitis
- Cocaine in pregnancy: Fetal infarctions in BG, ↑ rate of neural tube closure defects
- Amphetamine, cocaine, MDMA: ICH, SAH
- MDMA: Vasoconstriction in recent users, vasodilatation in ex-users, bilateral GP necrosis (secondary prolonged vasospasm)

Microscopic Features

- Amphetamines: Inflammatory vasculitis + vessel wall necrosis ("speed arteritis") similar to PAN
- Cocaine: Vasculitis affecting CNS
- Heroin: Vasculitis (rare), probably related to drug contaminants

CLINICAL ISSUES

Presentation

- Most common signs/symptoms
  - Cocaine, MDMA, amphetamines: Stroke, headache, seizures
  - Heroin: BG damage (Parkinsonism, hemiballismus)
    - Toxic leukoencephalopathy: Cerebellar, pyramidal, and pseudobulbar signs, spasms, death
  - Wernicke: Obtundation and ataxia
  - Subacute combined degeneration: Loss of proprioception
- Clinical profile
  - Cerebral infarcts, TIAs, ICH, SAH
    - Temporal proximity of stroke to drug use

Demographics

- Age
  - 85-90% of drug-related strokes in 4th through 5th decade
- Epidemiology
  - 30% of strokes in patients < 45 are drug-related
  - Estimated relative risk for stroke among drug abusers (after controlling for other stroke risk factors): 6.5 out of 10
  - Subacute combined degeneration
    - Individuals with access to medical NO_2
    - Abuse of NO_2 canisters (poppers)

Natural History & Prognosis

- Time interval between drug use and stroke onset: Up to 1 week
  - Stroke risk highest within 1st 6 hours after drug use
- IE-related strokes may be delayed
  - 20% mortality for IE-associated strokes, 67% mortality for hemorrhagic strokes
- Cocaine worsens presentation and outcome of aneurysmal SAH patients

Treatment

- Management of drug-related stroke largely supportive
- Antibiotics for embolic stroke due to IV-drug-induced IE ↓ risk of recurrent infarction
- Aggressive addiction rehabilitation
- Experimentally, magnesium reverses cocaine-induced vasospasm
- Wernicke: Supplementary thiamine
- Subacute combined degeneration: B12 injection

DIAGNOSTIC CHECKLIST

Consider

- Drug abuse in young/middle-aged patient with stroke

Image Interpretation Pearls

- Drug-related hemorrhages may indicate underlying vascular abnormality
- Vasculitis can be very difficult to distinguish from drug-related vasospasm

SELECTED REFERENCES

1. Gupta PK et al: Hippocampal involvement due to heroin inhalation--"chasing the dragon". Clin Neurol Neurosurg. 111(3):278-81, 2009
2. Renard D et al: Bilateral haemorrhagic infarction of the globus pallidus after cocaine and alcohol intoxication. Acta Neurol Belg. 109(2):159-61, 2009

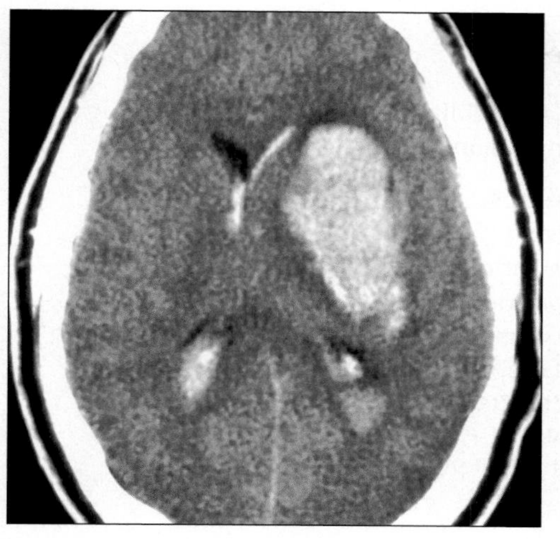

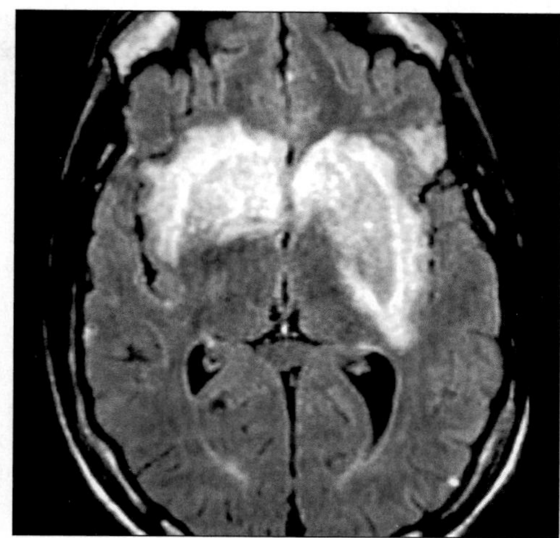

(Left) *Axial NECT shows a large left basal ganglia hemorrhage in a young patient with no vascular risk factors. Drug screen was positive both for cocaine and amphetamines. Imaging mimics a hypertensive hemorrhage. Note the extension of the hemorrhage into the ventricular system.* ***(Right)*** *Axial FLAIR MR in a patient with a history of amphetamine abuse shows bilateral basal ganglia edema related to vasculitis. Corresponding angiogram showed the typical beaded appearance of vasculitis.*

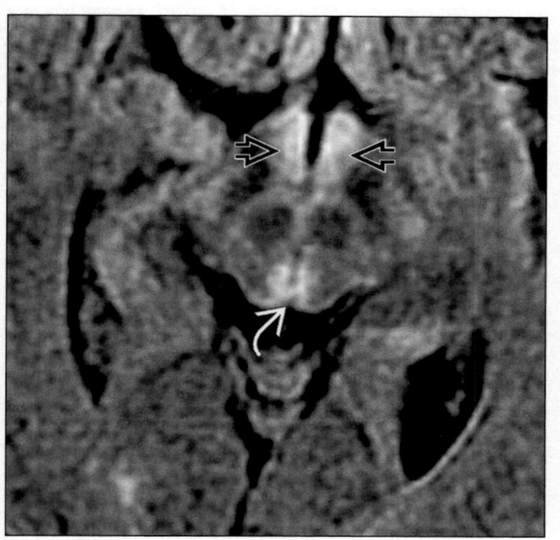

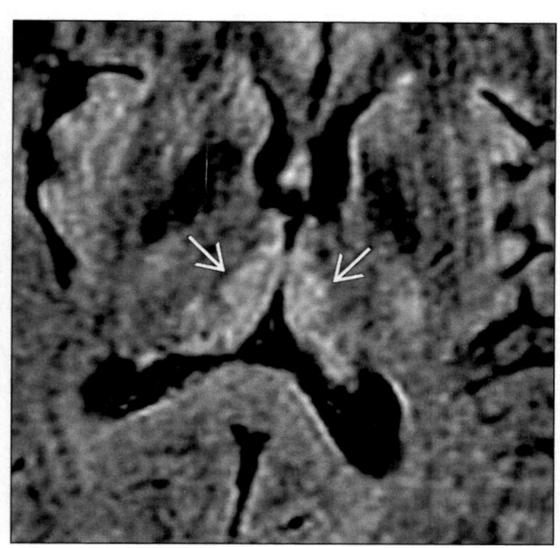

(Left) *Axial FLAIR MR in a patient with a history of alcohol abuse and thiamine deficiency shows focal symmetric hyperintensity involving the mammillary bodies and hypothalamus ➩ as well as the periaqueductal gray matter ➨.* ***(Right)*** *Axial FLAIR MR in the same patient shows symmetric FLAIR hyperintensity involving the medial dorsal thalami ➨ without focal mass effect. Wernicke encephalopathy including the triad of ataxia, oculomotor abnormalities, and confusion.*

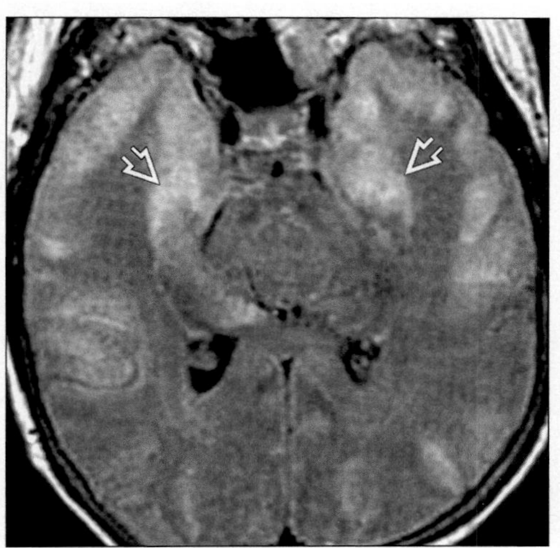

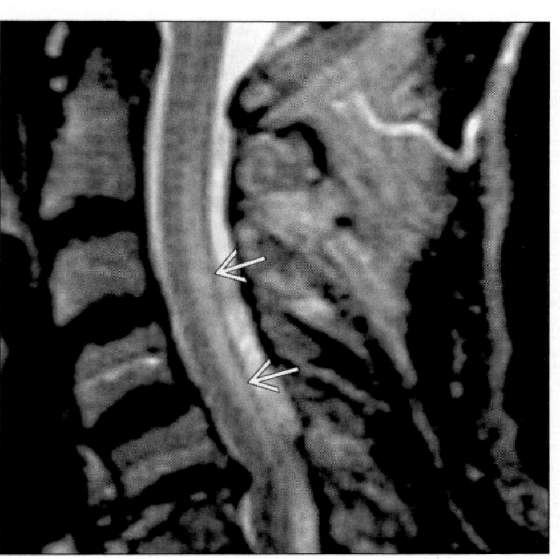

(Left) *Axial FLAIR MR in a patient with a history of fulminant hepatic encephalopathy related to Tylenol overdose shows diffuse cortical hyperintensities involving the medial and anterior temporal lobes as well as the hippocampi ➩ bilaterally.* ***(Right)*** *Sagittal T2WI MR shows hyperintensity within the dorsal column white matter related to subacute combined degeneration ➨. This may be seen in patients with a history of nitrous oxide (NO_2) abuse, which inactivates vitamin B12.*

METHANOL POISONING

Key Facts

Terminology
- Acute toxic effects of methanol on CNS

Imaging
- Bilateral hemorrhagic putaminal necrosis
- Putamen, hemispheric white matter
  - Caudate nuclei may be involved
  - Uncommon: Corpus callosum, brainstem, cerebellum
- DWI: Restriction in putamina ± white matter
- Protocol: MR (including GRE + DWI)

Top Differential Diagnoses
- Hypertensive intracranial hemorrhage
- Anoxic infarcts
- Carbon monoxide (CO) poisoning
- Osmotic demyelination syndrome
- Wilson disease
- Leigh disease
- Creutzfeldt-Jakob disease (CJD)
- Huntington disease

Pathology
- Methanol metabolized to formaldehyde, formic acid
- Causes "anion gap acidosis"

Clinical Issues
- Blurred vision
- Drowsiness, confusion, seizure, coma
- Nausea/vomiting, abdominal pain
- Respiratory arrest → death
- Untreated methanol poisoning
  - Visual deficits in ~ 1/3
  - Death rate of ~ 1/3
- Treatment: Fomepizole or ethanol

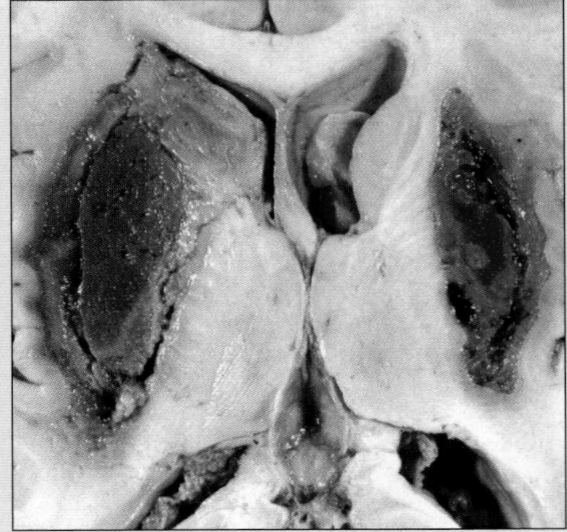

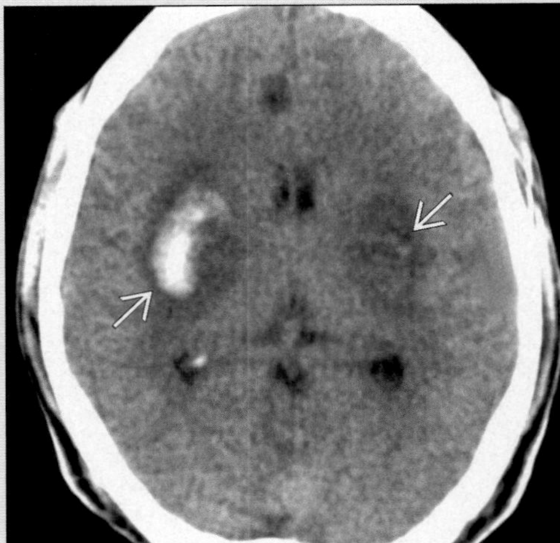

(Left) *Axial gross pathology specimen sectioned through the basal ganglia in a patient who died from methanol poisoning shows bilateral hemorrhagic necrosis of both basal ganglia and the right caudate. The putamina are most severely affected. Note sparing of the thalami. (Courtesy R. Hewlett, PhD.)* ***(Right)*** *Axial NECT shows mixed density lesions in the basal ganglia in a patient who had been drinking methanol. Note gross and petechial hemorrhage in the putamen ➔, typical of acute methanol toxicity.*

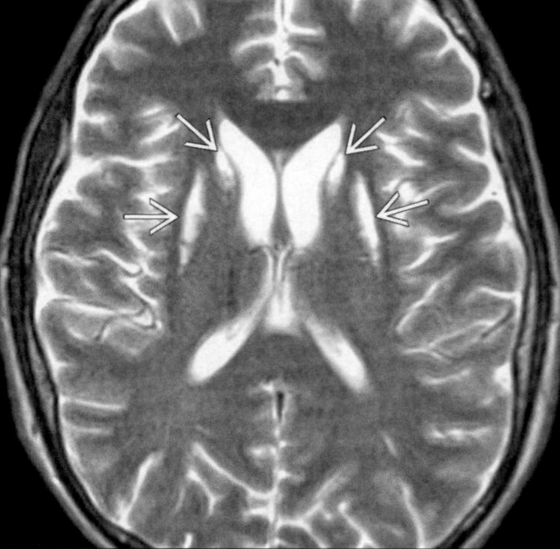

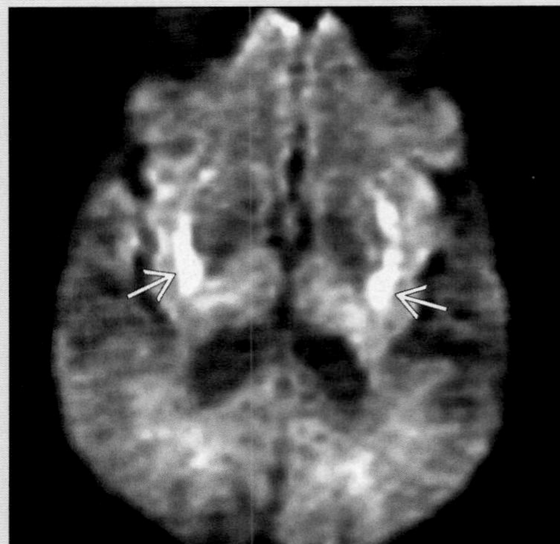

(Left) *Axial T2WI MR shows striking hyperintensities in the putamina and caudate nuclei ➔ in a 37-year-old man with longstanding abuse of both ethanol and methanol. Generalized volume loss is consistent with a history of chronic substance abuse.* ***(Right)*** *Axial DWI MR in a patient with acute methanol poisoning shows restricted diffusion in both putamina ➔. Follow-up NECT scans obtained 1 week later (not shown) demonstrated symmetrical low density in the putamina, as well as subcortical WM.*

METHANOL POISONING

TERMINOLOGY

Abbreviations

- Methanol (MtOH) encephalopathy

Definitions

- Acute toxic effects of MtOH on CNS

IMAGING

General Features

- Best diagnostic clue
  - Bilateral hemorrhagic putaminal necrosis
- Location
  - Putamen, hemispheric white matter
    - Caudate nuclei may be involved
    - Uncommon: Corpus callosum, brainstem, cerebellum

CT Findings

- NECT
  - Bilateral hemorrhagic putaminal necrosis
  - White matter hypodensity may be seen

MR Findings

- T1WI
  - Bilateral hemorrhagic putaminal necrosis is characteristic
  - Hemorrhagic subcortical necrosis
  - White matter hypointense lesions (confluent hemispheric ± optic nerves)
- T2WI
  - Lesions typically hyperintense
  - Acute hemorrhagic necrosis may cause hypointense foci
- FLAIR
  - Lesions all typically hyperintense
- T2* GRE
  - Hypointense foci in putamina
- DWI
  - Restriction (high signal) in putamina ± white matter
- T1WI C+
  - May see subtle enhancement

Imaging Recommendations

- Best imaging tool
  - NECT initially
- Protocol advice
  - MR (including GRE + DWI)

DIFFERENTIAL DIAGNOSIS

Hypertensive Intracranial Hemorrhage

- Usually unilateral

Anoxic Infarcts

- Most are nonhemorrhagic vs. hemorrhagic necrosis in MtOH
- Symmetric ↑ T2 in basal ganglia (BG) typical

Carbon Monoxide (CO) Poisoning

- ↑ T2 in globus pallidus (GP) > putamen typical ± hemispheric WM

Osmotic Demyelination Syndrome

- Extrapontine myelinolysis results in ↑ T2 in BG
- High signal in central pons common

Wilson Disease

- ↑ T2 in the BG, brainstem typical

Leigh Disease

- ↑ T2 lesions (brainstem, BG, and WM) with onset in infancy/early childhood

Creutzfeldt-Jakob Disease (CJD)

- Progressive ↑ T2 of BG (putamen and caudate > GP), thalamus, and cerebral cortex

Huntington Disease

- Caudate atrophy, ↑ T2 caudate/putamen

PATHOLOGY

General Features

- Etiology
  - Methanol metabolized to formaldehyde, formic acid
  - Causes "anion gap acidosis"
  - Select toxic effect on putamen, optic nerves
  - Commercial products containing methanol include antifreeze, paint remover, photocopying fluid

Gross Pathologic & Surgical Features

- Pallidal necrosis
- Optic nerve demyelination and atrophy

CLINICAL ISSUES

Presentation

- Most common signs/symptoms
  - Blurred vision
    - May progress to blindness
  - Drowsiness, confusion, seizure, coma
  - Nausea/vomiting, abdominal pain
  - Respiratory arrest → death

Natural History & Prognosis

- Latency period between ingestion and symptoms because of time required for enzymatic oxidation
- Untreated methanol poisoning
  - Visual deficits in ~ 1/3 of survivors
  - Death rate of ~ 1/3

Treatment

- Fomepizole or ethanol
  - Inhibit alcohol dehydrogenase
  - Prevents metabolism of methanol to formic acid

SELECTED REFERENCES

1. Ahsan H et al: Diffusion weighted image (DWI) findings in methanol intoxication. J Pak Med Assoc. 59(5):321-3, 2009
2. Brent J: Fomepizole for ethylene glycol and methanol poisoning. N Engl J Med. 360(21):2216-23, 2009
3. Bronstein AC et al: 2007 Annual Report of the American Association of Poison Control Centers' National Poison Data System (NPDS): 25th Annual Report. Clin Toxicol (Phila). 46(10):927-1057, 2008

CYANIDE POISONING

Key Facts

Terminology

- Anoxic encephalopathy caused by exposure to cyanide (CN)

Imaging

- Hemorrhagic striatal, cortical laminar necrosis
  - Basal ganglia (BG)
  - Cortex (especially sensorimotor)
- T2/FLAIR hyperintense foci in BG, cortex
- Restricted diffusion in BG, cortex
- May see T1 hyperintensity, enhancement in BG/ cortex

Top Differential Diagnoses

- Hypoxic-ischemic encephalopathy
- Toxic exposure, especially carbon monoxide (CO)
- Inherited/metabolic disease
- Infectious etiologies

Pathology

- Inhibits mitochondrial cytochrome c oxidase
  - Compromises aerobic oxidative metabolism, phosphorylation
  - Cellular hypoxia, lactic acidosis ensues

Clinical Issues

- Odor of bitter almond
- Tachypnea, tachycardia, hypertension
  - Cardiorespiratory collapse ensues
- Seizure ± coma ± death
- Often overlaps with signs/symptoms of CO exposure

Diagnostic Checklist

- May have overlapping features related to CN and CO poisoning, especially in smoke inhalation

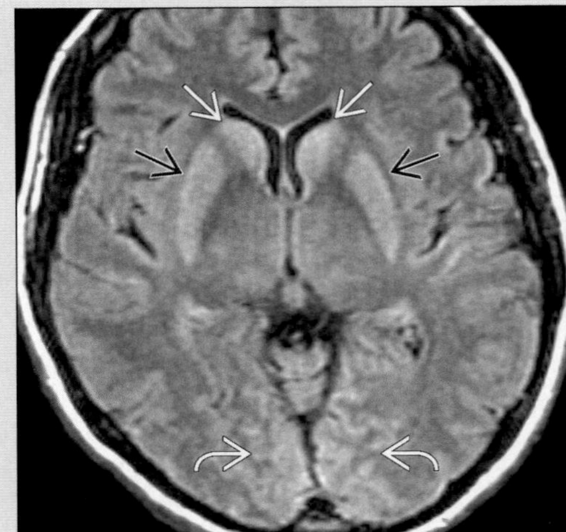

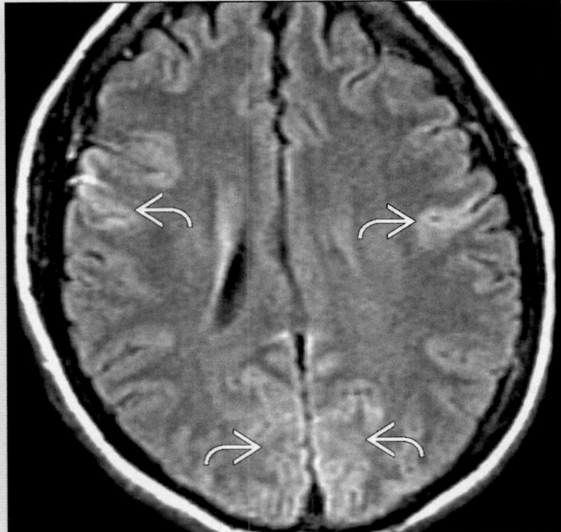

(Left) *Axial FLAIR MR demonstrates increased signal in the putamina ⇨, caudate nuclei ➡, and cortex ➦ in this patient who was found unconscious after smoke inhalation.* ***(Right)*** *Axial FLAIR MR in the same patient shows multiple areas of high signal in the cortex ➦.*

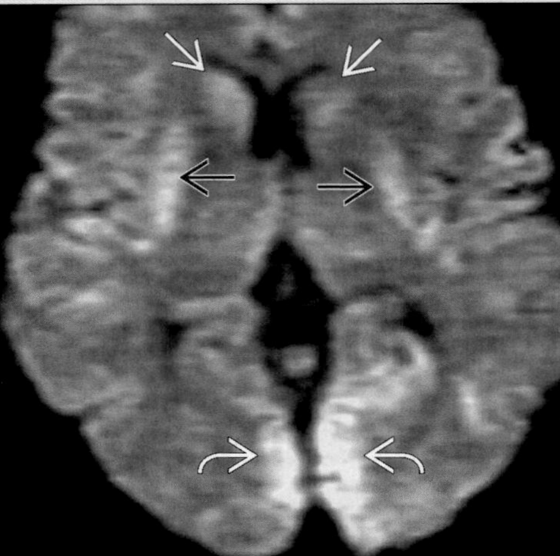

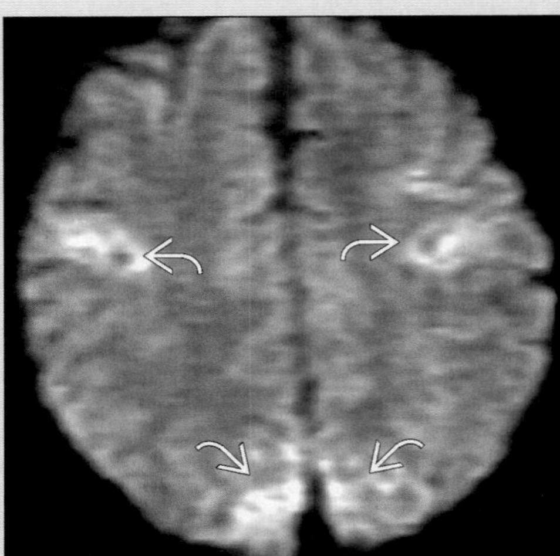

(Left) *Axial DWI demonstrates corresponding areas of high signal in the putamina ⇨, caudate nuclei ➡, and cortex ➦.* ***(Right)*** *Axial DWI at a higher level demonstrates multiple areas of increased signal in the cortex ➦, consistent with restricted diffusion and infarction. Although these imaging findings are nonspecific, the bilateral symmetric appearance should raise the possibility of a global hypoxic/ toxic/metabolic or infectious insult. Clinical correlation is required to confirm the diagnosis.*

CYANIDE POISONING

TERMINOLOGY

Abbreviations

- Cyanide (CN) poisoning

Definitions

- Anoxic encephalopathy caused by exposure to CN

IMAGING

General Features

- Best diagnostic clue
  - Hemorrhagic striatal, cortical laminar necrosis
- Location
  - Basal ganglia (BG)
    - Bilateral involvement typical
  - Cortex
    - Multifocal lesions, especially sensorimotor cortex
  - Cerebellum

CT Findings

- NECT
  - Hypodense foci in BG

MR Findings

- T1WI
  - Early: Hypointense BG foci
  - Late: Hyperintensity in BG, curvilinear cortical hyperintensity
- T2WI
  - Hyperintense foci in BG
  - Cortical hyperintensity
- FLAIR
  - Same as T2WI
- DWI
  - Restricted diffusion in BG, cortex
- T1WI C+
  - May see enhancement in BG, cortex

Imaging Recommendations

- Best imaging tool
  - MR with FLAIR, DWI

Nuclear Medicine Findings

- PET
  - 18F-fluorodopa: ↓ striatal uptake
  - 18F-FDG PET: ↓ metabolism in putamen, temporoparietooccipital, and cerebellar cortices

DIFFERENTIAL DIAGNOSIS

Hypoxic-Ischemic Encephalopathy

- Includes anoxia, hypoxia, near drowning, and cerebral hypoperfusion injury

Toxic Exposure

- Methanol, alcohol, carbon monoxide (CO), heroin

Inherited/Metabolic Disease

- Wilson disease, Leigh disease, Huntington disease

Infectious Etiologies

- Japanese encephalitis, Creutzfeldt-Jakob disease (CJD), etc.

PATHOLOGY

General Features

- Etiology
  - Inhibits mitochondrial cytochrome c oxidase
    - Compromised aerobic oxidative metabolism, phosphorylation
    - Cellular hypoxia, lactic acidosis ensue

Gross Pathologic & Surgical Features

- Hemorrhagic BG necrosis
- Cortical laminar necrosis

CLINICAL ISSUES

Presentation

- Most common signs/symptoms
  - Often overlaps with signs/symptoms of CO exposure
  - Odor of bitter almond
  - Tachypnea, tachycardia, hypertension
    - Cardiorespiratory collapse
  - Seizure, coma, death

Demographics

- Epidemiology
  - Residential fires (smoke inhalation)
  - Accidental exposure (work-related)
  - Nonaccidental exposure

Natural History & Prognosis

- Range of outcomes
  - From full recovery to death
  - Permanent neurological disability
    - Extrapyramidal syndromes and vegetative state

Treatment

- Decontamination, supportive
- Oxygen therapy: Normobaric and hyperbaric
- Cyanide antidotes

DIAGNOSTIC CHECKLIST

Consider

- May have overlapping features related to CN and CO poisoning, especially in smoke inhalation

SELECTED REFERENCES

1. Baud FJ: [Acute poisoning with carbon monoxide (CO) and cyanide (CN).] Ther Umsch. 66(5):387-97, 2009
2. Bronstein AC et al: 2007 Annual Report of the American Association of Poison Control Centers' National Poison Data System (NPDS): 25th Annual Report. Clin Toxicol (Phila). 46(10):927-1057, 2008
3. Baud FJ: Cyanide: critical issues in diagnosis and treatment. Hum Exp Toxicol. 26(3):191-201, 2007
4. Rachinger J et al: MR changes after acute cyanide intoxication. AJNR Am J Neuroradiol. 23(8):1398-401, 2002

OSMOTIC DEMYELINATION SYNDROME

Key Facts

Terminology
- Osmotic demyelination syndrome (ODMS)
  - Formerly called "central pontine myelinolysis" (CPM) &/or "extrapontine myelinolysis" (EPM)
- Acute demyelination from rapid shifts in serum osmolality
  - Classic setting: Rapid correction of hyponatremia
  - ODMS may occur in normonatremic patients!

Imaging
- Central pons T2 hyperintensity with sparing of periphery
- 50% in pons (CPM); 50% in extrapontine sites (EPM)
  - Central fibers involved; peripheral fibers spared
  - Basal ganglia (BG)
  - Cerebral white matter (WM)
- CPM + EPM = almost pathognomonic for ODMS
- Acute: Confluent hyperintensity in central pons with sparing of periphery and corticospinal tracts
- Subacute: Hyperintensity often normalizes
- Best imaging tool: MR > > CT

Top Differential Diagnoses
- Pontine ischemia/infarction
- Demyelinating disease
- Pontine neoplasm (astrocytoma, metastasis)
- Metabolic disease (Wilson, Leigh, diabetes, hypertensive encephalopathy)

Pathology
- Heterogeneous disorder with common etiology: Osmotic stress

Clinical Issues
- Alcoholic, hyponatremic patient with rapid correction of serum sodium

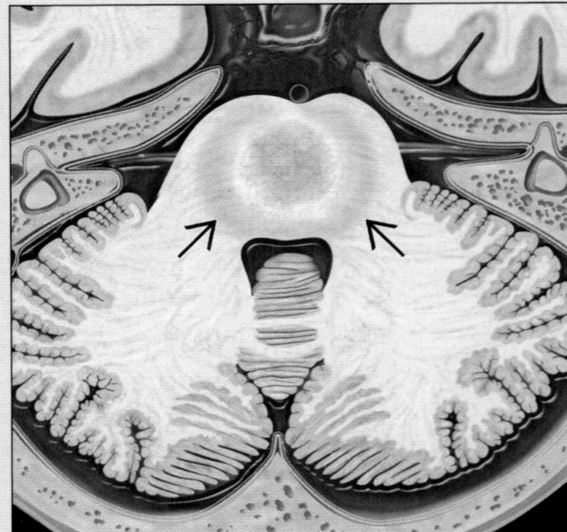

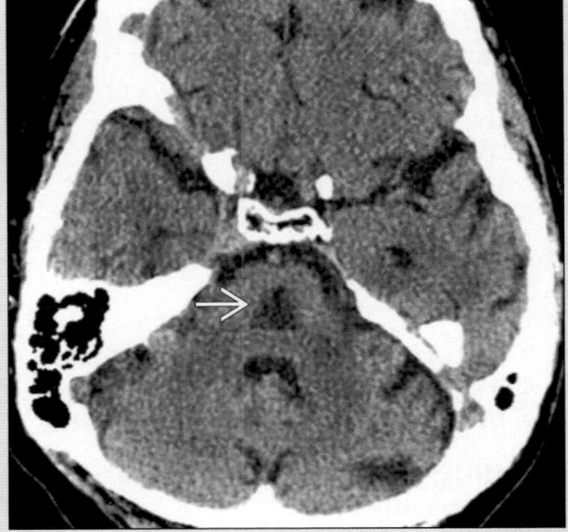

(Left) Axial graphic shows acute osmotic demyelination affecting the central pons ⇨. The pons is slightly swollen with mild mass effect on the 4th ventricle. (Right) Axial NECT demonstrates central pontine hypodensity ➡ in keeping with a remote osmotic insult in this chronic alcoholic patient.

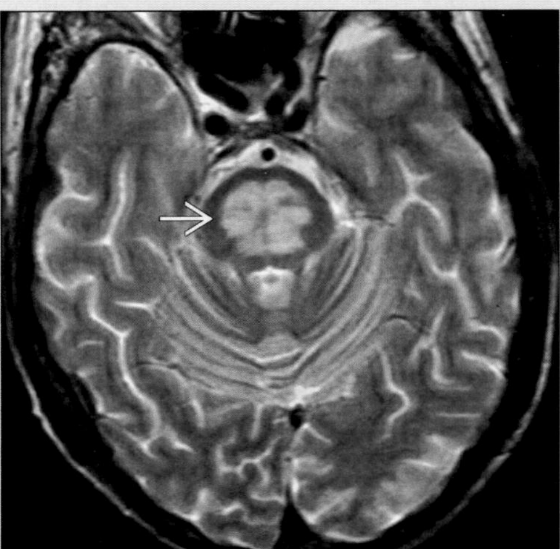

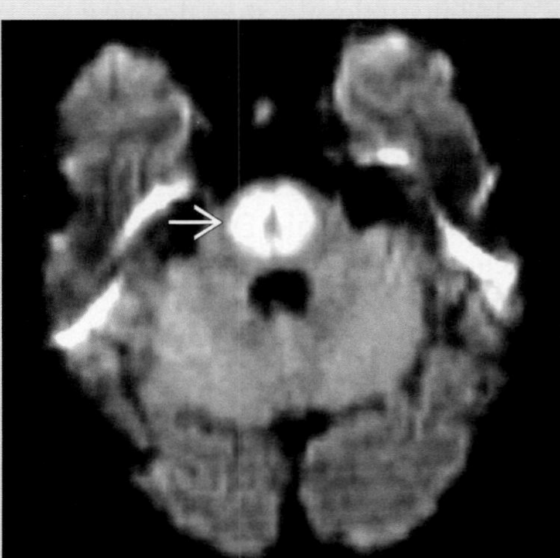

(Left) Axial T2WI MR shows a high signal area in the central pons ➡ that spares the peripheral white matter. (Right) Axial DWI MR in the same patient shows diffusion restriction, with a pattern that precisely matches the hyperintensity on the T2WI ➡.

OSMOTIC DEMYELINATION SYNDROME

TERMINOLOGY

Abbreviations

- Osmotic demyelination syndrome (ODMS)

Synonyms

- Formerly called "central pontine myelinolysis" (CPM) &/or "extrapontine myelinolysis" (EPM)

Definitions

- Acute demyelination caused by rapid shifts in serum osmolality
- Classic setting: Rapid correction of hyponatremia
  - ODMS may occur in normonatremic patients

IMAGING

General Features

- Best diagnostic clue
  - Central pons T2 hyperintensity with sparing of periphery
- Location
  - 50% in pons (CPM)
    - Central fibers involved; peripheral fibers spared
  - 50% in extrapontine sites (EPM)
    - Basal ganglia (BG)
    - Cerebral white matter (WM)
    - Uncommon: Peripheral cortex, hippocampi
    - Rare: Lateral geniculate bodies
  - CPM + EPM = almost pathognomonic for ODMS
- Morphology
  - Round or triangular (pons)
  - Regardless of site, demyelination often bilateral/ symmetric
  - Rare: Gyriform (cortical involvement)

CT Findings

- NECT
  - Low density in affected areas (pons, BG, etc.)
  - Look for other abnormalities (e.g., vermian atrophy)
  - No hemorrhage
- CECT
  - Classic: No enhancement
  - Early, acute/severe demyelination may enhance moderately strongly

MR Findings

- T1WI
  - Acute
    - Classic: Mildly/moderately hypointense
    - Less common: Can be isointense with surrounding normal brain
    - Findings may be transitory, resolve completely
    - Initial study may be normal
  - Subacute
    - May resolve completely
    - Less common: Hyperintensity at 1-4 months (coagulative necrosis)
- T2WI
  - Acute: Confluent hyperintensity in central pons with sparing of periphery and corticospinal tracts
    - Symmetric hyperintensity in BG, white matter (EPM)
  - Subacute: Hyperintensity often normalizes, may resolve completely
- PD/intermediate
  - Hyperintense
- FLAIR
  - Hyperintense
- T2* GRE
  - Hemorrhage, "blooming" rare
- DWI
  - Acute
    - DWI: Hyperintense (restricted); ↓ ADC
  - Delayed
    - DWI: Isointense
- T1WI C+
  - Common: Usually does not enhance
  - Less common: Moderate confluent enhancement
- MRS
  - Acute: ↓ NAA, ↑ choline

Nuclear Medicine Findings

- PET
  - Early metabolic stress = variable hypermetabolism
  - Late = hypometabolic areas in affected sites

Imaging Recommendations

- Best imaging tool
  - MR > > CT
- Protocol advice
  - FLAIR, DWI, T1WI C+
  - Repeat imaging as needed

DIFFERENTIAL DIAGNOSIS

Pontine Ischemia/Infarction

- Often asymmetric
- Usually involves both central, peripheral pontine fibers
- Caution: Perforating basilar artery infarct(s) may involve central pons; imaging can mimic CPM (including DWI)

Demyelinating Disease

- Look for typical lesions elsewhere
- "Horseshoe" (incomplete ring) enhancement pattern in acute multiple sclerosis common

Pontine Neoplasm (Astrocytoma, Metastasis)

- Primary neoplasm (e.g., pontine "glioma")
  - Typically pediatric/young adult patients
- Pons is rare site for solitary metastasis

Metabolic Disease

- e.g., Wilson, Leigh, diabetes, hypertensive encephalopathy
- Basal ganglia > pons in Wilson disease
- Basal ganglia, midbrain in Leigh disease
- Parietooccipital lobes = most common site in hypertensive encephalopathy
- Pontine hypertensive encephalopathy
  - Typically does not spare peripheral fibers
  - Other lesions common

OSMOTIC DEMYELINATION SYNDROME

PATHOLOGY

General Features

- Etiology
  - Heterogeneous disorder with common etiology: Osmotic stress
    - Osmotic stress: Any change in osmotic gradient
  - Most common: Iatrogenic correction of hyponatremia
  - Less common: Osmotic derangement with azotemia, hyperglycemia, hypokalemia, ketoacidosis
  - Precise mechanism of osmotic stress-related myelinolysis unknown
    - Osmotic insult, change in serum osmolality
    - Relative intracellular hypotonicity
    - Serum osmolality change causes endothelial damage
    - Organic osmolyte deficiency predisposes to endothelial breakdown
    - Endothelial cells shrink, causing blood-brain barrier breakdown
    - Accumulation of hypertonic sodium-rich fluid in extracellular fluid (ECF)
    - Hypertonic ECF, release of myelin toxins damages WM
    - Cell death ensues
- Associated abnormalities
  - Demyelination without associated inflammation

Gross Pathologic & Surgical Features

- Bilateral/symmetrical, soft, gray-tan discoloration

Microscopic Features

- Extensive demyelination, gliosis
- Macrophages contain engulfed myelin bits and fragments
- Axis cylinders, nerve cells preserved
- No inflammation

CLINICAL ISSUES

Presentation

- Most common signs/symptoms
  - Seizures, altered mental status
  - Often biphasic when hyponatremia present
    - ODMS symptoms emerge 2-4 days (occasionally weeks) after correction of hyponatremia
    - Changing level of consciousness, disorientation
    - Pseudobulbar palsy, dysarthria, dysphagia (CPM)
    - Movement disorder (EPM)
  - Symptoms may resolve with increase in serum osmolality
- Clinical profile
  - Alcoholic, hyponatremic patient with rapid correction of serum sodium
  - "Comorbid" conditions that may exacerbate ODMS
    - Hepatic, renal, adrenal, pituitary, paraneoplastic disease
    - Nutritional (alcohol, malnutrition, vomiting)
    - Burn, transplantation, other surgery

Demographics

- Age
  - Occurs at all ages
    - Most common: Middle-aged patients
    - Uncommon: Pediatric patients (diabetes, anorexia)
- Gender
  - M > F
- Epidemiology
  - Autopsy prevalence in alcoholic individuals varies from < 1% to 10%

Natural History & Prognosis

- Spectrum of outcomes
  - Complete recovery may occur
  - Minimal residual deficits
    - Memory, cognitive impairment
    - Ataxia, spasticity, diplopia
  - May progress to
    - Spastic quadriparesis
    - "Locked in," may progress to coma, death
- "Comorbid" conditions common, poorer prognosis

Treatment

- No consensus; no "optimal" correction rate for hyponatremia
- Self-correction (fluid restriction, discontinue diuretics) if possible
- Plasmapheresis, steroids, glucose infusions being studied

DIAGNOSTIC CHECKLIST

Consider

- Diagnosis of ODMS in alcoholic patient with basal ganglia, white matter disease (EPM)

Image Interpretation Pearls

- Classic CPM spares peripheral pontine fibers
- EPM can occur without CPM
- Repeat MR may be necessary as initial study may be normal

SELECTED REFERENCES

1. de Morais BS et al: Central pontine myelinolysis after liver transplantation: is sodium the only villain? Case report. Rev Bras Anestesiol. 59(3):344-9, 2009
2. Howard SA et al: Best cases from the AFIP: osmotic demyelination syndrome. Radiographics. 29(3):933-8, 2009
3. Mount DB: The brain in hyponatremia: both culprit and victim. Semin Nephrol. 29(3):196-215, 2009
4. Roh JH et al: Cortical laminar necrosis caused by rapidly corrected hyponatremia. J Neuroimaging. 19(2):185-7, 2009
5. Ruiz S et al: [Severe hyponatraemia and central pontine myelinolysis: be careful with other factors!.] Ann Fr Anesth Reanim. 28(1):96-9, 2009
6. Fong CS: [Neurological complications in uremia.] Acta Neurol Taiwan. 17(2):117-26, 2008
7. Hoshino Y et al: [Pontine hemorrhage in a patient with type 1 renal tubular acidosis associated with osmotic demyelination syndrome.] Brain Nerve. 60(9):1061-5, 2008
8. Laczi F: [Etiology, diagnostics and therapy of hyponatremias.] Orv Hetil. 149(29):1347-54, 2008
9. Guo Y et al: Central pontine myelinolysis after liver transplantation: MR diffusion, spectroscopy and perfusion findings. Magn Reson Imaging. 24(10):1395-8, 2006

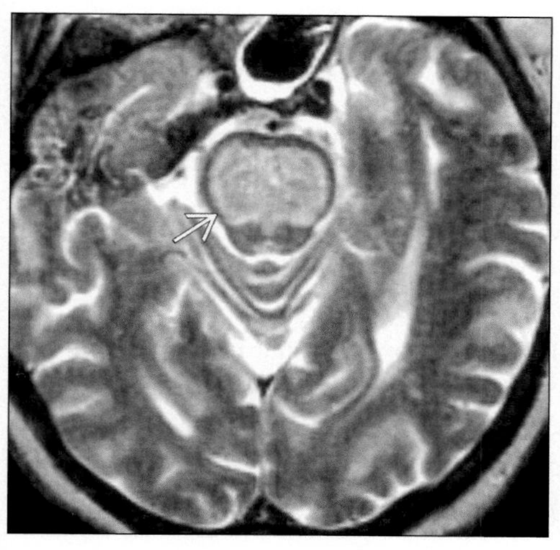

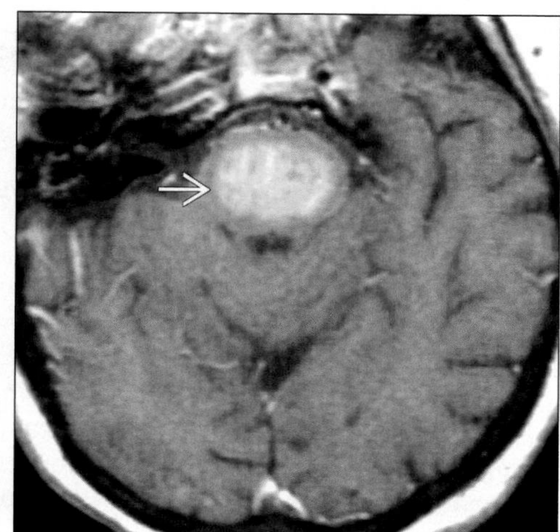

(Left) *Axial T2WI MR demonstrates striking hyperintensity within the central pons ➡, which is a classic finding in osmotic demyelination syndrome.* ***(Right)*** *T1WI C+ MR in the same patient shows enhancement of the acutely demyelinating area ➡.*

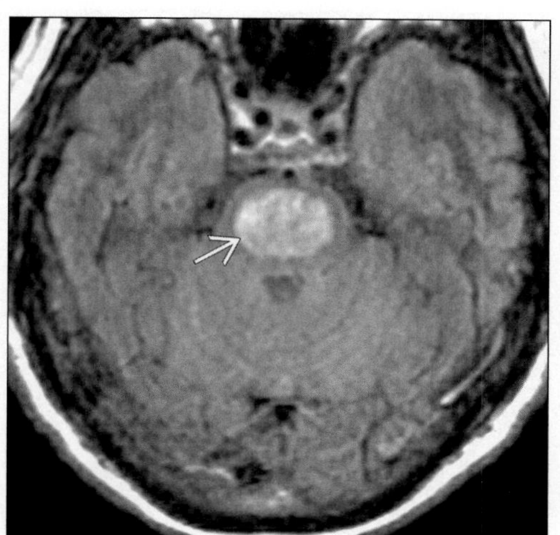

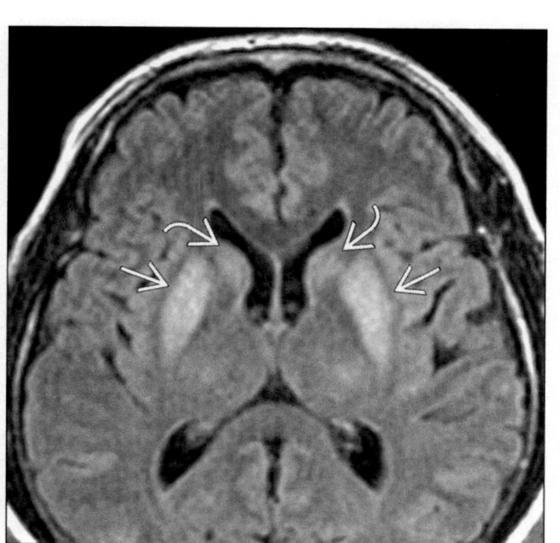

(Left) *Axial FLAIR MR shows abnormal signal intensity in the pons ➡.* ***(Right)*** *Axial FLAIR MR in the same patient demonstrates abnormal signal intensity in the putamina ➡ and in the caudate nuclei ↪. Osmotic demyelination syndrome may have manifestations of both central pontine and extrapontine myelinolysis.*

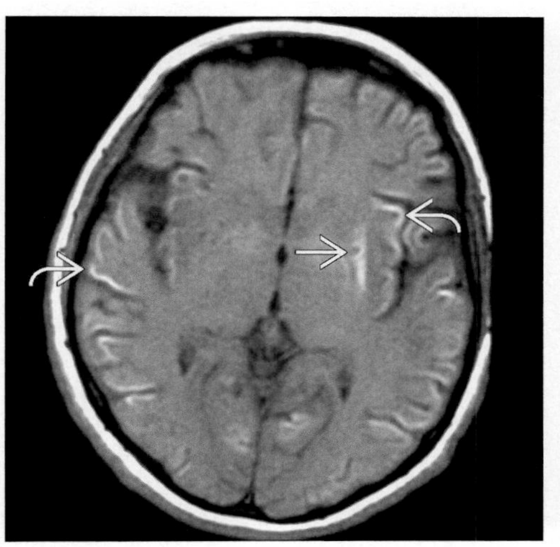

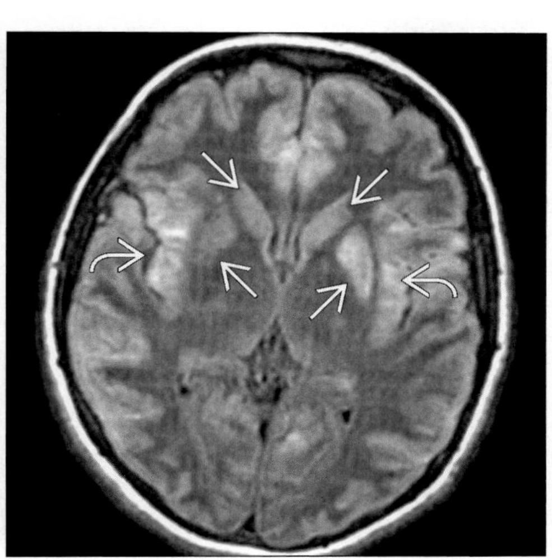

(Left) *Axial T1WI MR shows diffuse high signal in the cortex ↪ and left putamen ➡.* ***(Right)*** *Axial FLAIR MR in the same patient shows diffuse high signal in the cortex ↪ and striatum ➡. Frank cortical laminar necrosis is an atypical manifestation of osmotic demyelination syndrome. Some cases, such as this one, spare the pons (not shown) completely and affect only the basal ganglia &/or cortex. The hemispheric white matter is not involved in this case.*

RADIATION AND CHEMOTHERAPY

Key Facts

Terminology

- Radiation-induced injury may be divided into acute, early delayed injury, late delayed injury

Imaging

- **Radiation injury**: Mild vasogenic edema to necrosis
- **Radiation necrosis**: Irregular enhancing lesion(s)
  - MRS: Markedly ↓ metabolites (NAA, Cho, Cr), ± lactate/lipid peaks
  - Perfusion MR: ↓ rCBV compared with tumor
- **Leukoencephalopathy**: T2 WM hyperintensity, spares subcortical U-fibers
- **Mineralizing microangiopathy**: Basal ganglia (BG), subcortical WM Ca++, atrophy
- **Necrotizing leukoencephalopathy**: WM necrosis
- **PRES**: Posterior circulation subcortical WM edema
- MRS, MR perfusion, PET, or SPECT may help delineate recurrent tumor from radiation necrosis

Top Differential Diagnoses

- Neoplasm
- Abscess
- Multiple sclerosis
- Vascular dementia
- Progressive multifocal leukoencephalopathy

Pathology

- 2nd neoplasms: Meningiomas (70%), gliomas (20%), sarcomas (10%)
  - More aggressive tumors, highly refractory
  - Incidence: 3-12%
- Radiation-induced cryptic vascular malformations: Capillary telangiectasias ± cavernomas (CM)

Clinical Issues

- Overall incidence of radionecrosis: 5-24%
- Worse prognosis: Younger patient at treatment

__(Left)__ Axial NECT shows extensive calcification in the subcortical white matter in a 20-year-old patient. __(Right)__ Axial T1WI MR in the same patient shows extensive T1 shortening related to calcification in the subcortical white matter, basal ganglia, and thalami. There is mild diffuse atrophy, typical of mineralizing microangiopathy. Mineralizing microangiopathy usually results after a combination of radiation therapy and chemotherapy, 2 or more years after treatment.

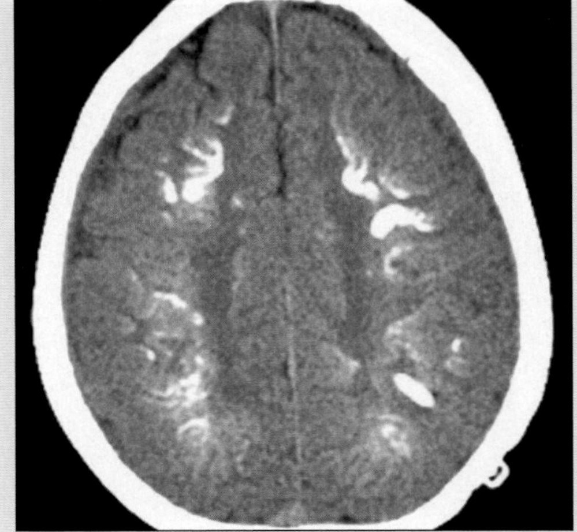

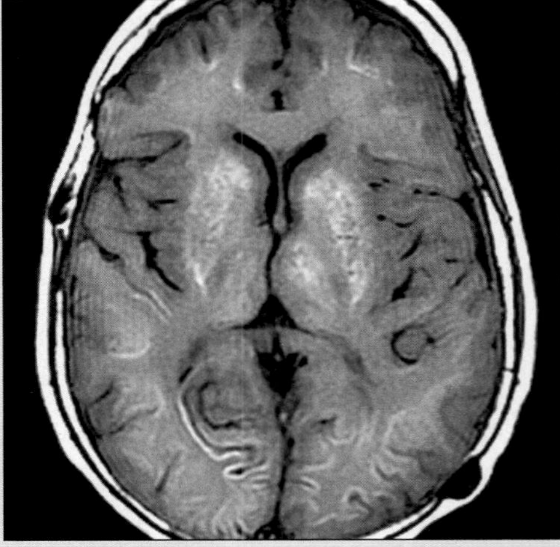

__(Left)__ Coronal T2WI MR in the same patient shows the typical features of a cavernoma as a mixed signal intensity mass with a dark hemosiderin rim ➔. Subtle T2 hypointensity is also noted ➔, related to calcification. Radiation-induced cryptic vascular malformations are most commonly capillary telangiectasias with or without a cavernoma. __(Right)__ Axial T1WI C+ MR shows an enhancing "mass" related to radiation necrosis in this patient who was treated with gamma knife for a vascular lesion.

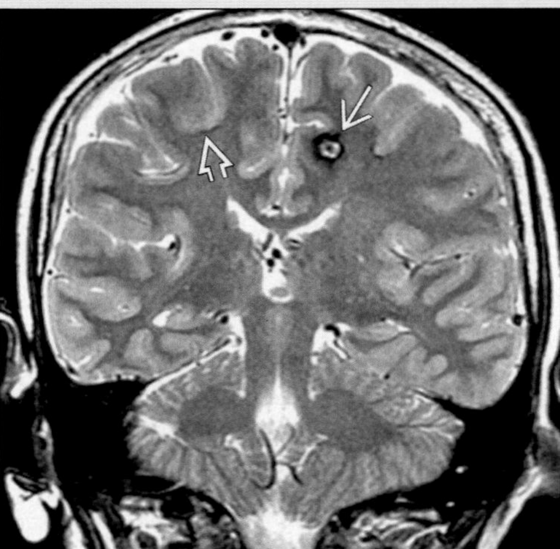

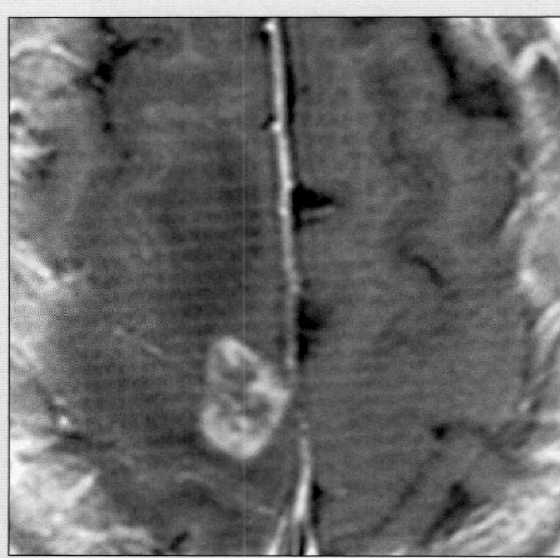

TERMINOLOGY

Synonyms

- Radiation-induced injury, radiation (XRT) changes, chemotherapy effects, treatment-related changes

Definitions

- Radiation-induced injury may be divided into acute, early delayed injury, and late delayed injury
- Includes radiation injury (edema, arteritis), radiation necrosis, leukoencephalopathy, mineralizing microangiopathy, necrotizing leukoencephalopathy, posterior reversible encephalopathy syndrome (PRES), radiation-induced tumors

IMAGING

General Features

- Best diagnostic clue
  - Radiation injury: Mild vasogenic edema to necrosis
  - Radiation necrosis: Irregular enhancing lesion(s)
  - Leukoencephalopathy: T2 white matter (WM) hyperintensity, spares subcortical U-fibers
  - Mineralizing microangiopathy: Basal ganglia (BG), subcortical WM Ca++, atrophy
  - Necrotizing leukoencephalopathy (NLE): WM necrosis ± Ca++
  - PRES: Posterior circulation subcortical WM edema
- Location
  - Radiation injury occurs in radiation port
  - Periventricular WM especially susceptible
  - Subcortical U-fibers and corpus callosum spared

CT Findings

- NECT
  - Acute XRT: Confluent WM low-density edema
  - Delayed XRT: Focal/multiple WM low density
  - **Leukoencephalopathy**: Symmetric WM hypodensity
  - **Mineralizing microangiopathy**: BG, subcortical WM Ca++, atrophy
  - **NLE**: Extensive areas of WM necrosis, Ca++
  - **PRES**: Subcortical WM edema, posterior circulation

MR Findings

- T1WI
  - Acute XRT: Periventricular WM hypointense edema
  - Delayed XRT: Focal or multiple WM hypointensities
  - **Leukoencephalopathy**: Diffuse, symmetric WM hypointensity; spares subcortical U-fibers
  - **Mineralizing microangiopathy**: Putamen hyperintensity, atrophy
  - **NLE**: Extensive areas of WM necrosis
  - **PRES**: Symmetric posterior WM hypointensity
  - **Cryptic vascular malformations**: Blood products
- T2WI
  - Acute XRT: Periventricular WM hyperintense edema
  - Early delayed XRT: Focal or multiple hyperintense WM lesions with edema, demyelination
    - Spares subcortical U-fibers and corpus callosum
  - Late delayed XRT: Diffuse WM injury or necrosis
    - Hyperintense WM lesion(s), ± hypointense rim
    - Mass effect and edema
  - **Leukoencephalopathy**: Diffuse, symmetric involvement of central and periventricular WM, relative sparing of subcortical U-fibers
  - **Mineralizing microangiopathy**: ↓ signal
  - **NLE**: Extensive WM necrosis
  - **PRES**: Confluent, symmetric hyperintensity in subcortical WM, ± cortex, posterior circulation
    - Occipital, parietal, posterior temporal lobes, cerebellum typical
    - May involve frontal lobes, BG, brainstem
  - **Cryptic vascular malformations**: Blood products
- T2* GRE
  - Radiation-induced cryptic vascular malformations: "Blooming" related to blood products
- T1WI C+
  - Acute XRT: No enhancement
  - Early delayed XRT: ± patchy enhancement
  - Late delayed XRT: Enhancement often resembles residual/recurrent tumor about resection cavity
    - May see nodular, linear, curvilinear, "soap bubble," or "Swiss cheese" enhancement
    - May have multiple lesions remote from tumor site
  - **NLE**: Marked enhancement, possibly ring
  - **PRES**: ± enhancement
- MRS: Markedly ↓ metabolites (NAA, Cho, Cr), ± lactate/lipid peaks in radiation necrosis
- Perfusion MR: Decreased rCBV in radiation necrosis

Angiographic Findings

- Radiation-induced vasculopathy: Progressive narrowing of supraclinoid ICA and proximal anterior circulation vessels; may develop moyamoya pattern

Nuclear Medicine Findings

- FDG PET: Radiation necrosis is hypometabolic
- Thallium-201 SPECT: Radiation necrosis is hypometabolic, decreased uptake

Imaging Recommendations

- Protocol advice
  - Enhanced MR ± MRS, MR perfusion, PET if question of XRT vs. recurrent neoplasm

DIFFERENTIAL DIAGNOSIS

Recurrent Glioblastoma Multiforme (GBM)

- Enhancing mass with central necrosis, mass effect
- T2/FLAIR WM signal, often follows WM tracts
- MRS shows ↑ Cho, ↓ NAA, ± lactate

Metastasis

- Typically multiple lesions at gray and white matter junctions, significant edema
- MRS shows ↑ Cho, ↓ NAA, ± lactate

Abscess

- Ring-enhancing mass, thinner margin along ventricle
- T2 hypointense rim, diffusion restriction characteristic
- MRS shows metabolites such as succinate, amino acids

Multiple Sclerosis

- Often incomplete, horseshoe-shaped enhancement, open toward cortex
- Other lesions in typical locations, young patients

RADIATION AND CHEMOTHERAPY

- Often lack significant mass effect

Vascular Dementia
- Large and small infarcts, WM disease
- Typically older patients, clinical diagnosis

Progressive Multifocal Leukoencephalopathy
- WM T2 hyperintensity, involves subcortical U-fibers
- May cross corpus callosum; usually no enhancement
- Immunosuppressed patients

Vasculitis
- Multiple small WM areas of T2 hyperintensity
- Gray matter involvement; enhancement may be seen

Foreign Body Reaction
- Granulomatous reaction (i.e., to gelatin sponge)
- Can mimic tumor recurrence, radiation necrosis

PATHOLOGY

General Features
- Etiology
  - **Radiation-induced vascular injury**
    - Permeability alterations, endothelial and basement membrane damage, accelerated atherosclerosis, telangiectasia formation
  - **Radiation-induced neurotoxicity**
    - Glial and WM damage (sensitivity of oligodendrocytes > > neurons)
  - **Radiation-induced tumor** (i.e., sarcoma)
    - Increased risk in patients with XRT ≤ 5 years old, those with genetic predisposition (NF1, retinoblastoma), bone marrow transplant survivors
  - **Radiation-induced cryptic vascular malformations**: Predominantly capillary telangiectasias ± cavernomas
  - **Mineralizing microangiopathy**: Common with chemotherapy and XRT, appears ≥ 2 years after XRT
  - **Necrotizing leukoencephalopathy**: Combined XRT and chemotherapy, progressive disease
  - **PRES**: Related to elevated blood pressure that exceeds autoregulatory capacity of brain vasculature
  - Many chemotherapy agents cause CNS effects: Methotrexate, cytarabine, carmustine, cyclophosphamide, cisplatin
  - XRT variables: Total dose, field size, fraction size, number/frequency of doses, adjuvant therapy, survival duration, patient age
    - Most XRT injury is delayed (months/years)

Staging, Grading, & Classification
- Neurotoxic reaction to radiation therapy divided into acute, early, and late delayed injury
  - **Acute**: Mild and reversible, vasogenic edema
  - **Early delayed** injury: Edema and demyelination
  - **Late delayed** injury: More severe, irreversible
- 2nd neoplasms: Meningiomas (70%), gliomas (20%), sarcomas (10%)

Gross Pathologic & Surgical Features
- XRT: Spectrum from edema to cavitating WM necrosis
- Demyelination: Sharp interface with normal brain
- Radiation necrosis: Coagulation necrosis that favors WM, may extend to deep cortex

Microscopic Features
- Acute XRT injury: WM edema from capillary damage
- Early delayed injury: Vasogenic edema, demyelination
  - Demyelination: Macrophage infiltrates, loss of myelin, perivascular lymphocytic infiltrates, gliosis
- Late delayed injury: WM necrosis, demyelination, astrocytosis, vasculopathy
  - Radiation necrosis: Confluent coagulative necrosis, Ca++, telangiectasias, hyaline thickening and fibrinoid necrosis of vessels, thrombosis
- Mineralizing microangiopathy: Hyalinization and fibrinoid necrosis of small arteries and arterioles with endothelial proliferation, Ca++ deposition

CLINICAL ISSUES

Presentation
- Most common signs/symptoms
  - Highly variable
- Radiation injury to brain is divided into 3 groups
  - Acute injury: 1-6 weeks after or during treatment
  - Early delayed injury: 3 weeks to several months
  - Late delayed injury: Months to years after treatment

Demographics
- Epidemiology
  - Overall incidence of radionecrosis: 5-24%
  - 2nd neoplasms: 3-12%

Natural History & Prognosis
- Younger patient at time of treatment: Worse prognosis
- Radiation necrosis is dynamic pathophysiological process; often progressive, irreversible

Treatment
- Biopsy if imaging does not resolve tumor vs. radionecrosis
- Surgery if mass effect, edema
- Acute radiation injury may respond to steroids

DIAGNOSTIC CHECKLIST

Consider
- Distinguishing residual/recurrent neoplasm from XRT necrosis difficult using morphology alone

Image Interpretation Pearls
- MRS, MR perfusion, PET, or SPECT may help delineate recurrent tumor from radiation necrosis

SELECTED REFERENCES

1. Chan KC et al: MRI of late microstructural and metabolic alterations in radiation-induced brain injuries. J Magn Reson Imaging. 29(5):1013-20, 2009
2. Burn S et al: Incidence of cavernoma development in children after radiotherapy for brain tumors. J Neurosurg. 106(5 Suppl):379-83, 2007
3. Kumar AJ et al: Malignant gliomas: MR imaging spectrum of radiation therapy- and chemotherapy-induced necrosis of the brain after treatment. Radiology. 217(2):377-84, 2000

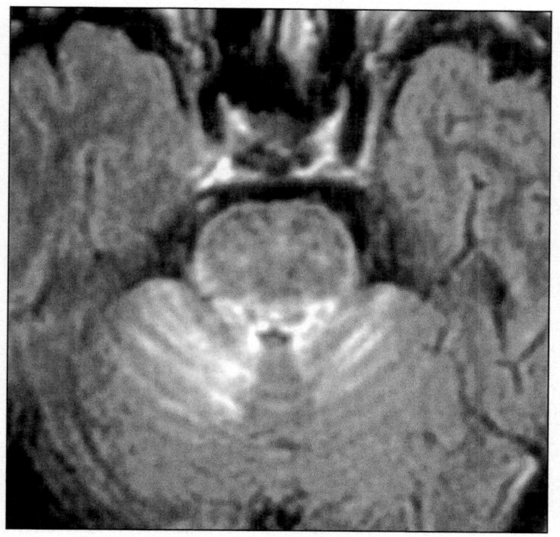

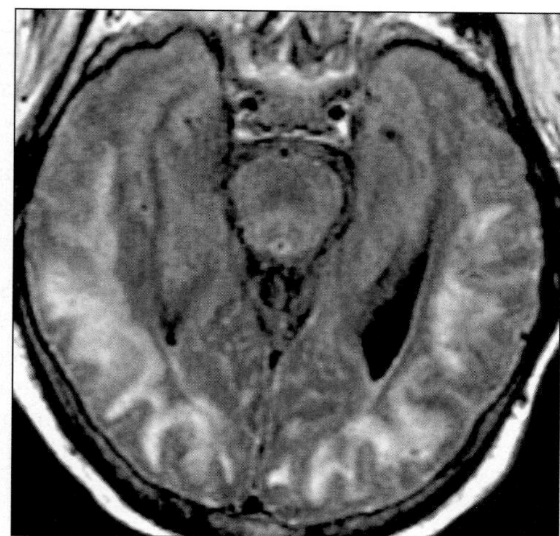

(Left) *Axial FLAIR MR shows bilateral cerebellar hyperintensity related to demyelination in a patient treated with chemotherapy. Treatment-related demyelination is often associated with radiation therapy and occurs 3 weeks to several months after treatment.* ***(Right)*** *Axial FLAIR MR shows confluent, symmetric hyperintense signal in the subcortical white matter of the posterior temporal and occipital lobes, related to posterior reversible encephalopathy syndrome (PRES).*

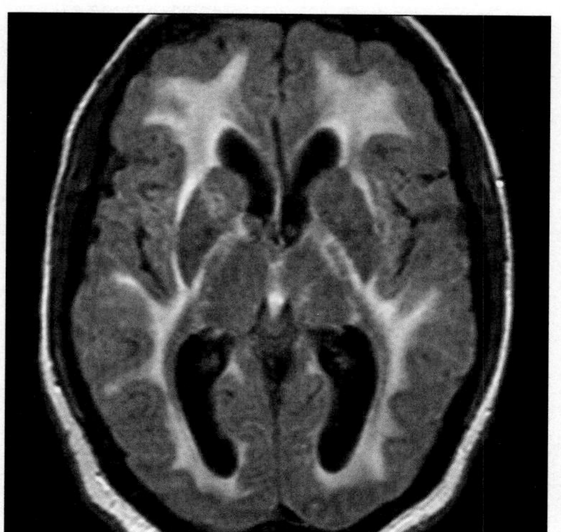

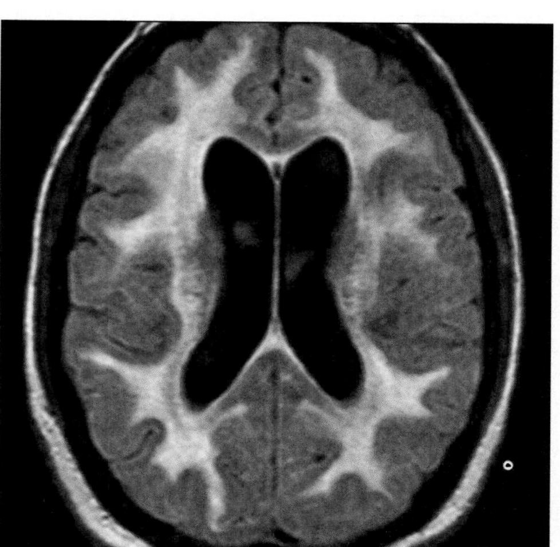

(Left) *Axial FLAIR MR in a patient treated with whole brain radiotherapy for lung cancer metastasis demonstrates extensive white matter hyperintensity with sparing of the subcortical U-fibers.* ***(Right)*** *Axial FLAIR MR in the same patient shows confluent white matter hyperintensity related to radiation-induced leukoencephalopathy, thought to be related to vascular injury with accelerated atherosclerosis. The patient's brain MR 6 months prior showed normal white matter.*

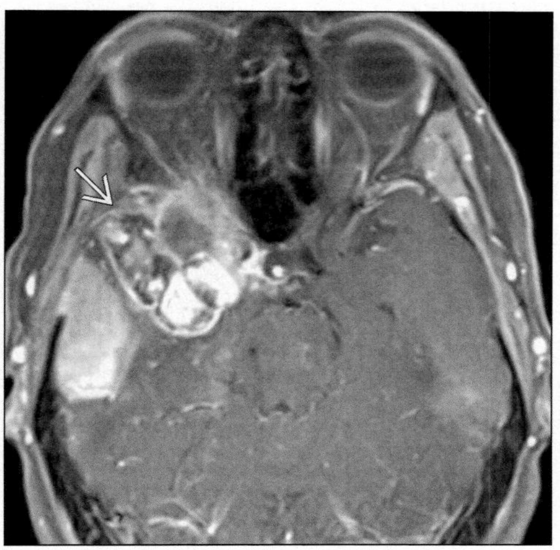

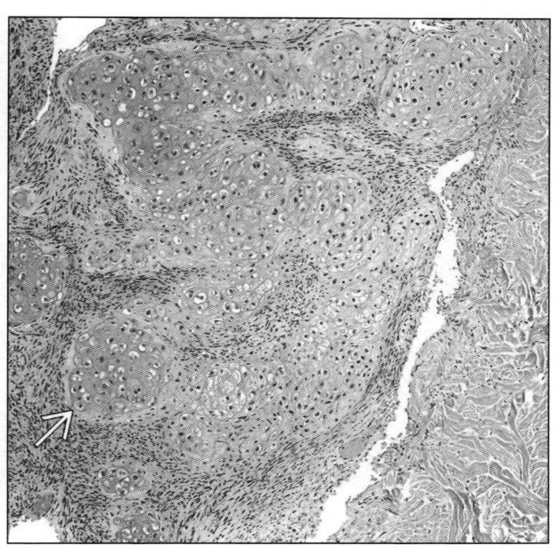

(Left) *Axial T1WI C+ FS MR shows a heterogeneous mass ➔ in the anterior middle cranial fossa in a patient with prior surgery and radiation therapy for a WHO grade I meningioma.* ***(Right)*** *High-power micropathology from the same patient shows chondrosarcoma elements ➔ at repeat resection. A 2nd neoplasm occurs in 3-12% of patients treated with radiation therapy. These are most commonly meningiomas (70%); gliomas (20%) and sarcomas (10%) are rare.*

MESIAL TEMPORAL SCLEROSIS

Key Facts

Terminology
- Seizure-associated neuronal loss and gliosis in hippocampus and adjacent structures

Imaging
- Primary determinants: Abnormal T2 hyperintensity, hippocampal volume loss/atrophy, obscuration of internal architecture
- Secondary signs: Ipsilateral fornix and mamillary body atrophy, enlarged ipsilateral temporal horn, and choroidal fissure

Top Differential Diagnoses
- Status epilepticus
- Low-grade astrocytoma
- Choroidal fissure cyst
- Hippocampal sulcus remnant

Pathology
- Prolonged febrile seizures may produce acute hippocampal injury → subsequent atrophy
- Coexistent 2nd developmental lesion in 15% of MTS patients

Clinical Issues
- Partial complex seizures, automatisms
- Often history of childhood febrile or medically intractable seizures

Diagnostic Checklist
- Most common cause of partial complex epilepsy in adult age group
- Low-grade neoplasms and cortical dysplasia more common causes of partial complex epilepsy than MTS in pediatric age group

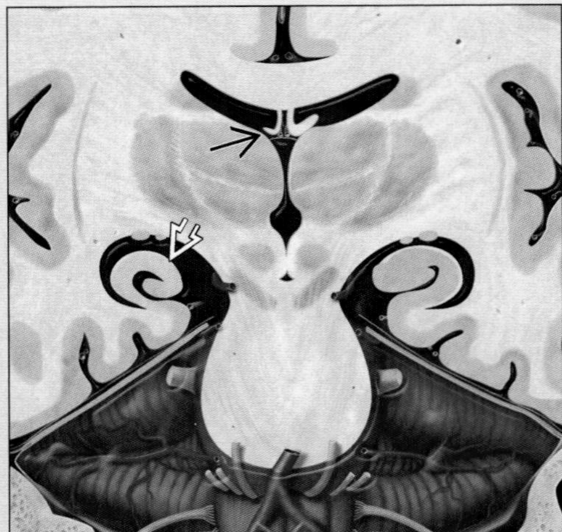

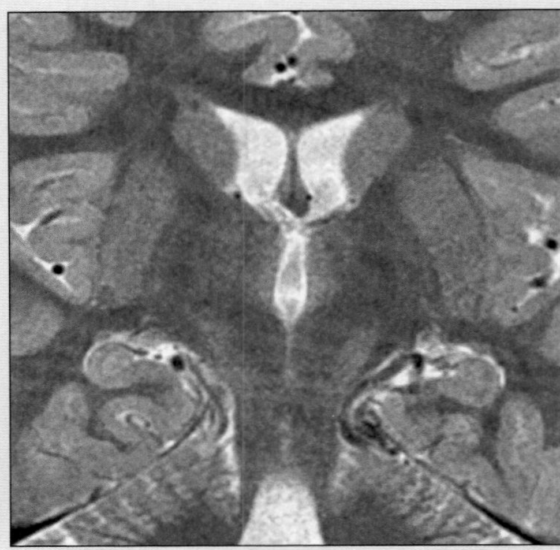

(Left) *Coronal graphic depicts a characteristic appearance of mesial temporal sclerosis (MTS). The right hippocampus ⇨ is small (atrophic) with loss of normal internal architecture reflecting neuronal loss and gliosis. Note concordant atrophy of the ipsilateral fornix → and widening of the ipsilateral temporal horn and choroidal fissure.* ***(Right)*** *Coronal STIR MR at 3.0 tesla in a normal nonepileptic patient imaged for headaches demonstrates normal bilateral hippocampal anatomy, size, and signal intensity.*

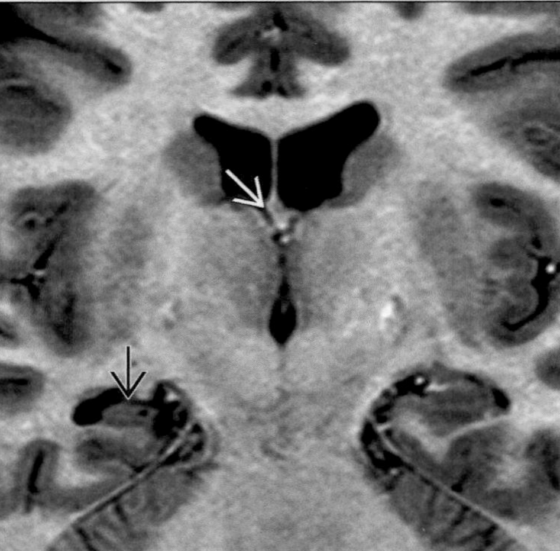

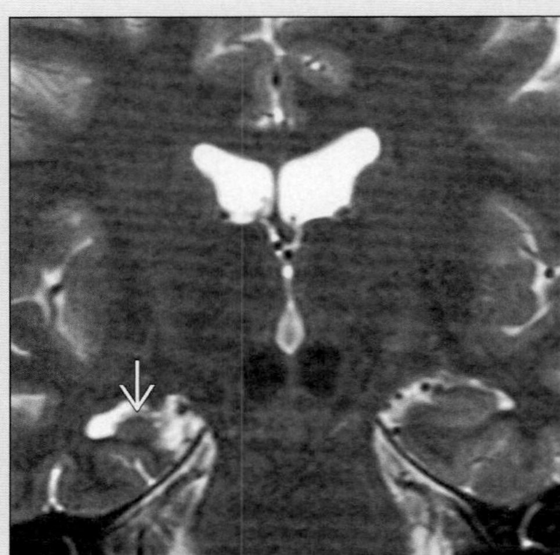

(Left) *Coronal T1-weighted true inversion recovery image at 3.0 tesla shows asymmetric right hippocampal volume loss → and obscuration of normal internal gray-white differentiation. The ipsilateral fornix → is smaller than the normal left fornix.* ***(Right)*** *Coronal T2WI MR at 3.0 tesla in the same patient with right hippocampal sclerosis → shows hippocampal volume loss and obscuration of normal internal architecture but normal T2 signal intensity. FLAIR better shows increase in signal intensity.*

MESIAL TEMPORAL SCLEROSIS

TERMINOLOGY

Abbreviations

- Mesial temporal sclerosis (MTS), febrile seizure (FS), temporal lobe epilepsy (TLE)

Synonyms

- Ammons horn sclerosis, hippocampal sclerosis (HS)

Definitions

- Seizure-associated neuronal loss and gliosis in hippocampus and adjacent structures

IMAGING

General Features

- Best diagnostic clue
  - Primary determinants: Abnormal T2 hyperintensity, hippocampal volume loss/atrophy, obscuration of internal architecture
  - Secondary signs: Ipsilateral fornix and mamillary body atrophy, enlarged ipsilateral temporal horn, and choroidal fissure
  - Additional findings: Loss of ipsilateral hippocampal head (pes) digitations, parahippocampal gyrus white matter atrophy, ↑ T2 signal in anterior temporal white matter
- Location
  - Mesial temporal lobe(s), 20% bilateral
  - Hippocampus > amygdala > fornix > mamillary bodies
- Size
  - Slight to marked ↓ in hippocampal volume
- Morphology
  - Abnormal shape, size of affected hippocampus

CT Findings

- NECT
  - Usually normal; CT insensitive to MTS

MR Findings

- T1WI
  - ↓ hippocampal size
  - Loss of normal hippocampal gray-white differentiation
  - ± ipsilateral fornix, mamillary body atrophy
  - Quantitative hippocampal volumetry: ↑ sensitivity of MTS detection (particularly bilateral MTS)
- T2WI
  - Hippocampal atrophy
  - Obscuration of normal internal architecture
  - ↑ hippocampal signal intensity
  - ± ipsilateral fornix, mamillary body atrophy, dilatation of ipsilateral temporal horn
  - ± abnormal hyperintensity, volume loss in ipsilateral anterior temporal lobe
- FLAIR
  - Hyperintense signal in abnormal hippocampus
- DWI
  - ↑ hyperintensity on DWI (T2 "shine through")
  - ↑ diffusivity on ADC
- T1WI C+
  - No enhancement
- MRS
  - ↓ NAA in hippocampus, temporal lobe
  - NAA/Cho ≤ 0.8 and NAA/Cr ≤ 1.0 suggests MTS
  - ± lactate/lipid peaks after 24 hours of continual seizure

Nuclear Medicine Findings

- FDG PET: Hypometabolism in abnormal mesial temporal lobe
- SPECT: Hypoperfusion (interictal) or hyperperfusion (ictal) in epileptogenic zone
  - Sensitivity of ictal > interictal

Imaging Recommendations

- Best imaging tool
  - High-resolution MR imaging
  - MRS, quantitative volumetry may help lateralize MTS in difficult cases
- Protocol advice
  - Thin section coronal T2WI and FLAIR (3 mm), angled perpendicular to long axis of hippocampus
  - Thin section coronal 3D SPGR (1-2 mm), angled perpendicular to long axis of hippocampus

DIFFERENTIAL DIAGNOSIS

Status Epilepticus

- Clinical history of multiple seizures or status epilepticus
- Temporary T2 hyperintensity ± gyriform enhancement in affected cortex, hippocampus

Low-Grade Astrocytoma

- Hyperintense temporal lobe white matter mass (usually nonenhancing)
- ± seizures, young adults typical

Choroidal Fissure Cyst

- Asymptomatic CSF signal cyst in choroidal fissure distorts normal hippocampus
  - Oval, parallels temporal lobe long axis on sagittal imaging
- No abnormal T2 hyperintensity in mesial temporal lobe

Hippocampal Sulcus Remnant

- Failure of normal hippocampal sulcus involution → asymptomatic cyst between dentate gyrus, cornu ammonis
- Common normal variant (10-15%)

Cavernous Malformation

- Heterogeneous hyperintense "popcorn" lesion with dark complete hemosiderin rim
- ± seizures

Dysembryoplastic Neuroepithelial Tumor (DNET)

- Demarcated "bubbly," variably enhancing cortical mass ± regional cortical dysplasia
- Partial complex seizures

Cortical Dysplasia

- Most common dual pathology associated with MTS
- T2 hyperintensity in anterior temporal white matter

MESIAL TEMPORAL SCLEROSIS

PATHOLOGY

General Features

- Etiology
  - Controversial whether acquired or developmental
    - Acquired: Follows prolonged febrile seizures, multiple early childhood seizures, status epilepticus, complicated delivery, ischemia
    - Developmental: 2nd developmental lesion identified in 15% ("double hit" theory for TLE)
    - Most likely MTS represents common outcome of both acquired and developmental processes
  - Febrile seizures (FS) most common childhood seizure disorder (2-5%)
    - Prolonged FS may produce acute hippocampal injury → subsequent atrophy
- Genetics
  - Familial cases of mesial TLE reported
  - Recent studies suggest relationship between FS and later epilepsy development may be genetic
  - Syndrome-specific genes for FS (channelopathies) account for small proportion of FS cases
- Associated abnormalities
  - Coexistent 2nd developmental lesion (15%)

Gross Pathologic & Surgical Features

- Mesial temporal lobe atrophy: Hippocampal body (88%), tail (61%), head (51%), amygdala (12%)
- Absence of hemorrhage or necrosis

Microscopic Features

- Chronic astrogliosis with fine fibrillary background of bland astrocytic nuclei and decreased residual neurons
- Ammons horn, cornu ammonis (CA), contains 4 zones of granular cells: CA1, CA2, CA3, CA4
  - CA1, CA4 pyramidal cell layers most susceptible to ischemia
  - All hippocampal regions may show varying neuronal cell loss

CLINICAL ISSUES

Presentation

- Most common signs/symptoms
  - Partial complex seizures, automatisms
    - Simple at younger ages and increasingly complex and discrete with age
- Other signs/symptoms
  - May progress to generalized tonic-clonic seizures
- Clinical profile
  - Often history of childhood febrile or medically intractable seizures
  - Surface electro- (EEG) or magneto- (MEG) encephalogram helpful for localization (60-90%)
  - Intracranial EEG (subdural or depth electrodes) may be indicated if noninvasive studies discordant

Demographics

- Age
  - Disease of older children, young adults
- Gender
  - No gender predominance
- Epidemiology
  - MTS accounts for majority of epilepsy patients undergoing temporal lobe seizure surgery

Natural History & Prognosis

- Anterior temporal lobectomy 70-95% successful if MR findings of MTS
- Success of anterior temporal lobectomy 40-55% if MR normal
- ↓ surgical success when amygdala involved (~ 50%)

Treatment

- Clinical management based on phenotypic features of initial febrile and subsequent seizures
- Medical treatment initial approach
- Surgical temporal lobectomy reserved for medically intractable seizures, intolerable drug side effects
  - Resection includes anterior temporal lobe, majority of hippocampus, variable portions of amygdala

DIAGNOSTIC CHECKLIST

Consider

- Most common cause of partial complex epilepsy in adults
- Bilateral in 20%; difficult to detect without quantitative volumetry unless severe
- MTS imaging findings not found in normal seizure-free patients (controversial)

Image Interpretation Pearls

- Coronal high-resolution T2WI, FLAIR MR most sensitive for MTS
- Dual pathology in 15%
- In pediatric age group, low-grade neoplasms and cortical dysplasia more common causes of partial complex epilepsy than MTS

SELECTED REFERENCES

1. Kröll-Seger J et al: Non-paraneoplastic limbic encephalitis associated with antibodies to potassium channels leading to bilateral hippocampal sclerosis in a pre-pubertal girl. Epileptic Disord. 11(1):54-9, 2009
2. Bote RP et al: Hippocampal sclerosis: histopathology substrate and magnetic resonance imaging. Semin Ultrasound CT MR. 29(1):2-14, 2008
3. Focke NK et al: Voxel-based diffusion tensor imaging in patients with mesial temporal lobe epilepsy and hippocampal sclerosis. Neuroimage. 40(2):728-37, 2008
4. Carne RP et al: 'MRI-negative PET-positive' temporal lobe epilepsy (TLE) and mesial TLE differ with quantitative MRI and PET: a case control study. BMC Neurol. 7:16, 2007
5. Ray A et al: Temporal lobe epilepsy in children: overview of clinical semiology. Epileptic Disord. 7(4):299-307, 2005
6. Cendes F: Febrile seizures and mesial temporal sclerosis. Curr Opin Neurol. 17(2):161-4, 2004
7. Van Paesschen W: Qualitative and quantitative imaging of the hippocampus in mesial temporal lobe epilepsy with hippocampal sclerosis. Neuroimaging Clin N Am. 14(3):373-400, vii, 2004

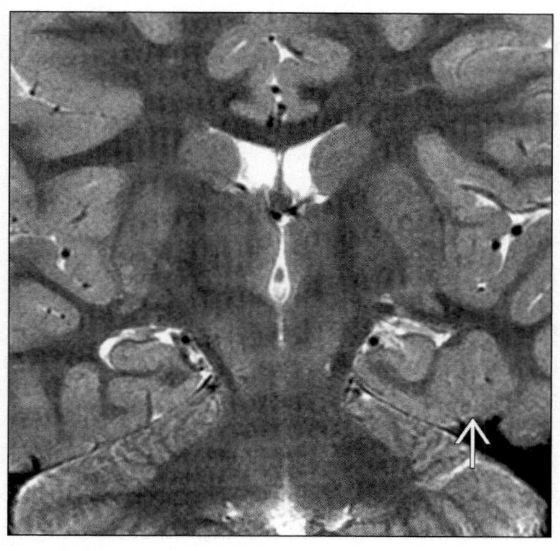

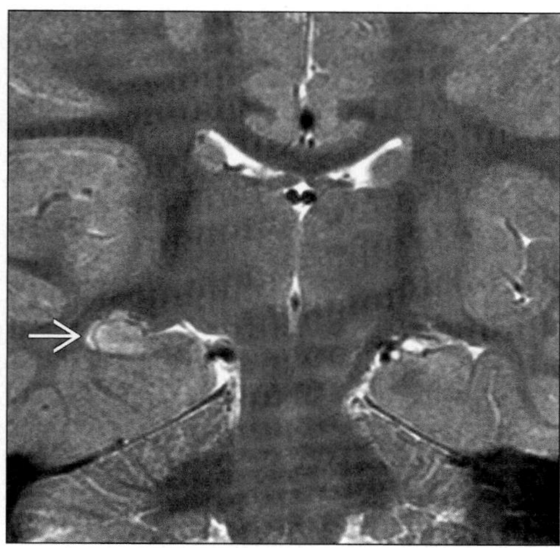

(Left) *Coronal STIR MR at 3.0 tesla in a normal nonepileptic patient shows a prominent left collateral sulcus ➡ that changes the morphology of the adjacent normal hippocampus. This common anatomical variant can be mistaken for hippocampal sclerosis.* ***(Right)*** *Coronal T2WI MR at 3.0T in a patient with prolonged febrile seizure shows abnormal enlargement and T2 hyperintensity in the right hippocampus ➡. DWI (not shown) revealed reduced diffusion. The patient later developed hippocampal sclerosis.*

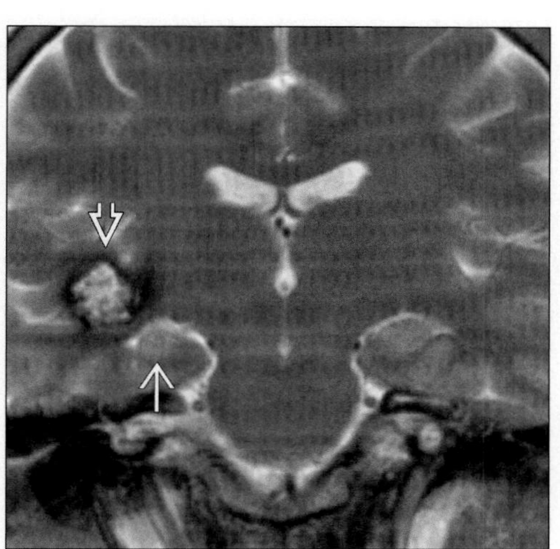

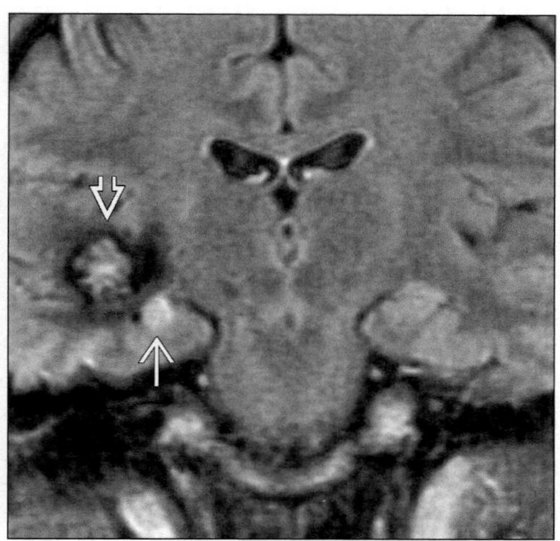

(Left) *Coronal T2WI MR in a chronic seizure patient with large right temporal lobe cavernous malformation ➡ demonstrates all 3 primary determinants of right hippocampal sclerosis ➡ (volume loss, T2 hyperintensity, and loss of internal architecture).* ***(Right)*** *Coronal FLAIR MR in the same patient with right temporal lobe cavernous malformation ➡ better shows hippocampal sclerosis ➡. Hyperintensity is usually more conspicuous on FLAIR, while T2 is better for depicting internal structure.*

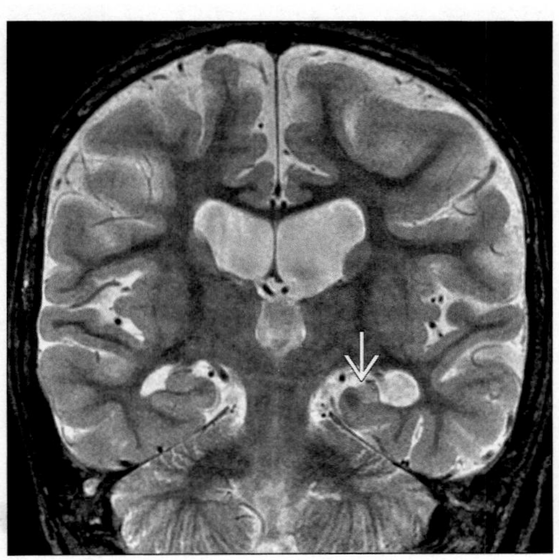

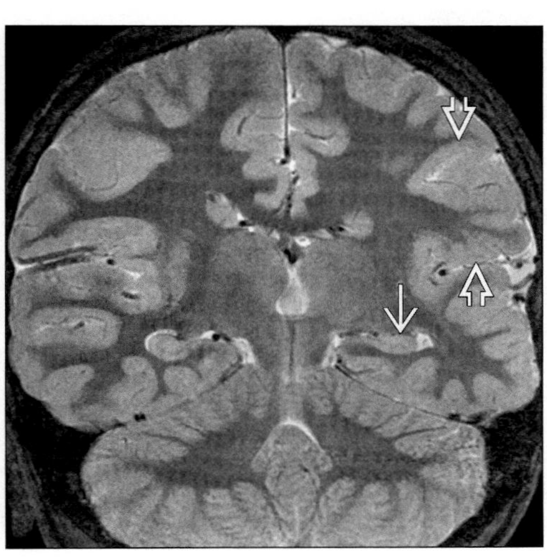

(Left) *Coronal STIR MR at 3.0 tesla in an individual who had been born prematurely with developmental delay shows diffuse white matter volume loss (left > right) and concordant left hippocampal volume loss with the abnormal T2 hyperintensity ➡ of hippocampal sclerosis.* ***(Right)*** *Coronal STIR MR at 3.0 tesla in a patient with chronic intractable epilepsy due to tuberous sclerosis demonstrates dual pathology, with left hippocampal sclerosis ➡ in addition to left frontal cortical dysplasia ➡.*

STATUS EPILEPTICUS

Key Facts

Terminology

- Status epilepticus: > 30 minutes of continuous seizures or ≥ 2 seizures without full recovery between seizures
  - MR changes associated with seizures likely related to transient cerebral edema
- Synonyms: Transient seizure-related MR changes, reversible post-ictal cerebral edema

Imaging

- Best diagnostic clue: T2 hyperintensity in gray matter &/or subcortical white matter (WM) with mild mass effect
  - Supratentorial, related to epileptogenic focus
  - Typically cortex &/or subcortical white matter
  - May involve hippocampus, corpus callosum
- Swelling and increased volume of involved cortex
- DWI: Restricted diffusion acutely
- T1WI C+: Variable enhancement, none to marked
- PWI: Marked hyperemia, ↑ rCBF and rCBV

Top Differential Diagnoses

- Cerebritis
- Cerebral ischemia-infarction
- Herpes encephalitis
- Astrocytoma

Diagnostic Checklist

- Acute seizures or status epilepticus may mimic other pathology, such as tumor progression or cerebritis
- Clinical information and follow-up imaging often differentiates from other etiologies
- Look for underlying mass that may have caused the seizures/status epilepticus
- Seizure-related changes usually resolve within days to weeks

__(Left)__ Coronal FLAIR MR performed shortly after a long episode of status epilepticus shows increased signal involving the left temporal lobe cortex and associated subcortical white matter. __(Right)__ Axial T1WI C+ FS MR in the same patient shows mild edema and vascular congestion in the left temporal lobe ⇨. Imaging 1 month later showed near complete resolution of the signal abnormalities. Status epilepticus may result in MR changes that are likely related to transient cerebral edema.

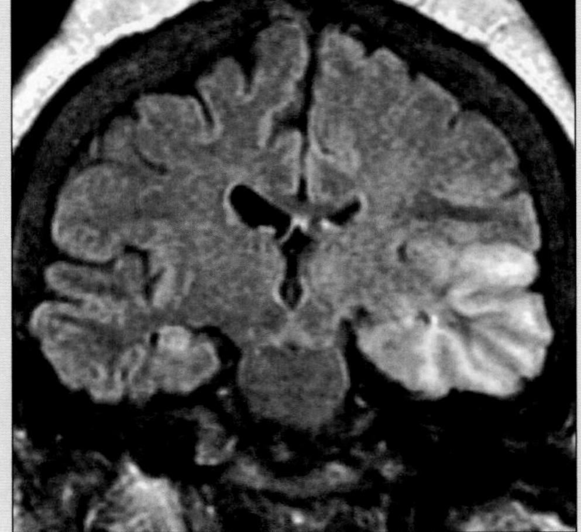

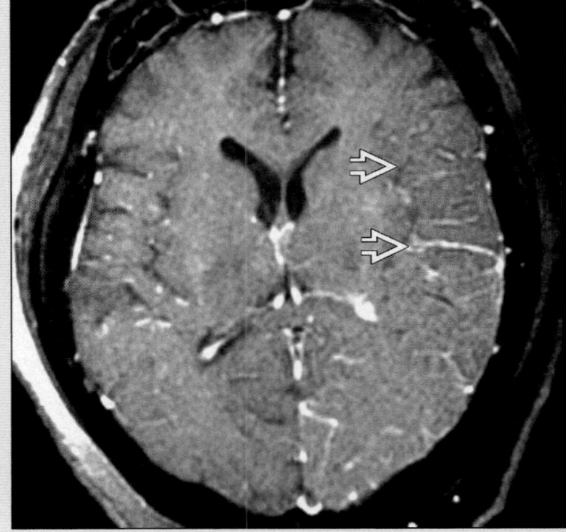

__(Left)__ Axial T1WI MR shows mild thickening of the temporal lobe cortex ➔ in a status epilepticus patient. Cortical and subcortical white matter involvement is characteristic. Follow-up imaging in such cases usually shows resolution of the acute imaging abnormalities in treated patients. Atrophy may be seen chronically. __(Right)__ Axial T2 MR in the same patient shows hyperintensity with mild mass effect in the temporal cortex ➔ and hippocampus ⇨. Imaging mimics that of infection, ischemia, and neoplasm.

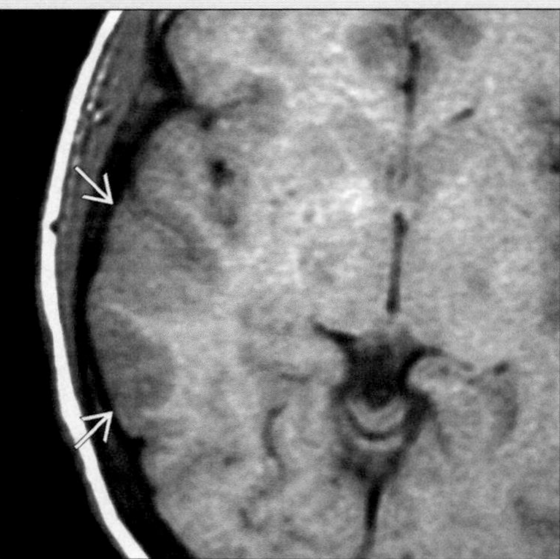

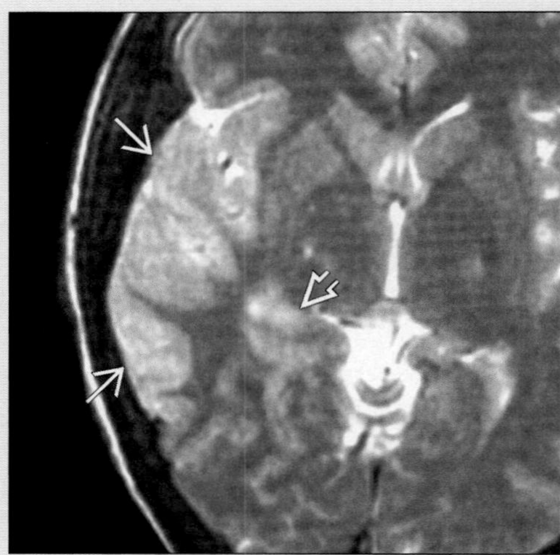

TERMINOLOGY

Synonyms

- Transient seizure-related MR changes, reversible post-ictal cerebral edema

Definitions

- Status epilepticus: > 30 minutes of continuous seizures or ≥ 2 without full recovery between seizures
- MR changes associated with seizures likely related to transient cerebral edema

IMAGING

General Features

- Best diagnostic clue
  - T2 hyperintensity in gray matter (GM) &/or subcortical white matter (WM) with mild mass effect
  - May focally involve hippocampus, corpus callosum
- Location
  - Supratentorial, related to epileptogenic focus
    - Typically cortex &/or subcortical white matter
  - May involve focal structures
    - Hippocampus (febrile or partial complex seizures)
    - Splenium of corpus callosum
  - Occasionally cerebellar involvement

CT Findings

- NECT
  - Hypodensity in cortex &/or subcortical WM
  - Blurring of corticomedullary junction
  - Hippocampus, splenium of corpus callosum may be involved
  - No hemorrhage
- CECT
  - Variable enhancement: None to marked

MR Findings

- T1WI
  - Hypointensity in cortex &/or subcortical WM
    - Swelling and increased volume of involved cortical gyri
  - Blurring of corticomedullary junction
  - Mild mass effect
  - Hippocampus, splenium of corpus callosum may be involved
  - Rarely cerebellar involvement seen
- T2WI
  - Hyperintensity in cortex &/or subcortical WM
    - Swelling and increased volume of involved cortical gyri
  - Mild edema and mass effect
  - Hippocampus, corpus callosum splenium may be involved
  - No hemorrhage
- FLAIR
  - Hyperintensity in cortex &/or subcortical WM
  - Mild edema and mass effect
  - Hippocampus, splenium of corpus callosum may be involved
- DWI
  - Restricted diffusion with decrease in ADC map acutely
  - ADC maps normal interictally, elevated in chronic seizures
- T1WI C+
  - Variable enhancement: None to marked
  - May see gyriform or leptomeningeal enhancement
- MRS
  - Lipids &/or lactate shown in hippocampi of temporal lobe epilepsy (TLE) patients within 24 hours of last seizure
  - Follow-up MRS after seizures under control show no lipids/lactate
- Perfusion imaging (PWI): Marked hyperemia on side of epileptic focus, elevated rCBF and rCBV maps

Nuclear Medicine Findings

- Seizures: Increased metabolism and perfusion
- PET: Increased glucose metabolism and metabolic rate
- HMPAO SPECT: High uptake in affected cerebral lobe during or immediately after a seizure

Imaging Recommendations

- Best imaging tool
  - MR is most sensitive
- Protocol advice
  - Contrast-enhanced MR with DWI
  - MRS may be helpful in TLE patients

DIFFERENTIAL DIAGNOSIS

Cerebritis

- T2 hyperintense "mass" with mass effect
- Typically DWI positive
- Patchy enhancement typical

Cerebral Ischemia-Infarction

- Typical vascular distribution (ACA, MCA, PCA)
- Acute/subacute DWI positive
- Wedge-shaped, involves GM and WM
- Gyriform enhancement in subacute ischemia

Herpes Encephalitis

- Confined to limbic system, temporal lobes
- Blood products, enhancement typical
- Acute onset, often with fever
- May present with seizures

Astrocytoma

- Infiltrating white matter mass
- May extend to involve cortex
- Variable enhancement in anaplastic (grade III)
- May cause epilepsy

MELAS

- Mitochondrial encephalopathy, lactic acidosis, and stroke-like episodes
- Multifocal bilateral T2 hyperintensities
- Predominantly GM involvement, may involve subcortical WM
- Ischemia in > 1 vascular territory
- MRS shows lactate peak

Mesial Temporal Sclerosis

- Abnormal T2 hyperintensity in mesial temporal lobe
- Hippocampal volume loss and architectural distortion

Vasculitis

- Multiple small areas of T2 hyperintensity in deep and subcortical WM, often bilateral, ± enhancement
- Gray matter involvement may be seen

Demyelination

- Multifocal white matter lesions, deep gray nuclei
- Incomplete rim or horseshoe-shaped enhancement
- Lesions often in typical locations

PATHOLOGY

General Features

- Etiology
  - MR signal abnormalities related to transient vasogenic &/or cytotoxic edema
    - Redistribution of intracellular and extracellular water, related to alteration in cell membrane permeability or cytotoxic edema
  - Hippocampus involvement by status epilepticus may result in mesial temporal sclerosis
  - Involvement of corpus callosum splenium, 2 theories
    - Transient focal edema related to transhemispheric connection of seizure activity
    - Reversible demyelination related to antiepileptic drugs
- Anatomic considerations
  - Portions of brain most vulnerable to damage from status epilepticus
    - CA1, CA3 and hilus of hippocampus, amygdala, piriform cortex, cerebellar cortex, thalamus, cerebral cortex

Gross Pathologic & Surgical Features

- Acutely
  - Swelling of cortex &/or subcortical WM or hippocampus
- Chronic
  - Atrophy of involved cortex &/or subcortical WM

Microscopic Features

- Acutely
  - Reactive astrocytes with swollen cytoplasm and neuropil, consistent with cytotoxic edema
- Chronic
  - Marked neuronal loss with intense astrocytic reaction; reactive astrocytes replacing absent neurons
- Gliosis and neuronal loss affecting gray-white matter junction with extension to cortex

CLINICAL ISSUES

Presentation

- Most common signs/symptoms
  - Active seizures &/or status epilepticus
  - Other signs/symptoms: Location dependent
- Clinical profile
  - EEG shows seizure activity

Demographics

- Age
  - Occurs at all ages, commonly young adults
- Gender
  - No gender predominance

Natural History & Prognosis

- Typically complete resolution with treatment of seizures
- May be complicated by infarction related to hypoxemia

Treatment

- Treatment of underlying seizure disorder
  - Antiepileptic medicines primary therapy
- Surgical resection in patients with intractable epilepsy

DIAGNOSTIC CHECKLIST

Consider

- Acute seizures or status epilepticus may mimic other pathology, such as tumor progression or cerebritis
- Clinical information and follow-up imaging often differentiates seizure-related MR changes from other etiologies

Image Interpretation Pearls

- Look for underlying mass that may have caused seizures/status epilepticus
- Seizure-related changes will usually resolve within days to weeks on follow-up imaging

SELECTED REFERENCES

1. Di Bonaventura C et al: Diffusion-weighted magnetic resonance imaging in patients with partial status epilepticus. Epilepsia. 50 Suppl 1:45-52, 2009
2. Goyal MK et al: Peri-ictal signal changes in seven patients with status epilepticus: interesting MRI observations. Neuroradiology. 51(3):151-61, 2009
3. Milligan TA et al: Frequency and patterns of MRI abnormalities due to status epilepticus. Seizure. 18(2):104-8, 2009
4. Buracchio T et al: Restricted diffusion on magnetic resonance imaging in partial status epilepticus. Arch Neurol. 65(2):278-9, 2008
5. Provenzale JM et al: Hippocampal MRI signal hyperintensity after febrile status epilepticus is predictive of subsequent mesial temporal sclerosis. AJR Am J Roentgenol. 190(4):976-83, 2008
6. Parmar H et al: Acute symptomatic seizures and hippocampus damage: DWI and MRS findings. Neurology. 66(11):1732-5, 2006
7. Calistri V et al: Visualization of evolving status epilepticus with diffusion and perfusion MR imaging. AJNR Am J Neuroradiol. 24(4):671-3, 2003
8. Castillo M et al: Proton MR spectroscopy in patients with acute temporal lobe seizures. AJNR Am J Neuroradiol. 22(1):152-7, 2001
9. Men S et al: Selective neuronal necrosis associated with status epilepticus: MR findings. AJNR Am J Neuroradiol. 21(10):1837-40, 2000
10. Kim SS et al: Focal lesion in the splenium of the corpus callosum in epileptic patients: antiepileptic drug toxicity? AJNR Am J Neuroradiol. 20(1):125-9, 1999

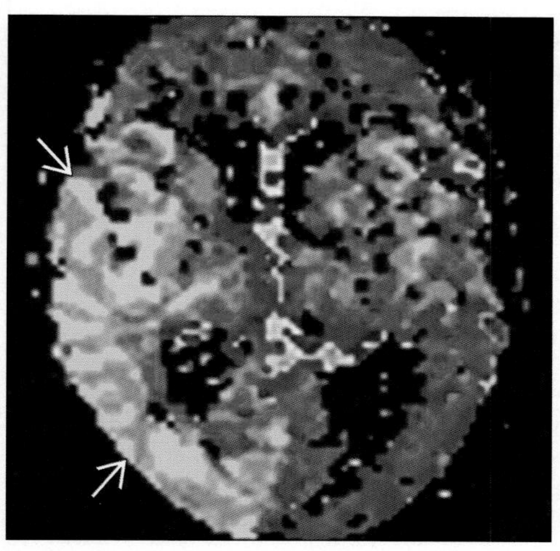

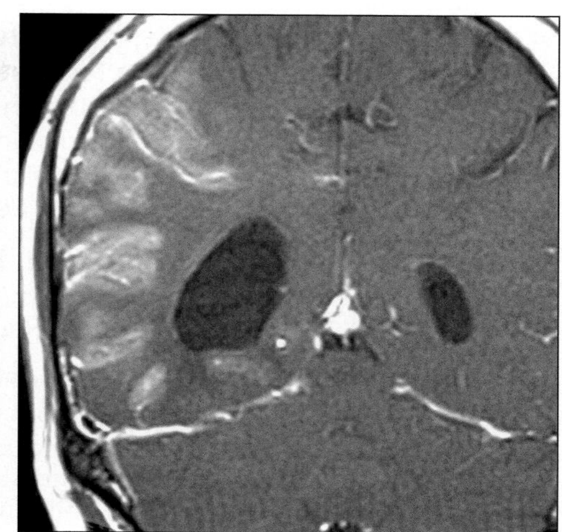

(Left) *Axial PWI MR in an elderly woman presenting with seizures shows markedly elevated perfusion in the right hemisphere ➔ compared to the normal left side. Cerebral hyperperfusion may occur after seizures, particularly with status epilepticus.* ***(Right)*** *Coronal T1 C+ MR shows gyriform and meningeal enhancement in the right parietal and occipital lobes related to status epilepticus. After treatment, the MR changes completely resolved. Involvement of the cortex and subcortical white matter is typical.*

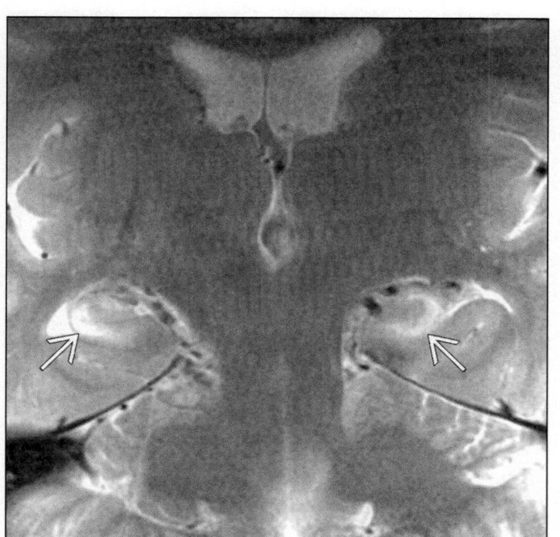

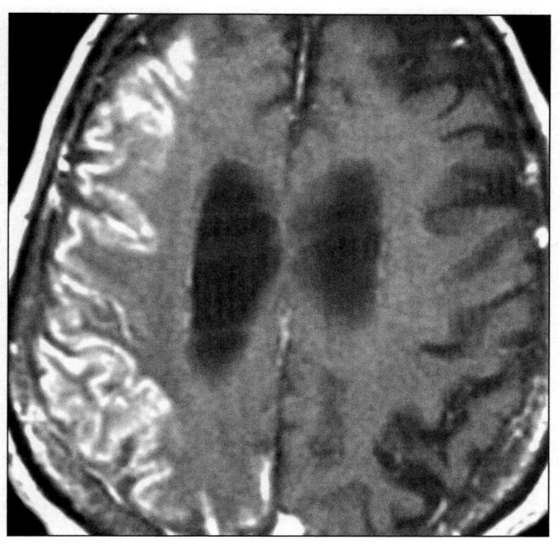

(Left) *Coronal T2WI MR shows abnormal hyperintensity in the hippocampi bilaterally ➔, related to temporal lobe status epilepticus. Imaging 1 year later showed mesial temporal sclerosis.* ***(Right)*** *Axial T1WI C+ MR in an elderly patient with seizures and a history of stroke shows extensive gyriform enhancement. This enhancement pattern is often seen in subacute stroke, encephalitis, and status epilepticus.*

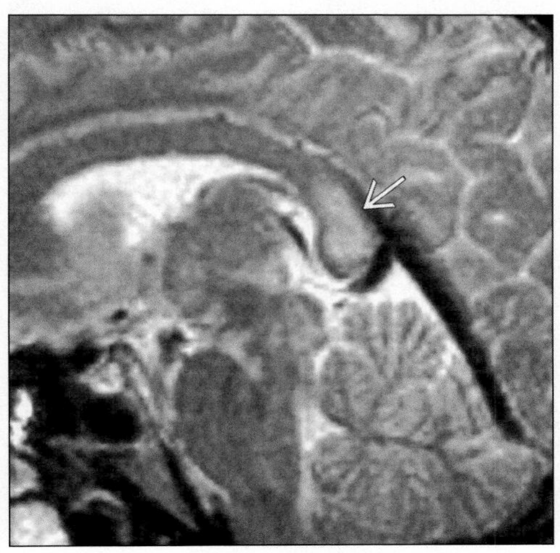

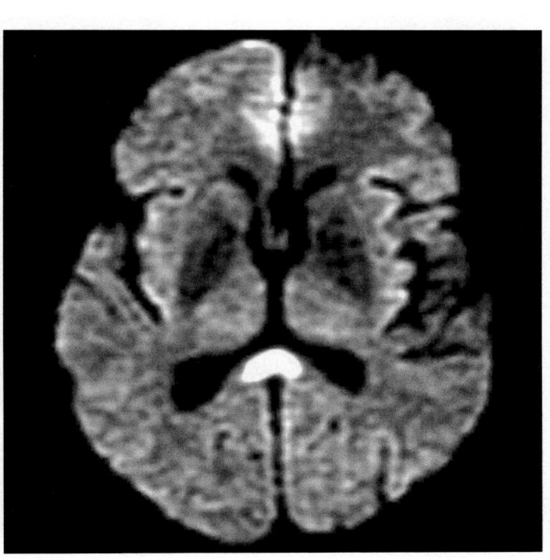

(Left) *Sagittal T2WI MR shows hyperintensity in the corpus callosum splenium ➔ caused by transient status epilepticus. Hyperintensity within the splenium may be caused by the seizures or by the antiepileptic medications.* ***(Right)*** *Axial DWI MR shows acute restriction in the splenium of the corpus callosum in a patient with status epilepticus. Restricted diffusion is often present acutely in these patients. Focal involvement of the corpus callosum splenium or hippocampus may be seen.*

NORMAL AGING BRAIN

Key Facts

Terminology

- ↓ overall brain volume with advancing age
  - Reflected in relative ↑ CSF spaces

Imaging

- Broad spectrum of "normal" on imaging in elderly
- "Successfully aging brain"
  - Smooth, thin, periventricular, high signal rim on FLAIR is normal
  - White matter hyperintensities (WMHs) absent/few
- Decreased total brain volume
  - Selective atrophy of white matter (not gray matter) predominates
- WMHs ↑ number/size after 50 years
  - ~ universal after 65 years
- GRE/SWI
  - Increasing mineralization of basal ganglia with age
  - "Black dots" > 60 years is **not** normal
- Age-related shift from anterior to posterior cortical metabolism

Top Differential Diagnoses

- Mild cognitive impairment
- Alzheimer disease
- Sporadic subcortical arteriosclerotic encephalopathy
- Vascular dementia
- Frontotemporal lobar degeneration (Pick disease)

Clinical Issues

- WMHs correlate with age, silent stroke, hypertension, female sex

Diagnostic Checklist

- Cannot predict cognitive function from CT/MR
  - Imaging only roughly correlates with cognitive function
  - Significant overlap with dementias

*(**Left**) Axial graphic depicts a normally aging brain in an 80-year-old patient. Note the widening of sulci and ventricles in the absence of any brain parenchymal abnormalities. (**Right**) Axial NECT demonstrates mild sulcal enlargement and mild ventriculomegaly in a 70-year-old patient. The white matter appears completely normal, without periventricular hypodensities or white matter lacunar infarcts.*

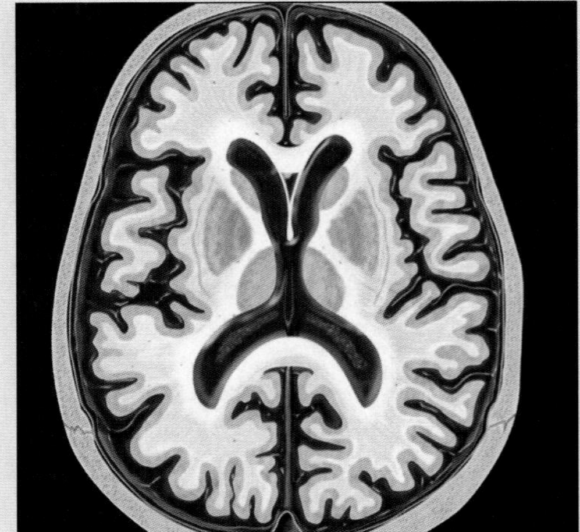

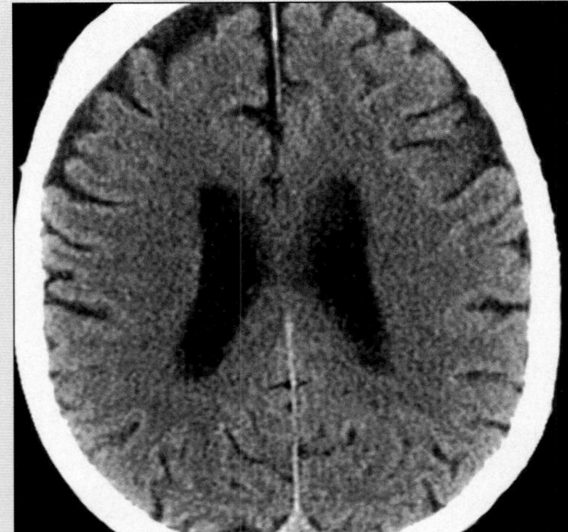

*(**Left**) Axial FLAIR shows mild periventricular hyperintensity ➡ and mild enlargement of the ventricles and sulci in a 65-year-old man. No focal hyperintensities are seen in the hemispheric white matter; cortical thickness and signal intensity are normal. (**Right**) Axial T2* SWI MR demonstrates hypointensity in the lentiform nuclei, particularly related to the globus pallidi ➡.*

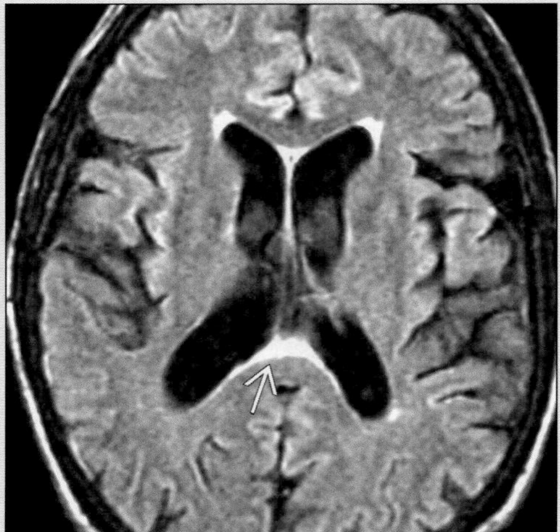

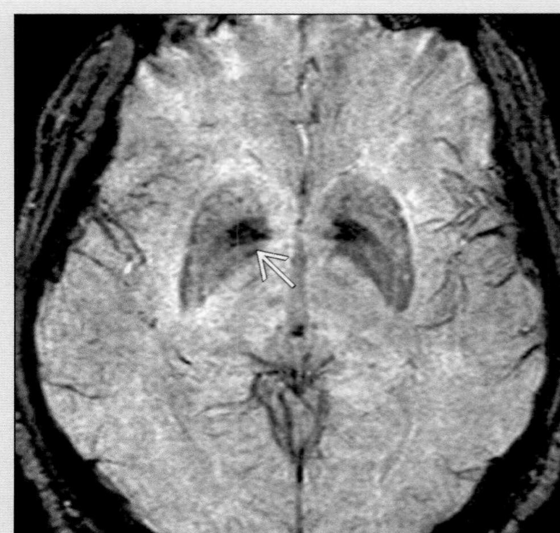

NORMAL AGING BRAIN

TERMINOLOGY

Definitions

- ↓ overall brain volume with advancing age
  - Reflected in relative ↑ CSF spaces

IMAGING

General Features

- Best diagnostic clue
  - "Successfully aging brain"
    - Thin, periventricular, high signal rim
    - Without white matter hyperintensities (WMHs)
    - Mild shrinkage of selected cerebellar regions normal
- Location
  - Selective atrophy of white matter (WM) predominates, not gray matter (GM)
  - Striatum (primarily caudate nucleus, putamen)
- Size
  - Decreased total brain volume
  - Absolute striatal size
    - Caudate decreases linearly with age
    - Putamen remains relatively stable
- Morphology
  - Brain tissue ↓, CSF volume ↑
    - Reflects overall WM volume loss > focal WM hyperintensities (WMHs)
    - Rounded appearance of dilated ventricles, sulci ↑
  - Strong correlation between WM volume and CSF volume: Measure of overall brain atrophy

CT Findings

- NECT
  - Enlarged ventricles, widened cortical sulci
  - Patchy/confluent periventricular low densities
  - ± symmetrical, punctate calcifications in globi pallidi (GP)
  - ± curvilinear vascular Ca++
- CECT
  - No parenchymal enhancement

MR Findings

- T1WI
  - Mild but significant age-related shrinkage of
    - Posterior vermis (lobules 6, 7, and 8-10)
    - Cerebellar hemispheres
  - Apparent age invariance of anterior vermis, ventral pons
  - Dilated perivascular Virchow-Robin spaces
    - Isointense to CSF on all sequences
    - Conform to course of penetrating arteries
    - Round/oval/curvilinear
    - Smooth, well-defined margins
    - Bilateral, often symmetrical; usually no mass effect
    - Increase in number, size (> 2 mm) with age
    - Can be found in most all areas
      - Tend to cluster around anterior commissure
      - Inferior 1/3 of putamen, external capsule
- T2WI
  - Focal/confluent periventricular WMHs
    - Number/size ↑ after 50 years; ~ universal after 65 years
    - Only rough correlation with cognitive function
    - Significant overlap with dementias
  - Infarct-like T2 hyperintense lesions
    - Seen in 1/3 of asymptomatic patients > 65 years
    - Mostly in basal ganglia (BG), thalami
    - Probably represent clinically silent lacunar infarcts
  - T2 shortening
    - "Black line" in visual, motor/sensory cortex
      - Common, normal in older patients
    - Ferric iron deposition
      - Normal in GP, abnormal in thalamus
    - With aging, hypointensity in caudate/putamen ↑
      - May equal GP in 8th decade
- FLAIR
  - Smooth, thin, periventricular hyperintense rim normal
  - BG and thalamic foci
    - Perivascular spaces suppress
    - Lacunar infarcts hyperintense
- T2* GRE
  - SWI: Increasing mineralization of BG with age
    - Can see linear "waves" or conglomerate mineralization in GP
  - "Black dots" in patients > 60 years is **not** normal
    - Longstanding hypertension
    - Amyloid angiopathy
- DWI
  - Small but significant increased water diffusibility
    - ADC increases
    - Decreased anisotropy on diffusion tensor imaging
- T1WI C+
  - Age-related WMHs do not enhance
  - If enhancing, consider acute lacunar infarct or metastases
- MRS
  - Metabolite distribution varies among different brain regions
    - Choline (Cho) content ↑ with aging
    - Creatine (Cr) ↑ with aging
    - N-acetyl aspartate (NAA) age-related change
      - ↓ in cortex, centrum semiovale, temporal lobes

Nuclear Medicine Findings

- PET
  - Metabolic alterations common
    - Global, regional changes in CBF
  - Gradual ↓ in regional cerebral blood flow (CBF) of GM, WM
    - Particularly in frontal lobes
  - Age-related shift from anterior to posterior cortical metabolism
    - Putamen receives primarily posterior cortical input
    - Caudate receives relatively more anterior cortical input
  - Relative glucose metabolic rate (rGMR) measured by FDG PET
    - With age, rGMR ↑ in putamen and ↓ in caudate
  - ↓ pre-/postsynaptic dopamine markers in BG
- Tc-99m-HMPAO SPECT, Xe-133 inhalation show regional, global reduction in CBF

NORMAL AGING BRAIN

Imaging Recommendations

- Best imaging tool
  - MR with FLAIR, DWI, T2* GRE/SWI

DIFFERENTIAL DIAGNOSIS

Mild Cognitive Impairment

- Overlap with normal on standard imaging studies
- ↓ NAA

Alzheimer Disease

- Parietal and temporal cortical atrophy
- Striking volume loss in hippocampi, entorhinal cortex
- ↓ NAA, ↑ myoinositol (mI)

Sporadic Subcortical Arteriosclerotic Encephalopathy

- Numerous WMHs (overlap with normal)
- Multiple lacunar infarcts

Vascular Dementia

- Hyperintense lesions on T2WI and focal atrophy suggestive of chronic infarcts

Frontotemporal Lobar Degeneration (Pick Disease)

- Asymmetric frontal, anterior temporal atrophy

PATHOLOGY

General Features

- Etiology
  - Previous conception of aging: Substantial cortical neuronal loss with age
  - New: Predominant neuroanatomic changes
    - White matter alterations, subcortical neuronal loss
    - Reduction in cell size > cell number
  - Neuronal dysfunction rather than loss of neurons/ synapses
    - ↓ neuronal viability or function associated with accelerated membrane degradation &/or ↑ glial cell numbers
    - Loss of synapses and dendritic pruning in selected areas rather than globally
  - Some investigators consider accumulation of neurofibrillary tangles (NFTs) may be responsible for memory loss associated with aging
- Genetics
  - Genetic factors clearly affect aging of brain
  - Contribution of ApoE allotype to age-dependent cognitive decline

Gross Pathologic & Surgical Features

- Widened sulci, large ventricles

Microscopic Features

- Decreased myelinated fibers in subcortical WM
- Increased extracellular space, gliosis
- Iron deposition in globus pallidus, putamen
- WM capillaries lose pericytes, have thinner endothelium
- Dilated perivascular spaces of Virchow-Robin
  - Extension of subarachnoid space that accompanies penetrating vessels into brain to level of capillaries
- Minimal loss of cortical neurons with age
- Neurofibrillary tangles (NFTs)
  - Tau phosphorylation, mitochondrial dysfunction may precede full NFT formation
  - NFTs appear in small numbers in entorhinal and transentorhinal cortices early in aging (patients ~ 60 years old)
  - NFTs may induce neural dysfunction, destruction of synapses, and, eventually, neuronal death

CLINICAL ISSUES

Presentation

- Most common signs/symptoms
  - Normal cognitive function
  - Mild cognitive impairment correlates with ↑ risk of Alzheimer disease

Demographics

- Age
  - > 60 years old
- Gender
  - Differences in striatal size
    - Relatively constant size across lifespan in men
    - Variable size across lifespan in women: Smaller size in women aged 50-70 years than in men
  - Differences in rGMR
    - Caudate: Higher rGMR in women than men
    - Putamen: Equal rGMR in women and men
  - Greater dopamine transporters in caudate in women
- Epidemiology
  - WMHs correlate with age, silent stroke, hypertension, female sex

Natural History & Prognosis

- Parenchymal volume ↓, CSF spaces ↑ progressively
- WMHs progressively ↑ with age

DIAGNOSTIC CHECKLIST

Consider

- Striatum may mediate age-associated cognitive decline
  - ↓ volume, functional activity with age

Image Interpretation Pearls

- Broad spectrum of "normal" on imaging in elderly
- Cannot predict cognitive function from CT/MR

SELECTED REFERENCES

1. Ni JM et al: Regional diffusion changes of cerebral grey matter during normal aging-A fluid-inversion prepared diffusion imaging study. Eur J Radiol. Epub ahead of print, 2009
2. Salat DH et al: Regional white matter volume differences in nondemented aging and Alzheimer's disease. Neuroimage. 44(4):1247-58, 2009
3. Gruber S et al: Metabolic changes in the normal ageing brain: consistent findings from short and long echo time proton spectroscopy. Eur J Radiol. 68(2):320-7, 2008

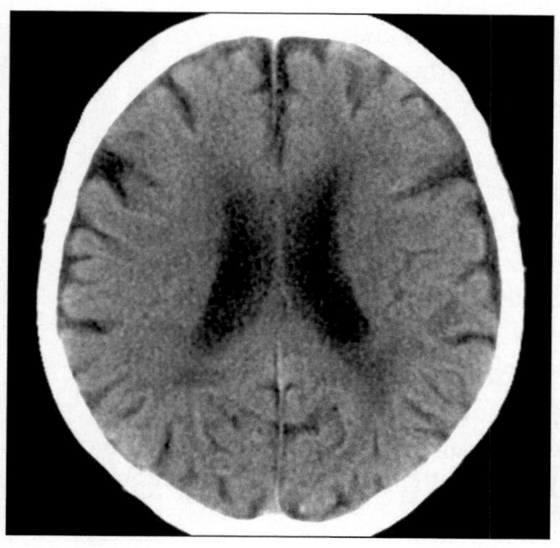

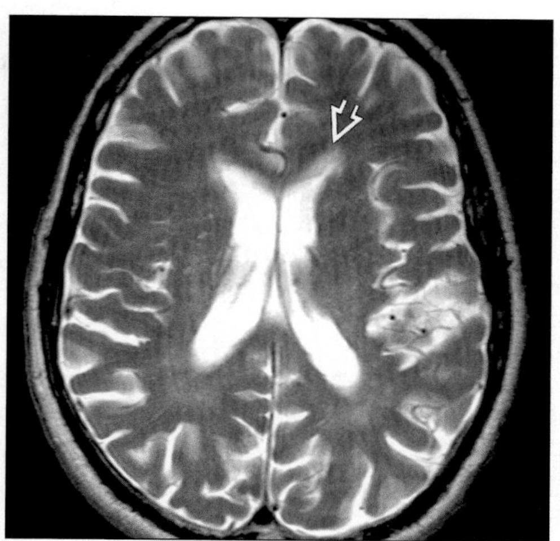

(Left) *Axial NECT in an 85-year-old patient without cognitive impairment shows wide sulci and lateral ventricles, as well as moderate periventricular hypodense white matter.* ***(Right)*** *Axial T2WI 3T MR in a 76-year-old patient shows mild periventricular hyperintensity ➔, mild ventriculomegaly, and mild sulcal enlargement.*

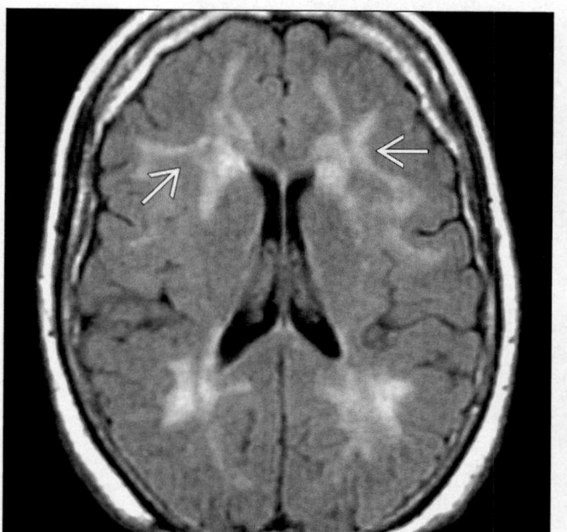

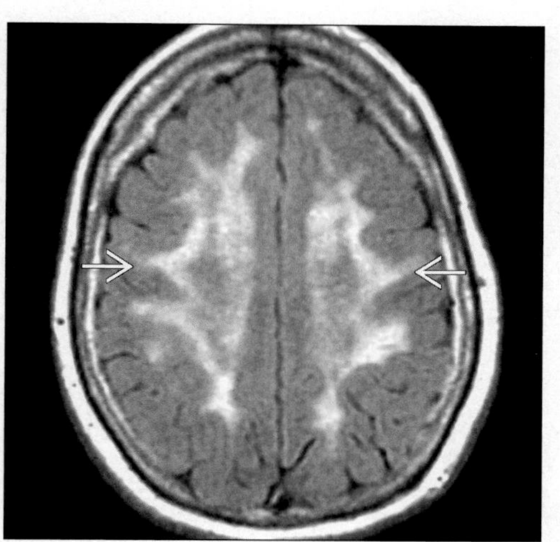

(Left) *Axial FLAIR MR demonstrates confluent hyperintense white matter changes ➔ that may occur during normal aging.* ***(Right)*** *Axial FLAIR MR in the same patient demonstrates prominent subcortical white matter hyperintensity ➔.*

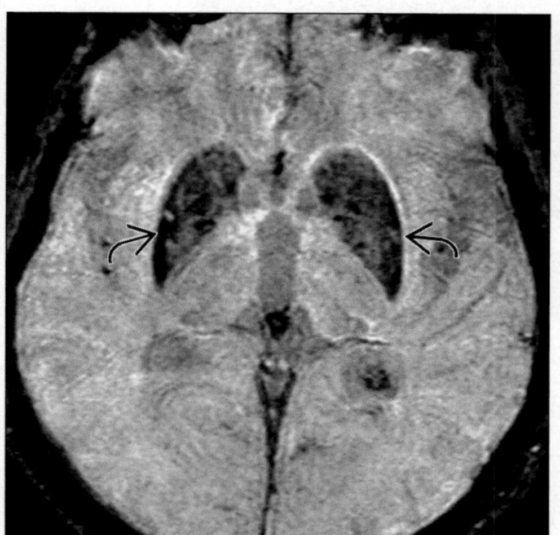

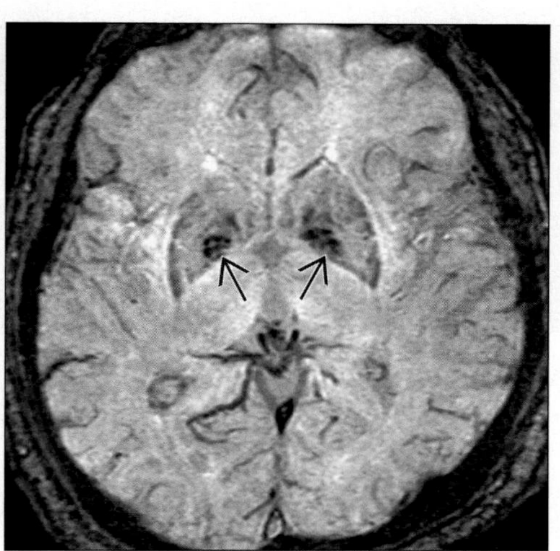

(Left) *Axial T2* SWI MR demonstrates marked hypointensity in the basal ganglia ➔ related to normal mineralization with age.* ***(Right)*** *Axial T2* SWI MR demonstrates horizontal linear "waves" of mineralization in the globus pallidi ➔, a normal finding in the aging brain.*

ALZHEIMER DISEASE

Key Facts

Terminology
- Alzheimer disease (AD)
  - Slowly progressive neurodegenerative disease

Imaging
- Current role of imaging in AD
  - Exclude other structural abnormalities
  - Evaluate degree, location of atrophic changes
  - Evaluate metabolic abnormalities (early disease)
  - Identify early AD for possible innovative therapy
- Best imaging = volumetric MR, FDG-18 PET
- MR to evaluate for presence of
  - Temporal/parietal cortical atrophy
  - Disproportionate hippocampal volume loss
  - Proportionate ventricular, sulcal enlargement
  - Coexisting microvascular disease
- FDG-18 PET to evaluate for
  - Regional ↓ glucose metabolism

Top Differential Diagnoses
- Frontotemporal lobar degeneration
- Dementia with Lewy bodies
- Normal pressure hydrocephalus
- Vascular dementia
- Normal aging

Clinical Issues
- Most common cause of dementia over age 65
- Age is biggest risk factor
  - 1-2% prevalence at age 65
  - Prevalence ↑ 15-25% per decade after 65

Diagnostic Checklist
- No masses, hemorrhage
- No evidence for ischemic stroke (probable AD) or with evidence of ischemic disease (possible AD)

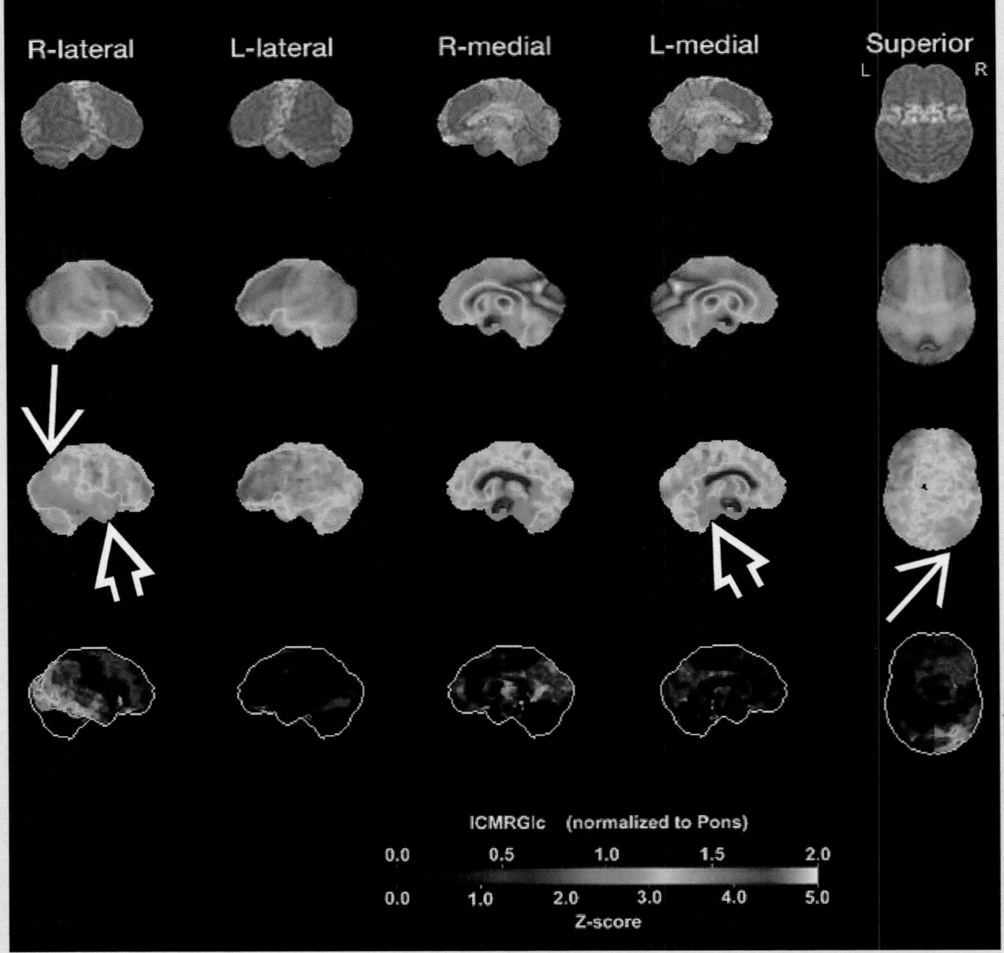

Sagittal FDG-18 PET with stereotaxic surface projections in a 70-year-old woman with possible AD. Standard MR (not shown) disclosed no definite abnormalities. Top row = reference map. 2nd row = glucose metabolism in normal elderly control group (n = 27). 3rd row = patient's glucose metabolism map. Note the decrease in medial temporal ⮕ and parietal lobes ➡ with sparing of the frontal, occipital lobes. Bottom row = Z-score map. (Courtesy N. Foster, MD.)

ALZHEIMER DISEASE

TERMINOLOGY

Abbreviations

- Alzheimer disease (AD)

Synonyms

- Senile/presenile dementia of Alzheimer type

Definitions

- Criteria for clinical diagnosis of AD
  - DSM-IV
    - Memory loss
    - At least 1 other area of impaired cognition
      - Aphasia, apraxia, agnosia, executive function
    - Causes impaired functioning
    - Gradual, continuous (no pathology required)
  - NINCDS-ADRDA
    - Clinical dementia confirmed by clinical rating
    - At least 2 areas of cognition involved
      - Definite AD: Requires clinical criteria and pathologic evidence
      - Probable AD: Clinical dementia without 2nd systemic brain illness present
      - Possible AD: Clinical dementia but with 2nd systemic brain illness present that is unlikely to account for AD alone

IMAGING

General Features

- Best diagnostic clue
  - MR: Temporal/parietal cortical atrophy
    - Disproportionate hippocampal volume loss
  - FDG PET: Regional ↓ glucose metabolism
    - Temporoparietal lobes, posterior cingulum
- Current role of imaging in AD
  - Exclude other structural abnormalities
  - Evaluate degree, location of atrophic changes
  - Evaluate metabolic abnormalities
    - When structural abnormalities absent/ uncharacteristic (i.e., early in disease course)
  - Identify early-onset AD for possible innovative therapy

CT Findings

- NECT
  - Preferential volume loss in temporal, parietal lobes

MR Findings

- T1WI (assess structure, atrophy patterns)
  - High resolution (MP-RAGE or SPGR)
  - ↑ ventricles, sulci
    - ↑ temporal horns (hippocampal, entorhinal volume loss)
  - Volumetric analysis of hippocampi/ parahippocampal gyri
    - Helps to distinguish patients with mild cognitive impairment (at risk for proceeding to AD) from normal elderly
  - Evidence of coexisting microvascular disease
    - May ↓ diagnosis from "probable" to "possible" AD
- T2* GRE for microhemorrhages, amyloid angiopathy
- pMR (↓ rCBV in temporal, parietal regions)

Nuclear Medicine Findings

- 18F-FDG PET
  - Regional hypometabolic areas
    - Correlate with severity of cognitive impairment
    - Helps distinguish AD from frontotemporal dementia
- SPECT
  - Perfusion deficits in hippocampus/temporoparietal regions
- Radiolabeled in vivo amyloid binding agents
  - Amyloid PET ligands
    - High sensitivity in detecting amyloid plaques and vascular amyloid in vivo
    - 11C-PIB binds to β-amyloid protein (not NFTs)

Imaging Recommendations

- Best imaging tool
  - Volumetric MR
  - 18F-FDG PET
- Protocol advice
  - MP-RAGE or SPGR for volumetric measurement

DIFFERENTIAL DIAGNOSIS

Causes of Reversible Dementia

- Alcohol abuse (thiamine deficiency)
- Endocrinopathies (e.g., hypothyroidism)
- Vitamin B12 deficiency
- Depression ("pseudodementia")
- Normal pressure hydrocephalus
- Mass lesions (chronic subdural hematoma, tumor, etc.)

Frontotemporal Lobar Degeneration

- Frontal &/or anterior temporal atrophy

Vascular Dementia

- 2nd most common dementia (15-30%)
- Parenchymal hyperintensities, focal atrophy (infarcts)

Dementia with Lewy Bodies

- Hypometabolism of entire brain

Corticobasal Degeneration

- Prominent extrapyramidal, cortical symptoms
- Asymmetric severe frontoparietal atrophy

Creutzfeldt-Jakob Disease

- Dementia + myoclonus, EEG abnormalities
- Hyperintensity in anterior basal ganglia, cortex

Cerebral Amyloid Angiopathy

- Often coexists with AD
- Microhemorrhages on T2*GRE/SWI

PATHOLOGY

General Features

- Etiology
  - Extracellular β-amyloid plaques
    - Located in cerebral cortex

- Intracellular accumulation of neurofibrillary tangles (NTs)
  - Initially around hippocampus, later spread to other cortical areas
- Genetics
  - Most cases spontaneous (5-10% familial)
  - Early-onset, familial, autosomal dominant AD
    - Mutations in amyloid precursor protein gene on chromosome 21
  - Late-onset familial/sporadic AD
    - 60-75% of patients carry at least 1 copy of apolipoprotein E (ApoE) ϵ4 allele on chromosome 19

Staging, Grading, & Classification

- Consortium to Establish a Registry for Alzheimer Disease (CERAD)
  - Semi-quantitative approach counting plaques/ tangles
  - Frequent, moderate, or infrequent
- Braak and Braak (B&B)
  - 6 levels of staging
    - Transentorhinal stage (1-2)
      - NTs develop in parahippocampal gyrus (clinically asymptomatic)
    - Limbic stage (3-4)
      - NTs dramatically increase in parahippocampal gyrus, begin to develop in hippocampus (mild cognitive impairment)
    - Neocortical stage (5-6)
      - NTs develop in temporal and parietal cortex, eventually spread to entire neocortex (severe dementia)
- NIA-Reagan
  - Likelihood high
    - CERAD frequent, B&B 5/6
  - Likelihood intermediate
    - CERAD moderate, B&B 3/4
  - Likelihood low
    - CERAD infrequent, B&B 1/2

Gross Pathologic & Surgical Features

- Shrunken gyri, widened sulci

Microscopic Features

- Neuritic plaques (NPs), NTs, astrogliosis
  - Hippocampus, neocortical/some subcortical areas
- Amyloid angiopathy
  - β-amyloid in NPs, blood vessels in AD

CLINICAL ISSUES

Presentation

- Most common signs/symptoms
  - Slowly progressive neurodegenerative disease
  - Initially affects episodic memory
    - Then at least 1 other area of cognition
- Clinical profile
  - Clinical subtypes
    - Mild cognitive impairment (amnestic): Early, mild memory impairment; no deficits in cognitive domains other than memory, not impairing daily function
    - Possible AD: Dementia features in presence of 2nd disease that could cause memory deficit but is not likely cause
    - Probable AD: Memory deficits on neuropsychological testing, progressive worsening of memory and ≥ 2 cognitive functions
    - Definite AD: Pathologic diagnosis

Demographics

- Age
  - Biggest risk factor
    - 1-2% prevalence at age 65
    - Prevalence increases by 15-25% per decade after age 65
- Gender
  - Women more commonly affected
- Epidemiology
  - AD most common neurodegenerative dementia
    - 50-75% of dementia cases
    - > 30 million people worldwide
- Other risk factors
  - Family history (20%)
  - Head trauma, metabolic syndrome

Natural History & Prognosis

- Chronic, progressive

Treatment

- May mildly improve cognitive function, delay decline in memory + cognitive functions by 9-12 months
  - Cholinesterase inhibitors, NMDA receptor antagonists

DIAGNOSTIC CHECKLIST

Consider

- Look for
  - Space-occupying lesions, intracerebral hemorrhage
  - Evidence of ischemic stroke (probable AD) **or** concurrent mild microvascular ischemic disease or stroke (possible AD)
  - Ventricular enlargement, sulcal widening proportionate
  - ↑ temporal horns of lateral ventricle
  - Hippocampal, entorhinal cortex volume loss

Image Interpretation Pearls

- MR volumetric analysis helps distinguish MCI at risk for AD from normal elderly subjects
  - Measure change hippocampus/parahippocampal gyri over time
- FDG-18 PET
  - Helps distinguish AD from frontotemporal dementia
  - May identify early AD when MR normal

SELECTED REFERENCES

1. Dai W et al: Mild cognitive impairment and alzheimer disease: patterns of altered cerebral blood flow at MR imaging. Radiology. 250(3):856-66, 2009
2. McEvoy LK et al: Alzheimer disease: quantitative structural neuroimaging for detection and prediction of clinical and structural changes in mild cognitive impairment. Radiology. 251(1):195-205, 2009

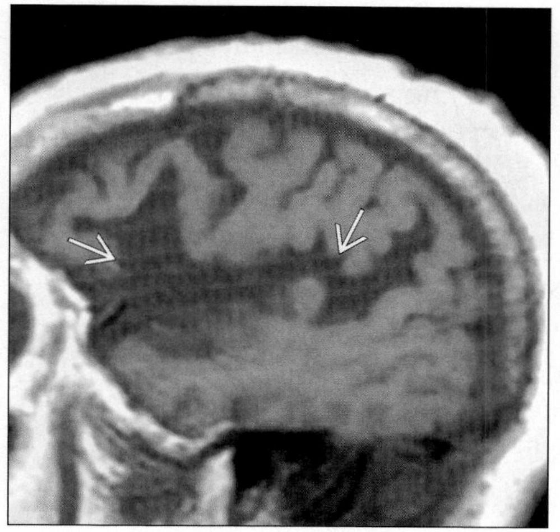

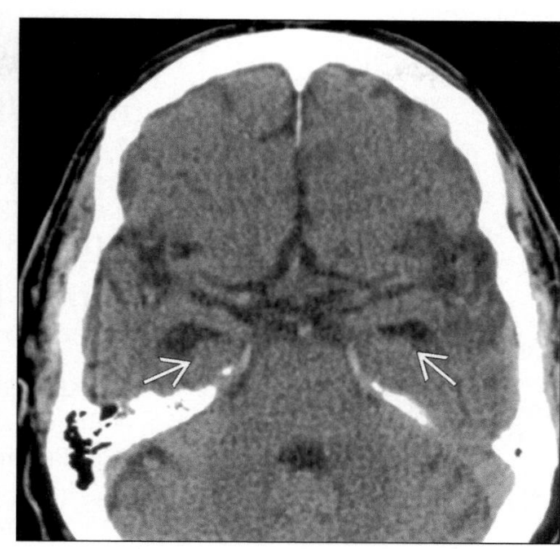

(Left) *Sagittal T1WI MR in a 72-year-old patient with suspected AD shows marked enlargement of the sylvian fissure ➔ compared to the other subarachnoid spaces. Cortical atrophy of structures around the sylvian fissures can be striking, as in this case.* ***(Right)*** *Axial NECT in a 59 year old with AD shows hippocampal atrophy is present as evidenced by temporal horn enlargement ➔. Both sylvian fissures are also very prominent. There was no evidence for intracranial mass lesion or ischemia/infarction.*

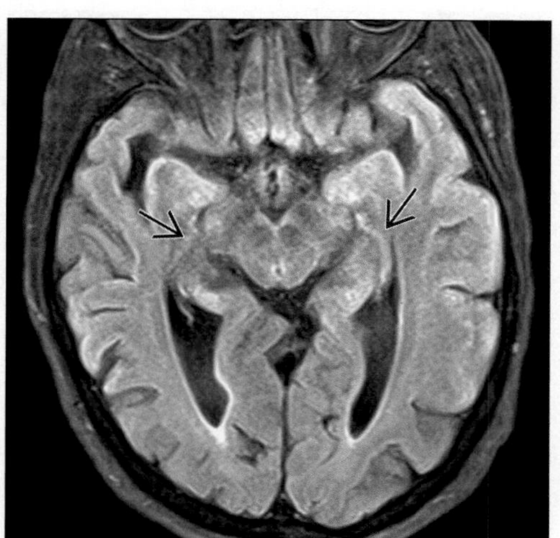

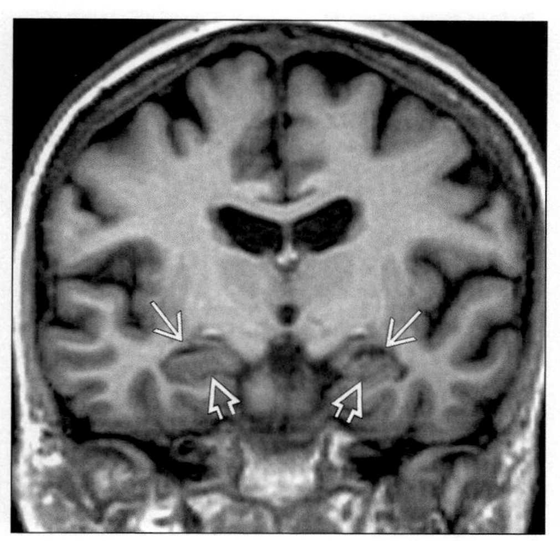

(Left) *Axial FLAIR scan in a 54-year-old woman with possible AD. While the sylvian fissures are slightly enlarged and the lateral ventricles are prominent for the patient's age, the hippocampi ➔ appear normal with no evidence for parenchymal ischemic lesions.* ***(Right)*** *Coronal MP-RAGE in same patient shows normal-appearing temporal horns ➔. Hippocampi ➲ show no evidence for volume loss. While volumetric analysis may have disclosed subtle abnormalities, the study was called normal.*

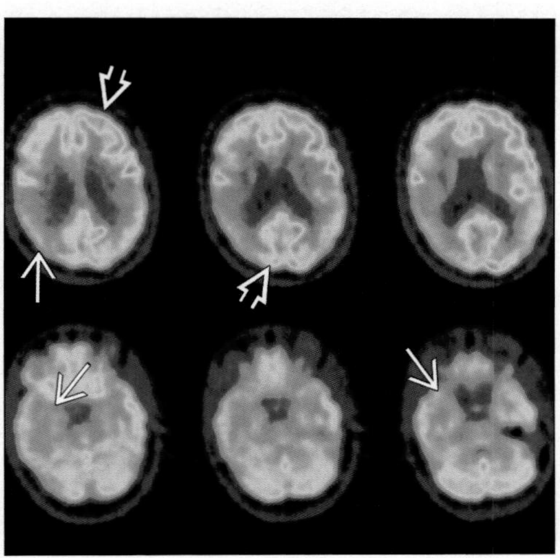

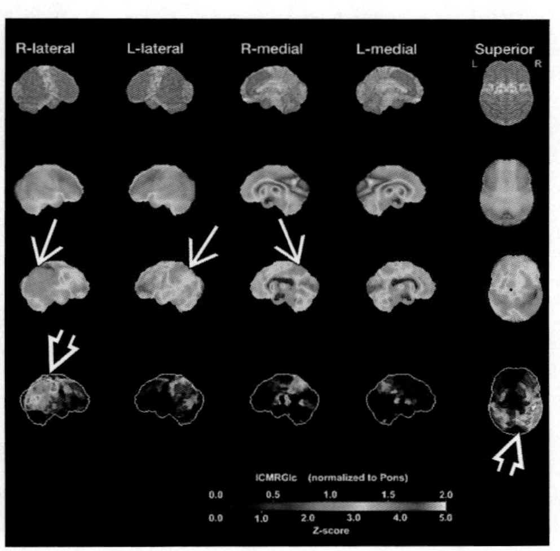

(Left) *Selected axial images from FDG-18 PET study in the same patient show a subtle decrease in glucose metabolism in the temporal and parietal lobes ➔ compared to the frontal and occipital lobes ➲.* ***(Right)*** *The stereotaxic surface projection in the same patient is dramatic. Mild hypometabolism is seen in the temporal lobes and especially diminished in the parietal lobes ➔. The Z-score map demonstrates the hypometabolism ➲ very well. (Courtesy N. Foster, MD.)*

VASCULAR DEMENTIA

Key Facts

Terminology

- Vascular dementia (VaD), multi-infarct dementia (MID)
- Stepwise progressive ↓ in cognitive function
- Heterogeneous group of disorders with varying etiologies, pathologic subtypes
  - VaD often mixed etiology
  - Can occur alone or in association with AD
  - MID secondary to repeated cerebral infarctions

Imaging

- General features
  - Multifocal infarcts (cortical GM, subcortical WM)
  - Basal ganglia (BG), pons
  - Territorial as well as lacunar lesions
  - Coexisting microvascular WM disease common
- CT
  - Multifocal infarcts
  - Single or multiple, lacunar to territorial
  - WM hypointensities (discrete to confluent)
- FDG PET
  - Multifocal regions ↓ metabolism in cortex, WM

Top Differential Diagnoses

- Alzheimer disease
- Frontotemporal lobar degeneration
- CADASIL
- Dementia with Lewy bodies

Clinical Issues

- 2nd most common dementia (after AD)

Diagnostic Checklist

- Report strategically placed infarcts
- Look for hemorrhage, DWI abnormalities

*(**Left**) Axial diagram of vascular dementia shows diffuse cerebral atrophy, focal volume loss due to multiple chronic infarcts ➡, an acute left occipital lobe infarct ➡, and small lacunar infarcts in the basal ganglia/thalami ➡. (**Right**) Axial NECT demonstrates periventricular white matter hypodensity, as well as bilateral MCA and right PCA infarcts, in a patient with vascular dementia. The clinical history plus findings of infarcts in multiple separate vascular distributions is consistent with VaD.*

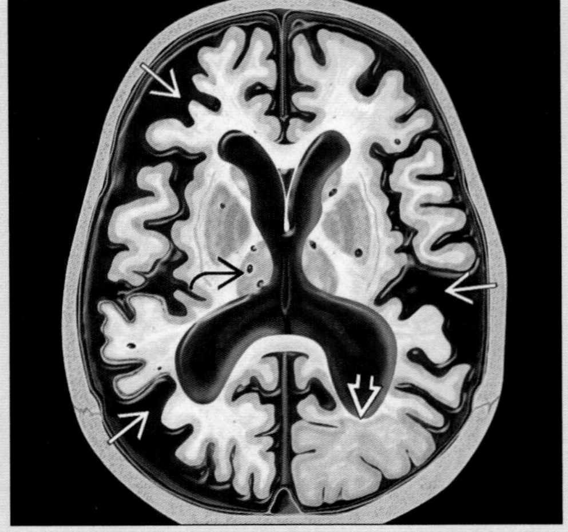

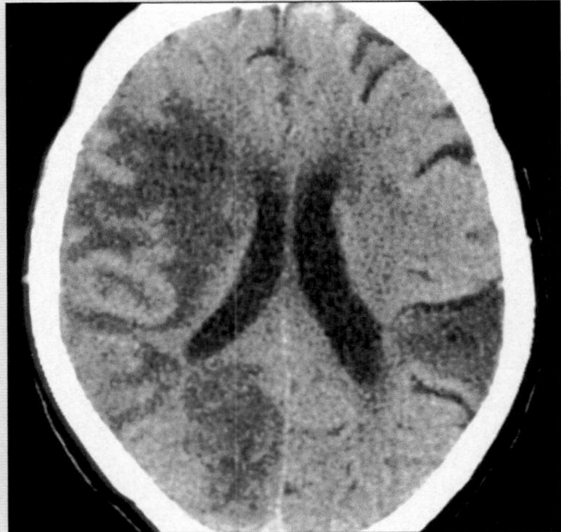

*(**Left**) Axial NECT in a patient with MID and numerous strokes shows diffuse atrophy with multiple old focal cortical infarcts ➡ and confluent periventricular white matter hypodensities ➡, consistent with arteriolosclerosis and lipohyalinosis. (**Right**) Axial FLAIR MR in the same patient shows changes of late acute/early subacute infarction in the right hemisphere ➡, old focal cortical infarcts in the left hemisphere ➡, and diffuse confluent white matter disease ➡ (arteriolosclerosis).*

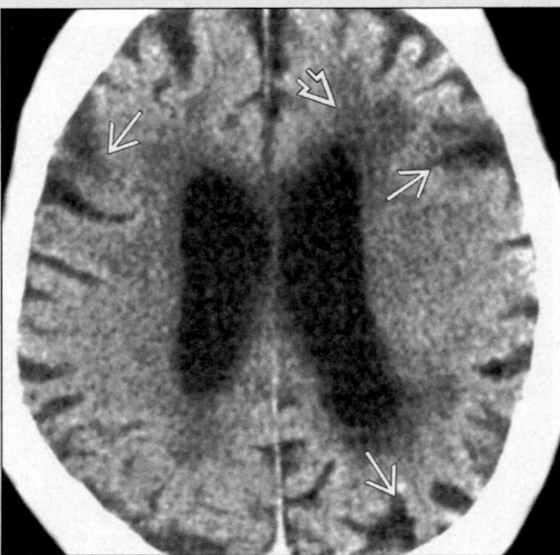

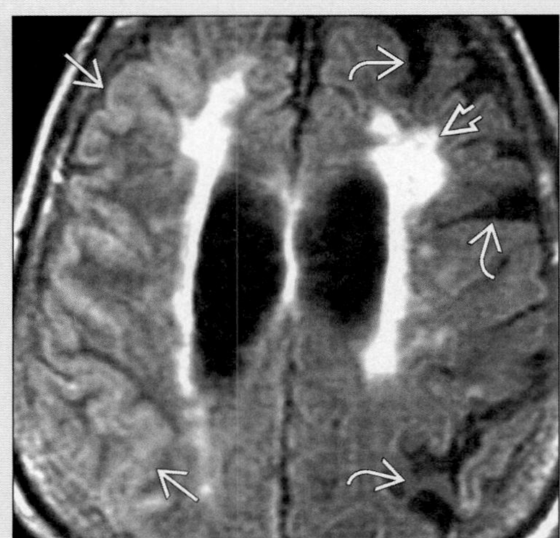

TERMINOLOGY

Abbreviations
- Vascular dementia (VaD)

Synonyms
- Multi-infarct dementia (MID)
- Vascular cognitive disorder (VCD)
- Vascular cognitive impairment (VCI)
- Alzheimer disease (AD)

Definitions
- Stepwise progressive deterioration of cognitive function
  - VaD = heterogeneous group of disorders with varying etiologies, pathologic subtypes
    - Often mixed etiology
  - Can occur alone or in association with AD
  - MID secondary to repeated cerebral infarctions

IMAGING

General Features
- Best diagnostic clue
  - Multifocal infarcts
    - Cortical gray matter (GM), subcortical white matter (WM)
    - Basal ganglia (BG), pons
    - Territorial as well as lacunar infarcts
    - Changes of microvascular WM ischemia common
- Location
  - Typically involve cerebral hemispheres and BG
  - Usually bilateral but may be unilateral
- Size
  - Vary from single to multiple, punctate to large/ confluent
- Morphology
  - Small infarcts are rounded or oval; large confluent abnormalities are ill defined

CT Findings
- NECT
  - Hypodensity in periventricular WM
  - Cortical, subcortical, BG infarcts
  - Generalized atrophy + focal cortical infarcts typical

MR Findings
- T1WI
  - Generally have hypointense BG lacunar infarcts
- T2WI
  - Central pontine infarcts
  - Punctate or confluent regions of hyperintense WM
  - Large areas of volume loss with widened sulci
- FLAIR
  - Hyperintense foci within BG, diffusely through WM, and in brain cortex
- T2* GRE
  - Many lesions have small hemorrhagic foci
- DWI
  - Diffusivity ↑ within lesions, normal-appearing WM (NAWM)
  - Increase in mean diffusivity of NAWM correlates with disability found on tests of executive function
- MRA
  - Most abnormalities in small arteries, generally not well seen on MRA
- MRS
  - ↓ NAA in both cortical and WM regions
  - Frontal cortex NAA negatively correlated with volume of WM signal hyperintensity

Ultrasonographic Findings
- Transcranial Doppler sonography: Pulsatility indices in large arteries are increased compared to AD

Nuclear Medicine Findings
- FDG PET
  - Severity of MID neuropsychiatric symptoms correlates with extent of ↓ metabolism in cortex and WM
- SPECT
  - Iodine-123 iodoamphetamine: ↓ frontal and BG CBF, which correlates with low cognitive scores
  - Technetium-99m hexamethyl propyleneamine oxime: CBF heterogeneity more prominent in anterior portion of brain
    - Unlike pattern in Alzheimer disease, in which posterior abnormalities predominate

Imaging Recommendations
- Best imaging tool
  - MR
  - PET or SPECT may also provide specificity
- Protocol advice
  - Axial FLAIR to detect white matter infarcts
  - Axial and coronal T2WI to assess regions of atrophy
  - T2* GRE to identify hemorrhage

DIFFERENTIAL DIAGNOSIS

Alzheimer Disease
- Striking hippocampus and amygdala atrophy
- PET: Bilateral temporoparietal hypoperfusion/ hypometabolism (BG spared)
- Often coexists with VaD

Frontotemporal Lobar Degeneration
- Characterized by early onset of behavioral changes with intact visual, spatial skills
- Frontal, temporal lobe atrophy
- Marked atrophy → knife-like gyri

Alcoholic Encephalopathy
- 3rd most common cause of dementia
- Generalized > focal atrophy; superior vermis atrophy

CADASIL
- Most common heritable cause of stroke, VaD in adults
- Earlier age of onset
- Imaging looks like "small vessel" disease

Dementia with Lewy Bodies
- Hypometabolism of entire brain
- Without infarcts or significant atrophy

VASCULAR DEMENTIA

PATHOLOGY

General Features

- Etiology
  - MID is usually due to multiple small infarctions
    - Infarcts involving entire major vessel territories are usually absent
    - Minority may be secondary to single or a few large infarctions
  - ~ 75% of all MID patients exhibit small vessel disease rather than thromboembolism
  - Growing evidence exists for involvement of cholinergic system in VaD
    - Cholinergic deficits well documented in VaD, independent of concomitant AD pathology
    - Cholinergic neuron loss in 70% of AD, 40% of VaD
- Genetics
  - Apolipoprotein E (*APOE*)
    - Serum protein involved in lipid metabolism
    - Encoded at single gene locus on chromosome 19 by 3 alleles: ϵ2, ϵ3, ϵ4
    - Frequency of ϵ4 allele significantly higher among patients with AD and VaD compared to controls
    - Odds of developing AD or VaD are 4.4x and 3.7x higher (respectively) in presence of even a single ϵ4 allele
  - Paraoxonase (*PON1*)
    - Component of high-density lipoproteins with antioxidative potential
    - 2 *PON1* polymorphisms (Gln192Arg associated with enzyme activity and T-107C associated with enzyme concentration) are independent risk factors for VaD particularly in *APOE* (ϵ4)

Staging, Grading, & Classification

- 8 subtypes of VaD
  - Multi-infarct dementias: Due to large cerebral emboli, usually readily identifiable
  - Strategically placed infarctions causing dementia
  - Multiple subcortical lacunar lesions: Develop VaD 5-25x more frequently than age-matched controls
  - Binswanger disease: Small vessel disease → widespread incomplete infarction of WM
  - Mixtures of 2 or more VaD subtypes
  - Hemorrhagic lesions causing dementia
  - Subcortical dementias due to other causes, e.g., cerebral autosomal dominant arteriopathy with subcortical infarcts and leukoencephalopathy (CADASIL)
  - Hybrid forms of Alzheimer dementia and VaD

Gross Pathologic & Surgical Features

- Multifocal infarctions with atrophy

Microscopic Features

- Myelin and axonal loss with astrocytosis
- Vessels display atheromata, lipohyalinosis, subintimal thickening, fibrinoid necrosis
- Infarcted tissue undergoes necrosis → gliotic wall surrounding CSF cavity

CLINICAL ISSUES

Presentation

- Most common signs/symptoms
  - Infarcts with transient focal neurologic deficits
    - Most deficits persist
  - Mood and behavioral changes
  - Severe depression is more common in VaD than AD
  - Deterioration of executive function and attention, changes in personality (rather than memory loss) predominate
- Clinical profile
  - Main risk factors
    - Advanced age, hypertension, diabetes, smoking
    - Hypercholesterolemia, hypercoagulable states

Demographics

- Age
  - Generally earlier age than AD
  - Incidence ↑ with age
- Gender
  - M > F
- Epidemiology
  - 10-30% of dementias
  - 2nd most common dementia (after AD)
  - Approximately 25% of elderly stroke patients meet VaD criteria

Natural History & Prognosis

- Progressive, episodic, stepwise downward course
- Intervals of clinical stabilization ± limited recovery
- 5-year survival with VaD ~ 50% of age-matched controls

Treatment

- Prevent further vascular insult
  - Control precipitating factors (e.g., HTN)

DIAGNOSTIC CHECKLIST

Image Interpretation Pearls

- Not a single entity, but a large group of conditions with variable clinical and imaging findings

Reporting Tips

- Report strategically placed infarcts, hemorrhagic components, DWI abnormalities, pattern of cortical volume loss if present

SELECTED REFERENCES

1. Dufouil C et al: Severe cerebral white matter hyperintensities predict severe cognitive decline in patients with cerebrovascular disease history. Stroke. 40(6):2219-21, 2009
2. Targosz-Gajniak M et al: Cerebral white matter lesions in patients with dementia - from MCI to severe Alzheimer's disease. J Neurol Sci. 283(1-2):79-82, 2009
3. Jellinger KA: Morphologic diagnosis of "vascular dementia" - a critical update. J Neurol Sci. 270(1-2):1-12, 2008

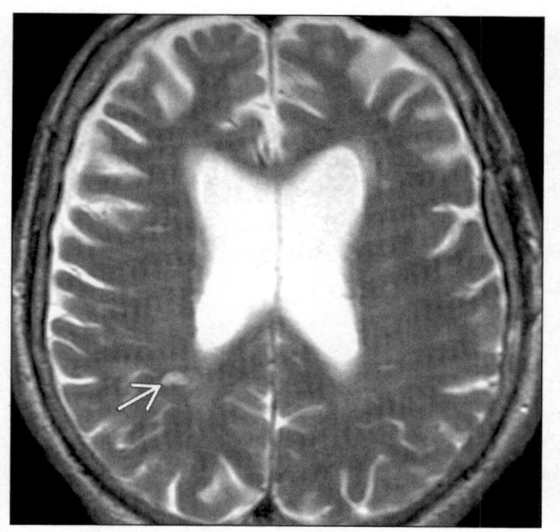

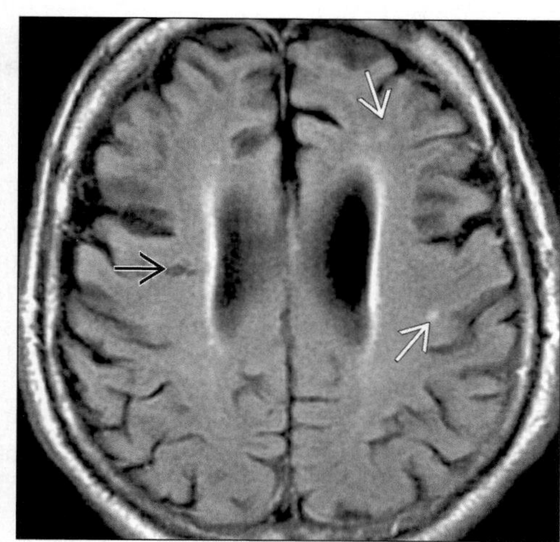

(Left) *Axial T2WI MR in an 82-year-old woman with clinical vascular dementia shows age-appropriate sulcal prominence, enlarged ventricles, and a focal right parietal lacunar infarct ➔.* ***(Right)*** *Axial FLAIR MR in the same patient shows another lacunar infarct in the right deep hemispheric white matter →. A few scattered white matter hyperintensities are present ➔ but within normal limits for the patient's age. MR images do not explain fully the extent of the patient's cognitive impairment.*

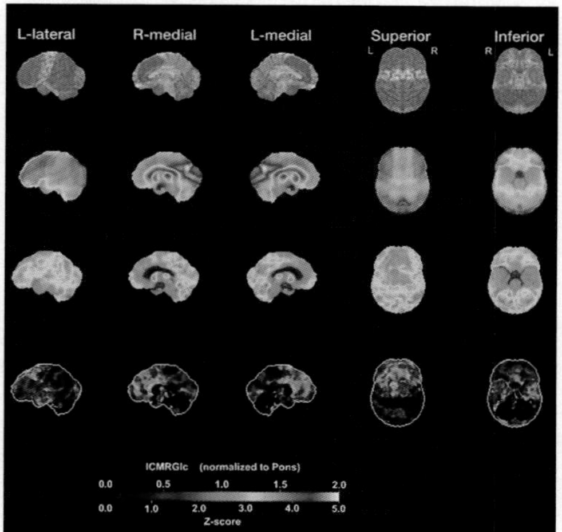

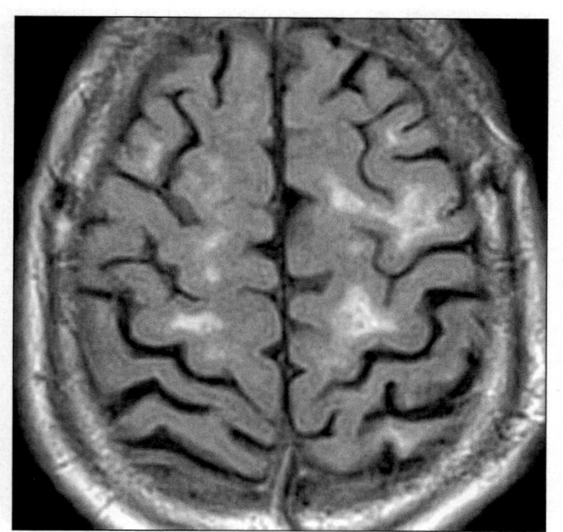

(Left) *PET scan in the same patient was performed. Stereotaxic surface projections show normal glucose metabolism in age-matched controls (2nd row). The patient's scan (3rd row) shows multifocal cortical areas of decreased glucose metabolism. Z-scores are shown on the bottom row. (Courtesy N. Foster, MD.)* ***(Right)*** *Axial FLAIR MR shows multiple subcortical hyperintensities in a 76-year-old normotensive man with clinical diagnosis of vascular dementia. No focal infarcts are seen.*

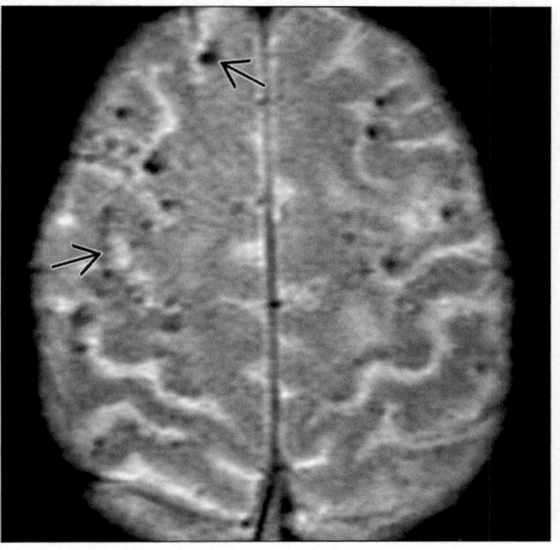

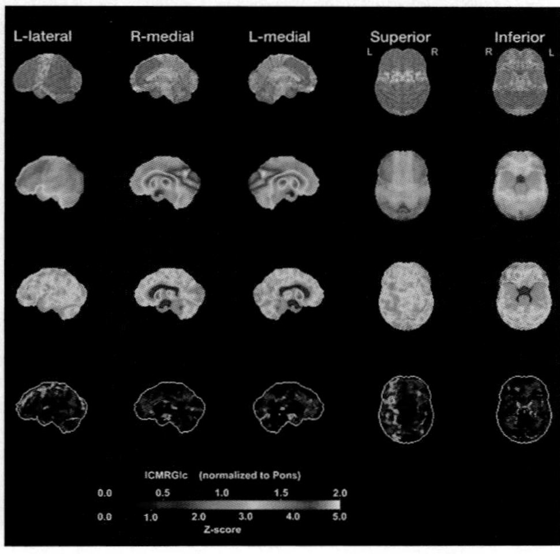

(Left) *Axial T2* GRE MR in the same patient shows multifocal cortical/subcortical blooming "black dots" →. The cerebellum and basal ganglia were spared, suggesting amyloid angiopathy as the most likely diagnosis.* ***(Right)*** *PET scan in the same patient shows multifocal areas of diminished glucose metabolism (3rd row) compared to normal age-matched controls (2nd row). Z-score maps (bottom row) confirm the multifocal, diffuse nature of this patient's vascular disease. (Courtesy N. Foster, MD).*

FRONTOTEMPORAL LOBAR DEGENERATION

Key Facts

Terminology

- Frontotemporal lobar degeneration (FTLD)
- Clinical subtypes
  - Frontotemporal dementia (FTD)
  - Semantic dementia (SD)
  - Nonfluent aphasia (NFA)

Imaging

- Early
  - PET shows frontotemporal ↓ glucose metabolism
- Late: Frontotemporal atrophy with knife-like gyri on MR
- Subtypes have characteristic cortical atrophy patterns
- Frontal vs. temporal, R vs. L help discriminate
  - FTD: Bilateral frontotemporal, R > L
  - SD: Predominately temporal atrophy
  - NFA: Bilateral frontotemporal, R < L

Top Differential Diagnoses

- Alzheimer dementia (AD)
- Vascular dementia
- Corticobasal ganglionic degeneration (CBD)
- Dementia with Lewy bodies (DLB)

Clinical Issues

- FTLD < 10% of primary degenerative dementias
  - 3rd most common cortical dementia
  - 2nd most common early-onset cortical dementia
- Onset usually < 70 years
  - Peak incidence 45-65 years
- Clinical syndromes (some overlap)
  - FTD: Early changes in personality; aphasia absent
  - SD: Fluent speech, progressive anomia/word comprehension
  - NFA: Progressive deficits in speech production

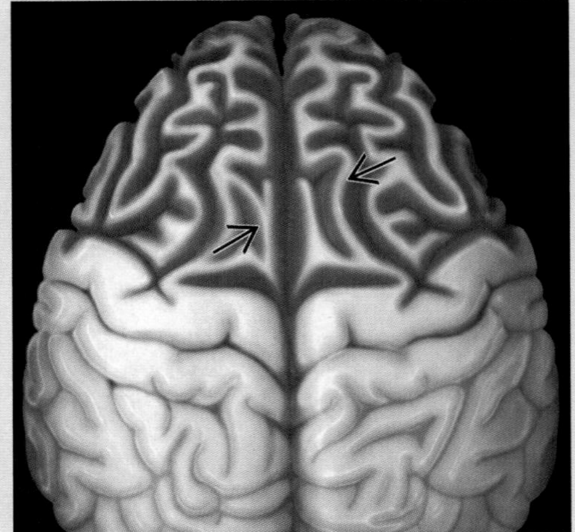

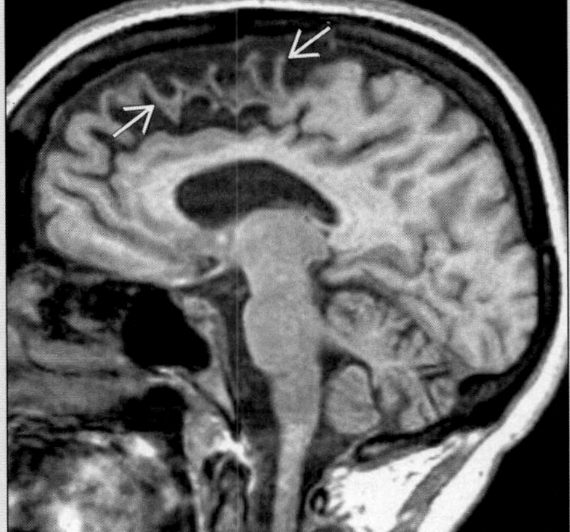

(Left) *Graphic depicts the classic disproportionate frontal lobe atrophy of late-stage frontotemporal dementia (FTD). The sulci are widened and gyri are knife-like →. Parietal occipital lobes are spared. Gyri around the central sulcus are normal.* ***(Right)*** *Parasagittal image (3D-MPRAGE) was obtained as part of the initial evaluation in a patient with suspected FTD. Note the frontal lobe knife-like gyri → with markedly widened sulci and preservation of the parietal and occipital lobes.*

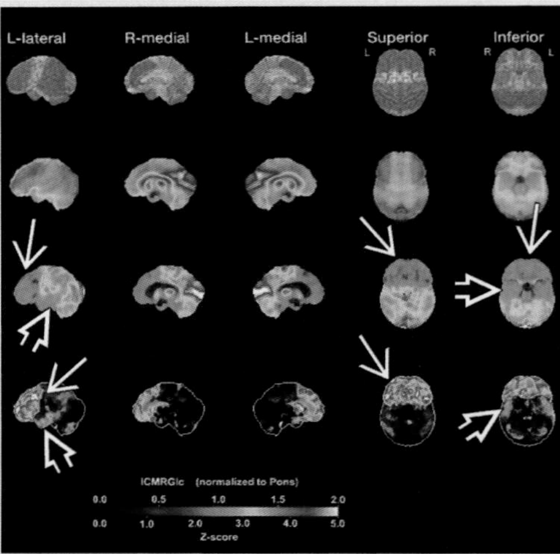

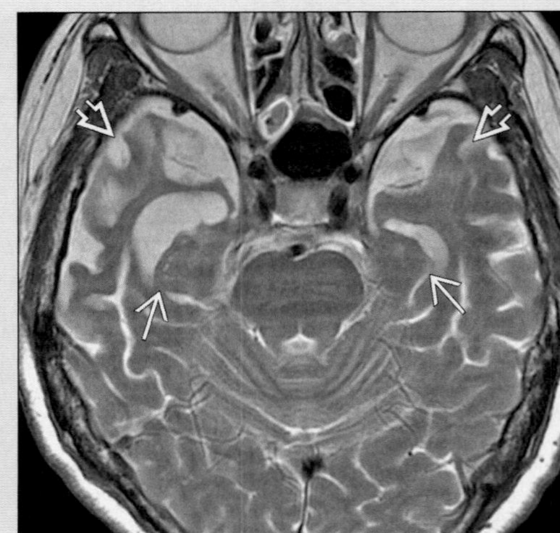

(Left) *Sagittal SSP FDG PET scan in a 72-year-old man with FTD shows a normal elderly control map (2nd row), the patient's glucose metabolism (3rd row), and Z-score statistical map (bottom row). The frontal lobes → are strikingly hypometabolic. The temporal lobes → are somewhat less severely affected.* ***(Right)*** *Axial T2WI MR in a patient with semantic dementia subtype of FTLD shows marked atrophy of anterolateral temporal lobes →. Note the relative preservation of the hippocampi →.*

FRONTOTEMPORAL LOBAR DEGENERATION

TERMINOLOGY

Abbreviations

- Frontotemporal lobar degeneration (FTLD)
- Clinical subtypes
  - Frontotemporal dementia (FTD)
  - Semantic dementia (SD)
  - Nonfluent aphasia (NFA)
- Frontotemporal dementia with extrapyramidal symptoms
  - Corticobasal degeneration (CBD)
  - Progressive supranuclear palsy (PSP)
- Frontotemporal dementia with motor neuron disease

Synonyms

- Pick disease no longer used
  - Referred to pathologic variant with Pick bodies

Definitions

- Degeneration with focal cortical atrophy involving frontal &/or temporal lobes

IMAGING

General Features

- Best diagnostic clue
  - PET scan showing frontotemporal ↓ glucose metabolism
  - Anterior frontotemporal atrophy with knife-like gyri
- Location
  - Anterior temporal/frontal lobes, orbital frontal lobe, medial temporal lobes
  - Relative sparing of
    - Posterior aspect of superior temporal gyrus
    - Pre- and postcentral gyri
    - Parietal, occipital lobes
- Morphology
  - "Knife blade" appearance of atrophic gyri
  - ± marked asymmetry
    - May have worst atrophy in dominant hemisphere

CT Findings

- NECT
  - Frontal lobe atrophy often most prominent feature
    - Increased size of frontal horns (larger than rest of lateral ventricles)
  - ± caudate atrophy (also reported)

MR Findings

- T1WI
  - Knife-like gyri with normal signal
  - Dilated frontal sulci reflecting atrophy
- T2WI
  - ± hyperintensity in frontotemporal WM
- FLAIR
  - ± hyperintensity in frontotemporal WM
- MRS
  - ↓ NAA and glutamate-plus-glutamine (neuronal loss), ↑ myoinositol (↑ glial content) in frontal lobes
    - ↓ NAA in posterior cingulate gyri
    - Reflects ↓ neuronal population, viability
  - ± lactate peak in frontal lobes
  - ↑ phosphomonoester, phosphodiester
- MR volumetry (3D MP RAGE)
  - Subtypes have characteristic cortical atrophy patterns
    - Frontal vs. temporal, L vs. R help discriminate
      - FTD: Bilateral frontotemporal, R > L
      - SD: Predominately temporal atrophy
      - NFA: Bilateral frontotemporal, R < L
- DTI
  - ↓ FA in frontal, temporal regions
    - Anterior corpus callosum
    - Anterior, posterior cingulum
    - Uncinate fasciculus

Nuclear Medicine Findings

- PET
  - FDG PET: ↓ metabolic activity in frontotemporal cortex
  - Amyloid imaging (11C-labeled Pittsburgh compound-B) helps differentiate FTLD from Alzheimer disease
- HMPAO-SPECT
  - Sensitive technique for early detection of FTD
    - Hypoperfusion in ventromedial frontal region
    - Occurs before atrophy is evident
  - Semantic dementia
    - Hypoperfusion of 1 or both temporal lobes
- SPECT perfusion deficits predominantly in frontal and anterior temporal lobes with preserved perfusion posteriorly
  - Helps distinguishes FTD from Alzheimer disease
- Reduced frontal perfusion is not specific to FTD but also occurs in some cases of schizophrenia, depression, HIV encephalopathy, Creutzfeldt-Jakob disease, Alzheimer disease

Imaging Recommendations

- Best imaging tool
  - PET; MR with volumetry
- Protocol advice
  - Routine T1WI, T2WI, coronal T2WI

DIFFERENTIAL DIAGNOSIS

Alzheimer Disease (AD)

- Parietal and temporal cortical atrophy with disproportionate hippocampal volume loss
- Increased rate of atrophy in FTD compared to AD
- Often coexisting microvascular disease, white matter hyperintensities
- Amyloid imaging (11C-labeled Pittsburgh Compound-B) helps to differentiate AD from other dementias when clinical diagnosis of AD is uncertain

Vascular Dementia

- 2nd most common dementia (15-30%)
- White matter and deep gray lacunae
- Hyperintense lesions on T2WI, hypodense areas on CT, and focal atrophy is suggestive of chronic infarcts

Corticobasal Degeneration

- Prominent extrapyramidal, cortical symptoms
- Severe frontoparietal atrophy
- Atrophy of paracentral structures

FRONTOTEMPORAL LOBAR DEGENERATION

Dementia with Lewy Bodies (DLB)
- Hypometabolism of entire brain, especially visual cortex
- Visual and auditory hallucinations, paranoid delusions

PATHOLOGY

General Features
- Etiology
  - Tau protein (hyperphosphorylated microtubular protein) or TDP-47 (TAR DNA-binding protein-43)
- Genetics
  - 25-40% of FTD is familial
  - Many genes involved in FTLD
    - Most common = microtubule-associated protein tau
      - Reported in up to 50% of FTLD patients

Staging, Grading, & Classification
- Classification of genotypes and proteotypes
  - Tauopathy (FTLD-τ)
    - "Pick disease" was 1st form of FTD described (1892)
    - Characterized by Pick body (argyrophilic inclusion in cortical layer 2/6)
  - Nontauopathy
    - FTLD with ubiquitin-positive neuronal inclusion (FTLD-U)

Gross Pathologic & Surgical Features
- Thin cortex, indistinct gray-white matter junction
- Firm cortical gray matter (gliosis)
- Soft, retracted subcortical white matter

Microscopic Features
- In affected brain areas: Almost complete loss of large pyramidal neurons, diffuse spongiosis, and gliosis
- Neuronal loss, gliosis in CA1 and subicular regions of hippocampus → hippocampal sclerosis
- Immunohistochemical stain
  - Tau positive (PiD) vs. ubiquitin positive (FTLD-U) vs. none (DLDH)

CLINICAL ISSUES

Presentation
- Most common signs/symptoms
  - Personality, behavior, and language changes
  - Memory loss, confusion, cognitive and speech dysfunction, apathy, and abulia
- Clinical profile
  - Frontal variant FTD (dementia of frontal type, 40%): Changes in social behavior and personality predominate
  - Semantic dementia (progressive fluent aphasia, 40%): Changes in social behavior and personality predominate
  - Progressive nonfluent aphasia (primary progressive aphasia): Nonfluent speech output, agrammatism, telegraphic speech

Demographics
- Age
  - Younger age group than Alzheimer disease
    - Onset usually < 70 years
    - Peak incidence 45-65 years
- Gender
  - Affects both genders equally
- Ethnicity
  - Familial forms of Pick-complex dementias particularly common in people of Scandinavian origin
- Epidemiology
  - < 10% of primary degenerative dementias; 3rd most common cortical dementia after Alzheimer disease and diffuse Lewy body disease

Natural History & Prognosis
- Insidious onset of behavioral and cognitive dysfunction
- Speech and language disturbance are often more profound than memory disorder
- Eventual loss of verbal and problem-solving skills
- Some patients develop artistic talents during course of dementia (disinhibition of "creative" brain areas)

DIAGNOSTIC CHECKLIST

Consider
- Other common forms of dementia (AD, DLB)

Image Interpretation Pearls
- Bilateral frontal lobe atrophy should cause diagnosis of FTD to be considered
- Bilateral asymmetric anterior temporal lobe atrophy: SD variant of FTD

Reporting Tips
- Report pattern of cortical volume loss

SELECTED REFERENCES

1. King RD et al: Characterization of atrophic changes in the cerebral cortex using fractal dimensional analysis. Brain Imaging and Behavior 3(2):154-66, 2009
2. Krueger CE et al: Longitudinal Rates of Lobar Atrophy in Frontotemporal Dementia, Semantic Dementia, and Alzheimer's Disease. Alzheimer Dis Assoc Disord. Epub ahead of print, 2009
3. Lindberg O et al: Cortical morphometric subclassification of frontotemporal lobar degeneration. AJNR Am J Neuroradiol. 30(6):1233-9, 2009
4. Moon WJ et al: Atrophy measurement of the anterior commissure and substantia innominata with 3T high-resolution MR imaging: does the measurement differ for patients with frontotemporal lobar degeneration and Alzheimer disease and for healthy subjects? AJNR Am J Neuroradiol. 29(7):1308-13, 2008

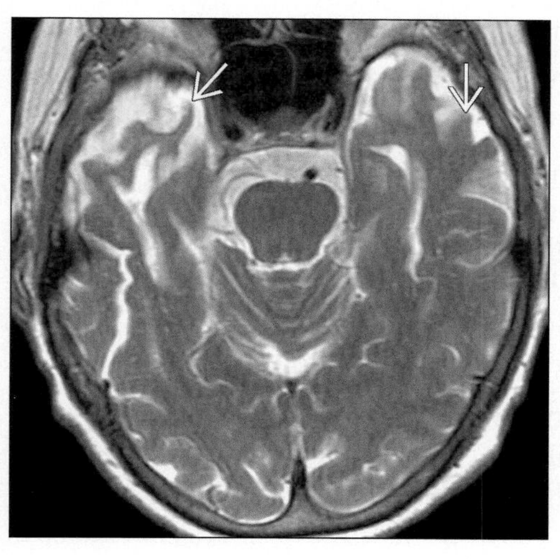

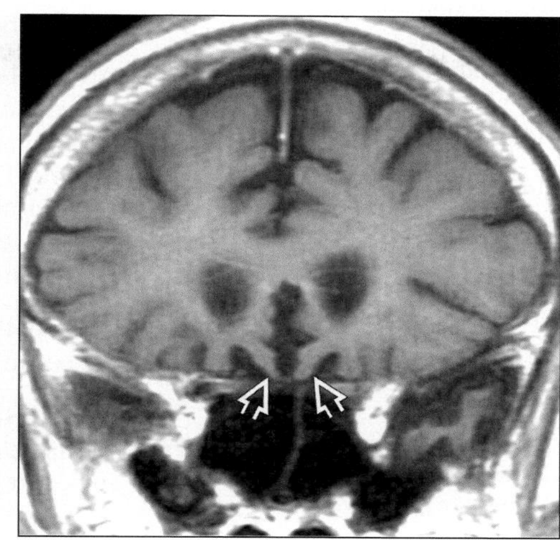

(Left) *Axial T2WI MR in a 57-year-old woman with probable FTD shows temporal lobe atrophy with knife-like gyri ➔. The parietal and occipital lobes are relatively well preserved.* ***(Right)*** *Coronal T1WI MR in the same patient shows focal atrophy of the olfactory gyri ➔. This finding was initially overlooked, and the patient was given the imaging diagnosis of Alzheimer disease. Review and subsequent clinical evaluation confirmed frontotemporal dementia.*

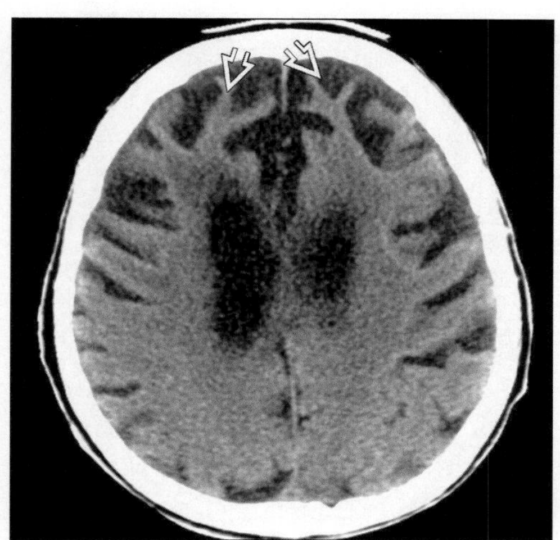

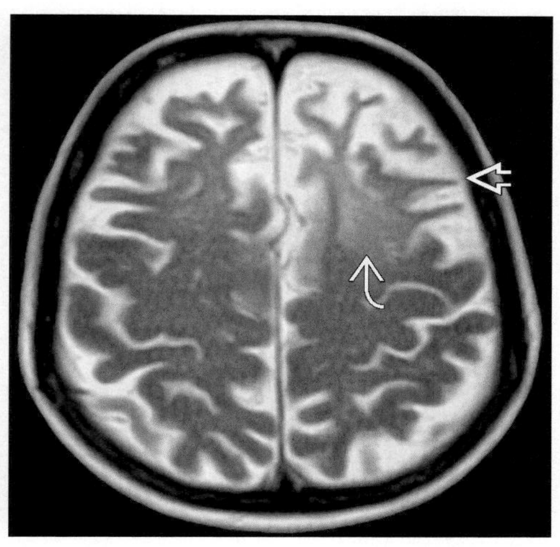

(Left) *Axial NECT in a 78-year-old patient diagnosed with late-stage FTD through the upper lateral ventricles shows striking frontal lobar atrophy, with classic knife-like gyri ➔ characteristic of FTD. In contrast, the parietal and occipital lobes appear relatively spared.* ***(Right)*** *Axial T2WI MR in a patient with classic FTD shows predominantly frontal lobar atrophy ➔. In this case, an associated region of hyperintense white matter ➔ is present.*

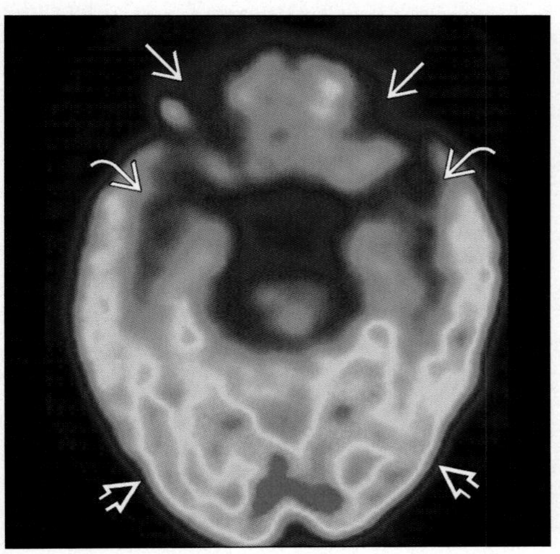

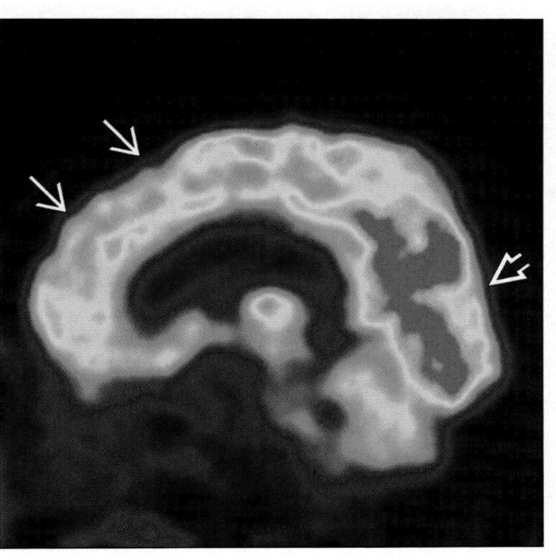

(Left) *Axial FDG PET in a patient with FTD shows decreased glucose metabolism in frontal ➔ and temporal lobes ➔. The parietal and occipital lobes ➔ are spared.* ***(Right)*** *Sagittal FDG PET in the same patient with FTD depicts glucose hypometabolism in the frontal lobes ➔. The occipital lobes ➔ are normal.*

DEMENTIA WITH LEWY BODIES

Key Facts

Terminology

- Progressive neurodegenerative dementia
  - Parkinsonism, visual hallucinations prominent
  - Caused by abnormal accumulation of α-synuclein protein

Imaging

- Difficult to appreciate on standard MR
  - MR helps ↓ likelihood of AD
  - Lobar atrophy less severe, slower than AD
- MR volumetry
  - DLB has less hippocampal atrophy than AD
  - Greater atrophy of putamen than AD
  - ± midbrain, substantia innominata, hypothalamus
- FDG PET
  - ↓ ↓ in glucose metabolism in occipital cortex, especially primary visual cortex
  - Sensitivity 86%, specificity 90%
- 18F-fluorodopa-PET
  - ↓ ↓ striatal dopamine uptake (sensitivity 86%, specificity 100% vs. AD)

Top Differential Diagnoses

- Parkinson disease-associated dementia (PDD)
  - Similar clinical, pathological, imaging features with DLB
- Alzheimer disease (AD)
- Frontotemporal lobar degeneration (FTLD)
- Vascular dementia

Pathology

- Accumulation of Lewy bodies (LB)

Diagnostic Checklist

- Unlike Alzheimer disease, medial temporal lobe atrophy not a prominent feature

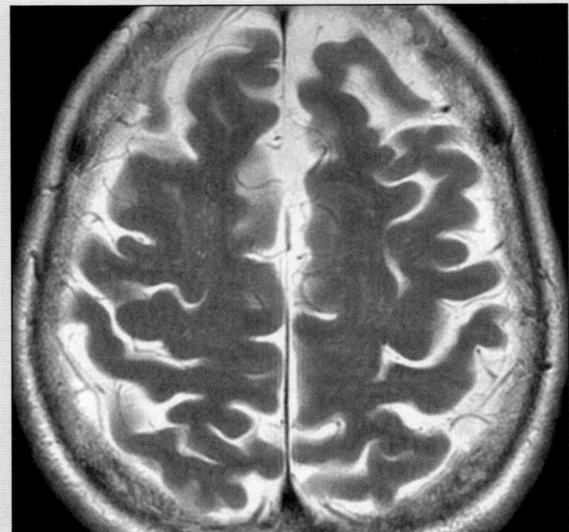

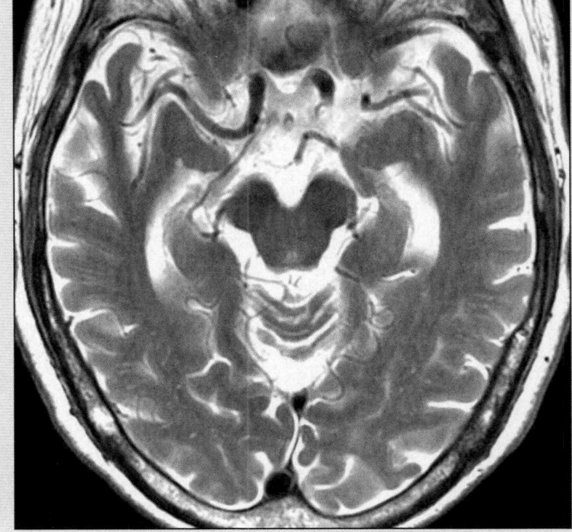

(Left) *Axial T2WI MR in a patient with cognitive decline, visual hallucination, and parkinsonism shows diffuse cortical atrophy, consistent with dementia with Lewy bodies.* ***(Right)*** *Axial T2WI MR in the same patient exhibits mild atrophy of the medial temporal lobes.*

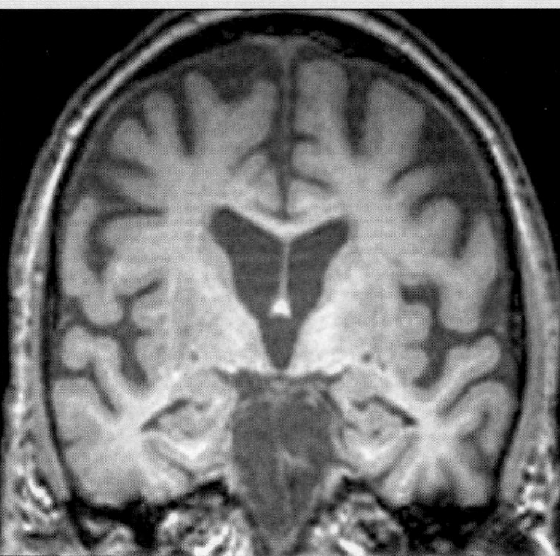

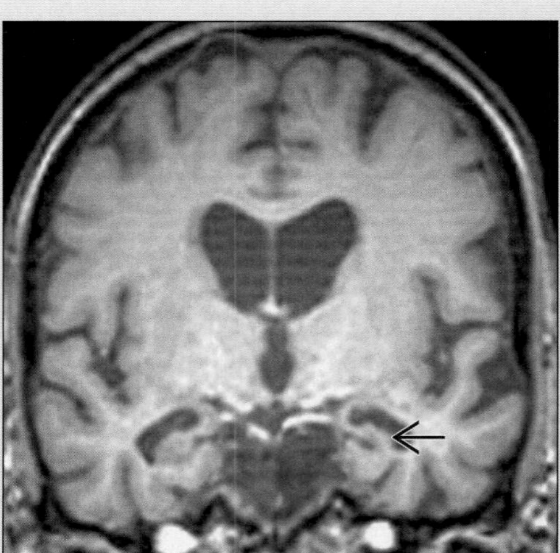

(Left) *Coronal T1WI MR in a patient with dementia with Lewy bodies shows prominent frontal lobe volume loss with relative sparing of hippocampal volume. (Courtesy M.J. Firbank, MD, and J.T. O'Brien, MD.)* ***(Right)*** *Coronal T1WI MR in a patient with Alzheimer disease shows marked hippocampal volume loss ⇒ and relative sparing of frontal lobes compared to the patient from the previous image with dementia with Lewy bodies. (Courtesy M.J. Firbank, MD, and J.T. O'Brien, MD.)*

DEMENTIA WITH LEWY BODIES

TERMINOLOGY

Abbreviations

- Dementia with Lewy bodies (DLB)

Definitions

- Progressive neurodegenerative dementia
  - Parkinsonism, visual hallucinations prominent features
  - Caused by abnormal accumulation of α-synuclein protein

IMAGING

General Features

- Best diagnostic clue
  - MR may differentiate Alzheimer disease (AD) from DLB
  - PET, SPECT most useful for DLB diagnosis

Imaging Recommendations

- Best imaging tool
  - Dopamine SPECT or PET

MR Findings

- T1WI
  - Ventricular enlargement
- T2WI
  - ± ischemic changes in cerebral white matter
- MRS
  - ↓ NAA/Cr, ↓ Glx/Cr, ↑ Cho/Cr in white matter
- MR volumetry
  - DLB has less hippocampal atrophy than AD
    - Greater atrophy of putamen than AD

Nuclear Medicine Findings

- PET
  - FDG PET: ↓ ↓ in glucose metabolism in occipital cortex, especially primary visual cortex (sensitivity 80%, specificity 90%)
- SPECT
  - Occipital lobe hypoperfusion, especially visual cortex

DIFFERENTIAL DIAGNOSIS

Parkinson Disease-Associated Dementia

- Dementia typically develops at least 12 months after onset of initial parkinsonian symptoms
- Similar clinical, pathological, imaging features to DLB

Alzheimer Disease (AD)

- Parietal/temporal cortical atrophy
  - Disproportionate hippocampal volume loss
- More severe, faster rate of progression than DLB

Frontotemporal Lobar Degeneration (FTLD)

- Asymmetric frontal, anterior temporal lobar atrophy

Vascular Dementia

- 2nd most common dementia (15-30%)
- Hyperintense lesions on T2WI, hypodense areas on CT, and focal atrophy suggestive of chronic infarcts

PATHOLOGY

General Features

- Etiology
  - Accumulation of Lewy bodies (LB)
- Genetics
  - Majority of DLB is sporadic; some are familial

Staging, Grading, & Classification

- 3 major forms: Brainstem dominant, limbic/transitional, diffuse neocortical

Microscopic Features

- LBs in substantia nigra, neocortex, limbic system
  - Intracellular protein aggregates
  - Mainly composed of α-synuclein protein

CLINICAL ISSUES

Presentation

- Most common signs/symptoms
  - Cognitive decline, fluctuations in level of alertness
  - Visual hallucinations, parkinsonian features

Demographics

- Age
  - 55-85 years; age is only risk factor
- Gender
  - Men more commonly affected
- Epidemiology
  - 20% of dementia cases
  - 3rd most common cause of dementia (after Alzheimer disease, vascular dementia)

Natural History & Prognosis

- Average survival after diagnosis = 8 years

DIAGNOSTIC CHECKLIST

Image Interpretation Pearls

- No characteristic features on standard MR

SELECTED REFERENCES

1. Burton EJ et al: Medial temporal lobe atrophy on MRI differentiates Alzheimer's disease from dementia with Lewy bodies and vascular cognitive impairment: a prospective study with pathological verification of diagnosis. Brain. 132(Pt 1):195-203, 2009
2. Schmidt SL et al: Value of combining activated brain FDG-PET and cardiac MIBG for the differential diagnosis of dementia: differentiation of dementia with Lewy bodies and Alzheimer disease when the diagnoses based on clinical and neuroimaging criteria are difficult. Clin Nucl Med. 33(6):398-401, 2008
3. Whitwell JL et al: Focal atrophy in dementia with Lewy bodies on MRI: a distinct pattern from Alzheimer's disease. Brain. 130(Pt 3):708-19, 2007

CREUTZFELDT-JAKOB DISEASE (CJD)

Key Facts

Terminology

- CJD: Rapidly progressing, fatal, potentially transmissible dementia caused by a prion

Imaging

- Best imaging clue: Progressive T2 hyperintensity of basal ganglia (BG), thalamus, and cerebral cortex
- Predominantly gray matter (GM): Caudate and putamen > GP
  - Thalamus: Common in variant CJD (vCJD)
  - Cerebral cortex: Frontal, parietal, and temporal
- Heidenhain variant: Occipital lobe
- 2 signs characteristic of vCJD
  - "Pulvinar" sign: Symmetric T2 hyperintensity of pulvinar of thalamus relative to anterior putamen
  - "Hockey stick" sign: Symmetric pulvinar and dorsomedial thalamic nuclear hyperintensity
- Best imaging tool: MR with DWI

Top Differential Diagnoses

- Hypoxic-ischemic injury
- Osmotic demyelination syndrome
- Other causes of dementia
  - Alzheimer, frontotemporal, multi-infarct dementia, dementia in motor neuron disease
- Leigh syndrome
- Corticobasal degeneration

Clinical Issues

- Definite CJD diagnosed by brain biopsy or autopsy
- Progressive dementia associated with myoclonic jerks & akinetic mutism; variable constellation of pyramidal, extrapyramidal, and cerebellar signs
- Incidence 1 per 1,000,000 (USA and internationally)
  - sCJD (85%), familial (15%), infectious/iatrogenic (< 1%) (includes vCJD)
- Death usually ensues within months of onset

*(**Left**) Axial FLAIR MR shows symmetric hyperintensity in the caudate and putamen, characteristic of sporadic CJD (sCJD). sCJD is the most common type of CJD, representing 85% of cases. (**Right**) Axial DWI MR shows asymmetric diffusion restriction in the caudate nuclei and putamen. Involvement of the anterior more than the posterior putamen is typical of CJD. There is also asymmetric hyperintensity in the frontal and temporal lobe cortical ribbons ➔, typical of sCJD. (Courtesy N. Fischbein, MD.)*

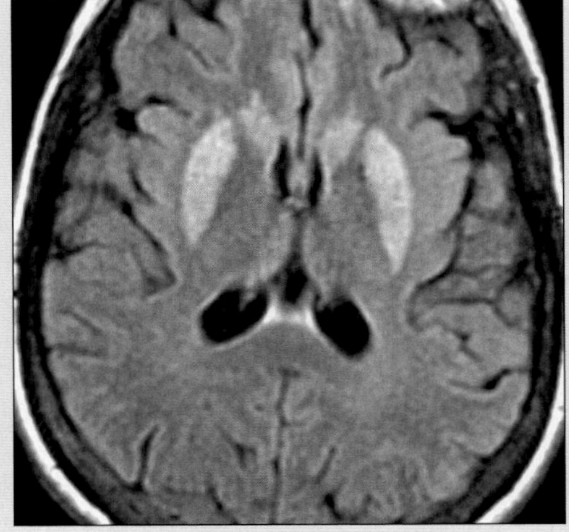

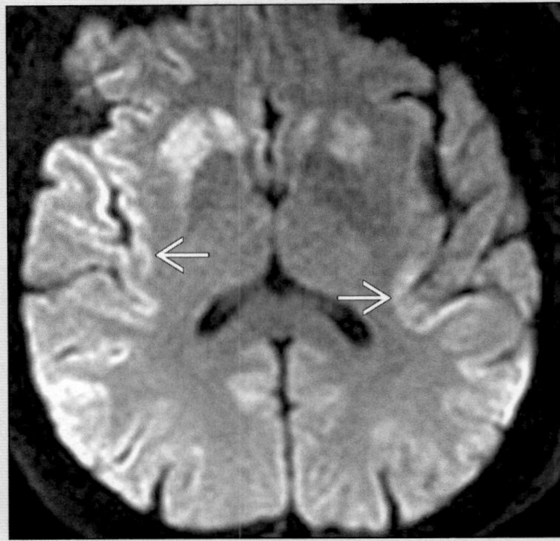

*(**Left**) Axial DWI MR shows classic sCJD with diffusion restriction in the caudate and putamen as well as throughout the cortex. Frontal, temporal, and parietal cortical involvement is most common. Relative sparing of the pre- and postcentral gyri is typical of CJD. (**Right**) Axial FLAIR MR shows bilateral, symmetric hyperintensities in the posterior thalami representing the "pulvinar" sign, which is characteristic of variant CJD. Another "pulvinar" sign is the T1 shortening seen in Fabry disease.*

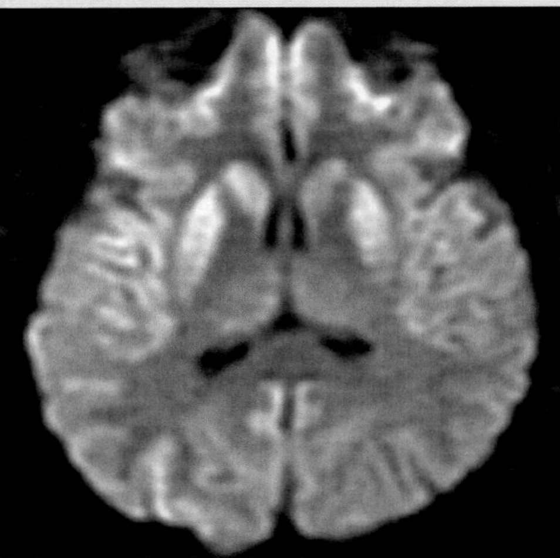

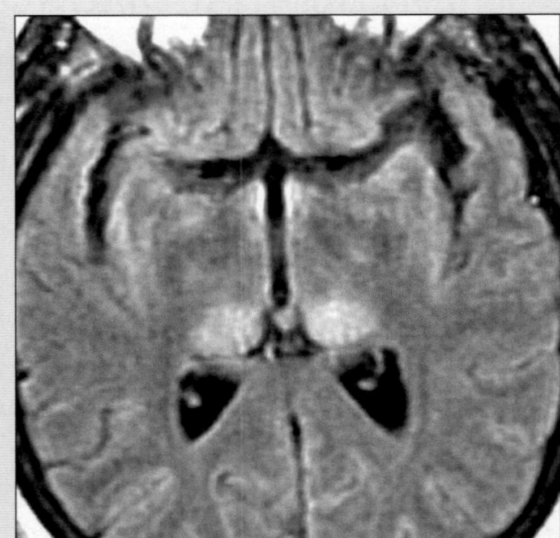

CREUTZFELDT-JAKOB DISEASE (CJD)

TERMINOLOGY

Abbreviations

- Creutzfeldt-Jakob disease (CJD)

Definitions

- Rapidly progressing, fatal, potentially transmissible dementing disorder caused by a prion (proteinaceous infectious particle devoid of DNA and RNA)
  - Transmissible spongiform encephalopathy

IMAGING

General Features

- Best diagnostic clue
  - Progressive T2 hyperintensity of basal ganglia (BG), thalamus, and cerebral cortex
- Location
  - Predominantly gray matter (GM)
    - BG: Caudate and putamen > globus pallidus (GP)
    - Thalamus (common in variant CJD)
    - Cerebral cortex (most commonly frontal, parietal, and temporal lobes)
      - Heidenhain variant: Occipital lobe
      - Brownell-Oppenheimer: Cerebellum
  - May involve only peripheral cortex
    - Cortical involvement often asymmetric
    - Primary sensorimotor cortex relatively spared
  - White matter (WM) usually not involved
- Size: Slight decrease (atrophy)
- Morphology: Hyperintense T2 signal conforms to outline of BG and gyriform pattern in cortex

CT Findings

- NECT: Usually normal (80%)
  - May show rapidly progressive atrophy and ventricular dilatation (20%)
  - Serial CT illustrates atrophy progression

MR Findings

- T1WI
  - Normal
  - GP hyperintensity reported in sporadic CJD (sCJD)
- T2WI
  - Hyperintense signal in BG and thalami
  - Hyperintense signal in cortical GM
  - Cerebral atrophy
  - With time, hyperintense foci may develop in WM
- FLAIR
  - 2 signs characteristic of variant CJD (vCJD)
    - "**Pulvinar**" sign: Bilateral symmetrical hyperintensity of **pulvinar** (posterior) nuclei of **thalamus** relative to anterior putamen
    - "**Hockey stick**" sign: Symmetrical **pulvinar and dorsomedial thalamic** nuclear hyperintensity
  - Periaqueductal GM hyperintensity
  - Cortical hyperintensity (common in sCJD)
- DWI
  - Progressive hyperintensity in striatum and cortex
  - Gyriform hyperintense areas in cerebral cortex
    - Correspond to localization of periodic sharp-wave complexes on EEG
  - DWI hyperintensity may disappear late in disease
- T1WI C+: No enhancement of lesions

Nuclear Medicine Findings

- PET: Regional glucose hypometabolism correlates with sites of neuropathologic lesions
- SPECT with N-isopropyl-p-(I-123) iodoamphetamine
  - ↓ uptake of tracer and ↓ absolute values of rCBF in various parts of cerebral cortex
    - Sometimes in asymmetrical pattern
    - Sensitive for diagnosis of early stage CJD

Imaging Recommendations

- Best imaging tool: MR with DWI and FLAIR

DIFFERENTIAL DIAGNOSIS

Hypoxic-Ischemic Injury

- BG and parasagittal cortical areas involved
- Hyperintense BG lesions on T1WI and T2WI
- DWI + symmetric GM involvement

Osmotic Demyelination Syndrome

- Extrapontine: T2 hyperintense putamen and caudate
- DWI positive acutely

Leigh Syndrome

- Primarily seen in pediatric patients
- T2 hyperintensity in putamen and GP

Other Causes of Dementia

- Alzheimer disease
- Dementia in motor neuron disease
- Frontotemporal dementia
- Multiinfarct dementia

Corticobasal Degeneration

- Neuronal loss in substantia nigra, frontoparietal cortex, and striatum (BG atrophy may be subtle)
- MR: Symmetric/asymmetric atrophy of pre- and postcentral gyri; prominent parasagittal involvement
- Subcortical gliosis: High intensity on T2WI

Wilson Disease

- WM and deep GM lesions (BG, dentate nucleus, brainstem); variably T2 hyperintense
- T1 hypointense (rarely hyperintense) lesions

Arteriolosclerosis

- BG involvement: Typically asymmetric and multifocal (rather than diffuse as in CJD)
- Focal hyperintensities in deep WM
- DWI negative, unless acute

PATHOLOGY

General Features

- Etiology
  - Prion protein is abnormal isoform (PrPSc) of normal host-encoded protein (PrPc)
    - PrPSc = conformationally modified form of PrPc
  - PrPSc introduced into healthy cells ⇒ initiates self-perpetuating vicious cycle: PrPc → PrPSc

CREUTZFELDT-JAKOB DISEASE (CJD)

- sCJD: Spontaneous PrPc → PrPSc or somatic mutation
- Familial CJD (fCJD): Mutations in *PRNP*
- Iatrogenic CJD: Infection from prion-containing material
  - Surgical instruments, dura mater grafts
  - EEG electrodes, corneal transplants
  - Human pituitary-derived gonadotrophins
  - Human-derived growth hormone
- vCJD: Bovine spongiform encephalopathy in cattle is transmitted to humans through infected beef
  - Primarily present in UK
  - Also known as new variant (nvCJD)
- Genetics
  - Can be inherited, sporadic, or acquired (infectious)
  - 10-15% of human prion disease cases associated with dominant mutations in autosomal prion protein (PrPc) gene (*PRNP*) on chromosome 20
  - PrPc is a normal host protein on surface of many cells, particularly neurons
- Associated abnormalities
  - EEG: Periodic high-voltage sharp waves on background of low-voltage activity

Staging, Grading, & Classification

- **Definite CJD**
  - Characteristic neuropathology (biopsy or autopsy)
  - Protease-resistant PrP by Western blot
- **Probable CJD**
  - Progressive dementia; typical findings on EEG
  - 14-3-3 protein in CSF
  - ≥ 2 of following: Myoclonus, visual impairment, cerebellar signs, pyramidal or extrapyramidal signs, or akinetic mutism
- **Possible CJD**
  - Progressive dementia; atypical findings on EEG
  - ≥ 2 of following: Myoclonus, visual impairment, cerebellar signs, pyramidal or extrapyramidal signs, or akinetic mutism
  - Duration < 2 years

Gross Pathologic & Surgical Features

- Mild cortical atrophy
- Ventricular enlargement

Microscopic Features

- Spongiform encephalopathy: GM most affected
  - Marked neuronal loss with reactive astrocytosis
  - Replacement gliosis
  - Neuronal vacuolation with spongiform changes
- 10% of patients with CJD have amyloid plaques in cerebellum or cerebral hemispheres
- Variable accumulation of PrPSc in brain tissue
  - PrPSc = abnormal, insoluble, protease-resistant amyloid form of PrPc
  - Diffuse (common in sCJD) or discrete plaques

CLINICAL ISSUES

Presentation

- Most common signs/symptoms
  - Rapidly progressive dementia associated with myoclonic jerks and akinetic mutism
  - Variable constellation of pyramidal, extrapyramidal, and cerebellar signs
- Clinical profile
  - **sCJD**: Cerebellar dysfunction (40%), rapidly progressive cognitive impairment (40%), both (20%)
    - 6 molecular subtypes: MM1, MM2, MV1, MV2, VV1, and VV2
      - Vary with respect to age at onset, disease duration, early symptoms, and neuropathology
  - **vCJD**: Psychiatric and sensory symptoms
    - **Heidenhain variant** of CJD
      - Isolated visual signs/symptoms (initially)
      - Predominantly occipital lobe degeneration
      - DWI/FLAIR may detect early cortical abnormalities
    - **Brownell-Oppenheimer**: Cerebellar signs/ symptoms
    - Extrapyramidal type of CJD
      - May show ↑ signal intensity in BG
    - Pyramidal involvement with disease progression

Demographics

- Age
  - Young in vCJD, older in sCJD (6th to 7th decade)
- Ethnicity
  - sCJD occurs throughout world, in all races
  - vCJD limited to Europe (almost all cases in UK)
- Epidemiology
  - Incidence 1 per million (USA and internationally)
  - SCJD (85%), familial (15%), infectious/iatrogenic (less than 1%)

Natural History & Prognosis

- Long incubation period but rapidly progressive once clinical symptoms begin
- Rapidly progressing dementia, with death usually ensuing within months of onset
  - Mean survival after diagnosis of sCJD is 8 months
  - vCJD has longer course (mean 16 months)
  - Familial CJD has mean survival of 26 months
- 10% 1-year survival

Treatment

- No effective treatment

DIAGNOSTIC CHECKLIST

Consider

- Heidenhain variant of CJD in patients with visual disorders of unclear origin and dementia

Image Interpretation Pearls

- Lack of BG findings does not rule out CJD

SELECTED REFERENCES

1. Manners DN et al: Pathologic correlates of diffusion MRI changes in Creutzfeldt-Jakob disease. Neurology. 72(16):1425-31, 2009
2. Fulbright RK et al: MR imaging of familial Creutzfeldt-Jakob disease: a blinded and controlled study. AJNR Am J Neuroradiol. 29(9):1638-43, 2008

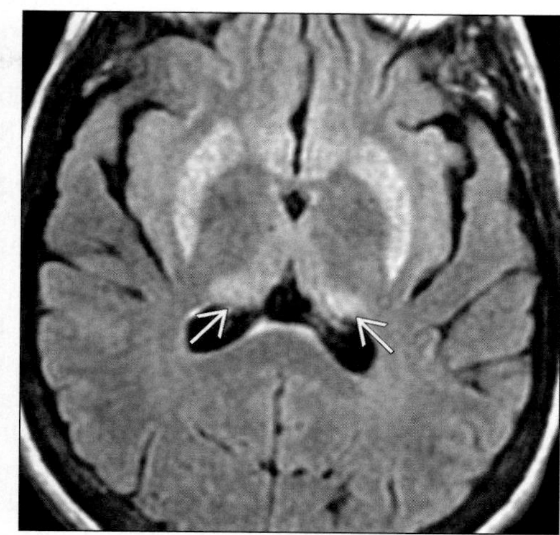

(Left) *Axial DWI MR shows symmetric hyperintensity in the basal ganglia and thalami bilaterally. The thalamic involvement shows the "hockey stick" sign, which is symmetric pulvinar and dorsomedial thalamus hyperintensity. This sign is most commonly seen in variant CJD but may also be present in sCJD, as in this case.* ***(Right)*** *Axial FLAIR MR shows symmetric hyperintensity in the putamen and thalami, particularly the pulvinar and the dorsomedial thalami ➔, which is more common in variant CJD.*

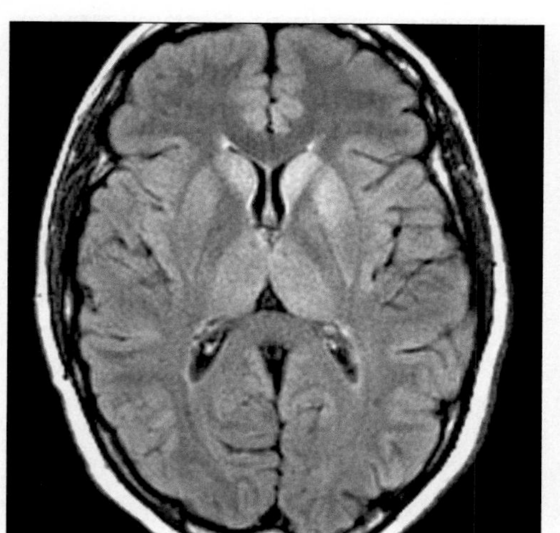

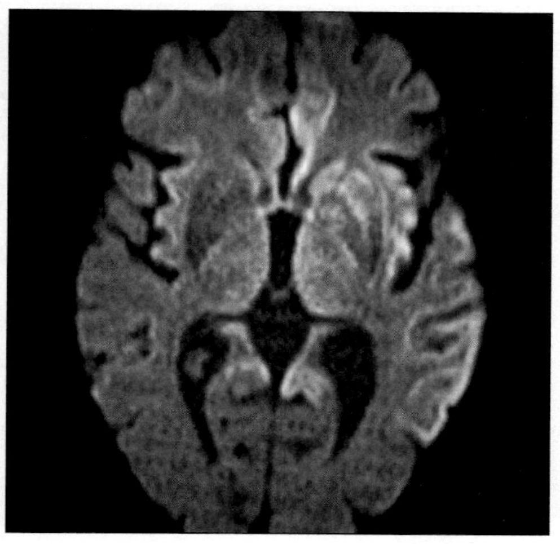

(Left) *Axial FLAIR MR shows asymmetric hyperintensity in the caudate heads, left greater than right, and the left putamen.* ***(Right)*** *Axial DWI MR in the same patient a few weeks later shows asymmetric hyperintensity in the basal ganglia, left greater than right, and the cerebral cortex. Asymmetric cortical involvement is more common than asymmetric basal ganglia involvement in CJD. This elderly man had rapidly progressive dementia and probable CJD, as EEG showed characteristic features.*

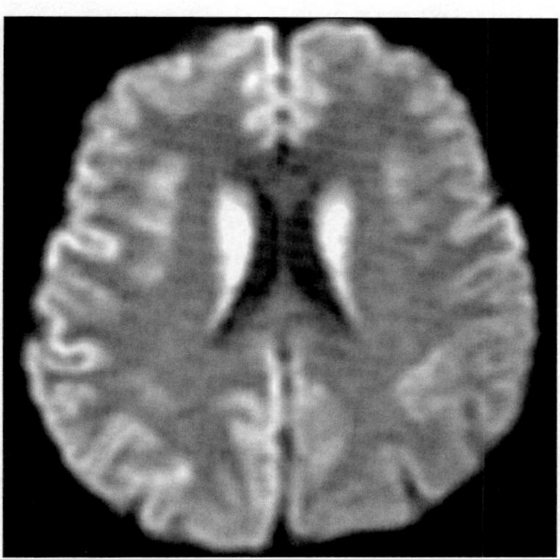

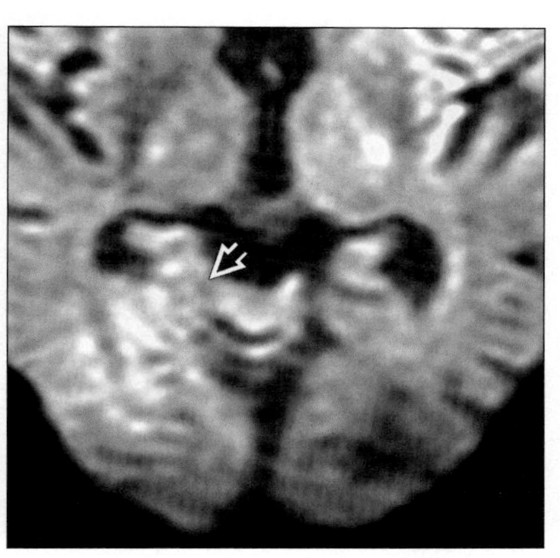

(Left) *Axial DWI MR shows marked hyperintensity related to decreased diffusivity in the caudate nuclei and cortex in this patient with CJD. DWI is the most sensitive sequence for diagnosis of CJD.* ***(Right)*** *Axial DWI MR shows marked hyperintensity in the right occipital lobe ➲ and left insula in a patient with primarily visual complaints. The Heidenhain variant of CJD is characterized by isolated visual signs and symptoms initially. Occipital lobe involvement predominates on imaging.*

PARKINSON DISEASE

Key Facts

Terminology

- Parkinson disease (PD)
  - Progressive neurodegenerative disease
  - Primarily affects pars compacta of substantia nigra (SNpc)

Imaging

- MR
  - SNpc narrowed/inapparent (T2WI)
  - SNpc progressively loses normal hyperintensity (from lateral to medial)
  - Border between SNpc, red nucleus blurred on PD
  - ↑ R2' relaxation at 3T in SNpc, caudal putamen (reflects ↑ iron content)
  - DWI may differentiate PD from PSP, MSA-P
  - ↑ ADC in both putamen, caudate nucleus
- PET/SPECT helpful for distinction from "Parkinson-plus" syndromes

Top Differential Diagnoses

- Multiple system atrophy (MSA)
  - Parkinsonian variant of MSA (MSA-P)
- Progressive supranuclear palsy
- Corticobasal ganglionic degeneration
- Dementia with Lewy bodies

Pathology

- Lewy bodies (eosinophilic intracytoplasmic inclusions with peripheral halos and dense cores), gliosis

Clinical Issues

- Resting tremor
- "Cogwheel" rigidity
- Bradykinesia
- Shuffling gate
- "Masked" facies

*(**Left**) Axial midbrain diagram shows narrowing and depigmentation of the substantia nigra ⇒ in Parkinson disease (upper) relative to normal anatomy (lower). (**Right**) Axial slice through the midbrain of a patient with severe Parkinson disease shows gross pathologic changes. Note the striking narrowing and depigmentation of the pars reticulata ⇒ of the substantia nigra. The pars compacta ⇒, which is the region between the pars reticulata and the red nucleus ⇒, is markedly narrowed.*

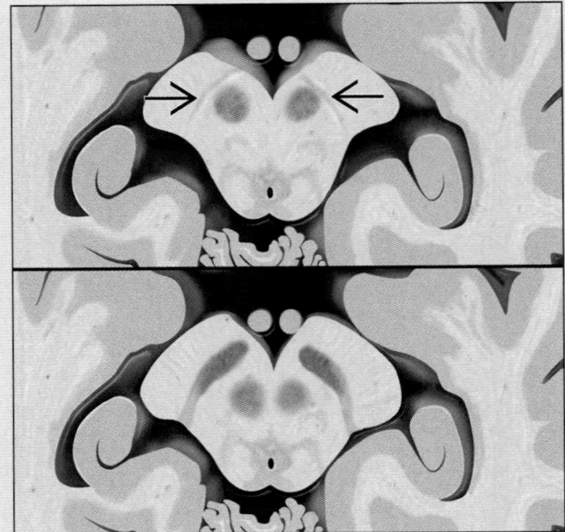

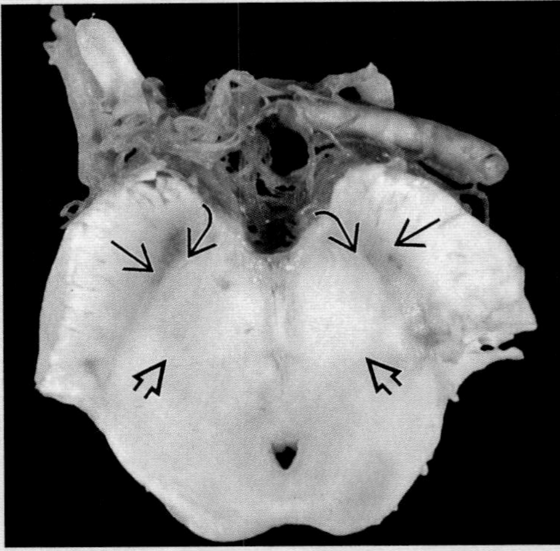

*(**Left**) Axial T2WI MR in a normal individual shows the appropriate width of the pars compacta ➡, a striking contrast to the abnormal findings seen in a patient with Parkinson disease. (**Right**) Axial T2WI MR in a patient with Parkinson disease shows classic midbrain findings. Note the "blurring" and thinning of pars compacta ➡ between 2 hypointense structures, i.e., the pars reticulata of substantia nigra and red nucleus. As a result, the red nuclei and substantia nigra are almost touching.*

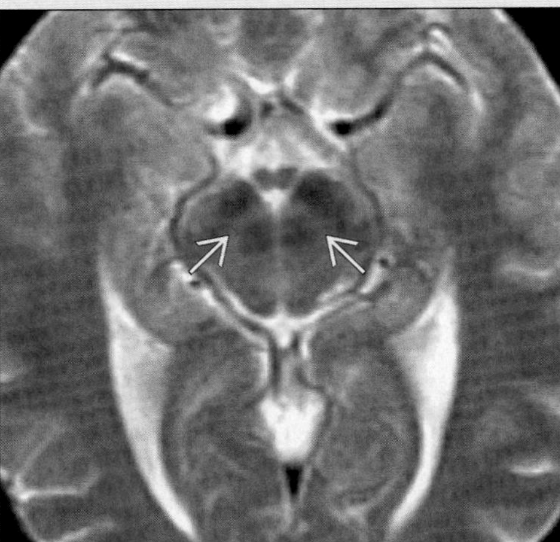

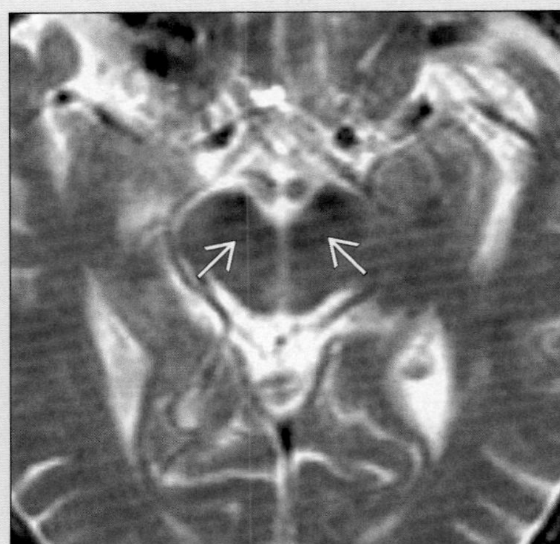

PARKINSON DISEASE

TERMINOLOGY

Abbreviations

- Idiopathic Parkinson disease (PD), paralysis agitans

Definitions

- Progressive neurodegenerative disease predominantly caused by primary disorder of pars compacta of substantia nigra (SNpc)
- Parkinsonism: Syndrome characterized by rigidity, tremor, bradycardia
  - Idiopathic PD (typically responsive to L-dopa therapy)
  - "Parkinson-plus" syndrome: Parkinsonism combined with other clinical signs
    - e.g., dementia with Lewy bodies, multiple system atrophy, progressive supranuclear palsy, corticobasal ganglionic disease

IMAGING

General Features

- Best diagnostic clue
  - Narrowing or absence of pars compacta of SNpc on T2WI
- Location
  - Substantia nigran (SN), caudate nucleus, and putamen
- Size
  - Decreased (atrophy)

CT Findings

- NECT
  - Nonspecific cerebral atrophy

MR Findings

- T1WI
  - Most commonly, generalized enlargement of sulci, ventricles, which is nonspecific
  - Volumetry
    - Helps to distinguish extrapyramidal multiple system atrophy (MSA-P) (15-30% volume decrease in pons and cerebellum) from PD
- T2WI
  - In normal subjects, SN is 2-layered gray matter (GM) structure at upper midbrain level
    - Hypointense area in posterior region of crus cerebri = pars reticulata of SN (SNpr)
    - Relatively hyperintense area between SNpr and red nucleus (RN) = pars compacta of SN (SNpc)
      - Some authors maintain this is best seen on PD images rather than T2WI
    - Hypointense area normally seen on axial T2WI corresponds to anterosuperior aspect of SN, adjacent crus cerebri (upper midbrain), anteromedial part of peduncular fibers (lower midbrain)
  - SNpc narrows in PD, difficult to distinguish from adjacent SNpr and RN
  - T2 hyperintense foci can be seen in putamen and globus pallidus (GP) in some PD patients; in addition, volume of putamen is decreased
  - At 3.0T imaging, increased R2 relaxation rates, indicative of increased iron content, are seen in SNpc and caudal portion of putamen in PD
- PD/intermediate
  - Axial intermediate-weighted SE images in normal subjects: Anatomic location of SN can be accurately identified
    - SN seen as area of hyperintense GM surrounded by hypointense RN and crural fibers at upper midbrain level
    - SNpr and SNpc cannot be distinguished
  - Axial intermediate TE images in PD
    - Progressive loss of normal signal of SNpc from lateral to medial; SNpc no longer appears hyperintense
    - Indistinct border between SNpr and RN, which reflects neuronal loss and iron deposition
- STIR
  - Fast STIR images: Same findings as proton density-weighted images
- DWI
  - ↑ ADC in putamen and caudate nucleus
    - vs. progressive supranuclear palsy (PSP) and Parkinson variant of multiple system atrophy (MSA-P), which have ↑ putaminal ADC values
- MRS
  - Normal spectra or ↓ NAA and ↑ lactate
  - Significantly ↑ lactate/NAA ratio, especially in PD patients with dementia
    - Impairment of oxidative energy metabolism
- DTI
  - ↓ ↓ FA in SN in PD: Greater reduction of FA in caudal SN than rostral SN
  - ↓ FA in frontal lobe (supplementary motor area, presupplementary motor area, cingulum)
- T2 or T2* mapping
  - Sensitive to iron content in brain; ↑ ↑ R2' relaxation rate in SN of PD correlates with patient's motor symptoms but not with disease duration

Ultrasonographic Findings

- Brain parenchyma sonography: Hyperechoic appearance of SN in PD
  - Hypointense appearance of putamen (iron accumulation) in Parkinson-plus syndromes (PSP, MSA), not in PD

Nuclear Medicine Findings

- PET
  - May be used to study functional status of dopaminergic neurons in SN, dopamine D2 receptors in basal ganglia, or opiate receptors in basal ganglia
  - Dopaminergic neurons in SN
    - 18F-fluorodopa PET: ↓ striatal uptake proportional to decreased number of dopaminergic neurons; correlated with clinical severity
      - May diagnose early/relatively asymptomatic PD but normal in 10% of PD patients
  - Dopamine D2 receptors in basal ganglia
    - 11C-raclopride PET; putaminal dopamine terminals are normal or increased in early stages of PD but normalize in advanced PD, reduced in MSA

- Opiate receptors in basal ganglia
  - 11C-diprenorphine; reduced uptake in putamen, thalamus, and anterior cingulate in PD patients with dyskinesias, normal in nondyskinetic PD patients
- SPECT: Like PET, may be used to study dopaminergic neurons in SN or dopamine D2 receptors in basal ganglia
  - Dopaminergic neurons in SN
    - B-CIT SPECT findings in putamen similar to those seen with 18F-fluorodopa PET
  - Dopamine D2 receptors in basal ganglia
    - I-123 SPECT findings similar to those seen with 11C-raclopride PET

Imaging Recommendations

- Best imaging tool
  - Proton density-weighted SE MR and PET
- Protocol advice
  - Proton density-weighted SE, fast STIR images allow direct visualization of SN as GM structure

DIFFERENTIAL DIAGNOSIS

Multiple System Atrophy (MSA)

- 85% of cases: Prominent T2 hypointensity in putamen and caudate nucleus (abnormal iron deposition)

Progressive Supranuclear Palsy (PSP)

- a.k.a. Steele-Richardson-Olszewski syndrome
- MR: ↓ width of SNpc, atrophy of superior colliculi, and high intensity to periaqueductal GM

Corticobasal Degeneration

- Thinning of pre-/postcentral gyri + central sulcus dilatation with marked parasagittal involvement

Dementia with Lewy Bodies

- Lewy bodies (LB) found diffusely in brain
- Brainstem, SN, and cortical atrophy

Parkinsonism-Dementia-Amyotrophic Lateral Sclerosis Complex

- Corticospinal tract abnormalities

PATHOLOGY

General Features

- Etiology
  - Various genetic markers are under study for increased susceptibility to developing PD
  - Environmental exposure: MPTP (1-methyl-4-phenyl-1,2,3,6-tetrahydropyridine); possibly pesticide exposure
  - Aging: Normal aging is associated with decrease of neurons in SNpc
- Genetics
  - Sporadic (10-20% of cases familial)
- Associated abnormalities
  - Increased iron content in SNpc

Gross Pathologic & Surgical Features

- Loss of pigmentation in SN and locus ceruleus
- Recent pathologic studies in PD: No significant ↓ in size of SNpc, despite remarkable neuronal cell loss

Microscopic Features

- Loss of dopaminergic neurons in SN (especially SNpc), locus ceruleus, dorsal vagal nucleus, and substantia innominata

CLINICAL ISSUES

Presentation

- Most common signs/symptoms
  - Resting tremor with frequency of 3-5 Hz (pill-rolling tremor), "cogwheel" rigidity, bradykinesia, shuffling gate, masked facies, later dementia in 40%
- Other signs/symptoms
  - Autonomic dysfunction, depression, sleep disturbance

Demographics

- Age
  - Onset typically between 50-60 years
- Gender
  - M:F = 1.5:1
- Epidemiology
  - Idiopathic PD is most common movement disorder
  - Prevalence: 150-200/100,000; 1% of population > 60 years old, 3% of population > 65 years old

Natural History & Prognosis

- Onset of PD is typically asymmetric
- Slowly progressive course of bradykinesia, rigidity, and gait difficulty → eventual disability after several years

Treatment

- Medical (favored for some younger patients): Levodopa, bromocriptine, amantadine, selegiline
- Surgical (for medically refractive cases): Stereotactic pallidotomy or deep brain stimulation for subthalamic nucleus, thalamus, globus pallidus

DIAGNOSTIC CHECKLIST

Consider

- Parkinson-plus syndromes

Image Interpretation Pearls

- Role of imaging in parkinsonism: Exclude treatable bradykinesia (tumor, hematoma, hydrocephalus)
- Minimal correlation between hypointense areas on T2WI and SN location on anatomical specimens/PD-weighted/fast STIR images

SELECTED REFERENCES

1. Wallis LI et al: MRI assessment of basal ganglia iron deposition in Parkinson's disease. J Magn Reson Imaging. 28(5):1061-7, 2008
2. Minati L et al: Imaging degeneration of the substantia nigra in Parkinson disease with inversion-recovery MR imaging. AJNR Am J Neuroradiol. 28(2):309-13, 2007
3. Oikawa H et al: The substantia nigra in Parkinson disease: proton density-weighted spin-echo and fast short inversion time inversion-recovery MR findings. AJNR Am J Neuroradiol. 23(10):1747-56, 2002

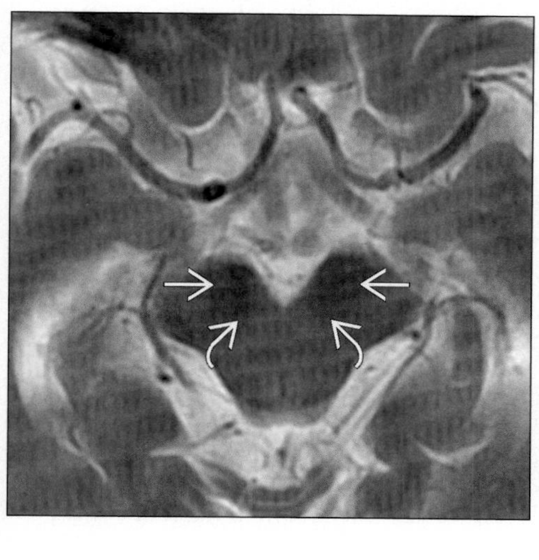

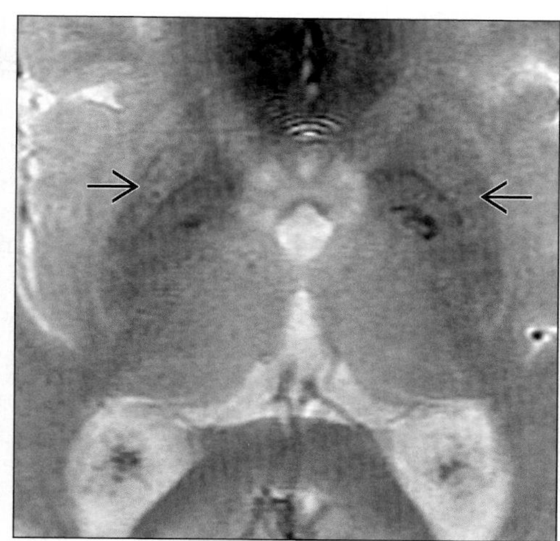

(Left) *Axial T2WI MR in 72-year-old man with idiopathic Parkinson disease shows loss of hyperintense band (i.e., pars compacta of substantia nigra) between the pars reticulata of substantia nigra ➔ and red nucleus ➔ due to abnormal iron accumulation in PD.* ***(Right)*** *Axial T2* GRE MR through the basal ganglia in the same patient shows that no decreased signal intensity, which would indicate abnormal iron deposition, is present in the putamen ➔ of this particular patient.*

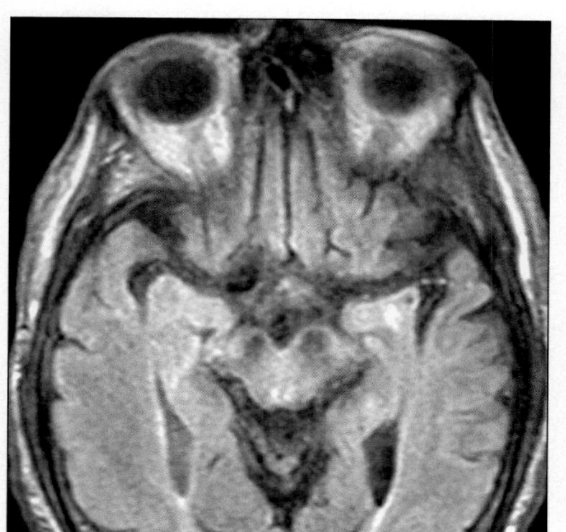

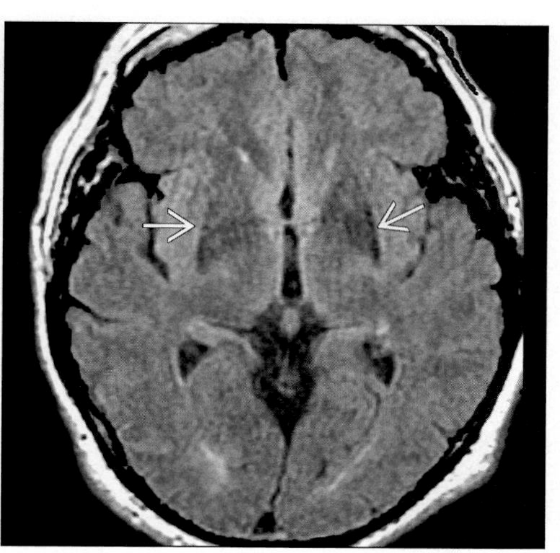

(Left) *Axial FLAIR MR in a 61-year-old patient with Parkinson disease shows enlargement of the sylvian fissures.* ***(Right)*** *Axial FLAIR MR shows abnormally decreased signal intensity of the posterior basal ganglia ➔, as well as mildly decreased volume of the putamina.*

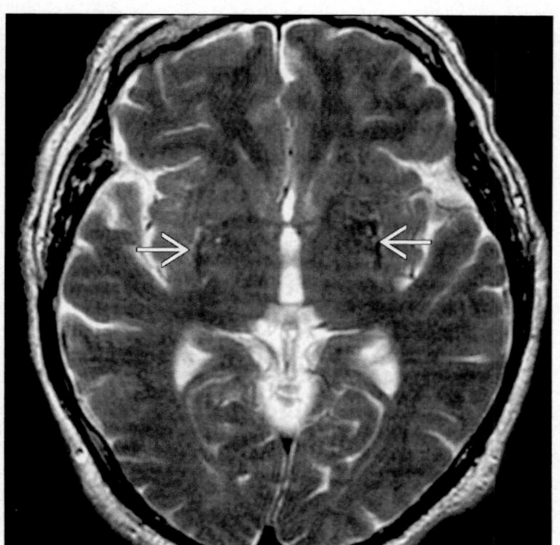

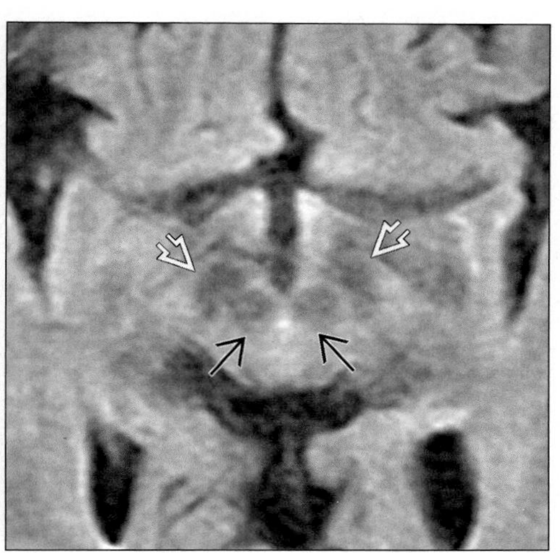

(Left) *Axial T2WI MR in a patient with Parkinson disease shows abnormal decreased signal intensity of the basal ganglia ➔.* ***(Right)*** *Axial FLAIR MR in the same patient shows the red nuclei ➔ and pars reticulata ➔ of the substantia nigra almost touching each other, indicating thinning of the pars compacta.*

MULTIPLE SYSTEM ATROPHY

Key Facts

Terminology

- Multiple system atrophy (MSA) has 3 clinical subtypes
- Cerebellar (MSA-C)
  - Sporadic olivopontocerebellar atrophy (sOPCA)
- Extrapyramidal (MSA-P)
  - Striatonigral degeneration (SND)
- Autonomic (MSA-A)
  - Shy-Drager syndrome (SDS)

Imaging

- General findings
  - ↓ ("flat") pons/medulla
  - Cerebellar vermis/hemispheres atrophic
- MSA-C
  - Pons, inferior olives, cerebellum atrophic
  - Cruciform pontine hyperintensity ("hot cross bun" sign)
- MSA-P
  - ↓ T2 signal in dorsolateral putamen
  - ± ↑ T1 signal in lateral putamen rim
- FDG PET shows ↓ metabolism in putamen

Top Differential Diagnoses

- Cerebelloolivary atrophy
- Friedreich ataxia (spinocerebellar ataxia)
- Progressive nonfamilial adult onset cerebellar degeneration
- Hereditary olivopontocerebellar atrophy
- Parkinson, Parkinson-plus syndromes

Diagnostic Checklist

- MR features may overlap
- All MR findings may be observed in every MSA subtype!

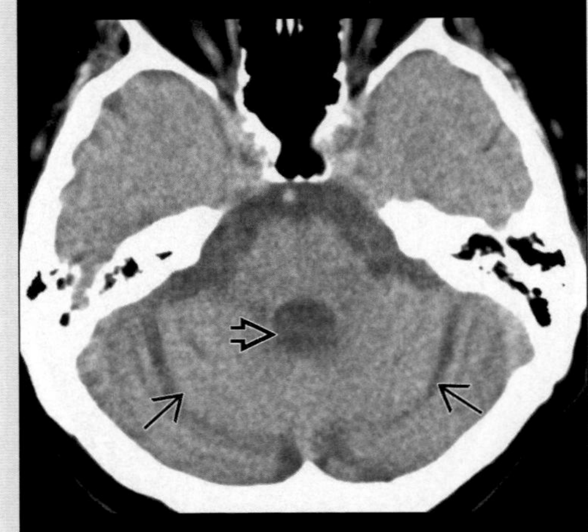

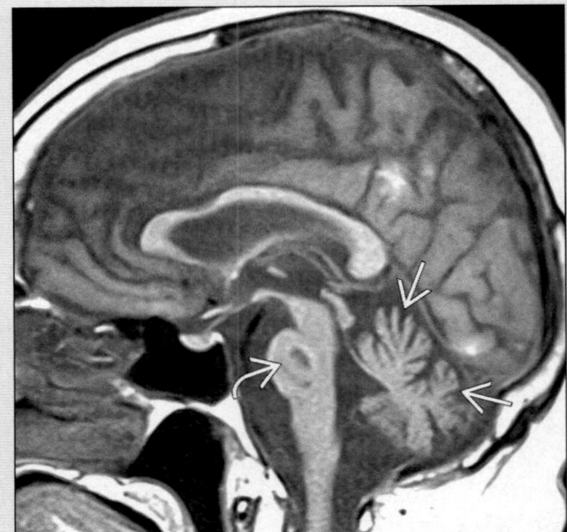

***(Left)** Axial NECT in a 62-year-old woman with multiple system atrophy of the cerebellar type shows cerebellar cortical atrophy, demonstrated by the prominence of the horizontal fissure → and enlargement of the 4th ventricle ⇨.* ***(Right)** Sagittal T1WI MR in the same patient shows that the pons is small and has a central region of hypointense signal ↪. Note vermian atrophy →.*

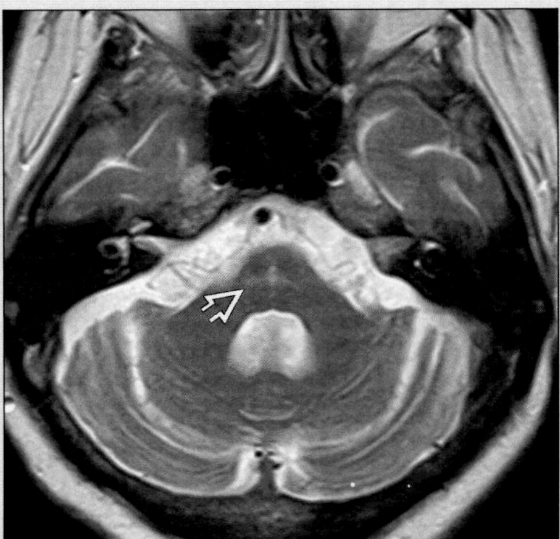

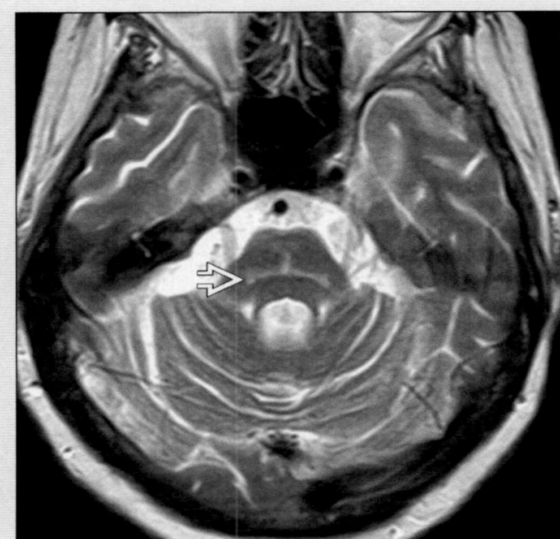

***(Left)** Axial T2WI MR through the lower pons in the same patient confirms cerebellar atrophy. The most striking feature is the cruciform region of hyperintense signal ⇨ within the atrophic pons, the "hot cross bun" sign.* ***(Right)** Axial T2WI MR nicely shows the "hot cross bun" sign ⇨ seen in patients with the cerebellar form of MSA (MSA-C). This is caused by loss of myelinated transverse pontocerebellar fibers in the pontine raphe with preservation of the pontine tegmentum and corticospinal tracts.*

MULTIPLE SYSTEM ATROPHY

TERMINOLOGY

Definitions

- Multiple system atrophy (MSA)
  - Sporadic progressive neurodegenerative disorder of adult onset, unknown etiology
  - Combination of cerebellar/pyramidal/extrapyramidal/autonomic disorders
    - Varying degrees of coexistence
- 3 clinical subtypes characterized by signs and symptoms
  - Predominantly cerebellar (MSA-C)
    - a.k.a. sporadic olivopontocerebellar atrophy (sOPCA)
  - Extrapyramidal (MSA-P)
    - a.k.a. striatonigral degeneration (SND)
  - Autonomic (MSA-A)
    - a.k.a. Shy-Drager syndrome (SDS)
- 2 distinct imaging subtypes: MSA-C and MSA-P

IMAGING

General Features

- Best diagnostic clue
  - MSA-C: Cruciform shape of hyperintense signal in pons on T2WI; atrophy of pons, inferior olives, and cerebellum
  - MSA-P: ↓ T2 signal in dorsolateral putamen ± ↑ T2 signal in lateral rim of putamen
- Location
  - Striatum (mainly putamen), middle cerebellar peduncles (MCP), base of pons, cerebellar white matter (WM), motor cortex
- Size
  - Decreased (atrophy)

CT Findings

- NECT
  - Pontine atrophy, enlarged 4th ventricle (4th V)
  - Cerebellar atrophy (hemispheres > vermis)
  - Cortical atrophy (especially frontal and parietal lobes)

MR Findings

- T1WI
  - On sagittal images
    - ↓ size of pons and medulla with flat ventral surface of pons
    - Atrophy of cerebellar vermis and hemispheres
  - On axial images
    - ↓ anteroposterior diameter of pons and midbrain
    - ↓ width of superior cerebellar peduncle and MCP
    - Enlargement of 4th V and cerebellopontine angle
  - Atrophy of MCP and cerebellum is greater in MSA-C than other MSA subtypes
- T2WI
  - Atrophy of brainstem and cerebellum
  - Hyperintense signal in MCP and in cruciform shape in pons ("hot cross bun" sign)
    - Reflects degeneration of pontine neurons and transverse pontocerebellar fibers (TPF)
  - ↓ signal in dorsolateral putamen ± ↑ signal in lateral rim of putamen
    - More frequent in MSA-P than other MSA subtypes
  - Atrophy of cerebral hemispheres
    - Especially frontal and parietal lobes
  - All MR findings may be observed in every MSA subtype!
- PD/intermediate
  - MSA-C: ↑ signal in TPF, MCP, and cerebellum
  - MSA-P: ↓ signal in dorsolateral putamen ± hyperintense lateral rim of putamen
- DWI
  - DWI of pons with transverse diffusion gradient
    - Normal individuals: TPF seen as low intensity bundles in base of pons on axial multishot
    - MSA-C: TPF not seen on DWI of pons
  - Diffusion tensor MR (DT-MR)
    - MSA-C: ↓ FA in MCP, TPF, and cerebellum
- MRS
  - ^{1}H-MRS: Significantly ↓ pontine and cerebellar NAA/Cr, Cho/Cr ratios in MSA-C
    - Pontine NAA/Cr ratio correlates with disability
  - Phosphorus MRS: ↓ phosphocreatine, ↑ phosphate
- MR volumetry: Significantly ↓ mean striatal and brainstem volumes

Ultrasonographic Findings

- Brain parenchyma sonography in MSA-P
  - Hyperechogenicity of lentiform nucleus; normal appearance of substantia nigra (SN)

Nuclear Medicine Findings

- PET
  - MSA-C: FDG uptake in cerebellar hemisphere, pons, and thalamus is moderately ↑ by walking
    - ↓ FDG uptake in cerebellar vermis during walking
    - PET activation ratio (FDG uptake during walking/ FDG uptake during resting) demonstrates cerebellar dysfunction in early phase of MSA-C
  - MSA-P
    - FDG PET shows ↓ metabolism in putamen
    - 11C-raclopride PET shows ↓ postsynaptic D2 receptor density in putamen
  - 11C-(R)-PK11195 PET in MSA
    - Microglia bind 11C-(R)-PK11195 when activated by neuronal injury
    - ↑ 11C-(R)-PK11195 binding in dorsolateral prefrontal cortex, putamen, globus pallidus (GP), pons, substantia nigra

Imaging Recommendations

- Best imaging tool
  - MR
- Protocol advice
  - Axial T2WI or FLAIR for "hot cross bun" sign

DIFFERENTIAL DIAGNOSIS

Cerebelloolivary Atrophy

- Cortical cerebellar degeneration
- Selective atrophy of lateral cerebellum ("fish-mouth deformity" on parasagittal sections) and superior vermis (especially declive, folium, and tuber)

MULTIPLE SYSTEM ATROPHY

Friedreich Ataxia (Spinocerebellar Ataxia)
- Severe atrophy of spinal cord (flat posterior aspect) and medulla oblongata
- Mild atrophy of vermian and paravermian structures

Progressive Nonfamilial Adult Onset Cerebellar Degeneration
- May occur in association with many conditions
  - Hashimoto thyroiditis (even in euthyroid state)
  - Paraneoplastic syndromes
  - Nutritional deficiency, alcohol abuse
  - Prolonged phenytoin/phenobarbital use
- Midline cerebellar atrophy on MR

Hereditary Olivopontocerebellar Atrophy (OPCA)
- Dominant OPCA
  - "Fine comb" type of cerebellar atrophy, involving hemispheres > vermis; atrophy of pons and MCP
- Recessive OPCA: Marked atrophy in lateral part of cerebellar hemispheres with "fish-mouth deformity"

Hereditary Cerebellar Atrophy
- Middle-aged patients; severe superior vermian atrophy

Parkinson Disease
- Thinned pars compacta

Other Parkinson-Plus Syndromes
- Progressive supranuclear palsy
- Corticobasal degeneration
- Dementia with Lewy bodies

PATHOLOGY

General Features
- Etiology
  - Unknown; environmental toxins are possibility
- Genetics
  - No genetic causes definitively identified

Staging, Grading, & Classification
- 3 histological grades of severity of MSA-P
  - SN pars compacta (SNpc) affected
    - Loss of pigmented neurons and gliosis: Caudal lateral > rostral and ventromedial
  - SNpc and posterior/dorsolateral putamen affected
    - SNpc: Severe neuronal loss, gliosis
    - Moderate neuronal loss and gliosis in putamen
  - SNpc, putamen, caudate nucleus, and GP affected
    - SNpc: Severe diffuse neuronal depletion
    - Putamen: Severe neuronal loss and gliosis (dorsolateral > ventromedial)
    - Mild-moderate degeneration of caudate nucleus and globus pallidus

Gross Pathologic & Surgical Features
- Atrophy of ventral pons, MCP, cerebellar cortex; secondary atrophy of inferior olive
- Frontal and parietal lobe atrophy

Microscopic Features
- Glial cytoplasmic inclusions localized in WM
  - Pallor or loss of myelin staining
- Loss of cerebellar Purkinje cells (vermis > hemispheres)
- Severe degeneration and gliosis in deep cerebellar WM
- Neuronal loss and proliferation of astroglia in putamen

CLINICAL ISSUES

Presentation
- Most common signs/symptoms
  - Parkinsonian features predominate in 80% of patients (MSA-P subtype)
    - Bradykinesia, rigidity, postural and rest tremor, unsteady gait, dysequilibrium
    - Differentiation from Parkinson disease is important
      - MSA-P more rapidly progressing, nonresponsive to L-Dopa
  - Cerebellar symptoms predominate in 20% of patients (MSA-C subtype)
    - Gait ataxia, limb akinetic ataxia, dysarthria, cerebellar oculomotor disturbance
  - Autonomic failure (MSA-A)
    - Symptomatic orthostatic hypotension
    - Erectile and urologic disturbance, constipation, hypo-/anhydrosis

Demographics
- Age
  - Onset of MSA: Usually 6th decade
- Gender
  - No gender preference
- Epidemiology
  - Prevalence of MSA in USA: 3-5/100,000
  - Incidence rate of MSA: 3/100,000 per year

Natural History & Prognosis
- Progressive neurodegenerative disease
- Death usually occurs within 10 years from onset

Treatment
- Options, risks, complications
  - 90% of MSA-P patients are unresponsive to L-dopa

DIAGNOSTIC CHECKLIST

Image Interpretation Pearls
- "Hot cross bun" sign (cruciform shape of hyperintense signal in pons on T2WI) suggests diagnosis of MSA-C

SELECTED REFERENCES

1. Lipp A et al: Prospective differentiation of multiple system atrophy from Parkinson disease, with and without autonomic failure. Arch Neurol. 66(6):742-50, 2009
2. Matsusue E et al: Cerebellar Lesions in Multiple System Atrophy: Postmortem MR Imaging--Pathologic Correlations. AJNR Am J Neuroradiol. Epub ahead of print, 2009
3. Köllensperger M et al: Red flags for multiple system atrophy. Mov Disord. 23(8):1093-9, 2008
4. Naka H et al: Characteristic MRI findings in multiple system atrophy: comparison of the three subtypes. Neuroradiology. 44(3):204-9, 2002

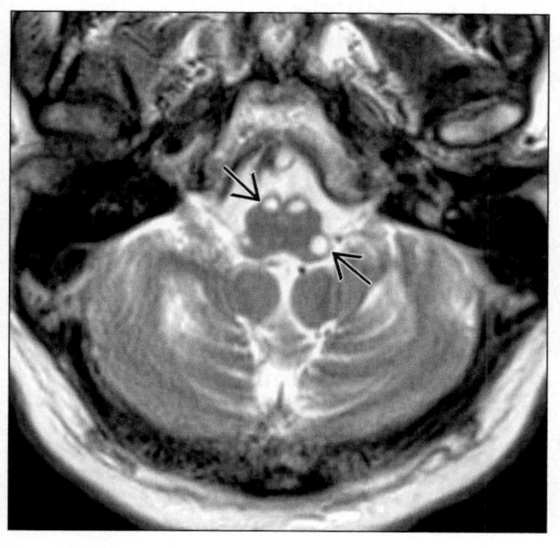

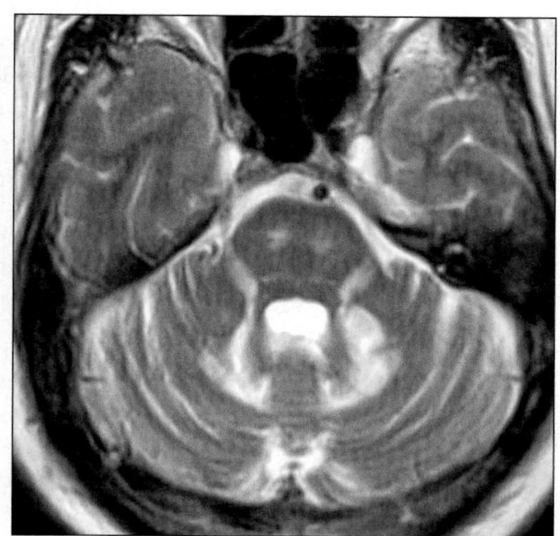

(Left) *Axial T2WI MR in a 55-year-old woman with sporadic olivopontocerebellar atrophy shows striking, symmetric high signal intensity in the pyramids and inferior cerebellar peduncles ➔.* ***(Right)*** *Axial T2WI MR in the same patient shows hyperintensity in the middle cerebellar peduncles, dentate nuclei, and pons. The cerebellum appears moderately atrophic for the patient's age. The basal ganglia and cerebral hemispheres (not shown) were normal.*

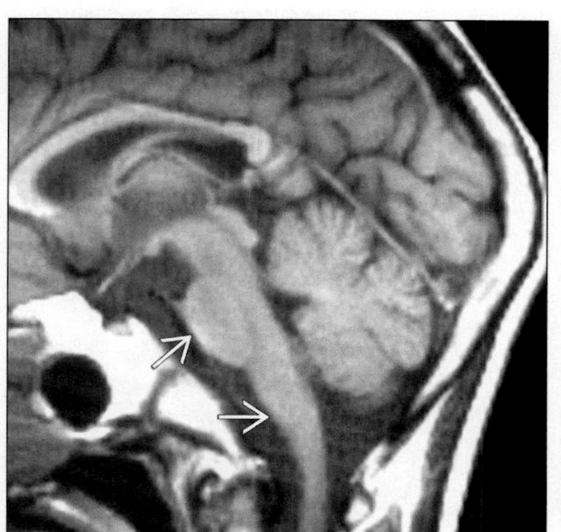

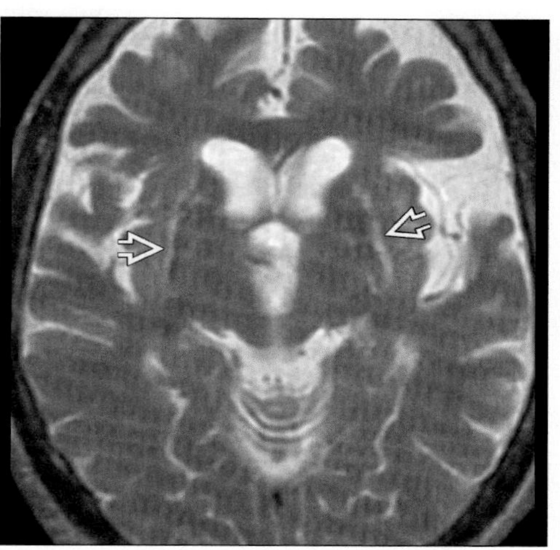

(Left) *Sagittal T1WI MR shows relatively "flat" pons and medulla ➔.* ***(Right)*** *Axial T2WI MR also demonstrates that the putamina appear small and hypointense, with a thin peripheral rim of high signal intensity ➔. The white matter appears quite normal compared to the overall degree of sulcal and ventricular enlargement.*

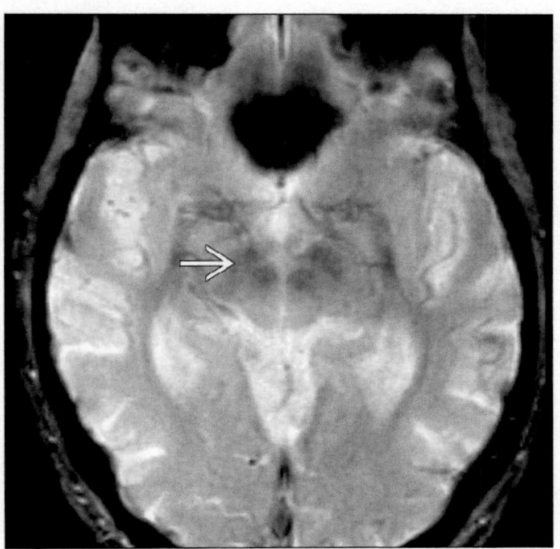

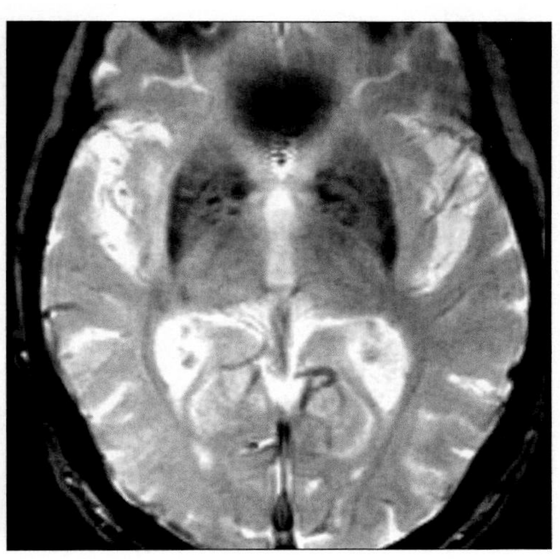

(Left) *Axial T2* GRE MR in a patient with multiple system atrophy (parkinsonian type) shows prominent hypointensity in substantia nigra ➔.* ***(Right)*** *Axial T2* GRE MR shows abnormal prominent hypointensity in the putamen and globus pallidus, which is characteristic of the parkinsonian type of multiple system atrophy and reflects iron accumulation due to striatonigral degeneration.*

CORTICOBASAL DEGENERATION

Key Facts

Terminology
- Corticobasal degeneration (CBD)
  - Progressive neurodegenerative disease
  - Presents with cognitive dysfunction, "asymmetrical" parkinsonism

Imaging
- Severe focal asymmetric cortical atrophy
  - Perirolandic (posterior frontal, parietal cortex)
  - Relative sparing of temporal, occipital regions
- ↑ signal intensity in frontal &/or parietal subcortical white matter
- Marked hypointensity
  - Putamen, globus pallidi
- PET
  - ↓ glucose metabolism in parietal cortex, BG
- SPECT
  - Asymmetric hypoperfusion
  - Frontoparietal lobes, BG, thalamus, cerebellum

Top Differential Diagnoses
- Progressive supranuclear palsy
- Frontotemporal lobar dementia/degeneration
- Alzheimer disease
- Dementia with Lewy bodies
- Amyotrophic lateral sclerosis (ALS)

Pathology
- Hyperphosphorylated tau/abnormal filamentous inclusions accumulate in neurons/glia

Clinical Issues
- Unilateral or asymmetrical parkinsonism
  - Dystonia, tremor
  - Ideomotor apraxia, "alien limb" phenomenon
- Cognitive decline

*(**Left**) Parasagittal T1WI MR through the right hemisphere in a 63-year-old man with corticobasal degeneration shows prominent volume loss in the posterior frontal and parietal cortex ➡. The anterior frontal lobe cortex is normal in appearance. (**Right**) Axial T2WI MR in the same patient shows prominent volume loss in both posterior frontal and parietal lobe cortices, slightly worse in the right hemisphere. Note the subcortical white matter hyperintensity ➡ and adjacent sulcal widening.*

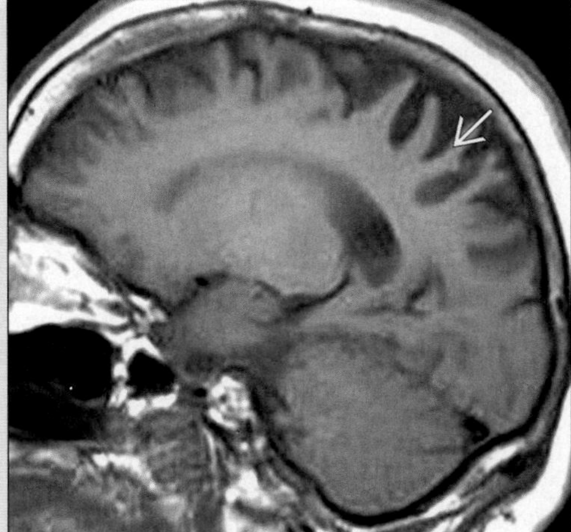

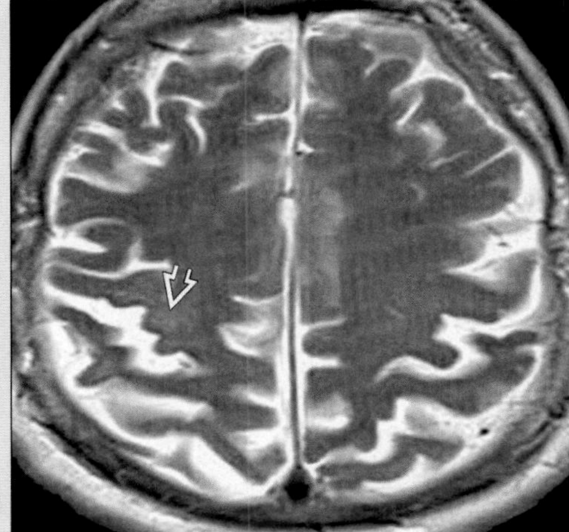

*(**Left**) Coronal FLAIR MR in the same patient shows asymmetric parietal atrophy, worse on the right ➡, with subcortical white matter hyperintensity ➡. (Courtesy A. Erbetta, MD.) (**Right**) Axial T2WI MR in a different patient with more subtle corticobasal degeneration shows asymmetric atrophy of the left perirolandic cortex ➡.*

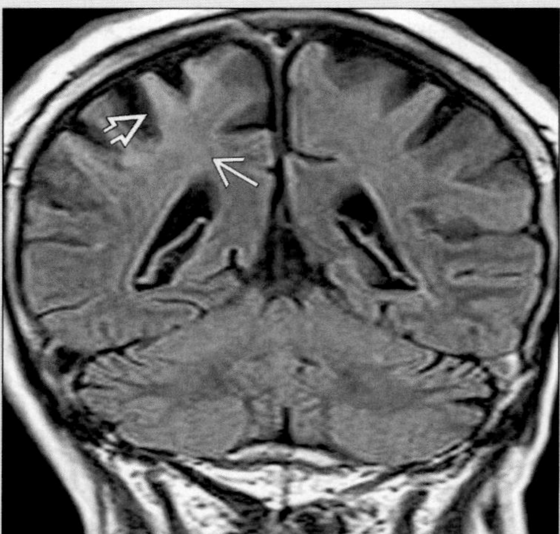

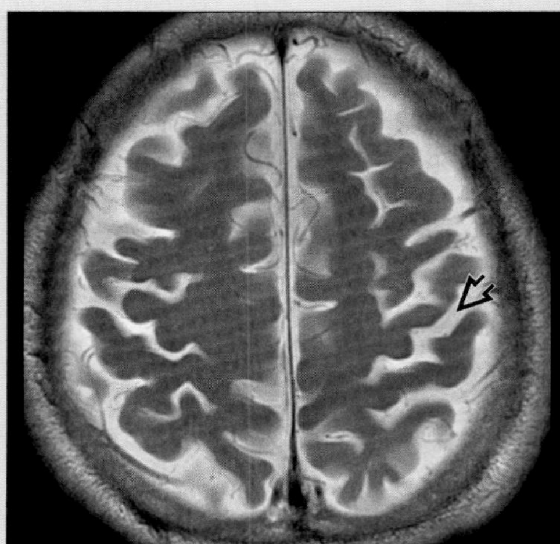

CORTICOBASAL DEGENERATION

TERMINOLOGY

Abbreviations

- Corticobasal degeneration (CBD)

Synonyms

- Corticobasal ganglionic degeneration
- Corticobasal degeneration syndrome
- Corticonigral degeneration with neuronal achromasia
- Cortical degeneration with swollen chromatolytic neurons

Definitions

- Progressive neurodegenerative disease
  - Presents with cognitive dysfunction, "asymmetrical" parkinsonism
  - Characterized pathologically by cortical and striatal tau protein accumulation

IMAGING

General Features

- Best diagnostic clue
  - Asymmetric cerebral atrophy (frontoparietal cortex ± cerebral peduncle)
- Size
  - Atrophy

Imaging Recommendations

- Best imaging tool
  - MR
- Protocol advice
  - Axial and coronal T2WI and FLAIR

CT Findings

- NECT
  - Asymmetric cerebral atrophy

MR Findings

- T1WI
  - Asymmetric cerebral atrophy
    - Posterior frontal, parietal cortex
    - ± cerebral peduncle, midbrain tegmentum, corpus callosum
- T2WI
  - Asymmetric hyperintensity in subcortical white matter (WM)
  - Marked hypointensity in putamen, globus pallidi
- FLAIR
  - ↑ signal intensity in frontal &/or parietal subcortical white matter
    - Seen more frequently in more cephalad brain regions
- DTI
  - Corticospinal tract atrophy with tractography
  - ADC
    - ↑ in motor thalamus, precentral/postcentral gyri (ipsilateral to affected frontoparietal cortex), bilateral superior mesenteric artery (SMA)
  - FA
    - ↓ in precentral gyrus, SMA, postcentral gyrus, cingulum

Nuclear Medicine Findings

- PET
  - ↓ glucose metabolism in parietal cortex, (to lesser extent) frontal cortex
  - 18F-dopa-PET: Decreased uptake in putamen, caudate
  - 11C-(R)-PK11195-PET: Assesses degree of microglial activation
    - ↑ ↑ binding in caudate nucleus, putamen, substantia nigra, pons, pre- and postcentral gyrus, and frontal lobe
- SPECT
  - Asymmetric hypoperfusion in frontoparietal lobes, basal ganglia (putamen), thalamus, and cerebellar hemispheres
  - Site of hypoperfusion is contralateral to side more severely affected clinically
  - I-123-FP-CIT or I-123-β-CIT: ↓ presynaptic dopamine transporter binding in striatum
  - I-123-IBZM: Relatively preserved D2 dopamine receptor activity in striatum

DIFFERENTIAL DIAGNOSIS

Progressive Supranuclear Palsy

- Prominent atrophy of midbrain ± pons ("penguin silhouette" sign)
- Postural instability, vertical gaze palsy
- Most common Parkinson-plus syndrome
- No subcortical hyperintense regions

Frontotemporal Lobar Degeneration

- Abnormalities of behavior and personality
- Bilateral frontal, anterior temporal lobar atrophy
- No subcortical hyperintense regions

Alzheimer Disease

- Parietotemporal lobar atrophy (entorhinal cortex, hippocampus)
- Major dysfunction in memory and cognition
- No subcortical hyperintense regions
- Amyloid PET: Uptake of radiotracer Pittsburgh compound-B (PiB) in temporoparietal cortex

Dementia with Lewy Bodies

- Mild diffuse brain atrophy
- No subcortical hyperintense regions
- PET: Hypometabolism in occipital cortex

Amyotrophic Lateral Sclerosis (ALS)

- No significant brain atrophy
- Abnormal high signal intensity of corticospinal tracts on T2WI/FLAIR

PATHOLOGY

General Features

- Etiology
  - Accumulation of hyperphosphorylated tau
  - Abnormal filamentous inclusions in neurons, glia
- Genetics
  - Tau gene is located on chromosome 17 (13 exons)

- Selective aggregation of 4R tau occurs in BG, cerebral cortex
- Tau haplotype H1 associated with both CBD, progressive supranuclear palsy
  - Suggests tau abnormality on chromosome 17 causes both diseases

Gross Pathologic & Surgical Features

- Severe focal cortical atrophy
  - Perirolandic (posterior frontal, parietal cortex)
  - Relative sparing of temporal and occipital regions

Microscopic Features

- Core features
  - Focal cortical neuronal loss, substantia nigra neuronal loss
  - Tau-positive neuronal, glial lesions
    - Astrocytic plaques and threads
    - In cortex, corpus striatum
- Supportive features
  - Cortical atrophy, commonly with superficial spongiosis
  - Ballooned neurons, typically mainly in atrophic cortices
  - Tau-positive oligodendroglial coiled bodies

CLINICAL ISSUES

Presentation

- Most common signs/symptoms
  - Unilateral or asymmetrical parkinsonism (typically in arm), dystonia, tremor
  - Ideomotor apraxia, "alien limb" phenomenon, cognitive decline
- Other signs/symptoms
  - Depression, apathy
- Proposed criteria for diagnosis of CBD
  - Core features
    - Insidious onset, progressive course
    - No identifiable cause (e.g., tumor, infarct)
    - Cortical dysfunction, including ≥ 1 of the following
      - Focal or asymmetric ideomotor apraxia, "alien limb" phenomena, cortical sensory loss, visual or sensory hemineglect, constructional apraxia, focal or asymmetric myoclonus, apraxia of speech or nonfluent aphasia
    - Extrapyramidal dysfunction as reflected by 1 of the following
      - Focal or asymmetric limb rigidity without marked and sustained l-dopa response
      - Focal or asymmetric limb dystonia
  - Supportive investigations
    - Varying focal or lateralized cognitive dysfunction
    - Relative preservation of learning, memory
    - Focal or asymmetric atrophy on CT or MR
      - Typically in perirolandic cortex
    - Focal or asymmetric hypoperfusion (SPECT, PET)
      - Typically maximal in frontoparietal cortex
      - Variable basal ganglia involvement

Demographics

- Age
  - Typically 50-70 years old
    - Mean age = 63 years
- Gender
  - No gender preference
- Epidemiology
  - True prevalence unknown (but likely ~ 5-7 per 100,000)
  - ~ 5% of cases of parkinsonism

Natural History & Prognosis

- Mean survival of 8 years after diagnosis
- Most common initial presentations: "Useless arm" (55%), gait disorder (27%) are common
- Subsequent development of unilateral limb rigidity or dystonia, bradykinesia, dementia

Treatment

- No curative treatment is available
- Motor symptoms: Levodopa and other dopaminergic drugs may help; botulinum toxin injections for dystonic clenched fist

DIAGNOSTIC CHECKLIST

Consider

- Consider CBD in case of asymmetric parkinsonism and cortical dysfunction

Image Interpretation Pearls

- Asymmetry atrophy of brain cortex and cerebral peduncle can be helpful MR findings

SELECTED REFERENCES

1. Erbetta A et al: Diffusion tensor imaging shows different topographic involvement of the thalamus in progressive supranuclear palsy and corticobasal degeneration. AJNR Am J Neuroradiol. 30(8):1482-7, 2009
2. Vitali P et al: Neuroimaging in dementia. Semin Neurol. 28(4):467-83, 2008
3. Koyama M et al: Imaging of corticobasal degeneration syndrome. Neuroradiology. 49(11):905-12, 2007
4. Klaffke S et al: Dopamine transporters, D2 receptors, and glucose metabolism in corticobasal degeneration. Mov Disord. 21(10):1724-7, 2006
5. Mahapatra RK et al: Corticobasal degeneration. Lancet Neurol. 3(12):736-43, 2004
6. Laureys S et al: Fluorodopa uptake and glucose metabolism in early stages of corticobasal degeneration. J Neurol. 246(12):1151-8, 1999
7. Hauser RA et al: Magnetic resonance imaging of corticobasal degeneration. J Neuroimaging. 6(4):222-6, 1996

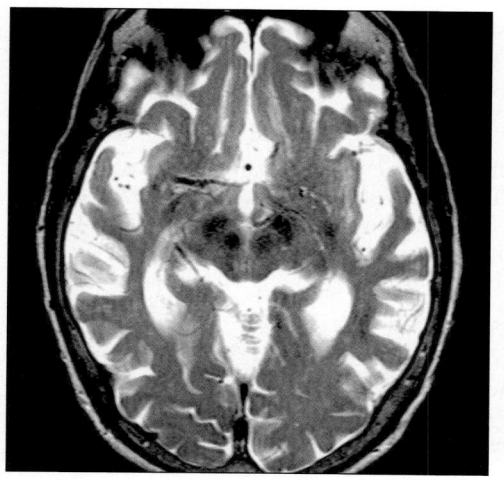

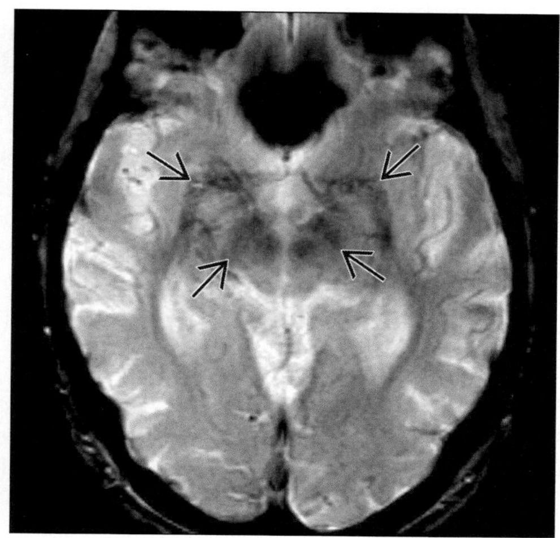

(Left) *Axial T2WI MR in a patient with corticobasal degeneration shows disproportionate enlargement of the basal cisterns and frontotemporal sulci. The red nucleus and substantia nigra are unusually hypointense.* ***(Right)*** *Axial T2* GRE MR in the same patient shows "blooming" in the heavily mineralized red nucleus, substantia nigra, and inferior basal ganglia →.*

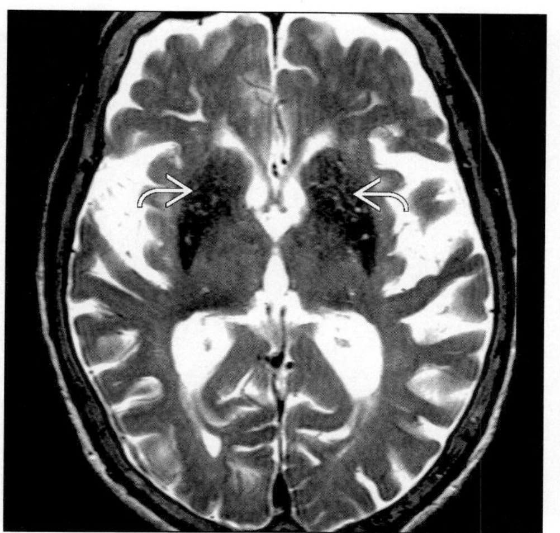

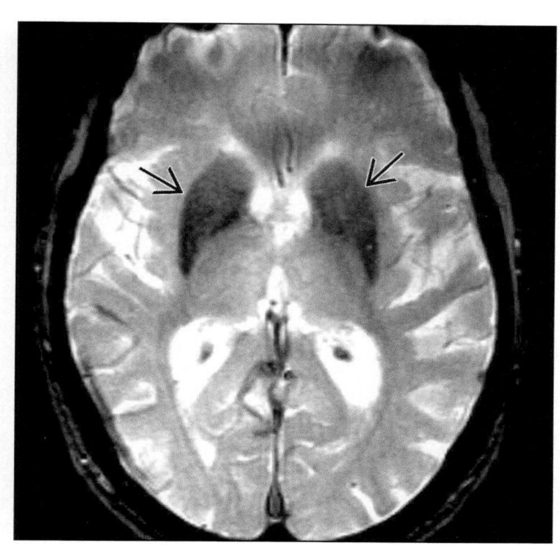

(Left) *Axial T2WI MR in the same patient shows prominent frontotemporoparietal atrophy. Both the putamen and the globus pallidi show prominent hypointense signal abnormality →.* ***(Right)*** *Axial T2* GRE MR in the same patient shows extensive mineralization of the putamen and globi pallidi →. This patient had progressive memory loss, limb dystonia, myoclonus, and the clinical diagnosis of corticobasal degeneration.*

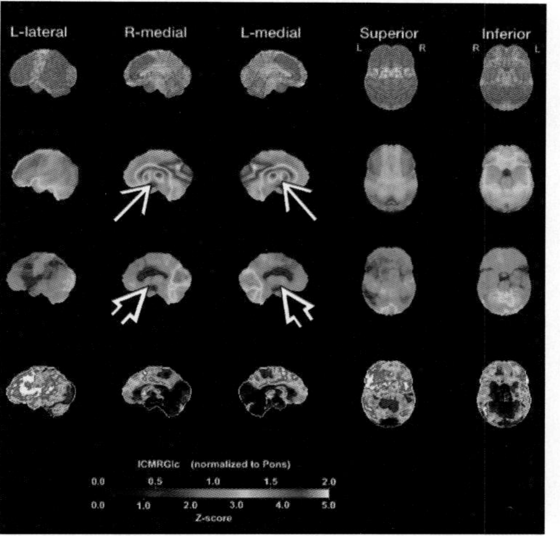

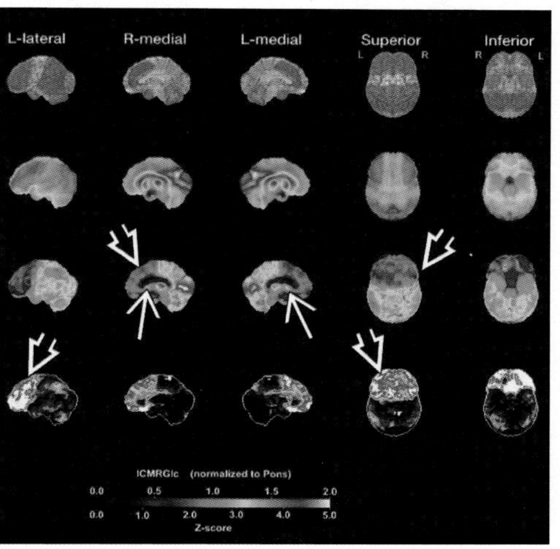

(Left) *SSP PET scan in a patient with severe CBD is illustrated. The 2nd row shows glucose metabolism in normal age-matched controls. Note the normal basal ganglia →. The 3rd row illustrates diffuse, severely diminished cortical metabolism, as well as markedly decreased glucose utilization, in the basal ganglia → compared to the normal control.* ***(Right)*** *SSP PET in another CBD patient shows less severely diminished glucose metabolism in the basal ganglia → and cortex →. (Courtesy N. Foster, MD.)*

PROGRESSIVE SUPRANUCLEAR PALSY

Key Facts

Terminology

- Neurodegenerative disease characterized by supranuclear palsy, postural instability, mild dementia

Imaging

- Midbrain atrophy ("penguin" or "hummingbird" sign)
  - Sagittal T1WI shows concave/flat upper border of midbrain (normally convex)
  - Axial images show abnormal concavity of lateral margins of midbrain tegmentum
  - Thinning of superior colliculus
- Mid-sagittal 3D-MPRAGE or FSPGR images
  - Voxel-based morphometry used to calculate ratio of midbrain to pons area
  - Midbrain area < 70 mm^2 (50% of normal)
  - Midbrain to pons ratio < 0.15 strongly suggests PSP

Top Differential Diagnoses

- Multiple system atrophy, parkinsonian type
- Corticobasal degeneration
- Dementia with Lewy bodies
- Parkinson disease

Pathology

- Neurofibrillary tangles and neuropil threads in globus pallidus, subthalamic nucleus, substantia nigra; cerebral cortex relatively preserved except for perirolandic cortex
- Neuronal loss, gliosis

Clinical Issues

- 2nd most common neurodegenerative cause of parkinsonism (after Parkinson disease)
- Characterized by down gaze palsy
- Progressive rigidity, imbalance → falls

(Left) *Sagittal T1WI MR in a patient with bradykinesia and suspected Parkinson disease shows the classic "penguin" or "hummingbird" sign of progressive supranuclear palsy (PSP). Note thinning of the midbrain ➡ with atrophy of the tectum ↪, also consistent with PSP. In contrast to the strikingly abnormal midbrain findings, here the pons appears normal.* ***(Right)*** *Axial T2WI MR in the same patient shows volume loss of the midbrain with thinned tectum → and concave lateral midbrain margins ⇨.*

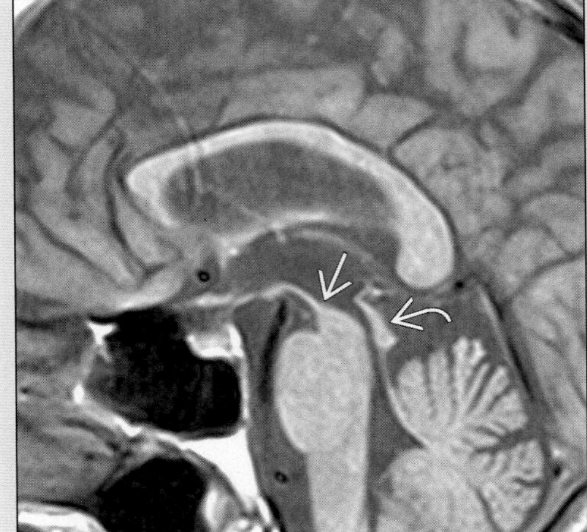

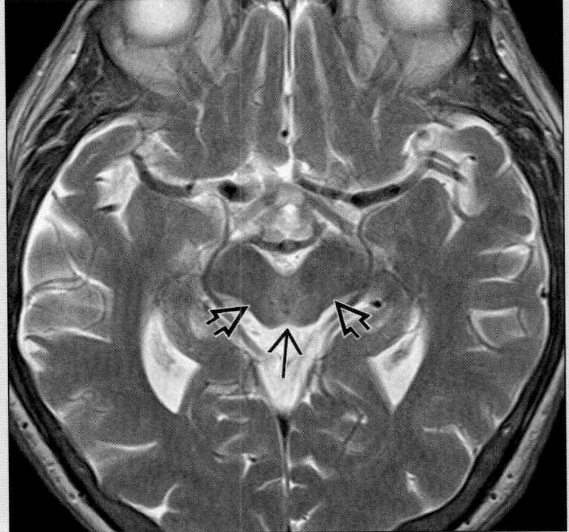

(Left) *Axial T2* GRE MR in the same patient shows no evidence for abnormal iron accumulation in the midbrain, which helps to distinguish PSP from Parkinson disease.* ***(Right)*** *Axial T2* GRE MR shows no evidence for abnormal iron accumulation in the striatum, another location in which iron is commonly found in Parkinson disease.*

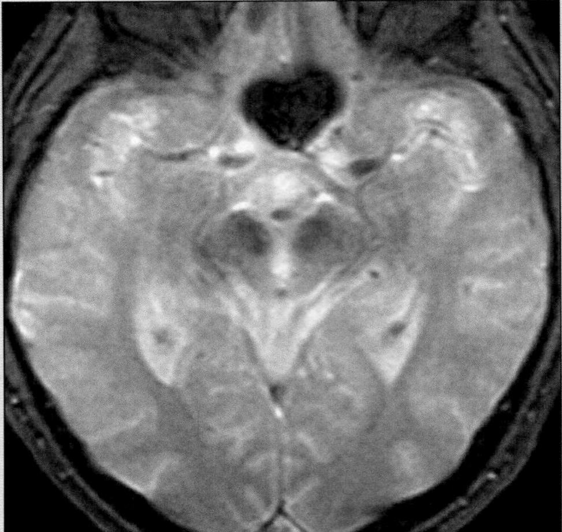

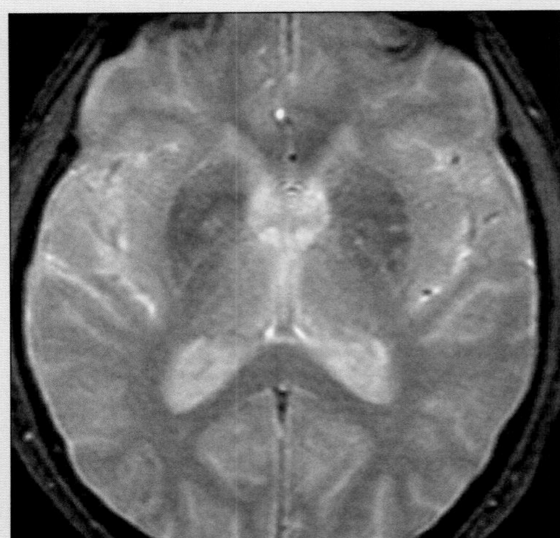

TERMINOLOGY

Abbreviations

- Progressive supranuclear palsy (PSP)

Synonyms

- Steele-Richardson-Olszewski syndrome

Definitions

- Neurodegenerative disease characterized by supranuclear palsy, postural instability, mild dementia

IMAGING

General Features

- Best diagnostic clue
  - Midbrain atrophy ("penguin" or "hummingbird" sign)
  - Most accurate = calculation of midbrain area/pons area ratio
    - Distinguishes PSP from other conditions
      - PSP vs. parkinsonian form of multi-system atrophy (MSA-P)
- Location
  - Midbrain
    - Tegmentum
    - Tectum (colliculi)
- Morphology
  - Prominent midbrain volume loss
    - Pons normal

Imaging Recommendations

- Best imaging tool
  - MR
  - PET
- Protocol advice
  - Mid-sagittal T1WI
  - 3D MP-RAGE or FSPGR images
    - Use voxel-based morphometry to calculate ratio of midbrain to pons area

CT Findings

- NECT
  - Atrophy of midbrain with cisternal and ventricular dilatation

MR Findings

- T1WI
  - Sagittal T1WI is helpful in detecting midbrain tectal atrophy ("penguin silhouette" sign)
    - Concave or flat profile of cephalad surface of midbrain (as opposed to normal convex superior profile)
    - Thinning of superior colliculus
  - Axial T1WIs show abnormal concavity of lateral margins of midbrain tegmentum
  - Midbrain area approximately 1/2 that of normal individuals
  - Significantly smaller ratio of midbrain-pons area (0.124) vs. Parkinson disease (0.208), multi-system atrophy (0.266), control (0.236)
  - Sagittal midbrain area < 70 mm^2, ratio of midbrain tegmentum to pons area < 0.15 → diagnostic of PSP
    - Sensitivity: 100%, specificity: 91-100%
  - Regional rates of brainstem atrophy > whole-brain atrophy in both PSP, MSA-P
- T2WI
  - Decreased AP diameter of midbrain on axial T2WI
  - Hyperintense signal in midbrain tegmentum
  - Occasionally abnormal hypointense signal in striatum
- DWI
  - Overlap of ADC values between PSP and Parkinson disease
- DTI
  - ↑ mean diffusivity in decussation of superior cerebellar peduncle

Nuclear Medicine Findings

- PET
  - Glucose hypometabolism in midline frontal regions and brain stem, caudate nucleus
  - Reduction of GABA receptors in cerebral cortex (anterior cingulate gyrus) but normal GABA activity in brain stem
  - Fluorodopa-PET: Reduction of F-dopa uptake in caudate, putamen (more severe than in PD)
- SPECT
  - I-123-IBZM SPECT: Reduced dopamine receptor binding in striatum

DIFFERENTIAL DIAGNOSIS

Multiple System Atrophy, Parkinsonian Type (MSA-P)

- T2 hypointensity in putamen without prominent midbrain atrophy
- Cerebellar atrophy
- Prominent cerebellar symptoms, autonomic dysfunction, parkinsonism

Corticobasal Degeneration

- Severe frontoparietal atrophy in asymmetrical pattern
- Unilateral parkinsonism
- "Alien limb" phenomenon, cortical sensory deficit

Dementia with Lewy Bodies

- Cortical atrophy without prominent midbrain atrophy
- Hallucinations, cortical dementia with aphasia, parkinsonism

Parkinson Disease

- No prominent midbrain atrophy
- Tremor-dominant clinical symptoms, good response to levodopa

PATHOLOGY

General Features

- Etiology
  - Abnormal accumulation of phosphorylated tau protein in brain
    - Pallidum, subthalamic nucleus, red nucleus, substantia nigra, pontine tegmentum, striatum, oculomotor nucleus, medulla, dentate nucleus
- Genetics
  - Associated with tau, *MTAP* gene on chromosome 17

PROGRESSIVE SUPRANUCLEAR PALSY

- Tau haplotype H1 is associated with both PSP and corticobasal degeneration
  - → suggests that gene on chromosome 17 for tau abnormality causes both diseases

Gross Pathologic & Surgical Features

- Atrophy of subthalamic nucleus and brainstem (midbrain tectum and superior cerebellar peduncle)
- Loss of pigmentation in substantia nigra → nigrostriatal dopaminergic degeneration

Microscopic Features

- Neuronal loss, gliosis
- Neurofibrillary tangles and neuropil threads in globus pallidus, subthalamic nucleus, substantia nigra; cerebral cortex relatively preserved except for perirolandic cortex
- Tau pathology is also noted in glia: Tufted astrocytes, coiled bodies of oligodendrocyte

CLINICAL ISSUES

Presentation

- Most common signs/symptoms
  - Postural instability and falls, bradykinesia, visual disturbance (e.g., diplopia)
  - Supranuclear ophthalmoplegia (vertical gaze palsy), pseudobulbar palsy (bilateral impairment of CN9-12 causing impairment of eating, swallowing, and talking), prominent neck dystonia
  - Personality change, memory problems, apathy
- Most common cause of atypical parkinsonian syndrome
  - 2nd most common neurodegenerative cause of parkinsonism overall
- Clinical criteria for PSP
  - Progressive akinetic-rigid syndrome starting after age 40
  - Progressive, prominent postural instability with falls in 1st year of illness
  - Slowing of vertical saccadic movements
  - Progressive vertical supranuclear gaze palsy
  - Supportive criteria
    - Axial rigidity out of proportion to appendicular rigidity, symmetric onset of symptoms, paucity of tremor, relative lack of levodopa therapy
  - Exclusion criteria
    - Evidence of AD, dementia with Lewy bodies disease, or lateralized corticobasal degeneration-type cognitive features

Demographics

- Age
  - Generally between 45-75 years
  - Mean approximately 65 years
- Gender
  - Slight male predominance
- Epidemiology
  - Prevalence: 7 cases per 100,000 population

Natural History & Prognosis

- Death usually within 6-12 years of diagnosis

Treatment

- No disease-modifying treatment has been developed as of yet

Variant PSP Syndrome

- PSP-parkinsonism
- PSP-pure akinesia with gait freezing
- PSP-corticobasal syndrome
- PSP-progressive nonfluent aphasia

DIAGNOSTIC CHECKLIST

Consider

- Consider PSP when MR shows marked midbrain atrophy in patients with atypical parkinsonism, vertical gaze palsy, and cognitive dysfunction

Image Interpretation Pearls

- Sagittal images are helpful in identifying "penguin silhouette" sign
- Minimal or no lobar atrophy

SELECTED REFERENCES

1. Williams DR et al: Progressive supranuclear palsy: clinicopathological concepts and diagnostic challenges. Lancet Neurol. 8(3):270-9, 2009
2. Quattrone A et al: MR imaging index for differentiation of progressive supranuclear palsy from Parkinson disease and the Parkinson variant of multiple system atrophy. Radiology. 246(1):214-21, 2008
3. Rizzo G et al: Diffusion-weighted brain imaging study of patients with clinical diagnosis of corticobasal degeneration, progressive supranuclear palsy and Parkinson's disease. Brain. 131(Pt 10):2690-700, 2008
4. Oba H et al: New and reliable MRI diagnosis for progressive supranuclear palsy. Neurology. 64(12):2050-5, 2005
5. Adachi M et al: Morning glory sign: a particular MR finding in progressive supranuclear palsy. Magn Reson Med Sci. 3(3):125-32, 2004
6. Righini A et al: MR imaging of the superior profile of the midbrain: differential diagnosis between progressive supranuclear palsy and Parkinson disease. AJNR Am J Neuroradiol. 25(6):927-32, 2004

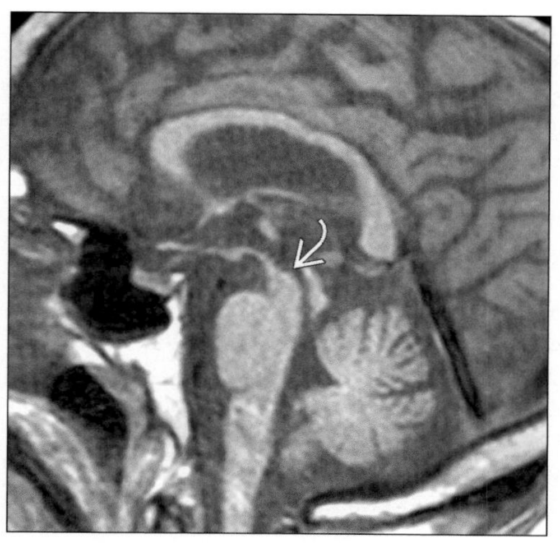

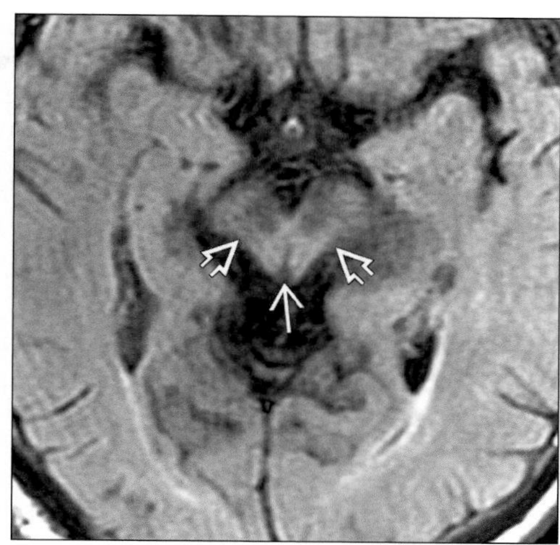

(Left) *Sagittal T1WI MR in a patient with progressive supranuclear palsy shows markedly diminished size of midbrain relative to pons. The cephalad surface of the midbrain appears concave ➔, in contrast to the normal convex superior profile.* ***(Right)*** *Axial FLAIR MR in the same patient shows striking atrophy of the midbrain tectum (colliculi) ➔ and concave margins of the midbrain tegmentum ➔.*

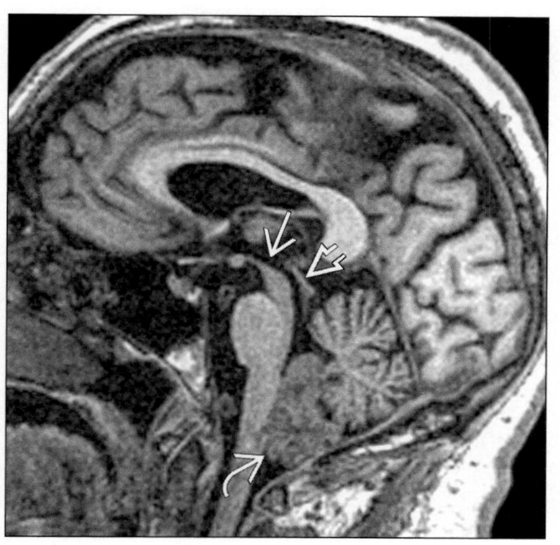

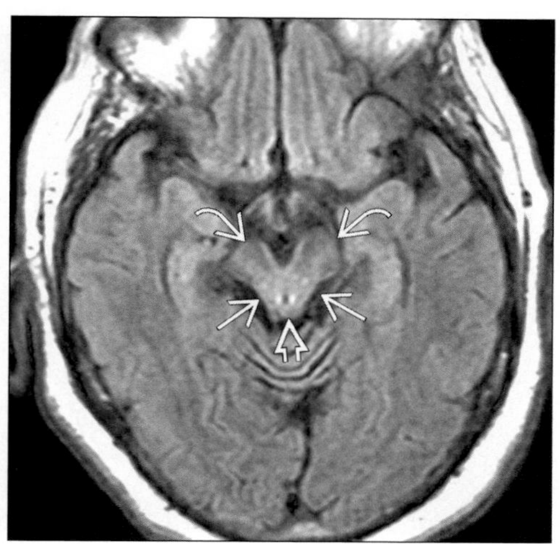

(Left) *Sagittal T1WI MR (3D MP-RAGE) in an 80-year-old woman with PSP shows striking midbrain volume loss, with "penguin" or "hummingbird" sign manifested by a concave upper border of the midbrain ➔. Note extreme thinning of the tectal plate ➔. An incidental subependymoma was found ➔.* ***(Right)*** *Axial FLAIR MR in the same patient shows the tectal plate is extremely thin ➔, the lateral aspects of the midbrain are concave ➔ ("morning glory" sign), and the cerebral peduncles ➔ are atrophic.*

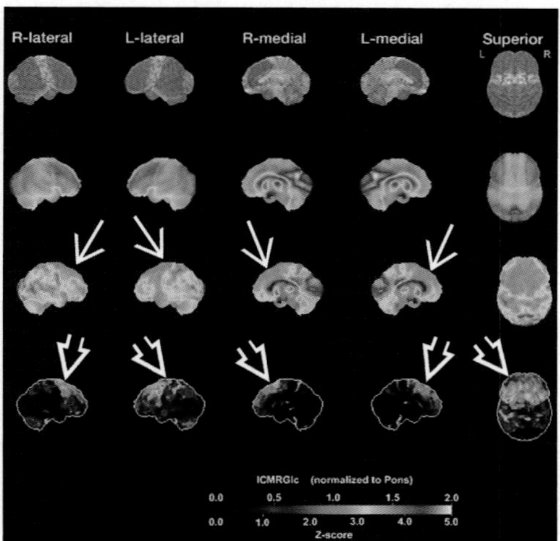

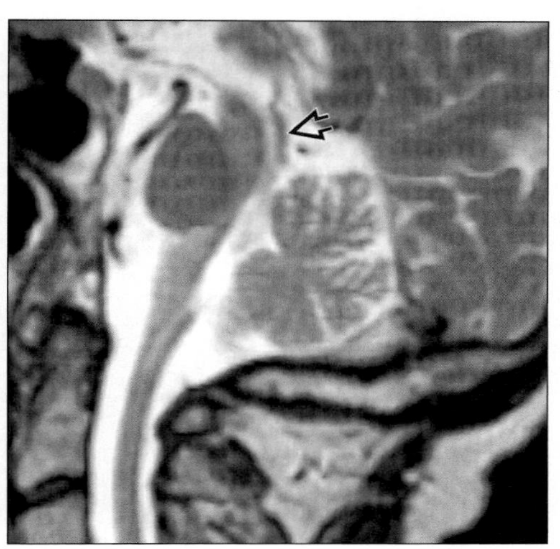

(Left) *PET scan with stereotaxic surface projections in the same patient. The top row is the reference map. The 2nd row illustrates glucose metabolism in elderly normal controls (n = 27). The 3rd row is the patient's glucose metabolism map. The 4th row is the Z-score map. The glucose metabolism ➔ and Z-score maps ➔ show markedly reduced metabolism in both frontal lobes. (Courtesy N. Foster, MD.)* ***(Right)*** *Sagittal T2WI MR in a patient with PSP shows diminished midbrain volume & thinned tectum ➔.*

AMYOTROPHIC LATERAL SCLEROSIS (ALS)

Key Facts

Terminology
- Amyotrophic lateral sclerosis (ALS)
- Selective degeneration of somatic motor neurons of brainstem/spinal cord and large pyramidal neurons of motor cortex
  - Eventual loss of corticospinal tract (CST) fibers

Imaging
- Bilateral hyperintensities along CST extending from corona radiata to brainstem on T2WI/PD/FLAIR
- Most specific finding is T2 hyperintensity in CST with corresponding PD hyperintensity
- DWI hyperintensity (↓ diffusivity) in CST
- Consider FLAIR and PD in all patients with clinically suspected ALS

Top Differential Diagnoses
- Primary lateral sclerosis
- Wallerian degeneration
- Hypertrophic olivary degeneration
- Metabolic diseases involving bilateral CSTs
- Demyelinating and inflammatory diseases
- Neoplasms: Brainstem glioma, malignant lymphoma
- CST can appear hyperintense on 3T MR normally

Pathology
- Majority of ALS cases are sporadic (sALS)
- 15-20% are familial (fALS)

Clinical Issues
- UMN signs: Babinski sign, spasticity, hyperreflexia
- LMN signs: Asymmetric muscle weakness, atrophy, fasciculations, hyporeflexia
- Bulbar signs: Slurred speech, dysphagia
- Onset usually between 4th-7th decades of life
- Complete disability and death within a decade

__(Left)__ Axial FLAIR MR shows increased signal in the precentral gyri ➔ in this ALS patient. There is also atrophy of bilateral motor cortices. __(Right)__ Coronal FLAIR MR shows linear hyperintensity ➔ along the corticospinal tract (CST) from the precentral gyrus to the cerebri crus. Right CST signal abnormality is out of this imaging slice. Hyperintensity of the precentral gyrus subcortical white matter on FLAIR is a potentially useful and specific sign of ALS that is not seen in healthy, asymptomatic patients.

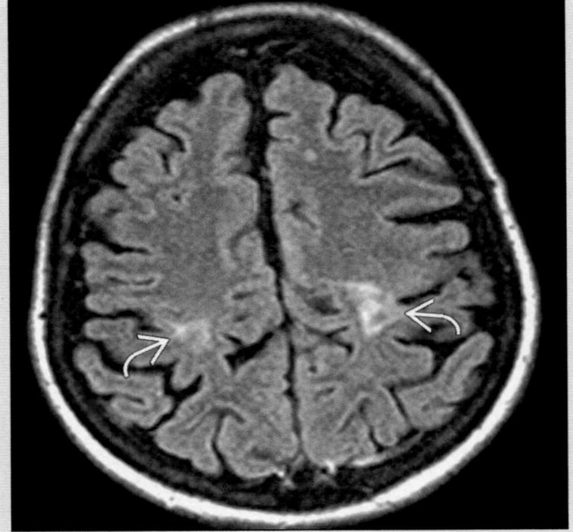

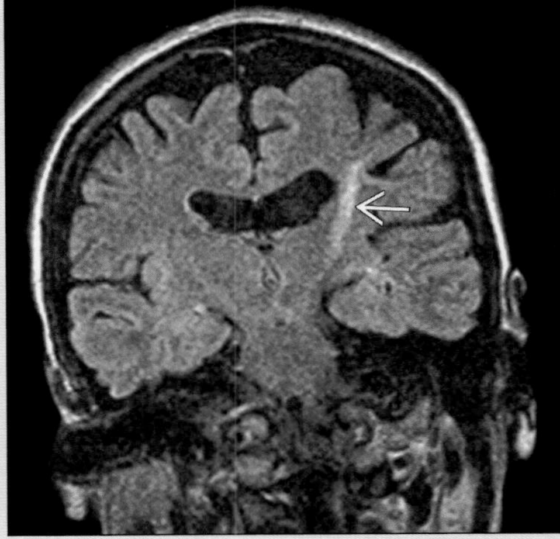

__(Left)__ Axial T2WI FS MR demonstrates ovoid hyperintensity along the CSTs bilaterally ➔. The atrophy and hyperintensity are due to myelin loss and gliosis. There is frequently involvement of the prefrontal motor neurons, which play a role in planning or orchestrating the work of the upper and lower motor neurons. __(Right)__ Axial DWI MR shows small foci of hyperintensity in the posterior limbs of bilateral internal capsules ➔ in this ALS patient.

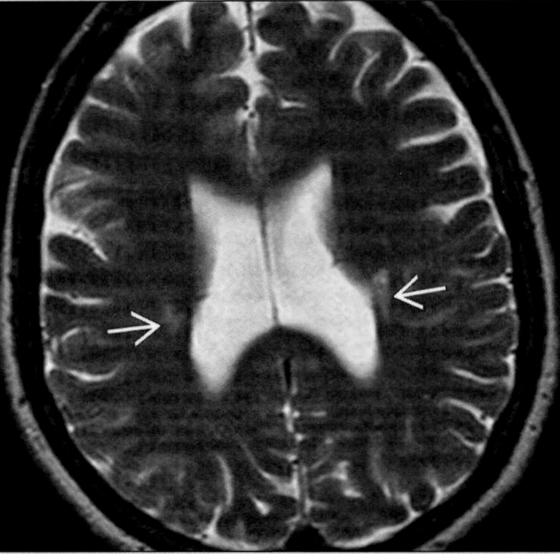

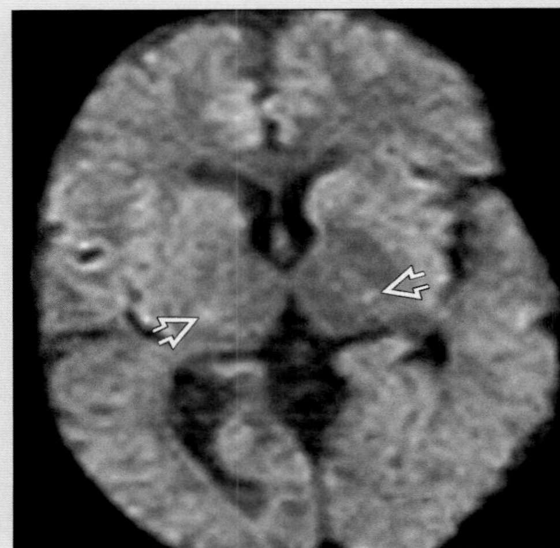

AMYOTROPHIC LATERAL SCLEROSIS (ALS)

TERMINOLOGY

Definitions

- Selective degeneration of somatic motor neurons of brainstem/spinal cord (lower motor neurons [LMN]) and large pyramidal neurons of motor cortex (upper motor neurons [UMN])
  - Eventual loss of corticospinal tract (CST) fibers

IMAGING

General Features

- Best diagnostic clue
  - Bilateral hyperintensities along CST extending from corona radiata to brainstem on T2WI/PD/FLAIR
- Location
  - Hallmark is CST and LMN degeneration
    - LMN in anterior horn of spinal cord and brainstem
    - Corticospinal UMN in precentral gyrus (motor cortex)
  - White matter (WM) and gray matter (GM)
- Size
  - Atrophy of motor system, particularly pyramidal tract, in advanced stages of ALS
- Morphology
  - Oval or thin curvilinear hyperintensities conforming to CST

CT Findings

- NECT
  - Serial CT exams may show progressive atrophy
    - Frontal, anterior temporal lobes → precentral gyrus → postcentral gyrus, anterior cingulate gyrus, corpus callosum, tegmentum

MR Findings

- T1WI
  - Different T1 appearances of CST
    - Isointensity (most common) may reflect ↑ content of free radicals
    - Hypointense or mild hyperintense signal
- T2WI
  - Diffuse hyperintensity following pyramidal tract
  - Hypointense GM in precentral gyrus (motor cortex)
    - Nonspecific; may be due to iron and heavy metals accumulation in cortex of aged patients
  - Symmetric, rounded foci of hyperintensity within caudal 1/3 of internal capsule (IC) posterior limb
    - Seen in ~ 50% of normal subjects
  - T2 hyperintense CST may be specific for ALS when seen on corresponding PD images
    - Most specific finding
- PD/intermediate
  - Hyperintense CST
- FLAIR
  - More sensitive and less specific than FSE for detecting hypointensity in precentral gyrus
  - Hyperintense CST
- DWI
  - Hyperintensity in CST
    - May be seen in the absence of T2 hyperintensity
- Diffusion tensor imaging (DTI)
  - Fractional anisotropy (FA) in CST is lower in ALS compared with normal individuals
    - ↓ fiber integrity in CST descending from motor and premotor cortex to IC and brainstem
  - ↓ FA in posterior limb of IC, more caudal CST (pons), underneath motor and premotor cortex, extramotor regions in frontal lobe
  - ↓ FA in thalamus and corpus callosum
  - Mean diffusivity (MD) is higher in ALS at level of IC
- ^{1}H-MRS useful for assessing UMN involvement
  - ↓ NAA/Cr, ↓ NAA, ↑ choline and myoinositol in precentral gyrus, perirolandic region, pons, and medulla
  - ↑ glutamate and glutamine, ↑ Glx/Cr in medulla
  - Longitudinal decline of cortical NAA and NAA/(Cr + Cho) ratios in motor cortex areas of both clinically more and less affected hemisphere
- Magnetization-transfer ratio (MTR) measurements
  - ↓ MTR in posterior limb of IC in ALS
  - CST hyperintensity on T1 MT contrast-enhanced images: 80% sensitivity, 100% specificity
  - May detect CST degeneration of ALS at early stage

Nuclear Medicine Findings

- PET, Tc-99m-HMPAO SPECT
  - Bilateral thalamic hypoperfusion, parietal and frontal hypoperfusion in familial ALS (fALS)
  - Hypoperfusion and oxygen hypometabolism in anterior cerebral hemispheres
    - Associated with progressive dementia in ALS
  - Metabolic and perfusion changes in cerebral cortex
  - Sensorimotor: Very mild ↓ rCBF, O_2 metabolism

Imaging Recommendations

- Best imaging tool: MR with T2, PD, FLAIR, DTI

DIFFERENTIAL DIAGNOSIS

Primary Lateral Sclerosis

- Neurodegeneration restricted to UMN
  - T2WI shows changes in motor pathways
- Autosomal recessive disease with juvenile onset

Wallerian Degeneration

- Dynamic signal intensities change along CST in patients with various cortical/subcortical lesions

Hypertrophic Olivary Degeneration

- Secondary degeneration of inferior olivary nucleus (ION), usually caused by primary lesions in dento-rubro-olivary pathway

Conditions with T2 Hyperintense Lesions along CST

- Metabolic diseases may involve CST bilaterally
  - X-linked adrenoleukodystrophy, Wilson disease
  - Hypoglycemic coma: Reversible CST changes
- Demyelinating and inflammatory diseases
  - Multiple sclerosis, ADEM, Behçet disease, AIDS, cervical myelopathy
- Neoplasms: Brainstem glioma, malignant lymphoma

AMYOTROPHIC LATERAL SCLEROSIS (ALS)

Normal Individuals

- CST can appear hyperintense on 3T MR (normal fully myelinated brain at any age) and mimic ALS

PATHOLOGY

General Features

- Etiology
  - Etiology of sporadic ALS (sALS) is largely unknown
  - Pathological hallmarks include loss of MNs with intraneuronal ubiquitin-immunoreactive inclusions in UMN and TDP-43 immunoreactive inclusions in degenerating LMN
  - Increased expression of cyclooxygenase-2 in spinal cord, frontal cortex, and hippocampus
  - Apoptosis, free radical-mediated oxidative stress, excessive glutamate-mediated excitotoxicity
  - Dopamine deficiency probably has important role
  - Biochemical studies have shown ↓ glutamate levels in CNS tissue and ↑ levels in CSF
- Genetics
  - Majority of ALS cases are sporadic (sALS)
  - 15-20% of ALS cases are familial (fALS)
    - 10-20% of fALS cases are caused by mutations in copper/zinc superoxide dismutase 1 gene (*SOD1*) on chromosome 21q
      - > 100 different mutations reported, majority are autosomal dominant
  - Rare autosomal recessive juvenile-onset ALS
    - *ALS2* gene on chromosome 2q encodes alsin
- Associated abnormalities
  - ALS-plus syndrome: Typical ALS phenotype associated with dementia, parkinsonism, or both
    - 2-3% of cases, ALS is accompanied by frontotemporal dementia
    - ~ 50% of cases show cognitive impairment
  - ALS-like motor neuron disease can occur as paraneoplastic syndrome

Gross Pathologic & Surgical Features

- Atrophic precentral gyrus in longer disease duration
- Degeneration of thalamus, corpus callosum atrophy

Microscopic Features

- Loss of cortical pyramidal motor neurons and astrocytosis
- Histologically uneven involvement of CST showing variable patterns of degeneration
- "Senescent changes" with lipofuscin pigment atrophy
- Proximal and distal axonopathy with axonal spheroids
- Surviving motor neurons are smaller and abnormal

CLINICAL ISSUES

Presentation

- Most common signs/symptoms
  - UMN signs: Babinski sign, spasticity, hyperreflexia
  - LMN signs: Asymmetric muscle weakness, atrophy, fasciculations, hyporeflexia
  - Bulbar signs: Slurred speech, dysphagia
  - Difficulty walking, unexplained weight loss
- Other signs/symptoms
  - El Escorial criteria diagnosis of ALS: Evidence of UMN findings, LMN findings, and progression
    - 4 regions or levels: Bulbar, cervical, thoracic, lumbosacral
- Clinical profile
  - Classic ALS: Both UMN and LMN affected
  - UMN-dominant ALS can be difficult to distinguish from primary lateral sclerosis
  - Predominantly bulbar form usually leads to more rapid deterioration and death
  - fALS associated with *SOD1* abnormality has mean age at 42 years limb onset, slow evolution

Demographics

- Age
  - Onset usually between 4th-7th decades of life
- Gender
  - M:F = 1.5:1
- Ethnicity
  - Caucasian to non-Caucasian ratio is 1.6:1 in USA
- Epidemiology
  - Incidence: 0.5-2 cases/100,000 persons
  - Prevalence: 5.2/100,000 persons

Natural History & Prognosis

- Progressive (distal to proximal)
  - Complete disability and death within a decade
  - 20% of patients survive > 5 years
- Some patients with familial, juvenile-onset ALS survive for longer periods (2-3 decades)

Treatment

- Riluzole (glutamate release inhibitor and insulin-like growth factor) may prolong survival
  - ↑ NAA/Cr in precentral gyrus and supplementary motor area after riluzole therapy

DIAGNOSTIC CHECKLIST

Consider

- FLAIR and PD in all patients with suspected ALS

Image Interpretation Pearls

- High signal intensity in posterior limb of IC is highly suggestive for ALS when also visible on PD
- T1- and PD-weighted images differentiate real degeneration from normal areas
- DTI can assess CST lesions before pyramidal symptoms

SELECTED REFERENCES

1. Wijesekera LC et al: Amyotrophic lateral sclerosis. Orphanet J Rare Dis. 4:3, 2009
2. Sage CA et al: Quantitative diffusion tensor imaging in amyotrophic lateral sclerosis. Neuroimage. 34(2):486-99, 2007
3. Unrath A et al: Brain metabolites in definite amyotrophic lateral sclerosis. A longitudinal proton magnetic resonance spectroscopy study. J Neurol. 254(8):1099-106, 2007
4. Kalra S et al: Rapid improvement in cortical neuronal integrity in amyotrophic lateral sclerosis detected by proton magnetic resonance spectroscopic imaging. J Neurol. 253(8):1060-3, 2006

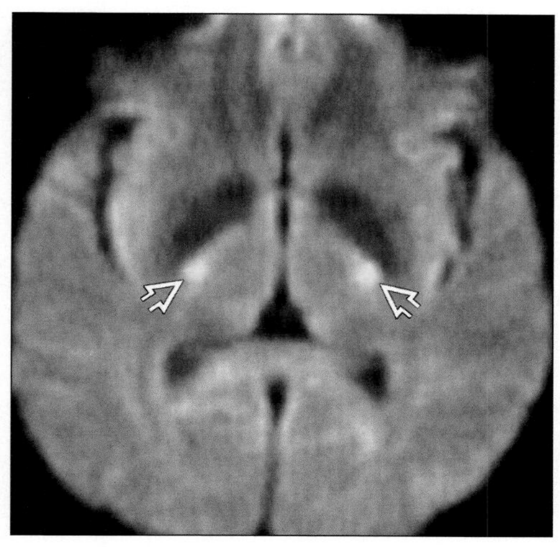

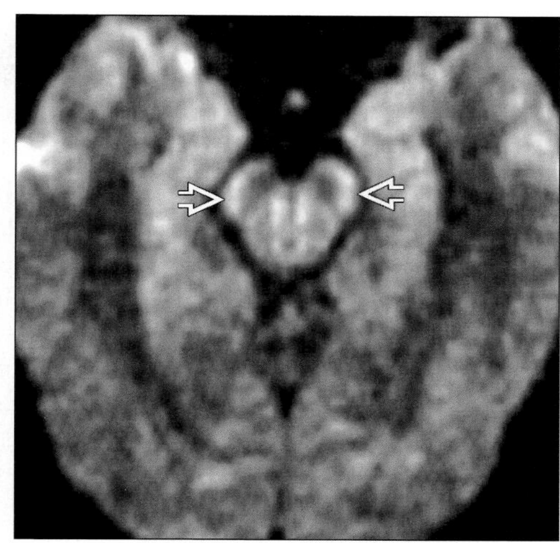

(Left) *Axial DTI trace image shows symmetric hyperintensity in the internal capsule posterior limbs ➡. Fractional anisotropy (FA) correlates with measures of disease severity and UMN involvement, whereas the mean diffusivity correlates with disease duration.* ***(Right)*** *Axial DWI MR shows round hyperintensities in bilateral cerebral peduncles ➡. Signal abnormality can be seen in the precentral gyrus, centrum semiovale, posterior 3rd of posterior limb of internal capsules, cerebral peduncles, and ventral brainstem.*

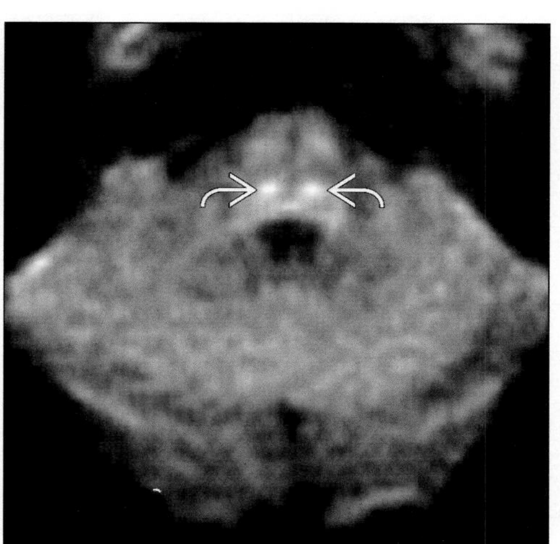

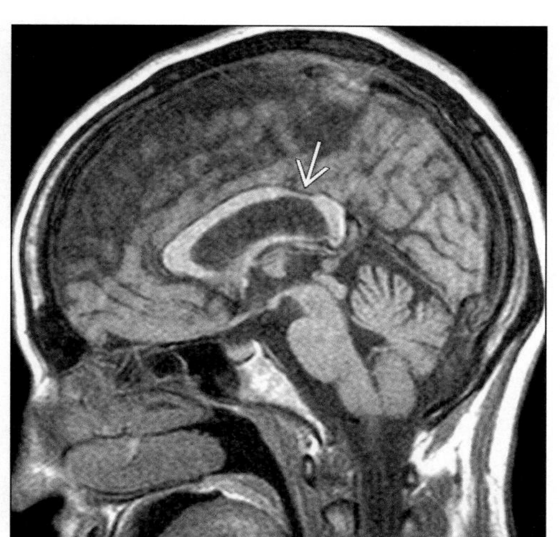

(Left) *Axial DWI MR shows oval hyperintensities corresponding to CSTs in the pons ➡. DWI/DTI can help differentiate progressive muscular atrophy (no change in FA or MD) from ALS (↑ MD, ↓ FA), which can be clinically difficult.* ***(Right)*** *Sagittal T1WI MR shows atrophy of the posterior corpus callosum body ➡. DTI also shows ↓ FA in the corpus callosum. Voxel-based morphometry has a high sensitivity in detecting local tissue atrophy in the motor cortex and along the corticospinal tracts.*

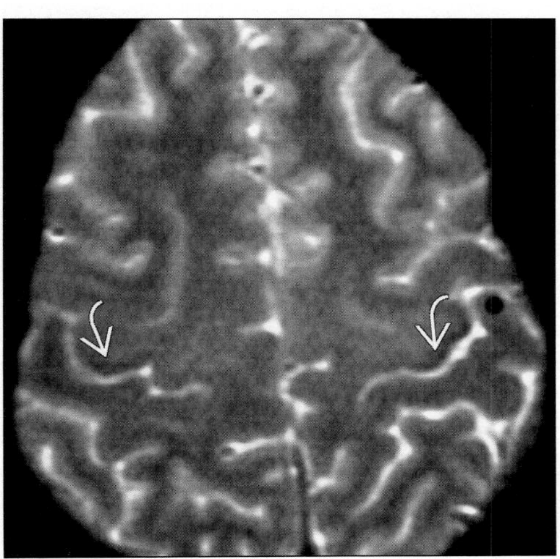

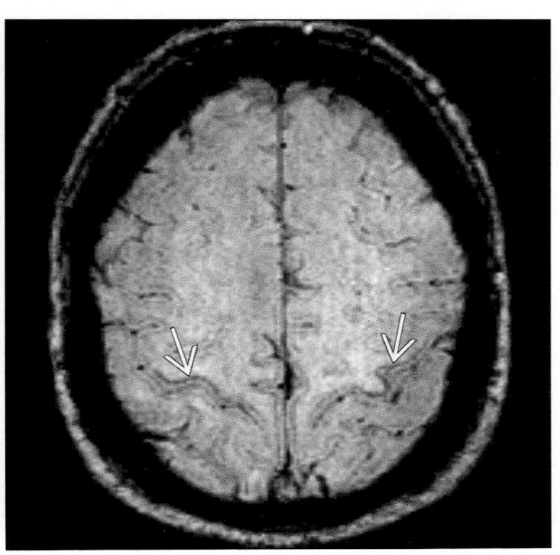

(Left) *Axial T2WI FS MR shows central cortical hypointense signal intensity ➡ in the precentral gyri due to iron deposition. While this is common in ALS patients, it is nonspecific and may be seen in aged patients due to iron and heavy metals accumulation.* ***(Right)*** *Axial T2* SWI MR demonstrates curvilinear hypointensity along the cortical gray matter of bilateral precentral gyri ➡. The T2* SWI technique accentuates the T2 hypointensity seen in the precentral gyrus gray matter of ALS patients.*

WALLERIAN DEGENERATION

Key Facts

Terminology

- Wallerian degeneration (WaD)
  - Secondary anterograde degeneration of axons and their myelin sheaths caused by proximal axonal or neuronal cell body lesions

Imaging

- Primary lesion is cortical or subcortical with WaD in descending white matter (WM) tracts ipsilateral to neuronal injury
  - WaD can be seen in fibers crossing the corpus callosum, fibers of optic radiations, fornices, and cerebellar peduncles
- CT is not sensitive for WaD in acute-subacute stages
  - Detects atrophy of CSTs in chronic stage
- Time-dependent changes in CSTs on MR
  - Strong correlation between WaD detected on T2WI and DWI and long-term morbidity
  - DWI findings precede development of WaD assessed by conventional MR
- DTI may distinguish between primary lesion and associated WaD
  - Reduced fractional anisotropy (FA) with increased mean diffusivity (MD) in infarct
  - Reduced FA with preserved MD in CST

Top Differential Diagnoses

- Neurodegenerative diseases
- Brainstem glioma
- Demyelinating and inflammatory diseases
- Hypertrophic olivary degeneration
- Metabolic diseases
- Intoxication (heroin inhalation)
- Normal appearance of hyperintensity on high field strength MR

*(**Left**) Axial NECT shows encephalomalacia in the left frontal and temporal opercula ➭ related to a chronic stroke. Hypodensity and volume loss in the thalamus ➭ is likely due to wallerian degeneration of the corticothalamic fibers. (**Right**) Axial NECT in the same patient shows atrophy of the left cerebral peduncle ➡ due to chronic wallerian degeneration of the corticospinal tracts. NECT is not sensitive for acute-subacute stages but detects atrophy of the pyramidal tracts in the chronic stage of wallerian degeneration.*

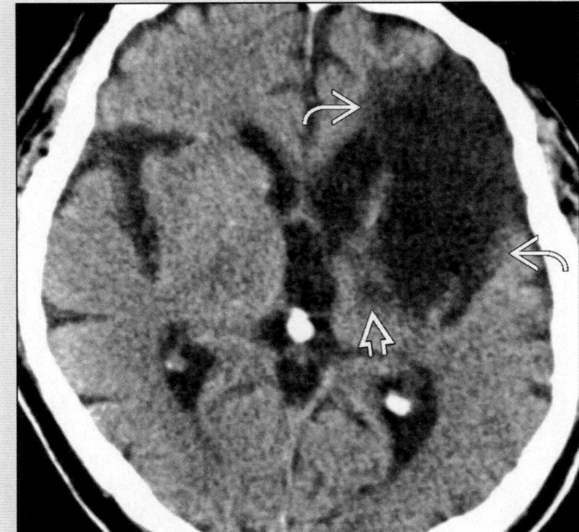

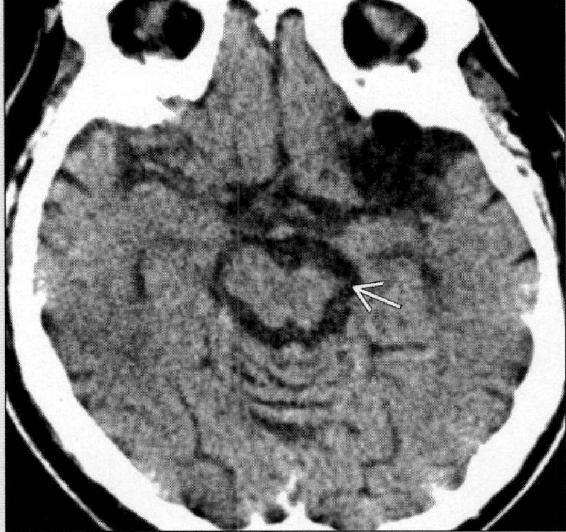

*(**Left**) Axial DTI trace image shows increased signal in the left corona radiata/corticospinal tract related to an acute infarct ➡. DTI may distinguish between the primary lesion and associated wallerian degeneration. Reduced fractional anisotropy may be seen in the affected corticospinal tract. (**Right**) Axial DTI trace shows increased signal in the central cerebral peduncle ➭ related to corticospinal tract wallerian degeneration. The lateral cerebral peduncle may show corticopontine tract involvement.*

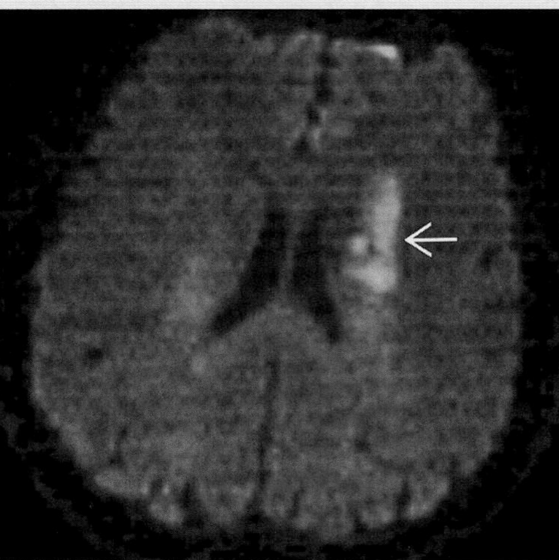

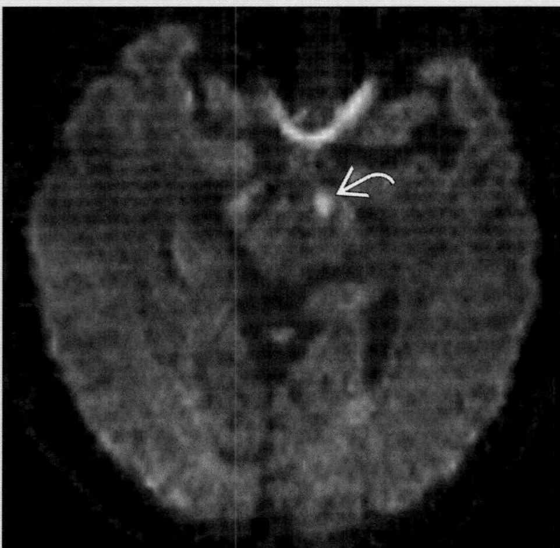

TERMINOLOGY

Abbreviations

- Wallerian degeneration (WaD)

Definitions

- Secondary anterograde degeneration of axons and their myelin sheaths caused by proximal axonal or neuronal cell body lesions

IMAGING

General Features

- Best diagnostic clue
  - Contiguous T2 hyperintensity along topographic distribution of corticospinal tract (CST) in internal capsule (IC) and brainstem in patients with various cerebral pathologies
- Location
  - Primary lesion: Cortical or subcortical
  - WaD: Descending white matter (WM) tracts ipsilateral to neuronal injury
    - CST, corticobulbar, corticopontine tracts
  - WaD can be seen in corpus callosum, optic radiations, fornices, and cerebellar peduncles
  - Corpus callosum has been shown to be susceptible to atrophy in Alzheimer disease mainly as correlate of wallerian degeneration of commissural nerve fibers of neocortex
  - Seizure-induced damage may cause secondary white matter degeneration along tapetum and through splenium of corpus callosum

CT Findings

- NECT
  - Not sensitive for WaD in acute-subacute stages
  - Detects atrophy of CSTs in chronic stage
    - ↓ size of corresponding aspect of brainstem

MR Findings

- T1WI
  - Time-dependent changes in descending WM tracts
    - Stage 1: No changes
    - Stage 2: T1 hyperintense
    - Stage 3: T1 hypointense
    - Stage 4: Ipsilateral brainstem atrophy ± hypointensity
- T2WI
  - Time-dependent changes in descending WM tracts
    - Stage 1: No changes in adult CNS
    - Stage 2: T2 hypointense
    - Stage 3: T2 hyperintense
    - Stage 4: Atrophy, best seen in brainstem
      - Sometimes, T2 hyperintense signal may persist
  - Neonates and infants: Identification of WaD by T2WI complicated by high water content and lack of myelination in immature WM
  - Adults: Strong correlation between T2WI detected WaD and long-term morbidity
- PD/intermediate
  - High intensity follows particular WM pathway
- FLAIR
  - Same as T2WI
- DWI
  - Neonates and infants: Indicates acute WM injury
    - DWI findings precede development of WaD assessed by conventional MR
    - May portend poor clinical outcome
  - Adults: Correlation of DW changes in descending motor pathways at presentation with long-term neurologic disability
  - Extent and severity of territorial ischemia is related to development of descending WM tract injury detectable by DWI
  - Hyperintense DW signal intensity and ↓ ADC values within territorial infarct and ipsilateral CST
    - DW and ADC time courses in region of territorial injury and CST injury may be different
      - Relatively delayed development of diffusion abnormality in descending WM tracts
  - Subacute period after territorial infarction in adults
    - Within infarct, WM ADC reduction > that in GM
  - DW signal intensity abnormality in descending WM tracts may persist, even as DW hyperintensity in ipsilateral cerebral hemisphere fades
- T1WI C+
  - No contrast enhancement of degenerated tracts
- MRS
  - ^{1}H-MRS enables in vivo assessment of axonal injury based on signal intensity of N-acetyl aspartate (NAA)
  - ↓ NAA concentration (< 3.0) in normal-appearing WM in pons and cerebellar peduncles in early stages of relapsing-remitting multiple sclerosis (MS)
    - Correlates best with disability, MS duration, and relapse rate
- Diffusion tensor imaging (DTI)
  - Myelin breakdown leads to ↓ diffusion anisotropy
  - Reduced FA with increased MD in infarct
  - Reduced FA with preserved MD in CST
  - In patients with motor pathway infarction, diffusion indices in degenerated CST stabilize within 3 months and early changes in CST FA may predict long-term clinical outcomes

Imaging Recommendations

- Best imaging tool
  - MR
- Protocol advice
  - DWI allows early detection (stage 1)
  - T2WI detects changes after 4 weeks

DIFFERENTIAL DIAGNOSIS

Neurodegenerative Diseases

- Amyotrophic lateral sclerosis (upper &/or lower motor neuron involvement)
  - Bilateral hyperintensities along CST extending from corona radiata to brainstem on T2WI/PD/FLAIR
- Primary lateral sclerosis and infantile-onset hereditary spastic paraplegia
  - Upper motor neuron degeneration only

Brainstem Glioma

- T2 hyperintense mass ± enhancement

Demyelinating and Inflammatory Diseases

- Multiple sclerosis: Periventricular T2 hyperintensity

- ADEM: Asymmetric T2 hyperintensity in white and gray matter after viral prodrome
- Behçet disease: Enlarged, T2 hyperintense brainstem ± thalamus

Hypertrophic Olivary Degeneration

- Secondary degeneration of inferior olivary nucleus (ION), usually caused by primary lesions in dentato-rubro-olivary pathway

Metabolic Diseases

- X-linked adrenoleukodystrophy: Enhancing peritrigonal demyelination
- Wilson disease: White and gray matter lesions involving basal ganglia, dentate nucleus, brainstem
- Hypoglycemic coma: Reversible CST changes

Heroin Inhalation

- Symmetric T2 hyperintensity in posterior WM, including posterior limb of internal capsule

Normal Individuals

- CST can appear hyperintense on 3T MR (normal fully myelinated brain)

PATHOLOGY

General Features

- Etiology
  - Infarction, hemorrhage, neoplasm, encephalitis
  - Demyelinating disease, trauma, AV malformations
  - Reported also in patients with movement disorder
- Genetics
  - Process of axonal degeneration is genetically regulated
- Associated abnormalities
  - Primary lesion/disorder that caused secondary WM tract degeneration

Staging, Grading, & Classification

- Stage 1 (0-4 weeks): Degradation of axon; mild changes in myelin
- Stage 2 (4-14 weeks): Myelin protein breakdown; lipids remain intact
- Stage 3 (> 14 weeks): Myelin lipid breakdown, gliosis, changes in water content and structure
- Stage 4 (after months to years): Atrophy of ipsilateral brainstem

Gross Pathologic & Surgical Features

- Brainstem asymmetry due to atrophy in chronic stage

Microscopic Features

- Stage 1: Beginning of myelin and axon breakdown
  - Myelin sheaths break up into ellipsoids and spheres but retain myelin staining properties
- Stage 2: Decreased protein:lipid ratio
- Stage 3: Increased edema and further lipid breakdown
- Stage 4: Atrophy due to volume loss; removal of axonal debris by microglia continues for 2 years (vs. completed in 3 weeks in peripheral nervous system)
- Expression of transcription factors ATF3 and c-Jun by nonneuronal cells during WaD
  - ATF3/c-Jun heterodimers may play role in regulating changes in gene expression necessary for preparing distal segments of injured peripheral nerves for axonal regeneration
  - Absence of ATF3 and c-Jun from CNS glia during WaD may limit their ability to support regeneration
- In CNS, astrocyte-dominated matrix fails to accommodate new axonal growth

CLINICAL ISSUES

Presentation

- Most common signs/symptoms
  - WaD in CST is associated with persistent hemiparesis

Demographics

- Age
  - Reported in all ages
- Gender
  - No gender preference
- Epidemiology
  - WaD commonly follows CNS lesions
    - WaD in pyramidal tract reported in 78.6% of cases of capsular infarct

Natural History & Prognosis

- WaD may begin within 1 week of fiber tract damage
- Demyelination can continue during next 6 months
- Signifies irreversible loss of neuronal function
- Extent of WaD is related to severity of motor deficit
  - Abnormal DWI signal in CST can be acute predictor of motor outcome in childhood infarction

Treatment

- No specific therapy

DIAGNOSTIC CHECKLIST

Image Interpretation Pearls

- In ischemic stroke: Important to differentiate DWI abnormality related to WaD from additional infarction
- Time-specific signal intensity changes of WaD → able to ascertain age of primary lesion

SELECTED REFERENCES

1. Domi T et al: Corticospinal tract pre-wallerian degeneration: a novel outcome predictor for pediatric stroke on acute MRI. Stroke. 40(3):780-7, 2009
2. Liang Z et al: Progression of pathological changes in the middle cerebellar peduncle by diffusion tensor imaging correlates with lesser motor gains after pontine infarction. Neurorehabil Neural Repair. 23(7):692-8, 2009
3. Oh MY et al: Ipsilateral wallerian degeneration of the distal optic radiations after infarction at their root. J Neuroophthalmol. 29(2):146-8, 2009
4. Yu C et al: A longitudinal diffusion tensor imaging study on Wallerian degeneration of corticospinal tract after motor pathway stroke. Neuroimage. 47(2):451-8, 2009
5. De Simone T et al: Wallerian degeneration of the pontocerebellar fibers. AJNR Am J Neuroradiol. 26(5):1062-5, 2005

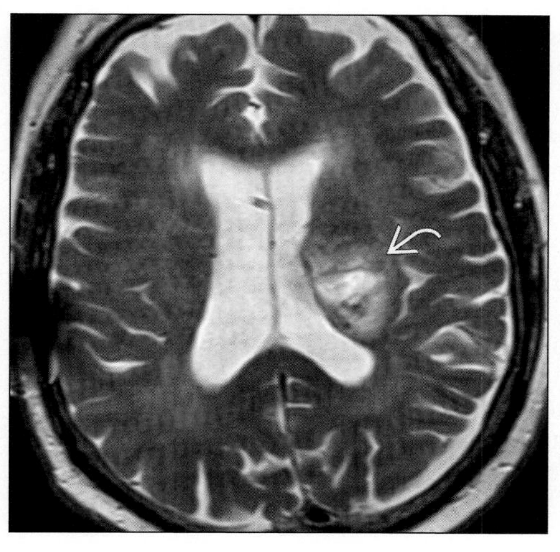

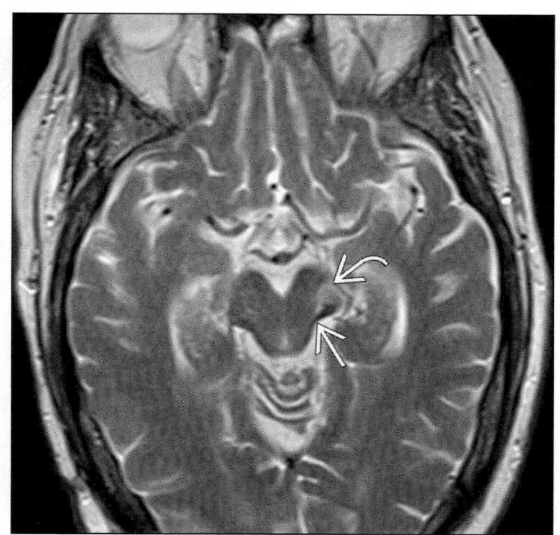

(Left) *Axial T2WI MR shows a heterogeneous hyperintense lesion involving the left corona radiata and corticospinal tract ➡ related to a glioblastoma. Note the internal curvilinear T2 hypointensity related to blood products or proteinaceous debris.* ***(Right)*** *Axial T2WI MR in the same patient shows cerebral peduncle hyperintensity ➡ due to corticospinal tract Wallerian degeneration from the tumor. There is slight volume loss with linear T2 hypointensity along the posterolateral margin ➡.*

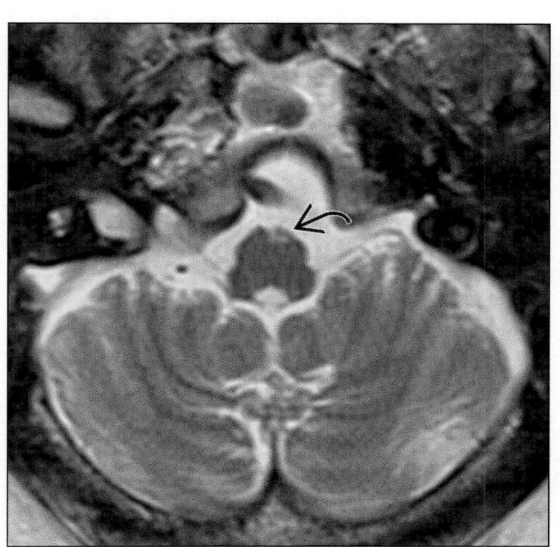

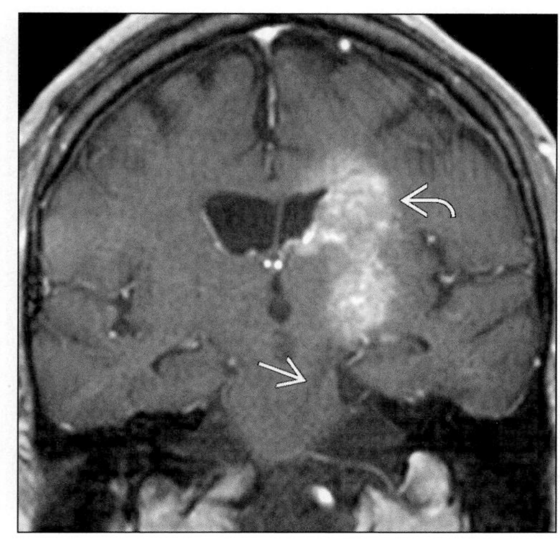

(Left) *Axial T2WI MR at the level of the medulla shows increased signal in the left pyramidal tract ➡ due to wallerian degeneration of the corticospinal tracts from a corona radiata tumor. T2 hyperintensity is due to myelin lipid breakdown and gliosis, as well as changes in water content and structure.* ***(Right)*** *Coronal T1WI C+ MR of the same patient shows an infiltrative, enhancing mass ➡. T1 hypointensity ➡ along the corticospinal tract is due to lipid breakdown and edema.*

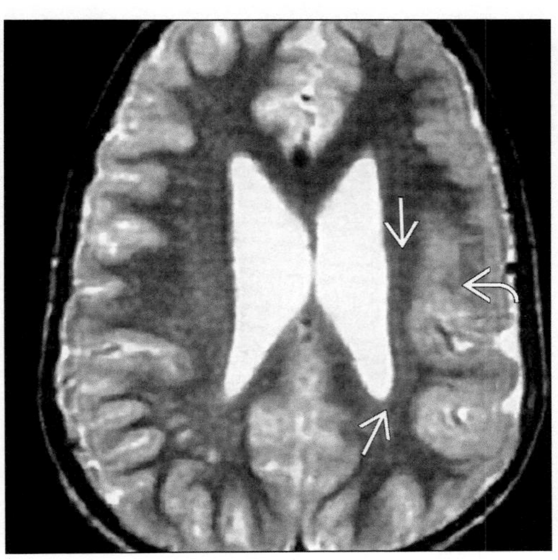

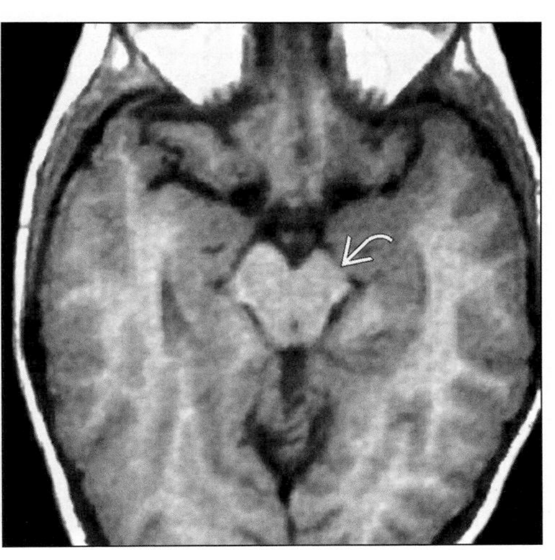

(Left) *Axial T2WI MR shows a left hemispheric lissencephaly with pachygyria ➡. When due to toxins or infections, as in this case, reactive gliosis with macrophage infiltration disturbs neuronal migration, resulting in abnormal cortex and sparse underlying white matter ➡.* ***(Right)*** *Axial T1WI MR in the same patient shows a diminutive left cerebral peduncle ➡. This neuronal migrational abnormality results in 4-layer cortex with sparse underlying white matter. There is consequent hypoplasia of the corticospinal tract.*

CROSSED CEREBELLAR DIASCHISIS

Key Facts

Terminology

- "Diaschisis" = sudden loss of function in brain connected to (but at distance from) damaged area
- CCD = decreased blood flow/metabolism in cerebellar hemisphere contralateral to supratentorial infarct

Imaging

- Acute: CT/MR perfusion shows ↓ CBF in cerebellar hemisphere opposite acute hemispheric infarct
  - ↑ TTP, ↓ CBF in cerebellum contralateral to infarct
  - Add DTI as subtle cases may show ↓ FA when conventional MR normal
  - (18)F-FDG PET/CT shows diffusely reduced uptake in contralateral cerebellar hemisphere
- Chronic: CT or MR shows atrophic cerebellar hemisphere opposite old hemispheric infarct

Top Differential Diagnoses

- Superior cerebellar artery infarct
  - CCD involves > just SCA territory
- Encephalomalacia
  - Trauma, infection, surgery
- Cerebellitis
  - Cerebellum swollen, hyperintense (not shrunken, atrophic)

Pathology

- Corticopontocerebellar (CPC) tract
  - Input to cerebellum via corticopontocerebellar tracts 40x all other afferent sources combined
  - Injury at any point along CPC can result in ↓ CBF, metabolism in contralateral cerebellar hemisphere
  - Most common cause = MCA infarct
  - Others: Neoplasm, trauma, surgery, epilepsy, etc.

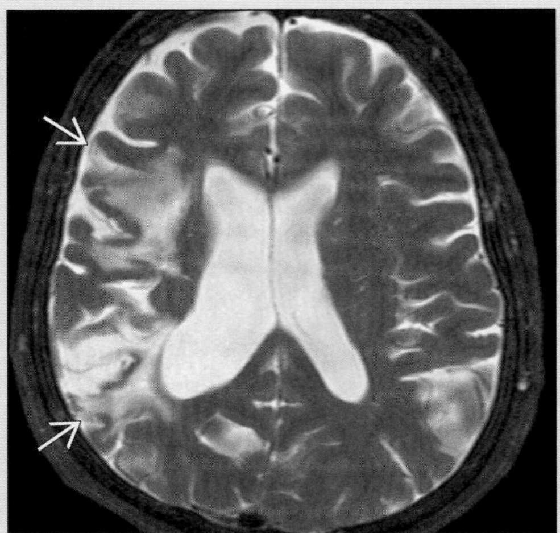

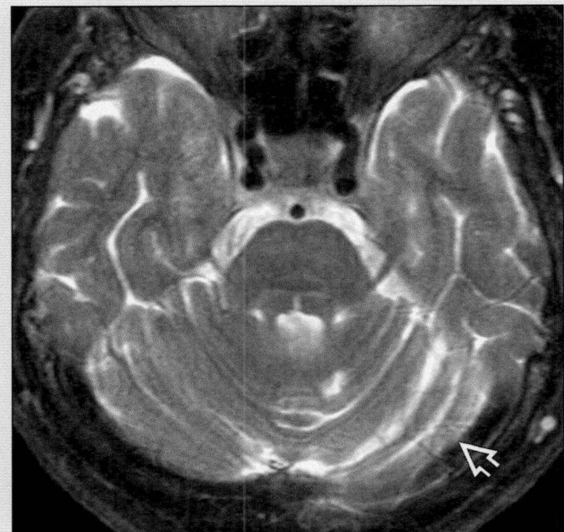

(Left) *Axial T2WI MR in a patient with a history of remote right middle cerebral artery infarct shows the typical changes of volume loss and hyperintensity in the cortex and subcortical white matter ➔. The ipsilateral ventricle is enlarged.* ***(Right)*** *Axial T2WI MR in the same patient shows volume loss with enlarged horizontal sulci in the contralateral cerebellar hemisphere ⇨. These findings are consistent with chronic crossed cerebellar diaschisis.*

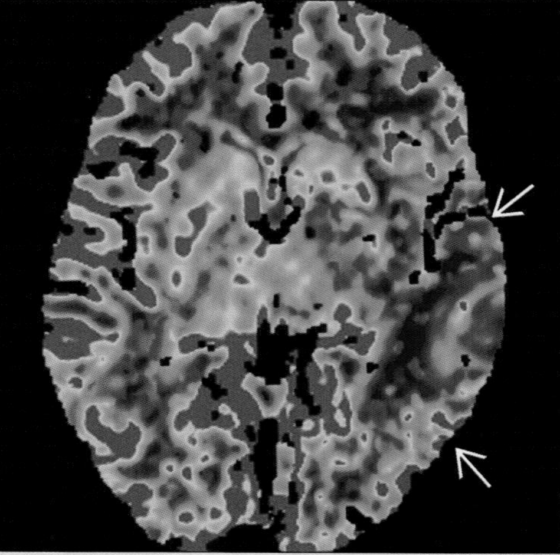

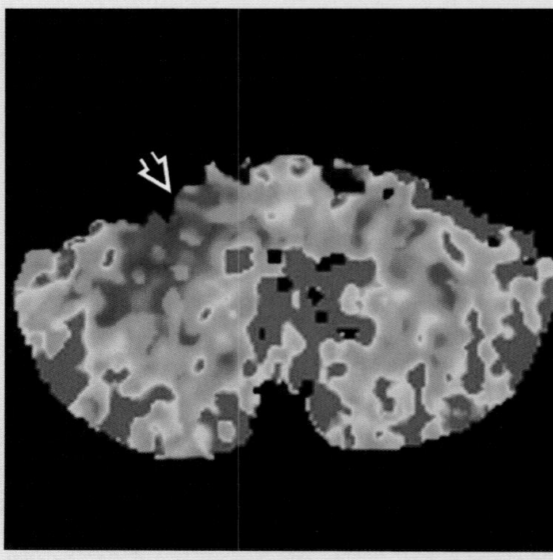

(Left) *Whole-brain CT perfusion study was obtained as part of an emergency stroke evaluation in patient with acute onset of right-sided weakness. CBF shows diminished blood flow ➔ (blue area) in the left MCA distribution.* ***(Right)*** *Section through the cerebellar hemispheres in the same patient shows acutely reduced CBF in the right cerebellar hemisphere ⇨. As afferent input to the cerebellum is reduced, regional metabolism diminishes and CBF falls. This is hyperacute crossed cerebellar diaschisis.*

CROSSED CEREBELLAR DIASCHISIS

TERMINOLOGY

Abbreviations

- Crossed cerebellar diaschisis (CCD)

Definitions

- "Diaschisis" = sudden loss of function in brain connected to (but at distance from) damaged area
- CCD = decreased blood flow/metabolism in cerebellar hemisphere contralateral to supratentorial infarct
  - Caused by interrupted input through corticopontocerebellar tract (CPC)
- CCD occurs in both acute and chronic phases
  - Acute CCD results from functional deafference
  - Subacute, chronic CCD reflects transneuronal degeneration

IMAGING

General Features

- Best diagnostic clue
  - Acute: CT/MR perfusion shows ↓ cerebral blood flow (CBF) in cerebellar hemisphere opposite acute hemispheric infarct
  - Chronic: CT or MR shows atrophic cerebellar hemisphere opposite old hemispheric infarct
- Location
  - Cerebellar hemisphere opposite hemispheric infarct

Imaging Recommendations

- Best imaging tool
  - Acute: CT or MR perfusion
    - PET/CT also effective but expensive; variable availability
  - Chronic: MR with T2WI, FLAIR, DTI
- Protocol advice
  - Add DTI as subtle cases may show ↓ fractional anisotropy when conventional MR normal

CT Findings

- NECT
  - Acute: Normal
  - Chronic: Cerebellar atrophy contralateral to supratentorial infarct
- CTA
  - MCA occlusion
  - Cerebellar vessels appear grossly normal
- CT perfusion
  - ↑ TTP, ↓ CBF in cerebellum contralateral to infarct

MR Findings

- T1WI
  - Unilateral cerebellar atrophy
- T2WI
  - Folia shrunken, fissures enlarged
- FLAIR
  - Except for atrophy, cerebellum usually normal
- MRA
  - Posterior fossa vasculature normal
- DTI
  - Shows ↓ FA in middle cerebellar peduncle
  - Visualizes altered CPC in chronic CCD that may not be seen on conventional MR

Nuclear Medicine Findings

- PET/CT
  - 18F-FDG PET/CT shows diffusely reduced uptake in contralateral cerebellar hemisphere
  - L-(methyl-11C) methionine (MET) uptake not reduced
- Tc-99m sulfur colloid
  - Tc-99m ECD, HMPAO SPECT can demonstrate distant areas of ↓ CBF, metabolism ("diaschisis")

DIFFERENTIAL DIAGNOSIS

Superior Cerebellar Artery Infarct

- CCD involves most of cerebellum, not just SCA territory
- Contralateral MCA infarct absent

Encephalomalacia

- No history of trauma, contralateral MCA infarct

Cerebellitis

- Cerebellum swollen, not shrunken

PATHOLOGY

General Features

- Etiology
  - Corticopontocerebellar tract (CPC tract)
    - Large afferent pathway derived from very extensive areas of cortex
    - Input to cerebellum via corticopontocerebellar tracts 40x all other afferent sources combined
      - 1st-order neurons arrive in ipsilateral pons
      - Synapse with 2nd-order neurons
      - Then cross to opposite cerebellar hemisphere via middle cerebellar peduncle
  - Injury at any point along CPC can result in ↓ CBF, metabolism in contralateral cerebellar hemisphere
    - Most common cause = MCA infarct
    - Others = neoplasm, trauma, surgery, epilepsy, migraine, Rasmussen encephalitis, etc.

CLINICAL ISSUES

Natural History & Prognosis

- CCD represents temporal continuum
  - Early, reversible functional hypometabolism
    - Cerebellum recovers (typical)
  - Irreversible degeneration in up to 20%
    - Cerebellar atrophy
    - Can be seen decades after initial insult

SELECTED REFERENCES

1. Garg G et al: Crossed cerebellar diaschisis demonstrated by (18)F- FDG-PET/CT. Hell J Nucl Med. 12(2):171-2, 2009
2. Lin DD et al: Crossed cerebellar diaschisis in acute stroke detected by dynamic susceptibility contrast MR perfusion imaging. AJNR Am J Neuroradiol. 30(4):710-5, 2009
3. Liu Y et al: Crossed cerebellar diaschisis in acute ischemic stroke: a study with serial SPECT and MRI. J Cereb Blood Flow Metab. 27(10):1724-32, 2007

HYPERTROPHIC OLIVARY DEGENERATION

Key Facts

Terminology

- Inferior olivary nucleus (ION) degeneration
  - Unique type of transneuronal degeneration
  - Olivary de-afferentation thought to be source of ensuing hypertrophic olivary degeneration (HOD)
- Usually caused by primary lesions in dento-rubro-olivary pathway (anatomical triangle of Guillain-Mollaret)
- Triangle of Guillain-Mollaret defined by 3 anatomic structures
  - Dentate nucleus (DN) of cerebellum
  - Contralateral red nucleus (RN)
  - ION ipsilateral to RN

Imaging

- ION initially hypertrophies rather than atrophies
- 3 distinct MR stages in HOD
  - Hyperintense signal without hypertrophy of ION: Within 1st 6 months of ictus
  - Increased signal + ION hypertrophy: Between 6 months and 3-4 years after ictus
  - Only ION hyperintensity: Begins when hypertrophy resolves (can persist indefinitely)

Top Differential Diagnoses

- Vertebrobasilar perforating artery infarct
- Demyelination (MS, microvascular disease)
- Amyotrophic lateral sclerosis
- HIV/AIDS
- Rhombencephalitis

Clinical Issues

- Palatal myoclonus (palatal "tremor")
- Usually develops 10-11 months after primary lesion

*(**Left**) Axial graphic of the upper medulla shows the medullary pyramids ➡ on each side of the ventral median fissure. The olives ➡ lie just posterior to the preolivary sulci ➡. (**Right**) Coronal graphic of the midbrain, pons, and medulla is sectioned to depict the Guillain-Mollaret triangle. The triangle of Guillain-Mollaret is composed of the ipsilateral inferior olivary nucleus (green), dentate nucleus (blue) of the contralateral cerebellum, and the ipsilateral red nucleus (red).*

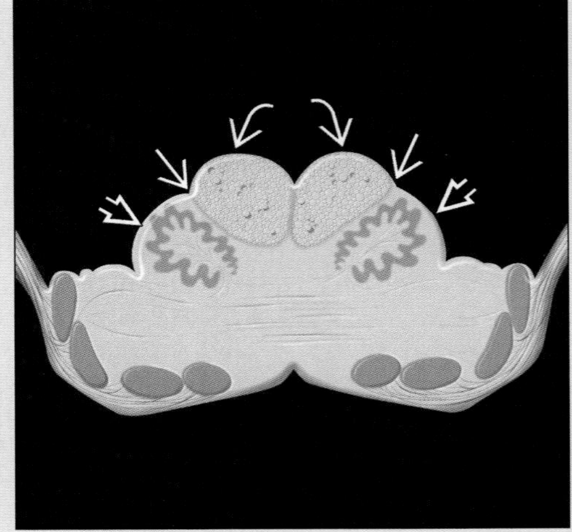

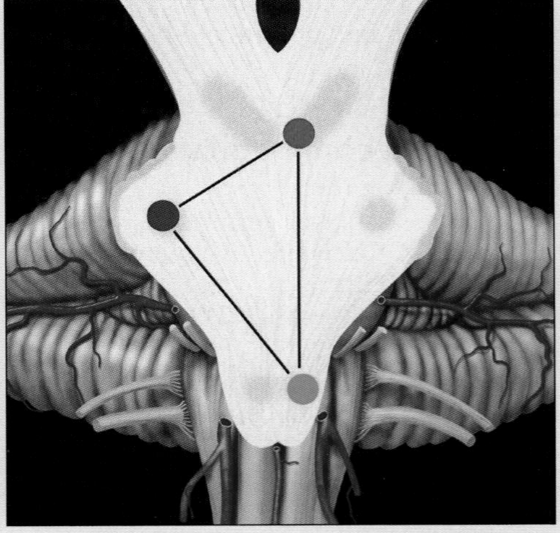

*(**Left**) Axial T2WI MR (CISS) shows the normal shape of the medullary olives ➡. (**Right**) Axial T2WI MR in a patient who developed palatal myoclonus approximately 6 months after resection of a midbrain cavernous malformation shows hyperintensity and enlargement of both olives ➡. This pattern is typical in the subacute stage of hypertrophic olivary degeneration, which typically appears between 6 months and 3-4 years after injury to the dento-rubro-olivary pathway.*

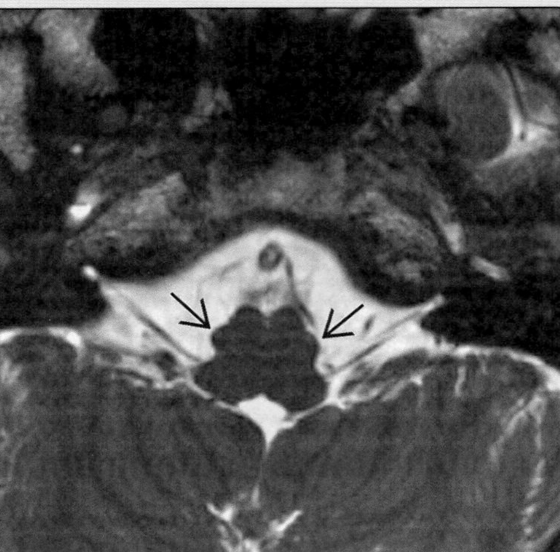

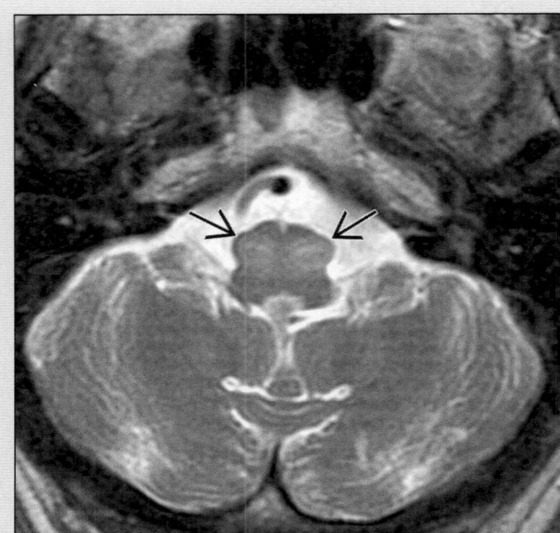

HYPERTROPHIC OLIVARY DEGENERATION

TERMINOLOGY

Abbreviations

- Hypertrophic olivary degeneration (HOD)

Synonyms

- Pseudohypertrophy of inferior olivary nucleus

Definitions

- Secondary degeneration of inferior olivary nucleus (ION), usually caused by primary lesions in dento-rubro-olivary pathway (anatomical triangle of Guillain and Mollaret)

IMAGING

General Features

- Best diagnostic clue
  - T2 hyperintense, nonenhancing enlargement of ION
- Location
  - Triangle of Guillain and Mollaret defined by 3 anatomic structures
    - Dentate nucleus (DN) of cerebellum
    - Contralateral red nucleus (RN)
    - ION ipsilateral to RN
  - Central tegmental tract connects RN to ipsilateral ION
  - Superior cerebellar peduncle (dentatorubral tract) connects DN to contralateral RN
  - Inferior cerebellar peduncle connects ION to contralateral cerebellar cortex and contralateral DN
  - 3 patterns of HOD in relation to primary lesion
    - Ipsilateral HOD: Primary lesion is limited to brainstem (central tegmental tract)
    - Contralateral HOD: Primary lesion is in cerebellum (DN or superior cerebellar peduncle)
    - Bilateral HOD: Primary lesion involves both central tegmental tract and superior cerebellar peduncle
- Size
  - Variable (time-dependent) size of affected ION
    - Normal in acute stage
    - Increased (hypertrophy) between 6 months to 3-4 years
    - Decreased (atrophy) in advanced stage (> 3-4 years)
- Morphology
  - Unique type of transneuronal degeneration
    - ION initially hypertrophies rather than atrophies

CT Findings

- NECT
  - May show acute primary injury (e.g., hemorrhage) in tegmentum
  - HOD typically not depicted on CT

MR Findings

- T1WI
  - Acute phase: Normal ION
    - Shows primary lesion in brainstem (cerebellum or tegmentum)
  - After HOD ensues
    - Enlargement confined to ION, isointense to slightly hypointense to gray matter
    - Slightly increased olivary T1 signal also reported
    - ± residual primary lesion
- T2WI
  - 3 distinct MR stages in HOD
    - Hyperintense signal without hypertrophy of ION: Within 1st 6 months of ictus
    - Both increased signal and hypertrophy of ION: Between 6 months and 3-4 years after ictus
    - Increased signal only in ION: Begins when hypertrophy resolves and can persist indefinitely
  - Axial MR: Disappearance of pre- and postolivary sulci in hypertrophic stage
  - MR also detects primary lesion located in ipsilateral central tegmental tract
    - Old hematomas: Low signal areas on T2WI revealing hemosiderin deposition
  - ± decreased size of contralateral ION, with higher than normal signal intensity
  - ± mild to severe atrophic changes of cerebellar cortex contralateral to HOD
- PD/intermediate
  - High signal intensity of ION better detected on PD images than on T2WI
- FLAIR
  - Similar to T2WI
- T1WI C+
  - No contrast enhancement of degenerated ION

Nuclear Medicine Findings

- PET
  - Hypermetabolism of glucose in medulla in patients with HOD

Imaging Recommendations

- Best imaging tool
  - MR imaging
- Protocol advice
  - T2WI (include coronal or sagittal sections)

DIFFERENTIAL DIAGNOSIS

Other Causes of High T2 Signal Intensity in Anterior Part of Medulla

- Demyelination related to multiple sclerosis
- Tumor (astrocytoma, metastasis, lymphoma)
- Lesions involving corticospinal tract
  - Wallerian degeneration, adrenoleukodystrophy
  - Amyotrophic lateral sclerosis
- Vertebrobasilar perforating artery infarct
  - Most medullary infarctions occur in posteroinferior cerebellar artery territory and involve posterolateral medulla (e.g., vertebral artery dissection)
  - Alternatively, medullary infarcts could be related to perforating branches of anterior spinal or vertebral arteries and have paramedial location
- Infectious/inflammatory processes
  - Tuberculosis
  - Sarcoidosis
  - HIV/AIDS
  - Rhombencephalitis

HYPERTROPHIC OLIVARY DEGENERATION

PATHOLOGY

General Features

- Etiology
  - Transsynaptic degeneration caused by interruption of pathways composing Guillain-Mollaret triangle
  - Olivary de-afferentation thought to be source of ensuing HOD
  - Primary lesions usually located in contralateral DN or ipsilateral central tegmental tract
  - Focal brainstem insults that may lead to dentatorubral-olivary pathway interruption
    - Ischemic infarction, demyelination
    - Hemorrhage (related to hypertensive disease, occult cerebrovascular malformation, or diffuse axonal injury following severe head trauma)
    - Cavernous hemangioma
- Associated abnormalities
  - Primary brainstem insult
    - Most commonly pontine hemorrhage from trauma (including surgery), hypertension, tumor, and infarction
- Olivary enlargement: Histologically unusual vacuolar cytoplasmic degeneration → hypertrophy related in part to ↑ number of astrocytes
- After onset of primary lesion
  - Vacuolar cytoplasmic degeneration in 6-15 months
  - Gliosis follows at 15-20 months

Staging, Grading, & Classification

- 6 phases of pathologic change
  - No olivary changes within 1st 24 hours
  - Degeneration of olivary amiculum (white matter capsule at olive periphery) at 2-7 days or more
  - Olivary hypertrophy (mild enlargement with neuronal hypertrophy, no glial reaction) at 3 weeks
  - Maximal olivary enlargement (hypertrophy of neurons and astrocytes) at 8.5 months
  - Olivary pseudohypertrophy (neuronal dissolution with gemistocytic astrocytes) after 9.5 months
  - Olivary atrophy (neuronal disappearance with olivary atrophy and prominent degeneration of amiculum olivae) after a few years

Gross Pathologic & Surgical Features

- Focal swelling of ION
- Unilateral HOD
  - Asymmetric enlargement of anterior medulla
  - "Pallor" in contralateral DN
  - Atrophy of contralateral cerebellar cortex
- Bilateral HOD: More difficult to observe
  - No left-right asymmetry

Microscopic Features

- Changes in hypertrophic degenerated ION
  - Hypertrophic, thickened neurites
  - Vacuolation of neurons
  - Fibrillary gliosis
  - Demyelination and astrocytic proliferation of WM
- In contralateral cerebellar cortex
  - Decreased number of Purkinje cells
- Contralateral DN reduced in size, possibly due to
  - Iron depletion secondary to axonal iron transport block
  - Loss of cells in nucleus

CLINICAL ISSUES

Presentation

- Most common signs/symptoms
  - Symptomatic palatal tremor/myoclonus
    - Rhythmic involuntary movement of soft palate, uvula, pharynx, and larynx
  - Severe myoclonus may also affect cervical muscles and diaphragm
  - ± dentatorubral tremor (Holmes tremor)
    - 2-5 Hz rest, postural, and kinetic tremor of upper extremity
    - May occur before onset of palatal tremor
  - Symptoms of cerebellar or brain stem dysfunction
    - Associated with acute lesion within triangle of Guillain-Mollaret
- Clinical profile
  - Palatal myoclonus (palatal "tremor")
    - Usually develops 10-11 months after primary lesion
    - Virtually all patients who develop palatal myoclonus after brain insult will have HOD
    - Not all HOD patients develop palatal myoclonus
    - May result from hypermetabolism of ION

Demographics

- Age
  - Rare; reported in all ages, both genders

Natural History & Prognosis

- After primary brainstem injury, olivary hypertrophy typically appears in delayed fashion
  - May occur between 3 weeks to 11 months (usually within 4-6 months)
- Maximum hypertrophy at 5-15 months
- Olivary hypertrophy typically resolves in 10-16 months
- Olivary hyperintensity on T2WI may persist for years after resolution of hypertrophy
- Finally ION undergoes atrophy
- Clinical symptoms (tremors) rarely improve

DIAGNOSTIC CHECKLIST

Image Interpretation Pearls

- Avoid misdiagnosis of tumor or multiple sclerosis
- Bilateral and symmetrical lesions in ION argue against subacute infarct and vertebral artery dissection

SELECTED REFERENCES

1. Lim CC et al: Images in clinical medicine. Pendular nystagmus and palatomyoclonus from hypertrophic olivary degeneration. N Engl J Med. 360(9):e12, 2009
2. Ogawa K et al: Pathological study of pseudohypertrophy of the inferior olivary nucleus. Neuropathology. Epub ahead of print, 2009
3. Hornyak M et al: Hypertrophic olivary degeneration after surgical removal of cavernous malformations of the brain stem: report of four cases and review of the literature. Acta Neurochir (Wien). 150(2):149-56; discussion 156, 2008

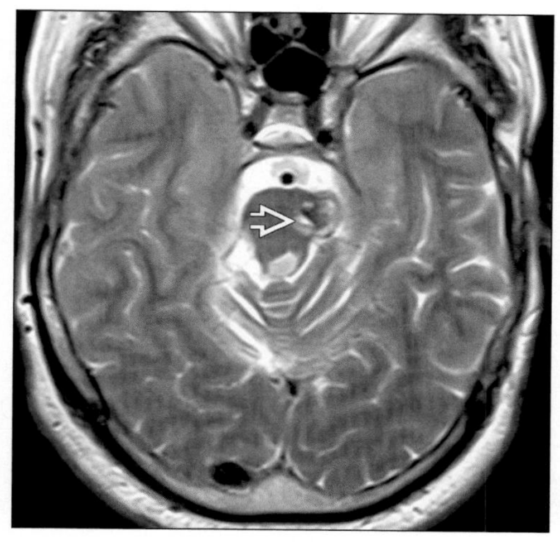

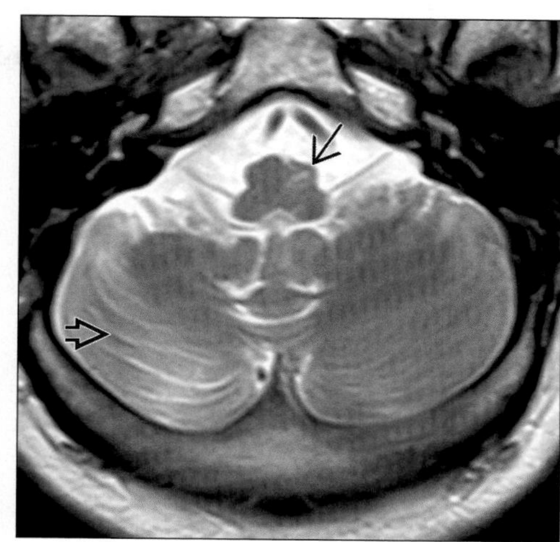

(Left) *Axial T2WI MR in a patient who developed palatal myoclonus several months following midbrain surgery for cavernous malformation. Imaging obtained 1 year later shows residual cavernous malformation ➡.* ***(Right)*** *Axial T2WI MR through the medulla shows that the ipsilateral olive is atrophic and hyperintense ➡. This patient also has crossed cerebellar atrophy ➡ due to interruption of the ponto-cerebellar pathway.*

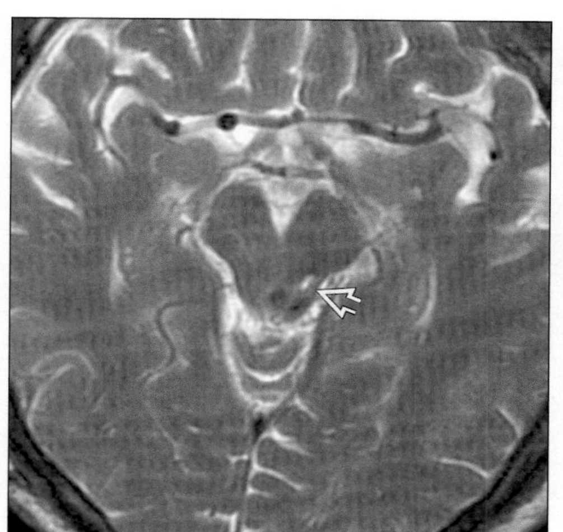

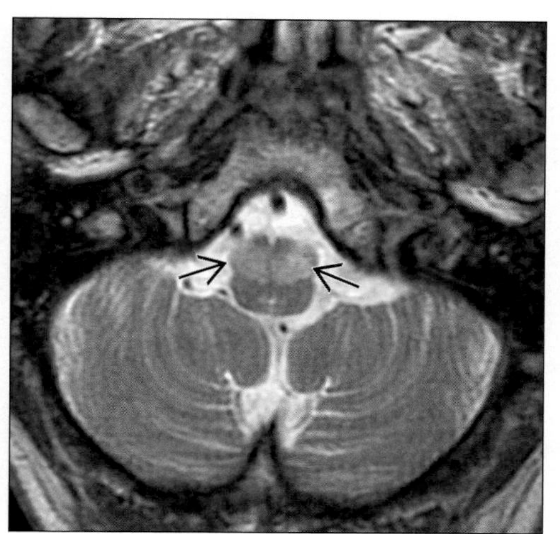

(Left) *Axial T2WI MR in a patient who developed onset of dysarthria and upper extremity dysmetria 15 months following stereotaxic XRT for midbrain AVM shows mixed hyper-/hypointensity in the residual vascular malformation ➡.* ***(Right)*** *Axial T2WI MR in the same patient shows bilateral inferior olivary hyperintensity and hypertrophy ➡.*

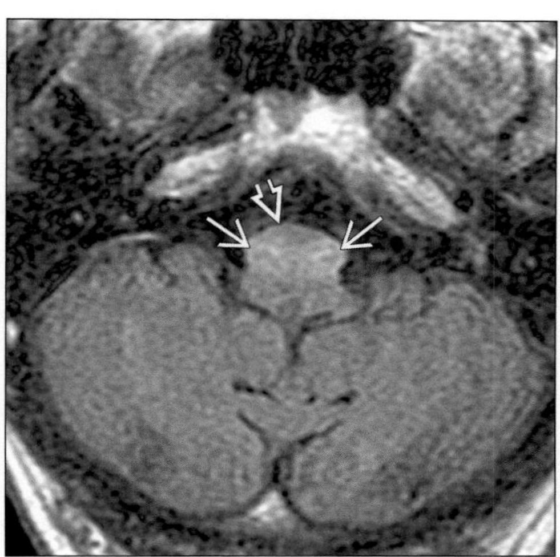

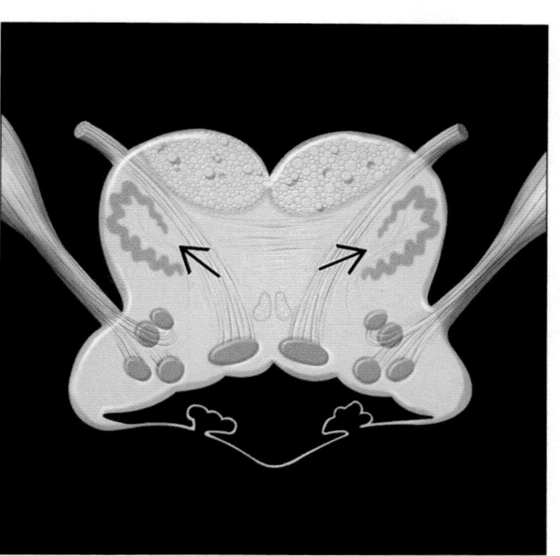

(Left) *Axial FLAIR MR in the same patient delineates the somewhat "wavy" appearance of the hyperintensity conforming to the configuration of the olives ➡. The pyramids ➡ are spared, helping differentiate hypertrophic olivary degeneration from perforating artery infarction.* ***(Right)*** *Axial graphic of the midbrain at the level of the hypoglossal nuclei shows the distinct "wavy" pattern of the olives ➡ corresponding to the FLAIR hyperintensity in the previous image.*

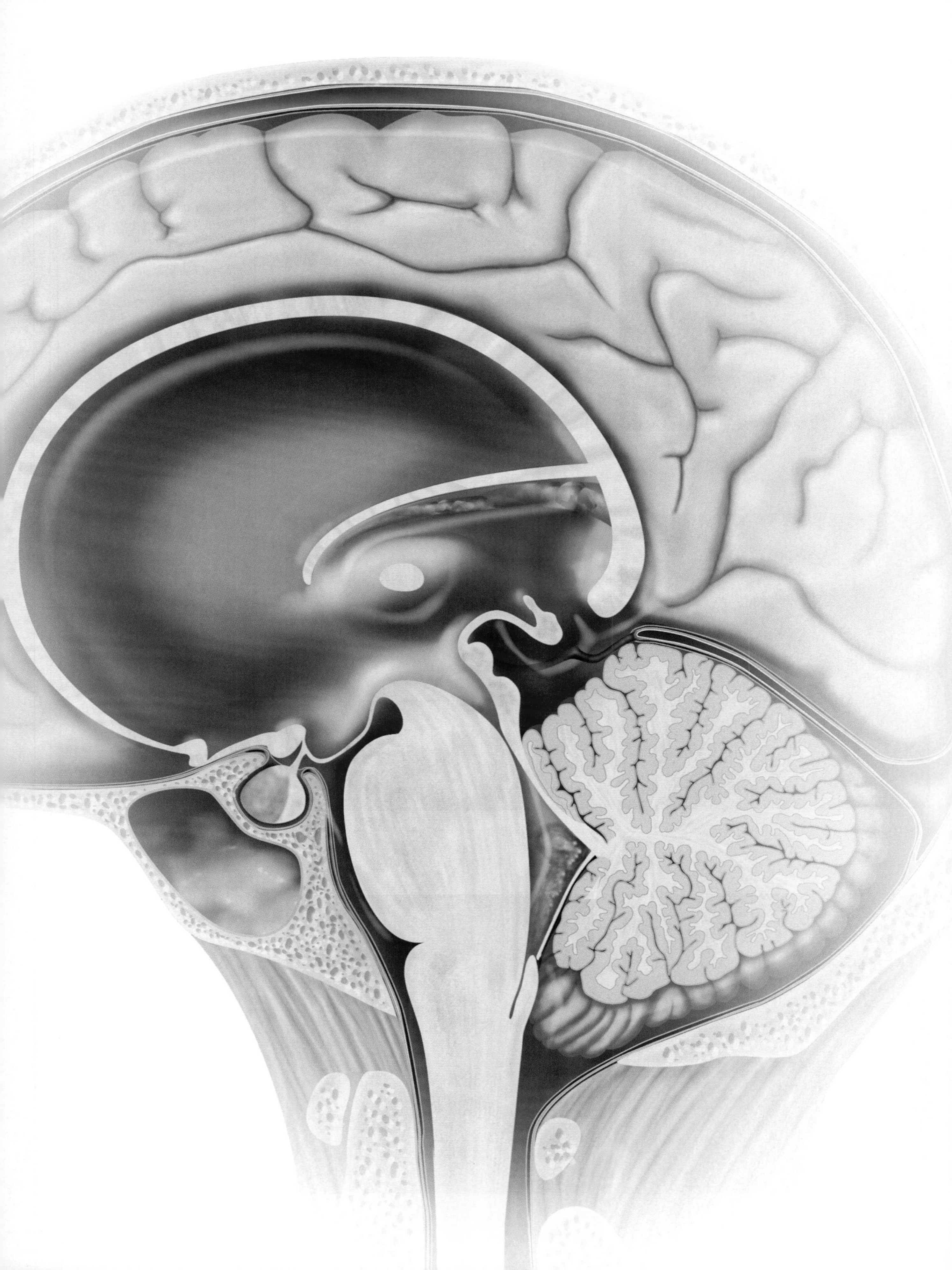

SECTION 1
Ventricles and Cisterns

Introduction and Overview

Normal Variants

Hydrocephalus

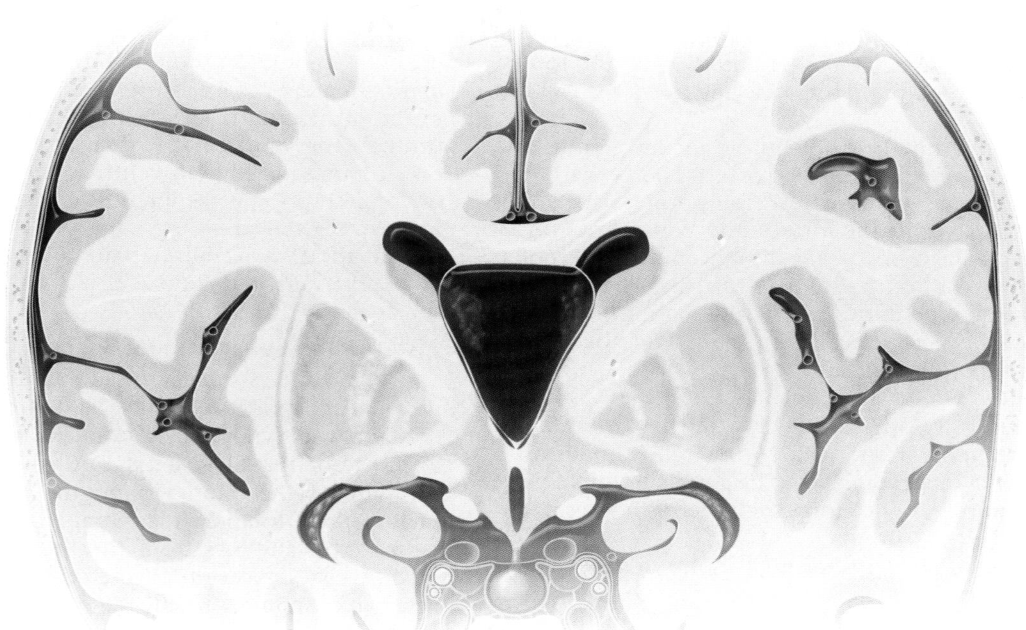

Gross and Imaging Anatomy

Ventricles and Choroid Plexus

Basic embryology. Early in embryonic development, the forebrain cavity divides into 2 lateral ventricles, which develop as outpouchings from the rostral 3rd ventricle and are connected to it by the interventricular foramen (a.k.a. foramen of Monro). In the coronal plane these form a central H-shaped "monoventricle." The 4th ventricle develops from a cavity within the hindbrain and merges caudally with the central canal of the spinal cord.

Anatomic overview. The brain CSF spaces include both the ventricular system and subarachnoid spaces (SAS). The ventricular system is comprised of 4 interconnected CSF-filled, ependymal-lined cavities that lie deep within the brain. The paired **lateral ventricles** communicate with the 3rd ventricle via the Y-shaped **foramen of Monro**. The **3rd ventricle** communicates with the 4th ventricle via the **cerebral aqueduct** (of Sylvius). In turn, the **4th ventricle** communicates with the SAS via its outlet foramina (the midline **foramen of Magendie** and the 2 lateral **foramina of Luschka**).

Lateral ventricles. Each lateral ventricle has a body, atrium, and 3 projections ("horns"). The roof of the **frontal horn** is formed by the corpus callosum genu. It is bordered laterally and inferiorly by the head of the caudate nucleus. The septum pellucidum, a thin sheet of tissue that extends from the corpus callosum genu anteriorly to the foramen of Monro posteriorly, forms the medial borders of both frontal horns.

The **body** of the lateral ventricle passes posteriorly under the corpus callosum. Its floor is formed by the dorsal thalamus and its medial wall is bordered by the fornix. Laterally, it curves around the body and tail of the caudate nucleus.

The **atrium** contains the choroid plexus glomus and is formed by the confluence of the body with the temporal and occipital horns. The **temporal horn** extends anteroinferiorly from the atrium and is bordered on its floor and medial wall by the hippocampus. Its roof is formed by the tail of the caudate nucleus. The **occipital horn** is surrounded entirely by white matter fiber tracts, principally the geniculocalcarine tract and the forceps major of the corpus callosum.

3rd ventricle. The 3rd ventricle is a single, slit-like, midline, vertically oriented cavity that lies between the thalami. Its roof is formed by the tela choroidea, a double layer of invaginated pia. The lamina terminalis and anterior commissure lie along the anterior border of the 3rd ventricle.

The floor of the 3rd ventricle is formed by several critical anatomic structures. From front to back these include the optic chiasm, hypothalamus with the tuber cinereum and infundibular stalk, mamillary bodies, and roof of the midbrain tegmentum.

The 3rd ventricle has 2 inferiorly located CSF-filled projections, the slightly rounded **optic recess** and the more pointed **infundibular recess**. Two small recesses, the **suprapineal and pineal recesses**, form the posterior border of the 3rd ventricle. A variably sized interthalamic adhesion (also called the **massa intermedia**) lies between the lateral walls of the 3rd ventricle. The massa intermedia is not a true commissure.

4th ventricle. The 4th ventricle is a roughly diamond-shaped cavity that lies between the pons anteriorly and the cerebellar vermis posteriorly. Its roof is covered by the anterior (superior) medullary velum above and the inferior medullary velum below.

The 4th ventricle has 5 distinctly shaped recesses. The **posterior superior recesses** are paired, thin, flat CSF-filled pouches that cap the cerebellar tonsils. The **lateral recesses** curve anterolaterally from the 4th ventricle, extending under the brachium pontis (major cerebellar peduncle) into the lower cerebellopontine angle cisterns. The lateral recesses transmit choroid plexus through the foramina of Luschka into the adjacent subarachnoid spaces. The **fastigium** is a triangular, blind-ending, dorsal midline outpouching that points towards the cerebellar vermis.

Choroid plexus and the production of CSF. The choroid plexus is comprised of highly vascular papillary excrescences with a central connective tissue core coated by an ependyma-derived secretory epithelium. The embryonic choroid plexus forms where the infolded tela choroidea contacts the ependymal lining of the ventricles, thus developing along the entire choroidal fissure.

The largest mass of choroid plexus, the **glomus**, is located in the atrium of the lateral ventricles. The choroid plexus extends anteriorly along the floor of the lateral ventricle, lying between the fornix and thalamus. It then dives through the interventricular foramen (of Monro) and curves posteriorly along the roof of the 3rd ventricle. The choroid plexus in the body of the lateral ventricle curls around the thalamus into the temporal horn, where it fills the choroidal fissure and lies superomedial to the hippocampus.

The choroid plexus epithelium secretes CSF at the rate of about 0.4 mL/minute. Total intracranial CSF volume is approximately 125 mL, with most (nearly 80%) contained in the subarachnoid spaces, not the ventricles. CSF flows through the ventricular system and passes through the exit foramina of the 4th ventricle into the SAS. The bulk of CSF resorption is through the arachnoid villi along the superior sagittal sinus.

Not all CSF is produced in the choroid plexus. Drainage of brain interstitial fluid is a significant extrachoroidal source.

Cisterns and Subarachnoid Spaces

Overview. The subarachnoid spaces (SAS) lie between the pia and arachnoid. The sulci are CSF-filled spaces between the gyral folds. Focal expansions of the SASs form the brain CSF cisterns. These cisterns are found at the base of the brain around the brainstem, tentorial incisura, and foramen magnum. Numerous pial-covered septae cross the SAS from the brain to the arachnoid. All SAS cisterns communicate with each other and the ventricular system, providing natural pathways for disease spread (e.g., meningitis, neoplasms).

The brain cisterns are conveniently grouped into supra-, peri-, and infratentorial cisterns. All contain numerous important critical structures such as vessels and cranial nerves.

Supratentorial/peritentorial cisterns. The **suprasellar cistern** lies between the diaphragma sellae and the hypothalamus. Critical contents include the infundibulum, optic chiasm, and circle of Willis.

The **interpeduncular cistern** is the posterior continuation of the suprasellar cistern. Lying between the cerebral peduncles, it contains the oculomotor nerves as well as the distal basilar artery and proximal segments of the posterior cerebral arteries. Important perforating arteries, the thalamoperforating and thalamogeniculate arteries, arise from the top of the basilar artery and cross the interpeduncular cistern to enter the midbrain.

The **perimesencephalic (ambient) cisterns** are thin wings of CSF that extend posterosuperiorly from the suprasellar cistern to the quadrigeminal cistern. They wrap around the midbrain and contain the trochlear nerves, P2 PCA segments, superior cerebellar arteries, and basal vein of Rosenthal.

The **quadrigeminal cistern** lies under the corpus callosum splenium, behind the pineal gland and tectal plate. It connects with the ambient cisterns laterally and the superior cerebellar cistern inferiorly. The quadrigeminal cistern contains the pineal gland, trochlear nerves, P3 PCA segments, proximal choroidal arteries, and vein of Galen. An anterior extension, the **velum interpositum**, lies below the fornix and above the 3rd ventricle. The velum interpositum contains the internal cerebral veins and medial posterior choroidal arteries.

Infratentorial cisterns. The unpaired posterior fossa cisterns that lie in the midline are the prepontine, premedullary, and superior cerebellar cisterns, as well as the cisterna magna. The lateral cisterns are paired and include the cerebellopontine and cerebellomedullary cisterns.

The **prepontine cistern** lies between the upper clivus and the "belly" of the pons. It contains numerous important structures including the basilar artery, the anterior inferior cerebellar arteries (AICAs), and the trigeminal and abducens nerves (CN5 and CN6).

The **premedullary cistern** is the inferior continuation of the prepontine cistern. It lies between the lower clivus in front and the medulla behind. It extends inferiorly to the foramen magnum and contains the vertebral arteries and branches (e.g., PICAs) and the hypoglossal nerve (CN12).

The **superior cerebellar cistern** lies between the straight sinus above and the vermis below. It contains the superior cerebellar arteries and veins. It connects superiorly through the tentorial incisura with the quadrigeminal cistern and inferiorly with the cisterna magna. The **cisterna magna** lies below the inferior vermis between the medulla and the occiput. It contains the cerebellar tonsils and the tonsillohemispheric branches of PICA. The cisterna magna merges imperceptibly with the SAS of the upper cervical spinal canal.

The **cerebellopontine angle cisterns** (CPAs) lie between the pons/cerebellum and the petrous temporal bone. Their most important contents are the trigeminal, facial, and vestibulocochlear nerves (CN5, CN7, and CN8). Other structures found here include the petrosal veins and AICAs. The CPA cisterns are contiguous inferiorly with the cerebellomedullary cisterns, sometimes termed the "lower" cerebellopontine angle cisterns.

The **cerebellomedullary cisterns** extend laterally around the medulla and are continuous with the cisterna magna below and the CPAs above. They contain the vagus, glossopharyngeal, and spinal accessory nerves (CN9, CN10, and CN11). A tuft of choroid plexus exits each foramen of Luschka into the cerebellomedullary cistern. The flocculus of the cerebellum that projects into this cistern can appear very prominent. The flocculus and choroid plexus are normal contents of the cerebellomedullary cisterns and should not be mistaken for pathology.

Imaging Recommendations

MR. Thin-section T2WI or CISS best detail CSF within the ventricular system, SASs, and basal cisterns and exquisitely delineates their contents. Whole brain FLAIR is especially useful for evaluating potential abnormalities in the SASs. Spin dephasing with pulsatile CSF flow is common and can mimic intraventricular pathology, especially in the basal cisterns and around the interventricular foramen. Incomplete CSF suppression with "bright" CSF can mimic pathologic SASs.

Differential Diagnosis Approach

Ventricles and Choroid Plexus

Overview. Approximately 10% of intracranial neoplasms involve the cerebral ventricles, either primarily or by extension. An anatomy-based approach is most effective, as there is a distinct predilection for certain lesions to occur in 1 ventricle or cistern and not others. Age is also a helpful consideration. Specific imaging findings such as signal intensity, enhancement, and the presence or absence of calcification are relatively less important than location and age.

Normal variants. Asymmetry of the lateral ventricles is a common normal variant, as is flow-related CSF pulsation artifact. A cavum septi pellucidi (CSP) is a common normal variant, seen as a CSF cleft between the 2 leaves of the septum pellucidum. An elongated, finger-like posterior continuation of the CSP between the fornices, a cavum vergae (CV), may be associated with a CSP.

Lateral ventricle mass. Choroid plexus cysts (xanthogranulomas) are a common, generally age-related, degenerative finding with no clinical significance. They are usually bilateral and calcified. They may be hyperintense on FLAIR and occasionally show reduced diffusivity on DWI. A strongly enhancing choroid plexus mass in a child is most likely a choroid plexus papilloma. With the exception of the 4th ventricle, a choroid plexus mass in an adult is usually meningioma or metastasis, not a choroid plexus papilloma.

Some lateral ventricle lesions display a distinct predilection for specific sublocations within the lateral ventricles. An innocent-appearing frontal horn mass in a middle-aged or older adult is most often a subependymoma. A "bubbly" mass in the body of the lateral ventricle is usually a central neurocytoma. Neurocysticercosis cysts can occur in all ages and in virtually every CSF space.

Foramen of Monro mass. The most common "abnormality" here is a pseudolesion caused by CSF artifact. Colloid cyst is the only relatively common pathology here. It is rare in children and typically a lesion of adults. Flow artifact can mimic a colloid cyst, but mass effect is absent. In a child with an enhancing mass in the interventricular foramen, tuberous sclerosis with subependymal nodule &/or giant cell astrocytoma should be a consideration. Masses such as ependymoma, papilloma, and metastasis are rare.

3rd ventricle mass. Again, the most common "lesion" in this location is either CSF flow artifact or a normal structure (the massa intermedia). Colloid cyst is the only common lesion that occurs in the 3rd ventricle; 99% are wedged into the foramen of Monro. Extreme vertebrobasilar dolichoectasia can indent the 3rd ventricle, sometimes projecting upward as high as the interventricular foramen, and should not be mistaken for colloid cyst.

Primary neoplasms in children are uncommon here but include choroid plexus papilloma, germinoma, craniopharyngioma, and a sessile-type tuber cinereum hamartoma. Primary neoplasms of the 3rd ventricle in adults are also uncommon, though an intraventricular macroadenoma and chordoid glioma are examples. Neurocysticercosis occurs here but is uncommon.

Cerebral aqueduct. Other than aqueductal stenosis, intrinsic lesions of the cerebral aqueduct are rare. Most are related to masses in adjacent structures (e.g., tectal plate glioma).

4th ventricle mass. Pediatric masses are the most common intrinsic abnormalities of the 4th ventricle. Medulloblastoma, ependymoma, and astrocytoma predominate. Atypical teratoid-rhabdoid tumor (AT/RT) is a less common neoplasm that may occur here. It usually occurs in children under the age of 3 years and can mimic medulloblastoma.

Metastases to the choroid or ependyma are probably the most common 4th ventricle neoplasm of adults. Primary neoplasms are rare. Choroid plexus papilloma does occur here, as well as in the CPA cistern. Subependymoma is a lesion of middle-aged adults that is found in the inferior 4th ventricle, lying behind the pontomedullary junction. A newly described rare neoplasm, rosette-forming glioneuronal tumor, is a midline mass of the 4th ventricle. It has no particular distinguishing imaging features and, although it may appear aggressive, it is a benign (WHO grade I) lesion. Hemangioblastomas are intraaxial masses but may project into the 4th ventricle. Epidermoid cysts and neurocysticercosis cysts can be found in all ages.

Subarachnoid Spaces and Cisterns

Overview. The subarachnoid spaces are a common site of pathology that varies from benign congenital lesions (such as arachnoid cyst) to infection (meningitis) and neoplastic involvement ("carcinomatous meningitis"). Anatomic location is key to the differential diagnosis, as imaging findings such as enhancement and hyperintensity on FLAIR are often nonspecific. Patient age is also helpful though generally of secondary importance.

Normal variants. CSF flow-related artifacts are common, especially in the basal cisterns on FLAIR imaging. Mega cisterna magna may be considered a normal variant, as is a cavum velum interpositum (CVI). A CVI is a thin, triangular-shaped CSF space between the lateral ventricles that lies below the fornices and above the 3rd ventricle. Occasionally a CVI may become quite large.

Suprasellar cistern mass. These are discussed more fully in the overview chapter of the sella and pituitary section. Common masses in adults are upward extensions of macroadenoma, meningioma, and aneurysm. The 2 most common suprasellar masses in children are astrocytoma of the optic chiasm/hypothalamus and craniopharyngioma.

Cerebellopontine angle mass. In adults, vestibular schwannoma accounts for almost 90% of all CPA-IAC masses. Meningioma, epidermoid cyst, aneurysm, and arachnoid cyst **together** represent about 8% of lesions in this location. All other less common entities such as lipoma, schwannomas of other cranial nerves, metastases, neurenteric cysts, etc., account for about 2%.

In the absence of neurofibromatosis type 2, vestibular schwannomas are very rare in children. CPA epidermoid and arachnoid cysts may occur in children. Extension of ependymoma laterally through the foramina of Luschka may involve the CPA.

Cystic-appearing CPA masses comprise their own special differential diagnosis. While vestibular schwannoma with intramural cysts can occur, it is less common than epidermoid and arachnoid cysts. Neurocysticercosis may occasionally involve the CPA. Large endolymphatic sac anomaly (IP-2) shows a CSF-like mass within the posterior wall of the temporal bone. Hemangioblastoma and neurenteric cysts are other less common cystic masses that occur in the CPA.

Cisterna magna mass. Tonsillar herniation, whether congenital (Chiari 1) or secondary to posterior fossa mass effect or intracranial hypotension, is the most common "mass" in this location. Nonneoplastic cysts (arachnoid, epidermoid, dermoid, neurenteric) may also occur here.

Neoplasms in and around the cisterna magna, such as meningioma and metastasis, are typically anterior to the medulla. Subependymoma of the 4th ventricle originates in the obex and lies behind the medulla.

FLAIR hyperintensity. Hyperintense sulci and subarachnoid spaces are seen with MR artifacts, as well as a variety of lesions. Pathologic FLAIR hyperintensity is typically related to blood (e.g., subarachnoid hemorrhage), protein (meningitis), or cells (pia-subarachnoid space metastases). Less commonly, gadolinium-based contrast agents in patients with blood-brain barrier leakage or renal failure can cause FLAIR hyperintensity.

Rare causes of FLAIR hyperintensity include ruptured dermoid cyst, moyamoya ("ivy" sign), and acute cerebral ischemia. Contrast enhancement helps distinguish meningitis and metastases from subarachnoid hemorrhage and CSF artifacts.

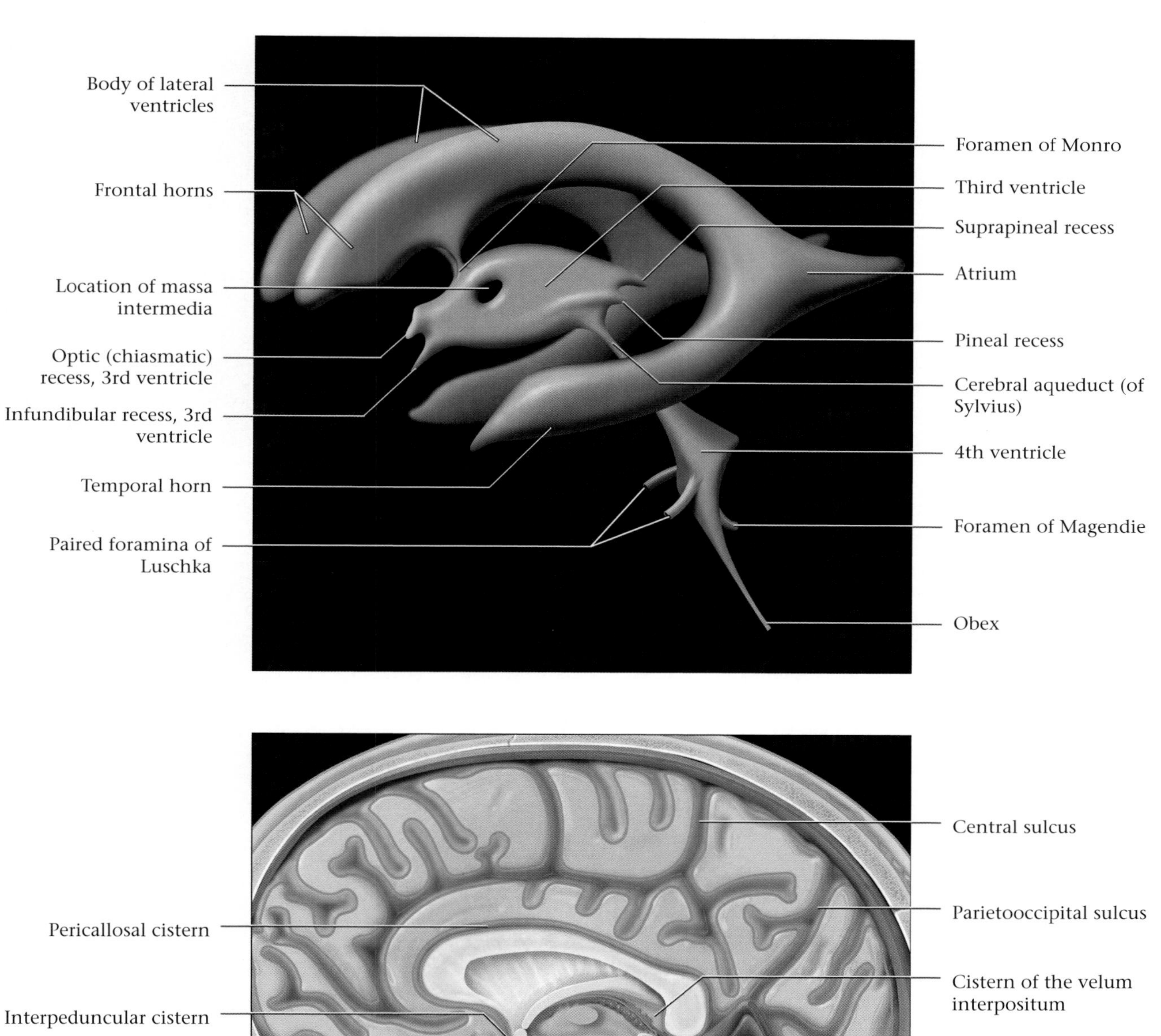

(Top) *Schematic 3D representation of the ventricular system, viewed in the sagittal plane, demonstrates the normal appearance and communicating pathways of the cerebral ventricles.* ***(Bottom)*** *Sagittal midline graphic through the interhemispheric fissure depicts SASs with CSF (blue) between the arachnoid (purple) and pia (orange). The central sulcus separates the frontal lobe (anterior) from the parietal lobe (posterior). The pia mater is closely applied to the brain surface, whereas the arachnoid is adherent to the dura. The ventricles communicate with the cisterns and subarachnoid space via the foramina of Luschka and Magendie. The cisterns normally communicate freely with each other.*

(Left) *Axial T1 C+ MR in an 18-month-old child with severe hydrocephalus shows a choroid plexus papilloma (CPP). The intensely enhancing frond-like projections ➔ and location in the atrium of the left lateral ventricle are both classic findings.* ***(Right)*** *Axial T1 C+ MR in a middle-aged woman shows a smoothly lobulated, intensely enhancing choroid plexus mass ➔. CPP in adults is rare, except for the 4th ventricle. Meningioma was found at surgery.*

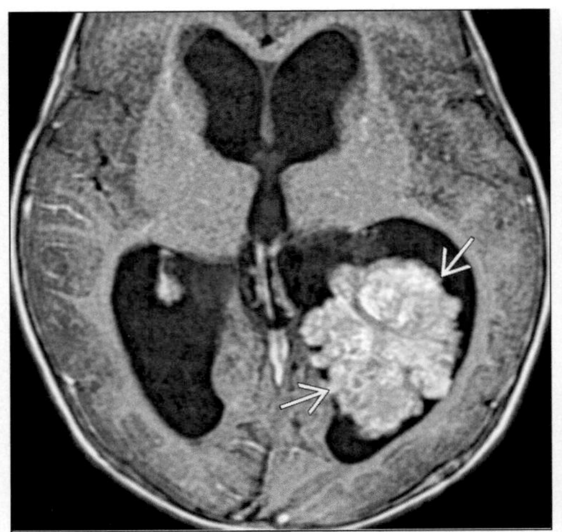

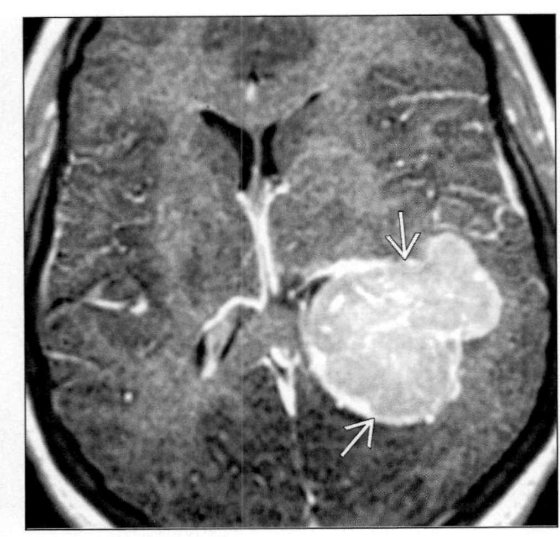

(Left) *Axial T1 C+ FS MR in a 72-year-old man with declining mental state shows a nonenhancing mass ➔ in the frontal horn of the left lateral ventricle. This is an incidental finding, most likely a subependymoma.* ***(Right)*** *Axial T1 C+ MR in a 33 year old with headaches shows an inhomogeneously enhancing "bubbly" lesion in the body of the left lateral ventricle. Appearance and location distinguish central neurocytoma from subependymoma and other possible lateral ventricular masses such as meningioma.*

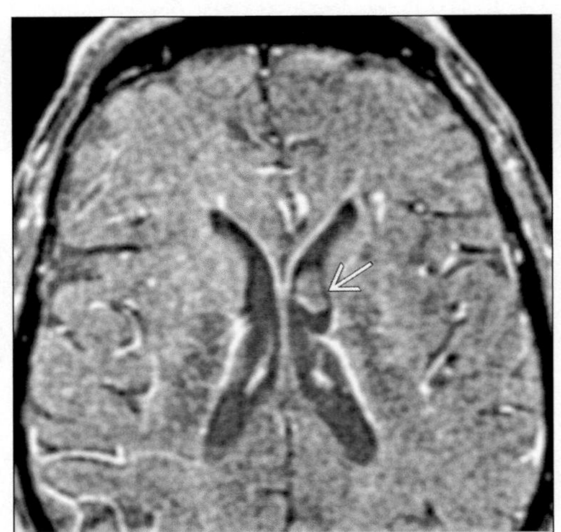

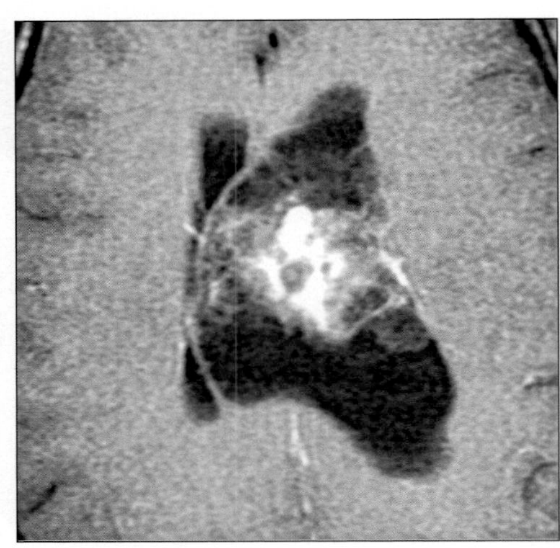

(Left) *Axial FLAIR MR in a 3 year old with seizures shows a hyperintense mass ➔ at the interventricular foramen. Note the flame-shaped subcortical hyperintensities ➔. Tuberous sclerosis with subependymal giant cell astrocytoma.* ***(Right)*** *Axial FLAIR MR in a 65 year old with "thunderclap" headache. This foramen of Monro mass ➔ is a colloid cyst. Other than CSF flow artifact, colloid cysts are the most common lesion found in this location. They are common in adults but relatively rare in children.*

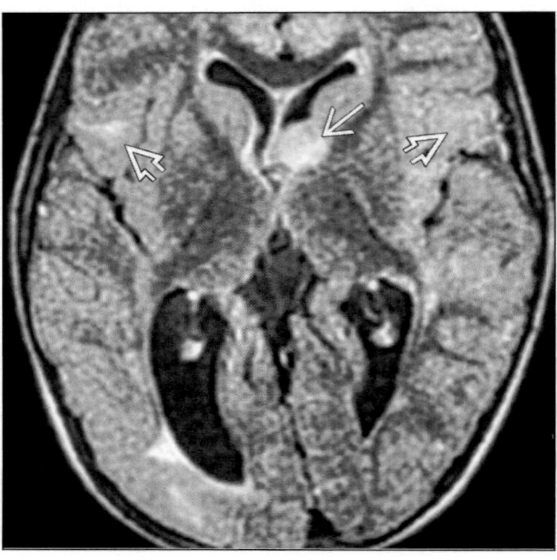

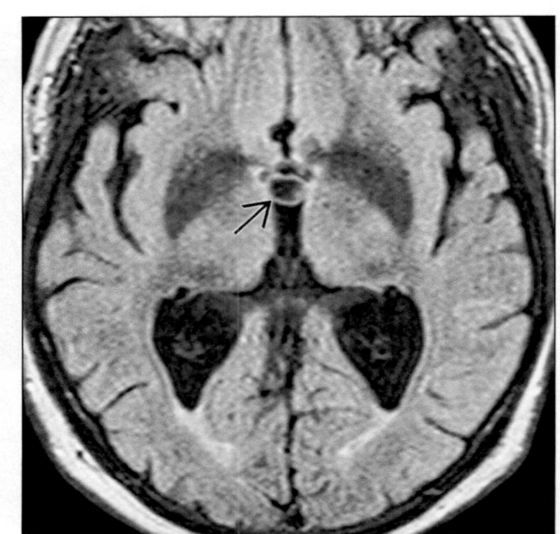

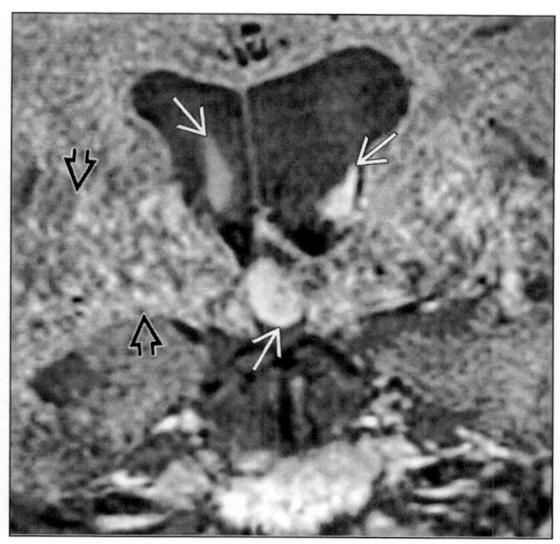

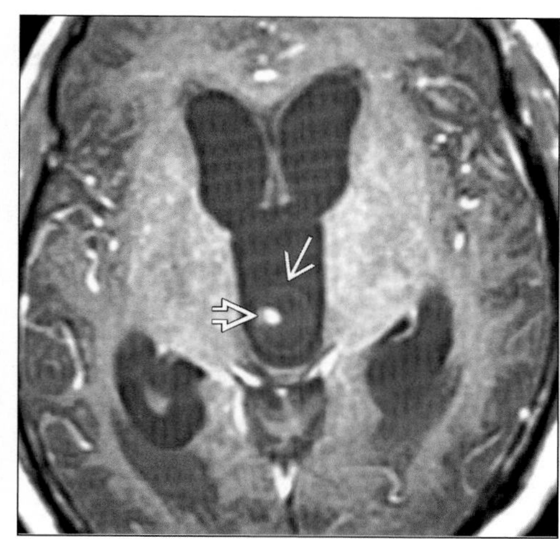

(Left) *Coronal T1WI MR shows prominent pseudomasses of the 3rd and lateral ventricles ➡ caused by pulsatile CSF in and around the interventricular foramen (of Monro). Note the propagation of phase artifact ⇨ across the image.* ***(Right)*** *Axial T1WI C+ MR shows large lateral 3rd ventricles with "blurred" margins from transependymal CSF flow. A cysticercus cyst ➡ with scolex ➡ causes obstructive hydrocephalus. Intrinsic 3rd ventricle masses are less common than lateral or 4th ventricular lesions.*

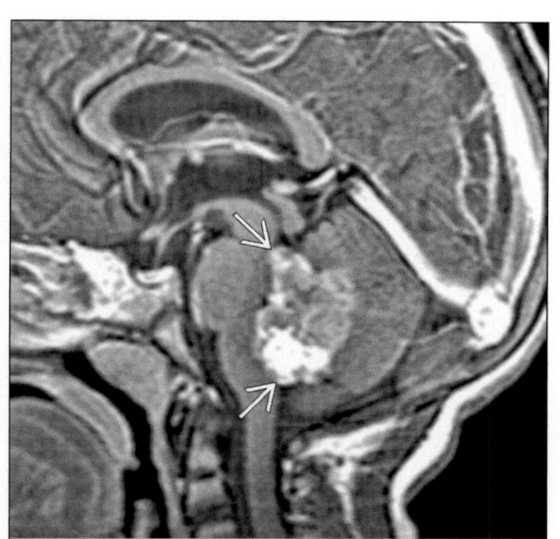

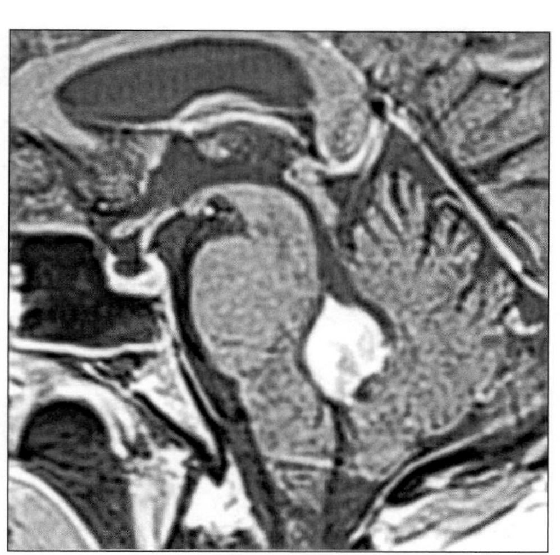

(Left) *Sagittal T1WI C+ MR in a 2 year old with ataxia, nausea, and vomiting shows a lobulated enhancing mass in the 4th ventricle ➡. Fourth ventricle masses in children are usually PNET or ependymoma, less often atypical teratoid-rhabdoid tumor. AT/RT was found at surgery.* ***(Right)*** *Sagittal T1WI C+ MR in a 52-year-old woman with episodic headaches, nausea, and vomiting shows an intensely enhancing 4th ventricle mass. This proved to be choroid plexus papilloma.*

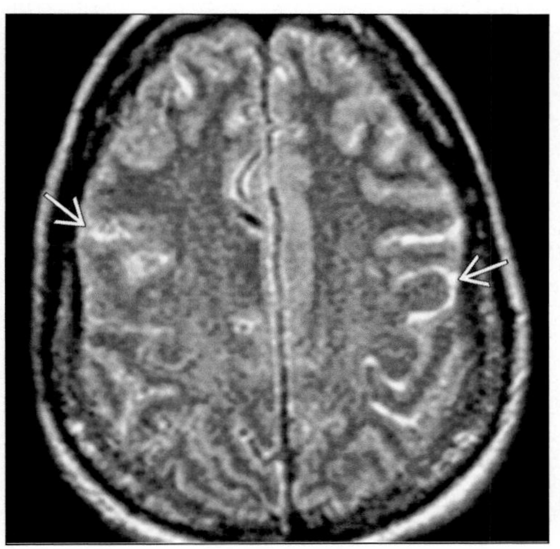

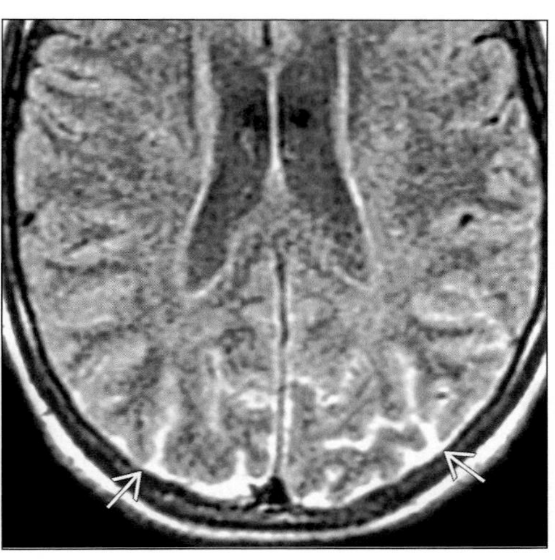

(Left) *Axial FLAIR MR shows multifocal sulcal hyperintensities ➡ caused by aneurysmal subarachnoid hemorrhage.* ***(Right)*** *Axial FLAIR MR shows artifactual hyperintensity in the occipital sulci ➡ secondary to incomplete CSF suppression. A repeat scan (not shown) was normal. Sulcal hyperintensity on FLAIR is nonspecific and can be caused by pia-subarachnoid metastases, blood, protein (meningitis), high oxygen content, retained contrast (renal failure), and artifact (as in this case).*

CAVUM SEPTI PELLUCIDI (CSP)

Key Facts

Terminology
- Cystic CSF cavity of septum pellucidum (SP)
  - Occurs ± cavum vergae (CV)

Imaging
- Elongated finger-shaped CSF collection between lateral ventricles
  - CSP: Between frontal horns of lateral ventricles
  - CV: Posterior extension between fornices
- Size varies from slit-like to several mm, occasionally > 1 cm
- SP invariably cystic in fetus
  - Width of fetal CSP increases between 19-27 weeks
  - Plateaus at 28 weeks
  - Gradually closes in rostral direction between 28 weeks and term
  - CSP present in 100% of premature, 85% of term infants
- CSP seen in up to 15-20% of adults

Top Differential Diagnoses
- Asymmetric lateral ventricles
- Cavum velum interpositum
- Ependymal cyst
- Absent septum pellucidum (SP)

Pathology
- CSP forms if fetal SP fails to obliterate
- Precise etiology of fluid accumulation unknown
- CSP is not the "5th ventricle"
- CV is not a "6th ventricle"

Clinical Issues
- Usually asymptomatic
- Usually not treated

*(**Left**) Coronal graphic with axial insert shows classic cavum septi pellucidi (CSP) with cavum vergae (CV) ➡. Note the finger-like CSF collection between the lateral ventricles. (**Right**) Axial T2WI MR shows cavum septi pellucidi as a CSF collection between the leaves of the septum pellucidum ➡.*

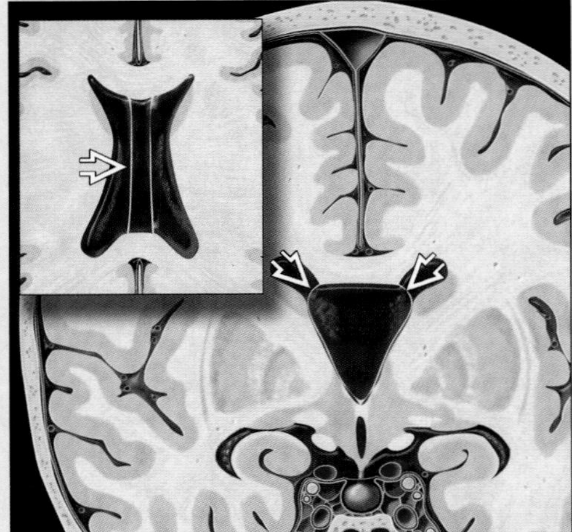

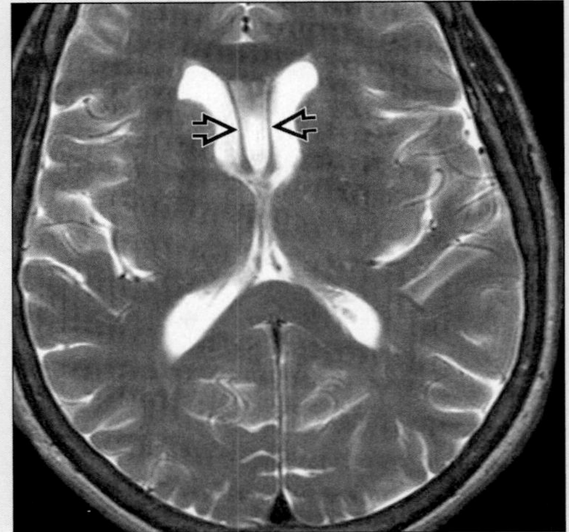

*(**Left**) Axial T1WI MR shows a small cavum septi pellucidi with cavum vergae ➡. Note the finger-like appearance of the CSF collection that lies between the frontal horns and bodies of the lateral ventricle. (**Right**) Axial T2WI MR shows a variant of a cavum septi pellucidi with cavum vergae. Note the large CSF collection between leaves of septum pellucidum ➡ continuing directly posteriorly with the CSF collection, splaying the fornices laterally →.*

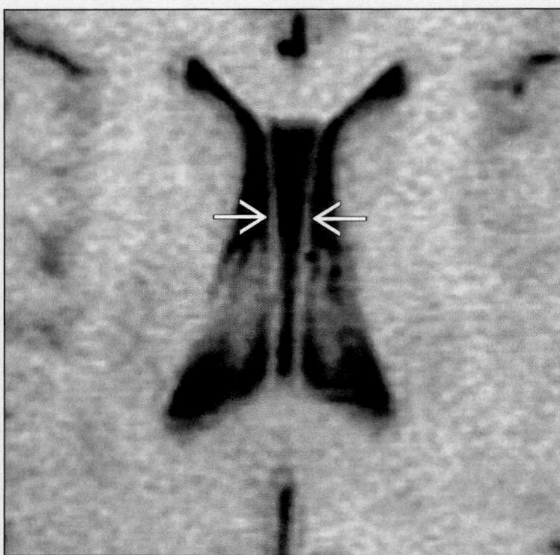

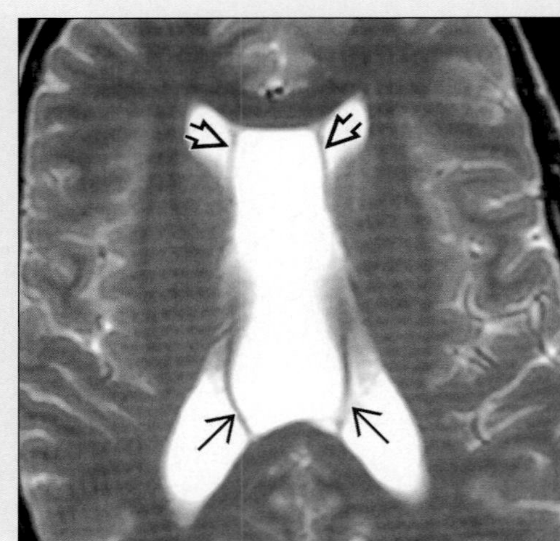

CAVUM VELUM INTERPOSITUM (CVI)

Key Facts

Terminology

- Cavum velum interpositum (CVI); cyst of velum interpositum (VI)

Imaging

- Triangular-shaped CSF space
  - Between lateral ventricles, over thalami
  - Apex points toward foramen of Monro
  - Elevates, splays fornices
  - Flattens, displaces internal cerebral veins inferiorly
- Size varies from slit-like linear to triangular to round/ovoid CSF collection
- Isodense/isointense with CSF
  - Suppresses completely
  - Does not restrict
  - Does not enhance
- US shows hypoechoic midline interhemispheric cyst

Top Differential Diagnoses

- Normal cistern of velum interpositum
- Cavum septi pellucidi (CSP), vergae (CV)
- Arachnoid cyst
- Epidermoid cyst

Clinical Issues

- Can be found at any age
  - Common in infants, rare in adults
- Symptoms
  - Usually asymptomatic, found incidentally
  - Headache (relationship to cyst unclear)

Diagnostic Checklist

- CSF-like "cyst" could be epidermoid
- Include FLAIR and DWI to distinguish between CVI, epidermoid cyst

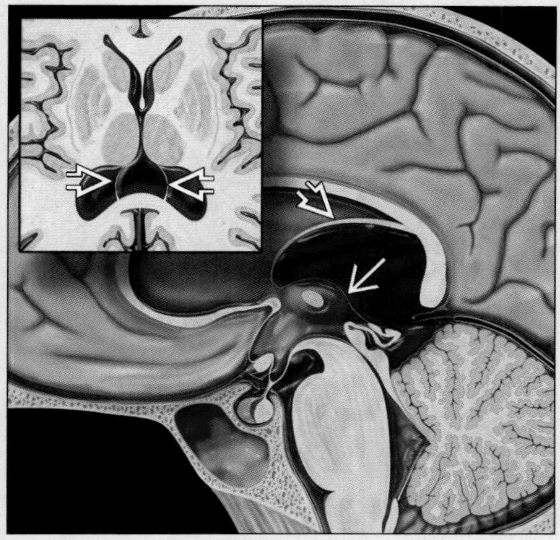

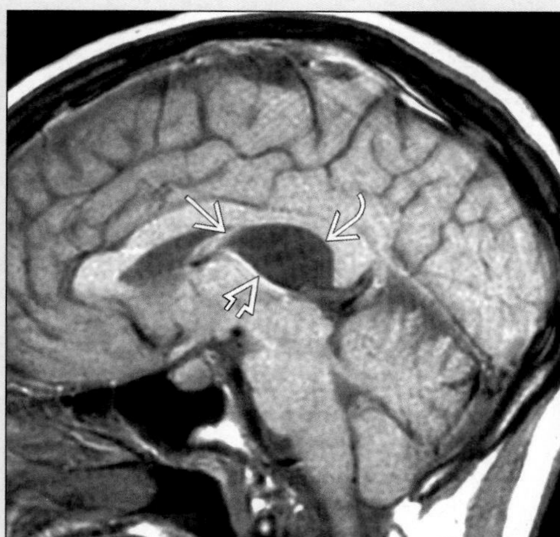

(Left) *Sagittal graphic with axial insert shows a CVI. Note the elevation and splaying of the fornices →. Also noted is the inferior displacement of the internal cerebral veins and 3rd ventricle →.* ***(Right)*** *Sagittal T1WI MR in a 40-year-old woman with headaches shows CSF-like enlargement of the velum interpositum → that elevates the fornix → and flattens and displaces the internal cerebral vein inferiorly →. This large CVI is probably unrelated to the patient's symptoms.*

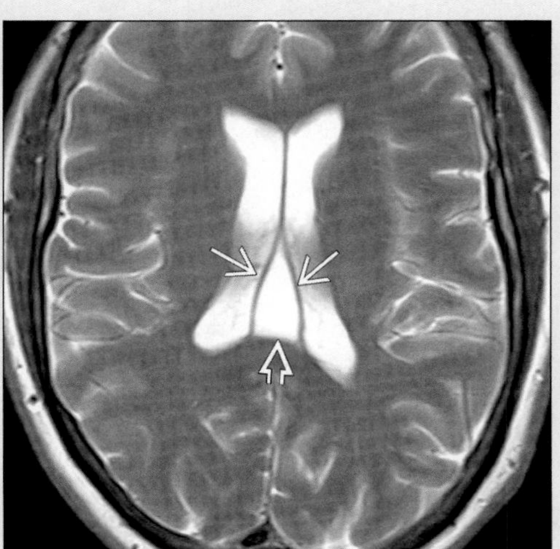

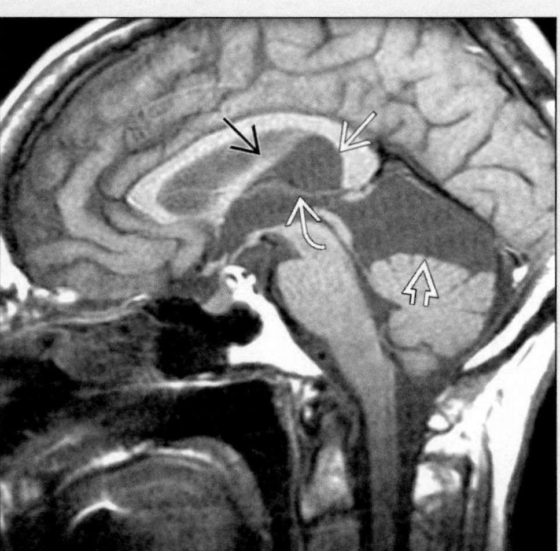

(Left) *Axial T2WI MR in a 46-year-old woman with headaches shows a classic CVI with a triangular-shaped CSF collection → spreading the fornices laterally →. The posterior location between the lateral ventricles is typical.* ***(Right)*** *Sagittal T1WI MR shows a variant CVI → that elevates the fornix →, flattens the internal cerebral vein →, and extends into the quadrigeminal and suprasellar cisterns →. This case probably represents an arachnoid cyst of the cavum velum interpositum.*

ENLARGED SUBARACHNOID SPACES

Key Facts

Terminology
- Idiopathic enlargement of SAS during 1st year of life

Imaging
- Enlarged SAS and ↑ head circumference (> 95%)
- CSF space follows (not flattens) gyral contour
- Right and left subarachnoid spaces are symmetric
- Macrocephaly, frontal bossing on radiography
- CECT demonstrates veins traversing SAS
- Spaces must follow CSF on all MR sequences and imaging

Top Differential Diagnoses
- Atrophy
- Acquired extraventricular obstructive hydrocephalus (EVOH)
- Nonaccidental trauma (NAT)

Pathology
- Immature CSF drainage pathways
- Family history of macrocephaly > 80%

Clinical Issues
- Increasing neurological signs or lack of development is not consistent with benign enlarged SAS
- No signs of elevated intracranial pressure; normal pressure on lumbar puncture
- Self-limited; SAS enlargement resolves without therapy by 12-24 months
- No treatment necessary

Diagnostic Checklist
- Consider nonaccidental trauma if enlarged SAS atypical in any way

*(**Left**) Axial graphic shows classic enlarged subarachnoid spaces in a macrocephalic infant with symmetric bifrontal enlargement, multiple bridging veins ➔, and mild ventriculomegaly. The craniocortical distance between the brain and calvarium is ≥ 5 mm. (**Right**) Axial CECT shows enlarged subarachnoid spaces with enhancing traversing veins ➔ and mildly enlarged ventricles in a macrocephalic infant. This benign condition usually peaks at 7 months and resolves spontaneously by 12-24 months of age.*

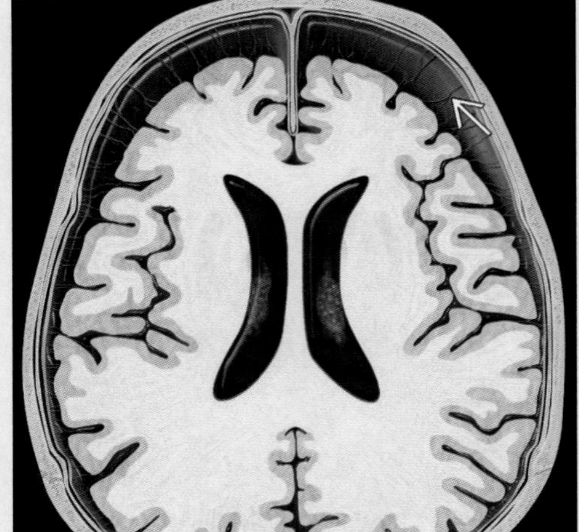

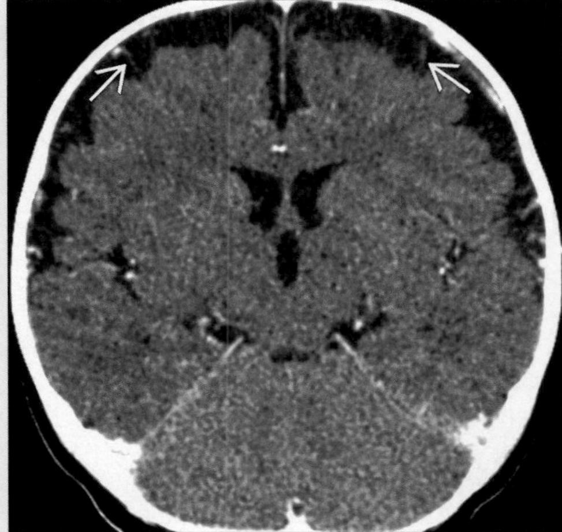

*(**Left**) Axial CECT shows markedly enlarged frontal subarachnoid spaces with traversing bridging veins ➔. The distance between the brain surface and the dura is 1.5 cm. (**Right**) Axial T2WI MR shows prominent frontal CSF spaces (craniocortical & interhemispheric) with mildly prominent ventricles in this macrocephalic infant. Note the squaring of the forehead, seen clinically as "frontal bossing." About 50% of cases have mild developmental delay (motor > > language), which nearly always resolves without therapy.*

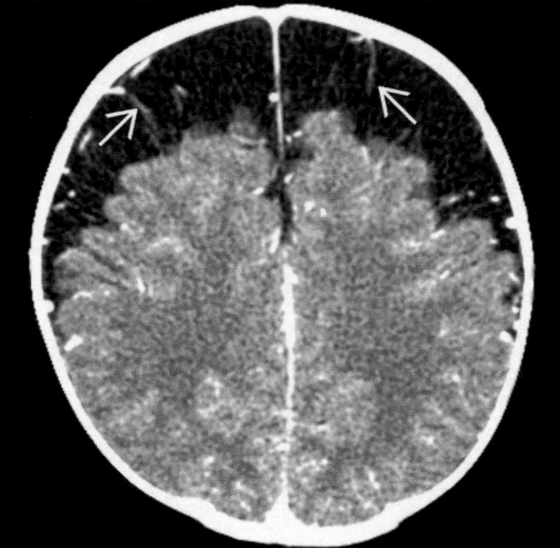

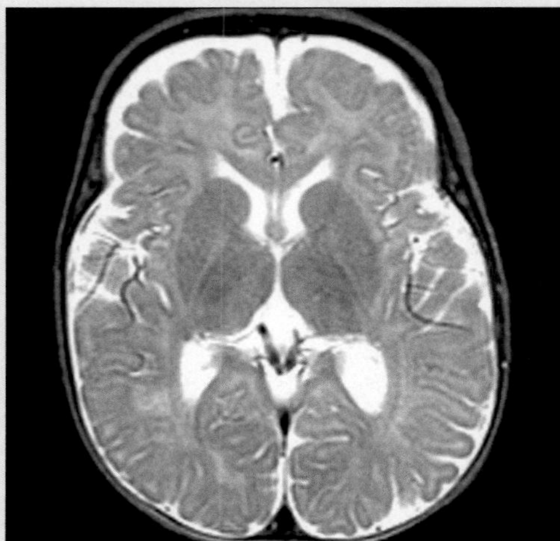

ENLARGED SUBARACHNOID SPACES

TERMINOLOGY

Abbreviations
- Physiologic subarachnoid space (SAS) enlargement

Synonyms
- Benign subarachnoid space enlargement
- Benign external hydrocephalus, benign extracerebral fluid collections of infancy
- Benign communicating hydrocephalus, physiologic extraventricular obstructive hydrocephalus

Definitions
- Idiopathic enlargement of SAS during 1st year of life

IMAGING

General Features
- Best diagnostic clue
  - Enlarged SAS and increased head circumference (> 95%)
- Location
  - SAS
    - Craniocortical width (CCW): Widest vertical distance between brain and calvarium
    - Sinocortical width (SCW): Widest distance between lateral wall of superior sagittal sinus and brain surface (SCW)
    - Interhemispheric: Widest distance between hemispheres
- Size
  - ≥ 5 mm widening bifrontal craniocortical/anterior interhemispheric SAS
  - **Note**: Normal maximum width peaks at 28 postnatal weeks (7 months) of life
- Morphology
  - CSF space follows (not flattens) gyral contour
  - Right and left subarachnoid spaces are symmetric

Radiographic Findings
- Radiography
  - Macrocephaly, frontal bossing

CT Findings
- NECT
  - ≥ 5 mm widening bifrontal/anterior interhemispheric SAS
  - Enlarged cisterns (especially suprasellar/chiasmatic)
  - Mildly enlarged ventricles (66%)
  - Sulci generally normal (especially posteriorly)
  - Postural unilateral lambdoid flattening is common
  - Posterior fossa normal
- CECT
  - Demonstrates veins traversing SAS
  - No abnormal enhancement of meninges

MR Findings
- T1WI
  - Similar to NECT
- T2WI
  - No abnormal brain tissue or signal abnormalities
  - Single layer of fluid (SAS) with traversing vessels
  - Normal flow void in aqueduct
- FLAIR
  - Homogeneous hypointense fluid in SAS (follows normal CSF signal)
- T2* GRE
  - No blood products
- DWI
  - No restriction, normal diffusivity
- T1WI C+
  - Enhancing veins traverse SAS
- Fetal MR: Distribution of fluid/ventricular prominence related to positioning of fetus
  - Usually frontal prominence after birth due to position of child lying on back for scan

Ultrasonographic Findings
- Grayscale ultrasound
  - Enlarged SAS ≥ 5 mm
  - Craniocortical width (CCW) and sinocortical width (SCW) < 10 mm in neurologically normal infants
  - Veins as "dots" floating in SAS
- Pulsed Doppler
  - Increased cerebral blood flow may identify "progressive" cases
- Color Doppler
  - Veins traverse SAS

Angiographic Findings
- Conventional
  - Widened space between skull and arteries of brain surface

Nonvascular Interventions
- Myelography
  - Cisternography confirms communication of SAS, but not necessary

Imaging Recommendations
- Best imaging tool
  - MR to exclude chronic subdural collections
- Protocol advice
  - Doppler sonography: Documents veins traversing SAS
  - MR or CECT: To exclude underlying etiology
  - MR: To exclude chronic subdural collections
    - SAS isointense with CSF on all sequences if benign
  - Phase-contrast MR shows normal intraventricular CSF flow
  - After diagnosis, best follow-up = tape measure and assess for normal development; not imaging!

DIFFERENTIAL DIAGNOSIS

Atrophy
- Small head circumference (HC)
  - Forehead "pointed" due to metopic fusion
- Patients with benign SAS enlargement have large head
  - Forehead "flat" due to frontal bossing
- Knowledge of HC critical for diagnosis

Acquired Extraventricular Obstructive Hydrocephalus (EVOH)
- Often hemorrhagic/postinflammatory/neoplastic
  - Density of extraaxial collection does not = CSF

- Achondroplasia and other skull base anomalies
  - Coarctation of foramen magnum (narrow)
- Intermittent intracranial pressure waves

Nonaccidental Trauma (NAT)

- Predisposition to bleed with minor trauma is controversial
  - Possible if SAS ≥ 6 mm
  - Venous "stretching" implicated

Glutaric Aciduria Type 1

- Enlarged sylvian fissures with delayed myelination
- T2 hyperintense basal ganglia

PATHOLOGY

General Features

- Etiology
  - Immature CSF drainage pathways
    - CSF primarily drained via extracellular space ⇒ capillaries
    - Pacchionian granulations (PGs) do not mature until 18 months
    - PGs are then displaced into veins (as Starling-type resistors)
    - PGs regulate pulse pressure/venous drainage CSF when fontanels close
    - Benign SAS enlargement usually resolves at that time
- Genetics
  - No documented genetic predisposition, although common in benign familial macrocrania families
    - Family history of macrocephaly > 80%
- Associated abnormalities
  - Possibility of increased risk for bridging vein injury and resultant subdural hematoma in absence of trauma

Staging, Grading, & Classification

- Danger signs
  - Elevated intracranial pressure (ICP)
  - Rapid enlargement of head circumference
  - Increasing lack of development or neurological signs
  - Onset or persistence > 1 year old

Gross Pathologic & Surgical Features

- Deep/prominent but otherwise normal-appearing SAS
- No pathologic membranes

Microscopic Features

- Ependymal damage not seen in benign SAS enlargement

CLINICAL ISSUES

Presentation

- Most common signs/symptoms
  - Macrocrania: Head circumference > 95%
  - Frontal bossing
  - No signs of elevated ICP; normal pressure on lumbar puncture
- Other signs/symptoms
  - Possible mild developmental delay (50%), which usually resolves
- Clinical profile
  - Family history of benign macrocephaly common
  - Male infants, sometimes late to walk

Demographics

- Age
  - Usually present at 3-8 months
- Gender
  - 80% male
- Epidemiology
  - Reported on 2-65% of neuroimaging for macrocrania < 1 year old

Natural History & Prognosis

- Enlarged SAS ⇒ ↑ suture/calvarial malleability/compliance ⇒ predisposes to posterior plagiocephaly
- Self-limited; SAS enlargement resolves without therapy by 12-24 months
  - Spontaneous resolution of spaces and symptoms
- Calvarium outgrows brain, brain eventually catches up
- Macrocephaly often persists

Treatment

- No treatment necessary
- Normal outcome (developmental delay resolves as prominent SAS resolves)

DIAGNOSTIC CHECKLIST

Consider

- Nonaccidental injury if enlarged SAS atypical in any way

Image Interpretation Pearls

- Crucial: Know head circumference
- Consider enhanced CT or MR to confirm veins traversing SAS and search for membranes or nonisointense fluid collections (chronic subdural)

SELECTED REFERENCES

1. Hellbusch LC: Benign extracerebral fluid collections in infancy: clinical presentation and long-term follow-up. J Neurosurg. 107(2 Suppl):119-25, 2007
2. Muenchberger H et al: Idiopathic macrocephaly in the infant: long-term neurological and neuropsychological outcome. Childs Nerv Syst. 22(10):1242-8, 2006
3. Fessell DP et al: Sonography of extraaxial fluid in neurologically normal infants with head circumference greater than or equal to the 95th percentile for age. J Ultrasound Med. 19(7):443-7, 2000
4. Papasian NC et al: A theoretical model of benign external hydrocephalus that predicts a predisposition towards extra-axial hemorrhage after minor head trauma. Pediatr Neurosurg. 33(4):188-93, 2000
5. Wilms G et al: CT and MR in infants with pericerebral collections and macrocephaly: benign enlargement of the subarachnoid spaces versus subdural collections. AJNR Am J Neuroradiol. 14(4):855-60, 1993
6. Maytal J et al: External hydrocephalus: radiologic spectrum and differentiation from cerebral atrophy. AJR Am J Roentgenol. 148(6):1223-30, 1987

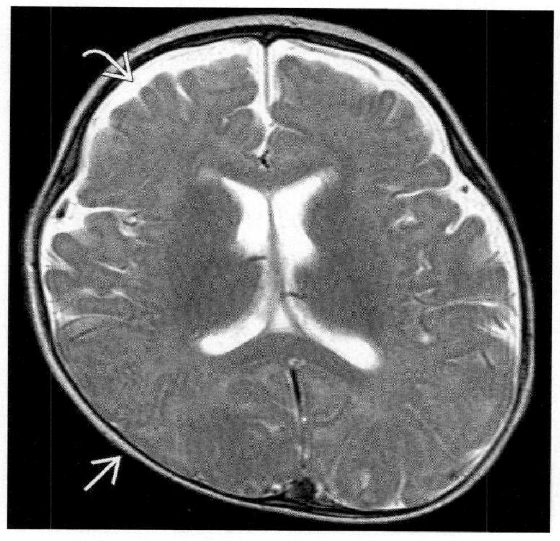

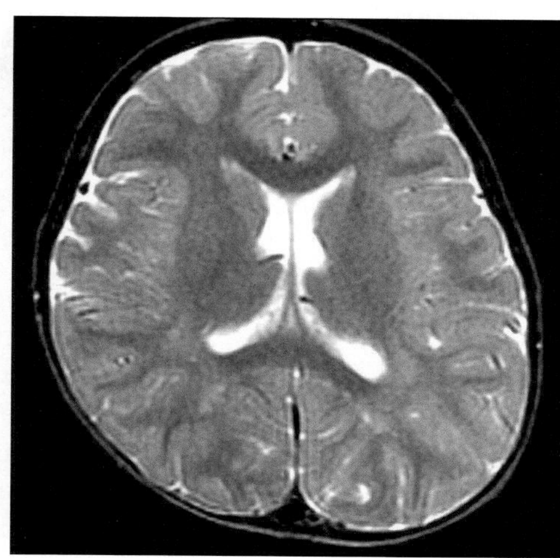

(Left) *Axial T2WI MR shows enlarged frontal and anterior interhemispheric pericerebral fluid spaces ⮫, mild ventriculomegaly, and right-sided posterior plagiocephaly ➡ in a 7-month-old male with macrocephaly.* ***(Right)*** *Axial T2WI MR follow-up of the same patient at 17 months of age shows that the pericerebral and anterior interhemispheric fluid spaces have normalized. A family history of benign macrocephaly is common in these patients.*

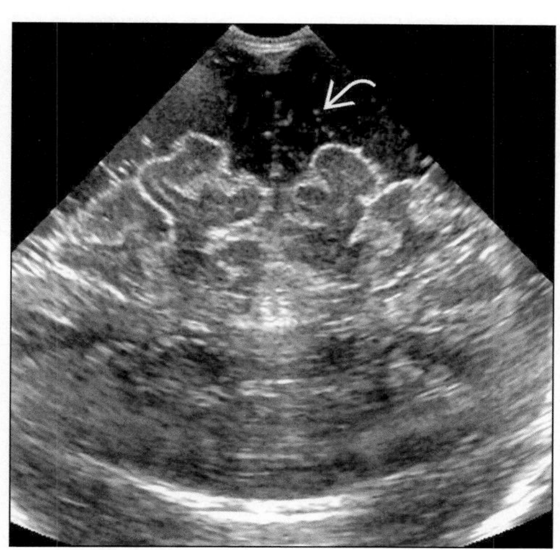

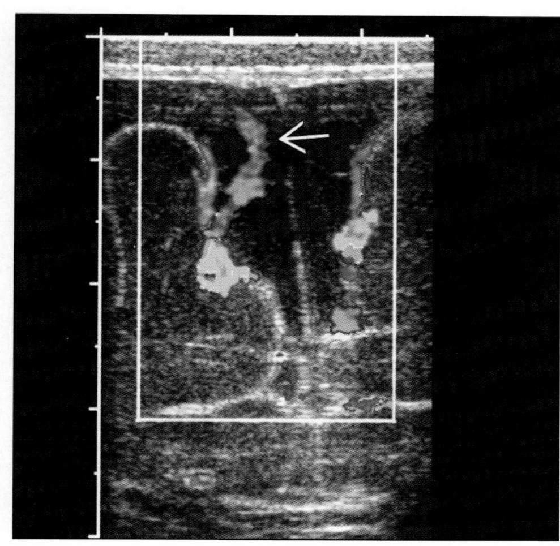

(Left) *Coronal brain ultrasound shows increased sinocortical distance in this case of markedly enlarged subarachnoid spaces in this young infant with macrocephaly. Echogenic foci within the CSF collection correspond to bridging veins ⮫. CSF spaces are most prominent at 7 months of life.* ***(Right)*** *Coronal color Doppler ultrasound demonstrates venous structures ➡ traversing the dilated subarachnoid space. Enlarged subarachnoid spaces are related to immature CSF drainage pathways.*

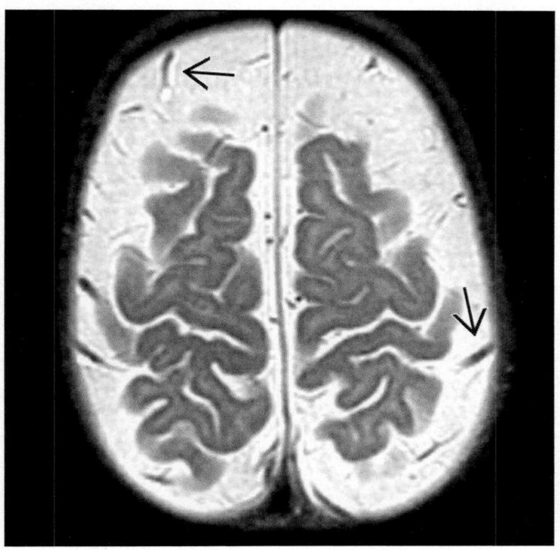

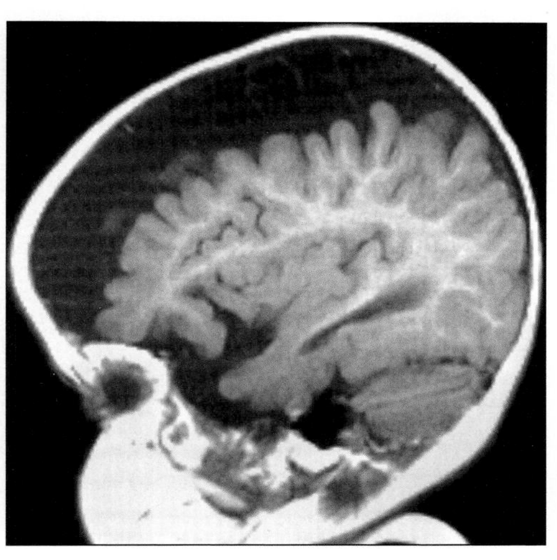

(Left) *Axial T2WI MR in a macrocephalic infant shows markedly prominent CSF spaces (craniocortical & interhemispheric) with normal flow voids of bridging veins ➡ traversing the CSF.* ***(Right)*** *Sagittal T1WI MR shows markedly enlarged subarachnoid spaces. Note the large calvarial size compared to the face, related to macrocephaly. Bridging veins traverse the enlarged subarachnoid spaces. It is important to ensure that the fluid follows CSF on all sequences to exclude nonaccidental trauma.*

INTRAVENTRICULAR OBSTRUCTIVE HYDROCEPHALUS

Key Facts

Terminology

- Intraventricular obstructive hydrocephalus (IVOH) = obstruction proximal to foramina of Luschka, Magendie
  - Acute (aIVOH)
  - Chronic "compensated" (cIVOH)

Imaging

- aIVOH = "ballooned" ventricles plus indistinct ("blurred") margins
  - "Fingers" of CSF extend into periventricular WM
  - Most striking around ventricular horns (periventricular "halos")
  - After decompression, corpus callosum may show hyperintensity
- cIVOH = "ballooned" ventricles without periventricular "halo"

Top Differential Diagnoses

- Ventricular enlargement 2° to parenchymal loss
- Normal pressure hydrocephalus
- Extraventricular obstructive hydrocephalus
- Choroid plexus papilloma
- Longstanding overt ventriculomegaly in adults

Pathology

- Intraventricular obstruction to CSF flow
  - CSF production continues, ventricular pressure ↑
- Ventricles expand, compress adjacent parenchyma
- Periventricular interstitial fluid increases
  - Leads to myelin vacuolization, destruction
- Pathology varies depending on obstruction etiology

Diagnostic Checklist

- Ventricle size generally correlates poorly with intracranial pressure

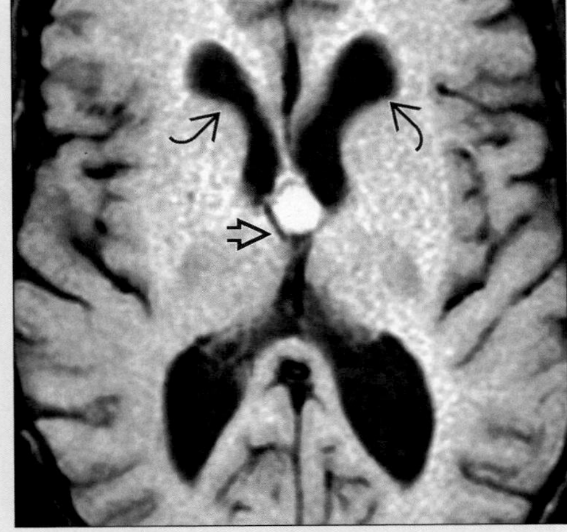

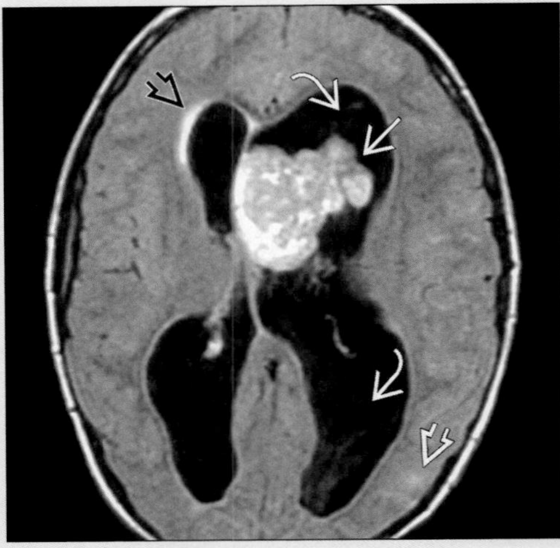

*(**Left**) Axial T1WI MR shows a well-defined, hyperintense lesion ⇨ at the foramen of Monro in a patient with headaches, most consistent with a colloid cyst. Note the enlargement of the lateral ventricles ↷ due to obstruction at the foramen of Monro. (**Right**) Axial FLAIR in a patient with tuberous sclerosis shows large subependymal giant cell astrocytoma ➡ causing obstructive hydrocephalus ↷ with mild periventricular edema ⇨. Note the subtle hyperintensity in the occipital lobe tuber ➡.*

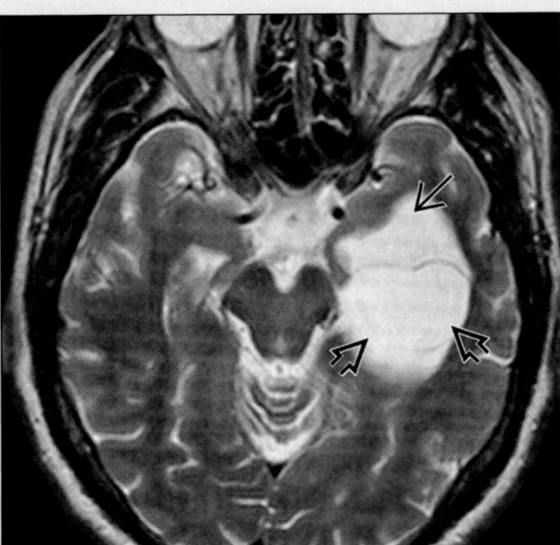

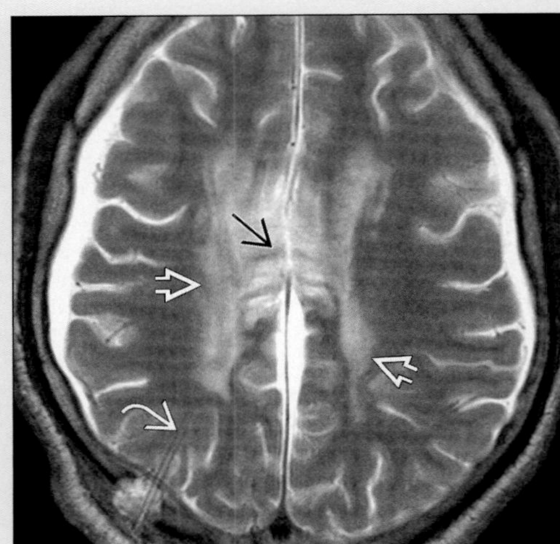

*(**Left**) Axial T2WI MR demonstrates a well-defined CSF intensity cyst with the left temporal horn most consistent with an ependymal cyst ⇨. Note the dilated and trapped left temporal horn →. (**Right**) Axial T2WI MR in a patient with corpus callosum impingement syndrome, after shunting for severe IVOH, shows a shunt tube ↷, bilateral subdural fluid collections, and peculiar "striated" hyperintensity in the corpus callosum → with somewhat less striking changes in the periventricular WM ⇨. (Courtesy S. Candy, MD.)*

INTRAVENTRICULAR OBSTRUCTIVE HYDROCEPHALUS

TERMINOLOGY

Abbreviations

- Intraventricular obstructive hydrocephalus (IVOH)
  - Acute IVOH (aIVOH)
  - Chronic "compensated" IVOH (cIVOH)

Synonyms

- "Noncommunicating" hydrocephalus

Definitions

- Enlarged ventricles caused by obstruction proximal to foramina of Luschka, Magendie

IMAGING

General Features

- Best diagnostic clue
  - aIVOH
    - "Ballooned" ventricles with indistinct ("blurred") margins
  - cIVOH
    - "Ballooned" ventricles without periventricular "halo"
- Size
  - Bifrontal horn to intracranial diameter ratio > 0.33
  - Temporal horn width > 3 mm
- Morphology
  - Varies with site, duration of blockage
  - Global/focally enlarged ventricle(s) ± elevated ICP
  - Ventricles proximal to obstruction enlarge, appear more rounded

CT Findings

- NECT
  - Large ventricles proximal to obstruction
    - aIVOH
      - "Ballooned" ventricles with periventricular low-density "halo"
    - cIVOH
      - "Ballooned" ventricles, periventricular "halo"
  - Basal cisterns, sulci compressed/obliterated

MR Findings

- T1WI
  - Lateral ventricles enlarged
  - Corpus callosum (CC) thinned, stretched upward
    - May be impinged against falx
    - Impaction may cause pressure necrosis
  - Fornix, ICV displaced downward
  - Enlarged 3rd ventricle often herniated into expanded sella
  - Funnel-shaped aqueduct of Sylvius in aqueductal stenosis
- T2WI
  - aIVOH
    - "Fingers" of CSF-like hyperintensity extend into periventricular WM, most striking around ventricular horns (periventricular "halos")
    - Disturbed/turbulent CSF flow
    - Absent aqueductal "flow void" common
    - CC may appear hyperintense
  - cIVOH
    - Large ventricles, normal CSF pressure
    - No periventricular "halo"
    - CC may show hyperintensity after decompression (15% of shunted IVOH cases)
- T1WI C+
  - Neoplasm causing IVOH may enhance
  - aIVOH may cause leptomeningeal vascular stasis, enhancement
    - Can mimic meningitis, metastases!

Other Modality Findings

- Contrast-enhanced ventriculography
  - MR/CT used to identify site of obstruction, status of 3rd ventriculostomies
  - MR can be used for assessing CSF flow
- Cardiac-gated cine MR
  - May show absent aqueductal CSF flow

Imaging Recommendations

- Best imaging tool
  - MR with contrast to evaluate cause of CSF obstruction
- Protocol advice
  - 3D constructive interference in steady state (CISS)
    - Decreases CSF flow artifact
    - Allows better delineation of ventricular contour, septa

DIFFERENTIAL DIAGNOSIS

Ventricular Enlargement Secondary to Parenchymal Loss

- Old term = "ex vacuo" hydrocephalus (not used)
- Age-related (ventricular volume increases 1.2-1.4 mL/ after 60 years)
  - Ischemia/infarction, trauma, infection, toxic
- Obtuse frontal angle (> 110°)
- Diffuse/focal enlargement of sulci, cisterns
- Normal lateral ventricles can be asymmetric (related to handedness, not gender)
- May correlate with some psychiatric disorders (e.g., schizophrenia)

Normal Pressure Hydrocephalus

- Progressive dementia, gait disturbance, incontinence
- Ventricular dilation with normal CSF pressure
- Sulci normal/minimally enlarged
- Increased CSF displacement through aqueduct
- MRS shows lactate peak

Extraventricular Obstructive Hydrocephalus (EVOH)

- Dilated ventricles due to mismatch between CSF formation, absorption
- Decreased CSF absorption through arachnoid villi
- Subarachnoid hemorrhage most common cause
  - Others: Meningitis, carcinomatosis, granulomatous disease

Choroid Plexus Papilloma

- Accounts for 2-5% of childhood intracranial tumors
- Child < 5 years with ↑ ICP
- Most lateral ventricle trigone

- May "overproduce" CSF
- Hemorrhage, tumor spread may cause IVOH

Longstanding Overt Ventriculomegaly in Adults

- Early childhood onset or longstanding progression of hydrocephalus into adulthood
- Markedly enlarged ventricles, high ICP

PATHOLOGY

General Features

- Etiology
  - Normal CSF production = 0.20-0.35 mL/min
    - Capacity of lateral, 3rd ventricles in adult = 20 mL
    - Total volume of CSF in adult = 120 mL
  - Intraventricular obstruction to CSF flow; as CSF production continues, ventricular fluid pressure ↑
  - Ventricles expand, compress adjacent parenchyma; stretching may rupture/open ependymal cell junctions
  - Periventricular interstitial fluid increases → myelin destruction
  - Etiology depends on site
    - Foramen of Monro
      - Colloid cyst
      - Subependymal nodule, tuberous sclerosis complex
      - Subependymal giant cell astrocytoma
    - 3rd ventricle
      - Pituitary macroadenoma
      - Craniopharyngioma
    - Aqueduct of Sylvius
      - Aqueductal stenosis
      - Tectal glioma
      - Pineal region tumors
    - 4th ventricle
      - Medulloblastoma, ependymoma
      - Glioma, pilocytic astrocytoma, hemangioblastoma
      - Congenital anomalies (Chiari malformations, Dandy-Walker malformations)
    - Metastasis, neurocysticercosis, or meningioma can occur at multiple intraventricular locations
- Genetics
  - Cell adhesion molecule L1 (*L1CAM*) only gene recognized to cause human hydrocephalus
    - Located on X chromosome (Xq28)

Gross Pathologic & Surgical Features

- Focal/generalized ventricular enlargement
- Ependyma, adjacent white matter are secondarily injured
- Variable pathology depending on causative factor

Microscopic Features

- Increased periventricular extracellular space
- Ependymal lining damaged or lost; surrounding white matter becomes pale and rarefied

CLINICAL ISSUES

Presentation

- Most common signs/symptoms
  - Headache, papilledema (aIVOH)
  - Nausea, vomiting, diplopia (6th nerve palsy)
- Clinical profile
  - Varies with etiology, severity, age of onset

Demographics

- Age
  - May be any age from in utero (congenital hydrocephalus) to adult
- Epidemiology
  - Epidemiological data varies widely, depending upon etiology and type of hydrocephalus
  - Most common neurosurgical procedure in children = CSF shunting for hydrocephalus

Natural History & Prognosis

- Usually progressive unless treated

Treatment

- Medical management to delay surgical intervention
- CSF diversion (shunt), endoscopic intervention, and ventriculostomy
- Surgery to alleviate primary cause of obstruction

DIAGNOSTIC CHECKLIST

Image Interpretation Pearls

- Size of ventricles generally correlates poorly with intracranial pressure
- Pulsatile CSF may create confusing signal intensity, even mimic intraventricular mass
- Ventricular asymmetry can be normal variant

SELECTED REFERENCES

1. Feng F et al: Evaluation of radionuclide cerebrospinal fluid scintigraphy as a guide in the management of patients with hydrocephalus. Clin Imaging. 33(2):85-9, 2009
2. Linninger AA et al: Normal and Hydrocephalic Brain Dynamics: The Role of Reduced Cerebrospinal Fluid Reabsorption in Ventricular Enlargement. Ann Biomed Eng. Epub ahead of print, 2009
3. Oertel JM et al: Endoscopic third ventriculostomy in obstructive hydrocephalus due to giant basilar artery aneurysm. J Neurosurg. 110(1):14-8, 2009
4. Stoquart-El Sankari S et al: Phase-contrast MR imaging support for the diagnosis of aqueductal stenosis. AJNR Am J Neuroradiol. 30(1):209-14, 2009
5. Yamada S et al: Visualization of cerebrospinal fluid movement with spin labeling at MR imaging: preliminary results in normal and pathophysiologic conditions. Radiology. 249(2):644-52, 2008
6. Sener RN: Callosal changes in obstructive hydrocephalus: observations with FLAIR imaging, and diffusion MRI. Comput Med Imaging Graph. 26(5):333-7, 2002

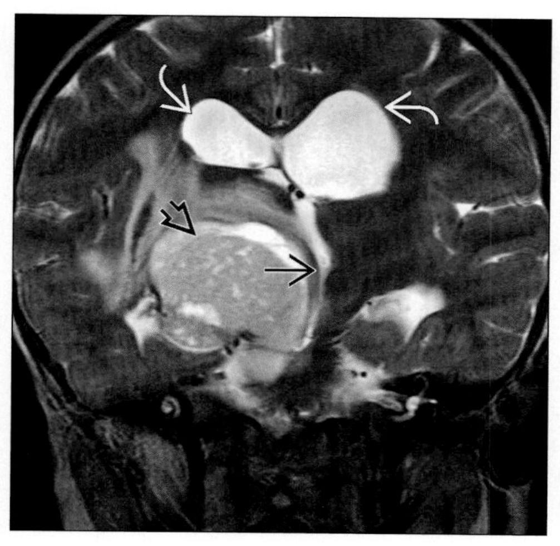

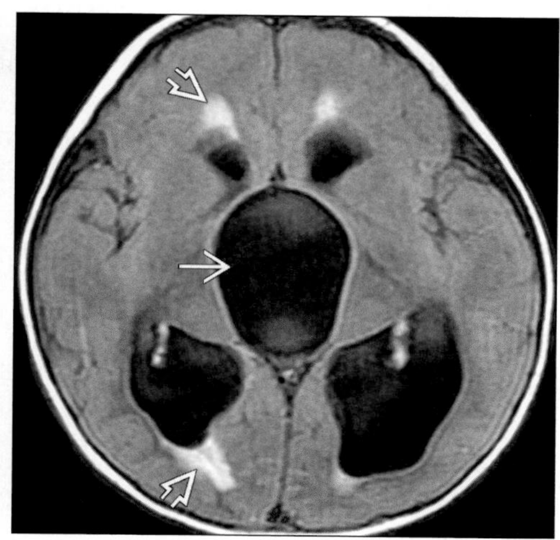

(Left) *Coronal T2WI MR shows a pilocytic astrocytoma centered in the right thalamus ⇨ causing severe mass effect on the 3rd ventricle → and resultant obstructive hydrocephalus ⮫.* ***(Right)*** *Axial FLAIR MR shows massive enlargement of the 3rd and lateral ventricles by what appears to be a CSF-like mass within the 3rd ventricle ➡. There is periventricular transependymal CSF flow ⇨. At surgery, an ependymal cyst of the 3rd ventricle was found and fenestrated.*

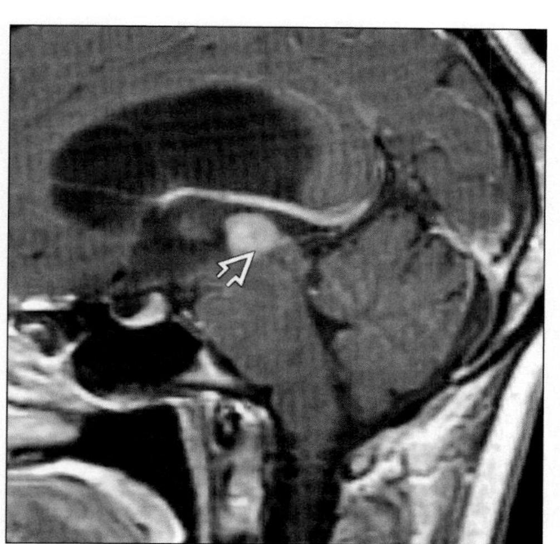

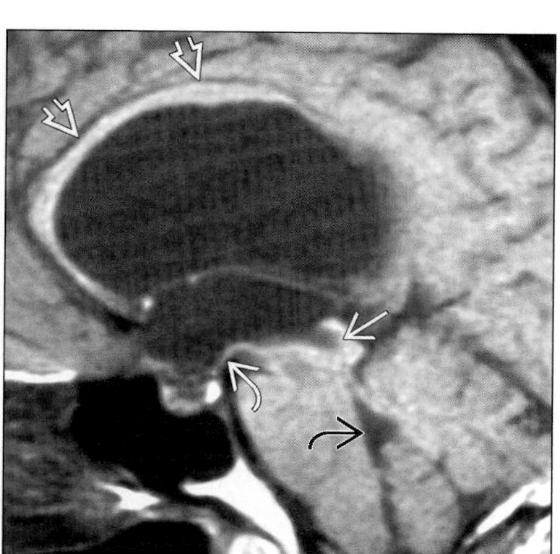

(Left) *Sagittal T1WI C+ MR shows a homogeneously enhancing mass in the posterior 3rd ventricle ⇨, which causes obstruction and dilatation of the lateral and 3rd ventricles. On pathology, this was an astrocytoma.* ***(Right)*** *Sagittal T1WI MR reveals typical findings in aqueductal stenosis: A funnel-shaped aqueduct of Sylvius ➡, normal 4th ventricle ⮫, thinned and stretched corpus callosum ⇨, and downward displacement of the floor of the 3rd ventricle ⮫.*

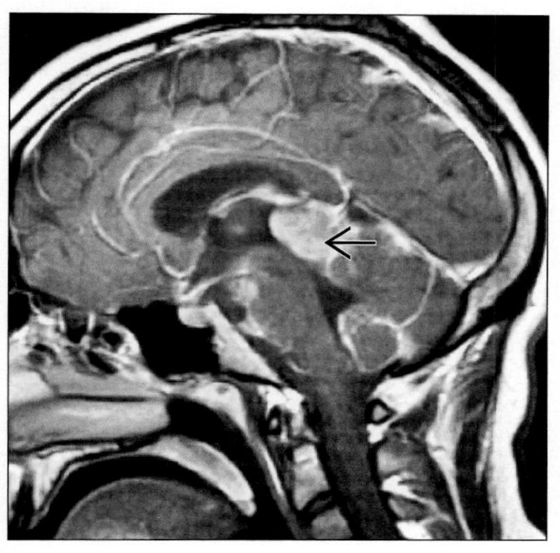

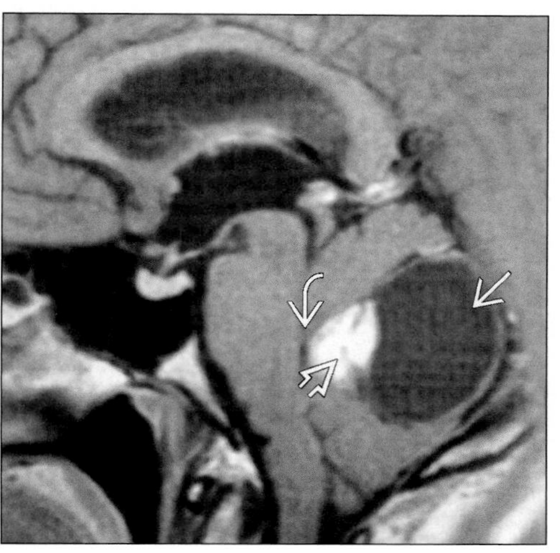

(Left) *Sagittal T1WI C+ MR shows an enhancing mass in the pineal region → causing mass effect on the tectal plate and aqueductal obstruction. Note the extensive leptomeningeal enhancement due to CSF spread of tumor. CSF cytology showed a primitive neuroectodermal tumor.* ***(Right)*** *Sagittal T1WI C+ MR shows a cyst ➡ with an enhancing mural nodule ⇨ of hemangioblastoma in the vermis, causing severe effacement of the 4th ventricle ⮫ and obstructive hydrocephalus.*

EXTRAVENTRICULAR OBSTRUCTIVE HYDROCEPHALUS

Key Facts

Terminology

- Extraventricular obstructive hydrocephalus (EVOH)
  - "Communicating" hydrocephalus
- Enlarged ventricles due to mismatch between CSF formation, absorption

Imaging

- Obstruction distal to 4th ventricle outlet foramina
- Size varies with duration of obstruction
- All ventricles enlarged with no intraventricular obstructive cause
- Lateral 3rd, 4th ventricles dilated
- ± abnormal density/intensity of cisternal CSF ± leptomeningeal enhancement

Top Differential Diagnoses

- Intraventricular obstructive hydrocephalus
- Ventricular enlargement secondary parenchymal loss
- Normal pressure hydrocephalus

Pathology

- Subarachnoid hemorrhage: Most common cause of EVOH
- Other etiologies include suppurative meningitis, neoplastic or inflammatory exudates
- SAH, exudates may fibrose/occlude subarachnoid space

Clinical Issues

- Headache, papilledema
- Nausea, vomiting, diplopia (cranial nerve palsy)

Diagnostic Checklist

- EVOH: Generalized ventricular enlargement with abnormal density/intensity in basal cisterns ± leptomeningeal enhancement

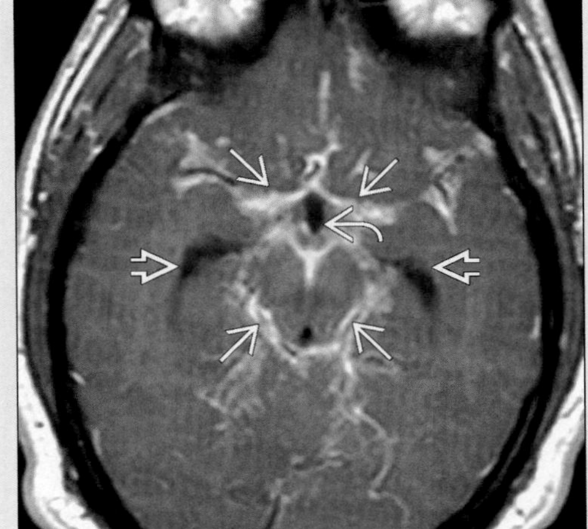

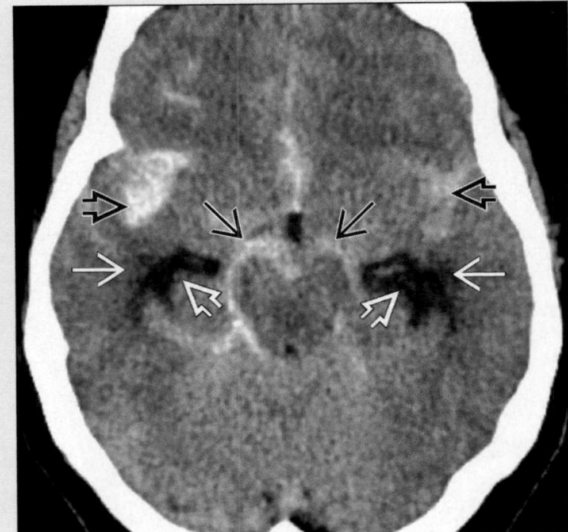

(Left) Axial T1WI C+ MR shows extensive leptomeningeal enhancement of the basal cisterns in neurosarcoidosis ➔. Notice the early communicating hydrocephalus with the dilated 3rd ventricle ➔ and temporal horns ➔. (Right) Axial NECT shows hyperdense material in the basal cisterns ➔ and sylvian fissures ➔ in acute subarachnoid hemorrhage. There is early dilatation of the ventricles ➔ with mild periventricular edema ➔ due to transependymal CSF leakage.

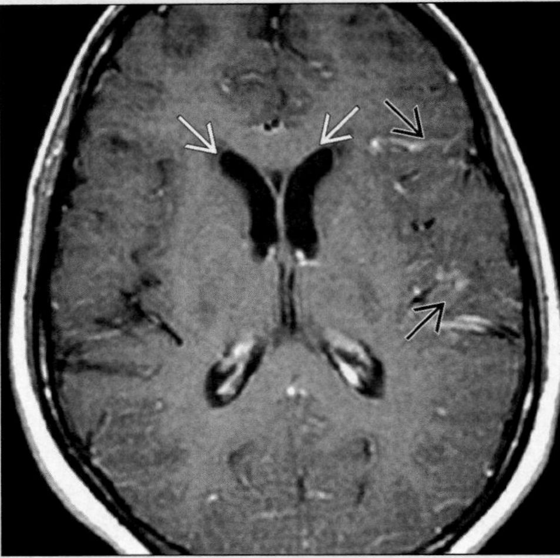

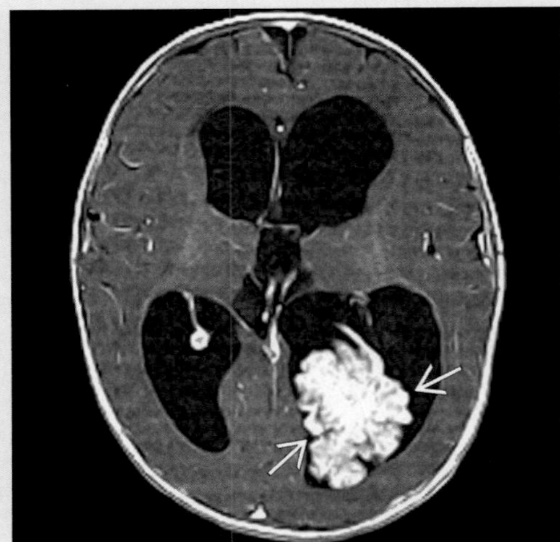

(Left) Axial T1WI C+ MR demonstrates subtle leptomeningeal enhancement in the left sylvian fissure ➔ in this patient with tuberculous meningitis. There is mild dilatation of the lateral ventricles ➔ due to EVOH. (Right) Axial T1WI C+ shows a lobulated choroid plexus papilloma arising from the glomus of the left lateral ventricle ➔ and hydrocephalus. In this case, the hydrocephalus although not obstructive, is likely secondary to CSF overproduction from the tumor.

EXTRAVENTRICULAR OBSTRUCTIVE HYDROCEPHALUS

TERMINOLOGY

Abbreviations

- Extraventricular obstructive hydrocephalus (EVOH)

Synonyms

- "Communicating" hydrocephalus

Definitions

- Enlarged ventricles due to mismatch between CSF formation, absorption

IMAGING

General Features

- Best diagnostic clue
  - Lateral, 3rd, 4th ventricles all dilated
  - ± abnormal density/intensity of cisternal CSF ± leptomeningeal enhancement
- Location
  - Obstruction distal to 4th ventricle outlet foramina
- Size
  - Bifrontal horn to intracranial diameter ratio > 0.33
  - Temporal horn width > 3 mm
- Morphology
  - All ventricles enlarged
    - Generally proportionate, symmetrical increase
    - No intraventricular obstructive cause

CT Findings

- NECT
  - Variable ventricular dilatation ± basal cisterns effaced
  - If subarachnoid hemorrhage (SAH), look for hyperdense CSF
- CECT
  - Look for sulcal/cisternal enhancement

MR Findings

- T1WI
  - "Dirty" CSF, ventricular dilatation
- T2WI
  - Dilated ventricles ± periventricular white matter hyperintensities
  - Hyperintense CSF-SAH, exudates
- T1WI C+
  - ± enhancement basal cisterns/sulci
    - Meningitis, carcinomatosis, etc.

Imaging Recommendations

- Best imaging tool
  - MR with T1WI C+

DIFFERENTIAL DIAGNOSIS

Intraventricular Obstructive Hydrocephalus

- Global/focal enlarged ventricles due to obstruction proximal to 4th ventricle outflow

Ventricular Enlargement Secondary Parenchymal Loss

- Age related
- Diffuse/focal enlargement of sulci, cisterns

Normal Pressure Hydrocephalus

- Ventricular enlargement with normal CSF pressure
- Sulci normal/minimally enlarged
- Progressive dementia, gait disturbance, incontinence

PATHOLOGY

General Features

- Etiology
  - Obstruction to CSF flow at level of basal cisterns or arachnoid villi
  - Rare: More CSF produced than can be absorbed ("overproduction" hydrocephalus; occurs with CPP, villous hyperplasia)
  - SAH: Most common cause of EVOH
  - Other etiologies include suppurative meningitis, neoplastic or inflammatory exudates

Gross Pathologic & Surgical Features

- SAH, exudates may fibrose/occlude subarachnoid space
- Generalized ventricular dilatation

CLINICAL ISSUES

Presentation

- Most common signs/symptoms
  - Headache, papilledema
  - Nausea, vomiting, diplopia (cranial nerve palsy)

Natural History & Prognosis

- Usually progressive unless shunted and primary cause treated

Treatment

- CSF diversion (shunt)
- Directed to primary cause

DIAGNOSTIC CHECKLIST

Consider

- EVOH: Generalized ventricular enlargement with abnormal density/intensity in basal cisterns ± leptomeningeal enhancement

SELECTED REFERENCES

1. Feng F et al: Evaluation of radionuclide cerebrospinal fluid scintigraphy as a guide in the management of patients with hydrocephalus. Clin Imaging. 33(2):85-9, 2009
2. Yamada S et al: Visualization of cerebrospinal fluid movement with spin labeling at MR imaging: preliminary results in normal and pathophysiologic conditions. Radiology. 249(2):644-52, 2008
3. ter Laan M et al: Improvement after treatment of hydrocephalus in aneurysmal subarachnoid haemorrhage: implications for grading and prognosis. Acta Neurochir (Wien). 148(3):325-8; discussion 328, 2006

AQUEDUCTAL STENOSIS

Key Facts

Terminology

- Focal reduction of cerebral aqueduct diameter

Imaging

- Ventriculomegaly of lateral and 3rd ventricles with normal-sized 4th ventricle
- ± periventricular interstitial edema (uncompensated hydrocephalus)

Top Differential Diagnoses

- Obstructing extraventricular pathology
  - Neoplasm
  - Vein of Galen malformation
  - Quadrigeminal cistern arachnoid cyst
- Obstructing intraventricular (aqueductal) pathology
- Postinflammatory gliosis (aqueductal gliosis)

Pathology

- Congenital AS is common cause of fetal hydrocephalus
- Aqueductal web and fork are pathological subsets

Clinical Issues

- Onset often insidious, may occur at any time from birth to adulthood

Diagnostic Checklist

- Consider postinflammatory gliosis (aqueductal gliosis), particularly if history of prematurity or meningitis
- Carefully scrutinize posterior 3rd ventricle, tectum, and tegmentum for obstructing neoplastic mass

*(**Left**) Sagittal graphic shows obstructive hydrocephalus with markedly enlarged lateral and 3rd ventricles, stretched (thinned) corpus callosum, and a funnel-shaped cerebral aqueduct ⇨ related to distal obstruction. Note the normal size of the 4th ventricle and herniation of the floor of the 3rd ventricle ⇨ from the hydrocephalus. (**Right**) Sagittal T1WI C+ MR demonstrates aqueductal web ➡ causing dilation of the proximal cerebral aqueduct and lateral/3rd ventriculomegaly. The 4th ventricle is normal.*

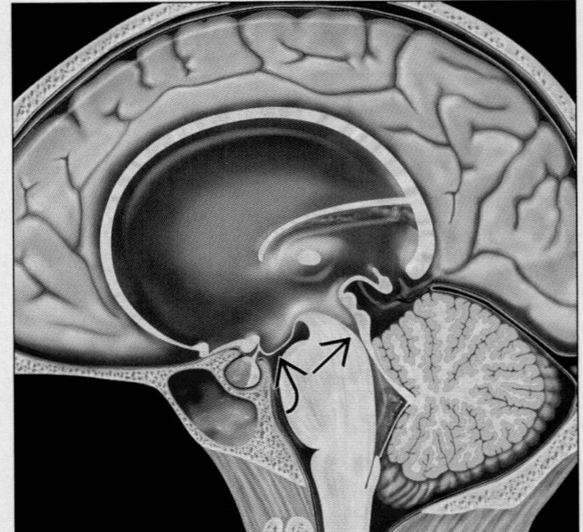

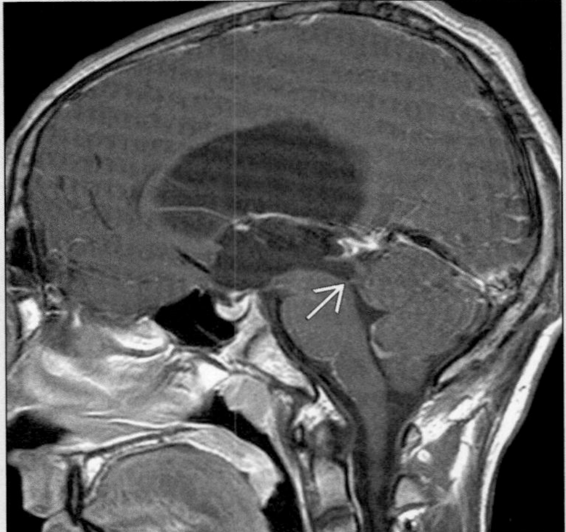

*(**Left**) Sagittal T1WI MR depicts proximal aqueductal stenosis ➡ producing enlargement of the lateral and 3rd ventricles with depression of the fornices ⇨ in conjunction with normal 4th ventricle size. Tectum is dysplastic, thickened with collicular fusion ➡. (**Right**) Sagittal T2WI MR reveals distal aqueductal stenosis with an enlarged, funnel-shaped cerebral aqueduct ➡ and mild abnormal tectal thickening. Note lateral and 3rd ventriculomegaly with normal size of the 4th ventricle.*

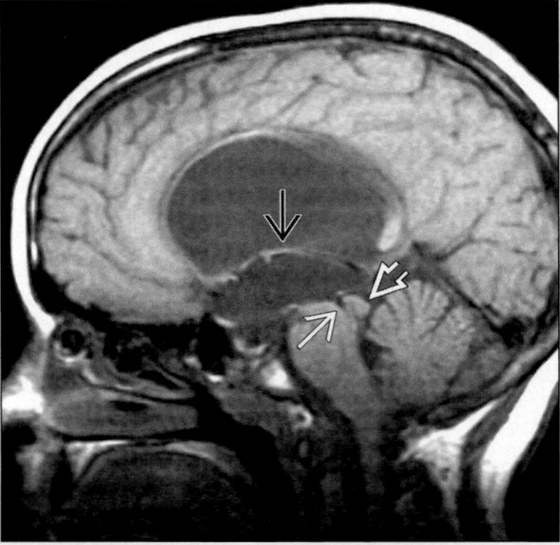

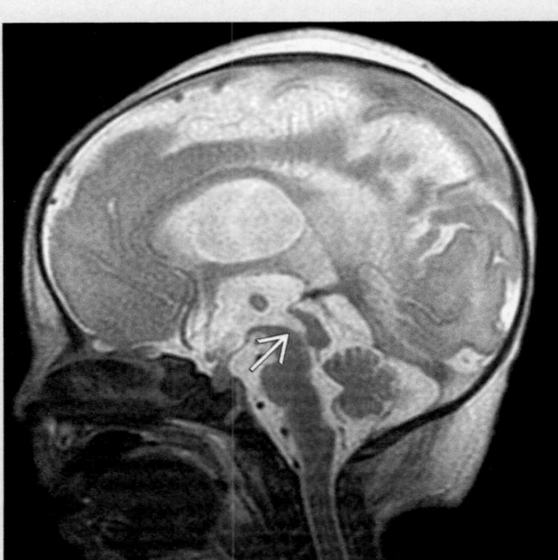

AQUEDUCTAL STENOSIS

TERMINOLOGY

Abbreviations

- Aqueductal stenosis (AS)

Definitions

- Focal reduction of cerebral aqueduct diameter with concomitant lateral and 3rd ventriculomegaly

IMAGING

General Features

- Best diagnostic clue
  - Ventriculomegaly of lateral and 3rd ventricles, foramina of Monro proximal to obstruction
  - Normal size of 4th ventricle, basilar foramina (Luschka, Magendie) distal to obstruction
- Location
  - Cerebral aqueduct; most commonly at superior colliculi or intercollicular sulcus level
- Size
  - Normal mean aqueductal cross-sectional area at birth is 0.2-1.8 mm^2
- Morphology
  - Funnel-shaped enlargement of proximal cerebral aqueduct or diffuse ↓ caliber of entire aqueduct

CT Findings

- NECT
  - Ventriculomegaly of lateral and 3rd ventricles, normal-sized 4th ventricle
    - Caveat: 4th ventricle is (near) normal size in many patients with communicating hydrocephalus
  - ± periventricular interstitial edema (uncompensated hydrocephalus)
  - No obstructing midbrain/thalamic mass
    - Tectal tumors may be occult on CT; asymmetry of posterior 3rd ventricle prompts MR imaging
- CECT
  - No pathologic brain enhancement
  - ± tectal tumor enhancement

MR Findings

- T1WI
  - Ventriculomegaly of lateral and 3rd ventricles, foramina of Monro
    - Corpus callosum (CC) thinned, stretched upward
    - Fornix, internal cerebral veins, 3rd ventricle floor displaced downward
  - Normal size of 4th ventricle, basilar foramina
  - Aqueductal narrowing commonly proximal in more severe hydrocephalus, distal in milder hydrocephalus
  - Aqueductal web: Thin tissue membrane separating dilated aqueduct from normal-sized 4th ventricle
- T2WI
  - Aqueductal "flow void" diminished or absent
  - Disturbed/turbulent CSF flow in lateral and 3rd ventricles
  - ± periventricular interstitial edema
- T1WI C+
  - Tumor enhancement differentiates neoplastic from benign AS
  - Hydrocephalus may induce leptomeningeal venous stasis → mimics meningitis or CSF metastases
- MRA
  - Upward displacement of anterior cerebral artery branches secondary to hydrocephalus
- MRV
  - Downward displacement of internal cerebral veins secondary to hydrocephalus
- MR cine
  - Absent or diminished CSF flow in aqueduct

Ultrasonographic Findings

- Grayscale ultrasound
  - Use mastoid (posterolateral) fontanelle window to supplement standard views in newborn
  - Obstetrical ultrasound may permit prenatal diagnosis

Imaging Recommendations

- Best imaging tool
  - Multiplanar MR with sagittal cardiac gated cine MR

DIFFERENTIAL DIAGNOSIS

Obstructing Extraventricular Pathology

- Neoplasm
  - Tectal astrocytoma
  - Pineal region tumor
  - Thalamic tumor
- Vein of Galen malformation
- Quadrigeminal cistern arachnoid cyst

Obstructing Intraventricular (Aqueductal) Pathology

- Neurocysticercosis with aqueductal cyst

Postinflammatory Gliosis (Aqueductal Gliosis)

- Destruction of aqueductal ependymal lining → fibrillary gliosis of adjacent tissue
- Perinatal infection or hemorrhage (ICH)
  - Increasing prevalence reflects improved neonatal survival following bacterial meningitis or ICH
- Difficult to distinguish congenital AS from aqueductal gliosis on imaging
  - GRE MR can detect hemosiderin deposition from previous interventricular hemorrhage

PATHOLOGY

General Features

- Etiology
  - Aqueductal stenosis
    - Common cause of fetal hydrocephalus
    - May be congenital or acquired, benign or neoplastic
    - AS pathologically obstructs CSF flow into 4th ventricle, basilar foramina

AQUEDUCTAL STENOSIS

- CSF production in choroid plexus continues → lateral/3rd ventricular fluid ↑ pressure, ventriculomegaly
  - Aqueductal web
    - Subset of aqueductal stenosis
    - Thin membrane of brain tissue within distal aqueduct restricts CSF flow into 4th ventricle
  - Aqueductal fork
    - Branching of aqueduct into dorsal and ventral channels
- Genetics
  - Cell adhesion molecule L1 (*L1CAM*) gene recognized cause of human hydrocephalus
    - Codes for neural cell adhesion molecule transmembrane glycoprotein in immunoglobulin superfamily of cell adhesion molecules
    - Gene located on X chromosome (Xq28)
    - *L1CAM* expression is essential during normal embryonic development of nervous system
    - Mutations in *L1CAM* gene responsible for 4 related disorders (X-linked hydrocephalus/HSAS, MASA, X-linked complicated spastic paraplegia type 1, and X-linked agenesis of corpus callosum)
      - Now collectively CRASH syndrome: **C**allosal hypoplasia, mental **r**etardation, **a**dducted thumbs, **s**pastic paraplegia, and X-linked **h**ydrocephalus)
      - Site of mutation within L1 protein correlates with disease severity
- Associated abnormalities
  - CRASH syndrome
    - Absence/diminution of corticospinal tracts, thalamic fusion, collicular fusion, absence of septum pellucidum, corpus callosum dysgenesis
    - Thin cerebral mantle, malformations of cortical development, hypoplastic white matter
  - Aqueductal fork
    - Fusion of quadrigeminal bodies and cranial nerve 3 nuclei, tectal molding (beaking)

Microscopic Features

- Malformations of cortical development with poor differentiation and maturation of cortical neurons on histology
- Aqueductal fork shows branching of aqueduct into dorsal and ventral channels
  - Dorsal channel usually divided into several ductules

CLINICAL ISSUES

Presentation

- Most common signs/symptoms
  - Symptoms depend upon patient age at time of diagnosis
  - Onset often insidious, may occur at any time from birth to adulthood
- Other signs/symptoms
  - Headache, papilledema, 6th nerve palsy, bulging fontanelles
  - Macrocrania, especially if sutures open
  - Parinaud syndrome (sun-setting eyes, lid retraction, and tonic downgaze)
  - Bobble-head doll syndrome (rare)

Demographics

- Age
  - Presentation age depends on severity of stenosis, hydrocephalus
- Gender
  - M:F = 2:1
- Epidemiology
  - 0.5-1 per 1,000 births, recurrence rate in siblings of 1-4.5%
  - AS responsible for approximately 20% of congenital hydrocephalus

Natural History & Prognosis

- Hydrocephalus usually progressive unless treated
  - May stabilize as "arrested" or compensated hydrocephalus
- Neonates with aqueductal stenosis and normal development ~ 24-86%

Treatment

- CSF shunt diversion
- Endoscopic 3rd ventriculostomy
- Cerebral aqueductoplasty for membranous and short-segment aqueductal stenoses (selected cases)

DIAGNOSTIC CHECKLIST

Consider

- Postinflammatory gliosis (aqueductal gliosis), particularly if history of prematurity or meningitis
- Carefully scrutinize posterior 3rd ventricle, tectum, and tegmentum for neoplastic mass

Image Interpretation Pearls

- Tectal astrocytomas large enough to obstruct aqueduct may be missed on routine CT scanning
  - MR more sensitive than CT for detecting obstructing mass lesion
  - Consider neurofibromatosis type 1 when tectal astrocytoma is identified

SELECTED REFERENCES

1. Stoquart-El Sankari S et al: Phase-contrast MR imaging support for the diagnosis of aqueductal stenosis. AJNR Am J Neuroradiol. 30(1):209-14, 2009
2. Bateman GA: Magnetic resonance imaging quantification of compliance and collateral flow in late-onset idiopathic aqueductal stenosis: venous pathophysiology revisited. J Neurosurg. 107(5):951-8, 2007
3. da Silva LR et al: Endoscopic aqueductoplasty in the treatment of aqueductal stenosis. Childs Nerv Syst. 23(11):1263-8, 2007
4. Tisell M et al: Neurological symptoms and signs in adult aqueductal stenosis. Acta Neurol Scand. 107(5):311-7, 2003
5. Castro-Gago M et al: Autosomal recessive hydrocephalus with aqueductal stenosis. Childs Nerv Syst. 12(4):188-91, 1996

AQUEDUCTAL STENOSIS

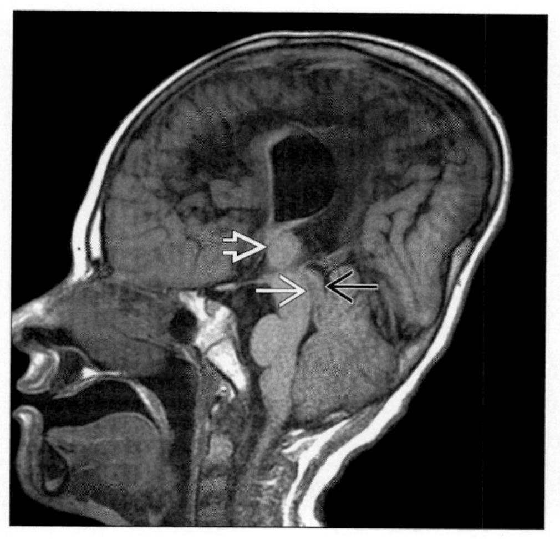

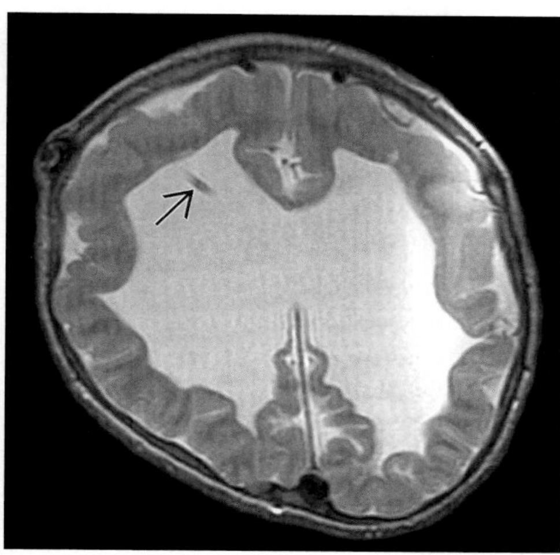

(Left) *Sagittal T1WI MR (CRASH syndrome) shows characteristic marked aqueductal stenosis → with small 4th ventricle size, dysplastic tectal thickening →, callosal dysgenesis, and large massa intermedia from thalamic fusion →.* ***(Right)*** *Axial T2WI MR (CRASH syndrome) confirms marked ventriculomegaly of the lateral ventricles with abnormal cortical sulcation, striking white matter volume loss, and absent septum pellucidum. A VP shunt → was placed for treatment of hydrocephalus.*

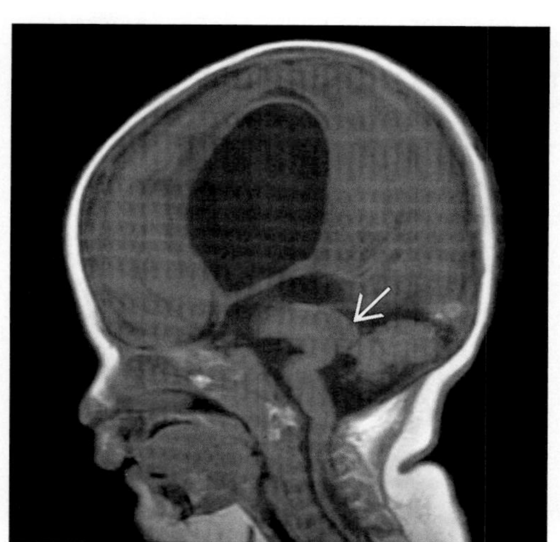

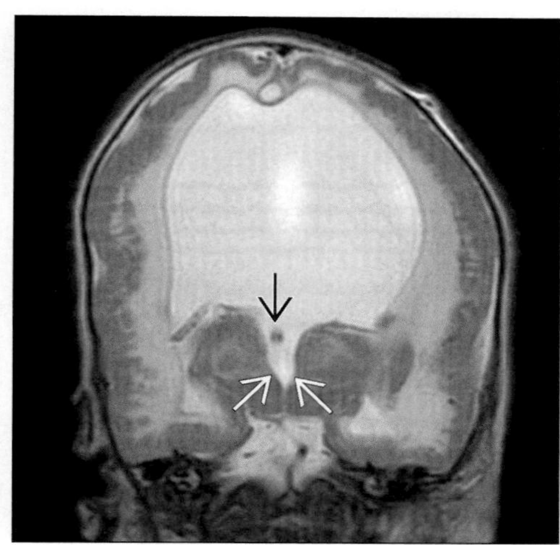

(Left) *Sagittal T1WI MR in a patient with Walker-Warburg syndrome shows severe tectal dysgenesis → with aqueductal occlusion. Marked enlargement of the lateral > 3rd ventricle is present. "Zigzag" brainstem and very small cerebellum are characteristic of this syndrome.* ***(Right)*** *Coronal T2WI MR in the same patient with Walker-Warburg syndrome confirms marked ventriculomegaly, funnel-shaped cerebral aqueductal stenosis →, fused fornices →, and classic cobblestone lissencephaly.*

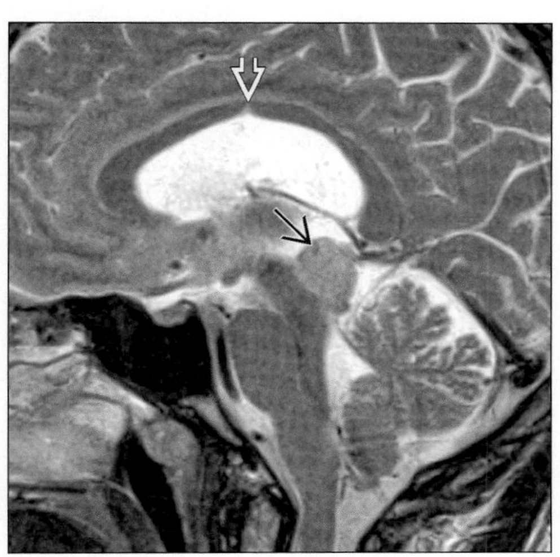

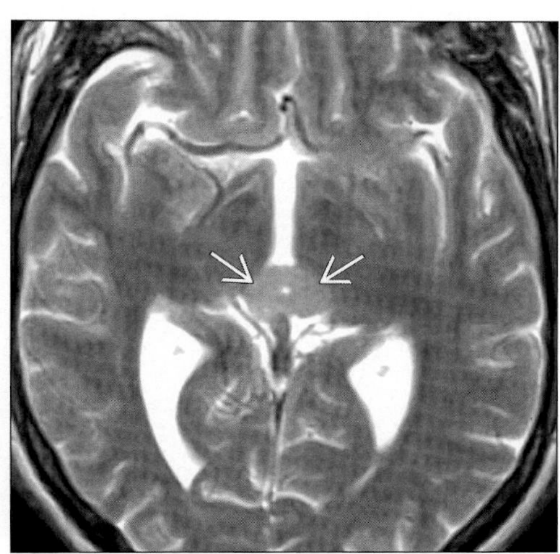

(Left) *Sagittal T2WI MR demonstrates acquired aqueductal stenosis secondary to a low-grade astrocytoma → of the quadrigeminal plate. The callosal defect → is the result of CSF diversion for hydrocephalus.* ***(Right)*** *Axial T2WI MR shows a heterogeneous, gray matter intensity, low-grade tectal astrocytoma → associated with mild lateral and 3rd ventriculomegaly. Ventricular size is only mildly enlarged because the patient has undergone CSF diversion for hydrocephalus.*

NORMAL PRESSURE HYDROCEPHALUS

Key Facts

Terminology
- Ventriculomegaly with normal CSF pressure, altered CSF dynamics

Imaging
- Ventricles/sylvian fissures symmetrically dilated
  - Out of proportion to sulcal enlargement
  - Hippocampus is normal (distinguishes from atrophy)
- ± aqueductal flow void
- Periventricular high signal transependymal CSF flow
- 50-60% periventricular & deep white matter lesions
- MRS: Lactate peaks in lateral ventricles in NPH
- Aqueduct stroke volume > 42 μL reported to correlate with good response to shunt

Top Differential Diagnoses
- Normal aging brain
- Alzheimer disease
- Multi-infarct dementia (MID)
- Subcortical arteriosclerotic encephalopathy

Pathology
- Leading theory: Poor venous compliance in superior sagittal sinus impairs CSF pulsations and CSF absorption through arachnoid granulations
- Pathogenesis of NPH poorly understood

Clinical Issues
- Heterogeneous syndrome (classic clinical triad = dementia, gait apraxia, urinary incontinence)

Diagnostic Checklist
- Is ventricular dilation solely due to atrophy?
- Diagnostic challenge = identify shunt-responsive NPH

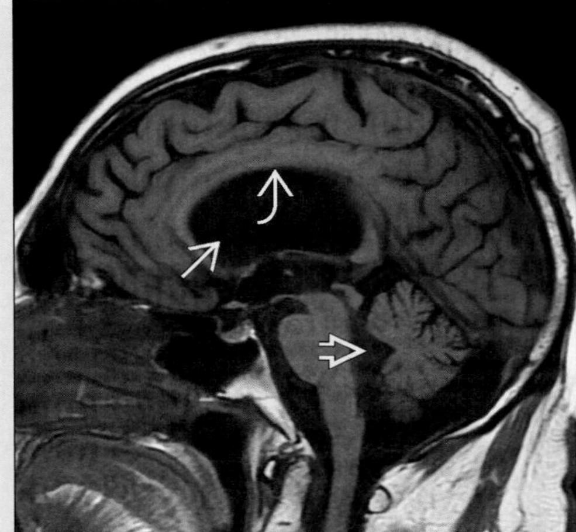
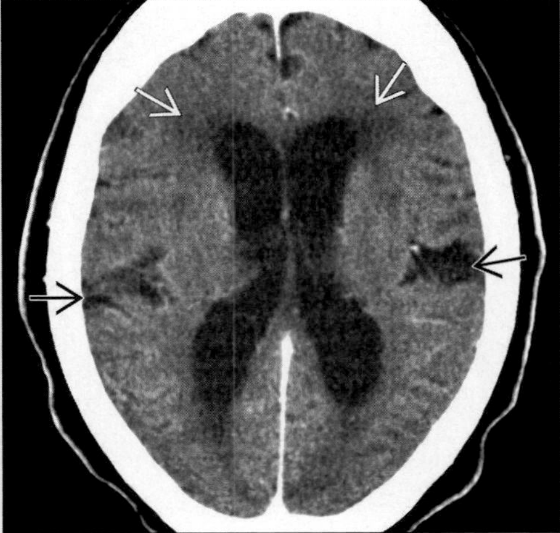

(Left) *Sagittal T1WI MR shows large lateral ventricles ➡, thinning of the corpus callosum ➡, and a relatively normal 4th ventricle ➡ in a patient with NPH.* ***(Right)*** *Axial CECT demonstrates typical findings suggestive of NPH. There is enlargement of the lateral ventricles and sylvian fissures ➡ out of proportion to the amount of general sulcal enlargement. The frontal horns show a characteristic rounded appearance. Periventricular hypodensities ➡ could reflect transependymal migration of CSF.*

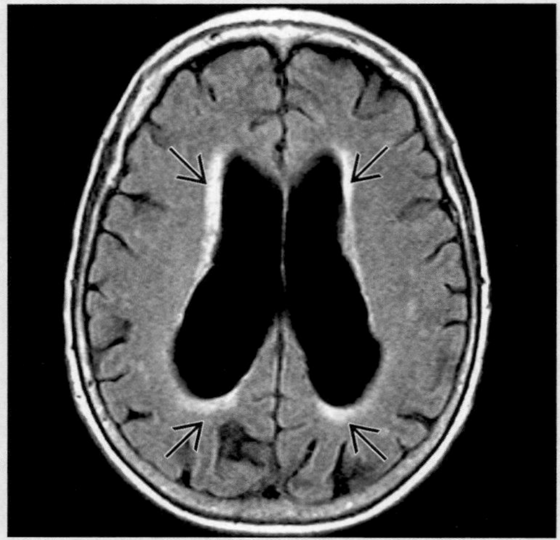
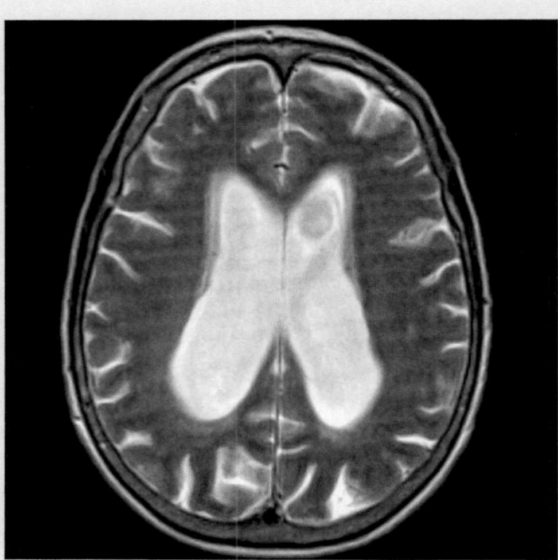

(Left) *Axial FLAIR MR shows enlarged ventricles out of proportion to the sulcal enlargement. Notice that periventricular hyperintensity is also present ➡.* ***(Right)*** *Axial T2WI MR in the same patient shows dilated ventricles.*

NORMAL PRESSURE HYDROCEPHALUS

TERMINOLOGY

Abbreviations

- Normal pressure hydrocephalus (NPH)

Synonyms

- Idiopathic adult hydrocephalus syndrome

Definitions

- Ventriculomegaly with normal CSF pressure, altered CSF dynamics

IMAGING

General Features

- Best diagnostic clue
  - Ventricles/sylvian fissures symmetrically dilated
    - Out of proportion to sulcal enlargement
    - Hippocampus is normal
      - Distinguishes NPH from atrophy
- Location
  - Ventriculomegaly involves all 3 horns of lateral ventricles plus 3rd ventricle
    - 4th ventricle relatively spared
- Size
  - Increased ventricular volume
- Morphology
  - Diffuse expansion of ventricles

CT Findings

- NECT
  - Ventriculomegaly with rounded frontal horns, out of proportion to sulcal atrophy (ventriculosulcal disproportion)
  - Frontal/occipital periventricular hypodensities (representing transependymal CSF flow) may be present
  - Corpus callosal thinning (nonspecific)

MR Findings

- T1WI
  - Lateral ventricles enlarge
  - ± aqueductal flow void
- T2WI
  - Periventricular high signal, primarily anterior to frontal horns or posterior to occipital horns of lateral ventricles (transependymal CSF flow)
  - 50-60% have periventricular and deep white matter (WM) lesions
    - More frequent, severe compared to age-matched controls
    - Correlates with poor outcome after shunting but should not exclude patients from surgery
- MRS
  - Proton chemical shift imaging (^{1}H-CSI): Lactate peaks in lateral ventricles in NPH patients, but not in those with other types of dementia
    - Reflects ischemic changes in periventricular regions despite normal CSF pressure in patients with NPH
    - May be key factor in differentiating NPH from other dementias
- Hypointense or absent signal in proximal 4th ventricle on T2WI, PD, FLAIR, with surrounding CSF appearing hyperintense
- Enlarged basal cisterns, sylvian fissures; normal sulci
- Dilatation of optic and infundibular recesses of anterior 3rd ventricle and downward displacement of hypothalamus
- Corpus callosum bowed upward (may be impinged by falx)
- Aqueductal flow void sign
  - Reflects increased CSF velocity through cerebral aqueduct
    - May be reduced if flow-compensation, FSE techniques used
  - Correlates with favorable outcome after shunt surgery
- Cortical and subcortical lacunar infarctions (basal ganglia, internal capsule)
- Diffusion tensor imaging
  - Abnormal or high diffusion values

Nuclear Medicine Findings

- PET
  - 18F-FDG PET shows decreased regional cerebral metabolism
  - O(15): Water PET shows decreased cerebral blood flow in cerebrum, cerebellum
- SPECT: Cerebral blood flow ↓ in patients with NPH

Other Modality Findings

- Phase-contrast cine MR imaging
  - Cardiac gated CSF flow studies to detect increased velocity ("hyperdynamic" flow)
  - Aqueduct stroke volume > 42 μL reported to correlate with good response to shunt
  - Some patients with normal CSF flow values also improve
- Indium-labeled CSF study with ventricular reflux, with no flow over convexities at 24-48 hours
- ICP monitoring: Wave amplitude > 9 mmHg correlates with post-shunt cognitive improvement

Imaging Recommendations

- Best imaging tool
  - MR with CSF flow studies
  - CT helpful

DIFFERENTIAL DIAGNOSIS

Normal Aging Brain

- Thin periventricular high signal rim is normal
- Few/no white matter hyperintensities ("successfully aging brain")

Alzheimer Disease

- Dementia out of proportion to gait disturbance
- Large parahippocampal fissures, small hippocampi, sulcal enlargement

Multi-Infarct Dementia (MID)

- Multiple infarcts on imaging

NORMAL PRESSURE HYDROCEPHALUS

Subcortical Arteriosclerotic Encephalopathy (Binswanger Disease)

- Continuous, irreversible ischemic degeneration of periventricular and deep white matter
- MR shows extensive periventricular and deep white matter hyperintensities, enlarged ventricles
  - Reflect microinfarctions and demyelination

PATHOLOGY

General Features

- Etiology
  - 50% idiopathic
  - 50% other (e.g., subarachnoid hemorrhage, meningitis, neurosurgery, or head trauma)
  - Age-related changes in CSF formation/absorption
    - Increased resistance to CSF outflow
    - May be exacerbated in NPH
  - Dysfunctional CSF dynamics
    - Reduced absorption through arachnoid villi
    - Compensatory CSF flow into periventricular white matter
    - Transcapillary CSF resorption
  - NPH: Reduced CBF, altered CSF resorption without increased CSF pressure
    - Brain expands in systole, causes CSF displacement
    - Loss of parenchymal compliance, altered viscoelastic properties of ventricular wall
    - Increased interstitial fluid
    - Pulsation pressure directed toward ventricles
    - "Water hammer" effect
    - May be further complicated by microangiopathy (including venous compromise), atrophy
  - Leading theory: Poor venous compliance in superior sagittal sinus impairs CSF pulsations and CSF absorption through arachnoid granulations
- Pathogenesis of NPH poorly understood

Gross Pathologic & Surgical Features

- Enlarged ventricles, normal CSF pressure
- Periventricular white matter stretched, dysfunctional
  - Inadequate perfusion without frank infarction

Microscopic Features

- Arachnoid fibrosis (50%)
- Periventricular tissue
  - Disruption of ependyma
  - Edema, neuronal degeneration, and gliosis
- Cerebral parenchyma
  - Almost 50% show no significant pathology
  - 20% neurofibrillary tangles, other Alzheimer disease changes
  - 10% arteriosclerosis, ischemic encephalomalacia

CLINICAL ISSUES

Presentation

- Most common signs/symptoms
  - Heterogeneous syndrome (classic clinical triad = dementia, gait apraxia, urinary incontinence)
  - Symptom severity related to CSF levels of neurofilament protein, a marker of neuronal degeneration
- Clinical profile
  - Reversible cause of dementia

Demographics

- Age
  - Most common in patients > 60 years
  - Idiopathic form of NPH tends to present in elderly
- Gender
  - M > F
- Ethnicity
  - No racial predilection
- Epidemiology
  - Accounts for approximately 0.5-5% of dementias

Natural History & Prognosis

- Continuing cognitive and motor decline, akinetic mutism, and eventual death
- Potentially reversible cause of dementia when shunted

Treatment

- Predictors of positive response to shunting
  - Absence of central atrophy or ischemia
  - Gait apraxia as dominant clinical symptom
  - Upward bowing of corpus callosum with flattened gyri and ballooned 3rd ventricular recesses
  - Prominent CSF flow void
  - Known history of intracranial infection or bleeding (nonidiopathic NPH)
- After shunt surgery, variable outcome
  - 1/3 of patients improve, 1/3 display arrest of symptom progression, and 1/3 continue to deteriorate
  - Irregular periventricular hyperintensities seem to be key reversible white matter change at MR imaging

DIAGNOSTIC CHECKLIST

Consider

- Whether ventricular dilation is solely due to atrophy
- Diagnostic challenge = identify shunt-responsive NPH

Image Interpretation Pearls

- Intraventricular lactate level may be useful in differentiating NPH from other types of dementia

SELECTED REFERENCES

1. Linninger AA et al: Normal and hydrocephalic brain dynamics: the role of reduced cerebrospinal fluid reabsorption in ventricular enlargement. Ann Biomed Eng. 37(7):1434-47, 2009
2. Scollato A et al: Changes in Aqueductal CSF Stroke Volume in Shunted Patients with Idiopathic Normal-Pressure Hydrocephalus. AJNR Am J Neuroradiol. Epub ahead of print, 2009

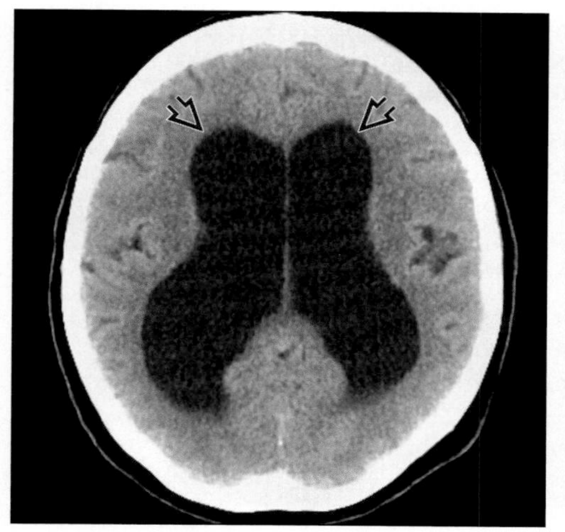

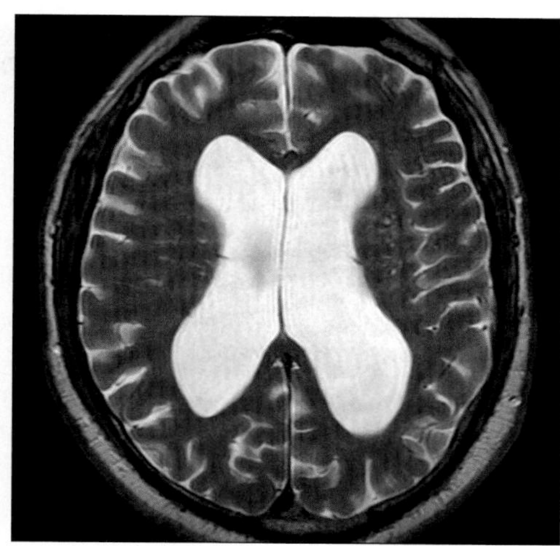

(Left) *Axial NECT shows large ventricles out of proportion to the sulcal prominence with a rounded appearance of the frontal horns ⇨.* ***(Right)*** *Axial T2WI MR in the same patient shows ventriculomegaly. The patient presented with the classic clinical triad of NPH: Dementia, gait apraxia, and urinary incontinence.*

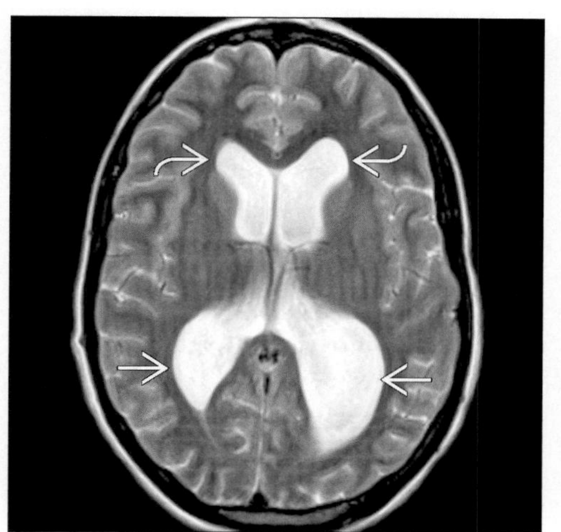

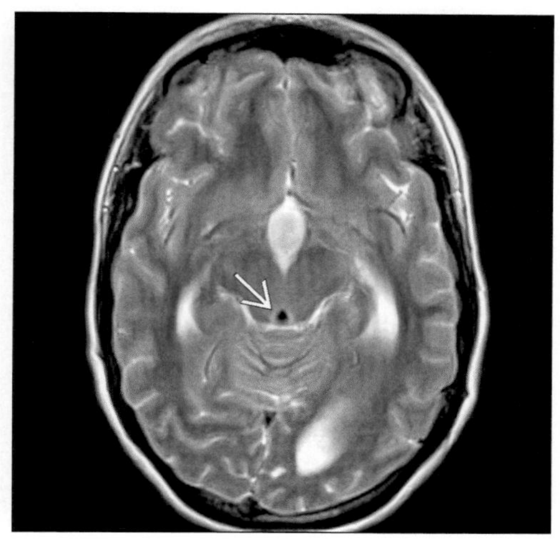

(Left) *Axial T2WI MR shows a typical case of normal pressure hydrocephalus. There is enlargement of the lateral ventricles ➡ with no sulcal enlargement. The frontal horns ➡ show a typical rounded configuration.* ***(Right)*** *Axial T2WI MR shows a hypointense signal flow void in the aqueduct ➡, supporting hyperdynamic flow of CSF in a patient with NPH.*

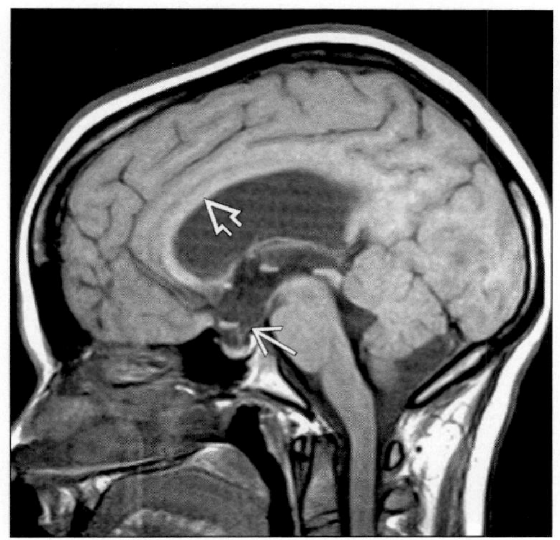

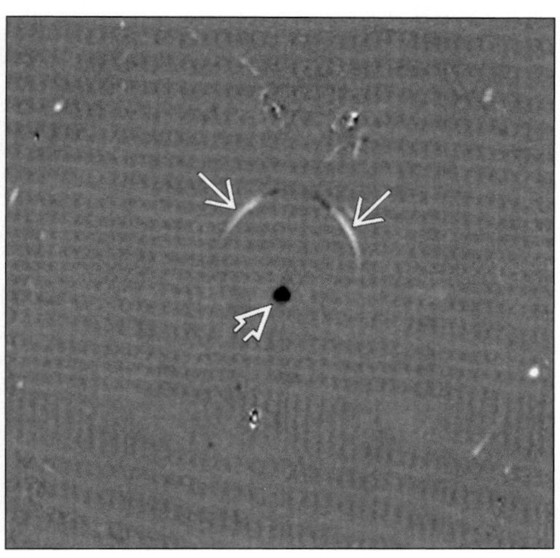

(Left) *Sagittal T1WI MR shows enlargement of the 3rd and lateral ventricles. The infundibular recess ➡ is enlarged and bulges downward. Note mild thinning of the corpus callosum ➡.* ***(Right)*** *Axial MR phase contrast cine CSF flow study shows increased velocity of CSF through the dilated aqueduct ➡. There is more hyperdynamic flow through the aqueduct than the cisterns, where no high velocity signal change is seen. Flow is incidentally noted in the posterior cerebral arteries ➡.*

CSF SHUNTS AND COMPLICATIONS

Key Facts

Terminology

- Hydrocephalus
  - Enlargement of cerebral ventricles secondary to abnormal CSF formation, flow, or absorption resulting in ↑ CSF volume

Imaging

- Shunt failure → dilated ventricles + edema around ventricles, along catheter and reservoir
- Use CT or MR to evaluate ventricle size, plain radiograph shunt series to identify mechanical shunt failure

Top Differential Diagnoses

- Shunt failure with normal ventricle size or lack of interstitial edema
- Noncompliant ("slit") ventricle syndrome
- Acquired Chiari 1 malformation/tonsillar ectopia

Pathology

- Obstructive hydrocephalus: Secondary to physical blockage by tumor, adhesions, cyst
- Communicating hydrocephalus: Secondary to ↓ CSF absorption across arachnoid granulations

Clinical Issues

- Older children/adults: Headache, vomiting, lethargy, seizure, neurocognitive symptoms
- Infants: Bulging fontanelle, ↑ head circumference, irritability, lethargy

Diagnostic Checklist

- Shunt + headache not always shunt failure!
- Confirm programmable shunt valve setting after MR
- Compare current CT with prior studies to detect subtle changes in ventricle size

__(Left)__ Lateral radiograph from a plain film shunt series in an infant with acute shunt failure demonstrates that the ventricular catheter has pulled out of the head and is laying along the distal catheter within the scalp (tip ➔). __(Right)__ Anteroposterior radiograph, in a patient with chest pain after ventriculopleural (VPL) shunt placement, depicts a moderate right pneumothorax (pleural margin, ➔) related to the shunt placement. Note the abandoned catheter fragment ➔ from a prior VP shunt system.

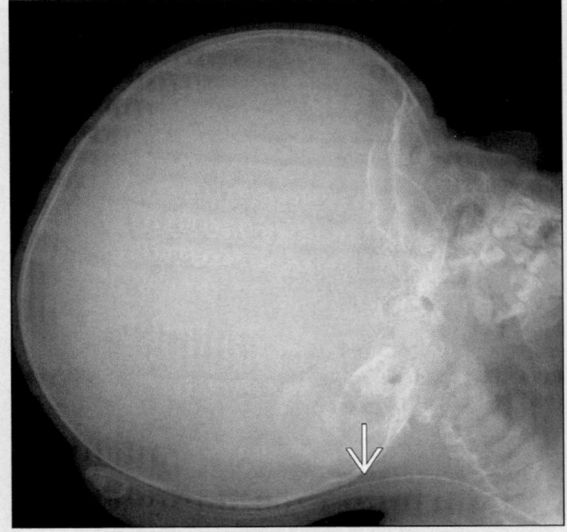

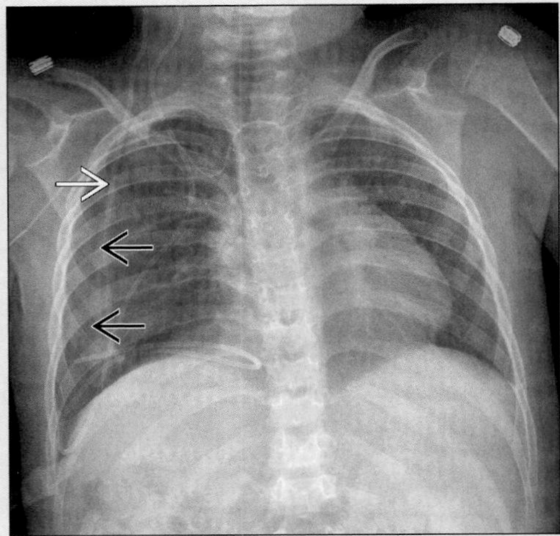

__(Left)__ Lateral skull radiograph of acute VP shunt failure from a plain radiograph shunt series demonstrates a mechanical shunt catheter disconnection ➔ between the programmable valve and the reservoir. __(Right)__ Axial bone CT in the same patient reveals the mechanical catheter disconnection ➔ between the reservoir and the programmable shunt valve. This finding had not appeared on the most recent comparison CT scan (not shown).

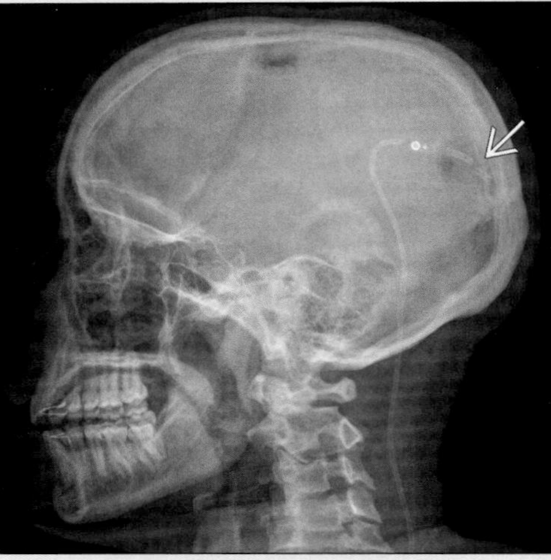

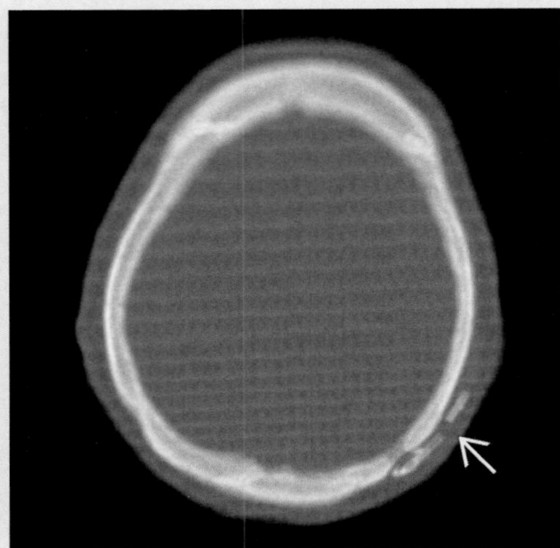

CSF SHUNTS AND COMPLICATIONS

TERMINOLOGY

Abbreviations

- Shunt types: Ventriculoperitoneal (VP), ventriculoatrial (VA), ventriculopleural (VPL), lumboperitoneal (LP)

Definitions

- Ventriculomegaly
  - General term for enlargement of cerebral ventricles
- Hydrocephalus (HCP)
  - Enlargement of cerebral ventricles secondary to abnormal CSF formation, flow, or absorption resulting in ↑ CSF volume
    - Onset over days (acute), weeks (subacute), or months to years (chronic)

IMAGING

General Features

- Best diagnostic clue
  - Shunt failure: Dilated ventricles + edema ("blurring") around ventricles and along catheter, reservoir
- Location
  - VP shunt common; VA and VPL used rarely unless VP contraindicated
- Size
  - Ventricular size is relative → ventriculomegaly may indicate shunt failure in 1 patient and be stable finding in another
    - Change in ventricular size in individual patient probably significant
    - Conversely, some patients manifest shunt failure with minimal to no change in ventricular size
- Morphology
  - Shunt system components
    - Proximal catheter in ventricles, subarachnoid space, syrinx cavity, or thecal sac
    - Unidirectional valve prevents reflux into ventricles
    - Reservoir used to sample CSF, acutely relieve pressure
    - Distal catheter tunneled through subcutaneous tissues → tip in peritoneal cavity, cardiac atrium, or pleural cavity

Radiographic Findings

- Radiography
  - Evaluate shunt catheter system integrity
    - Shunt fracture, separation, migration
    - Distal catheter may retract out of abdomen if significant somatic growth since shunt placement

CT Findings

- NECT
  - Ventricular dilatation (diffuse or loculated)
    - "Isolated" ventricle after infection, hemorrhage → interventricular synechia
    - Transependymal CSF flow ("blurred" ventricle margins) → acute hydrocephalus
  - Small, "slit" ventricles → noncompliant ventricle syndrome, chronic overdrainage
  - ± subdural hematoma (CSF overdrainage)

MR Findings

- T1WI
  - Assess ventricular size, characterize brain anatomy
- T2WI
  - ± transependymal CSF flow → acute shunt failure
- FLAIR
  - Transependymal CSF extension more conspicuous than on T1WI or T2WI
- T1WI C+
  - ± enhancement with ventriculitis, abscess, neoplasm
- MRA
  - Stretched, displaced arteries around dilated ventricles secondary to ventriculomegaly
- MRV
  - Venous thrombosis may precede hydrocephalus or follow shunting
    - → increased intraventricular/intracranial pressure (ICP)
- MR cine
  - Evaluate patency of normal CSF pathways, 3rd ventriculostomy

Ultrasonographic Findings

- Grayscale ultrasound
  - Useful in neonates for serial assessment of ventricular size (requires open fontanelle)

Nonvascular Interventions

- Interventricular contrast injection through shunt plus NECT→ detect ventricular isolation needing additional catheter

Nuclear Medicine Findings

- Shunt radionuclide studies
  - Radiotracer injected into shunt reservoir, serial imaging to document radiotracer egress from distal catheter tip
  - Used to confirm distal obstruction

Imaging Recommendations

- Protocol advice
  - Brain CT or MR to evaluate ventricle size
  - Plain film shunt series to identify mechanical shunt fracture or disconnection

DIFFERENTIAL DIAGNOSIS

Shunt Failure with Normal Ventricle Size or Lack of Interstitial Edema

- Look for fluid along shunt catheter or reservoir as only sign of malfunction
- May require diagnosis on clinical grounds

Noncompliant ("Slit") Ventricle Syndrome

- Usually older child (shunted in infancy)
- Small ventricles plus intermittent signs of shunt obstruction
- Ventricles normal/small even if shunt malfunctioning!

CSF SHUNTS AND COMPLICATIONS

Acquired Chiari 1 Malformation/Tonsillar Ectopia
- Functioning LP shunt produces tonsillar descent through foramen magnum
- More common with valveless systems

PATHOLOGY

General Features
- Etiology
  - Impairment of CSF circulation
    - Obstructive
      - Usually at narrowest points in CSF circulation (aqueduct, foramina of Monro)
      - Tumor, web/synechia, congenital aqueductal stenosis
    - Inadequate reabsorption across arachnoid granulations into venous sinuses
      - Arachnoid granulations "clogged" after hemorrhage, inflammation
      - Diminished gradient from subarachnoid space to venous sinuses secondary to venous hypertension
      - Impaired CSF absorption → CSF accumulation, ↑ ICP
  - CSF shunt establishes accessory drainage pathway to bypass obstructed natural CSF flow pathways
    - Restores or maintains normal intracranial pressure
  - Each shunt, valve, device carries own set of complications
    - All types → material degradation/fatigue, mechanical stress (especially craniocervical junction, inferior ribs)
    - VP → abdominal complications (CSF pseudocyst, ascites, bowel perforation)
    - VPL → symptomatic pleural effusion
    - VA → shunt nephritis, cor pulmonale, pulmonary embolus
    - LP → arachnoiditis, cerebellar tonsillar herniation, high catheter migration rate
    - Programmable shunt → unintentional re-program during MR imaging
- Associated abnormalities
  - Shunts placed with CSF blood/protein > 1 g/dL prone to early blockage, failure
  - Shunt infection rate 5-10%; especially infants < 6 months, failure ≤ 3 months after insertion
  - Ventricular loculation or isolation (6%)
  - Overshunting (3%)

Gross Pathologic & Surgical Features
- Ventricular ependymal adhesions ("scar")
- Extracranial shunt tubing calcification

Microscopic Features
- Gliosis along intracranial shunt tract

CLINICAL ISSUES

Presentation
- Most common signs/symptoms
  - Children, adults
    - Headache, vomiting, lethargy, seizure
    - Neuropsychologic, cognitive, or behavioral
  - Infants
    - Bulging fontanelle, increasing head circumference, irritability, lethargy

Demographics
- Epidemiology
  - 160,000 shunts implanted each year worldwide
  - CSF shunts in USA ≈ 125,000 total
    - 33,000 placed per year (≈ 50% revisions)

Natural History & Prognosis
- Acute shunt obstruction in shunt dependent patients may lead to death
- Majority of shunts eventually fail, complication rate 25-37%
  - ≤ 30% shunts fail in 1st year, 80% fail by 10 years
  - 50% of patients need multiple revisions, progressively shorter time interval to next failure

Treatment
- Shunt revision
  - Replace intraventricular component/valve for proximal obstruction
  - Alter valve pressure setting/type if over- or underdraining
    - Programmable shunt valves permit transcutaneous adjustment of pressure setting
  - Lengthen distal shunt as child grows
- 3rd ventriculostomy to avoid indwelling shunt
- Laparoscopic or open abdominal procedure for distal obstruction related to CSF pseudocyst

DIAGNOSTIC CHECKLIST

Consider
- Shunt + headache does not always mean shunt failure
- Confirm programmable shunt valve setting after MR

Image Interpretation Pearls
- Compare with prior studies to detect subtle ventricular size changes
- Poor ventricular compliance may prevent change in ventricular size despite florid clinical shunt failure

SELECTED REFERENCES

1. Willis B et al: Ventricular reservoirs and ventriculoperitoneal shunts for premature infants with posthemorrhagic hydrocephalus: an institutional experience. J Neurosurg Pediatr. 3(2):94-100, 2009
2. Dusick JR et al: Success and complication rates of endoscopic third ventriculostomy for adult hydrocephalus: a series of 108 patients. Surg Neurol. 69(1):5-15, 2008
3. Martínez-Lage JF et al: Acute cholecystitis complicating ventriculo-peritoneal shunting: report of a case and review of the literature. Childs Nerv Syst. 24(6):777-9, 2008
4. Winston KR et al: CSF shunt failure with stable normal ventricular size. Pediatr Neurosurg. 42(3):151-5, 2006
5. Salomão JF et al: Abdominal pseudocysts complicating CSF shunting in infants and children. Report of 18 cases. Pediatr Neurosurg. 31(5):274-8, 1999

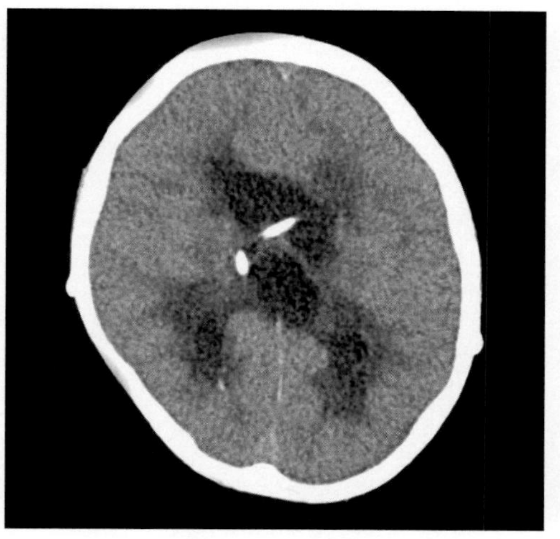

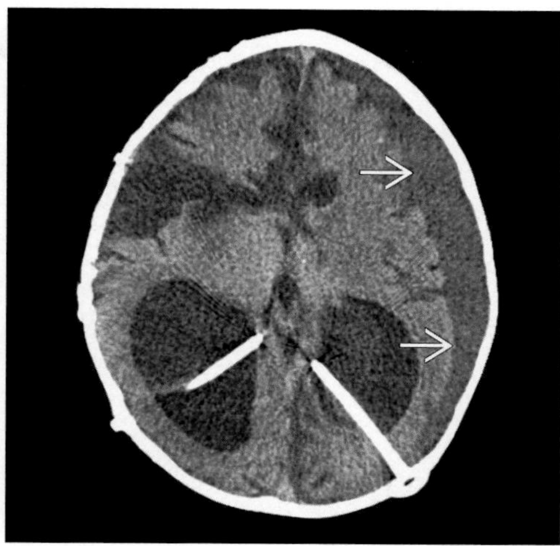

(Left) *Axial NECT in a patient with acute VP shunt failure shows symmetric interstitial edema within the periventricular white matter. Ventricular size is significantly larger than demonstrated on a prior CT (not shown), supporting the diagnosis of acute shunt failure.* ***(Right)*** *Axial NECT following bilateral ventricular catheter placement in a patient with severe hydrocephalus and concurrent brain atrophy shows development of a large left subdural hematoma ➔ following VP shunting.*

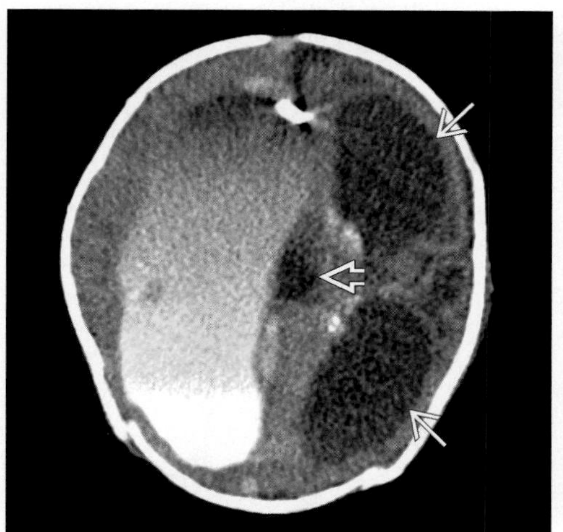

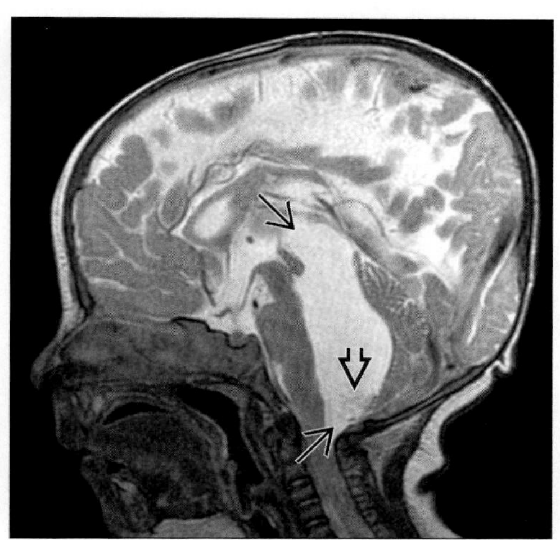

(Left) *Axial NECT in a patient with posthemorrhagic hydrocephalus following contrast injection through the right ventricular catheter shows contrast within the isolated right ventricle, but no contrast transit into either the left lateral ➔ or 3rd ventricle ➔.* ***(Right)*** *Sagittal T2WI MR depicts a dilated, isolated 4th ventricle in a patient with treated hydrocephalus. Septations are identified at the rostral and caudal ventricular margins ➔, with debris near the 4th ventricular outlets ➔.*

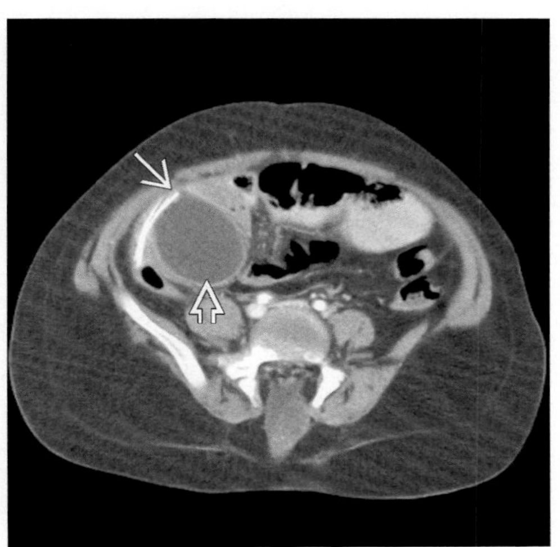

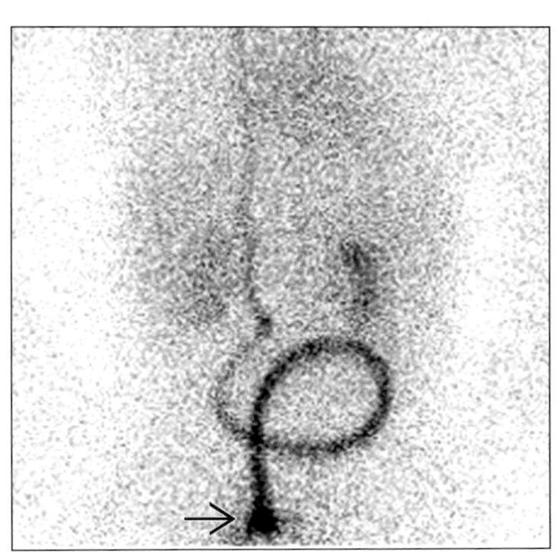

(Left) *Axial NECT in a hydrocephalic patient presenting with distal VP shunt failure shows the peritoneal catheter tip ➔ within a loculated pelvic fluid collection (CSF pseudocyst ➔).* ***(Right)*** *Frontal cisternogram-radionuclide shuntogram examination performed after injecting the shunt valve reservoir reveals no spillage from the distal catheter ➔ after 10 minutes. Further delayed imaging (not shown) confirmed absence of spillage from the catheter, substantiating distal shunt obstruction.*

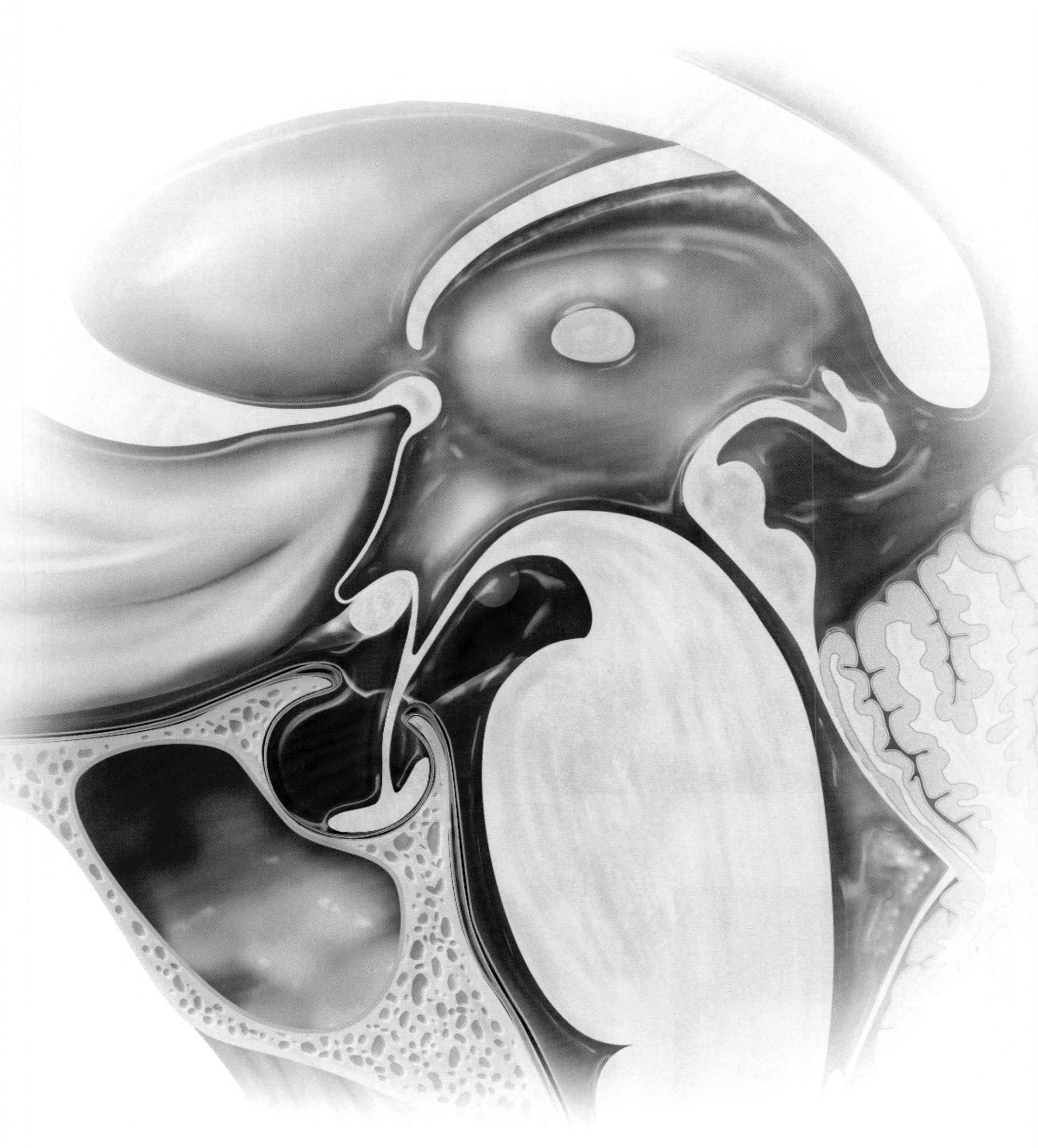

SECTION 2
Sella and Pituitary

Introduction and Overview

Congenital

Neoplasms

Miscellaneous

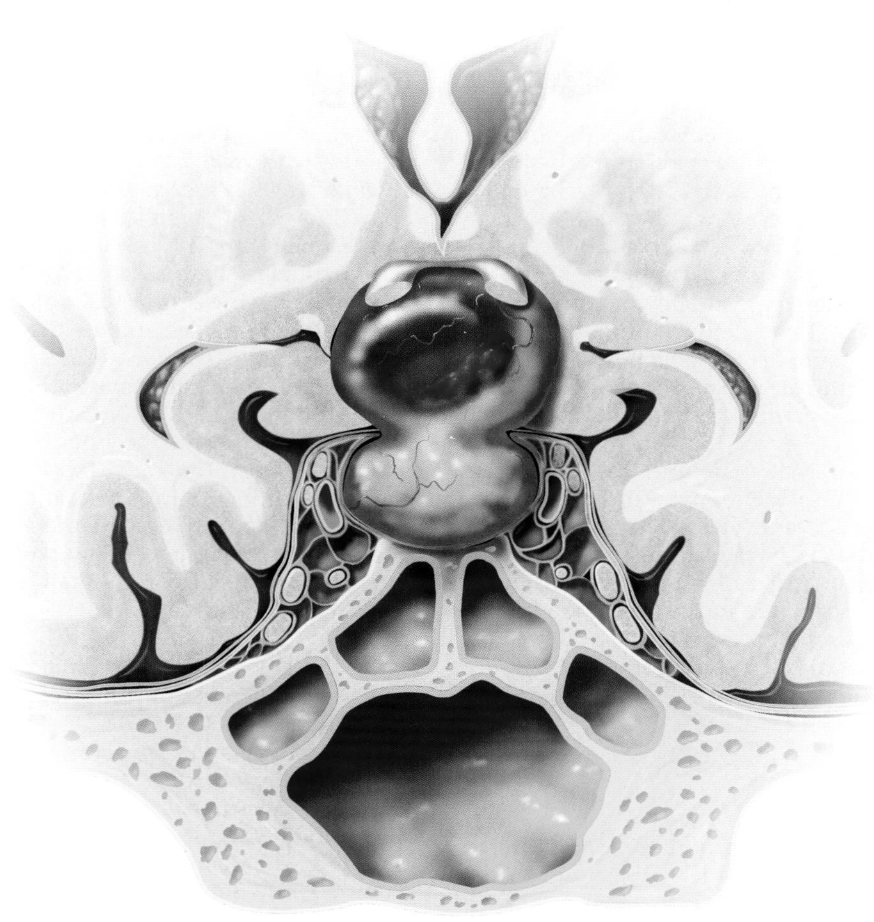

SELLA AND PITUITARY OVERVIEW

Gross Anatomy

Sella

Bony Anatomy. The sella turcica ("Turkish saddle") is a concave, midline depression in the basisphenoid that contains the pituitary gland (also called the hypophysis). The anterior borders of the sella are formed by the anterior clinoid processes of the lesser sphenoid wing while the posterior border is formed by the dorsum sellae. The top of the dorsum sellae expands to form the posterior clinoid processes, which in turn form the upper margin of the clivus. The floor of the sella is part of the sphenoid sinus roof, which is partially or completely aerated. The cavernous segments of the internal carotid artery lie in shallow grooves, called the carotid sulci, which are located inferolateral to the sella.

Meninges. The meninges in and around the sella turcica form important anatomic landmarks. Dura covers the bony floor of the sella itself. A thin dural reflection borders the pituitary fossa laterally and forms the medial cavernous sinus wall. A small circular dural shelf, the diaphragma sellae, forms a roof over the sella turcica that in most cases almost completely covers the pituitary gland. The diaphragma sella has a variably sized central opening that transmits the pituitary stalk. In some cases, this dural opening is large and gapes widely. In such cases, arachnoid with or without accompanying CSF may protrude from the suprasellar cistern inferiorly through the diaphragma sellae opening into the sella and cause the imaging appearance of an "empty sella."

Pituitary Gland

Overview. The pituitary gland, also called the hypophysis cerebri, consists of 3 major parts: The adenohypophysis (AH), the neurohypophysis (NH), and the pars intermedia (PI) plus the infundibulum (I), which are generally considered together as a unit.

Adenohypophysis. The AH, formerly called the anterior lobe, wraps anterolaterally around the NH in a U-shaped configuration. The AH contains acidophil, basophil, and chromophobe cells, as well as other cells, such as tanycytes. Cells of the AH secrete trophic hormones (TSH, ACTH, LH, and FSH) as well as growth hormone (GH). The AH forms 80% of the pituitary gland by volume.

Pars intermedia. The PI is derived from the buccal ectoderm of the embryonic Rathke pouch. It is relatively small (less than 5% of the pituitary volume). Axons from the hypothalamus carry granules of releasing hormones to the AH.

Neurohypophysis. The NH, sometimes called the pars nervosa, consists of the posterior lobe of the pituitary gland, infundibular stem, and median eminence of the hypothalamus. The NH is formed from the embryonic diencephalon (forebrain) as a downward extension of the hypothalamus. Vasopressin and oxytocin are formed within the hypothalamus, pass inferiorly along the hypothalamohypophysial tract, and are stored in the NH. The NH comprises approximately 20% of the pituitary gland.

Imaging Recommendations

MR

MR is generally the procedure of choice. Recommended sequences include precontrast thin-section, small FOV sagittal and coronal T1- and T2WIs followed by post-contrast sagittal and coronal T1WI C+ FS images. Whole-brain FLAIR is a useful sequence to add. T2* scans, especially SWI, may be helpful in detecting pituitary hemorrhage. If microadenoma is suspected, coronal thin-section T1WIs obtained at 10-15 second intervals following rapid bolus injection of contrast are recommended. At least 3 sections (3 mm or less with no interslice gap), sorted by slice, are typically obtained. Some 20-30% of microadenomas are detected only on dynamic contrast-enhanced MR imaging.

CT

Thin-section coronal 64- or 128-slice MDR CT with sagittal/coronal reconstruction is a useful imaging adjunct when lesions affecting the sella &/or cavernous sinus arise in the basisphenoid.

Imaging Anatomy

Size. The overall height of the pituitary gland varies with both gender and age. In prepubescent children, 6 mm or less is considered normal. Physiologic hypertrophy, with a normal height of up to 10 mm, is common in young menstruating females. An upwardly convex gland is common in these patients. Pregnant and lactating females can have an even larger gland with a height of 12 mm. The upward limit of normal in adult males and postmenopausal females is 8 mm.

Signal intensity. Pituitary gland signal varies. With the exception of neonates (in whom the AH can be large and very hyperintense), the AH is typically isointense to gray matter on pre-contrast T1WIs. A dark or "black" pituitary gland seen on T2* is found in iron overload states (thalassemia, hemochromatosis). A uniformly "white" pituitary gland on T1WI is uncommon and can be seen in liver failure.

The NH usually has a short T1 (posterior pituitary "bright spot" or PPBS) caused by vasopressin/oxytocin neurosecretory granules. The "bright spot" does not suppress with FS as it does not contain fat. Although the absence of a PPBS is common in central diabetes insipidus, up to 20% of normal imaged patients lack a PPBS.

Enhancement. The pituitary gland does not have a blood-brain barrier so it enhances rapidly and strongly following contrast administration. Enhancement is typically slightly less intense than that of venous blood in the adjacent cavernous sinuses.

Pituitary "incidentalomas" are common on T1WI C+ scans (found in 15-20% of cases). Seen as focal areas of hypointensity within the intensely enhancing pituitary gland, they can be caused by intrapituitary cysts as well as nonfunctioning microadenomas. Both are very common at autopsy. If a pituitary "incidentaloma" does not enhance at all, then a benign nonneoplastic cyst (such as a pars intermedia or Rathke cleft cyst) is more likely than microadenoma.

Differential Diagnosis Approach

Overview. Because the sellar region is anatomically very complex, at least 30 different lesions occur in and around the pituitary gland. They can arise from the pituitary gland or any adjacent structure (brain, 3rd ventricle, meninges, cavernous sinus, arteries, cranial nerves, etc.). At least 75-80% of all sellar/juxtasellar masses are in the "Big 5": Macroadenoma, meningioma, aneurysm, craniopharyngioma, and astrocytoma. All other lesions (e.g., Rathke cleft and arachnoid cysts, germinoma, lymphoma, metastasis, etc.) are each 1-2% or less.

Keys to diagnosis. Anatomic sublocation is the most important key to establishing an appropriate differential diagnosis. Initially dividing lesions into 3 categories, (1) intrasellar, (2) suprasellar, and (3) infundibular, is the 1st step.

The key to determining anatomic sublocation accurately is asking the question, "Can I find the pituitary gland separate from the mass?" If the gland **is** the mass, it is most likely a macroadenoma. Less likely pathologies that can enlarge the pituitary gland and sometimes appear indistinguishable from macroadenoma include infiltrating lesions, such as sarcoidosis, histiocytosis, hypophysitis, germinoma, and metastasis. If the mass can indeed be identified as separate from the pituitary gland, it is most likely not macroadenoma and arises from structures other than the hypophysis.

Clinical considerations. Patient age is an important consideration in differential diagnosis. Lesions that are common in children (craniopharyngioma and astrocytoma of the optic chiasm/hypothalamus) are less common in adults, in whom the most common masses are macroadenoma, meningioma, and aneurysm. Macroadenomas are very common in adults but, with the exception of adolescent females, are quite rare in children. Beware: A lesion in a prepubescent male that looks like a macroadenoma usually isn't; it is more often nonphysiologic nonneoplastic hyperplasia from end-organ failure.

Imaging appearance. Imaging appearance can be very helpful in evaluating a sellar/juxtasellar lesion. Is the lesion calcified? Does it appear cystic? Does it contain blood products? Is it focal or infiltrating? Does it enhance?

Intrasellar Lesions

Empty sella. "Empty sella" (ES) is seen in 5-10% of patients as an intrasellar CSF collection that flattens the pituitary gland against the sellar floor. Other than ES, most intrasellar masses are lesions of the pituitary gland itself.

Pituitary hyperplasia. Diffuse pituitary enlargement or hyperplasia is common and can be physiologic in young menstruating females and postpartum/lactating women. Less commonly, pituitary hyperplasia occurs as a result of end-organ failure, such as hypothyroidism. Rarely, intracranial hypotension and dAVFs cause pituitary enlargement, probably due to passive venous congestion.

Macro- and microadenomas. The most common "real" intrasellar masses are pituitary microadenomas (defined as < 10 mm) and macroadenomas. Macroadenomas may extend superiorly through the diaphragma sella opening into the suprasellar compartment. Occasionally macroadenomas can appear very aggressive and extremely invasive, extending into the cavernous sinus and eroding the skull base. Pituitary carcinoma is exceptionally rare.

Miscellaneous lesions. A number of neoplastic and nonneoplastic processes can infiltrate the pituitary gland and adjacent structures. Neurosarcoid, lymphoma, and metastases are examples.

Suprasellar Lesions

Children vs. adults. Once a lesion is defined as suprasellar, patient age is key to the differential diagnosis. Pediatric suprasellar masses are most often either pilocytic astrocytomas (hypothalamus, optic chiasm) or craniopharyngiomas. All other lesions, such as germinoma and histiocytosis, are much less common than neoplasm.

At least 1/2 of all suprasellar masses in adults are upward extensions of macroadenomas through the diaphragma sella. Meningioma and aneurysm are common in adults, accounting for approximately 10% each of all adult suprasellar masses. Both are rare in children.

Imaging appearance. Cystic-appearing suprasellar masses are often nonneoplastic (enlarged 3rd ventricle, Rathke cleft cyst, suprasellar arachnoid cyst, inflammatory cysts, such as neurocysticercosis). With the exception of craniopharyngioma, cystic-appearing neoplasms are rare in this location. Pilocytic astrocytoma is the overall most common pediatric neoplasm in this area. Pilocytic astrocytomas of the optic chiasm/hypothalamus are solid, not cystic (as they often are when they occur in the posterior fossa.)

The presence of calcification is helpful. In older patients, atherosclerosis (cavernous and supraclinoid internal carotid arteries), saccular aneurysm, and meningioma are common lesions that calcify. In children, a calcified suprasellar mass is most often a craniopharyngioma. Neurocysticercosis can calcify and may be found in both children and adults, but the suprasellar cistern is a rare location for NCC cysts. Look for lesions elsewhere as they are often multiple.

Hemorrhage into a sellar/suprasellar mass can be detected with T2* imaging. Hemorrhagic macroadenoma, pituitary apoplexy (which can also be nonhemorrhagic), and thrombosed aneurysm can show "blooming" on this sequence. The pilomyxoid variant of pilocytic astrocytoma is a rare but important cause of a hemorrhagic suprasellar mass in a child or young adult.

Infundibular Stalk Lesions

Infundibular stalk lesions are a distinct differential diagnosis. The normal infundibular stalk should be 2 mm or less in transverse diameter and taper gradually from top to bottom.

A "thick stalk" in a child is usually histiocytosis or germinoma. In an adult, neurosarcoid, lymphocytic hypophysis, lymphoma, and metastasis are more common. Enhancement is unhelpful as the normal infundibulum lacks a blood-brain barrier and enhances intensely following contrast administration.

SELLA AND PITUITARY OVERVIEW

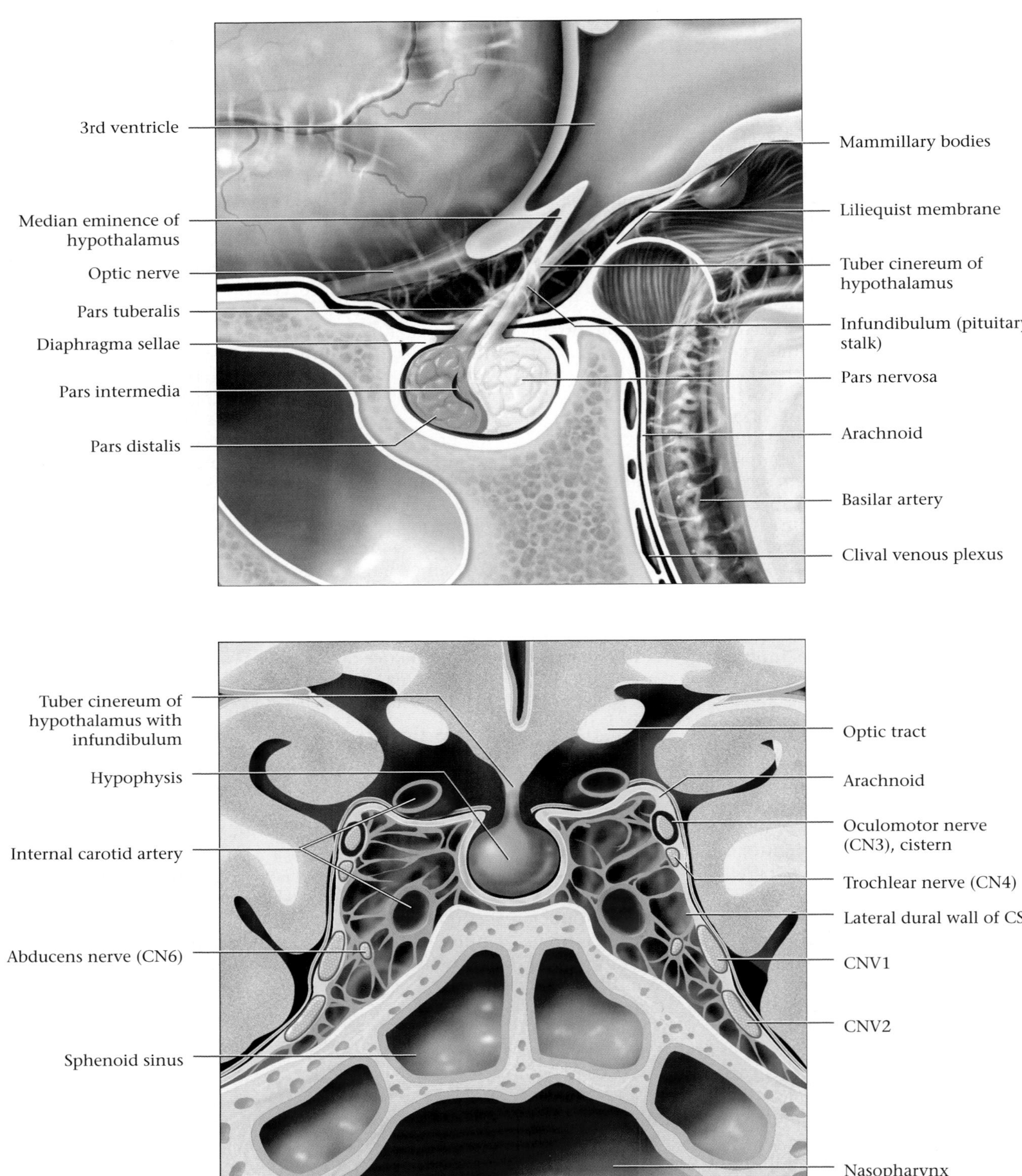

__(Top)__ Lateral graphic of a normal pituitary shows the adenohypophysis composed of the pars tuberalis, pars intermedia, and pars distalis. The neurohypophysis is composed of the median eminence of the hypothalamus, infundibulum, and pars nervosa. Periosteal dural layer covers the sellar floor. __(Bottom)__ Coronal graphic depicts the cavernous sinus contents. The cranial nerves that traverse the cavernous sinus within the lateral wall, from superior to inferior, are oculomotor (CN3), trochlear (CN4), and the 1st (ophthalmic or V1) and 2nd (maxillary or V2) divisions of trigeminal (CN5) nerves. The only cranial nerve actually within the venous sinusoids of the cavernous sinus is the abducens nerve (CN6).

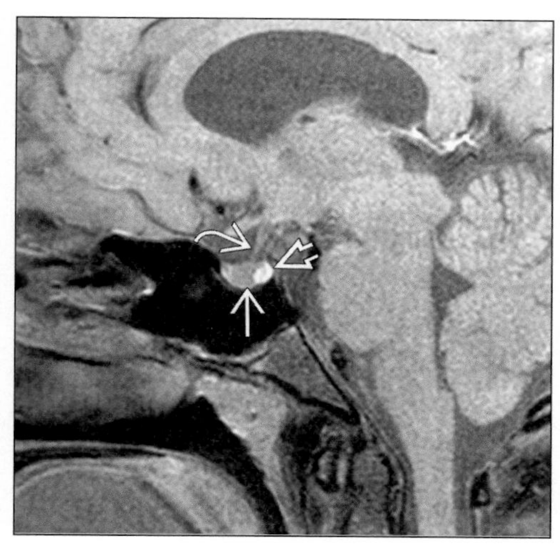

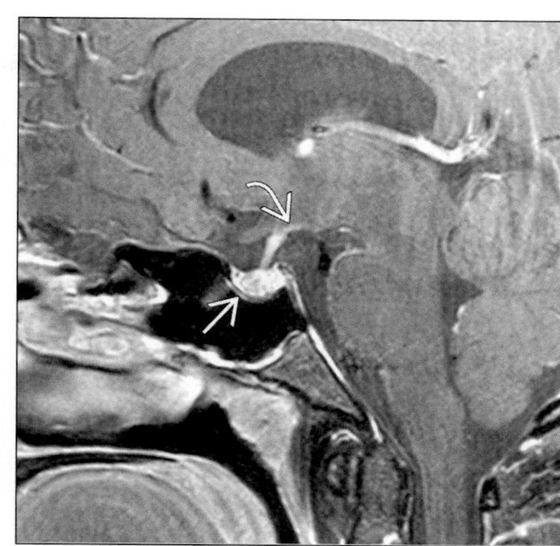

(Left) *Sagittal thin section 3T T1WI MR shows the normal adenohypophysis ➔ is isointense with gray matter; the posterior pituitary ➔ is hyperintense. This posterior pituitary "bright spot" does not suppress on fat-saturated sequences. Note the gradual top-to-bottom tapering of the infundibulum ➔.* ***(Right)*** *Sagittal T1WI C+ FS MR in the same case shows intense but slightly inhomogeneous enhancement of the pituitary gland ➔. The stalk enhances as does the tuber cinereum of the hypothalamus ➔.*

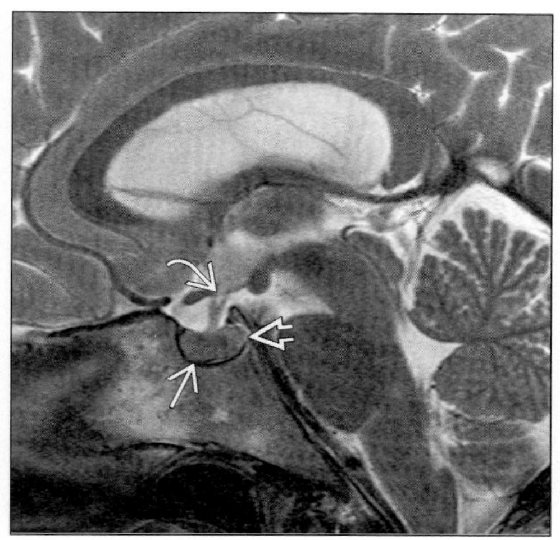

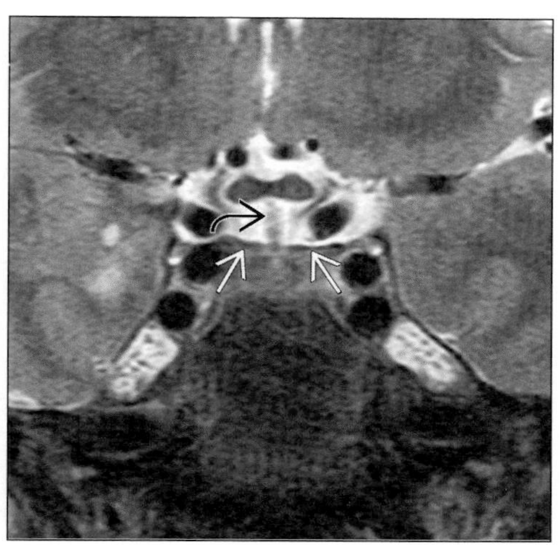

(Left) *Sagittal T2WI MR shows the adenohypophysis ➔ is isointense with brain. The neurohypophysis ➔ is slightly hyperintense compared to the AH. Note the infundibular recess of the 3rd ventricle ➔.* ***(Right)*** *Coronal T2WI MR shows the infundibular stalk ➔ passing inferiorly through a small discontinuity in the thin shelf of dura, the diaphragma sellae, seen here as thin black lines ➔ forming the roof of the pituitary fossa.*

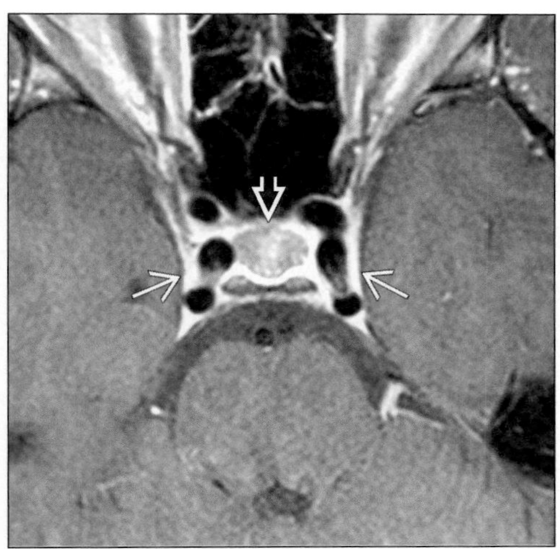

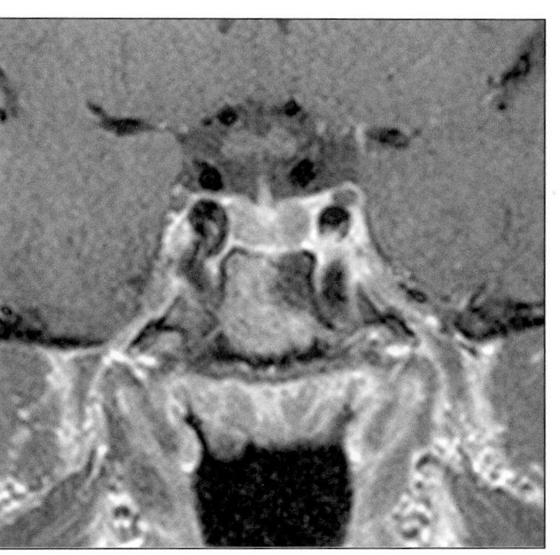

(Left) *Axial T1WI C+ FS MR through the sella shows the pituitary gland ➔ enhancing intensely but not as strongly as venous blood within the cavernous sinuses ➔.* ***(Right)*** *Coronal T1WI C+ FS MR in the same case shows the gland and infundibular stalk enhancement. The gland is bordered laterally by the intensely enhancing venous blood of the cavernous sinus. The medial dural wall is inapparent. Note that the right internal carotid artery appears to abut and slightly indent the pituitary gland.*

*(**Left**) Gross pathology of pituitary macroadenoma ⇒ shows a suprasellar mass arising from an enlarged pituitary gland ⇒. (Courtesy E.T. Hedley-Whyte, MD.) (**Right**) Coronal T1WI MR in a 46-year-old man with visual changes shows a large "snowman" suprasellar mass ⇒ with an enlarged pituitary gland ⇒ expanding the sella turcica and displacing the internal carotid arteries laterally. The mass and gland are indistinguishable from each other; the gland is the mass. Classic pituitary macroadenoma.*

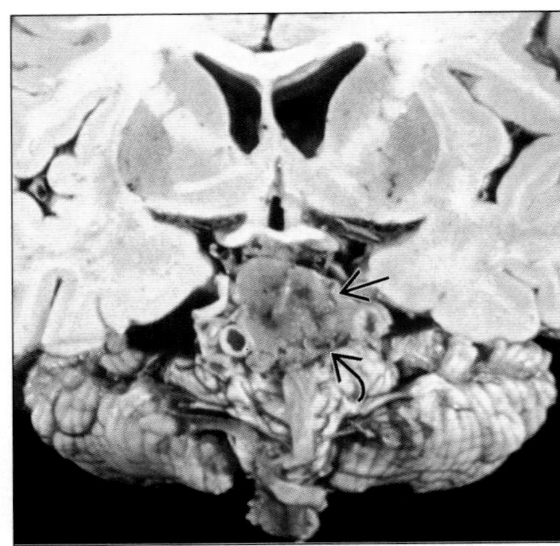

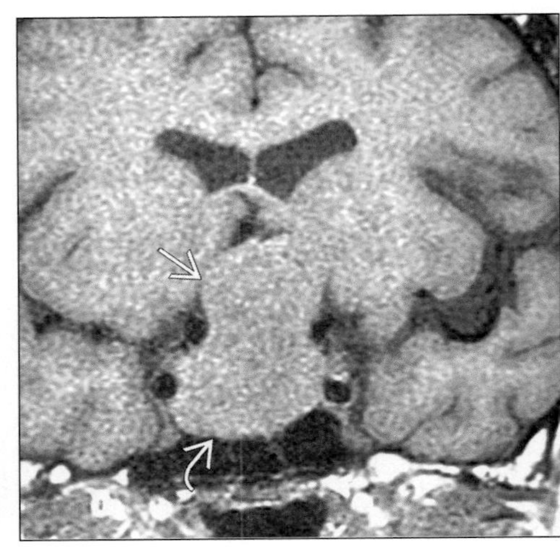

*(**Left**) Gross pathology from an autopsied case of meningioma illustrates typical findings of suprasellar mass. Note that the meningioma ⇒ is clearly separated from the pituitary gland ⇒ by the diaphragma sellae ⇒. (Courtesy J. Paltan, MD.) (**Right**) Coronal T1WI MR in a patient with "vision problems" illustrates the importance of identifying a suprasellar mass ⇒ that arises separately from the pituitary gland ⇒. Here the mass is separated from the gland by the diaphragma sellae ⇒.*

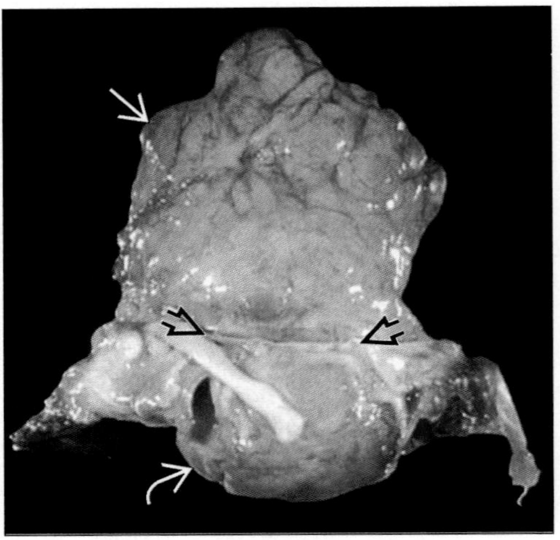

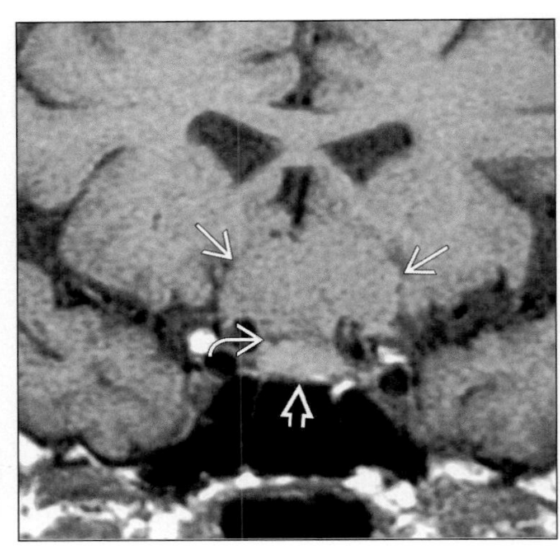

*(**Left**) Sagittal T1WI MR in the same patient shows the mass ⇒ and pituitary gland ⇒ are almost identical in signal intensity. (**Right**) Sagittal T1WI C+ MR in the same case shows the mass ⇒ and pituitary gland ⇒ both enhance strongly and quite uniformly. The diaphragma sellae is seen as a thin hypointense line ⇒ that clearly separates the mass, a meningioma, from the pituitary gland. Note the presence of dural "tails" along the planum sphenoidale and clivus ⇒ that enhance more strongly.*

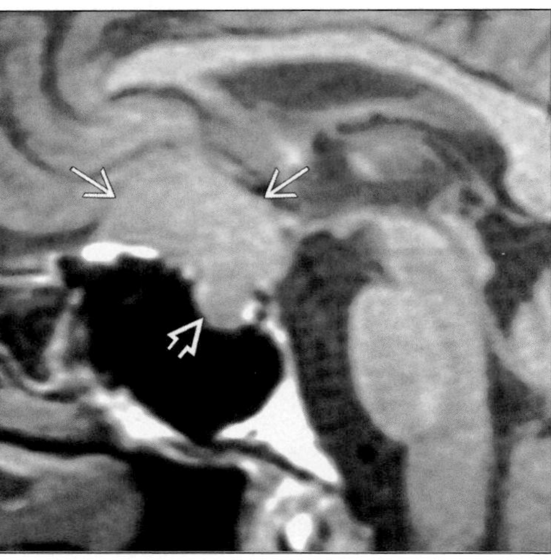

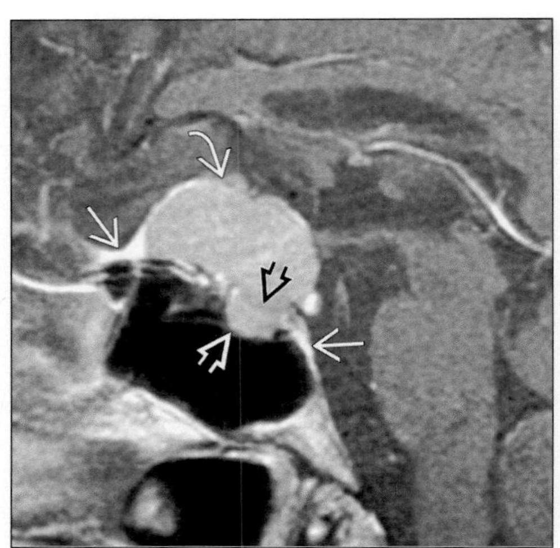

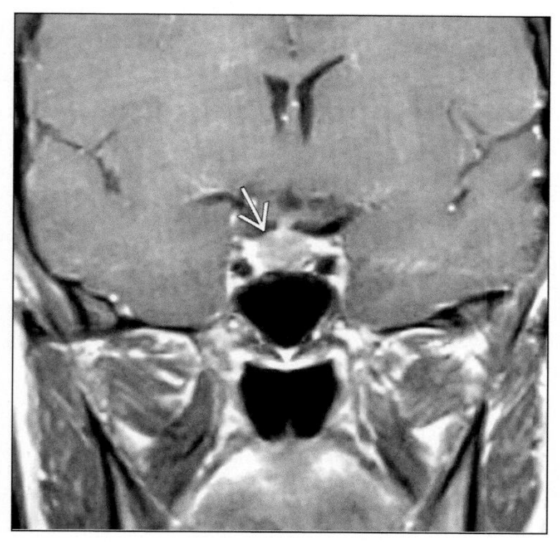

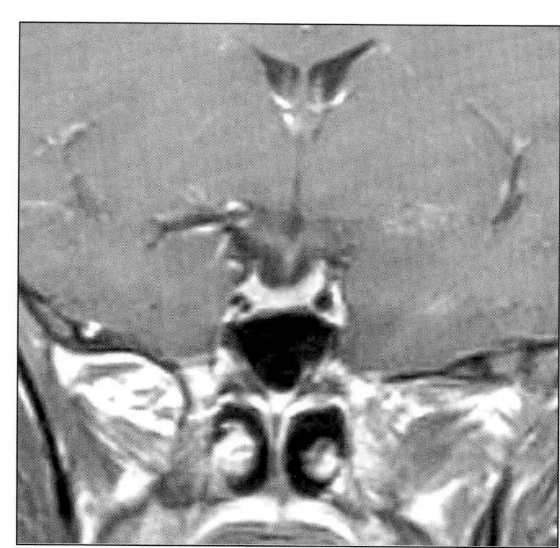

(Left) *Coronal T1WI C+ MR in a 28-year-old lactating, postpartum woman shows diffuse enlargement of the pituitary gland ➡. The gland measured 12 mm in height.* ***(Right)*** *Coronal T1WI C+ MR in the same patient 1 year later shows resolution of the physiologic enlargement. This case illustrates the importance of knowing gender, age, and clinical status in a patient with an intra- or suprasellar lesion. The enlarged gland seen on the left would be abnormal in a man or older woman, but was normal in this case.*

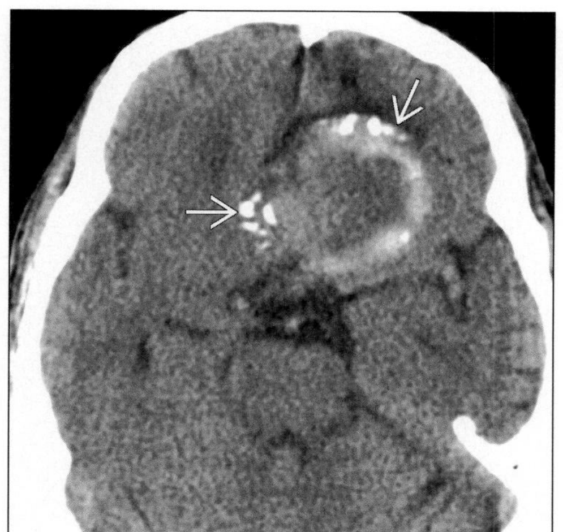

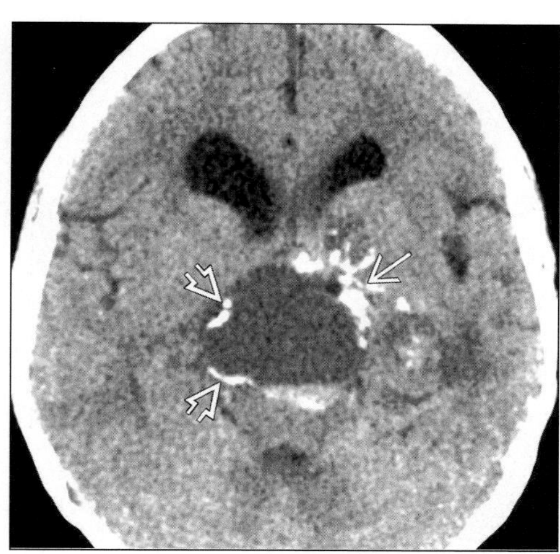

(Left) *Axial NECT in an older adult shows a hypodense suprasellar mass with globular and rim calcifications ➡. As calcified macroadenomas are uncommon, a calcified suprasellar mass in an adult is most often meningioma or, as in this case, saccular aneurysm.* ***(Right)*** *Axial NECT in a child shows a hypodense suprasellar mass with globular ➡ and rim ➡ calcifications. A calcified, cystic suprasellar mass in a child is typically a craniopharyngioma, less often an infectious cyst (neurocysticercosis).*

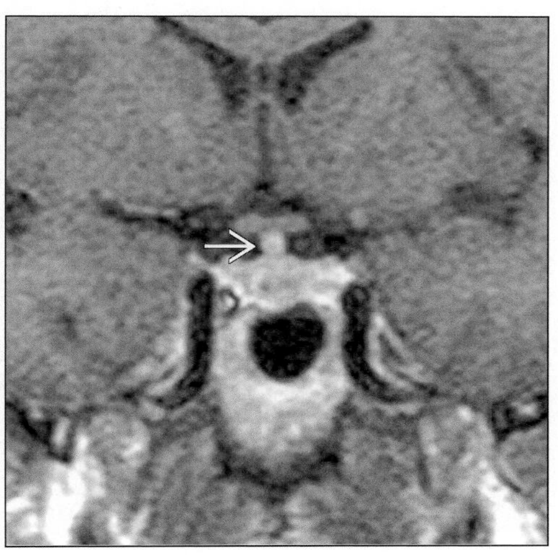

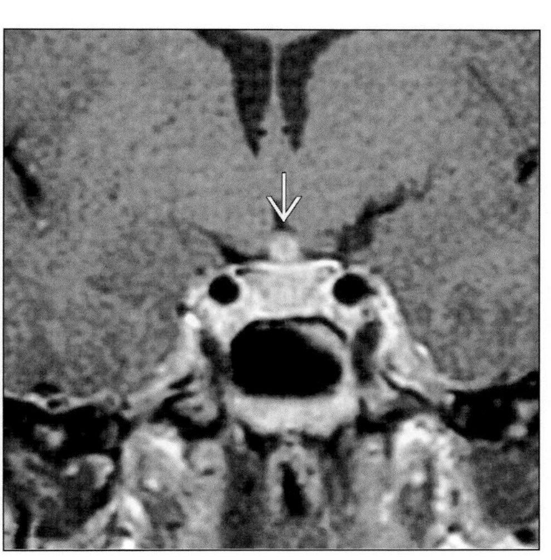

(Left) *Coronal T1WI C+ MR in a child with diabetes insipidus shows a thickened infundibular stalk ➡. Langerhans cell histiocytosis was subsequently diagnosed.* ***(Right)*** *Coronal T1WI C+ MR in an adult with diabetes insipidus shows a thickened, somewhat rounded infundibular stalk ➡. Proven neurosarcoidosis. Findings are basically identical with the imaging findings of histiocytosis on the previous image. As symptoms were identical, the only feature that distinguishes these 2 cases is patient age.*

PITUITARY ANOMALIES

Key Facts

Terminology
- Posterior pituitary ectopia (PPE)
- Duplicated pituitary gland/stalk (DP)
- Congenital anomalies of pituitary stalk → potential hypothalamic/pituitary axis malfunction

Imaging
- PPE: No (or tiny) pituitary stalk, ectopic posterior pituitary (EPP) on midline sagittal T1WI MR
- DP: 2 pituitary stalks on coronal view, thick tuber cinereum on midline sagittal view

Top Differential Diagnoses
- Surgical or traumatic stalk transection
- Central diabetes insipidus
- Lipoma
- Dilated infundibular recess of 3rd ventricle ("pseudoduplication")
- Tuber cinereum hamartoma

Pathology
- PPE: Genetic mutation → defective neuronal migration during embryogenesis
- DP: Gene mutation unknown; may constitute polytopic field defect due to splitting of notochord

Clinical Issues
- PPE: Short stature
- DP: Unsuspected finding on craniofacial imaging for other indications

Diagnostic Checklist
- PPE: Assess optic and olfactory nerves, frontal cortex
- DP: Oral tumors compromise airway patency

__(Left)__ Sagittal graphic demonstrates ectopia of the posterior pituitary gland ➡, located at the distal end of a truncated pituitary stalk. The sella turcica and adenohypophysis ↪ are both small. __(Right)__ Sagittal T1WI MR shows an ectopic posterior pituitary gland located at the median eminence ➡. The pituitary infundibulum is absent, the anterior pituitary gland ↪ is small, and the normal bright posterior pituitary gland is not identified.

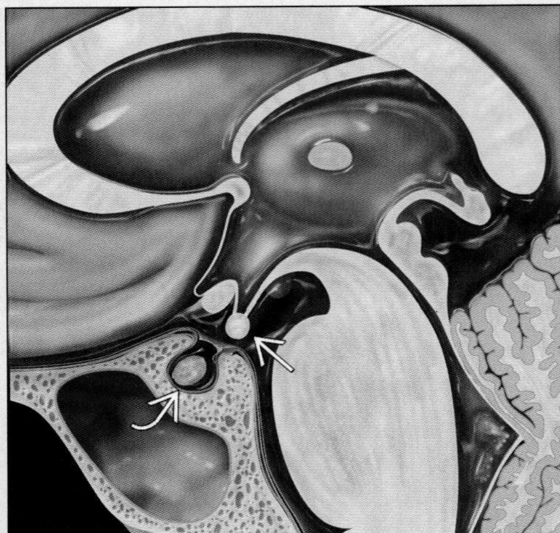

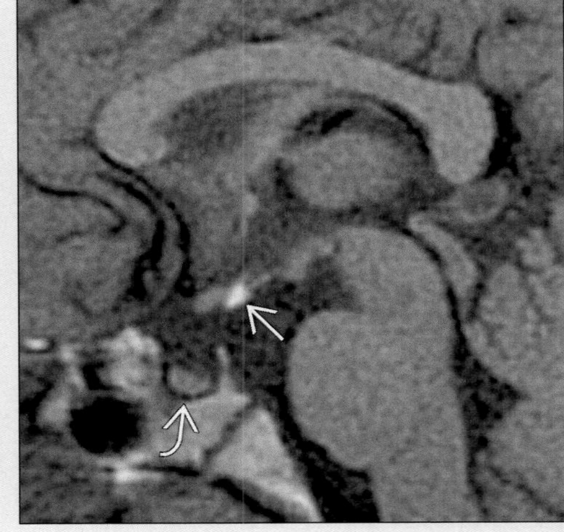

__(Left)__ Coronal T1WI MR depicts the ectopic posterior pituitary gland location at the median eminence ➡. A pituitary stalk is not visualized below the ectopic posterior pituitary. The septum pellucidum is present, and the optic tracts ↪ are of normal size. __(Right)__ Axial T1WI C+ MR confirms the ectopic position of the bright posterior pituitary gland ➡ at the median eminence in the expected location of the infundibular stalk base.

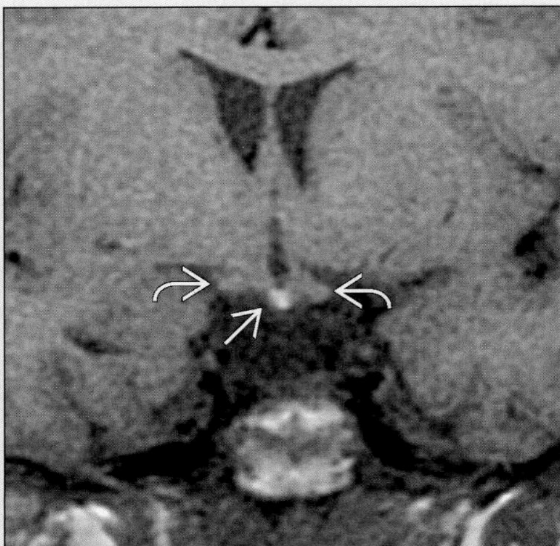

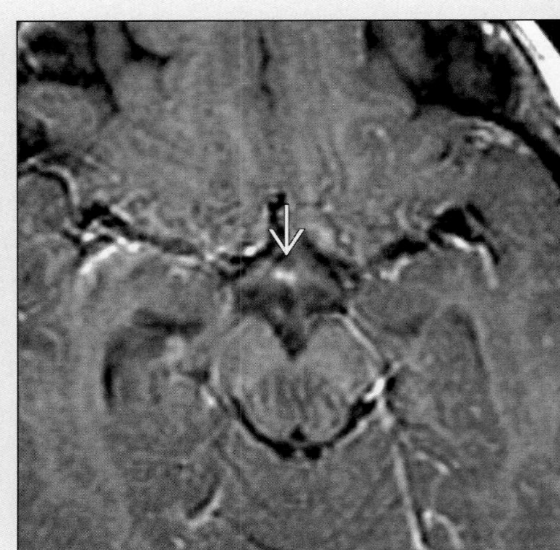

TERMINOLOGY

Abbreviations
- Posterior pituitary ectopia (PPE)
- Duplicated pituitary gland/stalk (DP)

Synonyms
- Ectopic pituitary bright spot

Definitions
- Congenital anomalies of pituitary stalk → potential hypothalamic/pituitary axis malfunction

IMAGING

General Features
- Best diagnostic clue
  - PPE: No (or tiny) pituitary stalk, ectopic posterior pituitary (EPP) on midline sagittal T1WI MR
  - DP: 2 pituitary stalks on coronal view, thick tuber cinereum on midline sagittal view
    - Tubo-mamillary fusion: Tuber cinereum/ mamillary bodies fused into single mass
- Location
  - PPE: EPP located along median eminence of tuber cinereum or truncated pituitary stalk
  - DP: Paired lateral stalks, pituitary glands, bony fossae
- Size
  - PPE: Anterior pituitary (adenohypophysis) small
  - DP: Each pituitary gland normal in size
- Morphology
  - PPE: Small adenohypophysis and osseous sella
  - DP: Each pituitary gland and osseous sella normal in morphology but laterally located

Radiographic Findings
- Radiography
  - PPE: Small sella turcica on lateral radiography
  - DP: Craniofacial/craniocervical anomalies common; may observe 2 fossae on AP view

CT Findings
- NECT
  - PPE: Narrow pituitary fossa & skull base structures and clivus, ± persistent sphenopharyngeal foramen
  - DP: 2 widely separated pituitary fossae, ± midline basisphenoid cleft or frontonasal dysplasia
- CTA
  - PPE: Medial deviation of juxtasellar/supraclinoid carotid arteries ("kissing" carotids)
  - DP: Duplicated basilar artery, ± widely separated juxtasellar/supraclinoid carotid arteries

MR Findings
- T1WI
  - PPE: Absent, truncated, or thread-like pituitary stalk; small adenohypophysis
    - EPP located along truncated stalk or median eminence of tuber cinereum
      - Usually ↑ signal on T1WI (phospholipids/ secretory granules)
      - Posterior pituitary may "dim" as patient outgrows available hormone levels
  - DP: Mass-like thickening of tuber cinereum on sagittal view portends duplicated pituitary axis
    - Mamillary bodies fused with tuber cinereum into thickened 3rd ventricle floor
    - 2 lateralized but otherwise normal pituitary glands/stalks
- T2WI
  - PPE: Variable signal of posterior pituitary
  - DP: Normal signal of glands, stalk, tubo-mamillary fusion mass
- T1WI C+
  - Both: Stalks and remnants enhance (absent blood-brain barrier)
  - PPE: Hyperintensity absent if multiple endocrine anomalies/diabetes insipidus; contrast enhancement helps find neurohypophysis
- MRA
  - PPE: Supraclinoid carotid arteries medially deviated, "kiss" in midline; rare absent carotid artery/canal
  - DP: Fenestration (common) or total duplication (rare) of basilar artery (BA); widely separated juxtasellar carotid arteries

Imaging Recommendations
- Best imaging tool
  - Multiplanar T1WI MR imaging
- Protocol advice
  - Both: Sagittal and coronal T1WI of hypothalamic/ pituitary axis
  - PPE: Assess olfactory nerves, anterior frontal lobes with coronal FSE T2WI
    - 3D T1WI SPGR can identify small posterior pituitaries, occult on conventional 2D sagittal T1WI
  - DP: 3D CT of skull base & face in selected patients

DIFFERENTIAL DIAGNOSIS

Posterior Pituitary Ectopia
- Central diabetes insipidus
  - Absent posterior pituitary bright spot, but normal location of stalk and gland
- Surgical or traumatic stalk transection
  - Permits build-up of neurosecretory granules along stump
- Lipoma
  - Posterior pituitary is not suppressed by fat saturation; lipoma is suppressed

Duplicated Pituitary Gland/Stalk
- Dilated infundibular recess of 3rd ventricle ("pseudoduplication")
  - Simulates duplicated stalk but only 1 gland and 1 pituitary fossa
- Tuber cinereum hamartoma
  - Round mass of 3rd ventricle floor but 1 midline pituitary stalk/gland

PATHOLOGY

General Features
- Etiology

PITUITARY ANOMALIES

- PPE: Genetic mutation → defective neuronal migration during embryogenesis
- DP: Congenital anomaly, presumed genetic duplication of stomodeal origin structures 2° to aberrant ventral induction

- Genetics
  - PPE: Mutations in genes encoding developmental transcription factors allow maldevelopment
    - *HESX1* (homeobox gene), *PIT1*, *PITX2*, *LHX3*, *LHX4*, *PROP1*, *SF1*, and *TPIT*
  - DP: Gene mutation unknown; may constitute polytopic field defect due to splitting of notochord
- Associated abnormalities
  - Duplicated pituitary gland/stalk
    - Midline tumors in oral, nasopharyngeal, palate
      - Epignathus, teratomas, dermoids, lipomas
    - Spinal anomalies include segmentation/fusion anomalies, schisms, hydromyelia, enteric cysts
    - Rib & cardiac anomalies, Pierre-Robin anomaly
  - **Both**: Common midline CNS anomalies
    - Posterior pituitary ectopia
      - ± anomalies of structures formed at same time (pituitary, forebrain, eyes, olfactory bulbs)
      - ± lobar holoprosencephaly, septooptic dysplasia, Joubert syndrome
    - Duplicated pituitary gland/stalk
      - Callosal dysgenesis, Dandy-Walker spectrum, frontonasal dysplasia
      - Craniofacial clefting and duplication anomalies: Frontonasal dysplasia; clefts/duplication of skull base, face, mandible, nose, palate

Gross Pathologic & Surgical Features

- PPE: Hypoplastic anterior lobe, stalk truncation or aplasia; sella may be covered over with dura
- DP: Tubo-mamillary fusion, 2 normal glands/stalks

Microscopic Features

- PPE: Ectopic pituitary cells in stalk or sphenoid bone
- DP: Normal (but duplicated) pituitary glands, tubo-mamillary fusion, incompletely migrated hypothalamic nuclear cells

CLINICAL ISSUES

Presentation

- Most common signs/symptoms
  - PPE: Short stature
  - DP: Unsuspected finding on craniofacial imaging for other indications
- Other signs/symptoms
  - PPE: Multiple pituitary hormone deficiencies common
  - DP: Rarely symptomatic from pituitary causes
- Clinical profile
  - PPE: Short stature (growth hormone deficiency), ± multiple endocrine deficiencies
    - Peak growth hormone levels < 3 g/L more likely to have abnormal MR
    - ± anosmia, poor vision, seizures (cortical malformations)
    - Neonatal hypoglycemia or jaundice, micropenis, single central incisor
  - DP: ± facial midline anomalies, oral mass
    - Face: ± hypertelorism or frontonasal dysplasia
    - Craniocervical segmentation & fusion anomalies
    - Airway or oral obstruction from pharyngeal tumor

Demographics

- Age
  - PPE: Early growth failure apparent in childhood
  - DP: Usually discovered in early infancy during imaging for complicated facial anomalies
- Gender
  - PPE: M > F
  - DP: M < F
- Epidemiology
  - PPE: Prevalence 1:4,000 to 1:20,000 births
  - DP: Extremely rare (reported in 20+ patients)

Natural History & Prognosis

- PPE: Stable if no pituitary/hypothalamic crises; growth may be normal for a while
  - Severity and number of hormone deficiencies predicted by degree of stalk and gland hypoplasia
- DP: Usually significant intracranial, upper airway, or cranio-cervical malformations (some lethal)
  - Clinical outcome unrelated to pituitary function

Treatment

- Assess/treat endocrine malfunction

DIAGNOSTIC CHECKLIST

Consider

- PPE: Assess optic and olfactory nerves, frontal cortex
- DP: Oral tumors compromise airway patency

Image Interpretation Pearls

- Both: Can miss findings/diagnosis if thick sections (MR) are used or osseous structures (bone CT) not evaluated

SELECTED REFERENCES

1. Kriström B et al: A novel mutation in the LHX3 gene is responsible for combined pituitary hormone deficiency, hearing impairment, and vertebral malformations. J Clin Endocrinol Metab. 6, 2009
2. Tajima T et al: OTX2 loss of function mutation causes anophthalmia and combined pituitary hormone deficiency with a small anterior and ectopic posterior pituitary. J Clin Endocrinol Metab. 94(1):314-9, 2009
3. Kelberman D et al: SOX2 plays a critical role in the pituitary, forebrain, and eye during human embryonic development. J Clin Endocrinol Metab. 93(5):1865-73, 2008
4. Loddenkemper T et al: Pituitary stalk duplication in association with moya moya disease and bilateral morning glory disc anomaly - broadening the clinical spectrum of midline defects. J Neurol. 255(6):885-90, 2008

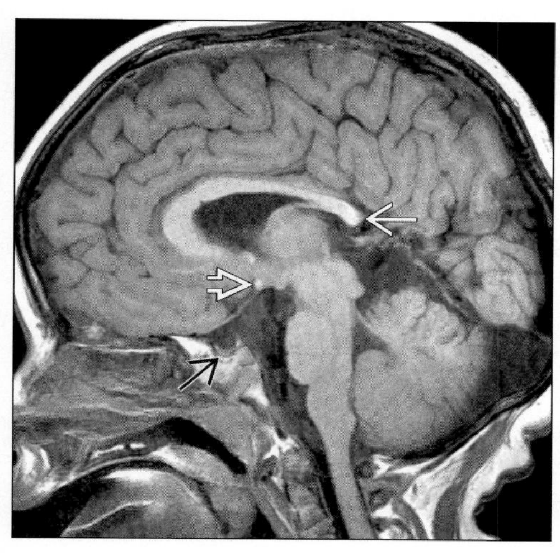

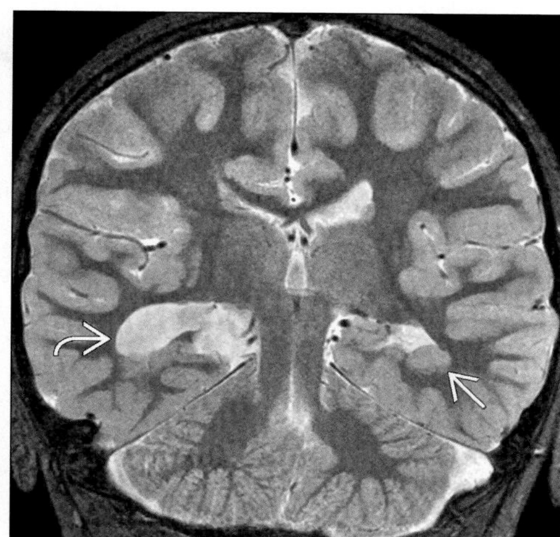

(Left) *Sagittal T1WI shows a small pituitary gland → and absent pituitary stalk. The hyperintense ectopic posterior pituitary gland → is located at the median eminence. The corpus callosum is also dysmorphic with characteristic small splenium →.* ***(Right)*** *Coronal T2WI MR in the same patient demonstrates associated left periventricular nodular gray matter heterotopia → and dysplastic inferior temporal lobe gray matter. Right choroid fissure cyst → is probably unrelated.*

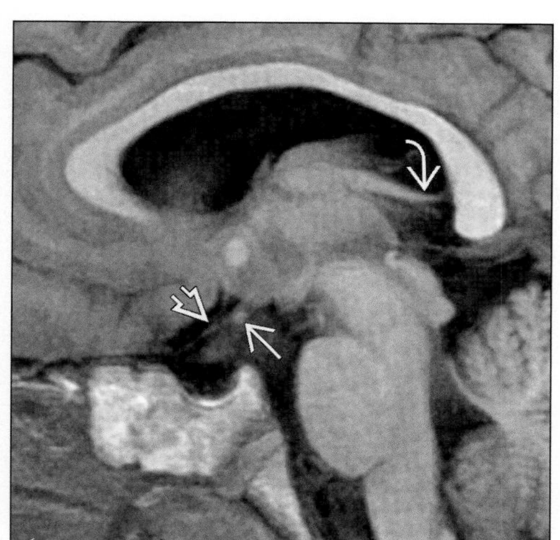

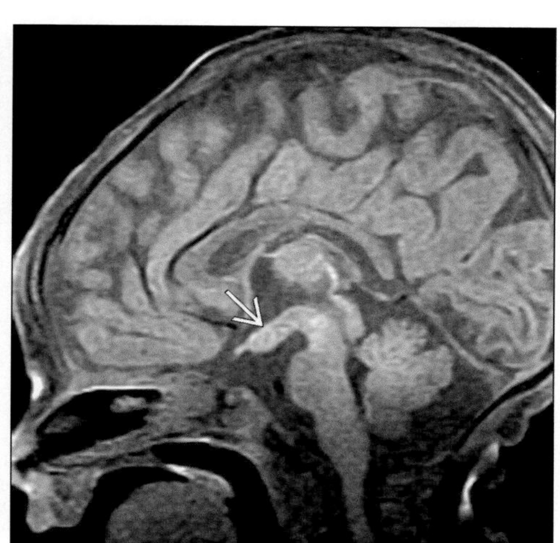

(Left) *Sagittal T1WI MR demonstrates a bright ectopic posterior pituitary gland → in a patient with septo-optic dysplasia. Note the small optic chiasm → and the low location of the fornices →.* ***(Right)*** *Sagittal T1WI MR in a patient with duplicated pituitary glands shows a thickened floor of sella and fusion of the tuber cinereum and mamillary bodies (tubo-mamillary fusion) →. Note the absence of a midline sella turcica and pituitary infundibulum.*

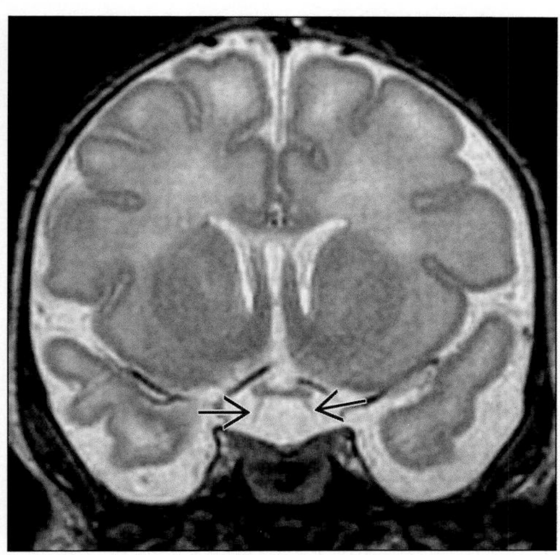

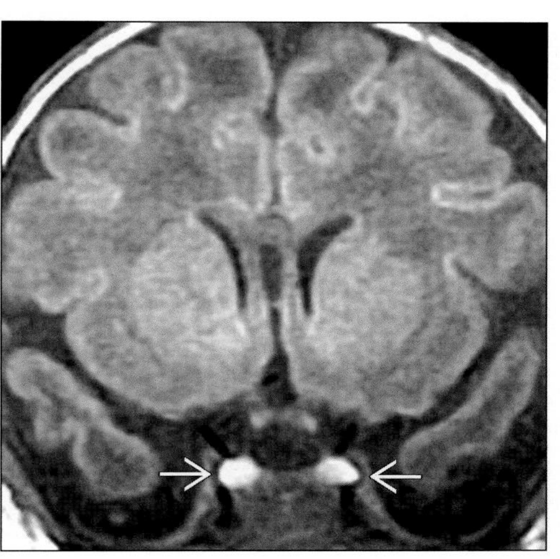

(Left) *Coronal T2WI MR in a newborn with midline skull base clefting reveals 2 pituitary stalks →. The normal-sized pituitary stalks project below the optic chiasm toward duplicated pituitary glands.* ***(Right)*** *Coronal T1WI MR demonstrates 2 normal-sized pituitary glands → laterally displaced within the abnormal skull base. The glands are uniformly hyperintense due to maternal hormonal influences. The pituitary gland is normally diffusely hyperintense on T1WI in newborns.*

TUBER CINEREUM HAMARTOMA

Key Facts

Terminology
- Nonneoplastic congenital gray matter heterotopia in region of tuber cinereum

Imaging
- Nonenhancing hypothalamic mass contiguous with tuber cinereum
- Sessile or pedunculated
- Mass located between mammillary bodies and infundibulum

Top Differential Diagnoses
- Craniopharyngioma
- Chiasmatic/hypothalamic astrocytoma
- Ectopic posterior pituitary
- Lipoma
- Germinoma
- Langerhans cell histiocytosis

Pathology
- Large sessile lesions ⇒ seizures
- Small pedunculated lesions ⇒ central precocious puberty
- Mature neuronal ganglionic tissue projecting from hypothalamus, tuber cinereum, or mamillary bodies
- Shape and size of hamartoma postulated to predict symptoms

Clinical Issues
- Infant with gelastic seizures or precocious puberty
- Older children with precocious puberty; tall, overweight, and advanced bone age

Diagnostic Checklist
- Hypothalamic mass identified during seizure imaging evaluation

(Left) Sagittal graphic shows a classic pedunculated tuber cinereum hamartoma ⇒ interposed between the infundibulum anteriorly and the mammillary bodies posteriorly. The mass resembles gray matter. ***(Right)*** Axial T2WI MR shows a mildly hyperintense (to gray matter) sessile mass ➡ in the tuber cinereum to the left of midline, posteriorly displacing the left mamillary body ➡ in comparison to the normally positioned right mamillary body ➡.

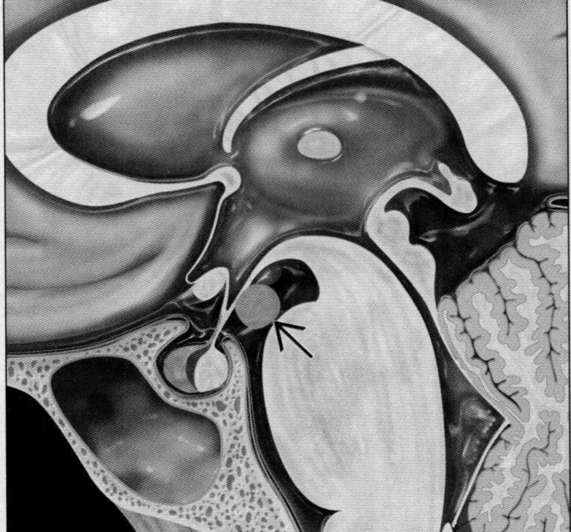

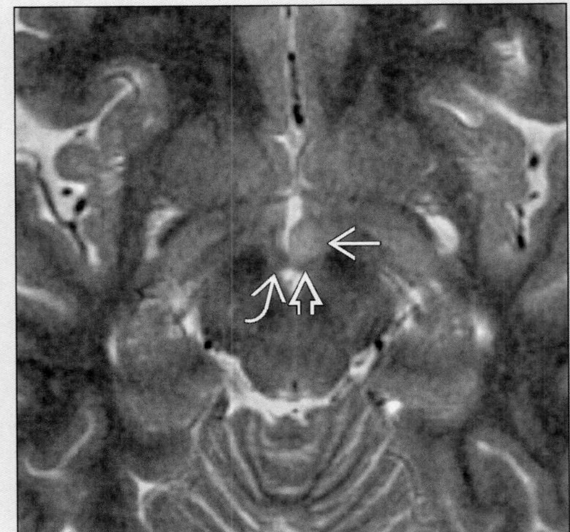

(Left) Sagittal T2WI MR in a patient presenting with precocious puberty reveals a pedunculated hypothalamic mass ➡ located between the median eminence and mamillary bodies. ***(Right)*** Sagittal T1WI C+ MR in a patient with precocious puberty reveals a pedunculated nonenhancing hypothalamic mass ➡ situated between the median eminence and mamillary bodies.

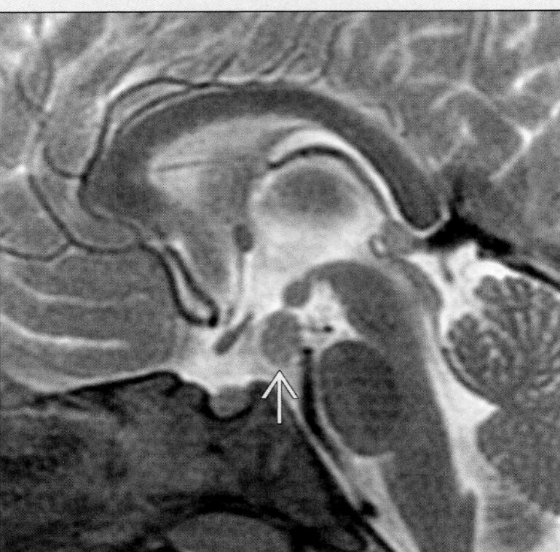

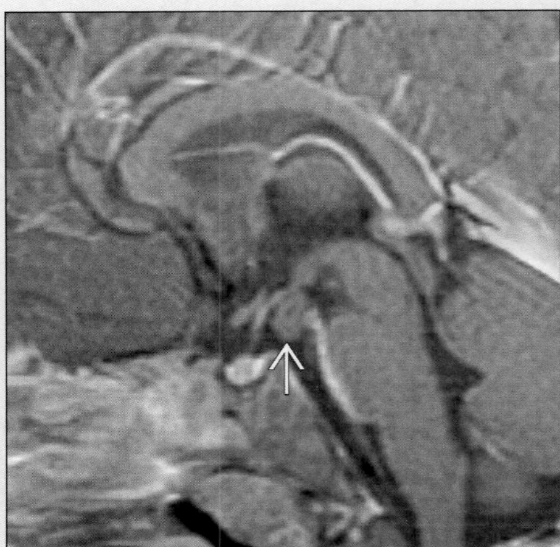

TUBER CINEREUM HAMARTOMA

TERMINOLOGY

Synonyms

- Hypothalamic hamartoma (HH), diencephalic hamartoma

Definitions

- Nonneoplastic congenital gray matter heterotopia in region of tuber cinereum

IMAGING

General Features

- Best diagnostic clue
  - Nonenhancing hypothalamic mass contiguous with tuber cinereum
- Location
  - Tuber cinereum of hypothalamus
  - Located between pons/mamillary bodies and hypothalamic infundibulum
- Size
  - Variable, few mm to giant (3-5 cm)
- Morphology
  - Sessile or pedunculated mass
  - Similar in density/intensity to gray matter

Radiographic Findings

- Radiography
  - ± suprasellar calcifications, eroded dorsum, enlarged sella (rare)

CT Findings

- NECT
  - Homogeneous suprasellar mass
    - Isodense → slightly hypodense
    - Cysts, Ca++ uncommon
    - ± patent craniopharyngeal canal (very rare)
- CECT
  - No pathologic enhancement

MR Findings

- T1WI
  - Mass located between mammillary bodies and infundibulum
  - Isointense → slightly hypointense to gray matter
- T2WI
  - Isointense → slightly hyperintense (2° to fibrillary gliosis)
- FLAIR
  - Isointense → slightly hyperintense to gray matter
- T1WI C+
  - Nonenhancing (if enhances, consider other diagnosis)
- MRS
  - ↓ NAA and NAA/Cr, mild ↑ choline (Cho) and Cho/Cr, ↑ myoinositol (mI) and mI/Cr
    - ↓ NAA and ↑ choline indicate reduced neuronal density and relative gliosis respectively compared to normal gray matter
    - ↑ mI/Cr correlates with ↑ glial component and lesion T2 hyperintensity

Imaging Recommendations

- Best imaging tool
  - Multiplanar MR imaging
- Protocol advice
  - Thin section sagittal and coronal T2, T1WI C+ MR

DIFFERENTIAL DIAGNOSIS

Craniopharyngioma

- Most common suprasellar mass in children
- Variable signal intensity cysts (90%), Ca++ (90%), enhancement (90%)
- Longstanding lesion, frequently with short stature and pituitary abnormalities

Chiasmatic/Hypothalamic Astrocytoma

- 2nd most common pediatric suprasellar mass (± NF1)
- Hyperintense on T2WI MR, ± contrast enhancement (heterogeneous, often vigorous)
- Optic pathway or hypothalamus ± optic tract extension

Ectopic Posterior Pituitary

- Ectopic hyperintense focus on T1WI MR
- No normal orthotopic posterior pituitary hyperintensity

Germinoma

- Thickening, abnormal enhancement of pituitary stalk rather than tuber cinereum
- Diabetes insipidus common
- ± multicentric: Suprasellar, pineal, thalamus, basal ganglia
- Early leptomeningeal metastatic dissemination

Langerhans Cell Histiocytosis

- Thickening, abnormal enhancement of pituitary stalk rather than tuber cinereum
- Diabetes insipidus common
- Look for lytic bone lesions in typical locations

Lipoma

- Hyperintense fat signal on T1WI MR
- Hypointense on STIR or fat-saturated sequences

PATHOLOGY

General Features

- Etiology
  - Neuronal migration anomaly (occurs between gestational days 33-41)
  - Affects normal hypothalamic regulation of autonomic, endocrine, neurological, behavioral functions
  - Shape and size of hamartoma postulated to predict symptoms
    - Large sessile lesions ⇒ seizures
    - Small pedunculated lesions ⇒ central precocious puberty (CPP)
    - Presentation with both seizures and CPP common
- Genetics

- Pallister-Hall syndrome (PHS): *GLI3* frameshift mutations, chromosome 7p13
  - Hamartoma or hamartoblastoma of tuber cinereum
  - Digital malformations (short metacarpals, syndactyly, polydactyly)
  - Other midline (epiglottis/larynx) and cardiac/ renal/anal anomalies
- Associated abnormalities
  - Holoprosencephaly; midline facial, extremity, cardiac, renal anomalies
  - Additional epileptogenic lesions described but rare

Staging, Grading, & Classification

- Valdueza classification
  - Pedunculated, central precocious puberty or asymptomatic
    - Originates tuber cinereum
    - Originates mamillary bodies
  - Sessile, hypothalamus displaced, seizures
    - More hypothalamic dysfunction and abnormal behavior

Gross Pathologic & Surgical Features

- Mature neuronal ganglionic tissue projecting from hypothalamus, tuber cinereum, or mamillary bodies
- Pedunculated or sessile, rounded or nodular

Microscopic Features

- Well-differentiated neurons interspersed with glial cells, myelinated/unmyelinated axons, variable amounts of fibrillary gliosis
  - Hamartoblastomas include primitive undifferentiated cells
- Rare reports of cysts, necrosis, calcifications, fat

CLINICAL ISSUES

Presentation

- Most common signs/symptoms
  - Luteinizing hormone-releasing hormone (LHRH) dependent central precocious puberty presenting at very young age
  - Refractory symptomatic mixed seizure types, including gelastic seizures
    - Gelastic seizures are recurrent automatic bursts of laughter without mirth
    - Rarely occur in conjunction with focal cortical dysplasia and hypothalamic astrocytoma in addition to HH
  - Other seizure types frequent, but only gelastic seizures originate in/near hamartoma
- Other signs/symptoms
  - Depression, anxiety common in adult HH patients
- Clinical profile
  - Infant with gelastic seizures or precocious puberty
  - Older children with precocious puberty; tall, overweight, and advanced bone age

Demographics

- Age
  - Usually present between 1-3 years of age
- Gender
  - No predilection; some reports M > F
- Ethnicity
  - No predilection
- Epidemiology
  - Of histologically verified lesions: 3/4 have precocious puberty, 1/2 seizures
  - Up to 33% of patients with central precocious puberty have HH

Natural History & Prognosis

- Size should remain stable; if growth detected, surgery/ biopsy indicated
- Symptomatic lesions: Sessile > pedunculated
  - Sessile lesions nearly always symptomatic
- Syndromic patients do poorly, may not survive other malformations

Treatment

- Medical: Hormonal suppressive therapy (LHRH-agonist therapy), treat seizures
- Surgical: Medical therapy failure or rapid lesion growth
  - Endoscopic or transcallosal surgical resection, stereotatic thermocoagulation, interstitial radiosurgery, Gamma knife surgery

DIAGNOSTIC CHECKLIST

Consider

- Hypothalamic mass identified during seizure imaging evaluation

Image Interpretation Pearls

- Classic imaging appearance is nonenhancing hypothalamic mass in tuber cinereum
  - Isointense to gray matter on T1WI, slightly ↑ signal on T2WI
  - Hypothalamic astrocytoma, histiocytosis, germ cell tumor all show some contrast enhancement

SELECTED REFERENCES

1. Beggs J et al: Hypothalamic hamartomas associated with epilepsy: ultrastructural features. J Neuropathol Exp Neurol. 67(7):657-68, 2008
2. Ng YT: Clarification of the term "status gelasticus" and treatment and prognosis of gelastic seizures. Pediatr Neurol. 38(4):300-1; author reply 301-2, 2008
3. Pleasure SJ et al: Hypothalamic hamartomas and hedgehogs: not a laughing matter. Neurology. 70(8):588-9, 2008
4. Castro LH et al: Epilepsy syndromes associated with hypothalamic hamartomas. Seizure. 16(1):50-8, 2007
5. Coons SW et al: The histopathology of hypothalamic hamartomas: study of 57 cases. J Neuropathol Exp Neurol. 66(2):131-41, 2007
6. Amstutz DR et al: Hypothalamic hamartomas: Correlation of MR imaging and spectroscopic findings with tumor glial content. AJNR Am J Neuroradiol. 27(4):794-8, 2006
7. Boudreau EA et al: Hypothalamic hamartomas and seizures: distinct natural history of isolated and Pallister-Hall syndrome cases. Epilepsia. 46(1):42-7, 2005
8. Freeman JL et al: MR imaging and spectroscopic study of epileptogenic hypothalamic hamartomas: analysis of 72 cases. AJNR Am J Neuroradiol. 25(3):450-62, 2004

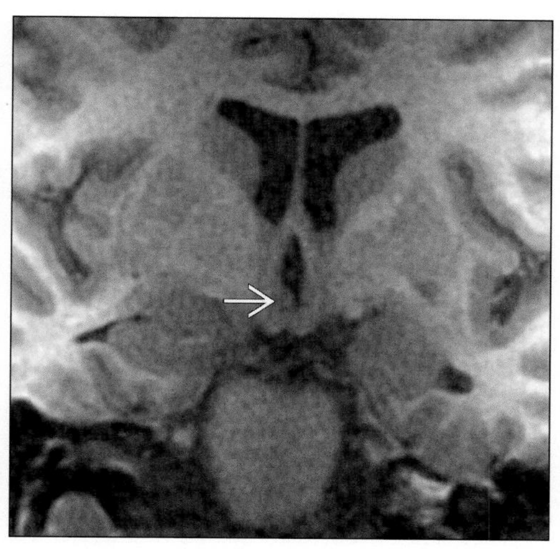

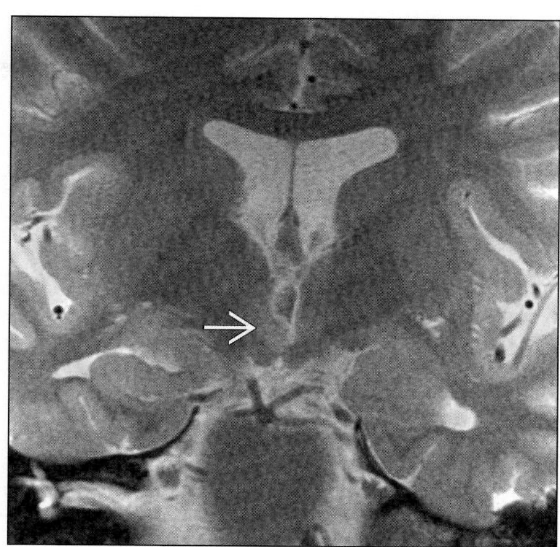

(Left) *Coronal T1WI MR of a patient with gelastic seizures demonstrates a slightly hypointense small hypothalamic mass* ➡ *extending from the right tuber cinereum adjacent to the mamillary bodies. The mass displaces the lateral wall of the 3rd ventricle.* ***(Right)*** *Coronal T2WI MR in a gelastic seizure patient demonstrates a small, sessile, slightly hyperintense, hypothalamic mass* ➡.

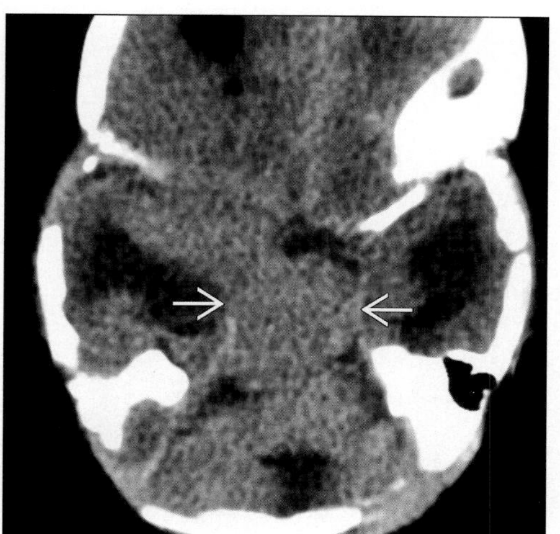

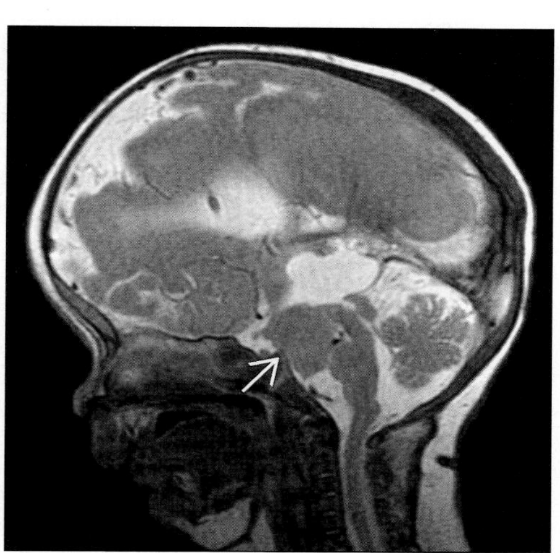

(Left) *Axial NECT in an infant imaged for congenital hydrocephalus demonstrates a large suprasellar mass* ➡ *that posteriorly displaces the brainstem and cerebellum. Note the dilated lateral ventricles.* ***(Right)*** *Sagittal T2WI MR of an infant with congenital hydrocephalus and macrocephaly reveals a large suprasellar and prepontine hamartoma* ➡ *with signal characteristics of the brain. Note the posterior displacement of the midbrain and pons.*

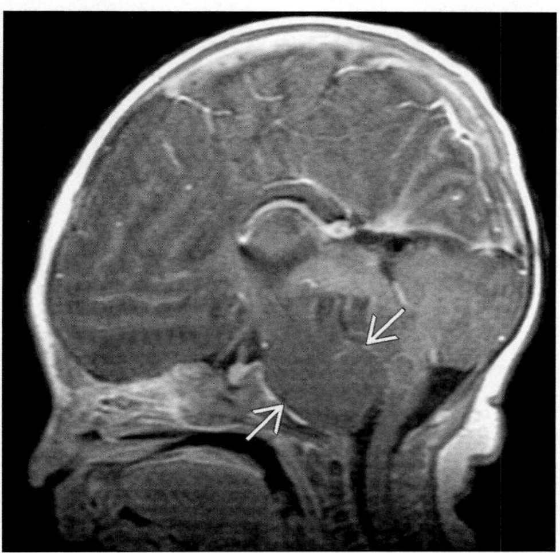

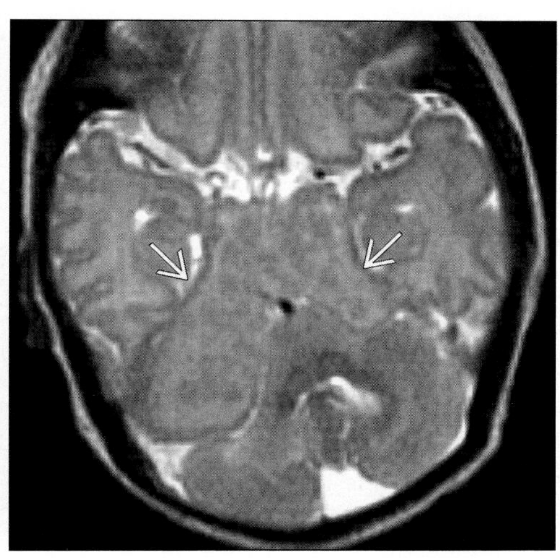

(Left) *Sagittal T1WI C+ MR of an infant reveals a giant pedunculated hypothalamic hamartoma* ➡ *that posteriorly displaces the cerebellum and brainstem. No incremental enhancement of the mass is identified.* ***(Right)*** *Axial T2WI MR shows that the large hypothalamic mass* ➡ *posteriorly displacing the cerebellum and brainstem has the signal intensity of gray matter, and at 1st glance has superficial resemblance to the cerebellum.*

RATHKE CLEFT CYST

Key Facts

Terminology

- Nonneoplastic cyst arising from remnants of embryonic Rathke cleft

Imaging

- Nonenhancing, noncalcified, intra-/suprasellar cyst with intracystic nodule
  - Completely intrasellar (40%), suprasellar extension (60%)
  - Density/intensity varies with cyst content (serous vs. mucoid)
- Most symptomatic RCCs: 5-15 mm in diameter
- Occasionally RCCs can become very large
- "Claw" sign = enhancing rim of compressed pituitary surrounding nonenhancing cyst

Top Differential Diagnoses

- Craniopharyngioma
  - Cytokeratin profile helps distinguish from RCC (RCCs express cytokeratins 8, 20)
- Cystic pituitary adenoma
- Other nonneoplastic cyst

Clinical Issues

- Most are asymptomatic, found incidentally at imaging or autopsy
- Headache (50%)
- Pituitary dysfunction (70%)
  - Amenorrhea/galactorrhea, diabetes insipidus, panhypopituitarism, hyperprolactinemia
- Rare but important: Apoplexy, cavernous sinus syndrome
  - Can be indistinguishable from pituitary apoplexy
  - Can occur ± intracystic hemorrhage!

(Left) Coronal graphic shows a typical suprasellar Rathke cleft cyst interposed between the pituitary gland ⇒ and the optic chiasm ➡. (Right) Axial gross pathology shows a mucinous-containing Rathke cleft cyst ⇒ found incidentally at autopsy. (Courtesy E. Hedley-Whyte, MD.)

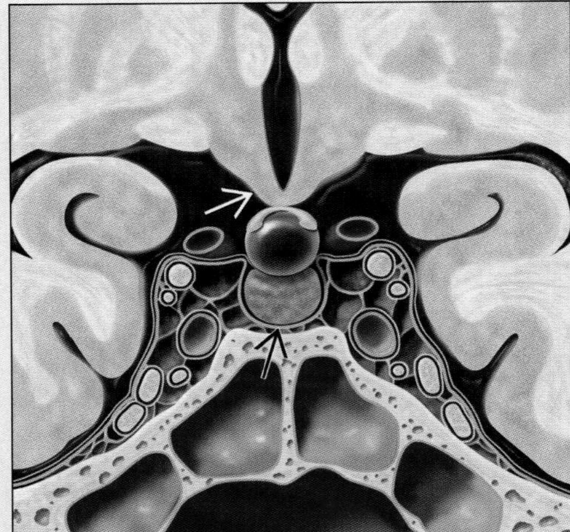

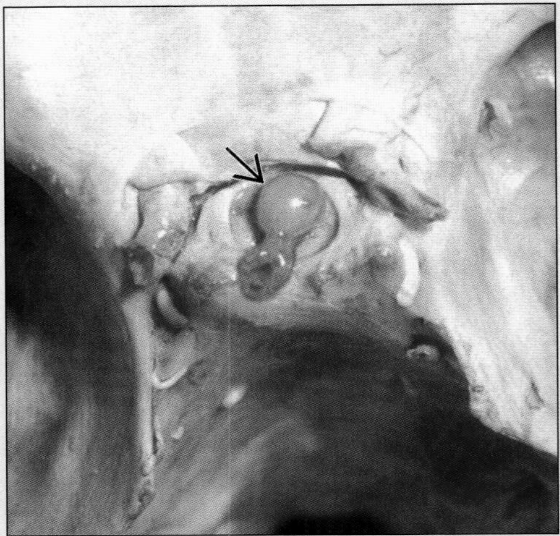

(Left) Coronal NECT in a patient with a headache shows a hyperdense intrasellar mass with minimal suprasellar extension ➡. (Right) Coronal T2WI MR in the same patient demonstrates that the cyst ➡ is primarily hypointense. Note the intracystic nodule ➡. Rathke cleft cyst was found at surgery.

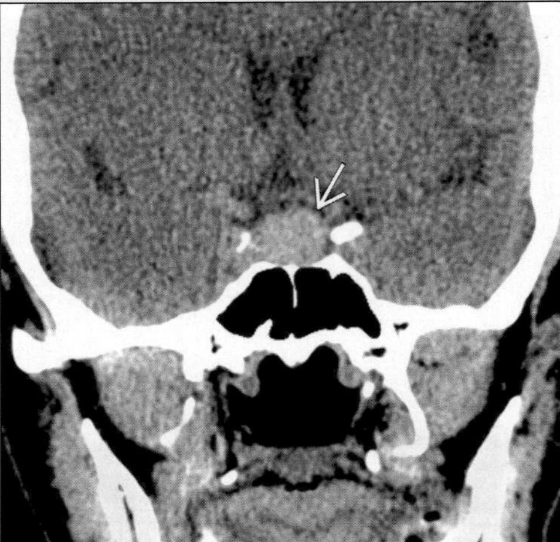

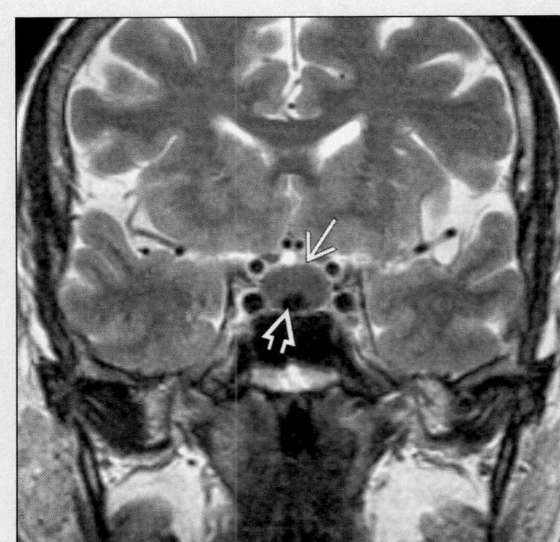

RATHKE CLEFT CYST

TERMINOLOGY

Abbreviations

- Rathke cleft cyst (RCC)

Definitions

- Nonneoplastic cyst arising from remnants of embryonic Rathke cleft

IMAGING

General Features

- Best diagnostic clue
  - Nonenhancing, noncalcified, intra-/suprasellar cyst with intracystic nodule
  - Uncommon but pathognomonic = "posterior ledge" sign
    - Upward extension through diaphragma sellae
    - Ledge of tissue overlies posterior lobe
- Location
  - Completely intrasellar (40%), suprasellar extension (60%)
  - Most Rathke cleft cysts are limited to sella
    - Between anterior, intermediate lobes
- Size
  - Most symptomatic Rathke cleft cysts are between 5-15 mm in diameter
  - Occasionally become very large
    - May cause expansile intra-/suprasellar mass
    - Rare: Erode skull base
  - Size usually constant, does not enlarge
    - Transient decrease reported in response to glucocorticoids
- Morphology
  - Well defined, round/ovoid

CT Findings

- NECT
  - Well-delineated, round/lobulated, intra/suprasellar mass
    - Hypo- (75%), mixed iso-/hypodense (20%)
    - Hyperdense (5-10%)
    - Ca++ (10-15%), curvilinear, in cyst wall
  - Rare: May cause sphenoid sinusitis
- CECT
  - Does not enhance

MR Findings

- T1WI
  - Varies with cyst content (serous vs. mucoid)
    - Hyper- (50%), hypointense (50%)
    - Hyperintense intracystic nodule (75%)
    - Mixed (5-10%), may have fluid-fluid level
- T2WI
  - Varies with cyst content
    - Hyper- (70%), iso-/hypointense (30%)
    - Hypointense intracystic nodule (75%)
- FLAIR
  - Hyperintense
- T2* GRE
  - Rarely blooms
- T1WI C+
  - No internal enhancement
    - "Claw" sign = enhancing rim of compressed pituitary surrounding nonenhancing cyst
    - Small nonenhancing intracystic nodule (75%)

Imaging Recommendations

- Best imaging tool
  - MR
- Protocol advice
  - Sagittal, coronal pre-contrast T1/T2WI
  - "Dynamic" contrast-enhanced coronal T1WIs through sella
  - Sagittal, coronal thin section T1WI C+

DIFFERENTIAL DIAGNOSIS

Craniopharyngioma

- Histologic continuum between Rathke cleft cyst, craniopharyngioma
- Floccular Ca++ common in craniopharyngioma, rare in Rathke cleft cyst
- Noncalcified RCC can be indistinguishable from craniopharyngioma on imaging
- Rim or nodular enhancement (90%)
- Cytokeratin profile helps distinguish from Rathke cleft cyst
  - RCCs express cytokeratins 8, 20

Cystic Pituitary Adenoma

- Ca++ rare
- Signal intensity often heterogeneous
- Rim or rim with nodular enhancement common

Other Nonneoplastic Cyst

- Arachnoid cyst
  - Signal identical to CSF, no intracystic nodule
- Dermoid cyst
  - May have short T1; Ca++; look for evidence of rupture
- Epidermoid cyst
  - Mild irregular enhancement, Ca++ (25%)
- Miscellaneous intrasellar cyst
  - Pars intermedia, colloid, dermoid, epidermoid cysts occur
- Rare: Sellar/hypophyseal neurocysticercosis

PATHOLOGY

General Features

- Etiology
  - 1 of spectrum of midline sellar/juxtasellar ectodermal cysts
  - Arises from embryonic remnants of Rathke pouch
- Genetics
  - No known heritable conditions
- Associated abnormalities
  - Sphenoid sinusitis (rare)
  - Compression of optic chiasm, hypothalamus
    - May cause hyperintensity on T2WI/FLAIR along optic chiasm, tracts
  - Embryology
    - Ectodermal origin (persistence of Rathke pouch)
    - Stomodeum (primitive oral cavity) invaginates

RATHKE CLEFT CYST

- Extends dorsally, forms ectodermal-lined craniopharyngeal duct
- Meets infundibulum (outgrowth of 3rd ventricle) by 11th fetal week, gives rise to hypophysis
- Anterior wall of pouch forms anterior lobe, pars tuberalis
- Posterior wall forms pars intermedia
- Lumen forms narrow cleft that normally regresses by 12th week of gestation
- Persistence, expansion gives rise to RCC
- Neuroepithelial or endodermal origin (less likely)

Gross Pathologic & Surgical Features

- Smoothly lobulated, well-delineated, intra-/suprasellar cystic mass
  - Content varies from clear CSF-like fluid to thick mucoid material

Microscopic Features

- Wall = single layer of ciliated cuboidal/columnar epithelium ± goblet cells
  - Changes of mixed acute, chronic inflammation may be present
- Variable cyst content
  - Clear or serous
  - ± hemorrhage, hemosiderin
  - Amorphous, inspissated, eosinophilic, mucicarmine(+) colloid ± cholesterol clefts
  - Firm, waxy, yellow, inspissated material
  - Rare: Hemorrhage (cyst apoplexy)
- Immunohistochemical stains positive for cytokeratin
  - Express cytokeratins 8, 20

CLINICAL ISSUES

Presentation

- Most common signs/symptoms
  - Most are asymptomatic, found incidentally at imaging or autopsy
  - Symptomatic Rathke cleft cyst
    - Pituitary dysfunction (70%)
      - Amenorrhea/galactorrhea, diabetes insipidus, panhypopituitarism, hyperprolactinemia
    - Visual disturbances (45-55%)
    - Headache (50%)
  - Other signs/symptoms
    - Head pain, visual disturbance (less common)
    - Hypopituitarism
    - Central diabetes insipidus
  - Rare but important: Apoplexy, cavernous sinus syndrome
    - Cyst apoplexy
      - Can occur ± intracystic hemorrhage!
      - Can be indistinguishable from pituitary apoplexy
    - Cavernous sinus syndrome
      - Caused by lateral extension of Rathke cleft cyst into cavernous sinus
- Clinical profile
  - Asymptomatic

Demographics

- Age
  - Mean age = 45 years
- Gender
  - Slight female predominance
- Epidemiology
  - Common intra-/suprasellar nonneoplastic cyst
  - Usually incidental, found in up to 1/3 of all autopsies

Natural History & Prognosis

- Most are stable, do not change in size/signal intensity
- Some cysts may shrink/disappear spontaneously
- Iso-/hyperintense cysts on T1WI more often cause symptoms
- Rathke cleft cysts do not undergo neoplastic degeneration

Treatment

- Conservative if asymptomatic
- Aspiration/partial excision if symptomatic
  - Persistent/recurrent cyst formation occurs in approximately 1/3 of patients
  - May occur many years after surgery

DIAGNOSTIC CHECKLIST

Consider

- Obtaining endocrine profile

Image Interpretation Pearls

- Look for hypointense intracystic nodule on T2WI

SELECTED REFERENCES

1. Kitajima M et al: Differentiation of common large sellar-suprasellar masses effect of artificial neural network on radiologists' diagnosis performance. Acad Radiol. 16(3):313-20, 2009
2. Binning MJ et al: Hemorrhagic and nonhemorrhagic Rathke cleft cysts mimicking pituitary apoplexy. J Neurosurg. 108(1):3-8, 2008
3. Glezer A et al: Rare sellar lesions. Endocrinol Metab Clin North Am. 37(1):195-211, x, 2008
4. Maruyama H et al: Rathke's cleft cyst with short-term size changes in response to glucocorticoid replacement. Endocr J. 55(2):425-8, 2008
5. Rao VJ et al: Imaging characteristics of common suprasellar lesions with emphasis on MRI findings. Clin Radiol. 63(8):939-47, 2008
6. Kunii N et al: Rathke's cleft cysts: differentiation from other cystic lesions in the pituitary fossa by use of single-shot fast spin-echo diffusion-weighted MR imaging. Acta Neurochir (Wien). 149(8):759-69; discussion 769, 2007
7. Kim JE et al: Surgical treatment of symptomatic Rathke cleft cysts: clinical features and results with special attention to recurrence. J Neurosurg. 100(1):33-40, 2004
8. Xin W et al: Differential expression of cytokeratins 8 and 20 distinguishes craniopharyngioma from rathke cleft cyst. Arch Pathol Lab Med. 126(10):1174-8, 2002
9. Byun WM et al: MR imaging findings of Rathke's cleft cysts: significance of intracystic nodules. AJNR Am J Neuroradiol. 21(3):485-8, 2000
10. Naylor MF et al: Rathke cleft cyst: CT, MR, and pathology of 23 cases. J Comput Assist Tomogr. 19(6):853-9, 1995

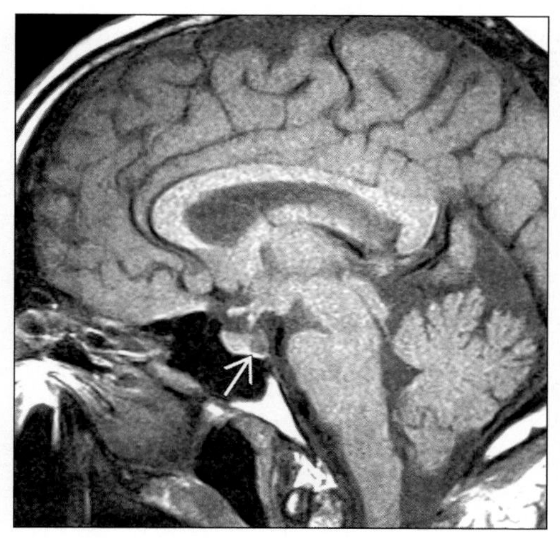

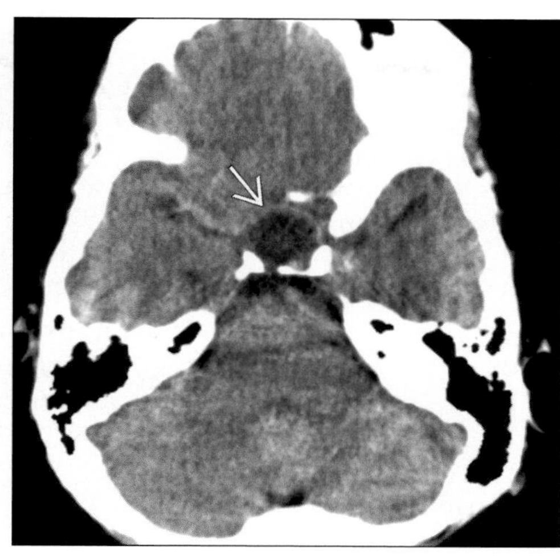

(Left) *Sagittal T1WI MR in a patient with a headache but no neurologic symptoms shows a small hypointense cyst ➡ that followed CSF on all sequences. It was an incidental finding and presumed to be a Rathke cleft cyst.* ***(Right)*** *Axial NECT shows a hypodense, CSF-like intra- and suprasellar mass ➡. Rathke cleft cyst was found at surgery.*

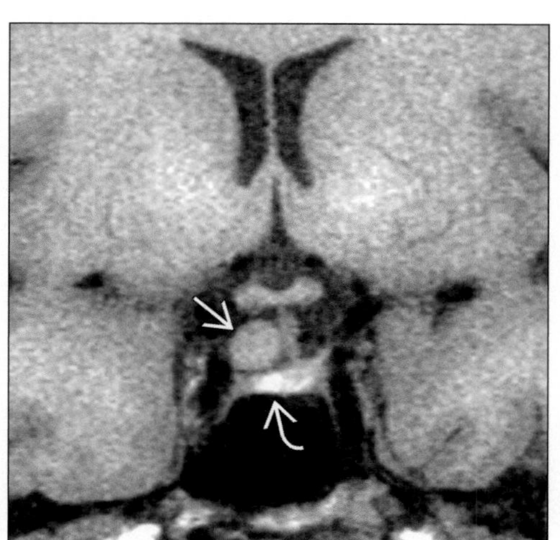

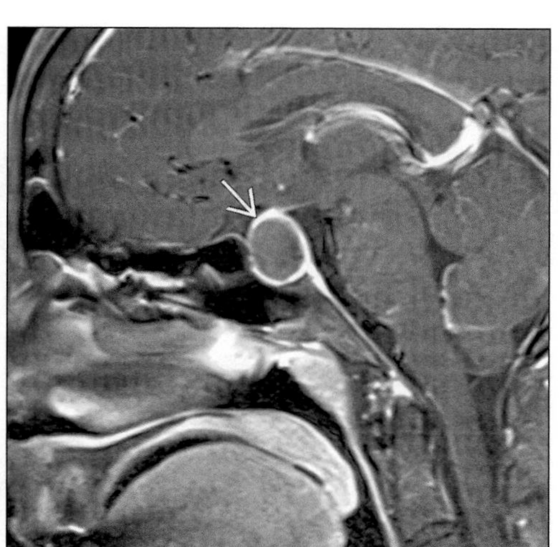

(Left) *Coronal T1WI MR in an asymptomatic patient shows a small suprasellar mass ➡ that is isointense with the brain clearly separate from the pituitary gland ➡. The infundibular stalk is slightly deviated to the left. This was presumed to be a Rathke cleft cyst.* ***(Right)*** *Sagittal T1 C+ FS MR shows a Rathke cleft cyst with a "claw" sign ➡ of residual enhancing pituitary gland draped around the large intra- and suprasellar cyst.*

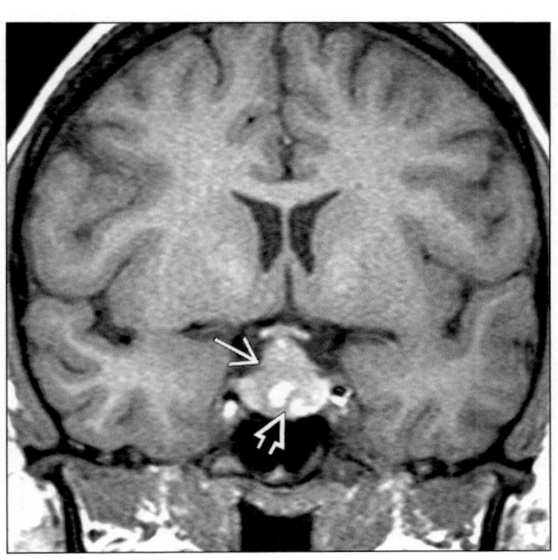

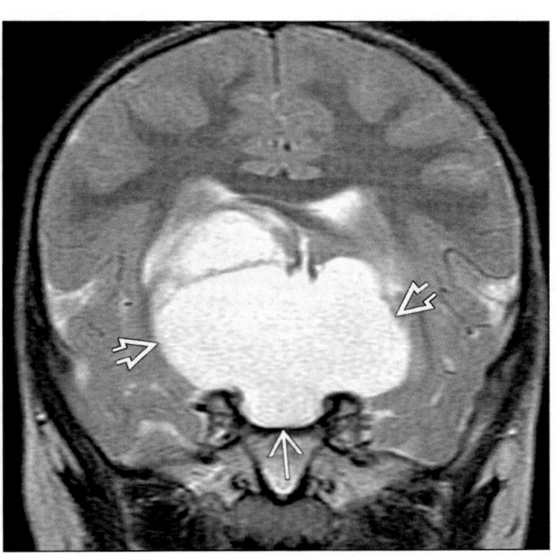

(Left) *Coronal T1WI MR in a 21-year-old woman, with sudden onset headache and decreased T4, shows a hyperintense mass ➡ with even more hyperintense intracystic nodules ➡. The preoperative diagnosis was pituitary apoplexy, and Rathke cleft cyst apoplexy was found at surgery.* ***(Right)*** *Coronal T2WI MR in 2-year-old child shows a huge cyst with intra- ➡ and suprasellar ➡ components. A large Rathke cleft cyst was found at surgery.*

PITUITARY MICROADENOMA

Key Facts

Terminology
- Microadenoma: < 10 mm in diameter

Imaging
- Intrasellar
  - Rare: Ectopic origin outside pituitary fossa
- Best technique = dynamic contrast-enhanced thin-section T1-weighted MR
  - Generally enhance but more slowly than adjacent normal pituitary
  - Beware: 10-30% can be seen only on dynamic contrast-enhanced scans!

Top Differential Diagnoses
- Rathke cleft
- Craniopharyngioma
- Pituitary hyperplasia
- Other nonneoplastic cyst (e.g., pars intermedia cyst)

Pathology
- Adenomas are almost always WHO grade I
  - Pituitary carcinoma exceedingly rare

Clinical Issues
- Symptoms of secreting tumors vary according to type
  - Asymptomatic/nonfunctioning most common
- 15-17% incidental finding at autopsy
- Pituitary "incidentaloma" seen in 6-27% of MR scans (common even in children)

Diagnostic Checklist
- Intrapituitary "filling defect" may be benign nonneoplastic cyst, as well as incidental microadenoma

*(**Left**) Coronal graphic shows a small microadenoma ➢ that slightly enlarges the right side of the pituitary gland and deviates the infundibulum toward the left. (**Right**) Coronal micropathology shows a normal pituitary gland surrounding a small nonfunctioning microadenoma ➢ that was found incidentally at autopsy. (Courtesy J. Townsend, MD.)*

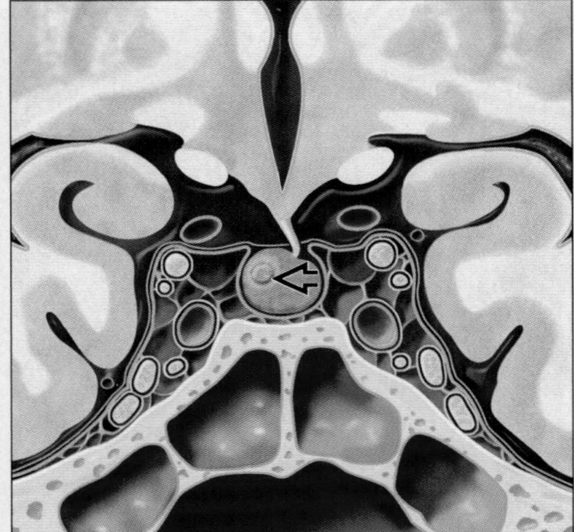

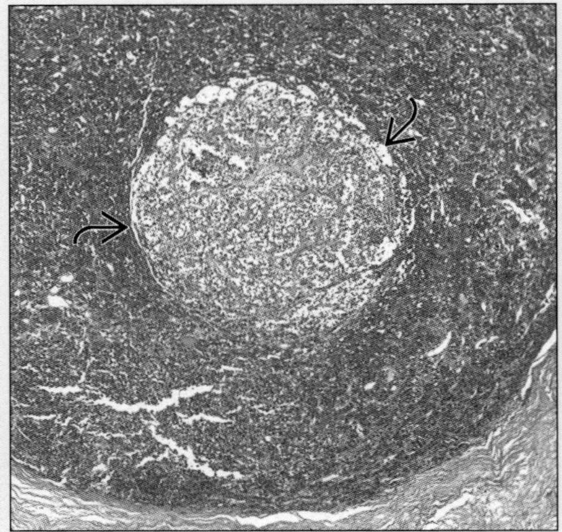

*(**Left**) Coronal T1WI C+ MR shows a focus of lesser enhancement ➔ within a mildly enlarged pituitary gland ➢. The patient was asymptomatic, and this was an incidental finding. Pituitary "incidentalomas" are common (seen in 15-20% of cases) and may represent nonfunctioning adenomas or nonneoplastic cysts (e.g., pars intermedia or Rathke cleft cyst). (**Right**) Coronal T1WI MR in a female with elevated prolactin shows an 8 mm mass ➔ in the left side of the pituitary gland. Most microadenomas are laterally located.*

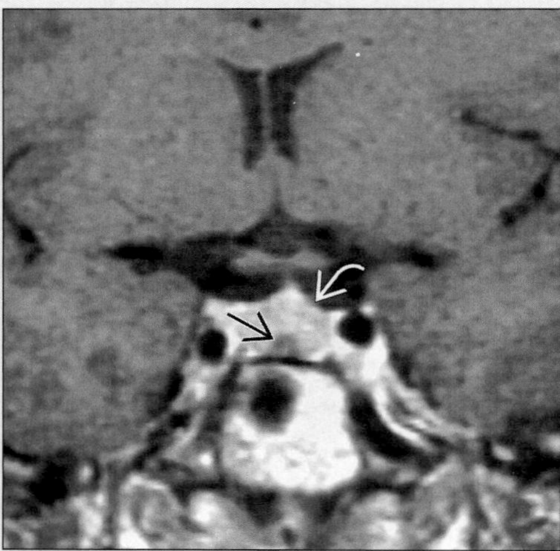

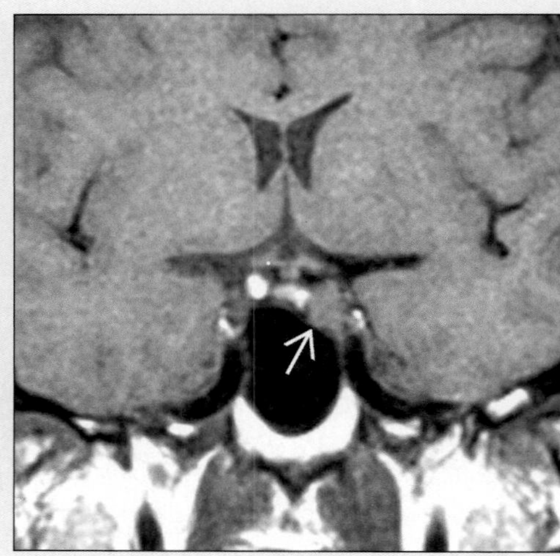

PITUITARY MICROADENOMA

TERMINOLOGY

Abbreviations

- Pituitary microadenoma

Synonyms

- Prolactinoma

Definitions

- Microadenoma: < 10 mm in diameter

IMAGING

General Features

- Best diagnostic clue
  - Intrapituitary lesion that enhances but less rapidly than surrounding normal gland
- Location
  - Intrasellar
  - Rare: Ectopic origin outside pituitary fossa
    - Sphenoid or cavernous sinus, clivus
    - Pituitary stalk, 3rd ventricle
    - Nasopharynx
- Size
  - By definition, microadenomas < 10 mm in diameter
- Morphology
  - Circumscribed, well-demarcated mass surrounded by crescentic rim of compressed anterior pituitary

CT Findings

- NECT
  - If uncomplicated (no hemorrhage, cyst), microadenomas are isodense, invisible
- CECT
  - 2/3 appear hypodense to normal pituitary on dynamic scans

MR Findings

- T1WI
  - Variable signal intensity
    - Usually isointense with normal pituitary gland
    - Can be hyperintense if hemorrhage, necrosis
- T2WI
  - Typically isointense to normal pituitary gland
- T2* GRE
  - May show "blooming" if hemorrhagic
- T1WI C+
  - 70-90% relatively hypointense compared to intensely enhancing pituitary gland, cavernous sinus
    - Generally enhance but more slowly than adjacent normal pituitary
  - Beware: 10-30% can be seen only on dynamic contrast-enhanced scans!

Other Modality Findings

- Cavernous/inferior petrosal sinus sampling (10% false-negative)

Imaging Recommendations

- Best imaging tool
  - Dynamic contrast-enhanced thin-section T1-weighted MR
- Protocol advice
  - Coronal thin-section T1WIs obtained during contrast infusion
    - Scans obtained at 10-15 second intervals following rapid bolus injection
    - At least 3 sections (3 mm or less, no interslice gap) through pituitary gland, sorted by slice
  - Time-signal intensity curves through normal, abnormal gland may be helpful

DIFFERENTIAL DIAGNOSIS

Rathke Cleft Cyst

- Hypo-/hyperintense to normal gland on T1-/T2WI
- No enhancement

Craniopharyngioma

- Completely intrasellar craniopharyngioma is uncommon
- May have Ca++
- Displaces/compresses normal pituitary
  - Microadenoma is contained within gland

Pituitary Hyperplasia

- Gland appears slightly, diffusely enlarged
- May appear slightly inhomogeneous, but usually no discrete foci of hypointensity seen on contrast-enhanced scans

Other Nonneoplastic Cyst (e.g., Pars Intermedia Cyst)

- Variable signal intensity
- Nonenhancing
- Indistinguishable from intrasellar Rathke cleft cyst

PATHOLOGY

General Features

- Etiology
  - 1 possible model of pituitary tumorigenesis
    - Hypophysiotrophic hormone excess, suppressive hormone insufficiency, or growth factor excess leads to hyperplasia
    - Increased proliferation predisposes to genomic instability; adenoma forms
  - 5 endocrine cell types in anterior pituitary (each secretes specific hormone, may develop into micro- or macroadenoma)
    - Lactotrophs: Prolactin (PRL)
      - 30% of adenomas
    - Somatotrophs: Growth hormone (GH)
      - 20% of adenomas
    - Corticotrophs: Adrenocorticotrophic hormone (ACTH)
      - 10% of adenomas
    - Thyrotrophs: Thyroid-stimulating hormone (TSH)
      - 1-2% of adenomas
    - Gonadotrophs: Gonadotropins, luteinizing hormone (LH), follicle-stimulating hormone (FSH)
      - FSH/LH (10%)
      - PRL/GH (5%)
  - Null cell: 20% of adenomas

PITUITARY MICROADENOMA

- Genetics
  - No consistent allelic losses or point mutations identified
    - 2 normal copies of POU transcription factor Pit-1 (*POU1F1*) gene necessary for normal anterior pituitary lobe function
  - Can occur as part of MEN type 1, Carney complex
    - MEN1-associated adenomas often plurihormonal, larger, more invasive
- Associated abnormalities
  - Growth hormone secreting adenoma
    - Acromegaly in adults
    - Gigantism in adolescents

Staging, Grading, & Classification

- Adenomas are almost always WHO grade I
- Pituitary carcinoma exceedingly rare
- Modified Kovacs and Horvath classification (cell type with tinctorial characteristics and hormones produced)
  - Growth hormone cell adenoma
    - Chromophobe or acidophil; growth hormone
  - Prolactin cell adenoma
    - Chromophobe or acidophil; prolactin
  - Mixed GH, prolactin cell adenoma
    - Variable; GH, prolactin
  - Acidophil cell adenoma
    - Chromophobe; GH and prolactin
  - Mammosomatotroph cell adenoma
    - Acidophil; GH and prolactin
  - Corticotroph cell adenoma
    - Basophilic or chromophobe; ACTH
  - Thyrotroph cell adenoma
    - Chromophobe; TSH
  - Gonadotroph cell adenoma
    - Chromophobe; FSH, LH, α subunit in varied combinations
  - Nonfunctioning adenoma
    - Chromophobe; scanty or no hormones
  - Plurihormonal adenoma
    - Variable; 2 or 3 hormones in variable combinations

Gross Pathologic & Surgical Features

- Small reddish-pink nodule

Microscopic Features

- Monotonous sheets of uniform cells
- Cell type varies, has variable trichrome staining, specific immunohistochemical stains

CLINICAL ISSUES

Presentation

- Most common signs/symptoms
  - Asymptomatic/nonfunctioning most common
  - Symptoms of secreting tumors vary according to type
    - Hyperprolactinemia, amenorrhea, galactorrhea, infertility
    - Symptoms can also occur with non-prolactin-secreting tumors ("stalk-section" effect, "macroprolactinemia" with "big prolactin")
- Clinical profile
  - Young female with primary or secondary amenorrhea and infertility, galactorrhea
- Noninvasive laboratory tests: Dexamethasone suppression, metyrapone stimulation, peripheral ovarian corticotropin-releasing hormone (CRH) stimulation

Demographics

- Age
  - Prolactinoma = 20-35 years, GH-secreting adenoma = 30-50 years
- Gender
  - Prolactinomas typically in females but can occur in males with delayed puberty, primary hypogonadism
  - Prolactinomas in men usually larger, more often cystic/hemorrhagic
- Epidemiology
  - 10-15% of all intracranial tumors (increasing due to improved imaging techniques)
    - 15-17% incidental finding at autopsy
    - 1% of microadenomas are multiple
  - Prolactin-secreting = 30-40% of symptomatic adenomas
  - Pathologically, microadenoma > > > macroadenoma
    - Most found incidentally (autopsy or imaging)
    - Pituitary "incidentaloma" seen in 6-27% of MR scans (common even in children)
    - 10-20% prevalence in general population (most are nonfunctioning)

Natural History & Prognosis

- Benign, slow growing
- Majority found incidentally

Treatment

- "Incidentaloma": Conservative (clinical, imaging follow-up unless change in size, ophthalmological/endocrinological evaluation)
- Functioning microadenomas
  - Medical (bromocriptine, other dopamine agonists, such as cabergoline) reduces PRL secretion to normal in 80%
  - Surgical (transsphenoidal) curative in 60-90%

DIAGNOSTIC CHECKLIST

Consider

- Intrapituitary "filling defect" may be benign nonneoplastic cyst, as well as incidental microadenoma

Image Interpretation Pearls

- Microadenomas **do** enhance but more slowly than normal pituitary, so dynamic studies are very helpful

SELECTED REFERENCES

1. Sonksen P et al: Pituitary incidentaloma. Clin Endocrinol (Oxf). 69(2):180, 2008

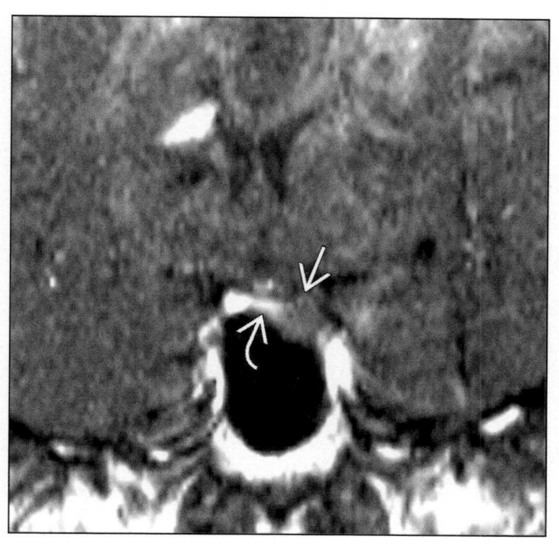

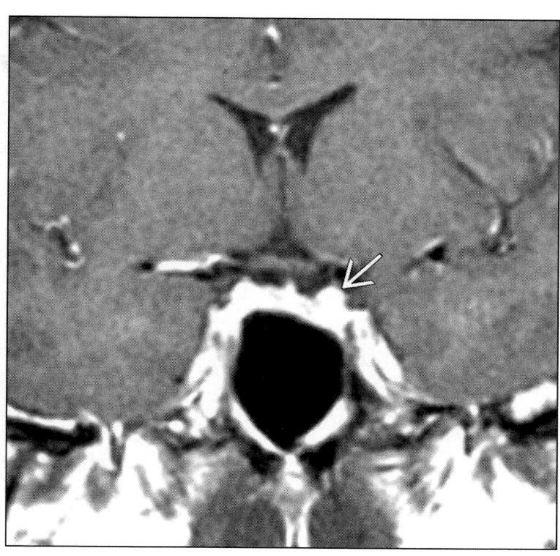

(Left) *Coronal dynamic T1WI C+ MR shows enhancement of a normal pituitary gland ➔. An 8 mm mass in the left side of the gland ➔ is well seen, because it is enhancing more slowly than the normal pituitary gland.* ***(Right)*** *After the dynamic enhanced sequence was complete, this coronal T1WI C+ MR shows the mass ➔ is now enhancing strongly on the delayed sequence. Were it not for the focal enlargement it is causing, the mass would be invisible on standard T1W C+ scan.*

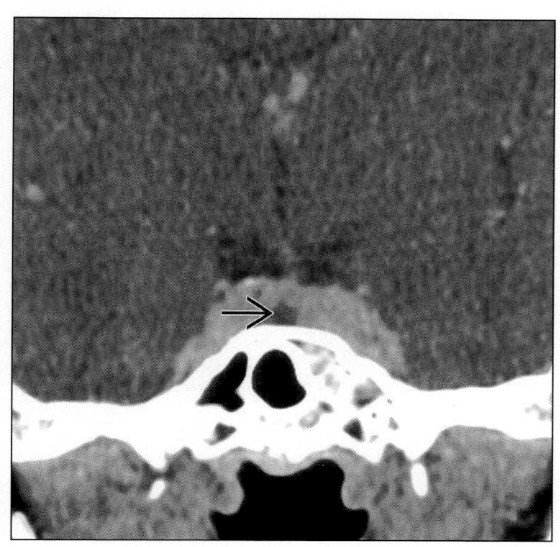

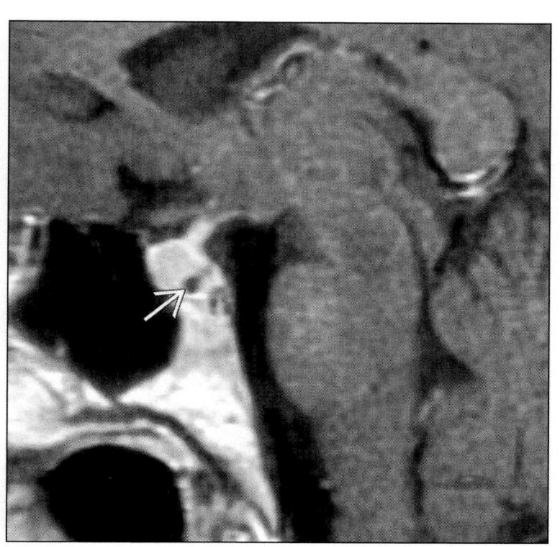

(Left) *Coronal CECT in an asymptomatic patient revealed a small nonenhancing focus ➔.* ***(Right)*** *Sagittal T1WI C+ MR in the same patient shows that the overall size of the gland is mildly enlarged and that the small lesion ➔ seen on the CT scan does not appear to enhance. Pituitary "incidentaloma" on contrast-enhanced CTs and MRs are common.*

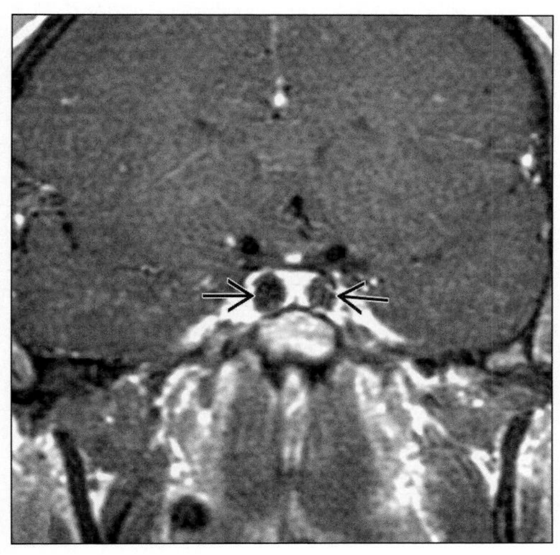

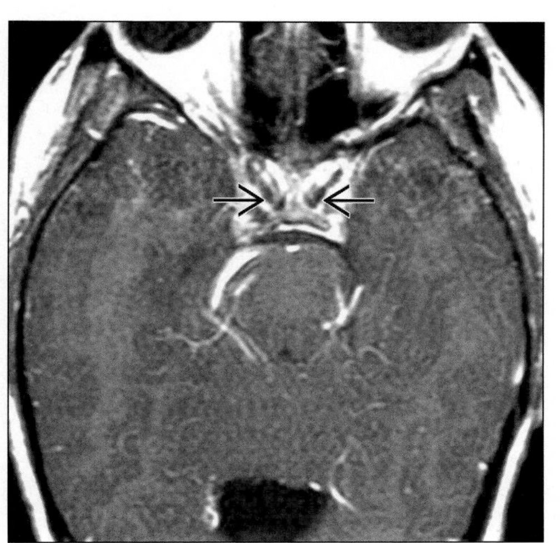

(Left) *Coronal T1WI C+ MR from an outside scan in a patient diagnosed with "pituitary microadenoma" shows paramedian ("kissing") internal carotid arteries (ICAs) ➔. These should not be mistaken for microadenomas, nor should upward displacement/bulging of the normal pituitary "squeezed" upward by the paramedian ICAs be misinterpreted as macroadenoma.* ***(Right)*** *Axial T1WI C+ MR in the same patient nicely demonstrates the paramedian ("kissing") ICAs ➔.*

PITUITARY MACROADENOMA

Key Facts

Imaging

- Upward extension of macroadenoma = most common suprasellar mass in adults
- Best imaging technique
  - MR with sagittal/coronal thin-section pre-contrast T1-/T2WI
- Findings
  - Sellar mass without separate identifiable pituitary gland
  - Mass **is** gland
  - Macroadenomas are usually isointense with gray matter
  - Cavernous sinus invasion difficult to determine (medial wall is thin, weak)
  - Enhance strongly, often heterogeneously

Top Differential Diagnoses

- Pituitary hyperplasia
- Saccular aneurysm
- Meningioma (diaphragma sellae)
- Metastasis
- Lymphocytic hypophysitis
- Craniopharyngioma

Pathology

- WHO grade I
- MIB-1 > 1% suggests early recurrence, rapid regrowth
- Invasive adenoma > > pituitary carcinoma (rare)

Clinical Issues

- Beware! "Adenoma-like" mass in adolescent/ prepubescent males may represent hyperplasia secondary to end-organ failure

Diagnostic Checklist

- No matter how aggressive/invasive it looks, pituitary tumors are almost never malignant

*(**Left**) Coronal graphic shows a snowman-shaped or "figure of eight" sellar/suprasellar mass ⇾. Small foci of hemorrhage → and cystic change ⇾ are present within the lesion. The pituitary gland cannot be identified separate from the mass; indeed, the gland IS the mass. (**Right**) Gross pathology shows a pituitary macroadenoma that extends upward through the diaphragma sellae into the suprasellar cistern → and laterally into the cavernous sinus ⇾, which is partially unroofed. (Courtesy R. Hewlett, PhD.)*

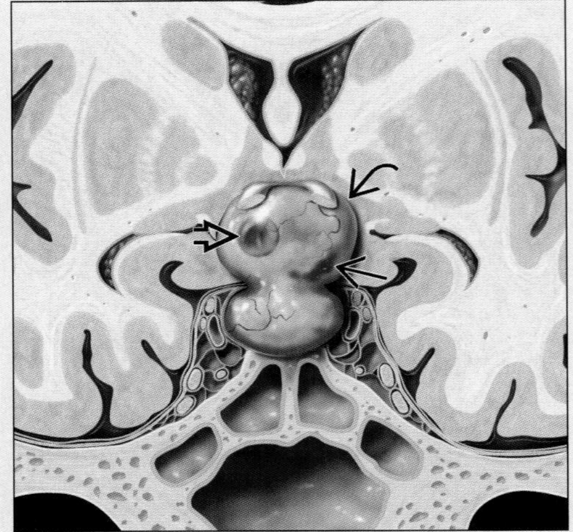

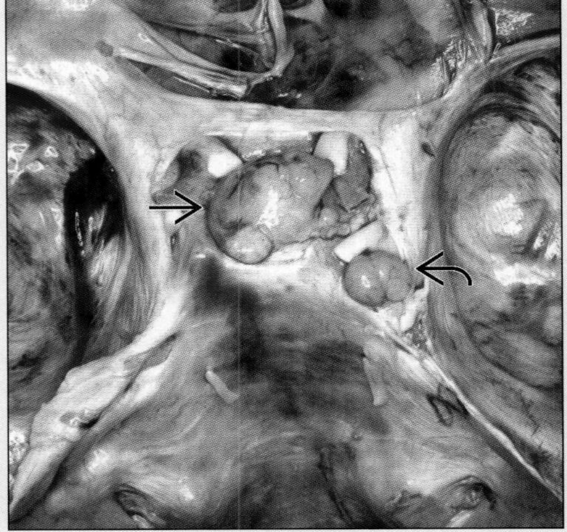

*(**Left**) Coronal T1WI MR shows the classic "figure of eight" or "snowman" appearance of pituitary macroadenoma ➔. The pituitary gland cannot be identified separate from the mass; the gland is the mass. (**Right**) Sagittal thin section T1WI FS MR in the same patient shows that the tumor ➔ expands and deepens the bony sella ➔. The tumor is isointense with gray matter.*

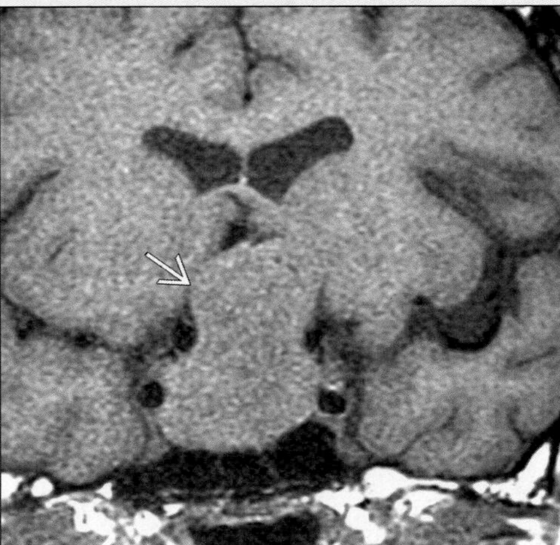

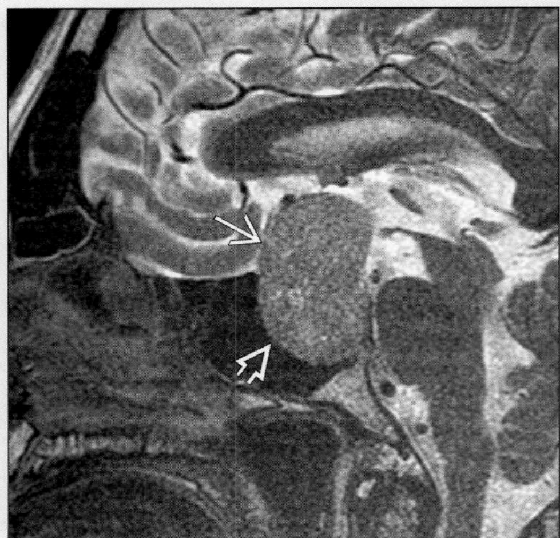

PITUITARY MACROADENOMA

TERMINOLOGY

Synonyms

- Macroadenoma, pituitary adenoma, prolactinoma

Definitions

- Benign neoplasm of pituicytes in adenohypophysis

IMAGING

General Features

- Best diagnostic clue
  - Sellar mass without separate identifiable pituitary gland; mass is gland
- Location
  - Most common: Intra- or combined intra-/suprasellar
    - Upward extension of macroadenoma = most common suprasellar mass in adults
  - Uncommon: Giant adenoma
    - May invade skull base, extend into anterior/ middle/posterior fossae
    - Can mimic metastasis or other malignant neoplasm
  - Rare: "Ectopic" pituitary adenoma
    - Sphenoid or cavernous sinus, clivus
    - 3rd ventricle, infundibulum
- Size
  - > 10 mm
  - "Giant": > 4 cm in diameter (< 0.5%)
- Morphology
  - Most common: "Figure of eight" or "snowman"
    - Indentation: Dural constriction caused by diaphragma sellae
  - Less common: Multilobulated margins

CT Findings

- NECT
  - Variable attenuation
    - Usually isodense with gray matter (typical)
    - Cysts, necrosis common (15-20%)
    - Hemorrhage (10%), Ca++ (1-2%)
- CECT
  - Moderate, somewhat inhomogeneous enhancement
- Bone CT
  - Large adenomas expand sella, may erode floor
  - Aggressive adenomas extend inferiorly, invade sphenoid, may destroy upper clivus

MR Findings

- T1WI
  - Usually isointense with gray matter
    - Subacute hemorrhage (T1 shortening)
    - Fluid-fluid levels may occur, especially with pituitary apoplexy
  - Posterior pituitary "bright spot" displaced into supradiaphragmatic level in 80% of cases
    - Posterior pituitary "bright spot" absent in 20% of large adenomas
  - Cavernous sinus invasion difficult to determine (medial wall is thin, weak)
- T2WI
  - Most common: Isointense with gray matter
  - Less common
    - Cysts (hyperintense), hemorrhage (signal varies with age)
    - Densely granulated, growth-hormone-producing adenomas often hypointense
  - Uncommon: High signal along optic tracts
    - Seen with 15-20% of adenomas that touch/ compress optic pathway
- FLAIR
  - Hyperintense to brain, gray matter
- T2* GRE
  - Blooms if hemorrhage present
- T1WI C+
  - Most enhance strongly but heterogeneously
    - Some macroadenomas (thyrotropin-secreting adenomas, necrotic adenomas) are hypoenhancing
    - Subtle/mild dural thickening ("tail") present in some cases
- MRA
  - Internal carotid arteries (ICAs) often displaced and encased (20%) but rarely occluded

Angiographic Findings

- Suprasellar extension splays supraclinoid ICAs, anterior choroidal arteries laterally
- Pituitary normally "blushes"
  - With macroadenoma, meningohypophyseal trunk may enlarge, causing prominent vascular staining

Other Modality Findings

- Cavernous/inferior petrosal sinus sampling may be helpful in evaluating ACTH-dependent Cushing syndrome

Imaging Recommendations

- Best imaging tool
  - Sagittal/coronal thin-section pre-contrast T1-/T2WI
  - T1WI C+ FS

DIFFERENTIAL DIAGNOSIS

Pituitary Hyperplasia

- 25-50% of females 18-35 years have upwardly convex pituitary
  - Usually < 10 mm unless pregnant, lactating
  - Homogeneous enhancement
  - Pituitary function normal
- Can occur with end-organ failure (e.g., ovarian, thyroid)
- If prepubescent female or young male has adenoma-looking pituitary, do endocrine work-up!

Saccular Aneurysm

- Usually eccentric, not directly suprasellar
- Pituitary gland visible, identified separate from mass
- "Flow void" common on MR
- Ca++ more common (rare in adenoma)

Meningioma (Diaphragma Sellae)

- Pituitary gland visible, can be identified **separate** from mass
  - Diaphragma sellae identifiable as thin, dark line between mass (above) and pituitary gland (below)
- Dural thickening more extensive than with adenoma

Metastasis

- Diffuse skull base invasion by adenoma may mimic more ominous disease
- Occasionally can see systemic metastases to stalk, pituitary gland

Lymphocytic Hypophysitis

- Can mimic adenoma clinically on imaging studies
- Most common in peripartum female

Craniopharyngioma

- Ca++, cysts; children > adults
- Rim/nodular > solid enhancement

PATHOLOGY

General Features

- Etiology
  - Same as microadenoma
- Genetics
  - Allelic loss of chromosome 11q in *MEN1* region
  - *MEN1* gene (probably tumor suppressor) involved in adenoma formation
- Associated abnormalities
  - Acromegaly, gigantism (growth-hormone-secreting macroadenomas)
  - MEN type 1 (parathyroid, pancreatic tumors with multicentric pituitary adenomas in 50%)

Staging, Grading, & Classification

- WHO grade I
- MIB-1 > 1% suggests early recurrence, rapid regrowth

Gross Pathologic & Surgical Features

- Reddish-brown, lobulated mass
- "Capsule" of macroadenoma is normal compressed pituitary gland
- Usual growth pattern: Bulges upward into suprasellar cistern
- Gross cavernous sinus invasion at autopsy in 5-10%, microscopic in 45%
- Invasive benign adenoma > > pituitary carcinoma (exceedingly rare)

CLINICAL ISSUES

Presentation

- Most common signs/symptoms
  - Endocrine abnormalities
    - 75% endocrinologically active (symptoms vary)
  - Visual field defect
    - 20-25% visual defect/cranial nerve palsy
    - Bitemporal hemianopsia
  - Rare: Nelson syndrome
    - Macroadenoma with elevated ACTH, MSH develops after bilateral adrenalectomy
- Clinical profile
  - Middle-aged female with bitemporal hemianopsia
  - Less common: Male with impotence, decreased libido, visual disturbance
  - Rare: Pituitary apoplexy (can be acute, life threatening)

Demographics

- Age
  - Peak age: 20-40 years
  - Uncommon: Presentation in childhood/adolescence
    - Pituitary adenomas account for < 6% of intracranial tumors in adolescents, even rarer in children
    - Approximately 60% are macro-, 40% are microadenomas
    - Beware! Adenoma-like mass in adolescent/prepubescent males may represent hyperplasia secondary to end-organ failure
- Gender
  - Varies with secretory type; prolactin-secreting tumors much more common in females
- Epidemiology
  - 10-15% of intracranial neoplasms
  - Prolactin-secreting: Most common (prevalence approximately 500 cases per 1,000,000)

Natural History & Prognosis

- Benign; usually slow but highly variable growth rate
  - Malignant transformation exceedingly rare
- "Giant" adenoma
  - Prolactin often > 1000 ng/mL
- Metastasizing pituitary adenoma
  - Occurs but very rare (both CSF, extra-CNS)
- Some adenomas (e.g., clinically silent corticotroph adenomas) behave in more aggressive manner with high recurrence rate
  - Apoptosis-related proteins (Bcl-2, BAX, p53) related to local control, recurrence

Treatment

- Resection (15% recurrence at 8 years, 35% at 20 years)
- Other: Medical, stereotaxic radiosurgery, conventional XRT

DIAGNOSTIC CHECKLIST

Consider

- Could sellar mass be nonneoplastic (e.g., hyperplasia, hypophysitis, etc.)?
- Check prolactin levels in male with giant invasive skull base mass; it may be a giant adenoma!

Image Interpretation Pearls

- No matter how aggressive/invasive it looks, pituitary tumors are almost never malignant

SELECTED REFERENCES

1. Kitajima M et al: Differentiation of common large sellar-suprasellar masses effect of artificial neural network on radiologists' diagnosis performance. Acad Radiol. 16(3):313-20, 2009

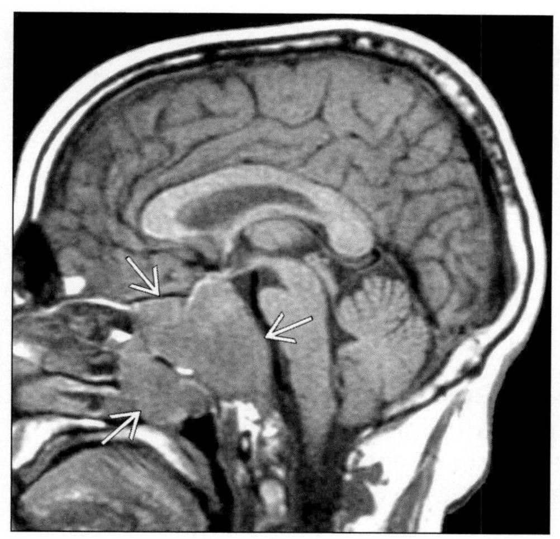

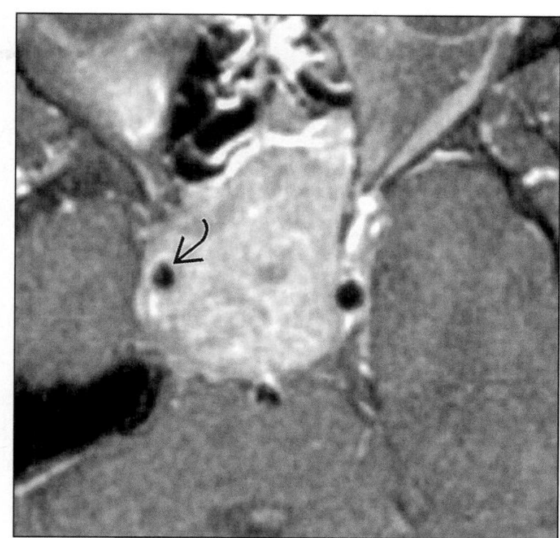

(Left) *Sagittal T1WI MR in a middle-aged man with gynecomastia and markedly elevated prolactin shows a huge invasive pituitary macroadenoma ➔ that has eroded the clivus, extending into the sphenoid sinus and nasopharynx.* ***(Right)*** *Axial T1WI C+ MR in the same patient shows the tumor invading and destroying the clivus. The tumor encases the right internal carotid artery ➔ but does not occlude it.*

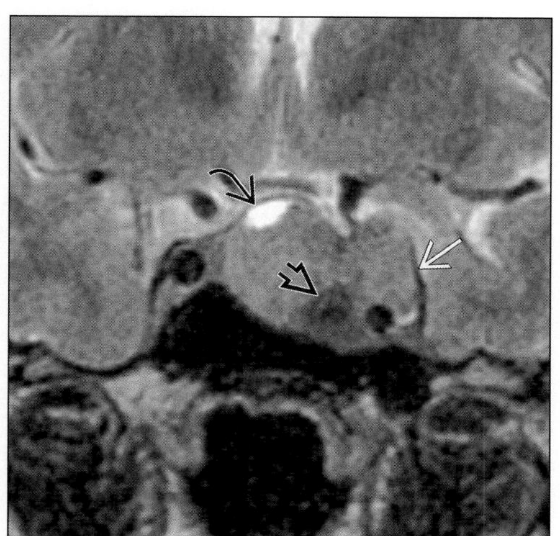

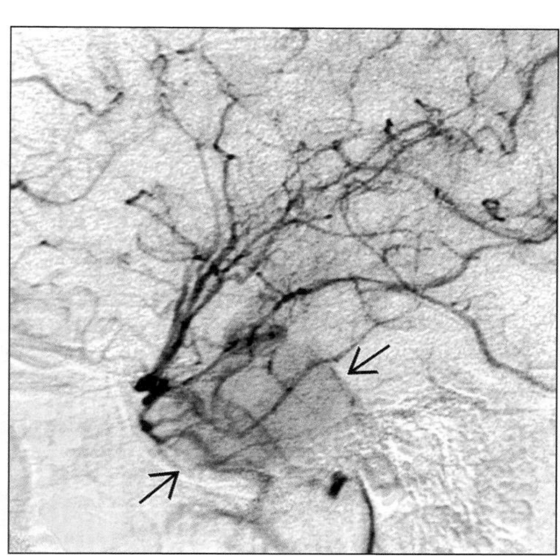

(Left) *Coronal T2WI MR of a pituitary macroadenoma shows a cyst ➔ and focus of hemorrhage ➔. The tumor invades the cavernous sinus ➔.* ***(Right)*** *Lateral early venous phase of selective internal carotid angiogram in a patient with a very large invasive macroadenoma shows striking tumor "blush" ➔. Macroadenomas are often very vascular.*

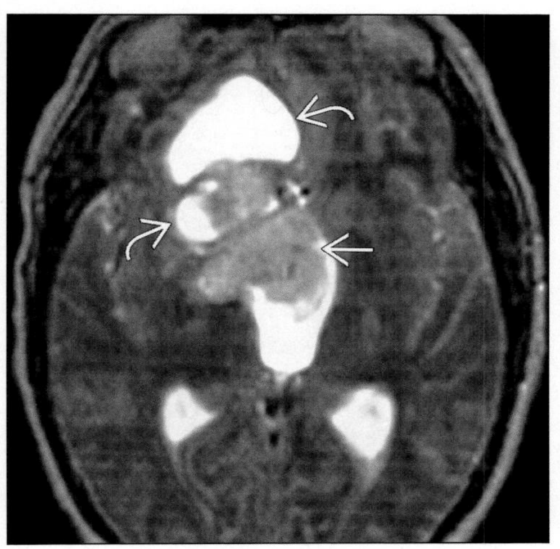

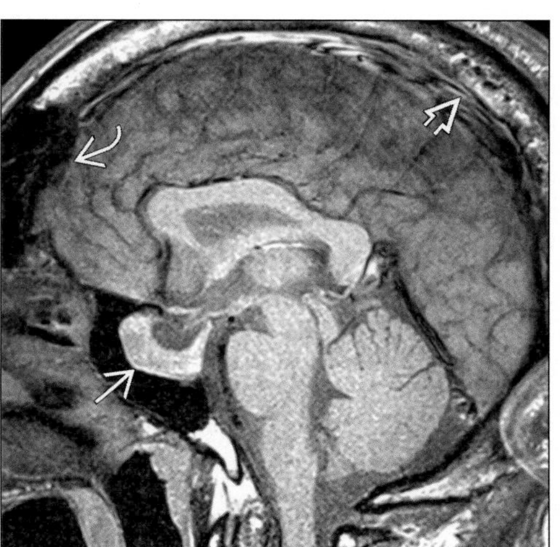

(Left) *Axial T2WI MR shows a macroadenoma ➔ with associated hyperintense cysts ➔. These probably represented trapped interstitial fluid in enlarged perivascular spaces.* ***(Right)*** *Sagittal T1WI MR in a 30-year-old man with longstanding acromegaly shows a pituitary macroadenoma invading the sphenoid sinus ➔. Note the thick skull ➔ and enlarged frontal sinuses ➔.*

PITUITARY APOPLEXY

Key Facts

Terminology

- Acute clinical syndrome with headache, visual defects/ophthalmoplegia, altered mental status, variable endocrine deficiencies
- Caused by either hemorrhage or infarction of pituitary gland
- Preexisting pituitary macroadenoma common

Imaging

- CT
  - Sellar/suprasellar mass with patchy or confluent hyperdensity
  - Peripheral enhancement, ± hemorrhage
  - May be associated with subarachnoid hemorrhage
- MR
  - Enlarged, hypointense (hemorrhagic) or hyperintense (nonhemorrhagic) pituitary on T2WI
  - "Blooming" if blood products present
  - Restricted diffusion within adenoma may be early sign of apoplexy
- Associated findings
  - Adjacent dural thickening, enhancement in 50%
  - Thickening of sphenoid sinus mucosa in 80%

Top Differential Diagnoses

- Pituitary macroadenoma (nonhemorrhagic)
- Craniopharyngioma
- Rathke cleft cyst
- Pituitary abscess
- Primary intrapituitary hemorrhage
- Giant thrombosed intrasellar aneurysm

Diagnostic Checklist

- Rim enhancement in snowman-shaped sellar/suprasellar mass may represent PA

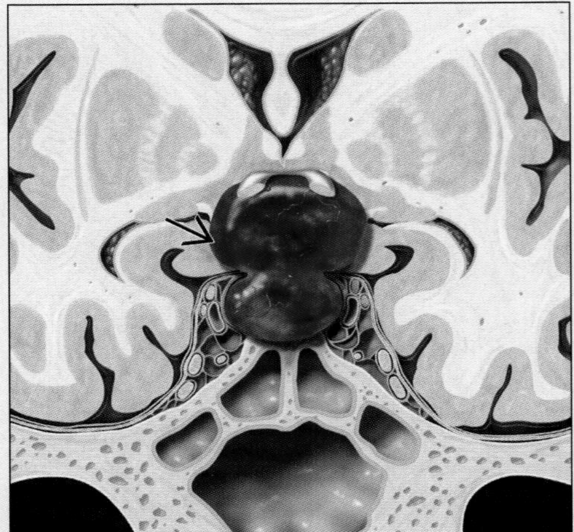

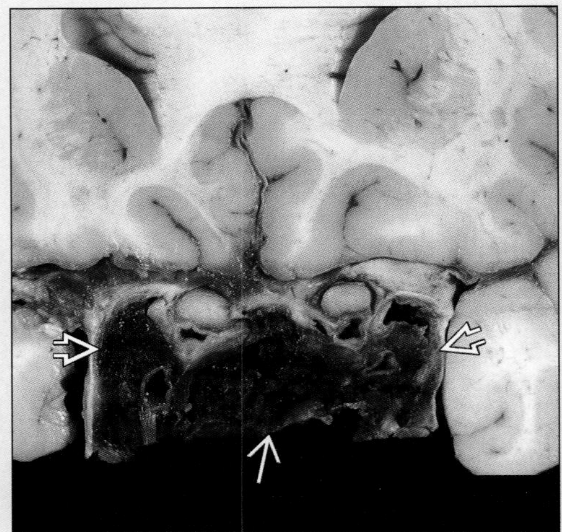

(Left) *Coronal graphic shows a macroadenoma with acute hemorrhage ⇨ causing pituitary apoplexy.* ***(Right)*** *Coronal gross pathology section through the sella turcica, in a patient who died from complications of pituitary apoplexy, shows hemorrhagic necrosis in the pituitary adenoma ➡ that extended into both cavernous sinuses ➡. (Courtesy R. Hewlett, PhD.)*

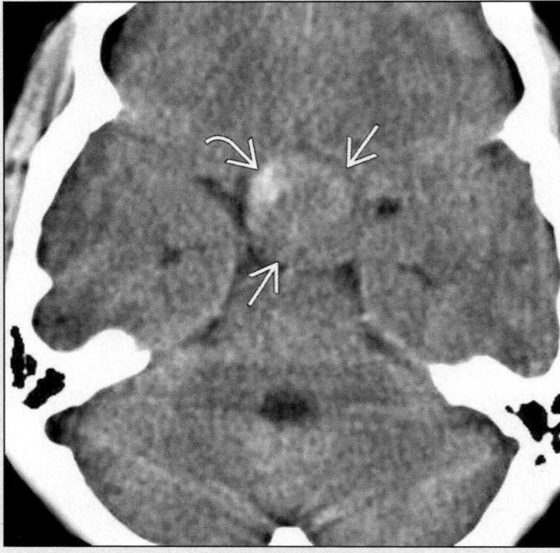

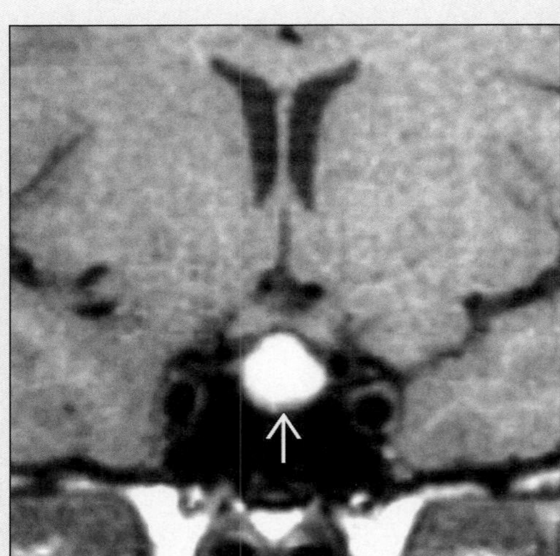

(Left) *Axial NECT in a patient with acute onset severe headache, bitemporal hemianopsia shows a mostly isointense mass in the suprasellar cistern ➡. Peripheral hemorrhage ➡ into large necrotic macroadenoma was found at surgery. (Courtesy S. Candy, MD.)* ***(Right)*** *Coronal T1WI MR in a patient with pituitary apoplexy shows subacute hemorrhage into a pituitary macroadenoma ➡.*

PITUITARY APOPLEXY

TERMINOLOGY

Abbreviations
- Pituitary apoplexy (PA)

Synonyms
- Pituitary necrosis

Definitions
- Acute clinical syndrome with headache, visual defects/ ophthalmoplegia, altered mental status, variable endocrine deficiencies
  - Caused by either hemorrhage or infarction of pituitary gland
  - Preexisting pituitary macroadenoma common

IMAGING

General Features
- Best diagnostic clue
  - Pituitary mass with peripheral enhancement, ± hemorrhage
- Location
  - Intra- or combined intra- and suprasellar
- Size
  - Variable but typically > 1 cm
- Morphology
  - "Snowman" or "figure of eight" intra- and suprasellar mass

CT Findings
- NECT
  - Acute
    - Sellar/suprasellar mass with patchy or confluent hyperdensity
    - May be associated with subarachnoid hemorrhage
  - Chronic: "Empty" sella
- CECT
  - Minimal or no enhancement
    - Rim enhancement suggestive (but not diagnostic) of pituitary apoplexy

MR Findings
- T1WI
  - Early acute: Enlarged gland, iso-/hypointense with brain
  - Late acute/subacute: Hyperintense
  - Chronic: Hypointense
    - "Empty" sella (filled with CSF)
    - Small isointense pituitary remnant
- T2WI
  - Acute
    - Enlarged, hypointense (hemorrhagic) or hyperintense (nonhemorrhagic) pituitary
    - Acute compression of hypothalamus, optic chiasm may cause hyperintensity along optic tracts
  - Subacute: Hyperintense
  - Chronic: Hyperintense ("empty" sella filled with CSF)
- FLAIR
  - Acute: Hyperintense
  - Chronic: Hypointense (CSF in "empty" sella suppresses)
- T2* GRE
  - "Blooming" if blood products present
- DWI
  - Restricted diffusion within adenoma may be early sign of apoplexy
  - ADC map: Markedly decreased signal intensity
- T1WI C+
  - Rim enhancement common
  - Adjacent dural thickening and enhancement in 50% of cases
  - Thickening of sphenoid sinus mucosa in 80% of cases

Angiographic Findings
- Conventional
  - Avascular or hypovascular mass effect

Imaging Recommendations
- Best imaging tool
  - MR
- Protocol advice
  - MR ± dynamic contrast-enhanced sequences; add GRE sequence, DWI

DIFFERENTIAL DIAGNOSIS

Pituitary Macroadenoma (Nonhemorrhagic)
- Clinical course usually subacute/chronic
- Predominately suprasellar, rather than intrasellar
- Cysts, small hemorrhagic foci may occur without necrosis

Craniopharyngioma
- Ca++, multiple cysts with variable contents, and mixed signal intensity common
- Can usually identify normal/compressed pituitary distinct from mass

Rathke Cleft Cyst
- Proteinaceous fluid may be hyperintense, mimic hemorrhage
- Cyst usually identifiable as separate from pituitary gland
- Minimal/no enhancement
- Clinical symptoms subacute/chronic

Pituitary Abscess
- Rare
- Clinical signs of infection may be absent
- May be difficult to distinguish from bland (ischemic) infarction on imaging studies
- T1 shortening along rim > center of mass
- Both apoplexy, abscess may restrict on DWI

Primary Intrapituitary Hemorrhage
- Hemorrhage into nonadenomatous tissue is rare
- Has been reported with infection (hantavirus), other neoplasms (germinoma)

Giant Thrombosed Intrasellar Aneurysm
- Acute thrombosis can present with panhypopituitarism, subarachnoid hemorrhage

PITUITARY APOPLEXY

- Patent aneurysm shows typical "flow void" on MR
- Partially/completely thrombosed aneurysm may show mixed-age laminated clot
- Rare

PATHOLOGY

General Features

- Etiology
  - Hemorrhagic or ischemic pituitary infarction
  - Preexisting macroadenoma common, but PA can occur with normal pituitary gland
- Genetics
  - Rare, MEN1 syndrome
- Associated abnormalities
  - Preexisting macroadenoma in 65-90% of PA cases
  - Multiple acute endocrine insufficiencies (pituitary, adrenal)
  - Both hemorrhagic and ischemic pituitary apoplexy typically occur in preexisting macroadenoma

Gross Pathologic & Surgical Features

- Hemorrhagic sellar/suprasellar mass
- Nonhemorrhagic (bland) pituitary infarction = swollen, edematous pituitary gland

Microscopic Features

- Pituicytes uniform but shrunken with dark pyknotic nuclei
- Most common adenoma = null-cell type

CLINICAL ISSUES

Presentation

- Most common signs/symptoms
  - Headache
    - 80% have panhypopituitarism
    - Visual impairment, ophthalmoplegia common
    - Occasionally can present with sudden onset ptosis, diplopia
  - Other signs/symptoms
    - Life-threatening pituitary insufficiency, acute adrenal crisis
    - Hypovolemia, shock, disseminated intravascular coagulation
  - Rare: Sheehan syndrome
    - Common: Loss of anterior pituitary hormone function long after index pregnancy (up to 15-20 years later)
    - Less common: Acute (peripartum) presentation
- Clinical profile
  - Male with pituitary adenoma or post-/peripartum female with hypovolemia, shock

Demographics

- Age
  - Mean age = 57 years
  - Rare < 15 years
- Gender
  - M:F = 2:1
- Epidemiology
  - PA occurs in approximately 1% of macroadenomas
  - Other reported clinical risk factors
    - Anticoagulation
    - Endocrinologic testing (dynamic pituitary function tests)
    - Radiation, bromocriptine therapy for existing macroadenoma
    - Trauma, surgery (especially cardiac)
    - Peri- or postpartum state
    - Elevated estrogen levels (pregnancy, exogenous hormones)
    - Diabetes

Natural History & Prognosis

- Varies from clinically benign event to catastrophic presentation with permanent neurologic deficits or death
- Long-term pituitary insufficiency common in survivors

Treatment

- Options, risks, complications
  - Early diagnosis, treatment of acute PA necessary to prevent morbidity/mortality
    - Best results with surgical decompression
    - Steroids, fluid/electrolyte replacement

DIAGNOSTIC CHECKLIST

Consider

- Could a high-density/hyperintense intrasellar mass represent something other than PA?
  - Giant intrasellar aneurysm
  - Craniopharyngioma or Rathke cleft cyst with high protein content

Image Interpretation Pearls

- Look for pituitary gland separate/distinct from mass (PA unlikely)
- Rim enhancement in snowman-shaped sellar/suprasellar mass may represent PA

SELECTED REFERENCES

1. Cho WJ et al: Pituitary apoplexy presenting as isolated third cranial nerve palsy with ptosis : two case reports. J Korean Neurosurg Soc. 45(2):118-21, 2009
2. Shirakawa J et al: Pituitary abscess with panhypopituitarism showing T1 signal hyperintensity of the marginal pituitary area: a non-invasive differential diagnosis of pituitary abscess and pituitary apoplexy. Intern Med. 48(6):441-6, 2009
3. Kaplun J et al: Sequential pituitary MR imaging in Sheehan syndrome: report of 2 cases. AJNR Am J Neuroradiol. 29(5):941-3, 2008
4. Semple PL et al: Pituitary apoplexy: correlation between magnetic resonance imaging and histopathological results. J Neurosurg. 108(5):909-15, 2008

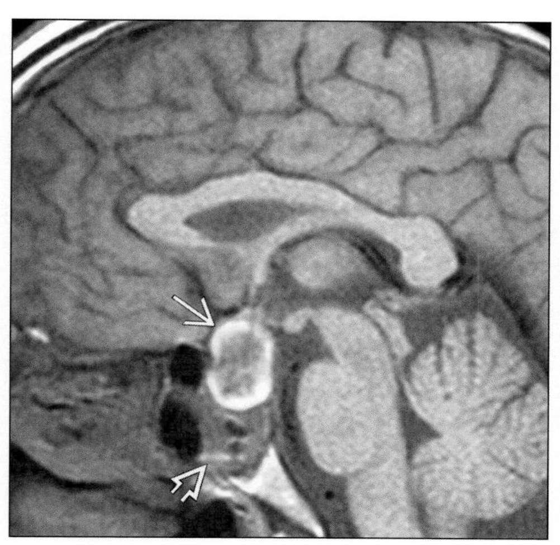

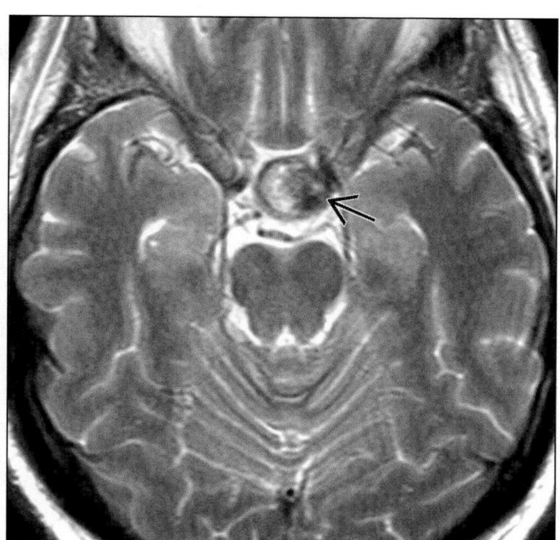

(Left) *Sagittal T1WI MR in a 53-year-old, hypertensive man with a 3-day history of lightheadedness, diaphoresis, nausea, and vomiting shows a mixed iso- and hyperintense intra- and suprasellar mass ➔. Note the associated acute sphenoid sinusitis ➔.* ***(Right)*** *Axial T2WI MR in the same patient shows very mixed signal intensity, with hypointense components predominating ➔. Hemorrhagic pituitary macroadenoma was found at surgery.*

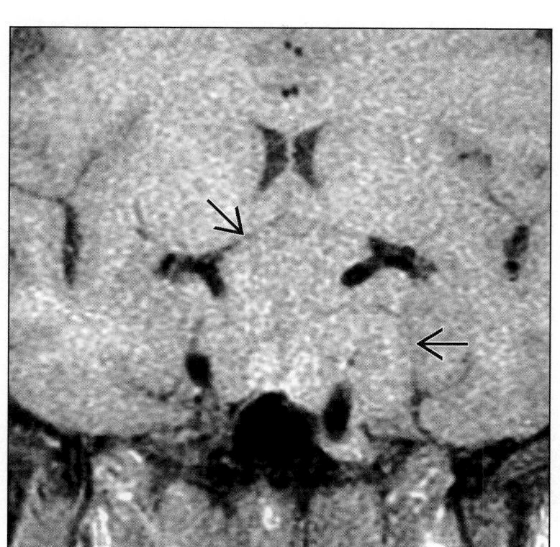

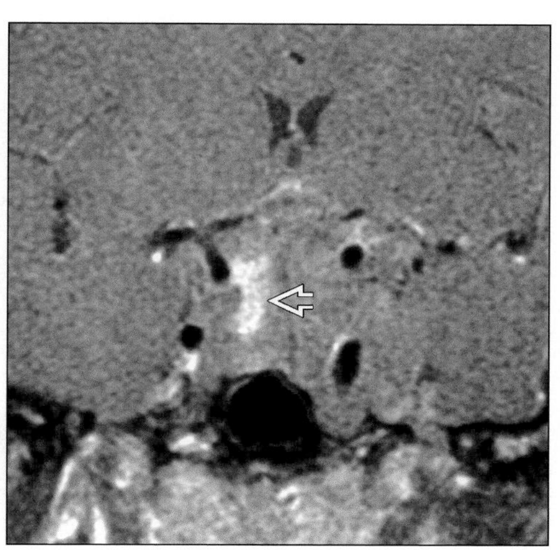

(Left) *Coronal T1WI MR in a 28-year-old man with sudden onset of headache and visual deficits, who was subsequently found to have panhypopituitarism, shows a large intra- and suprasellar mass ➔. The mass extends into both cavernous sinuses. Note the absence of T1 shortening, suggesting hemorrhage.* ***(Right)*** *Coronal T1WI C+ MR in the same patient shows very minimal enhancement of the mass ➔.*

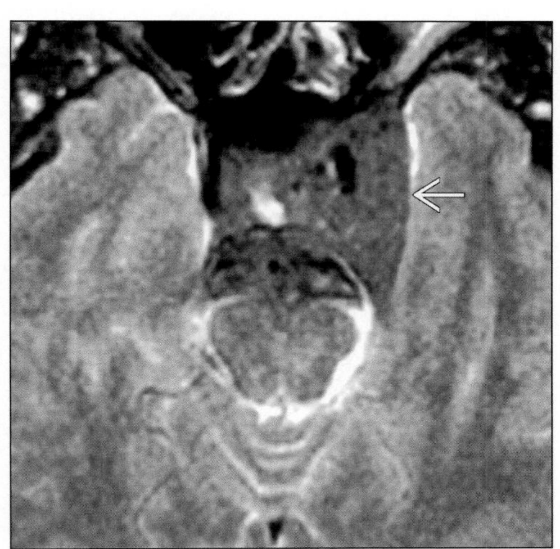

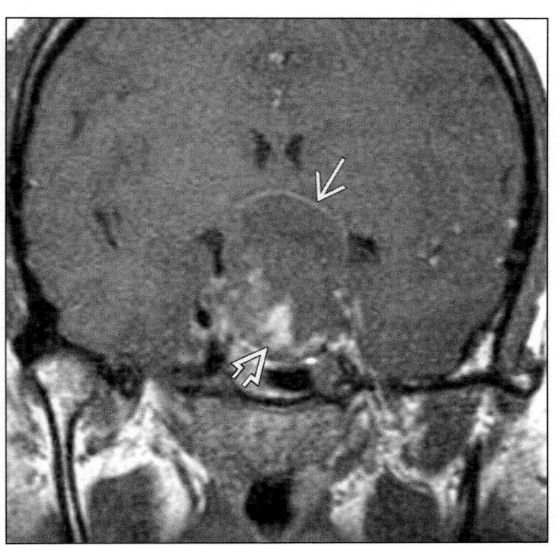

(Left) *Axial T2WI MR in the same patient shows that the mass appears strikingly hypointense. Extension into the left cavernous sinus ➔ is especially well appreciated on this sequence. Necrotic macroadenoma without hemorrhage was found at surgery.* ***(Right)*** *Coronal T1WI C+ MR in a young woman with sudden onset of headache and visual changes shows rim enhancement ➔ around a large intra- and suprasellar mass. Hemorrhage ➔ into a necrotic pituitary adenoma was diagnosed and confirmed at surgery.*

CRANIOPHARYNGIOMA

Key Facts

Terminology

- Benign, often partially cystic sellar region tumor derived from Rathke pouch epithelium
- 2 types
  - Adamantinomatous (cystic in childhood)
  - Papillary (solid in older adults)

Imaging

- General features
  - Multilobulated, often large (> 5 cm)
  - Occasionally giant, multi-compartmental
- CT
  - Cystic (90%), Ca++ (90%), enhance (90%)
- MR: Signal varies with cyst contents
  - Cysts variably hyperintense on T1-, T2WI
  - Solid portions enhance heterogeneously; cyst walls enhance strongly
  - Cyst contents show broad lipid spectrum (0.9-1.5 ppm)

Pathology

- Most common pediatric intracranial tumor of nonglial origin
- WHO grade I
- CPs arise from remnants of craniopharyngeal duct

Clinical Issues

- Bimodal age distribution
  - Peak 5-15 years; papillary CP > 50 years
- Pediatric patient with morning headache, visual defect, short stature
  - Endocrine disturbances include growth hormone (GH) deficiency
  - Others = hypothyroidism > adrenal failure > diabetes insipidus

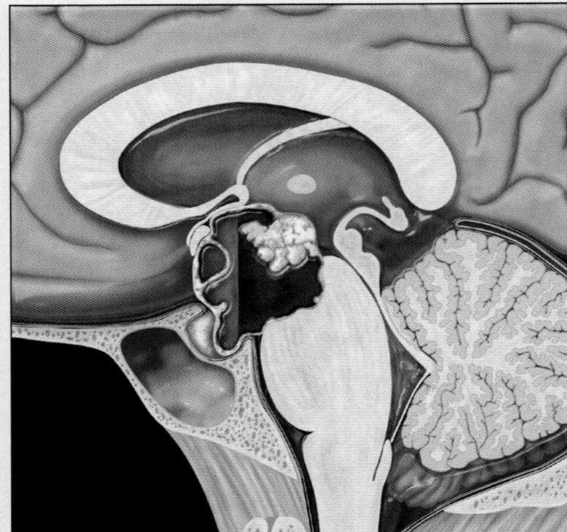

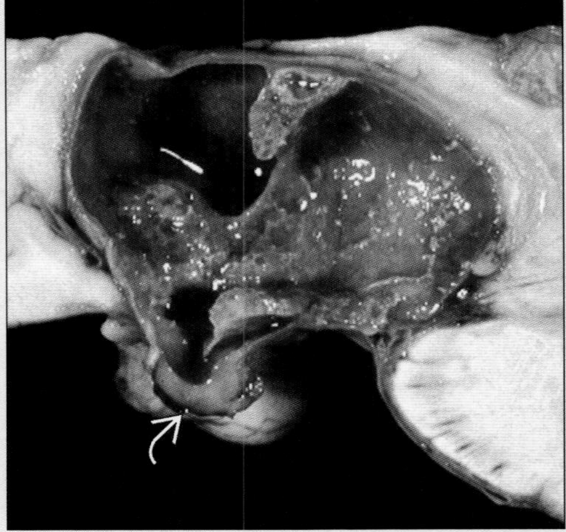

*(**Left**) Sagittal graphic shows a predominantly cystic, partially solid, suprasellar mass with focal rim calcifications. Note the small intrasellar component and fluid-fluid level. (**Right**) Sagittal gross pathology shows classic adamantinomatous craniopharyngioma with mixed solid, cystic components. Note the intrasellar extension ➔. (Courtesy R. Hewlett, PhD.)*

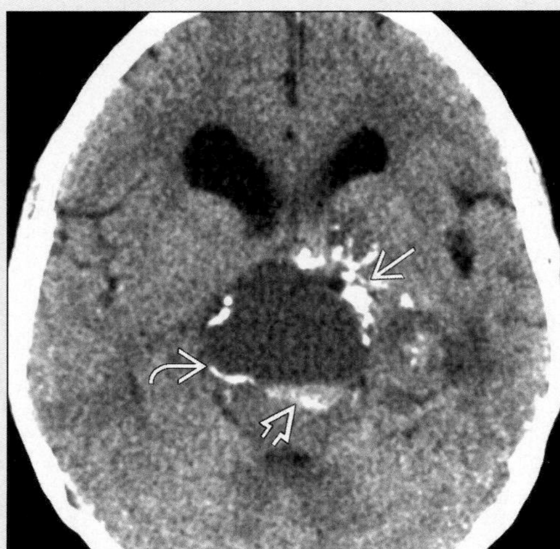

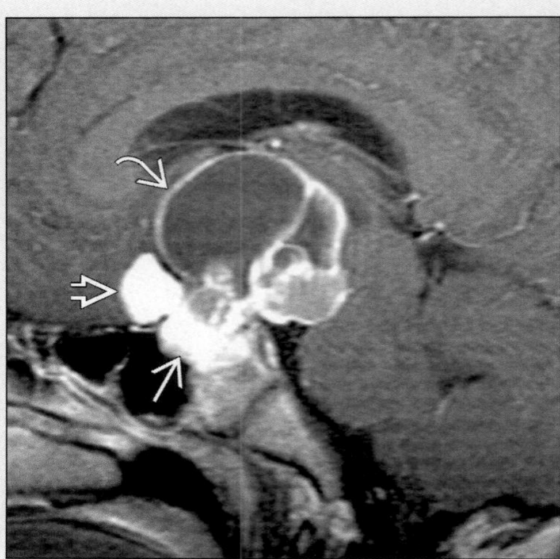

*(**Left**) Axial NECT shows classic findings of craniopharyngioma. Note the large suprasellar cyst with a fluid-fluid level ➔, rim ➔ and globular ➔ calcifications. (**Right**) Sagittal T1WI C+ MR shows a complex partially cystic suprasellar mass with an enhancing rim ➔ and solid components ➔. The multilobulated cysts contain fluid of different signal intensities. Note the large, suprasellar, smaller intrasellar ➔ components in this patient with classic craniopharyngioma.*

CRANIOPHARYNGIOMA

TERMINOLOGY

Abbreviations
- Craniopharyngioma (CP)

Synonyms
- Craniopharyngeal duct tumor, Rathke pouch tumor, adamantinoma

Definitions
- Benign, often partially cystic sellar region tumor derived from Rathke pouch epithelium
  - 2 types: Adamantinomatous and papillary

IMAGING

General Features
- Best diagnostic clue
  - CT: Partially Ca++ mixed solid/cystic suprasellar mass in child
  - MR: Complex signal intensity suprasellar mass
- Location
  - Surgical division of CPs into 3 groups
    - Sellar
    - Prechiasmatic
    - Retrochiasmatic
  - Imaging locations of CPs (adamantinomatous type)
    - Suprasellar (75%)
    - Suprasellar + intrasellar component (21%)
    - Entirely intrasellar (4%)
    - Often extends into multiple cranial fossae: Anterior (30%), middle (23%), posterior, &/or retroclival (20%)
  - Rare ectopic locations
    - Optic chiasm, 3rd ventricle
    - Other: Nasopharynx, paranasal sinuses, pineal gland, sphenoid (clivus), cerebellopontine angle
- Size
  - Variable; often large at presentation (> 5 cm)
    - Occasionally giant, multi-compartmental
- Morphology
  - Multilobulated, multicystic

CT Findings
- NECT
  - Adamantinomatous type
    - 90% mixed solid (isodense), cystic (hypodense)
    - 90% calcify
    - 90% enhance (solid = nodule; rim = capsule)
  - Papillary type: Often solid, isodense, rarely calcifies

MR Findings
- T1WI
  - Signal varies with cyst contents
    - Short T1 due to high protein content
    - Classic (adamantinomatous type)
      - Hyperintense cyst + heterogeneous nodule
    - Less common (papillary type)
      - Isointense solid component
- T2WI
  - Cysts are variably hyperintense
  - Solid component = heterogeneous (iso-/hyperintense, Ca++ portions hypointense)
  - Hyperintense signal in brain parenchyma adjacent to tumor may indicate
    - Gliosis, tumor invasion, irritation from leaking cyst fluid
    - Edema from compression of optic chiasm/tracts
    - Hypointense T2* = Ca++
- FLAIR
  - Cyst contents typically hyperintense
- DWI
  - Variable depending upon character of cyst fluid
- T1WI C+
  - Solid portions enhance heterogeneously; cyst walls enhance strongly
- MRA
  - Vascular displacement &/or encasement
- MRS
  - Cyst contents show broad lipid spectrum (0.9-1.5 ppm)

Imaging Recommendations
- Best imaging tool
  - MR with thin sagittal, coronal sequences
- Protocol advice
  - Pre-/post-contrast T1WI, T2, FLAIR, GRE, DWI, MRS

DIFFERENTIAL DIAGNOSIS

Rathke Cleft Cyst (RCC)
- Noncalcified, less heterogeneous
- Look for intracystic nodule
- Does not enhance
  - "Claw" sign (enhancing pituitary draped around cyst)
- Small RCC may be indistinguishable from rare intrasellar CP
- RCCs express cytokeratin 8, 20 (CPs generally do not)

Suprasellar Arachnoid Cyst
- No Ca++, enhancement

Hypothalamic/Chiasmatic Astrocytoma
- Solid or with small cystic/necrotic components
- Ca++ rare; robust enhancement common

Pituitary Adenoma
- Rare in prepubescent children
- Isointense with brain
- Enhances strongly
- Can mimic CP when cystic and hemorrhagic

(Epi-)Dermoid Tumors
- Minimal or no enhancement

Thrombosed Aneurysm
- Contains blood products
- Look for residual patent lumen, phase artifact

Germinoma or Mixed Germ Cell Tumor with Cystic Component(s)
- CSF spread common, Ca++ rare

CRANIOPHARYNGIOMA

PATHOLOGY

General Features

- Etiology
  - 2 proposed theories
    - CPs arise from remnants of craniopharyngeal duct
    - CPs arise from squamous epithelial cells in pars tuberalis of adenohypophysis
- Genetics
  - No known genetic susceptibility (rare reports of siblings, parent-child)
  - Small subset of CPs are monoclonal tumors, arise from oncogenes at specific loci
  - β-catenin gene mutations found in adamantinomatous CP (genetically distinctive)

Staging, Grading, & Classification

- WHO grade I
- MIB-1 labeling index > 7% predicts recurrence

Gross Pathologic & Surgical Features

- Solid tumor with variable cysts
- Adamantinomatous cysts often contain thick "crankcase oil" fluid
- Epithelial fronds penetrate adjacent hypothalamus/chiasm

Microscopic Features

- Adamantinomatous
  - Multi-stratified squamous epithelium with nuclear palisading
  - Nodules of "wet" keratin
  - Dystrophic Ca++
- Papillary
  - Sheets of squamous epithelium form pseudopapilla
  - Villous fibrovascular stroma
- Malignant transformation, distant metastases rare
  - May occur with varied histologies, resulting in poor prognosis

CLINICAL ISSUES

Presentation

- Most common signs/symptoms
  - Symptoms vary with location, size of tumor, age of patient
  - Visual disturbances
    - Bitemporal hemianopsia
- Other signs/symptoms
  - Endocrine disturbances
    - Growth hormone (GH) deficiency > hypothyroidism > adrenal failure > diabetes insipidus
    - Headaches
- Clinical profile
  - Pediatric patient with morning headache, visual defect, short stature

Demographics

- Age
  - Bimodal age distribution (peak 5-15 years, with smaller peak > 65 years)
    - Papillary CP > 50 years
- Gender
  - M = F
- Ethnicity
  - More common in Japanese children
- Epidemiology
  - Most common pediatric intracranial tumor of nonglial origin
  - Comprise 1.2-4% of all intracranial tumors across all ages
    - 6-9% of all pediatric intracranial tumors
    - Incidence = 0.5-2.5 new cases per 1,000,000 per year
  - ~ 54% of all pediatric sellar/chiasmatic region tumors are CPs

Natural History & Prognosis

- Typically slow-growing benign neoplasm
- Prognosis based upon size, extent of tumor at presentation
  - < 5 cm, recurrence rate (20%)
  - > 5 cm, recurrence rate (83%)
- Overall 10-year survival (64-96%)

Treatment

- Methods of primary treatment
  - Radical surgery = gross total resection
    - Complications = hypothalamic injury, endocrine symptoms, vasa vasorum injury, and pseudoaneurysm
  - Surgery may occur via craniotomy, transnasal, transorbital, or endoscopic routes
  - Limited surgery = subtotal resection, plus radiation therapy
  - Biopsy, cyst drainage, and radiation therapy
- Treatment for residual or recurrent tumor
  - Surgery, radiation therapy, or cyst aspiration
  - Cyst instillation with intracavitary radioisotopes, bleomycin, or other sclerosing agents

DIAGNOSTIC CHECKLIST

Consider

- Preoperative ophthalmologic and endocrine evaluations

Image Interpretation Pearls

- Use NECT to detect Ca++ if MR diagnosis is in question

SELECTED REFERENCES

1. Frangou EM et al: Metastatic craniopharyngioma: case report and literature review. Childs Nerv Syst. Epub ahead of print, 2009
2. Boongird A et al: Malignant craniopharyngioma; case report and review of the literature. Neuropathology. Epub ahead of print, 2008
3. Keil MF et al: Pituitary tumors in childhood: update of diagnosis, treatment and molecular genetics. Expert Rev Neurother. 8(4):563-74, 2008
4. Garrè ML et al: Craniopharyngioma: modern concepts in pathogenesis and treatment. Curr Opin Pediatr. 19(4):471-9, 2007

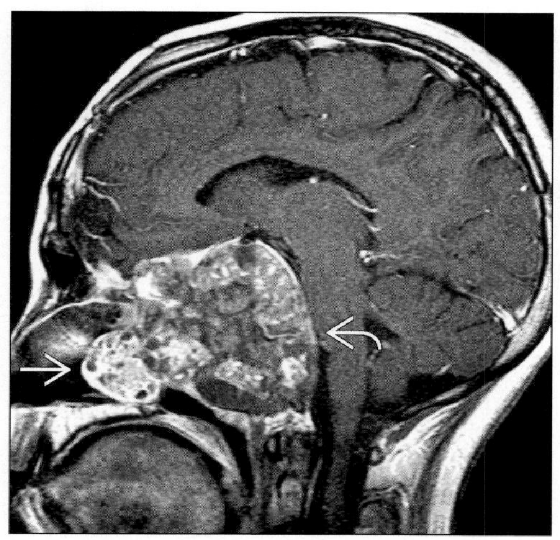

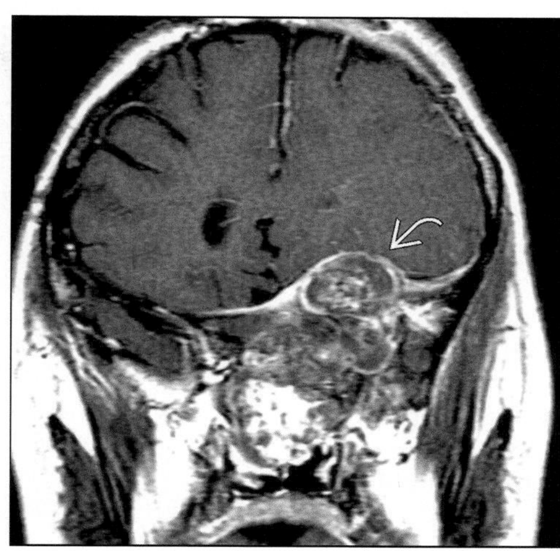

(Left) *Sagittal T1WI C+ MR of a large adamantinomatous craniopharyngioma in multiple compartments: Sella, suprasellar, nasopharyngeal ➔, & prepontine space ➔ with typical heterogeneous cystic & solid morphology. Note mass effect on optic chiasm and nerves, hypothalamus, & the circle of Willis, plus flattening of the belly of the pons. (Courtesy AFIP.)* ***(Right)*** *Coronal T1WI C+ MR in the same patient shows extension into the left anterior cranial fossa ➔. (Courtesy AFIP.)*

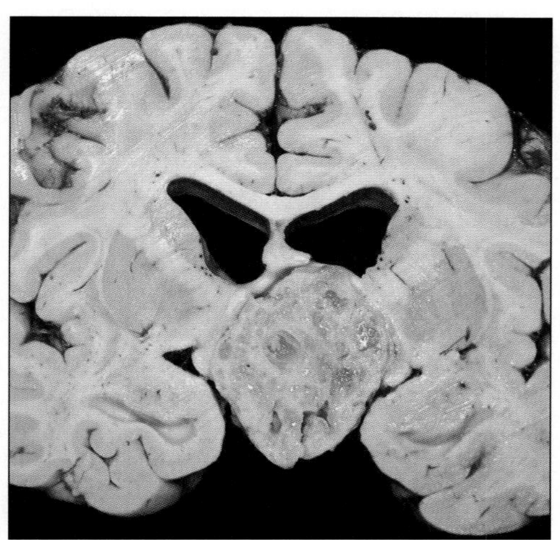

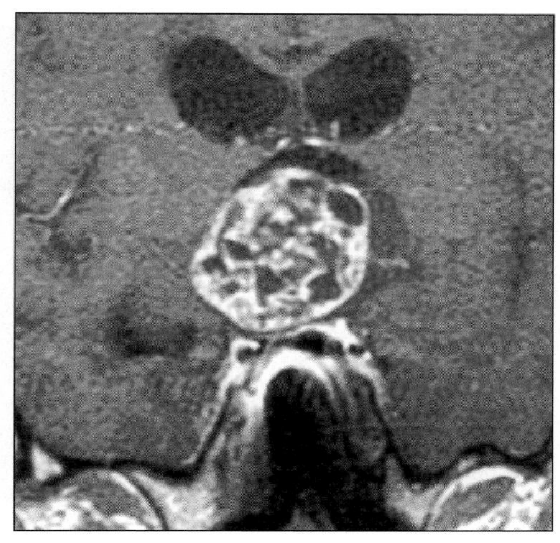

(Left) *Gross pathologic specimen displays a typical solid and cystic composition of an adamantinomatous craniopharyngioma. The cystic spaces contain a thick gelatinous material. In some cases of craniopharyngioma, the fluid is so dark brown that it is described by neurosurgeons as "crankcase oil." (Courtesy AFIP.)* ***(Right)*** *Post-contrast T1WI C+ MR in the same patient shows enhancing solid and nonenhancing cystic regions correlating well with the pathologic specimen. (Courtesy AFIP.)*

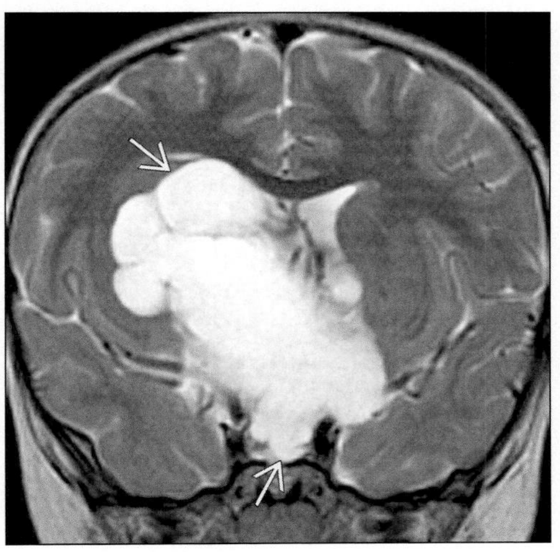

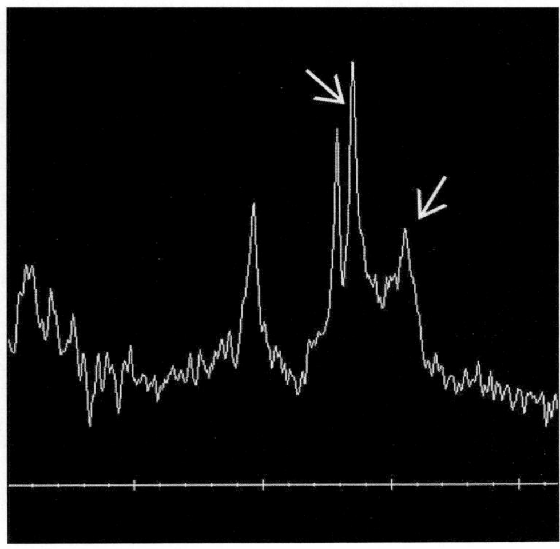

(Left) *Coronal T2WI MR in a 2 year old with a huge suprasellar mass shows multiple hyperintense cysts ➔. The intrasellar component is relatively small. The cyst fluid did not restrict on DWI (not shown).* ***(Right)*** *A short TE (35) H-MRS in the same patient acquired from the center of the cystic portion of the mass shows a large lipid-lactate peak ➔, characteristic of the cholesterol and lipid constituents found in craniopharyngiomas.*

PITUICYTOMA

Key Facts

Terminology

- Rare tumor arising from pituicytes, specialized glial cells in neurohypophysis and infundibulum

Imaging

- Enhancing sellar or suprasellar mass arising from neurohypophysis or infundibulum
- Isointense to hypointense solid mass
- Posterior pituitary "bright spot" often absent
- Variable enhancement, typically strong & uniform
- High-resolution MR of sella (2.5-3 mm slice thickness)
- Sagittal & coronal T1, coronal T2, post-contrast sagittal & coronal T1 with fat saturation
- Typically suprasellar (infundibular); pure intrasellar less common
- Well-demarcated, round or oval solid mass

Top Differential Diagnoses

- Pituitary adenoma
- Lymphocytic hypophysitis
- Pituitary hyperplasia

Pathology

- Distinct from granular cell tumor (WHO 2007)
- WHO grade I
- Hypervascular tumor at surgery

Clinical Issues

- Visual and endocrine dysfunction common

Diagnostic Checklist

- If mass is present posteriorly within gland or involves stalk, consider pituicytoma

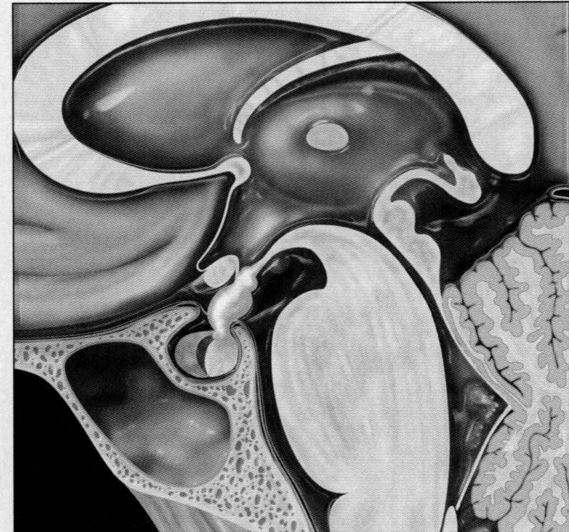

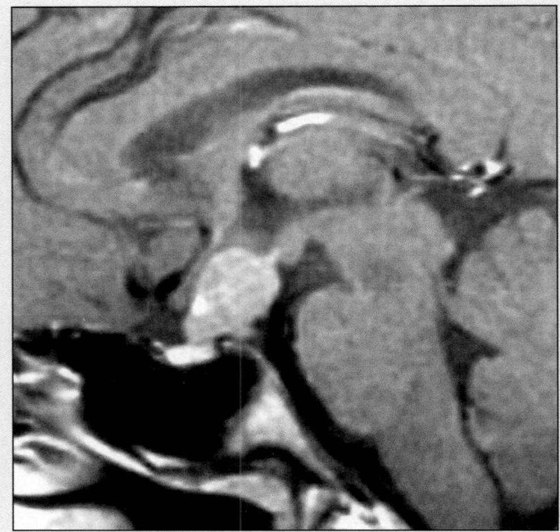

(Left) *Sagittal graphic shows a pituicytoma involving the infundibular stalk and neurohypophysis. A lobular suprasellar mass without significant compression of the adjacent structures is typical for this rare, low-grade, spindle cell glial neoplasm.* ***(Right)*** *Sagittal T1WI C+ MR shows a diffusely enhancing infundibular mass in this 22-year-old woman with delayed growth and hypopituitarism. After stable imaging over 5 years, this was presumed to be a pituicytoma.*

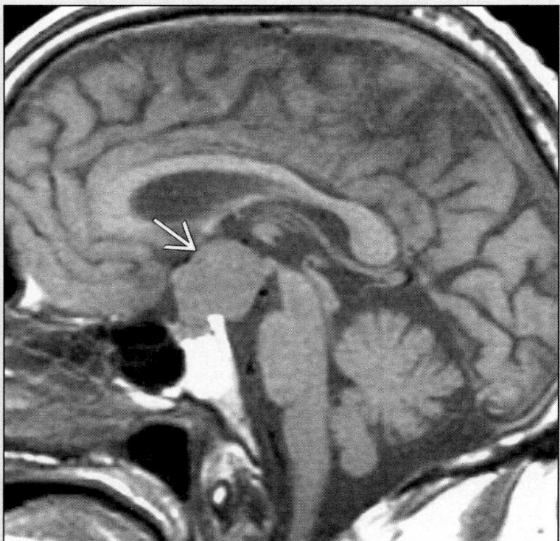

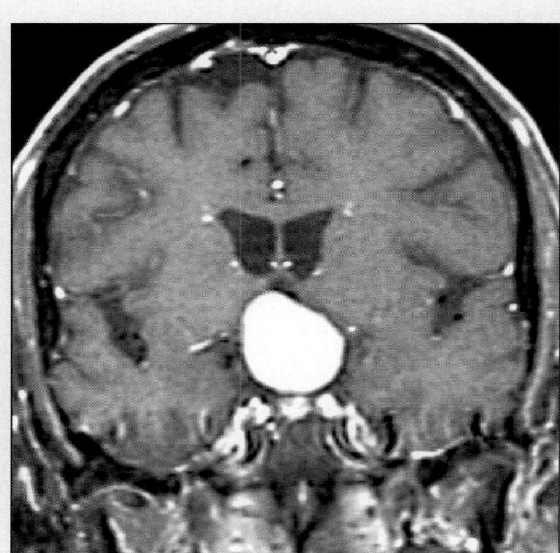

(Left) *Sagittal T1WI MR shows a well-delineated suprasellar mass ➡ extending into the posterior sella. Note the lack of a normal pituitary "bright spot," a common feature of pituicytoma.* ***(Right)*** *Coronal T1WI C+ MR in the same patient shows strong uniform enhancement of this large pituicytoma. Such enhancement is typical of these rare tumors of the neurohypophysis or infundibulum. These vascular tumors are WHO grade I. (Courtesy A.V. Hasso, MD.)*

Key Facts

Terminology
- Rare nonadenomatous, nonendocrine, nonfunctioning sellar tumor
- Thought to arise from folliculostellate cells of anterior pituitary

Imaging
- Indistinguishable from macroadenoma on imaging
- CT: Iso- to hyperdense sellar/suprasellar mass
- MR: Mostly isointense with white matter
  - Strong, typically uniform enhancement

Top Differential Diagnoses
- Pituitary macroadenoma
- Pituicytoma
- Granular cell tumor of neurohypophysis
- Metastasis

Pathology
- Gross appearance indistinguishable from macroadenoma
- Microscopic features
  - Interwoven fascicles of elongated spindled cells
  - Eosinophilic "oncocytic" cytoplasm
  - Mitotic rate typically low
- WHO grade I

Clinical Issues
- Tumor of adults (mostly 5th/6th decades)
- Symptoms indistinguishable from nonfunctioning pituitary macroadenoma
  - Visual defects
  - Panhypopituitarism
- Generally benign clinical course

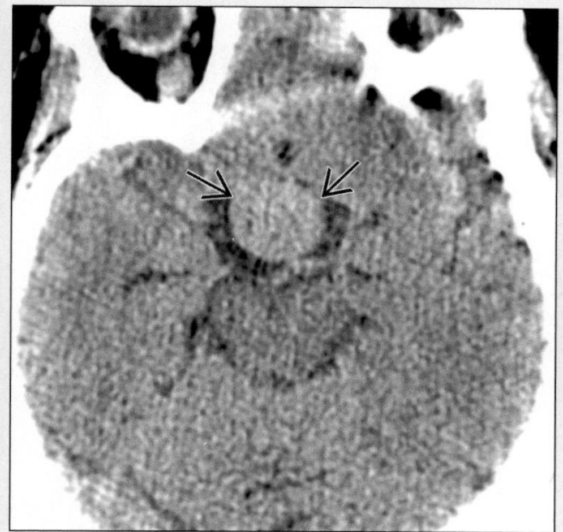

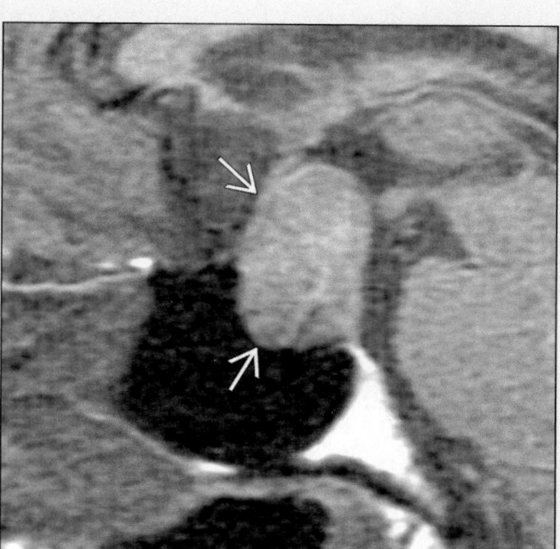

(Left) *Axial NECT in a 69-year-old woman with headaches and bitemporal hemianopsia shows a well-delineated, slightly hyperdense mass ➔ in the suprasellar cistern.* ***(Right)*** *Sagittal T1WI MR in the same patient shows an intra- and suprasellar mass ➔ that appears isointense with white matter. Note that the pituitary gland cannot be identified separate from the mass, nor can the infundibular stalk be distinguished from the rest of the lesion.*

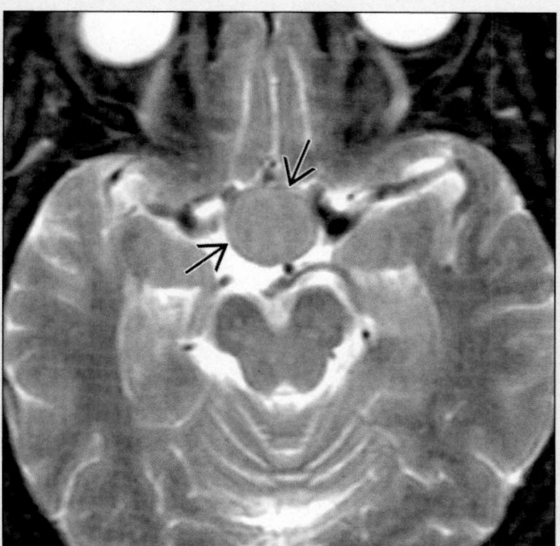

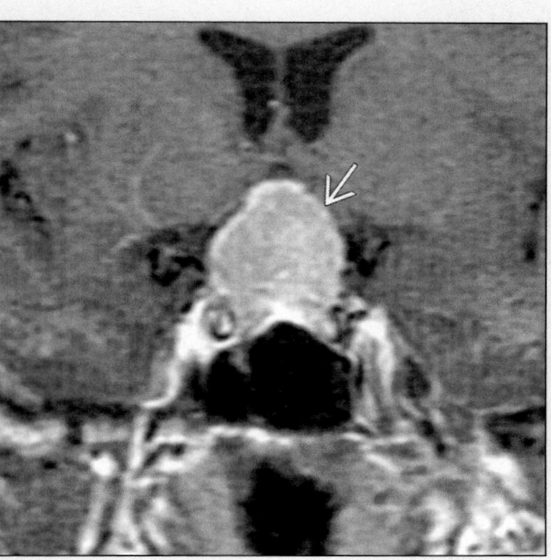

(Left) *Axial T2WI MR in the same patient shows that the mass ➔ is sharply circumscribed and remains isointense with white matter.* ***(Right)*** *Coronal T1 C+ MR shows the tumor ➔ enhances strongly and uniformly. Preoperative diagnosis was pituitary macroadenoma. Oncocytoma was found at surgery. Although imaging and clinical findings are indistinguishable from macroadenomas, oncocytomas are readily distinguished on histologic, immunohistochemical, and fine structural features.*

EMPTY SELLA

Key Facts

Terminology

- Sella partially filled with arachnoid-lined CSF collection
- Can be primary or secondary

Imaging

- Intrasellar CSF with pituitary gland flattened against sellar floor
  - Bony sella may be normal or moderately enlarged (secondary to pulsatile CSF)
  - Floor intact, not eroded/demineralized
  - Infundibular stalk, pituitary gland enhance normally
- Fluid exactly like CSF
  - Suppresses completely on FLAIR
  - Does not restrict on DWI

Top Differential Diagnoses

- Idiopathic intracranial hypertension
- Secondary intracranial hypertension
- Arachnoid cyst
- Pituitary apoplexy
- Pituitary anomalies
- Sheehan syndrome
- Epidermoid cyst

Pathology

- "Deficient" diaphragma sellae
  - Dural covering of sella is incomplete (widened)
  - Leaves large opening for infundibular stalk
  - Allows intrasellar herniation of arachnoid + CSF from suprasellar subarachnoid cistern above

*(**Left**) Sagittal graphic shows an empty sella. The extension of arachnoid with CSF through the diaphragma sellae ➔ flattens and displaces the pituitary gland ➲ posteroinferiorly against the sellar floor. (**Right**) Axial gross pathology shows a primary empty sella found incidentally at autopsy. Note the wide opening of the diaphragma sellae ➲ and CSF ➔ largely filling the bony sella. (Courtesy M. Sage, MD.)*

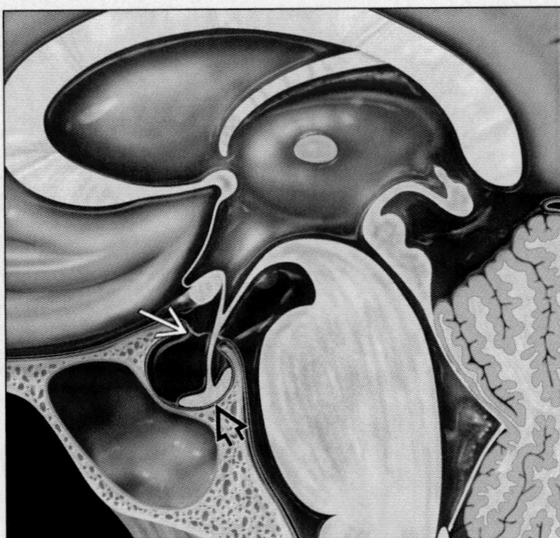

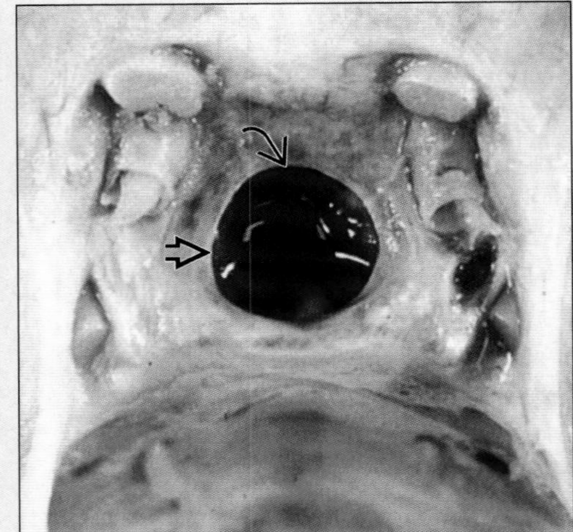

*(**Left**) Sagittal T1WI MR shows the incidental finding of a primary partially empty sella ➔, mostly filled with CSF. Note the absence of a posterior pituitary "bright spot," which is found in 15-20% of endocrinologically normal patients. (**Right**) Axial T2WI MR in the same patient shows the sella mostly filled with CSF ➔ from intrasellar herniation of the suprasellar subarachnoid space. Note that the infundibular stalk ➔ within the mostly empty sella is normally positioned.*

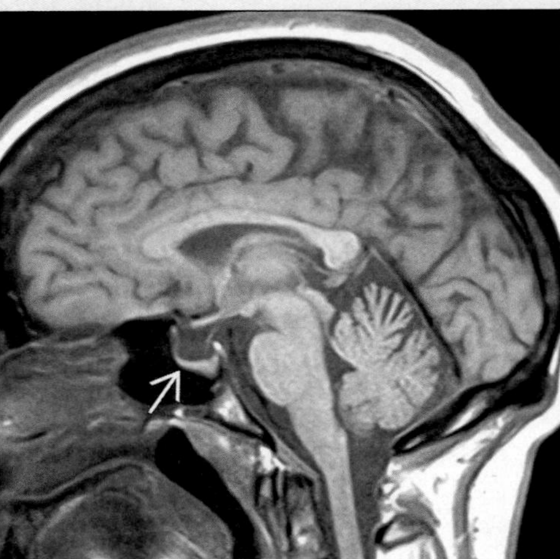

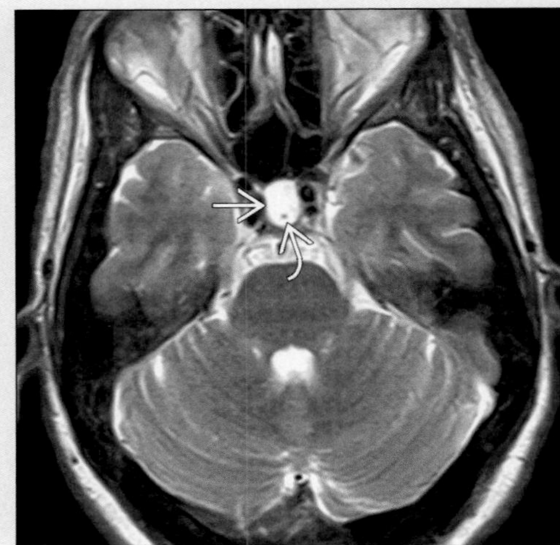

EMPTY SELLA

TERMINOLOGY

Abbreviations

- Empty sella (ES)

Definitions

- Arachnoid-lined, CSF-filled intrusion from suprasellar cistern through wide diaphragma sellae into bony sella turcica
- Sella turcica is partially filled with CSF
  - Rarely completely "empty"
  - Pituitary gland
    - Almost never completely absent
    - Thin, flattened rim of residual pituitary tissue
    - Generally at posteroinferior sellar floor
- Primary or secondary
  - Primary empty sella
    - Idiopathic
    - Normal variant
    - No history of trauma, surgery, radiation
    - Patients typically endocrinologically normal
  - Secondary empty sella
    - Many etiologies
      - Surgery
      - Radiation
      - Bromocriptine therapy
      - Trauma
      - Sheehan syndrome (postpartum pituitary necrosis)
      - Pituitary apoplexy
      - Pituitary abscess

IMAGING

General Features

- Best diagnostic clue
  - Intrasellar CSF with pituitary gland flattened against sellar floor
  - Bony sella may be normal or large
- Location
  - Intrasellar CSF
- Size
  - Variable

Imaging Recommendations

- Best imaging tool
  - Sagittal T1WI
  - Coronal T2WI

CT Findings

- NECT
  - CSF-like herniation of CSF into bony sella
    - Bony sella typically appears normal
  - May also be moderately enlarged (secondary to pulsatile CSF)
    - Floor intact, not eroded/demineralized
- CECT
  - Infundibular stalk and pituitary gland enhance normally
  - Occasionally intrasellar CSF collection may be asymmetric
    - Stalk may appear tilted to 1 side

MR Findings

- T1WI
  - Primary empty sella
    - Fluid looks exactly like CSF
    - Stalk usually midline
      - Stalk may be tilted to 1 side if intrasellar CSF herniation is asymmetric
    - 3rd ventricle, hypothalamus usually normal
      - Rare: Herniation of optic chiasm, anterior 3rd ventricle into sella
  - Secondary empty sella
    - Look for changes of transsphenoidal hypophysectomy
      - Defect in sellar floor
      - Fat packing
    - May cause distortion of stalk, chiasm
      - Stalk & pituitary remnant(s) may be scarred/ adhesed to side or bottom of sella turcica
- T2WI
  - Fluid exactly like CSF
- FLAIR
  - Intrasellar fluid suppresses completely on FLAIR
- DWI
  - No restriction
- T1WI C+
  - Primary empty sella
    - Stalk, gland enhance normally
    - No other abnormalities
  - Secondary empty sella
    - Gland and stalk may be adhesed/distorted

DIFFERENTIAL DIAGNOSIS

Idiopathic Intracranial Hypertension

- "Pseudotumor cerebri"
- Usually obese female, 20-40 years
- Headache, papilledema
- Enlarged optic nerve sheaths ± empty sella
- Ventricles may appear slit-like
- Subarachnoid spaces (cisterns, surface sulci) may be small

Secondary Intracranial Hypertension

- Increased intracranial pressure caused by
  - Obstructive hydrocephalus (intra-/extraventricular)
  - Mass (neoplasm, etc.)
- Dilated anterior recesses of 3rd ventricle herniate into sella
- Look for mass, evidence for transependymal CSF migration

Arachnoid Cyst

- Suprasellar arachnoid cyst may herniate into bony sella
  - Bony sella often enlarged, eroded/expanded
- Look for 3rd ventricle displaced/elevated over CSF-containing mass

Pituitary Apoplexy

- Acute: Pituitary gland usually enlarged, not small
  - Usually hemorrhagic
  - Look for rim enhancement around periphery of enlarged, nonenhancing gland

- Chronic: May cause empty sella

Pituitary Anomalies

- Ectopic posterior pituitary "bright spot"
  - May cause small pituitary gland
  - Infundibular stalk short, "stubby"
  - Bony sella often small, shallow-appearing
  - Sella can appear partially "empty"
- Persisting embryonal infundibular recess of 3rd ventricle
  - Can mimic empty sella (rare)
- Pituitary stalk duplication
  - Rare
  - Look for 2 thin stalks
  - Sella may appear partially empty

Sheehan Syndrome

- Original clinical description
  - Postpartum hemorrhage
  - Pituitary necrosis
  - Lactation failure
  - Hypopituitarism
- Anterior pituitary necrosis
  - Leaves small residual pituitary gland
  - Result = "empty sella"
- May occur years after pregnancy
- Slow clinical progression over years suggests factors other than ischemia may be involved
- Necrosis may be caused by antihypothalamus, antipituitary antibodies
- Pituitary autoimmunity may perpetuate hypopituitarism

Epidermoid Cyst

- True intrasellar epidermoid cyst very rare
  - Off-midline > midline
  - Usually extension from cerebellopontine angle epidermoid

PATHOLOGY

General Features

- Etiology
  - Primary empty sella
    - Deficient diaphragma sellae
      - Dural covering of sella is incomplete (widened)
      - Leaves widened dural opening for infundibular stalk
      - Allows intrasellar herniation of arachnoid + CSF from suprasellar subarachnoid cistern above
    - Pulsatile CSF may gradually enlarge sella
  - Secondary empty sella
    - Common: Surgery, bromocriptine therapy, radiation
    - Less common/rare: Pituitary apoplexy, pituitary abscess

Gross Pathologic & Surgical Features

- Diaphragma sellae appears widened, gaping
- Intrasellar herniation of arachnoid-containing CSF

CLINICAL ISSUES

Presentation

- Most common signs/symptoms
  - Incidental, asymptomatic
  - Headache, visual disturbances
  - Subtle endocrine disturbances in up to 80%

Demographics

- Age
  - Peak incidence between 40-49 years
- Gender
  - M:F = 1:5
- Epidemiology
  - 5-10% found incidentally on MR

Natural History & Prognosis

- Both primary and secondary empty sella usually benign, do not require treatment
- Hormonal replacement therapy may be required in some cases
- Surgery (rare)
  - "Chiasmapexy" to elevate optic chiasm if severe visual disturbances caused by inferior displacement of optic chiasm into empty sella
  - CSF rhinorrhea may require surgical intervention

DIAGNOSTIC CHECKLIST

Consider

- Look for endocrine abnormalities (e.g., panhypopituitarism, hypothyroidism)

Image Interpretation Pearls

- Intrasellar fluid follows CSF **exactly** on all sequences

SELECTED REFERENCES

1. González-Tortosa J. [Primary empty sella: symptoms et al:]. Neurocirugia (Astur). 20(2):132-151, 2009
2. Steno A et al: Persisting embryonal infundibular recess. J Neurosurg. 110(2):359-62, 2009
3. Pepene CE et al: Primary pituitary abscess followed by empty sella syndrome in an adolescent girl. Pituitary. Epub ahead of print, 2008
4. Schneider HJ et al: Pituitary imaging abnormalities in patients with and without hypopituitarism after traumatic brain injury. J Endocrinol Invest. 30(4):RC9-RC12, 2007

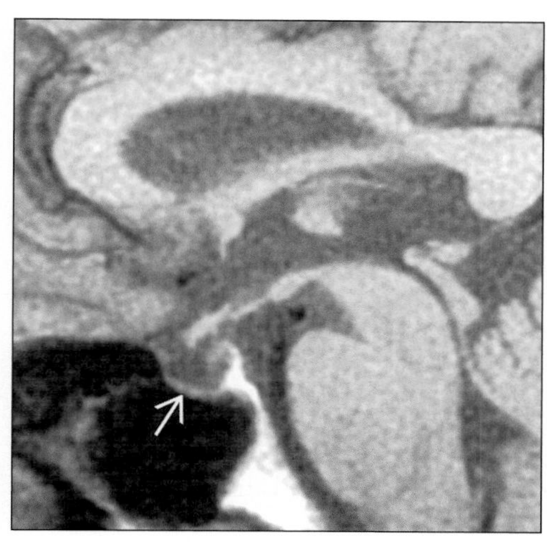

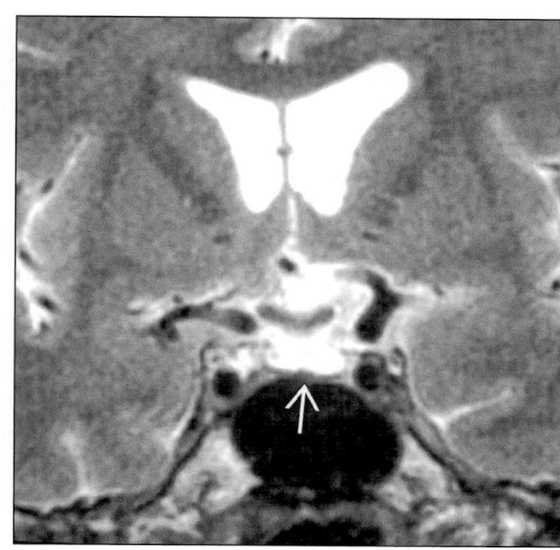

(Left) *Sagittal T1WI MR demonstrates a thinned pituitary gland ➔ along the floor of the mostly empty sella in a 34-year-old woman who had postpartum anterior pituitary gland necrosis (Sheehan syndrome) 10 years prior to imaging.* ***(Right)*** *Coronal T2WI MR in the same patient shows a thin, nearly inapparent pituitary gland remnant along the sellar floor ➔. The history distinguishes Sheehan syndrome from an incidental finding of partial empty sella.*

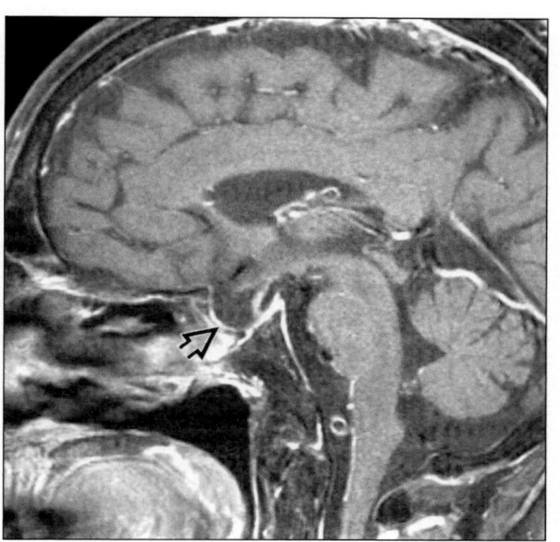

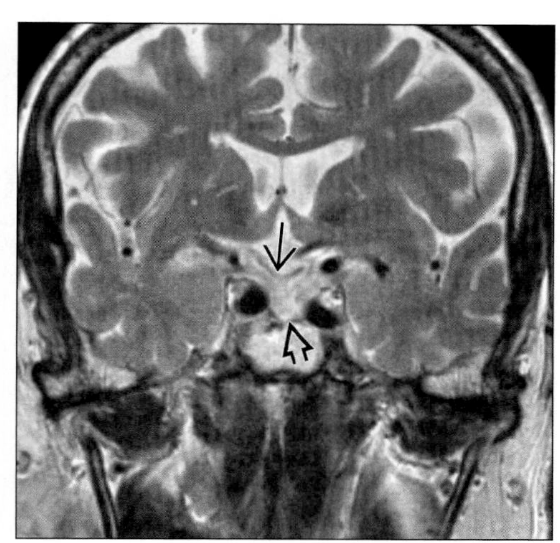

(Left) *Sagittal T1WI C+ FS MR shows an empty sella secondary to surgery for pituitary macroadenoma. Little pituitary tissue is apparent along the enlarged sellar floor ➔.* ***(Right)*** *Coronal T2WI MR of a secondary empty sella in the same patient demonstrates that the sella is filled with CSF ➔. Note the thinned optic chiasm ➔ retracted downward toward the sella.*

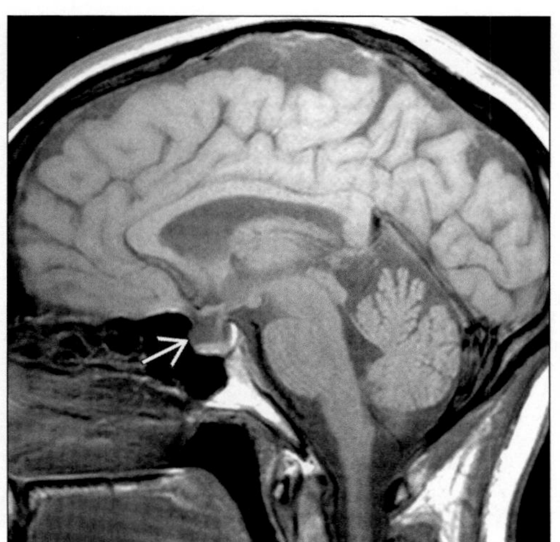

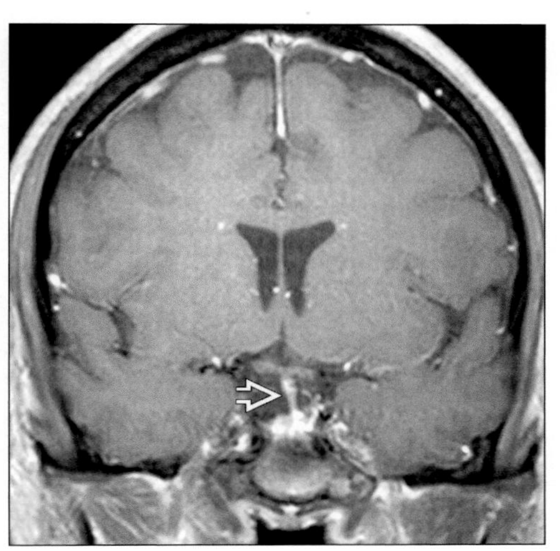

(Left) *Sagittal T1WI MR shows a partial empty sella ➔ in a 33-year-old, endocrinologically normal woman. The sella is largely, but not completely, filled with CSF.* ***(Right)*** *Coronal T1WI C+ MR in the same patient shows that the pituitary stalk tilts toward the left ➔. The pituitary gland appears normal; a somewhat off-midline infundibular stalk does not necessarily indicate pathology. Asymmetric intrasellar herniation of an arachnoid-lined CSF collection may cause this variant appearance.*

PITUITARY HYPERPLASIA

Key Facts

Terminology

- Upper limit of normal pituitary height varies with age, gender
  - Pregnant/lactating females: 12 mm
  - Young menstruating females: 10 mm
  - Males, postmenopausal females: 8 mm
  - Infants, children: 6 mm
- Nonphysiologic hyperplasia seen with
  - Hypothyroidism, Addison disease, or other end-organ failure
  - Some neuroendocrine neoplasms

Imaging

- Enlarged homogeneously enhancing pituitary gland with convex superior margin
- Best technique = high resolution MR
  - Sagittal/coronal T1; coronal T2
  - Dynamic coronal T1WI
  - Post-contrast T1 FS sagittal/coronal T1
  - 3-4 mm slice thickness

Top Differential Diagnoses

- Pituitary macroadenoma
- Pituitary microadenoma
- Lymphocytic hypophysitis
- Venous congestion

Pathology

- Growth hormone cell hyperplasia usually diffuse, occurs with neuroendocrine tumors
- Prolactin cell hyperplasia: Diffuse > nodular
- Corticotroph hyperplasia: Nodular or diffuse
- Thyrotroph hyperplasia
  - Longstanding primary hypothyroidism, may have associated prolactin hyperplasia
- Gonadotroph hyperplasia (e.g., Turner, Klinefelter)

*(**Left**) Coronal graphic shows physiologic pituitary hyperplasia. The gland is uniformly enlarged and has a mildly convex superior margin. (**Right**) Coronal T1WI C+ MR in a 27-year-old endocrinologically normal woman shows an upwardly convex pituitary gland that measures 10 mm in height. This is normal physiologic hyperplasia in a young menstruating female.*

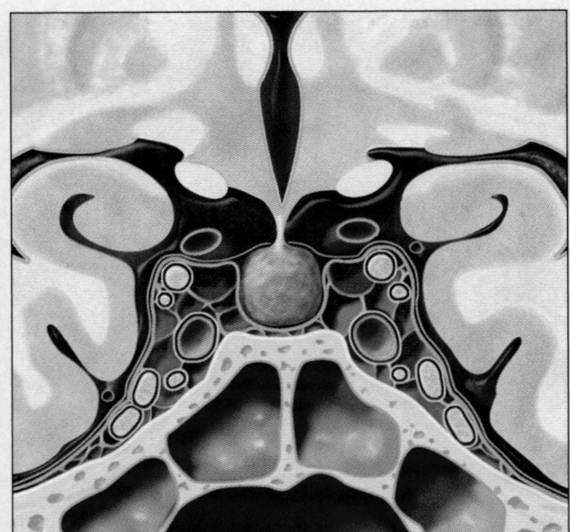

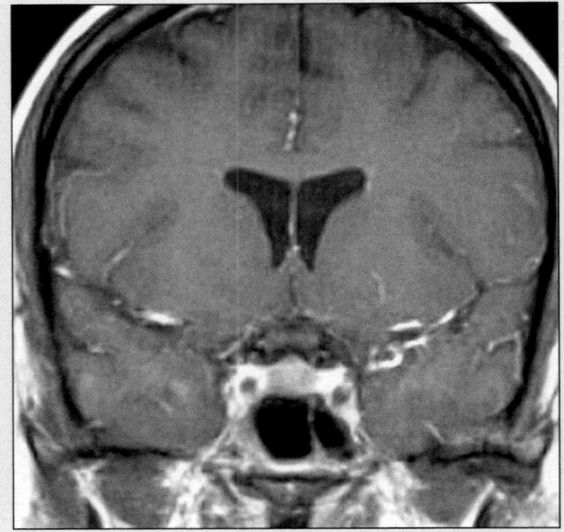

*(**Left**) Coronal T1WI C+ MR shows typical physiologic pituitary hyperplasia in a 28-year-old lactating woman. The gland has a mildly convex superior margin and measures nearly 14 mm in height. (**Right**) At follow-up 1 year later, coronal T1WI C+ MR reveals normal appearance to the pituitary gland with interval resolution of the postpartum physiologic enlargement.*

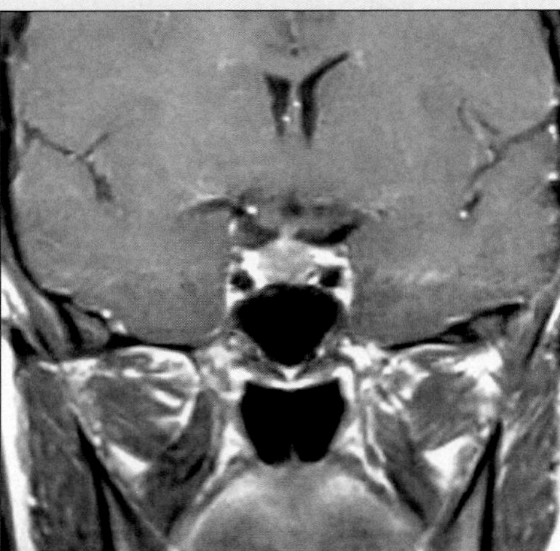

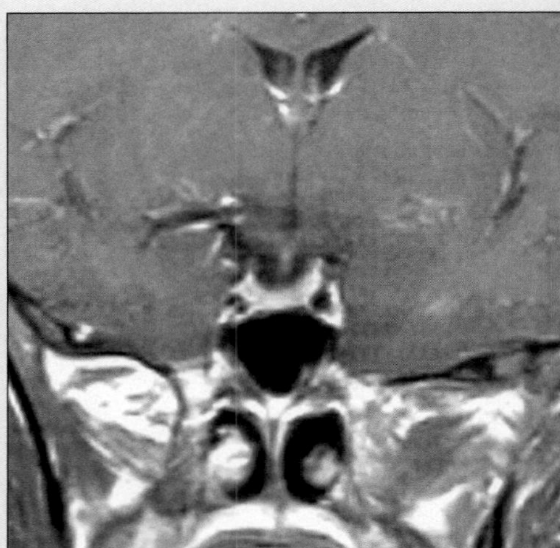

PITUITARY HYPERPLASIA

TERMINOLOGY

Definitions

- Upper limit of normal pituitary height varies with age, gender
  - Pregnant/lactating females: 12 mm
  - Young menstruating females: 10 mm
  - Males, postmenopausal females: 8 mm
  - Infants, children: 6 mm
- Nonphysiologic hyperplasia seen with
  - Hypothyroidism, Addison disease, or other end-organ failure
  - Some neuroendocrine neoplasms

IMAGING

General Features

- Best diagnostic clue
  - Enlarged homogeneously enhancing pituitary gland with convex superior margin
  - May be nodular, mimic pituitary adenoma
- Location
  - Sella; may extend into suprasellar region, compress adjacent structures
- Size
  - > 10 mm up to 15 mm

CT Findings

- NECT
  - Noncalcified pituitary gland enlargement
- CECT
  - Homogeneous enhancement

MR Findings

- T1WI
  - Isointense with remainder of pituitary gland
- T2WI
  - Isointense with remainder of pituitary gland
- T1WI C+
  - Diffusely enhancing gland is typical
  - May cause focal nodular enlargement
  - Dynamic MR: Enhances similar to remainder of gland

Imaging Recommendations

- Best imaging tool
  - MR with 3 mm slices, small FOV
- Protocol advice
  - Sagittal/coronal T1; coronal T2
  - Dynamic enhanced coronal T1WI
  - Post-contrast T1 FS sagittal/coronal

DIFFERENTIAL DIAGNOSIS

Pituitary Macroadenoma

- May be indistinguishable

Pituitary Microadenoma

- May be indistinguishable
- Enhances slower than normal gland on dynamic study

Lymphocytic Hypophysitis

- Enlarged gland &/or stalk
- Pregnant or postpartum females

Venous Congestion

- Can occur with intracranial hypotension
- Dural arteriovenous fistulas

PATHOLOGY

General Features

- Etiology
  - Response to endocrinologic stimulation by orthotopic or ectopic production of hypothalamic releasing hormones
    - Orthotopic: Response to end-organ failure
    - Ectopic: Related to neuroendocrine tumors
  - Physiologic hyperplasia occurs in pregnancy and lactation

Microscopic Features

- Nodular hyperplasia characterized by marked expansion of acini, architectural distortion
- Diffuse hyperplasia requires formal cell count
- Growth hormone cell hyperplasia usually diffuse, occurs with neuroendocrine tumors
  - Pancreatic islet cell tumor, pheochromocytoma, bronchial and thyroid carcinoid tumor
- Prolactin cell hyperplasia: Diffuse > nodular
  - May be seen with pregnancy and lactation, estrogen treatment, primary hypothyroidism, Cushing disease
- Corticotroph hyperplasia: Nodular or diffuse
  - Associated with Cushing disease, neuroendocrine tumors, untreated Addison disease, idiopathic
- Thyrotroph hyperplasia
  - Longstanding primary hypothyroidism, may have associated prolactin hyperplasia
- Gonadotroph hyperplasia (e.g., Turner, Klinefelter)

CLINICAL ISSUES

Treatment

- If related to hypothyroidism, regression after thyroid hormone therapy common
- Treat end-organ failure or neuroendocrine tumor

DIAGNOSTIC CHECKLIST

Consider

- Hyperplasia may mimic adenoma
  - Clinical information can help differentiate
- If imaging looks like adenoma in prepubescent male, consider end-organ failure!

SELECTED REFERENCES

1. Zhou J et al: Addison's disease with pituitary hyperplasia: a case report and review of the literature. Endocrine. 35(3):285-289, 2009

LYMPHOCYTIC HYPOPHYSITIS

Key Facts

Terminology

- Lymphocytic hypophysitis (LH), adenohypophysitis, primary hypophysitis, stalkitis
- Idiopathic inflammation of anterior pituitary

Imaging

- Thick stalk (> 2 mm + loss of normal "top to bottom" tapering)
- ± enlarged pituitary gland
- 75% show loss of posterior pituitary "bright spot"
- Enhances intensely, uniformly
- May have adjacent dural or sphenoid sinus mucosal thickening

Top Differential Diagnoses

- Pituitary hyperplasia
- Macroadenoma (prolactinoma)
- Metastasis
- Sarcoid
- Pituitary "dwarf"

Clinical Issues

- Peripartum female with headache, multiple endocrine deficiencies
- Middle-aged male with diabetes insipidus (lymphocytic infundibuloneurohypophysitis)
- Mean in females = 35 years, males = 45 years
- M:F = 1:8-9
- Often self-limited
- Unrecognized, untreated LH can result in death from panhypopituitarism
- Conservative care (steroids, hormone replacement)

Diagnostic Checklist

- LH can mimic adenoma

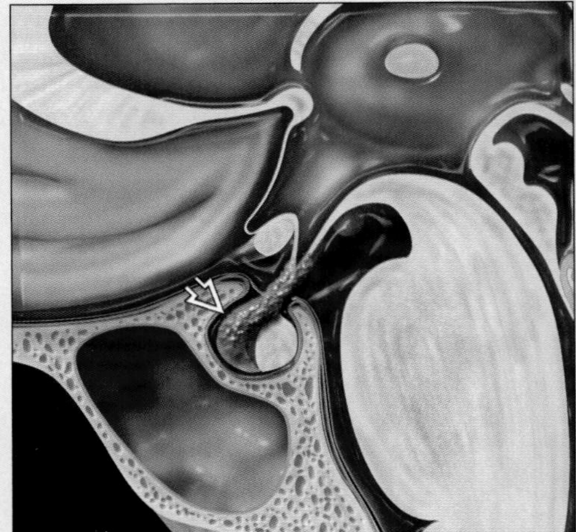

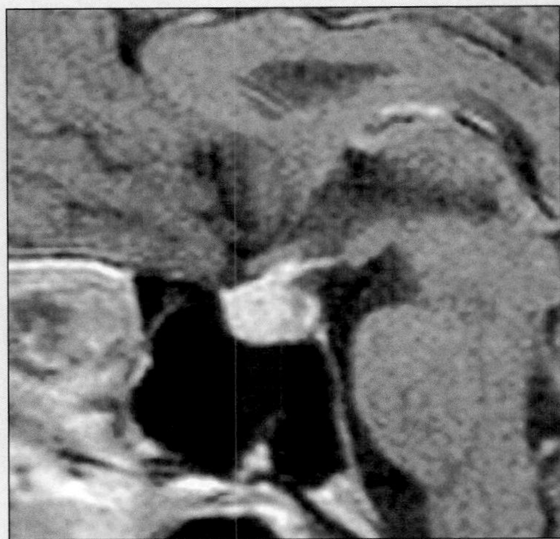

(Left) *Sagittal graphic shows lymphocytic hypophysitis. Note the thickening of the infundibulum as well as infiltration into the anterior lobe of the pituitary gland ➨.* ***(Right)*** *Sagittal T1WI C+ FS MR in a 41-year-old peripartum woman with headache and multiple endocrine deficiencies demonstrates enlargement of the pituitary gland and infundibular stalk, classic MR findings for lymphocytic hypophysitis. The lesion resolved with corticosteroids and endocrine replacement.*

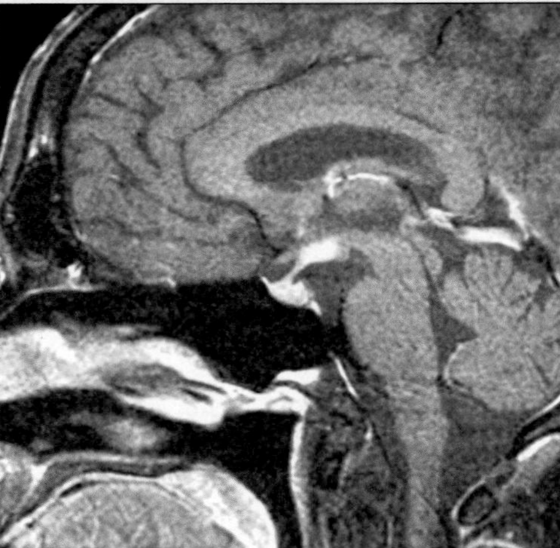

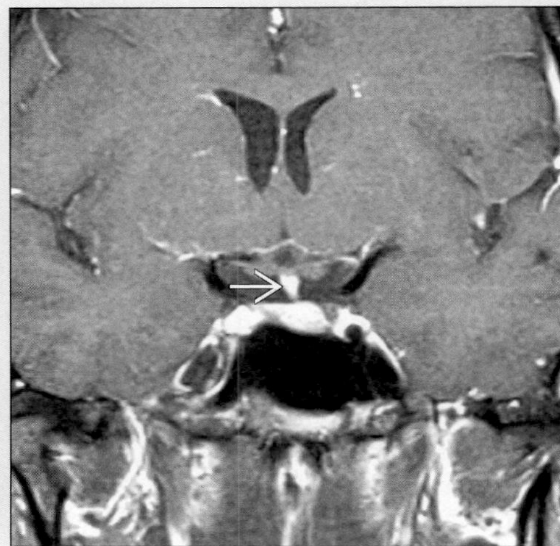

(Left) *Sagittal T1WI C+ FS MR in a middle-aged man who presented with diabetes insipidus shows a slightly thickened infundibular stalk and an infiltrating enhancing lesion in the hypothalamus. Imaging diagnosis was sarcoidosis vs. lymphocytic hypophysitis. Biopsy confirmed lymphocytic hypophysitis.* ***(Right)*** *Coronal T1WI C+ MR in a 50-year-old man with diabetes insipidus shows subtle bulbous enlargement of the upper stalk ➨. The diagnosis was lymphocytic infundibuloneurohypophysitis.*

LYMPHOCYTIC HYPOPHYSITIS

TERMINOLOGY

Abbreviations
- Lymphocytic hypophysitis (LH)

Synonyms
- Adenohypophysitis, primary hypophysitis, stalkitis

Definitions
- Idiopathic inflammation of anterior pituitary

IMAGING

General Features
- Best diagnostic clue
  - Thick nontapered stalk, ± pituitary mass
- Location
  - Supra-, intrasellar
- Size
  - Usually < 10 mm but may reach 2-3 cm
- Morphology
  - Rounded pituitary gland with infundibulum that appears thickened, nontapering, or bulbous

MR Findings
- T1WI
  - Thick stalk (> 2 mm + loss of normal "top to bottom" tapering)
  - ± enlarged pituitary gland
  - 75% show loss of posterior pituitary "bright spot"
- T2WI
  - Iso-/hypointense
- T1WI C+
  - Enhances intensely, uniformly
  - May have adjacent dural or sphenoid sinus mucosal thickening

Imaging Recommendations
- Best imaging tool
  - MR
- Protocol advice
  - Pre-contrast thin section (< 3 mm) sagittal, coronal T1- and T2WIs
  - Coronal "dynamic" T1WI C+ (may show delayed pituitary enhancement)

DIFFERENTIAL DIAGNOSIS

Pituitary Hyperplasia
- Stalk usually normal
  - In young females, late pregnancy/peripartum

Macroadenoma (Prolactinoma)
- Diabetes insipidus common in LH, rare with adenoma
- Posterior pituitary "bright spot" absent or displaced/deformed; sella enlarged/eroded

Metastasis
- Usually known primary (lung, breast, etc.)

Sarcoid
- Systemic disease often (**not** invariably) present
- Langerhans cell, Wegener, etc., can mimic LH

Pituitary "Dwarf"
- Stalk may appear short and "stubby"

PATHOLOGY

General Features
- Etiology
  - Uncertain; may be autoimmune

Gross Pathologic & Surgical Features
- Diffusely enlarged stalk/pituitary gland

Microscopic Features
- Acute
  - Dense infiltrate of B-, T-lymphocytes, plasma cells, occasionally eosinophils; ± lymphoid follicles
  - No granulomas, giant cells, or organisms; no evidence of neoplasm
- Chronic may demonstrate extensive fibrosis

CLINICAL ISSUES

Presentation
- Most common signs/symptoms
  - Headache, visual impairment
- Clinical profile
  - Peripartum female with headache, multiple endocrine deficiencies
  - Middle-aged male with diabetes insipidus (lymphocytic infundibuloneurohypophysitis)

Demographics
- Age
  - Mean in females = 35 years; males = 45 years
- Gender
  - M:F = 1:8-9
- Epidemiology
  - Rare (1-2% of sellar lesions)

Natural History & Prognosis
- Often self-limited
- Unrecognized, untreated LH can result in death from panhypopituitarism

Treatment
- Conservative (steroids, hormone replacement)

DIAGNOSTIC CHECKLIST

Image Interpretation Pearls
- LH can mimic adenoma!

SELECTED REFERENCES

1. Mirocha S et al: T regulatory cells distinguish two types of primary hypophysitis. Clin Exp Immunol. 155(3):403-11, 2009
2. Molitch ME et al: Lymphocytic hypophysitis. Horm Res. 68 Suppl 5:145-50, 2007

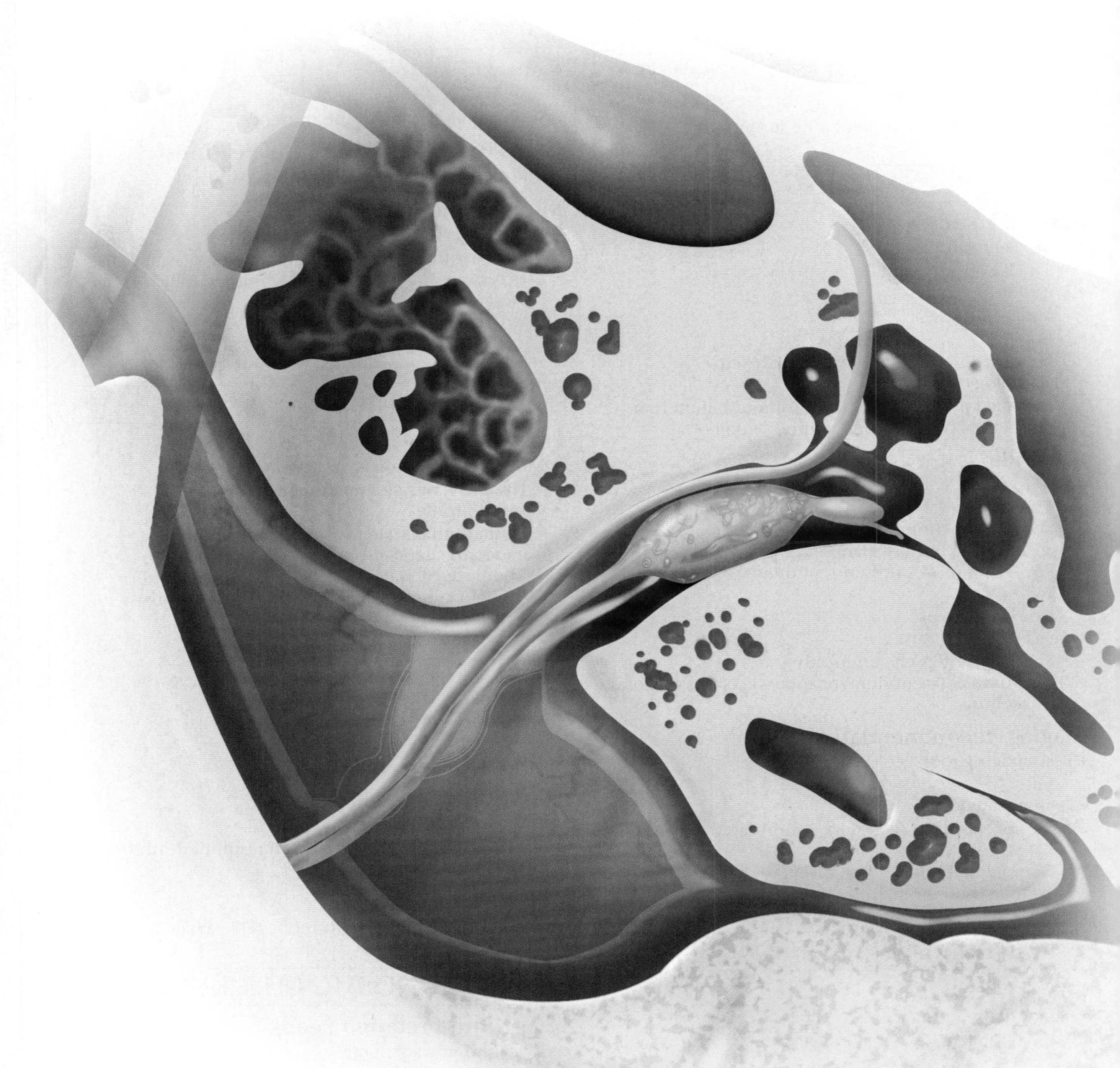

SECTION 3
CPA-IAC

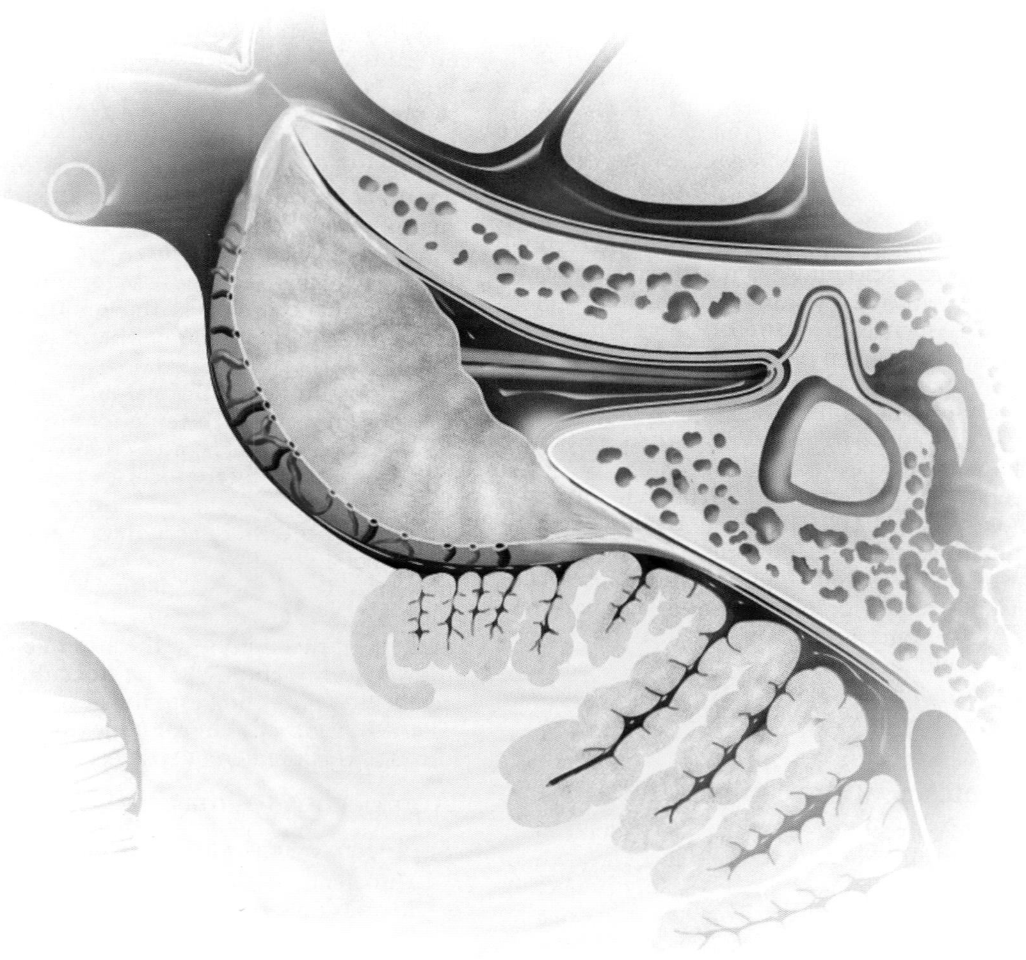

Embryology

The temporal bone forms as 3 distinct embryological events: 1) The external and middle ear, 2) the inner ear, and 3) the internal auditory canal (IAC). The practical implications of these 3 related but separate embryological events is that the IAC may be absent or present independent of inner, middle, or external ear development status.

The IAC develops in response to formation/migration of the facial and vestibulocochlear nerves through this area. IAC size depends on the number of nerve bundles migrating. The fewer the nerve branches, the smaller the IAC. If the IAC is very small and only 1 nerve is seen, it is usually the facial nerve.

Imaging Techniques & Indications

The principal imaging indication requiring radiologists to examine the CPA-IAC is **sensorineural hearing loss (SNHL)**. Three goals must be achieved when completing the MR study in SNHL: 1) Use contrast-enhanced T1 fat-saturated thin-section sequences through the CPA-IAC to identify lesions in this location, 2) utilize high-resolution T2-weighted sequences to answer presurgical questions when a mass lesion is found, and 3) screen the brain for intraaxial causes, such as multiple sclerosis.

The gold standard for imaging patients with SNHL is enhanced thin-section (≤ 3 mm) axial and coronal fat-saturated MR through the CPA-IAC. With these enhanced sequences it is highly unlikely that a lesion causing SNHL will be missed. Don't forget to obtain an axial or coronal precontrast T1 sequence and use fat-saturation when contrast is applied to avoid the rare but troublesome mistake of calling a CPA-IAC lipoma a vestibular schwannoma. In the absence of fat-saturation, the inherent high signal of lipoma will appear to "enhance," leading to the misdiagnosis of "vestibular schwannoma."

High-resolution T2-weighted thin-section (≤ 1 mm) MR sequences (CISS, FIESTA, etc.) in the axial and coronal plane can be used as a screening exam without contrast to identify patients with mass lesions in the CPA-IAC area. However, these sequences are currently more commonly used as supplements when vestibular schwannoma is found on the enhanced T1 sequences to answer specific surgically relevant questions. These questions include size of fundal cap and nerve of origin when vestibular schwannoma is small.

Whenever MR is ordered for SNHL, remember to include whole brain FLAIR, GRE, and DWI sequences. FLAIR will identify the rare multiple sclerosis patient presenting with SNHL as well other intraaxial causes. GRE will demonstrate micro- or macrohemorrhage within a vestibular schwannoma and may help with aneurysm diagnosis when blooming of blood products or calcium in an aneurysm wall is seen. When **DWI** shows restricted diffusion in a CPA mass, the diagnosis of **epidermoid** is easily made.

Imaging Anatomy of the Cochlea-IAC-CPA

The cochlear nerve portion of the vestibulocochlear nerve (CN8) begins in the modiolus of the cochlea where the bipolar **spiral ganglia** are found. Distally projecting axons reach the organ of Corti within the scala media. Proximally projecting axons coalesce to form the cochlear nerve itself within the fundus of the IAC.

CN8 in the CPA and IAC cisterns is made up of vestibular (balance) and cochlear (hearing) components. The cochlear nerve is located in the anterior-inferior quadrant of the IAC. In the region of the porus acusticus, the cochlear nerve joins the superior and inferior vestibular nerve bundles to become the vestibulocochlear nerve in the CPA cistern.

The vestibulocochlear nerve crosses the CPA cistern as the posterior nerve bundle (CN7 is the anterior nerve bundle) to enter the brainstem at the junction of the medulla and pons. The entering nerve fibers pierce the brainstem, bifurcate to form synapses with both the **dorsal and ventral cochlear nuclei**. These 2 nuclei are found on the lateral surface of the inferior cerebellar peduncle (restiform body). Their location can be accurately determined by looking at high-resolution T2 axial images and identifying the contour of the inferior cerebellar peduncle.

Remembering the normal orientation of nerves within the IAC cistern is assisted by the mnemonic "seven-up, coke down." CN7 is found in the anterosuperior quadrant while the cochlear nerve is confined to the anteroinferior quadrant. From there it is simple to remember that the superior vestibular nerve (SVN) is posterosuperior while the inferior vestibular nerve (IVN) is posteroinferior.

Other normal structures to be aware of in the IAC include the **horizontal crest** (crista falciformis) and the **vertical crest** ("Bill bar"). The horizontal crest is a medially projecting horizontal bony shelf in the IAC fundus that separates the CN7-SVN above from the cochlear nerve-IVN below. The vertical crest is found between CN7 and the SVN along the superior fundal bony wall. The horizontal crest is easily seen on both bone CT and high-resolution MR. The vertical crest can be visualized on bone CT only.

Openings from the IAC fundus into the inner ear are numerous. The largest is the anteroinferior **cochlear nerve canal** conveying the cochlear nerve from the modiolus to the IAC fundus. Anterosuperiorly the **meatal foramen** opens into the labyrinthine segment of CN7. The **macula cribrosa** is the multiply perforated bone separating the vestibule of the inner ear from the IAC fundus.

Other non-neural normal anatomy of interest in the CPA cistern includes the anterior inferior cerebellar artery (AICA loop), flocculus, and choroid plexus. **AICA** arises from the basilar artery, courses superolaterally into the CPA, and then into the IAC cistern. Within the IAC, the AICA feeds the internal auditory artery of the cochlea. AICA loop in the IAC or CPA cisterns may mimic a cranial nerve bundle on high-resolution T2WI MR. AICA vascular territory includes the cochlea, flocculus of the cerebellum, and anterolateral pons in the area of cranial nerve nuclei for CN5, CN7, and CN8. The **flocculus** is a lobule of the cerebellum projecting into the posterolateral CPA cistern. The 4th ventricle **choroid plexus** may normally pass through the foramen of Luschka in the CPA cistern.

Approaches to Imaging Issues of CPA-IAC

Approach to Sensorineural Hearing Loss in an Adult

Unilateral SNHL in an otherwise healthy adult is evaluated with enhanced thin-section fat-saturated T1WI

CPA Mass Differential Diagnosis

Pseudolesions
- Asymmetric cerebellar flocculus
- Asymmetric choroid plexus
- Marrow foci around IAC
- High jugular bulb
- Jugular bulb diverticulum

Congenital
- Epidermoid cyst
- Arachnoid cyst
- Lipoma
- Neurofibromatosis type 2

Infectious
- Meningitis
- Cysticercosis

Inflammatory
- Sarcoidosis
- Idiopathic intracranial pseudotumor

Vascular
- Aneurysm (vertebrobasilar, PICA, AICA)
- Arteriovenous malformation

Benign tumor
- Vestibular schwannoma
- Meningioma
- Facial nerve schwannoma
- IAC hemangioma
- Choroid plexus papilloma
- Hemangioblastoma, cerebellum

Malignant tumor
- Metastases, systemic or subarachnoid spread ("drop")
- Melanotic schwannoma
- Brainstem glioma, pedunculated
- Ependymoma

MR of the CPA-IAC area with high-resolution T2WI sequences providing help in surgical planning if a lesion is identified. Despite audiometric and brainstem-evoked response testing in the otolaryngology clinic, positive MR studies for lesions causing the SNHL are infrequent (< 5% even in highly screened patient groups). **Vestibular schwannoma** is by far the most common cause of unilateral SNHL (about 90% of lesions found with MR). It is important for the radiologist to become familiar with the wide range of appearances of vestibular schwannoma, including intramural cystic change, micro- and macroscopic hemorrhage, and associated arachnoid cyst.

Meningioma, epidermoid cyst, and CPA aneurysm are responsible for about 8% of lesions found in adult patients with SNHL. A long list of rare lesions, including otosclerosis, facial nerve, labyrinthine and jugular foramen schwannoma, IAC hemangioma, CPA metastases, labyrinthitis, sarcoidosis, lipoma, and superficial siderosis make up less than 2% of lesions found by MR causing unilateral SNHL in an adult.

Approach to Sensorineural Hearing Loss in a Child

When a child presents with unilateral or bilateral SNHL, the emphasis in the imaging workup veers away from the typical adult tumor causes. Instead, congenital inner ear and CPA-IAC lesions are sought as the cause of the hearing loss. Complications of suppurative labyrinthitis (labyrinthine ossificans) are also included in the differential diagnosis.

When the child's presentation is bilateral profound SNHL, the imaging is usually obtained as part of the workup for possible **cochlear implantation**. High-resolution T2 MR imaging is obtained in the axial and oblique sagittal planes to look for inner ear anomalies and labyrinthine ossificans as well as the presence or absence of a cochlear nerve in the IAC. If complex congenital inner ear disease is found, bone CT is often obtained to further define the inner ear fluid spaces and look for an absent cochlear nerve canal.

In reviewing the MR and CT in a child with sensorineural hearing loss it is important to accurately describe any inner ear congenital anomaly if present. If there is a history of meningitis, labyrinthine ossificans may be present. Look for bony encroachment on the fluid spaces of the inner ear. In particular, make sure the basal turn of the cochlea is open since occlusion by bony plaque may thwart successful cochlear implantation. Check the T2 oblique sagittal MR images for the presence of a normal cochlear nerve. If absent, cochlear implantation results may suffer. Finally, look carefully at the IAC and CPA for signs of epidermoid cyst (restricted diffusion on DWI), lipoma (high signal on T1 precontrast sequences) and neurofibromatosis type 2 (bilateral CPA-IAC vestibular or facial schwannoma).

References

1. Sheth S et al: Appearance of normal cranial nerves on steady-state free precession MR images. Radiographics. 29(4):1045-55, 2009
2. Trimble K et al: Computed tomography and/or magnetic resonance imaging before pediatric cochlear implantation? Developing an investigative strategy. Otol Neurotol. 28(3):317-24, 2007
3. Rabinov JD et al: Virtual cisternoscopy: 3D MRI models of the cerebellopontine angle for lesions related to the cranial nerves. Skull Base. 14(2):93-9; discussion 99, 2004
4. Daniels RL et al: Causes of unilateral sensorineural hearing loss screened by high-resolution fast spin echo magnetic resonance imaging: review of 1,070 consecutive cases. Am J Otol. 21(2):173-80, 2000
5. Schmalbrock P et al: Assessment of internal auditory canal tumors: a comparison of contrast-enhanced T1-weighted and steady-state T2-weighted gradient-echo MR imaging. AJNR Am J Neuroradiol. 20(7):1207-13, 1999
6. Held P et al: MRI of inner ear and facial nerve pathology using 3D MP-RAGE and 3D CISS sequences. Br J Radiol. 70(834):558-66, 1997

CPA-IAC OVERVIEW

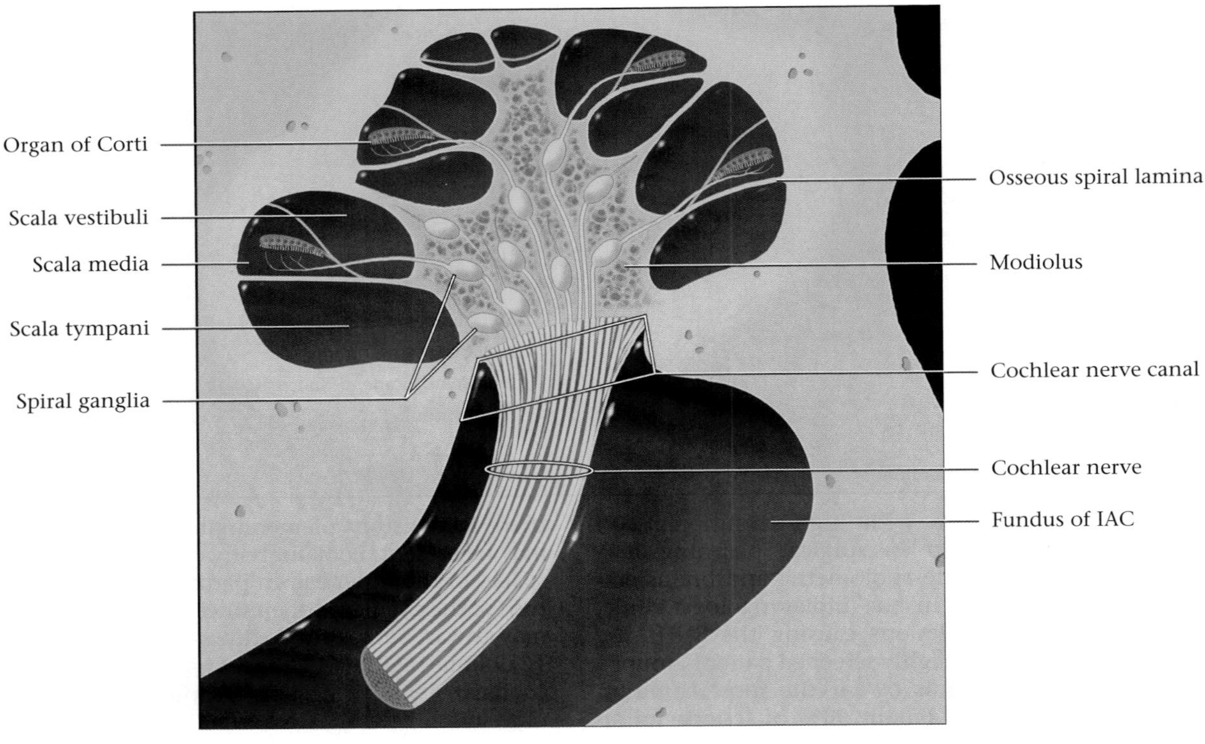

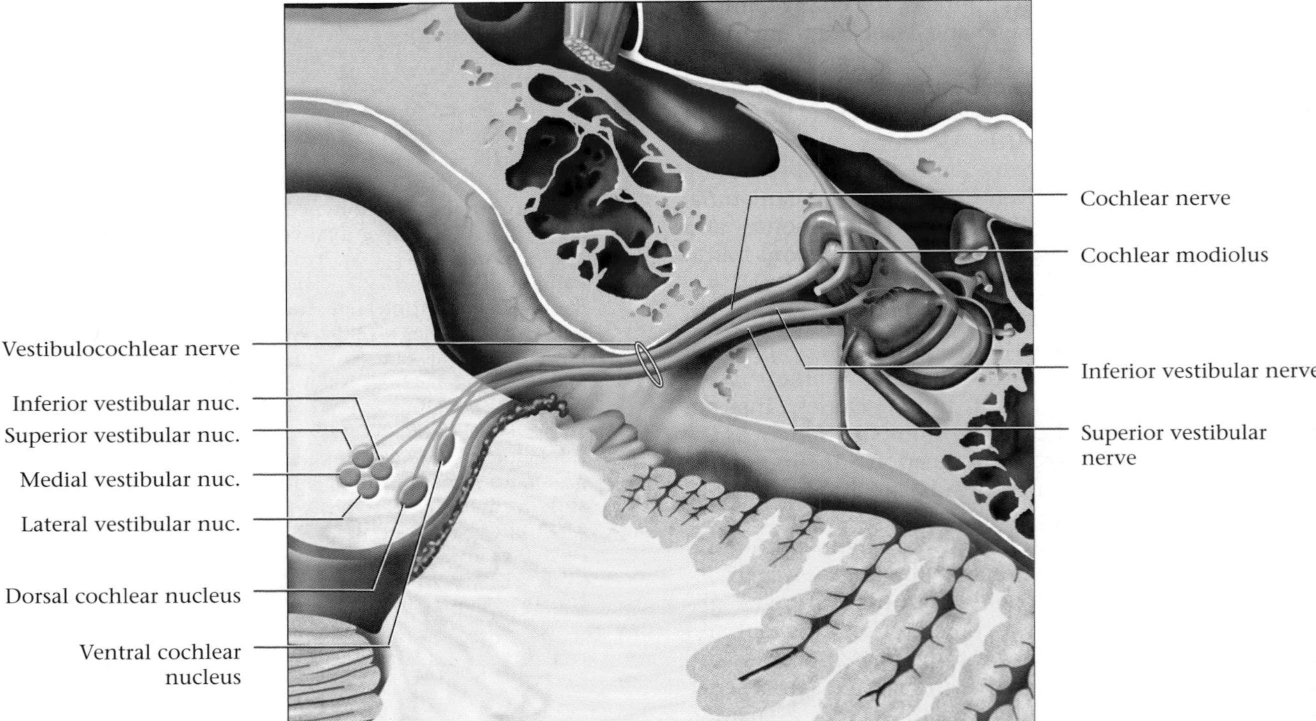

(Top) *The normal cochlear nerve is seen as a coalescence of proximal axons from the modiolar spiral ganglia. These axons pass through the cochlear nerve canal into the IAC fundus. Distally projecting axons from the spiral ganglia reach the organ of Corti in the cochlear scala media.* ***(Bottom)*** *Axial graphic of vestibulocochlear nerve (CN8). The cochlear component of CN8 begins in bipolar cells bodies within spiral ganglion in the modiolus. Central fibers run in the cochlear nerve to the dorsal & ventral cochlear nuclei on lateral margin of the inferior cerebellar peduncle. Inferior & superior vestibular nerves begin in cell bodies in vestibular ganglion, from there coursing centrally to 4 vestibular nuclei.*

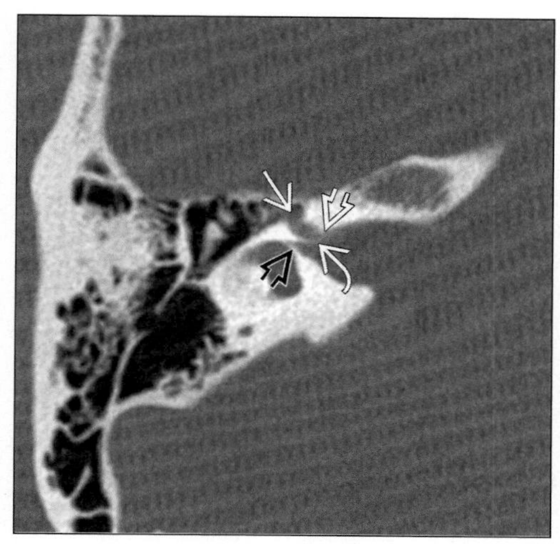

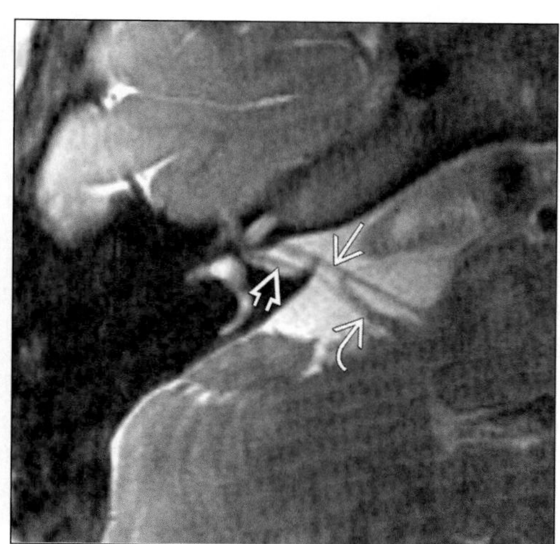

(Left) *Axial bone CT through the superior IAC reveals the labyrinthine segment of CN7, the meatal foramen, the vertical crest, and the superior vestibular nerve connecting the IAC to the vestibule through the macula cribrosa.* ***(Right)*** *Axial T2WI MR through the superior IAC shows the anterosuperior CN7, the superior vestibular nerve, and the vestibulocochlear nerve.*

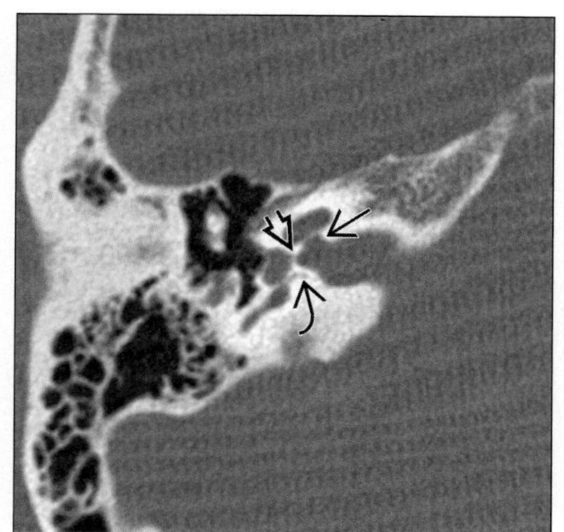

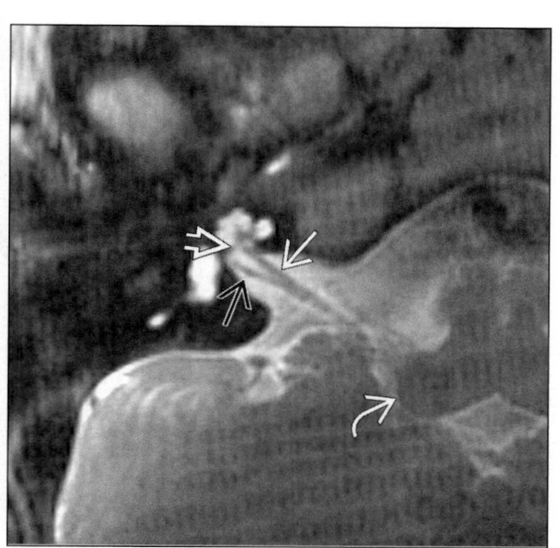

(Left) *Axial bone CT through the inferior IAC shows the cochlear nerve canal, inferior vestibular nerve leaving the fundus, and singular nerve canal containing the posterior branch of the inferior vestibular nerve.* ***(Right)*** *Axial T2WI MR through the inferior IAC reveals cochlear nerve projecting into cochlear nerve canal. Dorsal & ventral cochlear nuclei are not seen but known to reside in the lateral inferior cerebellar peduncle margin. Note the inferior vestibular nerve.*

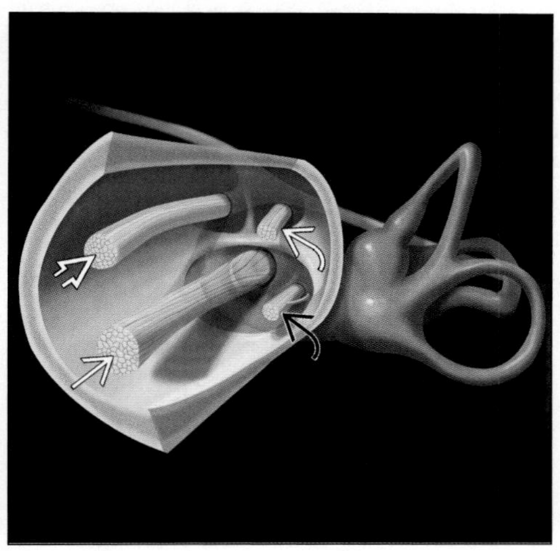

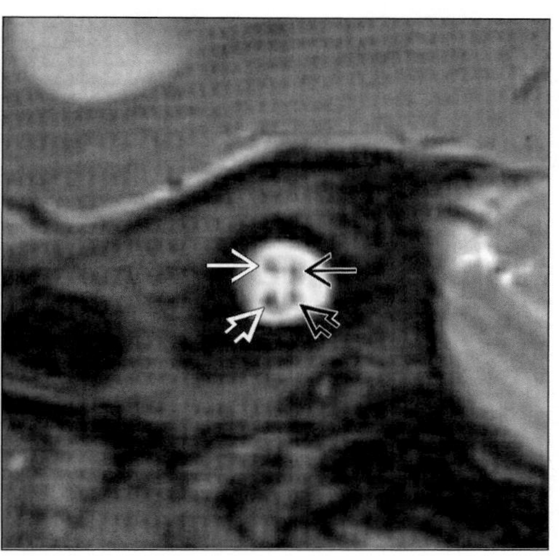

(Left) *Oblique sagittal graphic of the IAC shows all 4 nerves. Anterior superior is CN7, anterior inferior is the cochlear nerve, posterior superior is the superior vestibular nerve, and posterior inferior is the inferior vestibular nerve.* ***(Right)*** *Oblique sagittal T2WI MR shows the 4 nerve bundles of the mid-IAC cistern. CN7 is anterosuperior, cochlear nerve anteroinferior, while the superior and inferior vestibular nerves are posterosuperior and posteroinferior, respectively.*

LIPOMA, CPA-IAC

Key Facts

Terminology

- Lipoma, CPA-IAC: Nonneoplastic mass of adipose tissue in CPA-IAC area

Imaging

- Focal benign-appearing CPA-IAC mass, which follows fat density (CT) and intensity (MR)
- Concurrent intravestibular deposit may be seen in association with CPA-IAC lipoma
- MR: Hyperintense CPA mass (parallels subcutaneous and marrow fat intensity)
  - Becomes hypointense with fat saturation
  - Caveat: Fat-saturation MR sequences avoid mistaking lipoma for "enhancing CPA mass"

Top Differential Diagnoses

- Neurenteric cyst
- Ruptured dermoid cyst
- Hemorrhagic vestibular schwannoma
- Aneurysm, CPA-IAC

Pathology

- Persistence, maldevelopment of meningeal precursor tissue (embryonic meninx primitiva)

Clinical Issues

- Most common presentation: Adult presenting with unilateral sensorineural hearing loss
  - CN8 compression: Tinnitus (40%), vertigo (45%)
  - Compression of CN5 root entry zone: Trigeminal neuralgia (15%)
  - Compression of CN7 root exit zone: Hemifacial spasm, facial nerve weakness (10%)
  - May be found incidentally on brain CT or MR completed for unrelated reasons
- Treatment: No treatment is best treatment
  - Discontinue steroid treatment if present

*(**Left**) Axial graphic demonstrates a CPA lipoma ⇒ abutting the lateral pons. Notice that the facial nerve, vestibulocochlear nerve, and AICA loop all pass through the lipoma on their way to the internal auditory canal. (**Right**) Axial T1WI MR shows a right CPA lipoma ➡ projecting off the lateral pontine pial surface. Note the 2nd smaller lipoma ➡ along the lateral margin of the internal auditory canal. A portion of the AICA loop ➡ passes through the anterolateral lipoma.*

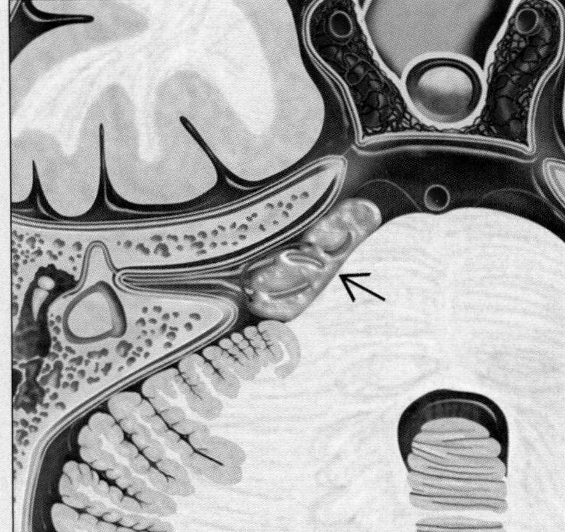

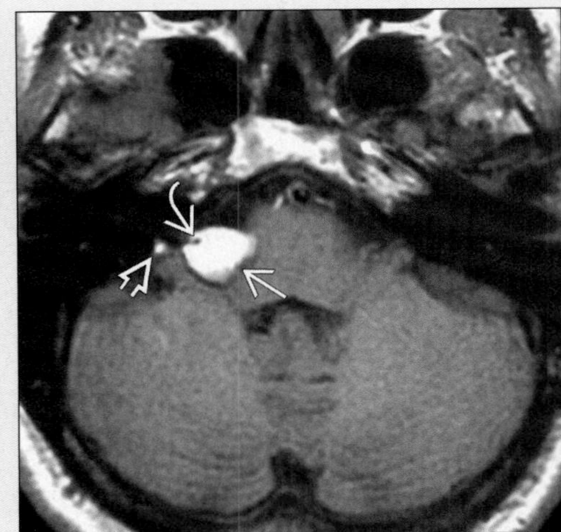

*(**Left**) Axial T1WI MR shows a hyperintense CPA lipoma ➡ abutting the lateral pons. Note the 2nd ➡ focus of T1 hyperintensity representing a small intravestibular lipoma. Other T1 hyperintense lesions include hemorrhagic or proteinaceous masses. (**Right**) Axial T1WI C+ FS MR in the same patient shows that the lesions disappear. Fat-saturation MR sequences are key to confirming the diagnosis of lipoma and to avoid mistaking a lipoma for an enhancing CPA mass.*

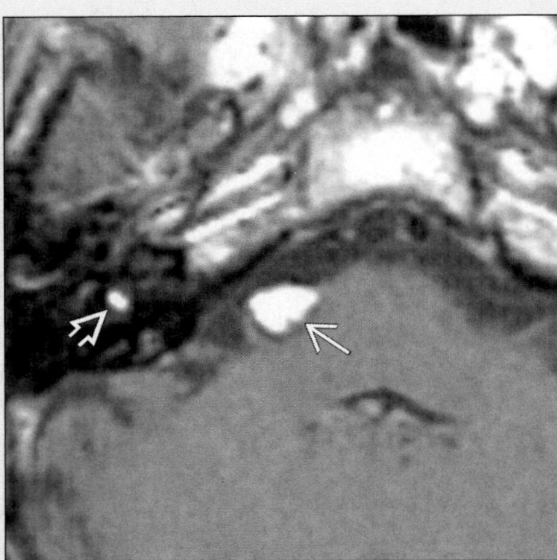

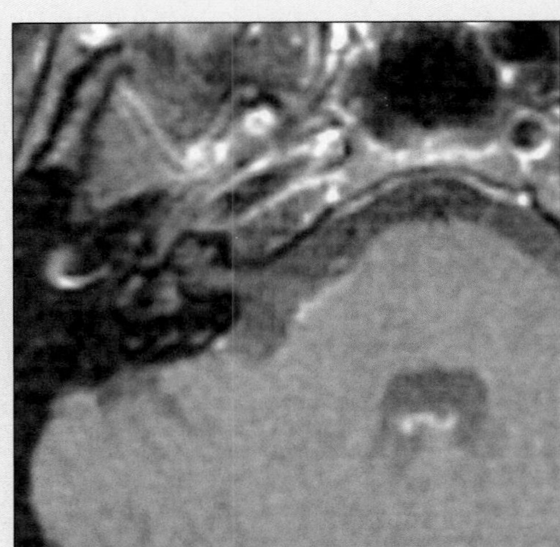

TERMINOLOGY

Synonyms

- Hamartomatous lipoma, lipomatous hamartoma

Definitions

- Lipoma, CPA-IAC: **Nonneoplastic** mass of adipose tissue in CPA-IAC area
  - Congenital malformation; not true neoplasm

IMAGING

General Features

- Best diagnostic clue
  - Focal benign-appearing CPA-IAC mass, which follows fat density (CT) and intensity (MR)
- Location
  - 20% of intracranial lipoma is infratentorial
  - Primary location = CPA cistern
    - May be in IAC only
    - Concurrent intravestibular deposit may be seen in association with CPA-IAC lipoma
- Size
  - 1-5 cm in maximum diameter
    - May be as small as a few millimeters
- Morphology
  - Lobulated pial-based fatty mass
    - May encase CN7, CN8, AICA loop
  - Small lesions
    - Linear along course of cranial nerves 7 and 8 in CPA
    - Ovoid within CPA cistern
  - Large lesions
    - Broad-based hemispherical shape adherent to lateral margin of pons

CT Findings

- NECT
  - **Low-density** CPA-IAC mass
  - Measure mass using HU if uncertain
    - Hounsfield unit range: **-50 to -100 HU**
  - Calcification rare in CPA-IAC lesions
- CECT
  - Lesion does not enhance

MR Findings

- T1WI
  - **Hyperintense** CPA mass (parallels subcutaneous and marrow fat intensity)
    - Inner ear (vestibule) noncontiguous 2nd fatty lesion may be present
  - Becomes hypointense with fat saturation
- T2WI
  - Intermediate "fat intensity" lesion
  - Conspicuous chemical shift artifact (frequency-encoding direction)
  - Signal parallels subcutaneous and marrow fat
- STIR
  - Hypointense due to STIR inherent fat saturation
- FLAIR
  - Hyperintense compared to cisternal CSF
- T1WI C+
  - Lesion already hyperintense on precontrast images
  - Use fat-saturated T1WI C+ sequence
    - Lesion "**disappears**" secondary to **fat saturation** aspect of this MR sequence
    - No enhancement in region of lesion is present

Imaging Recommendations

- Best imaging tool
  - **MR** is 1st study ordered when symptoms suggest possibility of CPA-IAC mass
  - CT can easily confirm diagnoses by measuring HU if some confusion on MR images persists
- Protocol advice
  - When T1WI C+ MR focused to CPA area is anticipated, need at least 1 precontrast T1 sequence
    - Precontrast T1 sequence helps distinguish fatty and hemorrhagic lesions from enhancing lesions
    - Fatty lesions include lipoma and dermoid
    - Hemorrhagic lesions with methemoglobin high-signal include aneurysm and venous varix
  - Once high signal is seen on precontrast T1 sequence, fat-saturated sequences distinguish fat from hemorrhage
    - **Caveat**: Fat-saturation MR sequences avoid mistaking lipoma for "enhancing CPA mass"

DIFFERENTIAL DIAGNOSIS

Hemorrhagic Vestibular Schwannoma

- Rare manifestation of common lesion
- Patchy intraparenchymal signal on precontrast T1WI MR
- Hyperintensities persist with fat-saturated sequences

Aneurysm, CPA-IAC

- CPA aneurysms from PICA > VA > AICA
- Rarely enters IAC (AICA)
- Ovoid CPA mass with calcified rim (CT) and complex layered signal (MR)
- MR signal complex with high-signal areas from methemoglobin in aneurysm lumen or wall

Neurenteric Cyst

- Most common in prepontine cistern
- Contains proteinaceous fluid (hyperintense on T1WI MR)

Ruptured Dermoid Cyst

- Ectodermal inclusion cyst
- Original location usually midline
- Rupture spreads fat droplets into subarachnoid space
- Rupture may lead to chemical meningitis

PATHOLOGY

General Features

- Etiology
  - Best current hypothesis for lesion formation
    - Persistence, maldevelopment of meningeal precursor tissue (embryonic meninx primitiva)
      - Normally develops into leptomeninges and cisterns
      - Maldifferentiates into fat instead
    - Hyperplasia of fat cells normally **within pia**

LIPOMA, CPA-IAC

- Genetics
  - No known defects in sporadic CPA lipoma
  - Epidermal nevus syndrome has CPA lipomas as part of complex congenital anomalies
- Associated abnormalities
  - 2nd fatty lesion may occur in inner ear vestibule

Gross Pathologic & Surgical Features

- Soft, yellowish mass attached to leptomeninges
  - Sometimes adherent to lateral pons
- May incorporate CN7 and CN8 with dense adhesions
  - AICA loop may also be engulfed

Microscopic Features

- Highly vascularized adipose tissue
- Mature lipocytes; mitoses rare

CLINICAL ISSUES

Presentation

- Most common signs/symptoms
  - Mild, unilateral sensorineural hearing loss (60%)
- Clinical profile
  - Adult presenting with slowly progressive unilateral sensorineural hearing loss
- Other signs/symptoms
  - May be found incidentally on brain CT or MR completed for unrelated reasons
  - CN8 compression: Tinnitus (40%), vertigo (45%)
  - Compression of CN5 root entry zone: **Trigeminal neuralgia** (15%)
  - Compression of CN7 root exit zone: **Hemifacial spasm**, facial nerve weakness (10%)

Demographics

- Age
  - Range at presentation: 10-40 years
- Epidemiology
  - Lipomas occur less frequently in CPA than epidermoid and arachnoid cysts
  - Epidermoid cyst > arachnoid cyst > > lipoma
  - CPA lipoma represents 10% of all intracranial lipomas
    - Interhemispheric (45%), quadrigeminal/superior cerebellar (25%), suprasellar/interpeduncular (15%), sylvian cisterns (5%)

Natural History & Prognosis

- Usually does not grow over time
- Stability confirmed with follow-up examinations
- Attempts at complete excision of CPA lipomas may result in injury to CN7 and CN8
- May enlarge if patient taking high-dose steroids
  - Compressive symptoms may result

Treatment

- No treatment is best treatment
  - Discontinue steroid treatment if present
- **Surgical removal** is **no longer recommended**
  - Cure often worse than disease due to entwined CN7 and CN8
  - Historically, 70% of postoperative patients had new postoperative deficits
- Surgical intervention only if cranial nerve decompression needed

DIAGNOSTIC CHECKLIST

Consider

- When high-signal lesion is seen in CPA on T1WI unenhanced MR, 3 explanations to consider
  - Fatty lesion
    - Lipoma most common (dermoid rare)
  - Hemorrhagic lesion
    - Aneurysm lumen clot or clotted venous varix (dural arteriovenous fistula)
    - Rare hemorrhagic acoustic schwannoma
  - Highly proteinaceous fluid
    - Neurenteric cyst (usually in prepontine cistern)

Image Interpretation Pearls

- Once high-signal lesion is seen in CPA on precontrast T1WI MR, use fat-saturation sequences to confirm diagnosis

Reporting Tips

- Report size and extent of lipoma
  - Check vestibule of inner ear for 2nd lesion
- Remind referring MD that CN7, CN8, and AICA loop often pass through CPA-IAC lipoma

SELECTED REFERENCES

1. Barajas RF Jr et al: Microvascular decompression in hemifacial spasm resulting from a cerebellopontine angle lipoma: case report. Neurosurgery. 63(4):E815-6; discussion E816, 2008
2. Vernooij MW et al: Intravestibular lipoma: an important imaging diagnosis. Arch Otolaryngol Head Neck Surg. 134(11):1225-8, 2008
3. Canyigit M et al: Epidermal nevus syndrome with internal carotid artery occlusion and intracranial and orbital lipomas. AJNR Am J Neuroradiol. 27(7):1559-61, 2006
4. Sade B et al: Cerebellopontine angle lipoma presenting with hemifacial spasm: case report and review of the literature. J Otolaryngol. 34(4):270-3, 2005
5. Gaskin CM et al: Lipomas, lipoma variants, and well-differentiated liposarcomas (atypical lipomas): results of MRI evaluations of 126 consecutive fatty masses. AJR Am J Roentgenol. 182(3):733-9, 2004
6. Dahlen RT et al: CT and MR imaging characteristics of intravestibular lipoma. AJNR Am J Neuroradiol. 23(8):1413-7, 2002
7. Tankéré F et al: Cerebellopontine angle lipomas: report of four cases and review of the literature. Neurosurgery. 50(3):626-31; discussion 631-2, 2002
8. Bigelow DC et al: Lipomas of the internal auditory canal and cerebellopontine angle. Laryngoscope. 108(10):1459-69, 1998
9. Kato T et al: Trigeminal neuralgia caused by a cerebellopontine-angle lipoma: case report. Surg Neurol. 44(1):33-5, 1995
10. Truwit CL et al: Pathogenesis of intracranial lipoma: an MR study in 42 patients. AJR Am J Roentgenol. 155(4):855-64; discussion 865, 1990
11. Dalley RW et al: Computed tomography of a cerebellopontine angle lipoma. J Comput Assist Tomogr. 10(4):704-6, 1986

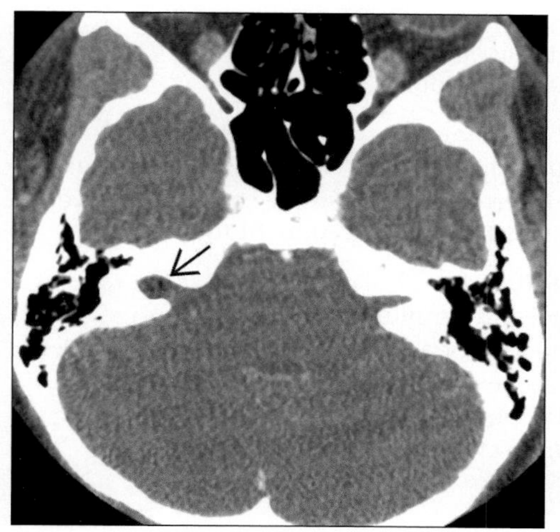

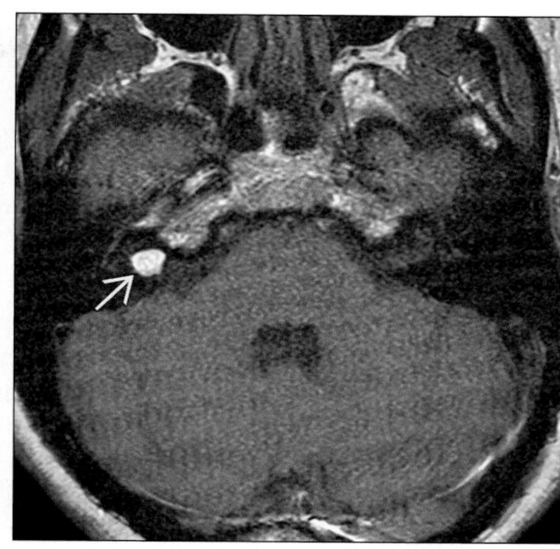

(Left) *Axial CECT reveals a fat-density lesion ➙ in the fundus of the right internal auditory canal. The bone shape in this area is bulbous in comparison to the opposite normal IAC suggesting a congenital origin of the lesion.* ***(Right)*** *Axial T1WI MR in the same patient shows the expected hyperintense fundal intracanalicular congenital lipoma ➙. Lipoma of the CPA-IAC area may be found in the CPA, IAC, and rarely, in the inner ear vestibule.*

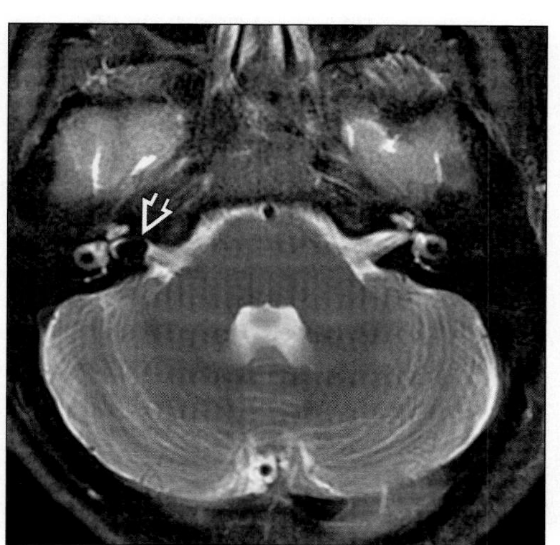

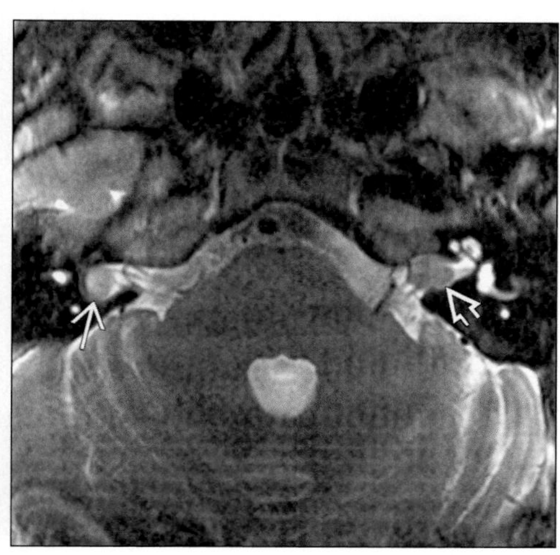

(Left) *Axial T2WI FS MR in the same patient shows that the lipoma ➙ in the IAC fundus has become hypointense.* ***(Right)*** *Axial T2WI MR without fat saturation shows a right intermediate-signal internal auditory canal mass ➙ as well as a left-sided ➙ mass. Initial suspicion based on T2 screening study was neurofibromatosis type 2. However, because the patient was 35 years old, further imaging was performed.*

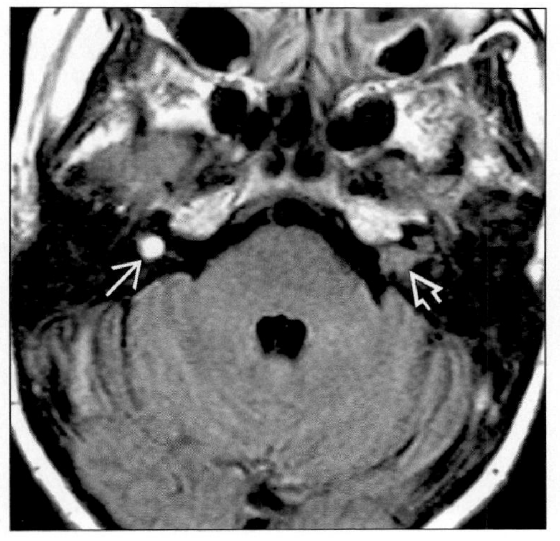

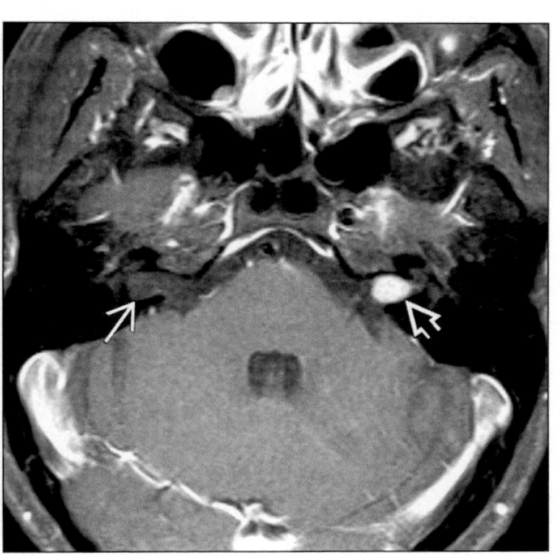

(Left) *Axial T1WI MR in the same patient shows that the right IAC lesion ➙ is hyperintense while the left lesion ➙ is intermediate brain intensity. Right IAC lipoma was diagnosed with probable left acoustic schwannoma.* ***(Right)*** *Axial T1WI C+ FS MR in the same patient confirmed a right IAC lipoma ➙ and left IAC vestibular schwannoma ➙. Fat-saturation sequence nulls fat signal so that lipoma is no longer visible while enhancing schwannoma is highly conspicuous.*

EPIDERMOID CYST, CPA-IAC

Key Facts

Terminology
- Congenital inclusion of ectodermal epithelial elements during neural tube closure

Imaging
- CPA cisternal insinuating mass with high signal on DWI MR
  - 90% intradural, 10% extradural
  - Margins usually scalloped or irregular
  - Cauliflower-like margins with "fronds" possible
- TI and T2: Isointense or slightly hyperintense to CSF
- FLAIR: Does not null (attenuate)
- DWI: Hyperintensity here makes diagnosis

Top Differential Diagnoses
- Arachnoid cyst, CPA
- Neurocysticercosis, CPA
- Neurenteric cyst
- Cystic neoplasm, CPA
  - Cystic vestibular schwannoma
  - Cystic meningioma, CPA
  - Infratentorial ependymoma
  - Pilocytic astrocytoma

Pathology
- Surgical appearance: Pearly white CPA cistern mass
- Cyst wall: Internal layer of simple stratified cuboidal squamous epithelium covered by fibrous capsule

Clinical Issues
- Principal presenting symptom: Dizziness
- Other symptoms depend on location, growth pattern
  - Cranial nerve 5, 7, 8 neuropathy possible
- Treatment: Complete surgical removal is goal
  - If recurs, takes many years to grow
  - DWI MR key to diagnosing recurrence

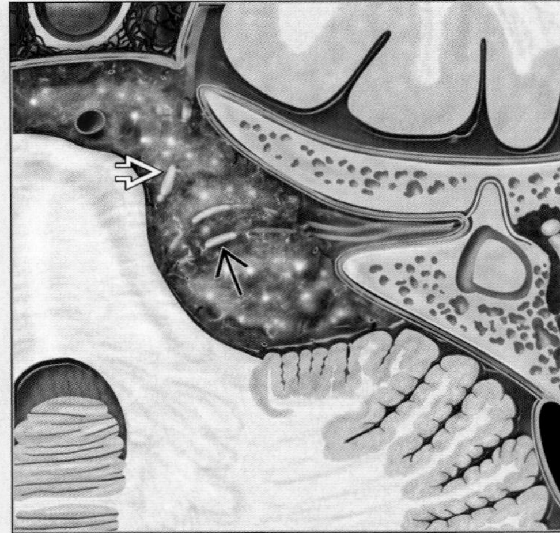

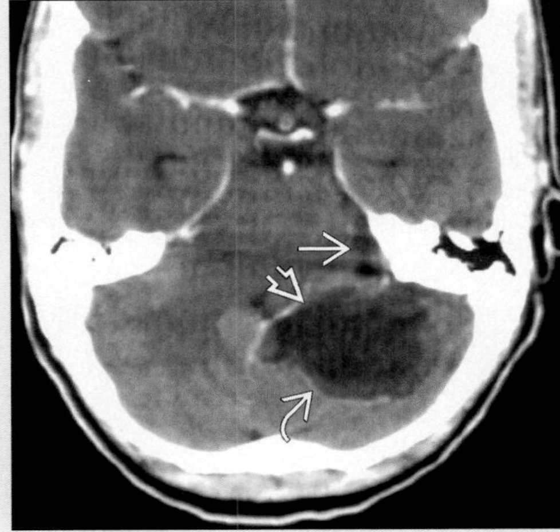

(Left) *Axial graphic shows a large CPA epidermoid cyst within a typical "bed of pearls" appearance. Note that the 5th ➡, 7th, and 8th cranial nerves ⇨ are characteristically engulfed by this insinuating mass.* ***(Right)*** *Axial CECT shows a large CPA epidermoid cyst ➡. Note that this low-density lesion appears to invade the left cerebellar hemisphere ➡. Minimal rim enhancement is visible along the posterior margin of the cyst ➡.*

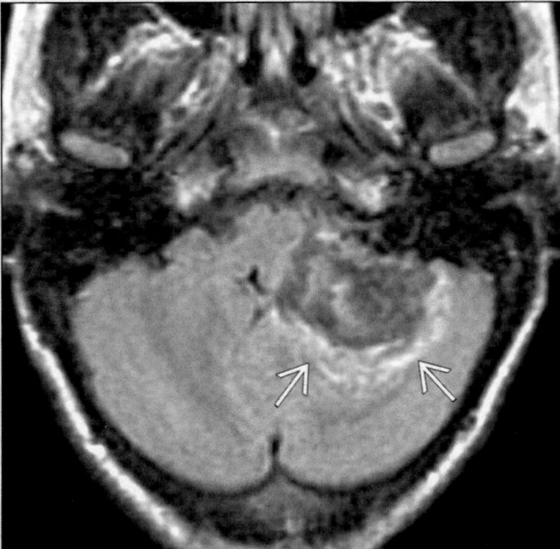

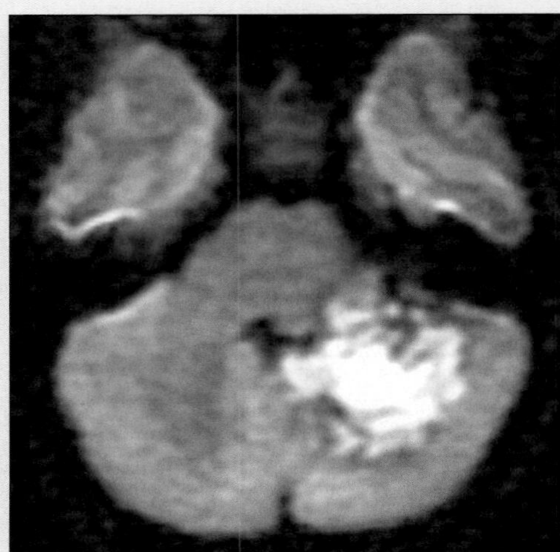

(Left) *Axial FLAIR MR of the same patient shows "incomplete" or partial nulling of the signal of this large epidermoid cyst. Associated high signal ➡ along the deep margins of the lesion is most likely due to gliosis of the cerebellar hemisphere.* ***(Right)*** *Axial DWI MR in the same patient reveals the expected high signal from epidermoid cyst diffusion restriction. DWI sequence allows differentiation of this epidermoid cyst from arachnoid cyst.*

EPIDERMOID CYST, CPA-IAC

TERMINOLOGY

Synonyms

- Epidermoid tumor, primary cholesteatoma, or epithelial inclusion cyst

Definitions

- Congenital **inclusion** of ectodermal epithelial elements during neural tube closure

IMAGING

General Features

- Best diagnostic clue
  - CPA cisternal **insinuating** mass with high signal on DWI MR
    - Engulfs cranial nerves (7th and 8th), vessels
- Location
  - 90% intradural, 10% extradural
    - Posterior fossa location most common
      - CPA ~ 40%; 4th ventricle ~ 20%
- Size
  - Wide range: 2-8 cm diameter
- Morphology
  - Insinuating mass in cisterns
  - Margins usually scalloped or irregular
    - Cauliflower-like margins with "fronds" possible
  - When large, compresses or invades brainstem ± cerebellum

CT Findings

- NECT
  - Similar density to cerebral spinal fluid (CSF)
  - Calcification in 20%, usually margins
  - Pressure erosion of T-bone and skull base may occur
  - Rare variant: "Dense epidermoid"
    - 3% of intracranial epidermoids
    - From protein, cyst debris saponification to calcium soaps or iron-containing pigment
- CECT
  - No enhancement is rule
    - Sometimes margin of cyst minimally enhances

MR Findings

- T1WI
  - Isointense or slightly hyperintense to CSF
  - If hyperintense, term "dirty CSF" has been applied
  - Rare variant: "White epidermoid" with high T1 compared to brain
    - Secondary to high triglycerides and unsaturated fatty acids
- T2WI
  - Isointense to hyperintense to CSF
  - "White epidermoid": Low T2 signal
- FLAIR
  - Does not null (attenuate)
    - Lack of any attenuation or "incomplete attenuation" on FLAIR suggests diagnosis
- DWI
  - **Hyperintensity** on DWI **makes diagnosis**
    - Secondary to high fractional anisotropy from diffusion along 2D geometric plane
      - Due to microstructure of parallel-layered keratin filaments and flakes
  - ADC = brain parenchyma
  - High-signal foci in surgical bed indicates recurrence
- T1WI C+
  - No enhancement is rule
  - Mild marginal C+ may occur (25%)
- MRA
  - Vessels of CPA may be displaced or engulfed
  - Artery wall dimension not affected
- MRS
  - Resonances from lactate
  - No NAA, choline, or lipid

Imaging Recommendations

- Best imaging tool
  - Brain MR with FLAIR, DWI, and T1WI C+ sequences
- Protocol advice
  - FLAIR and DWI sequences make diagnosis
  - If looking for recurrence, DWI best sequence

DIFFERENTIAL DIAGNOSIS

Arachnoid Cyst, CPA

- Displaces, does not engulf, adjacent structures
- Isointense to CSF on all standard MR sequences
  - T2 higher signal possible; if no CSF pulsations
- Completely nulls on FLAIR (low signal)
- Hypointense on DWI
  - Contains highly mobile CSF
  - ADC = stationary water

Cystic Neoplasm in CPA

- Cystic vestibular schwannoma
- Cystic meningioma, CPA
- Infratentorial ependymoma
  - Pedunculates from 4th ventricle
- Pilocytic astrocytoma
  - Pedunculate from cerebellum
- All show some areas of enhancement on T1WI C+ MR

Neurocysticercosis, CPA

- Partially enhances
- Density/signal intensity does not precisely follow CSF
- Adjacent brain edema or gliosis common

Neurenteric Cyst

- Most common prepontine cistern in location
- T1 high signal (might mimic "white epidermoid")
- T2 signal often low

PATHOLOGY

General Features

- Etiology
  - Congenital inclusion of ectodermal elements during neural tube closure
    - 3rd to 5th week of embryogenesis
  - CPA lesion derived from 1st branchial groove cells

Gross Pathologic & Surgical Features

- Pearly white mass in CPA

- Surgeons refer to it as "the beautiful tumor"
- Lobulated, cauliflower-shaped surface features
- Insinuating growth pattern in cisterns
  - Engulfs cisternal vessels and nerves
    - May become adherent
- Lesion filled with soft, waxy, creamy, or flaky material

Microscopic Features

- Cyst wall: Internal layer of simple stratified cuboidal squamous epithelium covered by fibrous capsule
- Cyst contents: Solid crystalline cholesterol, keratinaceous debris
  - No dermal appendages (hair follicles, sebaceous glands, or fat)
- Grows in successive layers by desquamation of squamous epithelium from cyst wall
  - Conversion to keratin/cholesterol crystals form concentric lamellae

CLINICAL ISSUES

Presentation

- Most common signs/symptoms
  - Principal presenting symptom: Dizziness
  - Other symptoms depend on location, growth pattern
    - Sensorineural hearing loss
    - Trigeminal neuralgia (tic douloureux)
    - Facial neuralgia (hemifacial spasm)
    - Headache
  - Symptoms usually present for > 4 years before diagnosis
- Clinical profile
  - 40-year-old patient with minor symptoms and large lesion discovered in CPA on MR

Demographics

- Age
  - Although congenital, presents in adult life
  - Broad presentation: 20-60 years
    - Peak age = 40 years
- Epidemiology
  - 3rd most common CPA mass
  - 1% of all intracranial tumors

Natural History & Prognosis

- Slow-growing congenital lesions that remain clinically silent for many years
- Smaller cisternal lesions are readily cured with surgery
- Larger lesions with upward supratentorial herniation are more difficult to completely remove
  - Larger lesions have more significant surgical complications

Treatment

- Complete surgical removal is goal
  - If large, near-total removal prudent surgical choice
    - Aggressive total removal may cause significant cranial neuropathy
    - Used when capsule is adherent to brainstem and cranial nerves
- If recurs, takes many years to grow
  - DWI MR key to diagnosing recurrence

DIAGNOSTIC CHECKLIST

Consider

- MR diagnosis based on
  - Insinuating CPA lesion
  - Low signal on T1, high on T2 (similar to, but not identical to CSF)
  - No or partial nulling on FLAIR
  - Hyperintense on DWI

Image Interpretation Pearls

- **Diffusion MR** imaging sequence is **key to correct diagnosis**

Reporting Tips

- Be sure to report prepontine or medial middle cranial fossa extension if present

SELECTED REFERENCES

1. Jolapara M et al: Diffusion tensor mode in imaging of intracranial epidermoid cysts: one step ahead of fractional anisotropy. Neuroradiology. 51(2):123-9, 2009
2. Schiefer TK et al: Epidermoids of the cerebellopontine angle: a 20-year experience. Surg Neurol. 70(6):584-90; discussion 590, 2008
3. Akhavan-Sigari R et al: Epidermoid cysts of the cerebellopontine angle with extension into the middle and anterior cranial fossae: surgical strategy and review of the literature. Acta Neurochir (Wien). 149(4):429-32, 2007
4. Ben Hamouda M et al: Atypical CT and MRI aspects of an epidermoid cyst. J Neuroradiol. 34(2):129-32, 2007
5. Osborn AG et al: Intracranial cysts: radiologic-pathologic correlation and imaging approach. Radiology. 239(3):650-64, 2006
6. Hakyemez B et al: Intracranial epidermoid cysts: diffusion-weighted, FLAIR and conventional MR findings. Eur J Radiol. 54(2):214-20, 2005
7. Dutt SN et al: Radiologic differentiation of intracranial epidermoids from arachnoid cysts. Otol Neurotol. 23(1):84-92, 2002
8. Kobata H et al: Cerebellopontine angle epidermoids presenting with cranial nerve hyperactive dysfunction: pathogenesis and long-term surgical results in 30 patients. Neurosurgery. 50(2):276-85; discussion 285-6, 2002
9. Dechambre S et al: Diffusion-weighted MRI postoperative assessment of an epidermoid tumour in the cerebellopontine angle. Neuroradiology. 41(11):829-31, 1999
10. Timmer FA et al: Chemical analysis of an epidermoid cyst with unusual CT and MR characteristics. AJNR Am J Neuroradiol. 19(6):1111-2, 1998
11. Ikushima I et al: MR of epidermoids with a variety of pulse sequences. AJNR Am J Neuroradiol. 18(7):1359-63, 1997
12. Kallmes DF et al: Typical and atypical MR imaging features of intracranial epidermoid tumors. AJR Am J Roentgenol. 169(3):883-7, 1997
13. Tien RD et al: Variable bandwidth steady-state free-precession MR imaging: a technique for improving characterization of epidermoid tumor and arachnoid cyst. AJR Am J Roentgenol. 164(3):689-92, 1995
14. Tsuruda JS et al: Diffusion-weighted MR imaging of the brain: value of differentiating between extraaxial cysts and epidermoid tumors. AJNR Am J Neuroradiol. 11(5):925-31; discussion 932-4, 1990

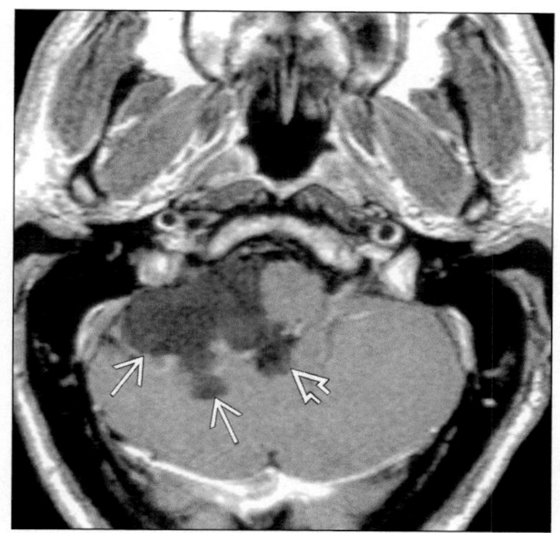

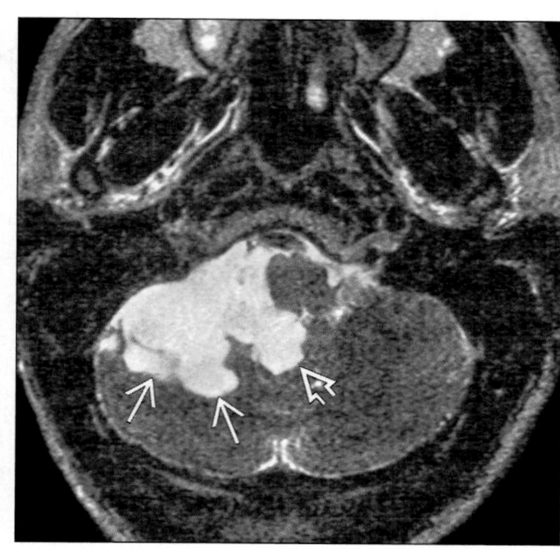

(Left) *Axial T1WI C+ MR demonstrates a large, invasive, right CPA cistern epidermoid cyst ➔. Note the low signal with lack of enhancement of the lesion. The cyst insinuates into the cerebellar hemisphere and foramen of Luschka ➔.* ***(Right)*** *Axial T2WI MR in the same patient reveals a large, insinuating epidermoid cyst with typical high T2 signal and invasion of the cerebellar hemisphere ➔ and foramen of Luschka ➔.*

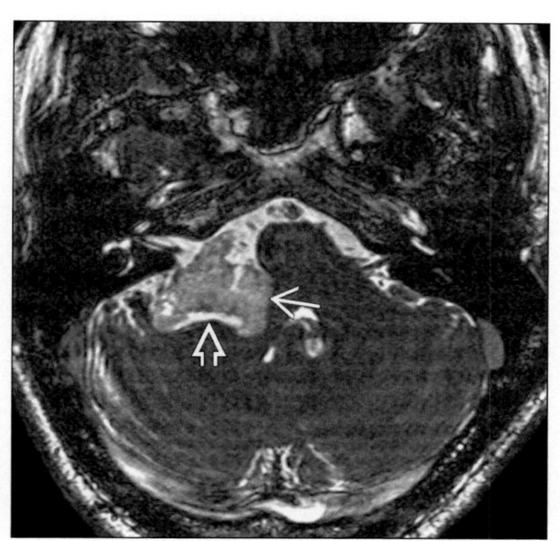

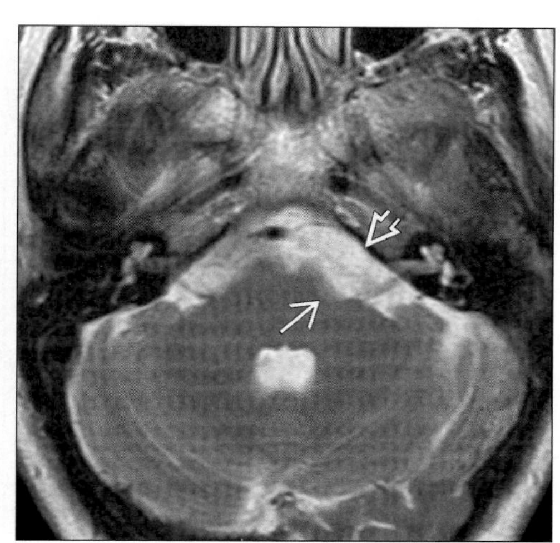

(Left) *Axial T2WI FS thin-section high-resolution MR shows a right CPA epidermoid cyst. Note the cauliflower-like surface architecture. This lesion is compressing the brachium pontis ➔ and adjacent cerebellar hemisphere ➔.* ***(Right)*** *Axial T2WI MR shows slight widening of the left CPA cistern ➔ with minimal mass effect on the brachium pontis ➔, but no definite lesion is visible. In a patient with left sensorineural hearing loss, arachnoid cyst or epidermoid cyst should be considered.*

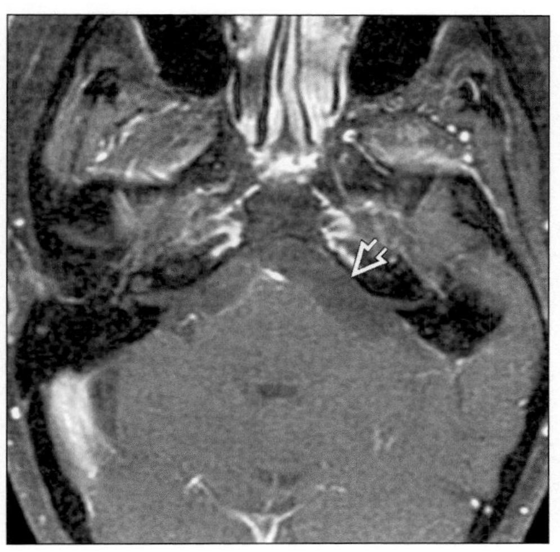

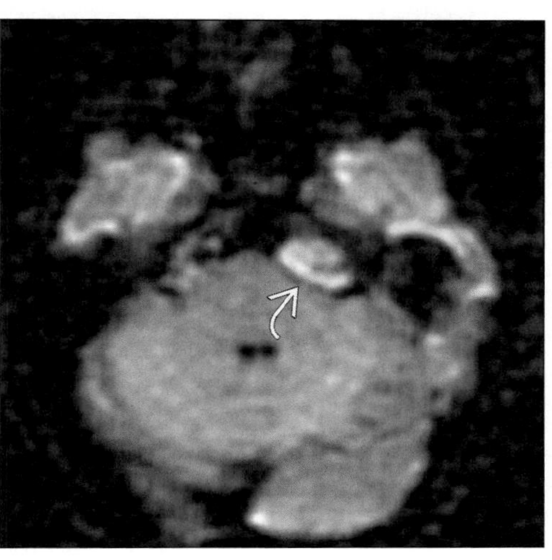

(Left) *Axial T1WI C+ FS MR in the same patient again reveals a widened CPA cistern ➔ but no evidence of enhancing tumor. Both FLAIR and DWI sequences are used at this point to differentiate an arachnoid cyst from epidermoid cyst.* ***(Right)*** *Axial DWI MR in the same patient demonstrates the characteristic restricted diffusion of the epidermoid cyst ➔ in the left CPA cistern. Without DWI information, the lesion could have been missed altogether.*

ARACHNOID CYST, CPA-IAC

Key Facts

Terminology
- Arachnoid cyst (AC): Developmental arachnoid duplication anomaly creating CSF-filled sac

Imaging
- Sharply demarcated round/ovoid extraaxial cisternal cyst with imperceptible walls with CSF density (CT) or intensity (MR)
- AC signal parallels CSF on all MR sequences
- Complete fluid attenuation on FLAIR MR
- No diffusion restriction on DWI MR imaging

Top Differential Diagnoses
- Epidermoid cyst, CPA-IAC
- Mega cisterna magna
- Cystic vestibular schwannoma
- Neurenteric cyst
- Cystic meningioma, CPA-IAC
- Cystic infratentorial ependymoma
- Cerebellar pilocytic astrocytoma

Clinical Issues
- Small AC: Asymptomatic, incidental finding (MR)
- Large AC: Symptoms from direct compression ± ↑ intracranial pressure
- Most AC do not enlarge over time
- Most cases require no treatment
- Surgical intervention is highly selective process

Diagnostic Checklist
- Differentiate AC from epidermoid cyst
- AC: No restriction on DWI = best clue
- Reporting tip: Since AC is usually not treated surgically, avoid offering any differential diagnosis when imaging findings diagnose AC

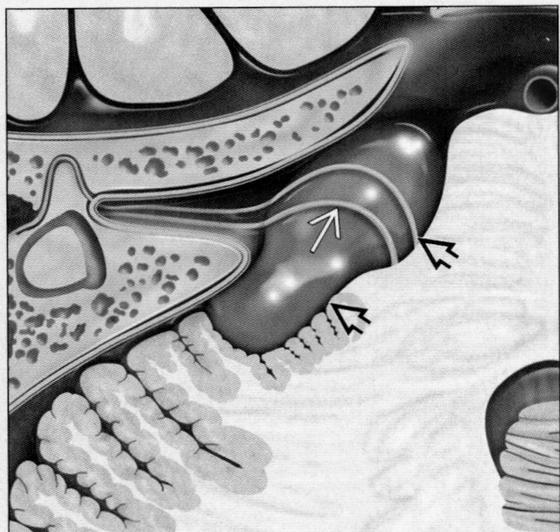

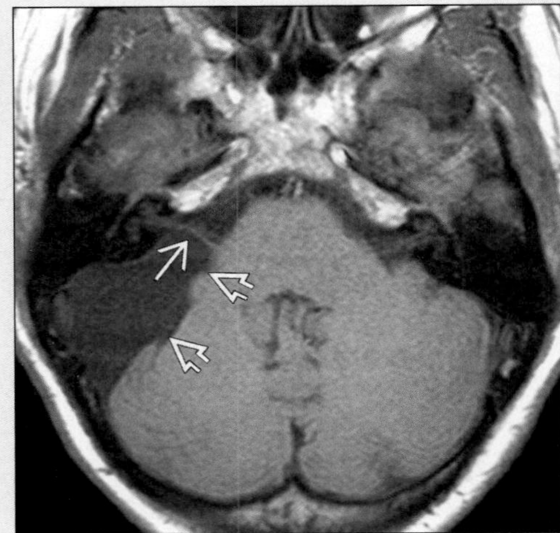

(Left) *Axial graphic of an arachnoid cyst in the CPA shows a thin, translucent wall. Notice the cyst bowing the 7th and 8th cranial nerves anteriorly ➡ and effacing the brainstem and cerebellum ⇨.* ***(Right)*** *Axial T1WI MR reveals a large right CPA arachnoid cyst causing bowing of the facial and vestibulocochlear nerves anteriorly ➡ and flattening of the lateral margin of the pons and cerebellar hemisphere ⇨. No restriction on DWI is characteristic of arachnoid cyst.*

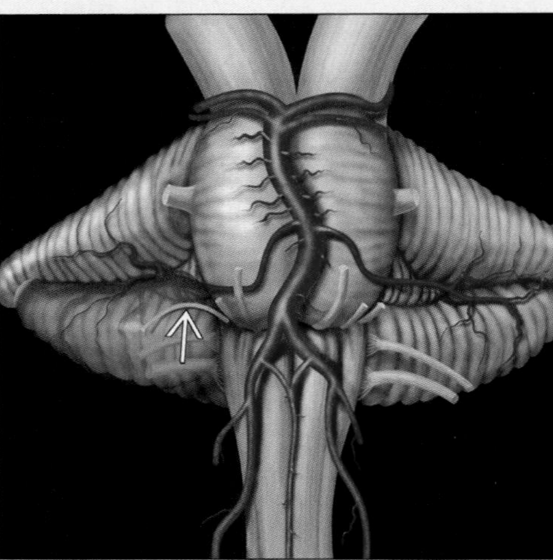

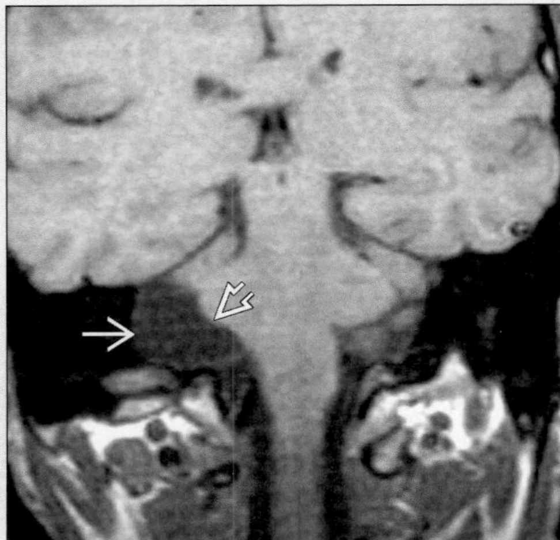

(Left) *Coronal graphic of a CPA arachnoid cyst depicts a typical translucent cyst wall. CN7 and CN8 are pushed by the cyst ➡ without being engulfed by it. In epidermoid cyst, cranial nerves are usually engulfed.* ***(Right)*** *Coronal T1WI MR demonstrates a small CSF intensity CPA arachnoid cyst ➡ with subtle mass effect on the adjacent brainstem ⇨. Complete fluid attenuation on FLAIR MR helps differentiate this lesion from an epidermoid cyst, which is the primary imaging differential diagnosis.*

ARACHNOID CYST, CPA-IAC

TERMINOLOGY

Abbreviations
- Arachnoid cyst (AC)

Synonyms
- Primary or congenital AC, subarachnoid cyst

Definitions
- Developmental arachnoid duplication anomaly creating CSF-filled sac

IMAGING

General Features
- Best diagnostic clue
  - Sharply demarcated round/ovoid extraaxial cisternal cyst with imperceptible walls with CSF density on CT or signal intensity on MR
  - AC signal parallels CSF on all MR sequences
    - **Complete fluid attenuation** on FLAIR MR
    - **No diffusion restriction** on DWI MR imaging
- Location
  - 10-20% of all AC occur in posterior fossa
    - CPA = most common infratentorial site
  - Spread patterns
    - Most remain confined to CPA (60%)
    - May spread dorsal to brainstem (25%)
    - Rarely spreads into IAC
- Size
  - Broad range: 1-8 cm
  - May be very large but asymptomatic
  - When large, will exert mass effect on adjacent brainstem and cerebellum
- Morphology
  - Sharply demarcated with broad-arching margins
  - Displaces, does not engulf, surrounding structures
  - Pushes cisternal structures but does not insinuate
    - Epidermoid cyst insinuates adjacent structures

CT Findings
- NECT
  - Density same as CSF
  - Rare high density from hemorrhage or proteinaceous fluid
- CECT
  - No enhancement of cavity or wall
- Bone CT
  - Rarely causes pressure erosion of adjacent bone
- CT cisternography
  - May show connection to subarachnoid space

MR Findings
- T1WI
  - Low signal lesion isointense to CSF
- T2WI
  - High signal lesion isointense to CSF
    - May have brighter signal than CSF
      - Cyst fluid lacks CSF pulsations
  - Well-circumscribed, pushing lesion compresses adjacent brainstem and cerebellum when large
    - Hydrocephalus seen with only larger CPA-IAC
- FLAIR
  - Suppresses (nulls) completely
- DWI
  - No restriction (low signal)
- T1WI C+
  - No enhancement seen
- Phase-contrast cine MR
  - Flow quantification can sometimes distinguish AC from subarachnoid space
  - May show connection between AC and cistern

Ultrasonographic Findings
- Grayscale ultrasound
  - Shows sonolucent AC in infants < 1 year of age

Imaging Recommendations
- Best imaging tool
  - MR ± contrast
- Protocol advice
  - Add FLAIR (suppresses)
  - Add DWI (no restricted diffusion)

DIFFERENTIAL DIAGNOSIS

Mega Cisterna Magna
- Prominence of retrocerebellar CSF space
- Large mega cisterna magna can extend into the CPA
- Not associated with cerebellar abnormalities

Cystic Vestibular Schwannoma
- Intramural or marginal cysts seen in larger lesions
- Foci of enhancing tumor always present on T1WI C+ MR
- Rarely larger lesions have associated AC

Epidermoid Cyst, CPA-IAC
- Major lesion of differential concern in setting of AC
- FLAIR: Incomplete fluid attenuation
- DWI: Restriction (high signal)
- Morphology: Insinuates adjacent CSF spaces

Cystic Meningioma, CPA-IAC
- Rare meningioma variant
- Dural "tails," asymmetry to IAC still present with mixed enhancement on T1WI C+ MR

Neurenteric Cyst
- Rare prepontine cistern near midline
- Often contains proteinaceous fluid (↑ on T1WI MR)

Cystic Infratentorial Ependymoma
- Ependymoma pedunculates from 4th ventricle via foramen of Luschka
- 50% calcified
- Cystic and solid enhancing components

Cerebellar Pilocytic Astrocytoma
- Cystic tumor in cerebellar hemisphere
- Enhancing mural nodule

PATHOLOGY

General Features
- Etiology

ARACHNOID CYST, CPA-IAC

- Embryonic meninges fail to merge
  - Remain separate as **duplicated** arachnoid
  - Split arachnoid contains CSF
- 2 types
  - Noncommunicating; most common type
  - Communicating with subarachnoid space/cistern
- Genetics
  - Usually sporadic; rarely familial
- Associated abnormalities
  - Acoustic schwannoma has AC associated in 0.5%

Gross Pathologic & Surgical Features

- Fluid-containing cyst with translucent membrane
- Displaces adjacent vessels or cranial nerves

Microscopic Features

- Thin wall of flattened but normal arachnoid cells

CLINICAL ISSUES

Presentation

- Most common signs/symptoms
  - Small AC: **Asymptomatic, incidental** finding (MR)
  - Large AC: Symptoms from direct compression ± ↑ intracranial pressure
- Other signs/symptoms
  - Defined by location and size
    - Headache
    - Dizziness, tinnitus ± sensorineural hearing loss
    - Hemifacial spasm or trigeminal neuralgia
- Clinical profile
  - Adult undergoing brain MR for unrelated symptoms

Demographics

- Age
  - May be initially seen at any age
    - 75% of AC occur in children
- Gender
  - M:F = 3-5:1
- Epidemiology
  - Accounts for 1% of intracranial masses

Natural History & Prognosis

- Most AC **do not enlarge** over time
  - Infrequently enlarge via CSF pulsation through ball-valve opening into AC
  - Hemorrhage with subsequent ↓ in size reported
- If surgery is limited to AC where symptoms are clearly related, prognosis is excellent
- Radical cyst removal may result in cranial neuropathy ± vascular compromise

Treatment

- Most cases require **no treatment**
- Surgical intervention is highly selective process
  - Reserved for cases where clear symptoms can be directly linked to AC anatomic location
  - Endoscopic cyst decompression via fenestration
    - Least invasive initial approach

DIAGNOSTIC CHECKLIST

Consider

- Differentiate AC from epidermoid cyst
  - AC: No restriction on DWI = best clue
- Determine if symptoms match location of AC before considering surgical treatment

Image Interpretation Pearls

- AC signal follows CSF on all MR sequences
  - Remember T2 signal may be higher than CSF from lack of CSF pulsation
- DWI sequence shows AC as low signal
- FLAIR sequence shows AC as low signal
- No enhancement of AC, including wall, is expected
  - If nodular C+, consider alternative diagnosis

Reporting Tips

- Since AC is usually not treated surgically, avoid offering any differential diagnosis when imaging findings diagnose AC

SELECTED REFERENCES

1. Boutarbouch M et al: Management of intracranial arachnoid cysts: institutional experience with initial 32 cases and review of the literature. Clin Neurol Neurosurg. 110(1):1-7, 2008
2. Marin-Sanabria EA et al: Evaluation of the management of arachnoid cyst of the posterior fossa in pediatric population: experience over 27 years. Childs Nerv Syst. 23(5):535-42, 2007
3. Helland CA et al: A population-based study of intracranial arachnoid cysts: clinical and neuroimaging outcomes following surgical cyst decompression in children. J Neurosurg. 105(5 Suppl):385-90, 2006
4. Osborn AG et al: Intracranial cysts: radiologic-pathologic correlation and imaging approach. Radiology. 239(3):650-64, 2006
5. Tang L et al: Diffusion-weighted imaging distinguishes recurrent epidermoid neoplasm from postoperative arachnoid cyst in the lumbosacral spine. J Comput Assist Tomogr. 30(3):507-9, 2006
6. Alaani A et al: Cerebellopontine angle arachnoid cysts in adult patients: what is the appropriate management? J Laryngol Otol. 119(5):337-41, 2005
7. Eskandary H et al: Incidental findings in brain computed tomography scans of 3000 head trauma patients. Surg Neurol. 63(6):550-3; discussion 553, 2005
8. Yildiz H et al: evaluation of communication between intracranial arachnoid cysts and cisterns with phase-contrast cine MR imaging. AJNR Am J Neuroradiol. 26(1):145-51, 2005
9. Dutt SN et al: Radiologic differentiation of intracranial epidermoids from arachnoid cysts. Otol Neurotol. 23(1):84-92, 2002
10. Ottaviani F et al: Arachnoid cyst of the cranial posterior fossa causing sensorineural hearing loss and tinnitus: a case report. Eur Arch Otorhinolaryngol. 259(6):306-8, 2002
11. Samii M et al: Arachnoid cysts of the posterior fossa. Surg Neurol. 51(4):376-82, 1999
12. Jallo GI et al: Arachnoid cysts of the cerebellopontine angle: diagnosis and surgery. Neurosurgery. 40(1):31-7; discussion 37-8, 1997
13. Higashi S et al: Hemifacial spasm associated with a cerebellopontine angle arachnoid cyst in a young adult. Surg Neurol. 37(4):289-92, 1992

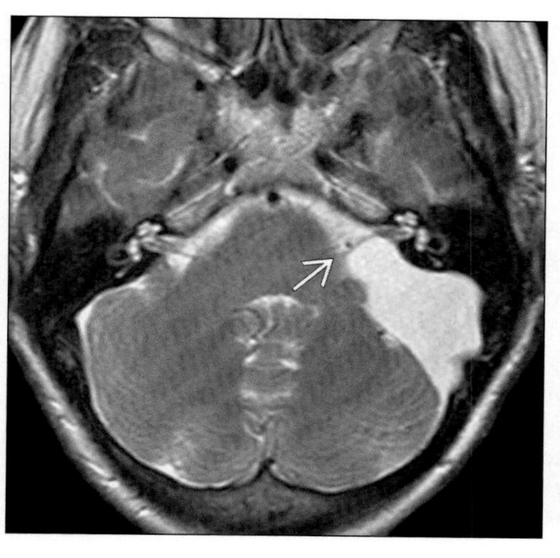

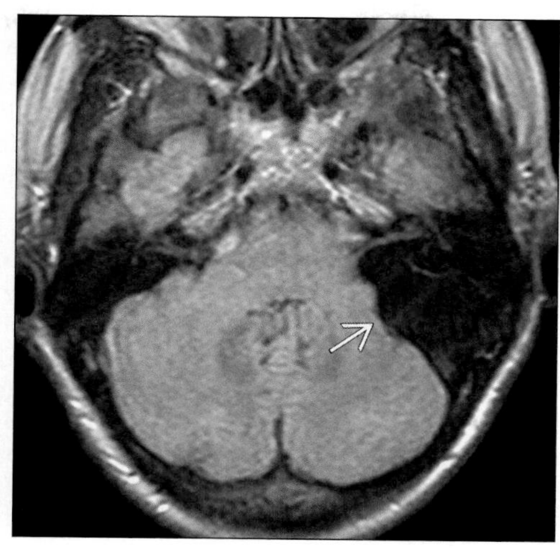

(Left) *Axial T2WI MR shows a high signal large arachnoid cyst enlarging the left cerebellopontine angle cistern. The facial and vestibulocochlear nerves are visible bowing over the anteromedial surface of the arachnoid cyst ➡.* ***(Right)*** *Axial FLAIR MR in the same patient shows the low signal arachnoid cyst ➡ and complete fluid attenuation. FLAIR suppression is expected as the arachnoid cyst is essentially CSF collecting between arachnoid layers.*

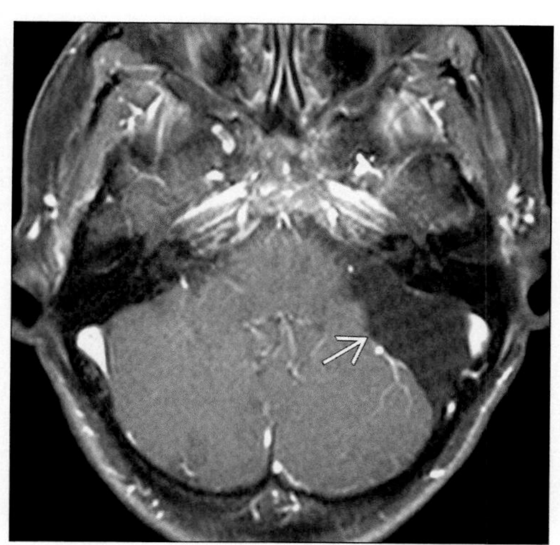

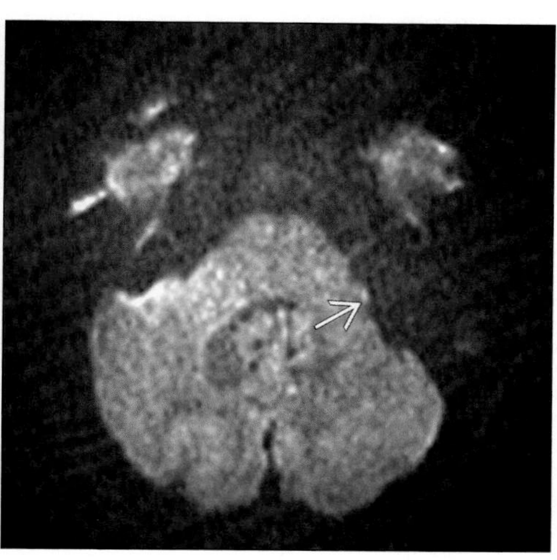

(Left) *Axial T1WI C+ FS MR in the same patient demonstrates that the CPA arachnoid cyst ➡ does not enhance.* ***(Right)*** *Axial DWI MR in the same patient shows the arachnoid cyst ➡ has no associated signal (no restricted diffusion). If this were an epidermoid cyst, high signal on DWI (restricted diffusion) would be present. DWI is the best way to differentiate an arachnoid cyst from an epidermoid cyst.*

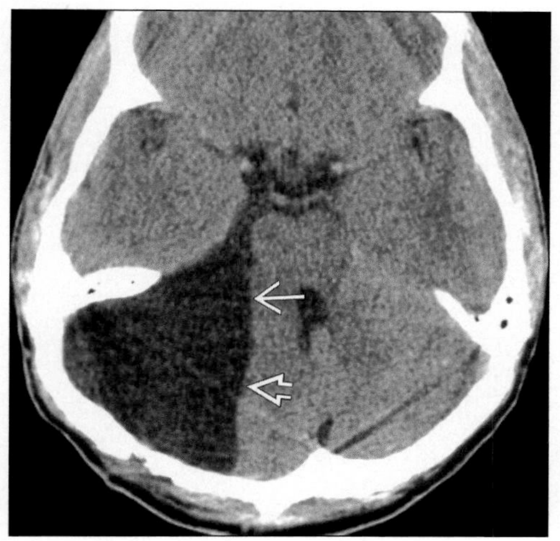

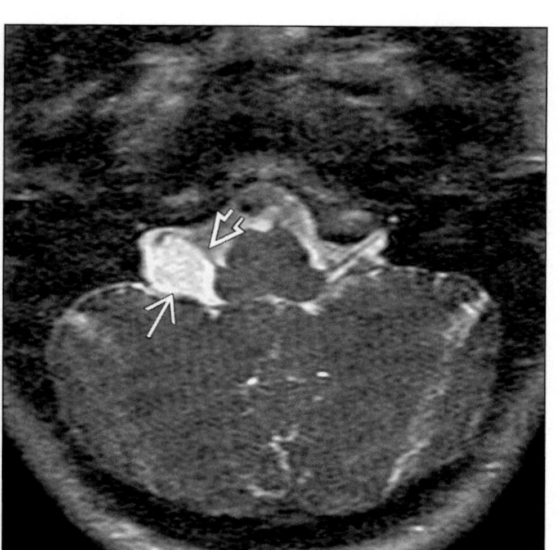

(Left) *Axial NECT through the upper CPA cistern shows a large low-density arachnoid cyst causing flattening of the lateral brachium pontis ➡ and cerebellar hemisphere ➡.* ***(Right)*** *Axial T2WI FS MR demonstrates an incidental hyperintense CPA arachnoid cyst ➡ found at the time of imaging for headache. This lenticular-shaped lesion displaces the glossopharyngeal nerve (CN9) anteriorly ➡. These small lesions require no additional imaging or treatment.*

BELL PALSY

Key Facts

Terminology

- Bell palsy (BP): Herpetic peripheral facial nerve paralysis secondary to herpes simplex virus

Imaging

- T1WI C+ fat-saturated MR: Fundal "tuft" and labyrinthine segment CN7 intense asymmetric enhancement
  - Entire intratemporal CN7 may enhance
- Imaging note: Classic rapid onset BP requires **no imaging** in initial stages
- If **atypical Bell palsy**, search with imaging for underlying lesion

Top Differential Diagnoses

- Normal enhancement of intratemporal CN7
- Facial nerve schwannoma
- Facial nerve hemangioma
- Perineural tumor from parotid

Pathology

- Etiology-pathogenesis (current hypothesis)
  - Latent herpes simplex infection of geniculate ganglion with reactivation and spread of inflammatory process along proximal and distal intratemporal facial nerve fibers

Clinical Issues

- Classic clinical presentation
  - Acute onset peripheral CN7 paralysis (36 hr onset)
- Medical therapy
  - Tapering course of prednisone; begin within 3 days of symptoms for best result
- Surgical therapy
  - Profound denervation (> 95%) treated with facial nerve decompression from IAC fundus to stylomastoid foramen

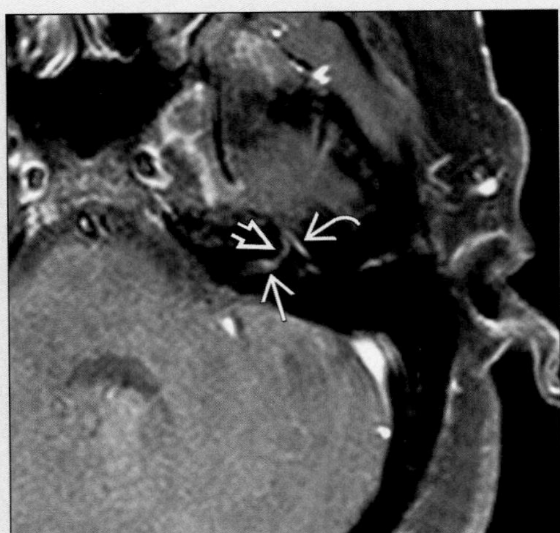

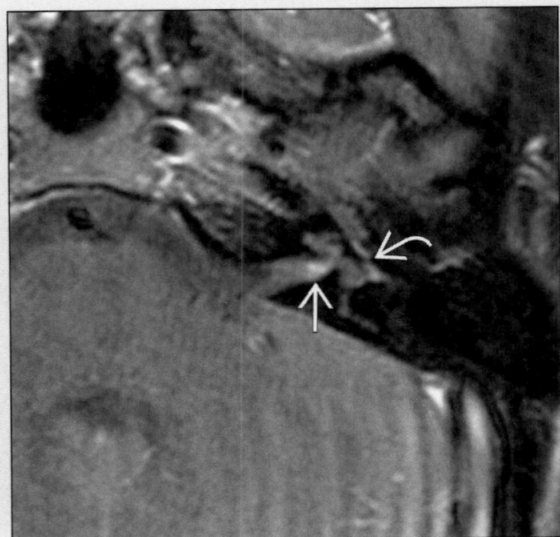

***(Left)** Axial T1WI C+ FS MR shows classic findings of Bell palsy with the fundal "tuft" sign →, labyrinthine ⇨, and tympanic ↪ facial nerve segment enhancement. **(Right)** Axial T1WI C+ FS MR in the same patient again shows the IAC fundal "tuft" sign → and tympanic segment of the facial nerve enhancement ↪. Remember that only the geniculate ganglion area of the facial nerve may normally enhance.*

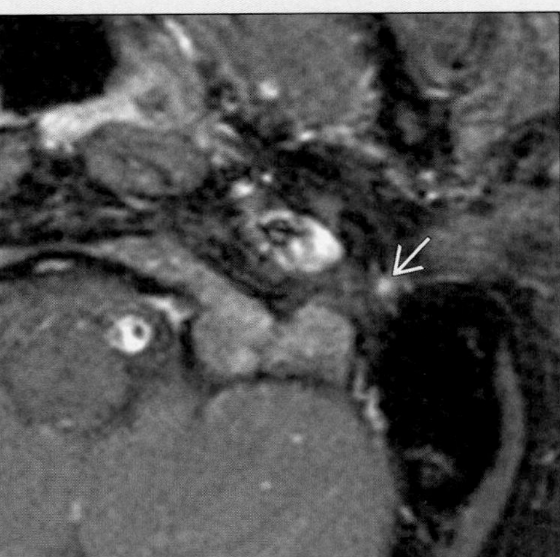

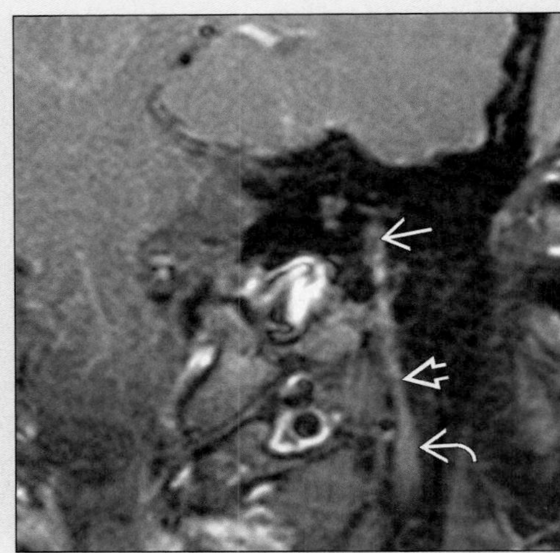

***(Left)** Axial T1WI C+ FS MR in the same patient through the stylomastoid foramen demonstrates an enhancing, slightly enlarged facial nerve →. Swelling of the facial nerve is possible outside the bony facial nerve canal within the temporal bone. **(Right)** Coronal T1WI C+ FS MR in the same patient reveals avid enhancement in the mastoid →, stylomastoid ⇨, and extracranial facial nerve ↪ in this patient with typical Bell palsy.*

BELL PALSY

TERMINOLOGY

Abbreviations

- Bell palsy (BP)

Synonyms

- Herpetic facial paralysis

Definitions

- BP (original definition): Idiopathic acute onset lower motor neuron facial paralysis
- BP (modern definition): Herpetic facial paralysis secondary to herpes simplex virus

IMAGING

General Features

- Best diagnostic clue
  - Fundal "tuft" and labyrinthine segment CN7 intense asymmetric enhancement on T1WI C+ MR
- Location
  - Fundal and labyrinthine segment CN7 most commonly affected
  - May involve entire intratemporal CN7
    - Intraparotid segment less commonly affected
- Size
  - CN7 swells within facial nerve canal

CT Findings

- CECT
  - No role for C+ CT in BP
- Bone CT
  - Normal facial nerve canal
    - If enlargement present, not Bell palsy

MR Findings

- T1WI
  - Intratemporal CN7 may be more conspicuous
- T2WI
  - Brain normal; no high signal lesions
  - High-resolution T2WI may show distal IAC CN7 enlargement
- T1WI C+
  - Uniform, contiguous CN7 enhancement
    - CN7: Normal in size within bony canal
    - CN7: Conspicuous high signal appears slightly enlarged
    - Enhancement pattern is linear, not nodular
  - Enhancement is usually present from distal IAC through labyrinthine segment, geniculate ganglion, and anterior tympanic segment
    - **Tuft** of enhancement in IAC fundus (premeatal segment) along with C+ of labyrinthine segment of CN7 are distinctive MR findings
    - Mastoid CN7 enhances less frequently
    - Enhancement of intraparotid CN7 infrequent
  - Holotympanic CN7 enhancement may be seen

Imaging Recommendations

- Best imaging tool
  - Thin-section fat-saturated T1WI C+ MR focused to IAC and temporal bone
  - T-bone CT: Only used if lesion found on MR
- Classic rapid onset BP requires no imaging in initial stages
  - 90% CN7 recover spontaneously in < 2 months
  - If decompressive surgery is anticipated, MR imaging warranted to ensure that no other lesion is causing CN7 paralysis
- If **atypical Bell palsy**, search for underlying lesion
  - Atypical Bell palsy
    - Slowly progressive CN7 palsy
    - Facial hyperfunction (spasm) preceding BP
    - Recurrent CN7 palsies
    - Unusual degrees of ear pain
    - BP with any other associated cranial neuropathies
    - Peripheral CN7 paralysis persisting or deepening > 2 months

DIFFERENTIAL DIAGNOSIS

Normal Enhancement of Intratemporal CN7

- Clinical: No facial nerve paralysis
- T1WI C+ MR: Mild, linear, discontinuous enhancement of anterior and posterior genus of intratemporal CN7
  - Premeatal and labyrinthine CN7 segments normal

Facial Nerve Schwannoma

- Clinical: Hearing loss more common than CN7 palsy
- T1WI C+ MR: Well-circumscribed, tubular, C+ mass within enlarged CN7 canal most commonly centered on geniculate ganglion

Facial Nerve Hemangioma

- Clinical: CN7 paralysis occurs when lesion is small
- Bone CT: May show intratumoral bone spicules
- T1WI C+ MR: Poorly circumscribed, enhancing mass commonly found in geniculate fossa

Perineural Tumor from Parotid

- Clinical: Parotid malignancy usually palpable
- Imaging: Invasive parotid mass is present
  - Tissue-filled sylomastoid foramen
  - CN7 is enlarged from distal to proximal with mastoid air cell invasion associated

PATHOLOGY

General Features

- Etiology
  - Etiology-pathogenesis (current hypothesis)
    - Latent herpes simplex infection of geniculate ganglion with reactivation and spread of inflammatory process along proximal and distal CN7 fibers
    - Pathophysiology: Formation of intraneural edema in neuronal sheaths caused by breakdown of blood-nerve barrier and by venous congestion in epineural and perineural venous plexus
    - CN7 swelling within bony canal causes ischemia
- Intratemporal CN7 normal anatomy
  - CN7 normal C+ at its anterior and posterior genus
  - C+ from robust circumneural arteriovenous plexus
  - Radiologist must be familiar with normal CN7 T1WI C+ MR enhancement

BELL PALSY

Brackman Facial Nerve Grading System

Grade	Description of Facial Paralysis	Measurement**	Function %	Estimated Function %
I	Normal	8/8	100	100
II	Slight	7/8	76-99	80
III	Moderate	5/8-6/8	51-75	60
IV	Moderately severe	3/8-4/8	26-50	40
V	Severe	1/8-/8	1-25	20
VI	Total	0/8	0	0

*** Facial nerve injury is measured the superior movement of the upper eyebrow mid-portion and the lateral movement of the oral commissure. For each 0.25 cm of upward motion for both eyebrow and oral commissure, a scale of 1 is assigned up to 1 cm. The points are then added together. A total of 8 points can be obtained if both the eyebrow and the oral commissure both move 1 cm. Adapted from House JW et al: Facial nerve grading system. Otolaryngol Head Neck Surg. 93(2):146-7, 1985.*

- ○ Familiarity with normal patterns of intratemporal CN7 C+ allows radiologist to identify abnormal C+ seen with BP

Gross Pathologic & Surgical Features

- CN7 edema peaks at 3 weeks after symptom onset

Microscopic Features

- Herpes simplex DNA recovered from BP CN7

CLINICAL ISSUES

Presentation

- Most common signs/symptoms
  - Acute onset peripheral CN7 paralysis (36 hour onset)
- Clinical profile
  - Healthy adult with acute unilateral CN7 paralysis
    - More common in diabetic patients
- Other signs/symptoms
  - Viral prodrome often reported before BP onset
  - 70%: Taste alterations days before CN7 paralysis
  - 50%: Pain around ipsilateral ear (not severe)
  - 20%: Numbness in ipsilateral face

Demographics

- Age
  - All ages affected; incidence peaks in 5th decade
- Epidemiology
  - Herpetic facial paralysis is responsible for > 50% of peripheral CN7 paralysis cases
  - Annual BP incidence: 15-30/100,000 persons

Natural History & Prognosis

- > 90% of patients spontaneously recover all or part of CN7 function without therapy in 1st 2 months

Treatment

- Test for diabetes and Lyme disease
- Medical therapy
  - Tapering course of prednisone; begin within 3 days of symptoms for best result
  - Acyclovir or valacyclovir (antivirals) out of favor
- Surgical therapy
  - Profound denervation (> 95%) treated with CN7 decompression, fundus to stylomastoid foramen
  - Decompression performed within 2 weeks of onset of total paralysis for maximal effect
- Intensity, pattern ± location of enhancement seen on T1WI C+ MR not helpful in predicting outcome for individual patient

DIAGNOSTIC CHECKLIST

Consider

- MR imaging reserved for atypical Bell palsy
- Abnormal CN7 C+ may persist well beyond clinical improvement or full recovery

Image Interpretation Pearls

- "Tuft" of IAC fundal C+ associated with labyrinthine segment CN7 C+ without associated focal lesion is highly suggestive of Bell palsy

Reporting Tips

- Remember to comment on parotid as normal
- Also note absence of focal CN7 lesions

SELECTED REFERENCES

1. Song MH et al: Clinical significance of quantitative analysis of facial nerve enhancement on MRI in Bell's palsy. Acta Otolaryngol. 128(11):1259-65, 2008
2. Sullivan FM et al: Early treatment with prednisolone or acyclovir in Bell's palsy. N Engl J Med. 357(16):1598-607, 2007
3. Kress B et al: Bell palsy: quantitative analysis of MR imaging data as a method of predicting outcome. Radiology. 230(2):504-9, 2004
4. Suzuki F et al: Herpes virus reactivation and gadolinium-enhanced magnetic resonance imaging in patients with facial palsy. Otol Neurotol. 22(4):549-53, 2001
5. Roob G et al: Peripheral facial palsy: etiology, diagnosis and treatment. Eur Neurol. 41(1):3-9, 1999
6. Engstrom M et al: Serial gadolinium-enhanced magnetic resonance imaging and assessment of facial nerve function in Bell's palsy. Otolaryngol Head Neck Surg. 117(5):559-66, 1997
7. Saatçi I et al: MRI of the facial nerve in idiopathic facial palsy. Eur Radiol. 6(5):631-6, 1996
8. Tien R et al: Contrast-enhanced MR imaging of the facial nerve in 11 patients with Bell's palsy. AJNR Am J Neuroradiol. 11(4):735-41, 1990

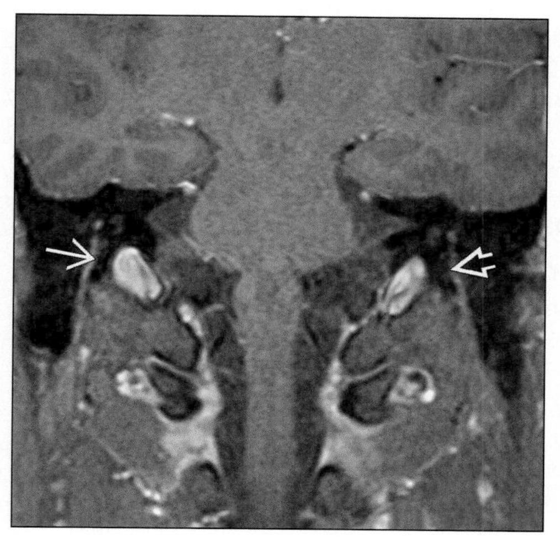

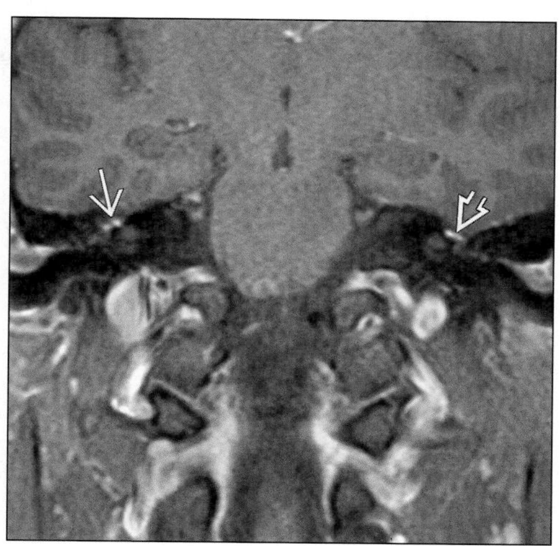

(Left) *Coronal T1WI C+ FS MR in a patient with right Bell palsy shows asymmetric right mastoid CN7 avid enhancement compared to the minimal enhancement on the left.* ***(Right)*** *Coronal T1WI C+ FS MR in the same patient shows similar enhancement of the right compared to the left geniculate ganglion. This can be explained by the fact that the geniculate ganglion is the area of normal intratemporal facial nerve enhancement.*

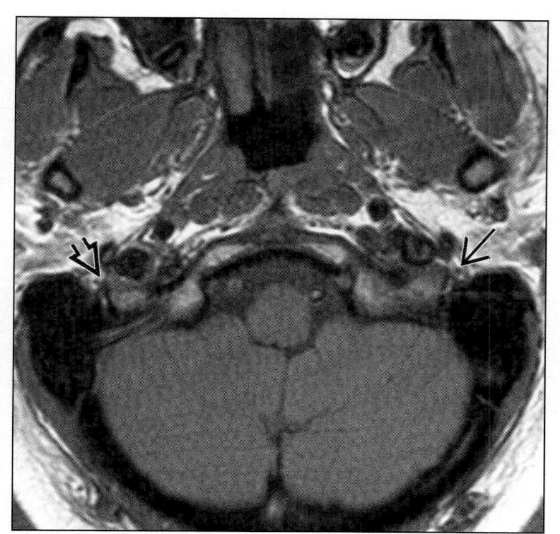

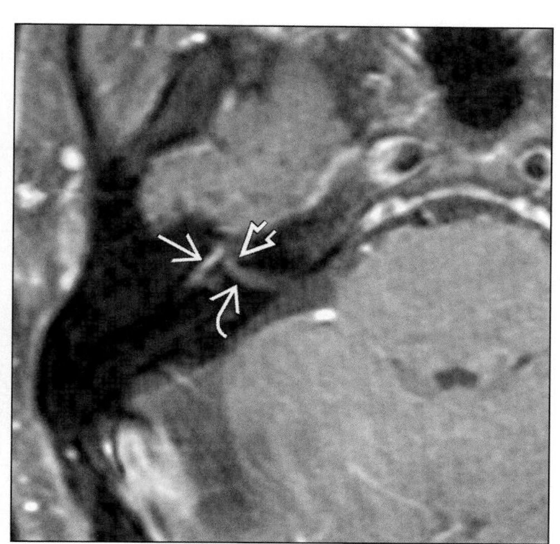

(Left) *Axial T1WI MR in a patient with left Bell palsy reveals the left facial nerve in the stylomastoid foramen is larger than the right. The injured left facial nerve swells when it is not confined by the intratemporal bony facial nerve canal.* ***(Right)*** *Axial T1WI C+ FS MR in a patient with right-sided Bell palsy demonstrates typical findings of enhancing tympanic and labyrinthine segments of the facial nerve. Notice the more subtle IAC fundus "tuft" sign.*

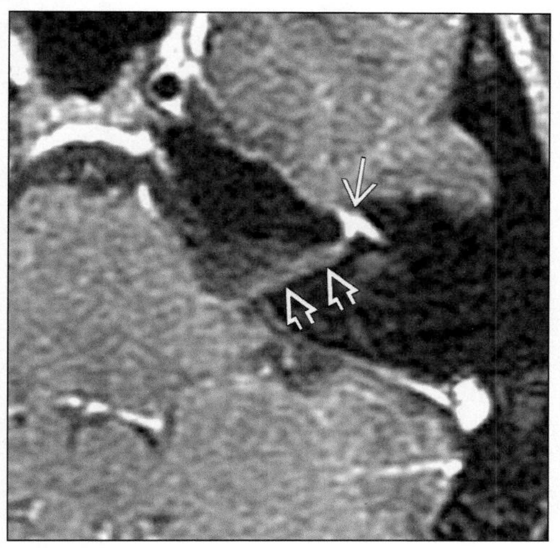

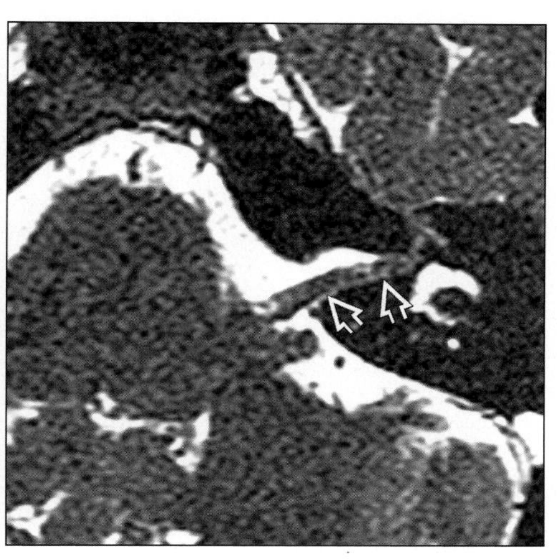

(Left) *Axial T1WI C+ FS MR in a patient with profound, unremitting Bell palsy shows intense enhancement of the labyrinthine, geniculate ganglion, and anterior tympanic portions of the facial nerve. The IAC "tuft" spreads along the IAC facial nerve as more subtle enhancement reaching the porus acusticus.* ***(Right)*** *Axial thin-section (1 mm) T2WI FS MR in the same patient reveals a swollen intracanalicular facial nerve through the internal auditory canal.*

Key Facts

Terminology
- Vascular loop compressing trigeminal nerve at its root entry zone (REZ) along lateral pontine surface

Imaging
- High-resolution T2WI MR shows serpiginous asymmetric signal void (vessel) in CPA CN5 REZ
- Offending vessels: Superior cerebellar artery > PICA > vertebral artery

Top Differential Diagnoses
- Aneurysm, CPA-IAC
- Arteriovenous malformation, CPA
- Venous angioma, posterior fossa

Pathology
- CN5 REZ experiences "irritation" from vessel

Clinical Issues
- Trigeminal neuralgia symptoms
  - Lancinating pain following V2 ± V3 distributions
  - May occur spontaneously or in response to tactile stimulation
- Treatment
  - Begin with conservative drug therapy
  - Gamma-knife therapy (70% success)
  - Microvascular decompression as needed

Diagnostic Checklist
- Look for multiple sclerosis and cisternal masses
- Follow CN5 distally into cavernous sinus and face
  - Exclude perineural tumor, malignancies of face
- Next view high-resolution thin-section T2WI MR images for offending vessel
- Negative MR does not preclude surgical therapy

*(**Left**) Axial T2WI MR in this patient with right trigeminal neuralgia shows the low signal superior cerebellar artery ➡ impinging on the root entry zone of the preganglionic segment ➡ of the trigeminal nerve. (**Right**) Coronal T1WI MR in the same patient reveals the superior cerebellar artery ➡ compressing and deforming the right proximal preganglionic segment of CN5 ➡. Notice the larger normal left preganglionic CN5 ➡ indicating that atrophy is a feature of the affected right side.*

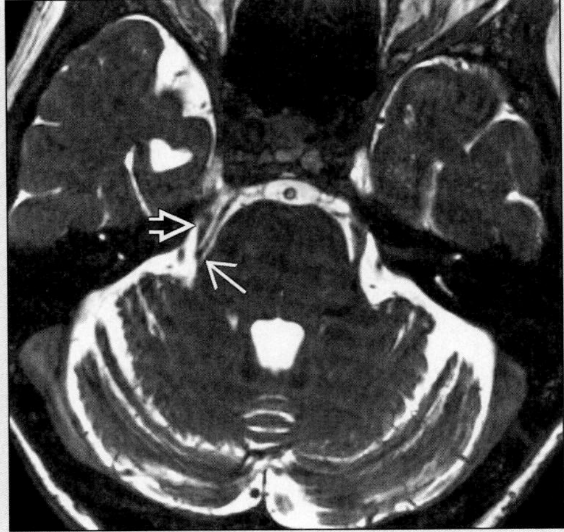

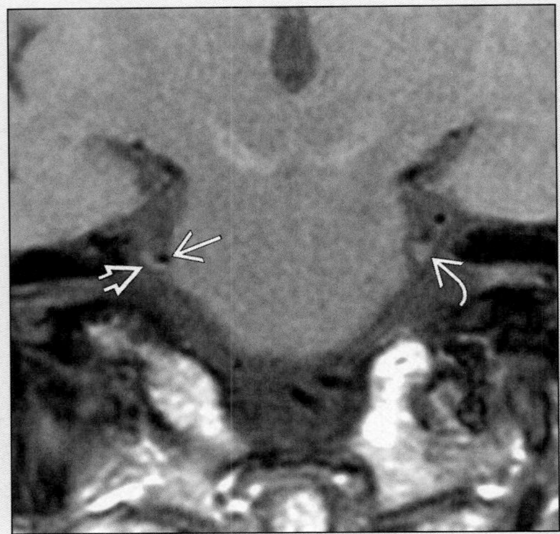

*(**Left**) Axial T2WI FS MR in patient with right trigeminal neuralgia reveals a multiple sclerosis lesion ➡ involving the lateral pons at the root entry zone of the trigeminal nerve ➡. Rarely cisternal masses or MS may present with trigeminal neuralgia. (**Right**) Axial T1WI C+ MR in a patient with right TN shows a development venous anomaly of cerebellum draining through lateral pons ➡ and root entry zone ➡ of CN5. Less than 5% of patients with TN have a venous explanation for their symptoms.*

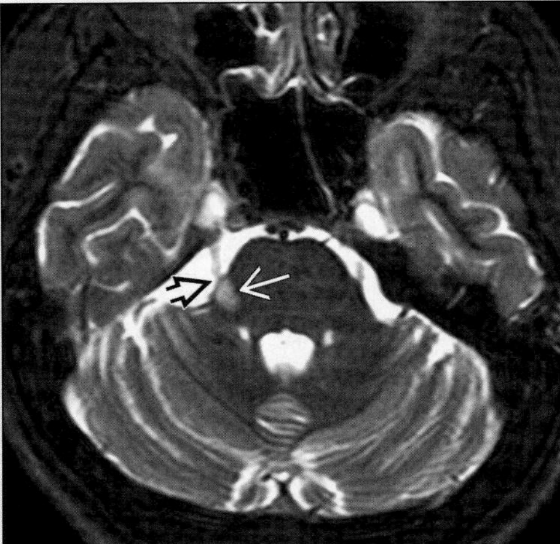

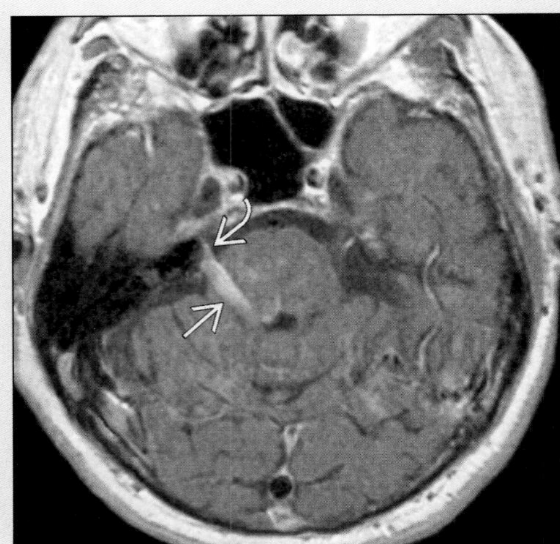

TRIGEMINAL NEURALGIA

TERMINOLOGY

Abbreviations

- Trigeminal neuralgia (TN)

Synonyms

- Tic douloureux, trigeminal nerve vascular loop syndrome, trigeminal nerve hyperactive dysfunction syndrome

Definitions

- Vascular loop compressing trigeminal nerve at its root entry zone (REZ) along lateral pontine surface

IMAGING

General Features

- Best diagnostic clue
  - High-resolution T2WI MR shows serpentine asymmetric signal void (vessel) in CPA CN5 REZ
- TN offending vessels: **Superior cerebellar artery** (SCA) > PICA > vertebral artery

CT Findings

- NECT: Most commonly normal

MR Findings

- T2WI
  - High-resolution T2 shows vessel compressing REZ of CN5 ± nerve atrophy
- FLAIR: Brainstem and brain are normal
  - Multiple sclerosis (MS) may present with TN
- MRA: Source images most helpful

Imaging Recommendations

- Best imaging tool
  - High-resolution T2 for imaging of vascular loop

DIFFERENTIAL DIAGNOSIS

Aneurysm, CPA-IAC

- PICA or vertebral artery aneurysm
- Oval complex signal mass
- Rarely causes TN

Arteriovenous Malformation, CPA

- Much larger vessels (arteries and veins) with nidus
- Rare in posterior fossa

Venous Angioma, Posterior Fossa

- Larger vessels (veins)
- CPA rare as venous drainage route
- Rarely causes venous compression-induced TN

PATHOLOGY

General Features

- Etiology
  - CN5 REZ vascular → **atrophy**
  - Atrophy secondary to structural abnormalities
    - Axonal loss and demyelination
  - Atrophy → abnormal contacts among nerve fibers
    - Abnormal contacts cause paroxysmal pain of TN

Gross Pathologic & Surgical Features

- Offending vessel compresses REZ CN5

Microscopic Features

- Myelin cover of proximal CN5 is breached

CLINICAL ISSUES

Presentation

- Most common signs/symptoms
  - Lancinating pain following V2 ± V3 distributions
  - Spontaneous or in response to tactile stimulation

Demographics

- Age
  - Older patients (usually > 65 years)
- Epidemiology
  - 5:100,000

Natural History & Prognosis

- Prognosis
  - 70% pain-free 10 years after surgery

Treatment

- Begin with conservative drug therapy
- Gamma-knife therapy (70% success)
- Microvascular decompression as needed

DIAGNOSTIC CHECKLIST

Consider

- Many normal vessels in CPA cistern

Image Interpretation Pearls

- Look for MS and cisternal masses
- Follow CN5 distally into cavernous sinus and face
  - Exclude perineural tumor, malignancies of face
- Next view T2 images for offending vessel
- Negative MR does not preclude surgical therapy

SELECTED REFERENCES

1. Fariselli L et al: CyberKnife radiosurgery as a first treatment for idiopathic trigeminal neuralgia. Neurosurgery. 64(2 Suppl):A96-101, 2009
2. Satoh T et al: Severity analysis of neurovascular contact in patients with trigeminal neuralgia: assessment with the inner view of the 3D MR cisternogram and angiogram fusion imaging. AJNR Am J Neuroradiol. 30(3):603-7, 2009
3. Sindou M et al: Microvascular decompression for primary trigeminal neuralgia: long-term effectiveness and prognostic factors in a series of 362 consecutive patients with clear-cut neurovascular conflicts who underwent pure decompression. J Neurosurg. 107(6):1144-53, 2007
4. Erbay SH et al: Nerve atrophy in severe trigeminal neuralgia: noninvasive confirmation at MR imaging--initial experience. Radiology. 238(2):689-92, 2006
5. Majoie CB et al: Trigeminal neuropathy: evaluation with MR imaging. Radiographics. 15(4):795-811, 1995

HEMIFACIAL SPASM

Key Facts

Terminology

- Vascular loop compressing facial nerve at its root exit zone within CPA cistern causing hemifacial spasm

Imaging

- High-resolution T2WI MR shows serpentine asymmetric signal void (vessel) in medial CPA
  - Offending vessels: AICA (50%), PICA (30%), VA (15%), vein (5%)

Top Differential Diagnoses

- Aneurysm, CPA-IAC
- Arteriovenous malformation, CPA
- Venous angioma, posterior fossa

Pathology

- CN7 bundle experiences "irritation" from vessel
- Multiple sclerosis has been reported to cause HFS
- Cisternal masses, such as epidermoid or meningioma, may cause HFS

Clinical Issues

- HFS: Unilateral involuntary facial spasms
  - Begins with orbicularis oculi spasms
  - Tonic-clonic bursts become constant over time

Diagnostic Checklist

- Positive MR findings present in ~ 50% HFS patients
- Look for cisternal mass lesions, multiple sclerosis
- Follow CN7 distally into T-bone and parotid
  - Exclude CN7 hemangioma, parotid malignancy
- Next determine if source images for MRA or high-resolution T2WI images identify offending vessel
  - Negative MR does not preclude surgical therapy

*(**Left**) Axial MRA source image in a patient with right hemifacial spasm shows a tortuous right vertebral artery ➔ and associated PICA ➔ pushing on the root exit zone of the facial nerve. The facial nerve is visible in the CPA cistern ➔. (**Right**) Axial CISS MR through the CPA cisterns in a patient with right hemifacial spasm demonstrates a PICA loop ➔ pushing the cisternal CN7 and CN8 posteriorly, causing them to drape over the posterior margin of the porus acusticus ➔.*

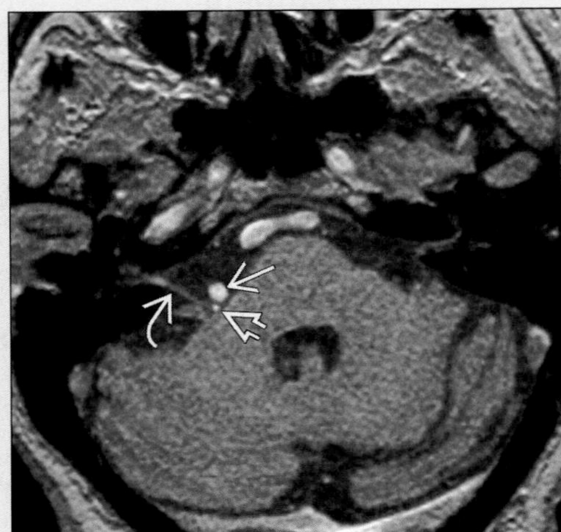

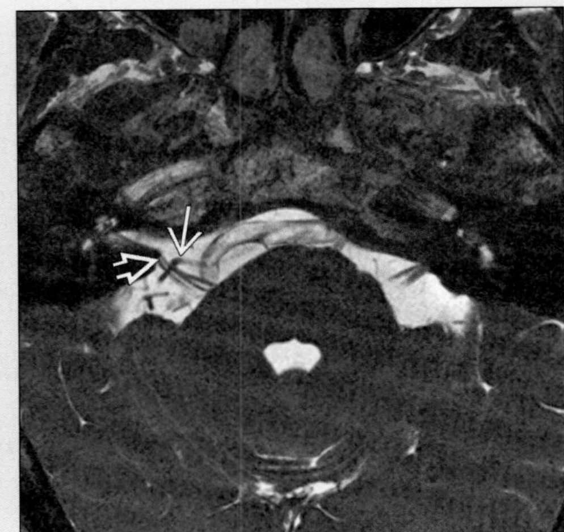

*(**Left**) Axial CISS MR in a patient with left hemifacial spasm reveals the left vertebral artery ➔ looping into the CPA cistern where it impinges on the proximal facial nerve ➔ at the root exit zone. (**Right**) Axial T2WI MR reveals a dolichoectatic vertebral artery ➔ impinging on the root exit zone ➔ of the facial nerve in the medial CPA cistern in this patient with hemifacial spasm. Approximately 50% of patients with hemifacial spasm have positive MR findings, typically on thin-section T2 or MRA sequences.*

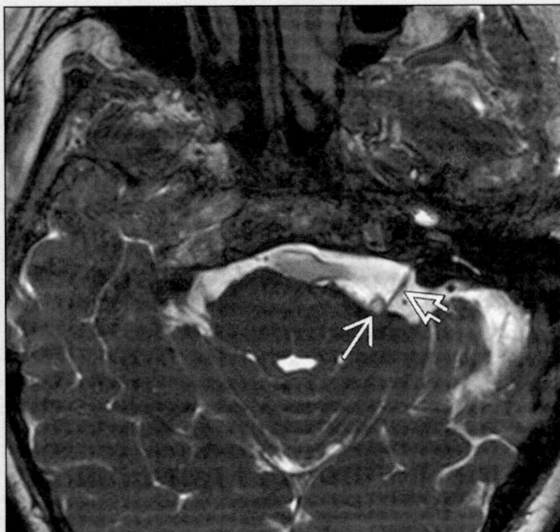

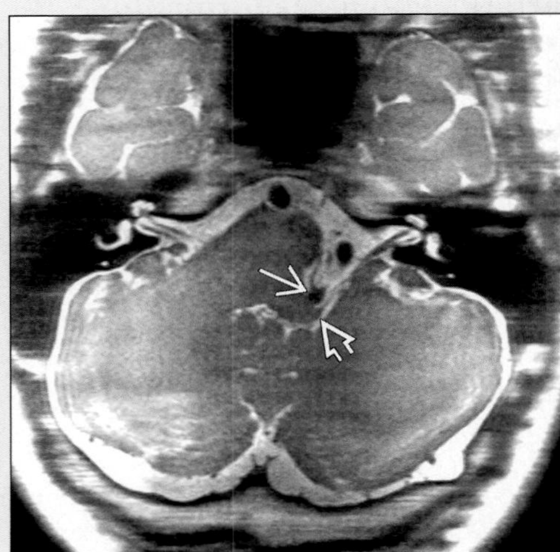

TERMINOLOGY

Abbreviations

- Hemifacial spasm (HFS)

Synonyms

- Facial nerve vascular loop syndrome, facial nerve hyperactive dysfunction syndrome

Definitions

- Vascular loop compressing facial nerve at its root exit zone within CPA cistern causing hemifacial spasm

IMAGING

General Features

- Best diagnostic clue
  - High-resolution T2WI MR shows serpentine asymmetric signal void (vessel) in medial CPA
- Location
  - Loop in medial CPA cistern at CN7 root exit zone
- HFS offending vessels: AICA (50%), PICA (30%), VA (15%), vein (5%)

CT Findings

- NECT: Most commonly normal

MR Findings

- T2WI
  - High-resolution T2WI: Vessel best seen as low-signal tube coursing through high-signal CSF
- FLAIR
  - Adjacent brain most commonly normal
  - Multiple sclerosis may present with HFS
- MRA: Source images most helpful

Imaging Recommendations

- Best imaging tool
  - Thin-section high-resolution T2WI MR of CPA allows best vascular loop visualization

DIFFERENTIAL DIAGNOSIS

Aneurysm, CPA-IAC

- PICA or vertebral artery aneurysm
- Oval complex signal mass

Arteriovenous Malformation, CPA

- Larger vessels (arteries and veins) with nidus
- Rare in posterior fossa

Venous Angioma, Posterior Fossa

- Larger vessels (veins)
- CPA rare as venous drainage route
- Rarely causes venous compression with HFS

PATHOLOGY

General Features

- Etiology
  - CN7 bundle experiences "irritation" from vessel
    - Brainstem nuclei secondarily affected
    - Abnormal brainstem response (ABR)

Gross Pathologic & Surgical Features

- Offending vessel compresses root exit zone of CN7

Microscopic Features

- Myelin cover on proximal CN7 breached

CLINICAL ISSUES

Presentation

- Most common signs/symptoms
  - HFS: Unilateral involuntary facial spasms
    - Begins with orbicularis oculi spasms
    - Tonic-clonic bursts become constant over time

Demographics

- Age
  - Older patients (usually > 65 years)
- Epidemiology
  - < 1:100,000

Natural History & Prognosis

- 90% symptom free for ≥ 5 years after surgery

Treatment

- Begin with conservative drug therapy
- Microvascular decompression as needed

DIAGNOSTIC CHECKLIST

Consider

- Positive MR findings present in ~ 50% of HFS patients

Image Interpretation Pearls

- Look for cisternal mass lesions, multiple sclerosis
- Follow CN7 distally into T-bone and parotid
  - Exclude CN7 hemangioma, parotid malignancy
- Next determine if source images for MRA or high-resolution T2WI images identify offending vessel
  - Negative MR does not preclude surgical therapy

SELECTED REFERENCES

1. Huh R et al: Microvascular decompression for hemifacial spasm: analyses of operative complications in 1582 consecutive patients. Surg Neurol. 69(2):153-7; discussion 157, 2008
2. Kakizawa Y et al: Anatomical study of the trigeminal and facial cranial nerves with the aid of 3.0-tesla magnetic resonance imaging. J Neurosurg. 108(3):483-90, 2008
3. Lee MS et al: Clinical usefulness of magnetic resonance cisternography in patients having hemifacial spasm. Yonsei Med J. 42(4):390-4, 2001
4. Yamakami I et al: Preoperative assessment of trigeminal neuralgia and hemifacial spasm using constructive interference in steady state-three-dimensional Fourier transformation magnetic resonance imaging. Neurol Med Chir (Tokyo). 40(11):545-55; discussion 555-6, 2000
5. Mitsuoka H et al: Delineation of small nerves and blood vessels with three-dimensional fast spin-echo MR imaging: comparison of presurgical and surgical findings in patients with hemifacial spasm. AJNR Am J Neuroradiol. 19(10):1823-9, 1998

VESTIBULAR SCHWANNOMA

Key Facts

Terminology

- VS: Benign tumor arising from Schwann cells that wrap vestibular branches of CN8 in CPA-IAC

Imaging

- High-resolution T2 or CISS: "Filling defect" in ↑ signal CSF of CPA-IAC cistern
  - Small VS: Ovoid filling defect in ↑ signal CSF
  - Large VS: "Ice cream on cone" shape in CPA-IAC
  - 0.5% associated arachnoid cyst
- FLAIR: ↑ cochlear signal from ↑ protein
- GRE/TSE: Microhemorrhage ↓ signal foci (common)
  - Not seen in meningioma
  - < 1%: Macroscopic intratumoral hemorrhage
- T1WI C+: Focal, enhancing mass of CPA-IAC cistern centered on porus acusticus
  - 15% with intramural cysts (low signal foci)

Top Differential Diagnoses

- Epidermoid cyst, CPA
- Aneurysm, CPA-IAC
- Meningioma, CPA-IAC
- Facial nerve schwannoma, CPA-IAC
- Metastases, CPA-IAC

Pathology

- Benign tumor arising from vestibular portion of CN8 at glial-Schwann cell junction

Clinical Issues

- Adults with unilateral sensorineural hearing loss
- Translabyrinthine resection if no hearing
- Middle cranial fossa approach for IAC VS
- Retrosigmoid approach when CPA or medial IAC component present
- Fractionated or stereotactic radiosurgery

*(**Left**) Axial graphic shows small intracanalicular vestibular schwannoma ➔ arising from the superior vestibular nerve. Notice the cochlear nerve canal is uninvolved ➔. (**Right**) Axial T2WI MR reveals a small intracanalicular vestibular schwannoma ➔ visualized as a tissue intensity mass surrounded by high intensity cerebrospinal fluid. The cochlear nerve canal ➔ is not involved, and an 8 mm fundal cap ➔ is present.*

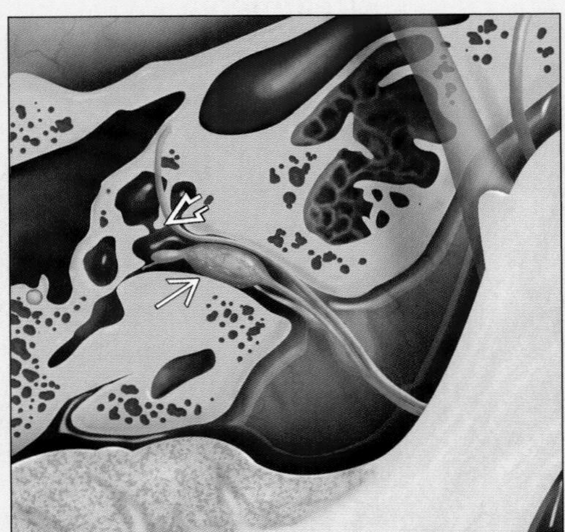

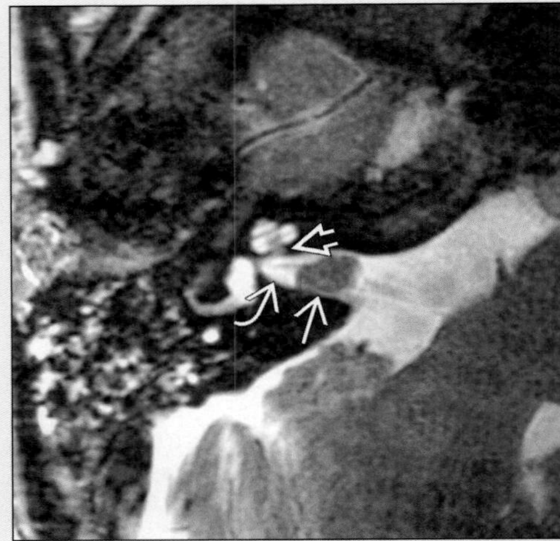

*(**Left**) Axial graphic of a large vestibular schwannoma reveals the typical "ice cream on cone" CPA-IAC morphology. Mass effect on the middle cerebellar peduncle ➔ and cerebellar hemisphere ➔ is evident. (**Right**) Axial T1WI C+ MR demonstrates a large CPA-IAC vestibular schwannoma compressing the middle cerebellar peduncle ➔ and cerebellar hemisphere ➔. Enhancement within the IAC and the large intramural cyst ➔ make the imaging diagnosis certain.*

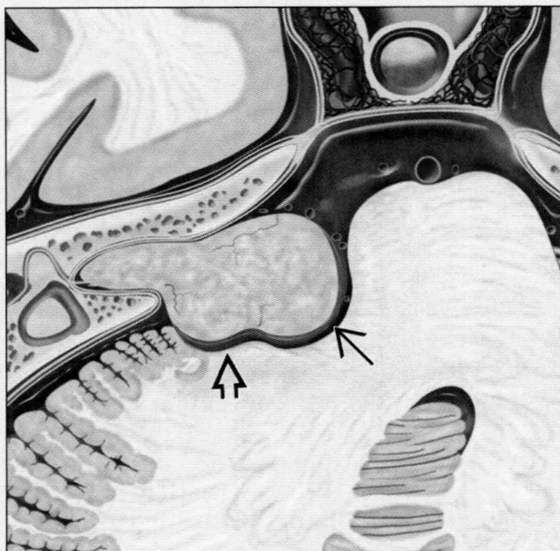

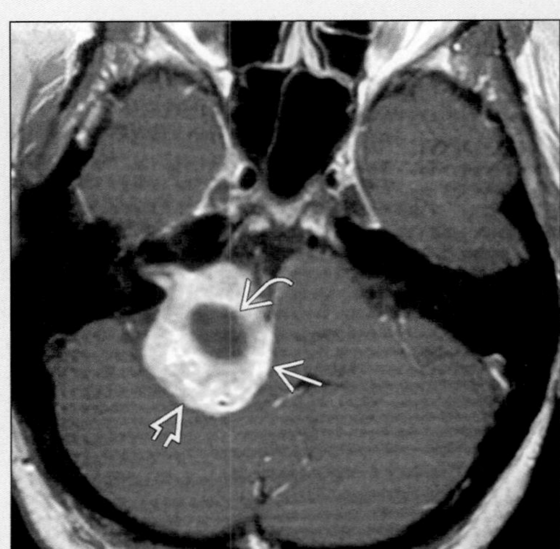

TERMINOLOGY

Abbreviations
- Vestibular schwannoma (VS)

Synonyms
- Acoustic schwannoma, acoustic neuroma, acoustic tumor
  - Uncommon names: Neurinoma, neurilemmoma

Definitions
- Benign tumor arising from Schwann cells that wrap vestibular branches of CN8 in CPA-IAC

IMAGING

General Features
- Best diagnostic clue
  - Avidly enhancing cylindrical (IAC) or "ice cream on cone" (CPA-IAC) mass
- Location
  - Small lesions: Intracanalicular
  - Large lesions: Intracanalicular with CPA cistern extension
- Size
  - Small lesions: 2-10 mm
  - Larger lesions: Up to 5 cm in maximum diameter
- Morphology
  - Small and intracanalicular VS: Ovoid mass
  - Large VS: "Ice cream (CPA) on cone (IAC)"

CT Findings
- CECT
  - Well-delineated, enhancing mass of CPA-IAC cistern
  - Calcification not present (compared to CPA meningioma)
  - May flare IAC when large
  - Smaller intracanalicular lesions (< 6 mm) may be missed with CECT

MR Findings
- T1WI
  - Brain signal most common
  - ↑ signal foci if rare hemorrhage present
- T2WI FS
  - High-resolution T2 or CISS: "Filling defect" in ↑ signal CSF of CPA-IAC cistern
    - Small lesion: Ovoid filling defect in ↑ signal CSF of IAC
    - Large lesion: "Ice cream on cone" filling defect in CPA-IAC
- FLAIR
  - ↑ cochlear signal from ↑ perilymph protein
- T2* GRE
  - Microhemorrhage low-signal foci common
    - Not seen in meningioma
- T1WI C+ FS
  - Focal, enhancing mass of CPA-IAC cistern centered on porus acusticus
  - 100% enhance strongly
  - 15% with intramural cysts (low-signal foci)
  - Dural "tails" rare (compared to meningioma)
- Other MR findings
  - < 1%: Macroscopic intratumoral hemorrhage
  - 0.5% associated arachnoid cyst

Imaging Recommendations
- Best imaging tool
  - Gold standard is full brain FLAIR MR with axial and coronal T1WI C+ FS MR of CPA-IAC
- Protocol advice
  - High-resolution T2 or CISS MR of CPA-IAC is only screening exam for VS
    - Used for uncomplicated unilateral SNHL in adult

DIFFERENTIAL DIAGNOSIS

Meningioma, CPA-IAC
- Intracanalicular meningioma may mimic VS (rare)
- CECT: Calcified dural-based mass eccentric to porus acusticus
- T1WI C+ MR: Broad dural base with associated dural "tails"

Epidermoid Cyst, CPA
- May mimic rare cystic VS
- Insinuating morphology
- T1WI C+ MR: Nonenhancing CPA mass
- DWI: Diffusion restriction (high signal)

Arachnoid Cyst, CPA-IAC
- Pushing CPA lesion that does not enter IAC
- Follows CSF signal on all MR sequences
- DWI: No restricted diffusion

Aneurysm, CPA-IAC
- Ovoid to fusiform complex signal mass in CPA

Facial Nerve Schwannoma, CPA-IAC
- When confined to CPA-IAC, may exactly mimic VS
- Look for labyrinthine segment "tail" to differentiate

Metastases, CPA-IAC
- May be bilateral meningeal involvement
  - Beware of misdiagnosing as NF2

PATHOLOGY

General Features
- Etiology
  - Benign tumor arising from vestibular portion of CN8 at glial-Schwann cell junction
    - Rare in cochlear portion CN8
- Genetics
  - Inactivating mutations of *NF2* tumor suppressor gene in 60% of sporadic VS
  - Loss of chromosome 22q also seen
  - Multiple or bilateral schwannomas = NF2
- Associated abnormalities
  - Arachnoid cyst (0.5%)

Staging, Grading, & Classification
- WHO grade I lesion

Gross Pathologic & Surgical Features
- Tan, round-ovoid, encapsulated mass

VESTIBULAR SCHWANNOMA

- Arises eccentrically from CN8 at glial-Schwann cell junction
  - Glial-Schwann cell junction most commonly near porus acusticus

Microscopic Features

- Differentiated neoplastic Schwann cells in collagenous matrix
- Areas of compact, elongated cells = Antoni A
  - Most VS comprised mostly of Antoni A cells
- Areas less densely cellular with tumor loosely arranged, ± clusters of lipid-laden cells = Antoni B
- Strong, diffuse expression of S100 protein
- No necrosis, instead intramural cysts
- < 1% hemorrhagic

CLINICAL ISSUES

Presentation

- Most common signs/symptoms
  - Adults with unilateral sensorineural hearing loss (SNHL)
- Clinical profile
  - Slowly progressive SNHL
  - Laboratory
    - Brainstem electric response audiometry (BERA) most sensitive pre-imaging test for VS
    - Screening MR could replace BERA
- Other symptoms
  - Small VS: Tinnitus (ringing in ear); disequilibrium
  - Large VS: Trigeminal ± facial neuropathy

Demographics

- Age
  - Adults (rare in children unless NF2)
  - Peak age = 40-60 years
  - Age range = 30-70 years
- Epidemiology
  - Most common lesion in unilateral SNHL (> 90%)
  - Most common CPA-IAC mass (85-90%)
  - 2nd most common extraaxial neoplasm in adults

Natural History & Prognosis

- 60% of VS are slow growing (< 1 mm/year)
- 10% of VS grow rapidly (> 3 mm/year)
- 60% of VS grow slowly; can be followed with imaging
  - Used in > 60 year olds, poor health, small tumor size, patient preference
- Successful surgical removal of VS will not restore any hearing already lost
- Negative prognostic imaging findings for hearing preservation
  - Size > 2 cm
  - VS involves IAC fundus ± cochlear aperture

Treatment

- **Translabyrinthine** resection if no hearing preservation possible
- **Middle cranial fossa** approach for intracanalicular VS
  - Especially lateral IAC location
- **Retrosigmoid approach** when CPA or medial IAC component present
- Fractionated or stereotactic radiosurgery
  - Gamma knife: Low dose, sharply collimated, focused cobalt-60 treatment
  - Used when medical contraindications to surgery and residual postoperative VS
  - Now used more commonly as 1st treatment

DIAGNOSTIC CHECKLIST

Consider

- Consider using high-resolution T2 unenhanced axial and coronal MR as "screening" for VS
- Thin-section, T1WI C+ axial and coronal MR is gold standard imaging approach

Image Interpretation Pearls

- Unilateral well-circumscribed IAC or CPA-IAC mass should be considered VS until proven otherwise
- Always make sure there is no labyrinthine "tail" on all VS to avoid misdiagnosing facial nerve schwannoma

Reporting Tips

- Comment on tumor size ± CPA involvement
- Does VS involve cochlear nerve canal or IAC fundus? How large in mm is "fundal cap"?
- Is hemorrhage, intramural cyst, or arachnoid cyst present within or associated with VS?
- When small, comment on nerve of origin as possible

SELECTED REFERENCES

1. Bakkouri WE et al: Conservative management of 386 cases of unilateral vestibular schwannoma: tumor growth and consequences for treatment. J Neurosurg. 110(4):662-9, 2009
2. Fukuoka S et al: Gamma knife radiosurgery for vestibular schwannomas. Prog Neurol Surg. 22:45-62, 2009
3. Bhadelia RA et al: Increased cochlear fluid-attenuated inversion recovery signal in patients with vestibular schwannoma. AJNR Am J Neuroradiol. 29(4):720-3, 2008
4. Ferri GG et al: Conservative management of vestibular schwannomas: an effective strategy. Laryngoscope. 118(6):951-7, 2008
5. Meijer OW et al: Tumor-volume changes after radiosurgery for vestibular schwannoma: implications for follow-up MR imaging protocol. AJNR Am J Neuroradiol. 29(5):906-10, 2008
6. Thamburaj K et al: Intratumoral microhemorrhages on T2*-weighted gradient-echo imaging helps differentiate vestibular schwannoma from meningioma. AJNR Am J Neuroradiol. 29(3):552-7, 2008
7. Okamoto K et al: Focal T2 hyperintensity in the dorsal brain stem in patients with vestibular schwannoma. AJNR Am J Neuroradiol. 27(6):1307-11, 2006
8. Darrouzet V et al: Vestibular schwannoma surgery outcomes: our multidisciplinary experience in 400 cases over 17 years. Laryngoscope. 114(4):681-8, 2004
9. Dubrulle F et al: Cochlear fossa enhancement at MR evaluation of vestibular Schwannoma: correlation with success at hearing-preservation surgery. Radiology. 215(2):458-62, 2000
10. Nakamura H et al: Serial follow-up MR imaging after gamma knife radiosurgery for vestibular schwannoma. AJNR Am J Neuroradiol. 21(8):1540-6, 2000
11. Allen RW et al: Low-cost high-resolution fast spin-echo MR of acoustic schwannoma: an alternative to enhanced conventional spin-echo MR? AJNR Am J Neuroradiol. 17(7):1205-10, 1996

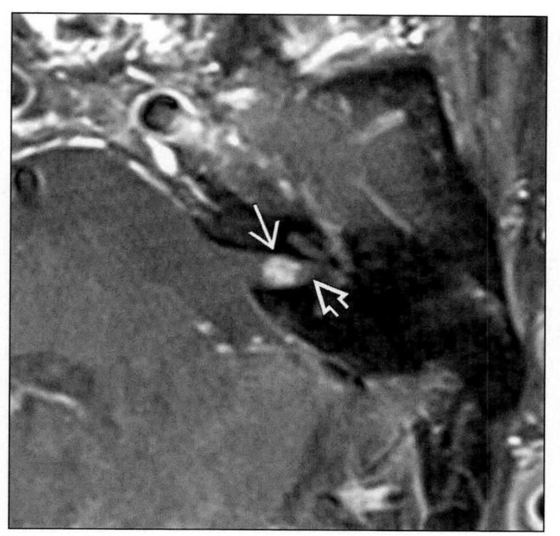

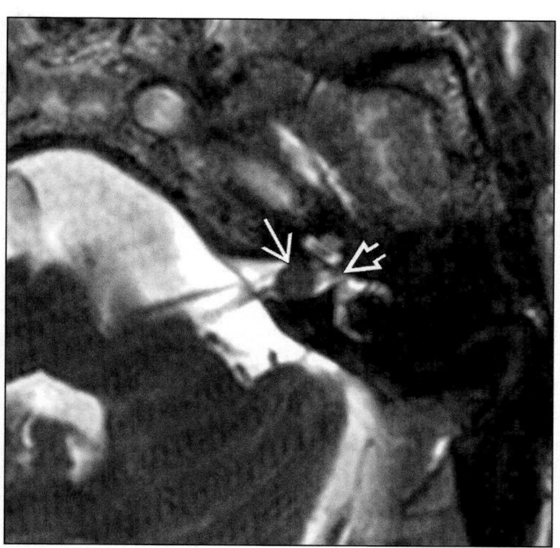

(Left) *Axial T1WI C+ FS MR in a patient with left sensorineural hearing loss shows a small enhancing vestibular schwannoma ➡ within the internal auditory canal with a 3 mm fundal CSF cap ➡ lateral to the tumor.* ***(Right)*** *Axial CISS MR in the same patient reveals a "filling defect" ➡ within the high-signal CSF in the IAC. The vestibular schwannoma is easily diagnosed with CISS imaging. The fundal CSF cap ➡ is more readily seen with T2 or CISS MR.*

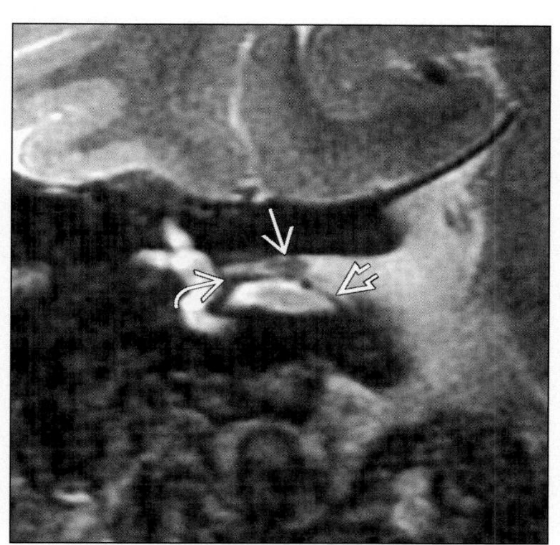

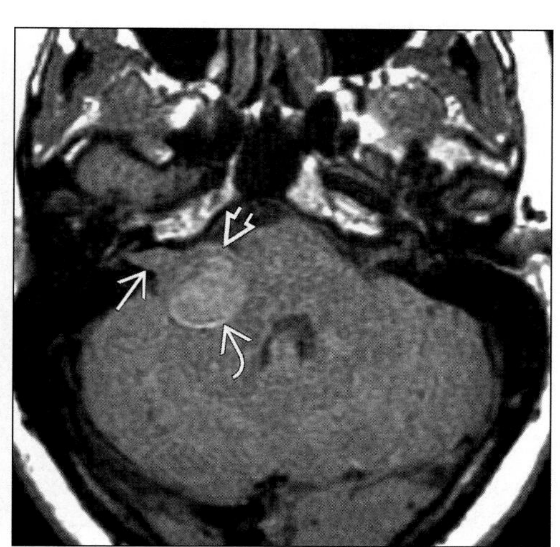

(Left) *Coronal high-resolution thin-section T2WI MR demonstrates a 2 mm superior vestibular schwannoma ➡. The lesion is seen superior to the crista falciformis ➡ with the anterior inferior cerebellar artery loop ➡ visible in the lateral IAC.* ***(Right)*** *Axial T1WI MR reveals the IAC ➡ and CPA ➡ components of a larger vestibular schwannoma. Increased signal in the medial CPA portion of this tumor ➡ is due to methemoglobin from subacute intratumoral hemorrhage.*

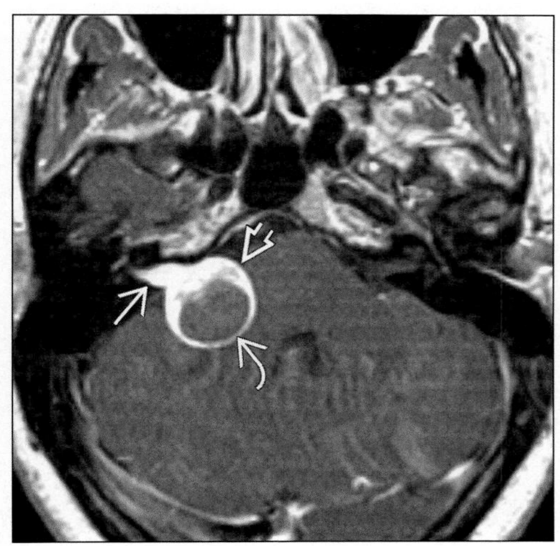

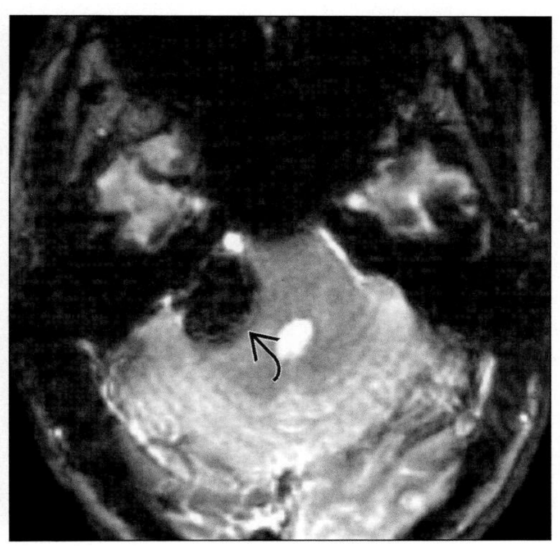

(Left) *Axial T1WI C+ MR in the same patient shows an enhancing vestibular schwannoma with IAC ➡ and CPA ➡ components. The medial CPA intramural cystic change ➡ is due to hemorrhage.* ***(Right)*** *Axial T2* GRE MR in the same patient demonstrates intense "blooming" ➡ of low signal in the CPA component of the vestibular schwannoma. This finding along with the high signal on the nonenhanced T1 image confirms intratumor hemorrhage.*

MENINGIOMA, CPA-IAC

Key Facts

Terminology

- Benign, unencapsulated neoplasm arising from meningothelial arachnoid cells of CPA-IAC dura

Imaging

- 10% occur in posterior fossa
- When in CPA, asymmetric to IAC porus acusticus
- NECT: 25% calcified; 2 types seen
  - Homogeneous, sand-like ("psammomatous")
  - Focal sunburst, globular, or rim pattern
- Bone CT: Hyperostotic or permeative-sclerotic bone changes possible (en plaque type)
- T2WI MR: Pial blood vessels seen as surface flow voids between tumor and brain
  - High-signal crescent from CSF ("CSF cleft")
- T1WI C+ MR: Enhancing dural-based mass with dural "tails" centered along posterior petrous wall

Top Differential Diagnoses

- Sarcoidosis, CPA-IAC
- Epidermoid cyst, CPA-IAC
- Idiopathic inflammatory pseudotumor, skull base
- Vestibular schwannoma
- Intracranial trigeminal schwannoma
- Metastases, CPA-IAC
- Primary CNS lymphoma

Clinical Issues

- Incidental brain MR finding
- < 10% symptomatic
  - Usually do not cause sensorineural hearing loss
- Treatment
  - Surgical removal if medically safe
  - Adjunctive radiation therapy with incomplete surgery

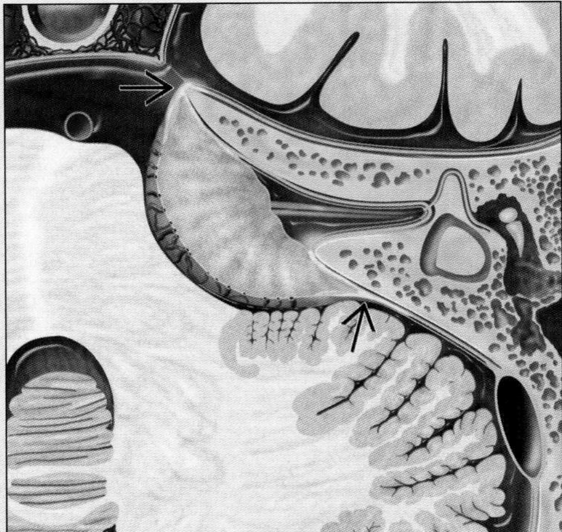

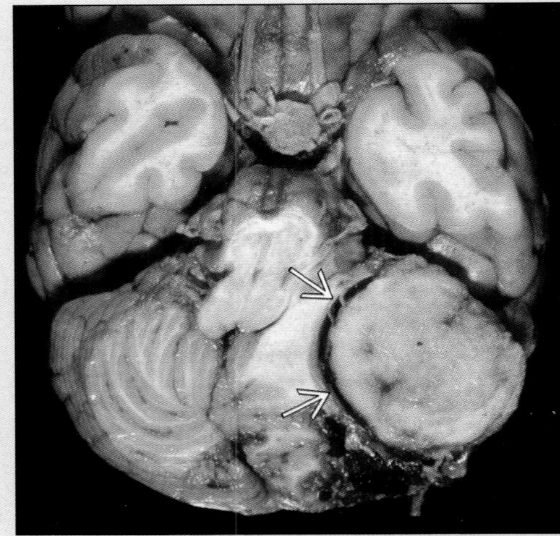

*(**Left**) Axial graphic at level of the IAC shows a large CPA meningioma causing mass effect on the brainstem and cerebellum. Notice the broad dural base creating the shape of a mushroom head. A dural "tail" ⇒ is present in approximately 60% of cases and typically represents reactive rather than neoplastic change. (**Right**) Gross pathologic section viewed from below shows a large CPA meningioma with a broad dural base compressing the cerebellum. The specimen demonstrates a CSF-vascular cleft ➡.*

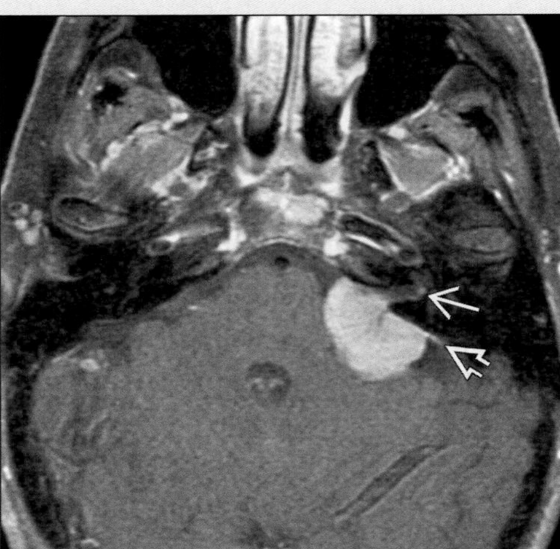

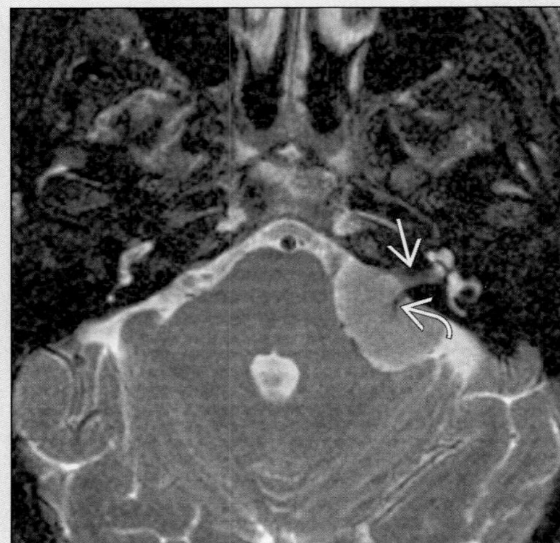

*(**Left**) Axial T1WI C+ FS MR through the IAC shows a meningioma overlying the porus acusticus. Note the dural "tail" ➡ extending along the temporal bone posterior wall. A dot of enhancement in the IAC fundus ➡ suggests the low signal area in the IAC is nonenhancing meningioma. (**Right**) Axial T2WI FS MR in the same patient reveals a high-velocity flow void ➡ representing a dural artery feeder penetrating the meningioma core. Low signal in IAC ➡ is intracanalicular meningioma.*

TERMINOLOGY

Synonyms

- Posterior fossa meningioma

Definitions

- Benign, unencapsulated neoplasm arising from meningothelial arachnoid cells of CPA-IAC dura

IMAGING

General Features

- Best diagnostic clue
  - CPA dural-based enhancing mass with **dural "tails"**
- Location
  - 10% occur in posterior fossa
  - When in CPA, **asymmetric** to IAC porus acusticus
- Size
  - Broad range; usually 1-8 cm but may be larger
  - Generally significantly larger than vestibular schwannoma at presentation
- Morphology
  - 3 distinct morphologies
    - "Mushroom cap" (hemispherical) with broad base towards posterior petrous wall (75%)
    - Plaque-like (en plaque), ± bone invasion with hyperostosis (20%)
    - Ovoid mass mimics vestibular schwannoma (5%)
  - Frequently (50%) herniates cephalad into medial middle cranial fossa

CT Findings

- NECT
  - 25% isodense, 75% hyperdense
  - 25% calcified; 2 types seen
    - Homogeneous, sand-like ("psammomatous")
    - Focal sunburst, globular, or rim pattern
- CECT
  - > 90% strong, uniform enhancement
- Bone CT
  - Hyperostotic or permeative-sclerotic bone changes possible (en plaque type)
  - IAC flaring is rare (cf. vestibular schwannoma)

MR Findings

- T1WI
  - Isointense or minimally hyperintense to gray matter
  - When tumor has calcifications or is highly fibrous, hypointense areas are visible
- T2WI
  - Wide range of possible signals on T2 sequence
    - Isointense or hypointense CPA mass (compared to gray matter) most likely meningioma
    - Focal or diffuse parenchymal low signal seen if calcified or highly fibrous
  - **CSF-vascular cleft**
    - Pial blood vessels seen as surface flow voids between tumor and brain
    - High-signal crescent from CSF
  - Tumor arterial feeders seen as arborizing flow voids
  - High signal in adjacent brainstem or cerebellum
    - Represents peritumoral brain edema
    - Correlates with pial blood supply
    - Signals problems with safe removal
- T2* GRE
  - Calcifications may "bloom"
- T1WI C+
  - Enhancing **dural-based mass** with **dural "tails"** centered along posterior petrous wall
    - > 95% enhance strongly
    - Heterogeneous enhancement when large
  - Dural "tail" in ~ 60%
    - Represents **reactive** rather than neoplastic change in most cases
    - When extending into IAC, may mimic IAC component of vestibular schwannoma
  - En plaque: Sessile thickened enhancing dura
- MRS
  - ↑ alanine at short TE
    - Triplet-like spectral pattern at 1.3-1.5 ppm (overlapping of alanine, lactate)
    - ↑ Glx alfa/glutationine

Angiographic Findings

- Digital subtraction angiography
  - Dural vessels supply tumor center, **pial vessels** supply **tumor rim**
  - "Sunburst" pattern: Enlarged dural feeders
  - Prolonged vascular "stain" into venous phase

Imaging Recommendations

- Best imaging tool
  - Enhanced MR focused to posterior fossa
  - Bone CT if bone invasion suspected on MR
- Protocol advice
  - Full brain T2 ± FLAIR shows brain edema best

DIFFERENTIAL DIAGNOSIS

Vestibular Schwannoma

- Intracanalicular 1st, then CPA extension
- Intracanalicular meningioma may mimic

Epidermoid Cyst, CPA-IAC

- Near CSF signal insinuating mass on MR
- DWI high signal characteristic

Metastases, CPA-IAC

- May be bilateral in CPA area
- Multifocal meningeal involvement

Sarcoidosis, CPA-IAC

- Often multifocal, dural-based foci
- Look for infundibular stalk involvement

Idiopathic Inflammatory Pseudotumor, Skull Base

- Diffuse or focal meningeal thickening
- CPA involvement is rare

Intracranial Trigeminal Schwannoma

- Ovoid, C+ mass centered in Meckel cave

Primary CNS Lymphoma

- Rare intracranial lymphoma
- Focal area enhancing, thickened meninges

MENINGIOMA, CPA-IAC

PATHOLOGY

General Features

- Etiology
  - Arises from arachnoid ("cap") meningothelial cells
- Genetics
  - Long arm deletions of chromosome 22 are common
  - *NF2* gene inactivated in 90% of sporadic cases
  - May have progesterone, prolactin receptors; may express growth hormone
- Associated abnormalities
  - Meningioma + schwannoma = NF2
  - Multiple meningiomas: 10% of sporadic cases

Staging, Grading, & Classification

- WHO grading classification (grades I-III)
  - Meningioma (classic, benign) = 90%
  - Atypical meningioma = 9%
  - Anaplastic (malignant) meningioma = 1%

Gross Pathologic & Surgical Features

- "Mushroom cap" (hemispherical) morphology most common (75%)
- En plaque morphology (20%) also seen in CPA
- Sharply circumscribed, unencapsulated
- Adjacent dural thickening (collar or "tail") is usually reactive, not neoplastic

Microscopic Features

- Subtypes (wide range of histology with little bearing on imaging appearance or clinical outcome)
  - Meningothelial (lobules of meningothelial cells)
  - Fibrous (parallel, interlacing fascicles of spindle-shaped cells)
  - Transitional (mixed; "onion-bulb" whorls and lobules)
  - Psammomatous (numerous small calcifications)
  - Angiomatous (↑ vascular channels), not equated with obsolete term "angioblastic meningioma"
  - Miscellaneous forms (microcystic, chordoid, clear cell, secretory, lymphoplasmocyte-rich, etc.)

CLINICAL ISSUES

Presentation

- Most common signs/symptoms
  - Incidental brain MR finding
  - < 10% symptomatic
- Clinical profile
  - Adult undergoing brain MR for unrelated indication

Demographics

- Age
  - Middle-aged, elderly; peak = 60 years old
  - If found in children, consider possibility of NF2
- Gender
  - M:F = 1:4
- Epidemiology
  - Accounts for ~ 20% of primary intracranial tumors
  - 1-1.5% prevalence at autopsy or imaging
  - 10% multiple (NF2; multiple meningiomatosis)
  - 2nd most common CPA-IAC mass

Natural History & Prognosis

- Slow-growing tumor
- Compresses rather than invades structures
- Negative prognostic findings on MR
  - Peritumoral edema in adjacent brainstem
  - Significant subjacent bone invasion

Treatment

- Surgical removal if medically safe
  - Complete surgical removal possible in 95% when tumor does not invade skull base
- Radiation therapy
  - Adjunctive therapy with incomplete surgery
  - Primary therapy if extensive skull base invasion

DIAGNOSTIC CHECKLIST

Consider

- Meningioma when MR shows hemispherical, dural-based enhancing CPA mass with dural "tails"
- Meningioma when CPA mass is large but asymptomatic

Image Interpretation Pearls

- Focal or diffuse hypointensity on T2 in CPA mass suggests meningioma
- Dural "tail" in IAC suggests meningioma

Reporting Tips

- Report extent of meningioma, including intraosseous component
  - Mention cranial nerves in area of involvement
  - Note any brainstem or brain edema indicating pia-arachnoid involvement

SELECTED REFERENCES

1. Takanashi M et al: Gamma knife radiosurgery for skull-base meningiomas. Prog Neurol Surg. 22:96-111, 2009
2. Thamburaj K et al: Intratumoral microhemorrhages on T2*-weighted gradient-echo imaging helps differentiate vestibular schwannoma from meningioma. AJNR Am J Neuroradiol. 29(3):552-7, 2008
3. Zeidman LA et al: Growth rate of non-operated meningiomas. J Neurol. 255(6):891-5, 2008
4. Nakamura M et al: Facial and cochlear nerve function after surgery of cerebellopontine angle meningiomas. Neurosurgery. 57(1):77-90; discussion 77-90, 2005
5. Roche PH et al: Cerebellopontine angle meningiomas. J Neurosurg. 103(5):935-7; author reply 937-8, 2005
6. Roser F et al: Meningiomas of the cerebellopontine angle with extension into the internal auditory canal. J Neurosurg. 102(1):17-23, 2005
7. Nakamura M et al: Meningiomas of the internal auditory canal. Neurosurgery. 55(1):119-27; discussion 127-8, 2004
8. Asaoka K et al: Intracanalicular meningioma mimicking vestibular schwannoma. AJNR Am J Neuroradiol. 23(9):1493-6, 2002
9. Roberti F et al: Posterior fossa meningiomas: surgical experience in 161 cases. Surg Neurol. 56(1):8-20; discussion 20-1, 2001
10. Ildan F et al: Correlation of the relationships of brain-tumor interfaces, magnetic resonance imaging, and angiographic findings to predict cleavage of meningiomas. J Neurosurg. 91(3):384-90, 1999

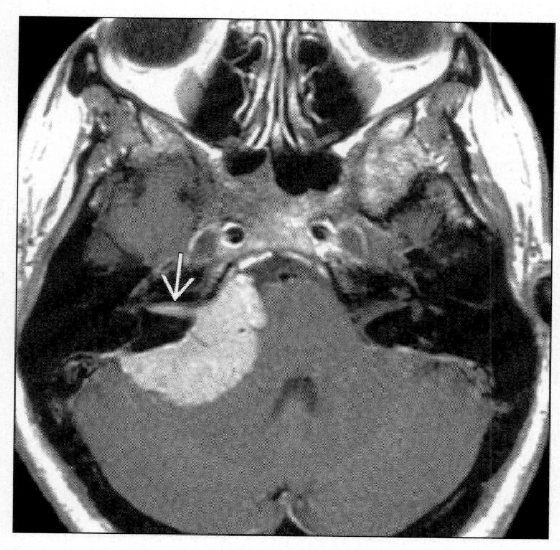

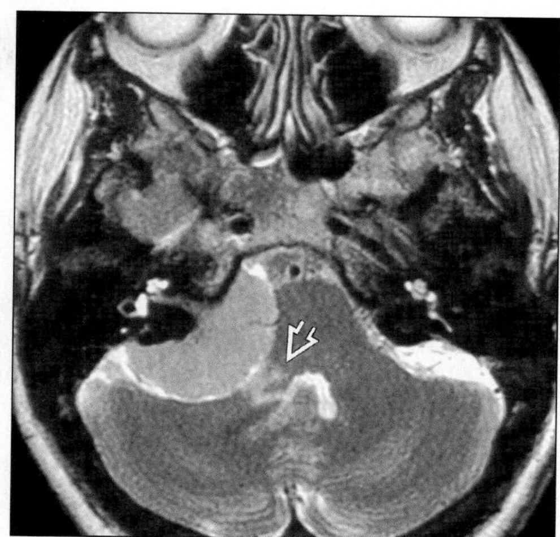

(Left) *Axial T1WI C+ MR demonstrates a large CPA meningioma with an IAC component ➡. This degree and depth of IAC enhancement usually signifies tumor rather than dural reaction.* ***(Right)*** *Axial T2WI MR in the same patient reveals high signal in the adjacent brachium pontis ➡. Pial invasion by the meningioma is likely. This MR finding is predictive of increased risk of complications when surgical removal occurs.*

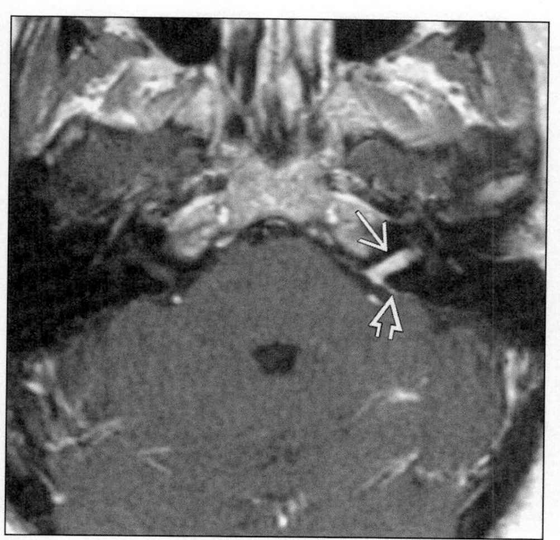

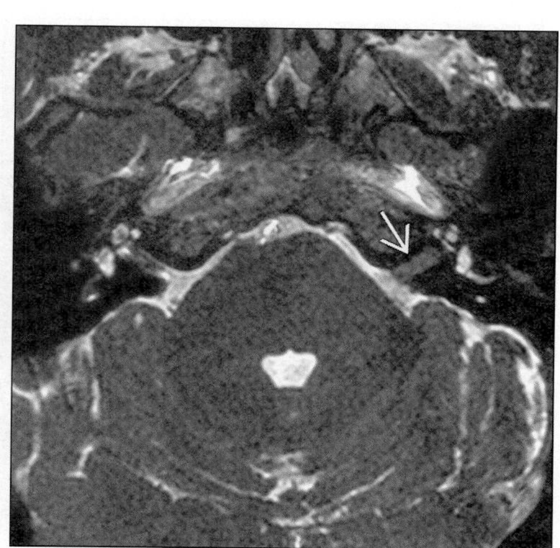

(Left) *Axial T1WI C+ MR shows an enhancing intracanalicular mass ➡. Dural "tails" ➡ along the posterior margin of the porus acusticus suggest but do not definitively diagnose meningioma.* ***(Right)*** *Axial T2WI MR in the same patient reveals the intracanalicular meningioma ➡ as low signal tissue filling the IAC. Often IAC meningioma cannot be reliably distinguished from IAC vestibular schwannoma, the most common lesion in this location.*

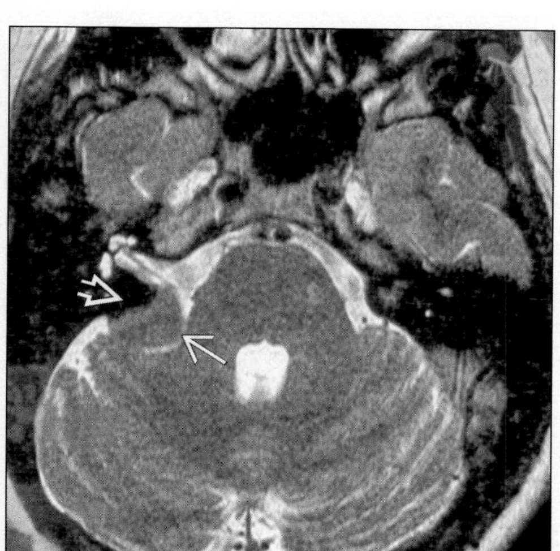

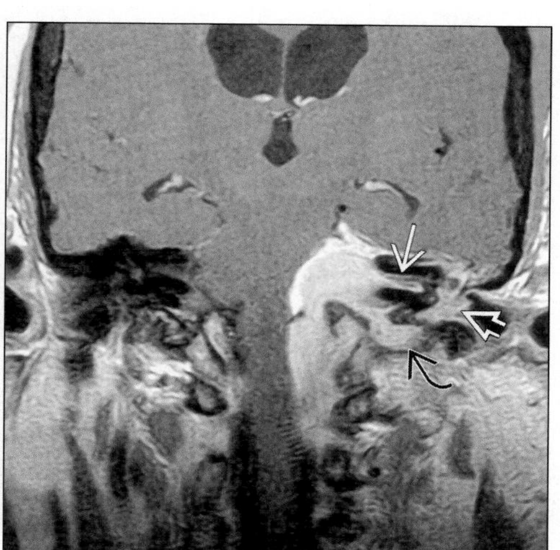

(Left) *Axial T2WI MR shows a parenchymal signal intensity meningioma ➡ abutting the posterior wall of the temporal bone. Note the underlying dark signal of bony hyperostosis ➡. Despite the tumor abutting CN7-8 along the posterior margin of the porus acusticus, the patient did not have hearing loss.* ***(Right)*** *Coronal T1WI C+ MR shows a large enhancing meningoma centered in the CPA. Note that the IAC ➡, middle ear ➡, and jugular foramen ➡ are filled with enhancing tumor.*

METASTASES, CPA-IAC

Key Facts

Terminology

- CPA-IAC metastases: Systemic or CNS neoplasia affecting area of CPA-IAC

Imaging

- 4 major sites: Leptomeningeal, dura, flocculus, and choroid plexus
- T1WI C+ MR
  - Leptomeningeal metastases: Diffuse thickening and enhancement of cranial nerves in IAC
  - Dural metastases: Thickened enhancing dura ± dural nodules
  - Floccular metastases: Enhancing floccular mass
  - Choroid plexus metastases: Enhancing nodular lesion along normal course of choroid plexus
  - Focal brain enhancing metastases may be present
- FLAIR MR
  - Parenchymal brain metastases usually high signal

Top Differential Diagnoses

- Bilateral vestibular schwannoma (NF2)
- Sarcoidosis, CPA-IAC
- Meningitis, CPA-IAC
- Ramsay Hunt syndrome

Clinical Issues

- Rapidly progressive unilateral or bilateral CN7 and CN8 palsies
- Patient with past history of treated malignancy

Diagnostic Checklist

- If trying to diagnose bilateral "vestibular schwannoma" in adult as NF2, probably CPA metastases instead
- Rapidly progressive 7th cranial nerve palsy + CPA mass suggests metastatic focus
  - Vestibular schwannoma rarely causes CN7 palsy

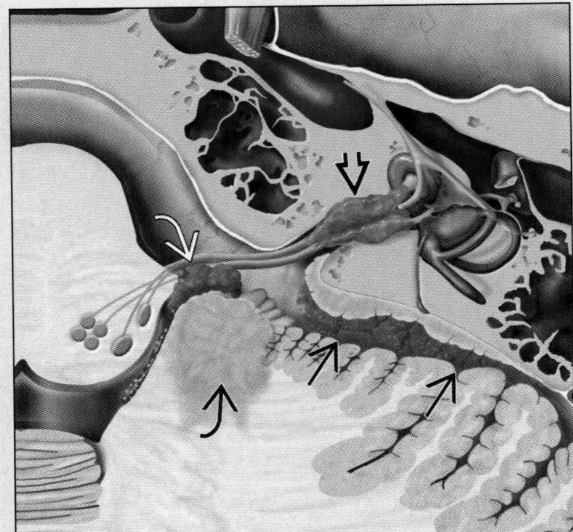

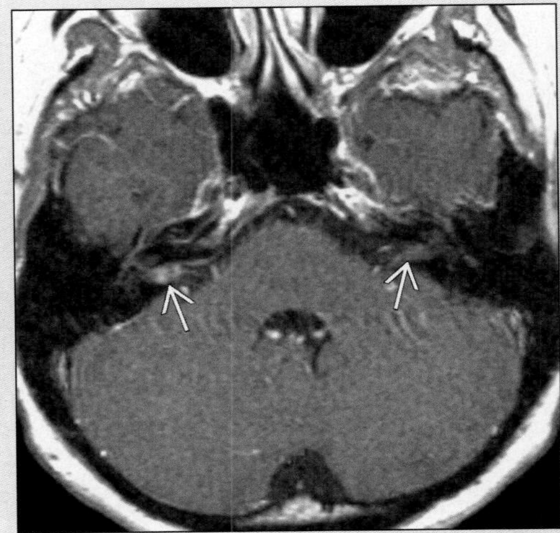

(Left) *Axial graphic depicts the 4 major types of CPA-IAC area metastases. Along the posterolateral margin of the IAC, thickened dural metastases ⇨ are visible. Within the IAC metastatic leptomeningeal (pia-arachnoid) ⇨ involvement is present. Choroid plexus ➩ and floccular ➩ metastases are also depicted.* ***(Right)*** *Axial T1WI C+ MR shows bilateral leptomeningeal breast carcinoma metastases ➡ within the internal auditory canals. The left-sided disease is more subtle than the right.*

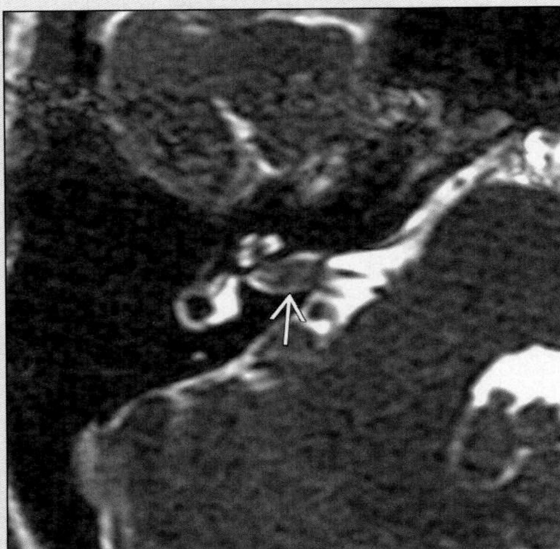

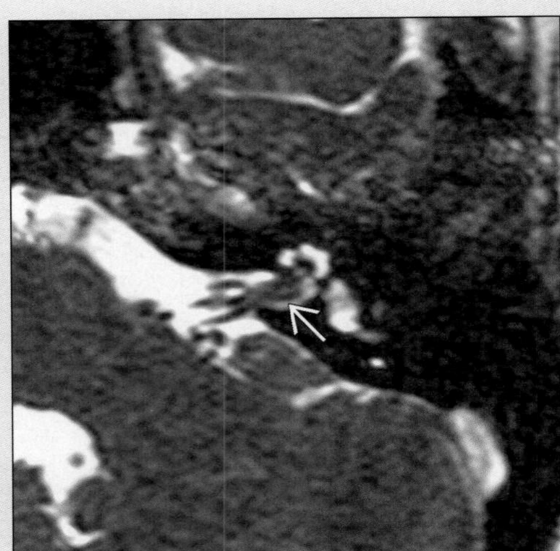

(Left) *Axial T2WI MR demonstrates right IAC leptomeningeal metastatic foci as thickening of the branches of CN7 and CN8 ➡ within the internal auditory canal.* ***(Right)*** *Axial T2WI MR reveals left IAC metastatic disease as subtle thickening of the branches of CN7 and CN8 ➡ within the internal auditory canal. In an adult patient with suspected "bilateral vestibular schwannoma," consider metastatic disease rather than NF2.*

METASTASES, CPA-IAC

TERMINOLOGY

Abbreviations

- Metastases (mets)

Synonyms

- Leptomeningeal carcinomatosis, meningeal carcinomatosis, carcinomatous meningitis
  - All of above terms are misnomers
    - 1st: Neoplasms are not always carcinomas
    - 2nd: Pachymeninges (dura) and leptomeninges (pia + arachnoid) are often both involved
    - 3rd: Usually does not contain inflammatory component (-itis suffix makes no sense)

Definitions

- CPA-IAC metastases: Systemic or CNS neoplasia affecting area of CPA-IAC

IMAGING

General Features

- Best diagnostic clue
  - Multiple enhancing masses on T1WI C+ MR
- Location
  - 4 major sites: Leptomeningeal (pia-arachnoid), dura, flocculus, and choroid plexus
  - Primary site locations
    - Primary tumors: Breast, lung, and melanoma
    - Meningeal lymphoproliferative malignancy
      - Lymphoma and leukemia
    - Primary CNS tumor seeds basal cisterns via CSF pathways: "Drop" metastases
- Size
  - Often small (< 1 cm)
    - Metastases cause symptoms early
- Morphology
  - Leptomeningeal: Thickened CN7 and CN8 in IAC
  - Dura: Diffuse dural thickening (pachymeninges)
  - Flocculus: Enlarged flocculus with associated brain edema
  - Choroid plexus: Nodular thickening

CT Findings

- CECT
  - Unilateral or bilateral dural enhancement along CPA and IAC
  - CT shows metastases only when larger ± multiple

MR Findings

- T1WI
  - Focal dural thickening isointense to gray matter
- T2WI
  - High-resolution T2 MR
    - Leptomeningeal metastases: CN7 and CN8 thickening
    - Floccular metastases: ↑ signal edema associated
- FLAIR
  - Larger CPA-IAC metastases may cause ↑ signal in adjacent brainstem ± cerebellum
  - Floccular metastases seen as ↑ signal
- T1WI C+
  - Leptomeningeal metastases: Diffuse thickening and enhancement of cranial nerves in IAC
    - Late findings shows plug of enhancing tissue in IAC
    - Unilateral or bilateral
  - Dural metastases: Thickened enhancing dura ± dural nodules
    - Associated with other dural or skull lesions
  - Floccular metastases: Enhancing floccular mass
  - Choroid plexus metastases: Enhancing nodular lesion along normal course of choroid plexus
    - Lateral recess 4th ventricle → foramen of Luschka → inferior CPA cistern
  - Focal brain enhancing metastases may be present

Imaging Recommendations

- Best imaging tool
  - T1WI C+ MR of posterior fossa is best imaging tool and sequence
  - Whole brain FLAIR and T1WI C+ for associated brain metastases
- Protocol advice
  - Axial and coronal planes recommended

DIFFERENTIAL DIAGNOSIS

Bilateral Vestibular Schwannoma (NF2)

- Younger patients; no history of malignancy
- T1WI C+ MR shows bilateral CPA-IAC enhancing masses
  - Mimics bilateral leptomeningeal metastases
- Other cranial nerve schwannoma possible

Sarcoidosis, CPA-IAC

- ↑ erythrocyte sedimentation rate (ESR) and serum angiotensin converting enzyme (ACE)
- T1WI C+ MR may be identical to metastases when multifocal meningeal type
  - May be bilateral CPA lesions mimicking NF2 or metastases
  - May be single, en plaque focus mimicking meningioma
- Look for infundibular stalk involvement

Meningitis, CPA-IAC

- Bacterial meningitis
- Fungal meningitis
- Tuberculous meningitis
- T1WI C+ MR may be identical to CPA-IAC metastases
- Clinical information and cerebrospinal fluid (CSF) evaluation are key

Ramsay Hunt Syndrome

- External ear vesicular rash
- T1WI C+ MR shows enhancement in IAC and inner ear ± 7th cranial nerve
  - Mimics unilateral leptomeningeal metastasis

PATHOLOGY

General Features

- Etiology

- Metastatic tumor involves leptomeningeal or dural surfaces of CPA-IAC
  - Leptomeningeal metastases follow CN7 and CN8 into IAC
- Metastatic tumor deposits in flocculus or choroid plexus
- Routes of spread
  - Extracranial neoplasm spreads hematogenously to meninges
  - CSF spread from intracranial or intraspinal neoplasm is less common
- Associated abnormalities
  - Multiple other pial or dural metastatic foci
  - Parenchymal brain metastases also possible
- Key anatomy: Meninges has 3 discrete layers
  - Dura (pachymeninges): Dense connective tissue attached to calvarium
  - Pia: Clear membrane firmly attaches to surface of brain; extends deeply into sulci
  - Arachnoid: Interposed between pia and dura
    - Pia + arachnoid = leptomeninges

Gross Pathologic & Surgical Features

- Diffuse, nodular ± discrete

Microscopic Features

- Common tissue types found
  - Solid tumors = breast, lung, and melanoma
    - All involve both leptomeninges and pachymeninges
  - Lymphoproliferative malignancy = lymphoma and leukemia
    - Involve both leptomeninges and pachymeninges
  - "Drop" metastases from CNS tumors
    - Medulloblastoma, ependymoma, glioblastoma multiforme

CLINICAL ISSUES

Presentation

- Most common signs/symptoms
  - Rapidly progressive unilateral or bilateral CN7 and CN8 palsies
- Other signs/symptoms
  - Vertigo and polycranial neuropathy
- Clinical profile
  - Patient with past history of treated malignancy

Demographics

- Age
  - Older adults
- Epidemiology
  - Increasingly more common neurologic complication of systemic cancer
    - Due to increase in survival rate of cancer patients

Natural History & Prognosis

- Meningeal metastases usually late-stage finding
- Poor prognosis as patients have advanced, incurable disease by definition

Treatment

- No curative treatments available
- Therapies aimed at preserving neurologic function and improving quality of life
- Treatments are same as for underlying neoplasm
  - Radiotherapy ± chemotherapy depending on tissue type
- Surgery will rarely play role at this stage
  - Solitary melanoma metastases may be exception
- If any question of diagnosis, excisional biopsy necessary

DIAGNOSTIC CHECKLIST

Consider

- If trying to diagnose bilateral "vestibular schwannoma" in adult as NF2, probably CPA metastases instead
- Rapidly progressive 7th cranial nerve palsy + CPA mass suggests metastatic focus
  - Vestibular schwannoma rarely causes CN7 palsy

Image Interpretation Pearls

- If suspect CPA-IAC metastasis from T1WI C+ MR appearance or history of known malignancy, make sure to review
  - Extracranial and calvarial structures for other lesions to confirm diagnosis
  - Look for involvement of other meningeal sites, such as parasellar, other basal meninges
  - Parenchymal brain for abnormal FLAIR high signal ± enhancing lesions on T1WI C+ sequences

SELECTED REFERENCES

1. Warren FM et al: Imaging characteristics of metastatic lesions to the cerebellopontine angle. Otol Neurotol. 29(6):835-8, 2008
2. Siomin VE et al: Posterior fossa metastases: risk of leptomeningeal disease when treated with stereotactic radiosurgery compared to surgery. J Neurooncol. 67(1-2):115-21, 2004
3. Soyuer S et al: Intracranial meningeal hemangiopericytoma: the role of radiotherapy: report of 29 cases and review of the literature. Cancer. 100(7):1491-7, 2004
4. Kesari S et al: Leptomeningeal metastases. Neurol Clin. 21(1):25-66, 2003
5. Krainik A et al: MRI of unusual lesions in the internal auditory canal. Neuroradiology. 43(1):52-7, 2001
6. Schick B et al: Magnetic resonance imaging in patients with sudden hearing loss, tinnitus and vertigo. Otol Neurotol. 22(6):808-12, 2001
7. Whinney D et al: Primary malignant melanoma of the cerebellopontine angle. Otol Neurotol. 22(2):218-22, 2001
8. Shen TY et al: Meningeal carcinomatosis manifested as bilateral progressive sensorineural hearing loss. Am J Otol. 21(4):510-2, 2000
9. Lewanski CR et al: Bilateral cerebellopontine metastases in a patient with an unknown primary. Clin Oncol (R Coll Radiol). 11(4):272-3, 1999
10. Swartz JD: Meningeal metastases. Am J Otol. 20(5):683-5, 1999
11. Kingdom TT et al: Isolated metastatic melanoma of the cerebellopontine angle: case report. Neurosurgery. 33(1):142-4, 1993
12. Mark AS et al: Sensorineural hearing loss: more than meets the eye? AJNR Am J Neuroradiol. 14(1):37-45, 1993

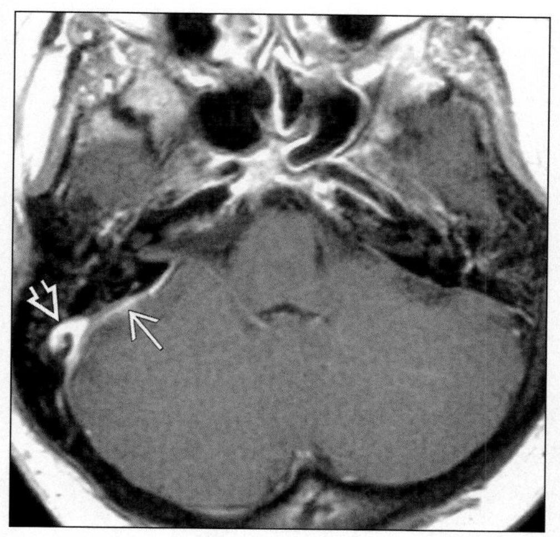

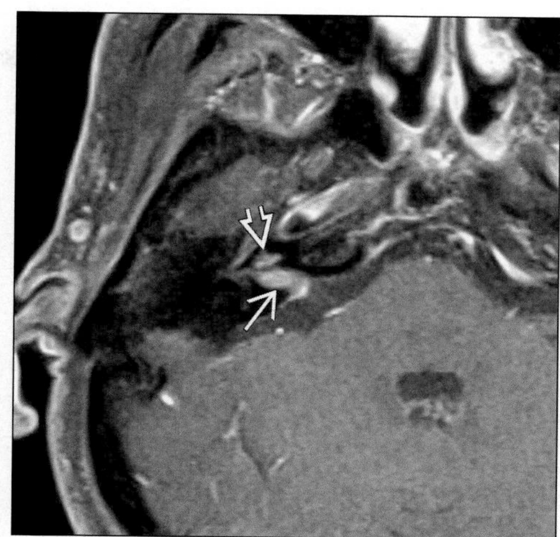

(Left) *Axial T1WI C+ MR reveals a dural lung carcinoma metastases ➡ in the CPA region. The enhancing, thickened dura should be distinguished from the enhancement in the normal sigmoid sinus ➡. CSF examination was positive for malignant cells.* ***(Right)*** *Axial T1WI C+ FS MR shows an enhancing metastasis in the right IAC ➡ with extension of enhancing tissue through the cochlear nerve canal, across the modiolus into the membranous labyrinth of the cochlea ➡.*

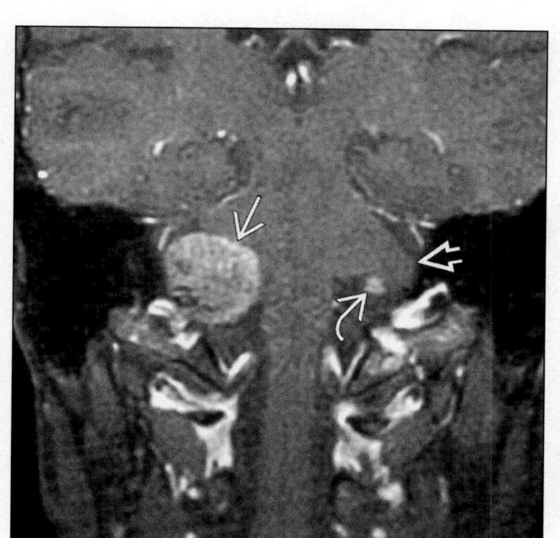

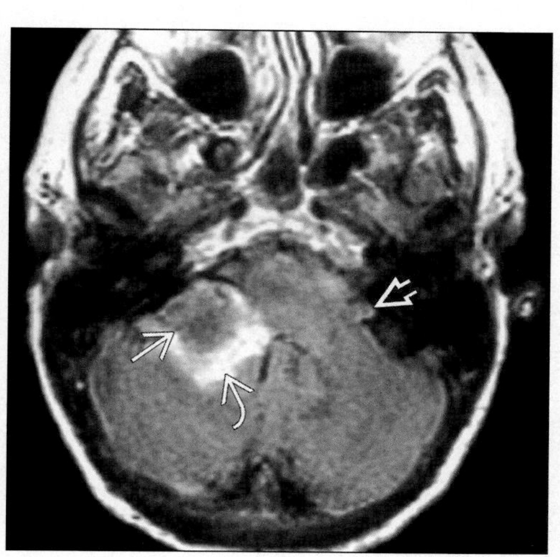

(Left) *Coronal T1WI C+ MR depicts an enhancing breast carcinoma metastasis ➡ centered within the right flocculus. Note the normal flocculus ➡ and cisternal choroid plexus ➡.* ***(Right)*** *Axial FLAIR MR in the same patient shows the mass ➡ to be slightly lower in signal than the adjacent gray matter. Vasogenic edema within the brachium pontis and cerebellum ➡ is seen as high signal. The left flocculus ➡ is normal.*

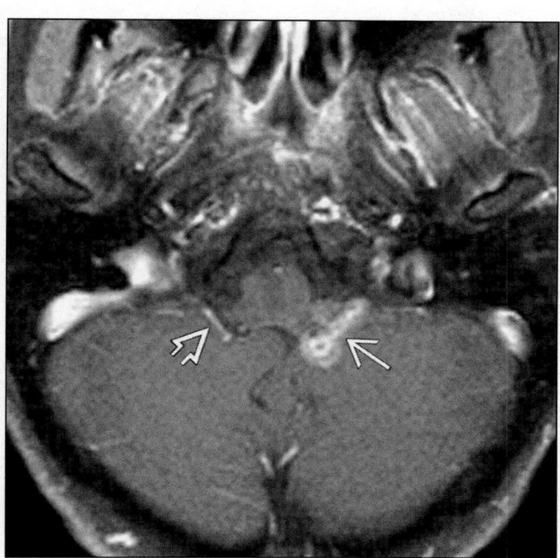

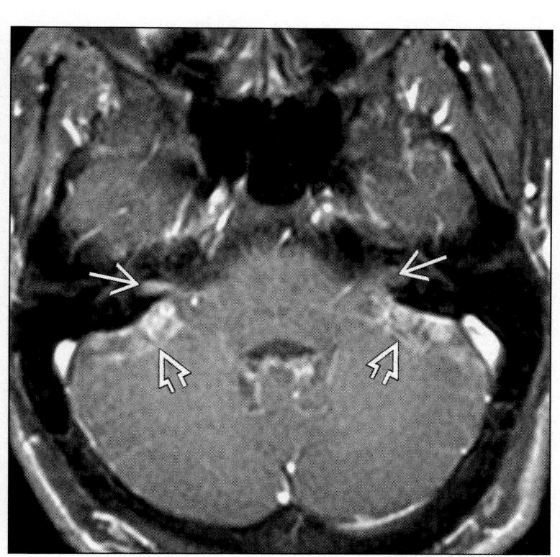

(Left) *Axial T1WI C+ FS MR in a patient with known metastatic rectal carcinoma shows an enhancing metastasis ➡ of the choroid plexus projecting into the low CPA cistern through the foramen of Luschka. The normal right choroid plexus ➡ is seen.* ***(Right)*** *Axial T1WI C+ FS reveals bilateral CPA-IAC "drop" metastases from a supratentorial glioblastoma multiforme. Bilateral IAC enhancing metastases ➡ are seen along with multiple leptomeningeal metastases on surface of the cerebellum ➡.*

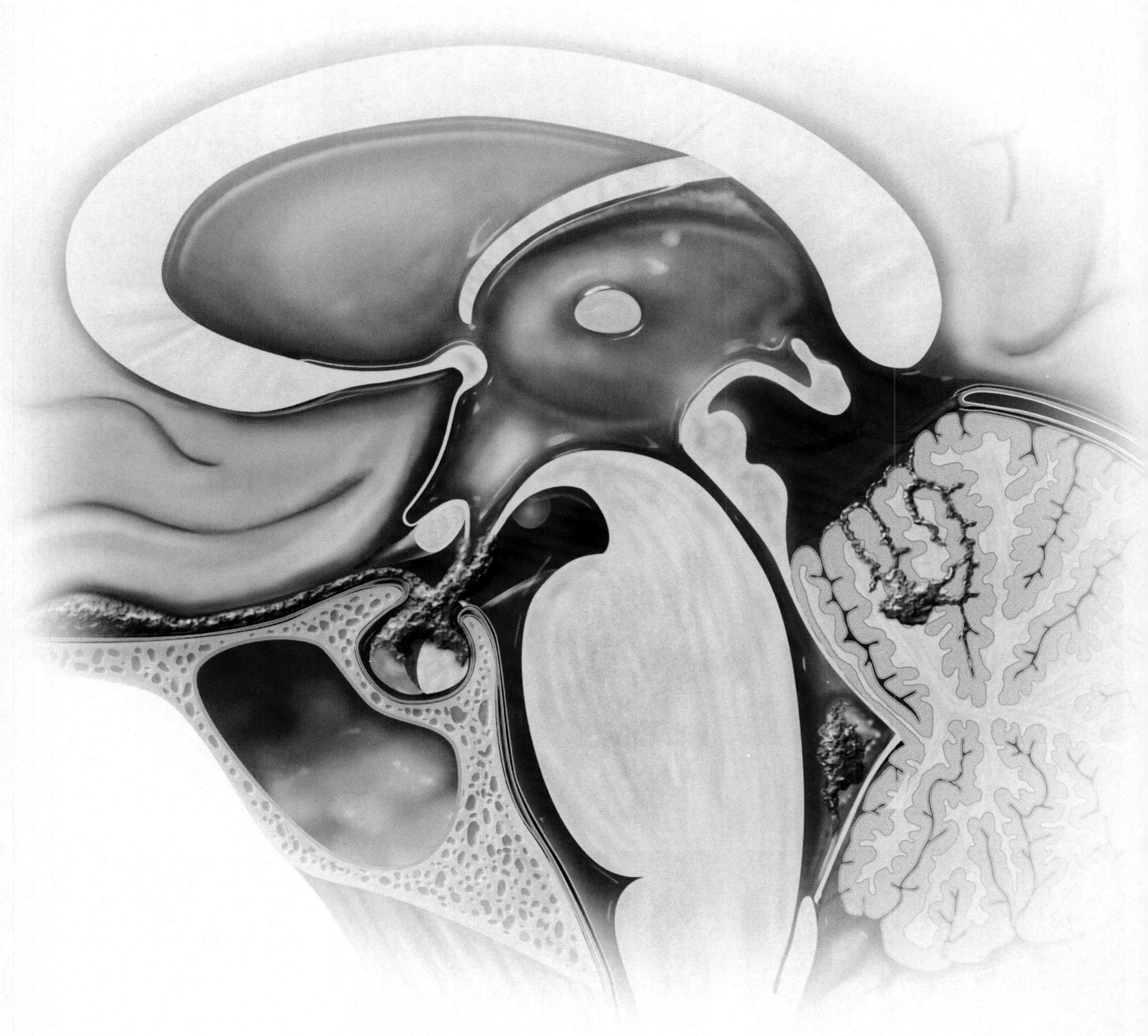

SECTION 4
Skull, Scalp, and Meninges

Introduction and Overview

Congenital

Trauma

Nonneoplastic and Tumor-like Disorders

Neoplasms

Overview

Understanding the anatomy of the skull, scalp, and meninges is key to formulating a correct imaging diagnosis. Several important differential diagnoses are based on location. Yet each of these locations requires a different imaging approach.

For example, CT is often the best imaging modality for lesions of the skull and scalp. When faced with a complex skull base lesion, a combination of bone CT and contrast-enhanced MR images is often required for optimal imaging. MR with contrast is the best imaging modality for meningeal processes.

Scalp

The scalp is made up of 5 layers including the dermis (skin), subcutaneous fibro-adipose tissue, epicranium and muscles, subaponeurotic areolar tissue, and pericranium. The 1st 3 layers are firmly connected and surgically act as a single layer.

The majority of scalp lesions are not imaged, as the area is easily accessible to both visual and manual inspection. Imaging becomes important when a scalp lesion is malignant or has a vascular component that could alter the surgical approach.

Skull Vault (Calvarium)

The calvarium is composed of 5 bones: Frontal, parietal, occipital, temporal, and sphenoid (greater wings) bones which are primarily connected by the major sutures, including the coronal, sagittal, and lambdoid sutures. The metopic suture is variably seen in adults.

There are many normal variants of the skull. These must be recognized to prevent misdiagnosis and unnecessary biopsy. Some of the most common skull normal variants include arachnoid granulations, vascular grooves from the meningeal arteries and veins, venous lakes, emissary veins, parietal thinning, asymmetric marrow (particularly in the petrous apex), aerated clinoid processes, and accessory sutures.

Meninges

Dura

The dura (or pachymeninges) is a thick, dense fibrous connective tissue that is made up of 2 layers: An outer (peri- or endosteal) and an inner (meningeal) layer. These outer and inner layers are closely adherent and apposed except where they separate to enclose the venous sinuses.

The outer layer forms the periosteum of the calvarium, tightly attached to the inner table, particularly at the sutures. The inner layer folds to form the falx cerebri, tentorium, and diaphragma sellae. It also divides the cranial cavity into compartments. On imaging, the dura usually shows smooth, thin enhancement (< 2 mm).

The dura forms 2 important potential spaces. First, the epidural space is located between the dura and the inner table of the calvarium. Important lesions of the epidural space include hemorrhage related to trauma and infection causing an empyema, a rare but potentially lethal complication of sinusitis. Second, the subdural space is the potential space between the inner layer of the dura and the arachnoid. A traumatic subdural hematoma is the most common process to affect the subdural space. The subdural space may also be affected by infection, either a subdural effusion related to meningitis or a subdural empyema related to meningitis in a child or sinusitis in an adult.

Leptomeninges

The leptomeninges are formed by the arachnoid and pia. Most pathologies affect both the arachnoid and pia together, and the 2 areas cannot be easily differentiated on imaging.

The arachnoid is a thin, nearly transparent layer of meninges closely applied to the inner (meningeal) dura. It forms the outer margin of the subarachnoid space (SAS). It does not enter the sulci or fissures except along the falx where it dips into the interhemispheric fissure. Trabeculae extend from the arachnoid across the SAS to the pia and are invested with a thin pia-like layer. The SAS is a CSF-filled space between the arachnoid and pia.

The pia is a thin, delicate membrane closely applied to the brain. It covers vessels and trabeculae in the SAS and lines the perivascular spaces.

Perivascular (Virchow-Robin) spaces are normal variants. They appear as interstitial fluid-filled, pial-lined spaces that accompany penetrating arteries and veins.

Arachnoid Granulations

Arachnoid granulations are normal extensions of the SAS and arachnoid through the dural wall and into the venous sinuses. They are covered with arachnoid cap cells and venous sinus endothelium. CSF drains through the endothelium into the venous sinus. The most common locations for arachnoid granulations are the superior sagittal sinus and transverse sinuses. These normal variants are important "pseudolesions" to recognize, as they may be misdiagnosed as pathology. They are CSF density or intensity on imaging and do not enhance. They are often associated with bone changes on CT, particularly in the occipital bone.

Differential Diagnosis

The following differential diagnosis lists are provided to help organize the most common scalp, skull, and meningeal lesions.

Scalp Masses

- Subgaleal hematoma, foreign body (most common)
- Sebaceous cyst
- Lipoma
- Dermoid
- Metastases (extension from calvarium)
- Vascular malformation
- Skin cancer (basal cell or squamous cell)

Calvarial Thickening

- Normal variant (most common)
- Chronic phenytoin (Dilantin) therapy
- Shunted hydrocephalus
- Paget disease
- Fibrous dysplasia
- Hyperparathyroidism
- Acromegaly
- Anemias

Calvarial Thinning

- Normal variants (parietal thinning) (most common)
- Arachnoid cyst
- Mega cisterna magna

Peripherally located tumors (oligodendroglioma, DNET)

"Hair on End"

Classic appearance of anemias: Thalassemia, sickle cell disease, hereditary spherocytosis

Skull hemangioma

Metastases (commonly neuroblastoma and prostate cancer)

Lytic Skull Lesion

Normal variant or surgical defects (most common)
Metastases
Epidermoid cyst
Eosinophilic granuloma
Hemangioma
Paget disease
Plasmacytoma
Osteomyelitis

Sclerotic Skull Lesion

Metastasis (most common)
Osteoma
Fibrous dysplasia
Meningioma-associated
Paget disease

Diffuse Dural Enhancement

Postoperative or post-procedure (i.e., lumbar puncture)
Chronic subdural hematoma
Meningitis (leptomeningeal enhancement common)
Neoplasm
Neurosarcoid
Intracranial hypotension (venous congestion)
Hypertrophic pachymeningitis
Dural sinus thrombosis

Leptomeningeal Enhancement

Meningitis (infectious or neoplastic)
Neurosarcoid

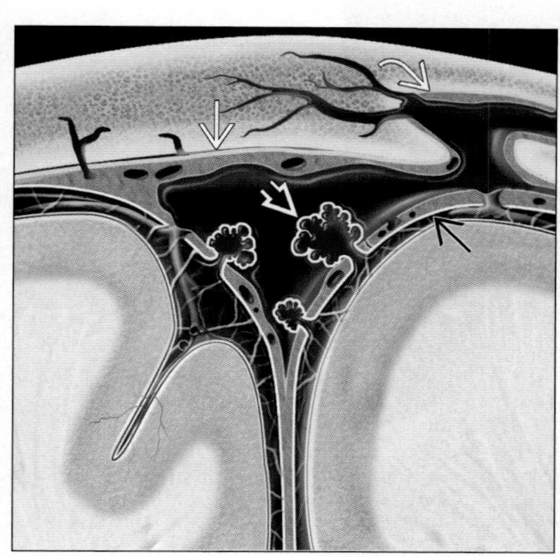

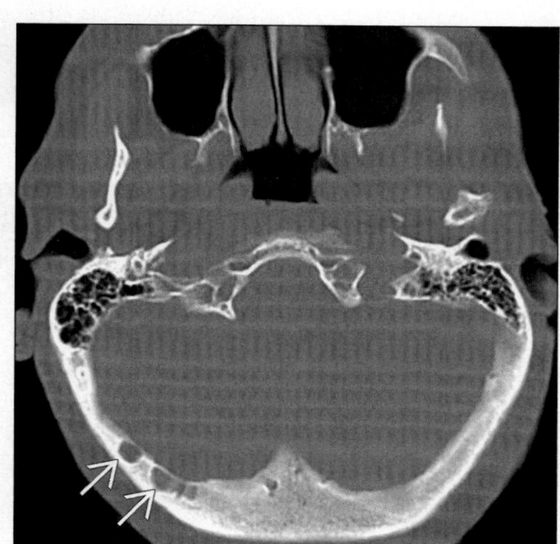

(Left) *Coronal graphic shows the calvarial apex with the superior sagittal sinus (SSS) and a venous lake ➲. The SSS is formed by 2 dural layers, an outer (periosteal) layer ➡ & inner (meningeal) layer. Arachnoid granulations ➡ extend from the arachnoid into the SSS. The arachnoid ➙ is closely applied to the inner layer of dura.* ***(Right)*** *Axial bone CT shows multiple sharply marginated, lucent, occipital bone lesions ➡ adjacent to the transverse sinus, characteristic of arachnoid granulations.*

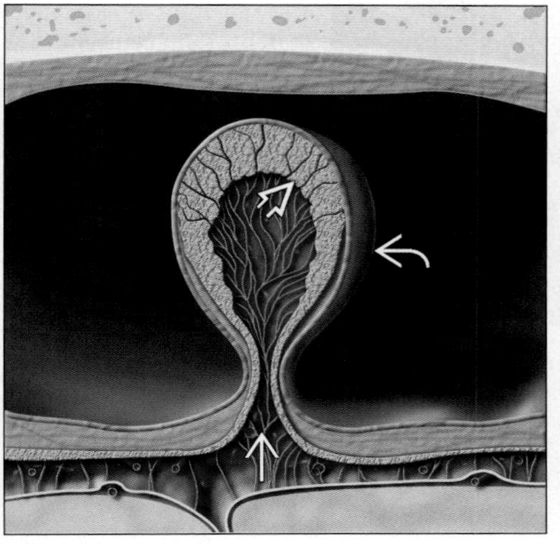

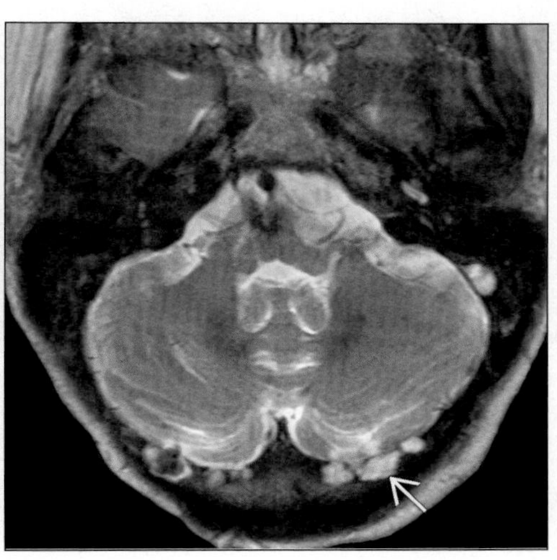

(Left) *Coronal graphic of an arachnoid granulation projecting from the subarachnoid space into the SSS. A CSF core ➡ extends into the arachnoid granulation and is separated by arachnoid cap cells ➡ from the venous sinus endothelium ➲. Arachnoid granulations allow drainage of CSF into the venous circulation.* ***(Right)*** *Axial T2WI FS MR shows multiple CSF signal intensity lesions representing arachnoid granulations ➡ in the occipital bone, a typical location.*

SKULL, SCALP, & MENINGES OVERVIEW

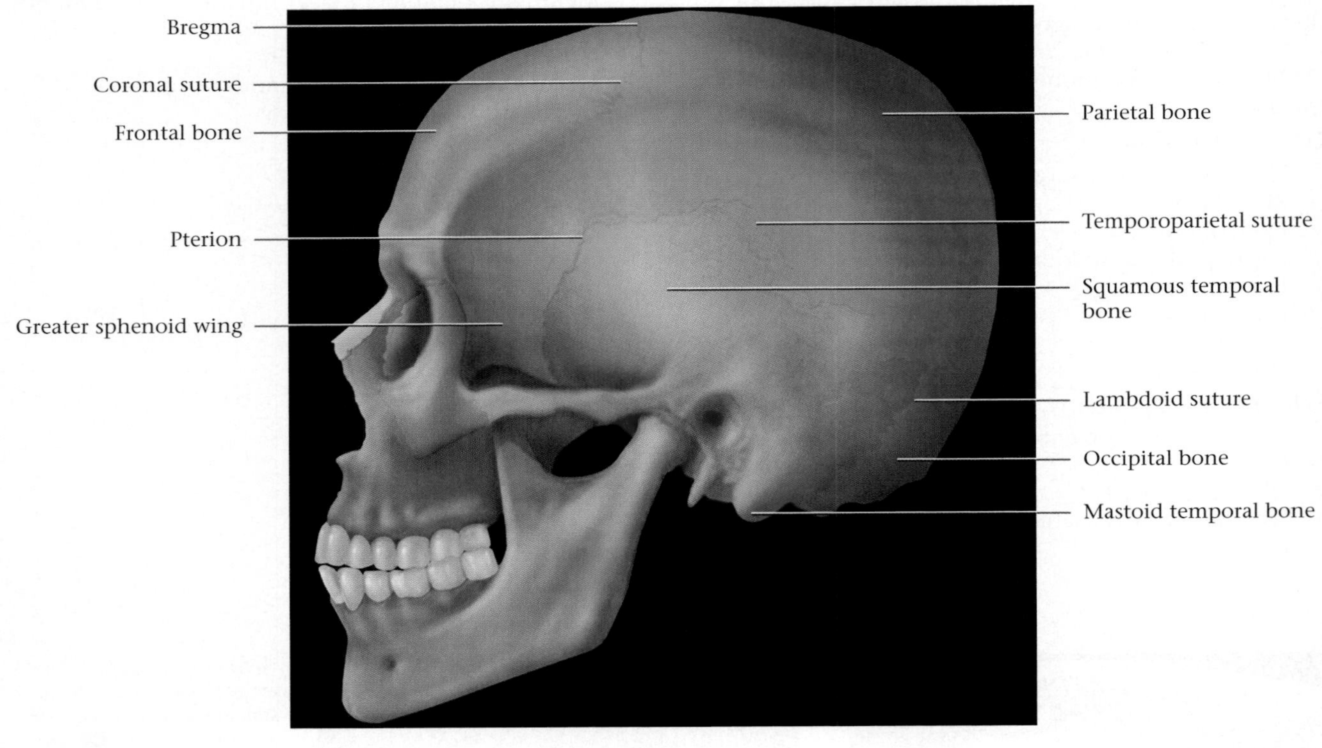

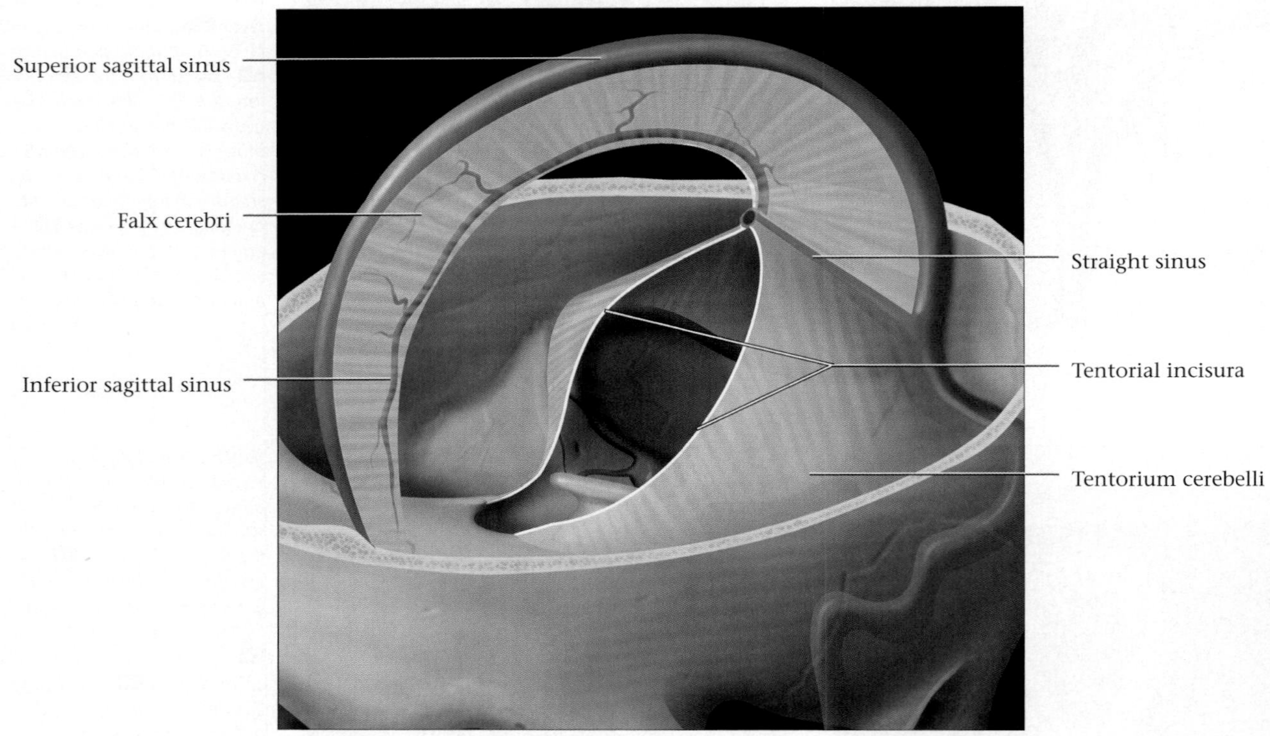

*(**Top**) Lateral view shows calvarial vault components. The pterion, an important surgical landmark, is a small area on the lateral skull at the intersection of the frontal, parietal, sphenoid, & squamosal temporal bones. (**Bottom**) Graphic shows the major dural sinuses as they relate to the falx cerebri & tentorium cerebelli. The falx inserts on the crista galli anteriorly & sweeps backwards in the midline to the straight sinus, becoming taller as it passes posteriorly. The tentorium meets the falx at the tentorial apex & curves downwards to contain the transverse sinuses. The leaves of the tentorium insert anteriorly on the petrous apex & fibers extend forward to the anterior clinoid processes.*

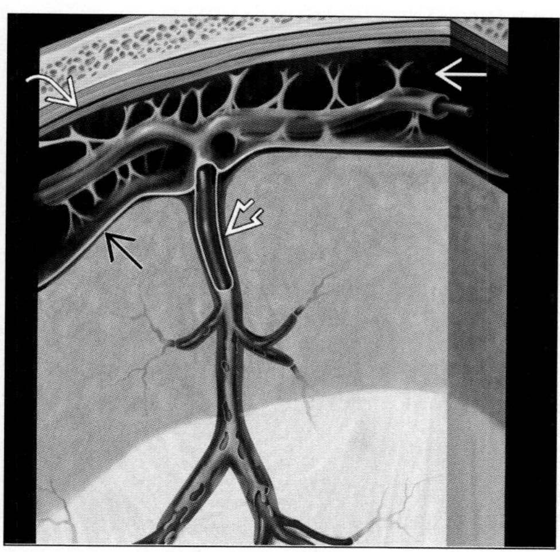

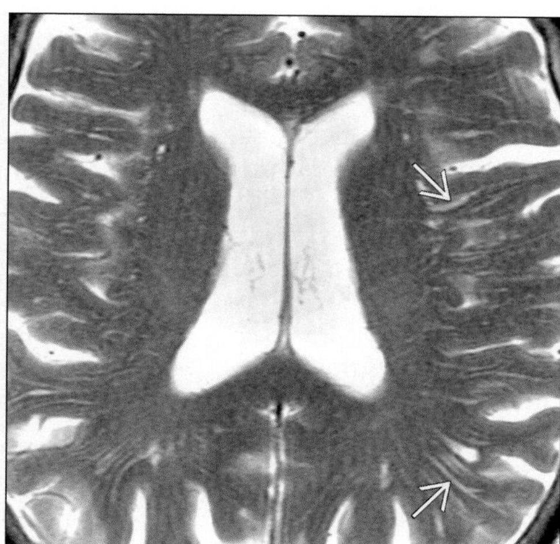

(Left) *Coronal graphic shows the cranial meninges and subarachnoid space (SAS) ➡. The pia is a thin delicate membrane that covers the brain ➡ as well as the vessels and trabeculae in the SAS. The pia also invaginates along a penetrating cortical artery to form a perivascular space ➡. The arachnoid ➡ forms the outer margin of the SAS and is loosely attached to the dura.* ***(Right)*** *Axial T2WI MR at 3T shows multiple normal perivascular spaces ➡ in the subcortical and deep white matter.*

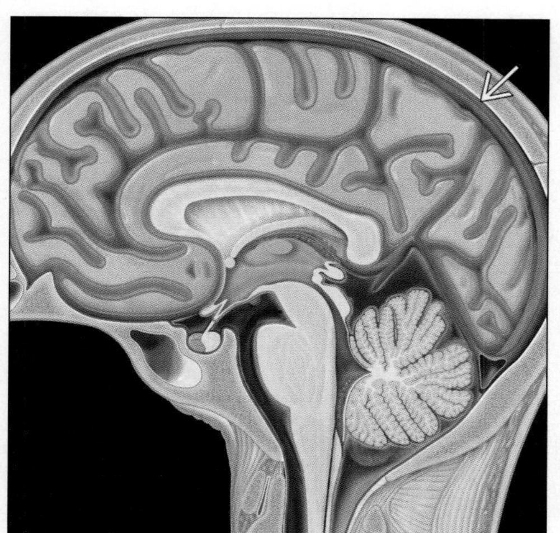

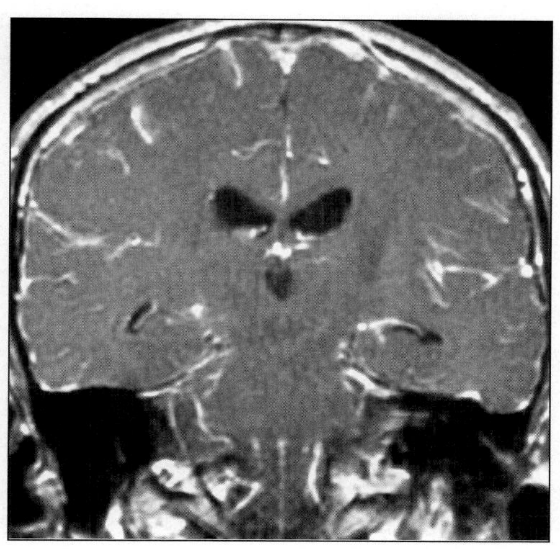

(Left) *Sagittal graphic depicts the cranial leptomeninges as they enclose the CSF cisterns, shown in blue. The arachnoid ➡ (purple) follows the dura around the inner calvarium but does not invaginate into the sulci. The pia (orange) is the innermost layer of leptomeninges and follows the brain surface and dips into the sulci. The subarachnoid space lies between the pia and arachnoid.* ***(Right)*** *Coronal T1 C+ MR shows extensive abnormal leptomeningeal enhancement related to infectious meningitis.*

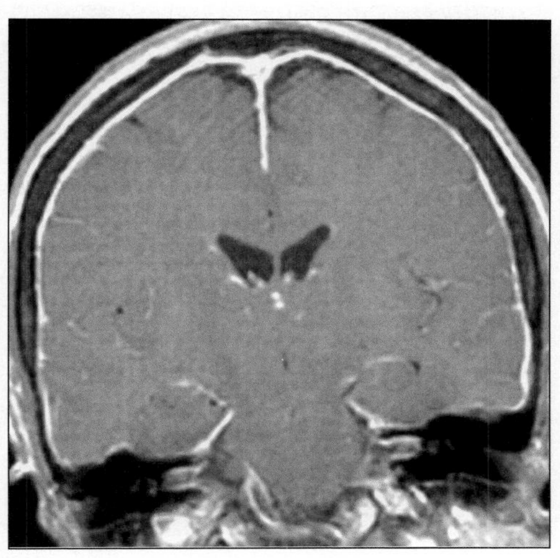

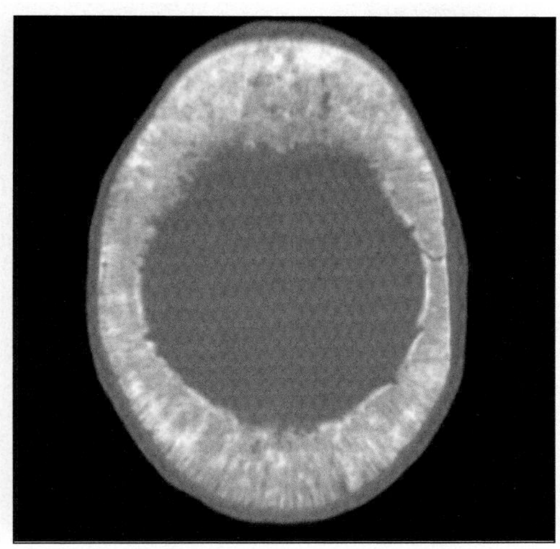

(Left) *Coronal T1 C+ MR shows diffuse dural enhancement related to intracranial hypotension in this patient with a CSF leak. Diffuse dural enhancement is commonly related to a prior procedure, infection, or inflammatory etiology. Venous congestion is the cause in intracranial hypotension.* ***(Right)*** *Axial bone CT shows diffuse calvarial thickening with widening of the diploic marrow resulting in a "hair on end" appearance. Thalassemia major is the most common cause of this classic imaging finding.*

CONGENITAL CALVARIAL DEFECTS

Key Facts

Terminology

- Parietal foramina
  - Nonossification of medial parietal bone embryonal rest
- Sinus pericranii
  - Abnormal communication between intracranial and extracranial venous systems through calvarial defect
- Aplasia cutis congenita
  - Congenital skin malformation; may have underlying skull defect
- Cleidocranial dysplasia
  - Defective membranous and endochondral bone formation → delayed skull ossification
- Amniotic band syndrome
  - Strands of amniotic sac (bands) from ruptured amnion entangle digits, limbs, or other fetal parts
- Cranium bifidum occultum

Imaging

- Symmetry, location best clues for diagnosis
- CT for calvarium, MR for underlying brain

Top Differential Diagnoses

- Epidermoid/dermoid
- Hemangioma
- Langerhans cell histiocytosis
- Metastasis
- Lacunar skull (Lückenschädel)

Clinical Issues

- Incidental finding on imaging or palpable scalp/ calvarial mass that may protrude with crying, ↑ ICP

Diagnostic Checklist

- Patients with EPF (> 5 mm) warrant imaging of brain parenchyma and vasculature

*(**Left**) Axial bone CT of the calvarium in a patient with a bilateral enlarged parietal foramina shows soft tissue extension through symmetrical, smooth, sharply demarcated osseous calvarial defects ➡. (**Right**) Axial NECT in the same patient shows soft tissue windows with bilateral enlarged parietal foramina and otherwise normal brain parenchyma ⇨ protruding through the large, well-demarcated bilateral calvarial defects.*

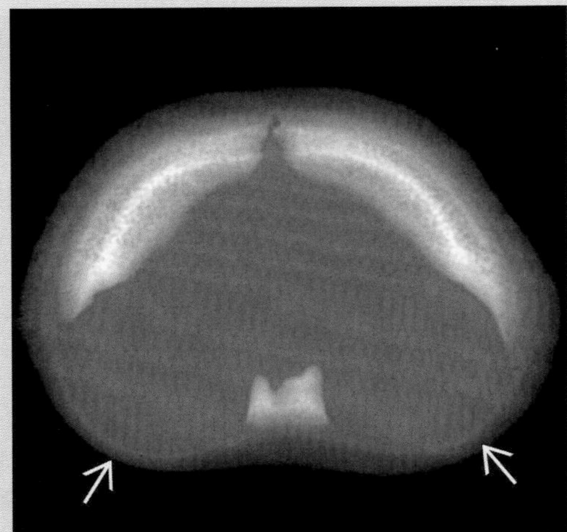

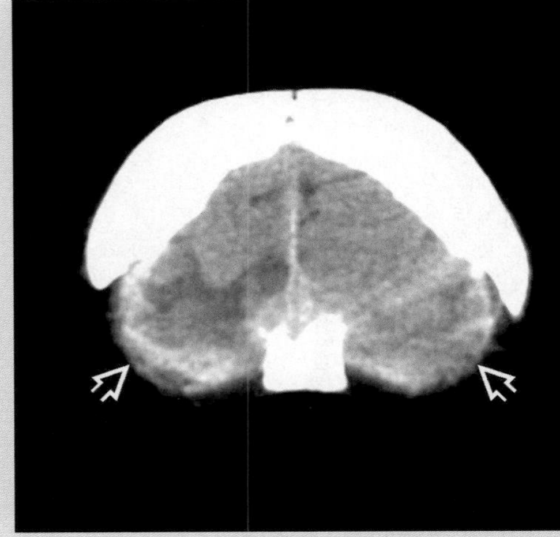

*(**Left**) Sagittal T1WI MR in a patient with sinus pericranii shows dilated parietal scalp veins ⇨ in contiguity with the superior sagittal sinus through a small calvarial defect ➡. (**Right**) Sagittal MRV MIP reconstruction in the same patient confirms the presence of large parietal scalp veins ⇨ in contiguity with the superior sagittal sinus ↪ via a small transcalvarial vein ➡. These are the classic imaging findings of sinus pericranii.*

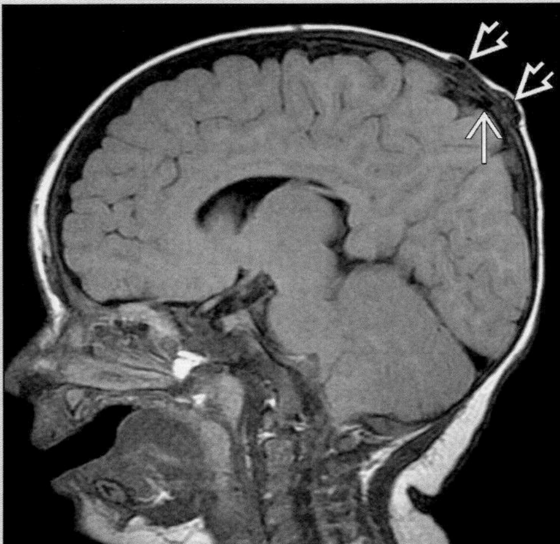

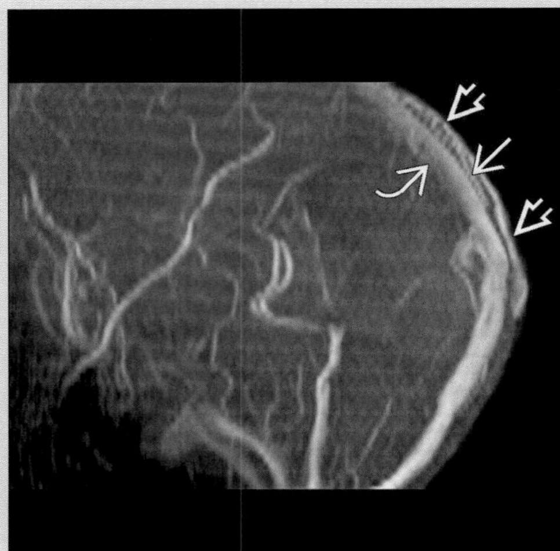

TERMINOLOGY

Abbreviations

- Enlarged parietal foramen (EPF), aplasia cutis congenita (ACC)

Definitions

- Parietal fissure (common)
  - Small, residual, "incomplete" medial parietal bone suture
- Parietal foramina (common; 60-70% of normal skulls)
  - Nonossification of medial parietal bone embryonal rest
  - Emissary vein portal between superior sagittal sinus and extracranial scalp veins
- Enlarged parietal foramina (rare; prevalence 1:15,000-25,000)
  - Delayed/incomplete ossification of membranous parietal bone → round or oval parietal bone defects
  - Calvarial defect may be large, palpable
- Sinus pericranii
  - Abnormal communication between intracranial, extracranial venous systems through calvarial defect
  - Soft (often red or blue) scalp mass near superior sagittal or transverse dural sinuses
  - ↑ size with ↑ ICP (Valsalva, dependent positioning)
- Craniolacunia (venous lakes)
  - Patulous calvarial diploic veins
  - Irregular, geographic, well-demarcated contour
  - Variable size and number
- Arachnoid (pacchionian) granulations
  - Located within 3 cm of superior sagittal sinus
  - Often multiple, irregular contour
- Abnormally large fontanelle
  - Secondary to ↑ intracranial pressure (suture spreading) or skeletal dysplasia
  - Search for ventriculomegaly, skeletal anomalies
- Cleidocranial dysplasia (uncommon)
  - Defective membranous and endochondral bone formation → delayed skull ossification
  - Enlarged sagittal and metopic sutures, wide anterior and posterior fontanelles, broad cranial diameter, multiple wormian bones along lambdoid sutures
- Cranium bifidum occultum ("cleft skull")
  - Delayed ossification of parietal bones → large midline skull defects
  - Progressive parietal bone ossification fills defects; may persist as parietal foramina
    - Persistence in adulthood rare (< 1%)
  - Brain covered by dura, intact scalp
- Amniotic band syndrome
  - Occurs when inner amnion membrane ruptures or tears without disruption of outer chorion
  - Strands of amniotic sac (bands) from ruptured amnion entangle digits, limbs, or other fetal parts
- Aplasia cutis congenita (uncommon)
  - Congenital skin malformation; may have underlying skull defect
  - Skin defects most frequent on midline scalp > trunk, face, limbs
- Acalvaria (rare)
  - Absent superior osseous cranial vault, dura mater
  - Normal skull base, facial bones, brain (usually)
- Acrania (rare)
  - Partial or complete absence of cranial vault bones, abnormal cerebral hemisphere development

IMAGING

General Features

- Best diagnostic clue
  - Symmetry, location best clues for diagnosis
- Size
  - Variable; small → large

CT Findings

- NECT
  - Variable soft tissue component
  - Intracranial extent may not be well demonstrated
- Bone CT
  - Characterize osseous margins as sharp or destructive, sclerotic or nonsclerotic, inner or outer table

MR Findings

- Variable; depends on composition of soft tissue component, size and etiology of calvarial defect

Imaging Recommendations

- Best imaging tool
  - Bone CT with 3D shaded surface reformats best demonstrates calvarial defect, bone margins
  - MR best demonstrates soft tissue component composition, intracranial extension, brain anomalies

DIFFERENTIAL DIAGNOSIS

Epidermoid/Dermoid

- Most common childhood benign calvarial tumor
- Sharp, slightly sclerotic osseous margins
- Most common along frontal, parietal bone sutures or adjacent to fontanelles

Hemangioma

- "Honeycomb" or "sunburst" pattern of bony spicules, avid enhancement
- Outer > inner table, nonsclerotic, nonbeveled margins
- ± prominent vascular grooves

Langerhans Cell Histiocytosis

- Lytic lesion(s) with nonsclerotic rim
- Beveled (outer > inner table)
- Predilection for calvarium, temporal bone

Metastasis

- Multiple poorly defined destructive osteolytic lesions
- Advanced leukemia, neuroblastoma most common
  - Neuroblastoma ± "hair on end" appearance
- Look for additional appendicular skeletal lesions, hepatosplenomegaly (leukemia)

Lacunar Skull (Luckenschadel) of Newborn

- Membranous bone dysplasia present at birth
- Well-defined calvarial lucencies = nonossified fibrous bone surrounded by normally ossified bone

CONGENITAL CALVARIAL DEFECTS

- Resolve spontaneously by ~ 6 months, unrelated to hydrocephalus severity
- Associated with myelomeningocele or encephalocele, Chiari II malformation

Leptomeningeal Cyst
- "Growing fracture" with adjacent encephalomalacia
- 0.6% of skull fractures (usually in child < 3 years)

Convolutional Markings
- True convolutional markings occur after sutural closure → differentiate from Lückenschädel

Osteomyelitis
- Lytic, poorly defined infiltrating margins, overlying soft tissue edema, fever or ↑ serum inflammatory markers

Cephalocele
- Osseous defect in characteristic location
- Brain anomalies, soft tissue component often clinically obvious

PATHOLOGY

General Features
- Etiology
  - Variable; many developmental and present early in life
  - Fortunately, majority of pediatric skull masses are histologically and clinically benign
- Genetics
  - Enlarged parietal foramina
    - Isolated autosomal dominant or syndromal
      - Chromosome 11p deletion with *ALX4* gene mutation
    - No causative mutation identified in nonsyndromic cases
  - Cleidocranial dysplasia
    - Autosomal dominant, locus on short arm of chromosome 6
    - Mutation in *CBFA1* gene coding for transcription factor activating osteoblastic differentiation
    - Variable expression, high penetrance
  - Cranium bifidum
    - Autosomal dominant, strong genetic heterogenicity
- Associated abnormalities
  - Enlarged parietal foramina
    - Scalp defects, cleft lip/palate, structural brain malformations
    - Vascular anomalies, including persistent falcine venous sinus ± adjacent focal encephalomalacia, occipital cortical infolding variations, atretic occipital encephalocele
  - Abnormally large fontanelles
    - Variable; depends on etiology or syndrome
  - Cleidocranial dysplasia
    - Absent/hypoplastic clavicles, small bell-shaped thorax, widened pubic symphysis, spinal anomalies, hypoplastic middle and distal phalanges, delayed deciduous dentition, hearing loss (38%)
  - Cranium bifidum
    - Midline neural tube malformations (myelomeningocele, meningoencephalocele, dermal sinus)
  - Amniotic band syndrome
    - ± constriction bands around limbs, congenital amputations, abdominal wall defects, and facial clefting
  - Acrania
    - Amniotic bands, anencephaly

CLINICAL ISSUES

Presentation
- Most common signs/symptoms
  - Palpable scalp or calvarial mass may bulge with crying, ↑ ICP
  - Incidental finding detected during imaging for other reasons
- Other signs/symptoms
  - Abnormally large anterior fontanelle (seen in osteogenesis imperfecta, cleidocranial dysplasia)

Natural History & Prognosis
- Dependent on severity of associated anomalies (especially orthopedic, neurological)

Treatment
- Surgical closure of calvarial defect with autologous bone or alloplastic material
- Multidisciplinary supportive care

DIAGNOSTIC CHECKLIST

Consider
- Patients with EPF (> 5 mm) warrant imaging of brain parenchyma and vasculature

Image Interpretation Pearls
- Confirm presence or absence of skull base, vascular, skeletal anomalies

SELECTED REFERENCES

1. Celik SE et al: Complete cranium bifidum without scalp abnormality. Case report. J Neurosurg Pediatrics. 1(3):258-60, 2008
2. Mavrogiannis LA et al: Enlarged parietal foramina caused by mutations in the homeobox genes ALX4 and MSX2: from genotype to phenotype. Eur J Hum Genet. 14(2):151-8, 2006
3. Glass RB et al: The infant skull: a vault of information. Radiographics. 24(2):507-22, 2004
4. de Heer IM et al: Parietal bone agenesis and associated multiple congenital anomalies. J Craniofac Surg. 14(2):192-6, 2003
5. Tubbs RS et al: Parietal foramina are not synonymous with giant parietal foramina. Pediatr Neurosurg. 39(4):216-7, 2003

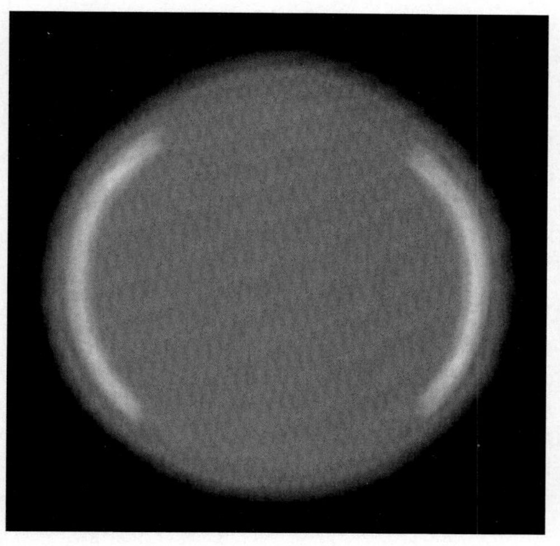

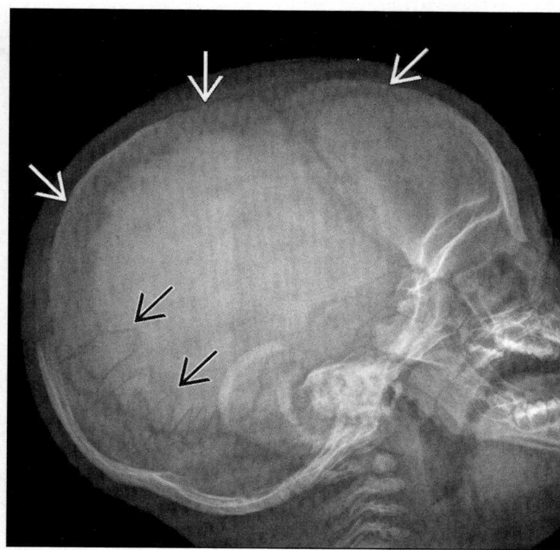

(Left) *Axial bone CT of the calvarium in a young patient with cleidocranial dysplasia demonstrates diminished midline bone structures, with abnormally large anterior and posterior fontanelles and wide sagittal suture.* **(Right)** *Lateral skull radiograph in a patient with cleidocranial dysplasia depicts large anterior/posterior fontanelles and a wide sagittal suture ➔. Note the numerous wormian bones ➔ characteristically distributed along the lambdoid sutures.*

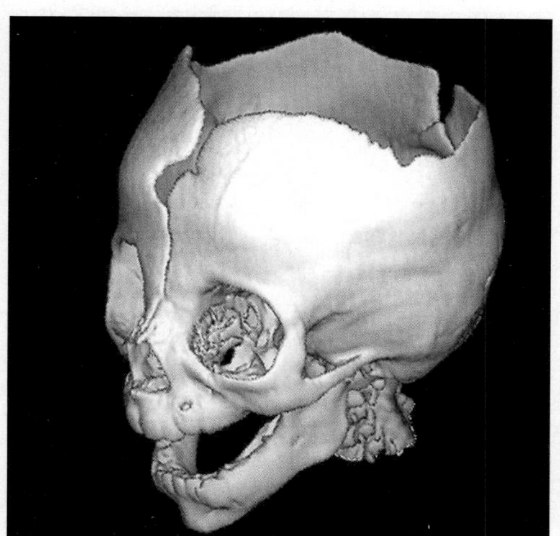

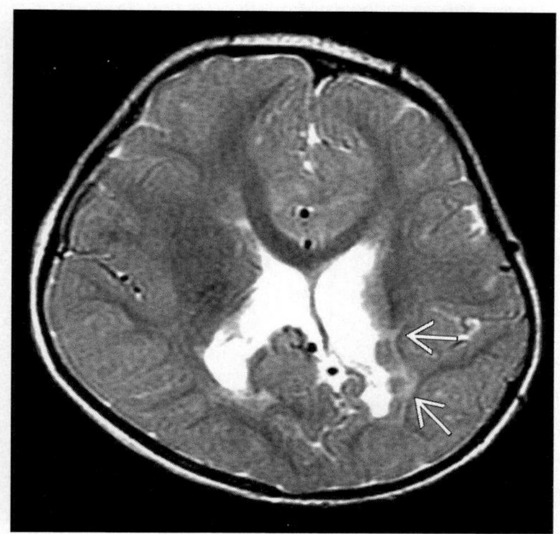

(Left) *Sagittal oblique 3D bone CT reconstruction of the head in a patient with a large calvarial defect resulting from amniotic band syndrome. Note the absence of the superior portions of the bilateral frontal and parietal bones. The superior cranial vault is "open."* **(Right)** *Axial T2WI MR in the same patient with amniotic band syndrome shows left parietal lobe white matter volume loss and ependymal irregularity with associated periventricular nodular gray matter heterotopia ➔.*

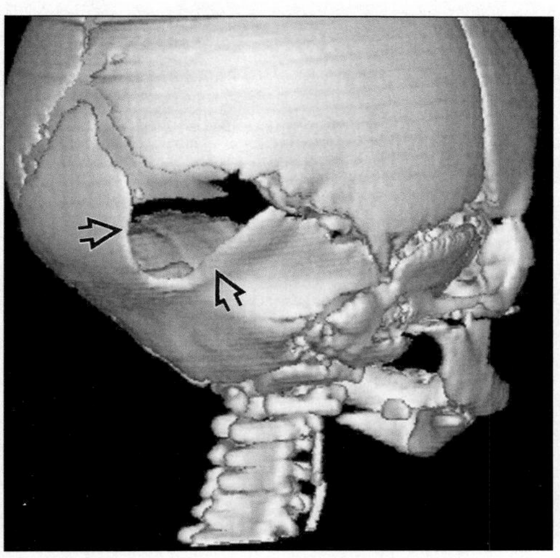

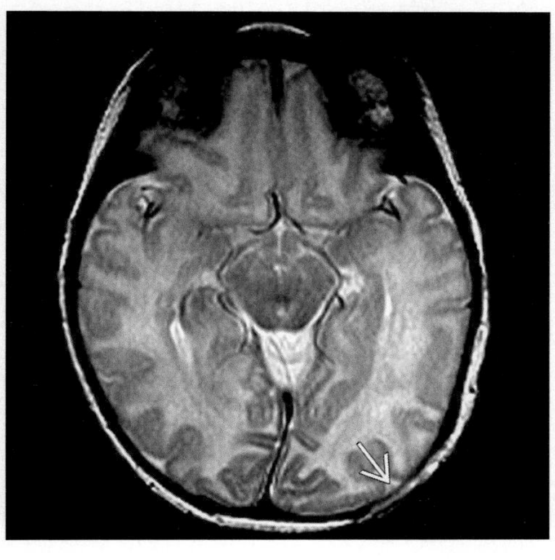

(Left) *Coronal oblique 3D bone CT reconstruction of the calvarium in a patient with focal cutis aplasia congenita of the scalp depicts a large calvarial defect ➲ subjacent to the region of cutis aplasia abutting the lambdoid suture.* **(Right)** *Axial T2WI MR in the same patient with focal cutis aplasia congenita and a left occipital calvarial defect demonstrates thinning of subcutaneous fat, but intact dura ➔, in the region immediately beneath the area of cutis aplasia.*

CRANIOSTENOSES

Key Facts

Terminology

- Synonyms: Craniosynostosis, sutural synostosis, cranial dysostosis, craniofacial dysostosis
- Heterogeneous group with abnormal head shape, premature sutural closure and fusion

Imaging

- Calvarial (and facial) distortion predictable based on suture(s) involved
- Fibrous or bony "bridging" ± "beaking" along suture

Top Differential Diagnoses

- Postural flattening or positional molding
- Secondary craniosynostosis

Pathology

- Premature upregulation of growth factors signaling sutural fusion → craniostenosis
- Head shape may be abnormal before osseous sutural changes detectable on imaging
- Some single sutural and nonsyndromic synostoses are genetic
- Syndromic synostoses usually autosomal dominant

Clinical Issues

- Asymmetric face/cranium, ↓ head growth, extremity anomalies, developmental delay
- Patients with more severe anomalies often present at time of birth

Diagnostic Checklist

- Nonsyndromic does not necessarily mean nongenetic; single sutural synostoses also governed by genes
- Look for venous drainage anomalies or occlusion (particularly with multisutural synostosis)

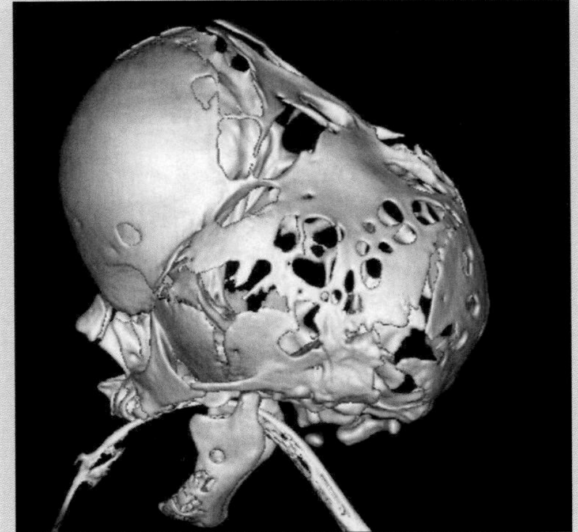

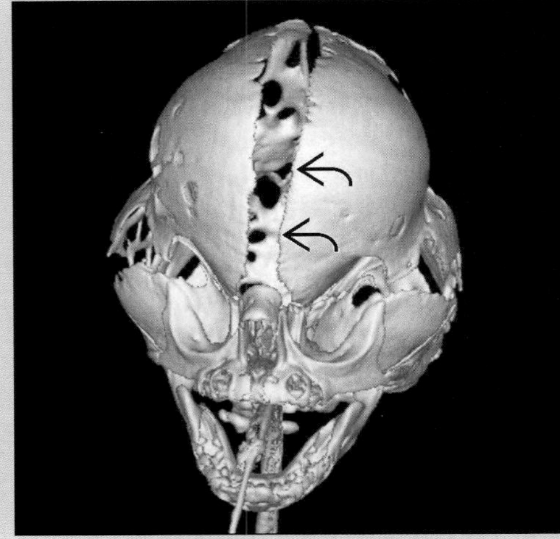

*(**Left**) Sagittal bone CT 3D shaded surface reformat of the calvarium in a 1 day old with Carpenter syndrome shows an abnormal head shape and frontal bossing with facial hypoplasia and premature closure of the squamosal, coronal, lambdoid, and sagittal sutures. (**Right**) Anterior coronal bone CT 3D shaded surface reformat in the same patient shows a very wide metopic suture → and anterior fontanelle with harlequin eyes and a small face due to premature closure of the facial sutures.*

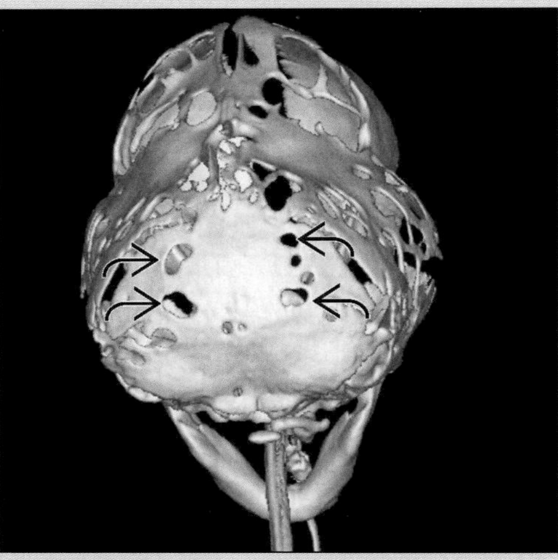

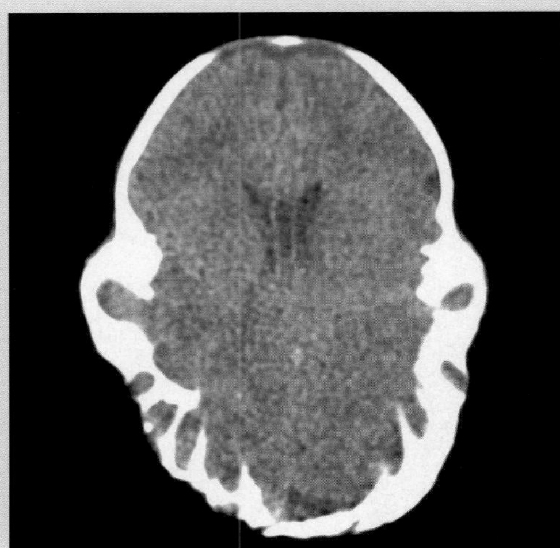

*(**Left**) Posterior coronal bone CT 3D shaded surface reformat in the same patient shows an abnormal head shape with occiput flattening, partial or complete closure of the lambdoid, sagittal sutures, and apparent "holes" → due to focal calvarial thinning. (**Right**) Axial NECT in the same patient reveals marked irregularity of the calvarium. The intracranial compartment is small, producing brain compression with posterior effacement of the convexity sulci.*

CRANIOSTENOSES

TERMINOLOGY

Synonyms

- Craniosynostosis, sutural synostosis, cranial dysostosis, craniofacial dysostosis

Definitions

- Heterogeneous group with abnormal head shape, premature sutural closure and fusion
  - Nonsyndromic (85%); isolated, classified according to involved suture(s)
    - Simple (single) suture (75-80%)
      - Abnormal head shape, (usually) normal intelligence
      - Usually sporadic, operated for cosmetic reasons
    - Multiple sutures (20-25%)
      - Oxycephaly (40-50%), brachycephaly (30-40%), unclassified (20%)
  - Syndromic (> 180 syndromes [15%]); multiple anomalies with (frequently) developmental delay
    - Association with craniofacial, skeletal, nervous system, other anomalies
    - Syndrome description based on clinical features
      - Acrocephalosyndactyly type 1 (Apert)
      - Acrocephalosyndactyly type 2 (Apert-Crouzon)
      - Acrocephalosyndactyly type 3 (Saethre-Chotzen)
      - Acrocephalosyndactyly type 4 (Waardenburg)
      - Acrocephalosyndactyly type 5 (Pfeiffer)
      - Acrocephalopolysyndactyly type 2 (Carpenter)

IMAGING

General Features

- Best diagnostic clue
  - Head shape predicts abnormal suture(s)
- Size
  - Part or all of abnormal suture may be fused
- Morphology
  - Classic imaging appearance: Calvarial (and facial) distortion predictable based on suture(s) involved
    - Scaphocephaly (dolichocephaly): ↓ transverse, ↑ AP, forehead bossing → sagittal synostosis
    - Trigonocephaly: Wedge-shaped forehead, hypotelorism → metopic synostosis
    - Plagiocephaly: Asymmetry → unilateral single or asymmetric multiple sutures
      - Unilateral coronal synostosis: Unilateral harlequin orbit, hemicalvarium shortened and pointed
      - Lambdoid synostosis: Trapezoid skull, ipsilateral posterior ear displacement, occipital flattening
    - Brachycephaly: ↑ transverse, ↓ AP → bicoronal or bilambdoid synostosis
      - Bilateral coronal synostosis: Bilateral harlequin orbit, brachycephaly, skull base and craniofacial aberrations
    - Turricephaly: "Towering skull" → bicoronal or bilambdoid synostosis
    - Oxycephaly: Coronal, sagittal, lambdoid sutures
    - Kleeblattschädel: "Cloverleaf skull," Bulging temporal bone, shallow orbits → bicoronal and bilambdoid synostosis
    - Unclassified: Multiple assorted sutural synostoses

Radiographic Findings

- Radiography
  - Skull: Dense suture; "bone bridge," inner table scalloping
  - Extremities: Many anomalies described, some specific
    - Apert: Hand/foot syndactyly
    - Pfeiffer: Wide, "stub" thumbs
    - Saethre-Chotzen: Duplicated distal phalanx, cone-shaped hallux epiphysis
    - Muenke-type mutations: Calcaneo-cuboid fusion
    - Crouzon: Hands/feet normal

CT Findings

- Bone CT
  - Fibrous or bony "bridging" ± "beaking" along suture
  - Head shape determined by involved suture(s)

MR Findings

- T1WI
  - Syndromic: Abnormal head shape ± cerebellar tonsillar ectopia, hydrocephalus, agenesis corpus callosum
  - Nonsyndromic: Abnormal head shape, brain (usually) normal
- T2WI
  - Same as T1WI
- MRV
  - ± congenital venous drainage anomalies
  - Postoperative dural venous occlusion

Imaging Recommendations

- Best imaging tool
  - Low-dose 3D bone CT reconstruction for sutural status
  - MR for brain abnormalities

DIFFERENTIAL DIAGNOSIS

Postural Flattening or Positional Molding

- Normal infants: Marked ↑ in incidence after 1994 pediatric "back to sleep" campaign
  - Parallelogram skull, ipsilateral anterior ear displacement
- Hypotonic infant: Lies on back → posterior flattening
- Premature infant: Lies on side → dolichocephaly

Secondary Craniosynostosis

- Brain growth arrest (myriad causes) → premature sutural fusion (especially metopic or universal craniosynostosis)

PATHOLOGY

General Features

- Etiology
  - Normal sutures permit skull growth perpendicular to long axis, close when brain growth slows
    - Order of closure: Metopic > coronal > lambdoid > sagittal

CRANIOSTENOSES

- Premature upregulation of growth factors signaling sutural fusion → anomalous skull base development, craniostenosis
  - Transforming growth factor (TGF), fibroblast growth factor/receptor (FGF/FGFR) mutations expressed in face, skull base, limb buds
- Abnormal head shape before osseous sutural changes apparent
  - Identifiable as early as 13 weeks gestation
  - Only part of suture needs to close → craniosynostosis
- ↓ growth of 1 suture compensated by ↑ growth of other sutures
  - Skull growth ↓ perpendicular, ↑ parallel to fused suture → abnormal head shape

- Genetics
  - Some single sutural and nonsyndromic synostoses are genetic
    - Gene expression often suture specific
  - Syndromic synostoses usually autosomal dominant
    - *FGFR1* (Pfeiffer syndrome)
    - *FGFR2* (Apert, Pfeiffer, Crouzon, Jackson-Weiss)
    - *FGFR3* (Thanatophoric dysplasia type 1 and 2, Crouzon)
    - *TWIST* (Saethre-Chotzen syndrome)
    - *MSX2* (Boston-type craniosynostosis)
- Associated abnormalities
  - Limb anomalies (syndactyly and polysyndactyly [30%], deficiencies [22%])
  - Neurological abnormalities/complications
    - ↑ intracranial pressure: Mechanical brain distortion, hydrocephalus, dural and collateral venous outflow obstruction at skull base
    - Tonsillar herniation ± syringohydromyelia
    - Exophthalmos, visual loss, mental retardation (secondary to ↑ ICP)

Gross Pathologic & Surgical Features

- Fibrous or osseous "bridging," "beaking" along suture

Microscopic Features

- ↑ osteoblastic cell differentiation/maturation

CLINICAL ISSUES

Presentation

- Most common signs/symptoms
  - Asymmetric face/cranium, ↓ head growth
  - Affected patients with more severe abnormalities often present at birth
- Other signs/symptoms
  - Extremity anomalies, developmental delay
- Clinical profile
  - Craniofacial asymmetry ± extremity anomalies
  - More common in twins (mechanical forces?)

Demographics

- Age
  - Usually present at birth or in infancy
- Gender
  - Overall (M:F = 4:1)
  - Scaphocephaly (M:F = 3.5:1)
  - Trigonocephaly (M:F = 2-3.3:1)
  - Coronal synostosis (M:F = 1:2)
  - Apert (M:F = 1:1)
- Epidemiology
  - Overall (1:2,500)
  - Sagittal (55-60%), coronal (20-30%), plagiocephaly (5-10%), metopic (1-2%)

Natural History & Prognosis

- Single suture → cosmetic only or secondary mandibular/maxillary deformities (suture dependent)
- Multiple suture → cosmetic with secondary mandibular/maxillary deformities, ↑ ICP, ↓ CBF; airway/aural/visual compromise
  - Craniofacial deformity socially stigmatizing
- Nonsyndromic → normal cognitive and motor development (debated)
- Syndromic ± midline brain anomalies → developmental delay

Treatment

- Mild deformity or positional molding
  - Aggressive physiotherapy, head repositioning, orthotic headband/helmet therapy
- Moderate to severe deformity
  - Surgical cranial vault reconstruction or cranial vault distraction osteogenesis

DIAGNOSTIC CHECKLIST

Consider

- Nonsyndromic does not mean nongenetic; single sutural synostoses also governed by genes
- Venous drainage anomalies (multisutural synostosis)

Image Interpretation Pearls

- Positional lambdoid flattening: Long axis of skull is oblique (forehead to contralateral occiput)
- Unilateral lambdoid synostosis: Long axis of skull remains unilateral A-P (forehead to ipsilateral occiput)

SELECTED REFERENCES

1. Blaser SI: Abnormal skull shape. Pediatr Radiol. 38 Suppl 3:S488-96, 2008
2. Dover MS: Abnormal skull shape: clinical management. Pediatr Radiol. 38 Suppl 3:S484-7, 2008
3. Slovis et al: Craniosynostosis, selected craniofacial syndromes, and other abnormalities of the skull. In Caffey's Pediatric Diagnostic Imaging. 11th ed. Amsterdam, Netherlands: Mosby-Elsevier. 471-500, 2008
4. Cunningham ML et al: Evaluation of the infant with an abnormal skull shape. Curr Opin Pediatr. 19(6):645-51, 2007
5. Kapp-Simon KA et al: Neurodevelopment of children with single suture craniosynostosis: a review. Childs Nerv Syst. 23(3):269-81, 2007
6. Kimonis V et al: Genetics of craniosynostosis. Semin Pediatr Neurol. 14(3):150-61, 2007
7. Sandberg DI et al: Anomalous venous drainage preventing safe posterior fossa decompression in patients with chiari malformation type I and multisutural craniosynostosis. Report of two cases and review of the literature. J Neurosurg. 106(6 Suppl):490-4, 2007

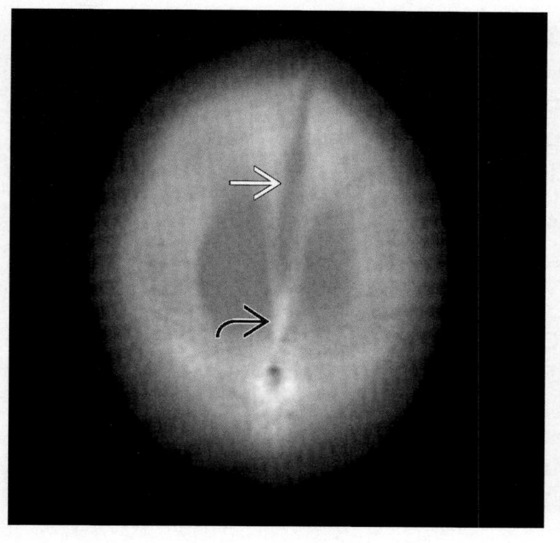

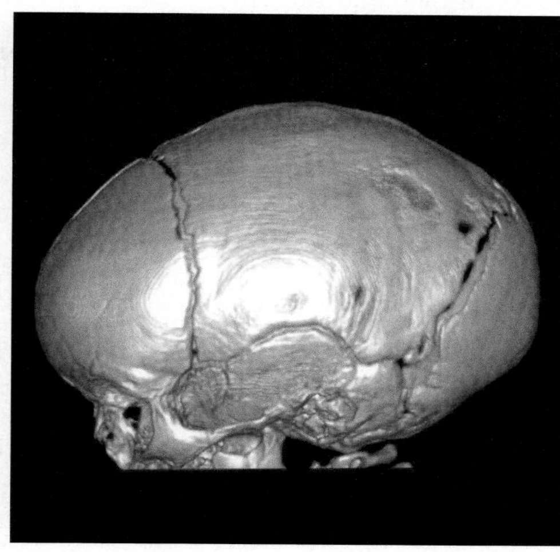

(Left) *Axial bone CT of the calvarium in a patient presenting with severe scaphocephaly shows sagittal synostosis. Note the straightening and narrowing of the sagittal suture ➡ with prominent ridges, osseous bridging, and bony fusion ➡ across the sagittal suture.* ***(Right)*** *Sagittal 3D bone CT of the calvarium in the same patient shows prominent dolichocephaly and confirms characteristic findings of isolated sagittal synostosis. The coronal, lambdoid, and squamosal sutures are normal.*

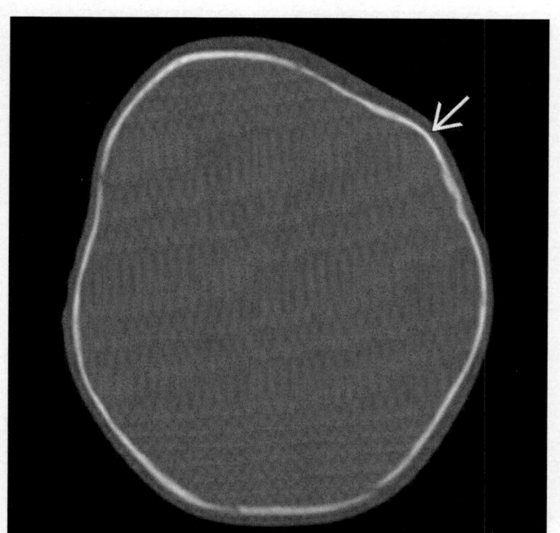

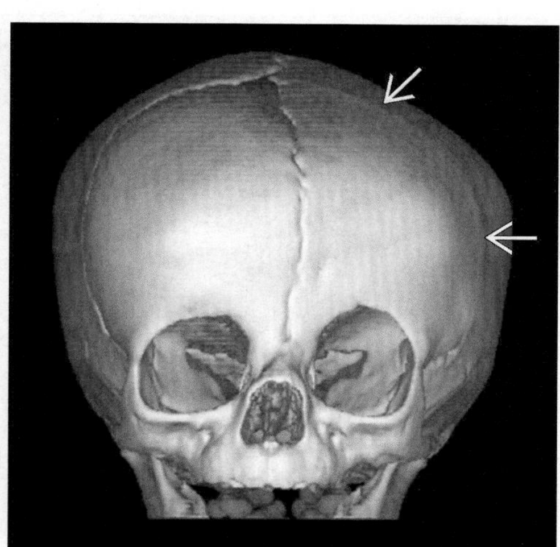

(Left) *Axial bone CT of the calvarium in a patient with plagiocephaly reveals abnormal flattening of the left forehead and pointed configuration ➡ at the left coronal suture from premature closure and fusion of the suture. The right coronal and lambdoid sutures are open.* ***(Right)*** *Coronal 3D bone CT reformat of the skull in the same patient confirms closure of left coronal suture ➡ with characteristic flattening of the ipsilateral forehead and retrusion of lateral superior orbit ("harlequin eye").*

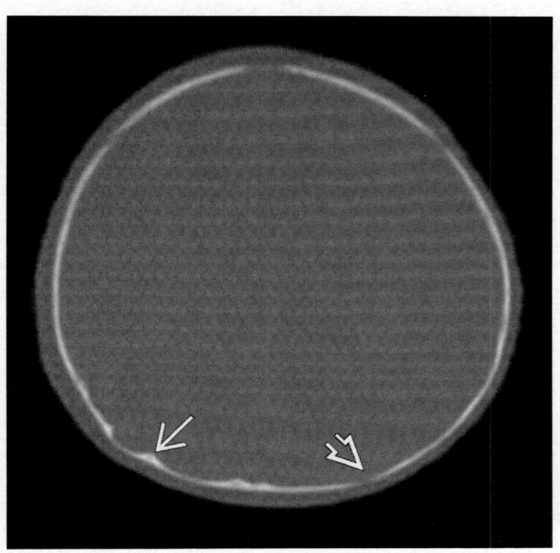

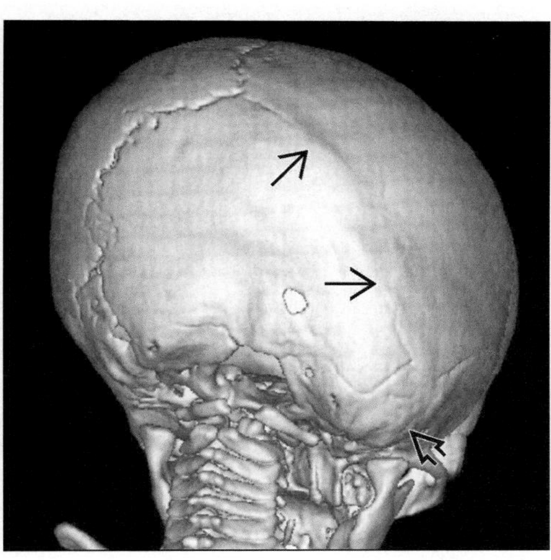

(Left) *Axial bone CT of the head in a patient with unilateral lambdoid synostosis demonstrates a fused right lambdoid suture ➡ producing asymmetric occipital flattening. The left lambdoid ➡ suture is normal.* ***(Right)*** *Coronal oblique 3D bone CT shaded surface reformat of the same patient confirms obliteration of the right lambdoid suture ➡ producing occipital flattening and protrusion of the right mastoid bone ("mastoid bump") ➡. The left lambdoid and sagittal sutures are open.*

CEPHALOCELE

Key Facts

Terminology

- Cephalocele is generic term for intracranial content protrusion through calvarial or skull base defect
  - Meningoencephalocele (encephalocele): Brain tissue, meninges, CSF
  - Meningocele: Meninges, CSF only
- Cephalocele types
  - Basal
  - Cranial vault
  - Frontoethmoidal (sincipital)
  - Nasopharyngeal
  - Occipital
  - Parietal
  - Temporal bone

Imaging

- Meninges ± brain tissue protruding through osseus skull defect
- Heterogeneous signal intensity reflecting brain tissue composition, CSF

Top Differential Diagnoses

- Atretic parietal cephalocele
- Nasal dermoid/epidermoid
- Nasal glioma (nasal cerebral heterotopia)
- Calvarial dermoid

Clinical Issues

- Most cephaloceles (except nasopharyngeal) present at birth

Diagnostic Checklist

- Location determines risk of associated anomalies, predicates prognosis
- Evaluation of cartilaginous nasofrontal region in infants using CT problematic; consider MR

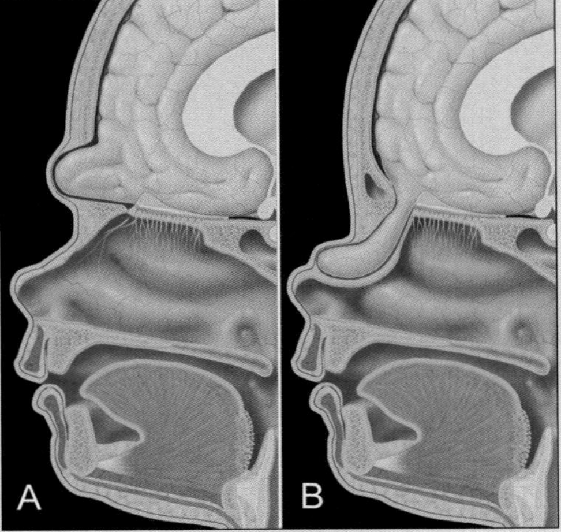

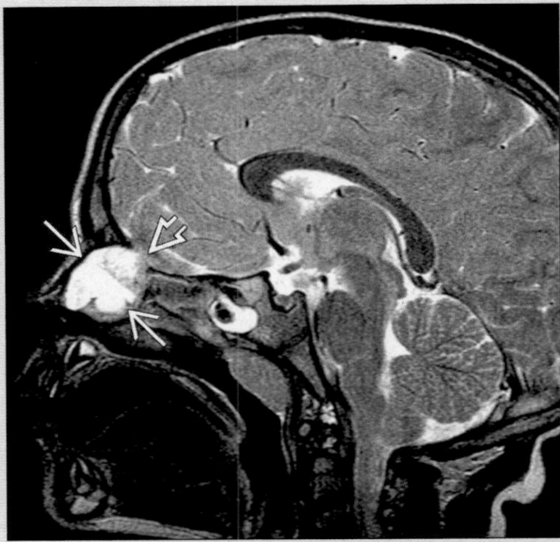

(Left) *Sagittal graphic show 2 variants of sincipital encephalocele. In the frontonasal type (A), the brain extends through the frontonasal suture into the glabellar region. In the nasoethmoidal type (B), the encephalocele extends through the foramen cecum into the nasal cavity.* ***(Right)*** *Sagittal T2WI MR demonstrates the nasoethmoidal type of sincipital encephalocele ➔ extending through the foramen cecum and anterior skull base defect ➔ into the nasal cavity.*

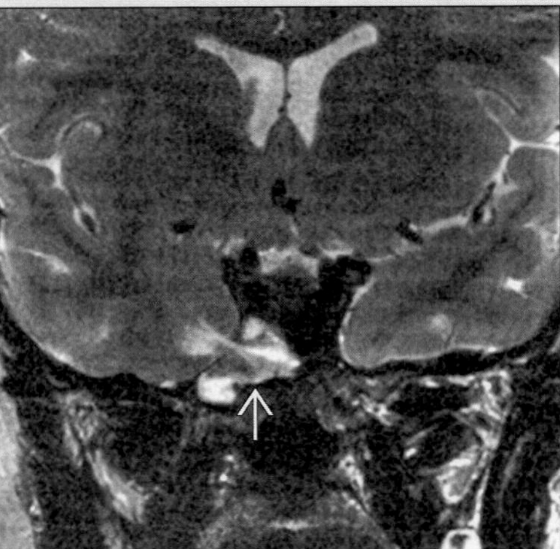

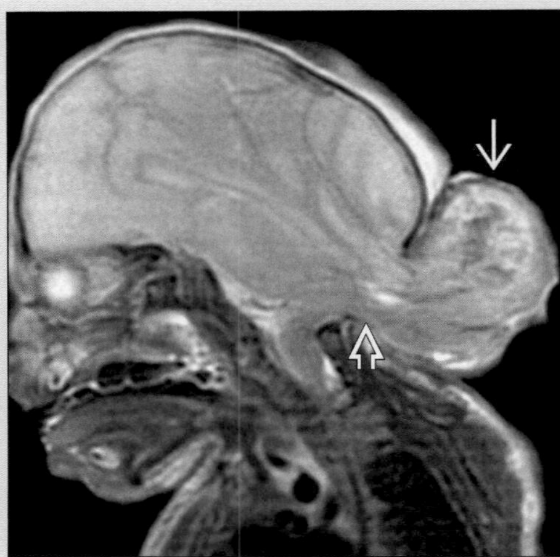

(Left) *Coronal T2WI MR shows a sphenoid encephalocele ➔ extending through a small right lateral sphenoid bone defect, identified during evaluation for temporal lobe epilepsy. EEG localized to the right mesial temporal lobe.* ***(Right)*** *Sagittal T2WI MR shows a low occipital cephalocele containing both occipital lobes ➔ and the cerebellum ➔ with severe traction distortion of the brainstem. Note the involvement of the foramen magnum. The herniated occipital lobe is dysmorphic and disorganized.*

TERMINOLOGY

Definitions

- Generic term for intracranial content protrusion through calvarial or skull base defect
  - Named for roof and floor of bone defect
  - Open or skin covered, dura attenuated or dehiscent
  - Congenital or post-traumatic
- Cephalocele contents
  - Meningoencephalocele (encephalocele): Brain tissue, meninges, CSF
  - Meningocele: Meninges, CSF only
- Cephalocele types
  - Basal (10%)
    - Midline basal cephalocele
      - Sphenopharyngeal: Sphenoid body
      - Sphenoethmoidal: Sphenoid, ethmoid bones
      - Transethmoidal: Cribriform plate
    - Lateral basal cephalocele
      - Sphenomaxillary: Maxillary sinus, orbital fissure into pterygopalatine fossa
      - Sphenoorbital: Sphenoid bone into orbit
    - May include pituitary gland, hypothalamus, optic nerves/chiasm, anterior 3rd ventricle
  - Frontoethmoidal (sincipital) (10-15%)
    - Midface, dorsum of nose, orbits, forehead
    - Subtypes (may be mixed 10%)
      - Frontonasal (40-60%): Foramen cecum, fonticulus frontalis into glabella
      - Nasoethmoidal (30%): Foramen cecum into nasal cavity
      - Nasoorbital: Maxilla, lacrimal bone into orbit
  - Nasopharyngeal (very uncommon)
    - Occult cephalocele through ethmoid, sphenoid, or basiocciput → nasal cavity or pharynx
  - Occipital (75%)
    - Occipitocervical: Occipital bone, foramen magnum, upper cervical posterior arches
    - Low occipital: With foramen magnum
    - High occipital: Without foramen magnum
  - Parietal (10%)
    - Usually associated with significant brain anomalies → poor prognosis
  - Temporal bone
    - Inferior extension through middle ear/mastoid, petrous apex
  - Cranial vault
    - Anterior fontanelle, interfrontal, lateral (coronal or lambdoid sutures), temporal, interparietal, posterior fontanelle

IMAGING

General Features

- Best diagnostic clue
  - Meninges ± brain tissue protruding through osseous skull defect

CT Findings

- NECT
  - Contrast resolution limits ability to distinguish encephalocele from paranasal sinus opacification
- Bone CT
  - Excellent delineation of bone margins
  - Nasofrontal lesions problematic in infants because of cartilaginous anterior skull base
    - By 24 months, 84% of anterior skull base ossified; CT more reliable
- CTA
  - CTV characterizes venous vascular anatomy and relationship to encephalocele

MR Findings

- T1WI
  - Heterogeneous signal intensity reflecting brain tissue composition, CSF
- T2WI
  - Heterogeneous signal intensity reflecting brain tissue composition, CSF
  - Best contrast resolution, signal properties for CSF, characterizing gliosis in dysplastic brain tissue
- MRV
  - Characterize venous vascular anatomy, relationship to encephalocele

Ultrasonographic Findings

- Grayscale ultrasound
  - Limited role reserved for neonates

Imaging Recommendations

- Best imaging tool
  - Multiplanar MR to delineate soft tissues and intracranial relationships
  - Bone CT to define osseous anatomy (except nasofrontal region in infants)
- Protocol advice
  - Multiplanar MR; contrast usually not necessary
  - Thin-section bone CT with multiplanar reformats

DIFFERENTIAL DIAGNOSIS

Atretic Parietal Cephalocele

- Small midline parietal mass, sharply marginated calvarial defect ± associated brain anomalies
- Cephalocele form fruste containing dura, fibrous tissue, dysplastic brain tissue

Nasal Dermoid/Epidermoid

- Failure of normal regression of dural projection through embryologic foramen cecum
- Small skin dimple or pit on external nose ± intracranial dermal sinus, (epi)dermoid cyst

Nasal Glioma (Nasal Cerebral Heterotopia)

- Congenital nonneoplastic heterotopia composed of dysplastic glial tissue
- Lack of normal regression of dural projection through embryologic foramen cecum
- Extranasal (60%), intranasal (30%), or mixed (10%)

Calvarial Dermoid

- Usually near sutures
- Signal intensity reflects ectodermal, skin elements

Chiari 3

- Chiari 2 malformation + cervical dysraphism, cephalocele

CEPHALOCELE

Exencephaly

- Absence of cranial vault bones, protrusion of brain tissue into amniotic cavity

PATHOLOGY

General Features

- Etiology
  - General theories for cephalocele formation
    - Membranous calvarium: Defective bone induction, focal dural dysgenesis, bone erosion by cephalocele, local failure of neural tube closure
    - Endochondral skull base: Faulty neural tube closure, failure of basilar ossification center unification
  - Specific cephaloceles
    - Occipital encephalocele
      - Abnormal primary neural tube closure failure
      - Association with other neural tube defects
    - Frontal encephaloceles
      - Cutaneous ectoderm, neuroectoderm at anterior neuropore fail to detach ~ 3rd week
      - Genetic, toxic, environmental causes
      - No relationship to neural tube defects
    - Basal encephaloceles
      - Developmental failure of skull base ossification → migration of neural crest cells, tissue herniation through defect
      - Persistent craniopharyngeal canal theory out of favor
- Associated abnormalities
  - Basal: Hypertelorism, optic nerve hypoplasia, coloboma, midline facial anomalies, cleft lip/palate
  - Frontoethmoidal: Microcephaly, hypertelorism, eye anomalies, hydrocephalus, seizures
  - Nasopharyngeal: Callosal dysgenesis, optic hypoplasia, hypothalamic-pituitary axis dysfunction
  - Occipital: Cerebellar and cerebral gray matter migrational anomalies, dural venous anomalies, callosal dysgenesis, Chiari II malformation, Dandy-Walker malformation
  - Parietal: Callosal dysgenesis, Chiari II malformation, Dandy-Walker malformation, Walker-Warburg syndrome, holoprosencephaly spectrum

Gross Pathologic & Surgical Features

- Bone dehiscence occurs at suture or synchondrosis
- Smoothly marginated rim of cortical bone

CLINICAL ISSUES

Presentation

- Most common signs/symptoms
  - Usually clinically obvious
  - Soft, bluish (skin covered) or moist red (nonskin covered) discoloration over soft tissue mass
- Other signs/symptoms
  - CSF rhinorrhea → meningitis
  - Airway obstruction, nasal stuffiness/mouth breathing (basal, nasopharyngeal)
  - Occult mass in oro-/nasopharynx → change in size with Valsalva (basal, nasopharyngeal)
  - Hypertelorism, broad nasal bridge (frontoethmoidal)

Demographics

- Age
  - Most cephaloceles present at birth
  - Nasopharyngeal present by end of 1st decade
- Gender
  - Frontoethmoidal (M = F)
  - Occipital (M:F = 1:2.4)
- Ethnicity
  - Occipital most common location in European, North American Caucasians
  - Frontoethmoidal most common location in South/Southeast Asia, Latin America
- Epidemiology
  - 1:4,000 live births

Natural History & Prognosis

- Variable depending on type and location
- Cephalocele relationship to dural venous sinuses important for operative planning

Treatment

- Complete surgical resection of dysplastic herniated brain tissue to prevent CSF leakage, meningitis

DIAGNOSTIC CHECKLIST

Consider

- Location determines risk of associated anomalies, predicates prognosis

Image Interpretation Pearls

- Evaluation of cartilaginous nasofrontal region in infants using CT problematic; consider MR
  - Absence of ossified bone in crista galli/cribriform plate region does not = cephalocele
- MR + MR venography best for operative planning

SELECTED REFERENCES

1. Sather MD et al: Large supra- and infra-tentorial occipital encephalocele encompassing posterior sagittal sinus and torcular Herophili. Childs Nerv Syst. Epub ahead of print, 2009
2. Valencia MP et al: Congenital and acquired lesions of the nasal septum: a practical guide for differential diagnosis. Radiographics. 28(1):205-24; quiz 326, 2008
3. Bui CJ et al: Institutional experience with cranial vault encephaloceles. J Neurosurg. 107(1 Suppl):22-5, 2007
4. Hedlund G: Congenital frontonasal masses: developmental anatomy, malformations, and MR imaging. Pediatr Radiol. 36(7):647-62; quiz 726-7, 2006
5. Rojas L et al: Anterior encephalocele associated with subependymal nodular heterotopia, cortical dysplasia and epilepsy: case report and review of the literature. Eur J Paediatr Neurol. 10(5-6):227-9, 2006
6. Lowe LH et al: Midface anomalies in children. Radiographics. 20(4):907-22; quiz 1106-7, 1112, 2000
7. Mernagh JR et al: US assessment of the fetal head and neck: a state-of-the-art pictorial review. Radiographics. 19 Spec No:S229-41, 1999
8. McComb JG: Spinal and cranial neural tube defects. Semin Pediatr Neurol. 4(3):156-66, 1997

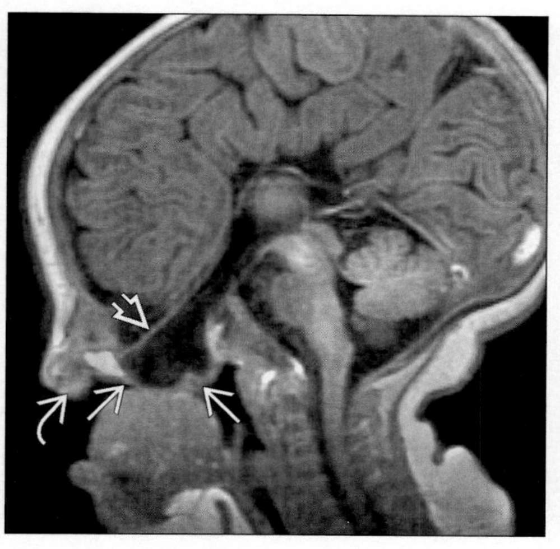
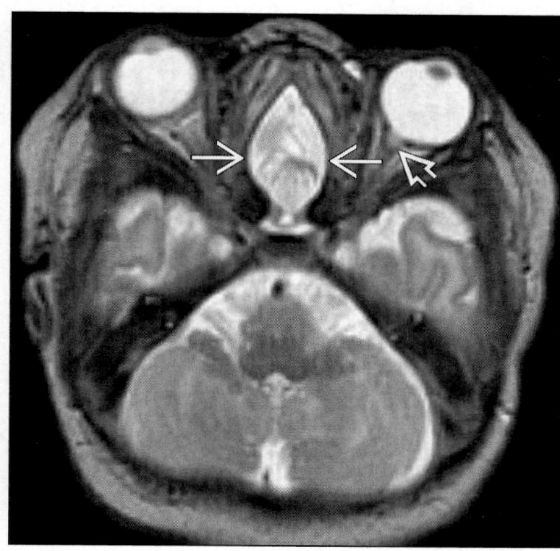

(Left) *Sagittal T1WI MR in an infant with nasal obstruction shows midline basal cephalocele ➡ containing CSF, meninges, & probably olfactory tracts ➡. Note the associated callosal agenesis, abnormal palate, & dysmorphic nose ➡.* ***(Right)*** *Axial T2WI MR in a newborn presenting with nasal obstruction reveals a large midline basal (sphenoethmoidal) encephalocele ➡. Note the associated marked hypertelorism & left ocular coloboma ➡, suggesting "morning glory" syndrome.*

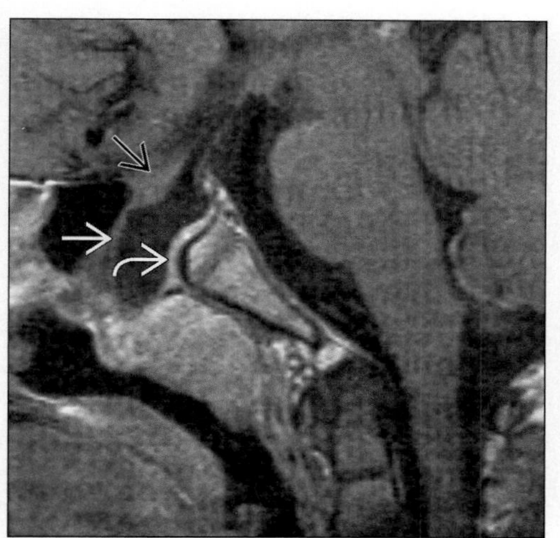
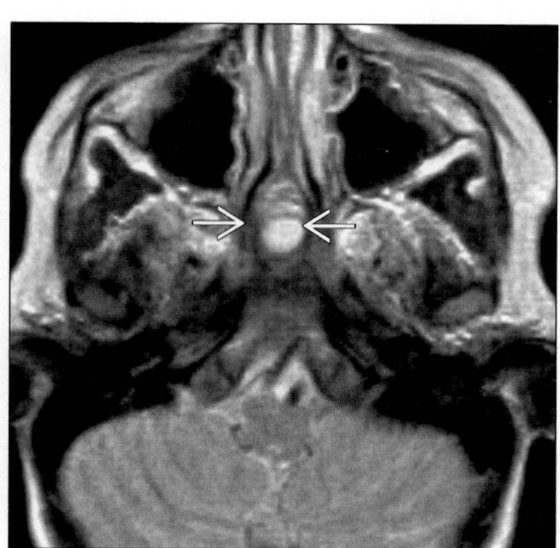

(Left) *Sagittal T1 C+ FS MR shows a large transsphenoidal cephalocele, with CSF and meninges extending through a large midline defect in the sphenoid bone. Optic chiasm ➡ is under traction, optic nerves ➡ are stretched, and pituitary ➡ is compressed.* ***(Right)*** *Axial T2WI MR depicts a midline sphenoidal cephalocele ➡. The cephalocele location in the midline anterior to the spheno-occipital synchondrosis suggests that it is extending through a residual patent craniopharyngeal canal.*

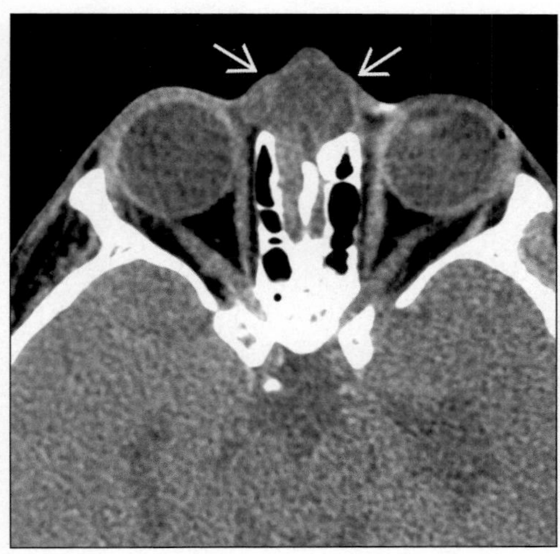
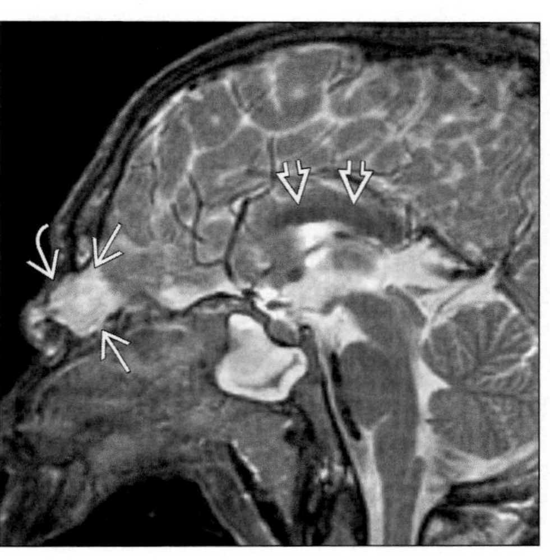

(Left) *Axial NECT in a boy with a glabellar mass (frontonasal cephalocele) shows absence of nasal bones and nasal processes of frontal bones and a fluid-intensity mass ➡ in the glabellar region. Mild hypertelorism is present. The left temporal horn is dilated.* ***(Right)*** *Sagittal T2WI MR in the same patient shows a bone defect ➡ near the frontonasal suture with a CSF-intensity mass ➡, findings compatible with a cephalocele protruding through the defect. The corpus callosum ➡ is dysmorphic.*

*(**Left**) Axial T2WI MR (frontonasal sincipital cephalocele) shows herniated brain ➔ extending through a large bone defect at the junction of the frontal and nasal bones. Signal intensity of the dysplastic herniated brain tissue is heterogeneous and slightly hyperintense to normal parenchyma. (**Right**) Coronal 3D bone CT (frontonasal sincipital cephalocele) demonstrates a large midline osseous defect ⇨ correlating with the abnormally wide fonticulus frontalis.*

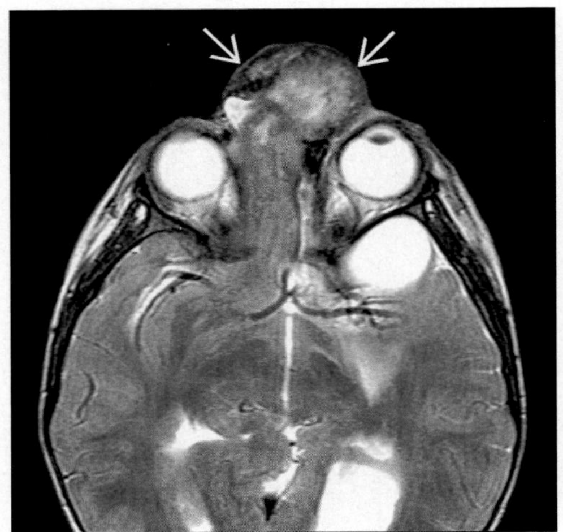

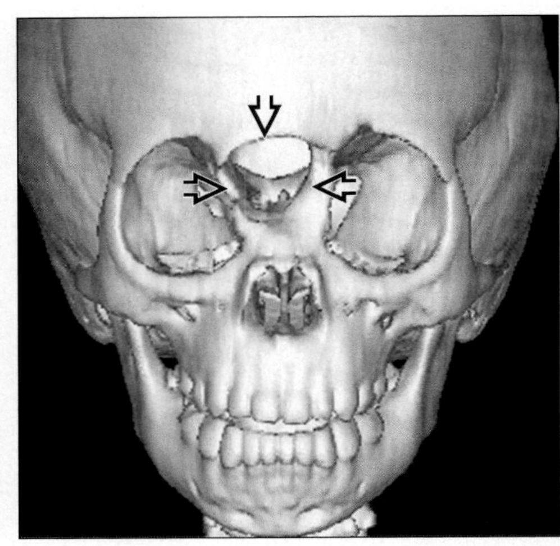

*(**Left**) Sagittal T2WI MR (acquired frontoethmoidal encephalocele) depicts extension of inferior frontal lobes ➔ through anterior skull base defect into the ethmoid sinuses. The initial injury was a bungee cord hook through the nose into the frontal fossa, treated nonsurgically. (**Right**) Coronal bone CT (acquired frontoethmoidal encephalocele) in a patient with post-traumatic CSF rhinorrhea reveals a midline osseous defect ➔ in the cribriform plate/frontal fossa.*

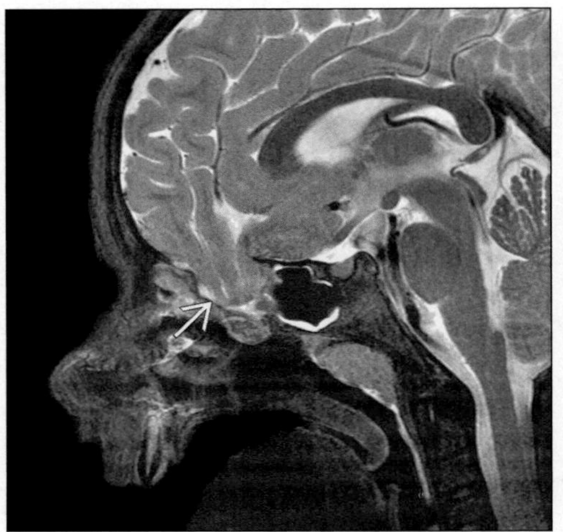

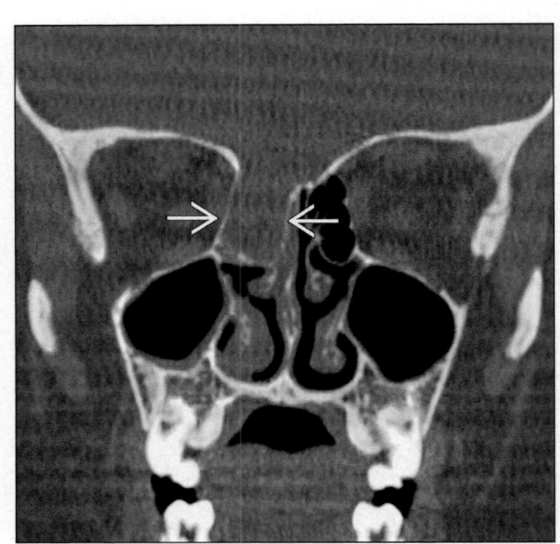

*(**Left**) Sagittal T1WI MR (occipital encephalocele) demonstrates extension of the dysplastic occipital lobes into the posterior cephalocele sac ➔. The cerebellum is distorted but not included within the sac. Bone defect sparing the foramen magnum indicates the high occipital variant. (**Right**) Axial T2WI MR in the same patient depicts displacement of both occipital lobes through the occipital bone defect into the cephalocele sac. The dysplastic brain in the cephalocele shows dysplastic cortex.*

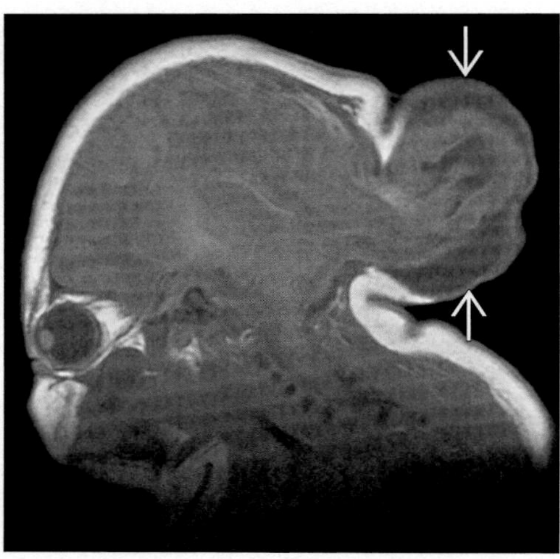

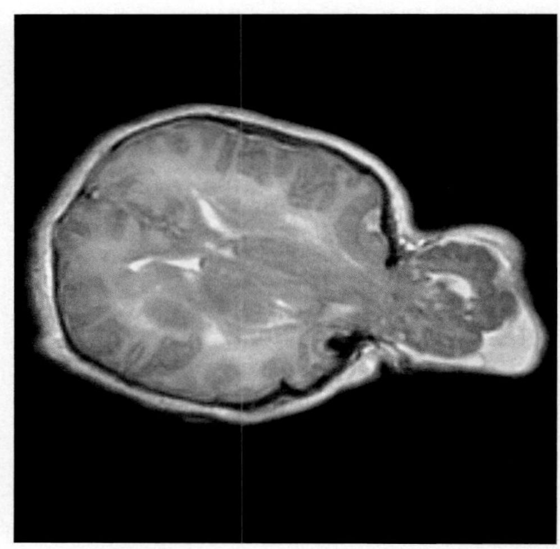

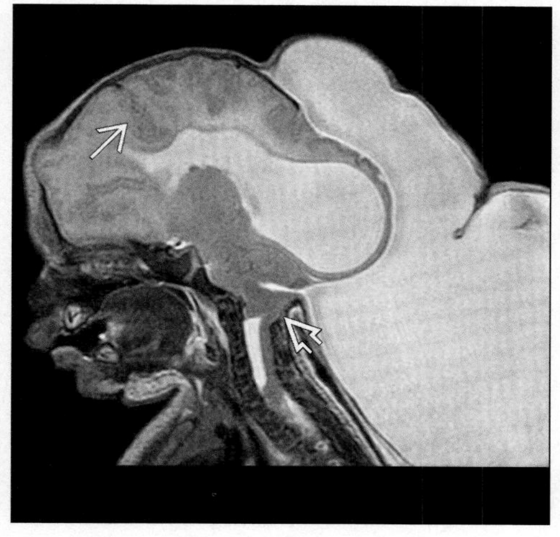

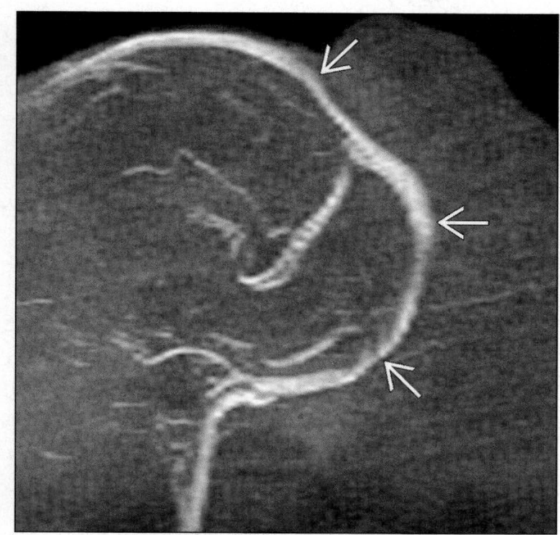

***(Left)** Sagittal T2WI MR (occipital encephalocele) shows extension of both the posterior parietal and occipital lobes as well as the cerebellum into the large fluid-filled cephalocele sac. Note traction deformity of the brainstem and upper cervical cord ➔ and associated frontal lobe cortical dysplasia ➔. **(Right)** Sagittal MRV in the same patient shows posterior displacement of the patent posterior superior sagittal sinus and venous confluence ➔ into the cephalocele sac.*

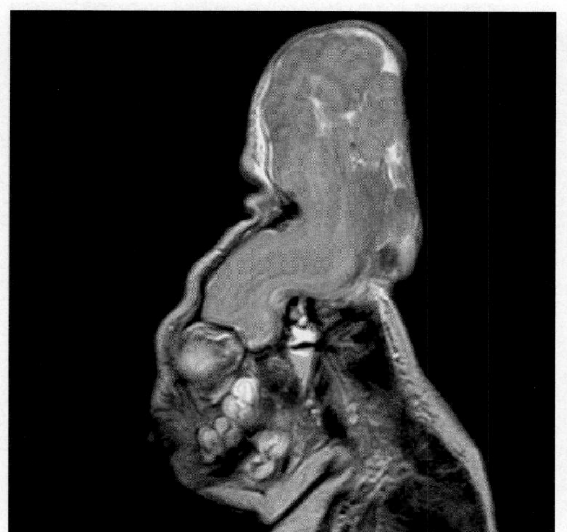

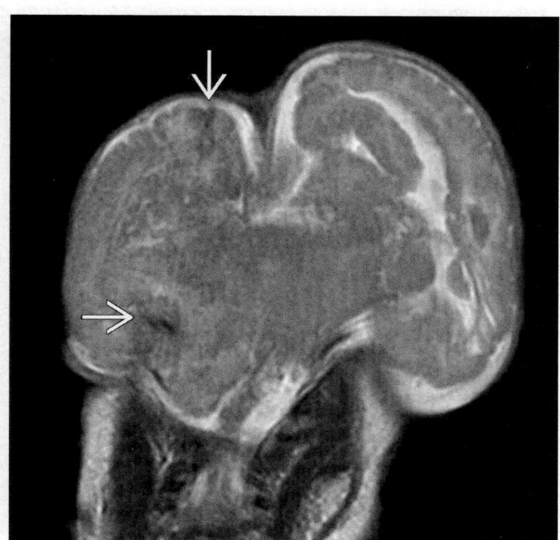

***(Left)** Sagittal T2WI MR in a newborn with parietal encephalocele and multiple severe congenital anomalies shows more brain parenchyma residing in the cephalocele than within the cranium. Brain tissue appears dysplastic within the cranium and the cephalocele. **(Right)** Coronal T2WI MR (parietal encephalocele) shows a combination of severe congenital brain malformation (bilateral cortical dysplasia) and acquired intraparenchymal hemorrhage ➔ within the cephalocele.*

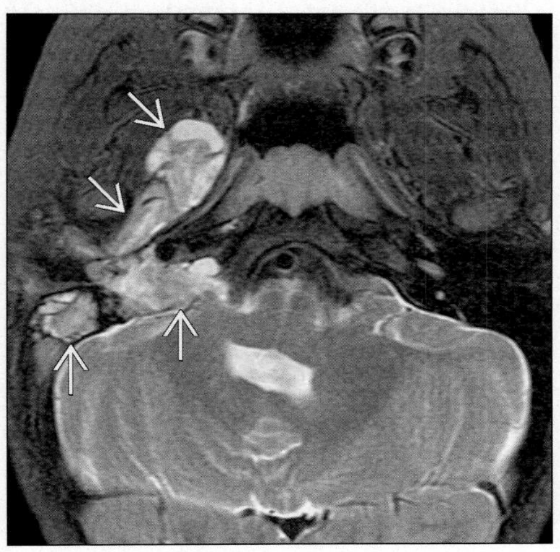

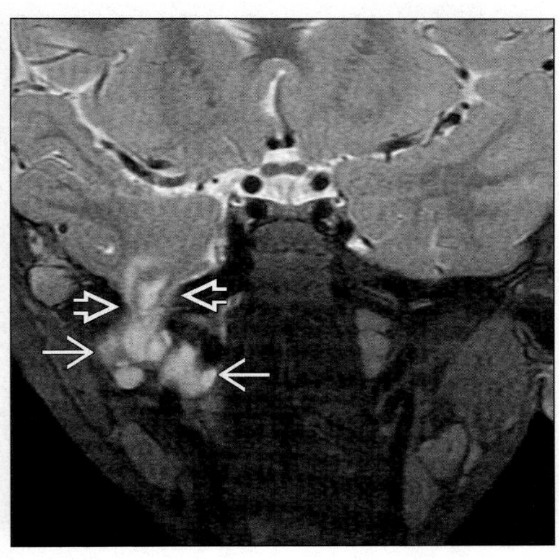

***(Left)** Axial T2WI FS MR shows a large right post-traumatic encephalocele with multiple areas of temporal bone osseous dehiscence ➔. The patient presented with right hearing loss and a remote history of head injury. Note the traction distortion of the medulla and cerebellum. **(Right)** Coronal T2WI FS MR of a post-traumatic temporal encephalocele reveals extension of the inferior right temporal lobe ➔ through a post-traumatic bone defect ➔ into the right middle ear and mastoid bone.*

ATRETIC CEPHALOCELE

Key Facts

Terminology
- Cephalocele "form fruste" consisting of dura, fibrous tissue, and dysplastic brain tissue

Imaging
- Heterogeneous subcutaneous scalp mass with intracranial extension
- Focal fenestration of superior sagittal sinus at APC
- CSF tract and vertical falcine vein "point" to subcutaneous scalp mass

Top Differential Diagnoses
- Dermoid or epidermoid cyst
- Proliferating (infantile) hemangioma
- Sinus pericranii
- Cephalohematoma or subgaleal hematoma
- Sebaceous cyst
- Metastasis

Pathology
- Considered involuted true cephalocele (meningocele or encephalocele) connected to dura mater via fibrous stalk
- Syndromic patients have increased incidence of associated intracranial anomalies

Clinical Issues
- Soft palpable interparietal subgaleal mass
- Usually identified in infants and young children
  - M ≤ F

Diagnostic Checklist
- Consider APC in differential diagnosis for child with midline parietal skin covered subgaleal mass
- Prognosis depends more on associated "occult" brain anomalies than existence of cephalocele itself

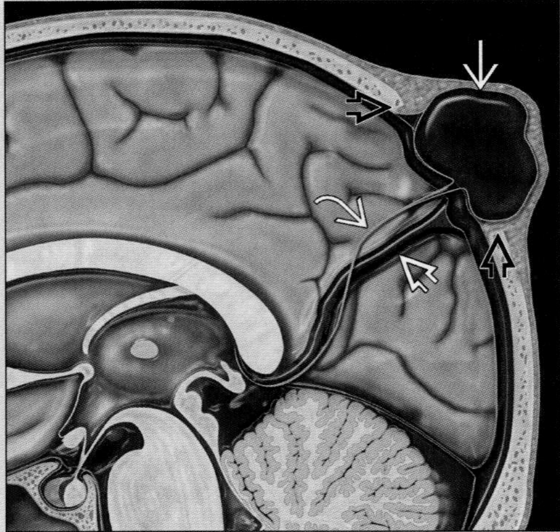

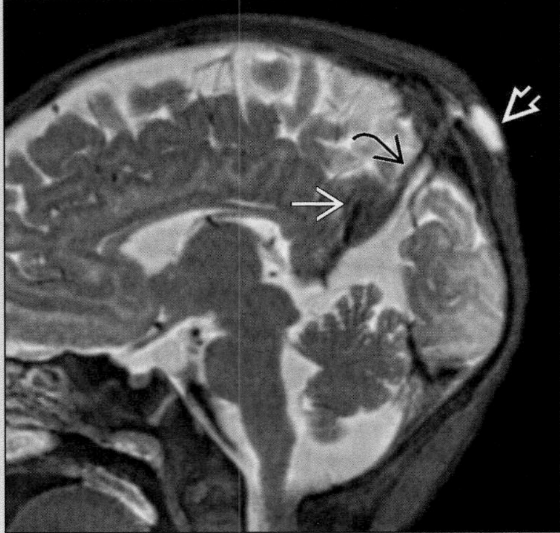

(Left) *Sagittal graphic shows a midline atretic parietal cephalocele with a cystic mass in the calvarial defect. Atretic cephaloceles are often associated with persistent primitive falcine veins. Note fibrous communicating stalk.* ***(Right)*** *Sagittal T1WI FS MR shows a classic atretic parietal cephalocele with falcine vein and fluid collection. The fibrous stalk connecting the cephalocele through the calvarial defect is difficult to distinguish from the venous flow void.*

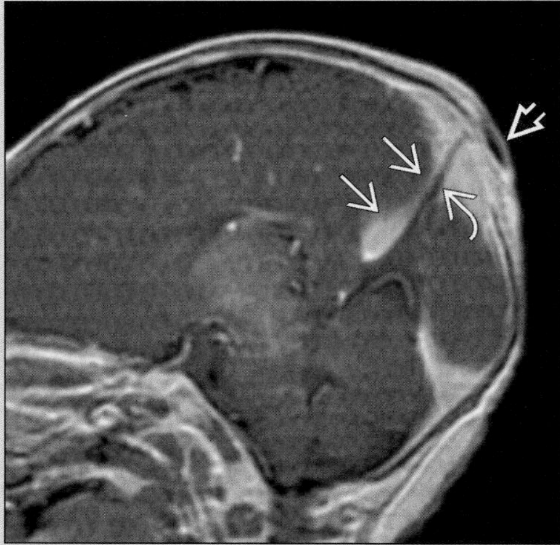

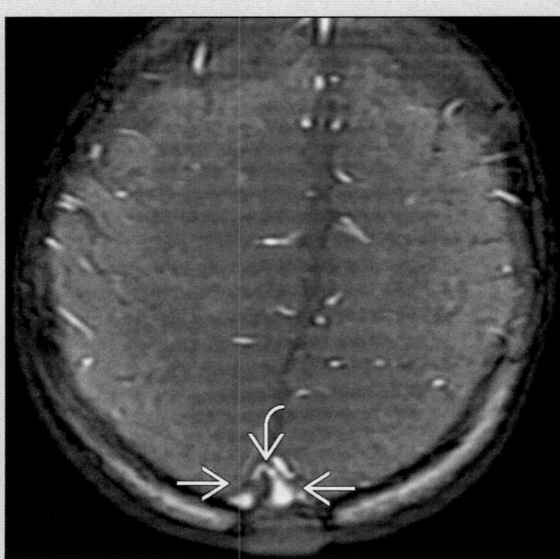

(Left) *Sagittal T1WI C+ MR in the same patient shows an atretic parietal cephalocele with a characteristic vertically oriented, persistent falcine vein and a fluid-filled, skin-covered cephalocele. The fibrous stalk connecting the cephalocele through the calvarial defect is clearly visible next to the enhancing falcine vein.* ***(Right)*** *Axial 2D time of flight MRV source image clearly demonstrates a focal split of the superior sagittal sinus surrounding the atretic cephalocele fibrous stalk.*

ATRETIC CEPHALOCELE

TERMINOLOGY

Abbreviations

- Atretic parietal cephalocele (APC)

Definitions

- Cephalocele "form fruste" consisting of dura, fibrous tissue, and dysplastic brain tissue

IMAGING

General Features

- Best diagnostic clue
  - Fibrous tract and vertical falcine vein "point" to subcutaneous scalp mass (APC)
- Location
  - Midline interparietal most common, occasionally occipital
- Size
  - Usually small (5-15 mm)
- Morphology
  - Skin-covered subgaleal mass with sharply marginated calvarial defect

Radiographic Findings

- Radiography
  - Cranium bifidum at obelion
    - May be difficult to appreciate

CT Findings

- NECT
  - Subgaleal soft tissue mass
  - Small cranium bifidum superior to lambda
  - "Spinning top" configuration of tentorial incisura (axial)
- CECT
  - Extension of subcutaneous scalp mass through dura delineated by enhancing veins
  - Fenestration of superior sagittal sinus, vertically oriented primitive falcine vein
- CTA
  - Vertical embryonic positioning of straight sinus equivalent (falcine sinus)
  - Fenestration of superior sagittal sinus

MR Findings

- T1WI
  - Heterogeneous subcutaneous scalp mass with intracranial extension
  - ± cigar-shaped CSF tract within interhemispheric fissure
  - Prominent superior cerebellar cistern and suprapineal recess
  - Characteristic appearance of tentorial incisura
    - "Spinning top" (axial) and "peaked" (coronal) configuration
- T2WI
  - Subcutaneous scalp mass representing APC is usually hyperintense
  - Other findings similar to T1WI
- STIR
  - Fat suppression better delineates subgaleal hyperintense cephalocele
- T1WI C+
  - Subcutaneous scalp mass usually shows heterogeneous enhancement
  - APC fibrous tract delineated by adjacent enhancing veins
- MRV
  - Vertically positioned straight sinus equivalent (persistent falcine vein)
  - Focal fenestration of superior sagittal sinus at APC

Ultrasonographic Findings

- Grayscale ultrasound
  - Scalp mass with heterogeneous echotexture
  - Cranium bifidum osseous defect usually too small to identify

Imaging Recommendations

- Best imaging tool
  - Multiplanar MR with intravenous contrast + MRV
- Protocol advice
  - MR: Thin section, small field of view, sagittal T1 and T2 with fat saturation
  - Intravenous contrast with fat saturation to define sagittal sinus and falcine vein; exclude sinus pericranii

DIFFERENTIAL DIAGNOSIS

Dermoid or Epidermoid Cyst

- Often located near sutures
- Scallops outer table of calvarium
- + marginal enhancement, no internal enhancement

Proliferating (Infantile) Hemangioma

- Lobulated soft tissue mass with internal flow voids
- + avid contrast enhancement

Sinus Pericranii

- Abnormal communication between intracranial and extracranial venous systems through osseous calvarial defect
- Soft red or blue scalp mass adjacent to superior sagittal or transverse dural sinuses
- ↑ size with ↑ intracranial pressure (Valsalva, dependent positioning)
- Internal venous flow, robust enhancement

Cephalohematoma or Subgaleal Hematoma

- Fluid in subgaleal space adjacent to intact calvarium
- Consider in newborn post trauma or following vaginal delivery

Sebaceous Cyst

- Dermal inclusion in scalp
- No calvarial defect or venous anomalies

Metastasis

- Destructive calvarial lesion + soft tissue mass
- Consider neuroblastoma in infant or toddler

Heterotopic Scalp Nodule

- Neuroectodermal malformation containing heterotopic leptomeningeal or glial tissue

- Focal alopecia surrounded by ring of long coarse hair ("hair collar" sign) ± surrounding capillary stain
  - May have rudimentary stalk with intracranial communication
- Clinically resembles dermoid cyst

PATHOLOGY

General Features

- Etiology
  - Considered involuted true cephalocele (meningocele or encephalocele)
  - Originates from overdistended rhombencephalic vesicle at 7-10 weeks of fetal life
  - Postulated link to folate deficiency, valproic acid exposure
- Genetics
  - Typically sporadic, some cases syndromic
  - Syndromic more likely to have associated intracranial anomalies
- Associated abnormalities
  - Variable incidence
    - Most APC are incidentally identified without additional intracranial anomalies
    - Holoprosencephaly, callosal agenesis, eye anomalies, and interhemispheric cyst most common

Gross Pathologic & Surgical Features

- Hamartomatous subgaleal mass with adjacent focal cranium bifidum
- Connects to dura mater via fibrous stalk terminating in falx or tentorium
- CSF tract to supracerebellar, suprapineal, and quadrigeminal cisterns

Microscopic Features

- Meningeal and vestigial neural tissue rests
- CSF tract ependymal lined

CLINICAL ISSUES

Presentation

- Most common signs/symptoms
  - Soft palpable interparietal subgaleal mass
- Other signs/symptoms
  - APC may enlarge with crying
- Clinical profile
  - Subgaleal mass identified incidentally or during imaging evaluation for other anomalies

Demographics

- Age
  - Infants and young children
- Gender
  - M ≤ F
- Epidemiology
  - APC 10x more common than large parietal cephalocele
  - More common in Western hemisphere

Natural History & Prognosis

- Outcome determined more by associated anomalies than presence of APC
  - Children with no associated intracranial anomalies usually have normal clinical outcome
  - Additional intracranial anomalies (more common in syndromic patients) → worse outcome

Treatment

- Surgical resection of cephalocele with dural repair

DIAGNOSTIC CHECKLIST

Consider

- APC in differential diagnosis for child with midline parietal skin-covered subgaleal mass
- Prognosis depends more on associated "occult" brain anomalies than existence of cephalocele itself

Image Interpretation Pearls

- Persistent falcine sinus points to cephalocele
- Lack of abnormally dilated scalp veins, absence of falcine vein, and characteristic fibrous tract distinguish from sinus pericranii

SELECTED REFERENCES

1. Morioka T et al: Detailed anatomy of intracranial venous anomalies associated with atretic parietal cephaloceles revealed by high-resolution 3D-CISS and high-field T2-weighted reversed MR images. Childs Nerv Syst. 25(3):309-15, 2009
2. Güzel A et al: Atretic parietal cephalocele. Pediatr Neurosurg. 43(1):72-3, 2007
3. Hunt JA et al: Common craniofacial anomalies: facial clefts and encephaloceles. Plast Reconstr Surg. 112(2):606-15; quiz 616,722, 2003
4. Abubacker S et al: Adult atretic parietal cephalocele. Neurol India. 50(3):334-6, 2002
5. Agthong S et al: Encephalomeningocele cases over 10 years in Thailand: a case series. BMC Neurol. 2:3, 2002
6. Aydin MD: Atretic cephalocele communicating with lateral ventricles. Childs Nerv Syst. 17(11):679-80, 2001
7. Yamazaki T et al: Atretic cephalocele--report of two cases with special reference to embryology. Childs Nerv Syst. 17(11):674-8, 2001
8. Brunelle F et al: Intracranial venous anomalies associated with atretic cephalocoeles. Pediatr Radiol. 30(11):743-7, 2000
9. Gulati K et al: Atretic cephalocele: contribution of magnetic resonance imaging in preoperative diagnosis. Pediatr Neurosurg. 33(4):208-10, 2000
10. Patterson RJ et al: Atretic parietal cephaloceles revisited: an enlarging clinical and imaging spectrum? AJNR Am J Neuroradiol. 19(4):791-5, 1998
11. Saatci I et al: An atretic parietal cephalocele associated with multiple intracranial and eye anomalies. Neuroradiology. 40(12):812-5, 1998
12. Martínez-Lage JF et al: The child with a cephalocele: etiology, neuroimaging, and outcome. Childs Nerv Syst. 12(9):540-50, 1996

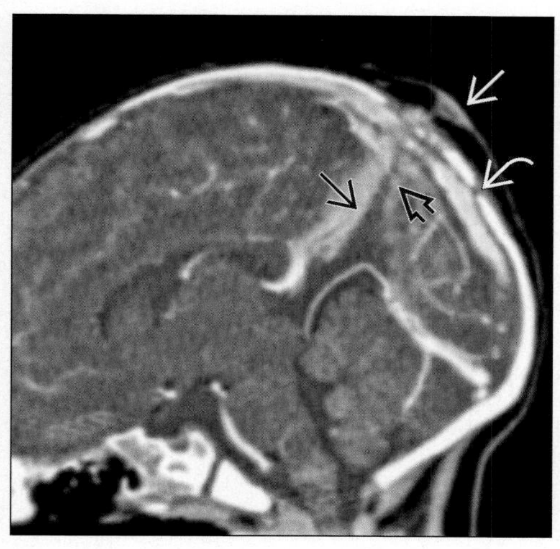

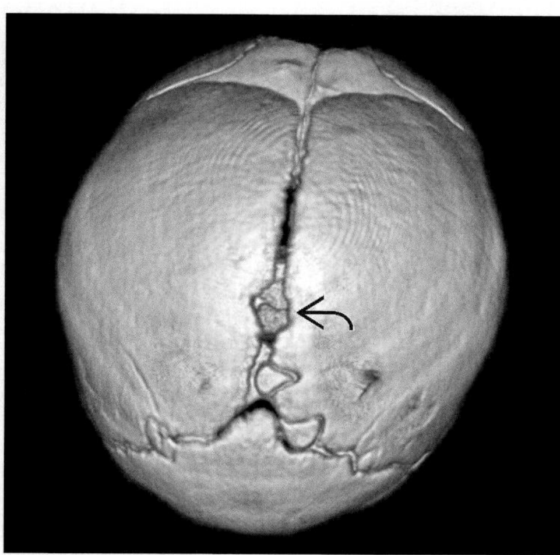

(Left) *Sagittal CECT shows the characteristic vertically oriented, enhancing falcine vein ⊳ and the close relationship between the atretic cephalocele ➡ and the superior sagittal sinus ➡. The hypodense fibrous stalk → is relatively inconspicuous.* ***(Right)*** *Axial 3D bone CT of the calvarium demonstrates a small, focal, midline, interparietal calvarial defect ↷ representing the focal cranium bifidum through which the cephalocele communicates intracranially via the fibrous stalk.*

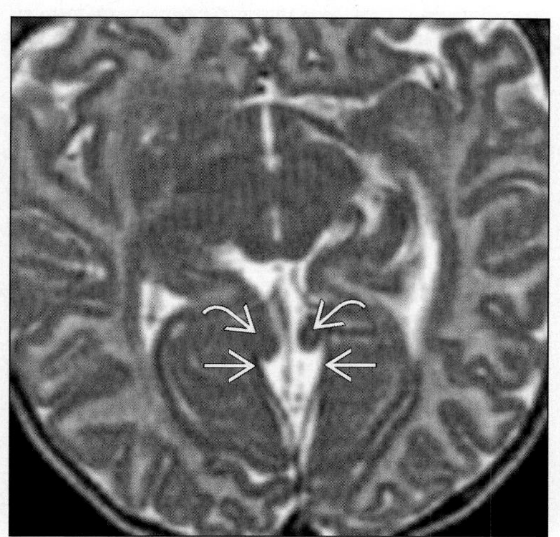

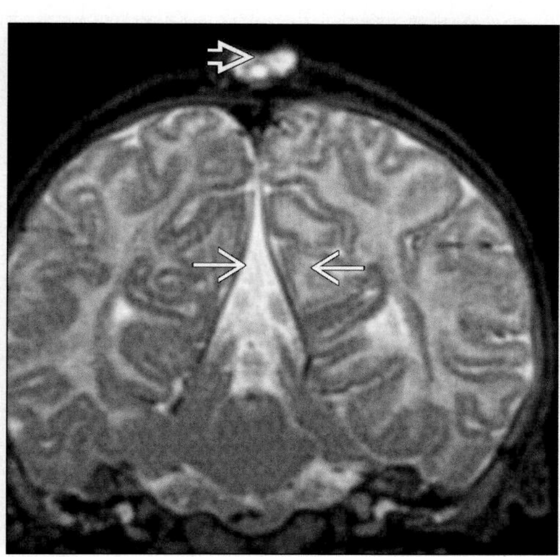

(Left) *Axial T2WI MR shows a superiorly deficient tentorium with medial temporal gyri ➡ extending into the tentorial incisura, giving a characteristic "spinning top" configuration ➡ of the incisura.* ***(Right)*** *Coronal T2WI FS MR confirms the characteristic "peaked" configuration of the tentorial leaves ➡, best seen in the coronal plane. Note the conspicuity of the hyperintense subgaleal atretic cephalocele ⊳ on fat-suppressed T2-weighted imaging.*

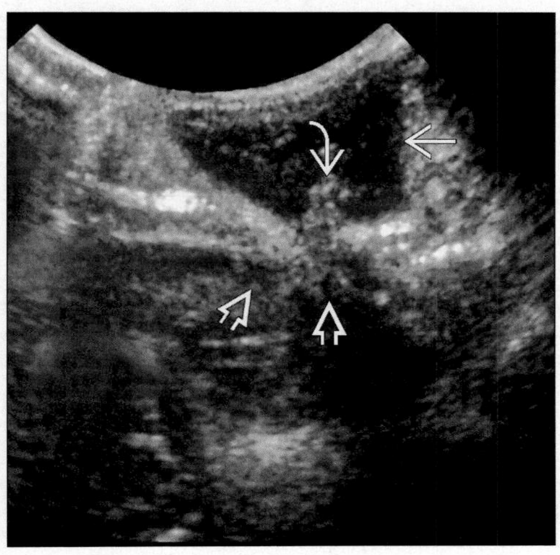

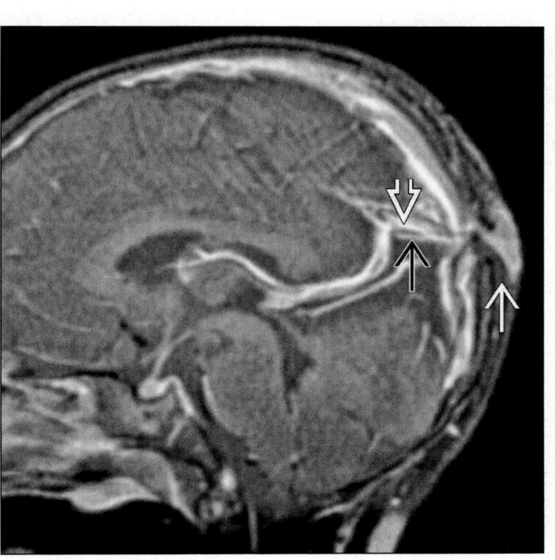

(Left) *Longitudinal grayscale ultrasound shows an anechoic, midline, parietal, subgaleal fluid collection ➡ containing a small plug of dysplastic fibrovascular neural tissue ➡. Margins of the cranium bifidum ⊳ are visible in this case.* ***(Right)*** *Sagittal T1WI C+ FS MR demonstrates the uncommon occipital variant of atretic cephalocele. As in the parietal variant, there is an aberrant vein ⊳ and fibrous tract → "pointing" to the atretic cephalocele ➡.*

CALVARIUM FRACTURE

Key Facts

Imaging

- Best diagnostic clue: Linear calvarial lucency
- Morphology: Linear, depressed, elevated; also comminuted, overriding, and closed or open
- Middle cranial fossa weakest with thin bones and foramina → at pterion look for epidural hematoma
- Bone CT: Sharply delineated lucent line
  - Depressed fx: Fragment(s) displaced inwards
  - Skull base fx → pneumocephalus common
  - Air in TMJ glenoid fossa may be only CT sign of inconspicuous skull base fx
- CTA quickly and easily evaluates for vascular injury
- Best imaging tool: CT; add MR if complicated

Top Differential Diagnoses

- Suture line
- Vascular groove
- Arachnoid granulation
- Venous lake

Pathology

- Raised suspicion of child abuse if multiple, complex, bilateral, depressed, without trauma

Clinical Issues

- Linear fx: Usually asymptomatic without LOC
- Symptoms often referable to epidural hematoma
- "Raccoon eyes" = periorbital ecchymosis
- "Battle" sign = mastoid ecchymosis
- Sequelae: CSF leak, delayed CN deficit(s), infarct
- Most skull fx, even depressed, do not require surgery

Diagnostic Checklist

- Sutures curvilinear, symmetric; fractures linear, asymmetric

*(**Left**) Axial bone CT shows a comminuted skull fracture with depressed fragments involving the right parietal bone near the vertex and a 2nd fracture involving the left parietal bone, an extension of the primary fracture across the vertex and sagittal suture. (**Right**) 3D CT shaded surface of the same patient shows depressed fragments, extension into the left parietal bone across the sagittal suture, extension into ipsilateral parietal bone, and coronal suture locations.*

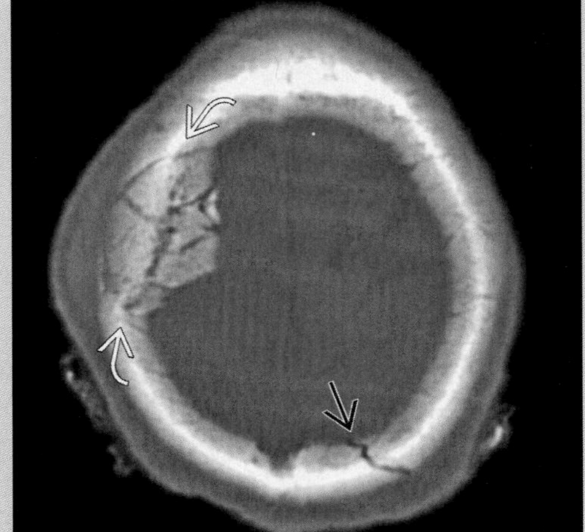

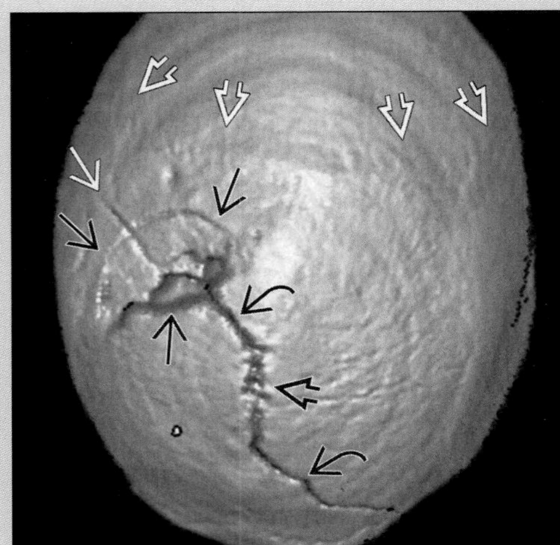

*(**Left**) Coronal bone CT displays a fracture of the right sphenoid; this affects the superior-lateral sphenoid sinus wall as well as the inferomedial right middle cranial fossa floor. The soft tissue density abutting the fracture represents CSF from a concomitant CSF leak. (**Right**) Axial bone CT demonstrates an impressive calvarial comminuted fracture that is elevated anteriorly as well as depressed posteriorly. Note the nondependent pneumocephalus.*

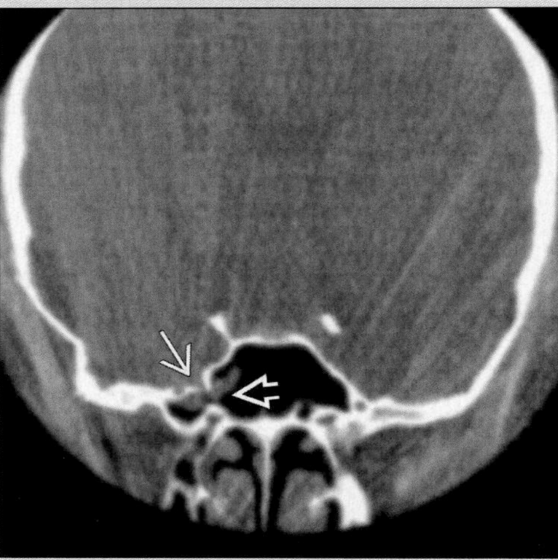

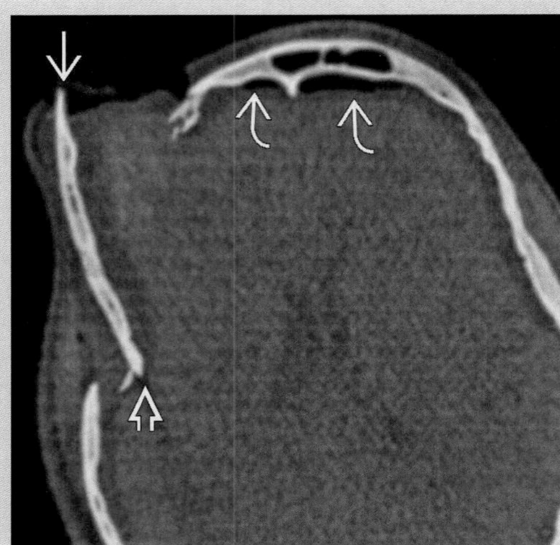

CALVARIUM FRACTURE

TERMINOLOGY

Synonyms

- Calvarial, skull, skull base, basilar skull fracture (fx)

IMAGING

General Features

- Best diagnostic clue
  - Linear calvarial lucency
- Location
  - Fracture anywhere involving skull
  - Middle fossa weakest (thin bones, multiple foramina)
  - Growing skull fracture (GSFx): Mostly parietal
- Morphology
  - Linear, depressed, elevated
  - Comminuted, overriding, closed or open

Radiographic Findings

- Radiography
  - Linear fx: Sharply defined linear lucent line
  - GSFx: Widening fx lines over time

CT Findings

- Bone CT
  - Linear fx: Sharply delineated lucent line
  - Depressed fx: Fragment(s) displaced inward
  - Elevated fx: Fragment(s) displaced outward
  - Skull base fx
    - Pneumocephalus common
    - Air-fluid level within adjacent air cell(s)
    - Nasal cavity fluid → CSF rhinorrhea
    - Ear cavity fluid from CSF otorrhea or blood density from hemotympanum
    - Air in TMJ glenoid fossa may be only CT sign of inconspicuous skull base fx
  - Temporal bone fx: Longitudinal or transverse
  - Occipital condyle fracture
  - GSFx: Herniation of CSF and perhaps brain tissue through widened fx defect
    - Intradiploic GSFx: Intact outer table, CSF-filled cyst, with defect of inner table and dura
- CTA
  - Quickly, easily evaluates for vascular injury

MR Findings

- T2WI
  - Best to delineate dural injury
- FLAIR
  - Hyperintense cerebral contusion
- T2* GRE
  - Foci of hemorrhage susceptibility
- MRA
  - For arterial injury (MRV for venous)

Imaging Recommendations

- Best imaging tool
  - NECT; add MR if depressed fx or GSFx
- Protocol advice
  - Thin-slice high-resolution NECT for skull base fx
    - Include sagittal/coronal reconstructions
- Trauma screen recommendations
  - Plain films have no role
  - CT scan for any clinical suspicion
  - Evaluate for vascular injury if carotid canal involved
    - CTA better than MRA
  - CTA or DSA if suspected traumatic carotid cavernous fistula

DIFFERENTIAL DIAGNOSIS

Suture Line

- < 2 mm width, same width throughout length
- At specific anatomic sites
- Not straight line, appears curvilinear
- Less distinct than fx, has dense sclerotic borders

Vascular Groove

- Corticated margins, nonlinear (branches like tree)
- Typical location (i.e., middle meningeal artery)

Arachnoid Granulation

- Corticated margins; typical location (i.e., parasagittal, transverse sinus)

Venous Lake

- Corticated margins; typical location (i.e., parasagittal)

PATHOLOGY

General Features

- Etiology
  - Linear fx: Low-energy blunt trauma over wide surface area of skull
  - Depressed fx: High-energy direct blow to small surface area with blunt object (e.g., baseball bat)
  - Elevated fx: Long, sharp wounding object elevates fragments (lateral pull, head rotation)
  - Occipital condylar fracture: High-energy trauma with axial load, lateral bending, or rotational injury
- Associated abnormalities
  - Linear fx: Associated with epi-/subdural hematoma
  - Depressed fx: Lacerated dura/arachnoid + parenchymal injury
  - Skull base fx: Cranial nerve (CN) injury, CSF leak
    - CN palsies may be immediate or delayed
  - Raised suspicion of child abused if multiple, complex, bilateral, depressed, and unexplained without trauma
  - Delayed intracranial hypertension from disturbance of superior sagittal sinus by depressed fx
  - Traumatic carotid cavernous fistula may accompany basilar skull fx

Gross Pathologic & Surgical Features

- Open fractures
  - Skin laceration over fracture
  - Fx results in communication between external environment, intracranial cavity
  - May be clean or contaminated/dirty
- Depressed fx
  - Comminution of fragments starts at point of maximum impact and spreads centrifugally
  - May compromise venous sinuses
- Elevated fx: Always compound

CALVARIUM FRACTURE

- CN deficits: Transection by bone fragments, arterial ischemia, nerve stretching, or nerve root avulsion
- GSFx: Progressively enlarging diastatic fracture with underlying dural laceration
  - Herniation of CSF, brain, or vessels through defect

Microscopic Features

- Skull fx: Extends through entire thickness of bone
- Intradiploic GSFx: Lined with arachnoid membrane

CLINICAL ISSUES

Presentation

- Most common signs/symptoms
  - Linear fx: Often asymptomatic without LOC
  - Depressed fx
    - Loss of consciousness (25% none, 25% < 1 hour)
    - Often symptoms referable to epidural hematoma
  - Skull base fx: Vernet/jugular foramen syndrome
    - Foraminal involvement → CN9, 10, and 11 deficits
    - Difficulty in phonation, aspiration
    - Ipsilateral paralysis: Vocal cord, soft palate, superior pharyngeal constrictor, sternocleidomastoid, and trapezius
  - Longitudinal temporal bone fx
    - **Conductive** hearing loss
    - 10-20% CN7 palsy from facial canal involvement
  - Transverse temporal bone fx
    - **Neurosensory** hearing loss, vertigo
    - 50% CN7 palsy from IAC fx
  - Mixed temporal bone fx: Signs/symptoms of both longitudinal and transverse fx
  - Occipital condylar fx
    - Coma, associated cervical spinal injuries, lower CN deficits, hemiplegia, quadriplegia
    - Collet-Sicard syndrome: CN9, 10, 11, 12 deficits
  - Traumatic carotid cavernous fistula: Vision impairment, limitation of ocular movements
- Clinical profile
  - Fx present in majority of severe head injury cases
  - Linear fx: Most common skull fx; swelling at impact site, skin often intact
  - Depressed fx: Often palpable abnormality
  - Skull base fx
    - "Raccoon eyes" = periorbital ecchymosis
    - "Battle" sign = mastoid ecchymosis
  - Sphenoid bone fx
    - CSF rhinorrhea/otorrhea, hemotympanum
  - Traumatic carotid cavernous fistula: Exophthalmos, bruit, chemosis

Demographics

- Age
  - GSFx: > 50% before 12 months, 90% before 3 years
- Epidemiology
  - Skull fx present in 80% of fatal injuries at autopsy
  - Skull base fx = 19-21% of all skull fractures
    - Sphenoid fx accounts for 15% of skull base fx
  - 75-90% of depressed fx are open fx
  - GSFx: 0.05-1.6% of pediatric skull fx
  - Traumatic carotid cavernous fistula in 3.8% of basilar skull fractures
    - Incidence with fx of anterior fossa (2.4%), middle fossa (8.3%), and posterior fossa (1.7%)

Natural History & Prognosis

- Sequelae: CSF leak, delayed CN deficit(s), infarct
- Healing process
  - Infants: Usually heals in 3-6 months without trace
  - Children: Heals within 12 months
  - Adults: Heals within 2-3 years, often residual lucency
- Transverse temporal bone fx
  - Permanent neurosensory hearing loss
  - Persistent vertigo, unrelenting CN7 palsy
- Growing fx ("post-traumatic encephalocele") can be late complication
  - Infants < 3 months with head injury and scalp hematoma are at high risk
  - Herniated brain matter may be damaged by fx edge
- Immediate CN palsies have lower rate of recovery than delayed deficits
- Traumatic carotid cavernous fistula: Untreated can lead to blindness

Treatment

- Most skull fx, even depressed, do not require surgery
- Contaminated open fractures: Broad spectrum of antibiotics and tetanus vaccination
- Indications for surgery
  - Depressed segment > 8-10 mm or > thickness of skull; cosmesis
  - Gross contamination, dural tear with pneumocephalus, underlying hematoma
  - Brain function difficulties related to pressure or injury of underlying brain
  - Correction of ossicle disarticulation
  - Occipital condylar type 3 fx (unstable) with atlantoaxial arthrodesis
  - Persistent CSF leak
  - Persistent intracranial hypertension secondary to superior sagittal sinus involvement and conservative treatment not effective
- Traumatic carotid cavernous fistula: Endovascular therapy

DIAGNOSTIC CHECKLIST

Consider

- Child abuse when trauma undocumented

Image Interpretation Pearls

- Sutures curvilinear, symmetric; fractures linear, asymmetric

SELECTED REFERENCES

1. Munoz-Sanchez MA et al: Skull fracture, with or without clinical signs, in mTBI is an independent risk marker for neurosurgically relevant intracranial lesion: a cohort study. Brain Inj. 23(1):39-44, 2009
2. Huang HH et al: Vagus nerve paralysis due to skull base fracture. Auris Nasus Larynx. 35(1):153-5, 2008
3. Zhao X et al: Basilar skull fracture: a risk factor for transverse/sigmoid venous sinus obstruction. J Neurotrauma. 25(2):104-11, 2008

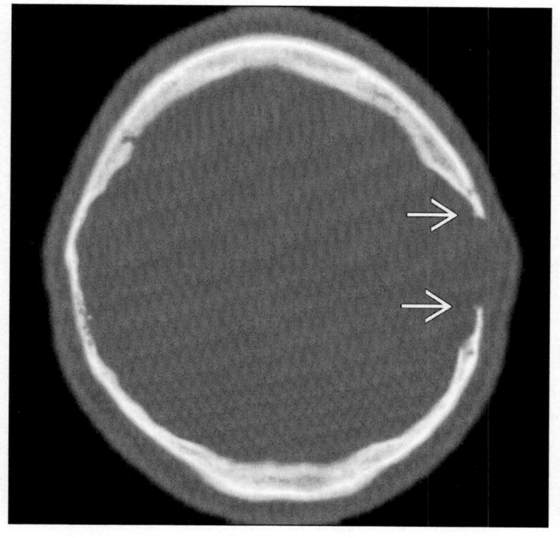

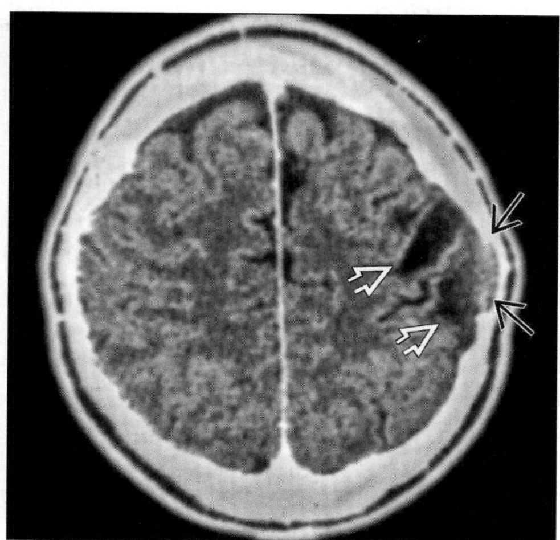

***(Left)** Axial bone CT demonstrates discontinuity of the left skull ➔ with scalloped edges and a lack of aggressive features from a growing skull fracture. **(Right)** Axial NECT in the same patient shows leptomeningeal, CSF, and early brain herniation into the calvarial defect ➔. Post-traumatic cortical encephalomalacia directly underlies the calvarial defect ➔.*

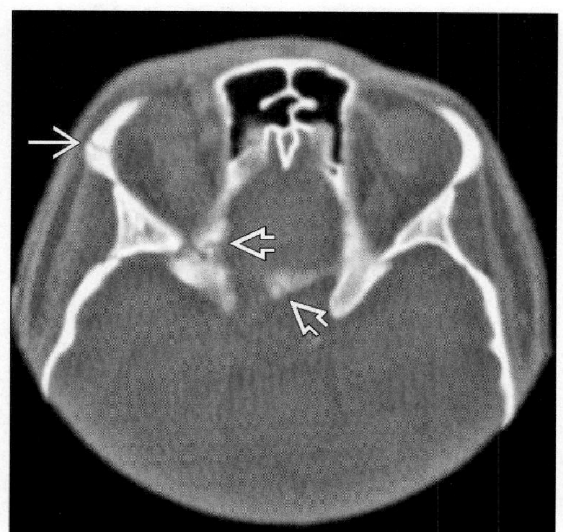

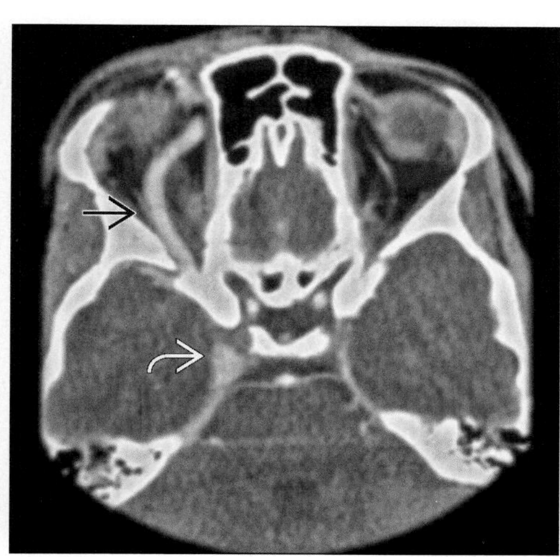

***(Left)** Axial bone CT shows a portion of comminuted and complex anterior and central skull base fractures involving the right lateral orbital wall ➔ and sphenoid bone ➔. **(Right)** Axial CECT in the same patient shows a distended right cavernous sinus ➔ and engorged right superior ophthalmic vein ➔ from a high-flow direct carotid cavernous fistula.*

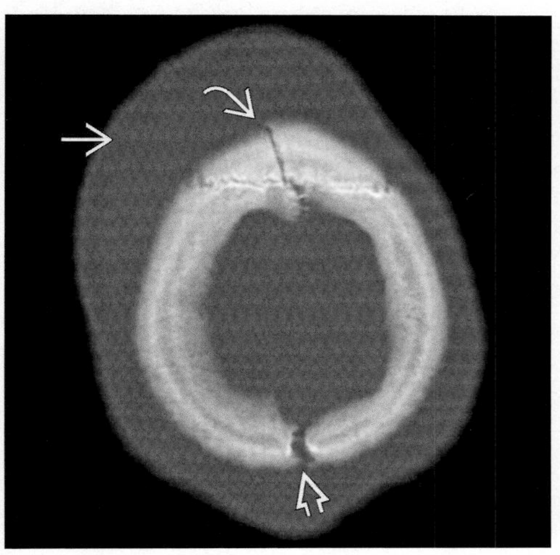

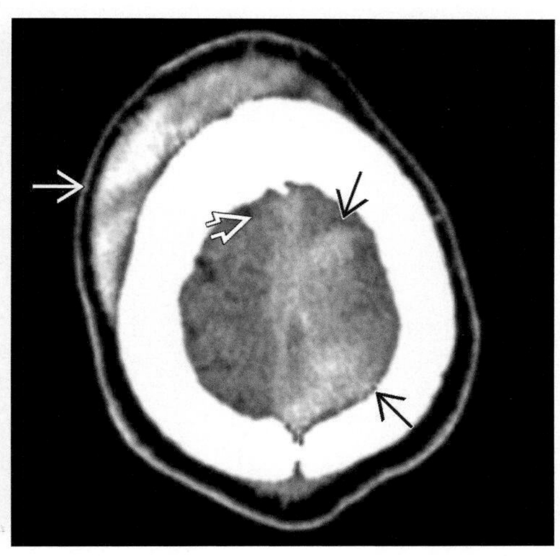

***(Left)** Axial bone CT demonstrates a linear, nondepressed skull fracture of the right paramedian frontal bone ➔, which involves the sagittal suture and results in diastasis ➔. There is also scalp injury with subgaleal hematoma ➔. **(Right)** Axial NECT in the same patient reveals an associated venous epidural hematoma ➔; on this image it begins to cross the sagittal suture and falx ➔. There is also scalp injury with subgaleal hematoma ➔.*

LEPTOMENINGEAL CYST ("GROWING FRACTURE")

Key Facts

Terminology
- Enlarging calvarial fracture adjacent to post-traumatic encephalomalacia

Imaging
- Linear lytic skull lesion with scalloped margins
- Brain tissue and cerebrospinal fluid (CSF) extending between bone edges acutely
- Subsequent development of encephalomalacia underlying fracture

Top Differential Diagnoses
- Epidermoid
- Parietal foramina/fissures
- Langerhans cell histiocytosis
- Calvarial metastasis
- Osteomyelitis

Pathology
- Scalloped fracture margins with differential erosion of inner, outer tables
- Absence of leptomeninges along inner surface of torn dura, over adjacent brain
- Brain necrosis, gliosis

Clinical Issues
- Infant or child: Enlarging palpable soft scalp mass
- Adults: Usually discovered as nontender, nonpulsatile, subcutaneous mass
- 90% occur in patients < 3 years

Diagnostic Checklist
- Consider diagnosis in all infants with radiographic skull defect or palpable scalp mass
- Increasing fracture diastasis over time rather than healing

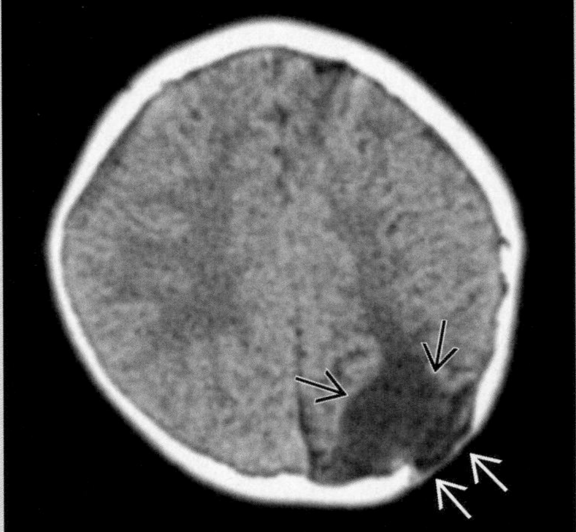
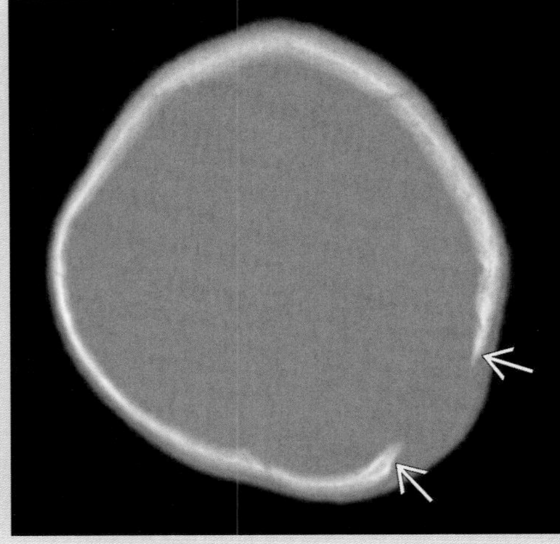

***(Left)** Axial NECT demonstrates left parietal encephalomalacia ⇨ with tissue and CSF seen extending into a post-traumatic parietal skull defect ➡. The patient has no history of prior craniotomy. **(Right)** Axial bone CT in the same patient confirms lytic bone defect with smooth margins in the left parietal bone. Note the beveled, scalloped margins of the edges of the bone defect ➡, with fluid and soft tissue extension through the calvarium.*

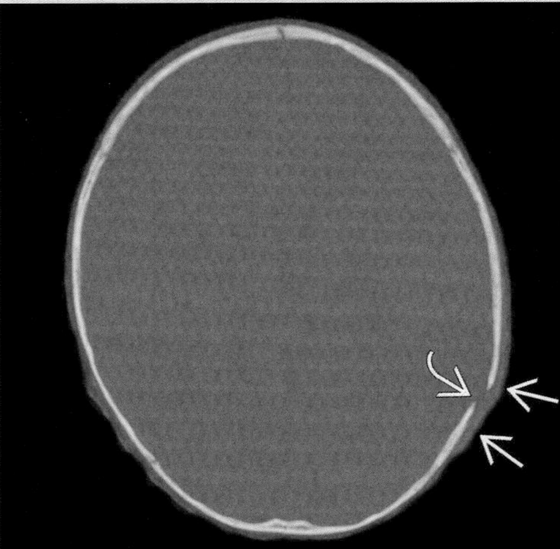
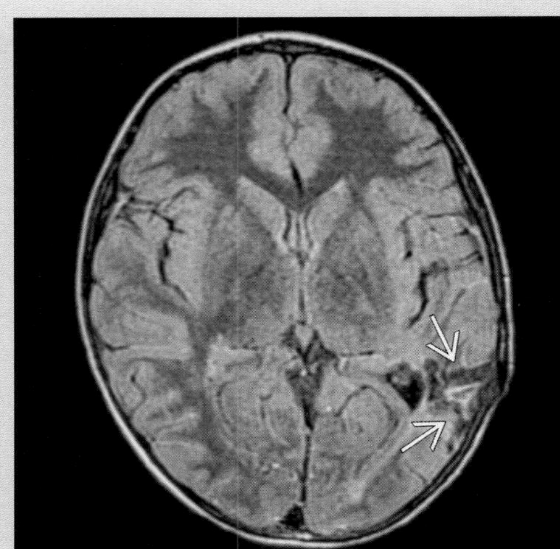

***(Left)** Axial NECT of head (bone algorithm) demonstrates a distracted left parietal bone fracture ➡ with smooth (not sharp) bone ends. The anterior parietal bone fragment is outwardly displaced with overlying scalp swelling ➡. **(Right)** Axial FLAIR MR of the same patient demonstrates the characteristic underlying parietal lobe encephalomalacia ➡ and CSF extending into the fracture site, preventing osteoblasts from migrating and healing the fracture.*

LEPTOMENINGEAL CYST ("GROWING FRACTURE")

TERMINOLOGY

Definitions

- Enlarging calvarial fracture adjacent to post-traumatic encephalomalacia

IMAGING

General Features

- Best diagnostic clue
  - Persistent or widening calvarial fracture line following head trauma
- Location
  - Parietal bone most common

Imaging Recommendations

- Protocol advice
  - Routine NECT viewed in brain and bone algorithm

Radiographic Findings

- Radiography
  - Linear lytic skull lesion with scalloped margins

CT Findings

- NECT
  - Brain tissue, cerebrospinal fluid (CSF) extending between bone edges acutely
  - Subsequent encephalomalacia under fracture

MR Findings

- T1WI
  - Cyst isointense with CSF, communicates with subarachnoid space
  - Subsequent development of encephalomalacia underlying fracture
- T2WI
  - Same as T1WI

DIFFERENTIAL DIAGNOSIS

Epidermoid Cyst

- Well-defined sclerotic margins, + diffusion restriction

Congenital Calvarial Defects

- Look for bilateral symmetry, characteristic location to suggest diagnosis

Langerhans Cell Histiocytosis

- Classic beveled edge appearance unusual in infants prior to development of diploic layer

Calvarial Metastasis

- Consider leukemia, neuroblastoma

Osteomyelitis

- Overlying soft tissue edema, poorly defined infiltrating destructive margins

PATHOLOGY

General Features

- Etiology
  - Skull fracture + dural tear → herniation of pia, arachnoid (leptomeninges) through dural tear
  - Leptomeninges disappear from inner surface of torn dura and over adjacent brain
  - CSF pulsations → progressive skull erosion around fracture
  - Interposition of brain tissue prevents osteoblast migration, inhibits fracture healing
  - Damaged brain becomes necrotic or gliotic → encephalomalacia

Gross Pathologic & Surgical Features

- Absence of leptomeninges along inner surface of torn dura, over adjacent brain

Microscopic Features

- Brain necrosis, gliosis

CLINICAL ISSUES

Presentation

- Most common signs/symptoms
  - Infant or child: Enlarging palpable soft scalp mass
    - Predisposing fracture may not have been clinically recognized
  - Adults: Usually discovered as nontender subcutaneous mass
    - History of childhood trauma rarely remembered or difficult to elicit

Demographics

- Age
  - 90% occur in patients < 3 years
- Epidemiology
  - Rare: 0.6% of pediatric skull fractures
  - Falling is most frequent injury mechanism

Natural History & Prognosis

- Increasing fracture diastasis over time
- ± progressive neurologic deficits (seizures, paresis), particularly in adult presentation

Treatment

- Surgical repair of dura, cyst resection

DIAGNOSTIC CHECKLIST

Consider

- Consider diagnosis in all infants with radiographic skull defect or palpable scalp mass

Image Interpretation Pearls

- Increasing fracture diastasis over time rather than healing

SELECTED REFERENCES

1. Slovis TL et al: Caffey's Pediatric Diagnostic Imaging, vol 1. 11th ed. Philadelphia: Mosby-Elsevier. 508, 2008
2. VandeVyver V et al: Multiple growing skull fractures. JBR-BTR. 90(1):52, 2007
3. Glass RB et al: The infant skull: a vault of information. Radiographics. 24(2):507-22, 2004

PNEUMOCEPHALUS

Key Facts

Terminology
- Presence of air or gas within skull

Imaging
- Can occur in any compartment: Extracerebral, intracerebral, intravascular
- CT: Very low density (-1,000 HU)
- MR: Foci of absent signal on all sequences, "blooms" on T2*
- Best imaging tool: NECT

Top Differential Diagnoses
- Traumatic vs. iatrogenic vs. infectious

Pathology
- Mechanism: Dural tear allows abnormal communication and air introduction
- Most common etiology: Trauma (74%)
  - Present in 3% of all skull fractures, 8% of paranasal sinus fractures

Clinical Issues
- Most common symptom: Headache
- Mortality (15%)
- Most common complication: CSF leak (50%)
- Infection (25%): Meningitis, epidural abscess, cerebritis, brain abscess
- Most often resolves on its own after removal of primary etiology

Diagnostic Checklist
- Pneumocephalus usually not problem: Find out what's causing it!
- Intravascular/cavernous sinus air without trauma or intracranial/intrathecal procedure generally of no clinical significance

__(Left)__ Axial NECT reveals diffuse post-traumatic pneumocephalus throughout the cisterns ➔ and subarachnoid spaces ➔. There are also right frontal lobe hemorrhagic contusions ➔. __(Right)__ Axial NECT demonstrates the "Mount Fuji" sign ➔ of tension pneumocephalus, in which subdural air separates and flattens the left frontal lobe and widens the interhemispheric space. Note the subdural air-fluid level ➔, a commonly associated finding.

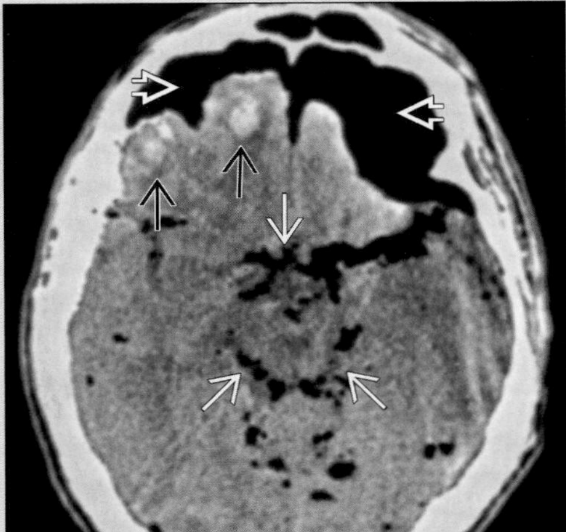

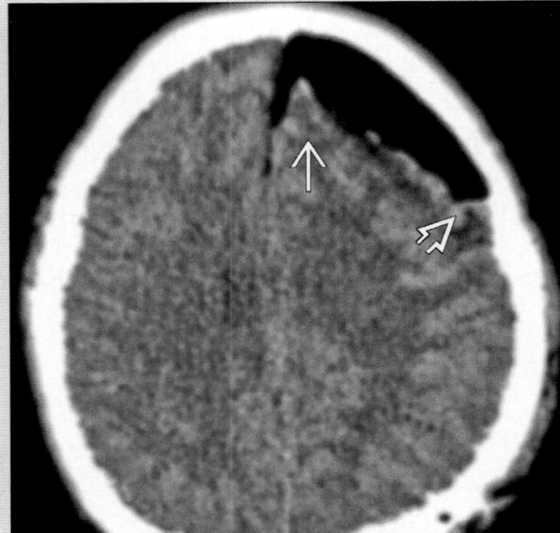

__(Left)__ Axial bone CT demonstrates a small collection of air within the nondependent aspect of the left lateral ventricle frontal horn following ventriculo-peritoneal shunt manipulation ➔. There is also air along the shunt track ➔ as well as mild global ventricular enlargement. __(Right)__ Axial NECT reveals a small focus of air within the left cavernous sinus ➔. Following a venous access procedure, there may be intravascular, cavernous sinus pneumocephalus, which is of no clinical significance.

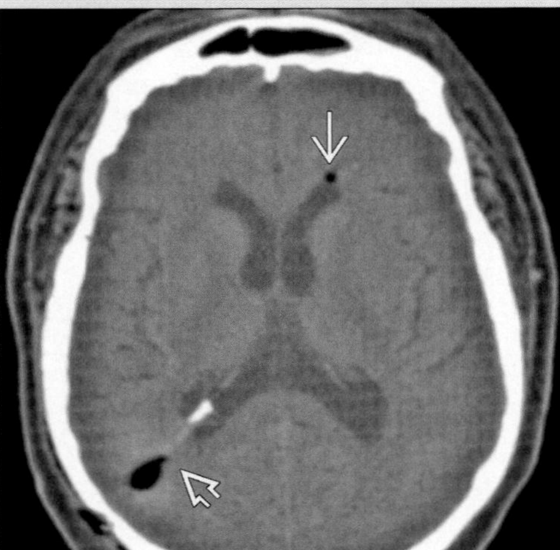

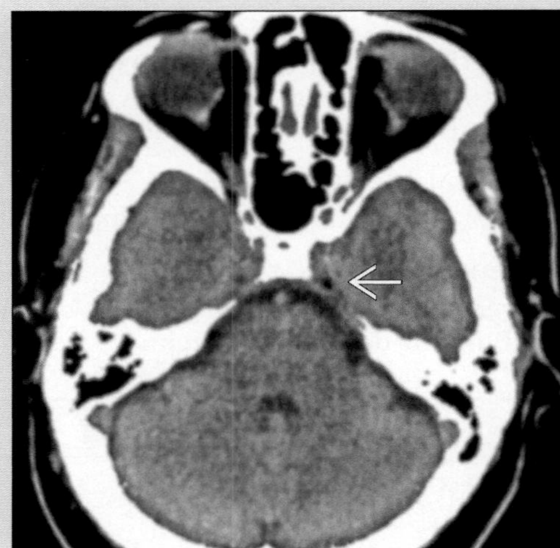

PNEUMOCEPHALUS

TERMINOLOGY

Synonyms

- Pneumatocele (when focal)

Definitions

- Presence of air or gas within skull

IMAGING

General Features

- Best diagnostic clue
  - Air anywhere within cranium
- Location
  - Can occur in any compartment
  - Extracerebral: Epidural, subdural, subarachnoid
  - Intracerebral: Brain parenchyma, cerebral ventricles
  - Intravascular: Arteries, veins, venous sinuses
- Size
  - Variable: Tiny to huge collection(s)
- Morphology
  - Focal to diffuse

CT Findings

- NECT
  - Very low density (-1,000 HU)
  - Epidural pneumocephalus
    - Remains localized
    - Does not move with changes of head position
  - Subdural pneumocephalus
    - Confluent, often forms air-fluid level(s)
    - Moves with changes of head position
    - May see cortical veins stretched within subdural air
  - Subarachnoid pneumocephalus
    - Multifocal, nonconfluent
    - Droplet-shaped, often within sulci
  - Intraventricular pneumocephalus
    - Rarely in isolation
  - Intravascular air most often venous
  - Tension pneumocephalus
    - "Mount Fuji" sign
      - Subdural air separates/compresses frontal lobes, creating widened interhemispheric space between frontal lobe tips, mimicking silhouette of Mount Fuji
    - "Air bubble" sign
      - Multiple, small air bubbles scattered throughout several cisterns
    - Associated chronic subdural hematoma(s)
  - Skull, skull base, paranasal sinus, mastoid fractures
  - Neoplasm invading sinus
    - Expansile or erosive; solid or cystic
  - Sinusitis, mastoiditis
  - Postoperative findings
    - Epidural, subdural, or subarachnoid air
    - Hyperdense hemorrhage
    - Craniotomy/-ectomy; sinus/sellar surgical defect
  - Iatrogenic
    - Ventriculostomy procedure
      - Intraventricular air common, especially after shunt manipulation
    - ICP monitor placement
    - Invasive subdural electrodes
- CECT
  - Any causative enhancing mass

MR Findings

- T2WI
  - Sinusitis, mastoiditis
- T1WI C+
  - Any causative enhancing mass
    - With erosive neoplasm often see dural involvement → thickening, occasionally breached
- MR: Foci of absent signal on all sequences, "blooms" on T2*
  - Any compartment
  - Iatrogenic
    - Ventriculostomy procedure: Also increased FLAIR signal along tract
    - ICP monitor placement
    - Invasive subdural electrodes

Imaging Recommendations

- Best imaging tool
  - NECT
- Protocol advice
  - Evaluate variable windows at PACS workstation

DIFFERENTIAL DIAGNOSIS

Traumatic

- Associated with other findings of trauma
- May also be found within any compartment

Iatrogenic

- Most often after surgical procedure
- Expected pneumocephalus seen in affected compartments and nondependent subarachnoid space
- May see intravascular, cavernous sinus following vascular access procedure; asymptomatic
- Susceptibility from hardware

Infectious

- Rare sequela of gas-producing infection

PATHOLOGY

General Features

- Etiology
  - Mechanism: Dural tear allows abnormal communication and air introduction via 2 possible events
    - Ball-valve mechanism from straining, coughing, sneezing, Valsalva
    - Vacuum phenomenon caused by CSF loss
  - Most common etiology = trauma
    - Blunt trauma produces skull &/or paranasal sinus fractures
    - Air cell involvement: Frontal > ethmoid > sphenoid > mastoid
    - Penetrating: GSW, knife, penetrable foreign bodies
  - Surgery (second most common)
    - Prevalence varies; almost universal with supratentorial surgery
    - Hypophysectomy

- Paranasal sinus surgery
  - Functional endoscopic sinus surgery (FESS) → cribriform plate
- Neoplasm invading into/from sinus
  - Osteoma: Frontal > ethmoid
  - Pituitary adenoma
  - Mucocele: Most often frontal
  - Epidermoid
  - Meningioma
- Infection from gas-forming organism
  - Extension from mastoiditis, sinusitis
  - Aerobic, anaerobic, or mixed infectious organisms
- Iatrogenic
  - Shunt placement/manipulation
  - ICP monitor placement
  - Invasive subdural electrodes for localization of seizure foci and functional mapping
- Tension pneumocephalus
  - Most commonly after neurosurgical evacuation of subdural hematoma
  - Lumbar drain placement, skull base surgery, paranasal sinus and posterior fossa surgery in sitting position
  - Use of nitrous oxide during anesthesia
- Rarely, open neural tube defect
- Associated abnormalities
  - CSF leak secondary to
    - Fracture: Cribriform plate, sphenoid sinus, mastoid air cells

Gross Pathologic & Surgical Features

- Air within skull
- Concomitant dural tear
- Direct communication outside ↔ inside established
  - Air is transmitted, forming pneumocephalus

CLINICAL ISSUES

Presentation

- Most common signs/symptoms
  - Headache
  - Acute: Most patients present within 4-5 days of inciting event
  - Chronic: Delay of several years reported
  - Tension: Headaches, ↓ level of consciousness, lateralizing deficits

Demographics

- Age
  - None; specific causes may have age prevalence
- Gender
  - None; specific causes may have gender prevalence
- Ethnicity
  - None; specific causes may have ethnic prevalence
- Epidemiology
  - Pneumocephalus present in 3% of all skull fractures, 8% of paranasal sinus fractures
  - 100% of patients undergoing supratentorial surgery have pneumocephalus in 1st 48 hours
  - Tension pneumocephalus: 2.5-16% prevalence following chronic subdural hematoma evacuation

Natural History & Prognosis

- Mortality (15%)
- Intravascular pneumocephalus
  - If trauma induced: Associated with mortal injury
  - If no history of trauma or intracranial/intrathecal procedure
    - Usually secondary to intravenous catheterization
    - Often seen within cavernous sinus
    - Patient will be asymptomatic
    - **Frequent** cause of consternation for on-call radiologists/residents
    - **Of no clinical concern**
- Tension pneumocephalus
  - Intracranial pressure rises as volume of air increases
  - Requires treatment
- Complications
  - Most common: CSF leak (50%)
  - Infection (25%): Meningitis, epidural abscess, cerebritis, brain abscess

Treatment

- Becomes an issue for air transport of trauma patients
  - Under normal flying conditions with ↓ cabin pressure, intracranial air volume will ↑ by ≈ 30% at normal maximum cabin altitude of 8,000 feet
  - ↑ in ICP dependent upon both initial air volume and rate of change in cabin altitude
  - Intracranial air volume of 30 cc = estimated worst case ↑ of ICP from sea level to max altitude = 10 mmHg → 31.8 mmHg
  - Sea-level pressure should be maintained during air transport of patients with suspected intracranial air
- Pneumocephalus most often resolves on its own after removal of etiology
- Administration of normobaric supplemental O_2 significantly ↑ rate at which pneumocephalus resolves after craniotomy
  - At room air (21% FiO_2): Resolves 31% per 24 hours
  - With nonrebreather mask delivering 68% FiO_2: Resolves 65% per 24 hours
- Tension pneumocephalus
  - Burr holes, craniotomy, needle aspirations, ventriculostomy, administration of 100% oxygen, and closure of dural defects
  - Mixed success rates

DIAGNOSTIC CHECKLIST

Image Interpretation Pearls

- Pneumocephalus usually not problem: Find out what's causing it!
- Intravascular/cavernous sinus air without trauma or intracranial/intrathecal procedure generally of no clinical significance

SELECTED REFERENCES

1. Choi YY et al: Pneumocephalus in the absence of craniofacial skull base fracture. J Trauma. 66(2):E24-7, 2009
2. Gore PA et al: Normobaric oxygen therapy strategies in the treatment of postcraniotomy pneumocephalus. J Neurosurg. 108(5):926-9, 2008

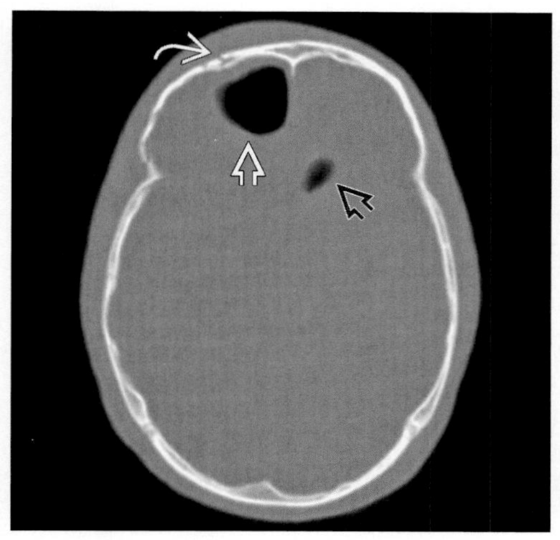

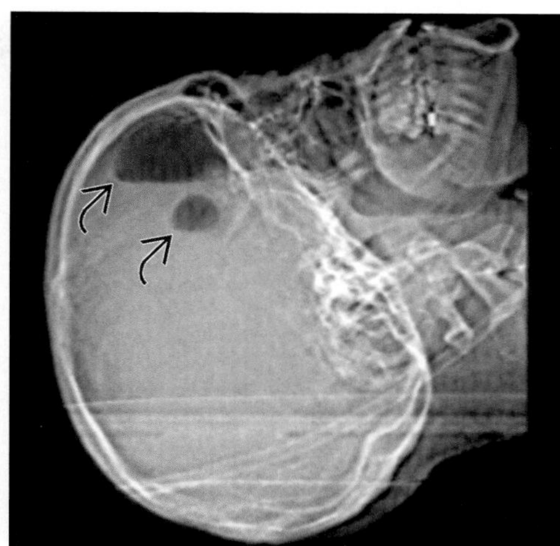

(Left) *Axial bone CT demonstrates a fracture of the right frontal bone ➡ with an associated underlying focal air collection ➡, as well as intraventricular air in the left frontal horn ➡. Pneumocephalus may be described as "pneumatocele" when focal.* ***(Right)*** *Lateral CT scout of the same case nicely shows focal air collections or "pneumatoceles" ➡ following skull fracture. Both pneumatoceles contain small air-CSF levels.*

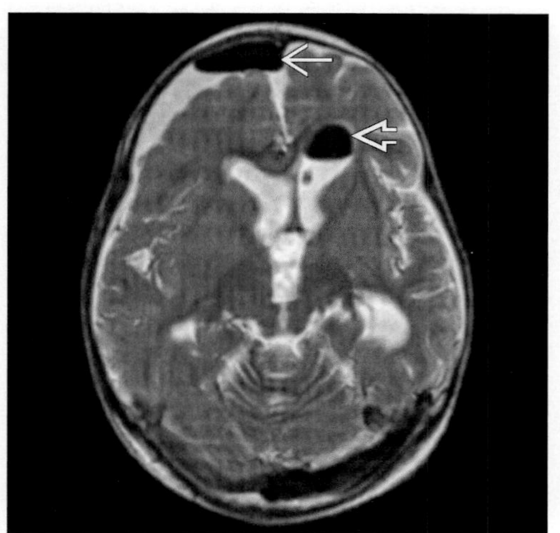

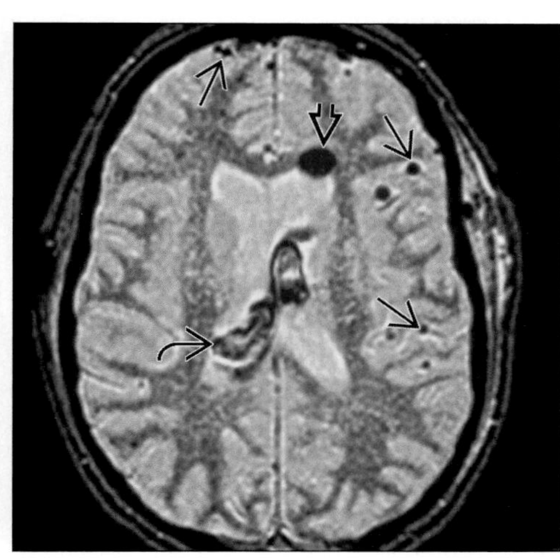

(Left) *Axial T2WI MR reveals a right frontal subarachnoid ➡ and a left lateral ventricle frontal horn ➡ pneumocephalus, both with air-CSF levels. Pneumocephalus is hypointense on all MR sequences.* ***(Right)*** *Axial T2* GRE MR obtained immediately after posterior fossa craniotomy shows air in the left frontal horn ➡, as well as multiple small "black dots" in the hemispheric sulci ➡. Some intraventricular blood ➡ is also present.*

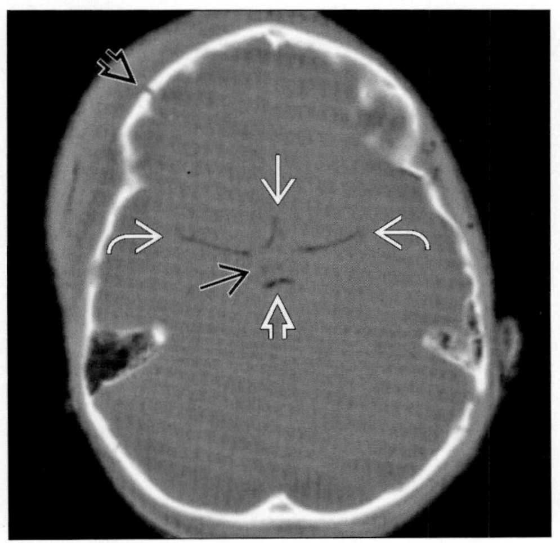

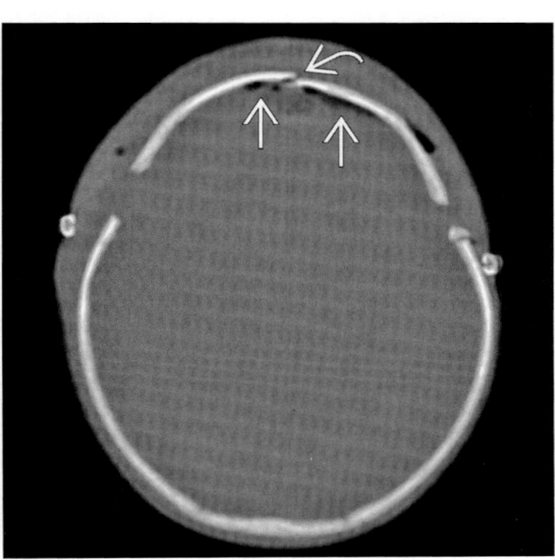

(Left) *Axial bone CT reveals impressive intravascular pneumocephalus within the circle of Willis arterial system, including bilateral MCA ➡ and ACA ➡, distal basilar artery with branch ostia and tip ➡, and right posterior communicating artery ➡. There is also a right frontal fracture ➡.* ***(Right)*** *Axial bone CT shows subarachnoid pneumocephalus ➡ underlying an iatrogenic skull fracture ➡ following metopic craniosynostosis repair. Pneumocephalus is common after neurosurgery procedures.*

INTRACRANIAL HYPOTENSION

Key Facts

Terminology
- Headache caused by ↓ intracranial CSF pressure

Imaging
- Classic imaging triad
  - Diffuse dural thickening/enhancement
  - Downward displacement of brain through incisura ("slumping" midbrain)
  - Subdural hygromas/hematomas
- Lack of 1 of 4 classic findings does not preclude diagnosis, however
- Dural enhancement is smooth, not nodular or "lumpy-bumpy"
- Veins, dural sinuses distended

Top Differential Diagnoses
- Meningitis
- Meningeal metastases
- Chronic subdural hematoma
- Dural sinus thrombosis
- Postsurgical dural thickening
- Idiopathic hypertrophic cranial pachymeningitis

Clinical Issues
- Severe headache (orthostatic, persistent, pulsatile, or even associated with nuchal rigidity)
- Uncommon: CN palsy (e.g., abducens), visual disturbances
- Rare: Severe encephalopathy with disturbances of consciousness

Diagnostic Checklist
- Frequently misdiagnosed; imaging is key to diagnosis
- Only rarely are **all** classic findings of IH present in the same patient!
- Look for enlarged spinal epidural venous plexi

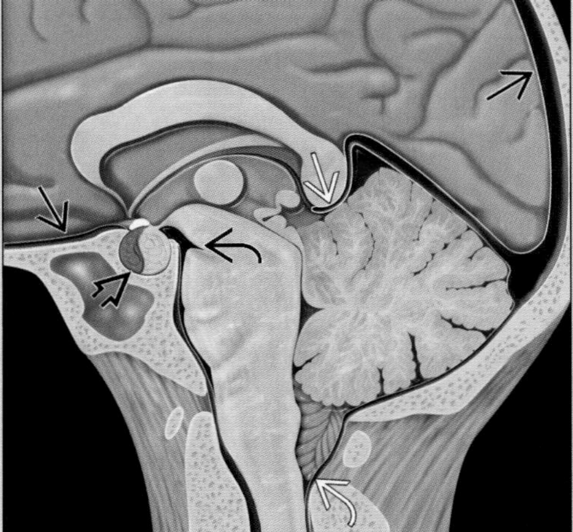

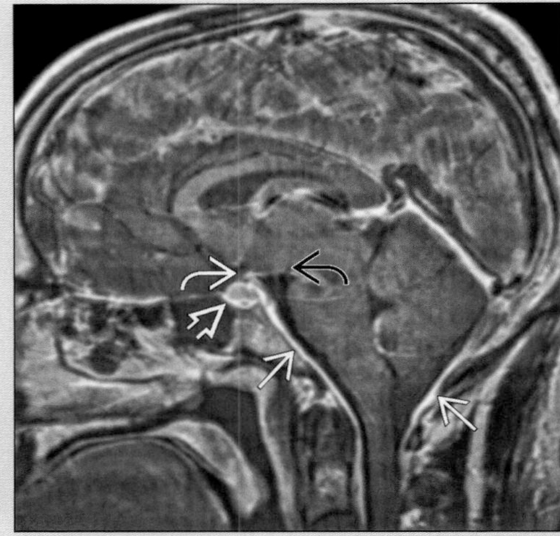

(Left) *Graphic shows IH with distended dural sinuses, enlarged pituitary, & herniated tonsils. Central brain descent causes midbrain "slumping," inferiorly displaced pons, "closed" pons-midbrain angle, & splenium depressing ICV/V of G junction.* ***(Right)*** *Sagittal T1WI C+ FS MR shows dura-arachnoid venous engorgement, enlarged pituitary, & suprasellar cistern effacement by inferior hypothalamus displacement. The angle between midbrain & pons is decreased.*

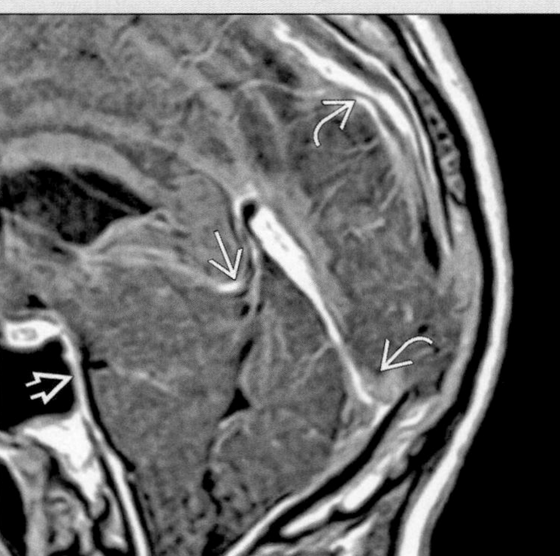

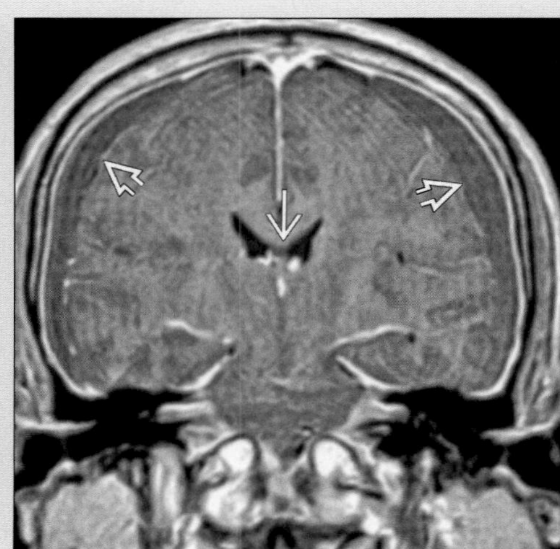

(Left) *Sagittal T1WI C+ MR in a patient with life-threatening ICH shows severely "sagging" midbrain, dural thickening/enhancement, distended torcular/superior sagittal/straight/transverse sinuses, and downward herniation of corpus callosum splenium causing acute angle between ICV/V of G.* ***(Right)*** *Coronal T1WI C+ MR in same patient shows subdural fluid, diffuse dural thickening/enhancement, and decreased angle between lateral ventricle roofs due to descent of central core brain structures.*

INTRACRANIAL HYPOTENSION

TERMINOLOGY

Abbreviations

- Intracranial hypotension (IH)

Definitions

- Headache caused by ↓ intracranial CSF pressure

IMAGING

General Features

- Best diagnostic clue
  - Classic imaging "quartet"
    - Downward displacement of brain through incisura ("slumping" midbrain)
    - Diffuse dural thickening/enhancement
    - Veins, dural sinuses distended
    - Subdural hygromas/hematomas
  - Lack of 1 of 4 classic findings does not preclude diagnosis, however
- Location
  - Pachymeninges (dura)
    - Both supra-, infratentorial
    - May extend into internal auditory canals
    - Spinal dura, epidural venous plexi may be involved
- Morphology
  - Dural enhancement is smooth, not nodular or "lumpy-bumpy"

CT Findings

- NECT
  - Relatively insensitive; may appear normal
  - ± thick dura
  - ± subdural fluid collections
    - Usually bilateral
    - CSF (hygroma) or blood (hematoma)
  - Suprasellar cistern may appear obliterated
  - Atria of lateral ventricles may appear deviated medially, abnormally close ("tethered") to midline
- CECT
  - Diffuse dural thickening, enhancement

MR Findings

- T1WI
  - Sagittal shows brain descent in 40-50% of cases
    - "Sagging" midbrain
      - Midbrain displaced inferiorly below level of dorsum sellae
      - Pons may be compressed against clivus
    - Decreased angle between peduncles, pons
    - Caudal displacement of tonsils in 25-75%
    - Optic chiasm, hypothalamus draped over sella
    - Pituitary enlarged above sella in 50%
    - Veins/dural sinuses distended (convex margins)
    - Decreased angle between ICVs, vein of Galen
  - Axial
    - Suprasellar cistern crowded/effaced
    - Midbrain, pons appear elongated ("fat" midbrain)
    - Temporal lobes herniated over tentorium, into incisura
    - Lateral ventricles small, often distorted
      - Atria pulled medially by downward displacement of midbrain
  - Coronal
    - Severe cases show decreased venous angle (< 120°) between roofs of lateral ventricles
  - Bilateral subdural fluid collections in 15%
    - 70% hygromas (clear fluid collects within dural border cell layer)
    - 10% hematomas (blood of variable signal intensity)
- T2WI
  - Thickened dura usually hyperintense
  - Subdural fluid (variable signal)
- FLAIR
  - Hyperintense dura, subdural fluid
- T2* GRE
  - May bloom if hemorrhage present
- T1WI C+
  - Diffuse, intense dural enhancement in 85%
  - Often extends into CPAs

Ultrasonographic Findings

- Color Doppler
  - Enlarged superior ophthalmic veins with higher mean maximum flow velocity

Angiographic Findings

- Cortical, medullary veins may be diffusely enlarged

Nonvascular Interventions

- Myelography
  - May demonstrate epidural contrast extravasation at precise site
    - Dynamic CT myelo may show extradural contrast
  - Caution: Myelography may facilitate CSF leak, worsen symptoms

Nuclear Medicine Findings

- Radionuclide cisternography (RNC)
  - Direct findings: Focal accumulation of radioactivity outside of subarachnoid space at leakage site
  - Indirect findings
    - Rapid washout from CSF space
    - Early appearance of activity in kidneys, urinary bladder
    - Poor migration of isotope over convexities

Imaging Recommendations

- Best imaging tool
  - Contrast-enhanced cranial MR for diagnosis
  - Radionuclide cisternography if localization required
- Protocol advice
  - Search for actual leakage site only if
    - 2 technically adequate blood patches fail
    - Post-traumatic leak is suspected

DIFFERENTIAL DIAGNOSIS

Meningitis

- Pia-subarachnoid enhancement > dura-arachnoid

Meningeal Metastases

- Enhancement usually thicker, irregular ("bumpy")

Chronic Subdural Hematoma
- Look for enhancing membranes with blood products

Dural Sinus Thrombosis
- Look for thrombosed sinus ("empty" delta sign, etc.)

Postsurgical Dural Thickening
- Look for other postoperative findings (e.g., burr holes)
- May occur almost immediately after surgery, persist for months/years

Idiopathic Hypertrophic Cranial Pachymeningitis
- Headache usually not orthostatic
- May cause bony invasion

PATHOLOGY

General Features
- Etiology
  - Dural thickening, enhancement due to venous engorgement
  - Common cause of IH = spontaneous spinal CSF leak
    - Weak dura ± arachnoid diverticulae common
    - Aberrant extracellular matrix with abnormalities of fibrillin-containing microfibrils
  - Reduced CSF pressure precipitated by
    - Surgery (CSF overshunting) or trauma (including trivial fall)
    - Vigorous exercise or violent coughing
    - Diagnostic lumbar puncture
    - Spontaneous dural tear, ruptured arachnoid diverticulum
    - Severe dehydration
    - Disc herniation or osteophyte (rare)
  - Pathophysiology = Monro-Kellie doctrine
    - CSF, intracranial blood volume vary inversely
    - In face of low CSF pressure, dural venous plexi dilate
- Associated abnormalities
  - Dilated cervical epidural venous plexus, spinal hygromas, retrospinal fluid collections
  - Low opening pressure (< 6 cm H_2O), pleocytosis, increased protein on lumbar puncture
  - Stigmata of systemic connective tissue disorder found in up to 2/3 of patients
    - Marfan, Ehlers-Danlos type 2
    - Clinical findings = minor skeletal features, small-joint hypermobility, etc.; may be subtle

Gross Pathologic & Surgical Features
- Surgical specimen generally unremarkable with grossly normal-appearing dura
- Spinal meningeal diverticula (often multiple), dural holes/rents common
- No specific leakage site identified at surgery in at least 50%

Microscopic Features
- Meningeal surface normal
  - No evidence for inflammation or neoplasia
- Inner surface
  - Layer of numerous delicate thin-walled dilated vessels often attached to inner surface
  - Nests of meningothelial cells may be prominent, should not be misinterpreted as meningioma
  - May show marked arachnoidal, dural fibrosis if longstanding

CLINICAL ISSUES

Presentation
- Most common signs/symptoms
  - Severe headache (orthostatic, persistent, pulsatile, or even associated with nuchal rigidity)
  - Uncommon: CN palsy (e.g., abducens), visual disturbances
  - Rare: Severe encephalopathy with disturbances of consciousness
- Clinical profile
  - Young/middle-aged adult with orthostatic headache

Demographics
- Age
  - Peak in 3rd, 4th decades

Natural History & Prognosis
- Most IH cases resolve spontaneously
  - Dural thickening, enhancement disappears; midline structures return (ascend) to normal position
- Rare: Coma, death from severe intracranial herniation

Treatment
- Aimed at restoring CSF volume (fluid replacement, bedrest)
  - Initial: Lumbar or directed epidural blood patch
  - Emergent intrathecal saline infusion if patient severely encephalopathic, obtunded
- Surgery if blood patch fails (usually large dural tear) or SDHs with acute clinical deterioration

DIAGNOSTIC CHECKLIST

Consider
- Frequently misdiagnosed; imaging is key to diagnosis

Image Interpretation Pearls
- Only rarely are **all** classic findings of IH present in the same patient!
- Look for enlarged spinal epidural venous plexi

SELECTED REFERENCES

1. Shankar JJ et al: The venous hinge-an objective sign for the diagnosis and follow-up of treatment in patients with intracranial hypotension syndrome. Neuroradiology. Epub ahead of print, 2009
2. Su CS et al: Clinical features, neuroimaging and treatment of spontaneous intracranial hypotension and magnetic resonance imaging evidence of blind epidural blood patch. Eur Neurol. 61(5):301-7, 2009
3. de Noronha RJ et al: Subdural haematoma: a potentially serious consequence of spontaneous intracranial hypotension. J Neurol Neurosurg Psychiatry. 74(6):752-5, 2003

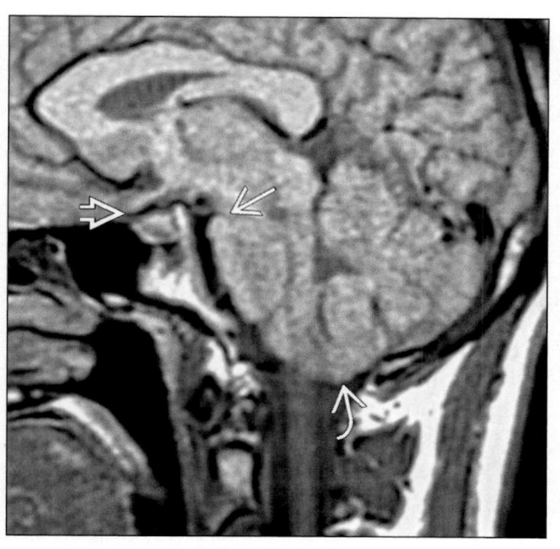

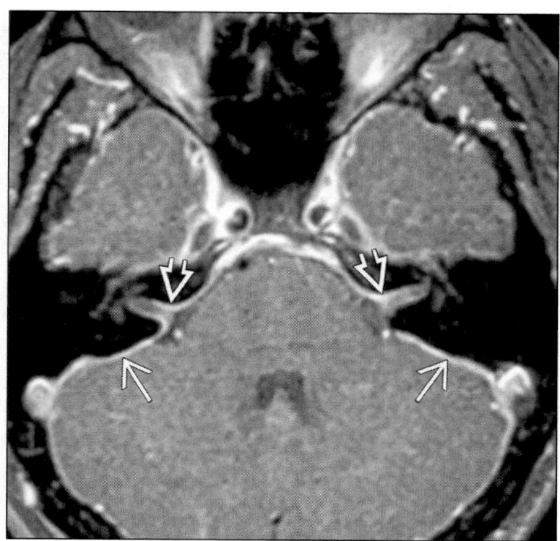

(Left) *Sagittal T1WI MR in a patient with intractable headache relieved in supine position. The tonsils ➡ are only mildly low, but the midbrain is definitely "slumping," with decreased pontine-midbrain angle ➡. The pituitary gland is somewhat rounded, & the suprasellar cistern ➡ is decreased by downward displacement of the optic chiasm/hypothalamus.* ***(Right)*** *Axial T1WI C+ FS MR in the same patient shows diffuse dura-arachnoid thickening ➡ from venous engorgement. Note extension into CPAs ➡.*

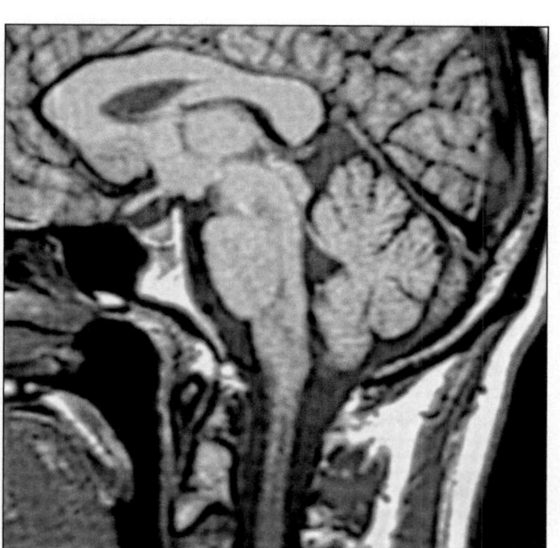

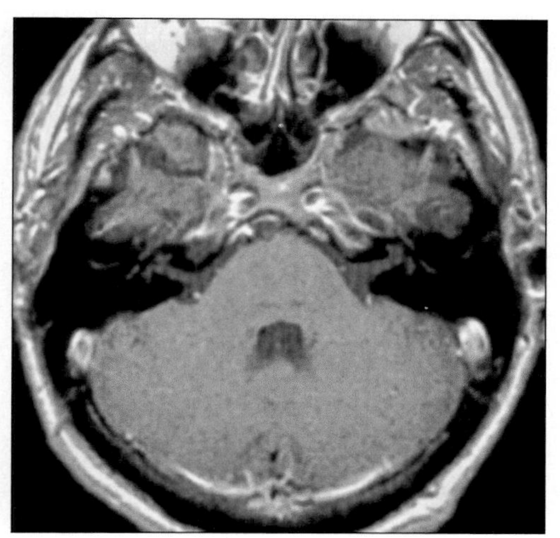

(Left) *Sagittal T1WI MR in the same patient following an epidural blood patch that relieved/resolved symptoms. Note the return of the pontine-midbrain angle to normal. The tonsils are no longer below the foramen magnum, the suprasellar cistern also appears normal, and the pituitary no longer appears rounded.* ***(Right)*** *Axial T1WI C+ MR in the same patient after the blood patch shows complete resolution of dura-arachnoid enhancement.*

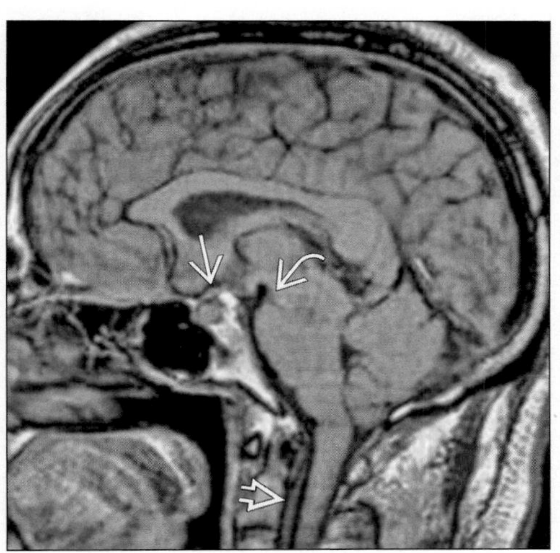

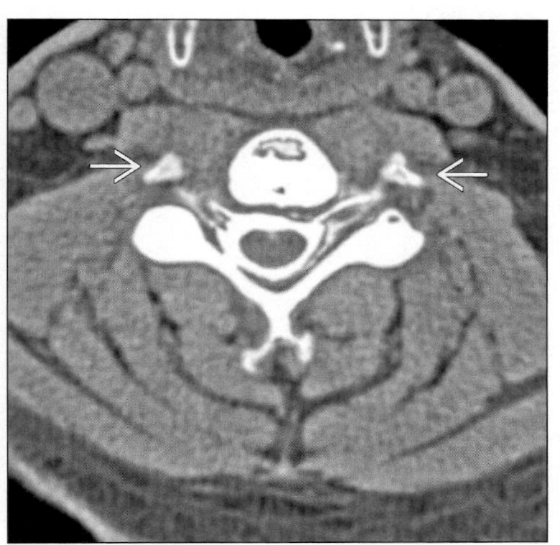

(Left) *Sagittal T1WI MR shows changes of severe IH. Note inferior displacement of the pons with decreased pontine-midbrain angle ➡. The optic chiasm is draped over the dorsum sellae, and the suprasellar cistern is effaced ➡. Note the venous engorgement in the upper cervical spine ➡.* ***(Right)*** *Axial post-myelographic CECT in a patient with IH shows contrast extending along the root sleeves and out into the cervical plexus ➡. The patient was successfully treated with an epidural blood patch.*

IDIOPATHIC INFLAMMATORY PSEUDOTUMOR, SKULL BASE

Key Facts

Terminology

- Nonspecific, nonneoplastic benign inflammatory process without identifiable local or systemic causes characterized by polymorphous lymphoid infiltrate with varying degrees of fibrosis

Imaging

- Intraorbital, cavernous sinus, meningeal, skull base, or nasopharyngeal enhancing infiltrating lesion
- T2: Iso- to hypointense infiltrating mass
  - ↑ ↑ fibrosis, ↑ ↑ hypointensity
- T1WI C+ MR: Diffusely C+ infiltrating mass with multiple appearances
  - Extends from orbit through superior orbital fissure to cavernous sinus, local meninges, Meckel cave
  - Extends through inferior orbital fissure to pterygopalatine fossa and nose
  - Involves deep spaces of nasopharynx
- MRA: When involves cavernous sinus, internal carotid artery narrowing often present

Top Differential Diagnoses

- Meningitis
- Neurosarcoid
- En plaque meningioma
- Metastases, skull and meningeal
- Meningeal non-Hodgkin lymphoma (NHL)
- Nasopharyngeal carcinoma

Clinical Issues

- Painful proptosis ± headaches ± cranial neuropathies
- Extracranial soft tissues: Focal or diffuse mass
- Diagnosis of exclusion; must be biopsied
- Treatment: High-dose systemic steroids

*(**Left**) Axial T1WI C+ FS MR through the orbits shows enhancing, infiltrating lesion in orbital apex ➡ and lateral rectus, cavernous sinus ➡ and Meckel cave ➡. The initial impression of adenoid cystic carcinoma gave way to biopsy-proven idiopathic inflammatory disease with both intraorbital and intracranial components. (**Right**) Axial T1WI C+ FS MR in the same patient shows the lesion invading inferiorly through the inferior orbital fissure into the pterygopalatine fossa ➡ and nose ➡.*

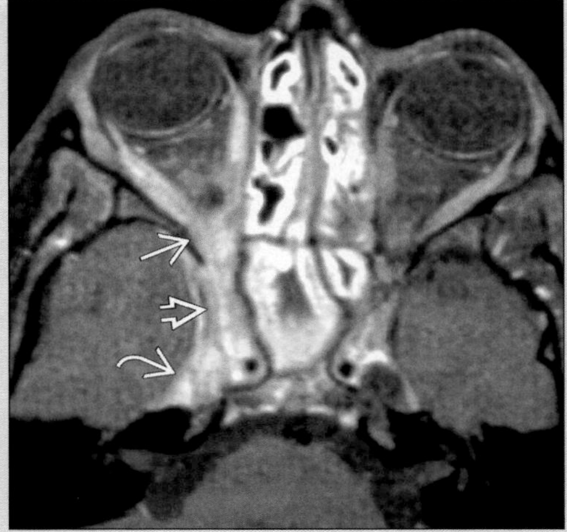

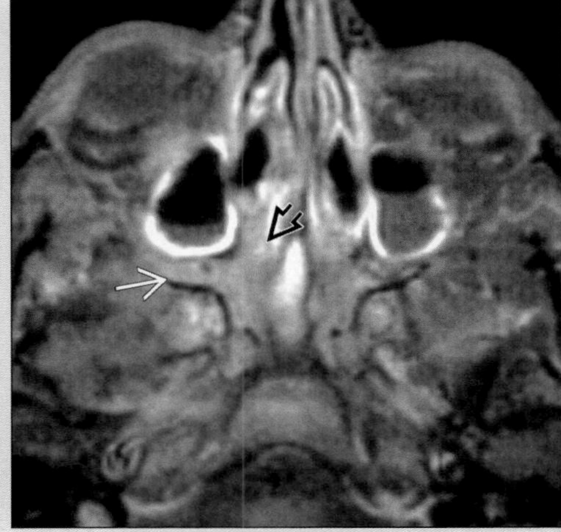

*(**Left**) Axial T1WI C+ FS MR demonstrates an enlarged, enhancing left cavernous sinus ➡ with subtle narrowing ➡ of the intracavernous internal carotid artery. (**Right**) Axial T2WI MR in the same patient reveals that the cavernous sinus lesion ➡ is strikingly low signal. Biopsy revealed an idiopathic inflammatory pseudotumor. No significant intraorbital disease was present. Imaging mimics a meningioma in this patient with cranial neuropathy.*

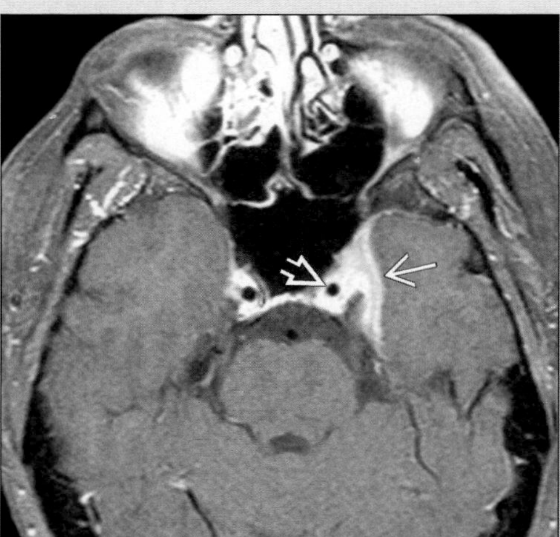

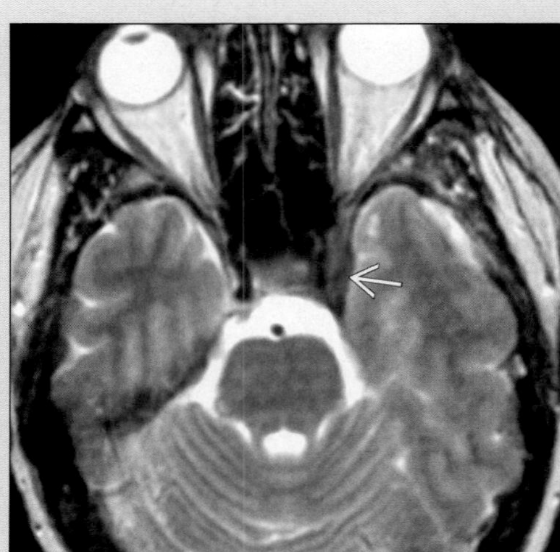

IDIOPATHIC INFLAMMATORY PSEUDOTUMOR, SKULL BASE

TERMINOLOGY

Abbreviations
- Idiopathic inflammatory pseudotumor (IIP)

Synonyms
- Idiopathic inflammatory disease, Tolosa-Hunt syndrome, hypertrophic cranial pachymeningitis, plasma cell granuloma

Definitions
- Nonspecific, nonneoplastic benign inflammatory process without identifiable local or systemic causes characterized by polymorphous lymphoid infiltrate with varying degrees of fibrosis

IMAGING

General Features
- Best diagnostic clue
  - Intraorbital, cavernous sinus, meningeal, skull base, or nasopharyngeal enhancing infiltrating lesion
- Location
  - Intracranial involvement
    - Meningeal surfaces
    - Cavernous sinus, Meckel cave area
    - Falx and tentorium are less often involved
  - Skull base and extracranial involvement
    - Central and anterior skull base
    - Pterygopalatine fossa and nose
    - Deep spaces of nasopharynx
- Size
  - May extensively involve meningeal surfaces and adjacent skull base
  - Focal meningeal thickening may range in thickness from few millimeters to > 2 cm
  - Skull base and extracranial soft tissue masses may be large (many centimeters)
- Morphology
  - Skull base and nasopharyngeal soft tissue infiltrating lesions mimic malignancy
  - Infiltrating mass along meningeal surfaces

CT Findings
- CECT
  - Enhancing, soft tissue mass
- Bone CT
  - Associated bone erosion unusual
- CTA
  - If cavernous ICA involved, often narrowed

MR Findings
- T1WI
  - Lesion isointense to gray matter
- T2WI
  - Iso- to **hypointense** infiltrating mass
    - ↑ ↑ fibrosis, ↑ ↑ hypointensity
- FLAIR
  - No adjacent brain edema
- T1WI C+
  - Diffusely enhancing infiltrating mass with multiple appearances
    - Extends from orbit through superior orbital fissure to cavernous sinus, local meninges, Meckel cave
    - Extends through inferior orbital fissure to pterygopalatine fossa
      - May affect posterior nose
    - Involves deep spaces of nasopharynx
  - Underlying bone is rarely invaded
    - Fat saturated T1WI C+ best sequence
- MRA
  - When involving cavernous sinus, **internal carotid artery narrowing** often present

Imaging Recommendations
- Best imaging tool
  - MR imaging intracranial & extracranial extensions
- Protocol advice
  - Begin with MR, including full brain FLAIR and enhanced T1WI C+ with fat saturation
  - Bone CT may help differentiate this lesion from en plaque meningioma

DIFFERENTIAL DIAGNOSIS

Neurosarcoid
- Systemic manifestations abound
- Increased erythrocyte sedimentation rate (ESR) and serum angiotensin converting enzyme (ACE)

Skull and Meningeal Metastases
- Nodular meningeal carcinomatosis less common than diffuse
- Cranial neuropathy occurs early
- CSF cellular analysis usually provides diagnosis, but meningeal biopsy may be necessary

En Plaque Meningioma
- Enhancing meningeal mass + dural "tails"
- Permeative-sclerotic invasive bone changes typical
- May exactly mimic intracranial IIP

Meningeal Non-Hodgkin Lymphoma (NHL)
- Usually more diffuse, multifocal with underlying bone involvement
- "Great pretender" (can mimic many intracranial diseases)

Nasopharyngeal Carcinoma
- Arises in nasopharyngeal mucosal space
- Invades cephalad into skull base, sinuses

Meningitis
- TB, fungal, or other infectious agent causes focal meningeal thickening
- CSF analysis may not make diagnosis
- Meningeal biopsy may be necessary

PATHOLOGY

General Features
- Etiology
  - Benign inflammatory process of unknown origin
  - Hypothesis 1: Immune-autoimmune pathophysiology

IDIOPATHIC INFLAMMATORY PSEUDOTUMOR, SKULL BASE

- Hypothesis 2: Low-grade fibrosarcoma with inflammatory (lymphomatous) cells
- Other pathologic features
  - IIP is "quasi-neoplastic" lesion; most commonly affects lung and orbit
    - Has been reported to occur in nearly every site in human body
  - Can involve meninges, cavernous sinus, skull base, extracranial soft tissues
  - Spectrum of idiopathic inflammatory lesions

Gross Pathologic & Surgical Features

- Surgical impression depends on histopathologic composition
  - Soft, compressible mass: Intracranial pseudotumor
  - Hard, fibrotic mass: Hypertrophic cranial pachymeningitis

Microscopic Features

- Histologic hallmarks
  - Mixed inflammatory infiltrate of lymphocytes (T and B cells) and plasma cells
  - Varying degrees of **fibrosis** present
- Terminology depends on mix during histopathologic evaluation
  - IIP-pseudotumor
    - Inflammatory meningeal mass with balanced mixture of lymphocytes, plasma cells, and fibrous tissue
  - Plasma cell granuloma
    - Inflammatory meningeal mass with predominance of plasma cells
  - Hypertrophic cranial pachymeningitis
    - Inflammatory meningeal mass with predominance of dense fibrous tissue

CLINICAL ISSUES

Presentation

- Most common signs/symptoms
  - Orbital lesion: Painful proptosis
  - Intracranial lesion only: Chronic headaches
  - Cavernous sinus: Cranial neuropathy (CN3, 4, 5, 6)
  - Extracranial soft tissues: Focal or diffuse mass
- Clinical profile
  - Adult presenting with painful proptosis, headaches, and cranial nerve palsies

Demographics

- Age
  - Intracranial IIP: Adults (40-65 years of age)
- Epidemiology
  - Extraorbital IIP: Intracranial or extracranial
    - Most commonly associated with orbital IIP
  - Can be seen without orbital IIP

Natural History & Prognosis

- Intracranial and extracranial IIP
  - May respond to steroid therapy
  - When extensive intra- & extracranial involvement present, may be resistant to all therapies
    - Such intractable disease may cause severe disability or death
- Orbital lesions
  - Treatment successes (65%)
  - Treatment failures (35%)

Treatment

- Options, risks, complications
  - **Diagnosis of exclusion**
    - Intra- or extracranial disease must be biopsied
    - Biopsy excludes infectious and neoplastic (NHL) causes of focal meningeal thickening
  - High-dose systemic steroids with slow taper is principal treatment option
  - Steroid resistant cases ± cases with extensive skull base involvement
    - Radiotherapy ± chemotherapy
    - Surgical resection as possible

DIAGNOSTIC CHECKLIST

Consider

- IIP is diagnosis of exclusion!
  - 1st exclude infection and malignancy with biopsy
  - Realize that intracranial IIP, plasma cell granuloma, and hypertrophic cranial pachymeningitis are all part of same disease spectrum

Image Interpretation Pearls

- If mass in orbit with proximal meningeal, cavernous sinus lesion, consider IIP
- IIP orbit alone > > orbit and intracranial > > orbit intracranial and extracranial

Reporting Tips

- If orbital lesion suggests IIP, report any associated intracranial or extracranial soft tissue lesions

SELECTED REFERENCES

1. Strasnick B et al: Inflammatory pseudotumor of the temporal bone: a case series. Skull Base. 18(1):49-52, 2008
2. Agir H et al: W(h)ither orbital pseudotumor? J Craniofac Surg. 18(5):1148-53, 2007
3. Mangiardi JR et al: Extraorbital skull base idiopathic pseudotumor. Laryngoscope. 117(4):589-94, 2007
4. Lee DK et al: Inflammatory pseudotumor involving the skull base: response to steroid and radiation therapy. Otolaryngol Head Neck Surg. 135(1):144-8, 2006
5. Lee EJ et al: MR imaging of orbital inflammatory pseudotumors with extraorbital extension. Korean J Radiol. 6(2):82-8, 2005
6. Narla LD et al: Inflammatory pseudotumor. Radiographics. 23(3):719-29, 2003
7. Yuen SJ et al: Idiopathic orbital inflammation: distribution, clinical features, and treatment outcome. Arch Ophthalmol. 121(4):491-9, 2003
8. Dehner LP: The enigmatic inflammatory pseudotumours: the current state of our understanding, or misunderstanding. J Pathol. 192(3):277-9, 2000
9. Tekkök IH et al: Intracranial plasma cell granuloma. Brain Tumor Pathol. 17(3):97-103, 2000
10. Bencherif B et al: Intracranial extension of an idiopathic orbital inflammatory pseudotumor. AJNR Am J Neuroradiol. 14(1):181-4, 1993
11. Clifton AG et al: Intracranial extension of orbital pseudotumour. Clin Radiol. 45(1):23-6, 1992

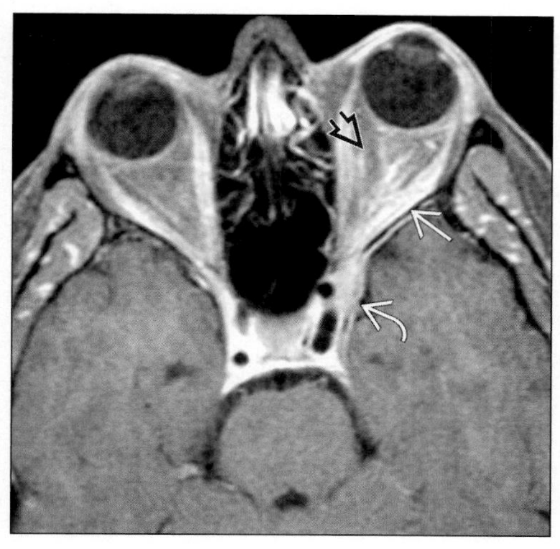

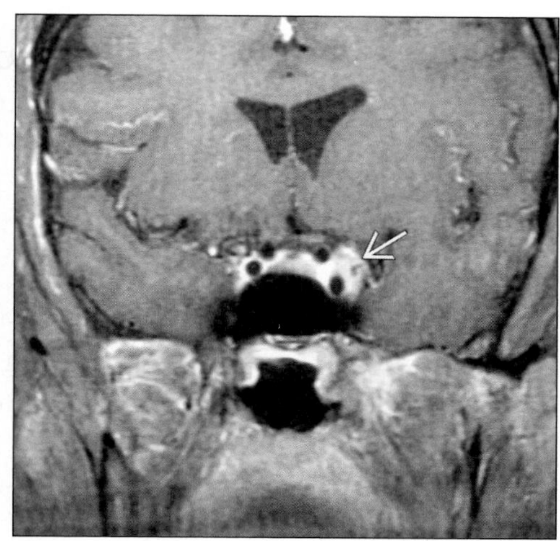

(Left) *In this patient with painful proptosis, an axial T1WI C+ FS MR shows an intraorbital lateral rectus ➡ & intraconal ⇨ lesion. Note the pseudotumor progresses through the superior orbital fissure to the anterior cavernous sinus ↪.* ***(Right)*** *Coronal T1WI C+ FS MR in the same patient shows the intracranial extension of the lesion into the left cavernous sinus ➡. Orbital pseudotumor extending into the cavernous sinus is the most common form of intracranial extension.*

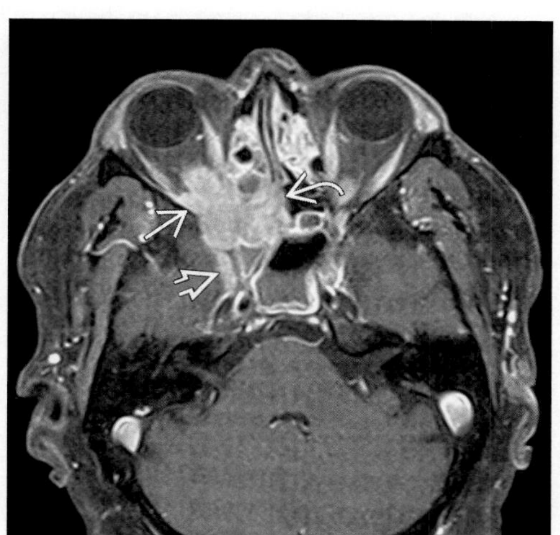

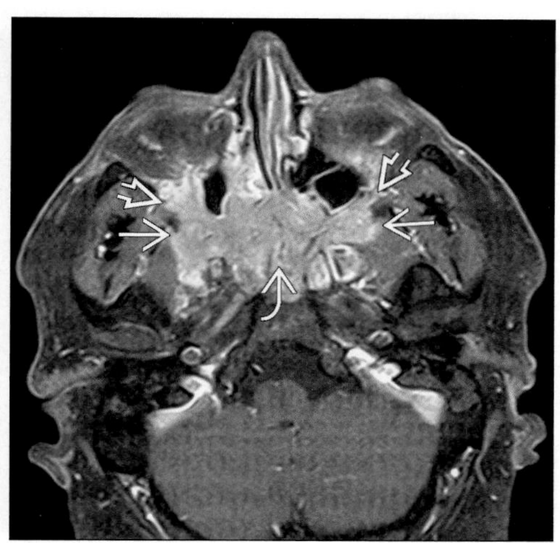

(Left) *Axial T1WI C+ FS MR shows extensive orbital apex ➡, ethmoid sinus ↪, and foramen rotundum ⇨ infiltrating enhancing idiopathic inflammatory pseudotumor.* ***(Right)*** *On a more inferior slice in the same patient, the axial T1WI C+ FS MR reveals bilateral pterygopalatine fossa ➡ involvement with continuous transnasal pseudotumor ↪. Both inferior orbital fissures are also affected ⇨. Imaging often mimics a neoplasm. A biopsy is necessary for diagnosis.*

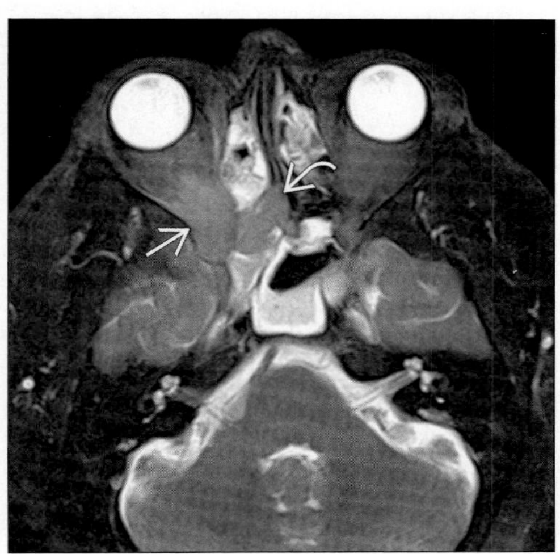

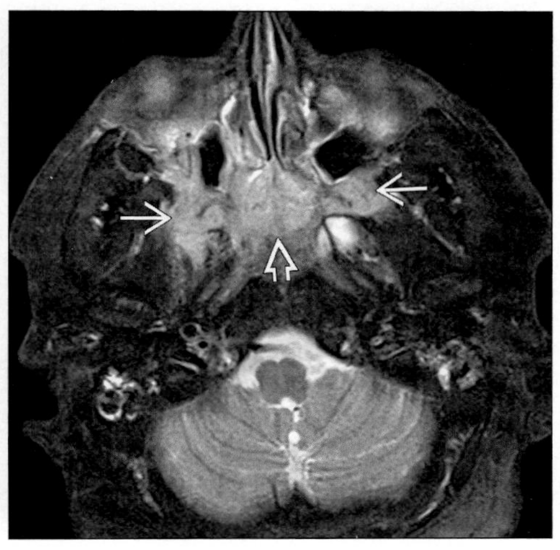

(Left) *Axial T2WI FS MR in the same patient shows an infiltrating pseudotumor in the orbital apex ➡ and ethmoid sinus ↪. Obstructed sinuses are easily differentiated from the pseudotumor. Isointensity of the pseudotumor results from greater cellular content in this lesion compared to fibrosis content.* ***(Right)*** *Axial T2WI FS MR in the same patient shows extensive pseudotumorous involvement of the pterygopalatine fossae ➡ and posterior nose ⇨.*

FIBROUS DYSPLASIA

Key Facts

Terminology

- Fibrous dysplasia (FD); craniofacial fibrous dysplasia (CFD); osteitis fibrosa; osteodystrophy fibrosa
- McCune-Albright syndrome (MAS)
  - 1 of most common FD syndromes
- Congenital disorder characterized by expanding lesion(s)
  - Defect in osteoblastic differentiation, maturation
  - Contains mixture of fibrous tissue, woven bone

Imaging

- Best diagnostic clue: Ground-glass matrix in bone lesion on CT
- CFD: Majority have > 1 bone involved
- MR: ↓ T2WI signal (if solid) or in rind (if "cystic")
  - Variable enhancement
  - Rim, diffuse, or none

Top Differential Diagnoses

- Paget disease
- Garré sclerosing osteomyelitis
- Jaffe-Campanacci (J-C) syndrome
- Craniometaphyseal dysplasia
- Meningioma

Clinical Issues

- Most common signs/symptoms: Painless swelling or deformity
- Rare progression to fibro-, osteo-, chondro-, and mesenchymal sarcoma

Diagnostic Checklist

- Monostotic and polyostotic FD likely on same spectrum of phenotypic expression; consider checking for gene to predict complications

*(**Left**) Axial graphic shows expansion of the lateral orbital rim, sphenoid wing, and temporal squamosa by fibrous dysplasia. Note the exophthalmos and stretching of the optic nerve on the ipsilateral side. (**Right**) Axial NECT of the mandible and maxilla demonstrates extensive multifocal bone expansion with a ground-glass appearance ➡, classic for fibrous dysplasia.*

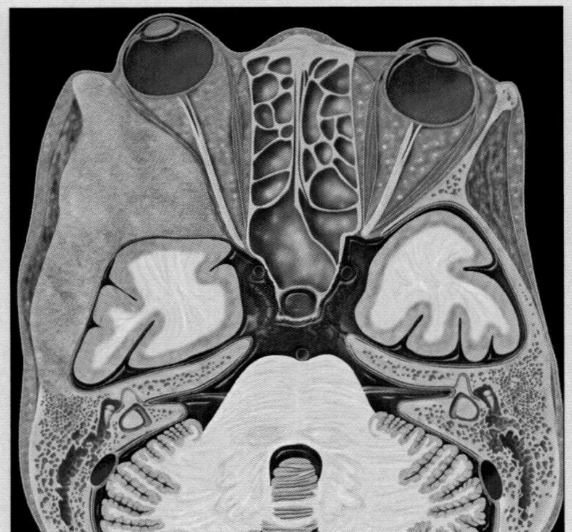

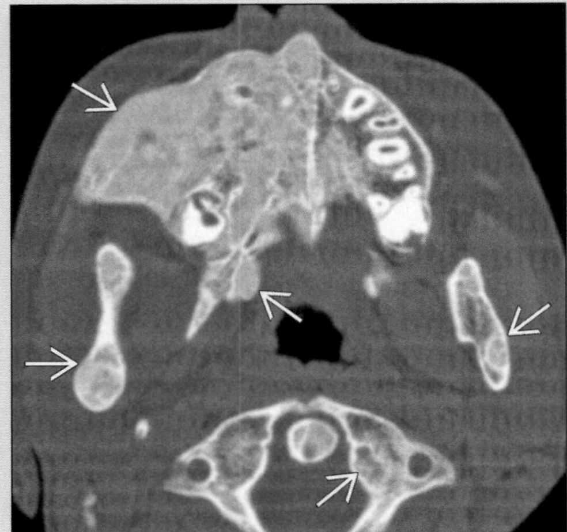

*(**Left**) Coronal 3D reconstruction demonstrates marked, asymmetric calvarial and facial bone thickening. Leontiasis ossea, named for its lion-like physiognomy, is caused by severe craniofacial osseous thickening. (**Right**) Axial T1WI C+ FS MR shows intense patchy enhancement within an expansile lesion ➡ without evidence for cortical breakthrough or abnormal dural enhancement.*

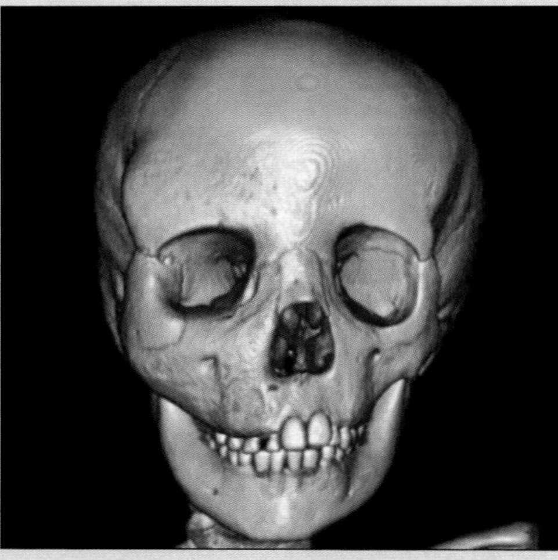

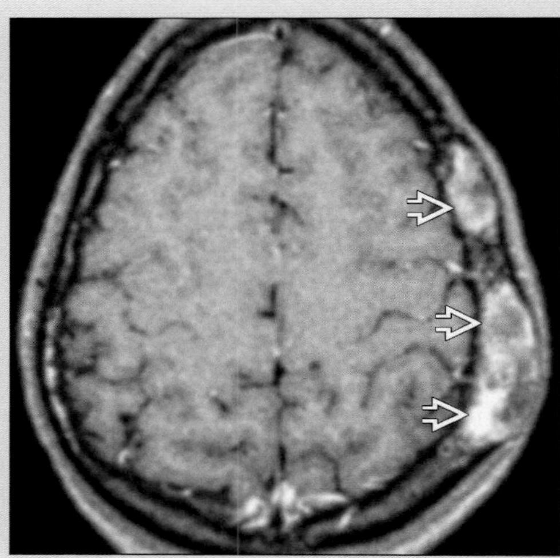

TERMINOLOGY

Abbreviations

- Fibrous dysplasia (FD)

Synonyms

- Craniofacial fibrous dysplasia (CFD); osteitis fibrosa; osteodystrophy fibrosa
- McCune-Albright syndrome (MAS): 1 of most common FD syndromes
- Jaffe-Lichtenstein dysplasia (monostotic FD)

Definitions

- Congenital disorder characterized by expanding lesions with mixture of fibrous tissue and woven bone
- Defect in osteoblastic differentiation and maturation
- 1 of most common fibroosseous lesions

IMAGING

General Features

- Best diagnostic clue
  - Ground-glass matrix in bone lesion on CT
- Location
  - May involve any aspect of skull
  - CFD: Majority have > 1 bone involved
    - Maxilla, orbit, and frontal bones most common in 1 series; ethmoids and sphenoids in another

Radiographic Findings

- Radiography
  - Expanded bone with ground-glass appearance
  - CFD: Dental malocclusions in 20%

CT Findings

- NECT
  - Imaging patterns relate to relative content of fibrous and osseous tissue
  - Expansile bone lesion, widened diploic space
  - CT shows "ground-glass," sclerotic, cystic, or mixed bone changes
    - If cystic may have thick sclerotic rind

MR Findings

- T1WI
  - Usual: ↓ T1WI signal
- T2WI
  - Usual: ↓ T2WI signal (if solid) or in rind (if cystic)
  - ↑ clinical-pathologic activity ⇒ ↑ signal
- T1WI C+
  - Variable enhancement depends on lesion pattern (rim, diffuse, or none)

Nuclear Medicine Findings

- Bone scan
  - Variable radionuclide uptake: Perfusion/delayed phases
  - Nonspecific; sensitive to extent of skeletal lesions in polyostotic FD
- PET
  - Accumulation of 11C-MET
  - Can be variably hot on FDG PET
    - Should not be mistaken for metastasis
    - Correlation with radiograph, CT helps

Imaging Recommendations

- Best imaging tool
  - Bone CT
- Protocol advice
  - CT or MR to define local extent
  - Bone scan to search for additional lesions

DIFFERENTIAL DIAGNOSIS

Paget Disease

- Pagetoid ground-glass FD mimics Paget disease
- Paget: Calvarium, not craniofacial; "cotton wool" CT

Garre Sclerosing Osteomyelitis

- Bony expansion, but inhomogeneous sclerotic pattern; ± dehiscent bone cortex; ± periosteal reaction

Jaffe-Campanacci (J-C) Syndrome

- Nonossifying fibromas, axillary freckling, and café-au-lait (lacks neurofibromas)
- Mimics polyostotic forms of FD
  - J-C café-au-lait: Coast of California (like neurofibromatosis 1)
  - McCune-Albright café-au-lait: Coast of Maine

Craniometaphyseal Dysplasia

- Hyperostosis and sclerosis of craniofacial bones ⇒ facial distortion, cranial nerve compression
- Abnormal modelling of long bone metaphyses; paranasal "bossing"

Meningioma

- Resulting hyperostosis mimics FD
- MR spectroscopy: Characteristic alanine peak

Other Disorders with Expanded Bone and Abnormal Bony Density

- Thalassemia: Maxillary sinus involvement typical; "hair on end" skull
- Osteopetrosis: Involvement of all bones
- Neurocutaneous disorders: Osteitis fibrosa cystica in
  - Tuberous sclerosis
  - Neurofibromatosis type 1
- Chronic renal failure: Renal osteodystrophy may simulate leontiasis ossea
- Morgagni syndrome of hyperostosis frontalis interna
  - Postmenopausal women, limited to frontal bone

PATHOLOGY

General Features

- Etiology
  - Mutation of Gsα protein in osteoblastic progenitor cells ⇒ ↑ proliferation; abnormal differentiation
- Genetics
  - Mutations in regulatory Gsα protein (encoded by *GNAS* gene) common to monostotic, polyostotic, and MAS

Staging, Grading, & Classification

- Monostotic vs. polyostotic

- Specific lesion type (pagetoid, sclerotic, cystic) relates to disease activity
  - Cystic, pagetoid, and sclerotic FD believed to represent (in order) most to least active
    - Cystic FD (11-21%): Hypodense (CT) except rind
    - Pagetoid mixed FD (56%): Ground-glass plus cystic change
    - Homogeneous sclerotic FD (23-34%)

Gross Pathologic & Surgical Features

- Fibrous, tan to gray gritty tissue
- Variable consistency depends upon fibrous vs. osseous components
- Woven bone immature, structurally weak, prone to fractures
- Hemorrhage, cystic change may be present

Microscopic Features

- Fibrous stroma, usually avascular, low cellularity
- Osseous metaplasia: Bone trabeculae made up of immature, woven bone seen as peculiar shapes floating in fibrous stroma
  - Looks like "Chinese letters" or "alphabet soup"

CLINICAL ISSUES

Presentation

- Most common signs/symptoms
  - Swelling &/or deformity, pain
- Clinical profile
  - Proptosis, cranial neuropathy (diplopia, hearing loss, blindness), atypical facial pain or numbness, headache
  - Multiple endocrine disorders typically with severe polyostotic FD
- Presentations: Monostotic, polyostotic, craniofacial (CFD), syndromic (many known syndromes)
  - Monostotic FD
    - 70% of all FD cases; single osseous site affected
      - Skull, face involved in 27%
      - Most common: Maxilla (especially zygomatic process), mandible (molar area)
      - Less common: Frontal > ethmoid, sphenoid > temporal > occipital bones
    - Older children/young adults (75% present < 30 years)
  - Polyostotic FD
    - 30% of all FD cases; involves ≥ 2 separate sites
    - Skull, face involved in 50%
    - Younger group, 2/3 have symptoms by age 10
  - CFD
    - Autosomal dominant, stabilizes with skeletal maturity
  - McCune-Albright syndrome (MAS)
    - Subtype of unilateral polyostotic FD: Clinical triad of polyostotic FD, hyperfunctioning endocrinopathies, café-au-lait spots
    - 5% of FD cases; appears earlier; affects more bones more severely
    - Renal phosphate wasting (50%) associated with elevation of circulating factor FGF-23; may result in rickets and osteomalacia
  - Mazabraud syndrome
    - Polyostotic FD, intramuscular myxoma
  - Cherubism: Familial bilateral FD of jaw
  - "Mulibrey" nanism: Severe, progressive growth failure; pericardial constriction; primarily Finland
    - **Mu**scle, **li**ver, **br**ain, **ey**e = triangular face; yellow ocular fundi pigment; hypoplastic tongue; peculiar high voice; nevae flammei 65%
    - FD of long bones in 25%

Demographics

- Age
  - < 6 years (39%), 6-10 years (27%), > 10 years (39%)
- Gender
  - MAS usually (but not exclusively) female
- Epidemiology
  - Actual incidence unknown
    - Monostotic FD is 6x more common than polyostotic FD
    - Calvarial involvement differs: Polyostotic FD (50%) > monostotic FD (25%)
    - Monostotic FD (75%): 25% found in skull, face
    - Polyostotic FD (25%): 50% found in skull, face

Natural History & Prognosis

- **Rare** progression to osteo-, fibrous-, chondro- and mesenchymal sarcoma
  - Usually polyostotic/syndromic forms
  - Nearly 1/2 arise following irradiation (marked increase in malignant potential)
- Monostotic craniofacial FD has excellent prognosis
- Most spontaneously "burn out" in teens, 20s

Treatment

- Aggressive resection reserved for visual loss, severe deformity ("vault" more accessible than skull base)
- No radiation therapy ⇒ malignant progression
- Bisphosphonate ameliorates course (pain, fractures) in polyostotic and monostotic forms

DIAGNOSTIC CHECKLIST

Consider

- Monostotic and polyostotic FD likely on same spectrum of phenotypic expression; consider checking for gene to predict complications

Image Interpretation Pearls

- Ground-glass appearance on plain films or CT, homogeneously decreased signal on T2WI characteristic

SELECTED REFERENCES

1. Dumitrescu CE et al: McCune-Albright syndrome. Orphanet J Rare Dis. 3:12, 2008
2. DiCaprio MR et al: Fibrous dysplasia. Pathophysiology, evaluation, and treatment. J Bone Joint Surg Am. 87(8):1848-64, 2005
3. MacDonald-Jankowski DS: Fibro-osseous lesions of the face and jaws. Clin Radiol. 59(1):11-25, 2004

FIBROUS DYSPLASIA

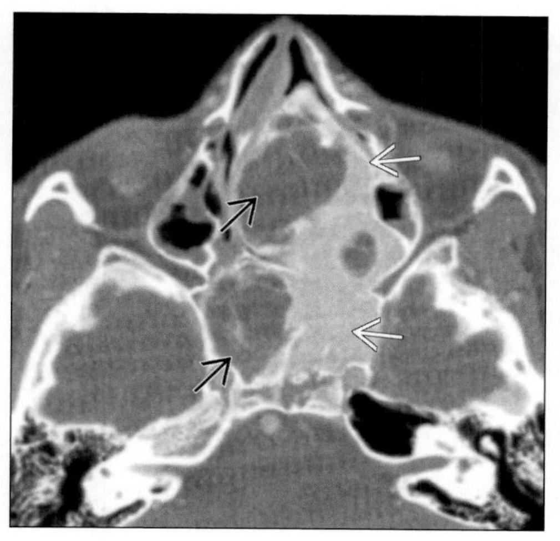

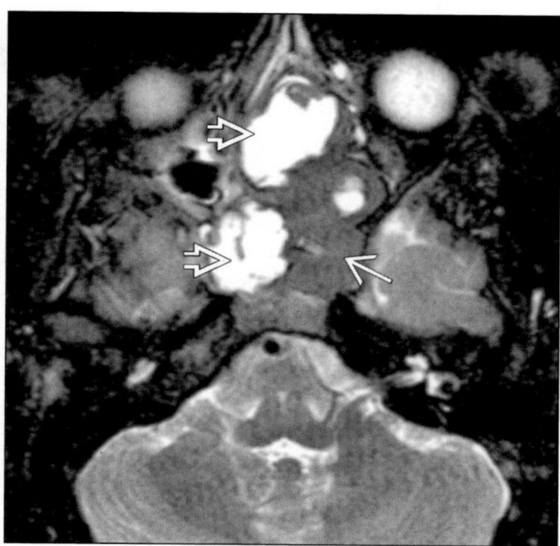

(Left) *Axial CECT demonstrates expansion of the sphenoid bone and turbinate by a complex mass consisting of cystic → and ground-glass solid → components. Note the obstruction of the left nasal cavity.* ***(Right)*** *Axial T2WI MR shows that the ground-glass components are quite low in signal → with high signal in the cystic component →. The cystic variant of fibrous dysplasia is the least common and likely represents the most active phase of the disease.*

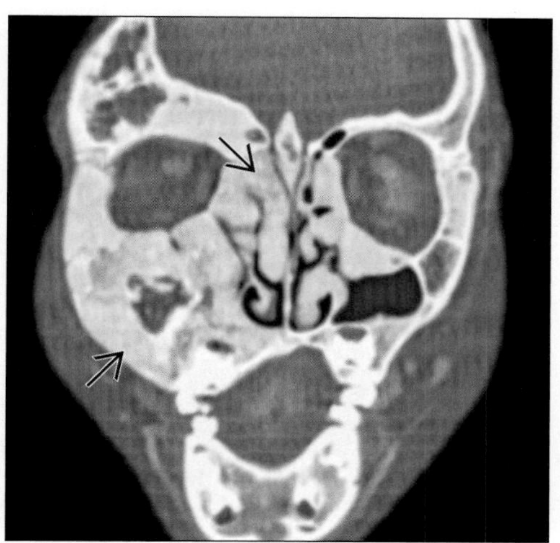

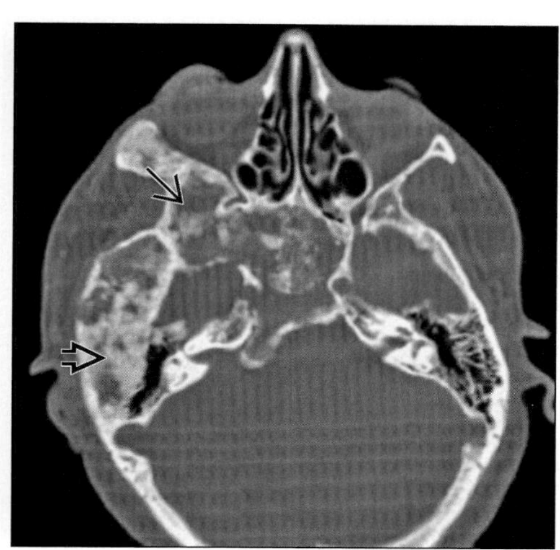

(Left) *Coronal NECT shows expansion of multiple facial bones with a classic ground-glass matrix encroaching and obliterating the maxillary and ethmoid sinuses →.* ***(Right)*** *Axial NECT shows a pagetoid mixed fibrous dysplasia with a ground-glass matrix → and cystic change → involving the sphenoid, zygomatic, and temporal bones.*

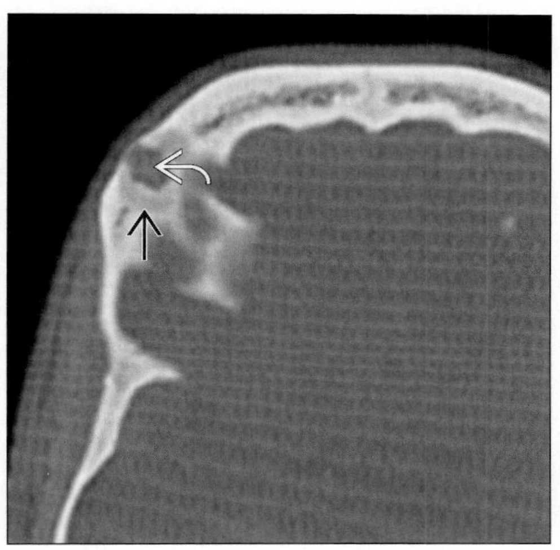

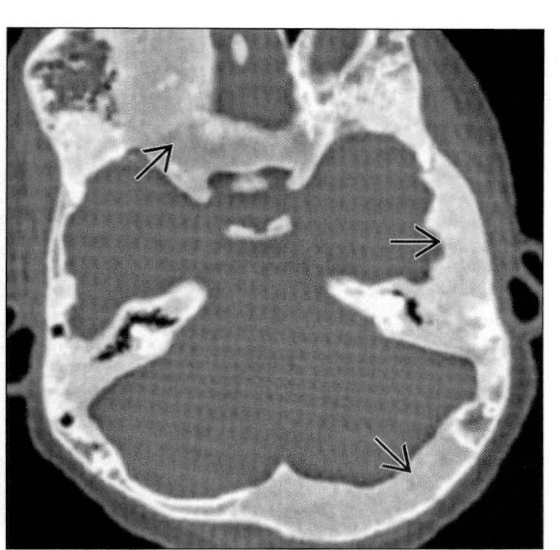

(Left) *Axial NECT shows a small cystic fibrous dysplasia of the superior orbital rim. Note the lucency → with a thick sclerotic "rind" →.* ***(Right)*** *Axial NECT shows classic fibrous dysplasia involving the calvarium and skull base with a homogeneous ground-glass matrix → and smooth bony expansion.*

PAGET DISEASE

Key Facts

Terminology

- Chronic metabolic skeletal disorder
- Characterized by bony expansion with variable destruction ± sclerosis

Imaging

- Well-circumscribed, sharply marginated defects &/or marked thickening + sclerosis
- Skull in 25-65% (may be isolated to skull base)
  - Diploic widening, coarse trabecula, thick cortices
  - "Tam-o'-shanter" skull: Marked ↑ diploic space, particularly inner table
  - "Cotton wool" skull: Focal sclerosis within previous areas of "osteoporosis circumscripta"
- Platybasia
- Typically "hot" throughout all bone scan acquisitions (blood flow, blood pool, static)
- Bone scans + radiographs abnormal in 56-86%

Top Differential Diagnoses

- Osteosclerotic metastases
- Osteolytic metastases
- Fibrous dysplasia
- Causes of calvarial thickening

Pathology

- Excessive and abnormal remodeling of bone, with both active and quiescent phases
- Individual sites progress at variable rates
  - Thus PD of differing phases may be seen within same patient

Clinical Issues

- 20% asymptomatic; pain, tenderness, ↑ hat size
- New pain/swelling → malignant transformation

*(**Left**) Coronal graphic illustrates diffuse Paget disease of the skull with severe diploic widening. (**Right**) Sagittal T1WI C+ MR in a patient with diffuse Paget disease of the calvarium shows markedly widened diploic space. Mostly maintained yellow marrow hyperintensity is seen within overall increased marrow fat ("atrophic marrow") →. Notice the platybasia deformity causing distortion of the brainstem →.*

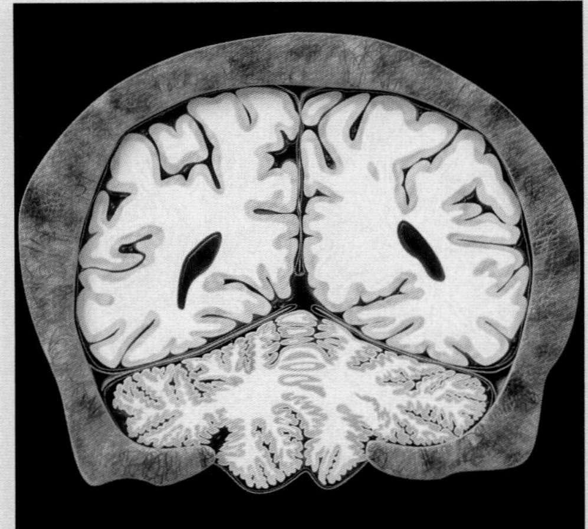

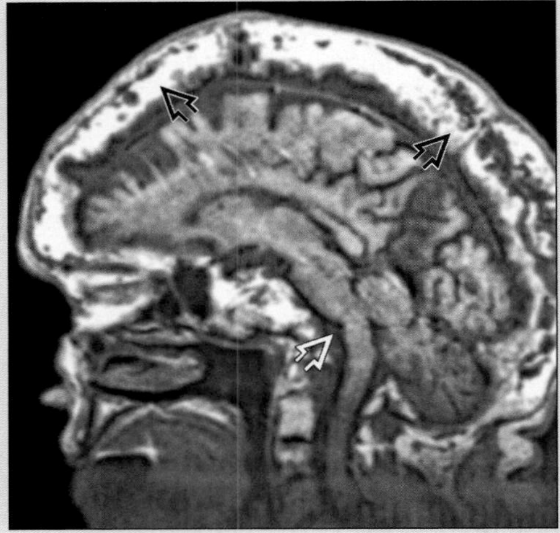

*(**Left**) Axial bone CT demonstrates both lytic and blastic Paget disease as evidenced by focal lysis → within a background of diffuse sclerotic diploic expansion and thickened cortices →, often adjacent to one another. (**Right**) Lateral radiograph shows the typical appearance of Paget disease with markedly thickened cortices →, diploic widening →, blastic lesions →, and platybasia.*

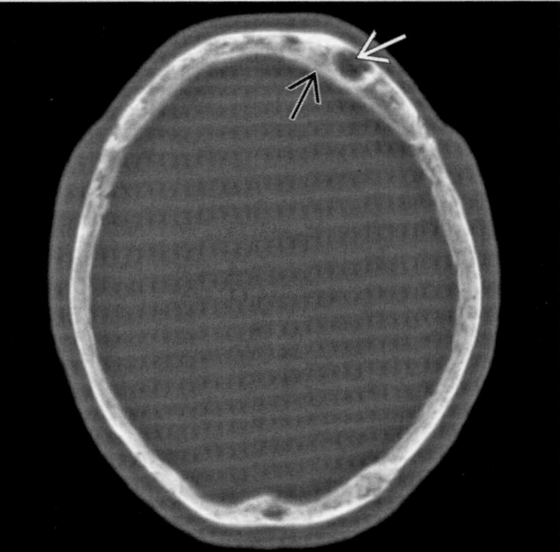

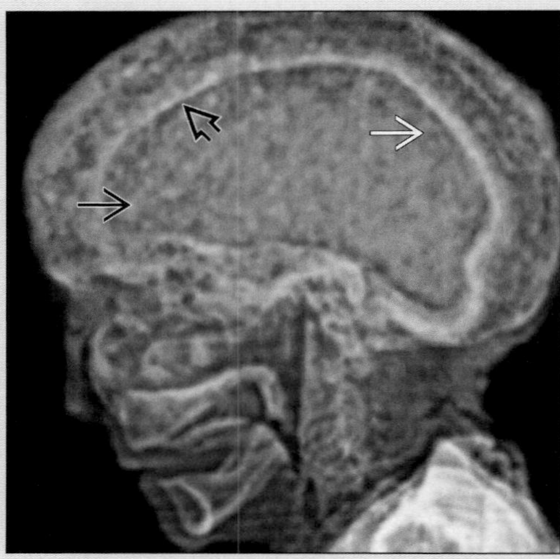

TERMINOLOGY

Abbreviations
- Paget disease (PD)

Synonyms
- Osteitis deformans

Definitions
- Chronic metabolic skeletal disorder
- Characterized by bony expansion with variable destruction ± sclerosis

IMAGING

General Features
- Best diagnostic clue
  - Well-circumscribed, sharply marginated defects &/or marked thickening + sclerosis
- Location
  - Monostotic (10-35%): Often axial skeleton
  - Polyostotic (65-90%)
  - Skull (25-65%): May be isolated to skull base

Radiographic Findings
- Radiography
  - Diploic widening, coarse trabecula, thick cortices
  - 3 phases identified
    - Early destructive phase
      - Well-defined lysis; commonly frontal > occipital
      - "Osteoporosis/osteolysis circumscripta"
      - Inner and outer tables involved; inner > outer
    - Intermediate phase
      - Both lytic and blastic lesions
      - Trabeculae & cortices coarsening & thickening
    - Late sclerotic phase
      - Blastic lesions, often crossing sutures
      - "Tam-o'-shanter" skull: Marked ↑ diploic space, particularly inner table
      - "Cotton wool" skull: Focal sclerosis within previous areas of "osteoporosis circumscripta"
  - Platybasia with variable basilar invagination

CT Findings
- NECT
  - Bones: 3 phases (same as radiography)
  - Platybasia with basilar invagination (BI)
  - Sarcomatous transformation
    - Aggressive osteolysis, cortical destruction, soft tissue mass, without periosteal reaction
  - Giant cell tumor (GCT) transformation
    - Lytic lesion without periosteal reaction or mass
    - Marrow replacement distinguishes from PD lysis
    - Cystic and hemorrhagic regions possible
  - PD pseudomass
    - "Soft tissue mass" 2° periosteal lifting by active PD
    - Significant absence of lysis
- CECT
  - ↑ enhancement reflecting pathologic ↑ vascularity
  - Sarcomatous transformation: Mass enhancement, often with central necrosis, aggressive lysis, cortical destruction
  - GCT transformation: Enhancing solid tumor areas

MR Findings
- T1WI
  - Yellow marrow hyperintensity usually maintained
    - Occasionally have more fat than uninvolved bone
  - Early destructive to early intermediate phase
    - ↓ marrow intensity 2° marrow replacement
    - Residual normal yellow marrow foci → excludes malignant transformation
  - Late sclerotic phase: Marrow hypointensity from sclerosis of coarse trabeculae and cortical thickening
  - PD pseudomass: Maintained areas of yellow marrow
- T2WI
  - Marrow changes with marrow replacement
- T1WI C+
  - ↑ enhancement reflecting pathologic ↑ vascularity
- MR findings of PD complications
  - Distortion and flattening of brain
  - Brainstem impingement from BI
  - Acquired Chiari 1 malformation
  - Sarcomatous transformation
    - Marrow replacement, focal bone destruction, soft tissue mass
  - GCT transformation
    - Lytic lesion without periosteal reaction/mass
    - Marrow replacement allows it to be distinguished from normal lytic phase of PD
    - Cystic and hemorrhagic regions possible

Nuclear Medicine Findings
- Bone scan
  - Marked uptake throughout all phases of PD
    - Typically "hot" throughout all bone scan acquisitions (blood flow, blood pool, static)
    - Findings may precede radiographic changes
  - Can be "cold" or normal in late sclerotic stage
  - Findings that suggest recurrence
    - New uptake, extension beyond initial boundaries
    - Cold foci in areas of ↑ activity of bone destruction
- Sulfur colloid scan: ↓ uptake = marrow replacement

Imaging Recommendations
- Best imaging tool
  - Radiography + bone scan
    - Bone scans + radiographs abnormal in 56-86%
    - Bone scan alone abnormal in 2-23%
    - Radiographs alone abnormal in 11-20%
  - NECT defines detail/extent, especially PD of skull base
  - MR for imaging PD complications
- Protocol advice
  - NECT: High-resolution, thin-cuts through skull base
  - MR
    - Coronal + sagittal sequences for BI
    - T1WI C+ to evaluate for malignant transformation

DIFFERENTIAL DIAGNOSIS

Osteosclerotic Metastases
- Classically prostate, breast, lymphoma

Osteolytic Metastases
- Most metastases, including lung, renal, thyroid

Fibrous Dysplasia

- Ground-glass appearance, outer > inner table involved

Causes of Calvarial Thickening

- Hyperostosis frontalis interna, meningioma, chronic calcified subdural hematoma

PATHOLOGY

General Features

- Etiology
  - Unknown
  - Viral theory
    - Probable chronic paramyxoviral infection, possibly measles
    - Intranuclear inclusion bodies found in osteoclasts
  - Genetic theory supported by findings listed above
  - Familial as well as geographic "foci" clustering support both environmental & genetic factors
- Genetics
  - Ashkenazi Jewish: ↑ prevalence of PD with associated ↑ frequency of HLA-DR2
  - North New Jersey patients with multifocal GCT and PD: Common ancestry to Avellino, Italy
  - "Hereditary hyperphosphatasia," a.k.a. "juvenile Paget disease": Rare; patients of Puerto Rican descent
  - ↑ expression of genes involved in inhibition of apoptosis, notably *Bcl-2*
  - Mutations in *p62* gene associated with PD
- Associated abnormalities
  - ↑ aortic stenosis, heart and bundle branch block

Gross Pathologic & Surgical Features

- Abnormally soft new bone causing deformity

Microscopic Features

- Early destructive phase: Giant osteoclasts with numerous nuclei show intense activity and aggressive bone resorption
  - Fibrovascular tissue with large vascular channels replaces normal yellow marrow
- Intermediate phase: ↓ osteoclastic and ↑ osteoblastic activity; gradual return of yellow marrow
- Late sclerotic phase: ↓ osteoblastic activity, bone turnover, and vascularity
- General histopathologic findings
  - Cement lines along coarsened/enlarged trabeculae characteristic; denotes bone resorption & formation
  - Trabecular thickening lacks normal interconnections and are weak; a.k.a. "pumice" bone
  - Cortices thickened, have most active bone turnover and repair
  - Areas of resorption and formation are hypervascular
  - Often ↑ in marrow fat ("atrophic marrow")

CLINICAL ISSUES

Presentation

- Most common signs/symptoms
  - 20% asymptomatic
  - Fatigue, pain, tenderness, ↑ hat size
  - Hyperthermia from hypervascularity
  - Cranial nerve deficit(s), pulsatile tinnitus
  - New pain/swelling → malignant transformation
- Clinical profile
  - Older patients
  - ↑ serum alk. phos. (mixed and blastic phase)
  - ↑ serum/urine hydroxyproline (lytic phase)

Demographics

- Age
  - > 40 years; unusual < 40 years
- Gender
  - M:F = 2:1, onset slightly younger in men
- Ethnicity
  - Caucasians > African-Americans > Africans
  - Ashkenazi Jewish have ↑ prevalence
- Epidemiology
  - 3-4% > 40 years; 10-11% > 80 years
- Geographic distribution
  - Overall ↑ prevalence in northern latitudes
  - ↑ in Great Britain: Lands settled by British (Australia, New Zealand, USA) share ↑ prevalence
  - Rare in Asia and Africa (excluding South Africa)

Natural History & Prognosis

- 10% develop secondary hyperparathyroidism from hypercalcemia related to aggressive bone remodeling
- Skull base thickening → CN deficit(s), sensorineural hearing loss (cochlear involvement), mixed hearing loss (stapes fixation to oval window)
- BI in up to 30%; more common in women → brainstem compression, syrinx, obstructive hydrocephalus
- Malignant transformation
  - Sarcomatous transformation (1% or less)
    - M:F = 2:1; 55-80 years
    - Osteosarcoma (50-60%), fibrosarcoma/malignant fibrous histiocytoma (20-25%), chondrosarcoma (10%)
    - Metastasizes frequently, most commonly to lung
  - GCT
    - Skull/facial GCT almost always associated with PD
    - M:F = 1.6:1; 32-85 years
    - Solitary or multiple; 91% in polyostotic PD
    - Rarely cause mortality; generally do not metastasize

Treatment

- Medical
  - Goal: Control, reduction, and alleviation of pain, rather than return to normal bone
    - Calcitonin, bisphosphonates, mithramycin
    - NSAIDs and acetaminophen for pain management
    - Radiography may or may not improve/normalize
- Biopsy with CT guidance needed to diagnose sarcomatous transformation

SELECTED REFERENCES

1. Cundy T et al: Paget disease of bone. Trends Endocrinol Metab. 19(7):246-53, 2008
2. Smith SE et al: From the archives of the AFIP. Radiologic spectrum of Paget disease of bone and its complications with pathologic correlation. Radiographics. 22(5): 1191-216, 2002

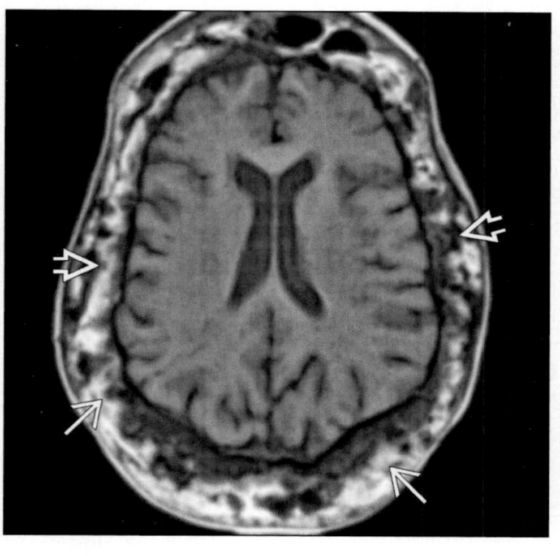

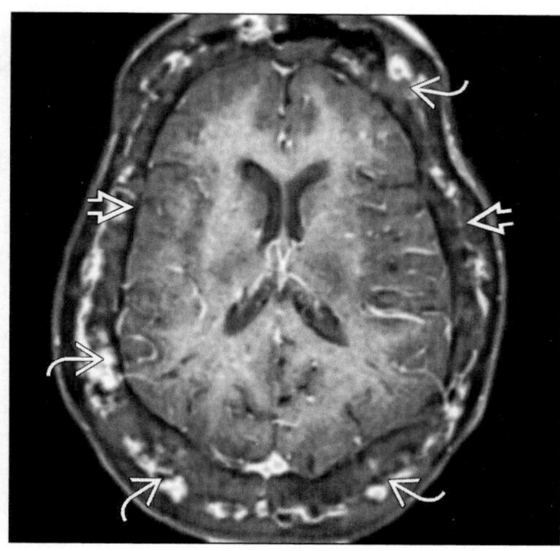

(Left) *Axial T1WI MR of diffuse, extensive skull Paget disease demonstrates diffuse calvarial diploic thickening with T1 heterogeneous marrow. Note the areas of fatty marrow* ➡ *with hypointense marrow replacement* ⇨*.* ***(Right)*** *Axial T1WI C+ MR of a patient with diffuse, extensive skull Paget disease reveals diploic widening, decreased intensity from marrow replacement* ⇨*, and scattered enhancement of abnormal vascularity* ↷*.*

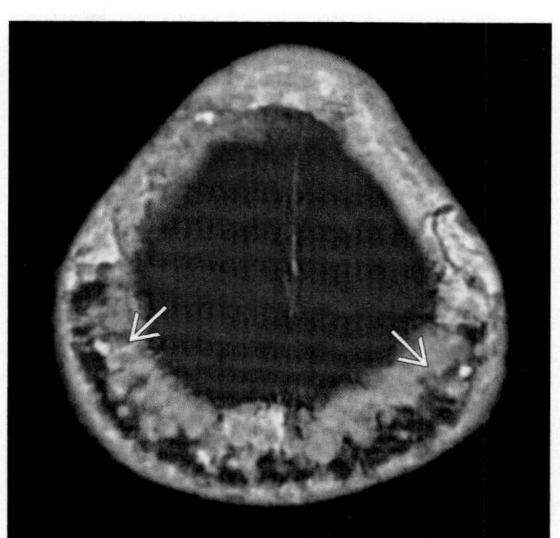

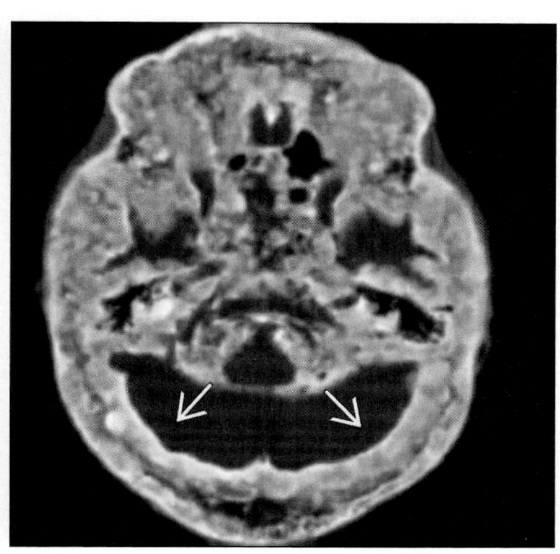

(Left) *Axial NECT shows the typical appearance of Paget disease, with patchy areas of calvarial thickening and multiple sclerotic areas* ➡ *in a background of osteolysis "cotton wool" appearance.* ***(Right)*** *Axial NECT demonstrates diffuse Paget disease of the skull base with diploic widening, coarsened trabeculae, and thick cortices* ➡*.*

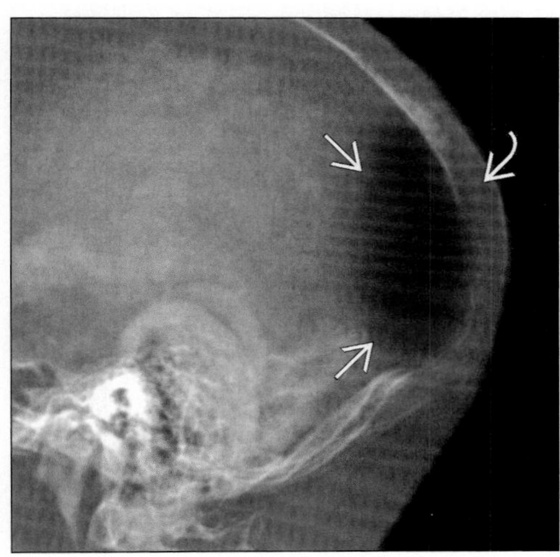

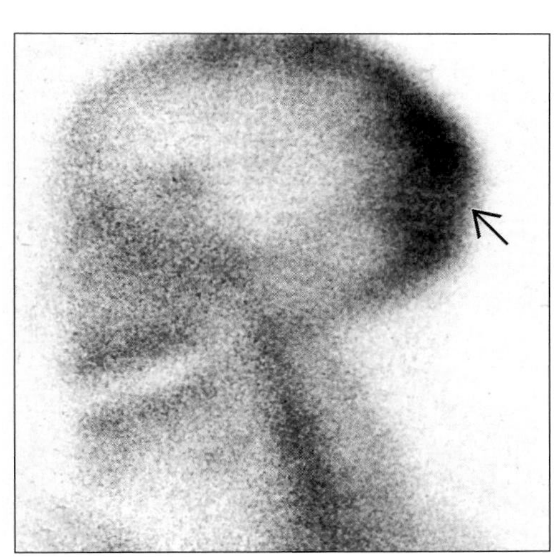

(Left) *Lateral radiograph shows a lytic phase "osteoporosis circumscripta"* ➡ *in the occipital bone, associated with calvarium thickening* ↷*. This appearance is virtually pathognomonic for Paget disease.* ***(Right)*** *Lateral bone scan demonstrates marked radiotracer uptake in the occipital region* ➡*, corresponding to the "osteoporosis circumscripta" seen on the skull radiograph.*

EXTRAMEDULLARY HEMATOPOIESIS

Key Facts

Terminology
- Extramedullary compensatory formation of blood elements due to decreased medullary hematopoiesis

Imaging
- Skull (epidural, dura matter, sinuses), spine (paraspinal, epidural)
  - Too thick or dense skull
  - May show findings of underlying disease
- Contrast-enhanced MR
  - Smooth juxtaspinal or cranial homogeneous masses in patients with chronic anemias or marrow depletion
- Look for local complication
  - Cranial foramina, nerves
  - Spinal nerve involvement
  - Cord compression

Top Differential Diagnoses
- Meningioma
- Metastases
- Subdural collections
- Intracranial hypotension

Pathology
- Primarily patients with congenital hemoglobinopathies
- "Trilineage" hyperplasia: Erythroid, myeloid, and megakaryocytic elements

Diagnostic Checklist
- EMH in unexplained extraaxial "collections" or perivertebral masses in child with congenital anemia or other hematological disorder
- EMH is dural &/or subdural hematoma mimic

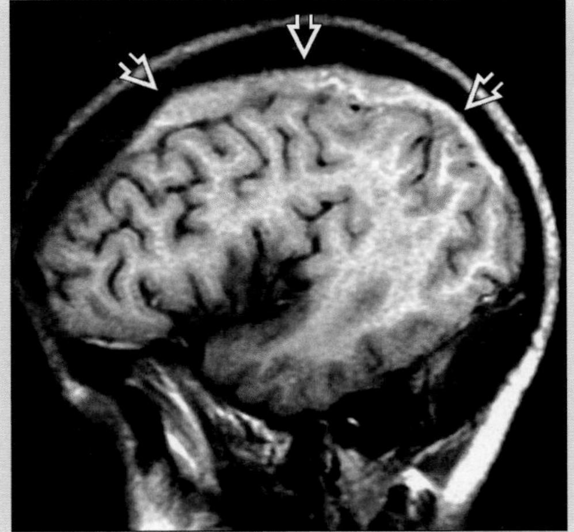
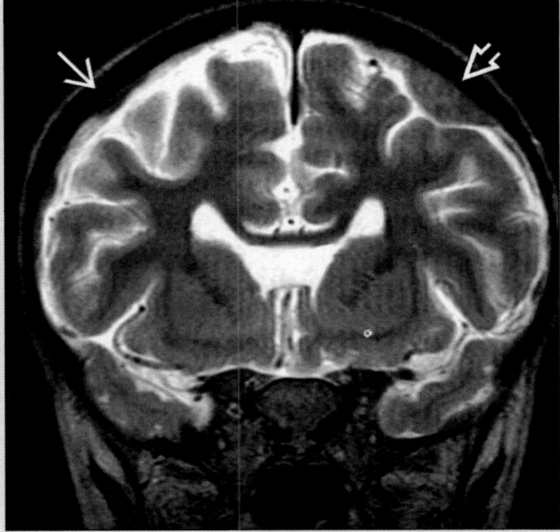

(Left) *Sagittal T1WI MR in an 8-year-old girl with myelosclerosis and callosal dysgenesis of an unknown cause. Slightly T1-hyperintense epidural tissue ⊡ overlies the hemisphere; the bone appears normal.* ***(Right)*** *Coronal T2WI MR demonstrates an extraaxial mass, likely epidural. The dura may be raised, over the left frontal lobe; the T2 signal ⊡ is identical to the brain. Mild dural thickening ➡ is seen on the right. The absent septum pellucidum is associated with the callosal dysgenesis.*

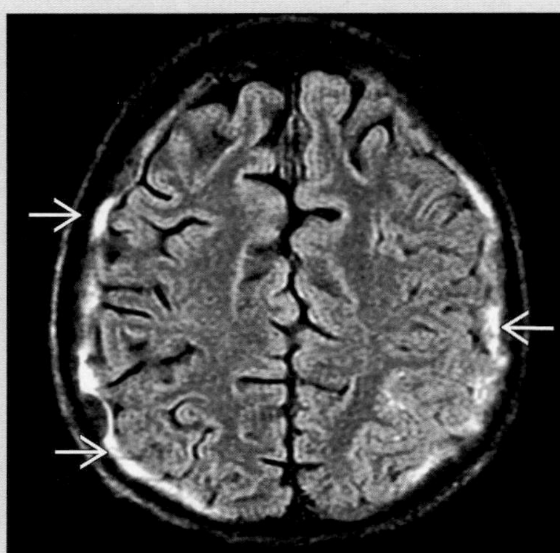
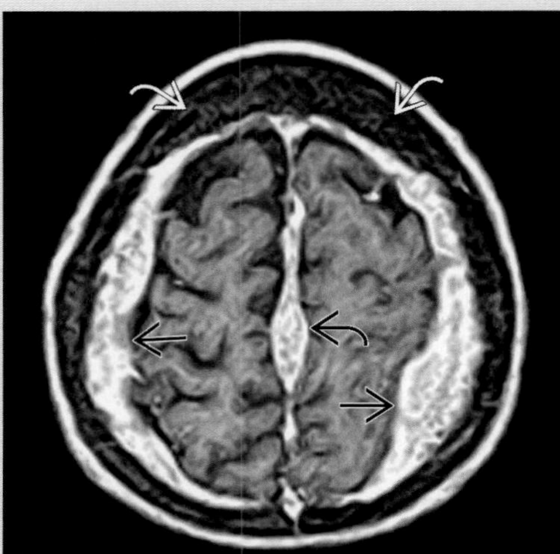

(Left) *Axial FLAIR MR in the same 8-year-old patient with myelosclerosis demonstrates heterogeneously bright FLAIR signal ➡ within the dural/epidural abnormal tissue that surrounds the brain.* ***(Right)*** *Axial T1WI C+ MR demonstrates avid enhancement in the dural/epidural lesions over the cerebral convexities ⇒ and along the falx cerebri ↪. The diagnosis of EMH was confirmed by a dural biopsy. Note the overlying calvarial thickening ↪.*

EXTRAMEDULLARY HEMATOPOIESIS

TERMINOLOGY

Abbreviations
- Extramedullary hematopoiesis (EMH)

Synonyms
- Extramedullary erythropoiesis

Definitions
- Extramedullary compensatory formation of blood elements due to decreased medullary hematopoiesis

IMAGING

General Features
- Best diagnostic clue
  - Smooth juxtaspinal or cranial homogeneous masses in patients with chronic anemia or marrow depletion
- Location
  - Skull (epidural, dura matter, sinuses), spine (paraspinal, epidural)
- Size
  - Variable, sometimes huge
- Morphology
  - Smooth, juxtaosseous circumscribed masses
  - Hypercellular tissue

Radiographic Findings
- Radiography
  - May show findings of underlying disease
    - Thalassemia → "hair-on-end" skull
    - Osteopetrosis → dense bone obliterating medullary space

CT Findings
- NECT
  - Smooth, homogeneous, isodense masses
    - May mimic subdural hematoma, lymphoma
    - Also simulates en plaque meningioma
  - May show osseous findings of underlying disease
    - Too thick or dense skull
    - Enlarged diploe
    - Changes of vertebral structure
  - Soft tissue filling paranasal sinus(es), orbits, juxtasellar
- CECT
  - Homogeneous enhancement

MR Findings
- T1WI
  - Iso- to slightly hyperintense to cortex
- T2WI
  - Slightly hypointense to cortex
- FLAIR
  - Hyperintense
  - No underlying parenchymal edema
- T1WI C+
  - Homogeneous enhancement
  - Simulates en plaque meningioma

Nuclear Medicine Findings
- Uptake by Tc-99m-sulfur colloid

Imaging Recommendations
- Best imaging tool
  - Contrast-enhanced MR
- Protocol advice
  - Investigate bone as well as soft tissue masses
    - Etiological context usually known
    - CT: Thickening of diploe, erosions, paranasal sinus disease
    - MR: Bone marrow changes in vertebral bodies
  - Look for local complication
    - Cranial foramina, nerves
    - Spinal nerve involvement
    - Cord compression

DIFFERENTIAL DIAGNOSIS

Meningioma
- Different context, different bony findings
- MRS (often impossible in masses adjacent to bone): Characteristic alanine peak

Metastases
- Often multifocal, infiltrative, skull invasion

Subdural Collections
- Trauma history
- Enhancement of limiting membranes, not diffuse

Intracranial Hypotension
- Thick skull, thick enhancing dura
- History of CSF diversion or leak
- Slit ventricles
- Tonsillar descent, bulging pituitary
- Enlarged venous dural sinuses

Neurosarcoid
- Abnormal chest radiograph, labs

Other Paraspinal Masses
- Spondylitis, abscesses: Bone, disk involved, peripheral abscesses
- Lymphoma

PATHOLOGY

General Features
- Etiology
  - Hematogenous stem cell spread to different organs
    - Liver and spleen
    - Kidneys
    - Lungs
    - Peritoneum
    - Juxtaosseous also common
      - Face
      - Skull
      - Spine
  - Primarily patients with congenital hemoglobinopathies
    - Thalassemia
    - Sickle cell disease
    - Hereditary spherocytosis
    - Hemorrhagic thrombocytopenia

EXTRAMEDULLARY HEMATOPOIESIS

- Leukemia
- Lymphoma
- Myeloid metaplasia
- Others
  - May be secondary to any depleted, infiltrated, or hyperactive bone marrow
    - Can be seen after granulocyte colony-stimulating factor therapy
  - May be seen in any myelosclerosis
    - Hematological disorders (e.g., polycythemia vera)
    - Bone diseases
    - Exposure to ionizing radiation, benzene
- Occasionally no etiology found
- Genetics
  - Genetics of causal disease
    - Congenital hemoglobinopathies
    - Genetic hemopathies
    - Myelosclerosis of genetic causes
- Associated abnormalities
  - Secondary subdural hemorrhage from EMH involvement of dura reported

Gross Pathologic & Surgical Features

- Peri-osseous soft tissue masses
- Epidural EMH may compress underlying neural tissue
- Associated bony changes

Microscopic Features

- "Trilineage" hyperplasia
  - Erythroid elements
  - Myeloid elements
  - Megakaryocytic elements

CLINICAL ISSUES

Presentation

- Most common signs/symptoms
  - Asymptomatic
  - Seizures
  - Cranial nerve deficit(s) at skull base
  - Increased intracranial pressure if compressing dural sinuses
- Clinical profile
  - Generally older adults with myelofibrosis
  - Younger patients with congenital hemolytic anemias

Demographics

- Age
  - Generally in older ages
  - But EMH has its own specific pediatric causes
- Gender
  - Equal
- Epidemiology
  - Rare

Natural History & Prognosis

- Evolution dependent on primary underlying disease
- Compensatory for bone marrow failure
- Uncommonly, local complications related to compression

Treatment

- Treat primary disease
- Low-dose radiotherapy treatment of choice
  - Remember that hematopoietic tissue is extremely sensitive to irradiation
- Surgical resection

DIAGNOSTIC CHECKLIST

Consider

- EMH in unexplained extraaxial "collections" or perivertebral masses in child with congenital anemia or other hematological disorder

Image Interpretation Pearls

- EMH is dural &/or subdural hematoma mimic

SELECTED REFERENCES

1. Debard A et al: Dural localization of extramedullary hematopoiesis. Report of a case. J Neurol. 256(5):837-8, 2009
2. Ashkzaran HR et al: Epidural extramedullary hematopoiesis. JBR-BTR. 91(3):82-3, 2008
3. Baehring JM: Cord compression caused by extramedullary hematopoiesis within the epidural space. J Neurooncol. 86(2):173-4, 2008
4. Meo A et al: Effect of hydroxyurea on extramedullary haematopoiesis in thalassaemia intermedia: case reports and literature review. Int J Lab Hematol. 30(5):425-31, 2008
5. Tun K et al: Meningeal extramedullary haematopoiesis mimicking subdural hematoma. J Clin Neurosci. 15(2):208-10, 2008
6. Ittipunkul N et al: Extra-medullary hematopoiesis causing bilateral optic atrophy in beta thalassemia/Hb E disease. J Med Assoc Thai. 90(4):809-12, 2007
7. Takahashi S et al: Paravertebral extramedulary hematopoiesis arising with osteopetrosis tarda. Intern Med. 46(18):1589-92, 2007
8. Tsitsopoulos P et al: Lumbar nerve root compression due to extramedullary hemopoiesis in a patient with thalassemia: complete clinical regression with radiation therapy. Case report and review of the literature. J Neurosurg Spine. 6(2):156-60, 2007
9. Collins WO et al: Extramedullary hematopoiesis of the paranasal sinuses in sickle cell disease. Otolaryngol Head Neck Surg. 132(6):954-6, 2005
10. Haidar S et al: Intracranial involvement in extramedullary hematopoiesis: case report and review of the literature. Pediatr Radiol. 35(6):630-4, 2005
11. Koch CA et al: Nonhepatosplenic extramedullary hematopoiesis: associated diseases, pathology, clinical course, and treatment. Mayo Clin Proc. 78(10):1223-33, 2003
12. Rizzo L et al: Extramedullary hematopoiesis: unusual meningeal and paranasal sinuses presentation in Paget disease. Case report. Radiol Med (Torino). 105(4):376-81, 2003
13. Chourmouzi D et al: MRI findings of extramedullary haemopoiesis. Eur Radiol. 11(9):1803-6, 2001
14. Aarabi B et al: Visual failure caused by suprasellar extramedullary hematopoiesis in beta thalassemia: case report. Neurosurgery. 42(4):922-5; discussion 925-6, 1998

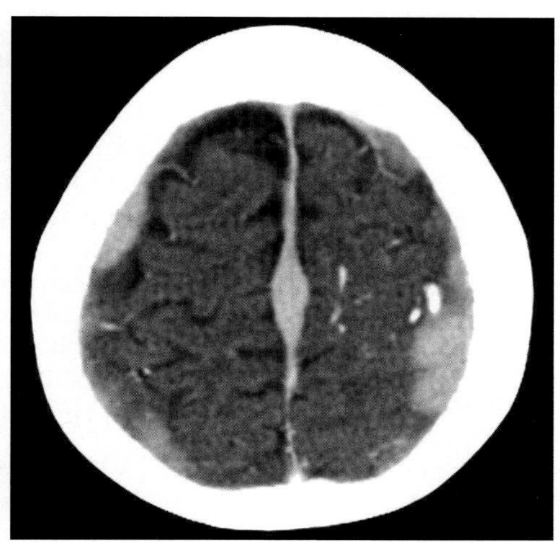

(Left) *Axial NECT in an 8-year-old girl with myelofibrosis shows multiple extraaxial masses, most likely due to dural, epidural, &/or subdural. Note the falx where the mass is shown on both sides of the dural layer. The masses are slightly denser than brain, with (probably) dural calcifications, consistent with EMH.* ***(Right)*** *Axial CECT in the same patient demonstrates diffuse, rather homogeneous enhancement of the lesions, again in keeping with EMH. This was confirmed by biopsy.*

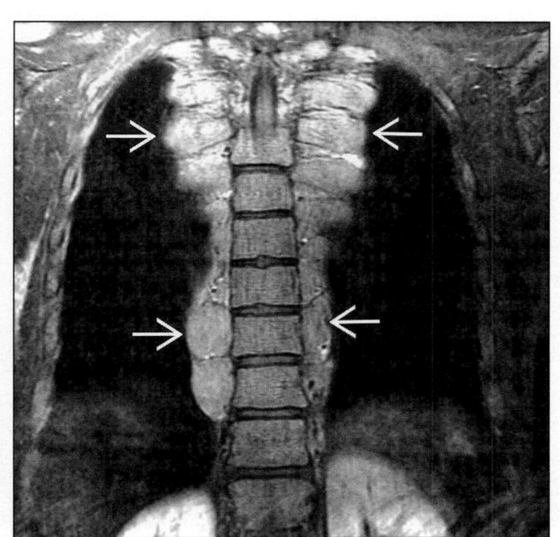

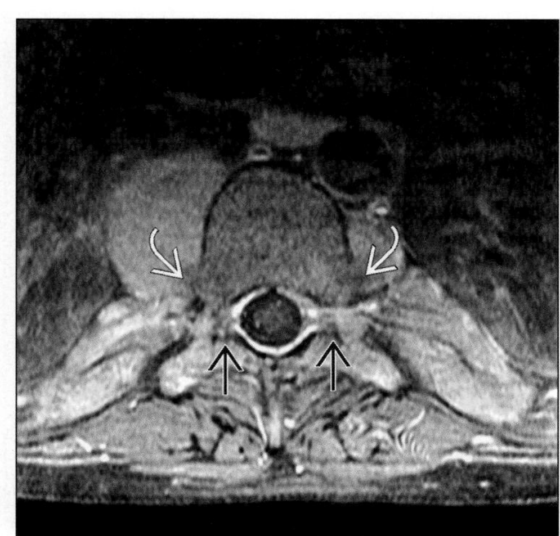

(Left) *Coronal T1WI C+ FS MR in a 17-year-old child with thalassemia. Multiple paravertebral masses are seen along the thoracic vertebral, extending into intercostal spaces. Given the context, appearances, and homogeneous enhancement, they likely represent EMH.* ***(Right)*** *Axial T1WI C+ FS MR demonstrates in-plane extension of the masses, especially into the intervertebral foramina bilaterally, where they involve the spinal nerves. Note the absence of cortical bone.*

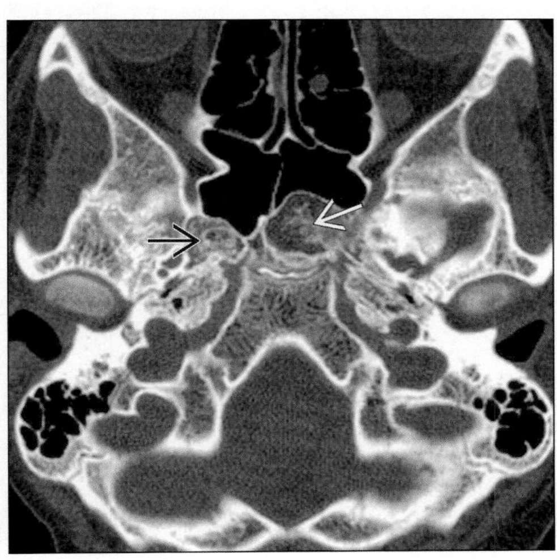

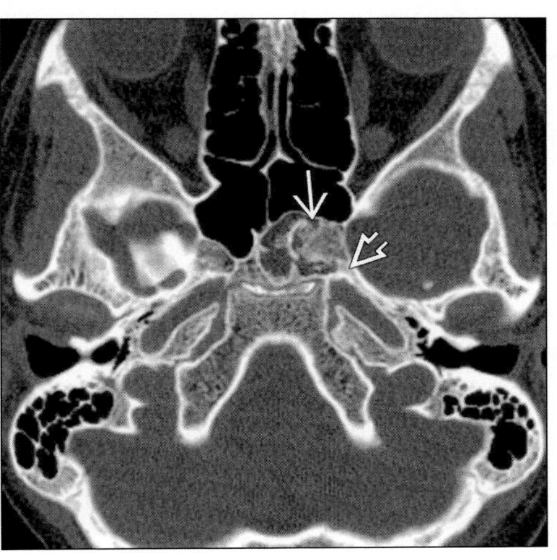

(Left) *Axial bone CT in a 13 year old with thalassemia. Asymptomatic masses within the body of the sphenoid and the base of the right pterygoid plate with bone expansion but preservation of the cortex, are suggestive of, but not specific for EMH.* ***(Right)*** *Axial bone CT at a higher level shows the proximity of the sphenoid body lesion to the carotid canal. This patient had multiple sites of proven EMH in other locations; thus, this is the most likely diagnosis.*

THICK SKULL

Key Facts

Terminology
- Skull thickening (ST)
  - Diploic space expanded ± thickened cortex

Imaging
- Widened calvarium (skull width)
  - Can be diffuse or focal
- NECT best for most causes of ST
  - Thin-section MDCT for detail skull base evaluation
- MR + contrast
  - If aggressive causes suspected (e.g, metastases)
  - Look for adjacent dural involvement

Top Differential Diagnoses
- Normal variation (most common cause)
- Hyperostosis interna
  - Bilateral, symmetric, usually frontal
- Paget disease
- Shunted hydrocephalus
  - With or without phenytoin
- Metastases (diffuse sclerotic)
- Microcephaly
- Chronic anemias

Clinical Issues
- Most often asymptomatic
- Patients with skull base ST
  - Look for foraminal/canal overgrowth/ encroachment
  - May cause cranial neuropathy
- Many tests can help discriminate among etiologies
- Skull findings often harbinger of underlying disease
- Therapy aimed at treating underlying etiology

Diagnostic Checklist
- What is underlying cause of skull thickening?

(Left) Axial bone CT demonstrates a diffusely thick skull, which is commonly seen as a normal variation. *(Right)* Axial T1WI MR shows typical focal skull thickening from bifrontal benign hyperostosis ➔, a commonly seen incidental entity.

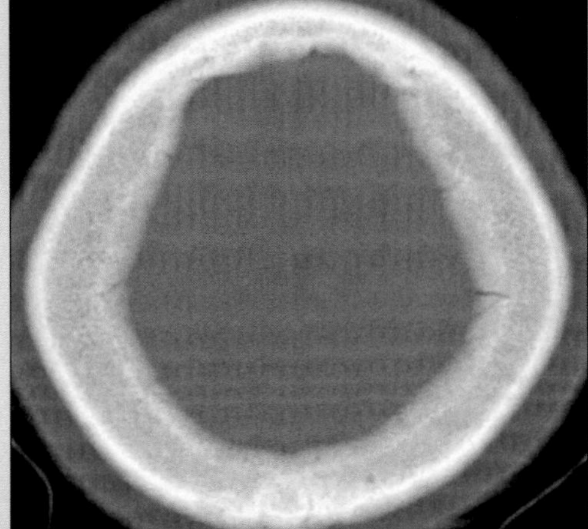

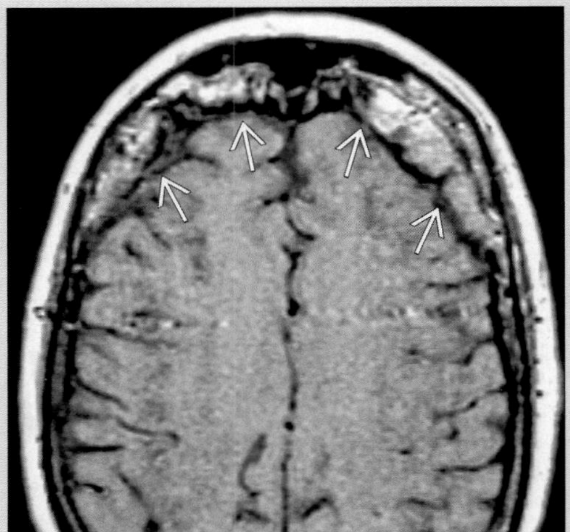

(Left) Axial T1WI MR shows the typical appearance of diffuse heterogeneous marrow with calvarial diploic thickening from extensive involvement by Paget disease ➔. Note the areas of hypointense marrow replacement ➔. *(Right)* Axial bone CT shows a diffuse thick skull with focal sclerotic regions ➔ in a patient with prostate metastasis.

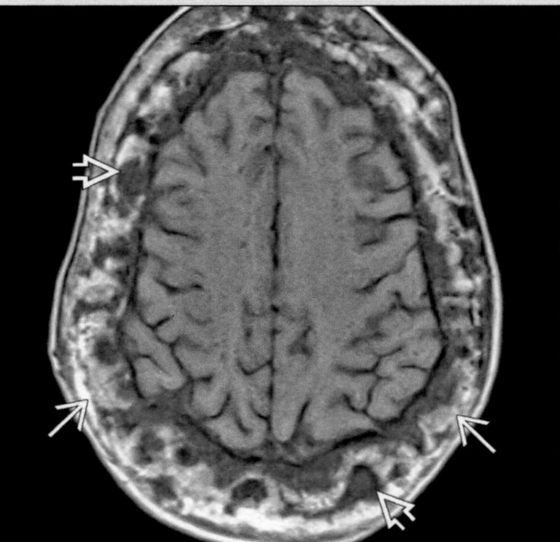

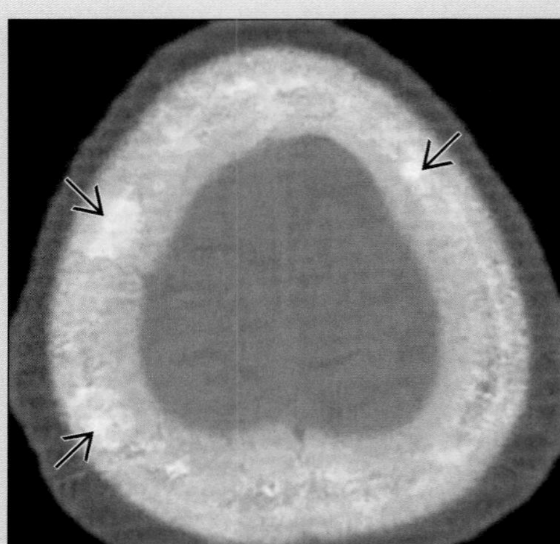

THICK SKULL

TERMINOLOGY

Abbreviations

- Skull thickening (ST)
- Calvarial thickening

Definitions

- Diploic space expansion ± adjacent cortical thickening

IMAGING

General Features

- Best diagnostic clue
  - Widened skull width, either diffuse or focal
- Location
  - Any bone can be involved
    - Frontal (older women), parietal bones most commonly affected
    - Calvarium > skull base
  - Occipital squamae do not contain marrow (usually spared)
- Size
  - Highly variable
    - Large/diffuse (involving nearly entire skull)
    - Small focal/regional involvement (any location)
- Morphology
  - Generalized
  - Regional or focal
    - Highly dependent on underlying etiology

Radiographic Findings

- Radiography
  - Insensitive for diffuse, although may be apparent when skull thickening is striking
  - Focal thickening more easily appreciated as subtle but definite increased density without defined borders
  - Some etiologies have dramatic and unique findings, which can quickly lead to cause
    - e.g., Paget disease → "cotton wool" skull
    - e.g., β-thalassemia → "hair on end" skull

CT Findings

- NECT
  - Thickened skull
    - Generalized or focal
    - Appearance can vary dependent on etiology
    - Inner table, outer table, diploic space involvement varies dependent on etiology
  - Findings may be classic/pathognomic
    - Dyke-Davidoff-Masson syndrome: Cerebral atrophy with ipsilateral compensatory osseous hypertrophy and hyperpneumatization of paranasal sinuses
    - β-thalassemia: "Hair on end" skull
    - Shunted hydrocephalus: Thick skull + shunt + chronic collapsed ventricles
    - Fibrous dysplasia: Medullary expansion with ground-glass appearance
- CECT
  - Some etiologies may show diploic enhancement

MR Findings

- T1WI
  - May show alterations in normal diploic space signal; varies with etiology
- T2WI
  - May show alterations in normal diploic space signal; varies with etiology
- T1WI C+
  - Some etiologies may show diploic enhancement

Nuclear Medicine Findings

- Bone scan
  - Variable, dependent on cause of skull thickening
    - May be cold or hot
    - Differences possible in early vascular vs. later bone uptake phases
- PET
  - 18F-fluoro-2-deoxyglucose (FDG) PET: May show uptake in aggressive etiologies

Imaging Recommendations

- Best imaging tool
  - NECT for most causes of skull thickening
  - MR + contrast if cellular or if aggressive causes are suspected (e.g., metastases)
- Protocol advice
  - Bone reconstruction algorithm
  - Thin-section, high-resolution MDCT for pathology at skull base
    - Coronal and sagittal reformats
    - Goal: Thoroughly evaluate foramina and canals

DIFFERENTIAL DIAGNOSIS

Normal Anatomic Variation

- Upper limits of normal
- Normal-appearing cortices and diploic space

Hyperostosis Interna

- Usually bilateral, symmetric
- Commonly predominant in frontal squama, may extend to parietal bones, orbital roof

Paget Disease

- Initial osteolytic change of skull is osteoporosis circumscripta
- Later osteosclerotic phase thickens bone
  - Abnormal architecture of primitive or woven bone
  - Increased vascularity and pronounced connective tissue reaction
  - Bones are enlarged and show increased radiodensity and accentuated trabeculae

Microcephaly

- Skull overgrowth occurs secondary to small brain
- Cause = developmental anomalies (e.g., lissencephaly) or result of very early brain damage

Many Others

- Shunted hydrocephalus
- Chronic anemias

THICK SKULL

PATHOLOGY

General Features

- Etiology
  - Etiologies more likely to cause generalized ST
    - Normal anatomic variation = most common
    - Drug therapy, e.g., phenytoin (Dilantin)
    - Microcephaly
    - Hyperparathyroidism
    - Acromegaly
    - Sclerosing bone dysplasias: Osteopetrosis
  - Etiologies more likely to cause regional or focal ST
    - Hyperostosis interna = most common
    - Hyperostotic meningioma
    - Hyperostosing en plaque meningioma
    - Osteoblastic metastases (usually prostate or breast)
    - Calcifying cephalohematoma
    - Osteoma
    - Dyke-Davidoff-Masson syndrome
    - Epidermal nevus syndrome
  - Etiologies causing both focal or generalized ST
    - Paget disease
    - Fibrous dysplasia
    - Calcified subdural hematoma
- Genetics
  - Some etiologies associated with genetic involvement/predisposition
- Associated abnormalities
  - Many causes are systemic, with plethora of associated abnormalities

Gross Pathologic & Surgical Features

- Skull thickening

Microscopic Features

- Inner/outer table cortical thickening ± diploic space involvement
- Specific histopathology varies greatly, dependent on underlying cause

CLINICAL ISSUES

Presentation

- Most common signs/symptoms
  - Most often asymptomatic
  - Without skull base disease: Most symptoms referable to disease affecting systems outside skull
  - Patients with skull base ST may be symptomatic from foraminal or canal encroachment
    - Manifests as cranial nerve (CN) deficit(s)
    - Sino-orbital and auditory complications
- Clinical profile
  - Many tests can help discriminate among etiologies
    - Phenytoin therapy: Phenytoin levels
    - Acromegaly: ↑ growth hormone and IGF-1
    - Sickle cell anemia: Hemoglobin electrophoresis and Sickledex test abnormal
    - Iron deficiency anemia: ↓ hematocrit and hemoglobin; small red blood cells; ↓ serum ferritin and iron; high iron binding capacity (TIBC)
    - β-thalassemia: Blood smear and hemoglobin electrophoresis abnormal
    - Hyperparathyroidism: ↑ serum calcium, ↑ parathyroid hormone, ↓ serum phosphorus
    - Osteopetrosis: Radiographic skeletal series diagnostic for diffusely dense bones
    - Engelmann disease: Radiographic skeletal series shows diaphyseal dysplasia
    - Prostate metastases: Abnormal prostate US; ↑ prostate specific antigen and alkaline phosphatase
    - Breast metastases: Abnormal mammogram; axillary adenopathy
    - Dyke-Davidoff-Masson syndrome: Pathognomic NECT with contralateral paresis
    - Epidermal nevus syndrome: Nevi (linear comedonicus, inflammatory linear verrucous epidermal, linear sebaceous, linear epidermal)
    - Paget disease: ↑ serum alk. phos. & serum/urine hydroxyproline; abnormal radiography

Demographics

- Age
  - Varies with etiology
- Gender
  - Hyperostosis interna: Female

Natural History & Prognosis

- Usually of no clinical concern
- Aggressive lesions, especially those involving skull base, have associated morbidity; usually CN deficit(s)

Treatment

- Usually no treatment required
  - Skull findings often harbinger of underlying disease
  - Therapy aimed at treating underlying etiology
- Indications for partial or total surgical excision
  - Cosmesis (most common)
  - Sino-orbital and auditive complications (less common)
  - Peripheral compressive cranial neuropathies (uncommon)
  - Compressive central neurological manifestations (rarest)

DIAGNOSTIC CHECKLIST

Consider

- What is underlying cause of skull thickening?

Image Interpretation Pearls

- Mnemonic "HIPFAM" to help remember some common causes of skull thickening
  - **H**yperostosis interna, **i**diopathic, **P**aget disease, **f**ibrous dysplasia, **a**nemia, **m**etastases/**m**eningioma

SELECTED REFERENCES

1. Lisle DA et al: Imaging of craniofacial fibrous dysplasia. J Med Imaging Radiat Oncol. 52(4):325-32, 2008
2. Waclawik AJ: Hyperostosis frontalis interna. Arch Neurol. 63(2):291, 2006
3. Smith SE et al: From the archives of the AFIP. Radiologic spectrum of Paget disease of bone and its complications with pathologic correlation. Radiographics. 22(5): 1191-216, 2002

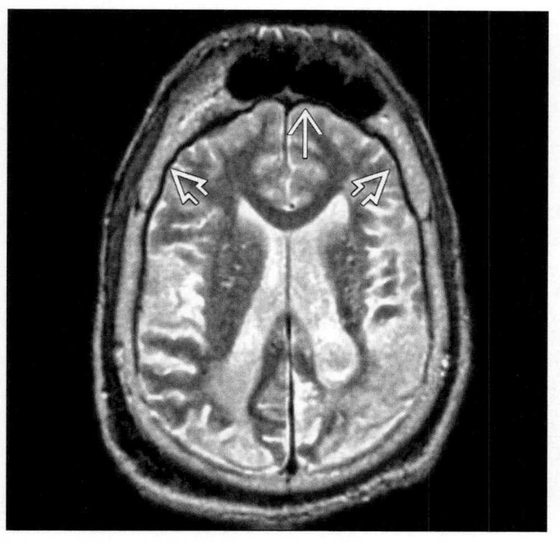

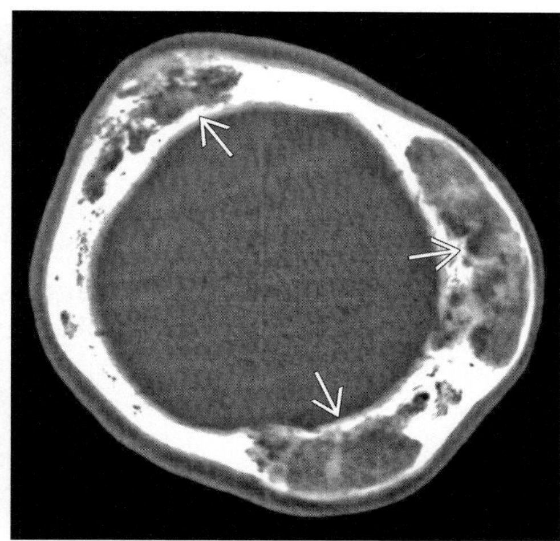

(Left) Axial T2WI MR shows diffuse skull thickening ⇨ and over-pneumatization of the frontal sinus ➡ in this patient with microcephaly. ***(Right)*** Axial bone CT shows multifocal areas of calvarial thickening with a ground-glass matrix of polyostotic fibrous dysplasia ➡.

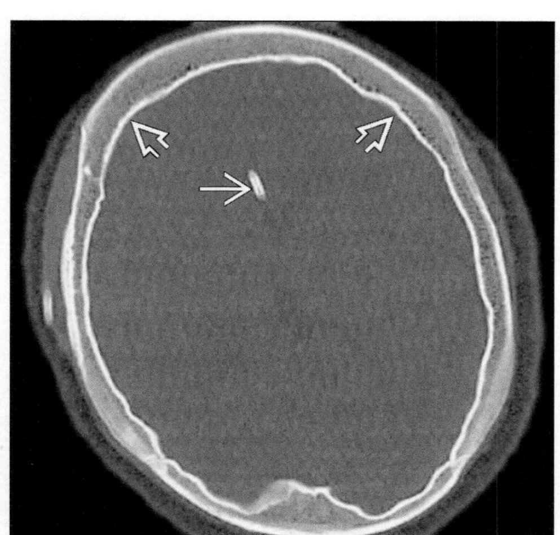

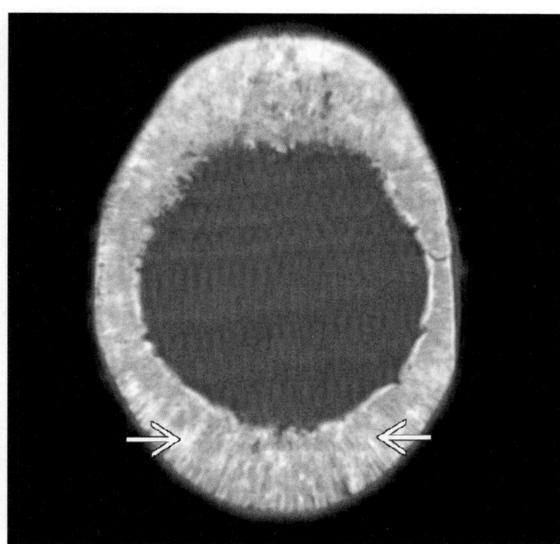

(Left) Axial bone CT demonstrates diffuse skull thickening in a patient with chronically shunted hydrocephalus ⇨. The shunt tube is partly visualized ➡. ***(Right)*** Axial bone CT demonstrates diffuse skull thickening with "hair on end" appearance of the diploic space, classic for severe hemolytic anemias like thalassemia, as in this case ➡.

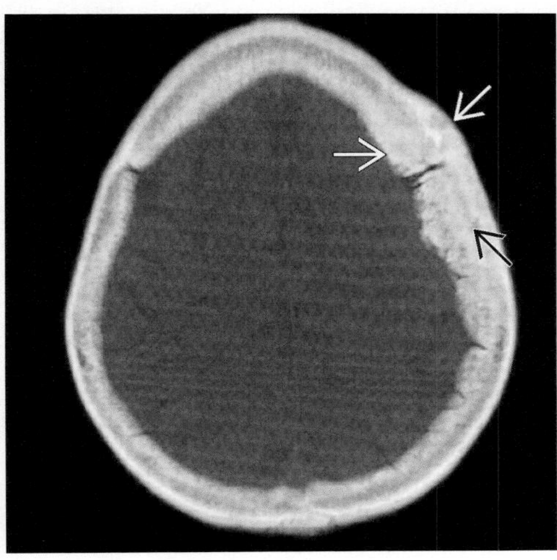

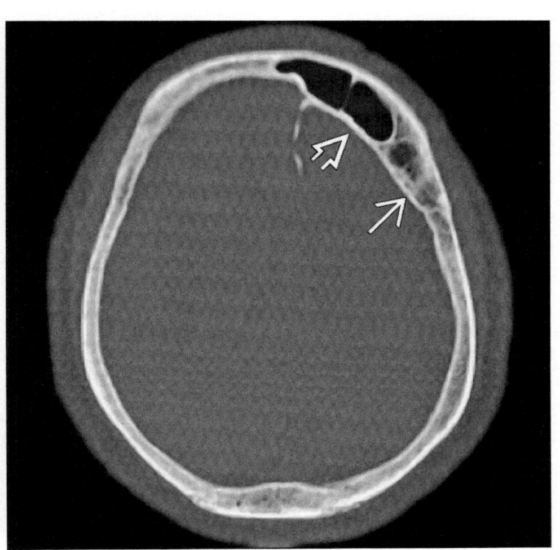

(Left) Axial bone CT shows localized hyperostotic skull thickening caused by an intradiploic meningioma. There is thickening of the inner and outer tables ➡ with sclerosis of the diploic space ⇒. ***(Right)*** Axial bone CT demonstrates over-pneumatization of the left frontal sinus ⇨ with ipsilateral calvarial thickening ➡ in Dyke-Davidoff-Masson syndrome. There is underlying left hemicerebral atrophy due to remote insult.

LANGERHANS CELL HISTIOCYTOSIS, SKULL AND BRAIN

Key Facts

Terminology

- Langerhans cell histiocytosis (LCH)
  - A.k.a. histiocytosis X (former)

Imaging

- Skull: Sharply marginated lytic skull defect with beveled margins
- Mastoid: Geographic destruction, soft tissue mass
- Brain: Thick enhancing infundibulum, absent posterior pituitary bright spot on T1WI

Top Differential Diagnoses

- Lytic calvarial lesions
- Surgical (burr hole, shunt, surgical defect)
- Epidermoid
- Dermoid
- Pituitary infundibular/hypothalamic thickening or masses
- Germinoma
- Glioma
- Metastasis

Clinical Issues

- Calvarial: Pain, subscalp mass, bony defect
- Mastoid destruction: Pain, chronic otitis externa, retroauricular subscalp mass
- Pituitary infundibular involvement: Central DI, ± visual disturbance, ± hypothalamic dysfunction

Diagnostic Checklist

- Skull is most frequent bony site involved by LCH
- Thick enhancing pituitary stalk is most common CNS manifestation of LCH
- CNS LCH for ataxic patient with choroid plexus masses and cerebellar WM demyelination

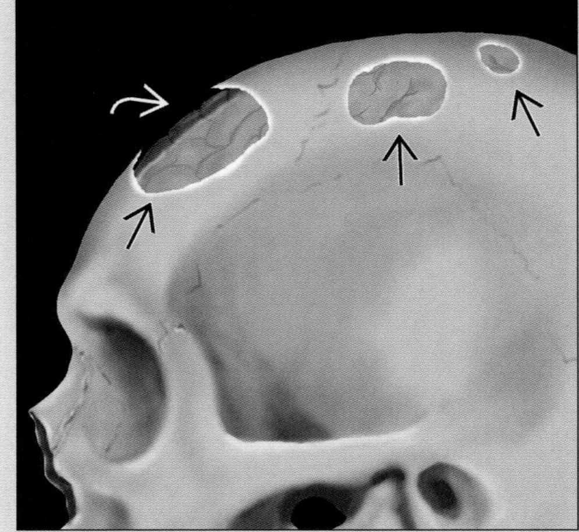

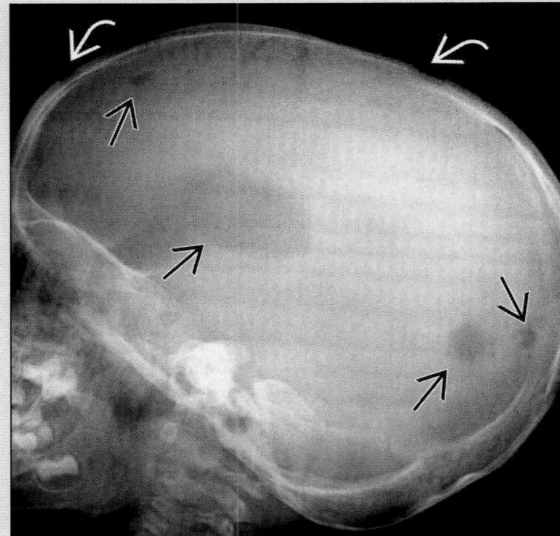

(Left) *Lateral graphic demonstrates 3 sharply defined lytic lesions ➔ of the membranous calvarium with geographic destruction. Note the beveled margins of the bony lysis ➔.* ***(Right)*** *Lateral radiograph in a 3-year-old boy with several subcutaneous masses and central diabetes insipidus demonstrates multiple lytic lesions of the skull ➔. Note the "cookie cutter" sharp pattern of bony lysis and the beveled edge pattern ➔ of differential inner and outer table calvarial involvement.*

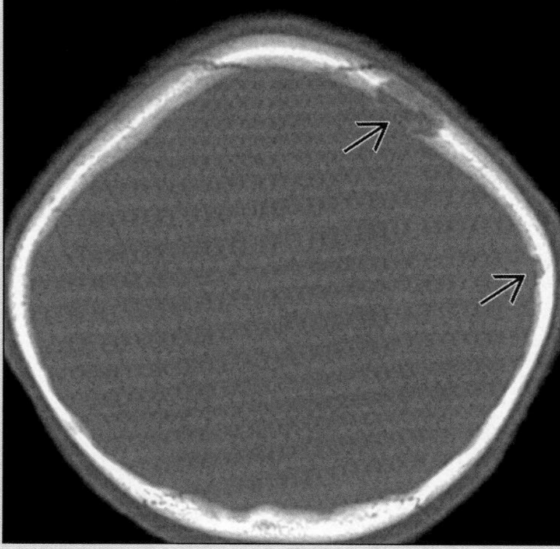

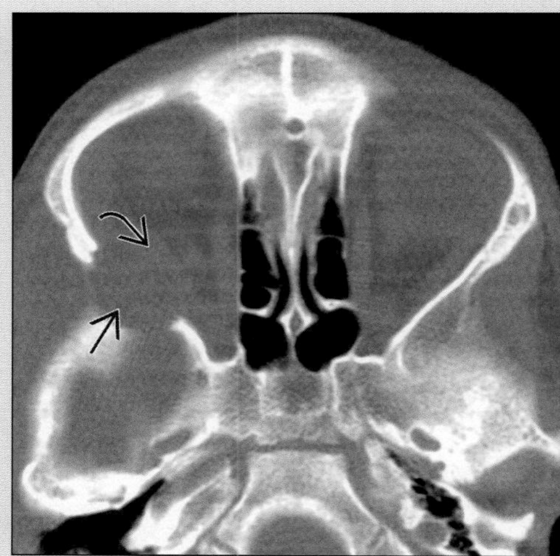

(Left) *Axial NECT in a 5-year-old girl with multiple scalp masses demonstrates 2 lytic lesions ➔ of the left frontal bone. Both lesions show the characteristic pattern of sharply defined geographic bony lysis. Note the unequal inner and outer table involvement creating a beveled edge appearance.* ***(Right)*** *Axial NECT in a proptotic 10-year-old boy shows a sharply defined lytic lesion of the lateral orbital wall ➔. Note the soft tissue mass displacing the lateral rectus muscle ➔.*

LANGERHANS CELL HISTIOCYTOSIS, SKULL AND BRAIN

TERMINOLOGY

Synonyms

- Langerhans cell histiocytosis (LCH)
  - A.k.a. histiocytosis X (former)

Definitions

- Proliferation of Langerhans cell histiocytes that form granulomas within any organ system

IMAGING

General Features

- Best diagnostic clue
  - Skull: Sharply marginated lytic skull defect with beveled margins
  - Mastoid: Geographic destruction, soft tissue mass
  - Brain: Thick enhancing infundibulum, absent posterior pituitary bright spot on T1WI
- Location
  - Skull
    - Calvarium most common bony site involved, especially prevalent in frontal, parietal bones
    - Also mastoid portion of temporal bone, mandible, orbit, facial bones
  - Brain: Pituitary infundibulum, hypothalamus
    - Rare: Choroid plexus, leptomeninges, basal ganglia, cerebellar white matter (WM), and brain parenchyma
- Size
  - Skull and facial bones: Lesions grow fast, moderate soft tissue mass common
  - Pituitary infundibulum: Small lesions due to early endocrine dysfunction (central DI)
- Morphology
  - Variable patterns of bony lysis
  - Soft tissue masses vary from discrete ↔ infiltrative

Radiographic Findings

- Radiography
  - Calvarium: Well-defined lytic lesion, beveled edge, lack of marginal sclerosis
    - ± button sequestra or sclerotic margins when healing
  - Mastoid: Geographic destruction, often bilateral, little regional adenopathy
  - Facial/orbital: More variable patterns of bony lysis, discrete ↔ permeative

CT Findings

- NECT
  - Calvarium
    - Lytic defect, beveled (inner table > outer table)
    - Small soft tissue mass
  - Mastoid
    - Bone destruction, often bilateral, soft tissue mass
- CECT
  - Calvarium/mastoid: Enhancing soft tissue in lytic defect
  - Brain: Enhancing, thick pituitary stalk, ± hypothalamic mass or enhancement

MR Findings

- T1WI
  - Soft tissue mass at site of bony lysis (± T1 shortening due to lipid-laden histiocytes)
  - Brain
    - Pituitary/infundibulum: Absent posterior pituitary bright spot, thick stalk, ± soft tissue mass
- T2WI
  - Skull, mastoid, orbital/facial lesions: Soft tissue masses show slight T2 hyperintensity
  - Brain
    - Infundibulum/hypothalamus: Slightly hyperintense
    - ± cerebellar white matter hyperintensity (autoimmune-mediated demyelination)
- FLAIR
  - Hyperintensity of rare cerebellar white matter demyelination
- T1WI C+
  - Skull, mastoid, orbital/facial: Enhancing soft tissue masses (defined or infiltrating)
  - Brain
    - Infundibulum: Vivid enhancement and stalk thickening
    - Rare enhancing masses in choroid plexus, leptomeninges, and basal ganglia

Nuclear Medicine Findings

- Bone scan
  - Tc-bone scan: Variable (cold ↔ warm)
- PET
  - 18-FDG: ↑ uptake in proliferating lesions, ↓ uptake for "burned-out" lesions

Imaging Recommendations

- Best imaging tool
  - Skull: NECT (CECT for mastoid disease)
  - Brain: MR with contrast
- Protocol advice
  - Skull: CT using bone algorithm; include coronal and sagittal reconstructions
  - Brain MR: Use in patient with neurologic signs or diabetes insipidus (DI); if initially "normal," repeat MR in 2-3 months
    - Pituitary MR: Small field of view, thin section, no gap, sagittal and coronal T1WI with contrast

DIFFERENTIAL DIAGNOSIS

Lytic Calvarial Lesions

- Surgical (burr hole, shunt, surgical defect)
- Epidermoid
- Dermoid
- Leptomeningeal cyst
- TB
- Metastases

Temporal Bone Destructive Processes

- Severe mastoiditis: Infection usually spares bony labyrinth
- Rhabdomyosarcoma: Often with large ipsilateral cervical nodes

LANGERHANS CELL HISTIOCYTOSIS, SKULL AND BRAIN

Pituitary Infundibular/Hypothalamic Thickening or Masses

- Germinoma
- Glioma
- Primitive neuroectodermal tumor
- Metastasis
- Lymphocytic hypophysitis
- Neurosarcoid
- Meningitis

PATHOLOGY

General Features

- Etiology
  - Uncertain: Inflammatory ↔ neoplastic
- Genetics
  - Familial cases documented
  - Monoclonality of pathologic Langerhans cell
  - T (7;12) translocation, involvement of tel gene on chromosome 12
- Associated abnormalities
  - ↑ risk of LCH: Family history of thyroid disease, underimmunization, penicillin use, solvent exposure

Staging, Grading, & Classification

- Formerly classified into 1 of 3 overlapping forms
  - Eosinophilic granuloma
    - Localized, calvarium most common (70%)
  - Hand-Schüller-Christian
    - Chronic disseminated form, multifocal (20%)
  - Letterer-Siwe
    - Acute disseminated form, onset at < 2 years of age, ± skeletal involvement (10%)
- Now classified according to risk factors: Young age, multifocal involvement, multiorgan dysfunction, relapse

Gross Pathologic & Surgical Features

- Yellow, gray, or brown tumor mass

Microscopic Features

- Monoclonality of Langerhans cells
  - Presence of CD1a and Birbeck granules needed to establish diagnosis

CLINICAL ISSUES

Presentation

- Most common signs/symptoms
  - Calvarial: Pain, subscalp mass, bony defect
  - Mastoid destruction: Pain, chronic otitis externa, retroauricular subscalp mass
  - Retroorbital mass: Exophthalmos, ± painful ophthalmoplegia
  - Pituitary infundibular involvement: Central DI, ± visual disturbance, ± hypothalamic dysfunction
- Clinical profile
  - Child < 2 years with diabetes insipidus, ± lytic calvarial lesion

Demographics

- Age
  - LCH typically presents at < 2 years
- Gender
  - M:F = 2:1
- Ethnicity
  - More common among Caucasians
- Epidemiology
  - Affects 4 in 1,000,000
  - Peak age at onset 1 year (isolated), 2-5 years (multifocal disease)
  - Inverse relation between severity of involvement and age
  - 50% of LCH cases are monostotic
  - Familial LCH < 2%
  - Bone lesions are most common manifestations of LCH (seen in 80-95% of children with LCH)

Natural History & Prognosis

- Variable depending on age of onset and extent of involvement
  - Multifocal and systemic LCH: Mortality may approach 18%
- Rarely, may spontaneously hemorrhage ⇒ epidural hematoma

Treatment

- Therapeutic options depend on symptoms, location, and extent of disease
  - Observation, excision/curettage, sclerotherapy/injection, radiation/chemotherapy
- Solitary eosinophilic granuloma has best prognosis with spontaneous remission common
  - Curettage if painful, observe asymptomatic
- LCH patients with DI: Oral or nasal vasopressin, ± chemotherapy and radiation

DIAGNOSTIC CHECKLIST

Consider

- CNS LCH for ataxic patient with choroid plexus masses and cerebellar WM demyelination

Image Interpretation Pearls

- Skull is most frequent bony site involved by LCH
- Thick enhancing pituitary stalk is most common CNS manifestation of LCH

SELECTED REFERENCES

1. Phillips M et al: Comparison of FDG-PET scans to conventional radiography and bone scans in management of Langerhans cell histiocytosis. Pediatr Blood Cancer. 52(1):97-101, 2009
2. D'Ambrosio N et al: Craniofacial and intracranial manifestations of langerhans cell histiocytosis: report of findings in 100 patients. AJR Am J Roentgenol. 191(2):589-97, 2008
3. Demaerel P et al: Paediatric neuroradiological aspects of Langerhans cell histiocytosis. Neuroradiology. 50(1):85-92, 2008
4. van der Knaap MS et al: Cerebellar leukoencephalopathy: most likely histiocytosis-related. Neurology. 71(17):1361-7, 2008

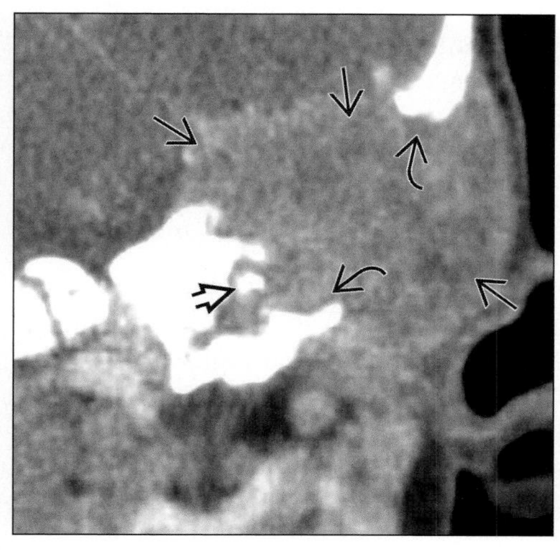

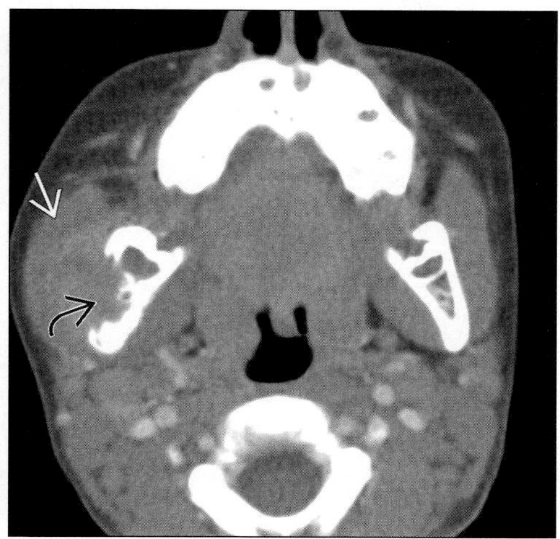

(Left) *Coronal CECT in a 5-year-old boy with chronic draining of left ear and conductive hearing loss shows a soft tissue mass → & bone destruction involving the mastoid segment of the temporal bone. Note sharply defined margins of bony destruction ↷ and displaced middle ear ossicle ⇒.* ***(Right)*** *Axial CECT in child with a slowly growing right cheek mass demonstrates the mass as soft tissue → in the lower masticator space. Note the associated lysis of the lateral mandibular ramus ↷.*

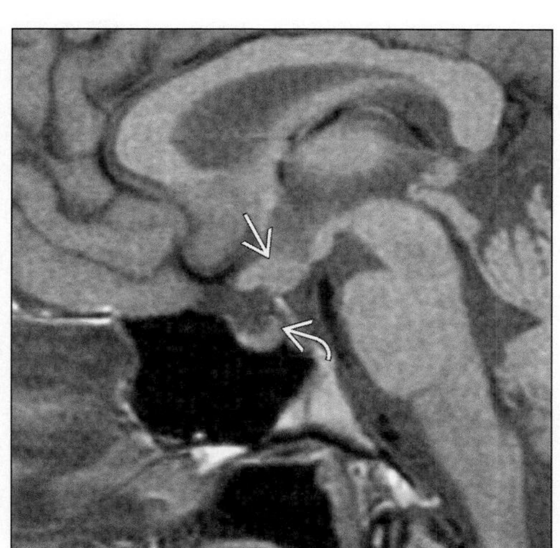

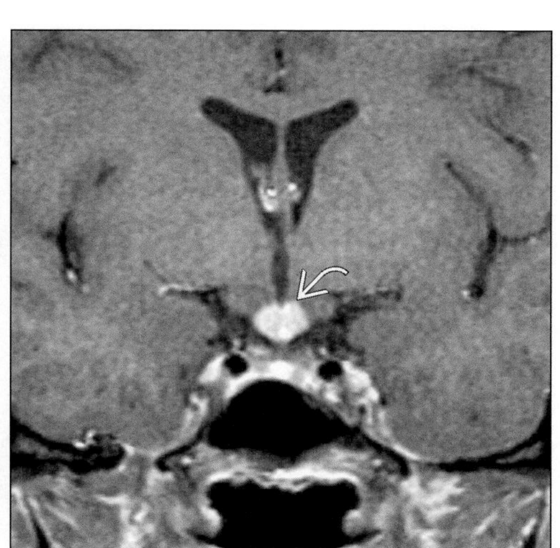

(Left) *Sagittal T1WI MR in a 7-year-old girl with central diabetes insipidus demonstrates a soft tissue mass → involving the hypothalamus. Note the absence of the normal posterior pituitary focus of T1 shortening ↷, a common finding in children with diabetes insipidus.* ***(Right)*** *Coronal T1WI C+ FS MR in the same patient shows enhancement of the hypothalamic nodule ↷. Pituitary stalk thickening is the most common finding with CNS involvement.*

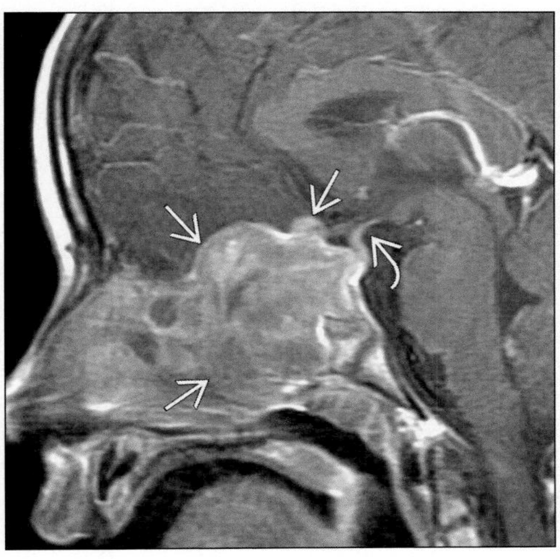

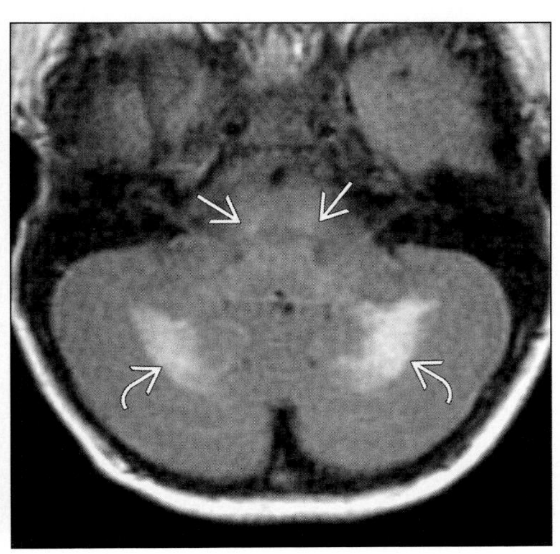

(Left) *Sagittal T1 C+ FS MR in a 5-year-old boy with chronic headaches and diabetes insipidus demonstrates a heterogeneously enhancing lesion → of the central skull base. Note the thickening and displacement of the pituitary infundibulum ↷.* ***(Right)*** *Axial FLAIR MR in a 6-year-old boy with behavior problems shows confluent regions of demyelination with FLAIR signal hyperintensity involving the cerebellar white matter ↷. Note the involvement of the abducens nuclei →.*

NEUROSARCOID

Key Facts

Terminology
- Multisystem inflammatory disease characterized by noncaseating epithelioid-cell granulomas

Imaging
- Solitary or multifocal CNS mass(es) + abnormal CXR
- Focal or diffusely infiltrating granulomas
- Chest x-ray abnormal in > 90% with NS
- May cause small vessel vasculitis/angiitis in white matter
- Wide spectrum of MR enhancement
- May coat CN, fill internal auditory canals
- Periventricular white matter disease

Top Differential Diagnoses
- Meningitis
- Meningioma
- Infundibular histiocytosis
- Metastases

Pathology
- Etiology remains unknown
- May infiltrate along perivascular spaces

Clinical Issues
- Neurologic manifestations frequently presenting symptoms of systemic sarcoid
- Most common symptom: CN deficit(s), most often facial nerve palsy
- CNS involved in 5% (clinical) to 27% (autopsy)
- Often indolent disease; up to 50% asymptomatic
- 67% with NS have self-limited monophasic illness; remainder have chronic remitting-relapsing course
- No known cure; goal to alleviate symptoms

Diagnostic Checklist
- Protean manifestations make NS a "great mimicker"

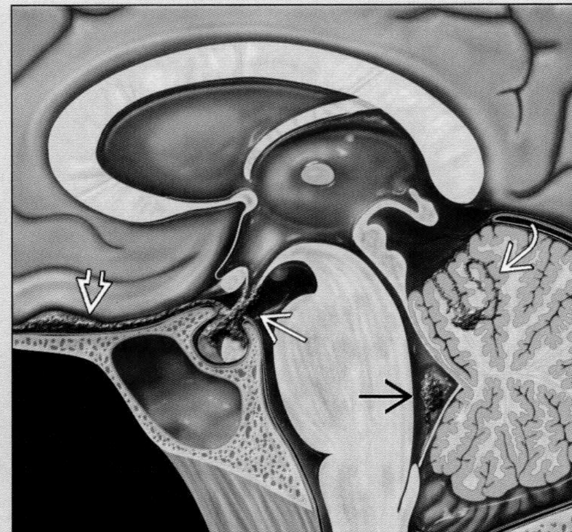

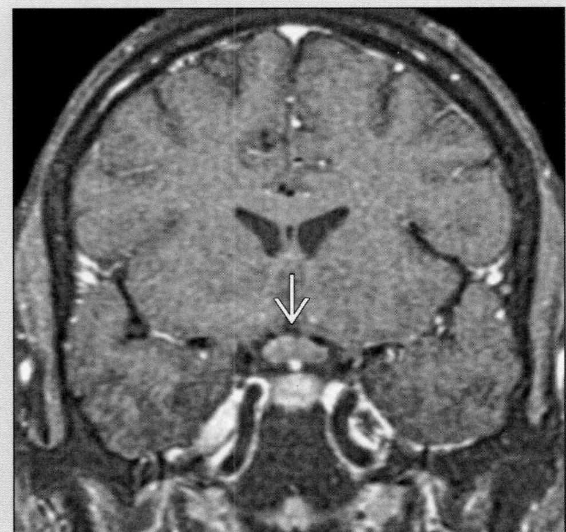

(Left) *Sagittal graphic illustrates common neurosarcoid locations: (1) enveloping the infundibulum and extending into the parasellar region; (2) contiguous disease wrapping the inferior frontal lobes; and (3) synchronous lesions of the superior vermis and 4th ventricle choroid plexus.* ***(Right)*** *Coronal T1WI C+ FS MR demonstrates significant thickening and mild enhancement of the optic chiasm. The next 2 images demonstrate the full extent of neurosarcoid in this patient.*

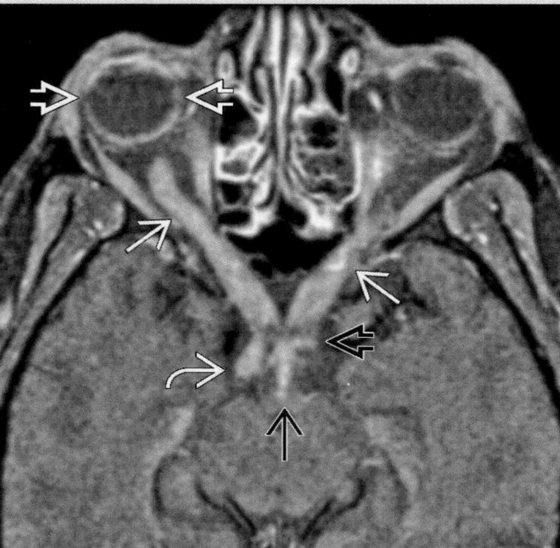

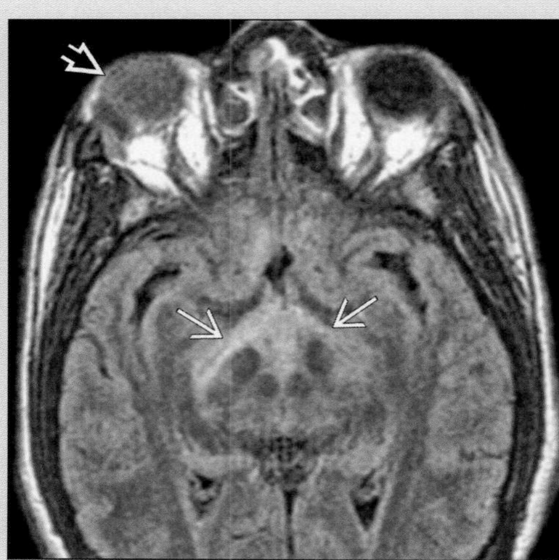

(Left) *Axial T1WI C+ FS MR of the same patient shows thickening and enhancement of both optic nerves, the chiasm, and the right proximal tract. The infundibulum is thickened, extending into the hypothalamus. The right globe demonstrates abnormal peripheral and vitreous enhancement.* ***(Right)*** *Axial FLAIR MR in the same patient shows T2 hyperintensity in both optic tracks and hypothalamus, as well as the right vitreous body.*

NEUROSARCOID

TERMINOLOGY

Abbreviations
- Neurosarcoid (NS)

Definitions
- Multisystem inflammatory disease characterized by noncaseating epithelioid-cell granulomas

IMAGING

General Features
- Best diagnostic clue
  - Solitary or multifocal CNS mass(es) + abnormal CXR
- Location
  - Dura (29-50%), leptomeninges (31%), subarachnoid/perivascular spaces
    - Preferential involvement of basal cisterns
    - Optic chiasm, hypothalamus, infundibulum
  - Cranial nerves (CNs) (34-50%); optic nerve (28%)
  - Brain parenchyma (22%): Hypothalamus > brain stem > cerebral hemispheres > cerebellum
  - Spine (25%)
- Morphology
  - Focal or diffusely infiltrating granulomas
  - Absence of pathological enhancement does not rule out diagnosis of neurosarcoid

Radiographic Findings
- Radiography
  - Chest x-ray abnormal in > 90% with NS
    - Hilar adenopathy ± parenchymal involvement

CT Findings
- CECT
  - May show basilar leptomeningeal enhancement

MR Findings
- T1WI
  - Hydrocephalus
  - Lacunar infarcts (brainstem, basal ganglia)
  - Isointense material within subarachnoid spaces
  - Isointense dural lesion(s)
- T2WI
  - Lacunar infarcts (brainstem, basal ganglia)
  - Hypointense material within subarachnoid spaces
  - Hypointense dural lesion(s)
  - Sellar disease may appear cystic
- FLAIR
  - ~ 50% have periventricular T2 hyperintense lesions
    - Can infiltrate perivascular (Virchow-Robin) spaces
    - May cause vasculitis/angiitis of white matter
- DWI
  - Distinguish restricted (acute ischemic cytotoxic edema) from nonrestricted NS (vasogenic) edema
- T1WI C+
  - Wide spectrum of MR enhancement
    - 10% seen as solitary intraaxial mass
    - Slightly > 1/3 have multiple parenchymal lesions
    - Slightly > 1/3 have leptomeningeal involvement; nodular &/or diffuse
    - 5-10% hypothalamus, infundibular thickening
    - 5% solitary dural-based extraaxial mass
    - Other: Vasculitic or ependymal enhancement
    - May coat CN, fill internal auditory canals

Nuclear Medicine Findings
- PET: FDG high pulmonary sarcoidosis uptake
- Gallium scan: ↑ uptake at systemic sites of inflammation, including NS (as high as 85%)

Imaging Recommendations
- Best imaging tool
  - MR + contrast
- Protocol advice
  - Multiplanar, fat saturation, T1WI C+

DIFFERENTIAL DIAGNOSIS

Dural, Leptomeningeal, Subarachnoid NS
- Meningitis: CSF shows infection/organism
- Meningioma: Not parenchymal or subarachnoid space
- Infundibular histiocytosis: Age of onset 6-14 years

Brain Parenchymal NS
- Metastases: Labs different, negative CXR
- Periventricular white matter disease: Different symptomatology and lab results, negative CXR

PATHOLOGY

General Features
- Etiology
  - Etiology remains unknown
    - Possibly stimulation of immune system by 1 or more antigens &/or abnormal immune response
  - DNA and RNA of *Mycobacterium*, *Propionibacterium* detected in some lesions, suggesting a possible cause
- Genetics
  - Sarcoidosis may occur in families
  - Genetic polymorphisms of MHC are associated with ↑ risk of disease or affect disease presentation
    - HLA-DRB1 (*11 & *14), HLA-DQB1*0201 alleles
    - Number of HLA genes involved unknown, but clear HLA region strongly implicated
  - Genetic polymorphisms of cytokines are associated with ↑ risk of disease or affect disease presentation
- Associated abnormalities
  - Löfgren syndrome (a.k.a. acute pulmonary sarcoid)
    - All: Fever, malaise, bilateral hilar adenopathy
    - Erythema nodosum and large joint arthralgia
    - May have uveitis, parotitis
  - Heerfordt syndrome (a.k.a. salivary gland sarcoidosis)
    - Fever, parotitis, uveitis, and facial nerve paralysis

Gross Pathologic & Surgical Features
- Granulomatous leptomeningitis (most common) or dural-based solitary mass (diffuse > nodular)
- May infiltrate along perivascular spaces

Microscopic Features
- Noncaseating granuloma: Compact, radially arranged epithelioid cells with pale-staining nuclei
- Large multinucleated giant cells in arc/circle around central granular zone

NEUROSARCOID

- Arterial wall invasion by epithelioid cell granuloma causing disruption of media and internal elastica
  - Tissue may then cause luminal stenosis or occlusion
- Fibrocollagenous tissue accumulates in dural lesions
  - Correlates with T2 hypointense lesions
- Inflammatory infiltration
  - Correlates with T2 hyperintense lesions

CLINICAL ISSUES

Presentation

- Most common signs/symptoms
  - Neurologic manifestations frequently presenting symptoms of systemic sarcoid
  - Imaging findings often do not have correlating symptoms at time of presentation
    - Nonetheless, post-therapy imaging shows excellent correlation with clinical improvement/ worsening
  - Most common symptom: CN deficit(s), most often facial nerve palsy
    - Bell palsy present 14x ↑ than general population
  - By imaging, optic nerve ± chiasm most affected
    - Clinical & imaging CN findings often disparate
  - Symptoms vary with location, size of granulomas
    - Other CN: Hearing loss, diplopia
    - Headache, fatigue, seizures, encephalopathy, dementia
    - Weakness, paresthesias
    - Pituitary/hypothalamic dysfunction
  - 5-10% occur without pulmonary/systemic sarcoid
  - Progressive encephalopathy, confusion, & dementia
    - Ascribed to longstanding microvascular changes of presumed granulomatous angiitis
  - Systemic involvement
    - Lung hilar nodes most often involved
    - Skin lesions 2nd (up to 1/3)
    - Eye (iritis, uveitis); polyarthritis
  - Children present differently
    - More likely: Seizures, space-occupying lesion
    - Less likely: Cranial nerve palsies
- Clinical profile
  - Kveim-Siltzbach skin test positive in 85%
  - Serum ACE levels elevated in < 50% of cases with NS
    - Normal CSF ACE levels do not rule out NS
  - Hypercalcemia + hypercalciuria in up to 15%
  - Serum CD4:CD8 ratio often ↓
  - ↑ CSF protein &/or cells insensitive, nonspecific

Demographics

- Age
  - Bimodal: Initial peak at 20-29 years, later peak in women > 50 years
- Gender
  - M:F = 2:1
- Ethnicity
  - In USA, lifetime risk in African-Americans is nearly 3x higher than Caucasians
  - In Europe, Caucasians mostly affected
- Epidemiology
  - In USA
    - Women: 6.3 per 100,000 person-years
    - Men: 5.9 per 100,000 person-years
  - CNS involved between 5% (clinical) and 27% (autopsy)
    - Primary, isolated CNS sarcoidosis < 1%
    - Imaging detects neurologic disease in 10% of all patients with sarcoidosis
- Geographic predilection
  - Temperate > tropical climates (< 10/100,000)
  - Swedes and Danes commonly affected
  - Rare in Chinese, Southeast Asians, Inuits, Canadian Indians, New Zealand Maoris, and Spanish

Natural History & Prognosis

- Often indolent disease; up to 50% asymptomatic
- 67% with NS have self-limited monophasic illness; remainder have chronic remitting-relapsing course
  - Most respond rapidly to steroids; others refractory
- Simultaneous expression of new and old granulomas suggest process may wax and wane
- Hydrocephalus
  - Direct obstruction (most common complication)
  - Also by loss/reduction of brain tissue compliance resulting from parenchymal infiltration
- Vasculitis may cause small vessel ischemia, lacunes, cortical infarcts
- Indicators of poor prognosis: Seizures; enhancing leptomeningeal, parenchymal, and spinal lesions
- Indicators of good prognosis: Nonenhancing dural, CN, and parenchymal lesions
- Death in 5%, mostly from pulmonary complications

Treatment

- No known cure; goal to alleviate symptoms
- Corticosteroids useful in most cases; immunosuppressive drugs occasionally
- In NS ~ 50% progress despite corticosteroid and immunosuppressive therapy
- MR imaging resolution lags clinical symptom resolution

DIAGNOSTIC CHECKLIST

Consider

- Look for abnormal CXR

Image Interpretation Pearls

- Protean manifestations make NS a "great mimicker"
- CN deficit(s) and pituitary dysfunction often have normal MR C+ imaging; conversely MR findings may be clinically silent

SELECTED REFERENCES

1. Shah R et al: Correlation of MR imaging findings and clinical manifestations in neurosarcoidosis. AJNR Am J Neuroradiol. 30(5):953-61, 2009
2. Westhout FD et al: Obstructive hydrocephalus and progressive psychosis: rare presentations of neurosarcoidosis. Surg Neurol. 69(3):288-92, 2008

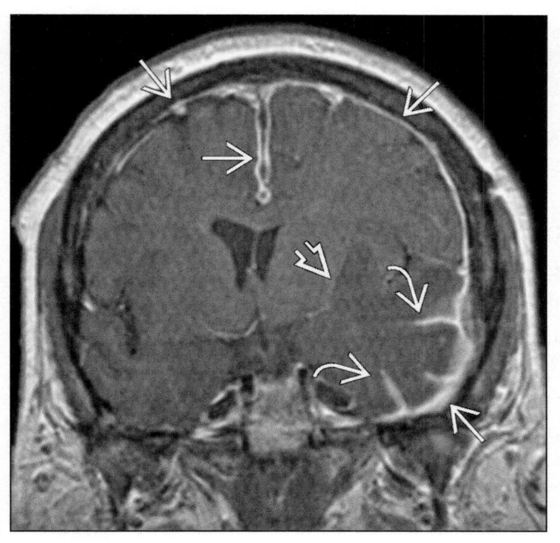

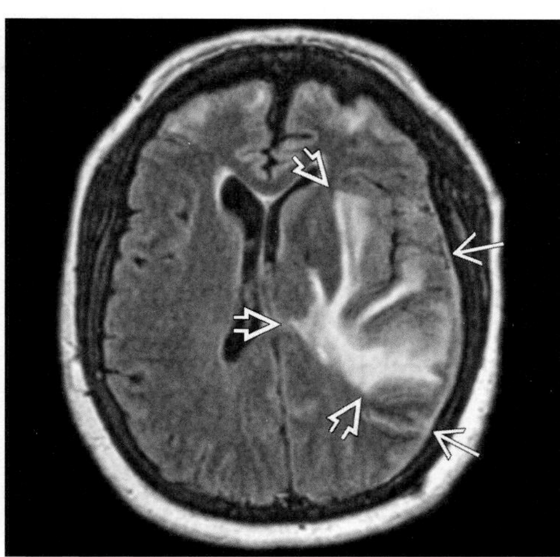

(Left) *Coronal T1WI C+ MR shows diffuse dural and leptomeningeal thickening with enhancement enveloping the temporal lobe extending over the convexity and into the falx* ➔*. Parenchymal extension is evident by contiguous enhancement* ➔*. Note the vasogenic edema* ➔ *& mass effect causing left-to-right shift.* ***(Right)*** *Axial FLAIR MR of the same patient shows diffuse dural & leptomeningeal abnormality* ➔*, as well as parenchymal T2 hyperintensity from vasogenic edema* ➔*.*

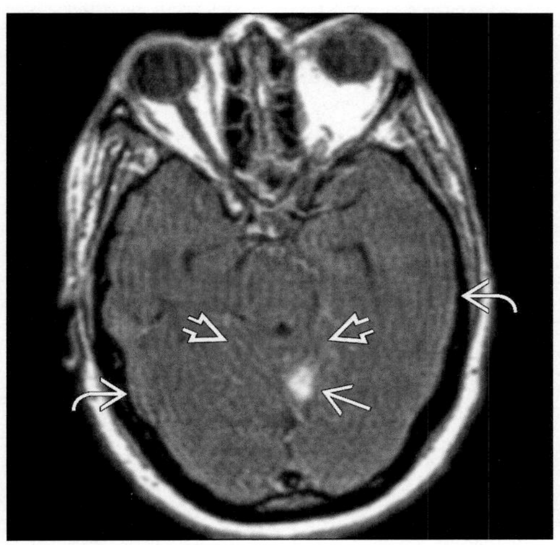

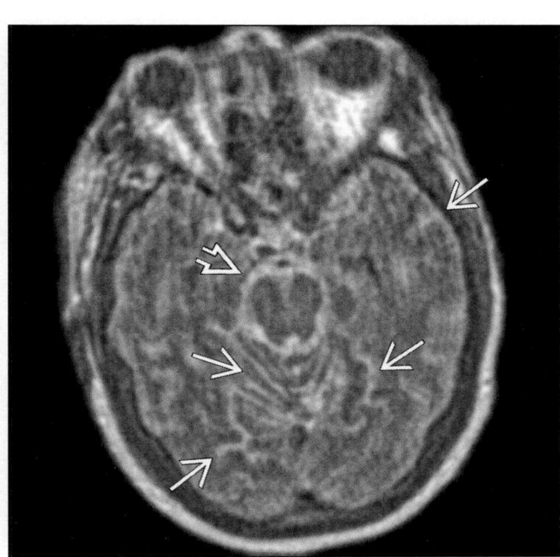

(Left) *Axial T1WI C+ MR demonstrates an enhancing parenchymal nodule of the left paramedian superior vermis* ➔*. There is also a suggestion of diffuse subarachnoid space abnormality by mild enhancement of dura* ➔ *and folial leptomeninges* ➔*.* ***(Right)*** *Axial contrast-enhanced FLAIR MR of the same patient reveals that there is diffuse and widespread subarachnoid/ leptomeningeal abnormality* ➔*, which extended from the basilar cisterns* ➔ *up to the vertex (not shown).*

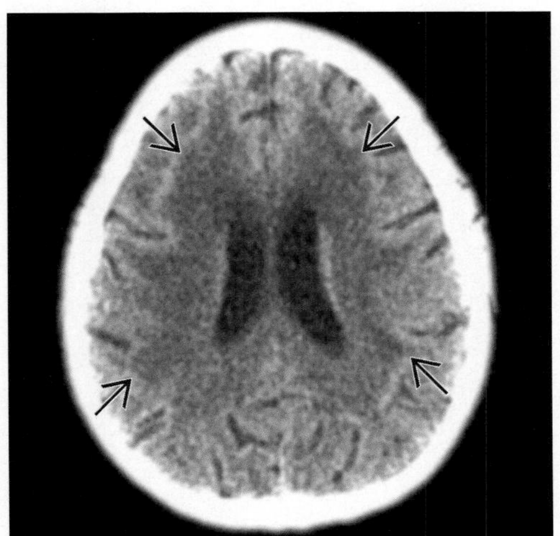

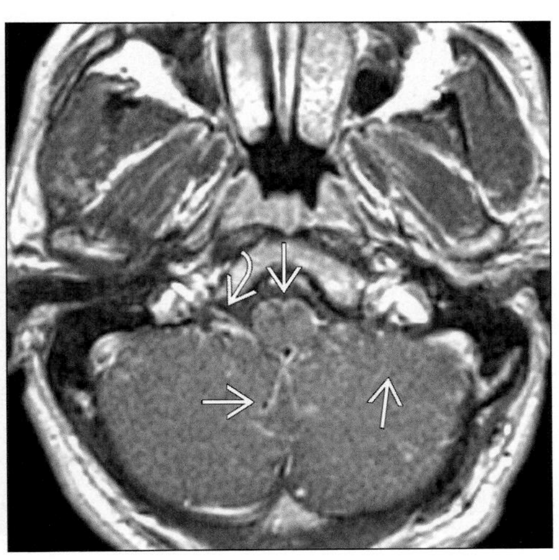

(Left) *Axial NECT demonstrates extensive white matter abnormality bilaterally from angiitis. The white matter is hypodense by CT* ➔ *and hyperintense on T2/ FLAIR (not shown).* ***(Right)*** *Axial T1WI C+ MR reveals a fine coating of abnormal enhancing material involving the medulla, cerebellar hemispheres, and vermis* ➔*. Also note the abnormal enhancement that coats the right hypoglossal cranial nerve* ➔*.*

MISCELLANEOUS HISTIOCYTOSES

Key Facts

Terminology

- Includes non-Langerhans cell histiocytoses (non-LCH)
  - Wegener granulomatosis (WG)
  - Rosai-Dorfman disease (RDD), a.k.a. sinus histiocytosis with massive lymphadenopathy (SHML)
  - Erdheim-Chester disease (ECD)
  - Hemophagocytic lymphohistiocytosis (HLH)

Imaging

- WG: Multiple cavitary lung nodules and large airway narrowing typical
  - CNS: Orbital masses with meningeal extension
  - Nasal and orbital masses; septal perforation
  - Sinus CT as initial study and consider MR to evaluate for intracranial involvement
- RDD: Massive, painless cervical lymphadenopathy in child or young adult
  - CNS: T2 hypointense orbital or dural masses
- ECD: Enhancing brainstem & cerebellar lesions
- HLH: Enhancing brain parenchymal lesions with leptomeningeal disease in infant or child
- Enhanced MR best for CNS manifestations

Clinical Issues

- WG: Sinus, lung, and renal disease (classic triad)
  - Mean age at diagnosis: 40-55 years
- RDD: Painless neck mass most common
  - Children and young adults
- ECD: Cerebellar and pyramidal syndromes most frequent manifestations
  - Older adults and elderly
- HLH: Seizures most common CNS presentation
  - Infants and children

(Left) Coronal NECT shows extensive paranasal sinus soft tissue thickening with contiguous disease into the left orbit ➔, characteristic of WG. Septal perforation is a classic feature of WG. When the disease is extensive, contrast-enhanced MR is helpful to evaluate for intracranial involvement. (Right) Axial T1WI C+ FS MR shows extensive sinonasal disease with infiltration of the left medial rectus muscle ➔ and orbital fat. Note the diffuse dural thickening ➔ in this patient with WG.

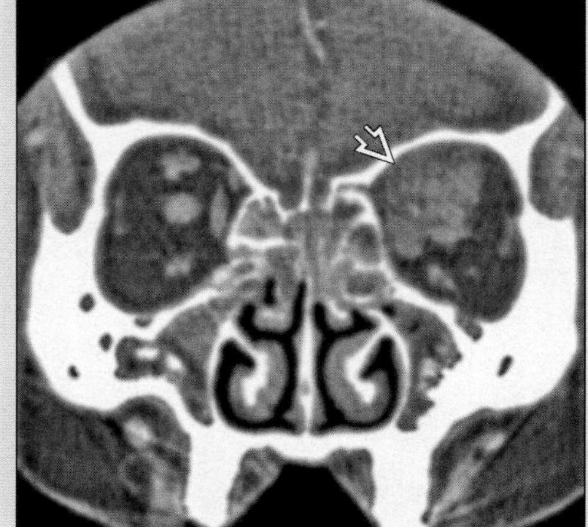

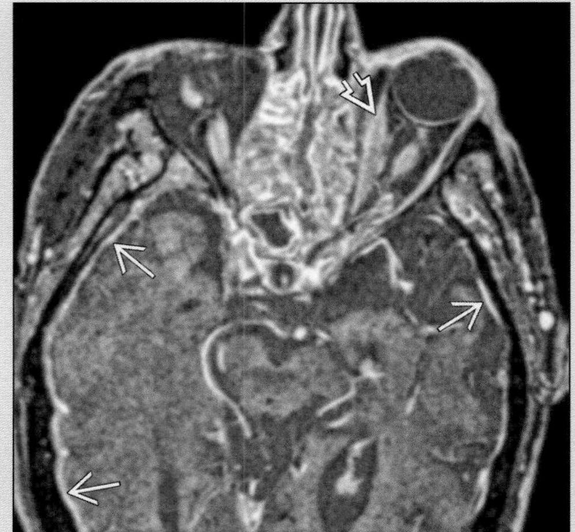

(Left) Axial CECT shows enlarged retropharyngeal lymph nodes ➔ in association with massive adenopathy in the deep cervical and spinal accessory nodal chains ➔. Non-Hodgkin lymphoma was suspected. Biopsy revealed Rosai-Dorfman disease. Painless adenopathy is the most common presentation of RDD. (Right) Axial T1WI C+ MR shows lobular dural masses along the falx in this male patient with RDD. These masses are typically T2 hypointense, which may help with an accurate preoperative diagnosis.

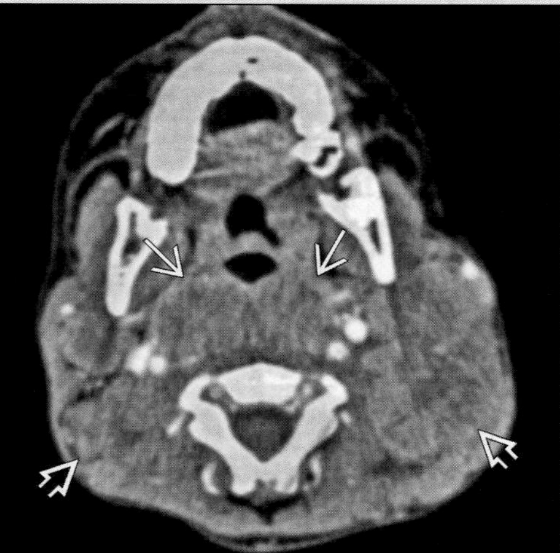

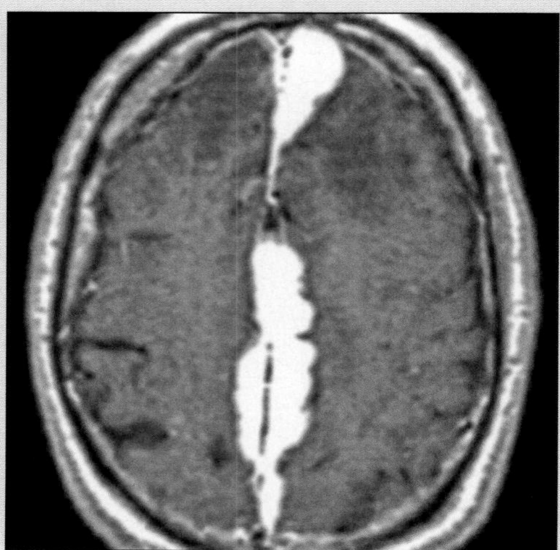

TERMINOLOGY

Abbreviations

- Includes non-Langerhans cell histiocytoses (non-LCH)
  - Wegener granulomatosis (WG)
  - Rosai-Dorfman disease (RDD)
    - a.k.a. sinus histiocytosis with massive lymphadenopathy (SHML)
  - Erdheim-Chester disease (ECD)
  - Hemophagocytic lymphohistiocytosis (HLH)

Definitions

- WG: Uncommon disease involving granulomatous inflammation, necrosis, & vasculitis; most frequently affects upper & lower respiratory tract & kidneys
- RDD: Rare, benign, idiopathic histioproliferative disorder usually manifesting as massive painless adenopathy
- ECD: Rare, non-Langerhans form of histiocytosis of unknown etiology that affects multiple organs
- HLH: Rare, nonmalignant disorder of immune regulation, with overproduction of cytokines and diminished immune surveillance
  - May affect multiple organs, including central nervous system (CNS)

IMAGING

General Features

- Best diagnostic clue
  - WG: Multiple cavitary lung nodules and large airway narrowing typical
    - CNS: Orbital masses with meningeal extension
      - Rarely causes parenchymal lesions
    - Nasal and orbital masses; septal perforation
  - RDD: Massive, painless cervical lymphadenopathy in child or young adult
    - CNS: T2 hypointense orbital or dural masses
  - ECD: Enhancing brainstem & cerebellar lesions
  - HLH: Enhancing brain parenchymal lesions with leptomeningeal disease in infant or child
- Location
  - WG: Paranasal sinuses, lungs, kidneys, joints, orbits, skin, peripheral nerves, meninges
  - RDD: Cervical lymph nodes, orbits, meninges, skin, paranasal sinuses, nasal cavity, bone, salivary glands
  - ECD: Bones, visceral organs, systemic fatty spaces
    - CNS: Cerebral hemispheres, hypothalamus, cerebellum, brainstem, orbits
  - HLH: Brain parenchyma, leptomeninges
- Morphology
  - WG, sinus: Nodular sinonasal masses with septal perforation
    - Orbits: Infiltrative masses; may involve lacrimal gland, extraocular muscles, retrobulbar fat
    - Meninges: Thickened
  - RDD: Homogeneous orbital mass; nodular dural mass
  - ECD: Parenchymal nodules or masses ± meningeal thickening or masses
  - HLH: Nodular parenchymal lesions

CT Findings

- NECT
  - WG: Nodular soft tissue thickening of paranasal sinuses ± bone erosion
    - Nasal septal perforation classic
  - RDD: Polypoid nasal mass ± bone erosion
  - ECD: Hypodense parenchymal lesions typical
    - Rarely see hyperdense lesions
  - HLH: Hypodense lesions
    - May become hemorrhagic
    - May see diffuse brain edema
- CECT
  - RDD: Cervical lymphadenopathy
    - Orbital mass with diffuse enhancement
    - Nodular dural mass with diffuse enhancement

MR Findings

- T1WI
  - WG: Nodular soft tissue thickening of paranasal sinuses and orbits
  - RDD: Isointense lesions
  - HLH: Ventriculomegaly; hypointense lesions
- T2WI
  - RDD: Marked hypointensity
  - ECD: Hyperintense lesions
  - HLH: Laminated, nodular hyperintense lesions; may become confluent
- T1WI C+
  - WG: Nodular soft tissue thickening of paranasal sinuses and orbits
    - Enhancing, thickened meninges (typically anterior cranial fossa)
    - Patchy parenchymal lesions (rare)
  - RDD: Diffuse, homogeneous enhancement
  - ECD: Enhancing parenchyma ± meninges
    - 3 patterns: Infiltrative (44%), meningeal (37%), or composite (infiltrative & meningeal lesions [19%])
  - HLH: Nodular or ring-enhancing lesions ± meningeal enhancement

Imaging Recommendations

- Best imaging tool
  - Enhanced MR best for CNS manifestations
  - WG: Sinus CT; consider MR to evaluate for intracranial involvement if disease is extensive

DIFFERENTIAL DIAGNOSIS

Wegener Granulomatosis

- Orbital mass: Lymphoma, orbital pseudotumor, sarcoid, RDD
- Nasal septal perforation: Trauma, cocaine necrosis, sarcoid, lymphoma, squamous cell carcinoma
- Meningeal thickening: Sarcoid, infectious etiologies, intracranial pseudotumor, metastases

Rosai-Dorfman Disease

- Orbital mass: Lymphoma, orbital pseudotumor, sarcoid, WG
- Meningeal masses: Meningiomas, sarcoid, lymphoma, extramedullary hematopoiesis, metastases
- Cervical lymphadenopathy: Lymphoma, reactive lymph nodes, tuberculosis

MISCELLANEOUS HISTIOCYTOSES

Erdheim-Chester Disease and Hemophagocytic Lymphohistiocytosis
- LCH: Sharply marginated, lytic skull lesion; thick enhancing infundibulum; parenchymal lesions rare
- TB: Meningeal & parenchymal enhancing lesions
- Metastases: Multiple enhancing nodules; primary tumor often known

PATHOLOGY

General Features
- WG: Combination of necrotizing granulomatous lesions of upper and lower respiratory tracts, generalized necrotizing vasculitis of arteries and veins, and glomerulonephritis
  - Involves CNS in up to 50% of patients
- RDD: Inflammatory infiltrate in absence of infectious agent, emperipolesis, S100(+) stain
- ECD: Non-Langerhans cell xanthogranulomas disseminated in cerebral hemispheres, hypothalamus, cerebellum, and brainstem
  - Touton giant cells characteristic
  - CD68(+), factor VIII(+), CD1a(-), S100(-)
- HLH: Starts as leptomeningeal process → perivascular infiltration with astrocytic proliferation affecting mainly white matter → areas of necrosis and focal demyelination

Staging, Grading, & Classification
- HLH: Consequence of uncontrolled, dysregulated cellular immune reactivity caused by number of different underlying diseases
  - 3 major risk groups of HLH identified
    - Familial HLH (FLH)
    - Epstein-Barr virus-associated HLH (EBV-HLH)
    - Life-threatening infection-associated or underlying disease; unknown HLH in infants

CLINICAL ISSUES

Presentation
- Most common signs/symptoms
  - WG: Sinus, lung, and renal disease (classic triad)
    - Orbital disease and meningeal involvement uncommon
    - Headache most common feature of CNS disease
    - Sinusitis, rhinitis, & otitis media (common triad)
  - RDD: Painless neck mass most common
    - Sinonasal disease: Progressive nasal obstruction
    - Orbit: Proptosis
    - CNS: Headache
  - ECD: Cerebellar (41%) and pyramidal (45%) syndromes most frequent manifestations
    - Seizures, headaches, neuropsychiatric or cognitive troubles, sensory disturbances, cranial neuropathy
    - Neurological manifestations always associated with other organ involvement, especially bones (86%) and diabetes insipidus (47%)
    - Systemic involvement: Long bones, retroperitoneal fibrosis, pulmonary fibrosis, orbital infiltration
  - HLH: Seizures most common CNS presentation
    - May see irritability, cranial nerve findings, coma

Demographics
- Age
  - WG: Mean age at diagnosis = 40-55 years
  - RDD: Children and young adults
  - ECD: Older adults and elderly
  - HLH: Infants and children

Natural History & Prognosis
- WG: Renal failure most common cause of death
- RDD: Benign, progressive disease
- ECD: Poor prognosis
- HLH: Generally poor outcome

Treatment
- WG: Systemic steroids and cyclophosphamide
- RDD: Radiation therapy, chemotherapy, steroids, surgery with varying success
  - Clinical observation without treatment when possible
- ECD: Corticosteroids, chemotherapy, radiotherapy, surgery
- HLH: Distinct therapeutic measures advised for each type; underlying cause must be established to allow prompt therapy
  - FLH: Immediate immunochemotherapy with combination of corticosteroids and etoposide together with brain MR, followed by stem cell transplantation (SCT)
  - EBV-HLH: Combination of corticosteroids and etoposide; aggressive or relapsed cases may require more intensive chemotherapy; SCT may be needed
  - Infection-associated or undetermined pathogen HLH in early infancy: Appropriate antiviral or antibacterial agents

DIAGNOSTIC CHECKLIST

Consider
- When destructive nasal septum lesion extends to involve orbits &/or meninges, consider WG!
- When orbital or dural mass has T2 hypointensity, consider RDD!
- Brainstem or cerebellar lesions in patient with bone lesions or diabetes insipidus, consider ECD!
- Infant or child with enhancing parenchymal and meningeal lesions, consider HLH!

SELECTED REFERENCES

1. Cannady SB et al: Sinonasal Wegener granulomatosis: a single-institution experience with 120 cases. Laryngoscope. 119(4):757-61, 2009
2. Horne A et al: Frequency and spectrum of central nervous system involvement in 193 children with haemophagocytic lymphohistiocytosis. Br J Haematol. 140(3):327-35, 2008
3. La Barge DV 3rd et al: Sinus histiocytosis with massive lymphadenopathy (Rosai-Dorfman disease): imaging manifestations in the head and neck. AJR Am J Roentgenol. 191(6):W299-306, 2008

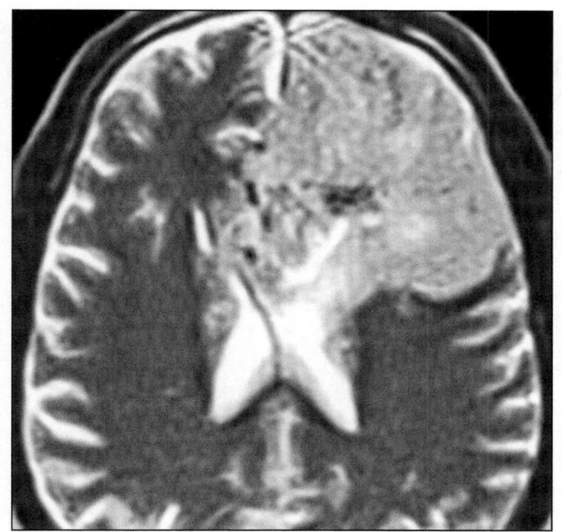

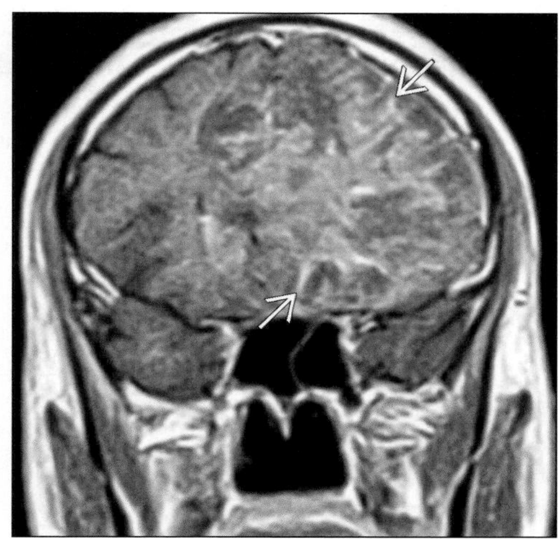

(Left) *Axial T2WI MR shows a heterogeneously hyperintense frontal lobe lesion with associated mass effect in this patient with nasal septal perforation.* ***(Right)*** *Coronal T1 C+ MR in the same patient with WG shows patchy, linear enhancement ➔, which helps differentiate this lesion from a primary brain tumor. Brain parenchymal involvement is a rare manifestation of this disease. Orbital and meningeal involvement are the typical CNS manifestations of WG.*

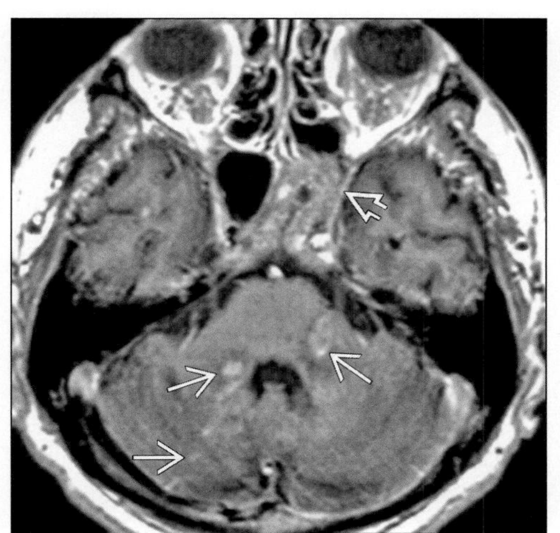

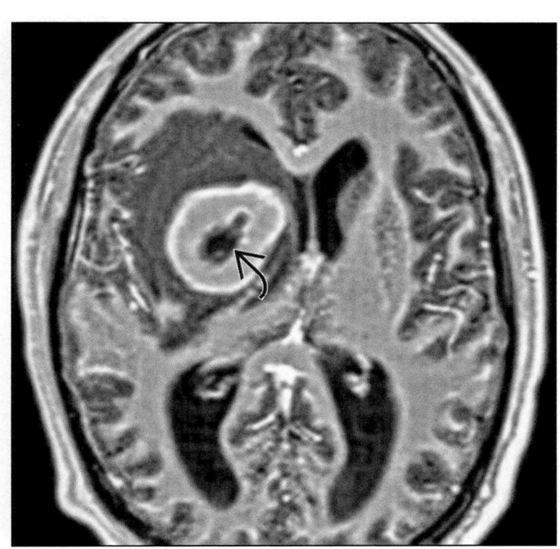

(Left) *Axial T1WI C+ MR shows patchy and nodular enhancement ➔ in the pons and cerebellum as well as the cavernous sinus ⇨. Biopsy proved non-Langerhans histiocytosis, consistent with Erdheim-Chester disease.* ***(Right)*** *Axial T1WI C+ MR shows an enhancing mass with central hypointensity ↷. Biopsy revealed ECD. ECD typically presents with brainstem or cerebellar lesions and may have meningeal enhancement. Long bone involvement is also typical. (Courtesy M. Warmuth-Metz, MD.)*

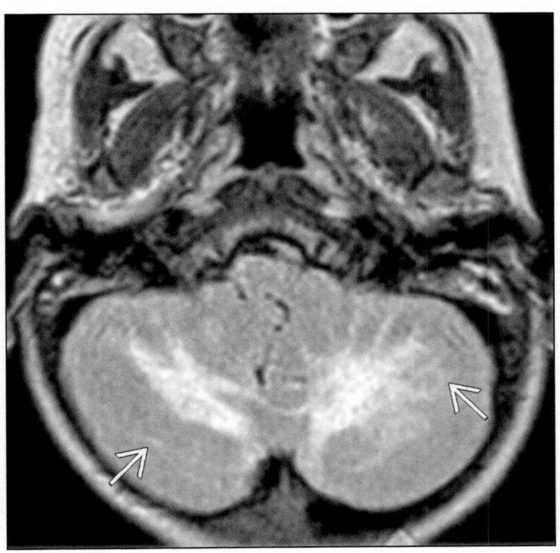

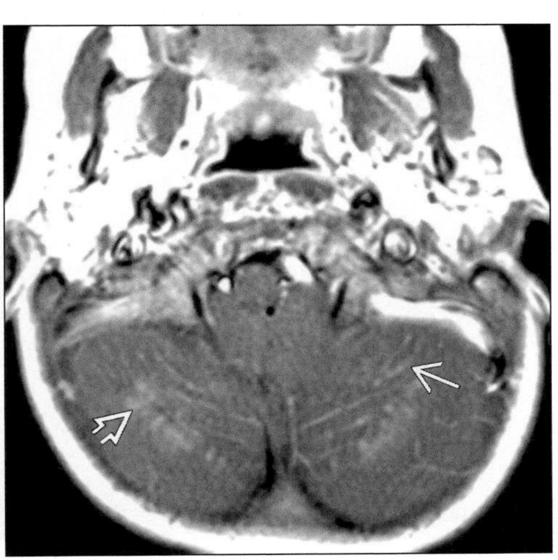

(Left) *Axial FLAIR MR shows abnormal hyperintensity in the cerebellar white matter & meninges ➔ of this young child. Abnormal white matter was also present in the cerebral hemispheres (not shown).* ***(Right)*** *Axial T1WI C+ MR in the same patient with HLH shows striking enhancement of both the parenchymal ⇨ and meningeal ➔ lesions. This rare immune disorder affects mostly infants and young children. Both familial (primary) and secondary forms are recognized.*

SEBACEOUS CYST

Key Facts

Terminology

- Trichilemmal cyst (TC) is preferred term
- Keratin-containing cyst
  - Lined by stratified squamous epithelium
  - Pathology looks like root sheath of hair follicle

Imaging

- General features
  - Most within dermis or subcutaneous tissue
  - Size varies from a few mm to several cm
  - Can become huge
  - Can be single or multiple
- CT
  - Round/ovoid, well-delineated scalp mass
  - Multifocal punctate/curvilinear/coarse Ca++
- MR
  - Isointense with brain, muscle on T1WI
  - Inhomogeneously hypointense on T2WI
  - Does not suppress on FLAIR
  - Multifocal "blooming" foci common on T2*
  - Simple sebaceous cysts usually do not enhance

Top Differential Diagnoses

- Basal cell, SCCa
- Dermoid cyst
- Epidermoid cyst
- Metastasis
- Cephalocele

Clinical Issues

- Classic presentation
  - Subepidermal scalp mass in woman > 60 years
  - Hairless, rubbery, nontender, mobile subcutaneous scalp mass(es)
  - Usually nonpainful

(Left) Axial NECT in a 63-year-old man was obtained for trauma evaluation. A superficial scalp mass ➡ that contained several hyperintense foci suggesting calcifications ⇨ was incidentally noted. (Right) Axial bone CT in the same patient shows that the scalp mass ➡ is sharply delineated. Multiple punctate and curvilinear calcifications ➡ within the mass can be seen. Note the lack of bone erosion or invasion. The remainder of the scalp appears normal. This was presumed to be a sebaceous cyst.

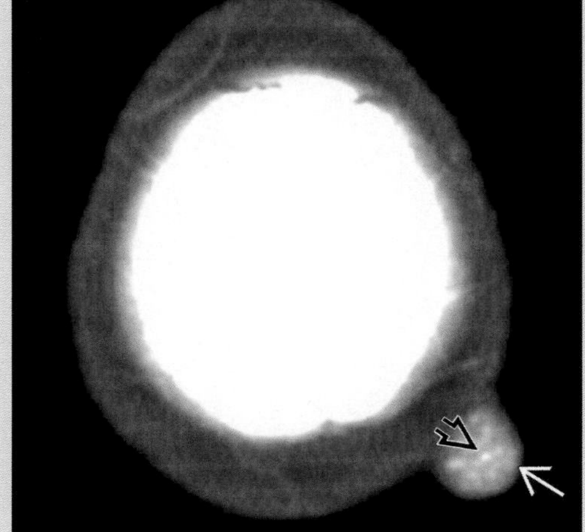

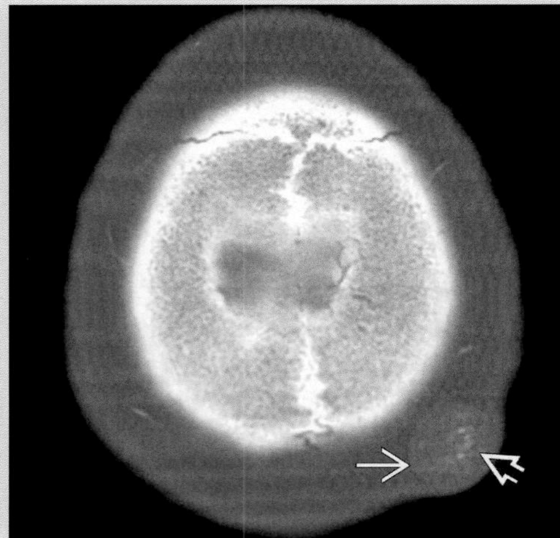

(Left) Sagittal T1WI MR in a 68-year-old woman with headaches shows 2 large but very well-circumscribed scalp masses ➡. The masses are incompletely surrounded by fat and isointense with brain and muscle. (Right) Axial T2WI MR in the same patient shows the mass ➡ to be inhomogeneously hypointense. Both lesions demonstrated some internal "blooming" on T2 that suggested calcifications. These lesions had been slowly enlarging over many years and are benign proliferating trichilemmal cysts.*

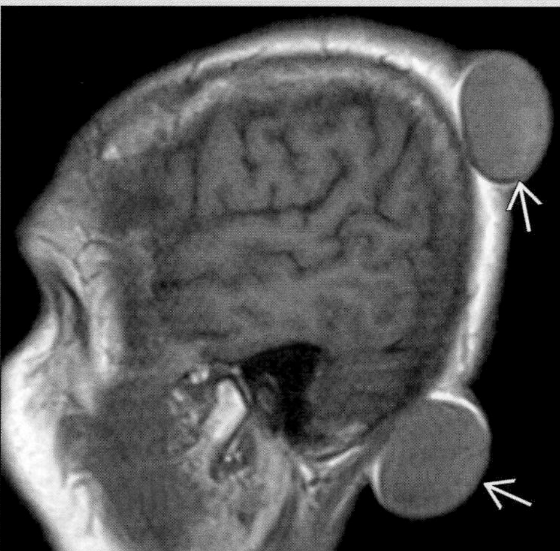

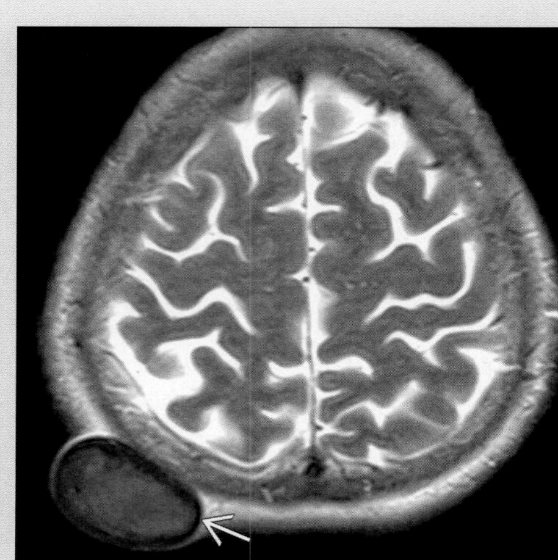

SEBACEOUS CYST

TERMINOLOGY

Abbreviations

- Sebaceous cyst (SC)
- Trichilemmal cyst (TC) is preferred term
- Variant = proliferating trichilemmal tumor (PTT)

Synonyms

- PTT also called "pilar" or "turban" tumor

Definitions

- Keratin-containing cyst
  - Lined by stratified squamous epithelium

IMAGING

General Features

- Best diagnostic clue
  - Nontender scalp mass in older woman
- Location
  - Soft tissues of scalp
    - Most within dermis or subcutaneous tissue
- Size
  - Varies from a few mm to several cm
  - Can be single or multiple
- Morphology
  - Round/ovoid, well delineated

Imaging Recommendations

- Best imaging tool
  - CT with soft tissue, bone windows

CT Findings

- NECT
  - Solid or cystic scalp mass(es)
  - Sharply delineated
  - Hyperdense to fat
  - Multifocal punctate, curvilinear, and coarse Ca++
    - May layer in dependent portion of larger cysts
- CECT
  - No enhancement

MR Findings

- T1WI
  - Isointense with brain, muscle
- T2WI
  - Inhomogeneously hypointense
- FLAIR
  - Does not suppress
- T2* GRE
  - Multifocal "blooming" foci common
  - Ca++, not hemorrhage
- T1WI C+
  - Simple sebaceous cysts usually do not enhance
  - PTTs may show significant enhancement with solid lobules, cystic cavities

DIFFERENTIAL DIAGNOSIS

Basal Cell, SCCa

- Basal cell carcinomas are ill defined, invade locally
- Primary scalp SCCas rare

Dermoid Cyst

- Skull > > scalp

Epidermoid Cyst

- Skull > > scalp

Hemangioma

- Skull > > scalp

Metastasis

- Ill-defined, invasive

Cephalocele

- Young patient
- Usually complex, containing brain/meninges/vessels

PATHOLOGY

Gross Pathologic & Surgical Features

- Elevated, slightly reddish scalp mass

Microscopic Features

- Resembles external root sheath of hair follicle
  - Lined by stratified squamous epithelial cells
- Cyst contents: Keratin, Ca++ frequent
- Malignant transformation rare

CLINICAL ISSUES

Presentation

- Most common signs/symptoms
  - Hairless, rubbery, nontender, mobile subcutaneous scalp mass
  - Usually nonpainful

Demographics

- Age
  - Any age
  - Proliferating trichilemmal cysts most common in elderly women
    - Classic is subepidermal scalp tumor in female > 60 years
- Gender
  - Female predominance

Natural History & Prognosis

- Usually slow growth
- May become locally aggressive
- Malignant transformation of trichilemmal cysts is rare
  - Proliferating trichilemmal cystic carcinoma (PTCC)

Treatment

- Surgical excision

SELECTED REFERENCES

1. Anolik R et al: Proliferating trichilemmal cyst with focal calcification. Dermatol Online J. 14(10):25, 2008
2. Kitajima K et al: Magnetic resonance imaging findings of proliferating trichilemmal tumor. Neuroradiology. 47(6):406-10, 2005

MENINGIOMA

Key Facts

Terminology
- Typical ("benign") meningioma (TM) = WHO grade 1

Imaging
- Supratentorial (90%)
  - Parasagittal/convexity (45%), sphenoid (15-20%)
  - Olfactory groove (5-10%), parasellar (5-10%)
- Infratentorial (8-10%) (CPA most common site)
- Rare: Paranasal sinuses, nose
- General features
  - Extraaxial mass with broad-based dural attachment
  - > 90% enhance homogeneously, intensely
- CT
  - Hyper- (70-75%), iso- (25%), hypodense (1-5%)
  - Hyperostosis, irregular cortex, ↑ vascular markings
  - Ca++ (20-25%) (diffuse, focal, sand-like, "sunburst," globular, rim)
  - Necrosis, cysts common; hemorrhage rare
- MR
  - Look for CSF/vascular "cleft" between tumor, brain
  - Dural "tail" (35-80% but nonspecific)
  - Use pMR to correlate with tumor grade

Top Differential Diagnoses
- Dural metastasis
- Granuloma (TB, sarcoid)
- Idiopathic hypertrophic pachymeningitis
- Extramedullary hematopoiesis
- Hemangioma, dura/venous sinuses

Clinical Issues
- Very common primary adult intracranial tumor (13-20%)
- TMs grow slowly, compress adjacent structures

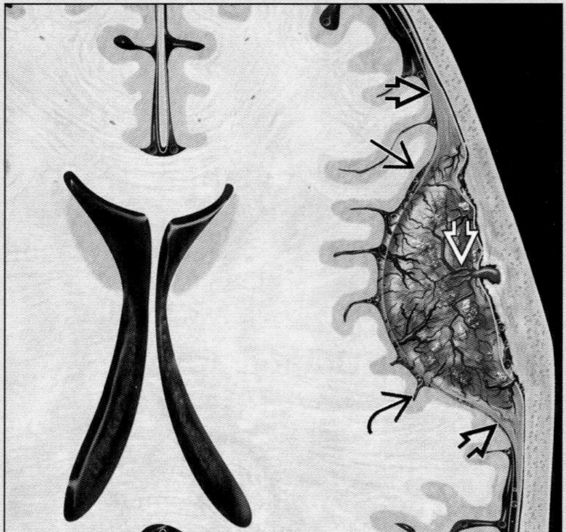

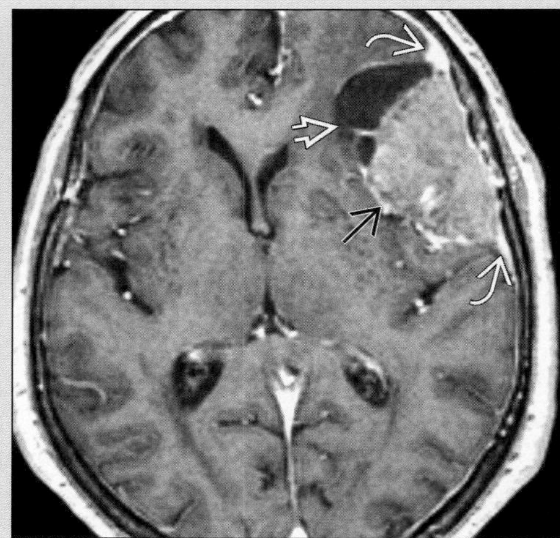

(Left) *Axial graphic shows a dural-based mass with Ca++ (white foci), inward cortical buckling, CSF/vascular "cleft" ➔, and dural "tail" ➔. Note the "sunburst" of dural vascular supply ➔. Intracranial arteries are becoming parasitized ➔, supplying the periphery.* ***(Right)*** *Axial T1WI C+ MR shows a dural-based extraaxial mass ➔ in the left frontal lobe with intense enhancement and dural "tail" ➔. Note the trapped pools of CSF around the tumor ➔.*

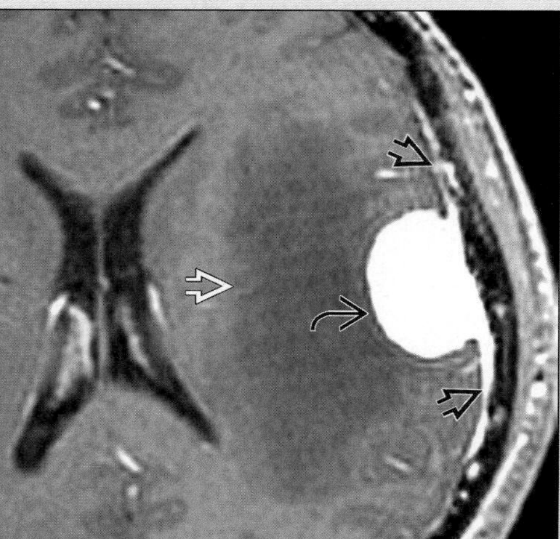

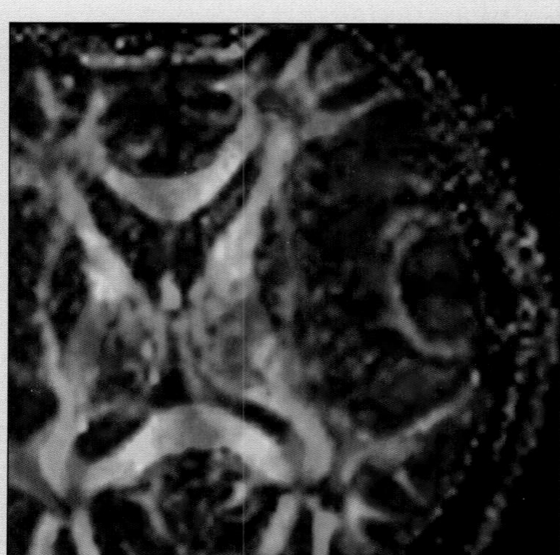

(Left) *Axial T1WI C+ MR shows a homogeneously, markedly enhancing extraaxial mass ➔ with a distinct dural "tail" ➔. Note the prominent hypointense perifocal edema ➔. A typical meningioma was found at surgery.* ***(Right)*** *Axial DTI (directional color map) demonstrates deviation of the adjacent white matter tracts nicely depicted with color diffusion tensor imaging.*

TERMINOLOGY

Abbreviations

- Typical meningioma (TM)
- Atypical meningioma (AM), malignant meningioma (MM)

Definitions

- TM = WHO grade 1 meningioma

IMAGING

General Features

- Best diagnostic clue
  - Dural-based enhancing mass → cortical buckling, trapped CSF/vessels in "cleft" between tumor and brain
- Location
  - Supratentorial (90%)
    - Parasagittal/convexity (45%), sphenoid ridge (15-20%)
    - Olfactory groove (5-10%), parasellar (5-10%)
    - Other (5%): Intraventricular, optic nerve sheath (ONSM), pineal region, intraosseous
    - Rare: Intraparenchymal without dural attachment
  - Infratentorial (8-10%): CPA most common
  - Extracranial (head/neck)
    - Most common: Paranasal sinuses
    - Less common: Nasal cavity, parotid, skin
  - Multiple meningiomas: Seen in 1-9% of cases
    - 16% at autopsy (M < F)
- Morphology
  - Extraaxial mass with broad-based dural attachment

CT Findings

- NECT
  - Sharply circumscribed smooth mass abutting dura
    - Hyper- (70-75%), isodense (25%)
      - Hypodense (1-5%), fat density (rare lipoblastic subtype)
    - Calcified (20-25%)
      - Can be diffuse, focal, sand-like ("psammomatous")
      - "Sunburst," globular, rim patterns
    - Necrosis, cysts, hemorrhage (8-23%)
  - Trapped CSF pools, cysts in adjacent brain common
  - Peritumoral hypodense vasogenic edema (60%)
  - Bone CT
    - Hyperostosis, irregular cortex, ↑ vascular markings
- CECT
  - > 90% enhance homogeneously, intensely
- CTA
  - May be helpful prior to DSA, embolization
  - Delineates arterial supply, venous drainage

MR Findings

- T1WI
  - Typically iso- to slightly hypointense with cortex
  - Necrosis, cysts, hemorrhage (8-23%)
  - Look for gray matter "buckling"
- T2WI
  - Variable ("sunburst" pattern may be evident)
  - 8-23% of intratumoral cysts (common; can be almost microcystic), hemorrhage (rare)
  - Best sequence for visualizing
    - CSF/vascular cleft between tumor, brain (80%)
    - Vascular flow voids (80%)
- FLAIR
  - Hyperintense peritumoral edema, dural "tail"
- T2* GRE
  - Ca++ common, hemorrhage rare
- DWI
  - DWI, ADC maps for TM variable in appearance
  - Lower ADC in MM and AM compared to TM
- T1WI C+
  - > 95% enhance homogeneously, intensely
  - Dural "tail" (35-80% of cases) nonspecific
    - Other neoplasms (schwannoma, adenoma, metastases), nonneoplastic dural-based masses
  - En plaque: Sessile thickened enhancing dura
- MRV
  - Evaluate sinus involvement
- MRS
  - Elevated levels of alanine at short TE
    - Triplet-like spectral pattern at 1.3-1.5 ppm (overlapping of Ala, Lac)
    - Elevated Glx alfa/glutationine
- Perfusion MR
  - rCBV and rMTE values of peritumoral edema differentiate TM and MM
    - High rCBV in peritumoral edema of anaplastic meningiomas

Angiographic Findings

- DSA
  - "Sunburst" or radial appearance
    - Dural vessels supply lesion core
    - Pial vessels may be parasitized, supply periphery
  - Prolonged vascular "stain"
  - Venous phase vital to evaluate sinus involvement
- Interventional: Preoperative embolization
  - Decreases operative time and blood loss
  - Particulate agents (e.g., polyvinyl alcohol) favored
  - Optimal interval between embolization & surgery is 7-9 days; allows for greatest tumor softening

Other Modality Findings

- Imaging predictors of difficult, extrapial surgical cleavage plane
  - Peritumoral edema on MR/CT → may obscure pial invasion by tumor
  - Tumor pial vascularization on DSA = pial invasion
  - Tumor/cortex interface is not reliable predictor

Imaging Recommendations

- Best imaging tool
  - MR + contrast
- Protocol advice
  - Consider MRS → look for alanine, glu:cr ratio

DIFFERENTIAL DIAGNOSIS

Dural Metastasis

- Skull often infiltrated; multifocal
- Breast most common primary

Granuloma
- Sarcoid
- TB

Idiopathic Hypertrophic Pachymeningitis
- Dural biopsy essential to confirm diagnosis

Extramedullary Hematopoiesis
- Known hematologic disorder
- Often multifocal

Hemangioma, Dura/Venous Sinuses
- Can be indistinguishable from TM
- Venous sinus (e.g., cavernous) > dural-based mass

PATHOLOGY

General Features
- Etiology
  - Arise from arachnoid meningothelial ("cap") cells
  - CM: 90% inactivation of *NF2* gene product "Merlin"
    - 1st event is 22 chromosomal loss → monosomy
    - "2nd hit theory": Remaining single *NF2* copy is mutated; vast majority are null mutations
    - Results in truncated nonfunctional protein
  - May be related to female sex hormones: M < F, correlate + with breast cancer, may ↑ in pregnancy, progesterone receptors identified
  - XRT predisposes: Most common radiation-induced tumor, latency 20-35 years
- Associated abnormalities
  - Neurofibromatosis type 2
    - Multiple inherited schwannomas, meningiomas, and ependymomas (MISME)
    - 10% with multiple meningiomas have NF2
  - Metastatic carcinoma to CM have been reported
    - CM are most common primary intracranial tumor to harbor metastases; majority are lung or breast
- Slow growing, benign

Gross Pathologic & Surgical Features
- 2 basic morphologies
  - Globose = globular, well-demarcated neoplasm with wide dural attachment
  - En plaque = sheet-like extension covering dura without parenchymal invagination
- Homogeneous reddish-brown translucent pale surface
- Soft to tough, occasionally gritty
  - Depends on fibrous tissue, Ca++ calcium content
- TMs usually invaginate into brain, do not invade it

Microscopic Features
- TM has wide range of subtypes
  - Meningothelial: Uniform tumor cells, collagenous septa, psammomatous calcifications (most common)
  - Fibrous: Interlacing fascicles of spindle-shaped cells, collagen/reticulin matrix
  - Transitional: Mixed; "onion-bulb" whorls, psammoma bodies
  - Lipoblastic: Metaplasia into adipocytes; large triglyceride fat droplets
  - Clear cell: Aggressive despite benign histology; metastasis & recurrence more than other subtypes
  - Others: Angiomatous, microcystic, secretory, chordoid, etc.

CLINICAL ISSUES

Presentation
- Most common signs/symptoms
  - < 10% of all meningiomas are symptomatic
  - Symptoms depend on tumor site
- Other signs/symptoms
  - Increased AQP4 in peritumoral edema

Demographics
- Age
  - Middle decades
- Gender
  - M:F = 1:1.5-3
- Ethnicity
  - More common in African-Americans
- Epidemiology
  - Very common 1° adult intracranial tumor (13-20%)
  - ~ 6/100,000 population; 1-1.5% autopsy prevalence
- Geographic predilection
  - Nearly 30% of adult 1° intracranial tumors in Africa

Natural History & Prognosis
- Generally grow slowly, compress adjacent structures
- Parasagittal often grow into and occlude superior sagittal sinus
- Metastases rare (0.1-0.2%): Histology, location do NOT correlate with metastases

Treatment
- Asymptomatic followed with serial imaging
- Surgical goals
- Radiotherapy infrequently utilized for CM

DIAGNOSTIC CHECKLIST

Image Interpretation Pearls
- Preoperatively define **entire** extent of tumor
- Could patient be syndromic (e.g., NF2)?

SELECTED REFERENCES

1. Sergides I et al: Utilization of dynamic CT perfusion in the study of intracranial meningiomas and their surrounding tissue. Neurol Res. 31(1):84-9, 2009
2. Nagar VA et al: Diffusion-weighted MR imaging: diagnosing atypical or malignant meningiomas and detecting tumor dedifferentiation. AJNR Am J Neuroradiol. 29(6):1147-52, 2008
3. Toh CH et al: Differentiation between classic and atypical meningiomas with use of diffusion tensor imaging. AJNR Am J Neuroradiol. 29(9):1630-5, 2008
4. Yue Q et al: New observations concerning the interpretation of magnetic resonance spectroscopy of meningioma. Eur Radiol. 18(12):2901-11, 2008
5. Zhang H et al: Perfusion MR imaging for differentiation of benign and malignant meningiomas. Neuroradiology. 50(6):525-30, 2008

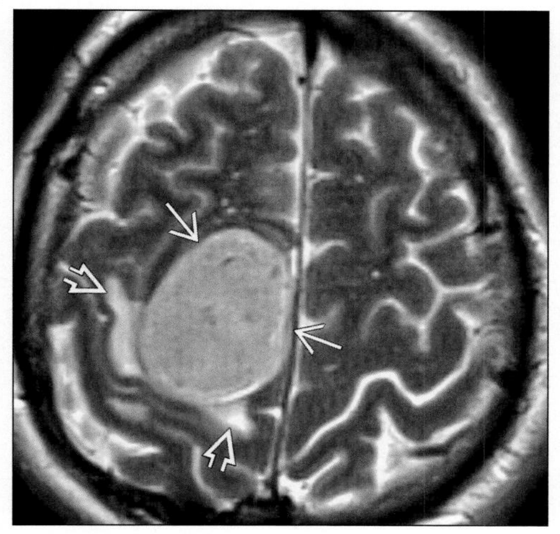

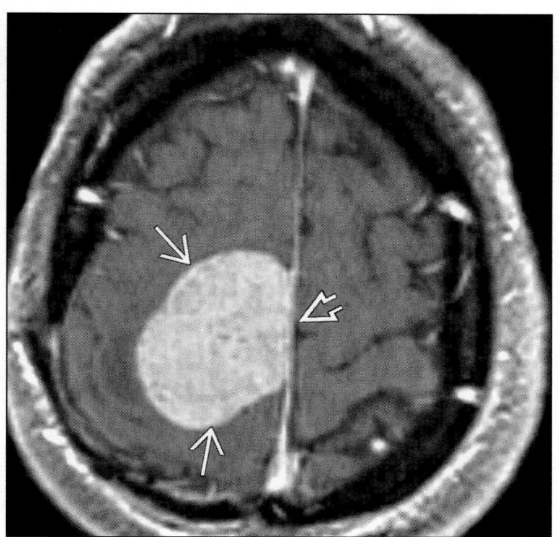

(Left) *Axial T2WI MR shows a homogeneous hyperintense mass attached to the falx ➡. Note the mild perifocal edema ➡.* ***(Right)*** *Axial T1WI C+ MR in the same patient shows intense, mostly homogeneous enhancement ➡. Note the broad base of attachment at the falx cerebri ➡ in this patient with typical meningioma.*

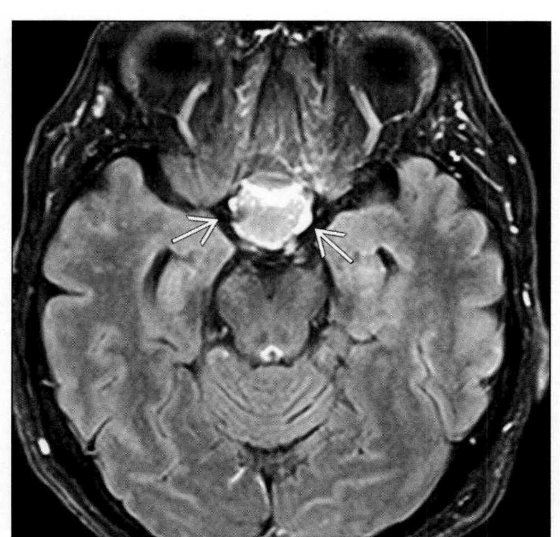

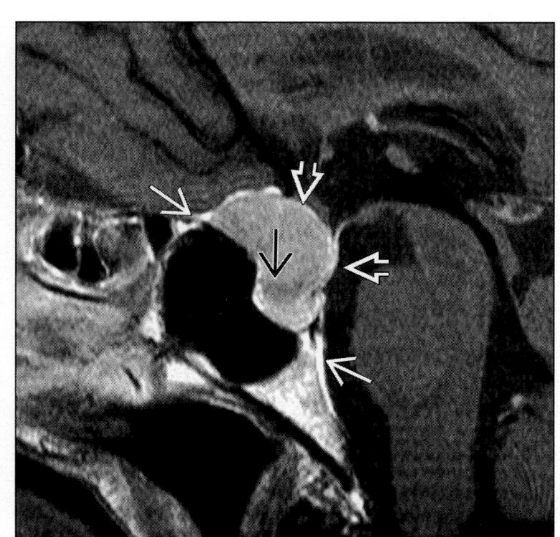

(Left) *Axial FLAIR MR shows a homogeneous high signal intensity mass ➡ projecting into the suprasellar cistern.* ***(Right)*** *Sagittal T1WI C+ MR in the same patient reveals a homogeneously enhancing meningioma ➡ arising from the limbus sphenoidale and diaphragma sellae, seen here as a faint, slightly hypointense area that slightly depresses the pituitary gland inferiorly ➡. Note the subtle dural "tails" ➡. Meningothelial meningioma was found at surgery.*

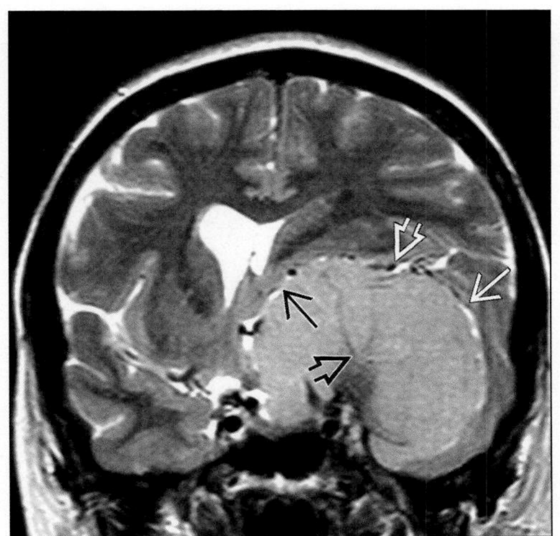

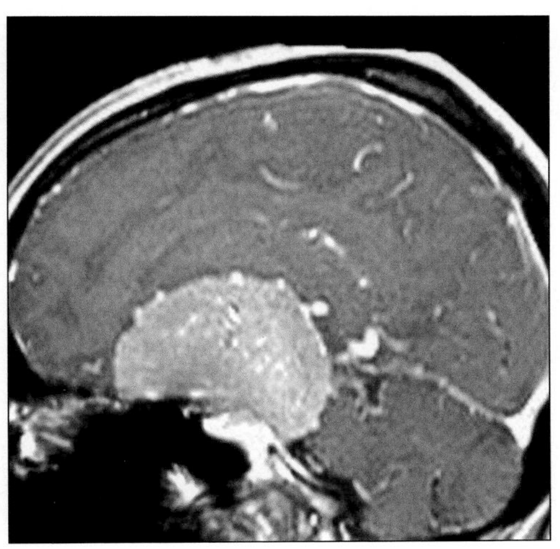

(Left) *Coronal T2WI MR demonstrates a mildly hyperintense mass in the left hemisphere with central "sunburst" appearance ➡. Note the inward "buckling" of the cortex ➡, indicating the extraaxial location of the mass. A thin CSF/vascular "cleft" ➡ with vascular flow voids ➡ is present at the periphery of the mass. No perifocal edema is seen.* ***(Right)*** *Sagittal T1WI C+ MR shows a meningioma of the sphenoid ridge with marked enhancement. Meningothelial (typical) meningioma was found at surgery.*

(Left) Axial T2WI MR shows a well-defined mass in the right cerebellopontine angle ➢ with extension into the right auditory canal ➡. (Right) Axial T1WI C+ MR demonstrates marked and homogeneous enhancement of the CPA meningioma.

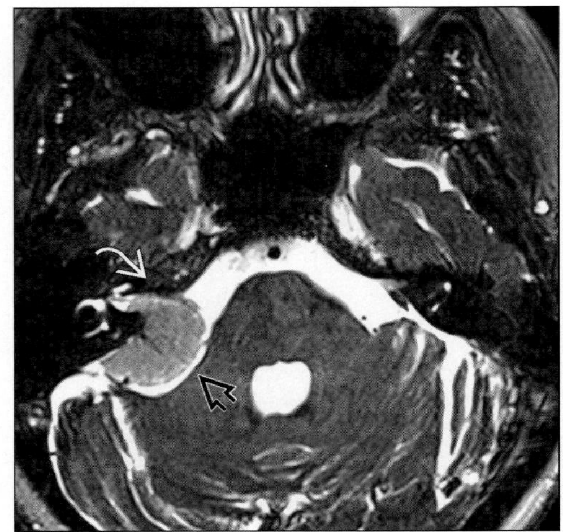

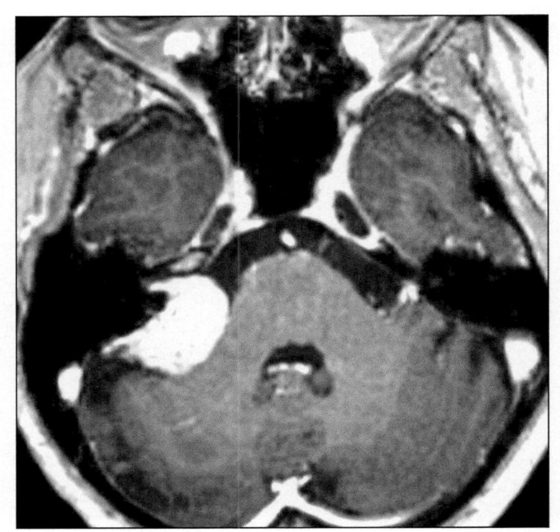

(Left) Coronal T2WI MR shows a cortex isointense mass ➢ in the region of the left olfactory bulb with perifocal edema ➡. (Right) Axial T1WI C+ MR shows marked and homogeneous enhancement of the mass ➢ representing olfactory meningioma.

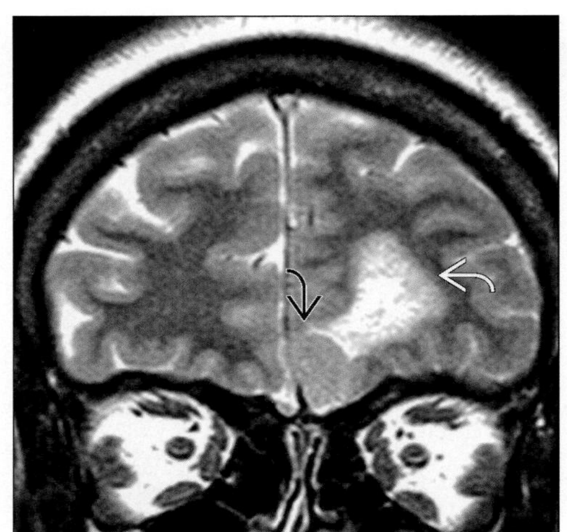

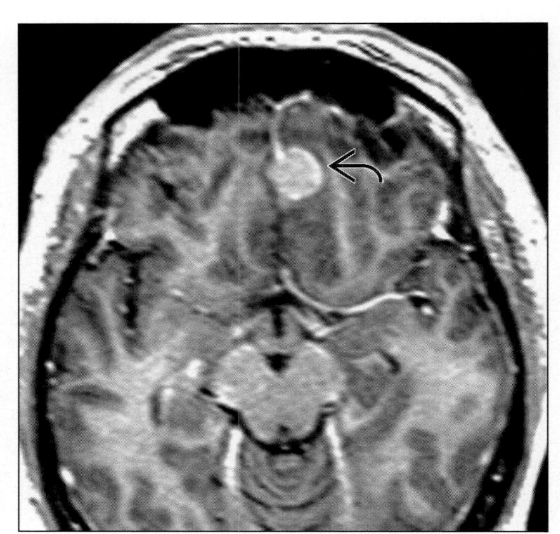

(Left) Axial CECT in a patient with primary optic nerve sheath meningioma shows marked enhancement along the left optic nerve, described as a "tram-track" sign ➢. (Right) Axial T1WI C+ MR in this patient with secondary optic nerve sheath meningioma shows meningioma arising from the sphenoid ridge around the anterior clinoid, narrowing the cavernous internal carotid, extending through the optic canal, and infiltrating the optic nerve sheath ➡.

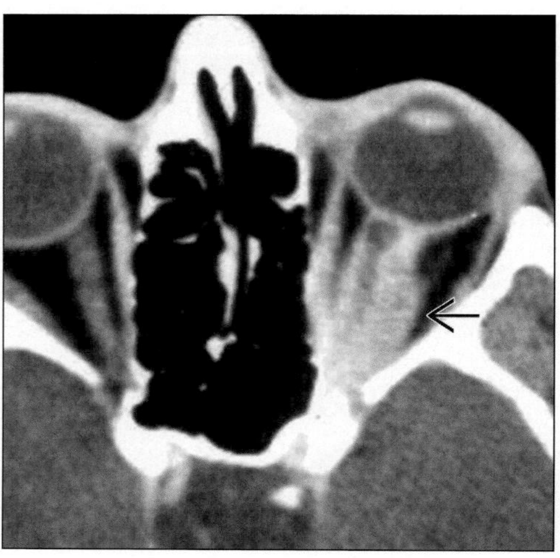

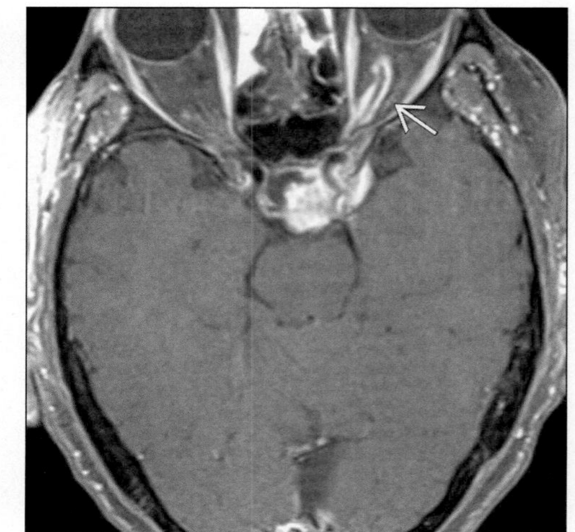

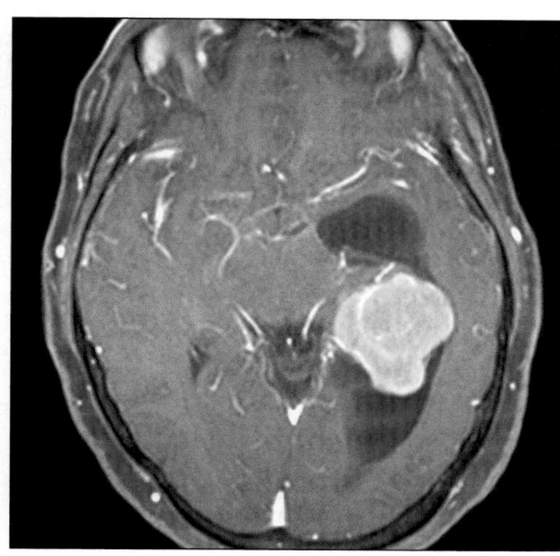

(Left) *Axial FLAIR MR shows a lobulated, mildly hyperintense intraventricular mass → arising from the choroid plexus glomus. Note the impressively enlarged temporal horn of left lateral ventricle with transependymal CSF migration →.* ***(Right)*** *Axial T1 C+ FS MR shows a strongly, uniformly enhancing mass. Intraventricular meningioma was found at surgery. About 1% of intracranial meningiomas are intraventricular; this is the most common location as arachnoid rests may persist within choroid plexus.*

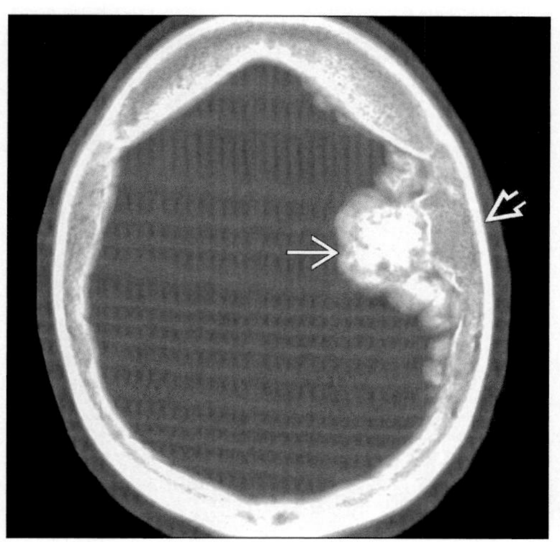

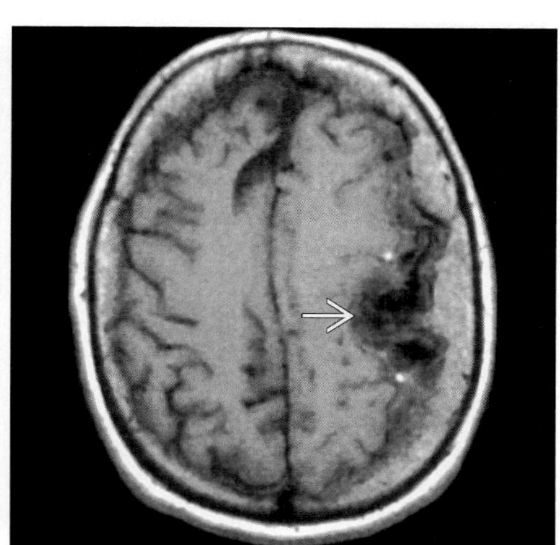

(Left) *Axial NECT shows marked hyperostosis → and calcification → in this plaque-like meningioma extending along the left inner table of the skull.* ***(Right)*** *Axial T1WI MR in the same patient demonstrates the characteristic hypointense appearance of calcification/ossification →.*

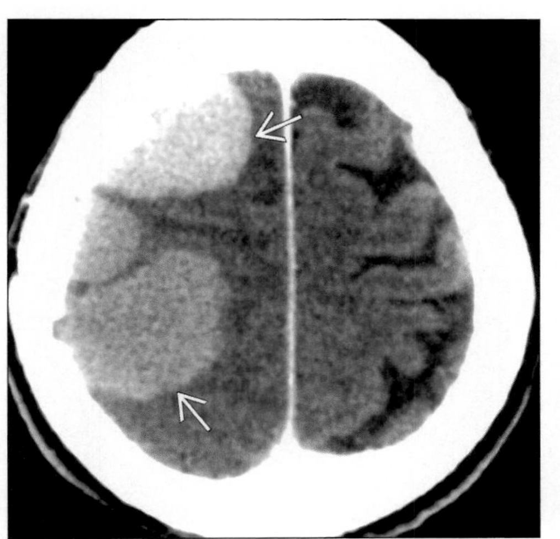

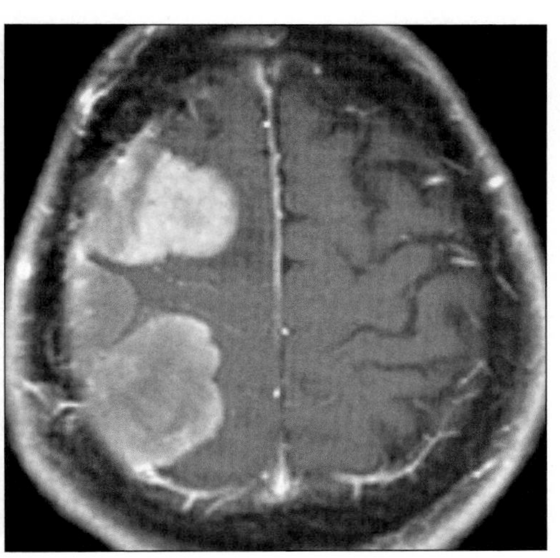

(Left) *Axial CECT shows multiple well-delineated, right-sided extraaxial masses → that are hyperdense on NECT and enhance strongly.* ***(Right)*** *Axial T1WI C+ MR shows strongly enhancing masses. Multiple meningiomas are more common in female patients and patients with NF2.*

ATYPICAL AND MALIGNANT MENINGIOMA

Key Facts

Terminology

- Typical ("benign") meningioma = WHO grade 1
- Atypical meningioma (AM) = WHO grade 2
- Malignant meningioma (MM) = WHO grade 3

Imaging

- CT "triad" of MM: Extracranial mass, osteolysis, intracranial tumor
- MR
  - Dural-based locally invasive lesion with areas of necrosis, marked brain edema
  - Indistinct tumor margins (tumor invades, interdigitates with brain)
  - Prominent tumor pannus extending away from mass = "mushrooming"
  - Marked peritumoral edema
  - DWI, ADC correlate with hypercellular histopathology (high signal on DWI, low ADC)

Top Differential Diagnoses

- Meningioma (typical)
- Dural metastasis
- Lymphoma
- Sarcoma (osteosarcoma, Ewing, gliosarcoma, etc.)

Pathology

- AM = high mitotic activity
- MM = AM features + findings of frank malignancy

Clinical Issues

- AM 29% recurrence (26% become MM)
- MM 50% recurrence

Diagnostic Checklist

- Typical imaging findings do not exclude atypical variants!

*(**Left**) Coronal graphic illustrates a malignant meningioma infiltrating the scalp, skull, and underlying brain. Extensive vasogenic edema (in gray) is present. Note osteolysis, invasion through dura/arachnoid, tumor "mushrooming" ➔, and interdigitation with the brain. (**Right**) Sagittal postcontrast T1WI MR of malignant meningioma shows enhancing tumor involving the scalp, skull, and underlying brain. Note "mushrooming" of tumor through the dura ➔, prominent hypointense brain edema ➔.*

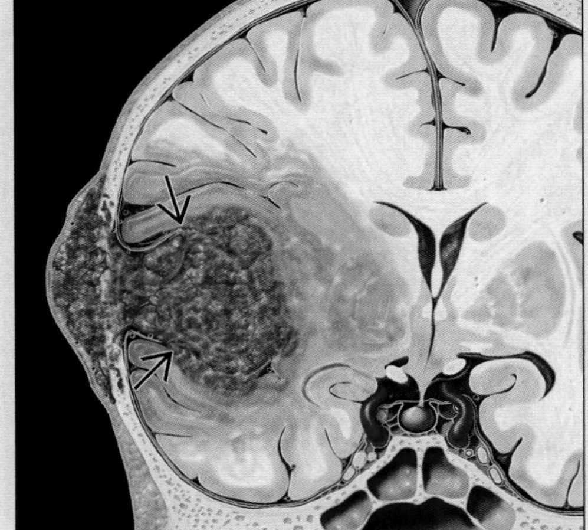

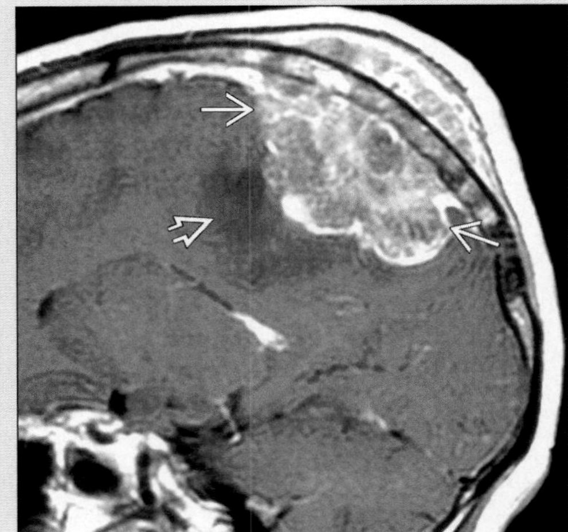

*(**Left**) MR was performed in a 60-year-old woman who presented with left-sided weakness and speech difficulties. Axial DWI MR shows a multilobulated high signal intensity mass ➔ in the left frontal lobe with low ADC values (not shown) suggesting high cellularity mass with restricted diffusion. (**Right**) Axial T1WI C+ MR in the same patient shows marked, homogeneous enhancement of the mass. MRS (not shown) demonstrated very high choline peak. Biopsy revealed clear cell meningioma.*

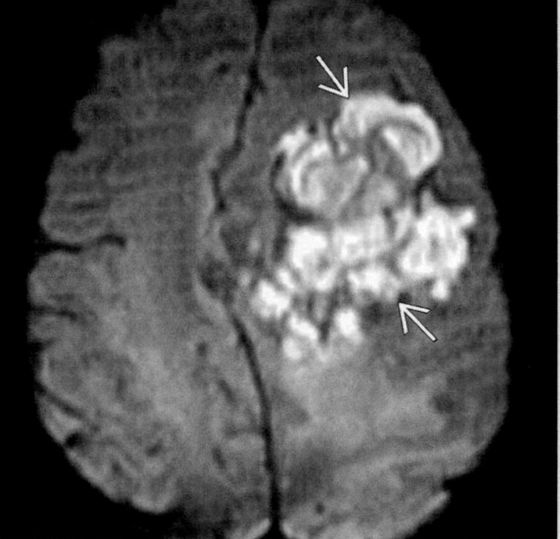

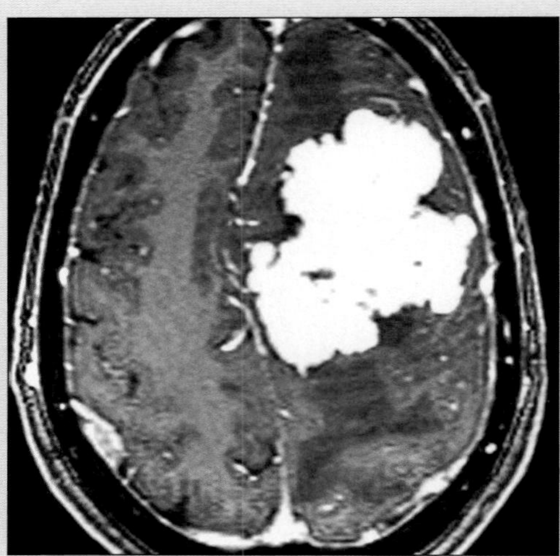

TERMINOLOGY

Abbreviations

- Atypical meningioma (AM), malignant (MM) meningioma

Definitions

- Typical (benign) meningioma = WHO grade 1
  - "Common" meningioma (CM)
- Atypical meningioma = WHO grade 2
  - Papillary, clear cell meningiomas (CCM)
- Malignant meningioma = WHO grade 3
  - Anaplastic meningioma

IMAGING

General Features

- Best diagnostic clue
  - Dural-based, locally-invasive lesion with areas of necrosis, marked brain edema
- Location
  - May occur anywhere in neuraxis (brain > > spine)
  - AM (clear cell variant)
    - Frequent in CPA , along tentorium
  - MM
    - Parasagittal (44%), cerebral convexities (16%) most common sites

CT Findings

- NECT
  - CT "triad" of MM: Extracranial mass, osteolysis, intracranial tumor
  - Hyperdense; minimal or no Ca++
    - Calcified = generally lower growth rate
  - Marked perifocal edema, bone destruction
- CECT
  - Enhancing tumor mass
  - Prominent tumor pannus extending away from mass = "mushrooming"

MR Findings

- T1WI
  - Indistinct tumor margins
  - Infiltrating tumor interdigitates with brain
- FLAIR
  - Marked peritumoral edema
- DWI
  - Markedly hyperintense on DWI, hypointense on ADC
- T1WI C+
  - Enhancing tumor mass
    - May extend into brain, skull, scalp
    - Often plaque-like ± "mushrooming"
- MRV
  - Look for dural sinus invasion
- MRS
  - Elevated levels of alanine at short TE (peak ranges from 1.3-1.5 ppm)
- Perfusion MR
  - Good correlation between volume transfer constant (K-trans), histologic grade

Angiographic Findings

- Conventional
  - Dural supply → central "sunburst" appearance
  - Intense vascular stain appears early, persists late
  - Venous phase vital to evaluate sinus involvement

Nuclear Medicine Findings

- PET
  - 18-FDG: AM, MM ↑ ↑ glucose utilization
  - High glucose metabolism present in radiation-induced meningiomas

Imaging Recommendations

- Best imaging tool
  - MR + contrast, ± MRS

DIFFERENTIAL DIAGNOSIS

Meningioma (Typical)

- Usually noninvasive but may need histology for definitive diagnosis

Dural Metastasis

- Often known extracranial primary neoplasm
- Osteolytic & destructive or osteoblastic & sclerotic

Lymphoma (Metastatic Intracranial)

- Lytic bone lesion with epidural and extracranial component

Osteosarcoma

- Osteolytic with soft tissue mass and poorly defined margins
- Tumoral calcification may be "sunburst"

Ewing Sarcoma

- Affects children
- CT: Laminated periosteal "onion skin" appearance

Primary Meningeal Sarcoma

- Extremely rare nonmeningothelial tumor of meninges

Gliosarcoma

- GBM with meningeal sarcoma

PATHOLOGY

General Features

- Etiology
  - CM: 90% inactivation of *NF2* gene product "Merlin"
  - AM & MM: After *NF2* inactivation, additional events occur and are related to greater aggressiveness
  - Occasionally no genetic defect found as etiology
- Genetics
  - Loss of 1 copy of chromosome 22 is most prevalent chromosomal change in meningioma
  - 2nd most frequent genetic abnormalities are 1p and 14q deletions, more aggressive behavior
  - Chromosome 10 abnormalities shared with nonmeningioma tumors
  - Chromosome 9p losses important in AM and MM
  - Multiple meningiomas
    - Many display expected *NF2* gene mutations

- Some have normal *NF2* genes: Suggests 2nd tumor-suppressor gene is also on chromosome 22
- Radiation associated meningiomas (RAM)
  - No significant differences between RAM and non-RAM in chromosome 1 and 22 losses
- Genetic effects on location and histology
  - Strong correlations found among anterior skull base location, intact 22q, and meningothelial; convexity location, disrupted 22q, transitional, fibrous
- **Summary**: Significant correlation between number of chromosomal imbalances and tumor grade
  - CM: 22q loss (47%), 1p deletion (33%)
  - AM: 1p (86%), 22q (71%), 10q (57%), 14q and 18q (43%) losses; 15q and 17q (43%) gains
  - MM: 1p loss (100%); also losses on 9p, 10q, 14q, 15q, 18q, and 22q and gains on 12q, 15q & 18p
  - Combined 1p/14q deletions in CM (13%), AM (43%), and MM (67%)

Staging, Grading, & Classification

- Immunohistochemical staining with MIB-1 antibody (Ki-67) correlates with recurrence
  - MIB-1 = nuclear, nonhistone protein expressed during cell-cycle proliferation but not resting
  - Staining with MIB-1 yields labeling index (LI) for quantification of number of dividing cells
    - LI < 4.4% → 82% recurrence free at 6 years
    - LI > 4.4% → 32% recurrence free at 6 years

Microscopic Features

- AM features (WHO criteria)
  - ↑ mitotic activity
- MM features (WHO criteria)
  - AM features with findings of frank malignancy

CLINICAL ISSUES

Demographics

- Age
  - Middle decades
  - AM occurs about 10 years earlier than typical meningioma
- Gender
  - M:F = 1:1.3-1.5
- Ethnicity
  - More common in African-Americans
- Epidemiology
  - Meningioma 1 of most common primary adult intracranial neoplasms (13-20%)
    - AM = 4.7-7.2% of all meningiomas
    - MM = 1-2.8% of meningiomas (rare)
  - ~ 6 in 100,000 population
  - Familial predilection for meningioma = *NF2*
- Geographic predilection
  - In Africa meningioma nears 30% of adult primary intracranial tumors

Natural History & Prognosis

- Recurrence-free survival, median time to recurrence longer for typical meningioma vs. AM vs. MM
  - Typical "benign" meningioma = only 9% recurrence
  - AM recurrence (28%)
  - MM recurrence (75%)

Treatment

- Preoperative embolization
  - Particulate agents (e.g., polyvinyl alcohol) favored
  - ↓ operative time, blood loss
- Surgical goals
  - Resection of tumor and involved dura/dural "tail" (with tumor-free margins) with duraplasty
  - Resection of involved or hyperostotic bone
  - Preoperative knowledge whether tumor is AM or MM may alter neurosurgery preoperative plan
    - More aggressive to achieve complete resection
    - Complication: CSF seeding
- Radiotherapy: Frequently used for AM, MM
  - Fractionated external beam irradiation
  - Stereotactic radiosurgery
- Recurrence treatments
  - Repeat surgery
  - External beam irradiation, stereotactic radiosurgery

DIAGNOSTIC CHECKLIST

Image Interpretation Pearls

- Preoperatively define **entire** tumor extent
- Typical imaging findings do not exclude atypical variants!

SELECTED REFERENCES

1. Aghi MK et al: Long-term recurrence rates of atypical meningiomas after gross total resection with or without postoperative adjuvant radiation. Neurosurgery. 64(1):56-60; discussion 60, 2009
2. Campbell BA et al: Meningiomas in 2009: controversies and future challenges. Am J Clin Oncol. 32(1):73-85, 2009
3. Norden AD et al: Advances in meningioma therapy. Curr Neurol Neurosci Rep. 9(3):231-40, 2009
4. Moradi A et al: Pathodiagnostic parameters for meningioma grading. J Clin Neurosci. 15(12):1370-5, 2008
5. Nagar VA et al: Diffusion-weighted MR imaging: diagnosing atypical or malignant meningiomas and detecting tumor dedifferentiation. AJNR Am J Neuroradiol. 29(6):1147-52, 2008
6. Pearson BE et al: Hitting a moving target: evolution of a treatment paradigm for atypical meningiomas amid changing diagnostic criteria. Neurosurg Focus. 24(5):E3, 2008
7. Toh CH et al: Differentiation between classic and atypical meningiomas with use of diffusion tensor imaging. AJNR Am J Neuroradiol. 29(9):1630-5, 2008
8. Jain D et al: Clear cell meningioma, an uncommon variant of meningioma: a clinicopathologic study of nine cases. J Neurooncol. 81(3):315-21, 2007
9. Ko KW et al: Relationship between malignant subtypes of meningioma and clinical outcome. J Clin Neurosci. 14(8):747-53, 2007
10. Modha A et al: Diagnosis and treatment of atypical and anaplastic meningiomas: a review. Neurosurgery. 57(3):538-50; discussion 538-50, 2005
11. Ma L et al: meningioma. Acta Neurochir (Wien). 2009 Mar 11. [Epub ahead of print] PubMed PMID: 19277460.

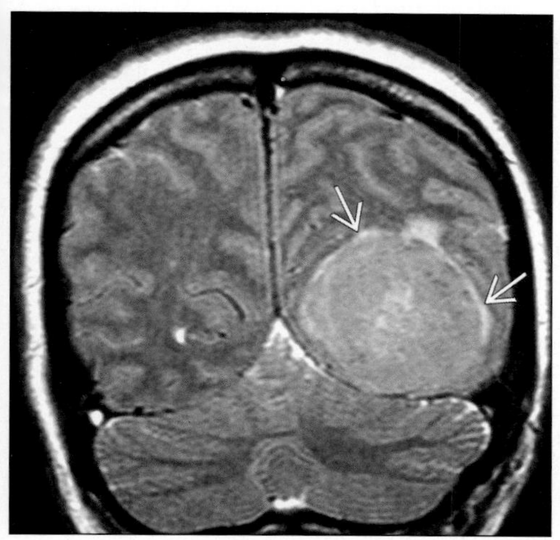

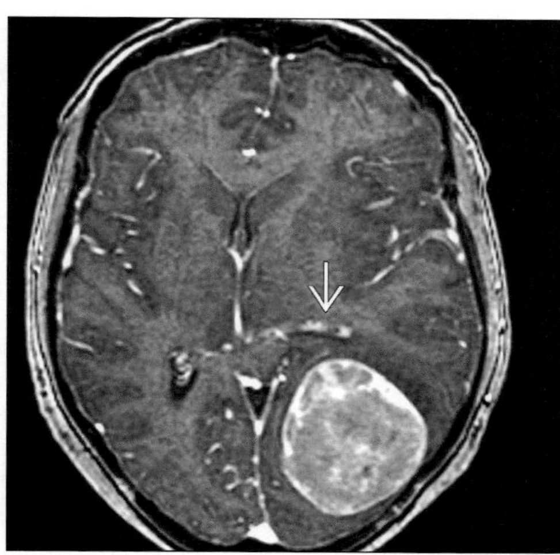

(Left) *Coronal T2WI MR in a 47-year-old man demonstrates a well-defined, homogeneous, extraaxial mass with minimal edema ➔.* ***(Right)*** *Axial T1 C+ MR in the same patient shows marked, relatively homogeneous enhancement. Note the compression of the left trigonum ➔. Surgical resection and histological evaluation revealed malignant meningioma despite the lack of aggressive features on imaging. Biopsy is necessary for definitive histologic type and grade of meningioma.*

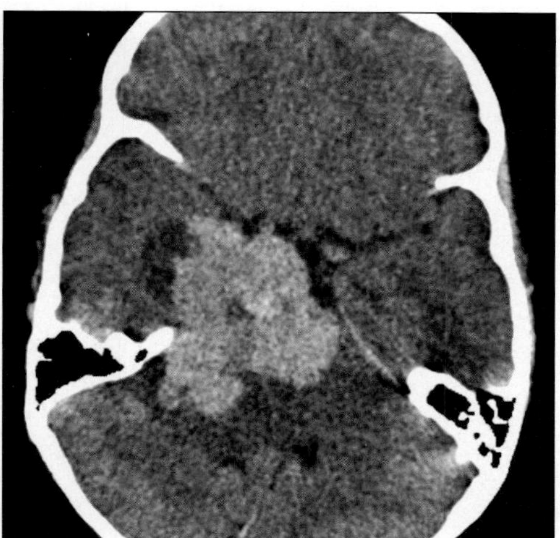

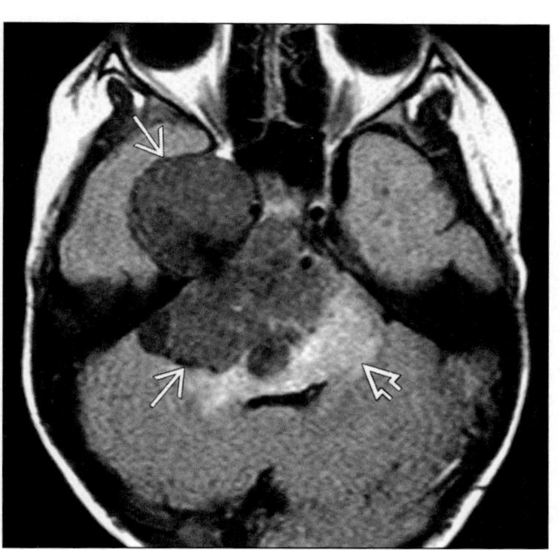

(Left) *Axial NECT demonstrates a lobulated hyperdense mass along the right tentorium.* ***(Right)*** *Axial FLAIR MR in the same patient shows a hypointense, multilobulated mass ➔ with perifocal edema ➔, and mass effect on the 4th ventricle.*

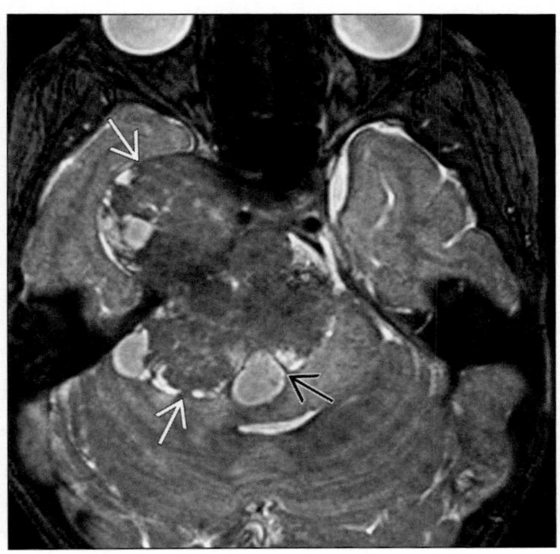

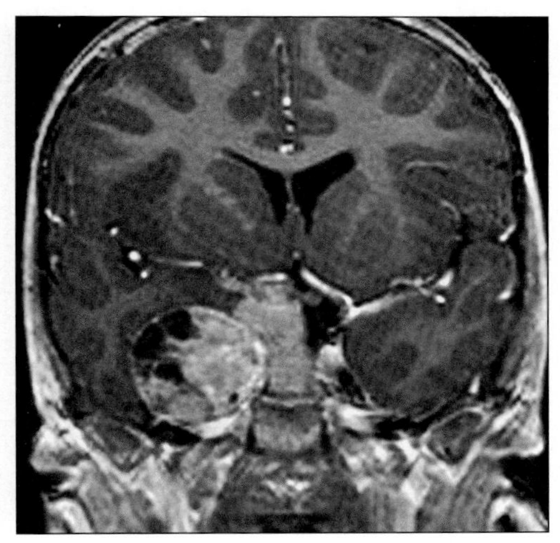

(Left) *High-resolution axial T2WI MR in the same patient nicely demonstrates a well-defined, low signal mass ➔ with cystic components ➔. Hypodensity indicates a high cellular matrix of the tumor.* ***(Right)*** *Coronal T1WI C+ MR shows enhancement of the solid tumor parts. Surgical removal was performed, and histological diagnosis was a mixture of clear cell meningioma and a whorling sclerosing variant of meningioma.*

MISCELLANEOUS BENIGN MESENCHYMAL TUMORS

Key Facts

Terminology
- Nonmenigotheliomatous benign mesenchymal tumor (BMT)
  - Typically dura, skull, &/or scalp lesion
  - Examples = chondroma, osteochondroma, osteoma, etc.

Imaging
- Lesion of dura, skull, skull base, scalp without malignant features
- Use NECT, bone CT for most
- T1WI C+ MR to image noncalcified cartilage, brain involvement, malignant transformation

Top Differential Diagnoses
- Benign meningothelial tumors
- Malignant meningothelial tumors
- Malignant nonmeningothelial tumors

Pathology
- Meninges contain primitive multipotential mesenchymal cells
  - May give rise to broad spectrum of nonmeningothelial neoplasms

Clinical Issues
- BMT are most often asymptomatic
- BMT are rare to very rare
- Asymptomatic lesions require no treatment
- Surgical indications: Relief of symptoms, cosmesis

Diagnostic Checklist
- Look for evidence of syndromic BMTs
  - Gardner syndrome: Multiple osteomas
  - Maffucci syndrome: Multiple enchondromas
  - Ollier disease: Enchondromatosis

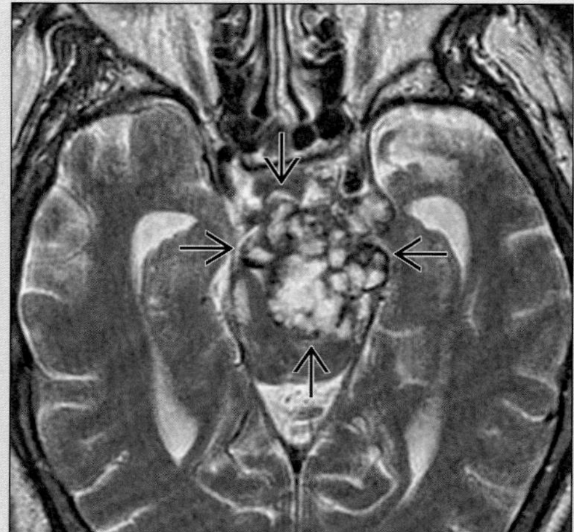
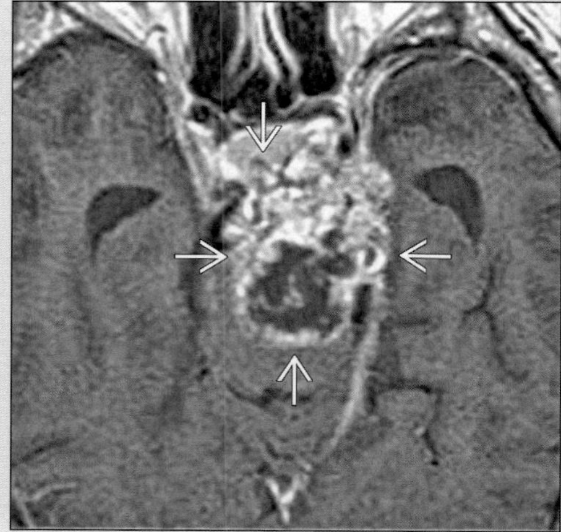

(Left) *Axial T2WI MR shows a well-delineated, mixed intensity mass in the left cavernous sinus and sella turcica extending into the suprasellar cistern and interpeduncular cistern ⇨. Note the hypointense arcs surrounding very hyperintense lobulations. Histopathology revealed typical enchondroma.* ***(Right)*** *Axial T1WI C+ MR of the same patient demonstrates enchondroma and reveals strong but inhomogeneous enhancement ➡. (Courtesy P. Sundgren, MD.)*

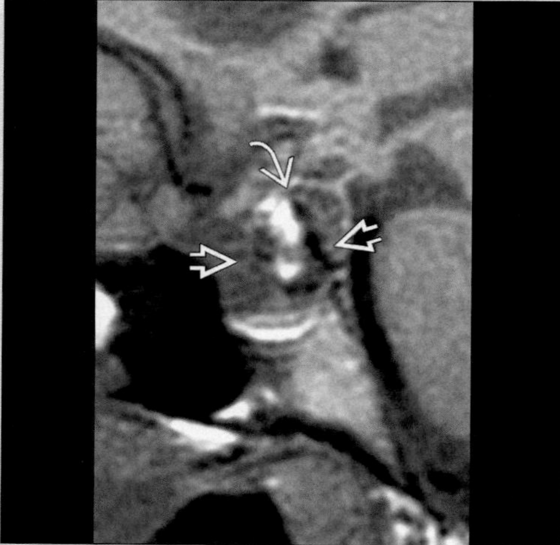
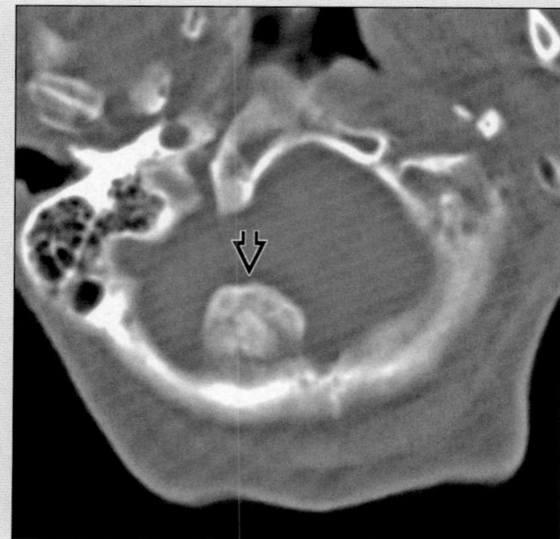

(Left) *Sagittal T1WI MR demonstrates an osteochondroma with heterogeneous matrix ➡ arising from the dorsum sella, contiguous with the parent cortex, with a mixed intensity cartilaginous cap ➡.* ***(Right)*** *Axial bone CT shows a benign osteoma ⇨ arising from the inner table of the occipital bone.*

MISCELLANEOUS BENIGN MESENCHYMAL TUMORS

TERMINOLOGY

Abbreviations

- Benign mesenchymal tumors (BMT)
  - Includes chondroma (CD), osteochondroma (OCD), osteoma (OST), and many others

Synonyms

- Benign nonmeningothelial tumors

Definitions

- Nonmenigotheliomatous mesenchymal benign neoplasm
  - Typically dura, skull, &/or scalp lesion

IMAGING

General Features

- Best diagnostic clue
  - Dura, skull, skull base, or scalp lesion without malignant features
- Location
  - BMT: Dura, skull, skull base, scalp
    - CD: Sellar/parasellar most common; dura/falx rare
    - OCD: Usually arises from skull base; dura/falx, rare
    - OST: Involves outer table; inner table rare

Radiographic Findings

- Radiography
  - CD: Expansile lesion containing matrix calcification with scalloped endosteum
  - OCD: Sessile or pedunculated bone-like projection
  - OST: Dense lesions without diploic involvement

CT Findings

- NECT
  - Chondroma
    - Expansile, lobulated, soft tissue mass
    - Contains curvilinear matrix calcification
    - Scalloped endosteal bone resorption → "saucerization"
    - No stalk or peduncle as in OCD
  - Osteochondroma
    - May see calcified matrix in cap atop cortical bone
    - Parent bone contiguous with cortex of OCD
  - Osteoma
    - Dense lesions without diploic involvement
- CECT
  - CD: May have slight enhancement
  - OCD: ± cartilaginous cap enhancement
  - OST: No enhancement

MR Findings

- T1WI
  - CD: Intermediate intensity
  - OCD: Mixed intensity; may see hypointense calcified matrix within cap atop cortical bone
  - OST: Hypointense
- T2WI
  - CD: Hyper- to hypointense
  - OCD: Mixed intensity; may see hypointense calcified matrix within cap atop cortical bone
  - OST: Variable intensity
- T1WI C+
  - CD: Enhancement of curvilinear septae (ring-and-arc pattern), scalloped margins
  - OCD: May have peripheral cartilaginous cap enhancement
  - OST: No enhancement

Nuclear Medicine Findings

- Bone scan
  - CD: Uptake if actively making bone
  - OCD: Varies
  - OST: Uptake during active growth phase, diminishing to background levels

Imaging Recommendations

- Best imaging tool
  - NECT + bone CT for most
  - MR + C for imaging noncalcified cartilage, affects on soft tissues, evaluating for malignant transformation
- Protocol advice
  - CT: Axial and coronal thin sections at skull base
  - MR: Fat saturation to confirm fat content or to optimize imaging of scalp lesions

DIFFERENTIAL DIAGNOSIS

Benign Meningothelial Tumors

- Common meningioma
  - Characteristic MR appearance with dural "tail"

Malignant Meningothelial Tumors

- Atypical/malignant meningioma
  - Infiltrative, destructive lesion

Malignant Nonmeningothelial Tumors

- Osteosarcoma
  - Osteolytic + soft tissue mass & ill-defined margins
  - Tumoral calcification may be "sunburst"
- Primary meningeal sarcoma
  - Extremely rare nonmeningothelial tumor of meninges
- Many other sarcomas

PATHOLOGY

General Features

- Etiology
  - Meninges contain primitive multipotential mesenchymal cells
    - May give rise to spectrum of nonmeningothelial neoplasms
  - CD
    - From clivus/skull base cartilage synchondroses
    - Ectopic embryologic cartilage cell rests; perhaps perivascular mesenchymal tissue metaplasia
  - OCD
    - Most common radiation-associated benign tumor
    - Arise from fragment of growth plate; in skull most likely from congenital defect
  - OST: Uncertain; found in auditory canals of cold water swimmers → may be inflammatory reaction
- Associated abnormalities

- Gardner syndrome: Multiple osteomas, skin tumors, colon polyps
- Maffucci syndrome: Multiple enchondromas associated with soft tissue hemangiomas
- Multiple hereditary exostoses: Multiple OCD
- Ollier disease: Enchondromatosis

Staging, Grading, & Classification

- 2007 WHO classification
  - Tumors of meninges
    - Tumors of meningothelial cells
      - Meningioma (15 subtypes listed)
    - Mesenchymal tumors
      - 23 subtypes listed
      - Includes both benign **and** malignant nonmeningothelial mesenchymal tumors
    - Primary melanocytic lesions (4 subtypes listed)
    - Other neoplasms related to meninges: Only hemangioblastoma listed

Gross Pathologic & Surgical Features

- General comment: Skull vs. skull base ossification
  - Skull develops by intramembranous ossification → origin of membranous tumors (e.g., OST)
  - Clivus and skull base develop by endochondral ossification → origin for cartilaginous tumors (e.g., CD and OCD)
- CD
  - Benign osteocartilaginous tumor
  - "Enchondroma" if within bone or cartilage
  - Multiple tumors = chondromatosis or enchondromatosis
  - No stalk or peduncle as in OCD
  - Gross path: Cartilage and ossified cartilage
- OCD
  - Benign osteocartilaginous tumor
  - Cartilage-capped bony exostosis; sessile or pedunculated
  - Gross path: Irregular bony mass with cartilage cap ± calcification
- OST: Benign membranous tumor
  - Gross path: Appears as mature lamellar bone

Microscopic Features

- CD
  - Benign chondrocytes in scattered lacunae
  - Abundant hyaline cartilage matrix
  - May exhibit cellular atypia
  - Immunohistochemical staining positive for vimentin and S100 protein
- OCD: Cartilaginous cap over bony excrescence with cortex, trabeculae, marrow identical to normal bone
- OST: 2 types
  - Compact or "ivory": Made of mature lamellar bone; no Haversian canals or fibrous components
  - Trabecular: Composed of cancellous trabecular bone with marrow surrounded by cortical bone margin

CLINICAL ISSUES

Presentation

- Most common signs/symptoms
  - BMT are most often asymptomatic
  - OCD and OST: May present as "bony lump"
  - CD and OCD: May have cranial nerve deficit(s) if at clivus/skull base; very rarely seizure

Demographics

- Age
  - CD: Occur at any age, peak in 2nd to 4th decades
  - OCD: Mean age for multiple = 21 years, solitary = 30 years
  - OST: Highest incidence in 6th decade
- Gender
  - CD: M:F = 1-2:1
  - OCD: M:F = 1.5-2.5:1
  - OST: M:F = 1:3
- Epidemiology
  - BMT are rare to very rare
  - CD: Most common benign osteocartilaginous tumor of clivus/skull base; 0.1-1% of intracranial tumors
  - OCD
    - Most common benign skeletal tumor (8-9% of primary bone tumors, 36% of those benign)
    - Most common cartilaginous tumor (12% multiple)
  - OST: Most common primary calvarial tumors → 0.4% of population

Natural History & Prognosis

- CD: Malignant transformation is rare
- OCD: Malignant transformation is rare
  - Sessile more likely to degenerate
  - Risk increases as number and size of OCD increases
  - Malignant transformation in osteochondromatosis 25-30% compared to ≈ 1% for solitary
- OST
  - Slow-growing lesions normally asymptomatic
  - Secondary mucocele invading intracranial vault

Treatment

- Asymptomatic lesions require no treatment
- Surgical indications: Relief of symptoms, cosmesis
- Surgical goals: Complete excision, curettage if tumors cannot be resected completely

DIAGNOSTIC CHECKLIST

Consider

- Patient may be syndromic

SELECTED REFERENCES

1. Fountas KN et al: Intracranial falx chondroma: literature review and a case report. Clin Neurol Neurosurg. 110(1):8-13, 2008
2. Ye J et al: Osteoma of anterior cranial fossa complicated by intracranial mucocele with emphasis on its radiological diagnosis. Neurol India. 56(1):79-80, 2008
3. Laghmari M et al: [Cranial vault chondroma: a case report and literature review.] Neurochirurgie. 53(6):491-4, 2007
4. Louis DN et al: The 2007 WHO classification of tumours of the central nervous system. Acta Neuropathol. 2007 Aug;114(2):97-109. Epub 2007 Jul 6. Review. Erratum in: Acta Neuropathol. 114(5):547, 2007

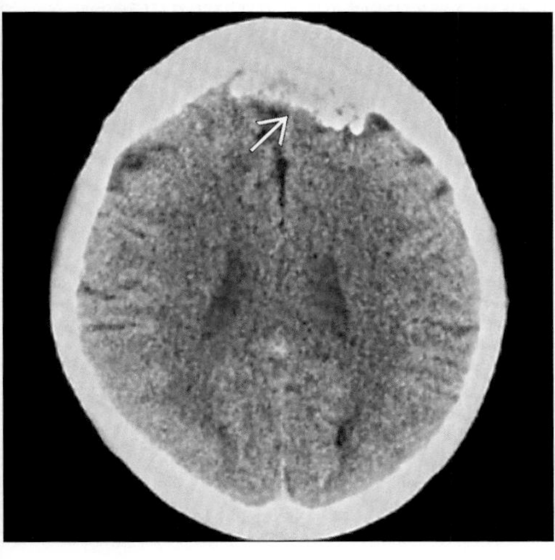

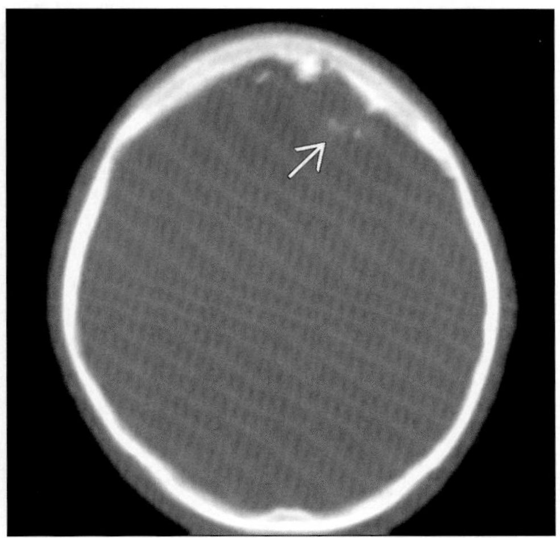

(Left) *Axial NECT demonstrates a chondroma as a lobulated, calcified, extraaxial mass in the left frontal region ➔.* ***(Right)*** *Axial bone CT of the same patient reveals slightly stippled, or flocculent, calcifications within the chondroma ➔. Curvilinear matrix calcifications such as these can help narrow the differential diagnosis.*

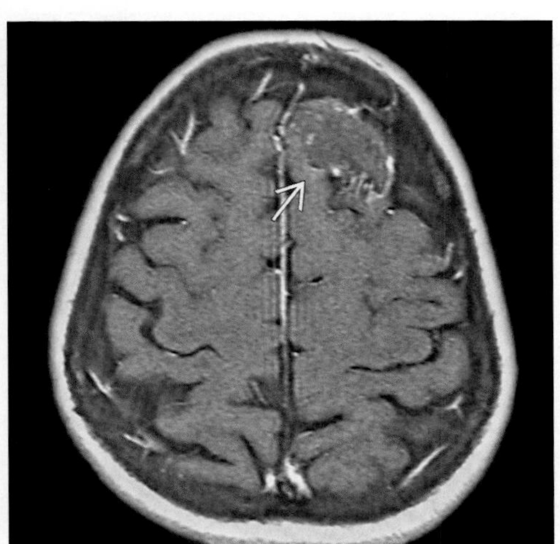

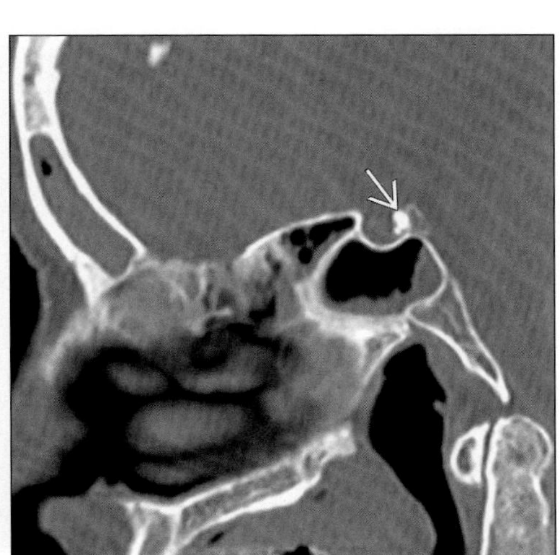

(Left) *Axial T1WI C+ MR of the chondroma in the same patient demonstrates minimal contrast enhancement, predominantly at the periphery of the lesion ➔.* ***(Right)*** *Sagittal bone CT reconstructed from axial source images shows a small, ossified intrasellar mass ➔ that appears to be projecting anteriorly from the dorsum sellae. A lesion was found incidentally on screening sinus CT and probably represents an osteoma of the dorsum sellae.*

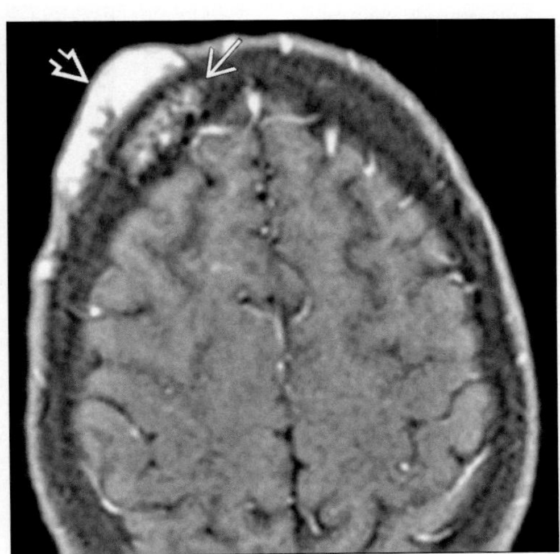

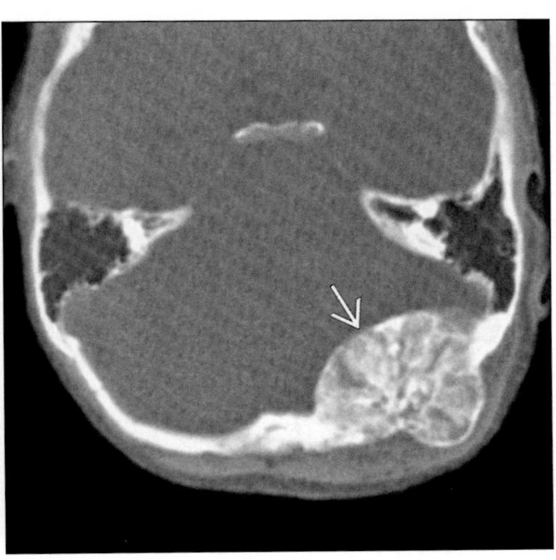

(Left) *Axial T1WI C+ FS MR of an enhancing benign scalp hemangioma ➔ shows that the lesion intercalates into the underlying calvarium ➔ but has no intracranial extension.* ***(Right)*** *Axial bone CT of a benign chondroblastoma in the left occipital bone reveals a large, expansile, hyperdense lesion with a chondroid matrix ➔ and a well-defined margin.*

MISCELLANEOUS MALIGNANT MESENCHYMAL TUMORS

Key Facts

Terminology

- Nonmenigotheliomatous malignant mesenchymal neoplasms
  - Correspond histologically to extracranial tumors of soft tissue or bone
  - Most are sarcomas

Imaging

- Highly aggressive dural, skull, skull base, scalp, lesions invading locally
- Amorphous, ill-defined, rapidly enlarging mass, often with both intra- and extraaxial components
- Best imaging tool: MR with T1WI C+ FS; CT for matrix

Top Differential Diagnoses

- Benign meningothelial tumors
- Malignant meningothelial tumors
- Metastases

Pathology

- Accepted theory: Meninges contain primitive multipotential mesenchymal cells capable of giving rise to different histological types of nonmeningothelial neoplasms

Clinical Issues

- Prognosis of MMT patients is generally very poor
- Biopsy is crucial to establish histiologic diagnosis and guide treatment plan
- Primary treatment: Wide radical surgical extirpation
- XRT: Prevent local recurrence, ↓ risk of metastasis
- Chemotherapy, brachytherapy often considered

Diagnostic Checklist

- No characteristic radiologic findings that distinguish from other neoplasms

(Left) Axial T1WI C+ MR in a patient with chondrosarcoma shows a lobulated dural-based mass with intense enhancement ➔ and minimal reaction within the underlying brain parenchyma. ***(Right)*** *Axial CECT demonstrates a very rare primary meningeal sarcoma as a strikingly infiltrative lesion with heterogeneous enhancement, skull destruction ➔, and scalp infiltration ➔.*

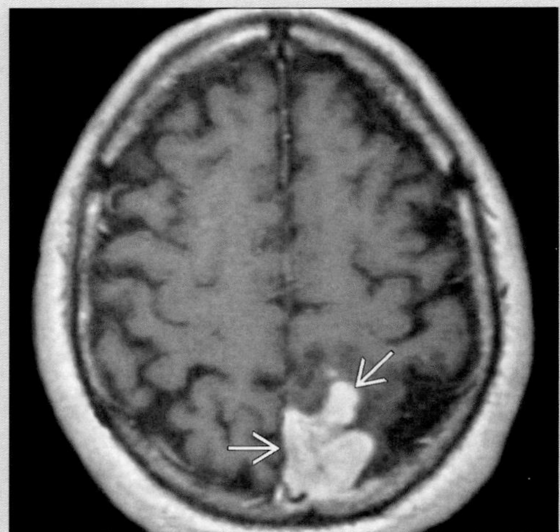

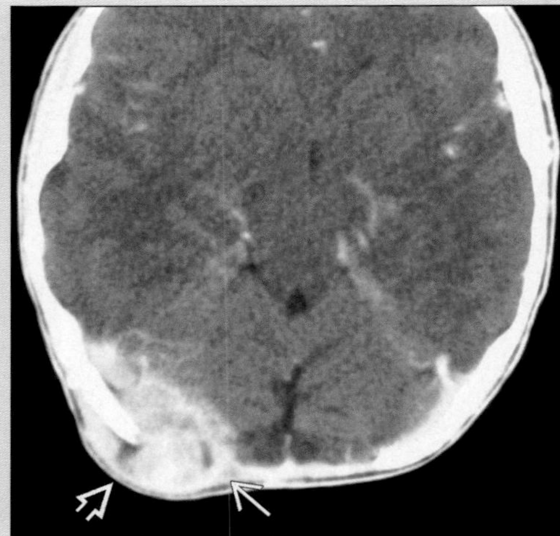

(Left) *Coronal T2WI MR in a patient with primary calvarial Ewing sarcoma shows a predominantly hypointense, extradural cellular mass with hyperintense cystic/necrotic components ➔, appearing to arise from the calvarium. Note the displaced dura ➔, transdural extension ➔, and large subgaleal component.* ***(Right)*** *Coronal T1WI C+ MR in the same patient reveals strong but inhomogeneous enhancement, better demonstrating the transdural component ➔.*

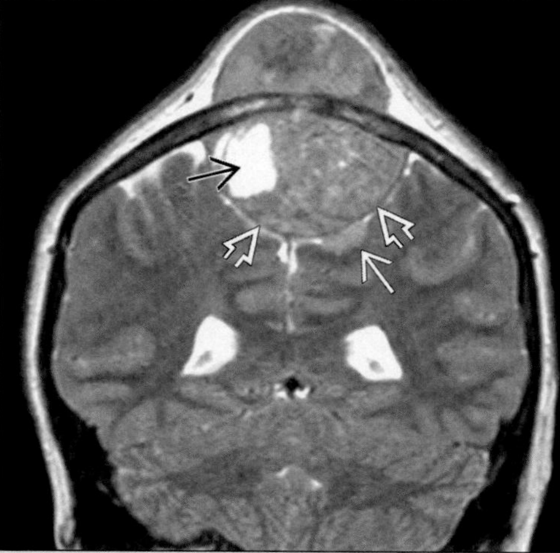

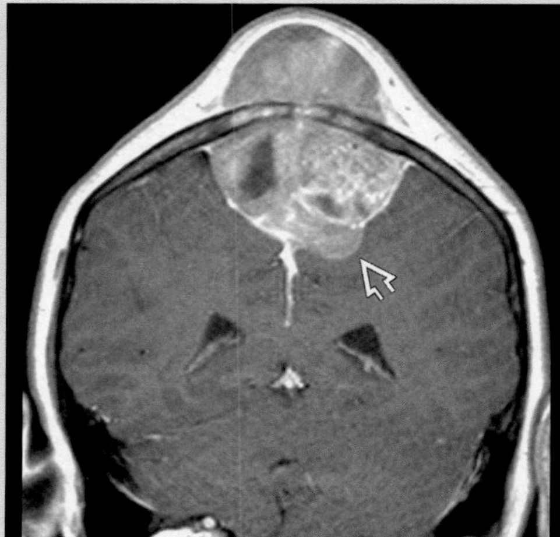

MISCELLANEOUS MALIGNANT MESENCHYMAL TUMORS

TERMINOLOGY

Abbreviations

- Malignant mesenchymal tumors (MMT)

Synonyms

- Malignant nonmeningothelial tumors

Definitions

- Nonmenigotheliomatous malignant mesenchymal neoplasms
  - Histologically correspond to extracranial tumors of soft tissue or bone
  - Most are sarcomas
    - Angiosarcoma (ANGIO), chondrosarcoma (CHON), fibrosarcoma (FIBRO)
    - Osteosarcoma (OSTEO), rhabdomyosarcoma (RHAB)
    - Meningeal sarcoma (MENSARC), Ewing sarcoma (EWING), etc.

IMAGING

General Features

- Best diagnostic clue
  - Highly aggressive dural, skull, skull base, scalp, lesions invading locally
- Morphology
  - Amorphous, ill-defined, rapidly enlarging mass, often with both intra- & extraaxial components

Radiographic Findings

- Radiography
  - Usually radiolucent lesions → ill-defined lytic borders, no periosteal reaction (except EWING)

CT Findings

- NECT
  - Usually radiolucent lesions → ill-defined lytic borders, no periosteal reaction (except EWING)
  - ANGIO: Reactive ossification, necrosis possible
  - CHON: May have stippled or rings & arcs Ca++
  - MENSARC: May be dense, biconvex, mimicking acute subdural hematoma
  - OSTEO: Calcified "sunburst" matrix possible
  - EWING: Often hyperdense (cellular)
- CECT
  - Most enhance
  - ANGIO: Very marked enhancement
  - EWING: Heterogeneous with periosteal reaction (but not "onion peel" for skull lesions)

MR Findings

- T1WI
  - Variably hypointense
  - Very hypointense (fibrous, chondroid, osteoid tissue)
  - Usually infiltrate brain
- T2WI
  - Most are predominantly hyperintense with heterogeneous signal and brain infiltration
  - May see extremely low signal from fibrous, chondroid, and osteoid tissue
  - EWING: Often hypointense (cellular)
- FLAIR
  - Best to evaluate edema, brain infiltration
- T1WI C+
  - Most enhance, often intensely
  - May have dural "tail," necrotic foci
  - ANGIO: Very marked enhancement
  - CHON: May show "honeycomb" pattern
  - EWING: Heterogeneous with necrosis

Angiographic Findings

- DSA
  - Most have high degree of neovascularity
  - Others show avascular mass effect
- Interventional: Preoperative embolization to ↓ operative time and bleeding

Imaging Recommendations

- Best imaging tool
  - MR with T1WI C+ FS; CT for matrix

DIFFERENTIAL DIAGNOSIS

Benign Meningothelial Tumors

- Common meningioma
  - Characteristic MR appearance
  - Not infiltrative

Malignant Meningothelial Tumors

- Atypical/malignant meningioma
  - Infiltrative, destructive lesion
  - Much more common than MMT

Metastases

- Often known extracranial malignancy
- Frequently multifocal
- Much more common than MMT

PATHOLOGY

General Features

- Etiology
  - Accepted theory: Meninges contain primitive multipotential mesenchymal cells capable of giving rise to different histological types of nonmeningothelial neoplasms
  - Exact cause is uncertain; 2 theories
    - Sarcomatous component may arise from mesenchymal elements of perivascular sheaths (fibroblasts, endothelium, smooth muscle, pericytes) or from arachnoid
    - Most likely from pluripotential meningeal mesenchymal cells
  - Radiation is known cause, most commonly FIBRO, with latency of 5-12 years
  - EWING: Uncertain histogenesis, belonging to family of neuroectodermal tumors
- Genetics
  - EWING: Cytogenetic translocation between chromosome 22 and 11 (80%)

Staging, Grading, & Classification

- 2007 WHO 4th edition classification
  - Tumors of meninges

MISCELLANEOUS MALIGNANT MESENCHYMAL TUMORS

- Tumors of meningothelial cells
  - Meningioma (15 subtypes listed)
- Mesenchymal tumors (23 subtypes listed)
  - Includes both benign **and** malignant nonmeningothelial mesenchymal tumors
- Primary melanocytic lesions (4 subtypes listed)
- Other neoplasms related to meninges: Only hemangioblastoma listed

Gross Pathologic & Surgical Features

- CHON: Bluish-white glistening external surface of homogeneous tan cartilaginous tissue
- FIBRO: Pinkish, meaty
- MENSARC: Diffuse leptomeningeal involvement (10%) or large discrete lesions
- OSTEO: Soft tissue with hemorrhage, Ca++, necrosis

Microscopic Features

- Given lack of clinical/radiologic findings specific for MMT, diagnosis nearly always made by histopathology
- ANGIO
  - Irregular anastomosing vascular channels lined by anaplastic endothelial cells and pericytes
  - Cytokeratin, vimentin, ulex europaeus agglutinin, antihuman endothelial cell marker CD31(+)
- CHON
  - Undifferentiated mesenchymal cells, islands of hyaline cartilage, vimentin, & S100 protein positive
  - Scant material mainly of monomorphic small round cells with granular cytoplasm and central round nuclei in a background of myxoid matrix
  - Occasional giant cells; periodic acid-Schiff(-)
- FIBRO
  - Highly cellular with spindle-shaped cells in sheets or interlacing fascicles with herring-bone pattern
  - Cells contain elongated nuclei with mild hyperchromasia and high mitotic activity
  - Bone, osteoid, cartilage are absent
- MENSARC
  - Polymorphocellular sarcoma
- OSTEO
  - Single or multinucleated atypical polygonal cells in lacunae surrounded by immature osteoid
  - Osteoblastic, chondroblastic, & small-cell subtypes
- RHAB
  - Malignant undifferentiated tumor
    - Foci of muscular differentiation
  - Electron microscopy: Intracytoplasmic filamentous striations of poorly formed myofibrils
  - Positive for actin, desmin, myoglobin, vimentin
- EWING
  - Small round-cell tumor
  - High nuclear:cytoplasmic ratio

CLINICAL ISSUES

Presentation

- Most common signs/symptoms
  - Highly variable dependent on tumor location
  - Convexity: Most commonly hemiparesis, seizure
  - Skull base: Cranial nerve deficit(s)
  - Often rapidly growing mass with swelling
  - Headache, pain, fever, malaise, emesis

Demographics

- Age
  - More highly differentiated tumors appear in childhood whereas poorly differentiated in adults
  - ANGIO: Any age
  - CHON: 2nd and 3rd decade, mean 37 years
  - FIBRO: Usually middle-aged adults
  - MENSARC: Children > adults
  - OSTEO: > 30 years; peak in 6th decade
  - RHAB: Children > > adults
  - EWING: 75% < 20 years; peak at 5-13 years
- Gender
  - Most have no sex predilection
  - FIBRO, MENSARC, and EWING: M > F
- Epidemiology
  - MMT: 0.5-2.7% of intracranial neoplasms
  - CHON: 0.15% of all intracranial tumors
  - MENSARC: 0.7-4.3% of pedi intracranial tumors
  - RHAB: < 1% of all intracranial tumors

Natural History & Prognosis

- Prognosis of MMT patients is generally very poor
  - CHON of dura & meninges have good prognosis; recurrence-free survival rate 65% after 5 years
  - EWING: Majority have good prognosis as can be fully or partially resected; 5-year survival (57.1%)
- Most have relentless tendency for local recurrence and metastases outside CNS
  - May recur years after diagnosis & initial treatment

Treatment

- Goal of treatment is to control disease locally
- Biopsy is crucial to establish histiologic diagnosis and guide treatment plan
- Primary treatment: Wide radical surgical extirpation
- Postoperative radiation therapy: Prevent local recurrence, ↓ risk of metastasis
- Chemotherapy, brachytherapy often considered

DIAGNOSTIC CHECKLIST

Image Interpretation Pearls

- No characteristic radiologic findings that distinguish MMT from other neoplasms

SELECTED REFERENCES

1. Dagcinar A et al: Primary meningeal osteosarcoma of the brain during childhood. Case report. J Neurosurg Pediatr. 1(4):325-9, 2008
2. Guilcher GM et al: Successful treatment of a child with a primary intracranial rhabdomyosarcoma with chemotherapy and radiation therapy. J Neurooncol. 86(1):79-82, 2008
3. Misra V et al: Cytodiagnosis of extraosseous mesenchymal chondrosarcoma of meninges: a case report. Acta Cytol. 52(3):366-8, 2008
4. Bricha M et al: [Primary Ewing sarcoma of the skull vault.] J Radiol. 88(12):1899-901, 2007

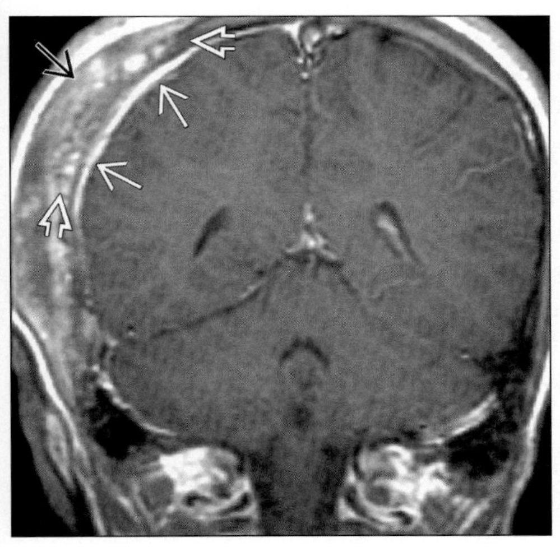

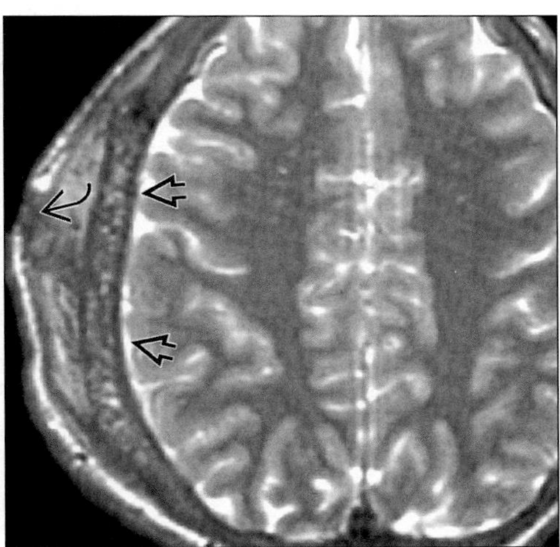

(Left) *Coronal T1WI C+ MR in a patient with primary calvarial Ewing sarcoma demonstrates striking scalp involvement* ⇒, *a mottled appearance of the expanded underlying calvarium* ➡, *and thickening of the underlying dura* ➡. ***(Right)*** *Axial T2WI MR in the same patient shows superficial ulceration, seen as disruption of the cutis* ⇒. *Note the expansion and mottled appearance of the underlying calvarium* ⇒.

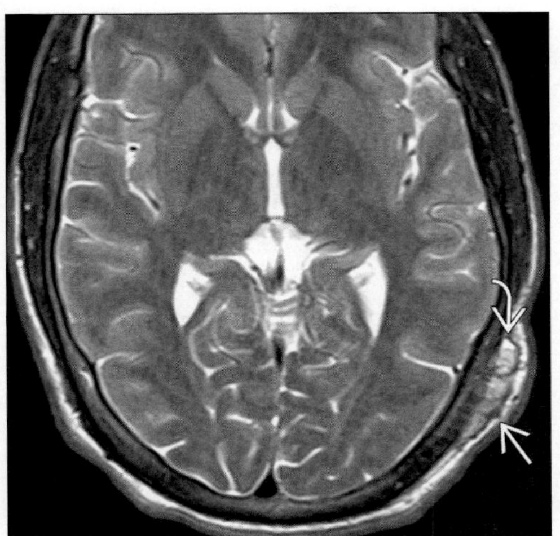

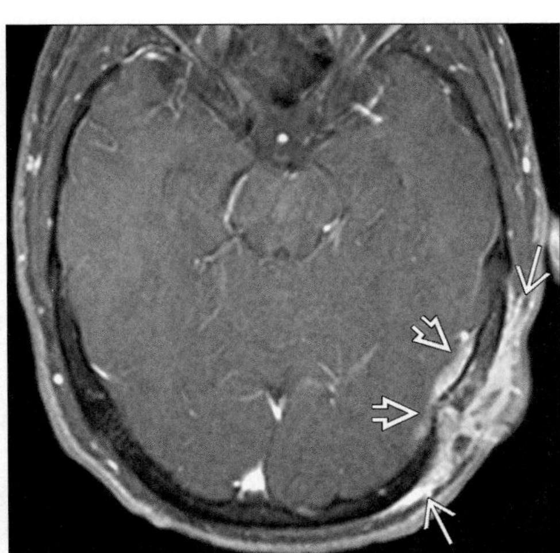

(Left) *Axial T2WI MR demonstrates a left parietal scalp mass* ➡ *infiltrating the underlying skull and containing a blood-fluid level* ➡. *Histology revealed a high-grade chondroblastic osteosarcoma (WHO III).* ***(Right)*** *Axial T1WI C+ FS MR in the same patient shows the true extent of the mass* ➡ *and more clearly delineates intracranial extension with calvarial penetration and dural infiltration* ➡.

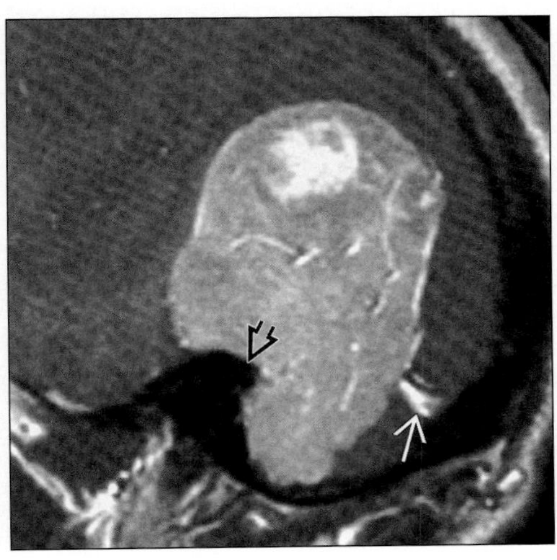

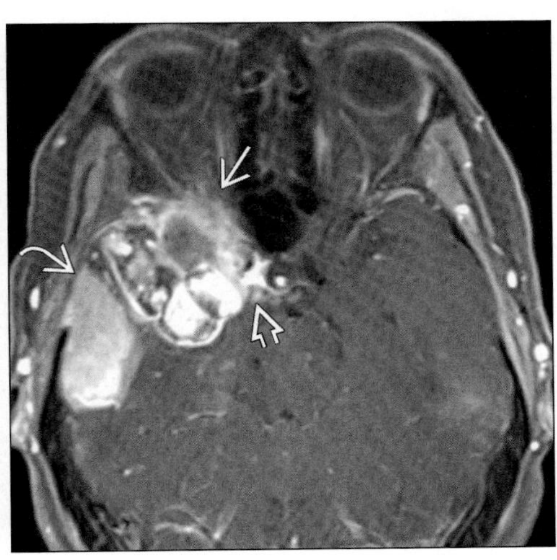

(Left) *Sagittal T1WI C+ MR shows a fibrosarcoma arising from the petrous apex* ⇒ *and occluding the transverse sinus* ➡. ***(Right)*** *Axial T1WI C+ FS MR shows an aggressive inhomogeneously enhancing mass invading the orbit* ➡ *and cavernous sinus* ➡, *extending through a craniotomy defect into the scalp* ➡. *Histology confirmed chondrosarcoma & osteosarcoma intermixed with atypical meningotheliomatous meningioma, arising as a complication from radiation therapy of a previously resected meningioma.*

CALVARIAL HEMANGIOMA

Key Facts

Terminology
- Benign intraosseous skull lesion with predominantly vascular and some avascular components

Imaging
- Best clue: Sharply marginated expansile skull lesion
- Frontal, temporal, parietal bone in decreasing order
- Most often solitary, but multiple in 15%
- Best imaging tool: Bone CT
  - Sharply marginated expansile lesion
  - Thin peripheral sclerotic rim in 1/3
  - Intact inner and outer table
  - Outer table often more expanded than inner table
  - Trabecular thickening with radiating spicules
- MR signal characteristics dependent on
  - Quantity of slow-moving venous blood
  - Ratio of red marrow to converted fatty marrow
  - Hypointense trabeculae

Top Differential Diagnoses
- "Holes in skull," solitary (common)
- "Holes in skull," solitary (uncommon)
- "Holes in skull," multiple (common)
- "Holes in skull," multiple (uncommon)

Pathology
- Classified on basis of dominant vessels: Capillary, cavernous, or mixed

Clinical Issues
- Most often asymptomatic
- Calvarial hemangiomas rare: 0.2% of bone tumors
- Rarely requires treatment

Diagnostic Checklist
- Hemangiomas are just 1 of large "holes in skull" diagnosis that require exclusion of others

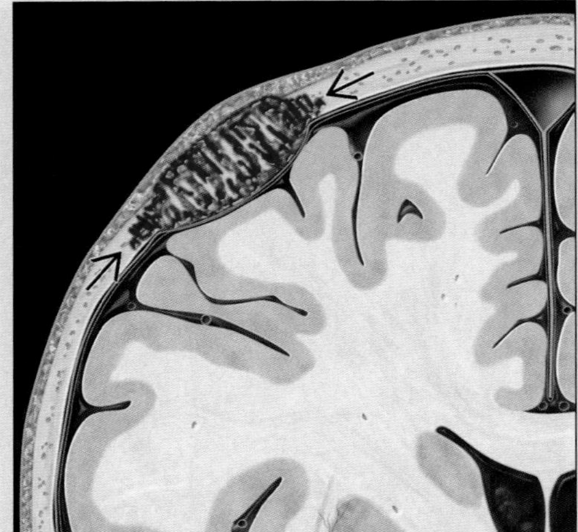

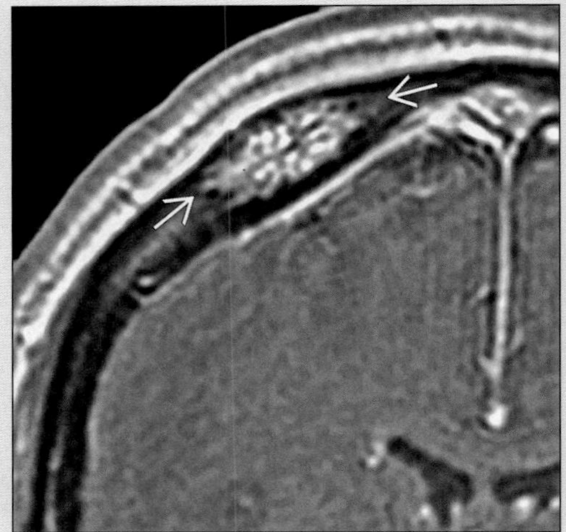

(Left) *Coronal graphic illustrates a sharply marginated expansile skull lesion → with a slight honeycomb-appearing pattern from intradiploic trabecular thickening.* ***(Right)*** *Coronal T1WI C+ MR shows diffuse yet heterogeneous enhancement of an expansile calvarial hemangioma →. Heterogeneity is a result of vascular enhancement combined with hypointense bony trabeculae.*

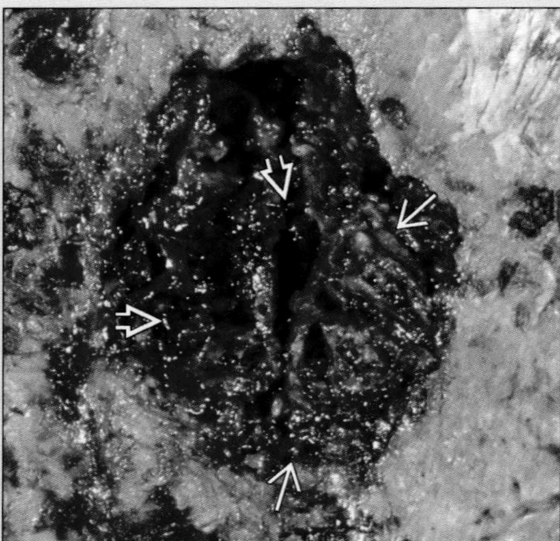

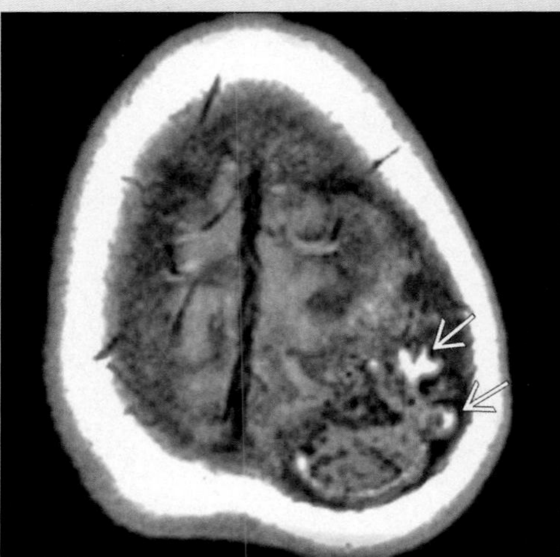

(Left) *Close-up view of resected calvarial hemangioma. Note the radiating spicules of lamellar bone → interspersed with vascular channels of varying sizes →.* ***(Right)*** *Axial T1WI MR demonstrates a variant case of hemorrhagic calvarial hemangioma containing hyperintense collections anteriorly from hemorrhage →. Note the otherwise classic findings of a sharply marginated expansile lesion involving the outer table more than inner, containing intradiploic trabecular thickening.*

CALVARIAL HEMANGIOMA

TERMINOLOGY

Synonyms

- Osseous hemangioma, intraosseous hemangioma

Definitions

- Benign intraosseous skull lesion with predominantly vascular and some avascular components

IMAGING

General Features

- Best diagnostic clue
  - Sharply marginated expansile skull lesion
- Location
  - Skull: 20% of intraosseous hemangiomas
    - Diploic space
    - Frontal, temporal, parietal in decreasing order
    - Less commonly occipital or sphenoid
  - Vertebra: 28% of intraosseous hemangiomas
- Size
  - 1-4 cm
- Morphology
  - Solitary but multiple in 15%; round or oval

Radiographic Findings

- Radiography
  - Sharply marginated expansile lesion
  - May have thin peripheral sclerotic rim
  - "Honeycomb" or "sunburst" pattern

CT Findings

- CECT
  - Enhances
- Bone CT
  - Sharply marginated expansile lesion
    - Thin peripheral sclerotic rim in 1/3
  - Intact inner and outer table
    - Outer table often more expanded than inner table
      - Erosion of both tables unusual (3%)
    - Scalloped nonsclerotic margins
  - "Spoke-wheel," "reticulated," or web-like pattern
    - Intradiploic trabecular thickening with radiating spicules
  - Also "soap bubble" or "honeycomb" appearance

MR Findings

- T1WI
  - Hypo- to isointense
    - Small lesions may appear hyperintense: Fatty tissue is main cause of T1WI hyperintensity
    - Larger lesions typically hypointense secondary to presence of thickened trabeculae
  - May be hemorrhagic
    - Signal dependent on hemoglobin stage
- T2WI
  - Usually heterogeneous
    - Often hyperintense: Slow flow or venous stasis is main cause of T2WI hyperintensity
    - May see hypointense spicules
  - May be hemorrhagic
    - Signal dependent on hemoglobin stage
- T1WI C+
  - Enhances diffusely and heterogeneously
  - Rarely may have dural "tail"
- MR signal characteristics dependent on
  - Quantity of slow-moving venous blood
  - Ratio of red marrow to converted fatty marrow
  - Hypointense trabeculae

Angiographic Findings

- DSA: Hypervascular, delayed persistent blush, "cluster of grapes" appearance
  - Middle meningeal artery, superficial temporal artery most commonly involved vessels
- Supraselective embolization → devascularize to ↓ intraoperative bleeding and procedural morbidity

Nuclear Medicine Findings

- Bone scan
  - From photopenia to moderate increased activity

Imaging Recommendations

- Best imaging tool
  - Bone CT defines trabecular and cortical detail
- Protocol advice
  - MR C+ to characterize interstices

DIFFERENTIAL DIAGNOSIS

"Holes in Skull," Solitary (Common)

- Normal anatomic variant: Fissure, foramen, canal, emissary venous channel, Pacchionian (arachnoid) granulation, parietal thinning
  - CT reveals normal anatomy
- Surgical: Burr holes, shunt, surgical defect
  - Surgical history
- Trauma, fracture
  - Fracture confirmed on CT
- Dermoid
  - Well-circumscribed unilocular cyst containing fat
- Eosinophilic granuloma
  - < 5 years; "beveled edge," "hole-within-a-hole," "button sequestrum"
  - Involves inner/outer tables
- Metastases
  - Older patients, often history of cancer
- Low-grade hemangioendothelioma
  - Can be indistinguishable

"Holes in Skull," Solitary (Uncommon)

- Osteoporosis circumscripta
  - Hypointense on T1WI and T2WI from cortical thickening, coarse trabeculation
- Epidermoid
  - Nonenhancing lesion with dense sclerotic borders
- Cephalocele
  - Very young; bony defect with tissue herniation
- Intradiploic arachnoid cyst
  - CSF isointensity on both T1WI and T2WI
- Intradiploic meningioma
  - Homogeneously enhances
  - May have inner/outer table destruction
- Leptomeningeal cyst
  - Appears as "growing fracture" on radiography/NECT
- Malignant mesenchymal tumors, miscellaneous

- Very rare, large, highly aggressive tumors

"Holes in Skull," Multiple (Common)
- Normal anatomic variants: Fissure, foramen, canal, emissary venous channel, Pacchionian (arachnoid) granulation, parietal thinning
  - CT reveals normal anatomy
- Surgical
  - Burr holes, surgical defects
- Metastases
  - Older patients, often history of cancer
- Lymphoma
  - History of systemic lymphoma
- Osteoporosis
  - Older; osteopenia, trabecular loss, cortical thinning

"Holes in Skull," Multiple (Uncommon)
- Hyperparathyroidism
  - "Salt and pepper" skull
- Myeloma
  - Multiple, well-circumscribed, lytic, "punched-out"
  - Involves both inner and outer tables
- Osteomyelitis
  - 2-12 years; M:F = 3:1; mixed lytic/proliferative lesion
  - Characteristically "moth-eaten"/permeative medullary and cortical destruction with new bone formation

PATHOLOGY

General Features
- Etiology
  - Congenital or related to previous trauma
- Genetics
  - Nearly all sporadic
  - In rare congenital hemangiomatosis, skull, vertebra, muscle, skin, and subcutaneous tissues may all be involved

Staging, Grading, & Classification
- Classified on basis of dominant vessels: Capillary, cavernous, or mixed

Gross Pathologic & Surgical Features
- Brownish-red, nonencapsulated, under periosteum

Microscopic Features
- 3 histopathologic types
  - Capillary (classically in spine)
    - Abundant vessels ≈ 10-100 microns in diameter with walls 1-3 cells thick
    - Vessels tend to run in parallel
  - Cavernous (classically in skull)
    - Large, dilated sinusoidal vessels separated by fibrous septi
    - Single layer of endothelial cells
    - Intravascular thrombosis with dystrophic calcification may be seen
  - Mixed capillary/cavernous
- There may be reactive new bone formation, which can appear similar to osteoblastoma
- Radiating, web-like, or "spoke-wheel" trabecular thickening caused by intramembranous bone formation adjacent to angiomatous channels

CLINICAL ISSUES

Presentation
- Most common signs/symptoms
  - Asymptomatic
  - Other signs/symptoms
    - Longstanding palpable lump, tender to pressure, spontaneous pain, deformity
    - Rarely epidural, subdural, or subarachnoid hemorrhage
- Clinical profile
  - Freely mobile skin above lump

Demographics
- Age
  - Usually adults: 4th-5th decade
  - Any age can be affected
- Gender
  - M:F = 1:2-4
- Epidemiology
  - Osseous hemangiomas: 0.7-1% of bone tumors
    - Calvarial hemangiomas (rare): 0.2% of bone tumors
  - 10% benign primary neoplasms of skull

Natural History & Prognosis
- Benign slow-growing neoplasms
- Increase in size may be due to repeated hemorrhage

Treatment
- Rarely requires treatment
- Indications for surgery include correction of mass effect, control of hemorrhage, cosmesis
  - En bloc surgical excision with rim of normal bone
  - Usually definitive treatment; recurrence is rare
- Radiotherapy may be considered when surgical access is difficult or as complement to subtotal resections
  - Complications may include scar formation, impairment of regional bone growth in children, rarely malignant transformation

DIAGNOSTIC CHECKLIST

Consider
- Hemangiomas are just 1 of large "holes in skull" diagnosis that require exclusion of others
- **Beware**: Routine bone biopsy and curettage may result in severe hemorrhage
  - Prior imaging diagnosis can prevent complications

Image Interpretation Pearls
- Intact inner/outer tables, thickened trabeculae, best aid in diagnosis

SELECTED REFERENCES

1. Cosar M et al: Intradiploic cavernous hemangioma of the skull in a child: a case report. Childs Nerv Syst. 24(8):975-7, 2008

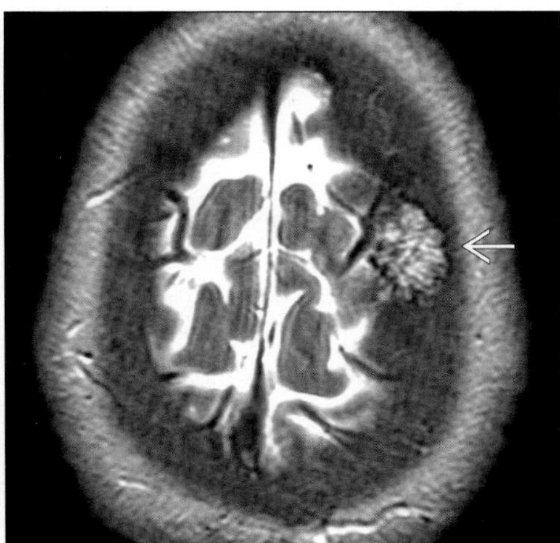

(Left) Axial bone CT demonstrates the benign appearance of a hemangioma as a sharply marginated expansile lesion with scalloped margins, a "honeycomb" or web-like pattern from thickened trabeculae, as well as intact inner and outer tables. **(Right)** Axial T2WI MR in the same case demonstrates hyperintense components, mainly the result of slow flow or venous stasis with a contribution from fat. Note the "honeycomb" or web-like hypointensities from thickened trabeculae.

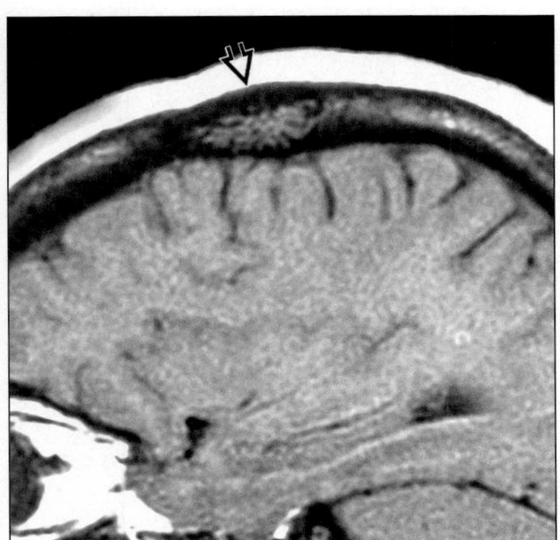

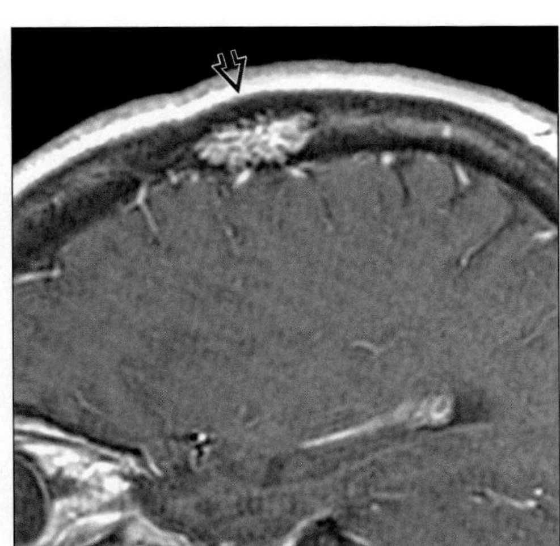

(Left) Sagittal T1WI MR in the same case shows the hemangioma as a mostly isointense lesion, which is less bright than the overlying fatty scalp. **(Right)** Sagittal T1WI C+ MR in the same case demonstrates diffuse yet heterogeneous enhancement, the latter a result of intense vascular enhancement combined with hypointense bony trabeculae.

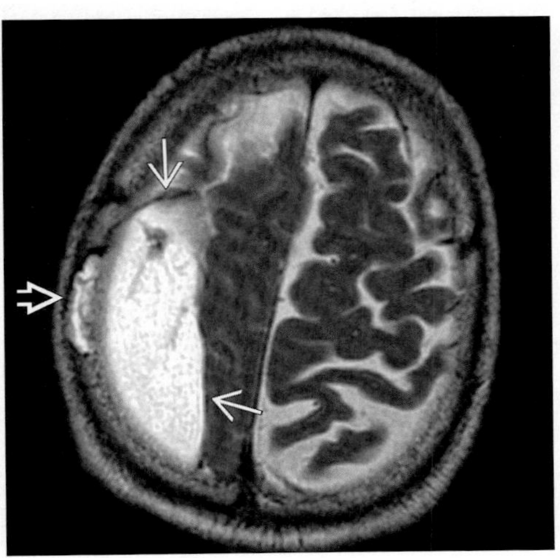

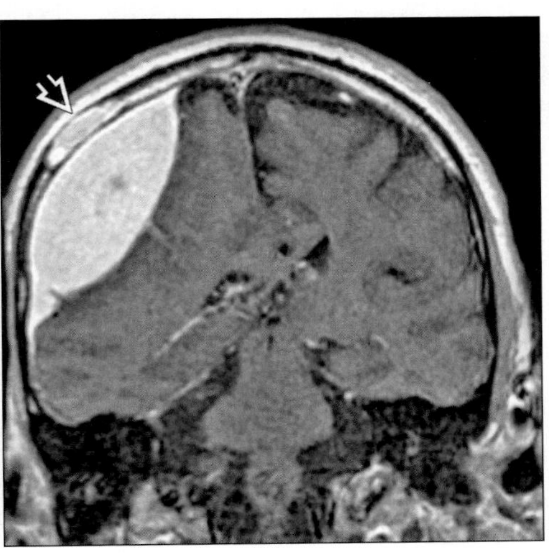

(Left) Axial T2WI MR shows a hyperintense septated subdural fluid collection, which is contiguous with a well-delineated hyperintense calvarial lesion. At surgery, a calvarial hemangioma was found that had eroded through the inner table of the skull, perforated the dura, and communicated with the subdural fluid collection. **(Right)** Coronal T1 C+ MR in the same case reveals strong enhancement. Hemangiomas are rarely associated with epidural, subdural, or subarachnoid hemorrhage.

Key Facts

Terminology

- Extraaxial vascular mass of dura &/or venous sinus

Imaging

- Best diagnostic clue: Marked T2 hyperintensity; delayed "filling in" with dynamic T1WI C+
- Location: Cavernous sinus, CPA, other dura
- Bone CT: Erosion or remodeling, not hyperostosis
- T1 C+: May be heterogeneous with slow centripetal "filling in" (analogous to liver hemangiomas)
- Best imaging tool: MR + dynamic T1WI C+

Top Differential Diagnoses

- Cavernous sinus: Meningioma, nerve sheath tumor, granuloma
- CPA: Schwannoma, meningioma, epidermoid
- Dural based: Meningioma, metastases, granuloma, mesenchymal tumor

Clinical Issues

- Very rare
- Nonneoplastic lesion that grows very slowly
- Dural-based treatment: Surgical resection, avoided unless tumor growth demonstrated
- Cavernous sinus treatment much more difficult
  - Complete resection difficult due to location, bleeding, and relationship to vital neurovascular structures
  - Complete resection rates as low as 16%; overall surgical mortality up to 25%
  - Preoperative radiation therapy has been used to reduce hemorrhage with doses up to 30 Gy

Diagnostic Checklist

- Frequently misdiagnosed preoperatively as meningioma on basis of imaging findings

*(**Left**) Axial T2WI MR demonstrates the characteristic marked hyperintensity of a dura/venous sinus hemangioma ➡, even brighter than CSF ➡. (Courtesy R. Hewlett, PhD.) (**Right**) Axial T1WI C+ FS MR obtained with dynamic protocol shows early enhancement of the normal cavernous sinus ➡ while the lesion ➡ remains unenhanced (left). The image obtained a few seconds later (right) shows lesional "filling in" ➡, characteristic for hemangioma.*

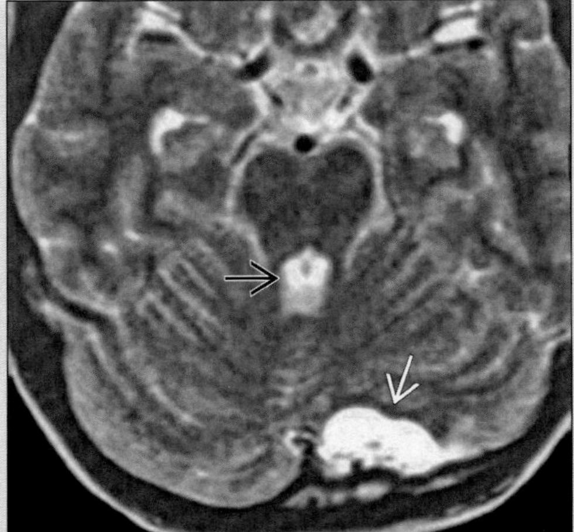

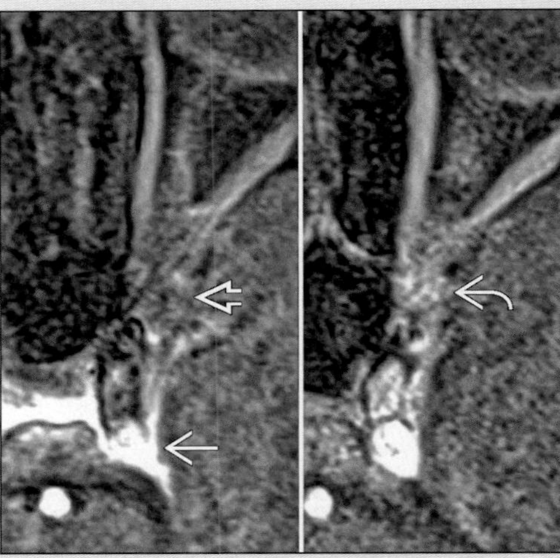

*(**Left**) Axial NECT of a giant cavernous sinus hemangioma ➡ obtained for head trauma shows the expanded left middle cranial fossa and thinned overlying calvarium ➡. The sella appears partly eroded and remodeled ➡. This patient had no symptoms referable to this lesion. (**Right**) Axial T1WI C+ FS MR in the same patient shows intense enhancement of the mass. The lesion originated in the cavernous sinus and was found to be a hemangioma at surgery.*

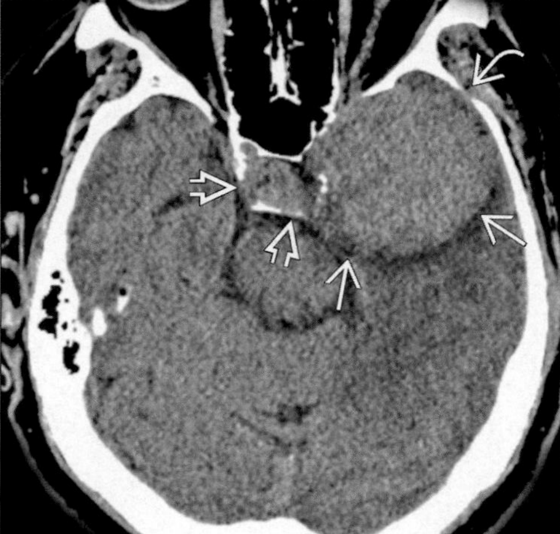

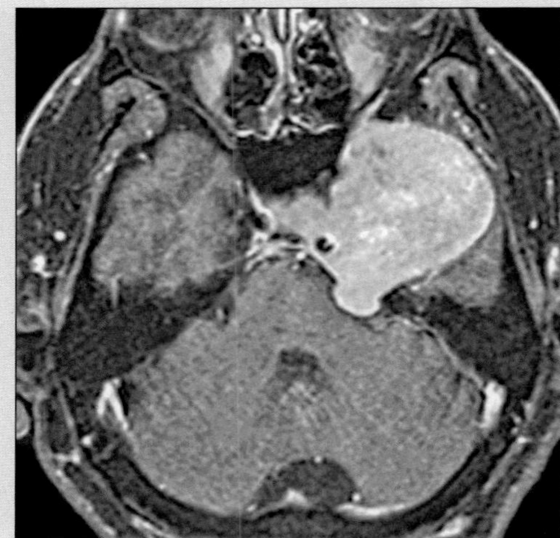

DURA/VENOUS SINUSES HEMANGIOMA

TERMINOLOGY

Definitions

- Extraaxial vascular mass of dura &/or venous sinus

IMAGING

General Features

- Best diagnostic clue
  - Marked T2 hyperintensity
  - Delayed "filling in" on dynamic contrast-enhanced MR
- Location
  - Cavernous sinus, CPA, other dura

CT Findings

- NECT: Iso- to hyperdense mass
- CECT: Marked homogeneous enhancement
- Bone CT: Erosion or remodeling, not hyperostosis

MR Findings

- T1WI
  - Hypo- to isointense
- T2WI
  - Marked hyperintensity
- T1WI C+
  - Dynamic may show slow centripetal "filling in"
  - Homogeneous enhancement if delayed
- MRV
  - Assess sinus &/or flow involvement

Angiographic Findings

- Variable: Avascular to staining with feeder arteries
- Consider preoperative embolization to decrease intraoperative blood loss

Nuclear Medicine Findings

- Tc-99m labeled red cell scintigraphy
  - Slow progressive accumulation
  - Persistent increased activity on delayed images

Imaging Recommendations

- Best imaging tool
  - MR with dynamic T1WI C+ for centripetal "filling in"

DIFFERENTIAL DIAGNOSIS

Cavernous Sinus

- Meningioma, nerve sheath tumor, granuloma

CPA

- Schwannoma, meningioma, epidermoid

Dural Based

- Meningioma, mets, granuloma, mesenchymal tumor

PATHOLOGY

Staging, Grading, & Classification

- Included within 2007 WHO "Tumors of the Meninges, Mesenchymal Tumors " subcategory

Gross Pathologic & Surgical Features

- Soft mass often with pseudocapsule formed by dura

Microscopic Features

- Honeycomb of multiple, thin-walled vascular channels
- Single endothelial cell layer with no elastic membrane or smooth muscle cells
- Contiguous walls of collagen & flattened endothelium
- Vascular channels separated by fibroconnective stroma

CLINICAL ISSUES

Presentation

- Most common signs/symptoms
  - Headaches, retro-orbital pain
- Other signs/symptoms
  - Cranial neuropathies, anisocoria, proptosis
  - Intracranial hypertension if sinus flow involved
  - Symptoms may appear or worsen during pregnancy or after hormone administration

Demographics

- Age
  - Cavernous sinus: Mean is 44 (range 22-64)
- Gender
  - Cavernous sinus: M:F = 1:7
- Ethnicity
  - Cavernous sinus: Japanese more often affected
- Epidemiology
  - Lesions very rare

Natural History & Prognosis

- Nonneoplastic lesion that grows very slowly

Treatment

- Dural based: Surgical resection, avoided unless tumor growth demonstrated
- Cavernous sinus much more difficult
  - Complete resection difficult due to location, bleeding, & relationship to neurovascular structures
  - Major intraoperative bleeding in 42%, massive or severe in 75% of these
  - Complete resection rates as low as 16%; overall surgical mortality up to 25%
  - Preoperative radiation therapy has been used to reduce hemorrhage with doses up to 30 Gy

DIAGNOSTIC CHECKLIST

Image Interpretation Pearls

- Frequently misdiagnosed preoperatively as meningiomas on basis of imaging findings

SELECTED REFERENCES

1. Jinhu Y et al: Dynamic enhancement features of cavernous sinus cavernous hemangiomas on conventional contrast-enhanced MR imaging. AJNR Am J Neuroradiol. 29(3):577-81, 2008

MYELOMA

Key Facts

Terminology
- Solitary = plasmacytoma (PC); multifocal = multiple myeloma (MM)
- Clonal B-lymphocyte neoplasm of terminally differentiated plasma cells

Imaging
- Osteolytic skull lesion
- "Punched-out" lytic lesion(s) (90%)
- Osteopenia/osteoporosis (10%)
- Meningeal myelomatosis: Uniform enhancement
- Bone scan → 74% patients, 24-54% sites
- Best imaging tool: Radiography (skeletal survey)
  - Detects 80% of sites in 90% of patients
- Up to 20% of radiographs & MR may be "normal"

Top Differential Diagnoses
- Surgical defect
- Lytic metastasis
- Hemangioma
- Hyperparathyroidism
- Many other causes of "holes in skull"

Pathology
- Durie-Salmon staging system
- Etiology remains unknown

Clinical Issues
- Most common symptom: Bone pain (68%)
- 2nd most prevalent blood cancer (1st = NHL)
- Incidence: ↑ with age
- Radiography significantly influences therapy

Diagnostic Checklist
- "Old fashioned" skeletal survey still highest sensitivity imaging modality

*(**Left**) Lateral radiograph of the skull shows multiple "punched-out" lytic lesions characteristic of multiple myeloma ➡. (**Right**) Axial bone CT demonstrates multiple lytic multiple myeloma lesions of the skull, some of which are indicated ➡. These are variable, ranging from tiny, innumerable lesions located diffusely to large "punched-out" foci.*

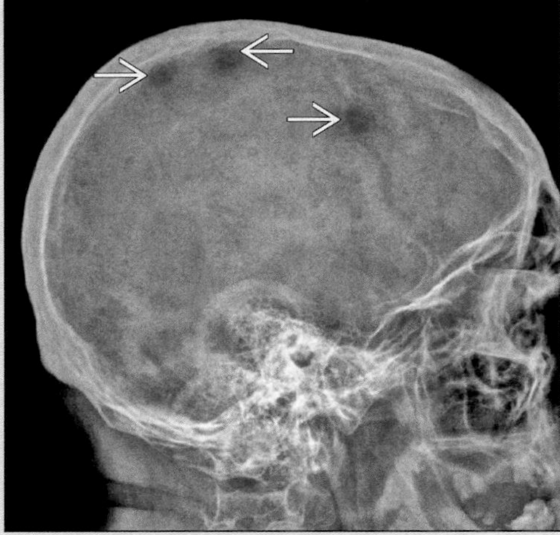

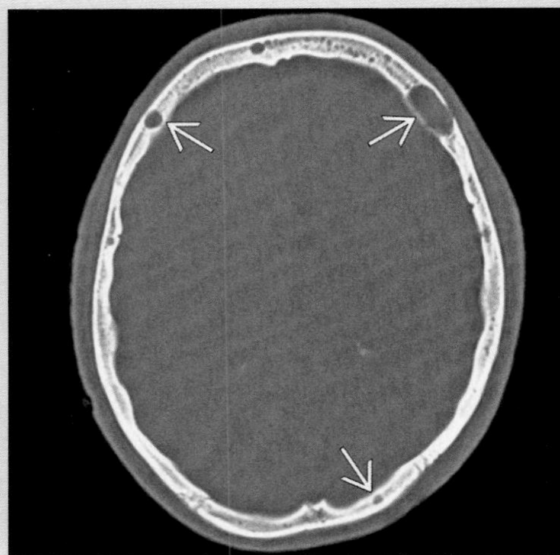

*(**Left**) Sagittal T1WI MR shows a typical case of plasmacytoma expanding the clivus ➡ and elevating the pituitary gland ➡. A normal-appearing pituitary gland argues against an invasive pituitary macroadenoma. (**Right**) Sagittal T1WI MR demonstrates a case of an osteolytic plasmacytoma, which mimics an epidural hematoma ➡.*

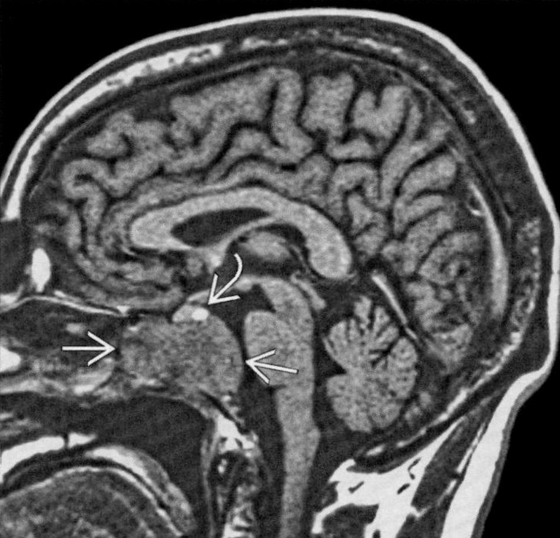

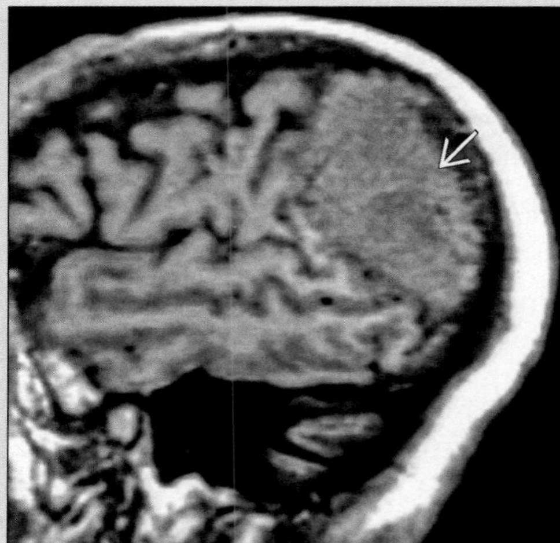

TERMINOLOGY

Abbreviations
- Solitary = plasmacytoma (PC)
- Multifocal = multiple myeloma (MM)

Definitions
- Clonal B-lymphocyte neoplasm of terminally differentiated plasma cells
- Intracranial MM rare
  - Usually **secondary** (extension from osseous lesions in calvarium, skull base, nose/paranasal sinuses)
  - **Primary** CNS disease (usually dural/leptomeningeal) is very rare
    - In Waldenström macroglobulinemia (a.k.a. Bing-Neel syndrome)

IMAGING

General Features
- Best diagnostic clue
  - Osteolytic skull lesion
- Location
  - MM: Vertebrae > skull; PC: Vertebrae > skull
  - Often widely disseminated at time of diagnosis
- Morphology
  - Focal, round or oval lesion(s)

Radiographic Findings
- Radiography
  - "Punched-out" lytic lesion(s) (90%)
  - Osteopenia/osteoporosis (10%)
  - Rarely sclerotic, except following therapy

CT Findings
- NECT
  - "Punched-out" lytic lesion(s)
  - Meningeal myelomatosis: Marked hyperdensity
- CECT
  - MM renal failure (RF) after contrast (0.6-1.25%)
    - 0.15% in general population
    - Thus, not 100% risk-free but may be performed if necessary and patient well hydrated
  - Meningeal myelomatosis: Uniform enhancement

MR Findings
- T1WI
  - Osseous lesions: Focal hypointensity (25%)
    - Diffuse marrow infiltration less common
  - Meningeal myelomatosis: Iso- to hyperintense
- T2WI
  - Osseous: Focal hyperintensity (53%)
  - Meningeal myelomatosis: Hypointense
- T1WI C+
  - Marked lesional enhancement
  - Meningeal myelomatosis: Uniform enhancement

Nuclear Medicine Findings
- Bone scan
  - Scintigraphy insensitive
- PET
  - 18-fluorodeoxyglucose (FDG) > bone scan
  - Conflicting reports of FDG PET vs. radiography
  - Residual or recurrent FDG activity after therapy is poor prognostic factor

Other Modality Findings
- Sensitivity of imaging detection for diagnosis
  - Radiography detects 90% of patients, 80% of sites
  - Bone scan detects 74% of patients, 24-54% of sites
  - Gallium scan detects 55% of patients, 40% of sites
- Up to 20% radiographs and MR may be "normal"
- MR → about 10% understaging of stage III disease
- Whole-body MDCT = lower detection rate and staging compared to whole-body MR

Imaging Recommendations
- Best imaging tool
  - Best imaging tool: Radiography (skeletal survey)
  - CT > MR for evaluation of specific lesion extent
  - MR best for delineating meningeal disease

DIFFERENTIAL DIAGNOSIS

Surgical Defects
- Burr hole, shunt, postoperative defect

Lytic Metastasis
- Commonly lung, breast, renal, thyroid

Hemangioma
- Sharply marginated expansile lesion often with "honeycomb" or "sunburst" appearance

Hyperparathyroidism
- Local destructive lesions ("brown tumor"), ↑ PTH

Other Causes of "Holes in Skull"
- Normal foramina, fissures, venous lakes

PATHOLOGY

General Features
- Etiology
  - Etiology remains unknown
  - Possible associations and supporting evidence
    - Immune system decline: More common in elderly
    - Genetic factors: Slight ↑ risk among children and siblings of MM patients; also definite ↑ racial risk
    - Certain occupations/chemicals: Agriculture, petroleum, leather industry, cosmetology, herbicides, insecticides, petroleum products, heavy metals, plastics, dusts (including asbestos)
    - Radiation: ↑ in Japanese atomic bomb survivors
    - Viral: Kaposi sarcoma-associated herpes virus found in marrow cells of some MM patients
- Genetics
  - 80-90% of patients have cytogenetic abnormalities
    - Chromosome 13 deletion is most common
- Associated abnormalities
  - "POEMS" syndrome: **P**olyneuropathy, **o**rganomegaly, **e**ndocrine abnormalities, **m**yeloma (usually sclerotic lesions!), **s**kin changes
  - PC = early/initial MM stage; precedes by 1-20 years
  - Underlying pathology is single plasma cell lineage expansion that replaces normal marrow and produces monoclonal immunoglobulins

MYELOMA

Staging, Grading, & Classification

- Durie-Salmon staging system
  - Stage I: All of following
    - Hemoglobin value < 10 g/dL
    - Serum calcium value normal or ≤ 12 mg/dL
    - No anemia, hypercalcemia, bone lesions
    - Low M-component: IgG value < 5 g/dL, IgA value < 3 g/dL, Bence Jones protein < 4 g/24 hours
    - Low myeloma cell mass: < 0.6 cells x 10^{12}/m2
  - Stage II: Fitting neither stage I nor stage III
    - Intermediate cell mass: 0.6-1.2 cells x 10^{12}/m2
  - Stage III: 1 or more of following
    - Hemoglobin value < 8.5 g/dL
    - Serum calcium value > 12 mg/dL
    - Advanced lytic bone lesions
    - IgG value > 7 g/dL, IgA value > 5 g/dL, Bence Jones protein > 12 g/24 hours
    - High myeloma cell mass: > 1.2 cells x 10^{12}/m2
  - Subclassification (either A or B)
    - A = relatively normal renal function
    - B = abnormal renal function

Gross Pathologic & Surgical Features

- Marrow replacement with gelatinous red-brown tissue

Microscopic Features

- Pleomorphic, enlarged plasma cells, often in sheets
  - Admixed with normal hematopoietic cells
  - Contain round/oval eccentric nuclei with clumped chromatin and perinuclear "halo" or pale zone
  - May have cytoplasmic inclusions: Mott, morula, or grape cells; Russell bodies
  - Cell clone produces excess monoclonal (M proteins) and free light-chain proteins
    - M proteins may be IgA, IgD, IgG, IgE or, IgM; depends on heavy chain class
    - Light-chain proteins may be κ or λ

CLINICAL ISSUES

Presentation

- Most common signs/symptoms
  - Most common symptom: Bone pain (68%)
  - Rare signs
    - Hyperviscosity syndrome: Shortness of breath, confusion, and chest pain
    - Cryoglobulinemia: Precipitating particles cause pain/numbness in fingers/toes during cold weather
    - Amyloidosis: Amyloid protein deposition, ↓ blood pressure, and kidney, heart, or liver failure
    - Bing-Neel syndrome: CNS involvement by lymphoplasmacytic lymphoma
- Clinical profile
  - Diagnosis often made with routine labs
  - Diagnosis confirmed by marrow aspirate/biopsy

Demographics

- Age
  - Peak onset = 65-70 years
  - Recent statistics: ↑ incidence and earlier age of onset
- Gender
  - Slight male predilection
- Ethnicity
  - African-Americans and Native Pacific Islanders have highest reported incidence; Asians lowest
- Epidemiology
  - 2nd most prevalent blood cancer (1st = NHL)
  - Incidence: ↑ with age
  - #1 primary bone malignancy in 4th-8th decades
    - Solitary PC without MM rare; solitary skull PC very rare (0.7% of all PC)

Natural History & Prognosis

- Solitary skull PC: No difference in prognosis between PC originating from bone vs. dura mater
- Multiple myeloma
  - Renal insufficiency frequent
  - Leukopenia leads to frequent pneumonias
  - Secondary amyloidosis (6-15%)
- 5-year survival (20%); death not from MM, but renal disease, infection, thromboembolism
  - Median survival is ~ 3 years with conventional chemotherapy
- Good prognosis indicators
  - Stage I or II disease
  - Normal chromosome 13
    - Abnormal cytogenetics is most important factor
    - Chromosome 13 or 11q deletions, or any translocation, predict poor prognosis
- Biphosphonate treatment related osteonecrosis of mandible

Treatment

- Radiography significantly influences therapy
  - 2 unequivocal rounded, "punched-out" lytic bone lesions indicates stage III → chemotherapy
  - Thus, important to radiographically assess osseous MM involvement at initial staging
- Treatment dependent on disease status

DIAGNOSTIC CHECKLIST

Image Interpretation Pearls

- "Old fashioned" skeletal survey still highest sensitivity imaging modality

SELECTED REFERENCES

1. Baur-Melnyk A et al: Multiple myeloma. Semin Musculoskelet Radiol. 13(2):111-9, 2009
2. Delorme S et al: Imaging in multiple myeloma. Eur J Radiol. Epub ahead of print, 2009
3. Dimopoulos M et al: International myeloma working group consensus statement and guidelines regarding the current role of imaging techniques in the diagnosis and monitoring of multiple Myeloma. Leukemia. Epub ahead of print, 2009
4. Cerase A et al: Intracranial involvement in plasmacytomas and multiple myeloma: a pictorial essay. Neuroradiology. 50(8):665-74, 2008

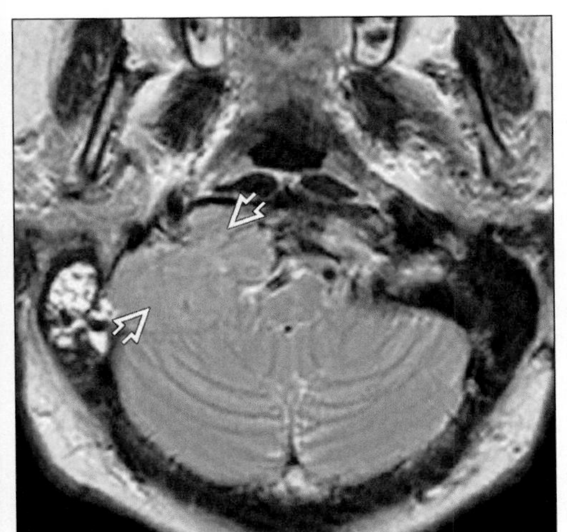

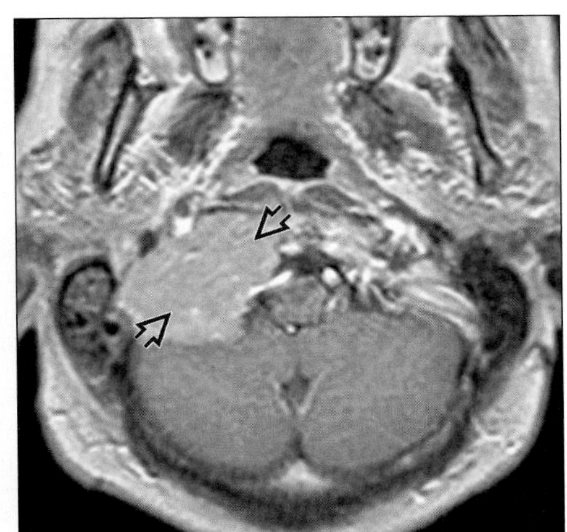

(Left) *Axial T2WI FS MR shows a large lobulated plasmacytoma involving the right aspect of clivus ➔, petrous bone, and occipital condyle. The mass is iso- to hyperintense to the brain parenchyma.* ***(Right)*** *Axial T1WI C+ MR in the same patient demonstrates homogeneous enhancement ➔, which is typical of plasmacytoma.*

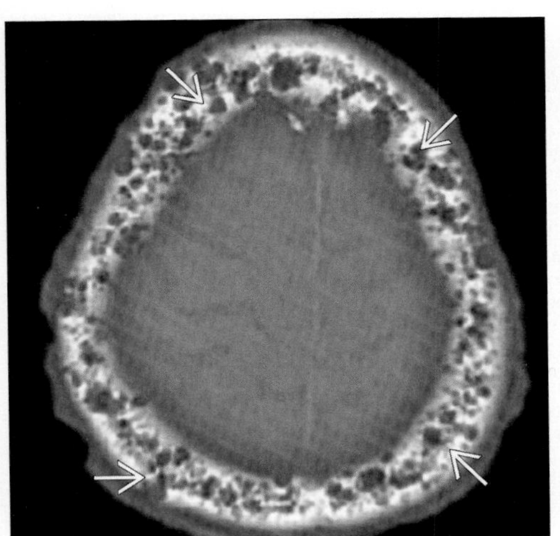

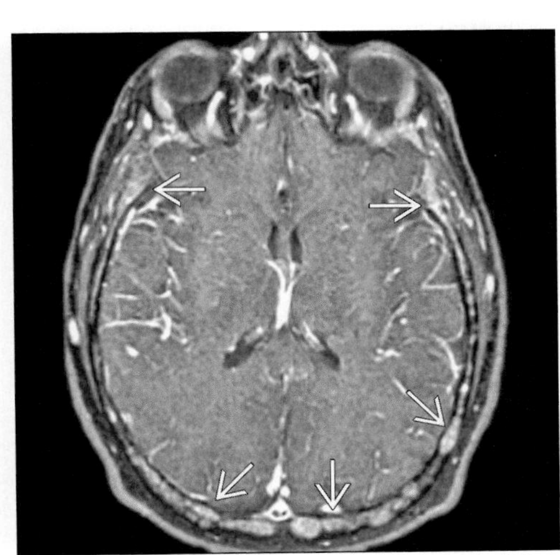

(Left) *Axial bone CT shows numerous "punched-out" lesions ➔ in the calvarium, typical of multiple myeloma.* ***(Right)*** *Axial T1WI C+ FS MR demonstrates a typical case of myeloma with extensive involvement of the skull. Multiple focal enhancing lesions are noted ➔ corresponding to lytic lesion on bone CT (not shown).*

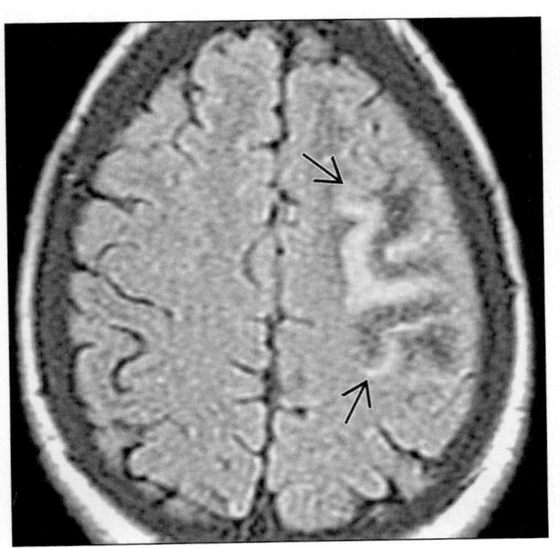

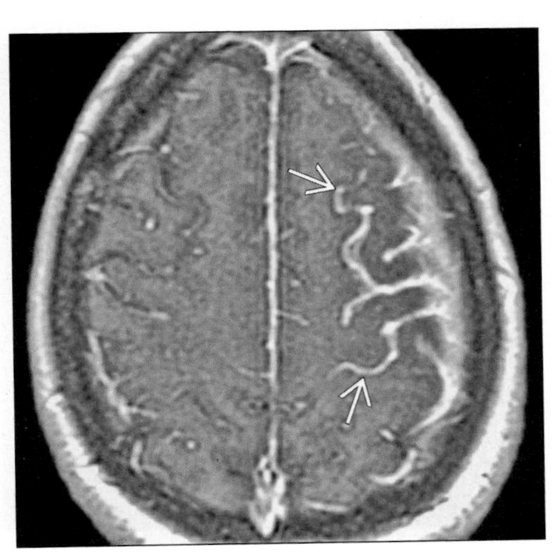

(Left) *A 48-year-old man with newly diagnosed Waldenström macroglobulinemia developed right hemiparesis. Axial FLAIR shows subtle effacement of left convexity sulci ➔ with hyperintensity in the affected sulci. Lymphoplasmatic cells were found in the CSF.* ***(Right)*** *Axial T1WI C+ MR shows diffuse dura-arachnoid thickening and sulcal involvement ➔. CNS symptoms with primary infiltration of the meninges (not 2° to osseous disease) is an uncommon presentation of plasmacytoma.*

SKULL AND MENINGEAL METASTASES

Key Facts

Imaging

- Enhancing lesion(s) with skull/meningeal destruction/infiltration
- Skull, dura, leptomeninges, arachnoid/subarachnoid, pia, and subgaleal
- Many manifestations: Smooth thickening, nodularity, loculation, lobulation, fungating masses

Top Differential Diagnoses

- SM: Surgical defect: Burr hole, craniectomy, myeloma
- DM: Epidural/subdural hematoma, meningioma
- LM: Subarachnoid hemorrhage, sarcoidosis, infectious meningitis

Clinical Issues

- 18% patients with extracranial and intracranial malignancies
- Primary tumor never identified in 2-4%
- All metastases: May be asymptomatic and unsuspected clinically
- Headache is most common symptom (50%)
- CSF cytology often falsely negative
- Accuracy of single lumbar puncture (LP) is 50-60% but 90% after 3 attempts
- Bimodal → children (medulloblastoma & leukemia); adults (breast, lung, melanoma, prostate)
- Average age ~ 50 years (relatively young secondary pediatric cancer and young women with breast cancer)
- Entire neuraxis must be treated as tumor cells are often widely disseminated throughout CSF

Diagnostic Checklist

- Both enhanced MR and LP should be performed, especially if initial test is negative

__(Left)__ Axial graphic illustrates a destructive skull metastasis ➡ expanding the diploic space and invading/thickening the underlying dura (light blue linear structure) ⇨. __(Right)__ Axial T1WI C+ MR shows skull metastasis with enhancement of the diploic space ➡. There is associated small subgaleal soft tissue ⇨ and extensive nodular dural thickening →.

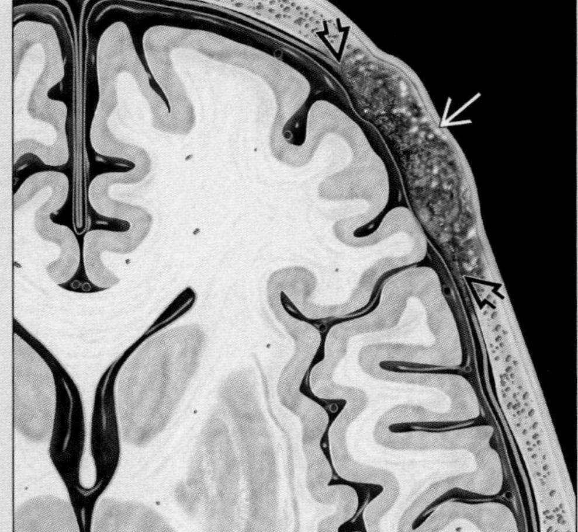

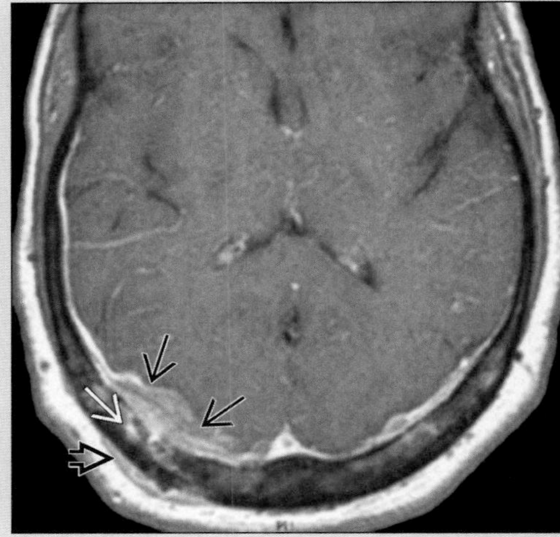

__(Left)__ Axial graphic illustrates diffuse leptomeningeal metastases (abnormal blue material →) coating the pial surface of the brain and filling the subarachnoid spaces between interdigitating sulci. __(Right)__ Axial T1WI C+ MR shows linear and nodular metastases extending throughout the cerebellar folia and basal cisterns →. Note the nodular thickening at the exit of both oculomotor nerves from the midbrain ➡.

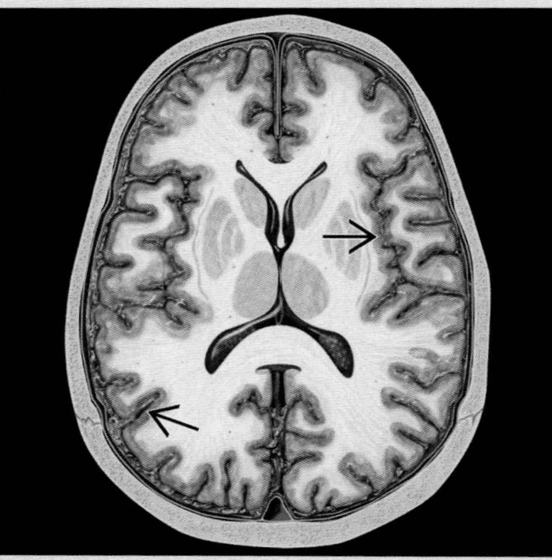

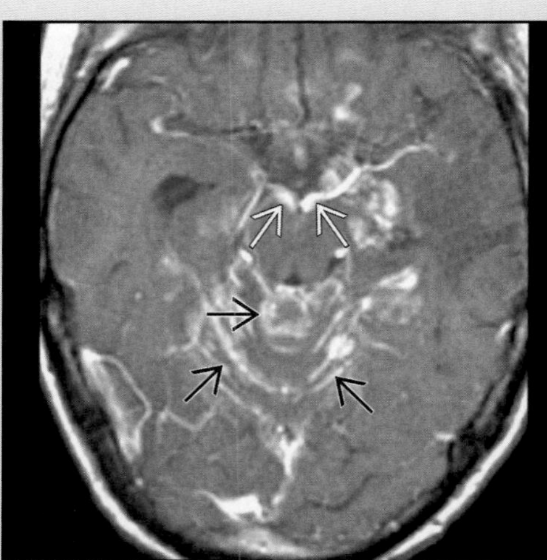

SKULL AND MENINGEAL METASTASES

TERMINOLOGY

Abbreviations

- Skull metastases (SM), dural metastases (DM), arachnoid/subarachnoid metastases (ASAM), pial metastases (PM), leptomeningeal (pia + arachnoid) metastases (LM)

Definitions

- Metastatic disease from extracranial primary tumor to tissues overlying brain

IMAGING

General Features

- Best diagnostic clue
  - Enhancing lesion(s) with skull/meningeal destruction/infiltration
- Location
  - Skull, dura, leptomeninges, arachnoid/ subarachnoid, pia, and subgaleal
- Morphology
  - Many manifestations: Smooth thickening, nodularity, loculation, lobulation, fungating masses

Radiographic Findings

- Radiography
  - SM: Focal lytic or blastic lesions lacking "benign" sclerotic border

CT Findings

- NECT
  - Any metastases: May find hemorrhagic hyperdensity
  - Subgaleal space: Relatively dense lesion
- CECT
  - SM: Enhancing mass centered in bone with osseous destruction, lacking "benign" sclerotic border
    - Most are lytic, though a few are sclerotic (e.g., prostate)
  - DM and LM: Both may appear as enhancing biconvex masses displacing brain
    - DM characterized by calvarial involvement
  - Carcinomatosis: CT is insensitive; however, hydrocephalus may be early sign

MR Findings

- T1WI
  - SM: Hypointense marrow lesion
  - DM and LM: Most masses hypointense to gray matter (GM)
  - Subgaleal space: Relative hypointense lesion
  - Any metastases: May find hemorrhagic signal
- T2WI
  - SM: Hyperintense marrow lesion; dura usually intact
  - DM between skull & elevated hypointense dura
  - DM and LM: Most hyperintense relative to GM
  - Any metastases: May find hemorrhagic signal
- FLAIR
  - LM and ASAM: Diffuse hyperintense CSF
  - ASAM infiltrating perivascular spaces (PVS): Loss of normal PVS-CSF suppression → hyperintensity
  - Carcinomatosis: Hyperintense thickening; affects adjacent sulcal nulling → hyperintensity
  - Brain infiltration: Hyperintense vasogenic edema
- DWI
  - Dural metastasis may show restricted diffusion due to high cellularity
  - DWI sensitive in picking subtle calvarial lesions
- T1WI C+
  - SM: Lesion may enhance to "normal" T1 marrow signal → requires fat saturation
    - Usually some dural thickening & enhancement
  - DM and LM: Both appear as enhancing biconvex masses displacing brain
    - DM often has calvarial involvement
    - LM often invades underlying brain
  - LM, ASAM, PM: Diffuse enhancing tissue ± nodularity
  - ASAM infiltrating perivascular spaces: Tiny enhancing nodules with miliary appearance
  - Carcinomatosis: Enhancing and thickened tissue ± nodules
    - May coat ependymal surfaces, cranial nerves
- MRV
  - May be helpful in evaluation of sinus displacement, compression, thrombosis

Nuclear Medicine Findings

- Bone scan
  - SM: Usually intensely positive
- PET
  - 18-fluorodeoxyglucose (FDG) PET may detect small calvarial metastases not seen by MR
  - Caveat: Adjacent activity from normal gray matter may limit detection of SM

Imaging Recommendations

- Best imaging tool
  - SM: NECT/bone algorithm for osseous evaluation
    - MR with contrast if dura, scalp involved
  - DM, ASAM, PM, LM: MR + gad, although sensitivity still only ~ 70%
    - 90% for extracranial solid tumor metastases
    - 55% when hematologic (lymphoma, leukemia)
- Protocol advice
  - Fat saturation necessary to distinguish enhancement from normal hyperintense marrow and scalp fat
  - FLAIR > T2WI; T1 C+ > FLAIR C+

DIFFERENTIAL DIAGNOSIS

Skull Metastases

- Surgical defect: Burr hole, craniectomy
- Myeloma: Characteristic labs

Dural Metastases

- Epidural hematoma: Distinctive MR
- Subdural hematoma: Distinctive MR
- Meningioma

Arachnoid/Subarachnoid Metastases

- Subarachnoid hemorrhage: Typical NECT appearance

Leptomeningeal Metastases (LM)

- Sarcoidosis: CXR → hilar adenopathy + Kveim-Siltzbach skin test
- Infectious meningitis: CSF → infection/organism

SKULL AND MENINGEAL METASTASES

PATHOLOGY

General Features

- Etiology
  - SM: Hematogenous (most commonly breast, lung, prostate, kidney) or by direct extension (SCCa)
  - DM: Hematogenous (most commonly breast > lymphoma > prostate > neuroblastoma)
  - LM, ASAM, PM: Hematogenous (most commonly lung, gastric, breast, ovary, melanoma, leukemia, lymphoma) or direct extension (primary CNS tumors)
- Associated abnormalities
  - Limbic encephalitis
- Dura and leptomeninges provide considerable barriers to contiguous spread of metastasis
  - General mechanisms of spread
    - Arterial hematogenous: Arterial transfer (e.g., breast, lung, melanoma, prostate)
    - Venous hematogenous: Via choroid plexus or through arachnoid vessels (classic for leukemia)
    - Direct extension: From primary brain tumors (e.g., GBM, PNET, ependymoma)
    - Perineural spread: H&N cancers (SCCa)
    - Iatrogenic: Following initial resection/debulking of primary brain tumors

Gross Pathologic & Surgical Features

- DM: Well-defined dural masses often invading skull
  - Necropsy → nodules on inner dura (subdural)
- LM, ASAM, PM: Gray-white or yellow thickening

Microscopic Features

- SM and DM: Metastatic cell infiltrates
- LM and ASAM: Metastatic cell infiltrates, often along perivascular spaces extending into brain

CLINICAL ISSUES

Presentation

- Most common signs/symptoms
  - All metastases: May be asymptomatic and unsuspected clinically
  - Headache is most common symptom (50%)
  - Less common signs/symptoms
    - N/V, pain, sensory deficit, weakness (33%)
    - Mental status change (25%)
    - Seizures (20%)
    - ↑ ICP from CSF obstruction
    - Cranial nerve deficit(s)
  - Symptoms from brain compression → highly dependent on locale
- Clinical profile
  - CSF cytology often falsely negative
    - Accuracy of single lumbar puncture (LP) is 50-60% but 90% after 3 attempts

Demographics

- Age
  - Bimodal → children (medulloblastoma and leukemia); adults (breast, lung, melanoma, prostate)
  - Average age ~ 50 years (relatively young 2° pediatric cancer and young women with breast cancer)
- Epidemiology
  - 18% patients with extra- and intracranial malignancies
  - 6-18% of CNS metastases also involve arachnoid/ subarachnoid space, pia, or both
  - Carcinomatosis in up to 25% of cancer patients
    - Primary tumor never identified in 2-4%
    - Occurs in breast (35%), lung small cell (25%), melanoma cancer (25%) patients

Natural History & Prognosis

- Dural sinus thrombosis from invasion or compression
- Obstructive hydrocephalus
  - Noncommunicating: Normal CSF flow obstructed, usually by cisternal metastases
  - Communicating: Normal CSF flow, ↓ arachnoid villi absorption, obstruction 2° tumor cells, blood, debris
  - Important to evaluate presence prior to LP to prevent downward herniation and death
  - Up to 70% of carcinomatosis patients have some degree of CSF obstruction
- Pachymeningitis interna hemorrhagica
  - Rare, usually bilateral, spontaneous, subdural hematomas from meningeal metastasis
  - Commonly from breast but also prostate, melanoma
- Untreated malignant meningeal metastases decreases survival time to 1-2 months

Treatment

- Early detection of meningeal metastases is crucial
  - MR often provides 1st clue
- Usually radiation with chemotherapy (intrathecal &/ or systemic) initiated to slow progression
  - Entire neuraxis must be treated as tumor cells are often widely disseminated throughout CSF
- Biopsy may be necessary if no evidence of primary tumor
- Ventriculoperitoneal shunt may be necessary in patients with symptomatic CSF obstruction

DIAGNOSTIC CHECKLIST

Image Interpretation Pearls

- Both enhanced MR and LP should be performed, especially if initial test is negative

SELECTED REFERENCES

1. Nayak L et al: Intracranial dural metastases. Cancer. 115(9):1947-53, 2009
2. Nemeth AJ et al: Improved detection of skull metastasis with diffusion-weighted MR imaging. AJNR Am J Neuroradiol. 28(6):1088-92, 2007
3. O'Meara WP et al: Leptomeningeal metastasis. Curr Probl Cancer. 31(6):367-424, 2007

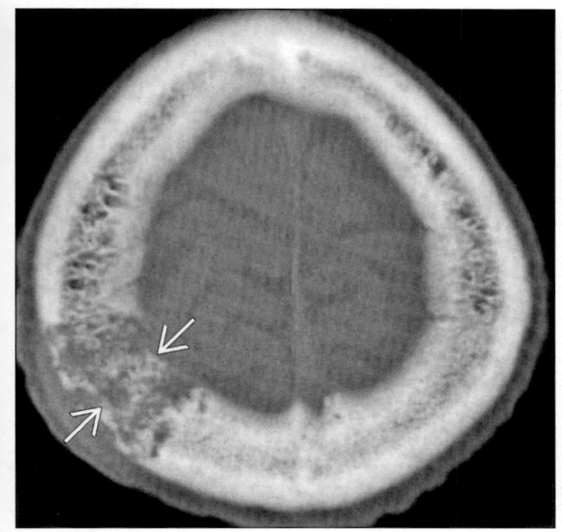

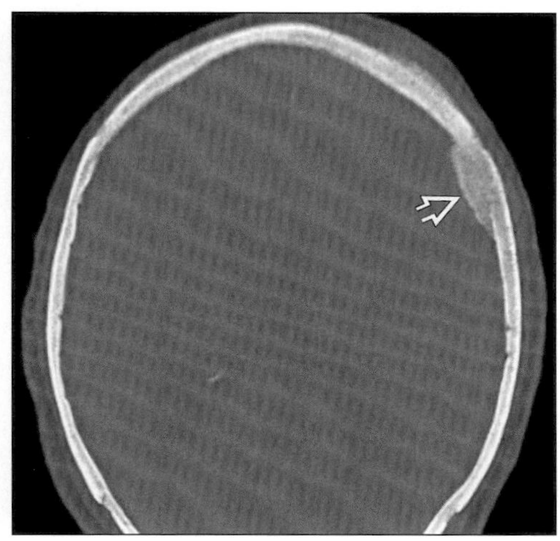

(Left) *Axial bone CT shows classic permeative skull destruction in a patient with metastatic lung carcinoma ➔.* ***(Right)*** *Axial bone CT demonstrates localized skull thickening with sclerotic prostatic metastasis ➔. Metastasis to the skull can be lytic, sclerotic, or mixed; prostate metastasis are commonly sclerotic.*

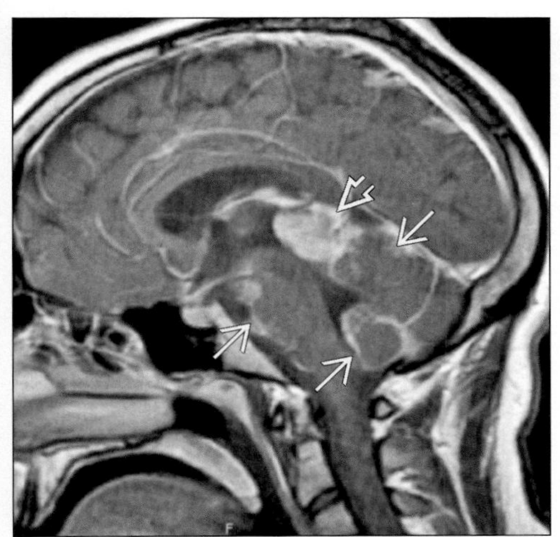

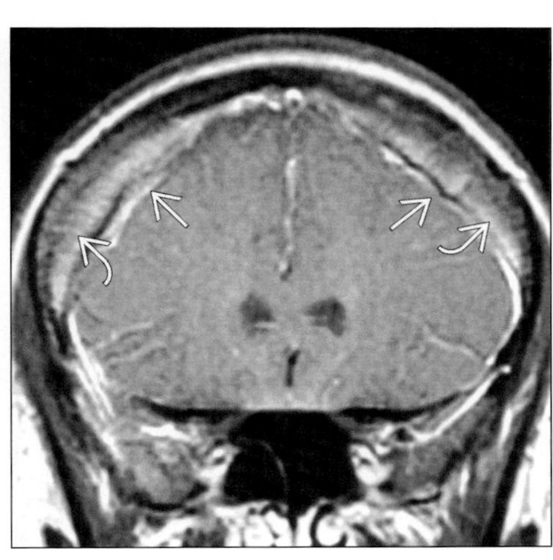

(Left) *Sagittal T1WI C+ MR shows a pineal region PNET ➔ with diffuse leptomeningeal enhancement coating the brainstem and cerebellum ➔, consistent with leptomeningeal metastasis.* ***(Right)*** *Coronal T1WI C+ MR shows markedly thickened dura ➔ with abnormal enhancement and marked expansion of the diploic space ➔ giving a "hair on end" pattern in a metastatic neuroblastoma.*

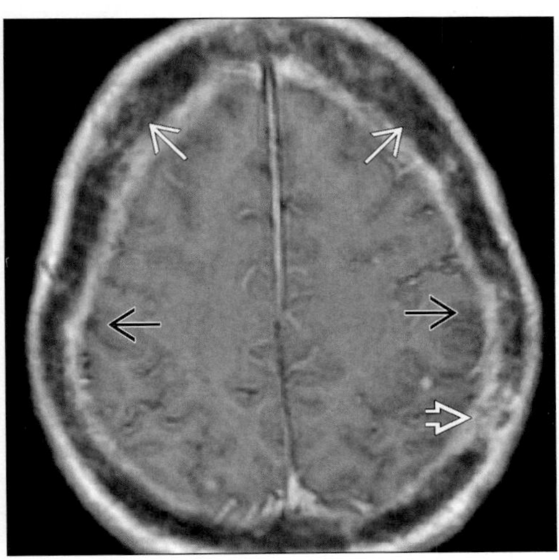

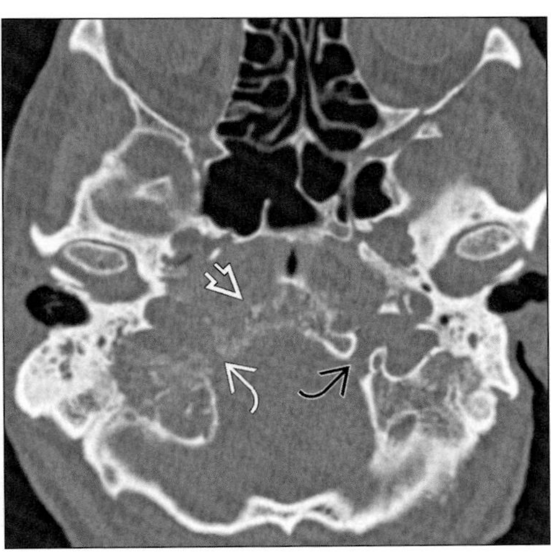

(Left) *Axial T1WI C+ MR shows diffuse low marrow signal ➔ due to breast carcinoma metastasis associated with focal areas of diploic enhancement ➔ and diffuse dural thickening ➔.* ***(Right)*** *Axial bone CT shows a large, permeative, destructive metastatic lesion in a patient with lung carcinoma and right hypoglossal palsy involving the skull base ➔. Note the involvement of the right hypoglossal canal ➔ with a normal-appearing left canal ➔.*

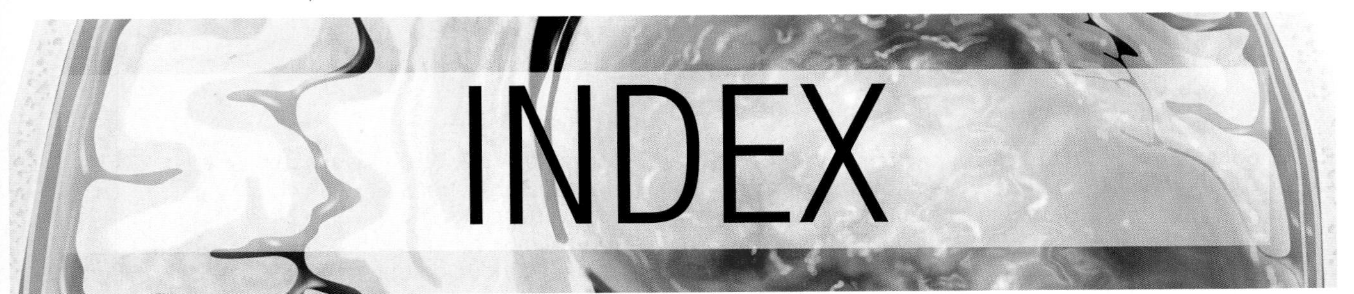

INDEX

A

INDEX

INDEX

INDEX

INDEX

INDEX

INDEX

Index

INDEX

INDEX

INDEX

INDEX

E

INDEX

INDEX

F

G

INDEX

H

INDEX

INDEX

INDEX

I

INDEX

J

K

INDEX

L

INDEX

M

INDEX

INDEX

N

INDEX

O

INDEX

P

INDEX

Q

R

S

INDEX

INDEX

INDEX

T

INDEX

U

INDEX

V

INDEX

W

X

Z